YOUMANS
Neurological Surgery

YOUMANS
Neurological Surgery

Fifth Edition

H. Richard Winn, MD
Professor of Neurological Surgery
and Neuroscience
Mount Sinai School of Medicine
New York, New York

VOLUME

4

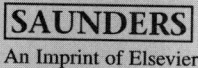
SAUNDERS
An Imprint of Elsevier

SAUNDERS
An Imprint of Elsevier

The Curtis Center
Independence Square West
Philadelphia, Pennsylvania 19106

YOUMANS NEUROLOGICAL SURGERY
Copyright 2004, Elsevier Inc. All rights reserved. ISBN 0-7216-8291-x.

Notice

Neurosurgery is an ever-changing field. Standard safety precautions must be followed, but as new research and clinical experience broaden our knowledge, changes in treatment and drug therapy become necessary or appropriate. Readers are advised to check the product information currently provided by the manufacturer of each drug to be administered to verify the recommended dose, the method and duration of administration, and the contraindications. It is the responsibility of the treating physician, relying on experience and knowledge of the patient, to determine dosage and the best treatment for each individual patient. Neither the publisher nor the editor assumes any responsibility for any injury and/or damage to persons or property arising from this publication.

The Publisher

First Edition 1973. Second Edition 1982. Third Edition 1990. Fourth Edition 1996.

Library of Congress Cataloging-in-Publication Data

Youmans neurological surgery / [edited by] H. Richard Winn.—5th ed.

p. cm.

Rev. ed. of: Neurological surgery / editor-in-chief, Julian R. Youmans; associate editors, Donald P. Becker . . . [et al.]. 4th ed. c1996.

Includes bibliographical references and index.

ISBN 0–7216–8291–X

1. Nervous system—Surgery. I. Title: Neurological surgery. II. Winn, H. Richard. III. Youmans, Julian R., 1928–
  [DNLM: 1. Neurosurgical Procedures. 2. Nervous System Diseases—surgery. 3. Neurosurgery—methods. WL 368 Y671 2003]

RE593 N4153 2003

617.4'8—dc21   2002017677

Vice President, Global Surgery: Richard Lampert

Developmental Editors: Anne Snyder, David Orzechowski

Project Manager: Jodi Kaye

Printed in the United States of America.

Last digit is the print number: 9 8 7 6 5 4 3 2 1

To my wife and family, and to my residents who have carried the message.

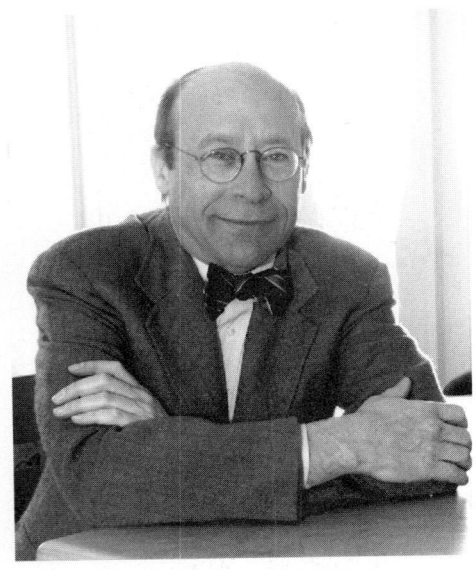
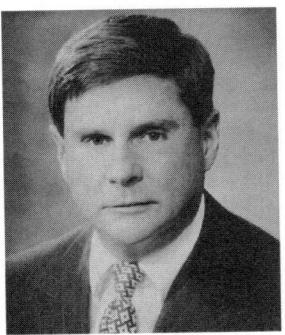

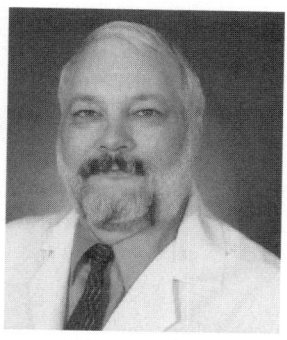

Roy A. E. Bakay, MD
Professor and Vice Chairman
Department of Neurosurgery
Rush Medical Center
Chicago, Illinois
Functional Neurosurgery, Volume 3

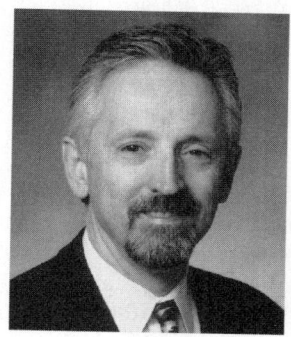

Kim J. Burchiel, MD
Professor and Chairman
Department of Neurological Surgery
Oregon Health & Science University
School of Medicine
Portland, Oregon
Functional Neurosurgery and Pain, Vol. 3

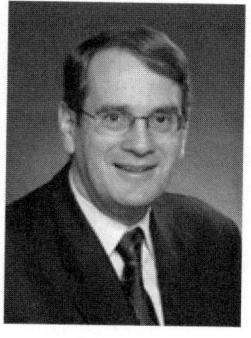

Henry Brem, MD
Harvey Cushing Professor of Neurosurgery,
Ophthalmology, and Oncology
Chairman, Department of Neurosurgery
Johns Hopkins University School of Medicine
Baltimore, Maryland
Oncology, Volume 1

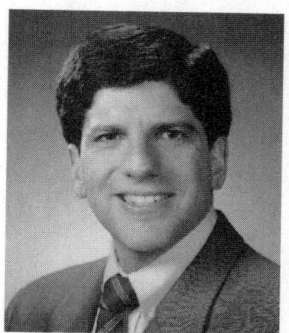

William A. Friedman, M.D.
Professor and Chair,
Department of Neurosurgery
University of Florida,
Gainesville, Florida
Radiation Therapy and Radiosurgery, Volume 4

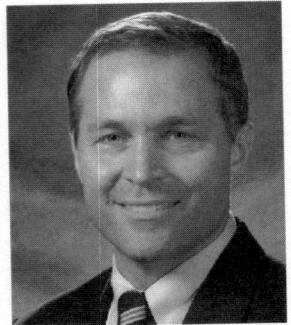

M. Sean Grady, MD

Charles Harrison Frazier Professor and Chair of the
Department of Neurosurgery
University of Pennsylvania School of Medicine
Philadelphia, Pennsylvania

Trauma, Volume 4

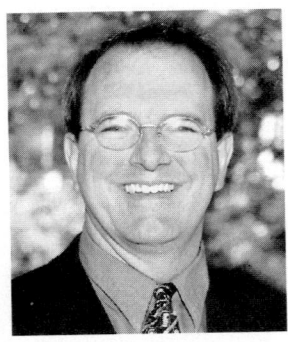

Joel D. MacDonald, MD

Assistant Professor of Neurosurgery
University of Utah Medical Center
Salt Lake City, Utah

Special Features

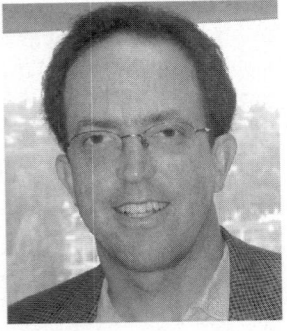

Michel Kliot, MD

Associate Professor of Neurosurgery
University of Washington School of Medicine
Seattle, Washington

*Introduction to Neurological Surgery, Volume 1; Peripheral
Nerve, Volume 4*

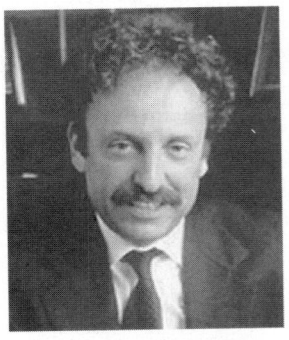

Lawrence F. Marshall, MD

Professor of Neurological Surgery
University of California, San Diego,
School of Medicine
San Diego, California

Trauma, Volume 4

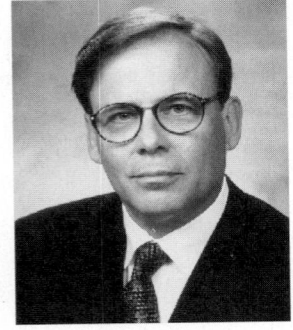

L. Dade Lunsford, MD

Lars Leksell Professor and Chairman of Neurological
Surgery, Radiology, and Radiology Oncology
University of Pittsburgh School of Medicine
University of Pittsburgh Medical Center
Pittsburgh, Pennsylvania

Radiation Therapy and Radiosurgery, Volume 4

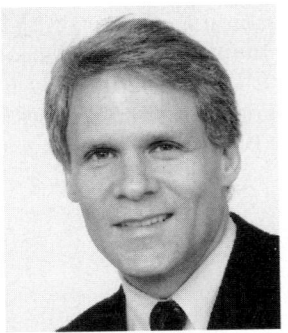

Marc R. Mayberg, MD

Chairman, Department of Neurosurgery
Cleveland Clinic Foundation
Cleveland, Ohio

Special Features

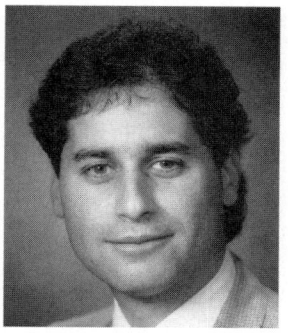

Fredric B. Meyer, MD
Professor of Neurosurgery
Mayo Medical School
Rochester, Minnesota
Vascular, Volume 2

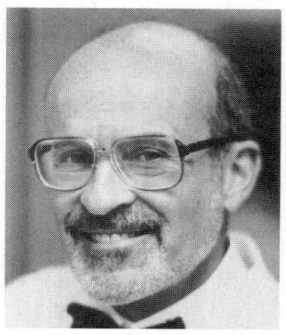

R. Michael Scott, MD
Professor of Neurological Surgery
Harvard Medical School
Boston, Massachusetts
Pediatric, Volume 3

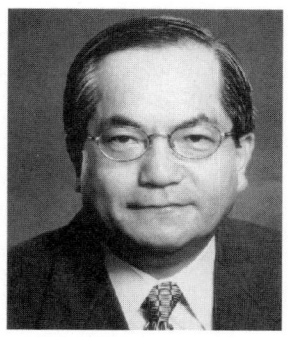

T. S. Park, MD
Shi H. Huang Professor of Neurosurgery and
Professor of Pediatrics and Anatomy and
Neurobiology
Washington University School of Medicine
St. Louis, Missouri
Pediatric, Volume 3

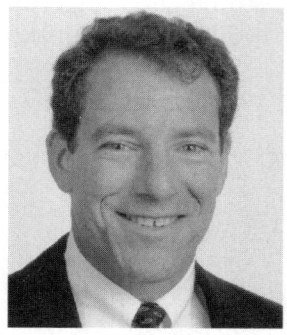

Daniel L. Silbergeld, MD
Associate Professor, Department of
Neurological Surgery
University of Washington School of Medicine
Seattle, Washington
Epilepsy, Volume 2

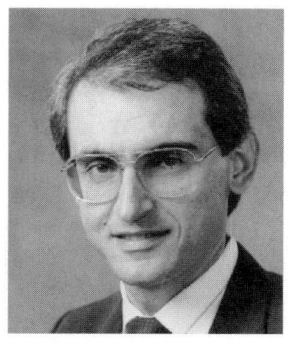

Raymond Sawaya, MD
Professor of Neurosurgery
University of Texas–Houston Medical School
Department of Neurosurgery
The University of Texas MD Anderson Cancer Center
Houston, Texas
Oncology, Volume 1

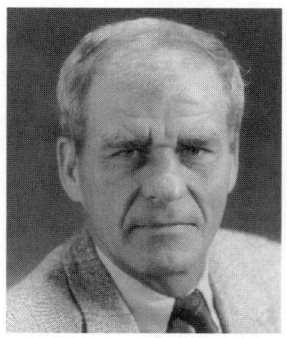

Volker K. H. Sonntag, MD
Clinical Professor of Neurosurgery
University of Arizona College of Medicine
Tucson, Arizona
Vice Chairman, Division of Neurological Surgery
Barrow Neurological Institute
Phoenix, Arizona
Spine, Volume 4

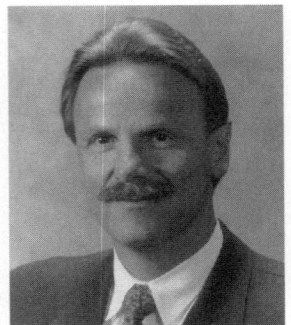

Robert F. Spetzler, MD

Professor, Department of Surgery,
Section of Neurosurgery
University of Arizona College of Medicine
Tucson, Arizona
Director and J. N. Harbor Chairman of
Neurological Surgery
Barrow Neurological Institute
Phoenix, Arizona

Vascular, Volume 2

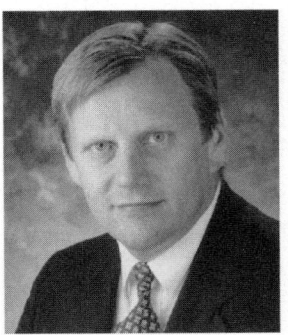

Dennis G. Vollmer, MD

Professor of Neurosurgery
University of Texas Health Science Center at Houston
Houston, Texas

Spine, Volume 4

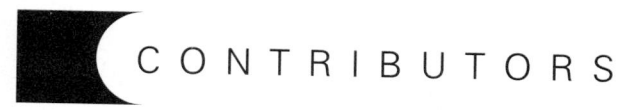

CONTRIBUTORS

Khaled M. Abdel Aziz, MD, PhD

Resident, Department of Neurosurgery, University of Cincinnati College of Medicine and University Hospital, Cincinnati, Ohio
Dorsal Rhizotomy and Dorsal Root Ganglionectomy

Muwaffak M. Abdulhak, MD

Clinical Instructor, Department of Neurosurgery, Medical College of Wisconsin, Milwaukee, Wisconsin
Bone Metabolism as It Relates to Spinal Disease and Treatment

Saleem I. Abdulrauf, MD

Assistant Professor, Neurological Surgery and Director, Cerebrovascular and Skull Base Surgery Program, Saint Louis University School of Medicine; Director, Cerebrovascular and Skull Base Surgery Program, Saint Louis University Hospital, St. Louis, Missouri
Meningiomas

Dima Abi-Said, MD

Attending, Department of Neurosurgery, The University of Texas M.D. Anderson Cancer Center, Houston, Texas
Metastatic Brain Tumors

John R. Adler, Jr., MD

Professor, Department of Neurosurgery, Stanford University School of Medicine, Stanford, California
General and Historical Considerations of Radiotherapy and Radiosurgery

Robin Albert, MD, MPH

Research Coordinator, Center for Endovascular Surgery, Institute for Neurology and Neurosurgery, Beth Israel Medical Center, New York, New York
Endovascular Management of Brain Arteriovenous Malformations

A. Leland Albright, MD

Professor of Neurosurgery, University of Pittsburgh School of Medicine; Chief, Pediatric Neurosurgery, Childrens Hospital of Pittsburgh, Pittsburgh, Pennsylvania
Patient Selection in Movement Disorder Surgery; Brainstem Gliomas

Felipe C. Albuquerque, MD

Staff Neurosurgeon and Assistant Director, Endovascular Neurosurgery, Barrow Neurological Institute, Phoenix, Arizona
Carotid Angioplasty and Stenting: Interventional Treatment of Occlusive Vascular Disease; Basilar Trunk Aneurysms

Kenneth Aldape, MD

Assistant Professor, Department of Pathology, Neuropathology Unit, University of California, San Francisco, School of Medicine, San Francisco, California
Low-Grade Gliomas: Astrocytoma, Oligodendroglioma, and Mixed Gliomas

Eben Alexander III, MD

Associate Professor of Surgery, Department of Surgery, Division of Neurosurgery, University of Massachusetts Medical School; Attending Neurosurgeon, University of Massachusetts-Memorial Hospitals, Worcester, Massachusetts
Linac Radiosurgery

Michael J. Alexander, MD

Assistant Professor, Department of Surgery, Divisions of Neurosurgery and Interventional Neuroradiology, Duke University School of Medicine, Durham, North Carolina
Nonatherosclerotic Carotid Lesions

Mir Jafar Ali, MD

Resident, Department of Neurosurgery, University of Michigan Hospital, Ann Arbor, Michigan
Basilar Apex and Posterior Cerebral Artery Aneurysms

Ahmed Alkhani, MD

Fellow in Functional Neurosurgery, University of Toronto Faculty of Medicine and Toronto Western Hospital, Toronto, Ontario, Canada
Pallidotomy for Parkinson's Disease

Cargill H. Alleyne, Jr., MD

Co-Director, Neurosurgery Residency Program, University of Rochester School of Medicine and Dentistry; Chief, Division of Stroke and Cerebrovascular Surgery, Department of Surgery, Rochester General Hospital, Rochester, New York
Carotid Angioplasty and Stenting: Interventional Treatment of Occlusive Vascular Disease; Traumatic Carotid Injury

Ossama Al-Mefty, MD
Professor and Chairman, Department of Neurosurgery, University of Arkansas for Medical Sciences, Little Rock, Arkansas
Meningiomas

Mahmoud Al-Yamany, MD
Department of Neurosurgery, Riyadh Medical Complex, King Saud University Affiliated Hospital, Riyadh, Saudi Arabia
Intracranial Internal Carotid Artery Aneurysms

Arun Paul Amar, MD
Clinical Instructor, Department of Neurosurgery, University of Southern California Keck School of Medicine; Staff, Children's Hospital of Los Angeles, Los Angeles, California
Ventricular Tumors; Vagus Nerve Stimulation for Intractable Epilepsy

Christopher Ames, MD
Assistant Professor, Department of Neurological Surgery, University of California, San Francisco, School of Medicine, San Francisco, California
Differential Diagnosis of Altered States of Consciousness

Sepideh Amin-Hanjani, MD
Instructor in Surgery, Harvard Medical School; Assistant Visiting Surgeon, Department of Neurosurgery, Massachusetts General Hospital, Boston, Massachusetts
Cerebral Lymphoma

Norberto Andaluz, MD
Clinical Fellow, Department of Neurosurgery, University of Cincinnati College of Medicine, Cincinnati, Ohio
Dorsal Rhizotomy and Dorsal Root Ganglionectomy

Peter Angevine, MD
Resident, Department of Neurological Surgery, Columbia-Presbyterian Medical Center, New York, New York
Anterior Lumbar Instrumentation

Ronald I. Apfelbaum, MD
Professor of Neurosurgery, University of Utah School of Medicine; Attending, University of Utah Hospital and Clinics, Salt Lake City, Utah
Treatment of Axis Fractures

Michael L. J. Apuzzo, MD
Edwin M. Todd/Treat M. Wells, Jr. Professor of Neurological Surgery and Professor of Radiation Oncology, Biology, and Physics, University of Southern California Keck School of Medicine; Staff, USC Care Medical Group, USC University Hospital, and USC/Norris Cancer Hospital, Los Angeles, California
Ventricular Tumors; Vagus Nerve Stimulation for Intractable Epilepsy

Claire Ardouin, MA
Psychologist, Hôpital Albert Michallon, Grenoble, France
Deep Brain Stimulation for Movement Disorders

E. Joy Arpin-Sypert, MD
Sypert Institute, Fort Myers, Florida
Evaluation and Management of the Failed Back Syndrome

James I. Ausman, MD
Professor of Neurosurgery, University of Illinois at Chicago, Chicago, Illinois; Editor, *Surgical Neurology*
Extracranial Vertebral Artery Disease

Issam A. Awad, MD, MSc
Ogsbury-Kindt Professor and Chairman, Department of Neurosurgery, and Professor of Neurosurgery, Neurology, and Pathology, University of Colorado School of Medicine, Denver, Colorado
Surgical Management of Supratentorial Cavernous Malformations

Julian E. Bailes, MD
Professor and Chairman, Department of Neurosurgery, West Virginia University School of Medicine, Morgantown, West Virginia
Carotid Endarterectomy

Roy A. E. Bakay, MD
Professor and Vice Chairman, Director of Movement Disorder Surgery, Rush-Presbyterian-St. Luke's Medical Center, Chicago Institute of Neurosurgery and Neuroresearch, Chicago, Illinois
History of Functional Neurosurgery; Cellular Transplantation in the Central Nervous System

Perry A. Ball, MD
Attending Neurosurgeon, Section of Neurosurgery, Dartmouth-Hitchcock Medical Center, Lebanon, New Hampshire
Treatment of Disk Disease of the Lumbar Spine

Gordon H. Baltuch, MD, PhD
Assistant Professor, Department of Neurosurgery, University of Pennsylvania School of Medicine; Attending Neurosurgeon, Hospital of the University of Pennsylvania, Pennsylvania Hospital, and Philadelphia Veterans Administration Medical Center, Philadelphia, Pennsylvania
Topectomy: Uses and Indications

Gene H. Barnett, MD
Professor of Surgery, Ohio State University College of Medicine and Public Health, Columbus; Chairman, Brain Tumor Institute, Cleveland Clinic Foundation, Cleveland, Ohio
Surgical Navigation for Brain Tumors

Stanley L. Barnwell, MD, PhD

Associate Professor of Neurological Surgery, Oregon Health & Science University School of Medicine; Staff, Dotter Interventional Institute, Portland, Oregon

Cerebral Venous and Sinus Thrombosis

Jean-Claude Baron, MD

Professor of Stroke Medicine, Department of Neurology, University of Cambridge Faculty of Medicine; Neurology Consultant, Addenbrooke's Hospital, Cambridge, England

Positron Emission Tomography in Cerebrovascular Disease

Daniel L. Barrow, MD

MBNA-Bowman Professor and Chairman, Department of Neurological Surgery, Emory University School of Medicine; Chief, Neurological Service, and Co-Director, Emory Stroke Center, Emory University Hospital, Atlanta, Georgia

Treatment of Lateral-Sigmoid and Sagittal Sinus Dural Arteriovenous Malformations

Juan Bartolomei, MD

Assistant Professor, Department of Neurosurgery, Yale University School of Medicine, New Haven, Connecticut

Anterior Approach including Cervical Corpectomy (Degenerative)

Jonathan J. Baskin, MD

Attending Neurosurgeon, Atlantic Neurosurgical Specialists, Chatham, New Jersey

Carotid Angioplasty and Stenting; Interventional Treatment of Occlusive Vascular Disease; Anterior Cervical Instrumentation; Occipitocervical Fusion

H. Hunt Batjer, MD

Professor and Chair, Department of Neurological Surgery, Northwestern University Feinberg School of Medicine; Chairman, Department of Neurological Surgery, Northwestern Memorial Hospital, Chicago, Illinois

Basilar Apex and Posterior Cerebral Artery Aneurysms

Thomas K. Baumann, PhD

Associate Professor, Department of Neurological Surgery and Department of Physiology and Pharmacology, Oregon Health and Science University School of Medicine, Portland, Oregon

Physiologic Anatomy of Pain

Andrew Beaumont, MD

Neurosurgical Fellow, Virginia Commonwealth University School of Medicine, Richmond, Virginia

Physiology of the Cerebrospinal Fluid and Intracranial Pressure

Joshua Bederson, MD

Professor, Department of Neurosurgery, Mount Sinai School of Medicine; Vice Chairman, Department of Neurosurgery, Mount Sinai Medical Center, New York, New York

Infectious Intracranial Aneurysms

Ghassan K. Bejjani, MD

Clinical Assistant Professor, Department of Neurosurgery, University of Pittsburgh School of Medicine; Neurosurgeon, Presbyterian University Hospital, Pittsburgh, Pennsylvania

Orbital Tumors

J. Brad Bellotte, MD

Resident, Department of Neurosurgery, Allegheny General Hospital, Pittsburgh, Pennsylvania

Brain Death; Diagnosis and Management of Seventh and Eighth Cranial Nerve Injuries due to Temporal Bone Fractures

Alim L. Benabid, MD, PhD

Professor of Biophysics, University Joseph Fourier Medical School; Head, Neurosurgery, and Director, INSERM U.318 Research Laboratory of Preclinical Neurosciences, Hôpital Albert Michallon, Grenoble, France

Deep Brain Stimulation for Movement Disorders

Eduardo E. Benarroch, MD

Professor of Neurology, Mayo Medical School; Consultant in Neurology, Mayo Clinic, Rochester, Minnesota

Cerebral Blood Flow and Metabolism

Abdelhamid Benazzouz, PhD

Research Fellow, University of Bordeaux School of Medicine; Director of Research, Neurophysiology Laboratory, University Victor Segalan, Bordeaux, France

Deep Brain Stimulation for Movement Disorders

Bernard R. Bendok, MD

Assistant Professor, Department of Neurological Surgery, Northwestern University Feinberg School of Medicine, Chicago, Illinois

Basilar Apex and Posterior Cerebral Artery Aneurysms

Gregory J. Bennett, MD

Clinical Assistant Professor of Neurosurgery, University of Buffalo; Clinical Director of Neurosurgery, Erie County Medical Center, Buffalo, New York

Spondylolysis and Spondylolisthesis

Alejandro Berenstein, MD

Professor of Radiology, Neurosurgery, and Neurology, Albert Einstein College of Medicine of Yeshiva University, Bronx; Director, Center for Endovascular Surgery, and Director, Institute for Neurology and Neurosurgery, Beth Israel Medical Center, New York, New York
Endovascular Management of Brain Arteriovenous Malformations

Mitchel S. Berger, MD

Professor and Chair, Department of Neurological Surgery, University of California, San Francisco, School of Medicine, San Francisco, California
Low-Grade Gliomas: Astrocytoma, Oligodendroglioma, and Mixed Gliomas; Hemangioblastomas of the Central Nervous System; Interstitial and Intracavitary Irradiation of Brian Tumors

Matt A. Bernstein, PhD

Assistant Professor of Radiologic Physics, Mayo Medical School; Senior Associate Consultant in Radiology, Mayo Clinic, Rochester, Minnesota
Magnetic Resonance Angiography

José Biller, MD

Professor and Chairman, Department of Neurology, Indiana University School of Medicine, Indianapolis, Indiana
Carotid Occlusive Disease: Natural History and Medical Management

Jeffrey R. Binder, MD

Professor, Department of Neurology, Medical College of Wisconsin, Milwaukee, Wisconsin
Functional Magnetic Resonance Imaging in Epilepsy Surgery

Barry D. Birch, MD

Attending, Department of Neurosurgery, Mayo Clinic Scottsdale, Scottsdale, Arizona
Anterior Thoracic Instrumentation

Rolfe Birch, MChir

Visiting Professor, University College and Imperial College, London University, London; Orthopaedic Surgeon, Peripheral Nerve Injury Unit, Royal National Orthopaedic Hospital, Stanmore, England
Management of Acute Peripheral Nerve Injuries

Peter M. Black, MD, PhD

Franc D. Ingraham Professor of Neurosurgery, Harvard Medical School; Neurosurgeon-in-Chief, Brigham and Women's Hospital and Children's Hospital, and Chief, Neurosurgical Oncology, Dana-Farber Cancer Institute, Boston, Massachusetts
Craniopharyngioma in the Adult

Miroslav P. Bobek, MD

Attending Surgeon, Providence Medford Medical Center, Medford, Oregon
Brain Edema and Tumor-Host Interactions

Anne Boulin, MD

Neuroradiologist, Hôpital Foch, Suresnes, France
Osseous Tumors

Blaise F. D. Bourgeois, MD

Director, Division of Epilepsy and Clinical Neurophysiology, Department of Neurology, Children's Hospital, Boston, Massachusetts
Antiepileptic Medications: Principles of Clinical Use

Guy Bouvier, MD

Professor of Neurosurgery, University of Montreal Faculty of Medicine, Montreal; Neurosurgeon, Hôpital Notredame, Montreal; Medical Advisor to the Vice President, Western Region, Workers' Compensation Board of Appeal, St. Lambert, Quebec, Canada
Selective Peripheral Denervation for Spasmodic Torticollis

Frank J. Bova, PhD

Professor of Neurosurgery, University of Florida College of Medicine; Staff, Shand's Hospital, Gainesville, Florida
Fractionated and Stereotactic Radiation, Extracranial Stereotactic Radiation, Intensity Modulation, and Multileaf Collimation

Robin Bowman, MD

Assistant Professor of Neurosurgery, Northwestern University Feinberg School of Medicine; Attending Neurosurgeon, Children's Memorial Hospital, Chicago, Illinois
Birth Head Trauma

Adam Brant, MD

Staff Neurosurgeon, St. Agnes Medical Center, Fresno, California
Traumatic Cerebrospinal Fluid Fistulas

Henry Brem, MD

Harvey Cushing Professor of Neurosurgery, Ophthalmology, and Oncology and Chairman, Department of Neurosurgery, Johns Hopkins University School of Medicine; Director, Hunterian Neurosurgical Laboratory, and Neurosurgeon-in-Chief, Johns Hopkins Hospital, Baltimore, Maryland
Brain Tumors: General Considerations; Basic Principles of Cranial Surgery for Brain Tumors

Steven Brem, MD

Professor and Chief, Neurosurgery Service/Director, Neuro-oncology Research Laboratory/NABTT; and Investigator/Program Leader, Neuro-oncology Program, H. Lee Moffitt Cancer Center and Research Institute, Tampa, Florida
Angiogenesis and Brain Tumors

Gavin W. Britz, MD

Assistant Professor, Department of Neurological Surgery, University of Washington School of Medicine; Attending Neurosurgeon, Harborview Medical Center, Seattle, Washington
The Natural History of Unruptured Saccular Cerebral Aneurysms; Traumatic Cerebral Aneurysms Secondary to Penetrating Intracranial Injuries; Endovascular Treatment of Spinal Cord Arteriovenous Malformations; Magnetic Resonance Imaging for Peripheral Nerve Disorders

Carolyn D. Brockington, MD

Attending, Department of Neurology, Herbert and Nell Singer Division, Beth Israel Medical Center, New York, New York
Acute Medical Management of Ischemic Disease and Stroke

Jason A. Brodkey, MD

Staff, Michigan Brain & Spine Institute, Michigan Orthopedic Center, Ypsilanti, Michigan
Glomus Jugulare Tumors

Richard A. Bronen, MD

Associate Professor of Diagnostic Radiology and Neurosurgery, Yale University School of Medicine, New Haven, Connecticut
Preoperative Evaluation for Epilepsy Surgery: Computed Tomography and Magnetic Resonance Imaging

David J. Brooks, MD, DSc

Hartnett Professor of Neurology, Imperial College Faculty of Medicine; Consultant Neurologist, Hammersmith Hospital, London, England
Positron Emission Tomography in Movement Disorders

Jeffrey A. Brown, MD

Professor, Department of Neurosurgery, Wayne State University School of Medicine, Detroit, Michigan
Percutaneous Techniques (Trigeminal Neuralgia)

Robert D. Brown, Jr., MD

Associate Professor of Neurology, Mayo Medical School and Mayo Graduate School of Medicine; Chair, Division of Cerebrovascular Diseases, and Consultant, Department of Neurology, Mayo Clinic, Rochester, Minnesota
Natural History of Intracranial Vascular Malformations

Jeffrey N. Bruce, MD

Associate Professor of Neurological Surgery, Colombia University College of Physicians and Surgeons; Associate Attending in Neurological Surgery, New York Presbyterian Hospital, New York, New York
Pineal Tumors

John M. Buatti, MD

Professor and Head, Department of Radiation Oncology, University of Iowa Roy J. and Lucille A. Carver College of Medicine; Attending, University of Iowa Hospitals and Clinics, Iowa City, Iowa
Radiobiology; Radiotherapy for Benign Skull Base Tumors; Fractionated and Stereotactic Radiation, Extracranial Stereotactic Radiation, Intensity Modulation, and Multileaf Collimation

Robert J. Buchanan, MD

Assistant Professor, Department of Psychiatry, University of California, San Diego, School of Medicine; Chief Resident, Division of Neurosurgery, UCSD Medical Center, San Diego, California
Traumatic Cerebrospinal Fluid Fistulas

Dennis E. Bullard, MD

Associate Clinical Professor, Department of Surgery, Division of Neurosurgery, University of North Carolina at Chapel Hill School of Medicine, Chapel Hill; Chief, Division of Neurosurgery, Rex Hospital, Raleigh, North Carolina
Caudalis Nucleus Dorsal Root Entry Zone Procedure for the Treatment of Intractable Facial Pain

M. Ross Bullock, MD, PhD

Virginia Commonwealth University School of Medicine, Richmond, Virginia
Surgical Management of Traumatic Brain Injury

Kim J. Burchiel, MD

Professor and Chairman, Department of Neurological Surgery, Oregon Health & Science University School of Medicine, Portland, Oregon
Pain: General Historical Considerations; Alternative Surgical Treatments for Trigeminal Neuralgia

Matthew V. Burry, MD

Resident in Neurosurgery, University of Florida College of Medicine, Gainesville, Florida
Vein of Galen Malformations

Richard W. Byrne, MD

Assistant Professor of Neurosurgery, Rush Medical College of Rush University; Attending Neurosurgeon, Rush-Presbyterian-St. Luke's Medical Center, Chicago, Illinois
Multiple Subpial Transection

Jeffrey W. Campbell, MD

Assistant Professor of Neurosurgery, University of South Carolina College of Medicine; Director, Pediatric Neurosurgery, MUSC Children's Hospital, Charleston, South Carolina
Cerebellar Astrocytomas in Children

Martin B. Camins, MD

Clinical Professor of Neurological Surgery, Mount Sinai School of Medicine; Attending Neurosurgeon, Mount Sinai Hospital, New York, New York
Tumors of the Vertebral Axis: Benign, Primary Malignant, and Metastatic Tumors

Michael E. Carey, MD, MS

Professor of Neurosurgery, Louisiana State University School of Medicine in New Orleans, New Orleans, Louisiana
Bullet Wounds to the Brain among Civilians

Carlos Carlotti, MD

Neurosurgeon, Da Universidade de São Paulo, São Paulo, Brazil
Encephaloceles

Thomas Carlstedt, MD, DM

Associate Professor, Karolinska Institute, Stockholm, Sweden; Visiting Professor, Imperial College, London University, London, England; Consultant Orthopaedic Surgeon, Royal National Orthopaedic Hospital, Peripheral Nerve Injury Unit, Stanmore, England
Management of Acute Peripheral Nerve Injuries

Peter Carmel, MD, DMedSci

Professor and Chairman Department of Neurological Surgery, University of Medicine and Dentistry of New Jersey—New Jersey Medical School; Attending, University Hospital, Newark, New Jersey
Craniopharyngiomas; Brain Tumors of Disordered Embryogenesis

Andrew L. Carney, MD

Clinical Associate Professor of Neurosurgery, Radiology, and Orthopedics, University of Illinois at Chicago College of Medicine, Chicago, Illinois
Extracranial Vertebral Artery Disease

Benjamin S. Carson, Sr., MD

Professor of Neurosurgery, Oncology, Plastic Surgery, and Pediatrics, Johns Hopkins University School of Medicine; Director, Pediatric Neurosurgery, Johns Hopkins Hospital, Baltimore, Maryland
Ependymoma; Achondroplasia and Other Dwarfism

L. Philip Carter, MD

Clinical Professor of Neurosurgery, University of Arizona School of Medicine; Private Practice, Western Neurosurgery, Ltd., Tucson, Arizona
Historical Considerations [Vascular]

Kenneth F. Casey, MD

Associate Professor of Neurosurgery, Drexel University School of Medicine, Philadelphia; Attending, Department of Neurosurgery, Allegheny Hospital, Pittsburgh, Pennsylvania
Ablative Surgery for Spasticity

Mauricio Castillo, MD

Professor of Radiology and Chief and Program Director of Neuroradiology, University of North Carolina School of Medicine, Chapel Hill, North Carolina

Webster K. Cavenee, PhD

Professor of Medicine, Cancer Genetics Program, University of California, San Diego, School of Medicine; Director, Ludwig Institute for Cancer Research, La Jolla, California
Molecular and Cytogenetic Techniques

C. Michael Cawley, MD

Assistant Professor, Department of Neurological Surgery, Emory University School of Medicine, Atlanta, Georgia
Treatment of Lateral-Sigmoid, and Sagittal Sinus Dural Anteriovenous Malformations

Stephan Chabardès, MD

Assistant Neurosurgeon, Hôpital Albert Michallon, Grenoble, France
Deep Brain Stimulation for Movement Disorders

Marc C. Chamberlain, MD

Professor of Neurology and Neurosurgery, University of Southern California Keck School of Medicine; Co-Director, Neuro-oncology Program, Norris Comprehensive Cancer Center and Hospital, Los Angeles, California
Neoplastic Meningitis: Diagnosis and Treatment

Amitabha Chanda, MD, MCh

Staff, AMRI-Apollo Hospitals, Kolkata, West Bengal
Chordoma and Chondrosarcoma

Chandrasekar Kalavakonda, MD

Anna Nagar, Chennai, India
Chordoma and Chondrosarcoma

Eric L. Chang, MD

Staff, Department of Radiation Oncology, The University of Texas M.D. Anderson Cancer Center, Houston, Texas
Metastatic Brain Tumors

Steven D. Chang, MD

Assistant Professor, Department of Neurosurgery, Stanford University School of Medicine, Stanford, California
Surgical and Radiosurgical Management of Giant Arteriovenous Malformations; General and Historical Considerations of Radiotherapy and Radiosurgery

Tailoi Chan-Ling, MOptom, PhD

Associate Professor and National Health and Medical Research Council, Senior Research Fellow, Department of Anatomy, University of Sydney Faculty of Medicine, Sydney, New South Wales, Australia
Astrocytes

Paul H. Chapman, MD

Professor of Surgery (Neurosurgery), Harvard Medical School; Neurosurgical Director, Proton Radiosurgery Group, Massachusetts General Hospital, Boston, Massachusetts
Proton Radiosurgery

Ali Charara, PhD

Post-Doctoral Fellow, Department of Neuroscience, University of Pittsburgh School of Medicine, Pittsburgh, Pennsylvania
Anatomy and Synaptic Connectivity of the Basal Ganglia

Fady T. Charbel, MD

Professor and Head, Department of Neurosurgery, University of Illinois at Chicago College of Medicine, Chicago, Illinois
Extracranial Vertebral Artery Disease

Thomas C. Chen, MD, PhD

Assistant Professor of Clinical Surgery, University of Southern California University Hospital, Los Angeles, California
Intradiskal and Percutaneous Treatment of Lumbar Disk Disease

Gopal Chopra, MD

Neurosurgeon, Department of Neurosurgery, St. John Regional Hospital, Saint John, New Brunswick, Canada
Surgical Approaches for Anterior Circulation Aneurysms

Cindy Christian, MD

Assistant Professor of Pediatrics, University of Pennsylvania School of Medicine; Chair, Child Abuse and Neglect Prevention and Director, Child Abuse Program, Children's Hospital of Philadelphia, Philadelphia, Pennsylvania
Child Abuse

Richard C. Clatterbuck, MD, PhD

Assistant Professor, Department of Neurosurgery, Johns Hopkins University School of Medicine; Attending, Johns Hopkins Hospital, Baltimore, Maryland
Surgical Positioning and Exposures for Cranial Procedures; Sarcoidosis, Tuberculosis, and Xanthogranuloma

Elizabeth B. Claus, PhD, MD

Associate Professor, Department of Epidemiology and Public Health, Yale University School of Medicine, New Haven, Connecticut
Scalp Tumors; Shunt Infection

Charles S. Cobbs, MD

Associate Professor of Neurological Surgery, Department of Surgery, University of Alabama School of Medicine; Attending, Kirklin Clinic, UAB Medical Center, Birmingham, Alabama
Meningeal Hemangiopericytoma

Kimberly Peele Cockerham, MD

Assistant Professor, Drexel University School of Medicine, Philadelphia; Director, Neuro-ophthalmology, Orbital Disease and Reconstruction, Allegheny General Hospital, Pittsburgh, Pennsylvania
Orbital Tumors

P. H. Cogen, MD

Chairman, Department of Neurosurgery, Children's National Medical Center, Washington, DC
Occult Spinal Dysraphism and the Tethered Spinal Cord

Alan R. Cohen, MD

Professor of Neurological Surgery and Pediatrics, Case Western Reserve University School of Medicine; Chief, Pediatric Neurosurgery, Rainbow Babies and Children's Hospital, Cleveland, Ohio
Myelomeningocele and Myelocystocele; Intervertebral Disk Disease in Children

Wendy A. Cohen, MD

Professor of Radiology and Neurosurgery, University of Washington School of Medicine; Chief, Neuroradiology, Harborview Medical Center, Seattle, Washington
Radiology of the Spine

Domingos Coiteiro, MD

Staff, Dobelle Institute, Lisboa, Portugal
Revascularization Techniques for Complex Aneurysms and Skull Base Tumors

Antony Colantonio, MD

Pain Fellow, Department of Anesthesiology, Oregon Health & Science University, Portland, Oregon
Management of Pain by Anesthetic Techniques

Andrew J. Cole, MD

Associate Professor of Neurology, Harvard Medical School; Associate Neurologist, Massachusetts General Hospital, Boston, Massachusetts
Identification of Candidates for Epilepsy Surgery

John J. Collins, MD

Assistant Professor of Neurosurgery, Loma Linda University School of Medicine; Chief, Pediatric Neurosurgery, Loma Linda University Children's Medical Center and Loma Linda University Medical Center, Loma Linda, California
Nonsyndromic Craniosynostosis and Abnormalities of Head Shape

Edward S. Connolly, MD

Attending, Ochsner Clinic Foundation, New Orleans, Louisiana
Metabolic and Other Nondegenerative Causes of Low Back Pain

E. Sander Connolly, Jr., MD

Irving Assistant Professor, Department of Neurological Surgery, Columbia University College of Physicians and Surgeons; New York, New York
Techniques for Deep Hypothermic Circulatory Arrest

Stephen W. Coons, MD

Staff, Division of Neuropathology, Barrow Neurological Institute, Phoenix, Arizona
Proliferation Markers in the Evaluation of Gliomas

James J. Corbett, MD

McCarty Professor and Chairman, Department of Neurology, and Professor of Ophthalmology, University of Mississippi School of Medicine, Jackson, Mississippi; Lecturer in Ophthalmology, Harvard Medical School, Boston, Massachusetts
Neuro-ophthalmology

Daniel M. Corcos, PhD

Professor, Department of Kinesiology, College of Associated Health Professions, University of Illinois at Chicago; Director, Clinical Motor Control Laboratory, Department of Neurological Sciences, Rush-Presbyterian-St. Luke's Medical Center, Chicago, Illinois
Management of Spasticity by Central Nervous System Infusion Techniques

G. Rees Cosgrove, MD

Associate Professor of Surgery, Harvard Medical School; Associate Visiting Neurosurgeon, Massachusetts General Hospital, Boston, Massachusetts
Identification of Candidates for Epilepsy Surgery; Neurosurgery of Psychiatric Disorders

Neil R. Crawford, PhD

Coordinator, Spinal Biomechanics, Barrow Neurological Institute, Phoenix; Adjunct Assistant Professor, Department of Bioengineering, Arizona State University, Tempe, Arizona
Basic Principles of Spinal Internal Fixation

Kerry R. Crone, MD

Associate Professor of Neurosurgery, Director of Graduate Education in Pediatric Neurosurgery, University of Cincinnati College of Medicine; Director, Department of Pediatric Neurosurgery, Cincinnati Children's Hospital Medical Center, Cincinnati, Ohio
Neuroendoscopy

Raimondo D'Ambrosio, PhD

Associate Professor of Neurosurgery, University of Washington; Seattle, Washington
Basic Science of Post-traumatic Epilepsy

Carlos A. David, MD

Director, Cerebrovascular and Skull Base Surgery, Lahey Clinic, Burlington, Massachusetts
Intracranial Occlusion Disease and Moyamoya

Arthur L. Day, MD

Professor of Neurosurgery, Program Director, and Associate Chairman, Department of Neurosurgery, Harvard Medical School; Director, Cerebrovascular Center, Brigham and Women's Hospital, Boston, Massachusetts
Surgical Treatment of Intracavernous and Paraclinoid Internal Carotid Artery Aneurysms

J. Diaz Day, MD

Associate Professor of Neurosurgery, Drexel University School of Medicine, Philadelphia; Director, Center for Cerebrovascular Surgery and Stroke, Allegheny General Hospital, Pittsburgh, Pennsylvania
Basilar Trunk Aneurysms; Cavernous Carotid Fistulas

A. Lee Dellon, MD

Professor of Plastic Surgery, Johns Hopkins University School of Medicine and University of Maryland School of Medicine, Baltimore, Maryland; Professor of Plastic Surgery and Neurosurgery, University of Arizona College of Medicine, Tucson, Arizona; Private Practice, Institute for Peripheral Nerve Surgery, Baltimore, Maryland, and Institute for Peripheral Nerve Surgery: Southwest, Tucson, Arizona
History of Peripheral Nerve Surgery

Mahlon R. Delong, MD

Professor and Chairman, Department of Neurology, Emory University School of Medicine, Atlanta, Georgia
Rationale for Surgical Interventions in Movement Disorders

Franco Demonte, MD

Associate Professor, Department of Neurosurgery, University of Texas–Houston Medical School; Clinical Associate Professor, Department of Neurosurgery, Baylor College of Medicine; Attending, The University of Texas M.D. Anderson Cancer Center, Houston, Texas
Neoplasms of the Paranasal Sinuses

Robert J. Dempsey, MD

Professor and Chair, Department of Neurosurgery, University of Wisconsin Medical School; Attending, University of Wisconsin Hospitals and Clinics, Madison, Wisconsin
Recurrent Carotid Stenosis

Milind Deogaonkar, MD

Department of Neurosurgery, University of Arizona Health Sciences Center, Tucson, Arizona
Historical Considerations [Vascular]

Antonio A. F. De Salles, MD, PhD

Professor, Division of Neurosurgery, Department of Surgery, David Geffen School of Medicine at UCLA; Co-Director, Epilepsy Surgery Program, West LA Veterans Administration Medical Center, Los Angeles, California
Molecular Imaging of the Brain with Positron Emission Tomography; Sympathectomy for Pain

Nicolas De Tribolet, MD

Professor, University of Geneva Faculty of Medicine; Attending, Department of Neurosurgery, University Hospital, Geneva, Switzerland
Aspects of Immunology Applicable to Brain Tumor Pathogenesis and Treatment

Paul W. Detwiler, MD, PhD

Staff, Tyler Neurosurgical Group, Tyler, Texas
Infratentorial Cavernous Malformations; Classification of Spinal Cord Vascular Lesions

Harel Deutch, MD

Instructor, Department of Neurosurgery, Emory University School of Medicine; Spinal Surgery Fellow, Department of Neurosurgery, Emory University Hospital, Atlanta, Georgia
Complication Avoidance in Neurosurgery

Paul T. Diamond, MD

Associate Professor, Department of Physical Medicine and Rehabilitation, University of Virginia School of Medicine, Charlottesville, Virginia
Rehabilitation and Prognosis after Traumatic Brain Injury

Mark S. Dias, MD

Staff, Department of Neurosurgery, Section of Neurosurgery, Milton Hershey Medical Center, Pittsburgh, Pennsylvania
Normal and Abnormal Embryology of the Spinal Cord and Spine

Curtis A. Dickman, MD

Associate Chief, Spine Section, and Director, Spinal Research, Division of Neurological Surgery, Barrow Neurological Institute, Phoenix, Arizona
Basic Principles of Spinal Internal Fixation; Anterior Cervical Instrumentation; Occipitocervical Fusion; Thoracoscopic Approaches to the Spine

Pierre-Yves Dietrich, MD

Associate Professor, University of Geneva Faculty of Medicine; Head, Laboratory of Tumor Immunology, Division of Oncology, University Hospital, Geneva, Switzerland
Aspects of Immunology Applicable to Brain Tumor Pathogenesis and Treatment

Francesco DiMeco, MD

Faculty Member, Department of Neurosurgery, Istituto Nazionale Neurologico, Milan, Italy
Brain Tumors during Pregnancy

Jacques E. Dion, MD

Professor of Neuroradiology and Neurosurgery, Department of Radiology, Emory University School of Medicine; Director, Interventional Neuroradiology, Emory University Hospital, Atlanta, Georgia
Treatment of Lateral-Sigmoid and Sagittal Sinus Dural Arteriovenous Malformations

Carl B. Dodrill, PhD

Professor, Departments of Neurology, Neurological Surgery, and Psychiatry and Behavioral Sciences, University of Washington School of Medicine; Associate Director, Regional Epilepsy Center, Harborview Medical Center, Seattle, Washington
Neuropsychological Assessment of the Neurosurgical Patient; The Intracarotid Amobarbital Procedure or Wada Test

Aclan Dogan, MD

Fellow, Division of Neurosurgery, Louisiana State University Health Sciences Center, Shreveport, Louisiana
Recurrent Carotid Stenosis

Vinko V. Dolenc, MD, PhD

Professor of Neurosurgery, Medical School at Ljubljana University; Head, Neurosurgical Department, University Hospital Center, Ljubljana, Slovenia
Skull and Skull Base Tumors

Egon M. R. Doppenberg, MD

Resident, Department of Neurosurgery, Medical College of Virginia Hospitals, Richmond, Virginia
Pediatric Head Injury

Zeena Dorai, MD

Resident, Department of Neurosurgery, University of Texas Southwestern Medical Center at Dallas, Dallas, Texas
Posterior Fossa Arteriovenous Malformations

Stephen E. Doran, MD

Clinical Assistant Professor of Neurosurgery, Department of Surgery, University of Nebraska College of Medicine; Neurosurgeon, University Medical Associates and Midwest Neurosurgery, Omaha, Nebraska

Brain Tumors: Population-Based Epidemiology, Environmental Risk Factors, and Genetic and Hereditary Syndromes

Catherine J. Doty, MD

Clinical Assistant Professor in Pediatrics, Washington University School of Medicine; Attending, St. Louis Children's Hospital, St. Louis, Missouri

Cerebral Palsy: An Overview

James M. Drake, MBBCh, MSc

Associate Professor, Division of Neurosurgery, University of Toronto Faculty of Medicine; Neurosurgeon, The Hospital for Sick Children, Toronto, Ontario, Canada

Physiology of Cerebrospinal Fluid Shunt Devices

Ann-Christine Duhaime, MD

Professor of Neurosurgery, Dartmouth Medical School; Director, Pediatric Neurosurgery, Dartmouth-Hitchock Medical Center, Lebanon, New Hampshire

Child Abuse

Christopher M. Duma, MD

Medical Director, Hoag Gamma Knife Program, Hoag Memorial Hospital Presbyterian, Newport Beach, California

Functional Radiosurgery

Charles Duncan, MD

Professor and Head, Section of Pediatric Neurosurgery, Department of Neurosurgery, Yale University School of Medicine; Chief, Pediatric Neurosurgery, Yale–New Haven Hospital, New Haven, Connecticut

Shunt Infection

Marc E. Eichler, MD

Clinical Instructor, Harvard Medical School; Associate Surgeon, Department of Neurosurgery, Brigham and Women's Hospital and Boston Children's Hospital, Boston, Massachusetts

Cervical Spine Trauma

F. J. Eismont, MD

Vice Chairman, Department of Orthopedics and Rehabilitation, University of Miami School of Medicine; Orthopedic Surgeon, Jackson Memorial Hospital, Miami, Florida

Diagnosis and Management of Thoracic Spine Fractures

Elizabeth A. Eldredge, MD

Instructor in Anesthesia, Harvard Medical School; Staff Anesthesiologist, Children's Hospital, Boston, Massachusetts

Neuroanesthesia in Children

Hikmat El-Kadi, MD, PhD

Clinical Associate Professor of Neurosurgery, University of Pittsburgh School of Medicine, Pittsburgh Pennsylvania

Brain Death

Richard G. Ellenbogen, MD

Associate Professor, Department of Neurological Surgery, University of Washington School of Medicine; Chief and Theodore S. Roberts Endowed Chair, Division of Pediatric Neurological Surgery, Children's Hospital and Regional Medical Center, Seattle, Washington

Diagnosis and Management of Juvenile Angiofibroma; Choroid Plexus Tumors; Craniofacial Trauma

J. Paul Elliott, MD

Assistant Professor, Department of Neurosurgery, University of Colorado School of Medicine; Chief, Neurosurgery, Denver Health Medical Center, Denver, Colorado

Traumatic Cerebrovascular Injury

Syed A. Enam, MD, PhD

Staff Physician, Department of Neurosurgery, Henry Ford Hospital, Detroit, Michigan

Invasion in Malignant Glioma

Fred J. Epstein, MD

Professor of Neurosurgery, Albert Einstein School of Medicine of Yeshiva University, Bronx; Attending Physician, Institute for Neurology and Neurosurgery, Beth Israel Medical Center, New York, New York

Intraspinal Tumors in Infants and Children

Nancy E. Epstein, MD

Clinical Professor of Neurological Surgery, Albert Einstein College of Medicine of Yeshiva University, Bronx; Adjunct Clinical Associate Professor of Surgery/Neurosurgery, Cornell University, Joan and Sanford I. Weill Medical College, New York; Attending Neurosurgeon, North Shore–Long Island Jewish Health System, Manhasset and New Hyde Park, and Winthrop University Hospital, Mineola, New York

Lumbar Spinal Stenosis

Joseph Eskridge, MD

Professor, Departments of Radiology and Neurosurgery, University of Washington School of Medicine, Seattle, Washington

Endovascular Treatment of Spinal Cord Arteriovenous Malformations

Matthew G. Ewend, MD

Assistant Professor of Neurosurgery and Section Chief of Neuro-oncology Clinical Research, University of North Carolina Lineberger Comprehensive Cancer Center, University of North Carolina, Chapel Hill, North Carolina
Meningeal Sarcoma

Gary G. Ferguson, MD, PhD

Professor of Neurosurgery, Department of Clinical Neurological Sciences (Neurosurgery), University of Western Ontario Faculty of Medicine; Attending Neurosurgeon, London Health Sciences Centre, London, Ontario, Canada
Distal Anterior Cerebral Artery Aneurysms

Richard G. Fessler, MD, PhD

Professor of Neurosurgery, Department of Surgery, University of Chicago, Division of the Biological Sciences, Pritzker School of Medicine; Chief, Section of Neurosurgery, University of Chicago Hospital and Clinics, Chicago, Illinois
Benign Extradural Lesions of the Dorsal Spine; Posterior Lumbar Instrumentation

Matthew E. Fewel, MD

Instructor, Department of Neurosurgery, University of Michigan Medical School, Ann Arbor, Michigan
Skull Tumors

Paul E. Fewings, MBBS

Consultant Neurosurgeon, Hull Royal Infirmary, Hull, England
Medical Management of Chronic Pain

J. Max Findlay, MD, PhD

Clinical Professor, Division of Neurosurgery, University of Alberta Faculty of Medicine; Neurosurgeon, University of Alberta Hospital, Edmonton, Alberta, Canada
Cerebral Vasospasm

Andrew D. Fine, MD

Staff, Neurological Associates, PA, Sarasota, Florida
Benign Extradural Lesions of the Dorsal Spine

Howard A. Fine, MD

Branch Chief, Neuro-Oncology, National Cancer Institute, National Institute of Health, Bethesda, Maryland
Principles of Chemotherapy

Jill B. Firszt, PhD

Assistant Professor and Director, Koss Cochlear Implant Program, Department of Otolaryngology and Communication Sciences, Medical College of Wisconsin; Attending, Froedtert & Medical College Hospital and Children's Hospital of Wisconsin, Milwaukee, Wisconsin
Neuro-otology

Michael T. Fitch, MD, PhD

Resident in Emergency Medicine, Carolina Medical Center, Charlotte, North Carolina
Cellular and Molecular Mechanisms Mediating Injury and Recovery in the Nervous System

James D. Fleck, MD

Clinical Assistant Professor, Department of Neurology, Indiana University School of Medicine, Indianapolis, Indiana
Carotid Occlusive Disease: Natural History and Medical Management

Ian G. Fleetwood, MD

Chief Resident, Department of Neurosurgery, Foothills Medical Centre, Calgary, Alberta, Canada
Hemorrhagic Disease: Arteriovascular Malformations

Kelly D. Flemming, MD

Assistant Professor, Mayo Graduate School of Medicine; Consultant in Neurology, Mayo Clinic, Rochester, Minnesota
Natural History of Intracranial Vascular Malformations

Susan Fletcher, MB

Acting Assistant Professor of Anesthesiology, University of Washington School of Medicine; Attending Anesthesiologist, Harborview Medical Center, Seattle, Washington
Anesthesia: Preoperative Evaluation

John C. Flickinger, MD

Professor of Radiation Oncology and Neurological Surgery, University of Pittsburgh School of Medicine, Pittsburgh, Pennsylvania
Fractionated Radiotherapy for Pituitary Tumors

Nancy Foldvary, DO

Staff Neurologist, Cleveland Clinic, Cleveland, Ohio
[Surgical Treatment of Epilepsy in Children] Recognition of Surgical Candidates and the Presurgical Evaluation

Kenneth A. Follett, MD, PhD

Professor, Department of Neurosurgery, University of Iowa College of Medicine, Iowa City, Iowa
Neurosurgical Management of Intractable Pain

Kelly D. Foote, MD

Assistant Professor, Department of Neurosurgery, University of Florida School of Medicine, Gainesville, Florida
Radiosurgery for Arteriovenous Malformations

Daryl R. Fourney, MD

Assistant Professor, Division of Neurosurgery, University of Saskatchewan Faculty of Medicine; Attending, Royal University Hospital, Saskatoon, Saskatchewan, Canada
Neoplasms of the Paranasal Sinuses

Valerie Fraix, MD, PhD

Assistant Neurologist, Hôpital Albert Michallon, Grenoble, France
Deep Brain Stimulation for Movement Disorders

Paul C. Francel, MD, PhD

Associate Professor, Department of Neurosurgery, University of Oklahoma College of Medicine, Oklahoma City, Oklahoma
Mild Brain Injury in Children, including Skull Fractures and Growing Fractures

Itzhak Fried, MD, PhD

Associate Professor of Neurosurgery and Psychiatry and Biobehavioral Sciences, David Geffen School of Medicine at UCLA, Los Angeles, California; Associate Professor of Neurosurgery, Sackler School of Medicine, Tel-Aviv University, Tel-Aviv, Israel; Director, of Epilepsy Surgery, and Co-Director, UCLA Seizure Disorder Center, UCLA Medical Center, Los Angeles, California; Director, Functional Neurosurgery Unit, Tel-Aviv Medical Center, Tel-Aviv, Israel
Surgery for Extratemporal Lobe Epilepsy

Jonathan A. Friedman, MD

Chief Resident, Department of Neurologic Surgery, Mayo Clinic, Rochester, Minnesota
Middle Cerebral Artery Aneurysms

William A. Friedman, MD

Professor and Chair, Department of Neurosurgery, University of Florida; Attending, Shand's Hospital, Gainesville, Florida
Radiobiology; Radiosurgery for Arteriovenous Malformations; Fractionated and Stereotactic Radiation, Extracranial Stereotactic Radiation, Intensity Modulation, and Multileaf Collimation

David M. Frim, MD, PhD

Assistant Professor of Surgery and Pediatrics, University of Chicago, Division of the Biological Sciences, Pritzker School of Medicine; Chief, Pediatric Neurosurgery, University of Chicago Children's Hospital, Chicago, Illinois
Benign Tumors of the Vertebral Column in Children

Michael J. Fritsch, MD

Fellow in Neurological Surgery, University of Miami School of Medicine, Miami, Florida
Surgical Management of Supratentorial Arteriovenous Malformation

Herbert E. Fuchs, MD, PhD

Associate Professor, Department of Surgery, Division of Neurosurgery, Duke University School of Medicine, Durham, North Carolina
Benign Tumors of the Skull, including Fibrous Dysplasia

Gregory N. Fuller, MD, PhD

Professor of Pathology, University of Texas–Houston Medical School; Chief, Section of Neuropathology, The University of Texas M.D. Anderson Cancer Center, Houston, Texas
Brain Tumors: An Overview of Histopathologic Classification

Aurelie Funkiewiez, MA

Staff, Department of Neurology, Centre Hospitalier Universitaire de Grenoble, Grenoble, France
Deep Brain Stimulation for Movement Disorders

Michael R. Gallagher, MD

Clinical Assistant Professor, Department of Surgery, University of Tennessee, Chattanooga, College of Medicine; Staff Neurosurgeon, Baroness Erlanger Hospital and Memorial Hospital, Chattanooga, Tennessee
Spondyloarthropathies, including Ankylosing Spondylitis

Ira M. Garonzik, MD

Neurosurgery Fellow, Department of Neurosurgery, Johns Hopkins Hospital, Baltimore, Maryland
Thalamotomy for Tremor

Hugh Garton, MD, MHSc

Assistant Professor, Department of Neurosurgery, University of Michigan Medical School, Ann Arbor, Michigan
Neurosurgical Epidemiology and Outcomes Assessment

Marilyn L. Gates, MD

Assistant Professor, Uniformed Services University of the Health Sciences, Medicine; Assistant Director, Complex Spine Surgery, National Naval Medical Center Hospital, Bethesda, Maryland
Bone Metabolism as It Relates to Spinal Disease and Treatment

Stephen S. Gebarski, MD

Professor, Department of Radiology, Division of Neuroradiology, University of Michigan Medical School, Ann Arbor, Michigan
Skull Tumors

Christopher C. Getch, MD

Assistant Professor, Department of Neurological Surgery, Northwestern University Feinberg School of Medicine, Chicago, Illinois
Basilar Apex and Posterior Cerebral Artery Aneurysms

Sanjay Ghosh, MD

Staff, Senta Clinic, Division of Skull Base Surgery, San Diego, California
Ventricular Tumors; Cavernous Carotid Fistulas

Steven L. Giannotta, MD

Professor of Neurological Surgery, University of Southern California Keck School of Medicine; Chief, Neurosurgery, and Medical Director, USC University Hospital, Los Angeles, California
Basilar Trunk Aneurysms

Philip L. Gildenberg, MD, PhD

Clinical Professor of Neurosurgery and Radiation Oncology, Baylor College of Medicine; Clinical Professor of Psychiatry, University of Texas–Houston Medical School, Houston, Texas
Brainstem Procedures for Management of Pain

Howard J. Ginsberg, MD

Senior Resident, University of Toronto, Division of Neurosurgery, Toronto, Ontario, Canada
Physiology of Cerebrospinal Fluid Shunt Devices

Ziya L. Gokaslan, MD

Clinical Assistant Professor, Department of Neurosurgery, University of Texas–Houston Medical School; Attending, The University of Texas M.D. Anderson Cancer Center, Houston, Texas
Treatment of Disk and Ligamentous Diseases of the Cervical Spine

Joel Goldwein, MD

Professor of Radiation Oncology, University of Pennsylvania School of Medicine; Chief, Pediatric Radiation Oncology, Children's Hospital of Philadelphia, Philadelphia, Pennsylvania
Intracranial Ependymomas

Robert Goodkin, MD

Associate Professor, Department of Neurological Surgery, University of Washington School of Medicine; Chief, Neurosurgical Section, Veterans Administration Puget Sound Health Care System, Seattle, Washington
Legal Issues; General Principles of Operative Positioning; Magnetic Resonance Imaging for Peripheral Nerve Disorders

James Tait Goodrich, MD, PhD

Professor of Clinical Neurological Surgery, Pediatrics, and Plastic and Reconstructive Surgery, Leo Davidoff Department of Neurological Surgery, Albert Einstein College of Medicine of Yeshiva University; Director, Division of Pediatric Neurosurgery, Montefiore Medical Center, Bronx, New York
Neurological Surgery in Childhood: General and Historical Considerations

John P. Gorecki, MD

Clinical Assistant Professor, The University of Kansas Medical School, Wichita, Kansas
Dorsal Root Entry Zone and Brainstem Ablative Procedures

M. Sean Grady, MD

Charles Harrison Frazier Professor and Chair of the Department of Neurosurgery, University of Pennsylvania School of Medicine, Philadelphia, Pennsylvania
Cellular Basis of Injury and Recovery from Trauma; Initial Resuscitation and Patient Evaluation; Modern Neurotraumatology: A Brief Historical Review

Sylvie Grand, MD, PhD

Assistant Professor of Biophysics and Radiology, University Joseph Fourier; Staff Neuroradiologist, Hôpital Albert Michallon, Grenoble, France
Deep Brain Stimulation for Movement Disorders

Gerald A. Grant, MD

Acting Instructor, Department of Neurological Surgery, University of Washington School of Medicine; Attending, Children's Hospital and Regional Medical Center, Seattle, Washington
The Blood-Brain Barrier; Diagnosis and Management of Juvenile Angiofibroma; General Principles in Evaluating and Treating Peripheral Nerve Injuries; Magnetic Resonance Imaging for Peripheral Nerve Disorders

B. A. Green, MD

Professor and Chairman, Department of Neurosurgical Surgery, University of Miami School of Medicine; Chief, Department of Neurosurgery, Jackson Memorial Medical Center, Miami, Florida
Diagnosis and Management of Thoracic Spine Fractures

Michael W. Groff, MD

Director, Spinal Surgery, Indiana University Hospital, Indianapolis, Indiana
Concepts and Mechanisms of Biomechanics

Andreas Gruber, MD

Professor, Department of Neurosurgery, University of Vienna Medical School, Vienna, Austria
Embolization of Arteriovenous Malformations as a Primary Treatment Modality

Joseph S Gruss, MBBCh

Professor, Department of Surgery; Adjunct Professor, Department of Neurosurgery; and Marlys C. Larson Professor and Endowed Chair in Pediatric Craniofacial Surgery, University of Washington School of Medicine; Chief, Division of Craniofacial, Plastic and Reconstructive Surgery, Children's Hospital and Regional Medical Center; Attending Surgeon, Harborview Medical Center, Seattle, Washington
Craniofacial Trauma

Michael Guarnieri, PhD, MPH

Research Associate, Johns Hopkins University School of Medicine, Baltimore, Maryland
Ependymoma

James D. Guest, MD, PhD

Assistant Professor of Neurological Surgery, University of Miami School of Medicine; Scientific Faculty, The Miami Project to Cure Paralysis; Attending Neurosurgeon, University of Miami Hospital and Clinics and Miami Veterans Administration Medical Center, Miami, Florida
Biologic Strategies for Central Nervous System Repair

Abhijit Guha, MSc, MD

Associate Professor, Division of Neurosurgery, University of Toronto Faculty of Medicine; Attending Neurosurgeon, University Health Network; Co-Director, Arthur and Sonia Labatts Brain Tumor Center, The Hospital for Sick Children, Toronto, Ontario, Canada
Management of Peripheral Nerve Tumors

Mary Kay Gumerlock, MD

Professor of Neurosurgery, University of Oklahoma, College of Medicine, Oklahoma City, Oklahoma
Epidermoid, Dermoid, and Neurenteric Cysts

Murat Gunel, MD

Assistant Professor of Neurosurgery, Yale University School of Medicine, New Haven, Connecticut
Surgical Management of Supratentorial Cavernous Malformations

Kern H. Guppy, MD, PhD

Assistant Professor of Neurosurgery, University of Illinois at Chicago College of Medicine, Chicago, Illinois
Extracranial Vertebral Artery Disease

Nalin Gupta, MD, PhD

Assistant Professor, Department of Neurosurgery, University of California, San Francisco, School of Medicine, San Francisco, California
Benign Tumors of the Vertebral Column in Children

Lee R. Guterman, MD, PhD

Assistant Professor, Department of Neurosurgery and Co-Director Toshiba Stroke Research Center, University at Buffalo; Neurosurgeon, Kaleida Health, Buffalo, New York
Endovascular Treatment of Aneurysms

Barton L. Guthrie, MD

Associate Professor of Neurological Surgery, Department of Surgery, University of Alabama School of Medicine; Co-Director, Health South/UAB Gamma Knife Program, Health South Medical Center, Birmingham, Alabama
Meningeal Hemangiopericytoma

P. W. Gutin, MD

Chief, Department of Neurosurgery, Memorial Sloan-Kettering Cancer Center, New York, New York
Interstitial and Intracavitary Irradiation of Brain Tumors

Eldad Hadar, MD

Assistant Professor, Department of Surgery, Division of Neurosurgery, University of North Carolina at Chapel Hill School of Medicine, Chapel Hill, North Carolina
General and Historical Considerations of Epilepsy Surgery

Georges F. Haddad, MD

Clinical Assistant Professor, Department of Neurosurgery, American University of Beirut, Beirut, Lebanon

Regis W. Haid, MD

Associate Professor, Department of Neurological Surgery, Emory University School of Medicine, Atlanta, Georgia
Spondyloarthropathies, including Ankylosing Spondylitis

Stephen J. Haines, MD

Professor and Chair, Department of Neurological Surgery, Medical University of South Carolina College of Medicine, Charleston, South Carolina
Neurosurgical Epidemiology and Outcomes Assessment

H. Bruce Hamilton, MD

Private Practice, Neurosurgery, Waco, Texas
Metabolic and Other Nondegenerative Causes of Low Back Pain

Mark G. Hamilton, MDCM

Associate Professor of Neurosurgery, Department of Clinical Neurosciences, University of Calgary Faculty of Medicine; Director, Pediatric Neurosciences, Alberta Children's Hospital, Foothills Medical Centre, Calgary, Alberta, Canada
Hemorrhagic Disease: Arteriovascular Malformations

Thomas A. Hammeke, PhD

Professor, Department of Neurology (Neuropsychology), Medical College of Wisconsin, Milwaukee, Wisconsin
Functional Magnetic Resonance Imaging in Epilepsy Surgery

Patrick P. Han, MD

Chief Resident, Division of Neurological Surgery, Barrow Neurological Institute, Phoenix, Arizona
Epidemiology and Natural History of Cavernous Malformations

Russell W. Hardy, Jr., MD

Professor of Neurological Surgery, Department of Surgery, Case Western Reserve University School of Medicine; Co-Director, University Hospitals Spine Center, Cleveland, Ohio
Treatment of Disk Disease of the Lumbar Spine

Raymond I. Haroun, MD

Instructor, Department of Neurosurgery, Johns Hopkins University School of Medicine, Baltimore, Maryland
Anterior Communicating Artery and Anterior Cerebral Artery Aneurysms; Achondroplasia and Other Dwarfism

Mark R. Harrigan, MD

Lecturer, Department of Neurosurgery, University of Michigan Medical School, Ann Arbor, Michigan
Pregnancy and Treatment of Vascular Disease

Griffith R. Harsh IV, MD

Professor, of Neurosurgery, Stanford University School of Medicine; Director, Stanford Brain Tumor Center, Stanford, California
Cerebral Lymphoma

Jaimie M. Henderson, MD

Associate Staff, Department of Neurosurgery, Cleveland Clinic, Cleveland, Ohio
Medical Management of Chronic Pain

Jeffrey S. Henn, MD

Assistant Professor, Department of Neurological Surgery, University of Florida College of Medicine, Gainesville, Florida
Giant Aneurysms

Roberto C. Heros, MD

Professor, Department of Neurological Surgery, University of Miami School of Medicine; Attending Neurosurgeon, Jackson Memorial Hospital, Miami, Florida
Surgical Management of Supratentorial Arteriovenous Malformation

Karl Herrup, PhD

Professor of Neurosciences and Neurology, Case Western Reserve University School of Medicine; Director, University Memory and Aging Center, University Hospitals of Cleveland, Cleveland, Ohio
Neurons and Neuroglia

Jason Heth, MD

Chief Resident, Department of Neurosurgery, University of Iowa Hospitals and Clinics, Iowa City, Iowa
Tumors of the Craniovertebral Junction

Julian T. Hoff, MD

Professor and Chair, Department of Neurosurgery, University of Michigan Medical School, Ann Arbor, Michigan
Brain Edema and Tumor-Host Interactions; Skull Tumors; Treatment of Intractable Vertigo

Dominique Hoffmann, MD

Staff Neurosurgeon, Hôpital Albert Michallon, Grenoble, France
Deep Brain Stimulation for Movement Disorders

Brian L. Hoh, MD

Clinical Fellow in Surgery, Harvard Medical School; Resident, Neurosurgical Service, Massachusetts General Hospital, Boston, Massachusetts
Vertebral Artery, Posterior Inferior Cerebellar Artery, and Vertebrobasilar Junction Aneurysms

Anna Depold Hohler, MD

Chief, Neurology Clinic, Madigan Army Medical Center, Tacoma, Washington
Approach to Movement Disorders

Eric C. Holland, MD, PhD

Staff, Departments of Surgery (Neurosurgery), Neurology, and Cell Biology, Memorial Sloan-Kettering Cancer Center, New York, New York
Molecular Genetics and the Development of Targets for Glioma Therapy

James P. Hollowell, MD

Associate Professor of Neurosurgery, Medical College of Wisconsin; Staff, Neuroscience Research Laboratory and Veterans Affairs Medical Center, Milwaukee, Wisconsin
Concepts and Mechanisms of Biomechanics; Bone Metabolism as It Relates to Spinal Disease and Treatment

Mark D. Holmes, MD

Associate Professor of Neurology, University of Washington School of Medicine; Director of EEG, Regional Epilepsy Center, Harborview Medical Center, Seattle, Washington
Approaches to the Diagnosis and Classification of Epilepsy

John Honeycutt, MD

Assistant Professor, Department of Neurosurgery, University of Oklahoma College of Medicine, Oklahoma City, Oklahoma
Mild Brain Injury in Children, including Skull Fractures and Growing Fractures

L. Nelson Hopkins, MD

Professor and Chairman, Department of Neurosurgery, and Professor of Radiology, School of Medicine and Biomedical Sciences, State University of New York at Buffalo, Buffalo, New York
Endovascular Treatment of Aneurysms

Frank P. K. Hsu, MD, PhD

Assistant Professor of Neurosurgery, Department of Surgery, Loma Linda University School of Medicine, Loma Linda, California
Cerebral Venous and Sinus Thrombosis

Sherwin E. Hua, MD, PhD

Resident and Fellow, Department of Neurosurgery, Johns Hopkins Hospital, Baltimore, Maryland
Sarcoidosis, Tuberculosis, and Xanthogranuloma; Thalamotomy for Tremor

Alan R. Hudson, MBChB

Professor, Department of Surgery, University of Toronto Faculty of Medicine, Toronto, Ontario, Canada
Management of Peripheral Nerve Tumors

Robin P. Humphreys, MD

Emeritus Professor, Department of Surgery, University of Toronto Faculty of Medicine, Division of Neurosurgery, The Hospital for Sick Children, Toronto, Ontario, Canada
Arteriovenous Malformations and Intracranial Aneurysms in Children

John Huston III, MD

Assistant Professor of Radiology, Mayo Medical School; Consultant in Neurologic Radiology, Mayo Clinic, Rochester, Minnesota
Magnetic Resonance Angiography

Mark Iantosca, MD

Assistant Clinical Professor, Department of Neurosurgery, University of Connecticut School of Medicine; Director, Pediatric Neurosurgery, Connecticut Children's Medical Center, Farmington, Connecticut
Encephaloceles

Koji Ihara, MD

Attending, Department of Neurosurgery, Toronto Western Hospital, University Health Network, Toronto, Ontario, Canada
Surgical Approaches for Anterior Circulation Aneurysms

Robert J. Jackson, MD

Department of Neurosurgery, Baylor College of Medicine; Attending, The University of Texas M.D. Anderson Cancer Center, Houston, Texas; Surgeon, Massoudi and Jackson Neurosurgical Medical Associates, Laguna Hills, California
Treatment of Disk and Ligamentous Diseases of the Cervical Spine

Deane B. Jacques, MD

Medical Director, The California Neuroscience Institute, Oxnard, California
Functional Radiosurgery

George I. Jallo, MD

Assistant Professor, Departments of Neurosurgery and Pediatrics, Albert Einstein School of Medicine of Yeshiva University, Bronx; Attending Physician, Institute for Neurology and Neurosurgery, Beth Israel Medical Center, New York, New York
Intraspinal Tumors in Infants and Children

C. David James, PhD

Professor of Laboratory Medicine, Mayo Medical School, Rochester, Minnesota
Molecular and Cytogenetic Techniques

John A. Jane, Sr., MD, PhD

Chairman, Department of Neurosurgery, University of Virginia School of Medicine, Charlottesville, Virginia
Esthesioneuroblastoma

Damir Janigro, PhD

Director, Cerebrovascular Center, Department of Neurosurgery, Cleveland Clinic, Cleveland, Ohio
The Blood-Brain Barrier; Electrophysiologic Properties of the Mammalian Nervous System

Peter J. Jannetta, MD

Professor of Neurosurgery, Drexel University College of Medicine, Philadelphia; Vice Chairman, Department of Neurosurgery, Allegheny General Hospital, Pittsburgh, Pennsylvania
Trigeminal Neuralgia: Microvascular Decompression of the Trigeminal Nerve for Tic Douloureux

Abel D. Jarell, MD

CPD Medical Corps, Department of the Army, Washington, DC
Growth Factors and Brain Tumors

Jeffrey G. Jarvik, MD, MPH

Associate Professor, Departments of Radiology and Neurosurgery, University of Washington School of Medicine; Adjunct Associate Professor, Department of Health Services, University of Washington School of Public Health; Director, Neuroradiology Fellowship, University of Washington Medical Center, Seattle, Washington
Radiology of the Spine; Magnetic Resonance Imaging for Peripheral Nerve Disorders

Kurt A. Jellinger, MD

Professor, University of Vienna Medical School, and Director, Ludwig Boltzmann Institute of Clinical Neurobiology, Vienna, Austria
Neuropathology of Movement Disorders

Arthur L. Jenkins III, MD, BA

Assistant Professor, Department of Neurosurgery, Mount Sinai School of Medicine, New York, New York

Complication Avoidance in Neurosurgery; Tumors of the Vertebral Axis: Benign, Primary Malignant, and Metastatic Tumors; Cervical Spine Trauma

Eric W. Johnson, MD

Chief, Molecular Genetics–Neurogenetics, Division of Neurology/Division of Neurosurgery, Barrow Neurological Institute, Phoenix, Arizona

The Genetics of Cerebral Cavernous Malformations

John Patrick Johnson, MD

Director, Cedars-Sinai Institute for Spinal Disorders, Los Angeles, California

Sympathectomy for Pain

Wayel Kaakaji, MD

Staff Neurosurgeon, Michigan Brain and Spinal Surgery Institute, Detroit, Michigan

Alternative Surgical Treatments for Trigeminal Neuralgia

Michael G. Kaiser, MD

Assistant Professor, Department of Neurological Surgery, Columbia University College of Physicians and Surgeons; Attending Neurosurgeon, New York Presbyterian Hospital, New York, New York

Anterior Thoracic Instrumentation; Anterior Lumbar Instrumentation

Iain H. Kalfas, MD

Head, Section of Spinal Surgery, Department of Neurosurgery, Cleveland Clinic, Cleveland, Ohio

Image-Guided Spinal Navigation

Paul M. Kanev, MD

Attending Neurosurgeon, Department of Surgery, Milton Hershey Medical Center, Hershey, Pennsylvania

Arachnoid Cysts

Yücel Kanpolat, MD

Professor and Chairman, Department of Neurosurgery, University of Ankara Faculty of Medicine; Ankara, Turkey

Cordotomy for Pain

Stuart S. Kaplan, MD

Assistant Professor of Neurosurgery, University of Cincinnati College of Medicine; Attending Neurosurgeon, Cincinnati Children's Hospital Medical Center, Cincinnati, Ohio

Birth Brachial Plexus Injury

Michael G. Kaplitt, MD, PhD

Assistant Professor, Department of Neurosurgery, Director, Center for Stereotactic and Functional Neurosurgery, Director, Laboratory of Molecular Neurosurgery, Cornell University Joan and Sanford I. Weill Medical College, New York, New York

Deep Brain Stimulation for Chronic Pain

Zvonimir S. Katusic, MD, PhD

Professor of Pharmacology, Mayo Medical School, Rochester, Minnesota

Cerebral Blood Flow and Metabolism

Bruce A. Kaufman, MD

Professor of Neurosurgery, Medical College of Wisconsin; Chief, Division of Pediatric Neurosurgery, Children's Hospital of Wisconsin, Milwaukee, Wisconsin

Medulloblastoma

Howard H. Kaufman, MD

Department of Neurosurgery, West Virginia University School of Medicine, Morgantown, West Virginia

Brain Death

Robert F. Keating

Associate Professor, Department of Neurosurgery, George Washington University School of Medicine; Chief, Children's National Medical Center, Washington; DC

Occult Spinal Dysraphism and the Tethered Spinal Cord

G. Evren Keles, MD

Assistant Professor, Department of Neurosurgery, University of California, San Francisco, School of Medicine; San Francisco, California

Low-Grade Gliomas: Astrocytoma, Oligodendroglioma, and Mixed Gliomas

John S. Kennerdell, MD

Professor of Ophthalmology, Drexel University Medical School, Philadelphia, and Adjunct Professor of Ophthalmology, University of Pittsburgh School of Medicine; Chairman, Department of Ophthalmology, Allegheny General Hospital, Pittsburgh, Pennsylvania

Orbital Tumors

Lawrence T. Khoo, MD

Department of Neurosurgery, University of Southern California Keck School of Medicine, Los Angeles, California

Intradiskal and Percutaneous Treatment of Lumbar Disk Disease

Vini G. Khurana, MD, PhD

Sundt Fellow, Departments of Neurologic Surgery and Molecular Pharmacology and Experimental Therapeutics, Mayo Clinic, Rochester, Minnesota

Cerebral Blood Flow and Metabolism

Monika Killer, MD

Attending, Christian Doppler Medical Center, Salzburg, Austria
Embolization of Arteriovenous Malformations as a Primary Treatment Modality

Jung Kim, MD

Professor, Department of Pathology, Yale University School of Medicine, New Haven, Connecticut
Unusual Gliomas

Thomas A. Kim, MD

Assistant Professor, Department of Radiology, University of Washington School of Medicine; Staff Neuroradiologist, Harborview Medical Center, University of Washington Medical Center, and Veterans Administration Puget Sound Medical Center, Seattle, Washington
Magnetic Resonance Imaging of Brain

Wesley A. King, MD

Associate Professor, Department of Neurosurgery, Mount Sinai School of Medicine; Attending Neurosurgeon, Mount Sinai Hospital, New York, New York
Neuro-otology

Gregory A. Kinney, PhD

Assistant Professor, University of Washington School of Medicine; Associate Director, Surgical Neuromonitoring University of Washington Medical Center and Harborview Medical Center, Seattle, Washington
Physiology of the Peripheral Nerve

Paul Klimo, MD

Resident, Department of Neurosurgery, University Hospital, Salt Lake City, Utah
Treatment of Axis Fractures

David G. Kline, MD

Boyd Professor and Chairman, Department of Neurosurgery, Louisiana State University School of Medicine at New Orleans; Visiting Staff, Medical Center of Louisiana at Charity Hospital and University Hospital; Academic Staff, Ochsner Foundation Hospital; Senior Staff, Touro Infirmary, S. Baptist and Mercy Hospitals; Consultant, Veterans Administration Hospital, New Orleans, Louisiana; and Keeslor AFB Hospital, Biloxi, Mississippi
Management of Peripheral Nerve Tumors

Michel Kliot, MD

Associate Professor of Neurosurgery, University of Washington School of Medicine; Attending Neurosurgeon, University of Washington Medical Center and Veterans Administration Puget Sound Health Care System, Seattle, Washington
Cellular and Molecular Mechanisms Mediating Injury and Recovery in the Nervous System; General Principles in Evaluating and Treating Peripheral Nerve Injuries; Magnetic Resonance Imaging for Peripheral Nerve Injuries; Carpal Tunnel Syndrome; Entrapment Syndromes of Peripheral Nerve Injuries

Douglas Kondziolka, MD, MSc

Professor of Neurological Surgery and Radiation Oncology, University of Pittsburgh School of Medicine, Pittsburgh, Pennsylvania
Patient Selection in Movement Disorder Surgery; Fractionated Radiotherapy for Pituitary Tumors; Gamma Knife Radiosurgery

Thomas A. Kopitnik, MD

Professor of Neurosurgery, University of Texas Southwestern Medical School; Director of Cerebrovascular Surgery, University of Texas Southwestern Medical Center at Dallas, Dallas, Texas
Posterior Fossa Arteriovenous Malformations

Oleg Kopyov, MD, PhD

Research Director, The California Neuroscience Institute, Oxnard, California
Functional Radiosurgery

Karl F. Kothbauer, MD

Assistant Professor, Department of Neurological Surgery, Albert Einstein College of Medicine of Yeshiva University, Bronx; Attending, Beth Israel Medical Center, New York, New York
Intraspinal Tumors in Infants and Children

Adnah Koudsié, MD

Staff Neurosurgeon, Hôpital Albert Michallon, Grenoble, France
Deep Brain Stimulation for Movement Disorders

Paul Krack, MD

Professor of Neurology, University Joseph Fourier Medical School; Staff Neurologist, Hôpital Albert Michallion, Grenoble, France
Deep Brain Stimulation for Movement Disorders

Michael A. Kraut, MD, PhD

Associate Professor of Radiology, Johns Hopkins University School of Medicine; Chief of Neuro–MRI, Johns Hopkins Hospital, Baltimore, Maryland
Radiologic Features of Central Nervous System Tumors

Lynda Kulawiak, RN

Research Associate, Department of Anesthesiology and Perioperative Medicine, Oregon Health & Science University, Portland, Oregon
Management of Pain by Anesthetic Techniques

V. G. R. Kumar, MBBS

Consultant Neurosurgeon, West Bank Hospital, Calcutta, West Bengal, India
Cervical Spondylotic Myelopathy

Lara J. Kunschner, MD

Assistant Professor, Department of Neurology, Drexel University College of Medicine, Philadelphia; Attending, Allegheny General Hospital, Allegheny Neurological Associates, Pittsburgh, Pennsylvania
Medulloblastoma

Charles Kuntz IV, MD

Assistant Professor of Neurosurgery, University of Cincinnati School of Medicine; Associate Director, Spine and Peripheral Nerve Surgery, The Maxfield Clinic and Spine Institute, and Director, Spine and Peripheral Nerve Research, Department of Neurological Surgery, The Neuroscience Institute, Cincinnati, Ohio
Approach to the Patient and Medical Management of Spinal Disorders

Inam Kureshi, MD

Department of Neurovascular Surgery, Hartford Hospital Stroke Center, Hartford, Connecticut
Revascularization Techniques for Complex Aneurysms and Skull Base Tumors

Arthur M. Lam, MD

Professor of Anesthesiology and Neurological Surgery, University of Washington School of Medicine; Head, Division of Neuroanesthesia, Harborview Medical Center, Seattle, Washington
Anesthesia: Preoperative Evaluation; Transcranial Doppler Ultrasonography

Lois A. Lampson, PhD

Associate Professor of Neurosurgery, Brigham and Women's Hospital, Harvard Medical School, Boston, Massachusetts
Basic Principles of Central Nervous System Immunology

Frederick F. Lang, Jr., MD

Attending, Department of Neurosurgery, The University of Texas M.D. Anderson Cancer Center, Houston, Texas
Medulloblastoma; Metastatic Brain Tumors

Guiseppe Lanzino, MD

Associate Professor, Department of Neurosurgery, University of Illinois College of Medicine at Peoria; Chief, Section of Cerebrovascular Surgery, Illinois Neurological Institute, Peoria, Illinois
Endovascular Treatment of Aneurysms

Donald Larsen, MD

Associate Professor, Department of Neurological Surgery, University of Southern California Keck School of Medicine; Director of Neuro-interventional Section, USC University Hospital, Los Angeles, California
Cavernous Carotid Fistulas

Sean D. Lavine, MD

Assistant Professor of Neurosurgery and Radiology, Columbia University, College of Physicians and Surgeons; Clinical Director, Endovascular Neurosurgery and Interventional Neuroradiology, Columbia-Presbyterian Medical Center, New York, New York
Basilar Trunk Aneurysms

Michael T. Lawton, MD

Tong-Po Kan Assistant Professor of Neurological Surgery, University of California, San Francisco, School of Medicine; Chief of Cerebrovascular Surgery, University of California, San Francisco Medical Center, San Francisco, California
Surgical Approaches for Posterior Circulation Aneurysms

Edward R. Laws, MD

Professor, Department of Neurosurgery, University of Virginia, Charlottesville, Virginia

Daniel A. Lazar, MD

Resident, Department of Neurological Surgery, University of Washington Hospitals, Seattle, Washington
Cellular and Molecular Mechanisms Mediating Injury and Recovery in the Nervous System

Jean F. Le Bas, MD, PhD

Professor of Biophysics and Radiology, University Joseph Fourier Medical School; Head, Division of Neuroradiology and MRI, and Director, Institut Federatif de Recherche eu IRM, Hôpital Albert Michallon, Grenoble, France
Deep Brain Stimulation for Movement Disorders

Chong C. Lee, MD, PhD

Resident, Department of Neurological Surgery, University of Washington, Seattle, Washington
Carpal Tunnel Syndrome; Entrapment Syndromes of Peripheral Nerve Injuries

Jang-Chul Lee, MD, PhD

Associate Professor, Department of Neurosurgery, Keimyung University School of Medicine, Taegu, Korea
Diagnostic Biopsy of Peripheral Nerves and Muscle

Jung-Il Lee, MD

Associate Professor, Department of Neurosurgery, Samsung Medical Center, Sungkyun Kwan University School of Medicine, Seoul, Korea
Thalamotomy for Tremor

Sunghoon Lee, MD

Administrative Chief Resident, Yale Neurosurgery Program, Yale–New Haven Medical Center, New Haven, Connecticut
Unusual Gliomas; Intracranial Monitoring

Elizabeth A. Leedom, JD

Lecturer, University of Washington School of Law, Seattle, Washington
Legal Issues

James W. Leiphart, MD, PhD

Resident in Neurosurgery, UCLA Medical Center, Los Angeles, California
Surgery for Extratemporal Lobe Epilepsy

G. Michael Lemole, Jr., MD

Private Practice, Huntingdon Valley, Pennsylvania
Giant Aneurysms

Frederick A. Lenz, MD

Professor of Neurosurgery, Johns Hopkins University School of Medicine; Attending Neurosurgeon, Johns Hopkins Hospital, Baltimore, Maryland
Thalamotomy for Tremor

Phillipp M. Lenzlinger, MD

Division of Trauma Surgery, Department of Surgery, University Hospital, Zuroch, Switzerland
Cellular Basis of Injury and Recovery from Trauma

Jeffrey R. Leonard, MD

Assistant Professor, Department of Neurosurgery, Washington University School of Medicine; Attending Neurosurgeon, St. Louis Children's Hospital, St. Louis, Missouri
Dandy-Walker Syndrome

Peter D. Le Roux, MB, ChB, MD

Associate Professor of Neurosurgery, University of Pennsylvania School of Medicine, Philadelphia, Pennsylvania
Surgical Decision Making for the Treatment of Cerebral Aneurysms

Allan D. O. Levi, MD, PhD

Assistant Professor, University of Miami School of Medicine; Chief, Section of Neurospinal Services, Jackson Memorial Hospital, Miami, Florida
Spine Trauma: Approach to the Patient and Diagnostic Evaluation

Elad I. Levy, MD

Neurosurgical Chief Resident, University of Pittsburgh Medical Center System, Pittsburgh, Pennsylvania
Trigeminal Neuralgia: Microvascular Decompression of the Trigeminal Nerve for Tic Douloureux

Michael L. Levy, MD, PhD

Associate Professor, Department of Neurosurgery, University of Southern California Keck School of Medicine, Los Angeles, California
Vagus Nerve Stimulation for Intractable Epilepsy

David H. Lewis, MD

Associate Professor of Radiology, University of Washington School of Medicine; Director, Division of Nuclear Medicine, Harborview Medical Center, Seattle, Washington
Single-Photon Emission Computed Tomography and Positron Emission Tomography

Patricia Limousin, MD, PhD

Senior Lecturer, Institute of Neurology, and Honorary Consultant Neurologist, National Hospital for Neurology and Neurosurgery, Queen's Square, London, England
Deep Brain Stimulation for Movement Disorders

E. Paul Lindell, MD

Attending Radiologist, Department of Radiology, Mayo Clinic, Rochester, Minnesota
Magnetic Resonance Imaging of Brain

Lawrence S. Liu, MD

Attending, Department of Neurosurgery, Kaiser-Permanente Los Angeles Medical Center, Los Angeles, California
Technical Aspects of Bone Graft Harvest and Spinal Fusion

Jay S. Loeffler, MD

Andreas Soriano Professor of Radiation Oncology, Harvard Medical School; Chair, Department of Radiation Oncology, Massachusetts General Hospital, Boston, Massachusetts
Proton Radiosurgery

Christopher Loftus, MD

Professor and Chairman, Department of Neurosurgery, University of Oklahoma College of Medicine, Oklahoma City, Oklahoma
Carotid Occlusive Disease: Natural History and Medical Management

William J. Logan, MD

Professor of Pediatrics and Medicine, University of Toronto Faculty of Medicine; Attending, Division of Neurology, The Hospital for Sick Children, Toronto, Ontario, Canada
Neurological Examination in Infancy and Childhood

Donlin M. Long, MD, PhD

Distinguished Service Professor of Neurosurgery, Johns Hopkins University School of Medicine; Active Staff, Johns Hopkins Hospital; Principal Staff, Applied Physics Laboratory, Johns Hopkins University, Baltimore, Maryland
Acoustic Neuroma

Luca Longhi, MD

Terapia Intensiva Neuroscienze, Padiglione Beretta Neuro II piano (Rianimazione), Ospedale Maggiore Policlinico IRCCS, Milano, Italy
Cellular Basis of Injury and Recovery from Trauma

James B. Lowe III, MD, MBA

Instructor in Surgery, Division of Plastic and Reconstructive Surgery, Washington University School of Medicine, St. Louis, Missouri
Ulnar Nerve Entrapment at the Elbow

Andres M. Lozano, MD, PhD

Professor of Neurosurgery and R. R. Tasker Chair in Functional Neurosurgery, University of Toronto Faculty of Medicine; Attending, Toronto Western Hospital, Toronto, Ontario, Canada
Pallidotomy for Parkinson's Disease; Deep Brain Stimulation for Chronic Pain

Mark Luciano, MD, PhD

Chief, Pediatric and Congenital Neurosurgery Section, and Director, Cleveland Clinic Hydrocephalus Project, Cleveland Clinic, Cleveland, Ohio
Infantile Posthemorrhagic Hydrocephalus

Jürgen Lüders, MD, PhD

Chairman, Department of Neurology, Cleveland Clinic Foundation, Cleveland, Ohio
General and Historical Considerations of Epilepsy Surgery

David Lundin, MD

Resident, Department of Neurological Surgery, University of Washington, Seattle, Washington
Spondylolisthesis

L. Dade Lunsford, MD

Lars Leksell Professor of Neurological Surgery, Radiology, and Radiology Oncology and Chairman, Department of Neurological Surgery, University of Pittsburgh School of Medicine; Director, Center for Image-Guided Neurosurgery, University of Pittsburgh Medical Center, Pittsburgh, Pennsylvania
Patient Selection in Movement Disorder Surgery; Radiosurgery of Tumors

W. David Lust, PhD

Professor of Neurological Surgery, Case Western Reserve University School of Medicine; Attending, Department of Neurological Surgery, and The Research Institute of University Hospitals of Cleveland, Cleveland, Ohio
Intraoperative Cerebral Protection

R. Loch MacDonald, MD, PhD

Professor, Department of Surgery, Division of the Biological Sciences, Pritzker School of Medicine University of Chicago; Attending Neurosurgeon, University of Chicago Medical Center, Chicago, Illinois
Perioperative Management of Subarachnoid Hemorrhage

Susan E. Mackinnon, MD

Shornberg Professor and Chief, Division of Plastic and Reconstructive Surgery, Department of Surgery, Washington University School of Medicine, St. Louis, Missouri
Ulnar Nerve Entrapment at the Elbow

Roger M. Macklis, MD

Professor of Radiology, Ohio State University College of Medicine and Public Health; Chairman, Department of Radiation Oncology, Cleveland Clinic, Cleveland, Ohio
Principles of Radiotherapy

Christopher Madden, MD

Clinical Assistant Professor, Ohio State University, Columbus, Ohio
Cervical Spondylotic Myelopathy

Parley W. Madsen III, MD, PhD

Staff, Department of Neurological Surgery, Conemaugh Memorial Medical Center, Johnstown, Pennsylvania
Diagnosis and Management of Thoracic Spine Fractures

Dennis J. Maiman, MD, PhD

Professor, Department of Neurosurgery, and Director, Spine Surgery Fellowship, Medical College of Wisconsin; Physical Medicine and Rehabilitation, Froedtert Hospital; Attending Neurosurgeon, Veterans Affairs Medical Center, Milwaukee, Wisconsin
Concepts and Mechanisms of Biomechanics

Allen Maniker, MD

Assistant Professor, Department of Neurological Surgery, University of Medicine and Dentistry of New Jersey, Newark; Attending Neurosurgeon, University Hospital, Newark, and Hackensack University Hospital, Hackensack, New Jersey
Peripheral Nerves

Scott C. Manning, MD

Professor, Department of Otolaryngology, University of Washington School of Medicine; Chief, Division of Pediatric Otolaryngology, Children's Hospital and Regional Medical Center, Seattle, Washington
Diagnosis and Management of Juvenile Angiofibroma

Timothy B. Mapstone, MD

Professor and Vice-Chairman, Department of Neurological Surgery, Emory University School of Medicine; Director, Pediatric Neurosurgery, Children's Health Care of Atlanta, Atlanta, Georgia
Intracranial Germ Cell Tumors

Kenneth Maravilla, MD

Professor of Radiology and Director of
Neuroradiology, Department of Neurological Surgery,
University of Washington School of Medicine;
Research Affiliate, Center on Human Development
and Disability, Seattle, Washington
*Magnetic Resonance Imaging for Peripheral Nerve
Disorders*

Douglas A. Marchuk, PhD

Associate Professor, Department of Genetics, Duke
University School of Medicine, Durham, North
Carolina
The Genetics of Cerebral Cavernous Malformations

Paul J. Marcotte, MD

Associate Professor of Neurosurgery, University of
Pennsylvania School of Medicine; Attending,
Department of Neurosurgery, Hospital of the
University of Pennsylvania, Philadelphia,
Pennsylvania
Technical Aspects of Bone Graft Harvest and Spinal Fusion

Anthony Marmarou, PhD

Professor and Vice Chairman, Director of Research,
Division of Neurosurgery, Virginia Commonwealth
University School of Medicine, Richmond, Virginia
*Physiology of the Cerebrospinal Fluid and Intracranial
Pressure*

Joseph C. Maroon, MD

Clinical Professor and Heindl Scholar, Department of
Neurosurgery, University of Pittsburgh School of
Medicine; Vice Chairman, Department of
Neurosurgery, UPMC-Presbyterian Hospital,
Pittsburgh, Pennsylvania
Orbital Tumors

Lawrence F. Marshall, MD

Professor of Neurological Surgery, University of
California, San Diego, School of Medicine; Chief,
Division of Neurosurgery, UCSD Medical Center, San
Diego, California
*Differential Diagnosis of Altered States of Consciousness;
Modern Neurotraumatology: A Brief Historical Review;
Traumatic Cerebrospinal Fluid Fistulas*

Sharon B. Marshall

Director of Clinical Research, Department of
Neurosurgery, University of California, San Diego,
San Diego, California
Modern Neurotraumatology: A Brief Historical Review

Neil A. Martin, MD

Professor and Chair, Department of Neurosurgery,
David Geffen School of Medicine at University of
California, Los Angeles, Los Angeles, California
*Revascularization Techniques for Complex Aneurysms and
Skull Base Tumors*

Timothy J. Martin, MD

Associate Professor of Surgical Sciences/
Ophthalmology, Department of Ophthalmology, Wake
Forest University School of Medicine; Attending,
Baptist Medical Center and Wake Forest University
Eye Center, Winston-Salem, North Carolina
Neuro-ophthalmology

Robert E. Maxwell, MD, PhD

Professor and Chair, Department of Neurosurgery,
University of Minnesota Medical School;
Neurosurgery Clinical Service Chief, Fairview
University Medical Center, Minneapolis, Minnesota
*Standard Temporal Lobectomy and Transsylvian
Amygdalohippocampectomy*

Nina A. Mayr, MD

Professor and Director, Radiation Oncology,
Oklahoma University Health Sciences Center,
Oklahoma City, Oklahoma
Radiobiology

Kevin McCarthy, MD

Assistant Professor and Director, Department of
Medicine, Nuclear Medicine Division, Louisiana State
University School of Medicine in New Orleans, New
Orleans, Louisiana
Intracranial Monitoring

Paul C. McCormick, MD, MPH

Professor of Clinical Neurosurgery, Department of
Neurological Surgery, Columbia University College of
Physicians and Surgeons; Attending Neurosurgeon,
New York Presbyterian Hospital, New York, New
York
*Anterior Thoracic Instrumentation; Anterior Lumbar
Instrumentation; Spinal Cord Tumors in Adults*

M. W. McDermott, MD

Assistant Professor, Department of Neurological
Surgery, University of California, San Francisco,
School of Medicine, San Francisco, California
Interstitial and Intracavitary Irradiation of Brain Tumors

Cameron G. McDougall, MD, FRCS(C)

Director, Division of Endovascular Neurosurgery,
Barrow Neurological Institute, Phoenix, Arizona
*Carotid Angioplasty and Stenting: Interventional
Treatment of Occlusive Vascular Disease*

Tracy K. McIntosh, PhD

Professor of Neurosurgery, Pharmacology, and
Bioengineering, Vice-Chair for Research and Director,
University of Pennsylvania Head Injury Center,
University of Pennsylvania, Philadelphia,
Pennsylvania
Cellular Basis of Injury and Recovery from Trauma

Guy M. McKhann II, MD

Assistant Professor, Department of Neurological Surgery, Columbia University College of Physicians and Surgeons; Staff, The Neurological Institute, and Attending, New York Presbyterian Hospital, New York, New York
Electrophysiologic Properties of the Mammalian Central Nervous System

David G. McLone, MD, PhD

Staff, Department of Pediatric Neurosurgery, Children's Memorial Hospital, Chicago, Illinois
Normal and Abnormal Embryology of the Spinal Cord and Spine

Max B. Medary, MD

Director, Orlando Neurosurgical Foundation, Celebration, Florida
Carotid Endarterectomy

Sanford L. Meeks, PhD

Associate Professor of Radiology, University of Iowa Roy J. and Lucille A. Carver College of Medicine; Director of Medical Physics, Department of Radiation Oncology, University of Iowa Health Care, Iowa City, Iowa
Radiobiology; Radiotherapy for Benign Skull Base Tumors; Fractionated and Stereotactic Radiation, Extracranial Stereotactic Radiation, Intensity Modulation, and Multileaf Collimation

Minesh P. Mehta, MBChB

Associate Professor, Department of Human Oncology, University of Wisconsin—Madison Medical School, Madison, Wisconsin
Fractionated Radiation Therapy for Malignant Brain Tumors

Vivek Mehta, MD, MSc

Assistant Professor, Department of Neurosurgery, University of Alberta Faculty of Medicine; Attending, Walter MacKenzie Health Sciences Center, Edmonton, Alberta, Canada
Craniopharyngioma in the Adult

William P. Melega, PhD

Associate Professor, Department of Molecular and Medical Pharmacology, David Geffen School of Medicine at UCLA, Los Angeles, California
Molecular Imaging of the Brain with Positron Emission Tomography

Arnold H. Menezes, MD

Professor and Vice Chairman, Department of Neurosurgery, University of Iowa College of Medicine; Attending Neurosurgeon, University of Iowa Hospitals and Clinics, Iowa City, Iowa
Developmental Abnormalities of the Craniovertebral Junction; Acquired Abnormalities of the Craniocervical Junction; Tumors of the Craniovertebral Junction

Robert A. Mericle, MD

Assistant Professor, Department of Neurosurgery, University of Florida College of Medicine; Staff, McKnight Brain Institute, Gainesville, Florida
Vein of Galen Malformations

Glen S. Merry, MD

Professor of Neurosurgery, University of Queensland Faculty of Medicine; Consultant Neurosurgeon, Royal Brisbane Hospital, Brisbane Queensland, Australia
Mild Head Injury in Adults

Ali Mesiwala, MD

Resident, University of Washington Hospitals, Seattle, Washington
General Principles of Operative Positioning

Fredric B. Meyer, MD

Professor of Neurosurgery, Mayo Medical School; Staff, Departments of Diagnostic Radiology and Neurological Surgery, Mayo Clinic, Rochester, Minnesota
Cerebral Blood Flow and Metabolism; Multimodality Management of Complex Cerebrovascular Lesions

Jeff Michalski, MD

Associate Professor, Department of Radiation Oncology, Washington University School of Medicine; Clinical Director, Department of Radiation Oncology, Barnes-Jewish Hospital, St. Louis, Missouri
Radiotherapy of Tumors of the Spine

J. Parker Mickle, MD

Professor, Department of Neurosurgery, University of Florida College of Medicine; Staff, McKnight Brain Institute, Gainesville, Florida
Vein of Galen Malformations

Rajiv Midha, MD, MSc

Associate Professor, Department of Surgery, Division of Neurosurgery, University of Toronto Faculty of Medicine; Staff Neurosurgeon, Sunnybrook and Women's College Health Sciences Centre, Toronto, Ontario, Canada
Peripheral Nerve: Approach to the Patient

Tom Mikkelsen, MD

Co-Director, Hermelin Brain Tumor Center, and Attending, Henry Ford Hospital, Detroit, Michigan
Invasion in Malignant Glioma

Andrew N. Miles, MBBS

Consultant Neurosurgeon, Western Australian Comprehensive Epilepsy Service and Department of Neurosurgery, Royal Perth Hospital, Perth, Western Australia, Australia
Tailored Resections for Epilepsy

John W. Miller, MD, PhD

Professor of Neurology and Neurological Surgery,
University of Washington School of Medicine;
Director, Regional Epilepsy Center, University of
Washington Medical Center, Seattle, Washington
Approaches to the Diagnosis and Classification of Epilepsy

Neil R. Miller, MD

Professor of Ophthalmology, Neurology, and
Neurosurgery and Frank B. Walsh Professor of Neuro-
Ophthalmology, Johns Hopkins University School of
Medicine, Baltimore, Maryland
Pseudotumor Cerebri

Pedro Molina-Negro, MD, PhD

Professor of Surgery (Neurosurgery), University of
Montreal Faculty of Medicine, Howick, Quebec,
Canada
Selective Peripheral Denervation for Spasmodic Torticollis

Jacques J. Morcos, MD

Associate Professor, Department of Neurosurgery,
University of Miami School of Medicine, Miami,
Florida
*Spontaneous Intracerebral Hemorrhage:
Non–Arteriovenous Malformation, Nonaneurysm*

Michael Kerin Morgan, MD

Professor of Neurosurgery, University of Sydney
Faculty of Medicine, Sydney, New South Wales,
Australia
*Classification and Decision Making in Treatment and
Perioperative Management, including Surgical and
Radiosurgical Decision Making*

Glenn Morrison, MD

Professor of Neurological Surgery, University of
Miami School of Medicine; Chief, Division of
Neurological Surgery, Miami Children's Hospital,
Miami, Florida
*Temporal and Extratemporal Lobe Resections for Childhood
Intractable Epilepsy*

Richard S. Morrison, PhD

Professor, Department of Neurological Surgery,
University of Washington School of Medicine, Seattle,
Washington
Growth Factors and Brain Tumors

Wade M. Mueller, MD

Associate Professor, Department of Neurosurgery,
Medical College of Wisconsin, Milwaukee, Wisconsin
*Functional Magnetic Resonance Imaging in Epilepsy
Surgery*

J. Paul Muizelaar, MD, PhD

Professor and Chair, Department of Neurological
Surgery, University of California, Davis, School of
Medicine, Davis; University of California, Davis,
Medical Center, Sacramento, California
Clinical Pathophysiology of Traumatic Brain Injury

Jenny Multani, MD

Resident, Department of Neurosurgery, West Virginia
University School of Medicine, Morgantown, West
Virginia
Occult Spinal Dysraphism and the Tethered Spinal Cord

Karin M. Muraszko, MD

Associate Professor of Neurosurgery and Pediatric
and Communicable Diseases, University of Michigan
Medical School; Director, Pediatric Neurosurgery
Program, C. S. Mott Children's Hospital, University of
Michigan Hospital and Health Centers, Ann Arbor,
Michigan
Primitive Neuroectodermal Tumors

Antonio C. M. Mussi, MD

Research Fellow, Department of Neurological Surgery,
University of Florida College of Medicine, Gainesville,
Florida
Surgical Anatomy of the Brain

Neal J. Naff, MD

Assistant Professor of Neurosurgery, Johns Hopkins
University School of Medicine, Baltimore, and
Uniformed Services University of Health Sciences,
F. Edward Hébert School of Medicine, Bethesda; Chief
of Neurosurgery, Sinai Hospital of Baltimore,
Baltimore, Maryland
Endovascular Techniques for Brain Tumors

Blaine S. Nashold, MD

Professor Emeritus, Department of Surgery, Division
of Neurosurgery, Duke University School of Medicine;
Director, Neurosurgical Stereotactic Laboratory and
Neuroprosthesis Laboratory, Duke University Medical
Center, Durham, North Carolina
*Caudalis Nucleus Dorsal Root Entry Zone Procedure for
the Treatment of Intractable Facial Pain*

Gary M. Nesbit, MD

Associate Professor, Department of Neurological
Surgery, Diagnostic Radiology, and Neurology,
Oregon Health & Science University School of
Medicine and Dotter Interventional Institute; Chief,
Neuroradiology and MRI, University Hospital,
Portland, Oregon
Cerebral Venous and Sinus Thrombosis

David W. Newell, MD

Professor, Department of Neurological Surgery, University of Washington School of Medicine; Attending Neurosurgeon, Harborview Medical Center, University of Washington Medical Center, Children's Hospital Medical Center, and Veterans' Hospital Medical Center, Seattle, Washington

Transcranial Doppler Ultrasonography; Traumatic Cerebral Aneurysms Secondary to Penetrating Intracranial Injuries; Traumatic Cerebrovascular Injury

Douglas A. Nichols, MD

Associate Professor, Departments of Radiology and Neurosurgery, Mayo Medical School, Rochester, Minnesota

Multimodality Management of Complex Cerebrovascular Lesions

Ajay Niranjan, MBBS, MS, MCh

Assistant Professor, Department of Neurological Surgery, University of Pittsburgh School of Medicine; Director, Radiosurgery Research, University of Pittsburgh Medical Center System, Pittsburgh, Pennsylvania

Radiosurgery of Tumors

Russ P. Nockels, MD

Associate Professor and Vice Chair, Departments of Neurological Surgery and Orthopedic Surgery, Loyola University Stritch School of Medicine, Loyola University Medical Center, Maywood, Illinois

Diagnosis and Management of Thoracolumbar and Lumbar Spine Injuries

Michael J. Noetzel, MD

Professor of Neurology and Pediatrics, Washington University School of Medicine; Director, Clinical Services, Division of Pediatric Neurology, Washington University Medical Center; Medical Director, Clinical and Diagnostic Neuroscience Services, St. Louis Children's Hospital, St. Louis, Missouri

Acute Pediatric Neurorehabilitation

Patrick Noonen, MD

Department of Radiology, National Naval Medical Center, Bethesda, Maryland

Endovascular Techniques for Brain Tumors

Richard B. North, MD

Professor of Neurosurgery, Anesthesiology, and Critical Care Medicine, Johns Hopkins University School of Medicine, Baltimore, Maryland

Spinal Cord and Peripheral Nerve Stimulation for Chronic, Intractable Pain

Eric Nottmeier, MD

Chief Resident, Division of Neurosurgery, University of Missouri Hospitals and Clinics, Columbia, Missouri

Intracranial Occlusion Disease and Moyamoya

W. Jerry Oakes, MD

Professor of Neurosurgery and Pediatrics, University of Alabama School of Medicine; Chief, Pediatric Neurosurgery, University of Alabama Hospitals, Birmingham Alabama

Chiari Malformations

Maureen O'Donnell, MD, MSc

Assistant Professor and Head, Division of Developmental Pediatrics, Department of Pediatrics, University of British Columbia Faculty of Medicine; Medical Director, Child Development and Rehabilitation Program, Children's and Women's Health Centre of British Columbia, Vancouver, British Columbia, Canada

Intrathecal Baclofen Infusion

Christopher S. Ogilvy, MD

Associate Professor of Surgery, Harvard Medical School; Visiting Neurosurgeon, Massachusetts General Hospital, Boston, Massachusetts

Vertebral Artery, Posterior Inferior Cerebellar Artery, and Vertebrobasilar Junction Aneurysms

George A. Ojemann, MD

Professor of Neurological Surgery, University of Washington School of Medicine; Staff, University of Washington Regional Epilepsy Center, Seattle, Washington

Tailored Resections for Epilepsy

Jeffrey G. Ojemann, MD

Assistant Professor of Neurosurgery, Department of Neurological Surgery, and Assistant Professor of Pediatrics, Anatomy, Psychology, and Neurobiology, Washington University School of Medicine; Attending Neurosurgeon, St. Louis Children's Hospital, St. Louis, Missouri

Dandy-Walker Syndrome

Michael S. Okun, MD

Assistant Professor of Neurology, University of Florida College of Medicine; Co-Director, Movement Disorders Center, Department of Neurology, McKnight Brain Institute, Gainesville, Florida

Surgery for Dystonia

Edward H. Oldfield, MD

Chief, Surgical Neurology Branch, National Institute of Neurological Diseases and Stroke, National Institutes of Health, Bethesda, Maryland

Spinal Arteriovenous Malformations

Alessandro Olivi, MD

Professor of Neurosurgery, Johns Hopkins University School of Medicine, Baltimore, Maryland

Brain Tumors during Pregnancy

Stephen L. Ondra, MD

Assistant Professor of Neurosurgery, Northwestern University Feinberg School of Medicine, Chicago, Illinois
Adult Thoracolumbar Scoliosis

Michael Ostad, MD

Clinical Adjunct Assistant Professor of Urology, Cornell University, Joan and Sanford I. Weill College of Medicine; Attending Urologist, New York Presbyterian Hospital, New York, and North Shore University Hospital, Manhasset, New York
Neurourology

Renatta J. Osterdock, MD

Pediatric Neurosurgery Fellow, University of Tennessee, Memphis, College of Medicine and Semmes-Murphy Clinic, Memphis, Tennessee
Lipomyelomeningocele

Jeffrey H. Owen, PhD

President and Owner, Sentient Medical Systems, Cockeysville, Maryland
Intraoperative Electrophysiologic Monitoring of the Spinal Cord and Nerve Roots

Dachling Pang, MD

Professor of Clinical Neurosurgery, University of California, Davis, School of Medicine, Davis; Chief, Regional Center for Pediatric Neurosurgery, Kaiser Permanente Hospital, Oakland, California
Pediatric Vertebral Column and Spinal Cord Injuries

T. S. Park, MD

Shi H. Huang Professor of Neurosurgery and Professor of Pediatrics and Anatomy and Neurobiology, Washington University School of Medicine; Neurosurgeon-in-Chief, St. Louis Children's Hospital, St. Louis, Missouri
Birth Brachial Plexus Injury; Selective Dorsal Rhizotomy for Spastic Cerebral Palsy

Andrew T. Parsa, MD, PhD

Assistant Professor, Department of Neurological Surgery, University of California, San Francisco, School of Medicine, San Francisco, California
Anterior Thoracic Instrumentation; Anterior Lumbar Instrumentation

Michael Partington, MD

Neurosurgeon, Department of Pediatrics, Gillette Children's Specialty Healthcare, St. Paul, Minnesota
Normal and Abnormal Embryology of the Spinal Cord and Spine

Naresh P. Patel, MD

Assistant Professor of Neurosurgery, Mayo Medical School Scottsdale; Assistant Attending, Mayo Clinic Scottsdale, Scottsdale, Arizona
Complication Avoidance in Neurosurgery

Jogi V. Pattisapu, MD

Clinical Faculty, Department of Molecular Biology and Microbiology and Department of Nursing, College of Health Sciences, University of Central Florida; Medical Director, Pediatric Neurosurgery, Arnold Palmer Hospital for Women and Children, Florida Children's Hospital, Wade's Center for Hydrocephalus Research, HRI, Orlando, Florida
Infantile Posthemorrhagic Hydrocephalus

Richard D. Penn, MD

Professor of Neurosurgery, University of Chicago, Division of the Biological Sciences, Pritzker School of Medicine; Attending, Neuroscience Institute, Neurosurgery Division, Rush-Presbyterian-St. Luke's Medical Center, and University of Chicago Hospitals, Chicago, Illinois
Management of Spasticity by Central Nervous System Infusion Techniques; Intrathecal Drug Infusion for Pain

Noel I. Perin, MD

Clinical Associate Professor of Neurosurgery, Columbia University College of Physicians and Surgeons; Attending Physician, St. Luke's Roosevelt Beth-Israel Hospital, New-York, New York
Sacral Fractures

Richard G. Perrin, MD, MSc

Associate Professor of Neurological Surgery, Division of Neurosurgery, University of Toronto Faculty of Medicine; Staff, St. Michael's Hospital, Toronto, Ontario, Canada
Tumors of the Vertebral Axis: Benign, Primary Malignant, and Metastatic Tumors

Jonathan R. Perry, MD

Professor, Department of Radiology, University of Washington School of Medicine, Seattle, Washington
Radiology of the Spine

John A. Persing, MD

Professor, Department of Neurosurgery, Yale University School of Medicine; Chief, Section of Plastic Surgery, Yale–New Haven Hospital, New Haven, Connecticut
Scalp Tumors; Craniofacial Syndromes

Michael E. Phelps, PhD

Norton Simon Professor and Chair, Department of Molecular and Medical Pharmacology, David Geffen School of Medicine at UCLA; Director, Crump Institute for Molecular Imaging; Associate Director, Laboratory of Structural Biology and Molecular Medicine and Chief, Division of Nuclear Medicine, UCLA Medical Center, Los Angeles, California
Molecular Imaging of the Brain with Positron Emission Tomography

Loi K. Phuong, MD

Resident, Department of Neurology, Mayo Clinic, Rochester, Minnesota
Pediatric Cerebral Hemispheric Tumors

David G. Piepgras, MD

Professor of Neurologic Surgery, Mayo Medical School; Chairman, Department of Neurologic Surgery, Mayo Clinic, Rochester, Minnesota
Middle Cerebral Artery Aneurysms

Joseph Piepmeier, MD

Nixdorff-German Professor and Vice Chairman for Clinical Affairs, Department of Neurosurgery, Yale University School of Medicine; Director, Neuro-oncology Unit, Yale Comprehensive Cancer Center, New Haven, Connecticut
Unusual Gliomas

Webster H. Pilcher, MD, PhD

Professor and Chair, Department of Neurological Surgery, University of Rochester School of Medicine and Dentistry and School of Nursing; Staff, Eastman Dental Center and Strong Memorial Hospital, Rochester, New York
Epilepsy Surgery: Outcome and Complications

Frank A. Pintar, PhD

Professor, Department of Neurosurgery, Medical College of Wisconsin; Adjunct Professor of Biomedical Engineering, Marquette University; Director, Neuroscience Research Laboratories, and Principal Investigator/Biomedical Engineer, Veterans Administration Medical Center, Milwaukee, Wisconsin
Concepts and Mechanisms of Biomechanics

Joseph D. Pinter, MD

Assistant Professor of Neurology, University of California, Davis, School of Medicine, Davis; Attending, UC Davis Medical Center, Sacramento, California
Neuroembryology

Serge Pinto, PhD

Hôpital Albert Michallon, Service de Neurologie Grenoble and University Joseph Fourier, Grenoble, France
Deep Brain Stimulation for Movement Disorders

Farhad Pirouzmand, MD

Assistant Professor of Neurosurgery, University of Saskatchewan Faculty of Medicine; Program Director, Division of Neurosurgery, Royal University Hospital, Saskatoon, Saskatchewan, Canada
Arteriovenous Malformations and Intracranial Aneurysms in Children

Ian F. Pollack, MD

Professor of Neurosurgery, University of Pittsburgh School of Medicine; Co-Director, University of Pittsburgh Cancer Institute Brain Tumor Center, Children's Hospital of Pittsburgh, Pittsburgh, Pennsylvania
Brainstem Gliomas

Pierre Pollak, MD, PhD

Professor of Neurology, University Joseph Fourier Medical School; Head, Movement Disorders Unit, Hôpital Albert Michallon, Grenoble, France
Deep Brain Stimulation for Movement Disorders

Bruce E. Pollock, MD

Associate Professor, Department of Neurological Surgery, Mayo Medical School, Rochester, Minnesota
Multimodality Management of Complex Cerebrovascular Lesions

Randall W. Porter, MD

Chief, Interdisciplinary Skull Base Section, Barrow Neurological Institute, Phoenix, Arizona
Infratentorial Cavernous Malformations; Classification of Spinal Cord Vascular Lesions

Kalmon D. Post, MD

Professor and Chairman, Department of Neurosurgery, Mount Sinai School of Medicine; Chairman, Department of Neurosurgery, Mount Sinai Medical Center, New York, New York
Complication Avoidance in Neurosurgery; Trigeminal Schwannomas

Sujit S. Prabhu, MD

Director, Department of Neurosurgery, M.D. Anderson Cancer Center, Houston, Texas
Surgical Management of Traumatic Brain Injury

Charles J. Prestigiacomo, MD

Assistant Professor of Cerebrovascular/Endovascular Surgery, Departments of Neurological Surgery and Radiology, University of Medicine and Dentistry of New Jersey—New Jersey Medical School; Attending, Neurological Institute of New Jersey, University Hospital, Newark, New Jersey
Neurosonology

Robert Prost, PhD

Assistant Professor of Radiology, Medical College of Wisconsin; Attending, Froedtert & Memorial Lutheran Hospital, Milwaukee, Wisconsin
Magnetic Resonance Imaging of Brain

Chad J. Prusmack, MD

Resident, Department of Neurosurgery, University of Miami Hospital and Clinics, Miami, Florida
Spontaneous Intracerebral Hemorrhage: Non–Arteriovenous Malformation, Nonaneurysm

Donald O. Quest, MD

Professor, Department of Neurological Surgery, Columbia University College of Physicians and Surgeons; Attending, Department of Neurological Surgery, Neurological Institute of New York Presbyterian Hospital, and New York Presbyterian Medical Center, New York, New York
Neurosonology

Corey Raffel, MD, PhD

Professor of Neurosurgery, Mayo Medical School, Rochester, Minnesota
Pediatric Cerebral Hemispheric Tumors

Ramesh Raghupathi, PhD

Assistant Professor, Department of Neurobiology and Anatomy, Drexel University College of Medicine, Philadelphia, Pennsylvania
Cellular Basis of Injury and Recovery from Trauma

Frank A. Raila, MD

Professor Emeritus, Department of Radiology, University of Mississippi School of Medicine, Jackson, Mississippi
Radiology of the Skull

Zvi Ram, MD

Associate Professor of Surgery, Division of Neurosurgery, Tel Aviv University Sackler School of Medicine, Tel Aviv; Deputy Chairman, Department of Neurosurgery, Chaim Sheba Medical Center, Tel Hashomer, Israel
Principles of Gene Therapy

Bruce R. Ransom, MD, PhD

Professor and Chairman, Department of Neurology, University of Washington School of Medicine, Seattle, Washington
Astrocytes

Robert A. Ratcheson, MD

Professor of Neurological Surgery, Department of Neurological Surgery, Case Western Reserve University School of Medicine; Director, Department of Neurological Surgery, and the Research Institute, University Hospitals of Cleveland, Cleveland, Ohio
Intraoperative Cerebral Protection

Peter Raudzens, MD

Anesthesiologist, Department of Neuroanesthesia, Barrow Neurological Institute, Phoenix, Arizona
Anesthesia in Cerebrovascular Disease

Shlomo Raz, MD

Professor of Urology, Head of Reconstructive and Female Urology, David Geffen School of Medicine at UCLA, Los Angeles, California
Neurourology

Gary L. Rea, MD, PhD

Private Practice, University Orthopedic Physicians, Columbus, Ohio

Alyssa T. Reddy, MD

Assistant Professor of Pediatrics and Neurology, University of Alabama School of Medicine; Pediatric Neurologist, The Children's Hospital of Alabama, Birmingham, Alabama
Intracranial Germ Cell Tumors

Patrick M. Reilly, MD

Assistant Professor of Surgery, University of Pennsylvania School of Medicine, Philadelphia, Pennsylvania
Initial Resuscitation and Patient Evaluation

Harold L. Rekate, MD

Clinical Professor of Surgery, Division of Neurosurgery, University of Arizona College of Medicine, Tucson; Chairman, Section of Pediatric Neurosciences, and Director, Pediatric Neurosurgical Research Laboratory, Barrow Neurological Institute, Phoenix, Arizona
Hydrocephalus in Children

Ali R. Rezai, MD

Associate Professor and Head, Section for Stereotactic and Functional Neurosurgery, Department of Neurological Surgery, The Cleveland Clinic Foundation, Cleveland, Ohio
Deep Brain Stimulation for Chronic Pain

Laurence D. Rhines, MD

Assistant Professor of Neurosurgical Oncology, Department of Neurosurgery, University of Texas–Houston Medical School; Director, Spine Program, Department of Neurosurgery, The University of Texas M.D. Anderson Cancer Center, Houston, Texas
Brain Tumors during Pregnancy; Sarcoidosis, Tuberculosis, and Xanthogranuloma

Albert L. Rhoton, Jr., MD

R.D. Keene Family Professor, Chairman Emeritus, Department of Neurosurgery, University of Florida College of Medicine, Gainesville, Florida
Surgical Anatomy of the Brain

Teresa Ribalta, MD, PhD

Associate Professor of Pathology, University of Barcelona Medical School; Consultant, Department of Pathology, Hospital Clinic of Barcelona, Barcelona, Spain
Brain Tumors: An Overview of Histopathologic Classification

Bernd Richling, MD

Professor of Neurosurgery, Private Medical University of Salzburg, Salzburg Austria
Embolization of Arteriovenous Malformations as a Primary Treatment Modality

Charles J. Riedel, MD

Assistant Professor of Neurosurgery, Columbia University College of Physicians and Surgeons; Attending, Department of Neurological Surgery, Columbia-Presbyterian Medical Center, New York, New York
Surgical Exposures and Positioning for Spinal Surgery

Daniele Rigamonti, MD

Professor, Department of Neurosurgery, Johns Hopkins University School of Medicine; Director, Skeletal Dysplasias and Genetics, Johns Hopkins Hospital, Baltimore, Maryland
Anterior Communicating Artery and Anterior Cerebral Artery Aneurysms; Achondroplasia and Other Dwarfism

Howard A. Riina, MD

Assistant Professor of Neurological Surgery, Neurology, and Radiology, Cornell University Joan and Sanford I. Weill Medical College; Attending Neurosurgeon, New York Presbyterian Hospital, New York, New York
Giant Aneurysms; Classification of Spinal Cord Vascular Lesions

Michael E. C. Robbins, PhD

Professor, Department of Radiology, Wake Forest University School of Medicine; Head, Radiation Biology Section, Wake Forest Baptist Medical Center, Winston-Salem, North Carolina
Radiobiology

Claudia Robertson, MD

Professor, Department of Neurosurgery, Baylor College of Medicine; Medical Director, Neurosurgical Intensive Care Unit, Ben Taub General Hospital, Houston, Texas
Critical Care Management of Traumatic Brain Injury

Jon H. Robertson, MD

Chairman, Department of Neurosurgery, University of Tennessee, Memphis, College of Medicine, Memphis, Tennessee
Glomus Jugulare Tumors

Lawrence Robinson, MD

Professor and Chair, Department of Rehabilitation Medicine, University of Washington School of Medicine; Director, Electrodiagnostic Laboratory, Harborview Medical Center, Seattle, Washington
Electrodiagnostic Evaluation of Peripheral Nerves: Electromyography, Somatosensory Evoked Potentials, Nerve Action Potentials

Shenandoah Robinson, MD

Assistant Professor, Department of Neurological Surgery, Case Western Reserve University School of Medicine; Pediatric Neurosurgeon, Rainbow Babies and Children's Hospital, Cleveland, Ohio
Myelomeningocele and Myelocystocele; Intervertebral Disk Disease in Children

Mark A. Rockoff, MD

Professor of Anesthesia, Harvard Medical School; Vice-Chairman, Department of Anesthesia, Children's Hospital, Boston, Massachusetts
Neuroanesthesia in Children

Mark L. Rosenblum, MD

Chairman, Department of Neurosurgery, and Co-Director, Hermelin Brain Tumor Center, Henry Ford Hospital, Detroit, Michigan
Invasion in Malignant Glioma

Walter Royal III, MD

Associate Professor, Departments of Neurology, Morehouse School of Medicine, Atlanta, Georgia
Multiple Sclerosis

Ronald Ruff, PhD

Clinical Professor, Department of Psychiatry, University of California, San Francisco, School of Medicine, San Francisco, California
Sequelae of Traumatic Brain Injury

James T. Rutka, MD, PhD

Professor and Chairman, Division of Neurosurgery, University of Toranto Faculty of Medicine; Staff Neurosurgeon, The Hospital for Sick Children, Toronto, Ontario, Canada
Encephaloceles

Kathryn E. Saatman, MD

Associate Professor, Department of Neurosurgery, University of Pennsylvania School of Medicine, Philadelphia, Pennsylvania
Cellular Basis of Injury and Recovery from Trauma

Oren Sagher, MD

Associate Professor, Section of Neurosurgery, University of Michigan Medical College, Ann Arbor, Michigan
Diagnosis and Nonoperative Management [Trigeminal Neuralgia]

Sean A. Salehi, MD

Chief Resident, Department of Neurological Surgery, Northwestern Memorial Hospital, Chicago, Illinois
Adult Thoracolumbar Scoliosis

Ali Samii, MD

Assistant Professor of Neurology and Neurological Surgery, University of Washington School of Medicine, Seattle, Washington
Approach to Movement Disorders

Madjid Samii, MD

Professor and Chairman, Department of Neurosurgery, International Neuroscience Institute, Hanover, Germany
Basic Principles of Skull Base Surgery

Prakash Sampath, MD

Assistant Professor of Neurosurgery and Assistant Professor of Clinical Neurosciences, Brown University School of Medicine; Director, Neurosurgical Oncology, and Chief of Neurosurgery, Roger Williams Hospital, Providence, Rhode Island
Acoustic Neuroma; Sarcoidosis, Tuberculosis, and Xanthogranuloma

Duke Samson, MD

Professor and Chair, Department of Neurosurgery, University of Texas Southwestern Medical School, Dallas, Texas
Posterior Fossa Arteriovenous Malformations

Paul Santiago, MD

Resident, Department of Neurological Surgery, University of Washington Hospitals, Seattle, Washington
Malignant Gliomas: Anaplastic Astrocytoma, Glioblastoma Multiforme, Gliosarcoma, Malignant Oligodendroglioma; Benign Extradural Lesions of the Dorsal Spine

Harvey B. Sarnat, MD

Professor of Pediatrics (Neurology) and Pathology (Neuropathology), David Geffen School of Medicine at UCLA; Director, Division of Pediatric Neurology, and Neuropathologist, Cedars-Sinai Medical Center, Los Angeles, California
Neuroembryology

Raymond Sawaya, MD

Professor of Neurosurgery, University of Texas–Houston Medical School; Director, Brain Tumor Center, and Chairman, Department of Neurosurgery, The University of Texas M.D. Anderson Cancer Center, Houston, Texas
Brain Tumors: General Considerations; Metastatic Brain Tumors

Paul D. Sawin, MD

Private Practice, Orlando, Florida
Biology of Bone Grafting and Healing in Spinal Surgery; Posterior Cervical Stabilization and Fusion Techniques

Wouter I. Schievink, MD

Assistant Clinical Professor, Department of Neurological Surgery, University of California, Irvine, School of Medicine, Irvine; Attending Neurosurgeon, Cedars-Sinai Medical Center, and Co-Director, Neurovascular Surgery Program, Cedars-Sinai Neurosurgical Institute, Los Angeles, California
Genetics of Intracranial Aneurysms

Jay J. Schindler, MD, MS

Assistant Professor, Department of Neurologic Surgery, Mayo School of Medicine; Resident, Mayo Clinic, Rochester, Minnesota
Multimodality Management of Complex Cerebrovascular Lesions

James M. Schuster, MD, PhD

Assistant Professor of Neurosurgery, University of Pennsylvania School of Medicine; Attending, Department of Neurosurgery, Hospital of the University of Pennsylvania, Philadelphia, Pennsylvania
Growth Factors and Brain Tumors; Motor, Sensory, and Language Mapping and Monitoring for Cortical Resections; Posterior Thoracic Instrumentation

Theodore H. Schwartz, MD

Assistant Professor of Neurosurgery, Cornell University Joan and Sanford I. Weill Medical College; Assistant Attending in Neurosurgery, New York Presbyterian Hospital, New York, New York
Spinal Cord Tumors in Adults

R. Michael Scott, MD

Professor of Neurological Surgery, Harvard Medical School; Director, Clinical Pediatric Neurosurgery, The Children's Hospital and Medical Center, Boston, Massachusetts
Choroid Plexus Tumors; Cerebellar Astrocytomas in Children

Raymond Sekula, MD

Resident, Department of Neurosurgery, Allegheny General Hospital, Pittsburgh, Pennsylvania
Ablative Surgery for Spasticity

Laligam N. Sekhar, MD

Private Practice, Annandale, Virginia
Chordoma and Chondrosarcoma

Warren R. Selman, MD

Professor of Neurological Surgery, Department of Neurological Surgery, Case Western Reserve University School of Medicine; Vice Chairman, Department of Neurological Surgery, and The Research Institute, University Hospitals of Cleveland, Cleveland, Ohio
Intraoperative Cerebral Protection

Chandranath Sen, MD

Chairman, Department of Neurosurgery, and Co-Director, Center for Cranial Surgery, St. Luke's-Roosevelt Medical Center, New York, New York
Trigeminal Schwannomas

Joel L. Seres, MD

Clinical Professor, Department of Neurosurgery, Oregon Health Sciences University School of Medicine; Director, Northwest Occupational Medicine Center, Portland, Oregon
Approach to the Patient with Chronic Pain

Franco Servadei, MD

Professor of Neurotraumatology, Post-Graduate Medical School, University of Catania, Ancona; Director, WHO Neurotrauma Collaborating Center, Division of Neurosurgery, Hospital M. Bufalini, Cesena, Italy
Mild Head Injury in Adults

Avi Setton, MD

Attending, Center for Endovascular Surgery, Institute for Neurology and Neurosurgery, Beth Israel Medical Center, New York, New York
Endovascular Management of Brain Arteriovenous Malformations

Christopher I. Shaffrey, MD

Professor, Department of Neurological Surgery and Department of Orthopaedic Surgery, University of Virginia School of Medicine, Charlottesville, Virginia
Spondylolisthesis; Approach to the Patient and Medical Management of Spinal Disorders; Posterior Approach to Cervical Degenerative Disease

David Shafron, MD

Neurosurgeon, Phoenix Children's Hospital, Phoenix, Arizona
Benign Extradural Lesions of the Dorsal Spine

William R. Shapiro, MD

Professor of Neurology, University of Arizona College of Medicine, Tucson; Chief, Neuro-oncology, Division of Neurology, Barrow Neurological Institute, Phoenix, Arizona
Clinical Features: Neurology of Brain Tumor and Paraneoplastic Disorders

Michael Shea, MD

Attending, Department of Radiation Oncology, Hoag Memorial Hospital Presbyterian, Newport Beach, California
Functional Radiosurgery

Jonas M. Sheehan, MD

Chief, Division of Neuro-oncology and Cranial Base Surgery, Department of Neurosurgery, Pennsylvania State University Hospitals, Hershey, Pennsylvania
Esthesioneuroblastoma

Joseph H. Shin, MD

Assistant Professor of Surgery, Section of Plastic Surgery, Department of Surgery, Yale University School of Medicine; Director, Yale Craniofacial Center, Yale–New Haven Hospital, New Haven, Connecticut
Craniofacial Syndromes

Raj K. Shrivastava, MD

Chief Resident, Department of Neurosurgery, Mount Sinai Medical School,, New York, New York
Trigeminal Schwannomas

David Sibell, MD

Assistant Professor, Department of Anesthesiology and Perioperative Medicine, Oregon Health & Science University, Portland, Oregon
Management of Pain by Anesthetic Techniques

Bo K. Siesjö, Md, PhD

Professor, Center for the Study of Neurological Disease, The Queen's Neuroscience Institute, Honolulu, Hawaii
Cerebral Metabolism and the Pathophysiology of Ischemic Brain Damage

Peter Siesjö, MD, PhD

Assistant Professor, Department of Neurosurgery, University of Lund School of Medicine; Consultant, University Hospital, Lund, Sweden
Cerebral Metabolism and the Pathophysiology of Ischemic Brain Damage

Daniel L. Silbergeld, MD

Associate Professor, Department of Neurological Surgery, University of Washington School of Medicine, Seattle, Washington
Malignant Gliomas: Anaplastic Astrocytoma, Glioblastoma Multiforme, Gliosarcoma, Malignant Oligodendroglioma; Motor, Sensory, and Language Mapping and Monitoring for Cortical Resections

Jerry Silver, Ph.D.

Professor, Department of Neurosciences, Case Western Reserve University School of Medicine, Cleveland, Ohio
Cellular and Molecular Mechanisms Mediating Injury and Recovery in the Nervous System

Scott L. Simon, MD, MPH

Resident, Department of Neurosurgery, Hospital of the University of Pennsylvania, Philadelphia, Pennsylvania
Posterior Thoracic Instrumentation

Ran Vijai P. Singh, MBBS

Resident, Department of Neurosurgery, University of Miami Hospital and Clinics, Miami, Florida
Spontaneous Intracerebral Hemorrhage: Non–Arteriovenous Malformation, Nonaneurysm

Ash Singhal, MD

Senior Resident, Department of Neurosurgery, University of Toronto Faculty of Medicine, Toronto, Ontario, Canada
Tumors of the Vertebral Axis: Benign, Primary Malignant, and Metastatic Tumors

Grant Sinson, MD

Associate Professor of Neurosurgery, Medical College of Wisconsin, Milwaukee, Wisconsin
Initial Resuscitation and Patient Evaluation [Moderate and Severe Traumatic Brain Injury]

Stephen L. Skirboll, MD

Assistant Professor, Department of Neurosurgery, Stanford University; Staff, Palo Alto Veterans Affairs Medical Center, Palo Alto, California
Monitoring and Mapping of Vision in the Neurosurgical Patient

Jefferson Slimp, PhD

Associate Professor, Department of Rehabilitation Medicine, University of Washington School of Medicine; Director, Neurophysiological Monitoring, University of Washington Medical Center, Seattle, Washington
Electrodiagnostic Evaluation of Peripheral Nerves: Electromyography, Somatosensory Evoked Potentials, Nerve Action Potentials

Yoland Smith, PhD

Professor of Neurology, Emory University School of Medicine; Staff, Yerkes National Primate Research Center, Atlanta, Georgia
Anatomy and Synaptic Connectivity of the Basal Ganglia

P. K. Sneed, MD

Professor in Residence, Department of Radiation Oncology, University of California, San Francisco, San Francisco, California
Interstitial and Intracavitary Irradiation of Brain Tumors

Robert A. Solomon, MD

Byron Stookey Professor and Chairman, Department of Neurological Surgery, Columbia University College of Physicians and Surgeons, New York, New York
Techniques for Deep Hypothermic Circulatory Arrest

Volker K. H. Sonntag, MD

Clinical Professor of Surgery (Neurosurgery), University of Arizona College of Medicine, Tucson; Vice Chairman, Division of Neurological Surgery, Director, Residency Program, and Chairman, Spine Section, Barrow Neurological Institute, Phoenix, Arizona
Anterior Approach including Cervical Corpectomy; Anterior Cervical Instrumentation; Basic Principles of Spinal Internal Fixation; Occipitocervical Fusion; Overview and Historical Considerations [Spine];

Sulpicio G. Soriano, MD, MSEd

Associate Professor of Anesthesia, Harvard Medical School; Associate in Anesthesia, Children's Hospital, Boston, Massachussetts
Neuroanesthesia in Children

Dennis D. Spencer, MD

Professor, Department of Neurosurgery, Yale University School of Medicine, New Haven, Connecticut
Intracranial Monitoring

Robert F. Spetzler, MD

Professor, Department of Surgery, Section of Neurosurgery, University of Arizona College of Medicine, Tucson; Director and J. N. Harbor Chairman of Neurological Surgery, Barrow Neurological Institute, Phoenix, Arizona
Anesthesia in Cerebrovascular Disease; Traumatic Carotid Injury; Surgical Approaches for Posterior Circulation Aneurysms; Giant Aneurysms; Infratentorial Cavernous Malformations; Classification of Spinal Cord Vascular Lesions

Brett Stacey, MD

Associate Professor, Department of Anesthesiology and Perioperative Medicine, Oregon Health & Science University, Portland, Oregon
Management of Pain by Anesthetic Techniques

Gary K. Steinberg, MD, PhD

Lacroute-Hearst Professor and Chairman, Department of Neurosurgery, Stanford University School of Medicine, Stanford, California
Surgical and Radiosurgical Management of Giant Arteriovenous Malformations; General and Historical Considerations of Radiotherapy and Radiosurgery

Paul Steinbok, MBBS

Professor, Department of Surgery, University of British Columbia Faculty of Medicine; Head, Division of Pediatric Neurosurgery, Children's and Women's Health Centre, Vancouver, British Columbia, Canada
Intrathecal Baclofen Infusion

Barney J. Stern, MD

Professor and Executive Vice Chairman, Department of Neurology, Emory University School of Medicine, Atlanta, Georgia
Sarcoidosis, Tuberculosis, and Xanthogranuloma

David A. Steven, MD

Chief Resident, Department of Clinical Neurological Sciences (Neurosurgery), University of Western Ontario Faculty of Medicine, London, Ontario, Canada
Distal Anterior Cerebral Artery Aneurysms

Kimberly J. Stewart, PhD

Clinical Neuropsychologist, Hampton Roads Neuropsychology, Inc., Virginia Beach, Virginia
Rehabilitation and Prognosis after Traumatic Brain Injury

Charles B. Stillerman, MD

Clinical Professor, Department of Surgery, University of North Dakota School of Medicine, Grand Forks; Director, Department of Neurosurgery, Trinity Medical Center, Minot, North Dakota
Intradiskal and Percutaneous Treatment of Lumbar Disk Disease

John H. Suh, MD

Clinical Director, Department of Radiation Oncology, Cleveland Clinic, Cleveland, Ohio
Principles of Radiotherapy

Peter P. Sun, MD

Assistant Clinical Professor, Department of Neurological Surgery, University of California, San Francisco, School of Medicine, San Francisco; Chief, Division of Neurosurgery, Children's Hospital and Research Center at Oakland, Oakland, California
Pediatric Vertebral Column and Spinal Cord Injuries

Leslie N. Sutton, MD

Professor of Neurosurgery, University of Pennsylvania School of Medicine; Chief, Neurosurgery, Children's Hospital of Philadelphia, Philadelphia, Pennsylvania
Intracranial Ependymomas

Phillip D. Swanson, MD, PhD

Professor of Neurology, University of Washington School of Medicine, Seattle, Washington
History and Physical Examination [Introduction: Approach to the Patient]

Sara J. Swanson, PhD

Associate Professor, Department of Neurology, Medical College of Wisconsin, Milwaukee, Wisconsin
Functional Magnetic Resonance Imaging in Epilepsy Surgery

George W. Sypert, MD

Sypert Institute, Fort Myers, Florida
Evaluation and Management of the Failed Back Syndrome

Derek A. Taggard, MD

Chief Resident, Division of Neurosurgery, University of Iowa Hospitals and Clinics, Iowa City, Iowa
Treatment of Occipital C1 Injury

Jamal M. Taha, MD

Taha Neurosurgical Clinic Kettering; Ohio
Dorsal Rhizotomy and Dorsal Root Ganglionectomy

Rafael J. Tamargo, MD

Associate Professor, Department of Neurosurgery and Otolaryngology, Division of Head and Neck Surgery, Johns Hopkins University School of Medicine; Director, Division of Cerebrovascular Neurosurgery, Department of Neurosurgery, Johns Hopkins Hospital, Baltimore, Maryland
Surgical Positioning and Exposures for Cranial Procedures; Anterior Communicating Artery and Anterior Cerebral Artery Aneurysms

Nitin Tandon, MD

Chief Resident, Center for Neurosurgical Sciences, University of Texas Health Science Center; Chief Resident, University Hospital, Audie L Murphy VA Hospital, San Antonio, Texas
Infections of the Spine and Spinal Cord

Ronald Tasker, MD

Emeritus Professor, Division of Neurosurgery, Department of Surgery, University of Toronto Faculty of Medicine, Toronto, Ontario, Canada
Deep Brain Stimulation for Chronic Pain

Marcos Tatagiba, MD, PhD

Professor and Chairman, Department of Neurosurgery, University of Tuebingen, Tuebingen, Germany
Basic Principles of Skull Base Surgery

Christopher L. Taylor, MD

Resident, Department of Neurological Surgery, University Hospitals of Cleveland, Cleveland, Ohio
Intraoperative Cerebral Protection

Steven A. Telian, MD

John L. Kemink Professor of Neurotology, Department of Otolaryngology–Head and Neck Surgery, University of Michigan Medical School; Director, Division of Otology, Neurotology and Skull Base Surgery, and Medical Director, Cochlear Implant Program, University of Michigan Hospitals, Ann Arbor, Michigan
Treatment of Intractable Vertigo

Kamal Thapar, MD

Assistant Professor, Department of Neurosurgery, University of Toronto Faculty of Medicine, Toronto, Ontario, Canada

Nicholas Theodore, MD

Chief, Section of Neurosurgical Trauma, Division of Neurosurgery, Barrow Neurological Institute, Phoenix, Arizona
Anesthesia in Cerebrovascular Disease; Thoracoscopic Approaches to the Spine

Philip V. Theodosopoulos, MD

Assistant Professor, Department of Neurological Surgery, University of Cincinnati College of Medicine; Director, Skull Base Surgery, Mayfield Clinic, Cincinnati, Ohio
Ossification of the Posterior Longitudinal Ligament and Other Enthesopathies

B. Gregory Thompson, MD

Associate Professor, Department of Neurosurgery, University of Michigan Medical School; Director, Cerebrovascular and Skull Base Section, University of Michigan Hospitals, Ann Arbor, Michigan
Spinal Arteriovenous Malformations; Pregnancy and Treatment of Vascular Disease

Todd P. Thompson, MD

Chief of Neurosurgery, Straub Clinic and Hospital, Honolulu, Hawaii
Patient Selection in Movement Disorder Surgery

William E. Thorell, MD

Resident, Department of Neurosurgery, University of Nebraska Medical Center, Omaha, Nebraska
Brain Tumors: Population-Based Epidemiology, Environmental Risk Factors, and Genetic and Hereditary Syndromes

Robert Tiel, MD

Associate Professor, Department of Neurosurgery, Louisiana State University School of Medicine at New Orleans; Attending Neurosurgeon, Charity Hospital and Ochsner Hospital, New Orleans, Louisiana
Management of Peripheral Nerve Tumors

Suzie C. Tindall, MD

Professor, Department of Neurosurgery, Emory University School of Medicine, Atlanta, Georgia
Carpal Tunnel Syndrome; Entrapment Syndromes of Peripheral Nerve Injuries

Paul Tolentino, MD

Resident, Department of Neurosurgery, University of Florida College of Medicine, Gainesville, Florida
Posterior Lumbar Instrumentation

Tadanori Tomita, MD

Yeager Professor of Pediatric Neurosurgery, Northwestern University Feinberg Medical School; Chairman, Division of Neurosurgery, Children's Memorial Hospital, Chicago, Illinois
Birth Head Trauma

Steven A. Toms, MD, MPH

Assistant Professor, Department of Neurological Surgery, and Head, Section of Neurosurgical Oncology, Oregon Health & Science University School of Medicine; Chief, Section of Neurosurgery, Portland VA Medical Center, Portland, Oregon
Tumor Suppressor Genes and the Genesis of Brain Tumors

Kathleen R. Tozer, MD

Resident, Department of Neurosurgery, University of Washington, Seattle, Washington
Monitoring and Mapping of Vision in the Neurosurgical Patient

Bruce D. Trapp, PhD

Professor, Department of Neurosciences, Case Western Reserve University School of Medicine, Cleveland; Professor, Department of Cell Biology, Neurobiology, and Anatomy, Ohio State University, Cleveland; Professor Department of Chemistry, Cleveland State University, Cleveland; Professor Department of Cellular and Molecular Biology, Kent State University, Kent; Chairman, Department of Neurosciences, Lerner Research Institute, Cleveland Clinic Foundation, Cleveland, Ohio
Neurons and Neuroglia

Vincent C. Traynelis, MD

Professor of Neurosurgery, Department of Surgery, University of Iowa College of Medicine; Staff Neurosurgeon, University of Iowa Hospitals and Clinics, Iowa City, Iowa
Tumors of the Craniovertebral Junction; Treatment of Occipital C1 Injury

R. Shane Tubbs, MS, PA-C

Instructor in Anatomy, University of Alabama School of Medicine; Physician Assistant, Pediatric Neurosurgery Section, Children's Hospital, Birmingham, Alabama
Chiari Malformations

Ramachandra Tummala, MD

Resident, Department of Neurosurgery, University of Minnesota Medical School, Minneapolis, Minnesota
Standard Temporal Lobectomy and Transsylvian Amygdalohippocampectomy

Michael Tymianski, MD, PhD

Assistant Professor, Department of Surgery, University of Toronto Faculty of Medicine; Staff Neurosurgeon, Toronto Western Hospital, University Health Network, Toronto, Ontario, Canada
Surgical Approaches for Anterior Circulation Aneurysms

Atsushi Umemura, MD

Fellow in Stereotactic and Functional Neurosurgery, Department of Neurosurgery, University of Pennsylvania School of Medicine, Philadelphia, Pennsylvania
Topectomy: Uses and Indications

G. Edward Vates, MD, PhD

Staff, Department of Neurological Surgery, Brigham and Women's Hospital, Boston, Massachusetts
Hemangioblastomas of the Central Nervous System; Surgical Approaches for Posterior Circulation Aneurysms

A. Giancarlo Vishteh, MD

Co-Director, Neurotrauma, John C. Lincoln North Mountain Hospital, Phoenix, Arizona
Anesthesia in Cerebrovascular Disease; Traumatic Carotid Injury; Anterior Cervical Instrumentation;

André Visot, MD

Chief, Neurosurgical Service, Hôpital Foch, Suresnes, France
Osseous Tumors

Jerrold L. Vitek, MD, PhD

Professor, Department of Neurology, Emory University School of Medicine, Atlanta, Georgia
Surgery for Dystonia

Kenneth P. Vives, MD

Assistant Professor, Department of Neurosurgery, Yale University School of Medicine; Neurosurgeon, Yale Neurovascular Surgery Program, Neurovascular-Neuroscience Intensive Care Unit, Yale–New Haven Hospital, and Backus Hospital, New Haven, Connecticut
Unusual Gliomas; Surgical Management of Supratentorial Cavernous Malformations; Intracranial Monitoring

Dennis G. Vollmer, MD

Professor of Neurosurgery, University of Texas Health Science Center at Houston; Director, Comprehensive Center for Cerebrovascular Surgery, Memorial Hermann Hospital, Houston, Texas
Overview and Historical Considerations [Spine]; Infections of the Spine and Spinal Cord; Cervical Spine Trauma

Jennifer Vookles, MD

Assistant Professor, Department of Anesthesiology and Perioperative Medicine, Oregon Health & Science University, Portland, Oregon
Management of Pain by Anesthetic Techniques

Phillip A. Wackym, MD

John C. Koss Professor and Chairman, Department of Otolaryngology and Communication Sciences, Medical College of Wisconsin; Chief, Otolaryngology–Head and Neck Surgery, Froedtert & Medical College Hospital, and Children's Hospital of Wisconsin, Milwaukee, Wisconsin
Neuro-otology

Tom Wagner, PhD

Instructor, Department of Oncology, Mayo Graduate School of Medicine, Mayo Clinic; Therapeutic Radiological Physicist, St. Luke's Hospital, Jacksonville, Florida
Fractionated and Stereotactic Radiation, Extracranial Stereotactic Radiation, Intensity Modulation, and Multileaf Collimation

Gregory R. Wahle, MD

Clinical Associate Professor of Urology, Indiana University School of Medicine, Indianapolis, Indiana
Neurourology

Marion L. Walker, MD

Professor of Neurosurgery and Professor of Pediatrics, University of Utah School of Medicine; Chairman, Division of Pediatric Neurosurgery, Primary Children's Medical Center/University of Utah Medical Center, Salt Lake City, Utah
Nonsyndromic Craniosynostosis and Abnormalities of Head Shape

Paul R. Walker, PhD

Private Docent, University of Geneva, Faculty of Medicine; Biologist, University Hospital Geneva, Geneva, Switzerland
Aspects of Immunology Applicable to Brain Tumor Pathogenesis and Treatment

M. Christopher Wallace, MD

Chief, Division of Neurosurgery, University of Toronto Health Network, Toronto, Ontario, Canada
Intracranial Internal Carotid Artery Aneurysms

John W. Walsh, MD, PhD

Professor of Neurosurgery and Pediatrics, Tulane University Medical School; Chief, Section of Pediatric Neurosurgery, Tulane University Hospital and Clinic, New Orleans, Louisiana
Lipomyelomeningocele

Paul P. Wang, MD

Attending, Department of Neurological Surgery, Johns Hopkins Hospital, Baltimore, Maryland
Glomus Jugulare Tumors

John D. Ward, MD

Professor and Vice Chairman, Division of Neurosurgery, Department of Surgery, Virginia Commonwealth University School of Medicine, Richmond, Virginia
Pediatric Head Injury

Benjamin C. Warf, MD

Formerly Professor of Neurosurgery, University of Kentucky College of Medicine, Lexington, Kentucky
Tethered Spinal Cord

Ronald E. Warnick, MD

Professor of Neurosurgery, University of Cincinnati School of Medicine, Cincinnati, Ohio
Surgical Complications and Their Avoidance

Katherine E. Warren, MD

Tenure-Track Clinician, Pediatric Neuro-oncology, National Cancer Institute, National Institutes of Health, Bethesda, Maryland
Principles of Chemotherapy

W. Lee Warren, MD

Chief Resident, Department of Neurosurgery, Allegheny General Hospital, Pittsburgh, Pennsylvania
Diagnosis and Management of Seventh and Eighth Cranial Nerve Injuries due to Temporal Bone Fractures

Kyle D. Weaver, MD

Department of Neurosurgery, University of North Carolina at Chapel Hill School of Medicine, Chapel Hill, North Carolina

Jon Weingart, MD

Associate Professor of Neurosurgery and Oncology, Johns Hopkins University School of Medicine; Attending Neurosurgeon, Johns Hopkins Hospital, Baltimore, Maryland
Basic Principles of Cranial Surgery for Brain Tumors

Philip R. Weinstein, MD

Professor of Neurosurgery, University of California, San Francisco, School of Medicine, San Francisco, California
Ossification of the Posterior Longitudinal Ligament and Other Enthesopathies

Bryce Weir, MD

Interim Dean, Biological Sciences Division, University of Chicago Medical Center, Chicago, Illinois
Perioperative Management of Subarachnoid Hemorrhage

Hung Tzu Wen, MD

Courtesy Assistant Professor, Department of Neurological Surgery, University of Florida College of Medicine, Gainesville, Florida; Clinical Instructor, Division of Neurosurgery Hospital Das Clínicas—University of São Paulo; Clinical Associate, Hospital Samaritanod, São Paulo, Brazil
Surgical Anatomy of the Brain

G. Alexander West, PhD, MD

Associate Professor, Department of Neurological Surgery, Oregon Health & Science University Portland, Oregon
Traumatic Cerebral Aneurysms Secondary to Penetrating Intracranial Injuries

Michael F. Whelan, MD, DDS

Assistant Professor, Department of Surgery, Division of Craniofacial Plastic and Reconstructive Surgery, University of Washington School of Medicine; Attending Plastic and Craniofacial Surgeon, Children's Hospital and Regional Medical Center and Harborview Medical Center, Seattle, Washington
Craniofacial Trauma

Walter W. Whisler, MD

Professor and Chairman Emeritus, Department of Neurosurgery, Rush Medical College; Attending Neurosurgeon, Rush-Presbyterian-St. Luke's Medical Center, Chicago, Illinois
Multiple Subpial Transection

Jonathan White, MD

Assistant Professor of Neurosurgery, University of Texas Southwestern Medical School, Dallas, Texas
Posterior Fossa Arteriovenous Malformations

Thomas Wichmann, MD

Associate Professor of Neurology, Emory University School of Medicine, Atlanta, Georgia
Rationale for Surgical Interventions in Movement Disorders

Agadha Wickremesekera, MBChB (Ontario),

Consultant Neurosurgeon, Wakefield Hospital, Wellington, New Zealand
Infantile Posthemorrhagic Hydrocephalus

Gregory C. Wiggins, MD

Staff Neurosurgeon, David Grant Medical Center, Travis AFB, California
Posterior Approach to Cervical Degenerative Disease

James C. Wilberger, MD

Chair, Department of Neurosurgery, Allegheny General Hospital, Pittsburgh, Pennsylvania
Diagnosis and Management of Seventh and Eighth Cranial Nerve Injuries due to Temporal Bone Fractures

David M. Wildrick, PhD

Attending, Department of Neurosurgery, The University of Texas M.D. Anderson Cancer Center, Houston, Texas
Metastatic Brain Tumors

Lorna Sohn Williams, MD

Assistant Professor, Department of Radiology, University of Florida College of Medicine, Gainesville, Florida
Vein of Galen Malformations

H. Richard Winn, MD

Professor of Neurological Surgery and Neuroscience, Mount Sinai School of Medicine, New York, New York

The Natural History of Unruptured Saccular Cerebral Aneurysms; Surgical Decision Making for the Treatment of Cerebral Aneurysms; Traumatic Cerebral Aneurysms Secondary to Penetrating Intracranial Injuries; Monitoring and Mapping of Vision in the Neurosurgical Patient

Diana Barrett Wiseman, MD

Spine Fellow, Department of Neurological Surgery, University of Washington School of Medicine, Seattle, Washington

Spondylolisthesis

Jeffrey H. Wisoff, MD

Associate Professor of Neurosurgery and Pediatrics, New York University School of Medicine; Director, Division of Pediatric Neurosurgery, New York University Medical Center, New York, New York

Optic Pathway and Hypothalamic Gliomas in Children

Timothy F. Witham, MD

Department of Neurological Surgery, University of Pittsburgh School of Medicine, Pittsburgh, Pennsylvania

Gamma Knife Radiosurgery

W. Putnam Wolcott, MD

Department of Neurological Surgery, University of Virginia School of Medicine, Charlottesville, Virginia

Approach to the Patient and Medical Management, of Spinal Disorders

Donald C. Wright, MD

Surgeon, Washington Brain & Spine Institute, Bethesda, Maryland

Elaine Wyllie, MD

Head, Pediatric Epilepsy Program, Cleveland Clinic, Cleveland, Ohio

Recognition of Surgical Candidates and the Presurgical Evaluation

Kevin Yao, MD

Resident, Department of Neurosurgery, Mount Sinai Medical Center, New York, New York

Infectious Intracranial Aneurysms

Narayan Yoganandan, PhD

Professor and Chair, Department of Biomedical Engineering, and Professor, Department of Neurosurgery, Medical College of Wisconsin; Adjunct Professor of Biomedical Engineering, Marquette University, Milwaukee, Wisconsin

Concepts and Mechanisms of Biomechanics

Howard Yonas, MD

Peter J. Jannetta Professor of Neurological Surgery, University of Pittsburgh School of Medicine; Vice Chairman, Neurological Surgery, and Chief, Cerebrovascular Surgery, and Co-Director, University of Pittsburgh Medical Center Stroke Institute, University of Pittsburgh Medical Center-Presbyterian, Pittsburgh, Pennsylvania

Xenon Computed Tomography

Julie E. York, MD

Instructor, Department of Neurosurgery, Loyola University of Chicago Stritch School of Medicine, Maywood, Illinois

Treatment of Axis Fractures; Diagnosis and Management of Thoracolumbar and Lumbar Spine Injuries

Andrew S. Youkilis, MD

Chief Resident, Department of Neurosurgery, University Hospital, Ann Arbor, Michigan

Primitive Neuroectodermal Tumors; Diagnosis and Nonoperative Management [Trigeminal Neuralgia]

George P. H. Young, MD

Associate Professor of Clinical Urology, Cornell University Joan and Sanford I. Weill Medical College; Associate Attending Urologist and Director, Female Urology, Neurourology, Urodynamics, and Reconstructive Urology Unit, New York Presbyterian Hospital, New York, New York

Neurourology

David M. Yousem, MD

Professor of Radiology, Johns Hopkins University School of Medicine; Director, Division of Neuroradiology, Johns Hopkins Hospital, Baltimore, Maryland

Radiologic Features of Central Nervous System Tumors

Eric C. Yuen, MD

Associate Director of Clinical Research, Department of Clinical Neuroscience, Merck Research Laboratories, West Point, Pennsylvania

Peripheral Neuropathies; Electrodiagnostic Evaluation of Peripheral Nerves: Electromyography, Somatosensory Evoked Potentials, Nerve Action Potentials

Joseph M. Zabramski, MD

Chairman, Section of Cerebrovascular Surgery, Division of Neurological Surgery, Barrow Neurological Institute, Phoenix, Arizona

Epidemiology and Natural History of Cavernous Malformations; The Genetics of Cerebral Cavernous Malformations

Alois Zauner, MD

Clinical Instructor, Department of Radiology; University of California, Los Angeles, California

Surgical Management of Traumatic Brain Injury

Seth M. Zeidman, MD

Assistant Professor of Neurosurgery, University of Rochester School of Medicine and Dentistry; Chief, Division of Complex Neurological Surgery, Strong Memorial Hospital, and Attending Neurosurgeon, Highland Hospital, Park Ridge Hospital, and Rochester Memorial Hospital; Private Practice, Rochester Brain and Spine Neurosurgery, Rochester, New York

Hyperextension and Hyperflexion Injuries of the Cervical Spine

Gregory J. Zipfel, MD

Resident, Department of Neurological Surgery, University of Florida School of Medicine, Gainesville, Florida

Surgical Treatment of Intracavernous and Paraclinoid Internal Carotid Artery Aneurysms

Justin A. Zivin, MD, PhD

Professor of Neuroscience, University of California, San Diego, School of Medicine, La Jolla, California

Acute Medical Management of Ischemic Disease and Stroke

Geoffrey Zubay, MD

Chief Resident, Division of Neurological Surgery, Barrow Neurological Institute, Phoenix, Arizona

Basic Principles of Spinal Internal Fixation

Alexander Y. Zubkov, MD, PhD

Resident, Department of Neurology, University of Mississippi Medical Center, Jackson, Mississippi

Radiology of the Skull

Marike Zwienenberg-Lee, MD

Resident in Neurosurgery, Department of Neurological Surgery, University of California, Davis, Medical Center, Sacramento, California

Clinical Pathophysiology of Traumatic Brain Injury

PREFACE

Neurological surgery is a dynamic field, but one that is built on and sustained by the broad shoulders of earlier scientific discoveries and clinical experiences. The fifth edition of *Neurological Surgery* reflects this ever-changing discipline and combines what is "new" with that which is not only "old," but enduring. Thus, this latest volume continues the original intent of the first[1] and subsequent texts edited by Julian Youmans. Reflecting the breadth and complexity of neurosurgery at the beginning of the 21st century, this new volume has had a long gestation period.

This edition has been radically restructured to reflect the ever-changing nature of our discipline. The initial section is focused on the key basic science areas and associated clinical disciplines, the knowledge of which is a necessity for the rational practice of neurosurgery. Subsequent sections reflect the mixture of time-tested information and new advances in the areas of oncology, vascular system, epilepsy, functional, pain, pediatrics, peripheral nerve, radiation therapy and radiosurgery, spine, and trauma. Each section begins with a consideration of general features and historical background that allows the reader to place in context the advances within each section. There then follow chapters dealing with basic scientific information and advances relevant to each area, whereas the subsequent topics within each section deal with clinical advances and surgical techniques. Thus, in all sections, we have added a wealth of new horizontally and vertically integrated information.

The overall aim of each section reflects the unifying goal of the entire book: to provide comprehensive knowledge of disorders and surgery of the nervous system to the student, whether that "student" is a junior resident or an experienced practitioner. Moreover, I hope that future physicians dealing with surgery of the nervous system, whether they are mechanical or biological surgeons,[2] will value the information contained in this text.

It is self-evident that these volumes represent the diligent work of many individuals. I enthusiastically express my appreciation to each of the Section Editors who contributed many long hours to the success of this effort: Roy Bakay (Functional), Henry Brem (Oncology), Kim Burchiel (Functional and Pain), Bill Friedman (Radiation Therapy and Radiosurgery), Sean Grady (Trauma), Michel Kliot (Introduction and Peripheral Nerve), Dade Lunsford (Radiation Therapy and Radiosurgery), Joel MacDonald (Special Features), Larry Marshall (Trauma), Marc Mayberg (Special Features), Fred Meyer (Vascular), T. S. Park (Pediatric), Ray Sawaya (Oncology), Michael Scott (Pediatric), Dan Silbergeld (Epilepsy), Volker Sonntag (Spine), Robert Spetzler (Vascular), and Dennis Vollmer (Spine). A special acknowledgement and thanks go to my long-time colleague, Ralph Dacey, Deputy Editor-in-Chief.

To bring to fruition a work of this magnitude requires a highly professional and disciplined editorial effort and for this I thank the members of the Saunders/Elsevier team: Publishing Directors, Richard Lampert and Richard Zorab (formerly); Developmental Editors, Anne Snyder and David Orzechowski (formerly); and Project Manager, Jodi Kaye. Most importantly, Margaret Connelly, my Editorial Assistant throughout this entire project, should be recognized for her vital and superb contributions.

A personal note of gratitude goes to my wife Debbie, our daughter Allison and her husband Adam, and our son Randy and his wife Tamara for their sustaining support and encouragement.

Lastly, matching the stellar quality of the Deputy Editor-in-Chief, the Section Editors, and the editorial team at Saunders/Elsevier, are the authors of the 335 chapters. With much enthusiasm, I thank them one and all. Their contributions are truly the broad shoulders upon which future care and advances in Neurosurgery will stand.

H. Richard Winn, MD
Editor-in-Chief
Professor of Neurological Surgery and Neuroscience
Mount Sinai School of Medicine New York, New York

1. Youmans JR: Neurological Surgery. Philadelphia, WB Saunders, 1973, pp xvii–xviii.
2. Winn HR, Howard MA: The next 100 years of neurosurgery. Lancet 354(Suppl):36, 1999.

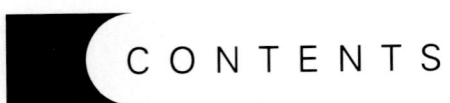

CONTENTS

VOLUME 1

VOLUME 2

VOLUME 3

VOLUME 4

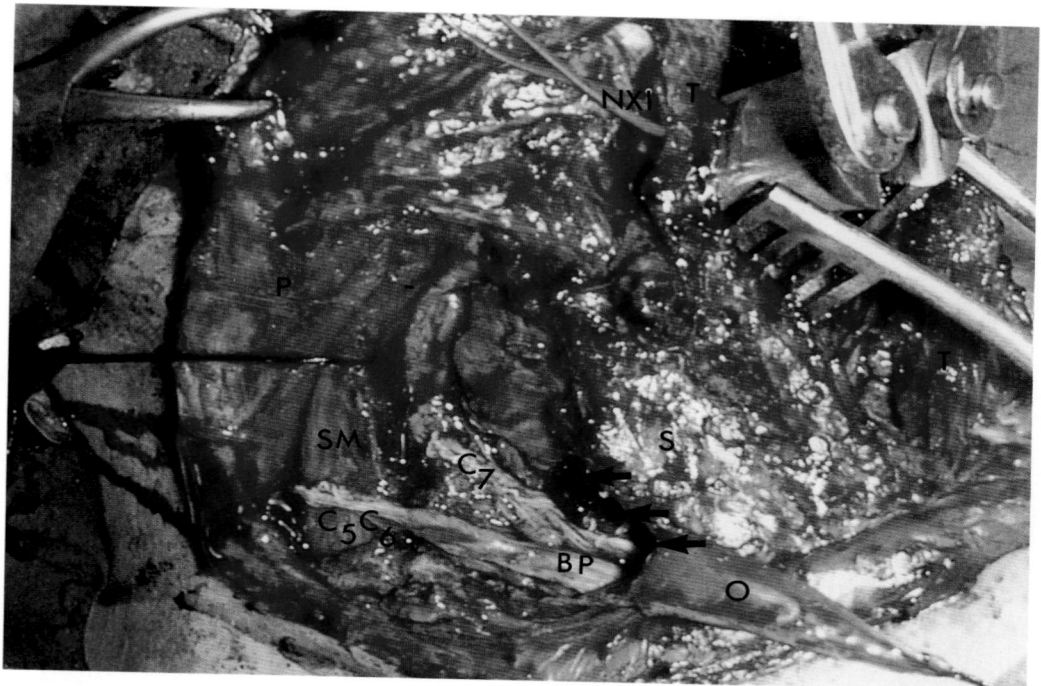

B

FIGURE 260-3. *B,* Intraoperative picture of an exploration of extraspinal parts of the brachial plexus (BP). C5, C6, and C7 spinal nerves are avulsed from the spinal cord. *Arrows* indicate the empty foramina through which endoscopic diagnosis of intraspinal lesions can be made (see Fig. 260-4). There is a sling around the accessory nerve (NXI). A retractor is placed in the posterior part of the wound for the lateral approach to the cervical spine. O, omohyoid muscle; P, platysma; S, scalenus muscles; SM, sternoecleidomastoid muscle; T, trapezius muscle.

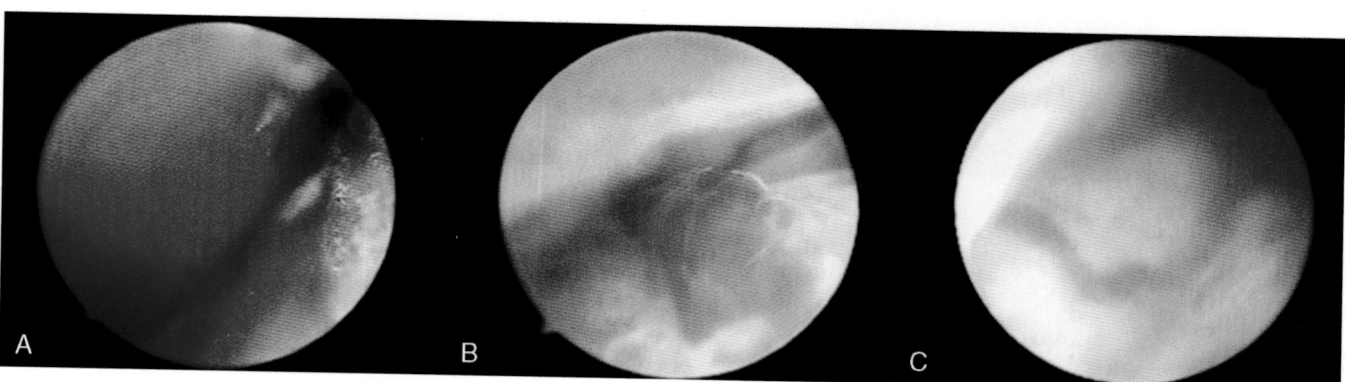

FIGURE 260-4. Intraspinal endoscopy. *A,* The endoscope is placed through the intervertebral foramen of C7. *B,* A vessel is visualized in the medial part of the canal, and a small part of the spinal cord can be seen. *C,* Close to the spinal cord, there are no remaining roots.

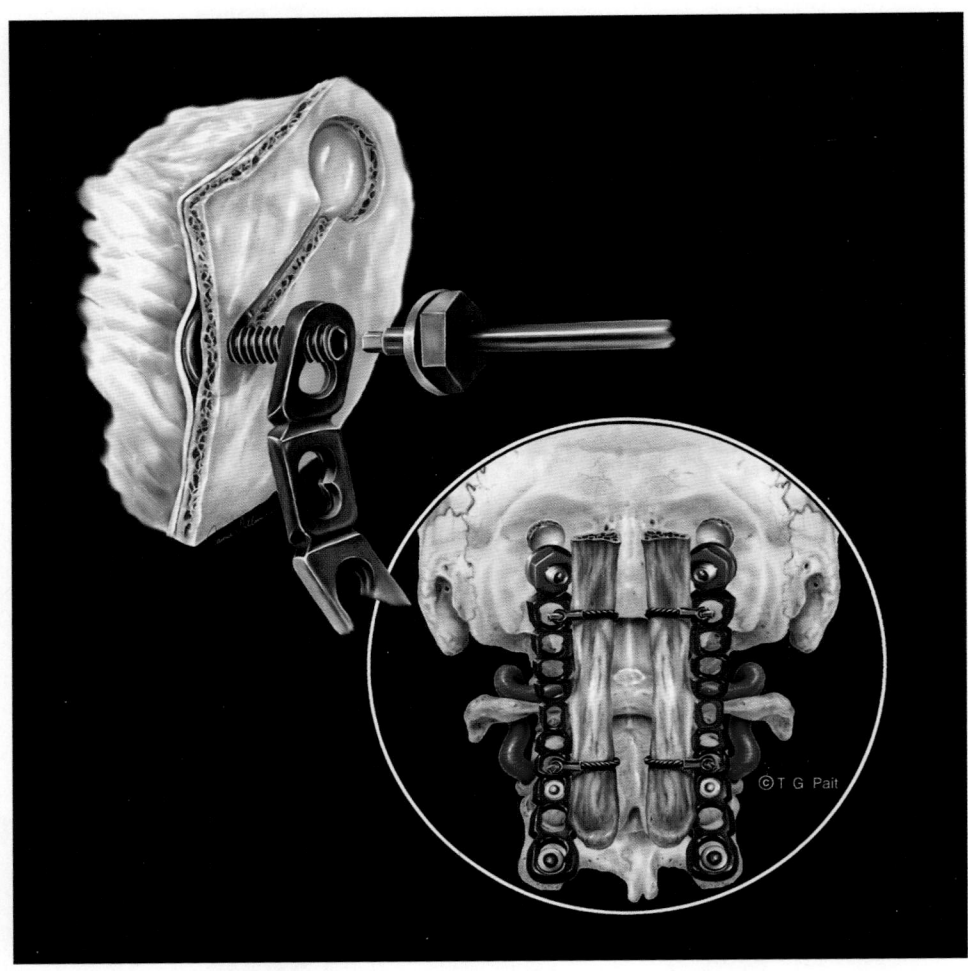

FIGURE 303-12. Illustration of the "inside-out" technique for occipital bone screw placement as described by Pait and associates.[15] (From Pait TG, Al-Mefty O, Boop FA, et al: Inside-outside technique for posterior occipitocervical spine instrumentation and stabilization: Preliminary results. J Neurosurg 90:1–7, 1999 [cover illustration].)

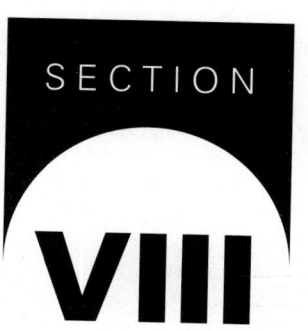

SECTION

VIII

Peripheral Nerve

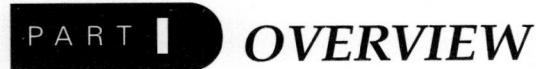

PART I OVERVIEW

MICHEL KLIOT

The section on peripheral nerve disorders tries to cover all clinical aspects of this field relevant to the surgeon. It is divided into chapters on the clinical examination, diagnostic workup, and surgical management of particular types of peripheral nerve problems. Peripheral nerve disorders constitute one clinical area for which the physical examination is the most important component of the patient's evaluation. Electrophysiologic techniques provide important additional information on the extent and location of the underlying nerve problem, its grade or severity, and whether it represents an acute or chronic process. Such information can often help to make a definitive diagnosis. An evolving area is the use of imaging techniques, particularly magnetic resonance imaging (MRI), in diagnosing and treating a variety or peripheral nerve disorders. Standard and evolving surgical approaches remain quite effective in dealing with many peripheral nerve problems, some of which are quite common. For example, the chapter on the surgical treatment of carpal tunnel syndrome describes open and endoscopic surgical approaches. It is hoped that the information provided in this volume will serve as a logical framework for evaluating and treating, medically or surgically, many peripheral nerve disorders.

CHAPTER 248

General Principles in Evaluating and Treating Peripheral Nerve Injuries

GERALD A. GRANT ■ MICHEL KLIOT

Acute and chronic trauma is by far the most frequent cause of peripheral nerve injury. An understanding of the biologic responses of peripheral nerves after injury and during recovery is critical to diagnosing and treating peripheral nerve injuries. Evaluation of peripheral nerve injuries has traditionally relied primarily on a thorough clinical history and physical examination supplemented by electrophysiologic studies (see Chapter 253), such as electromyographic and nerve conduction tests.[1] Improvements in MRI have added another important tool to the diagnostic armamentarium of the clinician dealing with peripheral nerve injuries (see Chapter 254).[2] This chapter describes how an understanding of the pathologic and clinical grades of peripheral nerve injuries guides the physician in formulating a rational treatment plan.

The mechanisms of peripheral nerve injury usually consist of acute or chronic compression, traction, and laceration. Most acute traumatic nerve injuries are caused by blunt, closed trauma, which may stretch and compress a nerve but which usually leaves it in continuity. An open laceration injury may be sharp or blunt and may produce complete or partial nerve injury. A peripheral nerve is also susceptible to chronic compressive and tensile forces, such as entrapment syndromes (e.g., carpal tunnel syndrome), which represent the most common type of chronic nerve injury. Mass lesions (e.g., tumors, cysts, traumatic pseudoaneurysms) can also secondarily damage adjacent nerves. Entrapment neuropathies represent anatomic sites where a peripheral nerve becomes chronically compromised through compression or tethering, or both, to the point where symptoms and clinical findings of nerve dysfunction result. The underlying pathophysiology represents a combination of direct mechanical distortion through compression or stretching and secondary ischemia.

The severity or grade of a peripheral nerve injury is determined to a large extent by the magnitude, duration, and type of applied forces of injury. Three pathologic grades of nerve injury (i.e., neurapraxia, axonotmesis, and neurotmesis) were defined by Seddon[3] during World War II and were based on the extent of injury to three specific structural or functional components of the nerve (Fig. 248–1): Schwann cells, which insulate axons in the peripheral nervous system; peripheral axons, which conduct signals to and from the central nervous system composed of the spinal cord and brain; and a surrounding peripheral nerve connective tissue matrix, which can serve as a "highway" for regenerating axons. Others, such as Sir Sydney Sunderland,[4] expanded this simple classification system by subdividing neurotmetic grades of injury. For most clinical situations, the three grades of Seddon are adequate in describing the pathophysiology of peripheral nerve injuries and are described in greater detail.

Neurapraxic injuries involve damage specifically to the Schwann cell myelin sheaths while preserving axonal continuity. Nerve conduction is slowed or absent across a neurapraxic lesion, although it is preserved proximal and distal to the lesion. These injuries are often quite localized and represent the mildest grade of nerve injury. They are reversible, with full recovery of function usually occurring within weeks to several months of the initial traumatic injury. *Axonotmetic injuries* are more severe and are characterized by interruption of the axons with preservation of the surrounding highways. Distal wallerian degeneration occurs, and recovery can only occur through axonal regeneration at a rate of approximately 1 mm per day (1 inch per month). *Neurotmetic injuries* represent the most severe grade of peripheral nerve injury. These injuries are characterized by disruption of the axon, myelin, and highway components of the nerve. Neurotmetic injuries may leave the nerve in physical continuity or discontinuity. Wallerian degeneration occurs, but regeneration cannot occur because of the disruption with intervening scar tissue (i.e., neurotmetic injury in continuity) or absence (i.e., neurotmetic injury in discontinuity) of the necessary axonal highways. These injuries therefore require surgical repair, often with interposition nerve grafts.[5]

On the basis of clinical symptoms and physical findings alone, it is often challenging to differentiate neurapraxic, axonotmetic, and neurotmetic grades of injury. Electrodiagnostic studies are particularly helpful

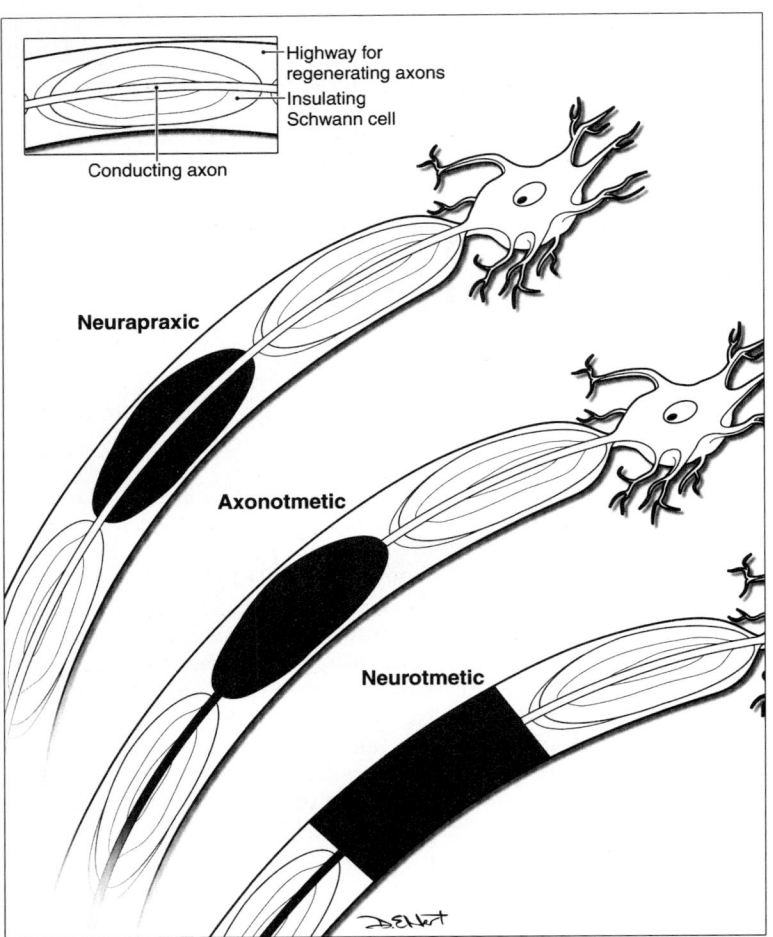

Highway for
regenerating axons
Insulating
Schwann cell
Conducting axon

Neurapraxic

Axonotmetic

Neurotmetic

FIGURE 248–1. The three pathologic grades of peripheral nerve injury are shown in the schematic drawing of the structural and functional components of a nerve (*upper left*). In neurapraxic injury, damage is confined to the insulating Schwann cells while preserving axonal continuity. Axonotmetic injury is characterized by damage to the axons and myelin. The most severe type, neurotmetic injury, involves damage to the axon, myelin, and molecules of the connective tissue matrix, which can serve as a highway for regenerating axons.

in differentiating neurapraxic from axonotmetic and neurotmetic injuries (see Chapter 253). MRI has proved to be a valuable diagnostic tool in the evaluation of nerve injuries by virtue of its ability to detect signal changes in denervated muscles earlier than electromyelography.[2, 6] Further improvements in MRI may eventually make it possible to correlate MRI signal changes in nerve and muscle with phases of axonal degeneration and regeneration, muscle denervation and reinnervation, and loss and recovery of function after peripheral nerve injury and thereby reduce the need for exploratory surgery.[7–9]

The clinical examination can provide important information in evaluating peripheral nerve injuries. These injuries can cause symptoms of pain, dysesthesias, and partial or complete loss of sensory, motor, or autonomic function. The strength of the individual muscles or muscle groups is graded, and a detailed sensory examination is performed that includes testing for light touch, pinprick, two-point discrimination, vibration, and proprioception. The investigation must be logical and systematic, going from proximal to distal, and it must be based on a thorough knowledge of peripheral nerve anatomy and function.[10] Pathology can be classified into one of three clinical grades based on the severity of clinical symptoms. *Mild* clinical

grade is characterized by intermittent sensory symptoms such as dysesthesias, pain, and numbness. *Moderate* clinical grade is characterized by constant symptoms but no evidence of axonal loss such as muscle atrophy and weakness or diminished two-point sensory discrimination. *Severe* clinical grade is characterized by constant symptoms with evidence of axonal loss marked by muscle atrophy, weakness, and diminished two-point discrimination.[11]

The pathologic and clinical grades of nerve injury previously described are useful in classifying nerve injuries and formulating a treatment plan. After an acute traumatic nerve injury, neurapraxic and axonotmetic nerve injuries should be left alone to heal on their own. Neurotmetic injuries, in continuity or discontinuity, require surgery to resect any intervening scar tissue and reestablish continuity of the damaged segment of nerve with nerve grafts.[1, 12] The clinical grading of chronic nerve injuries, such as entrapment neuropathies (e.g., carpal tunnel syndrome, ulnar nerve entrapment across the elbow) allows the physician to develop a rational medical and surgical treatment decision tree (Table 248–1). In general, chronic nerve entrapment injuries of a mild clinical grade can be followed and treated medically with a combination of physical therapy and avoidance of activities that exac-

TABLE 248–1 ■ Clinical Grades of Peripheral Nerve Injury

CLINICAL GRADE	CRITERIA
Mild	Intermittent symptoms
Moderate	Constant symptoms without evidence of axonal loss
Severe	Evidence of axonal loss as shown by muscle atrophy, abnormal two-point discrimination, or both

erbate symptoms. Chronic nerve entrapment injuries of a severe clinical grade should be strongly considered for a surgical decompression. Chronic nerve entrapment injuries of a moderate clinical grade can be treated with an initial trial of medical therapy followed by surgery if the response to treatment proves inadequate.

The basic principles described in this chapter should help guide the clinician in dealing with myriad peripheral nerve problems. These principles are simplifications and cannot substitute for a careful consideration of each patient's problems by astute clinicians calling on all of their clinical knowledge and experience.

REFERENCES

1. Grant GA, Goodkin R, Kliot M: Evaluation and surgical management of peripheral nerve problems. Neurosurgery 44:825–840, 1999.
2. Grant GA, Britz GW, Goodkin R, et al: The utility of magnetic resonance imaging in evaluating peripheral nerve disorders. Muscle Nerve 25:324–331, 2002.
3. Seddon HJ: Three types of nerve injury. Brain 66:237–288, 1943.
4. Sunderland S: A classification of peripheral nerve injuries producing loss of function. Brain 74:491–516, 1951.
5. Kline DG: Surgical repair of peripheral nerve injury. Muscle Nerve 13:843–852, 1990.
6. West GA, Haynor DR, Goodkin R, et al: Magnetic resonance imaging signal changes in denervated muscles after peripheral nerve injury. Neurosurgery 35:1077–1086, 1994.
7. Carlstedt T: Spinal nerve root injuries in brachial plexus lesions: Basic science and clinical application of new surgical strategies. Microsurgery 16:13–16, 1995.
8. Birch R, Bonney G, Parry CBW: Surgical Disorders of the Peripheral Nerves. London, Churchill Livingstone, 1998.
9. Dailey AT, Tsuruda JS, Filler AG, et al: Magnetic resonance neurography of peripheral nerve degeneration and regeneration. Lancet 350:1221–1222, 1997.
10. Omer GE Jr, Spinner M (eds): Management of Peripheral Nerve Problems. Philadelphia, WB Saunders, 1980.
11. Dawson DM, Hallet M, Millender LH: Entrapment Neuropathies. Boston, Little, Brown, 1983.
12. Mackinnon SE, Novak CB: Nerve transfers: New options for reconstruction following nerve injury. Hand Clin 15:643–666, 1999.

CHAPTER 249

History of Peripheral Nerve Surgery

A. LEE DELLON

The fundamental of nerve repair is to re-establish the proximal end to the distal end. That matter of re-establishment, from a surgical point of view, has gone through a multitude of processes. The first process that I knew about was to suture it together and then wrap it in Cargile membrane. Most of you never heard of Cargile membrane. It was pig's bladder. They used to wrap it around the nerve, and they thought they were doing a very good job.

The next we had was the English method of sticking it together with cockerel plasma made into some sort of glue. I believe it was necessary that they should be cockerels; the hens wouldn't do. . . . They put the ends together and they didn't suture them. They wiped the joint around much as a plumber wipes a joint, and they thought that was a swell job. I tried it and found that in the end my difficulty was in getting cockerel's plasma together in such a form that I could use it in the middle of the night when I was trying to sew up a nerve.

The next procedure was to do nothing. . . . This was Seddon's idea. This end here, nothing to it and it's raring to go! A nerve that is cut builds up a great big bundle of nerves that have no place to go, and there it sits and it hurts, and that is what you call a neuroma. The other end undergoes degeneration. This is the Seddon method, and I had disagreeable words with Dr. Seddon. He said afterwards they get some thickening of the neurolemma, so we tried it out in our cases. . . . Our cases that we sutured primarily were just as good as Dr. Seddon's.

Then after that came along a method of sewing it together and covering it with a tantalum wire. I have heard a lot about how clever the surgeons in this war were and how dumb we fellows were in the First World War, but we didn't suture it and put tantalum wire around it because it violated every principle of healing. It turned off all the blood, and the darned things just degenerated. After, it took them half of the war to learn that that was no good. They stopped doing it.

[After the war] following sound surgical principles, we put the nerve together, something like that, and we brought the other one up and mated it. We then sewed the neurolemma here, very carefully together. . . . We put the nerve ends together like this, and then we sutured it. Now that's an honest suture. You have to do an honest suture anyway, and if you don't do that, then you have a couple of neurolemma sticking out like this and another one like that, and when you get the job done you have a lateral neuroma and the patient has pain and he doesn't like it. That is the problem.

Now, here we come to the next step. . . . [If a microfilter sheath] will aid our honest suture, which will hold it together, but at the same time will supply it with oxygen, as

his pictures seem to show, then that is a step in advance. But if his system does not permit the introduction of extracellular fluids into that nerve, it is not good.

Experiments have shown us that to graft with large nerves you can't get blood into the center, so that we have had to reduce ourselves to using small nerves. In general, I have used the tibial nerve out of the middle of the back of the leg and used multiple cables, so that I had many cables, and into those the blood could get, it could furnish it with oxygen and get regeneration.

[Ensheathing a nerve repair with] material can aid that good surgical operation. This is not a shortcut, as I see it, for surgery. This is an aid to good surgery.
—HENRY C. MARBLE, M.D., 1960[1]

The quotation from Henry C. Marble, a neurosurgeon on the faculty of the Massachusetts General Hospital, represents a lifetime of experience in attempting to decide how to treat a divided peripheral nerve. Marble had just heard a neurosurgeon from Columbia University, James B. Campbell, review his group's basic science and clinical experience with neural regeneration through cellulose acetate (Millipore) used as a nerve wrap or conduit.[2] Marble's comments, given at a national meeting of trauma surgeons, emphasizes the critical points in the history of peripheral nerve surgery. This history of peripheral nerve surgery is a series of controversies over ideas related to neural regeneration in the setting of evolving technology.

As we know it today, peripheral nerve surgery had its origins in the mid-19th century, when scientists and surgeons were struggling to understand the neuron and its ability to regenerate. The first half of the 20th century was an attempt to guide nerve regeneration in a clinically meaningful way, gathering experience, as surgeons always did, from the World Wars. Investigators in the second half of the 20th century attempted to incorporate the expanding neuroscience universe within the scope of microsurgery, especially related to neural regeneration through conduits and nerve transplantation.

It is especially relevant to consider the history of peripheral nerve surgery at the beginning of the 21st century, because there now exists the American Society for Peripheral Nerve (ASPN), established in 1990. The ASPN approaches its 13th birthday in the year 2003, and it is composed of more than 200 members from 20 countries (Table 249–1). The subspecialty of peripheral nerve surgery is included. The ASPN members include

TABLE 249–1 ■ **Founding Members of the American Society for Peripheral Nerve**

Warren Breidenbach, M.D.	Michael Orgel, M.D.
David T. Chiu, M.D.	Elliott Rose, M.D.
A. Lee Dellon, M.D.	Joseph Rosen, M.D.
Richard Ehrlichman, M.D.	Brooke Seckel, M.D.
Nelson Goldberg, M.D.	Saleh Shenaq, M.D.
Roger Khouri, M.D.	Thomas Stevenson, M.D.
Howard Klein, M.D.	Julia K. Terzis, M.D., Ph.D.
Susan E. Mackinnon, M.D.	Allen Van Beek, M.D.
Wyndell Merritt, M.D.	H. Bruce Williams, M.D.

neurosurgeons, plastic surgeons, orthopedic surgeons, and hand surgeons. A few of these members devote themselves almost exclusively to surgery of the peripheral nerve (Table 249–2). To best understand the history of peripheral nerve surgery, it is necessary to consider the resolution of the various controversies that gave birth to this new specialty.

CONTROVERSIES

Reticular versus Neuron Theories

Reading early peripheral nerve research is intriguing when viewed from the vantage point of someone who was trained in the last quarter of the 20th century. Why would anyone take a piece of a sensory nerve and place it between two ends of a motor nerve to learn whether a sensory nerve could reinnervate a muscle? Today, we would neurotize the distal motor nerve with a proximal sensory nerve. Although Theodore Schwann described the cell that bears his name in 1839, he was interested in describing the cellular basis of tissues, and he did not describe a function for this particular cell. This cell appeared as if it might be an individual nerve cell, which was linked one to another such nerve cell to constitute the peripheral nerve.

One theory held that any piece of a nerve could be removed and transplanted into a new area, and this piece would regenerate a new nerve. Holders of this theory were called reticularists, peripheralists, or dualists. Alfred Vulpian,[3] who probably did the first nerve grafts, optic to hypoglossal and lingual in 1863 and lingual to hypoglossal in 1870, was a reticularist. He

TABLE 249–2 ■ **Presidents of the American Society for Peripheral Nerve**

1991	Julia K. Terzis, M.D., Ph.D.
1992	Julia K. Terzis, M.D., Ph.D.
1993	A. Lee Dellon, M.D.
1994	Berish Strauch, M.D.
1995	H. Bruce Williams, M.D.
1996	Susan E. Mackinnon, M.D.
1997	Wyndell Merritt, M.D.
1998	Allen Van Beek, M.D.
1999	Saleh Shenaq, M.D.
2000	David T. Chiu, M.D.

was a tenured professor on the Paris Faculty of Medicine, laureate of the Institute of Experimental Physiology, past president of the Philomatique Society, past vice-president of the Biology Society, and a member of the Anatomical Society (Fig. 249–1). When Vulpian obtained contraction of the tongue in a dog by galvanic stimulation of the hypoglossal nerve proximal to his lingual nerve graft, he rationalized that proximal hypoglossal fibers had grown over or around the sensory graft, interfering with the interpretation of the sensory graft's regenerative potential.[4]

In contrast, those who believed that neural regeneration began in the nerve cell nucleus, which was related to the spinal cord, were called holders of the neuron theory, centralists, or monistic. August Waller belonged to this latter group. Although he is most credited with his 1850 description of distal degeneration in a nerve (i.e., glossopharyngeal nerve of the frog) after its division,[5] he is credited by Ochs[6] as having demonstrated nerve fiber regeneration in the cat, with the distance of the regeneration increasing over time. Perhaps the earliest observation of the nerve fiber being the basic unit and of its ability to regenerate was made by Felice Fontana, about 70 years earlier. He was the Director of the Museum in Florence, physicist to the Court of the Medici, and professor at the University of Pisa.[7] From

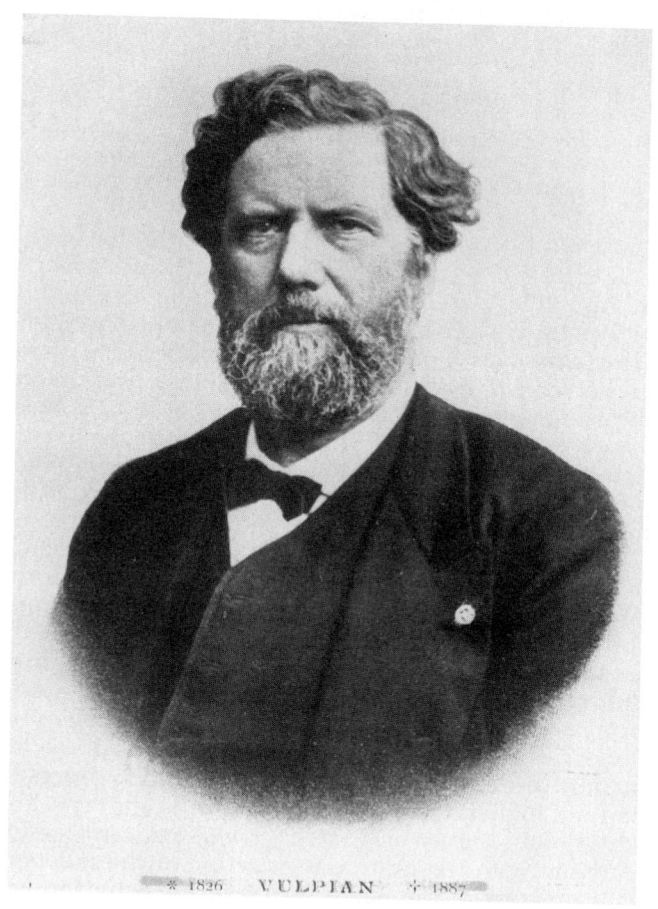

FIGURE 249–1. Alfred Vulpian, M.D. (1826–1887). (Courtesy of the National Library of Medicine, Bethesda, MD.)

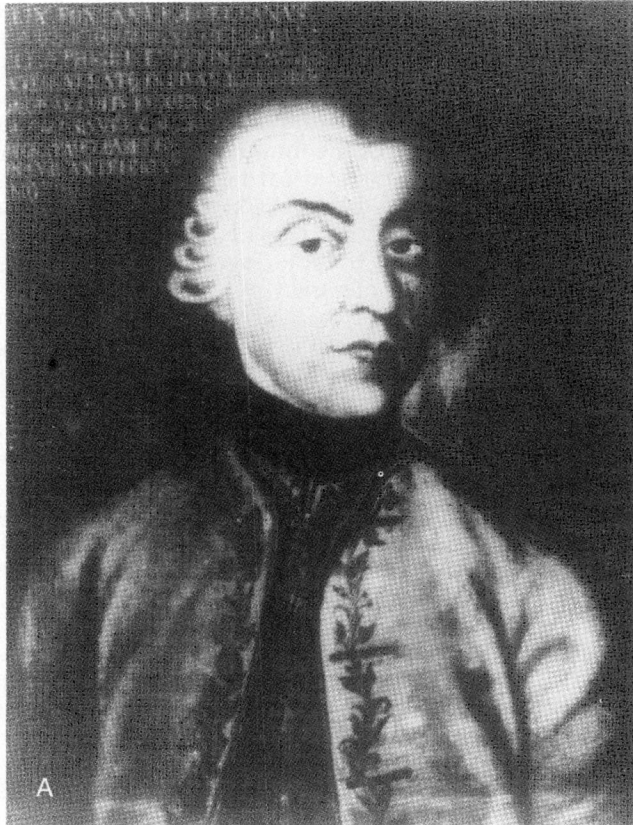

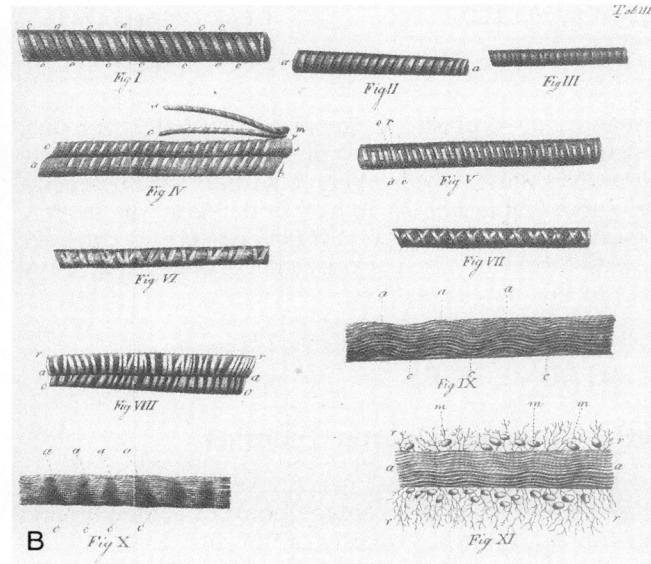

FIGURE 249–2. Felice Fontana (1730–1805). *A,* At about 50 years of age. *B,* Plate VII from his *Treatise* shows the nerve on the 29th day after a six-spiral length had been removed; plate III at a 3× magnification; and with a "strong lense" in plates V and VI. The narrowed region is the site of reconnection of the two ends by regeneration. (Courtesy of the Society di Studyi Trentini di Scienze Storiche.)

1776 to 1780, he took a sabbatical, studying primarily in Paris (Fig. 249–2). During this time, he also studied with John Hunter in London, using hand-held magnifying glasses to examine nerves. Although Fontana is most credited with describing the spiral bands along the peripheral nerve,[7] plate VII from his *Treatise on the Venom of the Viper*[8] in 1781 demonstrated the regeneration of nerve fibers distal to a site of excision of a small piece (six spirals) of a nerve from "the eighth pair of a middle sized rabbit" sciatic nerve (see Fig. 249–2).

During this period, Charles Bell (1774–1842) identified the motor function of the facial nerve and the origin of motor nerves in the ventral horn of the spinal cord. François Magendie (1783–1855) identified that sensory nerves originated in the dorsal root ganglion. Robert Remak (1815–1855) differentiated myelinated from unmyelinated nerve fibers, and Johannes von Purkinje (1787–1869) described the relationship of the neuron to the axon.[9] Joseph Boyes, Sterling Bunnel's partner in hand surgery in California and the first editor of the *Journal of Hand Surgery* (American), credits Harrison with the first demonstration of the independent function of the nerve fiber and the Schwann cell in 1904.[10]

With the controversy resolved and with a new level of scientific understanding, attempts to connect the two ends of a divided nerve began to receive appropriate attention.

To Connect or Not Connect the Injured Nerve Ends

Nerves could not be connected until they were identified and their purpose understood. Hippocrates of Cos (460–136 BC) did not differentiate nerves from tendons. It remained for Galen (31–201 AD), who dissected apes and humans, to make this distinction, as well as to identify 7 of the 12 cranial nerves. Because injured or divided nerves were thought responsible for "convulsions" and because it was believed that they never healed, regardless of treatment, connection of divided nerves was not done. For example, as late as 1551, Ambroise Paré (1510–1590), the French army surgeon, wrote, "The cut nerves retire themselves towards their origninall, and thereby cause a paine like to convulsions."[11]

Nevertheless, this dogma was challenged. In Bologna, William of Saliceto (1210–1277) was reported to have connected the two ends of a nerve by direct suture.[10] The Arabian physician, Avicenna, in his medical text, *Canon,* advocated nerve connection by direct suturing. Rhazes, an Arabian physician in Baghdad, sutured a nerve in 1511.[12] The first detailed account of an operative procedure for nerve connection was by Gabrielle Ferrara, who, in 1608, described splitting the tendons of a tortoise leg into fine filaments, dipping them into hot red wine as an antiseptic, threading them on to a needle, and then using them to connect the ends of severed nerves.[13]

Over the next two and one-half centuries, injured nerves generally were not connected. It was believed that the suture material would cause further infection and be a barrier to regeneration and that the sutured nerves might be the source of worse pain. Many assumed that spontaneous nerve growth would occur without ever touching the nerve. In 1846, Rudolf Virchow, the renowned pathologist stated that "nerve gaps over 10 cm long may not completely regenerate, but in time, function returns sometimes that is unbelievable."[12] This view was held as recently as 1858.[14]

In 1847, Sir James Paget (1814–1899), in England, reported the connection of the two divided ends of the median nerve in an 11-year-old child. The suture was done primarily and reportedly went on to an excellent functional result.[15] Similar results were reported for the median nerve by von Langenback[16] in Germany in 1854 and by Laugier[17] in France in 1864.

With this controversy resolved in favor of attempting to reunite the two ends of a divided nerve, there followed a wide variety of potential techniques to accomplish the connection. Clifford C. Snyder, Professor of Plastic Surgery Emeritus at the University of Utah, and a pioneer in microsurgery (perhaps the first to replant a limb on a dog), authored a chapter on the history of nerve repair. It offers a unique pictorial insight into some of the earliest approaches to connection of two nerve ends[11] (Fig. 249–3). These "drawing board techniques," Snyder states, "were as useless as cataracts in an artist's lens" and "as useless as shoes on a snake." They were, however, the beginning of a new series of controversies that would shape current surgery of the peripheral nerve. These new controversies considered *when* the nerve ends should be connected and *whether the entire nerve or its fascicles* should be connected.

To Connect Now or Later

If two ends of a divided nerve are to be connected, should this be done as soon after the injury as possible? Should the connection be delayed for a period until the metabolic processes of the nucleus are at their maximum efficiency and the epineurium has thickened sufficiently to hold the sutures? As Terzis and Smith[18] stated, "Logical arguments supporting two quite contradictory points of view abound in the literature . . . unfortunately, from the comparison of data on functional recovery of nerve lesions which were very different."

The largest peripheral nerve surgery experiences have been provided by war. In the setting of military conflict, the nerve is generally exposed to significant force, as is the surrounding tissue. The risk of infection is great. Any foreign body placed into the wound acutely increases the risk of infection. In World War I and the beginning of World War II, antibiotics were not available. It is not surprising that the experience of the military, reported by neurosurgeon Barnes Woodhall in the United States[19, 20] and mostly orthopedic surgeons under the direction of Sir Herbert Seddon in England,[21] concluded that primary nerve repair was not recommended. Wounds were explored secondarily at intervals depending on referral to base hospitals and on other injuries. Sometimes, the neuroma end-bulbs were sutured.[22] However, in general, resection of the damaged proximal and distal nerve ends was recommended and the nerves connected, almost always under tension. Motor end-organ atrophy was predictable. The generally poor results, regardless of timing, were not surprising.

By the end of the third quarter of the 20th century, the pendulum swung to the other pole of the controversy. Introduction of magnification into clinical peripheral nerve surgery and the basic science research laboratory, as well as the application of electrophysiologic and histomorphometric analysis to the evaluation of peripheral nerve regeneration, demonstrated that connection of two cleanly and sharply divided nerve ends at the time of the injury or shortly thereafter could result in good recovery of nerve function.[23–27]

Although this controversy has been resolved in favor of doing a primary connection of two nerve ends, if the initial wound is clean and the injury is sharp, the results of primary nerve repair still yield only a small percentage of excellent results, about 10% for digital nerves and 1% for median and ulnar nerves at the wrist.[28] Basic research has demonstrated that the surgeon evaluating these two freshly injured nerve endings cannot determine the extent of that injury on the neural tissue until about 3 weeks after the injury.[29] This inability limits the amount of tissue the surgeon can resect at the time of the primary repair. It is probably this failure to resect sufficient tissue initially that continues to limit the success of peripheral nerve surgery in this circumstance, because the nerve sprouts will regenerate into scar.[30] If the nerve is approached at a time interval that permits the distal neuroma to form, thereby allowing the surgeon to identify the appropriate proximal level for resection of damaged nerve, the resultant nerve gap cannot be closed without tension. Resolution of this problem created the controversy over nerve grafting.

Epineurial versus Perineurial Sutures

During the first half of the 19th century, basic science research, primarily related to the anatomy of the nervous system, initiated the next controversy. During this period, Camillo Golgi (1843–1926) in Italy and Ramon y Cajal (1852–1934) in Spain carried out studies that demonstrated the nervous system was a continuous neural network, composed of individual nerve cells with functional connections. They were awarded the Nobel Prize for these efforts in 1906.[10] Langley and

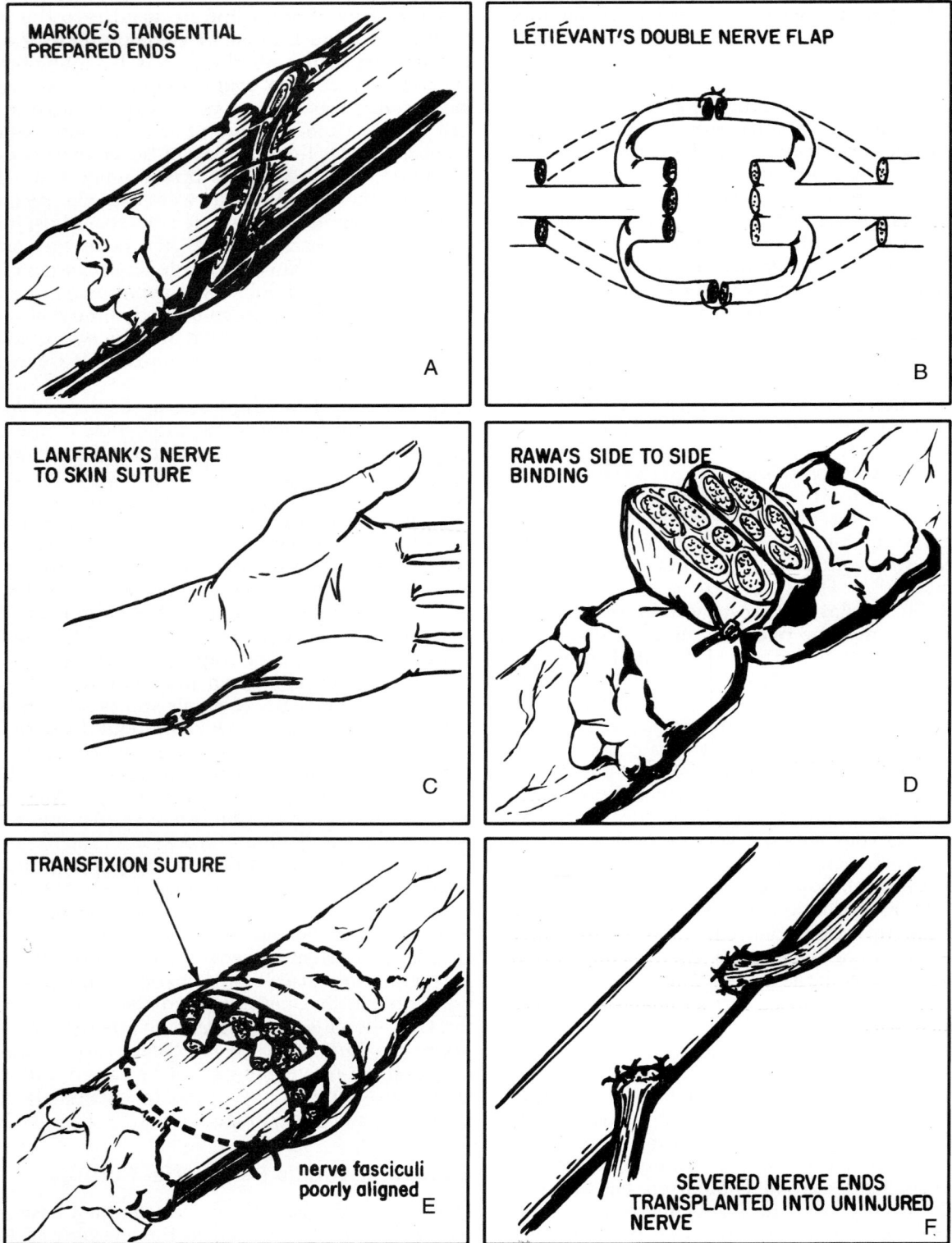

FIGURE 249–3.   Nerve connection techniques. *A,* Tangential cut to increase surface area (1885). *B,* Double nerve flap designed to bridge gaps (1873). *C,* Nerve-to-skin suture to abolish suture interference at the repair site (date unknown). *D,* Side-to-side binding (1885). *E,* Transfixion suture (date unknown). *F,* Implantation into adjacent nerve (date unknown). (Adapted from Terzis JK, Smith KL: The Peripheral Nerve: Structure, Function, and Reconstruction. Norfolk, VA, Hampton Press, 1990.)

Hashimoto[31] in Japan in 1917 and Sunderland[32] in Australia in 1945 laid the groundwork for understanding the fascicular structure of peripheral nerves. Sunderland's encyclopedic work on the peripheral nerve (1968) became the standard reference book for peripheral nerve surgery.[33] Unfortunately, the illustration of the intricate plexus formation within the musculocutaneous nerve discouraged many from doing interfascicular dissection. It was also believed that the intraneural dissection would create significant scarring that would impede regeneration. The controversy was formidable for about a decade.[34-36]

The dissections and insight provided by Jabaley[37] led to the resolution of this controversy. The intraneural plexus formation becomes progressively less distally. When function can be determined by known anatomic localization, by intraoperative electrical stimulation,[38, 39] or by histochemical staining techniques,[40, 41] perineurial sutures are indicated, where possible. Often, this takes the form of a grouped fascicular repair. At the most proximal level of the peripheral nerve, where this knowledge may not be applicable, an epineurial repair is indicated.

To Graft or Not to Graft

It was clear to pioneers in peripheral nerve surgery that a gap in a nerve should be filled with another nerve. In 1885, Albert[42] used a nerve from another human. In 1896, Mayo-Robertson[43] thought a nerve from another animal, such as the spinal cord of the rabbit, might be a good nerve source. Alternative sources of preparing nerves for grafting, such as freeze-drying were applied by Weiss[44] in 1943.

The nerve graft controversy was related to the analysis of autografts by Seddon in 1947 and continued in 1963.[45, 46] This analysis, unfortunately, demonstrated extremely poor results. In retrospect, we know that the problem came not with the concept of autogenous nerve grafting, but with the realization that large nerve grafts did not revascularize well. Many of the early procedures were done in patients with difficult, scarred wounds and were complicated by infection. The "failure" of nerve grafting caused further analysis of nerve repair, which was then being done for gaps that required the nerves to be sutured under tension, with closure often requiring joint flexion.

Today, the universally accepted value of nerve grafts has come through three decades of dedicated research, writing, and teaching by Hanno Millesi. In 1968, he began research that demonstrated that tension at the suture line caused failure of regeneration after a nerve suture and that tension should be avoided. To avoid tension, a nerve graft was to be used, but the caliber of the graft must be small enough that it could be revascularized.[47] The first clinical results for upper extremity nerves were published in 1972 with his coworkers Meissl and Berger.[48] Terzis, Faibisoff, and Williams[49] confirmed Millesi's observations on tension-induced nerve regeneration failure. Millesi's group published their follow-up series in 1976.[50] Interposition

interfascicular microsurgical nerve grafting became a significant part of peripheral nerve surgery.

Long nerve grafts required a long time for the nerve to regenerate to the distal target. It was hypothesized that, if the nerve graft could bring its own blood supply into the scarred region, perhaps more Schwann cells would remain viable, and perhaps neural regeneration would be faster. From 1976 through 1985, this hypothesis was confirmed by microsurgeons doing vascularized nerve grafts in Australia,[51] the United States,[52] France,[53, 54] and Japan.[55] This technique permits large-diameter nerve autografts, such as the ulnar nerve, to be used for brachial plexus reconstruction.

The remaining problem for reconstructing a large deficiency of peripheral nerve is a source for the nerve graft. This problem can be solved by going back to the earliest attempts to reconstruct the nerve gap with use of nerves that were not autografts. Mackinnon's group[56] pioneered this area since 1981, and they reported the first clinically successful human nerve allograft using immunosuppression with cyclosporin A in 1992.

Threshold versus Innervation Density

Underlying all the decisions about management of peripheral nerve problems is the assumption that peripheral nerve function can be measured. This has not been a problem for motor function, which can be measured directly in terms of force created by that muscle or the range of motion given to the joint crossed by the muscle. With loss of motor nerve fibers, muscle atrophies. Early in the course of nerve compression, for example, the ulnar nerve has measurable weakness in pinch strength and, with further loss of function, wasting of intrinsic muscles. In 1958, Erik Moberg[57] from Gotteborg, Sweden, introduced hand surgeons to static two-point discrimination measurement as the main correlate with the sensory function of the hand. This is a measurement of innervation density. In 1979, George Omer, an orthopedic surgeon who did pioneering work on sensory testing in the United States Army, introduced nylon monofilaments to hand surgeons.[58] These were used in 1962 by Josephine Semmes and Sidney Weinstein, both clinical psychologists at Bellevue Hospital in New York City, to measure the cutaneous pressure threshold in soldiers with intracranial injuries and to correlate certain hand and cortical functions.[59]

It was time for neurophysiology to enter the debate. In 1944, Joseph Erlanger and Herbert S. Gasser, both at Johns Hopkins University, were awarded the Nobel Prize for their description of the electrical properties of the sensory nerve fibers.[60] In 1967, Vernon B. Mountcastle and coworkers, in the same department of neurophysiology, described the relationship of quickly and slowly adapting fibers and the neurophysiologic basis of the sense of flutter and vibration.[61] In 1969, A. Lee Dellon, a medical student at Johns Hopkins University, after taking Mountcastle's course, correlated the clinical perceptions of moving and static touch and vibratory perception with recovery of function in patients who had a peripheral nerve repair.[62] It was Dellon's

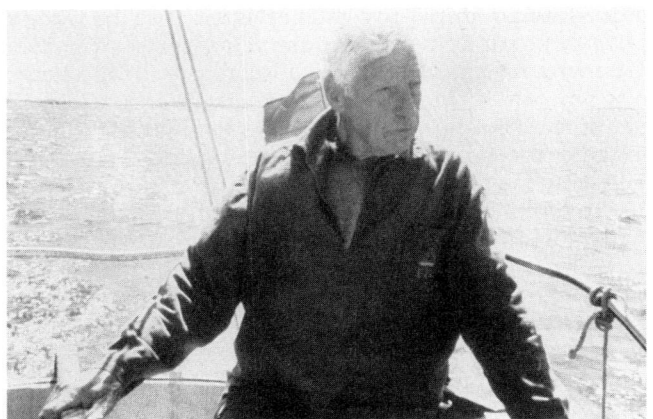

FIGURE 249–4. Erik Moberg, M.D., was a founding member of the American Society for Hand Therapy and founding editor of the *Journal of Hand Therapy*. The photograph was taken by Evelyn Mackin, C.H.T., on Dr. Moberg's boat while sailing in Scandinavia, shortly before his death in 1993.

introduction of vibratory perception testing (i.e., a threshold measurement)[63] and moving two-point discrimination testing[64] during his plastic surgery residency in 1978 that began the staging of chronic nerve compression. In 1988, these concepts were expanded in the textbook, *Surgery of the Peripheral Nerve*, by Mackinnon and Dellon,[65] for individual peripheral nerves. Translation of that text into Chinese and Japanese editions created a worldwide approach to analysis of peripheral nerve problems. A numeric grading system for peripheral nerve function was introduced that permitted better statistical evaluation of the results of peripheral nerve surgery.[66]

Erik Moberg (Fig. 249–4) remained concerned with two-point discrimination testing, because different individual examiners applied different amounts of force to the tips of the prongs used for testing. An instrument was needed to measure the pressure required to discriminate one from two touch stimuli. The Pressure-Specified Sensory Device, the instrument used to make this type of measurement, was introduced in 1992. Because it could measure the cutaneous pressure threshold for one-point moving or static touch and because it could measure the pressure required to distinguish one or two points, moving or static, this device was validated for measurement of hand function,[67] could identify all stages of chronic nerve compression,[68] and provided the final resolution to the threshold versus innervation density controversy because it could measure both.[69]

Neurotropism versus Contact Guidance

How do the regenerating neural sprouts find their way to their appropriate target end-organs? Are they guided by the material on which they regenerate (i.e., contact guidance), or are they attracted by some distant chemical signal (i.e., neurotropism)? The classic drawings of Ramon y Cajal[70] demonstrate regenerating nerve fibers traveling from the end of the proximal

nerve to a distal nerve fiber that is offset in space, giving origin to the neurotropism school. Some of the earliest attempts to connect the two ends of a divided nerve did so through a tube of one sort or another. Paul Weiss,[71] a neurosurgeon who was the leading proponent of the contact guidance school, reviewed the literature through 1943 on this subject. For example, in 1880, Gluck[72] united the two ends of the nerve through the marrow cavity of a bone. Other substances that have been used to unite two ends of nerves without sutures were artery, vein, a feather quill, gelatin, fascia, fat, epineurium, agar, trachea, casein, rubber, dura, muscle, and parchment.

Searching for a technique that would avoid the suture altogether, in 1940, Young and Medawar[73] used a nonmammalian glue prepared from a rooster's plasma and clotted by the addition of chick embryo extract. This is the reference made by Henry Marble to "cockerl glue."[1] The search for an ultimate tissue adhesive that would not interfere with neural regeneration was pursued by Tarlov,[74] who found, working in rabbits and with human plasma, that nerves regenerated well through plasma and that autologous plasma caused less tissue reaction than silk. A related technique, concerned that regenerating axons would "escape" or "wander off," placed a wrapper about the two ends, with or without suturing the two ends. This was the source of the reference Henry Marble made to Cargile membrane,[1] which was pig bladder used by Huber in 1895 for this purpose,[75] and to tantalum, used by Spurling as a wrap and as a tube.[76]

The contact guidance school dominated thinking through the 1960s, as continued attempts were made to identify methods to guide axons distally. For example, James B. Campbell, a neurosurgeon at Columbia University, worked with a group, including C. Andrew Bassett, an orthopedic surgeon, that studied regeneration through nonabsorbable microfilter sheaths, such as cellulose acetate (Millipore).[2] They were sufficiently encouraged to use this technique to repair a median nerve and documented the patient's functional improvement with a handwriting sample. They considered reinforcing the tube with stainless steel so that it would not collapse. Demonstrating dramatic clinical results, Bromley S. Freeman,[77] a plastic surgeon at Baylor University, wrapped a micropore tape (Steri-Strip) around the junctures of a median and ulnar nerve, a digital nerve, and a facial nerve reconstructed with cervical plexus grafts and demonstrated successful neural regeneration in 1965. Another important study from that time was by Richard M. Braun,[78] a hand surgeon in California who suggested that regeneration through a collagen tube, which could be placed without a microscope, gave as good regeneration as a nerve suture technique done through the microscope.

Continued research, such as that by Letorneau,[79] documented that neural sprouts were attracted to the negative charges on the molecules of fibronectin and laminin and confirmed unequivocally that contact guidance existed. However, advances in transplantation biology suggested that observations by Weiss and Taylor of their Y-shaped aortic homografts that discredited neurotropism were probably more the result of a foreign body tissue reaction than proof against neurotropism.

A Nobel Prize was awarded to Rita Levi-Montalchini in 1952 for the discovery of nerve growth factor.[80] During the next decade, surgeons began again to investigate the value of tubes as a means of connecting two ends of a divided nerve, using nonabsorbable tubes, such as silicone,[81] and absorbable tubes.[82] Regeneration through the silicone tubes would not proceed for more than 9 or 10 mm, until it was appreciated that a method for oxygen to enter the tubes—by diffusion through the tube—was required.[83] Silicone tubes were used, however, by Goran Lundborg, a hand surgeon, and his group in Sweden to demonstrate that, in rats, a regenerating sciatic nerve would cross a diagonal space if a nerve were placed at the diagonally opposite end of the space and that a regenerating nerve in a silicone Y-shaped tube would regenerate preferentially to a piece of nerve rather than a piece of tendon or muscle.[84, 85] Basic scientists combined with surgical scientists throughout the 1980s to demonstrate that nerves in rats could regenerate across a variety of absorbable tubes, and they confirmed that neurotropism existed.[86-89]

The controversy about neurotropism versus contact guidance was resolved by concluding that both mechanisms are critical to neural regeneration. A remaining question was how this conclusion would be applied to peripheral nerve surgery in humans. This was answered by Susan E. Mackinnon, Professor of Plastic Surgery at Washington University School of Medicine in St. Louis, and A. Lee Dellon, Professor of Plastic Surgery and Neurosurgery at Johns Hopkins University School of Medicine in Baltimore. In a series of studies from 1982, when Mackinnon was a Hand Surgery Fellow at Baltimore's Raymond M. Curtis Hand Center, through 1988, they demonstrated that the ulnar nerve at the elbow could regenerate 3 cm across a vascularized mesothelial lined tube in the baboon[90] and across a 3-cm bioabsorbable tube made of polyglycolic acid in the monkey[91] and could reinnervate the hand as well as an interposition interfascicular sural nerve graft. They also confirmed that the same ability to choose the correct distal target that Lundborg observed in the rat occurred in the monkey.[92] Mackinnon and Dellon[93] then demonstrated that neural regeneration occurred successfully through up to a 3-cm gap in the human digital nerve. The bioabsorbable tube used in that study, the Neurotube, has a corrugated series of ridges that prevent the tube from collapsing, a problem that has probably prevented clinical use vein grafts from achieving widespread use in areas of critical sensibility.[94]

In 1999, as a result of the first prospective, randomized clinical trial of nerve reconstruction in the United States,[95] the U.S. Federal Drug Administration approved the use of the Neurotube for peripheral nerve reconstruction. That cooperative study,[95] which included five centers, three of which included a past president of the American Society of Surgery of the Hand, demonstrated a statistically significant improved recovery of two-point discrimination for patients who underwent reconstruction using the tube for a minimal gap (<4 mm) (i.e., the type that had a primary repair as the control) or a larger gap (<30 mm) (i.e., the type that had an interposition nerve graft as the control).

THE FINAL CONTROVERSY?

Is there a surgical subspecialty entitled to be called peripheral nerve surgery? From these historical considerations, it is clear that a specific body of knowledge has developed. Are there surgeons who devote a considerable part of their practice to surgery of the peripheral nerve? Yes.

A case may be made for considering James R. Learmonth[96] as the first peripheral nerve surgeon (Fig. 249–5). This neurosurgeon began his peripheral nerve research with observations made early in his career, in 1918, in Glasgow, Scotland, and continued his work at the Mayo Clinic. His career culminated back in Scotland. His contributions to peripheral nerve surgery are given in Table 249–3. Early in the history of peripheral nerve surgery, neurosurgeons such as Barnes Woodhall in St. Louis and James B. Campbell in New York led the way. They were followed by the next generation of neurosurgeons, including Alan R. Hudson in Toronto and David Kline in New Orleans. Neurosurgery is

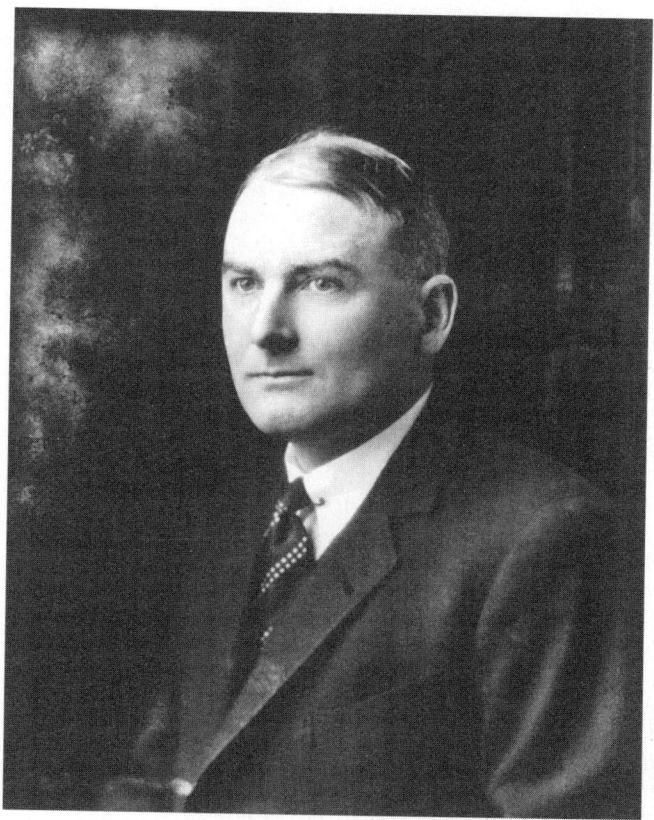

FIGURE 249–5. James R. Learmonth, M.D., neurosurgeon and the first peripheral nerve surgeon.

TABLE 249-3 ■ **Contributions of James R. Learmonth to Peripheral Nerve Surgery**

1920	Description of anomalous innervation of the dorsoradial forearm
1926	Approach to neuromas of the trigeminal nerve
1927	Critique of the literature on laryngeal and phrenic nerve paralysis
1929	Description of "lesions peripheral nerves" Investigation of lumbar sympathetic function and the levator ani October 15, submuscular transposition of the ulnar nerve
1930	Description of neural sheath tumor of the gasserian ganglion Description of spinal cord injuries Treatment of Hirschprung's disease and constipation by denervation July 22; release of the carpal tunnel
1931	Description of lesions of the optic nerve and chiasm
1932	Follow-up report of hypoglossal to facial nerve reconstruction Report of three cases of peripheral nerve tumor
1933	Denervation of the perineum for pruritus of the vulva Described "the principle of decompression in treatment of peripheral nerves," including cervical rib, meralgia paresthetica, carpal and cubital tunnels, and the posterior interosseous nerve
1940	Established a hospital for treatment of peripheral nerve injuries
1942	Pictorial essay on submuscular transposition of the ulnar nerve, including resection of the intermuscular septum
1943	Formulated principle of soft tissue coverage and muscular bed for secondary nerve repair
1953	Served on the Nerve Injuries Committee of the Medical Research Council

Adapted from Dellon AL, Amadio PC: James R. Learmonth: The first peripheral nerve surgeon. J Reconstr Microsurg 16(3):213–215, 2000.

represented in this "third generation" today by James C. Campbell and Alan Beltzberg in Baltimore and by Michel Kliot in Seattle. A few orthopedic surgeons, such as Sir Herbert Seddon in England and George Omer Jr. in New Mexico, devoted themselves to peripheral nerve surgery during the beginning of this subspecialty. Today, orthopedic surgery is represented by those who went on to hand surgery training, such as Richard H. Gelberman in St. Louis, Thomas M. E. Brushart in Baltimore, and A. Lee Osterman in Philadelphia. Peripheral nerve surgery is represented overwhelmingly by plastic surgeons, many of whom consider themselves to be hand surgeons and have held the position of president of the American Society for Peripheral Nerve (see Table 249-2).

A surgical subspecialty should be documented by texts written by these specialists. Consider the "classics": Sir Herbert Seddon's *Peripheral Nerve Injury* (1954)[21]; Woodhall and Beebee's *Peripheral Nerve Repair* (1956)[20]; Sir Sidney Sunderland's *Nerves and Nerve Injuries* (1968)[33]; Sir Herbert Seddon's *Surgical Disorders of the Peripheral Nerves* (1975)[97]; Morton Spinner's *Injuries to the Major Branches of the Peripheral Nerves of the Forearm* (1978)[98]; Hunter, Schneider, Mackin, and Callahan's *Rehabilitation of the Hand* (1978)[99]; Omer and Spinner's *Management of Peripheral Nerve Problems* (1980)[100]; and Dellon's *Evaluation of Sensibility and Reeducation of the Hand* (1981).[28] Since then, the following

textbooks on peripheral nerve surgery have appeared: Mackinnon and Dellon's *Surgery of the Peripheral Nerve* (1988)[65]; Lundborg's *Nerve Injury and Repair* (1988)[101]; Terzis and Smith's *The Peripheral Nerve: Structure, Function, and Reconstruction* (1990)[10]; Gelberman's *Operative Nerve Repair and Reconstruction* (1991)[102]; Hudson and Kline's *Nerve Injuries: Operative Results for Management of Nerve Injury, Entrapment, and Tumor* (1995)[103]; and Dellon's *Somatosensory Testing and Rehabilitation* (1997).[69] The classics are being revised and reissued, including Omer, Spinner, and Van Beek's *Management of Peripheral Nerve Problems* (1998)[104]; Birch, Bonney, and Wynn Parry's *Surgical Disorders of the Peripheral Nerves* (1998)[105]; and Osterman, Mackin, Callahan, and Skirven's *Rehabilitation of the Hand* (2000).[106]

A surgical subspecialty should have fellowship training, which now exists for surgery of the peripheral nerve in programs run by Julia K. Terzis in Norfolk, Virginia, and by Susan E. Mackinnon in St. Louis, Missouri.

With the establishment in 1990 of an organization that represents surgery of the peripheral nerve, the ASPN, it can be concluded that this is a legitimate surgical subspecialty.

EPILOGUE

Tube, or not tube . . . that is the question:
Whether 'tis nobler in the mind to suffer
The stings and shooting pains of neuroma formation,
Or to take our nerve after a divisive injury,
And oppose its ends within a tube? . . . To frustrate,
No more, and by entubulation will end
The pain and the thousand natural shocks
That nerve is heir to . . . 'tis a consummation
Devoutly to be wish'd. To regenerate,
To rehabilitate! Perchance to discriminate . . . ay,
There's the sense.

—*HamLeet*
Act III, Scene I[107]

REFERENCES

1. Marble HC: Discussion of the presentation of JB Campbell and colleagues at the Twentieth Annual Meeting of the American Association of Trauma, Coronado, California, October, 5–7, 1960. J Trauma 1:156–157, 1961.
2. Campbell JB, Bassett CA, Husby, J, et al: Microfilter sheaths in peripheral nerve surgery: A laboratory report and preliminary clinical study. J Trauma 1:139–155, 1961.
3. Dellon ES, Dellon AL: The first nerve graft, Vulpian and the nineteenth century neural regeneration controversy. J Hand Surg Am 18:369–372, 1993.
4. Philipeaux JM, Vulpian A: Note sur des essais de greffe d'un troncon du nerf dernier nerf. Arch Physiol Norm Pathol 3: 618–620, 1870.
5. Waller A: Experiments on the section of the glossopharyngeal and hypoglossal nerves of the frog, and observations on the alterations produced thereby in the structure of their primitive fibers. Philos Trans R Soc Lond 140:423–429, 1850.
6. Ochs S: Waller's concept of the trophic dependence of the nerve fiber on the cell body in the light of the early neuron theory. Clin Med 10:253, 1975.
7. Zachary LS, Dellon ES, Nicholar EM, Dellon AL: The structural basis of Felice Fontana's spiral bands and their relationship to nerve injury. J Reconstr Microsurg 9:131–138, 1993.

8. Fontana F: Traite sur le Venin de la Vipere sur Les Poisons Americains, vol 2. Florence, , 1781.
9. Boyes JH: On the Shoulders of Giants: Notable Names in Hand Surgery. Philadelphia, JB Lippincott, 1976, p 59.
10. Terzis JK, Smith KL: The Peripheral Nerve: Structure, Function, and Reconstruction. Norfolk, VA, Hampton Press, 1990, pp xiii–xiv.
11. Singer DW: Selections from the Works of Ambroise Paré, with a Short Biography. Oxford, John Bale Sons & Danielssohn, 1924.
12. Snyder CC: The history of nerve repair. In Omer GE Jr, Spinner M (eds): Management of Peripheral Nerve Problems. Philadelphia, WB Saunders, 1980, pp 353–365.
13. Ferrara G: Nuova Selva di Cirurgia Divisia in tre Parti. Venice, S Combi, 1608.
14. Adams J: The nervous system. Dublin Q J Med Sci 5:548, 1858.
15. Boyes JH: On the Shoulders of Giants: Notable Names in Hand Surgery. Philadelphia, JB Lippincott, 1976, p 65.
16. von Langenback B: . Verh Dtsch Ges Chir Kongress xx:111, 1876.
17. Laugier G: Seance de L'Academie des Sciences. Paris Gas Hop 37:297, 1864.
18. Terzis JK, Smith KL: The Peripheral Nerve: Structure, Function, and Reconstruction. Norfolk, VA, Hampton Press, 1990, p 117.
19. Woodhall B: Peripheral nerve injuries. II. Basic data from the Peripheral Nerve Registry concerning 7,050 nerve sutures and 67 nerve grafts. J Neurosurg 4:146–154, 1947.
20. Woodhall B, Beebee GW: Peripheral Nerve Repair: A Follow-up study of 3,656 World War II Injuries. Washington, DC, Veterans Administration Monograph, 1956.
21. Seddon HJ: Peripheral Nerve Injury. Medical Research Council special report series 282. London, Her Majesty's Stationery Office, 1954.
22. Kirklin JW, Murphey F, Berkson J: Suture of peripheral nerves. Factor affecting prognosis. Surg Gynecol Obstet 88:719–, 1949.
23. Sakellarides H: A follow-up study of 172 peripheral nerve injuries in the upper extremity in civilians. J Bone Joint Surg Am 44:1–, 1962.
24. Smith JW: Microsurgery of peripheral nerves. Plast Reconstr Surg 33:317–329, 1964.
25. Grabb WC: Median and ulnar nerve suture. An experimental study comparing primary and secondary repair in monkeys. J Bone Joint Surg Am 50:964–972, 1968.
26. Van Beek A, Glover JL: Primary versus delayed-primary neurorrhaphy in rat sciatic nerve. J Surg Res 18:335–339, 1975.
27. Kline DG, Hackett ER: Reappraisal of timing for exploration of civilian peripheral nerve injuries. Surgery 78:54–65, 1975.
28. Dellon AL: Evaluation of Sensibility and Re-education of Sensation in the Hand. Baltimore, Williams & Wilkins, 1981, pp .
29. Zachary LS, Dellon AL, Seiler WA IV: Relationship of intraneural damage in the rat sciatic nerve to mechanism of injury. J Reconstr Microsurg 5:137–140, 1989.
30. Dellon AL: Resection: Nerve repair's most neglected technique. Plast Surg Tech 1:191–199, 1995.
31. Langley JN, Hashimoto M: On the suture of separate bundles in a nerve trunk and on internal nerve plexuses. J Physiol 51:318–345, 1917.
32. Sunderland S: The interneural topography of the radial, median, and ulnar nerves. Brain 68:243–298, 1945.
33. Sunderland S: Nerves and Nerve Injuries. Edinburgh, Churchill Livingstone, 1968.
34. Cabaud HE, Rodkey WG, McCarroll HR, et al: Epineurial and perineurial fascicular nerve repairs: A critical comparison. J Hand Surg 1:131–137, 1976.
35. Kline D, Hudson AR, Bratton BR: Experimental study of fascicular nerve repair with and without epineurial closure. J Neurosurg 54:513–520, 1981.
36. Orgel MG: Epineurial versus perineurial repair of peripheral nerves. In Terzis JK (ed): Microreconstruction of Nerve Injuries. Philadelphia, WB Saunders, 1987, pp 97–100.
37. Jabaley ME, Wallace WH, Heckler FR: Internal topography of major nerves of the forearm and hand: A current view. J Hand Surg 5:1–18, 1980.
38. Hakstian RW: Funicular orientation by direct stimulation. J Bone Joint Surg Am 50:1178–1186, 1968.
39. Gaul JS Jr: Electrical fascicle identification as an adjunct to nerve repair. J Hand Surg 8:289–296, 1983.
40. Gruber H, Freilinger G, Holle J, Mandl H: Identification of motor and sensory funiculi in cut nerves and their selective reunion. Br J Plast Surg 29:70–73, 1976.
41. Engel J, Ganel A, Melamed R, et al: Choline acetyl-transferase for differentiation between human motor and sensory nerve fibers. Ann Plast Surg 4:376–380, 1976.
42. Albert E: Einge Operationen an Nerven. Wein, Med Presse, 1885, p 285.
43. Mayo-Robertson AW: A case in which the spinal cord of a rabbit was successfully used as a graft in the median nerve of man. Br Med J 2:1312, 1896.
44. Weiss P, Taylor AC: Repair of peripheral nerves by grafts of frozen dried nerves. Proc Soc Exp Biol 52:326, 1943.
45. Seddon HJ: The use of autogenous nerve grafts for the repair of large gaps in peripheral nerves. Br J Surg 35:151, 1947.
46. Seddon HJ: Nerve grafting. J Bone Joint Surg Am 45:447–461, 1963.
47. Millesi H: Zum Problem der Uberbruckung von Defkten peripherer Nerven. Wien Med Wochenschr xx:118–182, 1968.
48. Millesi H, Meissl G, Berger A: The interfascicular nerve grafting of the median and ulnar nerve. J Bone Joint Surg Am 54:727–750, 1972.
49. Terzis JK, Faibisoff B, Williams HB: The nerve gap: Suture under tension versus graft. Plast Reconstr Surg 56:166–170, 1975.
50. Millesi H, Meissl G, Berger A: Further experience with interfascicular grafting of median, ulnar, and radial nerves. J Bone Joint Surg Am 58:209–218, 1976.
51. Taylor GI, Ham F: The free vascularized nerve graft. Plast Reconstr Surg 57:413–426, 1976.
52. Breidenbach WC, Terzis JK: The anatomy of free vascularized nerve grafts. Clin Plast Surg 11:65–72, 1984.
53. Gilbert A: Vascularized sural nerve graft. Clin Plast 11:73–77, 1984.
54. Restrepo Y, Merle M, Michon J, et al: Free vascularized nerve grafts: An experimental study in the rabbit. Microsurgery 6:78–84, 1985.
55. Koshima I, Harri K: Experimental study of vascularized nerve grafts: Multifactorial analyses of axonal regeneration of nerves transplanted into an acute burn wound. J Hand Surg Am 10:64–72, 1985.
56. Mackinnon SE, Hudson AR: Clinical application of peripheral nerve transplantation. Plast Reconstr Surg 90:695–699, 1992.
57. Moberg E: Objective methods of determining functional value of sensibility in the skin. J Bone Joint Surg Br 40:454–466, 1958.
58. Werner JK, Omer GE Jr: Evaluating cutaneous pressure sensation in the hand. Am J Occup Ther 24:347, 1979.
59. Semmes J, Weinstein S, Ghent L, Teuber HL: Somatosensory Changes After Penetrating Brain Wounds in Man. Cambridge, MA, Harvard University Press, 1960.
60. Erlanger J, Gasser HS: Electrical Sings of Nervous Activity. Philadelphia, University of Pennsylvania Press, 1937.
61. Mountcastle VB, Talbot WH, Darian-Smith I, Kornhuber HH: Neural basis for the sense of flutter-vibration. Science 155:597–600, 1967.
62. Dellon AL, Curtis RM, Edgerton MT: Evaluating recovery of sensation in the hand after nerve injury. Johns Hopkins Med J 130:235–243, 1972.
63. Dellon AL: The moving two-point discrimination test: Clinical evaluation of the quickly-adapting fiber receptor system. J Hand Surg 3:474–481, 1978.
64. Dellon AL: Clinical use of vibratory stimuli to evaluate peripheral nerve injury and compression neuropathy. Plast Reconstr Surg 65:466–476, 1980.
65. Mackinnon SE, Dellon AL: Surgery of the Peripheral Nerve. New York, Thieme, 1988.
66. Dellon AL: A numerical grading scale for peripheral nerve function. J Hand Ther 6:152–160, 1993.
67. Dellon ES, Keller KM, Moratz V, Dellon AL: Validation of cutaneous threshold measurements for the evaluation of hand function. Ann Plast Surg 38:485–492, 1997.
68. Dellon AL, Keller KM: Computer-assisted quantitative sensory testing in carpal and cubital tunnel syndromes. Ann Plast Surg 38:493–502, 1997.
69. Dellon AL: Threshold versus innervation density. In Somatosensory Testing and Rehabilitation. Bethesda, MD, American Occupational Therapy Association, 1997.

70. Ramon y Cajal S: Degeneration and regeneration of the nervous system. May RM, translator. London, Oxford University Press, 1928.

71. Weiss P, Taylor AC: Further experimental evidence against "neurotropism" in nerve regeneration. J Exp Zool 95:233–257, 1944.

72. Weiss P: The technology of nerve regeneration: A review. Sutureless tubulation and related methods of nerve repair. J Neurosurg 1:400–450, 1944.

73. Young JZ, Medawar PB: . Lancet 2:126, 1940.

74. Tarlov IM, Benjamin B: Plasma clot and silk suture of nerves. I. An experimental study of comparative tissue reaction. Surg Gynecol Obstet 76:366–374, 1943.

75. Huber GC: A study of the operative treatment for loss of nerve substance in peripheral nerves. J Anat Morphol 11:629, 1895.

76. Spurling RG: Tantalum repair of peripheral nerves. Med Clin North Am 23:1491, 1943.

77. Freeman BS: Adhesive neural anastomosis. Plast Reconstr Surg 35:167–176, 1965.

78. Braun RM: Comparative studies of neurorrhaphy and sutureless peripheral nerve repair. Surg Gynecol Obstet 45:15–17, 1966.

79. Letorneau PC: Neurite extension by peripheral and central nervous system neurons in response to substratum bound fibronectin and laminin. Dev Biol 98:212–215, 1983.

80. Levi-Montalcini R, Hamburger V: Selective growth stimulating effects of sarcoma on sensory and sympathetic nervous system of the chick embryo. J Exp Zool 116:321–327, 1951.

81. Ducker T, Hayes GJ: Experimental improvements in the use of Silastic cuff for peripheral nerve repair. J Neurosurg 28:582–587, 1968.

82. Kline DG, Hayes GJ: The use of resorbable wrapper for peripheral nerve repair: Experimental studies in chimpanzees. J Neurosurg 21:737–750, 1967.

83. Jenq CB, Jenq LL, Coggeshall RE: Nerve regeneration changes with filters of different pore size. Exp Neurol 97:662–671, 1987.

84. Lundborg G, Hanson HA: Regeneration of peripheral nerve through a preformed tissue space: Preliminary observations on the reorganization of regenerating nerve fibres and perineurium. Brain Res 178:573–576, 1979.

85. Lundborg G, Dahlin LB, Danielsen N, et al: Nerve regeneration in silicone chambers: Influence of gap length and of distal stump components. Exp Neurol 76:361–375, 1982.

86. Rosen JM, Hentz VR, Kaplan EN: Fascicular tubulization: A cellular approach to peripheral nerve repair. Ann Plast Surg 11:397–411, 1983.

87. Seckel BR, Chiu TH, Nyilas E, Sidman RL: Nerve regeneration through synthetic biodegradable nerve guides: Regulation by the target organ. Plast Reconstr Surg 74:173–181, 1984.

88. Henry EW, Chiu TH, Nyilas E, et al: Nerve regeneration through biodegradable polyester tubes. Exp Neurol 90:652–676, 1985.

89. Brushart TME, Seiler WA IV: Selective reinnervation of distal motor stumps by peripheral motor axons. Exp Neurol 97:289–300, 1987.

90. Mackinnon SE, Dellon AL, Hudson AR, Hunter DA: Nerve regeneration through a pseudosynovial sheath in a primate model. Plast Reconstr Surg 75:833–839, 1985.

91. Dellon AL, Mackinnon SE: An alternative to the classical nerve graft for the management of the short nerve gap. Plast Reconstr Surg 82:849–856, 1988.

92. Mackinnon SE, Dellon AL, Lundborg G, et al: A study of neurotropism in a primate model. J Hand Surg 11:888–894, 1986.

93. Mackinnon SE, Dellon AL: Clinical nerve reconstruction with a bioabsorbable polyglycolic acid tube. Plast Reconstr Surg 85:419–424, 1990.

94. Chiu DT, Strauch B: A prospective clinical evaluation of autogenous vein grafts used a nerve conduit for distal sensory nerve defects of 3 cm or less. Plast Reconstr Surg 86:928–934, 1990.

95. Weber RA, Breidenbach WC, Brown RE, et al: A randomized prospective study of polyglycolic acid conduits for nerve reconstruction in humans. Plast Reconstr Surg 106:1036–1045, discussion 1046–1048, 2000.

96. Dellon AL, Amadio PC: James R. Learmonth, the first peripheral nerve surgeon. J Reconstr Microsurg 16:213–217, 2000.

97. Seddon HJ: Surgical Disorders of the Peripheral Nerves. Edinburgh, Churchill Livingstone, 1975.

98. Spinner M: Injuries to the Major Branches of the Peripheral Nerves of the Forearm. Philadelphia, WB Saunders, 1978.

99. Hunter JM, Schneider LH, Mackin EJ, Callahan A: Rehabilitation of the Hand. Philadelphia, CV Mosby, 1978.

100. Omer GE Jr, Spinner M: Management of Peripheral Nerve Problems. Philadelphia, WB Saunders, 1980.

101. Lundborg G: Nerve Injury and Repair. Edinburgh, Churchill Livingstone, 1988.

102. Gelberman RH: Operative Nerve Repair and Reconstruction. Philadelphia, JB Lippincott, 1991.

103. Kline D, Hudson AR: Nerve Injuries: Operative Results for Management of Nerve Injury, Entrapment, and Tumor. Philadelphia, WB Saunders, 1995.

104. Omer GE Jr, Spinner M, Van Beek A: Management of Peripheral Nerve Problems. Philadelphia, WB Saunders, 1998.

105. Birch R, Bonney G, Wynn Parry CB: Surgical Disorders of the Peripheral Nerves. Edinburgh, Churchill Livingstone, 1998.

106. Osterman AL, Mackin EJ, Callahan A, Skirven TM: Rehabilitation of the Hand, 5th ed. Philadelphia, CV Mosby, 2000.

107. Dellon AL: Tube or not tube. J Hand Surg Br 19:271–272, 1994.

CHAPTER 250

Physiology of the Peripheral Nerve

GREGORY A. KINNEY

The peripheral nervous system (PNS) is integral in maintaining autonomic function and providing sensory information and feedback to the central nervous system (CNS). The PNS is the primary channel through which the CNS physically interacts with the external environment. Injury or damage to the PNS through physical trauma, disease, or chemical exposure can result in partial to complete disruption of PNS function. The specific details underlying disturbances to the PNS can vary considerably, but all result in dysfunction of a common pathway: transmission through the peripheral nerve to or from the spinal cord. This chapter describes the anatomy of the peripheral nerve, the physiology underlying peripheral nerve transmission, and some of the causes and consequences of disruption of peripheral nerve transmission.

ANATOMY OF THE PERIPHERAL NERVE

The PNS is composed of numerous fiber types that convey electrical impulses to and from the CNS. These fiber types include large, myelinated fibers (type I, or Aα); small, myelinated fibers (type II, or Aβ); smaller, myelinated fibers (type III, or Aδ); and unmyelinated fibers (type IV, or C). The large, myelinated fibers are the fastest conducting, and the unmyelinated fibers are the slowest, with the type II and III fibers providing intermediate conduction velocities (Table 250–1). Although some important points about this system are provided in this chapter, a detailed description of the various subtleties of peripheral nerve anatomy and function is available elsewhere.[1–8]

Sensory nerve fibers arise from neurons located in the dorsal root ganglion of the spinal cord; the efferent endings terminate onto neurons within the spinal cord or the brainstem. The numerous types of sensory nerve afferent endings located in the periphery include mechanoreceptors (i.e., Aα and Aβ fibers), which provide the CNS with pressure and proprioceptive information, and nociceptors (i.e., Aδ and C fibers), thermoreceptors (i.e., Aδ and C fibers), and chemoreceptors (i.e., Aδ and C fibers), which together provide the CNS with temperature and pain information. Motor nerve fibers arise from neurons located in the anterior horn of the spinal cord. The afferent endings within the spinal cord receive input from the CNS (i.e., command and reflex information) and sensory input from the PNS (i.e., reflex information only), and the efferent endings of motor nerve fibers terminate on motor units within the periphery at the neuromuscular junction.

Peripheral Nerve Endings

Two important structures of peripheral nerve anatomy are the afferent endings of the sensory nerve fibers and the efferent endings of the motor nerve fibers. Sensory nerve fibers usually terminate subcutaneously (i.e., mechanical, pain, or thermal endings) or in muscle fibers and joint capsules (i.e., limb proprioception) as a bare nerve ending for nociceptors and thermoreceptors or an end-organ encasing the nerve terminal for mechanoreceptors. The various end-organs include the Meissner corpuscle, the Pacinian corpuscle, the Ruffini corpuscle, the Merkel receptor, and the muscle spindle (Fig. 250–1). Each of these end-organs is highly specialized to translate specific types of mechanical energy, temperature change, or chemical content into an electrical signal.

Motor nerve efferent terminals form a highly specialized structure, *the neuromuscular junction* (Fig. 250–2). At the neuromuscular junction, a motor nerve axon releases acetylcholine from the presynaptic terminal, which acts on acetylcholine receptors at the *end plates* on the muscle fibers to elicit depolarization and subsequent contraction of the motor unit. Although rarely a target of trauma-related dysfunction, the neuromuscular junction can be disrupted by toxins and immune system dysfunction.

T A B L E   2 5 0 – 1 ■ **Conduction Velocities of Primary Afferent Fibers in the Cat**

MUSCLE NERVE	CUTANEOUS NERVE	CONDUCTION VELOCITY (m/sec)	DIAMETER (μm)
Myelinated Nerves			
Group I	Aαβ	72–130	12–22
		35–108	6–18
Group II		36–72	6–12
Group III	Aδ	3–30	3–7
Unmyelinated Nerves			
Group IV	C	0.2–2	0.25–1.35

Adpted from Light AR, Perl ER: Peripheral sensory systems. In Dyck PJ, Thomas PK, Griffin JW, Low PA (eds):
Peripheral Neuropathy, vol 1, 3rd ed. Philadelphia, WB Saunders, 1993, pp 149–165.

Myelin Sheath

One of the most notable features of the peripheral nerve is the myelin sheath (see Fig. 250–2*A*). The myelin sheath is a fatty substance generated by nearby Schwann cells, and it surrounds and <u>insulates type I through III peripheral nerve axons.</u> The insulation provides better conducting velocity and signal preservation in myelinated neurons than in nonmyelinated neurons, and it may also be necessary for axonal regeneration after a traumatic injury, such as the crushing of a nerve.

<u>Axonal myelination is segmented</u> (see Fig. 250–2). A single Schwann cell forms concentric layers of myelin around a small segment of the axon, giving rise to one *internodal segment.* Multiple Schwann cells line up along the length of an axon to give rise to multiple internodal segments, each separated by a space of bare nerve known as a *node of Ranvier.* Nodes of Ranvier have a <u>high concentration of sodium ion (Na$^+$) channels,</u> which gives rise to the characteristic <u>saltatory conduction</u> observed in myelinated axons, whereas <u>potassium ion (K$^+$) channels are primarily located in the internodal region.</u> Destruction of the myelin sheath <u>through genetic</u> or acquired disorders has dramatic consequences on signal transmission through the peripheral nerve and can lead to severe disability and death.

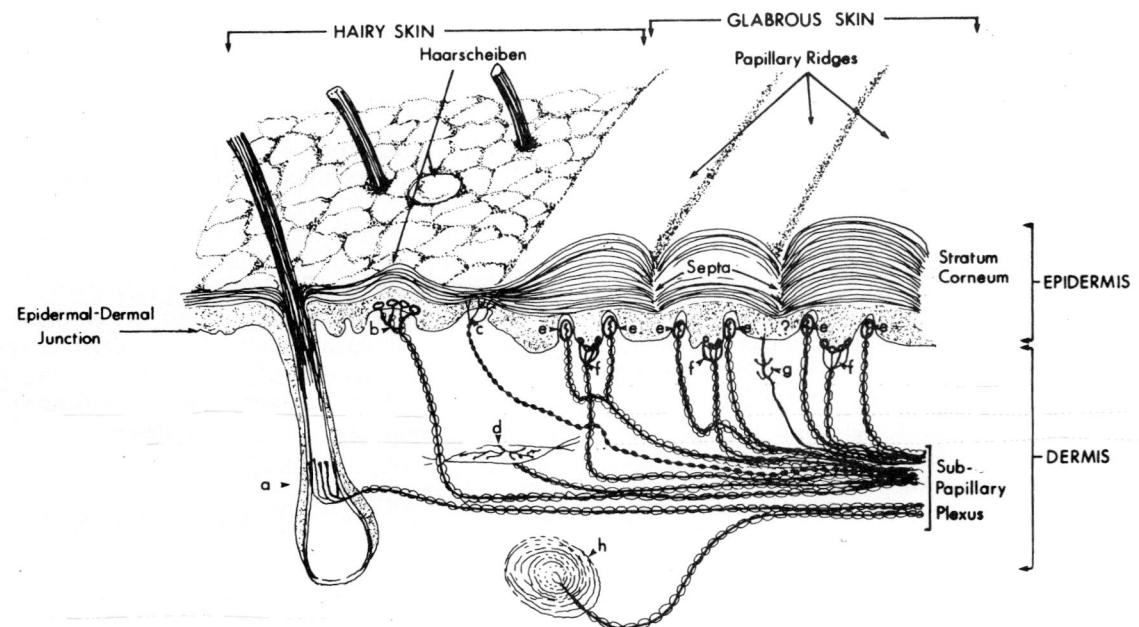

FIGURE 250–1. Various types of sensory receptors are located in the skin of primates. The receptors are located in the superficial skin, the dermis-epidermis junction, and deep within the dermis and subcutaneous tissue. Some of these receptors are the Meissner corpuscle (i.e., detecting flutter vibration), the Pacinian corpuscle (i.e., detecting vibration), and the Ruffini corpuscle and the Merkel receptor (i.e., detecting steady skin indentation). Hair receptors are responsible for flutter sensations, and bare nerve endings (not shown) are primarily responsible for pain and temperature sensations. (From Light AR, Perl ER: Peripheral sensory systems. In Dyck PJ, Thomas PK, Griffin JW, Low PA [eds]: Peripheral Neuropathy, vol 1, 3rd ed. Philadelphia, WB Saunders, 1993, p 153.)

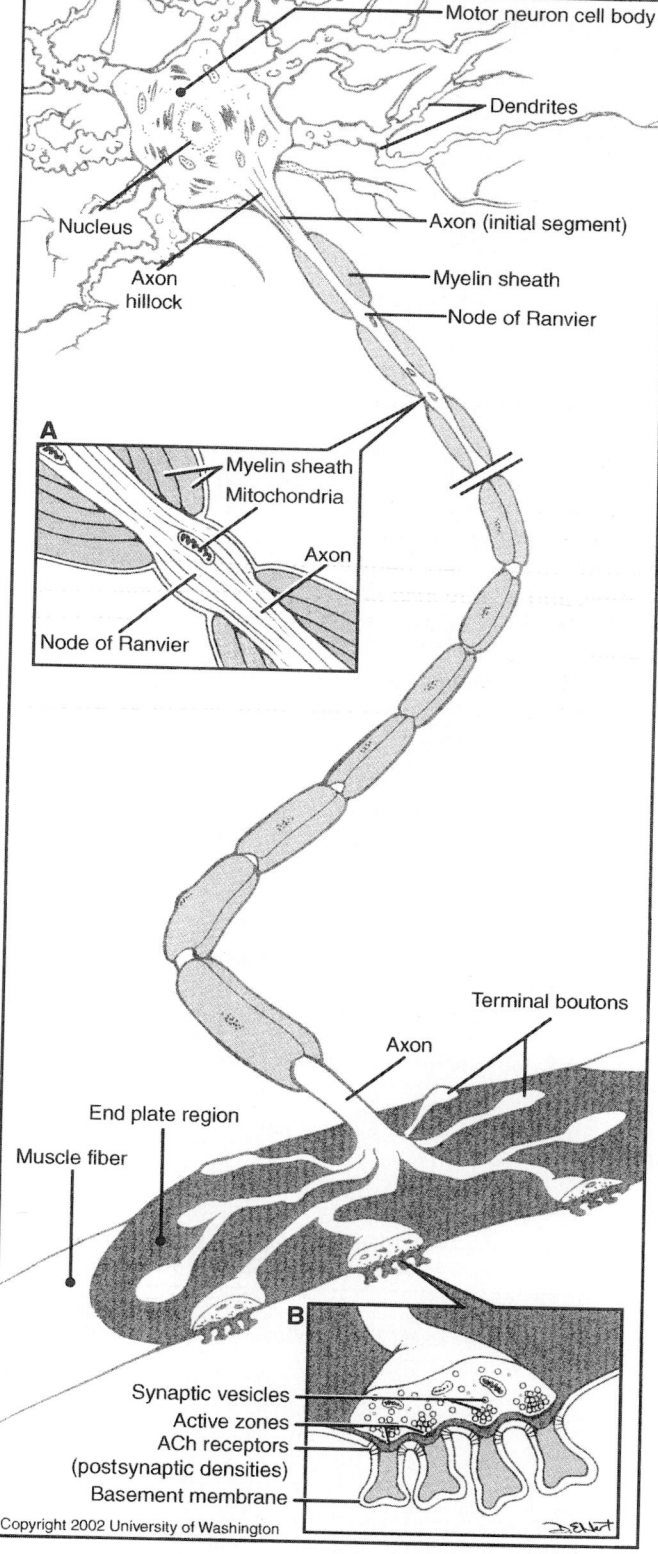

FIGURE 250–2. Schematic drawing of a peripheral motoneuron and motor nerve terminal. A motor nerve is a typical neuron consisting of a cell body, dendrites, and an axon. The cell body and dendrites are located in the ventral (anterior) horn of the spinal cord. The dendrites receive excitatory and inhibitory commands along with reflex input and send the resulting integrated signal out through the axon. An action potential in the neuron is initiated at the axon hillock, which contains a high concentration of voltage-dependent sodium channels. The motor nerve axon exits the spinal cord to form a ventral root, a collection of motor nerve axons from the same level in the spinal cord. Most motor nerve axons are sheathed by myelin, which insulates the neuron, providing more efficient signal transduction. *A,* The myelin sheath is broken up at regular intervals by the nodes of Ranvier, where a high concentration of voltage-dependent sodium channels ensures propagation of the action potential. The motoneuron terminates at the end-plate region on a muscle fiber, where terminal boutons form at multiple locations on a motor end plate. *B,* Within a terminal bouton, high densities of synaptic vesicles, or active zones, directly appose postsynaptic specializations on the muscle fiber known as junctional folds. Within a junctional fold, high concentrations of acetylcholine receptors line the top and sides, whereas acetylcholinesterase, located in the basement membrane, breaks down acetylcholine after synaptic release. (Data from references 5, 40, 41.)

PHYSIOLOGY OF PERIPHERAL NERVE TRANSMISSION

The physiology underlying neuronal transmission in the CNS is maintained in peripheral neurons. The generation of local ionic gradients at the cell membrane through the selective permeability of membrane ion channels results in an electrochemical potential difference between the inside and the outside of the cell. This electrochemical potential is the driving force behind signal transmission through a peripheral nerve. Detailed highlights of the physiology of neuronal transmission are provided in the following sections. More comprehensive reviews of the physiology and electrophysiology of neurons are available elsewhere.[5, 9–19]

Electrochemical Gradient

Every neuron has a potential difference between the inside and the outside of the cell, which is created by the distribution of ions across the cell membrane and the selective permeability of ion channels embedded in the cell membrane. This potential difference is defined as the *resting membrane potential*. Generation of the resting membrane potential depends on the concentrations of ions inside and outside the cell and on the permeability of the cell membrane for those ions. Neurons typically contain a high concentration of K^+ and anions (A^-) inside the cell and a high concentration of Na^+ and chloride ions (Cl^-) outside the cell (Table 250–2). The neuronal cell membrane contains a high concentration of passive K^+ channels that allow the free flow of K^+ ions across the cell membrane. However, the membrane is much less permeable to the other ions

present. As a consequence, K^+ ions are free to flow through the cell membrane, but the other ions are not.

K^+ ions flow out of the cell, moving down the K^+ concentration gradient. The result is an accumulation of cations outside the cell, accumulation of the nonpermeant anions inside the cell, and generation of an electrochemical potential difference across the cell membrane. By convention, the outside of the cell is defined as zero, and the inside of the cell is said to have a negative membrane potential with respect to the outside of the cell. As the charge separation between the inside and the outside of the cell increases, the electrical driving force for K^+ to enter the cell becomes strong and counteracts the chemical driving force of K^+ to move out of the cell. At some point, equilibrium between the electrical and chemical driving forces for K^+ is achieved. This is known as *equilibrium potential* for K^+ (E_K). E_K can be calculated by using the Nernst equation:

$$E_K = \frac{RT}{zF} \ln \frac{[K^+]_o}{[K^+]_i}$$

In Equation 1, R is the gas constant, T is the temperature in Kelvin, z is the variance of K^+, F is the Faraday constant, and $[K^+]_o$ and $[K^+]_i$ are the concentrations of K^+ on the outside and the inside of the cell, respectively. E_K is the value of the membrane potential at which there is no net (passive) movement of K^+ in or out of the cell. At 25°C, the value of RT/zF for K^+ is 26 mV, and E_K for a typical neuron is approximately -75 mV. The Nernst potential for any ion present on both sides of the membrane can be calculated using the Nernst equation, provided the concentrations of the ions are known. Generally, the Nernst potential for K^+ is a close approximation of the resting membrane potential of a neuron, because the permeability of the membrane for K^+ is much higher than any other ion. However, the actual resting membrane potential of a neuron is usually slightly positive compared with the K^+ Nernst potential, because the membrane is slightly permeable to Na^+ and because the electrical and chemical driving forces for Na^+ are toward the inside the cell.

A consequence of the slight permeability of the membrane to Na^+ is that Na^+ constantly flows into the cell. To counterbalance this influx of Na^+, K^+ steadily flows out of the cell to maintain a steady resting membrane potential. If allowed to continue unchecked for any appreciable length of time, the result of this situation would be depletion of $[K^+]_i$ and an increase in $[Na^+]_i$ over time, causing degradation of the resting membrane potential of the cell. To counteract the effects of the steady flux of Na^+ and K^+ into and out of the cell, neurons contain the electrogenic Na^+-K^+ pump, which is a transmembrane-bound protein that extrudes Na^+ from the cell and transports K^+ back into the cell through an ATP-dependent mechanism. This pump translocates 3 Na^+ ions out for every 2 K^+ ions in, resulting in one net positive charge outward for every pump cycle, which results in a slightly more

T A B L E   2 5 0 – 2 ■ **Ionic Distributions**

IONIC DISTRIBUTIONS IN THE SQUID GIANT AXON			
ION	**Cytoplasm (mM)**	**Blood (mM)**	**Seawater (mM)**
K^+	400	20	10
Na^+	50	440	460
Cl^-	40–150	560	540
Ca^{2+}	0.4	10	10

IONIC DISTRIBUTIONS AND EQUILIBRIUM POTENTIALS FOR MAMMALIAN SKELETAL MUSCLE		
	Extracellular (mM)	**Intracellular (mM)**	**Equilibrium Potential (mV)***
Na^+	145	12	+67
K^+	4	155	−98
Ca^{2+}	1.5	10^{-7} M	+129
Cl^-	123	4.2	−90†

* Calculated from Equation 1 at 37°C.
† Calculated assuming a −90 mV resting membrane potential for the muscle membrane and that Cl^- ions are at equilibrium at rest.
Top half adapted from Hodgkin AL: The conduction of the nervous impulse. Liverpool, UK, Liverpool University Press, 1964; bottom half adapted from Hille B: Ionic Channels of Excitable Membranes, 2nd ed. Sunderland, MA, Sinauer, 1992.

negative resting membrane potential than would be expected by diffusion alone.

Action Potential Generation

At rest, there is a strong electrical and chemical driving force for Na⁺ to move inside the cell, but such movement is restricted by the low permeability of the neuronal membrane to Na⁺. However, during the generation of an action potential, there is a brief but dramatic increase in the membrane permeability to Na⁺. This increase in membrane permeability is caused by the opening of voltage-gated Na⁺ channels, and it results in the rapid influx of Na⁺ (Fig. 250–3). For a brief instant, the membrane potential is determined primarily by E_{Na} (i.e., Nernst potential for the sodium ions), which is approximately +55 mV at 25°C, and the result is transient depolarization of the membrane to about +50 mV. In a neuron, the initial generation of this inward Na⁺ current occurs at the axon hillock (see Fig. 250–2), where very high numbers of voltage-gated Na⁺ channels are located. (By convention, a net influx of positive charge is called an *inward current*, which results in *depolarization*, whereas a net efflux of positive charge is called an *outward current*, which results in *hyperpolarization*.) These rapidly activating channels are designed to open only when the neuron depolarizes to a *threshold*, which usually is −45 to −50 mV. Depolarization can occur when dendritic receptors are stimulated by presynaptic inputs or sensory nerve endings are deformed by pressure.

For the neuron to be able to generate another action potential, the Na⁺ channels must be turned off, and the cell must be hyperpolarized back to near the resting membrane potential. The neuron accomplishes this task through two mechanisms: fast Na⁺ channel inactivation and voltage-gated K⁺ channel activation (see Fig. 250–3). Inactivation of voltage-gated Na⁺ channels occurs after a sustained depolarization and is a consequence of that depolarization; in this sense, the Na⁺

channels are self-regulating. The intensity and duration of the depolarization is limited by the inherent properties of the voltage-gated Na⁺ channels. After the depolarization, the cell then returns to its resting membrane potential. This repolarization of the cell membrane could occur by means of the Na⁺-K⁺ pump and passive diffusion. However, to decrease the *refractory period* (i.e., time the cell is unable to fire another action potential), the axonal membrane contains large numbers of voltage-gated K⁺ channels, which open after depolarization and rapidly (<1 msec) hyperpolarize the cell to the resting state through the outward movement of K⁺. Although there is a significant diversity of K⁺ channel types in neurons (unlike Na⁺ channels, which are very similar across different neurons and species), axonal membranes largely express the delayed rectifier K⁺ channel.[9] Like the voltage-gated Na⁺ channels, these voltage-gated K⁺ channels are designed to open only during depolarization, though on a slower time scale than the voltage-gated Na⁺ channels. The more slowly activating outward K⁺ current reverses the depolarization caused by the inward Na⁺ current and repolarizes the membrane (see Fig. 250–3) and relieves Na⁺ channel inactivation. The combination of fast Na⁺ channel inactivation coupled with a large K⁺ conductance after depolarization results in a neuron with the ability to fire action potentials repetitively for extended periods.

Action Potential Conduction

After an action potential is generated in the axon hillock, it propagates down the axon toward the nerve terminal. For the longer axons of the PNS, a high conduction velocity is necessary to make a physical action or sensation occur as quickly as possible. The PNS accomplishes this task by increasing the diameter of the conducting axon, thereby reducing axial resistance (r_a), and by the addition of myelin, which reduces membrane capacitance (c_m). Large-diameter, myelinated axons have the fastest conduction velocity. Conduction down a myelinated axon is referred to as *saltatory conduction* (from the Latin *saltare*, meaning *to leap*).

After generation in the unmyelinated axon hillock, the depolarization generated by the action potential travels down the axon toward the terminal. Because myelin provides high-electrical-resistance, low-capacitance insulation around the nerve fiber, only a small capacitance at the internodal region has to be charged, and there is little voltage attenuation in the signal as the action potential travels down the axon to the next node. The depolarization is well preserved between the nodes of Ranvier and is able to activate the voltage-gated Na⁺ channels located at the next node. The action potential rapidly jumps from node to node, down the axon to the nerve terminal. K⁺ channels in the internodal region then repolarize the membrane.

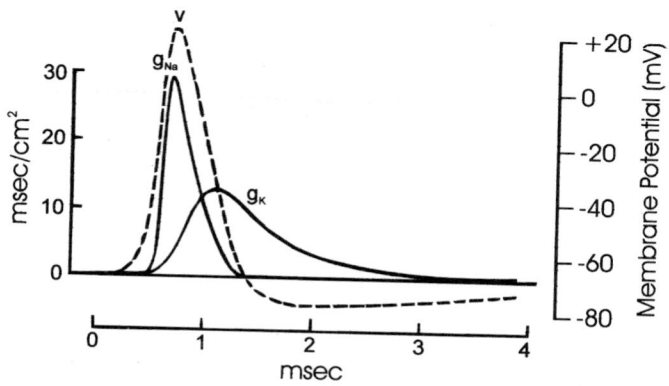

FIGURE 250–3. A theoretical action potential voltage trace was calculated from Na⁺ (g_{Na}) and K⁺ (g_K) conductance changes obtained from a voltage-clamp experiment. The *dashed line* represents the predicted voltage (V) change associated with the opening and closing of the Na⁺ and K⁺ channels in an axon. (From Hodgkin AL: The conduction of the nervous impulse. Liverpool, UK, Liverpool University Press, 1964, p 63.)

Transmission at the Motor Nerve Terminal

The motor nerve terminal is a highly specialized structure designed to provide signal transmission through

Ohm's Law and the Neuron as an Equivalent Circuit

Study of the electroohysiology of neurons and signal transduction requires an understanding of the physics of electricity. The neuron behaves much like an electrical circuit containing electromotive forces, fixed and variable resistors, a capacitor, and a current path (Fig. 250–4). The fundamentals of neuronal behavior in a variety of circumstances can be understood by application of the basic laws of physics. Perhaps the most important of these laws is Ohm's law:

$$V = IR$$

The units of the equation are volts (potential difference), amperes (current), and ohms (resistance). Ohm's law states that the potential difference (V) across a resistor is equal to the current flow (I) across the resistor multiplied by the resistance (R).

This law can be used to calculate the input resistance of a neuron, provided the membrane potential and the current flow are known; these measurements are obtained using voltage-clamp techniques on neurons. For example, if a −10 millivolt (mV) step from −70 to −80 mV results in a −0.2 nanoampere (nA) current, the input resistance of the cell is 50 megaohm (MΩ). If this is repeated in a condition that alters channel activity, a change in input resistance would be observed. An observed decrease in input resistance signifies the opening of membrane channels; an observed increase in input resistance signifies the closing of membrane channels. Put another way, if R decreases, I will increase by a proportional amount to generate the same V.

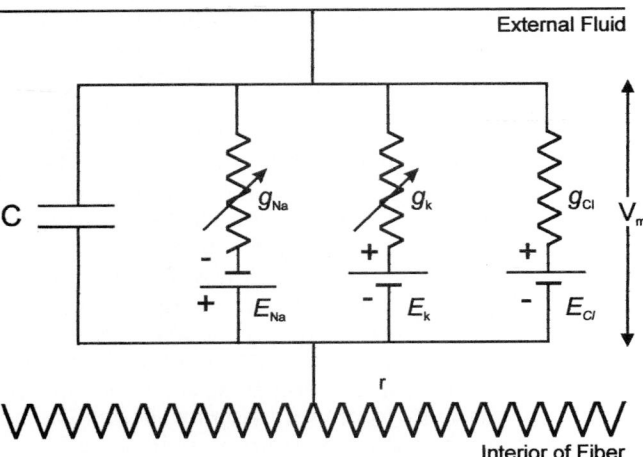

FIGURE 250–4. Equivalent circuit for a length of excitable membrane, such as an axon. E_{Na}, E_K, and E_{Cl} are Nernst potentials for the individual ions. Conductances are represented by resistors, which are variable for Na^+ and K^+ *(arrows)*. C_m is the membrane capacitance, and V_m indicates the membrane potential between the inside and outside of the cell. (From Hodgkin AL: The conduction of the nervous impulse. Liverpool, UK, Liverpool University Press, 1964, p 57.)

the release of a chemical neurotransmitter. The neuromuscular junction is composed of large synaptic contacts (i.e., synaptic boutons) of the presynaptic nerve terminal onto the muscle fiber (see Fig. 250–2*B*). At each of these boutons, a complex structure is developed at the presynaptic membrane and the postsynaptic muscle fiber. At the presynaptic terminal, clusters of synaptic vesicles containing acetylcholine (i.e., active zones) appose postsynaptic clusters of acetylcholine receptors at the *motor end plate*. These acetylcholine receptor clusters are located at the top of a fold of connective tissue known as the *basement membrane*, where the enzyme acetylcholinesterase is concentrated.

Invasion of the action potential into the nerve terminal elicits activation of voltage-gated Ca^{2+} channels, which are highly concentrated at the nerve terminal. Ca^{2+} channels located at the presynaptic terminal are highly voltage-dependent, generating a maximum current at +10 to +20 mV. When the depolarization invades the nerve terminal, these channels are activated, and they open to allow Ca^{2+} to flow into the nerve terminal by moving down the concentration gradient. There are several known subtypes of Ca^{2+} channels (i.e., L, P/Q, N, R, and T), each having distinctive activation and inactivation properties. Some are very fast activating and inactivating, whereas others are more slow to activate and do not readily inactivate. Generally, the combination of Ca^{2+} channel subtypes expressed at a nerve terminal results in a calcium transient that directly reflects the depolarization time course generated by the action potential; the longer the depolarization, the greater the Ca^{2+} entry and subsequent transmitter release.

In the nerve terminal, calcium triggers the fusion of the acetylcholine-containing presynaptic vesicles to the presynaptic membrane (i.e., exocytosis) at the active zone through a complex intracellular mechanism. Transmission of the nerve signal to the motor unit is completed by diffusion of acetylcholine from the presynaptic nerve terminal to postsynaptic acetylcholine receptors located on the muscle fiber membrane (i.e., the motor end plate) (see Fig. 250–2). Activation of these postsynaptic acetylcholine receptors results in the opening of the acetylcholine receptor channel, which is permeable to Na^+, K^+, and Ca^{2+}, and triggers an action potential in the muscle fiber. Termination of the signal is accomplished through degradation of acetylcholine in the nerve terminal by acetylcholinesterase.

PERIPHERAL NERVE PATHOLOGY

Impairment of peripheral nerve function can have significant consequences on the overall health and well-being of the patient. Loss of function through physical trauma, disease, or biochemical insult can result in partial or complete paralysis leading to a level of complete dependence. Understanding the cellular mechanisms underlying peripheral nerve impairment promotes successful treatment of the patient.

Physical Trauma

Forceful impact on a peripheral nerve can temporarily or permanently impair its function, depending on the level of trauma to the peripheral nerve unit. Crushing or severing of the axon results in the formation of two separate nerve segments—one peripheral and one distal to the injury—because the severed or crushed axons eventually close. Disruption in the continuity of the peripheral nerve axons leads to degeneration of the distal segment axons of the peripheral nerve, because they are separated from their metabolic supply center, the cell body. This type of degeneration is known as *wallerian degeneration*. In many cases, regeneration of the nerve can occur if the myelin nerve sheaths (i.e., bands of Bünger) are intact after the injury.

An important result of transecting a spinal sensory neuron is the observed increase in expression of certain Na+ channel subtypes after regrowth. The newly ex-pressed Na+ channels display a shorter refractory period after activation than the typical axonal Na+ channels (Fig. 250–5; see also Fig. 250–1), which leads to bursting behavior and hyperexcitability in the transected sensory neuron.[20] The resultant hyperexcitability contributes to paresthesias and chronic pain and is thought to underlie the formation of painful neuromas.[21, 22]

Genetic Diseases and Acquired Disorders

Numerous disease conditions adversely affect peripheral nerve function. Many of these diseases affect myelination of the peripheral nerve, channel function of the peripheral nerve axon, or the function of the peripheral nerve synapse.

Several well-known demyelinating diseases preferentially affect the peripheral nerve, including the various types of Charcot-Marie-Tooth disease (i.e., CMT

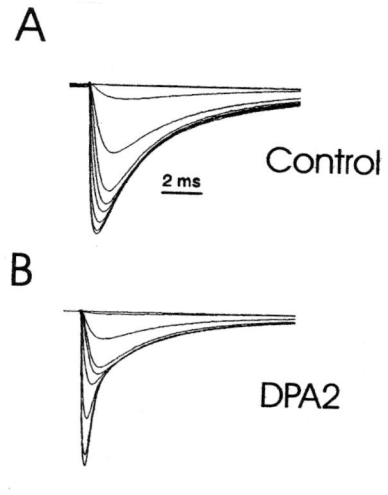

A

Control

2 ms

B

DPA2

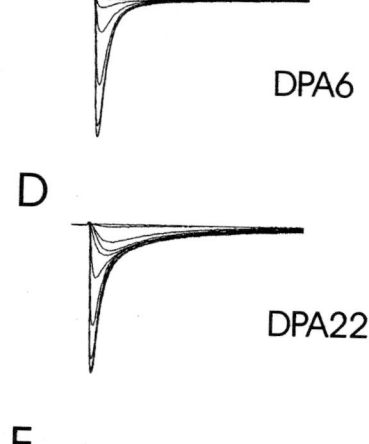

C

DPA6

D

DPA22

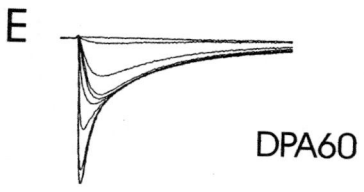

E

DPA60

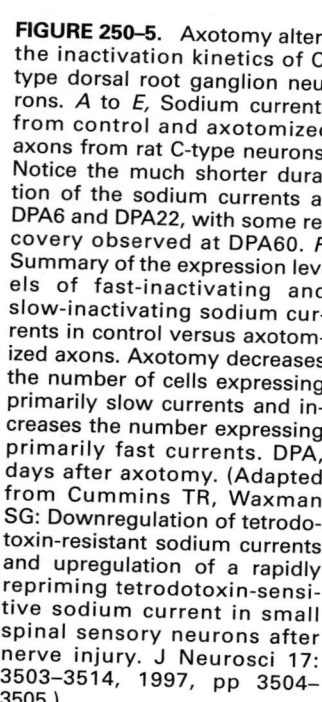

FIGURE 250–5. Axotomy alters the inactivation kinetics of C-type dorsal root ganglion neurons. *A* to *E,* Sodium currents from control and axotomized axons from rat C-type neurons. Notice the much shorter duration of the sodium currents at DPA6 and DPA22, with some recovery observed at DPA60. *F,* Summary of the expression levels of fast-inactivating and slow-inactivating sodium currents in control versus axotomized axons. Axotomy decreases the number of cells expressing primarily slow currents and increases the number expressing primarily fast currents. DPA, days after axotomy. (Adapted from Cummins TR, Waxman SG: Downregulation of tetrodotoxin-resistant sodium currents and upregulation of a rapidly repriming tetrodotoxin-sensitive sodium current in small spinal sensory neurons after nerve injury. J Neurosci 17: 3503–3514, 1997, pp 3504–3505.)

F

Summary Table
Effect of axotomy on sodium current kinetics

Cell Type	Fast	Mixed	Slow	Number of cells
Control	15	39	46	113
Axotomized				
PDA2	32	48	20	40
PDA6	71	29	0	31
PDA22	73	21	6	33
PDA60	50	35	15	54

types 1 through 5 and CMTX) and Guillain-Barré syndrome. Although the cause of demyelinating diseases may differ, the effect is the same: demyelination of the peripheral nerve leads to slowing or block of conduction in the affected nerve due to current loss through unmyelinated regions of the nerve. The consequences and severity of demyelination vary but include weakness; loss of vibration, pain, and temperature sensitivity; footdrop; loss of reflex; and paresthesias.

The mechanism of action of many demyelinating diseases appears to be an autoimmune attack on the myelination of the peripheral nerve. Some channel diseases (i.e., channelopathies) also have such a mechanism of action. Neuromyotonia (i.e., Isaacs syndrome) is a disorder that results in continuous motor unit activity of the peripheral nerve and target muscle. Autoantibodies against voltage-gated K^+ channels result in hyperexcitability of the affected peripheral nerves. K^+ channel antibodies appear to cause a reduction in surface expression of the delayed-rectifier K^+ channel, which results in impairment of the repolarization of the neuron after an action potential and produces overexcitation in the affected neuron and subsequent continuous muscle fiber activity.[23–25]

Autoimmune disorders also affect the nerve terminal. In Lambert-Eaton myasthenic syndrome, a disease characterized by muscle weakness, autoantibodies decrease presynaptic release of acetylcholine at the neuromuscular junction. Evidence indicates that reduction in expression of the N- and P/Q-type voltage-gated Ca^{2+} channels at the presynaptic terminal may be the mechanism of action of this disorder.[26–29] On the postsynaptic side of the synaptic terminal, antibodies produced against the acetylcholine receptor underlie the symptoms of myasthenia gravis, a disease that results in mild to severe muscle weakness.[30–32] This disease is frequently treated by the use of cholinesterase inhibitors, which prevent the breakdown of acetylcholine after synaptic release.

Chemical Interference of Nerve Function

Numerous nerve toxins have highly specific actions on ion channels or other aspects of nerve function. The list is too numerous to review here, but some of the more clinically useful toxins and antagonists deserve mention.

Tetrodotoxin, which comes from the puffer fish, and saxitoxin, which comes from the "red-tide" dinoflagellate, are highly specific and effective blockers of Na^+ channels. Saxitoxin has proved useful clinically to lengthen the effects of anesthesia,[33, 34] and tetrodotoxin has been an indispensable tool in basic scientific research.

Lidocaine, bupivacaine, and tetracaine, all of which block certain types of Na^+ and K^+ channels, are used as local anesthetics and have notable effects on dorsal root ganglia neurons.[35] Although most local anesthetics are more potent in blocking Na^+ channels than K^+ channels, the sensitivity of certain potassium channels is notable. For example, the ATP-sensitive K^+ channel found in heart muscle cells is sensitive to block by lidocaine and bupivacaine, which can lead to toxic side effects of these compounds.[36, 37]

ω-Conotoxin, from the marine snail *Conus* species, is a highly specific blocker of the neuronal N-type Ca^{2+} channel. It has been investigated for its clinical usefulness in relieving severe and intractable pain.[38, 39]

Curare, a plant alkaloid well known for its use as an arrow-dart poison by South American Indians, has as its site of action the neuromuscular junction, where it blocks acetylcholine receptors. It is commonly used as a muscle relaxant in operations and minor clinical procedures, and it has been used as a diagnostic tool for myasthenia gravis.

Botulinum toxin, produced by the bacterium *Clostridium botulinum*, interferes with vesicle fusion at the presynaptic terminal by cleaving proteins associated with this process. Referred to as the most potent neurotoxin known, botulinum toxin has been clinically useful for a variety of conditions, including strabismus, blepharospasm, dystonias, hemifacial spasms, hyperfunctional facial lines, and migraine headaches.

CONCLUSIONS

The PNS is a complex and structured extension of the CNS, providing sensory feedback from the surroundings and allowing the organism to act on the external environment. The physiology of the peripheral nerve is essentially the same as that of CNS neurons, with the cell generating electrical potential energy through ion-selective membrane channels and transmitting that energy by an action potential using voltage-gated ion channels. This electrical energy travels rapidly down a myelinated axon using saltatory conduction and is then transmitted into chemical energy at the neuromuscular junction through the release of acetylcholine into the synaptic cleft, where it binds to acetylcholine receptors at the motor end plate, eliciting muscular contraction. Interference in peripheral nerve function occurs through a variety of mechanisms, including direct damage to the integrity of the neuron or its myelin sheath, disruption in the function of one of the many ion-selective channels on the neuron, or interference with the process of release or binding of neurotransmitter.

REFERENCES

1. Birks RI: The fine structure of motor nerve endings at frog myoneural junctions. Ann N Y Acad Sci 135:8–19, 1966.
2. Bovie JJG, Perl ER: Neural substrates of somatic sensation. In Hunt CC (ed): MTP International Review of Science. Physiology, series 1. Neurophysiology, vol 3. Baltimore, University Park Press, 1975, pp 303–411.
3. Ramon Y Cajal S: Histology of the Nervous System [English translation], vol 1. New York: Oxford University Press, 1995.
4. Iggo A, Andres KH: Morphology of cutaneous receptors. Annu Rev Neurosci 5:1–31, 1982.
5. Kandel ER, Schwartz JH, Jessell TM: The Principles of Neural Science, vol 3. Norwalk, CT, Appleton and Lange, 1991.
6. Light AR, Perl ER: Peripheral sensory systems. In Dyck PJ, Thomas PK, Griffin JW, Low PA (eds): Peripheral Neuropathy, vol 1, 3rd ed. Philadelphia, WB Saunders, 1993, pp 149–165.

7. Waxman SG, Ritchie JM: Molecular dissection of the myelinated axon. Ann Neurol 33:121–136, 1993.
8. Waxman SG, Ritchie JM: Organization of ion channels in the myelinated nerve fiber. Science 228:1502–1507, 1985.
9. Hille B: Ionic Channels of Excitable Membranes, 2nd ed. Sunderland, MA, Sinauer, 1992.
10. Johnston D, Wu SM: Foundations of Cellular Neurophysiology. Cambridge, MA, MIT Press, 1994.
11. Nicholls JG, Wallace BG, Fuchs PA, Martin AR: From Neuron to Brain, 4th ed. Sunderland, MA, Sinauer, 2001.
12. Hodgkin AL: The ionic basis of electrical activity in nerve and muscle. Biol Rev 26:339–409, 1954.
13. Hodgkin AL: The conduction of the nervous impulse. Liverpool, UK, Liverpool University Press, 1964.
14. Hodgkin AL, Huxley AF: The components of membrane conductance in the giant axon of *Loligo*. J Physiol (Lond) 116:473–496, 1952.
15. Hodgkin AL, Katz B: The effect of sodium ions on the electrical activity of the giant axon of the squid. J Physiol (Lond) 108:37–77, 1949.
16. Hodgkin AL, Huxley AF, Katz B: Measurements of current-voltage relations in the membrane of the giant axon of *Loligo*. J Physiol (Lond) 116:424–448, 1952.
17. Goldman DE: Potential, impedance, and rectification in membranes. Gen Physiol 27:37–60, 1943.
18. Katz B, Miledi R: Membrane noise produced by acetylcholine. Nature 226:962–963, 1970.
19. Katz B, Miledi R: Further study of the role of calcium in synaptic transmission. J Physiol 207:789–801, 1970.
20. Cummins TR, Waxman SG: Downregulation of tetrodotoxin-resistant sodium currents and upregulation of a rapidly reprimimg tetrodotoxin-sensitive sodium current in small spinal sensory neurons after nerve injury. J Neurosci 17:3503–3514, 1997.
21. Waxman SG, Dib-Hajj S, Cummins TR, Black JA: Sodium channels and pain. Proc Natl Acad Sci 96(14):7635–7639, 1999.
22. Waxman SG: Acquired channelopathies in nerve injury and MS. Neurology 56(12):1621–1627, 2001.
23. Shillito P, Molenaar PC, Vincent A, et al: Acquired neuromyotonia: Evidence for autoantibodies directed against K⁺ channels of peripheral nerves. Ann Neurol 38:714–722, 1995.
24. Hart IK, Waters C, Vincent A, et al: Autoantibodies detected to expressed K⁺ channels are implicated in neuromyotonia. Ann Neurol 41:238–246, 1997.
25. Hart IK: Acquired neuromyotonia: A new autoantibody-mediated neuronal potassium channelopathy. Am J Med Sci 319:209–216, 2000.
26. Lennon VA, Kryzer TJ, Griesmann GE, et al: Calcium-channel antibodies in the Lambert-Eaton syndrome and other paraneoplastic syndromes. N Engl J Med 332:1467–1474, 1995.
27. Magnelli V, Grassi C, Parlatore E, et al: Down-regulation of non-L-, non-N-type (Q-like) Ca^{2+} channels by Lambert-Eaton myasthenic syndrome (LEMS) antibodies in rat insulinoma RINm5F cells. FEBS Lett 387:47–52, 1996.
28. Motomura M, Lang B, Johnston I, et al: Incidence of serum anti-PO-type and anti-N-type calcium channel autoantibodies in the Lambert-Eaton myasthenic syndrome. J Neurol Sci 147:35–42, 1997.
29. Engel AG: Review of evidence for loss of motor nerve terminal calcium channels in Lambert-Eaton myasthenic syndrome. Ann N Y Acad Sci 635:246–258, 1991.
30. Almon RR, Appel SH: Serum acetylcholine-receptor antibodies in myasthenia gravis. Ann N Y Acad Sci 274:235–243, 1976.
31. Grob D, Namba T: Characteristics and mechanism of neuromuscular block in myasthenia gravis. Ann N Y Acad Sci 274:143–173, 1976.
32. Kaminski HJ, Ruff RL: The myasthenic syndromes. In Physiology of Membrane Disorders, vol 1. New York, Plenum, 1996, pp 565–593.
33. Schantz EJ, Johnson EA: Properties and use of botulinum toxin and other microbial neurotoxins in medicine. Microbiol Rev 56:80–99, 1992.
34. Kohane DS, Lu NT, Gokgol-Kline AC, et al: The local anesthetic properties and toxicity of saxitoxin homologues for rat sciatic nerve block in vivo. Reg Anesth Pain Med 25:52–59, 2000.
35. Komai H, McDowell TS: Local anesthetic inhibition of voltage-activated potassium currents in rat dorsal root ganglion neurons. Anesthesiology 94(6):1089–1095, 2001.
36. Olschewski A, Olschewski H, Brau ME, et al: Effect of bupivacaine on ATP-dependent potassium channels in rat cardiomyocytes. Br J Anaesth 82:435–438, 1999.
37. Scholz A: Mechanisms of (local) anaesthetics on voltage-gated sodium and other ion channels. Br J Anaesth 89:52–61, 2002.
38. Malmberg AB, Yaksh TL: Effect of continuous intrathecal infusion of omega-conopeptides, N-type calcium-channel blockers, on behavior and antinociception in the formalin and hot-plate tests in rats. Pain 60(1):83–90, 1995.
39. Bowersox SS, Luther R: Pharmacotherapeutic potential of omega-conotoxin MVIIA (SNX-111), an N-type neuronal calcium channel blocker found in the venom of *Conus magus*. Toxicon 36(11):1651–1658, 1998.
40. Bunge RP: Glial cells and the central myelin sheath. Physiol Rev 48:197–251, 1968.
41. McMahan UJ, Kuffler SW: Visual identification of synaptic boutons on living ganglion cells and of varicosities in postganglionic axons in the heart of the frog. Proc R Soc Lond B Biol Sci 177:485–508, 1971.

Peripheral Nerve: Approach to the Patient

RAJIV MIDHA

The approach to the patient with a peripheral nerve problem is fundamentally clinical, resting on a thorough history and physical examination. A rigorous clinical approach allows the generation of an appropriate anatomic and differential diagnosis. In addition to providing an understanding of the mechanism of injury or neuropathy, the history gives an appreciation of the temporal progression of the problem. The neurological examination remains the cornerstone in evaluating a peripheral nerve condition and has not been easily supplanted by imaging advances, as has occurred with most pathologic conditions affecting the central nervous system (CNS). The ability to conduct an appropriate and systematic examination is well rewarded because the clinician can diagnose not only the anatomic confines of the lesion but also, in many cases, the severity of the underlying injury to the nerve element in question. Moreover, gaining expertise in a thorough peripheral nerve examination endows the physician with skills that can be used toward the clinical assessment of all neurosurgical patients.

In approaching the patient with a neurological condition, the clinician must first determine the anatomic location of the lesion. Is the lesion in the CNS (spinal cord, brainstem, or brain) or can it be localized to a nerve root, nerve element, or peripheral nerve distribution? A thorough history aided by a systematic neurological examination allows precise definition of the lesion location. Additional laboratory tests, such as electrodiagnostic studies and imaging modalities, provide corroborative evidence,[1] as discussed in subsequent chapters.

The mechanism and nature of nerve damage is sought. The clinical circumstances answer several important key questions that dictate further management. What is the precise diagnosis or mechanism of nerve injury? How severe is the injury? Are the mechanism and clinical findings consistent with a focal versus diffuse injury? Is the nerve element lacerated or in continuity? Is the damage to the nerve or nerve element complete or incomplete (sparing some aspect of autonomic, sensory, or motor function). Inherent to this determination is the attribution of an injury grade (neuropraxia, axonotmesis, and neurotmesis), which is discussed later.

The clinician next attempts to discern the evolution of the injury. Is the patient's condition static, improving, or deteriorating? The majority of peripheral nerve problems either improve or remain unchanged, whereas only a small minority of conditions worsen. Sometimes this is clear from the history, but there is no substitute for a thoroughly performed and well-documented initial examination, which serves as a baseline. Subsequent examinations easily allow the determination of progression to be made. If the patient is worsening, a prompt search and correction of a secondary ischemic or compressive complication (hematoma, compartment syndrome, or pseudoaneurysm) is needed to prevent irreversible nerve damage.

EMERGENCY ROOM EVALUATION

The emergency room management of a patient who is suspected of having sustained peripheral nerve injury differs greatly from that of the patient who is seen electively or even urgently in the clinical setting. In any trauma patient, attention to life-threatening airway, respiratory, circulatory, and CNS injuries always take first priority before limb injuries are addressed. In multitrauma victims, nerve injuries and brachial plexus injuries are relatively frequent, affecting 5% and 1% of trauma patients, respectively.[2] Moreover, these injuries can be diagnosed at the initial trauma encounter in more than 60% of cases.[2, 3] In patients with an altered level of consciousness (even the comatose patient), an asymmetrical neurological examination, with loss of function confined to one limb when accompanied by loss of deep tendon reflexes, can be suggestive of nerve injury.[2] Further confirmation of nerve or plexus injury can be provided by electrical studies, such as somatosensory evoked potential studies.[4] The precise distribution of nerve injury, even in the comatose patient, can also be ascertained by assessing the lack of autonomic function (sweating and loss of wrinkling after immersion of hand or foot in water), as suggested by Kline and Hudson.[5]

In approaching the patient, a high index of suspicion is required. Any patient with a soft tissue, tendon, bone, joint, or vascular injury in the limb should be examined for nerve damage. Conversely, patients with an obvious peripheral nerve injury should have careful assessment of their peripheral pulses and tendons, along with liberal use of radiologic imaging of the bones and joints adjacent to the area of nerve damage.

The rule of thumb to exclude a nerve injury is to verify that the most distal aspect of the nerve is functioning. For example, in considering a possible injury to the median nerve, normal function of the pronator teres, wrist flexors, and long finger flexors would not preclude damage to the more distal median nerve. Conversely, a normal motor evaluation of the thenar muscles, such as the abductor pollicis brevis, and preserved sensation to the volar aspect of the thumb and index finger establish that the median nerve is intact.

In addition to excluding nerve damage, the initial neurological examination serves several purposes. A baseline is provided. Worsening function spontaneously and from iatrogenic circumstances (such as open or closed fracture reduction) can be reliably diagnosed. The location and severity of nerves that are injured is determined. A key concern is the completeness of nerve injury. Preservation of *any* function (autonomic, sensory to autonomous distributions, and especially motor) in the distribution of the nerve or nerve element is noted. Such partial injuries are by their nature less likely to be severe and often exhibit spontaneous recovery over time.[6, 7] Conversely, complete injuries may or may not recover.

Open injuries deserve special consideration. Principles of tetanus prophylaxis, antibiotic administration, timely closure of lacerations, and débridement of contaminated and extensive wounds are adhered to. In sharp penetrating trauma (e.g., glass, knife, and razor blade injuries) with nerve injury, primary exploration and suture repair of the divided nerve, aided by microtechniques and magnification, in the operating room is best. At times, the nerve is found to be merely contused or bruised during exploration by the neurosurgeon or other surgeon repairing a lacerated tendon or vessel. In these situations, it is best to make a careful note of the location and degree of damage and then follow the patient clinically for evidence of recovery, as in the management of any patient with a known neuroma in continuity.[8] A similar approach is appropriate in the majority of patients with nerve damage from gunshot wounds or injuries from high-velocity missiles, as the injury is much more likely to have contused the nerve

than to have divided it.[9, 10] Finally, when the penetrating damage is from a more blunt object (such as wounds from industrial accidents and chainsaw injuries), the role of the initial exploration is débridement and identification of the nerve damage. The contused and divided nerve ends are sutured, using large nonabsorbable suture, to fascial tissue under some distraction (to minimize retraction) adjacent to each other. The definitive nerve repair is performed at a secondary exploration after several weeks have elapsed to allow the extent of longitudinal injury to declare itself.[11]

HISTORY

Patients with peripheral nerve problems, like those with most neurological conditions, present with one or more symptoms of pain, sensory and motor change or loss, and functional disability related to the injury. An additional mode of presentation is underactivity or overactivity of autonomic function, such as palmar hyperhidrosis.

Pain

Pain is a frequent presenting complaint of patients with peripheral nerve damage.[12] A common source of pain relates to disuse phenomenon (swelling, joint stiffness, muscle and tendon shortening, and fibrosis) that follows many nerve injuries in which the limbs are immobilized or are not adequately mobilized. Simple attention to positive encouragement for the patient, institution of adequate physiotherapy, and judicious use of analgesics, nonsteroidal anti-inflammatory medications, and other medications to treat neuropathic pain are often all that is necessary to prevent and overcome disuse-related problems.

In entrapment neuropathy, referred pain adjacent to and along the distribution of the compressed nerve is commonplace.[13] For example, the description of aching discomfort in wrist and forearm, nocturnal symptoms, and paresthesias in the median nerve distribution are so characteristic as to be virtually diagnostic of carpal tunnel syndrome. Serious damage to peripheral nerves often produces an even more profound neuritic pain syndrome, characterized by severe, sometimes burning, pain in the distribution of the injured nerve, accompanied by sensory changes (hypoesthesia and hyperesthesia).[14] In addition to the treatment principles outlined earlier, use of tricyclic antidepressants (such as amitriptyline) and anticonvulsants (particularly, carbamazepine and gabapentin)[15, 16] is often effective in decreasing neuropathic pain.

Pain after nerve injury may also arise secondary to multiple other pathophysiologic mechanisms.[14] Autonomic disturbance is characteristic of both true (or major) causalgia and minor causalgia (reflex sympathetic dystrophy).[17, 18] True causalgia typically occurs after significant damage (often from gunshot wounds) to a major mixed nerve (such as median, ulnar, and tibial).[19] A severe burning pain, the patient's careful attempts to protect the involved extremity from movement and manipulation, and evidence of autonomic overactivity are cardinal features.[20] This type of sympathetically mediated pain may benefit from a sympathectomy.[17, 18] Some patients exhibit features of deafferentation pain, resulting from nerve root avulsion, a condition that is well palliated by dorsal root entry zone ablation.[21] Regenerating nerves may also produce pain, often described as tingling, electric shocks, and dysesthesias along the course of the nerve.[22] Injured cutaneous peripheral nerves demonstrate a profound capacity to regenerate. When they do so into a scar or superficial area, painful neuroma formation is likely.[12] In this case, the patient usually describes a well-localized pain syndrome, along with a trigger point overlying the often palpable subcutaneous lesion that is exquisitely tender. Painful neuromas may respond to desensitization treatment and a series of local anesthetic and steroid blocks, but they often require wide surgical resection for effective therapy.[5, 12, 13, 23]

Sensory Loss

A description of the precise distribution and alteration of the sensory deficit is sought from the patient. The sensory deficit may be described in one or many ways. Some patients may describe complete loss of sensation (anesthesia) or an alteration of sensation, either decreased (hypoesthesia) or increased (hyperesthesia). Other patients may report dysesthesia, such as tingling, electric shocks sensations, and pins and needles. Light touch or other nonpainful stimuli may be perceived as painful (allodynia). Functional consequences may include accidental burning, injury, and even frank ulcer formation (Fig. 251–1). The evolution of sensory loss and change is sought, particularly to ascertain whether recovery is occurring and precisely in what distribution.

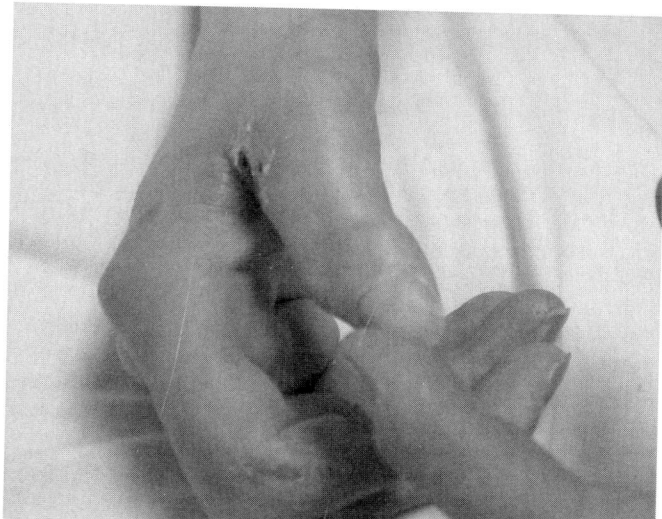

FIGURE 251–1. A swollen, cool, shiny and atrophic-appearing hand of a patient with chronic and complete pan plexus injury. The insensate limb is prone to accidental injury and ulcerative changes as demonstrated in the first dorsal web space and radial aspect of the index and middle fingers.

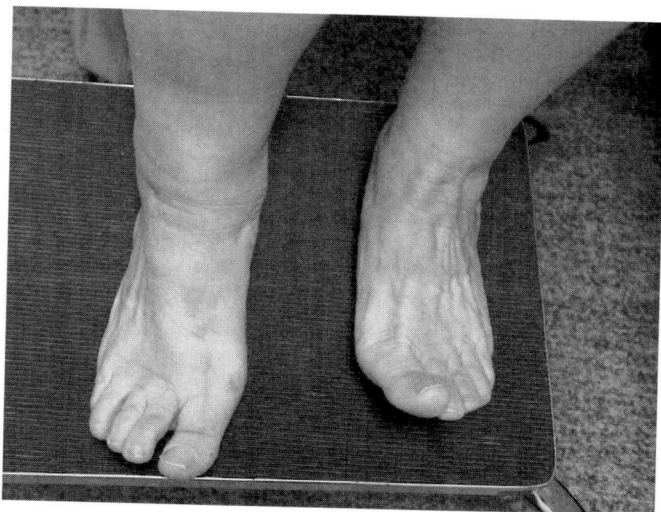

FIGURE 251–2. Early evidence of recovery in a right common peroneal nerve palsy, with long toe extensors (extensor digitorum longus) just having attained antigravity function (Medical Research Council [MRC] grade 3). Ankle eversion (not illustrated) graded 4, while extensor hallucis longus fails to contract (MRC grade 0). The patient still manifests a foot drop while standing, but when supine (gravity eliminated), contraction of the anterior tibialis was apparent 1 month before this examination (grade 1) and now results in some ankle dorsiflexion (grade 2).

Motor Deficit

The precise location, severity, and change in motor loss are key features of the patient's history. The majority of patients describe the deficit in terms of general movements and its impact on activities of daily living. If not provided, the latter information is important to obtain, as is the consequences on occupational and recreational performance. For example, a patient with a severe groin-level femoral nerve injury with complete denervation of the quadriceps may simply give the impression that the leg feels weak overall and is resulting in a limp.[24] Questions directed as to how the patient performs on stairs or on getting up from a sitting or squatting position leads to improved understanding of the nature of the functional deficit. In a similar manner, precise questions may provide important insight into the evolution of a neurological deficit. For instance, the patient with a complete peroneal nerve injury needs to be questioned about any dorsiflexion of the toes or foot while lying down, with gravity eliminated, to suggest early evidence of recovery (Fig. 251–2).

In certain circumstances, history from collateral sources is extremely helpful. An obvious scenario is the baby with a plexus injury in which information provided by the parents is particularly helpful. Much of this will simply reflect the day-to-day observations of the baby's behavior and play activity. Pertinent information related to the spontaneous range of movement and the relative strength of various muscle groups will be discerned. Another source of collateral information is the patient's physiotherapist. In addition to providing supervised range of movement activities, the therapist often performs serial examination and documentation of the patient's strength and movement of various muscle groups. Such a record gives an excellent profile of the evolution in the patient's condition.

Autonomic Dysfunction

Loss of sweating, coolness, some degree of cyanosis, and swelling result from the autonomic hypofunction that accompanies many major complete peripheral nerve injuries (see Fig. 251–1). In circumstances of sympathetic overactivity, particularly in sympathetically mediated pain syndromes, abnormal vasodilation and increased sweating may occur.

PHYSICAL EXAMINATION

General Principles

A rigorous neurological examination remains the cornerstone in approaching the patient with a peripheral nerve problem. Several general principles are paramount (Table 251–1). Full exposure of the limb being examined is recommended. The examination should be performed in a consistent and repeatable fashion so that findings are not overlooked. Starting from the proximal aspect of the limb, one works distally in a systematic fashion. In the upper extremity, this necessarily means first examining the posterior parascapular and shoulder girdle muscles before proceeding to the more distal arm and hand (Fig. 251–3). In the lower extremity, the preceding principles entail examining both the anterior and the posterior aspects of the patient up to and including the gluteal region. The clinician compares and contrasts findings from the affected to the unaffected limb in all situations. In assessing muscle strength, an attempt is made to discriminate given movement of a limb from specific actions of muscles, since the latter provide the precise information needed.[25] For example, lateral abduction of the shoulder over the first 30 degrees is produced by the supraspinatus, over the next 120 degrees it is supplied by the deltoid, and then is completed by medial rotation of the scapula by parascapular muscles such as the trapezius and rhomboids. Being aware of each of these actions, the clinician can direct the examination and attention to assessing the strength and contributions from each of the individual muscles in turn. Finally, one needs to be aware of "trick" or substitutive movements that the patient learns and adapts in order to overcome deficits. The unwary or inexperienced clinician will confuse these for recovery of muscle function, when in fact there is none. For example, a patient with a complete deltoid palsy may be able to laterally abduct the shoulder to 90 degrees simply by using a combination of strong supraspinatus action, clavicular head fibers of the pectoralis major and medial rotation of the scapula, using parascapular muscles. Careful visualization of the shoulder mechanics from above and behind and palpation of the deltoid allows the examiner to make an accurate assessment.

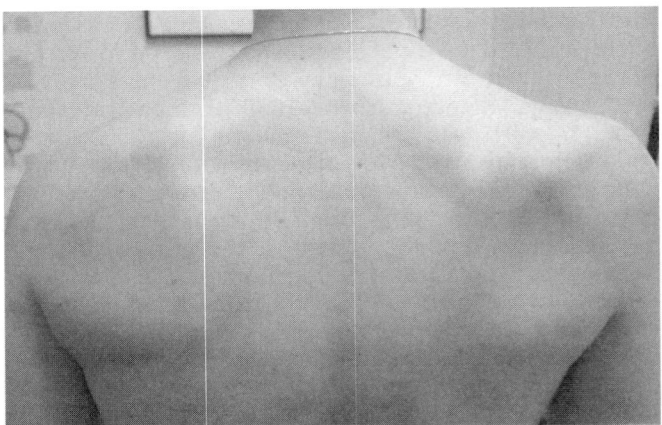

FIGURE 251–3. Posterior upper extremity photograph of a patient with Erb's palsy. At a simple glance, the atrophy of supraspinatus, infraspinatus, and deltoid muscles is apparent on the right side, in contrast to the normal appearance on the left.

Motor and Muscle Testing

Motor testing is undoubtedly the most important aspect of the physical examination in assessing a peripheral nerve problem. Adhering to the principles outlined previously, the examiner compares the involved and the unaffected extremities with respect to motor bulk and tone and then proceeds to a thorough evaluation of the strength of individual muscle groups. The latter are rated using a standard British Medical Research Council system.[25, 26] The scope of this chapter does not allow a detailed analysis of the key steps to testing each and every muscle. Instead, the reader is referred to the excellent techniques and photographic illustrations in the pertinent chapter and appendix in Kline and Hudson's textbook[5] and the monograph, *Aids to Investigation of Peripheral Nerve Injuries.*[25]

Muscle bulk asymmetry is usually obvious (Fig. 251–4). The specific muscle and compartments affected should be noted. When possible, an accurate assessment of muscle bulk using a tape measure should be performed. In performing the latter, one should first mark the extremity from a fixed bony landmark so that one compares comparable areas of the affected and the unaffected limbs (see Fig. 251–4).

Certain motor findings are so classic as to be almost diagnostic (Fig. 251–5). For example, consider the patient with an upper and middle trunk brachial plexus injury (or Erb's palsy). The typical "waiter's tip" posture is apparent, with the shoulder internally rotated

---

T A B L E   2 5 1 – 1 ■ **General Principles of Peripheral Nerve Examination**

Expose the limb or limbs fully
Compare one limb with the other
Use a systematic and orderly approach, from proximal to distal limb
Assess and grade individual muscles
Be aware of, and avoid being fooled by, trick movements

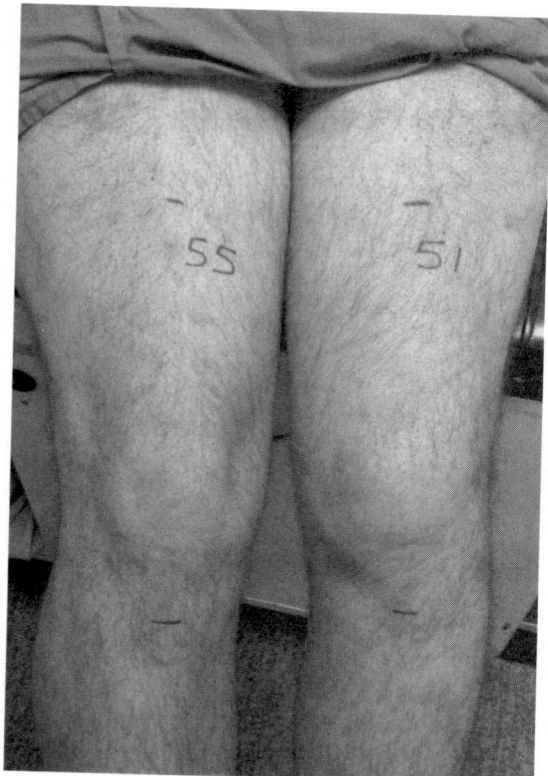

FIGURE 251–4. Quadriceps atrophy in a young man with femoral nerve injury is quantified, with a 4-cm disparity in muscle bulk. Thigh circumference is measured at equidistant levels from a common bony prominence, the tibial tuberosity, on each side.

and held tight against the body (because the deltoid and spinatei are absent), elbow extended (because the biceps is paralyzed) and forearm pronated, with the hand facing backward (because the supinator is paralyzed) and palm up (unopposed finger flexion from

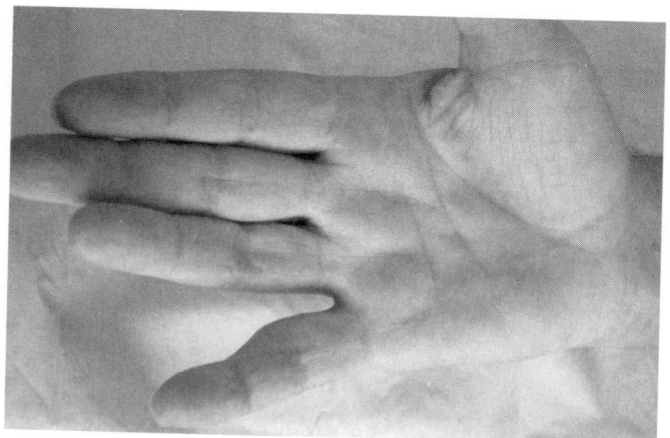

FIGURE 251–5. Several classic features of an elbow-level ulnar neuropathy are illustrated. Hypothenar muscle atrophy, clawing of ring (early) and little (more advanced) fingers, and virtual paralysis of volar interossei to the little finger and dorsal interossei to the ring finger, resulting in their wide separation, are all apparent.

extensor paresis). A radial nerve injury produces a typical wrist and finger drop, whereas posterior interosseous palsy produces a characteristic finger drop only, with wrist extension spared in a radial direction as extensor carpi radialis longus and brevis are spared.

An appreciation of hand function and deficits after upper extremity nerve injuries is especially important.[27] The patient with an anterior interosseous nerve palsy fails to make an "O" when the tip of the thumb and index finger are brought in apposition because flexor pollicis longus and flexor digitorum profundus to index finger are affected. Clawing of the fingers indicates loss of lumbricales muscle action, which normally flexes the fingers at the metacarpophalangeal (MCP) joints and extends them at the interphalangeal (IP) joints. Loss of this function and unopposed long extensors (acting as the MCP joint) and the long flexors (acting at the IP joint) bring the finger into a claw configuration. Thus, patients with an elbow-level ulnar nerve injury typically display the claw hand with the little and ring finger affected (see Fig. 251–5). Conversely, the more distal median nerve injury produces the "Benedictine hand" in which the index and middle fingers are similarly affected. Finally, the "ape hand," with all four fingers involved, is typical of patients with combined forearm level ulnar and median nerve injuries.

The preceding classic neurological findings, although characteristic, still require careful examination to localize the level of the lesion. Consider the example of a unilateral foot drop (see Fig. 251–2). An upper motor neuron lesion affecting the pyramidal tract, a cord lesion affecting the L5 motor neuron pool, a spinal lesion interfering with L5 outflow, or peripheral lesions affecting the L5 nerve root, lumbosacral trunk, the sciatic nerve peroneal division, or the peroneal nerve in exclusion may all result in foot drop. Careful attention to examining the limb for increased reflexes and tone helps distinguish upper from lower motor neuron pathology. Further attention to examining common L5 innervated muscles, such as gluteus and posterior tibialis (ankle inversion) helps distinguish radicular and more proximal lumbosacral plexus lesions from more distal sciatic or peroneal neuropathies. Moreover, assessment of the short head of the biceps femoris (innervated from contributions from the peroneal division of the sciatic nerve above the knee) may help distinguish a sciatic peroneal division lesion from the more typical common peroneal neuropathy. The preceding exercise demonstrates that armed with some appreciation of anatomy and a systematic examination technique, the clinician can often localize the lesion based on simple clinical findings.

It has already been stressed that motor strength should be assessed for individual muscles and not particular limb movements. For example, ankle dorsiflexion should not be recorded as such, but a grade should be given for the function of the anterior tibialis (see Fig. 251–2). The grading of strength itself is performed using a standard British Medical Research Council system (see Fig. 251–2).[26] A shortcoming of this system is the lack of discrimination. For example, strength somewhere between antigravity function (grade 3) and normal function (grade 5) would be graded at 4. Yet grade 4 may represent quite disparate levels of function so that for practical reasons many clinicians use a 4 minus, 4, and 4 plus grading system in an attempt to discriminate among severe, moderate, and mild weakness, respectively. However, such a grading system would likely have poor inter- and intrarater reliability. Kline and Hudson have devised a Louisiana State University Medical Center grading system for motor function.[5] This system addresses the deficiencies inherent in the British MRC scale by assigning grades 3, 4, and 5 to movements against gravity as well as mild, moderate, and maximal resistance (respectively). Unfortunately, grading systems such as this and other practical ones have not yet been validated or generally accepted. When testing a given muscle, it is important both to inspect and to be in a position to palpate the muscle being examined. This allows detection of even minimal or flickers of contraction, which perhaps may not even result in limb movement. Paretic muscles need to be tested both with and without the aid of gravity. To eliminate gravity, special maneuvers may be necessary. For example, having the patient lie supine while testing for lateral abduction of the shoulder eliminates gravity when testing the supraspinatus as well as the deltoid. Similarly, the supine patient can rest the arm on the chest wall and then be asked to flex the hand toward the head, thus allowing the biceps to be tested without the effects of gravity interfering.

Sensory Evaluation

After motor evaluation, the examiner tests sensation. Sensory examination includes testing for light touch, pinprick, two-point discrimination, vibration, and proprioception.[28] A common feature of a complete peripheral nerve injury is the loss of all modalities of sensation in the distribution of the nerve. However, in incomplete or partial injuries, some modalities may be affected more so than others. Nerve entrapment syndromes represent an example in which modalities of discriminative touch, which reflect receptor density, may be more sensitive.[29] Thus, loss of moving two-point discrimination may occur before loss of other modalities of sensation.[29]

To get a quick idea about an area of anesthesia or markedly altered localizing sensibility, the patient is directed to close the eyes and to point to areas that are stimulated by light touch from the end of a blunt object such as a dull pen tip. This simple technique readily allows one to map the area of poor or absent sensation. Having the patient compare simultaneous stimulation can allow the discernment of more subtle loss of sensation. One technique is to stroke the patient's affected finger or area of sensory alteration gently while simultaneously using the same force of finger stroke on an unaffected area and have the patient simply comment on the alteration of sensory touch.[5] Attempts to validate such a simultaneous sensory testing paradigm, using a 10-point analog scale developed by Strauch,

have been reported.[30] A more thorough sensory examination can be performed with the most rudimentary instrumentation, such as a fresh safety pin, cotton wool, a 128-Hz tuning fork (for vibration testing, as well as temperature testing using the cold metallic tuning fork), and paper clips, blunt tip calipers or a specially made device (Dellon-Mackinnon Disk-Criminator, NeuroRegen LLC, Lutherville, Md) for two-point discrimination.

The distribution of sensory loss is important to denote. The hysterical patient or the patient seeking secondary gain may be distinguished by the nonphysiologic and nonsensical anatomic sensory loss. A glove or stocking distribution of sensory loss would be compatible with a peripheral or metabolic neuropathy. The sensory findings may help discriminate between a radiculopathy and a peripheral neuropathy.

A key principle regarding sensory testing for peripheral nerve injuries is to examine autonomous zones of innervation, in which there is the least likelihood or no likelihood of sensory overlap from adjacent nerves. The standard autonomous zone for the ulnar nerve is the volar aspect beyond the IP joint of the little finger; that for the median nerve is the volar aspect beyond the distal IP joint of the index finger and the IP joint of the thumb. Note that although the anatomic snuffbox is considered the autonomous sensory distribution of the radial nerve, there can be variable overlap from other cutaneous nerves such as the lateral antebrachial cutaneous nerve. Indeed, the patient may not have any loss of sensation after a radial nerve injury. Hence, as a general rule, one should not use the lack of sensory findings as proof of absence of a complete peripheral nerve injury. For example, patients with axillary nerve palsy often initially have a zone of absent or decreased sensation in the lateral upper arm (Fig. 251–6). Over time, this zone of altered sensibility either decreases or becomes completely normal despite no motor reinnervation of the deltoid muscle and an ongoing severe axillary nerve palsy.

Reflexes and Other Tests

Deep tendon reflexes are examined next. Again, one endeavors to compare the affected to the unaffected side. Myotatic reflexes are extremely sensitive indicators of peripheral nerve pathology. For example, it is not uncommon to find loss or diminution of the ankle reflex in a patient with a buttock- or midthigh-level sciatic nerve injury who has complete peroneal division involvement clinically but no other findings (except an absent ankle reflex) with respect to the posterior tibial division.[31] Further, once lost, myotatic reflexes often do not return even though peripheral sensation and function in the muscle might.

A general inspection of the limb discloses evidence of autonomic activity. The limb and digits are examined for their color, temperature, sweating behavior (or lack of), and atrophic changes in skin organs and nail beds (see Fig. 251–1).

An injured nerve often exhibits an overlying mechanical hypersensitivity. First discovered by Tinel, the

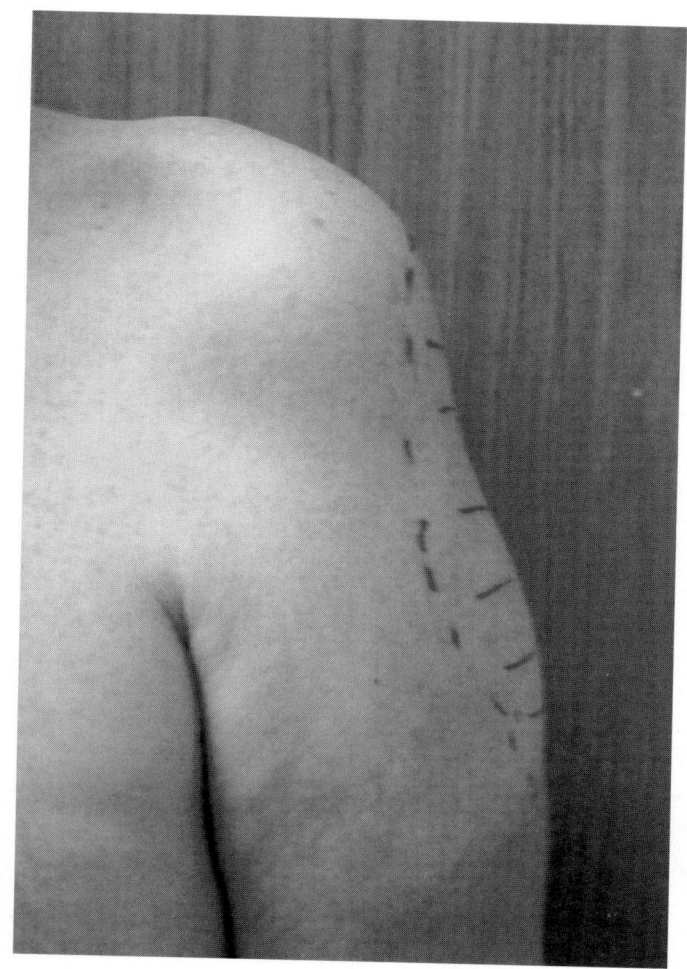

FIGURE 251–6. Axillary nerve palsy results in the squared off appearance in the anterior shoulder, reflecting atrophy of the anterior deltoid muscle, in addition to variable loss of sensation in the upper lateral arm *(hatched zone).*

inch a month, this provides evidence of ongoing regeneration. Although an *advancing* Tinel sign may be a positive indicator of regeneration, it was associated with subsequent muscle reinnervation with functional recovery in only approximately half of patients in one study.[32] Hence, patients need to be followed closely, even in the presence of an advancing Tinel sign. Conversely, the lack of an advancing Tinel sign is a strong negative finding, suggesting complete neural interruption or poor regeneration.[5]

In addition to the preceding physical examination findings, there are special tests that can be performed to provoke symptoms with presumed nerve entrapment. For instance, a Phalen test is an excellent provocative test for carpal tunnel syndrome.[13] In contrast, many tests for thoracic outlet syndrome such as the modified Adson, Roos, and other tests have not been validated and have questionable significance.[33]

A special circumstance of physical examination relates to the patient suspected of having a nerve sheath tumor. In such patients, a careful history and physical examination of the skin for stigmas of neurofibromatosis is important. With regard to the lesion itself, if it is palpable, the mobility of the lesion with respect to the underlying nerve is sought. Specifically, nerve sheath tumors are usually mobile in a side-to-side manner but not up and down along the nerve.

NERVE INJURY GRADING AND TIMING OF SURGERY

One important goal of the history and physical examination is to gain an appreciation of the severity of injury to the affected nerve element. In doing so, one essentially determines and ascribes a probable injury grade. Seddon's elegant three-grade (neuropraxia, axonotmesis, and neurotmesis) classification scheme, based on clinicopathologic correlation, remains useful given its brevity and relevance in predicting natural history and outcome.[34] The modification of the Seddon scale to the five-point grading system by Sunderland provides a somewhat more accurate anatomic appreciation of the damage to the internal nerve structure (Table 251–2).[35]

In *neuropraxia* (Sunderland grade 1), the mildest form of injury, there is a reversible conduction block, manifested clinically as loss of function, which persists for hours to days.[34] Typical mechanisms that produce neuropraxia include direct mechanical compression, is-

finding of shocklike electrical sensations or paresthesias evoked in the nerve distribution by percussing over the injured nerve is called a *Tinel sign.*[32] This sign is often present overlying the nerve in an area of entrapment neuropathy and can remain present for long periods, sometimes indefinitely, overlying the area of previous nerve injury. When a Tinel sign is found to be advancing along the anatomic distribution of the nerve, particularly if it does so at the expected rate of nerve regeneration, approximately 1 mm a day or an

TABLE 251–2 ■ **Nerve Injury Grading (Sunderland Grading Scale)**[35]

INJURY GRADE	MYELIN	AXON	ENDONEURIUM	PERINEURIUM	EPINEURIUM
I (Neuropraxia)*	+/−				
II (Axonotmesis)*	+	+			
III	+	+	+		
IV	+	+	+	+	
V (Neurotmesis)*	+	+	+	+	+

*Seddon grading system.[34]
+, anatomical structures affected by injury.

chemia, mild blunt trauma or stretch, some metabolic derangements, and toxins or disease that result in demyelination.[1, 36] There is either minimal or no discernible histopathologic alteration in nerve structure, or in some (more severe) neuropraxic injuries, axons have localized thinning and mild segmental demyelination.[35] The initial clinical examination often shows incomplete loss, with disproportionate motor over sensory loss and sparing of autonomic function.[36] In patients exhibiting complete loss, an initial single clinical assessment cannot distinguish neuropraxia from more severe injuries; rather the distinction is made retrospectively because grade 1 injuries are characterized by excellent spontaneous recovery over days to weeks and rarely over some months.

In an *axonotmetic* (Sunderland grade 2) lesion, axon continuity is disrupted but with relative sparing of the connective tissue structure of the nerve.[35] Importantly, the fascicular integrity is maintained, as is the fine endoneurial network, with minimal endoneurial edema and fibrosis. After division of the nerve fiber, wallerian degeneration occurs in the distal axon.[37] Degeneration of the axon also occurs for a variable distance proximal to the site of nerve division.[38–40] After this period of degeneration, myelinated and unmyelinated fibers from the proximal stump will sprout, forming regenerating units that attempt to reinnervate the distal stump.[41, 42] The elongating tips of regenerating axons are guided toward the end-organ by the intact endoneurial basement membrane. The rate of regeneration averages approximately 1 mm a day or an inch per month, parameters that are useful in serial clinical evaluation of the patient while awaiting possible return of function.[38–40] Grade 2 injuries often recover effectively without the need for operative intervention, although the completeness of recovery is governed by additional factors such as the location of the injury and the specific nerve or nerve element involved.[34]

Unfortunately, many injured nerves exhibit both loss of axonal continuity and a disruption in the connective tissue structures. When the damage is confined to the membranous structures within the fascicle, a Sunderland grade 3 lesion is present, whereas additional involvement of extrafascicular connective tissue denotes a grade 4 injury (see Table 251–2).[35] A variable degree of intrafascicular fibrosis results, frustrating regenerating axons and leading to their aberrant regrowth, despite gross continuity of the nerve itself. The resulting *neuroma in continuity* contains a meshwork of connective tissue entwined with fine-caliber, poorly myelinated axons.[43] Depending on the degree of internal disruption, spontaneous recovery may or may not occur. A wide range of clinical outcomes is therefore possible, from no return to a very good return of function in grade 3 injuries. In contrast, the grade 4 injury represents the most severe pathology for a neuroma in continuity. Clinical recovery seldom occurs, unless operative resection and repair are undertaken.

In a grade 5 injury, there is anatomic severance (*neurotmesis*) of the entire nerve. Injury mechanisms include lacerations from sharp or blunt forces, some iatrogenic causes, and division from missiles. Grade 5 injuries almost always require repair, and the only important consideration is the timing of repair. For sharply divided nerves (e.g., laceration by glass or knife), acute repair within hours to a day or two is ideal. More bluntly lacerated nerves are repaired 3 to 4 weeks after injury. This delay allows the longitudinal extent of injury to be fully delineated and declared so that débridement of the nerve to healthy proximal and distal stumps can be performed before repair.

The preceding clinical and neuropathologic classification allows the rational management of nerve injuries. Nerves that are known to be severed (grade 5) are best managed with early surgical repair, as outlined earlier. However, the majority of nerve injuries leave the nerve in continuity.[8] A baseline clinical evaluation and serial clinical and electrical follow-up is imperative to distinguish patients with less severe grades of injuries who will have spontaneous recovery from those with more severe grades that require surgical intervention. Moreover, a significant subset of injuries manifests more than one grade of injury across the cross section of the involved nerve element.[13] This is critical because return of function over time depends to a great extent on the underlying neuropathologic condition of the nerve; those with a large neurotmetic component do not generally recover, whereas those with a neuropraxic or axonotmetic pathology, or both, may recover.[44]

The primary indication for operative exploration of the nerve injury in continuity is lack of clinical or electrophysiologic recovery. Another important consideration is the location of nerve injury. In proximal lesions (e.g., supraclavicular brachial plexus), the surgeon cannot afford the luxury of waiting too long for recovery to manifest, because the time needed may compromise the window of opportunity when a nerve repair will bring about a useful outcome. In practice, more proximal nerve injuries and distal injuries not exhibiting spontaneous recovery are candidates for exploration. The optimal timing for exploration of a nerve injury that is in continuity is greatly influenced by the mechanism of injury.[11, 45] Injuries that are relatively more focal such as those produced by gunshot wounds, iatrogenic causes, stab wounds, lacerations, and fracture-associated contusions are best explored 2 to 3 months after wounding, whereas lengthier lesions resulting from severe contusion or stretch are ideally explored 4 to 5 months after onset. Further details of the clinical characteristics and approach to specific nerve injuries are discussed in the next section.

MECHANISMS OF INJURY

The peripheral nervous system may be involved by a diverse number of disease processes. Common pathologic mechanisms can be grouped into the following categories: metabolic, entrapment, traumatic, and mass lesions. Because peripheral neuropathies, entrapment syndromes, and tumors are dealt with elsewhere, the focus of this section is traumatic mechanisms of nerve injury. Common mechanisms that damage nerves include stretch, traction and contusion, laceration, compression and ischemia, burns (thermal and electrical), and injection and iatrogenic injuries.[36] The pathophysiologic circumstances, with an emphasis on the clinical consequences and approach to management, are discussed for each of these injury mechanisms.

Traction, Stretch, and Contusion

Blunt forces imparted to nerve remain by far the most common mechanisms underlying nerve injury. The elastin- and collagen-rich perineurial layer endows tensile strength, whereas the normal gliding of peripheral nerves in limbs during physiologic motion (aided by the undulating course of nerve fibers in a longitudinal direction) underlies the inherent ability of nerves to withstand moderate stretch forces.[6] However, even 8% stretch leads to a disturbance in intraneural circulation and blood-nerve barrier function.[46] Stretch beyond 10% to 20%, especially if applied acutely, results in structural failure.[47–49] Failure of the axons, myelin sheath, and connective tissue layers occurs in variable amounts, typically leaving the nerve in continuity with a variable spectrum of internal disruption (see Table 251–1).[6, 50] Rarely, a stretch insult may be so great as to result in complete mechanical failure of the nerve such that the nerve is literally pulled apart. The most frequent examples of severe stretching injuries are the brachial plexus palsies, seen as obstetric complications in infants or after motorcycle and snowmobile accidents in adults. In approximately half of these severe stretch plexus injuries, one or more nerve roots are avulsed from the spinal cord.[2] In addition to nerve root avulsion or rarely disruption, the general pathology of these severe stretch injuries is a long segment of disrupted nerve. In addition to the brachial plexus, nerve elements that are prone to extensive and severe damage include the lumbosacral plexus from severe fractures and dislocations in the pelvis, the sciatic nerve with hip dislocation, the peroneal nerve with knee dislocation, and the axillary nerve with shoulder dislocation.[31, 36] Relatively more focal stretch and contusive injuries with somewhat better prognosis result from simple fractures adjacent to nerves.[51, 52] An illustrative example is the radial nerve palsy following a midhumeral fracture, which exhibits a tendency to recover spontaneously in between 70% and 80% of patients.[51, 53]

Since the vast majority of injuries resulting from blunt and stretch trauma remain in continuity, general principles of management are serial clinical and electrical evaluation with timely surgical exploration if no evidence of recovery ensues.[11] In this fashion, the less severe Sunderland grade 1 and grade 2 injuries will declare themselves to be recovering or regenerating, whereas the more severe grade 3 and grade 4 injuries will come to surgical attention. The timing of surgery continues to be somewhat controversial.[11] It is generally accepted, and is the author's contention, that most of these in-continuity lesions should be explored between 3 and 6 months from the onset of injury when they fail to improve spontaneously.[1, 5, 8, 11]

Laceration

Sharp or blunt instruments may lacerate nerves. Sharp objects include glass, scalpels, knives, and razor blades. Blunt causes of laceration include injuries from chainsaws, metal and automobile shrapnel, industrial accidents, propeller blades, and occasionally low- and high-velocity missiles, such as gunshot. Distinguishing a sharp laceration from a more blunt laceration to the nerve is critical because this determines the optimal form of management.[11, 36] As already discussed in the emergency room evaluation section of this chapter, sharp clean lacerations are best sutured primarily. Conversely, definitive surgical repair of bluntly lacerated nerves should wait (usually weeks) until the degree of damage has a chance to declare itself clearly and be demarcated so that repair can be performed between normal proximal and distal stumps.[11] In contrast, suturing of a bluntly lacerated nerve acutely may produce a neuroma in continuity, defeating the purpose of nerve repair. Occasionally, a nerve or nerve element is partially lacerated. Under such circumstances, there is no substitute for careful evaluation in the operating room with appropriate magnification and internal neurolysis to spare the nerve element that is in continuity and selectively repair the divided nerve elements selectively.

Missiles (Gunshot Wounds)

Gunshot wounds remain a relatively frequent cause of nerve injury. In the vast majority of situations, the missile or bullet does not actually divide the nerve but rather produces intraneural damage secondary to shock, blast, or cavitation effects.[10, 54] Other than the obvious need to attend to general principles of open wound tissue débridement,[55] the management of a gunshot wound–associated nerve injury essentially follows the principles of management of any neuroma in continuity. Using this approach in military practice, approximately 70% of Vietnam War casualties demonstrated spontaneous recovery of function over several months.[9] Hence, an expectant attitude toward recovery is advised, but with careful clinical and electrophysiologic follow-up to offer exploration and possible nerve repair for patients not exhibiting evidence of recovery over approximately 4 months.[36] With this approach, approximately 60% of patients with civilian gunshot wounds to the brachial plexus required nerve exploration, and many of them required nerve repair.[10] A baseline clinical examination is particularly important in the patient sustaining missile wounds because there is a somewhat higher incidence of concomitant vascular injury with pseudoaneurysm formation. Such patients exhibit progressive neurological loss and require urgent angiography to establish the diagnosis, followed by prompt repair of the aneurysm or expanding hematoma, or both, to prevent irreversible neurological deficit.

Compression and Ischemia

Although the pathophysiology of chronic nerve entrapment likely involves both compressive and ischemic mechanisms, acute nerve injury occurs infrequently under these types of pathophysiologic circumstances. Relatively focal compression usually results in reversible nerve injury, whereas diffuse compression and that of longer duration (exceeding 8 hours[56]) can lead to irreversible damage. Examples of focal compression include a tourniquet paralysis and a characteristic "Saturday night palsy," resulting from mechanical compression as well as likely ischemia of the radial nerve against the humerus.[57] In the latter condition, the patient presents with a complete radial nerve palsy, with sparing of the triceps. As the pathology in the nerve is typically neuropraxic (Sunderland grade 1), complete clinical recovery is the rule in the majority of these patients. Similar types of reversible grade 1 and occasionally grade 2 injuries are produced from anesthesia-related palsies and from improper applications of plaster casts and splints. It is important to recognize that the onset of the neurological deficit is related to the application of such devices so that their prompt discontinuation is performed. Under these circumstances, there is a good prognosis of spontaneous recovery.

Compression of nerves within a fascial compartment from hematoma with a progressive neurological deficit should also be urgently managed with a prompt search for the location of the hematoma using appropriate imaging studies, reversal of anticoagulation, and consideration for urgent surgery to decompress the nerve element. The prognosis of these patients is variable, depending on multiple factors such as the type and level of nerve involved, the age and overall medical condition of the patient, the degree of underlying nerve damage, and the timing of surgical decompression. A closed compartment syndrome presents another type of emergency situation, in which prompt attention to decompression with thorough fasciotomies is needed to prevent an irreversible ischemic infarction of muscle, nerve, and other soft tissues, leading to a devastating Volkmann's ischemic contracture.[36]

Thermal and Electrical Injuries

Fortunately, nerve injury from thermal and electrical causes is relatively infrequent because there can be severe and widespread damage to underlying nerve structures. In burns and electrical injuries, there exists a variable spectrum of damage to the nerves. Typically, burns produce a direct thermal injury, with neural damage ranging from transient neuropraxia to severe neurotmesis with extensive necrosis of neural and adjacent soft tissues.[58] With electrical injuries, the relatively low tissue resistance of neurovascular structures often produces deeply penetrating and variable severity of damage within nerve, with the median and ulnar nerves most commonly involved.[59] The prognosis with most low-voltage injuries is excellent, but it is quite variable for high-voltage injuries.[60] Initial management is directed toward treatment of the life-threatening circumstances and proper attention to wounds, with the nerve damage taking a much lower priority. Delayed deficits from compression by circumferential eschars can be avoided by prompt and thorough escharotomy.[58]

Generally, nerve grafting and repair carry poor results, given the often extensive length of the damaged nerve and the poor vascularity of the soft tissue bed.

Injection Injury

Injury to peripheral nerves secondary to injection is a serious complication of intramuscular drug administration.[61] Any nerve is at risk, but the proximal radial nerve and the sciatic nerve in the buttock are by far the most common ones injected. Damage may occur from the needle itself, but mostly it is secondary to the toxic effects of the drug or agent being instilled in the intraneural compartment.[62–65]

The history associated with nerve injection is characteristic. In the typical scenario, needle placement results in an immediate electric-like shock sensation down the extremity. Concomitantly, on injection of the agent, severe radiating pain and paresthesias result. The patient usually experiences a severe pain—described with adjectives such as burning, searing, electrical—or a numbing sensation along the course of the injected nerve occurs.[22] In approximately 10% of cases, a delayed onset of neuropathy occurs after injection injury.[61] In these cases, the symptoms are often less dramatic, described variously as a burning pain, a deep discomfort, or bothersome paresthesias down the limb and in the distribution of the affected nerve. The neurological deficit may be complete or incomplete in the distribution of the injected nerve. When incomplete, motor loss is usually greater than sensory loss.[65] Neuritic pain, of variable intensity, often accompanies the neurological deficit.

Management of the patient with a peripheral nerve injection injury essentially follows the guidelines established for any patient with a nerve lesion in continuity.[43] Electrophysiologic tests, along with the initial neurological examination, are useful as a baseline to assess the subsequent evolution of the neuropathy. Most partial injuries and some complete injuries recover without operative intervention, with early return of function appearing to be the most significant prognostic factor in these cases.[66] Patients not exhibiting spontaneous recovery over approximately 4 months, as well as the occasional patient with medically intractable neuritic pain syndrome, are candidates for surgical exploration of the injury site, with external and internal neurolysis and nerve repair, depending on intraoperative findings.[61]

Iatrogenic Injuries

The clinical approach to patients with suspected iatrogenic injuries is essentially no different from that for any other injury, except that medicolegal circumstances can cloud and sometimes interfere with evaluation.[67] It is of great importance to undertake a careful, detailed, and sequential history from the patient and to seek collateral forms of information from family members as well as medical notes and records and any other ancillary investigations that were performed. In many circumstances, it is not at all clear when the patient's nerve injury actually arose because of a decreased level of consciousness either from a concomitant head injury or from sedatives and large doses of analgesics that the patient was given. A relatively common situation is a fractured limb in which a delayed diagnosis of a neurological deficit is made. Was the deficit originally present but missed because of the patient's level of consciousness? Did the deficit result from an action of the treating physician, such as closed reduction, application of a plaster cast, or operative internal exploration and fixation? Only a good history and a reliable, documented initial and serial physical examination would allow this to be answered, but this is frequently unavailable. In nerve injuries associated with anesthesia, the mechanism of damage is also frequently unclear.[68]

In other circumstances, it is abundantly clear that the nerve damage occurred as a result of iatrogenic circumstances. A patient who awakens from an elective operative procedure with a new neurological deficit in the distribution of a nerve within the operative field represents this type of case. An all too frequent example is the postoperative accessory nerve palsy, with trapezius denervation, after exploration and removal of a lymph node through a small transverse incision in the posterior triangle. Other nerves at relatively high risk for iatrogenic surgical damage include the radial, posterior interosseous, and ulnar nerves during open wound exploration and orthopedic fracture fixation in the upper extremity.[69] In the lower extremity, the common peroneal, saphenous, and femoral nerves are at risk during vascular surgery procedures such as arterial surgery and varicose vein stripping.[23, 24, 70]

The management of the patient with the presumed iatrogenic injury depends on the mechanism of the nerve damage. If it is recognized that the nerve has sustained a sharp or clean laceration, early exploration and suture repair would be an optimal form of treatment. If the nerve damage arises and progresses after traction, limb lengthening, or the application of a plaster cast that may be causing external pressure, discontinuation of the offending apparatus is clearly indicated.[71] Often the nerve is damaged by an unknown mechanism of action, which can include retractor pressure or compression during surgery, injudicious use of suture or cautery used to control bleeding, injury from a prosthetic device (such as during arthroplasty or plate and screw application), or by heat from bone cement.[31] Many of these forms of injury leave the nerve in continuity and have a variable degree of pathology affecting the nerve. Hence, after exclusion of obvious lacerating-type mechanisms and ongoing compressive problems (such as external devices and hematoma), the majority of patients are followed in a careful fashion with the hope that they will demonstrate spontaneous clinical or electrophysiologic recovery, or both. In the absence of such recovery over 3 to 4 months, the nerve injury should be explored, with appropriate repair dictated by the findings at surgery.[1, 5, 8, 11]

REFERENCES

1. Grant GA, Goodkin R, Kliot M: Evaluation and surgical management of peripheral nerve problems. Neurosurgery 44:825–839, 1999.
2. Midha R: Epidemiology of brachial plexus injuries in a multitrauma population. Neurosurgery 40:1182–1189, 1997.
3. Noble J, Munro CA, Prasad VSSV, Midha R: Analysis of upper and lower extremity peripheral nerve injuries in a population of patients with multiple injuries. J Trauma 45:116–122, 1998.
4. Houlden DA, Schwartz ML, Klettke KA: Neurophysiologic diagnosis in uncooperative trauma patients: Confounding factors. J Trauma 33:244–250, 1992.
5. Kline DG, Hudson AR: Nerve Injuries: Operative Results from Major Nerve Injuries, Entrapments, and Tumors. Philadelphia, WB Saunders, 1995.
6. Sunderland S: Nerve and Nerve Injuries, 2nd ed. Edinburgh, Churchill-Livingstone, 1978.
7. Sunderland S: Nerve Injuries and their Repair: A Critical Appraisal. New York, Churchill Livingstone, 1991.
8. Midha R, Kline DG: Evaluation of the neuroma in continuity. In Omer GE, Spinner M, Van Beek AL (eds): Management of Peripheral Nerve Problems. Philadelphia, WB Saunders, 1998, pp 319–327.
9. Omer GE: Nerve injuries associated with gunshot wounds of the extremities. In Gelberman RH (ed): Operative Nerve Repair and Reconstruction. Philadelphia, JB Lippincott, 1991, pp 655–670.
10. Kline DG: Civilian gunshot wounds to the brachial plexus. J Neurosurg 70:166–174, 1989.
11. Hudson AR, Hunter D: Timing of peripheral nerve repair: Important local neuropathologic factors. Clin Neurosurg 24:392–405, 1977.
12. Burchiel KJ, Ochoa JL: Surgical management of post-traumatic neuropathic pain. Neurosurg Clin North Am 2:117–126, 1991.
13. Mackinnon SE, Dellon AL: Surgery of the Peripheral Nerve. New York, Thieme, 1988.
14. Devor M: The pathophysiology and anatomy of damaged nerve. In Wall PD, Melzack R, Bonica JJ (eds): Textbook of Pain. New York, Churchill Livingstone, 1984, pp 49–64.
15. Merren MD: Gabapentin for treatment of pain and tremor: A large case series. South Med J 91:739–744, 1998.
16. Hansen HC: Treatment of chronic pain with antiepileptic drugs: A new era. South Med J 92:642–649, 1999.
17. Hendler N: Reflex sympathetic dystrophy and causalgia. In Tollison CD (ed): Handbook of Chronic Pain Management. Baltimore, Williams & Wilkins, 1989.
18. O'Neill OR, Burchiel KJ: Role of the sympathetic nervous system in painful nerve injury. Neurosurg Clin North Am 2:127–136, 1991.
19. Mitchell SW: Injuries of Nerves and Their Consequences. Philadelphia, JB Lippincott, 1872.
20. Mitchell SW, Morehouse GR, Kern WW: Gunshot Wounds and Other Injuries of Nerves. Philadelphia, JB Lippincott, 1864.
21. Nashold BS Jr, Ostdahl RH: Dorsal root entry zone lesions for pain relief. J Neurosurg 51:59–69, 1979.
22. Ochs G: Painful dysesthesias following peripheral nerve injury: A clinical and electrophysiological study. Brain Res 496:228–240, 1989.
23. Midha R: Management of femoral, saphenous, and sural nerve injuries. Perspect Neurol Surg 9:67–81, 1998.
24. Kim DH, Kline DG: Surgical outcome for intra- and extrapelvic femoral nerve lesions. J Neurosurg 83:783–790, 1995.
25. Medical Research Council, Nerve Injuries Committee: Aids to Investigation of Peripheral Nerve Injuries. MRC War Memorandum No. 7, His Majesty's Stationery Office, 1943. London, Balliere Tindall, 1986.
26. Medical Research Council: Aids to the Examination of the Peripheral Nervous System. Memorandum No. 45, Her Majesty's Stationery Office, London, Balliere Tindall, 1976.
27. Bowden REM, Napier JR: The assessment of hand function after peripheral nerve injuries. J Bone Joint Surg Br 43:481–492, 1961.
28. Moberg E: Methods for examining sensibility of the hand. In Flynn J (ed): Hand Surgery. Baltimore, Williams & Wilkins, 1975, pp 295–304.
29. Dellon AL: Evaluation of sensibility and re-education of sensation in the hand. Baltimore, Williams & Wilkins, 1981.
30. Patel MR, Bassini L: A comparison of five tests for determining hand sensibility. J Reconstr Microsurg 15:523–526, 1999.
31. Kline DG, Kim D, Midha R, et al: Management and results of sciatic nerve injuries: A 24-year experience. J Neurosurg 89:13–23, 1998.

32. Henderson WR: Clinical assessment of peripheral nerve injuries: Tinel's test. Lancet 2:801–804, 1948.
33. Pang D, Wessel HB: Thoracic outlet syndrome. Neurosurgery 22:105–121, 1988.
34. Seddon HJ: Three types of nerve injury. Brain 66:238–288, 1943.
35. Sunderland S: A classification of peripheral nerve injuries producing loss of function. Brain 74:491–516, 1951.
36. Gentili F, Hudson AR, Midha R: Peripheral nerve injuries: Types, causes, and grading. In Wilkins RH, Rengachary SS (eds): Neurosurgery. New York, McGraw-Hill, 1996, pp 3105–3114.
37. Waller A: Experiments on the section of the glossopharyngeal and hypoglossal nerves of the frog, and observations of the alterations produced thereby in the structure of their primitive fibres. Phil Trans Roy Soc (Lond) 140:423–429, 1850.
38. Seddon HJ, Medawar PB, Smith H: Rate of regeneration of peripheral nerves in man. J Physiol 102:191, 1943.
39. Sunderland S: Rate of regeneration in human peripheral nerves. Arch Neurol Psychiatry 58:251, 1947.
40. Sunderland S: Rate of regeneration in human peripheral nerves: Analysis of interval between injury and onset of recovery. Arch Neurol Psychiatry 58:291, 1947.
41. Morris JH: An Electron Microscope Study of Degeneration and Regeneration in Mammalian Peripheral Nerves [thesis]. Oxford, England, University of Oxford, 1971, pp i–173.
42. Morris JH, Hudson AR, Weddell G: A study of degeneration and regeneration in the divided rat sciatic nerve based on electron microscopy. III: Changes in the axons of the proximal stump. Z Zellforsch Mikrosk Anat 124:131–164, 1972.
43. Kline DG, Nulsen FE: The neuroma in continuity: Its preoperative and operative management. Surg Clin North Am 52:1189–1209, 1972.
44. Seddon HJ: Surgical Disorders of the Peripheral Nerves. Baltimore, Williams & Wilkins, 1972.
45. Kline DG, Hackett ER: Reappraisal of timing for exploration of civilian peripheral nerve injuries. Surgery 78:54–65, 1975.
46. Lundborg G, Rydevik B: Effects of streching the tibial nerve of the rabbit: A preliminary study of the intraneural circulation and the barrier function of the perineurium. J Bone Joint Surg 55B:390–401, 1973.
47. Liu CT, Benda CE, Lewey FH: Tensile strength of human nerves: Experimental physiological and histological study. Arch Neurol Psychiatry 59:322–336, 1948.
48. Sunderland S, Bradley KC: Stress-strain phenomena in human peripheral nerves. Brain 84:102–119, 1961.
49. Lundborg G: Compression and stretching. In Lundborg G (ed): Nerve Injury and Repair. New York, Churchill Livingstone, 1988, pp 64–101
50. Haftek J: Stretch injury of peripheral nerve: Acute effects of stretching on rabbit nerve. J Bone Joint Surg Br 52:354–365, 1970.
51. Seddon HJ: Nerve lesions complicating certain closed bone injuries. JAMA 135:691–694, 1947.
52. Siegel DB, Gelberman RH: Peripheral nerve injuries associated with fractures and dislocations. In Gelberman RH (ed): Operative Nerve Repair and Reconstruction. Philadelphia, JB Lippincott, 1991, pp 619–633.
53. Omer GE: Results of untreated peripheral nerve injuries. Clin Orthop Related Res 163:15–19, 1982.
54. Suneson A, Hansson HA, Seeman T: Peripheral high-energy missile hits cause pressure changes and damage to the nervous system: Experimental studies on pigs. J Trauma 27:782–789, 1987.
55. Marcus NA, Blair WF, Shuck JM, Omer GE Jr: Low-velocity gunshot wounds to extremities. J Trauma 20:1061–1064, 1980.
56. Lundborg G: Structure and function of the intraneural microvessels as related to trauma, edema formation and nerve function. J Bone Joint Surg 57-A:938–948, 1975.
57. Gilliatt R: Physical injury to peripheral nerves, physiological and electrodiagnostic aspects. Mayo Clin Proc 56:361–370, 1981.
58. Salzberg CA, Salisbury RE: Thermal injury of peripheral nerve. In Gelberman RH (ed): Operative Nerve Repair and Reconstruction. Philadelphia, JB Lippincott, 1991, pp 671–678.
59. Di Vincenti FC, Moncrief JA, Pruitt BA: Electrical injuries: A review of 65 cases. J Trauma 9:497–507, 1969.
60. Grube BJ, Heimbach DM, Engrav LH, Copass MK: Neurological consequences of electrical burns. J Trauma 30:254–258, 1990.
61. Midha R, Guha A, Gentili F, et al: Peripheral nerve injection injury. In Omer GE, Spinner M, Van Beek AL (eds): Management of Peripheral Nerve Problems. Philadelphia, WB Saunders, 1999, pp 406–413.
62. Gentili F, Hudson AR, Hunter D, Kline DG: Nerve injection injury with local anesthetic agents: A light and electron microscopic, fluorescent microscopic, and horseradish peroxidase study. Neurosurgery 6:263–272, 1980.
63. Gentili F, Hudson AR, Hunter D: Clinical and experimental aspects of injection injuries of peripheral nerves. Can J Neurol Sci 7:143–151, 1980.
64. Mackinnon SE, Hudson AR, Gentili F, et al: Peripheral nerve injection injury with steroid agents. Plast Reconstr Surg 69:482, 1982.
65. Clark WK: Surgery for injection injuries of peripheral nerves. Surg Clin North Am 52:1325–1328, 1972.
66. Clark K, Williams PEJ, Willis W, McGravan WA: Injection injury of the sciatic nerve. Clin Neurosurg 17:111–125, 1970.
67. Hudson AR, Hunter GA, Waddell JP: Iatrogenic femoral nerve injuries. Can J Surg 22:62–66, 1979.
68. Kroll DA, Caplan RA, Posner K, et al: Nerve injury associated with anesthesia. Anesthesiology 73:202–207, 1990.
69. Birch R, Bonney G, Dowell J, Hollingdale J: Iatrogenic injuries of peripheral nerves. J Bone Joint Surg Br 73:280–282, 1991.
70. Kim DH, Kline DG: Management and results of peroneal nerve lesions. Neurosurgery 39:312–320, 1996.
71. Galardi G, Comi G, Lozza L, et al: Peripheral nerve damage during limb lengthening: Neurophysiology in five cases of bilateral tibial lengthening. J Bone Joint Surg Br 72:121–124, 1990.

Peripheral Neuropathies

ERIC C. YUEN

Peripheral neuropathy refers to dysfunction of the nerves in the peripheral nervous system, which leads to a variety of symptoms and signs. Diagnosis and treatment of peripheral neuropathies is complicated because of the large numbers of different causes (Table 252–1). As with disorders of the central nervous system, a systematic approach is required to evaluate peripheral neuropathies. The first step is to acquire an understanding of the basic anatomy and physiology of nerves. These topics have been discussed in other sections of this volume. The common theme of peripheral neuropathies is the dysfunction or absence of nerve action potentials. Abnormalities of nerve action potentials can occur because of conduction block, dysfunction of the myelin sheath, or degeneration of nerve axons. There are various mechanisms of nerve injury (Table 252–2). Nerve trauma is a frequent cause of peripheral neuropathy. Typically, only one or a few nerves are injured, leading to focal neurologic deficits. Acute and chronic traumatic neuropathies are discussed in other chapters. Further details of the other mechanisms of nerve injury are discussed later in this section. In particular, neurologic disorders that are of particular interest to the neurosurgeon are discussed later. Neuropathies that can mimic neurosurgical conditions are listed in Table 252–3 and are also discussed later.

SYMPTOMS AND SIGNS

Sensory Symptoms and Signs

Peripheral neuropathies cause a number of different symptoms and signs (Table 252–4). Injury to the sensory nerve fibers leads to loss of sensation, which is usually referred to as numbness. However, it is important to keep in mind that patients often do not complain of numbness when they have only loss of or decreased sensation. Furthermore, some patients with severe weakness of a limb due to loss of motor neurons complain of numbness even though they have normal objective sensory function by neurologic examination and electrophysiologic testing. Thus, it is important to ask the patient whether the symptom of numbness refers to the inability to sense cool or warm stimuli or

to the decreased ability to feel light touch or the textures of objects. Oftentimes, the first symptom that the patient experiences is tingling or paresthesias ("pins and needles"). These "positive" sensations are presumably due to aberrant nerve action potentials from dysfunctional sensory axons. Hyperesthesia—sensations that are more intense than would normally be elicited for the degree of stimulation—is another symptom. Allodynia is an extreme form of hyperesthesia whereby normally nonpainful sensory stimuli, such as light touch, causes pain. Some patients have spontaneous pain in the distribution of the injured nerve, referred to as *dysesthesia* or *neuropathic pain*. The pain is frequently described as burning, electrical shocks, or painful paresthesias. Aching, tightness, and a tight bandlike feeling can also be experienced. Neuropathic pain beyond the distribution of the injured nerve can occur and is called *causalgia*. The pain from causalgia is often debilitating and is most likely mediated through abnormalities of sympathetic nerve fibers. When loss of sensation is widespread and severe, patients can suffer sensory ataxia and incoordination resulting from the lack of sensory feedback necessary for normal motor control.

The sensory examination involves evaluation of the five primary sensory modalities: light touch, pain, temperature, vibration, and proprioception. Light touch is useful as a screening tool for sensory abnormalities. The function of the small diameter, unmyelinated sensory fibers is evaluated by testing pain or temperature sensation. The large diameter, myelinated fibers are evaluated by testing vibration sensation or proprioception. Pseudoathetosis—abnormal limb movements that mimic athetosis when the patient's eyes are closed—are due to the lack of sensory and visual feedback required for maintaining an outstretched limb stationary. The presence of pseudoathetosis is rare and is usually found only in pure sensory neuropathies or ganglionopathies. In typical sensorimotor polyneuropathies, the sensory loss that would normally be severe enough to result in pseudoathetosis would also be accompanied by severe weakness, thus preventing the demonstration of pseudoathetosis on examination.

Motor Symptoms and Signs

Abnormalities of motor nerve fibers result in weakness. Loss of motor axons leads to muscle atrophy after

TABLE 252–1 ■ Peripheral Neuropathies

Inflammatory or Immune-Mediated Neuropathies
Guillain-Barré syndrome
Chronic inflammatory demyelinating polyradiculoneuropathy
(CIDP)
Multifocal motor neuropathy
Neuralgic amyotrophy
Idiopathic lumbosacral plexopathy
Sensory ganglionopathy
Monoclonal gammopathy–associated neuropathy
Sarcoidosis

Infectious Neuropathies
HIV neuropathy
Cytomegalovirus polyradiculopathy
Herpes zoster
Herpes simplex
Hepatitis B or C
Lyme disease
Leprosy
Diphtheria
Chagas' disease

Endocrine Neuropathies
Diabetic neuropathy
Hypothyroidism
Acromegaly

Toxic Neuropathies
Alcohol
Medications
Chemicals

Nutritional Neuropathies
Vitamin B_{12} deficiency
Vitamin E deficiency
Pyridoxine (vitamin B_6) deficiency or toxicity
Thiamine (vitamin B_1) deficiency
Strachen's syndrome
After gastroplasty

Vascular Neuropathies
Vasculitic neuropathy
Peripheral vascular disease

Neoplastic and Paraneoplastic Neuropathies
Lymphoma
Focal mass lesions
Paraneoplastic sensory ganglionopathy
Paraneoplastic motor neuropathy
Paraneoplastic mononeuropathy multiplex
Monoclonal gammopathy (see Table 252–11)
Amyloidosis

Traumatic, Compressive, and Entrapment Neuropathies (see Chapters 255–258)
Hereditary Neuropathies (see Table 252–16)
Miscellaneous
Renal failure
Radiation
Critical care neuropathy
Cold
Electrical

Idiopathic Neuropathies
Sensorimotor polyneuropathy
Small fiber sensory polyneuropathy
Sensory neuropathy
Autonomic neuropathy (Shy-Drager syndrome)
Bell's palsy
Trigeminal neuralgia
Cranial or limb mononeuropathy

HIV, human immunodeficiency virus.

TABLE 252–2 ■ Mechanisms of Nerve Injury

Trauma
    Acute compression
    Chronic compression (entrapment)
    Laceration
    Stretch
    Percussion
Ischemia
Inflammatory or immune-mediated
Metabolic
Toxic
Infectious
Tumor
Electrical
Thermal (cold and heat)
Radiation
Genetic
Idiopathic

TABLE 252–3 ■ Peripheral Neuropathies and Other Peripheral Nervous System Disorders That Can Mimic Neurosurgical Disorders

NEUROLOGIC DISEASE	SIMILAR NEUROSURGICAL DISEASES
Neuralgic amyotrophy	Cervical radiculopathy, brachial plexopathy
Proximal diabetic neuropathy (diabetic amyotrophy)	Lumbosacral radiculopathy or plexopathy
Diabetic mononeuropathy and radiculopathy	Radiculopathy, entrapment neuropathy
Hereditary neuropathy with liability to pressure palsy	Entrapment neuropathy
Vasculitic neuropathy	Compressive neuropathy
Amyotrophic lateral sclerosis	Radiculopathy, entrapment neuropathy
Multifocal motor neuropathy	Radiculopathy, entrapment neuropathy
Idiopathic lumbosacral plexopathy	Lumbosacral radiculopathy or plexopathy
Cytomegalovirus polyradiculopathy associated with AIDS	Cauda equina or conus medullaris syndrome

AIDS; acquired immunodeficiency syndrome.

TABLE 252–4 ■ Symptoms and Signs of Peripheral Neuropathies

SENSORY	MOTOR	DEEP TENDON REFLEXES
Numbness	Weakness	Decreased or absent
Tingling	Muscle atrophy	
Paresthesias	Incoordination	
Hyperesthesia	Fasciculations	
Allodynia	Cramps	
Pain	Pes cavus	
Causalgia		
Sensory ataxia (pseudoathetosis)		

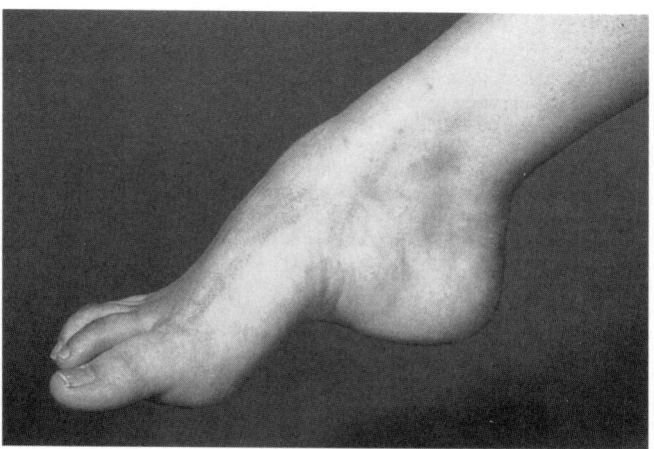

FIGURE 252–1. Pes cavus. (Courtesy of Thomas Bird, M.D., Department of Neurology and Medical Genetics, University of Washington.)

several weeks because of loss of muscle trophic factors supplied by motor axons to muscle fibers. In contrast, demyelination of motor nerves leads to weakness without muscle atrophy. When the condition is mild and insidious, patients may describe a loss of coordination. For example, patients with a loss of motor axons in the hand may complain of difficulties with buttoning, writing, and other fine motor hand tasks. Patients with an insidious onset of leg weakness may not realize that they are weak but instead may complain of twisting their ankles, tripping over their toes because of foot drop, or gait incoordination. Fasciculations and muscle cramps are frequent complaints with disorders of the motor neuron, and less often with peripheral neuropathies. Because fasciculations and cramps are frequently present in normal individuals and in a variety of metabolic conditions, they are a nonspecific finding that cannot be relied on as an indication of a peripheral neuropathy. Foot deformities (hammer toes and pes cavus) may occur, depending on the distribution of nerve damage and resulting imbalance of muscle tone on various foot joints (Fig. 252–1).

Deep Tendon Reflex Signs

Abnormalities of deep tendon reflexes are crucial in differentiating central from peripheral causes of motor and sensory loss. Abnormalities of either the motor or sensory nerve fibers interrupt the deep tendon reflex pathways and result in depressed or absent deep tendon reflexes. The pattern of reflex abnormality depends on the anatomic distribution of nerve injury. Thus, a peripheral neuropathy causing abnormalities of the distal nerves in the legs would result in depressed or absent ankle reflexes while knee and arm reflexes remain normal.

Patterns of Symptoms and Signs

Peripheral neuropathies can be subdivided into focal or generalized neuropathies. Both focal and multifocal

neuropathies produce sensory, motor, and reflex abnormalities in the distribution of the injured nerve or nerves. The patterns of neurologic deficits for the various common focal neuropathies are described elsewhere in this chapter. Generalized neuropathies, often referred to as *polyneuropathies,* are typically length-dependent, that is, the longer nerves are more severely injured compared with the shorter nerves. A number of factors may cause this phenomenon. First, in polyneuropathies with loss of nerve axons, the longer axons have greater metabolic requirements compared with the shorter axons, and thus are more likely to degenerate in response to an insult. Second, for demyelinating and axonal polyneuropathies, there is a higher probability of nerve injury in longer nerves than in shorter ones by virtue of their longer length. Thus, generalized, length-dependent peripheral neuropathies are usually symmetrical in onset and severity, with numbness beginning in the toes and feet. As the polyneuropathy becomes more severe, the numbness begins to affect the lower legs. By the time numbness reaches the knees, the fingers and hands are usually affected because the length of nerve from the lumbosacral dorsal root ganglia to the knees is about the same as the length from the cervical dorsal root ganglia to the hands. In severe cases, the distal ends of the intercostal nerves are affected, leading to numbness in the midline of the chest and abdomen (Fig. 252–2). Weakness of toe extensors and flexors are an early finding. Later, foot drop and ankle instability are common complaints due

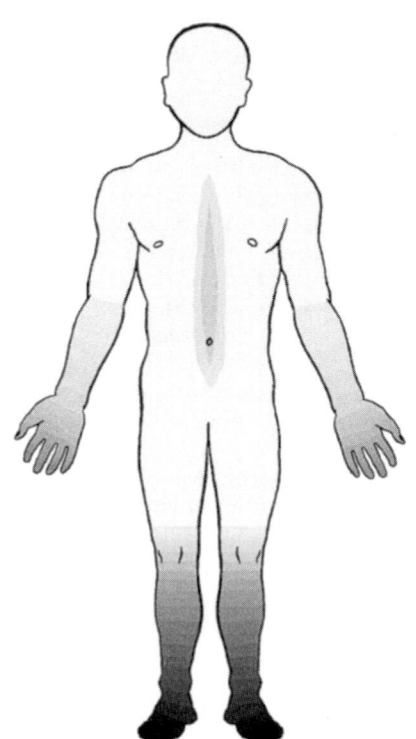

FIGURE 252–2. Distribution of numbness in a length-dependent peripheral neuropathy. Darker areas are affected earlier and more severely compared with lighter areas.

TABLE 252–5 ■ Steps to Diagnosing Peripheral Neuropathies

Localize the lesion
  Symmetrical and diffuse versus asymmetrical, focal, or multifocal
  Sensory versus motor
  Axonal versus demyelinating
Time course
Acquired versus hereditary
Associated present or past disorders
Ancillary tests

TABLE 252–7 ■ Mononeuropathy Multiplex

Ischemia: vasculitis, diabetes mellitus, rheumatoid arthritis, SLE, cryoglobulinemia, Sjögren's syndrome, emboli, hypercoagulopathy, hyperviscosity
Multiple focal lesions from trauma, tumors, cancer, hemorrhage, sarcoidosis, amyloidosis, porphyria
Multiple compressions and entrapments associated with polyneuropathy or rheumatic conditions
Infection: herpes zoster, leprosy, HIV, syphilis, tuberculosis
Multifocal demyelinating neuropathy
Sensory perineuritis
Migrant sensory neuritis of Wartenberg
Hereditary neuropathy with liability to pressure palsy

HIV, human immunodeficiency virus; SLE, systemic lupus erythematosus.

to weakness of the lower leg muscles, especially of the tibialis anterior and peroneus longus. Weakness and muscle atrophy of the hands are late findings. In long-standing polyneuropathies, the combination of hammer toes and high-arched feet (pes cavus; see Fig. 252–1) occurs because of greater weakness of the intrinsic foot muscles compared with the toe extensors and flexors in the lower leg by virtue of the difference in nerve lengths to those muscles. Ankle reflexes are depressed and later absent, with relative sparing of the knee and arm reflexes. Only when sensory or motor loss affects the proximal lower extremities or arms are the knee or arm reflexes depressed.

DIAGNOSING PERIPHERAL NEUROPATHIES

Localizing the Lesion

Symmetrical and Diffuse Versus Asymmetrical, Focal, or Multifocal. Because of the many hundreds of possible causes of peripheral neuropathy, a systematic approach to diagnosis is required. By using five steps, most peripheral neuropathies can be correctly categorized and diagnosed (Table 252–5). The first step involves localizing the lesion. Neuropathies can be divided into two broad categories: (1) symmetrical, diffuse, and length-dependent or (2) asymmetrical, focal, or multifocal (Table 252–6). This is an important distinction because the differential diagnoses of the two categories vary greatly. Further localization is possible depending on the anatomic distribution of neuro-

logic deficits. For example, a neuropathy affecting only one leg is asymmetrical and may be due to a focal neuropathy, lumbosacral plexopathy, or radiculopathy (see Table 252–6). Neurologic deficits in multiple focal nerve distributions fall under the category of *mononeuropathy multiplex* (sometimes referred to as *mononeuritis multiplex* or *multiple mononeuropathies*) and have a limited differential diagnosis (Table 252–7).

Sensory Versus Motor. Neuropathies can also be localized by whether sensory or motor abnormalities are equal or whether one or the other is more severe or is the only abnormality. For example, neuropathies affecting primarily the motor system may be the result of a disorder of the motor neurons (anterior horn cells) or other disorders (Table 252–8). If the sensory system is the predominant abnormality, further evaluation can determine if the small or large fiber sensory axons are affected. Large fiber sensory neuropathies result in a loss of vibration or proprioception; diabetes mellitus, renal failure, and monoclonal gammopathy are among the more common causes (Table 252–9). Small fiber

TABLE 252–6 ■ Distribution of Deficits in Peripheral Neuropathy

SYMMETRICAL AND DIFFUSE	ASYMMETRICAL, FOCAL (MULTIFOCAL)
Sensorimotor polyneuropathy	Mononeuropathy, single or multiple
Motor > sensory polyneuropathy	Radiculopathy, single or multiple
Sensory > motor polyneuropathy	Plexopathy, brachial or lumbosacral
Sensory neuropathy (large fiber versus small fiber)	Sensory ganglionopathy
	Motor neuropathy
	Motor neuron disease

TABLE 252–8 ■ Predominantly Motor Loss

Disorders of motor neurons
  Amyotrophic lateral sclerosis
  Spinal muscular atrophy
  Poliomyelitis
  Postpolio syndrome
  Kennedy's disease
Diabetic amyotrophy
Multifocal motor neuropathy
Hereditary motor and sensory neuropathy (HMSN) I and II
Hexosaminidase A deficiency
Subacute paraneoplastic motor neuropathy
Guillain-Barré syndrome
Chronic inflammatory demyelinating polyradiculoneuropathy (CIDP)
Infectious hepatitis
Infectious mononucleosis
Lymphoma
Porphyria
Toxicity
  Lead
  Mercury
  Organophosphates
  Nitrofurantoin
  Dapsone

TABLE 252–9 ■ **Predominantly Large Fiber Sensory Loss**

Diabetes mellitus
Monoclonal gammopathy
Paraneoplastic (anti-Hu antibody–associated)
Renal failure
Vitamin B_{12} or vitamin E deficiency
Connective tissue disorder (especially systemic lupus
  erythematosus, Sjögren's syndrome)
Toxicity
  Cisplatin
  Pyridoxine
  Nitrous oxide
  Glutethimide
Hereditary sensory and autonomic neuropathy (HSAN) II and IV
Idiopathic sensory ganglionopathy, most likely inflammatory

TABLE 252–11 ■ **Demyelinating Neuropathy**

Guillain-Barré syndrome
Diphtheria
Acute arsenic intoxication
Chronic inflammatory demyelinating polyradiculoneuropathy
Monoclonal gammopathy
  Monoclonal gammopathy of undetermined significance
  Multiple myeloma
  Cryoglobulinemia
  Waldenström's macroglobulinemia
  POEMS syndrome (osteosclerotic myeloma)
  Lymphoma
  Leukemia
N-hexane (slow nerve conduction velocity; mimics
  demyelination)
Hereditary
  Hereditary motor and sensory neuropathy (HMSN) I (Charcot-
    Marie-Tooth disease type I)
  Hereditary motor and sensory neuropathy III (Dejerine-Sottas
    disease)
  Refsum's disease (HMSN IV)
  Hereditary neuropathy with liability to pressure palsy
  Congenital hypomyelination neuropathy
  Metachromatic leukodystrophy
  Krabbe's disease
  Adrenoleukodystrophy

POEMS, polyneuropathy, organomegaly, endocrinopathy, M protein, skin changes.

sensory neuropathies lead to loss of pain or temperature sensation and are frequently accompanied by neuropathic pain. Early diabetes mellitus or human immunodeficiency virus (HIV) infection are frequent causes of a small fiber sensory neuropathy (Table 252–10).

Axonal Versus Demyelinating. Another step in localizing a neuropathy is to determine whether there is predominantly axonal degeneration or demyelination. This differentiation cannot be reliably determined by clinical examination and usually requires ancillary testing with either electromyography (EMG) and nerve conduction studies (NCS) or nerve biopsy. In the proper hands, EMG and NCS are accurate for differentiating the two possibilities, and nerve biopsy usually is not necessary. The demyelinating neuropathies are caused by a relatively limited number of different possibilities and are usually associated with good prognoses (Table 252–11). Conversely, the axonal, length-dependent polyneuropathies can be caused by a wide variety of causes (Table 252–12).

Tests to Aid Localization. The most important tests for evaluating a peripheral neuropathy are EMG and NCS (Table 252–13). They can help localize a lesion to the peripheral nerve, plexus, or root, or elsewhere in the peripheral nervous system, such as the anterior

TABLE 252–10 ■ **Predominantly Small Fiber Sensory Loss**

Early diabetic polyneuropathy
Human immunodeficiency virus
Renal failure
Amyloidosis
Leprosy
Toxicity
  Arsenic
  Thallium
  Metronidazole
  Chloramphenicol
Tangier's disease
Fabry's disease
Hereditary sensory and autonomic neuropathy (HSAN)
  I, III, and IV
Sensory perineuritis
Migrant sensory neuritis of Wartenberg

horn cell, neuromuscular junction, or muscle. Furthermore, they can determine whether there is axonal degeneration or demyelination, as well as the degree of sensory and motor involvement. EMG can determine the presence of motor axonal regeneration, which can help determine the cause and prognosis.

A lumbar puncture is sometimes helpful to determine whether the root or spinal cord is affected, usually by the presence of an elevated cerebrospinal fluid (CSF) protein concentration. Often, an elevated CSF protein level indicates a demyelinating radiculoneuropathy, that is, a neuropathy due to demyelination of the nerves and roots. Magnetic resonance imaging may help visualize mass lesions or edematous nerves resulting from inflammation. Somatosensory evoked potentials are occasionally helpful in differentiating peripheral from central causes of numbness. Autonomic testing may be helpful in that small fiber sensory neuropathies are often associated with autonomic abnormalities because of the similar small diameter, unmyelinated structure of autonomic nerve fibers. Quantitative sensory testing is not yet advocated for routine clinical testing but has been useful as a research tool to quantify loss of temperature or vibratory sensation. The utility of a nerve biopsy is discussed further on.

Time Course

The second step in diagnosing peripheral neuropathies involves obtaining a detailed history of the onset and time course of symptoms (Table 252–14). The differential diagnosis of acute-onset neuropathies is limited, with Guillain-Barré syndrome being the most common cause. Nerve infarction, usually from vasculitis, and compression are the most common acute causes of

TABLE 252–12 ■ **Acquired, Symmetrical, Length-Dependent, Axonal Polyneuropathy**

Endocrine	Diabetes mellitus, hypothyroidism, acromegaly
Drugs	Chemotherapeutic agents (vincristine, doxorubicin [Adriamycin], taxol), phenytoin (Dilantin), tricyclic antidepressants, isoniazid (INH), hydralazine, nitrofurantoin, amiodarone, disulfiram, metronidazole, dapsone
Toxins	Alcohol, arsenic, lead, mercury, thallium, industrial toxins, acrylamide, methylbutyl ketone, triorthocresylphosphate, carbon disulfide
Nutritional	Deficiency in vitamins B_1, B_6, B_{12}, E; vitamin B_6 intoxication
Metabolic	Renal failure, hyperglycemia or hypoglycemia, hypophosphatemia
Infectious	Hepatitis B, mononucleosis, HIV infection, Lyme disease, tick paralysis
Neoplastic/paraneoplastic	Lymphoma, leukemia, amyloidosis (acquired and hereditary)
Trauma	Mechanical, radiation, cold
Idiopathic	

TABLE 252–13 ■ **Tests to Aid Localization of Peripheral Neuropathy**

Nerve conduction studies and electromyography (EMG)
    Nerve versus plexus versus root versus combination
    Neuropathy versus neuromuscular versus myopathy
    Axonal versus demyelinating
    Motor versus sensory
    Regenerative activity
Lumbar puncture
Magnetic resonance imaging (MRI)
Somatosensory evoked potential
Autonomic testing
Quantitative sensory testing

multiple mononeuropathies. The differential diagnoses for subacute and chronic peripheral neuropathies are fairly broad. The most common cause of a monophasic peripheral neuropathy is Guillain-Barré syndrome or an episode of toxic exposure. Most causes of relapsing peripheral neuropathies are inflammatory or immune-mediated, especially chronic inflammatory demyelinating polyradiculoneuropathy (CIDP).

Acquired Versus Hereditary

The onset of most hereditary neuropathies occurs in childhood or in the young adulthood years, which differs from most acquired polyneuropathies, which usually begin in middle-aged or elderly individuals. However, some hereditary neuropathies are mild in onset and do not cause symptoms until later in life. In these instances, differentiating an acquired from a hereditary neuropathy can be difficult. Obtaining a detailed family history of peripheral neuropathy is the most important aspect of diagnosing hereditary neuropathy. Often, examination of the parents, siblings, and children of the patient is necessary, because affected members may overlook the insidious onset of symptoms. Other clues that are suggestive of a hereditary neuropathy include the failure to recognize major deficits, because of the insidious onset of symptoms, and the lack of paresthesias (Table 252–15). Features suggestive of an acquired peripheral neuropathy include an acute or subacute onset, the presence of paresthesias, a feeling of numbness as if a limb has "fallen asleep," and an asymmetrical or multifocal onset. The differential diagnosis of the hereditary neuropathies is shown in Table 252–16.

Associated Present or Past Disorders

Other present or past medical disorders can shed light on the cause of a peripheral neuropathy (Table 252–17). A detailed history and examination, focusing on the concurrent and past medical and social histories, review of systems, and general physical examination, often provides evidence for other medical problems.

TABLE 252–14 ■ **Onset and Time Course of Peripheral Neuropathy**

ACUTE ONSET (hours to days)	SUBACUTE ONSET (weeks to months)	CHRONIC (years)	MONOPHASIC	RELAPSING
Guillain-Barré syndrome	Inflammatory and immune disorders	CIDP	Guillain-Barré syndrome	Inflammatory and immune disorders (CIDP, MGUS, connective tissue disorders)
Ischemia	Infectious	Monoclonal gammopathy	Single toxic exposure	
Compression	Nutritional	Amyloidosis	Inflammatory ganglionopathy	Repeated toxic exposure
HIV	Toxic	Diabetes mellitus	Herpes zoster	Porphyria
Lyme disease	Metabolic	Hereditary neuropathy		Refsum's disease
Tick paralysis	Paraneoplastic			Hereditary neuropathy with liability to pressure palsy
Porphyria				
Diphtheria				
Arsenic poisoning				

CIDP, chronic inflammatory demyelinating polyradiculoneuropathy; HIV; human immunodeficiency virus; MGUS; monoclonal gammopathy of undetermined significance.

TABLE 252–15 ■ Inherited Versus Acquired Neuropathy

INHERITED	ACQUIRED
Family history	Sometimes acute or subacute in onset
Insidious onset over many years	Paresthesias
Failure to recognize major deficits	Limb has "fallen asleep"
No paresthesias	Asymmetrical or multifocal

TABLE 252–16 ■ Hereditary Neuropathies

Demyelinating (with secondary axonal degeneration)
   Hereditary motor and sensory neuropathy (HMSN) I (Charcot-Marie-Tooth [CMT] type I)
   HMSN III (Dejerine-Sottas disease)
   HMSN IV (Refsum's disease)
   Hereditary neuropathy with liability to pressure palsy
   Congenital hypomyelination neuropathy
   Metachromatic leukodystrophy
   Globoid cell leukodystrophy (Krabbe's disease)
   Adrenoleukodystrophy
Axonopathy
   HMSN type II (CMT type II)
   HMSN type V–VII
   Amyloidosis
   Kennedy's disease
   Hereditary sensory and autonomic neuropathy (HSAN) type I–IV
   Congenital indifference to pain
   Giant axonal neuropathy
   Hereditary ataxias—Friedreich's ataxia, ataxia telangiectasia, xeroderma pigmentosum
   Porphyria
   Abetalipoproteinemia (Bassen-Kornzweig disease)
   High-density lipoprotein deficiency (Tangier's disease)
   α-Galactosidase A deficiency (Fabry's disease)
   Chediak-Higashi disease
   Mitochondrial cytopathy
   Hereditary neuralgic amyotrophy

TABLE 252–17 ■ Associated Past or Present Disorders

   Endocrine disorders (e.g., diabetes mellitus)
   Malnutrition
   Vitamin deficiency
   Infection
   Cancer
   Hematologic disorders
   Connective tissue disorders
   Occupational history
   Toxic exposures (e.g., alcohol abuse, n-hexane exposure)
   Travel history

For example, symptoms of diabetes mellitus or a previous diagnosis of this disorder may suggest the cause of a peripheral neuropathy, especially in light of the fact that diabetes mellitus is one of the most common causes of peripheral neuropathy. Alcohol abuse is often another common cause of neuropathy that may be suggested by the history, examination, or the presence of liver abnormalities. Cancers and hematologic disorders can be associated with neuropathies through infiltration of the nerve or from a paraneoplastic syndrome, side effects from chemotherapy or radiation therapy, or a monoclonal gammopathy. Although leprosy is rare in developed nations, it is still the most common cause of neuropathy in developing countries and must be considered, especially in patients from regions where it is endemic. Most rheumatic diseases, especially systemic lupus erythematosus, can cause peripheral neuropathy.

Ancillary Tests

The decision as to which blood tests and ancillary tests to perform is complicated because of the wide variety available, which can often add up to thousands of dollars worth of tests. In general, the treatable neuropathies should be excluded, and patients with severe neuropathies should have more extensive testing compared with those with mild symptoms. Some of the tests that can be performed, depending on the four previous steps, including EMG and NCS, are listed in Table 252–18.

A nerve biopsy is usually performed only on selected patients with peripheral neuropathy. Usually, the biopsy involves a sensory nerve such as the sural, superficial peroneal, or superficial radial nerves. A nerve biopsy usually is not used to differentiate a demyelinating from an axonal neuropathy because EMG and NCS are more accurate, less invasive, and more cost effective. The indications for performing a nerve biopsy are listed in Table 252–19 and revolve around the possibility of one of several different causes. The most common indication is the possibility of vasculitis, because such a diagnosis involves risky treatment.

TREATMENT

Treatment of a peripheral neuropathy depends on the cause and such treatments are discussed in the sections on the specific neuropathies further on. In general, any endocrine, metabolic, nutritional, or toxic abnormality is reversed, and cancers or connective tissue disorders are treated. Inflammatory or immune-mediated neuropathies are treated with immunomodulating therapies. Occasionally, the cause of a peripheral neuropathy is uncertain, and inflammation, vasculitis, or an immune-mediated mechanism remains a possibility. In those cases, therapeutic trials of the appropriate immunomodulating therapy may be warranted both to treat the neuropathy and to determine the cause. If the peripheral neuropathy is severe enough to result in foot

TABLE 252–18 ■ **Blood and Other Ancillary Tests**

Acute Onset

CBC, metabolic panel (including Na^+, K^+, BUN, creatinine, glucose, liver function tests, Ca^{2+}, PO_4^-, Mg^{2+}), thyroid function tests, sedimentation rate, ANA, creatine kinase

Consider HIV, Lyme, serum and urine immunofixation, urine porphobilinogen and δ-aminolevulinic acid (for porphyria), urine for arsenic

Subacute or Chronic Onset

First set: CBC, metabolic panel, fasting glucose, hemoglobin A1C, thyroid function tests, sedimentation rate, VDRL, vitamin B_{12}, HDL

Second set: ANA, RF, serum and urine immunofixation, cryoglobulins

Consider HIV, Lyme, hepatitis B and C serologic tests

If Acquired, Symmetrical, Axonal Polyneuropathy

Vitamin E, urine for heavy metals, SS-A (anti-La), SS-B (anti-Ro), angiotensin-converting enzyme, chest radiograph, cancer screen

If Multiple Axonal Mononeuropathy

Consider vasculitis or leprosy (consider nerve biopsy)

Consider SS-A (anti-La), SS-B (anti-Ro), angiotensin-converting enzyme, chest radiograph, cancer screen

If Acquired Demyelinating Neuropathy

Anti-MAG (myelin-associated glycoprotein), anti-SGPG (sulfate-3-glucuronyl paragloboside), anti-GM1 (monosialoganglioside) antibodies

Hepatitis screen to differentiate CIDP from other immune-mediated neuropathy

Consider phytanic acid, tests for CMT1, HNPP, metachromatic leukodystrophy, Krabbe's disease, adrenoleukodystrophy, and other hereditary demyelinating neuropathies

If Monoclonal Gammopathy Is Present

Check anti-MAG and anti-GM1 to differentiate MGUS from other immune-mediated neuropathy

Workup for multiple myeloma, plasmacytoma (skeletal survey, bone marrow biopsy)

Workup for amyloidosis (C-reactive protein, urinalysis for proteinuria, DNA for transthyretin mutation, nerve biopsy)

If workup is normal, periodically repeat ANA, RF, serum and urine immunofixation, cryoglobulins, Lyme titer

---

ANA, antinuclear antibody; BUN, blood urea nitrogen; CBC, complete blood count; CIDP, chronic inflammatory demyelinating polyradiculoneuropathy; CMT1, Charcot-Marie-Tooth type 1; HDL, high-density lipoprotein; HIV, human immunodeficiency virus; HNPP, hereditary neuropathy with liability to pressure palsy; MGUS, monoclonal gammopathy of undetermined significance; RF, rheumatoid factor; VDRL, Venereal Disease Research Laboratory.

---

drop or gait imbalance, physical and occupational therapy is helpful, as is a cane or ankle-foot orthosis. Most peripheral neuropathies do not result in significant disabilities and are almost never life-threatening. Discussion of the generally good prognosis is often reassuring to patients, as they frequently fear the worst outcome.

TABLE 252–19 ■ **Indications for Nerve Biopsy**

Inflammation (vasculitis, sarcoidosis, ganglionitis, CIDP, antibody deposition)

Infiltration (amyloidosis, lymphoma, tumor)

Infection (leprosy)

Unique tissue abnormalities (e.g., excessive glycogen)

CIDP, chronic inflammatory demyelinating polyradiculoneuropathy.

Some patients develop severe neuropathic pain, often described as burning, painful paresthesias or electrical shocks. At times, neuropathic pain can be debilitating and needs to be treated aggressively. Treatment usually involves oral medications, although research suggests that topical medications may be effective. Usually, a single oral medication is started at a low dose and slowly increased until an effective dose is achieved, intolerable side effects occur, or the maximal safe dose is reached, whichever occurs first. If a medication is ineffective, it is discontinued and a different medication is tried. The tricyclic antidepressants amitriptyline, desipramine and nortriptyline have been used for many years and have been shown to be safe and effective.[1–3] If patients have insomnia, amitriptyline may be a good choice because of its significant sedating side effects. Elderly patients may be sensitive to the anticholinergic side effects and may benefit from desipramine. Most patients can tolerate nortriptyline. They all have in common side effects related to their anticholinergic effects, such as drowsiness, dry mouth, urinary retention, and confusion. Usually, a small dose is started, such as 25 mg PO once per day at night before sleep (QHS) in most individuals, and 10 mg PO QHS in the elderly. The dose is then slowly increased in 10- to 25-mg increments per week, continuing in a QHS dosing schedule, until effective or until side effects occur or the maximal dose of 150 mg QHS is reached, whichever happens first.

The next medication that can be attempted is the antiepileptic agent gabapentin. Gabapentin has been shown to be effective in painful diabetic neuropathy and postherpetic neuralgia.[4, 5] Its most significant side effect is drowsiness. It is started at 300 mg PO daily and then increased in 300-mg increments per week in a three times daily dosing schedule until it is effective or until side effects occur, whichever comes first. There does not appear to be an upper limit for the maximal safe gabapentin dose. Some children taking it for epilepsy can tolerate up to 10 g/day. Most adults have difficulty taking more than 3600 mg/day because of drowsiness.

Tramadol has been shown to be effective for the treatment of painful diabetic neuropathy.[6] The initial dose is 50 mg/day and gradually increasing in 50-mg increments every 3 days in an every 4- to 6-hour dosing schedule until it is effective, until side effects occur, or until a maximal dose of 400 mg/day (300 mg/day maximum for patients older than 75 years) is reached.

Mexiletine is an antiarrhythmic drug that has been shown to be effective for the treatment of neuropathic pain.[7, 8] It has many more potentially serious side effects than the other medications and cannot be used in patients with electrocardiographic evidence of conduction block, a history of myocardial infarction, congestive heart failure, or seizures. The initial dose is 150 mg PO twice daily, and increasing in 150-mg increments every week in a three times daily dosing schedule until effective, side effects occur, or a maximal dose of 900 mg/day is reached. Periodic monitoring with an electrocardiogram, complete blood count, and liver function tests is required.

The antiepileptic medications carbamazepine and phenytoin are usually helpful only for neuropathic pain that is brief, intermittent, and electrical shock-like in sensation. The dosage is similar to that used for the treatment of epilepsy.[3]

INFLAMMATORY OR IMMUNE-MEDIATED NEUROPATHIES

Guillain-Barré Syndrome

Guillain-Barré syndrome is a rapidly progressive paralytic illness that is caused by inflammatory demyelination of peripheral nerves and nerve roots.[9, 10] Typically, the first symptom is paresthesias of the feet. Leg weakness ensues within a few days, followed by rapid ascending weakness and numbness from the lower extremities to the arms and trunk. In severe cases, quadriplegia, bulbar weakness, and respiratory failure occur. Often, a patient experiences pain that is similar to sciatica, myalgias, or "charley horses."[11] The symptoms and signs are relatively symmetrical. On examination, there is limb weakness, with the lower extremities more severely affected than the arms. Deep tendon reflexes are usually absent or diminished. Despite early and significant paresthesias, sensory deficits on examination are usually mild and less severe than motor deficits. A third of patients may develop facial diplegia. In severe cases, patients may develop ophthalmoparesis, dysarthria, dysphagia, respiratory insufficiency, or autonomic instability. Occasionally, ataxia or sphincter dysfunction may be present.

Symptoms usually progress over days to weeks. Maximal deficits occur within 1 month, followed by plateau of deficits for days to weeks and rarely months. Gradual improvement occurs after the plateau phase. Prognosis is good, with a 5% mortality rate and 5% to 10% of patients with permanent disabilities, 65% to 75% with mild deficits, and 15% with no deficit. The annual incidence is one to two cases per 100,000 population. Guillain-Barré syndrome most often affects young and middle-aged adults. About 60% of cases are associated with an antecedent upper respiratory or gastrointestinal illness within 1 month of onset. The most common associated illness is *Campylobacter jejuni* enteritis. Viral infections from cytomegalovirus, Epstein-Barr virus, viral hepatitis, and HIV infection have also been implicated. Often, the pathogen causing the illness is unknown. Other associated antecedent or associated events include vaccinations, surgery, cancer, and pregnancy.

Ancillary tests should include blood tests to evaluate for other acute causes of peripheral nervous system abnormalities (see Table 252–18). A lumbar puncture is helpful in the diagnostic evaluation. CSF protein levels are abnormally elevated initially in 50% of patients, and eventually in 90%, with values ranging from 55 to 250 mg/dL. The CSF is usually acellular with normal pressure. If more than 10 white cells/mm^3 are present, an alternative diagnosis should be considered. EMG and NCS almost always show evidence of a polyneuropathy, with 69% demonstrating a demyelinating polyneuropathy, 3% demonstrating only axonal degeneration, 3% with inexcitable nerves, 2% with normal findings, and 29% with equivocal findings that can be consistent with either a demyelinating or an axonal process.[12] Nerve biopsy is rarely required to confirm the diagnosis.

Pathologically, there is usually inflammation of peripheral nerves with lymphocytes and macrophages surrounding endoneurial vessels and macrophage processes stripping myelin from axons.[13] Secondary axonal degeneration is sometimes apparent. The pathophysiology of Guillain-Barré syndrome is most likely an aberrant response to an immunologic stimulus that involves a lymphocytic T-cell mechanism.

There are several variants of Guillain-Barré syndrome.[14, 15] The most common variant, the Miller-Fisher syndrome, accounts for about 5% of all cases of Guillain-Barré syndrome. Patients develop the triad of ophthalmoplegia, ataxia, and areflexia, with no significant weakness or numbness. Other variants include (1) weakness without paresthesias or sensory loss, (2) pharyngocervicobrachial weakness, (3) paraparesis, (4) facial paresis with distal paresthesias, (5) pure ataxia, (6) acute pandysautonomia, and (7) rapid axonal Guillain-Barré syndrome. All these variants have in common absent or diminished reflexes, elevated CSF protein levels, and EMG and NCS abnormalities.

Treatment options are fairly limited and consist of plasmapheresis, intravenous immunoglobulin (IVIg), intensive care unit support, and physical and respiratory therapy. Since 1984, four clinical trials have unequivocally demonstrated that plasmapheresis is effective in improving short- and long-term neurologic function.[16–20] In addition, two large randomized clinical trials comparing IVIg and plasmapheresis demonstrated that they are equivalent in efficacy.[21, 22] The cost of plasmapheresis and IVIg is similar, and the relapse rate for IVIg is no different than that for plasmapheresis. The advantages of IVIg over plasmapheresis are that IVIg is associated with fewer complications such as hemodynamic fluctuations, is easier to administer, and is more readily available. In contrast, the advantage of plasmapheresis over IVIg is that IVIg can be given immediately after plasmapheresis if the patient has severe deficits. If a patient were given IVIg first and then continued to worsen, plasmapheresis after IVIg would remove the IVIg and negate its effects. The combination of plasmapheresis followed immediately by IVIg was found to be slightly better than IVIg alone.[22] Thus, using plasmapheresis first as a treatment would leave open the option of IVIg afterward in patients who develop severe Guillain-Barré syndrome.

Although corticosteroids were administered for 50 years, they are no longer used after having been proven not to be beneficial in two randomized, placebo-controlled clinical trials.[23, 24] Other immunosuppressant medications have not been sufficiently tested.

Chronic Inflammatory Demyelinating Polyradiculoneuropathy

CIDP is a chronic progressive polyneuropathy caused by inflammatory demyelination of peripheral nerves and nerve roots.[25-27] The clinical, electrodiagnostic, and pathologic features are similar to Guillain-Barré syndrome, except that the time course differs in that symptoms progress for a longer duration, often with relapses. Unlike Guillain-Barré syndrome, in which symptoms often peak within a month of onset and spontaneously improve days to weeks later, patients with CIDP continue to worsen beyond a month and often do not improve for many months. Symptoms and signs include progressive weakness, numbness, and paresthesias in the distal extremities (worse in the legs), and absent or diminished reflexes. Cranial nerves are occasionally affected. Lumbar puncture reveals an elevated CSF protein concentration with minimal to no pleocytosis. A monoclonal gammopathy is sometimes present. The laboratory evaluation is otherwise unremarkable. EMG and NCS reveal a demyelinating polyneuropathy with multifocal areas of conduction block and slowing. Nerve biopsy is occasionally performed and shows evidence of mononuclear infiltration of the nerve with demyelination, remyelination, and secondary axonal degeneration.

Treatment with corticosteroids, plasmapheresis, and IVIg have been proved beneficial in placebo-controlled clinical trials.[28-32] Further studies have demonstrated that plasmapheresis and IVIg are about equally effective.[33] Azathioprine, cyclosporine A, and cyclophosphamide are other immunosuppressive medications reported to be beneficial, but they have not been tested in controlled clinical trials. In one series, 95% of patients responded to treatment, but only 40% were in partial or complete remission and receiving no medications.[26]

Multifocal Motor Neuropathy

Multifocal motor neuropathy (also referred to as *multifocal motor neuropathy with conduction block*) is an immune-mediated, multifocal demyelinating neuropathy affecting motor nerves only and sparing sensory nerves.[34] It was first recognized in 1988 as a unique syndrome separate from motor neuron disease.[35-38] Since then it has become an increasingly recognized treatable disease. Patients develop asymmetrical weakness in multiple distal nerve distributions resulting from conduction block and axonal loss. Symptoms consist of the insidious onset of progressive focal or multifocal weakness and fasciculations predominantly in the distal limbs, but with no significant sensory symptoms. Proximal limb muscles are less commonly affected, and cranial nerves are usually spared. On examination, weakness is more prominent than the degree of muscle atrophy because the weakness results mainly from conduction block rather than axonal degeneration. Only after many months or years is there secondary motor axonal loss and subsequent denervation muscle atrophy. Sensation is normal, and reflexes are diminished only in weak muscles. EMG and NCS usually, but not always, reveal conduction block in motor nerves with normal sensory responses.[39, 40] Elevated antibody titers against the ganglioside GM1 are present in 50% to 85% of cases, depending on the laboratory that performs the test.[41] In early stages, the

diagnosis can be confused with motor neuron disease, such as amyotrophic lateral sclerosis (ALS), because the clinical presentation of insidious progressive weakness and fasciculations without sensory loss is the same in both conditions. Unlike with ALS, multifocal motor neuropathy is never associated with upper motor neuron signs, only rarely affects cranial nerves, and is not fatal. When multifocal motor neuropathy affects only one nerve, the presence of conduction block may mimic a nerve entrapment syndrome and lead to unsuccessful surgical decompression and neurolysis. Thus, this diagnosis should be considered in anyone presenting with progressive focal weakness in a nerve distribution, especially in an area not commonly associated with nerve entrapment.

Many immunomodulating treatments have been attempted. Cyclophosphamide was the first agent shown to be effective in reversing conduction block and weakness.[35, 42] Two placebo-controlled trials have demonstrated IVIg to be beneficial.[43, 44] There are also reports of cyclosporine A being effective. Corticosteroids, azathioprine, and plasmapheresis are considered ineffective. Many patients do not respond to treatment and are left with persistent weakness predominantly in the distal limbs.[40]

Neuralgic Amyotrophy

There are many synonyms for neuralgic amyotrophy, including *Parsonage-Turner syndrome, acute brachial neuritis, acute brachial plexitis, acute brachial neuropathy, shoulder-girdle syndrome,* and *brachial plexus neuralgia.* Patients present with acute onset of severe unilateral pain in the shoulder that typically lasts a few weeks.[45, 46] The pain is usually severe enough to cause insomnia. Because the pain worsens with movement of the affected arm, most patients minimize the use of that limb. Weakness often occurs within hours to days of onset but may not be apparent until the pain resolves or improves to the point of allowing use of the arm. Motor deficits, sometimes accompanied by muscle atrophy, most often occur in the distribution of single or multiple nerves. Any nerve of the upper limb can be affected, but the more commonly affected nerves include the long thoracic (causing winging of the scapula), suprascapular, axillary, and anterior interosseous nerves. Interestingly, there is usually only minor or no significant sensory symptoms or deficits, and reflexes may be normal or diminished. Most cases are sporadic, unilateral, and monophasic. However, up to a third can have minimal to significant involvement of the contralateral side. A small percentage are familial or recurrent.[45, 47] Men are affected more frequently than women in a 2.4:1 ratio.[45] The annual incidence is estimated to be about 1 to 3 per 100,000 population.

The cause is unknown, but an immune-mediated or inflammatory mechanism is proposed based on a pathologic study demonstrating inflammation on brachial plexus biopsy in four patients.[48] Episodes may be triggered by surgery, pregnancy, infections, and immunizations, suggesting the possibility of an event that up-regulates the immune system, similar to the proposed pathophysiologic events in Guillain-Barré syndrome. Prognosis is excellent, with 60% recovering completely within 1 year, and 80% within a few years.[45] There are no studies demonstrating that steroids, IVIg, or other immunomodulating agents are beneficial during an episode, and most patients recover fully without specific treatment. However, given the inflammatory mechanism of nerve injury, many patients are given a short course of corticosteroids. Aggressive treatment with narcotics should be undertaken because of the severity of the pain. Because of the clinical symptoms and signs, neuralgic amyotrophy can be confused with a cervical radiculopathy. Recognition of this syndrome is important to avoid unnecessary surgery.

Idiopathic Lumbosacral Plexopathy

Idiopathic lumbosacral plexopathy is most likely an under-recognized syndrome because of its misdiagnosis as lumbosacral radiculopathy. Patients develop acute or subacute onset of pain in the lower extremity, with weakness occurring immediately or within a few days. More often, the pain involves the lower back and proximal lower extremity, and the weakness is in the upper lumbar plexus distribution. Less often, the pain and weakness are in a lower lumbosacral plexus distribution. The pain often subsides after days to weeks, followed by gradual improvement in weakness over a few weeks to months. Sensation is usually affected less severely than the degree of weakness but may remain normal. Reflexes are usually decreased in weak muscles. The time course and distribution of symptoms have led many to suggest that this syndrome represents the lumbosacral plexus counterpart to neuralgic amyotrophy.[49] However, some patients develop a more chronic progressive presentation of pain, weakness, and muscle atrophy, often in the proximal lower extremity, that mimics proximal diabetic neuropathy (diabetic amyotrophy), but without evidence of diabetes mellitus.[50]

The age of affected patients ranges from 2 to 81 years, with approximately equal gender representation. A minority of patients have bilateral symptoms. The diagnosis is determined by localizing the lesion to the lumbosacral plexus by EMG and NCS and by excluding other causes of lumbosacral plexopathy, such as mass lesions or nerve infarction. Ancillary evaluation is generally unremarkable except for a number of cases associated with an elevated sedimentation rate. Vaccination, pregnancy, and IV heroin use have been implicated as a precipitating event in some cases. The cause is unknown but is postulated to be an inflammatory or immune-mediated disorder, similar to neuralgic amyotrophy.

Prognosis is usually excellent, with most patients experiencing spontaneous complete or nearly complete recovery of strength, especially patients with an acute or subacute clinical course. Recurrences are rare but have been reported. Some patients with the more chronic presentation were treated with corticosteroids or IVIg and experienced a temporally related improvement.[51]

Monoclonal Gammopathy

A monoclonal gammopathy, usually idiopathic but sometimes due to multiple myeloma, Waldenström's macroglobulinemia, osteosclerotic myeloma, lymphoma, or leukemia, can cause a chronic progressive polyneuropathy that is either demyelinating or axonal.[52] Some are associated with specific antibodies to myelin-specific proteins, such as myelin-associated glycoprotein (MAG), or gangliosides, such as GM1 or GD1b. The demyelinating polyneuropathies usually respond more readily to immunomodulating therapy than do the axonal polyneuropathies. Prognosis is good with treatment.

INFECTIOUS NEUROPATHIES

Human Immunodeficiency Virus Neuropathy

A number of different forms of peripheral neuropathy are caused by HIV infection.[53] The most common presentation is a chronic, distal, symmetrical, axonal sensorimotor polyneuropathy that affects the small fiber sensory axons most severely. It occurs in up to 30% of patients with HIV infection, most frequently in patients with acquired immunodeficiency syndrome (AIDS). There is no specific treatment other than anti-HIV viral agents. Neuropathic pain can be severe and is treated as discussed earlier.

HIV infection can cause Guillain-Barré syndrome, which occurs early in the infection, and CIDP appears later in the course of AIDS. Immunomodulating medications are helpful, as in the non-HIV causes of Guillain-Barré syndrome or CIDP. In late AIDS, HIV infection can cause mononeuropathy multiplex due to vasculitis, cytomegalovirus (CMV) infection, or infiltration from lymphoma or lymphocytosis. Treatment is often unsuccessful.

Cytomegalovirus Polyradiculopathy

CMV infection occurs opportunistically in late AIDS and can cause an acute or subacute lumbosacral polyradiculopathy.[54] Patients present with rapidly progressive flaccid weakness, numbness and areflexia in the legs, and urinary incontinence. This presentation mimics neurosurgical causes of cauda equina or conus medullaris syndrome. Magnetic resonance imaging may show enhancement of the cauda equina. Lumbar puncture reveals a significant CSF pleocytosis, usually with a predominance of polymorphonuclear cells despite the viral cause. The CSF protein level is elevated, and polymerase chain reaction (PCR) analysis reveals evidence of CMV infection. Treatment with foscarnet or ganciclovir can sometimes arrest progression or induce improvement if started early.

Other Neuropathies

Herpes zoster (shingles) is a recurrence of latent viral infection of the dorsal root ganglion after varicella infection (chickenpox). It often recurs with a decreased immune state, especially with increasing age. Patients develop sensory loss, pain, and vesicular eruption in a radicular distribution.[55] It is occasionally associated with weakness from loss of anterior horn cells due to myelitis. Postherpetic neuralgia is a frequent sequela, especially in the elderly. Treatment includes famciclovir or acyclovir during the early stages of infection, and medications for neuralgia, similar to those used for neuropathic pain.

Hepatitis B and C can cause a mononeuropathy multiplex or polyneuropathy due to vasculitis or deposition of immune complexes or cryoglobulins.[56]

As mentioned earlier, leprosy is a frequent cause of neuropathy in developing countries.[57] It is caused by infection of distal sensory nerves by *Mycobacterium leprae*. Patients develop sensory loss in patchy distributions, including the face and trunk. Treatment with dapsone, clofazimine, and rifampin usually prevents progression.

Lyme disease is caused by *Borrelia burgdorferi* spirochete infection spread by tick bites. The disease initially causes erythema migrans followed by arthritis. If untreated in the initial stages, 25% of patients develop single or multiple mononeuropathies of cranial or peripheral nerves.[58] Treatment with antibiotics is usually curative. Vaccination is also available for prevention.

ENDOCRINE NEUROPATHIES

Diabetic Neuropathy

One of the most common complications of diabetes mellitus is neuropathy. The neuropathy can present in a number of different distributions and time courses. One of the most common presentations is a chronic, progressive distal symmetrical polyneuropathy that most often affects the sensory and motor fibers equally but can at times present with predominantly large fiber or small fiber sensory or autonomic loss. An acute painful axonal polyneuropathy can occur in the setting of poor diabetes glucose control and weight loss, or with the institution of insulin. Proximal diabetic neuropathy, also referred to as *diabetic amyotrophy,* is an uncommon presentation that can mimic a neurosurgical problem. Single or multiple mononeuropathies are also common complications.

The prevalence of diabetic neuropathy is about 10% within the first year of diagnosis and approaches 50% by 25 years after diagnosis.[59] Length-dependent polyneuropathies account for about 50% of the diabetic neuropathies, and focal neuropathies account for about 40%.[60] The main risk factors are duration of diabetes mellitus, older age, male gender, and greater height.[61]

Sensorimotor or Sensory Polyneuropathy. The typical polyneuropathy begins insidiously in a distal, length-dependent, symmetrical distribution with slow progression. Sensory symptoms consist of tingling, paresthesias, numbness, or neuropathic pain. Often, sensory loss on examination precedes sensory symptoms. Weakness is not a frequent complaint and is a later finding on examination compared with sensory loss and absent ankle reflexes. Foot drop from ankle dorsiflexion weakness and foot ulcers are late sequelae.

Autonomic Neuropathy. Symptoms and signs usually begin insidiously and progress slowly. Patients can develop any number of autonomic abnormalities in isolation or in combination, including cardiovascular disturbances (postural hypotension, heart rate abnormalities), thermoregulatory disorders (distal anhidrosis, gustatory sweating, abnormal vasomotor responses to change in temperature), gastrointestinal disorders (gastrointestinal atony, diarrhea, anal sphincter weakness), genitourinary disorders (bladder atony, impotence, retrograde ejaculation), unawareness of hypoglycemia, respiratory control abnormalities, and pupillary and lacrimal gland dysfunction. Awareness of autonomic neuropathy is important because of the associated poor prognosis. The mortality rate of patients with autonomic neuropathy is 45% at 2.5 years and 55% at 5 years compared with about 10% and 20%, respectively, in a comparable diabetic population.[62]

Proximal Diabetic Neuropathy. This syndrome, also commonly referred to as *diabetic amyotrophy,* is estimated to account for about 1% of all diabetic neuropathies. Clinically, patients develop weakness and muscle atrophy of the pelvic and anterior thigh muscles in a unilateral, asymmetrical, or symmetrical distribution. There is usually only mild or no significant sensory loss. Reflexes are decreased in weak muscles, especially the knees. Pain is usually severe in the thigh and pelvis and sometimes the lower back, but occasionally is not present. Weight loss is often a prominent feature. The onset is usually subacute over weeks or months, but is sometimes acute and followed by slow progression. Onset occurs predominantly in patients with type II diabetes who are middle-aged or elderly. It is not uncommon that the disorder occurs before the diagnosis of diabetes mellitus is discovered. The scapulohumeral muscles are only rarely involved. Some patients may have concomitant mild diabetic distal polyneuropathy. If distal leg weakness is present, it is always less than the degree of pelvifemoral weakness. The weakness is monophasic, with spontaneous improvement in virtually all patients, possibly hastened by better glucose control.[63] Because proximal lower extremity weakness, muscle atrophy, and lower back and pelvic pain are the most prominent features, the disorder mimics a lumbar radiculopathy, and patients are occasionally subjected to unnecessary lower back surgery.

The pathophysiology of proximal diabetic neuropathy is the subject of intense debate. The two most commonly proposed mechanisms include metabolic and ischemic causes, similar to the mechanisms for the other types of diabetic neuropathies (see later). Inflammation and vasculitis have been proposed as mechanisms based on the results of four published studies of biopsies of the intermediate cutaneous nerve of the thigh. Many of the biopsy samples showed either inflammation of the nerve or vasonervorum.[64-67] Some of the patients improved with immunomodulating treatments, especially IVIg. However, since the natural history of the disease is one of spontaneous improvement, it is unclear whether treatment resulted in more substantial improvement and whether inflammation or vasculitis is a cause rather than an epiphenomenon. Placebo-controlled clinical trials are needed to answer those questions.

Focal Mononeuropathy and Radiculopathy. These disorders account for a large portion of diabetic neuropathies, especially the neuropathies that occur at common sites of entrapment. In one series of focal diabetic mononeuropathies, the median and ulnar nerves each accounted for 30% of the lesions, the peroneal nerve accounted for 16%, and the remainder of the lesions were in the sciatic and femoral nerves and cranial nerves III, VI, and VII.[68] Others have reported radiculopathies (including of the thoracic roots), lateral femoral cutaneous neuropathy, radial neuropathy, and other cranial neuropathies. The focal diabetic neuropathies can be divided into acute and chronic categories.

The acute mononeuropathies and radiculopathies are typically associated with an acute onset of pain and sensory and motor symptoms and deficits. They are caused by acute infarction of the nerve. They occasionally occur simultaneously in a mononeuropathy multiplex presentation. Radiculopathies caused by diabetes are often indistinguishable from those caused by structural lesions. The concomitant presence of other forms of diabetic neuropathies, as well as the lack of structural lesions on imaging tests, would support diabetes as a cause.

The chronic mononeuropathies are usually due to entrapment and present with signs and symptoms that are typical for other causes of entrapment neuropathy. The pathophysiology involves an increased susceptibility of diabetic nerves to compression injury.

Pathophysiology. The pathophysiology of the symmetrical diabetic polyneuropathies is uncertain. The two main proposed mechanisms include metabolic abnormalities and nerve ischemia from vascular insufficiency.[69] Evidence suggests that both mechanisms are involved. There are a number of metabolic abnormalities in diabetic nerves. Aldose reductase, which converts glucose to sorbitol, shows increased activity due to elevated intracellular glucose levels, thus leading to increased sorbitol and decreased myoinositol levels and Na^+-K^+-ATPase activity. Other mechanisms may include abnormalities in osmotic regulation, oxidative stress, abnormal carnitine and fatty acid metabolism, nonenzymatic protein glycation, and abnormal protein synthesis and axonal transport. All these metabolic abnormalities have been demonstrated in diabetic animal and human nerves, and some or all these mechanisms may be involved in the pathogenesis of diabetic neuropathy.

Besides a number of metabolic abnormalities, there is evidence for nerve ischemia that may also play a role in the development of neuropathy. In diabetic nerves, there is evidence of thrombosis and vessel wall thickening and decreased nitric oxide and prostacyclin production, leading to a decrease in vasodilation and nerve ischemia.

Treatment. The only definitive treatment and preventive measure for all the different types of diabetic neuropathies is tight glucose control. This treatment has been proved most definitively for the sensorimotor polyneuropathy in a randomized, prospective study whereby patients treated with intensive glucose control had 60% less polyneuropathies compared with those treated with conventional, less intensive therapy.[70] All other treatments to prevent or reverse diabetic polyneuropathy are experimental and include aldose reductase inhibitors, neurotrophic factors,[71] gamma-linolenic acid, gangliosides, uridine, and corticotropin analogs.[69] Symptomatic treatment of diabetic neuropathy consists of a number of approaches that are similar to the treatments outlined in the section "Treatment."

Other Endocrine Neuropathies. Hypothyroidism can cause a mild, painful, mixed demyelinating and axonal sensorimotor polyneuropathy that resolves with thyroid replacement.[72] Hypothyroidism also causes entrapment neuropathies, especially carpal tunnel syndrome.[72]

Acromegaly can cause entrapment neuropathies because of connective tissue hyperplasia and bony overgrowth.[73]

TOXIC NEUROPATHIES

Alcoholic Neuropathy

Alcoholism is a common cause of polyneuropathy.[74] Up to 30% of hospitalized alcoholics have a polyneuropathy. The neuropathy is typically symmetrical, distal, and length-dependent, with axonal degeneration of sensory and motor fibers. Symptoms occur insidiously, followed by gradual progression. Patients who drink several glasses of alcohol daily for several years are at risk. The pathophysiology may involve the direct toxicity of alcohol on peripheral nerves, with nutritional deficiency (e.g., thiamine deficiency) as a possible contributing factor. Treatment involves discontinuing alcohol consumption and reversing any vitamin deficiencies. Neurologic deficits can improve if treated early.

Medications and Chemical Toxins

Many medications, chemicals, and other toxins can potentially cause a subacute, progressive peripheral neuropathy that is usually symmetrical, distal, and length-dependent with sensory and motor axonal degeneration. When a patient presents with a peripheral neuropathy, a history directed toward medications and chemical exposures at work, at home, or encountered in hobbies often uncovers potential causative agents. Discontinuation of causative medications or removing exposure to chemical toxins is often attempted. Stabilization or improvement of symptoms usually occurs immediately or occasionally after a few days or weeks. However, symptoms can occasionally continue to worsen for a few days to weeks, a phenomenon referred to as *coasting*.[75] The more commonly implicated medications include amiodarone, chloramphenicol, cisplatin, colchicine, dapsone, dideoxycytidine (ddC), disulfiram, FK506, gold, isoniazid, nitrofurantoin, perhexiline, propafenone, pyridoxine, phenytoin, simvastatin, taxol, thalidomide, and vincristine. Potentially causative toxins include acrylamide, arsenic, carbon disulfide, hexacarbons, lead, mercury, organophosphates, platinum, and thallium.

NUTRITIONAL NEUROPATHIES

Vitamin B$_{12}$ (Cobalamin) Deficiency

Vitamin B$_{12}$ deficiency results from malabsorption due to pernicious anemia, gastrectomy or inflammatory bowel disease, or insufficient consumption resulting from the individual following a strict vegetarian diet, including the avoidance of eggs and dairy products. Vitamin B$_{12}$ deficiency leads to a number of neurologic conditions, including dementia, subacute combined degeneration of the spinal cord, and a symmetrical, length-dependent, axonal sensorimotor polyneuropathy.[76] Patients develop paresthesias or burning in the feet and hands, distal limb weakness and loss of sensation, and diminished or loss of ankle reflexes. There is axonal degeneration without demyelination seen on EMG and NCS and nerve biopsy. Laboratory abnormalities include a megaloblastic anemia and serum vitamin B$_{12}$ deficiency, although there are case reports of symptomatic vitamin B$_{12}$ deficiency without anemia or elevated mean corpuscular volume. Testing for elevations of serum homocysteine and methylmalonic acid levels is helpful when the vitamin B$_{12}$ level is borderline low. With early treatment, the paresthesias may improve, but loss of large fiber sensory axons is often permanent.

Thiamine (Vitamin B$_1$) Deficiency

Thiamine deficiency results from insufficient consumption related to alcoholism, starvation, gastric stapling, prolonged vomiting, or an unbalanced diet of carbohydrates without vitamins, protein, or fat. Three neurologic syndromes occur.[77] Dry beriberi consists of a painful, symmetrical, length-dependent axonal sensorimotor polyneuropathy. Patients develop pain, paresthesias, and numbness in the feet; weakness in the lower legs; and absent ankle reflexes. Sensory and motor axonal degeneration is demonstrated by EMG, NCS, and nerve biopsy. The polyneuropathy may improve with thiamine replacement.[2] Wet beriberi consists of the same polyneuropathy seen with dry beriberi along with congestive heart failure.[3] Wernicke-Korsakoff syndrome consists of the triad of confusion, ophthalmoparesis, and gait ataxia.

Vitamin E (Tocopherol) Deficiency

Vitamin E deficiency occurs from malabsorption states related to abetalipoproteinemia (Bassen-Kornzweig syndrome), cystic fibrosis or biliary atresia, or abnormal vitamin E metabolism from a genetic defect of the alpha-tocopherol transfer protein. Patients develop a large fiber sensory neuropathy and myelopathy, with progressive loss of vibration sensation and proprioception, absent ankle reflexes, limb and gait ataxia, and Babinski signs.[78] Pathologically, there is degeneration of sensory axons, dorsal root ganglia, posterior columns, and spinocerebellar tracts. On EMG and NCS, there is a symmetrical, length-dependent, axonal sensory neuropathy with no loss of motor axons or demyelination. Serum vitamin E levels are decreased, and treatment with vitamin E halts progression of symptoms but does not induce significant improvement.

Pyridoxine (Vitamin B$_6$) Deficiency or Toxicity

Pyridoxine deficiency or toxicity results in a sensory neuropathy with distal burning, paresthesias and numbness in the feet and hands, and sensory axonal degeneration demonstrated by EMG and NCS or nerve biopsy. The motor system is seen to be spared on examination and EMG and NCS. Pyridoxine deficiency most commonly results from isoniazid or hydralazine treatment but can also occur with polynutritional deficiency.[79] Pyridoxine is toxic at doses greater than 200 mg/day.[80] Reversal of the abnormalities results in improvement of symptoms.

VASCULAR NEUROPATHIES

Vasculitic Neuropathy

Vasculitis causes nerve infarction, leading to weakness, numbness, paresthesias, pain, and absent reflexes in the distribution of the infarcted nerve. Most patients present with infarction of a single nerve or in a mononeuropathy multiplex distribution. However, about 15% of patients develop a symmetrical, length-dependent polyneuropathy. When infarction occurs in a single nerve, it can mimic a compressive neuropathy. Vasculitic neuropathy can be isolated to the peripheral nervous system or can be associated with systemic vasculitis such as polyarteritis nodosa, Wegener's granulomatosis, Churg-Strauss syndrome, other connective tissue disorders, cancer, hypersensitivity reaction, hepatitis B or C infection, HIV infection, or Lyme disease.[81] Nerve biopsy is often performed to verify the diagnosis. Treatment consists of immunomodulating therapies such as corticosteroids, cyclophosphamide, or plasmapheresis. Prognosis is good for isolated peripheral nervous system vasculitis but is often poor for systemic vasculitis due to high mortality from other end-organ involvement.

NEOPLASTIC AND PARANEOPLASTIC NEUROPATHIES

Any mass lesion can cause compression or infiltration of the nerve and resulting motor, sensory, and reflex deficits. Details of clinical presentations and treatment are discussed elsewhere in this volume.

A paraneoplastic syndrome results in neurologic deficits from a remote effect of a neoplasm. The most common to affect the peripheral nervous system is a sensory ganglionopathy that is usually associated with small cell carcinoma of the lung and the anti-Hu antibody directed against sensory neurons in the dorsal root ganglion.[82] Patients present with subacute onset of numbness, sensory ataxia, and areflexia. The sensory ataxia is often severe and limits mobility and function. Muscle bulk and strength remains intact because motor axons are unaffected. Treatment involves immunosuppressive therapy and treatment of the underlying cancer. Prognosis is poor because of mortality associated with the cancer and because the sensory deficits persist despite treatment.

HEREDITARY NEUROPATHIES

Most of the hereditary neuropathies listed in Table 252–16 occur in childhood and are often associated with other neurologic or systemic abnormalities such as developmental delay, visual or hearing loss, spasticity, ataxia, or cardiac abnormalities. The most common hereditary neuropathies encountered by neurosurgeons are Charcot-Marie-Tooth disease type 1 (CMT1) hereditary neuropathy with liability to pressure palsy (HNPP), and hereditary neuralgic amyotrophy (see "Neuralgic Amyotrophy"), the latter two because they can mimic neurosurgical disorders.

Charcot-Marie-Tooth Disease Type 1

CMT1 is by far the most common hereditary neuropathy. There are different genotypes causing the same phenotype referred to as CMT1.[83] CMT1A is the most common and is due to a duplication of the peripheral myelin protein 22 *(PMP22)* gene on chromosome 17. CMT1B is due to a mutation in the peripheral myelin protein zero *(P0)* gene on chromosome 1. Mutations in the early growth response 2 *(EGR2)* gene can cause CMT1, Dejerine-Sottas syndrome, or congenital hypomyelination neuropathy, depending on the mutation within the gene. Most pedigrees in CMT1 follow an autosomal dominant inheritance pattern, including those caused by *PMP22* duplication, or *P0* or *EGR2* mutations. Occasional families have an autosomal recessive pattern in which the genetic abnormality is not yet known. Undoubtedly, other genetic abnormalities causing the same CMT1 phenotype will be discovered in the near future.

The CMT1 phenotype consists of a slowly progressive, symmetrical, length-dependent, demyelinating polyneuropathy.[83] The onset of symptoms is insidious and consequently often is not noticed in the earliest stages by the patient. Patients often learn to accommodate to their neurologic deficits and do not seek medical attention until another family member is diagnosed or until symptoms and signs are advanced. Sensory symptoms are often absent or minimal. Motor symp-toms usually manifest as a propensity to twist the ankle or run clumsily because of lower leg muscle weakness. Muscle cramps and leg pain are common presenting symptoms. The neurologic examination is remarkable for hammer toes and pes cavus deformities (see Fig. 252–1) and weakness and muscle atrophy in the feet, lower legs and, in advanced cases, the hands, forearms, and distal thighs. Because of muscle atrophy of the lower legs that spares the thighs, the lower extremities have the appearance of inverted champagne bottles. Muscle atrophy and weakness of the hands and forearm lead to a claw hand deformity. Ankle reflexes are typically absent or diminished early, with more proximal reflexes diminished later. Sensation is diminished or absent in a distribution that is typical for length-dependent polyneuropathies (see Fig. 252–2). Hypertrophy of the nerves, especially of the posterior auricular and ulnar nerves, can be palpated. In severe cases, skin ulcerations, cellulitis, or lymphangiitis can occur because of severe sensory and autonomic deficits. NCS reveal a uniform and symmetrical pattern of conduction slowing within an individual in the 15 to 35 m/sec range. Pathologically, there is loss of both the myelin and axons of large fiber sensory and motor axons, the latter presumably due to the loss of myelin with secondary axonal degeneration. Treatment consists of supportive care, such as ankle-foot orthoses for foot drop, and physical and occupational therapies to help the patient adapt to the neurologic deficits.

Hereditary Neuropathy with Liability to Pressure Palsy

HNPP is becoming more recognized because of the availability of a genetic test to confirm the disease. It is due to a deletion in the *PMP22* gene, the same gene that, when duplicated, causes CMT1A.[83] The most common presentation of HNPP is one of recurrent acute focal neuropathies due to nerve compression.[84] Nerves in the upper extremities and brachial plexus are commonly involved. Neurologic deficits improve or resolve in several weeks to months. However, different clinical presentations also occur, including chronic progressive sensorimotor or sensory polyneuropathy, recurrent brief positional numbness and paresthesias, progressive focal neuropathy, and relapsing polyneuropathy similar to CIDP. About 15% to 25% of carriers of the genetic abnormality are asymptomatic.[84] Bilateral carpal tunnel syndrome and other common entrapment neuropathies are common findings. Given the wide variety of presenting symptoms, any patient with unexplained focal polyneuropathy, especially in common entrapment sites, should be tested for HNPP through a commercially available genetic test. EMG and NCS reveal multiple areas of focal conduction slowing, especially in common entrapment sites, superimposed on a generalized demyelinating polyneuropathy. Pathologically, nerves reveal evidence of tomaculous lesions, a result of multiple cycles of demyelination and remyelination. There is no specific treatment for HNPP. Patients are advised to prevent compression palsies. There are few published data regarding the utility of surgical release of focal neuropathies at common entrapment sites, especially the carpal and cubital tunnels. One study found neurolysis to be beneficial at the carpal and cubital tunnels where there was significant and persistent conduction block on nerve conduction studies.[85] However, nerve transposition or other manipulation of the nerve may worsen neurologic deficits. Until more studies are available, it would appear that surgical release at the carpal and cubital tunnels without nerve transposition under conditions of persistent conduction slowing or block has a favorable reward-to-risk ratio.

MISCELLANEOUS

Renal Disease

Approximately half of patients with end-stage renal disease who are receiving dialysis develop a symmetrical, length-dependent, axonal, sensorimotor polyneuropathy.[86] The toxin or toxins causing the polyneuropathy are not known but are most likely a dialyzable toxin or metabolite that is normally excreted by the kidneys and that has a molecular weight greater than that of urea or creatinine. Men are affected twice as often as women. Patients experience distal dysesthesias, pain, numbness, muscle cramps, weakness, and absent ankle reflexes. Symptoms usually progress slowly but can rarely be rapid in onset. EMG, NCS, and nerve biopsy demonstrate axonal degeneration of sensory and motor fibers. Symptoms improve with more intensive dialysis or renal transplantation.

IDIOPATHIC NEUROPATHIES

The most common idiopathic neuropathy is distal, symmetrical, and length-dependent.[87] It often results in axonal degeneration of the sensory and motor axons. Symptoms usually begin insidiously with subsequent chronic progression. At times, the small fiber sensory axons are predominantly affected and can be associated with significant neuropathic pain. Onset often occurs between 50 and 70 years. The diagnosis is one of exclusion of known causes. Neurologic deficits are usually mild, and patients can be reassured that it is not life-threatening and rarely leads to significant weakness or gait instability.

AMYOTROPHIC LATERAL SCLEROSIS

ALS is a disorder of motor neurons and not a peripheral neuropathy. However, because of loss of motor neurons, many of the symptoms and signs are similar to peripheral neuropathies, and thus it is discussed in this section. Other disorders of the motor neurons include poliomyelitis, postpolio syndrome, spinal muscular atrophy, and Kennedy's disease (see Table 252–8). ALS is the most common of the adult disorders of motor neurons, with an annual incidence of 0.8 to 1.5 per 100,000 and a median age of onset of 60 years.[88]

Patients often present with an insidious onset of progressive weakness and muscle atrophy, initially in one or a few spinal segments before becoming more widespread. About 50% of patients develop symptoms in the arms, with the remainder having symptoms begin in the bulbar or lumbosacral regions. Weakness, muscle atrophy, fasciculations, and cramps are frequent symptoms and signs when there is anterior horn cell degeneration. Weakness, spasticity, gait imbalance, and emotional incontinence (inability to control emotions), are found with loss of the corticobulbar and corticospinal motor neurons. Onset of upper and lower motor neuron signs are often not simultaneous, but they are almost always present concurrently after the early stages of the disease. Other symptoms include dysarthria, dysphagia, shortness of breath, facial weakness, gait difficulties, or hand incoordination from loss of either the upper or lower motor neurons, or both. As motor neuron degeneration progresses in severity and spreads to the entire neuraxis, most or all these symptoms become apparent. However, neurons other than the motor neurons remain intact; hence, cognition, sensation, vision, and hearing remain normal. For unknown reasons, the motor neurons that control the extraocular muscles and sphincters are relatively unaffected, and those functions remain normal. Otherwise, all other upper and lower motor neurons that control voluntary movement are affected. Death usually occurs from respiratory depression or aspiration pneumonia, with a median time of survival of 3 to 4 years from the onset of symptoms.

Since neck or lower back pain and spondylosis are commonly found in older patients, it can occasionally be difficult to distinguish cervical or lumbosacral radiculopathy from early ALS. For example, a typical presentation is one of unilateral weakness and muscle atrophy of the hand. There may or may not also be concomitant hyperreflexia in the arms or legs. Magnetic resonance imaging of the cervical spine may reveal cervical spondylosis with neuroforaminal and central stenosis that could account for the upper and lower motor neuron signs. In such a presentation, one may be uncertain as to whether the patient has early ALS or a C8 radiculopathy and cervical myelopathy. The lack of sensory loss or bowel or bladder incontinence may help differentiate ALS from symptoms caused by cervical myelopathy. Normal somatosensory evoked potentials or the presence of denervation of thoracic paraspinal muscles or leg muscles also favors the diagnosis of ALS. Another presentation may be one of unilateral weakness and muscle atrophy of the leg, which can be difficult to distinguish from a lumbosacral radiculopathy.

Established risk factors for ALS include male gender (the male to female ratio is 1.5:1), older age, presence of familial ALS, and living in Guam.[88] For unknown reasons, there is a high incidence of ALS, Parkinson's disease, and dementia in the residents of Guam, western New Guinea, and the Kii peninsula in Japan. Pesticide and heavy metal exposures have also been suggested as risk factors.

Approximately 5% to 10% of cases are familial. Familial ALS is clinically and pathologically similar to sporadic ALS.[88] The inheritance pattern for almost all families is autosomal dominant with age-dependent penetrance. One of the biggest advances in ALS research has been the discovery that about 20% of familial ALS cases are due to mutations in Cu/Zn superoxide dismutase (SOD1). These mutations of SOD1 implicate oxidative stress in the pathogenesis of ALS. The remainder of the familial ALS genetic mutations are not yet known.

The diagnosis of ALS is made by demonstrating evidence for the typical symptoms and signs of progressive loss of upper and lower motor neurons and by excluding other diseases that could mimic ALS. Thus, other disorders of motor neurons or motor neuropathies (see Table 252–8) must be excluded, as must lesions of the spinal cord. EMG and NCS often play a key role in demonstrating widespread loss of motor neurons and excluding the motor conduction block that can be seen with multifocal motor neuropathy.

Pathologically, there is degeneration of upper and lower motor neurons, with relative sparing of the oculomotor and Onuf's nuclei. Nonmotor systems are affected to a much lesser degree and can include Clarke's column, the spinocerebellar tracts, and the posterior columns. Some have suggested occasional, late abnormalities of the dorsal root ganglion, thalamus, corpus callosum, superior colliculi, pontine tegmentum, and substantia nigra. The anterior horns of the spinal cord reveal degeneration primarily of the anterior horn cell bodies (neuronopathy) with a possible additional dying-back motor axonopathy. Gliosis surrounds the atrophied motor neurons. There are very few inflammatory cells and no chromatolysis or neuronophagia. Surviving but atrophied anterior horn cells contain neurofilament accumulation in the proximal axon and soma, as well as spheroids (10-nm neurofilaments) in proximal axons. Lipofuscin (residues of lysosomal digestion) and Bunina bodies (2- to 6-μm eosinophilic granules) have also been reported. About 30% of motor neurons have ubiquitin. Lewy body–like hyaline inclusions and Hirano bodies are less frequently present.

The pathogenesis of ALS is unknown, but tremendous progress has been made in the past several years. The two possible mechanisms that have been the subject of the most research are glutamate excitotoxicity and oxidative stress; they are reviewed elsewhere.[89] Neurofilament abnormalities and autoimmunity have also been studied, but the evidence for their involvement in the pathogenesis is less compelling.

Treatment strategies for ALS have centered on protecting against glutamate excitotoxicity and oxidative stress. Riluzole is the only medication proved in placebo-controlled clinical trials to prolong survival in ALS, possibly through diminished glutamate release.[90] Other medications are being developed that may further protect against glutamate excitotoxicity. Vitamin E, coenzyme Q10, and other antioxidants are being studied. Neurotrophic factors, administered by either injection or gene therapy, are also being actively tested and have the potential to be beneficial regardless of the cause of motor neuron degeneration.[71] Supportive

treatment of ALS is also important for improving quality of life and is best administered by physicians familiar with the complex requirements of the ALS patient.

REFERENCES

1. Max M, Culnane M, Schafer S, et al: Amitriptyline relieves diabetic neuropathy pain in patients with normal or depressed mood. Neurology 37:589–596, 1987.
2. Max M, Lynch S, Muir J, et al: Effects of desipramine, amitriptyline, and fluoxetine on pain in diabetic neuropathy. N Engl J Med 326:1250–1256, 1992.
3. Kingery W: A critical review of controlled clinical trials for peripheral neuropathic pain and complex regional pain syndromes. Pain 73:123–139, 1997.
4. Rowbotham M, Harden N, Stacey B, et al: Gabapentin for the treatment of postherpetic neuralgia: A randomized controlled trial. JAMA 280:1837–1842, 1998.
5. Backonja M, Beydoun A, Edwards K, et al: Gabapentin for the symptomatic treatment of painful neuropathy in patients with diabetes mellitus: A randomized controlled trial. JAMA 280:1831–1836, 1998.
6. Harati Y, Gooch C, Swenson M, et al: Double-blind randomized trial of tramadol for the treatment of the pain of diabetic neuropathy. Neurology 50:1842–1846, 1998.
7. Chabal C, Jacobson L, Mariano A, et al: The use of oral mexiletine for the treatment of pain after peripheral nerve injury. Anesthesiology 76:513–517, 1992.
8. Jarvis B, Coukell A: Mexiletine: A review of its therapeutic use in painful diabetic neuropathy. Drugs 56:691–707, 1998.
9. Asbury A, Cornblath D: Assessment of current diagnostic criteria for Guillain-Barré syndrome. Ann Neurol 27(Suppl):S21–4, 1990.
10. Hahn A: Guillain-Barré syndrome. Lancet 352:635–641, 1998.
11. Ropper A, Shahani B: Pain in Guillain-Barré syndrome. Arch Neurol 41:511–514, 1984.
12. Hadden R, Cornblath D, Hughes R, et al: Electrophysiological classification of Guillain-Barré syndrome: Clinical associations and outcome. Plasma Exchange/Sandoglobulin Guillain-Barré Syndrome Trial Group. Ann Neurol 44:780–788, 1998.
13. Asbury A, Arnason B, Adams R: The inflammatory lesion in idiopathic polyneuritis: Its role in pathogenesis. Medicine (Baltimore) 48:173–215, 1969.
14. Fisher M: An unusual variant of acute idiopathic polyneuritis (syndrome of ophthalmoplegia, ataxia and areflexia). N Engl J Med 255:57–65, 1956.
15. Ropper A: Unusual clinical variants and signs in Guillain-Barré syndrome. Arch Neurol 43:1150–1152, 1986.
16. Österman P, Fagius J, Lundemo G, et al: Beneficial effects of plasma exchange in acute inflammatory polyradiculoneuropathy. Lancet 2:1296–1299, 1984.
17. The Guillain-Barré Syndrome Study Group: Plasmapheresis and acute Guillain-Barré syndrome. Neurology 35:1096–1104, 1985.
18. French Cooperative Group on Plasma Exchange in Guillain-Barré syndrome: Efficiency of plasma exchange in Guillain-Barré syndrome: Role of replacement fluids. Ann Neurol 22:753–761, 1987.
19. French Cooperative Group on Plasma Exchange in Guillain-Barré Syndrome: Plasma exchange in Guillain-Barré syndrome: One-year follow-up. Ann Neurol 32:94–97, 1992.
20. The French Cooperative Group on Plasma Exchange in Guillain-Barré Syndrome: Appropriate number of plasma exchanges in Guillain-Barré syndrome. Ann Neurol 41:298–306, 1997.
21. van der Meche F, Schmitz P, Dutch Guillain-Barré Study Group: A randomized trial comparing intravenous immune globulin and plasma exchange in Guillain-Barré syndrome. N Engl J Med 326:1123–1129, 1992.
22. Plasma Exchange/Sandoglobulin Guillain-Barré Syndrome Trial Group: Randomised trial of plasma exchange, intravenous immunoglobulin, and combined treatments in Guillain-Barré syndrome. Lancet 349:225–230, 1997.
23. Hughes R, Newsom-Davis J, Perkin G, et al: Controlled trial prednisolone in acute polyneuropathy. Lancet 2:750–753, 1978.
24. Guillain-Barré Syndrome Steroid Trial Group: Double-blind trial of intravenous methylprednisolone in Guillain-Barré syndrome. Lancet 341:586–590, 1993.

25. Dyck P, Lais A, Ohta M, et al: Chronic inflammatory polyradiculoneuropathy. Mayo Clin Proc 50:621–637, 1975.

26. Barohn R, Kissel J, Warmolts J, et al: Chronic inflammatory demyelinating polyradiculoneuropathy: Clinical characteristics, course, and recommendations for diagnostic criteria. Arch Neurol 46:878–884, 1989.

27. Albers JW, Kelly JJ Jr: Acquired inflammatory demyelinating polyneuropathies: Clinical and electrodiagnostic features. Muscle Nerve 12:435–451, 1989.

28. Hahn AF, Bolton CF, Pillay N, et al: Plasma-exchange therapy in chronic inflammatory demyelinating polyneuropathy: A double-blind, sham-controlled, cross-over study. Brain 119(Pt 4):1055–1066, 1996.

29. Hahn AF, Bolton CF, Zochodne D, et al: Intravenous immunoglobulin treatment in chronic inflammatory demyelinating polyneuropathy: A double-blind, placebo-controlled, cross-over study. Brain 119(Pt 4):1067–1077, 1996.

30. van Doorn PA, Brand A, Strengers PF, et al: High-dose intravenous immunoglobulin treatment in chronic inflammatory demyelinating polyneuropathy: A double-blind, placebo-controlled, crossover study. Neurology 40:209–212, 1990.

31. Dyck PJ, Daube J, O'Brien P, et al: Plasma exchange in chronic inflammatory demyelinating polyradiculoneuropathy. N Engl J Med 314:461–465, 1986.

32. Dyck PJ, O'Brien PC, Oviatt KF, et al: Prednisone improves chronic inflammatory demyelinating polyradiculoneuropathy more than no treatment. Ann Neurol 11:136–141, 1982.

33. Dyck PJ, Litchy WJ, Kratz KM, et al: A plasma exchange versus immune globulin infusion trial in chronic inflammatory demyelinating polyradiculoneuropathy. Ann Neurol 36:838–845, 1994.

34. Pestronk A: Multifocal motor neuropathy: Diagnosis and treatment. Neurology 51(6 Suppl 5):S22–S34, 1998.

35. Pestronk A, Cornblath DR, Ilyas AA, et al: A treatable multifocal motor neuropathy with antibodies to GM1 ganglioside. Ann Neurol 24:73–78, 1988.

36. Parry GJ, Clarke S: Multifocal acquired demyelinating neuropathy masquerading as motor neuron disease. Muscle Nerve 11:103–107, 1988.

37. Krarup C, Stewart JD, Sumner AJ, et al: A syndrome of asymmetric limb weakness with motor conduction block. Neurology 40:118–127, 1990.

38. Pestronk A, Chaudhry V, Feldman EL, et al: Lower motor neuron syndromes defined by patterns of weakness, nerve conduction abnormalities, and high titers of antiglycolipid antibodies. Ann Neurol 27:316–326, 1990.

39. Chaudhry V, Corse AM, Cornblath DR, et al: Multifocal motor neuropathy: Electrodiagnostic features. Muscle Nerve 17:198–205, 1994.

40. Katz J, Wolfe G, Bryan W, et al: Electrophysiologic findings in multifocal motor neuropathy. Neurology 48:700–707, 1997.

41. Pestronk A, Choksi R: Multifocal motor neuropathy: Serum IgM anti-GM1 ganglioside antibodies in most patients detected using covalent linkage of GM1 to ELISA plates. Neurology 49:1289–1292, 1997.

42. Feldman EL, Bromberg MB, Albers JW, et al: Immunosuppressive treatment in multifocal motor neuropathy. Ann Neurol 30:397–401, 1991.

43. Van den Berg LH, Kerkhoff H, Oey PL, et al: Treatment of multifocal motor neuropathy with high dose intravenous immunoglobulins: A double blind, placebo controlled study. J Neurol Neurosurg Psychiatry 59:248–252, 1995.

44. Azulay JP, Blin O, Pouget J, et al: Intravenous immunoglobulin treatment in patients with motor neuron syndromes associated with anti-GM1 antibodies: A double-blind, placebo-controlled study. Neurology 44(3 Pt 1):429–432, 1994.

45. Tsairis P, Dyck P, Mulder D: Natural history of brachial plexus neuropathy: Report on 99 patients. Arch Neurol 27:109–117, 1972.

46. England J: The variations of neuralgic amyotrophy. Muscle Nerve 22:435–436, 1999.

47. Chance P, Windebank A: Hereditary neuralgic amyotrophy. Curr Opin Neurol 9:343–347, 1996.

48. Suarez G, Giannini C, Bosch E, et al: Immune brachial plexus neuropathy: Suggestive evidence for an inflammatory-immune pathogenesis. Neurology 46:559–561, 1996.

49. van Alfen N, van Engelen B: Lumbosacral plexus neuropathy: A case report and review of the literature. Clin Neurol Neurosurg 99:138–141, 1997.

50. Bradley W, Chad D, Verghese J, et al: Painful lumbosacral plexopathy with elevated erythrocyte sedimentation rate: A treatable inflammatory syndrome. Ann Neurol 15:457–464, 1984.

51. Triggs W, Young M, Eskin T, et al: Treatment of idiopathic lumbosacral plexopathy with intravenous immunoglobulin. Muscle Nerve 20:244–246, 1997.

52. Dalakas MC, Quarles RH, Farrer RG, et al: A controlled study of intravenous immunoglobulin in demyelinating neuropathy with IgM gammopathy. Ann Neurol 40:792–795, 1996.

53. Dalakas MC, Cupler EJ: Neuropathies in HIV infection. Baillieres Clin Neurol 5:199–218, 1996.

54. So YT, Olney RK: Acute lumbosacral polyradiculopathy in acquired immunodeficiency syndrome: Experience in 23 patients. Ann Neurol 35:53–58, 1994.

55. Cohen JI, Brunell PA, Straus SE, et al: Recent advances in varicella-zoster virus infection. Ann Intern Med 130:922–932, 1999.

56. Apartis E, Leger JM, Musset L, et al: Peripheral neuropathy associated with essential mixed cryoglobulinaemia: A role for hepatitis C virus infection? J Neurol Neurosurg Psychiatry 60:661–666, 1996.

57. Nations SP, Katz JS, Lyde CB, et al: Leprous neuropathy: An American perspective. Semin Neurol 18:113–124, 1998.

58. Halperin J, Luft BJ, Volkman DJ, et al: Lyme neuroborreliosis: Peripheral nervous system manifestations. Brain 113(Pt 4)):1207–1221, 1990.

59. Pirart J: Diabetes mellitus and its degenerative complications: A prospective study of 4,400 patients observed between 1947 and 1973. Diabetes Care 1:168–188, 1978.

60. Dyck PJ, Kratz KM, Karnes JL, et al: The prevalence by staged severity of various types of diabetic neuropathy, retinopathy, and nephropathy in a population-based cohort: The Rochester Diabetic Neuropathy Study. Neurology 43:817–824, 1993.

61. The Diabetes Control and Complications Trial Research Group: Factors in development of diabetic neuropathy: Baseline analysis of neuropathy in feasibility phase of Diabetes Control and Complications Trial (DCCT). Diabetes 37:476–481, 1988.

62. Ewing DJ, Campbell IW, Clarke BF: The natural history of diabetic autonomic neuropathy. Q J Med 49:95–108, 1980.

63. Barohn RJ, Sahenk Z, Warmolts JR, et al: The Bruns-Garland syndrome (diabetic amyotrophy): Revisited 100 years later. Arch Neurol 48:1130–1135, 1991.

64. Said G, Goulon-Goeau C, Lacroix C, et al: Nerve biopsy findings in different patterns of proximal diabetic neuropathy. Ann Neurol 35:559–569, 1994.

65. Krendel DA, Costigan DA, Hopkins LC: Successful treatment of neuropathies in patients with diabetes mellitus. Arch Neurol 52:1053–1061, 1995.

66. Said G, Elgrably F, Lacroix C, et al: Painful proximal diabetic neuropathy: Inflammatory nerve lesions and spontaneous favorable outcome. Ann Neurol 41:762–770, 1997.

67. Llewelyn JG, Thomas PK, King RH: Epineurial microvasculitis in proximal diabetic neuropathy. J Neurol 245:159–165, 1998.

68. Fraser DM, Campbell IW, Ewing DJ, et al: Mononeuropathy in diabetes mellitus. Diabetes 28:96–101, 1979.

69. Feldman EL, Stevens MJ, Greene DA: Pathogenesis of diabetic neuropathy. Clin Neurosci 4:365–370, 1997.

70. The Diabetes Control and Complications Trial Research Group: The effect of intensive treatment of diabetes on the development and progression of long-term complications in insulin-dependent diabetes mellitus. N Engl J Med 329:977–986, 1993.

71. Yuen EC, Mobley WC: Therapeutic potential of neurotrophic factors for neurological disorders. Ann Neurol 40:346–354, 1996.

72. Rao SN, Katiyar BC, Nair KR, et al: Neuromuscular status in hypothyroidism. Acta Neurol Scand 61:167–177, 1980.

73. O'Duffy JD, Randall RV, MacCarty CS: Median neuropathy (carpal-tunnel syndrome) in acromegaly: A sign of endocrine overactivity. Ann Intern Med 78:379–383, 1973.

74. Monforte R, Estruch R, Valls-Sole J, et al: Autonomic and peripheral neuropathies in patients with chronic alcoholism: A dose-related toxic effect of alcohol. Arch Neurol 52:45–51, 1995.

75. Berger AR, Schaumburg HH, Schroeder C, et al: Dose response, coasting, and differential fiber vulnerability in human toxic neuropathy: A prospective study of pyridoxine neurotoxicity. Neurology 42:1367–1370, 1992.

76. Hemmer B, Glocker FX, Schumacher M, et al: Subacute combined degeneration: Clinical, electrophysiological, and magnetic resonance imaging findings. J Neurol Neurosurg Psychiatry 65:822–827, 1998.

77. Takahashi K: Thiamine deficiency neuropathy, a reappraisal. Int J Neurol 15:245–253, 1981.

78. Jackson CE, Amato AA, Barohn RJ: Isolated vitamin E deficiency. Muscle Nerve 19:1161–1165, 1996.

79. Snider DE Jr: Pyridoxine supplementation during isoniazid therapy. Tubercle 61:191–196, 1980.

80. Schaumburg H, Kaplan J, Windebank A, et al: Sensory neuropathy from pyridoxine abuse: A new megavitamin syndrome. N Engl J Med 309:445–448, 1983.

81. Said G: Necrotizing peripheral nerve vasculitis. Neurol Clin 15:835–848, 1997.

82. Pourmand R, Maybury BG: AAEM case report #31: Paraneoplastic sensory neuronopathy. Muscle Nerve 19:1517–1522, 1996.

83. Keller M, Chance P: Inherited neuropathies: From gene to disease. Brain Pathol 9:327–341, 1999.

84. Mouton P, Tardieu S, Gouider R, et al: Spectrum of clinical and electrophysiological features in HNPP patients with the 17p11.2 deletion. Neurology 52:1440–1446, 1999.

85. Magistris M, Roth G: Long-lasting conduction block in hereditary neuropathy with liability to pressure palsies. Neurology 35:1639–1641, 1985.

86. Fraser CL, Arieff AI: Nervous system complications in uremia. Ann Intern Med 109:143–153, 1988.

87. Teunissen LL, Notermans NC, Franssen H, et al: Differences between hereditary motor and sensory neuropathy type 2 and chronic idiopathic axonal neuropathy: A clinical and electrophysiological study. Brain 120(Pt 6)):955–962, 1997.

88. Li TM, Alberman E, Swash M: Comparison of sporadic and familial disease amongst 580 cases of motor neuron disease. J Neurol Neurosurg Psychiatry 51:778–784, 1988.

89. Brown RH Jr: Amyotrophic lateral sclerosis: Insights from genetics. Arch Neurol 54:1246–1250, 1997.

90. Bensimon G, Lacomblez L, Meininger V: A controlled trial of riluzole in amyotrophic lateral sclerosis: ALS/Riluzole Study Group. N Engl J Med 330:585–591, 1994.

Electrodiagnostic Evaluation of Peripheral Nerves: Electromyography, Somatosensory Evoked Potentials, Nerve Action Potentials

ERIC YUEN ■ LAWRENCE ROBINSON ■ JEFFERSON SLIMP

ELECTROMYOGRAPHY AND NERVE CONDUCTION STUDIES

Electromyograms (EMGs) and nerve conduction studies (NCSs), also referred to as electrodiagnostic studies, are used to test the function of the nervous system.[1, 2] They are usually used to test the integrity of the peripheral nervous system (PNS) but can also be used to evaluate movement disorders, such as cervical dystonia (torticollis). EMGs and NCSs are best used as an extension of the neurological examination to help localize and define a lesion. They can help determine whether weakness or numbness is due to a lesion of the central nervous system (CNS) or the PNS. Once a lesion is determined to be in the PNS, EMG and NCS can localize the lesion to the anterior horn cell, nerve root, dorsal root ganglion, plexus, nerve, neuromuscular junction, or muscle. In addition, the degree of involvement of the sensory and motor nerves can be determined. Lesions can also be localized to the cell body, axon, or myelin. The pattern of abnormalities on EMG and NCS is used to provide a definitive diagnosis. These electrodiagnostic studies can also be used to determine the duration, severity, and prognosis of a lesion. Finally, they can provide an objective measure of improvement or worsening, which is often useful when determining response to treatment.

There are several limitations of EMG and NCS. Only the motor axons and large-diameter myelinated sensory axons that mediate vibration sensation, proprioception, and light touch can be evaluated. The small-diameter autonomic and sensory axons that control pain and temperature sensation cannot be tested by EMG and NCS, for reasons that are explained later. These tests cause discomfort and are often painful, but fortunately, there are minimal risks of bleeding or infection. The safety features of modern equipment prevent electrical injury.

Fundamentals of Electrodiagnostic Testing

EMG and NCS employ different means of measuring action potentials of nerve axons or muscle fibers. The physiology of an action potential is discussed elsewhere. Measurement of action potentials involves placing two recording electrodes along a nerve axon or muscle fiber (Fig. 253–1). The difference in electrical potentials between the two electrodes is amplified through a differential amplifier and plotted on a monitor for analysis. Because the recording electrodes are close to each other (usually within a few centimeters), in the absence of an action potential, there is no significant difference in electrical potential between them. As an action potential approaches one of the electrodes,

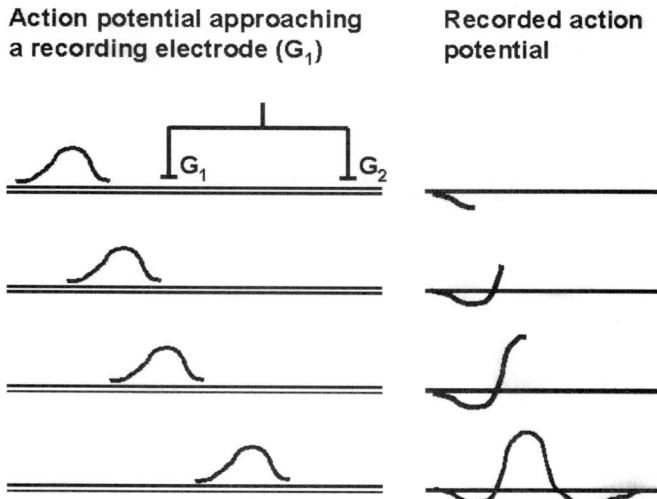

Action potential approaching a recording electrode (G₁)

Recorded action potential

FIGURE 253–1. The change in electrical potential as an action potential passes under a recording electrode. G_1 is the active recording electrode, and G_2 is the reference electrode. The instrument displays the voltage difference between the two electrodes.

this electrode measures an electrical potential that is not measured by the other electrode. A triphasic wave is recorded as the action potential passes under the first electrode. Most recordings during EMG and NCS involve the summation of a number of action potentials from nerve or muscle fibers. For example, a sensory NCS involves recording the summation of individual action potentials from all the hundreds or thousands of sensory axons of a particular nerve.

Sensory Nerve Action Potential

NCS of the sensory nerves generates a recording referred to as a *sensory nerve action potential* (SNAP). In this study, the sensory nerve is stimulated with sufficient electrical current such that all the large-diameter sensory axons are simultaneously depolarized (Fig. 253–2). This stimulation is referred to as *supramaximal stimulation*, because a higher electrical current than the minimum required for stimulation of all the axons is used to ensure that all the axons are depolarized. Action potentials of the depolarized axons immediately travel away from the site of stimulation at various velocities, depending on a number of factors. For instance, the conduction velocity increases with larger axon diameter, increased myelination, and higher nerve temperature. The action potentials travel along the axons and are recorded by the recording electrodes over the nerve (see Fig. 253–2). Each individual action potential generates a triphasic recording (see Fig. 253–1). A typical sensory nerve contains up to several hundred sensory axons, and an equal number of action potentials is recorded from the nerve. The SNAP is the sum of the individual action potentials recorded from each sensory axon. Under normal conditions, the action potentials of large-diameter sensory axons travel at similar velocities and thus pass under the recording

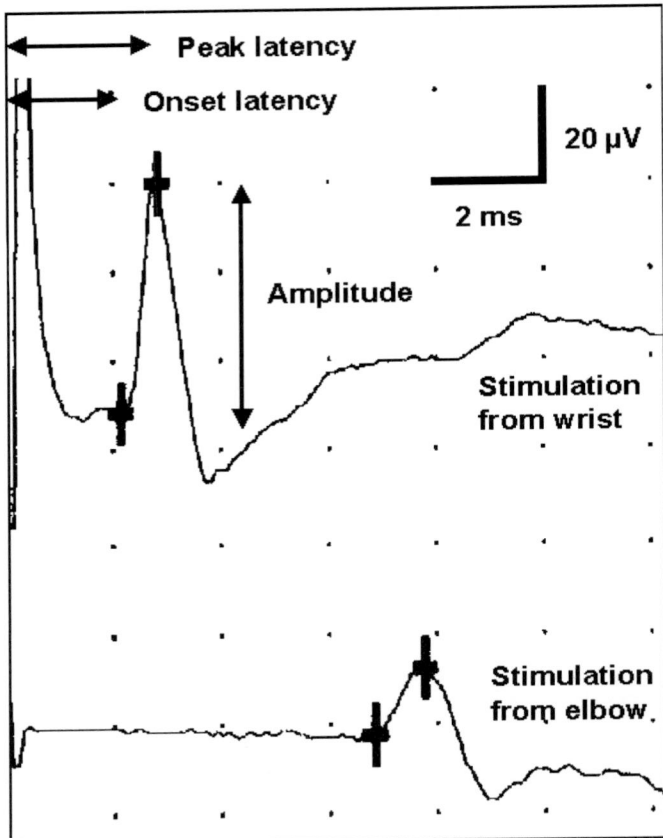

FIGURE 253–3. Sensory nerve action potential of a normal median nerve when recording at the index finger and stimulating at the wrist or elbow.

electrode nearly simultaneously. The sum of these action potentials results in the SNAP (Fig. 253–3). The action potentials of small-diameter myelinated and unmyelinated axons travel at slower and more variable velocities. Thus, these action potentials pass under the recording electrode at variable times and do not summate sufficiently to generate enough amplitude to be a visible waveform. The amplitude of the SNAP is calculated from the baseline, or first positive peak, to the negative peak (keeping in mind that negative is upward) and is a reflection of the number of normal large-diameter myelinated sensory axons. The conduction velocity is calculated by dividing the distance between the sites of stimulation and recording by the time the first action potentials reach the recording electrodes, which is represented as the beginning of the upward slope from the baseline or first positive peak. Under normal circumstances, a longer distance between the stimulation and recording sites results in less synchronized action potentials from the variety of slow- and fast-conducting axons. This phenomenon is referred to as *temporal dispersion* and results in a decreased SNAP amplitude and increased duration when recording over large distances (see Fig. 253–3).

In the presence of nerve injury or disease, there is often a change in the SNAP conduction velocity or amplitude. Changes in the SNAP depend on the site

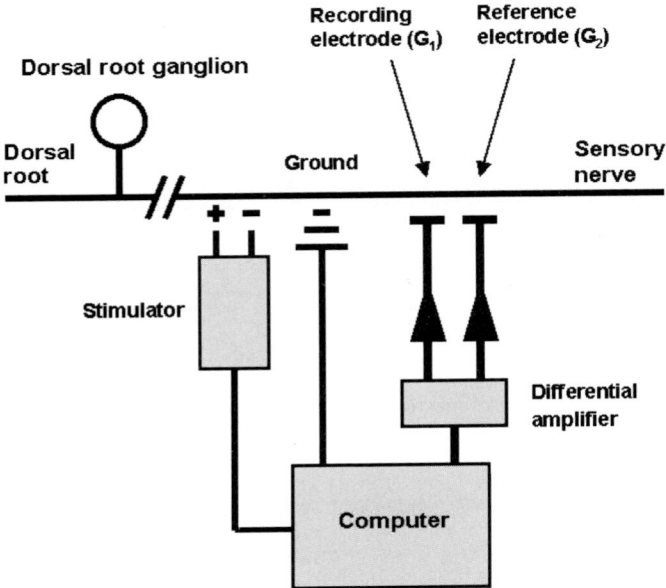

FIGURE 253–2. Typical setup of a sensory nerve action potential.

and mechanism of the lesion, but all such lesions cause numbness, paresthesias, and other sensory symptoms. Any lesion at or distal to the dorsal root ganglion that causes wallerian degeneration results in fewer sensory axons, fewer action potentials recorded by the electrodes, and a decreased SNAP amplitude (Fig. 253–4*A*). Conduction velocity is normal or near normal, because the remaining axons are myelinated and function normally. With marked axonal loss, conduction velocity may be slightly decreased owing to the loss of faster-conducting axons. Conduction velocity can be decreased to 80% of the lower limit of normal for mild axonal loss and to 70% of normal when the SNAP amplitude is less than 50% of the lower limit of normal.

Demyelination distally between the sites of nerve stimulation and recording leads to slowing of the individual action potentials and thus more markedly reduced conduction velocity or increased latency (time from stimulation to initial waveform) of the SNAP (see Fig. 253–4*B*). Typical clinical presentations include carpal tunnel syndrome with demyelination of the median sensory nerve at the carpal tunnel or a demyelinating polyneuropathy such as Guillain-Barré syndrome. Because acquired demyelinating lesions often result in varying degrees of slowing of the individual axons, there is often increased temporal dispersion. If the demyelination is severe enough, the action potential may be unable to continue propagating down the axon across the site of demyelination to the recording electrode, resulting in conduction block. Conduction block, which is almost always caused by demyelination, can result in a low-amplitude or absent SNAP. In most cases of conduction block, there is concomitant

conduction slowing, because some axons are demyelinated to the point of conduction block, but others are only partially demyelinated, causing conduction slowing. Thus, a low-amplitude SNAP with conduction slowing suggests a demyelinating lesion, whereas a low-amplitude SNAP without conduction slowing suggests a lesion causing axonal degeneration without primary demyelination.

A demyelinating lesion proximal to the point of nerve stimulation and recording leaves the distal nerve intact. A lesion causing axonal loss proximal to the dorsal root ganglion, such as at the root, results in wallerian degeneration of the proximal axon. However, the sensory axons distal to the dorsal root ganglion maintain their continuity to the cell body and thus remain normal. The SNAP remains normal under these circumstances (see Fig. 253–4*C*), even in the presence of anesthetic sensations. Thus, a normal SNAP in a patient with numbness suggests that the lesion is proximal to the dorsal root ganglion (root or CNS) or is a proximal demyelinating lesion.

Compound Muscle Action Potential

NCS of the motor nerves generates a recording referred to as the *compound muscle action potential* (CMAP). Unlike with a sensory NCS, the CMAP is recorded from the muscle and not the motor nerve. Similar to a sensory NCS, the motor nerve is stimulated with supramaximal stimulation, such that all the motor axons are simultaneously depolarized. Action potentials of the depolarized axons immediately travel away from the site of stimulation at nearly identical velocities. The action potentials travel along the axons to the neuromuscular junction. Each motor axon innervates up to several hundred muscle fibers. Because the typical motor nerve contains up to a few hundred motor axons, the amplitude of the CMAP—a summation of action potentials from muscle fibers—is 100 to 1000 times the magnitude of the SNAP. Compared with sensory nerves, the motor axons of motor nerves are much more similar in diameter and degree of myelination, resulting in more similar individual axonal conduction velocities and very little temporal dispersion (Fig. 253–5). Moreover, the duration of motor unit action potentials (MUAPs) is long enough so that the degree of overlap is affected relatively little by temporal dispersion.

Conduction velocity of the distal motor nerve segment cannot be calculated for the CMAP as it can for the SNAP, because the time from nerve stimulation to recording of muscle fiber action potentials includes the release of acetylcholine. Acetylcholine must diffuse across the neuromuscular junction and bind to the acetylcholine receptor before the muscle fiber action potential can be recorded. This process takes about 0.5 to 1 msec. Instead of calculating conduction velocity from a point of stimulation to the muscle, the time from stimulation at a distal point of the nerve to the onset of the CMAP—referred to as the *distal motor latency*—is compared with that in normal controls to determine whether there is distal conduction slowing.

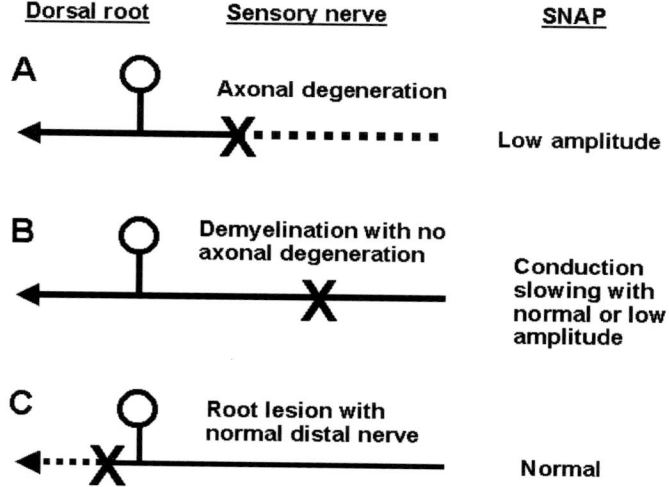

FIGURE 253–4. Numbness from different mechanisms and sites of lesions, and the corresponding sensory nerve action potential (SNAP). *A*, Axonal degeneration from a lesion distal to the dorsal root ganglion, such as a severed nerve or dying-back axonopathy, resulting in a low-amplitude SNAP with normal or near-normal conduction velocity. *B*, Distal demyelination between the site of nerve stimulation and recording, resulting in conduction slowing and possibly a low-amplitude SNAP, depending on the degree of temporal dispersion or conduction block. *C*, Proximal demyelination or radiculopathy leaving the distal axons and myelin intact, resulting in a normal SNAP.

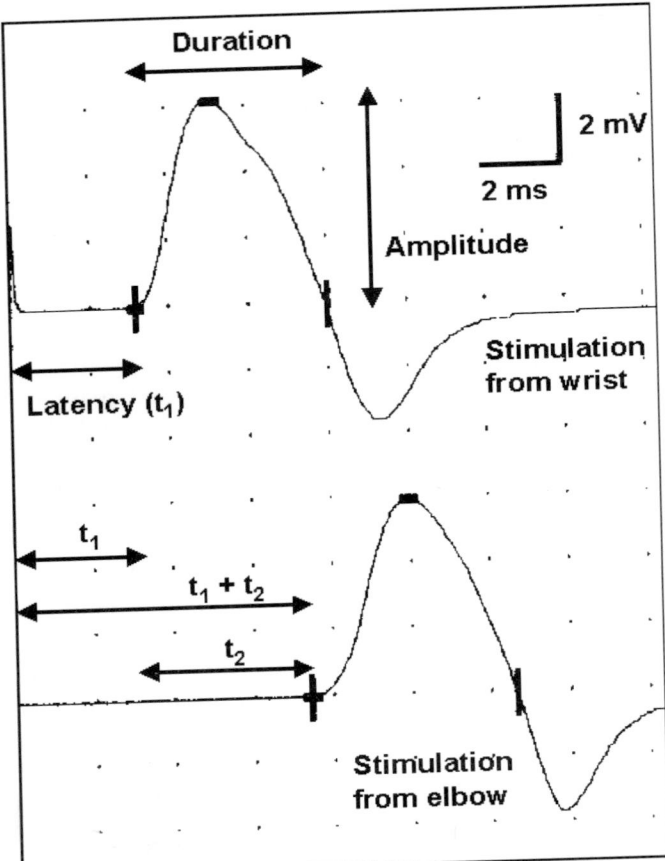

FIGURE 253–5. Compound muscle action potential (CMAP) of a normal median nerve when recording at the abductor pollicis brevis (APB) and stimulating at the wrist and elbow. The distal motor latency is the time from stimulation at the wrist (the most distal point of stimulation) to the onset of the CMAP at the APB; this time is called t_1, and in this case, it is 3.8 msec. The time from stimulation at the elbow to the onset of the CMAP at the APB is $t_1 + t_2$; in this case, it is 14.5 msec. Subtracting the two times (14.5 msec − 3.8 msec = 10.7 msec) is equivalent to $(t_1 + t_2) - t_1 = t_2$, which is the time for the action potential to travel from the elbow to the wrist. The distance between stimulation points at the elbow and wrist can be measured (d = 180 mm), and the conduction velocity can be calculated by dividing the distance by time (t_2/d = 180 mm/10.7 msec = 57 m/second).

Conduction velocity of the proximal portion of the motor nerve can be calculated as described in Figure 253–5. The three most important aspects of the CMAP are the amplitude, conduction velocity, and distal motor latency.

In the presence of injury or disease of the motor nerve or muscle, there is often a change in the CMAP conduction velocity, amplitude, or distal motor latency. Changes in the CMAP depend on the site and mechanism of the lesion, but all such lesions cause weakness and possibly muscle atrophy in the case of denervation. The more common scenarios are presented in Figure 253–6. For the sake of illustration, consider a motor nerve consisting of two motor axons, with each motor axon innervating two muscle fibers. Under conditions of normal PNS functioning, supramaximal stimulation of the motor nerve distally and proximally leads to

action potentials in both motor axons and all four muscle fibers. The CMAP recordings consist of the sum of the muscle action potentials from all four muscle fibers (see Fig. 253–6A).

When there is motor axonal degeneration from distal dying-back axonopathy, wallerian degeneration from a proximal lesion, or loss of motoneurons, only one of the two motor axons is present and can transmit an action potential to its two innervated muscle fibers (see Fig. 253–6B). The other two muscle fibers cannot be stimulated, leading to decreased CMAP amplitudes from both the distal and proximal stimulation sites.

In this model, conduction block between the distal and proximal sites of stimulation results in a characteristic CMAP abnormality (see Fig. 253–6C). A typical demyelinating lesion, such as from an entrapment neuropathy, may result in conduction block of one motor axon and conduction slowing of the other. Distal to the site of demyelination, the motor axons and myelin are normal. Thus, stimulation of the motor nerve distally results in activation of both motor axons and all four muscle fibers, yielding a normal CMAP amplitude and distal motor latency. Stimulation of the motor nerve proximal to the site of demyelination leads to action

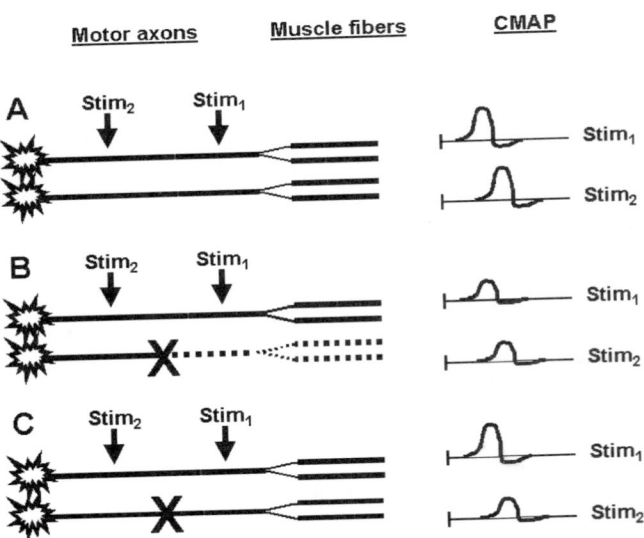

FIGURE 253–6. Various compound muscle action potential (CMAP) amplitude and velocity results, depending on the site of the lesion. *A,* Normal strength or a central nervous system cause of weakness. *B,* Axonal degeneration without reinnervation results in only one of the two motor axons and two of the four muscle fibers being able to generate action potentials. The CMAP amplitude is one half of normal when stimulating either distally (stim$_1$) or proximally (stim$_2$). *C,* Demyelination and conduction block between sites of stimulation result in no motor axonal loss. The CMAP amplitude is normal when stimulating distal (stim$_1$) to the site of the lesion, because the motor axons are normal there and all four muscle fibers are able to generate action potentials. When stimulating proximally, action potentials are generated in both motor axons. However, one of the action potentials is blocked at the site of demyelination and cannot proceed to the muscle fibers. Thus, only one of the motor axons can transmit the action potential to two muscle fibers, and the CMAP amplitude is one half of normal. The decline in CMAP amplitude from a point of distal stimulation to one of proximal stimulation is characteristic of conduction block.

potentials in both motor axons. However, because one of the action potentials is blocked at the site of demyelination, it is unable to proceed to activate the corresponding muscle fibers. The other action potential is slowed but can still activate two of the muscle fibers. Thus, the CMAP from the proximal point of stimulation is the sum of two muscle fiber action potentials; its amplitude and area are smaller than normal, and it is delayed because of conduction slowing. Thus, a scenario in which there is decreased CMAP amplitude and area at the proximal point of stimulation compared with the distal site is indicative of a conduction block between the two points of stimulation. If there is a decrease in CMAP amplitude but area is maintained, this suggests temporal dispersion. Unlike with sensory nerves, there is normally very little temporal dispersion of motor nerves, and its presence indicates an area of demyelination.

Demyelination between the point of distal stimulation and the muscle can lead to distal conduction slowing and result in prolonged distal motor latency. However, the proximal conduction velocity and CMAP amplitudes are normal, because all the muscle fibers are activated and the nerve is normal proximally.

Late Responses

SNAP and CMAP studies are best at evaluating distal nerves. Stimulation and recording from nerves at proximal sites, such as the root or plexus (e.g., Erb's point), are often unreliable. When stimulating proximally, it is often difficult to ensure supramaximal stimulation or to limit stimulation to one nerve. Alternatively, evaluation of the late responses can provide useful data regarding the proximal portions of nerves. The two most commonly evaluated late responses are the F wave and H-reflex (Fig. 253–7).

F waves result from the late response of a motor unit, defined as a single motoneuron and all the muscle fibers it innervates. The F-wave response is generated by stimulation of motor axons. Action potentials normally travel distally and proximally from the site of stimulation. The distally traveling action potential results in the CMAP, or M wave. The proximally traveling action potential reaches the motoneuron cell bodies in the anterior horn of the spinal cord. For unknown reasons, one or a few of the motoneurons often immediately generate an action potential that travels back from the cell body to the muscle, as if the action potential had bounced from the cell body back down the axon. The action potential from one or a few motoneurons activates the innervated muscle fibers, thus generating an F wave consisting of the sum of the action potentials from the motor unit. The most reliable value of the F-wave response is the latency, or the time it takes the action potential to travel from the site of stimulation proximally to the motoneuron cell body and then distally from the cell body to the muscle. Comparisons to normal controls or to the contralateral side are used to help identify conduction slowing anywhere along the motor axon. F-wave latencies are most sensitive for disorders causing generalized or multifo-

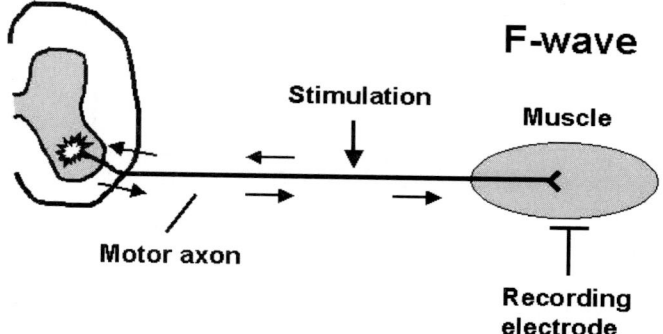

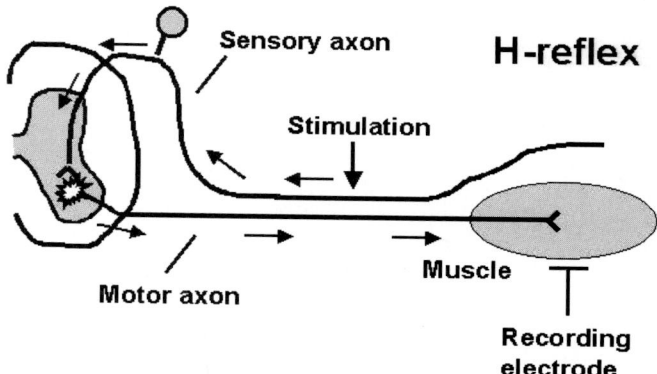

FIGURE 253–7. F-wave and H-reflex pathways.

cal demyelination, such as Guillain-Barré syndrome. They are less sensitive for focal demyelinating disorders such as a radiculopathy, because any focal conduction slowing is diluted by the normal conduction velocity over most of the F-wave pathway.

H-reflexes are equivalent to an electrophysiologic ankle reflex. In adults, the H-reflex can be elicited only in the soleus muscle. The tibial nerve is stimulated at the popliteal fossa. An action potential travels proximally along the sensory pathway of the tibial nerve, similar to the pathway of an action potential generated by stretching of the ankle tendon during testing of the ankle reflex. The action potential enters the spinal cord along the sensory axons, which synapse with the anterior horn cells. These sensory action potentials result in neurotransmitter release from the sensory end terminals and activation of the anterior horn cells and motor axons to the soleus muscle, similar to the sensory-to-motor monosynaptic ankle reflex pathway. The CMAP amplitude and latency generated by the soleus are recorded and compared with those of normal controls or the contralateral side. A delay in the latency or a diminished amplitude suggests a lesion anywhere along the H-reflex pathway.

Repetitive Stimulation

Repetitive stimulation is used to diagnose abnormalities of the neuromuscular junction, such as myasthenia gravis, botulism, Lambert-Eaton myasthenic syndrome, and congenital myasthenia. The technique involves rapid, repetitive CMAP recordings from 2 to 50 Hz. Defects in neuromuscular transmission, especially of the postsynaptic site, lead to successive decrements in CMAP amplitude with stimulation at low frequencies of 2 to 3 Hz. An increase in CMAP amplitude at high frequencies such as 50 Hz is indicative of a presynaptic neuromuscular transmission defect, such as Lambert-Eaton syndrome. The principles underlying these abnormalities can be found in other textbooks.[1, 2]

Needle Electromyography

EMG examination consists of inserting a recording needle into a muscle to measure the action potentials from muscle fibers. This information is used to determine the functioning of motoneurons and muscle. There are three aspects of an EMG examination: (1) assessment of spontaneous muscle fiber action potential activity; (2) measurement of MUAP duration, amplitude, and phases; and (3) recruitment and interference pattern of MUAPs.

SPONTANEOUS ACTIVITY

Under normal conditions, when a patient is relaxed, muscle fibers are electrically silent, with no significant spontaneous muscle fiber action potentials. Different types of abnormal spontaneous muscle fiber action potentials can be seen and indicate specific abnormalities of the PNS (Table 253–1). The most common and significant spontaneous activities consist of fibrillation potentials and positive sharp waves (Fig. 253–8*A* and *B*). These are spontaneous action potentials from individual muscle fibers in response to either acute denervation or acute muscle fiber injury. Muscle disorders associated with these discharges include muscle fiber necrosis from muscle trauma, muscular dystrophies or

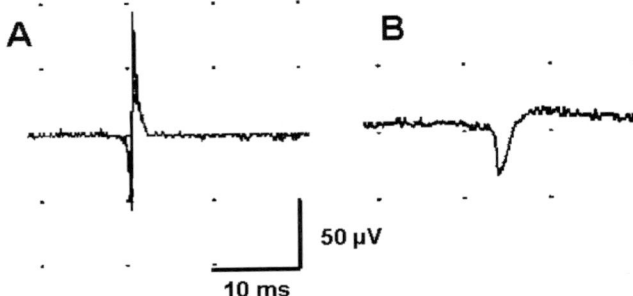

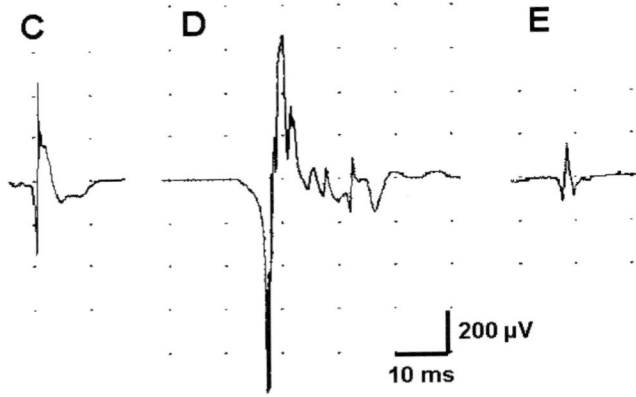

FIGURE 253–8. Fibrillation potentials *(A)*; positive sharp waves *(B)*; and motor unit action potentials of normal *(C)*, reinnervated *(D)*, and myopathic *(E)* motor units. The sensitivities are 50 μV/division for *A* and *B* and 200 μV/division for *C–E*.

inflammatory myopathies, and other muscle diseases such as acid maltase deficiency or hyperkalemic periodic paralysis. Because fibrillation potentials and positive sharp waves are caused by the same group of PNS abnormalities, they usually occur together. Denervation of muscle results in fibrillation potentials and positive sharp waves within 2 to 3 weeks. These findings persist until the muscle fiber is reinnervated, usually within 3 to 4 months in mild injuries, or until the denervated muscle fiber undergoes complete atrophy after up to a few years of persistent denervation without reinnervation.

Complex repetitive discharges are generated from muscle fibers that have been denervated for more than 2 months or from injured muscle fibers, usually associated with muscle fiber necrosis. The neurological disorders that cause complex repetitive discharges are similar to those associated with fibrillation potentials and positive sharp waves, except that complex repetitive discharges occur under chronic conditions. The other spontaneous abnormalities listed in Table 253–1 are seldom encountered in patients with neurosurgical conditions and are not discussed.

MOTOR UNIT ACTION POTENTIAL SIZE AND POLYPHASIC NATURE

The MUAP consists of the sum of action potentials from all the muscle fibers of a single motor unit (see

T A B L E   2 5 3 – 1 ■ **Abnormal Spontaneous Muscle Fiber Action Potentials and Associated Peripheral Nervous System Abnormalities**

MUSCLE FIBER ACTION POTENTIAL	ABNORMALITY
Fibrillation potential	Acute denervation; acute muscle fiber necrosis
Positive sharp wave	Acute denervation; acute muscle fiber necrosis
Complex repetitive discharge	Chronic denervation; chronic muscle fiber necrosis
Fasciculation potential	Normal finding; motoneuron disease; radiculopathy; neuropathy
Myotonic discharge	Myotonic dystrophy; myotonia congenita; paramyotonia
Myokymic discharge	Radiation plexopathy or myelopathy; multiple sclerosis; brainstem glioma with facial myokymia
Cramp discharge	Normal finding; motoneuron disease; radiculopathy; neuropathy
Neuromyotonic discharge	Isaac's disease; neuropathy

Fig. 253–8C). To evaluate MUAPs, an EMG recording needle is inserted into the muscle, and the patient contracts the muscle slightly so that one or a few motor units are activated and recorded. The size of the MUAP is related to the number of muscle fibers within the recording range of the EMG needle. If the MUAP is larger than normal (increased duration or amplitude), there must be an increased number of summated muscle fiber action potentials per motor unit (see Fig. 253–8D). An increased number of muscle fibers per motor unit can occur only through reinnervation, suggesting that there was denervation at least 2 months ago. If the MUAP is smaller than usual (decreased duration or amplitude), there are decreased numbers of muscle fibers per motor unit, which occurs in myopathies or neuromuscular junction disorders (see Fig. 253–8E).

A normal MUAP is usually triphasic (see Fig. 253–8C). An MUAP with five or more phases is polyphasic and results from increased temporal dispersion of the individual muscle fiber action potentials within a motor unit due to chronic denervation with reinnervation, myopathy, or neuromuscular junction disorder (see Fig. 253–8D).

RECRUITMENT AND INTERFERENCE PATTERN

Recruitment of motor units refers to the process of activation of additional motor units with increasing strength of muscle contraction. Under normal circumstances of EMG recording, minimal muscle contraction results in activation of a single motor unit at a slow frequency of 5 to 10 Hz. When the subject increases the strength of muscle contraction, two processes occur: (1) the single motor unit fires at a faster frequency of 10 to 15 Hz, and (2) a second motor unit is recruited and begins firing. As the strength of muscle contraction is further increased, additional motor units are recruited, and they all fire at a faster rate. The frequency of motor unit firing is directly proportional to the degree of activation from the upper motoneurons and can be decreased from any central cause of weakness, including any cause of upper motoneuron loss or decreased effort. Under normal recruitment, a specific number of MUAPs is activated for a given firing frequency. There are only two pathologic abnormalities of recruitment: decreased recruitment and early recruitment. If a neurological disorder has caused a decrease in motor units (e.g., loss of motor axons or conduction block), fewer motor units are available for recruitment, and the ones present fire faster than usual to make up for the decreased numbers. Thus, decreased recruitment of MUAPs indicates loss of motor axons or motor conduction block.

Early recruitment of MUAPs refers to a normal recruitment pattern for a given firing frequency, except that the recruitment and firing frequency generate less muscle strength than normally expected. When there are small motor units (i.e., fewer active muscle fibers per motor axon), early recruitment occurs because activation of a motor unit generates less force than normal. Small motor units result from myopathies or neuro-

muscular junction abnormalities. Thus, early recruitment indicates one or both of those abnormalities.

The interference pattern is the EMG recording seen with maximal voluntary contraction of the muscle. There are usually 20 to 40 MUAPs within the recording range of the EMG needle firing at about 40 Hz with maximal contraction. Any disorder causing loss of motor units, from either motor axon loss or motor conduction block, results in a decrease in the number of MUAPs with maximal contraction and thus a decreased interference pattern.

COMMON CLINICAL DISORDERS

An electrodiagnostic consultation can be helpful when assessing patients with a variety of lesions involving the peripheral nerves, brachial and lumbosacral plexus, roots, and CNS. This section discusses some of the more common problems routinely assessed by electrodiagnostic examination.

Carpal Tunnel Syndrome

NCSs are very sensitive for the diagnosis of median neuropathy at the wrist, such as carpal tunnel syndrome. Together with needle EMG, they are useful for making a diagnosis, differentiating among various possible causes of hand numbness (e.g., cervical radiculopathy, brachial plexopathy, distal entrapment), and delineating the extent of nerve demyelination or axon loss.

Most studies have shown that large-diameter, highly myelinated sensory fibers are affected before motor fibers in entrapment neuropathies. Hence, sensory conduction studies are more commonly affected than motor studies. There are a number of approaches for measuring sensory conduction of the median nerve across the wrist, most of which involve evaluating the sensory latency compared with "normal" (more appropriately called reference) values or compared with another nearby nerve that does not traverse the carpal tunnel (e.g., radial or ulnar nerve). The former approach—simply measuring the median sensory latency—is less satisfactory because of all the nonpathologic factors that can prolong sensory latencies, including cool limb temperature, increasing age, and greater height. Comparing the median latency with that of another nearby nerve avoids these factors, because both nerves will be equally affected.

Three conduction studies are most commonly performed to evaluate median sensory latency across the wrist.[3, 4]

1. Median-ulnar midpalmar latency comparison: Median nerve latency measurements are made by placing an electrode over the median nerve at the wrist and stimulating the median nerve in the palm, between the second and third metacarpal bones. Ulnar nerve latency measurements are made similarly, but with recordings over the ulnar nerve at the wrist and stimulation between the fourth and fifth metacarpal bones.

The latency difference is calculated as median latency minus ulnar latency, with an upper limit of normal of 0.3 msec difference.

2. Median-ulnar ring finger latency comparison: Median nerve latency measurements are made by placing ring electrodes over the ring finger and stimulating at the wrist over the median nerve. Ulnar nerve latency measurements are made similarly, but with stimulation over the ulnar nerve at the wrist. The latency difference is calculated as median latency minus ulnar latency, with an upper limit of normal of 0.4 msec difference.

3. Median-radial thumb latency comparison: Median nerve latency measurements are made by placing ring electrodes over the thumb and stimulating at the wrist over the median nerve. Radial nerve latency measurements are made similarly, but with stimulation over the radial nerve at the wrist. The latency difference is calculated as median latency minus radial latency, with an upper limit of normal of 0.5 msec difference.

Commonly, one or more of these studies are performed to evaluate patients referred for possible carpal tunnel syndrome. One should be aware, however, that the more studies one performs, the greater the chance of false-positive results.[5, 6] Recent studies have shown that performing all three studies and simply adding together the latency differences is more sensitive, specific, and reliable than performing a single study or performing multiple studies and considering them independently.[7, 8] When the three latency comparisons are added, a sum (referred to as the combined sensory index) of 1 msec or greater is considered abnormal and is suggestive of carpal tunnel syndrome.

Motor conduction studies are less commonly abnormal than sensory studies in carpal tunnel syndrome. When abnormalities are present, it likely represents more severe electrophysiologic abnormalities than sensory slowing alone. Median motor latencies also vary with age, temperature, and height, so comparison with the ulnar nerve is usually helpful. A median-ulnar motor latency difference greater than 1.5 msec is likely abnormal.

Needle EMG of the thenar muscles is sometimes useful for detecting motor axon loss in thenar muscles. Denervation is usually seen in more severe cases of entrapment or in traumatic median neuropathy at the wrist. Depending on the clinical presentation, needle EMG might not be needed (e.g., when NCSs show only mild sensory slowing), may be limited to thenar muscles, or might be used to examine a number of muscles in the limb to detect possible radiculopathy or plexopathy.

It should be noted that some improvement in latencies is usually expected after surgical release of the median nerve at the wrist. However, in many cases, latencies do not return to normal despite a good postsurgical clinical outcome.[3] Thus, in patients with persistent postoperative symptoms, it is important to compare results with preoperative conduction studies. If preoperative results are not available, postoperative testing separated by several months should be performed to see whether latencies are getting better or worse over time.

Ulnar Neuropathy at the Elbow

Motor NCSs are often the most useful technique for localizing the site of ulnar neuropathy at the elbow and determining the pathophysiology of the lesion. Recording from the abductor digiti minimi is the most common method. Some authors, however, have found that recording from the first dorsal interosseous muscle, the most distal muscle supplied by the ulnar nerve, is more sensitive.[9-11] A two-channel technique may be used to record from both muscles simultaneously so that extra stimulation is not required.

Stimulation is usually performed at the wrist, below the elbow, above the elbow, and sometimes at the axilla. Study of the across-elbow segment requires much care in technique and interpretation. The position of the elbow greatly influences the measured conduction velocity. When the elbow is extended, the ulnar nerve may become redundant in the ulnar groove, and surface measurements may not reflect the true distance of the underlying nerve. Flexing the elbow stretches the nerve to its full length, and measurement of the distance over the ulnar groove more closely reflects the distance along the nerve.

Because there is room for considerable error in measurement of the across-elbow conduction velocity owing to distance measurements and elbow position, most electromyographers allow up to 11 to 15 m/second difference between the across-elbow and forearm segments before calling the finding "abnormal."[12] Slowed conduction velocity is not the only finding that should be considered diagnostic of ulnar neuropathy at the elbow. Such patients may also have a drop in amplitude in the across-elbow segment. An amplitude reduction of more than 10% in the across-elbow segment is likely abnormal.[12]

It is often found that studying very short segments yields a higher sensitivity for focal lesions. With short-segment studies, the area of demyelination occupies a higher percentage of the distance studied, compared with longer segments in which normal nerve dilutes the measurement. Inching studies (or perhaps more appropriately called "centimetering" studies) can be performed by stimulating the nerve at 2-cm increments across the elbow.[13, 14] With this technique, a conduction delay of more than 0.7 msec across 2-cm segments is probably abnormal.[13] More impressive are focal changes in amplitude or waveform morphology across a segment.

Most of the aforementioned abnormalities require the presence of demyelination for localization. However, in many traumatic ulnar neuropathies in which there is only axon loss without demyelination, localization of ulnar neuropathy is far more difficult. In such cases, there is diffuse, mild slowing of conduction velocity without focal slowing or conduction block; there are no focal nerve conduction changes across the lesion. Therefore, despite one's best technique, localization cannot be precisely determined in a significant number of patients with traumatic or vasculitic lesions of the ulnar nerve (in which there is only axon loss present).

Sensory NCSs are often of less localizing value than motor studies. Nevertheless, sensory responses are often helpful for measuring the degree of sensory axon loss. A drop in amplitude of the ulnar SNAP is probably one of the more sensitive indicators of ulnar neuropathy at the elbow.[15]

Needle EMG of the ulnar-innervated muscle is critical, both to determine whether any axon loss has occurred and to help localize lesions that may be purely axonal in nature. Thus, even if NCSs are entirely normal, when ulnar neuropathy is clinically suspected, needle EMG should still be performed. The most helpful hand muscles to assess are the abductor digiti minimi and first dorsal interosseous, two muscles commonly involved in ulnar neuropathy at the elbow.[9] Study of the flexor carpi ulnaris and the ulnar half of the flexor digitorum profundus is marginally helpful. Although the branch to these muscles usually comes off distal to most entrapment sites at the elbow, the fascicles supplying these muscles are in a relatively protected position within the nerve, so these muscles are often spared.

Needle EMG of non-ulnar-innervated muscles is often useful to rule out other lesions that may mimic ulnar neuropathy. Examination of thenar muscles or the extensor indicis proprius offers the opportunity to compare C8-T1 muscles not innervated by the ulnar nerve. This can be useful to rule out lower cervical radiculopathies as well as lower brachial plexopathies.

Radiculopathies

In most cases, radiculopathies are a result of nerve root compression proximal to the dorsal root ganglion. Mild cases may have only demyelination or irritation of the nerve root, whereas more severe cases demonstrate motor and sensory axon loss.

The practitioner should keep in mind the relative sensitivity and specificity of various imaging and electrodiagnostic testing. Although magnetic resonance imaging (MRI) provides a very sensitive method for assessing nerve roots in the back and neck, it is a highly nonspecific technique. Many asymptomatic people have disk bulges and disk protrusions, and the frequency increasing with age. In one study, 61% of asymptomatic 40- to 49-year-olds had a disk bulge on MRI, and 33% had a disk protrusion; the incidence is considerably higher in older individuals.[16] Other studies have shown a specificity of only about 50%.[17, 18] Hence, there is about an equal chance that a disk abnormality will or will not correspond with clinical symptoms at that site. Electrophysiologic studies are somewhat less sensitive than MRI at detecting mild root compression, but their specificity is considerably higher—likely more than 85% to 90%. It is often useful to combine the highly sensitive but nonspecific imaging modalities with the more specific electrophysiologic testing when evaluating someone with possible radiculopathy.

Needle EMG is likely the best electrophysiologic test for detecting radiculopathy.[19] After the onset of radiculopathy, evidence of denervation can be seen in proximal muscles, such as the paraspinal muscles, in as little as 10 to 14 days. More distal muscles in the limb become abnormal later, taking up to 3 to 4 weeks to show evidence of denervation. For diagnosis of radiculopathy, at least two muscles in the same myotome, but supplied by different peripheral nerves, should show evidence of denervation (fibrillations, positive sharp waves). In chronic root lesions, evidence of reinnervation (long-duration, polyphasic, large-amplitude MUAPs) may be seen in a myotomal distribution; however, this is a softer finding than evidence of recent denervation.

It is helpful to demonstrate paraspinal muscle involvement as well as limb muscle abnormalities, although a significant proportion of patients with radiculopathies do not have abnormalities in paraspinal muscles. Needle EMG of paraspinal muscles has some specific limitations. False-positive findings can be seen after laminectomy and recent myelography, as well as in patients with some metabolic diseases (e.g., diabetes). Hence, abnormalities limited to the paraspinal muscles may be suggestive of some level of nerve root irritation but should not be considered diagnostic.

Sensory NCSs should usually be normal in patients with radiculopathies, because compression occurs proximal to the dorsal root ganglion and distal sensory axons remain in continuity with their cell bodies. Nevertheless, sensory conduction studies are often helpful to rule out a more distal lesion, such as plexopathy or entrapment neuropathy, both of which should affect sensory conduction studies in the appropriate distribution.

Motor NCSs are often normal unless there is severe axon loss. When severe motor axon loss is present and sufficient time has passed for axonal degeneration, the motor nerve response falls in amplitude, roughly in proportion to the degree of axon loss. For example, if half the motor axons in the L5 root were recently lost, the motor response from the extensor digitorum brevis (predominantly L5 root innervated) with stimulation of the peroneal nerve would be about half that of the other side.

Late responses can sometimes be helpful in assessing patients with possible radiculopathies. The F wave is usually normal or only mildly affected. The H wave, in contrast, is probably more sensitive than needle EMG for detecting S1 root lesions, because it can detect demyelination, whereas needle EMG detects primarily motor axon loss.

Somatosensory evoked potentials (SEPs) theoretically should be better at detecting root abnormalities affecting sensory fibers. However, data indicate that SEPs are not as good at detecting isolated radiculopathy as needle EMG is. This is likely due to the overlap of dermatomes, such that multiple roots are stimulated simultaneously during SEPs; normal roots can produce a normal result. In contrast, SEPs are probably better than EMG at detecting spinal stenosis, in which more than one root is involved.[20]

ASSESSMENT OF TRAUMATIC PERIPHERAL NERVE INJURY

Timing

The time course of electrodiagnostic changes after onset of a traumatic nerve lesion should always be considered when interpreting the electrophysiologic examination. Neurapraxia (conduction block), demyelination, and severe axon loss produce electrophysiologic changes immediately if one can stimulate proximal to the lesion to detect conduction block. More proximal lesions, in which one cannot easily stimulate proximal to the lesion, do not immediately produce changes on NCS or EMG. Moreover, distinction between neurapraxia and axonotmesis or neurotmesis cannot be made until time for wallerian degeneration has passed. Optimal timing of electrodiagnostic studies varies according to the clinical circumstances. When it is important to define a lesion early, initial studies 7 to 10 days after injury may be useful for localizing the lesion and separating conduction block from axonotmesis. When clinical circumstances permit waiting, studies performed 3 to 4 weeks after injury provide much more diagnostic information, because fibrillations will be apparent on needle EMG. Finally, when a nerve lesion is surgically confirmed and EMG is used primarily to document recovery, initial studies a few months after injury may be most useful.

Nerve Conduction Studies

In purely neurapraxic lesions, the motor response changes immediately after injury, assuming that one can stimulate both above and below the site of the lesion. When recording from distal muscles and stimulating distal to the site of the lesion, the response should always be normal, because no axonal loss and no wallerian degeneration have occurred. Moving the stimulation proximal to the lesion produces a small or absent motor response, as conduction in some or all fibers is blocked. In addition to conduction block, partial lesions often demonstrate concomitant slowing across the lesion. This slowing may be due to either loss of faster-conducting fibers or demyelination of surviving fibers.

Electrodiagnostically, complete axonotmesis and complete neurotmesis look the same; the difference between these lesions is in the integrity of the supporting structures, which have no electrophysiologic function. Thus, these lesions can be grouped together as axonotmesis for purposes of this discussion. Immediately after axonotmesis and for a few days thereafter, motor conduction studies look the same as those seen in a neurapraxic lesion. Nerve segments distal to the lesion remain excitable and demonstrate normal conduction, while proximal stimulation results in an absent or small response from distal muscles. Early on, this picture looks the same as conduction block and can be confused with neurapraxia. Hence, neurapraxia and axonotmesis cannot be distinguished until sufficient time for the occurrence of wallerian degeneration

in all motor fibers has passed, typically about 9 days after injury.[21]

After this time, the amplitude of the motor response elicited with distal stimulation falls. This starts at about day 3 and is complete by about day 9.[21] Thus, in complete axonotmesis, by day 9 the picture is very different from that of neurapraxia. There are absent responses both above and below the lesion. Partial-axon-loss lesions produce small-amplitude motor responses, with the amplitude roughly proportional to the number of surviving axons.

Lesions that have a mixture of axon loss and conduction block pose a unique challenge. These can usually be sorted out by carefully examining amplitudes of the CMAP elicited from stimulation both above and below the lesion and by comparing the amplitude with distal stimulation to that obtained from the other side. The percentage of axon loss is best estimated by comparing the CMAP amplitude from distal stimulation with that obtained on the contralateral side. Of the remaining axons, the percentage with conduction block is best estimated by comparing amplitudes, or areas, obtained with stimulation distal and proximal to the lesion.

Needle Electromyography

The needle EMG examination in purely neurapraxic lesions shows changes in recruitment but usually no abnormalities in spontaneous activity (i.e., no fibrillations or positive sharp waves).

After an axon-loss lesion (axonotmesis or neurotmesis), needle EMG demonstrates fibrillation potentials and positive sharp waves a number of days after injury. The time between injury and onset of fibrillation potentials depends in part on the length of the distal nerve stump. When the distal stump is short, it takes only 10 to 14 days for fibrillations to develop. With a longer distal stump (e.g., ulnar-innervated hand muscles in a brachial plexopathy), 21 to 30 days are required for full development of fibrillation potentials and positive sharp waves.[22]

Fibrillation and positive sharp wave density are usually graded on a 1-to-4 scale. This is an ordinal scale, meaning that as numbers increase, findings are worse. However, it is not an interval or ratio scale; that is, 4+ is not twice as bad as 2+ or four times as bad as 1+. Moreover, 4+ fibrillation potentials do not indicate complete axon loss and in fact may represent only a minority of axons lost.[9, 23] Evaluation of recruitment and particularly of distally elicited CMAP amplitude is necessary before one can decide whether complete axon loss has occurred.

When there are surviving axons after an incomplete axonal injury, remaining MUAPs are initially normal in morphology but demonstrate reduced or discrete recruitment. Axonal sprouting is manifested by changes in morphology of existing motor units. Amplitude increases, duration becomes prolonged, and the percentage of polyphasic MUAPs increases as motor unit territory increases.[24, 25]

In complete lesions, the only possible mechanism of recovery is axonal regrowth. The earliest needle EMG finding in this case is the presence of small, polyphasic, often unstable motor unit potentials previously referred to as *nascent potentials*. (This term is now discouraged because it implies a cause; it is preferable to simply describe the size, duration, and phasic nature of the MUAP.) Observation of these potentials is dependent on establishing axon regeneration as well as new neuromuscular junctions, and this observation represents the earliest evidence of reinnervation, usually preceding the onset of clinically evident voluntary movement.[25] These potentials represent the earliest definitive evidence of axonal reinnervation in complete lesions.

Localization

Localization of peripheral nerve injuries is usually straightforward but can be complicated by a variety of pitfalls. Localization is usually performed by two methods: detecting focal slowing or conduction block on NCSs, or assessing the pattern of denervation on needle EMG.

Localizing peripheral nerve lesions by NCSs usually requires that there be focal slowing or conduction block as one stimulates above and below the lesion. To see such a change, there must be focal demyelination, or the lesion must be so acute that degeneration of the distal stump has not yet occurred. Thus, lesions with partial or complete neurapraxia (due to demyelination) can be well localized with motor NCSs, as can very acute axonal injuries.

In pure axonotmetic or neurotmetic lesions, it is difficult if not impossible to localize the lesion using NCSs. In such cases, there is mild and diffuse slowing in the entire nerve due to loss of the fastest fibers, or there is no response at all. Conduction across the lesion site is no slower than that across other segments. In addition, if enough time for wallerian degeneration has elapsed (at least 9 days for motor fibers and 11 days for sensory fibers), there will be no change in amplitude as one traverses the site of the lesion. Thus, pure axon-loss lesions are not well localized along a nerve by NCSs.

Another indirect inference that can be made based on sensory NCSs is placement of the lesion at a pre- versus postganglionic location. Lesions that are proximal to the dorsal root ganglion—that is, at the preganglionic level (proximal root, cauda equina, spinal cord)—tend to have normal SNAP amplitudes, even if there is reduced or absent sensation.[26, 27] This is a particularly bad prognostic sign when seen in the setting of possible root avulsion. Conversely, lesions occurring distal to the dorsal root ganglion have small or absent sensory responses (when these are recorded in the appropriate distribution).

The other major electrodiagnostic method of determining the site of nerve injury is needle EMG. Conceptually, if one knows the branching order to various muscles under study, one can determine that the nerve injury is between the branches to the most distal normal muscle and the most proximal abnormal muscle. There are, however, a number of potential limitations to this approach. First, the branching and innervation

for muscles are not necessarily consistent from one person to another. Sunderland[28] demonstrated a great deal of variability in the branching order to muscles in the limbs, in the number of branches going to each muscle, and in which nerve or nerves supply each muscle. Thus, the typical branching scheme may not apply to the patient being studied, and the lesion site can be misconstrued.

Additionally, the existence of partial lesions can lead to misdiagnosis to more distal sites. In partial ulnar nerve lesions at the elbow, for example, the forearm ulnar-innervated muscles are often spared.[23] This is thought to be due at least partially to sparing of the fascicles in the nerve that are preparing to branch to the flexor digitorum profundus and flexor carpi ulnaris (i.e., they are in a relatively protected position). This finding could lead one to inadvertently localize the lesion distally to the distal forearm or wrist. Intraneural topography needs to be considered when making a diagnosis based on branching.[29]

Localization of brachial plexus lesions deserves special consideration. In such cases, it is important to differentiate injury to the root (e.g., avulsion) from plexus injuries and from multiple peripheral nerve injuries. Differentiation between root and plexus lesions is accomplished primarily by examination of the paraspinal muscles and sensory amplitudes. Both these methods are subject to the limitations mentioned earlier for needle EMG and sensory conduction studies. Distinguishing between plexus and peripheral nerve lesions is sometimes more complex. An intimate knowledge of brachial plexus anatomy is required to distinguish between a peripheral nerve distribution of abnormalities and a plexus distribution. Sampling of muscles from the cord and trunk levels of the plexus (e.g., latissimus dorsi, pectoralis major, infraspinatus) is often helpful. Even with this knowledge, however, multiple peripheral nerve lesions (e.g., axillary, radial) can be erroneously ascribed to a single plexus insult (e.g., posterior cord).

PROGNOSTICATION OF AWAKENING FROM COMA

A number of electrophysiologic methods have been studied for their ability to predict outcomes in comatose patients. Of these methods, median nerve SEPs have the strongest evidence for utility in predicting outcome after coma.[30] Specifically, bilateral absence of cortical responses to median nerve stimulation is usually associated with a very poor prognosis. Pathologic studies in small numbers of patients have shown that essentially complete cortical necrosis is required to obliterate the cortical response in patients with nontraumatic encephalopathy.[31]

It has been shown that for adult patients with coma due to hypoxic-ischemic encephalopathy, bilateral absence of cortical responses to median nerve stimulation confidently predicts nonawakening. Out of more than 200 patients with this finding, no one has awakened, with an upper 95% confidence interval (CI) of 1%.[30]

Whereas normal SEPs in this group do not necessarily predict a good outcome, they do suggest a better outcome than average.

SEPs are also useful but not quite as predictive in adults who are comatose from traumatic causes. Bilateral absence of cortical responses in this group predicts about a 5% chance of awakening (95% CI of 2% to 8%), but the great majority who have awakened had severe disability (unpublished literature review).

Children seem to form a separate prognostic group. While bilaterally absent responses still predict only a 7% chance of awakening (95% CI of 3% to 10%), many of these children have a better recovery than adults do, with less severe disability (unpublished literature review).

NEUROMONITORING OF PERIPHERAL NERVES

Preoperative and postoperative electrodiagnostic studies provide essential information about the functional status of individuals with peripheral nerve problems. These studies are important tools in the diagnostic process, for understanding the nature and extent of disease or injury, and when planning a surgical approach. The application of electrophysiologic techniques in the operating room has also become an integral part of the surgical treatment of peripheral nerve disorders and injuries.[32–34]

For the most part, neuromonitoring is considered a way to reduce the risk of intraoperative, iatrogenic injury to the nervous system. Certainly, this is true for the brain and spinal cord, but for peripheral nerves, neuromonitoring is more than simply a nerve monitor. By the judicious use of SEPs, CMAP recordings, NCSs, and free-running EMGs, neuromonitoring of peripheral nerves can serve several purposes. One of the main functions is the traditional role of monitoring both sensory and motor components. Additionally, neuromonitoring may be involved in more diagnostic-oriented pursuits, such as the evaluation of a nerve's functional status and identification and localization of functioning and nonfunctioning neural elements.

Given the variety of neurophysiologic techniques that may be applied[32–40] and their potential use at multiple points during surgery, it is obvious that a close and cooperative working relationship must exist between the neurophysiologist and the surgeon to maximize the benefit to the patient. The neurophysiologist must understand the surgical approach sufficiently to suggest appropriate uses of neurophysiologic techniques, and the surgeon should appreciate the purposes of neurophysiology and request or be receptive to its application. *Teamwork* is the operative word.

Neurophysiologic monitoring may be applied to a variety of procedures involving the peripheral nerve:

- Neurolysis or nerve graft following traumatic injury. Neuromonitoring may help identify nerves and distinguish functioning versus nonfunctioning elements of nerve.

- Excision of tumors. Neuromonitoring may protect functioning neural elements and locate nerve fibers within or on a tumor.
- Resection of cysts. Neuromonitoring may protect nerves and identify nerve fibers coursing across a cyst capsule.
- Entrapment or nerve transposition. During dissection, neuromonitoring can locate nerves, which takes on greater significance in cases of scarring from previous surgery.

Most peripheral nerves with a motor component are appropriate candidates for monitoring. Monitoring is most often used in cases involving the brachial plexus, lumbar plexus, and major nerves of the arms and legs, such as median, ulnar, radial, sciatic, peroneal, and tibial nerves.

It is important to point out that in all these applications, neuromonitoring must be interactive with the surgical technique and should be used throughout the procedure. For example, stimulation should be used to look for nerve fibers before dissecting tissue, not just to confirm their presence once they are visualized after dissection. In our experience, nerve fibers are often demonstrated electrophysiologically yet are not apparent by visual inspection.

Neuromonitoring Techniques during Peripheral Nerve Surgery

As mentioned, a combination of neurophysiologic techniques is used, including SEPs; triggered EMG; spontaneous, free-running EMG; and compound nerve action potentials (CNAPs). A brief description of these techniques and the responses recorded follows. Further discussion of these techniques may be found in other publications.[32–34]

Somatosensory Evoked Potentials. SEPs reflect sensory conduction along the somatosensory pathway. These signals are quite small (0.2 to 4 microvolts) and require averaging technology to resolve these signals from the surrounding electrical noise. SEPs may be recorded to stimulation of nerves distally (mixed nerve SEPs), of the skin (dermatomal SEPs), and even of proximal nerves or nerve roots. Recordings may be taken from the cervical spine, reflecting activity in the spinal cord; the mastoid, reflecting brainstem-level activity; or the scalp, reflecting cortical-level function. Because stimulation is usually distal to the surgical field, these centrally recorded SEPs reflect conduction through the surgical field and serve as a monitor of afferent fibers or as an assessment of nerve function.

Triggered Electromyography. A triggered EMG refers to the recording of CMAPs from a muscle either with surface electrodes or with needle electrodes placed in the muscle. The response is elicited by electrical stimulation of a nerve innervating that muscle at a point on the nerve proximal to the muscle, such as in the surgical field. Triggered EMG is the result of the response of a large number of motor units, rendering responses in the millivolt range.

Spontaneous, Free-Running Electromyography. Spontaneous EMG is the latent activity recorded from a muscle that is not specifically elicited by electrical stimulation but occurs spontaneously. This spontaneous activity may derive solely from the patient, reflecting some degree of central activation, such as when the patient awakes and begins contracting his or her muscles. But of more critical interest is activity that is correlated with actions in the surgical field. Iatrogenic, mechanical irritation of the nerve membranes may lead to generation of action potentials in motor fibers that conduct distally to a muscle, leading to activation of motor units and spontaneous EMG. These spontaneous EMG potentials are due to relatively few motor units with responses in the microvolt to millivolt range, depending on the distance between the recording electrode and the active muscle fibers. It should be noted that these potentials are normal MUAPs and are not the pathologic signals (fibrillation potentials and positive sharp waves) mentioned earlier. Their occurrence indicates contact or irritation of nerve fibers and can be used to guide a surgeon's actions. Caution must be used when predicting clinical outcome, because the amount of activity is not a good indicator. In other words, a brief burst of activity has the same chance of being associated with a postoperative motor deficit as does a large amount of activity.

Compound Nerve Action Potentials. CNAPs are recordings taken from a nerve to stimulation of the nerve either distally or centrally to the recording point. If a whole nerve is stimulated, CNAPs represent sensory and motor fiber conduction. A CNAP may represent sensory function (SNAP) if only sensory elements are stimulated, such as the digital nerves of the fingers or a cutaneous nerve such as the sural nerve. The peripheral nerve recordings that are often done in concert with SEPs may be considered a CNAP.

In general, these techniques are quite similar to those used clinically, but some adaptations of stimulation and recording electrodes and their placement are specific to the operating room.

STIMULATION TECHNIQUE

Electrodes. Stimulation in the operating room is done both outside of and within the surgical field. Outside the surgical field, stimulating electrodes may be either surface electrodes that are taped or stuck in position or 0.5-inch bare needle electrodes that are taped or stapled in position. For stimulation within the surgical field, which occurs routinely, stimulating electrodes must be sterile and fixed in position with sterile adhesive strips or stapled. Needle electrodes are better suited to sterile field application than surface electrodes are. The needles can be fixed in position and the leads passed off the sterile filed for connection to the neurophysiologic equipment.

Stimulation within the wound is often with a hand-held electrode but may be done with fixed electrodes such as needles or a cuff-type electrode. Hand-held electrodes may be monopolar or bipolar. The monopolar probes that are commercially available are excellent for probing tissue and locating nerve. Their stimulation area is quite focal, however. For stimulation of a larger area of the nerve or the whole nerve, bipolar hook electrodes are more appropriate.

Stimulation Parameters. Percutaneous stimulation of peripheral nerves is done in the same manner as in clinical tests. Stimulus durations are from 0.1 to 0.2 msec, with an intensity 1.5 times the twitch threshold, or about 10 to 30 mA. For direct stimulation of nerve, stimulus durations are reduced to 0.05 to 0.2 msec, and intensities are brought up carefully from zero until the threshold is found, usually 0.1 to 0.2 mA. If there is scarring or if the nerve is deeper in the tissue, larger amplitudes may be necessary.

The rate of stimulation depends on the signal recorded. SEPs use rates from 3 to 5 Hz for cortical recordings, but rates of 10 to 15 Hz may be used if only subcortical recordings are taken. Triggered EMG may be either a single stimulus or slow rates of 1 to 2 Hz.

RECORDING TECHNIQUE

Somatosensory Evoked Potentials. SEP recordings are generally taken from electrodes that are not in the surgical field, so either surface or needle electrodes can be used. However, for consistent quality of recording, good impedance matching, and ease of application, needle electrodes are preferred.

Peripheral nerve recordings are a required part of the SEP montage and should be distal to the surgical site. This recording serves to verify stimulation and conduction of activity in functional nerves. Occasionally, these recordings are taken from positions within the surgical field, necessitating a sterile electrode such as a 0.5-inch needle.

Cervical spine recordings are taken from the lower cervical spine, C5-7, and reflect activity generated by the spinal cord. Electrodes may be surface or 0.5-inch subcutaneous needles. Some benefit in response amplitude may be gained by using a long insulated needle inserted through the paraspinal muscles, with the tip of the electrode positioned near or on the lamina of a cervical vertebra. The reference electrode for any of these active electrodes may be placed on the low occipital region of the scalp or at the frontal scalp, for example, Fz of the International 10-20 system.

Recordings made with a surface or needle electrode placed on the mastoid or the ear reflect activity originating in the brainstem.[41–43] Our convention is to use Fz as an active electrode site and the mastoid lead as a reference, which renders a positive waveform that is distinct from the negative waveform of the cervical response.

Surface or needle electrodes placed on the scalp overlying the postcentral gyrus provide responses that reflect activity in the sensory cortex. For stimulation of the upper extremities, recordings are made from the lateral scalp (positions C_3', C_4'); for stimulation of the lower extremities, recordings are made from the midline (Cz'). Cortical-level signals are the largest and most easily obtainable of all the SEP recording sites, but they are the most susceptible to anesthetics and other conditions that can suppress and alter the signals.[44-46] More conduction block or axonal discontinuity is required to change cortical signals than to change subcortical signals.[47] Both cervical- and brainstem-level responses are less susceptible to these confounding factors and thus are more reliable and reproducible. Subcortical signals can, however, be more difficult to record, because these signals are often small in amplitude.

Electromyography. EMG recordings can be made with surface electrodes, 0.5-inch subcutaneous needles, or insulated EMG needles (monopolar or bipolar). Surface or 0.5-inch subcutaneous needles provide a quiet, noise-free recording that samples a broad area of muscle. In contrast, EMG needles are noisy, may cause bleeding, and sample a more restricted area of muscle. Because the objective is to provide qualitative rather than quantitative assessments of motor response, surface or 0.5-inch needles are adequate.

CONFIGURATION OF ELECTRODIAGNOSTIC TECHNIQUES

The techniques of SEP, CNAP, and EMG may be configured to form six different ways to monitor or assess nerve function during peripheral nerve surgery.

Somatosensory Evoked Potentials to Distal Nerve Stimulation. This technique is the conventional method of recording SEPs, analogous to that used in a clinical setting—that is, stimulation of a nerve at a location distal to the surgical field and recording SEPs from central locations. A typical example is a median nerve SEP with stimulation of the median nerve at the wrist and recording of SEPs at the cervical spine, mastoid, and scalp.

The afferent signal conducts through the surgical field from distal to proximal. These SEPs serve two functions: to monitor afferent nerve fiber conduction, and to assess the function of those nerves that are stimulated.

Somatosensory Evoked Potentials to Root or Proximal Nerve Stimulation. In this technique, centrally recorded SEPs are taken to stimulation of exposed nerves or nerve roots within the surgical field. Recordings may be taken at the cervical, brainstem, or cortical level but are probably most easily recorded at the cortical level, because the stimulus artifact is least at this location. The waveforms are similar in configuration to those recorded to stimulation of a nerve more distally, but the latencies are much shorter, commensurate with the shorter conduction distance to the brain. The only caution is to be aware that myogenic artifacts may be caused by such proximal stimulation. To resolve this problem, either the stimulation intensity is reduced below the twitch threshold, or a bolus of short-acting neuromuscular blockade can be administered. The latter method is preferred, as the former approach may be insufficient to activate the nerve.

This technique is useful for evaluating the state of conduction over proximal segments of nerve or nerve roots. This can be useful for assessing root avulsion or for determining the proximal border between the functional and damaged portions of a nerve (see Fig. 21–6 in reference 34).

Compound Nerve Action Potentials Recorded in the Surgical Field to Stimulation Outside the Surgical Field. CNAPs can be recorded with bipolar electrodes, such as a hook electrode, or with monopolar electrodes, such a ball-tip or needle electrode. The recordings reflect conduction of the distal portion of a nerve from its point of stimulation distally to the surgical field. Nerve conduction velocity can be determined if the conduction distance is measured carefully. Another valuable contribution of these recordings is location of a nerve's position in the surgical field by recording the CNAPs at several locations; the position with the largest amplitude is the point closest to the nerve. This information may facilitate the dissection process and localize the position of a nerve. Examples of this technique can be found in other publications (see Fig. 21–2 in reference 34 and Fig. 3 in reference 33).

Compound Nerve Action Potentials Recorded in the Surgical Field to Stimulation in the Surgical Field. For the best results, stimulation and recording should be done with hook electrodes to minimize stimulus artifact and to produce quiet, noise-free recordings. These recordings over short segments of nerve can be used to assess nerve conduction in cases of nerve regeneration or neuroma in continuity,[37, 40] to evaluate conduction in scarred or injured nerve, and to derive nerve conduction velocity (see Fig. 4 in reference 33).

Triggered Electromyography. The technique is to stimulate nerves of interest in the surgical field and observe the CMAPs generated in target muscles for the nerves under examination. Stimulation may be done with monopolar electrodes, such as a flush-tip or ball-tip probe, or with bipolar electrodes, such as a hook electrode. Monopolar electrodes make it easier to probe the surgical field and give fine responses, but one should remember that their stimulation is focal and is probably not activating all the fibers in a nerve. Full activation of a nerve is best done with hook electrodes.

CMAPs are recorded from an array of muscles that represent the target muscles for all the nerves that may come under investigation. By examining the pattern of responses, one can determine the identity of the nerve under consideration. For single nerves, interpretation is straightforward. For example, a CMAP in the deltoid indicates stimulation of the axillary nerve, whereas a CMAP in the biceps indicates stimulation of the musculocutaneous nerve. Stimulation of a component of the brachial or lumbar plexus or of nerve roots, however, leads to more complex patterns that require closer examination. Because of individual anatomic variation, patterns of responses may vary considerably.

Triggered EMG is useful for determining the overall function of motor fibers, identifying a nerve in question, and deriving motor nerve conduction velocities.

Spontaneous, Free-Running Electromyography. In most circumstances, a completely relaxed or well-anesthetized individual would not be expected to generate any EMG activity in a continuous, real-time recording from an array of muscle. The presence of low-level, continuous EMG activity in several muscles may indicate an increasing level of arousal and may help in the anesthetic management of the patient. Of greater significance to the surgeon is the presence of bursting EMG activity (i.e., short bursts of activity) or trains of EMG activity (i.e., activity that persists for periods of time). This spontaneous EMG activity in the free-running EMG record may indicate iatrogenic, mechanical irritation of nerves. This activity is a useful indicator of manipulation of motor fibers and may serve as a warning of possible damage to these fibers.

APPLICATION OF TECHNIQUES DURING SURGERY

Complete monitoring and analysis during peripheral nerve surgery require the application of all the techniques just described. These techniques may be applied at various times throughout a surgery to provide information about the function, location, and identification of nerves. To this end, neurophysiologic monitoring is more than simply the monitoring of nerve integrity; it involves the additional goals of guiding dissection, identifying and localizing nerves, and assessing nerve function.[32–34]

Monitoring the Approach and Manipulation of Nerves. Traditional monitoring of nerve function during the approach and manipulation of nerves is done during all phases of surgery, because functioning nerves are at continual risk for stretching during dissection and by vessel loops, compression due to retraction, or manipulation during examination of the tissue or neurolysis. For monitoring of sensory function, SEPs are typically used, whereas motor function is monitored with either spontaneous EMG or triggered EMG to stimulation at a point proximal to the surgical field (if available). Spontaneous EMG is particularly appropriate during manipulation of a nerve such as dissection or neurolysis, as it provides a rapid indication of distress to the nerve membrane.

Guiding Dissection. Visual inspection does not always reveal the presence of nerve fibers. Even in normal anatomic situations, dissection may be problematic, but in pathologic or traumatic situations, visual identification of nerve fibers is certainly compromised. Triggered EMG from an array of possible target muscles may be helpful in identifying the presence of motor fibers and distinguishing neural from non-neural tissue. For complete success in this regard, it is imperative that electrical stimulation be done before the dissection and as it proceeds. Stimulation after an area has been dissected may reveal only that a nerve was inadvertently transected or injured.

Triggered EMG is particularly useful in mapping the course of nerve fibers across a tumor capsule. Stimulation with a monopolar electrode, such as a flush-tip probe, and recording CMAPs from an array of target muscles can be an invaluable tool for determining which areas of a tumor capsule contain nerve fibers. For example, the nerve fibers of most schwannomas are spread over its capsule. Visualization of these fibers can be difficult, and the only sure way of identifying nerve fibers is through electrical stimulation before any dissection.

The converse of using stimulation to locate nerve fibers is recording the electrical response, a CNAP, within the surgical field to stimulation of a nerve distally. Recordings are made from several locations within the field, and the position of the largest-amplitude response indicates the location nearest to the nerve. This technique requires the presence of an intact distal component of a nerve, such as may occur with a preganglionic lesion. This technique can reduce the dissection time in cases of extreme scarring. (An example of this technique can be found in Figs. 21–2 and 21–3 in reference 34.)

Identifying and Localizing Nerves. The identity of a nerve may be uncertain in cases of extreme scarring because of altered anatomy. Electrophysiologic techniques can be used not only to identify a nerve's location within scarred tissue but also to help identify the nerve itself.

By analyzing the CMAPs from an array of possible target muscles to intrafield stimulation, the likely identity of a nerve can be determined. Nowhere is this more helpful than in a nerve plexus. Identification of the roots, trunks, divisions, and cords of the brachial plexus is much easier with electrical stimulation. A good understanding of functional anatomy is imperative for both the surgeon and the neurophysiologist.

Assessing Nerve Function. Some of the most salient information that neurophysiology can provide the surgeon concerns the functional status of the nerve in question. Electrophysiologic identification of the presence of functional nerve fibers in neuromas in continuity, in scarred tissue, or in traumatized nerve may suggest that the nerve should be left alone or treated with neurolysis but not grafted. To obtain this information, several techniques can be used.

Standard SEPs to distal stimulation provide information about the integrity of the sensory pathway. Stimulation is usually to major nerves to obtain information about the nerve itself or its path through a proximal plexus. Median and ulnar SEPs assess the integrity of each of these nerves and of the upper and lower trunks of the brachial plexus, respectively. Likewise, tibial and peroneal nerve SEPs can provide information about the integrity of these nerves or of the tibial and peroneal component of the sciatic nerve. Nerve root assessment by SEPs cannot be done by nerve stimulation, because of the multiroot innervation by most nerves, but it can be done by dermatomal stimulation. Thumb, middle finger, and little finger stimulation addresses the C6, C7, and C8 nerve roots, respectively.

SEPs to intrafield stimulation can be used to distinguish functional from nonfunctional portions of a nerve. In this situation, if the nerve proximal to an injury site is stimulated and demonstrates SEPs, stimulation can be carried successively distal until the response is lost to identify the distal extent of functioning nerve fibers (see Fig. 21–6 in reference 34). This information can be used to help determine the optimal place on the proximal stump to graft to.

CNAPs to intrafield stimulation are well suited for the assessment of regenerating nerve fibers in a neuroma in continuity.[36, 37, 40] The presence of a response is considered a good sign that regeneration is in progress.

CMAPs to intrafield stimulation can assess the integrity of the motor components, as mentioned earlier. Occasionally, CMAPs are detected in muscle that clinically shows no action. Two situations have been observed. One is small-amplitude CMAPs, which could indicate that a few motor fibers remain following an injury or that regeneration has just reached the muscle. The other is a larger, more normal-sized CMAP, which may indicate a neurapraxic injury in which the distal component of the nerve is intact and functional but conduction cannot proceed across the injury site.

These applications expand the traditional role of monitoring nerve function to that of an active partner in surgical treatment. With a close working relationship between neurophysiologist and surgeon, an injured nerve can be completely assessed, injury can be avoided, and optimal treatment can be provided.

CASE EXAMPLES

Two examples are presented to illustrate the techniques described earlier and their integration into the surgical procedure. The first case involves resection of a median nerve schwannoma and demonstrates the use of SEPs, spontaneous EMG, and triggered EMG to stimulation of the tumor capsule. The second case involves an individual with a severe brachial plexus injury and demonstrates the use of triggered EMG to root stimulation and SEPs to root stimulation as well as to distal nerve stimulation.

■ CASE HISTORY 1

A 29-year-old woman presented with a mass along the medial aspect of her right upper arm. Her clinical examination and electrodiagnostic evaluation demonstrated normal function in the right upper extremity. MRI revealed a mass located on the median nerve.

During surgery, the mass was easily localized and resected through an incision in the capsule of the tumor. Postoperatively, the woman recovered well, retaining normal sensory and motor function of the median nerve.

Intraoperative electrophysiologic monitoring consisted initially and throughout the surgery of SEPs recorded at Erb's point to median nerve and ulnar nerve stimulation at the wrist. Both nerves were monitored to ensure no incidental involvement of the adjacent ulnar nerve. The before and after resection waveforms are shown in Figure 253–9. The responses were clearly apparent and showed no changes in latency or amplitude.

Spontaneous EMG monitoring was done during the exposure and localization of the tumor and especially during resection of the mass. Spontaneous EMG was taken from 0.5-inch needles placed subcutaneously over the wrist flexors, thenar, hypothenar, and first dorsal interosseous muscles. During the dissection and isolation of the tumor, several bursts and a few occurrences of continuous EMG activity were noted in the thenar muscles. An example is shown in Figure 253–10. This activity was used by the surgeon as a guide for careful dissection of the tumor.

Once the tumor was isolated, as can be seen in Figure 253–11, the capsule of the tumor was probed for the presence of motor fibers. Stimulation was done with a monopolar, flush-tip probe. Triggered EMG was taken from the aforementioned muscle groups. As can be seen in Figure 253–11, stimulation at the top and bottom of the tumor capsule yielded prominent CMAPs in the wrist flexors and thenar muscles (upper left panel). Stimulation in an area in the middle of the tumor capsule, however, yielded no responses (upper right panel), providing an avenue for incision into the capsule. No spontaneous EMG activity was noted during debulking of the tumor.

Following debulking of the tumor (Fig. 253–12), stimulation of the median nerve both proximal and distal to the tumor elicited comparable CMAPs in the wrist flexors and

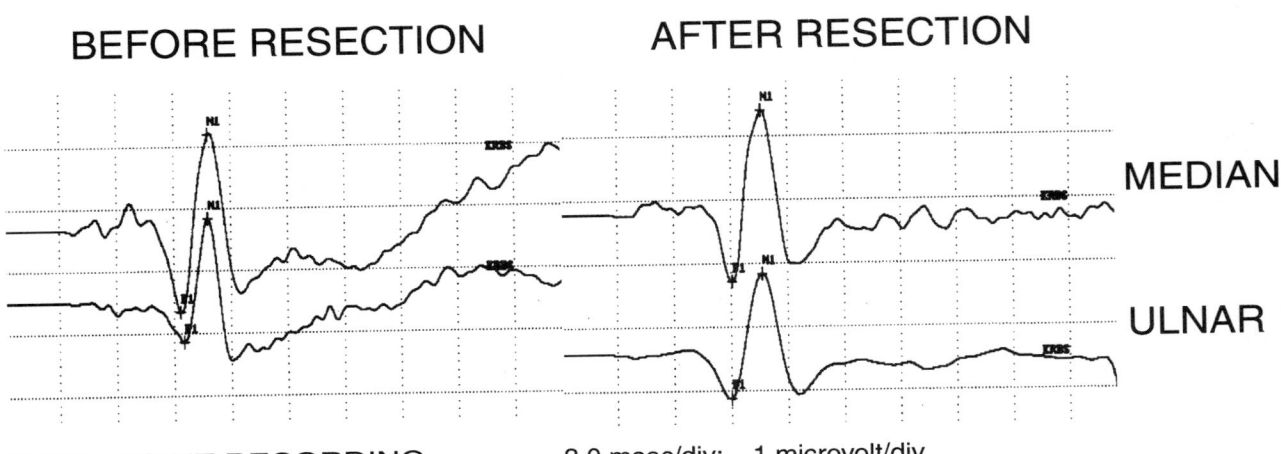

BEFORE RESECTION   **AFTER RESECTION**

MEDIAN

ULNAR

ERB'S POINT RECORDING   3.0 msec/div: 1 microvolt/div

FIGURE 253–9. Erb's point somatosensory evoked potentials to median and ulnar nerve stimulation taken before and after median nerve tumor resection.

SPONTANEOUS EMG

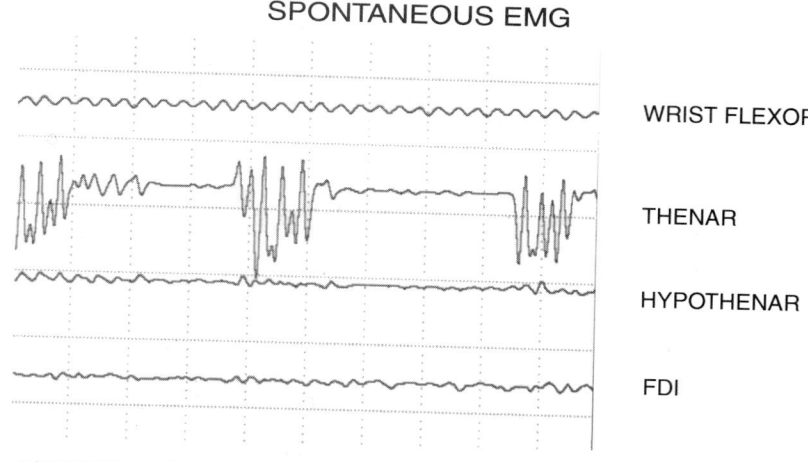

WRIST FLEXOR

THENAR

HYPOTHENAR

FDI

3 MSEC/DIV: 20 MICROVOLT/DIV

FIGURE 253–10. Spontaneous, free-running electography (EMG) records taken from wrist flexor, thenar, hypothenar, and first dorsal interosseous (FDI) muscles. Bursting EMG activity elicited during dissection was seen in the thenar muscle record.

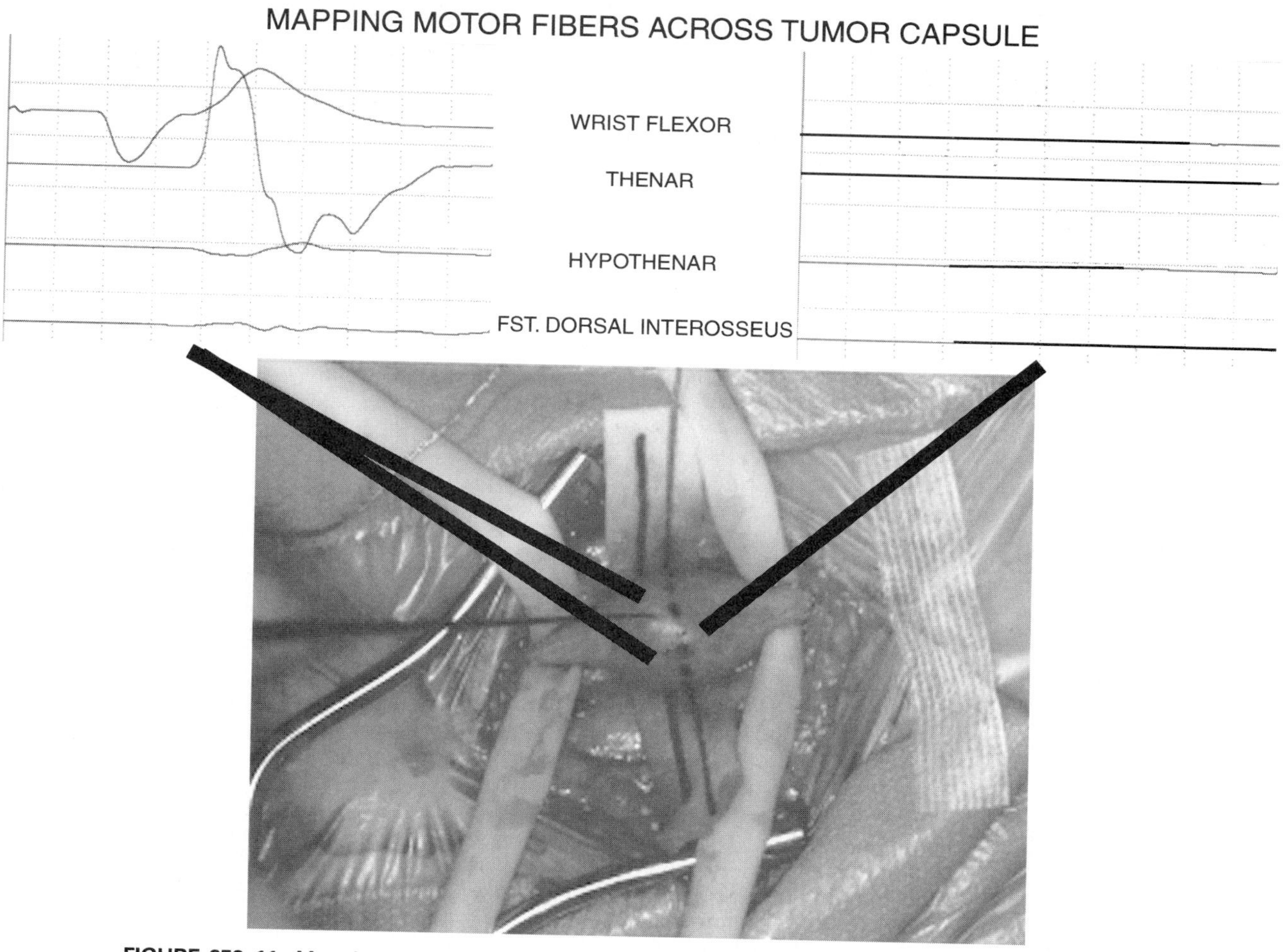

MAPPING MOTOR FIBERS ACROSS TUMOR CAPSULE

WRIST FLEXOR

THENAR

HYPOTHENAR

FST. DORSAL INTEROSSEUS

FIGURE 253–11. Mapping a tumor capsule for motor fibers. Stimulation of the capsule above and below the middle portion of the tumor elicited compound muscle action potentials in median nerve–innervated muscles *(left panel)*, whereas stimulation in the middle portion elicited no response, indicating an area devoid of motor fibers.

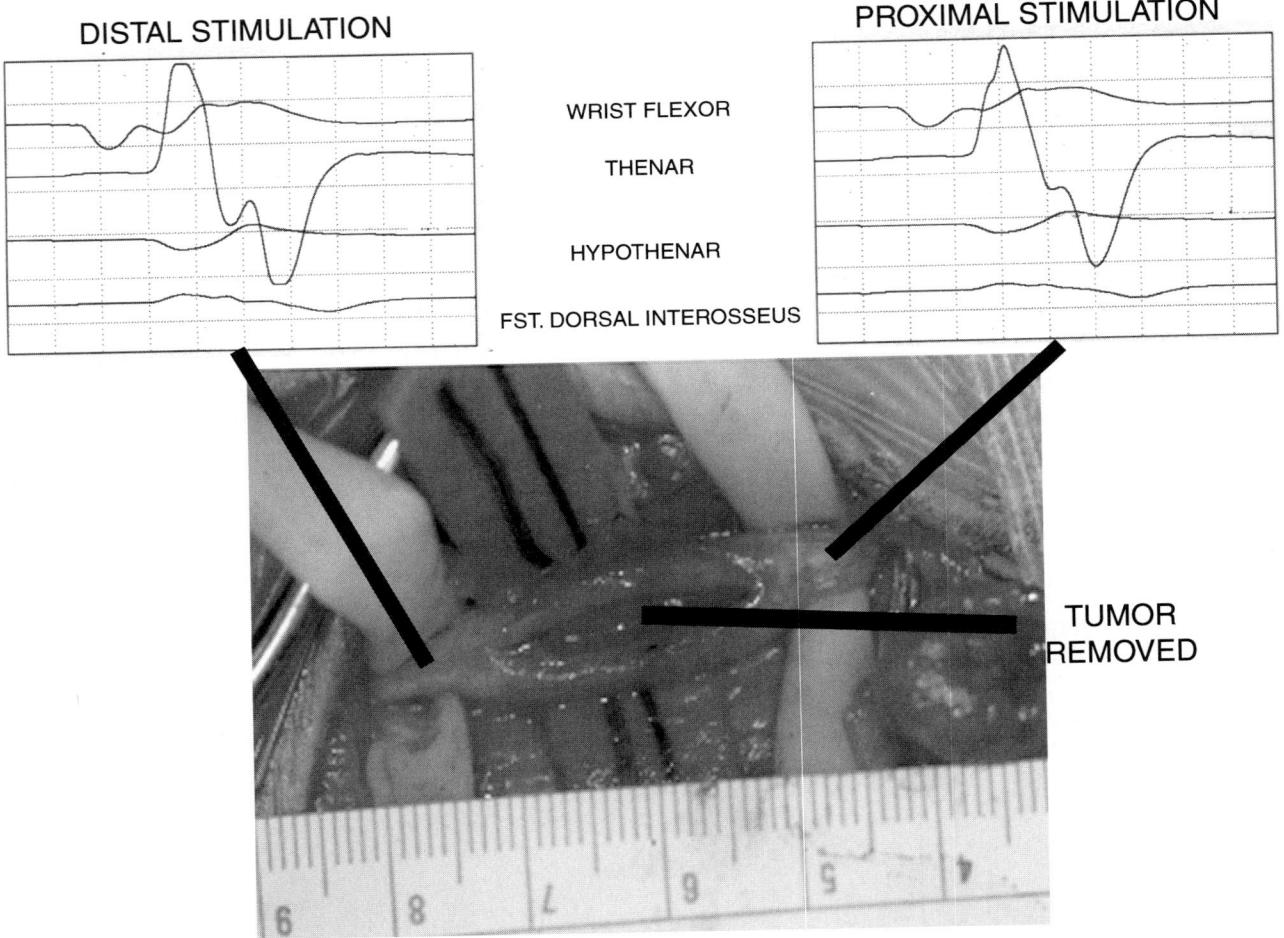

FIGURE 253–12. Following debulking of the tumor (see central portion of tumor), proximal and distal stimulation of the median nerve elicited comparable compound muscle action potentials, giving no indication of compromise of the median nerve.

thenar muscles (upper panels of Fig. 253–12), giving no indication of compromise to the motor component of the median nerve. This finding is in accord with the Erb's point SEPs shown in Figure 253–9.

■ CASE HISTORY 2

A 49-year-old woman had sustained a severe right brachial plexus injury in an automobile accident 5 months earlier. Clinically, she showed reduced sensation in the C4 through C6 distributions and a complete motor deficit in C5, C6, and the upper trunk distributions. MRI, computed tomography–myelography, and electrodiagnostic studies suggested the possibility of both preganglionic and postganglionic injury. At 5 months after injury there was no evidence of recovery, and she was brought to surgery.

Baseline SEPs taken after induction of anesthesia showed well-developed responses to right median and right ulnar nerve stimulation, as recorded at the cervical spine, mastoid, and scalp (Fig. 253–13). These responses were clearly present throughout the surgery, with no change in latency or amplitude. A C6 dermatomal SEP recorded at the scalp (not shown) was noted at baseline and continued to be present throughout the surgery as well.

Following exposure of the C4-7 nerve roots, during which no spontaneous EMG activity was noted, intrafield stimulation was conducted using a monopolar, flush-tip probe. Triggered EMG was taken from needles placed over the serratus anterior, rhomboid, supraspinatus-infraspinatus, deltoid, biceps, triceps, and wrist extensor muscles. Stimulation of the C4, C5, and C6 roots elicited no CMAPs, whereas stimulation of the C7 root elicited responses in the serratus anterior, biceps, triceps, and wrist extensor muscles (Fig. 253–14). The response seen in Figure 253–14 in the deltoid was considered questionable. The latency was too long for a deltoid response and, together with the absence of palpable twitch, was thought to represent a possible movement artifact response.

Analysis continued with SEPs recorded to stimulation of the C4-7 nerve roots. The results, shown in Figure 253–15, clearly demonstrated absent conduction centrally of the C4, C5, and C6 nerve roots in the presence of good conduction of the C7 nerve root. Thus, the C4-6 nerve roots showed no conduction either distally or centrally, while the C7 nerve root was intact for both sensory and motor conduction. Moreover, it was noted that the C4 nerve root divulged a large branch via an anastomosis to the C5 nerve root. Because of this prefixed condition and because of the evidence that C7 contributed to the muscu-

RIGHT MEDIAN N.   RIGHT ULNAR N.

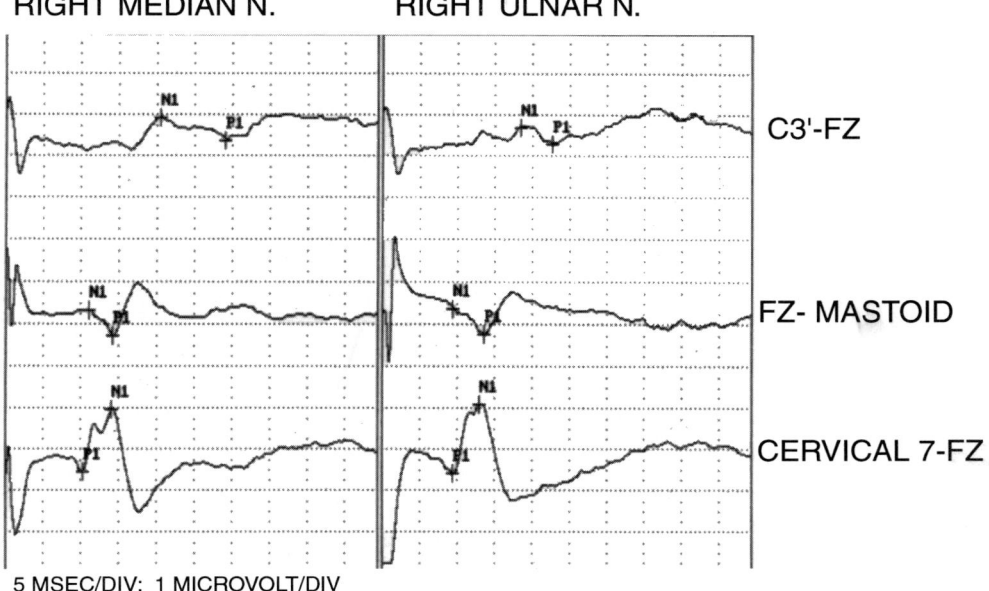

C3'-FZ

FZ- MASTOID

CERVICAL 7-FZ

5 MSEC/DIV: 1 MICROVOLT/DIV

FIGURE 253–13. Median and ulnar nerve somatosensory evoked potentials recorded at the contralateral scalp (C3'-Fz), the brainstem level (Fz-mastoid), and the cervical level (C7-Fz) were obtained throughout surgery.

C7 NERVE ROOT STIMULATION

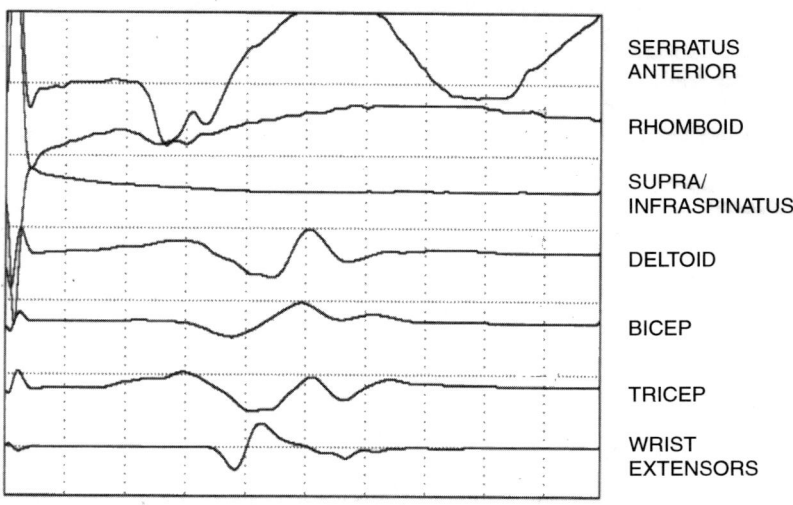

SERRATUS ANTERIOR

RHOMBOID

SUPRA/ INFRASPINATUS

DELTOID

BICEP

TRICEP

WRIST EXTENSORS

3 MSEC/DIV: 0.5 MVOLT/DIV

FIGURE 253–14. Compound muscle action potentials to stimulation of the C7 nerve root. Stimulation of the C7 root elicited activity in the serratus anterior, biceps, triceps, wrist extensor, and possibly the deltoid muscles. No responses were detected to stimulation of the C4, C5, or C6 roots.

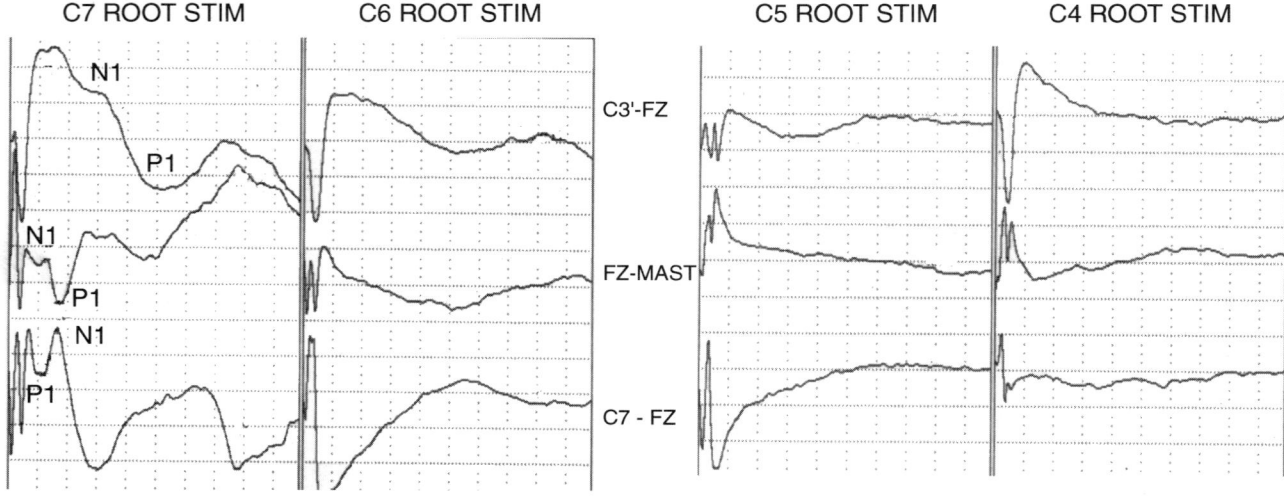

C7 ROOT STIM   C6 ROOT STIM   C5 ROOT STIM   C4 ROOT STIM

C3'-FZ

FZ-MAST

C7 - FZ

3 MSEC/DIV: 1 MICROVOLT/DIV

FIGURE 253–15. Somatosensory evoked potentials recorded at the contralateral scalp to stimulation of the C4-7 nerve roots. No responses were detected to C4, C5, or C6 root stimulation, whereas a clearly recognizable response was seen to C7 stimulation at the cervical, brainstem, and cortical levels.

locutaneous nerve and biceps, further neurotization or intercostal nerve transfer was not considered.

Postoperatively, the patient recovered with no changes in symptoms. Long-term follow-up has not yet been done.

As can be seen in these examples, neurophysiologic testing during peripheral nerve surgery is no longer the simple monitoring of nerve function to prevent intraoperative compromise. Through careful orchestration of SEPs, triggered EMG, spontaneous EMG, CNAPs, and nerve conduction, a comprehensive electrodiagnostic evaluation can be performed in the operating room. Not only can peripheral nerves be rescued from accidental injury, but information can be obtained that leads to an optimal postoperative outcome.

SUMMARY

Diseases and injuries affecting peripheral nerves, plexus, roots, and CNS are common causes for presentation to the electrodiagnostic medical consultant. Clinical assessment is critical to forming a reasonable list of differential diagnoses. The electrodiagnostic evaluation is helpful for localizing lesions, determining the extent of axon loss and prognosis, and following reinnervation over time in more complete injuries.

REFERENCES

1. Aminoff M: Electromyography in Clinical Practice: Clinical and Electrodiagnostic Aspects of Neuromuscular Disease, 3rd ed. Philadelphia, Churchill Livingstone, 1997.
2. Preston D, Shapiro B: Electromyography and Neuromuscular Disorders: Clinical-Electrophysiologic Correlations. Oxford Butterworth-Heinemann Medical, 1997.
3. Stevens J: AAEE minimonograph #26: The electrodiagnosis of carpal tunnel syndrome. Muscle Nerve 10:99–113, 1987.
4. Jablecki C, Andary M, So Y, et al: Literature review of the usefulness of nerve conduction studies and electromyography for the evaluation of patients with carpal tunnel syndrome. Muscle Nerve 16:1392–1414, 1993.
5. Rivner H: Statistical errors and their effect on electrodiagnostic medicine. Muscle Nerve 17:811–814, 1994.
6. Robinson L, Temkin N, Fujimoto W, et al: Effect of statistical methodology on normal limits in nerve conduction studies. Muscle Nerve 14:1084–1090, 1991.
7. Robinson L, Micklesen P, Wang L: Strategies for analyzing nerve conduction data: Superiority of a summary index over single tests. Muscle Nerve 21:1166–1171, 1998.
8. Lew H, Wang L, Robinson L: Test-retest reliability of combined sensory index: Implications for diagnosing carpal tunnel syndrome. Muscle Nerve 23:1261-1264, 2000.
9. Jabre J, Wilbourn A: The EMG findings in 100 consecutive ulnar neuropathies. Acta Neurol Scand 60(Suppl 73):91, 1979.
10. Payan J: Electrophysiological localization of ulnar nerve lesions. J Neurol Neurosurg Psychiatry 32:208, 1969.
11. Stewart J: The variable clinical manifestations of ulnar neuropathies at the elbow. J Neurol Neurosurg Psychiatry 50:252, 1987.
12. Kincaid J: AAEE minimonograph #31: The electrodiagnosis of ulnar neuropathy at the elbow. Muscle Nerve 11:1005–1015, 1988.
13. Kanakamamedala R, Simons D, Porter R, et al: Ulnar nerve entrapment at the elbow localized by short segment stimulation. Arch Phys Med Rehabil 69:959, 1988.
14. Miller R: The cubital tunnel syndrome: Diagnosis and precise localization. Ann Neurol 6:56, 1979.
15. Eisen A: Early diagnosis of ulnar nerve palsy: An electrophysiologic study. Neurology 24:256, 1974.
16. Jensen M, Brant-Zawadzki M, Obuchowski N, et al: Magnetic resonance imaging of the lumbar spine in people without back pain. N Engl J Med 331:69–73, 1994.
17. Nardin R, Patel M, Gudas T, et al: Electromyography and magnetic resonance imaging in the evaluation of radiculopathy. Muscle Nerve 22:151–155, 1999.
18. Robinson L: Electromyography, magnetic resonance imaging, and radiculopathy: It's time to focus on specificity. Muscle Nerve 22:149–150, 1999.
19. Wilbourn A, Aminoff M: AAEE minimonograph #32: The electrophysiologic examination in patients with radiculopathies. Muscle Nerve 11:1099–1114, 1988.
20. Snowden ML, Haselkorn JK, Kraft GH, et al: Dermatomal so-

matosensory evoked potentials in the diagnosis of lumbosacral spinal stenosis: Comparison with imaging studies. Muscle Nerve 15:1036–1044, 1992.

21. Chaudry V, Cornblath D: Wallerian degeneration in human nerves: Serial electrophysiological studies. Muscle Nerve 15:687–693, 1992.

22. Thesleff S: Physiological effects of denervation of muscle. Ann N Y Acad Sci 228:89–103, 1974.

23. Campbell W, Pridgeon R, Riaz G, et al: Sparing of the flexor carpi ulnaris in ulnar neuropathy at the elbow. Muscle Nerve 12:965–967, 1989.

24. Buchthal F: Fibrillations: Clinical electrophysiology. In Culp WJ, Ochoa J (eds): Abnormal Nerves and Muscle Generators. New York, Oxford University Press, 1982, pp 632–662.

25. Dorfman L: Quantitative clinical electrophysiology in the evaluation of nerve injury and regeneration. Muscle Nerve 13:822–828, 1990.

26. Brandstater M, Fullerton M: Sensory nerve conduction studies in cervical root lesions. Can J Neurol Sci 10:152, 1983.

27. Tackman W, Radu E: Observations of the application of electrophysiological methods in the diagnosis of cervical root compressions. Eur Neurol 22:397–404, 1983.

28. Sunderland S: Nerves and Nerve Injuries, 2nd ed. New York, Churchill Livingstone, 1978.

29. Wertsch J, Oswald T, Roberts M: Role of intraneural topography in diagnosis and localization in electrodiagnostic medicine. Phys Med Rehabil Clin N Am 5:465–475, 1994.

30. Zandbergen E, deHaan R, Stoutenbeek C, et al: Systematic review of early prediction of poor outcome in anoxic ischemic coma. Lancet 352:1808–1812, 1998.

31. Rothstein T, Thomas E, Sumi S: Predicting outcome in hypoxic-ischemic coma: A prospective clinical and electrophysiologic study. Electroencephalogr Clin Neurophysiol 79:101–107, 1991.

32. Kliot M, Slimp J: Techniques for assessment of peripheral nerve function at surgery. In Loftus C, Traynelis V (eds): Intraoperative Monitoring Techniques in Neurosurgery. New York, McGraw-Hill, 1994, pp 275–285.

33. Slimp J: Intraoperative Monitoring of nerve repairs. Hand Clin 16:25–36, 2000.

34. Slimp J, Kliot M: Electrophysiological monitoring: Peripheral nerve surgery. In Andrews R (ed): Intraoperative Neuroprotection. Baltimore, Williams & Wilkins, 1996, pp 375–392.

35. Kline D: Surgical repair of peripheral nerve injury. Muscle Nerve 13:843–852, 1990.

36. Kline D: Penfield lecture: A quarter century's experience with intraoperative nerve action potential recording. Can J Neurol Sci 20:3–10, 1993.

37. Kline D, Hudson A: Acute injuries of peripheral nerves. In Youmans J (ed): Neurological Surgery, 3rd ed. Philadelphia, WB Saunders, 1990, pp 2423–2510.

38. Kline D, Kim D, Midha R, et al: Management and results of sciatic nerve injuries: A 24-year experience. J Neurosurg 89:13–23, 1998.

39. Oberle J, Antoniadis G, Rath S, et al: Value of nerve action potentials in the surgical management of traumatic nerve lesions. Neurosurgery 41:1337–1342, 1997.

40. Tiel R, Happel L, Kline D: Nerve action potential recording method and equipment. Neurosurgery 39:103–108, 1996.

41. Delestre F, Lonchampt P, Dubas F: Neural generator of P14 far-field somatosensory evoked potential studied in a patient with a pontine lesion. Electroencephalogr Clin Neurophysiol 65:227–230, 1986.

42. Jacobson G, Tew J: The origin of the scalp recorded P14 following electrical stimulation of the median nerve: Intraoperative observations. Electroencephalogr Clin Neurophysiol 71:73–76, 1988.

43. Maugiere F, Courjon J, Schott B: Dissociation of early SEP components in unilateral traumatic section of the lower medulla. Ann Neurol 13:309–313, 1983.

44. Lam A, Sharar S, Mayberg T: Isoflurane compared with nitrous oxide anaesthesia for intraoperative monitoring of somatosensory-evoked potentials. Can J Anaesth 41:295–300, 1994.

45. Pathak K, Amaddio M, Scoles P: Effects of halothane, enflurane, and isoflurane in nitrous oxide on multilevel somatosensory evoked potentials. Anesthesiology 7:207–212, 1989.

46. Peterson D, Drummond J, Todd M: Effects of halothane, enflurane, isoflurane, and nitrous oxide on somatosensory evoked potentials in humans. Anesthesiology 65:35–40, 1986.

47. Slimp J, Stolov W, Wagner T: Spine and scalp recordings as a function of intensity: A model for changes during spinal cord monitoring. Spine 21:99–103, 1996.

Magnetic Resonance Imaging for Peripheral Nerve Disorders

GERALD A. GRANT ■ GAVIN W. BRITZ ■ ROBERT GOODKIN ■ JEFFREY G. JARVIK ■ KENNETH MARAVILLA ■ MICHEL KLIOT

Radiologic imaging techniques developed over the past 30 years have revolutionized the diagnosis and treatment of neurological disorders. These techniques, especially computed tomography (CT) and magnetic resonance imaging (MRI), were rapidly applied to regions of the central nervous system (CNS) in the brain and spinal cord. Seldom is a surgery performed on the CNS without a preoperative imaging study that serves as an essential roadmap for the surgeon. Until recently, imaging studies played a less important and integral role in the evaluation and treatment of patients with diseases involving the peripheral nervous system (PNS). In part, this diminished role resulted from technical difficulties in visualizing peripheral nerves and in distinguishing them from surrounding soft tissue structures. As these technical difficulties have been surmounted, especially using new and rapidly evolving MRI techniques, so has the potential usefulness of imaging studies grown in evaluating and treating a variety of peripheral nerve disorders.

In this chapter, we summarize some of the radiologic developments, particularly in the field of MRI, and provide examples of their growing clinical application and utility in diagnosing and treating a variety of peripheral nerve problems.[1] We discuss how rapidly evolving MRI techniques are helping to manage patients with peripheral nerve mass lesions, focal entrapment neuropathies, and traumatic nerve injuries.

IMAGING FOR PERIPHERAL NERVE DISORDERS

Radiologic imaging for peripheral nerve disorders was limited initially to the demonstration of secondary skeletal changes on x-ray films. Initially, CT and ultrasonography were of limited usefulness because of their relatively poor ability to visualize peripheral nerve structures.[2–5] Fine-cut CT-myelography has proved to be very accurate in predicting spinal nerve root avulsion in patients suffering from severe proximal brachial plexus injuries.[10] Advances in ultrasonography have enabled improved visualization of peripheral nerve structures.[4] However, MRI has proved to be more effective in resolving the fine anatomic detail of soft tissue structures such as peripheral nerves.[6, 7] Innovations in MRI have made it possible to identify nerves reliably when adjacent to lymph nodes, adipose collections, blood vessels, ligaments, and other structures and tissues of similar size, shape, and location. However, conventional MRI techniques suffer from spatial and contrast resolution limitations, as well as motion artifact.

Technical advances using phased-array surface coils and fast spin-echo (FSE) pulse sequences on a standard 1.5-T MRI system have made possible the development of magnetic resonance neurography (MRN). These developments have allowed MRI to become increasingly useful in diagnosing and treating a variety of peripheral nerve problems, ranging from masses arising from peripheral nerves, such as schwannomas and neurofibromas, to entrapment neuropathies, such as carpal and cubital tunnel syndromes, as well as peripheral nerve trauma.

TECHNICAL ASPECTS OF MAGNETIC RESONANCE NEUROGRAPHY

MRN, as originally described by Filler and colleagues,[8, 9] can be defined as tissue-selective imaging directed at identifying and evaluating characteristics of nerve morphology. This technique is based on enhancing the signal differences between peripheral nerves and the surrounding tissues using specialized diffusion pulse sequences on high-field-strength MR scanners. These diffusion pulse sequences capitalized on the unique anisotropic properties of nerves whereby water diffuses longitudinally along nerves more readily than in other directions. Another strategy has been to generate images with improved spatial resolution on standard 1.5-T MRI systems using custom-designed phased-array coils. These specialized MR coils have been developed and customized to optimize the visualization of anatomic structures within a particular body region. For example, data from four separate coils that constitute the array are combined to give a composite image. The resultant incremental increase in the signal-to-noise ratio over conventional coils can be used to optimize spatial resolution, and combining the field of view of the multiple coils in the array allows for a relatively larger field of view. We are able to obtain an in-plane spatial resolution as fine as 0.4 mm.

Standard MR pulse sequences are used to visualize different anatomic features of normal and abnormal peripheral nerves and the surrounding tissues. Image contrast depends on the "weighting" of the pulse sequences used to acquire the MR image data. T1-weighted pulse sequence images (i.e., short TR/short TE) are optimal for demonstrating fine anatomic detail such as the fascicular structure of nerves (Figs. 254–1 and 254–2). An important characteristic of this pulse

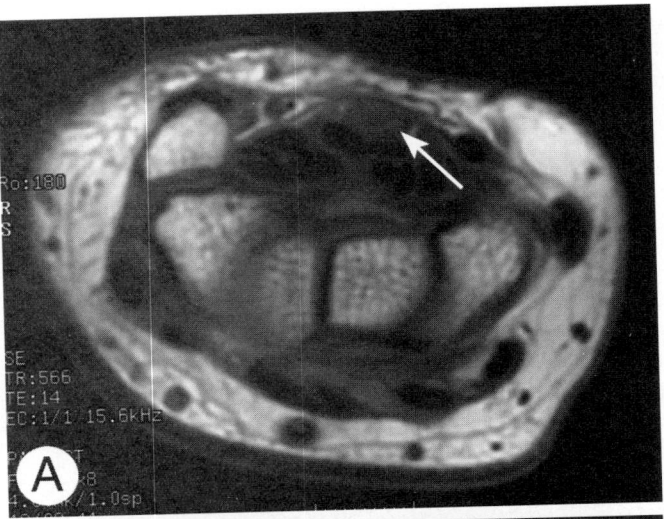

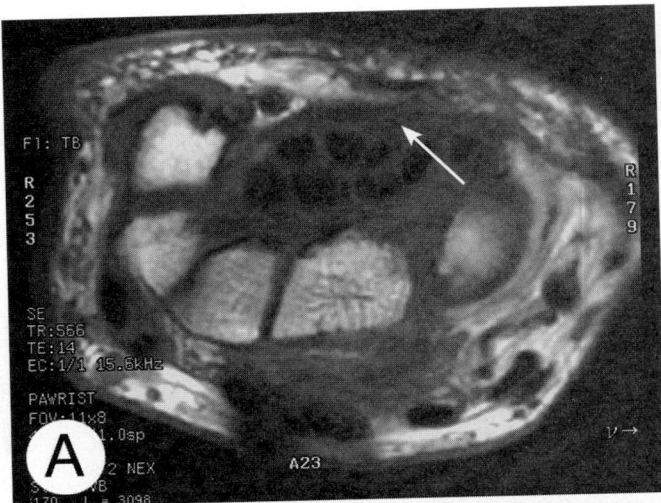

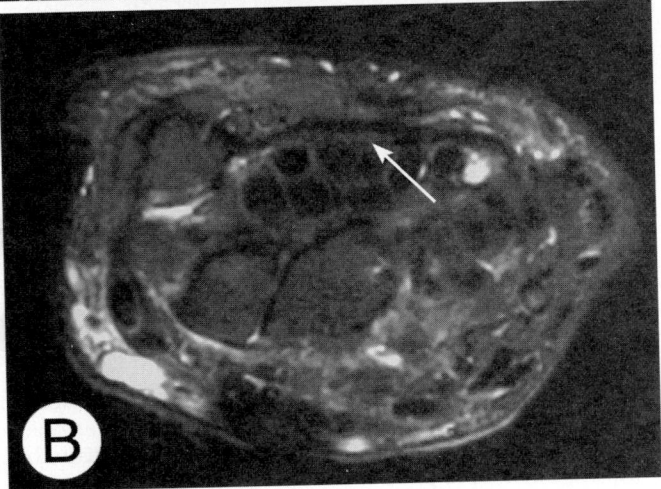

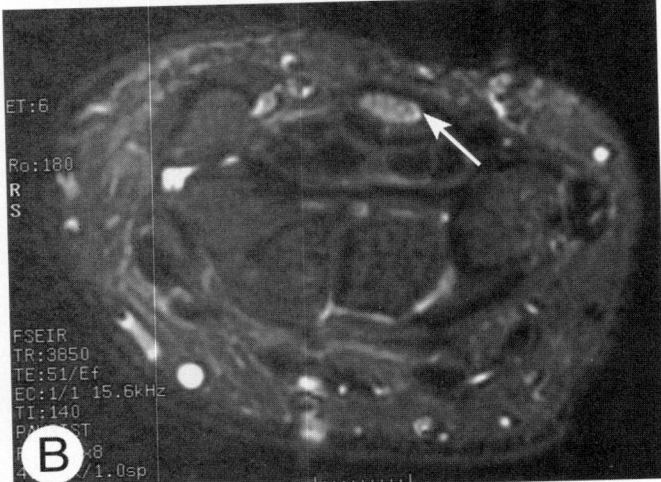

FIGURE 254–2. Axial magnetic resonance images through the palm of a patient with carpal tunnel syndrome at the level of the pisiform bone using T1-weighted *(A)* and short tau inversion recovery (STIR) *(B)* pulse sequences. The median nerve *(white arrows)* has an abnormally increased STIR signal *(B)* compared with the median nerve of an asymptomatic person (see Fig. 254–1*B*). Notice the prominent fascicular structure of the nerve, which is best seen in *B*. (From Grant GA, Goodkin R, Jarvik JG, et al: The utility of magnetic resonance imaging in evaluating peripheral nerve disorders. Muscle Nerve 25:314–331, 2002.)

FIGURE 254–1. Axial magnetic resonance images through the palm of a person with no symptoms of carpal tunnel syndrome at the level of the pisiform bone using T1-weighted *(A)* and short tau inversion recovery (STIR) *(B)* pulse sequences. The fascicular structure of the nerve is best seen in *B*. The median nerve *(white arrow)* has normal STIR signal intensity, which is isointense with normally innervated muscle. (From Grant GA, Goodkin R, Jarvik JG, et al: The utility of magnetic resonance imaging in evaluating peripheral nerve disorders. Muscle Nerve 25:314–331, 2002.)

sequence is that fat appears bright. A normal nerve on T1-weighted images appears as a smooth, round to ovoid structure that is isointense in signal compared with normal muscle. A rim of bright-signal fat tissue often surrounds peripheral nerves. Individual nerve fascicles, seen best in cross section, are demarcated by a thin rim of perineurium and internal epineurial tissue that is slightly brighter in signal by virtue of its fatty tissue content. The T1-weighted pulse sequence in combination with an intravenous contrast agent, such as gadolinium, can be useful in delineating the anatomic relationship of nerve fascicles to closely associated mass lesions, such as schwannomas and neurofibromas.[6] Gadolinium enhances tumors but not normal peripheral nerves.[10] The MR signal of normal peripheral nerves on T2-weighted images, such as T2-weighted FSE or short tau inversion recovery (STIR) pulse sequences, is isointense to mildly hyperintense relative to normal muscle. Prominent nerve fascicles seen in cross section can have a slightly higher signal intensity than the surrounding perineurium and internal epineurial tissue.

In the setting of acute nerve trauma or chronic nerve entrapment, the injured nerve remains isointense to normally innervated muscle on T1-weighted images but becomes hyperintense to muscle on pulse sequences sensitive to free water content, such as T2-weighted FSE and STIR sequences.[8, 9, 11] The STIR pulse sequence has two advantages. The bright signal from fat is suppressed with a larger field of view, and it has an increased sensitivity to water content compared with standard T2-weighted pulse sequences. Fat-saturated, FSE, T2-weighted sequences (i.e., long TR/long TE) may be used in place of STIR, with the advantage of increased spatial resolution. The increased signal intensity seen in injured peripheral nerves on T2-weighted and STIR pulse sequences may reflect changes in water content due to altered axoplasmic flow, endoneurial or perineurial edema as a result of changes in the blood-nerve barrier, or axonal and myelin degeneration.[10] In contrast to the evaluation of peripheral nerve tumors, gadolinium has not been very helpful in the study of acute traumatic nerve injury.

The ability of MRI to construct images in any plane allows the examiner to choose imaging planes that optimize the visualization of specific nerves in particular locations and orientations. Axial and coronal planes of section are most useful in visualizing the median, ulnar, and sciatic nerves, which are all longitudinally oriented within an extremity. The coronal and oblique sagittal planes of section are best for brachial plexus imaging in the neck. For imaging the cervical spinal nerves within the neck, the coronal plane combined with a straight sagittal or oblique axial plane is optimal.

MAGNETIC RESONANCE IMAGING IN THE EVALUATION OF PERIPHERAL NERVE MASSES

With the advent of CT, ultrasonography, and MRI, radiologic studies have played an increasingly important role in the preoperative evaluation of peripheral nerve mass lesions.[12, 13] Improvements in MRI, such as the use of phased-array coils, have made it possible to generate multiplanar images with higher resolution, thereby allowing for clearer visualization of nerves. The high-resolution imaging of the fascicular anatomy of normal peripheral nerves and its distortion by mass lesions (e.g., tumors, cysts) becomes useful for preoperative diagnosis and as a roadmap for surgical planning. A major surgical goal is the removal of the tumor from the nerve with maximal preservation of function. An important feature for the successful removal of tumors involving peripheral nerves is the relationship of the tumor to functioning nerve fascicles.

Normal peripheral nerve fascicles are isointense on T1-weighted sequences and slightly hyperintense on T2- and STIR-weighted sequences. Signs of peripheral nerve disease include gross changes in the nerve configuration, loss or distortion of the characteristic fascicular pattern, and swelling of individual fascicles with abnormally high signal intensity on T2-weighted and STIR sequences. The cause of the abnormally high signal intensity in pathologic fascicles remains unknown, although it has been speculated that it represents edema from increased endoneurial fluid or alterations in axoplasmic flow. Peripheral nerve masses usually appear as cylindrical, fusiform, spherical, or irregular enlargements along the course of the nerve. Three-dimensional reconstruction algorithms have made it possible to visualize a mass in relation to the nerve from which it is arising over some distance. Almost all tumors show enhancement on T1-weighted images after the administration of gadolinium.

Neurofibromas, Schwannomas, and Ganglion Cysts

The most common peripheral nerve tumors are schwannomas and neurofibromas, which originate from the supporting cells such as the nerve sheath cells that make up the myelin, also known as Schwann cells.[14] Most peripheral nerve sheath tumors are homogeneous or mildly inhomogeneous on MRI and have smooth and well-defined margins. These tumors display neutral to moderately bright signal on T1-weighted images and bright signal on T2-weighted images compared with adjacent muscle tissue. It is usually difficult, if not impossible, to reliably differentiate schwannomas from neurofibromas on the basis of MRI features despite their different pathologic characteristics.[15] Schwannomas can be surgically resected with little or no loss of sensory and motor function. Neurofibromas are more difficult to resect without loss of function. However, Kline and colleagues[14] showed that most neurofibromas could be resected with minimal loss of function when removed carefully and with the aid of intraoperative electrophysiologic monitoring.

High-resolution MRI using phased-array coils has made it possible to visualize the relationship of nerve fascicles to intraneural and extraneural tumors (Fig. 254–3). We have found these images to be particularly useful in preoperatively identifying, localizing, and assessing the surgical resectability of peripheral nerve tumors.[6] In our experience, preoperative high-resolution MR images have correlated well with the intraoperative findings of functioning nerve fibers and nonfunctioning tumor tissue identified on the basis of anatomic appearance and response to electrophysiologic stimulation.[6] These images have often allowed us to anticipate where to find functioning nerve fibers, which often become incorporated into portions of the tumor capsule, particularly when the tumor is large in relation to the peripheral nerve from which it is arising. On four occasions, we have encountered at surgery a hyperplastic lymph node close to a nerve that we mistakenly thought was a peripheral nerve tumor.

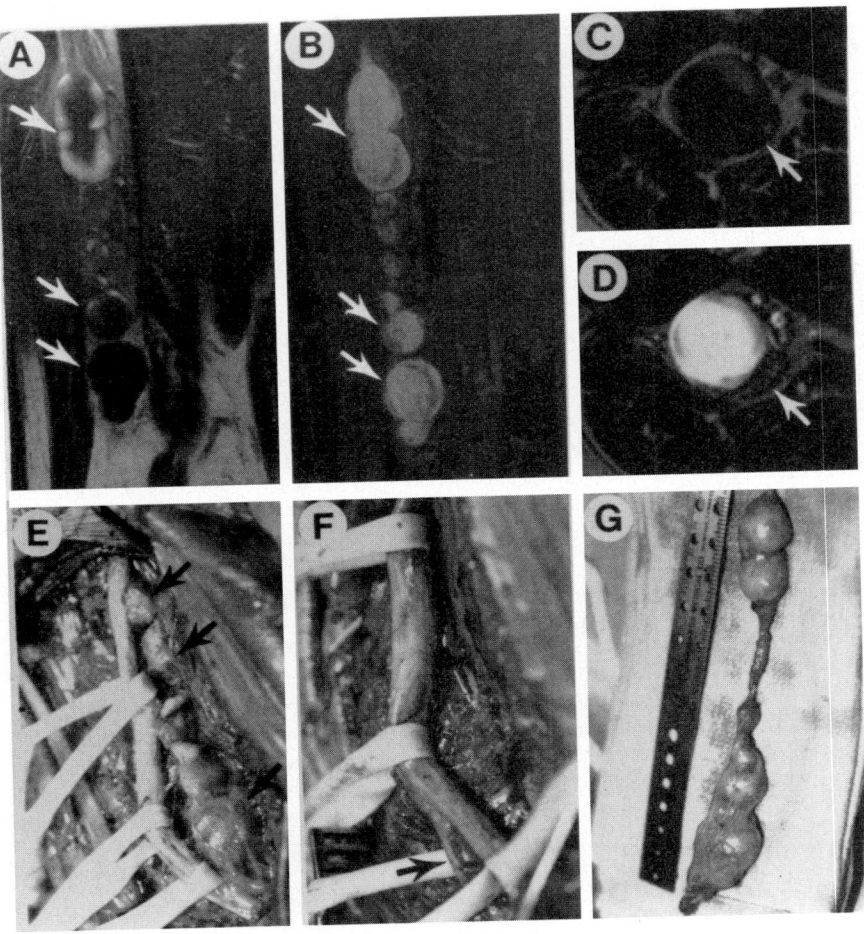

FIGURE 254–3. Magnetic resonance images of a 69-year-old woman with a right sciatic neurofibroma in the lower thigh. *A,* Coronal, fat-suppressed, T1-weighted image after administration of gadolinium shows heterogeneous enhancement of a multilobulated and cystic mass lesion *(white arrows)* in the posterior thigh. *B,* Coronal, short tau inversion recovery (STIR) image shows high signal intensity within the multilobulated lesion *(white arrows).* *C,* Axial, T1-weighted magnetic resonance image after administration of gadolinium. *D,* Axial, T2-weighted magnetic resonance image shows a discrete demarcation of the fascicular structure of the sciatic nerve *(white arrow)* along the posteromedial circumference of the tumor. *E,* Intraoperative photograph shows Penrose loops elevating the sciatic nerve from the multilobulated neurofibroma *(black arrows).* *F,* Intraoperative photograph after removal of the neurofibroma. Notice the splitting of the distal sciatic nerve into the common peroneal and tibial *(black arrow)* nerve branches. *G,* Photograph of the resected neurofibroma oriented as shown in *A* and *B.* (Adapted from Kuntz C, Blake L, Britz GW, et al: Magnetic resonance neurography of peripheral nerve lesions in the lower extremity. Neurosurgery 39:750–757, 1996.)

These masses showed abnormally bright signal on T2-weighted images and contrast enhancement on T1-weighted images. A relatively subtle feature that might help to distinguish these hyperplastic lymph nodes from tumor was their somewhat brighter than expected appearance on T1-weighted images, most likely reflecting their high fatty tissue content.

High-resolution MRI has also been useful in visualizing other types of masses, such as ganglion cysts. These cystic structures have characteristically low signal intensity on T1-weighted images and high signal intensity on T2-weighted images (Fig. 254–4).

Differentiating Radiation-Induced Plexitis from Tumor

High-resolution MRI has helped us to differentiate recurrent tumor from radiation-induced plexitis, as in patients who have undergone treatment for breast cancer. In the case of recurrent tumor, we expect to see focal and often irregular enlargement of the nerve associated with increased signal intensity on T2-weighted images and contrast enhancement on T1-weighted images (Fig. 254–5). In contrast, radiation-induced plexitis produces uniform enlargement or narrowing of the involved nerves with a diffuse pattern of increased signal intensity on T2-weighted images (Fig. 254–5). Unfortunately,

high-resolution MRI has not yet allowed us to differentiate malignant from benign peripheral nerve tumors. Ongoing work at our institution is demonstrating the ability of positron-emission tomography (PET) using glucose analogs to visualize increased metabolic activity in the more malignant tumors. The development and application of new magnetic resonance spectroscopic techniques may also help to make this clinically important distinction preoperatively in the future.

MAGNETIC RESONANCE IMAGING EVALUATION OF FOCAL PERIPHERAL NERVE ENTRAPMENT NEUROPATHIES

Entrapment neuropathies occur at anatomic sites where a peripheral nerve is chronically compromised through compression or tethering, or both, to the extent that symptoms and clinical findings of nerve dysfunction result.[16, 17, 18, 19, 20]

Carpal Tunnel Syndrome

Carpal tunnel syndrome (CTS) is the most commonly diagnosed entrapment neuropathy.[21, 22] The underlying pathophysiology is thought to be mechanical distortion of the median nerve within the fibro-osseus canal

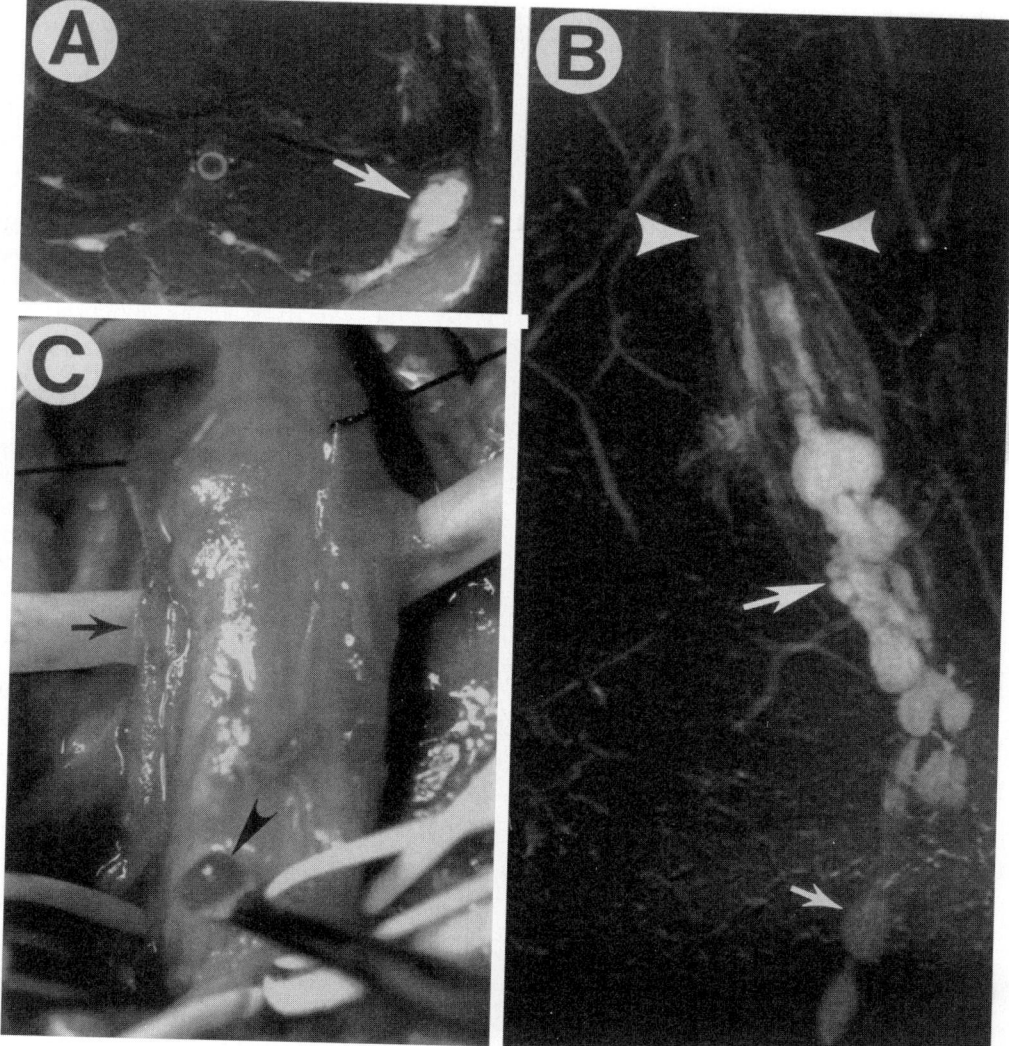

FIGURE 254–4. Magnetic resonance neurography of a 40-year-old man with multiple intraneural cysts involving the left common peroneal nerve and its deep peroneal nerve branch. *A*, Axial, T2-weighted, fast spin-echo (FSE) image shows high-signal-intensity cystic lesions *(white arrow)* within the common peroneal nerve. *B*, Coronal, T2-weighted, FSE multiplanar reconstruction shows multiple, high-signal-intensity intraneural cysts within the distal common peroneal nerve *(large white arrow)* that extend into the deep peroneal nerve branch *(small white arrow)*. Notice the abnormally bright nerve fascicles *(between white arrowheads)* splayed apart by the cysts. *C*, An intraoperative photograph demonstrates abnormal enlargement of the common peroneal nerve *(black arrow)*. Notice the extrusion of gelatinous material from a surgically ruptured cyst *(black arrowhead)*. (Adapted from Kuntz C, Blake L, Britz GW, et al: Magnetic resonance neurography of peripheral nerve lesions in the lower extremity. Neurosurgery 39:750–757, 1996.)

formed between the flexor retinaculum and the carpal bones at the wrist, a space also occupied by the superficial and deep flexor tendons of the fingers. Chronic compression or tethering, or both, of the median nerve is presumed to cause vascular compromise and mechanical damage, first to the myelin and later to the axons of the nerve.[20, 23] Clinical symptoms usually consist of tingling and numbness in a median nerve distribution, which are often worse at night and exacerbated by activity, combined with hand pain and weakness. Positive clinical signs consisting of a flick sign (i.e., shaking the hand to relieve symptoms), Tinel's sign (i.e., dysesthesias produced by tapping over the median nerve in the palm), and Phalen's sign (i.e., dysesthesias elicited by extreme wrist flexion) have sensitivities ranging from 20% to 70% and specificities ranging from 47% to 83%.[24–27] Objective findings on physical examination, such as reduced two-point discrimination and weakness of the thenar muscles, are usually seen only in more advanced cases of CTS.[26] Although patients with a clinical diagnosis of CTS can improve with medical therapy, such as modifying activities or

use of a splint, a significant number require further treatment, such as a surgical decompression.

To confirm the diagnosis of CTS and thereby optimize treatment decisions, electrodiagnostic studies are often performed, especially in patients who fail to improve after an initial course of medical therapy. Electrodiagnostic studies, specifically nerve conduction studies, have sensitivities and specificities of approximately 90%.[22, 28] However, the prevalence of electrodiagnostic abnormalities among asymptomatic workers has been found to range from 9% to 16%, resulting in positive predictive values (i.e., true positive studies/ all positive studies) as low as 30%.[29] Electrodiagnostic studies have not been able to predict reliably who will benefit from medical versus surgical treatment.[30, 31] Electrodiagnostic evidence for CTS can also be difficult to obtain in patients with diffuse nerve conduction abnormalities due to a superimposed peripheral neuropathy (e.g., diabetes), particularly if severe.[32]

The causes of CTS are multiple, but the most common include tenosynovitis of the flexor tendons due to repetitive trauma, systemic diseases, and hormonal

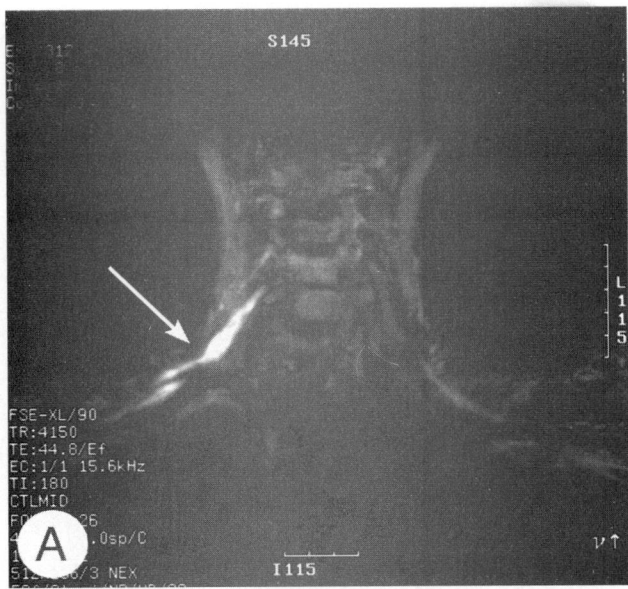

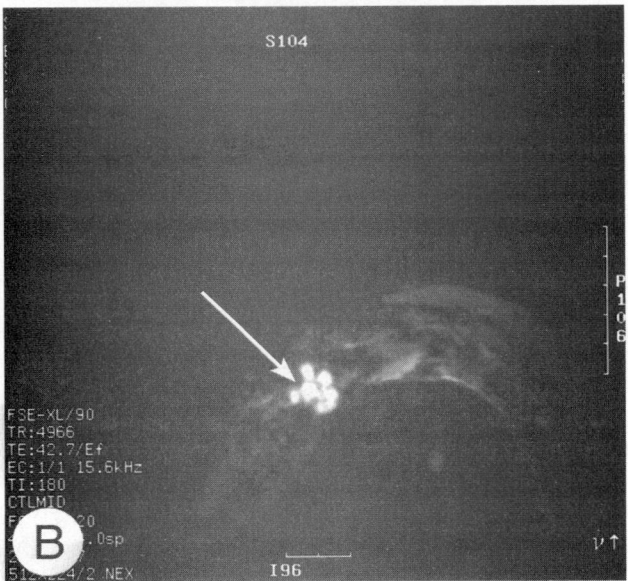

FIGURE 254–5. Coronal *(A)* and axial *(B)* short tau inversion recovery (STIR) magnetic resonance sequences were obtained through the brachial plexus in a patient with a radiation-induced right brachial plexopathy caused by treatment of breast cancer. The abnormal signal involves the spinal nerves and trunks *(white arrow in A)* and the divisions and cords more distally *(white arrow in B)*. No evidence of tumor recurrence was found. (Adapted from Grant GA, Goodkin R, Jarvik JG, et al: The utility of magnetic resonance imaging in evaluating peripheral nerve disorders. Muscle Nerve 25:314–331, 2002.)

changes (e.g., rheumatoid arthritis, diabetes, pregnancy, hypothyroidism); rarely, CTS is caused by space-occupying masses (e.g., ganglion cysts). All of these causes are thought to increase pressure within the canal. Whereas electrodiagnostic studies assess median nerve function, MRI visualizes anatomic features and abnormalities of the median nerve and surrounding tissues. MRI has been used to visualize a number of anatomic features in patients diagnosed with CTS, usu-

ally on the basis of clinical and electrodiagnostic criteria, and in control subjects. Such anatomic features have included median nerve configuration (i.e., an indicator of compression or swelling), signal (i.e., an indicator of intraneural edema), and location (i.e., in relation to the surrounding flexor tendons); mobility of the median nerve with changes in hand posture[33]; vascular circulation to the median nerve; thickening of the surrounding flexor tendon sheaths with widening of the interspaces; cross-sectional area of the carpal tunnel; bowing of the flexor retinaculum; and thenar muscle signal denervation changes.[9, 34–50]

Our group performed a study in which MRI findings were correlated with clinical and electrodiagnostic findings and with postoperative outcome for 43 hands of 32 patients with a clinical diagnosis of CTS.[34] Abnormal MR STIR signal or configuration changes involving the median nerve, or both, were found in all of the symptomatic patients. Such abnormalities were found in none of five asymptomatic control subjects. Nerve conduction abnormalities were found in 93% and electromyographic abnormalities in 33% of the symptomatic hands. A carpal tunnel release was performed on 27 hands, with a good or excellent outcome resulting in 74%. An abnormal nerve configuration on MRI was associated with an 83% chance of good or excellent outcome after surgery.

The diagnostic accuracy of MRI for CTS has been investigated in several studies.[37, 39, 40, 42, 45, 46, 48, 51–53] Jarvik and colleagues[54] designed a study to evaluate the reliability and diagnostic accuracy of MRI when used to image the median nerve in a large, prospectively assembled cohort of 120 subjects, 18 to 70 years old, with clinically suspect CTS.[55] All subjects were examined by a single study nurse who performed a standardized hand examination and administered a battery of questionnaires focused on their hand symptoms.[26, 56] All patients then underwent a standardized MRI study and a standardized nerve conduction study of their symptomatic hand to evaluate median nerve function and anatomy. Patients were considered to have CTS if they had a classic or probable hand diagram and a median minus ulnar nerve conduction peak latency of 0.3 msec or longer recorded across an 8-cm palm-to-wrist distance.[57] Two neuroradiologists graded the following MRI parameters on a four-point scale (i.e., normal, mild, moderate, and severe) with no knowledge of the clinical or electrodiagnostic findings: median nerve STIR signal intensity, degree of nerve compression, bowing of the flexor retinaculum, thickening of the flexor tendon interspace, signal within the palmar bursa, thenar muscle signal, and nerve fascicular prominence. A statistical analysis of the data to determine the diagnostic accuracy of MRI demonstrated that no single MRI parameter was extremely sensitive and specific. Sensitivity was greatest for the overall abnormality score of the MR images (96%), followed closely by increased median nerve signal (91%) when a rating of mild, moderate, or severe was counted as abnormal. An interesting finding was the strong correlation between length of abnormal median nerve signal on T2-weighted images and the median-ulnar nerve conduction latency abnormality. This finding provided strong evidence that T2-weighted MRI nerve signal abnormalities closely reflected nerve pathology.

Several conclusions can be drawn from this study. First, MRI can be used to identify reliably the median nerve and other structures within the carpal tunnel. Second, the diagnostic accuracy of MRI compared with electrodiagnostic studies is only moderate in evaluating patients with CTS. This finding may not be all that surprising, because the two methods are evaluating different aspects of this disease. It must be kept in mind that subjects were diagnosed as having CTS (i.e., the gold standard) on the basis of clinical and electrodiagnostic criteria. MRI could prove useful in helping to predict which patients will respond best to medical or surgical treatment. MRI may also be useful in diagnosing and guiding treatment of patients with clinical CTS who have normal electrodiagnostic studies, a group representing 10% of the subjects in this study. It is important to follow their clinical course in response to medical or surgical therapy. MRI may be helpful in diagnosing and treating patients with clinical CTS who have electrodiagnostic abnormalities that preclude localization of median nerve pathology to the carpal tunnel, such as patients with advanced CTS and those with a severe, superimposed peripheral diabetic neuropathy.

Ulnar Nerve Entrapment at the Elbow

Ulnar nerve entrapment at the elbow (UNEE) is the second most common entrapment neuropathy.[13, 58, 59] It is thought that UNEE is caused by mechanical compression or tethering of the ulnar nerve in the cubital tunnel, a connective tissue sleeve formed from the retinaculum that extends from the medial epicondyle to the olecranon process and then distally for about 3 cm.[60] Injury to the ulnar nerve can also occur when it subluxates over the medial epicondyle during elbow flexion in patients with an ill-formed cubital tunnel. In a few patients, identifiable structural abnormalities are found, such as fractures of the distal humerus, ganglion cysts in and around the elbow, an anomalous anconeus muscle, and rarely, a peripheral nerve tumor.

The diagnosis of UNEE is usually made on the basis of symptoms in an ulnar nerve distribution combined with evidence of ulnar nerve pathology localized to the elbow. Electrodiagnostic studies, consisting of nerve conduction measurements across long and short ("inching") segments of ulnar nerve, and electromyography are useful when they corroborate the diagnosis of UNEE. These studies have a reported diagnostic accuracy ranging from 20% to 100%.[8, 9, 15, 21, 41, 61–63] Other disease processes can mimic UNEE, such as cervical radiculopathy, brachial neuritis, or a lung apex tumor (e.g., Pancoast tumor) involving the C8 or T1, or both, spinal nerves, as well as ulnar nerve compression within the hand at Guyon's canal.

Treatment for UNEE can be broadly divided into two categories: medical and surgical. Medical treatment includes ergonomic measures such as splinting, using a protective elbow pad, avoidance of activities that contribute to symptoms, and nonsteroidal anti-

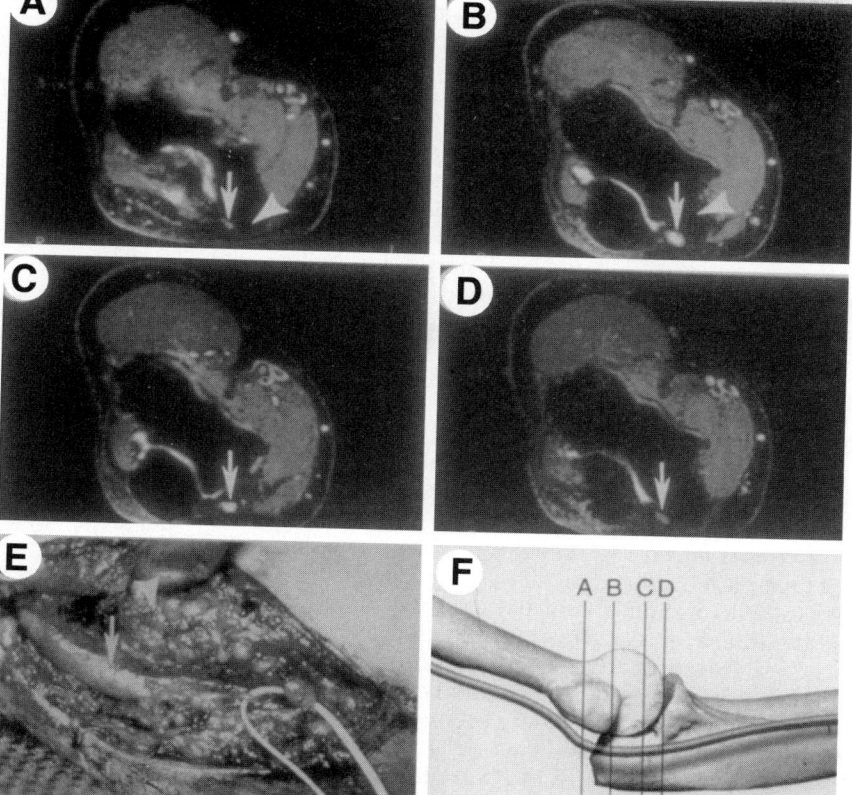

FIGURE 254–6. Magnetic resonance imaging axial sections were obtained using a short tau inversion recovery (STIR) pulse sequence across the elbow at levels demonstrated schematically in *F* in a patient with left ulnar nerve entrapment at the elbow. The ulnar nerve *(white arrow in A to E)* is posterior to the medial epicondyle *(white arrowhead in A and B)*. Notice the increased signal and size of the ulnar nerve across the cubital tunnel *(B and C)* and decreased signal and size proximally *(A)* and distally *(D)*. An intraoperative photograph *(E)* shows exposure of the enlarged segment of the left ulnar nerve *(white arrow)* posterior to the medial epicondyle *(white arrowhead)*. (Adapted from Britz GW, Haynor DR, Kuntz C, et al: Carpal tunnel syndrome: Correlation of MRI, clinical, electrodiagnostic, and intraoperative findings. Neurosurgery 37:1097–1103, 1995.)

inflammatory drugs. Indications for surgery are continued symptoms despite conservative treatment and evidence of intrinsic hand muscle weakness, atrophy, or denervation on electromyographic studies. Several types of surgical procedure have been developed: simple decompression of the ulnar nerve in the cubital tunnel; decompression and transposition of the ulnar nerve into a subcutaneous, intramuscular, or submuscular position; and medial epicondylectomy.[10, 44, 59, 64] An analysis of the literature over the past 27 years failed to demonstrate a clinically important difference between these strategies, and good or excellent outcomes were found for only 69% of patients.[65] A better method of diagnosing UNEE and selecting patients for surgery is needed.

We performed a prospective study of 31 symptomatic ulnar nerves in 27 patients with a clinical diagnosis of UNEE, correlating MRI, clinical, electrodiagnostic, and operative findings and outcomes.[34] Electrodiagnostic studies confirmed ulnar neuropathy in 24 (77%) of 31 nerves, with localization to the elbow in 21 nerves (68%). MRI using STIR sequences demonstrated increased signal in 30 (97%) ulnar nerves across the elbow, with enlargement of the ulnar nerve seen proximally in 23 (74%) nerves (Fig. 254–6). All 12 nerves demonstrated abnormally increased signal on MRI, but 2 (17%) had normal electrodiagnostic studies. A control group of 10 asymptomatic subjects demonstrated no MRI abnormalities of their ulnar nerves across the elbow.

We undertook a pilot study of 21 patients diagnosed clinically with UNEE, all of whom underwent surgery (unpublished results). In all patients, MRI was performed in the axial plane through the elbow region on a Phillips 1.5-T Gyroscan or a General Electric Signal 1.5-T MR imager. Spin-density (TR/TE = 2000–2500/17–20), T2-weighted (TR/TE = 2000–2500/80–100), and STIR pulse sequences (TR/TE/TI = 2000/20/160) were obtained for all patients. All patients also underwent preoperative nerve conduction studies across long and short segments of the ulnar nerve, as well as needle electromyography (EMG). Intraoperatively, the ulnar nerve was isolated and nerve conduction performed with electrodes applied directly to the nerve across short and long segments of exposed nerve. Preoperative electrodiagnostic studies showed ulnar nerve abnormalities in 15 (71%) of 21 patients, and 19 (90%) of the 21 had intraoperative electrodiagnostic abnormalities. All 21 (100%) subjects showed MRI signal abnormalities of the ulnar nerve across the elbow. Postoperatively, clinical improvement occurred in 17 (81%) patients, whereas 3 (14%) had no improvement and 1 (5%) experienced worsening symptoms.

Our pilot study indicated a high degree of sensitivity for MRI in identifying pathology of the ulnar nerve at the elbow, which was superior to electrodiagnostic studies. Intraoperative electrodiagnostic studies were shown to have a higher sensitivity for demonstrating ulnar nerve pathology than preoperative electrodiagnostic studies. Additional work is necessary to determine MRI's specificity and its ability to select patients who can benefit from surgery.

Several other peripheral nerve entrapment syndromes are rare and difficult to diagnose with confidence.[18, 20] As a result, the clinical and diagnostic criteria for characterizing these syndromes are not nearly as well defined as they are for CTS and UNEE. Our experience in performing MRI on patients suspected of having one of these syndromes is at best anecdotal.

Thoracic Outlet Syndrome

Neurogenic thoracic outlet syndrome (TOS) is thought to be caused by compression of the brachial plexus in

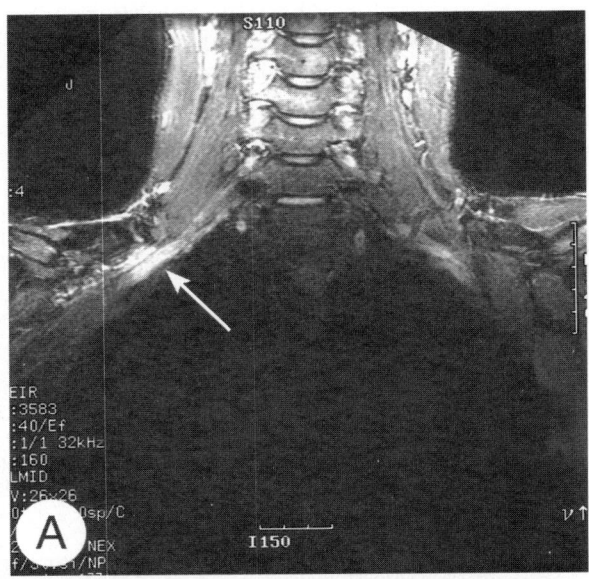

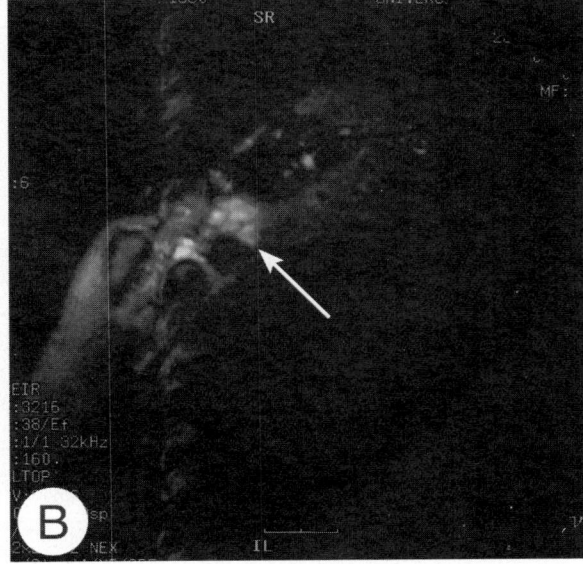

FIGURE 254–7. Coronal *(A)* and sagittal *(B)* short tau inversion recovery (STIR) magnetic resonance images through the brachial plexus of a patient with clinical and electrodiagnostic evidence of thoracic outlet syndrome. Increased signal intensity is visualized in peripheral nerve elements of the brachial plexus in both planes and is maximal in the lower trunk *(white arrows).* (Adapted from Grant GA, Goodkin R, Jarvik JG, et al: The utility of magnetic resonance imaging in evaluating peripheral nerve disorders. Muscle Nerve 25:314–331, 2002.)

the neck, usually lower trunk elements, among muscle (i.e., anterior and middle scalenes), bone (i.e., an anomalous cervical rib, enlarged transverse process, first thoracic rib, or the clavicle), and ligamentous or fascial tissues.[66] The diagnosis of TOS is often made primarily on the basis of symptoms (i.e., upper extremity pain, numbness, dysesthesias, and weakness) exacerbated by certain postures and activities (e.g., working with hands raised above the shoulder). Physical findings, such as Adson's sign (i.e., reduced radial arterial pulse with arm abduction at the shoulder above the horizon), muscle weakness, and muscle atrophy, when present, are not specific. Electrodiagnostic study findings are often normal. Over the past several years, we have used MRI for patients suspected of having TOS. We have seen signal abnormalities (increases on STIR or T2-weighted pulse sequences) involving portions of the brachial plexus, most often in patients who have had corroborative nerve conduction or electromyographic changes (unpublished results) (Fig. 254–7). Others have reported subtle changes in the configuration or trajectory of brachial plexus nerve elements.[10]

Piriformis Syndrome

Piriformis syndrome represents another difficult to diagnose entrapment neuropathy.[67, 68] This syndrome is characterized by painful symptoms in a sciatic nerve distribution, usually associated with sciatic notch tenderness, which cannot be accounted for by lumbosacral spine pathology. It is thought to be caused by compression of the sciatic nerve by the piriformis muscle just distal to the sciatic notch. Electrodiagnostic abnormalities are usually not present. Anatomic abnormalities of the piriformis muscle, such as fibrosis and hypertrophy and its relation to the sciatic nerve, have been reported.[67, 69] We have performed MRI on more than 20 patients suspected of having this syndrome. Only two patients showed abnormally increased T2-weighted signal involving their sciatic nerve just distal to the notch. One underwent a surgical decompression with no significant improvement in his symptoms. In the other, we were able to visualize an abnormal cystic mass arising from the sciatic nerve just distal to the notch, which at surgery proved to be a ganglion cyst

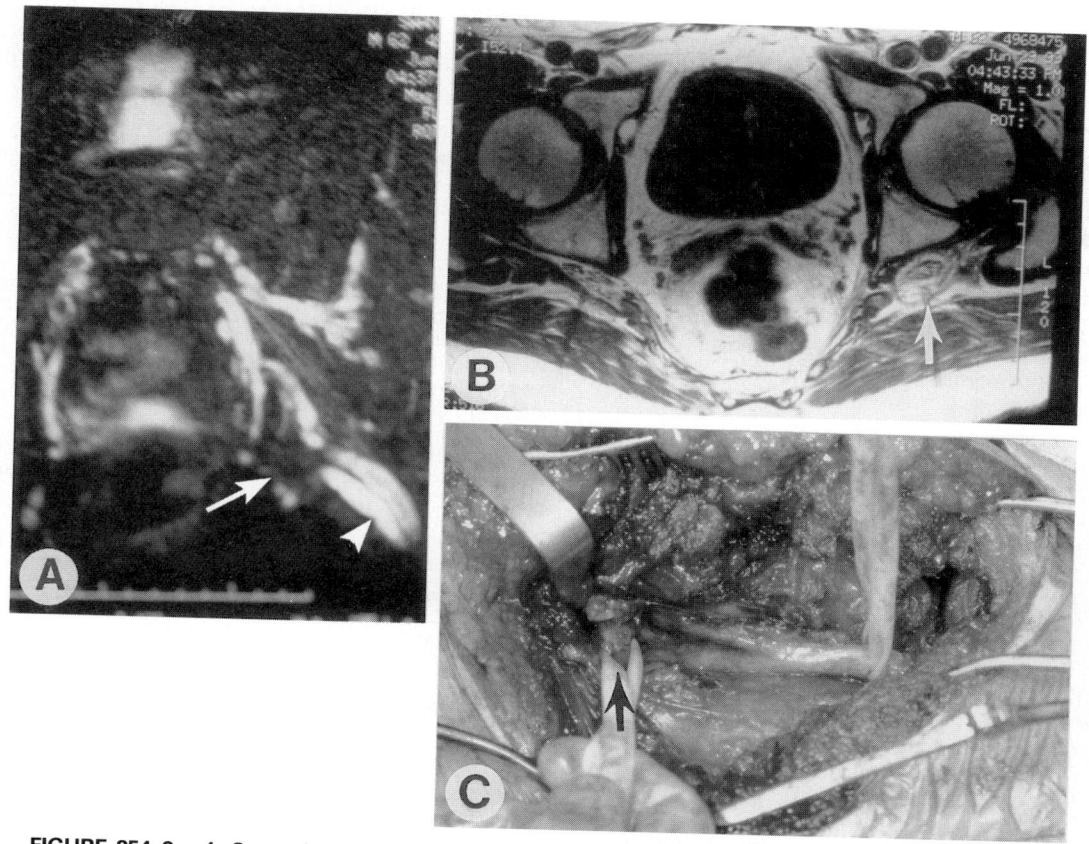

FIGURE 254–8. *A,* Coronal, short tau inversion recovery (STIR) sequence of the left lumbar sacral plexus demonstrates a cystic mass *(white arrow)* associated with increased signal intensity of the sciatic nerve as it exits from the sciatic notch *(white arrowhead). B,* Axial, T1-weighted magnetic resonance image through the pelvis demonstrates the cystic mass *(white arrow)* involving the proximal left sciatic nerve. *C,* Intraoperative photograph just distal to the sciatic notch demonstrates the ganglion cyst *(black arrow)* arising from the proximal sciatic nerve (encircled by vessel loops) at the level of the piriformis muscle. (Adapted from Grant GA, Goodkin R, Jarvik JG, et al: The utility of magnetic resonance imaging in evaluating peripheral nerve disorders. Muscle Nerve 25: 314–331, 2002.)

(Fig. 254–8). Others have reported more frequent MR signal or configuration abnormalities involving the proximal sciatic nerve in patients diagnosed with piriformis syndrome (unpublished results).

Radial Tunnel Syndrome

The radial tunnel syndrome is thought to be caused by compression of the deep branch of the radial nerve, the posterior interosseus nerve, most often as it passes under the tendinous arch of the supinator muscle (i.e., arcade of Fröhse).[64] We have MRI examples in which the posterior interosseous nerve is abnormally bright on T2-weighted and STIR pulse sequences in patients who have clinical evidence of this syndrome and may or may not have electrodiagnostic abnormalities (Fig. 254–9). This nerve can be particularly difficult to see on MRI because of its small size and frequent close association with adjacent blood vessels. Several patients have undergone a surgical decompression, with clinical improvement occurring in some instances.

Lower Extremity Entrapment Syndromes

In the lower leg, the peroneal nerve is particularly prone to injury or entrapment where it passes adjacent to the fibular head. In the clinical setting of a spontaneous footdrop, it is important to differentiate a distal peroneal nerve problem from the much more common radiculopathy of the fifth lumbar spinal nerve and its roots, which usually is caused by a herniated disk. We have found MRI to be particularly useful in localizing pathology of the peroneal nerve to the lower leg and in determining whether a surgical intervention might be of benefit (Fig. 254–10). We also have examples in which the distal tibial nerve in the lower leg displays signal abnormalities in patients suspected of having tarsal tunnel syndrome.

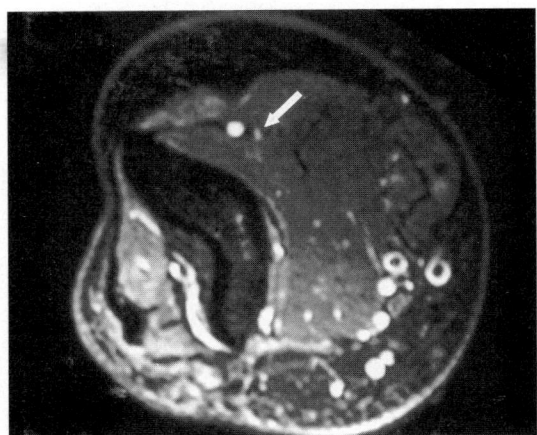

FIGURE 254–9. Axial, short tau inversion recovery (STIR) magnetic resonance image through the proximal forearm of a patient with clinical and electrodiagnostic evidence of a radial neuropathy. Notice the increased signal intensity of the radial nerve *(white arrow)*. (Adapted from Grant GA, Goodkin R, Jarvik JG, et al: The utility of magnetic resonance imaging in evaluating peripheral nerve disorders. Muscle Nerve 25:314–331, 2002.)

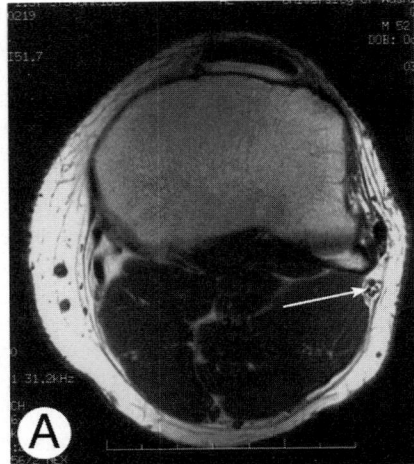

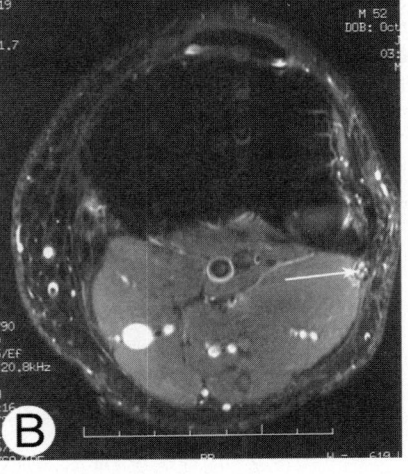

FIGURE 254–10. Axial magnetic resonance images were obtained through the lower extremity at the level of the fibular head in a patient with a traumatic peroneal neuropathy. *A,* The T1-weighted sequence visualizes the common peroneal nerve surrounded by fat *(white arrow)*. *B,* This nerve was found to display increased signal intensity on the short tau inversion recovery (STIR) sequence image. (Adapted from Grant GA, Goodkin R, Jarvik JG, et al: The utility of magnetic resonance imaging in evaluating peripheral nerve disorders. Muscle Nerve 25:314–331, 2002.)

Cervical Radiculopathy

Cervical radiculopathy is usually caused by compression of the proximal portion of a spinal nerve or its roots by soft tissue, such as a protruding or herniated disk, or bone, as in the case of an osteophyte. Although not considered an entrapment neuropathy in the traditional sense, cervical radiculopathy nevertheless shares a common underlying pathophysiology of peripheral nerve compromise caused by surrounding tissue compression or tethering. Because entrapped nerves demonstrate MRI signal abnormalities, we investigated whether similar signal changes could be found in patients with cervical radiculopathy.

MRI performed on standard coils has been used extensively in the evaluation of cervical and lumbosacral radiculopathy because of its sensitivity in visualizing degenerative changes of the spine, such as a disk or osteophyte disease. Its specificity, however, is limited because these changes are found in a large percentage of asymptomatic patients.[38, 70] A custom-designed, high-resolution, phased-array surface coil was used to visualize signal changes in the cervical spinal nerves of three patients with radicular signs and symptoms (Fig. 254–11).[71] Patients were positioned with moderate neck flexion so that the cervical spine appeared straight in a T1-weighted, sagittal-plane scout image. An oblique coronal image plane was then oriented to be parallel to the posterior longitudinal ligament, with additional slices proceeding anteriorly.[10] Using MR neurographic techniques, we observed abnormal hyperintensity on T2-weighted and STIR images in symptomatic spinal nerves compared with adjacent ipsilateral and contralateral control nerves. This abnormal spinal nerve signal was found to extend several centimeters distal to the point of spinal nerve compression by a disk or osteophyte. The increased spinal nerve signal was seen in symptomatic patients with or without electrodiagnostic abnormalities. If this MRI finding proves to be a reliable indicator of symptomatic spinal nerves, it may help to increase the specificity of this highly sensitive technique and thereby help in selecting patients who will benefit most from a surgical decompression.

Other Peripheral Nerve Diseases

Chronically compressed or tethered peripheral nerves can have abnormal signal and configuration characteristics on MRI. In most cases of CTS and UNEE, the underlying pathology represents a neurapraxic or demyelinating grade of nerve injury. It is therefore not surprising that MRI signal changes (i.e., increases on T2-weighted and STIR pulse sequences) have been seen in the nerves of patients with chronic inflammatory demyelinating polyneuropathy,[72, 73] certain types of Charcot-Marie-Tooth disease,[74] and brachial neuritis often involving the axillary and suprascapular nerves.

MAGNETIC RESONANCE IMAGING EVALUATION OF PERIPHERAL NERVE TRAUMA

Most serious peripheral nerve injuries do not lead to transection of the nerve; they instead leave the nerve in

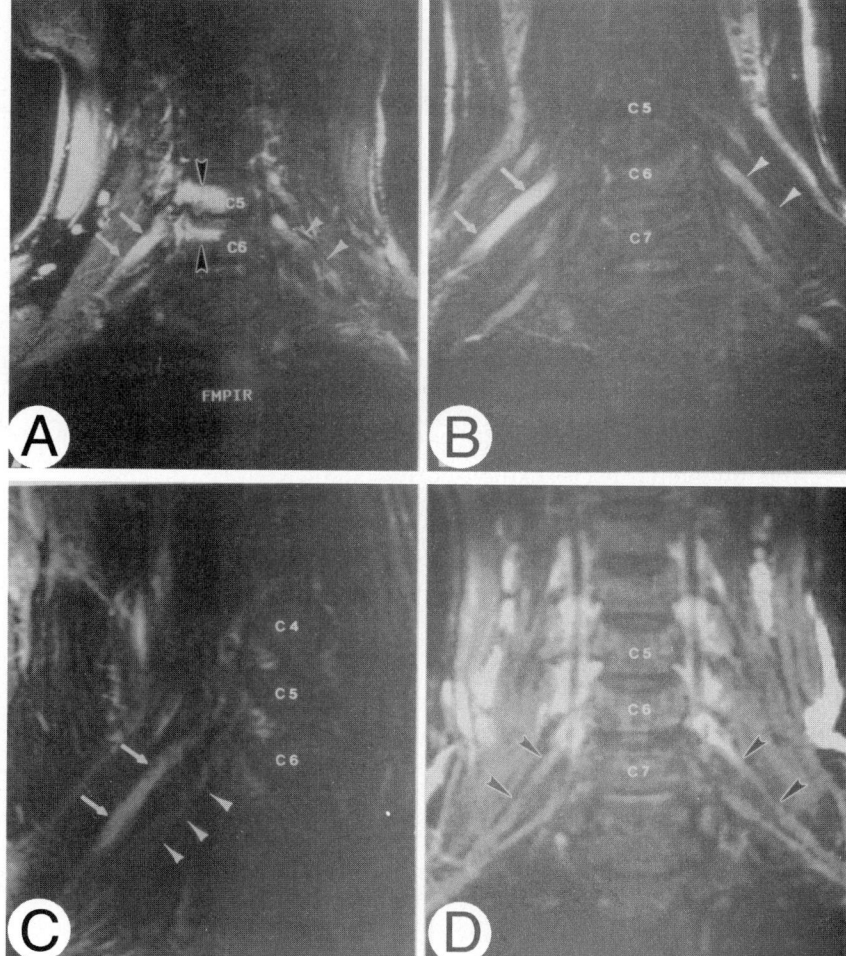

FIGURE 254–11. Coronal, short tau inversion recovery (STIR) and T2-weighted magnetic resonance images were obtained through the necks of three patients with symptoms of cervical radiculopathy *(A to C)* and in an asymptomatic, control subject *(D)*. *A,* Notice the markedly higher STIR signal in the right C6 spinal nerve *(white arrows)* compared with the left *(white arrowheads)* and the degenerative, reactive marrow changes in the C5 and C6 vertebral bodies *(black arrowheads)*. *B,* Notice the higher STIR signal in the right C6 nerve *(white arrows)* compared with the asymptomatic, left C6 spinal nerve *(arrowheads)*. *C,* Notice the higher T2-weighted signal in the right C5 spinal nerve *(white arrows)*, corresponding to the symptomatic spinal nerve with electromyographic abnormalities, compared with the adjacent, asymptomatic C6 spinal nerve *(white arrowheads)*. *D,* No difference in STIR signal intensity can be identified when comparing the right and left spinal nerves *(black arrowheads* point to the C6 spinal nerve bilaterally) in this asymptomatic control subject. (Adapted from Dailey AT, Tsuruda JS, Goodkin R, et al: Magnetic resonance neurography for cervical radiculopathy: A preliminary report. Lancet 38:488–496, 1996.)

continuity.[75] Initially, it may be difficult to differentiate closed nerve injuries that recover on their own (i.e., neurapraxic and axonotmetic grades) from those that do not (i.e., neurotmetic grade) and therefore require a surgical repair.[76] Serial clinical and electrodiagnostic evaluations, often over a period of months, have traditionally been the mainstay of decision making in the management of closed traumatic peripheral nerve injuries.[75–78] Clinical or electrodiagnostic evidence of recovering sensory-motor nerve function indicates an injury with a neurapraxic or axonotmetic component and dictates a more conservative, nonoperative approach. Failure to improve is evidence of a more severe injury that requires a surgical exploration and repair. Delaying exploratory surgery to determine whether recovery through axonal regeneration is occurring must be balanced against the diminishing chance of obtaining a good functional recovery if the muscles remain denervated for longer than 2 years.[75–77, 79] In the absence of recovering motor function or electrodiagnostic evidence of muscle reinnervation, an advancing Tinel sign is the only reliable noninvasive indicator of ongoing axonal regeneration.

MRI has been used to evaluate muscle signal changes in the clinical setting of a variety of peripheral nerve disorders (Fig. 254–12).[34, 35, 58, 59, 80] MRI was shown to detect increased signal in denervated muscle groups that is most prominently seen using STIR or T2-weighted pulse sequences.[80] The increased signal intensity correlates with the degree of muscle denervation seen on EMG and weakness found on the clinical examination. In general, the threshold for producing an increased STIR signal is weakness graded at 3 or less of 5 (i.e., at or below antigravity on the Medical Research Council [MRC] grading scheme) and conspicuous muscle denervation changes of 3+ or more seen on EMG.[34, 80, 81] The MRI muscle signal changes occur as early as 4 days after a traumatic nerve injury, in contrast to the 2 to 3 weeks required for electromyographic evidence of denervation to develop in muscle. These signal changes normalize with muscle reinnervation as assessed clinically and by electrodiagnostic studies.

In the setting of pure neurapraxic injuries (i.e., demyelination without axonal loss) or disuse muscle atrophy, the involved muscles exhibit normal signal characteristics on STIR and T2-weighted pulse sequences. In contrast, in severe axonotmetic and neurotmetic injuries, both of which involve loss of axons, increased STIR and T2-weighted signal appears in the affected muscles as a result of muscle denervation. MRI of muscle therefore can be useful in differentiating neurapraxic from the more severe axonotmetic and neurotmetic grades of injury early after trauma. In chronically denervated muscles, atrophic changes eventually occur with the development of fatty infiltration after several months, which is best visualized on T1-weighted images, along with the eventual normalization of signal on T2-weighted and STIR pulse sequences.

We have been attempting to determine whether MRI can be used to localize and determine the grade of a traumatic peripheral nerve injury and thereby help to determine whether surgery would be of benefit in a

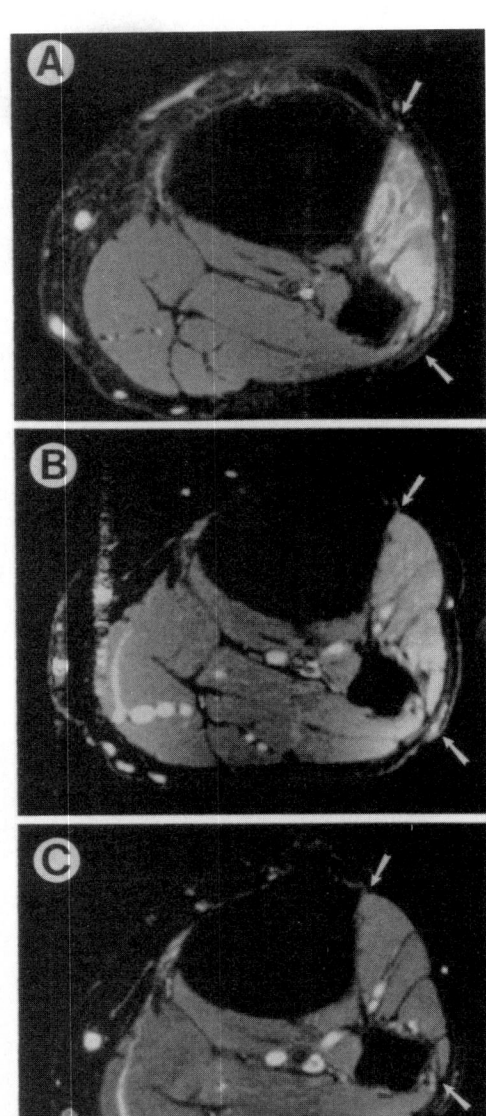

FIGURE 254–12. Axial, short tau inversion recovery (STIR) magnetic resonance images were obtained through the lower leg of a 40-year-old man who spontaneously developed a severe peroneal nerve palsy. *A,* STIR image of the right lower leg 2 weeks after the onset of symptoms shows bright signal in the peroneal-supplied muscles *(between white arrows in A to C).* Motor strength in these muscles was Medical Research Council grade 2. No denervation changes were identified on electromyography (EMG). *B,* At 8 weeks after the onset of symptoms, the STIR signal in the peroneal-supplied muscles remained increased but less so than in *A.* Motor strength had improved to grade 4 in the involved muscles. Denervation potentials were identified on EMG. *C,* At 20 weeks after the onset of symptoms, the STIR signal was normal in all muscles. Results of EMG and strength studies were normal as well. (Adapted from West GA, Haynor DR, Goodkin R, et al: Magnetic resonance imaging signal changes in denervated muscles after peripheral nerve injury. Neurosurgery 35:1077–1086, 1994.)

more expeditious manner. Soon after traumatic nerve injuries, electrodiagnostic testing can reliably identify neurapraxic injuries by virtue of the ability of such injured nerves to conduct nerve action potentials distal to the site of partial or complete conduction block.[82] Neurapraxic injuries also exhibit no electromyographic or MRI evidence of muscle denervation.[80, 83] In contrast, electrodiagnostic studies cannot distinguish between complete axonotmetic and neurotmetic grades of nerve injury soon after acute trauma.

Using high-resolution MRI techniques, we have found that traumatic injuries produce increased signal in nerves on T2-weighted and STIR pulse sequences that is usually greatest at the site of injury. These MRI signal changes have been useful to us in visualizing damaged nerve segments, such as in the setting of traumatic brachial plexus avulsion injuries. We have found that the absence of increased T2-weighted or STIR nerve signal changes in the clinical setting of severe trauma with complete loss of function is usually associated with the intraoperative finding of extensive fibrosis, which can make it difficult to distinguish between peripheral nerve elements and the surrounding tissues. These severe types of nerve injury are also characterized by the loss of nerve fascicular structure that is usually best seen on cross-sectional (i.e., axial) T1-weighted pulse sequences.

An important question is whether MRI of nerve can distinguish between axonotmetic and neurotmetic grades of nerve injury (Table 254–1). Both grades of injury are characterized by absent nerve conduction responses and muscle denervation seen on EMG and MRI.[80, 83] After traumatic nerve injuries of sufficient magnitude to produce distal loss of axons, increased signal on T2-weighted and STIR pulse sequences occurs in the nerve at and distal to the site of injury (Fig. 254–13). These nerve signal changes, however, can be transient. For example, increased nerve signal was shown to slowly normalize over a period of many months as axonal regeneration with concomitant recovery of function, confirmed clinically and electrodiagnostically, occurred in a patient after a nerve graft repair operation. In chronically and severely damaged nerves, we have seen examples where peripheral nerves retain increased T2-weighted and STIR signal for several years, such as after a preganglionic brachial plexus avulsion injury or in the nerve graft segments

of surgically repaired nerves. However, we have also seen clinical examples of chronically degenerated peripheral nerve for which the increased signal eventually normalizes over months, even in the absence of functional recovery.

In summary, MRI can be used to noninvasively evaluate recovery in the peripheral nervous system after axonal injury in a manner that confirms or supplements information gained from electrodiagnostic studies (see Table 254–1). MRI signal changes in nerve and muscle correlate with phases of axonal degeneration and regeneration, muscle denervation and reinnervation, and loss and recovery of function after peripheral nerve injury. Our results demonstrate MRI's *potential* to noninvasively visualize and differentiate traumatic peripheral nerve injuries that recover through axonal regeneration (i.e., an axonotmetic grade) from those that do not and therefore require a surgical repair (i.e., a neurotmetic grade). However, before MRI can do so in a clinically useful manner, we must develop techniques that can more reliably distinguish regenerating nerve and chronically degenerating nerve.

New and improved MRI techniques employing diffusion weighting, magnetization transfer, and MR spectroscopic pulse sequences, as well as new contrast agents that can label nerve, may make such an important goal possible. Such a noninvasive diagnostic modality would significantly improve the treatment of patients with traumatic peripheral nerve injuries by providing an earlier and more accurate diagnosis and prognosis and thereby reduce the need for exploratory surgery.

FUTURE DEVELOPMENTS IN MAGNETIC RESONANCE IMAGING FOR PERIPHERAL NERVE DISORDERS

MRI has revolutionized the imaging of soft tissues and has become the imaging modality of choice to evaluate the peripheral nervous system. Improvements in hardware, such as phased-array coils, and software, such as novel pulse sequences, have dramatically improved the visualization of normal and pathologic peripheral nerve structures and lesions in a variety of clinical settings. These MRI techniques are already proving to be clinically useful in diagnosing and treating mass

T A B L E 2 5 4 – I ■ Correlation of Magnetic Resonance Imaging Findings with Electrodiagnostic Test Results

DIAGNOSTIC MODALITY	NEURAPRAXIA	AXONOTMETIS	NEUROTMETIS
Nerve conduction study	Focal nerve conduction block or slowing	Initial absence of nerve conduction distal to injury followed by recovery through regeneration	Persistent absence of nerve conduction distal to injury
Electromyography MR neurography	Minimal to no denervation Focal signal increase	Denervation after 2–3 wk Transient signal increase distal to injury followed by normalization with axonal regeneration	Persistent denervation Signal increase distal to injury followed by delayed normalization
MRI of muscle	Normal	Transient signal increase, then normalization with muscle reinnervation	Transient signal increase, then reduction with atrophy and fatty infiltration

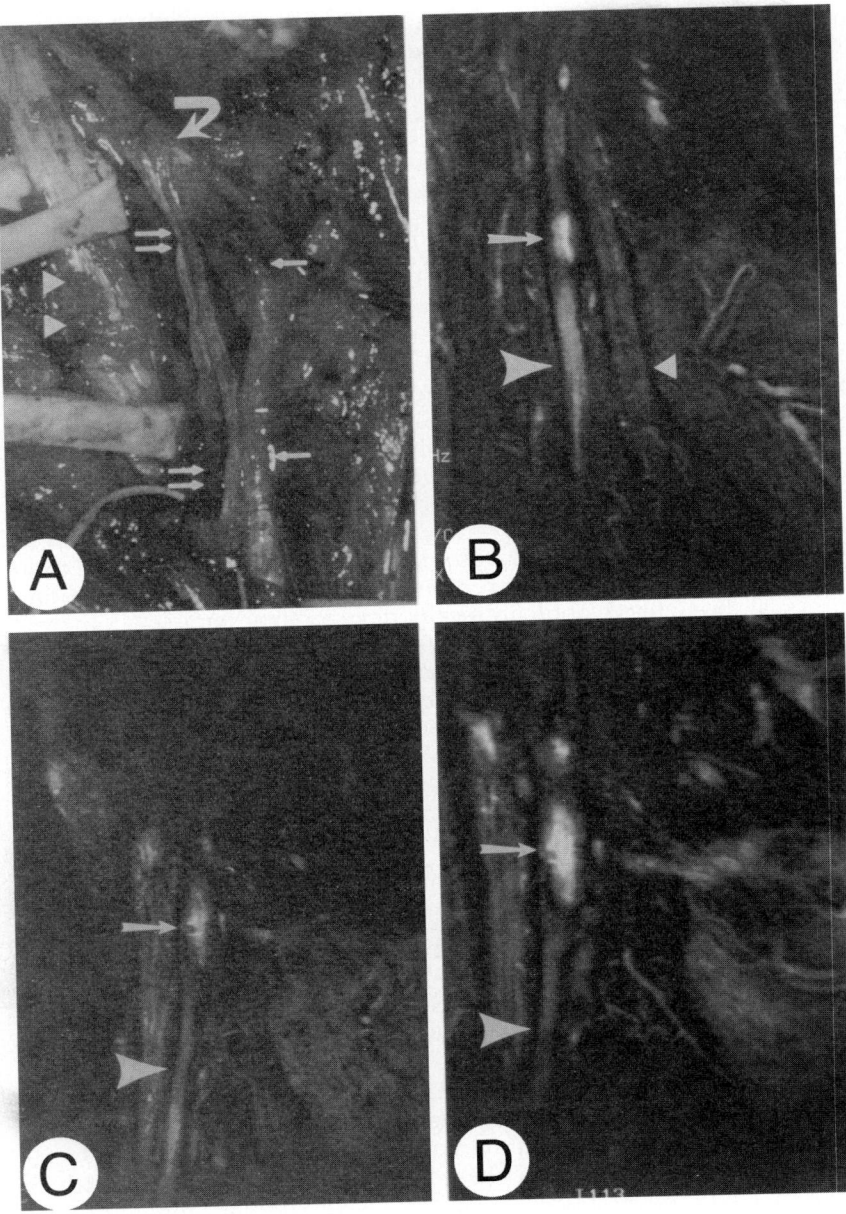

FIGURE 254–13. A 29-year-old man suffered a traumatic laceration to his right peroneal nerve just above the popliteal fossa that resulted in a complete footdrop that had been suture repaired. He failed to recover peroneal nerve function, and 6 months later, a coronal, T2-weighted magnetic resonance image *(B)* visualized high signal intensity in the nerve at the repair site *(white arrow)* and distal to the suture repair site *(white arrowhead).* At the second operation performed 8 months after the first, no nerve conduction response could be recorded across the scarred suture repaired segment of the peroneal nerve *(A).* This scarred segment was excised and the resultant gap bridged by two sural nerve grafts *(double white arrows in A),* leaving several sensory fascicles intact *(single arrows in A).* Eight months later, the patient began to show clinical and electromyographic evidence of muscle reinnervation, and a coronal, T2-weighted magnetic resonance image *(C)* showed partial return to normal of the bright signal in the distal peroneal nerve *(white arrowhead).* By 16 months, strength in peroneal-supplied muscles was near normal, the electromyographic findings confirmed additional muscle reinnervation, and coronal, T2-weighted magnetic resonance imaging showed further normalization of signal in the distal peroneal nerve *(white arrowhead),* although signal intensity remained high at the graft repair site *(white arrow in C and D).* (Adapted from Grant GA, Goodkin R, Jarvik JG, et al: The utility of magnetic resonance imaging in evaluating peripheral nerve disorders. Muscle Nerve 25:314–331, 2002.)

lesions involving peripheral nerves, nerve entrapment syndromes, and traumatic nerve injuries. Traditionally, the patient's symptoms, physical examination, and electrodiagnostic test results have been the mainstay in diagnosing peripheral nerve problems. As improvements in MRI continue to occur, we believe that it will play an increasingly important and useful role in diagnosing and treating peripheral nerve problems, just as MRI already has done in disorders involving the brain and spine.

ACKNOWLEDGMENTS

We are grateful to Paul Schwartz and Janet Schukar for their excellent assistance with photography. This work was supported by a Clinician Investigator Development Award from the National Institutes of Health (NIH) (M.K.), a Dana Foundation grant (M.K., K.M.), and an NIH training grant (T32NS-07144-15) to the Department of Neurological Surgery. Michel Kliot and Kenneth Maravilla are founders of UltraImage, a division of Pathway Medical Inc., which is a company involved in the commercial production of phased-array MRI coils similar to the ones used to generate the images shown in this chapter.

REFERENCES

1. Grant GA, Goodkin R, Jarvik JG, et al: The utility of magnetic resonance imaging in evaluating peripheral nerve disorders. Muscle Nerve 25:314–331, 2002.
2. Buchberger W, Judmaier W, Birbamer G, et al: Carpal tunnel syndrome: diagnosis with high-resolution sonography. AJR Am J Roentgenol 159:793–798, 1992.
3. Fornage BD: Peripheral nerves of the extremities with US. Radiology 167:179–182, 1988.

4. Lee D, Holsbeeck MT, Janevski PK, et al: Diagnosis of carpal tunnel syndrome: Ultrasound versus electromyography. Radiol Clin North Am 37:859–872, 1999.

5. Zucker-Pinchoff B, Hermann G, Srinivasan R: Computerized tomography of the carpal tunnel: A radioanatomical study. J Comput Assist Tomogr 5:525–528, 1981.

6. Kuntz C, Blake L, Britz GW, et al: Magnetic resonance neurography of peripheral nerve lesions in the lower extremity. Neurosurgery 39:750–757, 1996.

7. Stull MA, Moser RP, Kransdorf MJ: MR appearance of peripheral nerve sheath tumors. Skeletal Radiol 20:9–14, 1991.

8. Filler AG, Howe FA, Hayes CE, et al: Magnetic resonance neurography. Lancet 341:659–661, 1993.

9. Howe FA, Filler AG, Bell BA, et al: Magnetic resonance neurography. Magn Reson Med 28:328–338, 1992.

10. Filler AG, Kliot M, Howe FA, et al: Application of magnetic resonance neurography in the evaluation of patients with peripheral nerve pathology. J Neurosurg 85:299–309, 1996.

11. Roemer PB, Edelstein WA, Hayes CE, et al: The NMR phased array. Magn Reson Med 16:192–225, 1990.

12. Fornage BD: Peripheral nerves of the extremities: Imaging with ultrasound. Radiology 167:179–182, 1988.

13. Powers SK, Norman D, Edwards MSB: Computerized tomography of peripheral nerve lesions. J Neurosurg 59:131–136, 1983.

14. Donner TR, Voorhies RM, Kline DG: Neural sheath tumors of major nerves. J Neurosurg 81:362–373, 1994.

15. Cerofolini E, Landi A, DeSantis G, et al: MR of benign peripheral nerve sheath tumors. J Comput Assist Tomogr 15:593–597, 1991.

16. Birch R, Bonney G, Parry CBW: Surgical Disorders of the Peripheral Nerves. London, Churchill Livingstone, 1998.

17. Gelberman RH, Eaton RG, Urbaniak JR: Peripheral nerve compression. In Anonymous 31–51, 1999.

18. Hallett M: Electrophysiologic approaches to the diagnosis of entrapment neuropathies. Neurol Clin 3:531–541, 1985.

19. Mackinnon SE, Novak CB, Landau WM: Clinical diagnosis of carpal tunnel syndrome. JAMA 284:1924–1925, 2000.

20. Mackinnon SE: Surgery of the peripheral nerve. New York, Thieme Medical Publishers, 1988.

21. de Krom MCTFM, Knipschild PG, Kester ADM, et al: Carpal tunnel syndrome in Washington State, 1984–1988. J Clin Epidemiol 45:373–376, 1992.

22. Stevens JC, Sun S, Beard CM, et al: Carpal tunnel syndrome in Rochester, Minnesota. Neurology 38:134–138, 1988.

23. Lundborg G, Dahlin LB: Anatomy, function, and pathophysiology of peripheral nerves and nerve compression. Hand Clin 12:185–193, 1996.

24. D'Arcy CA, McGee S: Clinical diagnosis of carpal tunnel syndrome. JAMA 284:1924–1925, 2000.

25. Gellman H, Gelberman RH, Tan AM, et al: Carpal tunnel syndrome: An evaluation of the provocative diagnostic tests. J Bone Joint Surg 68:735–737, 1986.

26. Katz JN, Larson MG, Sabra A: The carpal tunnel syndrome: Diagnostic utility of the history and physical examination findings. Ann Intern Med 112:321–327, 1990.

27. Stewart JD, Eisen A: Tinel's sign and the carpal tunnel syndrome. Br Med J 2:1125–1127, 1978.

28. Jablecki CK, Andary MT, So YT, et al: Literature review of the usefulness of nerve conduction studies and electromyography for the evaluation of patients with carpal tunnel syndrome. Muscle Nerve 16:1392–1414, 1993.

29. Nathan PA, Takigawa K, Keniston RC, et al: Slowing of sensory conduction of the median nerve and carpal tunnel syndrome in Japanese and American industrial workers. J Hand Surg 19:30–34, 1994.

30. Concannon MJ, Gainor B, Petroski GF, et al: The predictive value of electrodiagnostic studies in carpal tunnel syndrome. Plast Reconstr Surg 100:1452–1458, 1997.

31. Glowacki KA, Green CJ, Schar K, et al: Electrodiagnostic testing and carpal tunnel release outcome. J Hand Surg 21:117–121, 1996.

32. Carter GT, Robinson LR, Chang VH, et al: Electrodiagnostic evaluation of traumatic nerve injuries. Hand Clin 16:1–12, 2000.

33. Greening J, Smart S, Leary R, et al: Reduced movement of median nerve in carpal tunnel during wrist flexion in patients with non-specific arm pain. Lancet 354:217–218, 1999.

34. Britz GW, Haynor DR, Kuntz C, et al: Carpal tunnel syndrome: Correlation of MRI, clinical, electrodiagnostic, and intraoperative findings. Neurosurgery 37:1097–1103, 1995.

35. Britz GW, Haynor DR, Kuntz C, et al: Ulnar nerve entrapment at the elbow: Correlation of magnetic resonance imaging, clinical, electrodiagnostic, and intraoperative findings. Neurosurgery 38:458–465, 1996.

36. Dalinka MK, Meyer S, Kricun ME, et al: Magnetic resonance imaging of the wrist. Hand Clin 7:87–98, 1991.

37. Horch RE, Allmann KH, Laubenberger J, et al: Median nerve compression can be detected by magnetic resonance imaging of the carpal tunnel. Neurosurgery 41:76–82, 1997.

38. Jarvik JG, Hollingworth W, Heagerty P, et al: The longitudinal assessment of imaging and disability of the back (LAIDBack) study: Baseline data. Spine , 2001.

39. Kleindienst A, Hamm B, Hildebrandt G, et al: Carpal tunnel syndrome: Staging of median nerve compression by MR imaging. Acta Neurochir 138:228–233, 1996.

40. Kleindienst A, Hamm B, Lanksch WR: Carpal tunnel syndrome: Staging of median nerve compression by MR imaging. J Magn Reson Imaging 8:1119–1125, 1998.

41. Mesgarzadeh M, Schneck CD, Bonakdarpour A, et al: Carpal Tunnel: MR imaging. Radiology 171:749–754, 1989.

42. Mesgarzadeh M, Schneck CD, Bonakdarpour A: Carpal tunnel: MR imaging. Part I. normal anatomy. Radiology 171:743–748, 1989.

43. Mesgarzadeh M, Triolo J, Schneck CD: Carpal tunnel syndrome. MR imaging diagnosis. Magn Reson Imaging Clin N Am 3:249–264, 1995.

44. Middleton W, Kneeland J, Kellman G, et al: MR imaging of the carpal tunnel: Normal anatomy and preliminary findings in the carpal tunnel syndrome. AJR Am J Roentgenol 148:307–316, 1987.

45. Murphy RX Jr, Chernofsky MA, Osborne MA, et al: Magnetic resonance imaging in the evaluation of persistent carpal tunnel syndrome. J Hand Surg 18:113–120, 1993.

46. Soccetti A, Carloni S, Giovagnoni M, et al: MR findings in post-traumatic carpal tunnel syndrome. Chir Organi Mov 78:233–239, 1992.

47. Sugimoto H, Miyaji N, Ohsawa T: Carpal tunnel syndrome: Evaluation of median nerve circulation with dynamic contrast-enhanced MR imaging. Radiology 190:459–466, 1994.

48. Timins ME, O'Connell SE, Erickson SJ, et al: MR imaging of the wrist: Normal findings that may simulate disease. Radiographics 16:987–995, 1996.

49. Weiss AP, Beltran J, Sharmam OM, et al: High-field MR surface-coil imaging of the hand and wrist. Radiology 160:143–146, 1986.

50. Zeiss J, Skie M, Ebraheim N, et al: Anatomic relations between the median nerve and flexor tendons in the carpal tunnel: MR evaluation in normal volunteers. AJR Am J Roentgenol 153:533–536, 1989.

51. Oneson SR, Scales LM, Erickson SJ, et al: MR imaging of the painful wrist. Radiographics 16:997–1008, 1996.

52. Pierre-Jerome C, Bekkelund SI, Husby G, et al: MRI of anatomical variants of wrist in women. Surg Radiol Anat 18:37–41, 1996.

53. Radack DM, Schwitzer ME, Taras J: Carpal tunnel syndrome: Are the MR findings a result of population selection bias? Surg Radiol Anat 18:37–41, 1997.

54. Jarvik JG, Yuen E, Haynor DR, et al: MR nerve imaging in a prospective cohort of patients with suspected carpal tunnel syndrome. Neurology 58:1597–1602, 2002.

55. Jarvik JG, Kliot M, Maravilla KR: MR nerve imaging of the wrist and hand. Hand Clin 15:13–24, 2000.

56. Levine DW, Simmons BP, Koris MJ, et al: A self administered questionnaire for the assessment of severity of symptoms and functional status in carpal tunnel syndrome. J Bone Joint Surg Am 75:1585–1592, 1993.

57. Rebpel D, Evanoff B, Armadio PC, et al: Consensus criteria for the classification of carpal tunnel syndrome in epidemiologic studies. Am J Public Health 88:1447–1451, 1998.

58. Fleckenstein JL, Watumull D, Conner KE, et al: Denervated human skeletal muscle: MR imaging evaluation. Radiology 187:213–218, 1993.

59. Shabas D, Gerard G, Rossi D: Magnetic resonance imaging examination of denervated muscle. Comput Radiol 11:9–13, 1987.

60. Ahern V, Soo YS, Langlands AD: MRI scanning in brachial plexus neuropathy. Australas Radiol 35:379–381, 1991.

61. Dailey AT, Tsuruda JS, Filler AG, et al: Magnetic resonance neurography of peripheral nerve degeneration and regeneration. Lancet 350:1221–1222, 1997.

62. Holmes W, Young JZ: Nerve regeneration after immediate and delayed suture. J Anat 77:63–106, 1942.

63. Maravilla KR, Aagaard BDL, Kliot M: MR Neurography. Magn Reson Imaging Clin N Am 6:179–194, 1998.

64. Beltran J, Rosenberg ZS: Diagnosis of compressive and entrapment neuropathies of the upper extremity: Value of MR imaging. AJR Am J Roentgenol 163:525–531, 1994.

65. Carvalho GA, Nikkhah G, Matthis C, et al: Diagnosis of root avulsions in traumatic brachial plexus injuries: Value of computerized tomography, myelography, and magnetic resonance imaging. J Neurosurg 89:69–76, 1997.

66. Roos DB: Historical perspectives and anatomic considerations. Thoracic outlet syndrome. Semin Thorac Cardiovasc Surg 8:183–189, 1996.

67. Mitzuguchi T: Division of the pyriformis muscle for the treatment of sciatica. Postlaminectomy syndrome and osteoarthritis of the spine. Arch Surg 111:716–722, 1976.

68. Synek VM: The pyriformis syndrome: Review and case presentation. Clin Exp Neurol 23:31–37, 1987.

69. Hopayian K: Sciatica in the community—not always disc herniation. Int J Clin Pract 53:197–198, 1999.

70. Jensen MC, Brant-Zawadzki MN, Obuchowski N, et al: Magnetic resonance imaging of the lumbar spine in people without back pain. N Engl J Med 331:69–73, 1994.

71. Dailey AT, Tsuruda JS, Goodkin R, et al: Magnetic resonance neurography for cervical radiculopathy: A preliminary report. Lancet 38:488–496, 1996.

72. Kuwabara S, Nakajima M, Matsuda S, et al: Magnetic resonance imaging at the demyelinative foci in chronic inflammatory demyelinating polyneuropathy. Neurology 48:874–877, 1997.

73. Midroni G, de Tilly LN, Gray B, et al: MRI of the cauda equina in CIDP: Clinical correlations. J Neurol Sci 170:36–44, 1999.

74. Ellegala DB, Lankerovich L, Haynor D, et al: Characterization of generically defined types of Charcot-Marie-Tooth neuropathies using magnetic resonance neurography [abstract]. Neurosurgery , 1998.

75. Kline DG, Hudson AR: Nerve injuries. In Operative Results for Major Nerve Injuries, Entrapments, and Tumors. Philadelphia, WB Saunders, 1995.

76. Grant GA, Goodkin R, Kliot M: Evaluation and surgical management of peripheral nerve problems. Neurosurgery 44:825–840, 1999.

77. Kline DG, Hudson AR: Acute injuries of peripheral nerves. In Youmans J (ed): Neurological Surgery. Philadelphia, WB Saunders, 1990, pp 2423–2510.

78. Spinner RJ, Kline DG: Surgery for peripheral nerve and brachial plexus injuries or other nerve lesions. Muscle Nerve 23:680–695, 2001.

79. Gordon T, Fu SY: Long-term response to nerve injury. Adv Neurol 72:185–199, 1997.

80. West GA, Haynor DR, Goodkin R, et al: Magnetic resonance imaging signal changes in denervated muscles after peripheral nerve injury. Neurosurgery 35:1077–1086, 1994.

81. British Medical Research Council: Aids to the Examination of the Peripheral Nervous System. London, Bailliere Tindall–WB Saunders, 1988.

82. Aminoff MJ, Olney RK, Parry GJ, et al: Relative utility of different electrophysiologic techniques in the evaluation of brachial plexopathies. Neurology 39:1136–1137, 1989.

83. Wilbourn AJ, Aminoff MJ: AAEE minimonograph #32: The electrophysiologic examination in patients with radiculopathies. Muscle Nerve 11:1099–1114, 1988.

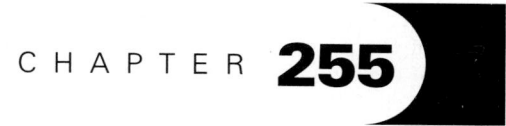

CHAPTER 255

Carpal Tunnel Syndrome

CHONG C. LEE ■ SUZIE C. TINDALL ■ MICHEL KLIOT

Entrapment of the median nerve at the wrist, or carpal tunnel syndrome (CTS), is the most common entrapment neuropathy in humans. CTS is estimated to occur in 125 of 100,000 people.[1] Because it occurs so frequently, it has been studied extensively and is the best-defined entrapment syndrome from clinical, electrophysiologic, and operative standpoints. It was first postulated as a clinical problem in 1913 by Marie and Foix, who observed the postmortem enlargement of the median nerve proximal to the transverse carpal ligament in a patient who had bilateral thenar atrophy.[2] Learmonth is credited with the first operative decompression of the median nerve in the carpal tunnel in 1933.[2]

ANATOMY

The carpal tunnel is bounded superficially by the transverse carpal ligament (the flexor retinaculum) and laterally and inferiorly by the carpal bones and their fibrous coverings and interosseous ligaments. Within the tunnel lie the flexor tendons of the fingers and the median nerve. The palmaris longus tendon, when present, and the palmaris brevis muscle lie superficial to the flexor retinaculum. The flexor retinaculum is a wide band of fibers that normally extends 1 cm or more proximal to the most distal wrist crease, where it merges with the medial antebrachial fascia and extends distally at least 3 to 4 cm below this crease into the palm.

Important aspects of median nerve anatomy in this area include the palmar cutaneous branch of the median nerve. This sensory branch exits the main trunk of the median nerve along its anterolateral or volar-radial quadrant about 3 to 4 cm above the distal wrist crease, at the point where the median nerve emerges from under the radial margin of the flexor digitorum superficialis tendon. It then passes superficial to the transverse carpal ligament in a radial direction to supply sensation to the proximal surface of the thenar eminence.[3] The median nerve is usually a solitary structure as it traverses the carpal tunnel; high division of this nerve is possible, however, so there may be two or more branches traversing the tunnel. This variation may be associated with a persistent median artery or an anomalous accessory lumbrical muscle between the two branches.[4] The thenar branch, also known as the recurrent motor branch, usually leaves the radial side of the nerve just distal to the flexor retinaculum and curves back around to enter the thenar muscle mass. However, there are multiple variations of this branching pattern that are of great importance to the surgeon. In about 31% of cases, the motor branch arises beneath the transverse carpal ligament but may come from the volar or ulnar side of the nerve. In slightly more than 20% of cases, the motor branch takes a transligamentous course, which may lead to difficulties at operation and predispose to solitary entrapment of this branch (see the later discussion).[4, 5] Small accessory branches may arise at the distal carpal tunnel and are most often sensory, although a true double thenar motor branch may occur. The proximity of the vascular arch to the distal retinaculum is of obvious importance to the surgeon.

CAUSE AND ASSOCIATED DISORDERS

CTS occurs more frequently in women than in men (ratio of 2.5:1) and is most common during middle age (40 to 60 years), although it may occur at any time during adult life.[6–8] It usually affects people who use their hands extensively in their jobs or in other daily activities. The dominant hand is most often involved, but the nondominant hand may be affected alone, and the condition is bilateral in at least 10% of patients. There is some evidence that a congenitally small carpal tunnel canal, as demonstrated by computed tomography, may predispose to the development of this syndrome.[9]

Any condition that increases the volume of the contents of the carpal tunnel and thereby compresses the median nerve may produce clinical CTS. Examples include a malaligned carpal fracture, a ganglion cyst or other benign mass, and amyloid infiltration in multiple myeloma or amyloidosis. Phalen believed that thickening or fibrosis of the flexor synovialis within the carpal tunnel was the most common cause of CTS.[7, 8] He cited data from pathologic flexor synovialis biopsy specimens and the frequent association of other rheumatic conditions, such as trigger finger, de Quervain's disease, tennis elbow, or periarthritis of the shoulder, in these patients to support his contention. About 15% of patients in most series have diabetes mellitus. This strong association is usually attributed to the fact that nerves mildly involved with a peripheral neuropathy are more prone to symptomatic entrapment. Rheumatoid arthritis is also a frequently associated illness and is thought to cause distal median nerve compromise within the carpal tunnel by synovial overgrowth and alterations in carpal bone alignment.

Up to one third of patients with acromegaly have electrical evidence of CTS, and many have symptoms of distal median nerve entrapment.[10, 11] Proper diagnosis and treatment of the acromegaly usually result in relief of the carpal tunnel symptoms. Both hyperthyroidism and hypothyroidism may be associated with carpal tunnel disorders.[12]

CTS is common during pregnancy, with approximately 62% of pregnant women reporting symptoms. The symptoms usually resolve completely following delivery.[13–15] CTS is so common that it may occasionally coexist with cervical radiculopathy or thoracic outlet syndrome, resulting in the so-called double crush syndrome.[16, 17] Recently, attention has been directed at the role of vibration exposure and repetitive motion activities in the workplace as precipitating factors for CTS.[18–20]

DIAGNOSIS

The diagnosis of CTS rests on symptoms in a distal median nerve distribution, with evidence of nerve entrapment at the level of the carpal tunnel in the hand. The most common symptom of CTS is numbness or tingling in the fingers or hand. Patients frequently refer to a "pins and needles" sensation in the whole hand, but when questioned carefully, they usually indicate that the little finger is not involved. Pain is also a frequent complaint. Patient may find the paresthesias painful or may complain of a deep, aching pain. Although this pain is most often in the fingers or the hand, it may be referred up the forearm into the elbow, upper arm, or, rarely, the shoulder.[21] Pain almost never occurs in the neck, however. Symptoms are frequently made worse by activities involving the hand or wrist, such as computer keyboard work.

The nocturnal occurrence of symptoms (so-called waking numbness) is a characteristic of CTS, and it and other positive clinical signs have a reported sensitivity and specificity ranging from 20% to 70% and 47% to 83%, respectively.[22] After a good deal of hand activity during the day (e.g., sewing, gardening), the patient wakes up several times during the night with a painful numbness of the involved hand that causes him or her to get up, shake the hand vigorously, and occasionally seek relief by running water over the hand. Sunderland believes that the hypotonia of movements during sleep results in venous stasis, which activates the symptoms; the patient obtains relief by shaking the hand and thus aiding venous return.[23] Weakness is a less common complaint, and the patient is often surprised when weakness or atrophy of the thenar muscle group is demonstrated during the examination. Patients often complain of difficulty in opening jars.

Physical examination usually shows decreased sensation in a median nerve distribution in the involved hand, frequently limited to a subjective hypesthesia or altered two-point discrimination (the latter usually occurs later with evidence of axonal loss). Light percussion over the median nerve just below the distal wrist crease may provoke tingling dysesthesias in the median nerve distribution (i.e., Tinel's sign); when present, this is a helpful diagnostic finding (sensitivity 20% to 70%; specificity 70% to 83%).[24–26] Reproduction of symptoms when the wrist is placed in complete flexion for 30 to 60 seconds (Phalen's sign) is positive in up to 80% of patients suspected of having CTS, with a sensitivity and specificity of 83%.[7, 8, 25] Inflating a blood pressure cuff to above systolic pressure for 60 seconds proximal to the involved hand may reproduce the symptoms.[27]

Some degree of thenar atrophy involving the opponens pollicis, abductor pollicis brevis, or flexor pollicis brevis muscle is observed in about 30% of patients. This atrophy is best appreciated by comparing the two hands carefully. Weakness of the abductor pollicis brevis muscle, which is invariably innervated by the median nerve, may be demonstrated by having the patient abduct the thumb from the plane of the palm against resistance. The opponens pollicis draws the thumb toward the center of the thumb and medially rotates it. The functional integrity of this muscle can be tested by asking the patient to touch the thumb to the small finger, so that the nails are parallel with each other. Weakness outside the thenar muscles should force the examiner to rethink the diagnosis of CTS or consider an additional peripheral nerve problem. It should be noted that there is a rare syndrome that may cause thenar weakness and atrophy in the absence of sensory disturbances as a result of compression limited to the recurrent motor branch of the distal median nerve.[5]

Electrical studies are accurate in confirming the diagnostic impression of CTS. In fact, they have become so reliable that we are reluctant to decompress the carpal tunnel in the absence of supportive electrodiagnostic data. The most sensitive electrical test is the palmar sensory conduction time and amplitude, determined by stimulating the median sensory fibers in the palm just below the transverse carpal ligament and recording over the wrist. Conduction times and amplitudes are compared between hands, with the ipsilateral ulnar nerve conduction response, and with the established normal values of the laboratory performing the study.[28] Recent studies suggest that a ratio greater than 0.4 to 0.5 for the conduction time of median nerve to ulnar nerve is diagnostic for CTS; however, in active workers, a ratio of 0.8 may be more appropriate for diagnosis.[29] Orthodromic sensory potentials recorded by stimulating the finger and recording over the wrist, and motor distal latency or conduction times obtained by stimulating at the wrist and recording over the abductor pollicis brevis muscle, are also helpful in establishing the diagnosis. Electromyography is usually not necessary. Relying on the findings of distal nerve conduction studies obviates any confusion resulting from a coexisting Martin-Gruber anastomosis.[30] The sensitivity and specificity of nerve conduction studies are reportedly 90% for patients with CTS. However, 10% of patients with CTS have normal electrical studies, and approximately 9% to 16% of asymptomatic people have abnormal conduction studies.[25] When electrodiagnostic studies do not corroborate the diagnosis, magnetic resonance imaging studies may be helpful in diagnosing and treating CTS[22, 25, 31](refer to Chapter 254).

By monitoring motor conduction times intraoperatively, it has been possible to show an immediate and dramatic reduction in the conduction latency across the carpal tunnel canal after decompression is accomplished.[32] Although conduction times can be expected to improve postoperatively, they do not always return to normal. This can be explained by permanent intraneural changes as a result of fibrosis in more severe cases.

TREATMENT

Some patients with CTS can be treated conservatively, particularly if the underlying problem is self-limited (as with pregnancy) or the symptoms are mild and are related to activities or positions of the hand that can be avoided or altered. For example, if the patient is exposed to vibration or repetitive motion activities in the workplace, a change in job description with cessation of such activities may result in relief from symptoms.[18-20] Wearing a wrist splint that maintains the wrist in slight extension, particularly during sleep, may help. Steroid injections into the carpal tunnel, with or without splinting, can be an effective temporizing maneuver.[33, 34] The technique of injecting steroids is quite important, because the physician must take great care to avoid intraneural injection.[35] These measures usually result in only transient relief, however, and are not recommended for patients with severe symptoms or signs.

Conventional Carpal Tunnel Release (Open Technique)

Continued or disabling symptoms in the presence of electrodiagnostically proven CTS, evidence of muscle weakness or atrophy, and increased two-point discrimination are all indications for surgical decompression. The surgery is done under loupe magnification, and most routine carpal tunnel procedures are performed with the patient under local anesthesia in an outpatient operating room setting. A single dose of intravenous antibiotics may be given preoperatively. Simple local anesthesia is used (a 50%-50% combination of lidocaine and marcaine without epinephrine diluted in a 1:10 ratio with sodium bicarbonate). Tourniquets and axillary blocks or Bier blocks may be used, but we do not find them necessary. Meticulous bipolar coagulation as one proceeds maintains hemostasis without injury to surrounding structures.

After sterile prepping of the extremity, an incision is outlined that begins proximally just ulnar to the palmaris longus tendon at the distal wrist crease and extends distally in a line of trajectory between the third and fourth fingers as far as the base of the thumb (approximately 4 cm). The line of proposed incision is then injected with local anesthetic subcutaneously (Fig. 255–1). As the proximal part of the skin incision is made, care is taken to avoid injuring or sectioning any branches of the palmar cutaneous nerve (sometimes these small branches are difficult to distinguish from subcutaneous fat or small vessels in the area). Tiny self-retaining Weitlaner retractors are used to aid in spreading the incision as the decompression progresses. Fibers of the palmar aponeurosis and of the palmaris brevis muscle may have to be sectioned to expose the underlying carpal tunnel. The transverse carpal ligament is identified, and an initial incision is made into the proximal flexor retinaculum with a no. 11 scalpel. A no. 4 Penfield dissector is then placed beneath the ligament, and the scalpel is used to cut the ligament distally until the fat pad pops out. A Senn retractor is then used to provide proximal upward traction on the incision so that fine Metzenbaum scissors can cut the proximal portion of the carpal tunnel as it passes under the wrist and merges with the distal medial antebrachial fascia, thereby allowing free passage of the no. 4 Penfield blunt dissector under the wrist.

Direct contact with the nerve is limited, and decompression is accomplished by section of and traction on surrounding tissues. Throughout the process of ligament section, a careful watch is maintained for an anomalous position of the motor branch, to avoid sectioning it. The no. 4 Penfield blunt dissector can be used to gently separate the median nerve from surrounding tissues it may be adherent to, such as the overlying carpal tunnel. In cases of severe CTS with thenar atrophy, the recurrent motor branch should be visualized to make sure it is decompressed.

In most instances, the maximal point of nerve entrapment is about 2 cm below the level of the distal wrist crease, and at this site, the nerve usually looks

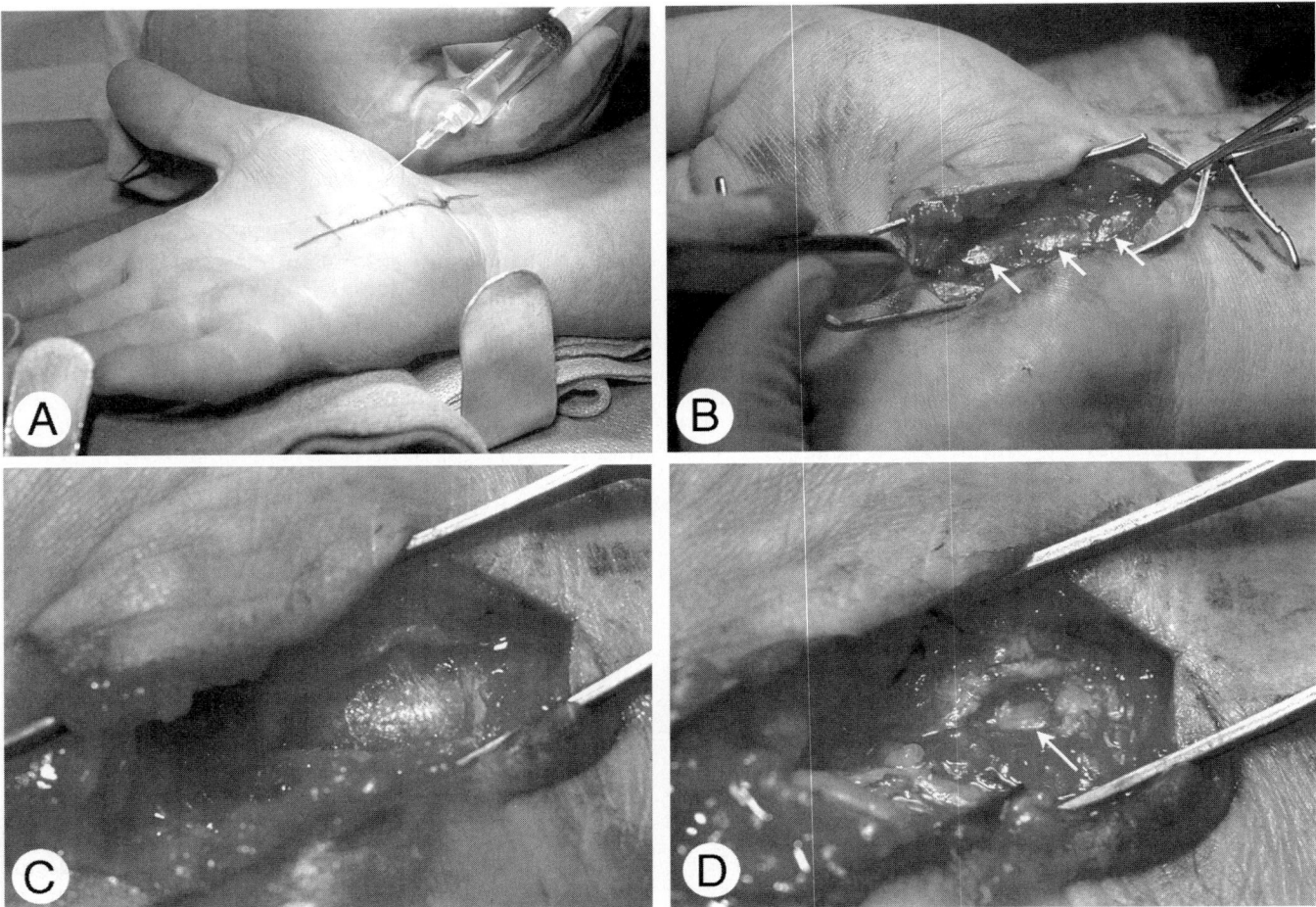

FIGURE 255–1.   Open carpal tunnel surgery. *A,* Marking of the incision on the palmar surface before the infiltration of local anesthetic. *B,* Exposure of the transverse carpal ligament *(arrows). C,* Close-up view of the transverse carpal ligament. *D,* After the transverse carpal ligament is identified, it is carefully incised, and the median nerve is identified *(arrow).*

hyperemic. Upon sectioning the most distal end of the ligament, a small fat pad is encountered, and the nerve is obviously free of entrapment. In this area, care should be exercised to avoid injuring the vascular arch as well as the sensory branches. We do not specifically seek out or individually decompress the motor branch unless motor weakness and atrophy are important parts of the clinical picture. The origin of the motor branch has many variations, and one must be on the lookout for this branch to avoid injuring it.[4, 5]

If this is the patient's first operation on the carpal tunnel, we do not perform internal neurolysis or flexor synovectomy. Studies comparing the efficacy of such adjuncts with simple decompression have failed to show a benefit, and those who vigorously advocate neurolysis do so without an adequate control group of patients and based on results that are no better than those of simple decompression in other series.[36–39] There is, however, a place for neurolysis in a repeat procedure in which fibrosis and scarring seem to be the reason for failure of the original procedure or for the return of symptoms.

Once the surgeon is certain of adequate decompres-

sion, the wound is closed in a single superficial layer of interrupted mattress sutures with a nonabsorbable monofilament suture material (e.g., 4–0 nylon). The sutures should be spaced far enough apart to make it easy to remove them 2 weeks later. An alternative strategy is to first place two absorbable 4–0 sutures superficially in the subcutaneous tissues in an inverted fashion before closing the skin in patients who do not have an allergy to suture material. A bulky hand bandage is then applied.

The patient is given a prescription for a mild oral analgesic and instructed to keep the hand moderately elevated for the first 48 hours postoperatively. Immediate gentle range-of-motion exercises about the finger and wrist joints are encouraged to reduce the chance of tethering adhesions forming around the decompressed median nerve. We advocate gently opening and closing the hand and partially flexing and extending the wrist 20 times an hour while awake. The bandage is changed in 7 days, and the incision is kept dry until the sutures are extracted at 2 weeks. The patient is instructed to avoid vigorous hand activities for 2 to 3 months to allow for optimal healing of the wound and recovery of median nerve function. The patient can then judiciously increase the level of hand activity while remaining within his or her comfort zone. Resumption of full work activities too soon can compromise the patient's long-term outcome.

The standard carpal tunnel release can be expected to result in good to excellent relief of symptoms in about 80% of patients, partial relief in about 10%, no change in 9%, and an exacerbation of the condition in less than 1%.[6, 8, 40] In those patients who present with motor atrophy, 84% have return of normal function, 9% have some improvement, and 7% show no improvement or become worse.[8]

Alternative methods of open surgical release are currently being used with success. The Paine retinaculatome, an instrument fashioned after a seam ripper with a flat footplate that rides over the nerve and a vertically oriented blade to section the ligament, has been used with success in large series of patients.[41, 42] The procedure performed with this instrument is relatively blind toward the distal retinaculum; thus, inadequate release or damage to an anomalous motor branch is a concern with this technique. Additionally, a limited incision technique has been described in which a 2- to 3-cm-long straight incision is made in line with the radial border of the ring finger, and the release is carried forward. We use neither of these techniques, although we do favor using the smallest incision necessary to fully decompress the nerve under direct vision.

Endoscopic Carpal Tunnel Release (Closed Technique)

Endoscopic carpal tunnel release is gaining popularity, and the techniques are evolving. The procedure was first described by Okutsu and coworkers and Chow in back-to-back articles in *Arthroscopy* in 1989.[43, 44] Since then, many techniques have been developed based on equipment and the number of ports used, and two of

these techniques have gained significant popularity in the United States: the two-portal method (Chow) and the single-portal technique (Agee).[45] Indications for using the endoscopic approach are similar to but more limited than those for the open technique. Patients with rheumatoid arthritis, significant tenosynovitis, recurrent CTS, concurrent ulnar tunnel syndrome, or a space-occupying lesion should not undergo an endoscopic release.

In the two-portal technique developed by Chow, two small transverse incisions are made. The proximal port incision is made 1 cm proximal and 1 cm radial to the pisiform bone. The second port is made along the distal edge of the transverse carpal ligament. An incision is made in the antebrachial fascia proximally, and the undersurface of the transverse carpal ligament is dissected free from the synovium. A trocar is placed through the proximal incision, under the ligament, and out through the distal incision. The endoscope is placed through the proximal incision, and the distal half of the transverse ligament is cut with a series of three separate knives. The camera is then transferred to the distal incision, and the proximal ligament is incised. The incisions are then visualized through the cannula.

In the one-portal method (Agee technique), a device that incorporates the endoscope and a disposable blade is used. A transverse incision (2 to 3 cm long) is made in the volar flexion wrist crease between the flexor carpi radialis tendon and the flexor carpi ulnaris tendon (Fig. 255–2A and B). The antebrachial fascia is incised and mobilized to expose the underside of the transverse carpal ligament. The device is inserted distally, and under endoscopic visualization, its tip is positioned under the fat pad at the end of the ligament (see Fig. 255–2C). The blade is then deployed, cutting the distal portion of the ligament first. The rest of the ligament is incised as the device is withdrawn proximally (see Fig. 255–2C).

Both these techniques require some practice before one becomes proficient. In early series, the mean time

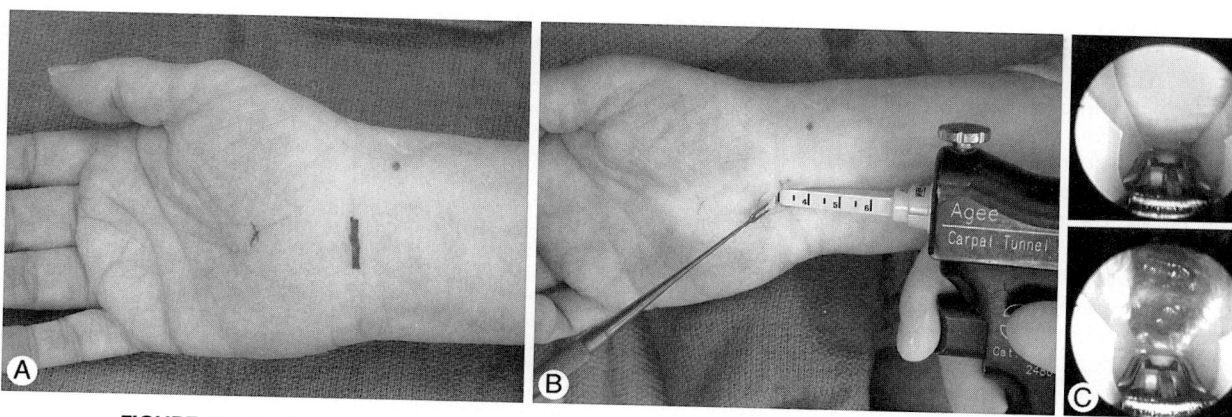

FIGURE 255–2. Endoscopic carpal tunnel surgery—single-portal (Agee) technique. *A*, Marking of the incision on the palmar surface before insertion of the endoscopic device. *B*, After the incision is made, the antebrachial fascia is incised and mobilized to expose the transverse carpal ligament, and the endoscopic device is inserted. *C*, Visualization of the underside of the transverse carpal ligament before and after it is incised to complete the carpal tunnel release. (Courtesy of Dr. Michael A. McClinton, Curtis National Hand Associates, Baltimore, MD.)

for return to work was less in patients undergoing endoscopic procedures than in those undergoing open procedures.[46–49] Postoperative pain seemed to be less in endoscopically treated patients, and grip and pinch strength improved earlier in this group. However, the results of more recent randomized studies directly comparing endoscopic and open techniques have been mixed. Some studies demonstrate some initial benefits of endoscopic carpal tunnel release,[50] but overall, there appears to be no significant benefit over open carpal tunnel release.[51–53]

The most common complications of endoscopic carpal tunnel release are incomplete release of the nerve, which may lead to a second open procedure; median nerve injuries; superficial vascular arch injuries; and tendon injuries. As with all surgical techniques, there is a learning curve before proficiency is reached, which affects the complication rate. However, the complications of endoscopic carpal tunnel release surgery do not appear to be significantly different from those associated with the open technique. The overall complication rate reported by the American Society of Surgery of the Hand in 1995 was 1.2% for endoscopic release and 0.8% for open release.[45]

COMPLICATIONS

Complications of carpal tunnel operations, either open or endoscopic, include (1) inadequate release of the ligament, resulting in persistence of symptoms; (2) postoperative fibrosis and scarring, resulting in a return of symptoms; (3) a tender neuroma of the palmar cutaneous branch of the median nerve; (4) tender or hypertrophic scars; (5) section of the recurrent motor branch of the median nerve, resulting in complete denervation and atrophy of the thenar muscle mass; (6) reflex sympathetic dystrophy; (7) bowstringing of the flexor tendons; and (8) wound infection.[2, 54–56] Most of these complications can be avoided if a thoughtful and careful operative procedure is performed.

Inadequate release of the ligament or an incorrect diagnosis should be suspected if the patient reports no relief of symptoms immediately after the operative procedure. An inadequate release can be avoided by visualizing complete section of the ligament at the time of operation through a longitudinal incision. Transverse incisions and methods that result in blind section of the ligament should be avoided.

Fibrosis and scarring may cause the return of symptoms after a symptom-free interval postoperatively. These complications can be avoided to a certain extent by maintaining meticulous hemostasis and by minimal handling of the nerve, as well as by encouraging early postoperative performance of range-of-motion exercises.

A tender neuroma of the palmar cutaneous branch of the median nerve is treated by section of the cutaneous branch at its origin from the median nerve in the lower forearm. It is possible to repair a sectioned recurrent motor branch by a secondary microscopic operative procedure, with good functional results. Sec-

ondary carpal tunnel surgery for the treatment of many of these complications was discussed by Mackinnon.[57] Different approaches to prevent extraneural scarring after surgery have been studied; wrapping the involved nerve with a graft, applying various chemical compounds such as ADCON-T/N (a bioabsorbable antiscar gel), and radiation have been used with varying degrees of success.[58]

Reflex sympathetic dystrophy is an unfortunate and poorly understood complication of peripheral nerve procedures but may have some relationship to the amount of nerve manipulation and trauma. Occasionally, it is responsive to sympathetic nerve blocks or to sympathectomy.

Overall, the judicious, meticulous, and careful evaluation and treatment of patients with CTS can be a rewarding experience both for the patient and the surgeon.

REFERENCES

1. Stevens JC, Sun S, Beard CM, et al: Carpal tunnel syndrome in Rochester, Minnesota, 1961 to 1980. Neurology 38:134–138, 1988.
2. Louis DS, Greene TL, Noellert RC: Complications of carpal tunnel surgery. J Neurosurg 62:352–356, 1985.
3. Taleisnik J: The palmar cutaneous branch of the median nerve and the approach to the carpal tunnel: An anatomical study. J Bone Joint Surg Am 55:1212–1217, 1973.
4. Lanz U: Anatomical variations of the median nerve in the carpal tunnel. J Hand Surg [Am] 2:44–53, 1977.
5. Bennett JB, Crouch CC: Compression syndrome of the recurrent motor branch of the median nerve. J Hand Surg [Am] 7:407–409, 1982.
6. Gainer JV Jr, Nugent GR: Carpal tunnel syndrome: Report of 430 operations. South Med J 70:325–328, 1977.
7. Phalen GS: Reflections on 21 years' experience with the carpal-tunnel syndrome. JAMA 212:1365–1367, 1970.
8. Phalen GS: The carpal-tunnel syndrome: Clinical evaluation of 598 hands. Clin Orthop 83:29–40, 1972.
9. Bleecker ML, Bohlman M, Moreland R, Tipton A: Carpal tunnel syndrome: Role of carpal canal size. Neurology 35:1599–1604, 1985.
10. O'Duffy JD, Randall RV, MacCarty CS: Median neuropathy (carpal-tunnel syndrome) in acromegaly: A sign of endocrine overactivity. Ann Intern Med 78:379–383, 1973.
11. Schiller F, Kolb FO: Carpal tunnel syndrome in acromegaly. Neurology 4:271–282, 1954.
12. Beard L, Kumar A, Estep HL: Bilateral carpal tunnel syndrome caused by Graves' disease. Arch Intern Med 145:345–346, 1985.
13. Gould JS, Wissinger HA: Carpal tunnel syndrome in pregnancy. South Med J 71:144–145, 154, 1978.
14. Massey EW: Carpal tunnel syndrome in pregnancy. Obstet Gynecol Surv 33:145–148, 1978.
15. Weimer LH, Yin J, Lovelace RE, Gooch CL: Serial studies of carpal tunnel syndrome during and after pregnancy. Muscle Nerve 25:914–917, 2002.
16. Eason SY, Belsole RJ, Greene TL: Carpal tunnel release: Analysis of suboptimal results. J Hand Surg [Br] 10:365–369, 1985.
17. Massey EW, Riley TL, Pleet AB: Coexistent carpal tunnel syndrome and cervical radiculopathy (double crush syndrome). South Med J 74:957–959, 1981.
18. Kirschberg GJ, Fillingim R, Davis VP, Hogg F: Carpal tunnel syndrome: Classic clinical symptoms and electrodiagnostic studies in poultry workers with hand, wrist, and forearm pain. South Med J 87:328–331, 1994.
19. Koskimies K, Farkkila M, Pyykko I, et al: Carpal tunnel syndrome in vibration disease. Br J Ind Med 47:411–416, 1990.
20. Miller RF, Lohman WH, Maldonado G, Mandel JS: An epidemiologic study of carpal tunnel syndrome and hand-arm vibration syndrome in relation to vibration exposure. J Hand Surg [Am] 19:99–105, 1994.

21. Cherington M: Proximal pain in carpal tunnel syndrome. Arch Surg 108:69, 1974.
22. Grant GA, Britz GW, Goodkin R, et al: The utility of magnetic resonance imaging in evaluating peripheral nerve disorders. Muscle Nerve 25:314–331, 2002.
23. Sunderland S: The nerve lesion in the carpal tunnel syndrome. J Neurol Neurosurg Psychiatry 39:615–626, 1976.
24. Gellman H, Gelberman RH, Tan AM, Botte MJ: Carpal tunnel syndrome: An evaluation of the provocative diagnostic tests. J Bone Joint Surg Am 68:735–737, 1986.
25. Jarvik JG, Yuen E, Haynor DR, et al: MR nerve imaging in a prospective cohort of patients with suspected carpal tunnel syndrome. Neurology 58:1597–1602, 2002.
26. Katz JN, Larson MG, Sabra A, et al: The carpal tunnel syndrome: Diagnostic utility of the history and physical examination findings. Ann Intern Med 112:321–327, 1990.
27. Fullerton PM: The effect of ischaemia on nerve conduction in the carpal tunnel syndrome. J Neurol Neurosurg Psychiatry 26:385–397, 1963.
28. Kimura J: The carpal tunnel syndrome: Localization of conduction abnormalities within the distal segment of the median nerve. Brain 102:619–635, 1979.
29. Werner RA, Andary M: Carpal tunnel syndrome: Pathophysiology and clinical neurophysiology. Clin Neurophysiol 113:1373–1381, 2002.
30. Iyer V, Fenichel GM: Normal median nerve proximal latency in carpal tunnel syndrome: A clue to coexisting Martin-Gruber anastomosis. J Neurol Neurosurg Psychiatry 39:449–452, 1976.
31. Jarvik JG, Kliot M, Maravilla KR: MR nerve imaging of the wrist and hand. Hand Clin 16:13–24, 2000.
32. Eversmann WW Jr, Ritsick JA: Intraoperative changes in motor nerve conduction latency in carpal tunnel syndrome. J Hand Surg [Am] 3:77–81, 1978.
33. Gelberman RH, Aronson D, Weisman MH: Carpal-tunnel syndrome: Results of a prospective trial of steroid injection and splinting. J Bone Joint Surg Am 62:1181–1184, 1980.
34. Green DP: Diagnostic and therapeutic value of carpal tunnel injection. J Hand Surg [Am] 9:850–854, 1984.
35. McConnell JR, Bush DC: Intraneural steroid injection as a complication in the management of carpal tunnel syndrome: A report of three cases. Clin Orthop 250:181–184, 1990.
36. Curtis RM, Eversmann WW Jr: Internal neurolysis as an adjunct to the treatment of the carpal-tunnel syndrome. J Bone Joint Surg Am 55:733–740, 1973.
37. Freshwater MF, Arons MS: The effect of various adjuncts on the surgical treatment of carpal tunnel syndrome secondary to chronic tenosynovitis. Plast Reconstr Surg 61:93–96, 1978.
38. Holmgren-Larsson H, Leszniewski W, Linden U, et al: Internal neurolysis or ligament division only in carpal tunnel syndrome—results of a randomized study. Acta Neurochir (Wien) 74:118–121, 1985.
39. Rhoades CE, Mowery CA, Gelberman RH: Results of internal neurolysis of the median nerve for severe carpal-tunnel syndrome. J Bone Joint Surg Am 67:253–256, 1985.
40. Cseuz KA, Thomas JE, Lambert EH, et al: Long-term results of operation for carpal tunnel syndrome. Mayo Clin Proc 41:232–241, 1966.
41. Pagnanelli DM, Barrer SJ: Carpal tunnel syndrome: Surgical treatment using the Paine retinaculatome. J Neurosurg 75:77–81, 1991.
42. Paine KW, Polyzoidis KS: Carpal tunnel syndrome: Decompression using the Paine retinaculotome. J Neurosurg 59:1031–1036, 1983.
43. Chow JC: Endoscopic release of the carpal ligament: A new technique for carpal tunnel syndrome. Arthroscopy 5:19–24, 1989.
44. Okutsu I, Ninomiya S, Takatori Y, Ugawa Y: Endoscopic management of carpal tunnel syndrome. Arthroscopy 5:11–18, 1989.
45. Schenck RR: The role of endoscopic surgery in the treatment of carpal tunnel syndrome. Adv Plast Reconstr Surg 11:17–43, 1995.
46. Agee JM, McCarroll HR Jr, Tortosa RD, et al: Endoscopic release of the carpal tunnel: A randomized prospective multicenter study. J Hand Surg [Am] 17:987–995, 1992.
47. Agee JM, Peimer CA, Pyrek JD, Walsh WE: Endoscopic carpal tunnel release: A prospective study of complications and surgical experience. J Hand Surg [Am] 20:165–171, discussion 172, 1995.
48. Erdmann MW: Endoscopic carpal tunnel decompression. J Hand Surg [Br] 19:5–13, 1994.
49. Roth JH, Richards RS, MacLeod MD: Endoscopic carpal tunnel release. Can J Surg 37:189–193, 1994.
50. Trumble TE, Diao E, Abrams RA, Gilbert-Anderson MM: Single-portal endoscopic carpal tunnel release compared with open release: A prospective, randomized trial. J Bone Joint Surg Am 84:1107–1115, 2002.
51. Muller LP, Rudig L, Degreif J, Rommens PM: Endoscopic carpal tunnel release: Results with special consideration to possible complications. Knee Surg Sports Traumatol Arthrosc 8:166–172, 2000.
52. Gerritsen AA, Uitdehaag BM, van Geldere D, et al: Systematic review of randomized clinical trials of surgical treatment for carpal tunnel syndrome. Br J Surg 88:1285–1295, 2001.
53. Ferdinand RD, MacLean JG: Endoscopic versus open carpal tunnel release in bilateral carpal tunnel syndrome: A prospective, randomised, blinded assessment. J Bone Joint Surg Br 84:375–379, 2002.
54. Langloh ND, Linscheid RL: Recurrent and unrelieved carpal-tunnel syndrome. Clin Orthop 83:41–47, 1972.
55. Lilly CJ, Magnell TD: Severance of the thenar branch of the median nerve as a complication of carpal tunnel release. J Hand Surg [Am] 10:399–402, 1985.
56. MacDonald RI, Lichtman DM, Hanlon JJ, Wilson JN: Complications of surgical release for carpal tunnel syndrome. J Hand Surg [Am] 3:70–76, 1978.
57. Mackinnon SE: Secondary carpal tunnel surgery. Neurosurg Clin N Am 2:75–91, 1991.
58. McCall TD, Grant GA, Britz GW, et al: Treatment of recurrent peripheral nerve entrapment problems: Role of scar formation and its possible treatment. Neurosurg Clin N Am 12:329–339, 2001.

CHAPTER 256

Ulnar Nerve Entrapment at the Elbow

JAMES B. LOWE III ■ SUSAN E. MACKINNON

Ulnar nerve entrapment at the elbow, or cubital tunnel syndrome, is the second most common nerve entrapment syndrome of the upper extremity.[1, 2] Although there is a high incidence of ulnar nerve entrapment at the elbow, there is no commonly accepted treatment strategy. A thorough understanding of the complexities of the condition is required to ensure the best clinical results. This chapter provides a historical review of ulnar nerve compression at the elbow and discusses its cause and diagnosis. A comparison of current treatment options, along with a rationale for their application, and our clinical recommendations and results are provided.

HISTORY

In 1816, Earle[3] described the excision of a segment of the ulnar nerve in the treatment of ulnar neuritis. The patient's severe neuralgia resolved following surgery. In 1833, Calder[4] treated another patient with severe neuralgia and confirmed Earle's results. Sunderland[5] reported that Andrae excised a portion of the ulnar nerve in the treatment of subluxation in 1889. In 1921, Sheldon[6] claimed that nerve excision in the treatment of ulnar neuropathy significantly increased morbidity.

In 1878, Panas[7] described the relationship of ulnar nerve compression at the elbow and clinical nerve palsy in three patients. Roux of Lausanne in 1897 reportedly described the anterior subcutaneous transposition of the ulnar nerve, which was unsuccessful.[8] Curtis[9] reported a case of "traumatic ulnar neuritis" treated with neurolysis and subcutaneous transplantation of the ulnar nerve in 1898. Most early reports of the treatment of ulnar nerve compression at the elbow favored anterior transposition of the ulnar nerve.[10, 11]

Throughout the early 1900s, ulnar neuropathy was generally thought to be the result of previous trauma in the region of the elbow and was referred to as *post-traumatic ulnar neuritis* or *tardy ulnar palsy*.[6, 8, 12] Treatment of the disorder originally focused on protecting the ulnar nerve from scarring or transposing it away from an area of trauma. Although most of the early studies of ulnar nerve compression at the elbow related the disease to trauma, the number of cases with no identifiable cause continued to increase.[6, 13, 14]

Anterior intramuscular transposition to treat ulnar nerve compression at the elbow was first described in 1918 by Adson at the Mayo Clinic.[13] In 1942, Learmonth[15] reported using an anterior submuscular transposition of the ulnar nerve. In 1959, King and Morgan[16] described medial epicondylectomy as yet another means of treating ulnar nerve compression at the elbow.

Osborne[17] in 1957 claimed that simple division of the tendinous edge of the flexor carpi ulnaris covering the ulnar nerve at the elbow would provide results similar to those of anterior transposition. Feindel and Stratford[18] first used the term *cubital tunnel* in 1958. They also believed that release of the cubital tunnel was the most important component in the treatment of ulnar nerve entrapment at the elbow. This provided the first explanation for idiopathic causes of the disease and generated support for simple decompression of the ulnar nerve.

Strong proponents of different surgical techniques remain, but no one surgical intervention has been fully embraced. Recently, we emphasized anterior transmuscular transposition of the ulnar nerve as a superior technique.[19] Knowledge of the rich history of this disease helps physicians understand the rationale for different surgical approaches (Table 256–1). Nevertheless, studies that compare different surgical techniques have failed to prove the benefit of one technique over another.

SURGICAL ANATOMY

General Anatomy

All potential anatomic compression points of the ulnar nerve must be understood to properly manage cubital tunnel syndrome. Nerve roots C7, C8, and T1 contribute to the ulnar nerve. The ulnar nerve is a terminal branch off the medial cord of the brachial plexus, and it runs posterior and medial to the brachial artery in the upper arm. At the midportion of the upper arm, the ulnar nerve travels between the brachialis and medial head of the triceps posterior to the intermuscular septum.

At the elbow, the ulnar nerve runs posterior to the

TABLE 256-1 ■ **History of Ulnar Nerve Surgery**

AUTHOR	YEAR	CONTRIBUTION
Earle[3]	1816	Described excision of segment of ulnar nerve
Panas[7]	1878	Described ulnar nerve compression at elbow with palsy
Curtis[9]	1898	Described anterior subcutaneous transposition of ulnar nerve
Adson[13]	1918	Described anterior intramuscular transposition of ulnar nerve
Learmonth[15]	1942	Described anterior submuscular transposition of ulnar nerve
Osborne[17]	1957	Described the ligament covering ulnar nerve
Feindel & Stratford[18]	1958	Described the "cubital tunnel"
King & Morgan[16]	1959	Described medial epicondylectomy to treat ulnar nerve compression at the elbow
Lowe et al[19]	2001	Described anterior transmuscular transposition of ulnar nerve

medial epicondyle in the postcondylar groove of the olecranon. At this level, the nerve is bounded medially and anteriorly by the medial epicondyle and laterally by the olecranon. Between these two bony prominences, a roof is formed over the ulnar nerve by dense fascia. The cubital tunnel begins with the fascia between the medial epicondyle and the olecranon and ends at the area between the two heads of the flexor carpi ulnaris muscle.

As the ulnar nerve passes into the cubital tunnel, it courses beneath the leading edge of Osborne's band. This is the fascia connecting the ulnar and humeral heads of the flexor carpi ulnaris. In the proximal forearm, the ulnar nerve travels deep to the flexor digitorum superficialis and the flexor carpi ulnaris and on top of the flexor digitorum profundus. At the wrist, the nerve is medial to the ulnar artery and runs beneath the flexor carpi ulnaris tendon, entering the hand through Guyon's canal.

Standard Innervation

The ulnar nerve provides sensation to the ulnar aspect of the hand, including the small finger and the ulnar half of the ring finger. In the distal forearm, the palmar branch of the ulnar nerve supplies the ulnar aspect of the palm, and the dorsal branch of the ulnar nerve supplies the ulnar aspects of the dorsal hand. Taleisnik[20] demonstrated that an incision 6 to 7 mm to the ulnar side of the thenar crease essentially separates ulnar and median cutaneous innervation of the palm.

The ulnar nerve innervates the ulnar artery by way of the nerve of Henle.[21] The nerve of Henle also provides sensory branches to the distal forearm and the hypothenar region; when the nerve of Henle is present, the palmar cutaneous branch of the ulnar nerve is not. McCabe and Kleinert[21] report that the nerve of Henle is absent in 43% of dissections.

In Guyon's canal, the ulnar nerve splits into superficial and deep branches. The superficial branch supplies sensation to the radial carpal joint, the small finger, and ulnar aspects of the ring finger. The deep branch supplies intrinsic motor function to the hand. Understanding the sensory distribution of the ulnar nerve aids the surgeon in diagnosing the specific level of ulnar nerve compression.

The ulnar nerve provides no motor branches to muscles in the upper arm, but there are motor branches that exit at the elbow en route to the forearm. In the proximal forearm, the ulnar nerve provides motor function to the flexor carpi ulnaris and the flexor digitorum profundus muscles to the small and ring fingers. The deep branch of the ulnar nerve provides motor function to the hypothenar, palmar and dorsal interosseous, third and fourth lumbrical, adductor pollicis, and deep head of the flexor pollicis brevis muscles.

Anomalous Innervation

Muscle innervation of the ulnar nerve can have anatomic variation. Sunderland[5] reported that innervation to the flexor digitorum profundus to the small and ring fingers is by the ulnar nerve in approximately 50% of cases. However, the median nerve can provide a portion of the innervation in the other 50%.

The ulnar nerve may have anomalous motor connections from the median nerve in the proximal forearm by way of a Martin-Gruber anastomosis.[22, 23] The Martin-Gruber anastomosis may also be present more distally, between the anterior interosseous nerve and the ulnar nerve. Leibovic and Hastings reported a 17% incidence of Martin-Gruber anastomoses.[24] Individuals with an injury or compression to the ulnar nerve proximal to a Martin-Gruber anastomosis have preservation of intrinsic motor function to the hand via the median nerve.

Anomalous motor connections known as Riche-Cannieu anastomoses are also noted in the palm between the ulnar and median nerves. Riche-Cannieu connections may occur in up to 70% of patients.[23] The significance of these anomalous motor innervations is that they may mask or confuse a potential injury to either the median or the ulnar nerve.

Vascular Anatomy

The blood supply to the ulnar nerve is provided by both intrinsic and extrinsic blood vessels.[25, 26] The extrinsic blood supply to the ulnar nerve is provided primarily through branches from the brachial and ulnar arteries. Prevel and coworkers[27] examined the extrinsic blood supply of the ulnar nerve in 18 cadavers after an intra-arterial injection of latex. They demonstrated that the two major pedicles to the ulnar nerve were the superior ulnar collateral artery proximally and the posterior ulnar recurrent artery distally. The superior ulnar collateral artery branched from the brachial artery approximately 16 cm above the elbow, and the posterior ulnar recurrent artery branched from the ulnar artery approximately 7 cm below the elbow. The inferior ulnar collateral artery was a minor pedicle seen in only 5 of 18 specimens.

Some authors have suggested that the vasa nervorum may be injured with mobilization of the ulnar nerve.[17, 28] The importance of preserving the extrinsic blood supply to the ulnar nerve was examined in 1988 by Sugawara.[29] In this study, 22 patients underwent treatment of cubital tunnel syndrome using a vascularized ulnar nerve transposition. Although Sugawara recommended preserving extrinsic blood supply during mobilization of the ulnar nerve, no clinically significant benefit could be demonstrated.

The intrinsic blood supply to the ulnar nerve is significant.[25, 30] The proximal and distal intrinsic blood vessels allow the ulnar nerve to be safely transposed over a long distance. Maki and colleagues[31] demonstrated experimentally the profound effect of the intrinsic blood supply to nerves. This study demonstrated in a rabbit model that the diameter-length ratio for bipedicled nerve survival was approximately 1:63.

A specific diameter-length ratio cannot necessarily be applied to nerves subject to ischemia caused by compression or trauma. Ogata and Naito[32] demonstrated that stretching and compressing peripheral nerves result in complete cessation of blood flow. In the canine model, Sugawara[29] showed that anterior transposition of the ulnar nerve resulted in 80% of normal flow when the extrinsic blood supply was preserved, but subsequent epineurolysis decreased blood flow by 45%. Ogata and associates[28] measured blood flow in the ulnar nerve of monkeys following anterior subcutaneous transposition and found a significant decrease in blood flow at 3 days, but the ischemia resolved by 7 days.

It is important to preserve as much of the blood supply to the ulnar nerve as possible. In most surgical cases in which complete ulnar nerve transposition is planned, the extrinsic blood supply to the ulnar nerve can be maintained to the level of the medial epicondyle. Sacrificing the extrinsic blood supply at this level during primary surgery for cubital tunnel syndrome carries no risk.

Medial Antebrachial Cutaneous Nerve

The medial antebrachial cutaneous (MABC) nerve is a terminal branch of the medial cord of the brachial plexus, and it has anterior and posterior branches that course both distal and proximal to the medial epicondyle. Both branches of the MABC nerve are at risk when an incision is made at the elbow.

In our experience, the MABC nerve has several main branches both proximal and distal to the medial epicondyle that cross the standard 6-cm surgical incision located over the postcondylar groove.[19] A proximal branch is present 60% of the time, located on average 3 cm (range, 1 to 5 cm) proximal to the medial epicondyle. The distal branch is present 100% of the time, located on average 3.5 cm (range, 1 to 5.5 cm) distal to the medial epicondyle. The MABC nerve often has a

complex distribution of branches that may be difficult to avoid during surgery (Fig. 256–1).

Persistent pain following surgery for ulnar nerve compression at the elbow may be due to injury to a branch or branches of the antebrachial cutaneous nerve.[33, 34] Leffert[35] was one of the first to strongly encourage surgeons to avoid injury to the MABC nerve. Dellon and Mackinnon[34] described the manifestations of injury to the MABC nerve, including hypesthesia, painful scarring, and hyperalgesia. The surgeon can identify an injury to the MABC nerve by gently tapping along the course of the brachial vein well proximal to the medial epicondyle. A positive Tinel's sign in this region with radiation into the distribution of the MABC nerve helps diagnose a painful neuroma.

COMPRESSIVE NEUROPATHY

Any discussion of nerve compression requires familiarity with the classification of peripheral nerve injuries (Fig. 256–2). In 1942, Seddon[36] described three types of nerve injury: neurapraxia, axonotmesis, and neurotmesis. In 1951, Sunderland[37] expanded Seddon's work by classifying nerve injuries into five different degrees.

First-degree injury is conduction block without evidence of wallerian degeneration. Histologically, there may be some areas of demyelination, and recovery is complete. Second-degree injury is axonal damage with wallerian degeneration distal to the site of injury. The injury is purely axonal, with intact endoneurial tubes, and full recovery is expected. Third-degree injury involves scarring of the endoneurium without injury to the perineurium. The basal laminae of the Schwann cells are injured, resulting in axonal regeneration, and recovery is incomplete. In fourth-degree injury, the nerve is in continuity, but without function secondary to complete scar block. A fifth-degree injury is complete nerve division. Mackinnon[38] described a sixth-degree injury that combines varying degrees of injury and may be associated with some normal fascicles.

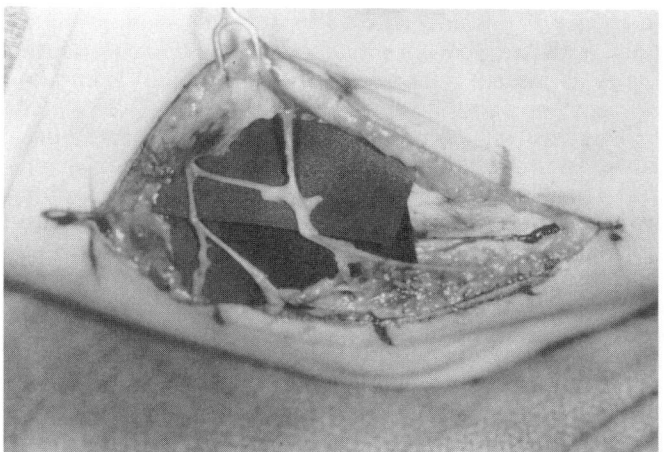

FIGURE 256–1. The branches of the medial antebrachial cutaneous nerve cross the ulnar nerve at the site of the standard surgical incision for repair of cubital tunnel syndrome.

Injured Nerve

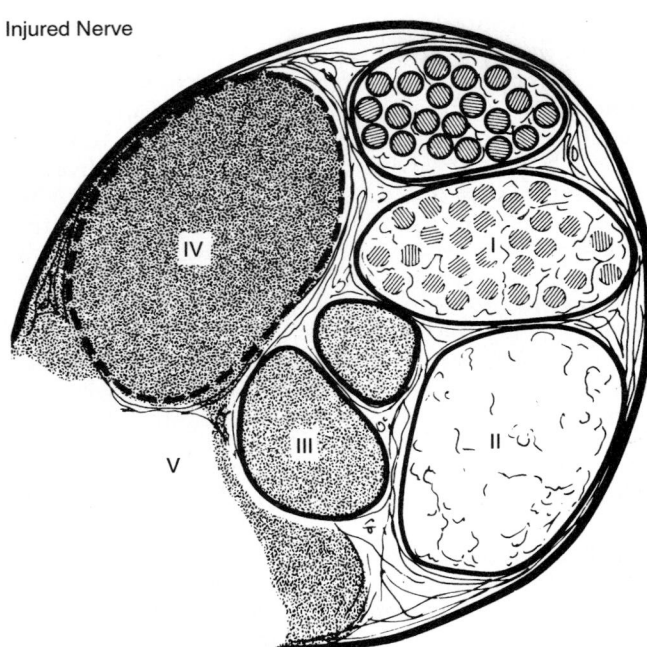

VI = any combination of I to V

FIGURE 256–2. Cross section of the peripheral nerve demonstrates a mixed, or sixth-degree, injury pattern. The fascicle at 1 o'clock is normal. Moving clockwise, the adjacent nerve demonstrates a first-degree injury (neurapraxia) with segmental demyelination. The next fascicle demonstrates a second-degree injury (axonotmesis). This injury involves both the axon and the myelin. The endoneurial tissue is not damaged. The central two fascicles demonstrate a third-degree injury, with injury to the axon, myelin, and endoneurium. The perineurium is intact and normal. The fascicle at 11 o'clock demonstrates a fourth-degree injury, with marked scarring across the nerve; only the epineurium is intact. The fascicle at 7 o'clock demonstrates a fifth-degree injury. In this injury pattern, the nerve is not in continuity but is transected. The surgeon will separate the fourth- and fifth-degree injury patterns, which requires reconstruction from the normal fascicles and the fascicles demonstrating first-, second-, and third-degree injury patterns. These latter patterns of injury require, at most, neurolysis. (From Mackinnon SE, Dellon AL: Surgery of the Peripheral Nerve. New York, Thieme-Stratton, 1988, p 36.)

Recovery is possible in fourth- and fifth-degree injury only with surgical repair. Recovery with sixth-degree injury is mixed, depending on the types of injury involved.

The greatest degree of injury within the nerve usually determines the clinical presentation. The peripheral fascicles are usually more susceptible to injury from compression. The combination of normal and abnormal fascicles seen in compression neuropathy explains patients with marked symptoms but normal electrodiagnostic studies. It is important to perform a complete examination to determine the innervation of all potential fascicles. This helps identify any clinically subtle evidence of nerve compression.

Entrapment neuropathy is a common clinical problem encountered by neurosurgeons. It is important to understand the pathogenesis of the disorder in order to properly treat patients.[39] The histopathologic changes associated with chronic nerve compression usually par-

allel the clinical progression of the disease. As the amount and duration of compression increase, so do connective tissue changes and nerve injury. The histopathology noted with nerve compression ranges from normal to severe wallerian degeneration (Fig. 256–3).

Chronic nerve compression can result in a spectrum of nerve injuries. There are some specific histologic and sensory changes that parallel the patient's clinical symptoms (Fig. 256–4). Certain extremity positions compress or stretch the nerve and result in slowly progressive histopathologic changes.[40] The histologic changes begin with injury to the blood-nerve barrier, resulting in subperineurial edema. The external and internal epineurium thickens. Renaut's bodies are usually noted in areas of compression following traction or repetitive motion. Large myelinated fibers demonstrate segmental demyelination, and unmyelinated fibers progressively degenerate; with long-standing compression, wallerian degeneration may occur. Clinically, patients at this point experience muscle atrophy and severe loss of sensation.

Patients with multiple nerve compression often present with diffuse or nonspecific clinical complaints that are difficult to diagnose on physical examination.[41] The double crush hypothesis first described in 1973 by Upton and McComas[42] should be understood when examining any patient with compressive neuropathies. Those authors hypothesized that one site of nerve compression might render other sites along the nerve less tolerant to compressive forces. They also noted an association between cubital tunnel syndrome and thoracic outlet and carpal tunnel syndromes. They referred to this as "multiple entrapment neuropathies" in the same extremity. Therefore, it is possible for more than one site of compression to produce the motor and sensory disturbances typical of cubital tunnel syndrome.

Other authors have suggested that systemic illness may make a nerve more susceptible to compression by acting like a "crush."[43, 44] A study in 1991 by Dellon and Mackinnon demonstrated that two separate sites of compression were worse than one of the same duration.[44] The mechanism of this disorder appears to be related to abnormal axoplasmic flow resulting in decreased transport of neurotrophic material.[45, 46]

Multiple sites of compression with different severities can cause symptoms ranging from minimal to severe, making diagnosis difficult. In the case of ulnar nerve entrapment at the elbow, other potential sites of compression must be excluded. If no single area of ulnar nerve compression explains the clinical symptoms, multiple sites of compression should be fully considered.

NORMAL ULNAR NERVE DYNAMICS

The exact point of pathologic ulnar nerve compression at the elbow is often unknown, and it may involve more than one area of compression. In normal situations, the ulnar nerve undergoes stretch, traction, and compression with repeated elbow flexion and extension.[2, 47, 48] Acute or chronic injury to the ulnar nerve

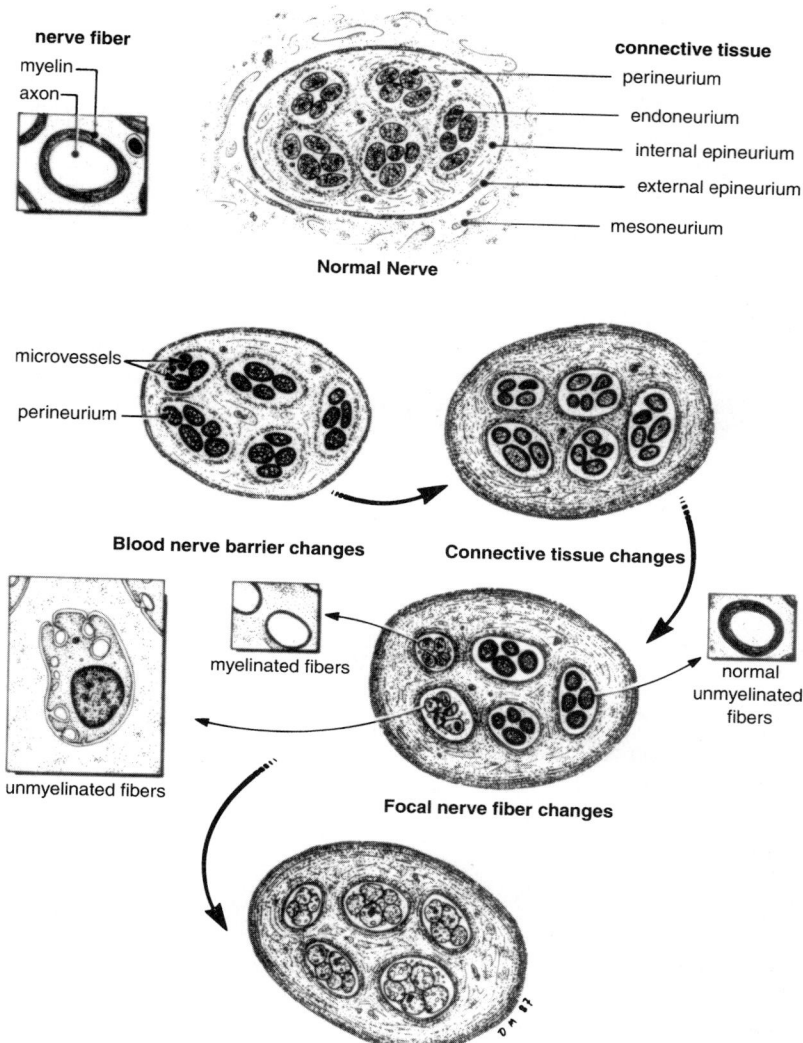

FIGURE 256–3. Histopathology associated with chronic nerve compression. The initial changes occur at the level of the blood-nerve barrier. These changes are followed by connective tissue changes and then focal nerve fiber changes. The large, myelinated fibers undergo segmental demyelination. The small, unmyelinated fibers demonstrate evidence of degeneration and regeneration, with the presence of a new population of very small, unmyelinated fibers. Thus, a bimodal rather than unimodal population of unmyelinated nerve fibers is noted. With progressive compression, diffuse wallerian degeneration is noted. (From Mackinnon SE, Dellon AL: Surgery of the Peripheral Nerve. New York, Thieme-Stratton, 1988, p 42.)

causes ischemic changes that eventually become symptomatic.

The physiologic stress placed on the ulnar nerve during normal activity demonstrates the resiliency of the human nervous system. Normal elbow flexion causes the fascia covering the cubital tunnel to tighten, increasing the pressure on the ulnar nerve. Elbow flexion decreases the area within the tunnel by up to 55%.[2] Pechan and Julius[47] demonstrated a 600% increase in intraneural pressure in the cubital tunnel with the wrist extended, elbow flexed, and shoulder abducted. The ulnar nerve also increased in length by 4.7 mm during elbow flexion. If the ulnar nerve does not elongate because of inflammation or scar, the intraneural pressure will increase even more with elbow flexion. Gelberman and coworkers[49] used magnetic resonance imaging and measured intraneural and extraneural pressures to determine the effect on the ulnar nerve in the cubital tunnel during elbow flexion. They found that the mean intraneural pressure within the cubital tunnel was significantly higher than the ex-

traneural pressure when the elbow was flexed beyond 90 degrees in human cadavers.

All these data demonstrate the extreme pressure changes that the ulnar nerve undergoes during normal activity. Therefore, it is not surprising that the ulnar nerve is particularly subject to disease at the elbow in the population at large. Repetitive trauma or activity can be tolerated for only a limited period of time in certain individuals. Symptoms of cubital tunnel syndrome will progress if patients do not modify activities that increase the pressure on the ulnar nerve at the elbow.

CAUSE OF ULNAR NERVE COMPRESSION AT THE ELBOW

The ulnar nerve is thought to have several points of compression in the region of the elbow.[50, 51] No surgery for cubital tunnel surgery is complete without fully addressing all potential points of compression. The

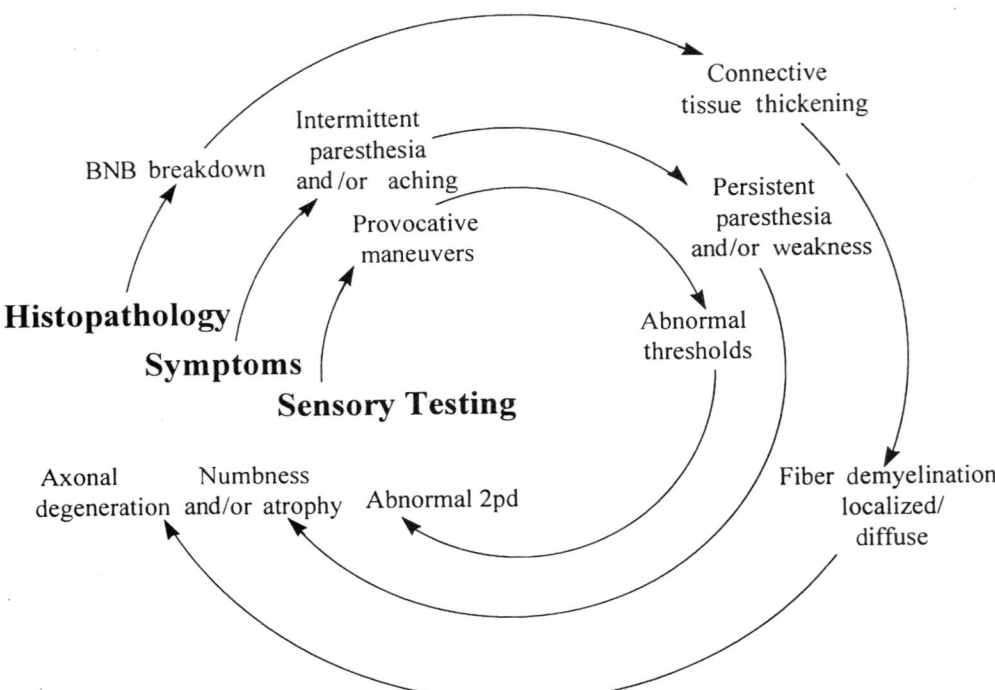

FIGURE 256–4. The histopathology of chronic nerve compression spans a broad spectrum from simple changes in the blood-nerve barrier (BNB) to wallerian degeneration. The patient's symptoms of chronic nerve compression similarly vary from intermittent paresthesia to persistent paresthesia to complete numbness. The motor analogy would be weakness to paralysis. The clinical findings parallel the histopathology and symptomatic complaints. Initially, the patient's symptoms are brought on only by positive pressure or positional provocative movements. Eventually, thresholds of vibration and pressure will be abnormal. Finally, the patient will demonstrate abnormal two-point discrimination. The motor component consists of weakness to muscle atrophy. (Modified from Mackinnon SE, Allieu Y: Nerve Compression Syndromes of the Upper Limb. Martin Dunitz, 2002.)

possible points of compression are discussed as they occur from proximal to distal on the arm (Fig. 256–5).

The arcade of Struthers has been described as a thick fascial structure spanning from the medial head of the triceps to the medial intermuscular septum, located approximately 8 cm proximal to the medial epicondyle.[52, 53] Spinner[54] reported the presence of the arcade of Struthers in up to 70% of cases of ulnar nerve compression at the elbow. Mackinnon and Dellon[55] believe that the arcade of Struthers simply represents the most proximal edge of previously undivided fascia seen primarily in the treatment of recurrent cubital tunnel syndrome.

The medial intermuscular septum is the next potential point of ulnar nerve compression. The ulnar nerve crosses the intermuscular septum after anterior transposition, and failure to remove it may result in a new point of compression. The cubital tunnel is where the ulnar nerve travels from superficial to deep within the flexor-pronator muscle mass. The two heads of the

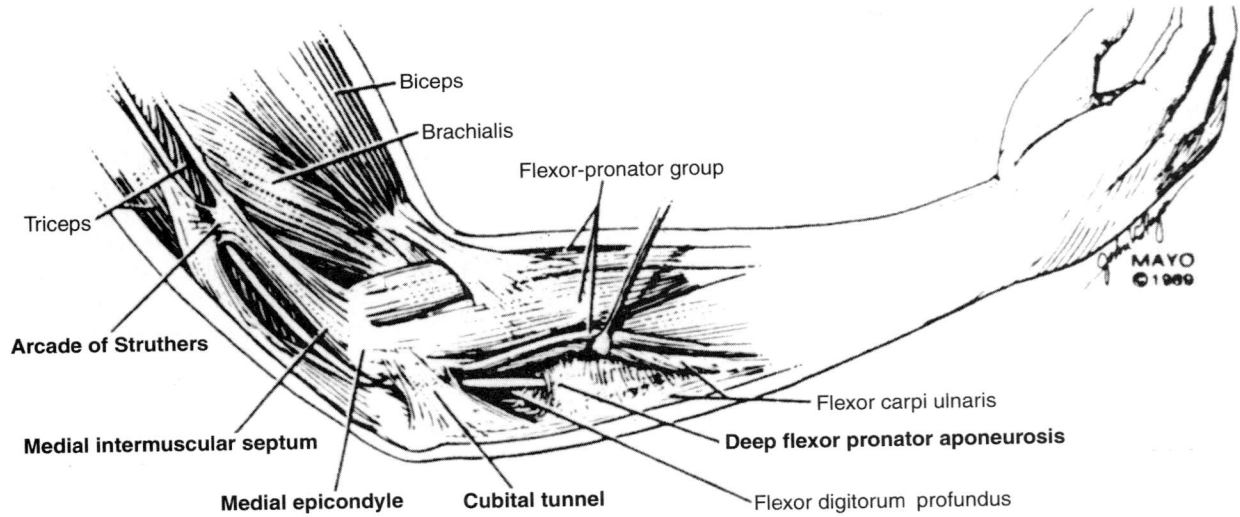

FIGURE 256–5. The five potential levels *(boldface)* of compression of the ulnar nerve in the region of the elbow. (From Amadio PC: Anatomical basis for a technique of ulnar nerve transposition. Surg Radiol Anat 8:158, 1986.)

flexor carpi ulnaris form the arcuate ligament of Osborne. These are common points of compression of the ulnar nerve at the elbow.

Finally, the nerve can be compressed as it passes through the flexor-pronator aponeurosis.[56] Once the ulnar nerve is transposed anteriorly, the deep fascia within the flexor carpi ulnaris may compress and "kink" the nerve. This fascia is very thin but strong, and it must be removed. Like the intermuscular septum, this fascia does not compress the ulnar nerve until it is transposed anteriorly.[51]

Instability of the ulnar nerve can result in subluxation of the nerve at the medial epicondyle. Childress[57] found a 16% incidence of ulnar nerve subluxation in the normal population. He classified subluxation into types A and B. Type A occurs when the ulnar nerve subluxes to the tip of the medial epicondyle, and type B occurs when the ulnar nerve subluxes beyond the medial epicondyle. All but one patient had type A subluxation, and all patients were asymptomatic.

Hypermobility of the ulnar nerve at the elbow appears to be associated with ulnar neuropathy. It may result in increased susceptibility of the ulnar nerve to trauma or a frictional type of injury.[2] Marked "snapping" of the ulnar nerve may represent a subluxing, prominent, or hypermobile triceps muscle and may be related to ulnar nerve compression at the elbow. In these situations, a portion of the tendinous insertion of the medial head of the triceps should be resected at the time of surgical treatment of the ulnar nerve. During surgery, the elbow is flexed and extended to ensure that enough triceps has been removed to prevent "snapping" of the ulnar nerve by the triceps.

The epitrochleoanconeus is an anomalous muscle thought to cause ulnar nerve compression in the region of the cubital tunnel. Hirasawa and associates[58] reported the muscle to be present in as many as 30% of patients. A more recent study showed the epitrochleoanconeus to be present bilaterally in approximately 12% of cadaver dissections.[59] This study also demonstrated that the epitrochleoanconeus muscle often presents with a prominent medial head of the triceps.

Space-occupying lesions, synovitis, and arthritis have all been implicated in the pathology of ulnar nerve compression. Trauma to the elbow, such as fracture, has long been described as a potential cause of the disorder.[6, 13, 14] Acute compression of the nerve at the elbow may result from improper positioning during surgery. Improper elbow padding and positioning during lengthy procedures are sometimes implicated, but there is little definitive evidence to show that poor intraoperative care results in ulnar neuropathy.[60] Nevertheless, ulnar neuropathy can occur after surgical procedures, even if great care was taken to protect the ulnar nerve. A report by Alvine and Schurrer noted that 17 patients in 6538 surgical procedures developed postoperative ulnar nerve palsy.[61] In a prospective study performed at the Mayo Clinic, 7 patients in 1502 surgical cases (0.5%) had compressive ulnar neuropathy postoperatively, with an average follow-up of 2 years.[62] The same group prospectively studied 986 patients admitted to the hospital for nonsurgical problems and noted that 2 patients (0.2%) developed ulnar neuropathy during a 7-day admission. It is likely that most of the patients in these two groups had a subclinical predisposition to this problem that was aggravated by bed rest or the supine position.[63]

Sunderland[64] described the internal topography of the ulnar nerve at the elbow in 1945. He noted that it consists of multiple fascicles connected by plexus formation. Some authors believe that the degree of plexus formation may affect the incidence of pseudoneuroma formation in the ulnar nerve.[55] A high degree of plexus formation is thought to inhibit the full movement of the nerve fascicles, resulting in fibrosis, Renaut's body formation, and scar within the nerve (pseudoneuroma). Sunderland[5] also found that the motor fibers to the intrinsic muscles of the hand are more superficial and therefore more susceptible to injury. However, Sunderland's description of the internal topography of the ulnar nerve is not consistent with the majority of clinical presentations.

CLINICAL DIAGNOSIS

The diagnosis of ulnar nerve entrapment at the elbow can usually be made with a brief clinical history; however, a thorough history and physical examination can help distinguish the subtle differences among the diagnostic possibilities. The differential diagnosis for cubital tunnel syndrome may include medial epicondylitis, but it is more commonly confused with cervical disk disease, thoracic outlet syndrome, or ulnar nerve compression at the wrist. Multiple nerve entrapments or double crush syndrome may cloud the definitive diagnosis of cubital tunnel syndrome. Patients presenting with profound motor but no sensory complaints must be considered for a motoneuron problem. Similarly, patients with no motor findings but severe sensory loss require a workup for a sensory polyneuropathy.

Patients with ulnar nerve compression at the elbow usually complain of numbness or tingling involving the small and ring fingers. Many patients report aching or pain in the medial forearm or elbow. These sensory changes are first noted during periods of prolonged elbow flexion, such as when the patient talks on the phone or sleeps. Sensory complaints usually precede any evidence of loss of motor function. There may be weakness or loss of fine motor skills in the affected hand, and patients may report difficulty writing, clumsiness, or dropping objects. Intrinsic muscle atrophy in the hand is usually noted later.

When evaluating any patient for suspected ulnar nerve compression at the elbow, all upper extremity compression should be ruled out. A simple form used in our office ensures that a full examination is performed in every patient (Fig. 256–6). Maneuvers such as Tinel's sign and positional or pressure provocation may identify points of nerve compression in the upper extremity. A positive response occurs when the patient reports "tingling," "electric shock," or alteration of sensation in the sensory distribution of the ulnar nerve.

Tinel's sign is one of the most accurate techniques

PERIPHERAL NERVE WORK SHEET
Dr. Susan MacKinnon

Patient Name _____   Date _____

TESTING:

X-rays: _____ C-Spine and Cervical Rib   _____ Hand   _____ Wrist

_____ Other _____   Date: _____

EMG: _____   Date: _____

NCS: _____   Date: _____

Bone Scan: Hands _____ Other _____   Date: _____

CT: _____   Date: _____

MRI: _____

EXAM:

	Right	Left		Right	Left
Pinch:	___	___	Forearm:		
Grip:	___	___	Tinel's	___	___
R.E.G.:			Provocative	___	___
2-Point: Median	___	___			
(M/S) Ulnar	___	___	Elbow:		
			Tinel's	___	___
Wrist:			Provocative	___	___
Tinel's	___	___	Pain:		
Provocative	___	___	Medial epicondyle	___	___
Atrophy:			Lateral epicondyle	___	___
Median	___	___			
Ulnar	___	___	TOS:		
Froment's sign	___	___	Tinel's	___	___
			Provocative	___	___
			Scalenes	___	___
Radial sensory:			Spurling's	___	___
Tinel's	___	___	Rotator Cuff/		
Provocative	___	___	Shoulder Impingement	___	___

SUPPLIES:

_____ Wrist Splint(s)
_____ Elbow Pad(s)
_____ Cervical Ruffs

BROCHURES:

_____ Carpal   _____ Tarsal Tunnel
_____ Cubital   _____ Radial Sensory
_____ TOS   _____ CTD
_____ Nerve Injury   _____ Pain Evaluation

CONSULTS:

_____
_____
_____

_____ Pain management _____
_____ MD referral _____
_____

FIGURE 256–6. The physical examination form used in our office when evaluating patients with possible nerve compression of the upper extremity.

used to identify axonal damage or regeneration. Patients with neurapraxia do not have Tinel's sign, because wallerian degeneration has not occurred. Patients with axonotmesis do have Tinel's sign. Tinel's sign often accurately demonstrates the level of regeneration and can be elicited by applying four to six manual taps on the ulnar nerve over Guyon's canal, the cubital tunnel, or the brachial plexus, depending on the anatomic level of compression.

Applying pressure over the nerve proximal to the distal wrist crease is the provocative test for ulnar nerve compression at the wrist. The most sensitive and specific provocative test for ulnar nerve entrapment at the elbow is the elbow flexion-pressure test with compression for 30 seconds.[65] The elbow is flexed, and the wrist and forearm are placed in neutral positions. Manual pressure is applied to the ulnar nerve just proximal to the cubital tunnel. A positive test results

in symptoms being reproduced in the distribution of the ulnar nerve within 1 minute (Fig. 256–7).

Brachial plexus nerve compression can be identified with abduction of the arms to increase the tension and compression on the brachial plexus.[66] Patients raise their arms overhead with the elbows extended and the wrists in a neutral position. A positive response occurs when the patient notices a sensory alteration in the hand. Spurling's test can identify patients with cervical nerve root impingement. The patient's head is placed to one side in slight extension, and axial compression is applied. This test should be repeated on the contralateral side, and a further cervical evaluation is required if this maneuver results in paresthesias or "electric shock" in the arms.

In 1950, McGowan[14] classified patients with ulnar neuropathy at the elbow to evaluate his clinical results. His classification system was based primarily on loss

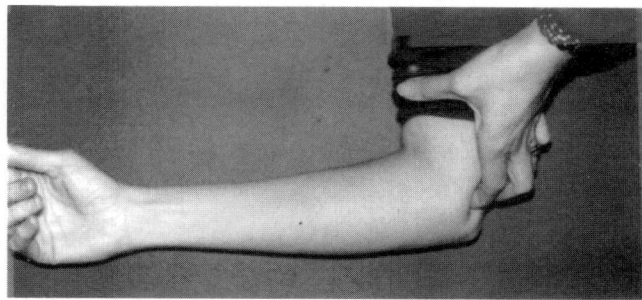

FIGURE 256–7. Elbow flexion test for the diagnosis of cubital tunnel syndrome.

of ulnar nerve motor function. Grade I lesions had no muscle weakness, grade II lesions had muscle weakness but no atrophy, and grade III lesions had muscle wasting. In 1988, a more complex classification of ulnar neuropathy was proposed based on the severity of motor and sensory deficits, along with Tinel's sign and the elbow flexion test[55] (Table 256–2). Unfortunately, no single classification system has been widely implemented to enable surgeons to accurately compare clinical results.

ELECTRODIAGNOSTIC EVALUATION

Electrodiagnostic studies can be a valuable tool to confirm the diagnosis of cubital tunnel syndrome. Elec-

T A B L E 2 5 6 – 2 ■ **Proposed Staging of Ulnar Nerve Compression at the Elbow**

Mild
Sensory
 Intermittent paresthesias
 Increased vibratory perception
Motor
 Subjective weakness, clumsiness, or loss of coordination
Tests
 Elbow flexion test, Tinel's sign, or both are positive

Moderate
Sensory
 Intermittent paresthesias
 Normal or decreased vibratory perception
Motor
 Measurable weakness in pinch or grip
Tests
 Elbow flexion test, Tinel's sign, or both are positive
 Finger crossing may be abnormal

Severe
Sensory
 Persistent paresthesias
 Decreased vibratory perception
 Abnormal two-point discrimination
Motor
 Measurable weakness in pinch and grip
 Muscle atrophy
Tests
 Positive elbow flexion test, Tinel's sign, or both may be present
 Finger crossing usually abnormal

From MacKinnon SE, Dillon AL: Surgery of the Peripheral Nerve. New York, Thieme-Stratton, 1988, p 246.

trodiagnostic studies may help determine disease severity, localize the area of compression, and rule out other sites of compression. They are helpful in patients who are difficult to examine or who cannot clearly communicate. Nevertheless, the clinical signs of disease for cubital tunnel syndrome are a prerequisite for diagnosis.[67]

Some authors do not perform electrodiagnostic studies before cubital tunnel surgery.[68–70] Other authors operate only on patients with electrodiagnostic evidence of disease.[71–74] Craven and Green suggest that a normal study is a contraindication for surgery.[72]

Several authors have operated on a significant number of patients with normal preoperative studies.[75, 76] Mackinnon and Dellon[55] state that a normal study does not necessarily exclude a patient from surgery for ulnar nerve entrapment at the elbow. Should an electrodiagnostic study be obtained if the results will not affect the surgeon's decision to operate? Some surgeons use the studies to aid in understanding the overall clinical picture and to help stage the severity of the compression. Many patients are referred with studies already in hand, and some insurance companies prefer to document the results. Nevertheless, surgeons should be cautious when proceeding with surgery on patients with normal nerve conduction studies.

A standard electrodiagnostic study includes sensory and motor evaluation. Raynor and coworkers[77] claimed that surface-recorded sensory and mixed nerve studies are more sensitive than motor studies. However, most investigators believe that motor conduction velocities across the elbow are most useful in confirming the diagnosis of ulnar nerve compression at the elbow.[55, 72, 78, 79]

Electrodiagnostic studies can be modified to directly localize points of compression along the course of the ulnar nerve.[78, 80–82] Eisen demonstrated that 80% of patients with mild symptoms and 47% of patients with severe symptoms had normal motor conduction across the elbow.[78] The most reliable electrical value was the motor conduction velocity from the elbow to the abductor digiti minimi. Electrodiagnostic studies may not correlate with clinical symptoms because of the differential fascicular injury mentioned earlier. Although nerve compression tends to be progressive, the severity of the injury may not correlate with the clinical complaints.

There is no decrease in motor nerve conduction that is diagnostic of cubital tunnel syndrome. Craven and Green[72] reported that motor conduction velocities less than 50 m/second at the elbow were abnormal. Eversmann[79] considered a 33% decrease in velocity at the elbow to be abnormal, and Eisen[78] considered a 10 m/second decrease in velocity from segments above and below the elbow to be abnormal. Electrodiagnostic studies can be modified to assist in identifying specific points of compression.[78, 80–82]

Improvement in electrodiagnostic study results may not be seen following cubital tunnel surgery. Wilson and Krout[83] found that postoperative studies did not correlate with patient outcome. Adelaar and associates[1] found that surgical success did not always result in improvements in motor conduction velocity. LeRoux and colleagues[84] reported that chronic nerve entrapment may be due more to axon loss than to demyelination, explaining why electrical study results fail to improve.

Electrodiagnostic studies often assist us in our clinical decision making. If there is clinical evidence of cubital tunnel syndrome and the symptoms are severe or fail to improve with nonoperative treatment, electrodiagnostic studies are routinely obtained. We find motor nerve conduction velocities across the elbow to be the most clinically relevant, and they are an integral part of our preoperative algorithm.

PREOPERATIVE EVALUATION

When patients are first evaluated for cubital tunnel syndrome, a complete history is taken and a physical examination is performed. A full upper extremity examination includes documentation of two-point discrimination, pinch and grip strength, and provocative nerve tests. Patients with complaints of pain are instructed to complete a pain evaluation score sheet (Fig. 256–8). Patients diagnosed with cubital tunnel syndrome are then further evaluated using our preoperative algorithm (Fig. 256–9).

Patients with mild to moderate symptoms of cubital

Pain Questionnaire

Name: _____   Date: _____

DOB: ___/___/___   Age: _____   Sex: Male _____ Female _____   Dominant Hand: Right _____ Left _____

Diagnosis: _____

1. Pain is difficult to describe. Circle the words that best describe your symptoms:

Burning	Throbbing	Aching	Stabbing	Tingling	Dull	Twisting
Cramping	Cutting	Shooting	Numbing	Vague	Stinging	Squeezing
Pulling	Smarting	Pressure	Coldness	Indescribable	Other _____	

2. Mark your average level of pain in the last month?

   No Pain ————————————————————————— Most Severe Pain

   Mark your worse level of pain in the last week?

   Right   No Pain ————————————————————— Most Severe Pain

   Left   No Pain ————————————————————— Most Severe Pain

3. Where is your pain? (Draw on diagram)

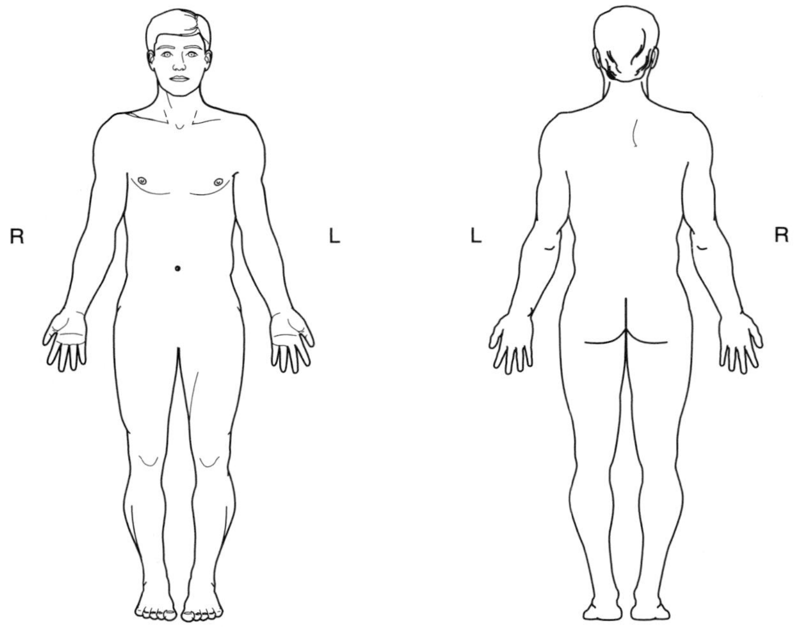

FIGURE 256–8. Pain evaluation score sheet. (From Novak CB, MacKinnon SE: Evaluation of the patient with thoracic outlet syndrome. Chest Surg Clin N Am 9:738–741, 1999.)

4. Mark your average level of stress in the last month?

At home   0 ——————————————————————— 10

At work   0 ——————————————————————— 10

5. How well are you able to cope with that stress?

At home   Very well ——————————————————— Not at all

At work   Very well ——————————————————— Not at all

6. Does movement have any effect on your pain?

    a. The pain is always worsened by use or movement
    b. The pain is usually worsened by use and movement
    c. The pain is not altered by use and movement

7. Does weather have any effect on your pain?

    a. The pain is usually worse with damp or cold weather
    b. The pain is occasionally worse with damp or cold weather
    c. Damp or cold weather have no effect on the pain

8. If you are retired, a student or homemaker, proceed to Question 8B

    8A. Are you still working?

        a. Works every day at the same pre-pain job
        b. Works every day but the job is not the same as the pre-pain job with
           reduced responsibility or physical activity
        c. Works occasionally
        d. Not currently working

    8B. Are you able to do your household chores?

        a. Does same level of household activities without discomfort
        b. Does same level of household activities with discomfort
        c. Does a reduced level of household chores
        d. Most household chores are now performed by others

9. Do you ever have trouble falling asleep or awaken from sleep?

    a. No - Proceed to Question 10   b. Yes - Proceed to Questions 9A and 9B

    9A. How often do you have trouble falling asleep?

        a. Trouble falling asleep every night due to pain
        b. Trouble falling asleep due to pain most nights of the week
        c. Occasionally having difficulty falling asleep due to pain
        d. No trouble falling asleep due to pain
        e. Trouble falling asleep which is not related to pain

    9B. How often do you awaken from sleep?

        a. Awakened by pain every night
        b. Awakened from sleep by pain more than 3 times per week
        c. Not usually awakened from sleep by pain
        d. Restless sleep or early morning awakening with or without being able to return to
           sleep, both unrelated to pain

10. Has your pain affected your intimate personal relationships?
    a. No   b. Yes

11. Are you involved in any legal action regarding your physical complaint?
    a. No   b. Yes

12. Is this a Workers' Compensation case?
    a. No   b. Yes

13. Have you ever thought of suicide?
    a. No   b. Yes   c. Previous suicide attempts

14. Are you presently receiving psychiatric treatment?
    a. No   b. Yes   c. Previous psychiatric treatment

FIGURE 256–8 *Illustration continued on following page*

15. Are you a victim of emotional abuse?

    a. No   b. Yes   c. No comment

16. Are you a victim of physical abuse?

    a. No   b. Yes   c. No comment

17. Are you a victim of sexual abuse?

    a. No   b. Yes   c. No comment

18. Are you presently a victim of abuse?

    a. No   b. Yes   c. No comment

19. How many surgical procedures have you had <u>in order to try to eliminate the cause of your pain</u>?

    a. None or one
    b. Two surgical procedures
    c. Three or four surgical procedures
    d. Greater than four surgical procedures

20. How did the pain that you are now experiencing occur?

    a. Sudden onset with accident or definable event
    b. Slow progressive onset
    c. Slow progressive onset with acute exacerbation without an accident or definable event
    d. A sudden onset without an accident or definable event

21. What medications have you used in the past month?

    a. No medications
    b. List medications _____

    _____

    _____

22. If you had three wishes for anything in the world, what would you wish for?

    1. _____

    2. _____

    3. _____

FIGURE 256–8 *Continued.*

tunnel syndrome undergo nonoperative treatment for approximately 8 weeks. If symptoms persist or are severe, an electrodiagnostic study is performed. Patients with motor conduction velocities across the elbow greater than 40 m/second undergo 8 weeks of nonoperative treatment even if they have failed previous nonoperative management. If symptoms improve, supportive care is continued, and regular follow-up is planned. If the patient does not obtain relief and clinical suspicion is high, elective surgery is scheduled.

Patients with persistent or severe symptoms of cubital tunnel syndrome who have motor conduction velocities across the elbow less than 40 m/second most likely require surgery. Patients with motor conduction velocities in the 30s undergo surgery electively, and those with velocities in the 20s undergo surgery as soon as it is convenient. Patients with motor conduction velocities across the elbow less than 20 m/second undergo surgery as soon as possible.

The preoperative treatment algorithm for cubital tunnel syndrome can be applied to patients being evaluated for primary or recurrent (redo) cubital tunnel syndrome. A review of our patients treated surgically demonstrated relative adherence to this algorithm.[85] We found that, on average, patients with motor conduction velocities in the 60s had surgery at 10 months, in the 40s and 50s at 5 months, in the 30s at 2 months, and in the 20s at 3 weeks.

NONOPERATIVE TREATMENT

Nonoperative treatment is initiated when the diagnosis of ulnar nerve entrapment at the elbow is first made. It involves patient education and physical activity modifications intended to improve symptoms and stop the progression of the disease. Patients with mild to moderate signs of compression are likely to benefit from conservative management.

Nonoperative treatment of ulnar nerve compression at the elbow starts with information about the basic anatomy of the ulnar nerve. Patients are taught that the ulnar nerve is surrounded by muscle in the upper arm and forearm, but it lies within a bony tunnel at the elbow that is protected only by overlying skin. Therefore, the ulnar nerve is most susceptible to pressure and trauma at the elbow.

Patients are taught to avoid positions that increase compression or stretch on the ulnar nerve. A simple demonstration can illustrate the importance of elbow position in the pathology of cubital tunnel syndrome (Fig. 256–10). The patient is shown that when the elbow

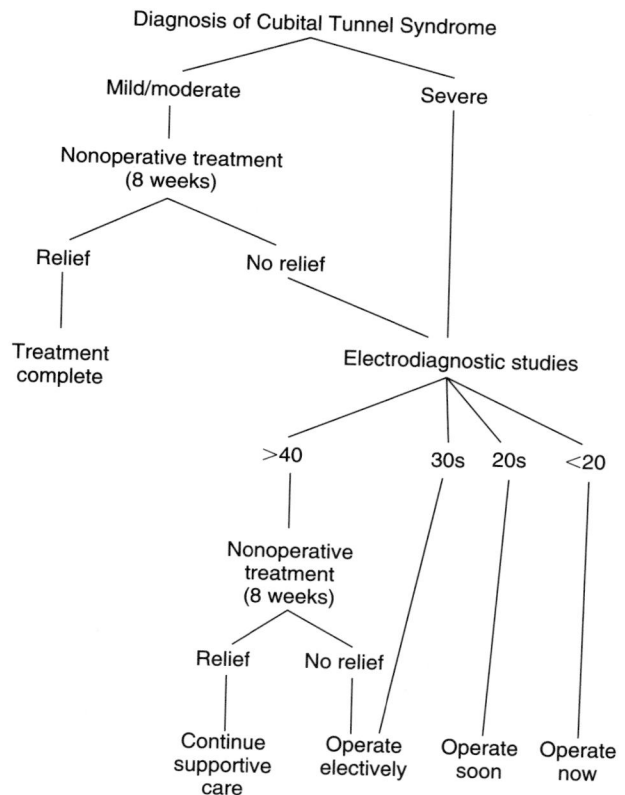

FIGURE 256–9. Treatment algorithm for cubital tunnel syndrome. (From Lowe JB, MacKinnon SE: Controversies in peripheral nerve surgery. Neurosurg Clin N Am 12:267–284, 2001.)

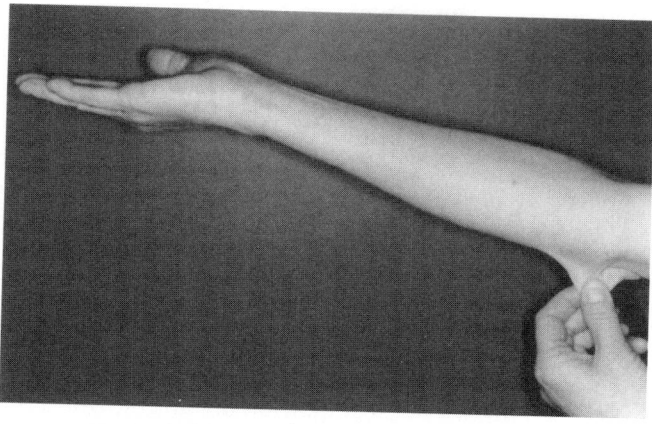

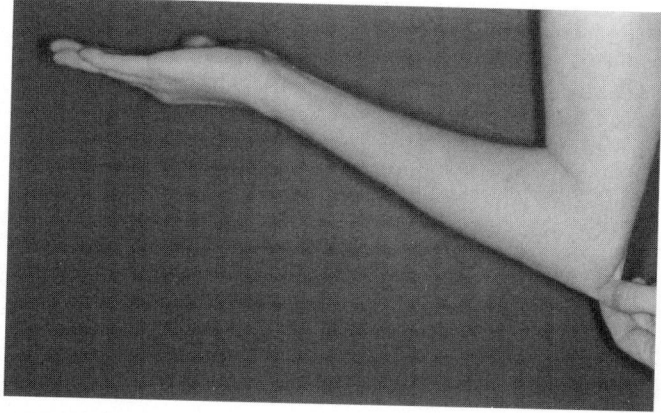

FIGURE 256–10. *Top,* The elbow extended, with loose skin overlying the ulnar nerve at the elbow. *Bottom,* The elbow flexed, with tight skin overlying the ulnar nerve at the elbow.

is straight, the ulnar nerve is loose, just like the overlying skin. In contrast, when the elbow is flexed, the ulnar nerve is tight, just like the overlying skin.

Patients are given specific physical activity modifications. Individuals who use the telephone a great deal are encouraged to use a headset. Patients who work at a desk place pads beneath the elbows to avoid pressure. Repositioning the chair or changing the angle of computer consoles may modify workstations so that patients can work with the elbows straighter and the shoulders lower. The best position is wrist in neutral, elbows slightly flexed at 30 degrees, and shoulders adducted. Patients who sleep with their elbows flexed experience more severe nighttime symptoms. They are instructed to straighten their elbows when they awake at night.

Rigid night splints can be used to maintain the elbows in extension, but they usually fail because of patient discomfort. Patients are more compliant with soft elbow pads, which are comfortable, protect the ulnar nerve from direct compression, and remind the patient to keep the elbows extended. Initially, the elbow pads are worn during the day and then primarily at night. The elbow pads we use are sold as "heel protectors" and resemble a light knee pad.

Patients are also instructed to perform stretching exercises focusing primarily on the flexor carpi ulnaris muscle. The stretching exercises are slowly increased, based on patient comfort.

Most patients with mild symptoms of ulnar nerve compression improve with conservative management, but patients with moderate to severe symptoms usually require further evaluation.

SURGICAL MANAGEMENT OF PRIMARY DISEASE

Controversy exists in the literature regarding the surgical management of cubital tunnel syndrome. In 1989, Dellon[86] concluded that personal bias was the primary factor in the choice of surgical techniques. Lundborg[87] advocated different surgical interventions based on the clinical situation and recommended anterior transposition of the ulnar nerve only in patients with significant ulnar neuropathy and poor local tissue beds. Although a review of the different surgical techniques can help define the controversy, it is unlikely to change the opinion of those with strong personal biases.

Simple Decompression

In 1957, Osborne[17] first described simple decompression of the ulnar nerve to treat entrapment at the elbow. Simple decompression involves the release of flexor carpi ulnaris fascia that spans the olecranon and the medial epicondyle.[73, 83, 88–91] The advantages of simple decompression are that it is minimally traumatic and easy to perform. The ulnar nerve branches and blood supply remain relatively undisturbed during surgery. The disadvantages include the possibility of incomplete release of all compression points, continued dynamic stress with elbow flexion, and dislocation of the ulnar nerve.[92, 93] Simple decompression of the ulnar nerve allows movement, and scar forms around the nerve with time.

Many authors claim that simple decompression of the ulnar nerve at the elbow is as good as any other surgery and has fewer complications and less postoperative morbidity.[73, 81, 94, 95] A review of the literature appears to support this claim. Nathan and coworkers[90] reported excellent to good results in 75% of 52 cases of simple decompression (average follow-up, 2.8 years). The authors claimed equal results, fewer complications, and more rapid rehabilitation with simple decompression compared with anterior transposition.

Steiner and associates[96] reported good results in 89% of 41 patients who underwent simple decompression of the ulnar nerve at the elbow. Three patients did not improve, but none were made worse at a mean follow-up of 2 years. Manske and colleagues[89] reported symptomatic relief in 22 of 27 patients following simple decompression of the ulnar nerve, with an average follow-up of 15.7 months. Four patients required revision using anterior transposition.

Some authors recommend simple decompression of the ulnar nerve at the elbow only in certain clinical situations.[2, 48, 56, 97] Dellon[86] found that 90% of mildly symptomatic patients with cubital tunnel syndrome improved with simple decompression alone.

Gellman and Campion[98] recommend simple decompression of the ulnar nerve when the site of compression is localized within the cubital tunnel. In 9 of 41 patients with isolated ulnar nerve compression, the authors were able to localize the site to 2 cm distal to the medial epicondyle. Eight of the nine patients had resolution of symptoms following simple decompression at an average follow-up of 18 months. Heithoff[99] recommends simple decompression of the ulnar nerve only after ulnar nerve subluxation has been excluded and the tissue bed is considered appropriate. Although ulnar nerve subluxation can be ruled out in most cases, the quality of the wound bed may not be as easy to determine.

The complication rate following simple decompression of the ulnar nerve at the elbow is extremely low.[51, 84, 88, 91] The most common complication is failure to relieve symptoms as a result of incomplete release of all points of compression.[98, 100] Simple decompression may produce more postoperative scarring around the nerve and increase the tendency for ulnar nerve subluxation. Given the probability of continued nerve compression following simple decompression, a particularly difficult revision can be expected.

Simple decompression of the ulnar nerve may be simple to perform, but correctly identifying patients who will benefit from it is difficult.[101] We do not recommend simple decompression of the ulnar nerve (or any

modification of the technique) in any clinical situation. It does not correct the problem of increased tension with elbow flexion, nor does it alter the potential exposure of the ulnar nerve to repeated trauma.

Medial Epicondylectomy

In 1959, King and Morgan[16] described medial epicondylectomy to treat ulnar nerve compression at the elbow. Many authors have reported success using a modification of the King and Morgan technique.[72, 99, 102–106] The ulnar nerve is transposed during a medial epicondylectomy without a formal dissection. Kuschner[106] claimed that the procedure also preserves the blood supply and proximal nerve branches to the ulnar nerve.

Craven and Green[72] reviewed 30 patients with cubital tunnel syndrome treated with medial epicondylectomy. All patients had improved at an average follow-up of 22 months. Froimson and colleagues[103] reported significant improvement in 97% of 66 cases of cubital tunnel syndrome following medial epicondylectomy, with an average follow-up of 4.5 years. Eighty-three percent of patients improved one or two McGowan grades. The best results were noted in patients with grade I and II lesions.

Froimson and Zahrawi[102] reported 30 cases of ulnar nerve compression at the elbow treated with medial epicondylectomy and neurolysis. All 30 patients showed no disease progression 2 years after surgery, but one patient developed medial elbow instability. Heithoff and Millender[105] reviewed 43 cases of medial epicondylectomy with an average follow-up of 2.3 years. Ninety-three percent of patients improved, and 72% had good or excellent results, but three postoperative flexion contractures and one painful cutaneous neuroma were reported. Nevertheless, the authors claimed that the major advantage of medial epicondylectomy over other techniques was safety.

The problem with medial epicondylectomy is the frequency and severity of reported complications. These complications include medial elbow instability, incomplete epicondylectomy, pain at the operative site, elbow flexion contracture, and persistent symptoms.[106] Preservation of the medial collateral ligament prevents medial elbow instability,[103] and some authors have suggested a partial epicondylectomy to protect the medial collateral ligament from injury.[99, 102] However, Heithoff and coworkers[104] reported incomplete removal of the medial epicondyle as a cause of recurrent cubital tunnel syndrome.

Postoperative elbow flexion contracture may be related to improper reattachment of the flexor-pronator muscle origin or prolonged postoperative elbow immobilization.[72, 106] Elbow pain is believed to be the result of the normal protection of the ulnar nerve by the medial epicondyle.[89, 107] Manske and colleagues[89] suggested that persistent elbow pain following medial epicondylectomy represents normal bone healing.

Heithoff and Millender[105] attributed the success of medial epicondylectomy in the treatment of cubital tunnel syndrome to a "mini-anterior transposition."

This may be one reason that it is not as successful as a full anterior transposition of the ulnar nerve. We believe that the ulnar nerve should be completely transposed, and medial epicondylectomy is unwarranted because of the significant risk of patient morbidity.

Subcutaneous Transposition

In 1898, Curtis[9] described subcutaneous transposition of the ulnar nerve for the treatment of ulnar nerve compression at the elbow. McGowan[14] performed the procedure with a more extensive dissection that included resection of the intermuscular septum. Many authors have reported success with a modification of the Curtis technique.[68, 86, 87, 108, 109] Some authors have expressed concern about this technique because of the potential exposure of the ulnar nerve to repeated trauma in its new superficial position.[16, 110]

Lugnegard and coworkers[69] reported that 84% of 25 cases of cubital tunnel syndrome improved after subcutaneous transposition, with a mean follow-up of 19 months. The results correlated with the severity and duration of symptoms, and 10 patients had improvement in motor conduction velocity. Two postoperative hematomas were noted, and one partial ulnar nerve paralysis. Richmond and Southmayd[109] reviewed 18 cases of subcutaneous transposition with a mean follow-up of 23 months. Eighty-three percent of patients had good to excellent results, 5% had satisfactory results, and 12% had unsatisfactory results.

Eaton and associates[75] described a modification of the subcutaneous technique. A fasciodermal sling harvested from the flexor-pronator mass was used to secure the nerve in the anterior position. Fifteen of 16 patients reported good relief after surgery, with an average follow-up of 18 months. There were no postoperative complications, and seven patients were baseball pitchers with no postoperative limitation in sports activities. Rettig and Ebben[111] reviewed 20 athletes who underwent subcutaneous transposition using a fascial sling, with an average follow-up of 19 months. Patients returned to full activity at an average of 12.6 weeks postoperatively, with 19 patients experiencing minimal or no symptoms after surgery.

Osterman and Davis[30] recommended subcutaneous transposition to treat cubital tunnel syndrome. They described plicating the subcutaneous layer directly to the flexor-pronator fascia to prevent subluxation of the ulnar nerve, and they warned of the possibility of compression from creation of a fascial sling. They claimed that their results were equal to those obtained with other techniques, and clinical failure was believed to be the result of technical error.

The success of subcutaneous transposition appears to be comparable to that of other techniques. Transposing the ulnar nerve into the subcutaneous space increases the risk of trauma to the nerve, however. We have found that recurrent cubital tunnel syndrome following subcutaneous transposition results from compression in areas where the nerve was not protected by overlying muscle and from scarring at the medial epicondyle. The ulnar nerve is often kinked at a right

angle at the distal end of the surgical site, where it travels from its subcutaneous position to deep within the flexor carpi ulnaris.

Submuscular Transposition

In 1942, Learmonth[15] described anterior submuscular transposition of the ulnar nerve. The procedure has been strongly advocated by many authors as the technique of choice.[35, 86, 97, 112–114] Siegel[115] recommended using the technique in previously failed procedures and in thin patients, where the nerve might be susceptible to trauma. Dellon[116] modified the Learmonth technique using Z-lengthening of the flexor-pronator mass. The superior success rate of submuscular transposition for ulnar nerve compression at the elbow has not been proved, but it is the technique of choice in the treatment of recurrent disease.[1, 35, 86]

Leffert[35] used the anterior submuscular transposition described by Learmonth in 38 patients, 14 of whom underwent surgery for recurrent disease. He concluded that patients with significant scarring from previous surgery or who were severely symptomatic tended to do worse. Complications included two patients with transient wrist pain and two patients with elbow contracture.

Nouhan and Kleinert[117] reported 33 cases of anterior submuscular transposition using the flexor-pronator Z-lengthening technique. The degree of nerve compression was classified preoperatively, and outcome was determined using a modification of the Bishop rating system. Ninety-seven percent of patients had good to excellent results at a mean follow-up of 49 months.

Pasque and Rayan[118] reviewed 50 cases of anterior submuscular transposition of the ulnar nerve using Z-lengthening of the flexor-pronator origin. Eighty-four percent of patients had good to excellent results at an average follow-up of 58 months. Seven complications were reported, including hematomas, flexor-pronator ruptures, cutaneous neuralgia, scarring, and one case of reflex sympathetic dystrophy.

Anterior submuscular transposition of the ulnar nerve is more technically demanding than simple decompression or anterior subcutaneous transposition. Proper performance of the procedure requires complete release of the ulnar nerve to transpose it anteriorly without tension, and division and repair of the flexor-pronator mass. Incomplete anterior mobilization of the ulnar nerve results in failed anterior transposition. When the flexor-pronator mass is placed over the ulnar nerve and reattached to the medial epicondyle (as in the traditional Learmonth procedure), the fascial bands within the flexor-pronator mass often act as a new point of ulnar nerve compression.

Intramuscular Transposition

In 1918, Adson[13] described anterior transposition of the ulnar nerve into the intramuscular bed of the flexor-pronator mass. Platt[119] modified the technique by placing the nerve deeper within the flexor-pronator mass. Many authors consider this technique the best choice to treat cubital tunnel syndrome.[88, 120–122] The intramuscular technique allows the ulnar nerve to be placed within the muscular bed without elevating or reattaching the flexor-pronator mass.

Gay and Love[120] reported that 70% of patients had satisfactory results with the Adson technique. The technique was used in 100 patients over a 25-year period at the Mayo Clinic. Internal neurolysis was performed in 54% of patients. Unfortunately, the authors failed to fully quantify results, distinguish between different techniques, and report the duration of follow-up.

Kleinmann and Bishop[121] reported 45 consecutive cases of ulnar nerve compression at the elbow treated with intramuscular anterior transposition. Eighty-seven percent of patients had excellent or good results, with an average follow-up of 28 months. However, four patients reported that they were worse after the procedure. Patients with abnormal electromyography or a work-related injury had a poorer prognosis.

The classic intramuscular placement of the ulnar nerve does not typically include release of the flexor-pronator mass, complete dissection of the nerve distally, or attempts at preventing subluxation of the nerve. Some authors are concerned about scar formation within the intramuscular bed.[112] Dellon and colleagues[123] demonstrated in a primate model that there was little scarring when a nerve was placed into a viable muscle bed. Placement of the ulnar nerve into a noncompressive intramuscular bed provides excellent clinical results with low morbidity when the tendinous bands of the flexor-pronator mass are fully resected and early postoperative mobilization is instituted.

Transmuscular Transposition (Authors' Preferred Technique)

Our technique is a modification of submuscular and intramuscular anterior transposition of the ulnar nerve. The procedure reached full maturity after 2 decades and has not been significantly modified in the last 5 years. We now refer to it as an *anterior transmuscular transposition* (Fig. 256–11). It is an attempt to apply the best components of each technique to achieve a consistently good clinical result.

The anterior transmuscular transposition has been described elsewhere,[19] but in general, it involves step lengthening of the flexor-pronator fascia, complete release and transposition of the ulnar nerve, creation of a transmuscular tunnel, and establishment of a loose fascial sling. A review of the technique by an independent observer demonstrated that 77% of 86 patients self-reported significant improvement after surgery. Eleven patients had no change, and none were made worse, with a mean follow-up of 38 months.[85]

Our preoperative algorithm is used to determine which patients are most likely to benefit from surgery (see Fig. 256–9). The procedure is usually performed with the patient under general anesthesia, but continuous intravenous regional or standard regional anesthesia is acceptable.[124] After the tourniquet has been inflated, intravenous bretylium (1.5 mg/kg, not to exceed 125 mg) is administered to the involved extremity to decrease the risk of postoperative pain syndromes. A longitudinal incision is made just posterior to the medial epicondyle approximately 6 to 8 cm in length.

The soft tissue is dissected to identify the branches of the MABC nerve. The branches of the MABC are freed for better exposure of the underlying flexor-pronator mass. If a branch of the MABC is inadvertently injured, the distal end is cauterized and transposed away from the surgical scar into the muscle bed above the elbow.

The skin and subcutaneous tissue are elevated to expose the proximal aspects of the flexor-pronator mass. The ulnar nerve is found posterior to the medial intermuscular septum, and the intermuscular septum is removed. The cubital tunnel is opened, Osborne's band is cut, and the fascia and muscle of the flexor carpi ulnaris are transected. The ulnar nerve is fully freed proximally and distally. The motor branches to the flexor carpi ulnaris are preserved, but they must be neurolysed to facilitate complete anterior transposition of the ulnar nerve. Watchmaker and coworkers[125] reported that an internal neurolysis of the proximal motor branches of the ulnar nerve can be performed up to 6.7 cm above the medial epicondyle.

Often a specific point of compression on the ulnar nerve is noted by a neuroma in continuity, or "dent," in the circumference of the nerve. During surgery for ulnar nerve compression, extreme motor activity in the hand during routine nerve dissection at the elbow may support the preoperative diagnosis of nerve compression. We believe that hypersensitivity of any nerve may provide physical evidence of compressive neuropathy, and we refer to this phenomenon as a *motor Tinel's sign.*

Next, a step-lengthening incision is made in the fascia of the flexor-pronator mass, and fascial flaps are elevated. A transmuscular tunnel is created through the flexor-pronator mass. Tendinous bands within the flexor-pronator mass are removed; otherwise, they would compress the nerve after it is transposed. Proximally, the tunnel is taken down to the brachialis muscle. Distally, where the muscle is much thicker, a portion of the flexor-pronator muscle is only partially divided. The ulnar nerve should be placed only within muscle and transposed anteriorly, avoiding any acute angles or curves. The intermuscular fascia within the flexor carpi ulnaris often kinks the ulnar nerve distally after anterior transposition. Therefore, the proximal and distal extents of the surgical dissection are checked to ensure that no points of compression have been created. The ends of the fascial flaps are then loosely reapproximated over the ulnar nerve.

Once hemostasis is obtained, a closed suction drain and bupivacaine (Marcaine) infusion pump are placed. Bupivacaine (0.5%) is also injected into the subcutaneous tissue before the skin is reapproximated. Patients are placed in a posterior splint with the elbow flexed at 90 degrees, the forearm in pronation, and the wrist in neutral. The drain is removed when the output is less than 30 mL in 24 hours.[126] The dressing and pain pump are removed by the third postoperative day, and patients are instructed on early range of motion for the hand, wrist, elbow, and shoulder.

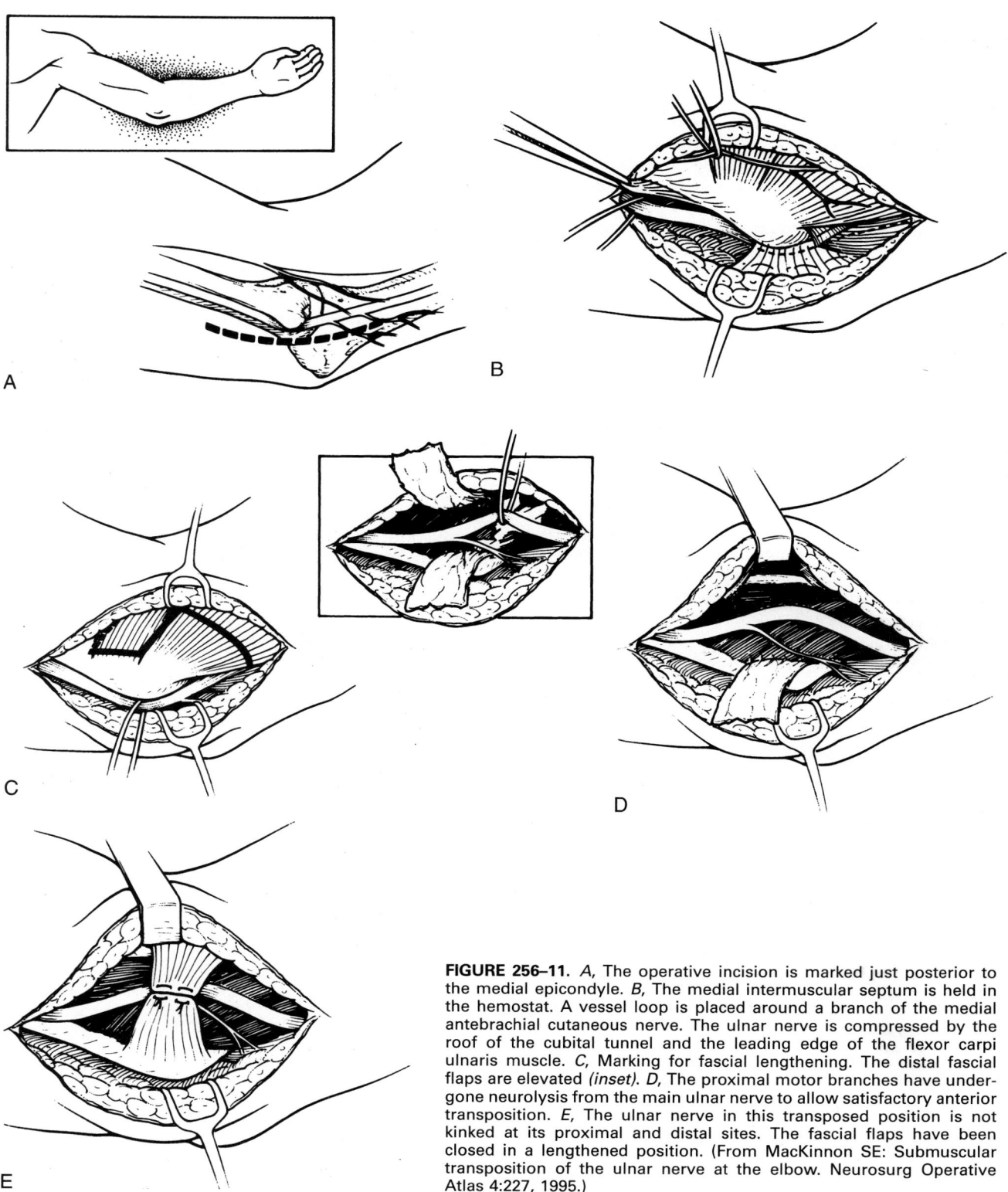

FIGURE 256–11. *A,* The operative incision is marked just posterior to the medial epicondyle. *B,* The medial intermuscular septum is held in the hemostat. A vessel loop is placed around a branch of the medial antebrachial cutaneous nerve. The ulnar nerve is compressed by the roof of the cubital tunnel and the leading edge of the flexor carpi ulnaris muscle. *C,* Marking for fascial lengthening. The distal fascial flaps are elevated *(inset)*. *D,* The proximal motor branches have undergone neurolysis from the main ulnar nerve to allow satisfactory anterior transposition. *E,* The ulnar nerve in this transposed position is not kinked at its proximal and distal sites. The fascial flaps have been closed in a lengthened position. (From MacKinnon SE: Submuscular transposition of the ulnar nerve at the elbow. Neurosurg Operative Atlas 4:227, 1995.)

COMPARISON OF SURGICAL RESULTS

It is difficult to compare various surgical treatments for cubital tunnel syndrome. Most studies lack a standardized preoperative or postoperative classification system, and no significant controlled, randomized trials have been performed. Most surgeons choose a surgical technique based on personal bias and training, and only a few studies have compared the results of different surgical techniques (Table 256–3). A limited review of several comparison studies is provided here.[1, 68, 88, 127, 128]

Chan and colleagues[88] compared simple decompression with anterior transposition in the treatment of cubital tunnel syndrome. They found full recovery or improvement in 82% of 235 patients in each group, with an average follow-up of 1.8 years. They noted that patients treated with simple decompression had a higher percentage of full recovery. Foster and Edshage[68] compared simple decompression with anterior subcutaneous transposition. They found no difference in results in 47 patients, with an average follow-up of 4.2 years. Although not statistically significant, patients with transposition reported better relief of paresthesias and muscle weakness.

Adelaar and associates[1] performed a prospective study of 32 patients with an average follow-up of 13 months. They found no significant difference between simple decompression and anterior transposition using either a submuscular or a subcutaneous technique. They concluded that anterior transposition of the ulnar nerve was indicated for anatomic compression, scarring in the cubital tunnel, or ulnar nerve hypermobility. Stuffer and coworkers[128] compared 33 cases of subcutaneous transposition with 17 cases of submuscular transposition, with an average 9.6-year follow-up. Satisfactory or good function was noted in 82% of subcutaneous transpositions and 62% of submuscular transpositions.

Geutjens and colleagues[127] performed a prospective, randomized study in 43 patients comparing medial-epicondylectomy with anterior submuscular transposition, with an average follow-up of 4.5 years. Patient satisfaction was better for medial epicondylectomy than for anterior submuscular transposition.

In 1989, Dellon[86] compared different authors' treatments for cubital tunnel syndrome. He reviewed nonoperative treatment, simple decompression, medial epicondylectomy, subcutaneous transposition, intramuscular transposition, and submuscular transposition. Dellon concluded that patients with moderate degrees of ulnar nerve compression at the elbow achieved the best results with submuscular transposition, and patients with severe disease did best with submuscular transposition and internal neurolysis. Dellon, an advocate of submuscular transposition, concluded that the procedure chosen appears to be based solely on the surgeon's preference.

The postoperative results may depend on the duration and severity of nerve compression.[68, 86, 87, 109] Osterman and Davis[30] found that patients with clinical symptoms for longer than 1 year and muscle atrophy did worse than patients with minimal symptoms present for less than 6 months. Age older than 50, revision surgery, diabetes, and muscle denervation are all thought to be poor prognostic indicators for ulnar nerve compression at the elbow.[1, 51, 76]

In our recent review of patients with cubital tunnel syndrome, we were unable to identify any specific prognostic indicators.[85] The surgical result was not significantly different in patients with workers' compensation, litigation, abnormal versus normal preoperative nerve conduction studies, obesity, smoking, or concomitant carpal tunnel syndrome or brachial plexus nerve compression.

RECURRENT DISEASE

Recurrent ulnar nerve entrapment at the elbow has many potential causes. Surgical failure may be related to the severity of the compressive neuropathy at the time of diagnosis and the success of decompression. Authors often report the number of redo operations they performed, but few articles have primarily addressed the issue of recurrent ulnar nerve compression at the elbow. The surgical technique most frequently used to treat patients with recurrent disease has been submuscular transposition with external or internal neurolysis.[35, 120, 129, 130]

Recurrent nerve compression is usually the result

T A B L E 2 5 6 – 3 ■ **Comparative Surgical Studies for the Treatment of Cubital Tunnel Syndrome**

AUTHOR	YEAR	SURGICAL TECHNIQUES COMPARED	TECHNIQUE FAVORED	AVERAGE FOLLOW-UP	NO. OF PATIENTS	STUDY
Chan et al[88]	1980	SD vs AT	SD	1.8 yr	214	Retrospective
Foster & Edshage[68]	1981	SD vs SQ	SQ	4.2 yr	47	Retrospective
Adelaar et al[1]	1984	SD vs SM vs SC	None	13 mo	32	Prospective
Stuffer et al[128]	1992	SM vs SQ	SQ	9.6 yr	51	Retrospective
Geutjens et al[127]	1996	ME vs SM	ME	4.5 yr	43	Prospective, randomized

AT, anterior transposition (includes both subcutaneous and submuscular techniques); ME, medial epicondylectomy; SD, simple decompression; SM, anterior submuscular transposition; SQ, anterior subcutaneous transposition.
From Lowe JB, MacKinnon SE: Current approach to cubital tunnel syndrome. Neurosurg Clin N Am 12:267–283, 2001.

of an incomplete release of the nerve. Broudy and associates[112] reviewed 10 failed anterior transposition procedures and found 9 instances of ulnar nerve compression at the medial intermuscular septum. All the patients improved following complete mobilization of the ulnar nerve with anterior submuscular transposition. Rogers and colleagues[131] reviewed 14 cases of failed cubital tunnel surgery. They reported failure to resect the intermuscular septum in 12 patients, injury to the antebrachial cutaneous nerve in 7, fibrosis in 5, and recurrent subluxation in 1. All patients improved following anterior submuscular transposition.

The operative technique most often associated with recurrent ulnar nerve compression at the elbow is not clear. Gabel and Amadio[51] operated on 30 patients with recurrent cubital tunnel syndrome. They reported 2 recurrences following medial epicondylectomy, 3 following submuscular transposition, 4 following simple decompression, 6 following internal neurolysis, 6 following intramuscular transposition, and 25 following subcutaneous transposition. They found an average of two sites of compression in each case. Most revisions were done using anterior submuscular transposition, and 75% of patients improved.

The treatment of recurrent cubital tunnel syndrome requires a consistent and thorough preoperative evaluation. Our preoperative algorithm can help with clinical decision making (see Fig. 256–9). The previous operative report can assist in the operative plan, and it may provide some insight on the path of the ulnar nerve. However, operative reports can be misleading, and no assumptions should be made about the course of the ulnar nerve. Extreme caution should be exercised during any surgical dissection in patients who have undergone prior surgery at the elbow.

Secondary Transmuscular Transposition (Authors' Preferred Technique)

In our experience, anterior transmuscular transposition with early postoperative range of motion achieves the best results for recurrent cubital tunnel syndrome. It provides a fresh muscular bed to decrease scarring around the ulnar nerve. Our technique for redo cubital tunnel surgery is essentially the same as our technique for primary surgery.

Intravenous bretylium is given through a sterile catheter in the affected arm after the tourniquet is inflated. Bretylium is important for patients who have significant pain before repeat surgical interventions. The incision is usually made through the previous scar, extending proximally and distally into normal tissue. The soft tissue is dissected, and the MABC nerve is carefully identified. If the MABC has been transected, the neuroma should be excised, and the nerve should be transposed proximally into a muscle bed in the upper arm. The end of the MABC is cauterized before the transposition to further inhibit regeneration. Step lengthening of the flexor-pronator mass allows for the transmuscular placement of the nerve as described previously.

All previous techniques for the treatment of ulnar nerve compression at the elbow are converted to an anterior transmuscular transposition if possible. If a previous subcutaneous transfer has been performed, the nerve usually lies in the soft tissue adherent to the underlying fascia. The ulnar nerve is released from all potential points of compression, and the intermuscular septum usually requires further resection. The distal portion of the ulnar nerve is often kinked where it travels from a subcutaneous to deeper position within the flexor carpi ulnaris.

The only time that a traditional transmuscular transposition of the ulnar nerve is not performed for recurrent disease is when there has been a previous submuscular transposition. Following a submuscular transposition, the nerve is usually found compressed by the tendinous bands within the flexor-pronator mass or kinked as the nerve travels under the flexor carpi ulnaris. The tendinous bands are excised, and the nerve is freed along its course. Some of the overlying muscle of the flexor-pronator mass is preserved.

Complete circumferential mobilization of the ulnar nerve should be avoided in patients who have undergone multiple surgical revisions, owing to the increased risk of ulnar nerve ischemia. To avoid excessive skeletization and devascularization, the posterior surface of the ulnar nerve is preserved at different intervals along its path. The nerve is often tethered at the elbow by scar or motor branches. Internal neurolysis of the branches to the flexor carpi ulnaris is usually required to allow for adequate anterior transposition of the ulnar nerve. Postoperative management should include early range of motion as described for primary surgery.

NEUROLYSIS

Controversy still exists regarding the efficacy of neurolysis during cubital tunnel surgery. In 1907, Babcock[132, 133] advocated the use of internal neurolysis when a nerve has evidence of compression secondary to a thickened nerve sheath. His technique was to separate the nerve bundles by opening the nerve sheath. In 1918, Adson[13] was the first to mention internal neurolysis for ulnar nerve compression at the elbow. More recently, Phalen[134] noted that internal neurolysis during carpal tunnel surgery results in permanent scarring to the nerve over time. However, a prospective, randomized trial showed no difference in outcome in carpal tunnel patients with or without internal neurolysis.[135]

Rydevik and coworkers[136] were among the first to perform basic research on the effects of internal neurolysis. They suggested that internal neurolysis be performed only when the preoperative intraneural fibrosis is more severe than the scarring that may be caused by the technique. They believed that internal neurolysis resulted in fibrosis of the nerve and permanent damage. Gentili and associates[137] carried out a study of internal neurolysis on rat sciatic nerve. This study showed that under experimental situations, it was possible to perform internal neurolysis without any ill effects. The authors noted the importance of handling all tissues gently to preserve the perineurium.

Mackinnon and Dellon[135] demonstrated in a primate model that median nerve decompression with microsurgical dissection was no better than decompression alone after 6 months. However, the internal neurolysis did not result in any significant scarring within the nerve. Clinically, it is difficult to prove any benefit of internal neurolysis. The problem lies in the inability to stage patients before and after surgery. Proper staging of chronic nerve compression could allow surgeons to differentiate results based on the severity of disease. Severe cubital tunnel syndrome suggests the presence of internal fibrosis that may benefit from internal neurolysis.[55]

It is often unclear what authors mean by *neurolysis*. In 1928, Platt[119] used the word in reference to anterior transposition of the ulnar nerve. Wadsworth[93] described neurolysis of the ulnar nerve as a movement of the ulnar nerve from its original position, but the term appears to be used differently later in the same text. Some authors use *neurolysis* as a synonym for *external neurolysis* or *decompression*. Leffert[35] pointed out that in all cases in which there was significant scarring of epineurium of the ulnar nerve, an "external neurolysis and epineurectomy" were carried out. He also stated that he never performed an internal neurolysis.

We describe *internal neurolysis* as a graded procedure progressing from external epineurotomy, external epineurectomy, internal epineurotomy, and internal epineurectomy. The technique is continued until the fascicles are freed from surrounding scar tissue. The reappearance of bands of Fontana suggests that the fascicles are decompressed and redundant and, therefore, a satisfactory neurolysis has been performed. We believe that internal neurolysis does not currently have a role in ulnar nerve compression, except when used to free and mobilize branches of the ulnar nerve that inhibit anterior transposition of the nerve. However, we typically perform epineurectomy of specific nerve segments that appear to be encased in scar after previous surgery. The benefit of this technique is not always clear, but anecdotal evidence seems to support its continued use in our patients.

NERVE STIMULATORS

Patients with chronic pain following injury to the ulnar nerve may be candidates for the placement of a peripheral nerve stimulator. These patients have usually failed previous medical and surgical interventions. A peripheral nerve stimulator has been recommended for patients with ongoing pain originating from a peripheral nerve and resistant to conventional treatments.[138–144]

The nerve stimulator provides pain relief by the direct application of continuous, high-frequency electrical stimulation to the peripheral nerve. The stimulation is thought to improve the symptoms of pain by the gate-control theory. The electrode is placed over the nerve and provides an alternative stimulation over

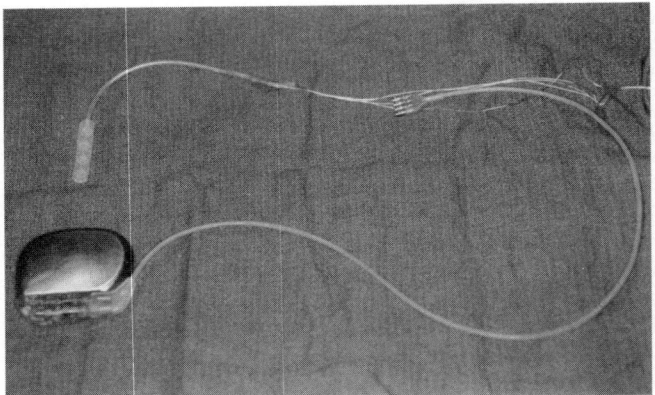

FIGURE 256–12. Standard equipment used for placement of a nerve stimulator.

the patient's distribution of pain. The nerve stimulator is usually placed proximal to the level of injury, and the entire system is shown in Figure 256–12. We place the electrode on the nerve and use an exterior power source in the hospital for 24 hours to examine the clinical benefit. If the patient experiences symptomatic relief, the battery is placed permanently beneath the skin at the second operative procedure.

Recently, we reviewed the usefulness of implanted nerve stimulators in 17 patients with pain following peripheral nerve injury.[145] A peripheral nerve stimulator was placed in the upper extremity in 12 cases. Eleven patients reported good to excellent pain relief, with a mean follow-up of 15 months. The peripheral nerve stimulator is useful for decreasing the level of pain in carefully selected patients, such as those with pain following ulnar nerve surgery at the elbow. Nevertheless, it is our practice to treat patients medically and surgically before placing a peripheral nerve stimulator on the ulnar nerve.

POSTOPERATIVE CARE

There is no consensus on the proper postoperative regimen after cubital tunnel surgery, but it involves a great deal more than dressing changes and patient reassurance. The type of physical therapy instituted is often dependent on the type of surgery performed. Early range of motion is one of the most important aspects of the successful management of patients who have undergone surgery for ulnar nerve compression at the elbow.

Various authors have advocated long periods of elbow immobilization following cubital tunnel release. Kleinmann[146] recommended that the patient be immobilized for 3 weeks after revision ulnar neuroplasty. Dellon[113] recommended 8 days of immobilization for successful management of ulnar nerve entrapment at the elbow.

Other authors advocate immediate range of motion following surgery for ulnar nerve entrapment at the elbow. Warwick and Seradge[147] reported the effects of

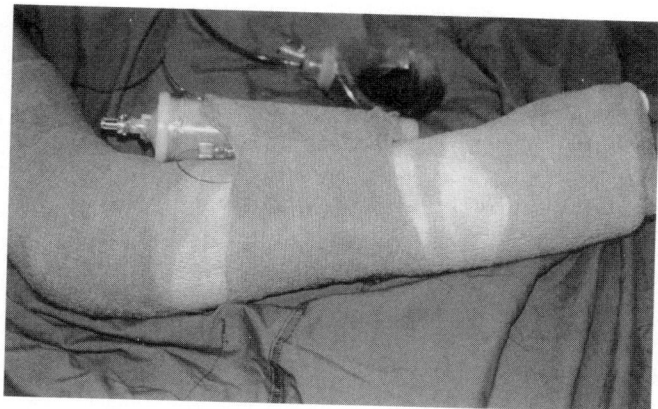

FIGURE 256–13. Postoperative dressing following surgery for ulnar nerve compression at the elbow.

early range of motion following medial epicondylectomy. Early range of motion at 3 days compared with 15 days postoperatively did not adversely affect grip strength and resulted in less flexion contracture. Nathan and colleagues[90] recommended early range of motion on postoperative day 1 for simple decompression of the ulnar nerve. We strongly believe that treatment failures following surgery for cubital tunnel syndrome can result from extended postoperative immobilization.

After surgery, our patients are placed in a splint that immobilizes the elbow flexed at 90 degrees, the forearm in pronation, and the wrist in neutral (Fig. 256–13). The splint and dressing are always removed 2 to 3 days after surgery, and the patient is immediately started on range-of-motion exercises for the hand, wrist, elbow, and shoulder. Patients are given a sling to wear at night for 3 weeks and during the day for comfort.

Patients are cautioned against heavy lifting and instructed to slowly stretch the forearm into supination and the elbow into extension. Often, stretching exercises cause some discomfort the first week. Patients achieve full range of motion by 3 weeks after surgery. At 1 month after surgery, patients may begin strengthening exercises. Early, aggressive range of motion prevents excessive scarring of the ulnar nerve in the surgical bed and ensures greater excursion of the nerve.

Surgical drains are usually removed on postoperative day 1, and a pain pump is left in place for approximately 48 hours. Once the dressing is removed on postoperative day 2 or 3, patients are encouraged to shower. Scar prevention techniques are begun at 3 weeks, with direct massage of the incision. Patients with preoperative complaints of pain are started on gabapentin (Neurontin) 300 mg orally three times a day, and a pain evaluation is performed. Often patients require reassurance that postoperative paresthesias are typical of nerve regeneration following surgery.

CONCLUSIONS

Neurosurgeons frequently evaluate patients for suspected ulnar nerve entrapment at the elbow. The diagnosis is dependent on a complete history and physical examination. Other associated disorders must be excluded or included to ensure an accurate diagnosis.

Many patients respond to nonoperative treatment, with no need for surgical intervention. The preoperative algorithm helps determine which patients are most likely to benefit from surgery.

The surgical technique used to treat cubital tunnel syndrome is dependent on the surgeon's preference. There has been no significant prospective, randomized trial to adequately compare the different surgical options. In the end, each surgeon must rely on his or her own personal experience and judgment. Our experience with various surgical techniques has convinced us of the efficacy of the transmuscular approach. Senior hand surgeons have often discarded their surgical techniques for cubital tunnel syndrome after being introduced to our technique, and they continue to report satisfaction with the results. The best results appear to be obtained with complete release of all potential points of compression, placement of the nerve in a muscular bed, removal of any acute angles to the nerve, and early postoperative mobilization.

REFERENCES

1. Adelaar R, Foster W, McDowell C: Treatment of cubital tunnel syndrome. J Hand Surg [Am] 9:90–95, 1984.
2. Apefelberg D, Larson S: Dynamic anatomy of the ulnar nerve at the elbow. Plast Reconstr Surg 51:76–81, 1973.
3. Earle H: Cases and observations illustrating the influence of the central nervous system in regulating animal heart. Med Chir Trans 7:173, 1816.
4. Calder F: Effects of a division of the ulnar nerve. Lancet 1:489–490, 1833.
5. Sunderland S: Nerve and Nerve Injuries. Baltimore, Williams & Wilkins, 1968.
6. Sheldon W: Tardy paralysis of the ulnar nerve. Med Clin North Am 5:499, 1921.
7. Panas P: Sur une cause peu connue de paralysie du nerf cubital. Arch Gen Med 5(ser 7), 1878.
8. Platt H: The pathogenesis and treatment of traumatic neuritis of the ulnar nerve in the post-condylar groove. Br J Surg 13:409–431, 1926.
9. Curtis B: Traumatic ulnar neuritis: Transplantation of the nerve. J Nerv Ment Dis 25:480–481, 1898.
10. Skillern P Jr: Surgical lesions of the ulnar nerve at the elbow. Surg Clin North Am 2:251–269, 1922.
11. Davidson A, Horwitz M: Late or tardy ulnar-nerve paralysis. J Bone Joint Surg 17:844–856, 1935.
12. Broca A, Mouchet A: Complications nervuses des fractures de l'extermite inferieure de l'humerus. Rev Chir (Paris) 19:701, 1899.
13. Adson A: The surgical treatment of progressive ulnar paralysis. Minn Med 1:455–460, 1918.
14. McGowan A: The results of transposition of the ulnar nerve for traumatic ulnar neuritis. J Bone Joint Surg Br 32:293–301, 1950.
15. Learmonth J: A technique for transplanting the ulnar nerve. Surg Gynecol Obstet 75:792–793, 1942.
16. King T, Morgan F: Late results of removing the medial humeral epicondyle for traumatic ulnar neuritis. J Bone Joint Surg Br 41:51–55, 1959.
17. Osborne G: The surgical treatment of tardy ulnar neuritis. J Bone Joint Surg Br 39:782, 1957.
18. Feindel W, Stratford J: The role of the cubital tunnel in tardy ulnar nerve palsy. Can J Surg 1:287–300, 1958.
19. Lowe J, Novak CB, Mackinnon SE: Current approach to cubital tunnel syndrome. Neurosurg Clin N Am 12:267–284, 2001.
20. Taleisnik J: The palmar cutaneous branch of the median nerve

and the approach to the carpal tunnel: An anatomic study. J Bone Joint Surg Am 55:1212–1217, 1973.

21. McCabe S, Kleinert J: The nerve of Henle. J Hand Surg [Am] 15:784, 1990.

22. Uchida Y, Sugioka Y: Electrodiagnosis of Martin-Gruber connection and its clinical importance in peripheral nerve surgery. J Hand Surg [Am] 17:54–59, 1992.

23. Matloub H, Yousif N: Peripheral nerve anatomy and innervation pattern. Hand Clin 8:201, 1992.

24. Leibovic S, Hastings H II: Martin-Gruber revisited. J Hand Surg [Am] 17:47, 1992.

25. Lundborg G: Structure and function of the intraneural microvessels as related to trauma, edema formation, and nerve function. J Bone Joint Surg Am 57:938–948, 1975.

26. Ogata K, Shimon S, Owen J, et al: Effects of compression and devascularization on ulnar nerve function. J Hand Surg [Br] 16:104–108, 1991.

27. Prevel C, Matloub H, Ye Z, et al: The extrinsic blood supply of the ulnar nerve at the elbow: An anatomic study. J Hand Surg [Am] 18:433–438, 1993.

28. Ogata K, Manske P, Lesker P: The effect of surgical dissection on regional blood flow to the ulnar nerve in the cubital tunnel. Clin Orthop Rel Res 193:195, 1985.

29. Sugawara M: Experimental and clinical studies of the vascularized anterior transposition of the ulnar nerve for cubital tunnel syndrome. J Jpn Orthop Assoc 62:755–765, 1988.

30. Osterman A, Davis C: Subcutaneous transposition of the ulnar nerve for the treatment of cubital tunnel syndrome. Hand Clin 12:421–433, 1996.

31. Maki Y, Firrell J, Breidenbach W: Blood flow in mobilized nerves: Results in a rabbit sciatic nerve model. Plast Reconstr Surg 100:627–633, 1996.

32. Ogata K, Naito M: Blood flow of the peripheral nerve: Effects of dissection, stretching and compression. J Hand Surg [Br] 11:10–14, 1986.

33. Dawson D, Hallet M, Millender L: Entrapment Neuropathies. Boston, Little, Brown, 1983.

34. Dellon A, Mackinnon S: Injury to the medial antebrachial cutaneous nerve during cubital tunnel surgery. J Hand Surg [Br] 10:33–36, 1985.

35. Leffert R: Anterior submuscular transposition of the ulnar nerve by the Learmonth technique. J Hand Surg 7:147–155, 1982.

36. Seddon H: Three types of nerve injury. Brain 66:237, 1943.

37. Sunderland S: A classification of peripheral nerve injuries producing loss of function. Brain 74:491, 1951.

38. Mackinnon SE: New directions in peripheral nerve surgery. Ann Surg 22:257–273, 1989.

39. Mackinnon SE, Dellon A: Experimental study of chronic nerve compression: Clinical implications. Hand Clin 2:639–650, 1986.

40. Mackinnon SE, Dellon A, Hudson A, et al: A primate model for chronic nerve compression. J Reconstr Microsurg 1:185–194, 1985.

41. Mackinnon SE: Double and multiple "crush" syndromes: Double and multiple entrapment neuropathies. Hand Clin 8:369–390, 1992.

42. Upton ARM, McComas AJ: The double crush in nerve entrapment syndromes. Lancet 2:359–362, 1973.

43. Dellon A, Mackinnon SE, Seiler W IV: Susceptibility of the diabetic nerve to chronic compression. Ann Plast Surg 20:117, 1988.

44. Dellon A, Mackinnon S: Chronic nerve compression model for double crush hypothesis. Ann Plast Surg 26:259–264, 1991.

45. Lundborg G: The reversed double crush syndrome. Am Soc Surg Hand Correspondence Newsletter 9, 1986.

46. Nemoto K, Matsumoto N, Ken-ichi T, et al: An experimental study on the "double crush" hypothesis. J Hand Surg [Am] 12:552–559, 1987.

47. Pechan J, Julius I: The pressure measurement in the ulnar nerve: A contribution to the pathophysiology of the cubital tunnel syndrome. J Biomech 8:75–79, 1975.

48. Vanderpool D, Chalmers J, Lamb D, Whiston T: Peripheral compression lesions of the ulnar nerve. J Bone Joint Surg Br 50:792–802, 1968.

49. Gelberman R, Yamaguchi K, Hollstien S, et al: Changes in interstitial pressure and cross-sectional area of the cubital tunnel

and of the ulnar nerve with flexion of the elbow: An experimental study in human cadavers. J Bone Joint Surg Am 80:492–501, 1998.

50. Amadio P, Gabel G: Treatment and complications of failed decompression of the ulnar nerve at the elbow. In Gelberman RH (ed): Operative Nerve Repair and Reconstruction. Philadelphia, JB Lippincott, 1991, pp 1107–1120.

51. Gabel G, Amadio P: Reoperation for failed decompression of the ulnar nerve in the region of the elbow. J Bone Joint Surg Am 72:213–219, 1990.

52. Kane E, Kaplan E, Spinner M: Observations on the course of the ulnar nerve in the arm. Ann Chir 27:470–496, 1973.

53. Spinner M, Spencer P: Nerve compression lesions of the upper extremity: A clinical and experimental review. Clin Orthop Rel Res 104:46–68, 1974.

54. Spinner M: Management of nerve compression lesions in the upper extremity. In Omer G, Spinner M (eds): Management of Peripheral Nerve Problems. Philadelphia, WB Saunders, 1980.

55. Mackinnon S, Dellon A: Surgery of the Peripheral Nerve. New York, Thieme Medical, 1988.

56. Amadio P, Beckenbaugh R: Entrapment of the ulnar nerve by the deep flexor-pronator aponeurosis. J Hand Surg [Am] 11:83–87, 1986.

57. Childress H: Recurrent ulnar-nerve dislocation at the elbow. Clin Orthop Rel Res 108:168–173, 1975.

58. Hirasawa Y, Sawamura H, Sakakida K: Entrapment neuropathy due to bilateral epitrochleoanconeus muscles: A case report. J Hand Surg 4:181–184, 1979.

59. Dellon A: Musculotendinous variations about the medial humeral epicondyle. J Hand Surg 11:175–181, 1986.

60. Idler R: General principles of patient evaluation and nonoperative management of cubital tunnel. Hand Clin 12:397–403, 1996.

61. Alvine F, Schurrer M: Post-operative ulnar-nerve palsy: Are there predisposing factors? J Bone Joint Surg Am 69:255–259, 1987.

62. Warner M, Warner D, Matsumoto J, et al: Ulnar neuropathy in surgical patients. Anesthesiology 90:54–59, 1999.

63. Warner M, Warner D, Harper C, et al: Ulnar neuropathy in medical patients. Anesthesiology 92:613–615, 2000.

64. Sunderland S: The intraneural topography of the radial, median, and ulnar nerve. Brain 68:243–253, 1945.

65. Novak C, Lee G, Mackinnon S, et al: Provocative testing for cubital tunnel syndrome. J Hand Surg [Am] 19:817–820, 1994.

66. Novak CB, Mackinnon SE, Patterson GA: Evaluation of patients with thoracic outlet syndrome. J Hand Surg [Am] 18:292–299, 1993.

67. Clark C: Cubital tunnel syndrome. JAMA 241:801–802, 1979.

68. Foster R, Edshage S: Factors related to the outcome of surgically managed compression ulnar neuropathy at the elbow. J Hand Surg 6:192, 1981.

69. Lugnegard H, Walheim G, Wennberg A: Operative treatment of ulnar neuropathy in the elbow region. Acta Orthop Scand 48:168–176, 1977.

70. Macnichol M: The results of operation for ulnar neuritis. J Bone Joint Surg Br 61:159–164, 1979.

71. Brown W, Yates S: Percutaneous localization of conduction abnormalities in human extremities. Can J Neurol Sci 9:391–400, 1982.

72. Craven P, Green D: Cubital tunnel syndrome: Treatment by medial epicondylectomy. J Bone Joint Surg Am 62:986–989, 1980.

73. Miller R, Hummel E: The cubital tunnel syndrome: Treatment with simple decompression. Ann Neurol 7:567–569, 1980.

74. Wright E, MacQuillen M: Hypoexcitability of ulnar nerve in patients with normal motor and nerve conduction studies. Neurology (Minneap) 23:78–83, 1973.

75. Eaton R, Crowe J, Parkes J: Anterior transposition of the ulnar nerve using a non-compressing fasciodermal sling. J Bone Joint Surg Am 62:820–825, 1980.

76. Paine K: Tardy ulnar palsy. Can J Surg 13:255–261, 1970.

77. Raynor E, Shefner J, Preston D, Logigian EL: Sensory and mixed nerve conduction studies in the evaluation of ulnar neuropathy at the elbow. Muscle Nerve 17:785–792, 1994.

78. Eisen A: Early diagnosis of ulnar nerve palsy: An electrophysiological study. Neurology 24:256–262, 1974.

79. Eversmann W: Entrapment and compression neuropathies. In

Green D (ed): Operative Hand Surgery, 2nd ed. New York, Churchill Livingstone, 1988, pp 1341–1385.

80. Eisen A, Danon J: The mild cubital tunnel syndrome, its natural history and indications for surgical intervention. Neurology 24: 608–613, 1974.

81. Miller R: The cubital tunnel syndrome: Diagnosis and precise localization. Ann Neurol 6:56–59, 1979.

82. Payan J: Electrophysiological localization of ulnar nerve lesions. J Neurol Neurosurg Psychiatry 32:208–220, 1969.

83. Wilson D, Krout R: Surgery of ulnar neuropathy at the elbow: 16 cases treated by decompression without transposition. J Neurosurg 38:780–785, 1973.

84. LeRoux P, Ensign T, Burchiel K: Surgical decompression without transposition for ulnar neuropathy: Factors determining outcome. Neurosurgery 27:709–714, 1990.

85. Novak C, Mackinnon S: Patient self reported outcome following anterior transposition of the ulnar nerve. Paper presented at the Annual Meeting of the American Association of Hand Surgery, Jan 4–6, 2000, Miami Beach, Florida.

86. Dellon A: Review of treatment results for ulnar nerve entrapment at the elbow. J Hand Surg [Am] 14:688–700, 1989.

87. Lundborg G: Surgical treatment for ulnar nerve entrapment at the elbow [editorial]. J Hand Surg [Br] 17:245, 1992.

88. Chan R, Paine K, Varughese G: Ulnar neuropathy at the elbow: Comparison of simple decompression and anterior decompression. Neurosurgery 7:545–550, 1980.

89. Manske P, Johnson R, Pruitt D, Strecker W: Ulnar nerve decompression at the cubital tunnel. Clin Orthop Rel Res 274:231–237, 1992.

90. Nathan P, Meyers L, Keniston R, Meadows K: Simple decompression of the ulnar nerve: An alternative to anterior transposition. J Hand Surg [Br] 17:251–254, 1992.

91. Thomsen P: Compression neuritis of the ulnar nerve treated with simple decompression. Acta Orthop Scand 48:164–167, 1977.

92. Folberg C, Weiss A, Akelman E: Cubital tunnel syndrome. Part II. Treatment. Orthop Rev 23:233–241, 1994.

93. Wadsworth T: The external compression syndrome of the ulnar nerve at the cubital tunnel. Clin Orthop Rel Res 124:198–204, 1977.

94. Assmuss H: New aspects of the pathogenesis and therapy of cubital tunnel syndrome. Adv Neurosurg 9:391–395, 1981.

95. Lavyne M, Bell W: Simple decompression without transposition for ulnar neuropathy: Factors determining outcomes. Neurosurgery 11:6–11, 1990.

96. Steiner H, von Haken M, Steiner-Milz HG: Entrapment neuropathy at the cubital tunnel: Simple decompression is the method of choice. Acta Neurochir (Wien) 138:308–313, 1996.

97. Amadio P: Anatomic basis for a technique of ulnar nerve transposition. Surg Radiol Anat 8:155–161, 1986.

98. Gellman H, Campion D: Modified in situ decompression of the ulnar nerve at the elbow. Hand Clin 12:405–410, 1996.

99. Heithoff S: Cubital tunnel syndrome does not require transposition of the ulnar nerve. J Hand Surg [Am] 24:898–905, 1999.

100. Ferlic D: Clinical assessment and conservative treatment of cubital tunnel syndrome. In Gelberman RH (ed): Operative Nerve Repair and Reconstruction. Philadelphia, JB Lippincott, 1991, pp 1055–1061.

101. Osborne G: Compression neuritis of the ulnar nerve at the elbow. Hand 2:10–13, 1970.

102. Froimson A, Zahrawi F: Treatment of compression neuropathy of the ulnar nerve at the elbow by epicondylectomy and neurolysis. J Hand Surg 5:391–395, 1980.

103. Froimson A, Anouchi Y, Seitz W, Winsberg D: Ulnar nerve decompression with medial epicondylectomy for neuropathy at the elbow. Clin Orthop Rel Res 265:200–206, 1991.

104. Heithoff S, Millender L, Nalebuff E: Medial epicondylectomy for the treatment of ulnar nerve compression at the elbow. J Hand Surg [Am] 15:22–29, 1990.

105. Heithoff S, Millender L: Medial epicondylectomy. In Gelberman RH (ed): Operative Nerve Repair and Reconstruction. Philadelphia, JB Lippincott, 1991, pp 1087–1096.

106. Kuschner S: Cubital tunnel syndrome: Treatment by medial epicondylectomy. Hand Clin 12:411–419, 1996.

107. Bednar M, Blair S, Light T: Complications of the treatment of cubital tunnel syndrome. Hand Clin 10:83–92, 1994.

108. Harrison M, Nurick S: Results of anterior transposition of the ulnar nerve for ulnar neuritis. BMJ 1:27–29, 1970.

109. Richmond J, Southmayd W: Superficial anterior transposition of the ulnar nerve at the elbow for ulnar neuritis. Clin Orthop Rel Res 164:42–44, 1982.

110. Jones R, Gauntt C: Medial epicondylectomy for ulnar nerve compression syndrome at the elbow. Clin Orthop Rel Res 139: 174–178, 1979.

111. Rettig A, Ebben J: Anterior subcutaneous transfer of the ulnar nerve in the athlete. Am J Sports Med 21:836–840, 1993.

112. Broudy A, Leffert R, Smith R: Technical problems with ulnar nerve transposition at the elbow: Findings and results of reoperation. J Hand Surg 3:85–89, 1978.

113. Dellon A: Techniques for successful management of ulnar nerve entrapment at the elbow. Neurosurg Clin N Am; 2:57–73, 1991.

114. Rayan G: Proximal ulnar nerve compression: Cubital tunnel syndrome. Hand Clin 8:325–336, 1992.

115. Siegel D: Submuscular transposition of the ulnar nerve. Hand Clin 12:445–448, 1996.

116. Dellon A: Operative techniques for submuscular transposition of the ulnar nerve. Contemp Orthop 16:17–24, 1988.

117. Nouhan R, Kleinert J: Ulnar nerve decompression by transposing the nerve and Z-lengthening the flexor-pronator mass: Clinical outcome. J Hand Surg [Am] 22:127–131, 1997.

118. Pasque C, Rayan G: Anterior submuscular transposition of the ulnar nerve for cubital tunnel syndrome. J Hand Surg [Br] 20: 447–453, 1995.

119. Platt P: The operative treatment of traumatic ulnar neuritis at the elbow. Surg Gynecol Obstet 47:822–825, 1928.

120. Gay J, Love J: Diagnosis and treatment of tardy paralysis of the ulnar nerve: Based on a study of 100 cases. J Bone Joint Surg Am 29:1087–1097, 1947.

121. Kleinmann W, Bishop A: Anterior intramuscular transposition of the ulnar nerve. J Hand Surg [Am] 14:972–979, 1989.

122. Kleinmann W: Anterior intramuscular transposition of the ulnar nerve. In Gelberman RH (ed): Operative Nerve Repair and Reconstruction. Philadelphia, JB Lippincott, 1991, pp 1069–1076.

123. Dellon A, Mackinnon S, Hudson A, Hunter D: Effects of submuscular versus intramuscular placement of ulnar nerve: Experimental model in the primate. J Hand Surg [Br] 11:117–119, 1986.

124. Glickman L, Mackinnon SE, Rao T, McCabe S: Continuous intravenous regional anesthesia. J Hand Surg 17:82–86, 1992.

125. Watchmaker G, Lee G, Mackinnon S: Intraneural topography of the ulnar nerve in the cubital tunnel facilitates anterior transposition. J Hand Surg [Am] 19:915–922, 1994.

126. Deune E, Mackinnon SE: Postoperative drainage is recommended in ulnar nerve transposition. Can J Plast Surg 6:201–203, 1998.

127. Geutjens G, Langstaff R, Smith N, et al: Medial epicondylectomy or ulnar nerve-transposition for ulnar neuropathy at the elbow? J Bone Joint Surg Br 78:777–779, 1996.

128. Stuffer M, Jungwirth W, Hussl H, Schmutzhardt E: Subcutaneous or submuscular transposition of the ulnar nerve? J Hand Surg [Br] 17:248–250, 1992.

129. Campbell J, Post K, Marantz R: A technique for relief of motor and sensory deficits occurring after anterior ulnar transposition. J Neurosurg 40:405–409, 1974.

130. Luch A: Ulnar nerve entrapment after anterior transposition at the elbow. N Y State J Med 75:75, 1975.

131. Rogers M, Bergfield T, Aulicino P: The failed ulnar nerve transposition: Etiology and treatment. Clin Orthop Rel Res 269:193–200, 1991.

132. Babcock W: Nerve disassociation: A new method for the surgical release of certain painful or paralytic afflictions of nerve trunk. Ann Surg 46:686–693, 1907.

133. Babcock W: A standard technique for operations on peripheral nerves, with special reference to the closure of large gaps. Surg Gynecol Obstet 45:365–378, 1927.

134. Phalen G: The birth of a syndrome, or carpal tunnel revisited. J Hand Surg 6:109–110, 1981.

135. Mackinnon SE, Dellon A: Evaluation of microsurgical internal neurolysis in a primate median nerve model of chronic nerve compression: Internal neurolysis versus decompression. J Hand Surg [Am] 13:345–351, 1988.

136. Rydevik B, Lundborg G, Nordborg C: Intraneural tissue reactions induced by internal neurolysis. Scand J Plast Reconstr Surg 10:3–8, 1976.

137. Gentili F, Hudson A, Kline D, Hunter D: Morphological and physiological alterations following internal neurolysis of normal rat sciatic nerve. In Gorio A, Millesi H, Mingrino S (eds): Posttraumatic Peripheral Nerve Regeneration: Experimental Basis and Clinical Implications. New York, Raven Press, 1981, pp 183–210.

138. Cooney W: Chronic pain treatment with direct electrical nerve stimulation. In Gelberman RH (ed): Operative Nerve Repair and Reconstruction. Philadelphia, JB Lippincott, 1991, pp 1551–1561.

139. Goldner J, Nashold B, Hendrix P: Peripheral nerve electrical stimulation. Clin Orthop Rel Res 163:33–41, 1982.

140. Law J, Swett J, Kirsch W: Retrospective analysis of 22 patients with chronic pain treated by peripheral nerve stimulation. J Neurosurg 52:482–485, 1980.

141. Nashold B, Goldner J, Mullen J, Bright D: Long-term pain control by direct peripheral nerve stimulation. J Bone Joint Surg Am 64:207–217, 1982.

142. Strege D, Cooney W, Woods M, et al: Chronic peripheral nerve pain treated with direct electrical nerve stimulation. J Hand Surg [Am] 19:931–939, 1994.

143. Sweet W: Control of pain by direct stimulation of peripheral nerves. Clin Neurosurg 23:103–111, 1976.

144. Waisbrod H, Panhans C, Hansen D, Gerbershagen H: Direct stimulation for painful peripheral neuropathies. J Bone Joint Surg Br 67:470–472, 1985.

145. Novak CB, Mackinnon SE: Outcome following implant of a peripheral nerve stimulator in patients with chronic nerve pain. Plast Reconstr Surg 105:1967–1972, 2000.

146. Kleinmann W: Revision ulnar neuroplasty. Hand Clin 10:461–477, 1994.

147. Warwick L, Seradge H: Early versus late range of motion following cubital tunnel surgery. J Hand Ther 8:245–248, 1995.

CHAPTER 257

Entrapment Syndromes of Peripheral Nerve Injuries

CHONG C. LEE ■ SUZIE C. TINDALL ■ MICHEL KLIOT

Peripheral nerve entrapment is common in humans. It should be suspected in any person who notices paresthesias, pain, progressive weakness, or muscle wasting in the distribution of a single peripheral nerve. Entrapment of the median nerve beneath the transverse carpal ligament in the hand (i.e., carpal tunnel syndrome) is the most common peripheral nerve entrapment syndrome and is the best defined clinically and diagnostically (see Chapter 255). It serves as the model with which all other nerve entrapments are compared. However, many other peripheral nerves may be subject to entrapment, and the mechanisms of entrapment vary according to the anatomic relationships of the nerve and the mechanical forces that come into play in the entrapment process. This chapter describes other peripheral nerve entrapment syndromes.

PATHOPHYSIOLOGY

Various mechanisms of nerve injury lead to the development of clinically apparent entrapment neuropathies. Physical forces resulting in injury, alone or in combination, include pressure, stretch, angulation, and friction. The amount of each force and the length of time over which it is applied, whether the force occurs over a short or a long segment, and how often it is applied are all variables in the final equation predicting the extent of nerve injury. Age and the presence of underlying systemic disease are also factors to be considered. Nerves lose some regenerative ability with increasing age and become more vulnerable to injury if underlying systemic diseases (e.g., diabetes) already compromise their metabolic processes. It has been difficult to control and duplicate all of these potential pathophysiologic factors in animal models of peripheral entrapment neuropathy.

In 1965, Fullerton and Gilliatt[1] reported an animal model of pressure neuropathy in the hind feet of guinea pigs that had been reared in small cages with wire-mesh floors. Their study of the posterior tibial nerves in these animals revealed electrophysiologic slowing of conduction in the distal parts of the motor fibers and histologic changes of segmental demyelination. The same group of investigators later documented the development of a spontaneous entrapment neuropathy in the median and ulnar nerves of older guinea pigs.[2, 3] Detailed histologic and physiologic studies of these lesions demonstrated some similarities to spontaneous median nerve entrapment in humans. Anatomically, the lesion occurred under the transverse cartilaginous bar that supports the footpad, and in severe cases, a neuromatous swelling was present proximal to the lesion. Electrophysiologically, there was slowing of nerve conduction or a complete conduction block. Conventional light and electron microscopy at the level of the lesion showed loss of large myelinated fibers, and the remaining fibers had disproportionately thin myelin sheaths or were demyelinated. Above and below the lesion, no changes were found in the nerves of animals that were only moderately affected, but in those with severe lesions, there was drop-out of large, myelinated fibers; segmental demyelination of other fibers proximal to the abnormality; and wallerian degeneration distal to the lesion.[2-4]

Another method of developing an animal model of chronic compression neuropathy has been to implant a constrictive device about the nerve and to study the preparation later. The spring clip used by Ranvier in the 1870s and later by Denny-Brown and Brenner in 1944 is such a device.[5-7] However, changes associated with initial application of the clip may make later histologic findings difficult to interpret. Aguayo and associates[8] applied siliconized rubber tubes to the sciatic nerves of 3- to 5-week-old rabbits. As the animals matured, there was increased slowing of motor nerve conduction across the constricted segment. Outer fibers of the compressed segment of the nerve showed segmental demyelination, whereas centrally located fibers were less affected. Animal models for acute peripheral nerve constriction have also been developed and usually consist of application of a tourniquet or a constrictive cord.[9-11]

Because peripheral nerve entrapment is not a life-threatening disorder and because operative treatment rarely involves neurectomy, there has been little human material for study. Thomas and Fullerton[12] reported studies of a patient who had a carpal tunnel syndrome documented before death from a malignant glioma. Findings were those of a striking reduction in fiber size and a lesser reduction in fiber number. Gilliatt and coworkers[7, 12] reported changes characteristic of acute constrictive entrapment in the median nerve of a man who died of an intracerebral hemorrhage and who had severe decorticate rigidity with flexion of the wrists for several hours before death.

Gelberman and coworkers[13, 14] studied the dynamic physiology of the carpal tunnel in humans by measuring the pressure in the tunnel with a wick catheter. Pressure in the canal of patients with carpal tunnel syndrome was elevated and was markedly increased when the wrist was flexed and extended.

Over the years, the debate regarding the pathophysiology of peripheral nerve entrapment has been about the relative roles of mechanical deformation versus ischemia or other vascular factors. From the current knowledge base, several conclusions can be drawn. First, the pathophysiologic changes of chronic nerve entrapment and acute compression are different. Second, in both situations, mechanical deformation is the initial insult, and vascular factors follow in the pathophysiologic cascade. Although much is known about the ultrastructural and microscopic changes in nerve compression, there is little information about the effect of compression on the basic metabolic processes within the parent nerve cell or axon.

In cases of chronic nerve compression, it appears that the earliest anatomic change is a distortion of the internodes of the myelinated fibers. In teased fiber preparations from spontaneous compressive lesions in the guinea pig, Ochoa and Marotte[15] showed that, proximal and distal to the entrapment site, the internodes were bulbous at one end and tapered at the other. In more advanced lesions, the end of the internode nearest the point of compression showed early demyelination. These changes were believed to represent movement of groups of inner myelin lamellae relative to the axon, and the direction of slippage was away from the site of entrapment.[15] Similar changes have been found in examination of specimens from patients with subclinical entrapment neuropathies.[16–18] Such changes are the result of mechanical compression. After they develop, a cascade of pathophysiologic changes takes place. Venous stasis occurs adjacent to the point of compression. Proximal and distal to the site of compression, swelling develops that consists of edema fluid located extra-axonally. The edema increases the intrafunicular pressure and produces ischemia. The long-term result is replacement of the contents of the funiculi by fibrous tissue.[19, 20] Fullerton[21] showed that nerves that have already undergone such changes develop alterations in electrical conductivity earlier than normal nerves when they are subjected to ischemia from a pneumatic tourniquet.

In the case of acute nerve compression, the morphologic changes in teased fiber preparations differ from those of chronic compression described previously. There is displacement of the nodes of Ranvier along the fibers away from the site of pressure. The nodes invaginate the myelin tube, and local demyelination occurs at the point of invagination.[10, 11, 22] Ischemia does not increase the susceptibility of the nerve to such damage.[23] After such changes occur, the pathophysiologic cascade described earlier takes over.[24] Mackinnon and colleagues[25] reviewed the pathophysiologic changes associated with nerve entrapment.

GENERAL CONSIDERATIONS

Patients presenting with entrapment of a peripheral nerve generally complain of paresthesias, pain, or motor weakness in the distribution of the nerve involved. The specific subset of symptoms depends to a large part on the location and anatomic makeup of the affected nerve, and for this reason, specific symptoms are discussed individually as each entrapment neuropathy is described. Signs of entrapment may include alteration of sensory thresholds, two-point discrimination, temperature or pain sensation, or motor atrophy or weakness in the distribution of the involved peripheral nerve. Symptoms may be reproduced or exacerbated by rendering the nerve relatively ischemic or increasing its entrapment by selected positional changes of parts of the extremity (e.g., Phalen's maneuver for carpal tunnel syndrome). Percussion over a nerve rendered irritable by entrapment may result in dysesthetic electric-like sensations radiating in the distribution of the nerve (e.g., Tinel's sign).

When peripheral nerve entrapment is suspected, confirmation is generally sought by the use of conventional nerve conduction and electromyographic techniques (see Chapter 253). These studies prove more advantageous in the evaluation of some entrapments than others, and the benefits and drawbacks of such studies are discussed in relation to each entrapment neuropathy. However, the following comments apply to their application in patients with peripheral nerve entrapments.

Orthodromically evoked sensory action potentials across relatively short segments of nerve usually are the most sensitive indicators of intervening entrapment. Prolonged motor distal latencies or a delay or block in motor conduction velocity (if this can be judged based on the nerve in question) is less sensitive but more reliable. In the later stages of entrapment neuropathy in which significant distal wallerian degeneration and denervation atrophy have occurred, electromyography shows fibrillation potentials. In many instances, however, electrical investigation of peripheral entrapment neuropathy need not include electromyography. The use of intraoperative stimulating and recording techniques to localize the specific point of entrapment and, in some instances, to verify complete decompression by virtue of a change in the amplitude or delay of an action potential may be helpful in selected cases.[26]

Newer modalities of evaluating nerve entrapment and aiding in localizing the entrapment sites have been developed. The use of magnetic resonance imaging

(MRI) has been increasing in evaluating the patient, planning surgery, and following recovery of the injured nerve. MRI has been useful in evaluating several nerve entrapment syndromes, including carpal tunnel syndrome, cubital tunnel syndrome or ulnar nerve entrapment across the elbow, thoracic outlet syndrome, and others.[27–29] This topic is extensively reviewed elsewhere in this textbook and in an article by Grant and colleagues.[29]

GENERAL SURGICAL APPROACH

The surgeon who chooses to operate on patients with peripheral nerve entrapments must have a reasonable knowledge of the anatomy of the extremities and be comfortable in managing an unexpected source of entrapment, such as ganglion or synovial cysts and soft tissue or bony masses. For the neurosurgeon, a fundamental knowledge of basic principles of general, vascular, orthopedic, and plastic surgery is essential for good results. On certain occasions, the help of a surgeon from one of these other specialties is indispensable. We prefer to operate on most patients with peripheral nerve problems without the use of a tourniquet. Generally, working without a tourniquet is safer because a nerve that is already ischemic is not rendered more so and because postoperative hemostasis is more satisfactory if the individual arteries and veins are appropriately coagulated or tied as they are initially encountered.

Operative techniques should avoid contact with or significant added trauma to the nerve in question. Dissection and traction should be on structures around the nerve, and the surgeon should avoid inserting instruments within an already tight compartment. Gentle, sharp dissection is carried out using short strokes with a long-handled knife with a no. 15 blade down through a retinaculum or band until it suddenly parts, exposing the epineurium of the compressed nerve. Inserting a scissors blade beneath a confining structure should be done with great care and after it has been bluntly cleared away from the underlying nerve. Bipolar coagulation is most helpful when working around the nerve, and we favor a small pair of straight Gerald bipolar forceps. Loupe magnification ($\times 2.5$) is employed when working around any nerve. The operating microscope is rarely necessary in dealing with peripheral nerve entrapment (see Chapter 28).

ENTRAPMENT NEUROPATHIES

Table 257–1 lists the most common points of entrapment of the peripheral nerves. The remainder of this chapter discusses each entrapment neuropathy on an individual basis. Entrapments are classified according to whether they occur in the upper or lower extremity. The most common entrapment neuropathy, carpal tunnel syndrome, is discussed only briefly here because it is described in great detail in Chapter 255.

T A B L E 2 5 7 – 1 ■ **Points of Entrapment of the Peripheral Nerves**

ANATOMIC PART	POINT OF ENTRAPMENT
Thoracic outlet	Cervical rib
	First rib
	Anomalous bands or muscles
Suprascapular nerve	Suprascapular notch
Musculocutaneous nerve	Elbow forearm fascia
Median nerve	Supracondylar process of the humerus (Struther's ligament)
	Lacertus fibrosis
	Pronator teres muscle
Anterior interosseous nerve	Tendinous origin of the flexor superficialis muscle
	Anomalous bands
Median nerve at wrist	Flexor retinaculum of wrist
Radial nerve	Anomalous bands of triceps
Posterior interosseous nerve	Arcade of Frohse in supinator muscle
Radial sensory nerve	Fascia or tendons at wrist
Ulnar nerve	Supracondylar process of the humerus (Struther's ligament)
	Aponeurotic sheath of flexor carpi ulnaris muscle
	Anomalous bands
	Bands or ganglion in Guyon's canal
Lateral femoral cutaneous nerve	Inguinal ligament
Sciatic nerve	Piriformis muscle
	Anomalous bands
Peroneal nerve	Tendinous bands at the fibular head
	Ankle fascia
	Foreleg fascia
Posterior tibial nerve	Anomalous bands
	Flexor retinaculum of ankle
Plantar digital nerve	Intermetatarsal ligament

Upper Extremity Peripheral Nerve Entrapment

Peripheral nerve entrapment may occur in the region of the brachial plexus and axilla, as well as in the upper extremity itself.

ENTRAPMENTS OF THE MEDIAN NERVE

Entrapment of the Median Nerve at the Wrist: Carpal Tunnel Syndrome

Entrapment of the median nerve at the wrist, called carpal tunnel syndrome, is the most common entrapment neuropathy in humans. The estimated incidence of carpal tunnel syndrome is 125 cases per 100,000 people.[30] Because it occurs so frequently, it has been studied extensively and is the best-defined entrapment clinically, electrophysiologically, and operatively. It was first postulated as a clinical problem in 1913 by Marie and Foix, who observed the postmortem enlargement of the median nerve proximal to the transverse carpal ligament in a patient who had bilateral thenar atrophy.[31] Learmonth is credited with the first operative decompression of the carpal tunnel in 1933.[31]

Carpal tunnel syndrome develops when the median

nerve is compressed between the carpal bones that surround the tunnel, the flexor retinaculum, and the deep or superficial tendons of the hand. Chronic compression of the nerve results in devascularization of the nerve, with additional direct damage to the nerve.[32, 33] The anatomy, evaluation, and treatment of carpal tunnel syndrome are discussed in Chapter 255.

Entrapments of the Median Nerve above the Wrist

The median nerve originates from the medial and lateral cords of the brachial plexus in proximity to the axillary artery and contains fibers derived from the C5 through T1 spinal nerve roots. It travels in the medial aspect of the upper arm, crosses the elbow anteriorly in the antecubital fossa, and then enters the forearm, where it gives off branches to the pronator teres, flexor digitorum sublimis, flexor carpi radialis, palmaris longus, and flexor digitorum profundus muscles. As it passes through the upper forearm, it penetrates the lacertus fibrosis (i.e., fascial band that extends from the biceps tendon to the deep forearm fascia medially) and, in most instances, passes between the two heads of the pronator teres muscle. As it gives off the anterior interosseous nerve, which supplies the flexor pollicis longus, flexor digitorum profundus, and pronator quadratus muscles, it dips under the sublimis bridge (i.e., tendinous arch of origin of the flexor digitorum sublimis). At the wrist, it gives off a palmar cutaneous branch and then enters the carpal tunnel deep to the flexor retinaculum of the wrist and palm. Within the hand, it supplies the first two lumbricales and all the thenar muscles except the adductor pollicis, and it provides sensation to the thumb, index, middle fingers, and the radial half of the ring finger.

High median nerve entrapments at the axilla are characterized by weakness in forearm pronation and radial wrist flexion, as well as by variable amounts of weakness of flexion of the proximal interphalangeal joints of all fingers and the distal interphalangeal joints of the thumb and index finger. The thenar musculature is weak, and sensory findings are related to the radial side of the palm in a typical median nerve distribution in the hand. Such entrapments unrelated to trauma are rare. The most common traumatic disorder is the so-called honeymoon palsy, in which symptoms of partial median nerve dysfunction are related to the effects of pressure of a partner's head on the patient's axilla during sleep.

Entrapments of the median nerve in the upper arm, across the elbow, and in the forearm can be divided into three categories, all of which are rare. The first is compression by a supracondylar process of the humerus, the second is compression in the region of the pronator teres muscle, and the third is isolated dysfunction of the anterior interosseous nerve as a result of entrapment in the region of the sublimis bridge. The most common entrapment neuropathy is distal median nerve entrapment at the wrist (i.e., the carpal tunnel syndrome).

Entrapment of the Median Nerve by the Supracondylar Process of the Humerus. Between 0.7% and 2.7% of the population has a small bony spicule on the medial side of the humerus above its supracondylar process. Occasionally, a dense band of connective tissue (i.e., Struthers' ligament) extends from this process to the medial epicondyle. Beneath this ligament pass the median nerve, brachial artery, and brachial vein. Entrapment of the median nerve at this point may result in elbow discomfort, paresthesias in the median distribution, and variable weakness in the median innervated musculature, particularly the pronator teres muscle. The bony spur is commonly palpable above the medial elbow, and a tangential x-ray study can confirm its presence. Excision of the bony process and release of the ligament result in relief of symptoms.[34]

Pronator Syndrome. There are three potential points of compression of the median nerve in the upper forearm: beneath the lacertus fibrosus, between the two heads of the pronator teres muscle or within the substance of the muscle itself, and beneath the tendinous origin of the flexor superficialis muscle.

Many patients with this disorder have work or recreational activities that require considerable muscular activity of the forearm and hand, especially forceful pronation accompanying finger flexion.[35] The most common complaint is aching pain in the proximal volar forearm, particularly after forceful pronation, and paresthesias of the hand. Numbness in the hand is rarely well localized, but most patients report that it involves the index finger and thumb. Although the complaints may suggest a carpal tunnel syndrome, the nocturnal symptoms often found in the latter disorder are not seen in the pronator syndrome. The most prominent physical finding is that of tenderness to palpation over the pronator teres muscle. Percussion or pressure in this area exacerbates the median paresthesias. The pronator muscle may appear to be unusually large or firm. Motor weakness is mild, if present at all, and the flexor pollicis longus and abductor pollicis brevis muscles are involved most prominently.

Electrodiagnostic studies are useful in ruling out other disorders, specifically carpal tunnel entrapment. In the pronator syndrome, the distal median nerve latency from the wrist is normal, but demonstration of slowing across the forearm may be difficult.

Conservative approaches to the problem are often effective, including pointing out to the patient activities that exacerbate the disorder and suggesting alternative methods of accomplishing the task. Some physicians advocate steroids injected within the substance of the pronator muscle.[35] Operative exploration in patients who fail to improve with conservative measures is appropriate. In the Mayo Clinic series of 36 operations, 16 patients had a hypertrophied pronator muscle or a tendinous band within the substance of the muscle, 15 had a thickened lacertus fibrosus, and 12 had a taut fibrous arch of the flexor digitorum superficialis (some patients were thought to have more than one abnormality). The operative results were excellent in 8, good in 20, and fair in 5 patients, and symptoms in 3 patients were unchanged.[36] The series of Johnson and associates[37] was similar and included a large number of patients who had entrapment by various fibrous bands. Only 4 of 51 patients operated on did not benefit from the procedure.

Anterior Interosseous Syndrome: Kiloh-Nevin Syndrome

Parsonage and Turner, in their classic paper on brachial neuritis, described one patient who manifested weakness only in the distribution of the anterior interosseous nerve, which they believed was caused by an anterior horn cell lesion. In 1952, Kiloh and Nevin[38] described two cases of isolated neuritis of the anterior interosseous nerve of spontaneous onset, and although they failed to recognize that this disorder often represented a distal entrapment neuropathy, the anterior interosseous syndrome is often referred to as the Kiloh-Nevin syndrome.[38, 39]

Anterior interosseous nerve palsy may follow forearm fractures or supracondylar fractures of the humerus.[40, 41] In the case of forearm fractures, the nerve may be involved directly but the mechanism in patients with supracondylar fractures appears to be traction on the nerve. The nerve may become spontaneously entrapped by fibrous bands or other anomalous structures within the forearm.[42–44] Symptoms may be related to a sudden strain or pull on the arm or may develop much more insidiously and include pain in the forearm and wrist and loss of hand dexterity. There is weakness of the long flexors of the thumb and index finger. This leads to a characteristic pinch attitude of the hand, with the index finger showing extension of the distal interphalangeal joint and increased flexion of the proximal interphalangeal joint, whereas the involved thumb has increased flexion of the metacarpophalangeal joint and hyperextension of the interphalangeal joint. Weakness of the pronator quadratus muscle is demonstrated by testing resistance to the forced supination of the forearm with the elbow flexed. There is no sensory deficit. Electromyography shows denervation in the muscles innervated by the anterior interosseous nerve, but demonstration of delayed motor velocities requires special techniques.[45]

In patients who do not show improvement with conservative measures, operative exploration is appropriate.[44, 46] Surgery usually reveals compression of the anterior interosseous nerve by the tendinous origin of the flexor superficialis muscles.

ENTRAPMENTS OF THE ULNAR NERVE

Entrapment of the Ulnar Nerve above the Wrist

The ulnar nerve is the most distal branch of the medial cord of the brachial plexus. Its fascicles are derived from the C8 and Tl spinal nerve roots. It travels along the medial aspect of the upper arm and approaches the elbow posterior to the medial intermuscular septum and in close association with the insertion of the medial head of the triceps muscle. As it passes around the elbow, it gives off a small articular branch

and a branch to the flexor carpi ulnaris muscle. Traveling in a groove between the medial epicondyle and the olecranon process, it then enters the cubital tunnel between the two heads of the flexor carpi ulnaris muscle. After passing through the forearm flexor-pronator muscle mass, about 6 to 8 cm above the wrist, it gives off the dorsal cutaneous branch that provides sensation over the dorsum of the medial hand and small finger. The main trunk of the nerve then enters the hand through Guyon's canal at the wrist, where it divides into a superficial and a deep branch. The superficial branch innervates the palmaris brevis muscle and supplies sensation to the volar surface of the ulnar hand, small finger, and ulnar half of the ring finger. The deep branch takes an abrupt turn about the hook of the hamate and innervates the most intrinsic muscles of the hand.

The ulnar nerve is most prone to entrapment at the elbow and then at the wrist. Rare cases of ulnar nerve entrapment in the middle forearm have been reported. This entrapment is most often at the level of takeoff of the dorsal cutaneous nerve, and isolated involvement of this nerve is possible.

Patients presenting with pain in the ulnar forearm or hand, paresthesias of the little and ulnar aspect of the ring finger, and weakness of the hand may have entrapment of the ulnar nerve across the elbow. Careful assessment should include questions about recent or remote sources of trauma to the nerve. The nerve should be carefully palpated throughout its course, and areas of fullness or swelling should be sought. A positive Tinel sign anywhere along the course of the nerve may give a clue about the anatomic site of entrapment. The ulnar nerve may also easily subluxate across the elbow, causing further irritation.

One of the earliest signs of ulnar nerve entrapment is weakness of the third palmar interosseous muscle, manifested by an abducted posture of the small finger (i.e., Wartenberg's sign). Clawing of the ring and small fingers occurs when the metacarpophalangeal joints are hyperextended and interphalangeal joints are flexed. Clawing occurs because the lumbrical and interosseous tendons (controlled by ulnar supplied muscles) no longer work, which destabilizes the metacarpophalangeal joints, resulting in wasting of the action of the extensor tendons (controlled by radial supplied muscles) and allowing the flexor tendons (controlled by median supplied muscles) to overpower the extensor tendons. Froment's sign occurs because the median supplied flexor pollicis muscle substitutes for the weakened ulnar supplied adductor pollicis muscle. In this sign, the metacarpophalangeal joint of the thumb is hyperextended, and the interphalangeal joint is flexed markedly when the patient attempts a pincer movement between the thumb and index finger. Function of the flexor carpi ulnaris muscle usually remains strong in ulnar nerve entrapment. However, all other ulnar-innervated muscles, including the flexor digitorum profundus (which flexes the fourth and fifth digits), the interosseous muscles, muscles of the hypothenar group (i.e., palmaris brevis, abductor, flexor, and opponens digiti minimi), and thenar group (i.e., adductor pollicis and flexor pollicis brevis), show various degrees of weakness and atrophy. An exception to these findings is the rare syndrome of isolated entrapment of sensory branches. Testing the first dorsal interosseous muscle by abducting the index finger against resistance is extremely valuable in assessment of ulnar nerve function. It is easily seen and palpated for bulk and compared with the muscle of the opposite side in the case of unilateral disease.

Sensory loss in ulnar nerve entrapments is quite variable because of anatomic variations and terminal sensory overlap. In most instances, the sensory disturbance begins below the wrist crease and involves the ulnar and volar sides of the hand and the small finger. Classically, numbness involves the ulnar half of the ring finger on the dorsal and volar surfaces. Because the dorsal cutaneous branch, which arises proximal to the wrist, is responsible for sensibility over the dorsal ulnar area of the hand and wrist, distal entrapment of the nerve at Guyon's canal spares this sensory territory. The earliest sensory abnormalities involve subtle alterations in tactile sensations; light touch (i.e., threshold test) is compromised early, and two-point discrimination (i.e., innervation density) is compromised later.

Entities that may be mistaken for entrapment neuropathies of the ulnar nerve include cervical radiculopathies, thoracic outlet syndrome, apical lung tumors, spinal cord diseases such as glioma or syrinx, and amyotrophic lateral sclerosis. These alternative diagnostic possibilities should be strongly considered if the patient's signs and symptoms do not strictly fit an ulnar nerve distribution. Bilateral symptoms, the presence of neck or shoulder pain, Horner's syndrome, weakness or sensory loss above the wrist, and long tract signs are not usually associated with ulnar nerve entrapment.

Entrapment of the Ulnar Nerve at the Elbow: Cubital Tunnel Syndrome

Compression of the ulnar nerve at the elbow is the second most common entrapment neuropathy (after carpal tunnel syndrome) seen in clinical practice. A complete description of cubital tunnel syndrome is found in Chapter 256. Panas, in 1878, is credited with the first description of this type of ulnar neuropathy in the literature.[47, 48] In this case, a man presented with progressive ulnar nerve dysfunction many years after an elbow fracture in childhood. Similar cases of ulnar nerve dysfunction appearing long after a fracture dislocation of the elbow and leading to a cubitus valgus deformity led Ramsay Hunt to coin the term *tardy ulnar palsy* in 1916. With current methods of proper alignment of elbow fractures, the classic tardy ulnar palsy has become a rarity.

The recognized causes of ulnar nerve entrapment at the elbow include direct trauma, recurrent subluxation of the nerve, compression from adjacent structures at the elbow, and the cubital tunnel syndrome. Because the ulnar nerve is located superficially at the elbow, it is vulnerable to direct trauma during the routine activities of daily living. Nerve dysfunction may follow a single blow, but it usually follows more chronic, repeated minor trauma. Ulnar nerve palsy may be seen when the nerve has been unprotected and traumatized during periods of prolonged unconsciousness as a result of anesthesia (see Chapter 256), intoxication, or other causes resulting in coma. Progressive palsy may be seen in bedridden patients who use their elbows for support and in people who chronically lean on their elbows. Examples of the latter are office workers who use the nondominant elbow for support while working at a desk or television fans who sit for prolonged periods in an easy chair with arm rests. The ulnar nerves of at least 16% of the normal population subluxate onto the tip of the humeral medial epicondyle or completely across the epicondyle when the elbow is flexed. Childress,[49] who studied this process in detail, believes that the condition is caused by congenital laxity of supporting ligaments. A few of these persons develop ulnar neuritis from direct trauma or frictional irritation.

As in the classic tardy ulnar palsy in which ulnar nerve dysfunction results from chronic stretch or compression of the nerve over a cubitus valgus deformity as a result of an improperly aligned fracture, other mechanical causes can be associated with progressive ulnar palsy. Osteophytes from arthritis or old fractures, chondromatosis of the elbow joint, overgrowth of rheumatoid synovium, a ganglion in the ulnar sulcus, an anomalous epitrochleoanconaeus muscle, or a prominent medial head of the triceps muscle may produce ulnar nerve compression and stretch.[48, 50]

Feindel and Stratford[51] first described the anatomy of the cubital tunnel and its relationship to motion at the elbow in 1958. Osborne[52, 53] emphasized the role of the cubital tunnel in causing progressive ulnar nerve dysfunction. The floor of the cubital tunnel is the medial collateral ligament, and the roof is the fibroaponeurotic triangular arcuate ligament that connects the two heads of the flexor carpi ulnaris muscle between the medial epicondyle and the olecranon. Chang and associates[54] described enlargement of the ulnar nerve just before it enters the cubital tunnel in about 50% of 400 specimens taken from 200 autopsy cadavers of Chinese subjects. Pathologic examination of this enlargement showed that it was caused by an increase in connective tissue.

The volume of the cubital tunnel is markedly reduced with elbow flexion, and as the tunnel constricts, the ulnar nerve is flattened and distorted. Forceful elbow flexion for at least 1 minute to elicit symptoms on examination is a useful provocative diagnostic test. The exact percentage of patients who present with progressive ulnar palsy due to cubital tunnel entrapment is unknown. It is possible that idiopathic or unexplained palsy in many patients is caused by this pathophysiologic mechanism.

The predominant symptoms of ulnar nerve entrapment at the elbow are paresthesias and weakness of the hand. In many patients the extent of weakness and muscle atrophy is much more pronounced than the sensory disturbance. This is particularly true in the case of the classic tardy ulnar palsy. Patients with extensive atrophy of the intrinsic hand muscles often report only minor disability. There may be aching pain in the elbow or medial forearm, but painful paresthesias are unusual and are most frequently seen in those patients with a distinct traumatic etiology.

McGowan[55] developed a functional classification of these lesions to assess the benefit derived from operation, and this classification has been used by others in evaluating their results:

Grade I: Minimal lesions with no detectable motor weakness of the hand

Grade II: Intermediate lesions with detectable motor weakness

Grade III: Severe lesions with paralysis of one or more of the ulnar intrinsic muscles

We use a somewhat different clinical grading system: mild (i.e., intermittent symptoms), moderate (i.e., continuous symptoms), and severe (i.e., loss of axons; abnormal two-point or muscle atrophy or weakness) (see Chapter 248).

Since Simpson initially showed in 1956 that measurement of ulnar nerve conduction could be useful in identifying an ulnar neuropathy at the elbow, a variety of electrophysiologic methods to evaluate such lesions have been described. Localization of the ulnar lesion to the elbow basically rests on demonstrating a block or slowing of motor or sensory nerve conduction across a segment of nerve at the elbow.[56] MRI is also proving to be very useful (see Chapter 254).

Some patients who present with progressive ulnar nerve entrapment at the elbow can be managed conservatively with benefit. This is particularly true if there is a definite traumatic cause that can be identified and eliminated. For instance, the habitual elbow rester may improve if educated to avoid leaning on his or her ulnar nerve. Most patients are treated operatively because of progression of symptoms despite medical measures or because of the extent of motor atrophy at the time of presentation.

The appropriate method of operative treatment is not established. There are three basic surgical approaches to the problem. The first is simple in situ decompression of the ulnar nerve within the cubital tunnel, originally popularized by Osborne.[52, 53] In this procedure, the nerve is exposed through an 8- to 10-cm incision overlying the ulnar nerve or an omega-shaped incision that courses partially anteromedial to the medial epicondyle. The nerve is freed throughout its course around the elbow, with particular attention to resection of the overlying aponeurosis between the heads of the flexor carpi ulnaris muscle (i.e., Osbourne's band). This procedure does not necessitate sectioning any nerve or vascular branches and can be easily accomplished under local anesthesia with mild sedation.

A second procedure is that of medial epicondylectomy, as originally advocated by King and Morgan in 1950.[57–61] This procedure is usually combined with in situ release of the nerve, as previously described. However, after the simple release is accomplished, a linear incision is made in the aponeurotic origin of the pronator teres and flexor muscles of the forearm over the front of the medial epicondyle, and

two leaves of fascia are raised from the bone subperiosteally. The epicondyle and 2 to 5 cm of the medial supracondylar ridge are removed with a drill or chisel. The bone is waxed, and the split aponeurosis is sutured to provide a smooth surface for the nerve. Because work on bone is needed, this procedure requires general or regional anesthesia.

The third operative approach involves the transposition of the ulnar nerve. The ulnar nerve is moved anterolateral to the medial epicondyle in an effort to shorten its course by providing a more linear course across the elbow joint. Three distinct types of ulnar nerve transposition can be performed surgically: superficial transposition within the subcutaneous tissues of the forearm, intermediate intramuscular transposition within a groove created in the flexor pronator muscle mass, or deep submuscular transposition beneath the fibers of the flexor-pronator muscle mass.[62–66] The skin incision is made somewhat longer than for the two previously described procedures; it directly overlies the nerve or has an omega configuration (we prefer the former type). The nerve must be freed circumferentially at least 4 to 8 cm above and below the elbow to permit unrestricted transposition. Careful attention must be given to sectioning the medial intermuscular septum proximal to the elbow. Adequate transposition virtually always requires sectioning of the small ulnar articular branches at the elbow, and the branches to the flexor carpi ulnaris muscle may need to be lengthened somewhat by internally neurolysing them away from the parent ulnar nerve. The nerve is secured in its transposed position by suturing the subcutaneous tissues laterally to the aponeurosis over the epicondyle medially in the case of a subcutaneous or intramuscular transposition. In the case of a submuscular transposition, a loose fascial sling is first fashioned using a Z-plasty incision in the superficial fascia of the flexor-pronator muscle mass. The entire aponeurotic attachment of the flexor-pronator muscles is then cut away from the medial epicondyle, creating a deep and wide groove into which the ulnar nerve can be transposed into its submuscular location. The two ends of the lengthened superficial fascia are then sutured together. The submuscular transposed nerve should be observed to ensure it is completely unencumbered while the arm is flexed and extended across the elbow through its entire range of movement. The complexity and duration of the operation dictates whether general or regional anesthesia is used.

There is no definite answer about which ulnar nerve surgical decompressive technique is superior. Studies attempting to resolve which technique is superior are flawed by retrospective analysis, failure to differentiate the various causes of the ulnar nerve entrapment being treated, and small numbers of procedures.[67–69] Our approach has been to tailor the operative procedure to the specific problem while attempting to do the least necessary to get a good result. Simple in situ decompression is considered if the ulnar nerve does not subluxate out of the ulnar groove when the elbow is fully flexed and the patient does not have a history of mechanically traumatizing the nerve, such as by leaning on the elbow. Epicondylectomy is rarely performed and reserved for patients who have a bony deformity of the medial epicondyle that prevents adequate nerve decompression. Transposition of the ulnar nerve is often used to create a smooth, linear, and unencumbered course of the ulnar nerve across the elbow.

The type of transposition performed is determined to some extent by each patient's anatomic findings at surgery and the surgeon's preference. Our approach has been to consider first performing a subcutaneous transposition. If such a transposition will not create a smooth, linear, and unencumbered course for the ulnar nerve, a submuscular transposition is performed.[63, 70] An intramuscular transposition combined with an extensive neurolysis of the ulnar nerve is reserved for patients who have undergone a submuscular transposition but then developed recurrent symptoms.

Regardless of the operative procedure employed, the outlook is not always good. In nonselective series employing the various procedures randomly, a good to excellent result can be expected in about 60% of patients, a fair result in about 25%, and a poor result (i.e., no improvement or increase in symptoms) in about 15%.[48, 64, 66–69]

Factors that may portend poor results include traumatic causes; symptoms persisting for more than 1 year preoperatively; presence of intraneural fibrosis at operation; severe preoperative atrophy, weakness, clawing, dysesthesia, or pain; alcoholism; and absence of an evoked sensory potential and large numbers of fibrillations by electromyography. However, none of these factors is a contraindication to surgery, because some patients with what seems to be end-stage disease show marked improvement postoperatively.

The largest number of complications has been reported with the various transposition procedures, probably because they have been performed much longer, have been used in greater numbers of patients, and require somewhat more operative expertise. Although many of the complications are caused by technical factors such as residual compression of the ulnar nerve at the intermuscular septum or at the entrance to the cubital tunnel or constriction by fascial slings, a number of cases have been reported in which the nerve has become densely fibrosed after intramuscular transposition.[71] There is much room for improvement in the diagnosis and treatment of ulnar nerve entrapment at the elbow.

Entrapments of the Ulnar Nerve at the Wrist and Hand

In 1861, Felix Guyon, a French urologist, first described the anatomy of the canal through which the ulnar nerve enters the hand. Guyon's canal, or the ulnar-carpal canal, is bounded by the pisiform bone proximally and medially and by the hook of the hamate laterally and distally. The floor is formed by the transverse carpal ligament and the roof by the volar carpal ligament.[72] At the distal end of the floor of this canal is the pisohamate hiatus, which is bounded superiorly by a concave musculotendinous arch and below by the pisohamate ligament.[73]

Within Guyon's canal course the ulnar artery and nerve. The nerve divides into a superficial branch, which is sensory to the palmar surface of the little finger and ulnar side of the ring finger and motor to the palmaris brevis muscle, and a deep motor branch, which innervates the hypothenar muscles and then passes through the pisohamate hiatus to innervate the third and fourth lumbricals, the interossei, the adductor pollicis, and the deep head of the flexor pollicis brevis muscles.

Shea and McClain[74] developed an orderly classification of distal ulnar nerve lesions into three categories. In the type I syndrome, there is motor weakness of all ulnar-innervated muscles in the hand and a sensory deficit to the palmar surfaces of the hypothenar eminence and of the fourth and fifth digits. Sensation over the dorsum of the hand is unaffected. This syndrome is caused by a lesion at the proximal part of Guyon's canal. The type II syndrome, which is the most common, spares sensation but results in weakness of muscles innervated by the deep branch of the ulnar nerve. The lesion is at the pisohamate hiatus or a more distal location, and the number of muscles involved depends on the site of compression along the deep branch. The type III syndrome involves a pure volar sensory deficit without motor findings and is caused by pathology solely affecting the superficial sensory branch at the most distal part of the canal. Electrophysiologic evaluation shows prolonged distal ulnar sensory action potentials in types I and III and a prolonged distal motor latency with a widened muscle action potential of diminished amplitude in types I and II. Denervation changes identified on electromyography spare the hypothenar muscles in type II.

Occupational or recreational neuritis and compression by ganglions lead the list of the lesions causing distal ulnar nerve syndromes in the hand. Examples of occupational trauma include compression in the ulnar palm in mechanics, pipe-fitters, and metal polishers.[50, 75] Recreational trauma includes handlebar pressure in long-distance cyclists and similar trauma in gymnasts.[76] Ganglions arising from the triquetrohamate joint or the triquetropisiform joints are the most common intrinsic masses causing distal ulnar nerve compression.[77, 78] Lipomas, anomalous muscles, and fractures of the carpal bones are other causes of these distal ulnar neuropathy syndromes.[36, 74]

In patients who have an obvious chronic, traumatic cause of the neuropathy, avoiding the precipitating trauma often results in a complete return of function. In patients who fail to respond to such measures or in cases of questionable origin, operative exploration is advisable. An incision over the hypothenar region that is carried laterally into the palm affords an excellent exposure of the contents of Guyon's canal. In cases of deep motor branch entrapment, the nerve should be followed well into the palm, and a careful inspection should be made for the presence of a ganglion.

ENTRAPMENTS OF THE RADIAL NERVE

The radial nerve originates from the posterior cord of the brachial plexus just distal to the axillary nerve. It gives off its first major branch to the triceps muscle just before it begins a curvilinear course around the humeral shaft in a posteromedial to posterolateral trajectory. The radial nerve then courses distally across the anterolateral aspect of the antecubital fossa into the forearm, where motor branches are given off to the brachioradialis and the extensor carpi radialis longus and brevis muscles just as the nerve enters the forearm between the biceps and brachioradialis muscles. Within the proximal forearm it divides into two main branches: the superficial sensory branch, which supplies sensation to the dorsum of the radial side of the hand (i.e., anatomic snuff box region), thumb, and index and middle fingers, and the posterior interosseous nerve. The posterior interosseous nerve enters the substance of the supinator muscle, where in 30% of the population it is bound anteriorly by a fibrous band called the arcade of Frohse. As this nerve continues its course in the dorsal forearm, it gives off multiple muscle branches to the remaining extensor muscles of the wrist and fingers.

Entrapments of the radial nerve may be divided into three major categories: those above the elbow, those at the posterior interosseous nerve, and those of the superficial sensory branch in the distal forearm and wrist.

Entrapment of the Radial Nerve above the Elbow

Injury to the radial nerve above the elbow results in paralysis of the brachioradialis muscle, complete wrist drop, digital extensor paralysis, and sensory deficit over the dorsum of the radial side of the hand. When testing finger extension, the clinician should passively extend the patient's wrist to avoid confusion with the mechanically mediated distal finger extension that occurs when the wrist is allowed to fall into flexion, causing passive tension on the digital extensor tendons. Involvement of the triceps muscles is unusual because of the proximal branches supplying these muscles.

The most common cause of a high radial nerve injury that involves the triceps is crutch palsy. The axillary nerve is also frequently involved or may be involved individually. Crutch palsies are distinctly unusual, because most patients requiring crutches are instructed in their proper use. Compression of the radial nerve above the elbow is usually caused by "Saturday night" palsy. In this syndrome, which frequently follows a drunken sleep during which the arm is allowed to hang off the bed or bench, triceps function is usually preserved. Prognosis for complete return of function is excellent in these cases, and a wrist dorsiflexion splint is usually prescribed to place the hand in a functional anatomic position (i.e., slight extension) until muscle strength returns, usually within several weeks. There are rare reports of compression of the radial nerve at the midhumeral shaft by anomalous insertions or fibrous bands of the triceps muscle.[79]

The other most common high entrapment of the radial nerve is that associated with displaced fractures of the humeral shaft. The paralysis may be complete or partial and may have occurred immediately at the time of fracture or may follow closed reduction. A partial lesion has a good prognosis and can be managed conservatively. Complete lesions, whether they occurred acutely or at the time of closed reduction, should be explored early. Findings at the time of exploration include a nerve trapped between bone ends or compressed or tented by bone spicules.[80] The nerve should be decompressed and then be appropriately repaired.

Entrapment of the Posterior Interosseous Nerve

The posterior interosseous nerve is most liable to entrapment just beyond its origin as it passes through the fibers of the supinator muscle in the upper forearm. At this point, a fibrotendinous band from which some of these muscle fibers originate (i.e., arcade of Frohse) is frequently found. Lipomas, ganglions, rheumatoid synovial overgrowth, and dislocations of the elbow may account for compression of the nerve at this site. Entrapment in the absence of such structural pathology does occur and is thought to result from compression of the nerve by the arcade of Frohse or by other vascular or fibrous structures in the area.[81, 82]

There are two distinct clinical syndromes for this disorder. The first is highly controversial, and many authorities are skeptical that it even exists. It is characterized mainly by pain and is the most difficult to diagnose. It is usually called the *radial tunnel syndrome* or *resistant tennis elbow*.[83] It was initially described by Roles and Maudsley in 1972 and has since gained wider recognition. Patients complain of lateral elbow pain, which is generally described as a dull ache located deep in the extensor muscle mass of the upper forearm. Night pain is common. On examination, tenderness is found not over the radial head but at a point about 5 cm distal over the extensor radialis longus muscle, just where the posterior interosseous nerve enters the supinator muscle mass. Pain is increased with forced supination. With the patient's elbow and wrist extended, resisted extension of the middle finger elicits the pain as well. This sign, called the middle finger test, is believed to be important by several surgeons.[83] The diagnosis is mainly a clinical one, although elaborate electrodiagnostic studies, in which radial nerve motor conduction is measured with the involved extremity in active resisted supination, are said to be reliable in some patients.[84] Those who have operated on patients with this syndrome report that, when the posterior interosseous nerve is explored in these cases, it is usually found to be compressed by fibrous bands from the radial head, a tethering vessel, the sharp tendinous margins of the extensor carpi radialis brevis muscle, or the arcade of Frohse. Operative decompression is reported to relieve the symptoms in most patients.

The second clinical syndrome is that of a gradually progressive or acute weakness of wrist and finger extension. Pain may be present at the onset but is usually not a prominent part of the syndrome. Sensory loss does not occur, and the weakness of wrist extension is never complete. The wrist deviates radially when wrist extension is checked. There is preservation of function in the brachioradialis, the extensor carpi radialis longus and brevis, and the supinator muscles, because branches to these muscles leave the nerve proximal to its point of entrapment. The anatomic basis for the electrophysiologic localization of this lesion by electromyography is obvious. This is the syndrome most often encountered when an anatomic mass lesion such as a lipoma is causing the compression, and it is also encountered in cases of compression by the arcade of Frohse.[50, 81, 85–87]

Operative release of the posterior interosseous nerve is best performed through an incision that begins above the elbow between the biceps and brachioradialis muscles and extends downward to the middle of the upper volar surface of the forearm.[88] Separating out the branches of the radial nerve and releasing the entrapment of the posterior interosseous branch should be done carefully and completely. We prefer general anesthesia for the procedure. Occasionally, a separate incision over the dorsum of the forearm through the supinator muscle may be necessary to completely decompress the small distal muscular branches of the posterior interosseous nerve. Excellent anatomic guides are provided in publications by Spinner[82] and by Kline and colleagues.[89]

Entrapment of the Superficial Sensory Branch of the Radial Nerve: Wartenberg's Syndrome

Tight casts, watch bands, athletic bands, and handcuffs may cause transient compression of the superficial sensory branch of the radial nerve, resulting in anesthesia, hypesthesia, or hyperesthesia over the dorsum of the radial side of the hand.[50, 90] Recognizing the causative agent and removing it are curative. DeQuervain's tenosynovitis often coexists with superficial radial sensory nerve entrapment. Blunt injury to this superficial branch that results in painful paresthesias is a much more difficult problem and may be resistant to all forms of treatment. Dellon and Mackinnon[91] reviewed 51 patients with entrapment of the superificial sensory branch of the radial nerve. Thirty-two of these patients underwent neurolysis, with the results judged to be excellent in 37%, good in 49%, fair in 6%, and not improved in 9%. Lanzetta and Foucher[92] reported 52 cases of superficial radial sensory entrapment. Thirty patients responded to conservative treatment, and 23 were operated on, with a good or excellent result for 74% of the patients. In some patients, a first extensor compartment release for treatment of DeQuervain's disease was done along with neurolysis of the superficial sensory branch of the radial nerve.

THORACIC OUTLET PERIPHERAL NERVE ENTRAPMENT

The topic of peripheral nerve entrapment at the thoracic outlet is a source of confusion for several reasons. Many patients with vague symptoms involving the upper extremity that cannot be attributed to any particular cause are sometimes given the diagnosis of thoracic outlet syndrome. The number of patients having clear-cut symptoms and physical findings of thoracic outlet syndrome is small. These patients tend to be referred to a variety of medical specialists, depending on the suspected underlying cause. For example, patients with vascular syndromes are cared for by vascular or thoracic surgeons, patients with neurogenic involvement by neurosurgeons, and patients with clavicular fractures by orthopedic surgeons. Consequently, most physicians see a very small and biased group of patients with this syndrome. The historical evolution of the concepts of the various clinical syndromes of the thoracic outlet has added to the confusion. Many patients included in early series of thoracic outlet syndromes probably suffered from carpal tunnel syndrome or cervical disk disease.

The evolution of this disorder is further clouded by concepts that at one time or another reached great popularity, only to fall into disfavor later. Examples include the use of Adson's maneuver to confirm entrapment by the loss of radial pulse with stretch of the scalenus anticus muscle, which is not considered a very accurate diagnostic test; the popularity of the procedure of simple scalenus anticus muscle section, which later proved ineffective in many circumstances; and the more recent reliance on the concept that electrical slowing of nerve conduction can be demonstrated reliably across the thoracic outlet using standard nerve conduction velocity techniques, a concept that has been difficult to replicate consistently. Although there are several specific classic clinical syndromes related to thoracic outlet entrapment, there is also a rather large body of literature based on great numbers of patients who have been diagnosed and treated as having thoracic outlet entrapment on the basis of subjective symptomatology and no objective means of documenting the problem preoperatively.

Criteria for the choice of the best operative approach (i.e., supraclavicular, posterior, or transaxillary) have not been well developed. The procedure used often depends on the specialty of the operating surgeon.

Anatomy of the Thoracic Outlet

Anatomically, the thoracic outlet can be thought of as a triangle, of which the posterior limb is the scalenus medius muscle, the anterior limb is the scalenus anticus muscle, and the base is the first rib. Through this triangle course the three trunks of the brachial plexus (i.e., upper, middle, and lower) and the subclavian artery. Compression of nerve structures traversing this triangle is usually caused by some sort of anatomic anomaly in the area. The most obvious abnormal structure that is occasionally present in this area is a cervical rib or an anomalous long transverse process of C7. Although the bony abnormality may be the source of compression, an anomalous fibrous band connecting the end of the cervical rib to the first rib is more often the etiologic agent when a cervical rib is present.[93] Some physicians believe that the most common anomalies associated with thoracic outlet syndrome are fibromuscular bands or scalene muscle abnormalities.[94, 95]

Clinical Syndromes of Thoracic Outlet Compression

Clinical syndromes of thoracic outlet compression are divided into vascular and neurogenic categories. It is unusual to see these two types of syndromes combined.

Vascular syndromes are rare and can result from aneurysmal dilatation of the subclavian artery, with or without thrombus and with or without embolization.[96, 97] Vascular compromise is often precipitated by certain postures, such as abduction of the arm at the shoulder. The patient complains of a cold, diffusely painful arm that becomes easily fatigued and develops cramps with effort. Signs are coldness, cyanosis, or paleness of the arm and hand with diminished or absent distal pulses and, in the later stages, gangrene of the digits. A supraclavicular mass or bruit may be present. Most of these cases are associated with cervical ribs. The diagnostic procedure of choice is angiography. Discussion of treatment is beyond the scope of this chapter.

The neurogenic syndrome is characterized by pain in the supraclavicular area that is aggravated by exercising the arm or certain postures involving abduction of the arm at the shoulder. Rest tends to diminish symptoms. The patient may complain of paresthesias on the medial side of the arm and hand that increase with exercise or arm abduction at the shoulder. These paresthesias are not nocturnal, as is so frequently the case in carpal tunnel syndrome, and they more often affect the ulnar side of the arm and hand. Muscle spasm of the shoulder girdle and neck frequently accompanies the pain, and some type of traumatic injury to the neck or upper arm may precipitate the symptoms. Most patients are women, and Swift and Nichols[98] noticed that these individuals might have a peculiar body habitus, with low-set, "droopy" shoulders and long necks.

Physical examination invariably shows reproduction of much of the syndrome with digital percussion over the medial supraclavicular area. In patients with later stages of the disease, the examiner may see wasting of the hand muscles, which is usually most marked in the thenar pad but may involve ulnar innervated intrinsic hand muscles as well. Sensory loss, when present, usually affects the inner side of the forearm and hand in a C8 and T1 dermatomal distribution.[93] Loss or diminution of the radial pulse with stretch of the scalenus anticus muscle (i.e., Adson's maneuver) or with hyperabduction of the arm may help to confirm the diagnosis, although some consider this to be a meaningless test because many normal individuals demonstrate this finding.

The diagnosis of a cervical rib or elongated C7 transverse process can be easily made by x-ray studies. However, clinical correlation is important even in the presence of a radiographically demonstrable cervical rib. All cervical ribs are not symptomatic. In the case of bilateral anomalous cervical ribs, the smaller of the two may be the symptomatic one because of an associated fibrous band. In the absence of x-ray evidence of a cervical rib or elongated C7 transverse process, it may be difficult to obtain objective evidence supporting a diagnosis of thoracic outlet syndrome.

Imaging studies such as MRI have been performed to detect abnormalities of the brachial plexus and surrounding structures. For example, signal abnormalities involving the brachial plexus in patients with thoracic outlet syndrome have been reported.[29, 99] However, much more work is necessary to demonstrate the diagnostic accuracy and utility of these techniques.

Urschel and Razzuk reported finding a conduction delay across the proximal brachial plexus using typical nerve conduction time recordings, but other investigators have been unable to duplicate these findings, and the original observations have now been shown to be artifactual.[100–102] In patients who are so severely affected that clinical evidence of muscle wasting is found in the hand, the ulnar sensory action potential amplitude may be reduced.[22] In most patients, however, the standard nerve conduction and electromyographic examination results are normal and best serve to rule out carpal tunnel syndrome (as a differential diagnosis or as an associated disorder), ulnar nerve entrapment at the elbow (i.e., so-called double crush syndrome when present in combination with thoracic outlet syndrome),[103] or cervical radiculopathy. Later work with somatosensory evoked responses recorded across the brachial plexus showed some promise in helping to delineate electrodiagnostic findings associated with this disorder, but no generally accepted and reliable standards are available.[104–106] Subclavian angiography is not indicated in the evaluation of patients with the neurogenic syndrome. Vascular constriction at the outlet does not necessarily indicate neurogenic constriction.

Because of the inability to demonstrate the presence of a clinically significant neurogenic thoracic outlet constriction objectively in the absence of x-ray evidence of a cervical rib, there is considerable controversy about the frequency with which this syndrome occurs.[107] The situation is complicated even further by the number of patients whose complaints may be more closely linked to emotionally related factors or issues of secondary gain such as workmen's compensation.[108–110] The question comes down to this: How common is the syndrome in the absence of a cervical rib? Purists say that it almost never occurs without a cervical rib, and they demand objective end-stage muscle wasting before a diagnosis is made.[111] Others believe that only 6% to 9% of patients with neurogenic thoracic outlet syndrome have demonstrable cervical ribs, and they have reported very large series of patients who were operated on based on subjective criteria only.[6, 94, 112–114]

Conservative treatment for thoracic outlet syndrome can take multiple forms.[112–114] Some physicians advocate weight reduction by women to reduce the pull of the breasts on the anterior chest wall. Several exercise programs are directed at strengthening the shoulder girdle and improving posture. In our experience, they are sometimes of benefit but may occasionally exacerbate symptoms. A major problem with this patient population is sorting out those with overriding depression or secondary gain who masquerade as having thoracic outlet compressive syndromes and who will therefore not improve with operative intervention. With changes in the health care environment, studies of reimbursement patterns and patient profiles are appearing. In one from Colorado, patients who did not have private insurance or worker's compensation were rarely diagnosed as having thoracic outlet syndrome, and Medicaid patients almost never underwent surgery for correction of this entity.[115]

Operative Approaches to Thoracic Outlet Syndrome

Three operative approaches to the thoracic outlet are described. Controversy exists regarding which is indicated and under what circumstances it should be performed.[116–118] We prefer the supraclavicular approach under most circumstances. A supraclavicular incision, usually in a neck crease just above and parallel to the clavicle, provides the best visualization of the anatomy of brachial plexus nerve elements and their relation to the scalenus muscles and compressive rib, transverse process, or fibromuscular band structures. In a review of results using this approach, Dellon[119] reported that, of 11 patients operated on, 5 had excellent results, 5 had good results, and only 1 had a poor result. The posterior approach has been advocated for use in bull-necked or very obese individuals in whom vascular pathology is not a factor or in cases of reoperation when the initial approach was anterior. Transaxillary removal of the first rib (essentially taking the bottom out of the triangle of the thoracic outlet) has been the most popular procedure among vascular and thoracic surgeons for treatment of the neurogenic syndrome. Although the results in reported series are generally good, there is a relatively high incidence of complications from this procedure, chief of which is brachial plexus injury. This injury may be caused by direct operative injury to the plexus elements, which are not well seen, or to a stretch injury of the plexus elements as a result of the marked hyperabduction of the arm required for adequate exposure.[6, 120]

Complications from operations for thoracic outlet syndrome are not unusual, regardless of the approach used. A French survey reported that complications were dramatic when they did occur and that they included vascular injury, partial or complete paralysis of brachial plexus elements, hemothorax, and chylothorax.[121] The risks inherent in performing thoracic outlet decompression should be carefully weighed when considering surgery.

ENTRAPMENT OF UPPER TRUNK NERVES

Suprascapular Nerve Entrapment

The suprascapular nerve arises as a large branch from the upper trunk of the brachial plexus lateral to the anterior scalene muscle, just above the clavicle. It courses posteriorly adjacent to the omohyoid muscle and winds over the superior border of the scapula, passing through the suprascapular notch and beneath the suprascapular ligament. The suprascapular artery, which travels nearby, passes over the suprascapular ligament and does not accompany the nerve through the notch, but it joins the nerve in the supraspinous fossa. Two branches are given off from the nerve to the supraspinatus muscle, and articular filaments are given off to the shoulder joint and the acromioclavicular joint. The nerve then curves around the lateral border of the spine of the scapula into the infraspinous fossa and gives off two branches to the infraspinatus muscle, as well as some filaments to the shoulder joint and the scapula.

The usual site of entrapment is within the suprascapular notch beneath the suprascapular ligament.[122–126] Entrapment may also occur at the lateral edge of the spine of the scapula in the spinoglenoid notch, in which case there is selective denervation of the infraspinatus muscle. Structures causing entrapment in such a location are a hypertrophied inferior transverse scapular ligament or ganglion arising from the shoulder joint.[127, 128]

Patients with entrapment of the suprascapular nerve complain of shoulder pain.[129] The pain is usually centered over the lateral scapula and posterior shoulder, is deep and aching, and is aggravated by shoulder motion, particularly abduction or external rotation of the upper arm. There may be a history of trauma to the shoulder. Atrophy of the supraspinatus and infraspinatus muscles is usually apparent on inspection. Supraspinatus weakness can be documented by demonstrating weakness in the first 15 degrees of abduction of the arm, and infraspinatus weakness is indicated when weakness of external rotation of the arm can be demonstrated with the elbow held in 90 degrees of flexion.

Electromyography reveals denervation potentials in the supraspinatus and infraspinatus muscles and is the best diagnostic test. It can be used to differentiate this entity from rotator cuff injuries, which may result in a similar pain syndrome and disuse atrophy of the spinatus muscles. In these situations, there is no electrical evidence of muscle denervation.[130, 131]

Conservative measures of care include shoulder exercises and local injections of steroids and analgesic agents. Operative decompression is usually necessary, particularly when atrophy and weakness are a prominent part of the picture. After placing the patient in the prone position, we prefer to approach the suprascapular notch through an incision that parallels the scapular spine and splits the fibers of the trapezius muscle. The notch can be felt by running the finger over the top edge of the scapula from medial to lateral. Sectioning the suprascapular ligament while sparing the overlying artery is satisfactory for nerve decompression in most cases, but some surgeons have advocated enlarging the notch by removal of extra bone.[132] The surgeon should probe beneath the surface of the supraspinatus muscle after sectioning the ligament to make sure a ganglion cyst is not lurking there. Shupech and Onofrio[133] described an alternative anterior approach that involved exposure of the brachial plexus and tracing the suprascapular nerve from anterior to posterior.

Musculocutaneous Nerve Entrapment

The musculocutaneous nerve originates from the lateral cord of the infraclavicular portion of the brachial plexus and supplies branches to the coracobrachialis, biceps, and brachialis muscles. It pierces the brachial fascia lateral to the biceps tendon at the level of the elbow, where it becomes subcutaneous and divides into the anterior and posterior cutaneous nerves of the forearm. Compression of the sensory branches of this nerve can occur at the point where it emerges from the fascia at the elbow crease.

Patients suffering from musculocutaneous nerve entrapment have pain in the anterolateral aspect of the elbow and burning dysesthesias along the radial aspect of the volar part of the forearm. Such symptoms are accentuated by repeated pronation and supination of the forearm. There is direct tenderness over the area of entrapment and a decrease in sensibility distally along the radial aspect of the forearm.

Treatment includes local injections of anesthetic and steroid preparations. If this fails to relieve the symptoms, operative release of the nerve at the free margin of the biceps aponeurosis may be required.[134]

Lower Extremity Peripheral Nerve Entrapment

The most common entrapment neuropathies of the lower extremities are those involving the lateral femoral cutaneous nerve, the peroneal nerve, the posterior tibial nerve, and the digital nerves. Less common entrapments are those of the proximal sciatic, the saphenous branch of the femoral nerve, and the sural nerve. Interest in entrapment neuropathies of the lower extremities has increased in recent years with several theories of entrapment as a possible exacerbating factor in diabetic neuropathy and as more emphasis has been placed on recreational and sports injuries.[135–138] Two excellent reviews can be consulted.[139–142]

The most common peripheral nerve entrapment of the lower extremity is that of the lateral femoral cutaneous nerve. The femoral nerve can be injured, stretched over a spontaneous hematoma in an adjacent muscle, or infarcted. The most common lesions that involve the obturator nerve alone or in combination with the femoral nerve are traumatic in origin. Pelvic fracture, iatrogenic injury during genitourinary or obstetric operations such as childbirth, and major trauma are examples. Retroperitoneal metastatic carcinoma may also damage these two nerves. A controversial entity is that of obturator nerve entrapment from obturator hernia. Dysfunction of the ilioinguinal or genitofemoral nerves, or both, is usually of traumatic origin from appendectomy or herniorrhaphy, although a chronic entrapment of the genitofemoral nerve has been described in women wearing tight jeans.[143]

MERALGIA PARESTHETICA

The lateral femoral cutaneous nerve has its origin from the second and third lumbar nerves high in the lumbar plexus. It courses from beneath the psoas muscle at the level of the crest of the ilium, travels across the surface of the iliacus muscle, and exits the pelvis just medial and inferior to the anterior superior iliac spine in a narrow tunnel between two slips of attachment of the inguinal ligament. As it emerges from the pelvis, a marked angulation of the nerve occurs. This angulation is increased by extension and lessened by flexion of the thigh because of pull on the inguinal ligament from contraction of the sartorius muscle.[144, 145] About 4 cm below the inguinal ligament, the nerve pierces the fascia lata. The nerve has an anterior branch and a posterior branch. The small posterior branch supplies the skin from the greater trochanter down to the area supplied by branches from the anterior division. The anterior branch supplies the skin of the lateral thigh down to the knee.

Stookey[146] was the first to emphasize the mechanical cause of meralgia paresthetica. He was impressed by the constant accentuation of the symptoms by standing and walking and by the sharp angulation of the lateral femoral cutaneous nerve as it left the pelvis.[146] Jefferson and Eames[16] examined this nerve at routine autopsy and found that 5 of 12 nerves showed pathologic changes in myelinated nerve fibers in the vicinity of the point of nerve contact with the inguinal ligament. These changes included local demyelination and wallerian degeneration in fibers with the largest diameters, the presence of polarized internodal swellings on single nerve fibers, and endoneurial and vascular thickening.

This disorder is more common in men than in women and usually manifests in middle age. It is associated with obesity and similar conditions that increase the abdominal girth, such as pregnancy and ascites. Local irritation from belts, corsets, and backpack harnesses is a frequent precipitating factor. Direct trauma to the nerve or compression by an adjacent hematoma, such as that after iliac bone graft removal, may also result in this syndrome. It has been reported as a complication of laparoscopic herniorrhaphy when staples were inadvertently placed through or around the nerve during hernia repair.[147] The disease is usually unilateral, although 20% of patients have bilateral symptoms. Right and left sides are affected with equal frequency.

Numbness along the lateral thigh is the most common and early symptom. Patients also complain of tingling, burning, and pain over the lateral thigh. Appreciation of touch, pain, and temperature sensations may be lost in the nerve distribution, but appreciation of pressure sensation is not lost. In long-standing cases, the skin of the lateral thigh may be thickened, the hair on the skin may be lost, a cutaneous rash may be seen, or small nodules in the subcutaneous tissue may be felt.

Diagnosis of this disorder is not always straightforward. Studies are occasionally necessary to rule out upper lumbar intraspinal pathology such as tumor, central or far lateral lumbar soft disk herniation, the lateral recess syndrome of lumbar spondylosis, or pelvic disorders. Confirmation of the pathology can sometimes be obtained from studies of sensory conduction velocity in the lateral femoral cutaneous nerve. These studies are done by stimulating the distal sensory branches of the nerve and recording beneath the inguinal ligament 1 cm medial to the anterior superior iliac spine with a needle electrode. Potentials are commonly absent on the involved side.[148, 149] In most instances, such a study is difficult to perform and not reliable. Injection of local anesthetic just medial to the anterior superior iliac spine can be useful to temporarily treat this neuropathy, aid in diagnosing the problem, and determine whether the patient would tolerate the anesthetic sensation produced by sectioning the nerve as subsequently described.

Treatment for this disorder is usually conservative. Inciting factors such as belts, trusses, corsets, and camping gear are removed and avoided. A switch to overalls or trousers with suspenders rather than a belt may be recommended. The obese patient is encouraged to lose weight. If the disorder persists and is considered a significant inconvenience by the patient, operative therapy can be recommended. Sectioning the nerve at its exit from the pelvis is a simple and effective procedure, provided the nerve can be found.[150] Such a procedure results in anesthesia over the lateral thigh. Some surgeons advocate release of the nerve at its point of entrapment beneath the inguinal ligament by sectioning the inferior slip of attachment of the inguinal ligament to the anterior superior iliac spine, allowing the nerve to move medially and reducing its angulation, but keeping the nerve intact.[145] However, in our experience, there is a significant incidence of failure of simple decompression, necessitating nerve sectioning at a later time.

ENTRAPMENTS OF THE SCIATIC, SAPHENOUS, AND SURAL NERVES

The syndrome of proximal entrapment of the sciatic nerve at the level of the piriformis muscle (i.e., piriformis syndrome) is controversial. Detailed anatomic studies of the relation of the sciatic nerve to the fibers of the piriformis muscle at this level have been done.[151] There are at least two well-documented cases of entrapment of the superior gluteal nerve by fibers of the piriformis muscle. These patients complained of chronic aching pain in the gluteal region, had a lurching gait due to weakness of the ipsilateral hip abductors, and had marked tenderness on palpation deep within the buttock in the region just lateral to the greater sciatic notch. Both improved after operative release of the piriformis muscle fibers.[50, 152] Most cases of pure sciatic nerve involvement at this level have been associated with antecedent trauma, such as intensive horseback riding or intramuscular injections in the area.[153] Most individuals are familiar with the usually transient "toilet seat palsy" manifested by paresthesias in the sciatic distribution. Cases of chronic sciatic nerve

entrapment due to a distinct myofascial band in the proximal thigh have been reported.[154, 155] Most patients with pain, numbness, and weakness in the sciatic distribution and depression or loss of an ankle jerk have pathology at the spinal level. Prominent weakness of the hamstring muscles and absence of denervation in the paraspinous muscles on electromyography should alert the clinician to consider a peripheral sciatic nerve lesion.

Standard electrical tests for accurate localization of a lesion along the course of the sciatic nerve are generally disappointing. Surgical exposure of the proximal sciatic nerve is usually achieved through a large question mark–shaped buttock incision and involves dissection through multiple deep layers of subcutaneous tissues and muscle. As the proximal sciatic nerve is exposed and the overlying pyriformis muscle sectioned, great care must be taken to avoid cutting the gluteal artery, which can retract into the pelvis and necessitate an anterior abdominal exploration to control the bleeding. Abnormal structures—a venous varix and an intraneural ganglion cyst—have been associated with the proximal sciatic nerve.

Spontaneous saphenous neuralgia is a well-recognized, although rare, clinical syndrome. The saphenous nerve is the most distal branch of the femoral nerve and is a purely sensory cutaneous nerve. Iatrogenic injury of the nerve can occur during medial arthrotomy and saphenous vein harvest. Spontaneous entrapment of the nerve is well recognized.[156, 157] Symptoms include pain localized to the medial aspect of the knee. The pain is aggravated by exercise, especially exercise that includes active knee extension, such as climbing stairs. Most of these patients are women. There is usually marked tenderness over the saphenous nerve in the thigh at the level of the subsartorial canal, about 10 cm above the knee, and sensory alterations may be found over the medial foreleg and foot. The diagnosis is confirmed by symptomatic relief with anesthetic blockade of the nerve. Treatment is usually decompression of the nerve in Hunter's subsartorial canal by release of a fascial band between the vastus medialis and the abductor magnus muscles.

Entrapment of the sural nerve posterior to the lateral malleolus has been reported, but in most cases, there has been preexisting trauma or compression by a ganglion arising from the adjacent joint.[158]

ENTRAPMENT OF THE PERONEAL NERVE

The peroneal nerve originates from the sciatic nerve in the popliteal fossa. It may be compressed at this point by abnormal depositions of fatty tissue or by the development of a Baker's cyst in the area. Under these circumstances, there are usually symptoms of combined dysfunction of the peroneal and the posterior tibial nerves. The nerve then travels laterally in the popliteal fossa and passes between the biceps femoris tendon and the lateral head of the gastrocnemius muscle. It wraps around the fibular neck and then passes through the peroneus longus muscle, where it divides into a small, recurrent branch; a deep branch; and a superficial branch. The common peroneal nerve may be trapped or compressed at the level of the fibular head, the deep branch at the ankle, and the superficial branch at its exit from the fascia of the anterior compartment about 10 cm above the ankle. Symptoms and signs from each of these entrapments may be easily confused with those of an L5 radiculopathy. Electrophysiologic studies may be helpful in localizing the probable peroneal nerve entrapment site.[159]

Common Peroneal Nerve Entrapment

Dysfunction of the common peroneal nerve is manifested by weakness and atrophy of the foot dorsiflexors and evertors and sensory alterations over the anterolateral foreleg and the dorsum of the foot. Pain in the lateral surface of the leg and foot is variable. Because of its superficial anatomic position at the fibular neck, the common peroneal nerve is prone to injury from pressure, traction, and penetration. A sudden flexion and inversion of the foot is the most common mechanism of injury. In the absence of a history of obvious trauma, the most common cause for minor dysfunction of this nerve is the cross-leg palsy found in women who habitually cross their legs or in cancer patients who have suffered a large weight loss and sit inactive with the legs crossed.[160, 161] A similar mechanism occurs in patients who are forced to squat or kneel for prolonged periods because of their occupation and in comatose or anesthetized patients who are poorly positioned. Ill-fitting, short leg casts are also offenders.

In all of these instances in which obvious compressive factors offer an explanation for the neurological deficit, eliminating the causative agent usually results in satisfactory recovery. However, if there are no precipitating factors or if the amount of trauma seems small for the extent of neurological deficit and if a generalized peripheral neuropathy or vasculitis predisposing to mononeuritis has been ruled out, the nerve should be explored. Compression of the nerve by a ganglion from the superior tibiofibular joint may be encountered.[162]

Entrapment of the Deep Branch of the Peroneal Nerve: Anterior Tarsal Tunnel Syndrome

Entrapment of the deep branch of the peroneal nerve is rare. It was first described by Kopell and Thompson.[163] The point of entrapment over the dorsum of the ankle is within the anterior tarsal tunnel, where the nerve and the anterior tibial vessels are bounded dorsally by the fascia overlying the talus and navicular bones and ventrally by the extensor hallucis longus muscle fibers and tendon, as well as by the inferior extensor retinaculum. Symptoms include aching or tightness about the ankle and dorsum of the foot. Numbness and paresthesias can be experienced in the first dorsal web space. The patient may hold the foot in a plantarflexed and inverted posture. Weakness and atrophy of the extensor digitorum brevis may be demonstrated, and hypesthesia is present in the first dorsal web space. Symptoms may be controlled by conserva-

tive measures such as a wedged orthosis for the shoe to correct over pronation, injection of steroids locally, or operative release of the entrapment.[164]

Entrapment of the Superficial Branch of the Peroneal Nerve

Henry first reported distal entrapment of the superficial branch of the peroneal nerve in 1949, and there have been scattered reports of this entity since then.[165, 166] The nerve usually is trapped or chronically injured, or both, at the point where it exits the fascia, about 10 cm above the ankle on the anterolateral aspect of the shin. Congenital fascial defects associated with small lipomas or muscle belly herniation may accompany the condition. There is frequently a history of ankle sprain. Patients complain of pain and occasionally of numbness over the outer border of the calf and the dorsum of the foot. There is usually no associated muscle weakness or sensory abnormality. The point at which the superficial branch exits the fascia is often quite tender to palpation. Diagnostic nerve block at this level may be helpful in confirming the diagnosis.

The entrapment is treated by incising the deep fascia at the point where the nerve exits until the nerve is thought to be lying freely between the peroneus longus and extensor digitorum longus muscles.

ENTRAPMENT OF THE DISTAL TIBIAL NERVE: TARSAL TUNNEL SYNDROME

The posterior tibial nerve may be involved by compression neuropathy at the level of the medial malleolus or in the medial foot. Predisposing factors include post-traumatic fibrosis due to fracture, an accessory or hypertrophied abductor hallucis muscle, tenosynovitis or compressive ganglion, varus heels and pronated splayed forefeet, compressive fat pads from obesity, diabetes, and the repetitive traumatic effects of jogging and running.[135, 138, 167–173] Many patients have none of these predisposing factors. Most patients with this disorder complain of burning pain localized along the plantar aspect of the foot. It may be in the region of the metatarsal heads or along the medial or lateral aspect of the foot. In many patients, the pain may radiate up the medial side of the calf. The pain is almost always increased by prolonged standing and may be exacerbated by walking. It usually has an insidious onset and an aching quality, although brief shooting pain is sometimes described. Nocturnal symptoms are not nearly as common as in patients with carpal tunnel syndrome. Physical examination invariably demonstrates a positive Tinel sign with percussion or pressure over the flexor retinaculum below the medial malleolus or, in the case of jogger's foot, at a point immediately posterior to the navicular tuberosity.[172] Hypesthesia in the distribution of the medial or lateral plantar nerves is occasionally present, and muscle weakness or atrophy is rare and difficult to demonstrate.

There are so many alternative possibilities when considering the diagnosis of tarsal tunnel syndrome that electrophysiologic investigation becomes a very important part of the decision-making process. Chief among the differential diagnostic possibilities are Achilles tendonitis and plantar fasciitis. Prolonged motor distal latency in the medial and lateral plantar nerves is a late finding and occurs in less than one half of the patients with tarsal tunnel syndrome. However, if present, it strongly supports the diagnosis. Sensory nerve conduction abnormalities, including slow nerve conduction velocities and dispersion phenomenon (i.e., prolonged duration and decreased amplitude of compound nerve action potentials recorded orthodromically) in the medial and lateral plantar nerves, particularly if recorded with a near-nerve needle electrode, are said to be much more sensitive indicators.[174, 175] The absence of such abnormalities in sensory conduction should make the clinician wary of the diagnosis. MRI of the foot and ankle may prove useful in evaluating patients with the tarsal tunnel syndrome.[29] MRI has demonstrated associated mass lesions, fracture or soft tissue injury, fibrous scar, flexor hallucis longus tenosynovitis, and abductor hallucis muscle hypertrophy in patients with tarsal tunnel–related symptoms.[29, 176]

Response to conservative measures such as shoe orthoses and local steroid injections is unusual in the patient with tarsal tunnel syndrome, with the exception of the syndrome of entrapment of the medial plantar nerve at the navicular tuberosity in joggers, which frequently responds to such measures.[172] Operative release of the entrapped distal tibial nerve, however, is not always as predictably beneficial as in the carpal tunnel syndrome. Pfeiffer and Cracchiolo[177] report that only 14 (44%) of 32 patients benefited markedly from the operative procedure. Decompression of the distal tibial nerve is accomplished under local anesthesia through a curvilinear incision posterior to the medial malleolus. The neurovascular bundle is isolated proximal to the tarsal tunnel, and the retinaculum overlying the nerve is sectioned. The nerve may be bound down within the tunnel, in which case it should be freed circumferentially. Care should be taken to avoid cutting the more proximal calcaneal branch, which may pierce the retinaculum. After the retinaculum is sectioned, the tibial nerve must be traced to its bifurcation into the medial and lateral plantar nerves, and each of these nerves is followed into the substance of the abductor hallucis muscle until relief of compression within this structure can be ensured.[141] The latter maneuver may be associated with some troublesome venous bleeding from a local venous plexus that encircles the nerve.

ENTRAPMENT OF THE DIGITAL NERVE IN THE FOOT: MORTON'S NEUROMA

Entrapment of the digital nerve in the foot is a relatively common form of peripheral nerve entrapment. The clinical symptoms and a rather crude form of operative therapy for the disorder were first described by Thomas G. Morton in 1876. The discomfort and disability from this disorder are so marked that the early medical literature is replete with graphic descriptions of the clinical syndrome, including several accounts from physicians who suffered from it themselves.[178] It is believed that the syndrome arises because of chronic entrapment and trauma to the digital nerve between the metatarsal heads. Usually, the nerve between the third and fourth metatarsals is involved, but the problem occasionally may arise at the second and third metatarsal junction. The syndrome is commonly seen in women who wear high-heeled shoes. The precipitating trauma may also be traced to foot positions during work or abnormalities of gait predisposing to abnormal metatarsal pressures. The syndrome may be seen in athletes and ballet dancers.[141, 173]

The symptoms occur much more frequently in women than in men and develop most commonly in midlife. The patient describes pain in the forefoot, particularly in the fourth toe, that is worse with walking. The pain frequently begins in the ball of the foot, runs down into the end of the toes, and later radiates up the dorsum of the foot. Most patients report removing their shoes when the pain strikes and may give the impression that they are exaggerating their symptoms. The physical examination is most marked by exquisite tenderness when the examiner squeezes the second or third intermetatarsal space between the thumb and index finger.

Some patients obtain significant improvement with conservative measures such as shoe modifications. Interdigital injection of local anesthetic and steroid combinations has been reported to provide long-term relief in a significant number of patients.[179] Operative therapy is beneficial in most instances. Under local anesthesia the interdigital "neuroma" is excised. A 2- to 3-cm dorsal incision is placed within the web space. The distal nerve is identified against the phalanx of the toes, cut, and held with a hemostat under gentle traction as the nerve is dissected proximal to the bifurcation and above the level of primary entrapment by the intermetatarsal ligament, where it is sectioned. The skin is closed with several interrupted stitches, and the patient avoids bearing weight on the foot for several days postoperatively. Results are generally gratifying. Infrequently, a patient may develop neuromas in contiguous common digital nerves. If adjacent neuromas are excised, the intervening toe will be rendered anesthetic. The patient must be forewarned to protect the toe.

Peripheral nerve entrapment disorders are quite common and diverse. They provide the interested neurosurgeon with the opportunity to treat a wide range of benign disorders in a variety of anatomic locations with the chance of often achieving good and long-lasting clinical outcomes.

REFERENCES

1. Fullerton PM, Gilliatt RW: Pressure neuropathy in the hind foot of the guinea-pig. J Neurol Neurosurg Psychiatry 30:18–25, 1967.
2. Anderson MH, Fullerton PM, Gilliatt RW, Hern JE: Changes in the forearm associated with median nerve compression at the wrist in the guinea-pig. J Neurol Neurosurg Psychiatry 33:70–79, 1970.

3. Fullerton PM, Gilliatt RW: Median and ulnar neuropathy in the guinea-pig. J Neurol Neurosurg Psychiatry 30:393–402, 1967.

4. Marotte LR: An electron microscope study of chronic median nerve compression in the guinea pig. Acta Neuropathol (Berl) 27:69–82, 1974.

5. Denny-Brown D, Brenner C: Lesion in peripheral nerve resulting from compression by spring clip. Arch Neurol Psychiatry 52:1–19, 1944.

6. Dale WA: Thoracic outlet compression syndrome. Critique in 1982. Arch Surg 117:1437–1445, 1982.

7. Gilliatt RW, Ochoa J, Rudge P, Neary D: The cause of nerve damage in acute compression. Trans Am Neurol Assoc 99:71–74, 1974.

8. Aguayo A, Nair CP, Midgley R: Experimental progressive compression neuropathy in the rabbit: Histologic and electrophysiologic studies. Arch Neurol 24:358–364, 1971.

9. Denny-Brown D, Brenner C: Paralysis of nerve induced by direct pressure and by tourniquet. Arch Neurol Psychiatry 51:1–26, 1944.

10. Ochoa J, Fowler TJ, Gilliatt RW: Anatomical changes in peripheral nerves compressed by a pneumatic tourniquet. J Anat 113:433–455, 1972.

11. Rudge P, Ochoa J, Gilliatt RW: Acute peripheral nerve compression in the baboon. J Neurol Sci 23:403–420, 1974.

12. Thomas PK, Fullerton PM: Nerve fiber size in the carpal tunnel syndrome. J Neurol Neurosurg Psychiatry 26:520–527, 1963.

13. Gelberman RH, Hergenroeder PT, Hargens AR, et al: The carpal tunnel syndrome: A study of carpal canal pressures. J Bone Joint Surg Am 63:380–383, 1981.

14. Lundborg G, Gelberman RH, Minteer-Convery M, et al: Median nerve compression in the carpal tunnel—functional response to experimentally induced controlled pressure. J Hand Surg Am 7:252–259, 1982.

15. Ochoa J, Marotte L: The nature of the nerve lesion caused by chronic entrapment in the guinea-pig. J Neurol Sci 19:491–495, 1973.

16. Jefferson D, Eames RA: Subclinical entrapment of the lateral femoral cutaneous nerve: An autopsy study. Muscle Nerve 2:145–154, 1979.

17. Neary D, Ochoa J, Gilliatt RW: Sub-clinical entrapment neuropathy in man. J Neurol Sci 24:283–298, 1975.

18. Neary C, Eames R: The pathology of ulnar nerve compression in man. Neuropathol Appl Neurobiol 1:69–88, 1975.

19. Sunderland S: The nerve lesion in the carpal tunnel syndrome. J Neurol Neurosurg Psychiatry 39:615–626, 1976.

20. Weisl H, Osborne GV: The pathological changes in rats' nerves subject to moderate compression. J Bone Joint Surg Br 46:297–306, 1964.

21. Fullerton PM: The effect of ischaemia on nerve conduction in the carpal tunnel syndrome. J Neurol Neurosurg Psychiatry 26:385–397 1963.

22. Gilliatt RW, Willison RG, Dietz V, Williams IR: Peripheral nerve conduction in patients with a cervical rib and band. Ann Neurol 4:124–129, 1978.

23. Williams IR, Jefferson D, Gilliatt RW: Acute nerve compression during limb ischaemia—an experimental study. J Neurol Sci 46:199–207, 1980.

24. Rydevik B, Lundborg G: Permeability of intraneural microvessels and perineurium following acute, graded experimental nerve compression. Scand J Plast Reconstr Surg 11:179–187 1977.

25. Novak CB, Mackinnon SE: Nerve injury in repetitive motion disorders. Clin Orthop 351:10–20, 1998.

26. Brown WF, Ferguson GG, Jones MW, Yates SK: The location of conduction abnormalities in human entrapment neuropathies. Can J Neurol Sci 3:111–122, 1976.

27. Jarvik JG, Kliot M, Maravilla KR: MR nerve imaging of the wrist and hand. Hand Clin 16:vii, 13–24, 2000.

28. Jarvik JG, Yuen E, Haynor DR, et al: MR nerve imaging in a prospective cohort of patients with suspected carpal tunnel syndrome. Neurology 58:1597–1602, 2002.

29. Grant GA, Britz GW, Goodkin R, et al: The utility of magnetic resonance imaging in evaluating peripheral nerve disorders. Muscle Nerve 25:314–331, 2002.

30. Stevens JC, Sun S, Beard CM, O'Fallon WM, Kurland LT: Carpal tunnel syndrome in Rochester, Minnesota, 1961 to 1980. Neurology 38:134–138, 1988.

31. Louis DS, Greene TL, Noellert RC: Complications of carpal tunnel surgery. J Neurosurg 62:352–356, 1985.

32. Mackinnon SE, Dellon AL, Hudson AR, Hunter DA: A primate model for chronic nerve compression. J Reconstr Microsurg 1:185–195, 1985.

33. Mackinnon SE, Novak CB, Landau WM: Clinical diagnosis of carpal tunnel syndrome. JAMA 284:1924–1925, discussion 1925–1926, 2000.

34. Laha RK, Dujovny M, DeCastro SC: Entrapment of median nerve by supracondylar process of the humerus: Case report. J Neurosurg 46:252–255, 1977.

35. Morris HH, Peters BH: Pronator syndrome: Clinical and electrophysiological features in seven cases. J Neurol Neurosurg Psychiatry 39:461–464, 1976.

36. Howard FM: Ulnar-nerve palsy in wrist fractures. J Bone Joint Surg Am 43:1197–1201, 1961.

37. Johnson RK, Spinner M, Shrewsbury MM: Median nerve entrapment syndrome in the proximal forearm. J Hand Surg Am 4:48–51, 1979.

38. Kiloh LG, Nevin S: Isolated neuritis of the anterior interosseous nerve. Br Med J 1:850–851, 1952.

39. Paine KW, Polyzoidis KS: Carpal tunnel syndrome: Decompression using the Paine retinaculotome. J Neurosurg 59:1031–1036, 1983.

40. Spinner M, Schreiber SN: Anterior interosseous-nerve paralysis as a complication of supracondylar fractures of the humerus in children. J Bone Joint Surg Am 51:1584–1590, 1969.

41. Warren JD: Anterior interosseous nerve palsy as a complication of forearm fractures. J Bone Joint Surg Br 45:511–512, 1963.

42. Fearn CB, Goodfellow JW: Anterior interosseous nerve palsy. J Bone Joint Surg Br 47:91–93, 1965.

43. Rask MR: Anterior interosseous nerve entrapment (Kiloh-Nevin syndrome): Report of seven cases. Clin Orthop 142:176–181, 1979.

44. Spinner M: The anterior interosseous-nerve syndrome, with special attention to its variations. J Bone Joint Surg Am 52:84–94, 1970.

45. Nakano KK, Lundergran C, Okihiro MM: Anterior interosseous nerve syndromes: Diagnostic methods and alternative treatments. Arch Neurol 34:477–480, 1977.

46. Lake PA: Anterior interosseous nerve syndrome. J Neurosurg 41:306–309, 1974.

47. Craven PR Jr, Green DP: Cubital tunnel syndrome: Treatment by medial epicondylectomy. J Bone Joint Surg Am 62:986–989, 1980.

48. Gay JR, Love JG: Diagnosis and treatment of tardy paralysis of the ulnar nerve. J Bone Joint Surg Am 29:1087–1097, 1947.

49. Childress HM: Recurrent ulnar nerve dislocation at the elbow. J Bone Joint Surg Am 38:978–984, 1956.

50. Dawson DM, Hallett M, Millender LH: Entrapment Neuropathies. Boston, Little, Brown, 1983.

51. Feindel W, Stratford J: Role of the cubital tunnel in tardy ulnar palsy. Can J Surg 1:287–300, 1958.

52. Osborne GV: The surgical treatment of tardy ulnar neuritis. J Bone Joint Surg Br 39:782, 1957.

53. Osborne G: Compression neuritis of the ulnar nerve at the elbow. Hand 2:10–13, 1970.

54. Chang KS, Low WD, Chan ST, et al: Enlargement of the ulnar nerve behind the medial epicondyle. Anat Rec 145:149–155, 1963.

55. McGowan AJ: The results of transposition of the ulnar nerve for traumatic ulnar neuritis. J Bone Joint Surg Br 32:293–301, 1950.

56. Kincaid JC, Phillips LH 2nd, Daube JR: The evaluation of suspected ulnar neuropathy at the elbow: Normal conduction study values. Arch Neurol 43:44–47, 1986.

57. Fannin TF: Local decompression in the treatment of ulnar nerve entrapment at the elbow. J R Coll Surg Edinb 23:362–366, 1978.

58. Froimson AI, Zahrawi F: Treatment of compression neuropathy of the ulnar nerve at the elbow by epicondylectomy and neurolysis. J Hand Surg Am 5:391–395, 1980.

59. Jones RE, Gauntt C: Medial epicondylectomy for ulnar nerve compression syndrome at the elbow. Clin Orthop 139:174–178, 1979.

60. King T, Morgan FP: The treatment of traumatic ulnar neuritis: Mobilization of the ulnar nerve at the elbow by removal of the medial epicondyle and adjacent bone. Aust N Z J Surg 20:33–42, 1950.

61. King T, Morgan FP: Late results of removing the medial humeral epicondyle for traumatic ulnar neuritis. J Bone Joint Surg Br 41:51–55, 1959.

62. Adson AW: The surgical treatment of progressive ulnar paralysis. Minn Med 1:455–460, 1918.

63. Dellon AL: Techniques for successful management of ulnar nerve entrapment at the elbow. Neurosurg Clin N Am 2:57–73, 1991.

64. Friedman RJ, Cochran TP: Anterior transposition for advanced ulnar neuropathy at the elbow. Surg Neurol 25:446–448, 1986.

65. Learmonth JR: A technique for transplanting the ulnar nerve. Surg Gynecol Obstet 75:792–793, 1942.

66. Leffert RD: Anterior submuscular transposition of the ulnar nerves by the Learmonth technique. J Hand Surg Am 7:147–155, 1982.

67. Adelaar RS, Foster WC, McDowell C: The treatment of the cubital tunnel syndrome. J Hand Surg Am 9A:90–95, 1984.

68. Foster RJ, Edshage S: Factors related to the outcome of surgically managed compressive ulnar neuropathy at the elbow level. J Hand Surg Am 6:181–192, 1981.

69. Macnicol MF: The results of operation for ulnar neuritis. J Bone Joint Surg Br 61:159–164, 1979.

70. Burchiel KJ, Ochoa JL: Pathophysiology of injured axons. Neurosurg Clin N Am 2:105–116, 1991.

71. Broudy AS, Leffert RD, Smith RJ: Technical problems with ulnar nerve transposition at the elbow: Findings and results of reoperation. J Hand Surg Am 3:85–89, 1978.

72. Kleinert HE, Hayes JE: The ulnar tunnel syndrome. Plast Reconstr Surg 47:21–24, 1971.

73. Uriburu IJ, Morchio FJ, Marin JC: Compression syndrome of the deep motor branch of the ulnar nerve (Piso-Hamate Hiatus syndrome). J Bone Joint Surg Am 58:145–147, 1976.

74. Shea JD, McClain EJ: Ulnar-nerve compression syndromes at and below the wrist. J Bone Joint Surg Am 51:1095–1103, 1969.

75. Hunt JR: Occupation neuritis of the deep palmar branch of the thenar nerve. J Nerv Ment Dis 35:673–689, 1908.

76. Noth J, Dietz V, Mauritz KH: Cyclist's palsy: Neurological and EMG study in 4 cases with distal ulnar lesions. J Neurol Sci 47:111–116, 1980.

77. Richmond DA: Carpal ganglion with ulnar nerve compression. J Bone Joint Surg Br 45:513–515, 1963.

78. Seddon HJ: Carpal ganglion as a cause of paralysis of the deep branch of the ulnar nerve. J Bone Joint Surg Br 34:386–390, 1952.

79. Manske PR: Compression of the radial nerve by the triceps muscle: A case report. J Bone Joint Surg Am 59:835–836, 1977.

80. Packer JW, Foster RR, Garcia A, Grantham SA: The humeral fracture with radial nerve palsy: Is exploration warranted? Clin Orthop 88:34–38, 1972.

81. Spinner M: The arcade of Frohse and its relationship to posterior interosseous nerve paralysis. J Bone Joint Surg Br 50:809–812, 1968.

82. Spinner M: Injuries to the Major Branches of Peripheral Nerves of the Forearm, 2nd ed. Philadelphia, WB Saunders, 1978.

83. Lister GD, Belsole RB, Kleinert HE: The radial tunnel syndrome. J Hand Surg Am 4:52–59, 1979.

84. Rosen I, Werner CO: Neurophysiological investigation of posterior interosseous nerve entrapment causing lateral elbow pain. Electroencephalogr Clin Neurophysiol 50:125–133, 1980.

85. Cravens G, Kline DG: Posterior interosseous nerve palsies. Neurosurgery 27:397–402, 1990.

86. Goldman S, Honet JC, Sobel R, Goldstein AS: Posterior interosseous nerve palsy in the absence of trauma. Arch Neurol 21:435–441, 1969.

87. Nielsen HO: Posterior interosseous nerve paralysis caused by fibrous band compression at the supinator muscle: A report of four cases. Acta Orthop Scand 47:304–307, 1976.

88. Mayer JH, Mayfield FH: Surgery of the posterior interosseous branch of the radial nerve: Analysis of 58 cases. Surg Gynecol Obstet 84:979–982, 1947.

89. Kline DG, Kim DH, Hudson AR. Atlas of Peripheral Nerve Surgery. Philadelphia, WB Saunders, 2001.

90. Massey EW, Riley TL, Pleet AB: Coexistent carpal tunnel syndrome and cervical radiculopathy (double crush syndrome). South Med J 74:957–959, 1981.

91. Dellon AL, Mackinnon SE: Radial sensory nerve entrapment. Arch Neurol 43:833–835, 1986.

92. Lanzetta M, Foucher G: Entrapment of the superficial branch of the radial nerve (Wartenberg's syndrome): A report of 52 cases. Int Orthop 17:342–345, 1993.

93. Gilliatt RW, Le Quesne PM, Logue V, Sumner AJ: Wasting of the hand associated with a cervical rib or band. J Neurol Neurosurg Psychiatry 33:615–624, 1970.

94. Roos DB: The place for scalenectomy and first-rib resection in thoracic outlet syndrome. Surgery 92:1077–1085, 1982.

95. Thomas GI, Jones TW, Stavney LS, Manhas DR: The middle scalene muscle and its contribution to the thoracic outlet syndrome. Am J Surg 145:589–592, 1983.

96. Banis JC Jr, Rich N, Whelan TJ Jr: Ischemia of the upper extremity due to noncardiac emboli. Am J Surg 134:131–139, 1977.

97. Scher LA, Veith FJ, Haimovici H, et al: Staging of arterial complications of cervical rib: Guidelines for surgical management. Surgery 95:644–649, 1984.

98. Swift TR, Nichols FT: The droopy shoulder syndrome. Neurology 34:212–215, 1984.

99. Filler AG, Howe FA, Hayes CE, et al: Magnetic resonance neurography. Lancet 341:659–661, 1993.

100. Relman AS: Responsibilities of authorship: Where does the buck stop? N Engl J Med 310:1048–1049, 1984.

101. Urschel HC Jr: Management of the thoracic-outlet syndrome. N Engl J Med 286:1140–1143, 1972.

102. Wilbourn AJ, Lederman RJ: Evidence for conduction delay in thoracic-outlet syndrome is challenged. N Engl J Med 310:1052–1053, 1984.

103. Daube JR: Nerve conduction studies in thoracic outlet syndrome. Neurology 25:347, 1975.

104. Glover JL, Worth RM, Bendick PJ, et al: Evoked responses in the diagnosis of thoracic outlet syndrome. Surgery 89:86–93, 1981.

105. Jerrett SA, Cuzzone LJ, Pasternak BM: Thoracic outlet syndrome. Electrophysiologic reappraisal. Arch Neurol 41:960–963, 1984.

106. Yiannikas C, Walsh JC: Somatosensory evoked responses in the diagnosis of thoracic outlet syndrome. J Neurol Neurosurg Psychiatry 46:234–240, 1983.

107. Sobey AV, Grewal RP, Hutchison KJ, Urschel JD: Investigation of nonspecific neurogenic thoracic outlet syndrome. J Cardiovasc Surg (Torino) 34:343–345, 1993.

108. Mayfield FH: Neural and vascular compression syndromes of the shoulder girdles and arms. Clin Neurosurg 15:384–393, 1968.

109. Mayfield FH: In Vinken PJ, Bruyn GW (eds): Handbook of Clinical Neurology. Amsterdam, North Holland Publishing, Amsterdam, 1970, pp 430–466.

110. Schlesinger EB: The thoracic outlet syndrome from a neurosurgical point of view. Clin Orthop 51:49–52, 1967.

111. Wilbourn AJ: Thoracic outlet syndromes: A plea for conservatism. Neurosurg Clin N Am 2:235–245, 1991.

112. Campbell JN, Naff NJ, Dellon AL: Thoracic outlet syndrome. Neurosurgical perspective. Neurosurg Clin N Am 2:227–233, 1991.

113. Leffert RD: Thoracic outlet syndromes. Hand Clin 8:285–297, 1992.

114. Luoma A, Nelems B: Thoracic outlet syndrome. Thoracic surgery perspective. Neurosurg Clin N Am 2:187–226, 1991.

115. Cherington M, Cherington C: Thoracic outlet syndrome: Reimbursement patterns and patient profiles. Neurology 42:943–945, 1992.

116. Hempel GK, Rusher AH Jr, Wheeler CG, et al: Supraclavicular resection of the first rib for thoracic outlet syndrome. Am J Surg 141:213–215, 1981.

117. Qvarfordt PG, Ehrenfeld WK, Stoney RJ: Supraclavicular radical scalenectomy and transaxillary first rib resection for the thoracic outlet syndrome: A combined approach. Am J Surg 148:111–116, 1984.

118. Sanders RJ, Monsour JW, Gerber WF, et al: Scalenectomy versus first rib resection for treatment of the thoracic outlet syndrome. Surgery 85:109–121, 1979.

119. Dellon AL: The results of supraclavicular brachial plexus neurolysis (without first rib resection) in management of posttraumatic "thoracic outlet syndrome." J Reconstr Microsurg 9:11–17, 1993.

120. Horowitz SH: Brachial plexus injuries with causalgia resulting from transaxillary rib resection. Arch Surg 120:1189–1191, 1985.

121. Melliere D, Becquemin JP, Etienne G, Le Cheviller B: Severe injuries resulting from operations for thoracic outlet syndrome: Can they be avoided? J Cardiovasc Surg (Torino) 32:599–603, 1991.

122. Clein LJ: Suprascapular entrapment neuropathy. J Neurosurg 43:337–342, 1975.

123. Hadley MN, Sonntag VK, Pittman HW: Suprascapular nerve entrapment: A summary of seven cases. J Neurosurg 64:843–848, 1986.

124. Rengachary SS, Neff JP, Singer PA, Brackett CE: Suprascapular entrapment neuropathy: A clinical, anatomical, and comparative study. Part 1. Clinical study. Neurosurgery 5:441–446, 1979.

125. Rengachary SS, Burr D, Lucas S, et al: Suprascapular entrapment neuropathy: A clinical, anatomical, and comparative study. Part 2. Anatomical study. Neurosurgery 5:447–451, 1979.

126. Rengachary SS, Burr D, Lucas S, Brackett CE: Suprascapular entrapment neuropathy: A clinical, anatomical, and comparative study. Part 3. Comparative study. Neurosurgery 5:452–455, 1979.

127. Aiello I, Serra G, Traina GC, Tugnoli V: Entrapment of the suprascapular nerve at the spinoglenoid notch. Ann Neurol 12:314–316, 1982.

128. Ganzhorn RW, Hocker JT, Horowitz M, Switzer HE: Suprascapular-nerve entrapment. J Bone Joint Surg Am 63:492–494, 1981.

129. Callahan JD, Scully TB, Shapiro SA, Worth RM: Suprascapular nerve entrapment: A series of 27 cases. J Neurosurg 74:893–896, 1991.

130. Donovan WH, Kraft GH: Rotator cuff tear versus suprascapular nerve injury: A problem in differential diagnosis. Arch Phys Med Rehabil 55:424–428, 1974.

131. Drez D Jr: Suprascapular neuropathy in the differential diagnosis of rotator cuff injuries. Am J Sports Med 4:43–45, 1976.

132. Rask MR: Suprascapular nerve entrapment: A report of two cases treated with suprascapular notch resection. Clin Orthop 123:73–75, 1977.

133. Shupeck M, Onofrio BM: An anterior approach for decompression of the suprascapular nerve. J Neurosurg 73:53–56, 1990.

134. Bassett FH 3rd, Nunley JA: Compression of the musculocutaneous nerve at the elbow. J Bone Joint Surg Am 64:1050–1052, 1982.

135. Aszmann OC, Kress KM, Dellon AL: Results of decompression of peripheral nerves in diabetics: A prospective, blinded study. Plast Reconstr Surg 106:816–822, 2000.

136. Dellon AL, Mackinnon SE, Seiler WA, et al: Susceptibility of the diabetic nerve to chronic compression. Ann Plast Surg 20:117–119, 1988.

137. Dellon AL: Treatment of symptomatic diabetic neuropathy by surgical decompression of multiple peripheral nerves. Plast Reconstr Surg 89:689–697, discussion 698–699, 1992.

138. Dellon AL, Dellon ES, Seiler WA, et al: Effect of tarsal tunnel decompression in the streptozotocin-induced diabetic rat. Microsurgery 15:265–268, 1994.

139. Lorei MP, Hershman EB: Peripheral nerve injuries in athletes: Treatment and prevention. Sports Med 16:130–147, 1993.

140. McCrory P, Bell S, Bradshaw C: Nerve entrapments of the lower leg, ankle and foot in sport. Sports Med 32:371–391, 2002.

141. Schon LC: Nerve entrapment, neuropathy, and nerve dysfunction in athletes. Orthop Clin North Am 25:47–59, 1994.

142. Touliopolous S, Hershman EB: Lower leg pain: Diagnosis and treatment of compartment syndromes and other pain syndromes of the leg. Sports Med 27:193–204, 1999.

143. O'Brien MD: Genitofemoral neuropathy. Br Med J 1:1052, 1979.

144. Ecker AD, Woltman HW: Meralgia paraesthetica. JAMA 110:1650–1652, 1938.

145. Keegan JJ, Holyoke EA: Meralgia paresthetica. J Neurosurg 19:341–345, 1962.

146. Stookey B: Meralgia paraesthetica. JAMA 90:1705–1707, 1928.

147. Eubanks S, Newman L 3rd, Goehring L, et al: Meralgia paresthetica: A complication of laparoscopic herniorrhaphy. Surg Laparosc Endosc 3:381–385, 1993.

148. Lysens R, Vandendriessche G, Van Mol Y, Rosselle N: The sensory conduction velocity in the cutaneous femoris lateralis nerve in normal adult subjects and in patients with complaints suggesting meralgia paresthetica. Electromyogr Clin Neurophysiol 21:505–510, 1981.

149. Sarala PK, Nishihara T, Oh SJ: Meralgia paresthetica: Electrophysiologic study. Arch Phys Med Rehabil 60:30–31, 1979.

150. Williams PH, Trzil KP: Management of meralgia paresthetica. J Neurosurg 74:76–80, 1991.

151. Pecina M: Contribution to the etiological explanation of the piriformis syndrome. Acta Anat 105:181–187, 1979.

152. Rask MR: Superior gluteal nerve entrapment syndrome. Muscle Nerve 3:304–307, 1980.

153. Gelmers HJ: Entrapment of the sciatic nerve. Acta Neurochir 33:103–106, 1976.

154. Banerjee T, Hall CD: Sciatic entrapment neuropathy: Case report. J Neurosurg 45:216–217, 1976.

155. Venna N, Bielawski M, Spatz EM: Sciatic nerve entrapment in a child: Case report. J Neurosurg 75:652–654, 1991.

156. Luerssen TG, Campbell RL, Defalque RJ, Worth RM: Spontaneous saphenous neuralgia. Neurosurgery 13:238–241, 1983.

157. Mozes M, Ouaknine G, Nathan H: Saphenous nerve entrapment simulating vascular disorder. Surgery 77:299–303, 1975.

158. Pringle RM, Protheroe K, Mukherjee SK: Entrapment neuropathy of the sural nerve. J Bone Joint Surg Br 56:465–468, 1974.

159. Singh N, Behse F, Buchthal F: Electrophysical study of peroneal palsy. J Neurol Neurosurg Psychiatry 37:1202–1213, 1974.

160. Nagler SH, Rangell L: Peroneal palsy caused by crossing the legs. JAMA 133:755–761, 1947.

161. Woltman HL: Crossing the legs as a factor in the production of peroneal palsy. JAMA 93:670–672, 1929.

162. Muckart RD: Compression of the common peroneal nerve by intramuscular ganglion from the superior tibio-fibular joint. J Bone Joint Surg Br 58:241–244, 1976.

163. Kopell HP, Thompson WA: Peripheral Entrapment Neuropathies. Baltimore, Williams & Wilkins, 1976.

164. Borges LF, Hallett M, Selkoe DJ, Welch K: The anterior tarsal tunnel syndrome: Report of two cases. J Neurosurg 54:89–92, 1981.

165. Banerjee T, Koons DD: Superficial peroneal nerve entrapment: Report of two cases. J Neurosurg 55:991–992, 1981.

166. Kernohan J, Levack B, Wilson JN: Entrapment of the superficial peroneal nerve: Three case reports. J Bone Joint Surg Br 67:60–61, 1985.

167. Edwards WG, Lincoln CR, Bassett FH 3rd, Goldner JL: The tarsal tunnel syndrome: Diagnosis and treatment. JAMA 207:716–720, 1969.

168. Jackson DL, Haglund BL: Tarsal tunnel syndrome in runners. Sports Med 13:146–149, 1992.

169. Linscheid RL, Burton RC, Fredericks EJ: Tarsal-tunnel syndrome. South Med J 63:1313–1323, 1970.

170. Mann RA: Tarsal tunnel syndrome. Orthop Clin North Am 5:109–115, 1974.

171. Radin EL: Tarsal tunnel syndrome. Clin Orthop 181:167–170, 1983.

172. Rask MR: Medial plantar neurapraxia (jogger's foot): Report of 3 cases. Clin Orthop 134:193–195, 1978.

173. Schon LC, Baxter DE: Neuropathies of the foot and ankle in athletes. Clin Sports Med 9:489–509, 1990.

174. Oh SJ, Sarala PK, Kuba T, Elmore RS: Tarsal tunnel syndrome: Electrophysiological study. Ann Neurol 5:327–330, 1979.

175. Oh SJ, Kim HS, Ahmad BK: The near-nerve sensory nerve conduction in tarsal tunnel syndrome. J Neurol Neurosurg Psychiatry 48:999–1003, 1985.

176. Kerr R, Frey C: MR imaging in tarsal tunnel syndrome. J Comput Assist Tomogr 15:280–286, 1991.

177. Pfeiffer WH, Cracchiolo A 3rd: Clinical results after tarsal tunnel decompression. J Bone Joint Surg Am 76:1222–1230, 1994.

178. Kite JH: Morton's toe neuroma. South Med J 59:21–25, 1966.

179. Greenfield J, Rea J Jr, Ilfeld FW: Morton's interdigital neuroma: Indications for treatment by local injections versus surgery. Clin Orthop 185:142–144, 1984.

Management of Peripheral Nerve Tumors

DAVID G. KLINE ■ ALAN R. HUDSON ■ ROBERT TIEL ■ AB GUHA

The nature and management of tumors originating in or involving nerve differ from those for nerve injuries and entrapments. These differences are best illustrated by the largest category of benign nerve tumors, the neural sheath tumors such as schwannomas and neurofibromas. Patients with these tumors usually present with pain and paresthesias or a mass, or both, but with minimal or no neurologic deficit, unlike the loss seen with injured or severely entrapped nerves. Nonetheless, such tumors are structurally intrinsic to nerves and can distort them greatly. As a result, tumor removal or even biopsy has the risk of producing serious neurologic deficits similar to those seen with traumatic injuries and severe entrapments on presentation. Extirpation of the tumor with the least risk to the nervous system is the usual initial goal for most nerve tumors, rather than correction of the deficit. Thus, the special challenge for the nerve tumor surgeon is to perform the removal as completely as possible to relieve pain, paresthesias, and other mass effects as well as to minimize recurrence, yet to do it in a fashion producing minimal neurologic deficit. In addition, the correct pathologic designations of tumorous lesions play an even greater role in their management than does histologic study for most entrapments and traumatic lesions. A number of texts have provided a good deal of information about peripheral nerve tumors but have not always emphasized the steps in their removal.[1–17]

INITIAL DIAGNOSIS

A nerve tumor is often suspected because of a discernible or palpable mass, or both, in an extremity. This is especially so if the mass is associated with pain of a radicular nature or with paresthesias, or both. Deficit may or may not be present but often is not except in malignancies or in some surgically biopsied benign lesions. Manipulation or tapping on the mass usually produces paresthesias, tingling, and "electric shocks" in the distribution of the nerve, and this maneuver is usually uncomfortable for the patient. In addition, the tumor associated with a nerve, especially if benign,

can frequently be displaced side to side but not in a longitudinal or up-and-down fashion. This is in contrast to malignancy involving a nerve, in which manipulation or tapping the mass gives severe pain and paresthesias, but the mass is relatively fixed and nonmobile as well as firm.

In some cases, tumor involving nerve becomes evident because of radiologic studies used to work up suspected differential diagnoses such as spinal disk disease and degenerative disease involving the spine, thoracic outlet syndrome, or arthritic disease involving joints. Plain radiographs can sometimes show apical pulmonary lesions with potential plexus involvement or neural foramen enlargement or bony erosion associated with paraspinal nerve tumors. Computed tomography and magnetic resonance imaging (MRI) may be useful in delineating the full extent of a tumor or associated lesions such as those seen with von Recklinghausen's disease (VRD) (Fig. 258–1).[18–21] Such studies are especially important with tumors close to or involving the spine.[22] In some special cases, myelography, angiography, or even ultrasonography may be useful.[23, 24] To date though, none of these studies is capable of differentiating a schwannoma from a neurofibroma or even diagnosing a neurogenic sarcoma with certainty.[25–27] Even when malignant transformation of a neural sheath tumor is suspected because of relatively rapid enlargement, radiologic criteria favoring malignancy are not definite enough, at least at this time. Such a diagnosis instead requires neuropathologic confirmation.

When a nerve tumor is suspected, evidence of other nerve tumors or the lesions associated with VRD should be sought. However, if there are no such findings, the tumor may still be of neural sheath origin because the majority of such tumors that are symptomatic are solitary and unassociated with more widespread disease such as neurofibromatosis.

When considering nerve tumors, it is convenient to classify them as either benign or malignant. The benign category can be divided into those designated as neural sheath in origin, such as schwannomas and neurofibromas, and those that are not, such as desmoids,

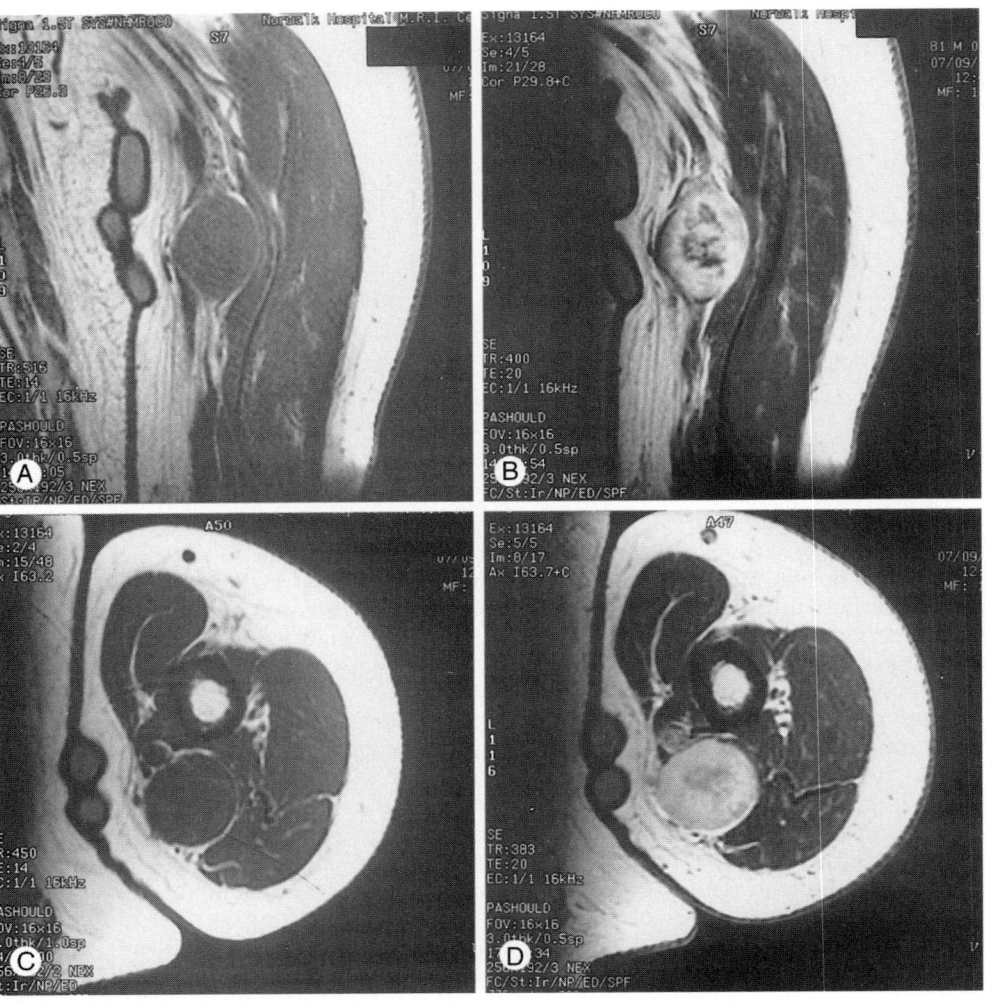

FIGURE 258–1. *A,* Sagittal magnetic resonance imaging (MRI) scan of a schwannoma at the axillary level involving the proximal ulnar nerve. Nerve entering and leaving the region of tumor and the shadows of vessels can be seen. *B,* MRI scan of same lesion after contrast with gadopentetate dimeglumine (Magnevist). *C,* Transverse section without contrast of proximal upper arm ulnar schwannoma. The tumor is isodense to adjacent muscles. *D,* Transverse section of same tumor after contrast injection.

ganglions and epidermoids, cysts, lipomas, and so on. The malignancies can, in turn, be divided into the neurogenic sarcomas and other tumors felt to be of neural origin and other non-neural sarcomas, such as fibrosarcomas and synovial sarcomas or carcinomas, which can involve nerve by either direct extension from the primary site or metastases.

BENIGN NEURAL SHEATH TUMORS

Schwannomas

Schwannomas are the most frequent and largest category of nerve tumors.[28] Their origin is from a cell with a basement membrane resembling a Schwann cell, so even though schwannoma is categorized as a neural sheath tumor, its origin is most likely from an intraneural supporting or glial cell.[29–31] The schwannoma tends to have both Antoni A and Antoni B tissue. Antoni A tissue is relatively cellular and compact with spindle-shaped cells that can form palisades or what is termed *Verocay bodies*.[32] Antoni B tissue is a loose arrangement of less compact spindle cells in a clear mucinous-like matrix. By comparison, the spindle-shaped cells of a

neurofibroma are usually separated by a more myxomatous stroma that tends to look somewhat like Antoni B tissue. S-100 stains can be positive in both schwannomas and neurofibromas but are more often positive and more intensely positive in the former. Alcian blue, which preferentially stains myxomatous tissue, will be more positive in neurofibromas than in schwannomas, as will reticulum stains such as provided by the Gridley technique.[33] Epithelial membrane antigen (EMA) studies are positive for perineurial cells but negative for Schwann cells and endoneurial fibroblasts.[34] In addition, neurofibromas are more likely than schwannomas to have some axons apparent on a Bodian or other silver stain. Research to identify factors specific to neural sheath tumors continues to hold interest for those studying more generalized mechanisms of tumor growth.[35–37]

Loss of function at the time of presentation of a schwannoma is rare unless removal or surgical biopsy of the tumor has been attempted previously or the tumor is massive. Instead, the lesion usually presents as a painless mass until it is manipulated or tapped, at which time paresthesias in the distribution of its origin may be evident. This tumor tends to spread apart or "basket" the fascicles and displace them to its periphery. Other schwannomas are more eccentrically or laterally located and tend to protrude or even "extrude" from a portion of the nerve's circumference. The fascicles may be elongated greatly by large lesions. This is, however, done so slowly that function usually is not lost but, of course, may occur with surgical intervention. There is usually one fascicle entering and leaving each pole of the tumor.[25] Schwannomas also tend to have a fairly well developed capsule that contains the majority of the fascicles.

REMOVAL OF SCHWANNOMAS

1. Surgical exposure of nerve and related structures well proximal and distal to the mass is mandatory (Fig. 258–2).
2. Other nerves or plexal elements are then dissected away, as are major vessels.
3. Nerve leading to and from the lesion is identified and encircled, usually with a narrow Penrose drain for gentle retraction.
4. An area on the circumference of the capsule with few or no fascicles is selected and then opened in a longitudinal fashion.
5. The capsule and accompanying "basketed" fascicles are gently dissected away and moved to one side or the other to expose the tumor itself (Fig. 258–3).
6. Some interfascicular dissection is often necessary at both poles of the tumor to identify the entering and leaving fascicles. Intraoperative stimulation and recording across entering and leaving fascicles at each pole of the tumor usually show the fascicles to be nonfunctional, and this permits their section. The tumor can usually be removed as a single mass, especially if after section of a nonfunctional entering or leaving fascicle it is lifted at one pole and dissected away from underlying and laterally reflected but retained fascicles. In this fashion, tumor is gradually elevated or lifted up and away from the residual nerve itself. The opposite pole's nonfunctional fascicle is then sectioned to complete the removal (Fig. 258–4).

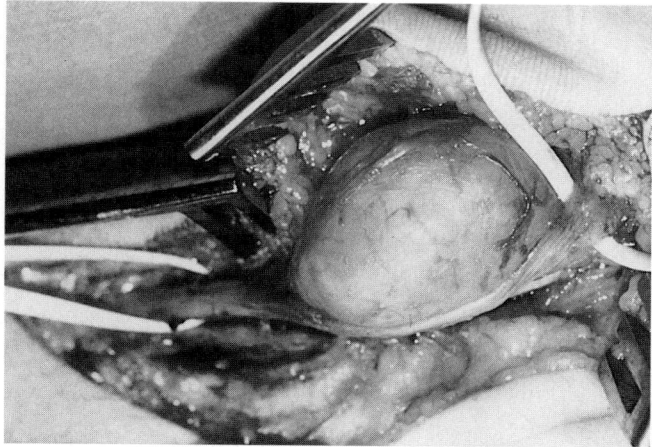

FIGURE 258–3. Typical gross appearance of a moderately large schwannoma after most of the fascicular structure has been dissected away from its upper surface.

7. The capsule can then be sharply trimmed or "sculpted" away from the remaining fascicles.
8. For large tumors, the capsule is opened over the length of the nerve. The tumor contents are then enucleated piecemeal, either by sharp resection or by use of the Cavitron ultrasonic aspirator (CUSA) and/or the bipolar coagulator, and suction.
9. As a large tumor is debulked, the capsule can gradually be pulled toward the center of the tumor to reduce the tension on "basketed" and badly stretched fascicles so that they can be dissected away and preserved as much as possible.

Massive schwannomas can be extremely difficult to remove totally even if significant functional loss is accepted.[25, 38] This is especially the case when brachial or pelvic plexus is involved by tumor. After surgery on such large lesions, recurrence or, probably more correctly, progression, can occur. Recurrence or progres-

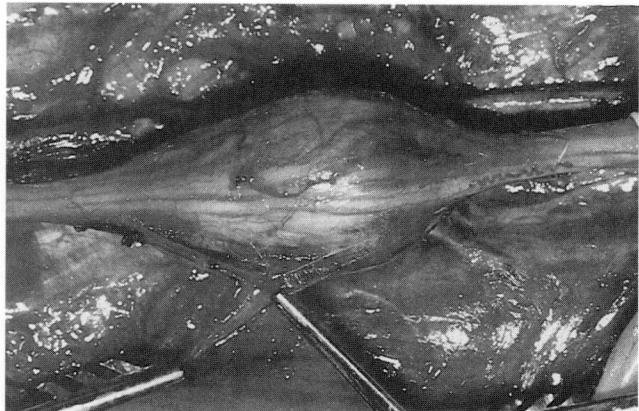

FIGURE 258–2. Typical gross appearance of a neural sheath tumor before fascicular dissection.

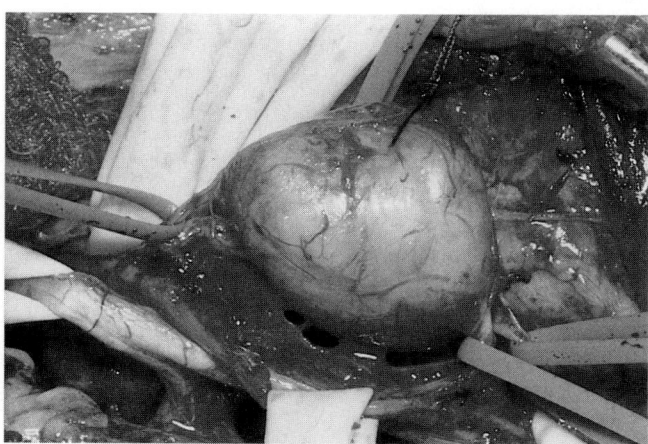

FIGURE 258–4. Most of the fascicles have been dissected away from this schwannoma and are located at the bottom of the field. Entering and leaving fascicles are marked by rubber loops. (From Kline D, Hudson A: Nerve Injuries. Philadelphia, WB Saunders, 1995.)

sion is less likely after resection of moderate-sized or even large lesions because they can usually be removed as a single mass or lump.

Neurofibromas

Although the cell of origin for neurofibromas has some similarities to a Schwann cell, such as having a basement membrane, it is probably more primitive. Such a cell might have origin from a stem cell such as a perineurial fibrocyte.[39, 40] There is more of a tendency for neurofibromas to arise from the motor portion of the nerve and schwannomas from its sensory portion. Although some fascicles are displaced to the periphery of the tumor, they are more likely to be clustered at the poles and more intrinsically involved in the peripheral portion of the tumor than in schwannomas. Compared with schwannomas, more than one fascicle usually enters and leaves the tumor at its poles.[25] Although it is not as well defined as in schwannomas, some capsule is usually present. Even though neurofibromas can be associated with café-au-lait spots, freckling, skin tags, and the other features of neurofibromatosis or VRD, the majority of peripheral nerve neurofibromas requiring surgery are solitary lesions unassociated with other neurofibromas or other signs of VRD.[25, 41] Solitary neurofibromas are likely to be fusiform rather than plexiform, are more likely to occur in females than in males and, as seen in our series, are more likely to be on the right side of the body than on the left (Fig. 258–5). Neurofibromas seen in patients with VRD have a more equal distribution between the sexes, no particular laterality, and are more likely, but not always, plexiform. Multiple tumors can be contiguous to each other and can be large to massive (Fig. 258–6). In addition, the VRD neurofibroma can be associated with other neurofibromas in other loci as well as a host of unique assorted findings.[32, 42, 43]

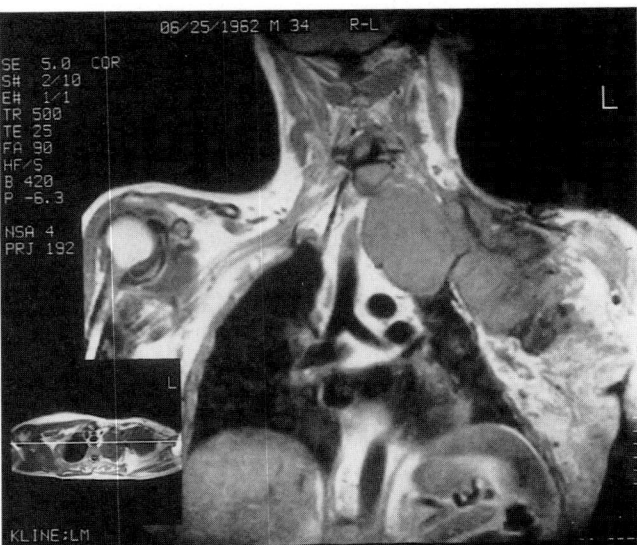

FIGURE 258–6. MRI scan of multiloculated neural sheath tumor, which is massive involving *(left)* brachial plexus.

REMOVAL OF NEUROFIBROMAS

1. The early steps involve wide exposure, isolation of the tumor poles, and dissection of adjacent structures as for schwannomas (Fig. 258–7).

2. Once again, fascicles on the surface need to be dissected away. Sometimes the dissection can proceed between what is usually a fine capsule and the surface fascicles, although in larger tumors any capsule is usually opened and a subcapsular dissection of tumor itself proceeds. Sometimes with large neurofibromas, tumor contents need to be debulked and removed piecemeal, but usually it is best to remove the tumor as a single mass.

3. It is most important to dissect the fascicles in the nerve just before it enters and leaves the mass at the

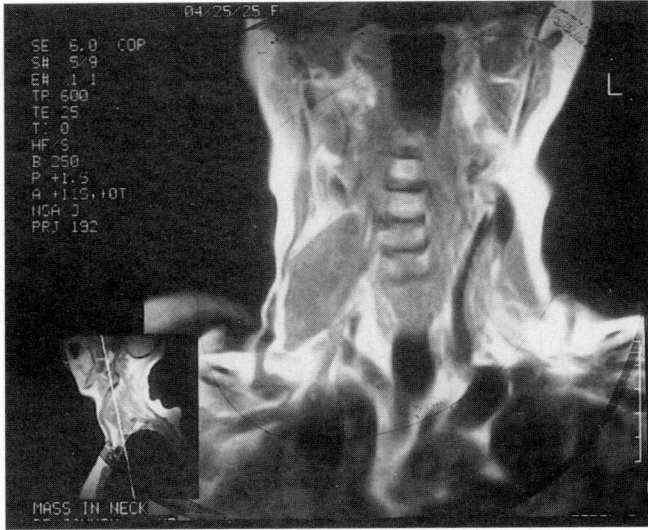

FIGURE 258–5. Neurofibroma involving *(right)* brachial plexus as viewed by MRI. Tumor arose from C5 but also had to be dissected away from C6 and C7 spinal nerves after mobilization of the carotid sheath and its contents.

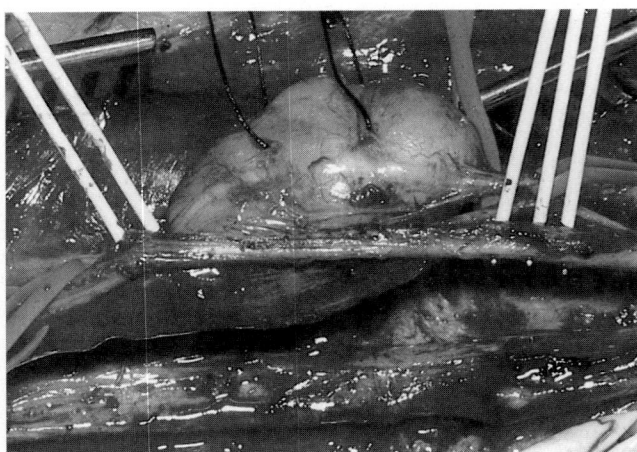

FIGURE 258–7. Stimulating *(right)* and recording *(left)* electrodes placed on the portion of the nerve cleared of tumor. (From Donner T, Voorhies R, Kline D: Neural sheath tumors of major nerves. J Neurosurg 81:362–373, 1994.)

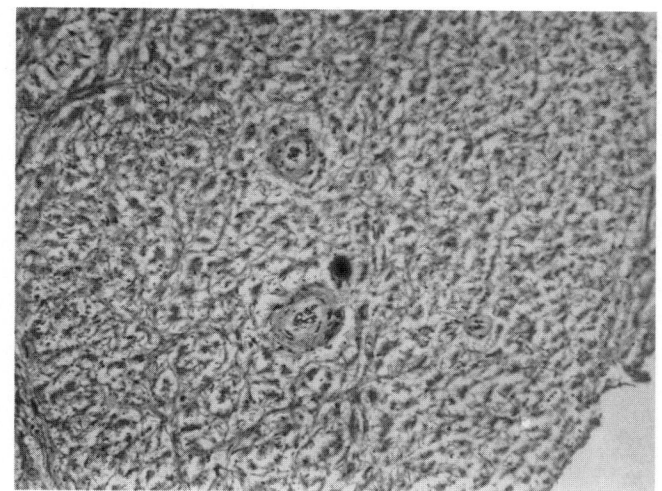

FIGURE 258–8. Bodian stain (×200) of exiting fascicle that had no nerve action potential activity. Most axons are fine or degenerated or failed to develop. Masson staining showed no myelinated axons. (From Donner T, Voorhies R, Kline D: Neural sheath tumors of major nerves. J Neurosurg 81:362–373, 1994.)

poles of the tumor so that entering and leaving fascicles can be carefully identified and tested. This usually means an interfascicular dissection at both the proximal and distal poles of the tumor.

4. If nerve action potential (NAP) traces are flat, fascicles going into and out of tumor can be sectioned and the tumor mass worked away from the more peripherally located fascicles. Such fascicles on histologic examination have poor structure (Fig. 258–8).

5. If NAPs are positive on entering and leaving fascicles (usually not the case with fusiform neurofibromas but often the case with plexiform lesions), these fascicles must be traced into and out of the tumor and if possible spared.

6. Fascicular defects may have to be replaced by grafts, but this can be difficult because of the length of the defects or tumorous involvement at more proximal or distal nerve levels, or both, especially in patients with VRD. In addition, donor nerves may be involved by neurofibromas in the patient with VRD, further complicating repair.

VRD-associated neurofibromas involving major nerves and requiring surgery are approached surgically in the same manner as are the solitary neurofibromas. Of course, the incidence of plexiform lesions is greater.[41] Plexiform lesions extend over a length of nerve and involve a different quadrant or cross section of nerve at different levels. This makes surgical removal difficult, although decompression is sometimes possible. One attempts to spare as much fascicular structure as possible. This type of lesion is quite characteristic in patients with regionalized VRD (Riccardi type V VRD). In these cases, multiple tumors are intrinsic to one or more nerves in a given region involving a length of the extremity as well as nerves in that area.[44–46] There are no tumors elsewhere in the body, and the cutaneous stigmata of VRD are usually re-

stricted to the area of the limb with the regionalized changes. Removal of plexiform lesions without production of deficit is most difficult. The surgeon then has to approach these extensive lesions as with other neurofibromas, yet work out as much tumor as possible. Sometimes, subtotal decompression or more total removal with resultant deficit is necessary because of severe pain or massive tumor size.

The surgical approach depends on the nerve or nerves involved, the level involved, the size of the lesion as well as involvement of vessels of other structures. Although most brachial plexus neural sheath tumors were approached by an anterior exposure at Louisiana State University Medical Center (LSUMC), 15 were operated on by a posterior subscapular approach.[47]

Surgical Results with Benign "Neural Sheath" Tumors

At the time of Donner and colleagues' publication in 1994, the LSUMC service had operated on 288 benign neural sheath tumors involving major nerves.[48] One hundred twenty-one involved the brachial plexus, 87 involved other upper extremity nerves, and 80 originated in lower extremity nerves, including 16 in the pelvic plexus (Fig. 258–9). Two hundred twenty-three of these 288 patients were available for follow-up.

Eighty-nine percent of 76 schwannomas were excised without residual significant loss of function. Fifteen patients did have mild (grade 4) functional loss, and eight more had serious loss (grade 3 or less). However, 31 of the schwannoma patients presented to us with weakness preoperatively, usually because of surgical biopsy or less frequently (3 cases) previous attempted removal of a huge lesion, or both. Of these 31 patients, 17 (55%) improved postoperatively, 10 (32%) were unchanged,

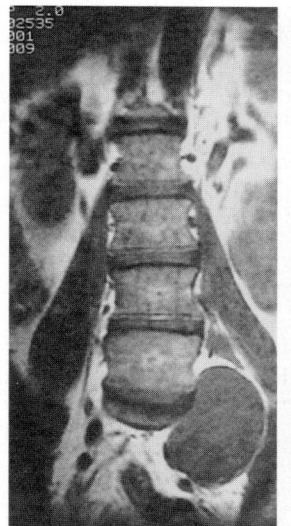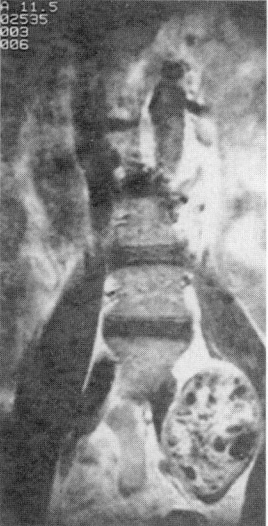

FIGURE 258–9. *Left,* Lumbosacral (pelvic) neurofibroma. This particular lesion required a transperitoneal exposure. (From Donner T, Voorhies R, Kline D: Neural sheath tumors of major nerves. J Neurosurg 81:362–373, 1994.)

TABLE 258-1 ■ **Surgical Outcomes* of Benign Neural Sheath Tumors of Major Nerves (n = 223)**

POSTOPERATIVE GRADES	PREOPERATIVE GRADES						
	5	4	3	2	1	0	TOTALS
5	83	33	11	1	0	0	128
4	15	15	17	2	2	0	51
3	0	6	9	2	0	1	18
2	0	2	4	5	3	1	15
1	0	0	1	2	4	0	7
0	0	0	0	0	1	3	4
Totals	98	56	42	12	10	5	223

*Preoperative versus postoperative motor grades for resected lesions. Overall 73 patients improved, 31 worsened, and 119 had unchanged motor function as a result of operation. Included were 76 schwannomas, 99 solitary neurofibromas, and 48 neurofibromas associated with von Recklinghausen's disease (VRD).

and 4 (13%) worsened. Among the 45 who had intact strength preoperatively, 41 (91%) maintained this, whereas 4 (9%) had a mild decrease to a grade 4 level.

Eighty percent of 99 solitary neurofibromas were excised without either loss of function or further loss of function. This was despite the fact that almost all the neurofibromas with substantial follow-up had had gross total excision. Six (5%) of these patients did require a graft repair. Fifty-eight neurofibroma patients presented with a motor deficit. Of these, 38 (60%) had improvement in motor function postoperatively, whereas 14 (24%) had no change, and 6 (10%) had some further decrease in function noted after operation. Of the 41 patients having normal function at presentation, 32 (78%) maintained this function, whereas 9 (22%) had postoperative weakness of some degree. Fifty-three of the 99 patients had had previous operations, including 11 prior attempts at removal. *Especially important was the fact that 7 of the 9 patients with new postoperative paresis and 12 of the 15 patients whose paresis worsened, and each of the 4 patients with new pain had had previous operations.*

Of the 48 patients with neurofibroma associated with VRD, 36 presented with some degree of weakness. Eighteen (50%) improved after tumor resection, 12 (33%) had no change, and 6 (17%) had increased deficit postoperatively. In the group with normal strength preoperatively (12 patients), only 2 had some degree of weakness postoperatively. Conversely, 16 of the 74 tumors operated on in this category could not be com-

pletely removed. When this was the case, usually small fragments had to be left attached to fascicles. There were two giant VRD-associated neurofibromas, one in the brachial plexus and one in the pelvic plexus, in which larger amounts of tumor had to be left behind.

Table 258-1 summarizes the preoperative and postoperative motor grades for all three types of benign neural sheath tumors. Overall, 73 patients improved, 31 worsened, and 119 had unchanged motor function as a result of operation.

Table 258-2 shows the outcomes referable to pain. Many of the patients who had worse or new pain had undergone previous biopsy or attempted removal of the tumor. A single definitive procedure, if possible, is best for benign neural sheath lesions because it preserves optimal function and also decreases the incidence of pain.

BENIGN NON–NEURAL SHEATH TUMORS

The casual observer or reader may feel that neural sheath tumors are so frequent that little attention needs to be paid to other more sporadic tumors involving nerve.[49] Nothing could be further from the truth because other tumors can and do present, and they have their own specific set of management challenges.[25, 50, 51] Table 258-3 lists benign tumors that are not schwannomas or neurofibromas but that either originate in nerve or are closely applied to nerve or plexus elements and that we have had operative experience with.

Desmoids, Myositis Ossificans, and Osteochondromas

Desmoids are felt to arise from muscle and are made up of a fibrous and infiltrative mesenchymal tissue. Although more common in the abdominal wall, they can occur in the neck, shoulder, or limbs.[52] They encase nerves as well as vessels and can be adherent to them or even infiltrate them (Fig. 258-10). As a result, they are extremely difficult to extricate. A careful and often tedious dissection of tumor away from neural elements is necessary but not always achievable without major deficit or other complications. Recurrence is common. For this reason and because desmoids *sometime* respond, irradiation has been used by some with limited success.

TABLE 258-2 ■ **Resolution of Pain after Operation on Benign Nerve Sheath Tumors**

	RESOLVED (%)	IMPROVED (%)	UNCHANGED (%)	WORSE PAIN (%)	NEW PAIN (%)
Schwannoma	15/20 (75)	2/20 (10)	1/20 (5)	2/20 (10)	4/52 (8)
Solitary neurofibroma	29/46 (63)	11/46 (25)	3/46 (6)	3/46 (6)	7/53 (13)
von Recklinghausen's neurofibroma	10/23 (43)	7/23 (31)	4/23 (17)	2/23 (9)	4/25 (16)

This table presents the outcome of patients with and without radicular pain syndromes preoperatively.
The first four columns represent results in patients who presented with pain syndromes.
The last column represents the number and percentage of patients who had no pain preoperatively but developed pain after surgery.

TABLE 258-3 ■ **Benign Non–Neural Sheath Tumor Affecting Nerve (Operated Cases at LSUMC)**

Desmoids (10)	*Myositis ossificans (4)*	*Osteochondromas (4)*	*Ganglion cysts (27)*
Brachial plexus, 6	Brachial plexus, 2	Radial, 1	Peroneal, 14
Median, 1	Radial, 1	Peroneal, 2	Suprascapular, 4
Radial, 1	Median, 1	Brachial plexus, 1	Median, 3
Peroneal, 1			Ulnar, 1
Sciatic, 1			Radial-PIN, 1
			Femoral, 1
(May behave in a malignant fashion although benign)			Sciatic, 1
			Post-tibial, 1
Cystic hygromas (2)	*Myoblastomas (2)*	*Lymphangiomas (2)*	Obturator, 1
Accessory, 2	Brachial plexus, 2	Median-ulnar, 1	*Lipomas (7)*
		Brachial plexus, 1	Median, 2
			PIN-radial, 1
			Ulnar, 1
			Sciatic, 1
Lipofibrohamartomas (4)			Brachial plexus, 2
Median, 4	*Ganglioneuromas (2)*	*Glomus tumors (2)*	*Epidermoid cysts (1)*
	Brachial plexus, 2	Peroneal branches, 1	Sciatic, 1
		Digital, 1	
Hemangiomas (3)	*Venous angiomas (4)*	*Hemangioblastomas (1)*	*Localized hypertrophic neuropathy (16)*
Ulnar, 2	Median, 1	Median, 1	Brachial plexus, 4
Peroneal, 1	Tibial, 1		Median, 3
	Femoral, 1		Ulnar, 2
	Sciatic, 1		Radial, 2
			Sciatic complex, 5

LSUMC, Louisiana State University Medical Center; PIN, Posterior interosseous nerve.

Myositis ossificans is a poorly defined disorder that may be related to previous, usually extensive soft tissue trauma or surgery or disorders such as chronic renal failure. Masses are firm to hard, calcified and, like desmoids, tend to incorporate and be adherent to neural elements, vessels, and sometimes tendons. It is necessary to develop a wide up-and-down exposure and to carefully dissect the tumorous mass away from neural and major vascular structures (Fig. 258–11). Complete removal may not be possible and is usually not indicated.

Osteochondromas that arise from bone can enlarge enough to compress or even incorporate nerve. In our series, this included one patient with bilateral peroneal

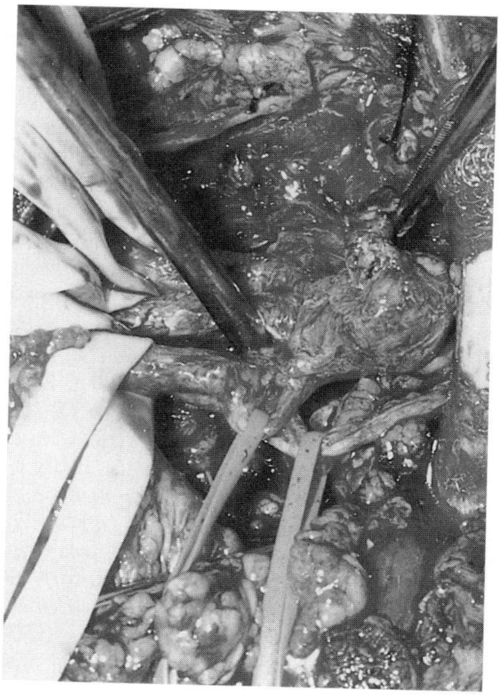

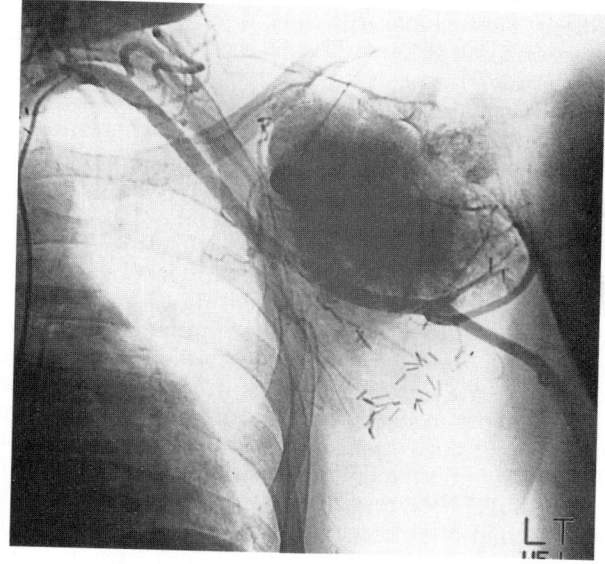

FIGURE 258–10. Desmoid tumor involving supraclavicular divisions. Supraclavicular nerve is encircled by a rubber loop. Clavicle has been pulled inferiorly by encircling it with strung-out 4 × 4 sponges.

FIGURE 258–11. Angiogram of large infraclavicular mass of myositis ossificans in a patient with chronic renal failure. This partially calcified mass encircled a portion of the axillary artery and the cords of the plexus. Clips from previous partial resection are seen below the mass.

involvement due to origin from both fibulas. Another lesion arising from humerus involved radial nerve, whereas in another patient the plexus was involved by a large osteochondroma arising from a cervical transverse process.

Ganglion Cysts

It is possible to separate ganglion cysts into two categories: (1) those that are extraneural but compressive to nerve or nerve branches and (2) those that are intraneural with absence of or a variable amount of extraneural cyst and with or without a connection to a joint.[53] Usually, ganglions arise and extend from a portion of a joint that does not involve nerve such as on the dorsum or side of the wrist or a non-neural portion of the knee, shoulder, or hip joint. Conversely, origin from the same joint at a different locus or projecting in a different direction can compress the thenar branch of the median, deep, or superficial branch of the ulnar nerve, the posterior interosseous nerve, the peroneal or tibial nerve, the suprascapular nerve, or even the sciatic or femoral nerve. Treatment for symptomatic lesions includes dissection of the involved nerve or elements away from the cyst, surgical isolation of the cyst, and ligation of its neck as close to the joint of origin as possible. Some of these lesions are quite aggressive, can reduce or remove function, are difficult to remove, and have a definite tendency to recur.

Ganglions that are intraneural include the fairly frequent peroneal ganglion and the surprisingly frequent suprascapular ganglion cyst. Involvement of either nerve can be due to either an intraneural or an extraneural cyst.[25, 54] It is presumed that even when a connection with a joint is not demonstrated operatively that at one time such a connection existed and then became closed. Computed tomographic and MRI studies, although excellent at demonstrating these cysts and their extent have difficulty demonstrating such a connection with a joint. This is especially so with the suprascapular nerve cysts in which the joint of origin is often unclear, even operatively. The intraneural cysts contain a mucinous material identical to that in a cyst at an extraneural locus. The cyst walls are made up of synovial cells similar to those in living joints. Removal without increasing or making complete any preexisting deficit is difficult but sometimes possible with the smaller, less extensive lesions. An internal neurolysis is necessary with cleaning or clearing of each fascicle of cyst wall so that recurrence is minimized. Any connection with the nearby joint should be sought and obliterated. In a published series of 27 cases, including 14 involving peroneal nerve, complete removal was possible in all but 1 case.[55] If the patient presented with mild deficit, good recovery was obtained in 83% of patients, but if the presentation was with severe deficit, only 50% had a good recovery after cyst excision with or without graft repair. Several large peroneal to sciatic cysts extended up the thigh to buttock level, and only a decompressive internal neurolysis could be performed for those cysts. One lesion at the knee level with extraneural extension has recurred twice, whereas

one cyst involving tibial nerve at the ankle level has recurred once. The knee lesion required an arthroscopic approach to the joint to attempt to obliterate the origin and thus minimize recurrence.

Even epidermoid cysts can involve nerve, and because of their somewhat inflammatory nature, nerve can be incorporated or adherent, or both. A careful dissection is necessary when these lesions are in loci close to major neural elements. The one case we had experience with involved sciatic nerve in the region of the sciatic notch.

Myoblastoma (Granular Cell Tumor) and Lymphangioma

Although of differing origin and histology, myoblastoma and lymphangioma behave toward nerve in a similar fashion. These lesions, like desmoids, incorporate nerve, especially plexus elements, but can sometimes be removed much more readily from them. Nonetheless, even though the myoblastomas are made up of plump cells having acidophilic granules and are compactly arranged and tend to layer on top of the nerve, the tumor sometimes takes on an invasive nature. Thus, one plexus lesion could be resected with little deficit, whereas the other could not, although fortunately in one sense the presentation was one of not only severe pain but also partial deficit, and resection at least relieved the former. Other, more common sites for myoblastomas include breast, peritoneum, tongue, bronchi, and gastrointestinal tract.

Lymphangiomas behave in a manner somewhat similar to that of myoblastomas in that they tend to spread as a sheet of tumor enveloping structures such as nerves and vessels rather than forming a fusiform or cylindrically shaped mass lesion within nerve. In our series, one lymphangioma involved proximal median and ulnar nerves in the upper arm, whereas the other involved the lower spinal nerves of a plexus and was removed by a posterior subscapular approach.

Lipomas and Lipofibrohamartomas

Lipoma is a common mass but does not usually compress or involve nerve. However, these benign lesions, although soft in nature, can grow in loci where, because of the anatomic confines of the area, nerves can be compressed by them. Examples of the latter have been seen by us in the carpal tunnel–involving median, near the olecranon notch involving the ulnar nerve, and in the forearm involving the PIN branch of the radial nerve. In the lower extremity, a lipoma near the fibular head compressed the peroneal nerve. These are anatomic areas where the tolerance or space available for nerve is less than at other sites. Removal of the lesions by definition included unroofing or opening up the snug region as well. Less frequently, a lipoma can be adherent to nerve or, on rarer occasions, appear to arise from it or even be intraneural.[56] We have seen two examples of the latter: one involving the sciatic nerve at the buttock level and one a plexus element at a supraclavicular level (Fig. 258–12). In these cases,

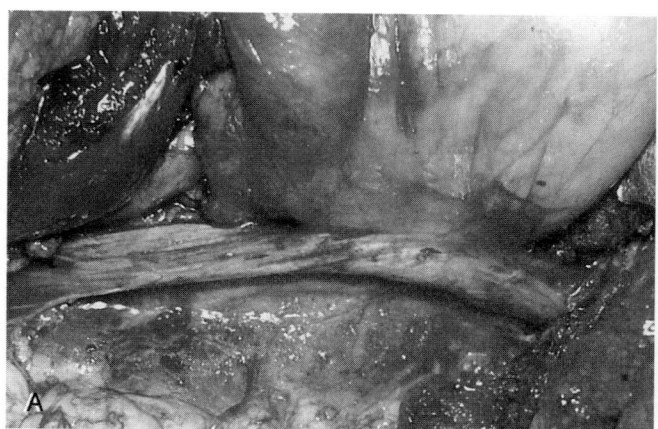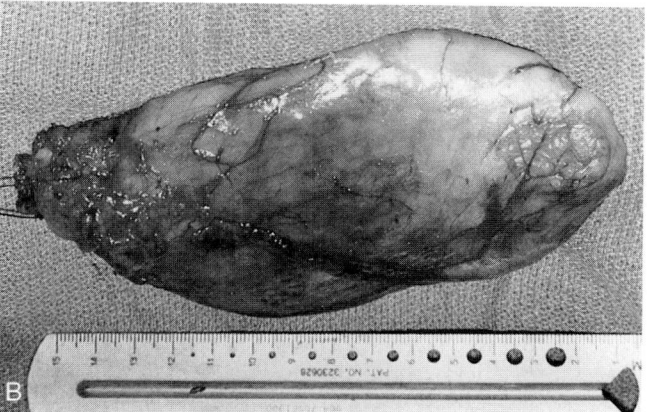

FIGURE 258–12. *A,* Large lipoma arising or adherent to posterior surface of buttock-level sciatic nerve. *B,* Lipoma specimen after resection.

some degree of intraneural dissection was necessary to remove the lipoma. Lipofibrohamartomas are fatty-fibrous masses of tissue intrinsic to nerve, although they can extrude or grow outside of nerve as well.[49, 57] They are congenital in nature and are most frequently seen in the median nerve at wrist and palmar levels. The usual initial management is to release the transverse carpal ligament and not attempt removal of the intrinsic mass. Conversely, because of size and progressive pain as well as decreased sensory and motor function, more extensive operations have been necessary in several of our patients. Internal neurolysis with thorough cleaning of each involved fascicle was attempted in one patient, which reduced the bulk but failed to preserve function. In the other case, the lipofibrohamartomatous mass and nerve were resected and a graft repair performed. There was limited sensory return probably related in part to the long length of the grafts necessary.

Meningiomas

Although associated almost exclusively with lesions in the head and spine, meningiomas can occur in the brachial plexus. In one of our two cases, the origin was paraspinal, which is understandable, but the other plexus lesion appeared to have a more peripheral origin. This was a massive lesion that required several operations. In both cases, plexus elements were incorporated by the tumor. In the latter case, extirpation without further damage to the plexus as well as complete excision was impossible. There had been four previous attempts at removal, and after we performed decompression, grafts from C6 to divisions and C7 to middle trunk were necessary. In addition, by 2 years after operation, there was evidence of recurrence localized to the lower plexus roots and the subscapular area.

Tumors of Vascular Origin

Trauma-induced hematomas, pseudoaneurysms and arteriovenous fistulas commonly involve nerve. Tu-

mors originating from vascular structures involving nerves are less common but do occur and are important.[58]

Hemangioma

Hemangiomas, which rarely involve nerve, can be intraneural or develop close enough to nerve to envelop it.[59, 60] Venous aneurysms may behave in the same fashion. In either case, when symptomatic and removal is indicated, an internal neurolysis is performed. Hemangioma or venous aneurysm is carefully dissected and stripped away from all involved fascicles in an attempt to spare as much function as possible. Recurrence is then possible and has been seen in both tumor categories in our experience. Total resection of the entire involved circumference of nerve is then performed, usually over a length of the nerve. Graft repair is then necessary. Of interest were two intraneural venous aneurysms, one involving the median nerve at the wrist level and the other the posterior tibial nerve at the level of the knee. In both cases, the size of the mass and paresthesias increased as the limb was placed in a dependent position; they then were ameliorated or disappeared as the limb was elevated. Because of progressive enlargement and pain, both required operative removal; the one on the median nerve then required reoperation and resection of nerve as well as its intraneural lesion and then graft repair.

Hemangioblastoma

Hemangioblastomas usually occur in the brain and spinal cord but can, on rare occasions, be present in nerve. The one we have had experience with was in the median nerve at the elbow.[61] Previous attempted biopsy elsewhere had led to heavy bleeding, and a subsequent angiogram showed a vascular stain similar to that seen with central nervous system hemangioblastoma. Again, internal neurolysis beginning above and below the lesion and extending through the lesion and clearing away as much tumor as possible was necessary. The tumor cells had an endothelial-like appearance and were interspersed with hemangiocytes and areas of hemorrhage.

Hemangiopericytomas

Hemangiopericytomas can begin in the mediastinum and grow superiorly to envelop brachial plexus, or they can envelop nerve elsewhere in an extremity. They are extremely difficult to remove, especially when plexus is involved, and have a malignant behavior with a high recurrence rate and a tendency to metastasize. The tumor bleeds easily and has a prominent blood supply. It is made up of a solid cellular background with densely packed polygonal cells with oval nuclei intermixed with vascular spaces that look like staghorns on microscopy. When a tumor similar to this involved meninges, it was felt to be an angioblastic hemangioma or meningioma. The lesion involving nerve has similar histologic features. It can have a malignant course just like a meningeal lesion and thus behave like a sarcoma. It is included in this portion of the discussion because it is of vascular origin.

Glomus Tumors

These exquisitely painful and tender lesions are usually found at a subungual site, but they can occur elsewhere.[62, 63] They are unusual tumors that are felt to arise from a glomerulus where an arteriole connects to an adjacent venule by way of a tiny canalicular system.[64] The histologic features are characteristic, with a canalicular-like arrangement of sheets of cells resembling glomus cells or pericytes. Special stains show a stroma with rich reticulum. The recurrence rate is high.

One of the lesions operated on by us was located over the anterior tibia and presented in a teenager who related it to ski boot compression several years before. It was reddish brown, vascular, and adherent to the periosteum. Resection relieved her pain and severe tenderness. The mass recurred and had to be re-resected 5 years later.[25]

Ganglioneuromas

There were two cases of ganglioneuroma in the LSUMC series and they both originated at a paraspinal locus and involved the brachial plexus. The ganglion-like cells and site suggest an origin from the sympathetic chain. Both lesions were in the superior mediastinum and involved lower elements of the plexus, so they were approached by a posterior subscapular operation. If the lesion is a large one, it is usually soft enough to be debulked with a CUSA. Neither of these tumors were secretors, and both patients have gone a number of years without recurrence.

Localized Hypertrophic Neuropathy ("Onion Whorl Disease")

Localized hypertrophic neuropathy is a strange, relatively infrequent disease of an unusual nature and unknown cause. Perhaps because of these features, localized hypertrophic neuropathy has generated a surprisingly large literature.[65-77] The lesion results in a swollen, thickened segment of nerve that gradually loses its function. Loci in the LSUMC series of 16 cases included the brachial plexus,[2] median nerve,[1] ulnar nerve,[78] radial nerve,[78] and sciatic complex, including the peroneal and tibial nerves.[79] Axons and their myelin coverings are reduced in size and appear strangulated by concentric rings of collagen. Thus, on cross section of the lesion and light microscopy, the nerve fibers that are left have the appearance of sectioned onions. There is, of course, a striking proliferation of perineurial cells leading some to term the lesion a *perineuroma*.[80, 81] There is compartmentation in which groups of axons are surrounded by fibrous tissue and their own proliferated perineurium.[4, 82] It is unclear whether these lesions are tumorous or traumatic in origin.[83] Although some of the histologic and behavioral features of the lesion favor a traumatic cause, a convincing history of this usually is not obtained. The disease usually affects one segment of one nerve but can involve several adjacent elements when it occurs in the brachial plexus. It often tends to present with a painless loss of motor function that is greater than the loss of sensory function in children or relatively young adults, although there certainly can be exceptions to this.

Computed tomographic and MRI scans are not characteristic for a neural sheath tumor but may show some nondescript thickening of the nerve or plexus elements. The T2 phase of the MRI may show a whitish streak in an enlarged nerve or plexus element. Involvement at levels where nerve is palpable may permit the examiner to feel a generalized thickening of a portion of the nerve. Differential diagnoses include other disorders that can enlarge nerve that are not tumorous. They include amyloidosis, Hansen's disease, Charcot-Marie-Tooth disease, and Refsum's disease.

In the past, we would operate on these lesions and record nerve action potentials that were usually greatly reduced in amplitude and velocity and because of this perform an external or sometimes internal neurolysis and submit a biopsy specimen for histologic analysis. This did not seem to improve function, and in at least one instance the biopsy reduced it further. Follow-up of those patients usually indicated a slow progression of loss and thus further disability. Hence, we now favor exploration, recordings and, when nerve action potential transmission is greatly decreased, resection and graft repair, even though loss is incomplete.[84] To do this, however, one has to be fairly certain of the lesion. Our pathologists fortunately have enough experience with the disease to spot it readily even on frozen section provided a cross-sectional rather than longitudinal specimen is submitted. In addition, it may not be advisable to perform a complete resection on nerves or elements for which outcomes with grafts, especially lengthy ones, are not good, such as the medial cord or lower trunk of the plexus, ulnar nerve, and proximal peroneal division of the sciatic nerve.

With the more aggressive approach described earlier,

a partial loss is converted to a complete loss, but outcome with some graft repairs, to date, seems to justify this. It is important to submit pathologic sections from either end to make sure the resection has extended beyond the proximal and distal extent of the disease.

MALIGNANT TUMORS OF NEURAL SHEATH ORIGIN (NEUROGENIC SARCOMAS)

In the LSUMC experience as well as in other series, malignant tumors of neural sheath origin are more frequently solitary tumors than malignancies associated with VRD (Table 258–4).[85, 86] However, their frequency is greater in the VRD population than in the population at large.[87, 88] Some investigators feel that a benign neural sheath tumor can undergo malignant transformation.[89] This likelihood appears greater in patients with VRD or with large benign tumors, or both, than in those with solitary, benign, small tumors.[90, 91] The exact pathogenesis and incidence of such transformations, if they do indeed occur, is not known, but research identifying abnormal regulation of metabolites offers promise.[92] Prior irradiation to a body area may also favor the development of a neurogenic sarcoma, as well as other types of sarcomas.[93]

Findings that might prompt a diagnosis of malignancy include a relatively rapid increase in the size of a mass over a period of weeks to months, large size of the mass on initial presentation or a relatively fixed, firm to hard lesion that is exquisitely painful to palpation.[94] Presentation is seldom because of metastasis to lung, bone, liver, or spleen, although such behavior is certainly a later feature of such sarcomas.[25] Either computed tomographic or MRI scans demonstrate these masses well and, as with more benign neural sheath tumors, these sarcomatous lesions are contrast-positive.[22, 95] However, at this time, these scans, as well as coil or special phase array scans, do not differentiate malignant tumors from benign ones. As a result, malignancy may not be suspected and is certainly not verified until biopsy or attempted surgical removal, or both, occur. In inexperienced hands, "simple biopsy" is even more likely to lead to deficit than it is in benign tumors because of the intrinsic nature of malignant tumors and their tendency to be adherent not only to adjacent nerves or plexus elements but also to muscle, tendons, vessels, and even bone. Also, as some of these lesions tend to be extensive, simple biopsy in one locus may lead to significant sampling error, reducing the likelihood of correct diagnosis. As with most other malignancies, these tumors show increased cellularity, nuclear pleomorphism, mitotic changes, and areas of necrosis. The dominant histologic feature is a spindle-like cell with a variable intensity of staining.[96] As a result, differentiation from other non-neurogenic sarcomas such as fibrosarcomas, synovial sarcomas, and rhabdomyosarcomas can be difficult. Even an ancient or very cellular schwannoma may have some features suggesting a sarcoma. Special studies such as for S-100, Leu-7, epithelial membrane antigen, and cytokera-tin and even electron microscopy can help evaluate or differentiate malignant tumors of neural sheath origin from other types of tumors but are not diagnostic in themselves.[93, 97, 98] As with other cancers, abnormality in DNA binding phosphoprotein such as p53 is found in neurogenic sarcomas. In addition, a few agents that seem to inhibit or slow growth have been identified.[99] As pointed out by Guha and others, oncogenes and tumor suppressor genes are most likely also involved in the pathogenesis of this tumor.[100, 101]

There is no fully accepted method of managing these difficult lesions.[25, 102, 103] Once identified as malignant, we favor as complete removal as possible, preferably a wide local resection (Fig. 258–13).[62, 104] This includes section of the nerve or element leading into and out of the tumor and provision of peripheral margins that are free of tumor.[105] Thus, wide local resection includes resection of adjacent soft tissue structures. Unfortunately, for neurogenic sarcomas that involve brachial or pelvic plexus or the proximal portion of the arm, this is not accomplished without paralysis or even limb loss from ischemia. Thus, wide local resection seems to work better for neurogenic sarcomas involving the more distal portions of the limb. Local resection or, if possible, wide local resection is usually followed by irradiation or chemotherapy, or both, provided that further workup shows no evidence of metastases to lungs, bone, or liver and spleen. In this regard, one must make sure these studies are negative before proceeding with amputation or forequarter resection or hip disarticulation. We have experience with several patients in whom that was not done. Amputation was performed even though studies carried out shortly after amputation showed metastatic disease. Local resection alone of neurogenic or other types of sarcomas, whether followed by radiation and chemotherapy or not, leads to a high rate of recurrence.[106] This recurrence rate is a number of times that of more aggressive therapy, such as amputation or proximal disarticulation or wide local resection followed by irradiation and chemotherapy.[107] Treatment of metastatic neurogenic sarcoma includes irradiation and chemotherapy but is as frustrating for these lesions as for other types of sarcoma.[108]

We present the option of amputation or more proximal disarticulation to relatively young patients with neurogenic sarcoma in whom metastatic disease has been cleared. Of course, amputation is not feasible for sarcomas involving the supraclavicular brachial plexus, pelvic plexus, or proximal femoral– or buttock-level sciatic nerve. In recent years, we have favored limb sparing surgery, including as wide a local resection as possible without paralysis beyond that of the nerve or element of origin, followed by radiation therapy.[109] The latter has sometimes been carried out by implantation of rods. Nonetheless, some of our longest survivors are patients who agreed to amputation, and this includes a small subset of patients with sarcomas who had either forequarter amputations or hip disarticulations. Usually, the major options are discussed with the patient's family as well as with the patient, and a conjoint decision is made favoring one approach or the other.

TABLE 258–4 ■ Management of Neurogenic and Other Sarcomas Involving Major Nerves (n = 33)

NEUROGENIC SARCOMAS	VON RECKLINGHAUSEN'S DISEASE	LOCAL RESECTION	LOCAL RESECTION WITH MARGINS	IRRADIATION PORTS/RODS	AMPUTATION	FOREQUARTER AMPUTATION OF SHOULDER AND ARM OR HIP DISARTICULATION	AVERAGE FOLLOW-UP (Mo)	DEATHS (AVERAGED POSTOPERATIVE SURVIVAL [Mo])
Brachial plexus (12)	5	9	3	8	1	4	46	6 (21)
Sciatic (4)	2	2	2	1	0	3	32	2 (16)
Peroneal (2)	1	0	2	2	0	0	48	0
Tibial (1)	1	1	0	1	1	0	50	1 (16)
Femoral (2)	1	0	2	1	1	0	46	1 (37)
Ulnar (2)	0	0	2	1	0	0	52	
OTHER SARCOMAS								
Brachial plexus (4)	0	4	0	4	0	0	47	2 (40)
Sciatic (2)	0	2	0	1	0	0	27	1 (12)
Femoral (1)	0	0	1	1	0	1	18	1 (18)
Peroneal (1)	0	0	1	0	0	0	28	0
Ewing's sarcoma								
Brachial plexus (1)	0	1	0	1	1	0	30	0
Peroneal (1)	0	1	0	1	0	0	72	0
Totals (33)	10	20	13	22	3	8	43	14 (29)

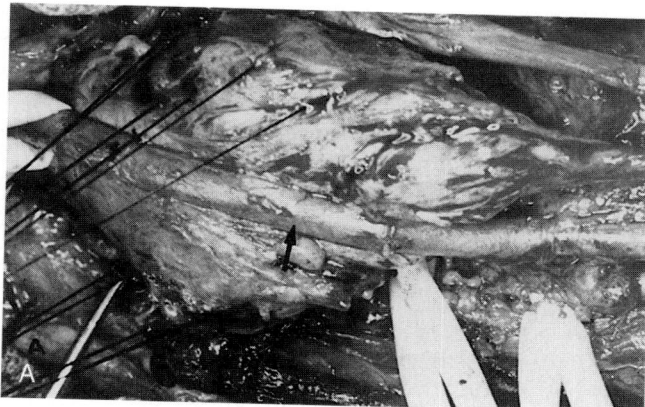
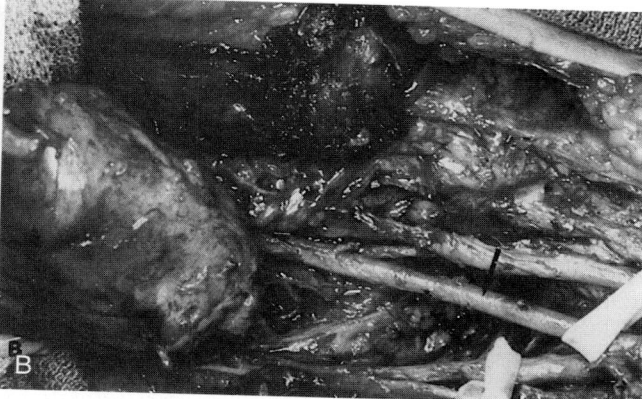

FIGURE 258–13. *A,* Neurogenic sarcoma of infraclavicular plexus. Tumor arose from medial cord and was adherent to axillary artery *(arrow).* (From Kline D, Hudson A: Nerve Injuries. Philadelphia, WB Saunders, 1995.) *B,* Tumor has been dissected away from lateral and posterior cords and artery *(arrow).*

Forequarter amputation for a distal brachial plexus lesion involving cords of the plexus or their proximal outflows involves removal of scapula and clavicle as well as shoulder and transection of subclavian vessels and plexus elements at a spinal nerve level.

Sarcomas not originating from nerve can compress or be adherent to plexus or other nerves and sometimes present because of a neuropathy. Wide local excision may not be possible, and response to irradiation and chemotherapy is variable. In the LSUMC series, non-neurogenic sarcomas at buttock, lateral shoulder, and elbow level involving nerves or plexus elements were excised as thoroughly as possible (see Table 258–4).

Neurogenic sarcoma associated with VRD has only a 16% to 18% 5-year survival after treatment as opposed to solitary neurogenic sarcoma in which 5-year survival is at a 50% level.[100, 110] Table 258–4 summarizes the LSUMC management of neurogenic sarcomas and other sarcomas with major nerve involvement. This series spans a period of about 24 years.

One of our cases was a teenage girl who presented with neck and shoulder pain and by MRI had a lesion in the C4–5 paraspinal region that appeared to be a neural sheath tumor. Instead, at operation this lesion was seen to be adherent to the paraforaminal structures and to the C4 and C5 spinal nerves (Fig. 258–14). Histologically, the lesion proved to be a primitive neuroectodermal (PNET) or extraosseous Ewing's tumor. Postoperatively, she received chemotherapy as well as irradiation. She is doing well, but it is only 2.5 years after operation. These lesions are malignant but radiosensitive and also responsive to some chemotherapeutic agents.[111] A second patient had wide local excision of an osseous Ewing's tumor arising from tibia and involving the tibial nerve. Excision was followed by radiation treatment and chemotherapy. The patient has remained disease free for a number of years. These lesions are infrequent, but four have been summarized by Birch and associates.[111]

Two other tumors that arise from nerve itself are the triton tumor and neuroblastomas. Both are rare tumors. Although usually benign histologically, the triton tu-

mor, like desmoids, can gradually take away function and behave as a more "malignant tumor."[112] The neuroblastoma is more clearly malignant. We have had experience with one triton tumor involving plexus and one neuroblastoma involving the sacral plexus. Triton tumors have an embryologic origin and can present in early life.[113] Such tumors are intrinsic to nerves. Muscle fibers are mixed with large myelinated nerve fibers. These histologic changes often coexist within fascicles. The best one can do is to decompress or debulk the tumor to try to prevent or retard progressive loss of function in involved elements. If seen early enough in life, total excision may be possible. Removal was the goal in a 36-year-old adult seen by us who presented with such a tumor involving the brachial plexus and had had subtotal excision as a child.[79] Our case of neuroblastoma involved a sacral nerve root for which

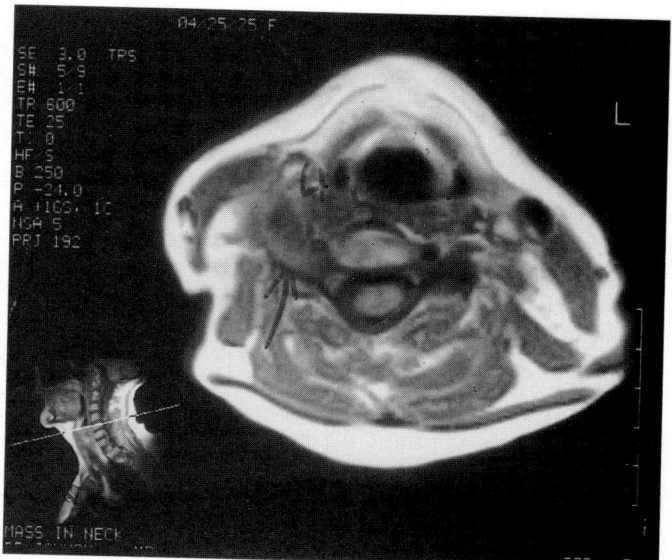

FIGURE 258–14. Transverse section of MRI scan at C5 level showing tumoral involvement of spinal nerve at that level on the right *(arrow).*

we performed gross total resection followed by irradiation.

MALIGNANT TUMORS OF NON–NEURAL SHEATH ORIGIN

These lesions can involve nerves either by direct extension or by metastasis via blood vessels or the lymphatic system. Mass effect from a cancer has to be differentiated from a carcinomatous neuromyopathy.[29] Operative indications for masses include pain that is usually severe, paresthesias, progression of deficits, and sometimes a palpable and tender mass. Good outcomes from surgery, let alone other therapy, are difficult to achieve. Incomplete excision, spread elsewhere, and eventually death from the cancer are the usual outcomes. Nonetheless, significant amelioration of severe pain can sometimes be achieved and, in some cases, operation on the secondary lesion helps identify the primary source or, in the case of breast carcinoma operated on years before, determine its estrogen sensitivity.

The largest category of carcinoma involving nerve operated on at LSUMC was breast carcinoma with spread to the brachial plexus. Each of these 12 patients had had prior mastectomy and irradiation. The differential diagnosis thus included carcinoma involving nerve or irradiation plexitis, or both. These diagnoses often cannot be resolved satisfactorily without multiple biopsies or, more likely, operative exposure and thorough biopsy of many areas, usually by removal of as much mass as possible.[78, 114]

Differentiation of metastatic cancer from irradiation plexitis remains difficult.[115–117] The following favor compression by carcinoma or tumoral invasion of plexus: (1) severe pain, especially in the distribution of specific elements; (2) absence of lymphedema; and (3) absence of myokymia on electromyographic sampling of plexus muscles. Unfortunately, many patients have involvement of plexus by both irradiation change and carcinomatous invasion, and lymphedema and myokymia may then be present. Presentation years after mastectomy and irradiation favors irradiation plexitis, whereas earlier presentation favors carcinoma. Unfortunately, there have been many exceptions to these temporal guidelines. Thus, we have seen three patients with brachial plexitis and without carcinoma who presented 3 to 9 months after mastectomy and irradiation. Conversely, we have seen several patients with metastatic breast carcinoma who presented 18 to 24 years after their initial treatment and who as a result were felt for years to be free of disease. In two of these cases, the tumor was found at an intraneural site within the lower trunk to medial cord portion of the plexus and not extraneural or elsewhere in the plexus.

Decompression of plexus has been attempted in the breast carcinoma cases and not en bloc removal of tumor and plexus elements as might be carried out for a neurogenic sarcoma. Dissections are especially difficult when there is both irradiation change and cancer. Most of the time, tumor was adherent to nerve but could be dissected away; however, as noted previously, there were exceptions when tumor was found in nerve. Operation usually reduced pain but not loss of function, especially if it was severe to begin with. As a matter of fact, further loss of function could and did result in some patients. Further treatment with irradiation and chemotherapy was individualized in consultation with the oncologist and radiotherapist. One of these patients with both radiographic change and tumor underwent subsequent amputation to try to help residual pain.

Fifteen patients with the preoperative diagnosis of irradiation plexitis were operated on. Radiation therapy had been carried out in these patients for a variety of lesions, including breast cancer, lung cancer, and Hodgkin's disease. In three of these patients, carcinoma was found at operation even though it was not suspected preoperatively. The principal indication for a decompressive operation was severe pain that could not be successfully managed pharmacologically or by other means. If predominant involvement and symptoms were in the distribution of the supraclavicular but lower plexus elements such as C8, T1, and the lower trunk, a posterior subscapular approach with resection of the first rib and decompression of plexus was carried out. The posterior approach does not permit dissection of scar or tumor extending distal to plexus divisions.[47] As a result, other patients underwent the more classic anterior supraclavicular and infraclavicular approach with as thorough neurolysis of plexus as possible. Although often successful at ameliorating the severe neuritic pain that afflicts these patients, it was often achieved at the expense of further neurologic loss of function. More than 100 other patients with presumed irradiation plexitis were seen and evaluated but were not felt to be candidates for operation. In the nine cases of pulmonary cancer involving plexus, the spread was usually by direct extension rather than true metastasis (Fig. 258–15). Operations were palliative with subtotal resection and decompression of plexus rather than total tumor resection. Five were performed by a posterior subscapular approach; in two cases this was carried out in conjunction with a laminectomy for tumor extending into the spinal canal. Fortunately, pain was ameliorated in most of these cases.

Lymphoma; bladder, head, and neck cancer; and metastatic melanoma were also seen and operated on because of severe pain and often progressive loss of function.[118] Several of the melanomas involved plexus, one at a divisional level, and two others at an infraclavicular cord to nerve level.[25] In one of the latter cases, postoperative difficulty with perfusion of an almost totally paralyzed limb led to amputation.

Twenty-five operative cancer cases involving nerve were summarized in 1995. Of importance, pain was significantly improved in 20 of these 25 cases. Fortunately, that trend has continued in cases added to the series since 1995. Local resection only was performed in almost all these cases, but despite this there was further loss of function in 10 cases, and in only 3 of these was any type of repair feasible. Fourteen of the

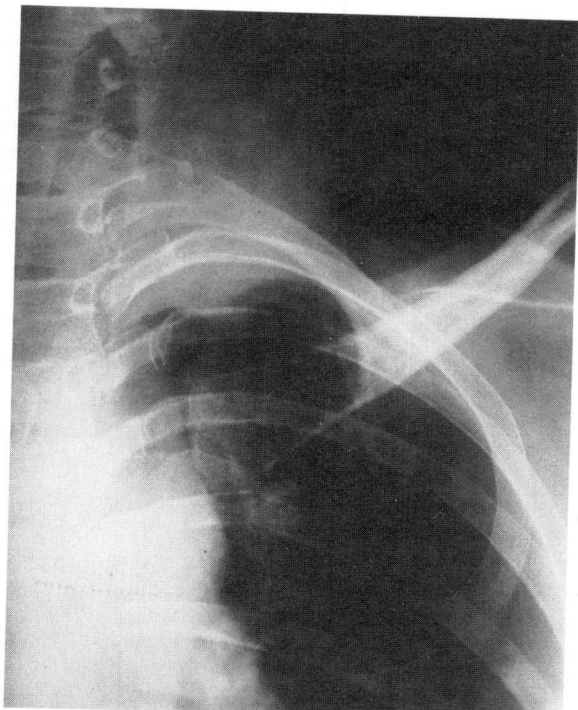

FIGURE 258–15. A Pancoast-like tumor is evident on this chest radiograph. (From Kline D, Hudson A: Nerve Injuries. Philadelphia, WB Saunders, 1995.)

25 patients reported in 1995 died with an average survival time after the decompressive operation of 15 months.

Complications

Although many operations for tumors involve peripheral nerves, complications other than those associated with loss of function and/or pain can and do occur. This is more likely for tumors involving the brachial or pelvic plexus than for those at more peripheral sites, but the latter are by no means free of such complications. They are also more frequent with the malignancies such as neurogenic sarcoma or cancer removal than with benign tumors, but again the latter are not free of complications. In our entire series of nerve tumors, including those performed more recently, there was one operative death, one postoperative brainstem infarct due to vertebral dissection, and several peripheral vascular complications requiring operative or postoperative repair. In addition to increased neurologic deficit, wound complications, and recurrence of tumor, which are always risks with this type of surgery, there are also further specific complications for each area of anatomy as well as tumor type. Examples of the latter are phrenic nerve paralysis associated with the anterior approach to plexus tumors and scapular winging associated with the posterior subscapular approach to the plexus. Lymph collections, the need for a chest tube, or major vascular involvement can also occur with either approach to the brachial plexus. Prolonged ileus, urinary retention, or even retroperitoneal clot can be associated with either transperitoneal or retroperitoneal approaches to pelvic tumors.

REFERENCES

1. Ariel IM: Current concepts in the management of peripheral nerve tumors. In Omer G, Spinner M (eds): Management of Peripheral Nerve Lesions. Philadelphia, WB Saunders, 1980, pp 669–693.
2. Asbury A, Johnson P: Pathology of Peripheral Nerves. Philadelphia, WB Saunders, 1978.
3. Batsakis JG: Tumors of the Head and Neck: Clinical and Pathological Considerations. Baltimore, Williams & Wilkins, 1974, pp 231–240.
4. Bigner D, McLendon R, Bruner J (ed): Russell and Rubenstein's Pathology of Tumors of the Nervous System, 6th ed. New York, Oxford University Press, 1998.
5. Brooks D: Clinical presentation and treatment of peripheral nerve tumors. In Dyck P, Lambert E, Thomas P, et al (eds): Peripheral Neuropathy. Philadelphia, WB Saunders, 1984, pp 2236–2251.
6. Burger PC, Vogel FS: Surgical Pathology of the Nervous System and Its Coverings, 2nd ed. New York, John Wiley & Sons, 1982, pp 649–699.
7. Byrne JJ: Nerve tumors. In Gelberman R (ed): Operative Nerve Repair and Reconstruction. Philadelphia, JB Lippincott, 1991.
8. Campbell R: Tumors of peripheral and sympathetic nerves. In Youmans JR (ed): Neurological Surgery, 3rd ed. Philadelphia, WB Saunders, 1990, pp 3667–3675.
9. Cravioto H: Neoplasms of peripheral nerves. In Wilkins R, Rengachary S (eds): Neurosurgery. Baltimore, Williams & Wilkins, 1988, pp 1894–1899.
10. Dart LH, MacCarty CS, Love JG, et al: Neoplasms of the brachial plexus. Minn Med 53:959–964, 1970.
11. Drake CG: Diagnosis and treatment of lesions of the brachial plexus and adjacent structures. Clin Neurosurg 11:110–127, 1963.
12. Lee DH, Dick HM: Management of peripheral nerve tumors. In Omer GE, Spinner M, Van Beek AL (eds): Management of Peripheral Nerve Problems, 2nd ed. Philadelphia, WB Saunders, 1998.
13. Russell DS, Rubinstein LJ: Pathology of Tumors of the Nervous System, 4th ed. Baltimore, Williams & Wilkins, 1977, pp 293–297.
14. Stout AP: The peripheral manifestations of the specific nerve sheath tumor (neurilemoma). Am J Cancer 24:751–796, 1935.
15. von Recklinghausen F: Ueber die Multiplen Fibrome der Haut und ihre Beziehung zu den Multiplen Neuromen. Berlin, A. Hirschwald, 1882.
16. Weller R, Cervos-Navarro J: Tumours of the peripheral nervous system. In Asbury AK, Johnson PC (eds): Pathology of Peripheral Nerves: Major Problems in Pathology. Philadelphia, WB Saunders, 1978, pp 206–249.
17. Woodhall B: Peripheral nerve tumors. Surg Clin North Am 34:1167–1172, 1954.
18. Cerofolini E, Landi A, DeSantis G, et al: MR of benign peripheral nerve sheath tumors. J Comput Assist Tomogr 15:593–597, 1991.
19. Filler A, Kliot M, Howe F, et al: Application of magnetic resonance neurography in the evaluation of patients with peripheral nerve pathology. J Neurosurg 85:299–309, 1996.
20. Kuntz C, Blake L, Britz G, Filler A, et al: Magnetic resonance neurography of peripheral nerve lesions in the lower extremity. Neurosurgery 39:750–757, 1996.
21. Thiebot J, Laissy JP, Delangre T, et al: Benign solitary neurinomas of the sciatic and popliteal nerves, CT study. Neuroradiology 33:186–188, 1991.
22. Stull M, Moser R, Kransdorf M, et al: Magnetic resonance appearance of peripheral nerve sheath tumors. Skeletal Radiol 20:9–14, 1991.
23. Abramowitz J, Dion JE, Jensen ME, et al: Angiographic diagnosis and management of head and neck schwannomas. AJNR Am J Neuroradiol 12:977–984, 1991.

24. Hughes DG, Wilson DJ: Ultrasound appearances of peripheral nerve tumours. Br J Radiol 59:1041–1043, 1986.

25. Kline D, Hudson AR: Nerve Injuries: Operative Results of Major Nerve Injuries, Entrapements and Tumors. Philadelphia, WB Saunders, 1995.

26. Suh J, Abenoza P, Galloway H, et al: Peripheral (extracranial) nerve tumors: Correlation of MR imaging and histological findings. Radiology 183:341–346, 1992.

27. Sundarem M, McGuire M, Herbold D: Magnetic resonance imaging of soft tissue masses: An evaluation of 53 histologically proven tumors. Magn Reson Imaging 6:237–248, 1988.

28. Das Gupta TK: Tumors of the peripheral nerves. Clin Neurosurg 25:574–590, 1978.

29. Dickersin G: The electron microscopic spectrum of nerve sheath tumors. Ultrastruct Pathol 11:103–146, 1987.

30. Erlandson RA: Peripheral nerve sheath tumors. Ultrastruct Pathol 9:113–122, 1985.

31. Fisher ER, Vusevski VD: Cytogenesis of schwannomas (neurilemoma), neurofibroma, dermatofibroma and dermatofibrosarcoma as revealed by electron microscopy. Am J Clin Pathol 49:141–154, 1968.

32. Harkin JC, Reed RJ: Tumors of the Peripheral Nervous System. Atlas of Tumor Pathology, Fascicle 3. Washington, DC, Armed Forces Institute of Pathology, 1969.

33. Lusk MD, Kline DG, Garcia CA: Tumors of the brachial plexus. Neurosurgery 21:439–453, 1987.

34. Perentes E, Nakagawa Y, Ross GW, et al: Expression of epithelial membrane antigen in perineural cells and their derivatives: An immuno-histochemical study with multiple markers. Acta Neuropathol 75:160–165, 1987.

35. Kawahara E, Oda Y, Ooi A, et al: Expression of glial fibrillary acidic protein (GFAP) in peripheral nerve sheath tumors. Am J Surg Pathol 12:115–120, 1988.

36. Kimura H, Fischer FW, Schubert D: Structure, expression and function of a schwannoma-derived growth factor. Nature 348:257–260, 1990.

37. Martuza R, MacLaughlin D, Ojemann R: Specific estradiol binding in schwannomas, meningiomas and neurofibromas. Neurosurgery 9:665–671, 1981.

38. Rizzoli HV, Horwitz NH: Peripheral nerve tumors. In Horwitz NH, Rizzoli HV (eds): Postoperative Complications of Extracranial Neurological Surgery. Baltimore, Williams & Wilkins, 1987, pp 283–298.

39. Erlandson R: The enigmatic perineural cell and its participation in tumors and in tumorlike entities. Ultrastruct Pathol 15:335–351, 1991.

40. Murray MR, Stout AP, Bradley CF: Schwann cell versus fibroblast as the origin of the specific nerve sheath tumor. Am J Pathol 12:303–323, 1940.

41. Seddon HJ: Surgical Disorders of the Peripheral Nerves. Baltimore, Williams & Wilkins, 1972, pp 153–170.

42. Heuly FH, Mekelatus CJ: Pheochromocytona and neurofibromatosis. N Engl J Med 258:540–543, 1958.

43. Schievink WI, Piepgras DG: Cervical vertebral artery aneurysms and arteriovenous fistulae in neurofibromatosis type 1: Case reports. Neurosurgery 29:760–765, 1991.

44. Friedman DP: Segmental neurofibromatosis (NF-5): A rare form of neurofibromatosis. AJNR Am J Neuroradiol 12:971–972, 1991.

45. Riccardi V: Neurofibromatosis: Phenotype, natural history, and pathogenesis. Baltimore, John Hopkins University Press, 1992.

46. Tang JB, Ishii S, Usui M, et al: Multifocal neurilemomas in different nerves of the same upper extremity. J Hand Surg [Am] 15:788–792, 1990.

47. Dubuisson A, Kline D, Weinshel S: Posterior subscapular approach to the brachial plexus: Report of 100 cases. J Neurosurg 79:319–330, 1993.

48. Donner T, Voorhies R, Kline D: Neural sheath tumors of major nerves. J Neurosurg 81:362–373, 1994.

49. Hudson A, Kline D: Peripheral nerve tumors. In Schmidek H, Sweet W (eds): Operative Neurosurgical Techniques, 3rd ed. New York, Grune & Stratten, 1998.

50. Enzinger FM, Weiss SW: Benign tumors of peripheral nerves. In Enzinger F, Weiss S (eds): Soft Tissue Sarcomas. St. Louis, CV Mosby, 1988.

51. Smith RJ, Lipke RW: Surgical treatment of peripheral nerve tumors of the upper limb. In Omer G, Spinner M (eds): Management of Peripheral Nerve Lesions. Philadelphia, WB Saunders, 1980, pp 694–711.

52. Chui M: Fibromatosis of the brachial plexus and shoulder girdle. Can Assoc Radiol J 40:28–31, 1989.

53. Tindall SC: Ganglion cysts of peripheral nerves. In Wilkins RH, Rengachary SS (eds): Neurosurgery. New York, McGraw-Hill, 1985.

54. Scherman B, Bilbao J, Hudson A, et al: Intraneural ganglion: A case report with electron-microscopic observations. Neurosurgery 8:487–490, 1981.

55. Harbaugh K, Tiel R, Kline D: Ganglion cyst involvement of peripheral nerve. J Neurosurg 87:403–408, 1997.

56. Morley G: Intraneural lipoma of the median nerve in the carpal tunnel. J Bone Joint Surg Br 46:734–735, 1964.

57. Silverman T, Enzinger F: Fibrolipomatous hamartoma of nerve: A clinicopathological analysis of 26 cases. Am J Surg Pathol 9:7–14, 1985.

58. Curtis RM, Clark GL: Tumors of the blood and lymphatic vessels. In Gelberman R (ed): Operative Nerve Repair and Reconstruction. Philadelphia, JB Lippincott, 1991.

59. Lusli EJ: Intrinsic hemangiomas of peripheral nerves: Report of 2 cases and review of the literature. Arch Pathol 53:266–270, 1952.

60. Pelerd J, Isosipovich A, Rousso M, Wexler MR: Hemangioma of the median nerve. J Hand Surg 5:363–365, 1980.

61. Kline DG: Discussion of Bradley J, Buchignari J, O'Brien T: Hemangioblastoma of the radial nerve: Case report. Neurosurgery 36:198–201, 1995.

62. Rosenberg A, Dick H, Botte M: Benign and malignant tumors of peripheral nerves. In Gelberman R (ed): Operative Nerve Repair and Reconstruction. Philadelphia, JB Lippincott, 1991, 1587–1625.

63. Smith K, Mackinnon S, Maccauley R, et al: Glomus tumor originating in the radial nerve: A case report. J Hand Surg 17:665–667, 1992.

64. Rosch JL: Soft tissue tumors of the hand. In Jupiter J (ed): Flynn's Hand Surgery. Baltimore, Williams & Williams, 1991.

65. Baker DK, Schoenberg F, Gullotta F: Localized hypertrophic neuropathy: A rare, clinically almost unknown syndrome. Clin Neuropath 3:226–230, 1984.

66. Hawke H, Jefferson JM, Jones EL, Smith WT: Hypertrophic mononeuropathy. J Neurol Neurosurg Psychiatry 37:76–81, 1974.

67. Imaginario JD, Coelho B, Tome F, Luis ML: Nevrite interssistinable hypertrophizive monosymplsloma tique. J Neurol Sci 1:340–367, 1964.

68. Iyer VG, Garretson H, Byrd R, Reiss S: Localized hypertrophic mononeuropathy involving the tibial nerve. Neurosurgery 23:218–221, 1988.

69. Ochoa J, Neary D: Localized hypertrophic neuropathy: Intraneural tumor or chronic nerve entrapment? Lancet 1:632–633, 1975.

70. Ohno T, Park P, Akai M, et al: Ultrastructural study of a perineuroma. Ultrastruct Pathol 12:495–504, 1988.

71. Peckham NH, O'Boynick PI, Menses A, Kepes JJ: Hypertrophic mononeuropathy: A report of two cases and review of the literature. Arch Pathol Lab Med 106:534–537, 1982.

72. Phillips LH, Persing JA, Vandenberg SR: Electrophysiological findings in localized hypertrophic neuropathy. Muscle Nerve 14:335–341, 1991.

73. Reyes RA, Chason JL, Rogers JS, Ausman JI: Hypertrophic neurofibrosis with onion bulb formation in an isolated element of the brachial plexus. Neurosurgery 4:66–70, 1979.

74. Richardson RR, Siqueira EB, Oi S, et al: Neurogenic tumors of the brachial plexus: Report of two cases. Neurosurgery 4:66–70, 1979.

75. Simpson DA, Fowler M: Two cases of localized hypertrophic neurofibrosis. J Neurol Neurosurg Psychiatry 29:80–84, 1966.

76. Snyder M, Cancilla PA, Batzdorf U: Hypertrophic neuropathy simulating a neoplasm of the brachial plexus. Surg Neurol 7:131–134, 1977.

77. Stanton C, Perentes E, Phillips L, Vandenberg SR: The immunohistochemical demonstration of early perineurial charge in the development of hypertrophic localized neuropathy. Hum Pathol 19:1455–1457, 1988.

78. Ampil F: Radiotherapy for carcinomatous brachial plexopathy: A clinical study of 23 cases. Cancer 56:2185–2188, 1985.

79. Awasthi D, Kline D, Beckman E: Neuromuscular hamartoma (benign "triton" tumor) of the brachial plexus. J Neurosurg 75: 795–797, 1991.

80. Bilbao JM, Briggs SJ, Hudson AR, et al: Perineurinoma (localized hypertrophic neuropathy). Arch Pathol Lab Med 108:557–560, 1984.

81. Mitsumoto H, Wilbourn A, Goren H: Perineuroma as the cause of localized hypertrophic neuropathy. Muscle Nerve 3:403–412, 1950.

82. Johnson PC, Kline D: Localized hypertrophic neuropathy: Possible focal perineurial barrier defect. Acta Neuropathol 77:514–518, 1989.

83. Urich A, Tien R: Tumors of the cranial, spinal and peritoneal nerve sheath. In Bigner D, McLendon R, Bruner J, (eds): Russell and Rubenstein's Pathology of Tumors of the Nervous System. New York, Oxford Press, 1998.

84. Gruen P, Mitchell W, Kline D: Resection and graft repair for localized hypertrophic neuropathy. Neurosurgery 43:78–83, 1998.

85. Cutler EC, Gross RE: Neurofibroma and neurofibrosarcoma of peripheral nerves, unassociated with von Recklinghausen's disease: A report of twenty-five cases. Arch Surg 33:733–779, 1936.

86. D'Agostino AN, Soule EH, Miller RH: Primary malignant neoplasm of nerves (malignant neurilemomas) in patients without manifestations of multiple neurofibromatosis (von Recklinghausen's disease). Cancer 16:1003–1014, 1963.

87. D'Agostino AN, Soule EH, Miller RH: Sarcomas of the peripheral nerves and somatic soft tissues associated with multiple neurofibromatosis (von Recklinghausen's disease). Cancer 16:1015–1027, 1963.

88. Hyse DG, Mulvihill JJ: Malignancy in neurofibromatosis. In Riccardi JM, Mulvihill JJ (eds): Advances in Neurology, vol 29. New York, Raven Press, 1981.

89. Robson D, Ironside J: Malignant peripheral nerve sheath tumor arising in a schwannoma. Histopathology 16:295–308, 1990.

90. Hosoi K: Multiple neurofibromatosis (von Recklinghausen's disease) with special reference to malignant transformation. Arch Surg 22:258–281, 1931.

91. Rogalski R, Louis D: Neurofibrosarcomas of the upper extremity. J Hand Surg 16A:873–876, 1991.

92. DeClue J, Papageorge A, Fletcher J, et al: Abnormal regulation of mammalian p21ras contributes to malignant tumor growth in von Recklinghausen (type 1) neurofibromatosis. Cell 69:265–273, 1992.

93. Foley KM, Woodruff JM, Ellis FT, Posner JB: Radiation-induced malignant and atypical nerve sheath tumors. Ann Neurol 7: 311–318, 1980.

94. Sordillo P, Helson L, Hajdu S, et al: Malignant schwannoma: Clinical characteristics, survival, and response to therapy. Cancer 53:2503–2509, 1981.

95. Chang AE, Matory YL, Swyer AJ, et al: Magnetic resonance imaging versus computed tomography in the evaluation of soft tissue saromas of the extremities. Ann Surg 205:340–348, 1987.

96. Thomas JE, Piepgras DG, Scheithauer B, et al: Neurogenic tumors of the sciatic nerve: A clinicopathologic study of 35 cases. Mayo Clin Proc 58:640–647, 1983.

97. Brodeur G, Morley J: Biology of tumors of the peripheral nervous system [review]. Cancer Metastasis Rev 10:321–333, 1991.

98. Wick M, Swanson P, Scheithauer B, et al: Malignant peripheral nerve sheath tumor: An immunohistochemical study of 62 cases. Am J Clin Pathol 87:425–433, 1987.

99. Lee J, Choi B, Sobel R, et al: Inhibition of growth and angiogenesis of human neurofibrosarcoma by heparin and hydrocortisone. J Neurosurg 73:429–435, 1990.

100. Guha A, Bilbao J, Kline D, Hudson A: Tumors of the Peripheral Nervous System. In Youmans J (ed): Neurological Surgery, 4th ed. Philadelphia, WB Saunders, 1996.

101. Hirose T, Hasegawa T, Kudo E, et al: Malignant peripheral nerve sheath tumors: An immunohistochemical study in relation to ultrastructural features. Hum Pathol 23:865–870, 1992.

102. Ducatman B, Scheithauer B, Peipgras D, et al: Malignant peripheral nerve sheath tumors: A clinical pathological study of 120 cases. Cancer 57:2006–2021, 1986.

103. Meis J, Enzinger F, Martz K, et al: Malignant peripheral nerve sheath tumors (malignant schwannomas) in children. Am J Surg Pathol 16:694–707, 1992.

104. Gentilli F, Rewcastle B: Malignant peripheral nerve tumors. Paper presented at the Eighth International Congress of Neurological Surgeons, July, 1985, Toronto, Canada.

105. Rosenberg SA, Tepper J, Glastein E, et al: The treatment of soft tissue sarcomas of the extremities: Prospective randomized evaluation of (1) limb sparing surgery plus radiation therapy compared with amputation and (2) the role of adjuvant chemotherapy. Ann Surg 196:305–315, 1982.

106. Collins CF, Friedrich C, Godbold J, et al: Prognostic factors for local recurrence and survival in patients with localized soft tissue sarcoma. Semin Surg Oncol 4:30–37, 1988.

107. Hruban R, Shiu M, Senie R, et al: Malignant peripheral nerve sheath tumors of the buttock and lower extremity. Cancer 66: 1253–1265, 1990.

108. Goldman R, Jones S, Hein Sinkweld RS: Combination chemotherapy of metastatic malignant schwannoma with vincristine, Adriamycin, cyclophosophamide, and imidazole carboxamide: A case report. Cancer 39:1955–1957, 1977.

109. Bolton J, Vauthey J, Farr G, Kline D: Is limb sparing surgery applicable to neurogenic sarcomas of the extremities? Arch Surg 124:118–121, 1989.

110. Sorensen S, Mulvhill J, Nielson A: Longterm follow-up of von Recklinghausen neurofibromatosis: Survival and malignant neoplasms. N Engl J Med 314:1010–1015, 1986.

111. Birch R, Bonney G, Parry CBW: Surgical Disorders of the Peripheral Nerves. London, Churchill Livingstone, 1998, pp 335–371.

112. Woodruff JM, Chernik NL, Smith MC, et al: Peripheral nerve tumors with rhabdomyosarcomatous differentiation (malignant "triton" tumors). Cancer 32:426–439, 1973.

113. Markel S, Enzinger R: Neuromuscular hamartoma: A benign "triton tumor" composed of mature neural and striated muscle elements. Cancer 49:140–144, 1982.

114. Kori SH, Foley FM, Posner JB: Brachial plexus lesions in patients with cancer: 100 cases. Neurology 31:45–50, 1987.

115. Lederman RJ, Wilbourn AJ: Brachial plexopathy: Recurrent cancer or radiation? Neurology 34:1331–1335, 1984.

116. Thomas JE, Colby MY: Radiation induced or metastatic brachial plexopathy? A diagnostic dilemma. JAMA 222:1392–1395, 1972.

117. Wilbourn AJ: Brachial plexus disorders. In Dyck PJ, Thomas PK, Griffin JW, et al (eds): Peripheral Neuropathy, 3rd ed. Philadelphia, WB Saunders, 1993.

118. Van Bolden J, Kline D, Garcia C, Van Bolden G: Isolated radial nerve palsy due to metastasis from a primary malignant lymphoma of the brain. Neurosurgery 21:905–909, 1987.

BIBLIOGRAPHY

Beech D: Soft tissue sarcoma. J La State Med Soc 151:33–41, 1999.

Croft P, Wilkinson F: Carcinomatous neuromyopathy: Its incidence in patients with carcinoma of the lung and carcinoma of the breast. Lancet 1:184–188, 1963.

Diagnostic Biopsy of Peripheral Nerves and Muscle

JANG-CHUL LEE

NORMAL STRUCTURE OF PERIPHERAL NERVES

Peripheral nerves consist of axons, ensheathing Schwann cells, and surrounding connective tissue matrix. Most peripheral nerves contain a mixture of myelinated and unmyelinated nerve fibers. Staining techniques that can be used to identify components of peripheral nerves are summarized in Table 259–1.

Connective Tissue Compartment

Cross section of a peripheral nerve reveals three separate histologic compartments; epineurium, perineurium, and endoneurium. Nerve fibers are embedded within a connective tissue compartment called the *endoneurium*. Nerve fibers are collected in fascicles, and each fascicle is surrounded by a perineurium. Nerve fascicles are embedded within a connective tissue compartment called the internal epineurium, which in turn, is encircled by several concentric layers of connective tissue and cells which form the external epineurium (Fig. 259–1).

The endoneurium contains myelinated or unmyelinated axons with ensheathing Schwann cells, collagen fibers, fibroblasts, endothelial cells of capillaries, rare macrophages, and a few mast cells. The endoneurial space is normally under a higher pressure than the surrounding tissue, which probably serves as a protective function of the nerve fibers.[1–3] Collagen fibers are oriented longitudinally in the outer endoneurial sheath and obliquely or circumferentially in the inner endoneurial sheath. The outer endoneurial sheath and the bands of Büngner, which represent the longitudinally oriented basal lamina lined tubes formed by Schwann cells during axonal degeneration, may play an important role in guiding regenerating axons after peripheral nerve damage.[4] Renaut bodies are occasionally found as acellular concentric whorls attached to the inner aspect of the perineurium, but their significance is not known.

The endoneurium, in turn, is ensheathed by the perineurium, which consists of concentric layers of spindle-shaped perineurial cells separated by layers of collagen. The perineurial cell is likely derived from fibroblasts[5] and surrounded on both sides by basement membrane. The perineurial cells are interlocked with each other by tight junctions that constitute the protective perineurial barrier.[6] The pinocytotic vesicles in the cytoplasm of the perineurial cell may provide selective and facilitated transport of nutrients and macromolecules across the protective perineurial diffusion barrier.[7] Immunocytochemically, perineurial cells are positive for epithelial membrane antigen (EMA) and are negative for S-100 protein and Leu-7.[8, 9]

The external epineurium encircles nerve fascicles and maintains the structural integrity of the entire nerve. This consists of longitudinally oriented collagen bundles and blends with the surrounding adipose tissues. The epineurial sheath of the nerve is continuous with the dura mater at the junction of spinal nerve roots, and the perineurium is continuous with the pia-arachnoid.

Myelinated Nerve Fiber

The axons function as an electrical impulse conduction system and as a chemical transport system. The cell bodies of sensory axons lie in the dorsal root ganglion, and those of motor axons lie in the anterior horn of the spinal cord. The myelinated nerve fiber consists of a single axon, and each Schwann cell enwraps the axon segment with the myelin sheath (Fig. 259–2A). Axons contain microtubules, neurofilaments, smooth endoplasmic reticulum, mitochondria, and various dense bodies and granules within the axoplasmic fluid. However, axons do not contain ribosomes or a Golgi complex, reflecting the absence of protein synthetic activity, so essential macromolecules must be transported from the cell body where they are made.[10] Nissl substances, a feature of the nerve cell body, are not present in the axon. The most prominent components of the axoplasm are the filamentous and tubular structures. Microtubules and neurofilaments form the cytoskeleton of the axon and are a fundamental component of the fast axonal transport system.[11] Immunocytochemistry for

TABLE 259-1 ■ **Histologic Methods Used Routinely for the Visualization of Specific Tissue Components of Peripheral Nerves**

ELEMENT	METHOD	RESULT
General	Hematoxylin and eosin	
	Toluidine blue	
Axon	Silver impregnations (Holms, Palmgren, Bodian, and Romanes techniques)	Axon: black
Myelin	Hematoxylin stains (Kultschitzky-Pal, Weil, Loyez, and so on)	Myelin: dark blue
	Luxol fast blue	Myelin: blue
	Gomori trichrome stain	Myelin: red; connective tissue: blue or green
	Osmium tetroxide-alpha-naphthylamine (OTAN)	For teased preparations
	Marchi technique	Normal myelin: unstained; degenerated myelin: black
Muscle fiber	Myosin ATPase preincubated at pH 9.4, 4.6, and 4.3	NADH tetrazolium reductase
Fat	Oil red O	
Amyloid	Congo red	
Immunocytochemical markers	Axons: neurofilaments	
	Myelin: myelin-associated glycoprotein (MAG)	
	Schwann cell: S-100, Leu-7, GFAP	
	Perineurium: epithelial membrane antigen	

ATPase: adenosine triphosphatase; NADH: nicotinamide adenine dinucleotide; GFAP: glial fibrillary acidic protein.

neurofilament protein is often valuable for detecting axons in normal nerves or in various pathologic conditions such as traumatic lesions or tumors. The axons are separated from the ensheathing Schwann cell membrane by a narrow gap, the periaxonal space of Klebs, which is in continuity with the extracellular space at the node of Ranvier through a narrow helical channel.[7] The full significance of the periaxonal space, however, is not clearly understood.

Two types of Schwann cells are recognized histologically: those associated with myelinated fibers and those with unmyelinated fibers. Schwann cells are derived from the neural crest.[10] These cells produce nerve growth factor, myelin, and sometimes collagen.[12, 13] The Schmidt-Lanterman cleft splits the cytoplasmic membranes at the major dense line and may form a route for the passage of substances from the outer cytoplasmic layer through the myelin sheath to the inner

cytoplasm. The Schwann cell cytoplasm contains intermediate filaments, microtubules, mitochondria, polyribosomes, Golgi cisterns, rough endoplasmic reticulum, and occasional multilayered membranous structures (Reich's pi granules). Schwann cells synthesize their own basement membrane.[14] Basement membrane, composed of laminin, type IV collagen, heparan sulfate, entactin, fibronectin, and other macromolecules, surrounds the entire external surface of the Schwann cell.[14-17] Schwann cells have positive immunoreactivity to S-100, the low affinity nerve growth factor receptor, and Leu-7 antibodies.[18, 19]

The myelin sheath derived from a Schwann cell acts as a biologic electrical insulator, resulting in conduction of action potentials along myelinated fibers proceeding in a discontinuous manner from node to node (saltatory conduction).[10] The three principal parameters that govern conduction in a myelinated fiber are axonal

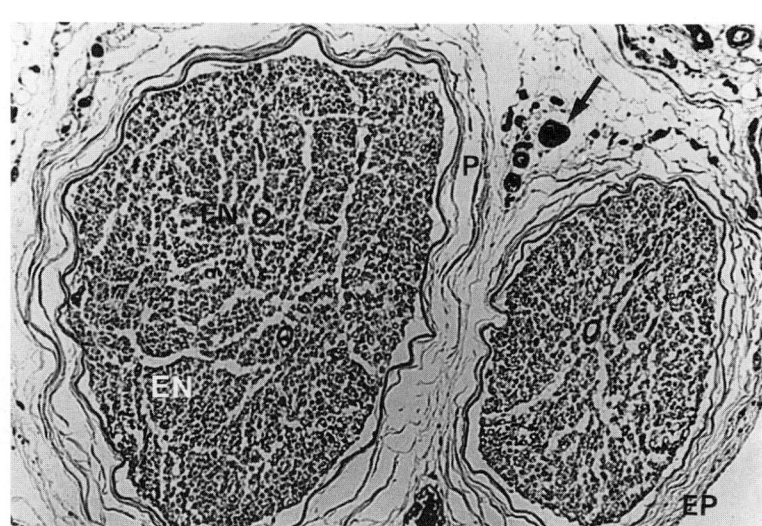

FIGURE 259-1. Transverse section of a normal sural nerve. Myelinated and unmyelinated nerve fibers are present in the endoneurial compartments (EN). The nerve fascicles are surrounded by perineurium (P) and are embedded in the connective tissue of the epineurium (EP). Epineurial blood vessels are also seen *(arrow)* (H & E stain, ×100).

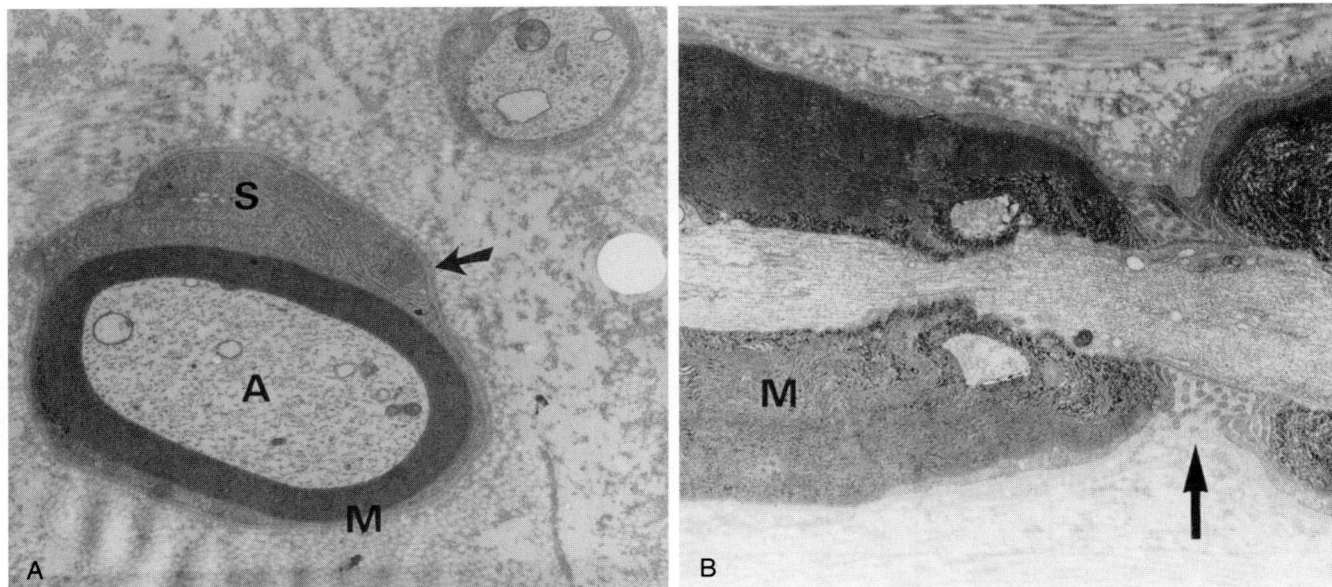

FIGURE 259–2. Myelinated nerve fiber. *A,* Transverse section in the perinuclear region. A small myelinated axon (A) is surrounded by a myelin sheath (M) with multiple lamellae, and both are encircled by a Schwann cell (S). The arrow denotes the basement membrane (×6000). *B,* Longitudinal section of a node of Ranvier. The node is identifiable as a cleft between neighboring myelin sheaths (M). In the midnodal region (*arrow*), processes of Schwann cytoplasm cover the axon (×8000).

diameter, myelin thickness, and internode length.[20] Myelin thickness is proportional to axon diameter.[21, 22] Ultrastructurally, the myelin sheath is characterized by a multilamellar structure that is alternately dark (the major dense lines) and light (the intermediate lines). Basement membrane and myelin-associated glycoprotein (MAG) play an important role in myelination.[23–25]

The axon is not covered by myelin at the meeting point of consecutive Schwann cells, which is known as the node of Ranvier (see Fig. 259–2B). However, Schwann cells from the two neighboring internodes extend interdigitating slender processes, and basement membrane is continuous over the nodal gap. At the paranodal regions of an internode, an axon loses its rounded contour and develops grooves that appear imposed by invagination of the overlying myelin. The Schwann cell nucleus is usually located around the middle of the internode. Internodal length is proportionate to the caliber of the fiber.

Unmyelinated Nerve Fiber

Unmyelinated fibers are more numerous than myelinated fibers in mixed peripheral nerves by a rate of 3:1 to 4:1.[26] One to several unmyelinated axons are ensheathed by one Schwann cell, sometimes referred to as a *Remak cell,* which is surrounded by a basement membrane (Fig. 259–3). The unmyelinated axons are not exposed at any point along their course because the adjacent Schwann cells are interlocked by flattened irregular, finger-like processes. Collagen fibers are frequently invaginated into the surface of the Schwann cell, called *collagen pockets,* and are separated from the surface of the Schwann cell by a basement membrane.

Although Schwann cells of myelinated and unmyelinated fibers may be regarded as originating from the same cell type,[27] those associated with unmyelinated axons are more likely to express glial fibrillary acidic protein (GFAP) and lack myelin-associated glycoprotein.[28, 29]

Nerve Barrier System

The peripheral nerve is protected from its surrounding environment by barrier systems analogous to but not

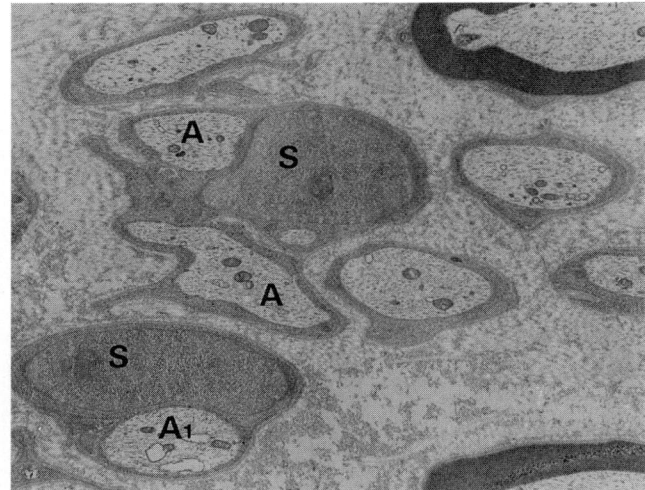

FIGURE 259–3. Transverse section of unmyelinated fibers. Several axons (A) lie within pockets of their ensheathing Schwann cell (S), whereas another axon (A1) is enclosed singly (×4000).

as tight as the blood-brain barrier.[30, 31] They include the perineurial diffusion barrier (tight junctions between the perineurial cells), the blood-nerve barrier (tight junctions between endothelial cells), and the paranodal barrier (tight junctions between myelin loops and paranodal axolemma). However, no such blood-nerve barrier exists in the dorsal root ganglia or in autonomic ganglia. The paranodal barrier serves not only as a diffusion barrier but also as an ion channel barrier because numerous sodium channels are present on the axolemma at the node of Ranvier, and potassium channels are present in the paranodal and internodal regions.[32]

GENERAL PATHOLOGY OF PERIPHERAL NERVE DISORDERS

The general pathologic features in positive peripheral nerve biopsy specimens are classified as (1) axonal degeneration and regeneration, (2) segmental demyelination and remyelination, and (3) secondary nerve changes due to pathologic conditions of the supporting tissues and blood vessels. In addition, some peripheral neuropathies reveal specific histopathologic features, such as amyloid deposition, the presence of lepra bacilli, abnormal lipids within the nerve, and vasculitis.[33, 34]

Axonal Degeneration and Regeneration

Axonal degeneration was first described by Augustus Waller in 1850 and the eponymous designation *wallerian degeneration* is still used.[10] Wallerian degeneration, strictly defined, represents the reaction of the nerve segment distal to a site of mechanical damage or transection. In general, the large myelinated axons are the most susceptible and degenerate first, although in amyloid neuropathy the reverse is true.[26] Most axonal neuropathies reveal axonal degeneration and regeneration simultaneously with secondary demyelination.[4]

The earliest axoplasmic changes are the accumulation of organelles at the nodes of Ranvier, especially on the distal side, which is followed by the disappearance of the microtubules, fragmentation of the neurofilaments, and swelling of the mitochondria. The axon then dissolves, and there is retraction of myelin from the nodes of Ranvier.

Transection of axons induces profound morphologic changes in the nerve cell body, including cell swelling, dissolution of the Nissl bodies, nuclear eccentricity, and nucleolar enlargement, which collectively are termed *chromatolytic changes*.[35] The nerve stump proximal to the lesion shows signs of "die-back" degeneration, usually up to the first node of Ranvier if the neuronal cell body survives.[36] Swelling of the proximal nerve stump probably occurs because cytoskeletal components, including organelles and proteins, which are normally transported continuously from the cell body via slow and fast axoplasmic transports, accumulate proximal to the site of transection.[36, 37]

Initially, myelin breakdown occurs within Schwann cells by lysosomal activity, so these cells contain multiple vacuoles.[38] These actions subsequently continue in hematogenously recruited macrophages, which engulf the debris (Fig. 259–4).[39–41]

While myelin breakdown is taking place, the Schwann cells start to proliferate within the basement membrane tube left behind by the degenerating axons. These form longitudinally continuous cell columns, the bands of Büngner (Fig. 259–5A). Nerve sprouts or neurites extend multiple finger-like processes from the growth cone and grow distally. As the neurites enter the bands of Büngner, they extend by attaching themselves to the inner surface of the basememt membrane or to the Schwann cell plasma membrane.[42–46] Schwann cells become myelinated with successful growth, whereas they may disappear and become replaced by fibrous tissue in cases of growth failure. Histologically, regeneration may be recognized by the presence of multiple, closely aggregated, small myelinated axons within a common basement membrane ("regenerating

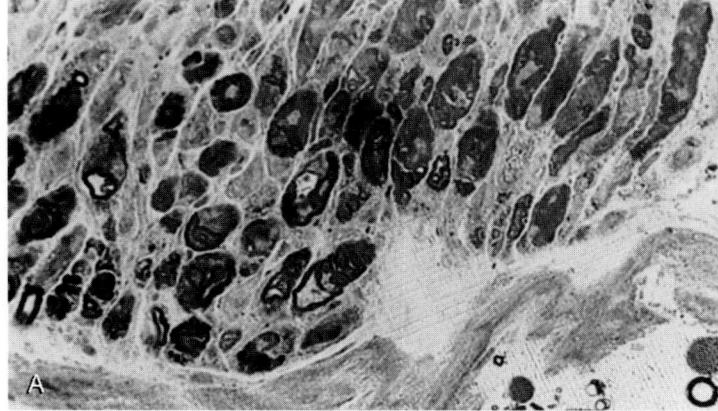
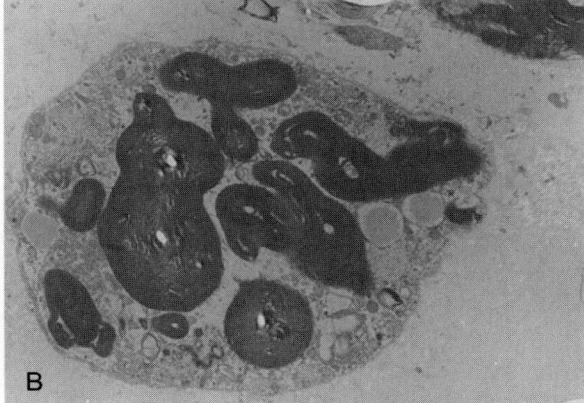

FIGURE 259–4. Axonal degeneration. *A,* A few macrophages are seen, and myelinated fibers show irregularly thickened myelin sheath and axonal degeneration (toluidine blue, ×200). *B,* Myelin debris is enclosed within a macrophage (×5000).

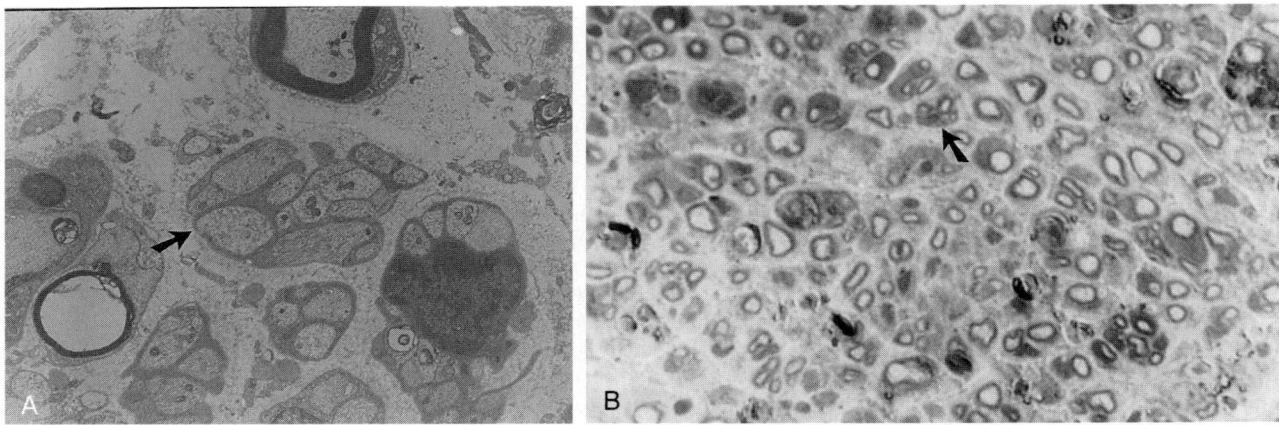

FIGURE 259–5. Axonal regeneration *A*, Bands of Büngner *(arrow)* (×4000). *B*, Several regeneration clusters *(arrow)* are visible as two to four thinly myelinated fibers surrounded by a common basement membrane (toluidine blue, ×200).

cluster"; see Fig. 259–5B).[47] As the regenerating clusters mature, they lose the common basement membrane, and some fibers may regress. In teased fiber preparations, short internodes in the distal part of the nerve indicate that axonal degeneration and regeneration have occurred in the past.

Unmyelinated axons undergo a degeneration process similar to that of myelinated axons. Loss of unmyelinated axons may result in the formation of numerous collagen pockets, and Schwann cell proliferation is less extensive than in myelinated axons.

Segmental Demyelination and Remyelination

Primary demyelination occurs as a consequence of Schwann cell dysfunction or direct damage to myelin itself. Demyelination has a segmental distribution with relative preservation of axonal integrity. The initial changes in demyelination are separation of terminal myelin loops, vesicular degeneration, myelin retraction, and a widening of the nodal gap at the node of Ranvier. The myelin sheath is broken down initially by Schwann cells and later by invading macrophages. The characteristic histologic feature of primary demyelination is myelin debris in the Schwann cell cytoplasm and myelin splitting or vacuolation, or both, with a denuded but otherwise normal axon. However, active myelin breakdown is rarely seen, since it occurs relatively rapidly.

The denuded axon provides a stimulus for remyelination. Initially, Schwann cell proliferation takes place, and only a layer of Schwann cells surround demyelinated segments of axons. A thin myelin sheath then forms within 3 to 5 days and progressively increases in thickness. Newly formed myelinated internodes are shorter than normal. Alternatively, remyelination after restricted paranodal demyelination may occur by extension of myelin from the neighboring intact internodes.

The typical changes of demyelination can also occur in primary axonal degeneration, which is termed *secondary demyelination.*[48, 49] In secondary demyelination, clustering of abnormal myelin segments occurs along certain abnormal axons, and in primary demyelination, the abnormal segments are spread randomly through the fibers. However, distinguishing axonopathy from demyelination may not be easy because the Schwann cells and axons are highly interdependent. An axonopathy results in the disturbance of Schwann cell metabolism and myelin structure, and myelin alterations affect axon morphology.

Sequential episodes of demyelination and remyelination are responsible for a concentric proliferation of Schwann cells surrounding the axon ("onion-bulb"), giving a distinctive histologic picture of hypertrophic neuropathy. It is a feature of chronic inflammatory demyelinating polyneuropathy and chronic hereditary neuropathies, such as Charcot-Marie-Tooth disease.[50, 51]

Vascular Pathologic Change

Vasculitis most commonly involves the epineurial vessels but can rarely affect the endoneurial vessels as well. The typical findings are perivascular or intramural infiltration of inflammatory cells, fibrinoid necrosis, disruption of the endothelium, and thrombosis. These changes are characteristic of several forms of systemic vasculitis with secondary peripheral neuropathy, including polyarteritis nodosa, rheumatoid arthritis, Sjögren's syndrome, and systemic lupus erythematosus (SLE).[52–54] However, these vasculitic changes may also occur as lesions confined to the peripheral nervous system.[55, 56]

NERVE BIOPSY

To diagnose peripheral neuropathies correctly, a detailed knowledge of the structure of the peripheral nerve and a clinicopathologic correlation is essential. Although not all patients with peripheral neuropathy need to undergo biopsy, nerve biopsy can often contribute valuable information that is not available from clinical data and electrophysiologic tests.[57, 58] If the cause of the neuropathy is readily apparent from clinical examination and laboratory tests, nerve biopsy is not indicated. Although the exact indications are difficult to state, nerve biopsy is usually indicated in two groups of patients: those suspected of having vasculitis and those with clinically significant peripheral neuropathy without known cause.[59–61] The nerve biopsy should not be performed if the nerve conduction is completely normal because the diagnostic yield is small. Most diagnostic nerve biopsies are taken from the sural nerve at the level of the lateral malleolus. The deep peroneal nerve, the obturator nerve, or the radial nerve may be appropriate when attempting to diagnose the more rare pure motor neuropathy by way of a fascicular biopsy.[62]

There are two types of nerve biopsy: fascicular biopsy and whole nerve biopsy. Although a few fascicles of nerve can be biopsied, in order to lessen permanent sensory loss and long-term dysesthesia, fascicular biopsy is not recommended because there is no significant difference in the areas of sensory loss compared with whole nerve biopsy.[63, 64] Furthermore, a fascicular biopsy may miss the vascular changes in the perineurial space in cases of vasculitis.

Procedure for the Sural Nerve Biopsy

Anticoagulants, including aspirin, must be discontinued before the procedure. The patient is placed in a comfortable lateral decubitus or prone position, and a pillow is placed under the ankle to be biopsied. Using local anesthesia (1% lidocaine or 1% bupivacaine [Marcaine]), the skin incision is made halfway between the posterior aspect of the Achilles tendon and the lateral malleolus and is extended proximally for 4 to 5 cm. The whitish, pearly sural nerve is identified medially under the lesser saphenous veins and superficial to the deep fascia. If the sural nerve is not found easily, usually the examiner has gone too deep. Sometimes a lesser saphenous vein is mistakenly identified as the sural nerve. This can be avoided by observing the broad angles at which the vein branches, in contrast to the narrow angles at which the nerve branches.[65] If a vein is cut, there is a tiny hole and bleeding in the center of the specimen. If the patient feels a shooting electrical pain when the nerve is transected, this finding confirms that the sural nerve has been cut.

Once the sural nerve is identified, the nerve is anesthetized with lidocaine a few millimeters proximal to the intended transection site before cutting in order to reduce the pain at the time of nerve cutting. However, the patient should be warned that he or she may experience a sharp pain at that time. A small amount lidocaine is injected slowly to avoid distorting nerve anatomy. The proximal portion of the nerve must be cut before the distal portion so that there is only one painful episode. The proximal nerve is pulled gently and cut with a sharp razor as high up in the incision as possible to reduce traumatic neuroma formation. At

least a 3-cm length of nerve should be obtained carefully without any unnecessary trauma to the nerve. The skin incision is closed using interrupted mattress skin sutures, and an elastic bandage is applied locally to reduce the accumulation of blood and fluid. The patient can move on the same day, but sitting with the leg in a dependent position for long periods or running is discouraged. Local pain is controlled with mild narcotics. Nonabsorbable sutures are removed in 7 to 10 days.

The surgeon should know the precise histologic methods to be performed in advance. Ideally, the nerve biopsy should be handled directly in the operating room by a histology technician. The specimen is not soaked in saline but is wrapped in moist gauze or polytef (Teflon) for transport. Four portions are prepared for investigation. One portion should be fixed in formalin for conventional staining and two portions in buffered 2.5% glutaraldehyde for electron microscopy and teased fiber analysis. The latter is most useful for detecting segmental demyelination and remyelination and for assessing whether axonal degeneration and regeneration have occurred within the nerve in the past.[66] One portion is frozen rapidly in liquid nitrogen for histochemical evaluation if immune-mediated neuropathy is suspected.

MUSCLE BIOPSY

In general, muscle biopsy is performed for the evaluation of muscle weakness, muscle cramps or discomfort, muscle fatigue with activity, and so on. However, diagnosis should always be based on a detailed history and clinical examination in conjunction with any special studies such as serum enzyme panels and electromyography. The biopsy should be performed only as the definitive confirmatory test of any underlying muscle pathologic condition. The diseases for which the muscle biopsy is indicated are classified as primary muscle disorders (e.g., myopathies, dystrophies), secondary muscle disorders (e.g., neurogenic, endocrine, or drug-induced), and systemic disorders (e.g., vasculitis).

For the best results, three factors are important: appropriate selection of the muscle, technique of the biopsy, and careful handling of the specimen. The selection of the muscle should be based on the distribution of the muscle weakness, as judged by detailed clinical assessment. Usually, the muscle for biopsy must be limited to certain well-characterized muscles such as the quadriceps femoris or gastrocnemius in the lower extremity or the biceps brachii or deltoid in the upper extremity. In a chronic disease such as muscular dystrophy, a muscle with only mild involvement may be the ideal site for biopsy, because fat or connective tissue will largely replace severely involved muscle. In an acute disease, a more severely involved muscle may be chosen because the process has not had time to progress to the point that extensive changes are present.[67] One should avoid sampling any muscles that have been the sites of either electromyography or injection, and sites of scar from previous surgery.[68] Areas of musculotendinous junction should also be avoided to minimize difficulty in fiber size evaluation.

It is essential to discuss the biopsy technique and specimen handling requirements with the requesting physician, the surgeon, and the neuropathologist before the biopsy to assess the need for special studies. There are three techniques available for muscle biopsy. Each has particular advantages and disadvantages, and it is important to be aware of these. Open biopsy technique offers the advantages of an adequate sample and proper orientation and length of the specimen fibers, but it has the disadvantage of causing unsightly scars. The advantages of needle biopsy are its simplicity, its speed, the small resultant incisional scar, and the ability to sample multiple sites in the muscle readily.[69-73] It has the disadvantage of producing a small sample and disoriented fibers. Another approach is a semi-open technique with an alligator-type forceps or conchotome, which can provide a slightly larger specimen than that available from needle biopsy.[74]

Procedure for Open Muscle Biopsy

Open muscle biopsy is usually performed with local anesthesia of the overlying skin. It is important not to infiltrate the muscle itself. An incision of 3 to 4 cm is made over the belly of the muscle in the direction of the fibers. A strip of muscle about 2.5 cm long × 0.5 cm wide can be isolated by placing a suture at either end and this cylinder of muscle can then be removed by cutting with sharp scissors while maintaining tension on the muscle by pulling on the sutures. The muscle may be stretched on a tongue blade after removal. The surgeon must be aware that clamping, stretching, squeezing, or drying the muscle tissue will produce unacceptable artifacts. After the muscle is removed, the fascia is sutured with absorbable material to prevent muscle herniation and the skin is then closed. Patients can use the limb normally immediately after the biopsy procedure. The muscle tissue should be wrapped in saline-moistened gauze and transported to the pathology laboratory as rapidly as possible. Four types of evaluation can be performed.[75] Slightly stretched pieces are needed for conventional histologic staining techniques after formalin fixation and for electron microscopy after fixation in 4% buffered glutaraldehyde. Part of the specimen is sent for genetic and protein analysis and part of the specimen is frozen rapidly in liquid nitrogen to preserve the enzymes and prevent artifacts for histochemical evaluation.

Procedure for Needle Muscle Biopsy

After Charriere and Duchenne introduced needle muscle biopsy in 1865, Bergström[76] reintroduced a similar percutaneous needle for the study of muscle change. The preparation and choice of the muscle in needle biopsy is similar to those in open muscle biopsy.[77] Using local anesthesia, a small stab incision is made over the belly of the muscle. After the biopsy needle, consisting of a cannula and sliding trocar with cutting blade, is inserted into the muscle, the sliding trocar is moved to and fro several times while pressing the muscle toward the window of the needle. Generally, three or four cores of muscle tissue are obtained. The needle is removed, and the biopsy sample is placed in saline-moistened gauze. Topical pressure is applied for several minutes to reduce the risk of hematoma formation.

REFERENCES

1. de la Motte DJ, Hall SM, Allt G: A study of the perineurium in peripheral nerve pathology. Acta Neuropathol (Berl) 33(3): 257–270, 1975.
2. Lundborg G, Dahlin LB: Anatomy, function, and pathophysiology of peripheral nerves and nerve compression. Hand Clin 12: 185–193, 1996.
3. McManis PG, Low PA, Lagerlund TD: Microenvironment of nerve: Blood flow and ischemia. In Dyck PJ, Thomas PK, Griffin JW, et al (eds): Peripheral neuropathy, 3rd ed. Philadelphia, WB Saunders, 1993, pp 453–473.
4. Ortiz-Hidalgo C, Weller RO: Peripheral nervous system. In Sternberg SS (ed): Histology for Pathologists. New York, Raven Press, 1992, pp 169–193.
5. Bunge MB, Wood PM, Tynan LB, et al: Perineurium originates from fibroblasts: Demonstration in vitro with a retroviral marker. Science 243:229–231, 1989.
6. Thomas PK, Bhagat S: The effect of extraction of the intrafascicular contents of peripheral nerve trunks on perineurial structure. Acta Neuropathol (Berl) 43:135–141, 1978.
7. Thomas PK, Berthold CH, Ochoa J: Microscopic anatomy of peripheral nervous system. In Dyck PJ, Thomas PK, Griffin JW, et al (eds): Peripheral Neuropathy, 3rd ed. Philadelphia, WB Saunders, 1993, pp 28–91.
8. Ariza A, Bilbao JM, Rosai J: Immunohistochemical detection of epithelial membrane antigen in normal perineurial cells and perineurioma. Am J Surg Pathol 12:678–683, 1988.
9. Perentes E, Nakagawa Y, Ross GW, et al: Expression of epithelial membrane antigen in perineurial cells and their derivatives: An immunohistochemical study with multiple markers. Acta Neuropathol (Berl) 75:160–165, 1987.
10. Thomas PK, Landon DN, King RHM: Diseases of the peripheral nerves. In Graham DI, Lantos PL (eds): Greenfield's Neuropathology. 6th ed. London, Arnold, 1997, pp 367–487.
11. Xu Z, Dong DL, Cleveland DW: Neuronal intermediate filaments: New progress on an old subject. Curr Opin Neurobiol 4:655–661, 1994.
12. Bunge RP: Expanding roles for the Schwann cell: Ensheathment, myelination, trophism and regeneration. Curr Opin Neurobiol 3: 805–809, 1993.
13. Church RL, Tanzer M, Pfeiffer SE: Collagen and procollagen production by a clonal line of Schwann cells. Proc Natl Acad Sci U S A 70:1943–1946, 1973.
14. Bunge MB: Schwann cell regulation of extracellular matrix biosynthesis and assembly. In Dyck PJ, Thomas PK, Griffin JW, et al (eds): Peripheral Neuropathy, 3rd ed. Philadelphia, WB Saunders, 1993, pp 299–316.
15. Bender BL, Jaffe R, Carlin B, Chung AE: Immunolocalization of entactin, a sulfated basement membrane component, in rodent tissues, and comparison with GP-2 (laminin). Am J Pathol 103: 419–426, 1981.
16. Cornbrooks CJ, Carey DJ, McDonald JA, et al: In vivo and in vitro observations on laminin production by Schwann cells. Proc Natl Acad Sci U S A 80:3850–3854, 1983.
17. Dziadek M, Edgar D, Paulsson M, et al: Basement membrane proteins produced by Schwann cells and in neurofibromatosis. Ann NY Acad Sci 486:248–259, 1986.
18. Perentes E, Rubinstein LJ: Recent applications of immunoperoxidase histochemistry in human neuro-oncology: An update. Arch Pathol Lab Med 111:796–812, 1987.

19. Weiss SW, Langloss JM, Enzinger FM: Value of S-100 protein in the diagnosis of soft tissue tumors with particular reference to benign and malignant Schwann cell tumors. Lab Invest 49:299–308, 1983.
20. Waxman SG: Determinants of conduction velocity in myelinated nerve fibers. Muscle Nerve 3:141–150, 1980.
21. Behse F: Morphometric studies on the human sural nerve. Acta Neurol Scand 82(Suppl 132):1–38, 1990.
22. Friede RL, Bischhausen R: How are sheath dimensions affected by axon caliber and internode length? Brain Res 235:335–350, 1982.
23. Filbin MT: Myelin-associated glycoprotein: A role in myelination and in the inhibition of axonal regeneration? Curr Opin Neurobiol 5:588–595, 1995.
24. Sternberger NH, Quarles RH, Itoyama Y, Webster HD: Myelin-associated glycoprotein demonstrated immunocytochemically in myelin and myelin-forming cells of developing rat. Proc Natl Acad Sci U S A 76:1510–1514, 1979.
25. Trapp BD, Quarles RH, Suzuki K: Immunocytochemical studies of quaking mice support a role for the myelin-associated glycoprotein in forming and maintaining the periaxonal space and periaxonal cytoplasmic collar of myelinating Schwann cells. J Cell Biol 99:594–609, 1984.
26. Schmidt RE: Diseases of the peripheral nervous system. In Nelson JS, Parisi JE, Schochet SS Jr (eds): Principles and Practice of Neuropathology. St. Louis, Mosby–Year Book, 1993, pp 561–595.
27. Mirsky R, Jessen KR: The biology of non–myelin forming Schwann cells. Ann NY Acad Sci 486:132–146, 1986.
28. Gray MH, Rosenberg AE, Dickersin GR, et al: Glial fibrillary acidic protein and keratin expression by benign and malignant nerve sheath tumors. Hum Pathol 20:1089–1096, 1989.
29. Jessen KR, Mirsky R: Non–myelin-forming Schwann cells coexpress surface proteins and intermediate filaments not found in myelin-forming cells: A study of Ran-2, A5E3 antigen and glial fibrillary acidic protein. J Neurocytol 13:923–934, 1984.
30. Londborg G: Intraneural microcirculation. Orthop Clin North Am 19:1–12, 1988.
31. Olsson Y, Reese TS: Permeability of vasa nervorum and perineurium in mouse sciatic nerve studied by fluorescence and electron microscopy. J Neuropathol Exp Neurol 30:105–119, 1971.
32. Black JA, Kocsis JD, Waxman SG: Ion channel organization of the myelinated fiber. Trends Neurosci 13:48–54, 1990.
33. Chimelli L, Freitas M, Nascimento O: Value of nerve biopsy in the diagnosis and follow-up of leprosy: The role of vascular lesions and usefulness of nerve studies in the detection of persistent bacilli. J Neurol 244:318–323, 1997.
34. Inoue S, Kuroiwa M, Saraiva MJ, et al: Ultrastructure of familial amyloid polyneuropathy amyloid fibrils: Examination with high-resolution electron microscopy. J Struct Biol 124:1–12, 1998.
35. Lundborg G: Nerve regeneration and repair: A review. Acta Orthop Scand 58:145–169, 1987.
36. Friede RL, Bischhausen R: The fine structure of stumps of transected nerve fibers in subserial sections. J Neurol Sci 44:181–203, 1980.
37. Smith RS: The short term accumulation of axonally transported organelles in the region of localized lesions of single myelinated axons. J Neurocytol 9:39–65, 1980.
38. Holtzman E, Novikoff AB: Lysosomes in the rat sciatic nerve following crush. J Cell Biol 27:651–669, 1965.
39. Brück W: The role of macrophages in wallerian degeneration. Brain Pathol 7:741–752, 1997.
40. Griffin JW, George R, Lobato C, et al: Macrophage responses and myelin clearance during wallerian degeneration: Relevance to immune-mediated demyelination. J Neuroimmunol 40:153–165, 1992.
41. Scheidt P, Friede RL: Myelin phagocytosis in wallerian degeneration. Properties of millipore diffusion chambers and immunohistochemical identification of cell populations. Acta Neuropathol (Berl) 75:77–84, 1987.
42. Clarke D, Richardson P: Peripheral nerve injury. Curr Opin Neurol 7:415–421, 1994.
43. Frostick SP, Yin QI, Kemp GJ: Schwann cells, neurotrophic factors, and peripheral nerve regeneration. Microsurgery 18:397–405, 1998.
44. Fu SY, Gordon T: The cellular and molecular basis of peripheral nerve regeneration. Mol Neurobiol 14:67–116, 1997.
45. Ide C: Peripheral nerve regeneration. Neurosci Res 25:101–121, 1996.
46. Thanos PK, Okajima S, Terzis JK: Ultrastructure and cellular biology of nerve regeneration. J Reconstr Microsurg 14:423–436, 1998.
47. Sima AAF, Blaivas M: Peripheral neuropathies. In Garcia JH (ed): Neuropathology: The Diagnostic Approach. St. Louis, Mosby–Year Book, 1997, pp 765–809.
48. Ballin RH, Thomas PK: Changes at the nodes of Ranvier during wallerian degeneration: An electron microscope study. Acta Neuropathol (Berl) 14:237–249, 1969.
49. Dyck PJ, Lais AC, Karnes JL, et al: Permanent axotomy, a model of axonal atrophy and secondary segmental demyelination and remyelination. Ann Neurol 9:575–583, 1981.
50. Harding AE, Thomas PK: The clinical features of hereditary motor and sensory neuropathy types I and II. Brain 103(Pt 2):259–280, 1980.
51. Prineas JW: Pathology of inflammatory demyelinating neuropathies. Baillieres Clin Neurol 3:1–24, 1994.
52. Chalk CH, Dyck PJ, Conn DL: Vasculitic neuropathy. In Dyck PJ, Thomas PK, Griffin JW, et al (eds): Peripheral neuropathy, 3rd ed. Philadelphia, WB Saunders, 1993, 1424–1436.
53. Hawke SHB, Davies L, Pamphlett R, et al: Vasculitic neuropathy: A clinical and pathological study. Brain 114(Pt 5):2175–2190, 1991.
54. McCombe PA, McLeod JG, Pollard JD, et al: Peripheral sensorimotor and autonomic neuropathy associated with systemic lupus erythematosus. Brain 110(Pt 2):533–549, 1987.
55. Davies L, Spies JM, Pollard JD, et al: Vasculitis confined to peripheral nerves. Brain 119(Pt 5):1441–1448, 1996.
56. Dyck PJ, Benstead TJ, Conn DL, et al: Nonsystemic vasculitic neuropathy. Brain 110(Pt 4):843–853, 1987.
57. David WS, Jones HR Jr: Electromyography and biopsy correlation with suggested protocol for evaluation of the floppy infant. Muscle Nerve 17:424–430, 1994.
58. Logigian EL, Kelly JJ Jr, Adelman LS: Nerve conduction and biopsy correlation in over 100 consecutive patients with suspected polyneuropathy. Muscle Nerve 17:1010–1020, 1994.
59. Chia L, Fernandez A, Lacroix C, et al: Contribution of nerve biopsy findings to the diagnosis of disabling neuropathy in the elderly: A retrospective review of 100 consecutive patients. Brain 119(Pt 4):1091–1098, 1996.
60. Oh SJ: Diagnostic usefulness and limitations of the sural nerve biopsy. Yonsei Med J 31:1–26, 1990.
61. Rappaport WD, Valente J, Hunter GC, et al: Clinical utilization and complications of sural nerve biopsy. Am J Surg 166:252–256, 1993.
62. Corbo M, Abouzahr MK, Latov N, et al: Motor nerve biopsy studies in motor neuropathy and motor neuron disease. Muscle Nerve 20:15–21, 1997.
63. Dyck PJ, Lofgren EP: Nerve biopsy: Choice of nerve, method, symptoms and usefulness. Med Clin North Am 52:885–893, 1968.
64. Pollock M, Nukada H, Taylor P, et al: Comparison between fascicular and whole sural nerve biopsy. Ann Neurol 13:65–68, 1983.
65. Asbury AK, Connolly ES: Sural nerve biopsy: Technical note. J Neurosurg 38:391–392, 1973.
66. Anthony DC, Vogel FS: Peripheral nervous system. In Damjanov I, Linder J (eds): Anderson's Pathology, 10th ed. St. Louis, Mosby–Year Book, 1996, pp 2799–2831.
67. O'Rourke KS, Ike RW: Muscle biopsy. Curr Opin Rheumatol 7:462–468, 1995.
68. Swash M, Schwartz MS: Biopsy pathology of muscle, 2nd ed. London, Chapman & Hall Medical, 1991, pp 15–37.
69. Campellone JV, Lacomis D, Giuliani MJ, et al: Percutaneous needle muscle biopsy in the evaluation of patients with suspected inflammatory myopathy. Arthritis Rheum 40:1886–1891, 1997.
70. Cote AM, Jimenez L, Adelman LS, et al: Needle muscle biopsy with the automatic Biopty instrument. Neurology 42:2212–2213, 1992.
71. Edwards RH: Percutaneous needle-biopsy of skeletal muscle in diagnosis and research. Lancet 2:593–595, 1971.
72. Magistris MR, Kohler A, Pizzolato G, et al: Needle muscle biopsy

in the investigation of neuromuscular disorders. Muscle Nerve 21:194–200, 1998.

73. O'Rourke KS, Blaivas M, Ike RW: Utility of needle muscle biopsy in a university rheumatology practice. J Rheumatol 21:413–424, 1994.

74. Henriksson KG: "Semi-open" muscle biopsy technique: A simple outpatient procedure. Acta Neurol Scand 59:317–323, 1979.

75. Pearl GS, Ghatak NR: Muscle biopsy. Arch Pathol Lab Med 119: 303–306, 1995.

76. Bergström J: Percutaneous needle biopsy of skeletal muscle in physiological and clinical research. Scand J Clin Lab Invest 35: 609–616, 1975.

77. Dubowitz V: Muscle Biopsy: A Practical Approach, 2nd ed. London, Baillière Tindall, 1985, pp 3–18.

Management of Acute Peripheral Nerve Injuries

THOMAS CARLSTEDT ■ ROLFE BIRCH

The success of regeneration after a peripheral nerve lesion is determined to a large extent by processes that take place immediately after the injury.[1] A delay in nerve regeneration conspires with atrophy and degeneration of denervated organs to increase the risk of permanent disability, emphasizing the importance of rapid and timely reconstruction to optimize organ viability.

Division of a peripheral nerve results in the unavoidable degradation and removal of the distal axon segment and associated myelin sheaths by wallerian degeneration.[2] This is a rather rapid process that is necessary for regeneration to occur as the Schwann cell phenotype changes to support axonal regrowth.[3–5]

Transection of the axon induces rapid metabolic and morphologic changes in the affected nerve cell bodies. Swelling, retraction of dendrites, and loss of synapses is accompanied by a decrease in transmitter production and up-regulation of the synthesis of neurotrophic proteins (Fig. 260–1A). Many neurons have an altered expression of neuropeptides in the acute phase after the lesion occurs. The amount of substance P and calcitonin gene–related peptide (CGRP) is decreased in injured primary sensory neurons; vasoactive intestinal peptide (VIP) is up-regulated.[6] Spinal motoneurons have an increased content of CGRP (see Fig. 260–1A). Some changes are transient, and others are reversible only if the neuron can successfully reestablish its contact with an appropriate target. Neurons that fail to regenerate become atrophic or die by retrograde degeneration. Axotomy-induced cell death represents a permanent impediment for reestablishment of function. The magnitude of neuron death depends on the proximity of the lesion and state of maturity. An injury close to the cell body, such as a brachial plexus lesion, may result in the death of neurons that would have survived a more distal lesion. In an immature individual, in whom nerve cells are most vulnerable, most neurons may die as a result of a proximal lesion (i.e., an obstetric brachial plexus lesion).[7]

There are considerable differences in the reactions of different types of neurons. Primary sensory neurons seem to be more susceptible to injury than motoneurons. The small, pain-transducing primary sensory neurons appear to be more vulnerable than larger sensory neurons. The gamma motoneurons, which innervate the muscle spindles, may die from retrograde cell death, whereas the larger alpha motoneurons usually resist the same type of lesion.[8] After a more proximal nerve injury, the root avulsion injury, there is time-dependent deterioration of all motoneurons in the pertinent spinal cord segment. The interruption of retrograde transport of neurotrophins such as brain-derived neurotrophic factor (BDNF), glia-derived neurotrophic factor (GDNF), and ciliary neurotrophic factor (CNTF) is of crucial importance. Within a few weeks after an avulsion lesion, all spinal cord motoneurons deprived of these neurotrophic substances have disappeared unless reconnection with a peripheral nerve is provided.[6, 7]

Multiple axonal sprouts emerge at the lesion site or from nodes of Ranvier in the proximal axon segment shortly after injury (see Fig. 260–1B). Growth cones at the front end of the sprouts elongate after sending out thin filopodia, which respond to environmental signals by retracting or dilating. Possible mechanisms for elongation and path finding include differential substrate adhesion abilities or activation of intracellular messengers through specific transmembrane receptors. Recognition molecules include cadherin, proteoglycans, fibronectin, and integrins (see Fig 260–1B). Signaling accomplished by punctate deposits of matrix proteins may include growth cone navigation.[9] The target-derived neurotrophins, which conceivably have an important function in maintaining neuronal survival, induce a powerful neurite outgrowth. These substances and their receptors show a dynamic regulation after nerve injury.

There is a rapid, transient, 15-fold increase in secretion of nerve growth factor (NGF) by Schwann cells and fibroblasts in the distal nerve segment. This is followed by a second increase that lasts several weeks and that depends on the interleukin-1 released from the recruited population of macrophages.[10]

The concentration of BDNF starts to increase 3 days after a nerve injury to reach a maximum level 3 to 4

Peripheral nerve injury

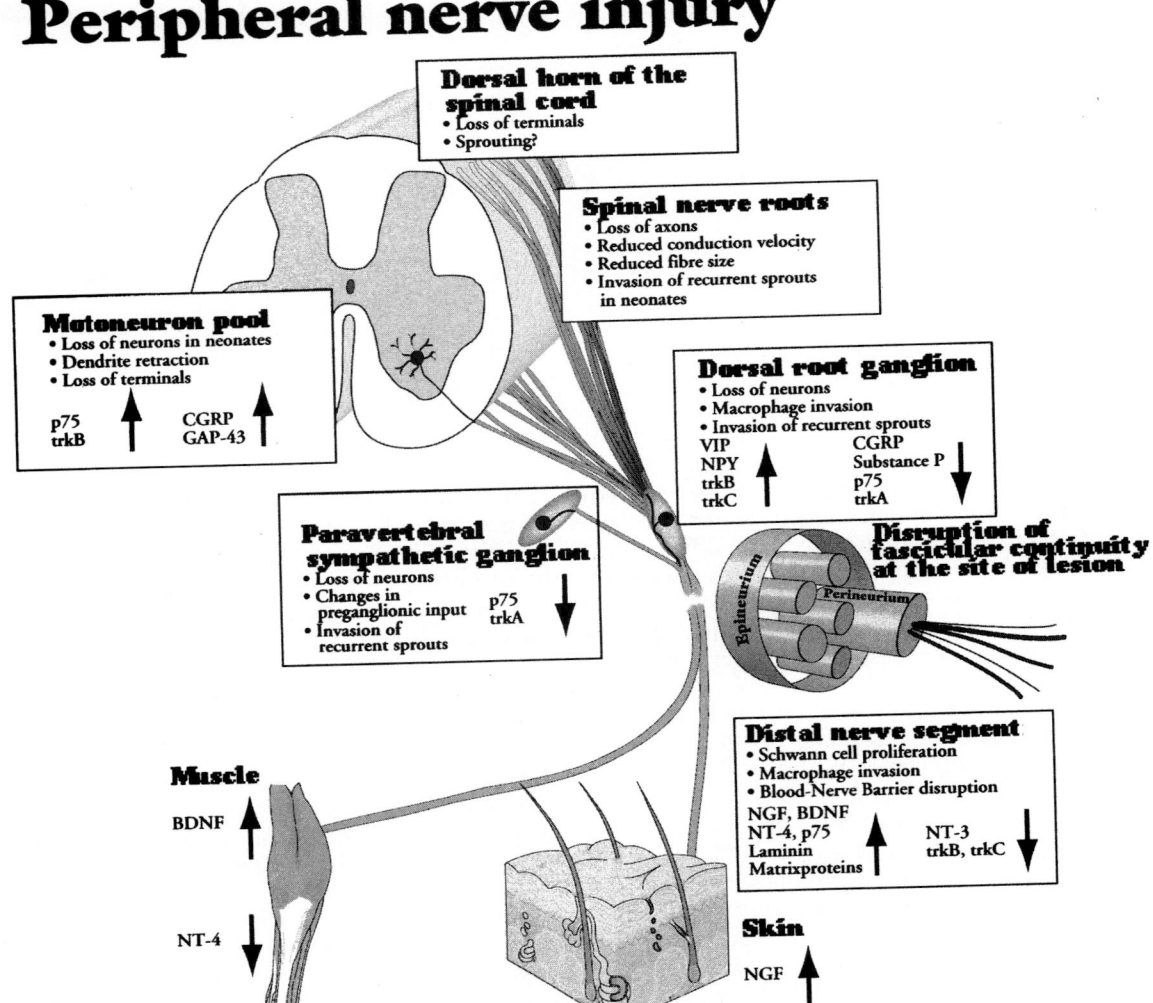

Dorsal horn of the spinal cord
• Loss of terminals
• Sprouting?

Spinal nerve roots
• Loss of axons
• Reduced conduction velocity
• Reduced fibre size
• Invasion of recurrent sprouts in neonates

Motoneuron pool
• Loss of neurons in neonates
• Dendrite retraction
• Loss of terminals

p75 ↑   CGRP ↑
trkB   GAP-43

Dorsal root ganglion
• Loss of neurons
• Macrophage invasion
• Invasion of recurrent sprouts

VIP   CGRP
NPY   ↑   Substance P ↓
trkB   p75
trkC   trkA

Disruption of fascicular continuity at the site of lesion

Epineurium   Perineurium

Paravertebral sympathetic ganglion
• Loss of neurons
• Changes in preganglionic input
• Invasion of recurrent sprouts

p75 ↓
trkA

Muscle

BDNF ↑

NT-4 ↓

Distal nerve segment
• Schwann cell proliferation
• Macrophage invasion
• Blood-Nerve Barrier disruption

NGF, BDNF
NT-4, p75   ↑   NT-3   ↓
Laminin   trkB, trkC
Matrixproteins

Skin

NGF ↑

A

FIGURE 260–1. *A,* Schematic drawing shows alterations in cell numbers, transmitter content, and immunoreactivity or mRNA levels for neurotrophins and neurotrophin receptors after peripheral nerve injury.

Illustration continued on following page

weeks later. Other substances, such as CNTF, show a 1000-fold increase during the first 24 hours after nerve injury,[11] and apolipoprotein E, which stimulates neurite outgrowth in vitro and is released by macrophages, shows an increased level in the immediate period after a nerve lesion occurs. There is also an immediate increase in the levels of insulin-like growth factor (IGF-1) and GDNF after nerve injury.[12] Based on the evidence accumulated on the distinct specificities of the different neurotrophins on sensory and motoneurons, a genetically engineered neurotrophin, panneurotrophin-1 (PNT-1), that combines the specific activities of the multiple neurotrophin family members has been used.[13] When applied immediately after nerve injury, there was an increase and acceleration in regeneration and functional recovery. The biologic response to nerve

injury demonstrates the urgency in nerve repair and shows that the optimal time for reconstruction after a nerve lesion is close to the time of injury.

The response to injury is quite different in the peripheral nervous system (PNS) compared with the central nervous system (CNS). Tissue components such as neurotrophic factors and extracellular matrix molecules of the PNS support nerve fiber regrowth, but these elements are not present in the CNS.[5] There is therefore a drastic difference in regeneration at the PNS-CNS interface in the spinal nerve root where growing nerve fibers are impeded.[14] At the PNS-CNS interface, the axon–Schwann cell units suspended in a collagen-containing extracellular space cross to an environment where the extracellular space is exceedingly small, collagen is lacking, and the axons are embedded in a

Outline of the cellular and molecular interaction at the site of lesion

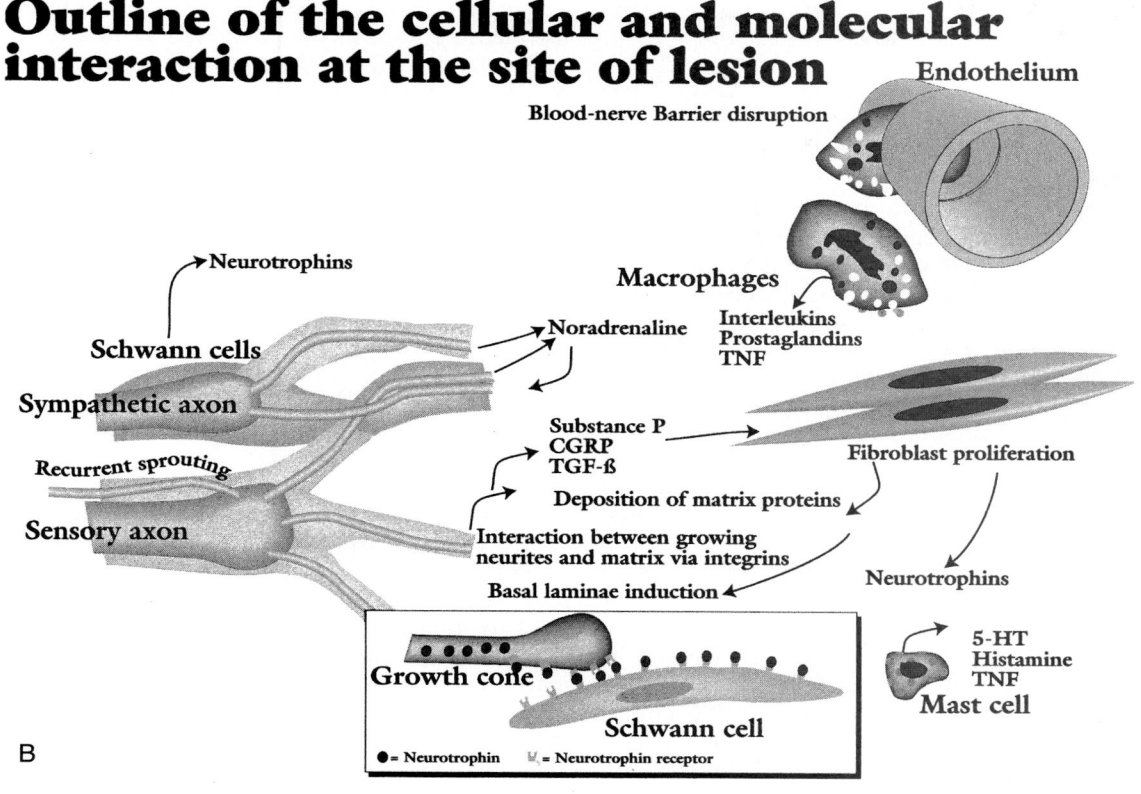

FIGURE 260–1. *Continued. B,* Schematic drawing shows possible interactions among neural mediators or transmitters, cytokines, growth factors, and matrix molecules at the site of a peripheral nerve injury. 5-HT, 5-hydroxytryptamine; BDNF, brain-derived neurotrophic factor; CGRP, calcitonin gene–related peptide; GAP-43, a growth-associated protein; LANR, low-affinity neurotrophin receptor; NGF, nerve growth factor; NT-3, neurotrophin 3; NT-4, neurotrophin 4; TGF, transforming growth factor; TNF, tumor necrosis factor; trkA, high-affinity receptor for NGF; trkB, high-affinity receptor for BDNF and NT-4; trkC, high-affinity receptor for NT-3; VIP, vasoactive intestinal peptide. (From Risling M, Carlstedt T, Cullheim S: Peripheral nerve injury and regeneration. In Glukman PD, Heymann MA (eds): Pediatrics and Perinatology: The Scientific Basis. Scarborough, Ontario, Arnold, 1996, pp 447–450.)

complex network of oligodendrocyte and astrocyte processes. This occurs in a specialized transitional region[15] at the attachment of spinal roots to the spinal cord, which contains elements of the PNS and CNS. The spinal nerve roots contain a proximal, short, cone-shaped CNS part and, distal to that, the longer PNS part. This arrangement is important in the root avulsion injury, which is a spinal cord (or CNS) lesion and therefore considered not amenable to treatment.[16]

ADULT NERVE PLEXUS INJURY

One of the most devastating nerve injuries is a lesion of the brachial or lumbosacral plexus. Restoration of limb function and control of pain after such injuries are formidable tasks. Prognosis for spontaneous recovery is often bleak, and several conditions can be recognized that make regeneration difficult. An injury such as this one—located in the most proximal part of the peripheral nervous system, close to the neuron cell body—can cause irreversible neuronal lesion. If regeneration takes place, the new neurites would have to elongate for long distances. They would have to find their appropriate targets and form functional contacts without being sidetracked in the complex intrafascicular communications along the peripheral nerves. In the most serious condition of severe plexus injury, one or several spinal nerve roots have ruptured or been avulsed (torn) from their attachments with the spinal cord.[17] Surgery of the brachial plexus, including intraspinal lesions, was introduced at the beginning of the 20th century,[18, 19] but it was later abandoned because of disappointing outcomes. Early amputation of the arm was recommended.

A more aggressive approach emerged about 25 years ago with the introduction of microsurgical and nerve-grafting techniques. Today, the outcome of surgery is so encouraging that it is no longer a question of what can be done but what should be done. However, the pioneering work of the brave surgeons during the early 1900s was not pursued. Much of the initially gained knowledge about the most common and most severe plexus lesions came to a long-lasting, unnecessary standstill.

Injury

The severity of the plexus lesion depends on the magnitude of the impact and can range from a temporary conduction block (i.e., neuropraxia), which recovers spontaneously, to a total severance (i.e., neurotmesis) or avulsion injury, for which recovery is possible only after surgical repair. Although open injuries from stabbing or missiles occur, the most frequent plexus lesion is the closed traction injury. A fall from a motorcycle at high speed can create a violent separation of the shoulder from the cervical spine with an elongation of the brachial plexus, causing a neurotmesis type of lesion. The injury is sometimes complicated by damage to the neighboring great vessels. They should be repaired by means of a reversed vein graft, even if there is collateral circulation.[20]

The nerve lesion may involve the entire brachial plexus, causing total impairment in arm and hand function, or it may be partial, sparing some activity in the limb. The injury is located supraclavicularly or infraclavicularly. The supraclavicular lesion is the most common type, and the infraclavicular injury occurs in about 30% of cases.[21] A lesion at both levels must be considered.[22] The infraclavicular injury is similar to a peripheral nerve trunk lesion and is often associated with fracture or fracture-dislocation of the proximal humerus and shoulder girdle and with vascular injury. In the supraclavicular type of brachial plexus injury, there may be one or several roots avulsed from the spinal cord, root ruptures, or spinal nerve injuries (Fig. 260–2).

Lumbosacral plexus injuries are relatively rare because of the protected position within the bony pelvis. In severe pelvic fractures, usually with dissociation of the sacroiliac joint together with fractures of the pubic bones, there also are traction lesions in the lumbosacral plexus[23, 24] or its spinal nerve roots, the cauda equina. These injuries can affect the lumbar part, with loss of function in hip flexors and knee extensors, and the sacral part, with loss of abduction and stability in the hip together with abolished function in knee flexors and all distal muscles. This injury occurs in more than 50% of patients with unstable pelvic fractures. Full recovery is rare. Many patients are left with classic burning dysesthesia and causalgia, for which management is difficult.

Diagnosis

Detailed anatomic knowledge of the nerve plexus and information about the nature of the trauma are the best means to accurately diagnose the site of the lesion, its extension, and the severity of the injury. Certain factors are considered favorable or unfavorable, and they should be taken into consideration when making decisions about surgery and considering the prognosis. A patient with brachial plexus palsy from dislocation of the shoulder has a very good chance of recovering completely, which means that the patient usually can be reassured about the prognosis. Similarly, an incomplete palsy (i.e., one muscle with an Medical Research Council [MRC] score of 1 or 2 in each myotome) can be regarded as a good sign. In contrast, a severe proximal lesion is indicated by a violent trauma. Serratus anterior muscle paralysis, the presence of Bernard-Horner syndrome, pain, and a medullary syndrome (i.e., Brown-Séquard syndrome) are bad signs. It is essential to discriminate between a spinal root and a spinal nerve lesion. Sympathetic paralysis is an indicator of spinal nerve rupture, as is the finding of a strong Tinel sign in the posterior triangle of the neck.[17] Spinal nerve root lesion of the upper roots of the plexus is suggested by the loss of sensation above the clavicle, with paralysis of the hemidiaphragm, serratus anterior, and the trapezius muscles. Bernard-Horner syndrome indicates a similar injury to the lower roots. In the lumbosacral plexus lesions the level of injury is much more difficult to appreciate clinically because this plexus is hidden, and there are few branches along its course. Laboratory assessments are therefore necessary.

The outcomes of magnetic resonance imaging (MRI), computed tomography (CT), myelography, and electrophysiologic tests are helpful in addition to the clinical examination. Based on this information, exploration of the injured plexus should be performed to reach a diagnosis and enable early repair.

Treatment

Swift intervention is important in optimizing the functional outcome of the injury. With early operation, exposure and nerve mapping by means of electrophysiology are particularly advantageous. Moreover, the biologic response to the trauma can be more easily exploited for regeneration in early intervention than after some time, when there is considerable nerve cell death, target cell death, and unfavorable concentrations of neurotrophins.[25]

For extraspinal lesions only, a standard repair is performed by means of excising the injured part of the plexus and reconstruction with excess amounts of nerve grafts. The superficial radial nerve and medial cutaneous nerve of the forearm are first choices for nerve grafts, but when in need of more grafts, the sural nerves are also used. The outcome should be close to normal except for intrinsic hand function. In most cases, however, there are also intraspinal injuries. If there is a partial lesion sparing hand function or a maximum of three root avulsions, nerve grafts and transfers offer excellent possibilities to regain close to normal function in the arm if the patient is operated on with urgency.[21] If one or two spinal nerves have been avulsed from the spinal cord (e.g., C5, C6), nerve transfers with accessory nerve and fascicles from the ulnar nerve and intercostal nerves can give quite useful functional return.[21] A good outcome can also be achieved when C5 through C7 have been avulsed from the spinal cord. In cases of isolated lower (e.g., C8, T1) brachial plexus spinal nerve root lesions or when four

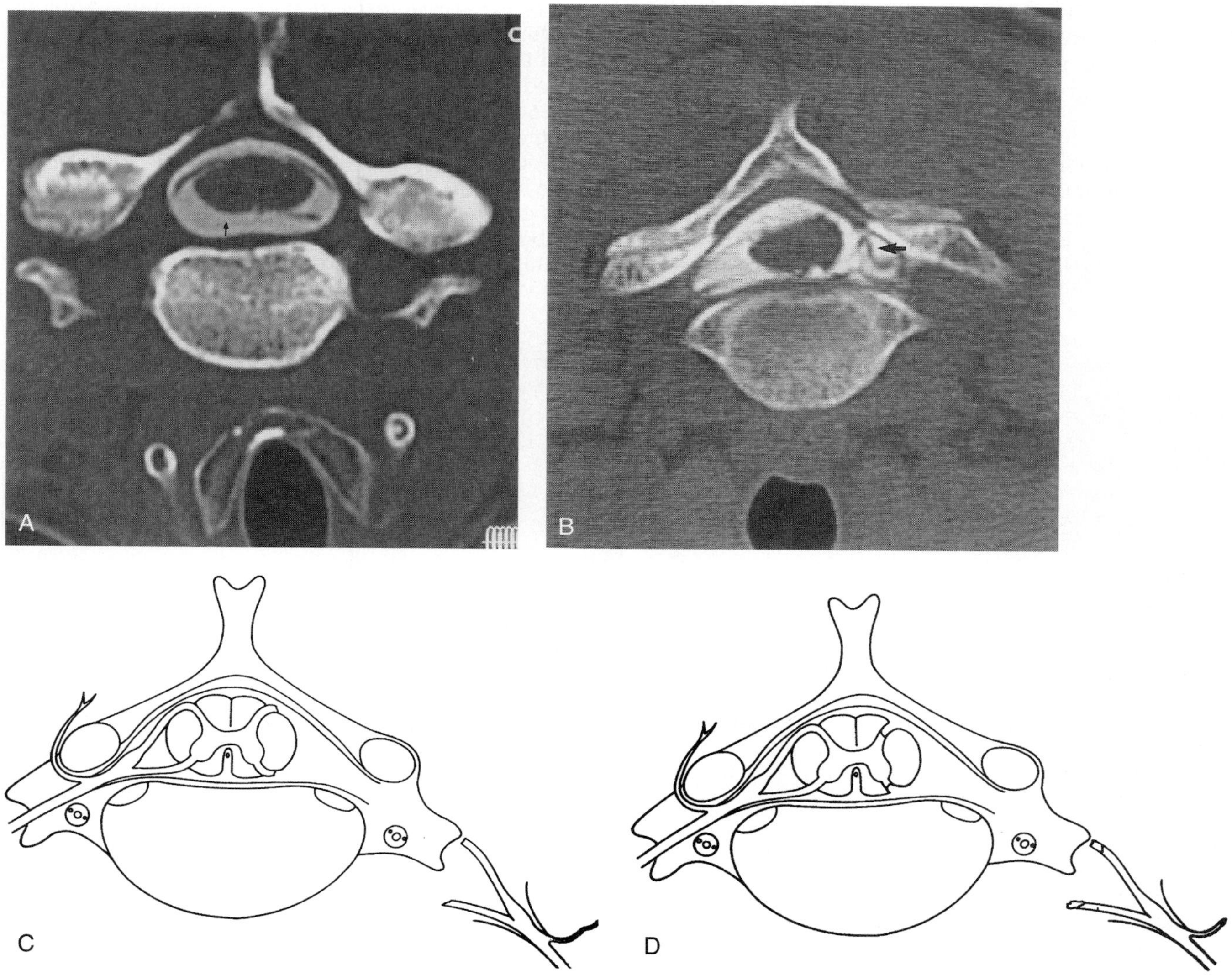

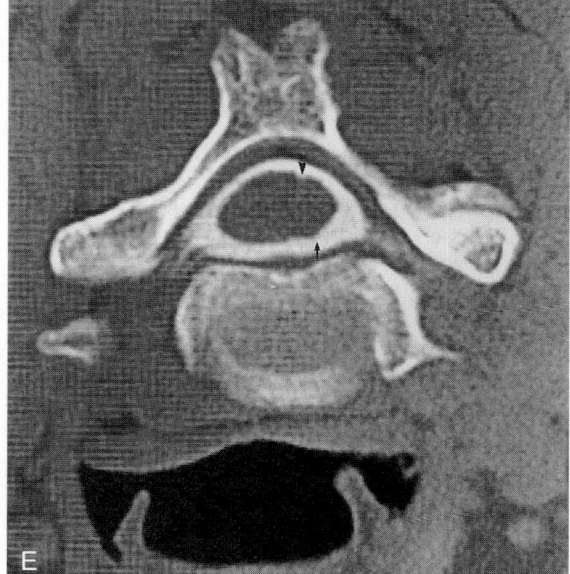

FIGURE 260–2. Computed tomographic myelograms (CT-myelograms). *A,* Avulsion of ventral root *(arrow)* and intact dorsal root. *B,* Dorsal and ventral root avulsion with roots in the meningocele *(arrow). C* and *D,* Diagrams show avulsions distal and central to transitional region (TR) (i.e., an intramedullary lesion). *E,* CT-myelogram shows ventral root avulsion distal to the TR, leaving a small stump *(arrow),* and dorsal root avulsion central to the TR, leaving a pit in the dorsal part of the cord *(arrowhead).*

or all five spinal nerves to the brachial plexus have sustained an intradural injury, the possibility to restore hand function is bleak. Still, shoulder and elbow function and relief of some pain can be achieved by early surgery.

In patients operated on within a short time after the accident, the surgical approach should enable simultaneous exploration of the intraspinal and extraspinal parts of the plexus. The extreme lateral approach to the cervical spine[26] gives easy access to all parts of the plexus (Fig. 260–3). In such cases, a view of and diag-

nosis of the intraspinal lesion can be obtained without performing a laminectomy. A small endoscope is introduced through the intervertebral canals for the already avulsed or ruptured and displaced roots and ganglia (Fig. 260–4). In most cases, the intraspinal plexus lesion is a mixture of various types of root ruptures and avulsions[14, 18] (Fig. 260–5; see Fig. 260–2).

The surgical strategy is to reinnervate the arm using nerve grafting for ruptures in the plexus, transfers of neighboring nerves (e.g., accessory, dorsal scapular, intercostal), and in selected cases, repair of intraspinal

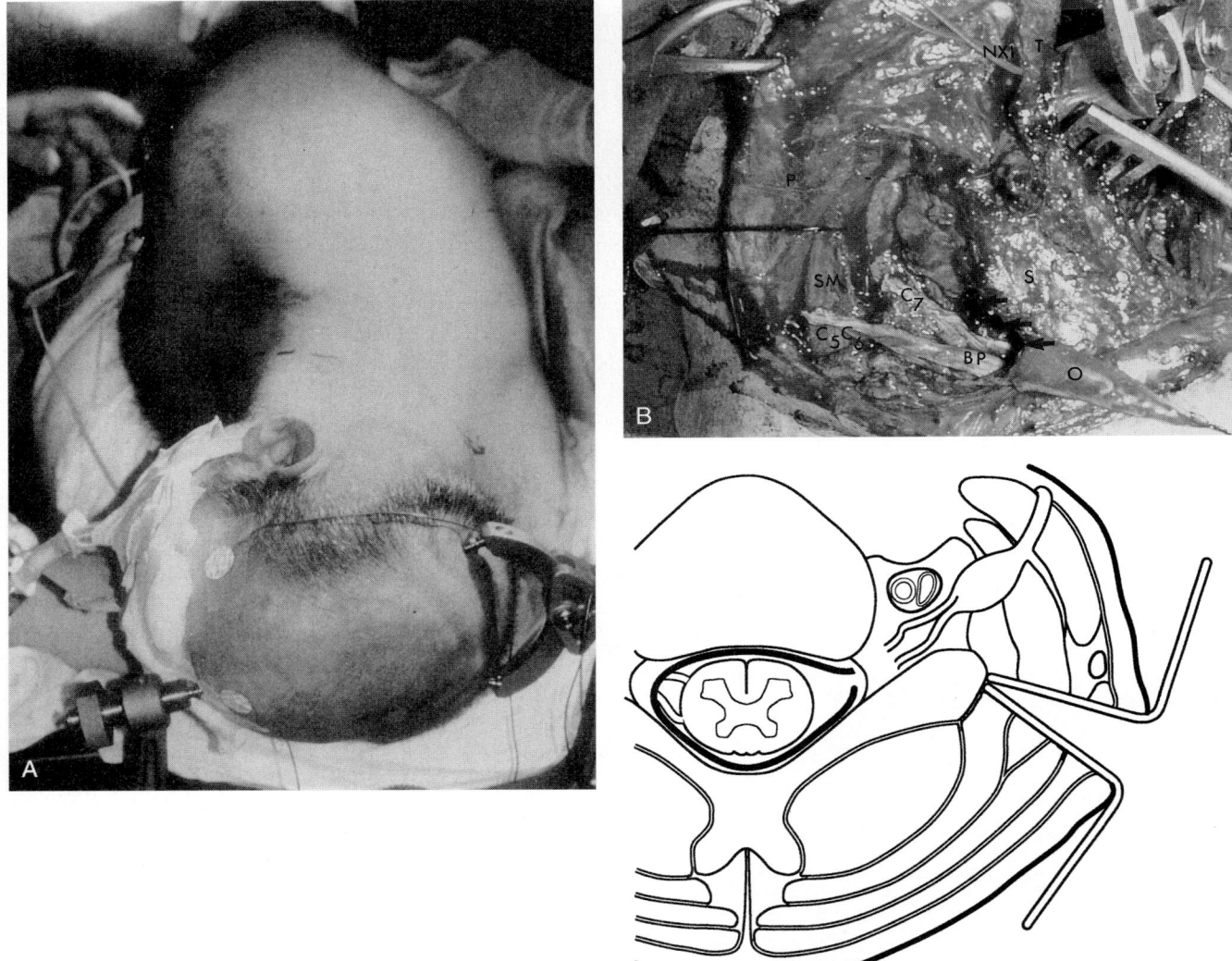

FIGURE 260–3. *A,* The patient is in a lateral position with the head fixed in a Mayfield clamp. The *dashed line* indicates the skin incision from the jugulum into the posterior triangle of the neck and toward the spinous process of C5. Scalp electrodes provide continuous spinal cord monitoring during the procedure. *B,* Intraoperative picture of an exploration of extraspinal parts of the brachial plexus (BP). C5, C6, and C7 spinal nerves are avulsed from the spinal cord. *Arrows* indicate the empty foramina through which endoscopic diagnosis of intraspinal lesions can be made (see Fig. 260–4). There is a sling around the accessory nerve (NXI). A retractor is placed in the posterior part of the wound for the lateral approach to the cervical spine. *C,* Schematic drawing of a transverse section through the lower part of the neck illustrates the far-lateral approach to the cervical spine. The spinal nerve roots have been avulsed from the spinal cord and the subdural space. Notice the relationship to the vertebral vessels. O, omohyoid muscle; P, platysma; S, scalenus muscles; SM, sternocleidomastoid muscle; T, trapezius muscle.

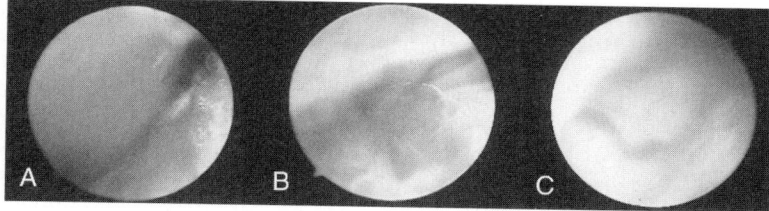

FIGURE 260–4. Intraspinal endoscopy. *A,* The endoscope is placed through the intervertebral foramen of C7. *B,* A vessel is visualized in the medial part of the canal, and a small part of the spinal cord can be seen. *C,* Close to the spinal cord, there are no remaining roots.

root ruptures and reimplantation of avulsed ventral roots into the spinal cord[27–29] (Fig. 260–6). The most devastating injuries are those with four or more intraspinal lesions. The patient has a totally flail and insensible arm with severe pain. The patient also has paralysis of the hemidiaphragm, Bernard-Horner syndrome, and occasionally weakening of the trapezius muscle. With no signs of compromised long fiber tracts in the spinal cord (i.e., Brown-Séquard syndrome) or severe vascular lesions, the patients would be candidates for intraspinal exploration and repair or implantation of avulsed roots if surgery could be performed within days of the accident. Together with appropriate nerve transfers, the intraspinal repair strategy has led to recovery of useful muscle function and to extra benefits, such as alleviating the sometimes excruciating pain and return of some degree of sensation.

The lumbar plexus lesion can be reached through an extraperitoneal approach, with the patient in a lateral position. The lumbosacral trunk situated in front of the sacroiliac joint, which is most susceptible to a traction lesion, can be reached through the transperitoneal route. The intrapelvic part of the sacral plexus can be accessed through a posterior approach after the gluteus maximus muscle has been detached medially.[30] The sacrum and the proximal part of the sciatic nerve are exposed. After the piriform muscle has been cut and the lower ipsilateral half of the sacrum is excised, most of the sacral plexus can be reached. The most proximal part of S1 and S2 is reached after their bony canals in the sacrum have been opened. If the lesion is irrepara-

ble, the lumbosacral plexus is accessible for nerve transfers from lower intercostal nerves[31] and by branches from an uncompromised femoral nerve. However, even in the case of intraspinal lesions, direct repair is sometimes possible. A traction lesion to the lumbosacral plexus rarely results in root avulsions, but rather in root ruptures.[24] A CT-myelogram is useful for tracing the roots of the cauda equina to find the site of rupture. Injured ventral roots can be repaired with functional gain.

Brachial and lumbosacral plexus lesions call for emergency treatment. Surgery should be performed as soon as possible to obtain the best functional outcome.

SPECIAL AND ANCILLARY INVESTIGATIONS

There are increasing numbers of tools at our disposal for exploration of the nervous system, but for the acute nerve injury, there are few diagnostic aids. An electrophysiologic examination must be interpreted expertly so as not to confuse the clinical observations. During the first 2 to 3 weeks, the severity of the nerve lesion can be underestimated by electromyography (EMG) because the trophic influence of the motor nerve on its muscle ceases in accordance with the rate of wallerian degeneration. The typical denervation potentials—positive sharp waves and fibrillations—are not apparent during the first weeks.[32] Even later, when denervation potentials have been established, it is not

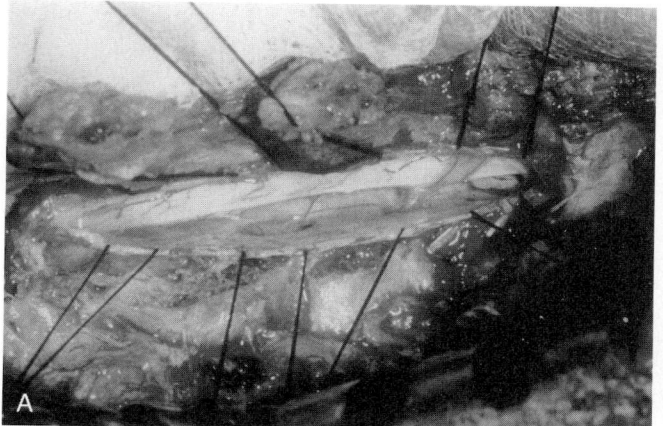

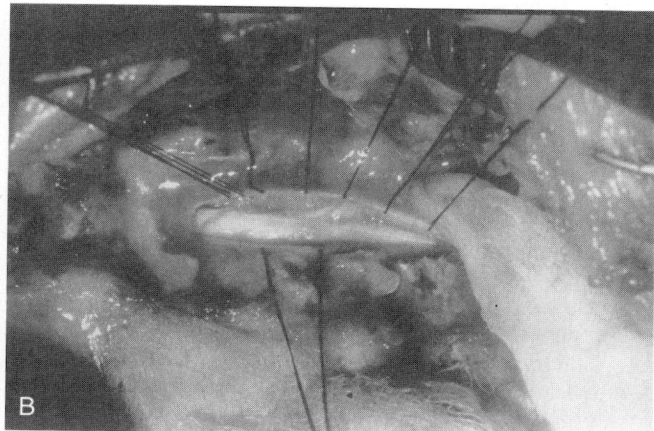

FIGURE 260–5. *A,* On the right side of the spinal cord, C5 to C8 are seen 6 months after a hemilaminectomy for an intradural lesion. There is a pseudomyelomeningocele in the middle part of the exposed cord. Notice the spinal cord atrophy at this level. *B,* The ventral root at C8 is intact, but there is central avulsion of the dorsal root.

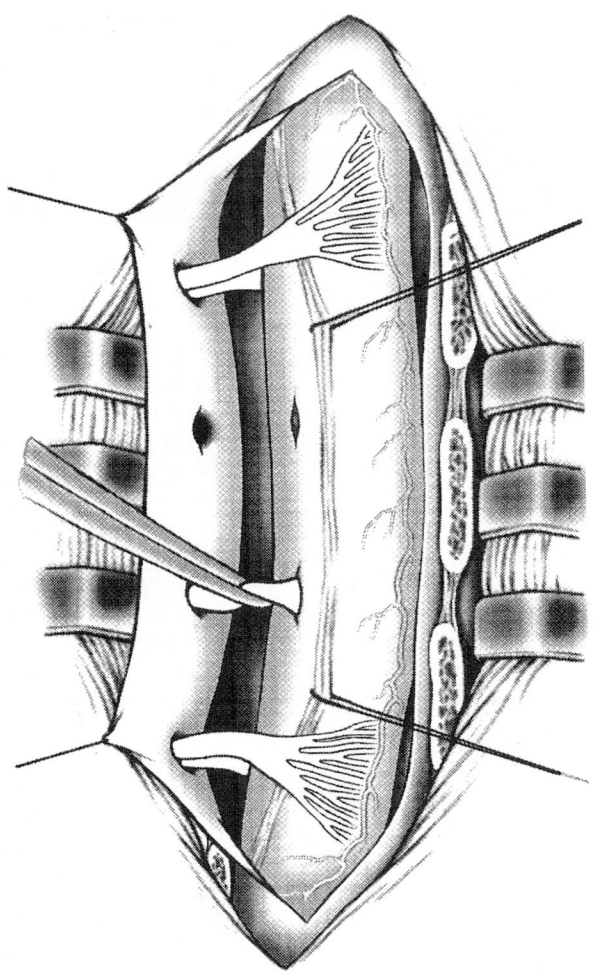

FIGURE 260–6. Schematic drawing depicts the exposed spinal cord after a lateral approach and a hemilaminectomy. The dura mater is opened, and by the stay sutures in the denticulata ligament, the spinal cord has been rotated slightly for access to its ventral part. Through slits in the pia mater and spinal cord surface, nerve grafts are implanted superficially into the spinal cord. (From Carlstedt T, Anand P, Hallin R, et al: Spinal nerve root repair and replantation of avulsed ventral roots into the spinal cord after brachial plexus injury. J Neurosurg 93[Suppl]: 237–247, 2000.)

clear from this test whether the nerve has been severed (i.e., neurotmesis) or has sustained a less severe conduction block (i.e., neuropraxia). Stimulating the nerve distal to the level of the lesion and observing the muscle reaction can be helpful. If there is a normal response in the muscle supplied by the injured nerve, the lesion may be a conduction block. If there is no motor response or if the response is weak, the lesion is probably more severe (i.e., axonotmesis-neurotmesis). This test is not applicable to the most proximal nerve injuries (i.e., brachial or lumbosacral plexus lesion) because it is difficult to stimulate proximal to such a lesion. The presence of a sensory nerve action potential (SNAP) with the simultaneous loss of sensation for the pertinent skin territory indicates that there is a lesion proximal to the ganglion. These severe injuries can be adequately diagnosed electrophysiologically by a normal

SAP together with preserved histamine response.[33] Demonstration of denervation potentials in the paraspinal muscles and absence of somatosensory evoked potentials together with fibrillations and absence of voluntary motor units are proof of the most proximal or intraspinal lesions.

Although the role of electrodiagnosis in adult brachial plexus lesions is limited because of the importance of early intervention, it has been of great value in obstetric brachial plexus lesions. The severity of this lesion is difficult to appreciate clinically. The infants are assessed by a protocol of a combination of mixed nerve action potential (NAP) recordings in the median and ulnar nerves, and electromyographic examination of several muscles. On the basis of these findings, the lesion can be characterized. A full description is offered by Smith.[34]

Preoperative scanning procedures can be useful even in early diagnosis. MRI can demonstrate changes in denervated muscles as early as 4 days after a nerve injury.[35] Magnetic resonance neurography can demonstrate the internal fascicular pattern of a nerve trunk[36] and reveal nerve lesions. This technique may substitute for the current strategy of exploring and intraoperative electrically stimulating a nerve lesion in continuity for assessment of the severity of the lesion. For intraspinal lesions in conjunction with brachial or lumbosacral injuries, CT-myelography has given the most reliable results[14] (see Fig. 260–2).

Intraoperative electrophysiologic assessments have brought advances in determining neural continuity across a lesion discriminating the site of a conduction block. The somatosensory evoked potential is particularly helpful in assessing the intraspinal conduction of an apparently intact part of the brachial plexus. However, an indirect test such as this cannot discriminate between a proximal dorsal root block in conduction and a rupture or avulsion. Moreover, the condition of the ventral root remains unknown. There are indications that the root avulsion injury is mostly a combination of avulsions and dorsal or ventral root ruptures. Only direct inspection by means of endoscopy or a straightforward laminectomy (indicated only in conjunction with intraspinal repair) can give the whole truth about intraspinal nerve plexus lesions.

IATROPATHIC INJURY

The occurrence of nerve injury in conjunction with medical treatment is probably more common than generally believed, and by no means are all cases reported. Mechanisms include direct and indirect injury. Nerves are acutely and directly injured by being impaled and injected, as well as injured in the field of operation by cutting, stretching, compression, and burning. Indirect injury occurs from incorrect positioning of the patient and by closed pressure from hematoma, tourniquet, and traction during general anesthesia.

Intraneural injection can cause mechanical disturbance of the nerve bundles, and the drug can have a direct harmful effect on the nerve fibers.[37] The site of injection is critical because intrafascicular injection produces damage.[38] Agents such as dexamethasone, penicillin, and diazepam are particularly harmful if injected intraneurally.[39] Large, myelinated fibers are more susceptible to damage than small fibers, and injury results in the loss of sensation and motor function. With time, there is often development of epineural fibrosis and intraneural scarring. Early intervention is advised, particularly if the substance injected is known to be neurotoxic, the injection instantly causes severe local and radiating pain, or there is complete paralysis.[21, 37]

The nerve should be widely exposed, and the epineurium should be opened and the nerve irrigated with a buffered physiologic solution. With delayed surgery, the nerve is most likely to develop fibrosis. If there is dense, intraneural fibrosis with loss of conduction and deranged internal fascicular anatomy, resection and repair with a nerve graft is indicated.

Hemorrhage into the neurovascular sheath after arterial puncture or intraneural bleeding in conjunction with the use of drugs that reduce the coagulability of blood (e.g., heparin, warfarin) can cause nerve damage. The onset is sudden, with paralysis and loss of sensation and usually with severe pain radiating down along the trajectory of the nerve. The chief indication for exploration is severe pain. Decompression with evacuation of the hematoma should be performed promptly. Surgery is less likely to be effective if postponed for more than 48 hours.[21, 40]

The most serious damage suffered by nerves is usually that inflicted in the field of operation. Insufficient knowledge of topographic and functional anatomy or pathology of tumors affecting nerves is the main reason for these mistakes. The nerves principally at risk are the brachial plexus, spinal accessory, radial, common peroneal, and ulnar nerves.[20] Two conditions that are most conspicuous are division of the accessory nerve and ignorance about the nature of the most common nerve sheath tumor, the schwannoma. The superficial position of the accessory nerve makes it vulnerable during a lymph node biopsy.[41] The consequence is often shoulder dysfunction in the form of an inability to fully abduct or lift the arm together with winging of the scapula[42] and persistent pain.[43] Delay is common in the diagnosis of this lesion.

The most common and disastrous mistakes are made with schwannomas. This tumor can be treated successfully with surgery, but it is too often misdiagnosed and removed with a part of the adjacent intact nerve.

Swift intervention is the best treatment for iatropathic nerve injuries. If there is loss of function and radiating pain from the site of intervention, a severe nerve lesion that needs to be explored should be suspected until proved otherwise.

Most important is the prevention of iatropathic injury. Minimization of risk depends on recognition of inadequate routines and on augmentation of skills and knowledge. The injury rate can be monitored by means of a registry of general complications.

OBSTETRIC BRACHIAL PLEXUS PALSY

Obstetric brachial plexus palsy (OBPP) in infancy is in many important respects so different from the adult form that lessons from one are not necessarily applicable to the other. Those engaged in this work are in danger of confusion because of the diversity of indications for operation, disagreement about the methods of investigation, continuing uncertainty about the prognosis and natural course, lack of agreement about methods of measuring outcome, and increasing doubts about the quality of results from many repair operations.

There are profound biologic differences between the effects of a proximal traction lesion of the brachial plexus at birth and those in an adult. In the infant, the spinal cord fills the cervical canal, and the spinal roots emerge at (or close to) a right angle to the cord; separation is more likely at the transitional zone than true avulsion. The posterior columns are not fully myelinated in the neonate. As Payan[44] points out, conduction velocity in the full-term neonate is about one half of that found in the normal adult, and normal motor conduction is achieved only by 3 years of age.

Alvares and Fitzgerald[45] summarized some of the immense changes in neurotrophins, neurotransmitters, ion channels, and receptors in the course of maturation from the embryo to adult. In the embryo, NGF is critical for survival of the sensory neurons; in the neonate, NGF regulates innervation density on peripheral targets. At maturity, NGF regulates substance P, CGRP, and other peptides in sensory neurons. Alvares and Fitzgerald[45] wrote that "the developing nervous system is more vulnerable to peripheral injury than the adult, presumably because of its greater dependence on retrograde signals from the periphery for survival." Experimental sectioning of the sciatic nerve of the rat showed 75% loss of neurons in the dorsal root ganglion in the neonate compared with 30% loss in the adult animal.[46] Neuronal death in the neonate is more rapid and involves other cell populations. Johnson and Yip[47] reported that sectioning of the dorsal root in neonatal rats provoked as much cell death as peripheral axonotomy, suggesting "an important role for central trophic support at this stage, although not all agree over this."

This is a striking argument for dealing with carefully selected, severe cases urgently. We next examine the very difficult matter of defining prognosis by means other than surgery.

Incidence, Risk Factors, and Natural History

Platt[48] described the birth lesion as "a vanishing condition," and Seddon[16] wrote that "the decline in the incidence of these injuries during the last forty years . . . is one indication of widespread improvement of the standard of obstetrics." Three large series of consecutive live births in U.S. hospitals found 113 cases in 58,000 births,[49–51] but there is some evidence that the incidence is increasing. Bager[52] surveyed one county in Sweden and found an incidence of 1.4 cases per 1000 births in 1980, which rose to 2.3 cases per 1000 births in 1994. The British Paediatric Surveillance Unit conducted a prospective study, and preliminary data, which has not yet been corrected, suggests 350 cases in more than 500,000 live births.

Workers in France and Italy defined the major risk factors more than 100 years ago. The heavy baby and the breech baby were especially at risk. Tan[53] found an incidence of 0.14 cases in 1000 vertex deliveries, increasing to 25.4 cases for breech deliveries. Boo[54] saw a similar increase complicating breech deliveries in Malaysian patients. The breech lesion in delivery is severe and often bilateral. Gilbert[55] found a high incidence of preganglionic injury. Slooff and Blaauw[56] reported 40 cases of OBPP in breech deliveries; at least one spinal nerve had been avulsed from the spinal cord in 35 of these cases. The lesion was bilateral in 11 cases, and phrenic palsy complicated 12 cases.

We studied risk factors in 230 consecutive cases.[57] There was no correlation with social class; there was a trend, which was not statistically significant, for the mother being shorter and heavier than the national average and for excessive weight gain during pregnancy. One factor of incontrovertible significance was the birth weight of the baby, with a mean of 4.5 kg compared with the mean for the North West Thames Region of 3.88 kg. Birth weight increased with the severity of the lesion. Shoulder dystocia was recorded as a complication in just over 60% of all cases of OBPP within the 230 cases analyzed. Power[58] provides an explanation for the apparent increase in OBPP in the United Kingdom, finding a 0.4% average increase in birth weight between 1981 and 1992 in Scotland and a mean annual increase of 0.35% in earlier years in England and Wales.

The direct physical cause of the lesion is the forced separation of the forequarter from the axial skeleton caused by obstruction at the narrowest point of the birth canal. When the shoulder is forward, separation is in the downward direction; when there is obstruction to breech delivery, it is in an upward direction.

Although the diagnosis is usually straightforward, fracture of the clavicle or humerus may cause immobility mimicking paralysis. Neonatal sepsis of the glenohumeral joint does the same, and we have seen cases

of cerebral palsy, arthrogryposis, and ischemic injury to the cord mimicking OBPP. The possibility of intrauterine causation is a factor in medicolegal disputes. Dunn and Engle[59] described cases of birth palsy from abnormal intrauterine posture. Jennett and colleagues[60] found marked differences between cases of OBPP born without shoulder dystocia compared with those born with dystocia; the latter were heavier babies born to older mothers and suggested possible intrauterine factors in the former. We have seen three cases in which ultrasound scanning showed the umbilical cord to be wrapped around the neck. These babies were born with complete lesions and Bernard-Horner syndrome. Despite these findings, recovery was full in one child at 6 months, and hand function was normal in the other two by 24 months, outcomes that were much more favorable than might have been expected. Occasionally, intrauterine causation must be admitted. Paradiso[61] found persuasive electromyographic evidence. There have been a handful of reports describing congenital aplasia of the spinal nerves.

It remains difficult to define the natural progress for recovery in any individual child, and no rational proposals for intervention can be made without such knowledge. An important contribution was the classification proposed by Narakas[62] (Table 260–1). It is widely used, and we commend it:

Group 1: The fifth and sixth cervical nerves are damaged. There is paralysis of deltoid and biceps. About 90% of babies proceed to full, spontaneous recovery, with clinical evidence of that recovery becoming plain at no later than 3 months.

Group 2: The fifth, sixth, and seventh cervical nerves are damaged; the shoulder, the elbow, and the wrist extensors are paralyzed. About 65% of these children make a full, spontaneous recovery; defects of function persist in the remainder. Recovery is generally slower, often delayed by 3 to 6 months.

Group 3: Paralysis is virtually complete, although there is some flexion of the fingers at or shortly after birth. Full, spontaneous recovery occurs in less than one half of these children; most are left with substantial impairment at the shoulder and

T A B L E 2 6 0 – 1 ■ **Clinical Classification of Obstetric Brachial Plexus Palsy**

GROUP	NERVES INJURED	PRESENTATION	LIKELY COURSE
Group 1	C5-6	Paralysis of shoulder, elbow flexion	Spontaneous recovery in >80%
Group 2	C5-6-7	As above with wrist drop	Good hand; good shoulder and elbow in about 60%
Group 3	All	Complete paralysis	Good hand in most; good shoulder and elbow in 30–50%
Group 4*	All	Complete paralysis, Bernard-Horner sign; limb may be atonic, marbled, and cold	Full recovery is rare; severe defects throughout the limb likely

* Shortening of the limb may be severe in group 4, with atrophy of the hand. Occasionally, the ipsilateral foot is smaller, suggesting an element of cord lesion.

Adapted from Narakas AO: Obstetrical brachial plexus injuries. In Lamb DW (ed): The Paralysed Hand. Edinburgh, Churchill Livingstone, 1987, pp 116–135.

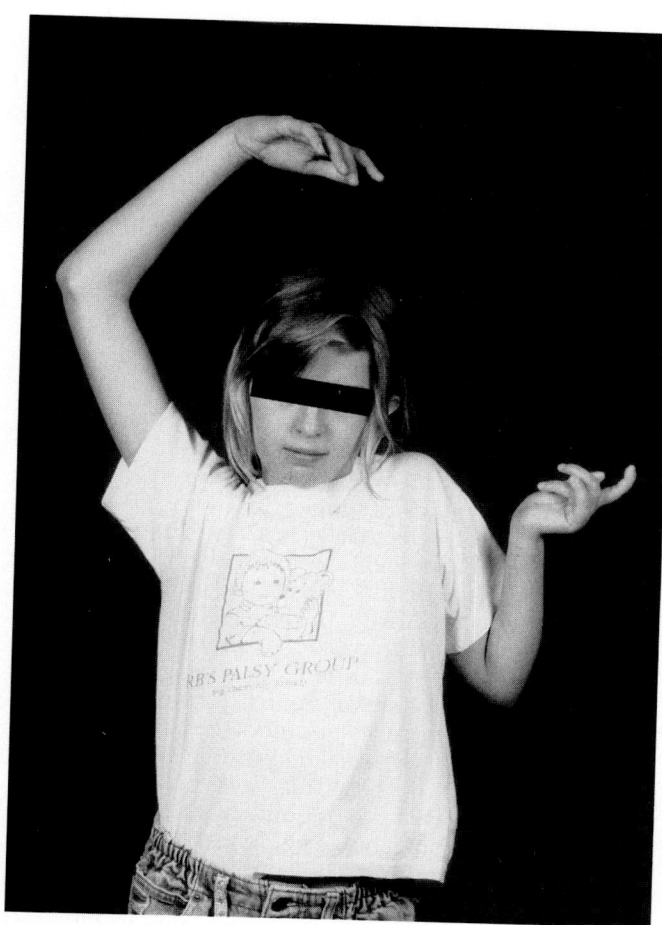

FIGURE 260–7. This 13-year-old girl has a group 4 lesion that was never treated. There was spontaneous recovery for the sixth cervical nerve, giving her elbow flexion and extension of the wrist, and some very limited recovery for C8, providing active flexion in the ring and middle fingers. Her shoulder was flail, the triceps muscle was paralyzed, the forearm lay in a supinated posture, the grasp was weak, and intrinsic function in the hand was absent. Sensation was good in the thumb and index finger, but it was defective elsewhere. She had no pain.

elbow, with defective rotation of the forearm. Wrist and finger extension does not recover in about one fourth of the children.

Group 4: The whole plexus is involved. Paralysis is complete. The limb is atonic, and the child has Bernard-Horner syndrome. Scarcely any child makes a full recovery; spinal nerves have been ruptured or avulsed from the spinal cord, and there is permanent and serious defect throughout the limb (Fig. 260–7).

The disparity of limb length ranges from up to 2% in group 1 to 20% in group 4. Damage to the spinal cord, which occurs in at least 2% of group 4 babies, manifests as delayed, unsteady walking and small size of the ipsilateral foot. The classification should be applied between 2 and 4 weeks, when lesions of simple conduction block have recovered or are beginning to recover. For the individual case, it cannot be taken as an accurate predictor of prognosis, and it is therefore

not an indication for operation. The classification does not recognize the true Klumpke lesion of isolated palsy of C8 and T1. It does not distinguish group 1 cases from breech delivery, for which the outlook is materially worse, nor does it recognize that a lesion in which the middle nerves, C7 and C8 in particular, are affected worse.[63]

We emphasize that the prognosis for group 4 lesions is not hopeless. We have seen 24 children born with Bernard-Horner syndrome and total paralysis, with only scanty evidence of recovery by 12 months from birth, who later regained good hand function. Bernard-Horner syndrome suggests avulsion but is not absolute proof.

What more can be done to predict the natural outcome? There have been many descriptions of the evolution of paralysis, some describing a favorable outcome for most cases. One such came from our late colleague, A. J. Harrold, a particularly astute clinician who recorded a favorable outcome in more than 80% of cases.[64] Equal weight must be given to the findings of investigators such as Sharrad,[65] who found that recovery was poor in at least one half of those born with a complete lesion. Eng and coworkers[66, 67] studied 135 children in particular detail, recording severe and persistent problems in about 30%. One notable finding was the demonstration of neurapraxia in eight of these children. Narakas,[62] in his original description of 490 children, found that few children with complete lesions recovered good function at the shoulder but that 90% regained useful hand function. Zancolli and Zancolli[68] found that one fifth of those with C8 to T1 lesions did not recover hand function. When there was no sign of hand function by 6 months, the outlook was especially poor.

The experience of Alain Gilbert is immense, and his recommendations command respect. Tassin[69] studied 44 of Gilbert's cases from birth to the age of 5 years and found that function at the shoulder was poor in children when recovery of the biceps and deltoid was delayed beyond 3 months. Gilbert and associates[70] defined indications for surgery, which should be recommended for patients with group 4 lesions; for patients in groups 1 and 2 who have no recovery by 3 months in the setting of unfavorable electromyographic evidence; and for those in group 1 if there is no clinical evidence of recovery of the biceps by 3 months. A more cautious approach was suggested by Michelow,[71] who devised a scoring system marking the recovery of different functions within the limb, including abduction at the shoulder, flexion at the elbow, extension of the wrist, and finger movements. A low score indicates poor or no recovery for a number of these functions, and it may be taken as an indication for operation. Laurent and colleagues[72] focus on recovery of three muscles—biceps, triceps, and deltoid—as measures of progression.

Recovery within 8 weeks is encouraging. In cases of children with favorable lesions, parents report powerful grasp at 2 weeks and flexion at shoulder and elbow between 2 and 8 weeks. Return of the grasp within 4 weeks virtually guarantees that the child will regain good hand function. We agree with Gilbert and Tassin[73] that progress for the fifth cervical nerve is monitored by the deltoid muscle and that function of the sixth cervical nerve is monitored by the biceps. Persistent paralysis at 3 months confirms a deep lesion of these two nerves. Pitfalls include spurious elevation of shoulder by the pectoralis major; the examiner should assess the child lying supine and observe true lateral elevation. Some children in groups 3 and 4 show recovery of the shoulder and arm by 3 to 6 months but never regain worthwhile hand function. They present later with supination deformity of the forearm, atrophy of the digits, and very limited flexion. In these cases, there has been useful recovery through C5 and very limited recovery for T1 with ruptures or avulsions of C6, C7, and C8. Another group of children show very good recovery for C5 and C6 injuries and present with good function at the shoulder, elbow control, and wrist extension, but they have no useful function in the hand. These have avulsions of C7, C8, and T1.

Persistent anesthesia is rare. Sympathetic function usually returns, and self-mutilation is distinctly uncommon. One child, who was 9 years old when we first saw her, had started to recover from a complete lesion at 8 months of age. Arm and forearm muscle function was good, but the distal extensors and flexors were powerful, and there was intrinsic balance. The Bernard-Horner syndrome persisted, and the child constantly chewed her fingers and had sustained unnoticed burns. Assessment of sensation showed remarkably good localization and proprioception; recognition of shapes and textures was present but impaired. The hand was dry. This suggests that the sympathetic outflow did not recover and that there was disproportionate impairment of Aδ and C fiber function, possibly indicating that there was damage to the anterolateral tract and descending autonomic fibers.

Supplementary Investigations

Gilbert[55] commended myelography for the detection of avulsion, finding 3 false-negative and 10 false-positive results in 395 roots examined by this technique. Sloof and Blaauw[56] described the advantages of CT-myelography and of MRI in showing hematoma within the spinal canal and identifying atrophy and denervation of muscles. Francel and associates[74] use fast spin-echo MRI, which provides high-speed, noninvasive imaging and permits clinicians "to evaluate pre-ganglionic nerve root injuries without the use of general anesthesia and lumbar puncture."

The place of neurophysiologic investigation remains controversial. Some clinicians with great experience have found the investigation unreliable because it offers unduly favorable evidence. It is only fair to say that electrophysiologic investigation must be done expertly and results must be interpreted expertly. Smith[34, 75] acquired great experience from analysis of more than 500 infants, assessing babies by combining mixed NAP recordings from the median and ulnar nerves of the forearm with EMG of appropriate muscles. The findings are described in Table 260–2. Smith sums up the role of electrodiagnosis as "firstly to determine the extent and level of involvement of the individual component of the plexus; secondly to identify root avulsion; and thirdly, to define the nature of the lesion in terms of neurapraxic, axonotmetic, and neurotmetic injury, to assist in making a prognosis." Kono matched these preoperative predictions with findings in 150 of our operated cases and showed a high level of accuracy (H. Kono, personal communication, 1999). At surgery, 138 of 145 roots classified as type C were found to be ruptured or avulsed, or both. Premature electrodiagnostic investigation shows evidence of a compete degenerative lesion, implying that the outlook is less favorable than it is; these tests seem to be most reliable from about 12 weeks of age. Ideally, intervention in the most severe cases can be done earlier than this.

The operative findings for children are less distinct than for adults. Fibrosis can be immense. Intraoperative neurophysiologic work is valuable. Sensory evoked potentials are recorded from each spinal nerve proximal and distal to the lesion, and the distal muscular response is noted. In postganglionic injury, there is always some distal muscular response; often, NAPs can be recorded across the lesion. In the neonatal injury, compete intradural rupture without displacement of the dorsal root ganglion is more likely; the spinal

T A B L E 2 6 0 – 2 ■ Classification of the Neurological Lesion by Electrodiagnostic Investigation

TYPE	NAP	EMG	LESION
Type A	Normal	No spontaneous activity; reduced number of normal motor units; increased firing rates	Conduction block
Type B (favorable)	Normal or >50% of uninjured side	Relatively good motor unit recruitment; mixture of normal units and potentials suggesting collateral reinnervation	Mild axonal (degenerative) lesion; axonotmesis
Type B (unfavorable)	Absent or <50% of uninjured side	Normal units few or absent; collateral reinnervation	Significant axonal lesion (neurotmesis)
Type C	Absent, occasionally present	Spontaneous activity; nascent units; poor recruitment	Severe axonal; injury (neurotmesis or intradural)

EMG, electromyography; NAP, nerve action potential.
Data from Smith SJM: The role of neurophysiological investigation in traumatic brachial plexus injuries in adults and children. J Hand Surg Br 21: 145–148, 1996, and from Smith SJM: Electrodiagnosis. In Birch R, Bonney G, Wynn Parry C (eds): Surgical Disorders of the Peripheral Nerves, 1st ed. Edinburgh, Churchill Livingstone, 1998, pp 467–490.

TABLE 260–3 ■ Classification of the Nerve Lesion by Electrophysiologic Evidence and Operative Findings

LESION	PREOPERATIVE NEUROPHYSIOLOGIC EVIDENCE	INTRAOPERATIVE NEUROPHYSIOLOGIC EVIDENCE			APPEARANCE OF NERVES AT OPERATION	COURSE OF SPONTANEOUS RECOVERY
		SEP from Spinal Nerve	Distal Muscle Response	SEP from Nerves Distal to Lesion		
Prolonged conduction block	Type A	Normal	Strong	Normal	Normal; perhaps some surrounding fibrosis	Normal
Recovering postganglionic rupture	B favorable	Normal	Strong	Usually present	Nerve thickened, fusiform swelling	Useful, possibly normal
Unfavorable postganglionic rupture	B unfavorable	Normal	Weak	Usually absent	Obvious neuroma, firm or hard, which may be "double humped"	Poor to fair; never normal
Unfavorable postganglionic rupture with some intradural lesion	B unfavorable or C	Abnormal	Very weak	Absent	Fibrosed, tortuous, elongated, attenuated or thickened.	Poor
Selective intradural lesion to ventral or dorsal roots	Variable: depends on whether ventral or dorsal roots are damaged	Present or absent	Weak or none	Present or absent	Normal or atrophic, surrounding fibrosis	Poor to fair, with defects in sensory or motor function
Complete intradural lesion without displacement of dorsal root ganglion	Type C	Absent	None	Absent	Atrophied	None
Complete intradural lesion, dorsal root ganglion displaced into posterior triangle of neck	Type C	Absent	None	Absent	Dorsal root ganglion with ventral and dorsal roots evident	None

SEP, sensory evoked potential.

nerves, when avulsed, are less frequently displaced distal to the scalenus anterior; and there is always some regeneration of fibers traversing the postganglionic rupture. Two lesions are particularly perplexing. In the first, an elongated and fibrosed nerve is displayed in which there is some conduction; recovery is poor in most cases. The second is the "silent nerve," which is apparently intact but shows no peripheral or central conduction. Although most of these patients do not recover, some do unexpectedly. Table 260–3 provides a classification of the types of injury to individual spinal nerves seen during surgery. Repair is indicated in type 3 and reinnervation by nerve transfer in types 4, 5, 6, and 7 (Fig. 260–8).

Simple clinical methods of recording recovery are described in Figures 260–9 and 260–10 and Tables 260–4 to 260–6. Full evaluation of hand function requires very much more than this. Anand[25] used quantitative assessment for the different modalities of sensation in a number of cases after repair of severe group IV lesions showing remarkable recovery of sensation. His demonstration of perfect localization of restored sensa-

tion in avulsed spinal root dermatomes, presumably routed through nerves that have been transferred from the distal spinal region, is evidence of CNS plasticity. Sensory recovery exceeded motor or sympathetic recovery in these cases.

Serial studies of limb function by appropriately skilled and experienced occupational therapists and physiotherapists are also valuable, but these must be modified to match the age of the child.

Recovery is slow. In some of our group IV cases, no evidence of recovery was seen in the hand until 3 years had passed, but the trophic state of the limb improved much earlier. Perhaps this prolonged course reflects the slow maturation of muscle spindles, proprioceptive function, and other afferent functions. In almost every case, the injured side becomes nondominant and stays so. It is rare to encounter cases of neuropathic pain.

The largest series of results comes from Gilbert,[55] who found that results for repairs of group I and group II lesions were generally good. In 54 children with total lesions, reinnervation of the lower trunk produced useful finger flexion in 75% of cases and useful intrinsic

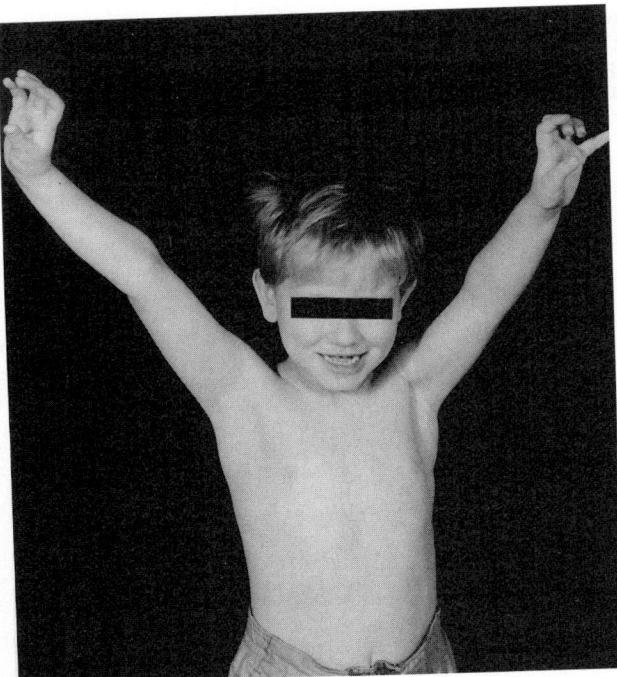

FIGURE 260–8. This 5-year-old boy had ruptures of C5 and C6 repaired at 6 months of age. Electrophysiologic assessment predicted that C6 would be classified as type C, and intraoperative work confirmed evidence of partial intradural injury. The result 4.5 years after the repair is shown. Elbow flexion was weak.

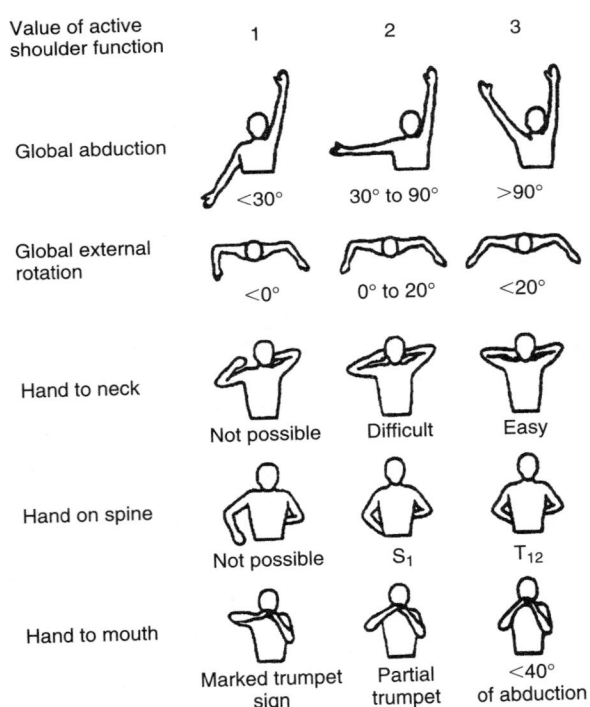

FIGURE 260–9. The Mallet system of measuring function is a simple system to use in clinics. Five functions are measured, and a score ranging from 1 to 3 is given. A score of 15 represents a good shoulder but by no means a normal one. A score of 11 or 12 indicates a shoulder in which there is useful function. A score of 10 or less is a poor shoulder.

TABLE 260–4 ■ **System for Grading Shoulder Function**

Stage 0	Flail shoulder
Stage I*	Abduction or flexion to 45 degrees; no active lateral rotation
Stage II	Abduction <90 degrees; lateral rotation to neutral
Stage III	Abduction = 90 degrees; weak lateral rotation
Stage IV	Abduction <120 degrees; incomplete lateral rotation
Stage V	Abduction >120 degrees; active lateral rotation
Stage VI	Normal

* The suffix + is added to indicate sufficient medial rotation permitting the hand to come against the opposite shoulder. Our convention restricts children with no lateral rotation beyond neutral to stage I, usually I+ because adequate medial rotation is maintained.

Data from Gilbert A: Evaluation of results in obstetrical brachial plexus palsy: Systems for shoulder. Presented at the International Meeting on Obstetric Brachial Plexus Palsy, 1993, Heerlen, Netherlands, and from Birch R, Bonney G, Wynn Parry C (eds): Surgical Disorders of the Peripheral Nerves. Edinburgh, Churchill Livingstone, 1998.

TABLE 260–5 ■ **Method for Evaluating Elbow Function**

FUNCTION	SCORE
Flexion	
Nil or some contraction	1
Incomplete flexion	2
Complete flexion	3
Extension	
No extension	0
Weak Extension	1
Good extension	2
Extension deficit	
0–30 degrees	0
30–50 degrees	−1
>50 degrees	−2

Data from Gilbert A, Raimondi P: A system of evaluation of elbow flexion. Presented at the International Meeting on Obstetric Brachial Plexus Palsy, 1993, Heerlen, Netherlands, and from Birch R, Bonney G, Wynn Parry C (eds): Surgical Disorders of the Peripheral Nerves. Edinburgh, Churchill Livingstone, 1998.

TABLE 260–6 ■ **Hand Evaluation Scale**

0	Complete paralysis or slight finger flexion of no use; useless thumb and no pinch; some or no sensation
I	Limited active flexion of fingers; no extension of wrist or fingers; possibility of thumb lateral pinch
II	Active flexion of wrist with passive flexion of fingers (tenodesis); passive lateral pinch of thumb
III	Active complete flexion of wrist and fingers; mobile thumb with partial abduction, opposition. Intrinsic balance with no active supination; good possibilities for palliative surgery
IV	Active complete flexion of wrist and fingers; active wrist extension; weak or absent finger extension. Good thumb opposition with active ulnaris intrinsics. Partial pronosupination
V	Hand grade IV with finger extension and almost complete pronosupination

Data from Raimondi P: Evaluation of the hand. Presented at the International Meeting on Obstetric Brachial Plexus Palsy, 1993, Heerlen, Netherlands, and from Birch R, Bonney G, Wynn Parry C (eds): Surgical Disorders of the Peripheral Nerves. Edinburgh, Churchill Livingstone, 1998.

Assessment Form: Royal National Orthopaedic Hospital
Peripheral Nerve Injury and Congenital Hand Unit
Shoulder Operations in Obstetric Brachial Plexus Palsy Patients

Name	Tassin	D.O.O.	X-rays	EMG	Operation	Surgical Pathology
					On BP: On shoulder:	Of plexus: Of shoulder: 1. Dislocation 2. Subluxation 3. Contracture 4. Flail
Seen by TO: Before opn: After opn:	Mallett Score Before opn: After opn:				Gilbert Grading (shoulder) Before opn: After opn:	Raimondi Grading (hand) Before opn: After opn:

Range of movement

FF		ER		GH angle		ABD		IR		Rotation forearm		FF		ER		GH angle		ABD		IR		Rotation forearm	
Ac	Pa	Ac	Pa	Ac	Pa	Ac	Pa	Ac	Pa	Ac	Pa	Ac	Pa	Ac	Pa	Ac	Pa	Ac	Pa	Ac	Pa	Ac	Pa

FIGURE 260–10. Our system records the active and passive range of movement in different axes of the shoulder joint. We now record the active and passive ranges of pronation and supination separately.

function in 50%. Gilbert proposed reinnervation of the hand in cases of avulsion of C7, C8, and T1 by transfer of adjacent spinal nerves that had been ruptured; he also conceived the idea of selective reinnervation of the avulsed ventral root by transfer of the spinal accessory nerve. Such methods provide the only chance of regaining any hand function in the most severe cases of multiple avulsions of the lower nerves. For the worst case, however, Tassin's[69] statement remains true: "Si seule persiste C5, le pronostie est effroyanle."

Further clarification of the indications for surgery is urgently needed. We need to know much more than we do about the natural course of spontaneous recovery, and there must be better definition of measurement of results. It can be said that repairs of severe ruptures are justifiable and that reinnervation of the limb by nerve transfer is better than nothing when there have been multiple avulsions. Gu's technique[76] of contralateral C7 transfer may be indicated when there has been avulsion of C5 and C6 or avulsion of the lower nerves of the plexus, although preferably by a technique that does not call for the use of the ulnar nerve. In severe cases, the earlier the repair is done, the better.

Medial Rotation Contracture and Posterior Dislocation of the Shoulder

Medial rotation contracture and posterior dislocation of the shoulder represent the most common and most significant secondary deformity in OBPP (Fig. 260–11). We found it necessary to operate on almost 500 children in our series of more than 1200. Delay in diagnosis is common. Fairbank[77] recognized that the subscapularis muscle was an important element in the contracture. Sever[78] described radiologic features, including "marked elongation of the coracoid process." Scaglietti,[79] reporting on Putti's work, thought that the deformity was caused by direct injury to the growing skeleton at birth: "The most constant and characteristic change is in the deformation of the angle of declination" (i.e., retroversion of the head of humerus on the shaft).

The controversy continued. Zancolli and Zancolli[68] thought that damage to the growth plate was the major factor, whereas Gilbert,[80] writing in the same volume, commented that "posterior subluxation and deformity of the humeral head permanently worsens the progno-

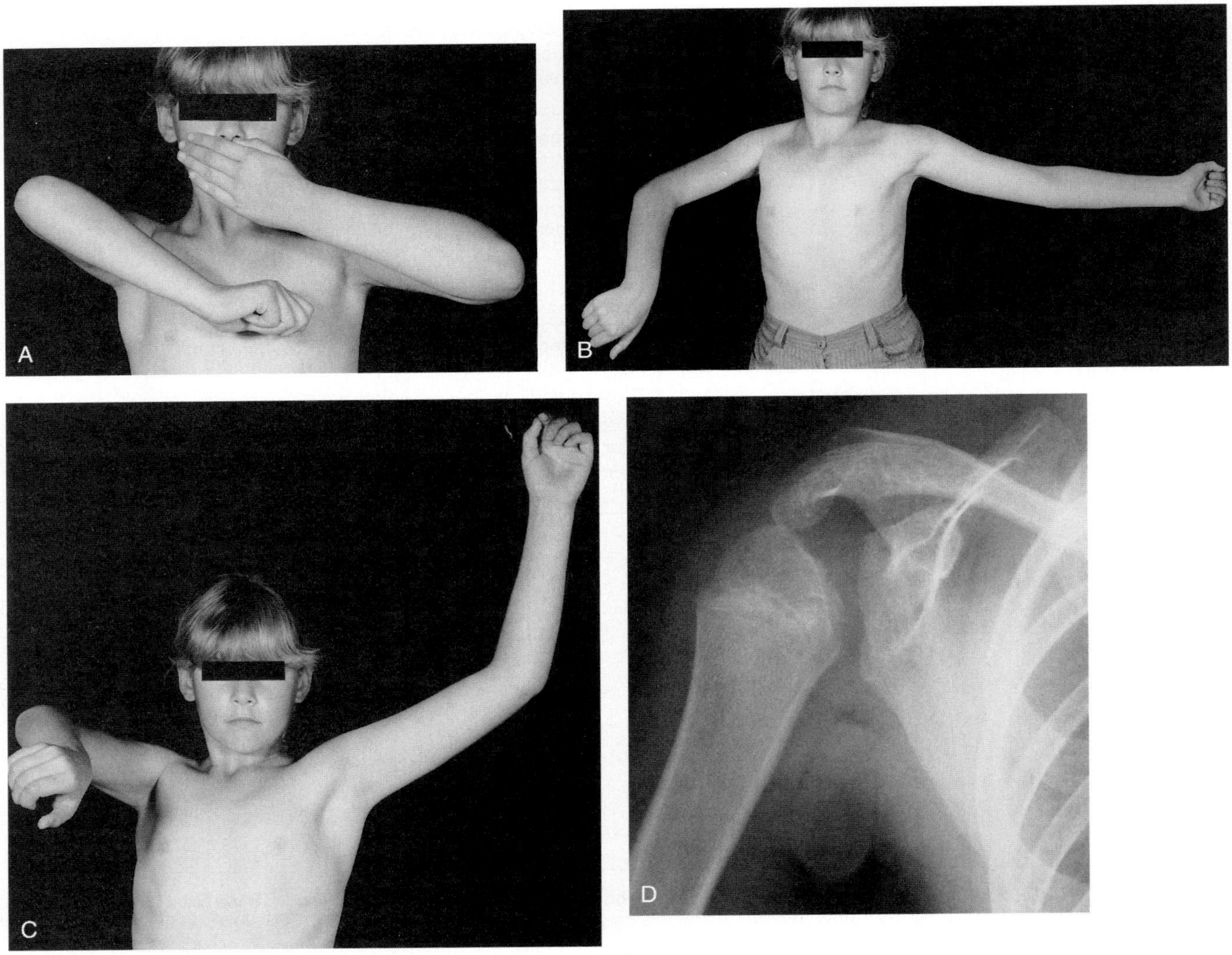

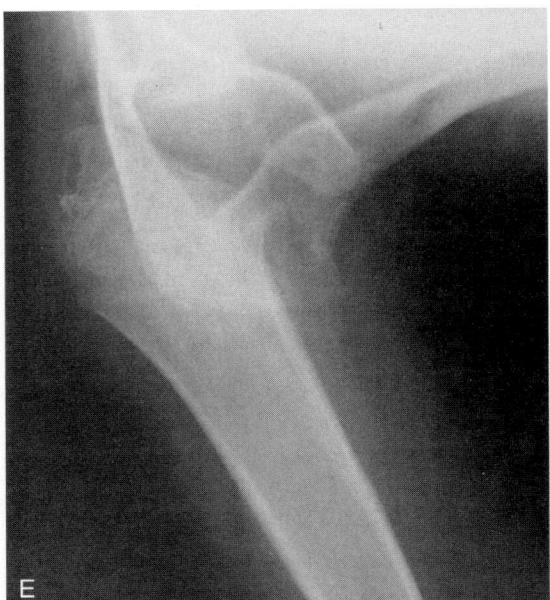

FIGURE 260–11. A through C, This 9-year-old girl had an untreated posterior dislocation of the head of the humerus. She had 100 degrees of elevation at the shoulder, a fixed medial rotation contracture exceeding 40 degrees, medial rotation of 90 degrees, and active pronation-supination of 90 degrees. D and E, The radiographs showed advanced changes, with deformity of the head of the humerus, overgrowth of the acromion, and a double facet appearance of the glenoid. The deformed head of the humerus articulated with the false glenoid.

sis. These anomalies, which have long been considered the results of obstetric palsy are in consequence of untreated contractures." These views are not incompatible. Our experience suggests that both are correct and represent important contributions.

Liang Chen studied a number of our cases, and classification of the deformity and summary of the outcomes in 60 cases rest on his work (Table 260–7). These children had good hand function and useful recovery for C5, C6, and C7 spontaneously or after repair. The dislocation probably occurred at birth in 11 babies. In most patients, the deformity developed or progressed while under observation, and in some, it occurred after repair of the upper trunk despite continuing observation and a rigorous course of exercises. In most cases, the primary cause is the neurological lesion. C5 and C6 are damaged, causing paralysis of the lateral rotator muscles. The medial rotators, particularly the subscapularis, innervated by the seventh and eighth cervical nerves are never paralyzed or are only weakened for a short time so that their action is unopposed. The tempo of progression is not related to age; marked secondary bone changes have been seen in children 3 years old or younger. However, dislocation in the presence of only minor deformity has been seen in children 11 or 12 years of age. The deformity is progressive, and there is a spectrum of injury from medial rotation contracture to full posterior dislocation of the shoulder. We have never encountered a case of anterior dislocation.

The diagnosis is made by clinical examination. The posture of the arm is characteristic; it lies in medial rotation with flexion and pronation at the elbow. The contour of the shoulder is abnormal; the head is prominent behind the glenoid, and palpation confirms abnormality of the coracoid and acromion. Measurements of the extent of contracture also indicate the extent of skeletal abnormality and soft tissue contracture. The difference between the active and passive ranges of motion gives an indication of the contribution to the observed defect from muscle weakness. In nearly every case, a clear impression of the diagnosis and the extent of secondary deformity can be achieved by physical examination and by plain anteroposterior and axial radiographs. The use of arthrography, MRI, and CT has been reported.[81, 82] The untreated deformity has severe consequences for function in the upper limb as a whole. By late adolescence or early adult life, movements of the shoulder girdle are greatly restricted. The upper limb lies in fixed medial rotation, there is pain from the disorganized glenohumeral joint, the flexion pronation posture of the elbow has become fixed, and there may be subluxation of the head of the radius. It is easy to miss the diagnosis in the first 12

T A B L E 2 6 0 – 7 ■ Clinical Classification of Shoulder Deformity

TYPE	RELATION OF HEAD OF HUMERUS TO GLENOID	CLINICAL EVIDENCE*	RADIOLOGIC EVIDENCE	SUPPLEMENTARY INVESTIGATIONS†
Medial rotation contracture	Congruent	Loss of passive lateral rotation of 30 degrees or more	Normal; coracoid may be elongated	Ultrasound—congruent; MR scan may show retroversion of head on shaft of humerus
Simple subluxation	Head of humerus in false glenoid	Lateral rotation to neutral; head palpable posteriorly	Incongruent; no other skeletal abnormality	Ultrasound, CT, and MR scans confirm incongruency; retroversion and "double facet" of glenoid may be seen
Simple dislocation	Head of humerus posterior to glenoid	Fixed medial rotation contracture at about 30 degrees, head evidently lying behind glenoid	Head of humerus behind glenoid; no other skeletal deformity	Ultrasound, CT, and MR scans confirm; retroversion may be seen
Complex subluxation	Head of humerus in false glenoid; secondary bone deformity	Lateral rotation to neutral or less; overgrowth of coracoid and acromion palpable	Extent of coracoid and acromion abnormality seen; "double facet" of glenoid	Confirms incongruency and skeletal abnormality but may mislead about glenoid shape
Complex dislocation	Head of humerus behind glenoid; secondary bone deformity	Fixed medial rotation contracture of 30 degrees or more; obvious secondary bone changes	Head of humerus behind glenoid; overgrowth of coracoid and acromion; abnormality of glenoid	Confirms dislocation and extent of skeletal abnormality

* In all cases, a flexion-pronation posture of elbow and forearm is seen. In advanced cases, this deformity becomes fixed, and may be associated with dislocation of head of radius.

† The extent of retroversion of the head on the shaft of the humerus cannot be measured accurately by any ancillary investigation, and it is best determined during an open reduction operation.

Data from Chen L: Results of reduction of the dislocated shoulder. In Birch R, Bonney G, Wynn Parry C (eds): Surgical Disorders of the Peripheral Nerves. Edinburgh, Churchill Livingstone, 1998.

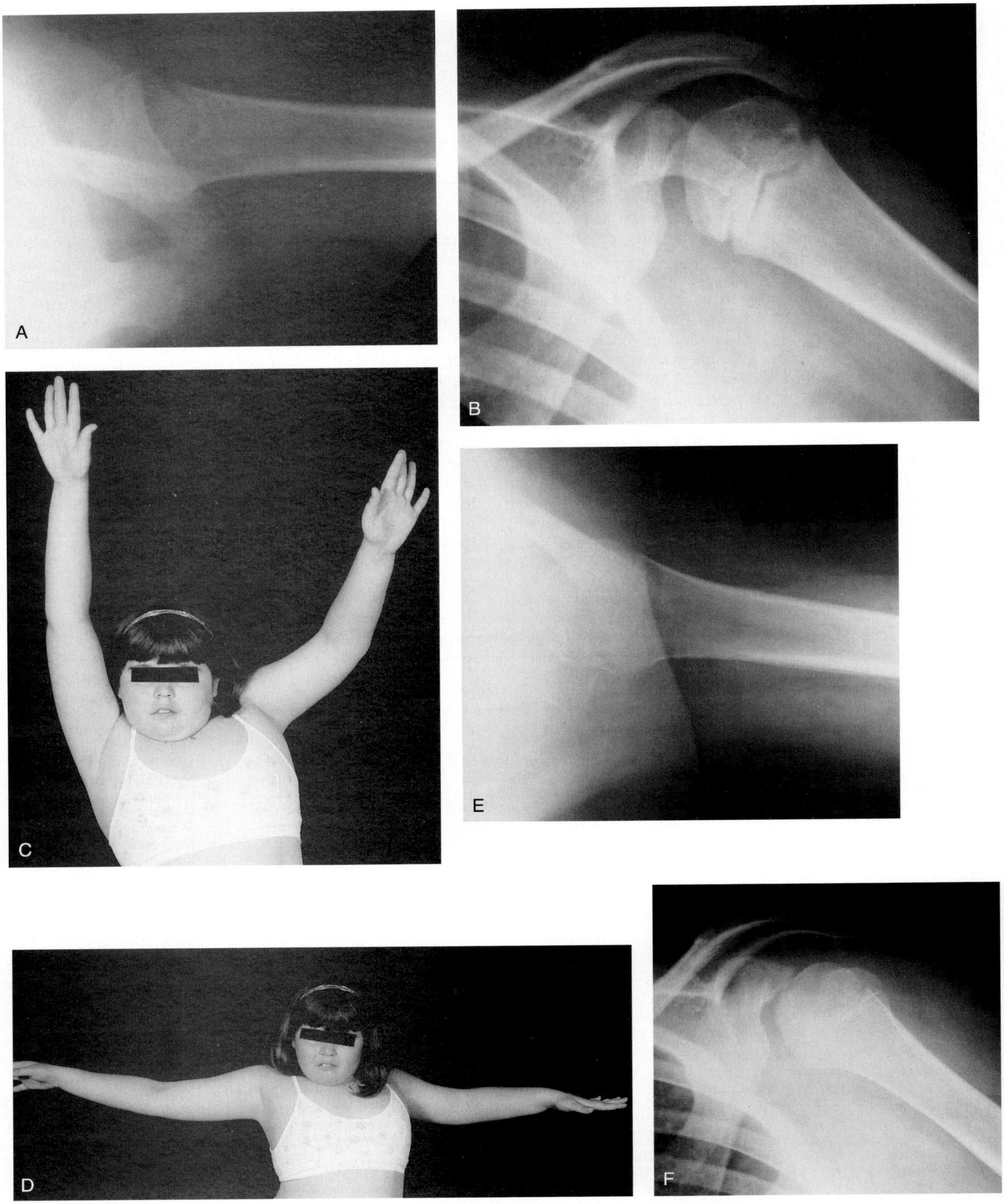

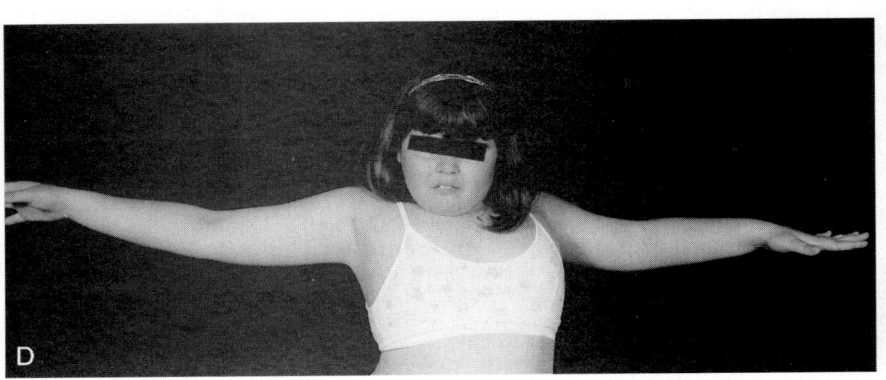

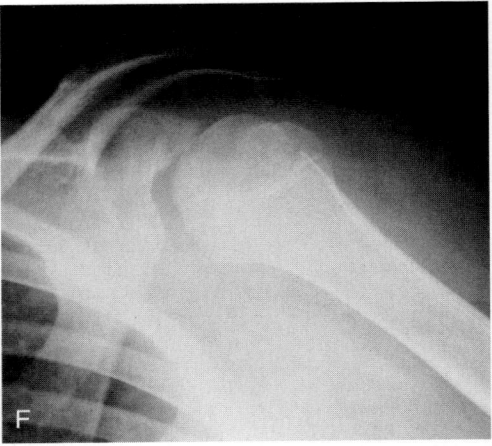

months of life, and preliminary findings suggest that ultrasound examination is a suitable aid to diagnosis at this age in cases for which the clinician has reason to suspect congruity of the shoulder.

CORRECTION BY SUBSCAPULARIS RECESSION

Subscapularis recession was described by Carlioz and Brahimi.[83] Gilbert[80] emphasized that the operation should be performed only if the shoulder is congruent. We performed 83 of these operations between 1986 and 1992, and although the initial results were promising, the deformity recurred in 41 of these cases. Each year witnesses further failures, and we think the operation of subscapularis recession has no place in the treatment of the deformity. It has been abandoned in our surgical unit.

CORRECTION BY THE ANTERIOR APPROACH

The principles of the anterior approach operation are as follows: removal of the impediments to lateral rotation or relocation of the head of the humerus into the glenoid; improving stability of the shoulder by correction of retroversion of the head on the shaft; and sound repair of subscapularis muscle, which is the most important medial rotator of the shoulder.

The shoulder is approached through the deltopectoral groove, displacing the cephalic vein medially. The coracoid is exposed. It is usually elongated and inclined dorsally. Flaps are elevated from the coracoid; the lateral flap contains the coracohumeral ligament and coracoacromial ligaments, and the medial flap contains coracoclavicular ligaments and pectoralis major. Improvement in the range of lateral rotation is usually evident after this. The coracoid is shortened to its base. The subscapularis muscle is exposed. The rotator interval is defined. If there is no doubt that the head of the humerus is congruent, the tendinous upper one third of the muscle is cut. If, as is usually the case, there is subluxation or dislocation, the subscapularis muscle is elongated in a Z-incision fashion. The superior flap, at least 2 cm long, is left attached to the lesser tuberosity. The inferior flap is prepared by detaching the tendon from the lower part of the lesser tuberosity. The capsule is preserved. The head relocates into the true glenoid, where it is grasped by the capsule and the labrum.

With the head of humerus reduced, it is possible to see the extent of deformity of its anterior part and the formation and depth of the true glenoid. The head of the humerus can be rotated from the true glenoid into the false glenoid by bringing the arm into medial rotation. There is almost always a clearly defined ridge of cartilage separating the two facets of the glenoid; only rarely have we found a glenoid that was flat or convex.

The extent of retroversion of the head of the humerus on the shaft is indicated by the instability of the reduction, and it can be estimated by placing the finger and thumb of one hand in the coronal plane of the head and the finger and thumb of the other hand on the epicondyle of the humerus. If the angle of retroversion exceeds 30 degrees (i.e., in about one half of cases), the appropriate derotation osteotomy of the shaft of humerus is necessary to enhance the ability to perform the reduction and permit a functional range of medial rotation. The osteotomy is done through an approach to the shaft of the humerus at the junction of the deltoid and brachialis muscles. A small four-hole plate is used, and the uppermost screws are inserted. A drill hole is placed in the distal fragment at the appropriate angle. The plate is then removed, the bone is cut, the distal fragment is rotated medially, and the plate is reapplied. The shoulder is reduced. There is a stable arc of rotation from about 40 degrees of lateral rotation to about 80 degrees of medial rotation. The subscapularis flaps are securely repaired; then the coracoid flaps are repaired.

The limb is immobilized in a plaster of Paris jacket with the arm in adduction, the elbow flexed to 90 degrees, and the forearm held in supination. The plaster is removed at 6 weeks. For the first 2 weeks after cast removal, exercises are done to regain and improve the range of elevation and lateral rotation; then more vigorous work is done to enhance medial rotation.

In earlier cases, medial rotation osteotomy was deferred until 1 year after reduction to improve the range of medial rotation and diminish winging of the scapula. Table 260–8 provides the results of 60 cases analyzed by Chen. These operations, which were done before 1994, did not regularly include derotation osteotomy of the humerus. Since that element was introduced, rehabilitation of the children and restoration of function have been consistently more reliable (Fig. 260–12).

In advanced cases, it may prove impossible to secure the location between the head of the humerus and the true glenoid. Glenoid osteotomy and bone grafting were done through a posterior approach in five of

FIGURE 260–12. Function was assessed 3 months after relocation of a complex dislocation in an 11-year-old girl. In her case, the deformity progressed in a slow, insidious manner. Derotation osteotomy of the humerus was unnecessary. *A* and *B,* Her preoperative scores were as follows: Mallett, 9; Gilbert, 1+; elbow, 4; and hand, 5. She had 180 degrees of elevation, 50 degrees of fixed medial rotation contracture, 90 degrees of active medial rotation, and 90 degrees of active pronation-supination. Radiographs showed a remarkably well-formed head of the humerus and an adequate glenoid. The coracoid was greatly prolonged and it was also inclined dorsally. *C* and *D,* Three months postoperatively, her scores were as follows: Mallett, 15; Gilbert, 5+; elbow, 4; and hand, 5. She had 160 degrees of abduction, 30 degrees of lateral rotation, 90 degrees of medial rotation, and 140 degrees of active pronation-supination. *E* and *F,* Radiographs show the head of the humerus is congruent within the glenoid. This case exemplifies the variable onset of secondary bone deformity, and it is an unusual result in a child presenting as late as this.

T A B L E 2 6 0 – 8 ■ **Subluxation or Dislocation: Outcome after Reduction in 60 Cases Operated, 1991 through 1994, with a Minimum Follow-up of 48 Months**

CASE STATUS	MALLET GRADE					GILBERT GRADE						RAIMONDI GRADE				
	5–6	7–8	9–10	11–12	13–15	1	2	3	4	5	6	1	2	3	4	5
Preoperative no. of cases	36	16	6	2	0	42	14	3	1	0	0	0	0	21	25	14
Postoperative no. of cases	0	4	18	16	22	0	6	15	20	16	3	0	0	10	10	40

Data from Chen L: Results of reduction of the dislocated shoulder. In Birch R, Bonney G, Wynn Parry C (eds): *Surgical Disorders of the Peripheral Nerves.* Edinburgh, Churchill Livingstone, 1998.

these children as a means of converting a dislocation into a subluxation after failed attempts at open reduction. By improving the anatomic relationship, subsequent arthrodesis or arthroplasty may be feasible. Only time will tell. We see no place for primary interventions on the dislocated shoulder through the posterior approach, nor we do we see any indication for the operation of lateral rotation osteotomy.

One half of the children studied by Chen regained full, active supination after relocation of the shoulder.

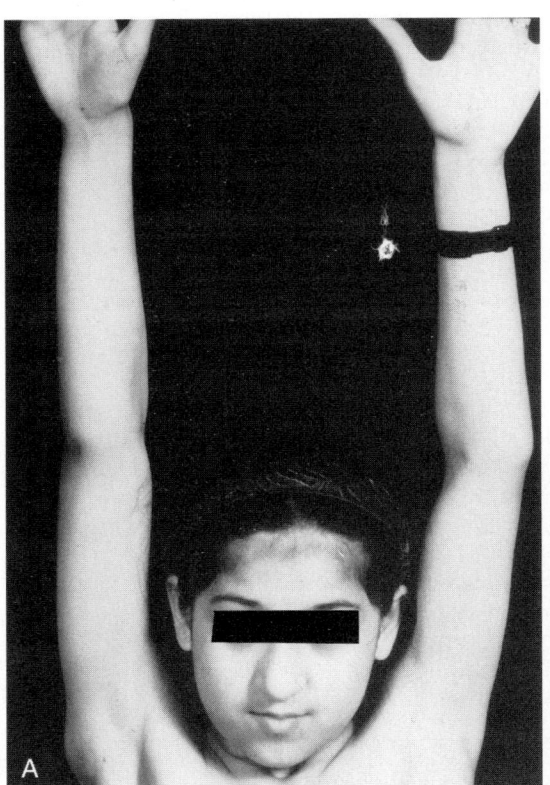

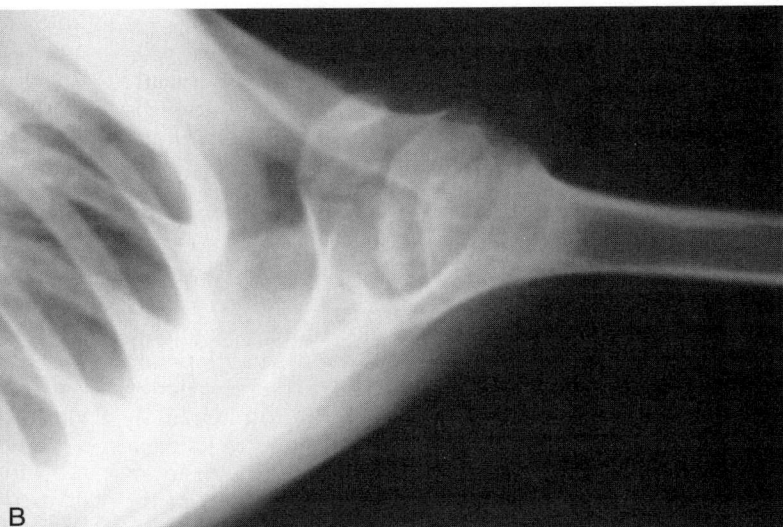

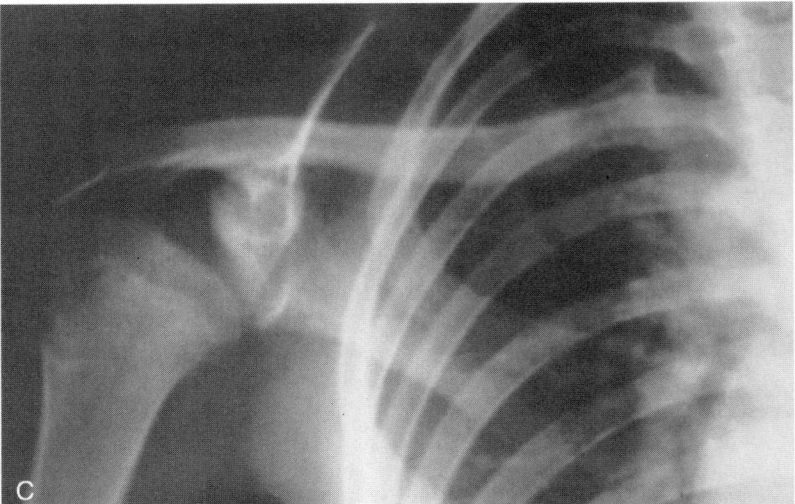

FIGURE 260–13. A 15-year-old girl 8 years after relocation of a complex dislocation. Her scores were as follows: Mallett, 15; Gilbert, 6; elbow, 5; and hand, 5. *A* to *C,* Radiographs show a persistent deformity of the head of the humerus, and enlargement of the head suggests an element of avascular necrosis in the early postoperative course.

There is often improvement in flexion contracture at the elbow. A small number of children showed marked improvement in active extension of the wrist. Functional assessments show that successful relocation of the shoulder brings about marked improvement at the shoulder and in hand function.

Prolonged study will be necessary to determine the long-term prognosis for the shoulder that has been reduced after a long-standing dislocation. It is possible that degenerative changes will occur in later decades in a number of these patients. However, the initial functional improvement is so great that it encourages us to pursue this method of treatment. The evidence shows that the outcome is substantially better than leaving the child with an untreated posterior dislocation (Fig. 260–13).

REFERENCES

1. Fu SY, Gordon T: The cellular and molecular basis of peripheral nerve regeneration. Mol Neurobiol 14:67–116, 1997.
2. Waller A: Experiments on the section of the glossopharyngeal and hypoglossal nerves of the frog, and observations of the alterations produced thereby in the structure of their primitive fibres. Philos Trans R Soc Lond B Biol Sci 140:423–429, 1850.
3. Stoll G, Griffins JW, Li Y, Trapp BD: Wallerian degeneration in the peripheral nervous system: Participation of both Schwann cells and macrophages in myelin degradation. J Neurocytol 18:671–683, 1989.
4. Griffin JW, Kidd G, Trapp BD: Interactions between axons and Schwann cells. In Dyck PJ, Thomas PK, Griffin JW, et al (eds): Peripheral Neuropathy, 3rd ed. Philadelphia, WB Saunders, 1993, pp 317–33.
5. Korsching S: The neurotrophic factor concept: A re-examination. J Neurosci 13:2739–2748, 1993.
6. Risling M, Carlstedt T, Cullheim S: Peripheral nerve injury and regeneration. In Glukman PD, Heymann MA (eds): Pediatrics and Perinatology: The Scientific Basis. Scarborough, Ontario, Arnold, 1996, pp 447–450.
7. Carlstedt T, Cullheim S: Spinal cord motoneuron maintenance, injury and repair. In Dunnett S, Bjorklund A (eds): Functional Neuronal Transplantation. II. Progress in Brain Research. Philadelphia, Elsevier (in press).
8. Takano K: Absence of gamma-spindle loop in the reinnervated hind leg muscles of the cat: "Alpha-muscle." Exp Brain Res 26:343–354, 1976.
9. Martini R: Expression and functional roles of neural cell surface molecules and extracellular matrix components during development and regeneration of peripheral nerves. J Neurocytol 23:1–28, 1994.
10. Brecknell JE, Fawcett JW: Axonal regeneration. Biol Rev 71:227–255, 1996.
11. Sendtner M, Stockli KA, Thoenen H: Synthesis and localization of ciliary neurotrophic factor in the sciatic nerve of the adult rat after lesion and during regeneration. J Cell Biol 118:139–148, 1992.
12. Trupp M, Ryden M, Jornvall H, et al: Peripheral expression and biological activities of GDNF, a new neurotrophic factor for avian and mammalian peripheral neurons. J Cell Biol 130:137–148, 1995.
13. Funakoshi H, Risling M, Carlstedt T, et al: Targeted expression of a multifunctional chimeric neurotrophin in the lesioned sciatic nerve accelerates regeneration of sensory and motor axons. Proc Natl Acad Sci U S A 95:5269–5274, 1998.
14. Carvalho GA, Nikkhah G, Matthies C, et al: Diagnosis of root avulsion in traumatic brachial plexus injuries: Value of computerized tomography myelography and magnetic resonance imaging. J Neurosurg 86:69–76, 1997.
15. Berthold C-H, Carlstedt T, Corneliusson O: The central-peripheral transitional zone. In Dyck PJ, Thomas PK (eds): Peripheral Neuropathy, 3rd ed. Philadelphia, WB Saunders, 1993, pp 73–91.
16. Seddon HJ: Surgical Disorders of Peripheral Nerves, 2nd ed. Edinburgh, Churchill Livingstone, 1975.
17. Bonney G: The value of axon response in determining the site of lesion of the brachial plexus. Brain 77:588–609, 1954.
18. Frazier CH, Skillern PG: Supraclavicular subcutaneous lesions of the brachial plexus not associated with skeletal injuries. JAMA 75:1957–1963, 1911.
19. Penfield W: Late spinal paralysis after avulsion of the brachial plexus. J Bone Joint Surg Br 31:40–41, 1949.
20. Birch R: Major neurovascular bundles. In Colton CL, Hall AJ (eds): Atlas of Orthopaedics: Surgical Approaches. Oxford, UK, Butterworth-Heinemann, 1991, pp 120–133.
21. Birch R, Bonney G, Wynn Parry CB: Iatropathic injury. In Birch R, Bonney G, Wynn Parry CB (eds): Surgical Disorders of Peripheral Nerves. Edinburgh, Churchill Livingstone, 1998, pp 293–334.
22. Alnot JY, Narakas A: Les Paralysies du Plexus Brachial, 2nd ed. Paris, Expansion Scientifique Français, 1996.
23. Huittinen VM: Lumbosacral nerve injury in fracture of the pelvis: A postmortem radiographic and patho-anatomical study. Acta Chir Scand 429(Suppl):7–43, 1972.
24. Huittinen VM, Slatis P: Nerve injury in double vertical pelvic fractures. Acta Chir Scand 138:571–575, 1972.
25. Anand P, Terenghi G, Warner G, et al: The role of nerve growth factor in human diabetic neuropathy. Nat Med 2:703–707, 1996.
26. Kratimenos P, Crockard AH: The far lateral approach for ventrally placed foramen magnum and upper cervical spine tumours. Br J Neurosurg 7:129–140, 1993.
27. Carlstedt T, Noren G: Repair of ruptured spinal nerve roots in a brachial plexus lesion. J Neurosurg 82:661–663, 1995.
28. Carlstedt T, Grane P, Hallin RG, Noren G: Return of function after spinal cord implantation of avulsed spinal nerve roots. Lancet 346:1323–1325, 1995.
29. Carlstedt T, Anand P, Hallin R, et al: Spinal nerve root repair and replantation of avulsed ventral roots into the spinal cord after brachial plexus injury. J Neurosurg 93(Suppl):237–247, 2000.
30. Roosen K: The trans-sacral, trans-coccygeal approach to prevertebral spinal tumors. Adv Neurosurg 14:111–115, 1986.
31. Zhao S, Beuerman RW, Kline DG: Neurotizations of motor nerves innervating the lower extremity by utilizing the lower intercostal nerves. J Reconstr Microsurg 13:39–45, 1997.
32. Weddell G, Feinstein B, Pattle RE: The electrical activity of voluntary muscle in man under normal and pathological conditions. Brain 67:178–252, 1944.
33. Bonney G, Gilliatt RW: Sensory nerve conduction after traction lesion of the brachial plexus. Proc R Soc Med 51:365–367, 1958.
34. Smith SJM: Electrodiagnosis. In Birch R, Bonney G, Wynn Parry C (eds): Surgical Disorders of the Peripheral Nerves, 1st ed. Edinburgh, Churchill Livingstone, 1998, pp 467–490.
35. West GA, Haynor DR, Goodkin R: Magnetic resonance imaging signal changes in denervated muscles after peripheral nerve injury. Neurosurgery 35:1077–1086, 1994.
36. Filler AG, Kliot M, Howe FA, et al: Application of magnetic resonance neurography in the evaluation of patients with peripheral nerve pathology. J Neurosurg 85,299–309, 1996.
37. Kline DG, Hudson AR: Injection injury. In Kline DG, Hudson AR (eds): Nerve Injuries. Philadelphia, WB Saunders, 1995, pp 46–50.
38. Gentili F, Hudson A, Kline DG, et al: Peripheral nerve injection injury: An experimental study. Neurosurgery 4:244–253, 1979.
39. Mackinnon SE, Dellon AL: Injection injury. In Mackinnon SE, Dellon AL (eds): Surgery of the Peripheral Nerve. New York, Thieme, 1988, pp 59–62.
40. Sedel L: Traitment palliatif d'un serie de 103 paralysis par elongation du plexus brachial: Evolution spontanee et resultats. Rev Chir Orthop 63:651–666, 1977.
41. Vastamaki M, Solonen KA: Accessory nerve injury. Acta Orthop Scand 55:296–299, 1984.
42. Narakas A: Examen du patient et de la fonction des divers groupes musculaires du membre supérieur. In Alnot JY, Narakas A (eds): Les Parlysies du Plexus Brachial. Paris, Expansion Scientifique Français, 1995, pp 52–67.
43. Olarte M, Adams D: Accessory nerve palsy. J Neurol Neurosurg Psychiatry 40:1113–1116, 1977.
44. Payan J: Clinical electromyography in infancy and childhood In Brett EM (ed): Paediatric Neurology. Edinburgh, Churchill Livingstone, 1991, p 829.

45. Alvares D, Fitzgerald M: Building blocks of pain: The regulation of key molecules in spinal sensory neurones during development and following peripheral axotomy. Pain 6(Suppl):571–585, 1999.

46. Himes BT, Tessler A: Death of some dorsal root ganglion neurones and plasticity of others following sciatic nerve section in adult and neonatal rats. J Comp Neurol 284:215–230, 1989.

47. Johnson EM, Yip HK: Central nervous system and peripheral nerve growth factor provide trophic support critical to mature sensory neuronal survival. Nature 314:751–752, 1985.

48. Platt H: Obstetrical paralysis: A vanishing chapter in orthopaedic surgery. Bull Hosp Joint Dis 34:4–21, 1973.

49. Greenwald AG, Schute PC, Shiveley JL: Brachial plexus palsy: a 10 year report on the incidence and prognosis. J Paediatr Orthop 4:639–692, 1984.

50. Levine MG, Holroyde J, Woods JR, et al: Birth trauma: Incidence and predisposing factors. Obstet Gynaecol 63:792–795, 1984.

51. Rubin A: Birth injuries: Incidence, mechanics and end results. Obstet Gynecol 23:218–221, 1964.

52. Bager B: Perinatally acquired brachial plexus palsy—a persisting challenge. Acta Paediatr 86:1214–1219, 1997.

53. Tan KL: Brachial palsy. J Obstet Gynaecol Br Commonw 80:60–62, 1973.

54. Boo NY, Lye MS, Kanchanala M, Ching CL: Brachial plexus injuries in Malaysian neonates: Incidence and associated risk factors. 37:327–330, 1991.

55. Gilbert A: Paralysie obstetricale du plexus brachial. In Alnot J-Y, Narakas A (eds): Les Paralysies du Plexus Brachial, 2nd ed. Monographie de la Société Français de Chirurgie de la Main. Paris, Expansion Scientifique Français, 1995, pp 270–281.

56. Slooff ACJ, Blaauw G: Aspects particuliers. In Alnot J-Y, Narakas A (eds): Les Paralysies du Plexus Brachial, 2nd ed. Monographie de la Société Français de Chirurgie de la Main. Paris, Expansion Scientifique Français, 1995, pp 282–284.

57. Giddins GEB, Birch R, Singh D, Taggart M: Risk factors for obstetric brachial plexus palsies. J Bone Joint Surg Br 76(Suppl II—III):156, 1994.

58. Power C: National trends in birth weight. BMJ 308:1270–1271, 1994.

59. Dunn DW, Engle WA: Brachial plexus palsy: Intrauterine onset. Paediatr Neurol 1:367–369, 1985.

60. Jennett RJ, Tarby TJ, Kreinick CJ: Brachial plexus palsy: An old problem revisited. Am J Obstet Gynaecol 166:1637–1677, 1992.

61. Paradiso G, Granana N, Maza E: Prenatal brachial plexus injury. Neurology 49:261–262, 1997.

62. Narakas AO: Obstetrical brachial plexus injuries. In Lamb DW (ed): The Paralysed Hand. Edinburgh, Churchill Livingstone, 1987, pp 116–135.

63. Brunelli GA, Brunelli GR: A fourth type of brachial plexus lesion: the intermediate (C7) palsy. J Hand Surg 16:492–494, 1991.

64. Bennet CC, Harrold AJ: Prognosis and early management of birth injuries to the brachial plexus. BMJ 1:1520–1521, 1976.

65. Sharrad WJW: Paediatric Orthopaedics and Fractures, 2nd ed. Oxford, UK, Blackwell, 1971.

66. Eng G: Brachial plexus palsy in newborn infants. Paediatrics 48:18–28, 1971.

67. Eng GD, Koch B, Smokvina MD: Brachial plexus palsy in neonates and children. Arch Phys Med Rehabil 59:458–464, 1978.

68. Zancolli EA, Zancolli ER: Palliative surgical procedures in sequelae of obstetrical palsy. In Tubiana R (ed): The Hand, vol IV. Philadelphia, WB Saunders, 1993, pp 602–623.

69. Tassin JL: Paralysies Obstétricales du Plexus Brachial: Evolution Spontanée, Résultats des Interventions Réparatrices Précoces [thesis]. Paris, Universite Paris VII, 1983.

70. Gilbert A, Razaboni R, Amar-Khodja S: Indications and results of brachial plexus surgery in obstetrical palsy. Orthop Clin North Am 19:91–105, 1988.

71. Michelow BJ, Clarke HM, Curtis CG, et al: The natural history of obstetrical brachial plexus palsy. Plast Reconstr Surg 93:675–680, 1994.

72. Laurent JP, Lee R, Shenaq S, et al: Neurosurgical correction of upper brachial plexus birth injuries. J Neurosurg 79:197–203, 1993.

73. Gilbert A, Tassin JL: Réparation chirurgicale de plexus brachial dans la paralysie obstétricale. Chirurgie (Paris) 110:70–75, 1984.

74. Francel PC, Koby M, Park TS, et al: Fast spin-echo magnetic resonance imaging for radiological assessment of neonatal brachial plexus injury. J Neurosurg 83:461–466, 1995.

75. Smith SJM: The role of neurophysiological investigation in traumatic brachial plexus injuries in adults and children. J Hand Surg Br 21:145–148, 1996.

76. Gu YD, Zhang GM, Chen DS, et al: Seventh cervical nerve root transfer from the contra-lateral healthy side for treatment of brachial plexus root avulsion. J Hand Surg Br 17:518–521, 1992.

77. Fairbank HAT: Subluxation of shoulder joint in infants and young children. Lancet 1:1217–1223, 1913.

78. Sever JW: Obstetrical paralysis: Report of eleven hundred cases. JAMA 85:1862–1865, 1925.

79. Scaglietti O: The obstetrical shoulder trauma. Surg Gynecol Obstet 66:868–877, 1938.

80. Gilbert A: Obstetrical brachial plexus palsy. In Tubiana R (ed): The Hand, vol 4. Philadelphia, WB Saunders, 1993, pp 576–601.

81. Waters PM, Smith GR, Jaramillo D: Glenohumeral deformity secondary to brachial plexus birth palsy. J Bone Joint Surg Am 80:668–677, 1998.

82. Pearl ML, Edgerton BW: Glenoid deformity secondary to brachial plexus birth palsy. J Bone Joint Surg Am 80:659–667, 1998.

83. Carlioz H, Brahimi L: La place de la déinsertion interne du sous-scapulaire dans le traitement de la paralysie obstétricale du membre supérieur chez l'enfant. Ann Chir Infant 12:159, 1986.

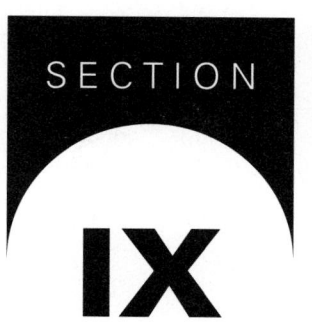

SECTION

IX

Radiotherapy and Radiosurgery

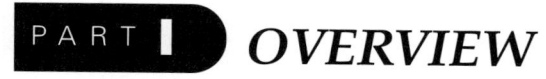

General and Historical Considerations of Radiotherapy and Radiosurgery

STEVEN D. CHANG ■ JOHN R. ADLER, JR. ■ GARY K. STEINBERG

The use of radiation as a treatment for disease is based on the concept that such energy has the capability to alter cellular function, primarily by interfering with cellular reproduction. Radiation results in the formation of free radicals as electrons are freed from their atoms, the presence of which results in disruption of normal cellular activity. The first therapeutic use of radiation in medicine began in the 1920s using low-voltage machines. Over the following decades, steady advances in the voltage (first orthovoltage, then megavoltage) of x-ray machines allowed the treatment of lesions at greater depths from the body surface. By the 1970s, fractionated radiotherapy delivered by medical linear accelerators (linacs) was a standard adjunctive treatment for a wide range of neoplasms, including those in the brain and spinal cord. At increasingly larger doses, radiotherapy achieved higher rates of cancer control and "cure." Unfortunately, these higher doses also carried increased risk of radiation injury. The development of stereotactic devices and high-speed computers over the past 2 decades has resulted in the advent of stereotactic radiosurgery, a method to deliver a single high dose (or a limited number of high doses) of focused radiation with very rapid falloff in the surrounding tissue. In this chapter, the historical background of both conventional fractionated radiotherapy and stereotactic radiosurgery is discussed.

RADIOTHERAPY

After the discovery of x-rays by Roentgen in 1895,[1] their biologic effects were rapidly recognized. By 1899, there was a report of the first patient with cancer to be cured with radiation.[2] Improvements in x-ray machines were achieved over the next several decades. By 1913, a 140-kilovolt (kV) machine had been developed, and a 200-kV machine became available in 1922.[2] The broad use of radiation to treat cancer began in 1922, when Coutard presented a case of laryngeal carcinoma treated with radiotherapy.[3] In 1934, Coutard first described the practice of fractionation.[4] His work remains the basis for present-day fractionation.

Before the 1950s, most conventional radiotherapy was delivered using x-rays generated with an energy of several hundred kilovolts by machines appropriately called kilovoltage units.[5] The primary drawback of these devices was the relatively low energy level of the emitted x-rays, which resulted in rapid energy loss and shallow depth penetration in most tissue. Although this was useful for the treatment of superficial lesions such as skin neoplasms, deep targets, including most intracranial lesions, could not be adequately irradiated without delivering a significantly higher dose at the surface. The development of even higher-energy machines, capable of producing radiation with megaelectron volts (MeV) of x-rays, allowed greater depth of penetration. This, combined with filtration (which removes much of the low-energy, poorly penetrating x-rays) has facilitated the treatment of deep-seated targets, including intracranial neoplasms. Van de Graaf generators were the first machines capable of producing x-rays with energy levels of several megaelectron volts.[5] However, these machines were soon replaced by cobalt-60 units and linacs, both of which were technologically better methods of producing high-voltage x-rays.

Linacs use electromagnetic waves to accelerate charged particles such as electrons to high energies through a linear tube.[5] The electrons emerge from the linac and strike a metal foil to produce x-rays through a process known as bremsstrahlung. The resulting x-rays exit the linac as a beam with diameters determined by primary and secondary collimators. Most linacs are constructed so that the source of radiation can rotate around a horizontal axis, while the treatment couch on which the patient lies rotates around a vertical axis. The point of intersection between the two axes is defined as the isocenter.

In contrast to linacs, cobalt-60 units use radioactive isotopes as a high-energy radiation source. These devices contain cobalt 60 produced in a reactor by irradiating stable cobalt with neutrons.[5] The cobalt-60 source is encapsulated and mounted on a gantry, a machine with a design similar to a linac. Unlike linacs, which deliver their maximal dose at a depth of more than 3 cm, cobalt-60 units administer their maximal dose at a depth of approximately 0.5 cm, making them much less useful for deep-seated targets. Given the relative lack of penetration by x-rays emitted by cobalt-60 units, linacs have emerged as the main method of delivering fractionated radiotherapy.

Patients with brain neoplasms treated with linac radiotherapy undergo fractionation, which involves division of the total dose of radiation into multiple smaller doses, typically given on a daily basis. This interval between radiotherapy doses allows the normal brain tissues within the radiation ports to recover from the effects of radiation. Current fractionated regimens vary based on the pathology, but they typically involve up to 30 treatments. Dose fractionation has several advantages, including (1) allowing repair of sublethal damage and potentially lethal damage in normal neural tissue; (2) reducing the acute effects of single high doses of radiation; (3) allowing for redistribution of cells within the cell cycle, so that there is a greater chance of individual target cells receiving some radiation during cell division, at which time cells are especially sensitive to radiation injury; and (4) allowing for improved oxygenation of tumor cells, which are more likely to respond to radiation than are hypoxic cells.[2] Ideally, the choice of optimal dose and fraction schedules for various tumors is individualized according to the particular cell kinetics of the target lesion and the clinical observations of patient response.

Extensive medical literature exists regarding the use of conventional fractionated radiotherapy to treat multiple brain metastases (symptomatic relief in 70% to 90% of patients),[6] pituitary neoplasms (10-year control rates of 77% to 87%),[7, 8] meningiomas (11% to 32% 4- to 8-year recurrence rate for irradiated tumors, versus 60% to 78% recurrence rate for nonirradiated tumors),[9–12] and gliomas (approximately 40-week mean survival for patients receiving 60 Gy after surgery, versus 20-week mean survival for those receiving surgery alone).[13, 14] Fractionated radiotherapy was used to treat arteriovenous malformations (AVMs) before the advent of stereotactic radiosurgery. Of 20 patients with angiographic follow-up after fractionated radiotherapy of 40 to 50 Gy for AVMs, 9 showed complete angiographic obliteration, and 5 showed a decrease in lesion size.[15]

STEREOTACTIC RADIOSURGERY

Although conventional radiotherapy of intracranial tumors has improved with respect to field shaping and optimal fractionation regimens, treatment typically involves irradiation of normal neural structures at a nearly full dose. Stereotactic radiosurgery, a method of delivering a single high dose of radiation to a well-defined target, has the advantage of a very steep dose gradient. As a result, it is possible to deliver a much larger, and presumably more efficacious, dose to a tumor without exceeding the radiation tolerance of adjacent normal tissues. In addition, several authors have hypothesized that a therapeutic gain may be achieved by treating slowly proliferating tumors, such as meningiomas, with larger-sized fractions, a treatment that is possible only by using radiosurgical principles.[16, 17]

Heavy-Particle Radiosurgery

Building on the stereotactic guiding device he had previously developed,[18] Leksell originated the concept of stereotactic radiosurgery and described his basic technique in 1951.[19] He developed a method for rotating an orthovoltage x-ray tube around the stereotactic instrument, thereby focusing its beam on a point at the center.[19] The first patients treated with this device had been diagnosed with trigeminal neuralgia. Leksell reported that most achieved long-term pain control.[20] Encouraged by this initial work, he began a long association with Larsson, a radiobiologist working at the cyclotron unit at the University of Uppsala. Together they developed a proton-based stereotactic radiosurgical system for the treatment of human brain malignancies (Fig. 261–1).[21–23] Over the next decade, Lawrence and Tobias at Lawrence Livermore Laboratory in Berkeley, California,[20, 24] and Kjellberg at Harvard University and the Massachusetts Institute of Technology[24] began treating pituitary tumors and AVMs, respectively, with this technology. Because therapies for these conditions were extremely limited at the time, radiosurgery substantially improved the options available to such patients. During the past 4 decades, charged-particle radiosurgery has been refined to treat a wide variety of lesions, largely due to advances in physics, computer planning, and modern imaging.

Charged particles (proton or helium ions) have a unique advantage over photons with respect to radiosurgery. When using photons, a significant dose of radiation is deposited along the entire path of the beam, including the points of entrance and exit to the head. To minimize irradiation of tissue other than the target lesion, photon-based radiosurgery systems crossfire beams from many directions. In contrast, charged particles produce a region of intermediate dose where the beam first enters the head, followed by a narrow zone of high dose (the Bragg ionization peak).[25] The exit dose is minimal. The depth in tissue at which the peak is maximal can be adjusted to strike a target (Fig. 261–2). Further, there is no limit to the size of the lesion being treated, and charged-particle radiosurgery can be precisely contoured to treat complex shapes. The drawbacks of charged-particle radiosurgery include (1) the great expense of constructing and maintaining these sites (there are currently only two centers in the United States); (2) some compromise in spatial accuracy, because instead of a frame attached to the skull,

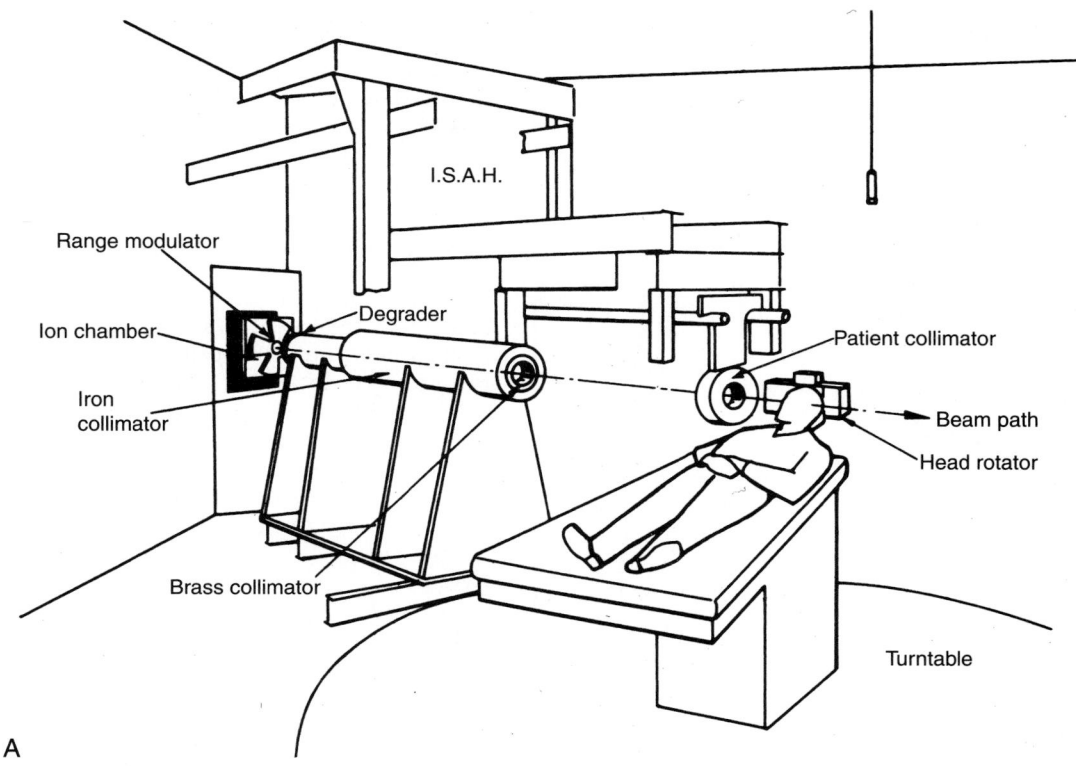

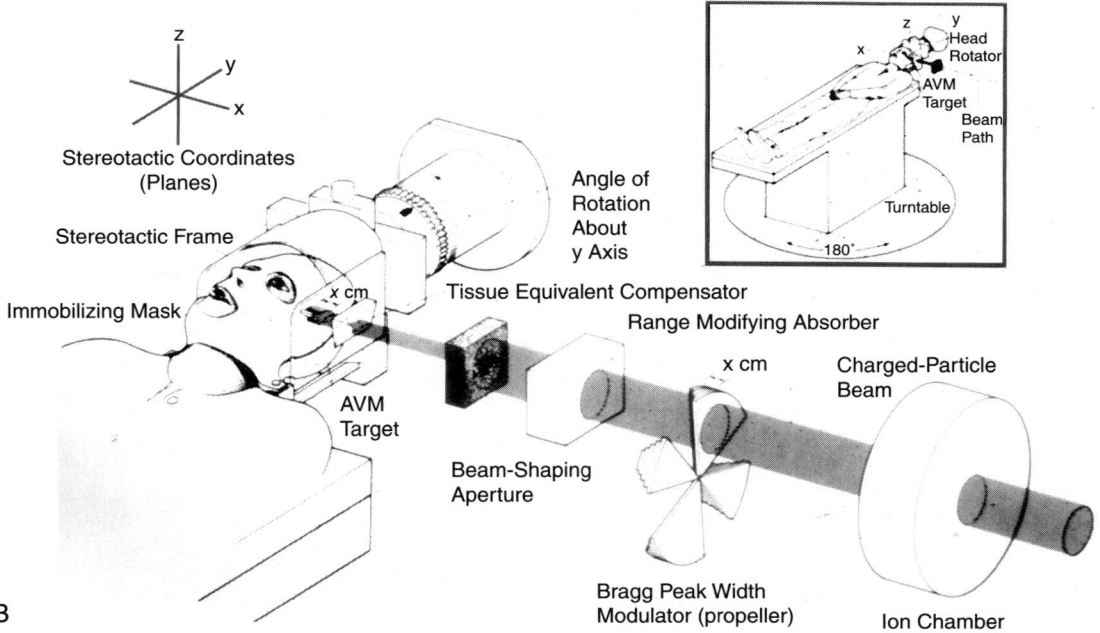

FIGURE 261–1. *A*, Schematic showing a typical heavy-particle stereotactic radiosurgery system. *B*, Close-up view of the charged particle beam delivery system. Beam shape is determined by the beam-shaping aperture, the range-modifying absorber, and the Bragg peak width modulator.

the patient wears an immobilizing plastic mask or bite block in the mouth to achieve fixation; (3) relatively time-consuming treatment planning; and (4) the need for beam-modifying devices that must be custom-made for each patient, thereby increasing the time and cost of treatment.

Heavy-particle radiosurgery has been shown to achieve a 94% obliteration rate for AVMs less than 4

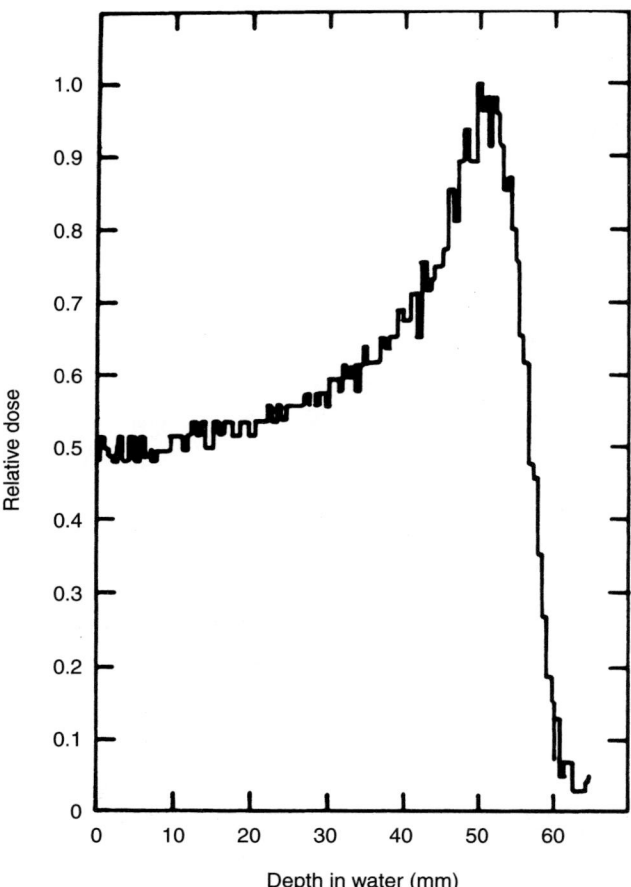

FIGURE 261–2. Example of the Bragg peak effect. The relative dose versus depth of penetration is shown for a target at a depth of 50 mm. Note that the exit dose is minimal.

spherical dose distributions (Fig. 261–3). A range of secondary collimators (within one of four helmets) provides 4-, 8-, 14-, or 18-mm-diameter openings. To avoid irradiation of a certain region, specific openings in the head shield are plugged.

The gamma knife treatment process begins by attaching a metal frame to the patient's skull under local anesthetic. A computed tomographic scan, magnetic resonance imaging scan, or angiogram (or a combination of these studies) is performed to locate the target and provide the three-dimensional image data used to develop a treatment plan for radiation delivery, which is calculated on a computer. Irregularly shaped targets are covered by using multiple isocenters and selectively plugging secondary collimator openings. Once the treatment plan is complete, radiosurgery is delivered by attaching the patient's head and stereotactic frame to the inside of the gamma knife helmet. The radiation dose to a specific target is determined primarily by the length of time a patient spends within the helmet.

Advantages of the gamma knife include rapid treatment time per isocenter, relatively simple treatment planning, and better field shaping than that obtainable with some linac units. Disadvantages of the gamma knife include high initial acquisition cost, the necessity of replacing the radiation source every 5 to 10 years, and difficulty with fractionation. Gamma knife radiosurgery has been shown to achieve 85% to 94% control or tumor shrinkage rates in metastatic tumors,[29, 30] 89% to 94% tumor stabilization rates in acoustic neuromas,[31–33] 89% to 96% tumor decrease or control in meningiomas,[33, 34] and 71% to 80% AVM obliteration rates (2 years after treatment) for malformations less than 4 cm in diameter.[35, 36]

Linear Accelerator Radiosurgery

As the number of applications for stereotactic radiosurgery increased, interest turned to modifying standard medical linacs to perform radiosurgery procedures; linacs that have the ability to emit high-energy photon beams are standard equipment in radiotherapy departments. This alternative to the gamma knife has proved to be efficacious and cost effective. Linac radiosurgery was developed in 1982 by two groups, led by Betti and Derechinsky[37] and Colombo.[38] Based on the success of these two groups, Winston and Lutz modified their linac in Boston in 1987 to treat neurosurgical patients.[39] Presently, in the United States, there are six times as many linac facilities performing stereotactic radiosurgery as gamma knife facilities. When adapted for radiosurgery, linacs crossfire a photon beam by moving in arc-shaped paths around the patient's head, thereby minimizing irradiation of normal tissue (Fig. 261–4).[39] The number, orientation, and length of arcs can be modified to optimize treatment of a target. Secondary collimators are used to select the optimal beam diameter for each isocenter. Patients treated with a linac generally wear a stereotactic head frame fixed to the skull. The process of treatment is in most ways comparable to that for the gamma knife.

cm³, a 75% obliteration rate for AVMs 4 to 25 cm³, and a 39% obliteration rate for AVMs greater than 25 cm³.[26] With respect to pituitary tumors, 65% to 90% of patients, depending on the type of adenoma, were clinically improved after radiosurgery, with normalization or near normalization of serum hormone values.[27]

Gamma Knife

Realizing that proton beams were extremely expensive and not practical for most radiosurgical applications, Leksell developed the gamma knife. The first gamma knife, which used cobalt 60 as the radiation source, was developed in 1967.[28] Because of its ease of use, it represented a significant improvement over the proton beam. The original gamma knife had oval openings in the metal head shield and was used primarily for functional neurosurgery cases.[20] However, the development of computed tomography and later magnetic resonance imaging eventually made it possible to treat tumors and vascular malformations with the gamma knife. To take advantage of this progress in imaging, the gamma knife was redesigned in 1975 to provide better treatment profiles.[20] Circular openings were incorporated in the head shield, thereby allowing for

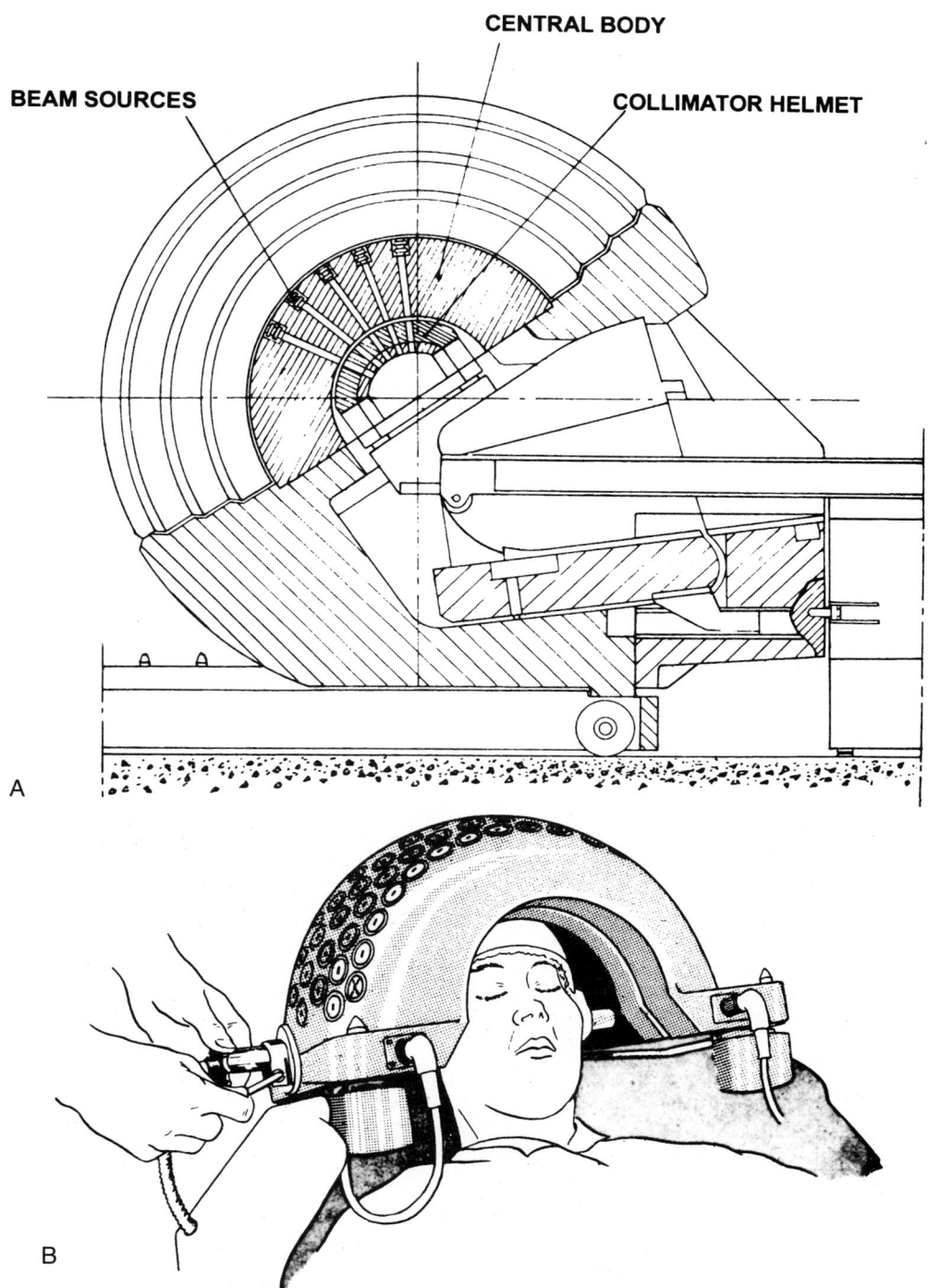

BEAM SOURCES

CENTRAL BODY

COLLIMATOR HELMET

A

B

FIGURE 261–3. *A*, Schematic of the gamma knife showing the cobalt-60 beam sources and the collimator helmet. Primary collimation is determined by the fixed collimator in the central body, and the secondary collimator size is determined by the collimator helmet. *B*, Illustration of the collimator helmet being attached to the stereotactic base ring before radiosurgery treatment.

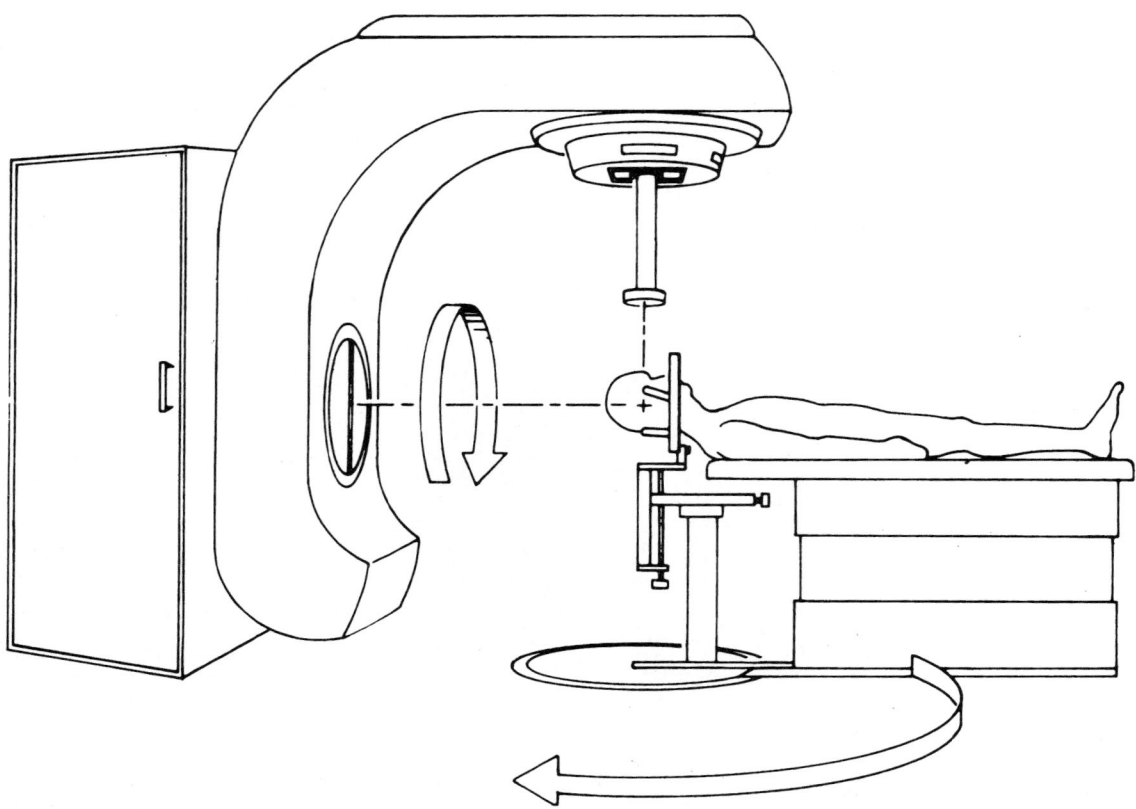

FIGURE 261–4. Schematic of a typical linear accelerator. The two axes of rotation are the gantry of the linear accelerator and the patient treatment table. A secondary collimator defines the shape of the x-ray beam.

The primary advantage of linacs over the gamma knife and cyclotron-based methods is that the cost of installation is low; only minor modifications are needed to standard medical linacs. Other advantages include great flexibility in photon delivery, lack of a field size limitation, and the possibility of fractionation. Disadvantages include longer treatment times compared with the gamma knife, especially for complex-shaped lesions, and more extensive quality-assurance procedures to ensure safety and reliability. Linac radiosurgery has been shown to achieve 85% to 96% control or tumor shrinkage rates for metastatic tumors,[40–42] greater than 90% tumor stabilization rates in acoustic neuromas,[43] 94% to 98% tumor decrease or control in meningiomas,[44, 45] and 80% to 87% AVM obliteration rates (2 years after treatment) for malformations less than 4 cm in diameter.[46, 47]

Frameless Image-Guided Radiosurgery

A novel method for performing precision irradiation, called the CyberKnife (Fig. 261–5), has recently been developed using image guidance instead of an external frame. The advantages of this instrument system include easier fractionation, the ability to treat young patients without general anesthesia, and the flexibility to treat lesions throughout the body.[48–51]

The CyberKnife combines a lightweight (130-kg)

6-MeV linac designed for radiosurgery and mounted to a highly maneuverable robotic manipulator, which can position and point the linac. Real-time image guidance eliminates the need to use skeletal fixation for either positioning or rigid immobilization of the target. This system acquires radiographs of skeletal features associated with the treatment site, uses image registration techniques to determine the treatment site's coordinates with respect to the linac and manipulator, and transmits coordinates of the lesion to the manipulator, which then directs the beam to the treatment site. If the target moves, the process detects the change and corrects the aim of the beam in near real time. Two fixed diagnostic fluoroscopes constitute the imaging hardware. They provide a stationary frame of reference for locating the patient's anatomy, which has a known relationship to the reference frame of the manipulator and linac.

The design of all conventional radiosurgical systems permits exclusively isocentric-based treatments, which results in a spherical region of high dose.[52–54] As a consequence, treatment of nonspherical lesions is problematic. Sphere packing, as is typically done with standard radiosurgical devices, inevitably produces some measure of both overtreatment in normal tissue and undertreatment within the target. The CyberKnife, however, enables the delivery of more complex treatments in which the beams originate at arbitrary points

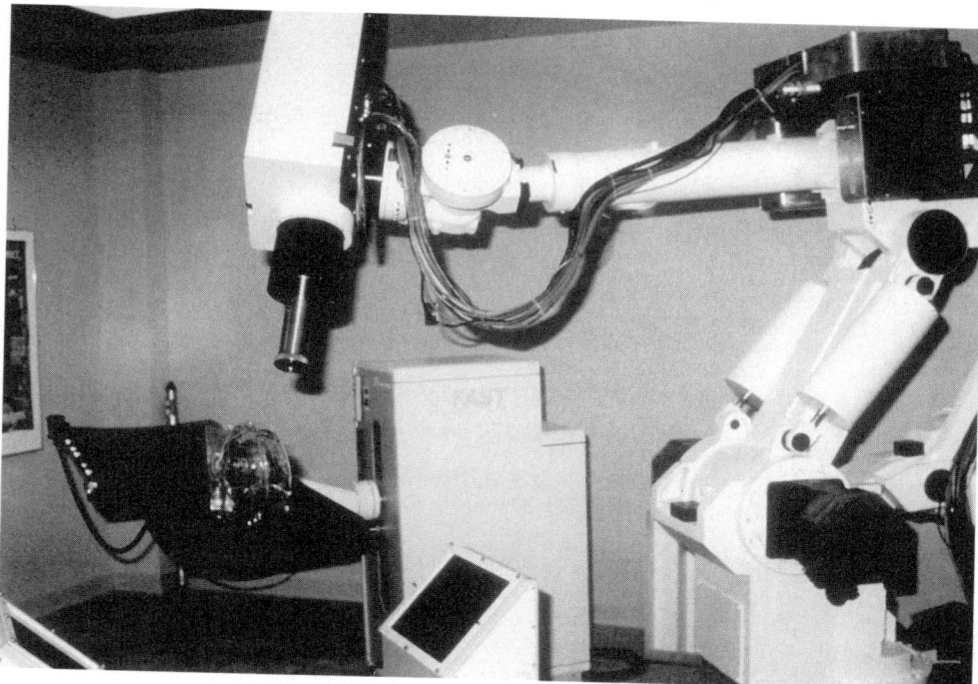

FIGURE 261–5. Photo of the CyberKnife showing a lightweight linear accelerator mounted to a robotic arm. The patient treatment table is also shown adjacent to the imaging cameras.

in the workspace and target arbitrary points within the lesion. The treatment beam is not limited to pointing at the center of the sphere; it can be aimed anywhere within a volume around the center. This allows delivery of nonisocentric beams that are aimed at points within the target that are not at the center of the sphere. Total treatment time depends on the complexity of the plan and delivery paths but is comparable to standard linac treatments. For complex-shaped lesions, the treatment time is frequently much shorter with the Cyber-Knife inverse treatment planning algorithm than it would be with other conventional radiosurgical systems. Further, because skeletal fixation is not required, fractionation is possible with minimal patient discomfort.

CONCLUSIONS

The last century has witnessed significant growth in our understanding and use of radiation to treat medical disorders. Conventional fractionated radiotherapy has evolved from low-voltage machines with wide ports of radiation delivery to megavoltage machines with increasingly refined collimation. Stereotactic radiosurgery represents a logical extension from conventional radiotherapy, in that highly focused stereotactic targeting allows the delivery of even greater doses of radiation, generally as a single fraction. Both radiotherapy and radiosurgery have become useful tools for neurosurgeons as they attempt to better treat and understand neurological diseases. Further advances in frameless image-guided delivery systems promise to expand the role of radiation treatment for these disorders.

REFERENCES

1. Roentgen WC: "On a new kind of rays (preliminary communication)." Translation of a paper read before the Physikalizchemedicinischen Gesellschaft of Wurzburg on December 28, 1895. Br J Radiol 4:32, 1931.
2. Perez CA, Brady LW: Overview. In Perez CA, Brady LW (eds): Principles and Practice of Radiation Oncology, 2nd ed. Philadelphia, JB Lippincott, 1992, pp 1–63.
3. Coutard H: Roentgentherapy of epitheliomas of the tonsillar region, hypopharynx and larynx from 1920 to 1926. AJR Am J Roentgenol 28:313–331, 1932.
4. Coutard H: Principles of x-ray therapy of malignant diseases. Lancet 2:1–8, 1934.
5. Khan FM: The Physics of Radiation Therapy. Baltimore, Williams & Wilkins, 1984.
6. Coia LR: The role of radiation therapy in the treatment of brain metastasis. Int J Radiat Oncol Biol Phys 23:229–238, 1992.
7. Hughes MN, Lamas KJ, Yelland ME, et al: Pituitary adenomas: Long-term results for radiotherapy alone and post-operative radiotherapy. Int J Radiat Oncol Biol Phys 27:1035–1043, 1993.
8. Tsang RW, Brierley JD, Panzarella T, et al: Radiation therapy for pituitary adenoma: Treatment outcome and prognostic factors. Int J Radiat Oncol Biol Phys 30:557–565, 1994.
9. Goldsmith BJ, Wara WM, Wilson CB, et al: Postoperative irradiation for subtotally resected meningiomas: A retrospective analysis of 140 patients treated from 1967 to 1990. J Neurosurg 80: 195–201, 1994; erratum in J Neurosurg 80:777, 1994.
10. Wilson CB: Meningiomas: Genetics, malignancy, and the role of radiation in induction and treatment. The Richard C. Schneider lecture. J Neurosurg 81:666–675, 1994.
11. Wara WM, Sheline GE, Newman H, et al: Radiation therapy of meningiomas. Am J Roentgenol Radium Ther Nucl Med 123: 453–458, 1975.
12. Taylor BW Jr, Marcus RB Jr, Friedman WA, et al: The meningioma controversy: Postoperative radiation therapy. Int J Radiat Oncol Biol Phys 15:299–304, 1988.
13. Chang CH, Horton J, Schoenfeld D, et al: Comparison of postoperative radiotherapy and combined postoperative radiotherapy and chemotherapy in the multidisciplinary management of malignant gliomas: A joint Radiation Therapy Oncology Group and Eastern Cooperative Oncology Group study. Cancer 52:997–1007, 1983.

14. Simpson JR, Horton J, Scott C, et al: Influence of location and extent of surgical resection on survival of patients with glioblastoma multiforme: Results of three consecutive Radiation Therapy Oncology Group (RTOG) clinical trials. Int J Radiat Oncol Biol Phys 26:239–244, 1993.

15. Johnson RJ: Radiotherapy of cerebral angiomas with a note on some problems in diagnosis. In Pia HW, Gleave JRW, Grok E, et al (eds): Cerebral Angiomas: Advances in Diagnosis and Therapy. Berlin, Springer-Verlag, 1975, pp 256–259.

16. Thames HD Jr, Withers HR, Peters LJ, et al: Changes in early and late radiation responses with altered dose fractionation: Implications for dose-survival relationships. Int J Radiat Oncol Biol Phys 8:219–226, 1982.

17. Withers HR, Thames HD Jr, Peters LJ: Biological bases for high RBE values for late effects of neutron irradiation. Int J Radiat Oncol Biol Phys 8:2071–2076, 1982.

18. Leksell L: A stereotactic apparatus for intracerebral surgery. Acta Chir Scand 99:229–233, 1949.

19. Leksell L: The stereotactic method and radiosurgery of the brain. Acta Chir Scand 102:316–319, 1951.

20. Lunsford LD, Alexander E, Loeffler JS: General introduction: History of radiosurgery. In Alexander E, Loeffler JS, Lunsford LD (eds): Stereotactic Radiosurgery. New York, McGraw-Hill, 1993, pp 1–4.

21. Larsson B, Leksell L, Rexed B, et al: The high energy proton beam as a neurosurgical tool. Nature 182:1222–1223, 1958.

22. Larsson B: On the application of a 185 MeV proton beam to experimental cancer therapy and neurosurgery: A biophysical study. Acta Univ Uppsala 9:7–23, 1962.

23. Larsson B: Radiobiological fundamentals in radiosurgery. In Steiner L, Lindquist C (eds): Radiosurgery: Baseline and Trends. New York, Raven Press, 1992, pp 3–14.

24. Kirn TF: Proton radiotherapy: Some perspectives. JAMA 259:787–788, 1988.

25. Lutz W: Radiation physics for radiosurgery. In Alexander E, Loeffler JS, Lunsford LD (eds): Stereotactic Radiosurgery. New York, McGraw-Hill, 1993, pp 7–15.

26. Steinberg GK, Fabrikant JI, Marks MP, et al: Stereotactic heavy-charged-particle Bragg-peak radiation for intracranial arteriovenous malformations. N Engl J Med 323:96–101, 1990; see comments.

27. Levy RP, Fabrikant JI, Frankel KA: Particle-beam irradiation of the pituitary gland. In Alexander E, Loeffler JS, Lunsford LD (eds): Stereotactic Radiosurgery. New York, McGraw-Hill, 1993, pp 157–165.

28. Leksell L: Stereotactic radiosurgery. J Neurol Neurosurg Psychiatry 46:797–803, 1983.

29. Kihlstrom L, Karlsson B, Lindquist C: Gamma knife surgery for cerebral metastases: Implications for survival based on 16 years' experience. Stereotact Funct Neurosurg 61(Suppl 1):45–50, 1993.

30. Flickinger JC, Kondziolka D, Lunsford LD, et al: A multi-institutional experience with stereotactic radiosurgery for solitary brain metastasis. Int J Radiat Oncol Biol Phys 28:797–802, 1994; see comments.

31. Flickinger JC, Lunsford LD, Linskey ME, et al: Gamma knife radiosurgery for acoustic tumors: Multivariate analysis of four year results. Radiother Oncol 27:91–98, 1993.

32. Noren G, Greitz D, Hirsch A, et al: Gamma knife surgery in acoustic tumours. Acta Neurochir Suppl (Wien) 58:104–107, 1993.

33. Lindquist C, Steiner L: Radiosurgery for tumors. In Wilkins R, Rengachary S (eds): Neurosurgery. New York, McGraw-Hill, 1995, p 185.

34. Kondziolka D, Lunsford LD: Radiosurgery of meningiomas. Neurosurg Clin N Am 3:219–230, 1992.

35. Steiner L, Prasad D, Lindquist C, et al: Gamma knife surgery in vascular, neoplastic, and functional disorders of the nervous system. In Schmidek HH, Sweet WH (eds): Operative Neurosurgical Techniques. Philadelphia, WB Saunders, 1994, pp 667–694.

36. Kondziolka D, Lunsford LD, Flickinger J: Gamma knife stereotactic radiosurgery for cerebral vascular malformations. In Alexander E, Loeffler JS, Lunsford LD (eds): Stereotactic Radiosurgery. New York, McGraw-Hill, 1993, pp 136–146.

37. Betti OO, Derechinsky VE: Hyperselective encephalic irradiation with a linear accelerator. Acta Neurochir Suppl (Wien) 33:385–390, 1984.

38. Colombo F: Linear accelerator radiosurgery: A clinical experience. J Neurosurg Sci 33:123–125, 1989.

39. Winston KR, Lutz W: Linear accelerator as a neurosurgical tool for stereotactic radiosurgery. Neurosurgery 22:454–464, 1988.

40. Alexander E, Moriarty TM, Davis RB, et al: Stereotactic radiosurgery for the definitive, noninvasive treatment of brain metastasis. J Natl Cancer Inst 87:34–40, 1995.

41. Engenhart R, Kimmig BN, Hover KH, et al: Long-term follow-up for brain metastases treated by percutaneous stereotactic single high-dose irradiation. Cancer 71:1353–1361, 1993.

42. Joseph J, Adler JR, Cox RS, et al: Linear accelerator–based stereotactic radiosurgery for brain metastases: The influence of number of lesions on survival. J Clin Oncol 14:1085–1092, 1996.

43. Mendenhall WM, Friedman WA, Bova FJ: Linear accelerator–based stereotactic radiosurgery for acoustic schwannomas. Int J Radiat Oncol Biol Phys 28:803–810, 1994; see comments.

44. Chang SD, Adler JR: The treatment of skull base meningiomas with linac radiosurgery. Neurosurgery 41:1022–1029, 1997.

45. Valentino V, Schinaia G, Raimondi AJ: The results of radiosurgical management of 72 middle fossa meningiomas. Acta Neurochir (Wien) 122:60–70, 1993.

46. Friedman WA, Bova FJ, Mendenhall WM: Linear accelerator radiosurgery for arteriovenous malformations: The relationship of size to outcome. J Neurosurg 82:180–189, 1995.

47. Colombo F, Pozza F, Chierego G, et al: Linear accelerator radiosurgery of cerebral arteriovenous malformations: An update. Neurosurgery 34:14–21, 1994.

48. Adler JR, Chang SD, Murphy MJ, et al: The CyberKnife: A frameless robotic system for radiosurgery. Stereotact Funct Neurosurg 69:124–128, 1998.

49. Adler JRJ, Cox RS: Preliminary clinical experience with the CyberKnife: Image-guided stereotactic radiosurgery. In Alexander E, Kondziolka D, Loeffler JS (eds): Radiosurgery 1995. Basel, Karger, 1996, pp 316–326.

50. Chang SD, Adler JR, Murphy MJ: Stereotactic radiosurgery of spinal lesions. In Maciunas RJ (ed): Advanced Techniques in Central nervous System Metastasis. Park Ridge, Ill, American Association of Neurological Surgeons, 1998, pp 269–276.

51. Chang SD, Murphy MJ, Tombropoulos R, et al: Robotic radiosurgery. In Alexander E, Maciunas R (eds): Advanced Neurosurgical Navigation. New York, Thieme, 1998, pp 443–449.

52. Lutz W, Winston KR, Maleki N: A system for stereotactic radiosurgery with a linear accelerator. Int J Radiat Oncol Biol Phys 14:373–381, 1988.

53. Podgorsak EB, Olivier A, Pla M, et al: Dynamic stereotactic radiosurgery. Int J Radiat Oncol Biol Phys 14:115–126, 1988.

54. Nedzi LA, Kooy HM, Alexander ED, et al: Dynamic field shaping for stereotactic radiosurgery: A modeling study. Int J Radiat Oncol Biol Phys 25:859–869, 1993.

CHAPTER **262**

Radiobiology

JOHN M. BUATTI ■ SANFORD L. MEEKS ■ NINA A. MAYR
MICHAEL E. C. ROBBINS ■ WILLIAM A. FRIEDMAN ■ FRANK J. BOVA

Radiotherapy has been used to treat cancers since 1895. Its application to brain tumors followed shortly thereafter. Since that time, radiation has been a standard treatment option after incomplete resection of malignant tumors, but its successful application to benign tumors has been more difficult to establish. The rationale for and radiobiology of radiation treatments are complex and involve both an understanding of the purely cellular effects of radiation and the physical characteristics of dose deposition in tissues. Together, these cellular and physical effects produce the radiobiology of radiation as applied through conventional radiotherapy, conformal three-dimensional radiotherapy, stereotactic radiotherapy, and stereotactic radiosurgery.

Radiotherapy uses ionizing radiation, which means that its energy is sufficient to remove an electron from the outer shell of an atom (>124 electron volts).[1] When this occurs, an atom becomes more reactive and hence more apt to interact with neighboring atoms and molecules. With this simple model of ionizing radiation, we can explain the effects of radiation on cells and its subsequent application for brain tumor treatment.

Within cells, the most abundant molecule is water. In addition, lipids, proteins, carbohydrates, and nucleotides are present at varying concentrations. When ionizing radiation interacts with a cell, it can interact with any of these molecules, but statistically, the most likely interaction is the ionization of water. This reaction creates reactive species that are apt to interact chemically with surrounding molecules. The most common of these reactive species are free radical derivatives of water.

Although radiation reactions with water are inconsequential alone, they give rise to events in which a reactive water derivative may interact with DNA. DNA is likely the most critical target for cellular radiation effects. Damage to DNA creates the potential for permanent cell injury or death, genetic mutation, or, conversely, repair of the cell's DNA. Radiation damage to DNA mediated through reactive species of water is called the indirect effect of ionizing radiation. More rarely, radiation interacts directly with DNA, and this is called the direct effect of radiation. In addition, injury to other intracellular molecules (such as lipids or proteins) is thought to play a role in the cellular effects of radiation. In particular, damage to lipids and the creation of free radicals outside of those directly damaging DNA may indirectly lead to cell death mediated by cellular apoptotic cascades or other damaging cellular events.[2, 3] Manipulation of the cells' normal capacity to handle metabolically derived free radicals is an area of active radiobiologic research.[4]

Much evidence indicates that DNA is the critical cellular target of radiation. Genetic damage and specific chromosomal abnormalities after irradiation have been correlated with cell death. Defects or proficiency in cellular DNA repair mechanisms increases or decreases radiosensitivity. Selective irradiation of the cell nucleus (where most DNA is located), as opposed to the cytoplasm, has mimicked the overall effect of radiation on cells.[1] This basic effect of radiation on DNA and subsequent repair underlies the principles of conventional fractionated radiotherapy treatment.

RADIOBIOLOGY OF CONVENTIONAL FRACTIONATED RADIOTHERAPY

The cellular effects of radiation occur in an unbiased way. In other words, radiation damages the DNA of tumor cells as well as the DNA of normal cells in its path. Therefore, to have a therapeutic effect, radiation must selectively injure tumor and not normal tissue.

Historically, radiotherapy has relied on physical examination of the patient, knowledge of the disease (spread patterns), and the technical ability to deliver the dose of radiotherapy to the tumor regions as determined by both the physical examination and the interpretation of two-dimensional images as defined by plain film radiographs.[5] A typical treatment planning session, called a *simulation*, approximately positions the patient in reference to the treatment machine for appropriate beam entrance and exit. The patient's position is recorded via the intersection of room lasers that emit thin red or green lines of light from the lateral walls and ceiling that intersect at the center point of the axis of rotation for the treatment machine, called the *isocenter*. The intersection of these laser lines with the patient's physical anatomy makes three points (one on each side and one at the intersection from the ceiling) that are marked or tattooed (permanent marks). Thus, the approximate position at the simulation is recorded permanently by the intersection of these isocenter-defining lasers with the patient's anatomy. This method of positioning is termed *triangulation*. The radiation oncologist can then manually map the patient's tumor from the examination or from other imaging methods such as computed tomography, and treatment portals are designed based on these transferred images.

In this paradigm, there is inherent recognition that the dose of radiation will not only treat the discrete tumor but also damage the normal surrounding tissue. Normal tissue, however, is generally more capable of DNA repair than are tumors. There are likely many reasons for this, but it is at least partly because of aberrant cell-cycle control mechanisms in tumors, as well as differences in genetic features that permit changes to the abnormal tumor phenotype.[6-8] Abnormal metabolic patterns may make tumors more susceptible to increases in oxidative stress compared with normal cells.[4] Therefore, the radiobiology of differential cellular repair is paramount for conventional radiotherapy, although the precise reasons for this are unclear.[9]

Cells require time to repair DNA damage, and the normal cell response to irradiation is to delay cell-cycle progression in the G1 and G2 phase.[6, 7] The length of G2 delay correlates with radiation resistance.[8] Another biologic observation is that more rapidly dividing, acutely responding normal tissues, such as skin, oral mucosa, and gastrointestinal mucosa, are more acutely sensitive to the effects of irradiation than are late-responding and slowly dividing or nondividing tissues, such as nervous system tissue.[9] This is especially true at low doses of irradiation, when repair of DNA damage is more likely. This is shown graphically on cell survival curves illustrating the difference in response to radiation doses between early- and late-responding tissues (Fig. 262–1).[1, 9, 10] Note that in the figure, a large single dose of radiation is capable of greater injury to late-responding normal tissue than to tumor, making it biologically undesirable. Therefore, to take advantage of the inherent ability of normal cells to repair sublethal doses of irradiation better than tumor cells, multiple small doses of radiation are recommended. This is particularly true for more malignant tumors.[11]

This principle has dominated the practice of radiation oncology for most of its history. Attempts at treatments using high doses were fraught with complica-

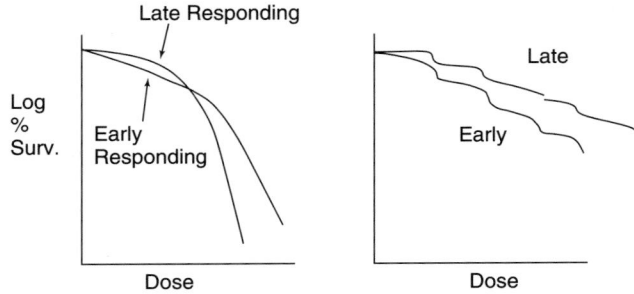

FIGURE 262–1. The radiation survival curve plots the log of the percentage of cell survival versus dose. In the initial curve, labeled late-responding tissue, there is relative resistance at low doses compared with the early-responding tissue. But at higher doses, the opposite is true. There is relatively greater sensitivity of the normal late-responding tissue (central nervous system). The second graph shows the advantage for the survival of normal late-responding tissue with repeated low doses of radiation compared with early-responding tissue.

tions. The initial inability to give high-energy treatments from multiple directions required high superficial doses of irradiation, which led to the perception that most treatments would lead to severe burns. Hence, early recognition that fractionated treatments could be tolerated and create a therapeutic advantage for the tumor was critical to the success of radiation oncology. The rationale for this approach is the biologic principle of differential cellular repair of normal tissues versus neoplastic disease.

The standard approach to radiotherapy includes the dose delivery simulation as described previously, followed by daily treatments. Dose is reported in the unit gray (Gy), which represents 1 joule of energy absorbed per kilogram of tissue. One centigray (cGy) is one hundredth of a gray and is equivalent to the older unit of dose, the rad. The most commonly prescribed unit of absorbed dose is 1.8 to 2 Gy, which has proved to be well tolerated at most areas of the body and can be repeated a specific number of times, depending on the region involved and the therapeutic target. For practical purposes, the tolerance of the whole brain is considered to be 45 to 50 Gy in 20 to 25 fractions, although it is recognized that this dose may yield substantial dementia and memory loss with time.[12] In children, it has been shown that tolerance is reduced in an age-dependent manner, such that whole-brain radiotherapy is seldom considered an option in those younger than 3 years of age.[13, 14] In addition, it has been shown that particular areas of the brain such as the optic apparatus, including the retina, optic nerve, and chiasm, may be more sensitive, particularly to larger doses greater than 1.9 Gy per fraction.[15] Hence, even in the most conventional treatment paradigm, it is clear that the radiobiology and the use of radiation as a clinical modality have much to learn from each other. The biology does not, strictly speaking, predict the clinical outcome reliably, and the clinical treatment may benefit from the knowledge that differential repair is a powerful therapeutic tool.[11]

The greatest interaction between radiobiology and clinical practice has occurred with efforts to change the standard fractionation schedules.[16, 17] Hyperfraction-ation is the division of a dose into two doses with an interval of time in between for repair. Practically speaking, doses of 1 to 1.5 Gy have been given two or more times daily with 4 to 6 hours between treatments. Accelerated fractionation involves giving the same dose over a shorter period of time. The ability to give more than 1 Gy at least twice daily not only yields hyperfractionation but also allows the total radiation dose to be reached more quickly than at doses of 2 Gy per day. Such altered fractionation schedules have been highly successful in improving the therapeutic out-come for head and neck cancers, but the applicability for brain tumors is unproved.[17] Despite this progress, conventional radiotherapy has proved to be most effec-tive as an adjunctive treatment for the majority of brain tumors.[18, 19]

RADIOBIOLOGY OF RADIOSURGERY

Therapeutic advantage may also be achieved by depos-iting more radiation dose in the tumor than in the normal tissue. A single radiation beam entering a pa-tient begins with a region of lower dose termed the *buildup region*.[20] The dose progressively increases until it reaches the depth of maximal dose that is characteris-tic of the radiation beam energy. This buildup region, in higher-energy situations, allows radiation beams to spare superficial areas (skin and subcutaneous tissue) from the highest doses of radiation. After the radiation beam reaches the depth of maximal dose, the dose decreases with depth because of attenuation of the beam by the intervening tissue. This is called the *fall-off region*.

To achieve selectivity of dose delivered to a tumor, several beams of radiation can be added from several directions (Fig. 262–2). A single beam of radiation en-tering a patient is shown in Figure 262–2*A*. Note that a characteristic group of same-dose, or isodose, lines is indicated. The numbers represent the percentage of maximal dose for that beam and also illustrate the buildup and falloff regions. If we put an imaginary tumor at the intersection of two beams of radiation oriented at right angles to each other, the isodose lines are shown in Figure 262–2*B*. Note that the tumor re-ceives the highest dose, and areas outside the tumor now receive progressively less radiation. This charac-teristic is commonly used in conventional radiotherapy, although the practical limits are two to four fields, and delivery accuracy is on the order of 1 cm or more in many anatomic sites. As 99 beams are added together, the isodose lines take on the configuration shown in Figure 262–2*C*. These examples of the physical charac-teristics of radiation beams illustrate the capacity of diligent radiation delivery to target a higher percentage of the radiation dose to the tumor, with progressively smaller areas of normal tissue receiving significant doses. This ability led Lars Leksell to describe the concept of radiosurgery in 1951.[21] He described the use of radiation as a means of replacing the scalpel or electrode for functional neurosurgery. In so doing, the biology of differential repair was discarded, and the

main biologic advantage became the ability to destroy focally identified areas and avoid the normal brain by physical means. This method required that the para-digm for radiation delivery be changed.

Stereotactic radiosurgery is the method that Leksell described. The application of stereotaxis to radiation delivery is the most important part of this treatment paradigm. It allows precise coidentification of an actual patient and a virtual patient as defined by a group of images in a computer, such that the two are linked with a robust system of fiducials. This is most commonly accomplished by attaching a rigid stereotactic head ring to the patient and using this ring as a frame of reference throughout the process. A system of three-dimensional fiducials is attached to the head ring dur-ing computed tomography acquisition, providing accu-rate spatial identification of each pixel within the image set. In essence, each pixel becomes a mathematical coordinate in reference to the head ring. After the treatment coordinates (pixels) have been identified in the treatment plan, they can be directly transferred to a mechanical system that provides accurate patient localization relative to the treatment unit. To use this paradigm optimally, mechanical error in the treatment delivery device and imaging inaccuracy defined by pixel size and slice thickness must be minimized.[20] This paradigm has become a standard treatment option for numerous benign and malignant central nervous sys-tem pathologies. The biologic principles of its use are completely different from those of standard radiother-apy.[11, 22] The method permits the development of ex-tremely conformal dose distributions that expose mini-mal volumes of normal brain to significant radiation, eliminating the need for differential repair to obtain a clinically relevant therapeutic advantage.

However, additional features of this nonfractionated therapy have relevance for biologic manipulation. It is recognized that although differential repair is advanta-geous if radiation therapy is used alone to treat a large volume of normal tissue, it is not an optimal way to take advantage of radiation-sensitizing agents or radioprotective agents. For example, in Figure 262–3, the therapeutic enhancement of the sensitizer at a dose of 2 Gy yields a 30% increase in cell kill. In contrast, at doses of 15 Gy, the enhancement is more than 3 logs of cell kill.[1] In addition, the single application of the sensitizer may reduce the side effects of the drug or biologic agent that, in a conventional pattern, would be required daily to produce the effect. Hence, the biology may favor the application of combined or con-current modality therapy, which has been often diffi-cult or ineffective with conventional radiation therapy delivery.

Finally, there may be poorly understood differences in biologic effects on the vasculature as well as the tumor at higher doses. The dose gradient in conven-tional treatment falls to less than half the dose over a number of centimeters, whereas the dose falloff occurs over 2 to 4 mm in a typical radiosurgical treatment. The differences in the dose characteristics have been incompletely described from a radiobiologic perspec-tive, and the clinical application has moved further than biology might explain. Again, both the clinical

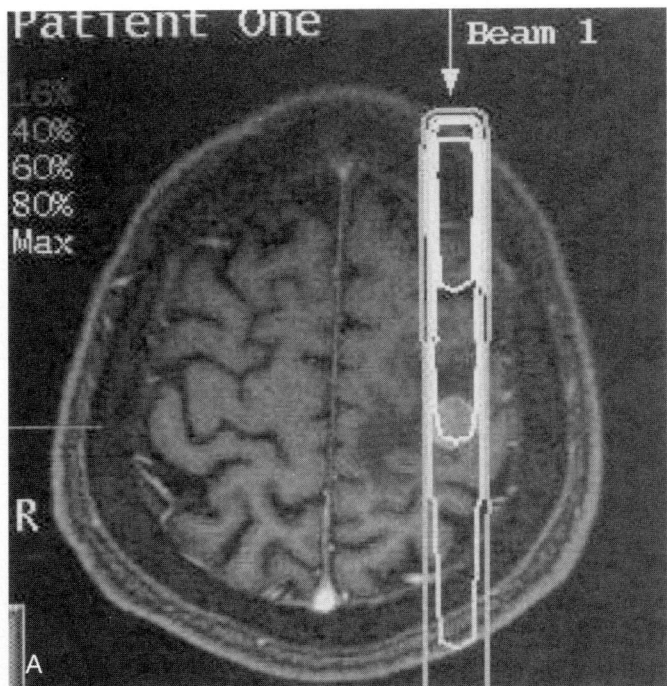

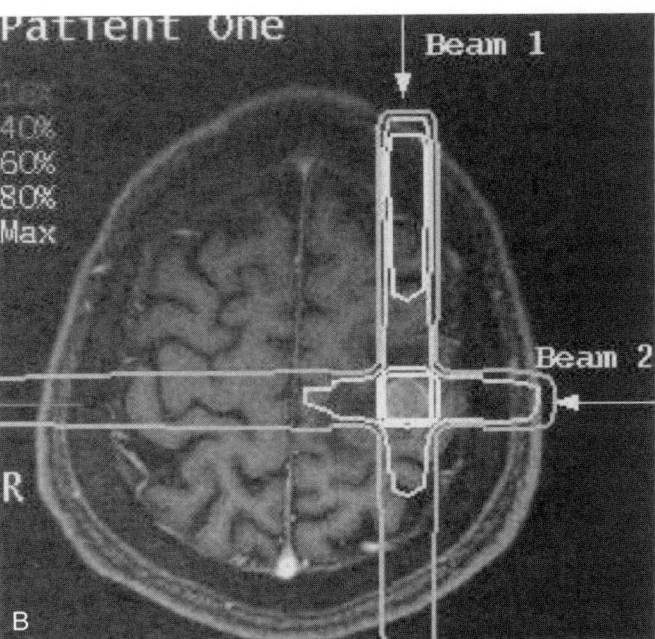

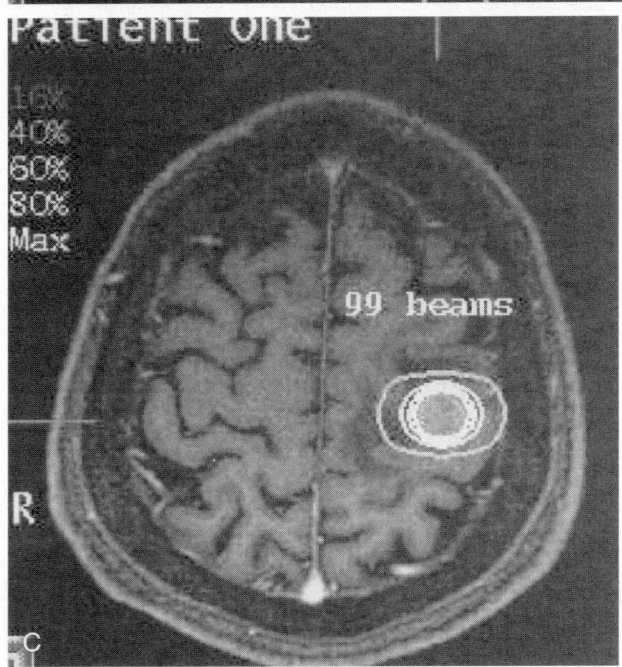

FIGURE 262–2. *A,* Single radiation field traversing the brain. This illustrates both the buildup region and the attenuation of the radiation beam. Same-dose, or isodose, lines are displayed. *B,* Effect of adding a second beam. Note that the isodoses show concentration of the high-dose region at the intersection of the two right-angled beams. The maximal dose is where there is least attenuation of the two beams and intersection. *C,* Effects of extending the concentrating ability to 99 beams of radiation, as in radiosurgery. By doing this, the dose falls off in 2 to 4 mm to less than half the dose.

application of radiation and the radiobiology have much to learn from each other regarding optimal application of the treatment.

RADIOBIOLOGY OF CONFORMAL AND STEREOTACTIC RADIOTHERAPY

From a practical perspective, conformal and stereotactic radiotherapy modalities lie between the extremes of conventional radiotherapy and radiosurgery, as does their biology. Clinically, these methods offer the capac-

ity to use fractionation to take advantage of differences in normal tissue repair. They enable the use of images and virtual simulation to make the doses more closely approximate the target lesion, but they do not achieve the precision or conformality of radiosurgery. These methods may alter fractionation patterns to somewhere between the conventional 1.8 to 2 Gy in many fractions and the 12.5 Gy or more used for the vast majority of radiosurgery treatments. The optimal use of three to six fraction regimens is an area of active clinical investigation, and it is unclear whether it will be better or worse than the more established methods of conven-

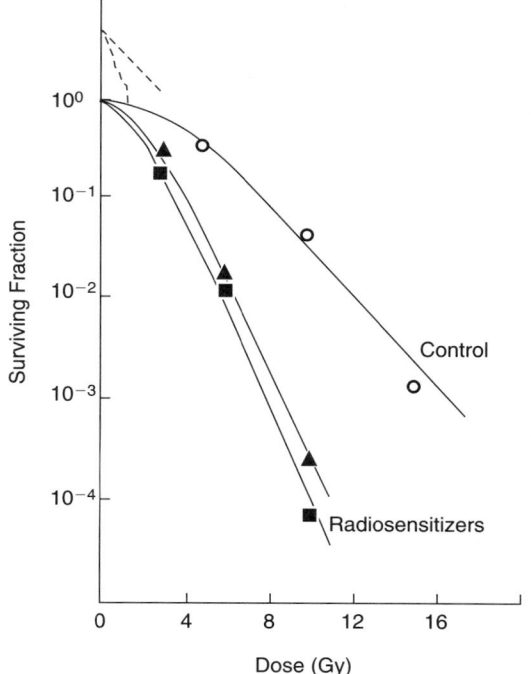

FIGURE 262–3. Effect of a radiosensitizer on a radiation survival curve. Note that the greatest effect is seen at higher single doses of irradiation. There are logs of difference in the range of ra diosurgical doses, compared with about a 30% advantage at conventional fractionated doses.

tional radiotherapy and radiosurgery.[23, 24] The radiobiology of such regimens is not clearly defined either.

FUTURE QUESTIONS

Although much is known about the radiobiology of radiotherapy in the central nervous system, there is even more that is unknown. The advent of stereotactic paradigms has provided the opportunity to precisely define the dose delivered to particular anatomic sites. The image-guided methods of conformal and stereotactic radiotherapy offer the same potential advantage in defining the biology of neurotolerance. In so doing, the possibility of defining radiation tolerance in far greater detail exists. Further, the ability to study radiation tolerance with noninvasive imaging methods such as functional imaging may be advantageous. Advances in neuroscience will undoubtedly improve our understanding of the biologic effects on a molecular level. This is important for both tumor and normal tissue interaction. The differences in response to large doses of radiation in focal areas versus large volumes treated with smaller doses will likely lead to different radiobiologic consequences. For example, it is known that certain radiation-induced genes do not become activated until doses in excess of conventional fractionation are given.[25] Hence, we have merely scratched the surface in discovering how radiation works and its potential use in treating disease.

REFERENCES

1. Hall EJ: Radiobiology for the Radiologist, 4th ed. Philadelphia, JB Lippincott, 1994, pp 1–13.
2. Hallahan DE, Virudachalam S, Kuchibhotla J, et al: Membrane-derived second messenger regulates x-ray–mediated tumor necrosis factor alpha gene induction. Proc Natl Acad Sci U S A 24:4897–4901, 1994.
3. Crompton NE: Programmed cellular response to ionizing radiation damage. Acta Oncol 37(suppl 11):129–142, 1998.
4. Spitz DR, Sim JE, Ridnour LA, et al: Glucose deprivation–induced oxidative stress in human tumor cells: A fundamental defect in metabolism? Ann N Y Acad Sci 899:349–362, 2000.
5. Khan FM: The Physics of Radiation Therapy, 2nd ed. Baltimore, Williams & Wilkins, 1994.
6. Yamada M, Puck TT: Action of radiation on mammalian cells. IV. Reversible mitotic lag in the S3 HeLa cell produced by low doses of x-rays. Proc Natl Acad Sci U S A 47:1181, 1961.
7. Little JB, Hahn GM: Life cycle dependence of repair of potentially-lethal radiation damage. Int J Radiat Biol 23:401–407, 1973.
8. Muschel RJ, Zhang HB, Iliakis G, et al: Cyclin B expression in HeLa cells during the G2 block induced by ionizing radiation. Cancer Res 51:5113–5117, 1991.
9. Fowler JF: Brief summary of radiobiological principles in fractionated radiotherapy. Semin Radiat Oncol 2:16–21, 1992.
10. Thames HD, Bentzen SM, Turesson I, et al: Fractionation parameters for human tissues and tumors. Int J Radiat Biol 56:701–710, 1989.
11. Hall EJ, Brenner DJ: The radiobiology of radiosurgery: Rationale for different treatment regimes for AVMs and malignancies. Int J Radiat Oncol Biol Phys 25:381–385, 1993.
12. Crossen JR, Garwood D, Glatstein E, Neuwelt EA: Neurobehavioral sequelae of cranial irradiation in adults: A review of radiation-induced encephalopathy. J Clin Oncol 12:627–642, 1994.
13. Dennis M, Spiegler BJ, Hoffman HJ, et al: Brain tumors in children and adolescents. I. Effects on working, associative and serial-order memory of IQ, age at tumor onset and age of tumor. Neuropsychologia 29:813–827, 1991.
14. Packer RJ, Sutton L, Atkins TE, et al: A prospective study of cognitive function in children receiving whole brain radiotherapy and chemotherapy: 2-year results. J Neurosurg 70:707–713, 1989.
15. Parsons JT, Bova FJ, Fitzgerald CR, et al: Radiation retinopathy after external-beam irradiation: Analysis of time-dose factors. Int J Radiat Oncol Biol Phys 30:765–773, 1994.
16. Fowler JF: The linear-quadratic formula and progress in fractionated radiotherapy. Br J Radiol 62:679–694, 1989.
17. Fu KK, Pajak TF, Trotti A, et al: A Radiation Therapy Oncology Group (RTOG) phase III randomized study to compare hyperfractionation and two variants of accelerated fractionation to standard fractionation radiotherapy for head and neck squamous cell carcinomas: First report of RTOG 9003. Int J Radiat Oncol Biol Phys 48:7–16, 2000.
18. Murray KJ, Scott C, Greenberg HM, et al: A randomized phase III study of accelerated hyperfractionation versus standard in patients with unresected brain metastases: A report of the Radiation Therapy Oncology Group (RTOG) 9104. Int J Radiat Oncol Biol Phys 39:571–574, 1997.
19. Stuschke M, Thames HD: Hyperfractionated radiotherapy of human tumors: Overview of the randomized clinical trials. Int J Radiat Oncol Biol Phys 37:259–267, 1997.
20. Friedman WA, Buatti JM, Bova FJ, Mendenhall WM: Linac Radiosurgery: A Practical Guide. New York, Springer Verlag, 1998.
21. Leksell L: The stereotaxic method and radiosurgery of the brain. Acta Chir Scand 102:316–319, 1951.
22. Buatti JM, Friedman WA, Meeks SL, Bova FJ: The radiobiology of radiosurgery and stereotactic radiotherapy. Med Dosim 23:201–207, 1998.
23. Lederman G, Lowry J, Wertheim S, et al: Acoustic neuroma: Potential benefits of fractionated stereotactic radiosurgery. Stereotact Funct Neurosurg 69(Pt 2):175–182, 1997.
24. Poen JC, Golby AJ, Forster KM, et al: Fractionated stereotactic radiosurgery and preservation of hearing in patients with vestibular schwannoma: A preliminary report. Neurosurgery 45:1299–1305, discussion 1305–1307, 1999.
25. Hallahan DE, Weichselbaum R: Role of gene therapy in radiation oncology. Cancer Treat Res 93:153–167, 1998.

Principles of Radiotherapy

JOHN H. SUH ■ ROGER M. MACKLIS

Until the 1950s, use of radiotherapy in the treatment of brain tumors was primarily palliative. Although certain types of tumors, such as medulloblastoma and pituitary adenoma, were known to be treatable and perhaps curable with radiotherapy, the great majority of primary glial tumors were thought to be too radioresistant to allow effective treatment without inordinate toxicity. The development of megavoltage radiotherapy in the 1950s and 1960s, coupled with the development of specialized imaging techniques such as computed tomography (CT) and magnetic resonance imaging (MRI), has led to a renaissance in brain tumor radiotherapy. The ability to deliver extremely high doses of focal radiation to specific anatomic regions means that highly conformal doses of radiation may be matched to biologically active target regions with minimal treatment of normal brain tissue. Parallel advances in the field of neurosurgery have also led to dramatic improvements in clinical success rates. These improvements in technical radiotherapy for the treatment of brain tumors and the development of specialized treatment devices and approaches specifically optimized for brain tumors make this aspect of radiation oncology one of the most interesting and dynamic in modern oncology.

BASIC PHYSICS

The physical basis of radiotherapy starts with the generation of radiation and the physical descriptions of the beams and particles used in modern radiotherapy. Briefly, radiotherapy can be divided into photon beams, such as x-rays and gamma rays, and energetic particle beams, such as electrons and protons. Gamma rays originate from inside a nucleus, and the energy of gamma rays produced by various radioisotopes, such as cobalt 60, have specific characteristic energies. In the case of cobalt 60, the gamma rays emitted have energies of 1.17 and 1.33 MeV.

X-rays result either when electrons shift to lower atomic orbits or when fast-moving electrons are made to collide with a target, resulting in rapid deceleration of the impinging electrons. In decelerating, the electrons must give up energy, and they give it up as x-ray photons. By varying the energy of the electrons, the material with which they collide, and the conditions of the collision, the frequency of the resultant spectrum of x-rays can be "tuned" to the energy characteristics desired for therapy. Most of modern radiotherapy uses photon energies between 6 and 25 MV. The most common energy range used for brain tumors is 4 to 6 MV.

Unlike photon beams, particle beams consist of rapidly moving bits of matter with known charge and mass. The utility of particle beams in tumor therapy relates to the limited range of these particles in tissue. For megavoltage electrons in the range of 6 to 25 MeV (the typical energies chosen for therapy), virtually all the beam energy is dissipated in the first 3 to 12.5 cm after contact with soft tissue. For protons, the range may be much more discrete. The characteristic Bragg peak, which describes a very narrow tissue width over which most proton energy is dissipated, is responsible for the interest in and recent enthusiasm for proton beam radiotherapy in the treatment of brain tumors.

RADIATION INTERACTIONS

The interaction of radiation beams with matter varies, depending on the type of beam, the energy, the atomic number, and the density of the material the beam is impacting. For purposes of this chapter, the most important interactions are those between photons and soft tissue. Three types of interactions are described: photoelectric effect, pair production, and Compton effect.

The *photoelectric effect* involves the transfer of all available photon energy to an inner-shell electron. Because all its energy is transferred, the photon disappears, and the electron is ejected from the atom carrying the transferred energy (minus binding energy), leaving an inner-shell vacancy. When an outer-shell electron fills this vacancy, a characteristic x-ray is released. The photoelectric effect is most important at low energies, and the probability that a photoelectric effect interaction will take place is proportional to the atomic number of the target material cubed, divided by the photon energy cubed.

A classic *pair production* interaction occurs with pho-

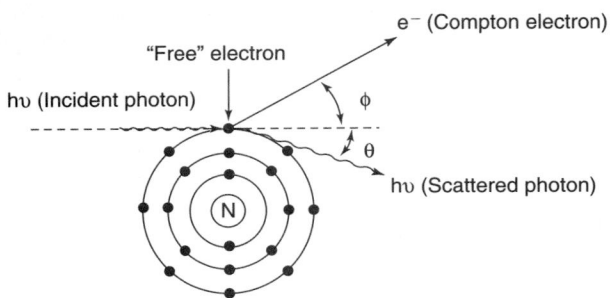

FIGURE 263–1. Schematic drawing illustrating the Compton effect. (From Purdy JA: Principles of radiologic physics, dosimetry, and treatment planning. In Perez CA, Brady LW [eds]: Principles and Practice of Radiation Oncology. Philadelphia, JB Lippincott, 1998, p 250.)

tons that have an energy greater than 1.02 MeV. When these high-energy photons approach the nucleus of a target atom, they transform into a pair of oppositely charged particles (electron and positron). All the energy originally possessed by the photon in excess of 1.02 MeV (the particle creation energy) is divided between the two new particles and appears as particle kinetic energy. The positron subsequently combines with an electron, and they annihilate each other, giving rise to low-energy (0.511 MeV) photons in the process. The probability of a pair production event is proportional to the atomic number of the target material and the initial photon energy.

The final mode of interaction between photons and matter is called the *Compton effect* (Fig. 263–1). In this interaction, an incoming photon knocks a loosely bound orbital electron out of its orbital shell, transferring a portion of its energy to the scattered Compton electron. Unlike in the other two modes of photon interaction, the probability of a successful Compton interaction is almost independent of the atomic number of the absorbing tissue energy range of 1 to 25 MV, but it does depend on electron density. The Compton effect is the dominant effect in the therapy range of photons.

BIOLOGIC EFFECTS OF RADIATION

For all these modes of interaction, a liberated unpaired electron is produced and is primarily responsible for biologic effects. When radiation interacts directly with biologically relevant molecules such as DNA, the instability caused by ionization results in damage to the molecule. In the case of DNA, the damage is often manifested as single-strand or double-strand breaks in the double-helix backbone. This is called the *direct action* of radiation. When radiation interacts with atoms or molecules that are not biologically critical but are positioned in close proximity to DNA (e.g., water molecules), the ionized water molecules may produce the same types of strand breaks in nearby DNA. In this case, the radiation acts through an intermediary molecule, and this type of interaction is termed *indirect action*.

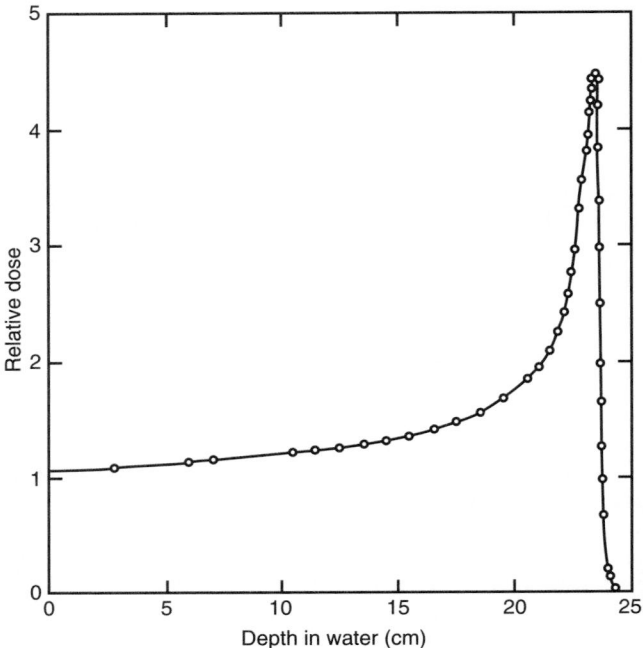

FIGURE 263–2. Depth-dose curve for 187-MeV proton. Note the sharp peak at about 23 cm. (Redrawn from Larsson B: Pre-therapeutic physical experiments with high energy photons. Br J Radiol 34:143–151, 1961.)

Some types of radiation, such as heavy particle beams, produce densely ionizing tracks as they pass through tissue. These densely ionizing forms of radiation are characterized by a high ability to transfer energy to the molecules with which they interact and are called high linear energy transfer beams. The amount of energy that a particle transfers is inversely proportional to the velocity with which the particle travels; thus, very fast moving particles may transfer little energy. As particles interact with matter and give up energy, they slow down and eventually reach a state in which large amounts of energy are transferred over a fairly short path length. This effect is responsible for the Bragg peak produced by protons and other particles (Fig. 263–2). Because the Bragg peak is produced at a specific and predictable depth in tissue, this sort of treatment seems ideal for targets located immediately adjacent to critical normal structures. For many applications, however, the focal location of the Bragg peak may be too restrictive to allow effective clinical treatment, and for that reason, some centers use physical means to spread the Bragg peak out over a wider area. Because proton beam therapy is used clinically in only a few centers worldwide, the optimal use of this modality is not yet clear.

ABSORBED DOSE AND UNITS OF RADIATION

The amount of energy absorbed per unit mass is the absorbed radiation dose. This, multiplied by a relative biologic effectiveness factor, represents the biologically significant effect of ionizing radiation on tissues. In the first step, energy from an impinging photon is transformed into kinetic energy of high-speed electrons. In the second step, the electrons produce a shower of additional electrons that decelerate and deposit their energy in the medium. Historically, the term *rad* was used as the unit of absorbed radiation dose.[1] The International System of Units (SI) now identifies the *gray* (Gy) as the unit of absorbed dose; it is equivalent to 1 joule per kilogram.[2] One hundred centigrays (cGy) or 100 rad is equivalent to 1 Gy. The *roentgen* (R) is based on the ability of gamma rays or roentgen rays to ionize air and represents a unit of exposure. For radioactive elements, the activity is expressed as the number of disintegrations per second. The *curie* (Ci) is equal to 3.7×10^{10} disintegrations per second. The parallel SI unit is the *becquerel* (Bq), which is 1 disintegration per second.

TYPES OF RADIOTHERAPY

Radiotherapy can be broadly divided into brachytherapy and external beam radiation therapy. Brachytherapy uses radioactive sources applied within or around a tumor. External beam radiation therapy (teletherapy) most commonly uses x-rays, gamma rays, or electrons, which are directed at specific anatomic targets. Both techniques have been proven effective in treating a variety of brain tumors, and they are often combined to take advantage of their specific dosimetric advantages.

Brachytherapy allows for high local doses of radiation. This technique has been used for many years and has proved to be effective against many different types of brain tumors.[3] The progressive decrease in radiation dose with distance of radiation is based on the inverse square law and is very rapid as one moves away from the source. Afterloading techniques with machines that automatically load the radioactive sources and the use of lower-energy isotopes have greatly increased radiation safety. The most commonly used isotopes in brachytherapy are iodine 125 and iridium 192.

Photon beam radiation represents the most common form of therapeutic radiation used in cancer treatment. It is broadly classified into orthovoltage (100 to 400 kV) or megavoltage, also called supervoltage (>1 MV). Before 1950, external beam radiation therapy consisted of kilovoltage units with energies up to 300 kV produced by accelerating electrons in an electric field. The sudden deceleration of electrons in a metal target produces x-rays. Examples of such units include contact, superficial, and orthovoltage units. Given the superficial depth of penetration, high doses are delivered to the cutaneous tissues, making treatment of deep tumors inadvisable. Thus this method is not used to treat brain tumors.

Megavoltage photons are emitted from a radioactive source such as cobalt 60 or produced by electrons accelerated along a microwave guide and decelerated by colliding with a tungsten target, causing the release of photons. The first commercial supervoltage machines were resonant transformers and Van de Graaf generators. These were superseded by the introduction of the linear accelerator (linac) and cobalt-60 teletherapy machines, which allowed for the routine use of megavoltage (>1 MV) beams. In 1951, the use of cobalt-60 units began in radiotherapy clinics.[4, 5] This provided much better penetration than orthovoltage units did and allowed for skin sparing.

The end of World War II brought the development of high-powered microwave generators. This allowed the use of microwave-accelerated electrons for megavoltage radiotherapy in modern linacs.[6] The linac uses high-energy electromagnetic waves to accelerate electrons to high energy through a microwave structure. When the electron strikes a target, x-rays are produced. The beam then goes through a primary collimator, flattening filter, secondary collimator, wedges, and blocks to shape the beam into its final form.

Linacs are the most commonly used machine for the clinical delivery of radiotherapy (Fig. 263–3). Most modern linacs are mounted on rotating gantries so that the system has a center of rotation. The treatment table also rotates about a center of rotation. The axis between the treatment table and the rotating gantry is the isocenter, or central point, of the beam. The table can be moved laterally, vertically, or horizontally to position the tumor at the isocenter.

The major components of a linac are illustrated in

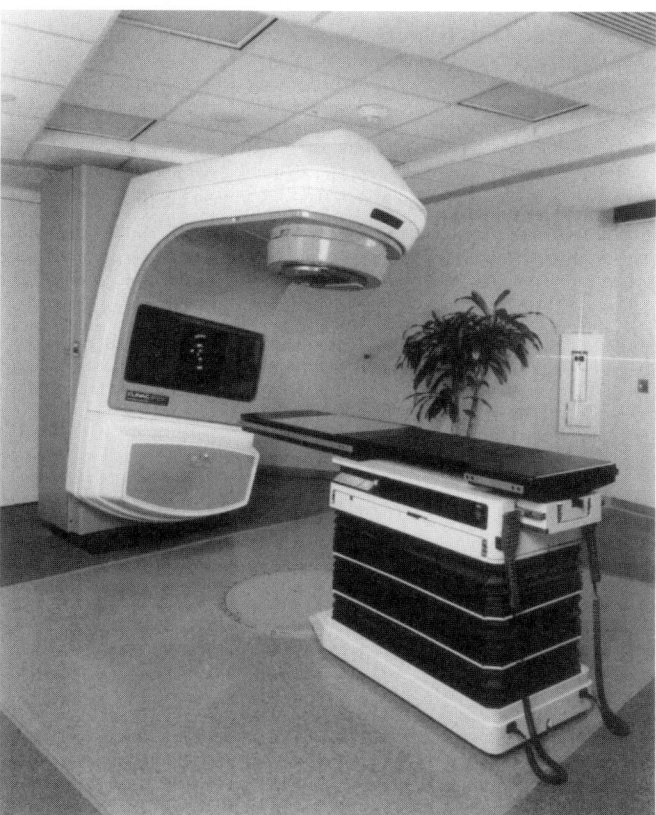

FIGURE 263–3. Linear accelerator. (Courtesy Varian Corp., Palo Alto, Calif.)

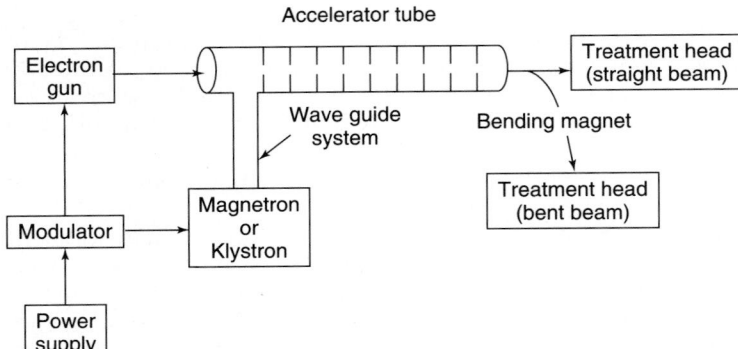

FIGURE 263–4. Major components of a linear accelerator. (From Khan FM: The Physics of Radiation Therapy, 2nd ed. Baltimore, Williams & Wilkins, 1994, p 51.)

Figure 263–4. Electron beams are also available from most modern linacs. Electron energies usually range from 5 to 20 MeV, and their limited tissue penetration makes them useful for the treatment of superficial tumors. Though some have used electron beam treatment to minimize the "exit dose" for medulloblastoma cases, the use of electrons is limited for most brain tumor patients.[7, 8]

Neutron therapy is also in clinical use at certain hospitals. Because they have no charge, neutrons cannot lose energy other than through direct nuclear interactions. Compared with photons, neutron radiobiology demonstrates less oxygen dependence and a higher radiobiologic effect. The falloff of neutron dose with depth mimics low-energy x-rays. To date, studies of neutron beam therapy for malignant gliomas have shown little benefit and greater toxicity compared with conventional radiotherapy.[9]

Protons and heavy particles are produced by cyclotrons or synchrotrons. These particles have a Bragg peak effect that allows for high dose localization at a discrete distance, with virtually no exit dose. If they can be targeted correctly, the use of heavy particles minimizes the dose to surrounding normal tissues, proving useful for patients with chordomas, pituitary adenomas, and ocular melanomas. Owing to the high cost of heavy particle therapy (tens of millions of dollars), only a few centers have established clinical treatment programs using this technology.

DEPTH-DOSE CURVES

The intensity of a photon beam decreases as it travels through an absorbing material. Thus, the beam loses intensity as it penetrates more deeply. The maximal dose occurs at varying positions below the surface, depending on the energy, and it falls gradually from this point, depending on the energy of the photon beam. The analysis of the penetration of various radiation beams once they impact clinically relevant tissue is referred to as *depth-dose analysis*. Characteristic depth-dose curves for various energies of x-rays and electrons are shown in Figure 263–5. Note that for high-energy photons, there is significant sparing of superficial tissues and a relatively greater depth of penetration. The radiation oncologist must use images

showing the position of the target tissue and have knowledge about the various penetration characteristics of different beams in order to optimize dose-deposition patterns.

TREATMENT PLANNING

Ideally, the radiation dose should be focused only on the tumor. This is difficult to achieve, and some radiation is always given to the surrounding normal tissues. Thus, the ability of surrounding normal tissues to absorb radiation without serious injury (tissue tolerance) has traditionally limited the dose that can be safely delivered. The goal of treatment planning is to maximize the dose to specified tumor volumes while minimizing the dose to normal tissues.

The use of multiple fields directed at a target allows for coverage of the tumor within a specified isodose line. In general, multiple fields lead to better conformality around the tumor while minimizing the dose to normal tissues. Wedges or compensators are used to provide dose homogeneity through beam shaping.

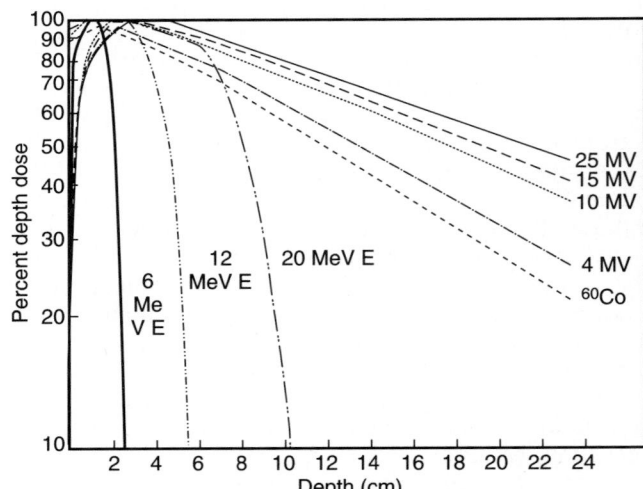

FIGURE 263–5. Examples of central axis depth-dose curves for megavoltage x-ray beams and electron beams. (From Purdy JA: The application of high energy x-rays and electron beams in radiotherapy. IEEE Trans Nucl Sci 26:1833–1837, 1979.)

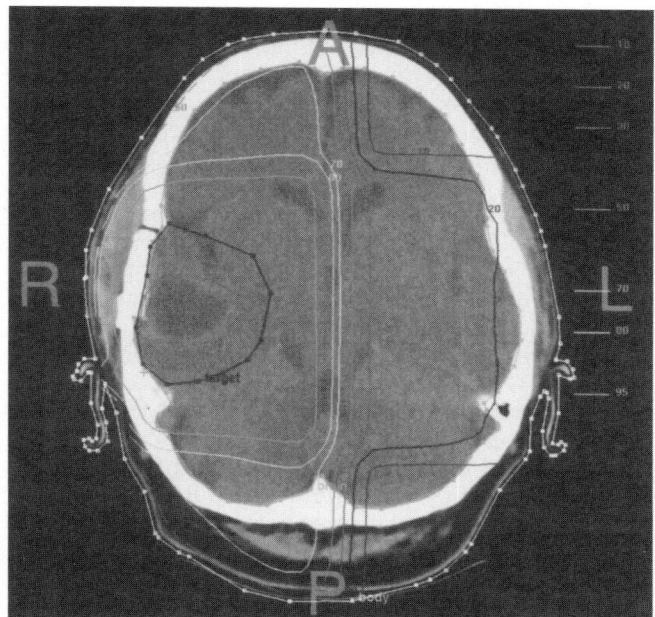

FIGURE 263–6. Single plane of isodose curves for a three-field arrangement for a patient with glioblastoma multiforme.

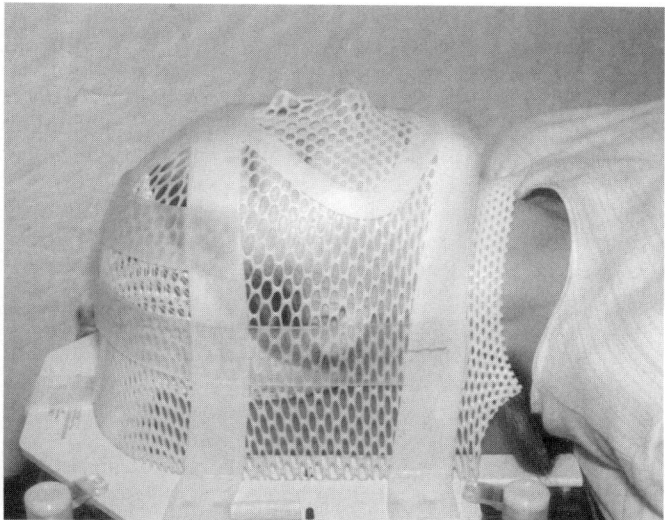

FIGURE 263–7. Thermoplastic mask used to help immobilize the patient's head to ensure reproducibility of the setup.

Points of equal dose are depicted using isodose lines. A set of these curves give a visual representation of the dose distribution in a single plane, similar to a topographic map depicting terrain elevation above sea level (Fig. 263–6). The shape of these curves can be modified by the source size, beam energy, flattening filters, field sizes, source-to-skin distance, and wedges.

SIMULATION

In devising treatment fields, the radiation oncologist must have a sound understanding of the areas at risk for tumor recurrence and must be able to localize the tumor's position relative to the treatment field. The simulator mimics the geometry of an isocentric treatment machine and reproduces the beam entry angles using low-energy diagnostic-quality x-rays to indicate beam trajectories. Simulation allows for visualization of beam direction and treatment fields and represents the first step in determining field arrangement, patient position, and immobilization device.

Immobilization is critical for proper simulation and daily treatment. For infants and young children, sedation or anesthesia may be needed. Devices such as head holders, chin supports, and thermoplastic masks may be used to maintain proper position. With a thermoplastic mask, target accuracy of approximately 5 mm may be achieved (Fig. 263–7). Marks on the mask and laser setup help ensure proper positioning. To improve on cranial fixation, repeat fixation methods that are invasive or noninvasive have been used.[10–13] An example of a simulation film is shown in Figure 263–8.

IMAGING: COMPUTED TOMOGRAPHIC AND MAGNETIC RESONANCE IMAGING SCANS

The introduction of CT in the late 1970s provided cross-sectional anatomic information for radiotherapy treatment planning. Computed tomographic images are now widely used in radiation oncology for the purpose

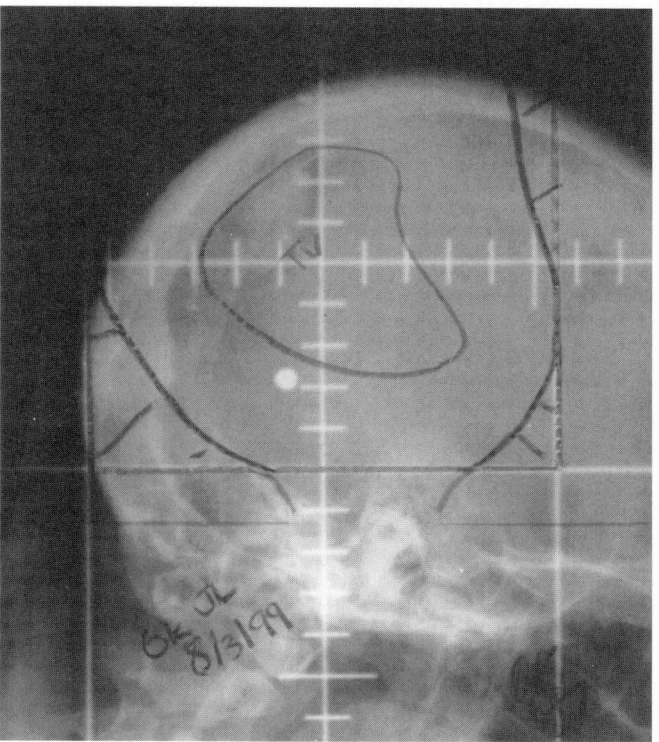

FIGURE 263–8. Simulation film. The quality of the film is similar to that of a diagnostic film.

of delineating target volume, assessing the relative geometry of critical structures to the tumor, determining beam placement and field shaping, and performing dose-distribution calculation and analysis.[14] CT-based planning has allowed radiation oncologists to visualize the tumor and thus minimize inaccuracy in defining treatment volumes.

Computed tomographic scanning is often done as an integral component of the simulation process. Scans are performed in the treatment position to help localize the target area and register this target position in relation to anatomic landmarks. In general, 0.5- to 1-cm cuts are taken from the top of the cranium to the neck. The images are then transferred to a treatment planning computer. From the treatment planning scan, various target volumes are defined by the physician in a process known as *contouring*. The critical structures of the brain, such as the optic chiasm, are contoured, with dose specification and margins given. Using clinical experience and trial and error, dosimetrists and physicists devise plans to optimize tumor coverage and minimize the radiation dose to normal tissues. Appropriate margins are selected, depending on tumor histology. In general, the initial treatment field encompasses tumor and edema, whereas the "boost" or "cone-down" fields encompass only the tumor and immediately adjacent tissue. In case of gross total resection, the tumor bed is generally used as the target. Normal tissue may be shielded from the direct beams through the use of shaped lead alloy blocks. Automated blocking may also be performed using computer-controlled multileaf collimation technology.

Patients usually undergo resimulation after treatment planning has been completed. The thermoplastic mask is re-marked with the planned fields. Films are taken at the various field positions to allow visualization of beam trajectory. During treatment, portal films or on-line portal images are obtained weekly and are compared with the simulation to verify accurate delivery (Fig. 263–9). Some centers are investigating the use of daily computed tomographic scans to verify internal anatomy and beam placement.

MRI provides greater anatomic and tumor detail compared with CT, but it may give less accurate geometric information. The fusion of CT and MRI provides a powerful planning technique, especially when correlation techniques are used. Postoperative MRI scans are optimally obtained within 72 hours after surgery to determine the extent of resection. At present, MRI scans are used more routinely for radiosurgery planning than for conventional radiotherapy.

COMPUTERIZED PLANNING

Computerized treatment planning provides an analysis of dose distribution within anatomic regions and has improved the ability to define tumor targets.[15, 16] Two-dimensional planning was considered state of the art until the development of more sophisticated computers capable of three-dimensional reconstructions. Three-dimensional radiation treatment planning can be viewed as a way of thinking about beam orientation from any arbitrary angle, allowing tremendous freedom in beam angle selection.[17] Cumulative dose distributions may be improved by varying the number of fields, entrance and exit of the beams, and beam energies. Multiple fields all centered on the target concentrate the high-dose region in the target tissue.

Radiation doses are prescribed to specified points, usually the intersection point of the central rays of all radiation beams. Isodose distributions depict the dose received in a given target volume. The process of optimizing the treatment plan calls for multistep improvement in the relative dose-delivery pattern using all the tools of beam shaping and delivery.

THREE-DIMENSIONAL CONFORMAL RADIOTHERAPY

The introduction of three-dimensional treatment planning allowed for better identification of target volumes in space and in relation to critical structures. Before the advent of MRI and CT, very large volumes of normal brain tissue received high doses of radiation based on the desire to prevent a geographic miss. Three-dimensional conformal radiotherapy allows for planning and delivery of the desired dose distribution to the entire target through the use of multiple static coplanar and noncoplanar fields or dynamic treatment modalities.

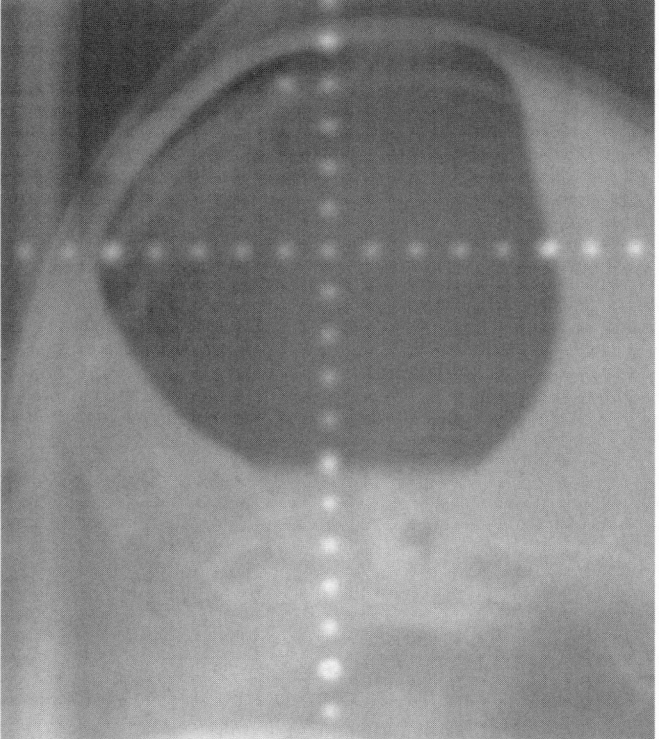

FIGURE 263–9. Portal films are compared with simulation films to verify the setup.

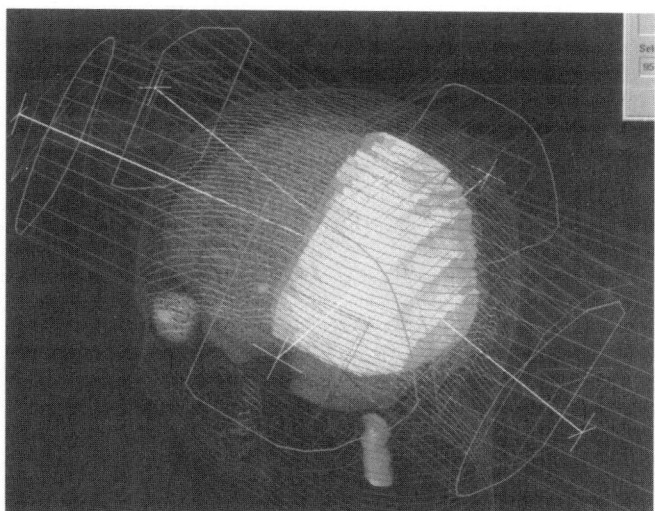

FIGURE 263–10. Beam's eye view (BEV) allows the arrangement of beams to produce conformal isodose distributions. This figure demonstrates the use of five fields.

ICRU Diagram for GTV, CTV, PTV

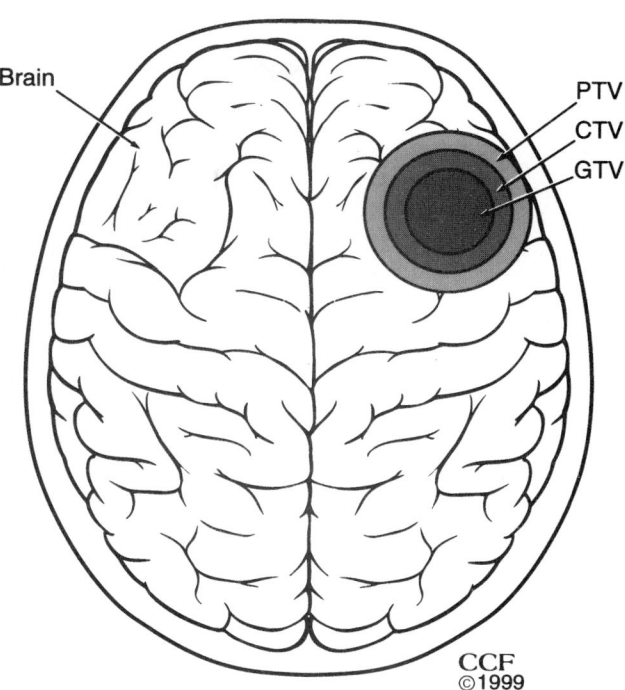

FIGURE 263–11. Gross tumor volume (GTV), clinical target volume (CTV), and planning target volume (PTV) are defined volumes that a physician determines for planning purposes.

In the 1980s, the development of computer-graphics technology applied to computed tomographic image sets allowed the three-dimensional display of anatomic information that had previously been presented in sequential two-dimensional slices.[18–20] Three-dimensional treatment planning offers several advantages over the two-dimensional approach. It allows more precise targeting of specified anatomic regions and allows adjacent normal tissues to receive less radiation. By excluding normal tissue from high-dose regions, this technique permits dose escalation without increasing the complications.[21] Dose escalation for brain tumor radiotherapy is currently being investigated in institutional and cooperative group trials in the hope of improving local control and perhaps survival.

Three-dimensional planning allows the delivery of more conformal radiation fields. Traditionally, customized cerrobend blocks were used to shape beams to reflect target profiles. Beam's-eye-view planning more accurately depicts the beam's shape, because block positions are determined on multiplanar target projections of each beam. The beam's eye view allows visualization of the fields that encompass a target from various angles while minimizing the radiation dose to normal tissues.[22] Thus the treatment team can plan and treat noncoplanar fields that intersect at the target volume (Fig. 263–10).

TARGET VOLUME DEFINITIONS

To help define and standardize target volumes, the International Commission on Radiation Units and Measurements published definitions of target volumes for photon radiation treatment.[23] These different volumes provide a framework for thinking about tumor coverage constraints. The *gross tumor volume* is defined as the volume of all known gross disease as delineated by postoperative CT or MRI. The *clinical target volume* is the gross tumor volume plus the area presumed to contain microscopic disease or thought to be at risk for microscopic extension. The clinical tumor volume is encompassed within a third volume, the *planning target volume*. The planning target volume adds an additional margin to compensate for geometric uncertainties in its shape and variation in location due to patient setup, organ motion, and organ deformation. Figure 263–11 illustrates the definitions of these treatment volumes.

DOSE-VOLUME HISTOGRAM

A dose-volume histogram provides a quantitative display of the portion of defined volume (tumor, brain, optic chiasm, and so forth) that will receive a given percentage of the prescribed dose.[24] This concept becomes particularly useful when comparing treatment plans. For example, treatment of pituitary adenomas can be performed with several different techniques. Figure 263–12 illustrates the dose-volume histogram for four different treatment techniques. Note that if the goal is to limit the percentage of temporal lobe receiving 20 Gy, a four-beam noncoplanar arc technique may be judged superior to a two- or three-field bilateral arc plan, based on dose-volume histogram analysis.[25]

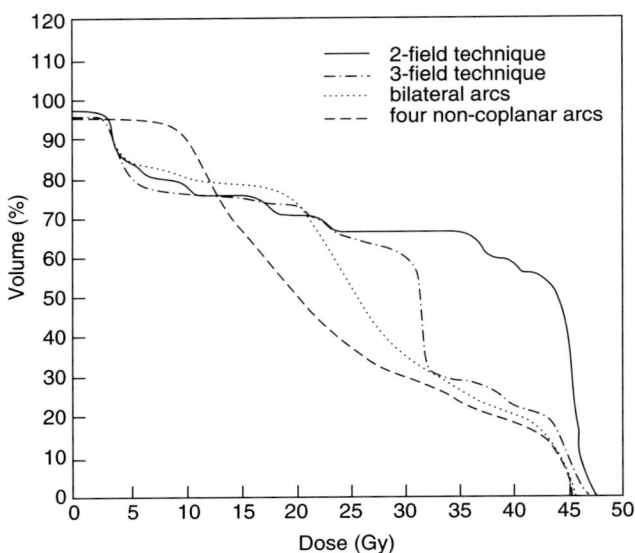

FIGURE 263–12. Dose-volume histogram (DVH) of the temporal lobe treated by four different techniques. (From Sohn JW, Dalzell JG, Suh JH, et al: Dose-volume analysis of techniques for irradiating pituitary adenomas. Int J Radiat Oncol Biol Phys 32:831–837, 1995.)

AUTOMATION AND MULTILEAF COLLIMATORS

The multileaf collimator and computer-controlled treatment machines have facilitated the use of complex three-dimensional treatment plans. The multileaf collimator contains multiple pairs of thin leaves that attenuate the beam. Each leaf can move independently of the others, and field shaping can be performed rapidly, thus eliminating the need to reenter the treatment room to insert customized blocks for each field. This can substantially improve treatment efficiency.[26, 27]

Other highly automated technologies are now being developed to enhance this flexibility in field design, and the use of "dynamic" multileaf collimation, in which the leaves are adjusted "on the fly," forms the core of some types of intensity modulation (see later).

RADIOSURGERY

Radiosurgery, like brachytherapy, allows for the delivery of highly focal doses of radiation with very sharp dose gradients. It uses many beams to conform the dose to the target and represents one of the most conformal three-dimensional techniques. A distinct advantage of stereotactic radiosurgery compared with brachytherapy is the minimal or noninvasive nature of the process. Radiosurgery radiation beams can be gamma rays, photons, or charged particles. Platforms for radiosurgery include specially adapted linacs, the gamma knife, and proton accelerators.

The gamma knife uses 201 individual cobalt-60 source capsules, whereas modified linac systems use multiple noncoplanar arcs to achieve target focus. Ra-

diosurgery has been shown to be clinically effective for benign tumors, malignant tumors, functional disorders, and vascular malformations. Stereotactic radiosurgery is, by definition, a single-treatment technique that uses multiple collimated beams directed stereotactically.[28] Given the sharp dose gradient beyond the target and the use of a frame affixed to the patient's skull, a large single dose of radiation can be delivered with minimal normal tissue effects.

In contrast, stereotactic radiotherapy implies the use of fractionated treatment. The implementation of multi-session stereotactic radiotherapy combines the precision of radiosurgery with the radiobiologic advantages of fractionation. Stereotactic radiotherapy may be particularly useful for neoplasms such as pituitary adenomas, meningiomas, and acoustic neuromas.[29]

INTENSITY-MODULATED RADIOTHERAPY

Intensity-modulated radiotherapy (IMRT) involves the delivery of radiation using nonuniform beams. Unlike conventional radiation treatments, IMRT uses many small beams of radiation, each of which can vary in intensity to provide a conformal dose distribution.[30-32] IMRT can be performed using static fields or dynamically collimated fields, which allows the rate of photon delivery to vary during irradiation of a single field.

One current IMRT system, the NOMOS Peacock system, uses arc therapy and a photon beam shaped by a collimator called the MIMiC (multivane intensity-modulating collimator), which attaches to the accessory tray of the linac.[33, 34] The MIMiC provides 40 separate beam apertures that can be opened and closed independently. Both treatment planning and treatment delivery must be computer controlled, because the beam options are too complex for conventional radiotherapy operational paradigms.

CONCLUSIONS

Technologic advances in imaging, computers, and radiation delivery have greatly enhanced brain tumor radiotherapy. These technologies now permit the delivery of precisely targeted radiation directed at sharply defined tumor targets. In the future, advances in the sequencing of radiation scheduling, the combined use of radiation and chemotherapy, the development of radiation sensitizers and protectors, new three-dimensional delivery systems, and further understanding of the cellular and molecular mechanisms for radiation response and resistance will continue to advance the effectiveness and safety of brain tumor radiotherapy.

REFERENCES

1. Harms WB, Purdy JA, Emami B, et al: Quality assurance for three-dimensional treatment planning. In Purdy JA, Fraass BA (eds): Syllabus: A Categorical Course in Physics. Oak Brook, Ill, Radiology Society of North America, 1994.

2. Bjarngard BE: Radiation therapy and SI units. Int J Radiat Oncol Biol Phys 7:283–285, 1981.
3. Suh JH, Barnett GH: Brachytherapy for brain tumor. In Crownover RL (ed): Brachytherapy. Hematol Oncol Clin North Am 13:635–650, 1999.
4. John HE, Bates LM, Watson TA: 1000 Curie cobalt units for radiation therapy. I. The Saskatchewan cobalt-60 unit. Br J Radiol 25:296–302, 1952.
5. Green ET, Errington RF: 1000 Curie cobalt unit for radiation therapy. III. Design of a cobalt-60 beam therapy unit. Br J Radiol 25:309–313, 1952.
6. Miller CW: Traveling-wave linear accelerator for x-ray therapy. Nature 171:278–279, 1953.
7. Gaspar LE, Dawson DJ, Tilley-Guilliford SA, et al: Long-term follow-up of patients treated with electron irradiation of the spinal field. Radiology 180:867–870, 1991.
8. Maor MH, Fields RS, Hogstrom KR, et al: Improving the therapeutic ratio of craniospinal irradiation in medulloblastoma. Int J Radiat Oncol Biol Phys 11:687–697, 1985.
9. Duncan W: An evaluation of the results of neutron therapy trials. Acta Oncol 33:299–306, 1994.
10. Simonova G, Novotny J, Novotny J Jr, et al: Fractionated stereotactic radiotherapy with the Leksell gamma knife: Feasibility study. Radiother Oncol 37:108–116, 1995.
11. Podgorsak EB, Souhami L, Caron JL, et al: A technique for fractionated stereotactic radiotherapy in the treatment of intracranial tumors. Int J Radiat Oncol Biol Phys 27:1225–1230, 1993.
12. Carol M, Grant WH III, Pavord D, et al: Initial clinical experience with the Peacock intensity modulation of a 3-D conformal radiation therapy system. Stereotact Funct Neurosurg 66:30–34, 1996.
13. Gill SS, Thomas DGT, Warrington AP, et al: Relocatable frame for stereotactic external beam radiation therapy. Int J Radiat Biol Oncol Phys 20:599–603, 1991.
14. Ling CC, Mohan R, Reinstein L, et al: Imaging in radiation oncology. In Leibel S, Phillips T (eds): Textbook of Radiation Oncology. Philadelphia, WB Saunders, 1998, pp 115–138.
15. Munzenrider JE, Pilepich M, Rene-Ferrero JB, et al: Use of body scanner in radiotherapy treatment planning. Cancer 40:170–179, 1977.
16. Goitein M: The utility of computed tomography in radiation therapy: An estimate of outcome. Int J Radiat Oncol Biol Phys 5:1799–1807, 1979.
17. Three-dimensional photon treatment planning: Report of the collaborative working group on the evaluation of treatment planning for external photon beam radiotherapy. Int J Radiat Oncol Biol Phys 21:1–265, 1991.
18. Lichter AS, Sandler HN, Robertson JN, et al: Clinical experience with three-dimensional treatment planning. Semin Radiat Oncol 2:257–266, 1992.
19. Rosenman J, Chaney EL, Sailer S, et al: Recent advances in radiotherapy treatment planning. Cancer Invest 9:465–481, 1991.
20. Mohan R, Barest G, Brewster LJ, et al: The comprehensive three-dimensional treatment planning system. Int J Radiat Oncol Biol Phys 15:481–495, 1988.
21. Lichter AS: Three-dimensional conformal radiation therapy: A testable hypothesis. Int J Radiat Biol Oncol Phys 21:853–855, 1991.
22. Goitein M, Abrams M, Rowell D, et al: Multi-dimensional treatment planning. II. Beam's eye-view, back projection, and projection through CT sections. Int J Radiat Oncol Biol Phys 9:789–797, 1983.
23. ICRU: Prescribing, Recording and Reporting Photon Beam Therapy (Report No. 50). Bethesda, Md, International Commission on Radiation Units and Measurements, 1993.
24. Dryzmala RE, Mohan R, Brewster L, et al: Dose-volume histograms. Int J Radiat Oncol Biol Phys 21:71–78, 1991.
25. Sohn JW, Dalzell JG, Suh JH, et al: Dose-volume histogram analysis of techniques for irradiating pituitary adenomas. Int J Radiat Oncol Biol Phys 32:831–837, 1995.
26. Powlis WD, Smith AR, Cheng E, et al: Initiation of multi-leaf collimator conformal radiation therapy. Int J Radiat Oncol Biol Phys 25:171–179, 1993.
27. Mohan R: Field shaping for three-dimensional conformal radiation therapy at multileaf collimation. Semin Radiat Oncol 5:86–99, 1995.
28. Leksell L: The stereotaxic method and radiosurgery of the brain. Acta Chir Scand 102:316–319, 1951.
29. Dunbar SF, Tarbell MJ, Kooy HM, et al: Stereotactic radiotherapy for pediatric and adult brain tumors: Preliminary experience. Int J Radiat Oncol Biol Phys 30:531–539, 1994.
30. Barth NH: An inverse problem in radiation therapy. Int J Radiat Oncol Biol Phys 18:425–431, 1990.
31. Brahme A, Roos JE, Lax I: Solution of an integral equation in rotation therapy. Phys Med Biol 27:1221–1229, 1982.
32. Webb S: Optimization by simulated annealing of three-dimensional conformal treatment planning for radiation fields defined by a multileaf collimator. Phys Med Biol 36:1201–1226, 1991.
33. Carol MP: Peacock: A system for planning and rotational delivery of intensity-modulated fields. Int J Imag Syst Technol 6:56–61, 1995.
34. Carol M, Grant WH, Bleier AR, et al: The field-matching problem as it applies to the Peacock three-dimensional conformal system for intensity modulation. Int J Radiat Oncol Biol Phys 34:183–187, 1996.

Fractionated Radiation Therapy for Malignant Brain Tumors

MINESH P. MEHTA

External beam radiation therapy plays a major role in the management of both primary and metastatic tumors of the brain. Four major delivery techniques of radiation therapy for brain neoplasms are commonly used, including fractionated external beam radiation therapy, radiosurgery, interstitial brachytherapy, and radioisotope instillation. The focus of this chapter is on the role of fractionated external beam radiation therapy in the management of primary and metastatic disease to the brain.

Primary malignant tumors of the brain are relatively uncommon neoplasms, accounting for less than 2% of all malignancies diagnosed in the United States; however, because of their extremely poor overall survival, they represent a significant cause of cancer mortality. In contrast, metastatic tumors to the brain are commonly encountered in clinical practice, and the annual estimated incidence of brain metastasis in the United States is probably in excess of 100,000 cases.[1] These patients have even poorer survival outcomes than those with primary brain tumors. In this chapter, the role of external beam radiation therapy in the management of both these disease processes is highlighted, and the outcomes as well as possible future avenues of investigation and clinical breakthroughs are emphasized.

BRAIN METASTASES

Of the more than 100,000 Americans who develop brain metastases annually, the vast majority die within a few months of diagnosis, making this one of the most common immediate causes of death in the United States.[1] Lung cancer accounts for more than half of all secondary tumors to the brain, but other primary tumors also contribute to this process, including breast cancer and melanoma, among others. Less commonly,

primary tumors of the gastrointestinal tract and kidney, gynecologic tumors, lymphomas, sarcomas, and prostate cancer also metastasize to the brain. The overall incidence of brain metastases in the United States is probably increasing because of better diagnostic techniques and also because of small gains in systemic therapeutic approaches, allowing patients with primary cancers to live longer and therefore have a greater likelihood of developing brain metastases. This is especially so because the brain has traditionally been thought to represent a sanctuary site that does not permit penetration by traditional chemotherapeutic agents when the blood-brain barrier is intact.

Medical Management

Older data from the 1970s suggest that the median survival time of untreated patients with brain metastases is approximately 1 month.[2, 3] The principal cause of this rapid mortality is uncontrolled peritumoral vasogenic edema, leading to herniation and rapid death.[4] As a consequence, measures to decrease vasogenic edema are commonly used in the initial management of patients with metastatic brain tumors. In particular, glucocorticoids have been shown to control vasogenic edema and result in minimal prolongation of median survival to approximately 2 months.[5-7]

External Beam Radiation

FRACTIONATION TRIALS

Chao and colleagues first reported the value of external beam radiation in brain metastases in 1954.[8] Subsequently, the Radiation Therapy Oncology Group (RTOG) conducted a series of sequential studies exploring a variety of fractionation schedules, evaluating their impact on outcome in patients with brain metasta-

T A B L E 2 6 4 – 1 ■ **Radiation Therapy Oncology Group Brain Metastases Dose/Schedule Trials**

YEAR	NUMBER	DOSE (Gy)	DURATION (wk)	MEDIAN SURVIVAL (wk)
1971–1973	227	40	4	16
	233	40	3	18
	217	30	3	18
	233	30	2	21
1973–1976	447	20	1	15
	228	30	2	15
	227	40	3	18
1976–1979	156	30	2	18
	153	50	4	17

ses. These trials were primarily conducted in the 1970s and focused on identifying the appropriate schedule and dose.[9, 10] Table 264–1 summarizes the outcome data from the first three RTOG brain metastases fractionation trials.

Based on more than 2000 patients enrolled in these three RTOG trials, it was apparent that no specific fractionation schedule was superior. The dose range that was explored was from 20 to 50 Gy, with median survival ranging from 15 to 21 weeks. The best median survival was seen in a group of 233 patients treated with a 30-Gy whole-brain radiation schedule delivered in 2 weeks. This cohort of patients exhibited a median survival of 21 weeks. As a consequence, this particular schedule has become the standard recommendation for most patients with brain metastases since the 1980s, and in a patterns of care palliation survey conducted from 1984 to 1985, this schedule was found to be the most commonly used in U.S. practice.[11]

SENSITIZER TRIALS

Because of the lack of clear efficacy of escalating the dose from 20 to 50 Gy, the RTOG strategy in the 1980s focused on exploring the use of radiation sensitizers to improve outcome in this group of patients. Two clinical trials were conducted using significantly different sensitizers—misonidazole, a hypoxic cell sensitizer, and bromodeoxyuridine (BudR), a halogenated pyrimidine—along with an S-phase sensitizer. In a four-arm trial evaluating misonidazole, no significant survival advantage was noted. Similarly, the BudR trial failed to show a significant survival advantage.[12] The data from these two sensitizer trials are presented in Table 264–2. These sensitizer trials unfortunately failed to show a significant impact on survival. In fact, the best survival was noted in the group of 36 patients on the control arm of the BudR trial with a median survival of 26 weeks.

IS THERE A DOSE-RESPONSE RELATIONSHIP?

The issue of a dose-response relationship continues to remain unclear because of conflicting data. It is of critical significance because in older RTOG studies,

50% or more of the patients died from neurologic deterioration, and it would be logical to assume that if such deterioration can be controlled, survival may be enhanced. To test this hypothesis, the RTOG conducted Study 8528, which evaluated the role of dose escalation using accelerated hyperfractionation (1.6 Gy twice daily to total doses ranging from 48 to 70.4 Gy). This trial demonstrated a significant advantage in survival and neurologic improvement with higher doses, therefore providing the first evidence that control of intracranial disease is related to dose and that such control actually translates to neurologic improvement and survival advantage.[13] However, the confirmatory trial RTOG 9104 failed to validate this observation.[14]

The relationship between local control and total dose has been well established in case-control analysis. Nieder and associates[15] treated a group of 164 patients with the standard whole-brain radiotherapy regimen of 30 Gy in 10 fractions and followed all patients with serial computed tomography and correlated local control and survival with various prognostic factors. Thereafter, 39 patients were treated to a total of 40 to 60 Gy and were compared with the cohort of 164 patients treated to 30 Gy using the matched cohort analysis method. The matching procedure produced absolutely equivalent groups of patients and showed a significant dose effect, with 30 Gy resulting in a local response rate of 50% compared with 77% for doses in the 40- to 60-Gy range. In this analysis, although local control improved from 50% to 77% by escalating the radiation dose, survival was not significantly altered. In a subsequent analysis from the same group, computed tomographic scans in 322 patients were analyzed, specifically to evaluate the impact of dose in the 25- to 50-Gy range on local control. The total dose was recalculated using the linear quadratic model and expressed as biologically effective dose (BED_{10}). The BED_{10} values ranged from 37.5 to 72 Gy, and the best local control was found to be a function of higher dose, the number of brain metastases, and the histologic features of the primary tumor. An increasing BED resulted in a significant decline in 1-year failure rates, with low BED values resulting in failure rates of 44% compared with 31% for high BED values. Once again, overall survival was not dependent on total dose.[16] In a 1999 analysis, Lagerwaard and colleagues identified prognostic factors in almost 1300 treated patients with brain metastases.[17] The single most important independent prognostic factor from this multivariate analysis

T A B L E 2 6 4 – 2 ■ **Radiation Therapy Oncology Group Brain Metastases Sensitizer Trials**

YEAR	NUMBER	Gy/FRACTIONS/WEEK	MEDIAN SURVIVAL (wk)
1979–1983	212	30/10/2	19
	216	+ misonidazole	17
	220	30/6/3	18
	211	+ misonidazole	13
1989–1993	36	37.5/15/3	26
	34	+ BudR	18

predicting for improved survival was treatment modality, suggesting that more aggressive therapy may improve survival.

How does one interpret these conflicting data? It is clear that a significant proportion of patients with brain metastases succumb to systemic diseases; therefore, enhancing the control of intracranial diseases is unlikely to provide a survival benefit to this group of patients. In clinical trials, whether prospective or retrospective, in which a significant majority of patients harbor considerable systemic disease that will dictate the outcome, survival improvement from more aggressive local control is unlikely to be demonstrated. However, in clinical situations in which patient selection identifies individuals who are less likely to succumb rapidly to systemic progression, local control does become critical. This has been best demonstrated in surgical trials in which resection and whole-brain radiation therapy are compared with whole-brain radiation therapy alone. Two such randomized trials by Noordijk and Patchell and their colleagues have validated this paradigm,[18, 19] showing improved survival for the more aggressive arm.

PROGNOSTIC FACTOR ANALYSIS

Although, studies such as those by Patchell and coworkers[19] and Noordijk and associates[18] have led to a paradigm shift, somewhat changing the nihilistic attitude toward patients with brain metastases, significant doubt remains whether more aggressive therapeutic approaches in patients with brain metastases truly produce survival advantage when outcomes are balanced by prognostic factors. Some of the seminal work in this area was done by the RTOG, which identified a set of prognostic criteria predictive of slightly improved survival. These included age less than 60, a Karnofsky performance score of greater than 70, a controlled primary tumor, absence of extracranial metastases, and three or fewer lesions.[9, 10, 20] In a 1997 evaluation, 1200 patients from three consecutive RTOG trials conducted from 1979 to 1993 were amalgamated into a single database, and a statistical methodology known as *recursive partitioning analysis* was used to identify subsets of patients based on prognostic factor evaluation. This analysis suggested that patients with brain metastases can be broadly categorized into three classes with different outcomes. The most favorable group of patients, class I, includes patients with a Karnofsky score of greater than 70, age less than 65, a controlled primary

tumor, and absence of extracranial metastases. These patients have a median survival of 7.1 months. Patients in the worst prognostic class, class III, were characterized by a Karnofsky score of less than 70, and their median survival was 2.3 months. The intermediate group, class II, had a median survival of 4.2 months.[21] These data, therefore, raise an important question regarding selection bias in studies that use more aggressive treatment modalities.

In order to evaluate the impact of these prognostic factors on the survival of patients with brain metastases, we performed a retrospective evaluation of 472 patients with brain metastases treated at nine institutions with whole-brain radiation therapy and stereotactic radiosurgery stratified by the RTOG recursive partitioning analysis classification. For each class, we found statistically significant survival benefit in median survival. For example, for class I, median survival improved from 7.1 to 13.6 months. For class II, the predicted median survival was 4.2 months, whereas the observed median survival was 9.4 months. Similarly for class III, survival shifted from 2.3 to 8.4 months. These data are presented in Table 264–3. Although not conclusive, such data suggest that for well-selected patients with brain metastases, a focus on improving local control is clearly merited. In order to broaden the application of improved local control, a number of clinical trials evaluating newer radiosensitizers are currently under way. A major, randomized phase III national effort is currently in place evaluating a unique radiosensitizer, gadolinium texaphyrin (Gd-Tex). Other sensitizers such as RSR13 are being tested in phase II trials.

ROLE OF WHOLE-BRAIN RADIATION THERAPY

With the emergence of a greater population of patients undergoing resection for brain metastases, significant questions regarding the role of postoperative whole-brain radiation therapy have arisen. Whole-brain radiation therapy has been used in this clinical situation with the rationale that micrometastatic disease in the brain needs to be controlled. The original data supporting this rationale came from nonrandomized evaluations of patients undergoing surgical resection with or without whole-brain radiation therapy. In these uncontrolled trials, significant reduction in intracranial failure with postoperative whole-brain radiation therapy was documented. A handful of other single institution reports emerged in the 1990s, some supporting postoper-

T A B L E 2 6 4 – 3 ■ Survival of Brain Metastases Patients by Radiation Therapy Oncology Group Recursive Partitioning Analysis Class

| Class | RTOG | | | RADIOSURGERY | | | P Value |
	No.	Median Survival	Confidence Interval	No.	Median Survival	Confidence Interval	
I	236	7.1	6.3–8.5	95	13.6	10.7–17.6	<.05
II	765	4.2	3.8–4.7	337	9.4	8.2–10.4	<.05
III	175	2.3	1.9–2.8	34	8.4	5.7–10.6	<.05

TABLE 264-4 ■ Role of Postoperative Whole-Brain Radiotherapy

	NO POSTOPERATIVE RADIATION THERAPY	POSTOPERATIVE RADIATION THERAPY
Number	46	49
Brain recurrence	70%	18%
Central nervous system death	44%	14%

ative radiation therapy, others demonstrating no significant value from it. In addition, with longer survival in these patients, the neurocognitive deficits seen in some patients are being ascribed to radiation therapy, and therefore the value of postoperative whole-brain radiation therapy has come under considerable scrutiny. A multi-institutional prospective randomized trial completed in 1998 evaluated the value of postoperative whole-brain radiation therapy in patients managed with surgical resection with or without postoperative whole-brain radiation therapy.[22] In this particular trial, 95 patients with single brain metastases were treated with complete surgical resection as verified by postoperative magnetic resonance imaging (MRI) and were subsequently randomized to postoperative whole-brain radiation therapy to 50.4 Gy in 28 fractions of 1.8 Gy each or to no postoperative whole-brain radiation therapy. Forty-nine patients were assigned to the whole-brain radiation therapy group and 46 to the observation group. Recurrence of tumor in the brain was significantly less frequent in the radiation therapy group (18%) than in the observation group (70%). Patients in the radiation therapy group (14%) were also less likely to die of neurologic causes than were those in the observation group (44%). There was, however, no significant difference in overall survival between the two groups (Table 264-4). This study therefore clearly demonstrated that postoperative whole-brain radiation therapy significantly diminishes intracranial relapse and neurologic death in well-selected patients with single brain metastases undergoing resection.

REIRRADIATION OF BRAIN METASTASES

The use of relatively moderate doses of whole-brain radiation therapy frequently results in a clinical situation requiring reirradiation of patients with progressive brain metastases. This is a frustrating experience because adequate doses of radiation cannot be delivered without significant risk to these patients. Several single-institution reports that used doses in the range of 20 to 25 Gy for the management of these patients are available in the literature, and in the majority of these reports, the outcome of patients reirradiated for brain metastases was uniformly poor. It is unclear whether reirradiation provided substantial benefit for these patients; therefore, when opting to reirradiate such patients, significant attention must be paid to the individual patient's history and clinical presentation to

determine whether there is any role for reirradiation and if so, whether it should be repeat whole-brain radiation therapy or limited-field radiation.

FUTURE DIRECTIONS

At present, it would appear that this entire field is moving in the direction of improving intracranial local control. For patients in whom surgical resection is feasible, resection followed by whole-brain radiation therapy remains a standard. In other patients, with limited disease, good performance status and three or fewer brain metastases, radiosurgery is frequently used in concert with whole-brain radiation therapy. Although retrospective data are appealing, prospective randomized trials remain to be completed. The RTOG is in the process of completing a major prospective randomized trial to answer the radiosurgery boost question. In yet other patients, whole-brain radiation therapy is being combined with radiosensitizers such as gadolinium texaphyrin or is being delivered in concert with chemotherapy. Finally, in selected patients with relatively radioresistant tumors, limited radiation to the observed brain metastases and delayed whole-brain radiation therapy is also being explored to limit the neurocognitive deficits encountered in long-term survivors.

MALIGNANT GLIOMA

Although malignant gliomas are relatively uncommon neoplasms (they account for only about 40% of the approximately 17,000 new annual cases of central nervous system [CNS] malignancies diagnosed in the United States every year), their clinical impact continues to far outweigh their incidence, principally because of their high fatality rate.[23] Glioblastoma multiforme, which accounts for about 80% of all malignant gliomas, has an annual U.S. incidence in excess of 5000 cases, and the median and 5-year survivals are typically 9 to 10 months and 5%, respectively.[23] The 5-year survival for anaplastic astrocytoma is typically less than 20%.[24]

Malignant gliomas rarely metastasize, and mortality is primarily attributed to nearly universal local failure. Hochberg and Pruitt demonstrated that more than 80% of failures occur within 2 cm of the primary tumor, with only 1 in 35 (3%) patients in their series having recurrence outside this 2-cm risk zone.[25] Similarly, in a trial of radiation therapy plus a nitroimidazole radiosensitizer, Urtasun and associates reported all recurrences within the initial target volume.[26] Autopsy studies, as well as stereotactic localization biopsy studies, have demonstrated that microscopic spread of tumor is present at the time of diagnosis beyond the zone of enhancement.[26, 27] Additionally, local control in these tumors is compromised by significant regions of hypoxia as well as a relative inability of chemotherapeutic drugs to perfuse through the blood-brain barrier into the tumor.[28, 29] These biologic observations provide a strong rationale for the investigation of aggressive modalities of local control in an attempt to improve the overall outcome in patients with malignant glioma.

Rationale for High-Dose Radiation Therapy in Malignant Glioma

Clinical trials conducted by the Brain Tumor Cooperative Study Group in the 1970s established improvement in local control and survival in patients with malignant glioma treated with postoperative radiation therapy compared with patients undergoing surgical resection alone. In addition, subsequent analysis of their serial trials demonstrated a possible dose-response survival relationship over a range from 45 to 62 Gy.[30] The median survival improved from 14 weeks at less than 45 Gy to 42 weeks at 60 Gy. These data are presented in Table 264–5. Further confirmatory data have become available from a Medical Research Council trial of two radiotherapy doses in the treatment of malignant glioma.[31] These trials formed the basic rationale for supporting the use of postoperative radiation therapy in the first place, and second for considering dose escalation. It would appear that based on these trials surgical resection alone, without postoperative radiation therapy, results in a median survival in the 14- to 18-week range, whereas high-dose radiation in the 60-Gy range improves the survival to approximately 42 weeks.

There is compelling evidence from in vitro studies that a dose-response relationship for malignant gliomas exists at doses greater than 60 Gy.[32] Unfortunately, the ability to escalate the external beam radiation dose is severely limited by the accompanying increase in neurotoxicity. For example, Marks and coworkers demonstrated that the risk of brain necrosis increases substantially with doses greater than 60 to 70 Gy.[33] Substantial clinical evidence indicating improved survival beyond 60 Gy is lacking. In an analysis of more than 600 patients treated in an intergroup RTOG/Eastern Cooperative Oncology Group (ECOG) study, 70 Gy did not result in increased survival compared with 60 Gy.[34] RTOG 83-02, a randomized phase I dose-escalation trial of twice daily radiation therapy accrued more than 700 cases from a dose range of 64.8 to 81 Gy, and although the 72-Gy arm had the best survival, toxicity beyond this dose resulted in worse survival.[35] In a prospective phase I/II dose-escalation study by Urtasun and colleagues, external beam doses of up to 80 Gy using a hyperfractionated regimen of 1 Gy three times daily were achieved without substantial toxicity or evidence of improved local control or survival.[36]

To determine whether higher doses affect quality of life, 786 patients with malignant glioma accrued to the RTOG phase I/II study 83-02 were analyzed using a modified quality-adjusted survival model. This allowed inclusion of both improvement and decline in neurologic functional status, and patients were scored by the presence or absence of 15 neurologic signs and symptoms during the study and at every follow-up. Within each category were included gradations of severity, with a quality of survival time adjusted according to any changes in these neurologic findings. The summation of all changes in signs and symptoms were weighted and incorporated into the model. Overall, the average quality-adjusted suvival time was 18.5 months for the study, with the best result of 20.8 months observed in the 72-Gy arm, which was significantly longer than that of all other groups.[37] Based on such data, accelerated hyperfractionation was pursued in the successor randomized trial RTOG 94-11. Unfortunately, this trial demonstrated no statistically significant survival advantage from dose escalation.

These clinical studies may be interpreted as representing a response ceiling at 60 Gy without substantial increase in local control or survival improvement, at least up to 80 Gy. This does not necessarily rule out the possibility of improved local control at doses beyond these levels. It is the latter argument that forms the primary rationale for delivering brachytherapy for malignant tumors of the brain. In fact, there are preliminary data from retrospective clinical trials suggesting that total cumulative doses with the use of brachytherapy or radiosurgery with external beam radiation therapy in excess of 100 Gy may in fact be necessary to achieve adequate tumor control for this highly malignant disease process. Brachytherapy and radiosurgery are not within the purview of this chapter and are not discussed.

Sensitizer Trials

Several different strategies for the radiosensitization of malignant gliomas have been used. One of the earliest agents tested was hydroxyurea, and although preliminary results of a phase III comparison study of carmustine (BCNU) and radiation appeared somewhat promising, the combination of carmustine and radiation has now become the gold standard.[38] Today, hydroxyurea has largely been abandoned in patients with malignant glioma.

Subsequently, attention was focused on the hypoxic cell sensitizer, misonidazole, and a randomized study was performed to evaluate its value in the treatment of malignant glioma. In the control arm of this RTOG study, patients received 60 Gy radiation therapy plus carmustine chemotherapy. In the experimental group, misonidazole was given once a week for 6 weeks, and the radiation schedule was adjusted to take into account the small number of fractions given concurrently with misonidazole. No significant benefit from misoni-

---

TABLE 264–5 ■ Glioblastoma Multiforme—Local Control Is a Function of Dose

DOSE (Gy)	MEDIAN SURVIVAL (wk)	TWENTY-FIFTH PERCENTILE SURVIVAL	P
0	18	N/A	N/A
<45	14	N/A	ns
50	28	52	<.001
55	36	57	<.001
60	42	68	<.001

Local control is a function of dose; median survival increases from 14 weeks at less than 45 Gy to 42 weeks at 60 Gy.
Data from Walker M, Strike G, Sheline G: An analysis of dose-effect relationship in the radiotherapy of malignant gliomas. Int J Radiat Oncol Biol Phys 5:1725–1731, 1979.

dazole was observed.[39] The median survival for radiation therapy plus carmustine was 55 weeks and for misonidazole plus radiation plus carmustine, the median survival was 46 weeks. The Brain Tumor Cooperative Group also evaluated misonidazole in their Study 77-02. In this particular clinical trial, 11 institutions randomized more than 600 patients with supratentorial malignant glioma to one of four treatment groups after surgery: conventional radiotherapy to 60 Gy with carmustine chemotherapy, radiation therapy plus streptozotocin, hyperfractionated radiotherapy (66 Gy in 60 fractions given twice daily) with carmustine, and conventional radiation therapy with misonidazole followed by BCNU. Median survival was 10 months with no statistically significant difference in survival among the four groups. In fact, among the nonglioblastoma patients, the misonidazole group appeared to have poorer survival.[40] Because of the lack of activity demonstrated by misonidazole, a newer imidazole compound etanidazole was tested in a phase I study given concurrently with external beam radiation therapy for patients with malignant glioma.[41] Unfortunately, etanidazole has not found a further role in the management of these tumors.

The RTOG has extensively evaluated halogenated pyrimidines as potential radiosensitizers in malignant glioma. A substantial amount of attention was focused on the use of iododeoxyuridine (IudR); to date, these clinical trials for glioblastoma multiforme have been inconclusive. Retrospective analyses, however, demonstrate consistent survival advantage for patients with anaplastic astrocytoma. In one such study, RTOG 86-12, toxicity and the survival benefit of iododeoxyuridine was evaluated, and no survival gain was identified for patients with glioblastoma. Twenty-one of the 79 patients entered in this study had anaplastic astrocytoma. These patients were treated with 60.16 Gy in 32 fractions with iododeoxyuridine delivered in a continuous intravenous infusion of long (96 hours) or short (48 or 24 hours) duration every week during radiation therapy. Median survival for anaplastic astrocytoma patients was 3.2 years, with 33% of patients surviving 5 years. These results compare favorably with the best results reported in the literature with postoperative external beam radiation plus chemotherapy. Previous RTOG experience with radiation therapy alone demonstrated a median survival time of 2 years.[42]

In 1998, Prados and colleagues reported on the effect of treatment using a different halogenated pyridimine, BudR, during radiation therapy. A retrospective analysis of patient data from several RTOG clinical trials as well as a single Northern California Oncology Group (NCOG) trial was conducted. In the entire cohort of 2077 patients, 1743 were treated without BudR, and 334 patients were treated with BudR. After adjusting for eligibility, a total of 1774 patients were eligible for survival evaluation. For patients with glioblastoma multiforme, the median survival was 9.8 months in the RTOG studies, and 18 months in the Northern California Oncology Group trial. For patients with anaplastic astrocytoma, the median survival was 35.1 months in the RTOG studies and 42.8 months in the Northern

California Oncology Group study. A univariate analysis demonstrated a survival advantage in favor of BudR. Using a proportional hazards regression model, BudR was found to influence outcome for patients with glioblastoma multiforme. The authors concluded that because of patient heterogeneity and treatment variation, absolute conclusions could not be derived, but a favorable treatment effect from BudR was observed in patients with glioblastoma multiforme.[43] Other evaluations of halogenated pyridimines are therefore under way. Preliminary results of a phase III randomized trial using BudR in anaplastic astrocytoma do not demonstrate a survival benefit from BudR, but a final analysis is pending. Other sensitizer approaches are being explored. Newer agents, such as gadolinium texaphyrin and RSR13, have just entered clinical testing. Other trials of taxanes and topoisomerase inhibitors have been completed, and data from these trials are pending.

Particle Beam Radiation

Because of the relatively poor results with dose escalation and sensitizers, particle beam radiation therapy has been explored in patients with malignant glioma. Castro and colleagues reported on 39 patients with primary recurrent glioma of the brain treated with heavy charged particle beam at the University of California–Lawrence Berkley Laboratory in a phase I/II clinical trial of the Northern California Oncology Group. These data did not show results superior to those obtained with standard therapies, and because of the limited availability of heavy charged particle, substantial investigation in this field is lacking.[44]

More attention has been focused on neutron beam radiation. Most commonly, a regimen of mixed photons and neutrons has been used, as neutrons alone have proved to be too toxic in terms of late radiation injury. In the mid-1980s, the RTOG conducted and completed a phase I trial in patients with malignant glioma, evaluating concomitant neutron boost. A total of 190 patients were randomized to six different neutron dose levels with no significant difference in overall survival among the six dose levels. For anaplastic astrocytoma, there was a suggestion that patients receiving higher dose levels had poorer overall survival compared with patients receiving the lower dose levels, suggesting a possible detrimental effect from neutrons.[45]

A second method of using neutron therapy in the management of patients with malignant brain tumors is a technique known as boron neutron capture therapy (BNCT). This method involves incorporating boron[10] into the tumor using an appropriate boronated pharmacologic agent followed by irradiation with thermal or epithermal neutrons. A review of the literature indicates that to date, more than 120 patients have been treated in this manner, principally by Japanese investigators. The Japanese reports have, for the most part, been relatively favorable, and an independent analysis of the Japanese data was conducted by Laramore and Spence.[46] In this particular analysis, the cohort of patients from the United States who received boron neutron capture therapy in Japan were compared with a matched cohort receiving conventional therapy in various RTOG studies. A total of 14 patients receiving boron neutron capture therapy were identified; of these, 12 were evaluable. When compared with a matched set of patients, median survival was 10.5 months in both groups, and no meaningful improvement in survival attributable to this form of therapy could be identified.[46] In conclusion, the data to date do not support the routine use of particle beam radiation in the management of patients with malignant glioma.

Prognostic Factor Analysis

Because few substantial gains have been made in the management of patients with malignant glioma through phase III trials, the current focus is on conducting a series of phase II trials with the expectation that if and when promising investigational agents or avenues are identified by such trials, they can rapidly be advanced to the phase III randomized trial mechanism. In order to facilitate such a process, it would be useful to ensure that comparable patients are treated in different phase II trials.

To facilitate this comparison, the RTOG used the recursive partitioning technique to analyze survival in 1578 patients entered in three RTOG malignant glioma trials from 1974 to 1989.[47] In this approach, a regression tree was created according to prognostic variables, and patients were classified into homogenous subsets by survival. Twenty-six pretreatment characteristics and six treatment-related variables were analyzed. This approach permitted the creation of six prognostic classes primarily using the variables of age, histologic appearance, mental status, performance status, symptom duration, and degree of resection. These classes are defined in Table 264–6. Table 264–7 shows survival stratified by prognostic class. This approach allows for stratification into appropriate subgroups, which can then be used for further prognostic analysis. It is obvi-

TABLE 264–6 ■ **Definition of Prognostic Classes from Radiation Therapy Oncology Group Recursive Partitioning**

PROGNOSTIC CLASS	DEFINITION
1	AA, age <50, normal mental status
2	AA, age ≥50, KPS ≥70, duration of symptoms >3 mo
3	AA, age <50, abnormal mental status, or GBM, age <50, KPS ≥90
4	AA, age ≥50, KPS ≥70, duration of symptoms ≤3 mo, or GBM, age <50, KPS <90, or GBM, age ≥50, KPS ≥70, partial or total resection, NFS = working
5	GBM, age ≥50, KPS ≥70, partial or total resection, NFS < working, or GBM, age ≥50, KPS ≥70, biopsy only, or GBM or AA, age ≥50, KPS <70, normal mental status.
6	GBM or AA, age ≥50, KPS <70, abnormal mental status

AA, anaplastic astrocytoma; GBM, glioblastoma multiforme; KPS, Karnofsky performance status; NFS, neurologic functional status.

TABLE 264–7 ■ **Survival of Malignant Glioma Patients Stratified by Radiation Therapy Oncology Group Prognostic Class**

CLASS	MEDIAN SURVIVAL (mo)	2-YEAR SURVIVAL %	NUMBER
1	58.6	76	139
2	37.4	68	34
3	17.9	35	175
4	11.1	15	457
5	8.9	6	395
6	4.6	4	263

ous that patients in classes 5 and 6 have the worst outcome, with 2-year survival of less than 6%, whereas patients in classes 1 and 2 have 2-year survival approaching and exceeding 70%. The 2-year survival of classes 3 and 4 is 35% and 15%, respectively.

ANAPLASTIC ASTROCYTOMA: IS MORE WORSE?

Historically, malignant glioma have been classified into two broad categories, glioblastoma multiforme or grade 4 astrocytoma, and anaplastic astrocytoma or grade 3 astrocytoma. Median survival for patients with glioblastoma typically has been in the 8- to 11-month range. The less common variant, anaplastic astrocytoma, has slightly better median survival, in the 2- to 3-year range. As alluded to earlier in this chapter, when more aggressive strategies are used, it appears that patients with anaplastic astrocytoma have a worse outcome with the more aggressive regimen. This phenomenon was initially identified by Laramore in an analysis of 163 patients with anaplastic astrocytoma treated in several RTOG and Eastern Cooperative Oncology Group trials. Three distinct patient groups were identified: those treated with standard photon radiation therapy in the 60- to 70-Gy range, those treated with radiation therapy and chemotherapy (either carmustine, [semustine MeCCNU] or [dacarbazine DTIC]), and those treated with photon radiation plus a neutron boost. The median survival of patients receiving radiation therapy alone was 3 years compared with 2.3 years for those receiving chemotherapy and radiation therapy, and 1.7 years for those receiving photon plus neutron therapy. For each subgroup of patients, further prognostic variable analysis using age and Karnofsky performance status was carried out. In each category, the median survival decreased with more aggressive therapy.[48]

A similar analysis was conducted in 149 patients with anaplastic astrocytoma treated with radiation therapy alone, radiation therapy and chemotherapy, or radiation therapy, chemotherapy, and misonidazole. The median survival of patients treated with radiation therapy alone was 3 years. The median survival of patients treated with chemotherapy and radiation therapy was 2.3 years, and 1.2 years for patients treated with chemotherapy and misonidazole. Both these reports suggest that the more aggressive modality, such as misonidazole sensitization and neutron boost, produce a decrease in survival in patients with anaplastic astrocytoma.[49] The one exception to this observation appears to be the use of halogenated pyrimidines, which in retrospective evaluations appear to yield a survival benefit, although the most recently completed prospective randomized trial does not appear to support this advantage on preliminary analysis.[50]

Being relatively rare, these tumors are extremely difficult to study in large clinical trials. The current international effort is focused on evaluating a new chemotherapy agent temozolomide, together with radiation therapy for these patients.

ANAPLASTIC OLIGODENDROGLIOMA: A SPECIAL CASE

Of the malignant gliomas, anaplastic oligodendroglioma represents one of the least common subtypes. This particular malignant neoplasm is characterized by its remarkable sensitivity both to radiation therapy and multiagent chemotherapy.[51] In addition, anaplastic oligodendrogliomas are also distinguished by a unique constellation of molecular genetic alterations, including loss of 1p and 19q in about 25% to 50% of these tumors. They also are typically characterized by relatively high rates of survival. For example, in an analysis of outcome of patients with oligodendroglioma based on grade and concomitant presence of astrocytic features, a group of Japanese investigators found the median survival time for anaplastic oligodendroglioma to be 12.7 years, but the presence of astrocytic features in this tumor (anaplastic oligoastrocytoma) decreased the median survival time to 4.8 years.[52] Because these tumors respond significantly well to both radiation and chemotherapy, a combination approach might logically produce substantial cures in this disease. A randomized clinical trial to evaluate this specific concept is currently under way. Until conclusive evidence from this trial is available, up-front combination chemotherapy and radiation therapy for this tumor remains investigational and should not be considered "standard-of-care."

PRIMARY CENTRAL NERVOUS SYSTEM LYMPHOMA

A variety of different distinct pathologic and clinical entities are included within the broad term of *primary CNS lymphoma*. In general, this term is meant to reflect lymphoma confined to the CNS, which occurs in less than 2% of all CNS tumors. The overall incidence of this disease has, in fact, been increasing, specifically because of an increase in the number of immunocompromised patients with acquired immunodeficiency syndrome (AIDS), as well as patients who have undergone organ transplantation, and so on. In general, for clinical trial purposes, patients are subdivided into AIDS-associated or non–AIDS-associated primary CNS lymphomas.

This disease is characterized by dissemination through the craniospinal axis as its natural history advances; it is a radiosensitive tumor with clinical response rates upward of 80%. In a report in the early 1970s, 83 patients with primary CNS lymphoma were followed with observation, surgical resection, or radiation therapy. In patients who were observed, median survival was 3.3 months; in those treated with surgical excision, median survival was 4.6 months; and in patients receiving external beam radiation therapy, the median survival was 15.2 months.[53] In other studies, median survival times between 14 and 40 months have been documented. In addition to prolonging survival, radiation therapy produces rapid responses and therefore quick and sustained clinical improvement.[54]

Unfortunately, cranial radiation alone does not result in significant long-term survival in spite of the high response rates. In a literature review, Leibel and Sheline noted that the 1-, 2-, and 5-year survival rates for this disease after radiation therapy were 66%, 43%, and 7% respectively.[55]

Significant controversy remains regarding the volume of radiation and the appropriate dose. In an attempt to define an appropriate dose, Murray and colleagues evaluated outcome in 198 patients treated with a dose range of less than 40 to greater than 50 Gy.[56] The median survival of 54 patients receiving more than 50 Gy was 17 months compared with 15 months for the 144 patients who received less than 50 Gy. More important, the actuarial 5-year survival for patients receiving greater than 50 Gy was 42% compared with 13% for those receiving less than 50 Gy. The latter survival value reached statistical significance, and their data would suggest that doses greater than 50 Gy should be used.

Another contentious issue regarding radiation therapy for CNS lymphomas is the volume to be treated. It has been estimated that the incidence of spinal relapse, as the first site of progression, occurs in up to half of patients with primary CNS lymphomas. It is, however, possible that these numbers may be exaggerated because of the inclusion of patients from older studies in which magnetic resonance imaging of the spine was not conducted before study entry. In the series by Murray and colleagues,[56] 7% of patients relapsed with positive cerebrospinal fluid cytologic findings or overt spinal disease. In addition, in their literature review of 308 patients, they identified 124 patients who received radiation to the whole brain, 16 patients who received radiation to the tumor bed alone, 16 patients who received treatment to the entire neuraxis, and 152 cases in which the treatment volume could not be assessed. They did not find a significant association between the volume treated and survival outcome. In contrast, the review by Leibel and Sheline[55] suggested that patients receiving radiation therapy to the primary tumor alone had a median survival of 39.4 months compared with 25.3 months for patients receiving whole-brain radiation therapy.

The current trend for using radiation therapy in this disease has recognized the role of chemotherapy. It appears that the use of intensive preradiation chemotherapy produces significant responses, and in the most recently completed phase II RTOG trial, significant survival benefit is suggested.[57] In the RTOG 93-10 study, 102 patients were treated with five cycles of high-dose methotrexate, vincristine, and procarbazine over 10 weeks, followed by 45 Gy whole-brain radiation therapy and high-dose cytarabine after radiation therapy. At 30 months of follow-up, median survival had not been reached, suggesting a possible doubling over historical controls. As a consequence, craniospinal radiation is not used in the absence of positive cytologic findings or gross disease in the spine. Typically, the whole brain is treated, with a boost to the original tumor site. The total dose and fractionation schedule remains a matter of some debate. As a word of caution, the Medical Research Council randomized trial of CHOP (cyclophosphamide, hydroxydaunomycin, Oncovin [vincristine], prednisone) chemotherapy failed to demonstrate a survival advantage, but this could be due to inadequate statistical power.[58]

MALIGNANT MENINGEAL TUMORS

Meningiomas are usually benign growths that rarely exhibit malignant features. However, at least two malignancies of meninges—hemangiopericytoma and atypical or malignant meningioma, including meningiosarcoma—do exhibit features characteristic of malignant neoplasms. These tumors in general are treated with aggressive surgical resection followed by postoperative radiation therapy to high doses.

Scheithauer has proposed a modification of the World Health Organization (WHO) classification of CNS neoplasms.[59] In this revised classification, he proposes grading meningiomas as typical meningiomas, atypical meningiomas, and malignant meningiomas. Malignant meningiomas frequently have histologic evidence of brain parenchymal invasion and rarely evidence of distant metastases. Histopathologically, these neoplasms show significant vascular proliferation, increased cellularity, high rates of mitosis, and frequent occurrence of necrosis. Under light microscopy, meningiosarcomas can be categorized as fibrosarcomas, spindle cell sarcomas, or mixed sarcomas. All these aggressive meningeal neoplasms have poor 5-year survival rates of less than 20%, and the majority of patients are treated with postoperative radiation therapy. Typically, doses in the 60-Gy range are used for these patients.

Hemangiopericytoma is a rare neoplasm arising from perivascular pericytes. Accounting for less than 1% of all brain tumors, these neoplasms are characterized by a high local response rate and metastatic potential. They tend to grow most frequently in the fifth decade of life. Nearly 300 cases of hemangiopericytoma have been described in the literature, arising from virtually every anatomic site. Overall, less than 100 cases of meningeal hemangiopericytoma have been reported. Surgical resection has been the historical and prevalent mode of therapy for these tumors. In 1992, we published a comprehensive review defining the role for radiation therapy in the management of this disease. A total of 80 patients with meningeal hemangiopericytoma were identified, and our analysis revealed a 90% 9-year actuarial risk for local recurrence after surgical resection only. Less than 33% of these recurrences were noted in the first 5 years, which may account for the false assumption that these tumors are highly curable with surgical resection alone. In our analysis, radiation therapy appeared to reduce this local recurrence rate, prolonging disease-free and overall survival. Radiation responses were noted to be dose-dependent with greater than 50 Gy providing superior long-term disease-free survival. Meningeal hemangiopericytomas are characterized by a slow but progressive radiographic response to ionizing radiation, not unlike other highly vascular brain lesions, such as arteriovenous malformations. These tumors also have significant metastatic potential, with the liver, lung, bone, and soft tissue being preferred sites for metastatic dissemination. Radiation therapy in doses greater than 50 Gy should be incorporated as primary or adjuvant therapy for patients being treated with a curative intent.[60]

OTHER MALIGNANT NEOPLASMS

Several other extremely rare malignant neoplasms are known to occur in adults. This category of tumors includes the primitive neuroectodermal tumors (previously classified as medulloblastoma or pineoblastoma, based on site of origin), germ cell tumors (both germinoma and nongerminoma), and other, rarer neoplasms.

Primitive Neuroectodermal Tumors

Primitive neuroectodermal tumors are exceptionally rare in adults, and are more frequently seen in the pediatric age group. Radiation therapy is frequently used in the management of these tumors. For primitive neuroectodermal tumors, a distinction into two prognostic categories is routinely made for patients in the pediatric age group, and craniospinal radiation is used for both subgroups. In the adult, such a prognostic division has not been validated. Craniospinal radiation remains the standard of care for the majority of these patients, with recommended doses of 36 Gy to craniospinal axis, and a 54-Gy posterior fossa boost. With the appropriate identification of the role of chemotherapy in the management of subsets of pediatric patients with primitive neuroectodermal tumors, this approach is now being increasingly used in adults as well.

Germ Cell Neoplasms

Historically, CNS germinomas have been managed with craniospinal radiation. The majority of these tumors occur in the pediatric age group, and because of growth impediment from radiation therapy, strategies to eliminate the spinal portion of the radiation or diminish the craniospinal dose have been aggressively pursued. Although single-institution studies suggest that spinal radiation may be deleted in some patients, this is not universally accepted. In a multicenter prospective trial reported in 1999, all 60 patients with intracranial germinoma treated with craniospinal radiation therapy without any chemotherapy achieved a complete remission. The 5-year relapse-free survival rate was 91%; of the five relapsing patients, four had recurrence outside the CNS.[61] Because growth considerations are not of significant concern in the adult population, the inclusion of chemotherapy in adult patients has taken on less significance. Outcome with craniospinal radiation in adult patients with germ cell neoplasms is excellent, with cure rates upward of 90%. For nonseminomatous germ cell tumors of the CNS, survival outcome is significantly poorer, and both surgical resection and chemotherapy are the primary modalities of treatment. For residual disease, radiation therapy may help in prolonging the disease-free survival.

COMPLICATIONS

In general, radiation reactions can be broadly classified into three temporal categories: acute, subacute, and delayed.[62] Acute reactions are those that occur during and immediately after completion of a course of external beam radiation therapy. Using current technologies, these reactions are usually rare and clinically readily manageable. They include acute skin reactions, typically dry desquamation and some degree of erythema, which are managed with local ointments. Temporary alopecia within the radiation field is a common sequela. Fatigue may be observed with radiation therapy but is often a function of several other variables such as age, performance status, underlying medical status, extent of brain being irradiated, and so on. Acute visual complications during radiation therapy are rare, but occasionally patients report seeing flashes of light while undergoing radiation therapy. This is believed to be caused by retinal stimulation, secondary to a phenomenon described as Cerenkov's radiation. If both ear canals are included in the radiation field, serous otitis media may develop toward the end of radiation therapy, sometimes producing muffled hearing. Nausea is uncommon unless the area postrema is treated to high doses or with large fractions. Increased intracranial pressure during radiation therapy is uncommon. It may, however, be masked because the vast majority of patients have been initiated on steroids before radiation therapy and are frequently maintained on steroids during radiation therapy.

Subacute reactions may occur several weeks or months after completion of radiation therapy. When large volumes of the brain are treated, especially in younger patients, lethargy and somnolence may be observed after approximately 3 months. In children, this is specifically described as an acute somnolence syndrome. Rarely, some patients may develop localized demyelination resulting in nausea, vomiting, ataxia, dysphasia, and cerebellar ataxia. This is usually self-limiting. If the lacrimal glands are included in the radiation portal, dry eye may result; similarly, keratoconjunctivitis may develop if the cornea is not protected.

Late complications of radiation therapy occur from several months to several years after completion of therapy. The exact incidence of these complications is unclear because a substantial proportion of patients are either short-term survivors only or have a component of both tumor progression and delayed radiation morbidity. Radiation necrosis in the absence of tumor progression is not commonly encountered when total doses are kept at less than 60 Gy. However, necrosis in concert with viable tumor is not uncommon especially in patients with malignant glioma. With sequential computed tomographic imaging, a mineralizing angiopathy can be identified, characterized by loss of white matter, enlarged ventricles, and microcalcifications. This occurs as a consequence of radiation injury to small vessels and clinically may result in impairment of intellectual function, especially memory and mathematical ability. In severe cases, this may result in significant dementia, ataxia, and confusion. Significant white matter atrophy may be an accompaniment on imaging studies. The clinical sequelae of these changes are frequently manifested as neurocognitive impairment. The exact incidence of such impairment remains inadequately quantified, as many patients with malignant neoplasms frequently succumb to the disease process before neurocognitive development is impaired; therefore, the true incidence of this phenomenon is probably greater than that reported in most clinical trials. Several factors have now been identified as contributory to overall neurocognitive decline in these patients, including the tumor itself, surgery, radiation, and chemotherapy. In addition, host factors such as underlying diseases, especially diseases characterized by microvascular changes, such as diabetes, hypertension, disease from smoking, stroke, cardiovascular insufficiency, and so on, also contribute. Specific radiation therapy parameters that influence the risk profile for neurocognitive decline include fraction size, total dose, and volume irradiated. Therefore, current radiation therapy paradigms, in general, avoid large-fraction irradiation, with radiosurgery representing an exception to this rule. More importantly, three-dimensional and conformal techniques are evolving and hold the promise of reducing the volume of normal brain irradiated. These approaches are of significance, since no effective therapy exists for the patient suffering neurocognitive decline after radiotherapy.

CONCLUSIONS

Radiation therapy plays a significant role in the management of most patients with malignant tumors of the brain. The most common malignant tumor of the brain is a secondary metastatic deposit, which is most often treated with radiation therapy, either singularly or in combination with surgical resection, or stereotactic radiosurgery. For malignant gliomas, radiation therapy is more frequently being used in concert with chemotherapeutic agents and aggressive surgical resection. The advent of technologic innovations will permit reduction of the volume of normal brain within the radiation field and thereby improve the radiotherapeutic ratio.

REFERENCES

1. Posner JB: Management of central nervous system metastases. Semin Oncol 4:81–91, 1977.
2. Hazra T, Mullins GN, Lott S: Management of cerebral metastases from bronchogenic carcinoma. Johns Hopkins Med J 130:377–383, 1972.
3. Posner JB: Diagnosis and treatment of metastases to the brain. Clin Bull 4:47–57, 1974.
4. Zimm S, Wampler GL, Stablein D, et al: Intracerebral metastases in solid tumor patients: Natural history and results of treatment. Cancer 48:384–394, 1981.
5. Kofman S, Garvin J, Nagamani D: Treatment of cerebral metastases from breast carcinoma with prednisolone. JAMA 163:1473–1476, 1957.
6. MacDonell A, Potter PE, Leslie RA: Localized changes in blood-brain barrier permeability following the administration of antineoplastic drugs. Cancer Res 38:2930–2934, 1978.
7. Weissman DE: Glucocorticoid treatment for brain metastases and epidural spinal cord compression: A review. J Clin Oncol 6:543–550, 1988.
8. Chao JH, Phillips R, Nickson JJ: Roentgen-ray therapy of cerebral metastases. Cancer 7:682–694, 1954.
9. Borgelt B, Gelber R, Kramer S, et al: The palliation of brain metastases: Final results of the first two studies by the Radiation Therapy Oncology Group. Int J Radiat Oncol Biol Phys 6:1–8, 1980.
10. Diener-West M, Dobbins TW, Phillips TL, et al: Identification of an optimal subgroup for treatment evaluation of patients with brain metastases using RTOG Study 7916. Int J Radiat Oncol Biol Phys 16:669–673, 1989.
11. Coia LR, Hanks GE, Martz K, et al: Practice patterns of palliative care for the United States 1984–1985. Int J Radiat Oncol Biol Phys 14:1261–1269, 1988.
12. Phillips TL, Scott CB, Leibel SA, et al: Results of a randomized comparison of radiotherapy and bromodeoxyuridine with radiotherapy alone for brain metastases: Report of RTOG trial 89-05. Int J Radiat Oncol Biol Phys 33:339–348, 1995.
13. Epstein BE, Scott CB, Sause WT, et al: Improved survival duration in patients with unresected solitary brain metastasis using accelerated hyperfractionated radiation therapy at total doses of 54.4 Gy and greater: Results of Radiation Therapy Oncology Group 85-28. Cancer 71:1362–1367, 1993.
14. Murray KJ, Scott CB, Greenberg HM, et al: A randomized phase III study of accelerated hyperfractionation vs. standard fractionation in patients with unresected brain metastases: A report of the Radiation Therapy Oncology Group (RTOG) 9104. Int J Radiat Oncol Biol Phys 39:571–574, 1997.
15. Nieder C, Berberich W, Nestle U, et al: Relation between local result and total dose of radiotherapy for brain metastases. Int J Radiat Oncol Biol Phys 33:349–355, 1955.
16. Nieder C, Nestle U, Walter K, et al: Dose/effective relationships for brain metastases. J Cancer Res Clin Oncol 124:346–350, 1998.
17. Lagerwaard FJ, Levendag BC, Nowak PJ, et al: Identification of prognostic factors in patients with brain metastases: A review of 1292 patients. Int J Radiat Oncol Biol Phys 43:795–803, 1999.
18. Noordijk EM, Vecht CJ, Haazma-Reiche J, et al: The choice of treatment of single brain metastasis should be based on extracranial tumor activity and age. Int J Radiat Oncol Biol Phys 29:711–717, 1994.
19. Patchell RA, Tibbs PA, Walsh JW, et al: A randomized trial of surgery in the treatment of single metastases to the brain. N Engl J Med 322:494–500, 1990.
20. Swift PS, Phillips T, Martz K, et al: CT characteristics of patients with brain metastases treated in RTOG study 79-16. Int J Radiat Oncol Biol Phys 25:209–214, 1993.
21. Gaspar L, Scott C, Rotman M, et al: Recursive partitioning analysis (RPA) of prognostic factors in three Radiation Therapy Oncology Group (RTOG) brain metastases trials. Int J Radiat Oncol Biol Phys 37:745–751, 1997.
22. Patchell RA, Tibbs PA, Regin W, et al: Post-operative radiotherapy in the treatment of single metastasis to the brain: A randomized trial. JAMA 280:1485–1489, 1998.
23. Landis S, Murray T, Bolden S, et al: Cancer statistics 1999. CA Cancer J Clin 49:8–31, 1999.
24. Mahaley M, Mettlin C, Natarajan N, et al: National survey of patterns of care for brain-tumor patients. J Neurosurg 71:826–836, 1989.
25. Hochberg F, Pruitt A: Assumptions in the radiotherapy of glioblastoma. Neurology 30:907–911, 1980.
26. Urtasun R, Feldstein M, Partington J, et al: Radiation and nitroimidazoles in supratentorial high grade gliomas: A second clinical trial. Br J Cancer 46:101–108, 1982.
27. Burger P: Pathologic anatomy and CT correlations in glioblastoma multiforme. Appl Neurophysiol 46:180–187, 1983.
28. Kelly P, Daumas-Dupont C, Kispert D, et al: Imaging-based stereotaxic serial biopsies in untreated intracranial glial neoplasms. J Neurosurg 66:865–874, 1987.
29. Groshar D, McEwan A, Parliament M, et al: Imaging tumor hypoxia and tumor perfusion. J Nucl Med 34:885–888, 1993.
30. Walker M, Strike T, Sheline G: An analysis of dose-effect relationship in the radiotherapy of malignant gliomas. Int J Radiat Oncol Biol Phys 5:1725–1731, 1979.
31. Bleehan N, Stenning S: A Medical Research Council trial of two radiotherapy doses in the treatment of grades 3 and 4 astrocytoma. Br J Cancer 64:769–774, 1991.
32. Taghian A, Suit H, Pardo F, et al: In vitro intrinsic radiation sensitivity of glioblastoma multiforme. Int J Radiat Oncol Biol Phys 23:55–62, 1992.
33. Marks J, Baglan R, Prassad S, et al: Cerebral radionecrosis: Incidence and risk in relation to dose, time, fractionation and volume. Int J Radiat Oncol Biol Phys 7:243–252, 1981.
34. Nelson D, Diener-West M, Horton J, et al: Combined modality approach to treatment of malignant gliomas—re-evaluation of RTOG 7401/ECOG 1374 with long-term follow-up: A joint study of the Radiation Therapy Oncology Group and the Eastern Cooperative Oncology Group. NCI Monographs 6:279–284, 1988.
35. Nelson D, Curran W, Scott C, et al: Hyperfractionated radiation therapy and bis-chlorethyl nitrosourea in the treatment of malignant glioma—possible advantage observed at 72.0 Gy in 1.2 Gy b.i.d. fractions: Report of the Radiation Therapy Oncology Group Protocol 8302. Int J Radiat Oncol Biol Phys 25:193–207, 1993.
36. Fulton D, Urtasun R, Scott-Brown I, et al: Increasing radiation dose intensity using hyperfractionation in patients with malignant glioma: Final report of a prospective phase I-II dose response study. J Neurooncol 14:63–72, 1992.
37. Murray KJ, Nelson DF, Scott C, et al: Quality adjusted survival analysis of malignant glioma patients treated with twice daily radiation and carmustine: A report of Radiation Therapy Oncology Group 83-02. Int J Radiat Oncol Biol Phys 31:453–459, 1995.
38. Prados MD, Larson DA, Lamborn K, et al: Radiation therapy and hydroxyurea followed by the combination of 6-thioguamine and BCNU for the treatment of primary malignant brain tumors. Int J Radiat Oncol Biol Phys 40:57–63, 1998.
39. Nelson F, Schoenfeld D, Weinstein A, et al: A randomized comparison of misonidazole sensitized radiotherapy plus BCNU and radiotherapy plus BCNU for treatment of malignant glioma after surgery: Preliminary results of an RTOG study. Int J Radiat Oncol Biol Phys 9:1143–1151, 1983.
40. Deutsch M, Green S, Strike T, et al: The results of a randomized trial comparing BCNU plus radiotherapy, streptozotocin plus radiotherapy, BCNU plus hyperfractionated radiotherapy, and BCNU following misonidazole plus radiotherapy in the postoperative treatment of malignant glioma. Int J Radiat Oncol Biol Phys 16:1389–1396, 1989.
41. Riese N, Loeffler J, Wen P, et al: A phase I study of etanidazole and radiotherapy in malignant glioma. Int J Radiat Oncol Biol Phys 29:617–620, 1994.
42. Urtasun R, Kinsella T, Farnan N, et al: Survival improvements in anaplastic astrocytoma combining external radiation with halogenated pyridimines: Final report of RTOG 86-12, phase I/II study. Int J Radiat Oncol Biol Phys 36:1163–1167, 1996.

43. Prados M, Scott C, Rotman M, et al: Influence of bromodeoxyuridine radiosensitization on malignant glioma patients' survival: A retrospective comparison of survival data from the Northern California Oncology Group and Radiation Therapy Oncology Group trials for glioblastoma multiforme and anaplastic astrocytoma. Int J Radiat Oncol Biol Phys 40:653–659, 1998.

44. Castro C, Saunders W, Austin-Seymourn N, et al: A phase I/II trial of heavy charged particle irradiation of malignant glioma of the brain: A Northern California Oncology Group Study. Int J Radiat Oncol Biol Phys 11:1795–1800, 1985.

45. Laramore G, Diener-West M, Griffin T, et al: A randomized neutron dose seeking study for malignant gliomas of the brain: Results of an RTOG study. Int J Radiat Oncol Biol Phys 14:1093–1102, 1988.

46. Laramore G, Spence A: Boron neutron capture therapy (BNCT) for high grade gliomas of the brain: A cautionary note. Int J Radiat Oncol Biol Phys 36:267–268, 1996.

47. Curran W, Scott C, Horton J, et al: Recursive partitioning analysis of prognostic factors in three Radiation Therapy Oncology Group malignant glioma trials. J Natl Cancer Inst 85:704–710, 1993.

48. Laramore G, Martz K, Nelson J, et al: Radiation Therapy Oncology Group survival data on anaplastic astrocytomas of the brain: Does a more aggressive form of treatment adversely affect survival? Int J Radiat Oncol Biol Phys 17:3057–3058, 1989.

49. Fischbach A, Martz K, Nelson J, et al: Long-term survival in treated anaplastic astrocytomas: A report of combined RTOG/ECOG studies. Am J Clin Oncol 14:365–370, 1991.

50. Prados M, Scott C, Phillips T, et al: Phase III randomized study of radiotherapy plus PCV with or without BudR for the treatment of anaplastic astrocytoma: RTOG 94-04. Proc Soc Neurooncol 2:112, 1997.

51. Cairncross G, Ueki K, Zlatescu N, et al: Specific genetic predictors of chemotherapeutic response and survival in patients with anaplastic oligodendroglioma. J Natl Cancer Inst 90:1473–1479, 1998.

52. Tamura M, Zama A, Kurihara H, et al: Clinical histological study of oligodendroglioma and oligoastrocytoma. Brain Tumor Pathol 14:35–39, 1997.

53. Henry J, Heffner R, Dillard S, et al: Primary malignant lymphomas of the central nervous system. Cancer 34:1293–1302, 1974.

54. Berry M, Simpson W: Radiation therapy in the management of primary malignant lymphomas of the brain. Int J Radiat Oncol Biol Phys 7:55–59, 1981.

55. Leibel S, Sheline G: Radiation therapy for neoplasms of the brain. J Neurosurg 66:1–22, 1987.

56. Murray K, Kun L, Cox J: Primary malignant lymphomas of the central nervous system: Results of treatment of 11 cases and review of the literature. J Neurosurg 65:600–607, 1986.

57. DeAngelis LM, Seiferheld SC, Schold B, et al: Combined modality treatment of primary central nervous system lymphoma: RTOG 93-10. Proc Am Soc Clin Oncol 18:140a, 1999.

58. Mead GM, Bleehen NM, Gregor A: Medical Research Council (MRC) randomized trial of adjuvant chemotherapy in primary CNS lymphoma (PCL)—BRO6. Proc Am Soc Clin Oncol 17:1547, 1998.

59. Scheithauer B: Tumors of the meninges: Proposed modifications of the World Health Organization classification. Acta Neurol Pathol 80:343–354, 1990.

60. Bastin K, Mehta M: Meningeal hemangiopericytoma: Defining the role for radiation therapy. J Neurooncol 14:277–287, 1992.

61. Bamberg M, Kortmann R, Calaminius G, et al: Radiation therapy for intracranial germinoma: Results of the German Cooperative prospective trials MAKEI 83/86/89. J Clin Oncol 17:2585–2592, 1999.

62. Goutin PH, Leibel S, Sheleine G (eds): Radiation Injury to the Central Nervous System. New York, Raven Press, 1991.

CHAPTER 265

Radiotherapy for Benign Skull Base Tumors

JOHN M. BUATTI ■ SANFORD L. MEEKS

Management of benign skull base tumors is complex. Decisions are best made with the close collaboration of a multidisciplinary team that includes neurosurgery, radiation oncology, neuro-ophthalmology, neuroradiology, and often neurology. The patient's symptoms and his or her ability to understand the alternative management approaches and the side effects of each are also important. Stereotactic radiosurgery and stereotactic radiotherapy (fractionated) are critical alternatives that should be available to all patients. In addition, the availability of multimodality imaging, with magnetic resonance imaging linked to computed tomographic simulation for treatment delivery, is important for high-quality radiation treatment planning.

Factors that complicate the treatment of these tumors include their slow growth potential[1, 2]; the difficulty of complete resection of skull base lesions without significant morbidity[3, 4]; the proximity to critical radiosensitive nervous tissue, including the optic nerve, optic chiasm, brainstem, cavernous sinus, vestibular apparatus, pituitary gland, and mesial temporal lobes; and the patient's often insidious symptoms. In addition, because a majority of these tumors are identified radiographically, obtaining tissue for diagnosis is only rarely an issue. Thus, in making the diagnosis, care must be taken to avoid mistaking a benign skull base tumor for a malignant one, such as from perineural spread of a skin cancer or another metastatic tumor. Non-neoplastic processes such as sarcoidosis, vascular anomalies, and infections must also be ruled out, because their radiographic appearance may be similar to that of some of these lesions. The expertise of a skilled neuroradiologist and skull base specialist is helpful in making these distinctions.

MANAGEMENT ALGORITHM

Fractionated radiotherapy (stereotactic) should be considered the fourth management alternative, following observation, neurosurgical resection, and stereotactic radiosurgery (single fraction). Conventional external beam therapy has been replaced by image-guided radiotherapy because of the former's tendency to treat a larger volume of tissue unnecessarily (Fig. 265–1).[5, 6] The large amounts of data compiled on the techniques and doses of external beam therapy are useful only for defining tumor control at a defined dose of fractionated treatment. Because radiosurgery uses no margin in defining the tumor target for treatment delivery and has shown equal control for virtually all types of benign tumors, there is no reason to treat larger volumes than necessary as defined by setup and imaging resolution errors.[7]

Observation

Some patients may have the incidental finding of a skull base tumor. If the lesion is small and the neurological examination is normal, there is no indication for treatment. It is important, however, to identify the lesion's proximity to the cranial nerves and to determine radiographically which nerves are most likely to be affected. If the optic or vestibular nerve is at risk, detailed neuro-ophthalmologic or auditory and vestibular testing is recommended, because it is common for radiographic progression to lag behind subtle neurological findings. Serial re-examination for both radiographic and neurological progression determines whether treatment is needed. If a patient presents with some neurological compromise, it is important to define its degree, because progression of the deficit, not its existence alone, determines the need for treatment. If a patient presents with acute deterioration, treatment is generally indicated. A final caveat is that it is reasonable to observe a patient with slow progression of a mild deficit or an asymptomatic radiographic finding who is otherwise a poor surgical and medical risk for radiotherapy.

Neurosurgical Resection

Surgery is an appropriate option if a benign lesion can be removed completely without significant risk of neurological deficit. In skull base tumors, this is the exception rather than the rule.

Surgery is the preferred option if the patient has an acute compressive neuropathy of the optic nerve or chiasm. In such cases, radiotherapy is unlikely to rapidly reverse the compression, limiting the possibility of recovering vision.[8] The probability of recovery is proportional to the length of time a neurological deficit has been present. Thus, it is important to initiate radiotherapy quickly if there is neurological compromise

and surgery is impossible because, for example, the patient is medically infirm.

A rare indication for surgery in skull base tumors is the presence of mass effect. Again, it is unlikely that radiation will rapidly correct this condition; therefore, a partial resection has great value in relieving the mass effect, as well as in limiting the volume of tissue that may require radiation if the lesion is subtotally re-

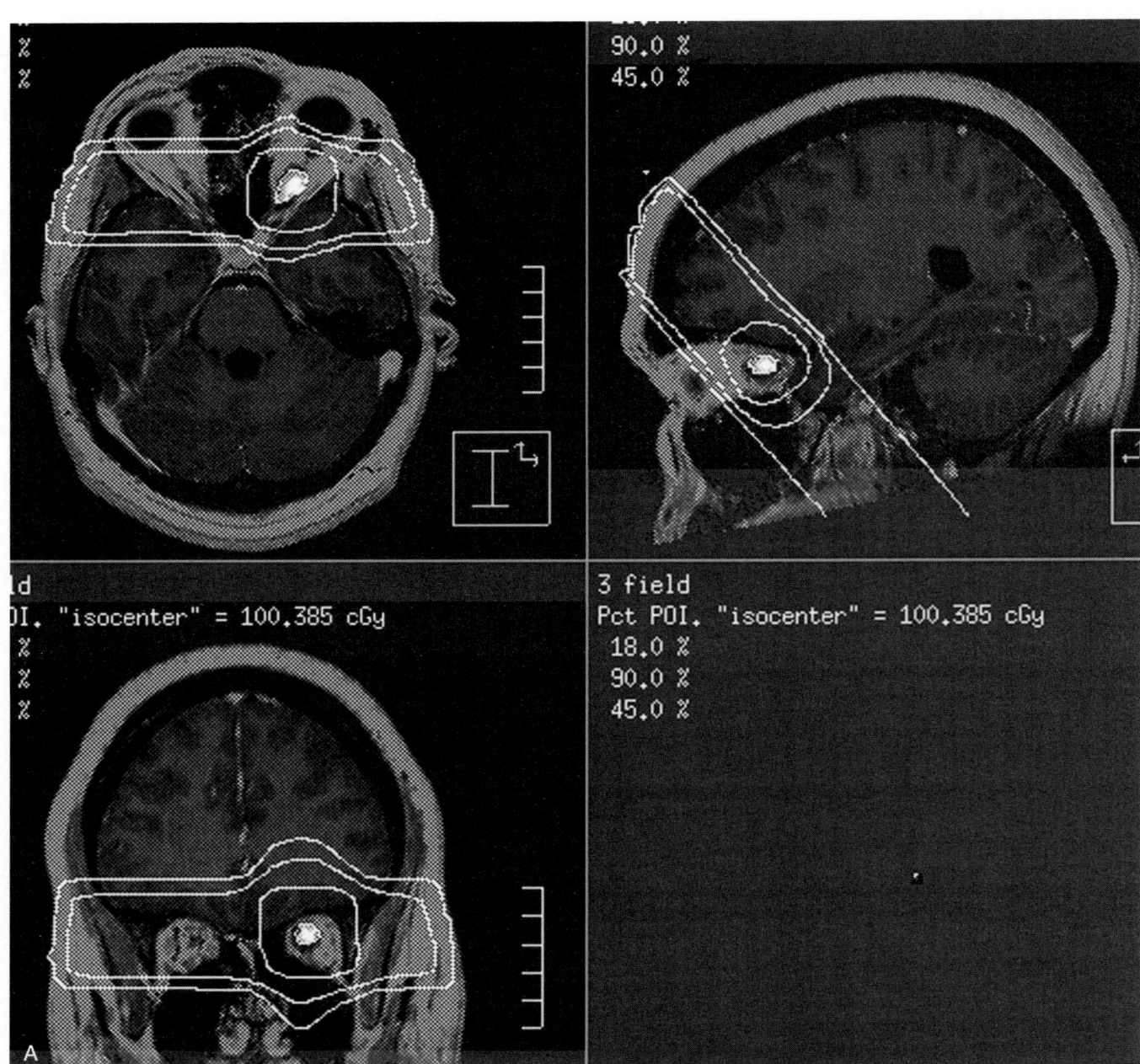

FIGURE 265–1. *A,* Conventional radiotherapy generally employed a three-field technique to deliver daily doses of radiation to benign skull base tumors. Fields were designed on plain x-ray films, transcribing the tumor based on bony anatomy. Daily delivery accuracy was on the order of 5 to 8 mm. This illustration reveals that the majority of brain in the region immediately around the tumor received near the prescription dose, and the entire brain through the region received more than half the dose. Note that the optic chiasm, pituitary gland, and mesial temporal lobes would all be treated with at least 50% of the prescription dose.

Illustration continued on following page

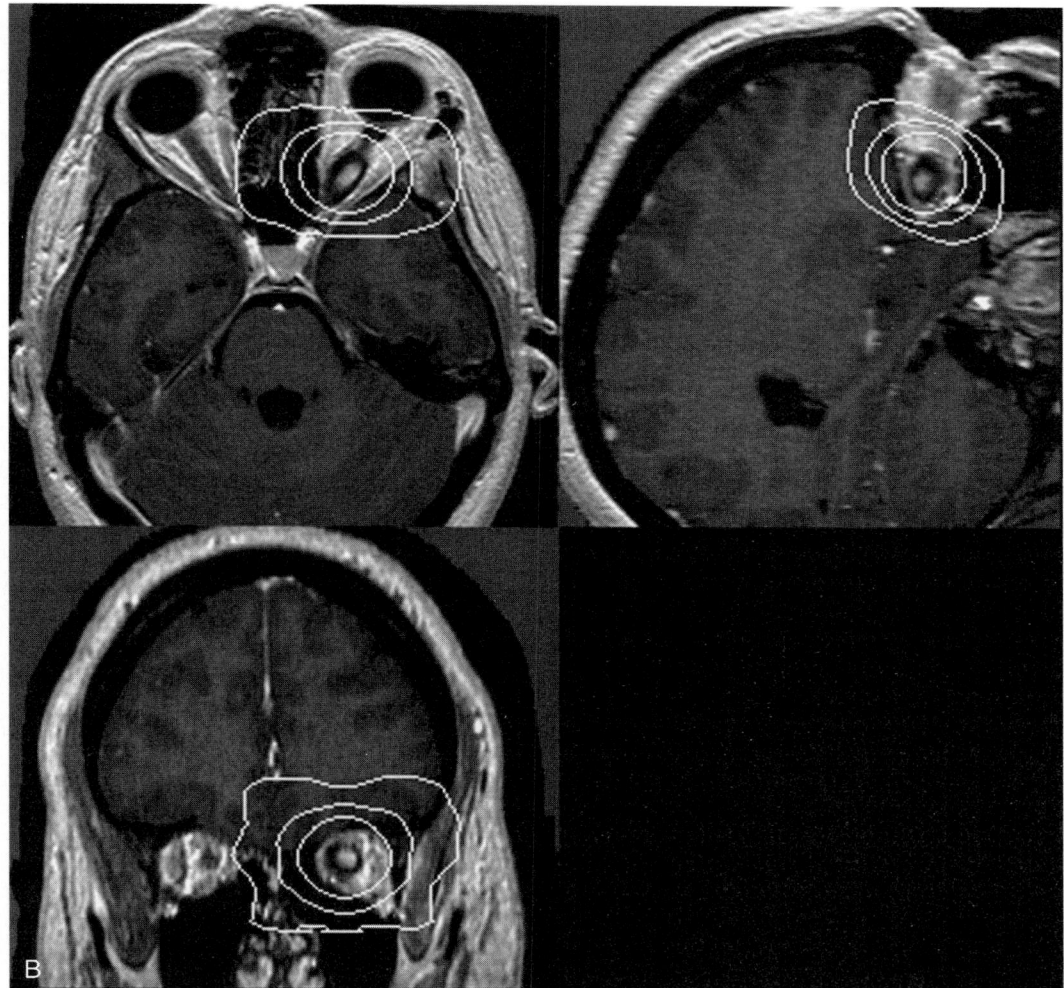

FIGURE 265-1. *Continued. B,* Stereotactic radiotherapy often allows the delivery of a conformal group of arcs or five or more coplanar fields directed at the tumor, with delivery accuracy of less than 1 mm. This allows reduction of the treatment margin so that less normal brain is treated unnecessarily.

moved. Partial resection can be advantageous when a lesion is too large for radiosurgery; decreasing the lesion's volume makes it more amenable to a limited radiotherapeutic approach.

Stereotactic Radiosurgery

Stereotactic radiosurgery is the preferred radiotherapeutic approach for benign skull base tumors because it exposes the least amount of normal surrounding brain to a significant dose of radiation, and it is at least as efficacious as fractionated therapy.[9] The main contraindications for radiosurgery are excessive tumor size and proximity to the optic nerve and chiasm.

Stereotactic Radiotherapy

Lesions that are larger than 3.5 cm or that are too close to the optic nerve and chiasm can be treated using stereotactic radiotherapy. The goal of treatment is to take advantage of the radiobiologic advantages of fractionation. These advantages are reviewed in detail in Chapter 262. In brief, because normal tissue is better able to repair DNA damage compared with tumor tissue, there is a selective advantage to treating the tumor and normal tissue with multiple small doses of radiation. At a dose of 54 Gy in 30 fractions (1.8 Gy/day), there is an extremely low risk of damage to the optic nerve and a high probability of obtaining local control of a benign tumor.[1, 10] Some tumors such as pituitary adenomas and glomus tumors require only 45 Gy for long-term control.[8, 11] Extensive experience using these doses has led to the recognition that fractionated therapy can control many benign skull base tumors.

Problems associated with the widespread use of conventional fractionated radiotherapy include the inconvenience of 25 to 30 daily treatments that take 30 to 60 minutes a day; acute side effects, including fatigue, hair loss, anorexia, and nausea, in many patients; and long-term sequelae such as recent memory deficit, pituitary dysfunction, and, rarely, more severe neurological deficits. Despite these shortcomings, fractionated therapy was an important advance, because many patients who suffer progressive symptoms and signs cannot undergo surgical resection without the risk of more substantial immediate morbidity.[1, 8, 12] Therefore, fractionated radiotherapy is an essential alternative in the management of many benign skull base tumors. Stereotactic radiotherapy and the enhanced use of multimodality imaging have eliminated many of the problems associated with standard fractionated radiotherapy. For instance, in some cases, there is no risk of hair loss, and fatigue, nausea, and anorexia can be ameliorated to a significant extent by more limited treatment volumes.[13] Although is seems logical that there would also be diminished neuropsychological sequelae, there is little objective evidence that this is the case. Fewer fractions have been proposed to improve the convenience of treatment for some skull base tumors,[3-6] although sequelae and late effects are significant concerns.[14, 15] It is unclear whether large tumors or those in proximity to the optic nerve would tolerate these regimens of hypofractionation; therefore, such regimens are not recommended outside of a study setting.

OUTCOME

Pituitary Tumors

The control rate for pituitary tumors treated with daily doses of 1.8 Gy to a total dose of 45 Gy exceeds 90% using conventional three-field or bicoronal arc radiotherapy techniques.[8, 16] These techniques produce hormone deficiency in more than 30% of cases. In addition, it is likely that the large volume of normal tissue receiving a significant radiation dose poses a risk of both neuropsychological deficits and secondary tumors.[8] Therefore, stereotactic radiotherapy or radiosurgery is preferable for the treatment of pituitary adenomas. Although radiosurgery has been reported to produce rapid hormonal decline and may, in the case of microadenomas, avoid normal pituitary dysfunction, the treatment of large tumors with single-fraction radiosurgery is not a safe option.[17, 18] We have treated 16 patients with stereotactic radiotherapy using circular collimators, and after a 2-year median follow-up, the progression-free survival is 100%. We anticipate that the long-term hormonal sequelae will be the same, and that neuropsychological sequelae and the risk of secondary malignancy will be less than with conventional techniques based on the volumes of tissue treated; however, definitive confirmation of this must await further study.

Meningiomas

Tumor control of benign meningiomas with postoperative radiotherapy exceeds 90%.[1, 10] The standard dose used with conventional radiotherapy is 54 Gy in 30 fractions. Radiosurgery has also been used and produces progression-free survival at least as good as that achieved with conventional radiotherapy.[12, 19, 20] Despite these promising results, a large number of tumors are not amenable to radiosurgery because of their large size or their proximity to radiosensitive structures. Our experience with 49 patients treated with stereotactic radiotherapy at doses between 52.7 and 54 Gy with both arced and fixed-field techniques reveals that progression-free survival is 100% at 2 years. Long-term follow-up will be required to establish definitive efficacy.

Vestibular Schwannomas

Although standard fractionated radiotherapy was used to treat incompletely resected acoustic schwannomas many years ago, the frequency of application was rare.[21, 22] Doses in excess of 45 Gy led to improved local control.[21] More recently, radiosurgery has achieved a high rate of local control, but with a significant risk of sequelae.[23, 24] Because of the early complications reported with radiosurgery, stereotactic radiotherapy was tried in an attempt to decrease cranial neuropathies. Different groups have used different regimens, ranging from conventional fractionation (50 to 54 Gy in 28 to 30 fractions) to three fractions of 7 Gy.[14, 15, 25] Each group reported hearing preservation in approximately 50% of patients and cranial nerve V and VII neuropathies in less than 1% of patients. More recent radiosurgery series using lower doses of radiation and multimodality imaging have produced results that are equivalent or superior to those obtained with radiotherapy.[26] Therefore, the use of stereotactic radiosurgery for vestibular schwannoma should be limited to tumors that are too large for radiosurgery.

Other Benign Neoplasms

Stereotactic radiotherapy is an ideal therapy for benign skull base neoplasms that were previously treated with conventional radiotherapy. These tumors include craniopharyngiomas, chemodectomas, low-grade glial tumors, hemangioblastomas, and nonacoustic schwannomas.[27-30] In each case, the control rate achieved with conventional radiotherapy is 90% or more, but this modality traditionally involves treating large volumes of normal brain tissue. All these tumors are well visualized and minimally invasive, so image registration should provide accurate targeting of the tumor. Limited experience is now accumulating and appears positive to date. No benign neoplasm had recurred in the group of more than 130 patients we treated with stereotactic radiotherapy techniques after 2 years' follow-up. These results, though encouraging, will require diligent follow-up, and experiences from numerous institutions will need to confirm the same.

REFERENCES

1. Condra KS, Buatti JM, Mendenhall WM, et al: Benign meningiomas: Primary treatment selection affects survival. Int J Radiat Oncol Biol Phys 39:427–436, 1997.

2. Strasnick B, Glasscock ME, Haynes D, et al: The natural history of untreated acoustic neuromas. Laryngoscope 104:1115–1119, 1994.
3. Sekhar LN, Lanzino G, Sen CN, et al: Reconstruction of the third through sixth cranial nerves during cavernous sinus surgery. J Neurosurg 76:935–943, 1992.
4. Sekhar LN, Sen CN, Jho HD, et al: Surgical treatment of intracavernous neoplasms: A four-year experience. Neurosurgery 24:18–30, 1989.
5. Lichter AS, Sandler HM, Robertson JM, et al: Clinical experience with three-dimensional treatment planning. Semin Radiat Oncol 2:257–266, 1992.
6. Buatti JM, Friedman WA, Meeks SL, et al: Radiation therapy and radiosurgery for brain tumors. In Kaye AH, Laws ER Jr (eds): Brain Tumors, 2nd ed. Philadelphia, WB Saunders, 2001, pp 357–374.
7. Friedman WA, Buatti JM, Bova FJ, et al: Linac Radiosurgery: A Practical Guide. New York, Springer Verlag, 1998.
8. McCord MW, Buatti JM, Fennell EM, et al: Radiotherapy for pituitary adenoma: Long-term outcome and sequelae. Int J Radiat Oncol Biol Phys 39:437–444, 1997.
9. Tome WA, Mehta MP, Meeks SL, et al: Fractionated stereotactic radiotherapy: A short review. Technology in cancer research and treatment. 1:153–172, 2002.
10. Goldsmith BJ, Wara WM, Wilson CB, et al: Postoperative irradiation for subtotally resected meningiomas: A retrospective analysis of 140 patients treated from 1967–1990. J Neurosurg 80:195–201, 1994.
11. Mendenhall WM, Parsons JT, Stringer SP, et al: Radiotherapy in the management of temporal bone chemodectoma. Skull Base Surg 5:83–91, 1995.
12. Hakim R, Alexander E III, Loeffler JS, et al: Results of linear accelerator based radiosurgery for intracranial meningiomas. Neurosurgery 42:446–454, 1998.
13. Buatti JM, Bova FJ, Friedman WA, et al: Preliminary experience with frameless stereotactic radiotherapy. Int J Radiat Oncol Biol Phys 42:591–599, 1998.
14. Poen JC, Golby AJ, Wertheim S, et al: Fractionated stereotactic radiosurgery and preservation of hearing in patients with vestibular schwannoma: A preliminary report. Neurosurgery 45:1299–1305, 1999.
15. Lederman GS, Wertheim S, Lowery J, et al: Acoustic neuromas treated by fractionated stereotactic radiotherapy. In Kondziolka D (ed): Radiosurgery 1997. Basel, Karger, 1998, pp 25–30.
16. Tsang RW, Brierley JD, Panzarella T, et al: Radiation therapy for pituitary adenoma: Treatment outcome and prognostic factors. Int J Radiat Oncol Biol Phys 30:557–565, 1994.
17. Mitsomuri M, Shreive DC, Alexander E, et al: Initial clinical results of Linac-based stereotactic radiosurgery and stereotactic radiotherapy for pituitary adenomas. Int J Radiat Oncol Biol Phys 42:573–580, 1998.
18. Witt TC, Kondziolka D, Flickinger JC, et al: Stereotactic radiosurgery for pituitary tumors. Radiosurgery 1:55–65, 1999.
19. Shaffron DH, Friedman WA, Buatti JM, et al: Linac radiosurgery for benign meningiomas. Int J Radiat Oncol Biol Phys 43:321–327, 1999.
20. Lunsford LD: Contemporary management of meningiomas: Radiation therapy as an adjuvant and radiosurgery as an alternative to surgical removal? J Neurosurg 80:187–190, 1994.
21. Wallner KE, Sheline GE, Pitts LH, et al: Efficacy of irradiation for incompletely excised acoustic neurilemomas. J Neurosurg 67:858–863, 1987.
22. Maire JP, Floquet A, Darrouzet V, et al: Fractionated radiation therapy in the treatment of stage III and IV cerebello-pontine angle neurinomas: Preliminary results in 20 cases. Int J Radiat Oncol Biol Phys 23:147–152, 1992.
23. Lunsford LD, Kondziolka D, Flickinger JC, et al: Acoustic neuroma management: Evolution and revolution. In Kondziolka D (ed): Radiosurgery 1997. Basel, Karger, 1998, pp 1–7.
24. Flickinger JC, Lunsford LD, Linskey ME, et al: Gamma knife radiosurgery for acoustic tumors: Multivariate analysis of four year results. Radiother Oncol 27:91–98, 1993.
25. Varlotto JM, Shrieve DC, Alexander E, et al: Fractionated stereotactic radiotherapy for the treatment of acoustic neuromas: Preliminary results. Int J Radiat Oncol Biol Phys 36:141–145, 1996.
26. Foote KD, Friedman WA, Buatti JM, et al: An analysis of risk factors associated with radiosurgery for vestibular schwannoma. J Neurosurg 95:440–449, 2001.
27. Loeffler JS, Dunbar SF, Tarbell N: Early experience with stereotactic radiation therapy in the management of intracranial lesions: The first 1200 treatments. Int J Radiat Oncol Biol Phys 27:154, 1993.
28. Delannes M, Daly NJ, Bonnet J, et al: Fractionated radiotherapy of small inoperable lesions of the brain using a noninvasive stereotactic frame. Int J Radiat Oncol Biol Phys 21:749–755, 1991.
29. Dunbar SF, Tarbell NJ, Kooy HM, et al: Stereotactic radiotherapy for pediatric and adult brain tumors: Preliminary report. Int J Radiat Oncol Biol Phys 30:531–539, 1994.
30. Mabanta SR, Buatti JM, Friedman WA, et al: Linear accelerator radiosurgery for nonacoustic schwannomas. Int J Radiat Oncol Biol Phys 43:545–548, 1999.

Fractionated Radiotherapy for Pituitary Tumors

JOHN C. FLICKINGER ■ DOUGLAS KONDZIOLKA

Conventional fractionated radiotherapy is a well-established treatment modality for pituitary adenomas. It has been in use since shortly after the development of radiotherapy as a treatment technique. Radiotherapy has been used either as an adjunct to surgery or as the primary therapy.[1-6] Other choices for managing pituitary adenomas have improved dramatically since the development and refinement of transsphenoidal microsurgery and dopamine agonist therapy. Currently, pituitary tumors are best managed in the setting of a multidisciplinary program with input from neurosurgery, radiation oncology, and endocrinology, with the assistance of pathology and diagnostic radiology.

TREATMENT TECHNIQUE

The last 5 decades saw dramatic improvements in radiotherapy treatment techniques. Radiotherapy equipment improved from 0.2- to 0.3-MeV orthovoltage x-ray beams to the first widely used megavoltage beam—1.25-MeV cobalt-60 gamma rays—in the 1950s to widespread use of 4- to 18-MeV medical linear accelerators in the 1960s. Cobalt-60 and linear accelerator beams allowed the use of simplified plans with right and left lateral fields, without causing moist skin desquamation. Unfortunately, this treatment technique delivers a dose to the temporal lobes that is higher than that at the tumor target, resulting in a small but unnecessary risk of temporal lobe necrosis. The addition of one other field from another direction (usually anteroposterior) can dramatically reduce this risk. Figure 266–1 shows a standard three-field (anteroposterior and right and left lateral) arrangement for treating pituitary tumors. Patients are usually treated with their heads held in position by custom-fitted plastic-mesh masks.

The development of computed tomography and, later, magnetic resonance imaging allowed radiotherapists to better define the tumor target for conformal radiation treatment that limits irradiation of surrounding normal tissue. Conformal treatment means that the radiation fields are shaped to match the tumor target, usually with a 10- to 15-mm margin from the beam edge (where the dose is 50%) to allow for setup uncertainties and dose falloff at the edge of the beam. Computerized three-dimensional beam's-eye-view tumor reconstruction from imaging data and three-dimensional treatment planning allow for conformal treatment from any direction. Stereotactic radiotherapy usually involves the use of a relocatable stereotactic head frame, usually with a custom bite block. This can allow the margin of the treatment field to be reduced to 2 to 3 mm (plus an additional 5 mm to the 50% beam edge). Normal tissue sparing with stereotactic radiotherapy can be improved if micro-multileaf collimators are used for conformal treatment portals rather than using standard circular collimators.

RADIOBIOLOGY AND DOSE SELECTION

Dose selection for radiotherapy requires consideration of what is known about both the dose responses for

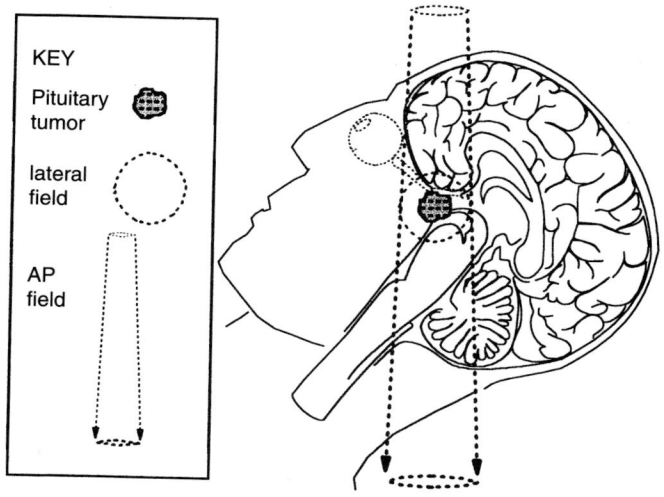

FIGURE 266–1. Standard three-field arrangement for conventional radiotherapy of pituitary adenomas with anteroposterior (AP), right lateral, and left lateral treatment portals.

KEY

Pituitary tumor

lateral field

AP field

tumor control and normal tissue injury. The consequences of tumor progression and radiation injury must also be considered. For a slow-growing tumor like a pituitary adenoma, for which there are multiple management options (pituitary surgery, drugs, adrenalectomy, repeat radiotherapy, or radiosurgery), and with blindness and brain necrosis as possible consequences of radiation injury, there is good reason to be conservative when choosing radiation doses.

The long natural history of these tumors and the relatively high tumor control rates with fractionated radiotherapy make them difficult to study, even in large series with long-term follow-up.[1-5] Evaluations of older treatment series can be biased by differences in imaging techniques available for treatment planning (with increased marginal misses before the advent of computed tomography) and in follow-up assessment (with later detection of tumor progression before computed tomography). Assessing tumor control is complicated by the different end points that could be studied. Tumor growth arrest is the only reasonable end point for nonfunctional pituitary adenomas. The main goal with functional tumors is to normalize elevated hormone levels. The rate at which this occurs varies among the different types of functional adenomas. Interpretation of follow-up hormone levels may be complicated by the success of different medical therapies. Because of these complexities, many questions about tumor control with radiotherapy have not been fully addressed. Tumor control dose-response curves have not been well defined within the range of doses explored for fractionated conventional radiotherapy of pituitary adenomas (40 to 65 Gy with 1.8- to 2.5-Gy fractions).[4-6] The seemingly flat dose-response function within this dose range may be due to heterogeneity in radiation dose response among these tumors. Most pituitary adenomas can be easily controlled with doses lower than those currently used, whereas unidentified subpopulations of more resistant tumors may require much higher doses.

Because of the long natural history of these patients, the risk of late radiation injury to the optic apparatus from pituitary irradiation has been well documented. Although there are rare case reports of optic neuropathy at doses as low as 45 Gy in 25 fractions, the risk of optic neuropathy does not become appreciable until a dose of 50 Gy in 25 fractions or 54 Gy in 30 fractions, when it is approximately 3%; it then rises to 13% when doses of 65 Gy are used.[4] Harris and Levene studied optic neuropathy after pituitary irradiation with different dose fractions.[7] They found that optic neuropathy (which developed with doses as low as 45 Gy with 2.5- and 3-Gy fractions) correlated more closely with the use of 2.5-Gy fractions than with total dose. Since this study, treatment with dose fractions greater than 2 Gy has not been explored. The biology and radiation response of these tumors suggest that higher dose-fraction schedules with lower total doses (such as 35 Gy at 2.5 Gy per fraction) might be just as safe and effective as smaller dose fractions.

The most commonly used dose schedule for irradiation of pituitary adenomas is 45 Gy in 25 fractions (at 1.8 Gy per fraction) over 5 weeks. Many radiotherapists use a slightly higher dose of 50 Gy in 28 fractions in treating functional adenomas, with the hope of achieving better hormone normalization. Improvement with higher doses has not been well documented for fractionated conventional radiotherapy.

NONFUNCTIONAL ADENOMAS

Patients with nonfunctional pituitary adenomas usually present with symptoms related to mass effect, such as visual field cuts, symptoms of hypopituitarism, or, rarely, cranial neuropathies related to cavernous sinus invasion. Cavernous sinus invasion may make complete surgical resection more difficult to achieve with these tumors (compared with functional adenomas, which usually present as smaller tumors).

Table 266–1 shows the long-term tumor control rates with fractionated radiotherapy of nonfunctional pituitary adenomas in several large, representative series. Tumor control in patients managed with radiotherapy alone (or with biopsy) appears to be similar to that in patients managed with incomplete surgical resection and subsequent radiotherapy. Long-term follow-up is essential in evaluating the results of radiotherapy and any other treatment modality used to manage these slow-growing tumors. Tumor control rates continued

TABLE 266–1 ■ **Long-term Control Rates for Pituitary Adenoma Radiotherapy in Representative Series**

INSTITUTION	TREATMENT	NO. OF PATIENTS	10 YEAR CONTROL (%)	20 YEAR CONTROL (%)
Royal Marsden Hospital[28]	S + RT	199	98	91
	RT alone	35	94	94
University of Florida[29]	S + RT	76	92	92
	RT alone	29	100	100
Princess Margaret Hospital[9]	S + RT or RT alone (n = 3)	160	87	83
University of Pittsburgh[5]	All patients	120	88	78
	S + RT	91	90	79
	RT alone	29	75	67

RT, radiotherapy; S, surgical resection.

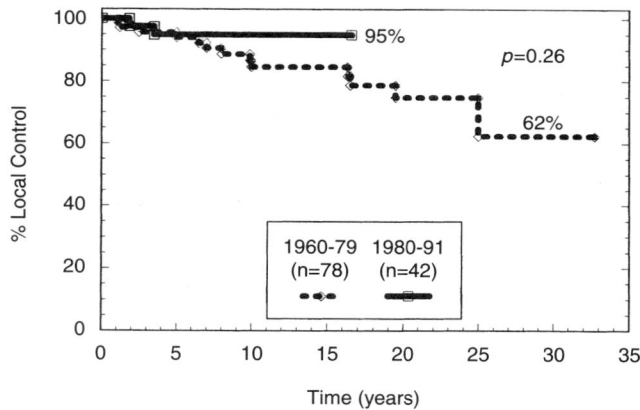

FIGURE 266–2. Comparison of actuarial tumor control curves for nonfunctional pituitary adenoma patients treated at the University of Pittsburgh before and after 1980.[5]

to drop in the University of Pittsburgh series, from 78% at 20 years to 65% at 30 years.[5] Figure 266–2 shows actuarial tumor control curves in the University of Pittsburgh series broken down by treatment date.[5] Continued late recurrences are seen in the patients treated in earlier years. It is uncertain whether further follow-up will prove that earlier detection of tumor progression and improved targeting of tumors with computed tomography and magnetic resonance imaging will lead to early flattening of the tumor control curve and a higher tumor control rate for more recently treated patients. Multivariate analysis in the University of Pittsburgh series found increased progression in patients with oncocytic tumors ($P = 0.04$) but no significant correlation with other factors such as dose. Figure 266–3 shows that higher equivalent total radiation doses did not lead to improved tumor control (tumor control was actually slightly poorer in the higher-dose group).[8] Multivariate analysis of tumor control in the series by Tsang and coworkers found correlations only with age and field size.[9] Multivariate analysis of 141 patients irradiated at the University of Florida with

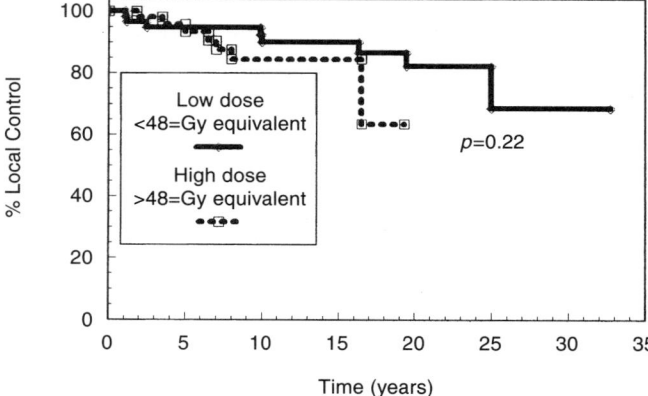

FIGURE 266–3. Comparison of actuarial tumor control curves in patients irradiated at the University of Pittsburgh with total doses above ($n = 57$) and below ($n = 63$) an equivalent total dose of 48 Gy at 1.8 Gy per fraction.[5, 8]

functional and nonfunctional pituitary adenomas found that significantly decreased tumor control was correlated only with young age.[10]

Some series make a reasonably strong case for routine postoperative radiotherapy in all patients with nonfunctional pituitary adenomas, because it appears to dramatically decrease tumor recurrence.[11] Lillehei and Kirschman reported achieving gross total resection in 38 of 45 patients with nonfunctional pituitary adenomas undergoing transsphenoidal surgery.[12] Tumor recurrence developed in 2 of 32 patients (6%) who did not undergo postoperative radiotherapy after a median follow-up of 5.5 years. They therefore advised against routine postoperative radiotherapy after gross total resection.

FUNCTIONAL ADENOMAS

In general, surgery has an advantage over conventional radiotherapy in the management of functional pituitary adenomas because successful tumor resection can reduce elevated hormone levels more quickly. With functional adenomas, radiotherapy must not only kill or inactivate the clonogenic cells responsible for tumor control but also decrease hormone oversecretion by either killing enough tumor cells or causing metabolic changes that decrease hormone oversecretion. It often takes 8 years for hormone levels to drop fully and level off after radiotherapy, with occasional cases showing continued hormone decline between 10 and 15 years after radiotherapy.

Tsang and colleagues analyzed the Princess Margaret Hospital experience.[6] From 1972 to 1986, 145 patients received radiotherapy for hormonally active pituitary adenomas: 52 with acromegaly, 64 with prolactinoma, and 29 with Cushing's disease. The median follow-up was 7.3 years. Radiotherapy (50-Gy median total dose at 2 Gy per fraction) was given as primary treatment in 17 patients, postoperatively in 65 patients, and for salvage therapy in 63 patients. The 10-year actuarial proportions of patients with persistent elevated hormone levels were 61% following radiotherapy alone and 44% with the addition of medical management. The progression-free rate was 96% at 10 years. Of 20 deaths, 3 were caused by uncontrolled pituitary adenoma, and 3 were the result of treatment complications. The actuarial 10-year overall and cause-specific survival rates were 86% and 97%, respectively. None of the factors examined predicted tumor control.

Cushing's Disease

Most centers that have evaluated the long-term results of radiotherapy for the management of Cushing's disease treated these patients before the refinement and popularization of microsurgical techniques for transsphenoidal resection. Remission rates in most series vary from 50% to 90%.[13–15]

Acromegaly

Rates of control and cure of acromegaly with radiotherapy differ in various reports, depending on the length of follow-up and the criteria used to define cure. Eastman and coworkers reported a 77% reduction in growth hormone levels among patients irradiated 5 to 10 years previously.[16] The percentage of patients with growth hormone levels less than 10 μg/L and less than 5 μg/L increased from 38% and 17%, respectively, at 2 years to 81% and 60%, respectively, at 10 years after radiotherapy. Caruso and colleagues' stricter criterion for cure was a fasting or suppressed growth hormone level less than 2 μg/L, with control defined as less than 5 μg/L.[17] They reported 6-year cure and control rates of 62% and 84%, respectively, in 53 patients undergoing transsphenoidal surgery and radiotherapy.

Improved hormone normalization (tumor control) has been correlated with lower pretreatment growth hormone levels. Reduction of growth hormone levels to less than 10 μg/L within 2 years was achieved in 100% versus 70% of patients with pretreatment growth hormone levels of less than 50 versus greater than 50 μg/L.[18] Werner and coworkers studied the effects of radiotherapy in 25 acromegalic patients who failed prior surgical resection and identified better results in patients with concomitant prolactin hypersecretion.[19]

Prolactinoma

The primary management of prolactinomas is medical, with radiotherapy reserved for patients who fail or are unable to tolerate medical therapy and surgical resection. Radiotherapy to the hypothalamus may lead to hypersecretion of prolactin in patients without prolactinoma through a reduction in the hypothalamic secretion of dopamine (which inhibits prolactin secretion). For this reason, radiosurgery or stereotactic radiotherapy may eventually lead to better results in treating prolactinomas.

Interpretation of the results of prolactinoma radiotherapy is difficult because of the success of dopamine agonist therapy. Series by Rush and Newell and Mehta and colleagues reported hormone normalization in 7 of 10 and 5 of 8 patients, respectively, 2 to 13 years after radiotherapy, before the availability of dopamine agonists.[20, 21]

Tsagarakis and associates updated the experience from St. Bartholomew's Hospital in irradiating 36 prolactinomas and using intermittent dopamine agonist therapy without surgery. Growth hormone levels normalized in 50% and fell to just above normal in another 28%.[22] Rush compared surgery and radiotherapy with surgery, radiotherapy, and dopamine agonist therapy in 19 patients with prolactin levels greater than 200 μg/L.[23] Although the 7 patients without dopamine agonist therapy had a 90% reduction in prolactin levels, none reached normal levels; in contrast, 12 of 12 patients undergoing surgery, radiotherapy, and dopamine agonist therapy reached normal levels (with a 99.5% reduction in prolactin levels).

SIDE EFFECTS OF RADIOTHERAPY

Potential late complications of radiotherapy include optic neuropathy, brain necrosis, hypopituitarism, stroke, and the development of secondary neoplasms. The risks of optic neuropathy and brain necrosis can be kept to less than 0.1% by limiting the total dose to no more than 45 Gy in 25 fractions, or its equivalent, and using a multiple-field treatment plan with a homogeneous radiation dose distribution.

In Tsang and coworkers' series of 128 functional tumors, the actuarial rates of radiation-induced hypopituitarism were 35%, 22%, and 22% at 10 years for thyroid, glucocorticoid, and gonadal functions, respectively.[6] Littley and associates studied radiotherapy effects in 165 patients with pituitary adenomas.[24] Preradiation growth hormone, gonadotropin, corticotropin reserve, and thyrotropin levels were normal in 18%, 21%, 57%, and 80% of patients, respectively, but these percentages dropped to 0%, 9%, 23%, and 58% 5 years after radiotherapy. Hyperprolactinemia (a mean of 63% over baseline) developed in 44% of patients 2 years after radiotherapy but then declined to baseline.

Page and colleagues compared 48 pituitary adenoma patients (18 who had radiotherapy) with 42 control patients who had mastoid surgery.[25] They found lower growth hormone levels in the pituitary adenoma patients but no significant difference in quality of life. The subset of 18 patients who received radiotherapy for pituitary adenoma had lower mental health scores and seemed more depressed and anxious than the other patients. McCord and associates reported that neurocognitive testing of their pituitary adenoma patients showed decreased memory in those undergoing both surgery and radiotherapy compared with patients undergoing either modality alone ($P = .005$).[10]

A trend toward an increased incidence of stroke (by a factor of 2.0) in 156 pituitary adenoma patients irradiated at the University of Pittsburgh was reported in 1989.[26] This observation was confirmed in a more convincing study of 331 irradiated pituitary adenoma patients by Brada and coworkers, who found that the relative risk of stroke was significantly elevated by a factor of 4.1 (21% risk at 20 years).[27] They found a significantly increased risk of stroke with greater radiation dose.

Second tumors may develop 10 to 30 years after fractionated radiotherapy in approximately 2% of patients.[4] The most common are meningiomas and gliomas.[4] The risks of developing stroke or second tumors should be reduced with the use of radiosurgery or, to a lesser degree, stereotactic fractionated radiotherapy.

SUMMARY

Fractionated conventional radiotherapy is an effective treatment modality that plays an important role in the multidisciplinary management of pituitary adenomas. Careful attention to treatment technique (proper dose selection and conformal treatment planning) is needed to optimize outcome, chiefly by minimizing late complications.

REFERENCES

1. Comtois R, Beauregard H, Somma M, et al: The clinical and endocrine outcome to transsphenoidal microsurgery of nonsecreting pituitary adenomas. Cancer 68:860–866, 1991.

2. Ebersold MJ, Quast LM, Laws ER, et al: Long-term results in transsphenoidal removal of nonfunctioning pituitary adenomas. J Neurosurg 64:713–719, 1986.
3. Flickinger JC, Nelson PB, Martinez AJ, et al: Radiotherapy of nonfunctional adenomas of the pituitary gland. Cancer 63:2409–2413, 1989.
4. Flickinger JC, Rush SC: Linear accelerator therapy of pituitary adenomas. In Landolt AM, Vance ML, Reilly PL (eds): Pituitary Adenomas. New York, Churchill Livingstone, 1996, pp 475–483.
5. Breen P, Flickinger JC, Kondziolka D, Martinez AJ: Radiotherapy for nonfunctional pituitary adenoma: Analysis of long-term tumor control. J Neurosurg 89:933–938, 1998.
6. Tsang RW, Brierley JD, Panzarella T, et al: Role of radiation therapy in clinical hormonally-active pituitary adenomas. Radiother Oncol 41:45–53, 1996.
7. Harris J, Levene MB: Visual complications following irradiation for pituitary adenomas and craniopharyngiomas. Radiology 120:167–171, 1976.
8. Flickinger JC, Kalend A: Use of normalized total dose to represent the biological effect of fractionated radiotherapy. Radiother Oncol 17:339–347, 1990.
9. Tsang RW, Brierly JD, Panzarella T, et al: Radiation therapy for pituitary adenoma: Treatment outcome and prognostic factors. Int J Radiat Oncol Biol Phys 30:557–565, 1994.
10. McCord MW, Buatti JM, Fennell EM, et al: Radiotherapy for pituitary adenoma: Long-term outcome and sequelae. Int J Radiat Oncol Biol Phys 39:437–444, 1997.
11. Gittoes NJ, Bates AS, Tse W, et al: Radiotherapy for non-function pituitary tumours. Clin Endocrinol 48:331–337, 1998.
12. Lillehei KO, Kirschman DL, Kleinschmidt-DeMasters BK, et al: Reassessment of the role of radiation therapy in the treatment of endocrine-inactive pituitary macroadenomas. Neurosurgery 43:432–438, 1998.
13. Grigsby PW, Sheline GE: Pituitary. In Perez CA, Brady LW (eds): Principles and Practice of Radiation Oncology. Philadelphia, JB Lippincott, 1992, pp 1108–1125.
14. Schteingart DE, Tsao HS, Taylor CL, et al: Sustained remission of Cushing's disease with mitotane and pituitary irradiation. Ann Intern Med 92:613–618, 1980.
15. Clarke SD, Woo SY, Buther EB, et al: Treatment of secretory pituitary adenoma with radiation therapy. Radiology 188:759–763, 1993.
16. Eastman RC, Gorden P, Roth J: Conventional supervoltage irradiation is effective treatment for acromegaly. J Clin Endocrinol Metab 48:931–940, 1979.
17. Caruso M, Shaw E, Davis D: Radiation treatment of growth hormone secreting pituitary adenomas. Int J Radiat Oncol Biol Phys 21:121–122, 1993.
18. Sheline GE, Wara WM: Radiation therapy of acromegaly and nonsecretory chromophobe adenomas of the pituitary. In Seydel HG (ed): Tumors of the Central Nervous System. New York, John Wiley, 1975, pp 119–131.
19. Werner S, af Trampe E, Palacios P, et al: Growth hormone secreting pituitary adenomas with concomitant hypersecretion of prolactin are particularly sensitive to photon irradiation. Int J Radiat Oncol Biol Phys 11:1713–1720, 1985.
20. Rush SC, Newell J: Pituitary adenoma: The efficacy of radiotherapy as the sole treatment. Int J Radiat Oncol Biol Phys 17:165–169, 1989.
21. Mehta AE, Reyes FL, Faihnern C: Primary radiotherapy of prolactinomas. Am J Med 83:59–68, 1989.
22. Tsagarakis S, Grossman A, Plowman PN, et al: Megavoltage radiotherapy in the management of prolactinomas: Long-term follow-up. Clin Endocrinol 34:399–406, 1991.
23. Rush S, Donahue B, Cooper P, et al: Prolactin reduction after combined modality therapy for prolactin macroadenomas. Neurosurgery 28:502–505, 1991.
24. Littley MD, Shalet SM, Beardwell CG, et al: Hypopituitarism following external radiotherapy for pituitary tumors in adults. Q J Med 70:145–160, 1989.
25. Page RC, Hammersley MS, Burke CW, et al: An account of the quality of life of patients after treatment for non-functioning pituitary tumours. Clin Endocrinol 46:401–406, 1997.
26. Flickinger JC, Nelson PB, Taylor FH, et al: Incidence of cerebral infarction after radiotherapy for pituitary adenoma. Cancer 63:2404–2408, 1989.
27. Brada M, Burchell L, Ashley S, et al: The incidence of cerebrovascular accidents in patients with pituitary adenoma. Int J Radiat Oncol 45:693–698, 1999.
28. Brada M, Rajan B, Traish D, et al: The long-term efficacy of conservative surgery and radiotherapy in the control of pituitary adenomas. Clin Endocrinol 38:571–578, 1993.
29. McCollough WM, Marcus RB, Rhoton A, et al: Long-term follow-up of radiotherapy for pituitary adenoma: The absence of late recurrence after greater than or equal to 4500 cGy. Int J Radiat Oncol Biol Phys 21:607–614, 1991.

CHAPTER 267

Radiotherapy of Tumors of the Spine

JEFF MICHALSKI

Spinal cord tumors are relatively rare, and few clinicians have an opportunity to treat a large number of patients with these lesions. Radiotherapy is an important modality in the management of both primary and metastatic tumors involving the spinal canal. Extradural and primary bone tumors are generally managed in a manner similar to tumors arising outside the vertebral column. For example, Ewing's sarcoma is often treated with a combination of systemic chemotherapy and radiotherapy; surgery is commonly avoided, because the tumors at this site are not amenable to an operation with wide negative margins. Osteosarcoma, in contrast, is considered a radioresistant neoplasm, and the risks of surgery are acceptable in this group of patients for whom there are no curative alternatives. Chondrosarcoma and chordoma are increasingly being treated with high-dose conformal radiotherapy or proton beam irradiation.[1]

EPIDEMIOLOGY

Primary tumors of the spinal canal are rare, occurring far less often than primary tumors of the brain. Primary spinal canal tumors constitute 15% of all primary central nervous system tumors.[2] Of the estimated 17,900 primary central nervous system tumors diagnosed in 1996, approximately 2700 arose from the spinal cord or its coverings.[3] The spine is frequently involved by metastatic cancer. Metastatic tumors can invade the vertebral bones, the epidural soft tissues, or even the spinal cord itself. Most extradural tumors are metastatic. True primary spinal cord neoplasms are typically intradural in location.

Primary tumors of the spinal canal affect a young population.[4, 5] More than half of pediatric patients are younger than 10 years.[6, 7] In a review of 872 children with intraspinal tumors, 36% had intramedullary tumors, 27% had intradural extramedullary tumors, and 24% had extradural tumors (13% were unclassified).[6] Nearly 75% of pediatric intramedullary tumors are astrocytomas, gangliogliomas, or ependymomas. The discovery of such tumors in this young population often limits the treatment options offered. Because young children are more sensitive to the harmful effects of radiotherapy, there is a strong desire to avoid

this potentially effective treatment. Skeletal growth in children can be arrested with radiation doses of 25 to 35 Gy. The morbidity of radiotherapy is most severe in small, young children in whom large lengths of the spinal column are treated.

NATURAL HISTORY AND PATHOLOGY

Radiotherapy treatment planning requires an understanding of the tumor's invasiveness and propensity to disseminate. Most primary tumors of the spinal canal are histologically low grade or benign. Despite their histologic character, they are often the cause of significant disability because they compress or invade the spinal cord and interfere with neurological function. Intramedullary tumors produce neurological damage by local invasion or cystic compression of the cord, whereas extramedullary lesions compress, stretch, or distort the cord or the spinal nerves. Local tumor progression is the dominant form of treatment failure in spinal cord tumors. Cerebrospinal fluid seeding has been reported in high-grade tumors and occasionally in pilocytic tumors; however, it is uncommon.[4, 8–10] The major causes of death in patients with spinal canal tumors are complications of paraplegia or quadriplegia, such as infection or respiratory compromise.

Primary spinal cord tumors may be focal or relatively localized, or they may involve nearly the entire length of the cord. In one report, 73% of affected children presented with widening of the entire spinal cord from the medulla or cervical medullary junction to the conus medullaris.[11] These "holocord" tumors are characterized by a discrete solid mass with an associated cystic component or syrinx that extends over a significant length of the spinal cord.

Primary tumors of the spinal cord are histopathologically similar to those found intracranially, but the distribution of the various tumor types depends on the relationship of the neoplasm to the spinal cord and dura.

INTRAMEDULLARY TUMORS

Most intramedullary tumors of the spinal cord are glial in origin, with astrocytomas and ependymomas accounting for the majority.

Astrocytoma

Astrocytoma is the most common intramedullary spinal cord tumor, accounting for 40% to 45% of all reported cases. In children, 75% to 90% of intramedullary spinal cord tumors are astrocytomas, and about 85% of these are low-grade fibrillary or juvenile pilocytic astrocytomas.[12–14] These low-grade tumors often have a low infiltrative nature. The recognition of this feature, along with advances in surgical techniques and intraoperative monitoring, has led to more radical resections.[13–15] In patients with good preoperative neurological function, stabilization or improvement in function often occurs. Even so, many astrocytomas are infiltrative, especially anaplastic astrocytomas and glioblastoma multiforme, and complete resection carries a significant risk of increased neurological disability. In these cases, a subtotal resection or biopsy may be the only safe surgical option. In patients with malignant astrocytomas or those with very poor preoperative function, aggressive resection generally does not improve the neurological function, and there is a risk of worsening the patient's status. Less than 10% of pediatric and 25% of adult spinal cord astrocytomas are malignant.[12, 16]

Astrocytomas are more likely to occur in the cervical and thoracic regions than are ependymomas. Ependymomas more often affect the lumbar spinal cord and cauda equina. Astrocytomas are frequently associated with cysts that can extend rostrally or caudally for a significant distance. The cystic component of a holocord astrocytoma can contribute to a neurological deficit.

Ependymoma

Ependymomas are usually histologically benign, and they may have a long and often indolent course. Poorly differentiated ependymomas are rare. Rostral tumors are more frequently cellular variants, whereas distal tumors (including those of the cauda equina) are more commonly a myxopapillary variant.[17–20] Approximately two thirds of ependymomas occur in the region of the cauda equina; these are discussed later. Ependymomas are more common in adults than in children.

INTRADURAL EXTRAMEDULLARY TUMORS

Most intradural extramedullary neoplasms are meningiomas, nerve sheath tumors, or myxopapillary ependymomas. They are usually amenable to complete surgical excision. Ependymomas arising in the region of the conus medullaris and filum terminale are not truly intramedullary and are therefore described in this section.

Nerve Sheath Tumor

Nerve sheath tumors arise from the Schwann cell, the specialized cell responsible for insulating peripheral nerves and contributing to their conduction function. Nerve sheath tumors have been called neurolemmomas, neurofibromas, schwannomas, neuromas, and neurilemomas in the past. Recently, a distinction between neurofibroma and schwannoma has been made. Although both tumors arise from Schwann cells, certain gross, microscopic, and clinical features help distinguish the two.[2] Neurofibromas produce plexiform enlargements of the involved spinal nerve that make it impossible to distinguish the nerve from the tumor tissue. Schwannomas, in contrast, are globoid and eccentrically attached to a nerve. The plexiform neurofibroma is associated with type 1 neurofibromatosis, and the presence of multiple tumors helps establish the diagnosis of this genetic condition.

Generally, nerve sheath tumors are solitary and may occur in any section of the spinal canal. They are evenly distributed in the cervical, thoracic, and lumbar regions; they are least common in the sacrum. They occur in males and females with equal frequency and are most commonly diagnosed in the fourth through sixth decades of life. Most of these tumors are completely intradural, although 10% to 15% may have an extradural component as well (so-called dumbbell tumors). Most nerve sheath tumors are benign, well-encapsulated lesions that are amenable to total surgical excision. The rare malignant nerve sheath tumors have a natural history similar to that of soft tissue sarcomas, and they should be treated as such.[21] This commonly includes wide excision followed by radiotherapy.

Ependymoma

About two thirds of all spinal canal ependymomas occur in the lumbosacral region, and 40% arise from within the filum terminale. Most intradural extramedullary ependymomas in the lumbosacral spine are of the myxopapillary type.[17–20, 22] They frequently can be completely excised. In many circumstances, these tumors tightly envelop the nerve roots of the cauda equina, making en bloc excision difficult. Gross total resection of these tumors often requires piecemeal removal. The myxopapillary variant may be biologically less aggressive than the cellular variant, but such tumors can recur even after complete gross excision; therefore, long-term follow-up of these patients is required.[20, 23–26]

EXTRADURAL TUMORS

Most extradural tumors are metastatic. The management of metastatic tumors is generally palliative, although some patients with chemotherapy-sensitive tumors can be controlled for long periods. Generally, radiotherapy is used in a palliative fashion to relieve painful or neurological symptoms caused by the metastasis. A variety of primary bone and soft tissue tumors may arise from an extradural location and involve the spinal canal. Bone tumors include osteosarcoma, chondrosarcoma, Ewing's sarcoma, and chordoma. Soft tissue tumors include soft tissue sarcoma, including malignant nerve sheath tumors; lymphoma; and neuroblastoma.

CLINICAL PRESENTATION

Pain is the presenting symptom in nearly 75% of patients with primary neoplasms of the spinal canal. Often the pain is confined to the region of involvement and may be present for a long time before the patient manifests localizing neurological signs. Radicular pain, a result of pressure on nerve roots, reflects the distribution of the involved root and indicates that conduction is intact. Extramedullary tumors can cause distention of the dura, with pain that is characteristically aggravated by recumbency because of venous congestion. Thus, pain is often worse at night.[11] Movement and Valsalva's maneuver may also worsen pain, which is most severe in the region of the tumor. Less commonly, pain is characterized as a burning sensation in one or more extremities. Numbness replacing pain is an advanced sign that indicates compromise of spinal nerves or nerve tract conduction.

Other symptoms of central nervous system involvement include weakness (75% of patients), sensory changes (65%), and sphincter dysfunction (15%).[4] Low-grade tumors generally have a more prolonged duration of symptoms than do high-grade tumors. Bladder and bowel dysfunction as a presenting symptom is relatively uncommon, except for tumors that involve the conus medullaris and filum terminale.

Lower extremity weakness often manifests as a disturbance in gait. In young children, there may be a history of failure to achieve milestones, such as ambulation and voluntary control of bladder and bowel, or of regression of acquired skills. With tumors of the cervical region, torticollis may occur in children, but adult patients may complain of nuchal pain and stiffness.

Tumors involving the lumbosacral spine can present with a cauda equina nerve root compression syndrome. These patients may have radicular pain in the anterior (L4), lateral (L5), or posterior (S1) thigh with corresponding paresthesias, followed by muscle wasting of the gluteus, hamstring, or tibialis anterior muscles. Saddle anesthesia, absent ankle reflexes (S1), or plantar responses (S2) may be present. Impotence and loss of anal or bulbar cavernous reflexes may also occur.

DIAGNOSTIC MAGNETIC RESONANCE IMAGING

Magnetic resonance imaging (MRI) has replaced myelography and computed tomography (CT) as the imaging study of choice in the evaluation of tumors of the spinal canal. It allows multiplanar evaluation of the spinal cord. Sagittal and axial images give the clinician a three-dimensional appreciation of the patient's anatomy and help in planning a therapeutic strategy. The various signal characteristics of the cerebrospinal fluid, white and gray matter, bone and bone marrow, fat, and flowing blood all facilitate the interpretation of the study. Some cystic tumors, vascular lesions, or lipomas can be diagnosed based on their characteristic signals on T1- and T2-weighted images without contrast injection. Intravenous administration of gadolinium-diethylenetriamine pentaacetic acid (Gd-DTPA) improves the sensitivity of MRI by enhancing the solid component of intramedullary tumors, differentiating them from surrounding edema or syrinx cavities. Unlike low-grade gliomas in the brain, nearly all spinal cord gliomas, regardless of grade, enhance with Gd-DTPA.[27] Sagittal T1-weighted images usually localize intramedullary mass neoplasms along with adjacent cysts. Intradural extramedullary lesions show considerable enhancement on T1-weighted images after the administration of Gd-DTPA. Gd-DTPA also increases the sensitivity of detecting leptomeningeal metastases.[27]

PROGNOSTIC FACTORS

The major prognostic factors in patients with primary spinal canal tumors are tumor type and grade, tumor extent and location, patient age, and presenting neurological function. Treatment-related factors that influence the outcome include tumor resectability and the use of radiotherapy in selected patients. Many of these factors are interdependent. For example, ependymomas occur most frequently in the distal spinal canal and are more likely to be resectable than are astrocytic tumors. Generally, patients with ependymomas survive longer without recurrence than do patients with astrocytomas.[9, 28–34]

Several authors have reported that patients with rostral tumors have a worse survival and neurological outcome than patients with more caudal tumors.[4, 28, 30, 35] Guidetti and associates[30] stated that patients with cervical lesions have a higher surgical risk and complication rate, which makes thorough resection of tumors in this location difficult and sometimes inadvisable. In a series of 62 patients with exclusively intramedullary ependymomas, patients with high cervical presentations (above C5) accounted for four of six postoperative deaths because of apneic respiratory complications.[35] In the Mallinckrodt Institute of Radiology experience, Garcia[4] reported that the primary tumor location is the most important prognostic feature. It was suggested that a greater concentration of function per unit volume of the upper spinal cord compared with that of the cauda equina accounts for the worse neurological outcome and survival in patients with rostral tumors. Chun and coworkers,[28] from the Medical College of Virginia, also reported that patients with cervical lesions have significantly worse outcomes than do patients with tumors in other sites. In both the Mallinckrodt Institute of Radiology and the Medical College of Virginia experience, tumors affecting the rostral or cervical spinal cord were more likely to be astrocytomas, and tumors in the caudal spinal cord, filum terminale, or cauda equina were more likely to be ependymomas. The anatomic dependence of various tumor types may contribute to the better prognosis seen in patients with tumors of the lower spinal canal.

High histopathologic tumor grade is associated with a high rate of disability and death. The median survival of patients with malignant astrocytomas is less than 6 months, with few patients living beyond 1 year.[36] Most series report no survivors among patients with malignant spinal cord astrocytomas.[9, 13, 37] As many as 58% of patients with malignant astrocytomas develop radiographic or autopsy evidence of tumor dissemination.[36] Merchant and colleagues[38] reported that patients with high-grade astrocytomas often have diffuse recurrence, extending outside the original tumor bed and even the radiation field. Most spinal cord ependymomas are low-grade tumors. High-grade ependymomas are associated with an increased recurrence rate and risk of death.[38–40] Myxopapillary ependymomas most commonly involve the cauda equina and are biologically less aggressive than cellular ependymomas.[20, 23, 24]

Extensive involvement of the spinal cord with ependymoma has been associated with a worse outcome. Linstadt and associates[9] reported a 93% 10-year disease-specific survival with localized ependymoma, compared with 50% survival for patients with diffuse tumors. Extensive tumors have a 50% local failure rate after surgery and radiotherapy, compared with only 20% for limited disease (one to three vertebral body segments).[19] Extent of disease has not been a prognostic factor in other series.[41] Encapsulated myxopapillary tumors of the cauda equina are frequently amenable to complete en bloc excision, and the recurrence rate is very low. Unencapsulated or adherent tumors are often removed piecemeal and are associated with a high local recurrence rate after surgery alone.[19, 20, 25, 42] Piecemeal excision of a cauda equina ependymoma may require adjuvant radiotherapy.

Neurological function at diagnosis is an important clinical prognostic factor. Generally, the fewer symptoms and the better the neurological function at presentation, the better the likelihood that the tumor will be controlled with few long-term adverse neurological sequelae.[4, 13, 30, 35, 43] Poor neurological function in patients with spinal cord tumors is often attributable to the disease process and a prolonged delay in diagnosis rather than the effect of surgery or radiotherapy.[7, 12, 16, 44–46]

Young age is associated with a good 5-year recurrence-free survival in patients with astrocytoma.[12, 47] It is unclear whether young age is an important factor in patients with ependymoma.[19, 35, 40, 43]

RADIOTHERAPY

Radiotherapy has been used postoperatively in the treatment of intramedullary astrocytomas and ependymomas. For tumors that are completely excised, the prognosis is excellent, and the patient should receive no adjuvant therapy. The frequency of complete excision varies from 33% to 94%.[48] For tumors that are incompletely excised, strong consideration should be given to the administration of adjuvant radiotherapy in an effort to provide durable local control and improve survival in these young adults and children.

It is important to note that uncontrolled local tumor is the major cause of death in patients with spinal cord gliomas. Although we advocate radiotherapy in the setting of subtotal resection, in some clinical circumstances, careful follow-up after surgery, with radiotherapy reserved until after a second operation for clinical recurrence, should be considered. Young children who are diagnosed before their pubertal growth spurt are at significant risk of developing radiation-induced bone growth delay with kyphoscoliosis or short stature, especially affecting their sitting height. This radiation-induced deformity is most severe in patients who have extensive tumors or holocord involvement of the spine. In these young children, if their neurological function is good or improved after subtotal resection, close follow-up without adjuvant therapy is a reasonable course of action. Most spinal cord tumors in young children are either low-grade astrocytomas or well-differentiated ependymomas that have a very slow growth rate. Delaying radiotherapy until recurrence or early tumor progression may allow the child to grow at a normal rate for several years before receiving radiotherapy. Even at the time of recurrence, the patient may be a candidate for re-resection. If this can be accomplished with minimal injury, the patient may be observed again without adjuvant therapy until progressive neurological signs or symptoms develop or radiographic evidence of inoperable tumor appears.

The data supporting the routine use of adjuvant radiotherapy in subtotally resected astrocytic tumors of the spinal cord are inconclusive. The prolonged natural history and slow growth of these neoplasms make it difficult to prove that radiotherapy is indeed beneficial. Most clinicians argue that the beneficial effects of radiotherapy in the management of subtotally resected astrocytomas of the cerebrum present reasonable evidence that these tumors are radioresponsive.[4] Despite this benefit in other sites, the spinal cord is a more radiosensitive structure, and even with treatment at radiation doses that are at or above the tolerance of the spinal cord, local recurrence remains the predominant pattern of treatment failure. Garcia[4] reported that radiation doses of greater than 40 Gy are associated with a lower rate of tumor progression, providing indirect evidence of the radioresponsiveness of these tumors in the range of spinal cord tolerance. The predominantly local pattern of treatment failure has led some investigators to treat spinal cord tumors beyond the tolerance of the spinal cord when the tumor is so advanced that no meaningful functional recovery can be expected. In these few cases of "radiocordectomy," some patients' disease has been controlled, albeit with permanent disability.[34]

Substantial evidence supports the use of postoperative radiotherapy in patients with ependymoma after incomplete or piecemeal excision. Guidetti and coworkers[30] first reported beneficial outcomes in patients receiving radiotherapy after incomplete excision of ependymomas. Some radiotherapy series have demonstrated that increasing doses of irradiation are associated with better tumor control in patients with ependymomas.[4, 19, 33] Shaw and colleagues[19] reported that the local failure rate was 35% in patients receiving 50 Gy or less, compared with only 20% in patients receiving more than 50 Gy. This dose response suggests that patients with incomplete resection or recurrent disease are appropriately managed with radiotherapy within the range of spinal cord tolerance.

Patients who have had complete excision of either astrocytoma[2, 13–15] or ependymoma[49–52] have an excellent local control rate without additional therapy. Patients who have undergone complete excision of cauda equina ependymoma by piecemeal removal have a local failure rate ranging from 20% to 43%.[19, 20, 42] The addition of radiotherapy in such patients produces a local recurrence rate equal to that of patients undergoing gross total resection.[19, 34, 42]

Nadkarni and Rekate[53] summarized the published literature on surgical and adjuvant therapy in the management of patients with intramedullary spinal cord gliomas. They pointed out that there are no class I data (randomized, controlled trials) on spinal cord tumors. The majority of existing data falls into class II (prospective reviews or retrospective data comparing two definable groups) or class III (everything else) studies.

Complete resection of ependymomas and low-grade astrocytomas is feasible and consistently achieved by several experienced neurosurgical groups, often without worsened postoperative neurological sequelae. Radical surgery in patients with high-grade astrocytomas has no impact on outcome and may contribute to poor postoperative neurological function. Despite the ability to safely remove low-grade astrocytomas, it is unclear that doing so improves survival in these patients, in contrast to the advantage demonstrated in patients with complete resection of ependymomas. Complete resection is more frequently achieved for ependymomas than for astrocytomas, and intraoperative assessment of tumor resection is more reliable in ependymomas than in astrocytomas. Ultrasonic aspirators, CO_2 surgical lasers, intraoperative ultrasonography, and evoked potential monitoring have contributed to improved postoperative outcomes for patients with intramedullary spinal cord tumors.

Nadkarni and Rekate[53] categorized treatment recommendations according to the level of available evidence supporting them. *Standards* represent principles of management that reflect a high degree of certainty and are supported by class I or strong class II data. Standards define a treatment program according to which clinicians must act. *Guidelines* represent a range of strategies that reflect moderate clinical certainty. These are based on class II or a preponderance of class III evidence. Guidelines offer a specific plan of therapy from which a clinician may deviate if there is sound clinical evidence that warrants this deviation. Treatment *options* are usually based on class III evidence. These are strategies that a physician may employ when standards or

guidelines do not exist for the particular clinical situation. Nadkarni's treatment recommendations for astrocytomas and ependymomas are summarized in Tables 267–1 and 267–2, respectively.

TABLE 267–1 ■ **Summary of Treatment Recommendations for Pediatric Spinal Cord Astrocytoma**

LEVEL OF RECOMMENDATION	TREATMENT RECOMMENDATION
Standards	No standards exist
Guidelines	Withhold radiotherapy if radical or total resection of low-grade astrocytoma is achieved
	Monitor somatosensory evoked potentials to improve safety of surgery
	Treat malignant astrocytomas with postoperative irradiation
Options	Attempt total resection if cleavage plane exists
	Reoperate for recurrences in ambulatory patients
	Use ultrasonic aspirator as surgical adjunct
	Monitor motor evoked potentials to improve safety of surgery
	Withhold radiotherapy for low-grade astrocytomas before tumor progression occurs
	Use osteoplastic laminotomy to decrease postoperative deformity

Modified from Nadkarni TD, Rekate HL: Pediatric intramedullary spinal cord tumors. Childs Nerv Syst 15:17–28, 1999.

TABLE 267–2 ■ **Summary of Treatment Recommendations for Pediatric Spinal Cord Ependymoma**

LEVEL OF RECOMMENDATION	TREATMENT RECOMMENDATION
Standards	Resect totally
	Reoperate if postoperative magnetic resonance imaging shows unexpected residual tumor
	Withhold radiotherapy if gross total resection achieved
Guidelines	Follow extent of resection with intraoperative ultrasonography
	Monitor somatosensory evoked potentials to improve safety of surgery
Options	Attempt total resection if cleavage plane exists
	Reoperate for recurrences in ambulatory patients
	Use ultrasonic aspirator as surgical adjunct
	Monitor motor evoked potentials to improve safety of surgery
	Use osteoplastic laminotomy to decrease postoperative deformity

Modified from Nadkarni TD, Rekate HL: Pediatric intramedullary spinal cord tumors. Childs Nerv Syst 15:17–28, 1999.

RADIOTHERAPY TECHNIQUES

Primary tumors of the spinal canal are easily treated with a direct posterior field. Some tumors of the lumbar region, including tumors of the cauda equina, may require opposed anteroposterior and posteroanterior portals because of the lumbar lordosis and the deep location of the vertebral bodies near the midline of the trunk. Other techniques in the treatment of spinal canal tumors have been described and should be considered when the exit dose to the anterior midline structures of the trunk would otherwise be excessive. Tumors exclusively involving the cervical spine may be treated with opposed lateral fields to avoid incidental irradiation of the hypopharynx and oral cavity. Similarly, tumors involving the thoracic and lumbar spinal canal can be treated with a paired set of oblique wedge fields to get a superior dose distribution compared with a single posterior field. The oblique paired field plan, although more complex, exposes the midline structures anterior to the spinal column to a lower cumulative irradiation dose. The high dose to the subcutaneous tissues delivered with a single posteroanterior field is also avoided. In female patients requiring treatment to the lumbosacral spine for cauda equina tumors, we have used a lateral technique to avoid exit irradiation to the pelvis and ovaries. This lateral beam technique may treat more of the pelvic bones, back musculature, and even some of the retroperitoneum, but it spares the more radiosensitive ovaries and uterus. Wedges may be required on these lateral lumbosacral fields to provide a homogeneous dose distribution. Care should be taken to avoid irradiating the kidneys at the L1 through L3 levels with this technique. Arm position should be appropriate to avoid entrance or exit irradiation from these lateral beams.

The width of posterior fields for treatment is typically 7 or 8 cm. Fields as small as 5 cm may be considered for young children. Traditionally, the superior and inferior borders encompass two vertebral bodies above and below the tumor defined by myelogram. This margin is generally adequate to avoid marginal miss. A more accurate definition of gross tumor on MRI may allow the tumor boost to encompass the lesion plus 2 cm. High-grade astrocytomas may require a more generous margin craniocaudally. Merchant and co-workers[38] described a diffuse failure pattern in children shortly after completing radiotherapy, suggesting that the tumor was not adequately covered within the irradiated volume. The field width should encompass the anterior vertebral foramina if tumor extension is suspected. In young children, the anterior vertebral bodies may be partially spared from irradiation by using posterior oblique wedge fields or opposed lateral fields. These techniques may spare the developing epiphyseal plates in growing children.

For small treated segments of spinal cord, the depth of the cord beneath the skin surface can be determined from CT or MRI, and this depth is used for dose prescription. The depth can also be determined by obtaining a lateral radiograph of the spine on the simulator, using a wire on the skin surface and calculating the spinal cord depth by employing the magnification factor used for the film.

If large segments of the spinal cord are irradiated, it is necessary to compute the spinal cord dose at multiple points because of the variation in curvature and depth of the spinal cord and the different source-to-skin distances below and above the central axis of the beam. A transverse and sagittal treatment plan using CT and MRI should be performed.

The treatment plan should reflect a homogeneous dose distribution. For small lesions of the cervical spinal cord, when lateral fields will be used, radiation beam energies of 4- to 6-MV photons achieve a homogeneous dose distribution. Lesions involving the thoracic and lumbar spine often require combinations of low-energy (4 to 6 MV) and high-energy (18 to 25 MV) x-rays to achieve a homogeneous dose distribution. Parallel opposed posterior and anterior fields or paired oblique wedge fields can give homogeneous dose distributions with x-ray energies as low as 4 or 6 MV. It has been suggested but not proved that conformal or intensity-modulated radiotherapy methods may reduce some of the risk of late radiation-induced effects in these patients.[54]

Craniospinal or spinal axis irradiation is generally not indicated in the treatment of spinal cord tumors. Local failure is a predominant cause of tumor recurrence at the original site.[4, 9, 19, 47] Patients with high-grade ependymomas[40] or malignant gliomas[36, 37] have a high rate of neuraxis dissemination. Consideration should be given to treating the spinal axis or even the entire craniospinal axis in patients with these high-grade neoplasms. Patients with neuraxis dissemination at the time of diagnosis should receive craniospinal axis irradiation.

Intramedullary ependymomas and astrocytomas should be irradiated to a total dose of 45 to 50 Gy, given in 1.5- to 2-Gy daily fractions. If more than half of the spinal cord is irradiated, the total tumor dose should probably not exceed 45 Gy, but small segments may safely tolerate 55 Gy. Ependymomas of the cauda equina should be irradiated to doses between 45 and 50 Gy in 1.8- to 2-Gy fractions. The treatment field should be extended to encompass the entire thecal sac, with the field widened inferiorly to the sacroiliac joints to ensure adequate coverage of the meningeal sleeves within the intervertebral foramina. Failure to adequately encompass the thecal sac has been associated with an increased rate of treatment failure.[42] The lateral beam technique described earlier for lumbosacral tumors adequately covers lateral cerebrospinal fluid extension of the thecal sac within the sacrum. In young children, the dose to the spinal cord should be limited to between 40 and 45 Gy in 1.5- to 1.75-Gy daily fractions, because the developing cord may have a lower tolerance for radiotherapy.

RESULTS OF TREATMENT

As described earlier, the outcome of patients treated for spinal cord tumors depends on the neurological function of the patient, the type of tumor and its differentiation, the anatomic compartment occupied by the tumor, and the extent of resection.

A summary of the results of therapy is complicated by the various natural histories and heterogeneous collection of tumor types that affect the spinal canal. Further, because of the rarity of even the more common histologic types, even the largest series consist of small numbers of patients affected by a single tumor type. Many of these series spanned several decades during which surgical and radiotherapy techniques underwent tremendous evolution. For surgery, the introduction of the operating microscope, Cavitron Ultrasound Aspirator (CUSA), intraoperative ultrasonography, laser coagulation, and evoked potential monitoring has meant that complete resection of many low-grade astrocytomas and ependymomas is now a frequent occurrence, with minimal neurological injury. In fact, most patients are stable or improved following today's aggressive surgeries for spinal cord tumors. Radiotherapy likewise has evolved. Better pretreatment imaging studies, such as MRI, have improved treatment targeting. Megavoltage linear accelerators have improved the radiation dose distribution and decreased the likelihood of severe or late sequelae. One of the most important factors contributing to improved outcomes among patients diagnosed with spinal cord tumors is our growing knowledge of the natural histories of these tumors after various surgical procedures. We can now select the group of patients most likely to benefit from radiotherapy and avoid or delay the use of this modality in many children and young adults.

Intramedullary Tumors

The 5- and 10-year overall survival rates for patients with primary ependymoma or astrocytoma of the spinal cord following surgery and radiotherapy are summarized in Table 267–3. Patients undergoing complete en bloc gross excision have an excellent prognosis after surgery alone, with cure rates sometimes exceeding 90%.[12, 13, 15, 22, 35, 50, 51] The survival of patients with ependymoma has changed little over the past 2 decades. The majority of these patients are cured with surgery or surgery and radiotherapy.

Patients with astrocytomas of the spinal cord have a worse survival and functional outcome than do patients with ependymomas.[4] Patients with spinal cord astrocytomas have had a gradual improvement in outcome over the past 2 decades, predominantly owing to better neurosurgical resection rates.[12, 45] Adults with astrocytomas may not benefit from radical excision as much as children do.[11, 29] Patients with malignant astrocytomas have an extremely poor prognosis, with few patients living longer than 1 to 2 years.[36–38]

Intradural Extramedullary Tumors

The prognosis is excellent for most patients with intradural extramedullary tumors. These tumors rarely re-

TABLE 267–3 ■ **Overall Survival after Surgery and Radiotherapy for Primary Spinal Cord Tumors**

AUTHOR	NO. OF PATIENTS	5-YEAR SURVIVAL (%)	10-YEAR SURVIVAL (%)
Ependymoma			
Kopelson et al[33]	12	100	
Garret & Simpson[43]	41	83	73
Garcia[4]	18	—	75
Shaw et al[19]	22	95	95
Linstadt et al[9]*	18	93	93
Linstadt et al[9]†	3	50	50
Chun et al[28]	16	87	67
Whitaker et al[40]	58	68	62
Wen et al[42]	20	95	86
Clover et al[17]	11	100	80
Waldron et al[39]	59	83	75
Hulschof et al[32]	34	—	91
Shirato et al[34]	22	96	—
Abdel-Whahab et al[94]‡	25	94	68
Astrocytoma			
Kopelson et al[33]	11	58	23
Garcia[4]	14	—	58
Reimer & Onofrio[95]‡	27	89	55
Linstadt et al[9]	15	91	91
Chun et al[28]	16	60	40
Sandler et al[47]	15	57	—
Hulschof et al[32]	13	—	43
Shirato et al[34]	7	50	—
Abdel-Whahab et al[94]‡	24	64	54
Jyothirmayi et al[96]‡	23	79	56

* Localized.
† Diffuse.
‡ Low grade.

cur after total excision, but subtotally resected meningiomas may recur 10 to 15 years after surgery.[55] Data supporting the use of postoperative radiotherapy in subtotally resected extramedullary spinal canal tumors are scarce. Some authors have suggested that postoperative radiotherapy is beneficial in this circumstance because of the favorable outcomes reported in patients with intracranial presentations of similar histologies.[56] Radiotherapy is beneficial to patients undergoing subtotal resection or piecemeal excision of intradural extramedullary ependymomas.[9, 19, 20, 42] Data supporting the routine use of radiotherapy in the management of patients with benign nerve sheath tumors, vascular malformations, lipomas, hemangiomas, teratomas, and dermoids are nonexistent.

SEQUELAE OF RADIOTHERAPY

Spinal Cord Myelopathy

One of the most feared complications following radiotherapy is irreversible spinal cord myelopathy. This injury is frequently disabling and generally untreatable.

A transient, reversible myelopathy can manifest itself 2 to 6 months after radiotherapy. Lhermitte's sign, characterized by shocklike sensations radiating to the hands and feet when the neck is flexed, is a classic finding in patients with transient myelopathy. It is believed that this phenomenon is related to transient demyelination of the treated length of the spinal cord.[57, 58] This syndrome generally lasts a few weeks, and no therapy is required. It is not associated with chronic progressive myelitis.

Chronic progressive or delayed myelopathy can occur months to years after radiotherapy. Permanent myelopathy is characterized by progressive neurological signs and symptoms, including paresthesias, motor weakness, and loss of pain or temperature sensation. Patients ultimately lose bowel and bladder control and develop complete sensory and motor function loss. Brown-Séquard syndrome or complete transection may occur. The latency period of chronic myelopathy is reportedly bimodal, with peaks of incidence occurring at 13 and 29 months.[59] The early peak may correspond to white matter injury with subsequent demyelination, and the latter peak may correspond to microvascular injury.[59] Diagnosis of radiation myelopathy requires that the dominant neurological abnormality be localized to a segment radiated and that all other causes be ruled out. MRI may assist in the diagnosis, with cord edema frequently being present in the early delayed phase. Within 8 months of the onset of symptoms, the T1-weighted image may show low intensity, while the T2-weighted image shows high intensity. The lesion may enhance with Gd-DTPA. Late changes in patients with permanent delayed myelopathy may include atrophy.[60]

The occurrence of chronic progressive myelopathy is dependent on total dose, fraction size, volume, and region irradiated.[56, 61, 62] Historically, radiation oncologists have limited the spinal cord dose to 45 to 50 Gy, with conventional fractionation schedules of 1.8 to 2.0 Gy/day. These estimates came from an era of inexact dose estimation, with a bias toward reporting injury in highly selected populations. More recently, data have been published from institutions treating large groups of patients in a systematic and reliable fashion. Marcus and Million[63] analyzed the outcomes of 1112 patients treated with radiation to the head and neck at doses greater than 30 Gy. They saw only two cases of myelopathy in patients receiving less than 50 Gy. They argued that the onset of permanent myelopathy in patients receiving less than 50 Gy was idiosyncratic. The actual incidence of myelopathy with these conventionally fractionated doses is less than 0.2% to 0.5% after 50 Gy and 1% to 5% after 60 Gy.[63, 64] The dose required to cause a 50% rate of myelopathy is 68 to 73 Gy.[59] The linear quadratic model of radiation effects has been applied to radiation myelopathy, with an α/β estimate of 2 providing a good fit with clinical observation. The linear quadratic model is as follows:

$$LQED = Nd \frac{(\alpha/\beta + d)}{(\alpha/\beta + 2)}$$

where N is the number of fractions, α/β is the ratio of the early and late biologic effect parameters, and d is the dose per fraction.[65, 66] As the dose per daily fraction increases, the maximal tolerated dose decreases.

When treating a patient with a spinal cord tumor, the radiation oncologist must weigh the risk of causing myelopathy against the risk of tumor progression resulting in severe neurological dysfunction. Indeed, after radiotherapy for spinal cord tumors, it is often difficult to determine whether progressive neurological symptoms are related to tumor progression or radiation-induced myelopathy. Irradiation doses of 45 to 50.4 Gy in 1.8-Gy fractions are generally used to treat spinal cord tumors. The cervical spinal cord may tolerate slightly higher doses of irradiation than the thoracic or lumbar spinal cord.

Late Effects in Children

Children diagnosed and treated for primary tumors of the spinal canal present special prognostic concerns and apprehensions because of the increased potential for treatment-induced morbidity. The spinal cord in children and adolescents may have a lower tolerance to irradiation; the recommended total tumor doses range from 40 to 45 Gy administered in fractions of 1.5 to 1.75 Gy/day.

Radiotherapy of the spine in a child may produce a spinal deformity (scoliosis or kyphosis) because of the retardation of bone growth from damage to epiphyseal plates of the vertebral bodies, as well as soft tissue fibrosis and contracture.[67] Other organs that may receive a significant irradiation dose in a preadolescent child include the thyroid, heart, bowel, and ovaries. Modifying the treatment technique, as described in previous sections, may minimize the radiation dose to these organs. Children should be followed long term for the development of any late radiation-induced sequelae.

Children are at greater risk than adults of developing complications after surgery. Prveious radiotherapy can increase the risk of wound complications.[6] Extensive laminectomy can produce severe kyphosis and scoliosis, which are typically accentuated during the adolescent growth spurt. The spinal deformity is more severe when higher vertebral levels are involved, many levels are involved, or radiotherapy has been administered. An osteoplastic laminotomy may be associated with a lower risk of spinal deformity.[68] Reconstructive procedures, such as Harrington rod or Cotrel-Dubousset system placement, may be necessary to prevent significant damage, and children must be followed closely by the neurosurgeon and a pediatric orthopedist to ensure early treatment of skeletal abnormalities.[6] In some cases, kyphosis can be so severe that it causes spinal cord compression and myelopathy.[6]

METASTATIC CANCER INVOLVING THE SPINAL COLUMN

Metastatic cancer may involve either the epidural space or the bones of the vertebral column itself. The most common primary cancers that involve the spinal column are those arising from the breast, lung, and prostate. Spinal cord compression can occur by direct extension from a metastatic lesion in the vertebral body, extension from a paraspinal metastasis through a neural foramen, or enlargement of an epidural mass. Rarely, intramedullary metastases can occur. At the time of diagnosis of spinal cord compression, the majority of patients have already been diagnosed with a malignancy. It is strongly encouraged that patients without a prior diagnosis of cancer undergo biopsy to establish the presence of malignancy before palliative radiotherapy is implemented. This recommendation is made because benign processes such as infection may mimic a malignant process. The administration of radiotherapy for nonmalignant disease is ineffective and causes an unnecessary delay in establishing the correct diagnosis and prescribing appropriate therapy. In addition, if the spinal cord lesion is the sole site of malignant disease, radiotherapy may prevent the accurate interpretation of subsequent pathology from this site. Appropriate systemic therapy may therefore be avoided or delayed without an accurate diagnosis.

The most common initial presenting symptom of spinal cord compression is pain; it often precedes other symptoms such as weakness, sensory loss, or autonomic dysfunction. Back pain can be localized to the metastatic lesion, or radicular pain may radiate along a dermatome caused by spinal nerve compression or invasion. It is important to recognize that once neurological deficits begin, rapid progression is common. Prompt therapy is important to minimize long-term neurological dysfunction.

When spinal cord compression is suspected, MRI with gadolinium contrast should be performed. Because metastatic cancer can involve multiple levels of the spinal column, it is our practice to obtain imaging of the entire spine. In patients who cannot tolerate MRI scanning, myelography with CT should be done.

Medical Management

Corticosteroids should be started as soon as the diagnosis of spinal cord compression is established. It is reasonable to begin this therapy even if cord compression is only suspected, while the diagnostic workup is being conducted. The exact starting dose of dexamethasone is controversial. In a randomized trial of high-dose dexamethasone (96 mg) compared with no steroids, Sorensen and colleagues[69] reported that 6 months after treatment, 59% of the patients in the dexamethasone group were still ambulatory, compared with 33% in the no-dexamethasone group. With this high dose of dexamethasone, clinical improvement of neurological function is no better than that achieved with more conventional doses (16 to 40 mg daily), and more side effects are seen.[70] It is our preference to administer 16 to 32 mg initially and then taper the dose near the end of radiotherapy.

Surgery

The traditional approach of decompressive laminectomy has recently been re-examined. Because many instances of spinal cord compression occur from anterior vertebral body metastases, posterior decompression may not always relieve the pressure exerted on the spinal cord. In some circumstances, laminectomy destabilizes the spine and worsens the neurological outcome. A randomized study of immediate radiotherapy versus decompressive laminectomy was conducted at the University of California–Los Angeles. In this small trial (29 patients), there was no difference in outcome between the two groups.[71] Increasingly, anterior vertebral body resection with stabilization or reconstruction has been used in patients with spinal cord compression. This is major surgery, and it carries significant operative and medical risks. A patient's overall performance status and prognosis should be taken into consideration when offering aggressive surgery.

Surgical decompression should be considered for the treatment of spinal cord compression when (1) the diagnosis of cancer has not been clearly established, (2) the patient has a relatively radioresistant neoplasm (e.g., melanoma), (3) the patient has been previously irradiated to tolerance doses at the site of the spinal cord compression, (4) the vertebral column is mechanically unstable, or (5) the patient progresses during radiotherapy.

Radiotherapy

Emergency initiation of radiotherapy is critical to relieve symptomatic spinal cord compression in patients who are not candidates for surgery. One of the most important prognostic factors affecting the recovery of neurological function is the extent of neurological impairment at the time therapy is begun.[72, 73] In a retrospective series from Memorial Sloan Kettering, patients who were ambulatory at the start of radiotherapy had a 79% chance of remaining ambulatory at the completion of therapy. Patients with paraplegia had only a 45% chance of remaining ambulatory, and patients with paralysis had less than a 3% chance of regaining an ambulatory state.[74]

Histology of the primary tumor may be a prognostic factor for neurological recovery. Radiosensitive tumors such as myeloma, lymphoma, small cell lung cancer, and seminoma have a rapid response to radiation, and recovery of neurological function occurs frequently. Unfavorable histologies such as non–small cell lung cancer and melanoma have a less favorable response.[75, 76]

Time to the development of motor deficits is another prognostic factor in spinal cord compression. Patients with a history of slowly progressive motor deficits have a better neurological prognosis than do those who present with a rapid decline in motor function. In a prospective study, Rades and associates[76] found that patients with more than 14 days of progressive motor symptoms had an 86% chance of neurological recovery, compared with only a 10% chance of recovery in those whose motor deficits progressed over less than 7 days. It has been suggested that patients with a rapid onset of paralysis may actually experience spinal cord ischemia or infarction. The antineoplastic effect of radiation is not likely to reverse such a vascular event.[76]

The fractionation schedule of radiotherapy plays a less critical role in the recovery of neurological function than does the timing of its initiation. Fractionation schedules of 200 cGy × 20 fractions, 300 cGy × 10 fractions, or 400 cGy × 5 fractions to cumulative doses of 4000 cGy, 3000 cGy, and 2000 cGy, respectively, all yield similar outcomes.[76] Generally, radiation oncologists prefer more prolonged regimens and higher total cumulative doses for patients with better prognoses and expected long-term survival. Shorter overall courses are most appropriate for patients with limited expected survival. In our department, we generally start with large fractions of 400 cGy for the first few fractions and then complete the course with 300-cGy fractions.

Radiation treatment volume should encompass the entirety of the lesion on the MRI scan, with a generous margin above and below the mass. Traditionally, the radiation portal encompassed two vertebral bodies above and below the level of the spinal cord compression. This two-vertebral-body margin dates to the era of myelography without CT or MRI. It ensured adequate coverage of disease visualized as a "complete block" on the myelogram.

PRIMARY TUMORS OF THE VERTEBRAL COLUMN

Chordoma

Chordomas are rare tumors arising from notochordal remnants in the axial skeleton. Nearly 50% of all chordomas arise from the sacrococcygeal region, another 35% arise from the clivus, and the remainder occur within the vertebral column.[77] These are slow-growing neoplasms that are locally invasive, destroy bone, and infiltrate soft tissues. Both radiographically and pathologically, chordoma may be difficult to distinguish from chondrosarcoma. Grossly, chordomas are soft, lobulated tumors that are frequently encapsulated, with areas of hemorrhage, calcification, or cystic change. Because of their location, chordomas are rarely completely resectable and have a very high local recurrence rate following surgery. Because of the high incidence of local recurrence, postoperative radiotherapy is generally recommended. Metastases are uncommon at presentation but have been reported in as many as 25% of patients with recurrent disease.[78]

The diagnostic workup for chordomas depends on the primary site. Patients with skull base tumors require laboratory investigation of pituitary and hypothalamic functions, and visual field testing should be done to document any impairment. CT is valuable for detailing bone invasion or destruction, and MRI is helpful in determining the extent of soft tissue invasion. These two imaging modalities are complementary in planning both surgery and radiotherapy.[77, 79]

Surgical excision is the primary treatment of choice. Surgery often relieves presenting symptoms while establishing the diagnosis. Complete gross tumor excision is associated with a lower rate of local recurrence than is either incomplete excision or biopsy.[80, 81] Tumors arising from the sacrum or vertebral column often require spine stabilization or reconstruction.

Postoperative radiotherapy can reduce the risk of local recurrence. Conventional radiotherapy with doses in the range of 50 to 60 Gy can offer palliation but seldom provides durable local control.[81–83] Because of chordomas' proximity to highly radiosensitive structures, conformal radiation techniques have been studied extensively in this disease. Because of its unique physical characteristics, proton therapy has been recommended for the postoperative management of patients with chordomas or chondrosarcomas of the skull base and vertebral column. Modern intensity-modulated radiotherapy with conventional x-ray beams may be able to achieve adequately conformal dose distributions to obtain the necessary local control without a high risk of complications. It appears that there is a radiation dose response to achieve maximal control of chordomas.[84] In a pattern-of-failure analysis in patients with clival chordomas treated with proton beam therapy for gross residual disease, Austin and coworkers[84] demonstrated that tumors often recur where the radiation dose was less than the intended prescription. A follow-up study by Terahara and colleagues[1] demonstrated that the "equivalent uniform dose" delivered to residual chordoma was an important factor in achieving optimal local control following surgery. When a higher equivalent uniform dose was delivered to the target volume, better local control was achieved. The actuarial rate of local control was 59% at 5 years with proton beam radiation. In that series, the prescribed radiation dose ranged from 66.6 cobalt-gray equivalent (CGE) to 79.2 CGE. Female gender was associated with a higher rate of local failure, and it was proposed that females require higher radiation doses for equal control. An updated report from Massachusetts General Hospital reported 73% 5-year local control with tumor doses ranging from 66 to 83 CGE.[85] The proton therapy experience from Loma Linda for skull base chordomas confirmed the effectiveness of high-dose conformal proton therapy. With a median follow-up of 33.2 months, the local control rate for patients with chordomas was 92% (23 of 25).[86] Noel and coauthors[87] reported favorable early results with proton beam therapy in a French series, with an 83.1% 3-year local control rate in 34 patients treated for chordoma with a median dose of 67 CGE.

Heavy charged particle radiotherapy has been explored in the management of chordoma. The high linear energy transfer of particle therapy is believed to offer a biologic advantage in chordoma and low-grade chondrosarcoma owing to the slow proliferative rate of these tumors. Berson and colleagues[88] reported the results of 45 patients with either chordomas or chondroscarcomas of the skull base and cervical spine treated with helium or neon ions. Radiation doses ranged from 36 to 90 CGE. The 5-year actuarial local control rate was 59%. Carbon ion radiotherapy has been used to treat chordomas in Darmstadt, Germany since 1997. Schulz-Ertner and coworkers[89] reported a 2-year local control rate of 83% using this modality. These 2-year results are encouraging but should be interpreted with caution, given the slow-growing nature of these neoplasms.

Stereotactic radiotherapy and radiosurgery have been evaluated in chordoma. Miller and associates[90] reported a multi-institutional retrospective analysis of patients treated with gamma knife radiosurgery for skull base tumors. In eight chordomas, they described 100% 2-year local control. Muthukumar and colleagues[91] reported local control in 11 of 15 patients treated with single-fraction gamma knife radiosurgery at tumor doses ranging from 12 to 20 Gy. This modality is practical for small tumor volumes. In that series, the mean tumor volume was only 4.6 cc. Fractionated stereotactic radiotherapy is applicable to larger tumor volumes. Debus and coworkers[92] reported 82% 2-year and 50% 5-year local control in chordomas treated with fractionated stereotactic radiotherapy. The median target volume was 56 cc (range, 17 to 215 cc). Radiotherapy was delivered at a median dose of 66.6 Gy in 1.8-Gy fractions using stereotactic guidance.[92] As mentioned earlier, 2-year results should be interpreted cautiously.

Chondrosarcoma

Chondrosarcomas arise from bone or cartilage. The most common sites of origin are the pelvis and femur. In the axial skeleton, they can be confused with chordomas. Surgery is the primary treatment of choice, but in the axial skeleton, gross total excision is difficult. Chondrosarcomas of the clivus or sacrococcygeal areas are often treated similarly to chordomas. Chondrosar-

comas generally have a better prognosis than do chordomas in the same location.[85–87] Like chordomas, they have been treated with high-dose conformal proton therapy. Munzenrider and Liebsch[85] reported 98% 5-year local control with proton therapy doses ranging from 66 to 83 Gy. The Loma Linda experience was similarly favorable, with 92% local control at 5 years.[86] The German experience with carbon ions achieved 100% 2-year local control for chondrosarcoma. With fractionated stereotactic radiotherapy, a local control rate of 100% was reported by Debus and associates.[92]

Osteosarcoma

Osteosarcoma is a primary bone sarcoma. It generally arises in the long bones of adolescents and young adults. The primary treatment for this tumor is surgical resection with adjuvant chemotherapy. Radiotherapy plays only a small role in the management of these tumors.

Ewing's Sarcoma

Ewing's sarcoma is an undifferentiated small, round, blue-cell tumor of childhood. It is most commonly diagnosed in adolescents and young adults. Nearly one third of children with Ewing's sarcoma have metastatic disease at the time of diagnosis. This tumor, unlike osteosarcoma, is both chemotherapy and radiation sensitive. Tumors arising in the appendicular skeleton are often treated with systemic chemotherapy and surgical resection. Patients with close or positive surgical margins are treated with postoperative radiotherapy. Unresectable tumors can be managed with primary radiotherapy. Although local control appears to be better with surgery than with primary radiotherapy, when corrected for bulk of disease and primary tumor site, the local control achieved by the two modalities may be similar.[93] Tumors of the axial skeleton, including the vertebral column, are often treated with combined chemotherapy and radiotherapy. Radiation doses to 55.8 Gy in conventional fraction sizes of 1.8 Gy/day are generally used. The spinal cord dose must be kept to less than 50 Gy to maintain acceptable tolerance and avoid paraplegia. Conformal radiotherapy techniques are highly recommended. Tumors below the level of L2 and the conus medullaris can be treated with less concern for spinal cord tolerance.

REFERENCES

1. Terahara A, Niemierko A, Goitein M, et al: Analysis of the relationship between tumor dose inhomogeneity and local control in patients with skull base chordoma. Int J Radiat Oncol Biol Phys 45:351–358, 1999.
2. McCormick PC, Stein BM: Spinal cord tumors in adults. In Youmans JR (ed): Neurological Surgery, 4th ed. Philadelphia, WB Saunders, 1996, p 3102.
3. Lenhard RE: Cancer statistics: A measure of progress. CA Cancer J Clin 46:3, 1996.
4. Garcia DM: Primary spinal cord tumors treated with surgery and postoperative irradiation. Int J Radiat Oncol Biol Phys 11: 1933, 1985.
5. Wood EH, Berne AS, Taveras JM: The value of radiation therapy

in the management of intrinsic tumors of the spinal cord. Radiology 63:11, 1954.

6. Constantini S, Epstein FJ: Intraspinal tumors in infants and children. In Youmans JR (ed): Neurological Surgery, 4th ed. Philadelphia, WB Saunders, 1996, p 3123.

7. deSousa AL, Kalsbeck JE, Mealey JM, et al: Intraspinal tumors in children. J Neurosurg 51:437, 1979.

8. Hely M, Fryer J, Selby G: Intramedullary spinal cord glioma with intracranial seeding. J Neurol Neurosurg Psychiatry 48:302, 1985.

9. Linstadt DE, Wara WM, Leibel SA, et al: Postoperative radiotherapy of primary spinal cord tumors. Int J Radiat Oncol Biol Phys 16:1397, 1989.

10. Vakili H: Spinal Cord. New York, Intercontinental Medical Book Corporation, 1967.

11. Epstein F: Spinal cord astrocytomas of childhood. Adv Tech Stand Neurosurg 13:135, 1986.

12. Epstein FJ, Farmer JP: Pediatric spinal cord tumor surgery. Neurosurg Clin N Am 1:569, 1990.

13. Epstein FJ, Farmer JP, Freed D: Adult intramedullary astrocytomas of the spinal cord. J Neurosurg 77:355, 1992.

14. Rossitch E, Zeidman SM, Buger PC, et al: Clinical and pathological analysis of spinal cord astrocytomas in children. Neurosurgery 27:193, 1990.

15. Epstein F, Epstein N: Surgical treatment of spinal cord astrocytomas of childhood. J Neurosurg 57:685, 1982.

16. Malis LI: Intramedullary spinal cord tumors. Clin Neurosurg 25:512, 1978.

17. Clover LL, Hazuka MB, Kinzie JJ: Spinal cord ependymomas treated with surgery and radiation therapy: A review of 11 cases. Am J Clin Oncol 16:350, 1993.

18. Schiffer D, Chio A, Giordana MT, et al: Histologic prognostic factors in ependymoma. Childs Nerv Syst 7:177, 1991.

19. Shaw EG, Evans RG, Scheithauer BW, et al: Radiotherapeutic management of adult intraspinal ependymomas. Int J Radiat Oncol Biol Phys 12:323, 1986.

20. Sonneland PRL, Sheithauer BS, Onofrio BM: Myxopapillary ependymoma: A clinicopathological and immunocytochemical study of 77 cases. Cancer 56:883, 1985.

21. Wanebo JE, Malik JM, Vandenberg SR, et al: Malignant peripheral nerve sheath tumors: A clinical pathologic study of 28 cases. Cancer 27:1247, 1993.

22. Rivierez M, Oueslati S, Phillipon J, et al: Ependymomas of the intradural filum terminale in adults: 20 cases. Neurochirurgie 36:96, 1990.

23. Chan HSL, Becker LE, Hoffman HJ: Myxopapillary ependymoma of the filum terminale and cauda equina in childhood: Report of seven cases and review of the literature. Neurosurgery 14:204, 1984.

24. Mork SJ, Loken AC: Ependymoma: A follow-up study of 101 cases. Cancer 40:907, 1977.

25. Ross DA, McKeever PE, Sandler HM, et al: Myxopapillary ependymoma: Results of nucleolar organizing region staining. Cancer 71:3114, 1993.

26. Schweitzer JS, Batzdorf U: Ependymoma of the cauda equina region: Diagnosis, treatment and outcome in 15 patients. Neurosurgery 30:202, 1992.

27. Sze G: Neoplastic disease of the spine and spinal cord. In Atlas SW (ed): Magnetic Resonance Imaging of the Brain and Spine. Philadelphia, Lippincott-Raven, 1996, pp 1339–1385.

28. Chun HC, Schmidt-Ullrich RK, Wolfson A, et al: External beam radiotherapy for primary spinal cord tumors. J Neurooncol 9:211, 1990.

29. Cooper PR: Outcome after operative treatment of intramedullary spinal cord tumors in adults: Intermediate and long-term results in 51 patients. Neurosurgery 25:855, 1989.

30. Guidetti B, Mercuri S, Vagnozzi R: Long-term results of the surgical treatment of 129 intramedullary spinal gliomas. J Neurosurg 54:323, 1981.

31. Hardison HH, Packer RJ, Rorke LB, et al: Outcome of children with primary intramedullary spinal cord tumors. Childs Nerv Sys 3:89, 1987.

32. Hulschof MC, Menten J, Dito JJ, et al: Treatment results in primary intraspinal gliomas. Radiother Oncol 29:294, 1993.

33. Kopelson G, Linggood RM, Kleinman GM, et al: Management of intramedullary spinal cord tumors. Radiology 135:473, 1980.

34. Shirato H, Kamada T, Hida K, et al: The role of radiotherapy in the management of spinal cord glioma. Int J Radiat Oncol Biol Phys 33:323, 1995.

35. Ferrante L, Mastronardi L, Celli P, et al: Intramedullary spinal cord ependymomas: A study of 45 cases with long term follow-up. Acta Neurochir (Wien) 119:74, 1992.

36. Cohen AR, Wisoff JH, Allen JA, et al: Malignant astrocytomas of the spinal cord. J Neurosurg 70:50, 1989.

37. Kopelson G, Linggood RM: Intramedullary spinal cord astrocytoma versus glioblastoma: The prognostic importance of histologic grade. Cancer 50:732, 1982.

38. Merchant TE, Nguyen D, Thompson SJ, et al: High-grade pediatric spinal cord tumors. Pediatr Neurosurg 39:1–5, 1999.

39. Waldron JN, Laperriere NJ, Jaakkimaninen L, et al: Spinal ependymomas: A retrospective analysis of 59 cases. Int J Radiat Oncol Biol Phys 27:223, 1993.

40. Whitaker SJ, Bessell EM, Ashley SE, et al: Postoperative radiotherapy in the management of spinal cord ependymomas. J Neurosurg 74:720, 1991.

41. Goh K, Velasquez L, Epstein F: Pediatric intramedullary spinal cord tumors: Is surgery alone enough? Pediatr Neurosurg 27:34–39, 1997.

42. Wen BC, Hussey DH, Hitchon PW, et al: The role of radiation therapy in the management of ependymomas of the spinal cord. Int J Radiat Oncol Biol Phys 20:781, 1991.

43. Garrett PG, Simpson WJK: Ependymomas: Results of radiation treatment. Int J Radiat Oncol Biol Phys 9:1121, 1983.

44. Fearnside MR, Adams CBT: Tumors of the cauda equina. J Neurol Neurosurg Psychiatry 41:24, 1978.

45. McCormick PC, Stein BM: Intramedullary tumors in adults. Neurosurg Clin N Am 1:606, 1990.

46. Nishio S, Morioka T, Fujii J, et al: Spinal cord gliomas: Management and outcome with reference to adjuvant therapy. J Clin Neurosci 7:20–23, 2000.

47. Sandler HM, Papadopoulos SM, Thornton AF, et al: Spinal cord astrocytomas: Results of therapy. Neurosurgery 30:490, 1992.

48. Hoshimaru M, Koyama T, Hashimoto N, et al: Results of microsurgical treatment for intramedullary spinal cord ependymomas: Analysis of 36 cases. Neurosurgery 44:264–269, 1999.

49. Epstein FJ, Farmer JP, Freed D: Adult intramedullary spinal cord ependymomas: The result of surgery in 38 patients. J Neurosurg 79:204, 1993.

50. Fischer G, Mansuy L: Total removal of intramedullary ependymomas: Follow-up study in 16 cases. Surg Neurol 14:243, 1980.

51. McCormick PC, Torres R, Post KD, et al: Intramedullary ependymoma of the spinal cord. J Neurosurg 72:523, 1990.

52. Rawlings CE, Giangaspero F, Burger PC: Ependymomas: A clinicopathologic study. Surg Neurol 29:271, 1988.

53. Nadkarni TD, Rekate HL: Pediatric intramedullary spinal cord tumors. Childs Nerv Syst 15:17–28, 1999.

54. Merchant TE, Kiehna EN, Thompson SJ, et al: Pediatric low-grade and ependymal spinal cord tumors. Pediatr Neurosurg 32:30–36, 2000.

55. Miraminoff RO, Dosoretz DE, Linggood RM, et al: Analysis of recurrence and progression following neurosurgical resection. J Neurosurg 62:18, 1985.

56. Larson DA: Radiation therapy of tumors of the spine. In Youmans JR (ed): Neurological Surgery, 4th ed. Philadelphia, WB Saunders, 1996, p 3168.

57. Fein DA, Marcus RB, Parsons JT, et al: Lhermitte's sign: Incidence and treatment variables influencing risk after irradiation of the cervical spinal cord. Int J Radiat Oncol Biol Phys 27:1029, 1993.

58. Jones A: Transient radiation myelopathy (with reference to Lhermitte's sign of electrical paresthesia). Br J Radiol 37:727, 1964.

59. Schultheiss TE, Higgins EM, El-Mahdi AM: The latent period in clinical radiation myelopathy. Int J Radiat Oncol Biol Phys 10:1109, 1984.

60. Rampling R, Symonds P: Radiation myelopathy. Curr Opin Neurol 11:627–632, 1998.

61. Phillips TL, Buschke F: Radiation tolerance of the thoracic spinal cord. AJR Am J Roentgenol 105:659, 1969.

62. Wara WM, Philips TL, Sheline GE, et al: Radiation tolerance of the spinal cord. Cancer 35:1558, 1975.

63. Marcus RB, Million RR: The incidence of myelitis after irradiation of the cervical spinal cord. Int J Radiat Oncol Biol Phys 19:3–8, 1990.

64. Schultheiss TE, Stephens LC, Jiang GL, et al: Radiation myelopathy in primates treated with conventional fractionation. Int J Radiat Oncol Biol Phys 19:935–940, 1990.
65. Macbeth FR, Wheldon TE, Girling DJ, et al: Radiation myelopathy: Estimates of risk in 1048 patients in three randomized trials of palliative radiotherapy for non–small cell lung cancer. Clin Oncol 8:176–181, 1996.
66. Fowler JF: The linear quadratic formula and progress in fractionated radiotherapy. Br J Radiol 62:6679–6694, 1989.
67. Mayfield JK: Postradiation spinal deformity. Orthop Clin North Am 10:829, 1979.
68. Abbott R, Feldstein N, Wisoff JH, et al: Osteoplastic laminotomy in children. Pediatr Neurosurg 18:153, 1992.
69. Sorensen S, Helweg-Larsen S, Mouridsen H, Hansen HH: Effect of high-dose dexamethasone in carcinomatous metastatic spinal cord compression treated with radiotherapy: A randomised trial. Eur J Cancer 30A:22–27, 1994.
70. Heimdal K, Hirschberg H, Slettebo H, et al: High incidence of serious side effects of high-dose dexamethasone treatment in patients with epidural spinal cord compression. J Neurooncol 12:141–144, 1992.
71. Young RF, Post E, King GA: Treatment of spinal epidural metastases: Randomized prospective comparison of laminectomy and radiotherapy. J Neurosurg 53:741, 1980.
72. Kim RY, Spencer SA, Meredith RF, et al: Extradural spinal cord compression: Analysis of factors determining functional prognosis—a prospective study. Radiology 175:279–282, 1990.
73. Turner S, Marosszeky B, Timms I, Boyages J: Malignant spinal cord compression: A prospective evaluation. Int J Radiat Oncol Biol Phys 26:141–146, 1993.
74. Gilbert RW, Kim JH, Posner JB: Epidural spinal cord compression from metastatic tumor: Diagnosis and treatment. Ann Neurol 3:40–51, 1978.
75. Kim RY, Smith JW, Spencer SA, et al: Malignant epidural spinal cord compression associated with a paravertebral mass: Its radiotherapeutic outcome on radiosensitivity. Int J Radiat Oncol Biol Phys 27:1079–1083, 1993.
76. Rades D, Heidenreich F, Karstens JH: Final results of a prospective study of the prognostic value of time to develop motor deficits before irradiation in metastatic spinal cord compression. Int J Radiat Oncol Biol Phys 53:975–979, 2002.
77. Sze G, Uichanco LS, Brant-Zawadski MN, et al: Chordomas: MR imaging. Radiology 166:187–191, 1988.
78. Saunders WM, Castro JR, Chen GT, et al: Early results of ion beam radiation therapy for sacral chordomas. J Neurosurg 64:243–247, 1986.
79. Oot RF, Melville GE, New PF, et al: The role of MR and CT in evaluating clival chordomas and chondrosarcomas. AJR Am J Roentgenol 151:567–575, 1988.
80. Forsyth PA, Cascino TL, Shaw EG, et al: Intracranial chordomas: A clinicopathological and prognostic study of 51 cases. J Neurosurg 78:741–747, 1993.
81. Keisch ME, Garcia DM, Shibuya RB: Retrospective long term follow-up analysis in 21 patients with chordomas of various sites treated at a single institution. J Neurosurg 75:374–377, 1991.
82. Catton C, O'Sullivan B, Bell R, et al: Chordoma: Long-term follow-up after radical photon irradiation. Radiother Oncol 41:67–70, 1996.
83. Pearlman AW, Friedman M: Radical radiation therapy of chordoma. AJR Am J Roentgenol 108:332–341, 1970.
84. Austin JP, Urie MM, Cardenosa G, Munzenrider JE: Probable causes of recurrence in patients with chordoma and chondrosarcoma of the base of skull and cervical spine. Int J Radiat Oncol Biol Phys 25:439–444, 1993.
85. Munzenrider JE, Liebsch NJ: Proton therapy for tumors of the skull base. Strahlenther Onkol 175(Suppl 2):57–63, 1999.
86. Hug EB, Loredo LN, Slater JD, et al: Proton radiation therapy for chordomas and chondrosarcomas of the skull base. J Neurosurg 91:432–439, 1999.
87. Noel G, Habrand JL, Mammar H, et al: Combination of photon and proton radiation therapy for chordomas and chondrosarcomas of the skull base: The Centre de Protontherapie D'Orsay experience. Int J Radiat Oncol Biol Phys 51:392–398, 2001.
88. Berson AM, Castro JR, Petti P, et al: Charged particle irradiation of chordoma and chondrosarcoma of the base of skull and cervical spine: The Lawrence Berkeley Laboratory experience. Int J Radiat Oncol Biol Phys 15:559–565, 1988.
89. Schulz-Ertner D, Haberer T, Jakel O, et al: Radiotherapy for chordomas and low-grade chondrosarcomas of the skull base with carbon ions. Int J Radiat Oncol Biol Phys 53:36–42, 2002.
90. Miller RC, Foote RL, Coffey RJ, et al: The role of stereotactic radiosurgery in the treatment of malignant skull base tumors. Int J Radiat Oncol Biol Phys 39:977–981, 1997.
91. Muthukumar N, Kondziolka D, Lunsford LD, Flickinger JC: Stereotactic radiosurgery for chordoma and chondrosarcoma: Further experiences. Int J Radiat Oncol Biol Phys 41:387–392, 1998.
92. Debus J, Schulz-Ertner D, Schad L, et al: Stereotactic fractionated radiotherapy for chordomas and chondrosarcomas of the skull base. Int J Radiat Oncol Biol Phys 47:591–596, 2000.
93. Dunst J, Jurgens H, Sauer R, et al: Radiation therapy in Ewing's sarcoma: An update of CESS 86 trial. Int J Radiat Oncol Biol Phys 32:919, 1995.
94. Abdel-Wahab M, Corn B, Wolfson A, et al: Prognostic factors and survival in patients with spinal cord gliomas after radiation therapy. Am J Clin Oncol 22:344–351, 1999.
95. Reimer R, Onofrio B: Astrocytomas of the spinal cord in children and adolescents. J Neurosurg 63:669, 1985.
96. Jyothirmayi R, Madhavan J, Nair MK, et al: Conservative surgery and radiotherapy in the treatment of spinal cord astrocytoma. J Neurooncol 33:205–211, 1997.

Radiosurgery of Tumors

AJAY NIRANJAN ■ L. DADE LUNSFORD

Stereotactic radiosurgery is usually used as an alternative to surgical removal of small to moderate-sized tumors. The goals of radiosurgery differ from those of conventional surgery because the target is not physically removed from the brain. The target is not destroyed immediately but instead is exposed to a high dose of radiation, which ultimately translates into a specific (toxic) radiobiologic response delivered to the target volume. Radiosurgery is based on the same fundamental principles that are used in stereotactic surgery. For neurosurgeons experienced in stereotaxy, radiosurgery is a logical replacement for more conventional surgical tools. The goals of tumor radiosurgery are to preserve neurologic function and to prevent further tumor growth. Intracranial tumors are the major indications for radiosurgery.

ROLE OF RADIOSURGERY AS A MANAGEMENT STRATEGY

Primary Radiosurgery

Radiosurgery is a reliable noninvasive strategy that can be used as either primary or adjuvant therapy in the management of brain tumors. It has become a definitive alternative to microsurgery for patients with newly diagnosed or recurrent benign tumors, especially those of the skull base. Most cranial base tumors, and those involving critical neural structures, cannot be completely removed without a high risk of additional neurologic deficits. Similarly, deep-seated metastatic brain tumors carry a higher risk of neurologic deficit if approached surgically. Primary radiosurgery can play a significant role for many tumors of the skull base whose diagnosis is determined by neuroimaging criteria alone.

Adjuvant Radiosurgery

Radiosurgery is used as an adjuvant in the multimodality management of malignant glial tumors. Adjuvant radiosurgery is also used for incompletely removed benign tumors that warrant tumor debulking because of symptoms of mass effect. Planned second-stage radiosurgery is an effective strategy to manage these residual tumors and to preserve neurologic function. Radiosurgery has been used for boost irradiation of patients with malignant glial tumors, in addition to conventional wide-margin fractionated radiotherapy. Because of its effectiveness in treating recurrent malignant gliomas, radiosurgery is being used increasingly as part of the initial management for newly diagnosed malignant gliomas in eligible patients. All patients also undergo fractionated external beam radiotherapy.

TECHNICAL CONSIDERATIONS

Imaging for Stereotactic Radiosurgery

The development of stereotactic radiosurgery has been closely linked with the evolution of imaging techniques. The highlights of stereotactic imaging include optimal contrast between normal and abnormal tissues in addition to high spatial resolution, short scan time, and thin slices so that accurate target localization can be achieved. The use of magnetic resonance imaging (MRI) in stereotactic planning has enhanced accurate targeting of lesions that usually are not adequately defined by any other modality. However, some physicians use fusion of MR and computed tomographic images for stereotactic guidance because they believe that in their setup, magnetic susceptibility artifacts and chemical shift artifacts may affect the accuracy of target localization in MRI.[1,2] For the initial 2 years, our group used both MRI and computed tomography (CT) for stereotactic planning. Significant target coordinate differences were not observed using the Leksell stereotactic system.[3] Since 1993, MRI alone has been used for stereotactic radiosurgery planning. Regular quality control checks of the MRI unit are necessary in order to be able to use MRI for radiosurgery planning. With a properly shimmed magnet, regular servicing, and strict quality assurance on the unit as well as the images, MRI provides high-resolution images with accurate target localization.

For stereotactic imaging of smaller targets (where millimeter accuracy is needed) a three-dimensional volume acquisition using fast spoiled-gradient recalled acquisition in steady state (SPGR) sequence at 512 × 256 matrix and 2 number of excitations (NEX) is preferred (28 slices × 1 mm or 1.5 mm). Additional sequences are used in specific situations to enhance the definition of target. For example in cases of nonenhancing tumors, a fluid-attenuated inversion recovery (FLAIR) sequence (TR 9002, TE 165, TI 2200) can be used in addition to the previously mentioned sequences to differentiate tumor from surrounding edema, which is helpful in radiosurgery planning to avoid radiation to normal tissue. Variable echo multiplanar (VEMP) sequence (TR 2200, TE 30/90) is helpful in demonstrating chordoma from surrounding normal tissue. A fat saturation sequence is helpful in differentiating pituitary tumor from fatty tissue used for packing during previous surgery.

Radiosurgical Dose Planning

Dose planning is the most important aspect of the entire radiosurgery treatment. Such planning is no different from surgical planning and requires a detailed knowledge of neuroanatomy and pathology. A variety of features are universal in treatment planning software. The program integrates the images with the isodose curves displayed on the monitor. A conformal plan is achieved using one or more radiation isocenters. Highlights of gamma knife radiosurgery planning include the use of multiple isocenters, beam weighting, and plug patterns. The experienced planner can achieve a conformal plan quickly. The success of benign tumor radiosurgery depends on high conformity to tumor margin. Recent versions of Gamma Plan (version 5.12 and 5.2) have facilitated the early use of inverse planning. With inverse planning, the surgeon defines the target volume three-dimensionally, after which the computer works to generate an initial conformal plan. The surgeon then adjusts and optimizes the final plan. Multileaf collimator systems as well as robotic systems (such as the Cyberknife system) also use inverse planning.

Tumors of the skull base, or those in critical brain locations such as the brainstem, are usually treated with multiple isocenter plans using small collimators in order to limit dose falloff to the surrounding normal tissue. Preservation of existing hearing and sharp dose falloff on the brainstem are important considerations in planning for acoustic tumors. The proximity of the optic apparatus may necessitate the use of beam blocking in radiosurgery planning for pituitary tumors or craniopharyngiomas. Similarly, the tolerance of cranial nerves is kept in mind when planning a meningioma involving the cavernous sinus.

Dose Prescription Influences

DOSE-VOLUME EFFECTS

Volume effects are commonly ignored in fractionated radiation therapy because there is little difference in volume from one patient to the other. In radiosurgery, however, target volumes may vary from 0.1 cc to 20 cc depending on the morphologic characteristics of the lesion. Because of such a wide range of volumes, the radiation tolerance of normal tissue varies from patient to patient, depending on the brain volume exposed to radiation. The target volume is one of the most important considerations in prescribing radiosurgery dose.

EFFECT OF PRIOR RADIOTHERAPY

Although there is no consensus about how to account for the effects of prior radiation therapy, some estimate that approximately 50% of the effect of a fractionated radiation therapy dose is repaired by 6 months.[4] Prior radiation therapy doses should be factored during radiosurgery planning, although the effects of the other factors (volume, location, and radiosurgery dose) outweigh the effects of prior radiation. To reduce risk to critical structures, however, the radiosurgery dose is reduced if radiation therapy has been performed previously.[4, 5]

EFFECT OF LOCATION ON RADIATION TOLERANCE

The chance of causing symptomatic radiation injury to the brain from radiosurgery is affected markedly by the location of the tumor. Cranial nerves appear to have differential radiation sensitivity. Special sensory nerves (optic, cochlear) are most sensitive, followed by somatic sensory nerves; the motor nerves are the least sensitive. Although differential radiation sensitivity of the brain's region has been hard to define, certain regions of brain are more likely to be associated with detectable symptomatic radiation injury than other relatively "silent" regions.

TUMOR DOSE-RESPONSE CURVES

Benign Tumors. No clear dose-response curves have been identified for radiosurgery of the different benign tumors managed by radiosurgery. We currently use 13 Gy as a margin dose for the acoustic tumors in which hearing preservation remains the prime concern. Benign meningiomas are treated with a margin dose ranging from 12 to 18 Gy depending on the volume treated and the tolerance of surrounding regions such as optic chiasm and brainstem. Our policy has been to treat tumor with doses as high as possible while limiting the optic nerve–chiasm dose to 8 Gy and brainstem dose to 10 to 12 Gy.

Malignant Tumors. Typical boost radiosurgery doses for metastatic tumors vary from 12 to 18 Gy depending on volume. For solitary brain metastases without prior radiation or malignant glioma recurrence after previous irradiation, a margin dose of 20 Gy is recommended. However, margin dose is often reduced because of large tumor volumes or surrounding eloquent brain regions.

Radiosurgery Techniques

Radiosurgery starts with rigid head fixation of an imaging-compatible stereotactic frame. Regional anesthetic scalp infiltration as well as mild intravenous sedation is used as needed. Images are acquired with a fiducial system attached to the stereotactic frame. Planning is performed on stereotactic images. After finalizing the plan, a maximal dose to the target is determined. The treatment isodose, maximal dose, and dose to the margin are jointly decided by a neurosurgeon, radiation oncologist, and medical physicist, keeping in view the goal of radiosurgery in an individual patient and the tolerance of the surrounding structures. Dose falloff to the critical structures is checked and kept below tolerable limits.

Radiosurgery is currently performed using the gamma knife or one of the linear accelerator–based systems or a heavy-charged particle beam. Morphologic gamma knife radiosurgery usually involves multiple isocenters of different beam diameters to achieve a dose plan that conforms to the irregular three-dimensional volumes of most mass lesions. The total number of isocenters may vary depending on the size, shape, and number of lesions. The most frequent range of isocenters varies from 5 to 10 for each patient. The recent version of the Gamma Knife (Model C) combines advances in dose planning with robotic engineering and reduces the need to set coordinates manually for each isocenter in selected cases. In LINAC-based radiosurgery, multiple radiation arcs are used to shoot photon beams in a crossfire pattern at a target defined in stereotactic space. Most of the currently functioning systems use nondynamic techniques in which the patient's couch is set at an angle and the arc is moved around its radius to deliver radiation that enters the skull through many different points. Different techniques have been developed to enhance conformity of dose planning and delivery using LINAC-based systems. These include beam shaping and intensity modulation. Newer developments include introduction of jaws, noncircular, and minileaf and microleaf collimators. Single isocenter radiosurgery is now possible with newer LINAC-based systems. The conformal beam can be delivered with the micromultileaf collimator or conformal blocks.

Heavy-charged particle beam radiosurgery systems use either the Bragg peak method, in which the charged particles stop within the target volume, or the plateau beam method, in which charged particles are projected at the target in a crossfire pattern. These facilities are available at only a limited number of centers because of their high cost.

RADIOSURGERY OF NONGLIAL TUMORS

Vestibular Schwannomas (Acoustic Tumors)

Vestibular schwannomas represent approximately 10% of all primary brain tumors and 80% of cerebellopontine angle tumors. Since the growth rate of acoustic tumors is unpredictable, there is no general consensus regarding the identification of candidates for therapeutic intervention. The management options include ob-

servation, microsurgery, and radiosurgery. In general, management outcomes are better for smaller tumors, regardless of the strategy chosen. Widespread availability of MRI and the advances in microsurgery techniques since the 1980s have reduced the morbidity and improved the results of surgery at the centers of excellence. The goals of acoustic tumor management have, however, shifted from complete tumor removal to preservation of neurologic function. Preservation of hearing has become the most challenging goal of acoustic tumor management. The rapid advances in radiosurgical techniques have resulted in a greatly improved outlook for patients with acoustic neuroma.

Acoustic tumor stereotactic radiosurgery using the gamma knife unit was first performed by Leksell in 1969.[6] In a review of their 20 years' experience with treatment of acoustic neuromas by radiosurgery, Norén and colleagues reported that more than 90% of patients had tumor growth control.[7] Acoustic tumor radiosurgery has evolved steadily since the early 1990s.[8–13] Advanced dose planning software, MRI guided dose planning, and gradual reductions of tumor margin dose over the years reflect the evolution of this technology. The results after radiosurgery of acoustic tumors have established it as an important, minimally invasive alternative to microsurgery.

EVALUATION BEFORE AND AFTER RADIOSURGERY

Patients with acoustic tumors are evaluated with high-resolution MRI and undergo clinical evaluation as well as audiologic tests, which include pure tone average (PTA) and speech discrimination score (SDS). Hearing is graded using the Gardner-Robertson modification of the Silverstein and Norell classification,[14] and facial nerve function is assessed according to the House-Brackmann grading system.[15] "Serviceable" hearing (class I and class II) is defined as a pure tone average or speech reception threshold (SRT) lower than 50 dB and a speech discrimination score better than 50%. After radiosurgery, all patients are followed with serial gadolinium-enhanced MRI scans, which are requested at 6-month intervals for 2 years. If there is no appreciable change in tumor size, subsequent MRIs are requested at 2-year intervals. All patients who have some preserved hearing are advised to obtain audiologic evaluation (pure tone average and speech discrimination score) near the time of their MRI follow-up.

TECHNICAL CONSIDERATIONS

Radiosurgical dose planning, the most critical aspect of the procedure, is similar to other image-guided surgical planning and requires a detailed knowledge of neuroanatomy and pathology. Preservation of cochlear and facial nerve function is the main concern during planning. For moderate-sized tumors, preservation of brainstem function is also a consideration. Acoustic tumor planning is usually performed using a combination of small beam diameter isocenters (4- and 8-mm collimators). Rarely, a 14-mm collimator is also used for larger tumors. Success of acoustic tumor radiosurgery depends on high conformity to the tumor margin. The facial and acoustic nerve complex usually courses along the anterior margin of the tumor, so the plan should be highly conformal in this region. For the extracanalicular tumor component, a combination of isocenters is used. A series of 4-mm isocenters is used to create a tapered isodose plan to conform to the lateral portion (intracanalicular) of the tumor. Hearing preservation rates are enhanced when a combination of only 4-mm collimators is used to irradiate intracanalicular portions of acoustic tumors.[13] The average diameter of the normal internal auditory canal is only 4 mm (range 2 to 8 mm). All four nerves (cochlear, facial, and superior and inferior vestibular) travel through this small space. The preservation of hearing associated with the exclusive use of the 4-mm collimator most likely is due to the sharp falloff of the radiation field at the tumor margin. Using the 4-mm collimators spares a substantial number of nerve fibers of the cochlear division, which likely is compressed and pushed anteriorly by the tumor. An 8-mm beam not only covers the tumor but also encompasses most of the cochlear and facial nerve fibers within the 50% isodose volume. Radiation injury to the cochlea may also lead to diminished postoperative hearing. Proximity to brainstem (large acoustic tumors) may sometimes necessitate the use of beam blocking to achieve sharper dose falloff. Dose prescriptions for acoustic tumors have changed significantly since 1988. During the earlier experience, higher tumor margin doses (average 16 Gy) were prescribed. Gradual reduction in doses has improved hearing preservation and reduced facial and trigeminal neuropathies. Currently, 13 Gy is recommended as the tumor margin dose. This dose is associated with reduced complications and yet maintains a high rate of tumor control.

MICROSURGERY VERSUS RADIOSURGERY

One stated goal of microsurgery is complete removal of tumor and avoidance of further surgery. With the current microsurgical techniques, complete tumor removal is often possible with low morbidity rates (Table 268–1).[16–20] Tumor recurrence rates of less than 1% have been reported by centers of excellence. Cerullo and colleagues, however, studied the risk of tumor recurrence in a series of surgically treated vestibular schwannoma patients in whom preservation of facial and cochlear nerve function was a routine objective.[21] These authors reported 18 recurrences in a series of 116 consecutive vestibular schwannoma patients. The Acoustic Neuroma Registry of 1579 patients reported incomplete resection in 8% of patients, and a recurrence rate of 8% to 10% after complete excision of the tumor.[22]

Immediate postoperative normal or nearly normal facial nerve function is maintained in approximately 65% to 70% of patients with small tumors (<3 cm in diameter), which improves to 78% to 96% at 1 year or more after surgery. Trigeminal dysfunction has been reported in up to 22% of patients.[23] Preservation of overall serviceable hearing (pure tone average, <50 dB;

speech discrimination score, >50%) has been reported in 27% to 47% (range 18% to 50%) of patients who are selected for hearing preservation surgery (see Table 268–1).[16–20] Preserved postoperative hearing function may further decline in as many as 18% to 56% of patients without tumor recurrence.[24] Although perioperative mortality and morbidity rates of surgery have declined significantly, mortality risks (1%) have not been eliminated. Postoperative cerebrospinal fluid leakage is the most common complication, occurring in 3% to 18% of patients; 2% of patients ultimately require reoperation to close the fistula.[17, 23] Wound infection, meningitis, lower cranial dysfunction, and postoperative hematomas account for 3% to 5% of the complications. Resumption of normal activity status after surgery is difficult to assess and is rarely reported. Wiegand and Fickel reported that approximately one third of 541 patients felt "normal" 4 months after surgery.[25]

The goal of radiosurgery is tumor growth control. Reports suggest a tumor control rate of 93% to 100% after radiosurgery (Table 268–2).[13, 26–30] Preradiosurgery hearing can be preserved in 60% to 70% of patients. Kondziolka and colleagues, in a review 162 patients, reported a 98% tumor control rate in a long-term (5- to 10-year) follow-up.[29] Sixty-two percent became smaller, 53% remained unchanged, and 6% became slightly larger. Only 2% of patients underwent tumor resection after radiosurgery. Some tumors initially enlarge 1 to 2 mm during the first 6 to 12 months after radiosurgery as they lose their central contrast enhancement. Such tumors invariably regress in volume compared with their preradiosurgery size (Fig. 268–1). Normal facial function was preserved in 79% of patients after 5 years, and normal trigeminal nerve function was preserved in 73%. The use of stereotactic MRI since 1993, instead of computed tomography, for radiosurgery planning has contributed to the reduction in the incidence of cochlear, facial, and trigeminal dysfunction after radiosurgery. Fifty-one percent of the patients had no change in hearing ability. Radiosurgery was found superior to microsurgery in preserving serviceable hearing in patients with intracanalicular tumors.[13, 29]

A direct comparison of patient outcome after microsurgery and radiosurgery in a randomized fashion is lacking, but in a retrospective matched cohort study involving 87 patients at the University of Pittsburgh, radiosurgery was found to be more effective in preserving normal facial function and serviceable hearing and had less treatment-related morbidity.[23] The hospital stay was shorter, charges were less, and patients were able to return to independent functioning sooner after radiosurgery. Ninety-three percent of the patients were either very satisfied or satisfied after radiosurgery, compared with 79% after microsurgery. Current results (since 1996) demonstrate that facial nerve function is preserved in 99% of patients and hearing can be preserved at preoperative levels in 50% to 70% of patients.

Meningiomas

The optimal treatment for meningioma is complete resection of tumor with its dural base. This result is

TABLE 268–1 ■ Modern Surgical Outcome after Acoustic Tumor Microsurgery

REFERENCE	TOTAL NO. OF PATIENTS	TUMOR SIZE	HEARING PRESERVATION	COMPLICATIONS				
				Facial Neuropathy	Cerebrospinal Fluid Leakage	Meningitis	Death	Other Complications
Nadol et al, 1992[16]	78	IC = 14 6–15 mm = 46 16–25 mm = 10 >25 mm = 8	32% overall 50% IC 37% small 31% for <25 mm	29% for IC 15% for small 40% for medium 25% for large	7%	0	0	Hemorrhage, 1.3%; stroke, 1.3%
Samii and Matthies, 1997[17]	1000	13.5	40% overall 47% in most recent 200 cases	36%	9.2%	3%	1.10%	Hemorrhage, 2%; lower cranial neuropathies, 2%; hemiparesis, 1%; tetraparesis, 0.2%
Gormley et al, 1997[18]	179	<2 cm = 67 2–4 cm = 84 >4 cm = 28	38% overall	4% for <2 cm 26% for 2 to 4 cm 62% for >4 cm	15%	3%	1.10%	Hydrocephalus, 3%; lower cranial neuropathies, 2%; brainstem injury with persistent ataxia, 0.6%
Fahlbusch, 1998[19]	61	20–30 mm >30 mm	27% overall 18% for 20 to 30 mm 21% for 30 mm	47.5%	Not reported	Not reported	0	
Colletti and Fiorino, 1999[20]	88	IC = 18, <25 mm = 70	40% overall 30% conventional 52% en bloc	40% (33.45% at 1 yr) 17.5% (10% at 1 yr)	8.3% 7.5%	0	0	Cerebellar edema, 2.1%; cerebellar infarct, 2.5%; sigmoid sinus phlebitis, 2.1%

IC, intracanalicular tumor.

T A B L E 2 6 8 – 2 ■ **Results of Radiosurgery for Acoustic Tumor**

REFERENCES	TOTAL NO. OF PATIENTS	PREVIOUS SURGERY	MEAN TUMOR VOLUME	MEAN MARGIN DOSE	MEAN FOLLOW-UP (Mo)	TUMOR VOLUME REDUCED	TUMOR VOLUME STABLE	TUMOR ENLARGED	TUMOR CONTROL RATE	SERVICEABLE HEARING PRESERVATION	COMPLICATIONS				
											Delayed Surgery	Facial Neuropathy	Trigeminal Neuropathy	Transient Imbalance	Hydro-cephalus
Kobayashi et al, 1994[26] (GK)	44	23%	6.2 cc	14.8	12 (3–20)	25%	75%	0%	100%	48%	0%	16% (4 of 7 resolved)	7% all resolved	4.5%	4.5%
Norén et al, 1998[27] (GK)	254	–	–	13.6 (8–20)	35 (10–67)	51%	42%	7%	93%	60% (2 yr)	1%	14% (none in last 55)	8% (none in last 55)	5%	
Lunsford et al, 1998[28] (GK)	402	24%	–	–	36 (88 >7 yr)	30%	63%	7%	93%	39% (CT) 68% (MRI)	2%	28% (CT) 8% (MRI)	34% (CT) 8% (MRI)		<3%
Kondziolka et al, 1998[29] (GK)	162	26%	22-mm diameter	16	5–10 yr	62%	33%	6%	98%	47%	2%	21%	27%	<1%	<1%
Foote et al, 1998[30] (LINAC)	101	27%	4.8 cc	14 (10–22.5)	34 (12–94)	55%	39%	7%	93%	–	5%	14% overall 5% after 1994	11% overall 0% after 1994	6%	7%
Niranjan et al, 1999[30] (GK)	29	1 patient	50–773 mm³ (IC)	13–17	33 (9–106)	21%	79%	0%	100%	Overall, 73% <14 Gy, 100%	0%	0%	0%	–	0%

CT, cases performed using CT-based planning before 1993; GK, gamma knife; IC, intracanalicular tumors only; LINAC, linear accelerator–based radiosurgery; MR, cases performed using MRI-based planning.

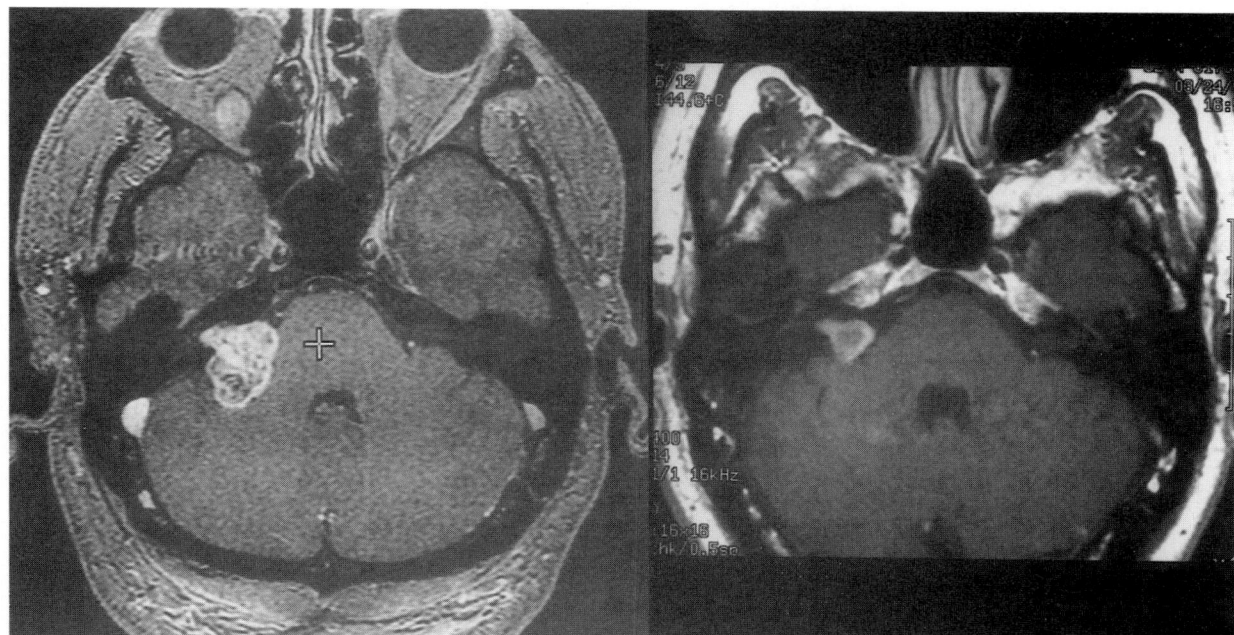

FIGURE 268–1. A 50-year-old man presented with tinnitus and diminished hearing in the right ear. An axial magnetic resonance imaging (MRI) scan *(left)* showed a right-sided acoustic tumor. He was treated with gamma knife radiosurgery using 14 Gy to the tumor margin. Two years later, significant tumor regression was noted *(right)*. His serial audiograms showed preservation of Gardner-Robertson class I hearing (pure tone average <30 dB and speech discrimination score of >70%) 2 years after radiosurgery.

associated with long-term disease-free survival.[31] However, in complex meningiomas, such as those attached to the skull base and the venous sinuses, complete resection may not be possible; multimodality management should then be considered. Morbidity and mortality from surgical resection are largely dependent on the location of the tumor, with an overall surgical mortality of 7% to 14%.[32] Age may also contribute to the risk of surgical resection.[33–35]

Although meningiomas are benign tumors, recurrence is not uncommon. Recurrence is related to the extent of its excision. Ten-year recurrence rates of 9%, 19%, 29%, and 40% were reported for grade I- through grade IV-type resection, respectively, by Simpson.[31] Recurrence rates are higher for meningiomas in critical locations where only subtotal resections are possible because of limited access and involvement of critical structures.

RATIONALE FOR MENINGIOMA RADIOSURGERY

Partial tumor resection is associated with a high recurrence rate. Condra and associates reported a 15-year tumor local control rate of 30% after subtotal resection alone, 87% after subtotal resection and radiation therapy, and 76% after total excision.[36] Table 268–3 shows results of meningioma radiosurgery from various institutions.[37–44] Tumor control rates ranged from 98% (at 2 years) to 75% (at 8 years), with regression of tumor volume occurring in 22% to 63% of the tumors in various reported series. Excellent outcomes of radio-

surgery for meningiomas of the skull base have been reported (Figs. 268–2, 3A and B).[45–51] Meningiomas attached to major venous sinuses, which pose difficult management challenges, can be successfully treated by radiosurgery.[52] Although the specific biologic response of radiosurgery on meningioma is not well understood, it is clear that the response occurs slowly and progressively. Tumor regression may occur for several years after radiosurgery. This modality can thus play a significant role in patients with meningiomas. Radiosurgery offers an attractive option for patients with residual or recurrent meningioma as well as for patients in whom complete resection of tumor is considered unattainable without acceptable morbidity. Radiosurgery provides long-term tumor control associated with a high rate of neurologic function preservation and patient satisfaction (Fig. 268–4). For meningiomas of convexity, anterior fossa, or lateral sphenoid ridge that can be easily approached, surgical excision is the preferred first-line approach. For meningiomas at all other intracranial locations, radiosurgery seems to be the preferred management approach unless the tumor needs debulking because of mass effect. Larger tumors, especially those involving critical locations such as the optic chiasm, need a combined approach. Malignant meningiomas, however, continue to require a multimodality management approach that includes resection, radiosurgery, and radiation therapy.

Pituitary Tumors

The primary aim of treatment for macroadenoma is tumor removal or tumor growth control in order to

TABLE 268–3 ■ Results of Radiosurgery for Meningioma

REFERENCES	TOTAL NO. OF PATIENTS	PRIOR SURGERY	MEAN TUMOR VOLUME (cc)	MEAN MARGIN DOSE (Gy)	MEAN FOLLOW-UP (Mo)	TUMOR VOLUME REDUCED	TUMOR VOLUME STABLE	TUMOR VOLUME ENLARGED	TUMOR CONTROL RATE	NEW NEUROLOGIC DEFICIT
Pendl et al, 1997[37] (GK)	97	55%	13.7 (0.8–82)	13.8 (7–25)	18.5 (6–46)	40%	56%	4%	96%	—
Chang and Adler, 1997[38] (LINAC)	55	69%	7.3 (0.5–28)	18.3 (12–25)	48 (17–81)	29%	69%	2%	98% (2 yr)	18% (7% permanent)
Lunsford et al, 1998[39] (GK)	141	60%	—	—	—	35%	60%	5%	95%	—
Shafron et al, 1998[40] (LINAC)	70	46%	10 (0.6–28.6)	12.7 (10–20)	23 (2–88)	44%	56%	0%	100%	3% (transient)
Hakim et al, 1998[41] (LINAC)	127	83%	4.1 (0.2–51)	15 (9–20)	31 (1–80)	—	—	—	89%	3% (permanent) Death 2 (1.65%)
Steiner et al, 1998[42] (GK)	151	69%	1–32	14 (10–20)	12–72	63%	26%	11%	89%	0%
Colombo and Francescon 1998[43] (LINAC)	74	64%	10 (1.7–55)	22.3 (18–23)	33.1 (4–144)	22%	68%	11%	75% (8 yr)	2% (permanent)
Kondziolka et al, 1999[44] (GK)	99	57%	4.7 (0.24–24)	16	5–10 yr	63%	32%	5%	93% (5–10 yr)	5%

GK, gamma knife; LINAC, linear accelerator–based radiosurgery.

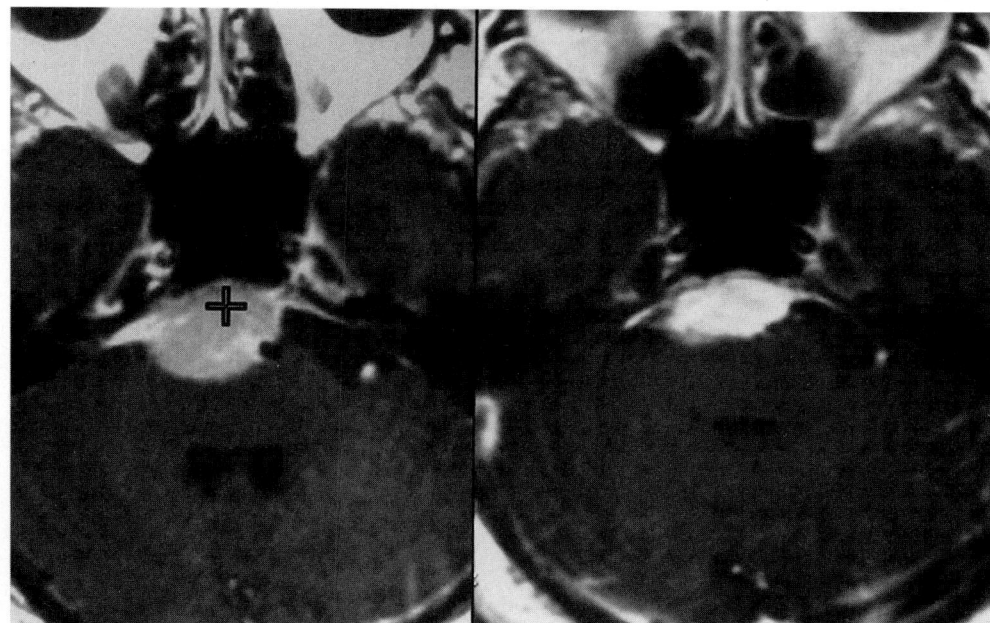

FIGURE 268–2. Axial MRI scan *(left)* of a 46-year-old man with a residual clival meningioma. He underwent multiple-isocenter gamma knife radiosurgery using a margin dose of 14 Gy and a maximal dose of 28 Gy. A 5-year follow-up axial MRI scan *(right)* showed regression of tumor.

regain or preserve visual function. Transsphenoidal radical resection is generally preferred. Adequacy of treatment is assessed by radiologic and visual evaluations.

Because microadenomas (<10 mm in diameter) are recognized because of endocrinopathy related to hyperactive tumor, the aim of treatment is to correct endocrine dysfunction. This usually requires radical tumor removal. The degree of urgency in correcting an endocrinopathy varies according to the type. The adequacy of treatment for hypersecreting tumors is defined by correction of endocrinopathy and preservation of normal pituitary function.

With current microsurgical techniques, the risk of serious complications is low, but the risk of residual or recurrent tumor is not insignificant. Failure to achieve remission occurs in at least 15% of patients, even in the hands of experienced microsurgeons.[53–55] The success and complication rates are significantly less favorable with a second surgery.[56] Fractionated radiation therapy has been the conventional method of treatment of unresectable pituitary adenomas. Rates of tumor control have been reported to vary from 76% to 97%.[57–59] Fractionated radiation therapy, however, has been less successful (38% to 70%) in reducing hypersecretion of hormones by the tumor. It may take years before a full therapeutic effect is exhibited. The complications of radiation therapy include a relatively high risk of hypopituitarism (12% to 100%) and a low but definite risk of optic neuropathy (1% to 2%).[57–59]

AIMS OF PITUITARY ADENOMA RADIOSURGERY

The aims of radiosurgery are the same as those of microsurgery with regard to endocrine dysfunction. However, regarding tumor volume, tumor control rather than tumor reduction has become a widely accepted indicator of successful treatment. For example,

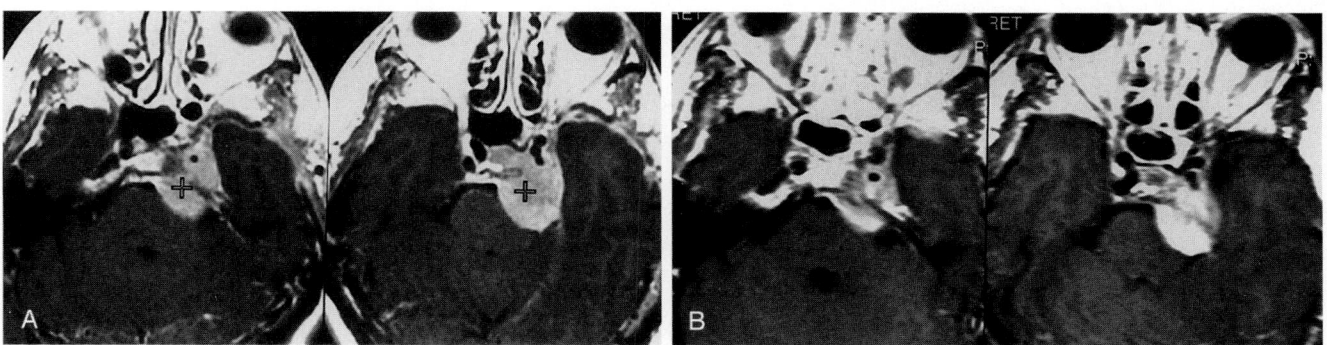

FIGURE 268–3. *A*, Axial MR images (*left* and *right*) of a 51-year-old woman with a left residual cavernous sinus meningioma. She underwent multiple-isocenter gamma knife radiosurgery using a margin dose of 12 Gy and a maximal dose of 24 Gy. *B*, A 5-year follow-up axial MRI scan (*right* and *left*) showed regression of tumor.

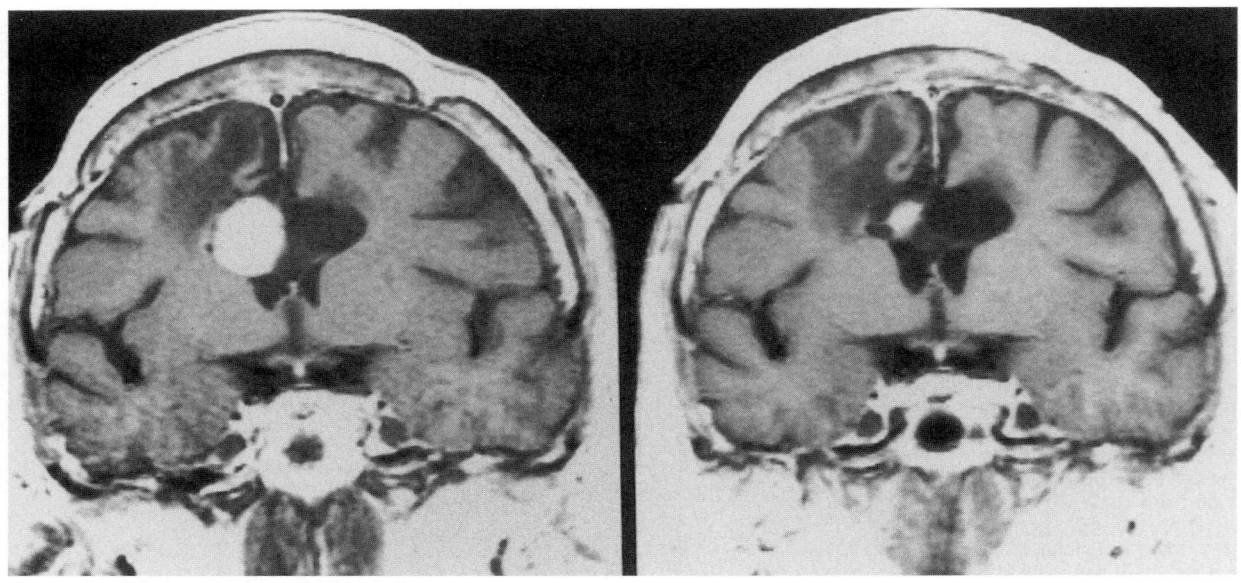

FIGURE 268–4. A 76-year-old man presented with an intraventricular meningioma *(left).* Gamma knife radiosurgery was performed using 18 Gy as tumor margin dose. A 20-month follow-up scan showed significant tumor regression *(right).*

Witt and coworkers reported 87 patients with pituitary adenomas who had gamma knife radiosurgery over a 10-year period.[60] The mean dose to the margin was 19.2 Gy (range 9.6 to 30 Gy). A 94% growth control rate was achieved at a median follow-up of 32 months (Fig. 268–5). Ganz and colleagues reported successful tumor control in 14 of the 15 patients treated by gamma knife.[61]

ACROMEGALY

Kjellberg and associates reported 551 patients treated by particle beam.[62, 63] The rate of normalization of growth hormone (defined then as <5 ng/mL) was 28%

at 2 years, 75% at 5 years, and 93% at 20 years. In a series of 318 patients reported by Levy and colleagues, the mean growth hormone level decreased by 70% within 1 year of radiosurgery.[64] Thoren and coworkers reported 10% cured and 38% improved in a series of 21 patients treated by gamma knife.[65] Lunsford and associates treated 14 patients and reported 64% cured or improved.[66] Voges and colleagues treated 12 patients with LINAC and reported a mean reduction in growth hormone level from 17 to 5 ng/mL.[67]

CUSHING'S DISEASE

Kjellberg and Abbe reported 163 patients with Cushing's disease.[63] Cure was achieved in 55% at 2 years,

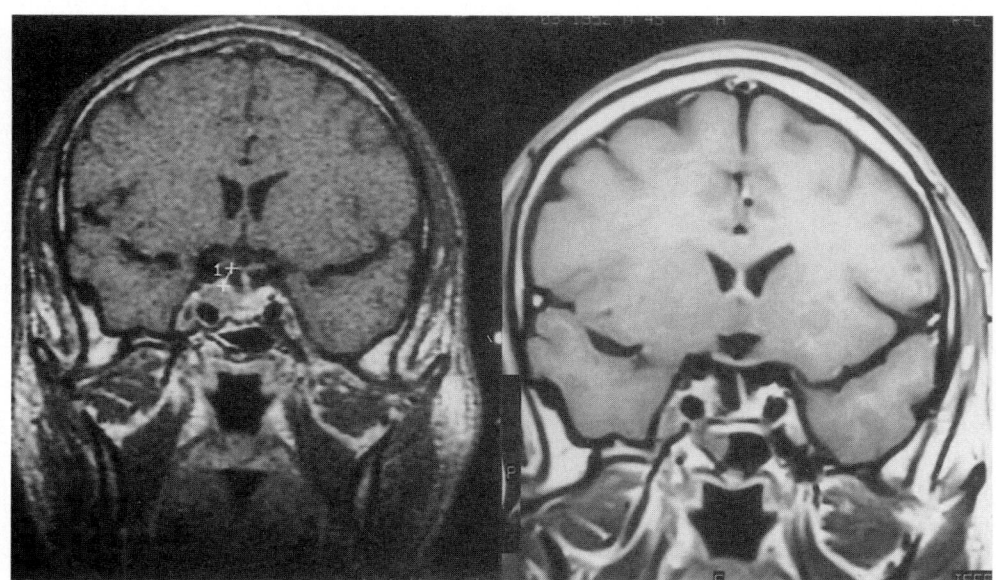

FIGURE 268–5. A coronal gadolinium-enhanced MRI scan *(left)* of a 35-year-old woman shows a pituitary adenoma Gamma knife radiosurgery was performed using 16 Gy as tumor margin dose. A 2-year follow-up MRI scan showed significant tumor regression *(right).*

80% at 5 years, and 90% at 20 years. Levy and associates reported an 86% cure rate within a year in 83 patients treated using a helium ion beam.[64] Rahn and colleagues reported an overall cure rate of 82% using multiple gamma knife procedures in a series of 59 patients.[68] Lunsford and associates treated 16 patients using gamma knife surgery and reported 62% cured or improved.[66]

PROLACTINOMAS

Levy and colleagues reported 23 patients with prolactinomas treated with heavy-particle radiosurgery using 50 to 150 Gy in three or four fractions over 5 days. Of the 20 patients followed 1 year after irradiation, 19 had a marked fall in prolactin levels (12 to normal levels).[64] Witt and coworkers reported the endocrine follow-up in 7 of 12 patients with prolactinoma treated with gamma knife radiosurgery. One had normal prolactin levels 4 months after radiosurgery, and levels dropped by 18% to 69% in five patients over 7 to 37 months (median 17 months).[60] Laws and associates reported 19 patients with prolactinoma treated using gamma knife radiosurgery. Of the 13 patients who had more than 6 months' follow-up, remission was achieved in 1 patient at 18 months.[69]

MORBIDITY

Complications of pituitary radiosurgery fall into three categories: hypopituitarism, visual deterioration, and hypothalamic damage. The incidence of hypopituitarism varies widely in different reported series using different modalities of radiosurgery (Table 268–4). The reported incidence of visual complications is generally less than 3%. However, Rocher and colleagues,[70] using LINAC radiosurgery, reported a 39% incidence of some visual compromise (6% of patients became blind). This complication can be avoided by conformal planning and accurate dose delivery. Lunsford and coworkers[66] reported one death due to hypothalamic tumor involvement in a patient who had multiple operations and radiation therapy. Voges and associates[67] reported one patient who developed severe hypothalamic syndrome.

At present, microsurgery remains the treatment of choice for macroadenomas compressing the optic apparatus or when a rapid reduction in excessive hormone level is required. For residual or recurrent tumors that are 2 to 3 mm away from the optic chiasm, however, radiosurgery provides growth control, and long-term endocrine control may be superior to that of repeat microsurgery. The risk of hypopituitarism is significantly lower with radiosurgery compared with fractionated radiation therapy.[66]

RADIOSURGERY OF GLIAL TUMORS

Malignant gliomas continue to represent one of the most serious challenges in neurosurgery. The natural history of untreated glioblastoma multiforme (GBM), which accounts for 80% of malignant gliomas, results in a median survival of 3 months.[71] Despite advances in surgical and radiation techniques, chemotherapy, gene therapy, and immunotherapy, the prognosis in these patients remains grim. A surgical cure cannot be achieved because of the infiltrative nature of the tumor. Although there has been some debate on the utility of extensive tumor resection in the management of malignant gliomas, debulking is often necessary in patients with significant mass effect. Radiation therapy has become the mainstay of treatment.[72] Although conventional fractionated local field radiation (1.8 Gy daily for 33 fractions, total dose 59.4 Gy, to fields extending 3 to 4 cm outside the region of enhancement) offers significant survival benefit, the effect for GBM patients is suboptimal, with mean survival improving from 6 to 9 months.[73] Conventional fractionated radiation (59.4 Gy) does not reliably achieve local control of enhancing tumor, and higher doses result in significant widespread necrosis.[74, 75] After surgery and radiation therapy for malignant gliomas, more than 80% of failures are because of local tumor recurrence (within the radiation field).[76] Increases in total radiation dose by conventional technique are limited by the tolerance of the surrounding normal brain.

The observation that local control and median survival can be improved through dose escalation is the basis for the application of radiosurgery to malignant gliomas.[73] A prospective, randomized trial by the Brain Tumor Cooperative Group has confirmed that interstitial brachytherapy boost results in prolonged survival (16-month versus 13-month median survival compared with controls) for patients with GBM.[77] Radiosurgery offers a similar ability to deliver a radiation boost but is noninvasive compared with brachytherapy.

Radiosurgery has been used for boost irradiation in addition to conventional wide-margin fractionated radiotherapy in patients with malignant glial tumors (Table 268–5).[78–87] It has been used mainly for patients with tumors less than 3.5 cm in diameter as part of a multimodality approach to malignant gliomas. Early radiosurgery reports varied widely in the outcomes for malignant gliomas, with a median survival for GBM patients ranging from 9.5[83] to 26 months.[81] These variations could result from patient selection biases and other prognostic factors.

T A B L E 2 6 8 – 4 ■ **Complications of Pituitary Radiosurgery**

REFERENCE	HYPOPITUITARISM	VISUAL DEFICITS
Kjellberg and Abbe[63]	10%	<1%
Levy et al[64] (heavy particle)	33%	<1%
Thoren et al[65] (GK)	24%	
Rocher et al[70] (LINAC)	33%	39% (6% blind)
Lunsford et al[66] (GK)	0%	1 patient
Voges et al[67] (LINAC)		1 patient

GK, gamma knife; LINAC, linear accelerator–based radiosurgery.

TABLE 268-5 ■ Results of Radiosurgery for Malignant Gliomas

REFERENCE	TOTAL NO. OF PATIENTS	HISTOLOGY	KARNOFSKY PERFORMANCE SCORE	MEDIAN TUMOR VOLUME (cc)	MEDIAN MARGINAL DOSE (Gy)	POSTRADIOSURGERY MEDIAN SURVIVAL (Mo)	ACTUARIAL SURVIVAL RATE	REOPERATION RATE (%)
Loeffler et al, 1992[81] (LINAC)	37	23 GBMs, 14 AAs	100% >70	4.8 (1.2–72)	12 (10–20)	GBM at 26, AA not reached	—	21
Coffey et al, 1993[82] (GK)	18	—	Mean, 83 (50–100)	—	15 (12–18)	10 (2–29)	—	—
Masciopinto et al, 1995[83] (LINAC)	31	GBMs	57% >70	16.4 (2.3–60)	11.5 (10–20)	9.5	37 (1-yr)	—
Sarkaria et al, 1995[84] (LINAC)	115	95 GBMs, 19 AAs	89% >70	10 (0.4–72)	12.2 (6–20)	GBM at 21, AA not reached	GBM, 38; AA 72 (2-yr)	29
Gannett et al, 1995[85] (LINAC)	30	19 GBMs, 11 AAs	97% >70	24 (2.1–115)	10 (5–18)	GBM at 13, AA at 28	GBM, 43; AA, 64.5 (1-yr) GBM, 8; AA, 53 (2-yr)	33
Hall et al, 1995[86] (LINAC)	35	26 GBMs, 9 AAs	57% >70	28 (2.4–98)	20 (7.5–40)	GBM at 8, AA at 12	GBM, 54; AA, 29 (1-yr) GBM, 6; AA, 0 (2-yr)	31
Kondziolka et al, 1997[80] (GK)	107	64 GBMs, 43 AAs	Mean, 90 (50–100)	6.5 (0.9–31)	15.5 (12–25)	GBM at 16, AA at 21	GBM, 38; AA, 49 (2-yr)	19
Alexander et al, 1998[87] (LINAC)	164	GBMs	—	10.1	13	19.9 at initial boost, 10.2 at recurrence	89 (1-yr); 37 (2-yr) at initial boost; 45 (1-yr); 19 (2-yr) at recurrence	22
Foote et al, 1998[30] (LINAC)	76	48 GBMs, 19 AAs	Mean, 84 (60–100)	12 (1.2–39)	13 (10–20)	GBM at 11.6, AA at 11.4	—	24

AA, anaplastic astrocytoma; GBM, glioblastoma multiforme; GK, gamma knife radiosurgery; LINAC, linear accelerator–based radiosurgery.

In an effort to control the prognostic factors and better evaluate the effect of radiosurgery on the survival of malignant glioma patients, a multicenter retrospective analysis was performed.[84] This study included 115 patients who were treated with a combination of surgery, fractionated radiation therapy, and radiosurgery boost using LINAC at three different centers under similar treatment protocols. Patients were assigned into six prognostic classes based on the recursive partitioning analysis of multiple prognostic factors. This classification (published previously by the Radiation Therapy Oncology Group [RTOG]) is based on the tumor's pathologic features, patient age, the patient's functional status using the Karnofsky performance score (KPS), duration of symptoms, and the extent of resection.[88] This stratification offers some control for the multitude of prognostic factors and allows more direct comparison of results. After a median follow-up of 91 weeks, the 2-year actuarial survival of the entire group was 45%. The GBM patients had a median survival of 21 months and a 2-year actuarial survival of 38%. For anaplastic astrocytomas, the median survival time was not reached in this study, and 2-year actuarial survival was 72%. In comparison to published RTOG results of similarly stratified malignant glioma patients treated without radiosurgery boost, radiosurgery resulted in a longer median survival of 4 to 20 months, depending on the prognostic class. The benefit was most pronounced for the patients in the moderate to poor prognostic classes.

This study strongly suggested that a radiosurgical boost is advantageous for patients with GBM, although no definite conclusion could be drawn regarding the utility of radiosurgery for patients with anaplastic astrocytomas. These results should be interpreted with some caution because the treatment in the RTOG study was performed before the advent of quality neuroimaging, and the average size of the tumor in the RTOG study was greater than in the radiosurgery cohort. However, on univariate analysis, the RTOG prognostic class and the Karnofsky performance score were found to be the only significant predictors of survival, excluding tumor size and the extent of surgery as potential factors. Furthermore, RTOG prognostic class was eliminated as an independent predictor of survival in multivariate analysis, leaving the Karnofsky performance score as the only significant independent prognostic factor. This study suggests that radiosurgery boost confers a survival advantage for GBM patients. It also suggests that patients in poor prognostic classes who had been excluded as candidates for radiosurgery in many series may actually benefit significantly from a radiosurgery boost.

We performed a retrospective study to evaluate the result of radiosurgery on 64 GBM and 43 anaplastic astrocytoma patients.[80] The median survival for the GBM group was 16 months after radiosurgery and 26 months after diagnosis. The 2-year survival rate was 51%. For patients with anaplastic astrocytomas, the median survival after radiosurgery was 21 months, and after diagnosis it was 32 months. The 2-year survival rate after diagnosis was 67%. The reported results of radiosurgical boost are summarized in Table 268-4.[30, 80–87] Other centers have reported survival rates that seem significantly improved as compared with the 9-month median survival and 10% 2-year actuarial rate reported for standard therapy.[89] There is a significant survival advantage using radiosurgery boost in patients with malignant glioma, especially if used appropriately with surgery and other adjuvant therapies.[80, 87, 90] However, a carefully designed prospective randomized trial is needed to reliably establish survival benefit from radiosurgical boost for malignant gliomas.

The acute complications that follow radiosurgery are unusual and limited to exacerbation of existing symptoms. The most frequently seen delayed complication of radiosurgical boost is radiation injury to the tumor or surrounding brain. The symptoms are usually controllable with steroid therapy. The reported incidence of necrosis ranges from 2% to 22%. Reoperation rates ranging from 21% to 33% have been reported after radiosurgery. Neither radiation necrosis nor reoperation is associated with diminished length of survival.[30] Current evidence suggests that radiosurgery boost is a safe and effective adjuvant therapy for malignant gliomas.

RADIOSURGERY OF METASTATIC TUMORS

The annual estimated incidence of brain metastases in the United States is in excess of 100,000 cases. The most frequent cause of brain metastases is lung cancer, which accounts for approximately half of all secondary tumors of the brain. The other major primary tumors include breast, melanoma, and renal cell cancer. Based on the RTOG trials, the standard recommendation for most patients with brain metastases since the early has been conventional fractionated whole brain radiation to 30 Gy administered in 10 to 12 fractions.[91, 92] However, conventional fractionated radiation therapy alone may not be adequate treatment in patients with good prognoses because of the possibility of regrowth of the brain metastases. Patchell and associates reported an actuarial recurrence rate exceeding 80% for whole-brain radiotherapy (36 Gy in 12 fractions) of solitary brain metastases.[93] The late sequelae after whole-brain radiation are another concern when it is used in patients with an otherwise good prognosis. The routine use of prophylactic cranial irradiation in patients with small cell lung carcinoma is controversial at present because of late effects on brain.[94]

Rationale for Use of Radiosurgery

There are several features that make brain metastases one of the ideal indications for radiosurgery. The majority of brain metastases are roughly spherical and therefore can easily be targeted by radiosurgery. Brain metastases are compact targets with frequent peritumoral microscopic spread, thus permitting the use of conformal radiosurgery, but providing some therapeutic benefit in the falloff zone of radiation outside the imaging defined margin. The common location of me-

TABLE 268–6 ■ Results of Radiosurgery for Brain Metastases

REFERENCE	TOTAL NO. OF PATIENTS	NUMBER OF LESIONS	WHOLE-BRAIN RADIATION THERAPY	MEAN MARGIN DOSE (Gy)	LOCAL CONTROL (%)	MEDIAN SURVIVAL (Mo)	CENTRAL NERVOUS SYSTEM DEATH
Kihlstrom et al, 1993[98] (GK)	160	235	—	29	94	NA	10%
Flickinger et al, 1994[96] (GK)	116	116	56	17.5	85	11	—
Alexander et al, 1995[95] (LINAC)	248	421	100	15	85	9.4	—
Valentino, 1995[99] (LINAC-multiple fractions)	139	139	—	50 (15–80)	92	13.5	—
Fukuoka et al, 1996[100] (GK)	130	>215	—	14–30	93	8	—
Gerosa et al, 1996[101] (GK)	225	343	—	21.1	88	9.3	19%
Joseph et al, 1996[102] (LINAC)	120	189	83	26.6 (10–35)	96	7.4	17%
Kim et al, 1997[103] (GK, lung carcinoma only)	77	115	92	16 (10–22.5)	88	11	—
Breneman et al, 1997[104] (LINAC)	84	177	96	16 (10–22)	25	11	—
Shiau et al, 1998[97] (GK)	100	219	83	18.5 (10–22)	77	12	—
Foote et al, 1999[30] (LINAC)	166	NA	>90%	15 (10–17.5)	86	9.3	—

GK, gamma knife radiosurgery; LINAC, linear accelerator–based radiosurgery.

tastases is the junction of gray and white matter, which is a relatively noneloquent area and permits the delivery of a relatively higher dose. Advances in neuroimaging have led to early diagnosis of metastases while they are still small and without significant mass effect and symptoms. Although a solitary brain metastasis without mass effect is the ideal indication for radiosurgery, multiple metastases have been treated by radiosurgery. Patients with multiple metastases (more than four or five) are ideally treated by conventional whole-brain radiation therapy rather than radiosurgery. Radiosurgery is not considered for patients with a large metastatic tumor causing significant mass effect. Such patients should undergo surgical excision.

Clinical Experience with Radiosurgery

There have been a number of reports on the effectiveness of radiosurgery in treating brain metastases. Table 268–6 lists several large representative series of patients treated by radiosurgery for brain metastases.[95–104] A variety of patients were included in these reports: those with newly diagnosed lesions, those with recurrent lesions, those with single or multiple lesions, those with varying performance statuses, and those with tumors with varying primary histologic appearances and those with a large range of sizes. Because of divergent definitions, response rates vary from 33% to 92%, local tumor control ranges from 25% to 97%, and median survival ranges from 6 to 15 months. The median response rate of 67% (range, 33% to 92%) appears superior to the local control rates after radiation therapy (50%), suggesting a possible increase in local control with the addition of radiosurgery. In the largest review to date, Alexander and colleagues reported a series of 421 lesions in 248 patients and indicated 1- and 2-year actuarial local control rates of 85% and 65%, respectively.[95] Similarly the Gamma Knife Users Group studied the outcomes of radiosurgery in 116 patients with solitary brain metastases.[96] Radiosurgery was part of the initial management in 71 patients, whereas 45 patients had recurrent tumors after previous whole-brain fractionated radiation therapy. In this study, an actuarial local control rate of 67% at 2 years was reported. Shiau and associates reported the radiosurgery experience with 219 brain metastases in 100 patients.[97] The actuarial tumor control, defined as freedom from progression, was 82% and 77% at 6 and 12 months, respectively. These data substantially validate the clinical observation of improved local control after radiosurgery (Fig. 268–6). Although local tumor control rates have improved, mortality is usually related to the uncontrolled primary tumor or metastatic spread to other organs.

Radiosurgery versus Surgery

Large tumors with significant mass effect usually require surgery to provide immediate palliation. Some neurosurgeons, however, select patients with single brain metastases for surgical resection as a common practice. Retrospective data suggest that a relapse rate of up to 85% is noted in patients treated by surgery alone.[105] Several retrospective series suggest that in highly selected patients, surgical resection followed by whole-brain radiation therapy may result in useful and prolonged survival ranging from a median of 16 to 26 months. Two studies comparing surgical resection plus whole-brain radiation therapy and radiation therapy alone for patients with single metastases demonstrated improvements in median survival to 43 and 40 weeks, reespectively.[93, 106] A more recent and relatively larger randomized trial addressing this issue failed to identify a survival benefit from the addition of surgery.[107] The median survival in the radiation alone group was 6.3 months compared with 5.6 months in the resection group. The role of surgery for brain metastases continues to remain controversial.

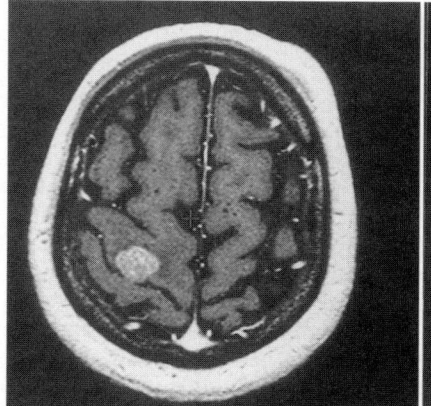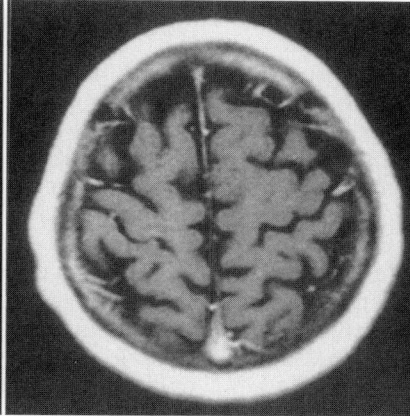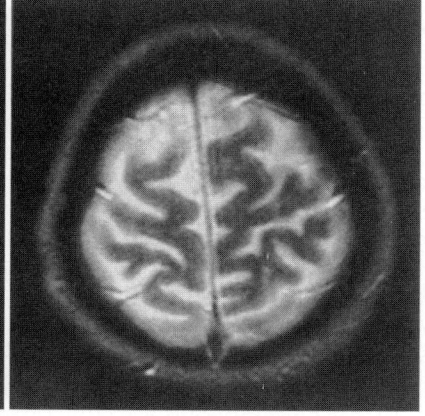

FIGURE 268–6. A 59-year-old man with a prior history of non–small cell carcinoma of the lung presented with left hemiparesis. An axial MRI scan showed a metastatic tumor approximately 2 cm in diameter in the right posterior frontal lobe within the motor strip *(left)*. He underwent gamma knife radiosurgery using a margin dose of 19 Gy and a maximal dose of 38 Gy. T1-weighted contrast-enhanced MRI *(middle)* and T2-weighted MRI *(right)* 18 months after radiosurgery showed complete regression of tumor.

In general, the survival and morbidity results of radiosurgery are superior to those reported for surgical resection followed by whole-brain radiation therapy.[96] The results show that radiosurgery is associated with high local control and low morbidity compared with surgical resection. While interpreting radiosurgery results, one should also take into account the fact that patients in surgical series are selected for the suitable locations of their tumors and their good general condition, whereas no such selection is performed for radiosurgery. On the contrary, those who are not suitable candidates for surgery, either because of eloquent brain locations or poor medical condition, are included in the radiosurgery series. Rutigliano and associates performed a cost-benefit comparison of gamma knife radiosurgery and surgical resection for solitary brain metastases and concluded that radiosurgery had a lower uncomplicated procedure cost, a lower average complication per procedure, was more effective, and had a better incremental cost-effectiveness per life-year. Treatment-related mortality and morbidity were higher for surgery.[108]

The best initial treatment for each patient with brain metastases remains to be defined. Current options include fractionated radiation therapy alone, surgery alone, radiosurgery alone, surgery plus radiation therapy, or radiosurgery plus radiation therapy. Although radiosurgery has increasingly replaced surgery, it has no role after complete excision of metastases because an imaging-defined target is needed to deliver radiosurgery. The presumed tumor bed after surgery is not targeted by radiosurgery in order to avoid added neurologic deficit. However, after incomplete excision of metastatic tumor, radiosurgery with or without radiation therapy can be another strategy. Further randomized trials are necessary to determine the most effective treatment for metastatic lesions.

RADIOSURGERY FOR OTHER TUMORS

Chordomas and Chondrosarcomas of the Skull Base

Chordomas are uncommon tumors that arise from notochordal remnants. They represent 0.1% to 0.2% of intracranial tumors and 2% to 4% of bone tumors. Almost one third of chordomas arise from the skull base. Chondrosarcomas are also rare neoplasms that often arise from the skull base and are presumed to originate from primitive mesenchymal cells or from cartilaginous matrix of the cranium. Both these tumors infiltrate adjacent tissues, which makes complete resection difficult. These tumors often recur locally. Traditionally, they have been considered to be radioresistant to standard fractionated radiation doses (<70 Gy).[109] To improve the radiobiologic effect, fractionated irradiation with charged particles or radiosurgery has been reported with encouraging results. In a report Hug and associates analyzed 58 patients with chordomas and chondrosarcomas of the skull base treated with fractionated proton-photon radiation therapy.[109] A custom-made mask or vacuum-assisted bite was used for immobilization and a proton-photon radiation therapy fraction of 1.8 Gy was administered once a day, 5 days per week, to a total mean target dose of 70.7 Gy. The target volume included an envelope of at least 5 mm around the gross tumor volume. All patients experienced a varying degree of temporary epilation, headaches, loss of appetite, fatigue, occasional nausea, and vomiting, which were symptomatically controlled. Delayed morbidity included grade 3 or grade 4 toxicity in four patients (medial temporal lobe enhancement, single seizure, bilateral hearing impairment, and bilateral loss of vision) and grade 1 or grade 2 toxicity in eight patients (partial pituitary insufficiency in four and unilateral hearing deficit in four). At a mean follow-up of 33 months, local control rates of 92% and 76% were reported for chondrosarcomas and chordomas, respectively. Four patients died and a total of 10 patients experienced local failure (17%).

Radiosurgery is a potent radiobiologic therapy for these lesions. The aim of radiosurgery for these tumors is to deliver a tumoricidal radiation dose in a single session, to spare critical brain structures, and to reduce treatment-related morbidity associated with fractionated radiation therapy. We have treated 15 patients (9 patients with chordomas and 6 patients with chondrosarcomas) between 1987 and 1997 with radiosurgery.[110] A median margin dose of 18 Gy (range 12 to 20 Gy) was delivered in a single session. No patient developed acute (nausea, vomiting, or new neuropathy) or delayed (cranial nerve, vascular or endocrine deficit) effects after radiosurgery. At a median follow-up of 40 months overall, 73% of patients either improved clinically or remained stable after radiosurgery, two thirds either showed reduction or stabilization of the tumor size on follow-up imaging, and four patients died. Although experience with these tumors is limited, we believe that small chordomas and chondrosarcomas can be controlled effectively with radiosurgery. For larger tumors, surgical debulking followed by radiosurgery appears to be a logical approach.

Nonacoustic Schwannomas

Trigeminal schwannomas are rare neoplasms that account for 0.07% to 0.36% of all intracranial tumors and 0.8% to 8% of intracranial schwannomas. These tumors are difficult to approach surgically because of their strategic location. Although surgical mortality and morbidity have been reduced considerably with the advent of modern techniques, complete excision is still difficult to achieve. Radiosurgery is an attractive option for these tumors. Only a few radiosurgical series with a small number of patients have been reported, suggesting a high rate of tumor control. Sixteen patients with trigeminal schwannomas were treated at our institution between 1987 and 1998.[111] Fifteen of the 16 patients presented with trigeminal sensory dysfunction. Six patients had undergone one or more previous resections. Ten underwent radiosurgery as the first procedure. The mean tumor volume was 5.3 cc (range, 1 to 17.8 cc). The mean tumor margin dose was 15.3 Gy (range, 12 to 20 Gy). During the average imaging follow-up of 44 months (range, 8 to 116 months), the tumor control rate was 100% (regression in nine patients and no further tumor growth in seven patients). Five patients had improvement of clinical symptoms, and 11 remained unchanged. No new cranial nerve deficit developed in any patient.

Schwannomas arising from the glossopharyngeal, vagus, or accessory nerve are uncommon and represent only 2.9% to 4% of all intracranial schwannomas. Surgical resection is difficult and is often associated with significant morbidity. Radiosurgery offers safe and effective treatment to these patients. At our institution, 17 patients were treated between 1987 and 1997.[112] Eight of 17 patients showed a decrease in tumor size; 8 showed a stable, unchanged appearance; and one showed tumor progression on follow-up imaging. No complications were noted. Six patients improved, and 10 others retained their preradiosurgery clinical status. One patient needed microsurgery because of unrestrained tumor growth. Radiosurgery seems a safe primary or adjuvant management approach for patients with trigeminal schwannomas and jugular foramen schwannomas.

Pineal Tumors

Management of pineal region tumors remains a significant challenge because of the anatomic complexity of the area and the presence of critical brain and vascular structures. Microsurgical techniques are often successful in obtaining a tissue diagnosis; however, the likelihood of curative resection remains low. There are only a few published reports on radiosurgery for pineal tumors. At our institution, 14 patients with parenchymal pineal tumors were treated between 1989 and 1997.[113] Local tumor control was achieved in 13 patients, whereas one died of tumor progression despite chemotherapy and craniospinal irradiation before radiosurgery. Neuroimaging follow-up showed complete disappearance of tumor in three patients, a decrease in tumor size in seven patients, no change in tumor size in three patients, and tumor growth in one patient.

SPINAL AND BODY RADIOSURGERY

Extracranial radiosurgery is a new concept. The mobility of extracranial targets with respiration has been the main concern for radiation delivery. Since the early 1990s, researchers have targeted spine as well as body tumors by radiosurgery. Lax and colleagues in 1994 described a vacuum pad stabilizer for fractionated delivery of radiation to extracranial soft tissue tumors.[114] Between 1991 and 1996, 50 patients with various soft tissue tumors were treated using one to five fractions of 15 to 45 Gy per fraction. The indications included primary and secondary hepatic and thoracic tumors. In 1995, Hamilton and colleagues devised a skeletal fixation frame for spinal radiosurgery. Their group reported treatment of 12 patients with spinal tumors (mostly metastatic) using LINAC radiosurgery.[115]

Frameless stereotactic localization appears ideal for spine and body radiosurgery. In this regard, the Cyberknife seems to be a promising radiosurgery system. A limited number of patients of spine and soft tissue tumors have been treated with the Cyberknife.[116] The concept of extracranial radiosurgery seems promising. More studies, however, are needed to study the long-term effect of radiosurgery on the spinal cord.

FUTURE DEVELOPMENTS

Rapid developments in neuroimaging, stereotactic techniques, and robotic technology in the 1990s contributed to improved results and wider applications of radiosurgery. The indications of radiosurgery are expanding, leading to the observation that more and more patients opt for radiosurgery rather than microsurgery. Radiosurgery has become a preferred management modality for many intracranial tumors. The desirable outcome of radiosurgery is dependent on the surgeon's ability to differentiate the target from the normal tissue. This is, however, not always possible. The development of cell-specific radiation response modifiers in the future may enhance the radiation response of the target cells and at the same time protect the normal tissue. Approaches like this would be especially helpful in treating small functional pituitary adenomas effectively without causing panhypopituitarism. Similarly, small, well-circumscribed tumors located in deep and critical brain locations would be treated more effectively in the future. Although radiosurgery provides survival benefits in diffuse malignant brain tumors, cure still is not possible. Microscopic tumor infiltration into surrounding normal tissue is the main cause of recurrence. Viral vector–based gene transfer in combination with chemotherapy and radiosurgery may prove to be a promising strategy. In the future, gene transfer to sensitize malignant tumor cells to radiosurgery may provide better tumor control and improve survival. Basic research will continue to enhance our understanding of the differential radiobiologic effect of radiosurgery on different tissues. Multicenter trials in the future will establish the role of radiosurgery compared with other treatment modalities in controlling intracranial tumors.

REFERENCES

1. Alexander E 3rd, Kooy HM, Herk MV, et al: Magnetic resonance image–directed stereotactic neurosurgery: Use of image fusion with computerized tomography to enhance spatial accuracy. J Neurosurg 83:271–276, 1995.
2. Burchiel KJ, Nguyen TT, Coombs BD, et al: MRI distortion and stereotactic neurosurgery using the Cosman-Robert-Wells and Leksell frames. Stereotact Funct Neurosurg 66:123–136, 1996.
3. Kondziolka D, Dempsey PK, Lunsford LD, et al: A comparison between magnetic resonance imaging and computed tomography for stereotactic coordinate determination. Neurosurgery 30:402–407, 1992.
4. Flickinger JC, Kondziolka D, Lunsford LD: Dose selection in stereotactic radiosurgery. Neurosurg Clin North Am 10:271–280, 1999.
5. Flickinger JC, Deutsch M, Lunsford LD: Repeat megavoltage

irradiation of pituitary and suprasellar tumors. Int J Radiat Oncol Biol Phys 17:171–175, 1989.

6. Leksell L: A note on the treatment of acoustic tumors. Acta Chir Scand 137:763–765, 1971.

7. Norén G, Greitz D, Hirsch A: Gamma knife radiosurgery in acoustic neurinoma. In Steiner L, Lindquist C, Forester D, Backlund EO (eds): Radiosurgery: Baseline and Trends. New York, Raven Press, 1992, pp 141–148.

8. Flickinger JC, Kondziolka D, Pollock BE, et al: Evolution in technique for vestibular schwannoma radiosurgery and effect on outcome. Int J Radiat Oncol Biol Phys 36:275–280, 1996.

9. Norén G: Long-term complication following gamma knife radiosurgery of vestibular schwannomas. Stereotact Funct Neurosurg 70(Suppl 1):65–73, 1998.

10. Linskey ME, Flickinger JC, Lunsford LD: Cranial nerve length predicts the risk of delayed facial and trigeminal neuropathies after acoustic tumor stereotactic radiosurgery. Int J Radiat Oncol Biol Phys 25:227–233, 1993.

11. Lunsford LD, Kondziolka D, Flickinger JC: Stereotactic radiosurgery as an alternative to microsurgery for the treatment of acoustic neurinomas. Clin Neurosurg 38:619–634, 1991.

12. Thomassin JM, Epron JP, Regis J, et al: Preservation of hearing in acoustic neuromas treated by gamma knife surgery. Stereotact Funct Neurosurg 70(Suppl 1):74–79, 1998.

13. Niranjan A, Lunsford LD, Flickinger JC, et al: Dose reduction improves hearing preservation rates after intracanalicular acoustic tumor radiosurgery. Neurosurgery 45:753–765, 1999.

14. Gardner G, Robertson JA: Hearing preservation in unilateral acoustic neurinoma surgery. Ann Otol Rhinol Laryngol 97:55–66, 1988.

15. House JW, Brackmann DE. Facial nerve grading system. Otolaryngol Head Neck Surg 93:146–147, 1985.

16. Nadol JB Jr, Chiong CM, Ojemann RG, et al: Preservation of hearing and facial nerve function in resection of acoustic neuroma. Laryngoscope 102:1153–1158, 1992.

17. Samii M, Matthies C: Management of 1000 vestibular schwannomas (acoustic neuromas): Hearing function in 1000 tumor resections. Neurosurgery 40:248–262, 1997.

18. Gormley WB, Sekhar LN, Wright DC, et al: Acoustic neuromas: Results of current surgical management. Neurosurgery 41:50–60, 1997.

19. Fahlbusch R, Neu M, Strauss C: Preservation of hearing in large acoustic neurinomas following removal via suboccipito-lateral approach. Acta Neurochir 140:771–777, 1998.

20. Colletti V, Fiorino FG: Retrosigmoid-transmeatal en bloc removal of small to medium-sized acoustic neuromas. Otolaryngol Head Neck Surg 120:122–128, 1999.

21. Cerullo L, Grutsch J, Osterdock R: Recurrence of vestibular (acoustic) schwannomas in surgical patients where preservation of facial and cochlear nerve is the priority. Br J Neurosurg 12:547–552, 1998.

22. Wigand DA, Ojemann RG, Fickel V: Surgical treatment of acoustic neuroma (vestibular schwannoma) in the United States: Report from the Acoustic Neuroma Registry. Laryngoscope 106:58–66, 1996.

23. Pollock BE, Lunsford LD, Kondziolka D, et al: Outcome analysis of acoustic neuroma management: A comparison of microsurgery and stereotactic radiosurgery. Neurosurgery 36:215–229, 1995.

24. Shelton C, Hitselberg WE, House WE, et al: Hearing preservation after acoustic tumor removal: Long-term results. Laryngoscope 100:115–119, 1990.

25. Wiegand DA, Fickel V: Acoustic neuroma: The patient's perspective—subjective assessment of symptoms, diagnosis, therapy, and outcome in 541 patients. Laryngoscope 99:179–187, 1989.

26. Kobayashi T, Tanaka T, Kida Y: The early effects of gamma knife on 40 cases of acoustic neuroma. Acta Neurochir Suppl (Wien) 62:93–97, 1994.

27. Norén G: Gamma knife radiosurgery for acoustic neurinomas. In Gildenberg PL, Tasker RR (eds): Textbook of Stereotactic and Functional Neurosurgery. New York, McGraw-Hill, 1998, pp 835–844.

28. Lunsford LD, Kondziolka D, Flickinger JC: Acoustic neuroma management: Evolution and revolution. In Kondziolka D (ed): Radiosurgery, vol 2. Basel, Karger, 1998, pp 1–7.

29. Kondziolka D, Lunsford LD, McLaughlin M, et al: Long-term outcome after radiosurgery for acoustic neuromas. N Engl J Med 339:1426–1433, 1998.

30. Foote KD, Friedman WA, Buatti JM, et al: Linear accelerator radiosurgery in brain tumor management. Neurosurg Clin North Am 10:203–242, 1999.

31. Simpson D: The recurrence of intracranial meningiomas after surgical excision. J Neurol Neurosurg Psychiatry 20:22–39, 1957.

32. Black PM: Meningiomas. Neurosurgery 32:643–657, 1993.

33. McDermott MW, Wilson CB: Meningiomas. In Yomans JR (ed): Neurological Surgery: A Comprehensive Reference Guide to the Diagnosis and Management of Neurological Problems, 4th ed. Philadelphia, WB Saunders, 1996, pp 2782–2825.

34. Awad IA, Kalfas I, Hahn JF: Intracranial meningioma in the aged: Surgical outcome in the era of computed tomography. Neurosurgery 24:557, 1989.

35. Djindjian M, Caron JP, Athayde AA, et al: Intracranial meningioma in the elderly (over 70 years old): A retrospective study of 30 surgical cases. Acta Neurochir (Wien) 90:121–123, 1988.

36. Condra K, Buatti J, Mendenhall WM, et al: Benign meningiomas: Primary treatment selection affects survival. Int J Radiat Oncol Biol Phys 37:427–436, 1997.

37. Pendl G, Schrottner O, Eustacchio S, et al: Stereotactic radiosurgery of skull base meningiomas. Minim Invasive Neurosurg 40:87–90, 1997.

38. Chang SD, Adler JR: Treatment of cranial base meningiomas with linear accelerator radiosurgery. Neurosurgery 41:1019–1025, 1997.

39. Lunsford LD, Kondziolka D, Flickinger JC: Deep brain surgery using the gamma knife. In Gildenberg PL, Tasker RR (eds): Textbook of Stereotactic and Functional Neurosurgery. New York, McGraw-Hill, 1998, pp 763–803.

40. Shafron DH, Friedman WA, Buatti JM, et al: Linac radiosurgery for benign meningiomas. Int J Radiat Oncol Biol Phys 43:321–327, 1999.

41. Hakim R, Alexander E 3rd, Loeffler JS, et al: Results of linear accelerator-based radiosurgery for intracranial meningiomas. Neurosurgery 42:446–453, 1998.

42. Steiner L, Prasad D, Lindquist C, et al: Clinical aspects of gamma knife stereotactic radiosurgery. In Gildenberg PL, Tasker RR (eds): Textbook of Stereotactic and Functional Neurosurgery. New York, McGraw-Hill, 1998, pp 763–803.

43. Colombo F, Francescon P: Clinical linear accelerator radiosurgery. In Gildenberg PL, Tasker RR (eds): Textbook of Stereotactic and Functional Neurosurgery. New York, McGraw-Hill, 1998, pp 757–762.

44. Kondziolka D, Levy EI, Niranjan A, et al: Long-term outcomes after meningioma radiosurgery: Physician and patient perspectives. J Neurosurg 91:44–50, 1999.

45. Liscak R, Simonova G, Vymazal J, et al: Gamma knife radiosurgery of meningiomas in the cavernous sinus region. Acta Neurochir 141:473–480, 1999.

46. Chang SD, Adler JR, Martin DP: LINAC radiosurgery for cavernous sinus meningiomas. Stereotact Funct Neurosurg 71:43–50, 1998.

47. Pendl G, Schrottner O, Eustacchio S, et al: Cavernous sinus meningiomas. What is the strategy: Upfront or adjuvant gamma knife surgery? Stereotact Funct Neurosurg 70(Suppl 1):33–40, 1998.

48. Muthukumar N, Kondziolka D, Lunsford LD, et al: Stereotactic radiosurgery for anterior foramen magnum meningiomas. Surg Neurol 51:268–273, 1999.

49. Lunsford LD: Contemporary management of meningiomas: Radiation therapy as an adjuvant and radiosurgery as an alternative to surgical removal? J Neurosurg 80:187–190, 1994.

50. Subach BR, Lunsford LD, Kondziolka D: Management of petroclival meningiomas by stereotactic radiosurgery. Neurosurgery 42:437–443, 1998.

51. Morita A, Coffey RJ, Foote RL, et al: Risk of injury to cranial nerves after gamma knife radiosurgery for skull base meningiomas: Experience in 88 patients. J Neurosurg 90:42–49, 1999.

52. Kondziolka D, Flickinger JC, Perez B, et al: Judicious resection and/or radiosurgery for parasagittal meningiomas: Outcomes from a multicenter review: Gamma Knife Meningioma Study Group. Neurosurgery 43:405–413, 1998.

53. Ciric I, Mikhail M, Stafford T, et al.: Transsphenoidal microsurgery of pituitary adenomas with long-term follow-up results. J Neurosurg 59:395–401, 1983.

54. Tindall GT, Herring CJ, Clark RV, et al: Cushing disease: Results of transsphenoidal microsurgery with emphasis on surgical failures. J Neurosurg 72:363–369, 1990.

55. Tindall GT, Oyesiku NM, Watts NB, et al: Transsphenoidal adenomectomy for growth hormone secreting adenomas in acromegaly: Outcome analysis and determination of failures. J Neurosurg 78:205–215, 1993.

56. Laws ER Jr, Fode NC, Redmond MJ: Transsphenoidal surgery following unsuccessful prior therapy. J Neurosurg 63:823–829, 1985.

57. Flickinger JC, Nelson PB, Martinez AJ, et al: Radiotherapy of nonfunctional adenomas of pituitary gland. Cancer 63:2409–2414, 1989.

58. Salinger DJ, Brady LW, Miyamoto CT: Radiation therapy in the treatment of pituitary adenomas. Am J Oncol 15:467–473, 1992.

59. Zeirhut D, Flentje M, Adolph J, et al: External radiotherapy of pituitary adenomas. Int J Radiat Oncol Biol Phys 33:307–314, 1995.

60. Witt TC, Kondziolka D, Flickinger JC, et al: Gamma knife radiosurgery for pituitary tumors. In Lunsford LD, Kondziolka D, Flickinger JC (eds): Gamma Knife Brain Surgery, vol 14. Basel, Karger, 1998, pp 114–127.

61. Ganz JC, Backlund EO, Thorsen FA: The effects of gamma knife surgery of pituitary adenomas on tumor growth and endocrinopathies. Stereotact Funct Neurosurg 61(Suppl 1):30–37, 1993.

62. Kjellberg RN, Kliman B: Lifetime effectiveness—a system of therapy for pituitary adenomas, emphasizing Bragg peak proton hypophysectomy. In Linfoot JA (ed): Recent Advances in the Diagnosis and Treatment of Pituitary Tumors. New York, Raven Press, 1979, pp 269–288.

63. Kjellberg RN, Abbe M: Stereotactic Bragg peak proton therapy. In Lunsford LD (ed): Modern Stereotactic Neurosurgery. Boston, Martinus-Nijhoff, 1988, pp 463–470.

64. Levy RP, Fabricant JI, Frankel KA, et al: Heavy charged particle radiosurgery of pituitary gland: Clinical results of 840 patients. Stereotact Funct Neurosurg 57:22–35, 1991.

65. Thoren M, Rahn T, Guo WY, et al: Stereotactic radiosurgery with the cobalt-60 gamma unit in the treatment of growth hormone–producing pituitary tumors. Neurosurgery 29:663–668, 1991.

66. Lunsford LD, Witt TC, Kondziolka D, et al: Stereotactic radiosurgery of anterior skull base tumors. Clin Neurosurg 42:99–118, 1995.

67. Voges J, Sturm V, Deuss U, et al: LINAC radiosurgery in pituitary adenomas: Preliminary results. Acta Neurochir 65(Suppl): 41–43, 1996.

68. Rahn T, Thoren M, Werner S: Stereotactic radiosurgery in pituitary adenomas. In Faglia G, Beck-Peccoz P, Ambrosi B, et al (eds): Pituitary Adenomas: New Trends in Basic and Clinical Research. New York, Excerpta Medica, 1991, pp 303–312.

69. Laws ER, Vance ML: Radiosurgery for pituitary tumors and craniopharyngiomas. Neurosurg Clin North Am 10:327–336, 1999.

70. Rocher FP, Sentenac I, Berger C, et al: Stereotactic radiosurgery: The Lyon experience. Acta Neurochir Suppl (Wien) 63:109–114, 1995.

71. Salcman M: Survival in glioblastoma: Historical perspective. Neurosurgery 7:435–439, 1980.

72. Alexander E 3rd, Loeffler JS. The role of radiosurgery for glial neoplasms. Neurosurg Clin North Am 10:351–358, 1999.

73. Mehta MP: Radiosurgery of malignant brain tumors. In de Salles AAF, Lufkin RB (eds): Minimally Invasive Therapy of the Brain. New York, Thieme, 1997, pp 213–224.

74. Sheline DC, Wara WM, Smith V: Therapeutic irradiation and brain injury. Int J Radiat Oncol Biol Phys 6:1215, 1980.

75. Gaspar LE, Fisher BJ, MacDonald DR, et al: Malignant glioma: Timing of response to radiation therapy. Int J Radiat Oncol Biol Phys 25:877–879, 1993.

76. Wallner KE, Galicich JH, Krol G, et al: Patterns of failure following treatment for glioblastoma multiforme and anaplastic astrocytoma. Int J Radiat Oncol Biol Phys 16:1405–1409, 1989.

77. Green SB, Shapiro WR, Burger PC, et al: A randomized trial of the interstitial brachytherapy boost for newly diagnosed malignant glioma: Brain Tumor Cooperative Group Trial 8701. Proc Am Soc Clin Oncol 13:174, 1994.

78. Shafman TD, Loeffler JS. Novel radiation technologies for malignant gliomas. Curr Opin Oncol 11:147–151, 1999.

79. Flickinger JC, Kondziolka D, Lunsford LD: Clinical applications of stereotactic radiosurgery. Cancer Treat Res 93:283–297, 1998.

80. Kondziolka D, Flickinger JC, Bissonette DJ, et al: Survival benefit of stereotactic radiosurgery for patients with malignant glial neoplasms. Neurosurgery 41:776–785, 1997.

81. Loeffler JS, Alexander E, Shea WM, et al: Radiosurgery as part of the initial management of patients with malignant gliomas. J Clin Oncol 10:1379–1385, 1992.

82. Coffey RJ: Boost gamma knife radiosurgery in the treatment of primary glial tumors. Stereotact Funct Neurosurg 61(Suppl 1): 59–64, 1993.

83. Masciopinto JE, Levin AB, Mehta MP, et al: Stereotactic radiosurgery for glioblastoma: A final report of 31 patients. J Neurosurg 82:530–533, 1995.

84. Sarkaria JN, Mehta MP, Loeffler JS, et al: Radiosurgery in the initial management of malignant gliomas: Survival comparison with the RTOG recursive partitioning analysis. Int J Radiat Oncol Biol Phys 32:931–944, 1995.

85. Gannett D, Baldassarre S, Lulu B, et al: Stereotactic radiosurgery as an adjunct to surgery and external beam radiotherapy in the treatment of patients with malignant gliomas. Int J Radiat Oncol Biol Phys 33:461–468, 1995.

86. Hall WA, Djalilian HR, Sperduto PW, et al: Stereotactic radiosurgery for recurrent malignant gliomas. J Clin Oncol 13:1642–1648, 1995.

87. Alexander E III, Loffler JS: Radiosurgery for primary malignant brain tumors. Semin Surg Oncol 14:43–52, 1998.

88. Curran WJ, Scott CB, Horton J, et al: Recursive partitioning analysis of prognostic factors in three Radiation Therapy Oncology Group malignant glioma group trials. J Natl Cancer Inst 85:704–710, 1993.

89. Shrieve DC, Alexander E 3rd, Black PM, et al.: Treatment of patients with primary glioblastoma multiforme with standard postoperative radiotherapy and radiosurgical boost: Prognostic factors and long-term outcome. J Neurosurg 90:72–77, 1999.

90. de Crevoisier R, Pierga JY, Dendale R, et al: Radiotherapy of glioblastoma. Cancer Radiother 1:194–207, 1997.

91. Borgelt B, Gelber R, Kramer S, et al: The palliation of brain metastases: Final results of the first two studies by the Radiation Therapy Oncology Group. Int J Radiat Oncol Biol Phys 6:1–8, 1980.

92. Diener-West M, Dobbins TW, Phillips TL, et al: Identification of an optimal subgroup for treatment evaluation of patients with brain metastases using RTOG Study 7916. Int J Radiat Oncol Biol Phys 16:669–673, 1989.

93. Patchell RA, Tibbs PA, Walsh JW, et al: A randomized trial of surgery in the treatment of single metastases to the brain. N Engl J Med 322:494–500, 1990.

94. Lishner M, Feld R, Payne DG, et al: Late neurological complications after prophylactic cranial irradiation in patients with small-cell lung cancer: The Toronto experience. J Clin Oncol 8: 215–221, 1990.

95. Alexander E 3rd, Moriarty TM, Davis RB, et al: Stereotactic radiosurgery for the definitive, noninvasive treatment of brain metastases. J Natl Cancer Inst 87:34–40, 1995.

96. Flickinger JC, Kondziolka D, Lunsford LD, et al: A multi-institution experience with stereotactic radiosurgery for solitary brain metastases. Int J Radiat Oncol Biol Phys 28:797–802, 1994.

97. Shiau CY, Sneed PK, Shu HK, et al: Radiosurgery for brain metastases: Relationship of dose and pattern of enhancement to local control. Int J Radiat Oncol Biol Phys 37:375–383, 1997.

98. Kihlström L, Karlsson B, Lindquist C: Gamma knife surgery for cerebral metastases: Implications for survival based on 16-year experience. Stereotact Funct Neurosurg 61(Suppl):45–55, 1993.

99. Valentino V: The results of radiosurgery management of 139 single cerebral metastases. Acta Neurochir Suppl (Wien) 63: 95–100, 1995.

100. Fukuoka S, Seo Y, Takanashi M, et al: Radiosurgery of brain metastases with the gamma knife. Stereotact Funct Neurosurg 66(Suppl 1):193–200, 1996.

101. Gerosa M, Nicolato A, Severi F, et al: Gamma knife radiosurgery for intracranial metastases: From local tumor control to increased survival. Stereotact Funct Neurosurg 66(Suppl 1):184–192, 1996.
102. Joseph J, Adler JR, Cox RS, et al: Linear accelerator based stereotaxic radiosurgery for brain metastases: The influence of number of lesions on survival. J Clin Oncol 14:1085–1092, 1996.
103. Kim YS, Kondziolka D, Flickinger JC, et al: Stereotactic radiosurgery for patients with nonsmall cell lung carcinoma metastatic to brain. Cancer 80:2075–2083, 1997.
104. Breneman JC, Warnic RE, Albright RE, et al: Stereotactic radiosurgery for treatment of brain metastases. Cancer 79:551–557, 1997.
105. Smalley SR, Schray MF, Laws ER Jr, et al: Adjuvant radiation therapy after surgical resection of solitary brain metastases: Association with pattern of failure and survival. Int J Radiat Oncol Biol Phys 13:1611–1616, 1987.
106. Noordijk EM, Berberich W, Nestle U, et al: The choice of treatment of single brain metastases should be based on extracranial tumor activity and age. Int J Radiat Oncol Biol Phys 29:711–717, 1994.
107. Mintz AH, Kestle J, Rathbone MP, et al: A randomized trial to assess the efficacy of surgery in addition to radiotherapy in patients with single cerebral metastases. Cancer 78:1470–1476, 1996.
108. Rutigliano M, Lunsford LD, Kondziolka D, et al: The cost effectiveness of stereotactic radiosurgery versus surgical resection in the treatment of solitary metastatic brain tumors. Neurosurgery 37:445–455, 1995.
109. Hug EB, Loredo LN, Slater JD, et al: Proton radiation therapy for chordomas and chondrosarcomas of the skull base. J Neurosurg 91:432–439, 1999.
110. Muthukumar N, Kondziolka D, Lunsford LD, Flickinger JC: Stereotactic radiosurgery for chordoma and chondrosarcoma: Further experiences. Int J Radiat Oncol Biol Phys 41:387–392, 1998.
111. Huang CF, Kondziolka D, Flickinger JC, et al: Stereotactic radiosurgery for trigeminal schwannomas. Neurosurgery 45:11–16, 1999.
112. Muthukumar N, Kondziolka D, Flickinger JC, et al: Stereotactic radiosurgery for jugular foramen schwannomas. Surg Neurol 52:173–178, 1999.
113. Subach BR, Lunsford LD, Kondziolka D: Stereotactic radiosurgery in the treatment of pineal region tumors. In Lunsford LD, Kondziolka D, Flickinger JC (eds): Gamma Knife Radiosurgery, vol 14. Basel, Karger, 1998, pp 175–194.
114. Lax I, Blomgren H, Naslund I, et al: Stereotactic radiosurgery of malignancies in the abdomen: Methodological aspects. Acta Oncol 33:677–683, 1994.
115. Hamilton AJ, Lulu BA, Fosmire H, et al: LINAC-based spinal stereotactic radiosurgery. Stereotact Funct Neurosurg 66:1–9. 1996.
116. Chang SD, Murphy M, Geis P, et al: Clinical experience with image-guided robotic radiosurgery (the Cyberknife) in the treatment of brain and spinal cord tumors. Neurol Med Chir 38:780–783, 1998.

Radiosurgery for Arteriovenous Malformations

WILLIAM A. FRIEDMAN ■ KELLY D. FOOTE

The most devastating presentation associated with arteriovenous malformations (AVMs) of the brain is intracerebral hemorrhage. Numerous natural history studies have demonstrated a substantial (3% to 4% per year) risk of hemorrhage in patients harboring AVMs.[1-5] There are several treatment modalities (microsurgery, radiosurgery, or endovascular therapy) available that may eliminate the lesion before a hemorrhage can occur—or recur in the case of a hemorrhagic presentation. When an AVM is amenable to safe microsurgical resection, this therapy is preferred because it offers immediate cure and elimination of hemorrhage risk. When the surgical morbidity is judged to be excessive, radiosurgery offers a reasonable expectation of delayed cure.

Stereotactic radiosurgery is the application of a single, high dose of radiation to a stereotactically defined target volume. It is a unique hybrid of surgery and radiation therapy and has become an important tool for the treatment of various intracranial lesions. When an AVM is treated with radiosurgery, a pathologic process appears to be induced that is similar to the response-to-injury model of atherosclerosis. Radiation injury to the vascular endothelium is believed to induce the proliferation of smooth muscle cells and the elaboration of extracellular collagen, which leads to progressive stenosis and obliteration of the AVM nidus,[6-10] thereby eliminating the risk of hemorrhage.

The advantages of radiosurgery, compared with microsurgical and endovascular treatments, are that it is noninvasive, has a minimal risk of acute complications, and is performed as an outpatient procedure requiring no recovery time for the patient. The primary disadvantage of radiosurgery is that cure is not immediate. Although thrombosis of the lesion is achieved in the majority of cases, it commonly does not occur until 2 or 3 years after treatment. During the interval between radiosurgical treatment and AVM thrombosis, the risk of hemorrhage remains. Another potential disadvantage of radiosurgery is the possible long-term adverse effects of radiation. Finally, radiosurgery has been shown to be much less effective for lesions greater than 10 cc in volume. For these reasons, selection of an appropriate treatment modality is dependent on multiple variables, including perceived risks of surgery and predicted likelihood of hemorrhage for a given patient.

RADIOSURGERY TECHNIQUE

The technical methods of radiosurgery have been described at length in other publications,[11] but a brief description of radiosurgical techniques—with emphasis on points specifically applicable to AVM treatment—is in order. The fundamental elements of a successful radiosurgical treatment are the same regardless of the system (i.e., modified linear accelerator, gamma knife, or particle beam) being used to deliver the stereotactically focused radiation. They include:

- Appropriate patient selection
- Application of stereotactic fiducial markers that are fixed in position relative to the skull (most commonly via a head ring and stereotactic frame-localizer)
- Acquisition of quality three-dimensional stereotactic images and transfer of this image database to a dose planning computer
- Use of the computer to formulate an optimal plan (dose distribution) for radiation delivery
- Selection of an appropriate treatment dose
- Precision radiation delivery that faithfully executes the plan
- Careful clinical and radiographic patient follow-up

All these elements are critical, and the poor performance of any step will result in suboptimal results.

Patient Selection

Open surgery is generally favored if an AVM is amenable to low-risk resection (e.g., low Spetzler-Martin grade; young, healthy patient) or is felt to be at high risk for hemorrhage during the latency period between radiosurgical treatment and AVM obliteration (e.g., associated aneurysm, prior hemorrhage, large AVM with diffuse morphologic features, venous outflow obstruction).

Radiosurgery is favored when the AVM nidus is small (<3 cm) and compact, when surgery is judged to carry a high risk or is refused by the patient, and when the risk of hemorrhage is not felt to be extraordinarily high.

Endovascular treatment, although rarely curative alone, may be useful as a preoperative adjunct to either microsurgery or radiosurgery.

The history, physical examination, and diagnostic imaging of each patient are evaluated, and the various factors outlined previously are weighed in combination to determine the best treatment approach for a given case.

Head Ring Application

Current stereotactic radiosurgical methodology requires attachment of a stereotactic head ring. The rigidly attached ring enables the acquisition of spatially accurate information from angiography, computed tomography (CT), and magnetic resonance imaging (MRI). The images obtained with the ring (and an attached stereotactic localizer) in place establish fixed relationships between the ring and the target lesion. These spatial relationships provide the substrate for computer-based treatment planning and are later translated from radiographic (virtual) space into real space so that the treatment target can be placed accurately at the precise isocenter of the radiation delivery device. Because the stereotactic head ring is bolted to the treatment delivery device, it also immobilizes the patient during treatment.

In general, patients are premedicated with 10 mg of oral diazepam approximately 0.5 hour before ring application. Premedication is optional. No skin shaving or scalp preparation is required. The ring and posts are assembled and positioned to fit the patient, taking care to avoid accidental placement of pins into a burr hole, over a shunt path, or onto a bone flap from a prior craniotomy. The pin sites are anesthetized with a local injection of lidocaine plus bupivacaine, and the aluminum-tipped (CT-compatible) pins are hand-tightened with a dedicated wrench that is then attached to the ring to ensure its ready availability for ring removal. At the conclusion of this procedure, the patient is transferred to a wheelchair and transported to the radiology department for the next step (imaging) in the radiosurgery process.

Stereotactic Image Acquisition

The most problematic aspect of AVM radiosurgery is target identification. In some series (see further on), targeting error is listed as the most frequent cause of radiosurgical failure. The problem lies with imaging. Although angiography effectively defines blood flow (feeding arteries, nidus, and draining veins), it does so in only two dimensions. Using the two-dimensional data from stereotactic angiography to represent the three-dimensional target results in significant errors of both overestimation and underestimation of AVM ni-

dus dimensions (Fig. 269–1).[12, 13] Underestimation of the nidus size may result in treatment failure, whereas overestimation results in the inclusion of normal brain within the treatment volume. This can cause radiation damage to normal brain, which—when affecting an eloquent area—may result in a neurologic deficit. To avoid such targeting errors, a true three-dimensional image database is required. Contrast-enhanced CT and MRI are commonly used for this purpose.

Diagnostic (nonstereotactic) angiography is used to characterize the AVM, but because of its inherent inadequacies as a treatment planning database, stereotactic angiography has been largely abandoned at our institution. We use contrast-enhanced, stereotactic CT as a targeting image database for the vast majority of AVMs. Our CT technique uses rapid infusion (1 mL/sec) of contrast while scanning through the AVM nidus with 1-mm slices. The head ring is bolted to a bracket at the head of the CT table, ensuring that the head-ring-localizer complex remains immobile during the scan (Fig. 269–2). This technique yields a clear three-dimensional picture of the nidus (Fig. 269–3). Alternative approaches use MRI–magnetic resonance angiography (MRA) instead of CT. Attention to optimal image sequences in both CT and MRI is essential for effective AVM radiosurgical targeting.

Once the stereotactic scans are completed, the images are transferred via Ethernet to the treatment planning computer. The fiducial markers on the stereotactic localizer are automatically identified in each image, and the dose planning software uses these reference points to define a three-dimensional Cartesian coordinate system relative to the head ring. Spatial coordinates are assigned to each point (pixel) in each computed tomographic slice. Because the ring remains fixed relative to the patient's skull during treatment, any point in the virtual volume defined by the computed tomographic scan (including the entire head, and, most importantly, the AVM nidus) can be mapped precisely to a point in real space.

Treatment Planning

Once the necessary stereotactic images have been acquired and transferred to the treatment planning computer, the next step is to plan the precise delivery of radiation. This is accomplished through the use of a computer workstation and specialized treatment planning software "tools." The methodology of treatment planning varies somewhat depending on the radiosurgery system and software used, but the objectives and basic principles of radiosurgery dose planning are universal.

The fundamental principle of radiosurgery is the delivery of focal, high-dose radiation to a designated intracranial target—in this case the nidus of the AVM—while sparing the surrounding normal brain tissue. This is accomplished by focusing hundreds of nonparallel radiation beams on a stereotactically defined target. When the effect of these beams is aver-

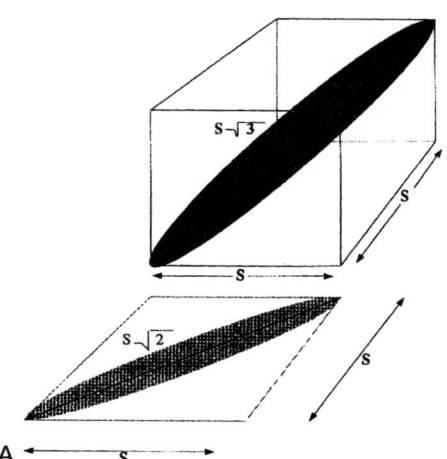

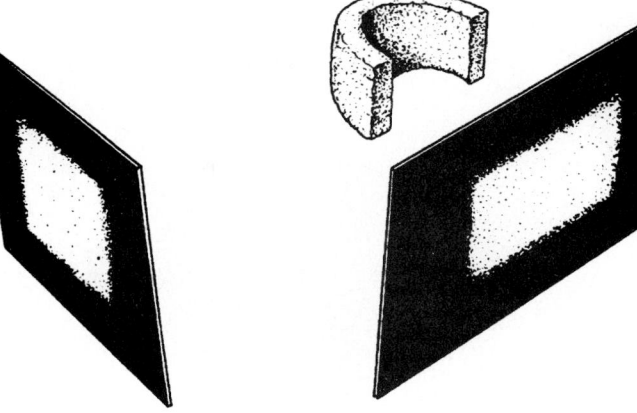

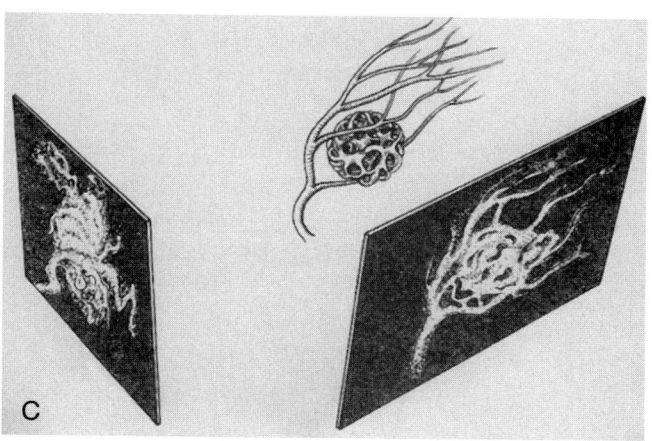

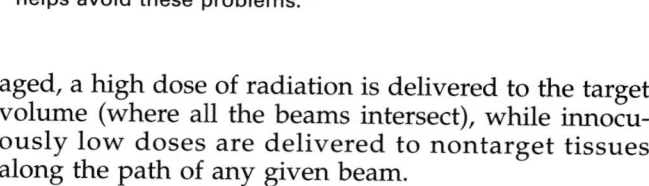

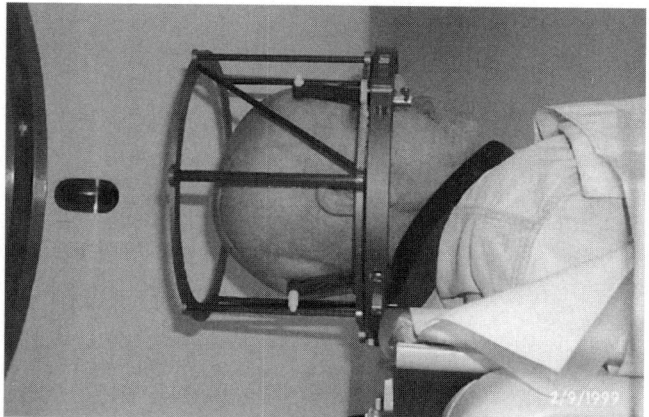

FIGURE 269–1. The use of stereotactic angiography as an image database for radiosurgery dose planning can result in inaccurate target identification. *A,* Underestimation of the nidus occurs when the nidal axis is not parallel to either anteroposterior (AP) or lateral angiographic projections. This can result in exclusion of part of the nidus from the target volume, which is a common cause of radiosurgical failure. *B,* Overestimation of the nidus occurs when angiographic projections fail to represent concave regions of the nidal contour. This can result in the irradiation of normal brain tissue interposed in the concavities of the nidus, increasing the risk of neural injury and radiation induced complications. *C,* Identification of the nidus can also be difficult on angiography because of the presence of overlying feeding arteries and draining veins. This spherical nidus is difficult to discern clearly on AP and lateral angiographic projections. Use of a truly three-dimensional image database (e.g., stereotactic computed tomography [CT] or magnetic resonance imaging [MRI]) helps avoid these problems.

aged, a high dose of radiation is delivered to the target volume (where all the beams intersect), while innocuously low doses are delivered to nontarget tissues along the path of any given beam.

FIGURE 269–2. This patient is ready for stereotactic CT scanning. The head ring is bolted to a bracket at the head of the CT table, and the stereotactic localizer is attached to the ring. The positions of the vertical and diagonal localizer rods in each computed tomographic image are used to locate each pixel in three-dimensional space relative to the head ring.

The primary goal of AVM radiosurgery treatment planning is to develop a plan with a target volume that conforms closely to the surface of the AVM nidus while maintaining a steep *dose gradient* (the rate of change in dose relative to position) away from the nidal surface in order to minimize the radiation dose to surrounding brain. A number of treatment planning tools can be used to tailor the shape of the target volume to fit even highly irregular nidus shapes. Regardless of its shape, the entire nidus—not including the feeding arteries and draining veins—must lie within the target volume (the "prescription isodose shell"), with as little normal brain included as possible (see Fig. 269–3).

Another goal of dose planning is to manipulate the dose gradient so that critical brain structures receive the lowest possible dose of radiation to avoid disabling complications. In addition, many radiosurgeons strive to produce a treatment dose distribution that maximizes uniformity (homogeneity) of dose throughout the entire target volume. A detailed discussion of the methodology of dose planning is beyond the scope of this chapter but can be found elsewhere.[11] Figure 269–4 illustrates a general approach to linear accelerator (LINAC)–based treatment planning. Dose planning is ideally a team effort, with the treating neurosurgeon,

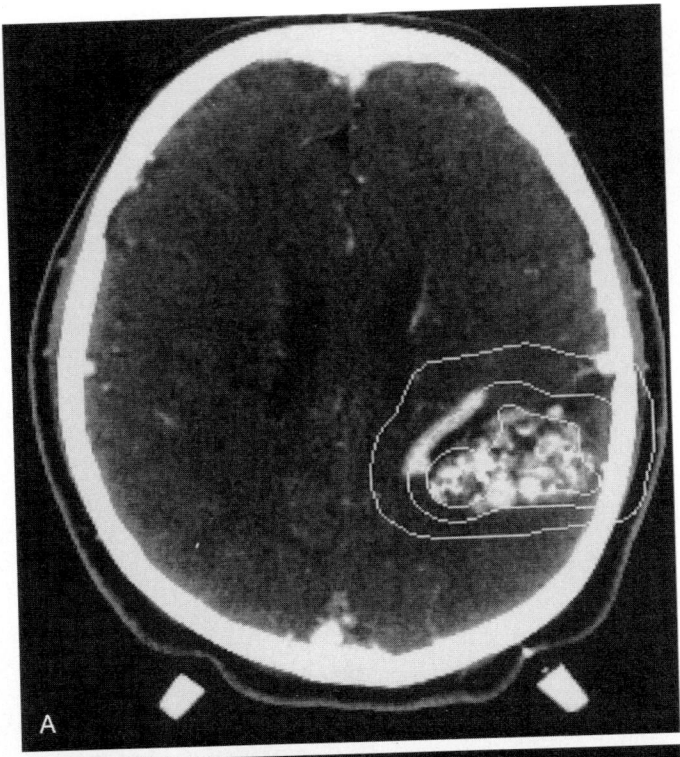

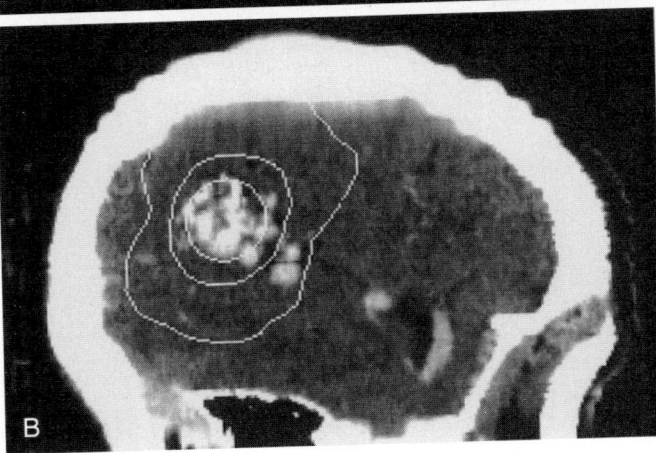

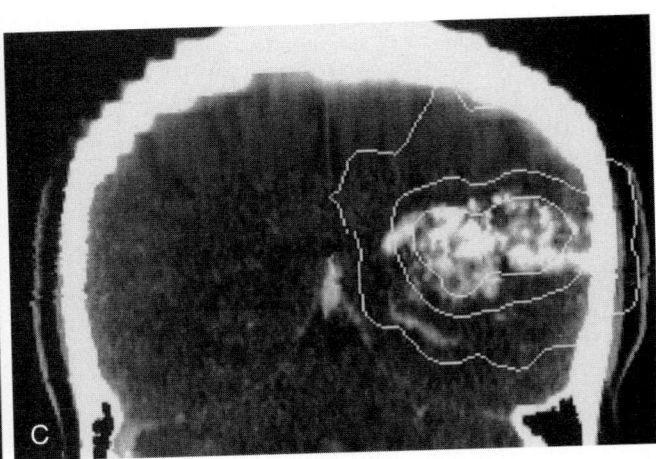

FIGURE 269–3. This 43-year-old male presented with seizures and refused surgical intervention in favor of radiosurgery. His treatment plan, based on a contrast-enhanced computed tomographic database, is shown here (*A*, axial; *B*, sagittal; *C*, coronal). Note the conformality of the innermost (70%) isodose line to the AVM nidus in all planes. The 35% and 14% isodose lines are also shown. This seven-isocenter plan delivered 15 Gy to the 70% isodose shell. The total AVM nidus volume treated was 12 cc.

radiation oncologist, and medical physicist contributing to the development of an optimal plan.

Dose Selection

Once a satisfactory treatment plan has been developed, a dose must be selected. By convention, radiosurgical doses are prescribed to the *isodose shell* (the set of all points in a dose plan that receive the same selected dose) that has been tailored to conform to the surface of the target. Isodose shells are commonly designated as percentages of the maximal dose delivered. For example, a typical AVM dose prescription may read "17.5 Gy to the 70% isodose line." In this case, the 70% isodose shell has been tailored to conform closely to the surface of the AVM nidus and the minimal target

dose of 17.5 Gy is delivered to the periphery of the nidus. Higher doses are delivered within the nidus to a maximum of 25 Gy (17.5 = 70% of 25).

Various analyses of AVM radiosurgery outcomes (described further on) have elucidated an appropriate range of doses for the treatment of AVMs. Minimal doses to the nidus of less than 15 Gy have been associated with a significantly lower rate of AVM obliteration, whereas doses greater than 20 Gy have been associated with a higher rate of permanent neurologic complications. We prescribe doses ranging from 15 Gy to as high as 22.5 Gy to the margin of the AVM nidus, nearly always at the 70% or 80% isodose line. The selection of a dose within this range is made based on the volume of the nidus, as well as the eloquence and radiosensitivity of surrounding brain structures. Lower doses are prescribed for larger lesions and lesions in eloquent areas.

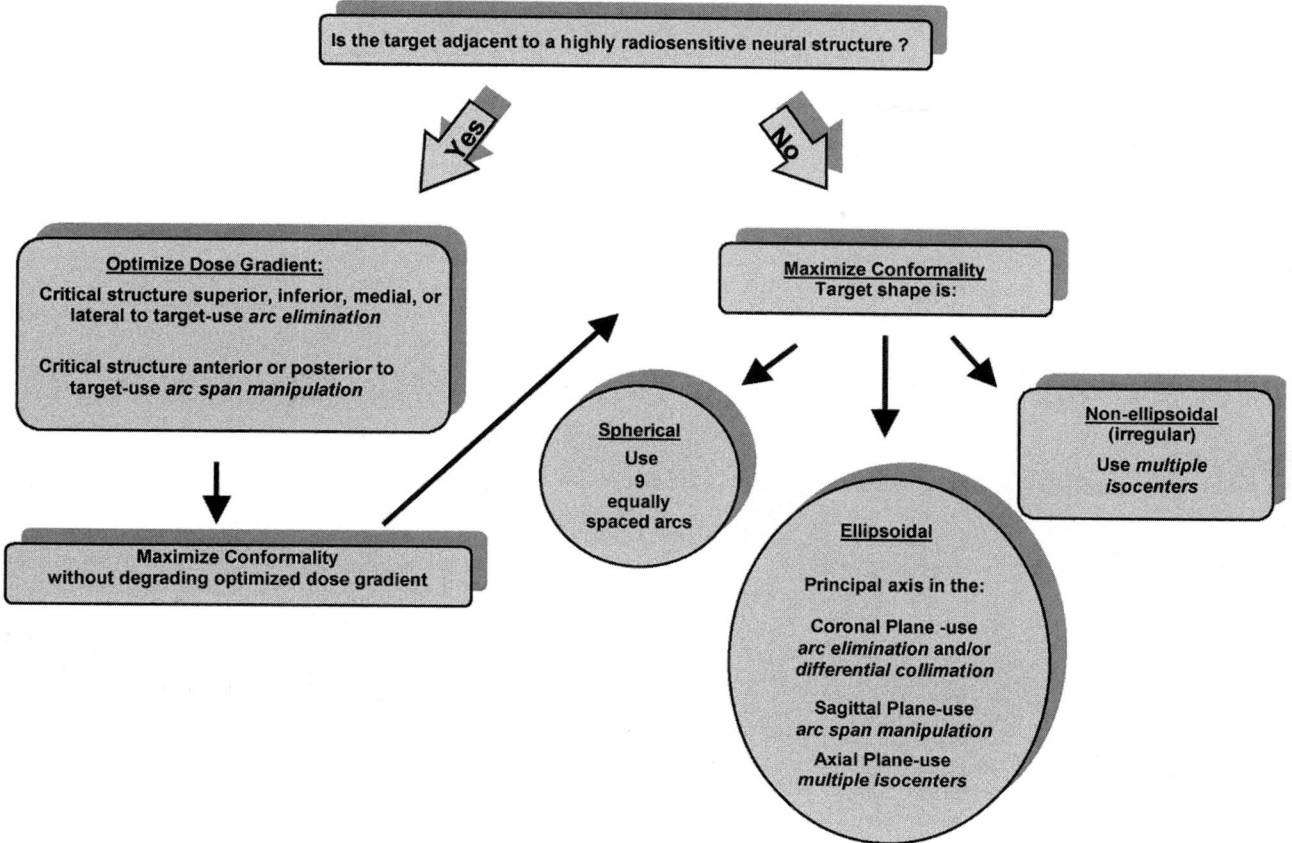

FIGURE 269–4. This algorithm, used at the University of Florida for stereotactic radiosurgery treatment planning, orders the use of various software tools available to LINAC-based radiosurgeons for tailoring the dose distribution to conform optimally to a target lesion.

Radiation Delivery

The next step in the process is the execution of the treatment plan. The patient is placed supine on the couch of the treatment device and the head ring is secured to an immobilizing bracket. The patient's head is positioned so that the focal point of the radiation delivery device (modified LINAC or gamma knife) coincides with the first isocenter in the treatment plan. An appropriately sized collimator is installed to determine the diameter of the beams; many beams of radiation are then directed at the isocenter from various directions. In the case of a LINAC-based system, this is accomplished by rotating the radiation source in several concentric arcs around the isocenter. The gamma knife achieves the same result by exposing the target simultaneously to 201 intersecting radiation beams from independent cobalt sources that are precisely aligned in a hemispherical array around the isocenter.

If the treatment plan includes multiple isocenters, the patient's head is repositioned for each isocenter. The beam collimator is changed when dictated by the treatment plan, and the process is repeated until the entire plan has been executed. The process of radiation delivery is straightforward, but careful attention to de-

tail and the execution of various safety checks and redundancies are necessary to ensure that the prescribed treatment plan is delivered accurately and safely. When radiation delivery has been completed, the head ring is removed and the patient is observed for approximately 30 minutes and then discharged to resume normal activities.

Follow-Up

Standard follow-up after AVM radiosurgery typically consists of annual clinic visits with MRI-MRA to evaluate the effect of the procedure and monitor for neurologic complications. If the patient's clinical status changes, he or she is followed more closely at clinically appropriate intervals.

Each patient is scheduled to undergo cerebral angiography 3 years after radiosurgery, and a definitive assessment of the success or failure of treatment is made based on the results of angiography (see further on). If no flow is observed through the AVM nidus, the patient is pronounced cured and is discharged from follow-up. If the AVM nidus is incompletely obliterated, appropriate further therapy (most commonly repeat radiosurgery on the day of angiography) is prescribed, and the treatment and follow-up cycle is repeated.

REPORTED EFFICACY OF RADIOSURGERY FOR ARTERIOVENOUS MALFORMATIONS

Multiple series have systematically evaluated rates of AVM thrombosis by obtaining follow-up angiograms both 1 and 2 years after radiosurgery. Steiner and associates have published multiple reports on gamma knife radiosurgery for AVMs.[10, 14–27] They have reported 1-year occlusion rates ranging from 33.7% to 39.5% and 2-year occlusion rates ranging from 79% to 86.5%. However, these results were "optimized" by retrospectively selecting patients who received a minimal treatment dose. For example, in one report he stated, ". . . a large majority of patients received at least 20 to 25 Gy of radiation. . . . Of the 248 patients treated before 1984, the treatment specification placed 188 in this group."[18] The reported thrombosis rates in this article applied only to these 188 patients (76% of the total series).

Interestingly, Yamamoto and colleagues reported on 25 Japanese patients treated on the gamma unit in Stockholm, but followed in Japan.[10] The 2-year thrombosis rate in those AVMs that were completely covered by the radiosurgical field was 64%. Complete thrombosis occurred in one additional patient at the 3-year angiography procedure and in one patient the at 5-year angiography procedure, for a total cure rate of 73%. In another article,[19] these authors reported angiographic cures in 6 of 9 (67%) children treated in Stockholm or Buenos Aires and followed in Japan. Yamamoto and associates reviewed the long-term follow-up results of a group of 40 Japanese patients undergoing gamma knife radiosurgery for AVMs in three different countries (Argentina, Sweden, and the United States). In this group of patients, the mean lesion volume was only 3.7 cc. Twenty-six patients (65%) were subsequently found to have angiographically confirmed nidus obliteration 1 to 5 years after radiosurgery.[20]

Kemeny and colleagues reported on 52 AVM patients treated with gamma knife radiosurgery.[21] They all received 25 Gy to the 50% isodose line. At 1 year, 16 (31%) patients had complete thrombosis, and 10 (19%) patients had "almost complete" thrombosis. He found that the results were better in younger patients and in patients with AVMs in a relatively lateral location. There was no difference in outcome between small (<2 cc), medium (2 to 3 cc), and large (>3 cc) AVMs.

Lunsford and colleagues reported on 227 AVM patients treated with gamma knife radiosurgery.[22] The mean dose delivered to the AVM margin was 21.2 Gy. Multiple isocenters were used in 48% of the patients. Seventeen patients underwent 1-year angiography, which confirmed complete thrombosis in 76.5%. As indicated in the article, "this rate may be spurious since many of these patients were selected for angiography because their MR image had suggested obliteration."

Among 75 patients who were followed for at least 2 years, 2-year angiography was performed in only 46 (61%). Complete obliteration was confirmed in 37 of 46 (80%) patients. This thrombosis rate strongly correlated with AVM size, as follows: less than 1 cc, 100%; 1 to 4 cc, 85%; 4 to 10 cc, 58%. In 1994, this group reported on a group of 65 "operable" AVMs, treated with radiosurgery.[23] Of 32 patients who subsequently underwent follow-up angiography, 84% showed complete thrombosis. In 1994 publication from this group, Pollock and colleagues[24] reported on 313 AVM patients; an angiographic cure rate of 61% was achieved.

Karlsson and associates[14] reported on 945 AVMs treated with the gamma knife in Stockholm between 1970 and 1990. The overall occlusion rate was 56%.

Steinberg and coworkers,[25] in an analysis of 86 AVMs treated with a particle beam radiosurgical system, reported a 29% 1-year thrombosis, a 70% 2-year thrombosis, and a 92% 3-year thrombosis rate. The best results were obtained with smaller lesions and higher doses. Initially, a treatment dose of 34.6 Gy was used, but a higher than expected neurologic complication rate (20% for the entire series) led to the currently used dose range of 7.7 to 19.2 Gy. No patient treated with the lower dose range had complications.

Betti and colleagues reported on the results of 66 AVMs treated with a LINAC radiosurgical system.[26] Doses of "no more than 40 Gy" were used in 80% of patients. They found a 66% 2-year thrombosis rate. The percentage of cured patients was highest when the entire malformation was included in the 75% isodose line (96%) or the maximal diameter of the lesion was less than 12 mm (81%).

Colombo and coworkers reported on 97 AVM patients treated with a LINAC system.[27] Doses from 18.7 to 40 Gy were delivered in one or two sessions. Of 56 patients who were followed longer than 1 year, 50 underwent 12-month follow-up angiography. In 26 (52%) patients, complete thrombosis was demonstrated. Fifteen of 20 (75%) patients undergoing 2-year angiography had complete thrombosis. They reported a definite relationship between AVM size and thrombosis rate, as follows: Lesions less than 15 mm in diameter had a 1-year obliteration rate of 76% and a 2-year rate of 90%. Lesions 15 to 25 mm in diameter had a 1-year thrombosis rate of 37.5% and a 2-year rate of 80%. Lesions greater than 25 mm in diameter had a 1-year thrombosis rate of 11% and a 2-year rate of 40%. In a more recent report,[28] Colombo and colleagues reported follow-up on 180 radiosurgically treated AVMs. The 1-year thrombosis rate was 46%, and the 2-year rate was 80%.

Souhami and colleagues reported on 33 AVMs treated with a LINAC system.[29] The prescribed dose at isocenter varied from 50 to 55 Gy. A complete obliteration rate of 38% was seen at 1-year angiography. For patients whose arteriovenous malformation nidus was covered by a minimal dose of 25 Gy, the total obliteration rate was 61.5%, whereas none of the patients who had received less than 25 Gy at the edge of the nidus obtained a total obliteration.

Loeffler and associates reported on 16 AVMs treated

TABLE 269-1 ■ **Major Arteriovenous Malformation Radiosurgery Series***

REFERENCE	YAMAMOTO ET AL[20]	POLLOCK ET AL[24]	KARLSSON ET AL[60]	STEINBERG ET AL[25]	COLOMBO ET AL[27]	FRIEDMAN ET AL[11]
Radiosurgical Device	Gamma knife	Gamma knife	Gamma knife	Proton beam	LINAC	LINAC
Number of Patients	40	313	945	86	180	388
Angiographic Cure Rate	65%	61%	56%	92%	80%	67%
Complications Permanent Radiation-Induced	3 patients (7.5%)	30 patients (9%)	5%	11%	4 patients (2%)	7 patients (2%)
Hemorrhage	None	8 fatal	55 patients	10 patients	15 patients (5 fatal)	25 patients (5 fatal)

*When a group had multiple reports, the most recent results are listed.
LINAC, linear accelator.

with a LINAC system.[30] The peripheral prescribed dose was 15 to 25 Gy, typically to the 80 to 90% line. The total obliteration rate was 5 of 11 (45%) at 1 year and 8 of 11 (73%) at 2 years after treatment. The major radiosurgery AVM series are summarized in Table 269-1.

RESULTS OF RADIOSURGERY FOR ARTERIOVENOUS MALFORMATIONS AND THE UNIVERSITY OF FLORIDA

Between May 18, 1988 and July 27, 1999, 388 AVMs were treated on the University of Florida radiosurgery system. There were 182 men and 206 women in the series. The mean age was 39 years (range, 4 to 70 years). Patients presented with hemorrhage (131), seizure (160), headache (91), incidental findings (42), and progressive neurologic deficit (12). Twenty-nine patients had undergone previous subtotal microsurgical AVM excision. Thirty-seven patients had undergone at least one embolization procedure. Patients were screened by a vascular neurosurgeon before radiosurgery was considered.

The mean lesion volume was 9 cc (0.2 to 45.3 cc). The treatment volume was determined in all cases by performing a computerized dose volume histogram of the treatment isodose shell (which was constructed to conform closely to the AVM nidus). Lesion volumes were stratified as follow: A, less than 1 cc; B, 1 to 4 cc; C, 4 to 10 cc; D, greater than 10 cc. Spetzler-Martin grades were distributed as follows: grade I, 20 patients; grade II, 142 patients; grade III, 163 patients; and grade IV, 63 patients. The mean radiation dose to the periphery of the lesion was 15.4 Gy (range: 7.5 to 25 Gy). This treatment dose was delivered to the 80% isodose line when single isocenter plans were used, and to the 70% line when multiple isocenters were used. Two hundred thirty-six patients were treated with a single isocenter, 46 patients were treated with 2 isocenters, 42 patients were treated with 3 isocenters, 21 patients were treated with 4 isocenters, and 44 patients were treated with five isocenters or more (range 5 to 10).

Mean follow-up duration for the entire AVM group

was 28 months (0 to 127 months). Follow-up generally consists of clinical examination and MRI scanning at one-year intervals after treatment, unless clinical symptoms indicate more frequent follow-up. When possible, follow-up was performed in Gainesville, Florida; otherwise, scan and examination results were forwarded by the patient's local physician.

Initially, all patients were asked to undergo angiography at yearly intervals, regardless of the MRI findings. After the first 50 patients were treated, it was decided to defer angiography until MRI-MRA strongly suggested complete thrombosis. Furthermore, if complete thrombosis was not identified 3 years after radiosurgery, repeat radiosurgery was undertaken in an effort to obliterate any remaining nidus (see further on).

An angiographic cure required that no nidus or shunting remain on the study, as interpreted by a neuroradiologist and the treating neurosurgeon. Of the 144 follow-up angiograms performed to date, 96 (67%) have demonstrated complete AVM obliteration. Using this traditional method of reporting, the following angiographic cure rates were seen in the various size categories: A, 80%; B, 84%; C, 74%; D, 43%. Definitive outcome end points are angiographic occlusion (cure), retreatment (failure), and fatal hemorrhage (failure). Successful end points have thus far been attained in 80% of category A patients, 89% of category B patients, 64% of category C patients, and 34% of category D patients.

WHY DOES RADIOSURGERY FAIL?

In an effort to clarify the causes of radiosurgical failure, we examined 36 patients who underwent repeat radiosurgery after an initial failure to obliterate their AVMs and compared them to 72 patients who were cured during the same period.[31] An image fusion methodology was used to fuse the treatment plan created at the first treatment to the computed tomographic scan obtained at the time of retreatment. Two patients were excluded from the targeting error analysis because the nidus was too small to visualize on CT. Of the remaining 34 patients in whom the original treatment failed, 9 (26%) had a partial targeting error at the time of the first treatment.

The retreatment group had statistically significantly higher Spetzler-Martin grade, larger AVM size, and lower treatment dose when compared with the group of patients who were cured. Statistical analysis also demonstrated that patients treated with a peripheral dose less than 15 Gy had a much higher failure rate. In addition, patients with AVM volumes greater than 10 cc had a much higher failure rate.

Other radiosurgery groups have also published analyses aimed at identifying factors that might be predictive of radiosurgical success or failure. Pollock and colleagues[24] found that the following factors predicted success: lower AVM volume, fewer draining veins, younger age, and more superficial location. Prior embolization of the AVM was a negative predictor. This group also published a review of 45 patients who underwent repeat radiosurgical treatment after an initial treatment failed to obliterate their AVMs.[32] In this study, causes of radiosurgical failure were identified as follows: In five (11%) patients, the entire AVM was not visualized secondary to incomplete angiography (two vessels instead of four vessels) or inadequate angiographic technique (failure to perform superselective angiography). In three (7%) patients, the AVM recanalized after previous embolization. In four (9%) patients, the AVM nidus re-expanded after resorption of a prior hematoma that had compressed the vessels within the nidus. In 21 (46%) patients, the true three-dimensional shape of the AVM nidus was not appreciated secondary to reliance on biplanar angiography alone. In the remaining patients, a definite cause for failure could not be determined. The authors believed that the AVMs in these patients were exhibiting some form of "radiobiologic resistance," that is, failure to be obliterated despite proper planning and adequate dose delivery. In an earlier analysis by the same group,[33] the dose to the periphery (D_{min}) of the target was found to be the most significant predictor of success. In that analysis, neither volume nor maximal dose was found to be predictive. "Problems defining the complete AVM nidus" were cited as significant limitations to successful AVM obliteration.

Touboul and associates[34] published an analysis of 100 consecutive AVM radiosurgery patients with a five-year actuarial obliteration rate of 62.5 ± 7%. Their statistical analysis confirmed the importance of peripheral dose as the most significant predictor of success and echoed the Pittsburgh finding that peripheral dose and target volume were not significant predictors.

The Stockholm group also published an analysis aimed at defining predictive factors for radiosurgical obliteration of AVMs.[14] Analyzing a 945-patient subset of the 1319 AVM patients treated with the gamma knife from 1970 to 1990, they again identified peripheral dose as the most significant predictive factor. The higher the minimal dose, up to 25 Gy, the higher the obliteration rate. This rate in the 268 cases that received this minimal dose (25 Gy) was 81%. In their analysis, higher average dose and lower AVM volume were also found to predict success. A higher average dose was found

to shorten the latency to AVM obliteration. They proposed that the product of the cubed root of the AVM volume and the peripheral dose (the "K index") would serve as a good combined predictor of success and found that a K index of 27 was optimal. Obliteration rates increased with increasing K values up to 27, above which no further improvement was observed.

Yamamoto and associates[20] reviewed the long-term follow-up results of a group of 40 Japanese patients undergoing gamma knife radiosurgery for AVMs in three different countries (Argentina, Sweden, and the United States). In this group of patients, the mean lesion volume was only 3.7 cc. Twenty-six patients (65%) were subsequently found to have angiographically confirmed nidus obliteration at 1 to 5 years after radiosurgery. Thirteen (32.5%) patients failed radiosurgery based on follow-up angiography at 3 to 7 years after treatment. In their retrospective analysis, they discovered that the nidus had only partially been covered at the time of the first treatment in 6 of the 13 (46%) patients in whom treatment subsequently failed.

The importance of targeting error as a cause for radiosurgical failure merits brief discussion. In the Pittsburgh series, 67% of all failures were attributed to targeting error resulting from inadequate imaging or obscuration of the AVM nidus by a hematoma. In Yamamoto and colleagues' analysis, targeting error was responsible for 46% of all failures. A similar analysis by Gallina and coworkers[35] attributed 10 of 17 (59%) AVM radiosurgery failures to inadequate targeting. In our experience,[31] targeting error was a less important cause of failure, accounting for only 26% of failures. This may suggest the importance of using a three-dimensional database, such as contrast-enhanced CT, for targeting, as opposed to stereotactic angiography alone.

In summary, the dose delivered to the D_{min} is the most significant predictor of successful obliteration provided that the nidus is completely encompassed by the prescription isodose shell. Lesion volume and Spetzler-Martin grade are also predictors, although they are less significant than D_{min}. The importance of AVM location and patient age are unclear. Based on our experience, lower rates of AVM obliteration can be expected at peripheral doses less than 15 Gy, and for lesion volumes greater than 10 cc.

COMPLICATIONS

Natural History of Arteriovenous Malformations

Many studies have addressed the issue of the natural history of arteriovenous malformations. Unfortunately, most are tainted by selection bias, the use of a variety of therapeutic techniques, relatively short duration of follow-up, and the inclusion of only certain subgroups of AVM patients (i.e., patients presenting with hemorrhage). The follow-up analysis of Troupp's series,[36] performed by Ondra and colleagues[5] provides a fairly pure look at a series of 160 patients with AVMs. Forty percent of the patients experienced a hemorrhage during the 24-year follow-up period, for a 4% per year risk of hemorrhage after entry into the study. There was a 7.7-year mean interval to hemorrhage. They found a 2.7% yearly incidence of significant morbidity and mortality. Others have reported an annual hemorrhage rate for AVMs ranging from 2% to 4%.[1-4]

Some have suggested that a prior history of hemorrhage predisposes to an increased incidence of subsequent hemorrhages.[2] For example, Forster and associates noted that if a patient had one hemorrhage, there was a 25% risk of rebleeding over the next 4 years. If the patient had two hemorrhages, the risk of rebleeding was 25% over the next year.[37] Others, including Ondra and colleagues,[5] do not support this view and believe that after the first 6 months, the risk of hemorrhage reverts to baseline.

A number of investigators have identified a tendency for smaller AVMs to hemorrhage.[3, 38-41] Others feel that this is an artifactual observation resulting from the fact that smaller lesions are less likely than larger ones to present with seizures or vascular steal. Likewise, an increased risk of hemorrhage during pregnancy has been postulated but never proved.[42, 43]

Various angiographic abnormalities have been purported to increase the likelihood of AVM hemorrhage. Vinuela and associates evaluated the venous drainage of 53 deep-seated AVMs, 41 of which presented with hemorrhage.[41] They found irregularity, stenosis, or absence of the vein of Galen in 11 cases. Willinsky and colleagues reviewed 178 patients and found that arterial aneurysms or venous stenosis were present is 73% of those presenting with hemorrhage.[44] Marks and co-workers found a statistically significant association of periventricular location, intranidal aneurysm, and central venous drainage with the occurrence of AVM hemorrhage.[45]

Hemorrhage after Radiosurgery

The issue of AVM hemorrhage after radiosurgical treatment was first discussed by investigators using particle beam methodology. Kjellberg and colleagues initially reported two deaths from hemorrhage in the first year after treatment of their first 75 patients.[46] In a subsequent report of 389 patients followed for at least 2 years, 8 had died of hemorrhage in the first 2 years after treatment.[47] Only one had died thereafter, for a 0.27% mortality in those patients who had survived past 2 years after treatment. Initially, these investigators suggested that only patients presenting with hemorrhage were at risk for subsequent lethal rebleeding. Later reports, however, document fatal hemorrhage in patients presenting with seizure only. It should be emphasized that these authors reported a total hemorrhage rate of 2.4% per year (lethal and nonlethal) for patients more than 2 years post-treatment. Whether this differs from the natural history of the disease is debatable.

Other particle beam proponents have also addressed the hemorrhage question. Steinberg and associates reported 10 (12%) hemorrhages (2 fatal), occurring between 4 and 34 months after radiosurgical treatment in a series of 86 patients.[25] Two of these patients had hemorrhages in the third year after treatment, suggesting no protective effect unless complete obliteration was achieved. Seifert and colleagues analyzed a series of 68 patients treated with proton beam therapy in the United States.[48] Eighteen patients deteriorated neurologically. Five of them had hemorrhages, two of which were fatal.

Gamma knife radiosurgeons have studied this question as well. Lunsford and colleagues, in an initial report on AVM treatment with the Pittsburgh gamma knife, noted that 10 patients (4%) in a series of 227 patients had experienced hemorrhage.[22] Two of these patients died. Pollock and colleagues, in a study of 65 patients with "operable" AVMs, noted that 5 (7.7%) patients had a hemorrhage, all within 8 months of radiosurgery.[23] Two of these patients died. Steiner and colleagues statistically analyzed bleeding in 247 consecutive AVM cases.[49] The Kaplan-Meier approach demonstrated a risk of nearly 3.7% per year until 5 years after radiosurgery, at which point a plateau was reached. This plateau was felt likely to be due to the small number of data points for that period and not indicative of any true protective effect. Karlsson and associates reported an analysis of bleeding in 1565 patients treated with the Stockholm gamma knife.[50] They felt the risk of hemorrhage was decreased, even with incomplete obliteration. They also reported that increasing age and increasing AVM volume correlated with an increased risk of hemorrhage.

Betti and associates, in a pioneering report on LINAC radiosurgery for AVMs, documented hemorrhage in 5 of 66 (8%) of their patients.[26] These hemorrhages occurred at 12, 18, 22, 25, and 29 months after treatment. All had a prior history of hemorrhage. Two of these patients died. Colombo and colleagues also reported a detailed analysis of 180 patients.[28] Fifteen patients had hemorrhages and five of them died. When the AVM nidus was totally irradiated, the bleeding risk decreased from 4.8% during the first 6 months to 0% starting from the 12th month of follow-up. In partially irradiated cases, the bleeding risk increased from 4% in the first 6 months to 10% from the 6th through 18th month, and then down to 5.5% from the 18th to the 24th month. No bleeding was observed thereafter.

Our analysis of this issue did not reveal any post-radiosurgical alteration in the risk of bleeding from the expected rate of 3% to 4% per year based on natural history.[51] A similar study by the Pittsburgh group confirmed that "stereotactic radiosurgery was not associated with a significant change in the hemorrhage rate of AVMs during the latency interval before obliteration."[52]

It should be noted that there are significant pitfalls to be avoided in the analysis of hemorrhage risk after radiosurgery. First, because radiosurgery is usually successful, a large number of patients are eliminated from the "at-risk" pool (the denominator) during the first and second year after radiosurgery. Failure to account for this fact adequately leads to the false impression that the smaller number of hemorrhages occurring at greater than 1 year after treatment are due to some "protective" effect. In fact, the decreasing number of hemorrhages is statistically due to the decreasing number of patients at risk.

Second, because there are a significant number of patients presenting with hemorrhage in any radiosurgery series, and because these patients may have an increased risk of hemorrhage for the first 6 months after hemorrhage,[3, 4, 37] the incidence of bleeding in the first 6 months after treatment may appear, in some series, to be elevated. This is likely not a direct effect of radiosurgery but rather a reflection of the inclusion of this group of patients with a higher than normal risk of hemorrhage. Series that treat a larger percentage of patients presenting with hemorrhage (as opposed to seizures or headache) might be expected to have an elevated hemorrhage rate during the first 6 months after treatment for this reason.

Third, and most important, the incidence of hemorrhage in AVM patients is small. This means that the effect of a slight alteration in the number of hemorrhages over a given period may, without the benefit of statistical analysis, significantly skew the conclusions in this type of analysis. Assuming a constant baseline AVM occurrence rate of 3 per 100 person-years follow-up (or 3% per year) in untreated patients, 726 person-years of follow-up would be required to have a 95% chance of detecting a reduction in the AVM rate to 1 per 100 person-years of follow-up (or 1% per year) in treated patients at a 0.05 significance level. Given the relatively high cure rate of radiosurgery, a large number (thousands) of patients treated would be needed to generate a sufficient number of patient follow-up years in years 2, 3, 4, and so on, in order to yield statistically valid information. These factors must be kept in mind when interpreting some of the papers discussed earlier. Any attempt to elucidate the question of AVM bleeding after radiosurgery, without benefit of detailed statistics, must be viewed with some skepticism.

As mentioned previously, Karlsson and colleagues reported an increased risk of AVM hemorrhage with increasing AVM size.[50] Colombo and associates found a higher incidence in subtotally irradiated AVMs, most of which were presumably larger lesions.[28] They also reported a statistically increased risk in patients treated more inhomogeneously (to a lower isodose line). In a subsequent article, their group attributed this observation to the earlier thrombosis of the portion of the AVM receiving the highest dose of radiation, with shunting of blood into the remaining nidus, increasing the risk of hemorrhage.[53]

In our series,[51] a strong correlation between AVM volume and the risk of hemorrhage was also found. Ten of the 12 AVMs that bled were greater than 10 cc in volume. In addition, the correlation of hemorrhage with lower dose and lower isodose line treated was likely due to the deliberate use of lower doses and multiple isocenter treatments (to lower isodose lines) in larger AVMs. Of equal importance are those factors that were found not to statistically correlate with bleeding risk. In this study, neither age nor history of prior

hemorrhage correlated with the incidence of hemorrhage.

Ten of the 12 AVMs that bled also had associated "angiographic risk factors" for bleeding, including arterial aneurysms, venous aneurysms, venous outlet obstruction, and periventricular location. Although these angiographic factors were not subject to statistical analysis, one might certainly conclude that their absence might be associated with a decreased risk.

Pollock and associates[52] found a significant correlation between the incidence of postradiosurgical hemorrhage and the presence of an unsecured proximal aneurysm and recommended that such aneurysms be obliterated before radiosurgery. The same group also studied factors associated with bleeding risk of AVMs and found three AVM characteristics to be predictive of greater hemorrhage risk: (1) history of prior bleed, (2) presence of a single draining vein, and (3) diffuse AVM morphologic characteristics.[54] Based on the presence or absence of these risk factors, they stratified AVM patients into four hemorrhage risk groups, and recommended that predicted hemorrhage risk be used to help determine appropriate management of patients with AVMs. For example, patients with a high predicted hemorrhage risk would be considered less attractive candidates for radiosurgery because of the greater risk during the latency period between treatment and cure.

Radiation-Induced Complications

Acute complications are rare after AVM radiosurgery. Several authors have previously reported that radiosurgery can acutely exacerbate seizure activity. Others have reported nausea, vomiting, and headache occasionally occurring after radiosurgical treatment.[55]

Delayed radiation-induced complications have been reported by all groups performing radiosurgery. In 1984, Steiner reported symptomatic radiation necrosis in approximately 3% of his patients.[15] Statham described one patient who developed radiation necrosis 13 months after gamma knife radiosurgery of a 5.3-cc AVM with 25 Gy to the margin.[56] In 1991, Lunsford and associates reported that 10 patients in the Pittsburgh series (4.4%) developed new neurologic deficits that were thought to be secondary to radiation injury.[22] Symptoms were location-dependent and developed between 4 and 18 months after treatment. All patients were treated with steroids and all improved. Only two patients were reported to have residual deficits that appeared to be permanent. In this early analysis, the radiation dose and isodose line treated did not correlate with incidence of complication. As they noted, the failure of correlation of dose and complications likely related to the fact that doses had been selected to fall below Flickinger's computed 3% risk line. This is a mathematically derived line that prescribes lower doses for larger lesions and underpins the well-established correlation between increasing radiosurgical target volume and increasing incidence of radiation necrosis.[57, 58]

Flickinger and associates published an updated

analysis of complications from AVM radiosurgery that emphasized the importance of lesion location and dose.[59] The analysis, which includes outcome data from 332 Pittsburgh gamma knife AVM radiosurgery cases from 1987 to 1994, found that 30 (9%) patients developed some symptomatic sequelae after radiosurgery (any neurologic problem, including headache). Symptoms resolved in 58% of these patients within 27 months. Statistically, the likelihood of having a transient versus a permanent deficit was dose-dependent, with a difference noted at a peripheral dose of 20 Gy (D_{min}). When D_{min} was less than 20 Gy, 89% of patients who developed deficits experienced complete resolution of their symptoms, whereas only 36% of patients receiving minimal target doses less than 20 Gy recovered fully. The 7-year actuarial rate for developing a permanent radiation-induced neurologic deficit was 3.8%. The relative risks for various lesion locations were compared, and a "postradiosurgery injury expression (PIE)" score was assigned to various brain locations. In general, deeper locations had higher postradiosurgery injury expression scores, indicating a greater risk of radiation-induced complications. Multivariate statistical analysis identified only postradiosurgery injury expression location score and 12-cc volume as significant predictors of radiation-induced symptomatic sequelae. Variables analyzed, but found not to be significant predictors of complications, included previous neurologic deficit, previous hemorrhage, use of MRI-enhanced treatment planning, prescription isodose line, and number of isocenters.

The Stockholm group also published an analysis of factors associated with complications after AVM radiosurgery.[60] Their report confirms the predictive importance of AVM location and dose. They found that a history of previous hemorrhage was associated with a lower risk of complications in their series, and previous irradiation was associated with a higher risk of complications.

Steinberg reported a definite correlation among lesion size, lesion dose, and complications.[25] His initial treatment dose of 34.6 Gy led to a relatively high complication rate. Subsequently, patients were treated with a much lower dose and had no radiation induced complications. In an earlier report on 75 AVM patients treated with helium particles, at a dose of 45 Gy, 7 of 75 patients (11%) experienced radiation-induced complications.[61]

Kjellberg and coworkers,[46, 62] using a compilation of animal and clinical data, constructed a series of log-log lines, relating prescribed dose and lesion diameter. His 1% isorisk line is similar to Flickinger's mathematically derived 3% risk line.

In Colombo and associates' series, 9 of 180 (5%) patients experienced symptomatic radiation-induced complications.[28] Four (2.2%) were permanent. Loeffler and colleagues reported that 1 of 21 AVM patients developed a similar problem, which responded well to steroids.[30] Souhami and coworkers reported "severe side-effects" in 2 of 33 (6%) patients.[29] Marks and Spencer reviewed six radiosurgical series and found a 9% overall incidence of clinically significant radiation reac-

tions.[63] Seven of 23 patients received doses below Kjellberg's 1% risk line.

Others have reported that asymptomatic radiation-induced changes appear frequently (20% in the Pittsburgh series) on postradiosurgery MRI.[64–66] We have also observed this phenomenon. These changes tend to be asymptomatic if the lesion is located in a relatively "silent" brain area, and symptomatic if the lesion is located in an "eloquent" brain area. This is further evidence that lesion location is an important consideration in radiosurgical treatment planning and dose selection.

Most radiosurgical series report their radiation-induced complications as a percentage of the total patient population treated. It should be noted that since most radiation-induced complications do not appear until 12 to 18 months after treatment, this results in a systematic underestimate of the true complication rate.

Very Late Onset Complications

Yamamoto and colleagues published a series of papers describing radiation-related adverse effects observed on late neuroimaging after AVM radiosurgery.[67–69] In their study of 53 patients' status following gamma knife AVM radiosurgery, MRIs were performed up to 10 years after treatment. In this series, of the five (9.4%) patients who developed delayed neurologic symptoms, three presented at least 5 years after treatment. One patient with a midbrain AVM developed a hemi-Parkinson's syndrome 5.5 years after radiosurgery. Another patient developed gradual visual field narrowing accompanied by signs of increased intracranial pressure 7 years after treatment; MRI revealed a large cyst in the left parieto-occipital lobe at the site of the irradiated AVM, and surgery was required. The third patient presented 7 years after treatment with hemiparesis caused by a diffuse white matter necrotic lesion.

Also concerning was the late development of four additional *asymptomatic* radiologic abnormalities. One middle cerebral artery stenosis of the M1 segment was detected 3 years after radiosurgery. A dural AV fistula developed 7 years after treatment, and two delayed cysts had formed at 5 and 10 years after treatment.

The lesion volumes and treatment doses used in this series were not unusual (median volume 1.5 cc, mean peripheral target dose 21.5 Gy), and careful examination of the complicated cases revealed no obvious deviation from standard radiosurgical practice. Uncommonly meticulous radiologic follow-up may explain some of these unusual findings. Perhaps such abnormalities are not rare, but are simply going undetected, especially in asymptomatic patients.

Kihlstrom and colleagues also reported a series of late radiologic abnormalities after AVM radiosurgery.[65] MRI scans and follow-up angiography were performed on 18 patients at a mean interval of 14 years (8 to 23 years) after radiosurgical treatment. All patients had previous angiographic documentation of AVM obliteration, and all were clinically asymptomatic. Radiologic findings included cyst formation at the previous AVM site in five (28%) patients, contrast enhancement at the former lesion site (without AVM recanalization) in 11 (61%) patients, and an increased T2 MRI signal at the former lesion site in three (17%) patients. In this series, unlike the case reported by Yamamoto and colleagues, none of the observed cysts exceeded 2 cm in diameter, all were confined to the volume of the previous AVM nidus, and none caused any mass effect. Because treatment doses used in this study were higher than those currently administered, it is difficult to predict whether similar findings will be reproduced in more recent patient series. The absence of clinical symptoms in these patients may indicate that such late radiographic abnormalities will be of limited clinical importance.

Although the utility of routine, very late (after obliteration) MRI and angiography has not been determined, these findings alert radiosurgeons to the reality that very late complications can and do occur.

SALVAGE RETREATMENT FOR FAILED ARTERIOVENOUS MALFORMATION RADIOSURGERY

The Stockholm radiosurgery group is the only group that has reported specifically on the results of repeat radiosurgical treatment after an initial treatment has failed to obliterate an AVM.[70, 71] In their most recent report,[71] they analyzed 101 cases of such salvage retreatment. Obliteration was achieved in 62% of these cases, a rate almost identical to that currently reported by this group for primary AVM radiosurgery. The complication rate was 14%, which was significantly higher than that currently reported by this group for primary radiosurgery. The annual risk of hemorrhage during the first 2 post-treatment years was 1.8%, a value not statistically different from that associated with the natural history of this disease.

MULTIMODALITY TREATMENT FOR ARTERIOVENOUS MALFORMATIONS

When an AVM is amenable to safe microsurgical resection, this therapy is preferred because it offers immediate cure and elimination of hemorrhage risk. When the estimated morbidity of resection is excessive, radiosurgery offers a reasonable chance for delayed cure. However, some unresectable AVMs, by virtue of their large size, are not candidates for radiosurgery. These problematic lesions are often managed with presurgery or preradiosurgery embolization.

The most important role of embolization before radiosurgery is to reduce the size of the lesion. Potential secondary advantages of preradiosurgical embolization are that associated aneurysms may be treated, and high-flow arteriovenous fistulas—felt to be less sensitive to radiosurgery—may be identified and occluded.[72]

Dawson and colleagues[73] reported on seven patients with large AVMs who were treated with embolization followed by gamma knife radiosurgery. At 2-year follow-up, two AVMs were obliterated and two others

had a 98% reduction in volume. Lemme-Plaghos and colleagues[74] reported their results in 16 patients with high-grade AVMs who were treated with embolization and gamma knife radiosurgery. Four cures (25%) were reported. Mathis and associates[75] reported on a series of patients with large AVMs (volume >10 cc) who were treated with embolization and radiosurgery. Of the 56 patients treated, 24 were included in their analysis, and 12 were cured. Among the analyzed group, two patients (8%) experienced transient neurologic deficit after embolization, and one developed mild upper extremity weakness after radiosurgery. Recanalization of previously embolized, but not irradiated, regions of AVM nidus occurred in three patients. Guo and associates reported 46 patients treated with embolization and gamma knife radiosurgery.[76] In 16 cases, collateral vessels developed that made subsequent delineation of the nidus for radiosurgery difficult. In addition, nine patients had neurologic complications after embolization. Only 19 of 35 large AVMs were sufficiently reduced in size to be subsequently treatable with radiosurgery.

A larger series of patients, treated with a combination of embolization and LINAC radiosurgery, was reported by Gobin and colleagues.[72] Of the 125 AVMs treated with (usually multiple-session) endovascular treatment, 14 (11%) were completely occluded with embolization alone. Ninety-six AVMs (77%) were reduced in size by embolization enough to be considered for radiosurgery. Of those who underwent postembolization radiosurgery, complete occlusion was achieved in 65%. Embolization resulted in a mortality rate of 1.6% and a morbidity rate of 12.8%. No complications were associated with radiosurgery in this series. The post-treatment AVM hemorrhage rate was 3% per year. Despite the use of cyanoacrylate (the current standard in durable embolic material), a 12% revascularization rate was observed.

The results of combination therapy with embolization and radiosurgery are promising, and this technique appears to offer a reasonably good treatment option for patients with large, unresectable AVMs. Enthusiasm for the use of preradiosurgery embolization should be tempered, however, not only because of its non-negligible morbidity and mortality but also because embolic material can obscure the AVM nidus on planning images. Furthermore, delayed recanalization may occur in areas not targeted during radiosurgery. Embolization should be used as adjuvant therapy only when an AVM is too large to be treated safely with surgery or radiosurgery alone. Furthermore, exceptionally large, asymptomatic AVMs might be more prudently managed conservatively, given the significant morbidity associated with their treatment and their lower likelihood of cure.

Multimodality therapy is not limited to embolization. For example, radiosurgery can be used to obliterate a subtotally resected AVM or, conversely, surgery may be used to remove an AVM remnant when radiosurgery does not result in complete occlusion. Thus, embolization, surgery, and radiosurgery may occasionally all be used in a single patient.

CONCLUSIONS

Many reports indicate that approximately 80% of arteriovenous malformations in the "radiosurgery size range" will be angiographically obliterated 2 to 3 years after radiosurgical treatment. The likelihood of successful AVM obliteration decreases with increasing lesion volume and decreasing peripheral target dose. Accurate targeting is critical to successful AVM radiosurgery, and a three-dimensional image database (e.g., CT or MRI) is an indispensable element in the treatment planning process; stereotactic angiography alone is inadequate.

The major drawback of this treatment method is that patients are unprotected against hemorrhage during the 2- to 3-year latent period after treatment. Radiosurgery does not significantly alter the natural rate of AVM hemorrhage until the lesion has completely thrombosed. Increasing AVM volume appears to be associated with a higher risk for hemorrhage, as are certain angiographic findings such as proximal aneurysms, venous outflow restriction, and periventricular location.

Radiation-induced neurologic symptoms occur in 5 to 10% of patients, but the majority of these are transient and respond to steroid therapy. Permanent complications are rare (2% to 4%). The most significant predictors of radiation-induced complications are AVM volume, lesion location, and dose. Asymptomatic MRI changes are not uncommon. Long-term radiation complications have been reported but appear to be rare.

Preliminary results of salvage retreatment for failed AVM radiosurgery are encouraging.

Although radiosurgery is used primarily as a single modality treatment, it has been used increasingly as part of a multimodality treatment approach incorporating surgical and endovascular methods. Multimodality therapy carries the additive risks of each treatment modality used but has been used successfully to treat very large AVMs that were not candidates for surgical or radiosurgical monotherapy.

REFERENCES

1. Brown RD, Wiebers DO, Forbes G: The natural history of unruptured intracranial arteriovenous malformations. J Neurosurg 68: 352–357, 1988.
2. Crawford PM, West CR, Chadwick DW: Arteriovenous malformations of the brain: Natural history in unoperated patients. J Neurol Neurosurg Psychiatry 49:1–10, 1986.
3. Fults D, Kelly DL: Natural history of arteriovenous malformations of the brain: A clinical study. Neurosurgery 15:658–652, 1984.
4. Graf CJ, Perret GE, Torner JC: Bleeding from cerebral arteriovenous malformations as part of their natural history. J Neurosurg 58:331–337, 1983.
5. Ondra SL, Troupp H, George ED, et al: The natural history of symptomatic arteriovenous malformations of the brain: A 24-year follow-up assessment. J Neurosurg 73:387–391, 1991.
6. Chang SD, Shuster DL, Steinberg GK, et al: Stereotactic radiosurgery of arteriovenous malformations: Pathologic changes in resected tissue. Clin Neuropathol 16:111–116, 1997.
7. Ogilvy CS: Radiation therapy for arteriovenous malformations: A review. Neurosurgery 26:725–735, 1990.
8. Schneider BF, Eberhard DA, Steiner, LE: Histopathology of arte-

riovenous malformations after gamma knife radiosurgery. J Neurosurg 87:352–357, 1997.
9. Szeifert GT, Kemeny AA, Timperley WR, Forster DM: The potential role of myofibroblasts in the obliteration of arteriovenous malformations after radiosurgery. Neurosurgery 40:61–65; discussion 65–66, 1997.
10. Yamamoto M, Jimbo M, Kobayashi M, et al: Long-term results of radiosurgery for arteriovenous malformation: Neurodiagnostic imaging and histological studies of angiographically confirmed nidus obliteration. Surg Neurol 37:219–230, 1992.
11. Friedman WA, Buatti JM, Bova FJ, et al: LINAC Radiosurgery—A Practical Guide. Berlin: Springer-Verlag, 1998.
12. Bova FJ, Friedman WA: Stereotactic angiography: An inadequate database for radiosurgery? Int J Radiat Oncol Biol Phys 20: 891–895, 1991.
13. Spiegelmann R, Friedman WA, Bova FJ: Limitations of angiographic target localization in radiosurgical treatment planning. Neurosurgery 30:619–624, 1992.
14. Karlsson B, Lindquist C, Steiner L: Prediction of obliteration after gamma knife surgery for cerebral arteriovenous malformations. Neurosurgery 40:425–430; discussion 430–431, 1997.
15. Steiner L: Treatment of arteriovenous malformations by radiosurgery. In Wilson CB, Stein BM (eds): Intracranial Arteriovenous Malformations. Baltimore, Williams & Wilkins, 1984, pp 295–313.
16. Steiner L: Radiosurgery in cerebral arteriovenous malformations. In Fein JM, Flamm ES (eds): Cerebrovascular Surgery, vol 4. New York, Springer-Verlag, 1985, pp 1161–1215.
17. Steiner L, Leksell L, Greitz T, et al: Stereotaxic radiosurgery for cerebral arteriovenous malformations: Report of a case. Acta Chir Scand 138:459–464, 1972.
18. Lindquist C, Steiner L: Stereotactic radiosurgical treatment of malformations of the brain. In Lunsford LD (ed): Modern Stereotactic Neurosurgery. Boston: Martinus-Nijhoff, 1988, pp 491–506.
19. Yamamoto M, Jimbo M, Ide M, et al: Long-term follow-up of radiosurgically treated arteriovenous malformations in children: Report of nine cases. Surg Neurol 38:95–100, 1992.
20. Yamamoto M, Jimbo M, Hara M, et al: Gamma knife radiosurgery for arteriovenous malformations: Long-term follow-up results focusing on complications occurring more than 5 years after irradiation. Neurosurgery 38:906–914, 1996.
21. Kemeny AA, Dias PS, Forster DM: Results of stereotactic radiosurgery of arteriovenous malformations: An analysis of 52 cases. J Neurol Neurosurg Psychiatry 52:554–558, 1989.
22. Lunsford LD, Kondziolka D, Flickinger JC, et al: Stereotactic radiosurgery for arteriovenous malformations of the brain. J Neurosurg 75:512–524, 1991.
23. Pollock BE, Lunsford LD, Kondziolka D, et al: Patient outcomes after stereotactic radiosurgery for "operable" arteriovenous malformations. Neurosurgery 35:1–8, 1994.
24. Pollock BE, Flickinger JC, Lunsford LD, et al: Factors associated with successful arteriovenous malformation radiosurgery. Neurosurgery 42:1239–1247, 1998.
25. Steinberg GK, Fabrikant JI, Marks MP, et al: Stereotactic heavy-charged particle Bragg peak radiation for intracranial arteriovenous malformations. N Engl J Med 323:96–101, 1990.
26. Betti OO, Munari C, Rosler R: Stereotactic radiosurgery with the linear accelerator: Treatment of arteriovenous malformations. Neurosurgery 24:311–321, 1989.
27. Colombo F, Benedetti A, Pozza F, et al: Linear accelerator radiosurgery of cerebral arteriovenous malformations. Neurosurgery 24:833–840, 1989.
28. Colombo F, Pozza F, Chierego G, et al: Linear accelerator radiosurgery of cerebral arteriovenous malformations: An update. Neurosurgery 34:14–21, 1994.
29. Souhami L, Olivier A, Podgorsak EB, et al: Radiosurgery of cerebral arteriovenous malformations with the dynamic stereotactic irradiation. Int J Radiat Oncol Biol Phys 19:775–782, 1990.
30. Loeffler JS, Alexander EI, Siddon RL, et al: Stereotactic radiosurgery for intracranial arteriovenous malformations using a standard linear accelerator. Int J Radiat Oncol Biol Phys 17:673–677, 1989.
31. Ellis TL, Friedman WA, Bova FJ, et al: Analysis of treatment failure after radiosurgery for arteriovenous malformations. J Neurosurg 89:104–110, 1998.
32. Pollock BE, Kondziolka D, Lunsford LD, et al: Repeat stereotactic

radiosurgery of arteriovenous malformations: Factors associated with incomplete obliteration. Neurosurgery 38:318–324, 1996.

33. Flickinger JC, Pollock BE, Kondziolka D, et al: A dose-response analysis of arteriovenous malformation obliteration after radiosurgery. Int J Radiat Oncol Biol Phys 36:873–879, 1996.

34. Touboul E, Al Halabi A, Buffat L, et al: Single-fraction stereotactic radiotherapy: A dose-response analysis of arteriovenous malformation obliteration. Int J Radiat Oncol Biol Phys 41:855–861, 1998.

35. Gallina P, Merienne L, Meder JF, et al: Failure in radiosurgery treatment of cerebral arteriovenous malformations. Neurosurgery 42:996–1002, 1998.

36. Troupp H, Marttila I, Halonen V: Arteriovenous malformations of the brain: Prognosis without operation. Acta Neurochir (Wein) 22:125–128, 1970.

37. Forster DMC, Steiner L, Hakanson S: Arteriovenous malformations of the brain. J Neurosurg 562:570, 1972.

38. Itoyama Y, Uemura S, Ushio Y: Natural course of unoperated intracranial arteriovenous malformations: Study of 50 cases. J Neurosurg 71:805–809, 1989.

39. Parkinson D, Bachers G: Arteriovenous malformations: Summary of 100 consecutive supratentorial cases. J Neurosurg 53:285–299, 1980.

40. Spetzler RF, Hargraves RW, McCormick PW: Relationship of perfusion pressure and size to risk of hemorrhage from arteriovenous malformations. J Neurosurg 76:918–923, 1992.

41. Vinuela F, Nombela L, Roach MR: Stenotic and occlusive disease of the venous drainage system of deep brain AVMs. J Neurosurg 63:180–184, 1985.

42. Dias MS, Sekhar LN: Intracranial hemorrhage from aneurysms and arteriovenous malformations during pregnancy and the puerperium. Neurosurgery 27:855–866, 1990.

43. Horton Y, Chambers WA, Lyons SL: Pregnancy and the risk of hemorrhage from cerebral arteriovenous malformations. Neurosurgery 27:867–872, 1990.

44. Willinsky R, Lasjaunias P, Terbrugge K: Brain arteriovenous malformations. J Neuroradiol 15:225–237, 1988.

45. Marks MP, Lane B, Steinberg GK: Hemorrhage in intracerebral arteriovenous malformations: Angiographic determinants. Radiology 176:807–813, 1990.

46. Kjellberg RN, Hanamura T, Davis KR, et al: Bragg-peak proton-beam therapy for arteriovenous malformations of the brain. N Engl J Med 309:269–274, 1983.

47. Kjellberg RN: Stereotactic Bragg peak proton beam radiosurgery for cerebral arteriovenous malformations. Ann Clin Res 18(Suppl)47:17–19, 1986.

48. Seifert V, Stolke D, Mehdorn HM, et al: Clinical and radiological evaluation of long-term results of stereotactic proton beam radiosurgery in patients with cerebral arteriovenous malformations. J Neurosurg 81:683–689, 1994.

49. Steiner L, Lindquist C, Adler JR, et al: Clinical outcome of radiosurgery for cerebral arteriovenous malformations. J Neurosurg 77:1–8, 1992.

50. Karlsson B, Lindquist C, Kihlstrom L, et al: Gamma Knife Surgery for AVM Offers Partial Protection from Hemorrhage Prior to Obliteration. AANS Program Book. Rolling Meadows, IL, American Association of Neurological Surgeons, 1995, p 142.

51. Friedman WA, Blatt DL, Bova FJ, et al: The risk of hemorrhage after radiosurgery for arteriovenous malformations. J Neurosurg 84:912–919, 1996.

52. Pollock BE, Flickinger JC, Lunsford LD, et al: Hemorrhage risk after stereotactic radiosurgery of cerebral arteriovenous malformations. Neurosurgery 38:652–661, 1996.

53. Colombo F, Francescon P, Cora S, et al: Evaluation of linear accelerator radiosurgical techniques using biophysical parameters. Int J Radiat Oncol Biol Phys 31:617–628, 1995.

54. Pollock BE, Flickinger JC, Lunsford LD, et al: Factors that predict the bleeding risk of cerebral arteriovenous malformations. Stroke 27:1–6, 1996.

55. Alexander EI, Siddon RL, Loeffler JS: The acute onset of nausea and vomiting following stereotactic radiosurgery: Correlation with total dose to area postrema. Surg Neurol 32:40–44, 1989.

56. Statham P, Macpherson P, Johnston R, et al: Cerebral radiation necrosis complicating stereotactic radiosurgery for arteriovenous malformation. J Neurol Neurosurg Psychiatry 53:476–479, 1990.

57. Flickinger JC: An integrated logistic formula for prediction of complications from radiosurgery. Int J Radiat Oncol Biol Phys 17:879–885, 1989.

58. Flickinger JC, Schell MC, Larson DA: Estimation of complications for linear accelerator radiosurgery with the integrated logistic formula. Int J Radiat Oncol Biol Phys 19:143–148, 1990.

59. Flickinger JC, Kondziolka D, Maitz AH, Lunsford LD: Analysis of neurological sequelae from radiosurgery of arteriovenous malformations: How location affects outcome. Int J Radiat Oncol Biol Phys 40:273–278, 1998.

60. Karlsson B, Lax I, Soderman M: Factors influencing the risk for complications following gamma knife radiosurgery of cerebral arteriovenous malformations. Radiother Oncol 43:275–280, 1997.

61. Hosobuchi Y, Fabrikant JI, Lyman JT: Stereotactic heavy-particle irradiation of intracranial arteriovenous malformations. Appl Neurophysiol 50:248–252, 1987.

62. Kjellberg RN, Abbe M: Stereotactic Bragg peak proton beam therapy. In Lunsford LD (ed): Modern Stereotactic Neurosurgery. Boston, Martinus-Nijhoff, 1988, pp 463–470.

63. Marks LB, Spencer DP: The influence of volume on the tolerance of the brain to radiosurgery. J Neurosurg 75:177–180, 1991.

64. Flickinger JC, Kondziolka D, Pollock BE, et al: Complications from arteriovenous malformation radiosurgery: Multivariate analysis and risk modeling. Int J Radiat Oncol Biol Phys 38: 485–490, 1997.

65. Kihlstrom L, Guo WY, Karlsson B, et al: Magnetic resonance imaging of obliterated arteriovenous malformations up to 23 years after radiosurgery [see comments]. J Neurosurg 86:589–593, 1997.

66. Marks MP, Delapaz RL, Fabrikant JI, et al: Intracranial vascular malformations: Imaging of charged-particle radiosurgery. Part II: Complications. Radiology 168:457–462, 1988.

67. Yamamoto M, Ban S, Ide M, Jimbo MA: Diffuse white matter ischemic lesion appearing 7 years after stereotactic radiosurgery for cerebral arteriovenous malformations: Case report. Neurosurgery 41:1405–1409, 1997.

68. Yamamoto M, Hara M, Ide M, et al: Radiation-related adverse effects observed on neuro-imaging several years after radiosurgery for cerebral arteriovenous malformations. Surg Neurol 49: 385–397; discussion 397–398, 1998.

69. Yamamoto M, Ide M, Jimbo M, Ono Y: Middle cerebral artery stenosis caused by relatively low-dose irradiation with stereotactic radiosurgery for cerebral arteriovenous malformations: Case report. Neurosurgery 41:474–478, 1997.

70. Francel PC, Steiner L, Steiner M, et al: Repeat radiosurgical treatment in arteriovenous malformations following unsatisfactory results of initial single high-dose radiation. J Neurosurg 74: 352A, 1991.

71. Karlsson B, Kihlstrom L, Lindquist C, Steiner L: Gamma knife surgery for previously irradiated arteriovenous malformations. Neurosurgery 42:1–6, 1998.

72. Gobin YP, Laurent A, Merienne L, et al: Treatment of brain arteriovenous malformations by embolization and radiosurgery. J Neurosurg 85:19–28, 1996.

73. Dawson RCI, Tarr RW, Hecht ST, et al: Treatment of arteriovenous malformations of the brain with combined embolization and stereotactic radiosurgery: Results after 1 and 2 years. Am J Neuroradiol 11:857–864, 1990.

74. Lemme-Plaghos L, Schonholz C, Willis R: Combination of embolization and radiosurgery in the treatment of arteriovenous malformations. In Steiner L (ed): Radiosurgery: Baseline and trends. New York, Raven Press, 1992, pp 195–208.

75. Mathis JA, Barr JD, Horton JA, et al: The efficacy of particulate embolization combined with stereotactic radiosurgery for treatment of large arteriovenous malformations of the brain. AJNR Am J Neuroradiol 16:299–306, 1995.

76. Guo WY, Wikholm G, Karlsson B, et al: Combined embolization and gamma knife radiosurgery for cerebral arteriovenous malformations. Acta Radiol 34:600–606, 1993.

CHAPTER 270

Functional Radiosurgery

CHRISTOPHER M. DUMA ■ MICHAEL SHEA ■ DEANE B. JACQUES ■ OLEG KOPYOV

The use of stereotactic radiosurgery for functional disorders has enjoyed a renaissance based primarily on improved knowledge of neurophysiology and markedly improved imaging techniques using computer and magnetic resonance technology. Significant progress has been achieved since the pioneering efforts of Leksell.[1] Modern functional radiosurgery has been used most frequently for the treatment of trigeminal neuralgia, the tremor of Parkinson's disease, and essential tremor. Its use is also being explored for intractable epilepsy. This chapter reviews the use of radiosurgery in thalamotomy, pallidotomy, trigeminal neuralgia, and epilepsy.

RADIOSURGICAL THALAMOTOMY FOR PARKINSON'S TREMOR

The efferent pathway from the globus pallidus to the ventralis oralis anterialis of the thalamus was initially thought to be the prime target for surgical tremor elimination.[2] Since then, lesions have been moved posteriorly to the nucleus ventralis intermedialis for selective thalamotomy for tremor.[3] Tremor reduction rates using electrophysiologic monitoring and intraoperative physiologic feedback are as high as 70% to 90%, with minimal operative risk.[2-6] The introduction of deep brain stimulator implantation has had an enormous impact on the management of tremor. The high success rates and safety of these procedures make them the treatment of choice for tremor.

However, some Parkinson's patients have conditions that predispose them to higher risks of invasive stereotactic neurosurgery. These are patients who are taking anticoagulants, have respiratory or cardiac disease, are very elderly, or are generally poor candidates for invasive surgery. In addition, some patients may choose a less invasive alternative (Table 270–1). Because radiosurgery involves no incisions or opening of the cranium, the risks of hemorrhage and infection are eliminated. However, radiosurgery does not allow intraoperative physiologic feedback, and the indications for radiosurgery must be strict.

Patient Selection

We previously reported the largest series of patients with parkinsonian tremor treated with the gamma knife.[7] Patients with essential tremor were also included in the series, with similar entry criteria. Of more than 1300 patients treated with gamma knife radiosurgery over the past 8 years, gamma thalamotomies represented only 4% of the total cases. They also represented only 5% of the total number of Parkinson's cases treated. Our results in treating the tremor of Parkinson's disease using radiofrequency lesioning with unit cell recording and physiologic feedback consisted of 90% complete tremor relief, with less than 3% morbidity. Thus, this is usually our procedure of choice for this group of patients.

The same criteria used for radiofrequency thalamotomy may be used for radiosurgical thalamotomy. Patients with tremor-dominant Parkinson's disease and unilateral tremor are most appropriate. Bilateral symptoms may be treated with the same precautions one would use with deep brain stimulator implantation or radiofrequency lesioning, although we had no complications related to bilateral treatment using radiosurgery.

Sixty-seven patients (47 men and 20 women) with disabling tremor from Parkinson's disease and four patients with essential tremor recalcitrant to medical therapy underwent stereotactic radiosurgery using the 201-source cobalt 60 gamma knife at our institutions.[7] Eight patients had bilateral procedures, for a total of 79 lesions. Sixty lesions were left-sided for right-sided

TABLE 270–1 ■ **Clinical Conditions Predisposing a Patient to Radiosurgical Thalamotomy**

Patient choice
Essential anticoagulation
Advanced age
Severe cardiopulmonary disease
Inability to tolerate long intraoperative procedure
Mild dementia

tremor. No patients had undergone previous surgery for Parkinson's symptoms.

Patients were accepted for radiosurgery if they did not satisfy the criteria for invasive radiofrequency thalamotomy: poor surgical or anesthetic risk, advanced age, use of anticoagulants, or personal choice. The United Parkinson's Disease Rating Scale (UPDRS) was used to assess the patients pre- and postoperatively.[8] Only patients with UPDRS grade 3 or 4 tremor were chosen for treatment.

Target Localization

Target localization of the ventralis intermedialis nucleus of the thalamus was determined by coordinates based on the position of the nucleus relative to the anterior commissure–posterior commissure (AC-PC) line, anatomic information gathered from very high resolution magnetic resonance imaging, and subjective surgeon correlation with the Schaltenbrand atlas.[9] The 50% isodose line of the 4-mm collimator was placed at the edge of the contralateral internal capsule medially (Fig. 270–1A). At a level 4 mm above the AC-PC line, the 50% isodose line of the 4-mm collimator lies in the angle formed by a line drawn tracing the medial aspect of the posterior limb of the internal capsule and a line drawn between the posterior limits of the globus pallidus (see Fig. 270–1B). The average target coordinates for all thalamotomies in this series were X = 15 mm lateral to the AC-PC line, Y = 6 mm posterior to the midpoint of the AC-PC line, and Z = 4 mm superior to the AC-PC line. The same target was used for patients with essential tremor.

Dose Selection

Leksell and Lindquist and their colleagues described radiosurgical necrotic lesions from their early experience with functional radiosurgery.[1, 10–13] Doses of 160 to 200 Gy maximum were necessary to create a permanent necrotic lesion. Large collimator sizes (>4 mm) were to be avoided, based on complications encountered in their early experience. In our early experience, we tended to use smaller maximal doses for reasons of patient safety. Based on reports of the reliability of 4-mm collimator irradiation of the rat brain and its dose-response relationship for the parenchyma,[14] patients treated later in our experience tended to receive higher radiosurgical doses. These two groups served as an excellent dose-response comparison study.

Clinical and Radiologic Evaluation

Mild improvement was categorized as a change of one UPDRS grade per independent neurologist evaluation and a subjective patient response of 1% to 33% improvement. Good improvement was categorized as a change of two UPDRS grades and a subjective patient response of 34% to 66% improvement. Excellent improvement was categorized as a change of three UPDRS grades and a subjective patient response of 67% to 99% improvement. The UPDRS scoring system was used for evaluation of essential tremor as well.

Clinical and radiologic follow-up ranged from 2 to 84 months (average, 26 months). Changes in clinical tremor as determined by UPDRS scoring by neurologists and by subjective scoring by patients were highly correlative: 0.89 (Pearson correlation coefficient, P <.001).

Results

No change in tremor occurred in 18 gamma knife–treated patients (25%), mild or good improvement was seen in 25 (35%), and excellent improvement was seen

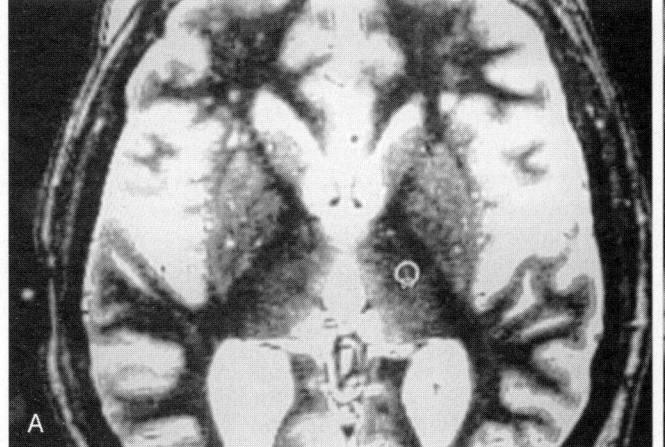
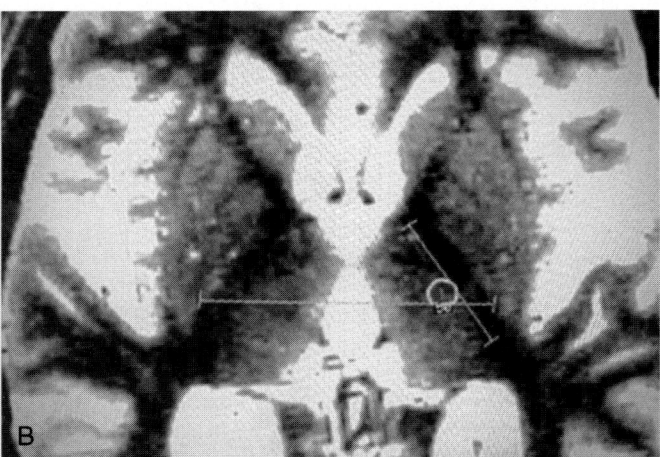

FIGURE 270–1. *A,* Target localization of the ventralis intermedialis nucleus. Average coordinates in the series of successfully treated patients: X = 15 mm lateral to the AC-PC line; Y = 6 mm posterior to mid–AC-PC line; Z = 4 mm superior to AC-PC line. B, "Duma's lines." Additional confirmatory information: 50% isodose line of the 4-mm collimator at the medial aspect of the contralateral posterior limb of the internal capsule. The target is at a point midway along the length of the posterior limb and just above a line joining the tips of the most posterior aspect of the globus pallidus (Duma's line).

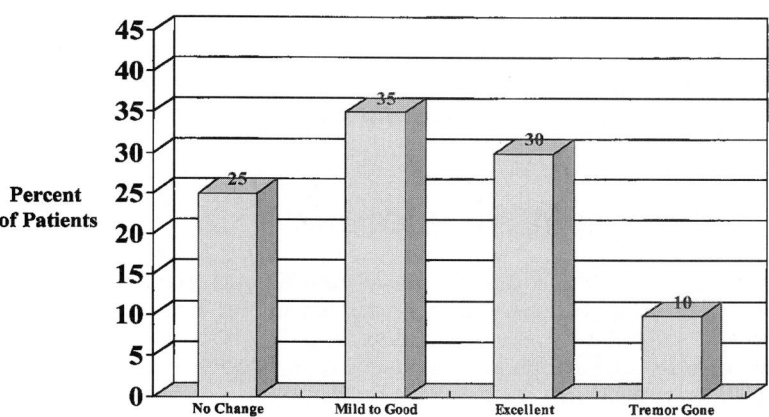

FIGURE 270–2. Clinical results of 71 patients treated for tremor using radiosurgical thalamotomy (percentage of patients vs. clinical result).

in 21 (30%). In seven patients (10%), the tremor was eliminated completely (Fig. 270–2). The high-dose (160 Gy mean maximal dose) thalamotomy lesion was more effective at reducing tremor (78% mean improvement) than was the low-dose (120 Gy mean maximal dose) lesion (56% mean improvement, P <.04, Wilcoxon nonparametric test).

Median time of onset of improvement was 2 months (range, 1 week to 8 months). Two patients who underwent unilateral thalamotomy had bilateral improvement of their tremors. Two patients who had initial improvement in their tremors but eventually returned to baseline during follow-up were included in the treatment failure group. All other patients maintained their level of improvement throughout the course of the follow-up. There were no neurologic complications.

Magnetic resonance imaging showed a circumscribed spherical lesion that enhanced with gadolinium on T1-weighted images at a median of 3 months after radiosurgical placement of the lesion. There was also a mildly diffuse T2 signal change, which usually followed white matter tracts, at a median of 4.5 months after treatment, representing edema.

The average T1-weighted, gadolinium-enhancing lesion size was no different for the low- and high-dose groups and ranged from 3 to 6 mm (mean, 5 mm) at a median follow-up of 6 months. This lesion was present on follow-up scans as long as 58 months after treatment.

The average T2-weighted lesion size was no different for the low- and high-dose groups and ranged from 6 to 22 mm (mean, 9.2 mm) at a median of 6 months' follow-up. This lesion also persisted on future scans (Fig. 270–3). Although not statistically different, there was a trend for the higher dose lesions to elicit a larger T2-weighted signal change or "streaking." This streaking may represent edema, radiation change, demyelination, or necrosis. It is unlikely that it represents necrosis, however, because the presence of streaking within the capsule or other thalamic nuclei never correlated with neurologic impairment. In addition, this streaking did not create mass effect. Only postmortem studies can elucidate the true nature of this finding on follow-up scans.

Clinical improvement in the higher dose group may be explained by *physiologically* larger lesions in this group correcting any target planning inaccuracies. Lack of complications related to bilateral lesions (as is reported in radiofrequency ablation series) may be due to the slow process of making lesions inherent in radiosurgery and the "neurologic healing" or "rerouting" of potentially affected peripheral tracts.

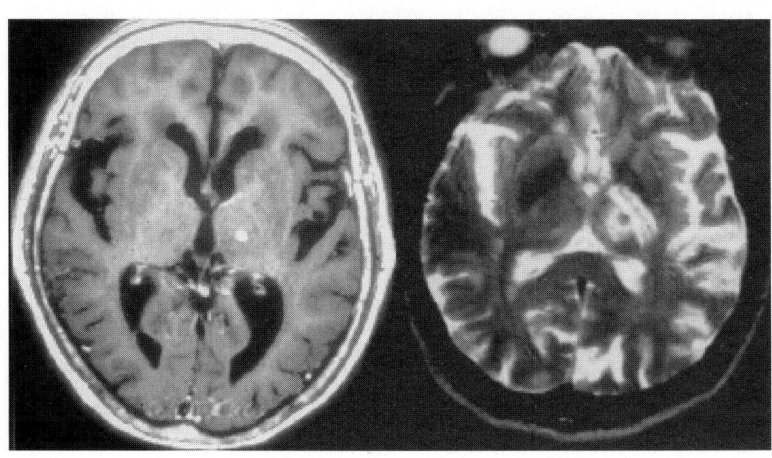

FIGURE 270–3. T1-gadolinium and T2-weighted magnetic resonance imaging sequences 6 months after gamma-thalamotomy. Note the white matter "streaking" on the T2 sequences. There were no clinical sequelae of such T2-weighted changes.

Conclusion

In a small subset of patients who might otherwise be unable to achieve surgical improvement of a disabling tremor, radiosurgical thalamotomy offers a safe and effective means of achieving that goal.

RADIOSURGICAL PALLIDOTOMY

As evidence emerged that the basal ganglia and thalamus control involuntary movement, surgeons strove for an operative cure for the disabling bradykinesia and rigidity of Parkinson's disease. Meyers' open pallidotomy procedures in the 1940s and Cooper's chemically generated lesions and anterior choroidal artery ligation of the 1950s were entrees into the world of stereotactically guided surgeries.[15-17] This, in turn, brought about the advent of cryosurgery and heat-lesioning techniques. Rigidity, bradykinesia, and dyskinesia that are recalcitrant to medical therapies have been improved using stereotactically directed radiofrequency lesioning of the posterior globus pallidus internus.[18-21] Success rates for amelioration of dyskinesia are as high as 90% in some studies and are in the range of 60% to 70% for rigidity and bradykinesia. Like the radiofrequency thalamotomy, it is a safe procedure, and the results can be enhanced using intraoperative electrophysiologic feedback.

There is little in the current or past literature on the treatment of rigidity, bradykinesia, and dyskinesia using a radiosurgically directed approach to pallidotomy. This is no doubt due to the safety and efficacy of radiofrequency lesioning. Friedman and coworkers described their results in four patients using gamma knife pallidotomy in advanced disease.[22] The selected target was the internal globus pallidus, as described by Laitinen and colleagues.[21] All four patients exhibited a response to levodopa before inclusion in the treatment. A single 4-mm collimator with a maximal dose prescription of 180 Gy was used to make the lesion in all patients. The results were disappointing. No patient improved in a significant manner during the follow-up of 18 months. One patient experienced an improvement in his dyskinesia but also became transiently psychotic and demented. The other three patients suffered no adverse effects. Follow-up magnetic resonance imaging scans at 1 year revealed accurately placed lesions, but with variable and unpredicted sizes.

Young and coworkers had more promising results.[23] Twenty-nine patients were treated with radiosurgical posteromedial pallidotomy for symptoms of bradykinesia, rigidity, and levodopa-induced dyskinesias. Eighty-five percent of the patients were relieved of dyskinesias; two thirds showed improvements in bradykinesia and rigidity but no objective improvement in their UPDRS scores. Only one patient had a complication of a homonymous field cut in the follow-up interval.

We treated 18 patients with medically intractable Parkinson's disease with gamma-pallidotomy.[24] Patients' ages ranged from 59 to 85 years at the time of treatment (median, 73 years). Fifteen patients were treated using a single 4-mm collimator with a median maximal prescription dose of 160 Gy (range, 90 to 165 Gy) aimed at the internal globus pallidus. Three patients were treated using a combination of two 4-mm shots with a dose of 160 Gy. Follow-up ranged from 6 to 40 months (median, 8 months).

The results were not good. Only six patients (33%) showed any improvement at all in rigidity and dyskinesia. Three patients (17%) were unchanged, and nine patients (50%) were worse after treatment (Table 270–2). Of the six patients with improvement, two exhibited visual field deficits. Overall, four patients had visual field deficits; three patients had speech or swallowing difficulties, or both; three had worsening of their gait; and one had numbness in the contralateral hemibody. Nine patients (50%) had one or more complications related to treatment (Figs. 270–4 and 270–5).

The explanation for the profoundly high complication rate of 50% in our series is no doubt the variability

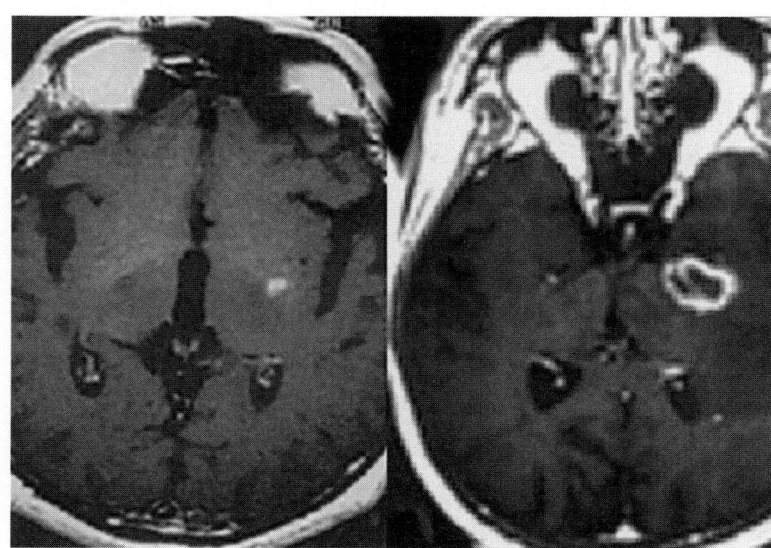

FIGURE 270–4. Variability in gadolinium-enhanced T1-weighted 8-month follow-up magnetic resonance images between two different patients who received the same 160-Gy maximal prescription dose to the globus pallidus.

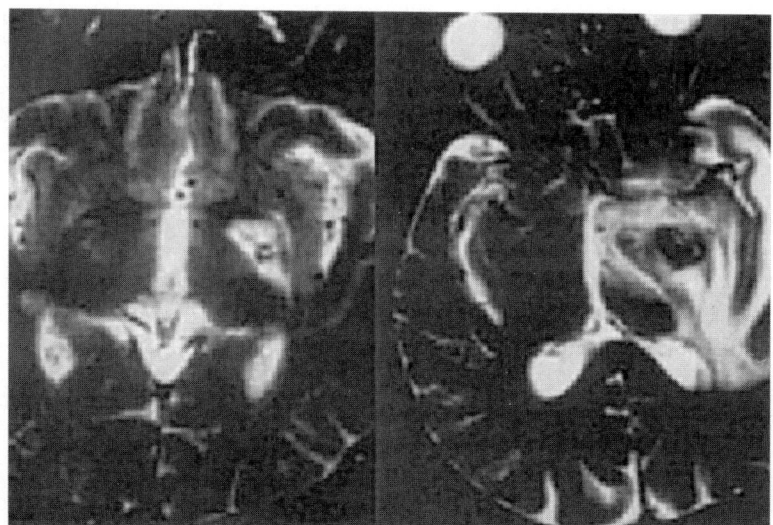

FIGURE 270–5. Extreme edema variability in T2-weighted 8-month follow-up magnetic resonance images between two different patients who received the same 160-Gy maximal prescription dose to the globus pallidus.

and unpredictability of the lesion size when the globus pallidus serves as the target. This degree of unpredictability and variability was not seen in the ventralis intermedialis thalamotomy series[7] and probably represents anatomic susceptibility to very small venous or arterial infarction in the area of the internal globus pallidus.

Because of our poor response rate and the high complication rate, we no longer perform radiosurgical pallidotomy. Patients are best served by radiofrequency lesioning with microelectrode recording and physiologic feedback. It is possible, however, that radiosurgical lesioning with a lower prescription dose could reduce or eliminate these complications and still be clinically effective.

RADIOSURGERY FOR DYSTONIA AND CHOREA

To date, there have been no publications on the radiosurgical treatment of dystonia or other movement disorders *unrelated* to Parkinson's disease, other than essential tremor.

RADIOSURGICAL TREATMENT OF TRIGEMINAL NEURALGIA

The history of radiosurgical treatment of trigeminal neuralgia dates to 1951, when the father of gamma knife radiosurgery, Lars Leksell, experimented by stereotactically aiming a beam of radiation from an x-ray tube to the gasserian ganglion.[1] By 1971, Leksell had reported two patients treated this way, with promising results. At a median follow-up of 17.5 years, both patients had complete relief of pain (Table 270–3).[12]

Lindquist and coworkers also reported their experience with radiosurgical management of trigeminal neuralgia using the 179-source gamma unit prototype and the more modern 201-source unit.[13] Forty-six patients were followed after radiosurgical treatment of the ganglion. In 59% of the patients, good to complete relief of pain was noted initially. Unfortunately, after a median of 2.5 years' follow-up, the success rate dropped to only 18%, a lower long-term rate than that reported in most surgical series.

Target Selection

These historical results from treatment of the ganglion prompted a number of investigators to resurrect the

TABLE 270–2 ■ Clinical Results of Gamma Knife Pallidotomy for Parkinson's Disease

PATIENT	FOLLOW-UP (Mo)	RIGIDITY, DYSKINESIA	COMPLICATIONS
1	8	No change	None
2	7	No change	None
3	35	No change	None
4	9	Improved	None
5	13	Improved	None
6	29	Improved	Homonymous visual field cut
7	40	Improved	None
8	7	Improved	Homonymous visual field cut
9	36	Improved	None
10	24	Worse	Homonymous visual field cut
11	6	Worse	None
12	7	Worse	Dysphagia, dysarthria, hemiparesis
13	7	Worse	Homonymous visual field cut, dysphagia
14	4	Worse	Hemianesthesia
15	12	Worse	None
16	12	Worse	Dysphagia, dysarthria
17	6	Worse	Worse gait
18	6	Worse	Worse gait

T A B L E   2 7 0 – 3 ■ **Results of Radiosurgical Treatment of Trigeminal Neuralgia**

STUDY	NUMBER OF PATIENTS	PERCENTAGE WITH 50–100% PAIN RELIEF	MEDIAN FOLLOW-UP (Yr)	PERCENTAGE WITH 50–100% PAIN RELIEF AT MEDIAN FOLLOW-UP
Gasserian Ganglion Targets				
Leksell (1971)[12]	2	100	17.5	100
Lindquist (1991)[13]	46	59	2.5	18
Proximal Nerve Root Targets				
Kondziolka (1996)[25]	50	94	1.5	88
Young (1998)[29]	110	95.5	4.1	91
Duma (results in this chapter)	65	85	3.5	73

radiosurgical treatment of trigeminal neuralgia. However, the target changed to the proximal portion of the nerve as it enters the pons. The selection of the proximal nerve target was based on a number of factors: (1) oligodendrocytes are more radiation-sensitive than are Schwann cells, (2) compared with the region of the ganglion, the axons are more compact for all three divisions at the root, and (3) targeting against a background of cisternal cerebrospinal fluid is easier.[25] Accuracy of the lesion was ensured with careful planning by magnetic resonance imaging scans and previous knowledge of the radiation effect of a single 4-mm collimator dose to the rat optic chiasm.[14, 26]

Dose Selection

The nerve bundle that makes up the trigeminal nerve is composed of pain fibers (C and A delta) and sensory fibers. The pain fibers are less myelinated than the sensory fibers. The anatomic lesion created by radiosurgery in the trigeminal nerve, based on rat experiments in the optic nerve, is one of demyelination and inflammation.[14] Thus, the ideal radiosurgical lesion would be powerful enough to affect only the pain fibers and be too weak to affect the heartier sensory fibers. Over the years, this "magic number" has been reported to be anywhere between 60 and 90 Gy in a single fraction with a 4-mm collimator and a dose factor of 0.8 using the gamma knife. Higher complication rates occur at doses greater than 90 Gy.

Results

As indicated in Table 270–3, Kondziolka and coworkers evaluated 50 patients treated at five centers by radiosurgery using a standard gamma knife technique for classic trigeminal neuralgia.[25] All patients received a maximum target dose between 60 and 90 Gy, with a single 4-mm collimator aimed at the proximal trigeminal nerve, approximately 2 to 4 mm from its entrance into the pons. The brainstem itself received maximum dose fall-off at the 20% isodose line. The median follow-up was only 18 months. Fifty-eight percent of patients were pain free, 36% of patients had good control of their pain (defined as 50% to 90% relief), and 6% failed. The median onset of pain relief was 1 month

(range, 1 day to 6.7 months). During follow-up, three patients had recurrence of their pain, but by 2 years, 88% of patients had 50% to 100% pain relief. Higher target doses were statistically more effective at eliminating pain than were lower doses. Only 6% of patients had any type of mild paresthesia, which improved with time in the majority of patients.

Regis and coworkers described their experience with the gamma knife in treating trigeminal neuralgia.[27, 28] Of the 20 patients in the series, only 5 had true idiopathic trigeminal neuralgia (the remainder had pain syndromes from tumors or arteriovenous malformations). The authors believed that follow-up was insufficient to make any assumptions.

Young and colleagues reported their series of 110 patients treated with the gamma knife to a single isocenter with a radiosurgical dose of 70 to 80 Gy (see Table 270–3).[29] Follow-up ranged from 4 to 49 months (mean, 19.8 months). Pain relief was achieved in 95.5% of patients with "typical" trigeminal neuralgia, and only 3.3% had recurrence of their pain in the follow-up period. Only three patients (2.7%) developed mild, delayed loss of facial sensation.

We reviewed the results of gamma knife radiosurgical treatment of 65 patients with trigeminal neuralgia over a period of 5 years at our institution (see Table 270–3). Median follow-up was 35 months (range, 11 to 55 months). Twenty-three patients were male and 42 were female. Ages ranged from 37 to 87 years (median, 73 years). Maximum target doses using a single 4-mm collimator ranged from 60 to 84 Gy (median, 82.5 Gy). The treatment isocenter was aimed at the proximal nerve 3 to 4 mm from its entrance into the pons, and the center of the nerve was targeted at the 80% isodose line (Fig. 270–6). Thirty-six patients (56%) had complete pain relief, and 29% rated their pain relief as good (50% to 90% improved). Fifteen percent failed therapy completely. The majority of improved patients were able to discontinue or markedly reduce their medications. Two patients had mild paresthesias that resolved with dexamethasone therapy. No patient experienced permanent paresthesias or anesthesia dolorosa. At the median follow-up of 3 years, seven patients (11%) had return of their pain, requiring repeat gamma knife treatments. Thus, our 3-year median success rate was approximately 73%.

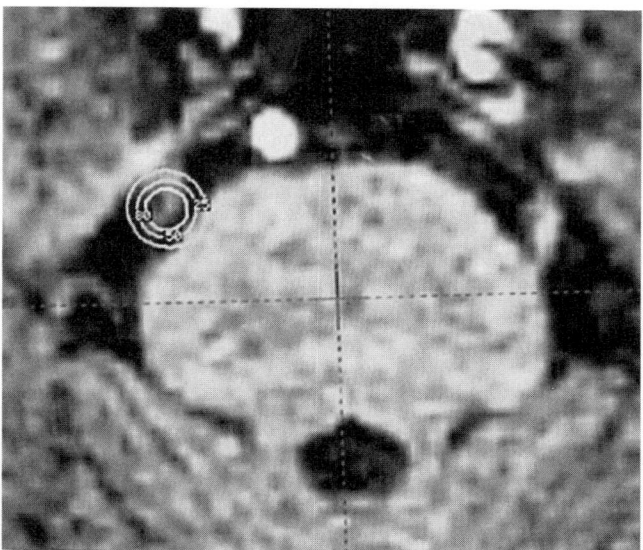

FIGURE 270–6. Target planning for gamma knife radiosurgery for trigeminal neuralgia. The 80% isodose line is used for targeting the entry zone region of the nerve, approximately 4 mm from its entry into the pons. Note the rapid falloff of radiation into the pons.

RADIOSURGERY FOR THE TREATMENT OF EPILEPSY

Barcia Salorio and coworkers described the use of gamma knife radiosurgery for the treatment of epilepsy as early as 1985.[30] These results led to further investigation into this controversial use of radiosurgery. Whang and Kwon reported their 5-year results in 31 patients using gamma knife radiosurgery for the treatment of medically intractable epilepsy.[31] Thirteen patients had generalized seizures, six patients had partial-complex seizures, and four had focal seizures. Electroencephalograms and magnetic resonance imaging scans were used to identify and localize the seizure focus. The radiosurgical lesions were less than 2 cm in diameter and described as nonprogressive. At follow-up, 12 patients had excellent results (Engel class I).[32] In five others, the results were described as class II or III. In the remaining nine patients, seizure frequency was unchanged. Whang and Kwon concluded that the indications for radiosurgery in intractable epilepsy are still limited. Regis and colleagues, however, had more promising results.[28] Fifteen of 16 patients in their series were completely free of seizures in their follow-up interval. One patient had only rare nondisabling seizures after gamma knife treatment.

Given the fact that radiation effects in the penumbra around radiosurgically treated tumors and arteriovenous malformations may themselves induce seizures, the usefulness and efficacy of placing radiosurgical lesions as a primary treatment of epilepsy remain to be elucidated.

SUMMARY

Based on the literature and our experience, radiosurgical thalamotomy should be reserved for only a very

small percentage of the patient population with functional disorders. Thalamotomy is an effective and useful alternative to invasive radiofrequency techniques for patients at high surgical risk. Higher radiosurgical doses are more effective than lower ones at eliminating or reducing tremors and are associated with low complication rates. Radiosurgical thalamotomy should be considered for patients who would otherwise have no surgical treatment options.

The results of radiosurgical pallidotomy, in contrast, have been disappointing. A 50% complication rate (homonymous field cuts, hemiparesis, and dysphagia), combined with a poor success rate (only 33% of patients showed any improvement in dyskinesia and rigidity), has led us to re-evaluate the indications for this procedure in the face of the excellent results of radiofrequency pallidotomy with physiologic monitoring. The high complication rate may be related to the special radiosensitivity of the globus pallidus tissue.

Radiosurgical treatment of trigeminal neuralgia has been encouraging, and some centers are now using it as their treatment of choice for the disease. Future studies are needed to define the dose tolerance of the nerve, but escalated prescription doses in the future may offer patients even more successful and lasting pain relief.

Radiosurgical treatment of epilepsy is in its earliest stages of development and needs more animal study and clinical experience.

REFERENCES

1. Leksell L: The stereotaxic method and radiosurgery of the brain. Acta Chir Scand 102:316–319, 1951.
2. Laitinen L: Brain targets in surgery for Parkinson's disease. J Neurosurg 62:349–351, 1985.
3. Tasker RR: Thalamotomy. Neurosurg Clin N Am 1:841–864, 1990.
4. Ohye C: Selective thalamotomy for movement disorders: Microrecording stimulation techniques and results. In Lunsford L (ed): Modern Stereotactic Neurosurgery. Boston, Martinus Nijhoff, 1988, pp 315–331.
5. Jankovic J, Cardoso F, Grossman RG, et al: Outcome after stereotactic thalamotomy for parkinsonian, essential and other types of tremor. Neurosurgery 17:680–687, 1995.
6. Ohye C, Hirai T, Miyazaki M, et al: VIM thalamotomy for the treatment of various kinds of tremor. Appl Neurophysiol 45:275–280, 1982.
7. Duma C, Jacques D, Kopyov O, et al: Gamma knife radiosurgery for thalamotomy in parkinsonian tremor: A five-year experience. J Neurosurg 88:1044–1049, 1998.
8. Fahn S, Elton RL, et al: Unified Parkinson's disease rating scale. In Fahn S, Marsden CD, Caine DB, Goldstein M (eds): Recent Developments in Parkinson's Disease, vol 2. Florham Park, NJ, Macmillan Healthcare Information, 1987, pp 153–163.
9. Schaltenbrand G, Wahren W: Atlas for Stereotaxy of the Human Brain, 2nd ed. Chicago, Georg Thieme, 1977, pp 124–126.
10. Lindquist C, Steiner L, Hindmarsh T: Gamma knife thalamotomy for tremor: Report of two cases. In Steiner L (ed): Radiosurgery, Baseline and Trends. New York, Raven Press, 1992, pp 237–243.
11. Leksell L, Backlund EO: Stereotactic gammacapsulotomy. In Hitchcock E, Ballantine H Jr, Meyerson B (eds): Modern Concepts in Psychiatric Surgery. Amsterdam, Elsevier, 1979, pp 213–216.
12. Leksell L: Stereotactic radiosurgery in TN. Acta Chir Scand 137:311–314, 1971.
13. Lindquist C, Kihlstrom L, Hellstrand E: Functional neurosurgery—a future for the gamma knife? Stereotact Funct Neurosurg 57:72–81, 1991.
14. Kondziolka D, Lunsford LD, Claasen D, et al: Radiobiology of

radiosurgery. Part I. The normal rat brain model. Neurosurgery 31:940–945, 1992.

15. Meyers HR: Surgical procedure for postencephalitic tremor with notes on the physiology of premotor fibers. AMA Arch Neurol Psychiatry 44:453–459, 1940.

16. Cooper IS, Bravo C-J: Implications of a five-year study of 700 basal ganglia operations. Neurology 8:701–707, 1958.

17. Cooper IS, Bravo G: Chemopallidectomy and chemothalamectomy. J Neurosurg 15:244–250, 1958.

18. Bakay RAE, DeLong MR, Vitek JL: Posteroventral pallidotomy for Parkinson's disease. J Neurosurg 77:487–488, 1992.

19. Iacono RP, Shima F, Louser R, et al: Results and mechanisms for pallidotomy for Parkinson's akinesia. Mov Disord 9:484–485, 1994.

20. Kelly PJ, Ahlskog JE, Goerss SJ, et al: Computer-assisted stereotactic ventralis lateralis thalamotomy with microelectrode recording control in patients with Parkinson's disease. Mayo Clin Proc 62:655–664, 1987.

21. Laitinen L, Bergenheim AT, Hariz MI: Leksell's posteroventral pallidotomy in the treatment of Parkinson's disease. J Neurosurg 76:53–61, 1992.

22. Friedman JH, Epstein M, Sanes JN, et al: Gamma knife pallidotomy in advanced Parkinson's disease. Ann Neurol 39:535–538, 1996.

23. Young RF, Vermeulen S, Posewitz A, et al: Pallidotomy with the gamma knife: A positive experience. Stereotact Funct Neurosurg 70(Suppl 10):218–228, 1998.

24. Duma C, Jacques D, Kopyov O: Gamma knife radiosurgery for the treatment of movement disorders. In Lunsford L, Kondziolka D, Flickinger J (eds): Gamma knife brain surgery. Prog Neurol Surg 14:195–211, 1998.

25. Kondziolka D, Lunsford LD, Flickinger JC, et al: Stereotactic radiosurgery for trigeminal neuralgia: A multiinstitutional study using the gamma unit. J Neurosurg 84:940–945, 1996.

26. Kondziolka D, Linskey ME, Lunsford LD: Animal models in radiosurgery. In Alexander E III, Loeffler J, Lunsford LD (eds): Stereotactic Radiosurgery. New York, McGraw-Hill, 1993, pp 51–64.

27. Regis J, Manera L, Dufour H, et al: Effect of the gamma knife on trigeminal neuralgia. Stereotact Funct Neurosurg 64(Suppl 1):182–192, 1995.

28. Regis J, Barotolomei F, Metellus P, et al: Radiosurgery for trigeminal neuralgia and epilepsy. Neurosurg Clin N Am 10:359–377, 1999.

29. Young RF, Vermulen S, Posewitz A: Gamma knife radiosurgery for the treatment of trigeminal neuralgia. Stereotact Funct Neurosurg 70(Suppl 10):192–199, 1998.

30. Barcia Salorio JL, Roldan P, Hernandez G, et al: Radiosurgical treatment of epilepsy. Appl Neurophysiol 48:400–403, 1985.

31. Whang CJ, Kwon Y: Long-term follow-up of stereotactic gamma knife radiosurgery in epilepsy. Stereotact Funct Neurosurg 66(Suppl 10):349–356, 1996.

32. Classification of epilepsy. In Engel J, Pedley TA (eds): Epilepsy: A Comprehensive Textbook, vol 1. Philadelphia, Lippincott-Raven, 1997, pp 518–519.

CHAPTER 271

Interstitial and Intracavitary Irradiation of Brain Tumors

M. W. MCDERMOTT ■ P. H. GUTIN ■ MITCHEL S. BERGER ■ P. K. SNEED

Brachytherapy is the practice of administering therapeutic irradiation by means of a source placed a short distance from, or within, the body part being treated, as opposed to teletherapy, in which the radiation source is outside the body, several feet away. The clinical practice of brain tumor brachytherapy began with Hirsch, who in 1912 inserted a radium probe into the sella of a woman with acromegaly, followed by Frazier, who in 1914 implanted radium into a malignant glioma tumor bed at the time of craniotomy.[1, 2] The development in the late 1940s and early 1950s of new radioisotopes, coupled with the development of frame-based stereotactic systems, brought about renewed interest in interstitial brachytherapy for the treatment of brain tumors. The early experience was with permanent interstitial implants for inoperable low-grade tumors and intracavitary therapy for cystic gliomas and craniopharyngiomas.[3–9] The first attempt at intracavitary brachytherapy for craniopharyngioma was made in 1950 by Leksell[6]; using phosphorus 32 (^{32}P) sodium phosphate solution, he treated a 40-year-old man with a recurrent cystic craniopharyngioma. In North America, intracavitary therapy has not caught on, but there is extensive experience with interstitial brachytherapy using iodine 125 (^{125}I), high- and low-activity implants, and iridium (Ir) 192 for malignant supratentorial gliomas.[10–36] At our institution, there has been a shift from high- (temporary) to low- (permanent) activity ^{125}I implants. The former delivers higher doses in shorter intervals, and the latter implant can be performed at the same debulking operation for first diagnosis or recurrence. Interstitial hyperthermia has been added to interstitial irradiation for malignant gliomas, with some encouraging results. At our institution, the first randomized phase III trial has been completed, indicating an added survival benefit.[32] Intracranial metastases, recurrent meningiomas, and skull base neoplasms are also suitable for temporary or permanent implantation using interstitial techniques.

Probably the biggest change affecting the practice of brachytherapy for gliomas and metastases has been the increased availability and use of radiosurgery. Radiosurgery has been used as a boost for small malignant gliomas at diagnosis and for tumors at recurrence. The results of randomized trials of radiosurgery boost for newly diagnosed patients, compared with standard therapy, have not yet been published. Retrospective data seem to indicate that for small-volume tumors there is probably some benefit, with improvements in tumor control and survival.[37] For large tumors with associated edema, mass effect, and clinical symptoms of increased intracranial pressure, tumor debulking with or followed by brachytherapy may be the preferred treatment option.

Interstitial and intracavitary brachytherapy attempts to improve the therapeutic ratio by using a modality that has the radiobiologic advantage of low-dose irradiation and allows for the delivery of high doses of radiation to localized volumes without significant irradiation of surrounding normal brain. For malignant glioma, it has been shown experimentally and clinically that radiotherapy is the single most effective form of treatment; however, significant improvements in median survival time have not been realized using external beam irradiation, in spite of manipulations of the total dose and fractionation schedule and the use of radiation sensitizers and particle beam therapy.[38–40] Although early clinical experience using interstitial brachytherapy for recurrent gliomas showed promise, prompting evaluation of its use in newly diagnosed patients, questions have been raised about using a focal form of therapy in a tumor that is clearly infiltrating.[41–44] Yet in several studies analyzing the pattern of recurrence after external beam irradiation, local recurrence within 2 cm of the primary tumor site was the most common pattern of failure.[12, 29, 45–50] Rates of tumor recurrence within the brain but removed from the primary site have varied from 0% to 10%, and systemic failures from 0% to less than 1%. Thus, the local control rate for malignant gliomas remains poor with conventional external beam radiation therapy alone, and it is this shortcoming that interstitial brachytherapy attempts to address.

The controversy surrounding the treatment of craniopharyngiomas continues, with clinical series supporting aggressive surgical resection, limited resection followed by external beam irradiation, intracavitary irradiation of cystic tumors, and radiosurgical treatment of small residual or recurrent solid tumors.[51-61] With cystic tumors, the target tissue is the cyst wall, only millimeters thick. The low energy and short depth of tissue penetration of several β-emitting radioisotopes allows the safe delivery of large doses of radiation to the walls of these tumor cysts. Pathologic specimens from patients treated in this manner demonstrate that the epithelial lining cells are destroyed and replaced largely by fibrous tissue.[62] Success with the technique has led some authors to suggest an algorithm that incorporates surgery and stereotactic intracavitary and radiosurgical therapies into the management of these tumors, depending on the relative proportions of solid and cystic tumor.[59]

RADIOBIOLOGY

Increases in the therapeutic ratio for interstitial and intracavitary brachytherapy, as compared with external beam teletherapy, are realized by placing the radioactive source or sources within the tumor volume and by the favorable radiation biology of continuous low-dose irradiation.

With the encapsulated sources used in interstitial brachytherapy, the dose rate falls off rapidly as one moves away from the radioactive source. The falloff in dose rate does not conform strictly to the inverse square law, because within the first centimeter or so from the radioactive source there is a buildup of dose from scattered secondary photons.[63] At greater distances from the source, the dose distribution depends on the number of radioactive sources within the implanted volume, their spatial relationship to one another, the density or absorbance of surrounding tissues, and the energy of the emitted irradiation.

The characteristics of the common isotopes used in brachytherapy are listed in Table 271–1. With the low-energy β-emitting sources used for intracavitary treat-

ment, most of the radiation dose is deposited in the first few millimeters of cyst wall or tumor, with little dose reaching normal tissues. "Plating" of some isotopes up against a cyst wall may occur, so one cannot assume a uniform distribution of isotope within the cyst, and the actual dose to the cyst wall may be higher than calculated. By comparing the activity of fluid aspirated a certain number of days after the instillation of isotope with the activity as measured on an isotope scintillation scan, Fig and colleagues showed that the larger the cyst, the higher the actual dose to the cyst wall.[64]

The type of ionizing radiation used, the total activity of the sources, and the dose rate are important determinants of the biologic effect of any radiation dose on tissue. In general, the lower the dose rate, the smaller the biologic effect of a given dose; this effect is observable particularly over the range of 0.01 to 1 Gy/minute.[1, 65-71] Dose rates from interstitial brachytherapy sources are commonly on the order of 0.4 to 0.6 Gy/hour, as compared with 1.8 to 2 Gy/minute with conventional linear accelerators. The effectiveness of low dose rates on a particular tumor and cell line has a lower limit below which tumor cell proliferation is not inhibited. One therapeutic advantage of continuous low-dose irradiation relates to differences in repair of sublethal damage between tumor and normal tissue, with normal tissue being more efficient in this regard.[67-69, 72] Experimentally, the higher the dose rate, the less this separation of effect, and the lower the total dose at which normal tissue damage is observed.[73] As radiation-sensitive cells are destroyed during continuous irradiation, other cells continuing through the cell cycle enter its more sensitive G_2M phase.[74] This redistribution of cells into the more radiation-sensitive phase of the cell cycle also accounts for the improved tumor cell kill. In addition, hypoxic cells, traditionally regarded as being resistant to conventional radiation, are relatively more sensitive to the effects of continuous low-dose irradiation.[75] Repopulation of tumor cells is also reduced with interstitial brachytherapy, because

T A B L E 2 7 1 – 1 ■ **Characteristics of Isotopes Used in Modern Interstitial and Intracavitary Brachytherapy**

		INTERSTITIAL BRACHYTHERAPY	
Isotope	**Half-Life**	**Energy Emitted—Gamma Rays (mean)**	**Half-Value in Tissue (mm)**
Iodine 125	60.2 days	28 keV	20
Iridium 192	74.2 days	380 keV	70
Cobalt 60	5.3 yr	1250 keV	111
Palladium 103	17.0 days	21 keV	0.008
Gold 198	2.7 days	412 keV	2.5
Calf 252	2.56 yr	1 MeV	98
		2.35 MeV neutrons	31
		INTRACAVITARY BRACHYTHERAPY	
Isotope	**Half-Life**	**Energy Emitted—Beta Rays (mean)**	**Half-Value in Tissue (mm)**
Phosphorus 32	14.2 days	0.69 MeV	0.8
Yttrium 90	2.7 days	0.93 MeV	1.1
Rhenium 186	3.7 days	0.36 MeV	0.4
Gold 198	2.7 days	0.32 MeV	0.4

during a standard course of clinical treatment, at least one cell cycle is irradiated with at least two to three times the dose necessary to inhibit mitosis (720 to 900 cGy).[11, 76] Assuming a dose rate of 0.4 to 0.6 Gy/hour, a cell-cycle time for malignant gliomas of anywhere from 24 to 120 hours, and a total implant duration of 4 to 6 days, the total dose delivered per cell cycle will be well above the critical value for inhibiting mitosis.[11]

The results of two clinical studies support the beneficial effects of low-dose irradiation on malignant gliomas. Siddiqi and coworkers evaluated the effects of ^{125}I brachytherapy on the histologic features of malignancy and the proliferating cell nuclear antigen (PCNA) index in patients with newly diagnosed glioblastoma randomized to brachytherapy boost or not.[77] Thirteen of the control group and 11 of the implant group underwent reoperation during follow-up. The mean histologic score (each feature graded 0 to 4) for cellularity, pleomorphism, vessel hyperplasia, mitosis, and necrosis with pseudopalisading was significantly less in the brachytherapy group at reoperation. PCNA indices were also significantly lower in the brachytherapy group. Within the tumor tissue removed at reoperation, radionecrosis was increased by brachytherapy. The authors concluded that the data indicated that ^{125}I brachytherapy can have additional effects in reducing the proliferative potential of glioblastomas treated by conventional therapy. Kunisho and associates looked at the MIB-1 labeling index in 30 patients before and after interstitial brachytherapy.[78] In the 12 patients with histologic evidence of radionecrosis at reoperation, the MIB-1 index was $7.6 \pm 5.5\%$, compared with $17.0 \pm 11.2\%$ in the same tumors at first operation ($P < 0.05$). Although morphologically viable tumor cells were found in specimens with radionecrosis, brachytherapy reduced the proliferative potential of these cells as measured by the MIB-1 index.

For ^{125}I, the energy of emitted gamma rays is in the range of 27 to 35 keV, compared with 300 to 610 keV for Ir192. For permanent ^{125}I implants, sources of 0.5-mCi strength are used, and 97% of their total dose is delivered over 5 half-lives of the isotope. The total dose delivered using any isotope depends on the number of sources, total activity, and duration of the implant. The higher tissue attenuation of the low-energy photons accounts for the reduced irradiation of normal tissue surrounding the target and improved radiation safety with the use of [125]I.[1] The relative biologic effectiveness of ^{125}I has also been found to be slightly better than that of Ir192.[79–82] Low-energy photons of ^{125}I also have a predominance of photoelectric absorption dependent on the atomic number of the interposed tissue.[83] Therefore, the absorption in tissue such as bone is four to five times that of soft tissue, contributing again to the improved radiation safety of ^{125}I compared with Ir192.

Dempsey and colleagues described a new method for interstitial brachytherapy.[84] The device consists of an inflatable silicone balloon reservoir attached to a positionable catheter that is placed in a glioma resection cavity and filled postoperatively with liquid ^{125}I radionuclide solution. Using a dosimetric modeling system, the authors showed that compared with ^{125}I seed implants, the balloon–liquid isotope method produced a more conformal dose, with no target underdosing and no hot spots. Homogeneity of dose within the target volume was superior, as expected, but there was an increased volume of normal tissue receiving 50% to 75% of the prescribed target tissue dose.

For intracavitary treatment of craniopharyngioma cysts, where the epithelial cell-cycle time is longer, effective doses of 200 to 250 Gy are delivered over 5 half-lives of the isotope, or approximately 71 days for [32]P.[51–54] The mean energy of the emitted β particles is 0.69 MeV, with a half-value in tissue of only 0.8 mm. At this time, ^{32}P is the only isotope licensed in the United States for intracavitary therapy.

PATIENT SELECTION

Interstitial Brachytherapy

Patients must be in good neurological condition with a Karnofsky performance score (KPS) greater than or equal to 70. They must be able to understand the potential benefits and risks of interstitial brachytherapy and be available for the recommended interval of follow-up. For patients with cerebral metastases, the solitary nature of the metastasis is first confirmed with a triple-dose contrast magnetic resonance imaging (MRI) scan, and the patient must have stable systemic disease. All patients must have a life expectancy greater than 3 months.

Factors of tumor size, location, radiographic appearance, and histologic type also determine whether the patient has an implantable lesion. For temporary high-activity implants, tumors less than 6 cm in maximal diameter are the largest acceptable size, and because of the fear of brainstem injury, only supratentorial, subcortical locations are implanted. For permanent low-activity implants inserted stereotactically, deeper ganglionic and brainstem locations seem to tolerate the low-dose irradiation. Permanent low-activity sources can also be used for newly diagnosed and recurrent malignant glioma and for skull base and dural lesions that are subtotally resected and exposed at open operation.[18, 85, 86] Patients with diffuse intra-axial tumors, tumors that appear to be multicentered, or those with involvement of the corpus callosum or ependymal lining of the ventricles are not appropriate candidates for interstitial brachytherapy.

Based on our experience, patients with newly diagnosed glioblastoma multiforme (GM) benefit most from combined interstitial brachytherapy and hyperthermia. We are currently evaluating the use of permanent low-activity implants in combination with hyperfractionated external irradiation in a phase II study for newly diagnosed malignant glioma. Patients with recurrent GM or anaplastic astrocytoma and selected skull base tumors may also benefit from interstitial brachytherapy.[18–20, 27, 33] Image-guided surgical systems are particularly helpful in defining the contrast-enhancing margin in recurrent gliomas, because the goal with permanent implants is to place sources within 1 cm of this enhancing margin. Patients with skull base, dural, and paraspinal lesions considered for permanent low-activity ¹²⁵I implants must have lesions that can be debulked at open operation, and they should be at least 1 cm away from sensitive neural structures (optic nerve, chiasm, and tract; brainstem; spinal cord). In some situations, gold foil has been used to protect the spinal cord and brainstem from the emitted radiation.

Intracavitary Brachytherapy

Intracavitary brachytherapy has been used successfully for cystic craniopharyngiomas and for treating recurrent cystic low-grade gliomas. All patients with lesions adjacent to the optic nerve, chiasm, and tract and the hypothalamus require formal neuro-ophthalmologic evaluation of visual acuity and fields, as well as assessment of the hypothalamic-pituitary axis, before treatment. For craniopharyngiomas, a significant portion of the tumor should be cystic, and gliomatous cysts should be refractory to standard therapy and the primary cause of recurrent neurological symptoms. Patients with malignant glioma cysts are not appropriate candidates for this treatment, and only those with low-grade tumor cysts should be selected.

IMPLANTATION TECHNIQUE

Interstitial Brachytherapy

HIGH-ACTIVITY IMPLANTS

Our technique for temporary high-activity implants strives to encompass all enhancing tumor within a given isodose surface (40 to 60 cGy/hour) while attempting to achieve a smooth dose distribution at the margin of the tumor, thus limiting the dose to surrounding normal brain. We attribute less importance to dose inhomogeneity within the tumor volume, which is consistent with the notion that the enhanced therapeutic ratio for brachytherapy lies partly in its ability to selectively deliver high doses of radiation to the tumor volume while sparing the surrounding normal brain. Others have developed systems that attempt to produce a homogeneous dose distribution within the target volume by means of rigid templates that create a fixed spatial pattern for catheter placement.[87, 88] Based on the results of our phase III randomized trial, we now combine high-activity implants with hyperthermia for patients with small, localized, enhancing, newly diagnosed glioblastoma after resection and the completion of external irradiation.[32] A previous publication describes the treatment planning and surgical technique for temporary high-activity implants in detail.[89]

LOW-ACTIVITY IMPLANTS

Treatment Planning

Preoperative computed tomographic or MRI scans are used to determine the approximate surface area and volume of tumor that must be implanted after surgical resection. The radiation oncologist then calculates the number of seeds and total activity required to deliver 6000 cGy over the lifetime of the permanent sources, assuming a 1-cm spacing on the walls of the resection cavity. Volumetric image-guided MRI data sets are collected preoperatively and used as navigational systems intraoperatively.[90] Unless otherwise instructed, the radiation oncologist assumes that the surgeon will resect all the contrast-enhancing tissue and uses the maximal diameter of the lesion for calculations. Contrast-enhancing tumor that is more than 1 cm away from implanted sources is not assumed to be adequately treated, and in such settings, adjuvant chemotherapy may be recommended. Dosimetry is calculated postoperatively based on computed tomographic scans and can be superimposed on MRI sets (Fig. 271–1). The minimal tumor dose is defined by the isodose line that surrounds all residual tumor administered over 5 half-lives of the isotope (half-life = 60 days). Unlike temporary implants afterloaded in nylon catheters, there is no opportunity to adjust spacing or source strength after the implant. Some comparisons of permanent and temporary implants are presented in Table 271–2. In contrast, permanent sources that are implanted at the margin of the lesion have very conformal dose distributions at a depth of 0.5 cm (Fig. 271–2).

Surgical Technique

An open craniotomy for tumor resection is carried out using modern techniques, including image-guided surgical systems and intraoperative electrophysiology for motor, sensory, and speech mapping. After resection and hemostasis, the surgeon and radiation oncologist dress in radioprotective garments. In most cases, free, individual 0.67-mCi ¹²⁵I seeds are placed lining the walls of the resection cavity by the surgeon. Sterile lead pegs containing the sources are emptied, and the total number of sources is counted by the radiation oncologist. Sources in groups of 10 are placed within a multichamber holder; then individual sources are counted and placed on a Mayo stand connected to the surgical field by a sterile drape (Fig. 271–3). The sources are placed at approximately 1 cm² spacing on the walls of resection cavities, covered by squares of absorbable hemostatic gauze, and glued in position with fibrin glue. Sources embedded in polyglactin su-

TABLE 271–2 ■ **Comparison of Temporary and Permanent Iodine-125 Implants**

	TEMPORARY	PERMANENT
Activity per source	0.67 mCi	10–20 mCi
Dose rate	11 cGy/hr	40–60 cGy/hr
Median number of sources	80	8
Hospital cost per case	$2720	$3200
Total dose	25,000 cGy	5300 cGy
Time to total dose	Infinity	4–5 days

Data from University of California–San Francisco.[85]

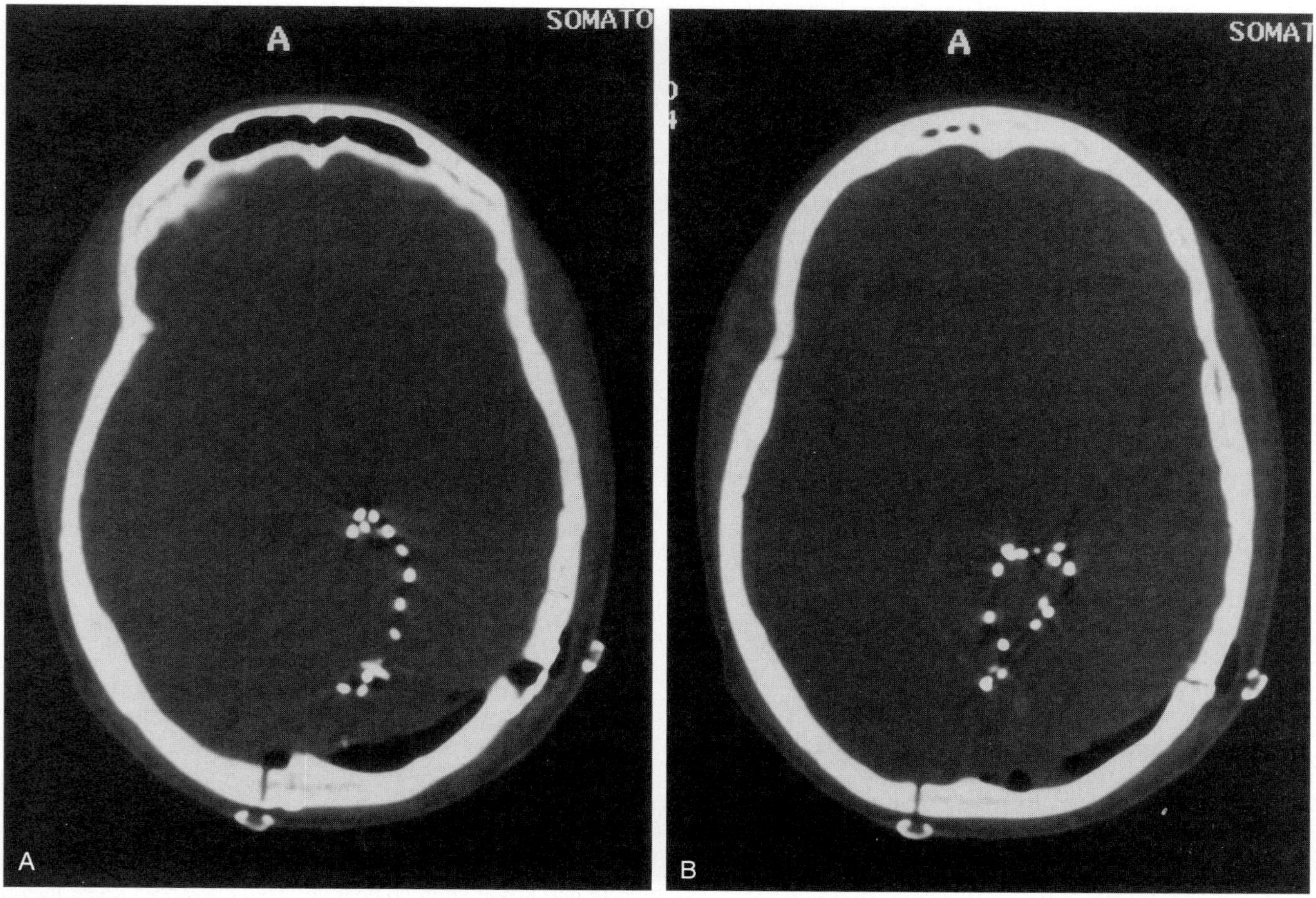

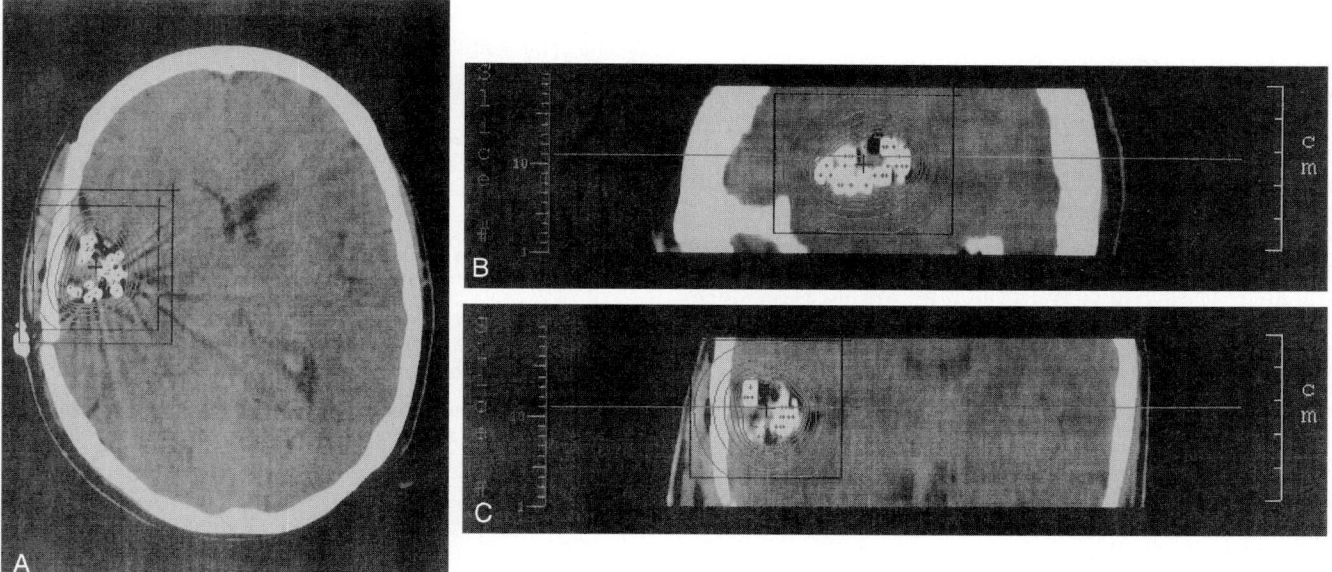

FIGURE 271–1. Postoperative computed tomographic scans of a patient with a low-activity implant for recurrent medial left occipital malignant glioma. Bone window settings on inferior *(A)* and superior *(B)* aspects of the resection cavity were used to digitize the seed location for dosimetry.

FIGURE 271–2. Axial *(A)*, sagittal *(B)*, and coronal *(C)* computed tomography with 10,000- to 60,000-Gy isodose lines displayed, calculated assuming an infinite time of decay.

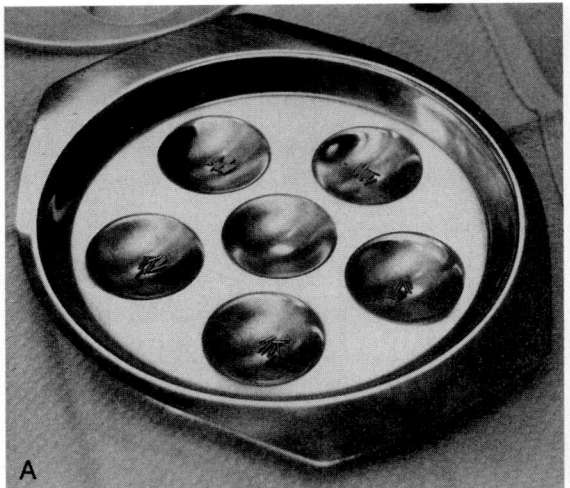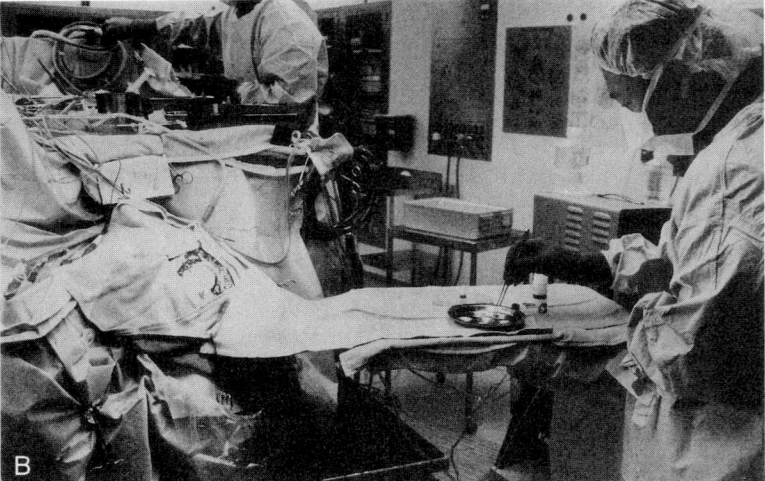

FIGURE 271–3. *A,* Five-well dish holding iodine-125 seeds. Each well around the edge of the dish contains 10 seeds. *B,* Operating room setup, with the radiation oncologist standing to one side and wearing protective gloves and thyroid and chest lead-lined shields. A sterile drape extends from the Mayo stand to the operative field to prevent seeds from falling to the floor.

ture can also be used for permanent implants and are preferred in cases of dural lesions such as recurrent malignant meningioma.

At the completion of implantation, the number of sources implanted is totaled and confirmed. At the completion of surgery, metered readings of radiation output are taken 1 m from each side of the patient's head. Patients wear a lead-lined cap back to the recovery room or intensive care unit, and on the second day after surgery, they are given an instruction sheet (Fig. 271–4).

Intracavitary Brachytherapy

TREATMENT PLANNING

The methods of intracavitary brachytherapy for cystic tumors have been well described by Lunsford and associates.[91] The patient is placed in the Cosman-Roberts-Wells (CRW) base ring (a target-centered system). An intravenous contrast-enhanced computed tomographic scan using 3-mm-thick slices is performed, covering the entire volume of the cyst. The margin of the cyst on sequential axial slices is marked with the computed tomographic console trackball, and the area of the cyst on each slice is determined. The volume of the cyst is then calculated as the sum of all the areas of each slice multiplied by the slice thickness. This method is just as accurate as the isotope dilution technique using technetium 99m.[91] For cysts larger than 1.5 cm in diameter, surgical navigation systems can be used that do not require the application of a stereotactic frame. A series of 128 contiguous 1.5-mm-thick slices is obtained for volumetric image reconstruction of the skin surface; the same images can be used to measure the area of interest and derive the volume of the cyst. The amount of ^{32}P necessary to deliver 200 Gy to the cyst wall can then be calculated, as well as the dose at any other point from the cyst wall, with the method of Kobayashi and colleagues.[92]

<u>**RADIOACTIVE IMPLANT: INSTRUCTIONS FOR PATIENT AND FAMILY**</u>

1. Please observe the following instructions from _____ to _____ . During this time, family members 45 years and older should stay 3 feet or more from the patient as much as is practical. Spouses may share sleeping accommodations but should maintain a 3-foot distance most of the time. Adult visitors and family members under 45 years may spend up to an hour per day at distances closer than 6 feet from the patient. Pregnant women should visit no more than a few minutes per day within a distance of 9 feet.

These restrictions apply only when on the patient's left side. There are no limitations necessary on the right side.

2. After _____ no restrictions in patient contact are required.

3. There are no restrictions with the lead cap on.

Details of Implant

Seed Type:	Mediphysics Model 6711
Radionuclide	Iodine-125
Amount administered:	23.2 mCi
Number of seeds:	42 seeds (0.552 mCi each)
Site:	Brain
Date:	Jan. 6, 2003

Initial average exposure rate at 1 meter:	0.133 mr/hr
Initial maximum exposure rate at 1 meter:	0.3 mr/hr

Medical and rehabilitation personnel may provide therapy but should limit contact closer than 3 feet to 33 hours per week on the left side. There are no limitations necessary on the right side.

If any questions arise regarding radiation safety or in the event of a medical emergency, we can be reached at the phone number listed above.

_____   _____
Fellow   Professor

FIGURE 271–4. Instruction sheet given to patients who undergo permanent low-activity implants. (Courtesy of University of California–San Francisco.)

SURGICAL TECHNIQUE

Using a stereotactic frame, a target for cyst puncture is selected within the midportion of the cyst as measured in the vertical plane; then the anteroposterior, lateral, and vertical coordinates are measured directly from the computed tomography console using the CRW localizer. When image-guided systems are used, the center of target is defined in the operating room using the trajectory view.

In the operating room, using a frame-based system, the anteroposterior, lateral, and vertical coordinates for the cyst target are entered into the phantom base and the CRW arc ring system. The trajectory to the target is confirmed, and the stereotactic needle is set to the target depth on the phantom base. A bur hole is then fashioned 2 to 3 cm from the midline just anterior to the coronal suture for lesions in the suprasellar region, or over the brain harboring a gliomatous cyst. The dura is opened in a cruciate fashion, a small cerebrotomy is made, and the CRW arc ring is returned to the patient base ring. With image-guided frameless systems, the cyst is visualized on the trajectory view, and the trajectory is fixed with a needle guide that is screwed into the outer table of the skull. A two-way stopcock is attached to a fine 20-gauge needle, with a blunt and sharp inner stylet available. The needle with a blunt stylet is advanced to the target. If resistance is felt a short distance from the final target position, this usually represents the cyst wall. At this point, the blunt stylet is exchanged for a sharp-tipped stylet, and the wall is penetrated, advancing to the center of the cyst. The central stylet is removed, and a small volume of fluid is removed into a syringe and measured. The precalculated volume of isotope is then drawn into a tuberculin syringe. Through one stopcock, the ^{32}P is injected and repeatedly aspirated back and forth using the same tuberculin syringe. Through the other stopcock, a volume of saline equal to the amount of cyst fluid withdrawn on the initial puncture, minus the volume of colloidal solution, is injected to flush the remaining isotope out of the needle into the cyst and to restore the original cyst volume. The needle is withdrawn. The needle and the syringes used in the procedure are collected by a radiation technologist. The wound is closed in the usual manner.

FOLLOW-UP

Neurological examinations and follow-up computed tomographic or MRI scans are performed at 2-month intervals for the first year. Craniopharyngioma cyst patients are seen at 2 and 4 weeks postoperatively to assess for worsening symptoms due to mass effect or signs of optic pathway compression. At each follow-up, clinical symptoms, dexamethasone dose, neurological status, KPS, and results of imaging studies are recorded. Those patients treated in the hypothalamic-pituitary area must have annual endocrine and neuro-ophthalmologic assessments as well. For patients with malignant gliomas who have had high-activity tempo-

rary implants and in whom there is a question of tumor recurrence versus radiation necrosis, magnetic resonance spectroscopy, positron emission tomography, or single photon emission computed tomography is used to attempt to differentiate radiation necrosis from recurrent tumor.[93, 94] Artifact from permanent ^{125}I sources makes magnetic resonance spectroscopy technically difficult to perform and interpret. After brachytherapy, reoperation is considered for neurological deterioration in patients with recurrent tumor by magnetic resonance spectroscopy or positron emission tomography or when there is an expanding contrast-enhancing mass and symptoms are not controlled by increasing doses of steroids. Patients with symptoms referable to local mass effect from a treated cyst can have the cyst contents aspirated by stereotactic means. In the experience of many authors, virtually no radioactivity is recovered in cyst fluid aspirated several weeks after injection.[51–54, 64, 91, 95, 96]

RESULTS

Interstitial Brachytherapy

NEWLY DIAGNOSED MALIGNANT GLIOMA

Up until 1998, most of the information from prospective trials of high-activity brachytherapy for newly diagnosed malignant gliomas was based on the results of phase II studies. Scharfen and colleagues[27] analyzed the entire University of California–San Francisco experience of 307 patients with gliomas treated between December 1979 and June 1990.[27] They found median survivals of 88 weeks in 106 patients with GM, 142 weeks in 52 patients with NGM, and 226 weeks in 16 patients with low-grade NGM. Postimplant chemotherapy resulted in no difference in survival, so we no longer use adjuvant chemotherapy following brachytherapy for newly diagnosed GM patients. In the entire brachytherapy patient population, 40% required reoperation, and there was no association between the total activity of the implant or the implant volume and the reoperation rate. Of the 124 patients who had reoperations, 5% had necrosis only, 29% had tumor only, and 66% had both tumor and necrosis; the median survivals for these three pathologic groups were not significantly different. The total acute complication rate for the 307 patients was 7.8%, and the mortality was 0.7%. Two patients died within 30 days of the implant, but neither death was related to an intracranial event (one from sepsis; one from pulmonary embolism).

Florell and coworkers reminded us that some of the improved survival in these series is related to patient selection.[17] In their review of consecutive patients referred to a regional cancer center, they found that only about 30% of patients were considered eligible for brachytherapy based on imaging studies and KPS alone. Eligible patients tended to be younger, had better KPSs, had more extensive surgical resection, and survived longer than noneligible patients when both groups were treated in the same manner. Videtic and colleagues applied the RTOG recursive partitioning analysis to attempt to determine the impact of selection bias on the results of permanent ^{125}I brachytherapy in newly diagnosed patients.[35] Compared with the data from the RTOG database, they found improved survival in the poorest prognostic categories (classes II to VI) in their retrospective review (Table 271–3). They suggested that with these criteria taking into account age, pathology, KPS, and other factors, selection alone may not account for the improved survival seen.

Sneed and associates analyzed the results of brachytherapy boost in 159 patients with GM over an 11-year period and found that on multivariate analysis, only age was a significant independent predictor of outcome.[30] As expected, the younger the patient, the better the outcome, but some of the results were impressive in terms of long-term survival. For the age groups 18 to 29.9, 30 to 39.9, 40 to 49.9, 50 to 59.9, and 60 years and older, the 2-year survival figures were 78%, 58%, 44%, 25%, and 18%, respectively, with median survivals of "not reached," 109, 96, 77, and 76 weeks, respectively.

In 1998, the results of two prospective, randomized trials using high-activity temporary brachytherapy implants were reported. Sneed and associates reported the results of a trial using adjuvant hyperthermia in patients with glioblastoma undergoing brachytherapy after conventional radiotherapy.[32] The scientific background for adding hyperthermia is that it kills cells exponentially as a function of temperature above 41°C and inhibits the repair of sublethal and potentially lethal radiation damage.[97] Heat is particularly effective against cells that tend to be resistant to radiation, such as S-phase cells and low-pH, nutrient-deprived hypoxic cells.[97] The hyperthermia goal was to attain steady-state temperatures within 5 to 10 minutes of turning the power on and to heat as much of the tumor as possible to at least 42.5°C for 30 minutes, without exceeding 50°C, immediately before and after brachytherapy.[32] From 1990 to 1995, 39 patients were randomized to brachytherapy without heat and 40 patients to brachytherapy with heat. By intent to treat, the time to tumor progression and median survival were longer for heat than for no heat ($P = 0.04$ and $P = 0.04$). A comparison between groups that actually received the randomized treatment revealed the same results, with median and 2-year survivals of 95 weeks and 31% for the hyperthermia group ($n = 35$) versus 76 weeks and 15% for the nonhyperthermia group ($n = 33$). The rate of reoperation was similar in the no-heat and heat groups, at 58% and 69%, respectively. Pathologic findings were also similar in the two groups, with tumor and necrosis the most common finding at reoperation in 48% of the no-heat and 51% of the heat groups. Toxicity of the hyperthermia itself was acceptable, and there were no therapy-related deaths within 30 days of treatment in either treatment arm. There was a trend for an increased incidence of neurological changes and seizures in the heat group. Multivariate analysis also revealed that after adjusting for age and KPS, improved survival was significantly associated with randomization to hyperthermia ($P = 0.008$). This was the first prospective clinical trial to show an added benefit for hyperthermia in addition to brachytherapy for any body site or tumor.

Laperriere and colleagues reported the results of their trial randomizing 140 patients with GM between 1986 and 1996 to high-activity brachytherapy implants after operation and external irradiation.[22] Of the 71 patients randomized to receive an implant, only 63 actually did, although the final analysis of data was performed on an intent-to-treat basis. Review of the brachytherapy treatment data revealed that these tumors were large, with a median prescription dose volume of 42.3 cc, clearly a treatment volume inappropriate for consideration of radiosurgery. Most implants (85.7%) were performed using one or two catheters. There was no significant difference in median survival for the nonimplant and implant arms: 13.2 and 13.8 months, respectively ($P = 0.24$). For the 63 patients who actually received the implant, the median survival was 15.7 months. Multivariate analysis revealed a trend for improved survival in the implant arm ($P = 0.07$) and, significantly, for KPS of 90 or greater ($P = 0.007$) and treatment at recurrence (chemotherapy or reoperation) ($P = 0.004$). At 6 and 12 months after randomization, there was no difference in the KPS of the nonimplant and implant groups (at 6 months, 80 and 80; at 12 months, 70 and 60, respectively), but there was a significant increase in the median dexamethasone dosage for patients in the implant arm of the study (at 6 months, 4 versus 8 mg; at 12 months, 8 versus 16 mg). Reoperation rates were the same in both groups (33% versus 31%), and 24% of the implant group suffered significant complications attributable to the implant. Recurrence at the original site occurred in 93% and 82% of nonimplant and implant patients, respectively,

TABLE 271–3 ■ Survival of Patients with Newly Diagnosed Malignant Glioma Treated with Permanent Iodine-125 Implant Based on RTOG Class

RTOG CLASS	MEDIAN SURVIVAL (MO)	2-YEAR SURVIVAL (%)
I/II*		
Iodine 125	37	68
RTOG I	58.6	76
RTOG II	37.4	68
III		
Iodine 125	31	74
RTOG	17.9	35
IV		
Iodine 125	16	34
RTOG	11.1	15
V/VI*		
Iodine 125	11	29
RTOG V	8.9	6
RTOG VI	4.6	4

*Classes combined for permanent iodine-125 group
Adapted from Videtic GMM, Gaspar LE, Zamarano L, et al. Use of the RTOG recursive partitioning analysis to validate the benefit of iodine-125 implants in primary treatment of malignant gliomas. Int J Radiat Oncol Biol Phys 45:687–692, 1999.

TABLE 271–4 ■ **Results of Brachytherapy Boost for Malignant Glioma since 1995**

AUTHOR	YEAR	NO. OF PATIENTS	PATHOLOGY	MEDIAN SURVIVAL (MO)
Sneed et al[30]	1995	159	GM	19
		52	AA	36
Fernandez et al*[16]	1995	18	GM	>23
		40	AA	>31
Sneed et al[32]	1998	33	GM	17.5 (no heat)
		35	GM	19.6 (heat)
Videtic et al*[35]	1998	53	GM	17
		22	AA	38
Laperriere et al[22]	1998	69	GM	13.2 (no implant)
		71	GM	13.8 (implant)

*Permanent low-activity implant.
AA, anaplastic astrocytoma; GM, glioblastoma multiforme.

with an increased incidence of multifocal recurrence in the implant arm. The Brain Tumor Cooperative Group trial has been published only in abstract form, suggesting a survival benefit for implant patients ($P = 0.05$); the final results of the 272 patients randomized through September 1993 have not been published.[98] Based on the results of our own trial and that of the Toronto group, we no longer use temporary high-activity implants alone for newly diagnosed glioblastoma but continue to explore it in combination with hyperthermia in selected cases. Newly diagnosed patients are also eligible for a phase II study of permanent low-activity implants in combination with hyperfractionated external irradiation. The results of clinical series since 1995 are summarized in Table 271–4.

RECURRENT MALIGNANT GLIOMA

Most of the initial clinical trials with brachytherapy were in patients with recurrent malignant glioma. Table 271–5 contains the results of several series published since 1995. In one of the earliest studies to support continued work with brachytherapy, Gutin and co-workers found that reoperation was necessary in 41% of patients, and despite the presence of apparently viable tumor cells in the surgical specimens, more than half the patients were alive more than 2 years after reoperation.[73] Bernstein and colleagues reoperated on 27.8% of their recurrent patients, with a median survival of 16.5 weeks.[13] In an analysis of the largest group of patients from the University of California–San Francisco, the reoperation rate for necrosis varied from

36% to 47%, depending on the original diagnosis, and reoperation significantly prolonged survival.[27] Shrieve and associates compared the rates of reoperation and survival in well-matched series of retrospectively reviewed patients treated with either temporary high-activity brachytherapy implants or radiosurgery.[28] The median survivals were comparable in the two groups: 11.5 months for brachytherapy, and 10.2 months for radiosurgery. The actuarial risk for reoperation was lower in the radiosurgery group—33% at 12 months, compared with 54% in the brachytherapy group. However, the volumes of treatment were three times greater in the brachytherapy group (29 cc) than in the radiosurgery group (10.1 cc).

In contrast to the experience with high-activity implants, low-activity permanent sources seem to be better tolerated and can be placed during the operation for tumor debulking. Larson and coworkers reported on the use of permanent gold 198 in recurrent grade 3 and 4 tumors; the median survivals after implantation were 17 and 9 months, respectively.[23] No patient required reoperation for radiation necrosis in this series. Fernandez and colleagues used permanent ^{125}I implants for 58 patients with newly diagnosed malignant glioma, 40 with anaplastic astrocytoma, and 18 with GM.[16] Although 45% of the patients underwent reoperation, in only 11% was the pathologic material consistent with necrosis alone during a median 22-month follow-up. Halligan and associates reoperated and implanted 18 patients with GM and achieved a median survival of 64 weeks.[21] None of their patients required reoperation for symptomatic radiation necrosis. Suplica

TABLE 271–5 ■ **Results of Brachytherapy Implant for Recurrent Glioma Since 1995**

AUTHOR	YEAR	NO. OF PATIENTS	DIAGNOSIS	MEDIAN SURVIVAL (MO)
Chamberlain et al[14]	1995	16	MG	9.5
Shrieve et al[28]	1995	32	GM	11.5
Halligan et al*[21]	1996	22	MG	15.0
Perez-de la Torre et al*[26]	1999	59	MG	16.0
Suplica et al*[33]	1999	38	GM	11.8
Patel et al*[86]	2000	40	GM	10.8

*Permanent low-activity implant.
GM, glioblastoma multiforme; MG, malignant glioma.

and colleagues reported on 38 patients with recurrent GM implanted with permanent ^{125}I sources, and in no case was a second reoperation necessary for necrosis.[33] Median follow-up from time of the implant was 46.4 weeks, and median survival was 51.3 weeks. Perez-de la Torre and coworkers reported the results of permanent low-activity ^{125}I sources for recurrent malignant glioma and found similar control rates and limited toxicity.[26] With a median follow-up of 40 months, the survival for recurrent GM patients was 0.9 year; it was 2.04 years for those with non-GM recurrent malignant glioma. Factors predicting a poor outcome were GM histology, target volume of more than 17 cc, and tumor location within the corpus callosum or thalamus. Only three patients (5%) underwent reoperation for necrosis. A recent paper reporting the results for permanent ^{125}I implants by Patel and coworkers found a median time to tumor progression of 25 weeks and a median survival of 47 weeks.[86] Multivariate analysis revealed that time to progression was influenced significantly only by gross total resection ($P < 0.05$). Ninety percent of patients had a local component to their failure, indicating that the predominant problem remains local recurrence. No patient in this series developed symptoms attributable to radiation necrosis or injury.

Thus it appears that the toxicity of high-activity implants is greater than that of low-activity implants, with comparable survivals in retrospective series.

PERMANENT IMPLANTS AS SOLE TREATMENT FOR MALIGNANT GLIOMA

Mundinger has published extensively on the use of permanent implants alone, but mainly for low-grade astrocytomas.[7, 99–101] Median survival figures for the combined treatment of malignant glioma (grades 3 and 4) using permanent implants and external irradiation were not given in these papers. Etou and colleagues, reporting on a 10-year follow-up for patients younger than 10 years old with malignant diencephalic tumors, found a median survival of approximately 6 months with permanent Ir192 for grade 4 tumors ($n = 6$) and a 33% 1-year survival for grade 3 tumors treated with ^{125}I or Ir192 ($n = 9$).[102] Ostertag and Kreth used permanent ^{125}I implants alone as the primary treatment for 73% of grade 3 and 79% of grade 4 tumors.[103] Temporary implants in the remaining patients were left in place for 20 to 30 days, delivering a mean dose of 6000 cGy at 10 cGy/hour. The median survival was 8 months for grade 3 patients and 6 months for grade 4 patients. Clearly, these results are inferior to those of conventional external beam therapy.

PERMANENT IMPLANTS AS SOLE TREATMENT FOR LOW-GRADE ASTROCYTOMA

European centers have extensive experience with permanent implants for low-grade astrocytomas, especially in children. As pointed out by Bernstein and Laperriere, one must view the results in light of the variable natural history of these slow-growing neoplasms.[104] Etou and colleagues reported 3-year survivals of 58% to 70% in 69 patients younger than 18 years of age treated with permanent implants for grade 1 astrocytomas.[102] For 27 grade 2 patients, the 3-year survivals were 36% to 38%, depending on the isotope used. Mundinger and coworkers reported the long-term outcome for 89 patients with low-grade brainstem gliomas after interstitial irradiation as the primary form of treatment.[99] The 5-year survival rates were 54.8% in the ^{125}I group, 26.9% in the Ir192 group, and 14.7% in the biopsy-only group. Mortality was 2.4%, and morbidity 6.2%. There was a trend toward more favorable outcomes using ^{125}I as opposed to Ir192.

Ostertag and Kreth treated 430 patients with low-grade tumors using interstitial brachytherapy as the primary therapy.[103] The 5-year survival rates were 77% for pilocytic astrocytoma, 65% for grade 2 astrocytoma, 80% for oligoastrocytoma, and 58% for oligodendroglioma. No patients in this series required reoperation for radiation necrosis.

METASTASIS

With the proliferation of radiosurgical facilities, brachytherapy for solitary intracranial metastases has declined. It is still an alternative therapy for solitary metastases that recur after surgery and external beam irradiation, or for patients with superficial, large, solitary metastases who require operation for relief of mass effect or reduction of intracranial pressure. In both cases, permanent low-activity sources can be placed at operation, avoiding the need for a second procedure.

Our last review of high-activity implants revealed 30 patients treated in total, 25 of those at recurrence.[105] The median survival for the entire group was 14.7 months; it was 13.9 months for those treated for recurrence. Multivariate analysis revealed that KPS was the only factor significantly influencing outcome ($P = 0.007$). The median survival for those with a KPS less than 70 was 8.5 months, compared with 34.8 months for those with a KPS of 80 or greater. Schulder and associates reported their experience with permanent low-activity implants in combination with whole-brain radiation for solitary brain metastases.[106] One patient received a second implant at operation for recurrence. The median survival was 9 months, but 4 of 13 patients (31%) were alive 27 to 94 months after the implant. Three of these patients had a KPS of 70 or more, and two were no longer on steroids. Bogart and coworkers recently reported on the use of permanent low-activity ^{125}I implants without whole-brain irradiation in patients with solitary brain metastases from non–small cell lung cancer.[107] Median survival was 14 months, and 30% of patients had failure in the brain: two adjacent to the original site, two with multiple metastases outside the primary site, and one with a combined pattern of failure. The clinical series from 1989 to 1999 are summarized in Table 271–6.

As for patients with brain metastases selected for radiosurgery, the status of systemic disease, life expectancy, KPS, and presence of leptomeningeal metastases are important determinants of the suitability of patients for brachytherapy of solitary brain metastases.

T A B L E   2 7 1 – 6 ■ **Results of Brachytherapy for Brain Metastases**

AUTHOR	YEAR	NO. OF PATIENTS	MEDIAN SURVIVAL (MO)
Prados et al[108]	1989	14	18.3
Zamorano et al[36]	1992	16	10.2
Bernstein et al[109]	1995	10	10.5
McDermott et al[105]	1996	30	14.7
Schulder et al[106]	1997	13	9
Bogart et al[107]	1999	15	14

SKULL BASE TUMORS

Permanent implants have been used most commonly for skull base tumors and meningiomas. Kumar and colleagues treated 15 patients with primary and recurrent skull base meningiomas with permanent ^{125}I implants delivering doses ranging from 100 to 500 Gy at 5 to 25 cGy/hour.[110] With a median follow-up of 29 months, the authors reported a remarkable complete radiographic response rate of 73%, partial responses in the remaining patients, and no early or late delayed complications. The results of our experience with skull base tumors and meningiomas were published previously.[85] At last review, there were 26 patients: 10 with malignant meningioma; 3 with recurrent benign meningioma; 5 with chordoma; 3 with paraspinal metastatic lesions; and 1 each with meningeal sarcoma, malignant schwannoma, pituitary adenoma, chondrosarcoma, and glomus jugulare tumor. All patients received permanent low-activity implants; in some cases, thin strips of gold foil were placed between the implant cavity and spinal cord or brainstem to protect the central nervous system tissue. Of the 13 patients with malignant or recurrent meningiomas, 8 patients were stable at a median follow-up of 10.5 months (range, 5 months to 6.5 years). Three of these patients had recurrence at 9, 13, and 14 months; one developed a radiation-induced sarcoma; and one died of pulmonary emboli 2 months after implantation. Of the five patients with chordomas, three had recurrence at 10 months, 19 months, and 2 years after implantation; the same three were alive with disease at 17 months, 2 years, and 4 years. One patient died of medical complications 4 months after surgery with stable disease, and the fifth had stable disease at 19 months. Of the remaining skull base tumor types implanted, three patients died of recurrent disease at 5, 14, and 19 months after implantation. Two patients are alive, one without and one with disease progression, at 18 and 10 months, respectively.

PEDIATRIC INTERSTITIAL BRACHYTHERAPY

Brachytherapy for childhood central nervous system neoplasms presents several challenges. If temporary sources are used, the stereotactic procedure must be done under general anesthesia, and the child must be protected from the accidental removal of sources. There is a wide variety of tumor types, and most pediatric gliomas occur in sites not traditionally considered for implantation.

Several groups have reported their experience with brachytherapy for childhood tumors, two of them using temporary high-activity implants. Chuba and co-workers treated 28 patients with permanent ^{125}I implants, 10 of these with stereotactic implantation into brainstem gliomas.[111] No complications occurred related to catheter placement. Brachytherapy was carried out after completion of standard external irradiation. The planned implant dose was 82.9 Gy at 4 cGy/hour. Half the patients died 7 to 9 months after diagnosis, and four remained alive at a median of 10 months after diagnosis. One patient treated with implant alone for a low-grade astrocytoma was found to have radiation necrosis 36 months after the implant and was salvaged with hyperbaric oxygen. Sneed and associates completed a long-term follow-up on 28 patients who had high-activity implants between 1980 and 1991.[31] There were 4 GMs, 11 malignant gliomas, 10 low-grade gliomas, 2 choroid plexus carcinomas, and 1 rhabdomyosarcoma. All patients had external irradiation, and brachytherapy doses ranged from 31.2 to 83.8 Gy. Twenty patients had no complications in the first months after discharge, and those that did experienced minor side effects. However, 79% of patients underwent reoperation at a median of 10 months after the brachytherapy implant. The median follow-up for 13 living patients was 8.9 years (range, 4.6 to 12 years) from the date of implant. All GM patients expired. The mean KPS was 88 ± 9 at the time of the implant, 87 ± 7 at 3 years, and 87 ± 9 in 11 patients alive at 6 to 12 years. The authors concluded that the aggressive surgical management of radiation necrosis rather than prolonged steroid use contributed to a favorable outcome in these patients.

Intracavitary Brachytherapy

CRANIOPHARYNGIOMA

Stereotactic drainage of a craniopharyngioma cyst was first performed by Leksell, followed several years later by an attempt at a more permanent solution using intracavitary brachytherapy with [32]P.[6, 51–54, 57, 112] The practice of irradiating the cyst walls of these histologically benign, frequently cystic (60% to 80%), but locally recurrent tumors has continued using β-emitting isotopes. These isotopes, with their very short half-values in tissue, are ideally suited to the treatment of a tumor located close to sensitive structures such as the hypothalamus, optic apparatus, pituitary stalk, and circle of Willis.

In 1990, Coffey and Lunsford summarized the experience with intracavitary brachytherapy up to 1986 at nine centers.[54] In the clinical series published to that time, there were 102 patients, 89 of whom were available for follow-up at 4 to 156 months after treatment. Eighty-one patients (91%) had a documented reduction in cyst size, and three (3.7%) an increase. Fifty-seven of the 89 patients had visual function follow-up, and in 84.2% it was stable or improved. Three studies provided sufficient information about endocrine follow-up; in these 47 patients, anterior lobe function remained stable in 38 (81%) and improved in 8 (17%). There were two fatalities in the entire group, and the recurrence rate was 12.7%. Doses to the cyst wall of less than 100 Gy were associated with early failure and recurrence, whereas a dose greater than 400 Gy caused radiation injury. In current practice, the usual calculated dose is 200 to 300 Gy, 95% delivered over 5 half-lives of the isotope in use.

Long-term results from a single-center were published by Pollack and coworkers in 1995.[113] The series included 30 patients treated between 1981 and 1993. Intracavitary irradiation with ^{32}P resulted in cyst regression in 88% of cases. Visual acuity and fields improved or remained stable in 63% of patients. In a comparison of the 13 patients who had intracavitary irradiation as a primary treatment versus the 17 who had treatment for recurrence after surgery, external irradiation, or both, the authors found no difference with respect to cyst control, visual deterioration, or preservation of endocrine function.

Voges and associates published the largest single-institution experience with intracavitary brachytherapy.[114] Papers in the English language since 1995 with more than three patients and more than 12 months' follow-up are listed in Table 271–7. Voges's group analyzed 62 patients harboring 78 craniopharyngioma cysts treated with intracavitary irradiation. The median follow-up was 11.9 years, and 41 of the 62 patients had been followed for more than 10 years. Twenty-one patients had solitary cysts, and cyst volume ranged from 2.2 to 330 cc (median, 18.5 cc). Thirty-four of the 62 patients had received prior external irradiation at standard doses, and 5 patients had received stereotactic radiosurgery. The overall response rate was 79.5%, which included those with complete or partial responses. Stabilization of cyst size was achieved in 15.4%, and no response was seen in 5.1%. Leakage of the radionuclide was documented in 10.2% of cases but was not thought to cause any complications. There were four patients with visual deterioration after treatment, three of whom were blinded, and there were three patients with deterioration in pituitary-hypothalamic function. All complications observed 6 to 12 months after treatment occurred exclusively with yttrium and not with ^{32}P or rhenium 186.

One of the concerns with intracavitary treatment is the proximity of the optic chiasm to the cyst wall being treated. Even though the emitted beta irradiation has a very short track in tissue (half-value in tissue), in many cases, craniopharyngioma cysts are immediately opposed to the front or back of the chiasm. Van den Berge and colleagues published detailed follow-up results with respect to visual function in 31 patients.[61] In 26 of 31 patients, intracavitary brachytherapy (^{90}yttrium) was the primary form of treatment. Ninety-one percent of cysts were the same size or smaller after treatment. Visual acuity was improved in 29%, stabilized in 13%, and deteriorated in 58% of eyes studied. Visual field defects improved in 28%, remained stable in 20%, and deteriorated in 52%. Visual deterioration occurred especially when optic atrophy was present before brachytherapy, and vision worsened in some cases in spite of decreased cyst size. Tumor-related mortality was 16%. Among the surviving patients, 65% lead active, independent lives. The authors concluded that although there was substantial visual morbidity, there were few other side effects and good tumor control, making it a reasonable alternative to craniotomy for attempted gross total resection.

Craniopharyngioma cysts are difficult to manage clinically, and intracavitary irradiation remains an option when these cysts recur after operation or external irradiation. Other techniques with intracavitary chemotherapy require further evaluation before they can be compared to the previously described results.

CYSTIC GLIOMA

Intracavitary treatment of gliomatous cysts has met with some success in patients with low-grade astrocytomas but not in those with malignant tumors.[116–119] Szikla and coworkers, using rhenium 186, treated 17 patients with low-grade glioma cysts (21 cysts) and 8 patients with malignant gliomas (8 cysts).[118] They reported success with all low-grade astrocytoma cysts: 10 stabilized, 5 retracted, and 6 disappeared over a mean follow-up of 34.5 months. Three recurred at 1, 2, and 4.5 years after treatment, with "good results" after a second treatment. With malignant glioma cysts, any benefit in controlling cyst size was negated by progression of the solid tumor. In this group, an initial response was evident in six of eight patients, although the mean survival was only 5 months. The mean calculated dose to the cyst wall for gliomas was 580 Gy, and one third of those receiving more than 400 Gy

T A B L E   2 7 1 – 7 ■ **Results of Intracavitary Brachytherapy for Cystic Craniopharyngiomas since 1995**

AUTHOR	YEAR	NO. OF CYSTS TREATED	ISOTOPE	CYST CONTROL RATE (%)	VISION IMPROVED OR STABLE (%)
Pollack et al[113]	1995	30	Phosphorus-32	88	63
Voges et al[114]	1997	66	Yttrium-90	97	94
		8	Phosphorus-32	100	N/A
		4	Rhenium-186	50	N/A
Blackburn et al[115]	1999	7	Yttrium-90	72*	100

*Success with single treatment; 100% success with two cases requiring second treatment.
N/A, not applicable.

experienced "minor white matter edema at 1–2 months."

Musolino and associates reported the largest single series of intracavitary treatment of glioma cysts.[117] Fifty cysts in 45 patients were treated, 11 with malignant glioma. Again, the benefits in the malignant group were offset by tumor progression, but in the low-grade group, more than 50% of the cysts disappeared, and 25% shrank to one third of their original volume. The prescribed dose to the cyst wall was 400 to 500 Gy using rhenium 186. In 17 cases of grade 1 astrocytoma, the cyst was aspirated at the end of the treatment period, with only 27% of the theoretically activity being recovered, related to adsorption of radionuclide to the cyst wall. Hood and McKeever used intracavitary irradiation for three cystic brainstem gliomas using ^{32}P, and although all three patients improved postoperatively, survival was only 7 (low grade), 8, and 10 (malignant) months.[116]

CONCLUSION

Interstitial brachytherapy has been used extensively in North America for newly diagnosed and recurrent malignant gliomas. The toxicity of temporary high-activity implants is not insignificant, and to date, only one prospective phase III trial combining interstitial hyperthermia with this type of brachytherapy has shown a survival advantage compared with brachytherapy alone. Although the Toronto brachytherapy trial showed no benefit for high-activity temporary brachytherapy implants, results from one other phase III trial have yet to be published. Permanent low-activity implants have been reported in a number of nonrandomized series and appear to have results comparable to those of high-activity implants, without the same degree of radiation toxicity. These implants have the advantage of being placed at the time as debulking surgery, avoiding the second stereotactic procedure necessary for high-activity temporary implants. We await the results of prospective trials using these low-activity sources to help define their role in the management of patients with newly diagnosed and recurrent malignant gliomas.

Intracavitary brachytherapy for cystic craniopharyngiomas has been used extensively in European centers but has not caught on elsewhere. Clearly, the data show that the treatment is effective for cysts related to craniopharyngiomas, but there is a small risk of significant visual toxicity. This treatment modality should be considered an option for craniopharyngioma cysts, in addition to open operation, simple aspiration, or intracavitary chemotherapy.

REFERENCES

1. Bernstein M, Gutin PH: Interstitial irradiation of brain tumors: A review. Neurosurgery 9:741–750, 1981.
2. Frazier CH: The effects of radium emanations upon brain tumors. Surg Gynecol Obstet 31:236–239, 1920.
3. Drake CG, Pfalzner PM, Linell EA: Intracavitary irradiation of malignant brain tumors. J Neurosurg 20:428–434, 1963.
4. Frank F, Gaist G, Frank G, et al: Stereotactic radioisotope implantations in the treatment of inoperable low malignancy neoplasms. J Neurosurg Sci 33:119–121, 1989.
5. Godano U, Frank F, Fabrizi AP, Ricci RF: Stereotactic surgery in the management of deep intracranial lesions in infants and adolescents. Childs Nerv Syst 3:85–88, 1987.
6. Leksell L: The stereotactic method and radiosurgery of the brain. Acta Chir Scand 102:316–319, 1951.
7. Mundinger F, Hoefer T: Protracted long term irradiation of inoperable midbrain tumors by stereotactic curie-therapy using iridium-192. Acta Neurochir Suppl (Wien) 21:93–100, 1974.
8. Szikla G, Musolino A, Miyahara S, et al: Colloidal rhenium-186 in endocavitary beta irradiation of cystic craniopharyngiomas and active glioma cysts: Long term results, side effects and clinical dosimetry. Acta Neurochir Suppl (Wien) 33:331–339, 1984.
9. Talairach J, Ruggiero G, Aboulker J, David M: A new method of treatment of inoperable brain tumors by stereotaxic implantation of radioactive gold—a preliminary report. Br J Radiol 28: 62–74, 1955.
10. Agbi CB, Bernstein M, Laperriere N, et al: Patterns of recurrence of malignant astrocytoma following stereotactic interstitial brachytherapy with iodine-125 implants. Int J Radiat Oncol Biol Phys 23:321–326, 1992.
11. Arbit E, Shapiro JR, Fiola M, et al: The significance of morphologically viable glioma cells found at the time of operation after interstitial brachytherapy. Neurosurgery 32:105–110, 1993.
12. Bashir R, Hochberg F, Oot R: Regrowth patterns of glioblastoma multiforme related to planning of interstitial brachytherapy radiation fields. Neurosurgery 23:27–30, 1988.
13. Bernstein M, Laperriere N, Leung P, McKenzie S: Interstitial brachytherapy for malignant brain tumors: Preliminary results. Neurosurgery 26:371–380, 1990.
14. Chamberlain MC, Barba D, Kormanik P, et al: Concurrent cisplatin therapy and iodine 125 brachytherapy for recurrent malignant brain tumors. Arch Neurol 52:162–167, 1995.
15. Coffey RJ, Friedman WA: Interstitial brachytherapy of malignant brain tumors using computed tomography–guided stereotaxis and available imaging software: Technical report. Neurosurgery 20:4–7, 1987.
16. Fernandez PM, Zamarano L, Yakar D, et al: Permanent iodine-125 implants in the upfront treatment of malignant gliomas. Neurosurgery 36:467–473, 1995.
17. Florell RC, MacDonald DR, Irish WD, et al: Selection bias, survival, and brachytherapy for glioma. J Neurosurg 76:179–183, 1992.
18. Gutin PH, Leibel SA, Hosobuchi Y, et al: Brachytherapy of recurrent tumors of the skull base and spine with iodine-125 sources. Neurosurgery 20:938–945, 1987.
19. Gutin PH, Leibel SA, Wara WM, et al: Recurrent malignant gliomas: Survival following interstitial brachytherapy with high-activity iodine-125 sources. J Neurosurg 67:864–873, 1987.
20. Gutin PH, Phillips TL, Wara WM, et al: Brachytherapy of recurrent malignant brain tumors with removable high-activity iodine-125 sources. J Neurosurg 60:61–68, 1984.
21. Halligan JB, Stelzer KJ, Rostomily RC, et al: Operation and permanent low activity ^{125}I brachytherapy for recurrent high grade astrocytomas. Int J Radiat Oncol Biol Phys 35:541–547, 1996.
22. Laperriere NJ, Leung PMK, McKenzie S, et al: Randomized study of brachytherapy in the initial management of patients with malignant astrocytoma. Int J Radiat Oncol Biol Phys 41: 1005–1011, 1998.
23. Larson GL, Wilbanks JH, Dennis S, et al: Interstitial radiogold implantation for the treatment of recurrent high-grade gliomas. Cancer 66:27–29, 1990.
24. Loeffler JS, Alexander E III, Hochberg FH, et al: Clinical patterns of failure following stereotactic interstitial irradiation for malignant gliomas. Int J Radiat Oncol Biol Phys 19:1455–1462, 1990.
25. Lucas GL, Luxton G, Cohen D, et al: Treatment results of stereotactic interstitial brachytherapy for primary and metastatic brain tumors. Int J Radiat Oncol Biol Phys 21:715–721, 1991.
26. Perez-de la Torre R, Zamarano L, Gaspar LE, et al: Brachytherapy with 125-iodine implants for recurrent malignant gliomas: Analysis of results and complications. In Proceedings of the

Congress of Neurological Surgeons Meeting, Oct. 1999, Boston, p 649.

27. Scharfen CO, Sneed PK, Wara WM, et al: High activity iodine-125 interstitial implant for gliomas. Int J Radiat Oncol Biol Phys 24:583–591, 1992.

28. Shrieve DC, Alexander E III, Wen PY, et al: Comparison of stereotactic radiosurgery and brachytherapy in the treatment of recurrent glioblastoma multiforme. Neurosurgery 36:275–284, 1995.

29. Sneed PK, Gutin PH, Larson DA, et al: Patterns of recurrence of glioblastoma multiforme after external irradiation followed by implant boost. Int J Radiat Oncol Biol Phys 29:719–727, 1994.

30. Sneed PK, Prados MD, McDermott MW, et al: Large effect of age on the survival of patients with glioblastoma treated with radiotherapy and brachytherapy boost. Neurosurgery 36:898–904, 1995.

31. Sneed PK, Russo C, Scharfen CO, et al: Long-term follow-up after high-activity 125-I brachytherapy for pediatric brain tumors. Pediatr Neurosurg 24:314–322, 1996.

32. Sneed PK, Stauffer PR, McDermott MW, et al: Survival benefit of hyperthermia in a prospective randomized trial of brachytherapy boost ± hyperthermia for glioblastoma multiforme. Int J Radiat Oncol Biol Phys 40:287–295, 1998.

33. Suplica JM, Berger MS, McDermott MW, et al: Total resection and permanent high-dose I-125 brachytherapy for recurrent or progressive glioblastoma. Int J Radiat Oncol Biol Phys 45(Suppl):321, 1999.

34. Thomson ES, Afshar F, Plowman PN: Pediatric brachytherapy. Br J Radiol 62:223–229, 1989.

35. Videtic GMM, Gaspar LE, Zamarano L, et al: Use of the RTOG recursive partitioning analysis to validate the benefit of iodine-125 implants in the primary treatment of malignant gliomas. Int J Radiat Oncol Biol Phys 45:687–692, 1999.

36. Zamorano L, Yakar D, Dujovny M, et al: Permanent iodine-125 implant and external beam radiation therapy for the treatment of malignant brain tumors. Stereotact Funct Neurosurg 59:183–192, 1992.

37. McDermott MW, Chang SM, Keles GE, et al: Gamma knife radiosurgery for primary brain tumors. In Germano IM (ed): Linac and Gamma Knife Radiosurgery. Park Ridge, Ill, American Association of Neurological Surgeons, 2000, pp 189–202.

38. Castro JR, Saunders WM, Austin-Seymour MM, et al: A phase I–II trial of heavy charged particle irradiation of malignant glioma of the brain: A Northern California Oncology Group study. Int J Radiat Oncol Biol Phys 11:1795–1800, 1985.

39. Deutsch M, Green SB, Strike TA, et al: Results of a randomized trial comparing BCNU plus radiotherapy, streptozocin plus radiotherapy, BCNU plus hyperfractionated radiotherapy, and BCNU following misonidazole plus radiotherapy in the postoperative treatment of malignant glioma. Int J Radiat Oncol Biol Phys 16:1389–1396, 1989.

40. Walker MD, Alexander E, Hunt WE, et al: Evaluation of BCNU and/or radiotherapy in the treatment of anaplastic gliomas. J Neurosurg 49:333–343, 1978.

41. Burger PC: Pathologic anatomy and CT correlations in glioblastoma multiforme. Appl Neurophysiol 46:180–187, 1983.

42. Burger PC, Dubois PJ, Schold SC, et al: Computerized tomographic and pathologic studies of the untreated, quiescent, and recurrent glioblastoma multiforme. J Neurosurg 58:159–169, 1983.

43. Halperin EC, Burger PC, Bullard DE: The fallacy of the localized supratentorial malignant glioma. Int J Radiat Oncol Biol Phys 15:505–509, 1988.

44. Kelly PJ, Daumas-Duport C, Scheithauer BW, et al: Stereotactic correlations of computed tomography and magnetic imaging–defined abnormalities in patients with glial neoplasms. Mayo Clin Proc 62:450–459, 1987.

45. Choucair AK, Levin VA, Gutin PH, et al: Development of multiple lesions during radiation therapy and chemotherapy in patients with gliomas. J Neurosurg 65:654–658, 1986.

46. Gaspar LE, Fisher BJ, MacDonald DR, et al: Supratentorial malignant glioma: Patterns of recurrence and implications for external beam local treatment. Int J Radiat Oncol Biol Phys 24:55–57, 1992.

47. Hochberg FH, Pruitt A: Assumptions in the radiotherapy of glioblastoma. Neurology 30:907–911, 1980.

48. Liang BC, Thornton AF Jr, Sandler HM, Greenberg HS: Malignant astrocytomas: Focal tumor recurrence after focal external beam radiation therapy. J Neurosurg 75:559–563, 1991.

49. Massey V, Wallner KE: Patterns of second recurrence of malignant astrocytomas. Int J Radiat Oncol Biol Phys 18:395–398, 1990.

50. Wallner KE, Galicich JH, Krol G, et al: Patterns of failure following treatment for glioblastoma multiforme and anaplastic astrocytoma. Int J Radiat Oncol Biol Phys 16:1405–1409, 1989.

51. Backlund EO: Studies on craniopharyngiomas. Acta Chir Scand 139:237–247, 1973.

52. Backlund EO: Colloidal radioisotopes as part of a multi-modality treatment of craniopharyngiomas. J Neurosurg Sci 33:95–97, 1989.

53. Backlund EO, Axelsson B, Bergstarnd CG, et al: Treatment of craniopharyngiomas—the stereotactic approach in a ten to twenty-three years' perspective. I. Surgical, radiological and ophthalmological aspects. Acta Neurochir (Wien) 99:11–19, 1989.

54. Coffey RJ, Lunsford LD: The role of stereotactic techniques in the management of craniopharyngiomas. Neurosurg Clin N Am 1:161–172, 1990.

55. Fischer EG, Welch K, Shillito J Jr, et al: Craniopharyngiomas in children: Long term effects of conservative surgical procedures combined with radiation therapy. J Neurosurg 73:534–540, 1990.

56. Hoffman HJ, De Silva M, Humphreys RP, et al: Aggressive surgical management of craniopharyngiomas in children. J Neurosurg 76:47–52, 1992.

57. Kodama T, Matsukado Y, Uemura S: Intracapsular irradiation therapy of craniopharyngiomas with radioactive gold: Indication and follow-up results. Neurol Med Chir (Tokyo) 21:49–58, 1981.

58. Saaf M, Thoren M, Bergstrand CG, et al: Treatment of craniopharyngiomas—the stereotactic approach in a ten to twenty-three years' perspective. II. Psychological situation and pituitary function. Acta Neurochir (Wien) 99:97–103, 1989.

59. Stephanian E, Lunsford LD, Coffey RJ, et al: Gamma knife surgery for sellar and suprasellar tumors. Neurosurg Clin N Am 3:207–218, 1992.

60. Strauss L, Sturm V, Georgi P, et al: Radioisotope therapy of cystic craniopharyngiomas. Int J Radiat Oncol Biol Phys 8:1581–1585, 1982.

61. van den Berge JH, Blaauw G, Breeman WAP, et al: Intracavitary brachytherapy of cystic craniopharyngiomas. J Neurosurg 77:545–550, 1992.

62. Szeifert GT, Julow J, Slowik F, et al: Pathological changes in cystic craniopharyngiomas following intracavital ^{90}yttrium treatment. Acta Neurochir (Wien) 102:14–18, 1990.

63. Schultz RJ, Chandra P, Nath R: Determination of the exposure rate constant for ^{125}I using a scintillation detector. Med Phys 7:355–361, 1980.

64. Fig LM, Shapiro B, Taren J: Distribution of (^{32}P)-chromic phosphate colloid in cystic brain tumors. Stereotact Funct Neurosurg 59:166–168, 1992.

65. Armour E, Wang ZH, Corry P, Martinez A: Equivalence of continuous and pulse simulated low dose rate irradiation in 9L gliosarcoma cells at 37: and 41:C. Int J Radiat Oncol Biol Phys 22:109–114, 1992.

66. Fu KK, Phillips TL, Kane LJ, Smith V: Tumor and normal tissue response to irradiation in vivo: Variation with decreasing dose rates. Radiology 114:709–715, 1975.

67. Hall EJ: The biological basis of endocurietherapy. Endocurie Hyperthermia Oncol 1:141–152, 1985.

68. Hall EJ: The promise of low dose rate: Has it been realized? Int J Radiat Oncol Biol Phys 4:749–750, 1978.

69. Hall EJ: Radiation dose rate: A factor of importance in radiobiology and radiotherapy. Br J Radiol 45:81–97, 1972.

70. Ling CC, Chui CS: Stereotactic treatment of brain tumors with radioactive implants or external photon beams: Radiobiophysical aspects. Radiother Oncol 26:11–18, 1993.

71. Schultz CJ, Geard CR: Radioresponse of human astrocytic tumors across grade as a function of acute and chronic irradiation. Int J Radiat Oncol Biol Phys 19:1397–1403, 1990.

72. Fowler JF: Why shorter half-times of repair lead to greater damage in pulsed brachytherapy. Int J Radiat Oncol Biol Phys 26:353–356, 1993.

73. Kim JH, Alfieri AA, Rosenblum M, et al: Low dose rate radiotherapy for transplantable gliosarcoma in the rat brain. J Neurooncol 9:9–15, 1990.

74. Knox SJ, Sutherland W, Goris M: Correlation of tumor sensitivity to low-dose-rate irradiation with G_2/M-phase bloc and other radiobiological parameters. Radiat Res 135:24–31, 1993.

75. Ling CC, Spiro IJ, Mitchell J, Stickler R: The variation of OER with dose rate. Int J Radiat Oncol Biol Phys 11:1367–1373, 1985.

76. Gutin PH, Bernstein M, Sano Y, Deen DF: Combination therapy with 1,3-bis(2-chloroethyl)-1-nitrosourea and low dose rate radiation in the 9L rat brain tumor and sphenoid models: Implications for brain tumor brachytherapy. Neurosurgery 15:781–786, 1984.

77. Siddiqi SN, Provias J, Laperriere N, Bernstein M: Effects of iodine-125 brachytherapy on the proliferative capacity and histopathological features of glioblastoma recurring after initial therapy. Neurosurgery 40:910–918, 1997.

78. Kunisho K, Matsumoto K, Higashi H, et al: Proliferative potential of malignant glioma cells before and after interstitial brachytherapy. Neurol Med Chir (Tokyo) 39:341–349, 1999.

79. Da Silva VF, Gutin PH, Deen D, Weaver KA: Relative biologic effectiveness of ^{125}I sources in a murine brachytherapy model. Int J Radiat Oncol Biol Phys 10:2109–2111, 1984.

80. Freeman ML, Goldhagen P, Sierra E, Hall EJ: Studies with encapsulated ^{125}I sources. II. Determination of the relative biological effectiveness using cultured mammalian cells. Int J Radiat Oncol Biol Phys 8:1355–1361, 1982.

81. Marchese MJ, Goldhagen PE, Zaider M, et al: The relative biological effectiveness of photon radiation from encapsulated iodine-125, assessed in cells of human origin. 1. Normal diploid fibroblasts. Int J Radiat Oncol Biol Phys 18:1407–1413, 1990.

82. Marchese MJ, Hall EJ, Hilaris BS: Clinical, physical and radiobiological aspects of encapsulated iodine-125 in radiation oncology. Endocurie Hyperthermia Oncol 1:67–82, 1985.

83. Krishnaswamy V: Dose distribution around an ^{125}I seed source in tissue. Radiology 126:489–491, 1978.

84. Dempsey JF, Williams JA, Stubbs JB, et al: Dosimetric properties of a novel brachytherapy balloon applicator for the treatment of malignant brain-tumor resection cavity margins. Int J Radiat Oncol Biol Phys 42:421–429, 1998.

85. McDermott MW, Sneed PK, Gutin PH: Interstitial brachytherapy for malignant brain tumors. Semin Surg Oncol 14:79–87, 1998.

86. Patel S, Breneman JC, Warnick RE, et al: Permanent iodine-125 interstitial implants for the treatment of recurrent glioblastoma multiforme. Neurosurgery 46:1123–1130, 2000.

87. Beach L, Young AB, Patchell RA: A template for rigid stereotaxic afterloading brachytherapy of the brain. Int J Radiat Oncol Biol Phys 26:347–351, 1993.

88. Lulu BA, Lutz W, Stea B, Cetas TC: Treatment planning of template-guided stereotaxic brain implants. Int J Radiat Oncol Biol Phys 18:951–955, 1990.

89. McDermott MW, Gutin PH, Larson DA, Sneed PK: Interstitial brachytherapy. Neurosurg Clin N Am 1:801–824, 1990.

90. McDermott MW: Image guided surgery. In Bernstein M, Berger MS (eds): Neuro-Oncology: The Essentials. New York, Thieme Medical, 2000, pp 135–147.

91. Lunsford DL, Levine G, Gumerman LW: Comparison of computerized tomographic and radionuclide methods in determining intracranial cystic tumor volumes. J Neurosurg 63:740–744, 1985.

92. Kobayashi T, Kageyama N, Ohara K: Internal irradiation for cystic craniopharyngioma. J Neurosurg 55:896–903, 1981.

93. Schwartz RB, Carvalho PA, Alexander E, et al: Radiation necrosis vs high-grade recurrent glioma: Differentiation by using dual-isotope SPECT with ^{201}Tl and ^{99m}Tc-HMPAO. AJNR Am J Neuroradiol 12:1187–1192, 1991.

94. Valk PE, Budinger TF, Levin VA, et al: PET of malignant cerebral tumors after interstitial brachytherapy. J Neurosurg 69:830–838, 1988.

95. Netzeband G, Sturm V, Georgi P, et al: Results of stereotactic intracavitary irradiation of cystic craniopharyngiomas: Comparison of the effects of yttrium-90 and rhenium-186. Acta Neurochir Suppl (Wien) 33:341–344, 1984.

96. Pan DHC, Lee LS, Huang CI, Wong TT: Stereotactic internal irradiation for cystic craniopharyngiomas: A 6 year experience. Stereotact Funct Neurosurg 54–55:525–530, 1990.

97. Dewey WC, Freeman ML, Raaphorst GP, et al: Cell biology of hyperthermia and radiation. In Meyn RE, Withers HR (eds): Radiation Biology in Cancer Research. New York, Raven Press, 1980, pp 589–621.

98. Green SB, Shapiro WR, Burger PC, et al: A randomized trial of interstitial radiotherapy boost for newly diagnosed malignant glioma. Brain Tumor Cooperative Group Trial 8701. Proc Am Soc Clin Oncol 13:174, 1994.

99. Mundinger F, Braus DF, Krauss JK, Birg W: Long-term outcome of 89 low grade brain-stem gliomas after interstitial radiation therapy. J Neurosurg 75:740–746, 1991.

100. Mundinger F, Weigel K: Indication and results of stereotactic curietherapy with iridium-192 and iodine-125 for non-resectable tumors of the hypothalamic region. Acta Neurochir Suppl (Wien) 33:323–330, 1984.

101. Mundinger F, Weigel K: Long term results of stereotactic interstitial curietherapy. Acta Neurochir Suppl (Wien) 33:367–371, 1984.

102. Etou A, Mundinger F, Mohadjer M, Birg W: Stereotactic interstitial irradiation of diencephalic tumors with iridium 192 and iodine 125: 10 years follow-up and comparison with other treatments. Childs Nerv Syst 5:140–143, 1989.

103. Ostertag CB, Kreth FW: Iodine-125 interstitial irradiation for cerebral gliomas. Acta Neurochir (Wien) 119:53–61, 1992.

104. Bernstein M, Laperiere NJ: A critical appraisal of the role of brachytherapy for pediatric brain tumors. Pediatr Neurosurg 16:213–218, 1990.

105. McDermott MW, Cosgrove GR, Larson DA, et al: Interstitial brachytherapy for intracranial metastases. Neurosurg Clin N Am 7:485–495, 1996.

106. Schulder M, Black PM, Shrieve DC, et al: Permanent low-activity iodine-125 implants for cerebral metastases. J Neurooncol 33:213–221, 1997.

107. Bogart JA, Ungureanu C, Shihadeh E, et al: Resection and permanent I-125 brachytherapy without whole brain irradiation for solitary brain metastases from non–small cell lung carcinoma. J Neurooncol 44:53–57, 1999.

108. Prados MD, Leibel S, Barnett CM, Gutin PH: Interstitial brachytherapy for metastatic brain tumors. Cancer 63:657–660, 1989.

109. Bernstein M, Cabantog A, Laperriere N, et al: Brachytherapy for recurrent single brain metastasis. Can J Neurol Sci 22:13–16, 1995.

110. Kumar PP, Patil AA, Syh HW, et al: Role of brachytherapy in the management of the skull base meningioma. Cancer 71:3726–3731, 1993.

111. Chuba PJ, Zamarano L, Hamre M, et al: Permanent I-125 brain stem implants in children. Childs Nerv Syst 14:570–577, 1998.

112. Leksell L, Backlund EO, Johansson L: Treatment of craniopharyngiomas. Acta Chir Scand 133:345–350, 1967.

113. Pollack BE, Lunsford LD, Kondziolka D, et al: Phosphorus-32 intracavitary irradiation of cystic craniopharyngiomas: Current technique and long term results. Int J Radiat Oncol Biol Phys 33:437–446, 1995.

114. Voges J, Sturm V, Lehrke R, et al: Cystic craniopharyngioma: Long term results after intracavitary irradiation with stereotactically applied colloidal β-emitting radioactive sources. Neurosurgery 40:263–270, 1997.

115. Blackburn TP, Doughty D, Plowman PN: Stereotactic intracavitary therapy of recurrent cystic craniopharyngioma by instillation of 90-yttrium. Br J Neurosurg 13:359–365, 1999.

116. Hood TW, McKeever PE: Stereotactic management of cystic gliomas of the brain stem. Neurosurgery 24:373–378, 1989.

117. Musolino A, Merckaert P, Munari C, et al: Stereotactic endocavitary treatment of cysts and pseudocysts of glioma. J Neurosurg Sci 33:107–114, 1989.

118. Szikla G, Schlienger M, Blond S, et al: Interstitial and combined interstitial and external irradiation of supratentorial gliomas: Results in 61 cases treated 1973–1981. Acta Neurochir Suppl (Wien) 33:355–362, 1984.

119. Zeng-min T, Zong-hui L, Gui-quan K, et al: CT-guided stereotactic injection of radionuclide for treatment of brain tumors. Stereotact Funct Neurosurg 59:169–173, 1992.

Linac Radiosurgery

EBEN ALEXANDER III

For the first half of its 5-decade life span, stereotactic radiosurgery (SRS) required specialized and expensive equipment to allow the precise delivery of single high-dose radiation to well-defined targets. The heavy-particle facilities in Boston, Berkeley, and Uppsala were extraordinarily expensive, and these techniques were used by only a handful of investigators. The advent of the gamma knife in 1967 was a definite step toward expanding the availability of SRS techniques. The gamma knife, though expensive, cost only a small fraction of the price of heavy-particle machines. The second phase of expansion, which allowed use of the gamma knife worldwide, occurred in August 1987 when Lunsford opened the gamma knife unit at the University of Pittsburgh.[1] That event marked the turning point in the availability of radiosurgery to neurosurgeons.

It was the adaptation of linear accelerators (linacs) to SRS, however, that provided the impetus for the performance of SRS on a large scale. These devices revolutionized the world of radiation oncology and were in widespread use, but the machines available in the 1970s did not offer sufficient stability and precision (<4 mm) for SRS. The pioneering efforts by Betti in South America,[2] Columbo in Italy,[3] and Winston, Lutz, and Saunders[4, 5] at the Brigham and Women's Hospital in Boston in the early 1980s culminated in the techniques and methods that allowed linacs to be converted for use in precise, high-dose SRS.[6]

EARLY INDICATIONS: VASCULAR, BENIGN TUMORS

Leksell originally developed the gamma knife in 1967 to create small, precise, functional lesions deep in the critical pathways and nuclei of the brain for the treatment of movement disorders, behavioral abnormalities, and chronic refractory pain syndromes.[7] As indications for its use moved from functional lesions to arteriovenous malformations and benign intracranial tumors

(mainly acoustic neurinomas, meningiomas, and pituitary adenomas), certain targets were encountered in which the overall treatment diameter was 4 to 6 cm, much larger than the collimator sizes of the gamma knife (maximal diameter of a single isocenter, 1.8 cm). Although modern, three-dimensional treatment planning software allows gamma knife treatment of multiple-isocenter targets, the linac provides a natural solution for SRS fields in the 3- to 6-cm diameter range.

Basic parameters that allow complex field shaping with the linac include the patient couch angle, gantry arc angle, isocenter position, and collimator size. Additional factors include beam weighting and the tissue depth through which various arc segments are delivered. Manipulation of these simple elements provides significant flexibility in the conformal three-dimensional dose distribution for a single isocenter. By also using multiple isocenters, one can construct elaborate field shaping to treat a given lesion optimally and safely, with maximal dose to the target volume, rapid dose falloff just outside the target, and control of the dose to adjacent critical structures.

Additional parameters that can be manipulated using modern treatment-planning software involve the position of the four "jaws" or vanes present in most linacs. They can be positioned so that the exiting beam at a given gantry angle is shaped to conform to the irregular projection of the target from that specific direction. For nonspherical targets (or when minimizing the dose to an adjacent critical structure at that border), this feature provides significant enhancement of the overall conformity of the three-dimensional shape of the radiation field to maximize target dose and minimize dose to adjacent normal structures. We reported a significant advantage (close to that of an "ideal" collimator) by using these vane manipulations to yield a very conformal three-dimensional treatment field.[6]

Meningiomas

We reported the outcomes in patients treated with linac-based radiosurgery for intracranial meningiomas at our institution. We reviewed 127 patients with 155 meningiomas treated with SRS between October 1988 and December 1995.[8]

There were 86 female and 41 male patients (median age, 61.5 years; range, 19.9 to 87.9 years). The median follow-up period was 31 months (range, 1.2 to 79.8 months). The median tumor volume was 4.1 mL (range, 0.16 to 51.2 mL), and the median marginal dose was 15 Gy (range, 9 to 20 Gy). The tumor locations were as follows: convexity, 31 tumors; parasagittal-falcine, 39 tumors; cranial base, 82 tumors; and ventricular-pineal, 3 tumors. There were 106 benign, 26 atypical, and 18 malignant meningiomas and 5 cases of meningiomatosis. SRS was performed on 48 lesions as the initial treatment and on 107 lesions as adjunct therapy.

Freedom from progression was observed in 107 patients (84.3%) at a median of 22.9 months (range, 1.2 to 79.8 months). Twenty patients (15.7%) had disease progression (16 marginal [12.6%], and 4 local [3.1%]) at a median of 19.6 months (range, 4.1 to 69.3 months); the median time for freedom from progression for benign, atypical, and malignant meningiomas was 20.9, 24.4, and 13.9 months, respectively. Actuarial tumor control for patients with benign meningiomas was 100%, 92.9%, 89.3%, 89.3%, and 89.3% at 1, 2, 3, 4, and 5 years, respectively. Six patients (4.7%) had permanent complications attributable to SRS (median time, 10.3 months; range, 4.3 to 18.0 months); 13 patients died of causes related to the meningioma (median, 17.5 months; range, 4.3 to 37.3 months).

The 1-, 2-, 3-, 4-, and 5-year survival probability for the entire group of patients was 90.3%, 82.6%, 73.6%, 70.5%, and 68.2%, respectively; for patients with benign meningiomas, excluding death resulting from intercurrent disease, the survival probability was 97.6%, 94.8%, 91.0%, 91.0%, and 91.0%, respectively. The 1-, 2-, 3-, and 4-year survival probability for patients with atypical meningiomas was 91.7%, 83.3%, 83.3%, and 83.3%, respectively; for those with malignant meningiomas, it was 92.3%, 64.6%, 43.1%, and 21.5%, respectively. Even though complications from SRS are expected more frequently with large tumors near critical structures, SRS is a safe and effective means of treating selected meningiomas.[9]

Vestibular Schwannomas

Microsurgery and SRS for vestibular schwannomas are associated with a relatively high incidence of sensorineural hearing loss. We started a comparison of SRS and stereotactic radiotherapy in 1992, and it is ongoing.[10, 11] Meijer and coworkers in Amsterdam recently published their comparison of SRS and stereotactic fractionated radiation for vestibular schwannomas. They assessed the local control and toxicity in 37 vestibular schwannoma patients treated with linac-based radiosurgery and fractionated stereotactic radiotherapy. All patients had progressive tumors, progressive symptoms, or both. The mean tumor diameter was 2.3 cm (range, 0.8 to 3.3 cm) on magnetic resonance imaging (MRI) scan. Dentulous patients were given a

dose of 5×4 Gy or 5×5 Gy, and edentulous patients were given a dose of 1×10 Gy or 1×12.5 Gy prescribed to the 80% isodose surface. All patients were treated with a single isocenter. With a mean follow-up of 25 months (range, 12 to 61 months), the actuarial local control rate at 5 years was 91% (only one patient failed). The actuarial rate of hearing preservation at 5 years was 66% in previously hearing patients. The actuarial rate of freedom from trigeminal nerve toxicity was 97% at 5 years. No patient developed facial nerve toxicity or other complications. These investigators concluded that fractionated stereotactic radiotherapy and linac-based radiosurgery resulted in excellent local control in vestibular schwannomas. They demonstrated a high rate of preservation of hearing and a very low rate of other toxicities, although the follow-up was relatively short.[12]

Poen and colleagues at Stanford reported their hypofractionated stereotactic radiotherapy results.[13] A prospective trial of fractionated SRS was undertaken in an attempt to preserve hearing and minimize incidental cranial nerve injury. Thirty-three patients with vestibular schwannomas were treated with 2100 cGy in three fractions during a 24-hour period using conventional frame-based linac radiosurgery. The median tumor diameter was 20 mm (range, 7 to 42 mm). Baseline and follow-up evaluations included audiometry and contrast-enhanced MRI. End points were tumor progression, preservation of serviceable hearing, and treatment-related complications. Thirty-one patients (32 tumors) were assessable for tumor progression and treatment-related complications, and 21 patients were assessable for preservation of serviceable hearing, with a median follow-up of 2 years (range, 0.5 to 4.0 years). Tumor regression or stabilization was documented in 30 patients (97%), and tumor progression occurred in 1 patient (3%). The patient with tumor progression remains asymptomatic and has not required surgical intervention. Five patients (16%) developed trigeminal nerve injury at a median of 6 months (range, 4 to 12 months) after SRS; two of these patients had preexisting trigeminal neuropathy. One patient (3%) developed facial nerve injury (House-Brackmann class 3) 7 months after SRS. Preservation of useful hearing (Gardner-Robertson class 1 to 2) was 77% at 2 years. All patients with pretreatment Gardner-Robertson class 1 to 2 hearing maintained serviceable (class 1 to 3) hearing as of their last follow-up examination. These investigators concluded that three-fraction SRS with a conventional stereotactic frame was feasible and well tolerated in the treatment of vestibular schwannoma. They showed a high rate of hearing preservation and few treatment-related complications among a relatively high-risk patient cohort (tumors >15 mm or neurofibromatosis type 2). Longer follow-up is required to assess the durability of tumor control.[13]

LINAC RADIOSURGERY FOR MALIGNANT TUMORS

Linacs are well suited to the demands of radiosurgery for both benign and malignant tumors, given their ability to readily treat volumes up to the biologic limits of radiosurgery (5 to 6 cm diameter). Large quasi-spherical targets are especially well suited to the linac; in such cases, the gamma knife might require 15 or 20 separate isocenters to equal the large field of a 5- to 6-mm diameter collimator on a linac.

Malignant Astrocytomas

Despite the ability of surgery, radiotherapy, and chemotherapy to prolong survival in patients with glioblastoma multiforme (GBM), most patients succumb to their disease, usually as a result of local tumor persistence or recurrence. SRS allows a substantial increase in total dose at sites of greatest tumor cell density while sparing most of the normal brain, resulting in significantly improved survival. SRS was designed to deliver a large single dose of radiation to a small, focal target; two of its hallmarks are the focal distribution of dose and the inverse relationship between dose and volume.

Acute complications of SRS are related to edema and manifest as a worsening of preexisting symptoms: seizures, aphasia, and motor deficits. These are treatable with steroids and are transient in the majority of cases. The actuarial risk of undergoing reoperation is 33% at 12 months and 48% at 24 months following SRS. Patterns of failure are similar following brachytherapy or SRS as treatment for recurrent GBM, with most patients experiencing marginal failure outside the original treatment volume.

Patients with small (<30 mm diameter), radiographically distinct, and focally recurrent GBM should be considered for SRS. Larger lesions (>30 mm diameter), especially those adjacent to eloquent cortex or critical white matter pathways, must be evaluated with caution. The potential for acute toxicity associated with SRS increases substantially for larger lesions. There is a significant survival advantage of using SRS in many patients with gliomas, especially if it is used appropriately with surgery and other adjuvant therapy.[14]

RADIOSURGERY IN THE INITIAL MANAGEMENT

We reported our experience using radiosurgery as part of the initial management of GBM.[8] Between June 1988 and January 1995, 78 patients underwent SRS as part of their initial treatment for GBM. All patients had undergone initial surgery or biopsy to confirm the diagnosis of GBM and received conventional external beam radiotherapy. SRS was performed using a dedicated 6-MV stereotactic linac.

Thirteen patients were alive at the time of analysis, with a median follow-up of 40.8 months. The median length of actuarial survival for all patients was 19.9 months. Twelve- and 24-month survival rates were 88.5% and 35.9%, respectively. Patient age and Radiation Therapy Oncology Group (RTOG) class were significant prognostic indicators according to univariate analysis ($P < 0.05$). Twenty-three patients younger than 40 years had a median survival time of 48.6 months, compared with 55 older patients who survived 18.2

months ($P < 0.001$). Patients in this series fell into RTOG classes III (27 patients), IV (29 patients), or V (22 patients). Class III patients had a median survival time of 29.5 months following diagnosis; this was significantly longer than the median survival for classes IV and V, which was 19.2 and 18.2 months, respectively ($P = 0.001$). Only patient age (younger than 40 years) was a significant prognostic factor according to multivariate analysis.

Acute complications were unusual and were limited to exacerbation of existing symptoms. There were no new neuropathies secondary to SRS. Thirty-nine patients (50%) underwent reoperation for symptomatic necrosis or recurrent tumor. The rate of reoperation at 24 months after SRS was 54.8%.

The addition of a radiosurgery boost appears to confer a survival advantage to selected patients.[8]

IMAGING INTERPRETATION AFTER RADIOSURGERY

Imaging assessment after radiosurgery is challenging, and we often use adjuncts such as dynamic enhanced MRI and dual-isotope thallium-technetium single photon emission computed tomography (SPECT) to help discriminate among radiation change, necrosis, and active tumor.

Dual-Isotope Thallium-Technetium Single Photon Emission Computed Tomography

We reported our assessment of the association between dual-isotope SPECT scanning and histopathologic findings of tumor recurrence and survival in patients treated with high-dose radiotherapy for GBM.

SPECT studies with thallium 201 (Tl-201) and technetium 99m–hexamethylpropylene amine oxime (Tc-99m–HMPAO) were performed 1 day before reoperation in 47 patients with GBM who had previously been treated by surgery and high-dose radiotherapy. Maximal uptake of Tl-201 in the lesion was expressed as a ratio to that in the contralateral scalp, and uptake of Tc-99m–HMPAO was expressed as a ratio to that in the cerebellar cortex. Patients were stratified into groups based on maximal radioisotope uptake values in their tumor beds. The significance of patient gender, histologic characteristics of tissue at reoperation, and SPECT uptake group with respect to 1-year survival was elucidated using the chi-square statistic. Comparisons of patient age and time to tumor recurrence as functions of 1-year survival were made using the t-test. Survival data at 1 year were presented according to the Kaplan-Meier method, and the significance of potential differences was evaluated using the log-rank method. The effects of different variables (tumor type, time to recurrence, and SPECT grouping) on long-term survival were evaluated using Cox proportional models that controlled for age and gender.

All patients in group I (Tl-201 ratio <2 and Tc-99m–HMPAO ratio <0.5) showed radiation changes in their biopsy specimens; they had an 83.3% 1-year survival rate. Group II patients (Tl-201 ratio <2 and Tc-

99m–HMPAO ratio $\geq$0.5, or Tl-201 ratio between 2 and 3.5 regardless of Tc-99m–HMPAO ratio) had predominantly infiltrating tumors (66.6%); they had a 29.2% 1-year survival rate. Almost all the patients in group III (Tl-201 ratio >3.5 and Tc-99m–HMPAO ratio $\geq$0.5) had solid tumors (88.2%); they had a 6.7% 1-year survival rate. Histologic data were associated with 1-year survival ($P < 0.01$); however, SPECT grouping was more closely associated with 1-year survival ($P < 0.001$) and was the only variable significantly associated with long-term survival ($P < 0.005$).

Dual-isotope SPECT data correlate with histopathologic findings at reoperation and with survival in patients with malignant gliomas after surgical and high-dose radiation therapy.[15]

Dynamic Enhanced Magnetic Resonance Imaging

In patients with malignant astrocytomas or metastatic brain disease treated with high-dose radiotherapy, conventional imaging methods may not adequately distinguish recurrent tumor from radiation change. We used a fast spoiled gradient refocusing technique in the open-configuration intraoperative MRI system to assess the rate of regional enhancement of the treated tumor bed and to localize specific sites for pathologic sampling to determine whether gadolinium uptake correlated with histologic data. Twenty-four patients were studied. Fourteen of 15 patients with areas of early enhancement had recurrent tumor present in histologic samples, and 8 of the remaining 9 patients had only reactive changes. Dynamic MRI was predictive of recurrent tumor ($P < 0.0005$, Fisher's exact test; $P < 0.002$, Student's t-test). Dynamic MRI in the open-bore magnet is a promising method for localizing potential sites of active tumor growth in patients treated for malignant astrocytomas and metastatic brain lesions.[16]

Brain Metastases

Brain metastases represent a significant health care problem, with almost 200,000 patients a year in the United States suffering from symptomatic parenchymal lesions. Lung, breast, renal, and gastrointestinal cancers and melanoma contribute the majority of lesions that come to clinical attention. Although median survival once brain metastases are diagnosed is less than a year, timely therapy can restore neurological function and can often prevent further neurological complications for the duration of a patient's survival.[17]

Metastases are ideal lesions for SRS treatment, for a variety of reasons: (1) they are usually quasi-spherical in shape; (2) they are usually less than 3 cm in diameter at the time of diagnosis; (3) they often grow rapidly and respond quickly with shrinkage after treatment; (4) commonly, they are efficiently cleared from the brain after necrosing, without major toxic metabolites and vasogenic edema; and (5) they are radiographically distinct targets, without significant cellular infiltration.

Important prognostic features associated with improved survival include the absence of extracranial disease progression, young age, high pretreatment neurological status, one to three versus more than three lesions, and long interval from primary disease diagnosis to development of brain metastases.

The need to treat brain metastases aggressively is becoming increasingly important as advances in treatment result in an increasing number of patients developing brain metastases in the setting of limited systemic disease. For many such patients, surgery provides the best therapy, but results are still not encouraging. Even patients with the best prognostic indicators often die within 18 to 24 months. Until superior treatment modalities are developed, the judicious use of available techniques provides the best opportunity for palliation and extended survival.

Perhaps the most significant development in the treatment of patients with brain metastases during the last decade is the increasing use of radiosurgery. For patients with a single lesion, local control and survival rates after radiosurgery compare well with those produced by surgical resection. Radiosurgery remains an important treatment modality and, when used promptly, can reverse neurological deficits, often for the remainder of a patient's life. There is compelling evidence that aggressive local therapy (surgery or radiosurgery) in patients with a single brain metastasis produces superior survival and quality of life compared with whole-brain radiotherapy alone. However, surgery should be restricted to the minority of patients for whom brain metastases represent the life-threatening site of their disease. For asymptomatic or mildly symptomatic patients with lesions smaller than 3 cm in diameter, radiosurgery is an excellent alternative to surgery. Although radiosurgery is a noninvasive procedure, the same selection criteria should be used as for patients undergoing surgical resection.[17]

RESURGENCE OF FUNCTIONAL RADIOSURGERY

In the early 1990s, Laitinen published his results using stereotactic lesioning in the globus pallidus to treat Parkinson's disease.[18] His techniques were largely the conventional electrode lesioning methods originally described by Leksell and used by many neurosurgeons in the 1950s and 1960s.[7] However, Laitinen's report rekindled a major interest in the neurosurgical management of movement disorders and in functional neurosurgery overall. With this renewed interest came a major impetus to redevelop SRS for the creation of lesions in the central nervous system. Functional lesioning was SRS's original raison d'être, so it is fitting that there is finally a renewed interest in this pursuit.

The last 5 years have witnessed a prodigious growth in neurosurgical experience using radiosurgery for the treatment of movement disorders (including targets in both the thalamus and the globus pallidus, especially for the treatment of Parkinson's disease), pain syndromes (especially trigeminal nerve entry zone lesions for trigeminal neuralagia), and behavioral disorders (e.g., capsulotomy).

Although the linac offers significant advantages in the administration of radiosurgery to the large target volumes needed to treat tumors and vascular malformations, special attention to technical detail is critical in verifying the stability and accuracy of a given linac when treating the small volumes of functional targets. Collimators in the 5- to 10-mm range (comparable to the 4- and 8-mm collimators used with the gamma knife for functional work) are commonly used to treat small targets in the thalamus and globus pallidus and adjacent to the internal capsule or cingulate gyrus. Although most commercial linac SRS systems routinely provide setup accuracy in the 2- to 3-mm range, these small targets necessitate an additional level of precision in verifying linac gantry and couch positions and the stability of these isocentric foci during routine system movement.

The doses used for functional radiosurgery are usually higher than those used for tumors and arteriovenous malformations. Thus, treatment times are approximately four to six times longer than the normal treatment period to deliver doses in the range of 120 to 140 Gy.

An issue critical for all practitioners of functional SRS is the verification of imaging accuracy, especially the use of MRI for stereotactic planning. Localization errors up to 6 mm between the fiducially defined stereotactic coordinates and the real spatial position of a given point are easily encountered due to various sources of potential shift.[19] One must fully comprehend the errors and limitations inherent in the MRI-stereotactic system and know how to detect and correct them before proceeding with functional SRS.

Linacs for Stereotactic Fractionated Radiotherapy

SRS allows significant dose escalation, with dramatic improvement in the control of arteriovenous malformations and benign and malignant tumors. However, there are practical radiobiologic limits to the use of these large single fractions (~1500 cGY and higher) when an excessive volume of normal tissue, or even a small volume of a very radiosensitive structure (e.g., optic nerve, chiasm, acoustic nerve), receives a high dose. There is a growing literature on the use of conventional fractions[10–12] as well as fewer, larger fractions (hypofractionation) compared with stereotactic guidance[13] and convergent arcs to combine the biologic advantage of fractionation with the geometric advantage of SRS. However, for most small and medium-sized lesions (up to 5 cm diameter) that are not intimately involved with the brainstem or cranial nerves, SRS (single fraction) is the treatment of choice over fractionated schemes.

Linac, Gamma Knife, or Protons?

The realm of SRS has grown tremendously in the last decade, and the combined experience of its prac-

titioners allows some substantial conclusions to be made regarding the relative merits of the available technologies.

The linac is the most widely available SRS technology. Commercial turnkey systems have been available worldwide for several years. These systems allow the conversion of standard linacs into devices capable of applying SRS in a wide variety of clinical scenarios. These systems demand a dedicated team of health care professionals, including a neurosurgeon, a radiation oncologist, and a medical physicist. Rigorous quality control and assurance programs are an essential part of these turnkey packages. Although these modern software-hardware packages have turned the flexibility of the linac into an asset, improper attention to the many degrees of freedom and technical variables involved in the performance of linac radiosurgery can turn this flexibility into more of a liability. The variability in quality and technique among linac centers is expected to result in significant differences in outcome.

The gamma knife, as in the case of the linac, is widely available. Designed for the precise delivery of radiosurgical doses for functional work, it excels at the expeditious delivery of small treatment fields for functional neurosurgery and for the treatment of small to moderate-sized tumors and vascular lesions. Targets with diameters greater than 3 cm involve increasingly cumbersome combinations of multiple isocenters, although current treatment software expedites this complicated process.

Heavy particles (e.g., protons, helium and carbon nuclei) involve very expensive technologies—cyclotrons and synchrocyclotrons—which are available at only a few centers around the world. However, certain radiosurgical targets, especially those whose surface is adjacent to a very radiosensitive structure (e.g., optic nerves or chiasm, brainstem, spinal cord), may be especially well suited to heavy-particle radiosurgery. The Bragg peak is a physical property of these heavy particles that allows one to deposit much of the radiation energy within the target and then have the distant edge of the target volume be the end of traversal of the beam. Various technical maneuvers allow the shaping of that distant beam edge to conform to the three-dimensnional shape of the target. One disadvantage is the deposition of approximately 30% of the beam energy on the entry pathway to the target, but that is often acceptable if one can "stop" the beam at the other edge of the tumor, which is designed to be the edge adjacent to the most radiation-sensitive neural structure. Control of the entry vector is somewhat unwieldy, given the limited setup flexibility of the patient localization systems and the massive machinery used to generate heavy-particle beams, so one can often obtain a better overall volumetric dose distribution using the cross-firing of photons (with linac or gamma knife) over a significantly large steradian distribution. However, heavy particles have an advantage in trimming the dose adjacent to one critical tumor margin. One other problem is the physical limitation of Bragg peak use in small targets, where the beam diameter is less than 7 to 8 mm. In such situations, one is less able to use the Bragg peak, which is important in the treatment of functional targets, which are often in the small size range.

Generally, the experience of the treating team is the most important variable in providing quality patient care. Experience and attention to detail are critical for a successful clinical radiosurgery program. Many centers are now using multiple technologies, choosing the treatment that best suits a given patient. This enables us to push the frontiers beyond simplistic approaches based solely on the availability of a given technology.

REFERENCES

1. Lunsford LD, Flickinger JC, Linder G, Maitz A: Stereotactic radiosurgery of the brain using the first United States 210-cobalt-60 source gamma knife. Neurosurgery 24:151–159, 1989.
2. Betti OO, Munari C, Rosler R: Stereotactic radiosurgery with the linear accelerator: Treatment of arteriovenous malformations. Neurosurgery 24:311–321, 1989.
3. Columbo F, Benedetti A, Pozza F, et al: Radiosurgery using a 4MV linear accelerator: Technique and radiobiologic implications. Acta Radiol Suppl 369:603–607, 1986.
4. Winston KR, Lutz W: Linear accelerator as a neurosurgical tool for stereotactic radiosurgery. Neurosurgery 22:454–464, 1988.
5. Loeffler JS, Alexander E III, Siddon RL, et al: Stereotactic radiosurgery for intracranial arteriovenous malformations using a standard linear accelerator. Int J Radiat Oncol Biol Phys 17:673–677, 1989.
6. Nedzi LA, Kooy HM, Alexander E III, et al: Dynamic field shaping for stereotactic radiosurgery: A modeling study. Int J Radiat Oncol Biol Phys 25:859–869, 1993.
7. Leksell L: The stereotaxic method and radiosurgery of the brain. Acta Chir Scand 102:316–319, 1951.
8. Shrieve DC, Alexander E III, Black PM, et al: Treatment of patients with primary glioblastoma multiforme with standard postoperative radiotherapy and radiosurgical boost: Prognostic factors and long-term outcome. J Neurosurg 90:72–77, 1999.
9. Hakim R, Alexander E III, Loeffler JS, et al: Results of linear accelerator–based radiosurgery for intracranial meningiomas. Neurosurgery 42:446–453, 1998.
10. Dunbar SF, Tarbell NJ, Kooy HM, et al: Stereotactic radiotherapy for pediatric and adult brain tumors: Preliminary report. Int J Radiat Oncol Biol Phys 30:531–539, 1994.
11. Shrieve DC, Tarbell NJ, Alexander E III, et al: Stereotactic radiotherapy: A technique for dose optimization and escalation for intracranial tumors. Acta Neurochir Suppl (Wien) 62:118–123, 1994.
12. Meijer OW, Wolbers JG, Baayen JC, Slotman BJ: Fractionated stereotactic radiation therapy and single high-dose radiosurgery for acoustic neuroma: Early results of a prospective clinical study. Int J Radiat Oncol Biol Phys 46:45–49, 2000.
13. Poen JC, Golby AJ, Forster KM, et al: Fractionated stereotactic radiosurgery and preservation of hearing in patients with vestibular schwannoma: A preliminary report. Neurosurgery 45:1299–1305, 1999.
14. Alexander E III, Loeffler JS: Radiosurgery for primary malignant brain tumors. Semin Surg Oncol 14:43–52, 1998.
15. Schwartz RB, Holman BL, Polak JF, et al: Dual-isotope single-photon emission computerized tomography scanning in patients with glioblastoma multiforme: Association with patient survival and histopathological characteristics of tumor after high-dose radiotherapy. J Neurosurg 89:60–68, 1998.
16. Schwartz RB, Hsu L, Kacher DF, et al: Intraoperative dynamic MRI: Localization of sites of brain tumor recurrence after high-dose radiotherapy. J Magn Reson Imaging 8:1085–1089, 1998.
17. Alexander E III, Loeffler JS: The case for radiosurgery. Clin Neurosurg 45:32–40, 1999.
18. Laitinen LV, Bergenheim AT, Hariz MI: Leksell's posteroventral pallidotomy in the treatment of Parkinson's disease. J Neurosurg 76:53–61, 1992.
19. Alexander E III, Kooy HM, van Herk M, et al: MRI-directed stereotactic neurosurgery: Use of image fusion with CT to enhance spatial accuracy. J Neurosurg 83:271–276, 1995.

Gamma Knife Radiosurgery

TIMOTHY F. WITHAM ■ DOUGLAS KONDZIOLKA

DEVELOPMENT OF THE TECHNOLOGY

Stereotactic radiosurgery is a noninvasive, closed-skull method that uses precisely targeted beams of ionizing radiation for the treatment of intracranial neoplasms, vascular malformations, and functional disorders. In 1906, Horsley and Clarke developed a technique for stereotactic localization in which anatomic coordinates could be registered with reference to a coordinate frame attached to the skull.[1] In 1951, Leksell combined the technique of stereotaxy using a guiding device with a radiotherapeutic modality and both defined the term *stereotactic radiosurgery* and initiated the technique.[2] His initial research efforts involved the use of orthovoltage x-ray tubes, proton beams, and linear accelerators to generate radiation.[3] In 1967, Leksell and Larsson installed the first gamma knife stereotactic radiosurgical unit at the Sofiahemmet in Stockholm.[4, 5] Leksell's first report on the use of gamma knife radiosurgery described the treatment of intractable pain in two patients by "gammathalamotomy," although the first patient in 1967 had radiosurgery for a craniopharyngioma.[4] The prototype unit contained 179 cobalt-60 sources and was designed mainly for functional procedures. The dose profile of the first unit was slender rather than semispherical.

The second-generation gamma unit, which was used extensively at the Karolinska Institute beginning in 1975, was designed for the treatment of vascular malformations and tumors. Using round collimators (4, 8, and 14 mm) rather than slotted ones, the dose profile was more spherical and better suited to the irradiation of mass lesions.

BASIC UNIT DESIGN

After a 30-year experience with gamma knife radiosurgery, the fundamental unit design remains almost unchanged and employs 201 separate cobalt-60 sources focused at a single point. The focal distance from radiation source to target is 40.3 cm. The cobalt sources are loaded into the central body (Fig. 273–1). Three models exist: model U uses a hemispherical array of radiation sources, and models B and C use a circular array. The radiation dose profile created varies slightly between the two designs. In the hemispherical array, the dose profile is slightly greater in the superior-inferior extent. With the circular array, the profile is greater in the left-right extent. This design facilitates irradiation of sellar or parasellar lesions by reducing the radiation falloff upward toward the optic chiasm. A multicollimator system design ensures the exact alignment of the radiation sources with the desired target. Strict quality control is observed when machining the unit so that the alignment of the sources with the final helmet collimator is ensured. Final collimator helmets are exchangeable and exist in four sizes: 4-, 8-, 14-, and 18-mm diameter. This variation in final collimator diameter allows for the treatment of intracranial lesions of different conformations and sizes. The new model C unit contains an automatic positioning system (Fig. 273–2). This system provides robotic control of stereotactic coordinate localization to facilitate multiple-isocenter radiosurgery.

RADIOSURGERY TECHNIQUE

The technique of radiosurgery is similar for all Leksell units.[6–8] After the administration of local anesthetic, pin fixation is used to attach the Leksell frame to the patient's head. This stereotactic system relies on a frame center that is designated in three planes by the following values: $x = 100$, $y = 100$, and $z = 100$. Ideally, the aim is to place the frame such that the lesion to be treated is located as close to the three-dimensional frame center as possible. Following frame application, imaging is performed, and the images are interfaced with a computer software treatment planning system. The Leksell GammaPlan is the current software program for treatment planning. Once a treatment plan has been acquired, the coordinates on the frame are set. First the y (anterior-posterior) and z (inferior-superior) coordinates are set. The patient is then positioned such that the attached frame can be secured to the trunnions of the final collimator helmet. Each coordinate is checked three times to minimize mechanical errors. The trunnions (x-coordinate bars that hold the stereotactic frame to the collimator helmet) are then adjusted to set

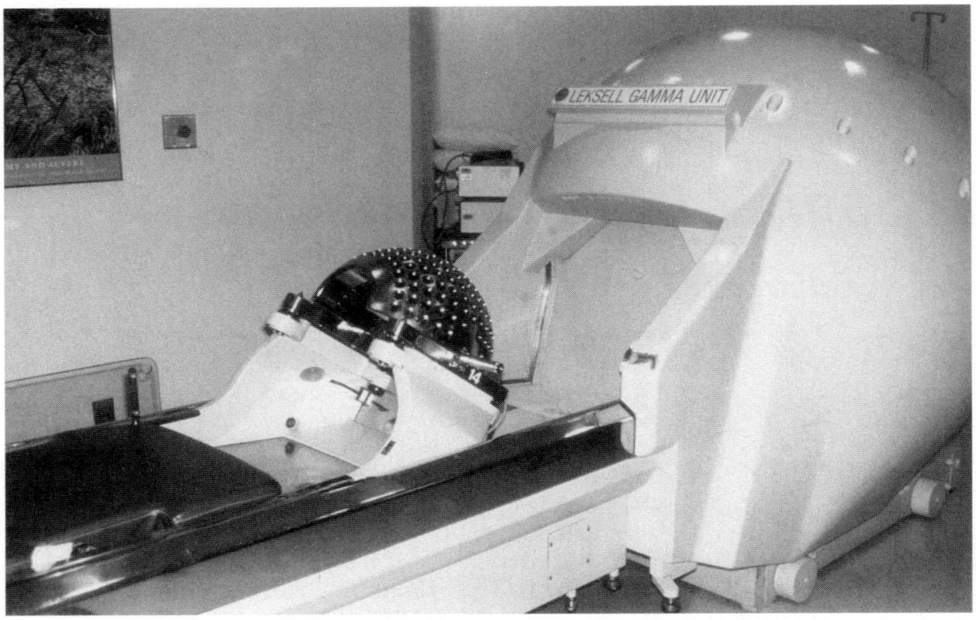

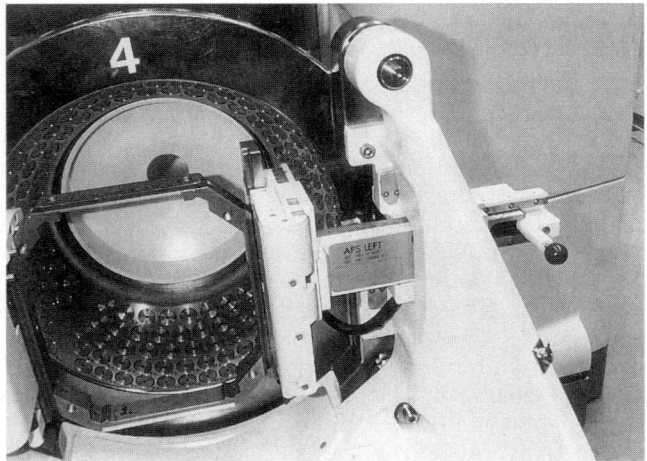

FIGURE 273–1. The model U gamma knife.

the *x* (right-left) coordinate. As treatment commences, the patient is advanced on the couch through the shielding door into the central body of the unit, where the helmet docks. The central body contains the 201 cobalt-60 sources, and as the helmet docks, these sources are aligned with the helmet collimators; then radiation commences (Fig. 273–3). When treatment is complete, the couch automatically moves the patient from the central body, and the shielding door closes.

TREATMENT PLANNING

As outlined by Leksell, radiosurgery is a procedure of precise and complete destruction of tissues at the tar-

FIGURE 273–2. The model C gamma knife with a robotic automatic positioning system attached to the side of the stereotactic frame.

get, whether they are pathologic or not.[3] Complete destruction aptly defines functional parenchymal radiosurgery. Significant concomitant or late radiation damage to tissues adjacent to the target is avoided. Therefore, the treatment planning concept of gamma knife radiosurgery is to achieve a destructive effect within the targeted volume. A sharply defined radiation treatment volume should perfectly match the target tissue and spare the surrounding tissue (Fig. 273–4). This precise destruction of targeted tissue is aided through the use of magnetic resonance imaging (MRI) and angiographic data that define the specific target location. Imaging data are directly linked to or may be scanned into the planning computer. Imaging inadequacies may result in imperfect treatment planning.

The ability to create irregularly shaped radiosurgical volumes is important to achieve conformal irradiation of the target tissue. Several techniques may be used to create an irregular-shaped plan. First, multiple isocenters of irradiation (of the same or different collimator sizes) may be combined in different planes (Fig. 273–5). For example, a series of 4-mm isocenters is often used to tailor radiation into the porus acusticus in the management of vestibular schwannoma. Second, the individual isocenters can be weighted variably to change their relative shape. Third, individual radiation beams can be blocked to restrict the dose away from critical structures, such as the optic chiasm.

Because the GammaPlan software is able to reconstruct coronal and sagittal images from axial acquisition images, the patient is required to undergo only high-resolution, thin-slice, axial acquisition sequences with MRI-obtained data. We use a volume acquisition, contrast-enhanced sequence divided into 1-mm slices. Quality-assurance measurements are made on the axial imaging sequences to assess the accuracy of the images.

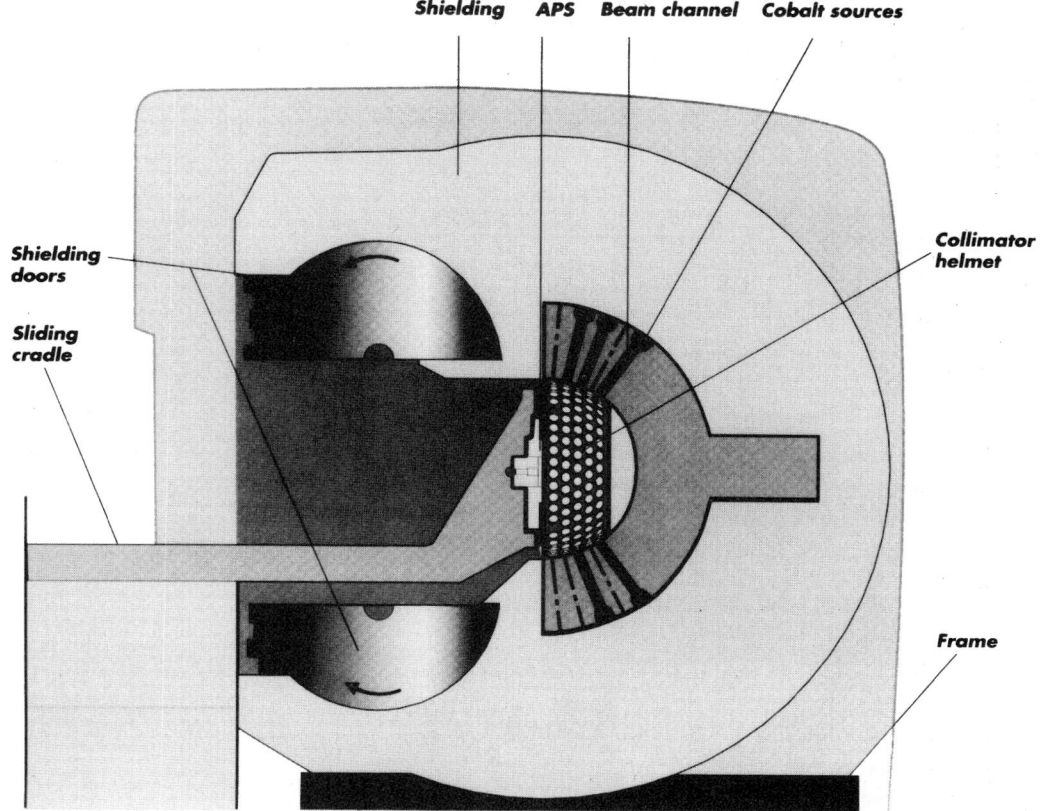

FIGURE 273–3. Cross-sectional diagram of the model C gamma knife. The collimator helmet is aligned with the cobalt sources when the patient is being treated.

Reimaging is performed for those images that are not within the acceptable range of error. Properly obtained imaging sequences are then interfaced with GammaPlan software through an ethernet connection for dose prescription and configuration planning.

In the case of planning for radiosurgery of vascular malformations, digital or biplane angiography using high-resolution magnification and photographic subtraction techniques are used. The angiogram films can then be scanned directly into the dose-planning computer using GammaPlan. It is now routine to have a direct network connection of stereotactic MRI data with the dose-planning computer in vascular cases. Because the treatment of certain vascular lesions may be quite complex, the ability to correlate angiographic and MRI data instantaneously at the time of targeting and dose planning is advantageous. Planning is rendered more conformal and safer, especially when targeting lesions situated in proximity to cranial nerves and other brainstem structures. Inverse dose planning is possible with current software. Functional parenchymal radiosurgery is facilitated by fast inversion recovery MRI sequences.

DOSE PRESCRIPTION

The basic tenet of a paired dose-response curve and a curve for complications that is applicable to conventional fractionated radiotherapy also applies, with some limitations, to radiosurgery. Therefore, the choice of an optimal dose relies on the balance between these two curves. In addition, the type of lesion being treated and the type of complication must be considered in this paradigm. For example, for lesions in which incomplete obliteration may result in disease progression and rapid death (malignant primary tumor), increasing the dose is probably desirable if the severity of the complication is not too great (temporary neurological deficit).

In radiosurgery, the risk of a complication is more dependent on treatment volume than it is with conventional radiotherapy. Because of this fact, separate complication curves are needed for each volume treated by radiosurgery. In addition, complication curves and dose-response curves vary less with dose changes and are therefore less steep than with conventional radiotherapy. A flattened dose-response curve is particularly evident with neoplasms.

Recent gamma knife dose prescriptions have been based on volume-dependent projected risks of radiation necrosis in normal brain tissue. Standard guidelines for dose prescription are derived from risk predictions of Kjellberg's 1% isoeffect line and from the integrated logistic formula of Flickinger.[9–11] Although both dose prescription models have inherent limitations, we recommend their continued use as a guide-

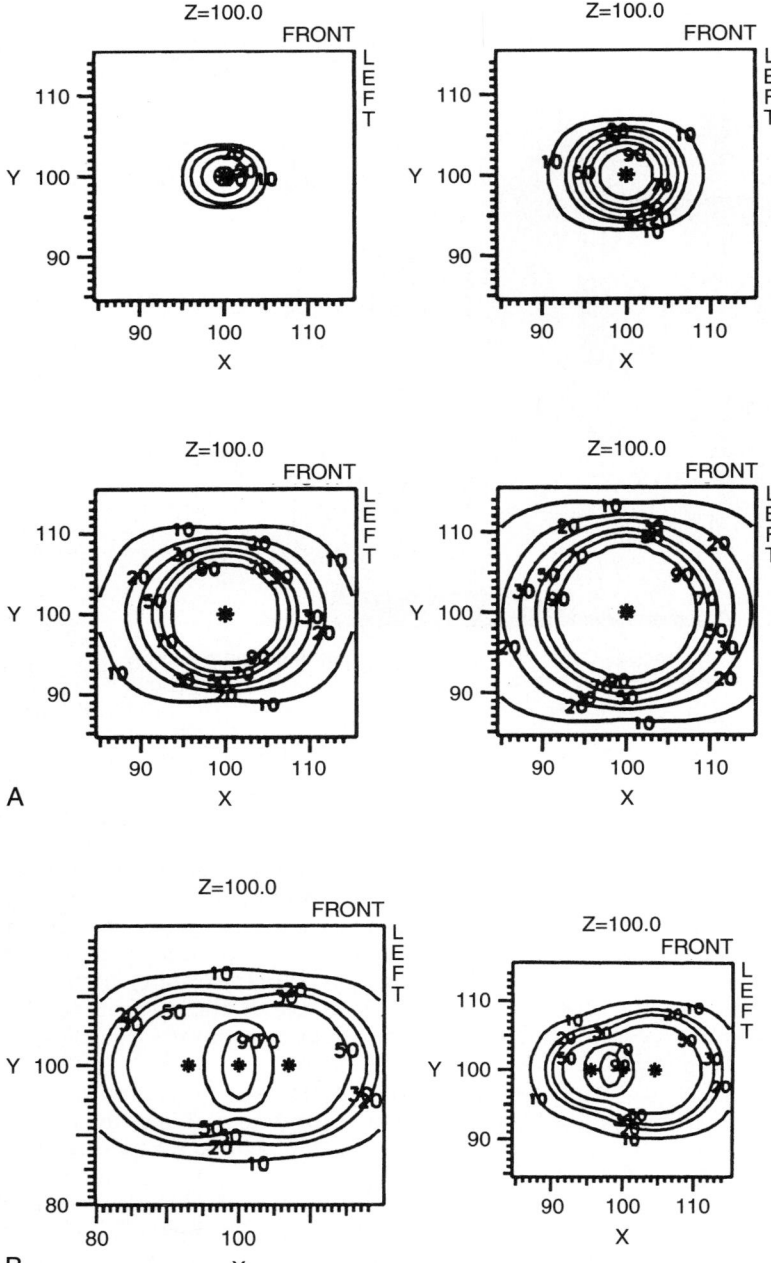

FIGURE 273–4. *A,* Dose profiles for the 4-, 8-, 14-, and 18-mm collimators of the model U unit. *B,* Multiple isocenters *(asterisks)* are used to create nonspherical radiosurgical volumes.

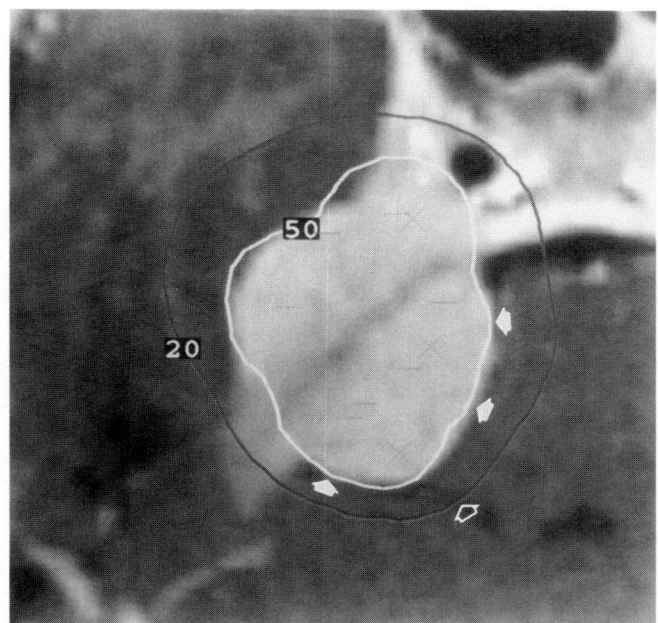

FIGURE 273–5. Axial contrast-enhanced magnetic resonance imaging scan showing the radiosurgical plan for a petrous apex meningioma with extension into the posterior cavernous sinus. Multiple irradiation isocenters were used to tailor the 50% line to the tumor margin *(solid arrows)*. The 20% isodose line *(open arrow)* indicates the falloff in the radiation dose.

line for dose prescription, except for lesions that are intimate with cranial nerves. In particular, special sensory nerves (optic and auditory) are more sensitive than somatic sensory nerves and motor nerves to radiation injury.[12] In the case of acoustic neuromas, it appears that the length of nerve (facial, trigeminal, or auditory) irradiated correlates positively with postoperative dysfunction.[12, 13] The length of nerve irradiated, in turn, correlates with the size of the tumor. Conse-

quently, small tumors adjacent to cranial nerves are less risky to treat than are larger tumors.

Careful attention to patient selection, use of imaging, dose planning, and dose selection helps ensure the proper use of the device. Refinements in the technology over the past 3 decades have been followed by improvements in reported clinical outcomes.

REFERENCES

1. Horsley V, Clarke RH: The structure and functions of the cerebellum examined by a new method. Brain 31:45, 1908.
2. Leksell L: The stereotactic method and radiosurgery of the brain. Acta Chir Scand 102:316–319, 1951.
3. Larsson B, Leksell L, Rexed B, et al: The high-energy proton beam as a neurosurgical tool. Nature 182:1222–1223, 1958.
4. Leksell L: Cerebral radiosurgery. I. Gammathalamotomy in two cases of intractable pain. Acta Chir Scand 134:585–595, 1968.
5. Rand RW, Khonsary A, Brown WJ, et al: Leksell stereotactic radiosurgery in the treatment of eye melanoma. Neurol Res 9: 142–146, 1987.
6. Walton L, Bomford CK, Ramsden D: The Sheffield stereotactic radiosurgery unit: Physical characteristics and principles of operation. Br J Radiol 60:897–906, 1987.
7. Lunsford LD, Flickinger J, Lindner G, et al: Stereotactic radiosurgery of the brain using the first United States 201 cobalt-60 source gamma knife. Neurosurgery 24:151–159, 1989.
8. Lunsford LD, Kondziolka D, Flickinger JC: Introduction. In Gamma knife brain surgery. Prog Neurol Surg 14:1–4, 1998.
9. Flickinger JC: The integrated logistic formula and prediction of complications from radiosurgery. Int J Radiat Oncol Biol Phys 17:879–885, 1989.
10. Kjellberg R, Hanamura T, Davis K, et al: Bragg-peak proton-beam therapy for arteriovenous malformations of the brain. N Engl J Med 309:269, 1983.
11. Loeffler JS, Alexander E, Siddon R, et al: Stereotactic radiosurgery for intracranial arteriovenous malformations using a standard linear accelerator. Int J Radiat Oncol Biol Phys 17:915–917, 1989.
12. Flickinger JC, Kondziolka D, Lunsford LD: Dose and diameter relationships for facial, trigeminal, and acoustic neuropathies following acoustic neuroma radiosurgery. Radiother Oncol 41: 215–219, 1996.
13. Linskey ME, Flickinger JC, Lunsford LD: The relationship of cranial nerve length to the development of delayed facial and trigeminal neuropathies after stereotactic radiosurgery for acoustic tumors. Int J Radiat Oncol Biol Phys 15:227–234, 1993.

Proton Radiosurgery

PAUL H. CHAPMAN ■ JAY S. LOEFFLER

HISTORICAL PERSPECTIVE

Proton beam irradiation has played a central role since the earliest conceptualization and practice of radiosurgery. The medical use of protons for focal irradiation of tissues was first proposed by Robert Wilson of the Research Laboratory of Physics, Harvard University, in 1947.[1] An early problem was the inability to control the beam's depth of penetration in tissue precisely to take advantage of the region of highest energy release at the Bragg peak. Initial work was therefore restricted to using a cross-fire technique in which the plateau region of several beams that completely traversed the head was aimed at a target at their point of intersection. This is the same principle that was later used for gamma knife and x-ray (linac) radiosurgery, both of which use beams of photons that lack a Bragg peak.

In 1954, the cross-fire technique was first put to use at the Lawrence Berkeley Laboratory in California for the therapeutic suppression of normal pituitary function.[2] The treatment was initially delivered in six to eight fractions over 2 to 3 weeks. Several years earlier, in 1951, Leksell had introduced the term (and concept of) *radiosurgery*. In 1958, he and colleagues began to use this method with the proton beam to make functional brain lesions in patients.[3] Until 1961, the clinical use of protons was still limited to cross-fire irradiation using the plateau region of the beam, although animal experiments had shown the feasibility of controlling the depth of the Bragg peak using energy-absorbing material.[4] At that time, Kjellberg and colleagues, working at the Harvard Cyclotron Laboratory, devised a technique that allowed precise control of the beam's depth of penetration in tissue and was practical for patient treatment.[5] Following this, the first Bragg peak radiation treatment of an intracranial tumor was carried out in 1961, and of an arteriovenous malformation in 1965.[6] Since then, Bragg peak therapy, whether radiosurgical or fractionated, has become standard therapy at all facilities using charged particles. Since the first treatments in 1954, this technique has been used for approximately 29,000 patients. Worldwide, there are 21 cyclotron facilities treating patients, 19 of which use protons and 2 of which use nonproton heavy ions.

PHYSICAL PRINCIPLES

Ionization and Photon Irradiation

Radiation causes alterations in biologic materials through the process of ionization.[7] At the cellular level, this produces chromosomal changes that ultimately manifest themselves as nonviability of either the affected cell or its progeny. This principle is valid, regardless of the specific type of ionizing radiation used. The distribution of energy deposition within tissue depends not only on the type of radiation (particulate or photon) but also on the beam energy. These differences have important clinical implications. Today, photon irradiation uses high energies called megavoltage radiation (>1 million electron volts, or MeV). Linear accelerators (4 to 20 MeV) predominate in current radiation therapy practice. In these devices, electrons are accelerated to very high energies to strike a target and produce x-rays. The resulting x-ray beam contains photons of varying energies up to the peak energy of the accelerated electrons. As the energy of a photon beam increases, the dose of radiation deposited at a specific depth relative to the maximal dose increases as well (Fig. 274–1). This property of radiation deposition in the high-energy range results in relative skin sparing, reduced absorption in bone, deeper penetration in tissue, and a sharper edge to the radiation beam. For example, the maximal dose occurs at 1, 2, and 3 cm with 4-MeV, 8-MeV, and 15-MeV linear accelerators, respectively. In spite of these advantages of using megavoltages for photon radiation, for targets deeper than 1 to 3 cm, a substantial dose is delivered to normal tissues proximal to the target, as well as an exit dose beyond it. It is important to understand this principle to appreciate the essential difference between the dose distribution of photons and charged particle radiation in tissue.

Charged Particle Irradiation

A number of charged and uncharged particles have been used for medical treatments, including protons, heavier charged particles such as helium and carbon

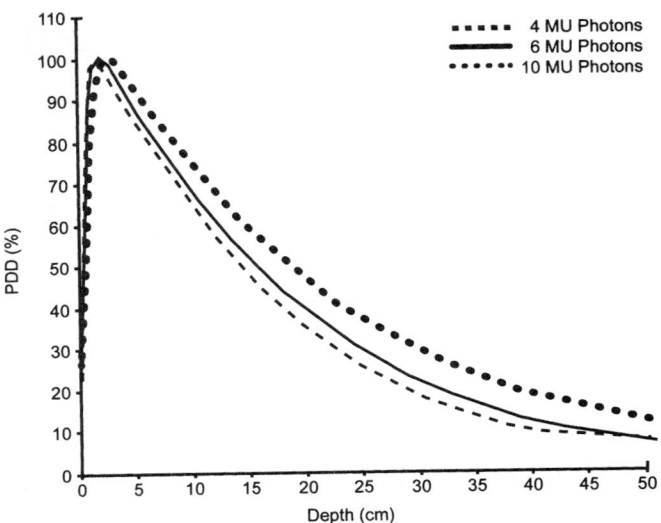

FIGURE 274–1. Depth-dose distribution for 4-, 6-, and 10-MeV x-ray beams. Note that the maximal dose (100% of depth dose or PDD) is delivered several centimeters below the surface. At greater depths, there is an exponential falloff in the dose received by the irradiated tissue.

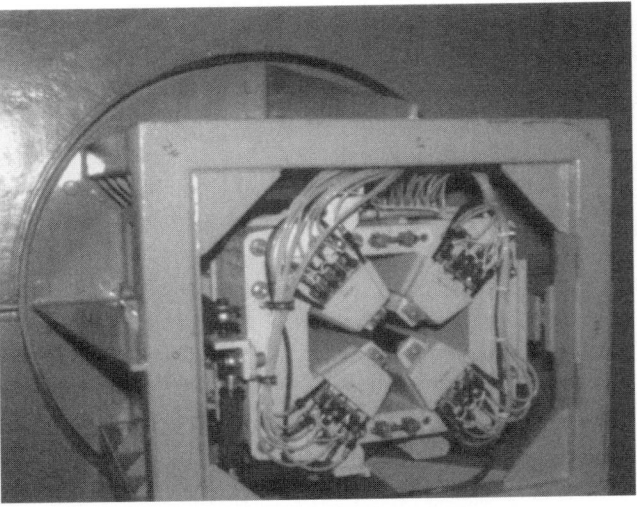

FIGURE 274–3. One of the quadripole steering magnets used to direct the protons after they exit the NPTC cyclotron.

nuclei, neutrons, and pions. Protons are most commonly used. Protons are produced by stripping the electron from a hydrogen atom. These positively charged particles are accelerated outward in a spiraling fashion by the magnetic field of a cyclotron or synchrocyclotron (Fig. 274–2). By the time they reach the outer perimeter of the accelerating magnets, they have attained kinetic energy in the range of 150 to 350 MeV, depending on the size of the accelerator. An extracting magnet then directs a beam of monoenergetic protons away from the accelerator. Further redirection of the beam can be achieved by means of steering and bend-

ing magnets (Figs. 274–3 and 274–4). Final magnets, collimators, and scatterers ensure that all the protons have the same kinetic energy and travel parallel to one another before entering the patient. These physical characteristics of the beam are essential for precise control of radiation deposition in the target tissue.

Most protons lose their energy in tissue by interactions with electrons in the constituent atoms of the material through which they pass. A smaller amount of energy is lost through collisions with the nuclei themselves. In quantitative terms, the amount of energy transferred to tissue per unit path length traversed by the protons is inversely proportional to the square of the proton velocity. The energy loss per unit of path length (linear energy transfer, or LET) through tissue is small and relatively constant until near the end of the proton's range. At that point, the residual kinetic energy is completely dissipated over a short distance (approximately 7 mm at 80% of the maximal dose), and the proton is absorbed. This results in a distinctive sharp rise in radiation dose to the target tissue, which is known as the *Bragg peak.* Because the proton travels no further, there is virtually no radiation dose beyond the target (Figs. 274–5 and 274–6). The low-dose region between the point of entrance into tissue and the Bragg peak is called the *dose plateau.* The dose in this region is 30% to 40% of the maximal dose delivered at the Bragg peak.

The range of protons in tissue is energy dependent. Because the protons are monoenergetic—that is, they have the same kinetic energy—they all penetrate to the same depth in tissue. The initial energy of the beam is specific for a given cyclotron and depends largely on the radius of the magnets used to generate the beam. To control the protons' depth of penetration precisely so that the Bragg peak falls within the desired target volume, the energy of the beam incident at the scalp is altered or modulated. This is done by interposing some absorbing material, such as water, in the beam path, which decreases the proton energy. An energy is cho-

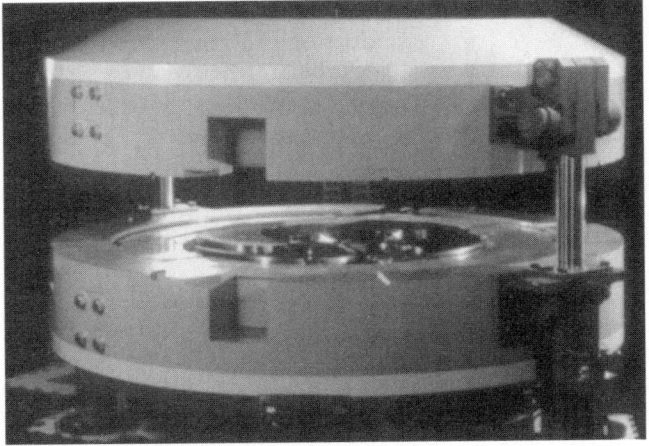

FIGURE 274–2. The cyclotron at the Northeast Proton Therapy Center (NPTC). Its diameter is 14 feet, and the combined weight of the two halves is 220 tons. The accelerating magnets of the lower half of the device are visible in this view. During operation, the upper half is lowered onto its counterpart so that the two are in contact, leaving an internal space where the protons are accelerated as they spiral outward toward the periphery.

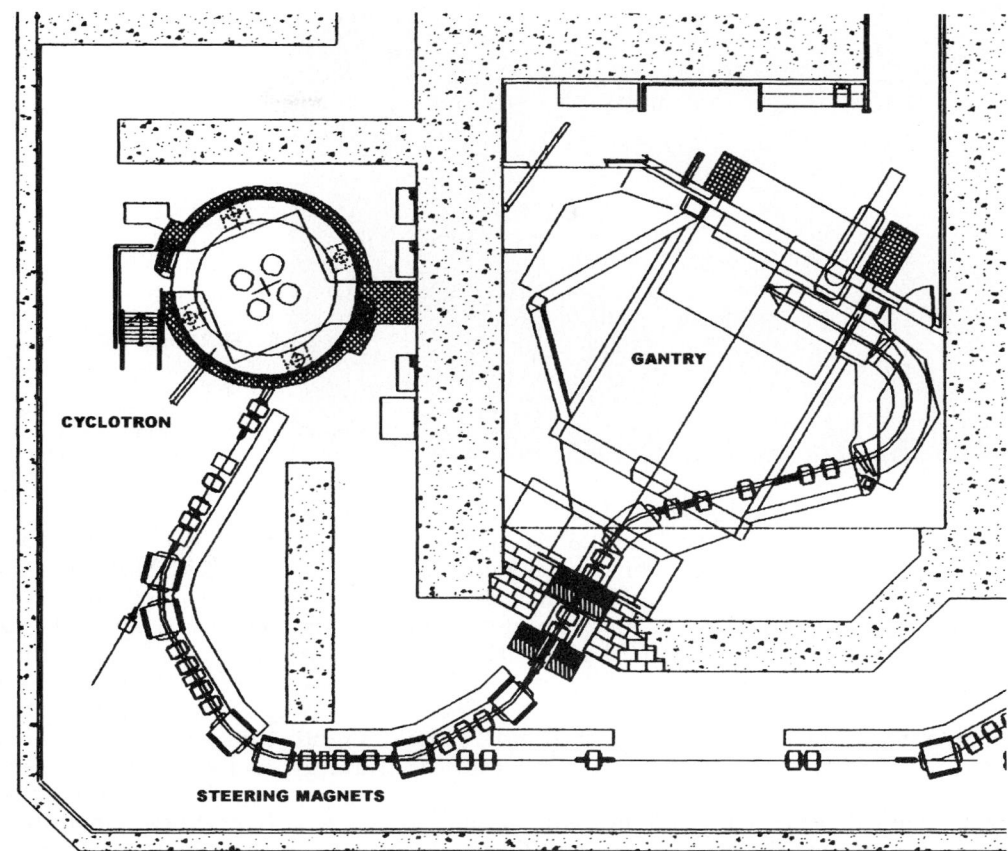

FIGURE 274–4. Overhead diagram of the beam delivery system at the NPTC. The 14-foot-diameter cyclotron, which generates a 231-MeV proton beam, is shown at the left. The beam is directed away, along a U-shaped path, to the adjacent gantry treatment room on the right. From there, it is redirected within the rotating gantry to emerge along a radius of the axis of gantry rotation toward the patient.

Pristine Bragg Peak NPTC

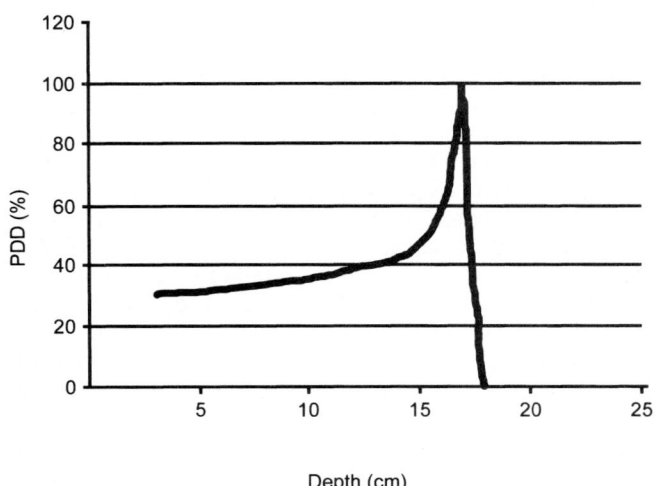

FIGURE 274–5. Depth-dose distribution for the monoenergetic 231-MeV proton beam at the NPTC. Note the lower dose received by tissue proximally in the dose plateau. The Bragg peak is characteristically narrow, requiring modulation to allow it to bracket the target.

sen so that the distal edge of the dose falls just beyond the deepest margin of the target. A single Bragg peak is too narrow to irradiate any but the smallest target, such as the normal pituitary or a very small ocular tumor. For larger lesions, which represent the majority of treatments, the beam energy is incrementally modulated or spread out to bracket the target. Two to six beams of closely spaced energies (ranges) are superimposed along the same axis to create a region of uniform dose over the depth of the target. This extended region of uniform dose is called the *spread-out Bragg peak* (Fig. 274–7). As with photon irradiation, treatment beams are directed along more than one axis to converge on the target volume.

Relative Biologic Effectiveness

The relative biologic effectiveness (RBE) of a specific type of ionizing radiation quantitates the efficiency of that particular radiation in producing a defined biologic effect. It is the ratio of the dose of a reference radiation (historically, cobalt 60) required to produce a biologic effect to the dose of another radiation required to produce that same effect.[8] For example, if the dose required to kill 50% of a population of irradiated cells were 55 Gy for cobalt and 50 Gy for protons, the RBE for protons would be 1.1. By definition, the proton RBE depends on the biologic system being studied. RBE values for the medical effects of proton beams are

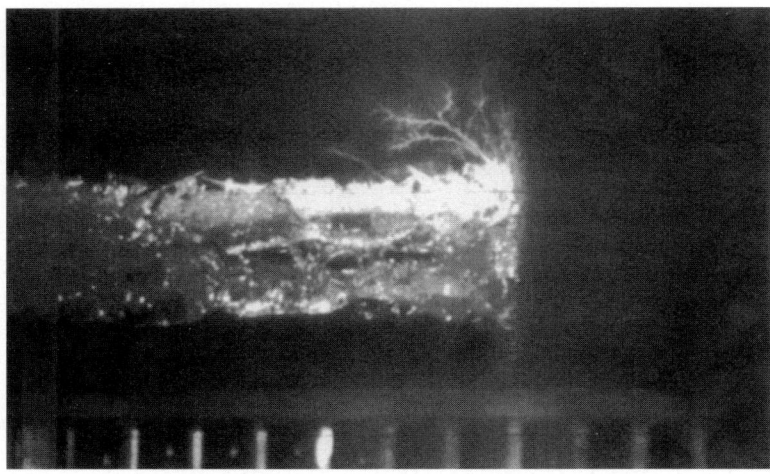

FIGURE 274–6. Plexiglas block after irradiation with 10 million rad of 160-MeV protons at the Harvard Cyclotron Laboratory. The beam enters from the left. Depth is indicated by the millimeter scale. Despite the enormous dose delivered, there is no radiation dose beyond the sharp cutoff at the Bragg peak.

reported variously between 0.9 and 1.3. Most values are in the range of 1.0 to 1.25. For clinical purposes, accurate estimates of the proton RBE are extremely important for determining the proper treatment dose of radiation compared with standard photon therapy. For an RBE of 1.1, the equivalent dose for cobalt 60 photons is the proton dose multiplied by 1.1. This is designated the cobalt gray equivalent (CgyE) dose, which is used for prescribing proton treatment doses.

For ionizing photon radiation such as gamma rays or x-rays, the RBE is equal to 1.0 and is invariable in clinical use. In reality, the issue of proton RBE is more complex. Laboratory studies of even a single biologic system yield RBE values that vary depending on pro-

ton energy, dose or fraction, and position in the spread-out Bragg peak. Moreover, there are no well-defined RBE values derived from studies of a single human tissue. Because a spectrum of normal tissues is included in the treatment volume, RBE values for human xenografts cannot be directly extrapolated to a given clinical application. Each of these presumably has a slightly different RBE and is dependent on dose, proton energy, and so forth. Although these RBE differences may be small, they are unlikely to be zero. This is especially pertinent when there is only a narrow margin between the dose that gives the desired therapeutic effect and the dose that causes complications (the therapeutic ratio). A range of RBE values from 1 to 1.25 is uncomfortably broad when small errors in estimation of the RBE could result in either a higher than expected rate of complications or an ineffective treatment outcome. Despite these unresolved issues, in clinical use, one must rely on an RBE value for protons that most closely approximates the combined results of laboratory studies and empirical clinical observations. In practice, a single value is used for all tissues, dose levels, and position in the spread-out Bragg peak.

The proton RBE generally accepted for clinical use is 1.1. This conservative value, at the lower end of the range of potential values, was chosen so that if the estimated value were in error, the RBE used would be low rather than high. In this case, the true radiation dose would be higher than intended, reducing the likelihood of undertreatment. Future studies of RBE that will be of the greatest clinical benefit are those that define the relationship of RBE to dose or fraction and its variation within the spread-out Bragg peak for a range of relevant tissues. Clinical trials comparing radiation effects in specific tissues for patients receiving equivalent doses of protons and photons may also yield valuable data. From such analyses, estimates of the RBE for human tissues irradiated in situ may be possible.

An equally powerful and more immediate means of determining appropriate proton doses for radiosurgery is to examine outcomes for the large body of patients treated with this method over many years. This can be

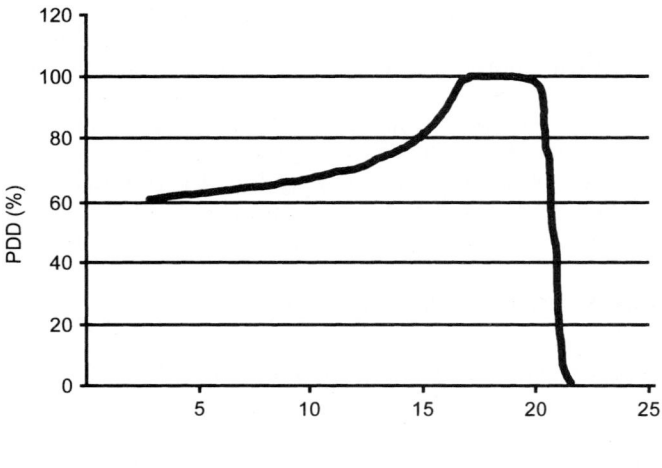

FIGURE 274–7. Depth-dose distribution for a spread-out Bragg peak generated with the 231-MeV proton beam. Seven Bragg peaks of slightly differing energies were combined to span a target measuring 4.4 cm along the beam axis. Note the high degree of dose homogeneity within the spread-out Bragg peak. There is also an increase in dose received in the plateau region resulting from the additive effects of the separate beams.

done for specific pathologic entities in order to account for differences in the biologic responses of these abnormalities. We analyzed the results for more than 1300 arteriovenous malformations treated at the Harvard Cyclotron Laboratory between 1965 and 1991.[9] This allowed us to modify existing risk prediction curves to accommodate this experience. The same type of analysis has been carried out for proton treatment of cavernous malformations.[10]

TREATMENT PRINCIPLES

Because radiosurgical treatments involve delivering a large single dose of radiation to the target tissue, the most important considerations are (1) accuracy in targeting and (2) a highly conformal distribution of radiation corresponding to the margins of the target, which spares adjacent normal tissue. Regardless of the type of radiation, the techniques of radiosurgical localization are all stereotactic. For proton radiosurgery at the Harvard Cyclotron Laboratory, three 1-mm-diameter stainless steel spheres are implanted percutaneously in the outer table of the skull before treatment. When the planning computed tomographic scan is performed later, these fiducial markers are registered and then used to localize the target volume at the time of treatment. Both contrast and noncontrast computed tomographic scans are necessary for treatment planning. The contrast scan is used to identify the lesion to be treated. A noncontrast scan is necessary to calculate the amount of proton energy that will be absorbed by all the tissues along the path of the treatment beam from the skin surface to the target. This allows one to determine the precise depth at which the Bragg peak occurs. The x-ray density of these tissues is measured in Hounsfield units and can be used to calculate the corresponding proton density of the same tissues. Although computed tomographic scanning is a necessary component of treatment planning, if the lesion is better seen with magnetic resonance imaging or angiography, image fusion is used.

Another universal feature of all types of radiosurgery is the use of multiple radiation portals whose point of convergence is the target volume. This minimizes the radiation dose to tissues that lie outside the target along the path of the treatment beam. For photon sources (gamma rays or x-rays), it is necessary to use many portals because the radiation dose deposited along the beam path for any single portal is considerably greater than the dose to the target. Tissues beyond the target also receive a substantial amount of radiation. For x-rays, the dose distribution has been improved somewhat by the introduction of progressively higher energy radiation sources. As the energy of an x-ray beam increases, the radiation dose deposited at a specific depth relative to the maximal dose increases proportionately. This results in deeper tissue penetration, relative skin sparing, reduced absorption in bone, and a sharper edge (penumbra) to the radiation beam. In spite of this, there is no inherent biologic advantage conferred by these high-energy sources, and the prob-

lem remains of high tissue dose along the radiation path outside the target.

Because protons deposit most of their radiation energy at the Bragg peak, only a few (two to four) treatment portals are needed to minimize the amount of radiation received by normal tissues proximal to the target along the radiation path. At the Harvard Cyclotron Laboratory, the beam of protons generated by the cyclotron has a fixed, horizontal orientation in the treatment room. To overcome this limitation and to enable easy alignment of the patient for any desired beam orientation, a specialized patient positioning couch is used that allows the supine patient to be rotated freely around horizontal and vertical axes. The point of intersection of these two axes corresponds to the position of the Bragg peak in space. The patient positioner—in reality, a large, target-centered stereotactic device called STAR (stereotactic alignment for radiosurgery)—allows the patient to be moved along x, y, and z axes to adjust the intracranial target to the isocenter of the axes of rotation of the device. Once that has been done, the patient can be rotated freely around these axes while the target remains fixed at a point in space represented by the Bragg peak (Figs. 274–8 and 274–9). Newer proton treatment facilities such as that at Loma Linda in California and the Northeast Proton Therapy Center at Massachusetts General Hospital in Boston overcome the limitations of a fixed beam by using enormous gantries that rotate the proton beam isocentrically around the patient. Although these impressive devices are much more versatile than fixed beams and allow treatment of other body sites such as the spine, they are expensive. This limits their application for general use.

Another important consideration for any type of radiosurgery is that the volume of tissue receiving the prescribed dose of radiation (*treatment volume*) conforms as closely as possible to the three-dimensional contours of the targeted lesion (*target volume*). Ideally, the treatment volume would correspond precisely to the target volume. In practice, this cannot be achieved; rather, one strives to make the treatment as conformal as possible. The larger and more complex the target volume, the more difficult this becomes, especially with gamma ray or x-ray treatments. Because the gamma knife is limited to treating relatively small, spherical volumes for any single isocenter, it is necessary to use multiple overlapping treatment volumes to approximate the target contours. For large lesions, in addition to the problem inherent to other photon sources of unavoidably increasing radiation to normal brain, there is the problem of prolonging the time required for treatment and creating substantial dose inhomogeneities within the treated volume. With linear accelerator radiosurgery, fewer isocenters are required to treat large lesions, because larger diameter beams are possible. In addition, new techniques such as intensity modulation and micromultileaf collimation are being designed and implemented to achieve more conformal treatments.[11, 12] These efforts have led to optimism that even higher doses of linear accelerator–generated x-

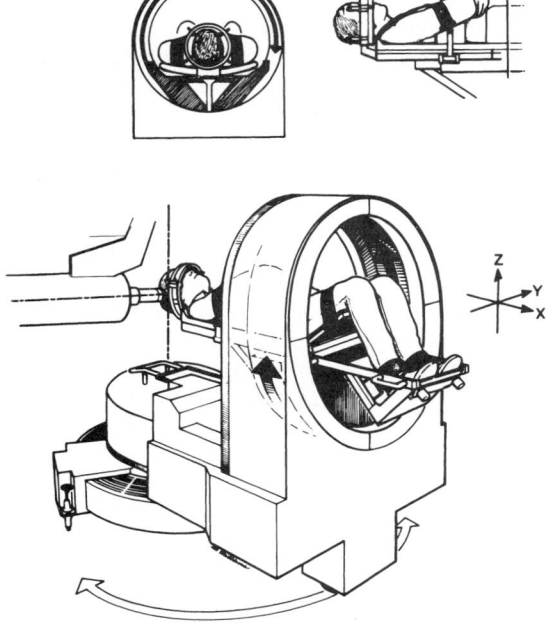

FIGURE 274–8. Diagrammatic representation of the STAR (stereotactic alignment for radiosurgery) patient positioning device used at the Harvard Cyclotron Laboratory. The patient is moved along x, y, and z axes until the intracranial target is at the intersection of the horizontal and vertical axes of rotation of the device. The patient can then be rotated freely around these axes while the target remains in the same position. The proton beam passes through the collimating system toward the patient from the left side. The smaller diameter collimator next to the patient's head is an adjustable water telescope, which allows the protons to be variably modulated so that the Bragg peak always occurs at the isocenter of the axes of rotation of the positioner. (From Chapman P, Ogilvy C, Butler W: A new stereotactic alignment system for charged-particle radiosurgery at the Harvard Cyclotron Laboratory, Boston. In Alexander E III, Loeffler J, Lunsford D [eds]: Stereotactic Radiosurgery. New York, McGraw-Hill, 1993, p 106.)

rays can be delivered with equal or reduced normal tissue complications.

With proton radiosurgery, it is less problematic to achieve a close approximation between the contour of a lesion and the volume actually treated by a prescribed dose. It is, in fact, with larger lesions that the advantages of proton over photon radiosurgery can be fully realized.[13] Two techniques, collimation and compensation, are used to accomplish this. For each treatment portal, the beam cross section is collimated with a custom aperture that corresponds to the silhouette of the lesion. In addition, the depth of penetration of the Bragg peak can be controlled over the cross-sectional area of the beam so that the contour of the deepest penetration of the protons matches the contour of the distal surface of the target. This is achieved by interposing a custom-milled bolus of material (*compensator*) in the beam path, which attenuates the energy of the protons incrementally across small areas of the beam cross section. This causes the protons that pass through the area of the compensator to penetrate to a depth corresponding to the deepest part of the lesion along the flight path of those protons. Finally, the entire beam is modulated to produce a series of Bragg peaks—the spread-out Bragg peak, which spans the lesion from its most proximal to distal surface. The fluctuation of dose within the spread-out Bragg peak is plus or minus 5%. In addition, beams with a cross-sectional diameter up to 50 mm can be used. This means that there is virtually no dose inhomogeneity in this dimension as well. As a result, a high degree of dose uniformity is achieved within the entire treatment volume.

TREATMENT TECHNIQUE

Treatment techiques for proton radiosurgery necessarily differ, depending on the facility. At the Harvard Cyclotron Laboratory, treatment planning is based on computed tomographic imaging. A frameless stereotac-

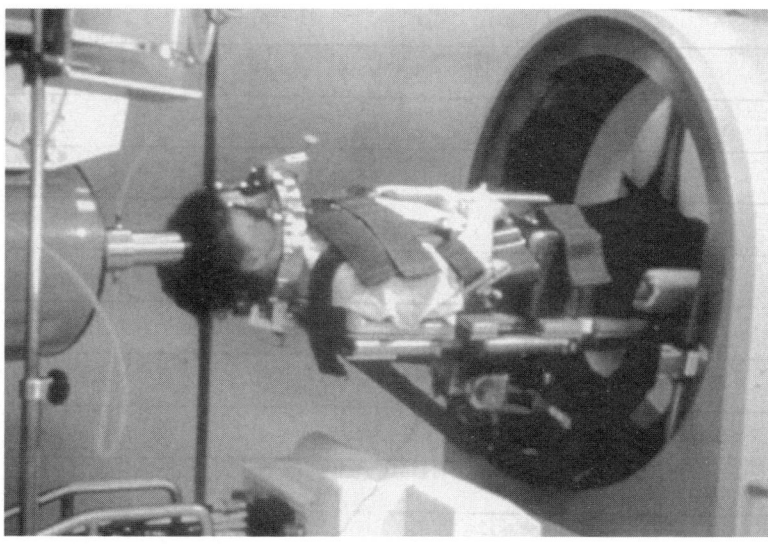

FIGURE 274–9. The patient is positioned in the STAR device for treatment with a vertex beam portal.

tic technique is used with implanted skull fiducial markers. Depending on the lesion to be treated, supplemental magnetic resonance imaging scans or angiographic images may be fused with the computed tomographic images. At the time of treatment planning, the implanted fiducial markers are registered spatially in relation to the lesion. Once the target volume has been three-dimensionally constructed, beam portals are selected that optimize the match between the target and treatment volumes. Depending on the size, location, and configuration of the target, two to four portals are chosen. For each of these beams, a so-called beam's-eye view of the target is constructed. This allows one to create a silhouette of the target, from which the template for a customized brass collimator is made. This same beam's-eye view is used to generate an image of the three radiopaque fiducial markers for later x-ray localization. At the time of treatment, the patient is placed supine in the STAR positioner. The head is immobilized using four-point skeletal fixation. Local anesthesia is supplemented by intravenous sedation. Orthogonal radiographs are taken to identify the previously implanted skull fiducial markers. Using these for stereotactic reference, the patient's position is adjusted in the x, y, and z directions to bring the target to the isocenter of the axes of rotation of the STAR device. This corresponds to the position of the Bragg peak. Localizing radiographs are repeated to identify the fiducial markers and confirm proper patient alignment before treatment. A water-filled telescope is positioned along the beam path in contact with the patient's scalp. During treatment, the length of this water column is varied incrementally to modulate the beam for a spread-out Bragg peak. Using the horizontal and vertical rotational axes of the positioner, the patient is sequentially repositioned for each of the planned beam portals. A typical treatment session requires 30 to 60 minutes.

EVOLVING TECHNOLOGY IN PROTON RADIOSURGERY

The implication of using protons as opposed to gamma rays or x-rays for radiosurgery is that for treatments using an equal number of beams, beam weights, and beam portals, the high-dose treatment volume is smaller than that achieved with these other modalities. This should lead to a lower probability of complications related to the irradiation of normal tissues. Within the treatment volume, dose uniformity is also greater. As improvements in dose distribution with photons are realized, efforts are also under way to increase the effectiveness and safety of proton treatments. The use of rotating gantries is already a reality in a limited number of facilities worldwide. This technology greatly simplifies the optimal use of beam portals, without the problems associated with patient repositioning during treatment. Gantries also widen the scope of body sites that can be treated with proton radiosurgery, in particular, the spine. In the future, different beam technologies will appear. For example, there is interest in very

small diameter scanning beams that paint a target, much like the electron beam in a cathode ray tube. If such a "pencil beam" were continuously modulated during its sweep to accommodate different depths within a complex target, a remarkable improvement in technical versatility and conformal dose delivery could be achieved.

Finally, the use of protons for radiosurgery cannot be viewed in isolation from their other applications in radiotherapy. One of the most fully exploited and successful uses of proton radiotherapy relates to the treatment of skull base chordomas and chondrosarcomas.[14] An exciting new application relates to the potential use of fractionated proton therapy for the treatment of central nervous system tumors in very young children, for whom the morbidity of conventional x-ray therapy is prohibitive. The superior dose distribution of protons, with relative sparing of normal tissues, offers the possibility of effective, safe radiation treatment. A particularly promising use in pediatric patients is the treatment of disseminating tumors, especially medulloblastoma, for which craniospinal as well as local treatment is indicated.[15, 16] Considering proton radiosurgery in the context of its fractionated counterpart is important, because it emphasizes that the use of protons is rapidly expanding beyond radiosurgery. In this wider view, significant innovations are in progress that will become available for radiosurgical applications. The expanding role of protons will make the establishment of larger numbers of medical cyclotrons more realistic, despite the initial expense for such facilities.

REFERENCES

1. Wilson WR: Radiological use of fast protons. Radiology 47:487–491, 1947.
2. Tobias C, Roberts J, Lawrence J, et al: Irradiation hypophysectomy and related studies using 340-MeV protons and 190-MeV deuterons with high-energy proton beams. In Proceedings of the International Conference on the Peaceful Uses of Atomic Energy, vol 10. Geneva, United Nations, 1955, pp 95–106.
3. Larsson B, Leksell L, Rexed B: The use of high-energy protons for cerebral surgery in man. Acta Chir Scand 125:1, 1963.
4. Malis LI, Baker CP, Kruger L, Rose JE: Effects of heavy, ionizing monoenergetic particles on the cerebral cortex. I. Production of laminar lesions and dosimetric considerations. J Comp Neurol 115:219–242, 1960.
5. Kjellberg R, Koehler A, Preston W, et al: Intracranial lesions made by a proton beam. In Haley T, Snider R (eds): Response of the Nervous System to Ionizing Radiation. Boston, Little, Brown, 1964, pp 36–53.
6. Kjellberg RN, Davis KR, Lyons S, et al: Bragg peak proton beam therapy for arteriovenous malformation of the brain. Clin Neurosurg 31:248–290, 1984.
7. Johns HE, Cunningham JR: Physics of Radiology. Springfield, Ill, Charles C Thomas, 1969.
8. Raju MR: Proton radiobiology, radiosurgery and radiotherapy. Int J Radiat Biol 67:237, 1995.
9. Barker FG II, Butler WE, Lyons S, Chapman PH: Dose-volume prediction of radiation-related complications after proton beam radiosurgery in 1250 AVM patients [abstract]. J Neurosurg 41:719, 1997.
10. Amin-Hanjani S, Ogilvy CS, Candia GJ, et al: Stereotactic radiosurgery for cavernous malformations: Kjellberg's experience with proton beam therapy in 98 cases at the Harvard Cyclotron. Neurosurgery 42:1229–1238, 1998.
11. Carol MP: Integrated 3-D conformal planning/multivane inten-

sity modulating delivery system for radiotherapy. In Purdy JA, Emami B (eds): 3-D Radiation: Treatment Planning and Conformal Therapy. Madison, Wis: Medical Physics Publishing, 1993.

12. Shiu AS, Kooy HM, Ewton JR, et al: Comparison of miniature multileaf collimation (MMLC) with circular collimation for stereotactic treatment. Int J Radiat Oncol Biol Phys 37:679–688, 1997.

13. Serago CF, Thornton AF, Urie MM, et al: Comparison of proton and x-ray conformal dose distributions for radiosurgery applications. Med Phys 22:2111–2116, 1995.

14. Munzenrider JE, Crowell C: Charged particles. In Mauch PM, Loeffler JS (eds): Radiation Oncology Technology and Biology. Philadelphia, WB Saunders, 1994, p 34.

15. Miralbell R, Lomax A, Bortfeld T, et al: Potential role of proton therapy in the treatment of pediatric medulloblastoma/primitive neuroectodermal tumors: Reduction of the supratentorial target volume. Int J Radiat Oncol Biol Phys 38:477, 1977.

16. Miralbell R, Lomax A, Russo M: Potential role of proton therapy in the treatment of pediatric medulloblastoma/primitive neuroectodermal tumors: Spinal theca irradiation. Int J Radiat Oncol Biol Phys 38:805, 1997.

Fractionated and Stereotactic Radiation, Extracranial Stereotactic Radiation, Intensity Modulation, and Multileaf Collimation

FRANK J. BOVA ■ SANFORD L. MEEKS ■ THOMAS WAGNER ■ WILLIAM A. FRIEDMAN ■ JOHN M. BUATTI

The field of stereotactic therapy started with the publication of Horsley and Clarke in 1908.[1] Their objective was to enable a surgeon to guide an electrode to a specified target. This target and other tissues were defined within a Cartesian coordinate system. Although the idea of stereotactic targeting was sound, the imaging available to Horsley and Clarke did not allow them to appreciate the anatomic variability of each patient. Since this initial attempt to use stereotactic guidance, many individuals have worked to advance stereotactic approaches. The development of technology to merge computed tomography (CT) and magnetic resonance imaging (MRI) to stereotactic localization has resulted in high spatial resolution of patient-specific information. These images allow the targeting of therapies with submillimeter precision and accuracy. This key advance has catapulted stereotactic techniques into the mainstream of neurosurgery.

RADIOSURGERY

The ability to administer a radiation beam through stereotactic targeting was first conceived by Leksell.[2] As initially described by him in 1951, radiosurgery is a single-fraction application of a radiation beam to a stereotactically defined intracranial target. The treatment technique that Leksell described required the use of a minimally invasive rigid reference frame. This clinical success led to the use of this therapy for extracranial applications and the development of noninvasive reference systems. The radiosurgery paradigm has also provided a methodology for the economical practice of virtual simulation.[3]

The application of conformal dose targeting and steep dose gradients to fractionated radiotherapy combines their respective advantages. However, the rapid clinical incorporation of radiosurgery into the mainstream of neurosurgery and radiation oncology has not always allowed sufficient time for clinicians to fully reflect on and appreciate the nuances of this new treatment tool. Unfortunately, this has often led to confusion between the art and the science of radiosurgery.

Radiosurgery and stereotactic surgery are similar image-based treatment techniques. In the standard application of stereotactic surgery, the surgeon has the ability to supplement the stereotactic database. In the case of a stereotactic biopsy, the surgeon can biopsy along a linear path to compensate for a misalignment of target tissue to the stereotactic reference frame. The surgeon can also target the center of a larger area of enhancement, thereby allowing for small alignment and targeting errors. When the objective of the stereotactic surgical procedure is lesion generation, the surgeon can use stimulation to validate target location or avoid critical tissues.

The radiosurgeon does not have these same tools available during radiosurgical therapy. A radiosurgeon cannot supplement the imaging database. Consequently, radiosurgery places added requirements on the spatial accuracy of image coordinates. In other words, the coordinates of the radiosurgical target are absolute. This requires higher precision and greater accuracy in all phases of the procedure (i.e., image acquisition, planning, treatment delivery). These added demands are met through increased quality assurance and an understanding of the pitfalls in data acquisition, targeting, planning, and treatment delivery. In an operative procedure, once the tissues have been removed, they cannot be replaced; in a radiosurgical procedure, once the radiation is delivered, it cannot be taken away.

Gamma Knife Radiosurgery

Leksell's early work involved x-ray apparatus as well as particle beam accelerators for radiosurgical application, but the development of the gamma knife allowed the efficient and economical practice of single-fraction stereotactic radiation delivery. The gamma knife has 201 tightly focused cobalt-60 sources. These sources are arranged so that the radiation beam resulting from each source intersects at an exact point within the treatment unit. The manufacturing tolerance requires the center of each of these 201 sources to come within 0.2 mm of the defined focal point. This manufacturing tolerance ensures that each unit produces nearly identical isodose patterns. The point at which the sources intersect is known as the *isocenter* of the device.

The gamma knife has a limited number of dose planning tools. The primary tool is to vary the size of the radiation collimator. This provides the treatment planning team with a limited variety of spherical dose patterns. For spherical targets less than approximately 3 mL, a single 18-mm-diameter isocenter placement is usually the plan of choice. For targets up to approximately 7.5 mL (i.e., approximately 24-mm-diameter targets), lower isodose curves can be used for prescribing the peripheral target dose. The second tool involves using multiple spherical dose distributions (i.e., setting multiple isocenters within the target volume) to provide a plan that conforms to the target volume. This planning technique is sometimes referred to as *sphere packing*. Using the various spherical dose distributions available, the clinician "packs" the treatment volume with these spheres, placing each distribution at the appropriate location relative to all other spherical distributions. Typically, the spheres are positioned approximately inside the target volume by the clinician. The treatment planning software has automated tools that then modify the shot locations and relative weights to provide the best plan. The goal is to provide a plan that is conformal to the target volume using a minimal number of individual dose spheres. The third tool available to the users of the gamma knife is to "plug"

or eliminate some of the 201 beams from an individual dose pattern. This tool is invoked when setting the patient at the appropriate isocenter results in the beam traversing a critical organ, such as part of the optic process, or when the planning team desires to alter the gradient of the nominal dose pattern. In practice, the plugging tool has a practical limitation. The dose rate delivered to the patient is directly related to the number of sources focused on the isocenter. As the sources are plugged, the dose rate decreases. For this reason, significant tilting of the dose pattern (described later for linear accelerator systems) is seldom attempted.

The downside is that the gamma knife (1) is applicable only to intracranial targets, (2) has a limited range of collimators (i.e., a limited range of spherical dose distributions) available, and (3) has a limited number of tools available for plan optimization. The upside of the gamma knife is that it allows a high degree of standardization in treatment planning. The dose distribution used to treat a 12-mm spherical target by one gamma knife site is identical to the distribution used at every gamma knife site. The planning tools available to optimize the plan are likewise identical at each site. Although this standardization does not extend to clinicians' identification of target tissues or dose selection, it does provide a significant level of standardization.

Linear Accelerator–Based Radiosurgery

Several groups around the world pioneered linear accelerator (linac)–based radiosurgery. Betti annd Derechinsky[4] in Argentina, Colombo and colleagues[5] in Italy, and Winston and Lutz[6] in the United States were all early contributors to linac-based radiosurgery. In each of these systems, the linac was used to obtain a dose pattern similar to that of the gamma knife. This dose distribution was achieved by applying multiple noncoplanar arcs at each isocenter (Fig. 275–1). The develop-

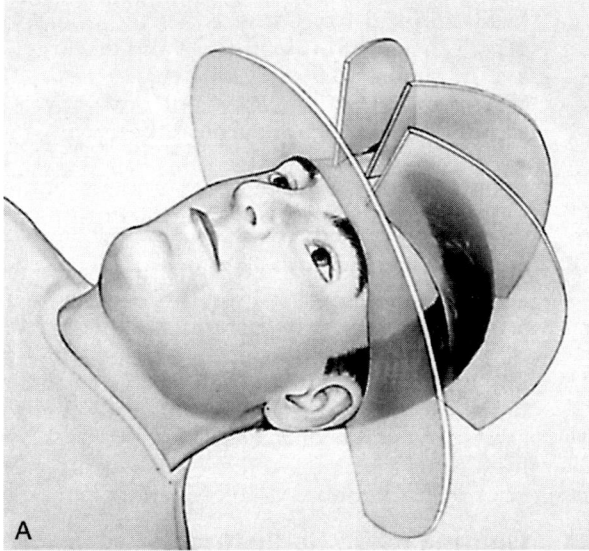
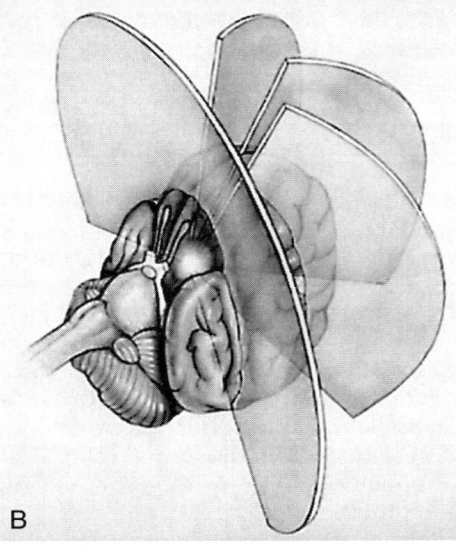

FIGURE 275–1. Four arcing beams shown in relation to their placement. All beams are focused on a unique point known as the *isocenter*.

ment of linac-based radiosurgical treatment units made radiosurgery more widely available. Once it was demonstrated that linacs were capable of executing stereotactic treatments, hundreds of radiation oncologists and neurosurgeons found that their facilities could purchase the necessary hardware and software to upgrade their linacs, making them radiosurgery ready. Within a few years, the number of radiosurgical units worldwide went from less than half a dozen to hundreds. Unfortunately, the proliferation of different approaches to the technology has led to a lack of standardization in the field, and the practice of radiosurgery varies widely among various academic, clinical, and commercial groups.

LINEAR ACCELERATOR SYSTEM REQUIREMENTS

One of the largest variables in linac radiosurgery is the overall system accuracy achieved. When considering the accuracy and precision necessary in a radiosurgical system, it is important to distinguish between the addition of a margin to ensure the inclusion of microscopic disease and the necessity of adding a margin because of system uncertainty. If the lack of system accuracy requires the clinician to include a margin of normal tissue in all stereotactic targets to ensure that the identified target is included in the selected isodose volume, normal tissues will be exposed to radiation unnecessarily. For example, adding a margin of 2 mm to a 24-mm clinical target volume increases the volume irradiated from 7.2 to 11.5 mL, an increase of 60%. Because all inaccuracies are cumulative, it is extremely important not to confuse margins required for target definition uncertainty with margins required for setup uncertainty. The fact that the edge of the target volume cannot be accurately defined is little justification for being unable to precisely predict a prescribed dose distribution. Further, the avoidance of critical structures is often as important as the inclusion of target tissues. Often, the presence of adjacent critical structures (whose locations are known exactly) places constraints on the prescribed dose. Inaccurate targeting and treatment delivery can just as easily include critical structures as it can exclude target tissues. Knowing the position of the high-isodose volumes as well as the location of the dose gradient to within a pixel of its true position is an absolute necessity.

Another aspect of stereotactic treatment that affects the accuracy requirements of a radiosurgery system is its general incompatibility with conventional radiotherapy verification techniques. Most radiosurgical targets and their surrounding normal anatomy cannot be imaged through conventional simulation and portal verification. The majority of radiosurgical targets can be visualized only during angiography or from a three-dimensional data set assembled from CT or MRI. The ability to generate a treatment plan through the manipulation of a three-dimensional diagnostic database is termed *virtual simulation.*[7] Radiosurgery and stereotactic radiotherapy differ from many other proposed applications of virtual simulation in two important aspects. The first is that these treatments consist of a large number of noncoplanar beams, and the second is the previously mentioned inability to determine the accuracy of treatment delivery through routine verification techniques. This remains true even if digitally reconstructed radiographs are available. The quality-assurance procedures necessary to guarantee system accuracy under these conditions make up a large part of each radiosurgical treatment.

As one would anticipate, a wide spectrum of linac-based radiosurgery systems have been proposed and are available commercially. The initial challenge in adapting a linac to a radiosurgery-ready treatment device is producing a system to guarantee absolute targeting to the stereotactic reference system (i.e., the stereotactic ring system). This involves creating a system that allows the mounting of the patient and the rigid fixing of the stereotactic ring to the linac. The coordinates of the target must then be set precisely over the linac's isocenter. It should be remembered that the treatment requires that multiple noncoplanar beams be applied to each isocenter. This requires that the isocenter for the linac's gantry as well as for the patient support system be evaluated and considered in the overall assessment of system accuracy. Typically, linacs must meet a nominal ± 1 mm isocentric tolerance for gantry rotation and patient support rotation. These two isocenters are seldom the same point in space. If one examines the total tolerance, it is often found to exceed the individual tolerance for each subsystem. It is therefore not uncommon to find systems that allow beam target inaccuracies to exceed 2 mm. When one looks at the smaller range of radiosurgery collimators, which are usually 5 mm in diameter, an error of 2 mm is not acceptable. Many systems attempt to correct for these inaccuracies by intertreatment adjustments, correcting for alignment inaccuracies based on test films. This, however, significantly slows down the treatment process, reducing the number of isocenters that can be treated and therefore the conformality of the treatment plan.

To stabilize the combined linac gantry–patient support system rotational accuracy, a device has been designed to stabilize the linac-based stereotactic system.[8] This approach enables a linac system to achieve treatment accuracy that equals that of the gamma knife system. The stabilization system can be applied to the linac in less than 10 minutes and enables a linac with greater than 2 mm inaccuracy to deliver radiosurgical treatment with an accuracy better than 0.2 mm (Fig. 275–2). Besides providing accuracy, the system eliminates the need for readjustments during the treatment of an individual isocenter, allowing each isocenter to be treated in 10 to 15 minutes, depending on the prescribed dose.

STEREOTACTIC IMAGING AND LOCALIZATION

As mentioned earlier, first radiosurgery and later stereotactic radiotherapy accounted for the first widespread applications of virtual simulation. Although various schemas have been proposed to carry out the virtual simulation process, the limiting factor is the

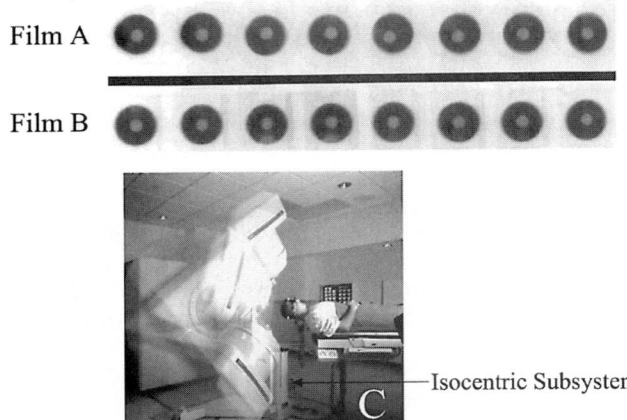

Film A

Film B

—Isocentric Subsystem

FIGURE 275–2. *A*, Upper set of films taken on a 6-MV linear accelerator. This unit has a gantry-table combined isocentric accuracy of 1.5 mm. *B*, Lower set of films taken on the same unit, but with the addition of an isocentric beam stabilization system. C, Stabilization system in a time-lapse picture showing progression through a single arc.

inability to guarantee replication of the initial simulation and planning geometry at the time of therapy. Radiosurgery overcomes this obstacle through the use of a rigidly fixed reference system in the form of a stereotactic frame.[9] The first step of each stereotactic procedure is application of the reference frame to the patient's skull. Once applied, this frame remains rigidly attached to the patient's skull throughout the procedure. Several frames have been developed for general stereotactic applications, and many of these have been adapted for radiosurgical use. Each of these systems has unique advantages and disadvantages, as well as its own coordinate system. They all, however, have one common feature: once the frame is fixed to the patient's skull, a rigid relationship between that patient's intracranial anatomy and the frame's coordinate system is established. Although there is often an optimal orientation for the frame relative to an individual patient's anatomy, the most important issue is the rigidity of the patient-frame relationship throughout the entire radiosurgical procedure.

Once the frame has been applied and this rigid relationship established, the diagnostic examinations necessary for target localization and treatment planning are performed. Each examination provides unique information about the target volume and its position relative to normal, nontarget tissues. The three most common diagnostic procedures used for stereotactic localization are angiography, CT, and MRI. Angiography provides unique information concerning vascular structures; CT and MRI provide information about both target tissues and normal anatomy and allow a full three-dimensional model of the patient's intracranial anatomy to be reconstructed. For each examination type, a special reference device is attached to the stereotactic frame.[10] This reference allows the spatial position of the tissues being imaged to be related to the frame's coordinate system.

Stereotactic imaging systems can be separated into two categories. The first includes systems that produce images containing all the information necessary to compute the stereotactic coordinates of all tissues contained within that image. These systems are equipment independent. Embedded in each image is a description of the stereotactic coordinate system. Using such a system places no special requirements on the image systems. For example, an independent system does not require biplanar angiographic images to be absolutely orthogonal. The fiducial marker on each image allows the trajectory of the x-ray beam relative to the stereotactic coordinate system to be computed. In the case of CT, the axial sections are not required to be absolutely parallel to the plane of the stereotactic reference system. The plane of the scan relative to the reference system can be computed with the information provided by the fiducial points within each transaxial image.

The second type of stereotactic system, a dependent system, does require special knowledge of the imaging conditions. For biplanar imaging, either orthogonality or exact knowledge of the angle between image planes is required. In the case of CT, the angle of the gantry must be known, and often the stereotactic frame's coordinate system must be specially aligned to the CT scanner's coordinate system.

When an independent system is used, the stereotactic application can be designed so that all necessary quality assurance can be carried out on the images used in each procedure. This is usually accomplished through defined fiducial systems or by verifying the geometry of fixed fiducial markers. When a dependent system is used, the quality assurance of the stereotactic procedure must be linked to the quality assurance of the diagnostic equipment at the time of image acquisition. Such quality-assurance issues may include the precision of the indexing of the CT table, the orthogonality of the CT gantry to the axis of the stereotactic system, the alignment of the laser alignment system within the CT gantry, or the orthogonality of plain film images within a biplanar angiographic procedure. Although it is feasible to use dependent reference systems, there appears to be little to gain and a great deal to lose in terms of the potential for error and increased time needed for quality assurance. It is thus recommended that an independent system be used whenever possible.

LINEAR ACCELERATOR–BASED RADIOSURGICAL DOSE PLANNING

This linac-based technique provided several planning tools not previously available in radiosurgery.[10] First, the entrance and exit pathways can be spread over a larger area. This allows the dose distribution to obtain a more spherical shape than the lower-isodose shells (Fig. 275–3). The second is an increased range of available spherical dose distributions. The maximal target volume applicable to the single-fraction dose in a radiosurgical treatment is the only limit to the collimator sizes available in linac-based systems. This has typi-

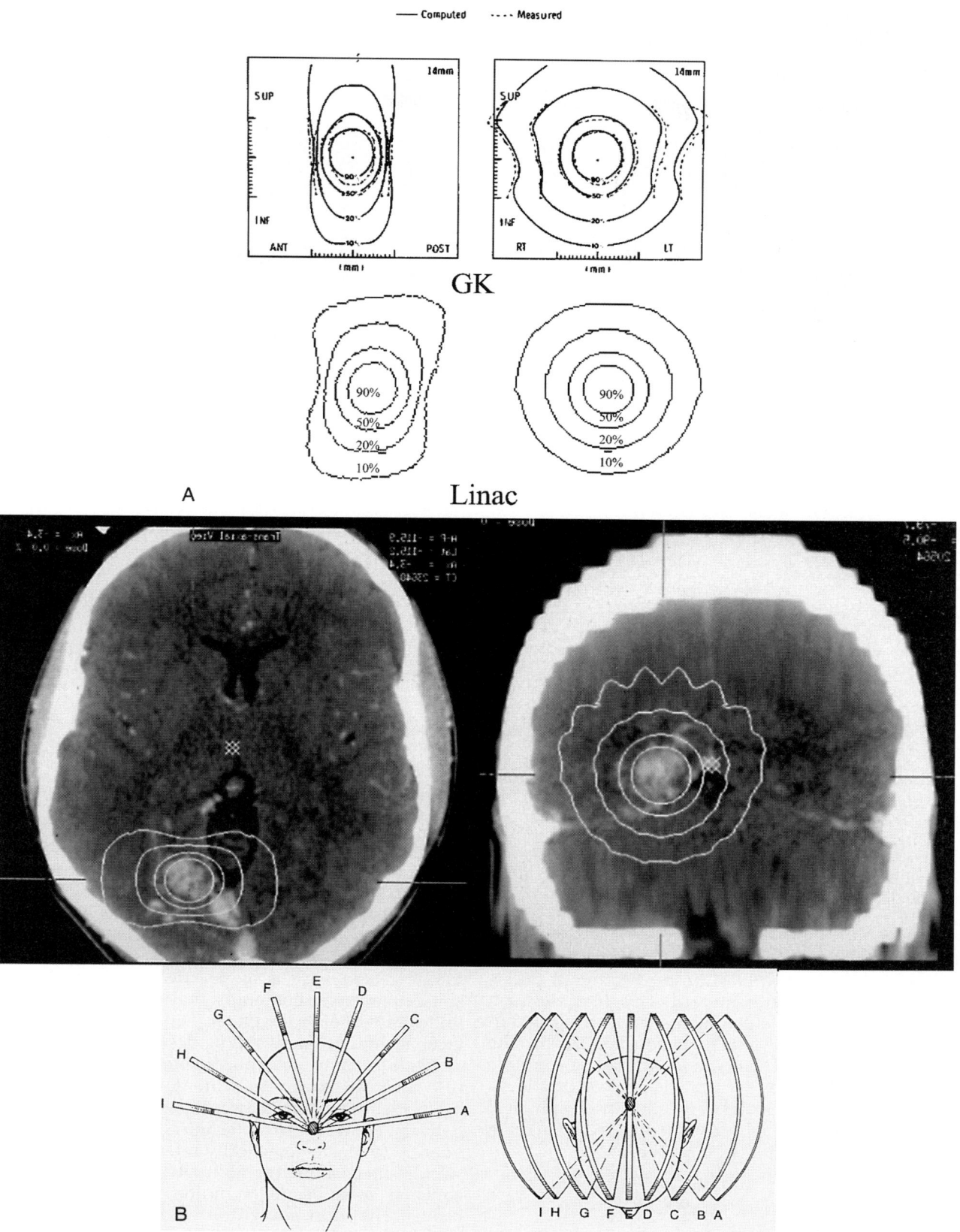

FIGURE 275–3. *A,* Dose distribution produced by a gamma knife unit *(top)* fitted with 14-mm collimators.[32] Dose distribution produced by a linear accelerator system *(bottom)* using a 14-mm collimator. *B,* Dose distribution and arc placement of nine evenly spaced arcs, with each arc spanning 100 degrees.

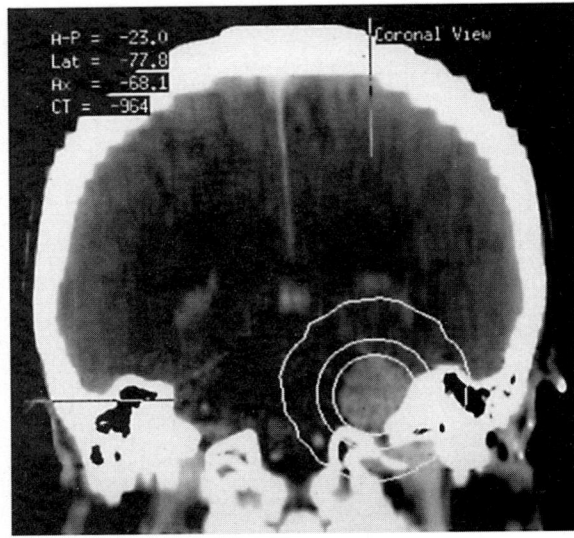
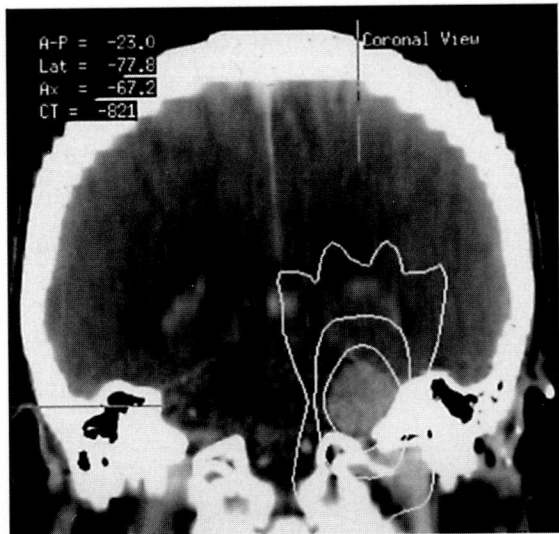

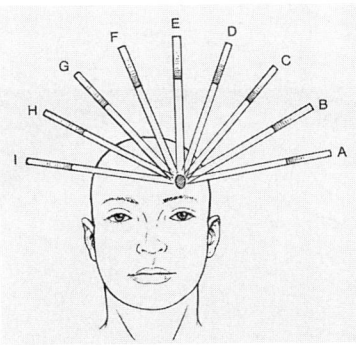
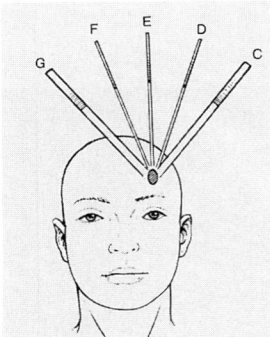

FIGURE 275–4. *Right,* Set of nine evenly spaced beams and the resulting dose distribution targeting an acoustic schwannoma. *Left,* Set of five arcs, with four of the most horizontal arcs eliminated, applied to the same target to reduce the radiation dose to the brainstem.[10]

cally been set between a 30-mm-diameter distribution (14 mL) and a 40-mm-diameter distribution (33 mL). The third tool is the ability to significantly alter the shape of both the high- and low-isodose volumes. This is achieved by limiting the placement and spacing of noncoplanar arcs (Fig. 275–4). A fourth tool used by linac-based systems involves the application of different collimators for different arcs. This tool allows a dose distribution to be either elongated or truncated in the superior-inferior or lateral plane (Fig. 275–5). The linac-based system also has the ability to use multiple isocentric planning (i.e., sphere packing) to provide a dose pattern to targets that are either not spherical or elliptical, which can be easily planned using the previously mentioned tools[10] (Fig. 275–6).

FRACTIONATED STEREOTACTIC RADIOTHERAPY

As previously defined, the radiosurgery procedure delivers the entire prescribed dose of radiation in a single treatment setting. There are, however, clinical situations in which a single fraction of radiation cannot be safely delivered. Examples include targets that either incorporate or are immediately adjacent to critical structures, such as the optic processes or the brainstem, and targets whose volume exceeds that which can be safely treated with a single effective dose. Although single-fraction radiotherapy may be inappropriate for these cases, the improved targeting provided by stereotactic techniques may still be desirable.

The ability to incorporate stereotactic techniques into a radiotherapy treatment allows noncoplanar beam delivery and increased accuracy in treatment delivery. However, it is technically challenging to deliver 30 to 45 stereotactically referenced treatment sessions, with each treatment involving five to seven noncoplanar static beams or multiple noncoplanar arcing beams. The most straightforward approach would be to design a reference ring that would remain in place for the entire course of treatment.[11] This approach, though a logical extension of the single-fraction technique, has met with limited success. The need for daily

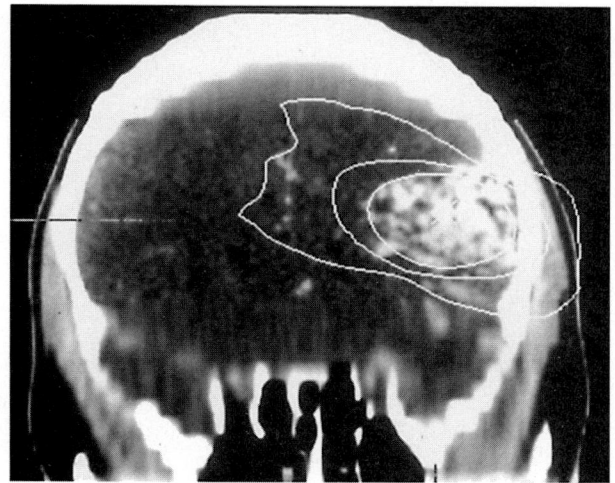

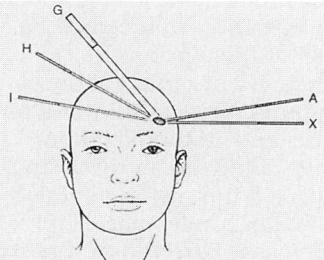

FIGURE 275–5. Set of five arcs targeting an arteriovenous malformation (AVM). The arc set is oriented along the long axis of the AVM, with a 35-mm collimator being used for the most vertically oriented arc and 28-mm collimators being used for the remaining four arcs.[10]

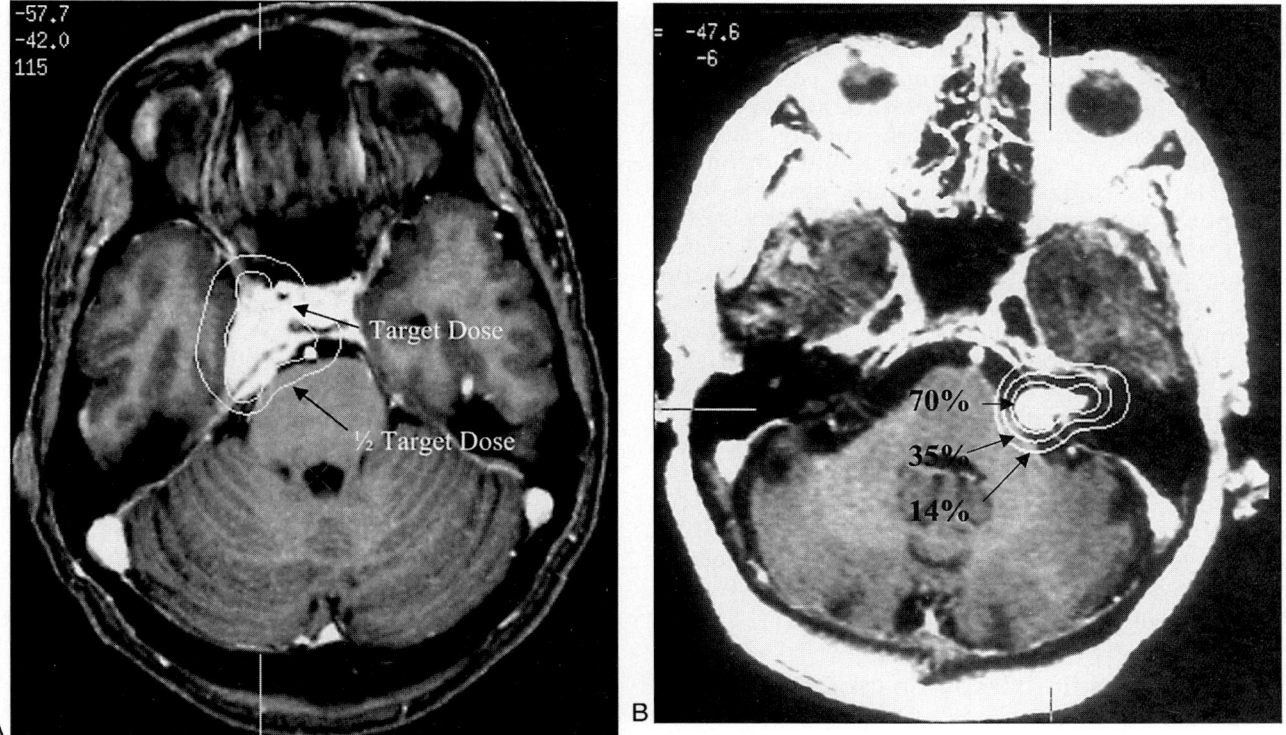

FIGURE 275–6. *A*, Meningioma treated using 11 isocenters. *B*, Acoustic schwannoma treated using two isocenters.

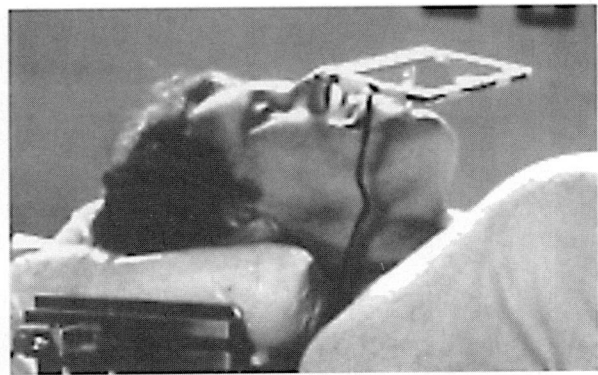
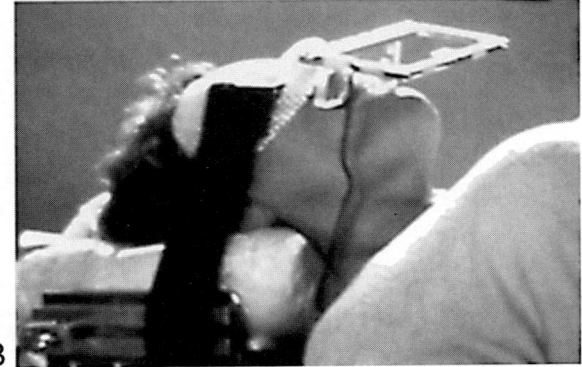

A

B

FIGURE 275–7. *A*, Patient with biteplate in place. *B*, Patient with biteplate and separate immobilization system added.

revalidation of the ring's alignment, infection at the pin sites, and patient reluctance have all reduced the effectiveness of this approach.

Within the field of radiation oncology, mask immobilization systems have been used for many years for patient setup and immobilization.[12] Historically, these systems have allowed repositioning and beam alignment to within 5 mm of a previously defined position, usually based on a reference plain x-ray film. Systems that measure and correct for this misalignment have also been suggested.[13] However, these approaches require too much time and have not gained clinical acceptance. It has also been determined that using only portal alignment films makes it difficult to measure absolute alignment to better than 5 mm in the plane perpendicular to the central axis of the treatment beam.[14] Misalignments that are along the path of the beam or rotations not perpendicular to the central axis are even more difficult to determine.

New systems have been introduced to improve on the mask-based approach by constructing masks of new materials and attempting to tighten the mask-patient fit.[15, 16] Unlike previous mask systems, these new approaches attempt to link the mask to the system used for stereotactic referencing. A biteplate system has been manufactured that provides a means of fabricating a custom biteplate and securing it to a stereotactic reference system.[17] The system also provides a method of determining the gross alignment of the skull relative to the reference system.

Another commercially available system attempts to separate the function of patient immobilization from the function of patient alignment.[18] This system uses a biteplate and infrared tracking to determine the patient's alignment to the isocenter of the linac (Fig. 275–7). This system has been shown to reset the stereotactic reference system to an average accuracy of 0.15 mm, with a standard deviation of 0.1 mm.[19]

Stereotactic Radiotherapy Beam Delivery Systems

The use of these systems allows multiple arc treatments, multiple static beam treatments, dynamic arc-

ing, or intensity-modulated radiotherapy treatments. Each of these beam delivery techniques has advantages and disadvantages.

Multiple arc treatments, similar to those used in radiosurgery, can be used for stereotactic radiotherapy. Unlike radiosurgery, only single-isocenter plans are applicable in fractionated cases. As discussed earlier, the primary requirement in radiosurgery is conformality and steep dose falloff; target homogeneity is not considered to be of extreme importance. The clinical setting in which stereotactic radiotherapy will be applied must be considered. In a large percentage of cases, the reason that the dose cannot be delivered in a single setting is the target's proximity to critical, radiosensitive tissues. In these cases, the fractionated dose that must be delivered repeatedly to the target tissues is very close to the tolerance dose of the critical tissues. If a multiple-isocenter plan were used and the prescription dose to the 70% line was 1.7 Gy per fraction, tissues within the distribution would be receiving in excess of 2.4 Gy per fraction. This is typically not acceptable for stereotactic radiotherapy. The clinical settings in which stereotactic radiotherapy is indicated usually coincide with a requirement for dose homogeneity. A typical example is treatment of an optic nerve meningioma. Because the target tissues are immediately adjacent to critical normal optic tissues, a single-fraction radiosurgery treatment cannot be safely administered.[10] Stereotactic radiotherapy treatment also has associated dose restrictions. Although it is advantageous to treat the target tissues using conventional fractionation of approximately 1.7 to 2 Gy per fraction, it is also advantageous to restrict the fraction dose to the optic nerve to less than 1.9 Gy per fraction.[20] This means that the prescription isodose level cannot be less than 90% of the maximal dose when 1.7 Gy is prescribed.

Although fractionated therapy places some restrictions on dose homogeneity, it simultaneously relaxes the criterion of absolute target conformality. The radiobiologic advantage of fractionated therapy is that a degree of normal tissue can be included in the prescribed radiation volume. To cover the tissues at risk of harboring microscopic disease, significant volumes of normal tissue are often included in the prescription dose volume. The criteria for fractionated dose planning are significantly different from those for radiosurgical dose planning, and the isodose prescriptions should be more similar to those selected in routine radiotherapy; the prescription isodose is usually between 90% and 98% of the maximal dose.

The advantage of applying multiple arcs in the stereotactic radiotherapy setting is the relatively steep dose gradient. However, when large collimators (>40 mm) are used, this advantage can be lost. The disadvantage of the spherical distributions is that unless the target is spherical, there will be poor conformality.

Multiple conformal static fields are often used for stereotactic radiotherapy. In this approach, multiple radiation portals are set, and each is tailored to the silhouette of the beam as viewed from the source of radiation to the target volume. The beams are spaced in an attempt to provide the best divergence possible and to ensure that the least amount of normal tissue is irradiated by more than one beam. The result of such an approach is usually a relatively conformal dose distribution.

A hybrid between the static conformal beam and the arcing circular beam is dynamic conformal arcing. In this technique, multiple arcs are used, but instead of a single circular beam shape, the beam is continuously adjusted to match the target's projected shape. This technique usually provides slightly improved conformality over the static conformal approach and also provides an improved dose gradient, with a more rapid falloff of the dose as a function of distance from the surface of the target volume.

Static conformal and dynamic conformal techniques are best applied to targets that are convex and have slowly or smoothly varying surfaces. When targets are concave or have highly irregular surfaces, radiation beams that depart from the nominal flat, open beam or the single-gradient wedged beam are required to maintain a high conformality and a steep dose gradient. These techniques that vary the beam's intensity within a given radiation portal are referred to as *intensity modulation*.

CIRCULAR COLLIMATORS AND MULTILEAF COLLIMATION

Historically, radiosurgical distributions have been created through the use of circular collimators. These collimators were designed to produce a relatively small radiation beam, ranging from 4 to 30 mm. When these collimators were used either to define the radiation beam for the 201 sources of a gamma knife or to define the beam that was arced through multiple hundred degrees, a spherical dose distribution was produced. The approximate size of the 80% isodose shell resulting from a collimator of X-mm diameter is usually close to X-mm in diameter (Fig. 275–8). As previously discussed, these distributions have very sharp edges, decreasing from the target dose of 80% to half the target dose in 3 to 4 mm.

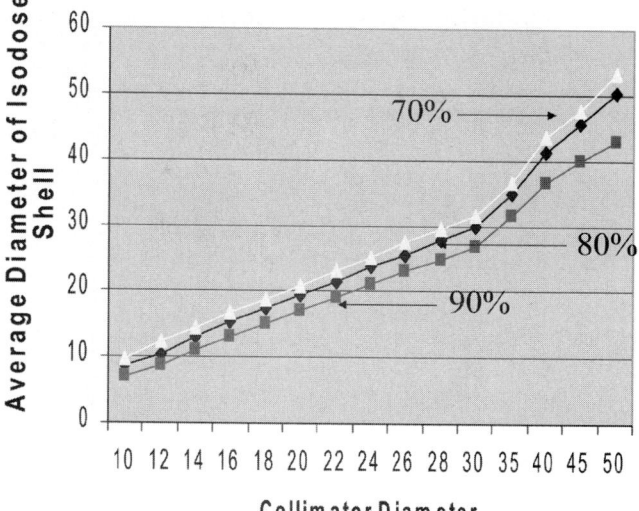

FIGURE 275–8. Diameter of the isodose shell (90%, 80%, and 70% of maximal dose) resulting from various collimator diameters. Each distribution contained five evenly spaced arcs, each spanning 100 degrees.

When stereotactic radiotherapy targets become very elongated or larger than 40 mm in diameter, it is often more appropriate to treat the volume with static irregular beams. In this planning technique, usually four to seven beams are focused at the target volume, with each radiation portal shaped to fit that projection of the target along the beam's central axis (Fig. 275–9). For the past 2 decades, the method of choice to produce these irregular beams was to cast the shape from a low-melting alloy.[21] Recently, however, new collimation devices known as *multileaf collimators* (MLCs) have been introduced and are becoming common on new linacs. The first MLCs used relatively coarse leaves, usually 10 mm at the isocenter, to approximate the shape of the radiation portal. New devices known as micro-multileaf collimators (mMLCs) have now been introduced. These devices usually have a maximal field size of 100 to 150 mm, with leaf widths of 1.5 to 5 mm at the isocenter. Although it was often difficult to approximate the shape of a small stereotactic radiotherapy beam with the initial 10-mm leaf systems, it is relatively easy to perform this task with the 1.5- to 5-mm leaf systems (Fig. 275–10).

MLCs also give the planner the option of using dynamic conformal planning. In this technique, arcing therapy, similar to the standard radiosurgical technique, is combined with conformal collimation. In some clinical settings, this combination produces conformal and homogeneous distributions. In other settings, the mMLC can be used to modulate the radiation beam's intensity, allowing intensity-modulated radiotherapy to be administered. This is usually achieved either by dragging the leaves across the radiation aperture, using temporal modulation to produce a unique intensity pattern, or by using multiple static beams to build up a unique dose profile.

The use of mMLC units for static beam stereotactic

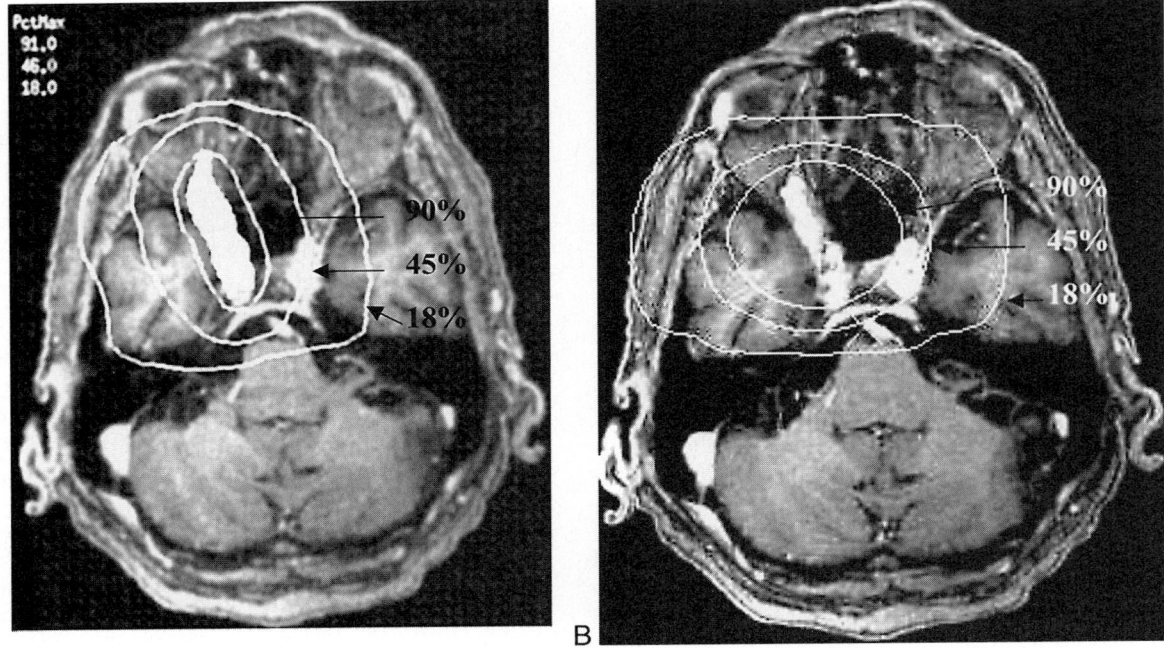

FIGURE 275-9. *A*, Optic nerve meningioma treated with a set of five static conformal beams. *B*, Same target treated using four evenly spaced arcs spanning 100 degrees, with each arc using a 40-mm collimator.

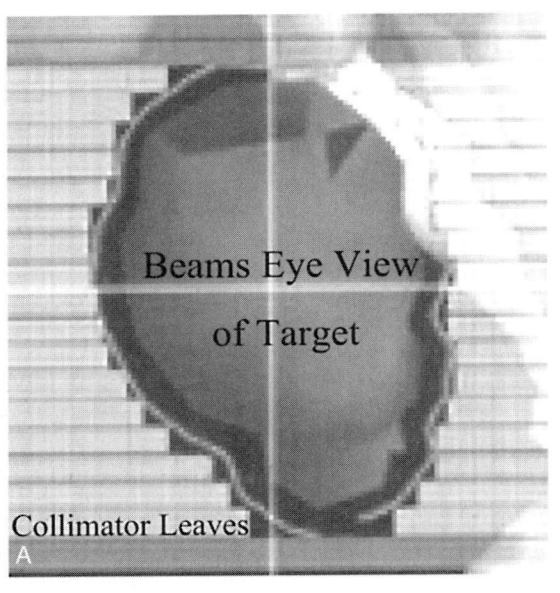

FIGURE 275-10. *A*, Beam's-eye view of an irregular target being approximated by a multileaf collimator. *B*, Beam's-eye view of a target being approximated by varying leaf widths (10, 5, and 1.5 mm).

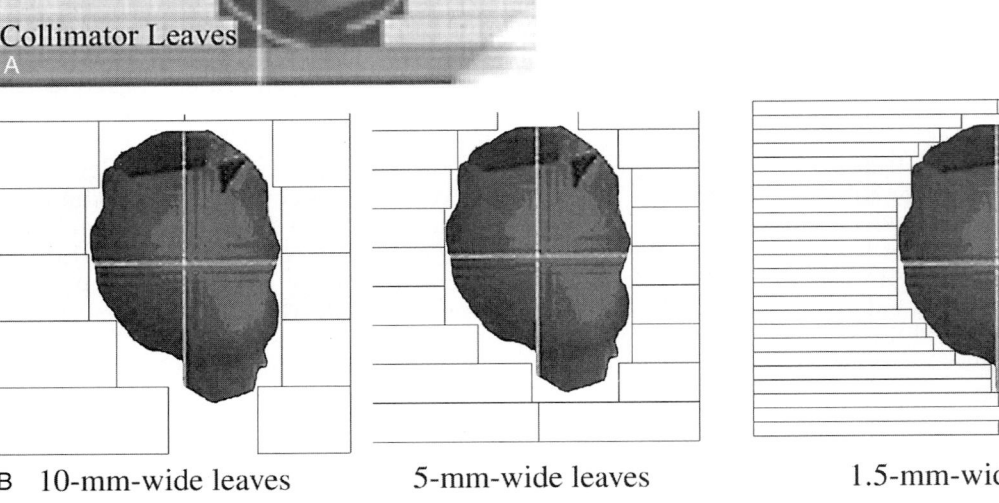

B 10-mm-wide leaves   5-mm-wide leaves   1.5-mm-wide leaves

radiotherapy has the same criteria as for the older conformal fields produced from low-melting alloys. The transmission through the block is usually held below 5% of the open, unblocked portion of the beam. Because the inclusion of some normal tissues is acceptable in stereotactic radiotherapy, the clinician has the luxury of widening the beam apertures to include small, irregular extensions of the planning target volume. This technique of aperture alteration, though common in radiotherapy treatment planning, can perform very poorly when used for radiosurgical planning. Although it appears to produce a conformal plan, the end result can be a significant decrease in the ability of the distribution to reduce to a fraction of the target dose within a few millimeters, which has been the historical norm for radiosurgical treatments. The 5-mm-wide leaves of an mMLC unit can easily accommodate the larger field sizes usually required for stereotactic radiotherapy. Although one can always show anecdotal cases that demonstrate an advantage of smaller leaves, the ability to conform to the required shapes

begins to plateau at a leaf width of approximately 5 mm.

The use of mMLC units for radiosurgery requires an entirely different set of planning criteria. The radiosurgery technique depends on a significant number of radiation beams focused on a single point. The ability to restrict the dose when using this technique requires that the arcing beam have a very sharp edge with very low leakage (Fig. 275–11). The allowable 5% static beam radiotherapy leakage for blocked fields may not be acceptable[22] for radiosurgical treatment techniques. This change in criteria also applies to the technique of aperture opening to include irregular target extensions. The ability to produce an intensity-modulated beam appears to hold the most promise for using mMLC approaches in radiosurgery.

A simple example of this approach, and the associated problems of mMLC leakage, can be seen in Figure 275–12. The initial approach to treating this target involved multiple isocenters. With a five-beam static field approach with a 0-mm margin, the 70% isodose shell

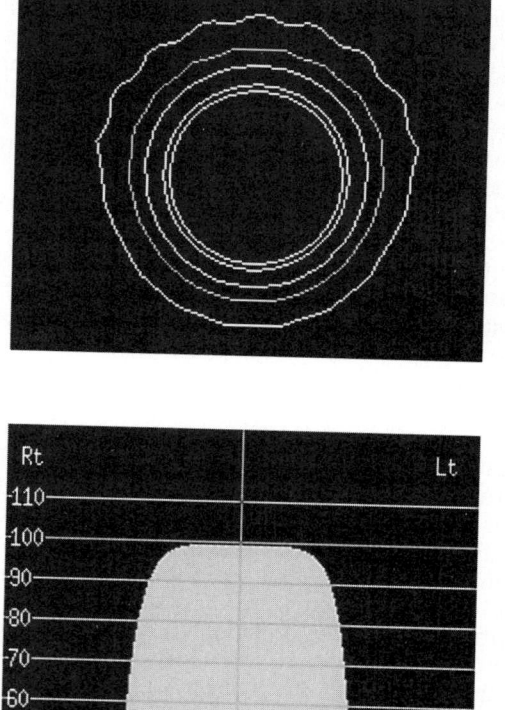

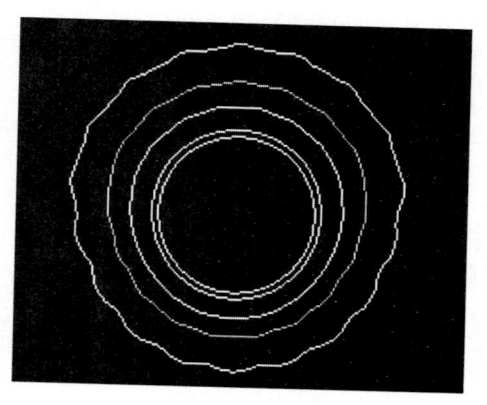

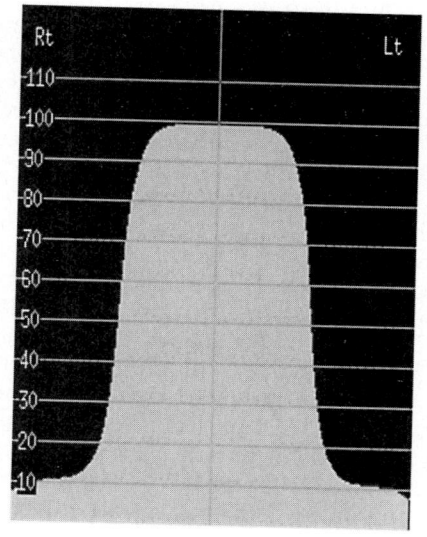

A Collimator Leakage at 0.5%

B Collimator Leakage at 5%

FIGURE 275–11. *A,* Coronal dose distribution from nine evenly spaced arcs using a 24-mm collimator with 0.5% leakage. *B,* Same arc set, but with 5% leakage.

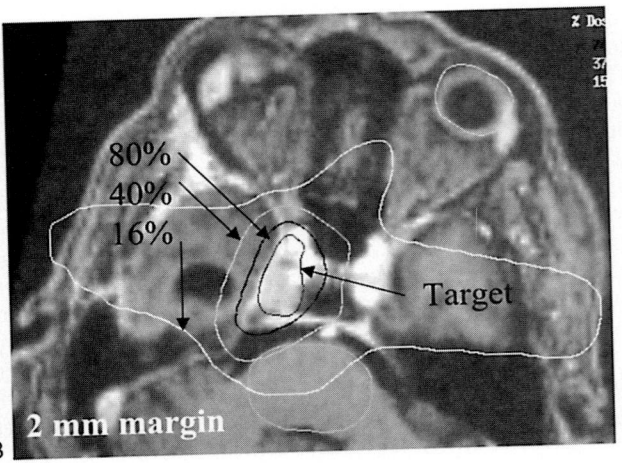

FIGURE 275–12. *A*, Nine-isocenter plan prescribing the target dose at the 70% isodose level. *B*, Seven-beam conformal plan using a 0-mm margin plus an annular boost *(left)*. Same seven-beam plan, but using a 2-mm margin *(right)*.

does not include all the target volume. When the beams are broadened, the target is covered, but a significant amount of normal tissue is now included in the target isodose shell. When each radiation portal is modulated by producing a high-intensity, 2-mm rim around the inside of each beam, however, the coverage of the target isodose shell remains conformal, and the gradient at the beam edge remains steep.

INTENSITY-MODULATED RADIOTHERAPY

Although BEV collimation schema can provide conformal dose distributions to many targets, they require sufficient geometric separation between the target and critical structures to be effective. Further, BEV conformal therapy does not work well when applied to concave targets. One of the latest developments in radiotherapy is the use of fields in which the beam intensity, or fluence, is varied across the radiation beam. This approach, termed *intensity-modulated radiotherapy* (IMRT), is capable of generating highly conformal dose distributions while simultaneously avoiding the irradiation of nearby critical structures. Conceptually, one can think of IMRT as a method in which the beam intensity is weighted to be proportional to the target thickness from each beam's-eye view. In other words, thinner target shapes require less radiation intensity than do thicker target shapes, and intensity modulation is a mechanism for providing different intensities to account for thickness variation across the target.

Physically, the required intensity patterns are most often achieved temporally through use of an MLC. The Peacock system (Nomos Corporation, Sewickley, PA), for example, uses the multivane intensity-modulating compensator (MIMIC) for treatment execution.[24] The MIMIC consists of 20 independent vanes, each of which projects a 1- by 1-cm block at the machine isocenter. The MIMIC attaches directly to a linac and temporally modulates the intensity of a slit-collimated

radiation beam. Intensity-modulated slit irradiation, in conjunction with gantry rotation about the patient, treats a slice of the patient with a radiation dose that conforms to the shape of the target volume within the slice. In a system analogous to axial computed tomographic scan acquisition, the treatment table is indexed, and each slice is treated in turn until all slices within the targeted volume have been treated. Other systems exist that provide intensity modulation using a conventional MLC.[25]

Variation of the beam intensity dramatically increases the number of options available to the treatment planner, thereby increasing the complexity of the treatment planning process. Therefore, IMRT relies on a planning technique called *inverse planning*. Inverse planning allows the user to specify the target volume and all critical structures of interest, and then specify the desired target dose and acceptable dose limits for each critical structure. The treatment planning system then determines the fluence patterns required to satisfactorily achieve the desired result. In the most comprehensive scenario, the computer determines not only the fluence patterns for each beam but also the optimal beam orientations and weights. This method entirely avoids the conventional manual, iterative planning method. Two general approaches exist for determining the optimal intensity patterns.[26] Explicit (analytic) methods typically involve target–beam delivery geometry simplifications or dosimetry algorithms excluding secondary particle transport, but they have the advantage of speed. Implicit (iterative) methods permit a wide range of target–beam delivery options and more easily incorporate advanced dosimetry algorithms, but they require significant processing time.

Regardless of the algorithm used, it is interesting to note that a good degree of conformity can be achieved for irregular targets with a moderate number of intensity-modulated beams. For radiosurgery, however, it is important to consider not only dose conformity but also the dose gradient outside the target volume. Owing to the exponential attenuation of photons, the only way to achieve a steep dose gradient is through the intersection of multiple noncoplanar beams on a single focus. Therefore, most IMRT systems use either arc therapy or multiple noncoplanar static beams.

Several groups have investigated the potential efficacy of IMRT applied to intracranial targets.[27–29] The results of these studies are mixed, partially because the quality of conventional radiosurgery plans is highly dependent on the experience of the treatment planner. Second, inverse radiotherapy treatment planning algorithms are still under development. As the algorithms become more sophisticated, the quality of the treatment plans produced will increase. However, it can be stated unequivocally that IMRT currently provides an advantage over conventional radiotherapy planning techniques as the size and irregularity of the treatment volume increase, and also as the distance to critical structures decreases. As is well known, target size and proximity to critical structures are two indicators for fractionated stereotactic radiotherapy; for this reason, IMRT has most commonly been implemented in this setting, where it has provided extremely conformal dose distributions and excellent clinical results.[30, 31] Overall, the efficacy and convenience of inverse radiotherapy and radiosurgery planning can be expected to continue to increase significantly over the coming years.

EXTRACRANIAL STEREOTACTIC RADIOTHERAPY

Although much progress has been made in radiotherapy planning and beam delivery systems, relatively few gains have been made in patient immobilization and localization. Representative studies of repositioning errors in the literature show that uncertainties in patient localization for head and neck treatments range from 2.5 to 4 mm,[33, 34] whereas for pelvis and abdomen treatments, the uncertainties range from 3 to 9 mm.[34, 35] It should be stressed that these numbers are derived from the assessment of bony anatomy and do not account for internal structure motion due to breathing, heartbeat, bowel gas, and so on. Therefore, although the bony anatomy may be positioned to within 3 to 9 mm, the precision of the actual target localization may be significantly worse.

Although virtual simulation is a significant improvement over conventional radiotherapy, its accuracy is clearly limited by the lack of a robust fiducial system. Recognizing the benefits of stereotaxy, several groups have designed stereotactic systems for the localization of extracranial targets. The University of Arizona system is designed to employ spinal or other skeletal osseous fixation to immobilize the treatment region.[36, 37] In phantom, this frame was shown to provide an overall treatment accuracy of 1.4 to 2 mm for the treatment of spinal lesions. The Karolinska system uses a body frame with a pressure fixation system.[38, 39] Although this system is less invasive than the first, the accuracy is also degraded; repeat CT studies determined a reproducibility for localization of liver and lung tumors of 5

to 8 mm for 90% of the patient setups, and the pressure fixation system reduced diaphragmatic movements to 5 to 10 mm. It is important to understand that these numbers represent the actual shift of the internal target, not just the reproducibility of positioning bony anatomy.

From these studies, it is apparent that high-precision extracranial radiotherapy requires real-time imaging at the time of treatment. The Nomos Corporation (Sewickley, PA) introduced the first such commercial system, which is an ultrasound-based targeting system marketed under the trade name BAT. This system uses an articulating arm to determine the location of the two-dimensional ultrasound image relative to the linac isocenter. Initial clinical investigations of this unit for prostate localization showed an absolute magnitude difference between CT and ultrasound localization of 3 ± 1.8 mm in the anteroposterior direction, 2.4 ± 1.8 mm in the lateral direction, and 4.6 ± 2.8 mm in the axial direction.[40]

The thrust of the research at the University of Florida and the University of Iowa is to extend our system for fractionated stereotaxy to extracranial targets that are localized using optic guidance of three-dimensional ultrasound images. We believe that our system has several advantages over other systems for extracranial stereotactic localization. The first is the ability to quantify the patient's alignment in each of six degrees of freedom. Because we are optically tracking the ultrasound image set, we can provide this feedback in real time. This allows the patient to be quickly and efficiently realigned relative to the treatment machine. Further, optic tracking allows the patient to be monitored during treatment. Any patient motion during treatment can therefore be detected and corrected. Last, rather than relying on an image plane, we are tracking a three-dimensional ultrasound volume. The quality of two-dimensional ultrasound images makes their interpretation difficult, and the outcome of a two-dimensional ultrasound-guided procedure depends on the skill and expertise of the operator in manipulating the transducer and in forming a correct mental impression of the three-dimensional anatomy. Techniques that rely on two-dimensional ultrasound targeting are variable owing to their reliance on inferior image quality, and we believe that these techniques can be significantly improved by using optic-guided three-dimensional ultrasonography as the targeting modality.

REFERENCES

1. Horsley V, Clarke RH: The structure and function of the cerebellum examined by a new method. Brain 31:45–124, 1908.
2. Leksell L: The stereotactic method and radiosurgery of the brain. Acta Chir Scand 102:316–319, 1951.
3. Sherouse GW, Mosher C, Novins K, et al: Virtual simulation: Concept and implementation. In Proceedings of the 9th ICCR, 1987, pp 433–436.
4. Betti OO, Derechinsky VE: Hyperselective encephalic irradiation with linear accelerator. Acta Neurochir Suppl 33:385–390, 1984.
5. Colombo F, Benedetti A, Pozza F, et al: Stereotactic radiosurgery utilizing a linear accelerator. Appl Neurophysiol 48:133–145, 1985.
6. Winston KR, Lutz W: Linear accelerator as a neurosurgical tool for stereotactic radiosurgery. Neurosurgery 22:454–464, 1988.

7. Sherouse GW, Borland JD, Reynolds KL, et al: Virtual simulation in the clinical setting: Some practical considerations. Int J Radiat Oncol Biol Phys 19:1059–1065, 1990.

8. Friedman WA, Bova FJ: The University of Florida radiosurgery system. Surg Neurol 32:334–342, 1989.

9. Gildenberg PL: The history of stereotactic neurosurgery. Neurosurg Clin N Am 11:765–780, 1990.

10. Friedman WA, Buatti JM, Bova FJ, et al: Linac Radiosurgery: A Practical Guide. New York, Springer-Verlag, 1997.

11. Houdek PV, Fayos JV, Van Buren JM, et al: Stereotactic radiosurgery technique for small intracranial lesions. Med Phys 12:469–479, 1985.

12. Bova FJ: Treatment planning for irradiation of head and neck cancer. In Million RR, Cassisi NJ (eds): Management of Head and Neck Cancer: A Multidisciplinary Approach. Philadelphia, JB Lippincott, 1984, pp 209–230.

13. Gildersleve J, Dearnaley DP, Evans PM, et al: A randomised trial of patient repositioning during radiotherapy using a megavoltage imaging system. Radiother Oncol 31:161–168, 1994.

14. Perera T, Moseley J, Munro P: Subjectivity in interpretation of portal films. Int J Radiat Oncol Biol Phys 2:529–534, 1999.

15. Hamilton RJ, Kuchnir FT, Pelizzari CA, et al: Repositioning accuracy of a noninvasive head fixation system for stereotactic radiotherapy. Med Phys 23:1909–1917, 1996.

16. Schlegel W, Pastry O, Bortfeld, et al: Stereotactically guided fractionated radiotherapy: Technical aspects. Radiother Oncol 29:197–204, 1993.

17. Gill SS, Thomas DG, Warrington AP, et al: Relocatable frame for stereotactic external beam radiotherapy. Int J Radiat Oncol Biol Phys 20:599–603, 1991.

18. Bova FJ, Friedman WA: The University of Florida frameless high-precision stereotactic radiotherapy system. Int J Radiat Oncol Biol Phys 38:875–882, 1997.

19. Butti JM, Bova FJ, Friedman WA, et al: Preliminary experience with frameless stereotactic radiotherapy. Int J Radiat Oncol Biol Phys 42:591–599, 1998.

20. Parsons JT, Bova FJ, Fitzgerald CR, et al: Radiation retinopathy after external-beam irradiation: Analysis of time-dose factors. Int J Radiat Oncol Biol Phys 30:765–773, 1994.

21. Henderson SD, Purdy JA, Gerber RL, et al: Dosimetry considerations for a Lipowitz metal tissue compensator system. Int J Radiat Oncol Biol Phys 13:1107–1112, 1987.

22. Pike B, Podgorsak EB, Peters TM, et al: Dose distributions in dynamic stereotactic radiosurgery. Med Phys 14:780–789, 1987.

23. Carol MP: Peacock: A system for planning and rotational delivery of intensity-modulated fields. Int J Imaging Syst Technol 6:56–61, 1995.

24. Galvin JM, Xuan-Gen Chen, Smith RM: Combining multileaf fields to modulate fluence distributions. Int J Radiat Oncol Biol Phys 27:697–705, 1993.

25. Harmon JF Jr, Bova FJ, Meeks SL: Inverse radiosurgery treatment planning through deconvolution and constrained optimization. Med Phys 25:1850–1857, 1998.

26. Woo SY, Grant WH III, Bellezza D, et al: A comparison of intensity modulated conformal therapy with a conventional external beam stereotactic radiosurgery system for the treatment of single and multiple intracranial lesions. Int J Radiat Oncol Biol Phys 35:593–597, 1996.

27. Meeks SL, Buatti JM, Bova FJ, et al: Potential clinical efficacy of intensity-modulated conformal therapy. Int J Radiat Oncol Biol Phys 40:483–495, 1998.

28. Kramer BA, Wazer DE, Engler MJ, et al: Dosimetric comparison of stereotactic radiosurgery to intensity modulated radiotherapy. Radiat Oncol Investig 6:18–25, 1998.

29. Cardinale RM, Benedict SH, Wu Q, et al: A comparison of three stereotactic radiotherapy techniques: ARCS vs noncoplanar fixed fields vs intensity modulation. Int J Radiat Oncol Biol Phys 42:431–436, 1998.

30. Carol M, Grant WHI, Pavord D, et al: Initial clinical experience with the Peacock intensity modulation of a 3-D conformal radiation therapy system. Stereotact Funct Neurosurg 66:30–34, 1996.

31. Grant WI, Cain RB: Intensity modulated conformal therapy for intracranial lesions. Med Dosim 23:237–241, 1998.

32. Walton L, Bomford CK, Ramsden D: The Sheffield stereotactic radiosurgery unit: Physical characteristics and principles of operation. Br J Radiol 60:897–906, 1987.

33. Hunt M, Kutcher GJ, Burman C, et al: The effect of setup uncertainties on the treatment of nasopharynx cancer. Int J Radiat Oncol Biol Phys 27:437, 1993.

34. Verhey LJ: Immobilizing and positioning patients for radiotherapy. Semin Radiat Oncol 5:100–114, 1995.

35. Hunt M, Schultheiss T, Desobry G, Hanks G: Convolving setup uncertainties with dose distributions. Med Phys 20:929, 1993.

36. Hamilton AJ, Lulu BA: A prototype device for linear-accelerator based extracranial radiosurgery. Acta Neurochir Suppl (Wien) 63:40–43, 1995.

37. Hamilton AJ, Lulu BA, Fosmire H, et al: Preliminary clinical experience with linear-accelerator based spinal stereotactic radiosurgery. Neurosurgery 36:311–319, 1995.

38. Lax I, Blomgren H, Naslund I, Svanstrom R: Stereotactic radiotherapy of malignancies in the abdomen: Methodological aspects. Acta Oncol 33:677–683, 1994.

39. Blomgrem H, Lax I, Naslund I, Svanstron R: Stereotactic high dose fraction radiation therapy of extracranial tumors using an accelerator: Clinical experience of the first thirty-one patients. Acta Oncol 34:861–870, 1995.

40. Lattanzi J, McNeeley S, Pinover W, et al: A comparison of daily CT localization to a daily ultrasound-based system in prostate cancer. Int J Radiat Oncol Biol Phys 43:719–725, 1999.

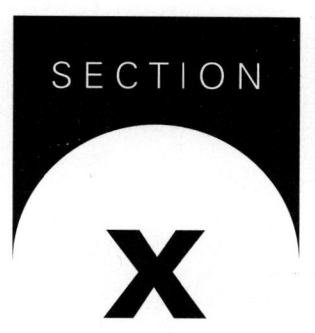

Spine

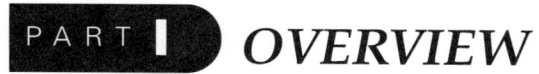

CHAPTER **276**

Overview and Historical Considerations

VOLKER K. H. SONNTAG ■ DENNIS G. VOLLMER

Spinal disorders have been recognized as a serious affliction of humans since ancient times. Early accounts of spinal disorders reflected the pessimism appropriate for the period, given the serious morbidity involved and the complexity of managing many of these conditions. The Hippocratic record was probably the first to describe active therapeutic intervention in the form of closed reduction of spinal injuries.[1] True surgical treatments for disorders of the spine were rare before the beginning of the 20th century. Surgical attempts with dismal results discouraged most surgeons,[2–4] but a few reports from remarkable pioneers described successful outcomes.[5–7]

In 1891, the ability to diagnose spinal disorders in vivo was revolutionized by the discovery of x-rays by Wilhelm Conrad Roentgen.[8] This new technology was rapidly incorporated into clinical problem solving.[9] Concurrently, neurologists and their surgical colleagues were gaining confidence in the concept of localizing lesions in the central nervous system on the basis of physical neurological examination.[10, 11] Emboldened by improvements in anesthesia and asepsis, the concepts of clinical localization, and the diagnostic power of radiology, 20th century surgeons began to address a broader spectrum of spinal lesions.

In the field of diagnostic imaging that emerged after Roentgen's discovery, several key developments enhanced the diagnosis of spinal conditions. Dandy's[12] use of gas instillation for ventriculography and myelography allowed visualization of the spinal cord and nerve roots and delineation of pathologic compression. The introduction of iodinated contrast material soon followed, with improved image quality.[13] The replacement of lipid-based media with water-soluble agents continued to refine the technique, further improving the images and obviating the need to manually remove the contrast through lumbar puncture. Diskography, which remains controversial, was described by Lind-

blom in 1948.[14] Epidural venography, performed through a transfemoral route, also enjoyed a period of use despite some difficulties with interpretation.[15]

Axial computed tomography (CT) revolutionized diagnostic imaging of the central nervous system. CT represents the synthesis of the work of numerous investigators into a tool for clinical problem solving. Although often credited to Hounsfield,[16, 17] numerous others played key roles in the theoretical background required for its development.[18–20] Further technical refinements for spinal imaging, including the combination with myelography, spiral acquisition, sagittal and coronal reformatted images, and three-dimensional reconstruction, continue to enhance its utility.[21–23]

Similar to the story for CT, the development of magnetic resonance imaging (MRI) was the result of numerous individuals building on the efforts of others. After years of basic investigations, Damadian[24] patented a device in 1972 for body imaging using the principles of magnetic resonance. Countless others have since contributed to the state of spinal imaging available today. MRI is the diagnostic imaging modality of choice for most clinical conditions involving the spine and spinal cord. Although CT remains superior for the evaluation of fine bony detail, the ability to image all tissues related to the spine in multiple planes gives MRI a clear advantage in many situations. The chief disadvantage of this modality is the time involved in performing the study, which may limit its use in trauma or emergency circumstances.

The armamentarium of diagnostic tools, including MRI, CT, three-dimensional reconstructions of the spine, high-resolution single photon emission computed tomography (SPECT), and numerous other modalities, has dramatically facilitated diagnosis in many cases, but judgment and skill remain as important as ever in deciding on surgical or medical treatments.

Historically, surgeons operated on the spine from a

posterior approach. This was logical because it was the most direct path to the bony elements, but the potential benefits of alternative approaches tailored to the offending pathology were soon realized. Posterolateral approaches first developed out of surgical treatment for Pott's disease. Menard[25] described an approach he called costotransversectomy in 1984. Menard's primary objective for this approach was the drainage of tuberculous paravertebral abscesses. Subsequent major modifications to the costotransversectomy were the lateral rhachotomy developed by Capener[26] and the lateral extracavitary approach of Larson and colleagues.[27] Both of these modifications achieved an even more lateral view, allowing direct decompression of the neural elements. These classic approaches continue to undergo modification, such as McCormick's[28] retropleural approach.

Anterior approaches to the spine were often developed in response to problems presented by tuberculous spondylitis. In 1956, Hodgson and Stock[29] reported their experiences with anterior decompressive operations. Cloward[30] and Smith and Robinson[31] are generally acknowledged for establishing the anterior approach to the cervical spine for the management of disk herniation. The transoral approach was described soon after and was also developed initially for treating tuberculosis.[32]

Hibbs[33] and Albee[34] independently described surgical treatments for Pott's disease, which are usually cited as the initial reports of fusion procedures for the spine. Subsequent surgeons applied similar techniques to other conditions, including fractures, degenerative disease, and spondylolisthesis.[35–38] Posterolateral intertransverse fusion techniques were further refined by Ghormley[39] and others. Unfortunately, many of the early methods of spinal fusion were flawed by relatively high rates of nonunion. Improved results, particularly in patients with prior instability, had to wait for the development of satisfactory spinal instrumentation. Anterior and posterior lumbar interbody fusion techniques were described by Burns[40] and Cloward,[41] respectively.

The use of metal implants to correct deformity and provide internal stabilization began in the late 19th century. Reviews often cite Wilkins'[42] use of a carbonized silver wire suture to stabilize T12-L1 in an infant as the first recorded use (1988) of internal fixation of the spine. Hadra[43] described placement of internal wire fixation in the cervical spine in 1891. Lange[44] and a few other surgeons reported attempts at internal fixation in the early 20th century, but further development of spinal instrumentation systems required advances in the art of spinal fusion, improved understanding of biomechanics, and noncorrosive metallic implants.

Harrington's distraction rod system was first used in the late 1940s.[45–47] Luque's L-rod with segmental sublaminar wires was developed in the 1970s.[48] A posterior, multiple hook–rod system was described by Cotrel and Dubousset in 1982.[49] Several other universal implant systems were introduced, including the Texas Scottish Rite Hospital (TSRH) and the Moss Miami spinal systems.[50, 51]

Screws placed into the facets were used by King[52] and others to promote fusion. The screw trajectory was later modified to provide fixation into the pedicle.[53] Transpedicular screw fixation was refined and clinically used in the 1960s and 1970s by Roy-Camille and colleagues[54] and by Louis[55] and was further developed and popularized in Europe in the 1980s. Pedicle fixation began to be widely used in North America as an adjunct to fusion in the 1980s and 1990s.[56]

Devices for anterior fixation of the spine in scoliosis were developed in part because of the early problems with Harrington's distraction rod. Dwyer and coworkers[57] described his device for the anterior correction of scoliotic deformity in 1969. Although drawbacks to this form of correction were soon recognized, the Dwyer device stimulated further development in anterior instrumentation systems.[58, 59]

Anterior plating of the cervical spine was a natural adjunct to the expansion of anterior approaches to this region and provided the surgeon with improved segmental immobilization compared with orthotic devices. Oroszco and Llovet[60] first applied plates to the anterior cervical spine, followed by Caspar[61] and others. During the 1970s and 1980s, implants for posterior cervical fixation using plates with screws inserted into the lateral masses were also undergoing development by several clinical investigators.[62, 63]

The continued dramatic expansion in the use of internal fixation for the gamut of spinal disorders is further testament to its utility. Today's spinal surgeons are continually challenged to adapt their techniques to newer instruments and techniques.

Over the past 100 years, progress in all areas relevant to the management of spinal disorders has been observed. In some areas, the growth has been steady; in others, it has been explosive. Through the chapters in this section of the textbook, we have sought to provide an overview of current neurosurgical spinal practice that reflects the recent and ongoing revolutionary changes in the field.

BASIC SCIENCE

Modern spinal surgery has been largely built on the foundation laid by clinical pioneers but must also draw on knowledge derived from laboratory and clinical investigations, including the biology of repair of the central nervous system, biomechanics, bone metabolism and its disorders, developmental biology of the spine and spinal cord, and clinical applications of electrophysiology. In each of these areas of study, key concepts emerge that directly impact the quality of surgical decision making.

Spinal cord injury is among the most devastating of injuries, robbing the individual of neurological function and offering limited prospect for recovery. Advances in basic neurobiology and neurophysiology have altered the historical view that the spinal cord has no potential for neural plasticity. Surgeons must acquaint themselves with promising strategies in this area to facilitate translational research and assist in the development of clinical applications.

In the introduction to their chapter on biomechanics (see Chapter 278), Maiman and colleagues state: "Although biomechanics is fundamentally a science designed to provide information for clinicians, it is not well understood or utilized by them." Increasingly, however, surgeons must address biomechanical concerns because they manage spinal conditions, and we hope that spinal surgeons are meeting this necessity with increased sophistication regarding biomechanics. This chapter provides an introduction to biomechanical concepts and basic research as it pertains to the spine.

As the surgical techniques for managing spinal disorders have become more powerful, the concept of intraoperatively monitoring the physiologic status of the neural elements during operative manipulation has become more important. Procedures that decompress the spinal cord or cauda equina, reduce fractures or subluxations, or correct deformity have the potential to alter neurological function. The goal of continuously assessing the status of the cord and nerve roots in real time will soon be attainable. Chapter 279 describes intraoperative physiologic monitoring as applied to spinal surgery and describes the reliability and validity of such measurements.

A surgeon who routinely performs spinal fusions or treats fractures must understand normal bone metabolism and its hormonal regulation. An appreciation of the effects of various physical and pharmacologic agents on bone deposition and resorption is imperative, as is an understanding of altered states of bone metabolism such as osteoporosis, Paget's disease, and osteomalacia.

A host of disorders occur as the result of derangements in the normal embryonic development of the spine and spinal cord, as outlined by Dias and colleagues in Chapter 281. Dysraphic states, congenital fusions, and certain deformities are examples that are best understood in the context of the normal developmental process. These problems are not confined to the pediatric age group. Frequently, adults become symptomatic from a congenital condition when it is compounded by superimposed traumatic injury or degenerative change.

APPROACH TO THE PATIENT

Low back pain is a problem that constantly confronts the spinal surgeon with diagnostic and therapeutic dilemmas. To succeed, the surgeon must maintain an organized, methodical, and individualized approach. Most patients referred to a spinal surgeon with complaints of low back pain are best treated by medical management, and it is therefore essential to remain abreast of current medical treatments. Patients who have failed prior operative interventions represent a particularly difficult group for which surgery must be considered only with extreme caution and attention to strict operative indications. In Chapters 282 and 283, Kuntz and colleagues and Sypert and Arpin-Sypert

give useful insights into evaluation and management of spinal patients in general and those with the failed back syndrome in particular. Surgeons must remain aware of a variety of other nondegenerative causes of low back pain, as described in Chapter 284 by Connolly and Hamilton, if they are to minimize the risk of surgical failure.

INFECTIONS

Spontaneous spinal infections are becoming increasingly common in clinical practice as a result of the prevalence of intravenous drug abuse and the greater incidence of patients in the population with immunoincompetence, diabetes, and other predisposing conditions. Improved diagnostic accuracy with magnetic resonance imaging has allowed earlier and often less extensive treatment in many cases. Nonetheless, surgical débridement and reconstruction is often indicated. Multimodality management typically is optimal, combining antimicrobial therapy with decompression of the neural elements, removal of necrotic tissue, and stabilization, followed by physical rehabilitation. Chapter 285 addresses these issues with respect to a number of infectious causes.

DEGENERATIVE DISEASE

Degenerative processes of the spine affect nearly everyone with time, but they achieve pathologic significance only when they produce clinical symptoms or loss of function. Disk degenerations or frank herniation, osteophyte formation, facet arthropathy, ligament hypertrophy or laxity, subluxation, decreased mobility, and deformity comprise the spectrum of changes that occur with aging. Surgery for this group of disorders is chiefly concerned with the decompression of neural elements and the stabilization of degenerative instability.

Several chapters in this section describe issues related to degenerative conditions of the cervical spine. Spondylosis and disk degeneration of the cervical spine usually manifest as radiculopathy, myelopathy, or both simultaneously. Therapeutic decisions must be individualized and take into account the patient's wishes, the natural history of the process, and the specific pathoanatomy. Chapters 286 through 289 review these topics and the various technical aspects of the surgical options.

Ankylosing spondylitis and other spondyloarthropathies pose unique problems for the surgeon, as does ossification of the posterior longitudinal ligament. The special issues related to these disorders are reviewed by Gallagher and Haid in Chapter 290 and Theodosopoulos and Weinstein in Chapter 291.

Despite the increased frequency with which thoracic disk herniations are visualized on MRI, the frequency of symptomatic lesions remains low. Nonetheless, these herniations can be associated with considerable neurologic morbidity. An expanding surgical armamentarium of open and thoracoscopic approaches is available to manage thoracic disk herniation. The chapters by Fine and colleagues and by Theodore and Dickman provide insights into these areas.

Degenerative conditions of the lumbar spine consist primarily of disk herniations, spondylosis and stenosis, spondylolisthesis of multiple origins, and deformity. Chapters 292 through 295 review the historical aspects, symptoms, physical findings, evaluation, and therapeutic options for these common conditions.

The topic of adult thoracolumbar scoliosis is not typically included in neurosurgical texts. With the trend toward subspecialization in spinal surgery, however, both neurosurgical and orthopedic spinal surgeons are increasingly being exposed to complex cases usually managed by the other specialty. As training and experience continue to converge in this area, it is expected that the borders of the parent specialty will continue to blur. Chapter 296 provides an overview of this interesting subject, the study of which offers many lessons for managing all forms of spinal disease.

ADULT CONGENITAL ABNORMALITIES

The craniocervical junction remains a challenging area for surgeons. Congenital abnormalities, tumors, and traumatic injuries each present problems with diagnosis and surgical management. Operative approaches to this area include anterior, lateral, anterolateral, posterolateral, and posterior procedures. Chapters 297 and 311 by Menezes and colleagues nicely illustrate these different options. Advances in instrumentation have expanded the options for occipitocervical stabilization. Multiple variations of screw-rod, hook-rod, and hybrid constructs are available for posterior fixation.

TECHNIQUES AND INSTRUMENTATION

Despite continued evolution in spinal implant systems, basic principles apply to their application. It is axiomatic that an instrumentation construct is only a means to a successful spinal fusion. In Chapter 298, Zubay and colleagues discuss the techniques of instrumenting the spine and the fundamental principles that must be considered for successful surgery. Nuances and technical aspects of autologous bone harvest and its employment in spinal fusion are reviewed by Marcotte and Sonntag in Chapter 299, and the basic biologic issues pertaining to bone grafting are outlined by Sawin in Chapter 300.

Chapters 306 through 307 on anterior and posterior spinal instrumentation review current concepts in the use of spinal implants as applied to these various regions and approaches.

The revolution in imaging technology coupled with advances in frameless stereotaxy resulted in the development of methods for intraoperative navigation in relation to the spine. In Chapter 308, Kalfas provides an overview of this rapidly evolving surgical tool and its use for the placement of pedicle fixation, tumor resection, and other applications.

Thoracoscopic approaches to the spine, first reported by Rosenthal in the 1990s, have become routine in some centers for a broad range of pathologies.[64] These techniques are thoroughly described by Theodore and Dickman in Chapter 309.

Intradiskal and percutaneous treatments for disk herniations and radiculopathy have sparked the imaginations of surgeons and patients for decades. The potential use of intradiskal proteolytic enzymes, called chemonucleolysis, was suggested by Hirsch[65] in 1959 and first performed by Smith[66] in 1963. Physical removal of nuclear material using a percutaneous approach was reported as early as 1975.[67] Continued interest in a less invasive treatment for symptomatic lumbar disk herniation has fueled ongoing investigation. The progress in this field and the current status of many of these modalities are reviewed by Chen and colleagues in Chapter 310.

TUMORS OF THE SPINE

Tumors affecting the spinal cord have been treated by neurosurgeons for decades, but more sophisticated techniques have recently been developed. These techniques, along with a number of postoperative pearls, are nicely described in Chapter 312 by Schwartz and McCormick. The management of benign and malignant vertebral tumors continues to evolve. Primary tumors of bone are much more effectively treated today as surgeons have become more adept at recognizing these lesions and applying an expanding array of approaches and reconstruction techniques. As oncologists continue to extend the life expectancy of patients with malignant disease, the frequency with which spinal metastases are encountered can also be anticipated to increase. MRI has dramatically facilitated the diagnosis of these lesions and greatly enhances surgical planning. Because metastases so commonly involve the vertebral body, greater familiarity with anterior and anterolateral techniques significantly improves the quality of canal decompression routinely achieved. Options for spinal reconstruction have also been expanded by the advances in surgical technique and implant design. Significant surgical obstacles remain to be overcome. Widespread multilevel disease, sacral lesions, and involvement of the cervicothoracic region tax our abilities to provide adequate palliation.

TRAUMA

Traumatic injuries to the vertebral column and spinal cord remain a serious problem for society at large and physicians in particular. It has been estimated that more than 100,000 unstable spinal injuries occur annually in the United States and at enormous costs in terms of medical care, rehabilitation, lost productivity, and human suffering. Although prevention strategies continue to deserve attention, advancement in the diagnosis and management of these injuries is a high priority for surgeons treating patients. Research into mechanisms of spinal cord injury and potential clinical strategies to maintain or even restore neurological function is also critical.

The highly mobile cervical spine is the region most vulnerable to traumatic injury and represents the most common site for spinal cord injury. In Chapter 315, Jenkins and colleagues provide an overview of the diagnosis and management of injuries to this region. The hyperflexion and hyperextension injuries discussed in Chapter 316 are among the most common spinal injuries seen in outpatient neurosurgical practice. The review by Zeidman offers insight into evaluation and management of these frustrating problems.

Occipitocervical injuries are more frequently encountered by neurosurgeons as a result of improvements in prehospital care and enhancements in diagnostic imaging. Occipital condylar and atlas fractures, which frequently can be missed on plain radiographs, are routinely seen on CT. Patients with occipitocervical dislocations, which once were considered to be almost uniformly fatal, are now arriving in emergency rooms in need of skilled management. In Chapter 317, Taggard and Traynelis discuss the management of these lesions.

The unique anatomic arrangement of the atlantoaxial complex produces distinct patterns of injury that require equally unique management. York and colleagues review the various treatment options in Chapter 318.

Injuries of the thoracic spine are usually the result of extreme physical force. As a result, the incidence of neurological involvement is high. Surgical approaches include standard posterior approaches, posterolateral trajectories, and anterior transthoracic approaches. The techniques and indications for each are presented in Chapter 319.

Fractures of the thoracolumbar junction are second in frequency only to those of the cervical spine because the junction represents a transitional zone between the rigid thoracic spine and the relatively mobile lumbar region. Compression fractures are common, especially with minor trauma and coexistent osteopenia. Burst fractures are the most frequent pattern necessitating treatment. A variety of approaches are available to treat fractures of the thoracolumbar and lumbar region, including standard posterior operations, the lateral extracavitary approach popularized by Larson and co-workers,[27] and anterolateral retroperitoneal approaches that facilitate anterior canal clearance and reconstruction of the anterior column.

Traumatic injuries of the sacrum are usually managed nonsurgically with success. In Chapter 321, Perin and colleagues describe the indications for surgical and nonsurgical treatments.

CHALLENGES

Spinal surgery at the dawn of the 21st century bears little resemblance to that practiced 100 years ago. The changes of the past 25 years have been especially profound. As in many areas of medicine, the pace of change continues to accelerate. It is difficult to envision the innovations that will evolve over the next quarter century, well within the practice life span of many of our readers.

Challenges for the future include a greater understanding of the degenerative process as it affects the spine. Biologic, nonsurgical solutions to degeneration of the disk, ligaments, and articular cartilage may allow reversal of some changes. Less invasive means to access the spine and deal with the affected segments will surely continue to progress. Spinal fusion, which clearly reflects a trade-off of greater stability for loss of joint function, will be perfected, perhaps through the use of agents such as the bone morphogenic proteins or through other osteoinductive agents or drugs.

Internal fixation will continue to change. Improvements in spinal fusion may render certain constructs unnecessary. Resorbable spinal implants may become feasible. Understanding the mechanisms of back pain and the role of surgical interventions will also progress.

Although prevention strategies will remain a priority for traumatic injuries of the spine and spinal cord, advances in basic and applied neuroscience research will build on the encouraging findings described in Chapter 277.

The editors and authors hope that the chapters in this section provide an overview of the current state of spinal surgery and a better understanding of diagnosis and management across the broad spectrum of spinal diseases.

REFERENCES

1. Hippocrates: The Genuine Works of Hippocrates. Adams F (trans). Baltimore, Williams & Wilkins, 1939, p 231.
2. Tyrell F: Compression of the spinal marrow from displacement of the vertebrae, consequent upon injury: Operation of removing the arch and spinous processes of the twelfth dorsal vertebra. Lancet 1:685–688, 1827.
3. Rogers DL: A case of fractured spine with depression of the spinous process and the operation for its removal. Am J Med Sci 16:91–94, 1835.
4. Church A, Eisendrath DW: A contribution to spinal cord surgery. Am J Med Sci 103:395–412, 1982.
5. Smith AG: Account of a case in which portions of three dorsal vertebrae were removed for the relief of paralysis from fracture, with partial success. North Am Med Surg J xx:94–97, 1829.
6. Macewen W: An address on the surgery of the brain and spinal cord. Br Med J 2:302–309, 1888.
7. Gowers WR, Horsley VA: A case of tumour of the spinal cord: Removal, recovery. Med Chir Trans 53(Suppl 2):379–428, 1888.
8. Roentgen WC: Uber eine neue Art von strahlen: Vorlaufige Mitteilung. Sitz Ber Phys Med Ges (Wurzburg) 137:132–141, 1895.
9. Keen WW: Application of the Roentgen rays in surgical diagnosis. Am J Med Sci 111:256–261, 1986.
10. Charcot JM: Lecons sur le localisations dans les maladies du cerveau et de la moelle epiniere. Paris, VA Delahaye, 1876.
11. Gowers WR: A Manual of the Diseases of the Nervous System. Philadelphia, Blakiston, 1888.
12. Dandy WE: Ventriculography following the injection of air into the cerebral ventricles. Ann Surg 68:5–11, 1918.
13. Sicard JA, Forestier J: Methode radiographique d'exploration de la cavité epidurale par le lipoidol. Rev Neurol 37:1264, 1921.
14. Lindblom K: Diagnostic puncture of intervertebral discs in sciatica. Acta Orthop Scand 17:231–239, 1948.

15. Miller MH, Handel SF, Coan JD: Transfemoral lumbar epidural venography. AJR Am J Roentgenol 126:1003–1009, 1976.

16. Hounsfield GN: Computerized transverse axial scanning (tomography). Part 1. Description of system. Br J Radiol 46:1016–1022, 1973.

17. Ambrose J: Computerized transverse axial scanning (tomography). II. Clinical application. Br J Radiol 46:1023–1046, 1973.

18. Oldendorf WH: Isolated flying spot detection of radiodensity discontinuities: Displaying the internal structural pattern of a complex object. Trans Biomed Elect 8:68–72, 1961.

19. Cormack AM: Representation of a function by its line integrals, with some radiological applications. J Appl Phys 34:2722–2727, 1963.

20. Cormack AM: Representation of a function by its line integrals, with some radiological applications. II. J Appl Phys 35:2908–2913, 1964.

21. Ahn HS, Rosenbaum AE: Lumbar myelography with metrizamide: supplementary technique. AJR Am J Roentgenol 136:547–551, 1981.

22. Rabassa AE, Guinto FC Jr, Crow WN, et al: CT of the spine: Value of reformatted images. AJR Am J Roentgenol 161:1223–1227, 1993.

23. Cacayorin ED, Kieffer SA: Applications and limitations of computed tomography of the spine. Radiol Clin North Am 20:185–206, 1982.

24. Damadian R: Tumor detection by nuclear magnetic resonance. Science 171:1151–1153, 1971.

25. Menard V: Causes de la paraplegie dans le mal de Pott. Son traitement chirurgical par ouverture direct du foyer tuberculeux des vertebras. Rev Orthop 5:47–64, 1984.

26. Capener N: The evolution of lateral rhachotomy. J Bone Joint Surg Br 36:173–179, 1954.

27. Larson SJ, Holst RA, Hemmy DC, Sances A Jr: Lateral extracavitary approach to traumatic lesions of the thoracic and lumbar spine. J Neurosurg 45:628–637, 1976.

28. McCormick PC: Retropleural approach to the thoracic and thoracolumbar spine. Neurosurgery 37:908–914, 1995.

29. Hodgson AR, Stock FE: Anterior spinal fusion: A preliminary communication on the radical treatment of Pott's disease and Pott's paraplegia. Br J Surg 44:266–275, 1956.

30. Cloward RB: The anterior approach for removal of ruptured cervical disks. J Neurosurg 15:602–617, 1958.

31. Robinson RA, Smith GW: Anterolateral cervical disc removal and interbody fusion for cervical disc syndrome. Bull Johns Hopkins Hosp 96:223–224, 1955.

32. Fang HSY, Ong GB: Direct anterior approach to the upper cervical spine. J Bone Joint Surg Am 44:1588–1594, 1962.

33. Hibbs RA: An operation for progressive spinal deformities. N Y Med J 93:1013–1016, 1911.

34. Albee FH: Transplantation of a portion of the tibia into the spine for Pott's disease: A preliminary report. JAMA 57:885–886, 1911.

35. Campbell WC: An operation for extra-articular fusion of sacroiliac joint. Surg Gynecol Obstet 45: 218–219, 1927.

36. Mackenzie-Forbes A: Techinque of an operation for spinal fusion as practiced in Montreal. J Orthop Surg 2:509–514, 1920.

37. Jenkins JA: Spondylolisthesis. Br J Surg 24:80–85, 1936.

38. Mercer W: Spondylolisthesis: With description of new method of operative treatment and notes of 10 cases. Edinb Med J 43:545–572.

39. Ghormley RK: Low back pain with special reference to the articular facets with presentation of an operative procedure. JAMA 101:1773–1777, 1933.

40. Burns BH: An operation for spondylolisthesis. Lancet 1:1233–, 1933.

41. Cloward RB: The treatment of ruptured lumbar intervertebral discs by vertebral body fusion. I. Indications, operative technique, after care. J Neurosurg 10:154, 1953.

42. Wilkins WF: Separation of the vertebra with protrusion of hernia between the same; operation and cure. St Louis Med Surg J 54:340–341, 1988.

43. Hadra BE: Wiring of the spinous processes in injury and Pott's disease. Trans Am Orthop Assoc 4:206–210, 1891.

44. Lange F: Support for the spondylitic spine by means of burred steel bars attached to the vertebrae. Am J Orthop 8:344–361, 1910.

45. Harrington PR: Treatment of scoliosis: Correction and internal fixation by instrumentation. J Bone Joint Surg Am 44:591–610, 1962.

46. Harrington PR: Technical details in relation to the successful use of instrumentation in scoliosis. Orthop Clin North Am 3:499–567, 1972.

47. Harrington PR: The history and development of Harrington instrumentation. Clin Orthop 93:110–112, 1973.

48. Luque ER: The anatomical basis and development of segmental spine instrumentation. Spine 7:256–259, 1982.

49. Cotrel Y, Dubousset J: Nouvelle technique d'osteosynthese rachidienne segmentaire par voie posterieur. Rev Chir Orthop Rep Appar Mot 70:489–494, 1984.

50. Richards BS, Herring JA, Johnston CE, et al. Treatment of adolescent idiopathic scoliosis using Texas Scottish Rite Hospital (TSRH) instrumentation. Spine 19:1598–1605, 1994.

51. Richardson AB, Taylor ML, Murphree B: TSRH instrumentation: Evolution of a new system. Part 1. Texas Scottish Rite Hospital. Orthop Nurs 9:15–21, 1990.

52. King D: Internal fixation for lumbosacral fusion. J Bone Joint Surg Am 30:560–565, 1948.

53. Boucher HH: A method of spinal fusion. J Bone Joint Surg Br 41:248–258, 1959.

54. Roy-Camille R, Roy-Camille M, Demeulenaere C: Osteosyntheses of dorsal, lumbar and lumbosacral spine with metallic plates screwed into vertebral pedicles and articular apophyses. Presse Med 78:1447–1448, 1970.

55. Louis R: Fusion of the lumbar and sacral spine by internal fixation with screw plates. Clin Orthop 203:18–33, 1986.

56. Steffee A: Segmental spine plates with pedicle screw fixation. Clin Orthop 203:45–51, 1986.

57. Dwyer AF, Newton NC, Sherwood AA: An anterior approach to scoliosis: A preliminary report. Clin Orthop 62:192–202, 1969.

58. Zielke K, Pellin B: Neue Instrumente und Implantate zur Erganzung des Harrington Systems. Z Orthop Chir 114:218–224, 1976.

59. Kaneda K, Abumi K, Fujiya K: Burst fractures with neurologic deficits of the thoraco-lumbar spine: Results of anterior decompression and stabilization with anterior instrumentation. Spine 9:788–795, 1984.

60. Orozco R, Llovet J: Osteointerior en las fracturas del raquir cervical. Rev Ortop Traumatol 14:285–288, 1970.

61. Caspar W: Anterior cervical fusions and interbody stabilizations with the trapezoidal osteosynthetic plate. Technique, 7th ed. Tittlingen, Aesculap Werke, 1986.

62. Magerl F, Seeman PS: Stable Posterior Fusion of the Atlas and Axis by Transarticular Screw Fixation. In Kehr P, Weidner A (eds): Cervical Spine. Berlin, Springer-Verlag, 1986, pp 322–327.

63. Roy-Camille R: Early fixation of the unstable cervical spine by posterior osteosynthesis with plates and screws. In The Cervical Spine Research Society (eds): The Cervical Spine. Philadelphia, JB Lippincott, 1985, pp 390–403.

64. Rosenthal D, Rosenthal R, de Simeone A: Removal of a protruded thoracic disc using microsurgical endoscopy: A new technique. Spine 19:1087–1091, 1994.

65. Hirsch C: Studies on the pathology of low back pain. J Bone Joint Surg Br 41:237–243, 1959.

66. Smith L: Chemonucleolysis. Clin Orthop 67:72–80, 1969.

67. Hijikata S: Percutaneous nucleotomy, a new concept: Technique and 12 years' experience. Clin Orthop 238:9–23, 1989.

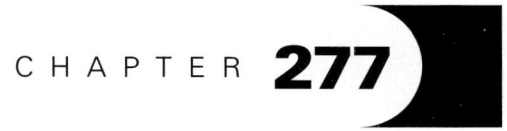

CHAPTER 277

Biologic Strategies for Central Nervous System Repair

JAMES D. GUEST

The investigator should have a robust faith—and yet not believe.

—CLAUDE BERNARD, FRENCH PHYSIOLOGIST (1813–1878)

There are no such things as applied sciences, only applications of science.

—LOUIS PASTEUR

Brain and spinal cord injuries cause enormous suffering, and advances in therapy are urgently needed. The quest to repair the injured brain and spinal cord is one of the most compelling of our generation. In the past decade, several discoveries have increased our confidence that it will eventually be possible to partially repair injuries of the central nervous system (CNS).

This chapter summarizes some of the evolving strategies for CNS repair after traumatic or ischemic injury. These strategies define a new field known as restorative neurobiology or cellular and molecular neurosurgery.[1] This field holds immense promise that neurosurgery will eventually become a specialty that emphasizes reconstruction of the CNS. This chapter focuses on the use of cells and molecules as tools to elicit repair; it does not focus on acute strategies to reduce secondary injury. However, there are points at which the protection of CNS tissue from secondary injury and the implementation of repair strategies are contingent and cannot be meaningfully distinguished. No strategy is conceivably more beneficial than preserving CNS tissue from the effects of progressive injury. Further, the injury process and its sequelae may persist into a period considered optimal for repair efforts, potentially hindering those efforts.[2] Dealing with secondary injury is further complicated by the evolving recognition that aspects of the inflammatory response to injury may support repair. Despite the importance of acutely implemented strategies to preserve functional CNS tissue, in some situations, the primary injury is of such magnitude that "reconstruction" is still necessary to restore function.

Although this chapter focuses on acute destructive injuries, the evolution of neural transplantation for neurodegenerative disease—the first fruit of the restorative neurobiology approach and an ongoing source of important principles and models—is reviewed briefly. I draw attention to some of the major unsolved problems that currently limit progress toward clinical applications. This review is weighted toward spinal repair paradigms.

CNS repair might be achieved by several mechanisms: improved *survival* of injured neurons and their connections; enhanced *plasticity* of remaining neurons; *regeneration* of injured axons, with formation of effective synapses; *replacement* of lost neurons; and *restoration* of glial function (e.g., repair of segmental *demyelination*). The basic techniques to effect these mechanisms are pharmacotherapy; cell and tissue transplantation; delivery of biologic molecules to maximize endogenous repair; and physical methods such as hypothermia, radiation,[3, 4] electric fields,[5, 6] and conditioning lesions.[7]

Optimism about the potential of restorative neurobiology is based on the discovery and clarification of previously unknown or misunderstood biologic principles, new technologies, and advances in key scientific fields such as molecular and developmental neurobiology. Advances in neuroimaging have greatly improved our ability to define injuries within the neuraxis. Several key principles are emerging: (1) the adult mammalian CNS contains a population of undifferentiated, self-renewing cells that can migrate, adopt glial or neuronal phenotypes, and form new connections; (2) components of adult CNS myelin that inhibit the elaboration of new axonal processes can be blocked by the delivery of specific molecules; (3) the "glial scar" that forms after CNS injuries contains specific extracellular matrix (ECM) molecules that can be modified or blocked to render the scar more permissive for regenerating axons; (4) the apoptotic death of some injured CNS cells might be interrupted pharmacologically; and (5) olfactory ensheathing glia are unique glial cells within the CNS that have characteristics of both astrocytes and Schwann cells, and they appear to circumvent the inherent limitations of either of those cells to support regeneration.

Progress in key fields has included the biology of neurotrophic molecules, neuroimmunology and cytokine biology, clinical CNS transplantation for neurodegenerative disease, and developmental neurobiology. Important evolving technologies include ex vivo and in vivo gene therapy, novel gene regulatory strategies, neural lineage analysis, differential display, and other powerful gene expression studies, such as gene arrays, that can enhance our understanding of cellular responses to injury and interventions.

Optimism is clearly justified, but significant problems remain, and their resolution is essential if we are to advance toward clinical application. It is unclear when the reparative strategies discussed here will reach the threshold of clinical application, but limited human trials have been initiated,[8] and others are anticipated in the coming decade.

SEQUELAE TO INJURY

When the CNS is subjected to a traumatic insult, the primary (instantaneous) injury causes immediate disruption of axons and their connections, massive shifts in membrane potential and ionic concentrations, disruption of blood vessels and the blood-brain barrier, and some instantaneous cellular death. These events cause sequelae, including ischemia, edema, additional ionic fluxes, apoptotic and necrotic cellular death, and inflammation.[9] Local microglial cells are activated, inflammatory cells are recruited, regions of necrosis are eventually cleared by macrophages, boundary zones demarcated by reactive astrocytes evolve, and wallerian degeneration ensues.

Local disruption of CNS connections is followed by multiple changes throughout the neuraxis that can seriously affect repair strategies. These changes include transneuronal degeneration, retrograde neuronal degeneration, segmental sprouting, plasticity, and alterations in neuronal excitability. Associated clinical sequelae include spasticity, autonomic dysreflexia, and neuropathic pain. These changes involve the formation of new local connections that may present obstacles to strategies designed to replace the original connections. These neuronal changes may be influenced by other pathologic sequelae, such as syringomyelia, myelomalacia, and spinal cord tethering.

The distinction between regeneration and plasticity is important for restorative neurobiologists. *Plasticity* refers to changes that occur within existing CNS connections. Reactive synaptogenesis is a form of plasticity that may underlie some chronic clinical problems. After descending inputs are lost, vacated synapses on local neurons may be occupied by new terminals that sprout from local neurons.[10, 11] One result of this plastic change is hyperactivity of local reflexes, which may also be due to a relative increase in excitatory neurotransmitters such as glutamate.[12] Postinjury reorganization can lead to other unusual phenomena caused by unmasking or strengthening synapses that are usually silent.[13] Axonal sprouting from the dorsal horn after peripheral nerve injury plays a role in the development of neuropathic pain.[14] Collateral sprouting from uninjured descending fibers, another form of plasticity, may underlie the recovery of ipsilateral leg function observed after spinal cord hemisection in primates.[15] Collateral sprouting from uninjured fibers in adult rats increases markedly when antibodies that block inhibitory sites on adult myelin are delivered.[16] In fact, such inhibitory molecules may protect the adult CNS from excessive plasticity.

Regeneration refers to the restoration of functional connections through regrowth of injured neuronal processes and de novo synaptogenesis. I do not adhere to the strictest definition, which requires restoration of the original connection. I believe that the CNS has sufficient plasticity and redundancy that novel connections can affect function.

Replacement refers to the restoration of a functional connection through integration of a transplanted or endogenous neuronal cell, de novo process formation, synaptogenesis, and neurotransmitter function. Myelinating cells can also be replaced.

Acute Sequelae to Injury: Gene Expression

A key concept in restorative neurobiology is that during the course of mammalian evolution, regeneration has been maintained for the peripheral nervous system (PNS) but lost for the CNS. Most tissue responses to injury can be understood as changing patterns of cellular and molecular interaction mediated through altered gene expression. It seems intuitive that repair strategies could be improved if the differences in gene expression when regeneration does or does not occur were understood. The advent of powerful molecular techniques such as differential display,[17] gene arrays,[18] and laser capture microdissection[19] may allow comparisons of the responses of key cells within regenerating and nonregenerating microenvironments.

Meaningful comparisons of postinjury gene expression have included PNS versus CNS, immature versus mature animals, regenerating nonvertebrates versus mammals, and neuronal populations that respond to a peripheral nerve graft versus those that do not.[20, 21] It is also valuable to study gene expression during the development of the nervous system[22]; interestingly, not all the molecular events observed during development are recapitulated in regeneration.[23] Most studies have used in situ hybridization of regeneration-associated genes necessary for axonal elongation after axotomy, such as the cytoskeletal elements actin, tubulin, and growth-associated protein-43. Such molecular observations can be correlated with neuroanatomic, electrophysiologic, or behavioral observations and might serve as assays of treatment.[24, 25] For example, a spinal cord lesion leads to sustained expression of c-jun in rubrospinal but not in corticospinal neurons,[26] and facial nerve lesions lead to an even more sustained expression of regeneration-associated genes than do rubrospinal lesions.[27] Likewise, axotomy of the poorly regenerating central dorsal root ganglion (DRG) process is followed by a less sustained expression of regeneration-associated genes than is axotomy of the regenerative peripheral process.[28] In general, regeneration-associated genes' observed expression in specific types of neurons has paralleled their observed regenerative capacity.

We need to know which systems are most responsive to specific regeneration-promoting interventions. Some experimenters have observed that axotomized rubrospinal axons grow into spinally transplanted peripheral nerve grafts, whereas axotomized corticospinal fibers do not. The response to peripheral nerve grafts is apparently influenced by several variables. Richardson and colleagues[29] showed that the response of injured rubrospinal fibers to peripheral nerve grafts depends on the distance from the graft insertion site to the neuronal cell body. More recent studies substantiate this "distance" concept.[24] Subsequent studies tested the hypothesis that injured neurons could be induced to respond to more distally located peripheral nerve grafts when provided with exogenous brain-derived neurotrophic factor (BDNF).[25] Similar studies are in progress for other systems.

Central Nervous System Inflammation and Neuroimmunology

The complex, rapidly evolving field of neuroimmunology focuses on immune cellular and cytokine responses within the CNS. The concept of the brain as an immunologically privileged site evolved from the observation that allograft transplants are not rejected.[30] The observation that constitutive expression of histocompatibility antigens is usually very limited[31] was generalized to characterize the brain as "immunologically inert." Other unique features that support this concept are the brain's lack of a lymphatic system to capture and concentrate antigens and its protection from most blood-borne constituents by the blood-brain barrier. The concept of inflammation after brain injury or spinal cord injury (SCI) has been greatly oversimplified and emphasizes the removal of cellular debris and unfavorable effects such as free radical liberation and lipid peroxidation.

Differences in the success of PNS and CNS regeneration have focused interest on the different responses to injury between the two compartments. Because of the significant dissimilarities in CNS and PNS inflammatory responses, the hypothesis that PNS inflammation may support repair has recently emerged.[32]

Several experiments have now compared PNS and CNS inflammatory responses. For example, Streit and coworkers[33] compared the cytokine profile of the lesioned facial nerve to that of the contused spinal cord. Sustained production of interleukin-6 (IL-6) in the facial nerve nucleus but not in the spinal cord correlated with regeneration. Neuroglial responses to injury were impaired in IL-6–deficient mice[34]; therefore, this inflammatory cytokine may play a role in regeneration.

Cytokines are receptor-binding protein molecules that regulate cellular functions. Inflammatory cytokines such as transforming growth factor-β are normally produced at minimal levels within the CNS, but their production is up-regulated after injury[35] or stimulation with other cytokines such as IL-1.[36] Cytokine release into injury sites influences cellular migration,[37] regulates the production of ECM molecules[38] such as tenascin,[39, 40] and can influence regeneration.[41] IL-1β may regulate reformation of the glia limitans after injury,[42] and ECM production is increased in mice that overproduce transforming growth factor-β after injury.[43]

Macrophages may be an important source of cytokines[44] and trophic factors. Macrophages recruited to the injured PNS release IL-1, which increases the production of nerve growth factor (NGF) and appears to be necessary for effective regeneration.[45] The CNS environment may have an inherently suppressive effect on inflammation. Zeev-Brann and associates[46] found that exposure of peripheral macrophages or brain-derived microglia to optic or peripheral nerves had opposing effects on phagocytic activity, suppressing or augmenting it, respectively. Lazarov-Spiegler and colleagues[47] found that macrophages exposed to injured peripheral nerves and subsequently transplanted to the optic nerve were distributed widely and enhanced the removal of myelin debris.

Macrophages and activated microglia around penetrating brain injury sites produce BDNF and glia-derived neurotrophic factor (GDNF), which can induce neuronal sprouting.[48] Macrophage cytokine production may also influence the behavior of astrocytes at injury sites. Astrocytes have a wide repertoire of responses and can produce trophic factors[48, 49] that influence axon growth.[50] Astrocytes have cytokine receptors, and interferon-γ, tumor necrosis factor-α, and IL-1 enhance both astrogliosis and astrocytic production of NGF. Evidence exists that the response of different CNS regions to proinflammatory cytokines varies. Breakdown of the spinal cord–blood-brain barrier and monocyte recruitment were significantly greater after injection of IL-1β or tumor necrosis factor-α into the spinal cord compared with injection into brain parenchyma.[51]

Cell Death by Apoptosis

After traumatic CNS injury, some neuronal and glial cells die by apoptosis.[52] Apoptosis may persist into the postinjury periods that are believed to be favorable for cellular and molecular repair strategies. Proximal axotomy of the optic nerve leads to apoptotic death of retinal ganglion neurons. Whether other neurons with cell bodies remote to sites of axotomy die by apoptosis has not been determined, but this is an important consideration for regeneration strategies. The caspase-3 family of cysteine proteases is associated with neuronal apoptosis[53]; their activation follows traumatic brain injury,[54, 55] axotomy,[56] and SCI.[57] Inhibition of caspase can spare injured neurons.[56] Other mechanisms associated with the induction of apoptosis, including activation of N-methyl-D-aspartate receptors and calpain-mediated cytoskeletal disruption, may also be amenable to pharmacologic inhibition.[58, 59]

Neurotrophin infusion can reduce apoptotic neuronal death in some paradigms.[60] A key unresolved issue in preventing apoptosis is determining the effective time window for therapy.

Chronic Responses to Injury

Our ability to design effective CNS repair strategies depends on a clear understanding of the distributed effects of an injury within the neuraxis. Changes such as transneuronal degeneration, retrograde degeneration, cell death, and atrophy may make CNS repair more difficult.

Transneuronal Degeneration. Transneuronal degeneration refers to the death of neurons subsequent to the loss of sustaining connections. In humans, transneuronal degeneration has been identified in the olivary and corticopontine nuclei after brain insults.[61, 62] Loss of gray matter interneurons has been described after the amputation of upper extremities.[63] However, loss of anterior horn cells does not appear to follow loss of cortical neurons after stroke[64] or thoracic spinal cord transection,[65] and quantitative losses of spinal cord tissue are modest above and below human lesion epicenters.[66] Preganglionic sympathetic neurons shrink after the loss of descending input but may survive owing to new local connections.[67] After a midcervical SCI, the number of thenar motor units appears to be normal in some patients.[68] Thus, spinal cord neuronal losses subsequent to transneuronal degeneration appear to be modest.

Retrograde Changes in Injured Neurons. Axons and dendrites can occupy many times the volume of their cell bodies, providing a vast membrane surface over which signals can be generated. The normal movement of molecules and vesicles between the neuronal soma and extensive processes depends on anterograde and retrograde transport. When the cell body's connection with its terminals is interrupted by axotomy, retrograde changes are rapid and distinct. These changes include cell body responses ranging from chromatolysis to atrophy and cell death, local gliosis, and microglial activation.[69] Experimental spinal cord lesions lead to significant retrograde changes in brainstem neurons that are important for supraspinally regulated movement, including the red[70, 71] and vestibular nuclei.[72] Retrograde changes have also been described in intrinsic neurons of the human spinal cord.[73]

Retrograde axonal degeneration after injury leads to retraction of terminals away from the injury site for significant distances. This process has been observed in corticospinal axons in both animal models[74] and human autopsy specimens.[75, 76] Neurotrophin delivery may partially prevent retrograde axonal degeneration.[77, 78] However, chronically injured neurons may lose their ability to transport proteins retrogradely.[79]

Wallerian Degeneration. Wallerian degeneration is a precondition for PNS regeneration[80, 81]; therefore, some investigators have studied whether CNS tissue that has undergone wallerian degeneration is more permissive of axon growth.[82, 83] Myelin-stimulated macrophages release trophic factors during PNS wallerian degeneration,[84] but macrophage activities that are important for PNS regeneration appear to be lacking in the CNS.[85] Wallerian degeneration in the spinal cord results in large gliotic areas devoid of axons and myelin and depleted of oligodendrocytes. Wallerian degeneration plays a role in supporting the plastic reorganization after incomplete SCI[86, 87] but does not appear to enhance CNS regeneration.

REASONS FOR OPTIMISM ABOUT THE POTENTIAL FOR CENTRAL NERVOUS SYSTEM REPAIR

Nonmammalian Species

Regeneration of the injured adult spinal cord occurs in species such as fishes and amphibians,[88, 89] but not in mammals. Differences in the structure of CNS tracts and the response to injury between these regenerative species and mammals may be instructive if a few clear differences account for the success or failure of regeneration.[90]

Immature Mammals

Some regeneration of CNS tracts can be observed after injuries in immature mammals. In general, the extent of repair correlates inversely with age. The neonatal opossum is an example of a mammal capable of functional spinal cord repair.[91]

Lessons from Development

Appropriately guided extension of nerve growth cones through the three-dimensional matrix of the CNS is necessary during both development and regeneration. Insight into the molecular interactions during development should contribute to our understanding of how to enhance regeneration. Key mechanisms include cell-cell contacts, cell-ECM contacts, and gradients of attractant or repulsive molecules. The observation that embryonic neurons are capable of extensive growth on adult white matter,[92] which is inhibitory to adult axons, indicates that the molecular state of the axonal growth cone is critical to allowing axonal elongation.

Cell adhesion molecules (CAM) (e.g., N-CAM, N-cadherin [N-CAD], and the glycoprotein L1) are present on both the axonal growth cone and their substrates and regulate secondary messenger cascades within the growth cone. For example, substrate-bound L1 acts together with basic fibroblast growth factor (FGF) to stimulate growth cone FGF receptors to open calcium channels.[93] Signal transduction by second messenger systems, including phospholipase C and diacylglycerol,[94] results in directional changes by modifying the growth cone cytoskeleton. Second messenger activation and cytoskeletal response appear to be linked through growth-associated protein-43.[95, 96]

During regrowth in vitro, rodent retinal ganglion axons differ from primarily growing axons during development because polysialylated N-CAM, but not N-CAD and L1, is expressed.[97] The lack of N-CAD expression on these regenerated axons could interfere with remyelination. During PNS regeneration, Schwann cells express N-CAD, N-CAM, and L1 on their surfaces.[98]

An example of cell-ECM contact is the interaction between laminin, an ECM molecule, and growth cone integrins.[99] The interaction leads to protein kinase C activation, which increases the speed at which the growth cone advances.[100] Maturational changes in the CNS of the developing chick that are correlated with the transition from regeneration permissive to nonpermissive include a transition from the predominance of heparan sulfate proteoglycan to chondroitin sulfate proteoglycan in the ECM[101] and the onset of myelination.[102] Secreted molecules within the extracellular space, such as netrins and semaphorins,[103, 104] can exert both attractant and inhibitory effects in different contexts.

Residual Function with Extensive but Incomplete Injuries

Windle and colleagues[105] incompletely transected the thoracic spinal cord of rats in progressive increments. Ten percent of intact ventral spinal cord axons was sufficient for significant locomotor function to be retained. These findings were validated in similar experiments by Eidelberg and coworkers[106] and Blight,[107] who demonstrated a threshold number of residual intact myelinated fibers below which obvious supraspinally mediated function was absent. Residual vestibulospinal and reticulospinal fibers were needed for locomotion.[108] Subsequent experiments by Fehlings and Tator[109] correlated preserved rubrospinal, vestibulospinal, and reticulospinal inputs with retained lower extremity function after compressive SCI. Nathan[110] correlated residual leg function after destructive surgical procedures for pain in cancer patients with subsequent autopsy specimens. Surprisingly good leg function persisted after complete bilateral interruption of the anterior spinal cord. This observation emphasizes the redundant organization of locomotor systems in the spinal cord.

These studies indicate that even small numbers of intact axons can support significant motor function. This observation has been extended to the hypothesis that a small number of regenerated axons might support meaningful function.

Organization of Mammalian Lower Extremity Function

Modern neurophysiologic studies indicate that brainstem systems interact with locally organized spinal cord central pattern generators to exert substantial control over lower extremity gait function in many species.[111, 112] Identification of a mesencephalic locomotor region in the mammalian brainstem has focused increased attention on ventral brainstem motor systems, particularly the reticulospinal tract, as important for walking.[113, 114] Central pattern generators coordinate patterned movement through reciprocal inhibitory and excitatory local interactions and are capable of autonomous function. Their activity can be provoked in spinalized animals by reflexive stimulation such as treadmill walking.[111] This activity is more difficult to elicit in primates,[115] but there is some evidence that central pattern generators exist in humans.[116, 117] Because spinal cord centers can pattern movement, the idea that regeneration of a few ventral brainstem axons might be sufficient to activate the central pattern generators has many proponents.[118]

MODELS OF CENTRAL NERVOUS SYSTEM INJURY AND REPAIR

The CNS consists of complex cellular and molecular patterns existing in concert with the metabolic, hormonal, and immune systems of the body. This complexity creates both distinct advantages and limitations for in vitro experimentation. Ultimately, in vitro experimental findings require in vivo validation. Experimentation tells us what is possible, often in unique and novel situations, but these concepts are not necessarily valid when applied to human clinical problems. Great care must be exercised in extrapolating experimental results to clinical situations. Further, the inherent variability in biologic systems makes it essential that important experimental findings be replicated by other investigators. Some scientists argue that direct application of experimental findings from rodents to humans may be inappropriate, and that promising experiments should be reproduced in higher nonhuman species. This argument is supported by descriptions of unique anatomic,[119] cellular, and molecular features in humans and primates.[120]

Several advances have improved the ability to compare experimental data among different investigators. First, the rodent has become the most popular experimental animal in spinal cord and brain injury. This uniform choice has assisted in the development of well-standardized injury and assessment methodologies that allow interinvestigator replication of data. The development of the New York University spinal cord impactor[121] created a high degree of reproducibility in modeling spinal injuries,[122, 123] and contusion is a more relevant injury model than sharp transection.[124] Using similar methodologies, however, carries a risk of limiting the opportunity for unique observations, and a balance between novel and widely used models should be encouraged. The clip compression SCI model has also demonstrated good reproducibility and correlation among grades of compression, axonal sparing, and behavioral recovery.[109]

METHODS OF EVALUATION

The efficacy of repair strategies can be assessed by anatomic, electrophysiologic, and behavioral methods. A number of studies have shown evidence of behavioral recovery in adult rodents after SCI.[125, 126] As of yet, none of these spinal cord repair strategies has been replicated successfully in primates.

The transected or contused rodent thoracic spinal cord is the most common model in SCI research. After severe thoracic SCI or complete spinal cord transection, adult rats do not recover weight-bearing ambulation, but they do recover after modest grades of contusion. The open-field assessment developed at Ohio State University[127] integrates several aspects of locomotion and is widely used. Although originally designed to evaluate outcome during recovery from incomplete injury, its use has been extended to transection paradigms.[128, 129] Twenty-one specific grades are assigned to recovery after injury. Scores are linearly correlated with the quantity of preserved spinal tissue.[130] The large number of grades apparently provides a greater degree of sensitivity than did the original Tarlov score,[131, 132] increasing the potential to demonstrate small but significant benefits. Other scoring systems, such as the inclined plane, have also demonstrated a linear correlation with axonal preservation.[109, 133] The optimal behavioral evaluation methods for assessing regeneration are likely to be established only when consistent regeneration can be achieved.

A key issue in behavioral testing after experimental therapy for thoracic SCI is the distinction between recovery related to intrinsic reorganization in the isolated spinal segment and that related to long-tract function with supraspinal input. These two possibilities can be distinguished by retransecting the spinal cord.[126] Some grafts can enhance locomotor activity generated from the isolated lumbar cord in the absence of regenerated descending input.[134, 135]

Anatomic assessment methods are essential to evaluate the behavior of injured axons after experimental injury and intervention, especially if little obvious behavioral change occurs. Reliable retrograde and anterograde neuronal tracing methods are essential techniques in regeneration studies and must be carefully standardized in each laboratory setting. The introduction of the biotinylated dextran amine family of tracing molecules has greatly enhanced the visualization of exquisite detail of small sprouts and growth cones.[136, 137]

STRATEGIES FOR REPAIR: TISSUE AND CELLULAR TRANSPLANTATION

Most biologic repair strategies involve manipulation of the injury environment. The strategy must address the spatial distribution of the injury, which may be diffuse in the brain but is often focal in the spinal cord, although there are consequent changes in multiple levels of the neuraxis. Whereas strategies to reduce secondary injury often involve systemic delivery, tissue repair strategies are directed focally and involve chiefly transplantation, local delivery of molecules, or both.

Embryonic Tissue Transplantation for Focal Neurodegenerative Lesions in the Brain

Embryonic tissues consist of cellular elements that have not attained maturity and have the capacity to survive and interact with adult neural and glial cells after transplantation. These tissues have been used in many restorative neurobiology experiments and clinical applications.

Lesions of the dopaminergic system cause defined neurological defects, simulating Parkinson's disease, in which the replacement of dopaminergic cellular function can be assessed through readily quantifiable responses. This research led to the first successful human trials in restorative neurobiology and numerous valuable observations. Olson and Malmfors[138] first demonstrated the potential for embryonic neurons to survive transplantation and establish new connections. Subsequently, Freed and colleagues[139] grafted embryonic dopaminergic neurons into parkinsonian rats. Ingestion of 1-methyl-4-phenyl-1,2,3,6-tetrahydropyridine (MPTP) causes a defined basal ganglia lesion and provides a good model for Parkinson's disease in relevant primate species[140]; Sladek and coworkers[141] demonstrated neuronal engraftment after fetal tissue transplantation into MPTP-lesioned parkinsonian primates. Kordower and associates[142] confirmed histologic survival of transplanted neurons for as long as 18 months after implantation in humans. Together with accumulated clinical and positron emission tomography data, this paradigm provides evidence that a restorative neurobiology approach is clinically feasible.[143] Complications can follow transplantation of human embryonic tissue.[144]

The brain's immune response to transplanted fetal tissue is modest and apparently nonspecific,[145] but it is more robust to adult-derived tissues.[146] Prior brain injury increases the survival of neurons owing to increased local production of neurotrophins,[49] but it significantly decreases both the extension of cell processes out of the graft and the extension of host cell processes toward the injured area.[147] Unresolved questions concerning fetal tissue transplantation paradigms include the optimal site of transplantation and age of donor tissue, how to enhance survival of grafted cells, and how to optimize their function. Exposure of grafts to neurotrophic molecules can enhance survival.[148] Mehta and colleagues[149] found that the survival of E14 ventral mesencephalic tissue increased after pretransplant exposure to GDNF, and Eaton and Whittemore[150] found that transfection of raphe precursor cells to cause autocrine BDNF production enhanced both graft survival and integration.

Intraspinal Transplantation of Embryonic Tissue

Embryonic tissue has been transplanted into the injured spinal cord to support axonal regeneration, to enhance plasticity, to replace lost neurons, and to establish neuronal "relays." The behavioral and anatomic effects of such transplants on both acute and chronic injuries have been assessed. Anatomic studies support the premise that transplanted embryonic neurons[151] can extend processes into the host spinal cord, establish synapses, and relay signals from descending or ascending regenerated neurons synapsing within the graft. However, the observed degree of motor recovery in transplanted spinal cord–injured animals has been too modest to justify human clinical trials.

Extensive studies by Bregman and coworkers[152] demonstrated that a greater degree of motor recovery occurs after fetal tissue transplantation into immature animals compared with adult animals.[153, 154] In adult rats with SCIs, the combination of embryonic tissue transplants and exogenous neurotrophins more effectively increased axonal growth and reduced retrograde loss of neurons in the red nucleus than did either treatment alone.[155, 156] Mori and colleagues[157] implanted fetal spinal tissue after spinal cord hemisection in adult rats. Injured rubrospinal neurons that usually die were preserved, and axons from the transplant extended up to two segments into the host spinal cord.

Stokes and Reier[158] demonstrated that delayed transplantation of fetal tissue into spinal cord contusion cavities led to a modest, stable improvement in some aspects of gait. Anderson and associates[159] placed fetal grafts into chronic cavities in the cat spinal cord. Grafts from embryonic spinal cord or brainstem (homotypic) were more effective than embryonic cortical (heterotypic) grafts. In the study by Giovanini and colleagues,[160] suspension grafts were more effectively integrated into both acute and chronic injuries than were solid grafts. Theele and coworkers[161, 162] determined that fetal allografts into rodent spinal cords were eventually rejected, although rejection could be significantly reduced by immunomodulation.

Iwashita and colleagues[163] found a remarkable degree of improved motor function after transplanting fetal spinal cord segments into neonatal rats. In their experiment, correct longitudinal orientation of the transplanted segment was essential. Subsequently, Ito and associates[164] found apparent regeneration of the vestibulospinal tract after intraspinal transplantation of embryonic brain tissue in adult rats.

Gimenez y Ribotta and collaborators transplanted embryonic monoaminergic neuronal suspensions into the lumbar region after complete spinal cord transection.[134] This strategy enhances functional recovery of the lower extremities by substituting the need for regeneration of lengthy descending brainstem neurons with new, local, short-distance connections.[135] Improved stepping was correlated with immunohistochemical evidence of de novo transplant-derived synapses. In general, transplant strategies have been most effective when the distance over which the new connections must be established is minimal.

Syringomyelia involves progressive enlargement of a cavity; it has been hypothesized that obliterating the cavity by filling it with embryonic tissue might arrest progression of the disease. A human clinical trial has been initiated, with promising initial results.[8]

What is the future for fetal tissue transplantation? The supply of fetal tissue is limited, and its transplantation is associated with ethical issues. The tissue is not homogeneous, and it is rather difficult to work with in culture. Novel techniques for selective enrichment of specific neuronal types may allow grafts to be more effective.[165] Stem cells and multipotent precursors, however, offer more extensive possibilities for ex vivo genetic manipulation and possibly for more complete integration with the host.[166]

Undifferentiated, Renewable Cells for Neuronal Replacement within the Central Nervous System

Until recently, it was widely believed (despite earlier suggestive studies)[167] that the adult mammalian CNS had no potential for endogenous replacement of lost neurons. The system of terminally differentiated, integrated neurons could respond to injury with limited plasticity, but functional replacement did not occur. Recent studies challenge this view. We now know that subventricular zone neurons are continuously born and migrate substantial distances within the rodent brain to replace olfactory bulb neurons.[168] In the past decade, multipotential endogenous "progenitor" cells were discovered in brain regions such as the subventricular zone and spinal cord of mammals.[169] These cells can give rise to neurons, astrocytes, and oligodendrocytes.

There is debate about the appropriate definition of stem cells, but self-renewal and multipotency are the essential characteristics. Initially, it was thought that true multipotential stem cells capable of forming tissues of all three germ layers could be derived only from blastocystic cells.[170, 171] Recent data, however, indicate that progenitor cells derived from the adult neuroepithelium have the capacity to differentiate into cells of other primary tissues, such as blood.[172, 173] Interestingly, adult bone marrow also contains cells with the potential to develop along neuroepithelial lineages after transplantation into the brains of adult rats.[174] Derivation of autologous neural precursors from readily accessible adult bone marrow means that autotransplantation, obviating immune rejection, may be possible. Several other types of precursor cells that are further differentiated or lineage committed are being actively investigated; these cells usually lack self-renewal unless they are specifically transformed into cell lines. Most experiments employ embryonic stem cells, neuroepithelial precursor cells, or neuronal cell lines. Altogether, these discoveries have led to the exciting new field of stem cell neurobiology.

Embryonic stem cells have been obtained from fetal or embryonic tissues of brain or spinal cord, including from humans.[175] Human neuroepithelial precursor cells have been derived from the adult subventricular zone,[176, 177] the hippocampus,[178, 179] and the spinal cord.[180] Such cells can be maintained in a dividing, nondifferentiating state for lengthy periods by chronic exposure to the growth factors basic FGF or epidermal growth factor (EGF),[181] and they differentiate in response to neurotrophins such as BDNF after the withdrawal of mitogens.[169] Human embryonic stem cells maintained in cell culture under nondifferentiating conditions for 5 months were still capable of differentiating to derivatives of all three germinal layers.[171] A primate stem cell line also has the capacity to differentiate into neural tissue.[170] The potential for a single clone of cells to produce neurons, astrocytes, and oligodendroglia has been shown in culture.[182] Even precursors derived from aged mammalian brains maintain responsiveness to neurotrophic factors.[183] BDNF produced by ependymal cells appears to play a key role in normally supporting the survival of precursors and may account for their locations.[184]

The goal of stem cell therapy is structural repair of CNS regions rendered dysfunctional by trauma, ischemic injury, or chronic disease. The anticipated necessary steps are (1) successful harvest, culture, and preparation of stem cells; (2) transplantation and survival; (3) appropriate migration; (4) appropriate phenotypic expression; (5) integration into existing neuronal circuits; (6) functional synapse formation; and (7) lack of harmful side effects. These steps also need to occur within injured regions lacking complete structural cues. The immunology of stem cell transplants is incompletely understood, but allotransplantation may be possible, because tolerance to the stem cells may be induced.[185]

The ideal CNS repair strategy would involve activation of the endogenous progenitor population to divide, migrate, and replace lost cells. Provision of exogenous trophic factors is one strategy to activate self-repair. Intraventricular infusion of EGF in the adult mouse brain led to an increase in nestin-positive cells; migration into parenchyma; and differentiation into astrocytes, oligodendrocytes, and neurons.[186] Such strategies have potential utility in neurodegenerative diseases and modest CNS injuries that do not involve massive disorganization. After highly selective apoptotic lesioning of cortical neurons, a local up-regulation of developmental cues may facilitate migration and integration of a transplanted progenitor cell line.[187] Magavi and associates[188] recently demonstrated that endogenous neurogenesis, migration, and integration can occur in adult mice after similar lesions.

Active areas of investigation in clinically oriented stem cell neurobiology include methods to optimize differentiation, migration, and integration after transplantation. Some authors have suggested that substantial differences in the ability of progenitor cells to migrate and differentiate may depend on the growth factor exposure used to maintain them in culture.[189] Vescovi and coworkers[190] required both EGF and FGF-2 to propagate brain-derived fetal human stem cells, which were passaged up to 2 years with maintenance of nestin expression and no visible differentiation. Multipotentiality was exhibited even after lengthy passage. After striatal transplantation of the cells into adult rats, both astrocytic and neuronal phenotypes were detected. In this experiment, both cortex- and thalamus-derived cells could give rise to tyrosine hydroxylase–positive neurons in the striatum. Human precursor cells derived from fetal spinal cord had a relatively low level of expansion to EGF and basic FGF and were restricted to astrocytic lineage after four passages.[191, 192] Factors within the culture media can restrict the phenotypic fate of progenitor cells.[193, 194] Ciliary neurotrophic factor (CNTF) exposure leads to astrocytic differentiation, triiodothyronine (T3) exposure leads to oligodendrocytic differentiation, and exposure to retinoic acid causes mouse stem cells to differentiate into γ-aminobutyric acid (GABA) neurons.[195] EGF-maintained neurospheres contain heterogeneous precursor cells (even if derived from a single cell). Some cells differentiate only into glia, while others differentiate into all three cell types, including astrocytes, oligodendrocytes, and neurons.[181, 196] Therefore, several partially determined precursor states may exist in a progenitor cell culture. Other strategies to purify neural precursors from heterogeneous embryonic stem cells include transfection and expression of a lineage-selecting gene.[197]

The signals that direct the migration and differentiation of progenitor cells are still largely unknown and are of profound importance in understanding how these cells could be used in CNS repair. Techniques such as lineage analysis can elucidate the interactions that normally direct the location and phenotype of identified multipotent progenitor cells during development.[198] Transgenic animals allow us to determine the effect of specific molecular perturbations on neural development. For example, fetal mice overexpressing the molecule "sonic hedgehog" exhibit prolonged germinal matrix proliferation and failure to differentiate, suggesting that this molecule can block differentiation.[199] Brustle and coworkers[200] generated chimeric brains by transplanting human neural stem cells into developing rats. The human cells could be identified and differentiated into a variety of well-integrated phenotypes and integrated widely. This chimeric model provides another method to study key developmental interactions that influence human progenitor cells. Auerbach and colleagues[201] recently confirmed that transplanted stem cells can form functional synapses.

Factors that influence migration of transplanted precursor cells include maturity of the host, location of the transplant, and whether the transplanted cell is already lineage committed. Herrera and associates[202] found that transplanted precursor cells that became neurons migrated only into the olfactory bulb. Cells that migrated into other regions became glia. Fricker and coworkers[203] found that transplanted progenitor cells that became neurons also migrated into the dentate region of the hypothalamus and into the striatum. Svendsen and coauthors[204, 205] found that the capacity of transplanted stem cells to migrate is substantially greater for those developing a glial as opposed to a neuronal phenotype. Zigova and colleagues[206] found that subventricular zone cells derived from neonatal rats and transplanted into the striatum exhibited local migration and integration but formed neurons characteristic of the olfactory bulb, not of the striatum, indicating a lack of multipotentiality. Jankovski and associates[207] found that the precursor cells derived from postnatal mice were already committed and did not respond to local epigenetic cues when transplanted to a heterotopic location. Takahashi and coworkers[208] performed intravitreal (heterotopic) transplantation of hippocampus-derived neural progenitor cells into developing rats. Cell survival was excellent with retinal integration, but phenotypic expression was incomplete. McDonald and colleagues[209] transplanted embryonic stem cells into the spinal cord 9 days after contusive SCI. Migration and differentiation into both glia and neurons were observed, as well as behavioral improvements in some animals. Although some foci of abnormal hamartomatous differentiation were also observed, this study is encouraging, because transplantation involved a region of significant injury in the chronic stage. Current evidence indicates that embryonic stem cells have a wider repertoire of potential phenotypic responses than do adult-derived progenitor cells.

Promising results have been obtained using neuronal cell lines. Cells of a neural progenitor line transplanted into neonatal mouse cerebellum integrated and formed synapses visible by electron micrography.[210] Similar progenitors could migrate across the corpus callosum and replace cortical neurons that had undergone targeted apoptosis.[187] The retrovirally transduced embryonic neuronal precursor cell line RN33B has been useful for examining integration and differentiation. When transplanted into uninjured adult and neonatal rat hippocampi, RN33B cells integrated and showed evidence of the induction of mature neuronal properties.[211] The cells assumed the morphology of hippocampal neurons, expressed appropriate neuronal markers, and also received synapses. However, cells transplanted into severely lesioned areas did not differentiate into region-specific neurons.[212] When RN33B was transplanted into normal spinal cord,[213] some cells assumed motoneuron-like morphology, whereas cells transplanted into injured spinal cord did not appear to differentiate. Therefore, the cells show phenotypic plasticity, and the intact adult CNS has the ability to direct their differentiation. Local epigenetic signals (cell-cell interactions), however, appear essential, and such signals appear to be lacking after SCI and destructive brain lesions. These authors found that each neuronal cell line exhibited different responses to in vitro and in vivo conditions.

Pluripotentiality in vitro does not necessarily predict the same capacity in vivo; the ability to control the phenotypic expression of transplanted stem cells remains incomplete. If neural progenitors are transplanted into the brain early in development, appropriate integration is excellent,[214] but it decreases substantially as development proceeds.[215] Successful and appropriate differentiation and integration have also been observed after stem cell or precursor transplantation into animals with well-defined cellular deficits or very limited lesions. However, examples of successful adult-derived precursor cell integration into the CNS of severely lesioned adult animals are lacking. Alternative phenotype-directing strategies to select for specific phenotypes from embryonic stem cells, including transfection with tissue-specific regulatory molecules, are being explored.[195]

A teratocarcinoma cell line is being transplanted into patients with established brain infarcts.[216] These cells, derived from an undifferentiated human embryonal teratocarcinoma, undergo differentiation to a mature neuronal phenotype after in vitro treatment with retinoic acid. Following transplantation of such cells into the rodent caudate nucleus 1 month after ischemic injury, behavioral improvement was sustained[217] and was correlated with the number of surviving transplanted cells.[218] Behavioral recovery in this paradigm is not necessarily linked to the replacement of lost neurons and the formation of new connections; it could reflect the release of trophic factors from the engrafted cells.

Glial Cellular Transplants to Support Long-Tract Regeneration

DORSAL ROOT ENTRY ZONE

Injured axons of the adult mammalian PNS normally regenerate, and some types of injured CNS axons can respond to implanted peripheral nerve grafts with substantial regenerative elongation. Interest in the use of peripheral nerve grafts to promote CNS regeneration has therefore been great. However, a central problem with using peripheral nerve grafts in spinal cord applications is that axons that readily regenerate within the grafts usually cannot reenter the CNS for significant distances.[128, 219] Whereas many types of axons enter a peripheral nerve graft and are inhibited at reentry, some, such as corticospinal axons, appear to be unable to even enter the graft.[220, 221]

The interface between a peripheral nerve graft and the spinal cord is analogous to the dorsal root entry zone (DREZ), or transition zone, the normal adult interface between the PNS and CNS. The DREZ provides a useful model of the barrier function of reactive CNS glia. During development, the central processes of DRG sensory neurons enter the spinal cord and synapse. In adult animals, however, if the central (DRG) process is injured by a crush, regeneration occurs only up to the delimiting astrocytes of the transition zone. At this point, axonal growth cones either turn back or form stable synaptoid terminations, indicating that the region is nonpermissive for axonal growth.[222, 223]

Other studies have demonstrated that the DREZ is also inhibitory to regeneration of other types of neurons grafted into the root,[224] including motor axons[225] and catecholaminergic fibers.[226] The DREZ stop signal does not occur in immature animals.[227] The transition from a regeneration-permissive to a nonpermissive DREZ zone appears to involve the establishment of a boundary of ECM molecules that includes chondroitin sulfate proteoglycans and tenascin expressed by astrocytes.[228] Peripheral nerve grafts or Schwann cell grafts placed into contact with CNS tissue form DREZ-like interfaces,[219] and the deposition of chondroitin sulfate proteoglycans is believed to inhibit axonal elongation.[128] Chondroitin sulfate proteoglycans are also believed to play an important role in the glial scar, as discussed later.[229]

A number of strategies have been employed to overcome the DREZ barrier, including depopulation of local barrier-forming astrocytes with radiation,[230, 231] transplantation of growth-supportive embryonic astrocytes,[232] and transplantation of ensheathing glia (discussed later). Gilmore and Sims[233] showed that an intact astrocytic DREZ barrier is needed to prevent spontaneous invasion of the spinal cord by Schwann cells.

Recent studies indicate that the DREZ may be only a relative barrier. This issue is of great importance in CNS regeneration. When unusually high levels of neurotrophins are present in the dorsal gray matter, some regenerating sensory processes can extend through the DREZ.[234, 235]

PERIPHERAL NERVE GRAFTS, SCHWANN CELLS, AND ENSHEATHING GLIA

The minimal necessary conditions for regenerative elongation of injured CNS axons are adequate neurotrophic support and a permissive substrate with favorable surface molecules such as laminin, N-CAM, and L1. Peripheral nerve grafts are regeneration-permissive substrates for many types of injured axons, whereas the grafted optic nerve, a model CNS tract, is not.[236, 237] A key difference between the CNS and peripheral nerve grafts is the presence of Schwann cells, which produce neurotrophic factors and surface adhesion molecules. Several studies have explored the possibility that transplanted peripheral nerve grafts might allow reconnection of injured axons to their CNS targets. This idea was based on observations by Tello,[238] a student of Ramon y Cajal. During the 1940s and 1950s, the idea was controversial,[239] and defining the paradigms in which effective CNS repair can be achieved with peripheral nerve grafts remains controversial.

Among the most elegant and successful experimental models employing this technique are peripheral nerve grafts from the transected optic nerve to the tectum in hamsters. In this model, the axons of retinal ganglion cells regenerate and form stable connections on denervated tectal neurons[240]; the function of the light reflex partially recovers.[241] Importantly, in this strategy, the distance from the graft's contact with the tectal surface to the target neurons is short, less than 1 mm. Similar successful regeneration has been observed when peripheral nerve grafts are used in other paradigms, such as the septohippocampal model, in which the distance to the target neurons is also small.[242]

The report by Cheng and colleagues[125] of significant regeneration across a complete adult spinal cord transection focused renewed attention on the prospects for peripheral nerve regeneration strategies. These investigators combined elements of current neurosurgical practice, such as autologous nerve grafts, spinal fixation, fibrin glue, and growth factors. The potential for

translation into humans was evident. They routed multiple grafts from white matter tracts into the more permissive gray matter.[243, 244] The spinal column was rigidly immobilized, and the spinal cord stumps and grafts were encased in a fibrin glue cast.[245] Fibrin glue was mixed with acidic FGF-1 to facilitate a sustained, slow release. FGF-1 is a known angiogenic factor that lacks a signal sequence for normal secretion and is released after neuronal injury.[246] FGF-1 can enhance regeneration of the PNS[247] but had not previously been known to influence regeneration of the CNS. The outstanding recovery observed by Cheng's group has not yet been obtained by others using similar strategies. The concept of sustained local delivery of trophic factors[248] is being explored in a variety of paradigms, including bioartificial substrates[249] and gene therapy.

No primate study has yet shown significant regeneration mediated by peripheral nerve grafts spanning injured regions of the spinal cord. However, functional reinnervation of muscles[250, 251] has been demonstrated after grafting peripheral nerves or roots into the spinal cords of primates and humans.[252]

Schwann cells can be purified from autologous peripheral nerves, and they reliably expand in culture, support the regeneration of large numbers of axons, and myelinate axons.[253, 254] However, as with peripheral nerve grafts, the axons that regenerate into these grafts show very little reentry into the CNS, and functional reconnection does not occur. The key explanation for this failure to regenerate appears to be the formation of an unfavorable molecular environment between the Schwann cells and the host spinal cord cells at the interface where axons are poised to reenter the spinal cord.

In a recent study, a Schwann cell–seeded guidance channel was placed to span a hemisection cavity.[255] In this model of incomplete SCI, some fibers regenerated distally into the gray matter. The smaller injury, with consequent incomplete glial scarring and some remaining intact tissue, may permit more favorable axon-glia interactions.

Another interesting technique for grafting Schwann cells is the creation of a stereotactic tract of Schwann cells into the distal spinal cord. This technique is still limited by the substantial astrocytic reaction to the presence of the Schwann cell graft. A potential advantage is that regenerating fibers are brought much closer to their potential target neurons.[256] However, axons within Schwann cell grafts are fasciculated, as in peripheral nerve grafts. This arrangement may limit the potential for regenerating axons to interact with local spinal cord neurons.

OLFACTORY ENSHEATHING GLIA

Recently, marked interest has developed in transplantation of olfactory ensheathing glial cells for CNS repair.[257] This interest derives from the unique properties of the mammalian olfactory system. Neurons within the olfactory epithelium of mammals undergo continuous turnover; newly generated primary sensory axons extend into the CNS environment of the olfactory bulb to connect specifically with target neurons. Because this phenomenon can occur in adult primates after section of the fila olfactoria, it is a unique natural paradigm of neuronal reconnection through a transition zone.[258, 259] The olfactory nerve has the only PNS-CNS transition region that lacks an astrocyte-derived glial limiting membrane.[260, 261] Remarkably, even if the olfactory bulb is removed, the primary sensory axons can reestablish functional contacts with the basal cortex.[262] Glia ensheathe large numbers of closely packed, small-diameter axons within their cytoplasm from the olfactory mucosa to the glomerulus of the olfactory bulb, where they synapse. A thin ensheathing glial membrane segregates the olfactory neuron from all other cell types, including astrocytes, from the receptor specialization to the synapse. Schwann cell ensheathment, however, involves the enfolding of each individual axon within a substantial furrow of cytoplasm, and basal lamina is present over the entire surface of the Schwann cell. The membranes of ensheathing glia are covered by basal lamina, except within the nerve fiber layer of the olfactory bulb.

Ensheathing glia share characteristics with both astrocytes and Schwann cells. They produce growth-permissive ECM molecules such as laminin and surface receptor molecules for neurons such as L1 and N-CAM (including embryonic N-CAM).[263] Expression of the central isoform of glial fibrillary acidic protein (GFAP) apparently distinguishes them from Schwann cells,[264] although many of their molecular characteristics are similar to those of nonmyelinating Schwann cells.[265] Other properties of ensheathing glia that appear to be important in supporting regeneration are their ability to migrate, lack of formation of inhibitory basal lamina, and production of soluble factors, including neurotrophic molecules.[266] Other unique glial subtypes, such as hypothalamic tanycytes, may have similar regeneration-supporting properties.[267]

When ensheathing glia and astrocytes meet, they do not establish inhibitory boundaries like Schwann cells and astrocytes do. Therefore, olfactory ensheathing glia are excellent candidate cells to provide a substrate to support regeneration of injured CNS tracts. Transplants of olfactory ensheathing glia can render the nonpermissive DREZ permissive[268] and facilitate restoration of a spinal reflex (providing evidence of functional reconnection) after a nerve root crush.[269] After focal injury to the corticospinal tract, transplants of unpurified cultures containing ensheathing glia support regeneration,[270] with evidence of functional recovery of upper extremity function.[271] Because Schwann cell grafts are associated with significant intragraft regeneration but poor reentry of axons into the CNS, placing ensheathing glia at the Schwann cell graft–host interface may enhance the permissiveness of the interface.[272] After transplantation, ensheathing glia initially form an elongated cellular bridge in the direction of their delivery tract,[273] a feature reminiscent of Schwann cells.[274] Recent evidence suggests that ensheathing glia may support functional regeneration of motor and sensory axons after complete spinal cord[275] or dorsal column

transection.[276] However, ensheathing glia may not support regeneration of all classes of neurons.[277]

Myelination of large-diameter regenerated axons is necessary for biophysical efficacy. Ensheathing glia do not normally form myelin around primary olfactory sensory axons, although aberrant myelin formation in the olfactory bulb may occur.[278] The potential for transplanted ensheathing glia to myelinate has been studied in chemically demyelinated lesions.[279, 280] A recent study supports the theory that human-derived ensheathing glia have the capacity to myelinate demyelinated axons in vivo.[281]

Bioartificial Regeneration Environments

Thus far, we have considered cellular and molecular manipulation of injury environments to foster axonal regeneration. A cell's external environment consists of soluble factors, other cell membranes, and ECM. ECM modulates the cytoskeleton, differentiation, and spatial architecture of cells and tissues.[282] The CNS microenvironment after injury is extremely complex, and another repair strategy is to replace the injury milieu with a simplified composite of cells, molecules, and polymers to support axonal regeneration.[283] Guidance channels can be engineered to release growth factors and to organize growing neuronal processes spatially[284] by having fragments of cell attachment molecules integrated into their surfaces.[285] Channels and other polymers can deliver neurotrophic factors within the cerebrospinal fluid.[286, 287] Another strategy is to optimize the regeneration of selected target populations by using several separate channels or polymer tracts containing selected ECM components, neurotrophins, and cells.[288] Transplantation of bioartificial constructs such as artificial skin is already well established in clinical practice.[289]

Bridging materials that have been employed to span CNS lesions include human amnion,[290] polymerized collagen,[291, 292] Matrigel (Fisher Scientific, Pittsburgh),[253] carbon filaments,[293] and polyglycolitic acid.[294] Enclosure of cells by channels or capsules can provide protection from immune rejection. Beneficial cell-biomaterial interactions can occur (e.g., Schwann cells seeded into polyacrylonitrile-polyvinylchloride guidance channels spontaneously organize their cytoplasmic processes along the axis of the channel). Because these constructs permit the combination of well-defined constituents, valuable experiments are possible. As an example, a transplanted, cell-free peripheral nerve graft (essentially a basal lamina tube) was unable to support regeneration of lesioned cholinergic septal axons. However, if it was presoaked in NGF, the axonal ingrowth was equivalent to that of normal peripheral nerve grafts, demonstrating that the Schwann cell function can apparently be replaced by a single molecule.[295] It is possible that isolated, simplified microenvironments could incorporate microchip technology.[296] A chip could serve as an input-output relay if axons regenerated and formed connections on its surface.

Transplantation of Inflammatory Cells

Macrophages support PNS regeneration, but macrophage activity within the injured CNS appears to be depressed, possibly by an intrinsic factor.[46, 297] Recent studies assessed the impact of modifying CNS macrophage activity after SCI. Rapalino and coworkers[126] exposed homologous macrophages to peripheral nerve segments to "activate" them and injected them into the spinal cord distal to a transection. After 3 months, a modest but significant motor recovery was observed in the treated animals. Cortically evoked lower extremity electromyography, neuroanatomic tracing, and spinal cord retransection supported the belief that behavioral recovery was partially mediated by reconnection from regenerating supraspinal axons. The observed recovery plateaued at 5 months and was stable for 1 year. In contrast, and illustrating the complexity of CNS inflammation, Popovich and colleagues[298] reported that depletion of hematogenous macrophages after contusive SCI significantly improves behavioral and histologic outcomes. This study concluded that the net effect of macrophage activity after contusive SCI increases the severity of injury. The explanation for these differing observations may depend on variables such as the state of macrophage activation, timing of intervention, site of delivery, and so on. Our current understanding of inflammation associated with CNS injury is incomplete.

Cellular Transplantation to Repair Myelin

After contusive SCIs, some axons remain in continuity but may fail to transmit impulses because of demyelination. Human studies indicate that such axons may remain unmyelinated for several years (Bunge and Guest, unpublished observations).[299, 300] The cause of chronic post-traumatic demyelination remains unclear but may be due to loss of local oligodendrocytes, possibly caused by apoptosis.[52] Evidence that restoration of transmission across focally demyelinated axons can enhance function derives from animal and human studies in which improved conduction followed blockade of abnormally exposed potassium ion channels with 4-aminopyridine.[301, 302] Experimental studies of the transplantation of myelinating cells following chemically induced demyelination have demonstrated substantial recovery of axonal transmission after remyelination. Several cell types have been explored for their myelinating ability in a variety of animal models: human embryonic oligodendrocytes,[303] oligodendrocyte cell lines,[304] O2-A progenitor cells,[305] Schwann cells,[306] mixed glial cells,[307] stem cells,[308, 309] and ensheathing glia.[279]

Autologous Schwann cell transplantation seems an obvious treatment to repair damaged myelin. However, transplanted Schwann cells exhibit remyelination only in regions not populated by astrocytes.[310] Schwann cells together with transplanted type 1 astrocytes promote remyelination over a broader area[311] than do Schwann cells alone.

STRATEGIES FOR REPAIR: AUGMENTATION OF INTRINSIC REGENERATIVE CAPACITY

Physical Methods and Conditioning Lesions

Neuronal regeneration is affected by both the tissue environment at the growth cone and the activation state at the neuron's cell body. These concepts have been nicely demonstrated using predegenerated nerve grafts and "conditioning lesions." Nerve grafts lesioned several days before transplantation support more robust axonal regeneration. This response is likely due to up-regulation of Schwann cell neurotrophin production[312] and infiltration with cytokine-secreting macrophages, which lead to a more favorable environment for growth cone extension.

A conditioning lesion is a "priming" injury to the axons of a peripheral nerve that up-regulates the neuron's regenerative "machinery" so that a second injury elicits a more robust regenerative response.[313, 314] A conditioning response follows injury to the peripheral nerve processes of DRG neurons but is not induced by injury to the central process in the absence of peripheral injury.[27] Conditioning lesions enhance the regeneration of the optic nerve in goldfish[315] but not in rats.[316] Whether adult mammalian CNS neurons can be conditioned is unknown, although suggestive data exist.[128] Stimulation of inflammation in the vicinity of DRG cell bodies can also enhance peripheral nerve regeneration by a "conditioning effect" on cell body activation.[317]

Neumann and Woolf[7] demonstrated that the glial scar in an incompletely injured spinal cord is a relative barrier. They lesioned the sciatic nerve and transected the dorsal columns simultaneously. In the absence of a sciatic nerve lesion, there was minimal sprouting, and all ascending sensory fibers stopped at the scar. If, however, a conditioning sciatic nerve lesion was performed, regeneration occurred rostral to the scar. Fibers that regenerated often did not enter the degenerated dorsal columns or the gray matter but took aberrant routes along the spinal cord surface. This finding demonstrates that the neuron's intrinsic regeneration potential is increased by a lesion in its PNS process and that the degenerated tracts are less permissive than the spinal cord surface. Chong and associates[318] demonstrated that a peripheral conditioning lesion substantially increases the ability of regenerating proximal sensory fibers to traverse the DREZ.

Trophic Molecules

Neurotrophic factors are protein molecules that bind to specific cell surface receptors and elicit biologic effects on neurons (or other cells). More than 30 proteins that can elicit neurotrophic function have been described. The intracellular signals generated by receptor binding can influence cell survival, maintenance and regeneration of cellular processes, phenotype (including neurotransmitter production), synaptogenesis, and plasticity. Molecular cloning techniques have allowed many of these molecules to be produced in quantities sufficient for potential therapeutic use. NGF was the first neurotrophin discovered and is the best characterized.[319] Neurotrophins generally support cellular growth, as opposed to growth factors (e.g., EGF, FGF), which influence cell division. NGF, BDNF, neurotrophin-3, and neurotrophin-4/5 constitute a family of similar molecules, all of which can bind to a single low-affinity (p75) receptor but also bind specifically to the tyrosine kinase–linked receptors trkA (NGF), trkB (BDNF and neurotrophin-4/5), and trkC (neurotrophin-3). CNTF is a cytokine similar to leukemia inhibitory factor and IL-6. GDNF is a member of the transforming growth factor-β family. Whereas native neurotrophic molecules may have a complex molecular structure of multiple chains, only the active "subunit" is usually cloned and synthesized for experimental and clinical purposes.

During PNS development, the quantity of neurotrophins is limited, and cellular survival is correlated with their abundance. For many years it was believed that neurotrophin functions were restricted to the immature nervous system. However, the observation that exogenous NGF could prevent the death of septal neurons in adult rats after transection of the fornix[320] indicated that neurotrophins are present in suboptimal quantities after the fornix is injured. The neurotrophic factors to which a neuron responds can change under different conditions,[321] and the response of an adult neuron may differ from that of an immature neuron of the same class.[322] Traditionally, it was believed that most neurotrophins were secreted from targets and transported retrogradely. Evidence now suggests that some neurotrophins may be transported anterogradely for release at presynaptic terminals.[323] NGF may also have a *neurotropic* function, providing directional guidance for growth cones through concentration gradients.[324, 325]

Most major neurotrophic factors can be produced within the CNS by either neurons or glia.[326] The normal levels appear to be regulated by activity and hormonal levels.[327] The use of trophic factors in CNS repair is attractive because of the multiple potential methods of delivery: systemic, local injection; slow local release; production by genetically modified, transplanted cells; or transfection of endogenous cells by vectors containing neurotrophin genes. In addition, the use of trophic molecules is readily combined with other strategies. Because neurotrophins are large proteins that do not readily cross the blood-brain barrier, the efficacy of systemic delivery to the CNS has been limited. Intraventricular cerebrospinal fluid delivery has been associated with some undesirable side effects,[328] including sprouting of sympathetic fibers in the DRG.[329] After parenchymal delivery, the diffusion distance varies substantially among types of neurotrophins. The site of action of neurotrophic factors has important implications for therapeutic delivery because of the unique geometry of many neurons with large distances from their cell bodies to axonal terminals. Some neurons have neurotrophin receptors on their dendrites or cell bodies and may use autocrine or paracrine mechanisms.[330] Whether neurotrophin delivery is more effective at the cell body or at the injured terminals remains controversial.[25, 331]

After CNS trauma, the levels of several neurotrophins are increased transiently.[246, 332, 333] Increases in NGF production by reactive astrocytes have been linked to cytokine secretion by inflammatory cells[334] and also to injury-associated growth factors.[335] Therefore, cytokines may also be useful for modulating the production of CNS neurotrophins.

The lesioned septohippocampal system has been a rich source of experimental observations on the differential effects of the delivery of various neurotrophins. NGF is normally produced in the hippocampus and retrogradely transported to septal neurons, a classic demonstration of the "neurotrophin hypothesis." After axotomy of the fimbria or fornix, septal cell bodies atrophy; many die, and key neurotransmitters cease to be produced. Intraventricular delivery of NGF can completely prevent these changes and preserve the choline acetyltransferase phenotype in rodents[336] and primates.[337] The effect is specific because the death of GABA neurons is not prevented. CNTF can prevent the death of the cholinergic neurons but does not preserve the choline acetyltransferase phenotype.[338] Alternative delivery methods that have achieved similar protective effects on septal neurons include transplantation of NGF-transfected fibroblasts[339] and the slow release of NGF from implanted polymer rods.[249]

Nigrostriatal dopaminergic neurons express the trkB and trkC receptors and retrogradely transport BDNF and neurotrophin-3 from the striatum. Eighty percent of nigrostriatal neurons die after axotomy. Exogenous delivery of CNTF, BDNF, neurotrophin-3, neurotrophin-4, or GDNF enhances neuronal survival. CNTF is the most potent survival factor but does not maintain the axodendritic arbor or tyrosine hydroxylase phenotype; BDNF, neurotrophin-4, and GDNF also enhance survival but do not maintain the tyrosine hydroxylase phenotype.[340] Neurotrophin-3 was less effective for survival but did maintain the tyrosine hydroxylase phenotype. Therefore, the effects of neurotrophins on injured systems are difficult to predict and must be assessed experimentally in each model.

Neurotrophin delivery creates the potential for significant modification of the CNS environment and possible undesirable effects (e.g., do sprouts from injured axons extend abnormally into normal parenchyma, or do normal axons sprout aberrantly in response to exogenous neurotrophins?). He and coworkers[341] examined patterns of sprouting in the septum and hippocampus after partially lesioning the fornix; inappropriate sprouting from nonlesioned neurons did not occur in the septum, but appropriate sprouting did occur in the partially denervated hippocampus. In a similar paradigm, NGF led to hypertrophy of unlesioned striatal cholinergic neurons, a potentially detrimental effect.[342]

Strategies that combine neurotrophins and cellular grafts are more complex and make local gradients of growth factors an important consideration. For example, when ventricular infusion of NGF was combined with a septohippocampal peripheral nerve graft, cholinergic sprouts occurred close to the site of infusion but did not enter the graft, presumably because it had lower levels of NGF.[325] Thus, NGF infusion interfered with the intended graft function. However, when NGF was infused into the dorsal hippocampus distal to the peripheral nerve graft, reinnervation was enhanced,[343] demonstrating the importance of the site of neurotrophin release. Maintenance of the new sprouts in the NGF septohippocampal model depended on the ongoing provision of trophic factor. Unless new contact with hippocampal neurons was established, the sprouts regressed. The observation that regenerated fibers regress unless a stable synapse is formed is believed to be true for most CNS systems.

Oudega and Hagg[344] infused NGF 4 mm rostral to a peripheral nerve graft placed within the lesioned dorsal column. A conditioning lesion was required to see substantial regeneration into the graft. In the absence of the exogenous neurotrophins, the regenerating sensory fibers did not extend beyond the peripheral nerve–dorsal column interface. NGF delivery resulted in extension of regenerating sensory fibers into the region of the degenerating dorsal columns. This study demonstrated that the glial scar formed at a peripheral nerve graft–spinal cord interface is a relative, not an absolute, barrier. Therefore, neurotrophins can be used to stimulate regeneration through glial barriers. Local delivery of trophic factors also reduces axonal dieback of corticospinal[78, 345] and retinal ganglion axons.[77]

Attempts to foster regeneration by simply providing high local concentrations of growth factors are rather simplistic approaches to enhancing regeneration. Such experiments have been highly instructive and, under certain well-defined conditions, successful. However, the reconstruction of complex CNS tracts and connections is likely to require a substantially more sophisticated program of regulated gene expression.

Completed human clinical trials have employed growth factors such as NGF and CNTF delivered primarily via subcutaneous or intraventricular access. Major benefits have not been observed in these initial attempts at systemic or cerebrospinal fluid delivery,[346, 347] and some unacceptable side effects have occurred.

Gene Therapy

Because of the complexity of CNS organization and the inadequacy of endogenous repair mechanisms, the ideal therapeutic methods should create minimal additional injury. Gene therapy approaches are most suitable for diseases that involve a single gene defect. In mice, for example, transplanted immortalized neural progenitor cells that were transformed to produce stable, high levels of β-glucuronidase or β-hexosaminidase were able to correct lysosomal storage disease[348] or the gene defect of Tay-Sachs disease.[349] Complex biologic phenomena such as regeneration, however, involve the activation of many genes and are not immediately amenable to strategies that change the local concentration of a single gene product. However, as discussed in the previous section, several experiments have demonstrated a beneficial response of injured

neurons to purified, exogenous trophic factors. Gene therapy approaches can facilitate the local production of molecules such as trophic factors via transduced native CNS cells or transplanted cells. Thus, the earliest CNS regeneration gene therapy experiments involved augmentation of concentrations of local trophic factors to study their effects on neuronal survival or axonal regeneration. These strategies are similar to the slow release of molecules such as neurotrophins from polymer matrix carriers[249] or fibrin glue.[248]

Vector-based gene delivery strategies offer the potential advantages of infecting specific target cells, providing stable levels of gene expression, and possibly achieving gene regulation. Among the available delivery vectors, viruses and transfected cells have been studied most extensively in CNS applications. Viral vectors are attractive because they have evolved specialized mechanisms for cellular entry and control. An especially useful feature may be the capacity for retrograde axonal transport of the vector from axonal terminals to the neuronal cell body.

Cell lysis is the usual result of the virus life cycle. Lysis may be useful in tumor therapy but not for repair applications. Therefore, viruses have been modified to minimize their toxicity, to optimize gene expression, and to prevent completion of their life cycle. Plasmid vectors consist of the gene of interest with an appropriate regulatory sequence and a minimal cassette of viral genes, such as a packaging signal, within the virus coat. Such vectors can efficiently infect cells and lead to transgene expression without provoking significant immune system activation or expressing other viral genes.[350, 351] Neurotrophic viruses such as herpes simplex (HSV) and rabies use retrograde transport to reach the cell nucleus, and HSV is capable of entering a lifelong latent state within some neurons. Thus, viral vectors may be employed to deliver genes selectively to specific CNS neurons from their axonal terminals. Gene expression in neurons with terminals outside the CNS (motor, sensory, autonomic) that could be infected by such vectors might have beneficial effects in states such as motoneuron disease. Alternatively, infection and transduction of these neurons could increase the concentration of locally secreted molecules, such as growth factors, thereby influencing the activity of cells or processes entirely within the CNS. The potential to regulate transgene expression may be useful to optimize effects on regeneration or injury.

Desirable vectors for CNS gene delivery require the following features: low toxicity, minimal host response, high transduction efficiency, cell specificity of transduction, stable transgene expression, large transgene capacity, and safe, reproducible production methods. An additional feature necessary for delivery by retrograde transport is efficient uptake from muscle or skin. Concerns about viral vectors include possible recombination and reversion to wild type, insertional mutagenesis with possible neoplasia, and potential adverse effects on normal cellular functioning.

Viruses used in current investigational strategies for in vivo transfer to the CNS include adenovirus, HSV, adenoassociated virus (AAV), and lentivirus; retroviruses have established efficacy for ex vivo gene transfer. Molecular biologic techniques allow the combination of useful features of distinct virus types into unique hybrids.[352]

Because motor and sensory neurons extend outside the CNS, they are logically accessible targets for experimental manipulation. Haase and associates[353] treated experimental motoneuron disease by intramuscular injection of neurotrophin-3–encoding adenovirus. Watabe and colleagues[354] demonstrated that injection of GDNF-encoding adenovirus into the nerve root foramen after root avulsion reduced motoneuron death and preserved phenotype. Zhang and coworkers[234] injected neurotrophin-3–encoding adenovirus into dorsal spinal cord gray matter after proximal root transection and reanastomosis. Sensory axons were able to regrow through the normally inhibitory DREZ toward the neurotrophin-3–producing cells. Wilson and coauthors[355] demonstrated that after skin inoculation of HSV-encoding enkephalin, DRG expression occurred, and responses to pain were attenuated. Another strategy to promote regeneration is to transduce adult neurons to express genes necessary to initiate the regenerative process. Interestingly, injection of growth-associated, protein-43–expressing adenovirus into adult substantia nigra was associated with aberrant plasticity.[356]

AAV is associated with minimal host immune response and long-term transgene expression; however, brain injections of AAV show very restricted diffusion,[357] and AAV does not appear to undergo retrograde transport from muscle to spinal neurons. One interesting viral construct is an AAV-HSV hybrid produced under helper virus–free conditions.[358] AAV sequences that direct site-specific DNA integration have been combined with the HSV packaging signal and a transgene for green fluorescent protein. Site-specific integration of the transgene is believed to extend its expression.[352] Because helper virus is not used to produce this vector, contamination with wild-type revertants is obviated. With no other HSV genes incorporated into the construct, cellular toxicity appears to be minimal. Use of this hybrid vector achieved highly efficient transfer from peripheral nerves into motoneurons, with no detectable host immune response at 6 weeks. Use of an earlier-generation HSV replication-deficient vector resulted in a marked host immune response and loss of gray matter neurons.[351] Costantini and coworkers[350] also observed minimal host response, good transduction efficiency, and stable gene expression after striatal injection of this vector.

Few CNS repair gene therapy experiments have been reported in primates. Choi-Lundberg and colleagues[359] demonstrated that stereotactically injected adenovirus-GDNF could prevent striatal neurons from undergoing degeneration after 6-OHDA ingestion. When a similar vector was injected into the primate striatum, substantial transfection occurred,[360] with gene expression for up to 2 months. However, the effect was titer dependent. Higher titers led to a marked immune response and limited gene expression.

Site-specific delivery of neurotrophins can also be achieved by transplantation of cells engineered in tissue culture (ex vivo) to secrete quantities of trophic factors. Fibroblasts have been employed in several paradigms because they can be obtained easily and handle well in cell culture.

The advantages of ex vivo gene transfer include stable gene expression, because retroviruses cause transgene integration into the genome. Retroviruses, however, infect only dividing cells, whereas other viruses, such as HSV, adenovirus, AAV, and lentivirus, can infect both dividing and nondividing cells. HSV and adenovirus are associated with transient gene expression because the transfected gene is not integrated.

Transfected fibroblasts or Schwann cells have been transplanted in several paradigms.[361] BDNF-transfected Schwann cells transplanted to the rat spinal cord were associated with an improved regenerative response after spinal cord transection.[256] Grill and associates[362] transplanted retrovirally transfected neurotrophin-3–secreting fibroblasts into the thoracic spinal cord after dorsal hemisection and observed regeneration of corticospinal fibers and behavioral recovery. Similar effects were obtained by transplantation of fibroblasts transfected to produce the cytokine leukemia inhibitory factor.[363] Liu and coauthors[364] transplanted BDNF-transfected fibroblasts into cervical lesions that damaged the rubrospinal tract. Rubrospinal axons regenerated through the transplant into the distal gray matter. Some functional recovery occurred, but it was lost after retransection of the regenerated axons.

Recently, CNS progenitor cells have been transduced to produce specific molecules such as neurotrophins.[365] Stem cells used for directed gene or neurotransmitter delivery[366, 367] offer the potential for integration into the existing neuronal circuits. Adenovirus neurotrophin-3–transfected neurons produce biologically significant quantities of trophic factor.[368] Liu and colleagues[367] determined that neurotrophin-3 retroviral-transduced neural stem cells produced 90 ng/10^6 cells per 24 hours in vitro. When these cells were transplanted into the spinal cord, they migrated, and some differentiated into neurons and astrocytes. Neurotrophin-3 production was inferred from ingrowth of host axons into the graft.

Reduction of Inhibition, Glial Scarring, and Extracellular Matrix

A long-standing concept to explain the failure of CNS regeneration has been that injury is followed by formation of a glial scar that blocks regenerating axons. Glial scarring is a ubiquitous phenomenon after almost all CNS injuries, including the placement of grafts. Observations by Ramón y Cajal[368a] and others established a correlation between reactive CNS glia and failure of regeneration. During the 1950s, Windle[369] showed that axons of regenerating peripheral nerves placed into CNS tissue did not appear to penetrate the graft-CNS interface. The subsequent observation that CNS axons can grow extensively within peripheral nerve grafts[370] proved that adult CNS axons have regenerative capacity in a permissive environment. The CNS is normally delimited by an astrocytic glia-limiting membrane, which may serve to prevent the entry of non-CNS cells. Basal lamina is deposited at the surface of this membrane, which normally opposes pia mater. This type of structure is reconstituted after a variety of CNS injuries.[371]

The main cells that participate in the formation of scars at sites of CNS injury are astrocytes, microglia, oligodendrocytes, oligodendrocyte precursors, and meningeal cells. Meningeal cells interacting with astrocytes form a new glia limitans at sites of CNS injury; this "scar" is a poor substrate for axonal growth.[372]

After an injury, astrocytic processes become hypertrophied. They fill with large quantities of GFAP[373, 374] and are interwoven and bound by tight and gap junctions.[375] GFAP up-regulation extends for a substantial distance from the injury site. Astrocytic release of CNTF after injury is associated with induction of the reactive phenotype.[376, 377] Macrophage and microglial cytokines also play a role in astrogliosis.[378] Astrocytes near the area of injury also up-regulate the intermediate filaments nestin and vimentin. For many years, tightly interwoven GFAP-containing processes were believed to constitute a mechanical barrier. However, axonal glial scars are not inhibitory in Amphibia,[379] and even large, disorganized scars in the *Xenopus* visual system do not inhibit regenerating axons.[380] Alternatively, the absence of glial scar components is insufficient to allow regeneration.[381, 382]

Astrocytes are very plastic, displaying growth-promoting or growth-inhibiting properties under different circumstances. Newborn astrocytes produce N-CAD, N-CAM, and laminin, which support axonal growth. Transplanted embryonic astrocytes can support regeneration through the normally inhibitory DREZ.[232] However, reactive astrocytes are not a good substrate for axonal growth[383] and express truncated neurotrophin receptors that can bind neurotrophic molecules, reducing their effective concentration and possibly reducing their biologic effectiveness.[384]

Microglia are activated by injury. They degrade myelin inhibitory molecules[44] and can make astrocytes more permissive to axonal growth.[385] A massive microglia-macrophage response may support optic nerve regeneration in *Xenopus*.[386] Therefore, microglial cells are unlikely to contribute to inhibition and, together with invading macrophages, probably support axonal sprouting.

The ECM produced by local cells after CNS injury appears to play a key role in blocking regeneration.[387, 388] Chondroitin sulfate proteoglycans produced by astrocytes, oligodendrocytes, oligodendrocyte precursors, and meningeal cells within glial scars are strongly implicated in regeneration failure.[229, 388] During CNS development, chondroitin sulfate proteoglycans are important in segregation of axonal bundles,[389, 390] and they may serve to stabilize the connections of the mature nervous system.[391] Chondroitin sulfate proteoglycans up-regulated at injury sites include neurocan, phosphocan, NG-2, and brevican.[392] Neurocan and phosphocan are produced by astrocytes and are found in chronic glial scars.[393] Neurocan is secreted into the ECM and inhibits axonal growth mediated by N-CAM and L1.[394] Its production has been linked to injury cytokines such as transforming growth factor-β.[395] Phosphocan is membrane bound and also appears to interfere with N-CAM function.[396]

Oligodendrocyte precursors are extensively recruited to injury sites and express large quantities of the proteoglycan NG-2 on their surface. NG-2 may be released and binds to other ECM components. NG-2 can also be produced by astrocytes and is highly inhibitory to axonal extension.[397] IL-1 is a potent stimulus for NG-2 production (Fawcett, personal communication, 1999). Specific blockade of NG-2 can increase neurite growth.[398] CNS myelin contains the chondroitin sulfate proteoglycans versican and brevican, which are inhibitory to axonal growth in vitro. The production of these chondroitin sulfate proteoglycans by oligodendrocytes can be inhibited by inhibitors of proteoglycan synthesis.[399]

Tenascin is a large molecule up-regulated by astrocytes and meningeal cells after CNS injury. Tenascin R exerts an inhibitory effect on axonal growth through an interaction with the neuronal receptor F3/11 and also has several binding sites for inhibitory chondroitin sulfate proteoglycans.[400]

Enzymatic removal of chondroitin sulfate proteoglycans from glial scars makes them more permissive.[401] Chondroitinase cleaves the side chains of chondroitin sulfate proteoglycans, promoting regeneration that may be mediated by laminin within the glial scar.[402] Spinal cord irradiation can increase regeneration, apparently in concert with decreased glial scarring.[4, 231]

Reduction of Inhibition and Myelin

An important neurobiologic discovery of the past decade was that adult CNS myelin inhibits the growth of neuronal processes.[403] Multiple independent lines of evidence now support this principle. Initial observations on cultured spinal cord slices showed that neurites failed to attach to white matter.[404] Cultured neurons failed to enter optic nerves[236] but readily regenerated into sciatic nerves. Increased regeneration was observed in spinal cords rendered myelin free by neonatal irradiation.[405] Extraction and fractionation of CNS myelin led to the identification of two inhibitory protein fractions, NI-35 and NI-250.[406] A monoclonal antibody (IN-1) raised against one of these fractions blocked inhibitory epitopes on CNS myelin in vitro[407] and in vivo,[408] permitting some functional recovery.[409] The protein to which IN-1 binds is called nogo A, and it was recently cloned.[410] In vitro studies have demonstrated that contact between elongating neuronal growth cones and oligodendrocyte membranes leads to a specific stop reaction[411] that is accompanied by markedly increased intracellular calcium[412] and collapse of the local cytoskeleton, presumably mediated through a second messenger pathway. This response could be inhibited by prebinding of oligodendrocytes with the antibody IN-1, and it could be induced by contact with NI-35–containing liposomes. Another molecule with inhibitory activity in certain contexts is myelin-associated glycoprotein.[413, 414] Myelin-associated glycoprotein function is complex and is influenced by concomitant trk receptor expression and exposure to neurotrophic factors.[415]

Myelin-associated inhibition may serve to restrict plasticity in the adult CNS and to define boundaries during development.[16, 416, 417] The permissive period for CNS regeneration can be extended by experimentally delaying the onset of myelination,[102, 418] and immunologic disruption of myelin increases axonal regeneration in the adult rat spinal cord.[419] Myelin, however, is not inhibitory to neuronal processes under all conditions[420]; immature neuronal cells can grow extensively in spinal cord white matter tracts.[92, 421] Recent studies demonstrate that adult DRG axons can grow extensively on white matter if they are transplanted with minimal trauma.[422] These observations focus attention on the role of neuronal surface receptors and the intrinsic state of the neuron to mediate growth or inhibition.

Removal of myelin debris is rather slow, especially in humans. Myelin debris within the glial scar is inhibitory.

Clinical application of myelin-blocking antibodies has not yet been attempted. The hybridoma tumors used to produce antibodies in experiments are infeasible. Intrathecal delivery of engineered Fab fragments leads to increased axonal sprouting, but adverse effects were encountered (Schnell, personal communication, 1999). Further, application of anti-inhibitor antibodies might lead to aberrant plasticity in uninjured systems.[423]

Recently, Huang and colleagues[424] demonstrated that vaccination with homogenized spinal cord delivered in incomplete Freund's adjuvant can elicit effects similar to those seen with IN-1 antibody in a mouse model of corticospinal injury. The authors presented evidence that increased regeneration was due to blockade of inhibition by serum antibodies; however, the immunization protocol was started before injury. These authors saw no evidence of increased CNS inflammation, but it remains a concern, because slightly different vaccination strategies can cause a multiple sclerosis–like pathology in rodents.

Chronic Injury

A critical issue is the timing of intervention after injury. The initial hospital course of injured patients, particularly those with multiple traumatic injuries, is often complicated. It is difficult to be absolutely certain that an injury is complete unless there is radiologic evidence of complete transection or significant hemorrhage. Thus, the appropriate selection of patients for major restorative interventions, such as grafting, may be problematic soon after injury. Therefore, it is important to know the window for efficacy of an intervention. Of course, interventions associated with minimal morbidity rates can be implemented in a less stringently selected group of patients.

Only a relatively small number of studies of chronic injuries have been performed. Neurotrophic factors can augment responses from chronically injured neu-

rons.[425, 426] Von Meyenburg and associates[427] assessed the ability of the IN-1 antibody and neurotrophin-3 to support regeneration and sprouting of chronically injured corticospinal fibers 2 and 8 weeks after injury. At both times, corticospinal sprouting could be elicited by neurotrophin-3, but long-distance regeneration occurred only when the strategy was applied 2 weeks after injury. Only minimal behavioral improvement followed these chronic treatments. The impression from a broad review of the experimental literature is that regenerative strategies are more likely to be effective if they are initiated within the first few days after injury.

SUMMARY

The objective of restorative neurobiology is to learn how to achieve meaningful functional recovery in the context of CNS injury. Major advances have been made in the past decade. Dramatic results often raise hopes of immediate clinical applicability, but it has been difficult to reproduce some of the most promising observations. Successful strategies are likely to be those that exhibit robust effects in several different laboratories. Effective therapies will likely evolve in proportion to the depth of our understanding of CNS injury and regeneration at the molecular level. There also may be important biologic differences between humans and the animals from which experimental data are derived. As we enter the era of human trials, unexpected observations and controversies may arise. I am convinced, however, that meaningful brain and spinal cord repair is possible.

REFERENCES

1. Zlokovic BV, Apuzzo ML: Cellular and molecular neurosurgery: Pathways from concept to reality. Part 1. Target disorders and concept approaches to gene therapy of the central nervous system. Neurosurgery 40:789–804, 1997.
2. Houle JD, Ye JH: Survival of chronically-injured neurons can be prolonged by treatment with neurotrophic factors. Neuroscience 94:929–936, 1999.
3. Kalderon N, Fuks Z: Structural recovery in lesioned adult mammalian spinal cord by x-irradiation of the lesion site. Proc Natl Acad Sci U S A 93:11179–11184, 1996.
4. Ridet JL, Pencalet P, Belcram M, et al: Effects of spinal cord x-irradiation on the recovery of paraplegic rats. Exp Neurol 161:1–14, 2000.
5. Fehlings MG, Tator CH, Linden RD: The effect of direct-current field on recovery from experimental spinal cord injury. J Neurosurg 68:781–792, 1988.
6. Borgens RB: Electrically mediated regeneration and guidance of adult mammalian spinal axons into polymeric channels. Neuroscience 91:251–264, 1999.
7. Neumann S, Woolf CJ: Regeneration of dorsal column fibers into and beyond the lesion site following adult spinal cord injury. Neuron 23:83–91, 1999.
8. Falci S, Holtz A, Akesson E, et al: Obliteration of a posttraumatic spinal cord cyst with solid human embryonic spinal cord grafts: First clinical attempt. J Neurotrauma 14:875–884, 1997.
9. Amar AP, Levy ML: Pathogenesis and pharmacological strategies for mitigating secondary damage in acute spinal cord injury. Neurosurgery 44:1027–1040, 1999.
10. Beattie MS, Leedy MG, Bresnahan JC: Evidence for alterations of synaptic inputs to sacral spinal reflex circuits after spinal cord transection in the cat. Exp Neurol 123:35–50, 1993.

11. de Groat WC, Araki I, Vizzard MA, et al: Developmental and injury induced plasticity in the micturition reflex pathway. Behav Brain Res 92:127–140, 1998.

12. Shapiro S: Neurotransmission by neurons that use serotonin, noradrenaline, glutamate, glycine, and gamma-aminobutyric acid in the normal and injured spinal cord. Neurosurgery 40:168–177, 1997.

13. Calancie B: Interlimb reflexes following cervical spinal cord injury in man. Exp Brain Res 85:458–469, 1991.

14. Woolf CJ, Shortland P, Coggeshall RE: Peripheral nerve injury triggers central sprouting of myelinated afferents. Nature 355:75–78, 1992.

15. Aoki M, Fujito Y, Satomi H, et al: The possible role of collateral sprouting in the functional restitution of corticospinal connections after spinal hemisection. Neurosci Res 3:617–627, 1986.

16. Thallmair M, Metz GA, Z'Graggen WJ, et al: Neurite growth inhibitors restrict plasticity and functional recovery following corticospinal tract lesions. Nat Neurosci 1:124–131, 1998.

17. Livesey FJ, Hunt SP: Differential display cloning of genes induced in regenerating neurons. Methods 16:386–395, 1998.

18. Iyer VR, Eisen MB, Ross DT, et al: The transcriptional program in the response of human fibroblasts to serum. Science 283:83–87, 1999.

19. Luo L, Salunga RC, Guo H, et al: Gene expression profiles of laser-captured adjacent neuronal subtypes. Nat Med 5:117–122, 1999; erratum in Nat Med 5:355, 1999.

20. Vaudano E, Campbell G, Hunt SP, et al: Axonal injury and peripheral nerve grafting in the thalamus and cerebellum of the adult rat: Upregulation of c-jun and correlation with regenerative potential. Eur J Neurosci 10:2644–2656, 1998.

21. Anderson PN, Campbell G, Zhang Y, et al: Cellular and molecular correlates of the regeneration of adult mammalian CNS axons into peripheral nerve grafts. Prog Brain Res 117:211–232, 1998.

22. Aubert I, Ridet JL, Gage FH: Regeneration in the adult mammalian CNS: Guided by development. Curr Opin Neurobiol 5:625–635, 1995.

23. Fawcett JW, Mathews G, Housden E, et al: Regenerating sciatic nerve axons contain the adult rather than the embryonic pattern of microtubule associated proteins. Neuroscience 61:789–804, 1994.

24. Fernandes KJ, Fan DP, Tsui BJ, et al: Influence of the axotomy to cell body distance in rat rubrospinal and spinal motoneurons: Differential regulation of GAP-43, tubulins, and neurofilament-M. J Comp Neurol 414:495–510, 1999.

25. Kobayashi NR, Fan DP, Giehl KM, et al: BDNF and NT-4/5 prevent atrophy of rat rubrospinal neurons after cervical axotomy, stimulate GAP-43 and T alpha 1-tubulin mRNA expression, and promote axonal regeneration. J Neurosci 17:9583–9595, 1997.

26. Tetzlaff W, Kobayashi N, Giehl K, et al: Response of rubrospinal and corticospinal neurons to injury and neurotrophins. In Seil F (ed): Progress in Brain Research. New York, Elsevier Science, 1994, pp 271–286.

27. Tetzlaff W, Alexander SW, Miller FD, et al: Response of facial and rubrospinal neurons to axotomy: Changes in mRNA expression for cytoskeletal proteins and GAP-43. J Neurosci 11:2528–2544, 1991.

28. Wong J, Oblinger MM: A comparison of peripheral and central axotomy effects on neurofilament and tubulin gene expression in rat dorsal root ganglion neurons. J Neurosci 10:2215–2222, 1990.

29. Richardson PM, Issa VM, Aguayo AA: Regeneration of long spinal axons in the rat. J Neurocytol 13:165–182, 1984.

30. Medawar P: Immunity of homologous grafted skin. III. The fate of skin homografts transplanted to the brain, to subcutaneous tissue and to the anterior chamber of the eye. Br J Exp Pathol 29:58–69, 1948.

31. Wong GH, Bartlett PF, Clark-Lewis I, et al: Inducible expression of H-2 and Ia antigens on brain cells. Nature 310:688–691, 1984.

32. Schwartz M, Moalem G, Leibowitz-Amit R, et al: Innate and adaptive immune responses can be beneficial for CNS repair. Trends Neurosci 22:295–299, 1999.

33. Streit WJ, Semple-Rowland SL, Hurley SD, et al: Cytokine mRNA profiles in contused spinal cord and axotomized facial nucleus suggest a beneficial role for inflammation and gliosis. Exp Neurol 152:74–87, 1998.

34. Klein MA, Moller JC, Jones LL, et al: Impaired neuroglial activation in interleukin-6 deficient mice. Glia 19:227–233, 1997.

35. Pitossi F, del Rey A, Kabiersch A, et al: Induction of cytokine transcripts in the central nervous system and pituitary following peripheral administration of endotoxin to mice. J Neurosci Res 48:287–298, 1997.

36. da Cunha A, Vitkovic L: Transforming growth factor-beta 1 (TGF-beta 1) expression and regulation in rat cortical astrocytes. J Neuroimmunol 36:157–169, 1992.

37. Fok-Seang J, DiProspero NA, Meiners S, et al: Cytokine-induced changes in the ability of astrocytes to support migration of oligodendrocyte precursors and axon growth. Eur J Neurosci 10:2400–2415, 1998.

38. Giulian D, Li J, Li X, et al: The impact of microglia-derived cytokines upon gliosis in the CNS. Dev Neurosci 16:128–136, 1994.

39. Meiners S, Marone M, Rittenhouse JL, et al: Regulation of astrocytic tenascin by basic fibroblast growth factor. Dev Biol 160:480–493, 1993.

40. Mahler M, Ferhat L, Gillian A, et al: Tenascin-C mRNA and tenascin-C protein immunoreactivity increase in astrocytes after activation by bFGF. Cell Adhes Commun 4:175–186, 1996.

41. DiProspero NA, Meiners S, Geller HM: Inflammatory cytokines interact to modulate extracellular matrix and astrocytic support of neurite outgrowth. Exp Neurol 148:628–639, 1997.

42. Scripter JL, Ko J, Kow K, et al: Regulation by interleukin-1-beta of formation of a line of delimiting astrocytes following prenatal trauma to the brain of the mouse. Exp Neurol 145(Pt 1):329–341, 1997.

43. Wyss-Coray T, Feng L, Masliah E, et al: Increased central nervous system production of extracellular matrix components and development of hydrocephalus in transgenic mice overexpressing transforming growth factor-beta 1. Am J Pathol 147:53–67, 1995.

44. David S, Bouchard C, Tsatas O, et al: Macrophages can modify the nonpermissive nature of the adult mammalian central nervous system. Neuron 5:463–469, 1990.

45. Lindholm D, Heumann R, Meyer M, et al: Interleukin-1 regulates synthesis of nerve growth factor in non-neuronal cells of rat sciatic nerve. Nature 330:658–659, 1987.

46. Zeev-Brann AB, Lazarov-Spiegler O, Brenner T, et al: Differential effects of central and peripheral nerves on macrophages and microglia. Glia 23:181–190, 1998.

47. Lazarov-Spiegler O, Solomon AS, Schwartz M: Peripheral nerve–stimulated macrophages simulate a peripheral nerve–like regenerative response in rat transected optic nerve. Glia 24:329–337, 1998.

48. Batchelor PE, Liberatore GT, Wong JY, et al: Activated macrophages and microglia induce dopaminergic sprouting in the injured striatum and express brain-derived neurotrophic factor and glial cell line–derived neurotrophic factor. J Neurosci 19:1708–1716, 1999.

49. Nieto-Sampedro M, Lewis ER, Cotman CW, et al: Brain injury causes a time-dependent increase in neuronotrophic activity at the lesion site. Science 217:860–861, 1982.

50. Lucius R, Young HP, Tidow S, et al: Growth stimulation and chemotropic attraction of rat retinal ganglion cell axons in vitro by co-cultured optic nerves, astrocytes and astrocyte conditioned medium. Int J Dev Neurosci 14:387–398, 1996.

51. Schnell L, Fearn S, Schwab ME, et al: Cytokine-induced acute inflammation in the brain and spinal cord. J Neuropathol Exp Neurol 58:245–254, 1999.

52. Crowe MJ, Bresnahan JC, Shuman SL, et al: Apoptosis and delayed degeneration after spinal cord injury in rats and monkeys. Nat Med 3:73–76, 1997; erratum in Nat Med 3:240, 1997.

53. Martinou JC, Sadoul R: ICE-like proteases execute the neuronal death program. Curr Opin Neurobiol 6:609–614, 1996.

54. Rink A, Fung KM, Trojanowski JQ, et al: Evidence of apoptotic cell death after experimental traumatic brain injury in the rat. Am J Pathol 147:1575–1583, 1995.

55. Yakovlev AG, Knoblach SM, Fan L, et al: Activation of CPP32-like caspases contributes to neuronal apoptosis and neurological dysfunction after traumatic brain injury. J Neurosci 17:7415–7424, 1997.

56. Kermer P, Klocker N, Labes M, et al: Inhibition of CPP32-like proteases rescues axotomized retinal ganglion cells from secondary cell death in vivo. J Neurosci 18:4656–4662, 1998.

57. Springer JE, Azbill RD, Knapp PE: Activation of the caspase-3 apoptotic cascade in traumatic spinal cord injury. Nat Med 5:943–946, 1999.

58. Springer JE, Azbill RD, Kennedy SE, et al: Rapid calpain I activation and cytoskeletal protein degradation following traumatic spinal cord injury: Attenuation with riluzole pretreatment. J Neurochem 69:1592–1600, 1997.

59. Wada S, Yone K, Ishidou Y, et al: Apoptosis following spinal cord injury in rats and preventative effect of N-methyl-D-aspartate receptor antagonist. J Neurosurg 91(Suppl):98–104, 1999.

60. Sinson G, Perri BR, Trojanowski JQ, et al: Improvement of cognitive deficits and decreased cholinergic neuronal cell loss and apoptotic cell death following neurotrophin infusion after experimental traumatic brain injury. J Neurosurg 86:511–518, 1997.

61. Suzuki M, Takashima T, Ueda F, et al: Olivary degeneration after intracranial haemorrhage or trauma: Follow-up MRI. Neuroradiology 41:9–12, 1999.

62. Smith MC: Histological findings after hemicerebellectomy in man: Anterograde, retrograde and transneuronal degeneration. Brain Res 95:423–442, 1975.

63. Suzuki H, Oyanagi K, Takahashi H, et al: Evidence for transneuronal degeneration in the spinal cord in man: A quantitative investigation of neurons in the intermediate zone after long-term amputation of the unilateral upper arm. Acta Neuropathol (Berl) 89:464–470, 1995.

64. Terao S, Li M, Hashizume Y, et al: Upper motor neuron lesions in stroke patients do not induce anterograde transneuronal degeneration in spinal anterior horn cells. Stroke 28:2553–2556, 1997.

65. Bjugn R, Nyengaard JR, Rosland JH: Spinal cord transection—no loss of distal ventral horn neurons: Modern stereological techniques reveal no transneuronal changes in the ventral horns of the mouse lumbar spinal cord after thoracic cord transection. Exp Neurol 148:179–186, 1997.

66. Tuszynski MH, Gabriel K, Gerhardt K, et al: Human spinal cord retains substantial structural mass in chronic stages after injury. J Neurotrauma 16:523–531, 1999.

67. Krassioukov AV, Bunge RP, Pucket WR, et al: The changes in human spinal sympathetic preganglionic neurons after spinal cord injury. Spinal Cord 37:6–13, 1999.

68. Yang JF, Stein RB, Jhamandas J, et al: Motor unit numbers and contractile properties after spinal cord injury. Ann Neurol 28:496–502, 1990.

69. Gould DJ, Goshgarian HG: Glial changes in the phrenic nucleus following superimposed cervical spinal cord hemisection and peripheral chronic phrenicotomy injuries in adult rats. Exp Neurol 148:1–9, 1997.

70. Padel Y, Angaut P, Massion J, et al: Comparative study of the posterior red nucleus in baboons and gibbons. J Comp Neurol 202:421–438, 1981.

71. Prendergast J, Stelzner DJ: Changes in the magnocellular portion of the red nucleus following thoracic hemisection in the neonatal and adult rat. J Comp Neurol 166:163–171, 1976.

72. Shamboul KM: Lumbosacral predominance of vestibulospinal fibre projection in the rat. J Comp Neurol 192:519–530, 1980.

73. Smith MC: Retrograde cell changes in human spinal cord after anterolateral cordotomies: Location and identification after different periods of survival. In Bonica JJ (ed): Proceedings of the Third World Congress on Pain, Advances in Pain Research and Therapy, vol 5. New York, Raven Press, 1976, pp 91–98.

74. Pallini R, Fernandez E, Sbriccoli A: Retrograde degeneration of corticospinal axons following transection of the spinal cord in rats: A quantitative study with anterogradely transported horseradish peroxidase. J Neurosurg 68:124–128, 1988.

75. Bronson R, Gilles FH, Hall J, et al: Long term post-traumatic retrograde corticospinal degeneration in man. Hum Pathol 9:602–607, 1978.

76. Yamamoto T, Yamasaki M, Imai T: Retrograde pyramidal tract degeneration in a patient with cervical haematomyelia. J Neurol Neurosurg Psychiatry 52:382–386, 1989.

77. Weibel D, Kreutzberg GW, Schwab ME: Brain-derived neuro-

78. trophic factor (BDNF) prevents lesion-induced axonal die-back in young rat optic nerve. Brain Res 679:249–254, 1995.

78. Guest JD, Hesse D, Schnell L, et al: Influence of IN-1 antibody and acidic FGF-fibrin glue on the response of injured corticospinal tract axons to human Schwann cell grafts. J Neurosci Res 50:888–905, 1997.

79. Tseng GF, Shu J, Huang SJ, et al: A time-dependent loss of retrograde transport ability in distally axotomized rubrospinal neurons. Anat Embryol (Berl) 191:243–249, 1995.

80. Stoll G, Muller HW: Nerve injury, axonal degeneration and neural regeneration: Basic insights. Brain Pathol 9:313–325, 1999.

81. Aldskogius H, Kozlova EN: Central neuron-glial and glial-glial interactions following axon injury. Prog Neurobiol 55:1–26, 1998.

82. Frisen J, Haegerstrand A, Fried K, et al: Adhesive/repulsive properties in the injured spinal cord: Relation to myelin phagocytosis by invading macrophages. Exp Neurol 129:183–193, 1994.

83. Davies SJ, Goucher DR, Doller C, et al: Robust regeneration of adult sensory axons in degenerating white matter of the adult rat spinal cord. J Neurosci 19:5810–5822, 1999.

84. Hikawa N, Takenaka T: Myelin-stimulated macrophages release neurotrophic factors for adult dorsal root ganglion neurons in culture. Cell Mol Neurobiol 16:517–528, 1996.

85. Avellino AM, Hart D, Dailey AT, et al: Differential macrophage responses in the peripheral and central nervous system during wallerian degeneration of axons. Exp Neurol 136:183–198, 1995.

86. Zhang Z, Guth L, Steward O: Mechanisms of motor recovery after subtotal spinal cord injury: Insights from the study of mice carrying a mutation (WldS) that delays cellular responses to injury. Exp Neurol 149:221–229, 1998.

87. Fruttiger M, Schachner M, Martini R: Tenascin-C expression during wallerian degeneration in C57BL/Wlds mice: Possible implications for axonal regeneration. J Neurocytol 24:1–14, 1995.

88. Stuermer CA, Bastmeyer M, Bahr M, et al: Trying to understand axonal regeneration in the CNS of fish. J Neurobiol 23:537–550, 1992.

89. Lurie DI, Selzer ME: Axonal regeneration in the adult lamprey spinal cord. J Comp Neurol 306:409–416, 1991.

90. Bastmeyer M, Bahr M, Stuermer CA: Fish optic nerve oligodendrocytes support axonal regeneration of fish and mammalian retinal ganglion cells. Glia 8:1–11, 1993.

91. Varga ZM, Bandtlow CE, Erulkar SD, et al: The critical period for repair of CNS of neonatal opossum (*Monodelphis domestica*) in culture: Correlation with development of glial cells, myelin and growth-inhibitory molecules. Eur J Neurosci 7:2119–2129, 1995.

92. Wictorin K, Bjorklund A: Axon outgrowth from grafts of human embryonic spinal cord in the lesioned adult rat spinal cord. Neuroreport 3:1045–1048, 1992.

93. Archer FR, Doherty P, Collins D, et al: CAMs and FGF cause a local submembrane calcium signal promoting axon outgrowth without a rise in bulk calcium concentration. Eur J Neurosci 11:3565–3573, 1999.

94. Doherty P, Walsh FS: CAM-FGF receptor interactions: A model for axonal growth. Mol Cell Neurosci 8:99–111, 1996.

95. Meiri KF, Saffell JL, Walsh FS, et al: Neurite outgrowth stimulated by neural cell adhesion molecules requires growth-associated protein-43 (GAP-43) function and is associated with GAP-43 phosphorylation in growth cones. J Neurosci 18:10429–10437, 1998.

96. Walsh FS, Meiri K, Doherty P: Cell signaling and CAM-mediated neurite outgrowth. Soc Gen Physiol Ser 52:221–226, 1997.

97. Bates CA, Becker CG, Miotke JA, et al: Expression of polysialylated NCAM but not L1 or N-cadherin by regenerating adult mouse optic fibers in vitro. Exp Neurol 155:128–139, 1999.

98. Fu SY, Gordon T: The cellular and molecular basis of peripheral nerve regeneration. Mol Neurobiol 14:67–116, 1997.

99. Schmidt CE, Dai J, Lauffenburger DA, et al: Integrin-cytoskeletal interactions in neuronal growth cones. J Neurosci 15(Pt 1):3400–3407, 1995.

100. Kuhn TB, Schmidt MF, Kater SB: Laminin and fibronectin guideposts signal sustained but opposite effects to passing growth cones. Neuron 14:275–285, 1995.

101. Dow KE, Ethell DW, Steeves JD, et al: Molecular correlates of

spinal cord repair in the embryonic chick: Heparan sulfate and chondroitin sulfate proteoglycans. Exp Neurol 128:233–238, 1994.

102. Keirstead HS, Hasan SJ, Muir GD, et al: Suppression of the onset of myelination extends the permissive period for the functional repair of embryonic spinal cord. Proc Natl Acad Sci U S A 89:11664–11668, 1992.

103. Tear G: Molecular cues that guide the development of neural connectivity. Essays Biochem 33:1–13, 1998.

104. Hong K, Nishiyama M, Henley J, et al: Calcium signaling in the guidance of nerve growth by netrin-1. Nature 403:93–98, 2000.

105. Windle W, Smart J, Beers J: Residual function after subtotal spinal cord transection in adult cats. Neurology 8:518–521, 1958.

106. Eidelberg E, Straehley D, Erspamer R, et al: Relationship between residual hindlimb-assisted locomotion and surviving axons after incomplete spinal cord injuries. Exp Neurol 56:312–322, 1977.

107. Blight AR: Cellular morphology of chronic spinal cord injury in the cat: Analysis of myelinated axons by line-sampling. Neuroscience 10:521–543, 1983.

108. Eidelberg E, Story JL, Walden JG, et al: Anatomical correlates of return of locomotor function after partial spinal cord lesions in cats. Exp Brain Res 42:81–88, 1981.

109. Fehlings MG, Tator CH: The relationships among the severity of spinal cord injury, residual neurological function, axon counts, and counts of retrogradely labeled neurons after experimental spinal cord injury. Exp Neurol 132:220–228, 1995.

110. Nathan PW: Effects on movement of surgical incisions into the human spinal cord. Brain 117(Pt 2):337–346, 1994.

111. Barbeau H, Rossignol S: Recovery of locomotion after chronic spinalization in the adult cat. Brain Res 412:84–95, 1987.

112. Rossignol S, Chau C, Brustein E, et al: Locomotor capacities after complete and partial lesions of the spinal cord. Acta Neurobiol Exp (Warsz) 56:449–463, 1996.

113. Grillner S, Shik ML: On the descending control of the lumbosacral spinal cord from the "mesencephalic locomotor region." Acta Physiol Scand 87:320–333, 1973.

114. Steeves JD, Jordan LM: Localization of a descending pathway in the spinal cord which is necessary for controlled treadmill locomotion. Neurosci Lett 20:283–288, 1980.

115. Eidelberg E, Walden JG, Nguyen LH: Locomotor control in macaque monkeys. Brain 104(Pt 4):647–663, 1981.

116. Dietz V, Colombo G, Jensen L: Locomotor activity in spinal man. Lancet 344:1260–1263, 1994.

117. Calancie B, Needham-Shropshire B, Jacobs P, et al: Involuntary stepping after chronic spinal cord injury: Evidence for a central rhythm generator for locomotion in man. Brain 117(Pt 5):1143–1159, 1994.

118. Barbeau H, McCrea DA, O'Donovan MJ, et al: Tapping into spinal circuits to restore motor function. Brain Res Brain Res Rev 30:27–51, 1999.

119. Maier MA, Illert M, Kirkwood PA, et al: Does a C3-C4 propriospinal system transmit corticospinal excitation in the primate? An investigation in the macaque monkey. J Physiol (Lond) 511(Pt 1):191–212, 1998.

120. Dzuris JL, Sidney J, Appella E, et al: Conserved MHC class I peptide binding motif between humans and rhesus macaques. J Immunol 164:283–291, 2000.

121. Gruner JA: A monitored contusion model of spinal cord injury in the rat. J Neurotrauma 9:123–128, 1992.

122. Stokes BT: Experimental spinal cord injury: A dynamic and verifiable injury device. J Neurotrauma 9:129–134, 1992.

123. Behrmann DL, Bresnahan JC, Beattie MS, et al: Spinal cord injury produced by consistent mechanical displacement of the cord in rats: Behavioral and histologic analysis. J Neurotrauma 9:197–217, 1992.

124. Metz GA, Curt A, van de Meent H, et al: Validation of the weight-drop contusion model in rats: A comparative study of human spinal cord injury. J Neurotrauma 17:1–17, 2000.

125. Cheng H, Cao Y, Olson L: Spinal cord repair in adult paraplegic rats: Partial restoration of hind limb function. Science 273:510–513, 1996.

126. Rapalino O, Lazarov-Spiegler O, Agranov E, et al: Implantation of stimulated homologous macrophages results in partial recovery of paraplegic rats. Nat Med 4:814–821, 1998.

127. Basso DM, Beattie MS, Bresnahan JC: A sensitive and reliable locomotor rating scale for open field testing in rats. J Neurotrauma 12:1–21, 1995.

128. Guest JD, Rao A, Olson L, et al: The ability of human Schwann cell grafts to promote regeneration in the transected nude rat spinal cord. Exp Neurol 148:502–522, 1997.

129. Jakeman LB, Wei P, Guan Z, et al: Brain-derived neurotrophic factor stimulates hindlimb stepping and sprouting of cholinergic fibers after spinal cord injury. Exp Neurol 154:170–184, 1998.

130. Basso DM, Beattie MS, Bresnahan JC: Graded histological and locomotor outcomes after spinal cord contusion using the NYU weight-drop device versus transection. Exp Neurol 139:244–256, 1996.

131. Tarlov I, Klinger H: Spinal cord compression studies. II. Time limits for recovery after acute compression in dogs. Arch Neurol Psychol 71:271–290, 1954.

132. Wrathall JR, Pettegrew RK, Harvey F: Spinal cord contusion in the rat: Production of graded, reproducible injury groups. Exp Neurol 88:108–122, 1985.

133. Rivlin A, Tator C: Objective clinical assessment of motor function after experimental spinal cord injury in the rat. J Neurosurg 47:577–581, 1977.

134. Gimenez y Ribotta M, Orsal D, Feraboli-Lohnherr D, et al: Recovery of locomotion following transplantation of monoaminergic neurons in the spinal cord of paraplegic rats. Ann N Y Acad Sci 860:393–411, 1998.

135. Feraboli-Lohnherr D, Orsal D, Yakovleff A, et al: Recovery of locomotor activity in the adult chronic spinal rat after sublesional transplantation of embryonic nervous cells: Specific role of serotonergic neurons. Exp Brain Res 113:443–454, 1997.

136. Veenman CL, Reiner A, Honig MG: Biotinylated dextran amine as an anterograde tracer for single- and double-labeling studies. J Neurosci Methods 41:239–254, 1992.

137. Li Y, Raisman G: Schwann cells induce sprouting in motor and sensory axons in the adult spinal cord. J Neurosci 14:4050–4053, 1994.

138. Olson L, Malmfors T: Growth characteristics of adrenergic nerves in the adult rat: Fluorescence histochemical and 3H-noradrenaline uptake studies using tissue transplantations to the anterior chamber of the eye. Acta Physiol Scand (Suppl) 348:1–112, 1970.

139. Freed WJ, Perlow MJ, Karoum F, et al: Restoration of dopaminergic function by grafting of fetal rat substantia nigra to the caudate nucleus: Long-term behavioral, biochemical, and histochemical studies. Ann Neurol 8:510–519, 1980.

140. Lindvall O: Update on fetal transplantation: The Swedish experience. Mov Disord 13(Suppl 1):83–87, 1998.

141. Sladek JR Jr, Collier TJ, Haber SN, et al: Survival and growth of fetal catecholamine neurons transplanted into primate brain. Brain Res Bull 17:809–818, 1986.

142. Kordower JH, Goetz CG, Freeman TB, et al: Dopaminergic transplants in patients with Parkinson's disease: Neuroanatomical correlates of clinical recovery. Exp Neurol 144:41–46, 1997.

143. Remy P, Samson Y, Hantraye P, et al: Clinical correlates of (18F)fluorodopa uptake in five grafted parkinsonian patients. Ann Neurol 38:580–588, 1995.

144. Mamelak AN, Eggerding FA, Oh DS, et al: Fatal cyst formation after fetal mesencephalic allograft transplant for Parkinson's disease. J Neurosurg 89:592–598, 1998.

145. Bakay RA, Boyer KL, Freed CR, et al: Immunological responses to injury and grafting in the central nervous system of nonhuman primates. Cell Transplant 7:109–120, 1998.

146. Borlongan CV, Stahl CE, Cameron DF, et al: CNS immunological modulation of neural graft rejection and survival. Neurol Res 18:297–304, 1996.

147. Sladek J, Collier T, Elsworth J, et al: Fetal grafts in Parkinson's disease. In Tuszynski M, Kordower J (eds): CNS Regeneration: Basic Science and Clinical Advances. San Diego, Calif, Academic Press, 1999, pp 321–364.

148. Zhou J, Bradford HF, Stern GM: Influence of BDNF on the expression of the dopaminergic phenotype of tissue used for brain transplants. Brain Res Dev Brain Res 100:43–51, 1997.

149. Mehta V, Hong M, Spears J, et al: Enhancement of graft survival and sensorimotor behavioral recovery in rats undergoing transplantation with dopaminergic cells exposed to glial cell line–derived neurotrophic factor. J Neurosurg 88:1088–1095, 1998.

150. Eaton MJ, Whittemore SR: Autocrine BDNF secretion enhances the survival and serotonergic differentiation of raphe neuronal precursor cells grafted into the adult rat CNS. Exp Neurol 140: 105–114, 1996.

151. Jakeman LB, Reier PJ: Axonal projections between fetal spinal cord transplants and the adult rat spinal cord: A neuroanatomical tracing study of local interactions. J Comp Neurol 307: 311–334, 1991.

152. Bregman BS, Kunkel-Bagden E, Reier PJ, et al: Recovery of function after spinal cord injury: Mechanisms underlying transplant-mediated recovery of function differ after spinal cord injury in newborn and adult rats. Exp Neurol 123:3–16, 1993.

153. Diener PS, Bregman BS: Fetal spinal cord transplants support growth of supraspinal and segmental projections after cervical spinal cord hemisection in the neonatal rat. J Neurosci 18: 779–793, 1998.

154. Diener PS, Bregman BS: Fetal spinal cord transplants support the development of target reaching and coordinated postural adjustments after neonatal cervical spinal cord injury. J Neurosci 18:763–778, 1998.

155. Bregman BS, McAtee M, Dai HN, et al: Neurotrophic factors increase axonal growth after spinal cord injury and transplantation in the adult rat. Exp Neurol 148:475–494, 1997.

156. Bregman BS, Broude E, McAtee M, et al: Transplants and neurotrophic factors prevent atrophy of mature CNS neurons after spinal cord injury. Exp Neurol 149:13–27, 1998.

157. Mori F, Himes BT, Kowada M, et al: Fetal spinal cord transplants rescue some axotomized rubrospinal neurons from retrograde cell death in adult rats. Exp Neurol 143:45–60, 1997.

158. Stokes BT, Reier PJ: Fetal grafts alter chronic behavioral outcome after contusion damage to the adult rat spinal cord. Exp Neurol 116:1–12, 1992.

159. Anderson DK, Howland DR, Reier PJ: Fetal neural grafts and repair of the injured spinal cord. Brain Pathol 5:451–457, 1995.

160. Giovanini MA, Reier PJ, Eskin TA, et al: Characteristics of human fetal spinal cord grafts in the adult rat spinal cord: Influences of lesion and grafting conditions. Exp Neurol 148: 523–543, 1997.

161. Theele DP, Schrimsher GW, Reier PJ: Comparison of the growth and fate of fetal spinal iso- and allografts in the adult rat injured spinal cord. Exp Neurol 142:128–143, 1996.

162. Theele DP, Reier PJ: Immunomodulation with intrathymic grafts or anti-lymphocyte serum promotes long-term intraspinal allograft survival. Cell Transplant 5:243–255, 1996.

163. Iwashita Y, Kawaguchi S, Murata M: Restoration of function by replacement of spinal cord segments in the rat. Nature 367: 167–170, 1994.

164. Ito J, Murata M, Kawaguchi S: Regeneration of the lateral vestibulospinal tract in adult rats by transplants of embryonic brain tissue. Neurosci Lett 259:67–70, 1999.

165. Wang S, Wu H, Jiang J, et al: Isolation of neuronal precursors by sorting embryonic forebrain transfected with GFP regulated by the T alpha 1 tubulin promoter. Nat Biotechnol 16:196–201, 1998; erratum in Nat Biotechnol 16:478, 1998.

166. Liu Y, Himes BT, Solowska J, et al: Intraspinal delivery of neurotrophin-3 using neural stem cells genetically modified by recombinant retrovirus. Exp Neurol 158:9–26, 1999.

167. Altman J, Das GD: Autoradiographic and histological evidence of postnatal hippocampal neurogenesis in rats. J Comp Neurol 124:319–335, 1965.

168. Lois C, Alvarez-Buylla A: Long-distance neuronal migration in the adult mammalian brain. Science 264:1145–1148, 1994.

169. Weiss S, Dunne C, Hewson J, et al: Multipotent CNS stem cells are present in the adult mammalian spinal cord and ventricular neuroaxis. J Neurosci 16:7599–7609, 1996.

170. Thomson JA, Kalishman J, Golos TG, et al: Isolation of a primate embryonic stem cell line. Proc Natl Acad Sci U S A 92:7844–7848, 1995.

171. Thomson JA, Itskovitz-Eldor J, Shapiro SS, et al: Embryonic stem cell lines derived from human blastocysts. Science 282: 1145–1147, 1998; erratum in Science 282:1827, 1998.

172. Moore MA: "Turning brain into blood"—clinical applications of stem-cell research in neurobiology and hematology. N Engl J Med 341:605–607, 1999.

173. Kuhn HG, Svendsen CN: Origins, functions, and potential of adult neural stem cells. Bioessays 21:625–630, 1999.

174. Keene C, Reyes M, Zhao L, et al: Phenotypic expression of transplanted human bone marrow–derived multipotent adult stem cells into the rat CNS. Paper presented at the Seventh Annual Meeting of the American Society for Neural Transplantation and Repair, April 2000, Clearwater, Fla.

175. Svendsen CN, Caldwell MA, Ostenfeld T: Human neural stem cells: Isolation, expansion and transplantation. Brain Pathol 9: 499–513, 1999.

176. Pincus DW, Harrison-Restelli C, Barry J, et al: In vitro neurogenesis by adult human epileptic temporal neocortex. Clin Neurosurg 44:17–25, 1997.

177. Kirschenbaum B, Nedergaard M, Preuss A, et al: In vitro neuronal production and differentiation by precursor cells derived from the adult human forebrain. Cereb Cortex 4:576–589, 1994.

178. Eriksson PS, Perfilieva E, Bjork-Eriksson T, et al: Neurogenesis in the adult human hippocampus. Nat Med 4:1313–1317, 1998.

179. Kukekov VG, Laywell ED, Suslov O, et al: Multipotent stem/progenitor cells with similar properties arise from two neurogenic regions of adult human brain. Exp Neurol 156:333–344, 1999.

180. Shihabuddin LS, Ray J, Gage FH: FGF-2 is sufficient to isolate progenitors found in the adult mammalian spinal cord. Exp Neurol 148:577–586, 1997.

181. Reynolds BA, Tetzlaff W, Weiss S: A multipotent EGF-responsive striatal embryonic progenitor cell produces neurons and astrocytes. J Neurosci 12:4565–4574, 1992.

182. Davis AA, Temple S: A self-renewing multipotential stem cell in embryonic rat cerebral cortex. Nature 372:263–266, 1994.

183. Goldman SA, Kirschenbaum B, Harrison-Restelli C, et al: Neuronal precursors of the adult rat subependymal zone persist into senescence, with no decline in spatial extent or response to BDNF. J Neurobiol 32:554–566, 1997.

184. Leventhal C, Rafii S, Rafii D, et al: Endothelial trophic support of neuronal production and recruitment from the adult mammalian subependyma. Mol Cell Neurosci 13:450–464, 1999.

185. van der Kooy D, Weiss S: Why stem cells? Science 287:1439–1441, 2000.

186. Craig CG, Tropepe V, Morshead CM, et al: In vivo growth factor expansion of endogenous subependymal neural precursor cell populations in the adult mouse brain. J Neurosci 16:2649–2658, 1996.

187. Snyder EY, Yoon C, Flax JD, et al: Multipotent neural precursors can differentiate toward replacement of neurons undergoing targeted apoptotic degeneration in adult mouse neocortex. Proc Natl Acad Sci U S A 94:11663–11668, 1997.

188. Magavi S, Leavitt B, Macklis J: Induction of neurogenesis in neocortex of adult mice. Paper presented at the Seventh Annual Meeting of the American Society for Neural Transplantation and Repair, April 2000, Clearwater, Fla.

189. Ray J, Plamer T, Shihabuddin L, et al: The use of neural progenitor cells for therapy in the CNS disorders. In Tuszynski MH, Kordower J (eds): CNS Regeneration: Basic Science and Clinical Advances. San Diego, Calif, Academic Press, 1999, pp 183–201.

190. Vescovi AL, Gritti A, Galli R, et al: Isolation and intracerebral grafting of nontransformed multipotential embryonic human CNS stem cells. J Neurotrauma 16:689–693, 1999.

191. Whittemore SR: Neuronal replacement strategies for spinal cord injury. J Neurotrauma 16:667–673, 1999.

192. Quinn SM, Walters WM, Vescovi AL, et al: Lineage restriction of neuroepithelial precursor cells from fetal human spinal cord. J Neurosci Res 57:590–602, 1999.

193. Raff MC, Miller RH, Noble M: A glial progenitor cell that develops in vitro into an astrocyte or an oligodendrocyte depending on culture medium. Nature 303:390–396, 1983.

194. Kilpatrick TJ, Bartlett PF: Cloned multipotential precursors from the mouse cerebrum require FGF-2, whereas glial restricted precursors are stimulated with either FGF-2 or EGF. J Neurosci 15(Pt 1):3653–3661, 1995.

195. Dinsmore J, Ratliff J, Deacon T, et al: Embryonic stem cells differentiated in vitro as a novel source of cells for transplantation. Cell Transplant 5:131–143, 1996.

196. Reynolds BA, Weiss S: Generation of neurons and astrocytes from isolated cells of the adult mammalian central nervous system. Science 255:1707–1710, 1992.

197. Wang S, Roy NS, Benraiss A, et al: Promoter-based isolation

and fluorescence-activated sorting of mitotic neuronal progenitor cells from the adult mammalian ependymal/subependymal zone. Dev Neurosci 22:167–176, 2000.

198. Turner DL, Cepko CL: A common progenitor for neurons and glia persists in rat retina late in development. Nature 328:131–136, 1987.

199. Rowitch DH, St-Jacques B, Lee SM, et al: Sonic hedgehog regulates proliferation and inhibits differentiation of CNS precursor cells. J Neurosci 19:8954–8965, 1999.

200. Brustle O, Choudhary K, Karram K, et al: Chimeric brains generated by intraventricular transplantation of fetal human brain cells into embryonic rats. Nat Biotechnol 16:1040–1044, 1998.

201. Auerbach JM, Eiden MV, McKay RD: Transplanted CNS stem cells form functional synapses in vivo. Eur J Neurosci 12:1696–1704, 2000.

202. Herrera DG, Garcia-Verdugo JM, Alvarez-Buylla A: Adult-derived neural precursors transplanted into multiple regions in the adult brain. Ann Neurol 46:867–877, 1999.

203. Fricker RA, Carpenter MK, Winkler C, et al: Site-specific migration and neuronal differentiation of human neural progenitor cells after transplantation in the adult rat brain. J Neurosci 19:5990–6005, 1999.

204. Svendsen CN, Clarke DJ, Rosser AE, et al: Survival and differentiation of rat and human epidermal growth factor–responsive precursor cells following grafting into the lesioned adult central nervous system. Exp Neurol 137:376–388, 1996.

205. Svendsen CN, Caldwell MA, Shen J, et al: Long-term survival of human central nervous system progenitor cells transplanted into a rat model of Parkinson's disease. Exp Neurol 148:135–146, 1997.

206. Zigova T, Pencea V, Betarbet R, et al: Neuronal progenitor cells of the neonatal subventricular zone differentiate and disperse following transplantation into the adult rat striatum. Cell Transplant 7:137–156, 1998.

207. Jankovski A, Rossi F, Sotelo C: Neuronal precursors in the postnatal mouse cerebellum are fully committed cells: Evidence from heterochronic transplantations. Eur J Neurosci 8:2308–2319, 1996.

208. Takahashi M, Palmer TD, Takahashi J, et al: Widespread integration and survival of adult-derived neural progenitor cells in the developing optic retina. Mol Cell Neurosci 12:340–348, 1998.

209. McDonald JW, Liu XZ, Qu Y, et al: Transplanted embryonic stem cells survive, differentiate and promote recovery in injured rat spinal cord. Nat Med 5:1410–1412, 1999.

210. Snyder EY, Deitcher DL, Walsh C, et al: Multipotent neural cell lines can engraft and participate in development of mouse cerebellum. Cell 68:33–51, 1992.

211. Shihabuddin LS, Hertz JA, Holets VR, et al: The adult CNS retains the potential to direct region-specific differentiation of a transplanted neuronal precursor cell line. J Neurosci 15:6666–6678, 1995.

212. Shihabuddin LS, Holets VR, Whittemore SR: Selective hippocampal lesions differentially affect the phenotypic fate of transplanted neuronal precursor cells. Exp Neurol 139:61–72, 1996.

213. Onifer SM, Cannon AB, Whittemore SR: Altered differentiation of CNS neural progenitor cells after transplantation into the injured adult rat spinal cord. Cell Transplant 6:327–338, 1997.

214. Winkler C, Fricker RA, Gates MA, et al: Incorporation and glial differentiation of mouse EGF-responsive neural progenitor cells after transplantation into the embryonic rat brain. Mol Cell Neurosci 11:99–116, 1998.

215. Olsson M, Bjerregaard K, Winkler C, et al: Incorporation of mouse neural progenitors transplanted into the rat embryonic forebrain is developmentally regulated and dependent on regional and adhesive properties. Eur J Neurosci 10:71–85, 1998.

216. Thompson TP, Lunsford LD, Kondziolka D: Restorative neurosurgery: Opportunities for restoration of function in acquired, degenerative, and idiopathic neurological diseases. Neurosurgery 45:741–752, 1999.

217. Borlongan CV, Tajima Y, Trojanowski JQ, et al: Transplantation of cryopreserved human embryonal carcinoma-derived neurons (NT2N cells) promotes functional recovery in ischemic rats. Exp Neurol 149:310–321, 1998.

218. Saporta S, Borlongan CV, Sanberg PR: Neural transplantation of human neuroteratocarcinoma (hNT) neurons into ischemic rats: A quantitative dose-response analysis of cell survival and behavioral recovery. Neuroscience 91:519–525, 1999.

219. Richardson PM, McGuinness UM, Aguayo AJ: Axons from CNS neurons regenerate into PNS grafts. Nature 284:264–265, 1980.

220. Hiebert G, McGraw J, Steeves J, et al: BDNF applied to the motor cortex promotes sprouting of corticospinal axons but not regeneration into a peripheral nerve transplant. Soc Neurosci Abstr 193:4, 1999.

221. Sonntag VKH, Gibson A, Guest JD: Tropic and trophic effects of FGF-1 and peripheral nerve grafts on injured CST fibers with and without grey matter sparing lesions. Soc Neurosci Abstr 194:18, 1999.

222. Stensaas L, Partlow LM, Burgess PR, et al: Inhibition of regeneration: The ultrastructure of reactive astrocytes and abortive axon terminals in the transition zone of the dorsal root. Prog Brain Res 71:457–468, 1987.

223. Carlstedt T: Regenerating axons form nerve terminals at astrocytes. Brain Res 347:188–191, 1985.

224. Fraher JP: The transitional zone and CNS regeneration. J Anat 194(Pt 2):161–182, 1999.

225. Carlstedt T: Regrowth of anastomosed ventral root nerve fibers in the dorsal root of rats. Brain Res 272:162–165, 1983.

226. Carlstedt T: Regrowth of cholinergic and catecholaminergic neurons along a peripheral and central nervous pathway. Neuroscience 15:507–518, 1985.

227. Carlstedt T, Dalsgaard CJ, Molander C: Regrowth of lesioned dorsal root nerve fibers into the spinal cord of neonatal rats. Neurosci Lett 74:14–18, 1987.

228. Pindzola RR, Doller C, Silver J: Putative inhibitory extracellular matrix molecules at the dorsal root entry zone during development and after root and sciatic nerve lesions. Dev Biol 156:34–48, 1993.

229. Lemons ML, Howland DR, Anderson DK: Chondroitin sulfate proteoglycan immunoreactivity increases following spinal cord injury and transplantation. Exp Neurol 160:51–65, 1999.

230. Sims TJ, Gilmore SA: Regeneration of dorsal root axons into experimentally altered glial environments in the rat spinal cord. Exp Brain Res 99:25–33, 1994.

231. Sims TJ, Durgun MB, Gilmore SA: Transplantation of sciatic nerve segments into normal and glia-depleted spinal cords. Exp Brain Res 125:495–501, 1999.

232. Kliot M, Smith GM, Siegal JD, et al: Astrocyte-polymer implants promote regeneration of dorsal root fibers into the adult mammalian spinal cord. Exp Neurol 109:57–69, 1990.

233. Gilmore SA, Sims TJ: Glial-glial and glial-neuronal interfaces in radiation-induced, glia-depleted spinal cord. J Anat 190(Pt 1):5–21, 1997.

234. Zhang Y, Dijkhuizen PA, Anderson PN, et al: NT-3 delivered by an adenoviral vector induces injured dorsal root axons to regenerate into the spinal cord of adult rats. J Neurosci Res 54:554–562, 1998.

235. Ramer MS, Priestley JV, McMahon SB: Functional regeneration of sensory axons into the adult spinal cord. Nature 403:312–316, 2000.

236. Schwab ME, Thoenen H: Dissociated neurons regenerate into sciatic but not optic nerve explants in culture irrespective of neurotrophic factors. J Neurosci 5:2415–2423, 1985.

237. Hall S, Kent AP: The response of regenerating peripheral neurites to a grafted optic nerve. J Neurocytol 16:317–331, 1987.

238. Tello F: La influencia del neurotrophismo en la regeneracion de los centros nerviosos. Trabajos Lab Invest Biol Univ Madrid 9:123–159, 1911.

239. Sugar O, Gerard R: Spinal cord regeneration in the rat. J Neurophysiol 3:1–19, 1940.

240. Vidal-Sanz M, Bray GM, Villegas-Perez MP, et al: Axonal regeneration and synapse formation in the superior colliculus by retinal ganglion cells in the adult rat. J Neurosci 7:2894–2909, 1987.

241. Sauve Y, Sawai H, Rasminsky M: Functional synaptic connections made by regenerated retinal ganglion cell axons in the superior colliculus of adult hamsters. J Neurosci 15(Pt 2):665–675, 1995.

242. Hagg T, Vahlsing HL, Manthorpe M, et al: Septohippocampal cholinergic axonal regeneration through peripheral nerve bridg-

es: Quantification and temporal development. Exp Neurol 109: 153–163, 1990.

243. Nygren LG, Fuxe K, Jonsson G, et al: Functional regeneration of 5-hydroxytryptamine nerve terminals in the rat spinal cord following 5,6-dihydroxytryptamine induced degeneration. Brain Res 78:377–394, 1974.

244. Crutcher KA: Tissue sections from the mature rat brain and spinal cord as substrates for neurite outgrowth in vitro: Extensive growth on gray matter but little growth on white matter. Exp Neurol 104:39–54, 1989.

245. Cheng H, Olson L: A new surgical technique that allows proximodistal regeneration of 5-HT fibers after complete transection of the rat spinal cord. Exp Neurol 136:149–161, 1995.

246. Koshinaga M, Sanon HR, Whittemore SR: Altered acidic and basic fibroblast growth factor expression following spinal cord injury. Exp Neurol 120:32–48, 1993.

247. Cordeiro PG, Seckel BR, Lipton SA, et al: Acidic fibroblast growth factor enhances peripheral nerve regeneration in vivo. Plast Reconstr Surg 83:1013–1021, 1989.

248. Cheng H, Fraidakis M, Blomback B, et al: Characterization of a fibrin glue–GDNF slow-release preparation. Cell Transplant 7: 53–61, 1998.

249. Hoffman D, Wahlberg L, Aebischer P: NGF released from a polymer matrix prevents loss of ChAT expression in basal forebrain neurons following a fimbria-fornix lesion. Exp Neurol 110: 39–44, 1990.

250. Emery E, Horvat JC, Tadie M: Motor reconnection between the damaged cervical cord and the denervated biceps muscle using an autologous peripheral nerve segment in the adult marmoset. [French]. Chirurgie 122:252–259, 1997.

251. Hallin RG, Carlstedt T, Nilsson-Remahl I, et al: Spinal cord implantation of avulsed ventral roots in primates: Correlation between restored motor function and morphology. Exp Brain Res 124:304–310, 1999.

252. Carlstedt T, Grane P, Hallin RG, et al: Return of function after spinal cord implantation of avulsed spinal nerve roots. Lancet 346:1323–1325, 1995.

253. Guenard V, Kleitman N, Morrissey TK, et al: Syngeneic Schwann cells derived from adult nerves seeded in semipermeable guidance channels enhance peripheral nerve regeneration. J Neurosci 12:3310–3320, 1992.

254. Xu X, Guenard V, Kleitman N, et al: Axonal regeneration into Schwann cell–seeded guidance channels grafted into transected adult rat spinal cord. J Comp Neurol 351:145–160, 1995.

255. Xu XM, Zhang SX, Li H, et al: Regrowth of axons into the distal spinal cord through a Schwann-cell-seeded mini-channel implanted into hemisected adult rat spinal cord. Eur J Neurosci 11:1723–1740, 1999.

256. Menei P, Montero-Menei C, Whittemore S, et al: Schwann cells genetically modified to secrete human BDNF promote enhanced axonal regrowth across adult rat spinal cord. Eur J Neurosci 10: 607–621, 1998.

257. Ramon-Cueto A, Avila J: Olfactory ensheathing glia: Properties and function. Brain Res Bull 46:173–187, 1998.

258. Monti Graziadei GA, Karlan MS, Bernstein JJ, et al: Reinnervation of the olfactory bulb after section of the olfactory nerve in monkey (*Saimiri sciureus*). Brain Res 189:343–354, 1980.

259. Barber PC: Neurogenesis and regeneration in the primary olfactory pathway of mammals. Bibl Anat 23:12–25, 1982.

260. Raisman G: Specialized neuroglial arrangement may explain the capacity of vomeronasal axons to reinnervate central neurons. Neuroscience 14:237–254, 1985.

261. Doucette R: PNS-CNS transitional zone of the first cranial nerve. J Comp Neurol 312:451–466, 1991.

262. Wright JW, Harding JW: Recovery of olfactory function after bilateral bulbectomy. Science 216:322–324, 1982.

263. Miragall F, Kadmon G, Husmann M, et al: Expression of cell adhesion molecules in the olfactory system of the adult mouse: Presence of the embryonic form of N-CAM. Dev Biol 129:516–531, 1988.

264. Barber PC, Lindsay RM: Schwann cells of the olfactory nerves contain glial fibrillary acidic protein and resemble astrocytes. Neuroscience 7:3077–3090, 1982.

265. Gudino-Cabrera G, Nieto-Sampedro M: Schwann-like macroglia in adult rat brain. Glia 30:49–63, 2000.

266. Kafitz KW, Greer CA: Olfactory ensheathing cells promote neurite extension from embryonic olfactory receptor cells in vitro. Glia 25:99–110, 1999.

267. Prieto M, Chauvet N, Alonso G: Tanycytes transplanted into the adult rat spinal cord support the regeneration of lesioned axons. Exp Neurol 161:27–37, 2000.

268. Ramon-Cueto A, Nieto-Sampedro M: Regeneration into the spinal cord of transected dorsal root axons is promoted by ensheathing glia transplants. Exp Neurol 127:232–244, 1994.

269. Navarro X, Valero A, Gudino G, et al: Ensheathing glia transplants promote dorsal root regeneration and spinal reflex restitution after multiple lumbar rhizotomy. Ann Neurol 45:207–215, 1999.

270. Li Y, Field P, Raisman G: Regeneration of adult rat corticospinal axons induced by transplanted olfactory ensheathing cells. J Neurosci 18:10514–10524, 1998.

271. Li Y, Field P, Raisman G: Repair of adult rat corticospinal tract by transplants of olfactory ensheathing cells. Science 277: 2000–2002, 1997.

272. Ramon-Cueto A, Plant GW, Avila J, et al: Long-distance axonal regeneration in the transected adult rat spinal cord is promoted by olfactory ensheathing glia transplants. J Neurosci 18:3803–3815, 1998.

273. Perez-Bouza A, Wigley CB, Nacimiento W, et al: Spontaneous orientation of transplanted olfactory glia influences axonal regeneration. Neuroreport 9:2971–2975, 1998.

274. Brook GA, Lawrence JM, Raisman G: Morphology and migration of cultured Schwann cells transplanted into the fimbria and hippocampus in adult rats. Glia 9:292–304, 1993.

275. Ramon-Cueto A, Cordero MI, Santos-Benito FF, et al: Functional recovery of paraplegic rats and motor axon regeneration in their spinal cords by olfactory ensheathing glia. Neuron 25: 425–435, 2000.

276. Imaizumi T, Lankford KL, Kocsis JD: Transplantation of olfactory ensheathing cells or Schwann cells restores rapid and secure conduction across the transected spinal cord. Brain Res 854:70–78, 2000.

277. Gudino-Cabrera G, Pastor AM, de la Cruz RR, et al: Limits to the capacity of transplants of olfactory glia to promote axonal regrowth in the CNS. Neuroreport 11:467–471, 2000.

278. Valverde F, Lopez-Mascaraque L: Neuroglial arrangements in the olfactory glomeruli of the hedgehog. J Comp Neurol 307: 658–674, 1991.

279. Franklin RJ, Gilson JM, Franceschini IA, et al: Schwann cell–like myelination following transplantation of an olfactory bulb–ensheathing cell line into areas of demyelination in the adult CNS. Glia 17:217–224, 1996.

280. Imaizumi T, Lankford KL, Waxman SG, et al: Transplanted olfactory ensheathing cells remyelinate and enhance axonal conduction in the demyelinated dorsal columns of the rat spinal cord. J Neurosci 18:6176–6185, 1998.

281. Kato T, Honmou O, Uede T, et al: Transplantation of human olfactory ensheathing cells elicits remyelination of demyelinated rat spinal cord. Glia 30:209–218, 2000.

282. Fernandez-Valle C, Gorman D, Gomez AM, et al: Actin plays a role in both changes in cell shape and gene-expression associated with Schwann cell myelination. J Neurosci 17:241–250, 1997.

283. Xu XM, Guenard V, Kleitman N, et al: A combination of BDNF and NT-3 promotes supraspinal axonal regeneration into Schwann cell grafts in adult rat thoracic spinal cord. Exp Neurol 134:261–272, 1995.

284. Bellamkonda R, Ranieri JP, Bouche N, et al: Hydrogel-based three-dimensional matrix for neural cells. J Biomed Mater Res 29:663–671, 1995.

285. Ranieri JP, Bellamkonda R, Bekos EJ, et al: Neuronal cell attachment to fluorinated ethylene propylene films with covalently immobilized laminin oligopeptides YIGSR and IKVAV. II. J Biomed Mater Res 29:779–785, 1995.

286. Aebischer P, Schluep M, Deglon N, et al: Intrathecal delivery of CNTF using encapsulated genetically modified xenogeneic cells in amyotrophic lateral sclerosis patients. Nat Med 2:696–699, 1996; erratum Nat Med 2:1041, 1996.

287. Deglon N, Heyd B, Tan SA, et al: Central nervous system delivery of recombinant ciliary neurotrophic factor by polymer

encapsulated differentiated C2C12 myoblasts. Hum Gene Ther 7:2135–2146, 1996.

288. Teng Y, Lavik E, Qu X, et al: Transplantation of neural stem cells seeded in biodegradable polymer scaffold ameliorates long-term functional deficits resulting from spinal cord hemisection in adult rats. Paper presented at the Seventh Annual Meeting of the American Society for Neural Transplantation and Repair, April 2000, Clearwater, Fla.

289. Suzuki S, Matsuda K, Isshiki N, et al: Clinical evaluation of a new bilayer "artificial skin" composed of collagen sponge and silicone layer. Br J Plast Surg 43:47–54, 1990.

290. Davis GE, Blaker SN, Engvall E, et al: Human amnion membrane serves as a substratum for growing axons in vitro and in vivo. Science 236:1106–1109, 1987.

291. Joosten EA, Bar PR, Gispen WH: Collagen implants and corticospinal axonal growth after mid-thoracic spinal cord lesion in the adult rat. J Neurosci Res 40:481–490, 1995.

292. Houweling DA, Lankhorst AJ, Gispen WH, et al: Collagen containing neurotrophin-3 (NT-3) attracts regrowing injured corticospinal axons in the adult rat spinal cord and promotes partial functional recovery. Exp Neurol 153:49–59, 1998.

293. Khan T, Dauzvardis M, Sayers S: Carbon filament implants promote growth across the transected rat spinal cord. Brain Res 541:139–145, 1991.

294. Kiyotani T, Teramachi M, Takimoto Y, et al: Nerve regeneration across a 25-mm gap bridged by a polyglycolic acid–collagen tube: A histological and electrophysiological evaluation of regenerated nerves. Brain Res 740:66–74, 1996.

295. Hagg T, Gulati AK, Behzadian MA, et al: Nerve growth factor promotes CNS cholinergic axonal regeneration into acellular peripheral nerve grafts. Exp Neurol 112:79–88, 1991.

296. Lundborg G, Drott J, Wallman L, et al: Regeneration of axons from central neurons into microchips at the level of the spinal cord. Neuroreport 9:861–864, 1998.

297. Hirschberg DL, Schwartz M: Macrophage recruitment to acutely injured central nervous system is inhibited by a resident factor: A basis for an immune-brain barrier. J Neuroimmunol 61:89–96, 1995.

298. Popovich PG, Guan Z, Wei P, et al: Depletion of hematogenous macrophages promotes partial hindlimb recovery and neuroanatomical repair after experimental spinal cord injury. Exp Neurol 158:351–365, 1999.

299. Dimitrijevic MR, Dimitrijevic MM, Faganel J, et al: Suprasegmentally induced motor unit activity in paralyzed muscles of patients with established spinal cord injury. Ann Neurol 16:216–221, 1984.

300. Bunge RP, Puckett WR, Becerra JL, et al: Observations on the pathology of human spinal cord injury: A review and classification of 22 new cases with details from a case of chronic cord compression with extensive focal demyelination. Adv Neurol 59:75–89, 1993.

301. Blight AR, Toombs JP, Bauer MS, et al: The effects of 4-aminopyridine on neurological deficits in chronic cases of traumatic spinal cord injury in dogs: A phase I clinical trial. J Neurotrauma 8:103–119, 1991.

302. Nashmi R, Jones OT, Fehlings MG: Abnormal axonal physiology is associated with altered expression and distribution of Kv1.1 and Kv1.2 K$^+$ channels after chronic spinal cord injury. Eur J Neurosci 12:491–506, 2000.

303. Gumpel M, Lachapelle F, Gansmuller A, et al: Transplantation of human embryonic oligodendrocytes into shiverer brain. Ann N Y Acad Sci 495:71–85, 1987.

304. Tontsch U, Archer DR, Dubois-Dalcq M, et al: Transplantation of an oligodendrocyte cell line leading to extensive myelination. Proc Natl Acad Sci U S A 91:11616–11620, 1994.

305. Groves AK, Barnett SC, Franklin RJ, et al: Repair of demyelinated lesions by transplantation of purified O-2A progenitor cells. Nature 362:453–455, 1993.

306. Honmou O, Felts PA, Waxman SG, et al: Restoration of normal conduction properties in demyelinated spinal cord axons in the adult rat by transplantation of exogenous Schwann cells. J Neurosci 16:3199–3208, 1996.

307. Utzschneider DA, Archer DR, Kocsis JD, et al: Transplantation of glial cells enhances action potential conduction of amyelinated spinal cord axons in the myelin-deficient rat. Proc Natl Acad Sci U S A 91:53–57, 1994.

308. Brustle O, Jones KN, Learish RD, et al: Embryonic stem cell–derived glial precursors: A source of myelinating transplants. Science 285:754–756, 1999.

309. Learish RD, Brustle O, Zhang SC, et al: Intraventricular transplantation of oligodendrocyte progenitors into a fetal myelin mutant results in widespread formation of myelin. Ann Neurol 46:716–722, 1999.

310. Blakemore WF: Remyelination by Schwann cells of axons demyelinated by intraspinal injection of 6-aminonicotinamide in the rat. J Neurocytol (Berl) 4:745–757, 1975.

311. Blakemore WF, Crang AJ: The relationship between type-1 astrocytes, Schwann cells and oligodendrocytes following transplantation of glial cell cultures into demyelinating lesions in the adult rat spinal cord. J Neurocytol 18:519–528, 1989.

312. Danielsen N, Kerns JM, Holmquist B, et al: Predegeneration enhances regeneration into acellular nerve grafts. Brain Res 681:105–108, 1995.

313. Oblinger MM, Lasek RJ: A conditioning lesion of the peripheral axons of dorsal root ganglion cells accelerates regeneration of only their peripheral axons. J Neurosci 4:1736–1744, 1984.

314. Richardson PM, Issa VM: Peripheral injury enhances central regeneration of primary sensory neurones. Nature 309:791–793, 1984.

315. McQuarrie IG, Grafstein B: Effect of a conditioning lesion on optic nerve regeneration in goldfish. Brain Res 216:253–264, 1981.

316. Kiernan JA: A conditioning lesion does not induce axonal regeneration in the optic nerve of the rat. Exp Neurol 87:181–184, 1985.

317. Lu X, Richardson PM: Inflammation near the nerve cell body enhances axonal regeneration. J Neurosci 11:972–978, 1991.

318. Chong MS, Woolf CJ, Haque NS, et al: Axonal regeneration from injured dorsal roots into the spinal cord of adult rats. J Comp Neurol 410:42–54, 1999.

319. Levi-Montalcini R, Hamburger V: A diffusable agent of mouse sarcoma, producing hyperplasia of sympathetic ganglia and hyperneurotization of viscera in the chick embryo. J Exp Zool 123:233–288, 1953.

320. Hefti F: Nerve growth factor promotes survival of septal cholinergic neurons after fimbrial transections. J Neurosci 6:2155–2162, 1986.

321. Molliver DC, Wright DE, Leitner ML, et al: IB4-binding DRG neurons switch from NGF to GDNF dependence in early postnatal life. Neuron 19:849–861, 1997.

322. Yasuda T, Sobue G, Ito T, et al: Nerve growth factor enhances neurite arborization of adult sensory neurons: A study in single-cell culture. Brain Res 524:54–63, 1990.

323. Conner JM, Lauterborn JC, Gall CM: Anterograde transport of neurotrophin proteins in the CNS—a reassessment of the neurotrophic hypothesis. Rev Neurosci 9:91–103, 1998.

324. Meiri KF, Burdick D: Nerve growth factor stimulation of GAP-43 phosphorylation in intact isolated growth cones. J Neurosci 11:3155–3164, 1991.

325. Hagg T, Varon S: Neurotropism of nerve growth factor for adult rat septal cholinergic axons in vivo. Exp Neurol 119:37–45, 1993.

326. Dreyfus CF, Dai X, Lercher LD, et al: Expression of neurotrophins in the adult spinal cord in vivo. J Neurosci Res 56:1–7, 1999.

327. Lindholm D, Castren E, Berzaghi M, et al: Activity-dependent and hormonal regulation of neurotrophin mRNA levels in the brain—implications for neuronal plasticity. J Neurobiol 25:1362–1372, 1994.

328. Winkler J, Ramirez GA, Kuhn HG, et al: Reversible Schwann cell hyperplasia and sprouting of sensory and sympathetic neurites after intraventricular administration of nerve growth factor. Ann Neurol 41:82–93, 1997.

329. Nauta HJ, Wehman JC, Koliatsos VE, et al: Intraventricular infusion of nerve growth factor as the cause of sympathetic fiber sprouting in sensory ganglia. J Neurosurg 91:447–453, 1999.

330. Hayashi M, Mitsunaga F, Ohira K, et al: Development of full-length Trk B–immunoreactive structures in the hippocampal formation of the macaque monkey. Anat Embryol (Berl) 199:529–537, 1999.

331. Sawai H, Clarke DB, Kittlerova P, et al: Brain-derived neurotrophic factor and neurotrophin-4/5 stimulate growth of axonal

branches from regenerating retinal ganglion cells. J Neurosci 16: 3887–3894, 1996.

332. Asada H, Kaseloo PA, Lis A, et al: Traumatized rat striatum produces neurite-promoting and neurotrophic activities in vitro. Exp Neurol 139:173–187, 1996.

333. Hayashi M, Ueyama T, Nemoto K, et al: Sequential mRNA expression for immediate early genes, cytokines, and neurotrophins in spinal cord injury. J Neurotrauma 17:203–218, 2000.

334. Gadient RA, Cron KC, Otten U: Interleukin-1 beta and tumor necrosis factor-alpha synergistically stimulate nerve growth factor (NGF) release from cultured rat astrocytes. Neurosci Lett 117:335–340, 1990.

335. Yoshida K, Gage FH: Fibroblast growth factors stimulate nerve growth factor synthesis and secretion by astrocytes. Brain Res 538:118–126, 1991.

336. Hagg T, Fass-Holmes B, Vahlsing HL, et al: Nerve growth factor (NGF) reverses axotomy-induced decreases in choline acetyltransferase, NGF receptor and size of medial septum cholinergic neurons. Brain Res 505:29–38, 1989.

337. Tuszynski MH, Uy HS, Amaral DG, et al: Nerve growth factor infusion in the primate brain reduces lesion-induced cholinergic neuronal degeneration. J Neurosci 10:3604–3614, 1990.

338. Hagg T, Quon D, Higaki J, et al: Ciliary neurotrophic factor prevents neuronal degeneration and promotes low affinity NGF receptor expression in the adult rat CNS. Neuron 8:145–158, 1992.

339. Kawaja MD, Rosenberg MB, Yoshida K, et al: Somatic gene transfer of nerve growth factor promotes the survival of axotomized septal neurons and the regeneration of their axons in adult rats. J Neurosci 12:2849–2864, 1992.

340. Lu X, Hagg T: Glial cell line–derived neurotrophic factor prevents death, but not reductions in tyrosine hydroxylase, of injured nigrostriatal neurons in adult rats. J Comp Neurol 388: 484–494, 1997.

341. He Y, Yao Z, Gu Y, et al: Nerve growth factor promotes collateral sprouting of cholinergic fibers in the septohippocampal cholinergic system of aged rats with fimbria transection. Brain Res 586:27–35, 1992.

342. Vahlsing HL, Hagg T, Spencer M, et al: Dose-dependent responses to nerve growth factor by adult rat cholinergic medial septum and neostriatum neurons. Brain Res 552:320–329, 1991.

343. Hagg T, Vahlsing HL, Manthorpe M, et al: Nerve growth factor infusion into the denervated adult rat hippocampal formation promotes its cholinergic reinnervation. J Neurosci 10:3087–3092, 1990.

344. Oudega M, Hagg T: Nerve growth factor promotes regeneration of sensory axons into adult rat spinal cord. Exp Neurol 140: 218–229, 1996.

345. Fernandez E, Pallini R, Lauretti L, et al: Spinal cord transection in adult rats: Effects of local infusion of nerve growth factor on the corticospinal tract axons. Neurosurgery 33:889–893, 1993.

346. ALS CNTF Treatment Study Group: A double-blind placebo-controlled clinical trial of subcutaneous recombinant human ciliary neurotrophic factor (rHCNTF) in amyotrophic lateral sclerosis. Neurology 46:1244–1249, 1996.

347. Eriksdotter Jonhagen M, Nordberg A, Amberla K, et al: Intracerebroventricular infusion of nerve growth factor in three patients with Alzheimer's disease. Dement Geriatr Cogn Disord 9:246–257, 1998.

348. Snyder EY, Taylor RM, Wolfe JH: Neural progenitor cell engraftment corrects lysosomal storage throughout the MPS VII mouse brain. Nature 374:367–370, 1995.

349. Lacorazza HD, Flax JD, Snyder EY, et al: Expression of human beta-hexosaminidase alpha-subunit gene (the gene defect of Tay-Sachs disease) in mouse brains upon engraftment of transduced progenitor cells. Nat Med 2:424–429, 1996.

350. Costantini LC, Jacoby DR, Wang S, et al: Gene transfer to the nigrostriatal system by hybrid herpes simplex virus/adeno-associated virus amplicon vectors. Hum Gene Ther 10:2481–2494, 1999; see comments.

351. Guest JD, Bakowska J, Breakefield X, et al: HSV/AAV hybrid amplicon vector surpasses recombinant HSV ICP 6 in gene delivery from peripheral nerve to spinal motor neurons. Soc Neurosci Abstr 735:9, 1999.

352. Johnston KM, Jacoby D, Pechan PA, et al: HSV/AAV hybrid amplicon vectors extend transgene expression in human glioma cells. Hum Gene Ther 8:359–370, 1997.

353. Haase G, Kennel P, Pettmann B, et al: Gene therapy of murine motor neuron disease using adenoviral vectors for neurotrophic factors. Nat Med 3:429–436, 1997.

354. Watabe K, Ohashi T, Sakamoto T, et al: Rescue of lesioned adult rat spinal motoneurons by adenoviral gene transfer of glial cell line–derived neurotrophic factor. J Neurosci Res 60:511–519, 2000.

355. Wilson SP, Yeomans DC, Bender MA, et al: Antihyperalgesic effects of infection with a preproenkephalin-encoding herpes virus. Proc Natl Acad Sci U S A 96:3211–3216, 1999.

356. Klein RL, McNamara RK, King MA, et al: Generation of aberrant sprouting in the adult rat brain by GAP-43 somatic gene transfer. Brain Res 832:136–144, 1999.

357. Lo WD, Qu G, Sferra TJ, et al: Adeno-associated virus-mediated gene transfer to the brain: Duration and modulation of expression. Hum Gene Ther 10:201–213, 1999.

358. Fraefel C, Jacoby DR, Lage C, et al: Gene transfer into hepatocytes mediated by helper virus-free HSV/AAV hybrid vectors. Mol Med 3:813–825, 1997.

359. Choi-Lundberg DL, Lin Q, Chang YN, et al: Dopaminergic neurons protected from degeneration by GDNF gene therapy. Science 275:838–841, 1997.

360. Bohn MC, Choi-Lundberg DL, Davidson BL, et al: Adenovirus-mediated transgene expression in nonhuman primate brain. Hum Gene Ther 10:1175–1184, 1999.

361. Tuszynski MH, Weidner N, McCormack M, et al: Grafts of genetically modified Schwann cells to the spinal cord: Survival, axon growth, and myelination. Cell Transplant 7:187–196, 1998.

362. Grill R, Murai K, Blesch A, et al: Cellular delivery of neurotrophin-3 promotes corticospinal axonal growth and partial functional recovery after spinal cord injury. J Neurosci 17:5560–5572, 1997.

363. Blesch A, Uy HS, Grill RJ, et al: Leukemia inhibitory factor augments neurotrophin expression and corticospinal axon growth after adult CNS injury. J Neurosci 19:3556–3566, 1999.

364. Liu Y, Kim D, Himes BT, et al: Transplants of fibroblasts genetically modified to express BDNF promote regeneration of adult rat rubrospinal axons and recovery of forelimb function. J Neurosci 19:4370–4387, 1999.

365. Martinez-Serrano A, Lundberg C, Horellou P, et al: CNS-derived neural progenitor cells for gene transfer of nerve growth factor to the adult rat brain: Complete rescue of axotomized cholinergic neurons after transplantation into the septum. J Neurosci 15:5668–5680, 1995.

366. Park KI, Liu S, Flax JD, et al: Transplantation of neural progenitor and stem cells: Developmental insights may suggest new therapies for spinal cord and other CNS dysfunction. J Neurotrauma 16:675–687, 1999.

367. Liu Y, Himes BT, Solowska J, et al: Intraspinal delivery of neurotrophin-3 using neural stem cells genetically modified by recombinant retrovirus. Exp Neurol 158:9–26, 1999.

368. Dijkhuizen PA, Hermens WT, Teunis MA, et al: Adenoviral vector-directed expression of neurotrophin-3 in rat dorsal root ganglion explants results in a robust neurite outgrowth response. J Neurobiol 33:172–184, 1997.

369. Windle W: Regeneration of axons in the vertebrate central nervous system. Physiol Rev 36:427–440, 1956.

370. David S, Aguayo A: Axonal elongation into peripheral nervous system "bridges" after central nervous system injury in adult rats. Science 214:931–933, 1981.

371. Bernstein JJ, Getz R, Jefferson M, et al: Astrocytes secrete basal lamina after hemisection of rat spinal cord. Brain Res 327: 135–141, 1985.

372. Ness R, David S: Leptomeningeal cells modulate the neurite growth promoting properties of astrocytes in vitro. Glia 19: 47–57, 1997.

373. Bignami A, Dahl D: The astroglial response to stabbing: Immunofluorescence studies with antibodies to astrocyte-specific protein (GFA) in mammalian and submammalian vertebrates. Neuropathol Appl Neurobiol 2:99–110, 1976.

374. Bunge RP, Puckett WR, Hiester ED: Observations on the pathology of several types of human spinal cord injury, with emphasis on the astrocyte response to penetrating injuries. Adv Neurol 72:305–315, 1997.

375. Reier P, Houle J: The glial scar: Its bearing on axonal elongation and transplantation approaches to CNS repair. Adv Neurol 47: 87–130, 1988.

376. Winter CG, Saotome Y, Levison SW, et al: A role for ciliary neurotrophic factor as an inducer of reactive gliosis, the glial response to central nervous system injury. Proc Natl Acad Sci U S A 92:5865–5869, 1995.

377. Kahn MA, Ellison JA, Speight GJ, et al: CNTF regulation of astrogliosis and the activation of microglia in the developing rat central nervous system. Brain Res 685:55–67, 1995.

378. Rostworowski M, Balasingam V, Chabot S, et al: Astrogliosis in the neonatal and adult murine brain post-trauma: Elevation of inflammatory cytokines and the lack of requirement for endogenous interferon-gamma. J Neurosci 17:3664–3674, 1997.

379. Wolburg H, Neuhaus J, Mack A: The glio-axonal interaction and the problem of regeneration of axons in the central nervous system—concept and perspectives. Z Naturforsch (C) 41:1147–1155, 1986.

380. Reier PJ: Penetration of grafted astrocytic scars by regenerating optic nerve axons in *Xenopus* tadpoles. Brain Res 164:61–68, 1979.

381. Guth L, Barrett CP, Donati EJ, et al: Histopathological reactions and axonal regeneration in the transected spinal cord of hibernating squirrels. J Comp Neurol 203:297–308, 1981.

382. Weidner N, Grill RJ, Tuszynski MH: Elimination of basal lamina and the collagen "scar" after spinal cord injury fails to augment corticospinal tract regeneration. Exp Neurol 160:40–50, 1999.

383. Le Roux PD, Reh TA: Reactive astroglia support primary dendritic but not axonal outgrowth from mouse cortical neurons in vitro. Exp Neurol 137:49–65, 1996.

384. Fryer RH, Kaplan DR, Kromer LF: Truncated trkB receptors on nonneuronal cells inhibit BDNF-induced neurite outgrowth in vitro. Exp Neurol 148:616–627, 1997.

385. Rabchevsky AG, Streit WJ: Grafting of cultured microglial cells into the lesioned spinal cord of adult rats enhances neurite outgrowth. J Neurosci Res 47:34–48, 1997.

386. Wilson MA, Gaze RM, Goodbrand IA, et al: Regeneration in the *Xenopus* tadpole optic nerve is preceded by a massive macrophage/microglial response. Anat Embryol (Berl) 186:75–89, 1992.

387. Fok-Seang J, Smith-Thomas LC, Meiners S, et al: An analysis of astrocytic cell lines with different abilities to promote axon growth. Brain Res 689:207–223, 1995.

388. McKeon RJ, Hoke A, Silver J: Injury-induced proteoglycans inhibit the potential for laminin-mediated axon growth on astrocytic scars. Exp Neurol 136:32–43, 1995.

389. Grumet M, Friedlander DR, Sakurai T: Functions of brain chondroitin sulfate proteoglycans during development: Interactions with adhesion molecules. Perspect Dev Neurobiol 3:319–330, 1996.

390. Margolis RU, Margolis RK: Chondroitin sulfate proteoglycans as mediators of axon growth and pathfinding. Cell Tissue Res 290:343–348, 1997.

391. Hockfield S, Kalb RG, Zaremba S, et al: Expression of neural proteoglycans correlates with the acquisition of mature neuronal properties in the mammalian brain. Cold Spring Harb Symp Quant Biol 55:505–514, 1990.

392. Fawcett JW, Asher RA: The glial scar and central nervous system repair. Brain Res Bull 49:377–391, 1999.

393. McKeon RJ, Jurynec MJ, Buck CR: The chondroitin sulfate proteoglycans neurocan and phosphacan are expressed by reactive astrocytes in the chronic CNS glial scar. J Neurosci 19:10778–10788, 1999.

394. Friedlander DR, Milev P, Karthikeyan L, et al: The neuronal chondroitin sulfate proteoglycan neurocan binds to the neural cell adhesion molecules Ng-CAM/L1/NILE and N-CAM and inhibits neuronal adhesion and neurite outgrowth. J Cell Biol 125:669–680, 1994.

395. Asher RA, Morgenstern DA, Fidler PS, et al: Neurocan is upregulated in injured brain and in cytokine-treated astrocytes. J Neurosci 20:2427–2438, 2000.

396. Milev P, Friedlander DR, Sakurai T, et al: Interactions of the chondroitin sulfate proteoglycan phosphacan, the extracellular domain of a receptor-type protein tyrosine phosphatase, with neurons, glia, and neural cell adhesion molecules. J Cell Biol 127(Pt 1):1703–1715, 1994.

397. Dou CL, Levine JM: Inhibition of neurite growth by the NG2 chondroitin sulfate proteoglycan. J Neurosci 14:7616–7628, 1994.

398. Fidler PS, Schuette K, Asher RA, et al: Comparing astrocytic cell lines that are inhibitory or permissive for axon growth: The major axon-inhibitory proteoglycan is NG2. J Neurosci 19: 8778–8788, 1999.

399. Niederost BP, Zimmermann DR, Schwab ME, et al: Bovine CNS myelin contains neurite growth-inhibitory activity associated with chondroitin sulfate proteoglycans. J Neurosci 19:8979–8989, 1999.

400. Pesheva P, Gennarini G, Goridis C, et al: The F3/11 cell adhesion molecule mediates the repulsion of neurons by the extracellular matrix glycoprotein J1-160/180. Neuron 10:69–82, 1993.

401. McKeon RJ, Schreiber RC, Rudge JS, et al: Reduction of neurite outgrowth in a model of glial scarring following CNS injury is correlated with the expression of inhibitory molecules on reactive astrocytes. J Neurosci 11:3398–3411, 1991.

402. Zuo J, Ferguson TA, Hernandez YJ, et al: Neuronal matrix metalloproteinase-2 degrades and inactivates a neurite-inhibiting chondroitin sulfate proteoglycan. J Neurosci 18:5203–5211, 1998.

403. Schwab ME, Kapfhammer JP, Bandtlow CE: Inhibitors of neurite growth. Annu Rev Neurosci 16:565–595, 1993.

404. Savio T, Schwab ME: Rat CNS white matter, but not gray matter, is nonpermissive for neuronal cell adhesion and fiber outgrowth. J Neurosci 9:1126–1133, 1989.

405. Savio T, Schwab M: Lesioned corticospinal tract axons regenerate in myelin-free rat spinal cord. Proc Natl Acad Sci U S A 87: 4130–4133, 1990.

406. Caroni P, Schwab ME: Two membrane protein fractions from rat central myelin with inhibitory properties for neurite growth and fibroblast spreading. J Cell Biol 106:1281–1288, 1988.

407. Caroni P, Schwab ME: Antibody against myelin-associated inhibitor of neurite growth neutralizes nonpermissive substrate properties of CNS white matter. Neuron 1:85–96, 1988.

408. Schnell L, Schwab ME: Axonal regeneration in the rat spinal cord produced by an antibody against myelin-associated neurite growth inhibitors. Nature 343:269–272, 1990.

409. Bregman BS, Kunkel-Bagden E, Schnell L, et al: Recovery from spinal cord injury mediated by antibodies to neurite growth inhibitors. Nature 378:498–501, 1995.

410. Chen MS, Huber AB, van der Haar ME, et al: Nogo-A is a myelin-associated neurite outgrowth inhibitor and an antigen for monoclonal antibody IN-1. Nature 403:434–439, 2000.

411. Bandtlow C, Zachleder T, Schwab ME: Oligodendrocytes arrest neurite growth by contact inhibition. J Neurosci 10:3837–3848, 1990.

412. Bandtlow CE, Schmidt MF, Hassinger TD, et al: Role of intracellular calcium in NI-35-evoked collapse of neuronal growth cones. Science 259:80–83, 1993.

413. McKerracher L, David S, Jackson D, et al: Identification of myelin-associated glycoprotein as a major myelin-derived inhibitor of neurite growth. Neuron 13:805–811, 1994.

414. Mukhopadhyay G, Doherty P, Walsh FS, et al: A novel role for myelin-associated glycoprotein as an inhibitor of axonal regeneration. Neuron 13:757–767, 1994.

415. Ming G, Song H, Berninger B, et al: Phospholipase C-gamma and phosphoinositide 3-kinase mediate cytoplasmic signaling in nerve growth cone guidance. Neuron 23:139–148, 1999.

416. Kapfhammer JP, Schwab ME: Inverse patterns of myelination and GAP-43 expression in the adult CNS: Neurite growth inhibitors as regulators of neuronal plasticity? J Comp Neurol 340: 194–206, 1994.

417. Kapfhammer JP: Myelin-associated neurite growth inhibitors: Regulators of plastic changes of neural connections in the central nervous system. Prog Brain Res 108:183–202, 1996.

418. Keirstead HS, Dyer JK, Sholomenko GN, et al: Axonal regeneration and physiological activity following transection and immunological disruption of myelin within the hatchling chick spinal cord. J Neurosci 15:6963–6974, 1995.

419. Dyer JK, Bourque JA, Steeves JD: Regeneration of brainstem-spinal axons after lesion and immunological disruption of myelin in adult rat. Exp Neurol 154:12–22, 1998.

420. Wictorin K, Brundin P, Gustavii B, et al: Reformation of long axon pathways in adult rat central nervous system by human forebrain neuroblasts. Nature 347:556–558, 1990.

421. Li Y, Raisman G: Long axon growth from embryonic neurons transplanted into myelinated tracts of the adult rat spinal cord. Brain Res 629:115–127, 1993.

422. Davies SJ, Fitch MT, Memberg SP, et al: Regeneration of adult axons in white matter tracts of the central nervous system. Nature 390:680–693, 1997.

423. Buffo A, Zagrebelsky M, Huber AB, et al: Application of neutralizing antibodies against NI-35/250 myelin-associated neurite growth inhibitory proteins to the adult rat cerebellum induces sprouting of uninjured Purkinje cell axons. J Neurosci 20:2275–2286, 2000.

424. Huang DW, McKerracher L, Braun PE, et al: A therapeutic vaccine approach to stimulate axon regeneration in the adult mammalian spinal cord. Neuron 24:639–647, 1999.

425. Ye JH, Houle JD: Treatment of the chronically injured spinal cord with neurotrophic factors can promote axonal regeneration from supraspinal neurons. Exp Neurol 143:70–81, 1997.

426. Houle JD, Schramm P, Herdegen T: Trophic factor modulation of c-Jun expression in supraspinal neurons after chronic spinal cord injury. Exp Neurol 154:602–611, 1998.

427. von Meyenburg J, Brosamle C, Metz GA, et al: Regeneration and sprouting of chronically injured corticospinal tract fibers in adult rats promoted by NT-3 and the mAb IN-1, which neutralizes myelin-associated neurite growth inhibitors. Exp Neurol 154:583–594, 1998.

CHAPTER 278

Concepts and Mechanisms of Biomechanics

DENNIS J. MAIMAN ■ FRANK A. PINTAR ■ MICHAEL W. GROFF ■
NARAYAN YOGANANDAN

This chapter presents considerations in the study of spinal biomechanics, with an emphasis on the clinical relevance of the study of pathologic forces on the spine. Spinal disorders present multiple problems in evaluation and treatment. For example, degenerative spinal disease is one of the most common causes of disability in the United States, yet it is one of the least understood. In addition, there are at least 100,000 unstable spine fractures annually, at a cost of $600 million to society, as well as immense human suffering.

Although biomechanics is fundamentally a science designed to provide information for clinicians, it is not well understood or used by them. Indeed, there are few areas in neurosurgery where experimental data are as valuable and readily applicable as in the management of spinal disorders.

Spinal biomechanics is the study of the consequences of the application of external forces to the spinal column.[1] Such forces may be normal (i.e., physiologic) or pathologic. Both can injure the structure and functional relationships of spinal structures and thus may be associated with degenerative disorders as well as trauma.

In analyzing the effects of these external forces, we not only look at the spine as a series of motion segments but also consider the relationships between the components of the spine and the column as a whole. In addition, we consider the physiologic forces that eventually lead to changes known as "degenerative," which are important not only for prescribing treatment but also for understanding the pathophysiology.

The spine can be analyzed in different ways, and each way provides unique information. Micromodels examine specific spinal structures such as ligaments, intervertebral disks, or vertebral bodies, emphasizing local effects and the contributions of individual structural components on the overall behavior of the spine.[2–7]

The smallest structure on which meaningful functional research can be performed is the motion segment (Fig. 278–1). Investigators have extrapolated motion segment data, considering the spine to be a group of motion segments functioning in series. This, however, assumes a linear superposition principle that may not apply to the nonlinearities of the human spinal column. Many investigators believe that the spinal column cannot be considered the sum of its parts. Instead, it is composed of nonlinear, heterogeneous materials and asymmetrical curves.[8–11] Therefore, the response of the spinal column is somewhat variable in different parts of the spine, even when they are subjected to the same load. Thus, investigation of the macromodel (the spinal column itself) becomes critical. Last, although rarely done, investigations of the spinal column in its investing structures (i.e., the entire torso) are particularly edifying when examining the relationships between the head and the spine and between the spinal cord and the spine.[12–14]

SPINAL STABILITY

The definition of spinal stability may be the most difficult concept in biomechanics. The classic definition of *clinical instability* by White and Panjabi[15] is "loss of the ability of the spine under physiologic loads to maintain its pattern of displacement so that there is no initial or additional neurological deficit, no major deformity, and no incapacitating pain." This is a general definition that lends itself to individual interpretation and expansion. Protection of the spinal cord is a primary consideration, and abnormalities that do not produce major deformity or neurological deficit are not necessarily unstable. Although this clinical definition can be used on a daily basis, it is not necessarily based on experimental biomechanical criteria. There are less dramatic biomechanical abnormalities that are mechanically significant, representing subclinical failure of multiple components of the spine.[16–18] For example, injuries to the posterior ligaments in conjunction with minor compression fractures can lead to cervical deformity, even if the spine appears relatively normal initially.[12, 19, 20]

Although theoretical concepts are popular among those in the laboratory, clinicians tend to favor absolute

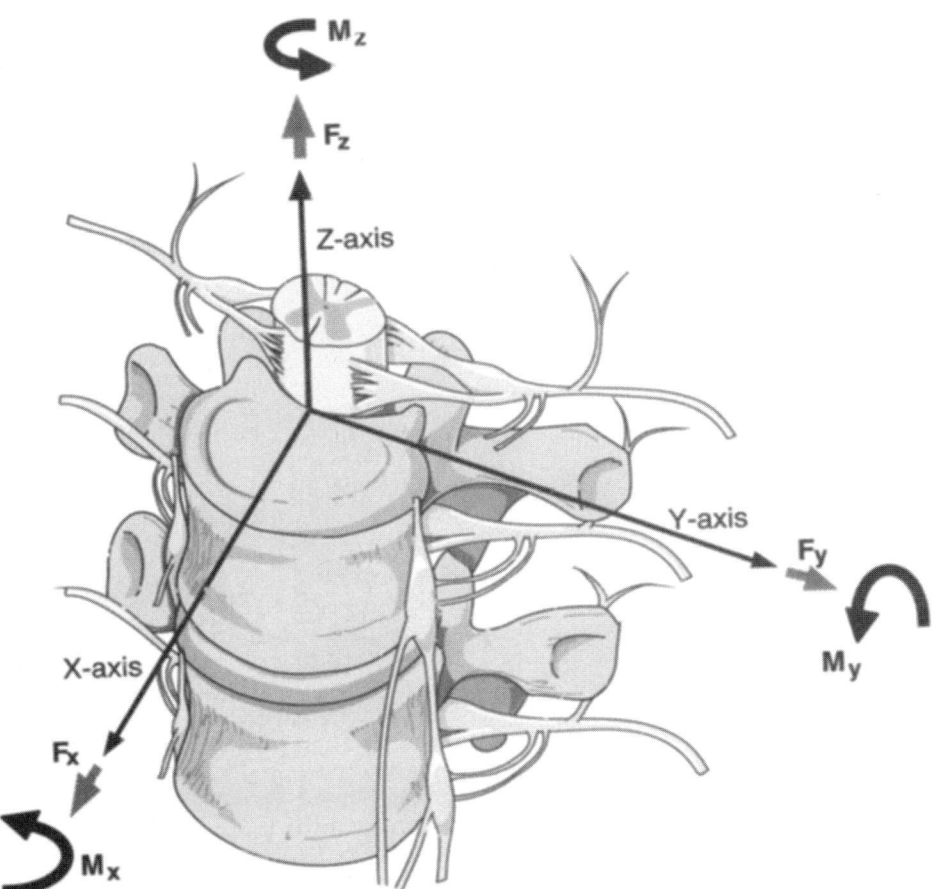

FIGURE 278–1. The motion segment. Three-dimensional coordinate axes are identified. Linear forces are designated Fx (posterior to anterior), Fy (right to left), and Fz (inferior to superior). Corresponding positive moments include Mx (right lateral bending), My (flexion), and Mz (left axial rotation).

concepts of stability that can be applied directly to the clinical situation. The clinical definitions of spinal stability have changed over the years, and at any one time, several different definitions may have existed. The question is not only whether the patient requires surgery but also, if there is surgical intervention, what procedure should be done. The classic definitions of stability are the simplest, and they treat the spine as consisting of subsets of "columns." These include the two-column and three-column theories.

Two-Column Concept

The original concept of describing stability in terms of two columns stems from a 1963 article by Holdsworth.[21] He based his definition on his own clinical experience as well as that of Nicoll[22] and experimental work done by Roaf.[23] In this two-column definition, the posterior column consists of the "posterior ligament complex," namely, the interspinous and supraspinous ligaments, the ligamenta flava, and the apophyseal joints. The anterior column consists of the vertebral body, disk, and anterior and posterior longitudinal ligaments (Fig. 278–2). Holdsworth contended that the stability of the spine largely depends on the integrity of the posterior ligament complex. A simple wedge fracture of the vertebral body with no posterior ligament involvement would be stable. A compression

burst fracture with intact posterior ligaments would also be stable. Unstable fractures involve loss of integrity of the posterior ligament complex and at least one component of the anterior column.[21] Although instabil-

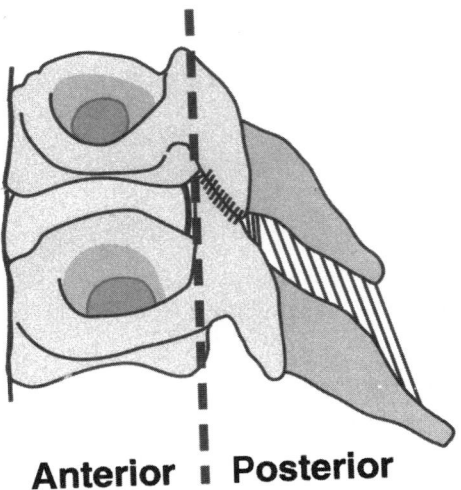

Anterior ┊ Posterior

FIGURE 278–2. Two-column theory. The anterior column *(left)* includes the vertebra, disk, and anterior and posterior longitudinal ligaments. The posterior column *(right)* includes the posterior elements and ligaments.

ity is said to result from injury to the posterior ligament complex, others assume instability to require significant injury of either column and partial injury of the other. The two-column concept is validated by significant amounts of clinical and experimental data.[1, 20, 24–28]

In actual clinical practice, the determination of stability using the two-column theory may be inaccurate. Theoretically, a 50% or greater compression fracture with normal posterior ligaments is stable; however, in reality, such a spine is at risk (as described later in this chapter). In defense of the two-column concept, the spine is unlikely to have a significant anterior column injury without posterior element compromise.[9, 29–32] Although clinically useful, from a biomechanical standpoint, this theory is contradicted by some studies. Experimental data have demonstrated that transection of the posterior ligament complex alone does not produce instability.[17, 18, 33–35] When the posterior longitudinal ligament and posterior disk are also transected, biomechanical instability may result. These findings led to more support of the three-column theory.

Three-Column Concept

One theory of spinal stability that has generated tremendous support among clinicians and biomechanists in recent years is the three-column theory first proposed by Denis.[36] He defined a "middle" column because of experimental studies that demonstrated that transection of the entire posterior ligament complex alone is not sufficient to produce instability. However, when the posterior longitudinal ligament and posterior portion of the disk annulus are also transected, instability results. Therefore, in the three-column concept, the middle column consists of the posterior longitudinal ligament, the posterior annulus fibrosus, and the posterior wall of the vertebral body; the anterior column consists of the anterior longitudinal ligament, the anterior annulus, and the anterior wall of the vertebral body; the posterior column is the same as in the two-column approach (Fig. 278–3).[36] Of the "major spinal injuries" defined by Denis, only minimal and moderate compression fractures with an intact posterior column are considered stable. Thus, classification of burst fractures is where the two- and three-column theories differ in terms of stability. Denis classifies the burst fracture under "neurological instability" because both the anterior and middle columns are affected. All the fractures and fracture-dislocations categorized under "instability" by Denis demonstrate trauma in at least two of the three columns.

There is evidence, however, that the most common type of thoracolumbar spine loading (i.e., flexion-compression of the anterior spine and distraction of the posterior elements) produces posterior ligament injury before vertebral body compression in many instances and is often unstable.[26, 37–39] In these compression-flexion injuries, an additional load is placed on both the vertebrae and the middle column. Also, the forces required to disrupt the posterior longitudinal ligament may not injure the disk, and vice versa.[29, 40–43]

The determination that there has or has not been

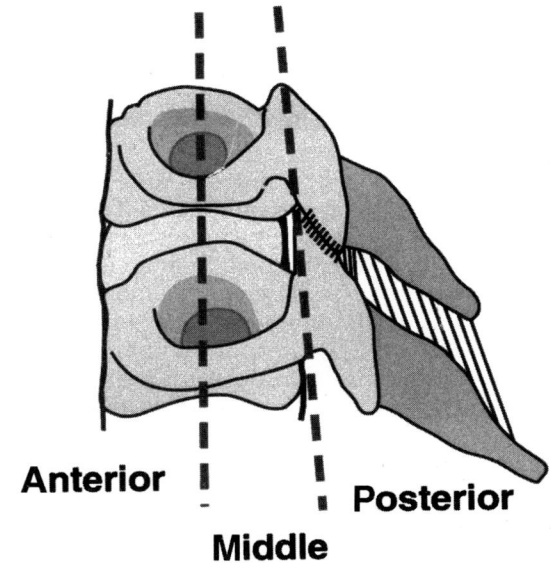

Anterior **Posterior**

Middle

FIGURE 278–3. Three-column theory. The anterior column *(left)* includes the anterior longitudinal ligament, anterior disk, and vertebra. The middle column incorporates the posterior vertebra and disk, posterior longitudinal ligament, and perhaps the pedicle. The posterior column includes the posterior elements and ligaments.

ligamentous injury based on static radiography is difficult. Studies of kinematics during spinal loading and fracture have shown significant variability in injuries produced with similar forces. As discussed later, partial injuries to structures such as the disk and body, as well as spinal ligaments, may allow a pathologic amount of motion, even if gross failure is not evident. Individuals with these injuries may be at significant risk for neurological deterioration as well as late deformity.

Continuum Concept and Microtrauma

We prefer to consider spinal stability as a continuum, with anatomic changes typically present before the occurrence of physiologic abnormalities (i.e., pathologic motion).[39, 44–48] In addition to severe injury of specific structures, partial injury to multiple structural elements of the spine, particularly the ligaments, can produce instability. Of particular concern is that over the spectrum of physiologic loading, one often reaches the margins of safe loading, defined as the physiologic loading region in Figure 278–4. During repeated loading in this region, microtrauma to spinal structures may occur that is not grossly visible radiographically but produces pain because of abnormal motion or alignment. This, in turn, increases the stresses on other spinal structures, leading to progressive anatomic changes over time.

As can be observed from a representative force-deformation curve (see Fig. 278–4), the traumatic loading zone does not represent the failure point of the spine: while anatomic injury is occurring, the spine is still resisting externally applied loads, although less effectively than in the linear part of the curve. For

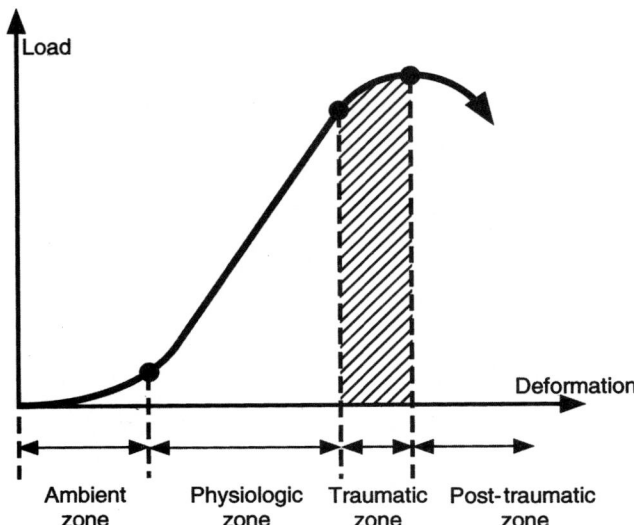

FIGURE 278–4. The continuum concept as described by Yoga-nandan and colleagues.[63] This idealized force-deformation curve demonstrates four phases of loading. During the physiologic zone, load-deformation behavior is almost linear. The critical phase is the traumatic zone, or the area of microtrauma. Here, although not grossly pathologic, injury to components of the column occurs, which is often not visible on radiographs.

Figure labels: Load; Deformation; Ambient zone; Physiologic zone; Traumatic zone; Post-traumatic zone

example, as a ligament experiences failure, initially a few strands may tear, but the rest of the strands are still resisting load. The initial tearing occurs at the beginning of the traumatic zone. This leads to the concept of microtrauma.

Gross failure, defined as the point at which further loads are poorly resisted with increasing deformations, is relatively easily determined. It is more difficult to determine the point at which microtrauma occurs, which may be more important in the area of degenerative diseases. A principal issue becomes defining the threshold at which subclinical injury becomes significant. For disk injury, our studies suggest that this point is reached when the end plates are injured.[46] However, even in trauma, the definition of instability must address the integrity of each spinal component. A second important issue in the area of spinal instrumentation is its purpose vis-à-vis stability: are we attempting to produce the maximal stiffness possible, or are we attempting to reduce the motion of the injured spine into a more physiologic range?

In attempting to define spinal stability, several factors need to be considered, including the force and mechanism of injury, the radiographic appearance of the lesion and the structures involved, and, according to some, the neurological status. Neurological injury may be a particularly useful consideration in initial stabilization of an injury, and it is appropriate for paramedical and medical staff providing early stabilization to assume an unstable spinal injury in any patient with neurological impairment. However, in the definitive determination of spinal stability, neurological status is not of significant value. Instead, results of biomechanical studies should be incorporated into the decision-

making process, along with information based on retrospective clinical observation.

Clinical Evaluation of Stability

One important consideration is the degree of compression of the vertebral body. Vertebral body compressions of more than 50% are commonly considered unstable, although instability may be seen even with minimal compression.[2] The degree of cord compression caused by the fractured vertebral body cannot be predicted from plain radiographs, because the central part of the body can compress the cord with only minimal loss in height. Evaluation of the posterior elements should include an overall view of spinal alignment and spinal curves. Increased distance between spinous processes often indicates disruption of the posterior ligament complex, presumably as a result of posterior distraction during flexion-compression loading. Again, this picture suggests instability. Fracture of the pedicles and separation of the facets are of similar concern. Indeed, the presence of thoracic and lumbar spine instability may best be determined by evaluation of the pedicle status (interpedicular distance, fracture) from the anteroposterior view, as well as by evidence of lateral translation. Posterior element trauma can easily be missed on plain films because of the direction of the fracture line and because its ligamentous nature may not produce spinal dislocation at rest. In addition, the severity of ligament injury cannot be predicted from changes in the integrity of the osseous spine.[49] Unfortunately, dynamic radiography such as that used in the cervical spine cannot be performed. Thus, one must evaluate the components of the fracture individually, as well as consider the biomechanics of the injury in making the determination of stability. Assuming that a given injury is unstable until proved otherwise may be prudent. Significant cord compression even in the absence of neurological deficit may be considered a surgical indication to prevent late cord injury following the development of even a minor post-traumatic kyphosis.

ANATOMIC SUBSTRUCTURES OF THE SPINE

Nowhere in the human body is anatomy translated into biomechanics more directly than in the spine.

Vertebrae

Anatomy of the vertebral elements varies in the different regions, reflecting the functional requirements of each area. However, several common characteristics are seen throughout. Outside the first two levels of the spine, the movable vertebrae consist of the ventral vertebral body, which is primarily load bearing, and the dorsal arch. The end plates are composed of centrally roughened cortical bone and bind the fibrocartilaginous intervertebral disks. In an ongoing study in our laboratory, we have found that the end plate is thickest at the periphery and weakest at the center.

The importance of the end plate in interbody fusion, however, has been called into question.[50] The sides of the body are concave in the thoracic and lumbar regions.

The outer case of the vertebra is composed of dense, strong, compact bone. The inner core, in constrast, is composed of cancellous bone that is aligned in vertical lamellae that resist compression. The average cross-sectional areas of the body range from 305 to 1000 mm² in the cervical region and 1055 to 2561 mm² in the lumbar spine.[15, 49, 51–53]

The vertebral body itself resists tension better than compression.[2, 53, 54] With tension loading, failure is routinely observed at the disk end plate rather than in the body. In studies performed in our laboratory, thoracic and lumbar vertebral segments were subjected to compression to 50% of original height; the values increased at lower levels.[55] Compressive strength is a consequence of the orientation of the trabeculae and bone density.[54, 56] Compressive strength of the vertebral body has decreased by about 50% at age 50.[51, 53, 57]

The arch is composed of the laminae and paired pedicles, as well as the articulating surfaces (facets) and spinous processes. The pedicles are stout bars of bone extending posterolaterally from the superior aspect of the vertebral body. Extending dorsomedially from the pedicles, the laminae fuse in the midline to form the dorsal wall of the spinal canal. The spinous processes arise from the junction of the laminae; their directions change, depending on the region of the spine. The transverse process arises from each side of the vertebral body near the junction of the pedicle and vertebral body. Both the transverse and spinous processes serve as attachment points for muscles and ligaments.

The articular processes are oriented to allow judicious motion of the spine and vary by region. In the cervical spine, they have largely a cranial-caudal orientation, upward 45 degrees. In the thoracic spine, from T1 to T10 they are almost coronal in orientation but are sagittally directed at lower thoracic levels and in the lumbar spine. The particularly abrupt changes in the orientation of the facets occurring at T1 and T11 render these transitional regions susceptible to dislocation. They provide resistance to anterior translation from T1 to T10, but in the lower thoracic region they acquire a more lumbar pattern, limit rotation, and have less effect on translation.

The facets are important in normal loading of the spine, accepting more than 20% of axial compression loads and perhaps more than 50% of extension and torsional loads in the cervical spine.[58, 59] There is an effective distribution of load across the facets and across the vertebral body in the resting position; however, when loads are moved anteriorly by 5 mm in front of the center of the vertebra, strains increase in the vertebra as the facets are unloaded.[48] Therefore, it is reasonable to assume that posterior element injury—often purely ligamentous—occurs with anterior loading. Even in the case of degenerative changes associated with abnormal long-term loading, posterior element changes can be expected.

Intervertebral Disks

The intervertebral disks are fibrocartilaginous structures attaching to the vertebrae centrally at the end plates and peripherally via the spinal ligaments and fibers of the annulus fibrosus. Although composition is consistent, heights vary by region and form the spinal curves by varying anterior-posterior height. Disks support bending loads, absorb compression, and, to a lesser extent, resist tension and shearing forces during physiologic movement. In loading of the cervical and lumbar spine, they carry more than 60% of compressive loads; in the thoracic spine, the figure may be greater.[40, 60]

The peripheral annulus fibrosus is composed of fibrous tissue arranged in concentric rings, the fibers aligning obliquely. Some fibers of the annulus blend into the anterior and posterior longitudinal ligaments. Others, known as Sharpey's fibers, attach to the rim of the vertebral body. The central nucleus pulposus is composed of a loose network of fibrous strands in a mucoprotein gel, with a water content of 88% at birth. By the seventh decade, this has decreased to 64%, with a corresponding drop in spinal mobility. Gradually, the annulus thickens, the disk space narrows, and ossification often follows.[61]

The biomechanics of the disk has been studied extensively, especially in compression. Many studies have suggested that end plate failure precedes disk failure; some have suggested that disk failure due to axial compression never occurs. This is partially because the normal nucleus pulposus acts hydrostatically during direct compression, and pressures are uniformly distributed. The initiation of damage can be identified biomechanically by the first decrease of stiffness. Diskography preformed as this occurs has demonstrated herniation of the nucleus pulposus through the end plate.[62] Actual failure in direct compression does not often occur without prior injury of the vertebra.[63] However, injury of the disk without gross bony failure certainly does occur.[15, 34, 40]

During all loads but direct compression, a portion of the disk is subjected to tension forces, under which the disk is less stiff. Torsion and bending loads are more dangerous to the disk than is compression, with failure due to torsion occurring with as little as 15 degrees of axial twist. Roaf noted that bulging of the annulus occurs only on the concave side (away from the bending).[23] During torsion, shear stresses are seen principally at the peripheral aspect of the disk, with horizontal shear stiffness of 260 newtons/mm at failure.[64–66] This high load requirement suggests that disk failure due to pure shear loads is unlikely; instead, bending or torsion is necessary.[34] Finite-element modeling has corroborated the biomechanical responses of the intervertebral disk and added to the understanding of disk pathogenesis.[67, 68]

As important as actual disruption of the disk may appear, degeneration of the disk as a function of repetitive loading may be a more significant phenomenon. Studies have shown that the disk is at its stiffest during physiologic elastic loading. However, as loads increase, trauma to the disk occurs gradually, with microfailure—not often discernible on radiography—and yielding of the disk. This is the point at which initiation of trauma occurs. Eventually, with continued loading, stiffness decreases to zero, and gross failure occurs. The recognition that initiation of disk trauma can occur without visible changes is important clinically, representing the stage at which mechanical pain and osteophyte formation may begin. In addition, disk microtrauma may be related to decreased effectiveness in buffering other spinal components from loading, leading to changes within facet joints and increased mobility; thus, clinical instability will develop.[46, 69]

Spinal Ligaments

The spinal ligaments and joint capsules preserve the articulated nature of the spine, allowing a restrained amount of movement. They are typically multilayered and may connect adjacent vertebrae or extend over several segments. The ligaments are composed of elastin, which provides the elastic nature of the ligaments, and collagen, which provides tensile strength. They are uniaxial; that is, they carry loads most effectively along the directions of their fibers. Because of the orientation of ligaments, they experience only tensile forces during spine motion. During physiologic movement, only small forces are required to produce stretch, and stiffness values and energy absorption of the ligaments are low. During movement beyond the physiologic range but before actual disruption, ligament stiffness dramatically increases. In the latter range, therefore, a great deal more energy is absorbed, providing protection to the cord during trauma.

Age-associated changes in ligaments have been analyzed. As is the case for the intervertebral disk, an increase in the amount of fibrous tissue is typically seen with age. These changes are more prominent in the more elastic ligaments, such as the ligamenta flava.[70]

ANTERIOR LONGITUDINAL LIGAMENT

The anterior longitudinal ligament, extending from the occiput to the sacrum, is composed primarily of longitudinally arranged collagen fibers aligned in interdigitating layers. The deepest of its three layers attaches to the edges of adjacent intervertebral disks, the middle layer binds to the bodies and disks over three levels, and the superficial fibers extend four to five layers. The ligament is thickest at the concavity of the vertebra, blending into the periosteum. Because of its high proportion of collagen and its firm, bony attachments, the primary action of the anterior longitudinal ligament is to prevent hyperextension and overdistraction.

Studies have been carried out in our laboratories evaluating the tensile strength of this ligament. Overall, mean breaking loads ranged from 50 newtons in the cervical spine to 600 newtons in the lumbar spine.[4, 6] Generally, the ligament becomes stronger as one moves down the thoracic spine to the thoracolumbar junction, being three times stronger at T11 than at T1. Although

the breaking load values for the anterior longitudinal ligament are approximately double those for other ligaments (particularly the posterior longitudinal ligament), when one considers the values as a function of cross-sectional area, breaking stresses are similar.[6, 71] As is the case in most other studies of biologic tissue, strength increases with loading rate.[7]

POSTERIOR LONGITUDINAL LIGAMENT

The posterior longitudinal ligament is located on the dorsum of the vertebral body, running from the axis to the sacrum. This ligament also consists of several layers, with the deep fibers extending only to adjacent vertebrae and the stronger superficial fibers spanning several levels. The ligament closely adheres to the disk annulus, but only marginally to the vertebral body. This ligament is much thinner over the vertebral body than over the disk, and it is thickest overall in the thoracic region. It is substantially smaller in diameter (one fourth to one tenth) than the anterior longitudinal ligament.[6, 71]

The posterior longitudinal ligament functions primarily to limit hyperflexion of the spine; in our clinical and experimental experience, it allows less deformation than the anterior longitudinal ligament. The tensile strength of the posterior longitudinal ligament in the thoracic spine ranges from 67 to 138 newtons and is somewhat stronger in the midthoracic region.[4, 72] Reliance on this relatively weak ligament to push bone fragments out of the spinal canal and back into the vertebral body during distraction may thus be unrealistic.

LIGAMENTA FLAVA

The ligamenta flava are broad, paired ligaments that connect the spinal laminae. These ligaments arise from the ventral surface of the lower lamina and attach to the dorsal border of the more cephalad lamina. Thus, they are discontinuous at midvertebral levels and in the midline. They extend laterally to the joint capsules and become confluent with them. The name of the ligament reflects its yellow color, which results from an approximately 80% elastin content. Indeed, this ligament is one of the most elastic tissues in the human body.[70] It has its largest cross-sectional diameter in the midthoracic and lumbar regions.[6] Tensile strength of the ligamenta flava is greatest at lower thoracic levels (mean, 300 newtons). Resting forces ranged from 18 newtons in the young to 5 newtons in subjects older than 70 years in studies conducted by Nachemson and Evans. The amount of extension created by the ligament was shown to decrease from 70% to 30% in older subjects, presumably as a result of age-related replacement of the elastic fibers by fibrosis.[70] In addition, certain types of degenerative pathology of the spine (i.e., lumbar stenosis, kyphosis) may increase the thickness of the ligament.[6]

The composition of the ligament and its mechanical characteristics have functional and clinical implications. The purpose of the ligamenta flava is to allow flexion of the spine with separation of the laminae and to encourage return of the laminae to their normal position upon release of the load. Because of both the elasticity of the ligament and the extension seen in the resting state, a significant amount of extension can occur without permanent deformation of the ligament. White and Panjabi suggested that this characteristic is particularly important in preventing impingement on the spinal cord when the spine goes from flexion to extension (during which the ligament is relaxed).[15]

CAPSULAR LIGAMENTS

The capsular ligaments attach to the vertebrae adjacent to the articular joints. Because the facet synovium has inherent strength, the ligaments and joint capsules are usually studied together. The fibers tend to be longer and more slack in the cervical than in thoracic and lumbar regions, and they are perpendicular to the plane of the facets. Thus, they serve primarily to limit joint distraction and, to a lesser degree, prevent translation.[73] During anterior eccentric axial loading, these ligaments may be subjected to stretch. Few investigations have been done on the strength of this ligament and its associated structures. Preliminary studies examining the breaking loads for the joint capsule in tension gave values of 150 to 270 newtons for bilateral failure in the thoracic region. It appears to be weakest in the upper thoracic spine.[4, 73]

INTERTRANSVERSE LIGAMENTS

The intertransverse ligaments are seen only in the thoracic and upper lumbar spine. They pass between the transverse processes and attach to the deep muscles of the back. Because of their large lever arms in lateral bending and axial rotation, these ligaments may have a disproportionate effect on the normal mechanics of the spine.[74]

INTERSPINOUS AND SUPRASPINOUS LIGAMENTS

The interspinous and supraspinous ligaments connect adjacent spinous processes. The former attach from the base to the tip of each spinous process, and the latter attach at their tips. The former ligament is most prominent in the lumbar region. These ligaments serve to limit hyperflexion.[74] We found that the interspinous ligament fails in tension at 20 to 150 newtons, approximately one third to one half the values for the anterior longitudinal ligament.[4, 6] The ligament is weakest in the cervical region and becomes progressively stronger as one moves caudally.

Failure patterns have been shown to differ significantly between ligaments. Indeed, the same ligaments may have different patterns at different levels. To some degree, these differences relate to the geometry of the spine at different regions (the posterior elements are subjected to more tension during flexion than are the anterior ligaments). In addition, the nature of the attachment of the ligament to the spine is important; that

is, some ligaments are most likely to fail by avulsion from their bony insertions. The amount of deflection is related not only to the proportion of elastic fibers composing the ligament but also to the distance of the ligament from the vertebral center of rotation.[4, 6] As a result, for a given ligament, the strength tends to be greater on the convex side of curves (such as the posterior ligaments in the midthoracic spine) than on concave surfaces.

These differences in failure patterns are of importance when determining spinal stability. Although it is safe to assume that ligament rupture requires pathologic tension applied to the ligament itself, the same may not be true if failure is produced by avulsion from the spinal attachment. Similarly, patterns in which ligaments are grouped, such as the posterior ligaments, may vary.

In addition, not all ligament injury consists of failure; there may be attenuation, or partial disruption of single layers or regions that causes weakening. Nachemson and Evans showed that there is linear deformation of ligaments, but there is a point at which they begin to fail and their curves become nonlinear.[70] Particularly in cervical dislocations, there is little doubt that ligaments will be stretched if not disrupted, losing the ability to maintain alignment of the spine.[75]

FUNCTIONAL BIOMECHANICS OF THE SPINE

Atlantoaxial Region

The unique anatomy and biomechanics of this region serve its functions well. Although this region is discussed elsewhere in this book, a brief presentation of some of the structural substrates is valuable. The modified ring of C1 serves primarily as a motion limiter for the odontoid and as a locus of attachment for various ligaments, including the anterior longitudinal ligament (anterior tubercle), ligamentum nuchae and muscles (posterior tubercle), and rotational muscles (transverse processes). Medially, tubercles for the transverse atlantal ligament exist. Thus, functionally as well as structurally, it can be considered the "atlas" of the cervical spine.

Ligament relationships are similarly unique. The apical ligament, which attaches at the tip of the odontoid process and foramen magnum, maintains alignment and resists both hyperextension and hyperflexion; the alar ligaments, which are lateral of the apical ligament, have similar functions and also may resist hyperrotation.[76] The most important and unique ligament is the transverse atlantal ligament. Besides being extremely strong, it has little elastic component.[72, 77] It limits motion of the odontoid process, to which it is attached.

Normal Motion of the Cervical Spine

Because pathology both produces and is produced by spinal injury, establishing normal motion values is important. Active motions are facilitated and inhibited by the musculature. Typically, several muscle groups are simultaneously activated and often counterbalance to provide posture. Although the importance of the muscles in the biomechanics of the spine has been mentioned,[78, 79] little work has been done on their effect. Work using motion segments, which ignores muscles' effects, must be considered somewhat suspect if extrapolated to the entire spine.

The primary motions of flexion-extension are more or less evenly distributed throughout the cervical spine, for a total of 60 to 75 degrees. Flexion-extension is greatest at the atlanto-occipital junction, at 13 degrees; it is next highest between C5 and C7, presumably explaining the high degree of degenerative problems at those levels. Translation is limited throughout (about 2 to 3 mm): at C1-2, by the dens, arch of C1, and transverse atlantal ligament; in the rest of the spine, by the ligaments, facet orientation, and disk annulus.[15] Axial rotation and lateral bending are most prominent at C1-2 (the former being 50 degrees). Although no axial rotation occurs at the occiput to C1, 8 degrees of lateral bending can occur at the latter. From C2 to C5, coupled lateral bending-rotation is 10 to 12 degrees and decreases to 4 to 8 degrees below C6, related to facet changes; this accounts for the high incidence of facet dislocation at C7.[80]

Coupling occurs throughout; for instance, lateral bending in the lower cervical spine is in a direction opposite to axial rotation at a given vertebra. Similarly, motions are coupled across levels: lateral bending occurs in the upper cervical spine before any action occurs in the mid and lower cervical region.

Clinical Biomechanics of Cervical Spine Injury

ATLANTOAXIAL INJURIES

At C1, the most common injuries are related to direct axial loading of the spine, due to the broad articulating surfaces and the large amount of flexion-extension that is considered physiologic. These fractures may be manifested as arch fractures or as linear fractures through the facets. Similar fractures can also occur at C2, although they are less common because of the thickness of the lamina. The common Jefferson's fracture represents a lateral explosion of C1, including bilateral fractures through the anterior and posterior arch, as well as disruption of the lateral masses. Jefferson's fractures were once believed to be unstable, but recent biomechanical and clinical data suggest instability only if the lateral masses are dislocated more than 5 mm, implying disruption or avulsion of the transverse atlantal ligament.[13, 81]

Fractures of the odontoid process can occur in flexion or extension across the stronger transverse atlantal ligament or arch of C1, respectively. They are best classified functionally. Type I fractures of the tip are probably due to bone avulsion related to tension applied by the apical and alar ligaments; these are stable. Type II fractures, which occur across the base of the odontoid, are most common; these are typically unstable, in that increased dislocation of the process can occur with movement.[82] Of course, as is commonly the case with other types of fractures, considerations other than stability may influence the decision for fusion versus nonoperative therapy, such as tolerance for nonoperative therapy, age, and general health. Type III fractures are C2 body fractures, produced by flexion or compression forces or both. These should be treated like vertebral fractures elsewhere, and in the absence of posterior element or major ligament injury, they are usually stable.

An unusual but biomechanically significant disorder of C2 is traumatic atlantoaxial dislocation.[19, 80, 82] Following cervical trauma, occasionally an increase in the atlantoaxial distance of more than 3 mm is seen on radiographs, due to rupture of the transverse atlantal ligament. Some investigators[12, 82] have been able to produce such injuries in flexion, with the ligament rupturing across a stronger odontoid process. In studies from our laboratory, atlantoaxial dislocation was produced in both flexion and extension.[12] It appears that there is variability in the strength of the transverse atlantal ligament, particularly in individuals with spinal variants such as congenital block vertebra and occipitalization of the atlas.

Fractures of the arch of C2 can also occur in flexion and extension. Because of the significant muscular attachments to C2, flexion can produce avulsion of the tip of the spinous process, the "clay shoveler's" fracture.[1, 83] By themselves, these are trivial fractures, although there may be signs of significant underlying ligamentous injury, necessitating careful evaluation.

Hyperextension injuries at C2 are common, occurring most frequently in high-speed motor vehicle accidents.[19, 80] The hyperextension of the head on the neck is thought to load the facets and pedicles, causing fractures most often through the latter. The resulting fracture causes disruption of the continuity of the arch and a resultant spondylolisthesis of the arch. Classically, these are unstable fractures, but they have an excellent chance of healing satisfactorily in external orthoses. The instability of these fractures is actually a consequence of coexisting ligament injury. Our studies indicate that disruption of the anterior longitudinal ligament can occur readily in hyperextension, producing a highly unstable injury.[84]

LOWER CERVICAL SPINE INJURIES

Most cervical fractures causing spinal cord injury, as well as unstable fractures as a group, are in part related to compression forces. These may occur with direct vertical (axial) loading or, more commonly, with additional flexion or extension. In a recent epidemiologic effort, 289 cervical fractures produced in automobile accidents were reviewed. The majority of fractures of the cervical spine from C3 downward were presumed—on review of radiographs, associated trauma, and available accident reports—to be due to compression forces. The most common levels of injury were C5 and C6. The most common mechanism of injury was flexion-compression, followed by axially loaded burst fractures, followed by extension injuries with compression.[19, 80]

BURST FRACTURES

The true burst fracture is produced primarily by direct axial loading. Several classic reports suggest that as the forces are directed through the vertebra, the intervertebral disk is traumatized, with fragments pushed into the vertebral body. More commonly, however, the end plate is injured by bulging of the disk, followed by vertebral body fracture.[12, 41, 84, 85] With continuing compression, these bone fragments are pushed into the spinal canal. In some instances, disk injury occurs, but not until after vertebral body fracture. This is contrary to work on motion segments as reported by other groups.[23] Theoretically, the true burst fracture is a stable construct, because ligaments are not injured in compression. In biomechanical studies, however, disruption of the anterior and posterior longitudinal ligaments by disk herniation through the annulus was occasionally observed. The mechanism of this disk injury is uncertain; it is possible that intermediate column buckling, with production of a flexion or extension bending moment and ligament injury, may occur.[12, 86]

In our studies, injuries thought to be produced by axial loading typically included some flexion, often localized to the injured levels.[12, 41] In addition, kinematic studies have shown that some element of shear force occurs during loading.[47, 87] In true experimental burst fractures, kinematic studies showed little movement of the targets in any direction; up to 80% compression of the vertebral body can occur in as little as 2 to 5 msec.[85]

These findings are important in the management of cervical fractures producing cord compression. Considered independently, anterior decompression-fusion is often destabilizing, in that it removes more vertebra than was typically fractured and disrupts potentially viable posterior and anterior ligaments. In the face of posterior ligament instability, performance of anterior procedures alone might be unwise, particularly if rigid orthoses are not employed. In addition, the use of anterior fixation devices alone, in the face of posterior instability, might prove fruitless because of the excess motion generated by the nonfixated posterior elements.[32, 52, 82, 88] Some recent clinical and experimental data suggest that the role of the posterior elements may be minimal if cervical spine alignment is maintained by anterior grafting and fixation; this needs substantiation. Meanwhile, posterior fusion and fixation may be an appropriate adjunct to anterior decompression in burst fractures, as well as fractures with obvious posterior ligament injury.

FLEXION-COMPRESSION INJURIES

Because pure axial loading of the lower cervical spine is unusual and other forces are generally applied in combination, subcategories of the burst fracture, in-

cluding flexion-compression and extension-compression, have been created.[89] In the former, the forces are directed primarily to the anterior aspect of the vertebral body and disks in the lower cervical spine. As a result, anterior wedging of the vertebral body and splaying of the spinous processes and facet joints are typically seen. Dislocation occurs as a result of column buckling secondary to the spinal curves, as well as any shear forces that may be present. In addition, there may be a rotational component to the trauma forces, causing further injury to the ligaments. In early work with spinal columns, early rupture of the posterior ligaments was typically observed. Dislocation of the cervical spine was found to be a consequence of ligament injury.[12] This is contrary to what has been published based on motion segment testing, which suggests that ligaments are disrupted as the spine dislocates.[23]

Dynamic loading studies suggest that spinal injuries are a direct consequence of the order of the force vectors applied to the spine. For instance, if enough preload is present, such that there is some shear loading before compression, dislocation will be particularly prominent; the same type of compression forces that produce significant compression fracture in other circumstances may produce only minor anterior vertebral wedging.[41, 75]

Forces required to produce fractures of the cervical spine in flexion-compression are less than those required to produce failure with axial loading. This phenomenon is predictable from mathematical modeling and on an anatomic basis, as the facets are unloaded in flexion preloading.[43, 90] Because of the anterior compression load applied to the vertebra and the equal amount of increased tension applied to the posterior ligament complex, anterior vertebral wedging becomes likely. Disk bulging and herniation, both anteriorly and posteriorly, are commonly observed with flexion-compression loading. The anterior component is produced by direct compression of the disk, whereas posterior disk protrusion may be related to the development of an incompetent annulus due to tension during flexion-compression.[12, 91]

Common modifications of flexion-compression loading add either shear or rotational forces. Locking of the cervical facets is an extreme example of this phenomenon, seen in about 5% of cervical fractures. Evidence suggests that this is produced by a combination of hyperflexion (but with compression loading) and shear forces, as may be seen in motor vehicle accidents or in falls with the head flexed maximally.[1, 82] More recently, it has been hypothesized that locked facet injury may be the result of hyperflexion and post-traumatic muscle contractions.[75] Dislocation is, to a major degree, the result of ligamentous instability.[75, 82] Total disruption of all ligaments in cervical dislocation is not uncommon, particularly the posterior complex and the anterior longitudinal ligament. The implications of this for clinical management, including efforts at closed reduction, are significant. For example, traction may be dangerous if larger weights are used; further, closed treatments such as the halo device are much more likely to fail when used with ligament failure rather than bone failure with intact ligaments.

ROTATION INJURIES

Rotation injuries produced by exaggerated normal motion (i.e., hyperrotation or lateral bending) are often manifested as unilateral locked or fractured facets, commonly with minimal malalignment of the vertebrae. Several recent clinical papers declare these injuries to be stable. In our experience, this is often the case for an isolated rotation injury. However, it must be emphasized that ligament injury cannot be predicted on the basis of radiographic demonstration of bone injury. Severe ligament and annulus fibrosus injury may be produced during the loading event, because rotation itself may injure ligaments by avulsing them from bony attachments or disrupt them as a result of tension applied to them.[4, 12, 41]

EXTENSION INJURIES

Compression forces are typically part of these injuries, commonly directed through the facet to the posterior elements. Multilevel pathology usually occurs, including pedicles, facets, laminae, and spinous processes.[15] If the forces are sagittal, injuries are bilateral. More commonly, because of the "whipping" of the head-neck complex, rotation or asymmetrical loading occurs. Most clinical reports and experimental studies using motion segments suggest that anterior ligament injury can occur after fracture of the posterior elements.[15] However, work from our laboratories has shown that the anterior longitudinal ligament can be injured before fracture of the posterior elements.[20] These results are consistent with the biomechanical properties of the facet, which is able to absorb a significant amount of any compressive load, decreasing the likelihood of arch fracture. Thus, experimental studies using entire cervical columns are likely to demonstrate more clinically applicable pathology.

Although radiographs may appear normal, cryosections of spines injured in extension often demonstrate several levels of disk injury and anterior longitudinal ligament disruption.[85, 92] Classic flexion-extension radiographs may also appear normal, but there is a potential for instability and subsequent deformity as a result of progressive disk degeneration and the ligament injury that has occurred. Experimentally, motion analysis is particularly helpful in demonstrating exaggerated but subpathologic motion that occurs at multiple levels, which may have significant long-term clinical implications.

Normal Motion of the Thoracic and Lumbar Spine

Physiologic motion of the spine is both facilitated and inhibited by the musculature (anterior and posterior, as well as lateral). Anterior muscle groups flex the spine. In addition, oblique muscles such as the abdominal obliques cause spine rotation. Others, such as the psoas group, participate in lateral bending as well as rotation. Similarly, both superficial and deep posterior muscles are concerned with extension of the spine; most muscles are also involved with rotation (semispinalis, rotators) or lateral bending (splenius group). In the posterior group, superficial muscles are more prominent in bending, and deeper muscles are more prominent in rotation of the spine. The muscles found lateral to the spinal column are involved in lateral rotation (sternocleidomastoid and scalenus group) as well as bending (trapezius, quadratus).

When considering the role of muscles in motion of the spine, one must recognize that typically several groups are simultaneously activated. For example, maintenance of posture requires support of the weight of the torso. If the center of gravity of the torso is shifted, a counterbalancing force is required on the other side. Here, the longissimus dorsi muscles are generally active during standing. During rotation of the lumbar spine, the ipsilateral erector spinae and contralateral short rotators actively contract.[93]

The rib cage serves to restrict motion and add stiffness to the spine. Andriacchi and associates predicted that the compression tolerance of the spinal column in the presence of the rib cage is increased by a factor of four.[94] It is likely that all physiologic movements of the ligamentous spine are decreased by the rib cage; for extension, this reduction may be as high as 70%. Rib-cage effects are less prominent in flexion and lateral rotation. Removal of one or two ribs, commonly performed during spinal surgery, does not similarly affect the stiffness of the spine–rib cage complex unless a portion of the sternum is also removed.[28, 93]

To accurately represent the characteristics of the thoracic spine, the coupled motions must be measured simultaneously. Although this can be done with functional segments, analyzing coupling associated with normal spine curvatures is difficult at best. Panjabi and coworkers analyzed the coupling phenomenon, using physiologic moments as the loads.[35] They found that in the thoracic spine with ribs removed, all sagittal plane movements are strongly coupled, including translation and rotation.

The extent of normal motion within the thoracic spine is determined partially by the rib cage and the orientation of the facets.[15] In part, the fixed ribs limit flexion-extension from T1 to T9; this is also a function of the spinal ligaments.[93] The bony components of the spine also have an effect on the motion in the thoracic region. White and Hirsch[95] and Panjabi and coworkers[35] analyzed the effects of removing the posterior elements on the stability of the thoracic spine. Extension was increased substantially following such removal, presumably because the intervertebral joints and spinous processes limit extension in the area, particularly in the mid and lower thoracic regions. The degree of rotation occurring about the horizontal plane also increased. Indeed, they emphasized that because of the alignment of the facets, resistance to axial rotation due to bone does not occur. They suggested that the major structures resisting rotation in addition to the rib cage and its musculature include the ligamenta flava, facet capsules, and anterior and posterior longitudinal ligaments.

Studies on the effects of laminectomy on the thoracic spine have recently been conducted in our laboratories. In isolated columns (with the ligaments intact but the rib cage removed), two-level laminectomy had a significant effect on the stiffness of the column, as well as on the amount of motion allowed. Loads to failure of the column, which typically occurred at the cephalad extent of the laminectomy, were reduced by almost 50%; motion was also increased at the more cephalad level, particularly at the posterior elements. Thus, it appears that even in axial loading, forces are transmitted eccentrically through the thoracic spine, particularly affecting the facets. Repetitive loading, which occurs continuously in vivo, may lead to deformities as a result.[96]

The effect of the disk on axial rotation would seem to be prominent, but this has not been assessed experimentally. The facets appear to provide stability primarily against anterior translation, especially between T1 and T8. Where the facets change in orientation to the more lumbar pattern, typically at T9 or T10, more anterior translation can occur, and axial rotation is more limited.

Other structures also limit hyperflexion in the thoracic region. The annulus of the disk, the well-developed posterior longitudinal ligament, and the thick ligamenta flava prevent hyperflexion. This again emphasizes the importance of the posterior elements and ligaments in the maintenance of stability of the thoracic spine. As is the case elsewhere in the spine, the anterior longitudinal ligament resists excess extension.

Generally, the extent of flexion and extension is approximately 65 to 80 degrees (with respect to the horizontal plane) in the thoracic spine.[15, 93] In the upper thoracic region, from Tl to T5, this averages 3 degrees per level. Values are increased slightly in the midthoracic region from T5 to T10 and reach a maximum in the lower thoracic spine for anatomic reasons already discussed. Gregerson and Lucas found that as much as 10 degrees of axial rotation per level is commonly seen in the upper and middle thoracic region.[97] Maximal rotation in their studies was from T4 to T9. Facet orientation in the upper thoracic region limits the amount of anterior translation possible. In the lower thoracic region, where the facets have acquired a lumbar pattern, axial rotation is extremely limited.

Lateral bending is fairly consistent throughout the upper and middle thoracic spine, at approximately 4 to 5 degrees per level. It increases substantially below the fixed rib cage to 5 to 10 degrees per level. There is a significant degree of coupling between lateral bending and axial rotation. Typically, it is seen to the extent that spinous process motion is toward the convexity of the curvature of the thoracic spine. This may have clinical significance in the pathophysiology of scoliosis. The extent of this coupling is variable, with strongest associations seen in the upper thoracic spine; from T5 to T10, the coupling pattern may be reversed.

The extent of normal range of motion in the lumbar spine is of critical importance because of the extensive coupling, as well as the strong relationship between motion and the development of degenerative changes. Flexion-extension increases caudally, from 12 to 14 degrees at L1 to 18 degrees at L5-S1, under normal circumstances. Lateral bending changes little, averaging 7 to 9 degrees throughout the lumbar spine. Similarly, rotation is consistent and extremely limited, averaging 3 degrees per level. In considering the little-studied area of translation (which is extremely important when diagnosing degenerative instability of the lumbar spine), 2 mm is probably normal for the lumbar spine.[98]

Coupling is an important phenomenon in the lumbar spine. The most clinically relevant pattern is that of axial rotation and lateral bending, which has strong relevance in the development of degenerative disk disease.[15, 98] As discussed earlier, this pattern is paradoxical: the spinous process is directed in the same direction as the lateral bending; this is the opposite of that seen in the rest of the spine.

Clinical Biomechanics of Thoracic and Lumbar Spine Injury

FLEXION-COMPRESSION INJURIES

Laboratory studies and clinical experience suggest that the majority of thoracic and lumbar vertebral fractures are related to both compression of the vertebral body and multilevel distraction injuries of the posterior elements.[9, 24, 26, 29, 30, 93, 99, 100] Thus, this is the emphasis of our discussion. However, other types of loading patterns are sometimes seen in the thoracic spine. In particular, compression fractures due to minor trauma in the presence of underlying bone disease (i.e., osteoporosis, tumor) may occur with trivial forces and be related to axial loads.

In what we call flexion-compression loading, referring to what happens biomechanically rather than anatomically, a load is developed over the dorsum of the upper thoracic spine or through the base of the pelvis, with a lever arm developed at the eventual level of failure. The injury typically produced by this type of loading has also been termed the type C burst fracture, or sometimes flexion-distraction injury.[31, 36] The bending moment developed as a result of the spinal loading reflects both the length of the column and the distance between the centrum of the vertebra and a line dropped from the top of the load point of the column. In the lower thoracic spine (T10-12), this flexion bending moment is created by anatomic factors, including the termination of the rib cage and the normal thoracic kyphosis, the initiation of the lumbar lordosis, and the orientation of the facets.

Normally, the center of mass at the level of the thoracolumbar spine is 4 cm anterior to the vertebra (in the sitting position).[101] When loads are applied to the dorsum of the back (as in a fall) or through the pelvis (as in motor vehicle or toboggan accidents), a significant amount of flexion occurs during impact, along with the transmitted compression forces. The eccentricity of a delivered load is increased even more during forward motion, further flexing the spine. Thus, the distraction loads transmitted to the posterior elements may be more pronounced than the compression loads applied to the vertebrae, depending, to some degree, on the location of the loading vector. In intact cadaver and spinal column studies using quasi-static loading, early disruption of the posterior elements was a consistent finding. Indeed, posterior ligamentous instability almost always occurs before vertebral fracture.[26] Injury of the posterior disk and posterior longitudinal ligament typically is the third part of the sequence, occurring after the vertebral fracture, although failure of the joint capsule occurs shortly after posterior ligament complex injury.[65]

CHANCE FRACTURES

Chance fractures may actually represent modifications of flexion-compression loading in which the predominant force is flexion, often incorporating an element of shear. The axis of loading is anterior to the spine, and progressive disruption of the posterior elements, the disk, and the posterior longitudinal ligament occurs. Typically, however, the load stops short of major compression of the vertebral body. In the compression-flexion fracture, with its more prominent vertebral fracture, a measure of vertical loading occurs simultaneously with the flexion moment, producing the combined injury. In the seat-belt injury, in contrast, the top part of the torso, which is unrestrained, flexes over the fixed pelvis. Chance fractures are unusual in the thoracic spine, although a few have been seen related to improper use of restraints. In addition, they can be produced by high-speed motor vehicle accidents when the lower half of the torso (i.e., the section caudal to the fracture) is relatively fixed.[9, 65]

BURST FRACTURES

The distinction between a burst fracture and one due to flexion-compression is not an academic one, because the true burst fracture (produced by axial loading) is probably biomechanically stable.[15, 102] Indeed, studies suggest that a symmetrical fracture of the vertebral body, even if there is fracture of a pedicle, may not be mechanically unstable. Atlas and colleagues retrospectively looked at 75 burst fractures.[29] Only 15% had no posterior element involvement on polytomography. Unilateral fractures were evident in 29 cases (39%), and bilateral injuries in 35 cases (47%). Interpedicular distances were above normal in 81% of cases.

The flexion-compression fracture is typically unstable, presenting risks to the integrity of the spinal cord. The stability of the spine following other less common types of fractures, such as the Chance fracture, is also a function of the trauma produced on each of the spinal elements.

It should be emphasized that similar forces and directions do not always produce similar injuries, so stability cannot necessarily be predicted from static radiographs. This has implications for surgical technique if surgery is required. Therefore, a thorough understanding of the biomechanics of injury is important in planning management.

BIOMECHANICS OF TREATMENT

Subjecting treatment concepts to biomechanical scrutiny has become increasingly important and popular in recent years. In particular, the emphasis has been on the effects of spinal instrumentation on the stiffness of the spine. This emphasis is unfortunate, because even ordinary types of treatment may have biomechanical implications. For example, little if any work has been done on the in vivo effects of aggressive rehabilitation programs on spinal stability; instead, the emphasis has been on symptomatic relief. Studies investigating resulting spinal motion, resistance to externally applied loads, and internally measured forces (using perhaps thin-wire pressure transducers or fluoroscopy) will be of value in measuring these parameters.

Surgical manipulations have a biomechanical impact as well. Pediatric neurosurgeons have long known that laminectomy—particularly cervical laminectomy—has an adverse mechanical effect on spinal alignment and may lead to the development of kyphosis and deformity. Recent studies, discussed later, suggest that the same may be true in the thoracic spine.

Biomechanics Research Techniques

Because the spine is best considered from the perspective of its components, typically the most basic unit of biomechanics research is the motion segment. The segment includes two vertebral bodies and their intermediate disk and ligaments (see Fig. 278–1). It can be used to study the characteristics of the disk and ligaments between them. However, results from these studies cannot substitute for column studies, because the spine is inhomogeneous, and thus the results of testing are nonlinear. In addition, many structures, such as the spinal ligaments, extend for more than two segments; therefore, such limited biomechanical trials should be considered merely a starting point.

Many biomechanical laboratories favor the use of macromodels, or spinal columns, in their studies. These allow more physiologic analysis, along with the consideration of treatment for spinal disorders, such as fusion. Unfortunately, the use of more physiologic models makes experimentation less well controlled and more subject to biologic variation.

Loading patterns also affect the physiologic nature of the studies conducted. The simplest method of spinal loading is to use pure moments—that is, to apply unidirectional forces around a single axis. These pure forces can be applied for each of the six possible moments (flexion, extension, right and left lateral bending, and right and left axial rotation), and loads to deformation (nondestructive loading) or injury can be measured. A more complex way of loading includes combining the various forces, such as compression and flexion, to obtain compression-flexion loading.

Although both pure moment and complex loading

techniques have value, the former have become more accepted in biomechanics research.[27, 30, 32, 48, 103, 104] Studies incorporating pure moment loading are more controllable but not necessarily as physiologic; for example, most clinical studies, and several experimental ones using cadavers, emphasized that thoracolumbar fractures are typically produced by combined flexion-compression loading (i.e., multimoment loading).[12, 29–31, 39, 105] When pure moment loading is used, the latest techniques that offer higher accuracy and more reproducible data include the use of an integrated six-axis load cell and automated three-dimensional imaging techniques.[106]

Loading rates can also be varied. The spine generally behaves as a viscoelastic structure and therefore responds differently to quasi-static loading (bodies at rest or being loaded at slow rates) and dynamic loading.[7, 27, 47, 105] As in the case of other parameters in biomechanics research, the most controllable type of loading (quasi-static) is not always the most physiologic. More rapid dynamic techniques are necessary when evaluating most common injury-producing scenarios. The spine is stiffer during dynamic loading, not unlike a shock absorber whose compression is altered by the speed of loading.[27, 105] There are interactive elements, however, such as age, which our laboratory has demonstrated can influence the effect of loading rate.[27]

It is difficult to control the effects of free-moving specimens in the absence of sophisticated computerized actuators, and it is also difficult to monitor the effects of loading without high-speed optics. However, the data thus generated have much more direct application to clinical injury. Thus, quasi-static loading can be used for nondestructive loading and provide valuable information about properties of the spine; if failure mechanics is being studied, dynamic loading becomes more valuable.

In quasi-static loading studies, the sequence of injury in the cervical and thoracolumbar spine subjected to flexion-compression is posterior element injury, followed by vertebral body compression.[12] In dynamic loading, however, although the net injuries may be similar, the sequence is altered, with vertebral compression often occurring earlier than posterior element injury.[85, 87]

Similarly, preloading (i.e., aligning the spinal column in a given direction or with a small load on it before the major force application) is very important in quasi-static loading. If the spine is preloaded in flexion, for example, the major injury vector tends to be flexion, although intermediate column buckling may alter this phenomenon. In dynamic loading, the effects of preloading are relatively unknown.[31, 47, 107]

In traditional biomechanical studies, the two characteristics measured are the forces required to produce changes in the structures loaded and the displacement of the column or components in response to those loads. Information derived from these two characteristics includes the structure's stiffness, which measures the structure's ability to resist deforming forces and is an important measure of the effectiveness of spinal instrumentation. Displacement can also be studied

without regard to forces (kinematics). In these studies, the spine is marked at multiple points, and movements of targets are tracked optically. The assumptions are that there are rigid elements between the spinal soft tissue components and that target motion can be measured as a function of time during a loading sequence.

The study of spinal kinematics has greatly expanded our understanding of the nature of spinal trauma. For instance, in studies of pedicle fixation in thoracolumbar spine trauma, motion at the posterior vertebra has been found to be significantly decreased within the fixation points but is largely unaffected at the anterior aspect of the vertebra.[108, 109] Such information is unobtainable from force-deformation data, and in conjunction with stiffness data, it has suggested further ideas for investigation, including the effects of anterior grafting on spinal alignment, as well as the role of restoration of vertebral body height in preventing late deformity.[110]

Cervical Spine Research

Devices proposing to stabilize the cervical spine need to be considered in light of some of the biomechanical principles presented earlier. The most important principle is that, at least in trauma, vertebral compression or dislocation in association with disruption of the posterior ligaments is common; therefore, stabilization techniques need to stiffen the "columns" of the spine.

FACETECTOMY AND FUSION

Fundamental studies have been carried out by Cusick and coworkers on the effects of partial and complete facet injury—whether traumatic or iatrogenic—on the stability of the cervical spine.[111] Motion segments were subjected to flexion-compression at low rates and subfailure loads, and kinematic testing was performed. Specimens then underwent unilateral or bilateral facetectomy and were retested. Fixation with facet-facet or facet–spinous process wiring was then accomplished, and testing was performed again.

Unilateral facet injury decreased strength by 31.6%, and bilateral facetectomy was responsible for a 53% decrease in strength. In the latter case, loading of the injured specimen was associated with 36% compression at the vertebra and 31% distraction at the spinous processes, both highly significant. Both wiring constructs restored at least 20% of the strength of the motion segments and reduced spinal motion.

In a follow-up study using a validated cervical finite-element computer model, this same group identified 50% removal of the facet joint as the critical point of strength decrease.[45] These additional modeling tools offer greater precision in determining the cutoff points where spinal stability can be affected.

These data are important in validating the importance of the facets in maintaining stability of the cervical spine in flexion-compression loads. The direct clinical implication of these data is that unilateral injury or dislocation of a facet, whether traumatic or iatrogenic, may be associated with decreased strength of the spine, even in the absence of other injury. The corollary is that appropriate stabilization of the cervical spine must incorporate fixation of the injured facets. Other studies, with similar results, have been performed in the lumbar spine by the same group.[17, 18]

CERVICAL FIXATION

The oldest and most effective means of stabilizing the cervical spine continues to be wiring of intact posterior spinal components, incorporating bone grafting as part of the construct. Several studies have compared the effectiveness of wiring and bone and plating systems, some of which are discussed here.

In studies using cadaver cervical spines, Coe and coworkers compared the effects of Caspar plates, as well as posterior fixation techniques (lateral mass plates, AO hook plates, posterior wiring), on spines injured at C5-6, using cyclic loading.[112] In flexion loading, all the posterior constructs, as well as the anterior-posterior construct, significantly reduced posterior strains to preinjury values. Caspar plates did not effectively reduce posterior strains or increase the stiffness of the cervical spine.

Spinal stiffness with extension loading was no better with Caspar plating alone than with posterior fixation. Indeed, there is evidence that even in extension, the posterior columns—especially the facets—have an important role in resisting pathologic forces.[112] Combination fixation, with anterior plating and posterior wiring or plating, as is commonly used in severe dislocation and ligament disruption, appears to be most effective in reducing anterior strains. It has been shown that anterior plating alone shifts the axis of rotation of the fused segment abnormally far forward. The result is paradoxical, with the interbody graft experiencing extreme compression in extension and becoming relatively unloaded in flexion.[113]

In pure axial and torsion loading, combination fixation was the most valuable for reducing anterior strains, followed by posterior fixation alone. Anterior plates were not effective in reducing posterior strains. In torsion, combination anterior-posterior plating and posterior plates were best, although not significantly so. Results of static cyclic loading were similar. By the end of 100 cycles, the Caspar-instrumented spines became less rigid because of loosening at the screw-plate junction; however, the bone-metal interface was not studied.

Available biomechanical studies suggest that posterior wiring and grafting are biomechanically equivalent to posterior plating for highly unstable injuries, with the possible exception of rotation. To the best of our knowledge, no studies have been performed testing cervical spine instrumentation using continuous motion analysis, which allows measurement of intermediate vectors. From the clinician's perspective, the choice of technique must be weighed against the potential risks. For instance, most authors note that sublaminar wiring carries a risk of neurological injury; because its biomechanical performance is not superior to that of spinous process wiring, it may be difficult to justify the risks. Similarly, posterior plating requires placing screws in the region of nerve roots and the vertebral artery. In the absence of evidence that plates are superior to wiring in terms of stiffening the spine, it may be prudent to reserve plating for cases in which clinical circumstances preclude wiring. Last, anterior plating alone does not stabilize the severely injured spine.[46] Its use should be limited to situations in which the purpose is to reduce motion in a spine with intact posterior elements, for protection of bone grafts, or in conjunction with posterior fixation or a rigid external orthosis.

We have not dealt at length with one of the most significant issues related to the biomechanics of spinal instrumentation: its ultimate status. As was shown in cyclic loading of the Caspar plates, repetitive loading produces changes at the bone-implant interface, which may decrease the effectiveness of any of these devices. Obtaining solid bone fusion, usually requiring grafting, is important in reaching that goal.

Thoracolumbar Spine Research

Biomechanical considerations in the thoracolumbar spine are different from those in the cervical spine. First, according to Denis,[36] the middle column acquires prominence. Second, loading factors are somewhat different, with much larger bending moments delivered.[26, 39, 100] This section is not all-inclusive; we emphasize work on transpedicular fixation, which has become increasingly popular among neurosurgeons for the treatment of tumor, trauma, and degenerative disease.[110, 114–118] Theoretical advantages of pedicle fixation include excellent fixation into the pedicle and vertebral body, which represents a biomechanically stiff construct, as well as the ability to produce stability by fixating a shorter spinal segment. Although most surgeons advocate instrumenting two levels above and below the fracture, others place screws at levels adjacent to the fracture and report reduction of deformity and maintenance of normal lordosis.[28, 101, 109, 114, 118] The question of the biomechanical stability of short-segment versus longer-segment fixation remains unanswered.

THORACIC LAMINECTOMY

Studies have been conducted to determine whether thoracic laminectomy increases the risk of injury to the thoracic spine acutely.[96] Fifteen thoracic columns, including seven controls and eight laminectomized spines, were studied. Strength and localized kinematic data were obtained. Load-deflection behavior indicated nonlinear sigmoidal characteristics typical of spinal columns. Failure forces and stiffness were higher for normal than laminectomized specimens; deflections were similar, however. Thus, the spinal column, irrespective of pathologic alteration, is deformation sensitive. The extent of anterior vertebral compression and posterior element distraction was greater in the laminectomized specimens. Decreases in strength (by as much as 45%) and increases in flexibility may add to the instability of the spine under pathologic or repeated loading. This has implications for the use of laminectomy as an isolated procedure in disorders that can involve the vertebral body (e.g., metastatic disease). It also appears that with repetitive motion incorporating subclinical but pathologic motion (i.e., microtrauma), accelerated degeneration and clinical instability may occur.

LONG-SEGMENT INSTRUMENTATION

Several early studies investigated the biomechanics of Harrington rodding, usually in distraction.[37, 38] Jacobs and associates determined that a "tension band" is the best replacement for the incompetent posterior ligaments in flexion injuries,[37] a principle that remains valid today. Most investigators have found that Harrington distraction rods are effective in reducing dislocation but often disengage in flexion. White and Panjabi compared compression and distraction rods using three-point bending.[15] They found distraction rods five times stiffer and therefore (in three-point loading) five times more effective than compression rods. They recommended that distraction rods be used to reduce deformities and that compression rods be used to improve stability.

Jacobs and associates also used flexion loading to compare Harrington distraction and compression rods and Roy-Camille plates fixed to facets or pedicles.[37] The unstable preparation included vertebral wedging and posterior ligament disruption. Distraction rods did not reduce deformities well and failed at low loads. Compression rods placed in the lamina and plates that were fixed segmentally both performed well, failing at moments of 80 Nm with fractures at the fixation points. Roy-Camille plates provided a more rigid construct. McAfee and colleagues evaluated Harrington distraction rods and Luque rods in axial compression and rotation.[119] The Luque rods were found to provide the greatest stiffness and resistance to rotation. In our own studies, Harrington distraction rods failed at low loads in flexion and were less stiff than sublaminar-wired Luque rods.[38] Other unpublished studies suggest that spinous process wiring improves the stiffness of Harrington rods, but the hooks are still likely to fail in flexion.

UNIVERSAL INSTRUMENTATION

In the early 1980s, a major development occurred in spinal instrumentation: the Cotrel-Dubousset "universal instrumentation" system, allowing maximal flexibility in hook choices and effective spinal stabilization. Developed primarily for patients with scoliosis, it soon found applications in those with trauma, tumors, and degenerative diseases. The biomechanics of universal instrumentation has been widely studied, and the characteristics of the different products available appear to be similar; any differences are related to the configuration of the construct.

An early biomechanical study of the Cotrel-Dubousset system compared it with the more traditional segmentally wired Harrington distraction rods and segmentally wired Luque rods.[120] Harrington rods demonstrated the lowest axial and torsional stiffness

in the cadaver model. In calf spines, the single-level Cotrel-Dubousset system was no stiffer in axial loading than the other devices tested, but it was much more stable in torsion. However, as we noted previously, because most fractures are related to flexion-compression, the forces that must be resisted for effective instrumentation are related primarily to axial configurations. The axial stability of two-level Cotrel-Dubousset instrumentation was four times greater than that of Harrington distraction rods or single-level Cotrel-Dubousset instrumentation. Our clinical series of Cotrel-Dubousset instrumentation corroborates many of the biomechanical data available. Patients were surgically corrected an average of 13 degrees. At 1 year, average loss of correction was 3.4 degrees. As a consequence of the construct's rigidity, more than 60% of our patients complained of painful stiffness; we removed instrumentation in 29 patients, with improvement in pain in all, but loss of alignment in two patients who had underlying nonunion. Another 60 patients have undergone long-segment Isola instrumentation, with similar results. Such long-term considerations may be as important as biomechanical considerations in many circumstances, and this has created interest in the use of pedicle fixation in stabilization following trauma.

PEDICLE FIXATION IN TRAUMA

In recent years, there has been increasing interest in the use of pedicle fixation in trauma patients, as well as to stabilize the spine in cases of subfailure instability resulting from degenerative disease and its treatment. Pedicle screw placement may provide three-column fixation, thereby allowing fewer segments to be incorporated.[36, 115, 121] This would maintain spinal range of motion and presumably decrease back pain in patients.

Biomechanical validation of the procedure exists. Most investigators have reported adequate stabilization with improved resistance to certain pathologic motion (compared with rod systems), particularly rotation and translation.[108–110, 114, 122] More recently, investigators examined the effect of depth of screw insertion into the vertebral body, finding that depth was significantly related to pullout strength.[121]

In an early clinical series, Whitesides and Shaw reported poor results in four of five patients with thoracolumbar fractures.[42] These patients suffered screw breakage, with recurrence of their deformities. Unfortunately, no information was provided as to the number of levels fixed. The authors suggested that these failures could have been prevented with the use of anterior grafting, recognizing the failure of rigid short-segment instrumentation to provide stability of the anterior column. Other investigators have obtained satisfactory fusion, but with more deformity than seen with anterior column reconstruction.[28, 123] Successful application of pedicle screw fixation requires recognition of the distinction between a cantilever beam and a construct in which the screws are not rigidly attached to the intervening rod or plate transmitting the vertical loads. Examples include the older Luque plates and the Steffee plate. The advantage of the cantilever system—namely, support of the anterior column—is the motivation for its current widespread use, particularly in the context of unstable thoracolumbar fractures. Unfortunately, it is also the reason for its failure when it is used without respect for the biomechanical principles at play. One series reported a 41% rate of screw fracture when a cantilever beam construct was used without an anterior graft.[124] Reconstruction of the anterior column reestablishes the load sharing of the anterior column and protects the cantilever beam from failure, which most often manifests as proximal screw breakage. When this construct is used in combination with an appropriate graft anteriorly, a short construct sparing motion segments can be successful.[125]

Gurr and associates measured rigidity produced by pedicle fixation versus hook-rod systems in a calf model.[126] Vertebrectomy and iliac crest grafting were performed with both posterior and anterior instrumentation systems. Anterior column stiffness associated with axial, flexion, or axial-flexion loading was measured. The amount of displacement allowed with pedicle screw systems was essentially the same as that in the intact spine and with fixation with a rod system in axial loading. They suggested that the excellent resistance to pathologic forces resulting from pedicle fixation was related to the anterior column fixation produced by the pedicle screw, as opposed to true posterior fixation. Unfortunately, the study did not examine the failure biomechanics of pedicle fixation over one level or without anterior strut grafting. Anteriorly placed Harrington rods and the Kaneda device were compared in a model not including posterior element instability, as is commonly seen in trauma. Indeed, there may be little indication for any kind of spinal instrumentation in the absence of posterior element instability.[28, 38] The anterior devices resisted axial loading as well as posterior pedicle fixation did. In rotation, anterior fixation was the most efficient, followed by long-segment (i.e., four-level) pedicle fixation.

In the studies of Chang and colleagues, five-level posterior instrumentation was more effective in resisting rotational loads than was a three-segment rod-screw system.[122] Three-segment fixation was more effective than other methods in resisting pure axial loads, which are uncommon. In flexion, which may represent the most frequent load responsible for failure of spinal instrumentation devices, the shorter system was not as effective as five-segment instrumentation, presumably as a result of the longer lever arm. Another study compared plate and rod systems in a corpectomy model using cyclic loading, measuring biomechanical strength characteristics for Zielke and AO internal fixator rods and Steffee, Luque, and AO notched plates.[114] Axial and torsional stiffness values were similar for all. However, stresses were beyond the material endurance of the Steffee plate and the AO internal fixator. Thus, there may be a risk of screw fatigue and fracture at the screw base in the two tested fixed-plate systems.

We have been investigating the biomechanics of pedicle fixation for several years.[108–110, 117, 125] In a recent clinical series with 1-year minimal follow-up, 34 patients underwent short-segment transpedicular fixation

for thoracolumbar fractures, with corpectomy via the extracavitary approach included in patients with spinal canal compromise. Length of time in spinal orthoses averaged 12 weeks. Average loss of correction during the follow-up period was 6.2 degrees, with successful fusion in all cases. These results are better than most of those reported in the American literature and are statistically similar to those of our Cotrel-Dubousset series. This may be because "load sharing" with the anterior graft occurs; another logical conclusion based on biomechanical data presented later is that the anterior graft, by better maintaining vertebral body height, allows loads to be more effectively transmitted though the instrumentation and normal vertebral loading paths.

Our series of patients undergoing pedicle fixation and fusion for degenerative instability and spondylolisthesis of the lumbar spine now numbers about 2500.[28] We have found that transpedicular fixation is effective in decreasing motion and enhancing fusion rates; however, we have inferred the possibility of accelerated degenerative changes at adjacent segments, as suggested later.

Methods in Pedicle Fixation Studies

Studies have typically been carried out in thoracolumbar spinal segments incorporating T11 to L5.[108–110] Three-dimensional motion analysis is an important component of instrumentation testing and has been used in all recent biomechanical studies. To injure the spine, a small amount of the anterior cortex of the vertebra in the middle of the spinal column is fractured using an osteotome to ensure fracture at an appropriate level. Each specimen is placed on a six-axis load cell, which is capable of measuring forces along the three anatomic directions and the three respective moments (flexion, lateral flexion, and axial twist). The column is then positioned in an electrohydraulic servosystem in the lateral position, with a slight flexion bending moment, and the spine is loaded to failure at a quasi-static rate of 2.5 mm/second under compression-flexion forces. Piston excursion is terminated at failure of the spinal column. With the spine still under load, a lateral radiograph is obtained. The specimen is then reloaded (injury cycle) by applying compression to the maximal deflection achieved at failure during the intact cycle. Following repeat radiography, Steffee pedicle screw-plate fixation is carried out with screws one level proximal and distal to the level of injury. The spine is then repositioned in the frame and—following repeat radiography—reloaded (stabilized cycle) to the deformation experienced during the first run.

Results of Pedicle Fixation Studies

In our first investigation of pedicle fixation in the injured thoracolumbar spine, we determined that stiffness of the construct is quite high. Following Steffee fixation, failure forces averaged 70% of control values, and deformations were 166% higher than control values, indicating that the specimen did not fail at the same level of deformation as in the intact spine. In other words, although the overall strength of the column appeared to be increased, the ductility of the fixated spine also appeared to be increased.

The stabilization provided by the system, as measured at the posterior vertebral body, was statistically significant.[108] However, we observed insignificant changes in the final stiffness between the stabilized and the injured configurations, demonstrating that the fixated column responds the same as the injured spine beyond a certain strain level. Because the instability of the injured spine is dictated principally by the decreased load-carrying capacity of the fractured vertebral body, this final stiffness corresponds to the load shared by the anterior column. Therefore, it can be hypothesized that the device has an initial stiffening effect on the posterior columns, enhancing the strength of the injured spine, after which the anterior column must absorb a higher portion of the external load. Above this threshold, little stiffness is added to the lumbar spine. Consequently, to further increase the strength of the structure, it may be necessary to reinforce the anterior column as well.[110] This observation has been made by others who noted deformity after pedicle fixation alone in trauma patients.

Increased motion at the proximal and distal disks was seen, indicating increased flexibility at these levels and the potential for instability at adjacent segments. This observation has been made clinically but has not been demonstrated biomechanically. We typically observed that motion in the bodies was similar for nonfixated and fixated spines, suggesting that fixation fails to maintain spinal integrity. In addition, the data suggest that repetitive loading might affect the integrity of such posterior fixation.[109]

Anterior Grafting Studies

In a series of experiments, the effects of anterior grafting on the strength of the pedicle-fixated spine, in conjunction with partial corpectomy, were investigated.[110] Two questions were addressed: Does anterior grafting improve the biomechanics of pedicle fixation? How does corpectomy affect the fixated spine?

Following the experimental sequence described earlier, partial vertebrectomy at the fractured level was accomplished, similar to that seen in the extracavitary approach to the spine.[25, 28] A tricortical iliac crest graft, taken from that cadaver, was introduced. The specimens were then reloaded to the failure deformation value. The anterior height of the fractured vertebra and Cobb angles were measured before, during, and after loading in each run. Stiffness of the structure was computed using the linear phases of the force-deformation plot. Force, deformation, stiffness, and energy were used to assess the strength characteristics of the specimen under the different configurations. The localized kinematics of the specimen for each configuration were obtained.

The differences in stiffness and load between the control and injury runs were highly significant. Stiffness in the intact column was higher than in any of the other conditions; the degree of stiffness in fixated spines was next. Maximal loads for the strut runs were higher than those for the injured spine but lower than those for the intact spinal column. In addition, they were lower than the values for the fixated column at the termination of loading.

Spinal alignment was altered by trauma. In all instances, differences between preloading and postloading angles were significant. An average of 12 degrees of forward flexion was seen in the initial failure group. Cobb angles in the initial injury group increased from a preload value of 4 to 16 degrees. Final Cobb angles in spines with pedicle fixation alone were not significantly different from those with anterior struts and pedicle fixation. However, the anterior heights of the fractured vertebrae were significantly different, with maintenance of body height in the anterior graft group.

Compared with the injured (destabilized) specimens, fixated specimens showed decreased motion at the posterior element targets. Decreases in anterior vertebral target motion were also seen. Motions were altered in the vertebral bodies by anterior grafting when measured from the bodies immediately proximal and distal to the fracture. Paradoxically, posterior vertebral motion was reduced by grafting in the midvertebral level as measured from the anterior-posterior direction. On gross observation, some collapse of the bicortical grafts into the adjacent vertebrae occurred during the strut-graft run.

In the companion clinical report discussed earlier, we hypothesized that "load sharing" with the anterior graft occurs; another logical conclusion from the present data is that the anterior graft, by better maintaining vertebral body height, allows loads to be more effectively transmitted through the instrumentation and normal vertebral loading paths. However, motion at the levels of the posterior intervertebral disk and anterior vertebra was decreased, but not to the extent observed in the posterior elements.[109, 123] Thus, some concern still exists that pedicle fixation alone may be inadequate for stabilization. Whether anterior strut grafting is associated with better alignment long term also remains a question.

The studies discussed here, though useful, have a significant problem: the single-cycle nature of the loading. Cyclic loading studies, as well as multiaxis loading studies, are critical in determining the clinical utility of instrumentation devices.

Ideal Geometry of Pedicle Fixation

As important as studies on the effects of instrumentation are, surgeons require information on ideal geometry to assist them in developing constructs for individual patients. These need to be configured for optimal stiffness and alignment, to promote bone growth, and to allow maximal patient comfort. Controlling costs by eliminating nonessential components is also increasingly important.

Studies were conducted to investigate the optimal geometry of pedicle fixation.[117, 123] The Isola system was subjected to in vitro evaluation to determine the effect of transverse fixation on rotational stability and to compare the stiffness produced by Steffee plates versus Isola rods. Pedicle screws were mounted in polymethyl methacrylate molded to mimic lumbar vertebrae. Rod lengths of 6, 12, and 18 cm were used, and loads were applied. In the rotation studies, 20 cycles were applied at loads of up to 15 newton meters. Constructs were tested with medial or lateral rod placement and with none, one, or two transverse fixators. In the flexion studies, loads of 120 newtons at 15 cm were applied to similar-length constructs incorporating Steffee plates or Isola rods.

With no transverse fixators, lateral rod placement was 20% stiffer in rotation than was medial placement, particularly at the longer rod lengths. Although transverse fixators stiffened the medial rod constructs, they were less stiff than the lateral rods, except at 18 cm. Except at the longest lengths, in rotation, one transverse fixator placed in the middle of the construct was equivalent to two fixators placed near the ends. Flexion studies failed to show any increased stiffness for any particular configuration. These preliminary studies further demonstrated that most rotation occurs at the screw-vertebra interface, and such rotation is not decreased by placement of transverse fixators at the point of the screw. We concluded that lateral rod placement with a single transverse fixator may be the optimal configuration for short-segment fixation of the traumatized thoracolumbar spine. As always, it is important to evaluate factors other than biomechanics in clinical decision making, such as device fit, area for bone graft, and so forth.

PEDICLE FIXATION IN DEGENERATIVE DISEASE

The preceding considerations may not be as critical for nontraumatic instability. It is safe to assume that a spine rendered unstable owing to degeneration has not failed, and some structural integrity is preserved. Single-cycle phenomena are not as critical as the impact of cyclic (i.e., continuous) loading on the spine. Thus, the characteristics of the systems used are very different. First of all, of course, they should provide increased stiffness. The question remains, how much stiffness is enough to maintain alignment and enhance bone healing (which is the desired outcome in all instrumentation)? Particularly in the absence of failure, dramatic increases in stiffness are not only unnecessary but may actually be clinically undesirable. Additionally, the question of micromotion across a bone graft and its impact on early fusion must be considered.

There have been few biomechanical studies of pedicle fixation in the lower lumbar spine. One group of investigators used an instability model consisting of removal of the posterior ligaments and injury of the disk at L5-S1.[127] Three-dimensional vertebral motion was measured using a marker on each vertebra. Stereoradiographs and multiple photographs were taken during loading. Flexion, extension, lateral bending, and axial torque moments were applied to a maximum of 10 Nm to multiple commonly used systems. They found that flexion was reduced 50% from the intact state. Stiffness values were higher than those in the

intact spine for all the devices. With extension loading, all the devices restored at least normal stiffness. In pure axial loading, all devices reduced motion to 50% to 75% of intact values, a statistically significant phenomenon.

To summarize, a great deal of work remains to be done to provide neurosurgeons a rational, scientific basis for the use of spinal instrumentation. The costs, risks, and added technical difficulties of newer instrumentation systems require biomechanical justification; they must be subject to the same careful scrutiny as that given to drugs and other medical devices. Adequate studies on the fundamental properties of a given device, its effectiveness, and the long-term biomechanics should be performed, disseminated, and examined before marketing and use by responsible surgeons. This area offers neurosurgeons the opportunity to incorporate objective information into the process of clinical decision making.

CONCLUSIONS AND FUTURE CONSIDERATIONS

Currently, there is a high level of interest in spinal biomechanics among neurosurgeons because of their recognition of its importance in treatment. Although much of the interest relates to the mechanics of fixation, exciting work is being done in other areas as well. More investigation, particularly in trauma causation, will be done using dynamic loading as we develop improved loading and measurement techniques. Research on the biomechanics of the spinal cord itself also needs to be done, because this may have significant implications for our understanding of the pathophysiology of even common disorders such as cervical myelopathy, lumbar stenosis, and spinal cord compression due to tumors.

An increasing emphasis on studies of spinal degeneration is necessary. We need a scientifically rational basis for treatment, because little is understood about the effects of chronic loading on the spine and the development and progression of cervical and lumbar spondylosis.

Traditional biomechanics studies are carried out on spinal components as discussed earlier. However, an artificial spine is under development in several centers, which may allow internal consistency (a significant problem in biomechanics research), as well as consistency in physiologic loading and injury patterns.

In spite of the difficulties involved, it is imperative that our questions about the structure, function, and pathology of the spine be answered in the laboratory and that new treatments be subjected to biomechanical scrutiny. Although it is tempting to hypothesize based on clinical experience and logic, it is unacceptable. Biomechanics is an experimental science, and its principles cannot be deduced. Theories and hypotheses must be studied and validated in the laboratory and then applied in the clinic and operating room. The neurosurgeon's obligation is to ask the questions and use the information obtained for the benefit of his or her patients.

REFERENCES

1. Yoganandan N, Pintar FA, Larson SJ, et al (eds): Frontiers in Head and Neck Trauma: Clinical and Biomechanical. Amsterdam, IOS Press, 1998.
2. Kazarian L, Graves G: Compression strength characteristics of human vertebral centrum. Spine 2:1–14, 1977.
3. Maiman DJ, Pintar FA, Yoganandan N, et al: Pull-out strength of Caspar cervical screws. Neurosurgery 31:1097–1101, 1992.
4. Myklebust J, Pintar F, Yoganandan N, et al: Tensile strength of spinal ligaments. Spine 13:526–531, 1988.
5. Pintar FA, Myklebust JB, Yoganandan N, et al: Biomechanical properties of human intervertebral disc in tension. ASME Adv Bioeng 2:38–39, 1986.
6. Pintar F, Yoganandan N, Myers T, et al: Biomechanical properties of human lumbar spine ligaments. J Biomech 25:1351–1356, 1992.
7. Yoganandan N, Pintar F, Butler J, et al: Dynamic response of human cervical spine ligaments. Spine 14:1102–1110, 1989.
8. Lucas D, Bresler B: Experimental and theoretical study of spine stability. J Bone Joint Surg Am 37:411–412, 1955.
9. Maiman D, Sypert G: Management of trauma of thoracolumbar junction. Parts I and II. Contemp Neurosurg 11:1–6, 1989.
10. Maiman D: Anatomy and clinical biomechanics of thoracic spine. Clin Neurosurg 38:296–324, 1992.
11. Pintar F, Yoganandan N, Voo L: Dependence of age and loading rate on cervical spine compression tolerance. In CDC Injury Prevention through Biomechanics Symposium. Detroit, CDC, 1996.
12. Maiman DJ, Sances A Jr, Myklebust JB, et al: Compression injuries of cervical spine: Biomechanical analysis. Neurosurgery 13:254–260, 1983.
13. Yoganandan N, Sances A Jr, Maiman D, et al: Experimental spinal injuries with vertical impact. Spine 11:855–860, 1986.
14. Yoganandan N, Pintar F, Maiman D, et al: Human head-neck biomechanics under axial tension. Med Eng Phys 18:289–294, 1996.
15. White A III, Panjabi M: Clinical Biomechanics of Spine, 2nd ed. Philadelphia, JB Lippincott, 1990, p 722.
16. Abumi K, Panjabi M, Kramer K, et al: Biomechanical evaluation of lumbar spinal stability after graded facetectomies. Spine 15:1142–1147, 1990.
17. Cusick J, Yoganandan N, Pintar F, et al: Biomechanics of sequential lumbar posterior surgical alteration. J Neurosurg 76:805–811, 1992.
18. Pintar FA, Cusick JF, Yoganandan N, et al: Biomechanics of lumbar facetectomy under compression-flexion. Spine 17:804–810, 1992.
19. Yoganandan N, Maiman D, Pintar F, et al: Cervical spine injuries from motor vehicle accidents. J Clin Eng 15:505–513, 1990.
20. Cusick J, Yoganandan N, Pintar F, et al: Cervical spine injuries from high-velocity forces: Pathoanatomical and radiological study. J Spinal Disord 9:1–7, 1996.
21. Holdsworth H: Fractures, dislocations and fracture-dislocations of spine. J Bone Joint Surg Br 45:6–20, 1963.
22. Nicoll EA: Fractures of the dorso-lumbar spine. J Bone Joint Surg Br 31:376–394, 1949.
23. Roaf R: Study of mechanics of spinal injuries. J Bone Joint Surg Br 42:810–823, 1960.
24. Bedbrook G: Treatment of thoracolumbar dislocation and fractures with paraplegia. Clin Orthop 112:27–43, 1975.
25. Larson S: Unstable thoracic fractures: Treatment alternatives and role of neurosurgeon. Clin Neurosurg 27:624–640, 1980.
26. Maiman D, Sances A Jr, Myklebust J, et al: Experimental trauma of thoracolumbar spine. In Sances A Jr, Thomas DJ, Ewing CL, et al (eds): Mechanisms of Head and Spine Trauma. Goshen, New York, Aloray, 1986, pp 489–504.
27. Pintar F, Yoganandan N, Voo L: Effect of age and loading rate on human cervical spine injury threshold. Spine 23:1957–1962, 1998.
28. Larson SJ, Maiman DJ: Surgery of the Lumbar Spine. New York, Thieme, 1999.
29. Atlas S, Regenbogen V, Rogers LF, Kim KS : The radiographic characterization of burst fractures of the spine. Am J Radiogr 147:575–582, 1986.
30. Frederickson B, Edwards W, Rauschning W, et al: Vertebral burst fractures: Experimental, morphologic and radiographic study. Spine 17:1012–1021, 1992.
31. McAfee P, Yuan H, Lasda N: The unstable burst fracture. Spine 7:365–373, 1982.
32. Ching R, Watson N, Carter J, et al: Effect of post-injury spinal position on canal occlusion in a cervical spine burst fracture model. Spine 22:1710–1715, 1997.
33. Hollowell J, Maiman D: Management of thoracic and thoracolumbar spine trauma. In Rea GL, Miller CA (eds): Spinal Trauma: Current Evaluation and Treatment. Rolling Meadows, IL, American Association of Neurological Surgeons, Joint Section on Disorders of Spine and Peripheral Nerves, 1993, pp 180–197.
34. King A, Vulcan A: Elastic deformation characteristics of spine. J Biomech 4:413–429, 1971.
35. Panjabi M, Hausfeld J, White A: Biomechanical study of ligamentous stability of thoracic spine in man. Acta Orthop Scand 52:315–326, 1981.
36. Denis F: Spinal instability as defined by the three-column spine concept in acute spinal trauma. Clin Orthop 189:65–76, 1984.
37. Jacobs R, Nordwall A, Nachemson A: Stability and strength provided by internal fixation systems for dorso-lumbar spinal injuries. J Biomech 13:802–807, 1980.
38. Maiman D, Sances A Jr, Larson S, et al: Biomechanical analysis of spinal fixation devices. Neurosurgery 17:574–580, 1985.
39. Yoganandan N, Pintar F, Sances A Jr, et al: Biomechanical investigations of human thoracolumbar spine. SAE Trans 97:676–684, 1989.
40. Nachemson A: Load on lumbar discs in different positions of the body. Clin Orthop 45:107–122, 1966.
41. Pintar F, Yoganandan N, Voo L, et al: Dynamic characteristics of human cervical spine. SAE Trans 104:3087–3094, 1995.
42. Whitesides T, Shaw S: On management of unstable fractures of thoracolumbar spine: Rationale for use of anterior decompression and fusion and posterior stabilization. Spine 1:99–107, 1976.
43. Yoganandan N, Pintar F, Sances A Jr, et al: Strength and motion analysis of human head-neck complex. J Spinal Disord 4:73–85, 1991.
44. Kumaresan S, Yoganandan N, Pintar F: Posterior complex contribution on compression and distraction cervical spine behavior: Finite element model. J Musculoskel Res 2:257–265, 1998.
45. Kumaresan S, Yoganandan N, Pintar F, et al: Finite element analysis of cervical laminectomy with graded facetectomy. J Spinal Disord 10:40–46, 1997.
46. Yoganandan N, Maiman D, Pintar F, et al: Microtrauma in the lumbar spine: A cause of low back pain. Neurosurgery 23:162–168, 1988.
47. Yoganandan N, Pintar F, Sances A Jr, et al: Strength and kinematic response of dynamic cervical spine injuries. Spine 16:511–517, 1991.
48. Pintar F, Yoganandan N, Pesigan M, et al: Cervical vertebral strain measurements under axial and eccentric loading. J Biomech Eng 117:474–478, 1995.
49. Rauschning W: Anatomy of normal and traumatized spine. In Sances A Jr, Thomas DJ, Ewing CL, et al (eds): Mechanisms of Head and Spine Trauma. Goshen, NY, Aloray, 1986, pp 531–564.
50. Hollowell J, Vollmer D, Pintar F, et al: Biomechanical analysis of thoracolumbar interbody constructs: How important is the endplate? Spine 21:1032–1036, 1996.
51. Evans F: Mechanical Properties of Bones. Springfield, Ill, Charles C Thomas, 1973.
52. Gallagher M, Maiman D, Reinartz J, et al: Biomechanical evaluation of Caspar cervical screws: Comparative stability under cyclical loading. Neurosurgery 33:1045–1051, 1993.
53. Yamada H: Strength of Biological Materials. Baltimore, Williams & Wilkins, 1970.
54. Galante J, Rostoker W, Ray R: Physical properties of trabecular bone. Calcif Tissue Res 5:5236–5246, 1970.
55. Sances A Jr, Myklebust JB, Maiman DJ, et al: Biomechanics of spinal injuries. CRC Crit Rev Bioeng 11:1–76, 1984.
56. Yoganandan N, Myklebust J, Wilson C, et al: Functional bio-

mechanics of thoracolumbar vertebral cortex. Clin Biomech 3: 11–18, 1988.

57. Carter D, Hayes W: Bone compressive strength: Influence of density and strain rate. Science 194:1174–1176, 1976.

58. Prasad P, King A, Ewing C: Role of articular facets during +Gz acceleration. J Appl Mech 41:321–326, 1974.

59. Pal GP, Sherk HH: Vertical stability of cervical spine. Spine 13:447–449, 1988.

60. Pal G, Routal R: Transmission of weight through lower thoracic and lumbar regions of vertebral column in man. J Anat 152:93–105, 1987.

61. Markolf K, Morris J: Structural components of intervertebral disc. J Bone Joint Surg Am 56:675–687, 1974.

62. Yoganandan N, Larson S, Pintar F, et al: Intravertebral pressure changes caused by spinal microtrauma. Neurosurgery 35:415–421, 1994.

63. Yoganandan N, Ray G, Pintar F, et al: Stiffness and strain energy criteria to evaluate threshold of injury to intervertebral joint. J Biomech 22:135–142, 1989.

64. Berkson M, Nachemson A, Schultz A: Mechanical behavior of human lumbar spine motion segments. Part II. Responses in compression and shear; influences of gross morphology. J Biomech Eng 101:53–57, 1979.

65. Farfan H: Torsional injury of lumbar spine. Spine 9:53–59, 1984.

66. Myers BS, McElhaney JH, Doherty BJ, et al: Role of torsion in cervical spine trauma. Spine 16:870–874, 1991.

67. Langrana N, Lee C, Yang SW: Finite element modeling of the synthetic intervertebral disc. Spine 16(6 Suppl):S245–S252, 1991.

68. Spilker R, Jacobs D, Schultz A: Material constants for a finite element model of intervertebral disc with fiber composite annulus. J Biomech Eng 108:1–11, 1986.

69. Natarajan RN, Ke JH, Andersson BJ: Model to study the disc degeneration process. Spine 19:259–265, 1994.

70. Nachemson A, Evans J: Some mechanical properties of third lumbar interlaminar (ligamentum flavum) ligament. J Biomech 1:211–220, 1968.

71. Tkaczuk H: Tensile properties of human lumbar longitudinal ligaments. Acta Orthop Scand 115(Suppl 1):1–69, 1968.

72. Pintar F, Myklebust J, Yoganandan N, et al: Biomechanics of human spinal ligaments. In Sances A Jr, Thomas DJ, Ewing CL, et al (eds): Mechanisms of Head and Spine Trauma. Goshen, NY, Aloray, 1986, pp 505–527.

73. Cyron B, Hutton W: Tensile strength of the capsular ligaments of apophyseal joints. Anatomy 132:145–150, 1981.

74. Chazal J, Tanguy A, Bourges M, et al: Biomechanical properties of spinal ligaments and a histological study of supraspinal ligament in traction. J Biomech 18:167–176, 1985.

75. Pintar F, Voo L, Yoganandan N, et al: Mechanisms of hyperflexion cervical spine injury. Paper presented at the 16th IRCOBI Conference, 1998, Goteborg, Sweden.

76. Panjabi M, Dvorak J, Crisco JI, et al: Flexion, extension, and lateral bending of upper cervical spine in response to alar ligament transections. J Spinal Disord 4:157–167, 1991.

77. Fielding J, Cochran G, Lawsing J, et al: Tears of the transverse ligament of the atlas. J Bone Joint Surg Am 56:1683, 1974.

78. Panjabi M: Stabilizing system of spine. Part I. Function, dysfunction, adaptation and enhancement. J Spinal Disord 5:383–389, 1992.

79. Wilke H, Wolf S, Claes LE, et al: Stability increase of the lumbar spine with different muscle groups. Spine 20:192–198, 1995.

80. Yoganandan N, Haffner M, Maiman D, et al: Epidemiology and injury biomechanics of motor vehicle related trauma to human spine. SAE Trans 98:1790–1807, 1990.

81. Benson D, Anderson D: Fractures, dislocations, infections and tumors of atlas and axis. In Chapman M, Madison M (eds): Operative Orthopaedics. Philadelphia, Lippincott, 1988, pp 1883–1892.

82. Maiman D, Yoganandan N: Biomechanics of cervical spine trauma. Clin Neurosurg 37:543–570, 1990.

83. Sances A Jr, Thomas D, Ewing C, et al (eds): Mechanisms of Head and Spine Trauma. Goshen, NY, Aloray, 1986.

84. Yoganandan N, Sances A Jr, Pintar F, et al: Injury biomechanics of human cervical column. Spine 15:1031–1039, 1990.

85. Pintar FA, Sances A Jr, Yoganandan N, et al: Biodynamics of total human cadaveric cervical spine. Paper presented at the 34th Stapp Car Crash Conference, 1990.

86. Nightingale RW, McElhaney JH, Richardson WJ, et al: Dynamic responses of the head and cervical spine to axial impact loading. J Biomech 29:307–318, 1996.

87. Pintar F, Yoganandan N, Sances A Jr, et al: Kinematic and anatomical analysis of human cervical spinal column under axial loading. Paper presented at the 33rd Stapp Car Crash Conference, 1989.

88. Bozic K, Keyak J, Skinner H, et al: Three-dimensional finite element modeling of a cervical vertebra: Investigation of burst fracture mechanism. J Spinal Disord 7:102–110, 1994.

89. Myers BS, Winkelstein B: Epidemiology, classification, mechanism and tolerance of human cervical spine injuries. Crit Rev Biomed Eng 23:307–409, 1995.

90. Camacho DL, Nightingale RW, Robinette JJ, et al: Experimental flexibility measurements for the development of a computational head-neck model validated for near-vertex head impact. Paper presented at the 41st Stapp Car Crash Conference, Lake Buena Vista, Fla, 1997, pp 473–486.

91. Pintar F, Yoganandan N, Schlick M: Biodynamics of cervical spine injury. Paper presented at IRCOBI Conference on Biomechanics of Impacts, 1995, Brunnen, Switzerland.

92. Pintar F, Yoganandan N, Sances A Jr, et al: Kinematic and anatomical analysis of human cervical spinal column under axial loading. SAE Trans 98:1766–1789, 1990.

93. Maiman D, Pintar F: Anatomy and clinical biomechanics of thoracic spine. In Selman W (ed): Clinical Neurosurgery. Baltimore, Williams & Wilkins, 1990, pp 296–324.

94. Andriacchi T, Schultz A, Belytschko T, et al: Model for studies of mechanical interactions between the human spine and rib cage. J Biomech 7:497–507, 1974.

95. White A, Hirsch C: Significance of vertebral posterior elements in mechanics of thoracic spine. Clin Orthop 81:2–14, 1971.

96. Yoganandan N, Maiman D, Pintar F, et al: Biomechanical effects of laminectomy on thoracic spine stability. Neurosurgery 32:604–610, 1993.

97. Gregerson G, Lucas D: In vivo study of axial rotation of human thoracolumbar spine. J Bone Joint Surg Am 49:247–262, 1967.

98. Pearcy M, Tibrewal S: Axial rotation and lateral bending in normal lumbar spine measured by three-dimensional radiography. Spine 9:582–591, 1984.

99. Dick W, Kluger P, Magerl F, et al: New device for internal fixation of thoracolumbar and lumbar spine fractures: The "fixateur interne." Paraplegia 23:225–232, 1985.

100. Goel V, Voo L, Weinstein J, et al: Response of ligamentous lumbar spine to cyclic bending loads. Spine 13:294–300, 1988.

101. Katonis P: Treatment of unstable thoracolumbar spine injuries using Cotrel-Dubousset instrumentation. Spine 24:2352–2357, 1999.

102. Pintar FA, Maiman DJ, Yoganandan N: Clinical and experimental biomechanics of the spine. In Tindall GT, Barrow DL (eds): The Practice of Neurosurgery. Baltimore, Williams & Wilkins, 1996, pp 2347–2356.

103. Cusick J, Pintar F, Yoganandan N, et al: Wire fixation techniques of cervical facets. Spine 22:964–969, 1997.

104. Hollowell J, Kumaresan S, Yoganandan N, et al: Biomechanics of human cervical spinal column under physiologic loads. ASME Adv Bioeng 43:289–290, 1999.

105. Tran N, Watson N, Tencer A, et al: Mechanism of the burst fracture in thoracolumbar spine: Effect of loading rate. Spine 20:1984–1988, 1995.

106. Baisden J, Voo L, Cusick J, et al: Evaluation of cervical laminectomy and laminoplasty: Longitudinal study in goat model. Spine 24:1283–1289, 1999.

107. Yoganandan N, Pintar F, Arnold P, et al: Continuous motion analysis of head-neck complex under impact. J Spinal Disord 7:420–428, 1994.

108. Yoganandan N, Larson S, Pintar F, et al: Biomechanics of lumbar pedicle screw/plate fixation in trauma. Neurosurgery 27:873–881, 1990.

109. Yoganandan N, Pintar F, Maiman D, et al: Kinematics of lumbar spine following pedicle screw plate fixation. Spine 18:504–512, 1993.

110. Maiman DJ, Pintar FA, Yoganandan N, et al: Effects of anterior vertebral grafting on traumatized lumbar spine following pedicle screw-plate fixation. Spine 18:2423–2430, 1993.

111. Cusick J, Yoganandan N, Pintar F, et al: Biomechanics of cervical spine facetectomy and fixation techniques. Spine 13:808–812, 1988.
112. Coe J, Warden K, Sutterlin C III, et al: Biomechanical evaluation of cervical spinal stabilization methods in a human cadaveric model. Spine 14:1122–1131, 1989.
113. Foley K: The in vitro effects of instrumentation of multi-level strut graft mechanics. Spine 24:2366–2376, 1999.
114. Ashman R, Galpin R, Corin J, et al: Biomechanical analysis of pedicle screw instrumentation systems in a corpectomy model. Spine 14:1398–1405, 1989.
115. Esses S: AO spinal internal fixator. Spine 14:373–388, 1989.
116. Gwon J, Chen J, Lim T, et al: In vitro comparative biomechanical analysis of transpedicular screw instrumentation in lumbar region of lumbar spine. J Spinal Disord 4:437–443, 1991.
117. Pintar F, Maiman D, Yoganandan N, et al: Rotational stiffness of a lumbar spinal pedicle screw/rod system. J Spinal Disord 8:49–55, 1995.
118. Carl A, Tromanhauser S, Roger D: Pedicle screw instrumentation for thoracolumbar burst fractures and fracture-dislocations. Spine 17:S317–S324, 1992.
119. McAfee P, Werner F, Glisson R: Biomechanical analysis of spinal instrumentation systems in thoracolumbar fractures. Spine 10:204–216, 1985.
120. Farcy J, Weidenbaum M, Michelsen C, et al: Comparative biomechanical study of spinal fixation using Cotrel-Dubousset instrumentation. Spine 12:877–881, 1987.
121. Krag M, Beynnon B, Pope MH, et al: Depth of insertion of transpedicular vertebral screws into human vertebrae: Effect upon screw-vertebra interface strength. J Spinal Disord 1:287–294, 1989.
122. Chang K, Dewei Z, McAfee P, et al: Comparative biomechanical study of spinal fixation using the combination spinal rod-plate and transpedicular screw fixation system. J Spinal Disord 1:257–266, 1989.
123. Maiman DJ, Pintar FA, Yoganandan N, Reinartz J: Effects of anterior vertebral grafting on the traumatized lumbar spine following pedicle screw-plate fixation. Spine 18:2423–2430, 1993.
124. Daniauz H, Seykora P, Genelin A, et al: Application of posterior plating and modifications in thoracolumbar spine injuries: Indication, techniques, and results. Spine 16:125–133, 1991.
125. Hollowell JP, Yoganandan N, Benzel EC: Spinal implant attributes: Cantilever beam fixation. In Benzel EC (ed): Spine Surgery. New York, Churchill Livingstone, 1999, pp 979–990.
126. Gurr K, McAfee P, Shih C: Biomechanical analysis of anterior and posterior instrumentation systems after corpectomy. J Bone Joint Surg 70:1182–1191, 1988.
127. Panjabi M, Yamamoto I, Oxford T, et al: Biomechanical stability of five pedicle screw fixation systems in a human lumbar spine instability model. Clin Biomech 6:97–105, 1991.

CHAPTER 279

Intraoperative Electrophysiologic Monitoring of the Spinal Cord and Nerve Roots

JEFFREY H. OWEN

Intraoperative monitoring (IOM) is the general term used to describe the various monitoring procedures administered during operations that place the central and peripheral nervous systems at risk. Traditionally, IOM procedures have been electrophysiologic and include evoked potentials, electroencephalography (EEG), and electromyography (EMG). Although newer applications of Doppler and other procedures are being developed, this chapter reviews only the traditional applications of IOM as they pertain to the spine.

There are three major purposes for IOM: to detect the onset of a surgically induced insult to the nervous systems, to provide the surgeon with information that can be used to modify surgical techniques and reverse the effects from an insult, and to monitor the efficacy of interventional strategies. By administering IOM procedures, surgical outcomes are improved and short- and long-term costs associated with the surgery are decreased.

This chapter reviews the various electrophysiologic procedures used to monitor the spinal cord and nerve roots and information regarding the methodology of each monitoring procedure, acquisition parameters, and methodologic validity and reliability. To help convey this information, several case studies demonstrating the use of IOM are presented.

Compared with other clinical and surgical procedures, IOM is unusual in that it attempts to provide the surgeon with information regarding the effects of the surgical technique on the nervous system. IOM detection of the onset of a surgically induced neurological insult allows reversal of its effects. Because of the medical and legal ramifications associated with IOM, the use of these procedures has taken on increased importance and relevance for neurological and orthopedic surgeons. The medicolegal aspects of IOM are briefly reviewed.

HISTORICAL REVIEW

The earliest use of electrophysiologic tests during surgery that involved the spine (i.e., spinal cord or nerve roots, or both) was reported by Dawson.[1] Although the use of electrocautery devices to stimulate nerve roots has been anecdotally referenced, these methods were uncontrolled and provided, at best, only gross information regarding nerve root function. In the Dawson study, somatosensory evoked potentials (SEPs) were used to actually determine and monitor the functional integrity of the spinal cord.

The growth of IOM, relative to the spine, was limited until the reports of Tamaki[2] and Brown and Nash.[3] In these two studies, SEPs were used to monitor spinal cord function during surgery for the correction of scoliosis. Although the emphasis of this application was orthopedic, results demonstrated that SEPs could be reliably recorded and that they provided valuable information regarding the status of spinal cord function throughout surgery. These study results were soon extrapolated to include operations for space-occupying lesions within the spinal cord.

Although the use of SEPs during spinal surgery was increasing, it soon became evident that this sensory-based response was not the ideal method for monitoring the function of spinal cord motor tracts. Although SEPs provided direct information regarding the status of spinal cord sensory tracts, they provided only indirect information regarding motor tract function. Because of the limitations associated with the SEP, it became apparent that a direct measure of motor tract that demonstrated the operational advantages of the SEP was needed. This resulted in the development procedures that acquired motor evoked potentials (MEPs).[4]

In addition to developing methods to monitor spinal cord function, a significant amount of effort has been expended in developing tests that monitor nerve root function. Initial efforts resulted in the development and use of procedures that acquired dermatomal somatosensory evoked potentials (DSEPs).[5, 6] DSEPs were used primarily during operations that placed nerve roots at risk, such as surgery for spinal stenosis or spondylolisthesis. Although DSEPs provided fairly reliable and valid information regarding the level of nerve root involvement and adequacy of decompression,[7, 8] they were found to be inappropriate for protecting nerve roots during the placement of pedicular instrumentation.

Because of the increased use of pedicular instrumentation and the limitations of the DSEP, two new procedures were developed for use during operations that used pedicular instrumentation. Both procedures recorded an electromyographic response in response to electrical or mechanical stimulation of the nerve root. Based on the method for eliciting the electromyographic response, the procedures became known as electrically elicited electromyography (E-EMG)[9] and mechanically elicited electromyography (M-EMG).[10] Compared with DSEPs, the two electromyographic procedures are essentially 100% accurate in detecting the presence of pedicle wall breakthrough by pedicular instrumentation or by nerve root irritation.

In addition to using electromyographic procedures during operations for spinal degeneration, this response is also acquired during surgery within the cauda equina.[11] By using appropriate stimulation and recording techniques, it is possible for the surgeon to discriminate between neural and non-neural tissue and to determine the location of tumors, neuromas in continuity, or other disorders.

METHODOLOGIC OVERVIEW

The IOM procedures reviewed in this chapter are limited to evoked potentials and electromyographic techniques. Based on the neurological structures that are at surgical risk, these procedures are divided into two categories: spinal cord and nerve root. These two categories are convenient because they allow classification of test procedures according to the structure at risk rather than using differences in test methodology as the classification determinant. This classification also enables the surgeon to more easily determine which procedure should be used when ordering IOM.

Electrophysiologic measures of the spinal cord (e.g., SEPs, MEPs) or nerve roots (e.g., DSEPs, E-EMG, M-EMG) provide information regarding the functional integrity of these structures. These tests do not provide information regarding anatomy, nor do they provide prognostic information regarding the structure's eventual return of function. These procedures provide information regarding the effects from an insult on neurological function rather than providing direct information about the insult. Although electrophysiologic procedures do not provide direct information regarding the specific type of insult that has occurred, these tests can provide information about the probable cause. For example, it has been shown that the rate at which an evoked potential is lost after the onset of an insult depends on whether the insult was mechanical or ischemic.[12] By determining when the loss of data began and reviewing their surgical notes, monitoring personnel can provide the surgeon with a fairly good idea about whether any surgical maneuver occurred that could have produced the insult. This type of information is helpful to the surgeon when deciding which interventional strategy should be administered first.

SPINAL CORD MONITORING

To monitor spinal cord function, it is necessary to ascertain which neurological structures are at direct and indirect surgical risk. After this is determined, the appropriate monitoring procedures can be chosen and administered. For example, during an operation for lumbosacral spinal degeneration, the lumbosacral nerve roots are at direct surgical risk. The brachial plexus is at indirect surgical risk because of the position of the patient on the operating table. By monitoring the nerve roots and brachial plexus, additional protection is provided for the patient.

Case Study 1 is an excellent example of the limitations associated with using the surgical approach as the basis for determining which neurological structures are at risk. The patient in Case Study 1 underwent a posterior decompressive cervical laminectomy. This patient had mild myelopathic symptoms preoperatively. The surgeon ordered spinal cord monitoring but, based on the surgical approach, obtained only mixed nerve SEPs. The surgeon believed that the surgical approach was simple and placed only the posterior aspects of the spinal cord at direct risk. Because SEPs directly measure the status of the dorsal medial tracts, they appeared to be the method of choice for monitoring this case. During surgery, the SEP data did not change, and the patient's sensory function was grossly unchanged postoperatively. However, the patient postoperatively had paraplegia in both lower extremities and significant weakness in the upper extremities. Based on clinical and imaging studies, it was determined that this patient had an anterior cord syndrome resulting from compromise of the anterior spinal artery.

Case Study 1 demonstrates that the IOM procedures administered during a surgery should be based on the neurological structures that are at direct and indirect risk during surgery. The patient's motor tracts were indirectly at risk, but the anterior cord syndrome evidenced after surgery could have been detected and probably prevented by administering some measure of motor tract function (i.e., the Stagnara wake-up test or MEP procedures) in conjunction with the SEPs.[4]

This section on spinal cord monitoring presents information regarding the use of SEPs and MEPs during neurological or orthopedic surgery that involves the spinal cord. Some combination of sensory and motor tract tests should be administered to provide total protection to the spinal cord. Although clinical procedures such as the Stagnara wake-up test can provide information regarding motor tract function, their use is not always feasible or practical.[4] Consequently, some combination of SEPs and MEPs should be administered.

Somatosensory Evoked Potentials

SEPs are used to monitor the functional integrity of the dorsal medial tracts during operations involving the spinal cord, such as surgery for scoliosis, kyphosis, or space-occupying lesions. SEPs are elicited by stimulating a peripheral mixed nerve with a repetitive electric shock. The elicited activity is propagated rostrally and enters the spinal cord through the dorsal roots.[13] Once within the spinal cord, the activity ascends to the contralateral sensory cortex through the dorsomedial tracts of the spinal cord.

To monitor spinal cord function, data are recorded at sites rostral and caudal to the levels of surgery. Based on the pattern of results (i.e., data are present or absent at a particular recording site), it is possible to determine whether the assessed neural network is intact; if not, it is possible to determine where the interruption of transmission occurred and whether the interruption was caused by surgical or perioperative variables.

SEPs are appropriate for administration during any operation that places the spinal cord at risk. Applications include operations for spinal deformity, space-occupying lesions, and aortic abdominal aneurysms.

STIMULATION SITES

The specific site of stimulation must take into consideration several important factors. First, evoked potentials are tests of continuity and therefore require that the elicited action potential propagate through the area at surgical risk. Although it is assumed that the relationship between the level of surgery and site of stimulation is understood, studies have reported the use of inappropriate stimulation relative to the level of surgery.[14] Second, the patient's preexisting neurological condition must be considered. This includes symptoms resulting directly from the abnormality and the patient's overall medical condition. For example, peripheral neuropathy in an 80-year-old person with diabetes significantly affects the reliability and morphology of an SEP elicited by stimulating the posterior tibial nerve at the medial malleolus. By decreasing the length of the peripheral nerve segment stimulated, the quality and reliability of the elicited waveform improve dramatically.

The surgeon needs to take into consideration the effects of surgery on neurological structures that are not at direct surgical risk. In the area of spinal surgery, major concerns are the indirect effects on the brachial plexus and other nerves from improper positioning of the patient on the operating table[15] or rotation of the patient's head.[16] For example, the functional integrity of the plexus can be degraded if the patient's shoulders are excessively distracted during positioning for an anterior or posterior cervical fusion or if the patient's shoulders are improperly positioned on a frame. By stimulating the ulnar nerve, in addition to the nerves used to monitor the neurological structures that are at direct surgical risk, it is possible to avoid the onset of a positioning-induced brachial plexopathy.

RECORDING SITES

To record the SEP, recording electrodes should be placed at sites that are caudal and cephalad to the

surgical levels. Each recording site has its own particular function and purpose. For example, the peripheral site allows the examiner to determine whether the eliciting stimulus has been neurologically encoded and whether this elicited activity has traveled rostrally. The more rostral recording sites allow the examiner to determine whether the impulse has traveled through the surgical site. Based on the pattern of responses (Table 279–1), it is possible to determine the probable causes for any changes that occur in the data and recommended courses of action.

How many recording sites are needed? Nuwer[17] found that, in normal patients, the use of more than one recording site increased the redundancy of the test. By increasing test redundancy, the effects from perioperative variables such as mean arterial pressure (MAP) or anesthesia on the SEP were more easily ascertained and controlled.

Owen and colleagues[18] investigated the need for using multiple recording sites during operations in which patients demonstrated preexisting neurological conditions. If only one cortical recording site was used, no reliable response could be recorded in 26% of the patients. Using three cortical and one cervical recording electrode recorded a reliable SEP in 92% of the patients. These data were in agreement with previous studies.[19, 20] By using multiple recording sites rostral to the level of surgery, the probability of recording a reliable response is significantly increased. Based on experience and what has been reported in the literature, a minimum of three cortical sites and one cervical recording site should be used during spinal surgery. The cortical recording electrodes should be placed over the sensory homunculus associated with the stimulation site; the cervical recording site should be placed over a cervical vertebra rostral to the level of surgery. If the surgery involves a posterior cervical approach, the cervical recording electrode can use a nasopharyngeal placement or an anterior placement. These active recording sites should be referenced to the Fpz site (i.e., International 10-20 System).[21]

Cortical signals are larger and more reliable than cervical data (Fig. 279–1). However, cortical data are more easily affected by anesthesia and other perioperative variables,[22] which reduce their reliability. Although the cervical response is more resistant to the same

TABLE 279–1 ■ Relationship between a Combination of Response Pattern and Probable Cause for the Pattern

RECORDING SITE			
Peripheral	Cervical	Cortical	PROBABLE CAUSE
Present	Present	Present	Normal
Present	Present	Absent	Technical/anesthesia
Present	Absent	Present	Technical/anesthesia
Absent	Present	Present	Technical
Present	Absent	Absent	Surgical
Absent	Absent	Present	Technical
Absent	Absent	Absent	Technical

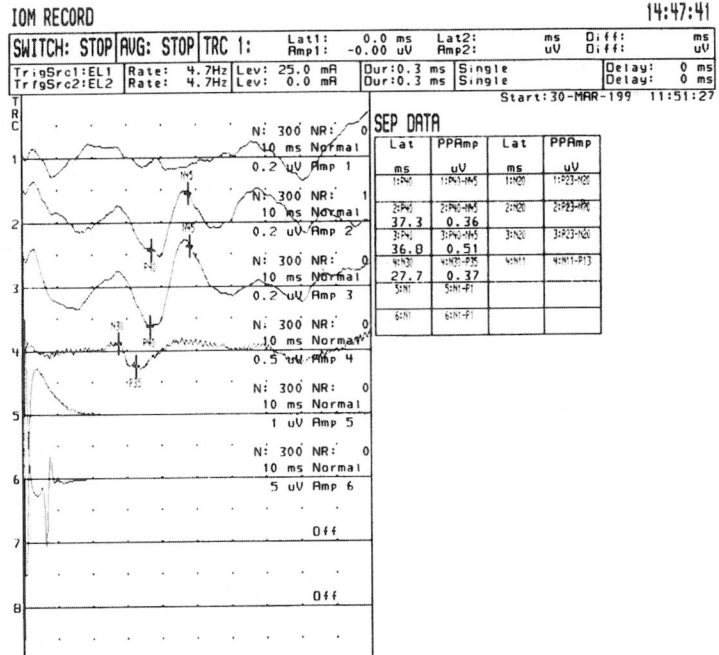

FIGURE 279–1. Normal somatosensory evoked potentials (SEPs), demonstrating cortical *(top three traces),* cervical *(fourth trace),* and peripheral *(fifth and sixth traces)* responses.

perioperative variables that affect the cortical response, the cervical response tends to be smaller and slightly more difficult to read. By using a combination of cortical and cervical recording sites, it is possible to take advantage of the strengths of these two types of responses, which provides more reliable monitoring to the surgeon.

ACQUISITION PARAMETERS

To acquire the SEP, appropriate parameters must be used (Table 279–2). When using evoked potentials, the goal is to glean the elicited neurological response from ongoing biologic (i.e., EEG) and electrical (e.g., 60-Hz) noise. To achieve this goal, it is necessary to use signal-averaging techniques and to adjust the acquisition parameters to provide the best signal-to-noise ratio. Five

general guidelines should be considered when determining the acquisition parameters. First, the frequency response of the elicited activity determines the bandwidth and frequency emphasis of the filters used. In general, the shorter the duration of the response, the broader is its frequency composition. For example, a peripheral response is much shorter in duration than a cortical SEP (see Fig. 279–1). Consequently, the frequency composition of the peripheral response is wider, which necessitates that the bandpass settings of the filter need to be widened. In addition to adjusting the width of the filter to correspond to the width of the frequency composition of the response, the filter needs to be centered over the major frequency components of the response. For example, the frequency response of a cortical SEP is narrower in its width and lower in its emphasis than those same characteristics of a cervical or peripheral response. When recording the cortical response, the width of the bandpass filters is set to reject unwanted noise, but the bandpass of the filter is centered to a lower frequency range.

Second, set the sensitivity of the amplifiers to reject the input signal approximately 10% of the time. This ensures that the artifact rejection system is adequately sensitive to reject unwanted, low-amplitude noise but not too sensitive, which would increase the time needed to collect a response.

Third, the stimulus presentation rate is adjusted to be an uneven multiple of the electrical line current. If the presentation rate is set to an even multiple of the line current, there is the probability that components of this cyclical noise will be averaged into the response. This could result in inappropriate labeling of data and inaccurate interpretation of a purported response.

Fourth, the number of stimuli presented and averaged should be adequate to obtain a reliable response

T A B L E 2 7 9 – 2 ■ **Parameters Used to Acquire a Mixed Nerve Somatosensory Evoked Potential**

ACQUISITION PARAMETER	VALUE
Filter	
Cortical recordings	30–250 Hz
Cervical recordings	30–1500 Hz
Peripheral recordings	30–3000 Hz
Stimulus rate	2.2–4.7/s
Sensitivity	10% rejection rate
Stimulus intensity	Saturation
Stimulus duration	200–300 μsec
Time base	100 msec (lower extremity SEPs)
	50 msec (upper extremity SEPs)

SEPs, somatosensory evoked potentials.

but not too large, which would prolong the testing time. In the diagnostic setting, large numbers of stimuli are presented before a response is interpreted. Although this method is appropriate when neurological structures are not at risk, it is not appropriate for the operating room. If too large of a sample size is collected during surgery, the information will not be updated frequently enough, which reduces the sensitivity of the response to the onset of an insult.

Fifth, the stimulus is given at an intensity that ensures stimulation of all the fibers within the nerve being stimulated. This *saturation level* also ensures greater synchronicity of neural firing.

INTERPRETATION

SEPs, as do all electrophysiologic data, consist of a series of positive and negative waves that propagate through peripheral nerves and the neural axis (see Fig. 279–1). Based on the distance between the stimulating and recording sites and on the conduction velocity of the neural impulse, each waveform demonstrates a certain time of occurrence, or latency, which is measured in milliseconds, and a certain amplitude, usually measured in microvolts. The amplitude of the waveform is determined by several factors, including the number of neurons firing, the synchrony of firing, and the impedance of the recording medium.

Interpretation of SEP data is based on changes in response latency or in amplitude relative to baseline values, or both. Baseline data should be acquired after the skin incision.[22] Establishing this baseline allows the examiner to control the effects from perioperative variables (e.g., anesthesia, temperature, MAP) on the response. After baseline data are acquired, they should be labeled and printed. Data should be continuously collected during the remainder of the operation. The latency and amplitude of all subsequently recorded data are then compared with baseline values to determine whether a significant change has occurred.

According to Keith and colleagues[23] and Nuwer and associates,[24] the most common criterion used to determine whether data have changed significantly is a 10% increase in latency or a 50% or larger diminution in response amplitude. These are only warning criteria; they do no necessarily indicate that the patient's neurological status has been compromised.[25] However, if changes in latency or amplitude meet warning criteria, they do indicate that the functional status of the monitored neural structures may be under duress and that the causes for these changes need to be addressed. If the probable cause for the changes is determined to be surgical in origin (see Table 279–1), appropriate steps must be initiated.

Latency and amplitude are used to interpret evoked potential data. However, latency and amplitude are not equally sensitive to the onset of a neurological insult. Although latency and amplitude are equally sensitive to the onset of mechanical insult to the spinal cord,[26] amplitude is more sensitive than latency to the effects of ischemia on neurological function. Because amplitude is sensitive to mechanical and ischemic insults, it

has always been considered the more sensitive of two response measures. Both criteria should be used to interpret evoked potential data during surgery.

Several perioperative variables affect SEP data, especially responses recorded over the somatosensory cortex.[22] Variables include anesthetic agents, muscle relaxants, amnesic agents, hypotension, and temperature. If an inadequate number of recording channels is used or if the recording sites are inappropriate, it can be very difficult to differentiate surgical from perioperative changes in SEP data. Because the recommended course of action after a degradation in data depends on the origin of the degradation, multiple and appropriate recording sites are strongly recommended. Table 279–1 lists the various combinations of test results that can occur during a surgery and the recommended course of action for the examiner. By using multiple recording sites, it is possible to identify the probable cause for the degradation of a response, which facilitates initiation of appropriate intervention.

If data have degraded to the point of meeting warning criteria and if it has been ascertained that the change in data is not caused by a perioperative variable, one or more interventional strategies should be administered. The interventional strategies used during a surgery depend on the type of surgery being performed and include stopping the surgical maneuvers for a few minutes and waiting for data to improve, administering the Stagnara wake-up test, removing spinal instrumentation, increasing MAP, and administering high-dose steroids.[4] Each of these strategies has certain strengths and weaknesses that determine its efficacy.[4] For example, the Stagnara wake-up test provides absolute information regarding spinal cord motor tract function. However, it requires awakening the patient from anesthesia and behavioral demonstration of motor function, which can be difficult, especially more than once during an operation. The efficacy of any interventional strategy depends on when it is administered relative to the time of onset of the insult.[27] After an interventional strategy has been decided, it must be administered as quickly as possible.

Although it is not realistic to expect a surgeon to become an expert in IOM, the surgeon should become familiar with reading data and knowledgeable about the strengths and weaknesses of each test modality. This allows the surgeon to become an active member of the IOM team.[24] To achieve this goal, the surgeon must understand how to read and interpret an evoked potential. Although the SEP data are used as an example, the following information is pertinent to all evoked potential data.

Figure 279–1 depicts an SEP elicited by stimulating the posterior tibial nerve at the ankle and recorded over the somatosensory cortex and cervical spine. These data were acquired from a neurologically normal patient undergoing surgery for idiopathic scoliosis. Figure 279–1 depicts four SEP traces. Reading from the top of the figure, the first three traces were recorded from the somatosensory cortex at the following sites: trace 1 (top), C1'; trace 2 (second trace), Cz'; trace 3 (third trace), C2'; and trace 4 (fourth trace), fourth to fifth cervical vertebrae. All four recording sites were referenced to Fpz, which is an electrode site on the forehead. C1′ is from the left side of skull; Cz′ is at the very top of the head; and C2′ is from the right side of the skull. The horizontal axis is the time of acquisition and, in this case, represents 100 msec. This time base is the same for all four traces. The horizontal axis is used to help determine the latency or time of occurrence of a response in milliseconds. The vertical scale is used as an index of the amplitude or height of each trace in microvolts. To the right of these traces is a table that lists the latencies and amplitudes of each trace. Cursors are used to determine the absolute latency and amplitude of a response. Inspection of this table indicates that the top trace (C1′) demonstrates a latency of 36.1 msec and amplitude of 0.75 μV. The latencies and amplitudes for the data recorded at Cz′ and C2′ were similar. The latency and amplitude of trace 4 (cervical) were 25.8 msec and 0.54 μV, respectively.

Interpretation of all evoked potential data is based on pattern recognition and the relationship between current data and baseline data. If significant changes in the latency and amplitude of current data relative to baseline data have occurred, it is necessary to determine the cause for the changes and, if surgical in nature, to inform the surgeon. Unlike the diagnostic setting, in which normative data are collected and used for interpretation, the patient acts as her or his own control in the operating room. The data depicted in Figure 279–1 are typical in latency, amplitude, and morphology for a neurologically normal patient. If, however, the patient demonstrated a preexisting neurological condition (e.g., peripheral neuropathies, myelopathies, numbness), changes in all three components of the response can be expected.

RELIABILITY AND VALIDITY

The SEP has been used for spinal cord monitoring for more than 25 years. During that period, a number of studies have described the reliability and validity of this response. The reliability of the SEP is determined by a number of variables, including anesthesia, temperature, and MAP. The probability of recording a reliable response can be increased if redundant recording sites are used. If the effects from perioperative variables on the SEP are controlled and if multiple sites are used to record the response, SEPs demonstrate a test-retest reliability of more than 98%.[4, 28] This means that SEPs demonstrated a false-positive rate of less than 2% for patients without a preexisting neurological condition. Reliable SEPs have been recorded in more than 93% of patients with preexisting neurological conditions,[18] for a false-positive rate of less than 7%.

The validity of the SEP is influenced by the purpose for which it was administered. If SEPs are administered to detect the onset of surgically induced sensory deficit, the response demonstrates a very high validity. According to a study by Dawson and coworkers,[29] SEPs correctly identified 100% of surgically induced neurological deficits in patients undergoing surgery for the correction of scoliosis if that insult resulted in a sensory deficit. However, if the insult produced only a motor deficit, the SEPs failed to detect the insult in 31% of the patients.

SUMMARY

SEPs are a reliable and valid measure of monitoring the functional integrity of the dorsal medial tracts within the spinal cord. They are not a direct measure of motor tract function and should not be used for this purpose. Because a number of perioperative variables affect the SEP, it is recommended that a minimum of four recording sites be used when administering this procedure. By continuously recording these data during surgery and using appropriate interpretation criteria, it is possible to determine the onset of an insult to the dorsal medial tracts in a timely manner that is efficacious to the initiation of intervention.

CASE STUDIES

Two case studies are presented that depict the relative sensitivity of SEPs to ischemic and mechanical insults to the spinal cord. During surgery, data need to be collected, labeled, and stored continuously. Although not all data need to be printed out during an operation, data should be printed at least every 15 minutes for each modality. In these two case studies, not all data that were recorded are depicted; only those that convey the purpose for the case study are shown.

■ CASE STUDY 1

The patient underwent posterior cervical decompression for cervical stenosis from C2 to C4. The patient demonstrated mild myelopathy in the upper extremities.

Intraoperative monitoring consisted of administering SEPs to ulnar, median, and posterior tibial nerves using normal acquisition parameters. Because none of the SEP data changed during this surgery, only ulnar nerve responses were demonstrated. Data were recorded before positioning the patient on the operating table, after positioning, and continuously throughout surgery. MEPs were not recorded during this operation at the request of the surgeon.

Baseline data (Fig. 279–2A and B) were normal and reliable. At no time during surgery were data lost, nor was it necessary to inform the surgeon of significant changes in the SEPs. At closure, data remained unchanged (see Fig. 279–2C and D). On awakening from anesthesia, the patient demonstrated grossly normal sensory function but had paraplegia in the lower extremities and significant weakness in the upper extremities. Subsequent imaging and surgical re-exploration failed to reveal the cause for the motor deficit.

■ CASE STUDY 2

The patient was an 11-year-old boy undergoing surgery for correction of neuromuscular scoliosis. In addition to the scoliosis, the patient had cerebral palsy and dysarthria. Surgery consisted of posterior spinal fusion with Luque

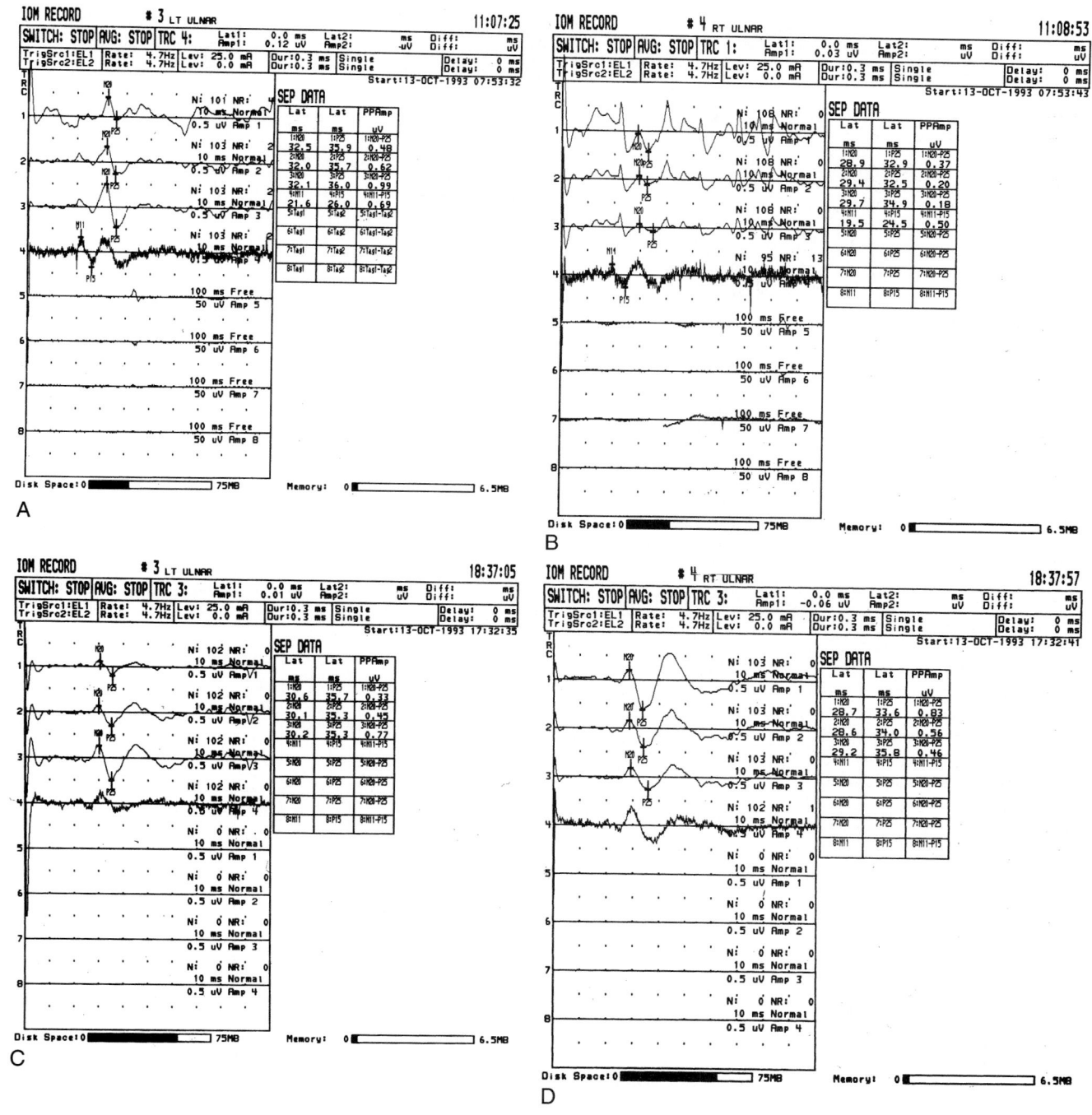

FIGURE 279–2. *A*, Baseline left ulnar response from the patient described in Case Study 1. *B*, Baseline right ulnar response from the patient described in Case Study 1. *C*, Closing left ulnar response from the patient described in Case Study 1. *D*, Closing right ulnar response from the patient described in Case Study 1.

instrumentation (rectangles) to the pelvis and sublaminar wires.

SEPs were used to monitor spinal cord function during this surgery. SEPs were elicited by stimulating the ulnar and posterior tibial nerves, and responses were recorded cervically and cortically using routine acquisition parameters. Ulnar nerve data were used to monitor brachial plexus function; posterior tibial nerve data were used to monitor spinal cord function.

To avoid confusion, only results after stimulation of the left posterior tibial nerve are shown. Data elicited by stimulation of the right posterior tibial nerve were equivalent to left leg data and demonstrated the same characteristics before and after the spinal cord insult as the left leg data. Ulnar nerve data did not demonstrate any significant changes as a function of positioning and are not shown.

Figure 279–3*A* shows the baseline data acquired at 11:

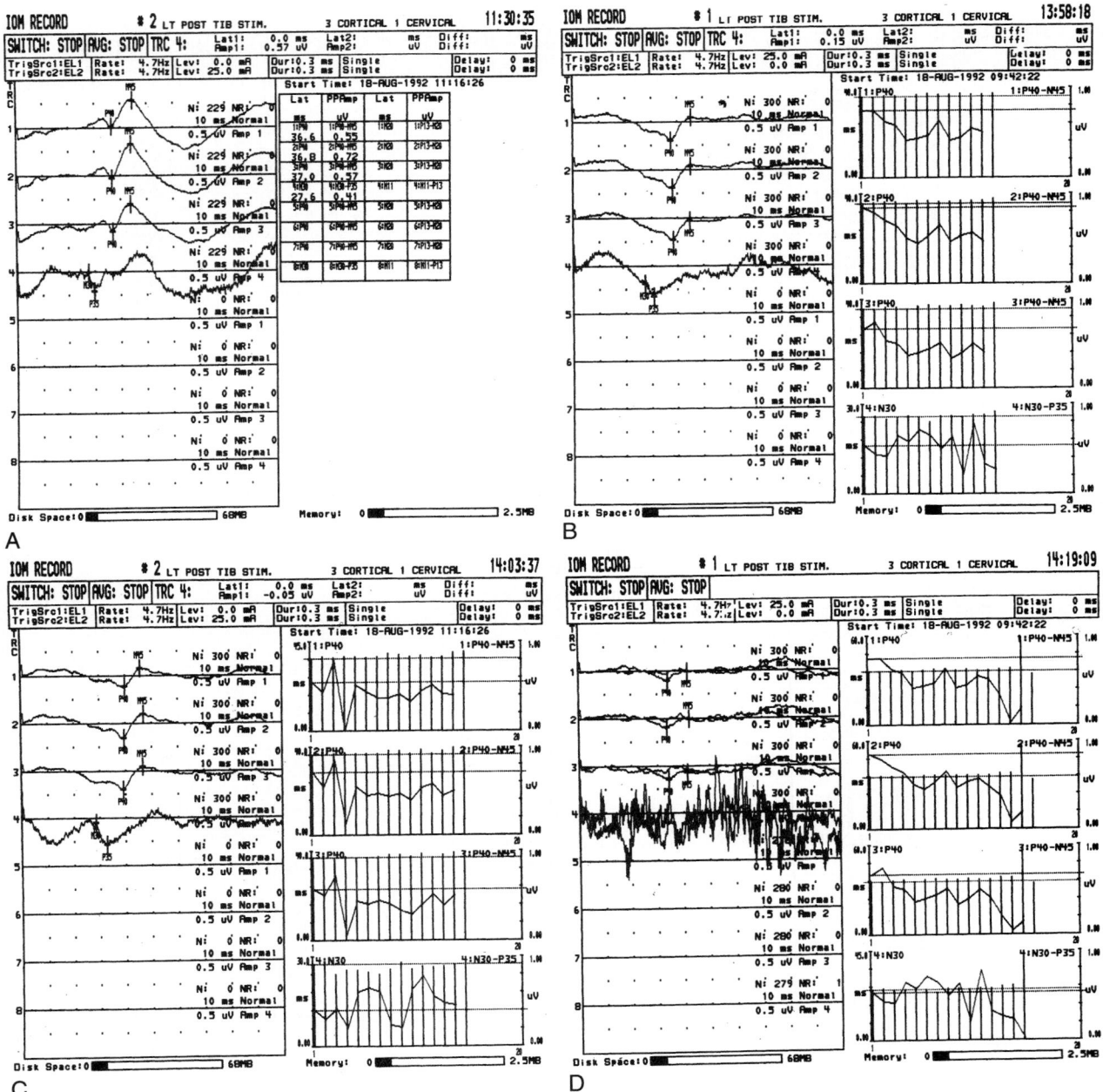

FIGURE 279–3. *A,* Baseline left posterior tibial somatosensory evoked potential from the patient described in Case Study 2. *B,* Normal SEP data from Case Study 1, recorded at 13:58. *C,* Normal SEP data from Case Study 1, recorded at 14:03. *D,* Loss of SEP data from Case Study 1, recorded after onset of the insult.

Illustration continued on following page

30 AM. These data were considered to be well formed, reliable, and within normal limits. Data continued to be normal and unchanged at 13:58 (see Fig. 279–3*B*), at 14:03 (see Fig. 279–3*C*), and until approximately 14:19. At that time, the surgeon was placing the fourth sublaminar wire. Data demonstrated an immediate degradation, as depicted in Figure 279–3*D*. The surgeon was immediately informed of the change, and blood pressure was increased and high-dose steroids administered. From 14:25 (see Fig. 279–3*E*) until slightly past 14:45 (see Fig. 279–3*F*), data continued to demonstrate a prolonged latency and sig-

nificantly reduced amplitude and morphology. By 14:54 (see Fig. 279–3*G*), the data began to improve so that by closure the latency of the responses was equivalent to baseline values, although amplitude remained reduced. Because of the patient's preexisting condition, it was not possible to administer a Stagnara wake-up test during surgery. After closure of the surgical site, the patient was awakened in the operating room and demonstrated grossly unchanged motor function. Subsequent clinical testing revealed a mild dysesthesia and weakness in both lower extremities.

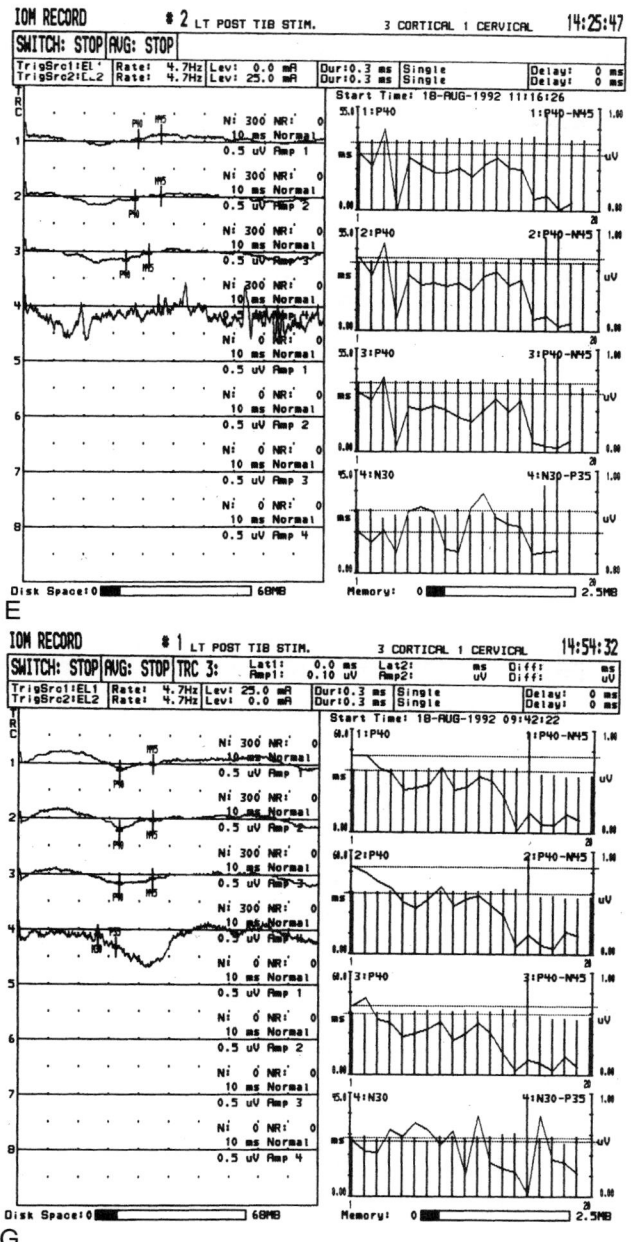

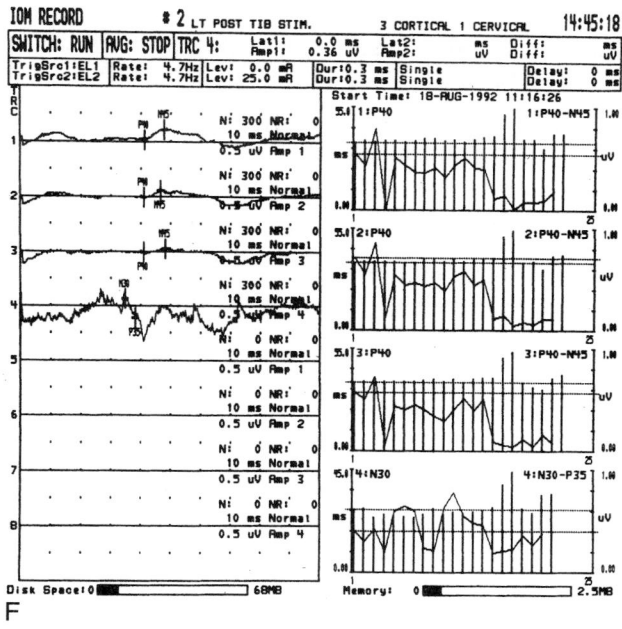

FIGURE 279–3. *Continued. E,* Absent SEP data from Case Study 1, recorded at 14:25. *F,* Absent SEP data from Case Study 1, recorded at 14:45. *G,* Start of improvement of SEP from Case Study 1, recorded at 14:54.

Case Study 1 and Case Study 2 were chosen to depict the relative sensitivity of SEPs to the effects of an ischemic or mechanical insult, respectively. In Case Study 1, an anterior cord syndrome occurred, but the patient's SEPs and gross sensory function remained unchanged. However, the patient demonstrated a significant motor deficit immediately postoperatively. This indicates that SEPs are not a direct measure of spinal cord motor tract function and that additional measures of motor tract function (i.e., Stagnara wake-up test, MEPs) need to be administered in conjunction with the SEP.

Case Study 2 depicts a patient in whom a severe mechanical insult to the spinal cord occurred. The SEPs detected the onset of the insult and were effective in monitoring the effects of the interventional strategies (i.e., increasing MAP and administering steroids) on spinal cord function. The time to data loss was very soon after the insult. By correlating the time of loss onset with the examiner's notes, it was possible to determine the probable cause for the insult. Although the patient demonstrated a mild sensory and motor deficit postoperatively, SEPs correlated with the clinical sensory examination.

Motor Evoked Potentials

The primary purpose for monitoring spinal cord function during surgery is to prevent the onset of surgically induced neurological deficit. Comparatively, a postoperative motor deficit demonstrates a greater debilitation and cost to the patient and society than a sensory deficit.[4] A postoperative motor deficit has always been of greater concern to the surgeon than a sensory deficit.

Originally, only SEPs were used to monitor spinal cord function during surgery. Although it was known that this sensory test provided only indirect information regarding motor tract function, it was reasoned that, if the motor tracts were surgically insulted, the sensory tracts would also be involved. This rationalization was based primarily on the proximity of the sensory to motor tracts. Although this rationalization has proved to be true if the insult is mechanical in origin, it is apparently incorrect if the insult is purely vascular.[12] Because of the differential perfusion patterns of the spinal cord, compromise of the anterior spinal artery can result in a postoperative motor deficit with grossly intact sensory function (see Case Study 1). To detect the onset of an insult to the motor tracts, methods have been developed that elicit an MEP.

STIMULATION SITES

The motor cortex or the spinal cord can be stimulated to elicit an MEP. The site used depends on the type and method of stimulation used (i.e., magnetic or electrical) and the preference of the examiner. Each has its strengths and weaknesses (Table 279–3). To stimulate the motor cortex using magnetic stimulation, the magnetic coil is positioned over the motor cortex, and a high-intensity stimulus (measured in tesla) is applied to the coil. This generates a large magnetic field that stimulates the underlying motor cortex. Stimuli are presented unilaterally and are recorded from muscles or mixed nerves in the contralateral limbs.

Electrical stimulation of the motor cortex requires that a pair of stimulating surface electrodes be placed over the motor cortex. A high-voltage electrical stimulus is then applied to the electrodes, which results in stimulation of the underlying motor cortex.

Electrical stimulation to the spinal cord is delivered in several ways. A pair of stimulating electrodes can be placed within the epidural space, or a pair of needle electrodes can be placed within the bone of the spine. Regardless of the site of stimulation, an electrical stimulus is presented to the spinal cord at an adequate intensity to stimulate the motor tracts.

If the motor cortex is stimulated, changes in the anesthetic regimen need to be made.[22, 30, 31] Regardless of the method of stimulation (i.e., magnetic or electrical), if inappropriate agents are used, amplitude, morphology, and reliability of the response will be significantly degraded. The effects that anesthesia has on the MEP are more deleterious if magnetic stimulation of the motor cortex is used rather than electrical stimulation.

If the spinal cord is stimulated, no significant changes in anesthetic protocol need to be made. Consequently, the same anesthetic protocols used for acquiring SEPs can be used to record the MEPs elicited by electrical stimulation of the spinal cord. Magnetic stimulation of the spinal cord cannot be used to elicit MEPs[32] because of the influence of the shape of the spinal canal and presence of cerebrospinal fluid on the transmission of the magnetic pulse to the spinal cord.

RECORDING SITES

To record the MEP, it must first be decided which type of response is going to be acquired: myogenic or neurogenic. The myogenic response is the compound muscle action potential (CMAP), and the neurogenic response is the compound nerve action potential (CNAP). The CMAP is recorded from muscles as an electromyographic response, and the CNAP is recorded from a mixed peripheral nerve as a neurogenic motor evoked potential (NMEP).

To record the electromyographic response, electrodes are placed over muscle groups distal to the site of surgery. Two recording electrodes are used at each site. To increase the probability of recording a response, large muscle groups are typically used and include the biceps, triceps, quadriceps, anterior tibialis, and medial gastrocnemius.[33] Surface or needle electrodes can be used to record the response. Figure 279–4 provides an example of electromyographic data elicited by electrical stimulation of the contralateral motor cortex.

To record a neurogenic response, recording electrodes are placed over a peripheral mixed nerve. Typical recording sites include the ulnar and median nerves in the upper extremities and at the popliteal fossa in the lower extremities.[32] A pair of needle or surface electrodes is used at each recording site. Figure 279–5 depicts a series of eight NMEPs that were elicited by stimulating the spinal cord at C5 and C6 and that were recorded from the left and right popliteal fossa.

T A B L E 2 7 9 – 3 ■ **Relationship between Perisurgical Variables and Type of Stimulation Used to Elicit a Motor Evoked Potential**

| | TYPE OF STIMULATION | | |
| | Magnetic | Electrical | |
VARIABLE			
Site of stimulation	Motor cortex	Motor cortex	Spinal cord
Stimulator	Coil	Surface electrodes	Needle electrodes
Anesthetic considerations	Significant	Minimal	None
Ease of testing	Difficult	Fairly easy	Easy
Cost	High	Fairly high	Minimal
Reliability	Fair	Good	Excellent

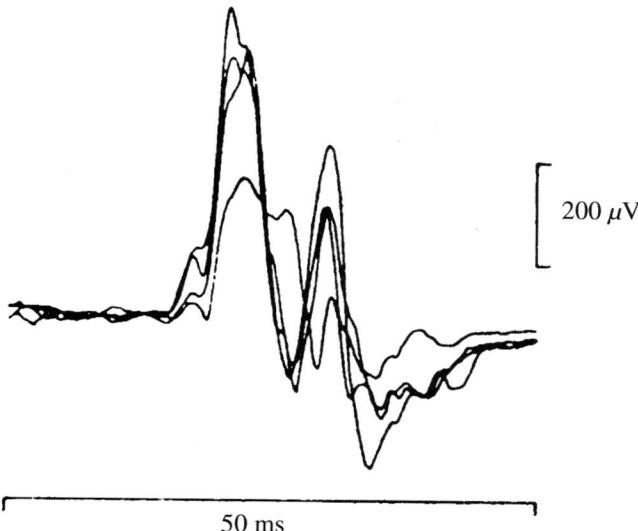

FIGURE 279–4. Test-retest reliability of the myogenic motor evoked potential elicited by cortical stimulation.

ACQUISITION PARAMETERS

Table 279–4 lists the parameters used to acquire MEPs as a function of method and type of response. The parameters for acquiring MEPs are very similar, regardless of whether a CMAP (electromyographic) or CNAP (neurogenic) response is recorded. The parameters are determined by the location of stimulation (i.e., cortical or spinal cord) and the type of response recorded. If the motor cortex is stimulated, a train of stimuli will produce a larger and more reliable response at lower intensity levels than a single impulse.[30] This is achieved because of the summation effect that a train of stimuli has on the excitability of the motor cortex compared with a single impulse. Electrical stimulation can achieve the necessary train of stimuli because they do not require recharging of the capacitors, which is the situation when a magnetic stimulator is used. Although later models of magnetic stimulators can recharge more quickly, which enables a faster presentation rate, they still are limited compared with electrical stimulators.

A second characteristic of the MEP that affects the

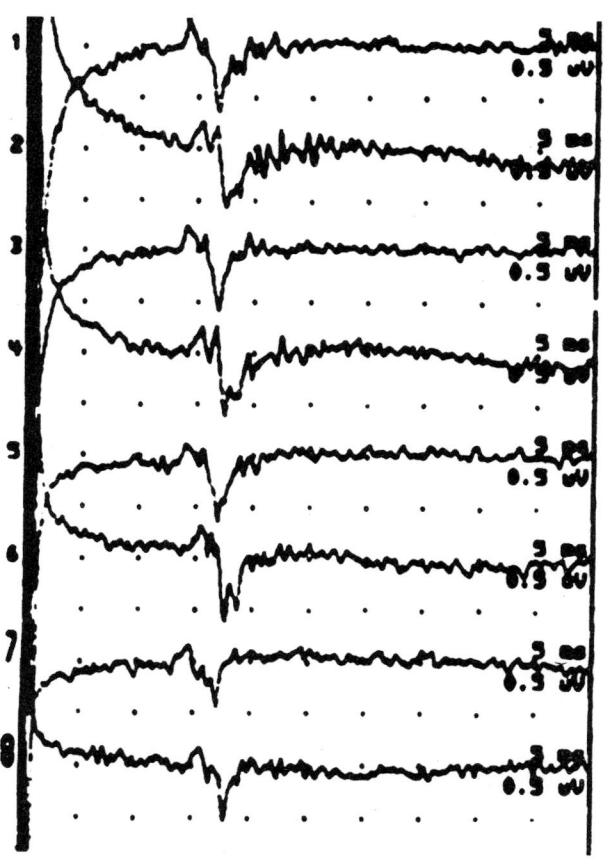

FIGURE 279–5. Eight traces of the neurogenic motor evoked potentials recorded from the left and right popliteal fossa.

acquisition parameters is whether a myogenic or neurogenic response is recorded. If a myogenic (electromyographic) response is recorded, the presentation rate cannot be too fast, or the response will fatigue. The level of muscle relaxation must be kept to a minimum. Typical levels of muscle relaxation are two to three twitches of a train of four. If the presentation rate is too fast or if too much muscle relaxant has been used, the electromyographic response will be smaller and demonstrate unreliable amplitude and morphology (see Fig. 279–4). If amplitude and morphology are un-

TABLE 279–4 ■ Parameters Used to Acquire a Motor Evoked Potential as a Function of Method of Stimulation

	METHOD OF STIMULATION		
PARAMETER	**Magnetic Cortex**	**Electrical Cortex**	**Electrical Spinal Cord**
Filter setting	10–10,000 Hz	10–10,000 Hz	30–1500 Hz
Presentation rate	400 Hz	1/sec	4.7 stimuli/sec
Sample size	4	4	100
Time base	15–105 msec	15–100 msec	50–100 ms
Intensity level	90% of peak power (2 tesla peak power)	500–1000 V	<400 V
Stimulus duration	Unknown	Unknown	300 μsec
Type of response	Myogenic	Myogenic	Myogenic/neurogenic

reliable, they cannot be used to interpret the response. This requires an alteration in the interpretative criteria to include the less sensitive measures of latency and the presence or absence of the response compared with the more sensitive measure of amplitude.

An alternative to recording the electromyographic response is to record its neurological precursor. This consists of recording an NMEP. The NMEP[34] is recorded in the presence of complete muscle relaxation, which results in the response being more reliable. This increased reliability facilitates interpretation and allows the examiner to use amplitude and latency to interpret the response. By recording the response during complete muscle relaxation, the patient does not move on the operating table in response to stimulation, which is the case when an electromyographic response is elicited and recorded and which is very distracting to the surgeon.

INTERPRETATION

The criteria used to interpret the MEP depend on whether an electromyographic or CNAP response is recorded. If an electromyographic response is recorded, the interpretation criteria are limited primarily to latency and to the presence or absence of the response.[31] Of these two criteria, the presence or absence of the response is most widely used.

Figure 279–3 reveals the test-retest reliability of the electromyographic response elicited by electrical stimulation of the right motor cortex. As indicated by the data in Figure 279–3, the amplitude and morphology of these four responses are very unreliable and cannot be used for interpretation. The latency of the four responses appears to be more reliable than the amplitude and morphology, but it is not as sensitive to the onset of an ischemic event. Because of their unreliability, interpretation of electromyographic data in the operating room is limited to the presence or absence of the response.

If an NMEP is recorded, interpretation is based on changes in latency (10% increase) or amplitude (60% decrease) relative to baseline values. Because the CNAP is very reliable, it is possible to use specific quantified criteria to interpret the response. By using these types of interpretative criteria, compared with the presence or absence of the response, the CNAP is more sensitive to the onset of an insult than an electromyographic response.

Figure 279–5 depicts eight traces of NMEP data. The data were elicited by electrically stimulating the spinal cord and were recorded at the left popliteal fossa (i.e., odd traces) and right popliteal fossa (i.e., even traces). The actual NMEP response consists of the large biphasic waveform that occurs at approximately 15 msec (three divisions in Fig. 279–5). The latency of the response is measured at the upward-tending peak, and the amplitude is based on the microvolt difference between the first upward-tending peak and the following downward-tending peak. As is evident in these eight traces, the test-retest reliabilities of response amplitude, latency, and morphology are very dependable.

RELIABILITY AND VALIDITY

MEP reliability depends on the type of response recorded and the method of stimulation. If an electromyographic response is recorded, the reliability of the amplitude and morphology is poor. Consequently, interpretation is based primarily on the presence or absence of the response and whether significant changes in response latency occur. Of these two characteristics, the presence or absence of the response is typically used as the primary interpretative criterion.[30]

MEPs elicited by electrical stimulation of the motor cortex are more reliable than those elicited by magnetic stimulation. In a study by Calancie and associates,[35] MEP data were recorded from 34 patients undergoing a variety of spinal operations. Data were elicited using traditional single-pulse electrical stimulation of the motor cortex and were recorded as an electromyographic response from 8 to 12 muscle groups. Baseline data were recorded in at least one muscle group in 32 of the 34 patients. However, responses were not present in all muscle groups in all patients. Calancie and colleagues concluded that traditional single-pulse stimulation techniques did not elicit a response that was reliable enough for routine clinical use.

In the same study, Calancie and associates[35] used a stimulation method that was a slight modification of traditional techniques. In traditional techniques, a single, high-intensity stimulus is presented, and an electromyographic response is recorded. Although multiple stimuli are used to elicit the responses, which are subsequently averaged, this method of stimulation can result in diminution of the response. In the second technique used by Calancie and colleagues,[35] the threshold of the electromyographic response was determined. Based on the intensity level associated with threshold, it was possible to improve the reliability of the response. However, reliability statistics were not presented. This method was experimental and is not yet clinically applicable.

To determine the reliability of electromyographic data elicited by magnetic stimulation of the motor cortex, MEPs were recorded from 29 patients undergoing surgery.[35] Of the patients tested, six failed to demonstrate a reliable response from any muscle group. In the remaining 23 patients, EMG demonstrated a coefficient of variation of 29% for amplitude and 5% for latency.

The reliability of the NMEP has been extensively investigated in neurologically normal patients and patients with preexisting neurological conditions. Padberg and coworkers[36] assessed the reliability of the NMEPs that had been recorded from 466 neurologically normal patients undergoing surgery for idiopathic scoliosis. A reliable baseline NMEP was recorded for 100% of the patients, and a reliable NMEP was present for 98.7% of the patients throughout surgery.

Wilson-Holden and coworkers[37] described the response in 38 patients undergoing surgery for correction of spinal deformity. All of these patients had a preexisting neurological condition that included weakness and numbness. A reliable SEP and NMEP were recorded in 87.2% and 76.6%, respectively, of the patients throughout surgery. There was good agreement between the patient's preexisting neurological condition and the reliability of the SEP and NMEP.

In addition to the reliability of the MEP, studies have investigated the validity of these procedures. In their report of electrical stimulation of the motor cortex, Calancie and associates[35] also discussed its validity. Based on data elicited using the threshold technique, there was 100% agreement between the patient's postoperative motor deficit and MEP results.

Gugino and colleagues[31] also investigated the validity of MEPs elicited by magnetic stimulation of the motor cortex. Two methods of stimulation—single pulse and trains of pulses—were administered to a total of 89 patients. Regardless of the method of stimulation, there were no false-negative results. There were three true-positive results, and there were two false-positive results.

Of the various MEP procedures developed, the validity of the NMEP has been most thoroughly investigated.[15, 26, 27, 36–38] In animals and humans, the NMEP always correlated with postoperative motor status. If the NMEP procedure is administered correctly, in more than 600 patients reported in the literature, there has not been one case in which the patient demonstrated a surgically induced motor deficit and the NMEP remained unchanged.

SUMMARY

MEP procedures demonstrate various degrees of reliability and validity. Because of normal fluctuations in amplitude and morphology, these two characteristics cannot be used to interpret the electromyographic response. However, it appears that threshold electromyographic data may be more reliable than data acquired at suprathreshold levels. NMEP data are more reliable than electromyographic data.

MEP data elicited by magnetic or electrical stimulation of the motor cortex demonstrate a high validity if appropriate stimulation and anesthetic techniques are used. However, significant modification in the anesthetic regimen is needed. NMEP data demonstrate a very high correspondence with postoperative motor deficit.

MEP procedures are not administered as routinely as SEP procedures. Because of the inherent limitations of the SEP and the goal of the surgeon to avoid a postoperative motor deficit, some type of MEP procedure needs to be administered. Which specific MEP technique is used depends on the availability of appropriate instrumentation, anesthetic considerations, and personnel and their skills. As with any testing procedure, there are advantages and disadvantages of each. The NMEP appears to be the method of choice for recording an MEP.

CASE STUDIES

■ CASE STUDY 3

A patient underwent surgery for the correction of severe kyphoscoliosis. Figure 279–6 depicts magnetic resonance imaging (MRI) of the patient's spine preoperatively. The

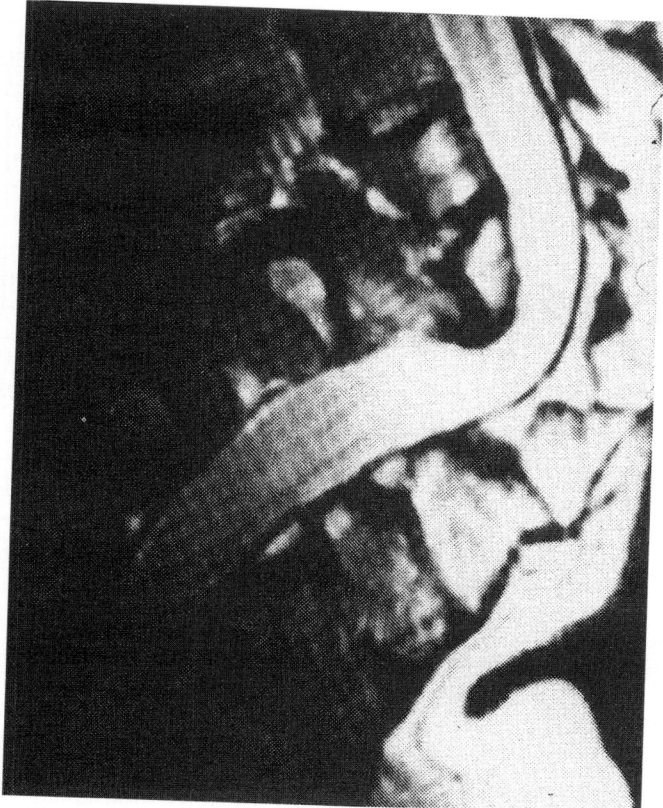

FIGURE 279–6. Preoperative magnetic resonance imaging of the patient described in Case Study 3.

patient underwent an anterior and posterior spinal fusion with instrumentation. Monitoring consisted of MEPs and SEPs with stimulation of the ulnar and posterior tibial nerves. Ulnar data were used to monitor brachial plexus function and to act as a point of reference in determining whether changes in the posterior tibial nerve were caused by surgical or nonsurgical insults. MEPs were recorded as an NMEP. SEPs and MEPs were acquired with standard acquisition parameters.

During the anterior spinal fusion, SEPs and MEPs remained unchanged. Figure 279–7 depicts baseline SEPs, and Figure 279–8 depicts baseline MEPs acquired during the posterior spinal fusion. After correction of the spine, SEPs remained unchanged (Fig. 279–9), but NMEPs were lost (Fig. 279–10). The surgeon was immediately informed of the loss of the MEPs, and a Stagnara wake-up test was administered. Results from the wake-up test were positive for paraplegia. Instrumentation was removed, but MEPs did not demonstrate any improvement. SEPs remained unchanged. On awakening from anesthesia, the patient demonstrated grossly intact SEPs and paraplegia.

Case Study 3 further demonstrates the necessity of administering SEPs and MEPs during any surgery that involves the spinal cord. The MEP procedure administered during this surgery demonstrated a differential sensitivity to motor tract function even though they have a small antidromic composition.

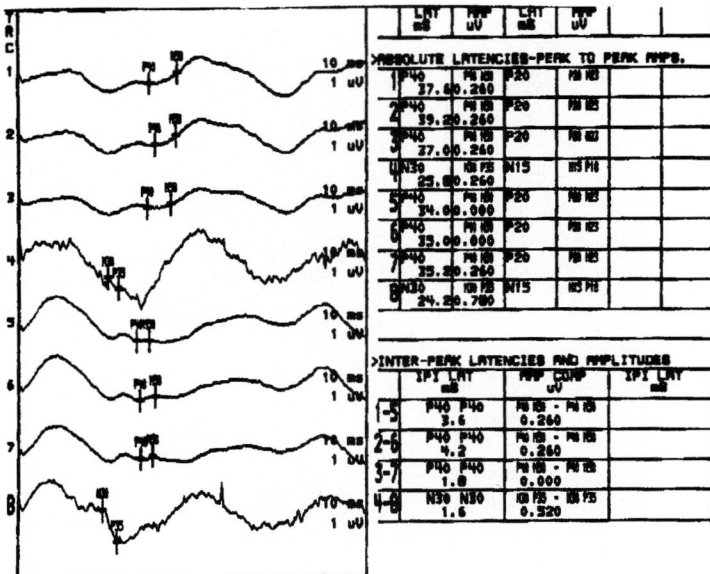

FIGURE 279–7. Baseline somatosensory evoked potentials after stimulation of the left *(top four traces)* and right *(bottom four traces)* posterior tibial nerves, acquired from the patient described in Case Study 3.

NERVE ROOT MONITORING

The purpose for monitoring spinal cord function is to detect the onset of a surgically induced sensory or motor deficit. However, during operations involving nerve roots, monitoring is used to determine levels of nerve root involvement, to determine the adequacy of decompression, to protect nerve roots during the placement of pedicular instrumentation, and to protect nerve roots during the removal of space-occupying lesions.

The methods my colleagues and I use to monitor the spinal cord usually are relatively insensitive and nonspecific to individual nerve roots. Spinal cord monitoring procedures use evoked potentials, which require a significant amount of signal processing (e.g., stimulus elicitation, signal averaging, large sample sizes) and time to acquire before the data can be interpreted. Because evoked potential procedures using mixed nerve or motor tract stimulation are not appropriate for nerve root monitoring, three different methods have been used during operations involving nerve roots: DSEP, E-EMG, and M-EMG.

Dermatomal Somatosensory Evoked Potentials

DSEPs are sensory-based evoked potentials that are elicited by stimulating a peripheral dermatomal field, and they are recorded cortically. In 1987, Herron and associates[39] reported the use of DSEPs to monitor individual nerve root function during surgery. This was followed by numerous reports about the methodology,[40] validity,[6, 41] and reliability[42] of the response.

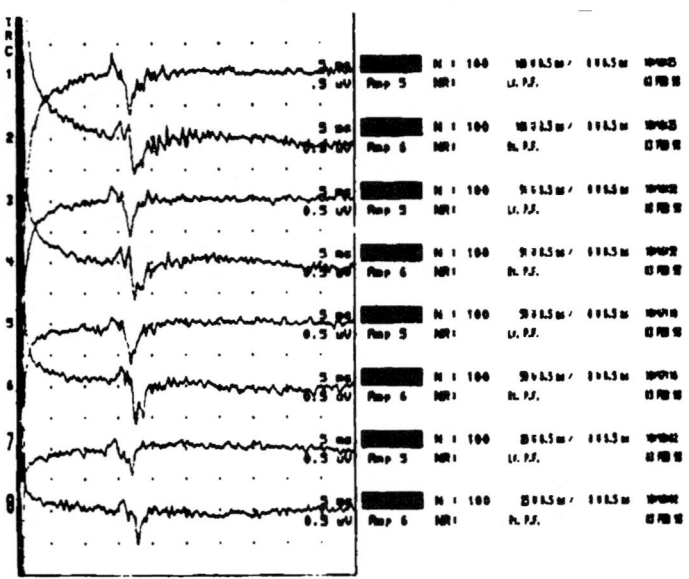

FIGURE 279–8. Baseline neurogenic motor evoked potentials from Case Study 3.

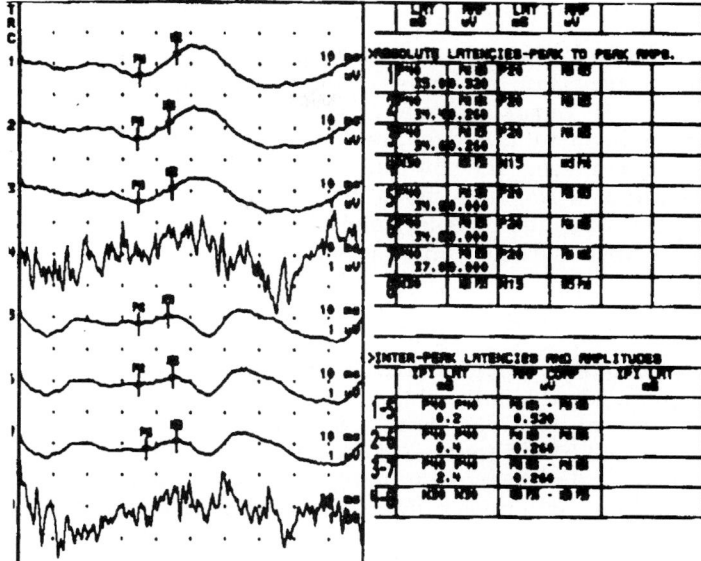

FIGURE 279–9. Unchanged somatosensory evoked potentials from Case Study 3 at the time of neurogenic motor evoked potential loss.

For IOM applications, DSEPs provide information regarding the levels of nerve root involvement and adequacy of nerve root decompression. However, they are not adequately sensitive to protect nerve roots during the use of pedicular instrumentation or during operations that involve the identification and removal of space-occupying lesions.

STIMULATION SITES

DSEPs are elicited by stimulating a peripheral dermatomal field. Cohen and associates[41] provided an excellent description of the dermatomal fields and the methods used to determine the most appropriate site of stimulation relative to each dermatomal field. One problem with dermatomal fields is that they are extremely variable, especially in the lower extremities. If DSEPs are going to be acquired and used during surgery, careful preoperative planning is required, which includes identifying the various dermatomal fields and collecting preoperative data.

DSEPs are elicited by stimulating receptors within the skin rather than subcutaneous receptors.[43] Large-area surface electrodes elicit a more reliable DSEP than responses elicited using subdermal needle electrodes.

RECORDING SITES

To record the DSEP, only cortical recording sites are used. Recording electrodes are placed over the sensory homunculus that is associated with the site of stimulation. The same type of electrodes used to record the mixed nerve SEP are used to record the DSEP.

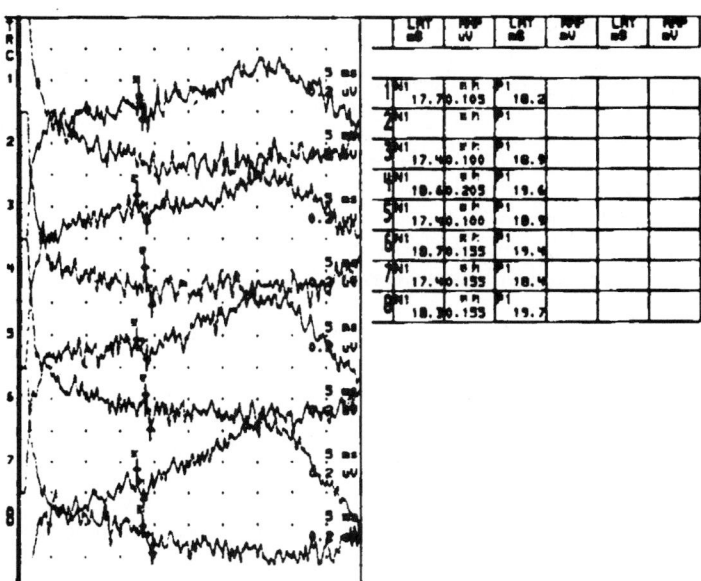

FIGURE 279–10. Loss of neurogenic motor evoked potentials after onset of the spinal cord insult in Case Study 3.

ACQUISITION PARAMETERS

Essentially the same parameters used to elicit and record a cortical mixed nerve SEP are used to acquire the DSEP. The major difference is the intensity level at which the DSEP is elicited. In the mixed nerve SEP, the goal is to present the stimulus at an intensity adequate to stimulate the underlying nerve. However, during DSEP testing, the receptors are more superficial, and a lower intensity level can be used.

INTERPRETATION

Interpretation of mixed nerve SEPs is based on the amplitude and latency of the response. However, interpretation of the DSEP uses only latency. Interpretation of the DSEP is based on comparing the latencies of responses elicited by stimulating adjacent dermatomal fields from within each limb and comparing between-limb data acquired at the same segmental level. For example, the latency of the left L5 DSEP can be compared with the left L4 and the S1 response about the right L5 response. For within-limb data, the latency of the L4 response should be 3 to 5 msec shorter than the L5, and the latency of L5 is typically comparable with the S1. The between-limb latencies should be within 10% at each segmental level. For example, the latency of the left L5 should be within 10% of the right L5 response. Any prolongation of latency within or between limbs is consistent with a compressed or involved nerve root. Latency is the primary interpretative criteria for DSEPs. Amplitude is not used to interpret these responses.

RELIABILITY AND VALIDITY

The reliability of the DSEP is poorer than that of the mixed nerve SEP. This reduction in reliability is caused by several factors. Only a cortical site is used to record the DSEP. Any changes in anesthetic regimen, MAP, or other factors can seriously affect the reliability of the response. Because a cervical recording site is not used during DSEP testing, it can be very difficult to control for the effects from these variables on the response. Consequently, it is extremely important that an appropriate anesthetic regimen be used during surgery. Owen and colleagues[40] found that, if the anesthetic regimen typically used to record a mixed nerve SEP was used during DSEP testing, a reliable DSEP could be obtained in only 69% of cases. However, use of a ketamine-based regimen ensured a reliable DSEP in 100% of cases.

One purpose for administering DSEPs is to determine the levels of nerve root involvement. The validity of the DSEP in achieving this goal is influenced by variations of innervation patterns of dermatomal fields. Owen and colleagues[42] investigated the relationship between the level of nerve root involvement and the preoperative and intraoperative DSEPs. The level of involvement was based on surgical confirmation. The specificity of the DSEP was found to vary as a function of segmental level and by whether data were acquired

TABLE 279–5 ■ **Correlation between Segmental Level and Positive Indication of Nerve Root Involvement as Indicated by Preoperative and Intraoperative Dermatomal Somatosensory Evoked Potentials**

SEGMENTAL LEVEL	DSEP CORRELATION	
	Preoperative	Intraoperative
L4	69%	89%
L5	81%	91%
S1	74%	Did not test

DSEP, dermatomal somatosensory evoked potential.

preoperatively or intraoperatively. Table 279–5 lists the degree of correlation between preoperative and intraoperative DSEPs and the level of surgically confirmed nerve root involvement. As shown, the level of correlation was greater at each segmental level for data acquired intraoperatively than for preoperative data. The correlation between DSEPs and surgically confirmed nerve root compromise varied as a function of the segmental level. In general, the percentage agreement was poorest at low lumbar levels and was best at L5 and S1. Based on normal variability of the location of dermatomal fields,[42] it was concluded that the correlation and, therefore validity, between DSEPs and levels of nerve root involvement could never be 100%.

Another purpose for administering DSEPs is to determine the adequacy of nerve root decompression. This purpose is based on work reported by Herron and coworkers.[39] They postulated that, if a nerve root was adequately decompressed, the intraoperative DSEPs should improve and be consistent with postoperative relief from pain as reported by the patient. If the DSEPS did not improve during surgery, it was reasoned that this result indicated inadequate nerve root decompression, which would be associated with continued pain postoperatively. Owen and associates[40] found that the improvement of intraoperative DSEPs was not based solely on the adequacy of decompression but included the duration of symptoms. If the patient had symptoms for less than 1 year, improvement of the DSEP could occur in the operating room, which correlated with adequate nerve root decompression and postoperative relief from pain. However, if the symptoms persisted for more than 1 year, there was very poor correlation between intraoperative improvements of the DSEP and the presence or absence of postoperative pain. DSEPs could not be reliably used as a method for determining adequacy of nerve root decompression during surgery in cases of chronic nerve root compression.

SUMMARY

DSEPs are sensory-based responses that are elicited by stimulating a dermatomal field, and they are recorded over the somatosensory cortex. DSEP procedures are typically administered during operations for the correction of spinal degeneration and nerve root involvement. DSEP procedures are used to obtain information about the levels of nerve root involvement and to determine the adequacy of nerve root decompression. Because the response is recorded only from the somatosensory cortex, its reliability is influenced by a number of perioperative variables, including anesthesia and MAP. If these variables are controlled, the response has good reliability.

The validity of the DSEP has been investigated and reported in the literature. DSEPS are fairly accurate in determining the levels of nerve root involvement. If the duration of symptoms is short, DSEPs can help in determining the adequacy of nerve root decompression. However, several studies have shown that DSEPs never demonstrate 100% accuracy in identifying the levels of nerve root involvement or adequacy of nerve root decompression.

CASE STUDIES

At one time, DSEPs were a very common method used to monitor individual nerve root function during surgery for spinal degeneration and degenerative disk disease. However, the use of this response has diminished significantly, and consequently, no case studies are presented for this response.

Electromyographic Responses

In the late 1980s and early 1990s, surgeons began to use pedicular instrumentation as points of fixation during operations for spinal degeneration and spinal stenosis. It was soon realized that this type of instrumentation posed a significant risk to adjacent nerve roots. Although intraoperative radiographs and fluoroscopy could be used to identify pedicles and aid in the placement of pedicle screws, the incidence of nerve root compromise was considered to be unacceptably high. To protect nerve roots during the use of pedicular instrumentation, traditional monitoring techniques (i.e., mixed nerve SEPs and DSEPs) were initially administered. However, because of their lack of sensitivity and specificity, they were not ideal methods for monitoring nerve roots that were at risk from pedicular instrumentation.

In response to this new need, two new monitoring procedures that used an electromyographic response were developed: E-EMG[9, 44] and M-EMG.[10] Each procedure has its own specific application. E-EMG is the method of choice when determining the integrity of the pedicle walls, and M-EMG should be used when the goal is to protect the nerve roots during the use of pedicular instrumentation.

STIMULATION SITES

Calancie and associates[9, 44] reported the first use of electromyographic responses during operations that used pedicular instrumentation. Based on the method of electrically eliciting the electromyographic response, the procedure became known as E-EMG. Their work focused on whether responses elicited by electrically stimulating the walls of a pedicle hole by a pedicle tap or finder or by stimulating the pedicle screw provided information about the integrity of the wall. They reasoned that, if the pedicle wall were intact, it would demonstrate high impedance that would prevent the flow of current of a low-intensity stimulus. If the wall were fractured, the wall's impedance would be reduced, which would allow current to flow through the fracture site and stimulate an adjacent nerve root at a very low intensity. By determining the minimum intensity (i.e., threshold) at which a nerve root could be stimulated, it was possible to ascertain whether the pedicle wall was intact or fractured.

The procedure consists of stimulating the walls of the pedicle hole and the head of the pedicle screw after it has been placed by the cathode pole of a bipolar stimulator. The anode pole of the stimulator consists of a subdermal needle electrode that has been placed in the surgical field. If pedicle wall breakthrough had occurred, an electromyographic response would be elicited; if intact, no response would occur.

A limitation of E-EMG is that data are collected only after the pedicle hole has been made or after the pedicle screw has been placed. However, during tapping of the pedicle and during placement of the screw, pedicle wall breakthrough may occur that can result in nerve root damage. During these more dynamic stages of surgery, M-EMG is administered.[10]

Using M-EMG, the response is elicited by mechanical irritation of a nerve root by pedicular instrumentation (i.e., pedicle finder, tap, or screw). If one of these instruments breaks through the pedicle wall, it can mechanically irritate the adjacent nerve root. Irritation of the root results in the elicitation of an electromyographic response, which can be seen on the examiner's monitoring instrument and heard as a popping noise.

RECORDING SITES

Regardless of the method of elicitation, electromyographic responses are recorded from muscles that are innervated by nerve roots that are at surgical risk. Pairs of recording electrodes are placed in each myotome, with one electrode placed over the belly of the muscle and the remaining electrode over the tendon. Although needle electrodes can be used to record the response, surface electrodes are as sensitive and are not invasive.

ACQUISITION PARAMETERS

To acquire the electromyographic response, appropriate acquisition parameters must be used. The patient cannot have completely relaxed muscles. The anesthesiologist needs to maintain a relaxation level of two to three twitches in a train of four. During intubation or other manipulations, complete muscle relaxation is permissible; however, the level of relaxation needs to be less when testing with EMG is initiated.

T A B L E   2 7 9 – 6 ■ **Parameters Used to Acquire an Electromyogram**

	PROCEDURE	
PARAMETER	**E-EMG**	**M-EMG**
Filter	5–5000 Hz	5–5000 Hz
Sensitivity	100 μV	50 μV
Time base	50 msec	1–2 sec
Stimulus intensity	<30 V	NA
Stimulus duration	100–200 μsec	NA
Presentation rate	1.1/sec	NA

E-EMG, electrically elicited electromyogram; M-EMG, mechanically elicited electromyogram; NA, not applicable.

Table 279–6 provides the parameters typically used to acquire responses with E-EMG and M-EMG during surgery. The parameters used to acquire responses with E-EMG and M-EMG are essentially identical, except for the type of stimulation used and the longer time base for M-EMG. E-EMG requires that the eliciting stimulus be presented at a fairly slow rate and at a starting intensity level equal to or less than 30 V. If a constant current stimulus is used, a starting intensity level of 7 mA should be used. The pedicle hole is stimulated at the bottom, approximately halfway up the walls, and the head of the pedicle screw is stimulated after it has been placed. If no response is elicited, it is assumed that the pedicle wall is intact. If a response is elicited, the intensity level of the stimulus is attenuated until threshold is determined. If the threshold is between 5 and 7 mA, no innervation is necessary. If threshold is less than 5 mA, the surgeon needs to consider reorienting the hole or screw.[45–47]

M-EMG does not require the surgeon's participation and is essentially continuous during the use of any pedicular instrumentation. The test is administered continuously, and the surgeon is kept informed about whether nerve root irritation has occurred. If a nerve root is irritated, an electromyographic response is elicited that is heard as a popping sound and that can be seen on the monitoring instrumentation. Many surgeons prefer to hear the firing patterns associated with nerve root irritation, which is easily achieved by increasing the volume of the monitor's loudspeaker.

INTERPRETATION

The criteria used to interpret the results of E-EMG are different from those used to interpret the results of M-EMG. Interpretation of data from E-EMG is based on the threshold intensity at which a response is elicited. If the pedicle wall is intact, no response is elicited at the starting intensity level. If pedicle wall breakthrough has occurred, the threshold of the response is significantly lower. If the threshold of the electromyographic response is at or below 5 mA, intervention should be considered. If threshold is between 5 and 7 mA, the surgeon should inspect the hole to determine the magnitude and location of breakthrough before initiating

intervention. Intervention consists of reorienting the pedicle hole or screw and retesting.[45] If, on retesting, threshold has increased to a normal level, that point of fixation should be used. If the threshold has not increased, an alternative site of fixation should be considered. Elevation of the threshold after intervention is attributed to sealing of the site of breakthrough by cancellous bone.

The criteria used to interpret the results of M-EMG are based on the presence or absence of electromyographic activity. If no activity is elicited, it can be assumed that the nerve root has not been irritated. If activity has been elicited, nerve root irritation has occurred. There is a sliding scale in terms of the amount of electromyographic activity compared with the degree of irritation. An occasional "pop" of electromyographic activity is not considered to be pathologic. However, a large burst of electromyographic activity or sustained firing is considered to be pathologic, and intervention should be initiated immediately. Intervention consists of immediately stopping the offending surgical maneuver and waiting until data return to normal. The site of irritation should then be examined.

RELIABILITY AND VALIDITY

The reliability and validity of E-EMG and M-EMG have been extensively studied. Calancie and coworkers[44] investigated the reliability and the validity of E-EMG. When a positive result for E-EMG was elicited, it was found to be 100% reliable and accurate for the presence of pedicle wall breakthrough. However, pedicle wall breakthrough did not correlate with nerve root irritation. If a positive result for E-EMG occurred, only 87% of the patients demonstrated nerve root involvement. This means that E-EMG is excellent for determining the integrity of the pedicle walls, but it is not the method of choice for protecting nerve roots.

To protect nerve roots, M-EMG should be used in conjunction with E-EMG. Two studies have investigated the reliability and validity of M-EMG.[44, 48] An irritated nerve root always elicits an electromyographic response; the response has a 100% reliability rate. However, it was also found that, in the initial applications of this procedure, there was a false-positive rate of 6% to 8%. This meant that the cause for EMG was not pathologic irritation of the nerve root by pedicular instrumentation but was probably irritation of the root by perioperative variables. These variables included cold irrigating fluid, patient movement on the operating table, and a lack of experience with the procedure by the monitoring team. After these variables were eliminated, the false-positive rate was reduced to 0%.

SUMMARY

E-EMG and M-EMG have been shown to be reliable and valid procedures for determining pedicle wall status and monitoring nerve roots during operations that use pedicle instrumentation. With E-EMG, responses are elicited by electrical stimulation of the pedicle hole or screw. With M-EMG, responses are elicited by mechanical irritation of the nerve roots. For both procedures, the electromyographic response is recorded from myotomes that are innervated by nerve roots that are at surgical risk.

E-EMG should be used to determine the presence of pedicle wall breakthrough, and M-EMG is the method of choice for protecting nerve roots. Because of their respective applications, both procedures should be administered during operations that use pedicular instrumentation. M-EMG is applied during the use of a pedicle finder and tap and when a pedicle screw is being placed. E-EMG is used to determine whether pedicle walls are intact after the pedicle hole has been made and after the pedicle screw has been placed.

CASE STUDIES

■ CASE STUDY 4

Case Study 4 reviews a patient who underwent surgery for the correction of spondylolisthesis at L5-S1. Preoperatively, the patient was neurologically normal. Surgery consisted of a posterior spinal fusion with pedicular instrumentation at L4, L5, and S1.

E-EMG and M-EMG were used to monitor the nerve roots. Mixed nerve SEPs (ulnar and posterior tibial nerves) were used to monitor brachial plexus and spinal cord function. Ulnar nerve data are not presented, and posterior tibial nerve data are presented but not extensively discussed.

Figure 279–11 depicts six traces of free-run activity (i.e., top six lines on graph) and two traces of posterior tibial

nerve SEPs (i.e., bottom two lines on graph). The six traces correspond to the following myotomes:

Trace 1: left quadriceps (L4)
Trace 2: left anterior tibialis (L5)
Trace 3: left medial gastrocnemius (S1)
Trace 4: right quadriceps
Trace 5: right anterior tibialis
Trace 6: right medial gastrocnemius

The seventh trace is a cortical SEP, and the eighth (bottom) trace is a cervical SEP. My colleagues and I always record mixed nerve SEP data during all operations involving the spine to ensure that no injury to the spinal cord goes undetected. In the first six traces, no evidence of electromyographic activity is evident.

Figure 279–12 depicts the same eight traces, but mechanically elicited electromyographic activity is present in the left anterior tibialis myotomes. The activity was elicited by mechanical irritation of the nerve root during the surgery. The surgeon heard and was informed of the popping noise associated with the irritating maneuver, which resulted in a cessation of the electromyographic activity.

Figure 279–13 depicts the same eight traces but also demonstrates an electrically mediated electromyographic response in the right L5 myotome. This activity was elicited when the surgeon electrically stimulated the head of a pedicle screw placed at that level. Based on the intensity level at which the threshold of this response was obtained (5 V), the surgeon visually inspected the area and found pedicle wall breakthrough at this level. The screw was removed, reoriented, and reinserted. The patient demonstrated normal neurological function during surgery.

The purpose of Case Study 4 was to demonstrate the type of electromyographic activity that can occur during surgery for spinal degeneration, spondylolis-

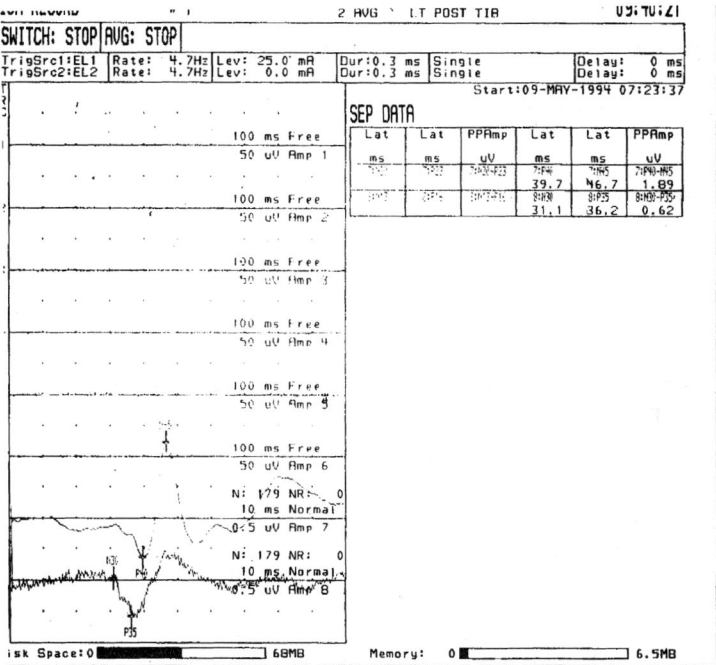

FIGURE 279–11.   Free-run electromyograms recorded from the patient described in Case Study 4.

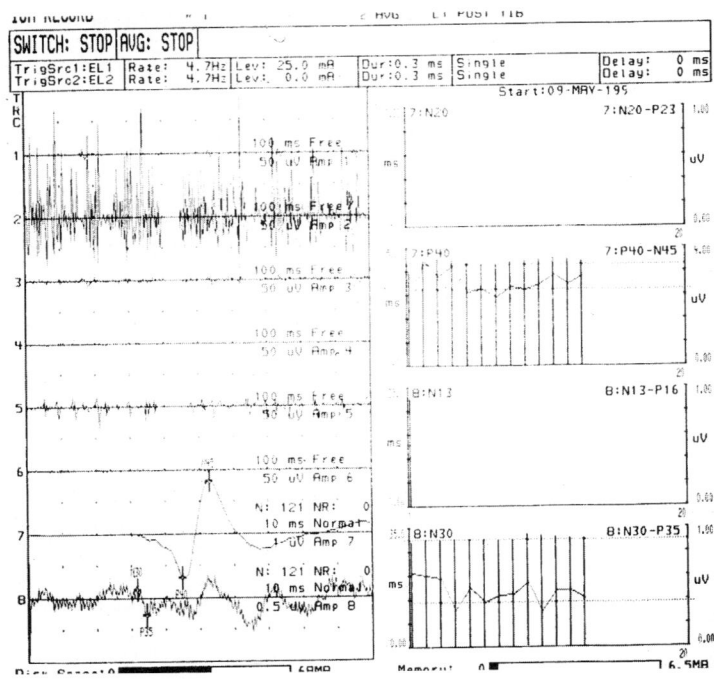

FIGURE 279–12. Mechanically elicited electromyograms after irritation of the left L5 nerve root in the patient described in Case Study 4.

thesis, or other disorders and the corrective maneuvers that are available to the surgeon. By initiating these maneuvers, more appropriate points of fixation can be achieved, and the incidence of nerve root irritation is decreased.

MONITORING FOR TETHERED CORDS AND SPACE-OCCUPYING LESIONS

The methods previously described can be used to monitor spinal cord or nerve root function. However, these same methods may not be appropriate during operations for a tethered cord or the removal of a space-occupying lesion within the cauda equina. During operations for these types of abnormalities, it is necessary to provide the surgeon with information regarding the type of tissue in the surgical field. By using electrical stimulation of tissue and recording an electromyographic response, it is possible to discriminate between neural and non-neural tissue.

These techniques are similar to E-EMG in that an electromyographic response is elicited by electrical

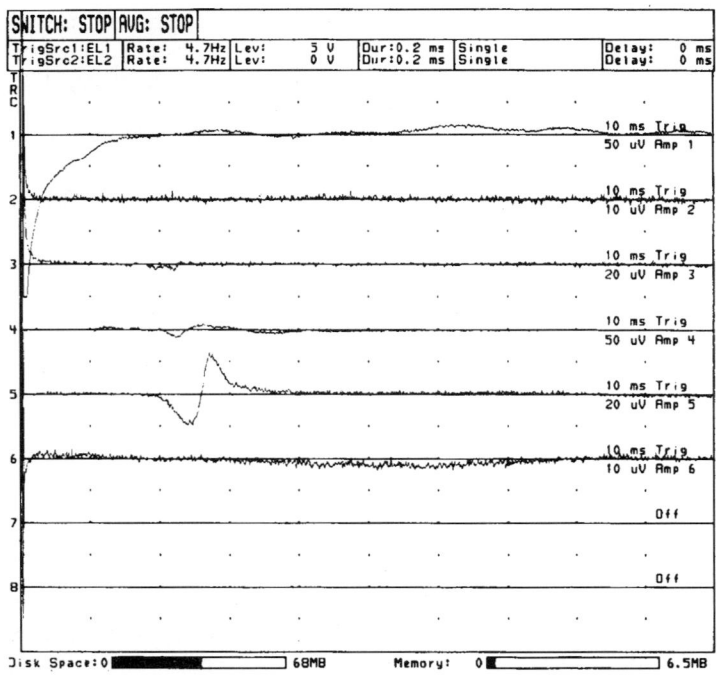

FIGURE 279–13. Electrically elicited electromyograms after stimulation of the right pedicle screw at L5.

stimulation and is recorded from peripheral myotomes. However, the manner of elicitation is different from the E-EMG used to ascertain the status of a pedicle wall.

Electrical Stimulation and Electromyographic Recording

STIMULATION SITE

To elicit the electromyographic response during operations for a tethered cord or removal of a tumor within the cauda equina, the suspected tissue is electrically stimulated using a hand-held bipolar stimulator. If appropriate stimulation parameters are used on neural tissue, an electromyographic response will be elicited. If the tissue is not neural, no response will be elicited.

To ensure that a reliable and valid response is obtained, certain procedures must be followed. First, there must be a good point of contact between the stimulating electrodes and the tissue. Second, the intensity level must be great enough to elicit a response but not too great, which would cause damage to the tissue or result in current spread to adjacent tissue. Accurate records must be kept regarding the various sites of stimulation and the types of responses recorded from stimulating those sites.

In addition to recording an electrically elicited electromyographic response, it is possible to record a free-run response similar to that of the M-EMG. Free-run electromyographic responses are helpful when the surgeon is manipulating a tumor or tissue. If neural tissue is manipulated, an electromyographic response will be elicited. This type of information can provide meaningful feedback to the surgeon regarding the type of tissue in the surgical site.

RECORDING SITES

Electromyographic recording sites include major muscle groups in the lower extremities. If bowel or bladder function is of concern, recording electrodes can be placed in perianal musculature.

ACQUISITION PARAMETERS

The parameters used to acquire the electromyographic response are similar to those used to acquire responses with E-EMG. The biggest differences are the intensity level at which the stimulus is presented and the stimulation site. To elicit the electromyographic response during this application, a bipolar stimulating electrode is placed on the suspected tissue, and a stimulus is presented. The presentation rate of the stimulus should be very slow. The stimulus intensity is then increased from 0 mA in very small steps until a response is elicited. If the tissue is neural, a response will be elicited; if it is not neural, no response will be elicited. The response can be recorded as an electromyographic response or directly from the nerve.

One of the precautions that must be taken when administering this procedure is to ensure that the intensity level of the stimulus is not too high. If the stimulus

intensity is too high, it is possible to damage the stimulated tissue or cause the current to spread to adjacent neural tissue, which would result in an erroneous response. To determine the appropriate intensity of the stimulus, a section of nerve that is known to be neurologically normal should be stimulated. A response is then recorded from the nerve or from a muscle that is peripheral to the stimulation site. By stimulating a normal segment of nerve, it is possible to determine the threshold of a response, which is then used to determine the approximate level at which a response should be expected when stimulating tissue of unknown functional status.

Another concern associated with direct nerve stimulation is the presence of a stimulus artifact, which appears at the very beginning of the trace. The artifact is approximately 1 to 2 msec in duration and can overlap and obliterate a response if the distance between the stimulating and recording electrodes is less than a few centimeters. This is especially true if a nerve-to-nerve response is being recorded. To eliminate the artifact, a tripolar stimulator should be used.

INTERPRETATION

Interpretation of the data depends on the presence or absence of the response. Although it is possible to determine the latency, amplitude, and conduction velocity of the response, these measures vary significantly based on factors such as the site of stimulation and the distance between the stimulation and recording sites. The presence or absence criteria are of primary interpretative use. If no response is elicited and if proper acquisition parameters are used, it can be assumed that the tissue being stimulated is not neural or is functionally impaired. If a response is elicited, it can be assumed that the tissue stimulated is neural in origin and is functionally intact.

If mechanically elicited electromyographic responses are recorded, interpretation is also based on the presence or absence of activity. If the surgeon is manipulating nerve tissue, electromyographic firing will occur and alert the surgeon to the manipulation of this type of tissue.

RELIABILITY AND VALIDITY

Results for the reliability and validity of direct nerve stimulation have not been published. However, the procedure is simple to administer, and data are easy to interpret. If the procedure is properly administered, it typically demonstrates 100% reliability and validity rates for identifying nerve tissue and informing the surgeon that nerve tissue is being irritated.

SUMMARY

The removal or sectioning of non-neural tissue in the cauda equina can pose a difficulty for the surgeon. The primary difficulties during these procedures include identification of neural tissue and protecting neural tissue during the manipulation or removal of non-neural tissue. Two procedures are available to the surgeon to help avoid the difficulties associated with these types of operations. Both procedures record an electromyographic response or a direct nerve action potential. Stimulation techniques consist of stimulating suspected tissue and recording the response at sites distal or rostral to the site of the lesion. If proper precautions are taken, there are minimal risks to the patient. These two monitoring procedures are very effective in avoiding complications associated with these types of operations.

MEDICOLEGAL ASPECTS OF INTRAOPERATIVE MONITORING

One of the purposes of IOM is to prevent the onset of a surgically induced postoperative neurological deficit. If IOM procedures are properly administered, they have been found to be a cost-effective method for reducing the incidence and severity of these deficits.[49] Because of their effectiveness in reducing postoperative deficits, their use has become of major interest to attorneys involved with malpractice law.

Kiersh[50] described the medicolegal aspects of IOM. The major point pertaining to IOM and malpractice lawsuits involves the issue of *standard of care*. Is it the standard of care to perform IOM during operations affecting the spinal cord, nerve roots, or other components of the peripheral or central nervous systems? How is standard of care defined? If it is not the standard of care, does the administration of these procedures help protect the surgeon in the event that a postoperative deficit occurs? To understand the relationship between IOM and standard of care issues, a brief background regarding the concept of standard of care is presented.

The standard of care pertains to medical procedures and methods administered during surgery or during a diagnostic test session. It is typically a national standard rather than a local custom or practice. Defining a standard can be achieved through expert testimony in which the course of action of a reasonably prudent physician, with the defendant's specialty, would have pursued under the same or similar circumstances. The standard can also be reported in professional journals as position statements by a professional society.[51] Although there are various sources for the definition of the standard, they are all based on a set of guidelines developed by experts and supported by the issuing society or body.

If a patient demonstrates a surgically induced neurological deficit, it is the plaintiff's responsibility to demonstrate that there was a deviation from the standard of care and that this deviation was more than likely the cause of the injury. If a standard of care already exists, the plaintiff's attorneys make reference to that standard. If no standard exists, it is the plaintiff's responsibility to hire several individuals who are experts in this area of medicine and who, through testimony, can demonstrate that the surgeon's course of action

did cause the postoperative deficit and that there were ways to avoid this deficit if they had been employed. However, malpractice cannot be based solely on the personal opinion of the expert witnesses. It is necessary for the plaintiff's attorney to demonstrate that a pattern is followed nationally regarding a particular form of treatment.

What is the status of IOM in terms of a standard of care? Several groups have indicated that IOM is the standard of care for certain types of operations. In 1988, a symposium was held at the Alfred I. DuPont Institute of the de Nemours Foundation in Wilmington, Delaware.[52] This symposium brought together neurosurgeons, neurologists, neurophysiologists, and anesthesiologists to discuss the usefulness of IOM in the United States. Based on the materials presented, the participants issued the following statement about the use of IOM: "Electrophysiological monitoring techniques should be considered the standard of care for surgical procedures that place the central nervous system at risk for injury."

In addition to position statements, published data in peer-reviewed journals regarding the efficacy of monitoring can also be used to define a standard. Dinner and coworkers[53] reported that the false-negative rate associated with SEP monitoring of the spine was 1.87%. Nuwer and colleagues[24] and Dawson and associates[25] reported that the use of SEPs during spinal surgery always detected the onset of a sensory-based neurological deficit. If SEP data changed and the surgeon initiated intervention, only 0.42% of the patients demonstrated a postoperative deficit. However, it was also shown that there were instances in which the SEPs did not change and the patient demonstrated a motor deficit in the presence of grossly intact sensory function.

This brings us to the matter of whether MEPs for motor tract monitoring and electromyographic responses for nerve root monitoring should be considered the standard of care. If a plaintiff's attorney can demonstrate through expert testimony that MEP or electromyographic monitoring can prevent a surgically induced neurological deficit to the spinal motor tracts or nerve roots, they have begun to develop a standard for the use of these tests during these types of surgical procedures. For example, it has already been shown that electromyographic monitoring during the pedicular screws is 100% sensitive to the onset of pedicle wall breakthrough and more than 99% sensitive to the onset of nerve root damage. It is unknown whether malpractice suits regarding the use of electromyographic response during nerve root surgery have been presented, but it is probably only a matter of time before such lawsuits occur.

The relationship between malpractice lawsuits and IOM places the surgeon in a difficult situation. If monitoring is not available, should the surgeon require that it be provided by the hospital before certain types of operations are performed? If monitoring is available, should the surgeon request it even though the surgeon may not consider it to be the standard of care for that operation? How does the surgeon know whether the monitoring being provided is adequate?

Monitoring is not available at all hospitals. Because of cost considerations and the availability of trained and experienced personnel,[4] many hospitals do not provide IOM. In-house IOM programs are expensive and logistically difficult to develop, and they are typically limited to large medical centers. In lieu of in-house services, many hospitals contract with private companies to provide IOM. The hospital needs to develop guidelines based on peer-reviewed journal articles that are intended to apply to these private companies.

The surgeon must become more familiar with IOM procedures. Neurosurgeons are fortunate in that they typically receive heavy emphasis on neurophysiologic tests during their training. Regardless of the subspecialty, the surgeon needs to meet with the monitoring team to discuss the types of procedures that will be administered during surgery, the criteria used to interpret data, anesthetic requirements, and the interventional strategies before IOM is initiated.

CONCLUSIONS

IOM is the application of various procedures that are used to monitor the functional integrity of neurological structures that are at direct or indirect surgical risk. Traditionally, these procedures have been electrophysiologic in nature, but they can include measures such as perfusion. IOM is a cost-effective method for protecting the neurological structures at risk. Because of the litigious complications associated with surgically induced neurological deficits, the relationship between the administration of IOM and standard of care issues has received significant scrutiny during the past 10 years.

Neurosurgeons often inquire about the value of evoked potential monitoring during surgery for the removal of an intramedullary tumor within the spinal cord. In most cases, the surgical approach consists of a posterior incision in the midline of the spinal cord and the identification and removal of the tumor. Because of this approach, the spinal cord is mechanically manipulated, which can affect the data. Surgeons have had a reluctance to use monitoring in these situations because of a fear of a high false-positive rate and the necessity of removing as much of the tumor as possible. During this type of surgery, data fluctuate in response to manipulation of the spinal cord and possibly because of removal of the tumor. Although data fluctuation occurs quickly, the data also recover quickly. If the surgeon is attempting to realistically maintain as much spinal cord function as possible, IOM should be administered. However, if the goal is to remove as much tumor as possible and forego maintaining function, the value of IOM is limited.

For IOM procedures to be effective, certain criteria must be met. Appropriate tests must be administered, personnel must be well trained and experienced, the criteria used to interpret data must be sensitive to the onset of vascular and mechanical insults to the central nervous system, and appropriate intervention strategies must be developed before IOM procedures are administered. Because IOM procedures have been shown to be differentially sensitive to the onset of specific types of neurological insults, a multimodality approach to monitoring is necessary. For an IOM program to be effective, the entire monitoring team must be experienced. This means that the surgeon must be familiar with the procedures being administered and that strict guidelines regarding the training and experience of the individuals performing and interpreting test results must be developed before a monitoring program is implemented.

REFERENCES

1. Dawson GD: Investigations in a patient subject to myoclonic seizures after sensory stimulation. J Neurol Neurosurg Psychiatry 10:141–162, 1947.
2. Tamaki T, Yamashita T, Kobayashi H: Spinal cord monitoring [in Japanese]. Nouha Kindenzu 1:218–227, 1969.
3. Brown RH, Nash CL: Current status of spinal cord monitoring. Spine 4:466–470, 1979.
4. Owen JH: The application of intraoperative monitoring during surgery for spinal deformity. Spine 15:2649–2662, 1999.
5. Slimp JC, Rubner DE, Snowden ML, et al: Dermatomal somatosensory evoked potentials: Cervical, thoracic and lumbosacral levels. Electroenceophalogr Clin Neurophysiol 84:55–70, 1992.
6. Cohen BA, Hulzenger BA: Dermatomal monitoring for surgical correction of spondylolisthesis: A case report. Spine 13:1125–1130, 1988.
7. Owen JH, Padberg AM, Spahr-Holland L, et al: Clinical correlation between degenerative spine disease and dermatomal somatosensory evoked potentials in humans. Spine 16:201–205, 1991.
8. Owen JH, Bridwell KH, Lenke LG: Innervation pattern of dorsal roots and their effects on the specificity of dermatomal somatosensory evoked potentials. Spine 18:748–754, 1993.
9. Calancie B, Lebwohl N, Madsen P, Klose KJ: Intraoperative evoked EMG monitoring in an animal model. Spine 17:1229–1233, 1992.
10. Owen JH, Kostuik JK, Gornet M, et al: The use of mechanically elicited EMGs to protect nerve roots during surgery for spinal degeneration. Spine 19:1704–1710, 1994.
11. Moller AR: Intraoperative recordings that can guide the surgeon in the operation. In Moller AR (ed): Intraoperative Neurophysiologic Monitoring. Sydney, Australia, Harwood Academic Publishers, 1995.
12. Owen JH, Naito M, Bridwell KH: Relationship among level of distraction, evoked potentials, spinal cord ischemia and integrity and clinical status in animals. Spine 15:852–857, 1990.
13. Epstein N: Intraoperative evoked potential monitoring. In Benzel EC (ed): Spine Surgery: Techniques, Complication Avoidance, and Management. New York, Churchill Livingstone, 1999, pp 1249–1257.
14. Lesser RP, Raudzins P, Luders H, et al: Postoperative neurological deficits may occur despite unchanged intra-operative somatosensory evoked potentials. Ann Neurol 19:22–25, 1986.
15. O'Brien MF, Lenke LG, Bridwell KH, et al: Evoked potential monitoring of the upper extremities during thoracic and lumbar spinal deformity surgery: A prospective study. J Spinal Disord 7:277–284, 1994.
16. Padberg AM, Bridwell KH: Spinal cord monitoring: Current state of the art. Orthop Clin North Am 31:407–433, 1999.
17. Nuwer MR: Evoked Potential Monitoring in the Operating Room. New York, Raven Press, 1986, pp 51–75.
18. Owen JH, Sponseller PD, Szymanski J, et al: Efficacy of multimodality spinal cord monitoring during surgery for neuromuscular scoliosis. Spine 20:34–43, 1995.
19. Lubicky JP, Spadoro JA, Yuan HA, et al: Variability of somatosen-

sory evoked potential monitoring during spinal surgery. Spine 14:790–798, 1989.

20. Ashkenaze D, Mudiyan R, Boachie-Adjei O, et al: Efficacy of spinal cord monitoring in neuromuscular scoliosis. Spine 18: 1627–1633, 1993.

21. Jasper HH: Report of committee on methods of clinical examination in EEG. Appendix: The ten-twenty electrode system of the International Federation. Electroenceophalogr Clin Neurophysiol 10:371–384, 1958.

22. Sloan TB: Anesthesia during spinal surgery with electrophysiological monitoring. Semin Spine Surg 9:295–301, 1997.

23. Keith R, Stambough JL, Asender SH: Somatosensory evoked potentials: A review of 100 cases of intraoperative spinal surgery monitoring. J Spinal Disord 3:220–229, 1990.

24. Nuwer MR, Dawson EG, Carlson LG, et al: Somatosensory evoked potential spinal cord monitoring reduces neurologic deficits after scoliosis surgery: Results of a large multi-center survey. Electroencephalogr Clin Neurophysiol 96:6–11, 1995.

25. Dawson EG, Sherman JE, Kanim LEA, et al: Spinal cord monitoring: Results of the Scoliosis Research Society and the European Spinal Deformity Society survey. Spine 16(Suppl):S361–S364, 1995.

26. Kai Y, Owen JH, Allen BT, et al: Relationship between evoked potentials and clinical status in spinal cord ischemia. Spine 19: 1162–1168, 1995.

27. Kai Y, Owen JH, Lenke LG, et al: Use of sciatic neurogenic motor evoked potentials versus spinal potentials to predict early onset neurologic deficits when intervention is still possible during overdistraction. Spine 18:1134–1138, 1993.

28. McCaffrey MT: Somatosensory evoked-potential monitoring during spinal surgery. Semin Spine Surg 9:309–314, 1997.

29. Bridwell KH, Lenke LG, Baldus C, et al: Major intraoperative neurologic deficits in pediatric and adult spinal deformities patients: Incidence and etiology at one institution. Spine 23:324–331, 1998.

30. Linden D, Johnson JR, Shields CB, et al: Intraoperative spinal cord monitoring with motor evoked potentials elicited by transcranial magnetic stimulation. In Bridwell KH, DeWald RL (eds): The Textbook of Spinal Surgery, 2nd ed. Philadelphia, Lippincott-Raven Publishers, 1997.

31. Gugino LD, Aglio LS, Segal ME, et al: Use of transcranial magnetic stimulation for monitoring spinal cord motor paths. Semin Spinal Surg 9:315–336, 1997.

32. Konrad P, Owen JH, Bridwell KH: Magnetic stimulation of the spine to produce lower extremity EMG responses: Significance of coil position and the presence of bone. Spine 19:2812–2818, 1994.

33. Owen JH: Intraoperative stimulation of the spinal cord for prevention of spinal cord injury. In Devinsky O, Beric V, Dogali J (eds): Electrical and Magnetic Stimulation of the Brain and Spinal Cord. New York, Raven Press, 1993, pp 217–288.

34. Owen JH, Bridwell KH, Grubb R, et al: The clinical application of neurogenic motor evoked potentials to monitor spinal cord function during surgery. Spine 16(Suppl):S385–S390, 1991.

35. Calancie B, Harris W, Broton JG, et al: Threshold level multipulse transcranial electrical stimulation of motor cortex for intraoperative monitoring of spinal motor tracts: Description of method

and comparison to somatosensory evoked potential monitoring. American Society for Neurophysiological Monitoring 7:32–47, 1999.

36. Padberg AM, Wilson-Holden TJ, Lenke LG, et al: Somatosensory and motor evoked potential monitoring without a wake-up test during idiopathic scoliosis surgery: An accepted standard of care. Spine 23:1392–1400, 1998.

37. Wilson-Holden TJ, Padberg AM, Lenke LG, et al: Efficacy of Intraoperative monitoring for pediatric patients with spinal cord pathology undergoing spinal deformity surgery. Spine 24:1685–1692, 1999.

38. Owen JH, Laschinger J, Bridwell KH, et al: Sensitivity and specificity of somatosensory and neurogenic motor evoked potentials in animals and humans. Spine 13:1111–1118, 1991.

39. Herron LD, Trippi AC, Gonyea M: Intraoperative use of dermatomal somatosensory evoked potentials in lumbar stenosis surgery. Spine 12:379–383, 1987.

40. Owen JH, Padberg AM, Spahr-Holland L, et al: Clinical correlation between degenerative spine disease and dermatomal somatosensory evoked potentials in humans. Spine 16(Suppl):S201–S207, 1991.

41. Cohen BA, Major MR, Huisenga BA: Predictability of adequacy of spinal root decompression using evoked potentials. Spine 16(Suppl):S379–S384, 1991.

42. Owen JH, Bridwell KH, Lenke LG: Innervation pattern of dorsal roots and their effect on the specificity of dermatomal somatosensory evoked potentials. Spine 18:748–753, 1993.

43. Toleikis JR, Carlvin AO, Shapiro DE, et al: The use of dermatomal evoked responses during surgical procedures that use intra-pedicular fixation of the lumbosacral spine. Spine 18:2401–2403, 1993.

44. Calancie B, Madsen P, Lebwohl N: Stimulus evoked monitoring during transpedicular lumbosacral spine instrumentation: Initial clinical results. Spine 19:2780–2787, 1994.

45. Darden BV, Wood KE, Hatley MK, et al: Evaluation of pedicle screw insertion monitored by intraoperative evoked electromyography. J Spinal Disord 9:8–16, 1996.

46. Lenke LG, Padberg AM, Russo MH, et al: Triggered electromyographic threshold for accuracy of pedicle screw placement. Spine 29:1585–1591, 1995.

47. Holland NR, Lukacyzk TA, Riley LH, et al: Higher electrical stimulus intensities are required to activate chronically compressed nerve roots. Spine 23:224–227, 1998.

48. Holland NR, Kostuik JP: Continuous electromyographic monitoring to detect nerve root injury during thoracolumbar scoliosis surgery. Spine 22:2547–2550, 1997.

49. Daube JR: The role of intraoperative electrophysiological monitoring. Muscle Nerve 36:1151–1153, 1999.

50. Kiersh SR: Medical-legal aspects of intraoperative monitoring. Semin Spine Surg 9:337–340, 1997.

51. Nash CL, Brown RH: Spinal cord monitoring. J Bone Joint Surg Am 71:627–630, 1989.

52. Salzman SK (ed): Neural Monitoring: The Prevention of Intraoperative Injury. Totowa, NJ, Humana Press, 1990.

53. Dinner DS, Luders H, Lesser RP, et al: Invasive methods of somatosensory evoked potential monitoring. J Clin Neurophysiol 3:113–120, 1986.

CHAPTER 280

Bone Metabolism As It Relates to Spinal Disease and Treatment

MUWAFFAK M. ABDULHAK ■ MARILYN L. GATES ■ JAMES P. HOLLOWELL

Bone metabolism is a complex process involving many physiologic and pathologic factors. Bone turnover is critical to the regulation and maintenance of mineral homeostasis within the body. Ninety-nine percent of the body calcium is stored within bone. Access to that store for the maintenance of critical body functions and the ongoing processes of reformation and resorption within the skeleton requires the interaction of such substances as parathyroid hormone (PTH), vitamin D, and calcitonin. In addition, there is interplay among calcium, phosphorus, and sex hormones.

An understanding of bone metabolism and its abnormalities, such as osteoporosis and hyperthyroidism, is paramount for physicians involved in treating bone diseases. Back pain, spinal deformity, and impaired spinal function can result from alterations in vertebral bone metabolism. Vertebral fractures have a different pathophysiology in the context of derangements in bony metabolism. Surgical treatment of such conditions necessitates special considerations and often an alteration in usual practices. In this chapter we discuss normal bone metabolism, followed by an overview of diseases associated with altered metabolism as it relates to our current understanding of disease pathophysiology.

ANATOMY

Bone is a specialized connective tissue with the unique ability to calcify, thus forming the skeleton. Bone performs three functions in humans:

1. Metabolic
2. Protective, for visceral organs
3. Supportive, providing mechanical support and an anchor for the attachment of muscles

There are two major compartments in the skeletal system of adult humans: cortical and cancellous (or trabecular) bone. Woven bone is a third type that consists of randomly placed coarse fibers that are structurally weaker than either cortical or cancellous bone. It is usually seen in premature bone during fetal life and in fracture healing.

Cortical Bone

Cortical bone accounts for approximately 80% of the total mass of the adult skeleton.[1] It provides strength and rigidity to the system, as well as structural integrity. The volumetric ratio of cortical to cancellous bone is roughly 4:1 anywhere in the body except for the spine, where it is 1:2.[2] The rate of cortical bone turnover has been determined to be approximately 3% per year.[1]

Osteon is the principal structure seen in cortical or compact bone (Fig. 280–1). It is the basis for the haversian system of arterioles, venules, capillaries, and lymphatics, which is necessary for the transport of nutrients to support the metabolic processes that take place within bone. A haversian canal measures about 300 μm in diameter and is 3 to 5 mm long.[3, 4] Haversian canals are interrupted by transversely oriented canals called Volkmann's canals. These transverse structures are necessary for communication with the medullary compartment of bone. Microscopically, thin cement lines separate osteons from one another. Between osteons are tightly packed concentric layers of lamellar bone. This pattern is the result of the rigidly linear arrangement of collagen laid down with bone matrix. This unique structure of cortical bone provides resistance to torsional loads.

Cancellous Bone

Cancellous, or trabecular, bone makes up 20% of the overall skeletal mass in adults[1] and contributes more than 60% of the bony structure in the spine.[2] Trabeculae are sheets of bone with multiple perforations that form struts. These struts are organized along the axis subject to the greatest mechanical forces (Fig. 280–2). Trabeculae are interconnected by horizontal struts that aid in providing resistance to compressive loads.

Trabecular bone has a fast turnover rate, estimated to be eight times faster than that of cortical bone.[1] It also has a very high surface area, which promotes

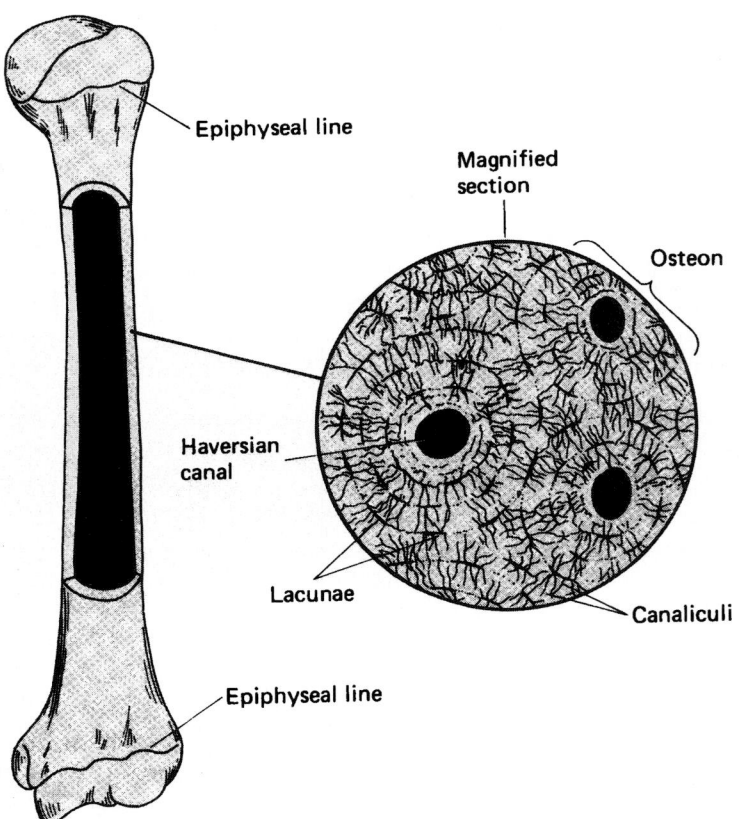

FIGURE 280–1. The structure of the bone. (From Guyton AC: Textbook of Medical Physiology. Philadelphia, WB Saunders, 1986.)

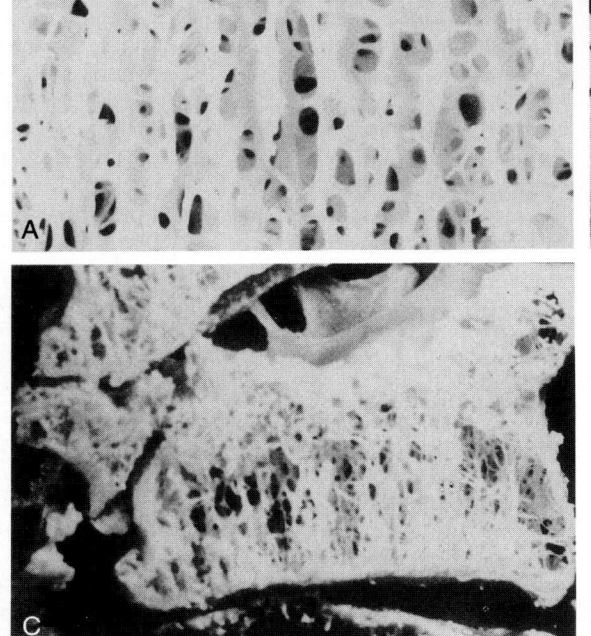

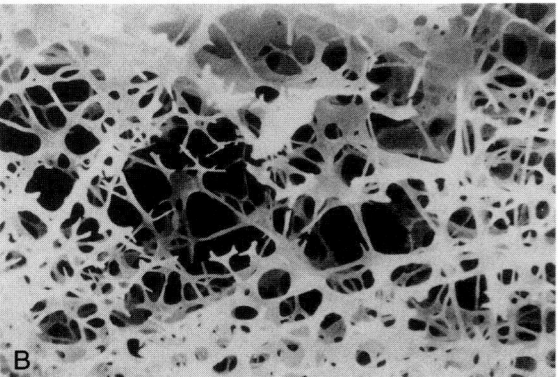

FIGURE 280–2. *A,* Microphotograph of the central portion of a normal T12 vertebral body demonstrating thick vertical trabeculae. Note the extensive interconnections of the horizontal cross-ties in relation to the vertical columns. *B,* Close-up view of the central portion of the T12 vertebral body from a 75-year-old osteoporotic woman. Note the loss of horizontal interconnections and the conversion of architectural components into thin trabecular spicules. *C,* Sagittal section of a T10 vertebra with a wedge compression fracture. Note the structural failure of the central portion of the body. (From Frymoyer JW: The Adult Spine: Principles and Practice, 2nd ed. Philadelphia, Lippincott-Raven, 1997.)

metabolic activity. This makes cancellous bone an important determinant of bone pathology and healing, especially in the spine, where cancellous bone is much more abundant.[5, 6]

HISTOLOGY OF BONE

The constituents of skeletal connective tissue are cells and matrix.

Cellular Structures

There are five major cell types seen in bone: osteoprogenitor, osteoblasts, osteoclasts, osteocytes, and bone lining cells.

Osteoprogenitor cells are preosteoblasts and preosteoclasts. Preosteoblasts arise from a stem cell line, and preosteoclasts are hematopoietic in origin. There is some evidence that differentiation of preosteoclasts to mature osteoclasts does not occur independent of the participation of osteoblasts.[7]

Osteoblasts are plump cuboid cells with large oval nuclei. They are responsible for the formation of bone and the calcification process,[1, 4] and they participate in regulating the movement of calcium and magnesium in and out of the cell. Structurally, osteoblasts are similar to any cell involved in the synthesis and secretion of protein substances. They secrete type I collagen, osteocalcin, osteonectin, growth factors, prostaglandins, collagenases, and tissue plasminogen activator.[8-10] Microscopically, osteoblasts contain large numbers of mitochondria, Golgi bodies, and rough endoplasmic reticulum. Externally, they express receptors for vitamin D and PTH, as well as estrogen.[11, 12] Presentation of these receptors allows the regulation of calcium, phosphorus, and magnesium within the extracellular and intracellular environment.[13, 14]

Osteoclasts develop from the granulocyte-macrophage line in the presence of osteoblasts.[1, 4, 6] These cells are responsible for the resorption of bone. They are large, highly polarized, multinucleated cells that exhibit a ruffled border and complex infolding within the cell membrane.[15] The ruffled border is essential to the resorptive function of osteoclasts, providing a large surface area for adherence. While active, these cells can be readily identified by their borders and a clear zone surrounding the cell.

Originally, it was thought that the osteoclast's multinucleated structure was the result of incomplete cleavage during cell development. However, studies have shown that these cells actually develop from fusion between developing cells. This action may be inhibited by calcitonin.[16]

Osteoclasts are responsible for the release of hydrogen ions (H$^+$) from the interface between cell and bone. This is done through the release of carbonic anhydrase via an adenosine triphosphatase (ATPase)–driven pump within the ruffled border.[15, 17] Hydrogen release causes a local decrease in pH, thereby facilitating degradation of the bony matrix at the leading edge and activating acid proteases that participate in this process as well.

Osteoclasts do not express receptors for vitamin D or PTH; thus, they do not respond directly to these substances. However, they do have receptors for direct interaction with interferon γ calcitonin, and colchicine (Fig. 280–3).

Osteocytes are the most abundant cells in the skeletal system, found within small lacunae in the osteon between concentric lamellae. They develop from osteoblasts. On microscopic examination, they exhibit few intracellular organelles and seem to participate in the maintenance and regulation of calcium and phosphorus within the cell and in the extracellular environment.[4, 6] Communication between osteocytes and osteoblasts takes place via long canals through which the cells are able to send long processes. It has been presumed that the fluid movement created in canaliculi and lacunae with loading is a physical signal to activate the cells to maintain strength and mass.[18-20]

Bone lining cells are flattened and elongated cells that line the edges of bone. They are presumed to participate in the regulation of calcium and phosphorus by controlling the movement of extracellular fluids across cell borders.

Bone Matrix

Osteoid, or bone matrix, is composed of organic and inorganic substances. The organic component is 90% type I collagen, along with noncollagenous substances and water. The inorganic portion contains 99% of the body's calcium stores in the form of hydroxyapatite crystals.[4, 6, 21-23] These crystals are composed mainly of calcium and phosphorus, with smaller contributions from magnesium and fluoride.[22, 24]

COLLAGEN

The human osteoblast synthesizes type I collagen, which provides the elastic stiffness property of bone.[25, 26] The strength of bone is largely dependent on the mineral content maintained within the collagen framework.[25] Collagen is secreted by the osteoblast as a pro-α-1 chain with a peptide attached, which prevents local aggregation from occurring until the substance is exported from the cell. Once exportation is complete, the peptide tail is removed, and the collagen molecules begin to line up end to end, forming a small gap junction at a point between lysine residues. These junctions serve as the basic structure for the initiation of mineral deposition.[24] There is a relationship between the onset of calcification of osteoid and the disappearance of calcium and phosphorus from the mitochondria of osteoblasts.

NONCOLLAGENOUS PROTEINS

The noncollagenous proteins account for 10% to 15% of total bone content. It is estimated that 50% of the protein-synthesizing activity of the osteoblast is related to the production of noncollagenous proteins.[4, 6, 22] Fol-

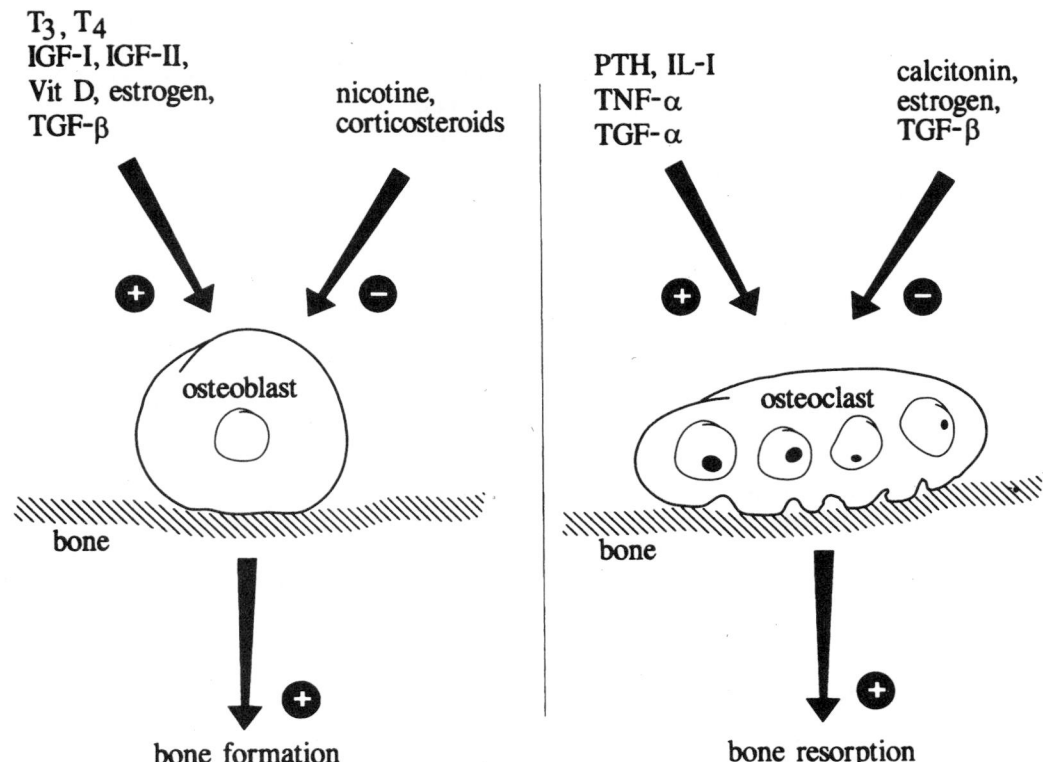

FIGURE 280–3. Control of osteoblast and osteoclast function. Stimulation of osteoblasts by thyroid hormone (T_3, T_4), insulin-like growth factor I (IGF-1), insulin-like growth factor II (IGF-II), vitamin D (Vit-D), estrogen, and transforming growth factor-β (TGF-β) leads to new bone formation. Nicotine and corticosteroids inhibit osteoblast function, decreasing the rate of new bone formation and promoting osteoporosis. Osteoclasts, which actively resorb bone, are stimulated by parathyroid hormone (PTH), interleukin-1 (IL-1), tumor necrosis factor-α (TNF-α), and transforming growth factor-α (TGF-α). Estrogen, calcitonin, and TGF-β inhibit osteoclast function, resulting in decreased bone resorption. (From Benzel EC, Stillerman CB: The Thoracic Spine. St Louis, Quality Medical Publishing, 1999.)

lowing are brief descriptions of some common protein subtypes.

Osteonectin, the most abundant noncollagenous protein in bone, has a high affinity for the binding of calcium and hydroxyapatite.[27] Although its exact function is unknown, it has been presumed that osteonectin plays a role in calcium regulation and bone resorption. Osteonectin is found in high concentrations in patients with prostate cancer.[28] This form of cancer is known to form destructive bony lesions, thereby reinforcing the idea that osteonectin is involved in the regulation of calcium and phosphorus. A sharp decline in osteonectin is associated with maturation of the osteoblast to the inactive osteocyte.[29]

Proteoglycans are presented in the bone in two main forms: chondroitin sulfate and heparan sulfate. Heparan sulfate is a facilitator of the interaction between osteoblasts and cell attachment proteins.[30]

Osteocalcin and matrix Gla protein are substances produced by osteogenic cells and are found only in bone and platelets. They are considered indicators of bone formation.[31] Matrix Gla protein is distributed throughout the system; osteocalcin is seen chiefly in mineralized bone. They are involved in structural re-

modeling activities that result from a chemotactic attraction between osteoclasts and osteocalcin. PTH is an inhibitor of osteocalcin.[6, 14]

Osteopontin is produced and secreted by osteoblasts and may also be a product of osteocytes and osteoclasts. It is an adhesion compound that acts as a substrate for osteoblasts and osteoclasts.[29] It is seen in the clear zone that develops between the ruffled border and leading edge of bone resorption. It is also found within the reverse lines that mark bone resorption sites. Within the cells, osteopontin interacts with integrins and steroid hormones.[14, 29, 32]

Bone sialoprotein is a glycoprotein found in bone, dentin, and hypertrophic cartilage. It binds to integrins within the cell. The function of bone sialoprotein is not clear.

Decorin and biglycan are noncollagenous substances that are seen in small amounts in bone matrix. Decorin is attached to a single chondroitin sulfate chain, and biglycan is attached to two such chains.[33] Biglycan is seen in the fetus and in newly developed woven bone and is characteristically found in the pericellular fluid. Decorin is widely distributed throughout the extracellular fluid and is seen in all stages of bone growth and development. These substances share a common ancestry but develop along divergent pathways.[33]

CALCIUM, MAGNESIUM, AND PHOSPHORUS

Ninety-nine percent of all the body's calcium, about 1000 g, is stored as hydroxyapatite crystals in the bone; the other 1% is found in the extracellular fluid and soft tissues.[24, 34] The major role of calcium within bone is to provide the basis for structural integrity and to maintain and regulate many important metabolic processes.[22]

Calcium occurs in three forms in serum: protein bound (40%), complexed with phosphate (10%), and ionized. The ionized fraction of calcium is maintained with both PTH and vitamin D, in conjunction with other less well represented substances.[14] The calcium fraction in skeletal stores is kept in the mitochondrial granules and matrix vesicles for release and integration into the dynamic remodeling and mineralization processes that take place on a continuous basis.[4, 6]

Phosphorus is an integral component of the hydroxyapatite crystal and is also partially responsible for maintenance of the structural integrity of the skeleton. Like calcium, phosphorus exists in three forms: ionized, protein bound, and complexed with sodium, calcium, and magnesium.[14] Bone remodeling causes phosphate to become available for formation and therefore contributes to phosphorus homeostasis. The ionized fraction of phosphate assists in the accumulation of minerals within the matrix and therefore plays a role in bone assimilation.

Magnesium is present mainly as part of the hydroxyapatite crystal, but in significantly lower volumes than calcium and phosphorus. Unlike the latter two minerals, magnesium is found on the surface of the crystal. Its function in metabolic processes may relate to its key role in enzymatic mediations similar to those required for the mobilization of calcium and phosphorus.

METABOLISM OF BONE

Bone remodeling is a process of both formation and resorption. It is regulated by local and systemic hormones and substances that affect recruitment, differentiation of cells, and replication to maintain mineral homeostasis and mechanical integrity of the skeleton.[6, 14, 23]

Bone formation is coupled with bone resorption. Pockets of resorption and formation may be considered the bone multicellular unit, which includes all the cells involved in the remodeling process.

There are four phases of bone remodeling to consider.[35] First, resting cells are activated to differentiate from osteoclastic stem cells to mature osteoclasts. In the resorptive phase, osteoclasts previously recruited form tight attachments to the bone surfaces to be resorbed. This is necessary to avoid loss of protons from the resorptive surface, which decreases the acidic environment required for this process. Hydroxyapatite

crystals of calcium and phosphorus are made soluble by the introduction of intracellular vacuoles, which release their acidic contents near the ruffled border. Some sources suggest that this process can be enhanced through the use of an ATPase proton pump of the ruffled border.[15, 17, 36]

The process of reversal is an interim process that connects the 1- to 2-week period between resorption and formation of bone. During this period, the lacunae are covered by a cement-like substance that forms the basis for the cement lines seen between osteons. At any time, approximately 15% of all osteoblasts are active, 20% are in transition from active to inactive forms, and 65% are at termination.[37–39]

The final step in bone turnover is formation (Fig. 280–4). During this phase, preosteoblasts are activated and begin migration to the lacunae and deposition of bone matrix. It usually takes about 10 days for newly laid down bone matrix to mineralize.

As discussed, multiple local and systemic hormones affect differentiation, replication, and recruitment of cells to regulate bone remodeling. Some of these substances are involved in both formation and resorption; others have specific actions (see Fig. 280–3).

Parathyroid Hormone

PTH and vitamin D are the principal regulators of calcium homeostasis.[4, 6, 14] PTH is an 84–amino acid peptide chain that is secreted by the chief cells of the

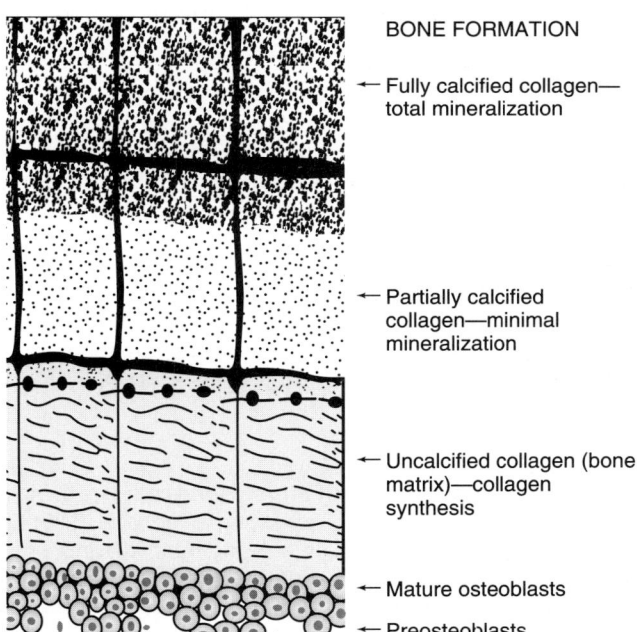

FIGURE 280–4. The process of bone formation. (1) Synthesis of collagen and its elaboration into the extracellular space to undergo maturation. (2) After maturation, the new collagen serves as the site of mineral nucleation. (3) After nucleation, mineralization proceeds rapidly at first; total mineralization is completed more slowly. (Modified from Krane SM: Calcium, phosphate and magnesium. In International Encyclopedia of Pharmacology and Therapeutics, sec 51, vol 1.)

parathyroid gland in response to decreased ionized calcium levels in serum. It also induces calcium reabsorption from the distal tubule of the kidney, whereas phosphate reabsorption in the proximal tubule is inhibited. In persons with renal failure, PTH action is affected because the kidney is unable to perform these functions as required.

PTH enhances osteoclastic activity and stimulates osteoclast progenitors; in addition, it activates mature osteoclasts indirectly by activating osteoblasts (see Fig. 280–3).[40] This causes an increase in osteoclast cell size and in their ruffled border surface area. The end result is a linear increase in bone resorption. PTH-related protein has an identical effect on these cells.

In the gut, one can see the indirect effect of PTH through the stimulation of 1,25-vitamin D.[41] There is a feedback effect on calcium that implicates both the kidney and the gut, owing to calcium-sensitive receptors on the parathyroid cells. These G protein–coupled receptors cause activation of phospholipase C and a resultant increase in phosphoinositol 3. The end result of this feedback system is the release of calcium into the system.

Whereas PTH causes calcium to mobilize from bone, it causes a transient decrease in serum calcium by improving bony uptake. The basis for this action is not clear.

Severe hypomagnesemia and hypocalcemia, either acute or chronic, may adversely affect the release of PTH. Acute hypocalcemia causes an increase in PTH release, whereas the chronic state causes the system to sense a continuous need for PTH, resulting in hyperplastic overdevelopment of the parathyroid gland.

Calcitonin

Calcitonin is released by the parafollicular cells of the thyroid gland and inhibits the resorptive activities of osteoclasts and the stabilization of calcium in bone matrix.[14, 23] The inhibition is dose dependent and direct.[38, 39]

Prolonged administration of calcitonin results in down-regulation of messenger RNA in the receptors; hence, the osteoclasts become refractory to treatment.[16] An increase in cyclic adenosine monophosphate may be the basis for this action.

Vitamin D

Vitamin D is a steroid derivative produced in an inactive form in the skin[11] or ingested in the diet. Its primary function is to stimulate bone resorption.[13, 42, 43] The biologically active form of vitamin D is the result of two hydroxylations. In the liver, inactive vitamin D is hydroxylated to become the hormone precursor of vitamin D, 25(OH)-vitamin D. This circulating, plasma-bound form of the vitamin travels to the kidney and undergoes a second hydroxylation to produce its active form, 1,25-dihydroxyvitamin D.[14, 41]

Vitamin D production may be improved in a hypocalcemic environment, and production is diminished in the presence of increased levels of phosphorus (Table

TABLE 280–1 ■ **Physiologic Factors Affecting the Vitamin D Activation Rate**

Increased Activation	Decreased Activation
Hypocalcemia	Hypercalcemia
Parathyroid hormone and hypocalcemia	Parathyroid hormone and hypercalcemia
Calcitonin	Hyperphosphatemia
Growth hormone	Vitamin D (feedback mechanism)
Prolactin	

280–1). In the presence of hypercalcemia, PTH diminishes the stimulatory effect of vitamin D on resorption. Additionally, vitamin D is affected by growth hormone, prolactin, calcitonin, and the substance itself.

In the bone, vitamin D works to stimulate bone resorption and remodeling,[9, 44] thereby mobilizing calcium from intracellular stores. This is a PTH-mediated effect on the bone to replenish calcium stores in times of decreased dietary intake.[4, 6, 13, 43] In elderly adults, the combination of hypovitaminosis and decreased dietary calcium intake may lead to chronic increases in PTH.[45]

Osteoblasts have both PTH and vitamin D receptors that allow direct activation of the cell with these substances. The effect on osteoclasts is, as mentioned previously, indirect and influenced by the activity and presence of osteoblasts.

Estrogen and Androgen

Both osteoblasts and osteoclasts carry special receptors for sex hormones.[46] The exact role of human sex hormones in bone maintenance and bone metabolism is still unclear.[47] Recent studies, however, suggest that estradiol stimulates osteoblast cell proliferation and bone matrix synthesis.[48] The hormone diffuses into the cells and interacts with cellular receptors. The receptor complexes then migrate to the nucleus and bind to DNA to activate the gene.[49] This, in turn, increases the efficacy of the cell receptor through nitric oxide and cyclic adenosine monophosphate second messengers.[50]

Estrogen influences calcium homeostasis. In postmenopausal women, aromatization of androgens to estradiol is the principal source of estrogen. Lack of circulating estrogen in this population affects calcium balance.[51] This, combined with decreased oral intake, causes a significant decline in calcium storage and a remarkable loss of bone mass after menopause. The accelerated loss of bone mass at the time of menopause is often attributed solely to ovarian failure. However, in premenopausal women, urinary excretion of calcium is kept to a minimum, while calcium absorption is enhanced. This way, calcium balance is maintained, and bone loss is inhibited.

Estrogen influences osteoclast activity, inhibiting bone resorption through certain cytokines and thus affecting the bone remodeling process.[52] It also activates transforming growth factor-β and enhances bone osteoblastic activity, increasing collagen synthesis and decreasing the differentiation of osteoclasts (see Fig. 280–3).[45, 50]

Men typically exhibit greater bone mass and less osteoporotic change than do women of the same age. The role of androgens in this process is suggested by studies such as that done by Vandershueren and coworkers, who reported that androgen-resistant male rats that were orchiectomized did not achieve normal adult trabecular bone volume. They also reported three men with estrogen or P450 aromatase gene defects who were all tall and eunuchoid and displayed low bone density. Once estrogen hormonal therapy was instituted, they demonstrated a significant increase in bone density.

Finkelstein and colleagues also reported on men with hypogonadism who demonstrated open epiphyseal plates.[53, 54] After treatment, bone mineral density increased 13% in 2 years, whereas those with closed epiphyseal plates showed no change.

These studies strongly suggest that the role of androgen in bone metabolism is to provide a substance for aromatization to estrogen, and that estrogen is the principal hormone required.

Steroid Hormones

In 1912, Cushing described a patient with adrenal hyperplasia and decalcification of bone.[55] This revelation prompted scientific inquiry into the role of steroids in bone metabolism.

Today, it is believed that glucocorticoids suppress osteoblast function and inhibit calcium absorption in the intestine. Glucocorticoid therapy is associated with osteopenia and is a risk factor for bone loss, not only through its direct effect on calcium and osteoblast activity but also through enhanced calcium secretion by the kidneys. The effect of glucocorticoids on the intestinal reabsorption of calcium was first thought to be caused by a defect in the transformation of vitamin D to its active form. However, it is now believed that decreased calcium absorption is a direct effect of glucocorticoids on intestinal mucosal cells.[56, 57] A daily dose of as little as 7.5 mg of prednisone is associated with significant bone loss, particularly trabecular bone.[58, 59] In postmenopausal women, the dose required for this effect is even smaller. This may be related to the cumulative effect of many physiologic changes related to menopause.

Crofton and associates showed that premature infants who are treated for bronchopulmonary dysplasia have a decrease in type I collagen peptides, which are necessary for bone development.[60] These infants also demonstrate aggravated weight loss and shrinkage of the lower extremities that improves after treatment is stopped.

Butler and coworkers demonstrated a decrease in bone mineral content in men and postmenopausal women with rheumatoid arthritis.[31] There was an increase in fractures in the steroid-treated population. They concluded that low-dose steroids increase the risk of fracture and bone loss in this population.

Finally, Adinoff and Hollister reported, in a study of 128 patients with asthma receiving steroid therapy for longer than 1 year, a greater number of fractures in the treated versus the not-treated group.[61]

Insulin

Insulin, produced in the beta cells of the pancreas, increases the synthesis of bone matrix. It is essential to normal bone mineralization. Patients with untreated diabetes therefore have abnormal bone mineralization.

Insulin causes an increased synthesis of insulin-like growth factor I in the liver. Whereas insulin increases the process of bone mineral synthesis, insulin-like growth factor I actually causes an increase in the number of cells involved in the process.[8]

Bisphosphonates

Bisphosphonates are pyrophosphonates with several different substitutions that increase the potency and reduce the degradation of various compounds. When tightly adherent to hydroxyapatite, bone becomes resistant to endogenous phosphatase activity, which inhibits remodeling by osteoclasts.[62–64]

Bisphosphonates have been successfully used to reduce bone loss in patients with metabolic bone diseases such as Paget's disease, as well as in paraplegics and those taking long-term supraphysiologic doses of steroids.[65, 66]

Other studies have demonstrated the successful use of etidronate in postmenopausal women, showing an improvement in bone mineral density and a reduction in vertebral fractures.[67–70] More recently, attention has been focused on alendronate (Fosamax), the only bisphosphonate approved by the Food and Drug Administration for the treatment of postmenopausal osteoporosis. Liberman and colleagues conducted a study on 994 postmenopausal women with osteoporosis who received alendronate 10 mg daily for 3 years.[71] They found that bone mineral density increased (compared with the placebo group) 8.8% in the spine, 5.9% in the femoral neck, 7.8% in the trochanter, and 2.5% in the total body. The study also showed a 48% reduction in new vertebral fractures and a reduction in the progression of vertebral deformities in the treatment group. The drug was well tolerated, although there was an increased incidence of serious gastrointestinal bleeding in about 34 of 450,000 patients. The exact role of alendronate has yet to be established.

FACTORS AFFECTING BONE HEALTH

Smoking

Studies have shown that individuals who are currently smoking have bone mineral density 1% to 3% lower than those who are not smoking.[72–76] The number of pack-years of smoking is a significant factor and a predictor of baseline bone mineral density.

Bernard showed that smokers, who tend to go through menopause slightly earlier than those who do not smoke, have a 50% faster overall loss of cortical bone than their nonsmoking counterparts.[77] In another study of women with osteoporosis and a first fracture before age 65, there was a clear association between the early onset of osteoporosis and postmenopausal cigarette consumption. In this study, lack of obesity was an additional risk factor.

In studies of postmenopausal bone mineral density, smokers tended to be younger, generally consumed less calcium, and had a higher alcohol intake.[78] A by-product of the Framingham Heart Study was to confirm that tobacco consumption was a significant factor in the overall effect on bone mineral density in this population.[78]

The mechanism of action of smoking and its by-products on bone health is not completely understood. However, it is proposed that smoking may cause subtle changes in local pH. This may occur as a result of changes associated with chronic respiratory disease or changes in PO_2 associated with increased lactic acid. Osteoclastic activity is reliant on an acidic environment. It may be that the amount of carbon monoxide in the bloodstream of chronic smokers reaches toxic levels and interferes with vital processes.

Alcohol Consumption

The long-term effects of chronic alcohol intake include osteopenia and an increase in bone loss in postmenopausal women and elderly men. Studies have demonstrated that alcohol is associated with decreased bone mass, particularly trabecular bone.[79]

Laitinen and coworkers suggested that acute and chronic alcohol ingestion may have an effect on bone health.[80–82] Acute alcohol intoxication may induce a transient hypoparathyroidism, with subsequent decreases in serum calcium and increases in serum magnesium. These minerals may be excreted in large quantities in urine as a result.

Chronic drinkers can be expected to have low vitamin D levels from both deficient diets and lack of exposure to direct sunlight. It is also likely that there is some malabsorption of vitamin D, decreased metabolism secondary to liver or biliary disease, or decreased reserves.[80, 81, 83]

Data on the effect of "moderate social drinking" on bone mineralization are conflicting. In a 15-year, prospective study of 449 upper-middle-class men and women, Holbrook and Barrett-Connor found that moderate social drinking correlated with increased bone mineral density.[84] This effect has been attributed to increased estrogen available from enhanced production of its adrenal precursor androstenedione.[85, 86] In contrast, Laitinen and associates demonstrated that social drinking involving a moderate intake of alcohol is not without some short-term effects.[83] There was an increase in PTH secretion in these patients. Additionally, they exhibited a 30% decrease in osteocalcin with alcohol intake.

In summary, although there is clear evidence in the literature that chronic alcohol consumption has a deleterious effect on bone mineralization, the effect of alcohol in small doses has not been fully established.

Caffeine

The effect of caffeine on bone density is also in dispute. Some studies suggested that caffeine induces a net urinary loss of calcium, resulting in a negative calcium balance in humans.[87]

Daniell showed that the association between high caffeine consumption and osteoporosis does not persist after correction for weight and smoking.[88] Holbrook and associates were unable to demonstrate a statistically significant association between high caffeine consumption and hip fractures in women.[89]

Kiel and coworkers evaluated 3170 patients as part of the Framingham study and demonstrated a strong association between high caffeine consumption (more than 22.5 cups of coffee per day) and hip fracture; lower caffeine consumption failed to demonstrate such a relationship.[90]

Based on these studies, it appears that moderate consumption of caffeine is unlikely to have a strong correlation with the development of osteoporosis, whereas higher levels of consumption may present an increased risk.

Exercise

Numerous studies have demonstrated that intense activity is associated with increased bone mass[91–98] unless calcium availability is restricted.[61]

Krolner and Toft studied loss of bone mineral density in 34 patients confined to bed rest for the treatment of low back pain.[93] They demonstrated a 0.9% loss of bone mineral density per week, which returned nearly to normal after 4 months of reambulation.

Marcus and colleagues found a significant reduction in bone mass in the spines of amenorrheic long-distance runners compared with age-matched nonrunner controls and menstruating long-distance runners.[100] The amenorrheic runners suffered increased stress-related fractures. When regular menses resumed, the previously amenorrheic women regained their lost bone density.

Dalsky and coworkers studied the effect of an active exercise program, including jogging and stair climbing, in postmenopausal women who received calcium supplementation to bring their total daily consumption to 1500 mg/day.[62] They found that the women's bone mineral density increased 5.2% after 9 months of training and 6.1% after 22 months. In contrast, there was a 1.4% loss of bone mineral density in the control group receiving calcium but not exercising. However, physically inactive time, such as hours spent watching television, did not negatively impact healthy children,[101] suggesting that aging necessarily results in consistent bone loss—a process that may be delayed by an active exercise program.

Body Weight

The PEPI trial[102] demonstrated less loss of bone mineral density in postmenopausal women with high body mass indexes (1.4% over 3 years) than in those with low body mass indexes (4.7% over 3 years). This may be related to the role of adipose tissue in maintaining higher estrogen levels.

CLINICAL CONDITIONS OF ALTERED BONE METABOLISM

Osteoporosis

Osteoporosis, the most prevalent metabolic bone disease,[42, 54] is estimated to affect 25 million Americans. It is a state characterized by abnormally low bone mass and architectural changes resulting in bone weakness and ultimately bone failure.

There are two types of involutional osteoporosis: postmenopausal (type I) and age related (type II).[103, 104] Postmenopausal osteoporosis involves predominantly cancellous bone and is typified by increased activity of osteoclasts deprived of the suppressive influence of estrogen[105, 106]; osteoblastic activity is near normal. Age-related osteoporosis occurs in older age groups and is almost evenly distributed between males and females. It is typified by reduced osteoblastic activity with near-normal osteoclasts.

As mentioned earlier, cancellous bone is composed of a meshwork of vertical trabecular struts, each of which is 200 µm thick, supported by thinner horizontal struts measuring 180 µm (see Fig. 280–2A). After menopause, osteoclastic disinhibition increases trabecular bone resorption and hence perforation proportional to the struts' thinness (see Fig. 280–2B). As more and more horizontal struts are perforated, the vertical struts begin to fail by buckling.[107] In addition, age-related thinness of the end plates reduces the vertebral load-carrying capacity by more than 10 times that of mature lumbar vertebrae. This makes osteoporotic vertebrae vulnerable to failure with physiologic loads (see Fig. 280–2C).

Steroid-Induced Osteoporosis

Prolonged exposure to high-dose endogenous or exogenous steroids results in significant loss of bone density.[108, 109] Loss of bone mineral density is more pronounced in the trabecular bone of the vertebrae than in bones with significant cortical content, such as the femur.[58, 59] When steroid excess is resolved, bone mineral density apparently returns to near normal.

A prospective study analyzed bone mineral density in the lumbar spine before, during, and after a 2-year period of steroid treatment and demonstrated a 15% loss of bone mineral density while on steroids. This returned to baseline 16.7 months after steroid use was discontinued.[110]

Multiple factors seem to interact to induce osteoporosis in steroid-treated patients. Steroids may decrease the proliferative function of osteoblasts[111] and increase the activity of osteoclasts, thus disturbing the balance of bone remodeling in favor of thinning of the trabeculae. Other factors include diminished intestinal absorption of calcium,[112] suppression of testosterone[113] and

circulating calcitonin, and indirect modulation of numerous cytokines and growth factors.[56, 114]

Paget's Disease

Paget's disease is a local disorder of bone remodeling that is usually asymptomatic and often does not come to medical attention. There is a higher incidence of Paget's disease in persons of northern European, North American, Australian, or New Zealand ancestry. The greatest incidence of Paget's disease occurs in Lancashire, England, where 6.3% to 8.3% of the population aged 55 and older has Paget's disease by radiograph.[115] The disease is rare in those younger than 25 years.

The cause of Paget's disease is not currently known. However, there is some evidence that it may be genetic, at least in part. Fifteen percent to 30% of patients with Paget's disease have a positive family history. There is a sevenfold increased incidence of the disease in those who have a first-degree relative with the disease. Recently, there have been reports that Paget's disease may be viral in origin.

Microscopic examination of osteoclasts in patients with Paget's disease demonstrates inclusion bodies that are similar to paramyxoviruses. Osteoclasts in Paget's disease are abnormal, and increased resorption of bone, coupled with accelerated formation, is the hallmark of the disease on a cellular level. Bone matrix becomes more random, with abnormal collagen patterns. The bone marrow exhibits an increase in connective tissue and blood vessels. As a result of increased resorption, there is an increase in the urinary excretion of hydroxyproline, a by-product of breakdown, and alkaline phosphatase. The rate of increase in these two by-products of bone metabolism is a measure of the extent and severity of the disease. An alkaline phosphatase level greater than 10 times normal is often an indicator of disease in the skull plus one other site, such as the femur, spine, or tibia.

Although most patients are asymptomatic, the most common presenting sign is bone pain. Radiographic studies show cortical thickening, coarsening of the trabecular markings, and lytic or sclerotic lesions. The area is often warm and tender, with obvious deformity and loss of range of motion, such as in the extremities, as a result of arthritic changes.

Treatment is aimed at the suppression of osteoclastic activity. Subcutaneous administration of human and salmon calcitonin may accomplish this. Salmon calcitonin is approximately 10 to 40 times more potent than that derived from human sources. Additional therapies may include bisphosphonate compounds such as etidronate, alendronate (which may be given orally),[116] and pamidronate; mithramycin; or bafilomycin, an osteoclast proton transport inhiibitor.[117]

Osteomalacia

Osteomalacia is a clinical condition consisting of soft bone that exhibits a failure to mineralize.[118, 119] This is now a rare condition and is seen most often in patients with renal disease or those who have intestinal malabsorption of calcium and vitamin D as a result of dietary restrictions or surgical procedures. Vegetarians who eschew milk and dairy products are particularly prone.

Osteomalacia is also associated with phosphate deficiency. This may be due to pharmacologic interventions, intestinal malabsorption, dietary deficiency, or failure of the renal tubular reabsorption of phosphate. Osteomalacia may also be associated with tumor toxins that cause phosphate wasting, such as in hemangiopericytoma, angiosarcoma, or hemangioma.[120]

Radiographic studies are remarkable for "milkman's lines." These are translucent areas running perpendicular to the long axis of bone and represent pseudofractures.

Treatment is typically replacement of vitamin D. The dose may range from 2000 to 200,000 U/day in patients with malabsorption.

CONCLUSION

A thorough understanding of normal bone metabolism and its disorders is paramount for the successful treatment of spinal abnormalities and fractures. Surgical treatment of patients with altered bone metabolism necessitates a complete understanding of the biochemical background of such disorders. The last decade has witnessed a great advance in our understanding of the biochemistry of bone disorders, which has led to more successful treatment outcomes.

REFERENCES

1. Einhorn TA.: Osteoporosis and metabolic bone disease. Adv Ortop Surg 8:175–184, 1984.
2. Hansson T, Roos B, Nachemson A: The bone mineral content and ultimate compressive strength of lumber vertebrae. Spine 5:46–55, 1980.
3. Prolo DJ: Biology of bone fusion. Clin Neurosurg 36:135–146, 1990.
4. Silver JJ, Majeska RJ, Einhorn TA: An update of bone cell biology. Curr Opin Orthop 1995.
5. McBroom RJ, Hayess WC, Goldbeerg RP, et al: Prediction of vertebral body fracture using quantitative computed tomography. J Bone Joint Surg Am 67:1206–1214, 1985.
6. Einhorn TA: Bone metabolism and metabolic bone disease. In Frymoyer JW (ed): Orthopedic Knowledge Update 4: Home Study Syllabus. Park Ridge, IL, American Academy of Orthopedic Surgeons, 1993, pp 69–88.
7. Masri L, Beneventi S, Tanini A, Brandi ML: Local regulation of bone metabolism. In McCarthy ID, Hughes SP (eds): Sciences Basic to Orthopaedics. London, WB Saunders, 1998, pp 28–32.
8. Gori F, Hofbauer LC, Conover CA, et al: Effects of androgens on the insulin-like growth factor system in an androgen-responsive human osteoblastic cell line. Endocrinology 140:5579–5586, 1999.
9. Hofbauer LC, Dunstan CR, Spelsberg TC, et al: Osteoprotegerin production by human osteoblast lineage cells is stimulated by vitamin D, bone morphogenetic protein-2, and cytokines. Biochem Biophys Res Commun 250:776–781, 1998.
10. Hofbauer LC, Lacey DL, Dunstan CR, et al: Interleukin-1-beta and tumor necrosis factor-alpha, but not interleukin-6, stimulate osteoprotegerin ligand gene expression in human osteoblastic cells. Bone 25:255–259, 1999.
11. Zerwekh JE, Reed BY, Heller HJ, et al: Normal vitamin D receptor concentration and responsiveness to 1, 25-dihydroxyvitamin D3 in skin fibroblasts from patients with absorptive hypercalciuria. Miner Electrolyte Metab 24:307–313, 1998.
12. Zerwekh JE, Hughes MR, Reed BY, et al: Evidence for normal

vitamin D receptor messenger ribonucleic acid and genotype in absorptive hypercalciuria. J Clin Endocrinol Metab 80:2960–2965, 1995.
13. Zerwekh JE: Vitamin D–dependent intestinal calcium absorption. Gastroenterology 76:404–411, 1979.
14. Norman AW, Roth J, Oric L: The vitamin D endocrine system: Steroid metabolism, hormone receptors and biology response. Endocr Rev 3:331–366, 1982.
15. Mattsson JP, Skyman C, Palokangas H, et al: Characterization and cellular distribution of the osteoclast ruffled membrane vacuolar H$^+$-ATPase B-subunit using isoform-specific antibodies. J Bone Miner Res 12:753–760, 1997.
16. Takahashi S, Goldring S, Katz M, et al: Downregulation of calcitonin receptor mRNA expression by calcitonin during human osteoclast-like cell differentiation. J Clin Invest 95:167–171, 1995.
17. Vaananen HK, Karhukorpi EK, Sundquist K, et al: Evidence for the presence of a proton pump of the vacuolar H(+)-ATPase type in the ruffled borders of osteoclasts. J Cell Biol 111:1305–1311, 1990.
18. Burger EH, Klein-Nulend J: Mechanotransduction in bone—role of the lacuno-canalicular network. FASEB J 13(Suppl):S101–S112, 1999.
19. Burger EH, Klein-Nulend J, van der Plas A, et al: Function of osteocytes in bone—their role in mechanotransduction. J Nutr 125(7 Suppl):2020S–2023S, 1995.
20. Burger EH, Klein-Nulend J, Veldhuijzen JP: Modulation of osteogenesis in fetal bone rudiments by mechanical stress in vitro. J Biomech 24(Suppl 1):101–109, 1991.
21. Vaes G: Cellular biology and biochemical mechanism of bone resorption: A review of recent development on the formation, activation, and mode of action of osteoclasts. Clin Orthop 231:239–271, 1988.
22. Boskey AL: Noncollagenous matrix proteins and their role in mineralization. Bone Miner 6:111–123, 1989.
23. Hurley DL, Tiegs RD, Wahneer HW, et al: Axial and appendicular bone mineral density in patients with long-term deficiency or excess of calcitonin. N Engl J Med 317:537–541, 1987.
24. In Hughes SP, McCarthy ID (eds): Sciences Basic to Orthopaedics. London, WB Saunders, 1998.
25. Burnstein A, Zilka HM, Eiple KG, et al: Contributions of collagen and mineral to the elastic properties of bone. J Bone Joint Surg Am 57:956–961, 1975.
26. Hall JC, Einhorn TA: Metabolic bone disease of the adult spine. In Frymoyer J (ed): The Adult Spine: Principles and Practice, 2nd ed. Philadelphia, Lippincott-Raven, 1997, pp 783–800.
27. Termine JD, Kleinman HK, Whitson SW, et al: Osteonectin, a bone-specific protein linking mineral to collagen. Cell 26(1 Pt 1):99–105, 1981.
28. Thomas R, True LD, Bassuk JA, et al: Differential expression of osteonectin/SPARC during human prostate cancer progression. Clin Cancer Res 6:1140–1149, 2000.
29. Riminucci M, Fisher LW, Shenker A, et al: Fibrous dysplasia of bone in the McCune-Albright syndrome: Abnormalities in bone formation. Am J Pathol 151:1587–1600, 1997.
30. Beresford JN, Fedarko NS, Fisher LW, et al: Analysis of the proteoglycans synthesized by human bone cells in vitro. J Biol Chem 262:17164–17172, 1987.
31. Butler RC, Davie MW, Worsfold M, et al: Bone mineral content in patients with rheumatoid arthritis: Relationship to low-dose steroid therapy. Br J Rheumatol 30:86–90, 1991.
32. Cheng SL, Lai CF, Fausto A, et al: Regulation of alphaVbeta3 and alphaVbeta5 integrins by dexamethasone in normal human osteoblastic cells. J Cell Biochem 77:265–276, 2000.
33. Bianco P, Fisher LW, Young MF, et al: Expression and localization of the two small proteoglycans biglycan and decorin in developing human skeletal and non-skeletal tissues. J Histochem Cytochem 38:1549–1563, 1990.
34. Krane SM: Calcium, phosphate and magnesium. In International Encyclopedia of Pharmacology and Therapeutics, sec 51, vol 1. pp 19–61.
35. Laitala-Leinonen T, Howell ML, Dean GE, et al: Resorption-cycle-dependent polarization of mRNAs for different subunits of V-ATPase in bone-resorbing osteoclasts. Mol Biol Cell 7:129–142, 1996.

36. Laitala-Leinonen T, Lowik C, Papapoulos S, et al: Inhibition of intravacuolar acidification by antisense RNA decreases osteoclast differentiation and bone resorption in vitro. J Cell Sci 112(Pt 21):3657–3666, 1999.

37. Klein-Nulend J, Veldhuijzen JP, de Jong M, et al: Increased bone formation and decreased bone resorption in fetal mouse calvaria as a result of intermittent compressive force in vitro. Bone Mineral 2:441–448, 1987.

38. Wallach S, Farley JR, Baylink DJ, et al: Effects of calcitonin on bone quality and osteoblastic function. Calcif Tissue Int 52: 335–339, 1993.

39. Farley JR, Tarbaux NM, Hall SL, et al: The anti-bone-resorptive agent calcitonin also acts in vitro to directly increase bone formation and bone cell proliferation. Endocrinology 123:159–167, 1988.

40. Finkelstein JS, Klibanski A, Schaefer EH, et al: Parathyroid hormone for the prevention of bone loss induced by estrogen deficiency. N Engl J Med 331:1618–1623, 1994.

41. Deluca HL: Vitamin D. In International Encyclopedia of Pharmacology and Therapeutics, sec 51, vol 1. 1970, pp 101–197.

42. Zerwekh JE, Marks SC Jr, McGuire JL: Elevated serum 1,25-dihydroxyvitamin D in osteopetrotic mutations in three species. Bone Mineral 2:193–199, 1987.

43. Breslau NA, McGuire JL, Zerwekh JE, et al: The role of dietary sodium on renal excretion and intestinal absorption of calcium and on vitamin D metabolism. J Clin Endocrinol Metab 55: 369–373, 1982.

44. Dawson-Hughes B, Harris SS, Krall EA, et al: Effect of calcium and vitamin D supplementation on bone density in men and women 65 years of age or older. N Engl J Med 337:670–676, 1997.

45. Hansen MA, Overgaard K, Riis BJ, Christiansen C: Potential risk factors for development of postmenopausal osteoporosis—examined over a 12-year period. Osteoporos Int 1:95–102, 1991.

46. Barger-Lux MJ, Heaney RP, Stegman MR: Effects of moderate caffeine intake on the calcium economy of premenopausal women. Am J Clin Nutr 52:722–725, 1990.

47. Hofbauer LC, Hicok KC, Khosla S: Effects of gonadal and adrenal androgens in a novel androgen-responsive human osteoblastic cell line. J Cell Biochem 71:96–108, 1998.

48. Fleisch HG, Francis RRG: Diphosphonates inhibit hydroxyapatite dissolution in vitro and bone resorption in tissue culture and in vivo. Science 1675:1262–1264, 1969.

49. Hofbauer LC, Khosla S, Dunstan CR, et al: Estrogen stimulates gene expression and protein production of osteoprotegerin in human osteoblastic cells. Endocrinology 140:4367–4370, 1999.

50. Gutin B, Kasper MJ: Can vigorous exercise play a role in osteoporosis prevention? A review. Osteoporos Int 2:55–69, 1992.

51. Krall EA, Dawson-Hughes B, Hirst K, et al: Bone mineral density and biochemical markers of bone turnover in healthy elderly men and women. J Gerontol A Biol Sci Med Sci 52: M61–M67, 1997.

52. Hofbauer LC, Khosla S, Dunstan CR, et al: The roles of osteoprotegerin and osteoprotegerin ligand in the paracrine regulation of bone resorption. J Bone Miner Res 15:2–12, 2000.

53. Finkelstein JS, Klibanski A, Neer RM, et al: Increases in bone density during treatment of men with idiopathic hypogonadotropic hypogonadism. J Clin Endocrinol Metab 69:776–783, 1989.

54. Finkelstein JS, Klibanski A, Neer RM, et al: Osteoporosis in men with idiopathic hypogonadotropic hypogonadism. Ann Intern Med 106:354–361, 1987.

55. Cushing H: The Pituitary Body and Its Disorders: Clinical States Produced by Disorders of the Hypophysis Cerebri. Philadelphia, JB Lippincott, 1912.

56. Hahn TJ, Halstead LR, Teitelbaum SL, et al: Altered mineral metabolism in glucocorticoid-induced osteopenia: Effect of 25-hydroxyvitamin D administration. J Clin Invest 64:655–665, 1979.

57. Hahn TJ, Halstead LR, Baran DT: Effects of short term glucocorticoid administration on intestinal calcium absorption and circulating vitamin D metabolite concentrations in man. J Clin Endocrinol Metab 52:111–115, 1977.

58. Reid IR, Heap SW: Determinants of vertebral mineral density in patients receiving long-term glucocorticoid therapy. Arch Intern Med 150:2545–2548, 1990.

59. Rizzato G, Montemurro L: The reversibility of exogenous corticosteroid-induced osteoporosis [abstract]. Bone Miner Res 17(Suppl 1):141, 1992.

60. Crofton PM, Stirling HF, Schonau E, et al: Biochemical markers of bone turnover. Horm Res 45(Suppl 1):55–58, 1996.

61. Adinoff AD, Hollister JR: Steroid-induced fractures and bone loss in patients with asthma. N Engl J Med 309:265–268, 1983.

62. Dalsky GP, Stocke KS, Ehsani AA, et al: Weight-bearing exercise training and lumbar bone mineral content in postmenopausal women. Ann Intern Med 108:824–828, 1988.

63. Dawson-Hughes B, Dallal GE, Krall EA, et al: Effect of vitamin D supplementation on wintertime and overall bone loss in healthy postmenopausal women. Ann Intern Med 115:505–512, 1991.

64. Hollowell J, Chen TC: The osteopenic patient. In Benzel E, Stillerman C (eds): The Thoracic Spine. St Louis, Quality Medical Publishing, 1999, pp 457–480.

65. Farley JR, Wergedal JE, Hall SL, et al: Calcitonin has direct effects on 3[H]-thymidine incorporation and alkaline phosphatase activity in human osteoblast-line cells. Calcif Tissue Int 48: 297–301, 1991.

66. Peck WA: The effects of glucocorticoids on bone cell metabolism and function. Adv Exp Med Biol 171:111–119, 1984.

67. Jacobson PC, Beaver W, Grubb SA, et al: Bone density in women: College athletes and older athletic women. J Orthop Res 2:328–332, 1984.

68. Soshi S, Shiba R, Kondo H, Murota K: An experimental study on transpedicular screw fixation in relation to osteoporosis of the lumbar spine. Spine 16:1335–1341, 1991.

69. Pfeifer BA, Krag MH, Johnson C: Repair of failed transpedicle screw fixation. Spine 19:350–353, 1994.

70. Heikkinen JE, Selander KS, Laitinen K, et al: Short-term intravenous bisphosphonates in prevention of postmenopausal bone loss. J Bone Miner Res 12:103–110, 1997.

71. Steinberg KK, Thacker SB, Smith SJ, et al: A meta-analysis of the effect of estrogen replacement therapy on the risk of breast cancer. JAMA 265:1985–1990, 1991.

72. Dawson-Hughes B: Smoking and bone loss among postmenopausal women. J Bone Miner Res 6:331–338, 1991.

73. Krall EA, Dawson-Hughes B: Heritable and life-style determinants of bone mineral density. J Bone Miner Res 8:1–9, 1993.

74. Krall EA, Dawson-Hughes B: Smoking increases bone loss and decreases intestinal calcium absorption. J Bone Miner Res 14: 215–220, 1999.

75. Krall EA, Dawson-Hughes B: Smoking and bone loss among postmenopausal women. J Bone Miner Res 6:331–338, 1991.

76. Valimaki MJ, Karkkainen M, Lamberg-Allardt C, et al: Exercise, smoking, and calcium intake during adolescence and early adulthood as determinants of peak bone mass. Cardiovascular Risk in Young Finns Study Group. BMJ 309:230–235, 1994.

77. Haddock L, Ortiz V, Vazquez MD, et al: The lumbar and femoral bone mineral densities in a normal female Puerto Rican population. P R Health Sci J 15:5–11, 1996.

78. Dawson-Hughes B, Krall EA, Harris S: Risk factors for bone loss in healthy postmenopausal women. Osteoporos Int 3(Suppl 1):27–31, 1993.

79. Moniz C: Alcohol and bone. Br Med Bull 50:67–75, 1994.

80. Laitinen K, Karkkainen M, Lalla M, et al: Is alcohol an osteoporosis-inducing agent for young and middle-aged women? Metabolism 42:875–881, 1993.

81. Laitinen K, Lamberg-Allardt C, Tunninen R, et al: Bone mineral density and abstention-induced changes in bone and mineral metabolism in noncirrhotic male alcoholics. Am J Med 93:642–650, 1992.

82. Laitinen K, Valimaki M: Alcohol and osteoporosis. Duodecim 107:1716–1718, 1991.

83. Laitinen K, Valimaki M, Lamberg-Allardt C, et al: Deranged vitamin D metabolism but normal bone mineral density in Finnish noncirrhotic male alcoholics. Alcohol Clin Exp Res 14: 551–556, 1990.

84. Ettinger B, Genant HK, Cann CE: Postmenopausal bone loss is prevented by treatment with low-dosage estrogen with calcium. Ann Intern Med 106:40–45, 1987.

85. Ginsburg ES, Mello NK, Mendelson JH, et al: Effects of alcohol ingestion on estrogens in postmenopausal women. JAMA 276: 1747–1751, 1996.

86. Cavanaugh DJ, Cann CE: Brisk walking does not stop bone loss in postmenopausal women. Bone 9:201–204, 1988.

87. Mamelle N, Dusan R, Martin JL, et al: Risk-benefit of sodium fluoride treatment in primary vertebral osteoporosis. Lancet 2: 361–363, 1988.

88. Bishop RC, Moore KA, Hadley MN: Anterior cervical interbody fusion using autogeneic and allogeneic bone graft substrate: A prospective comparative analysis. J Neurosurg 85:206–210, 1996.

89. Riis B, Thomsen K, Christiansen C: Does calcium supplementation prevent postmenopausal bone loss? A double-blind, controlled clinical study. N Engl J Med 316:173–177, 1987.

90. Ernst M, Heath JK, Schmid C, et al: Evidence for a direct effect of estrogen on bone cells in vitro. J Steroid Biochem 34: 279–284, 1989.

91. Pocock NA, Eisman JA, Hopper JL, et al: Genetic determinants of bone mass in adults. Am Soc Clin Invest 80:706–710, 1987.

92. Hanley EN, Harvell JC, Shapiro DE, Kraus DR: Use of allograft bone in cervical spine surgery. Semin Spine Surg 1:262–270, 1989.

93. Krolner B, Toft B: Vertebral bone loss: An unheeded side effect of therapeutic bed rest. Clin Sci 64:537–540, 1983.

94. Johnston CCJ, Miller JZ, Slemenda CW, et al: Calcium supplementation and increases in bone mineral density in children. N Engl J Med 327:82–87, 1992.

95. Speroff L, Rowan J, Symons J, et al: The comparative effect on bone density, endometrium, and lipids of continuous hormones as replacement therapy (chart study): A randomized controlled trial. JAMA 276:1397–1403, 1996.

96. Bernstein DS, Sadowsky N, Hegsted DM, et al: Prevalence of osteoporosis in high- and low-fluoride areas in North Dakota. JAMA 198:499–508, 1966.

97. Crawford RJ, Sell PJ, Ali MS, Dove J: Segmental spinal instrumentation: A study of the mechanical properties of materials used for sublaminar fixation. Spine 14:632–635, 1989.

98. Reginster JY, Albert A, Lecart MP, et al: One-year controlled randomised trial of prevention of early postmenopausal bone loss by intranasal calcitonin. Lancet 2:1481–1483, 1987.

99. Cummings SR, Kelsey JL, Nevitt MC, O'Dowd KJ: Epidemiology of osteoporosis and osteoporotic fractures. Epidemiol Rev 7:178–208, 1985.

100. Riggs BL, Hodgson SF, O'Fallon WM, et al: Effect of fluoride treatment on the fracture rate in postmenopausal women with osteoporosis. N Engl J Med 322:802–809, 1990.

101. Butler TE Jr, Asher MA, Jayaraman G, et al: The strength and stiffness of thoracic implant anchors in osteoporotic spines. Spine 19:1956–1962, 1994.

102. Mosekilde L, Mosekilde L: Normal vertebral body size and compressive strength: Relations to age and to vertebral and iliac trabecular bone compressive strength. Bone 7:207–212, 1986.

103. Riggs BL, Melton LJI: Involutional osteoporosis. N Engl J Med 314:1676–1686. 1986.

104. Melton LJI, Lane AW, Cooper C, et al: Prevalence and incidence of vertebral deformities. Osteoporos Int 3:113–119, 1993.

105. Heaney RP, Recker RR: Effects of nitrogen, phosphorus, and caffeine on calcium balance in women. J Lab Clin Med 99: 46–55, 1982.

106. Watts NB, Harris ST, Genant HK, et al: Intermittent cyclical etidronate treatment of postmenopausal osteoporosis. N Engl J Med 323:73–79, 1990.

107. Riggs BL, Melton LJI: Evidence for two distinct syndromes of involutional osteoporosis. Am J Med 75:899–901, 1983.

108. Meier DE, Orwoll ES, Jones JM: Marked disparity between trabecular and cortical bone loss with age in healthy men. Ann Intern Med 101:605–612, 1984.

109. Henderson BE: The cancer question: An overview of recent epidemiologic and retrospective data. Am J Obstet 161:1859–1864, 1989.

110. Gangi A, Kastler BA, Dietermann J-L: Percutaneous vertebroplasty guided by a combination of CT and fluoroscopy. AJNR Am J Neuroradiol 15:83–86, 1994.

111. Storm T, Thamsborg G, Steiniche T, et al: Effect of intermittent cyclical etidronate therapy on bone mass and fracture rate in women with postmenopausal osteoporosis. N Engl J Med 322: 1265–1271, 1990.

112. LeBlanc AD, Schneider VS, Evans HJ, et al: Bone mineral loss and recovery after 17 weeks of bed rest. J Bone Miner Res 5: 843–850, 1990.

113. Jung A, Bisaz S, Fleisch H: The binding of pyrophosphate and two diphosphonates by hydroxyapatite crystals. Calcif Tissue Res 11:269–280, 1973.

114. Hofbauer LC, Gori F, Riggs BL, et al: Stimulation of osteoprotegerin ligand and inhibition of osteoprotegerin production by glucocorticoids in human osteoblastic lineage cells: Potential paracrine mechanisms of glucocorticoid-induced osteoporosis. Endocrinology 140:4382–4389, 1999.

115. Barker DJ, Chamberlain AT, Guyer PB, et al: Paget's disease of bone: The Lancashire focus. BMJ 280:1105–1107, 1980.

116. Norman DA, Zerwekh JE, Pak CY: An apparent 1,25-dihydroxyvitamin D–independent stimulation of intestinal calcium absorption in patients with Paget disease of bone during a short-term diphosphonate therapy. Metabolism 30:290–292, 1981.

117. Sundquist K, Lakkakorpi P, Wallmark B, et al: Inhibition of osteoclast proton transport by bafilomycin A1 abolishes bone resorption. Biochem Biophys Res Commun 168:309–313, 1990.

118. Hruska KA, Rifas L, Cheng SL, et al: X-linked hypophosphatemic rickets and the murine Hyp homologue. Am J Physiol 268(3 Pt 2):F357–F362, 1995.

119. Zerwekh JE, Glass K, Jowsey J, et al: A unique form of osteomalacia associated with end organ refractoriness to 1,25-dihydroxyvitamin D and apparent defective synthesis of 25-hydroxyvitamin D. J Clin Endocrinol Metab 49:171–175, 1979.

120. Ryan EA, Reiss E: Oncogenous osteomalacia: Review of the world literature of 42 cases and report of two new cases. Am J Med 77:501–512, 1984.

Normal and Abnormal Embryology of the Spinal Cord and Spine

MARK S. DIAS ■ DAVID G. McLONE ■ MICHAEL PARTINGTON

Spinal cord and spinal malformations share a common embryogenesis as disorders of early development of the neural tube and surrounding structures. A working knowledge of normal embryology, as well as an appreciation of the ways in which normal development might go awry, is helpful for neurosurgeons to appreciate both the demographics and the surgical anatomy of these malformations. The usual classification schemes tend to lump all dysraphic malformations into simple categories such as open or closed, and they have done little to foster an understanding of the nature of these malformations or their embryogenesis. For example, confusion about early nervous system development has led to the erroneous use of terms such as *closed myelomeningocele* to refer to the skin-covered terminal myelocystocele. The misuse of these terms leads to improper identification and a poor understanding of the anatomy of both these malformations. A working knowledge of normal embryology would elucidate that a myelomeningocele, arising through a localized failure of primary neurulation, produces a placode that is still connected at its edges to the adjacent cutaneous ectoderm and therefore forms, by definition, an *open* malformation. In contrast, a terminal myelocystocele, likely arising through a localized disorder of secondary neurulation—a process occurring beneath a layer of intact cutaneous ectoderm—would be expected to form a closed malformation.

It is increasingly apparent that although dysraphic malformations share some common clinical features, the morphology, epidemiology, and natural history of these disorders suggest a diverse and heterogeneous embryologic origin.[1, 2] In our view, a classification of dysraphic malformations based on reputed embryonic mechanisms is much more helpful. In this chapter, we review the normal embryology of early neural tube and vertebral development and the embryonic mechanisms postulated to give rise to neural tube and vertebral malformations, with the intent of providing a mechanistic embryonic framework on which to hang these various disorders.

At the outset, it is important to understand that all the embryologic mechanisms discussed here for dysraphic malformations are putative—that is, there is no absolute proof that they are the cause of a particular human malformation. With the possible exceptions of the myelomeningocele and sacral agenesis, there are no adequate animal models to test our hypotheses about the origin of human malformations. However, we can gain considerable insight into the embryopathology of dysraphic states through the study of normal neural development. Throughout this chapter, we refer to human development in terms of both postovulatory days (PODs) and the embryonic staging system of O'Rahilly and Müller.[3]

NORMAL EARLY HUMAN NEURAL DEVELOPMENT

During the first 2 weeks after fertilization (PODs 1 to 13, stages 1 to 6), the human embryo undergoes a number of cell divisions and cellular rearrangements that ultimately form a blastocyst, which contains a two-layered embryo suspended between the amniotic and yolk sacs (Fig. 281–1). By stage 3 (POD 4), cells on the dorsal surface of the embryo, adjacent to the amniotic cavity, form the *epiblast*, whereas cells on the ventral surface, adjacent to the yolk sac, form the *hypoblast*.[3] By stage 6 (POD 13), the embryo thickens cranially to form the prochordal plate, the first morphologic feature of craniocaudal orientation.

By POD 13 (stage 6), the *primitive streak* first develops at the caudal end of the embryo and elongates cranially over the next 3 days (Fig. 281–2A). It reaches its full length by stage 7 (POD 16), at which time it occupies the midline in the caudal half of the human embryo; beyond this time, the primitive streak begins to regress—that is, it becomes shorter and moves back toward the caudal pole of the embryo.[3] At the cranial end of the primitive streak is *Hensen's node*. As the primitive streak develops, cells of the epiblast migrate toward the primitive streak and invaginate through a midline trough, the *primitive groove*, that runs the length of the primitive streak (see Fig. 281–2). The first cells to ingress (while the primitive streak is still elongating)

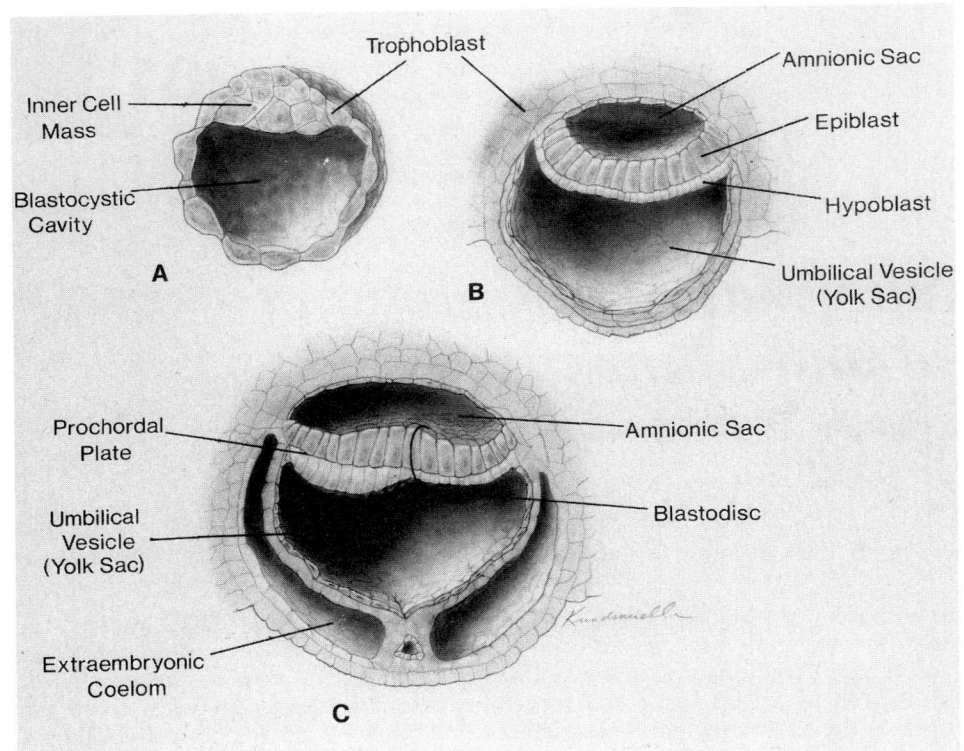

FIGURE 281–1. Development of the blastocyst; midsagittal illustrations. *A,* Continued proliferation of cells produces a sphere containing a blastocystic cavity surrounded by an eccentrically located inner cell mass and a surrounding ring of trophoblast cells. *B,* The inner cell mass develops further into a two-layered structure, the blastodisk, containing the epiblast adjacent to the amniotic cavity and the hypoblast adjacent to the yolk sac. *C,* With further development, the blastodisk thickens cranially to form the prochordal plate. (From Dias MS, Walker ML: The embryogenesis of complex dysraphic malformations: A disorder of gastrulation? Pediatr Neurosurg 18: 229–253, 1992.)

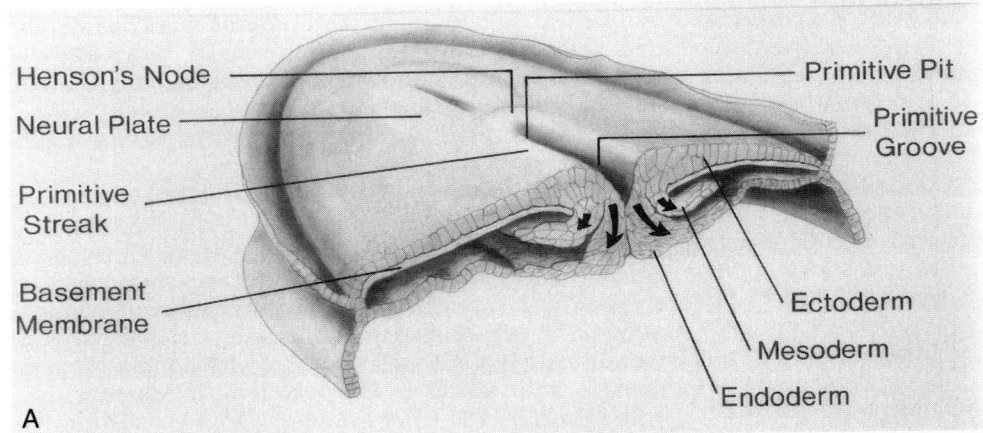

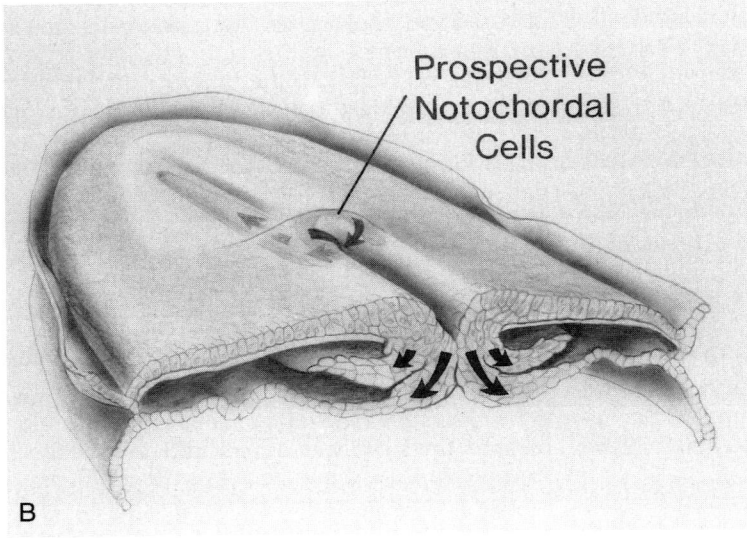

FIGURE 281–2. Normal human gastrulation. *A,* Prospective endodermal and mesodermal cells of the epiblast migrate toward the primitive streak and ingress (*arrows*) through the primitive groove to become the definitive endoderm and mesoderm. *B,* Prospective notochordal cells in the cranial margin of Hensen's node will ingress through the primitive pit during primitive streak regression to become the notochordal process. (From Dias MS, Walker ML: The embryogenesis of complex dysraphic malformations: A disorder of gastrulation? Pediatr Neurosurg 18:229–253, 1992.)

are endodermal cells that displace the hypoblast cells laterally (the displaced hypoblast cells ultimately form extraembryonic tissues) and form the endoderm (forming primarily the lining of the respiratory and gastrointestinal systems).[4-8] Later, as the streak regresses, mesodermal cells ingress through the primitive streak between the epiblast and the newly formed endoderm and become the mesoderm (including mesenchymal cells of the body wall and limbs, somites, and kidney).[7, 8] The remaining epiblast cells spread to replace the cells that have ingressed through the primitive groove and form the ectoderm (both neuroectoderm and surface ectoderm). Embryonic endoderm, mesoderm, and ectoderm are thus all derived from the epiblast. This process, referred to as *gastrulation*, transforms the embryo from a two-layered structure containing an epiblast and a hypoblast into a three-layered structure containing ectoderm, mesoderm, and endoderm.[9]

Hensen's node, located at the cranial end of the primitive streak, serves a special role as the "organizer" of the embryo. As the streak elongates, prospective endodermal cells migrate through the primitive pit (in the center of Hensen's node). By the time the streak is fully elongated and during its subsequent regression, mesodermal cells predominate[8, 9] and consist chiefly of prospective *notochordal cells* (see Fig. 281–2B), which ingress through Hensen's node and are laid down in the midline as the *notochordal process* (see later).

Localization of Prospective Neuroectoderm

Fate-mapping studies[10] have localized the prospective neuroectoderm to an area of the epiblast that surrounds and flanks Hensen's node and the cranial half of the primitive streak (Fig. 281–3). Earlier mapping studies[11] suggested that the prospective neuroectoderm is organized in a linear, craniocaudal sequence so that prospective forebrain cells are located more cranially than prospective midbrain cells, and so on. However, more recent studies suggest a different organization. Instead of contributing to a single neuraxial level, each region of the neuroepithelium contributes to multiple neuraxial levels. For example, marking the most cranial regions of the prospective neuroectoderm results in a strip of label that extends through all craniocaudal subdivisions of the neuraxis from forebrain to spinal cord; marking more caudal levels results in similar strips that, although beginning at more caudal levels, extend caudally through all subsequent levels of the neuraxis.[10]

Regression of the Primitive Streak and Formation of the Notochord

In humans, the formation of the notochordal process from cells invaginating through Hensen's node begins at stage 7 (POD 16), as the primitive streak begins to regress (Fig. 281–4).[3] To what extent does the notochordal process extend cranially from Hensen's node,

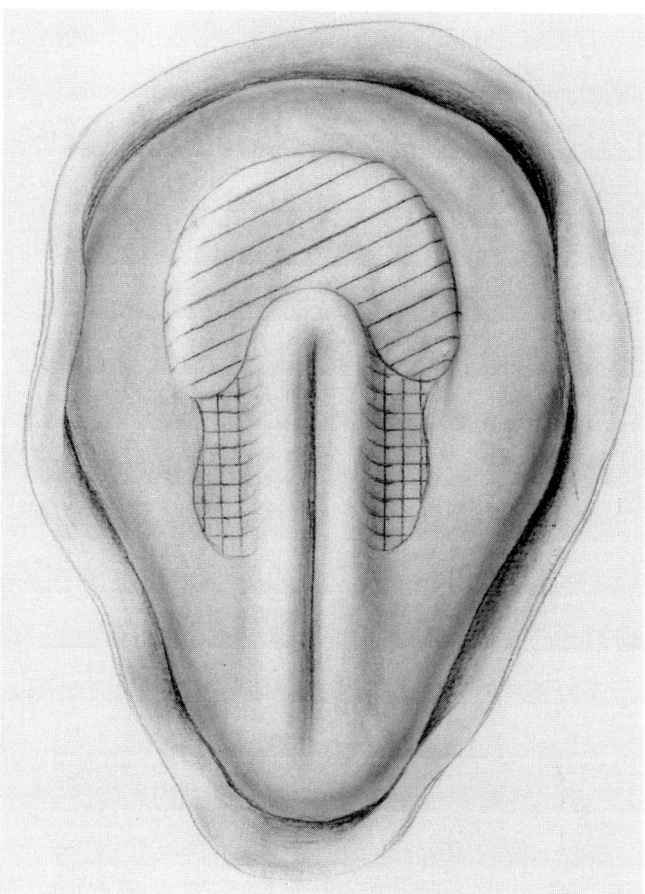

FIGURE 281–3. Location of prospective neuroepithelium. Dorsal view of an avian embryo during gastrulation. Striped region illustrates localization by earlier mapping studies that used carbon particles; hatched area illustrates additional caudal areas demonstrated by more recent mapping studies using horseradish peroxidase injections and chimeric transplantation. (From Dias MS, Walker ML: The embryogenesis of complex dysraphic malformations: A disorder of gastrulation? Pediatr Neurosurg 18: 229–253, 1992.)

and to what extent does it elongate caudally by addition of cells to its caudal end from the regressing Hensen's node? In the chick, the notochordal process grows largely by the latter mechanism.[11] In mammals, the available evidence suggests that the situation is much more complex and may involve both mechanisms.[12, 13] The mechanism of notochord elongation in humans is unknown.

The notochordal process at stage 7 consists of a median cord of cells, located between the ectoderm and endoderm cranial to Hensen's node[14]; in cross section, the cells of the notochordal process are radially arranged about a central lumen called the *notochordal canal* (Fig. 281–5).[3] The notochordal canal is continuous dorsally with the amniotic cavity through the primitive pit.[15] The notochordal canal is present in human[3] and nonhuman primate[16] embryos but has not been described in amphibian, avian, or nonprimate mammalian embryos. Its function is unknown.

The notochordal process continues to elongate dur-

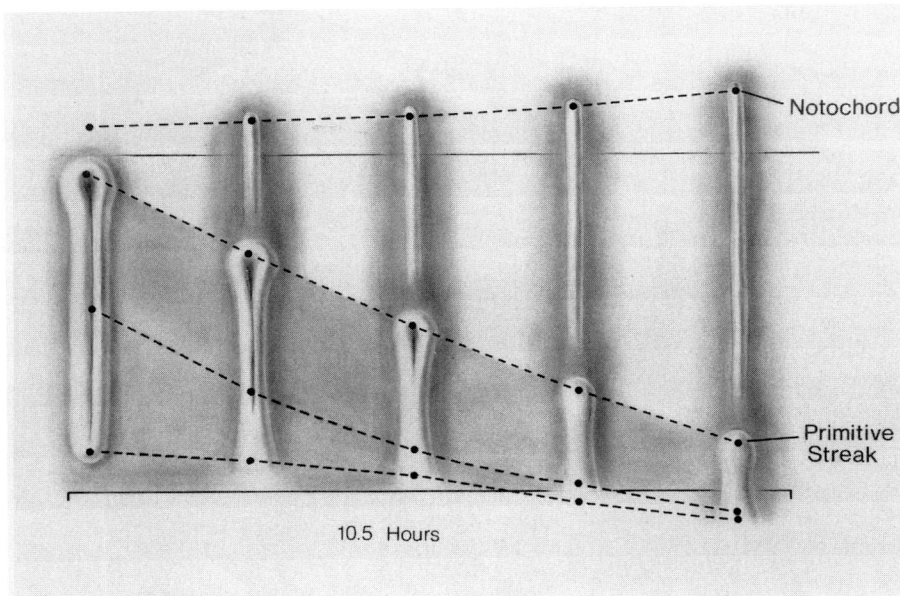

FIGURE 281–4. Formation of the notochord in avian embryos. The notochord is formed through the addition of cells to its caudal end as the primitive streak regresses; true cranial growth of the notochord is minimal. (Adapted from Spratt NT: Regression and shortening of the primitive streak in the explanted chick blastoderm. J Exp Zool 104:69–100, 1947.)

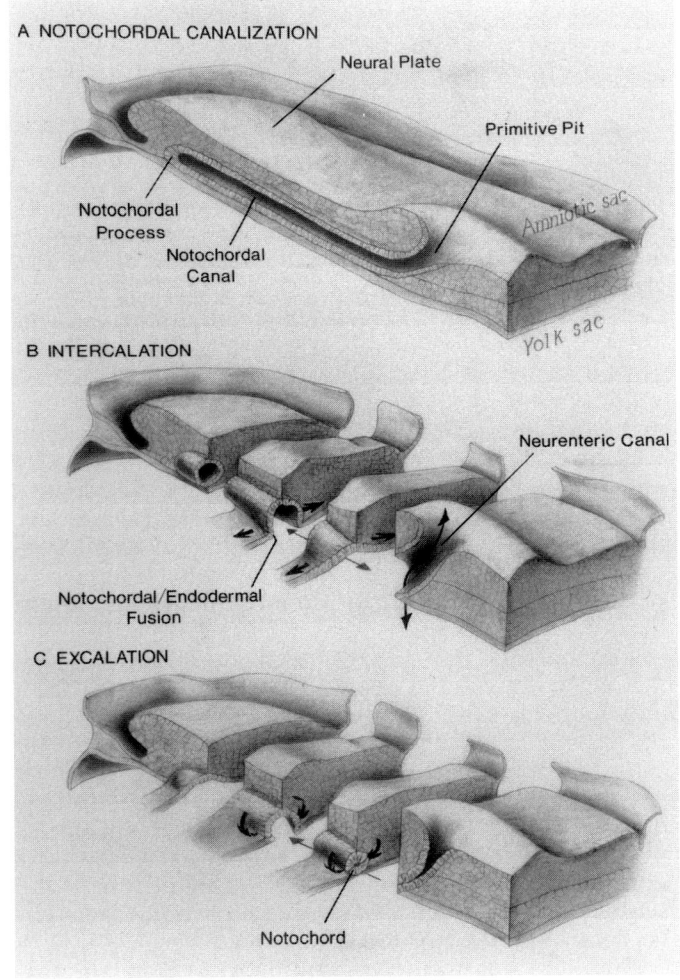

FIGURE 281–5. Notochordal canalization, intercalation, and excalation. *A*, The notochordal process contains a central lumen (the notochordal canal) that is continuous with the amniotic cavity through the primitive pit. *B*, During intercalation, the canalized notochordal process fuses with the underlying endoderm; the communication of the amnion with the yolk sac forms the primitive neurenteric canal. *C*, During excalation, the notochord rolls up and separates from the endoderm to become the definitive notochord; the primitive neurenteric canal becomes obliterated. (From Dias MS, Walker ML: The embryogenesis of complex dysraphic malformations: A disorder of gastrulation? Pediatr Neurosurg 18:229–253, 1992.)

ing stage 8 (PODs 17 to 19) and reaches its full length at stage 9 (PODs 19 to 21).[3, 17] Initially, it is rod shaped and lies between the neuroectoderm and the endoderm; however, during stage 8 (PODs 18 to 20) it fuses, or *intercalates*, with the underlying endoderm to form the *notochordal plate* (see Fig. 281–5). The notochordal plate is incorporated into the roof of the yolk sac, and the notochordal canal becomes continuous with the yolk sac. The most caudal portion of the notochordal canal is continuous both with the amnion through the primitive pit and with the yolk sac as a result of intercalation; this communication is called the *neurenteric canal*.[3]

The neurenteric canal first appears during stage 8 (PODs 17 to 19) and continues during stages 9 and 10 (PODs 19 to 23).[3, 17–19] During stage 10 (PODs 21 to 23), the notochordal plate begins to fold dorsoventrally and to separate (or *excalate*) from the endoderm. By stage 11 (PODs 23 to 25), it has completely separated once again from the underlying endoderm (see Fig. 281–5), obliterating the neurenteric canal and ending the communication between the amniotic and yolk sacs.[3, 18, 20] Thereafter, the *true notochord* exists as a solid rod of notochordal cells.[20]

Formation of the Neural Tube

The human neuroectoderm is first visible at stage 7 (POD 16) as a pseudostratified columnar epithelium overlying the midline notochord and contiguous laterally with the surrounding squamous epithelium of the cutaneous ectoderm.[21] By stage 8 (PODs 17 to 19), a shallow midline fold, the *neural groove*, forms a crease immediately above the midline notochord (Fig. 281–6A).[17] By stage 9 (PODs 19 to 21), the neural groove deepens considerably (see Fig. 281–6B), and neural folds develop laterally.[19] Further dorsal elevation and medial convergence of the neural folds continue during stages 9 and 10. The neural folds meet (see Fig. 281–6C) to form a closed neural tube during stage 10 (PODs 21 to 23). Closure usually involves the apposition and fusion of first the cutaneous ectoderm and then the neuroectoderm.[3, 18] In humans, the first part of the neural tube to close is the region of the caudal rhombencephalon or cranial spinal cord, usually when five pairs of somites are present.[18]

Closure of the neural tube takes place over 4 to 6 days. Although previously thought to close in a linear fashion, like a zipper extending cranially and caudally from the point of initial closure, neurulation in mammals (including humans) instead appears to extend from several initiation sites along its craniocaudal axis.[18, 22–24] The cranial neural tube closes from the coordinated interaction of at least four waves of discontinuous closure and is not described further.[18, 22–25] The spinal cord closes in a linear manner from a caudal wave of neurulation that extends from the point of initial contact, at the cranial end of the spinal cord, to the posterior neuropore.[23, 24]

The caudal neuropore closes during stage 12 (PODs 25 to 27).[26] At the time the caudal neuropore closes, approximately 25 somites have formed, but the caudal neuropore is located below the last visible somite. Therefore, the site of closure can only be estimated by measuring the space between the last visible somite and the caudal neuropore and by calculating the number of somites that would subsequently form in this space. Using this method, the site of closure has been estimated to be opposite somites 30–31,[26] which corresponds to both a spinal ganglion and a vertebral level of S2.[27] In humans, it appears that most of the spinal cord (as far caudal as the second sacral segment) forms by primary neurulation, and that the filum terminale and perhaps the lower sacral spinal cord form by secondary neurulation. Accordingly, one can deduce that all spinal malformations that arise cranial to S2, whether open or closed, involve regions of the neural tube formed from primary neurulation.

Formation of the Neural Crest

Neural crest cells in human,[20, 28] mouse,[29] and rat[30] embryos are thought to arise from the neural tube at the junction between the neural folds and adjacent surface ectoderm; in humans, however, a simultaneous origin for some neural crest cells from the adjacent surface ectoderm cannot be excluded.[18] The neural crest in human embryos first develops at stage 9 (PODs 19 to 21).[19]

The initial formation of the cranial neural crest in humans begins during neural fold elevation (stage 9; PODs 19 to 21), *before* the neural folds fuse, and continues from the closed neural tube at least until stage 14 (POD 32),[31] well after the neural folds have fused at stage 10 (PODs 21 to 23).[18, 20] More caudal neural crest cells arise only after neural tube closure.[3, 26] A similar sequence has been described in the rat.[30]

Spinal cord neural crest cells undergo terminal differentiation into a bewildering variety of cell types, including the melanocytes of the body wall and limbs, the Schwann cells investing the peripheral nerves, the dura of the spinal cord, and dorsal root and autonomic ganglion cells of the spinal nerves. In addition, these cells give rise to the adrenal medulla.[32] In both avian and mammalian (and presumably human) embryos, trunk neural crest cells choose either a dorsal or a ventral migratory pathway soon after they leave the neural tube. Neural crest cells that follow the dorsal, or subepidermal, migratory pathway form the melanocytes of the skin, whereas those that follow the ventral migratory pathway form the remaining neural crest derivatives.[33] The neural crest cells in the ventral migratory pathway advance between the neural tube and adjacent somites and traverse the rostral half of the sclerotomal portion of the somite. Some of the ventral neural crest cells remain near the neural tube and become dorsal root ganglion cells; others advance farther ventrally to become sympathetic ganglion and adrenal cells.[34] Further details regarding the control of migration and terminal differentiation of neural crest cells can be found in several reviews.[33, 35, 36]

Secondary Neurulation

With closure of the caudal neuropore at stage 12 (PODs 25 to 27), the entire nervous system is skin covered,

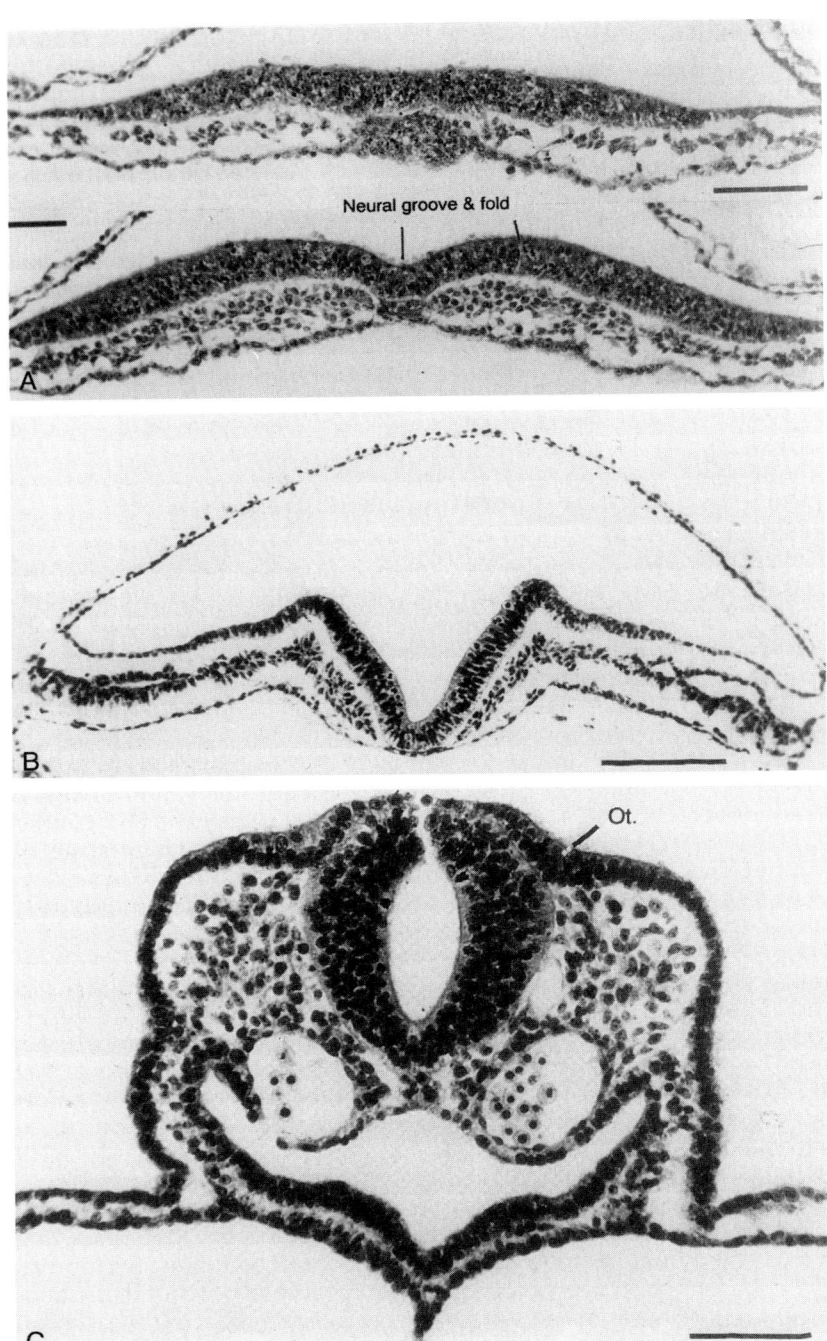

Neural groove & fold

Ot.

FIGURE 281–6. Neurulation in humans. *A,* Formation of the neural groove. Upper photomicrograph shows the neural plate overlying the prechordal plate in a stage 8 embryo. Lower photomicrograph from a more caudal area of the same embryo shows the neural groove and neural folds developing atop the notochordal plate. The notochordal plate is the roof of the notochordal canal after intercalation with the endoderm. Bar = 0.05 mm. *B,* Elevation of the neural folds at the rhombencephalon in a stage 9 embryo. Bar = 0.2 mm. *C,* Apposition and closure of the neural tube at the rhombencephalon in a stage 10 embryo. The otic placodes (Ot) are visible on either side. Bar = 0.15 mm. (From O'Rahilly R, Müller F: The Embryonic Human Brain. New York, Wiley-Liss, 1994.)

and more caudal neural development takes place by *secondary neurulation.*[26] The remnants of the primitive streak have regressed to the caudal embryonic pole and form a mass of pluripotent cells called the *tail bud* (Fig. 281–7), *caudal eminence,*[19] *end bud,*[37] or *caudal cell mass,* depending on the species. In humans, the term *caudal cell mass* (CCM) is most often used. By stage 12, the CCM extends from the posterior neuropore to the cloacal membrane. The cells of the CCM are multipotent and, at least in chick embryos, give rise to the neural tube and vertebrae caudal to S2 but not to the hindgut, which is derived from endoderm, nor to the

posterior notochord, which is derived from a posterior notochordal region located immediately anterior to the CCM and underlying the primary neural tube.[38]

The mechanism of secondary neurulation is species specific (Fig. 281–8). In the chick embryo, secondary neurulation results in the formation of a medullary cord from the dorsal cells of the CCM. Within the medullary cord, an outer layer of tightly packed cells surrounds an inner cluster of more loosely arranged cells. Cavitation between the two cell groups creates multiple tubules with the outer cells surrounding a central lumen, within which are the inner cells. The

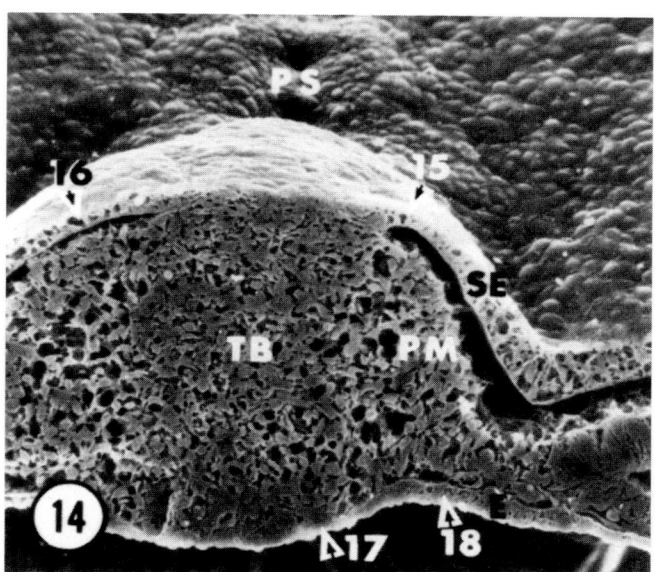

FIGURE 281–7. Electron micrograph of an axial section of a stage 15 chick embryo during secondary neurulation shows the relationships between the developing tail bud (TB) and the primitive streak (PS) cranially; the surface ectoderm (SE) dorsally; the endoderm (E) ventrally; and the caudal paraxial mesoderm (PM), which is derived from the tail bud and gives rise to the caudal somites, laterally. (From Schoenwolf GC: Histological and ultrastructural observations of tail bud formation in the chick embryo. Anat Rec 193:131–148, 1979.)

inner cells are eventually lost, and the outer cells then surround multiple empty lumina. Multiple smaller lumina coalesce to form larger cavities; eventually a single lumen is formed and is surrounded by the outer cell group. This secondary neural tube eventually fuses with the neural tube formed from primary neurulation in an area called the *overlap zone,* within which the primary neural tube is located dorsally and the secondary neural tube ventrally.[39]

Secondary neurulation in the mouse begins with the formation of a *medullary rosette,* a cluster of CCM cells radially arranged about a central lumen formed by cavitation. The cells of the medullary rosette are thought to be the homologue of the outer cell group in the chick embryo; the inner cell group seen in the chick is not present in the mouse. Caudal growth of the secondary neural tube occurs by additional cavitation of the medullary rosette and recruitment of additional cells from the CCM.[40]

Secondary neurulation in the mouse and chick differ in at least two respects. First, the secondary neural tube in the mouse is always directly continuous with the primary neural tube and develops caudally from the posterior neuropore. In contrast, the secondary neural tube in the chick develops independently and only later fuses with the primary neural tube. Second, the lumen of the secondary neural tube in the mouse is single and is always continuous with that of the primary neural tube. In contrast, multiple lumina are initially formed in the chick and only later communicate with one another and with the lumen of the primary neural tube.

Does secondary neurulation in humans more closely resemble that of the chick or the mouse? According to Müller and O'Rahilly,[26] human secondary neurulation more closely resembles that of the mouse. In their study, the neural cord was continuous with the primary neural tube, a single lumen was present and continuous with the central canal of the primary neural tube, and no overlap zone was present. In contrast, Lemire[41] and Bolli[42] described multiple independent secondary tubes having separate lumina and no discernible connection either with one another or with the primary neural tube, as occurs in the chick.[41] This issue is still unresolved.

Ascent of the Conus Medullaris

Beginning at about stage 18 to 20 (PODs 43 to 48) and continuing into later fetal development and perhaps even the first months of postnatal life, the position of the conus medullaris changes with respect to the adjacent vertebral column, a process termed the *ascent of the conus medullaris* (Fig. 281–9).[43, 44] As a result, the conus comes to lie opposite progressively more cranial vertebrae. This ascent involves at least two mechanisms. Before stage 22 (POD 54), the ascent is typically attributed to a process of *retrogressive differentiation,* in which the caudal neural tube loses much of its diameter and becomes thinner; fails to develop a distinct mantle zone; exhibits only a thin, rudimentary marginal zone; and generally appears less well developed than it did at earlier embryonic stages.[43] Beyond stage 22 (POD 54), the ascent of the conus is due primarily to a disparity between the growth rates of the vertebral column and the spinal cord.[43, 44]

The ascent of the conus medullaris during pre- and postnatal life has been examined by several investigators.[45–49] Most of the ascent occurs prenatally, between 8 and 25 weeks' gestation (see Fig. 281–9E); between 25 and 40 weeks, the rate of ascent slows.[48] Earlier studies of human cadavers by Barson[48] and others[49–51] suggested that the conus lies opposite the L2-3 disk space at birth and ascends further to its "adult" level, opposite or cranial to the L1-2 disk space, by 2 months of postnatal age. However, more recent studies using spinal ultrasonography and magnetic resonance imaging in newborn infants suggest that the conus medullaris has achieved its adult level opposite the L1-2 disk space at the time of birth and ascends no farther afterward.[45–47] Although as many as 2% of "normal" individuals have a more caudally positioned conus at or below the L3 vertebral body,[52] a conus that lies below the midbody of L2 is accepted by many as radiographic evidence of spinal cord tethering.

MECHANISMS OF PRIMARY NEURULATION

Neurulation is a complex morphogenetic process composed of several interdependent events, all of which overlap temporally to some degree. These include shaping of the neuroepithelium to form a neural plate;

Secondary Neurulation

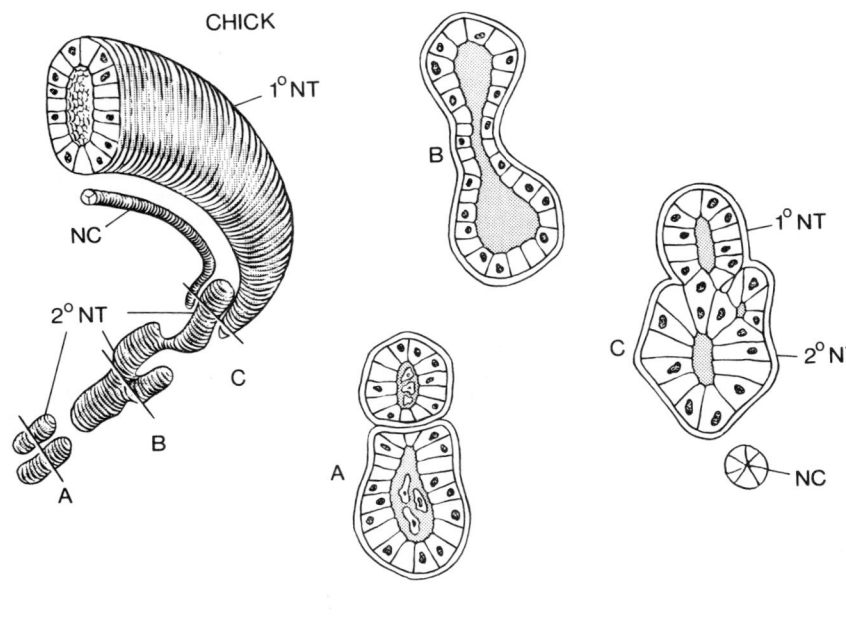

CHICK

1°NT

NC

2°NT

C

B

A

B

A

1°NT

C

2°NT

NC

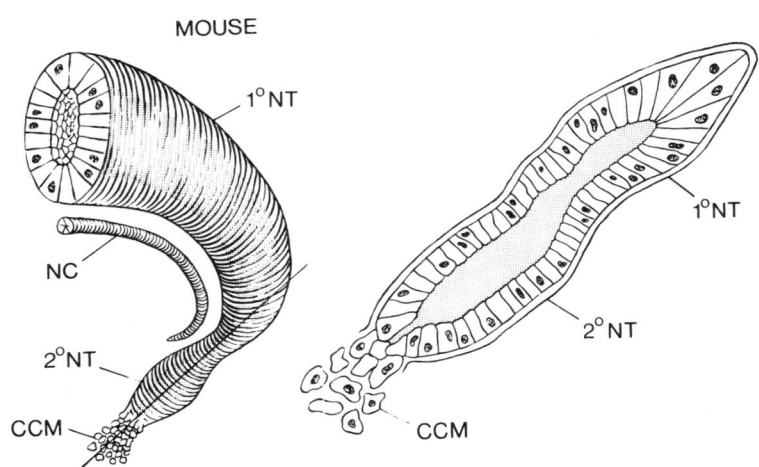

MOUSE

1°NT

NC

2°NT

CCM

1°NT

2°NT

CCM

FIGURE 281–8. Secondary neurulation. Upper illustration depicts secondary neurulation in avian embryos. *A*, The medullary cord consists of multiple lumina, each surrounded by an outer layer of tightly packed, radially oriented cells and containing an inner group of more loosely packed cells. *B*, Adjacent cords coalesce to form larger aggregates; simultaneously, the inner cells are lost. Eventually, a single structure is formed that has a single lumen, which is not yet in direct communication with the lumen formed by primary neurulation. *C*, Later, the neural tube formed by secondary neurulation (2° NT) fuses with that formed from primary neurulation (1° NT); at this point, the lumina of the two neural tubes communicate directly. Lower illustration depicts secondary neurulation in mouse embryos. A medullary rosette is composed of cells radially arranged about an empty central lumen. The lumen is always in communication with the central canal formed by primary neurulation. Growth of the secondary neural tube occurs by additional cavitation of the secondary lumen and by the recruitment of additional cells from the caudal cell mass (CCM). NC, notochord. (From McLone DG, Dias MS: Normal and abnormal embryology of the nervous system. In Cheek WR [ed]: Pediatric Neurosurgery: Surgery of the Developing Nervous System, 3rd ed. Philadelphia, WB Saunders, 1994, pp 3–39.)

bending of the neural plate, first in the midline neural groove and later along the lateral edges of the neural tube, resulting in elevation and apposition of the neural folds in the midline; and fusion of the neural folds to close the neural tube.[53] The mechanisms of normal neurulation are reviewed here; interested readers are referred to the monograph by Schoenwolf and Smith[53] for a more comprehensive discussion.

Shaping of the Neural Plate

The newly induced neuroepithelium undergoes a change in shape during which it thickens apicodorsally, narrows mediolaterally, and lengthens craniocaudally. These changes convert the neural plate from a relatively flat, oval structure to one that is narrower and more elongated. Three cellular mechanisms account for

this neural plate shaping: changes in neuroepithelial cell height, oriented cell divisions, and cell rearrangements.

The first visible feature of the newly formed neuroepithelium is an elongation of the neuroepithelial cells from a cuboidal to a columnar shape due to a reorganization of intracellular longitudinally (or paraxially) oriented microtubules. These microtubules are abundant in neuroepithelial cells of many species.[39, 40, 54–66] Moreover, neuroepithelium from embryos exposed to agents that depolymerize microtubules (e.g., colchicine, nocodazole, cold treatment) is not as fully elongated.[55, 57, 61, 67–69]

Although microtubules are important, they are probably not the only forces that play a role in neuroepithelial cell elongation. In chick embryos, microtubule depolymerization results in only a 25% loss of

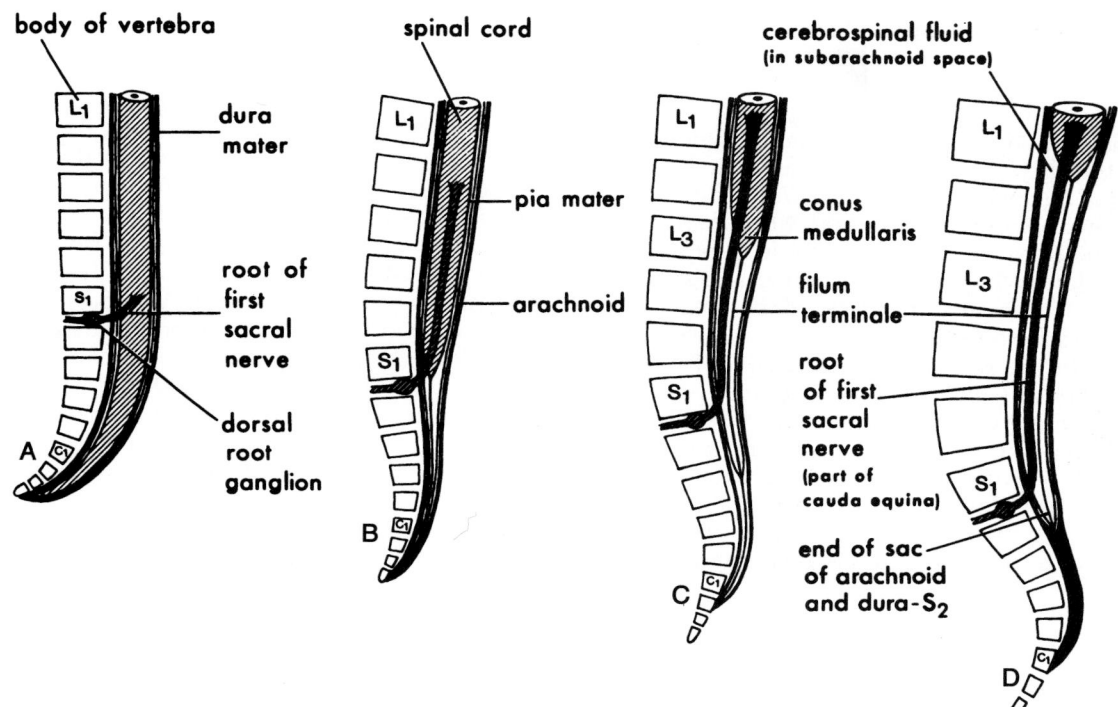

EMBRYOLOGY OF DYSRAPHISM

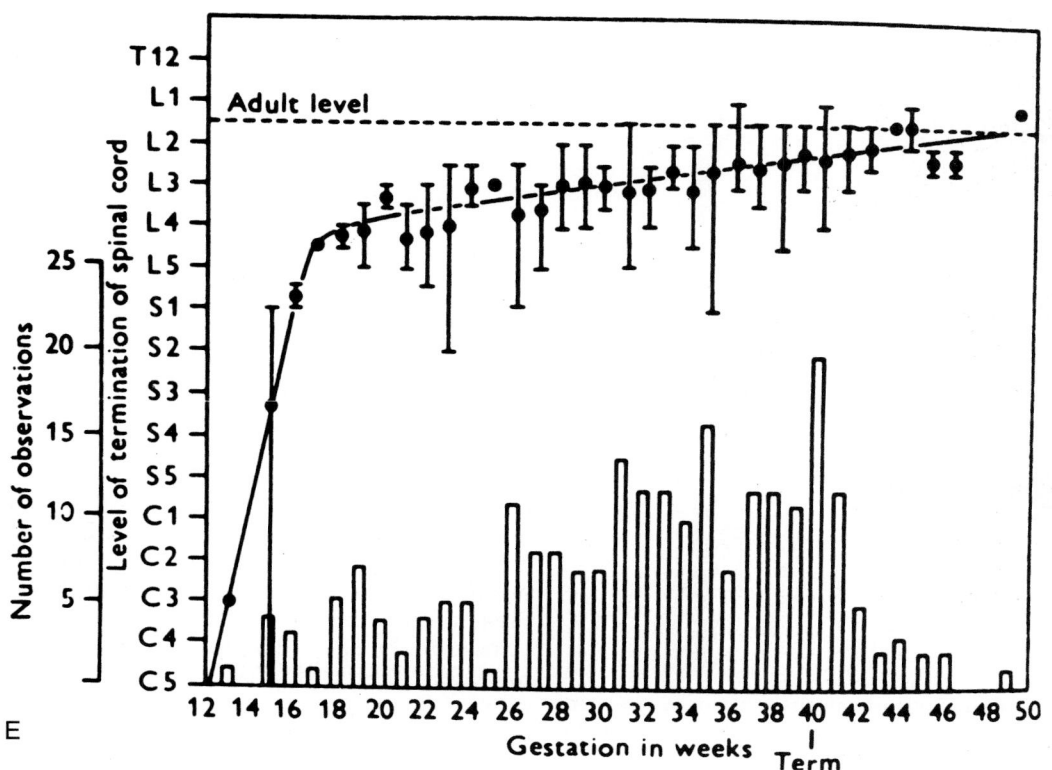

FIGURE 281–9. Ascent of the conus medullaris. *A–D,* Progressive ascent of the conus medullaris during embryogenesis and the immediate postnatal period. *A,* 8 weeks' gestation. *B,* 24 weeks' gestation. *C,* Newborn. *D,* Adult. *E,* Vertebral level of termination of the conus medullaris during fetal and early postnatal life. (*A–D,* From Moore KL: The Developing Human, 3rd ed. Philadelphia, WB Saunders, 1982. *E,* From Barson AJ: The vertebral level of termination of the spinal cord during normal and abnormal development. J Anat 106:489–497, 1970.)

neuroepithelial cell height.[63] Other mechanisms that may be important in neuroepithelial cell elongation include differential cell-cell adhesion[70, 71] and cortical tractoring.[72]

In addition to apicodorsal thickening, neural plate shaping involves two other morphologic changes: mediolateral narrowing and craniocaudal elongation (particularly in the caudal neural tube).[53] Although changes in neuroepithelial cell height account for some of the apicodorsal thickening of the neural plate, these changes can account for only 15% of the mediolateral narrowing and for none of the craniocaudal elongation that occurs during neural plate shaping.[73] Two other cellular events also contribute substantially to these morphologic changes: cell division (at least in avian and mammalian embryos) and cell rearrangement (intercalation). Computer modeling studies (Fig. 281–10) suggest that these three processes (cell elongation, cell division, and cell rearrangement-SC) can account for most of the changes in the shape of the avian neural plate.[73]

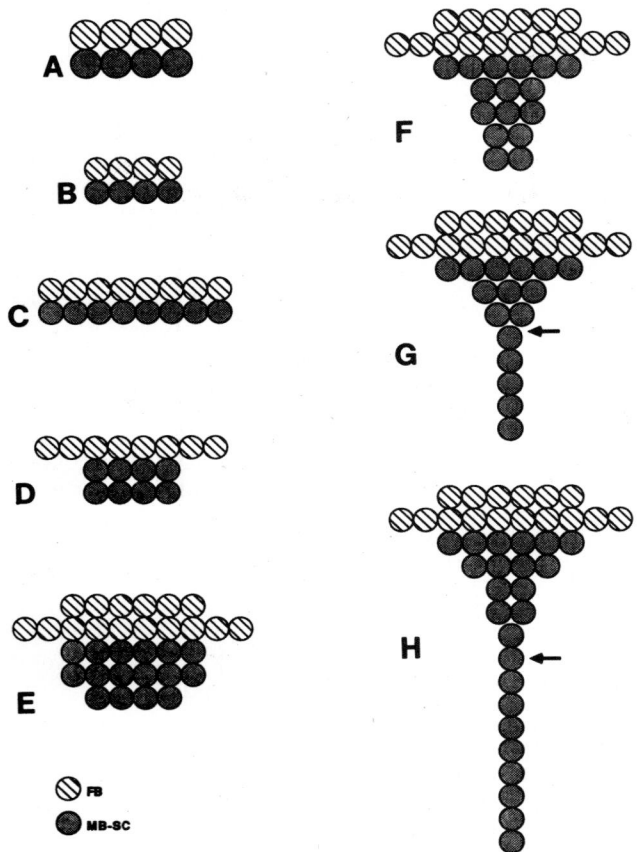

FIGURE 281–10. Contributions of cell shape changes, oriented cell division, and intercalation to shaping of the neuroepithelium. Computer simulation shows one possible mechanism by which neural plate shaping might be brought about by a 30% increase in neuroepithelial cell height (and a corresponding 15% decrease in cell diameter, leaving cell volume constant), two to three rounds of oriented cell divisions, and two rounds of cell rearrangement. FB, forebrain; MB-SC, midbrain–spinal cord. (From Schoenwolf GC, Alvarez IS: Roles of neuroepithelial cell rearrangement and division in shaping of the avian neural plate. Development 106:427–439, 1989.)

Bending of the Neural Plate

Standard embryology texts equate neurulation with neural plate bending, which converts the flat neural plate into a round neural tube. Neural plate bending in avian embryos has been extensively studied and involves several discrete steps (Fig. 281–11). First, specialized cells located in the midline of the neural plate and overlying the notochord change from a columnar to a wedge shape (by narrowing of the cell's apex or expansion of the base) to form a *median hingepoint*, or neural groove. Second, the neural folds elevate on either side of the median hingepoint to form a characteristic V shape. Third, similar cell shape changes develop later in discrete, bilaterally paired regions of the dorsolateral neural tube and are associated with the formation of the *dorsolateral hingepoints*, around which the neural folds converge toward the midline. Finally, the converging neural folds meet in preparation for neural fold fusion.[53] Similar morphologic changes have been observed in mammalian embryos,[74] but they have not been as well characterized as in the chick.

Traditional theories have espoused three fundamental concepts: (1) "all forces for neurulation are intrinsic to the neuroepithelium," (2) "neurulation is driven by changes in the shape of neuroepithelial cells," and (3) the "forces for cell shape changes are generated by the cytoskeleton of neuroepithelial cells."[53] However, each of these concepts has been challenged by more recent experimental evidence, and more recent theories have emphasized the importance of forces both intrinsic and extrinsic to the neuroepithelium during neural plate bending.

In 1885, Roux[75] first proposed that neurulation was a process intrinsic to the neuroepithelium; he demonstrated that the neural plate could roll up into a tube when cultured in isolation. However, the neural tubes in these experiments rolled up sooner than expected, did not undergo the characteristic shaping movements described earlier, and often rolled up backward—that is, with the apical side of the neuroepithelium on the outside of the neural tube.[53] Schoenwolf and Smith[53] argued that the bending movements of isolated neuroepithelium are nonspecific and do not represent neurulation.

More recent experimental evidence suggests that forces extrinsic to the neuroepithelium may play an important role in promoting neural tube bending.[76] A number of extrinsic forces have been identified that act on the neuroepithelium to assist neural plate bending: First, the medial convergence of the adjacent surface ectoderm "pushes" the neural folds together in the midline.[53, 76] Second, the accumulation of mesodermal cells or the expansion of the mesenchymal extracellular matrix beneath the neuroepithelium elevates the overlying neural folds.[77–86] Finally, the active elongation of the notochord or *notoplate* (the notochord plus the overlying median hingepoint cells of the neural tube) stretches the neural tube craniocaudally and, by simple mechanical deformation, draws the neural folds together, a process referred to as *eulerian buckling*.[87–90] The importance of these extrinsic forces in neural tube

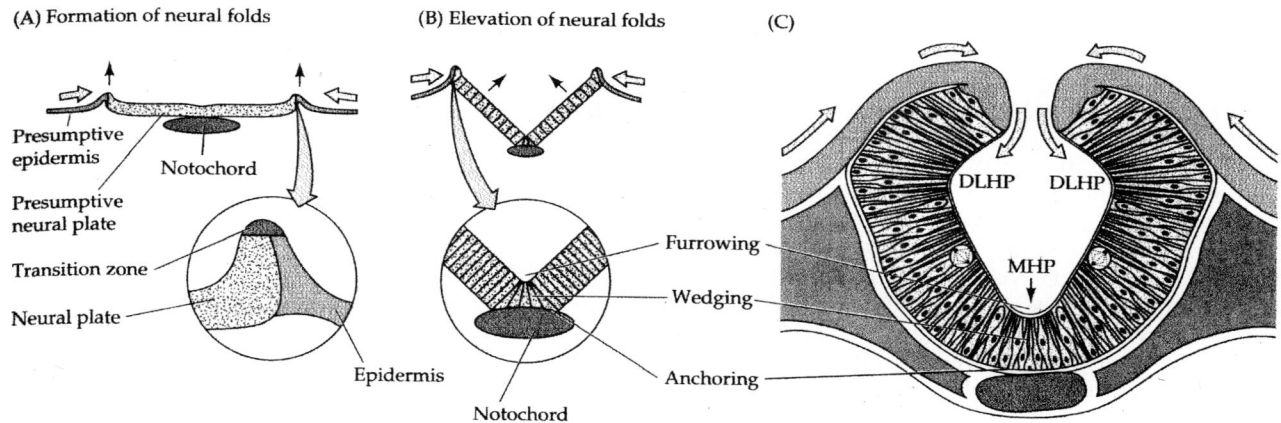

FIGURE 281–11. Illustration of the mechanisms of neural plate bending in chick embryos. *A,* The neural groove overlies the midline notochord. *Inset,* Transition between the neural folds and the surface ectoderm (the future epidermis). *B,* Apical constriction or basal expansion produces cell wedging in the median hingepoint (MHP) directly above the notochord, around which the neural folds elevate. *C,* Later, paired dorsolateral hingepoints (DLHP) form and further bend the neuroepithelium as the neural folds approach each other in preparation for neural fold fusion. (From Gilbert SF: Developmental Biology. Sunderland, MA, Sinauer Associates, 1997.)

formation has been debated by Gordon[90] and by Schoenwolf and Smith.[53]

The second traditional concept, that neural plate bending is driven by changes in neuroepithelial cell shape, was first proposed by His[91] in 1894. He suggested that if cells in a flat sheet were to become wedge shaped, through either apical constriction or basal expansion, the sheet would fold into a tube. Wedging of neuroepithelial cells during neural plate bending has been documented in a number of animals.[92–95] However, cell wedging appears to be restricted to the regions of the hingepoints in chick embryos.[94] Chick neuroepithelial cells are of four types, depending on their shape: (1) *spindle cells* have a wide waist and a tapering apex and base, (2) *wedge-shaped cells* have a wide base and a tapering apex, (3) *inverted wedge-shaped cells* have a wide apex and a tapering base, and (4) *globular cells* have a spherical shape. These cell shapes are determined by the location of the nucleus, which resides in the widest portion of the cell body; in the case of globular cells, the nucleus is in the mitotic phase of the cell cycle. Before neural plate bending begins, the distribution of the four cell types within the neural plate is random. However, as the neural groove forms, many of the median hingepoint cells change from spindle to wedge shaped. A similar shape change occurs slightly later in the dorsolateral hingepoint cells as the neural folds converge toward the midline. Most cells in the intervening regions of the neural tube remain spindle shaped. As a result of the cell shape changes in the hingepoint regions, the neural plate bends at these specific points.[94]

Although median hingepoint wedging may assist neural plate bending, experimental evidence suggests that it is neither necessary nor sufficient for neurulation to occur.[53] First, neural plate bending can occur in the absence of median hingepoint wedging. When prospective notochordal cells are destroyed by irradia-

tion[96, 97] or prevented from forming by excision of Hensen's node,[98] median hingepoint cells do not undergo wedging, yet neural plate bending occurs in many cases. Second, when the neural plate is experimentally isolated from more lateral tissues, median hingepoint cells still undergo wedging on schedule, but neurulation fails to occur.[76] It has been suggested that rather than *driving* neural plate bending, median hingepoint wedging may *direct* bending toward a specific site.[53] In this regard, the median hingepoint region may provide a "crease" on which neural plate bending may occur.

According to Schoenwolf and Smith,[53] the dorsolateral hingepoints may play a more important role in neural plate bending, at least in the chick. In one study, wedging of dorsolateral hingepoint cells did not occur in approximately one third of chick embryos treated with cytochalasin D (an agent that disrupts microfilaments). The neural folds in these embryos failed to converge about the dorsolateral hingepoints, and these embryos consequently were dysraphic.[99] A failure of neural fold convergence about the dorsolateral hingepoint region is also a common feature of many animal models of dysraphism (G. Schoenwolf, personal communication, 1990).

The third traditional concept is that cell wedging is the result of changes in cytoskeletal components within the neuroepithelial cells. We have already discussed the conversion of neuroepithelial cells from cuboidal to columnar during neural plate shaping due to the elongation of paraxially oriented microtubules. Similarly, neural plate bending is thought to be due to cell wedging brought about by the contraction of circumferentially oriented apical microfilaments.

A large body of observational and experimental evidence suggests an important role for apical microfilaments in neural plate bending. Apical microfilaments are present in the neuroepithelial cells of a number of animal embryos[54, 61, 65, 100–104] and are better seen during neural plate bending, suggesting a "sliding filament" action.[100] Actin and myosin are both localized to the apices of neuroepithelial cells,[105, 106] and the apical microfilaments bind heavy meromyosin,[102] a component of the actin-myosin complex. When embryos are treated with cytochalasins or vinblastine, agents known to disrupt microfilaments, neurulation often fails to occur.[55, 57, 61, 69, 107–118] Finally, calcium, a mediator of microfilament contraction, has been localized to coated vesicles in the apices of neuroepithelial cells[119] and is released during neurulation.[120] Neural plate bending is impaired by papaverine, which inhibits calcium release, and is promoted by the ionophore A23187, which enhances calcium release.[121, 122]

However, agents used to disrupt microfilament action may adversely affect many other cellular processes[115, 123–125] and may also interfere with many non-neuroepithelial cells that also contain microfilaments. In one study of embryos treated with cytochalasin D, neuroepithelial apical microfilaments were not demonstrable, yet two thirds of treated embryos underwent normal neurulation.[99] It is therefore unclear whether the effect of these agents on neurulation is due to a specific disruption of microfilament-mediated neuroepithelial cell apical constriction.

Alternatively, cells could become wedge shaped through the expansion of the cell base.[53, 55, 126, 127] Burnside[55] suggested that cytoplasm or subcellular organelles could be translocated toward the base of the neuroepithelial cell, expanding the base and producing cell wedging. In the chick, changes in neuroepithelial cell shape are closely correlated with the position of the cell nucleus.[126] The nuclear position varies with the cell cycle (due to interkinetic nuclear migration); nuclei of cells in both the DNA-synthetic (S) and non-DNA-synthetic (non-S) phases of the cell cycle are located near the cell base, whereas those in the mitotic (M) phase are located more centrally.[128–130] During cell wedging, the nucleus is translocated toward the cell base and is associated with a prolongation of both the S and the non-S phases of the cell cycle.[126] Moreover, this change in cell cycle appears to be induced, at least in the median hingepoint, by the notochord. When an accessory notochord is transplanted beneath a more lateral region of the neuroepithelium, a second hingepoint develops over the accessory notochord[98, 131] and exhibits a lower cell-cycle time than the corresponding contralateral region.[131] The stimulus for dorsolateral hingepoint formation is unknown. Finally, whether changes in neuroepithelial cell–cycle times are the cause or the result of changes in cell shape is unknown.

However intriguing, neither apical microfilament contraction nor changes in cell-cycle time have been proved to drive changes in neuroepithelial cell shape. Other cellular mechanisms of potential importance in neuroepithelial cell wedging include the cortical tractoring of adjacent neuroepithelial cells, as proposed by Jacobson and colleagues,[72] and interactions between adjacent neural fold and surface ectodermal cells at the point of divergence of the neural fold from cutaneous ectoderm, as proposed by Martins-Green.[74]

Neural Fold Fusion

Apposition and fusion of the converging neural folds are probably the least understood events in neurulation. The behavior of opposing neuroepithelial cells may involve molecule-molecule, molecule-cell, or cell-cell interactions.[132] At least three cellular mechanisms may contribute, alone or in combination, to neural fold fusion: (1) interactions of cell surface glycoproteins such as glycosaminoglycans (GAGs) or cell adhesion molecules (CAMs); (2) interdigitation of cell surface filopodia, or blebs; and (3) formation of intercellular junctions. All three processes may be involved at different times during neural fold fusion. Cell surface recognition may be the initial event that brings the neural folds into apposition. Interdigitating cell processes may aid further in establishing connections between opposing cell surfaces. Finally, intercellular junctions may serve to establish more permanent connections between adjacent neuroepithelial cells.[133]

Several lines of evidence suggest an important role for cell surface glycoproteins in neural fold fusion. A carbohydrate-rich surface coat material, which stains readily with ruthenium red and lanthanum (which bind to polyvalent anions) and with horseradish peroxidase–labeled concanavalin A (which binds to terminal glycosyl and mannosyl residues), has been demonstrated on the neural folds of amphibian,[134] chick,[135] and mouse[136] embryos. This surface coat material is largely composed of GAGs—complex glycoproteins that contain multiple carbohydrate residues. Both temporal and spatial distributions of cell surface glycoproteins change during neurulation. The labeling of cell surface glycoproteins is scant in early neural groove stages, progressively increases as the neural folds elevate and converge, reaches a maximum just before neural fold fusion, and declines thereafter.[133] Initially, labeling is present along the floor and walls of the neural plate but moves dorsally during neural fold elevation and becomes restricted to the prospective fusion areas of the neural folds.[133] The character of GAGs on the neuroepithelial cell surface also changes during neurulation. Hyaluronic acid is the predominant GAG before neural fold fusion is complete, whereas chondroitin sulfate predominates after neural fold fusion.[133]

Several experimental observations suggest that these cell surface glycoproteins participate in neural fold fusion. Exposing mouse embryos to phospholipase C, which removes surface coat glycoproteins[137]; treating rat embryos with heparatinase, which degrades heparan sulfate, or with β-D-xyloside, which interferes with chondroitin synthesis[80, 84]; and exposing chick embryos to concanavalin A, which binds to carbohydrate residues and interferes with GAG function,[138] all result in neural tube defects. Finally, GAG expression is defective in the splotch mouse (Sp/Sp) mutant; both hyaluronic acid and chondroitin sulfate are present in approximately equal amounts in the open neural tube of affected animals, whereas hyaluronic acid predominates in the normal open neural tube and chondroitin sulfate predominates in the normal closed neural tube.[133]

More recently, a 30-kDa GAG has been discovered on mouse neuroepithelium during neural tube closure and implicated in neural fold fusion. This glycoprotein binds with several exogenously administered carbohydrate-binding lectins. The pattern of lectin binding suggests that this molecule is a complex *N*-linked glycoprotein containing an *N*-acetyl-lactosamine oligosaccharide chain structure.[139] Following the maternal administration of vitamin A, mouse embryos with open neural tube defects exhibit decreased binding of the 30-kDa glycoprotein to carbohydrate-binding lectins compared with littermates with closed neural tubes.[140] A similar decrease in lectin binding of the 30-kDa glycoprotein occurs in the homozygous delayed splotch mouse mutant (Spd/Spd). Binding in the open region of the neural tube is decreased compared with closed regions of the neural tube of Spd/Spd mutants or with the neural tubes of control mice.[139]

Other cell surface molecules may also be important for neural fold fusion. In particular, the cell adhesion molecules N-CAM, E-CAM, and cadherin appear to be important for the separation of neuroectoderm from surface ectoderm. Before neurulation, both prospective epidermal and neuroectodermal cells express E-CAM. However, as neurulation proceeds, neuroepithelial cells stop expressing E-CAM and begin expressing N-CAM and cadherin. As a result, the two tissue types no longer adhere to each other and dissociate. Amphibian embryos in which surface ectodermal cells are made to express N-CAM have difficulty separating the neural tube from the surface ectoderm.[141, 142]

The second cellular mechanism that may contribute to neural fold fusion is the interaction of cell membrane processes. Variably described as filopodia, ruffles, or blebs, these processes have been described on the luminal surfaces of neuroepithelial cells in amphibian,[143] chick,[144–146] and mammalian[147, 148] embryos. Like cell surface glycoproteins, these processes become more prominent throughout neurulation, reach a peak at about the time of neural fold fusion, and decline thereafter. They are most conspicuous on the luminal surfaces of the converging neural folds.[143, 147] The temporal appearance and spatial distribution of these filopodia suggest a role in neural fold fusion, either by aligning the converging neural folds or by drawing the apposed surfaces together.[143, 145]

Eventually, intercellular connections are established between neuroepithelial cells of the apposed neural folds.[149–151] Neither the nature of these junctions (tight or gap) nor their function (cell adhesion, intercellular communication) is known with certainty. Much more work is needed to elucidate the roles of these intercellular junctions as well as the importance of cell surface glycoproteins and filopodia in promoting and maintaining neural fold fusion.

The forces underlying secondary neurulation are even less well understood than those underlying primary neurulation. In the chick, the outer cells of the medullary cord elongate during secondary neurulation to become columnar cells. These shape changes rely at least in part on microtubules, as do those that occur during primary neurulation.[63] The forces that drive

cavitation to form secondary lumina are not understood; however, at least in the chick, cavitation does not rely on hydrostatic pressure from the lumen of the primary neural tube, because these secondary lumina form without a direct connection with the lumen of the primary neural tube.[39] Moreover, when closure of the caudal neuropore is prevented in the chick, eliminating the hydrostatic pressure within the primary neural tube lumen, secondary neurulation occurs normally.[152]

MOLECULAR CONTROL OF EARLY NEURAL DEVELOPMENT

During the past decade, our understanding of the molecular and genetic control of early neural (and vertebral) development has exploded. Early embryonic development is highly controlled at the genetic level by certain *regulatory genes* that encode developmental regulatory proteins that either directly (by binding to regulatory sites on DNA) or indirectly (through inter- and intracellular signaling pathways) regulate the expression of developmental genes and their gene products, controlling the fate of cells and tissues within the embryo. This genetic control is highly conserved across species—both the expression of these regulatory genes and the intra- and intercellular signaling mechanisms by which they exert their control are almost identical, from the fruit fly *Drosophila* to the embryos of fish, amphibians, reptiles, birds, and mammals, including humans. Many of these regulatory proteins are expressed at numerous critical moments during embryogenesis to orchestrate early tissue interactions during gastrulation and neurulation as well as the later development of various organs. The result of these interactions is a tightly integrated and beautifully choreographed molecular "dance" that converts a single-celled zygote into a highly organized embryo. The molecules involved in this molecular control can be divided into two classes: signal transduction molecules and transcription factors.

Signal Transduction Pathways

Developmental regulatory genes all encode RNA or proteins that have, either directly or indirectly, a single function—regulation of DNA transcription, messenger RNA translation, or post-translational modification of gene products. Many are involved in the transfer of information from the cell surface to the genome through signal transduction pathways. Although the specifics of each pathway are different, all signal transduction pathways use common elements. A membrane-bound protein on the surface of the target cell interacts with an external ligand (usually a membrane-bound or secreted factor from another cell or group of cells). The membrane-bound protein on the target cell has an extracellular portion (the receptor) to which the ligand binds, a membrane-spanning region, and an intracellular portion. Receptor-ligand binding results in a conformational change in the receptor, thereby exposing or activating enzymatic sites on the intracellular portion of the molecule. Most commonly, the intracellular portion is a protein kinase of some sort, which uses adenosine triphosphate to phosphorylate a second intracellular messenger or cascade of messengers. Eventually, a transcription factor is activated, binds to regulatory regions of the DNA, and initiates or modulates the expression of multiple genes.

A number of signal transduction pathways have been studied, and their detailed descriptions can be found in Gilbert's textbook *Developmental Biology.*[153] The complexity within each pathway and the opportunity for cross-communication between pathways create numerous ways in which these pathways can be developmentally regulated. To understand the complexity of signal transduction pathways during development, consider the interaction of two *Drosophila* genes, *hedgehog* and *wingless*, which are expressed by cells in adjacent embryonic segments (Fig. 281–12).

Hedgehog, a signal transduction protein that is extremely important in the development of both the spinal cord and the vertebral column, is secreted from one cell and binds with the receptor *patched* on the surface of an adjacent cell. The binding of hedgehog to patched activates a third membrane-bound protein, *smoothened*. Activation of smoothened sets in motion a cascade of intracellular second messengers within the second cell, eventually activating the transcription of the gene *wingless* and the synthesis of the wingless protein. The wingless protein is secreted from the second cell and binds to a cell surface protein "frizzled" on the first. This interaction activates the intracellular protein *disheveled*, which then blocks the inhibiting action of Zw3kinase on β-catenin (also called *armadillo*), effectively activating β-catenin. β-catenin induces the tran-

scription of *engrailed*, a transcription factor that then activates the transcription of hedgehog. A positive feedback loop is thereby established between the two sets of cells, creating a distinct border between adjacent segments that have very different molecular expression. These borders are important in establishing segmentation in *Drosophila* as well as rostrocaudal metameric patterning in the vertebrate nervous system and spinal column.[153, 154]

Transcription Factors

A second class of regulatory developmental genes are the transcription factors—molecules that bind to DNA regulatory sites and modulate the transcription of other genes. These transcription factors are often the end products of the signal transduction pathways just described. Briefly, gene transcription is controlled by two types of regulators: *cis-regulators* and *trans-regulators*. Cis-regulators are specific DNA sequences that regulate the transcription of other genes only within the same strand of DNA. There are two types of cis-regulators: *promoters* and *enhancers*. Promoters are usually located immediately upstream from a gene and initiate transcription by binding RNA polymerase. Enhancers bind to the polymerase-promoter complex and control the efficiency of transcription by the promoter. Enhancers can either promote or suppress DNA transcription but can affect genes only within the same strand of DNA.[153]

In contrast, trans-regulators—also called transcription factors—are soluble molecules, including DNA sequences, RNA sequences, or peptides, that interact with promoters or enhancers on the same or different strands of DNA to modulate transcription. Most tran-

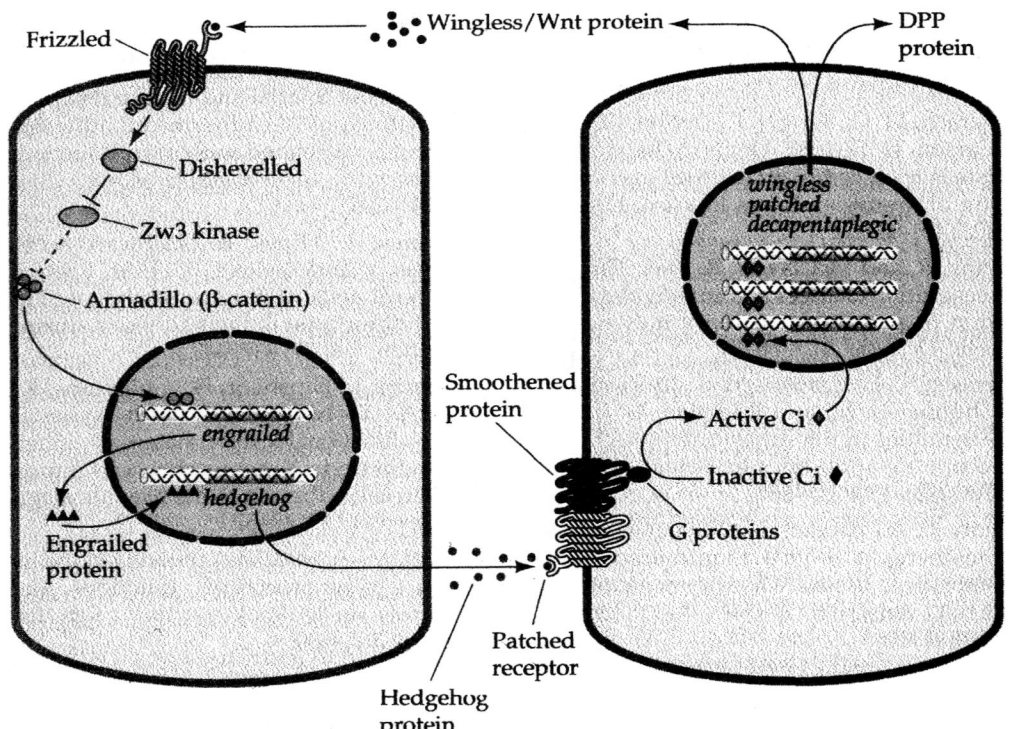

FIGURE 281–12. Reciprocal molecular interactions between adjacent cells establish segmentation patterns in *Drosophila* and are also responsible for metameric patterning in vertebrate embryos. (From Gilbert SF: Developmental Biology. Sunderland, MA, Sinauer Associates, 1997.)

scription factors have both a DNA-binding domain that binds with the promoter or enhancer region and other binding domains that interact with other DNA segments or regulators.

There are various classes of transcription factors, including the POU transcription class (the initials POU are derived from the first four proteins described with such domains: Pit-1, Oct-1, Oct-2, and Unc-86), the basic helix-loop-helix class, the basic leucine zipper class, the zinc finger class, the nuclear hormone receptor class, and the DNA bending class, each using a different mechanism to control DNA transcription. One large class of transcription factors are the *homeodomain proteins*, which are extremely important during development. These proteins have a DNA-binding region (the homeodomain) consisting of 60 amino acids arranged in a helix-turn-helix arrangement. The third helix in this arrangement extends into the major groove of the DNA at specific promoter sites, and other amino acids insert into the minor groove. Minor mutations (even a single amino acid substitution) can cause the homeodomain to recognize different promoters. The homeodomain proteins control the specification of metameric body patterning in all species from *Drosophila* to humans.[153]

One of the overriding principles governing embryonic assembly is the process of *embryonic induction,* whereby a particular group of embryonic cells controls the developmental fate of an adjacent group of cells. From the standpoint of the early nervous system and vertebral column, the most important inductive interactions are (1) the formation of an embryonic "organizer" through the interaction of specialized cells (the Nieuwkoop center in amphibians, and the posterior marginal zone in avian embryos) with adjacent, previously uncommitted cells; (2) the induction of midline mesoderm and neuroectoderm by the organizer during gastrulation and the subsequent control of neurulation; and (3) the rostrocaudal segmentation of the neural tube into various regions and the metameric patterning of each.[153] Each of these inductions involves the genetic control of cell fate in the responding tissues by signaling and transcription factors expressed by the inducing tissues.

Induction of the Organizer

A specialized area of dorsal cells in amphibian embryos, referred to as the Nieuwkoop center, performs a specific and highly important function—induction of the embryonic organizer. A homologous structure in chick embryos, the posterior marginal zone, is located at the caudal end of the embryo and appears to function in a similar manner. Both the Nieuwkoop center and the posterior marginal zone induce adjacent cells to become the embryonic organizer. Cells from both the Nieuwkoop center in amphibian embryos and the homologous posterior marginal zone in avian embryos express a number of common gene products, including β-catenin, Siamois, noggin, activin, goosecoid, and the activated form of Vg1.[153, 155] Experimental evidence suggests that these factors induce the adjacent cells to form

the organizer by repressing the ventralizing factor bone morphogenetic protein (BMP)–4 (which is expressed by the ventral cells of the embryo) in one of the earliest embryonic inductions. The formation of the organizer—referred to variously as the dorsal lip of the blastopore in amphibians, the embryonic shield in fish, and Hensen's node in birds and mammals—is critical to the formation of the notochord and the neuraxis.

Induction of Neuroectoderm by the Organizer

Gastrulation is initiated at, and organized by, the organizer. As prospective endodermal and chordamesodermal (notochordal and prochordal plate) cells migrate into the organizer, ingress, and come to underlie the midline dorsal ectoderm, molecular interactions between the future neuroectoderm and the organizer or its derivatives—the chordamesoderm and the endoderm—induce the formation of neuroepithelium. When the organizer is transplanted to the ventral side of a host amphibian embryo (or an uncommitted area of the chick embryo), the organizer can induce the formation of a secondary neuraxis from the ventral host structures.[156–159] The traditional view is that it is the chordamesoderm that induces the overlying neuroepithelium. However, other experimental evidence suggests that the endoderm may be important as well.[157] Moreover, induction may involve both "vertical" induction of the ectoderm from the underlying chordamesoderm or endoderm and "horizontal" or "planar" induction (within the plane of the ectoderm) from the organizer itself.[160] The inductive capacity of the organizer probably involves the secretion of a diffusible substance, because the organizer retains its inductive capacities even when separated from the responding tissue by a microfilter.[161–163]

The molecular mechanisms underlying this remarkable induction have been identified with the advent of molecular techniques.[153, 155, 160, 164] The organizer expresses a set of gene products. In amphibians, these include the homeodomain proteins Xlim1, Xnot, and goosecoid; the winged-helix (forkhead motif) protein HNF3β; the Brachyury transcription protein; and the secreted factors chondrin, noggin, and follistatin.[153, 165] In avian embryos, Hensen's node expresses the homologous homeodomain proteins goosecoid (and a related goosecoid protein, GSX), the homeodomain protein Otx2, HNF3β, hepatocyte growth factor–scatter factor, and the CNOT proteins CNOT1 and CNOT2. Several other homeodomain proteins are also expressed somewhat later.[160, 166] In mouse embryos, the node expresses goosecoid, Lim1, HNF3β, and the secreted proteins noggin and nodal; follistatin is not expressed.[13] Several of the secreted products of the organizer such as goosecoid, noggin, and follistatin antagonize the action of BMP-4 from the ventral cells, further promoting the recruitment and expression of dorsal cell types within the organizer. Thus, the regional expression of dorsal factors from the organizer and their antagonism of the ventralizing factor BMP-4 perpetuate the dorsal phenotype of cells within the organizer.[160, 164, 166] Many of these proteins are capable of inducing secondary neuraxes when added to indifferent regions of host embryos, and their misexpression in various mutants leads to deficiencies in the neuraxis.[13, 155, 160, 165, 167–169]

The ingressing chordamesoderm also expresses many of the factors secreted by the organizer.[166] Sonic hedgehog (shh) is expressed sequentially within the organizer, the developing notochord, and the midline floor-plate cells of the neural tube. The expression of shh is important for the development of the ventral neural tube, the sclerotome from the somite, and the spinal motoneurons.[154] In addition, goosecoid and Otx2 are expressed in the prochordal plate mesoderm, and CNOT1 is expressed in the notochord and tail bud.[160]

The molecular induction of the ectoderm to form neuroepithelium turns out to involve a somewhat indirect pathway. In the absence of any outside influence, isolated ectoderm forms neuroectoderm rather than epidermis. During normal development, this "default pathway" for ectoderm is inhibited by BMP-4 expressed by both ventral cells and the early ectoderm itself, thus inhibiting neuronal differentiation and promoting cutaneous ectodermal differentiation. Factors secreted by the organizer and its derivatives, such as noggin, follistatin, and chondrin, acting alone or in combination, suppress or antagonize the expression of BMP-4 and allow the ectoderm to follow its default pathway to form neuroectoderm (reviewed in references 165, 166, 169, 170). This "permissive interaction" is repeated often during early development; cellular determination is controlled by inhibiting a factor (or factors) that would otherwise produce an alternative cell fate.

A number of experimental observations support this view.[170] For example, follistatin, chondrin, and noggin have all been shown to bind to BMPs with high affinity and to suppress BMP activity, and both follistatin and noggin are capable of inducing secondary neuraxes from indifferent areas of host embryos. Other factors secreted by the organizer, such as hepatocyte growth factor–scatter factor in the chick, are also capable of inducing secondary neuraxes from isolated epiblast explants.[165] However, some of these interactions may be species specific. For example, the mouse node does not express follistatin yet is capable of inducing a neuraxis.[170] There are likely to be redundant mechanisms in place to ensure the fidelity of such an important embryonic process.

Primary Neurulation: Specification of Notochord and Floor Plate

The initial event in the bending of the neural plate to form the neural tube is the conformational cell shape change, from columnar to trapezoidal, among neuroepithelial cells overlying the notochord. This process, which results in the formation of a floor plate, or median hingepoint, is controlled by inductive interactions between the notochord and the floor-plate cells (reviewed in reference 53). Embryos in which the notochord is missing develop a neural tube but lack a floor plate. Conversely, transplanting a second notochord to

the lateral regions of the neural tube of a host embryo can induce an accessory floor plate.[98, 131] The expression of the homeodomain protein shh from the notochord is the molecular substrate for the formation of the median hingepoint. In addition, the expression of shh from the notochord or the induced floor-plate cells controls the differentiation of ventral horn motoneurons.[154, 171] Mutants that lack notochordal shh expression have neither a floor plate nor ventral horn motoneurons. Conversely, shh induces secondary floor-plate reactions and ectopic ventral horn motoneurons when placed adjacent to more lateral regions of the neural tube or in neural plate explants.[154, 165] In the mouse, loss of shh expression in the head mesenchyma and rostral neural tube can result in holoprosencephaly[154] and neural tube defects.[153] Point mutations in the human shh locus may be responsible for certain cases of familial holoprosencephaly.[154]

Sonic hedgehog is composed of a membrane-bound N-terminal peptide, responsible for both short- and long-range interactions of shh, and a freely diffusible C-terminal portion, which is cleaved from the parent molecule through internal autoproteolytic cleavage.[154] The N-terminal peptide spans the membrane and is bound intracellularly by cholesterol; drugs that inhibit cholesterol synthesis are potent teratogens and can produce both holoprosencephaly[154] and neural tube defects.[153] Sonic hedgehog is a signal transduction protein whose receptors include the transmembrane proteins patched and smoothened. Binding of shh with patched produces a conformational change in smoothened that initiates an intracellular cascade involving the zinc finger protein cubitus interruptus, costal, suppresser of fused, threonine kinase fused, and the cyclic adenosine monophosphate–dependent protein kinase A.[154]

The actions of shh on the neuroectoderm are concentration dependent. High concentrations of shh or even direct contact between notochordal and neuroectodermal cells is required to induce a floor-plate response, whereas a lower concentration of shh is required for ventral horn motoneuron differentiation.[154, 165] The type of ventral cell induced depends on its position along the rostrocaudal axis and is probably determined by interactions between shh and other rostrocaudal patterning cues. At more caudal levels, shh induces spinal cord motoneurons, whereas at midbrain and hindbrain levels, ventrolateral dopaminergic and cholinergic cell types form.[154]

The dorsoventral differentiation of the neural tube seems to be established through competitive interactions between shh (and perhaps also HNF3β) derived from the notochord and other "dorsalizing factors" derived from the cutaneous ectoderm and dorsal part of the neural tube. Both the cutaneous ectoderm and the dorsal neural tube express a number of neural dorsalizing factors, including BMP-4 and BMP-7, Pax3, msx-1, and dorsalin-1 (dsl-1), all of which promote the differentiation of dorsal cell types from the neural tube under experimental conditions. For example, application of dsl-1 protein to the neural plate inhibits the formation of ventral motoneurons and promotes the migration of neural crest cells.[165] Therefore, the dorsoventral polarity of the neural tube is established through competing interactions between these dorsalizing and ventralizing factors. Unfortunately, the molecular underpinnings of a more important process, the formation of the dorsolateral hingepoints, are unknown.

The final event in primary neurulation is the medial convergence and fusion of the neural folds. A number of observations suggest an important role for the homeobox gene *Pax3* in this process (reviewed in reference 172). The geographic and temporal expression of Pax3 in the dorsal neural tube precisely at the time of neural tube closure suggests that the Pax3 gene product might be important in neural fold fusion. Antisense oligonucleotides that block the function of Pax3 result in neural tube defects in mice. Moreover, the locus for the Sp mouse mutant, which exhibits neural tube defects (exencephaly and myelomeningocele), maps precisely to the *Pax3* locus. Last, the Sp mutant is the mouse homologue of the human Waardenburg's syndrome type I, and myelomeningoceles have been reported in at least one family with this disorder.[173]

Determination of Neural Crest Fate

Experimental evidence suggests that neural crest cells initially are multipotent but eventually become restricted to a particular cell type (terminal differentiation). At least three growth factors appear to be involved in the specification of neural crest cell fates: glial growth factor, which promotes glial differentiation; transforming growth factor-β, which promotes smooth muscle differentiation; and BMP-2 and -4, which promote autonomic differentiation. The temporal and spatial expression of these three growth factors suggests a direct role in neural crest determination. Moreover, targeted mutations of glial growth factor and transforming growth factor-β alter the terminal differentiation of neural crest cells to peripheral nerve cells and cardiac myocytes, respectively (reviewed in reference 174).

Other factors also influence neural crest determination. For example, the homeobox gene *MASH1* is expressed in autonomic (sympathetic and parasympathetic) but not sensory neurons, and a targeted mutation of *MASH1* blocks the development of autonomic neurons. *MASH1* is induced by BMP-2 (which itself is involved in autonomic determination). It is likely that a number of factors are involved, in a cascading fashion, in progressively specifying the fate of neural crest cells.[174, 175]

Rostrocaudal and Metameric Specification of the Neuraxis

In original experiments in which an organizer was transplanted to an indifferent site of a host embryo and a new neuraxis was induced, the age of the organizer determined the type of neuroepithelium that was induced in the host. Organizers from younger embryos induced rostral neuroepithelium, whereas organizers from slightly older embryos induced caudal neuroepi-

thelium.[156] This finding suggested that the organizer or its derivatives may emit at least two separate signals, which not only induce the neuroepithelium but also organize it along its rostrocaudal axis. According to this model, the interaction of two signals, one specifying a more rostral phenotype (forebrain, midbrain) and the second specifying more caudal structures (hindbrain, spinal cord), each expressed in different geographic patterns, could determine the craniocaudal pattern of the neuraxis.[156, 158, 165, 176, 177] More recent molecular approaches seem to support this view. For example, noggin, chondrin, follistatin, and Lim1 can induce rostral but not caudal neural tissue, whereas other factors such as retinoic acid and fibroblast growth factor induce more caudal regions of the neuraxis.[153, 164, 165, 168–170]

To properly understand the organization of the vertebrate neural tube, one must first understand the progressive specification of craniocaudal patterning in *Drosophila* in response to certain homeotic genes and their gene products. During normal development, the craniocaudal axis of *Drosophila* embryos is determined by the craniocaudal gradients of four proteins derived from the mother: bicoid, hunchback, nanos, and caudal. The highest concentrations of hunchback and bicoid are rostral, whereas the highest concentrations of nanos and caudal are caudal. Therefore, separate signals appear to specify rostral and caudal differentiation of the embryonic axis (reviewed in reference 153).

The gradients of these four proteins set in motion the sequential expression of sets of embryonic gap genes, pair-rule genes, and segment polarity genes, each set resulting in a progressively greater craniocaudal segmentation of the *Drosophila* embryo. Within each segment, specific collections of transcription factors are expressed, all having in common a DNA-binding segment called a homeodomain, which is encoded by a 180–base pair region of the DNA called the homeobox gene. The homeodomain binds to the promoter regions of other genes on the DNA, directs the transcription of many other gene products, and establishes a craniocaudal pattern within each segment. Interactions between homeodomain proteins from adjacent segments establish and maintain the segmental pattern of the embryo. "Homeotic" mutants, mutants that misexpress certain of the homeodomain proteins in various segments, can have bizarre phenotypes. For example, the misexpression of the *Antennapedia* gene within the head segment leads to legs rather than eyes growing out of the head.[153]

Homeobox genes are highly conserved across many species from *Drosophila* to humans (in whom they are referred to as *Hox* genes), and the transcription factors they encode control rostrocaudal patterning in higher vertebrates as well. For example, the homeobox genes *Lim1* and *Otx2* appear to be important in organizing head regions of the embryo. A knockout mutation of either of these genes produces mice lacking all neuraxial structures rostral to the otic vesicles but having normal trunk structures.[168, 178] Siamois may also play a role in rostral neural development; overexpression of siamois in *Xenopus* embryos results in the duplication of rostral neuraxial structures.[164] Another homeobox gene, *cerberus*, seems to specifically induce forebrain regions.[169] Other homeobox genes likely control more caudal neuraxial development but have not yet been characterized.

The earliest expression of these genes determines patterning in a more broad sense, such as the division of the neuraxis into prosencephalon, the mesencephalon-metencephalon border, and the myelencephalon, each having a distinct pattern of genetic expression.[179] Later, the expression of various homeobox genes controls the metameric segmentation *within* each segment.[169, 178–183] The metameric segmentation of the rhombencephalon into its constituent rhombomeres has been particularly well studied.[169, 178, 183] Various homeobox genes have been mapped to this region, and the boundaries of expression of various genes coincide with the boundaries of the rhombomeres, with a two-rhombomere periodicity.[169] The pattern and distribution of these various homeobox genes may determine the regional characteristics of each rhombomere,[169] although these interrelationships are complicated and not entirely defined. The expression of the homeobox genes of the rhombencephalon is controlled by other homeobox genes such as *Krox-20*, *kriesler*, and *c-maf*.[169] Metameric patterning in other segments of the neuraxis, including the spinal cord, is not as well worked out but is likely to be similarly controlled by homeobox genes.[169]

One of the most fascinating aspects of homeobox function is the discovery that these genes may provide cues for targeted axon outgrowth. For example, it has long been known that the growth of axons from the retina to the tectum of the midbrain is highly ordered, with nasal retinal axons projecting to the caudal tectum and temporal retinal axons projecting to the rostral tectum. If the tectum is experimentally rotated, retinal axons change direction and innervate their original tectal targets despite the new positions of the targets. A similar specificity exists in the outgrowth of spinal motoneurons to their target muscles in the limbs (reviewed in reference 170). Sperry[184] proposed the *chemoaffinity hypothesis* for directed axonal outgrowth. The theory states that both axons and their targets acquire specific positional information during embryonic life and that the nature of this information is chemical or molecular.

More recent studies have demonstrated that when the tectum is reversed, the expression gradient of En1 is also reversed. Moreover, when the En1 gradient is experimentally altered by misexpressing En1 in the rostral tectum, nasal retinal axons are redirected toward the rostral tectum.[169] En1 may, in turn, act by controlling the rostrocaudal expression of other proteins such as ligands for Eph-related receptor tyrosine kinases, RAGS, and ELF-1, which are also expressed in a rostrocaudal gradient and may function as growth inhibitors of temporal retinotectal axons that express a Mek-4 receptor.[169] Similarly, the differential expression of various Lim homeodomain transcription factors from various types of spinal motoneurons may guide their axons to specific muscle targets in the limb.[170]

Therefore, the homeobox genes, by controlling protein expression, may provide the chemical signal for directed axon outgrowth.

ABNORMAL EARLY NEURAL DEVELOPMENT

A large number of human neural malformations have been ascribed to disorders of early neural embryogenesis. As already discussed, the traditional classification scheme, which divides these malformations into open and closed types, is confusing at best and misleading at worst. We prefer a classification scheme based on reputed embryonic mechanisms (Table 281–1). However, it is important to recognize at the outset that all these embryogenetic theories are speculative, and none of them has been validated experimentally.

Failure of Neural Tube Closure: Neural Tube Defects

Myelomeningocele and anencephaly are thought to arise through one of two mechanisms. The nonclosure theory[185] proposes that neural tube defects (NTDs) represent a primary failure of neural tube closure. The overdistention theory, introduced in 1769 by Morgagni[186] and popularized by Gardner,[187–190] proposes that NTDs arise through overdistention and rupture of a previously closed neural tube. The nonclosure theory is more widely accepted; however, overdistention may contribute to some experimental NTD models, particu-

---

TABLE 281–1 ■ **Embryologic Classification of Dysraphic Malformations**

Disordered Midline Axial Integration during Gastrulation
  Split cord malformations
  Combined spina bifida
  Neurenteric cysts
  Some myelomeningoceles
  Some cervical myelomeningoceles
  Hemimyelomeningoceles
  Some examples of caudal agenesis and Klippel-Feil syndrome
  Complex dysraphic malformations

Localized Failure of Neurulation
  Myelomeningocele
  Anencephaly

Premature Ectodermal Dysjunction
  Lipomyelomeningoceles

Incomplete Ectodermal Dysjunction
  Dermal sinus tracts, dermoid or epidermoid tumors

Disordered Secondary Neurulation
  Terminal spinal lipomas
  Fatty filum terminale
  Myelocystoceles
  Currarino's triad

Postneurulation Disorders
  Encephaloceles
  Chiari II malformation

larly those caused by vitamin A[191] and the T-curtailed mouse mutant.[192]

Neural tube closure requires the complex interaction of multiple cellular processes. Consequently, it is not surprising that NTDs may result from a number of embryonic insults. NTDs have been produced experimentally using a number of teratogens (reviewed by Campbell and coworkers[2]), genetic mutations (reviewed by Copp and coworkers[192, 193]), and experimental manipulations (reviewed by Schoenwolf and Smith[53]). Although these all suggest a number of potential mechanisms whereby NTDs might arise, the cause of human malformations remains unknown. NTDs most likely have heterogeneous causes[1, 2, 192, 193] and are the result of a variety of embryonic disorders.

Genetic models of NTDs provide a means of identifying particular genes that might be involved in neural tube closure.[192, 193] Three examples illustrate the variety of ways genetic mutations can result in an NTD. The Sp mouse mutants are identified by a peculiar patch of white fur and exhibit both exencephaly and myelomeningoceles. The genetic locus for the Sp mutation is within the *Pax3* gene (discussed earlier). Although the Pax3 gene product appears to be involved in apposition and fusion of the neural folds, neither the mechanisms underlying the normal Pax3 gene product nor the mechanisms whereby the Sp mutation alters Pax3 function are known with certainty.

A second mouse mutant, curly tail, exhibits posterior NTDs and tail deformities associated with a delay in the closure of the caudal neuropore.[193] However, the delay is not the result of faulty neuroepithelial development, because isolated neuroepithelium from curly-tail mutants undergoes normal neurulation.[194] Rather, there is a delay in cell proliferation in the underlying notochord and hindgut endoderm, which causes an abnormal ventral curvature to the body axis and impedes posterior neuropore closure.[192, 193] If the ventral curvature is corrected by splinting the caudal curly-tail embryo with an eyelash[195] or by retarding neuroepithelial proliferation with retinoic acid,[196] the posterior neuropore closes normally, and the incidence of NTDs is reduced.

A third mouse mutant, T-curtailed, produces a lumbosacral myelomeningocele with dorsoventral forking of the caudal neural tube. However, rather than delayed or failed neural tube closure, the T-curtailed mutation causes rupture of the roof plate and reopening of a previously closed neural tube.[192]

A large number of environmental causes of NTDs have been identified and their underlying mechanisms studied. Recent attention has focused on the role of folate in the embryogenesis of NTDs. Maternal administration of folate antagonists such as aminopterin has long been known to produce NTDs.[197] Periconceptional administration of supplemental folate in randomized, placebo-controlled studies reduced both the recurrence rate of NTDs among women with previous affected pregnancies and the incidence among women without previous affected pregnancies.[198, 199] However, studies of maternal serum and red blood cell folate levels among mothers of infants with myelomeningocele

have produced inconsistent results (reviewed in Wald[200] and Seller[201]), and folate deficiency does not cause NTDs in mice or rat embryos (reviewed in Fleming and Copp[202]). These observations suggest that NTDs are seldom the result of an *absolute* folate deficiency.

More recent attention has focused on the possibility that NTDs are caused by abnormalities involving metabolic pathways (in either the mother or the fetus) that require folate[203]—abnormalities that predispose an individual to NTDs and might therefore be overcome by folate supplementation. Folate and its metabolites tetrahydrofolate and 5-methyltetrahydrofolate are important in a variety of mammalian metabolic reactions, including purine and pyrimidine (and therefore DNA) synthesis, and in the transfer of methyl groups during the metabolism of methionine and homocysteine (Fig. 281–13). In particular, the role of folate in methionine and homocysteine metabolism has generated considerable interest.[204–212]

The metabolism of homocysteine follows one of two pathways. One involves a trans-sulfuration to cystathionine, catalyzed by the enzyme cystathionine synthase. The second is the remethylation of homocysteine to methionine, catalyzed by the enzyme methionine synthase and requiring the donation of a methyl group from the folate metabolite 5-methyltetrahydrofolate (which, in turn, is converted to tetrahydrofolate), using vitamin B_{12} as a cofactor. Methionine is activated by adenosine triphosphate to produce S-adenosylmethionine, which is then used to donate a methyl group in a variety of cellular reactions involving protein, lipid, DNA, and RNA metabolism. Tetrahydrofolate is converted back to 5-methyltetrahydrofolate by the enzyme 5,10-methylenetetrahydrofolate reductase (see Fig. 281–13).

One hypothesis is that maternal or fetal mutations in either methionine synthase or 5,10-methylenetetrahydrofolate reductase may slow down this methylation cycle, drive the conversion of methionine to homocysteine, and lead to methionine deficiency or homocysteine excess. Ingestion of higher doses of folate may overcome this relative deficiency by restoring more normal homocysteine and methionine levels.[203, 211, 213] A number of observations support this view. For example, elevated maternal homocysteine levels have been identified in women carrying fetuses with NTDs, both in serum[212] and in amniotic fluid.[211] Disordered methionine metabolism has been demonstrated in nonpregnant women who had previously given birth to children with NTDs.[211, 213] Finally, mutations of the 5,10-methylenetetrahydrofolate reductase gene have been demonstrated in 18% of individuals with NTDs and in 13% of parents of children with NTDs, compared with 6% of controls.[209, 214] Abnormalities of cystathionine synthase have also been identified.[211]

A number of teratogens are known to act through a variety of cellular mechanisms to cause NTDs in animals and humans (see Copp and colleagues[192] for a review). One important teratogen, valproic acid, produces NTDs in both animal models and humans, probably by inhibiting neural fold fusion.[192] Although the

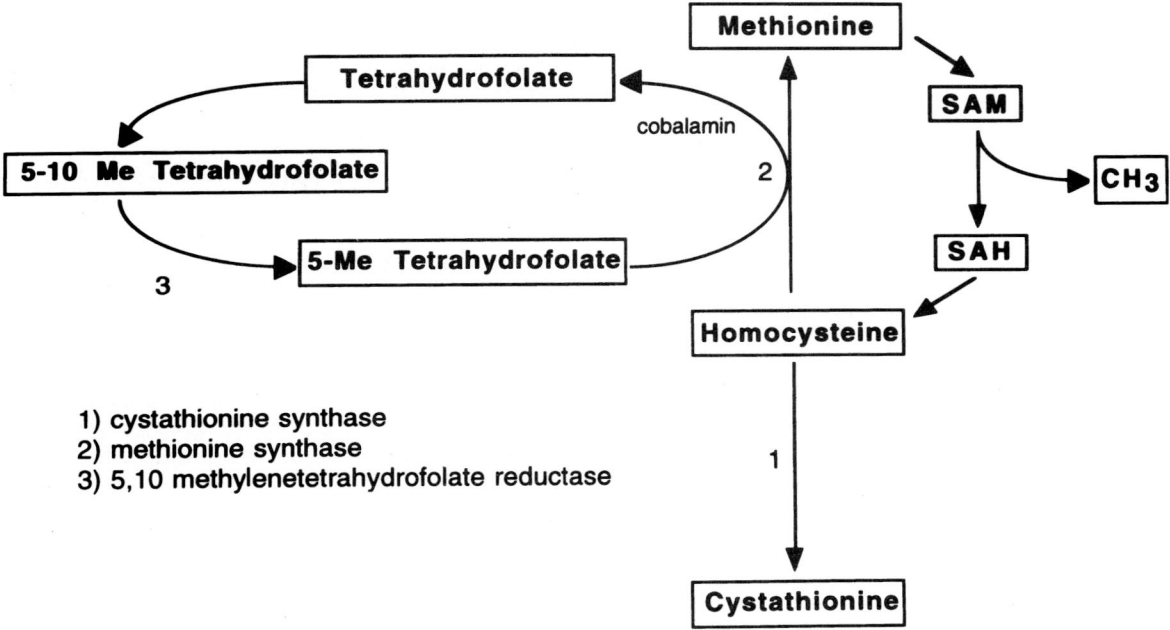

FIGURE 281–13. Metabolic pathways requiring folate that may be involved in the genesis of neural tube defects (myelomeningocele).

exact mechanism is unknown, valproic acid appears to disrupt folate metabolic pathways,[215] perhaps by interfering with the conversion of tetrahydrofolate to 5-formyltetrahydrofolate.[211] Maternal folate administration reduces the incidence of valproic acid–associated NTDs in some but not all studies,[215] and mouse strains that are susceptible to valproate-induced NTDs have significantly lower levels of 5,10-methylenetetrahydrofolate after valproate administration compared with resistant strains.[216] In addition, a number of developmental regulatory genes (such as transcription factors and cell-cycle checkpoint genes) may be altered in these susceptible strains.[217] One hypothesis is that valproic acid may act by changing folate-dependent methylation of regulatory proteins such as transcription factors.

Whatever the underlying causes of NTDs, the result is an open, unneurulated segment of neural tube, the nature and severity of which are determined by the location and length of the unneurulated segment. A failure of caudal neurulation produces a myelomeningocele. The term *myelomeningocele* has been used to refer to an open caudal neural tube in association with a fluid-filled sac, whereas *myeloschisis* has been defined as a completely open caudal neural tube having no evidence of a central canal[218] or investing meninges.[219] However, this classification is confusing and imprecise because in both cases, a portion of the neural tube has failed to close, the neural folds remain attached to the adjacent cutaneous ectoderm, and the placode is therefore exposed on the dorsal surface of the embryo. Because the exposed placode is attached to the cutaneous ectoderm, cerebrospinal fluid (CSF) can form only in the subarachnoid space beneath the placode. The extent to which the CSF displaces the placode dorsally

determines the characteristics of the malformation. In myelomeningocele, the accumulation of CSF displaces the neural placode to the top of a fluid-filled sac (Fig. 281–14). In myeloschisis, CSF does not accumulate beneath the placode (perhaps because it is vented through the central canal or through a tear in the attenuated surrounding tissues). Instead, the placode lies flush with the skin. Therefore, these two malformations likely share a common embryogenesis, with their morphologic differences reflecting only differences in subsequent development. We suggest that the term *myeloschisis* be discarded and that all such lesions be referred to as myelomeningoceles.

The embryogenesis of cervical and upper thoracic

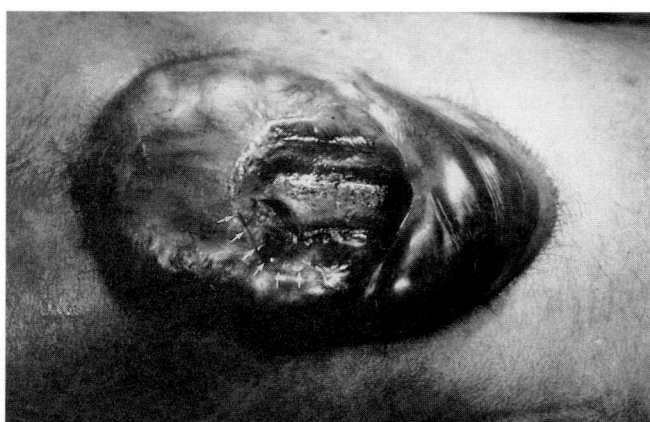

FIGURE 281–14. Human neural tube defect. Lumbosacral myelomeningocele in a newborn infant. The placode lies atop a cerebrospinal fluid–containing cystic sac and is attached *(arrows)* circumferentially to the adjacent surface ectoderm.

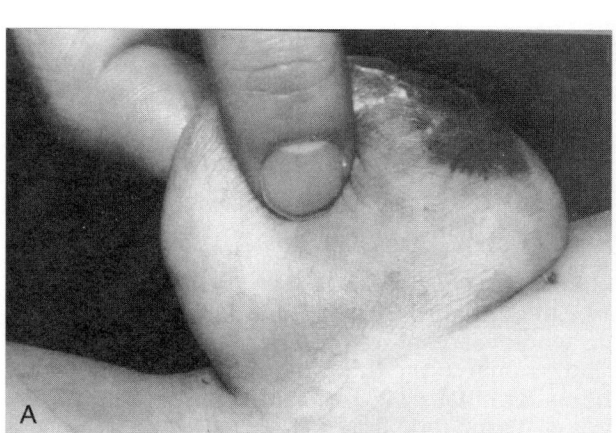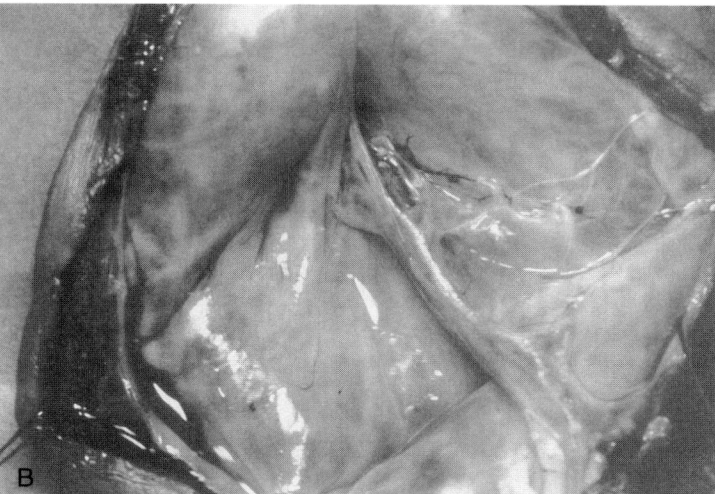

FIGURE 281–15. Cervical myelomeningocele. *A,* A full-thickness, skin-covered sac lies on the dorsum of the child's neck. The dome is violaceous and scarified. *B,* Once opened, the dome contains a small stalk of tissue that exits from the spinal canal through a tiny fascial defect.

myelomeningoceles deserves special mention.[220, 221] These cervicothoracic lesions are unique in several respects. First, cervicothoracic lesions are usually closed and have a tough covering of skin or a thick fibrous membrane and no exposed placode or CSF leakage (Fig. 281–15*A*). In contrast, lumbosacral myelomeningoceles are open and associated with an exposed placode and CSF leakage. Second, cervicothoracic lesions have only a limited fascial defect, and posterior bony dysraphism is minimal or absent. In contrast, lumbosacral fascial defects are larger, and posterior bony dysraphism is widespread. Third, cervicothoracic lesions contain only a small stalk of neural tissue, which arises *en passage* from the dorsum of the spinal cord, penetrates the small fascial defect, and ends along the inner surface of the sac (see Fig. 281–15*B*). There is an underlying split cord malformation in 45% of cases, and the stalk of neural tissue arises from the medial aspects of both hemicords.[221] In contrast, lumbosacral myelomeningoceles usually contain a large terminal placode, representing the unneurulated end of the neural tube. Fourth, cervicothoracic lesions are usually associated with normal or almost normal sensorimotor function caudal to the malformation, whereas lumbosacral lesions usually are associated with complete sensorimotor paralysis below the malformation.

Three embryogenetic mechanisms for cervicothoracic myelomeningoceles have been proposed. Single cord lesions may involve either a limited failure of dorsal closure, involving only the terminal stages of neural fold fusion and with minimal disruption of the surrounding mesenchyme,[221] or they may represent a form of myelocystocele in which the dorsal aspect of the neural tube, together with the surrounding dura and mesenchyma, expands into a posterior sac.[220] Lesions associated with an underlying split cord malformation may share a common embryogenesis with other forms of split cord malformations and complex dysraphic malformations (see later).[1, 221]

Finally, we should distinguish between myelomeningoceles, which arise through disordered neural tube closure, and the much more rare meningoceles, which are thought to be the products of a postneurulation disorder. In these malformations, neurulation has occurred relatively normally beneath the cutaneous lesion. However, the subsequent development of the overlying mesenchymal tissues and cutaneous ectoderm is aberrant and results in a cutaneous and mesenchymal defect that contains only CSF. The embryogenesis of meningoceles is unclear.

Incomplete Dysjunction: Dermal Sinus and Dermoid and Epidermoid Tumors

Dermal sinuses incorporate a tract of cutaneous ectoderm from the dorsal midline skin that extends for a variable distance into the underlying mesenchymal tissues and, in many instances, penetrates the dura to end within the thecal sac adjacent to or contiguous with the neural tube. Approximately 60% of dermal sinuses contain a dermoid or epidermoid tumor; conversely, approximately 30% of dermoid or epidermoid tumors occur in association with dermal sinus tracts.[222, 223] Cutaneous anomalies are frequently present and include skin dimples, hairy patches, and cutaneous nevi or hemangiomas.

The most widely accepted theory of embryogenesis for dermal sinus tracts proposes that they arise through faulty separation (dysjunction) of neuroectoderm from the overlying cutaneous ectoderm,[224] leaving a tongue of cutaneous ectoderm that becomes sequestered between the dorsal ectodermal (skin) surface and the neural tube (Fig. 281–16). Differentiation of this tract may produce a number of cutaneous ectodermal abnormalities, including epithelial-lined sinuses (dermal sinus tracts), epidermoid tumors (containing only ectodermal tissue, such as pseudostratified squamous epithelium), or dermoid tumors (containing both ecto-

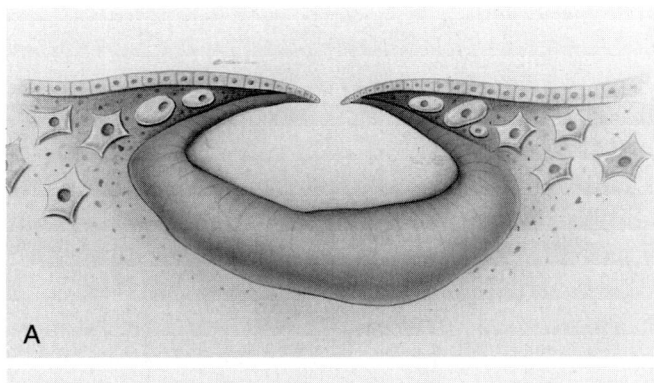

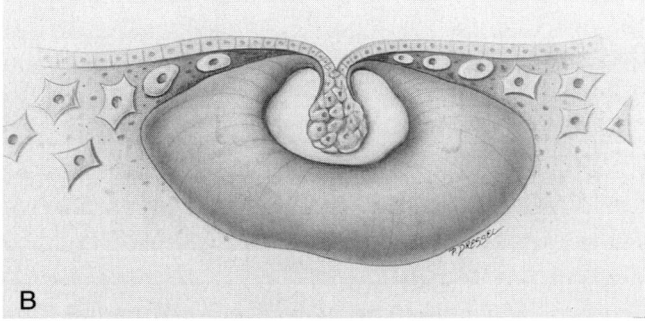

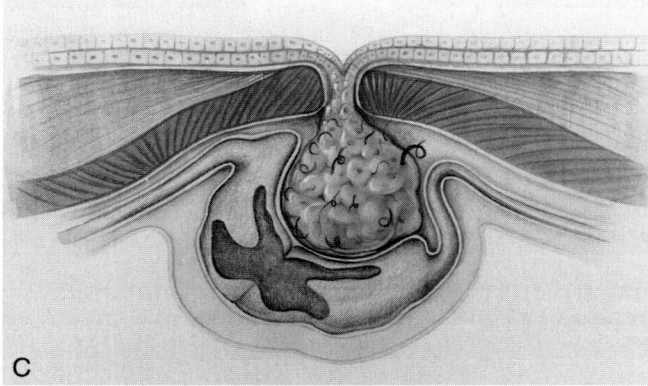

FIGURE 281–16. Embryogenesis of dermal sinus tracts. *A,* During early neurulation, the neural folds have elevated and approach each other in the midline, still connected to the adjacent cutaneous ectoderm. *B,* A failure of dysjunction of neuroectoderm from surface ectoderm drags a small tract of cutaneous ectoderm down beneath the skin surface, in association with the neural tube. *C,* The tract of epidermal cells produces a dermal sinus tract. An accumulating nest of cutaneous ectodermal and mesodermal cells adjacent to the spinal cord produces a dermoid tumor variably containing epidermal and dermal elements, adnexal structures, and hair.

dermal and mesodermal tissues, such as sebaceous glands and hair follicles), located anywhere between the skin and the neural tube (see Fig. 281–16). One way that abnormal dysjunction could arise is through the misexpression of CAMs or other molecular markers located on cutaneous ectoderm or neuroectoderm.

Dermal sinuses may involve any level of the neuraxis. Probably because of the complexities of neuropore closure, they exhibit a predilection for the lumbosacral region at the site of the caudal neuropore and the frontonasal region at the site of the cranial neuropore.

Lumbosacral dermal sinuses arise in the dorsal midline skin cranial to the intergluteal cleft. Some end blindly within the soft tissues superficial to the underlying lamina. Many penetrate the vertebral canal (usually between the laminae of two adjacent vertebrae or between bifid laminae), enter the dura near the level of the cutaneous lesion, and extend cephalad to a variable degree, ending as high as the conus medullaris. Those that reach the conus usually attach along the dorsal surface of the caudal neural tube just cranial to the tip of the conus, rather than to the end of the conus itself. A separate filum terminale is often present. This anatomic arrangement is predicted by the embryology of the region; dermal sinuses involving the posterior neuropore would be expected to arise from the S2 spinal segment, cranial to the tip of the conus medullaris and the filum terminale, both of which are derived from secondary neurulation.

It is important to distinguish between the lumbosacral dermal sinus, a pathologic malformation that can cause spinal cord tethering, bacterial or aseptic meningitis, or spinal cord compression from associated dermoid or epidermoid tumor growth, and the more common coccygeal dimple. The latter is an innocent and nonpathologic entity, present in 6% of the population, that likely represents a vestige of the primitive pit and cells of the surrounding CCM (Fig. 281–17*A*). The most important distinguishing feature is not the depth of the lesion but its craniocaudal location. Benign coccygeal dimples arise at or within a few millimeters cranial to the tip of the coccyx and therefore lie within the gluteal cleft. In contrast, dermal sinuses arise more cranially, at the second sacral level, and are therefore located on the "flat" portion of the sacrum, cranial to the gluteal cleft (see Fig. 281–17*B*). Dermal sinuses are usually larger, more complex cutaneous anomalies with uneven margins; associated skin dimples, hemangiomas, or tufts of hair; and often an abnormally formed intergluteal cleft. In contrast, coccygeal dimples are usually simple blind sinuses with no associated cutaneous abnormalities and a normally formed gluteal cleft.

Premature Dysjunction: Spinal Lipomas

Spinal lipomas are the most common occult dysraphic malformations, and they most frequently involve the lumbosacral spinal cord, conus medullaris, and filum terminale; rarely, they may involve more cranial regions of the spinal cord. Most lipomas span the dura and lie both intra- and extradurally. In 85% of cases, there is a visible subcutaneous mass that is contiguous, between bifid laminae and a dural defect, with the thecal space and caudal spinal cord.[225–228] Rarely, a lipoma may be purely intradural.

The involved spinal cord is dorsally dysraphic. The lipoma arises from within this area of dysraphism, occupying the central canal of the involved spinal cord and occasionally extending cephalad within the central canal to a variable degree (Fig. 281–18*A*). Ventrolateral to the lipoma are the displaced neural folds, from which the dorsal nerve roots emerge (see Fig. 281–18*B*).

Lipomas have been divided into three types—

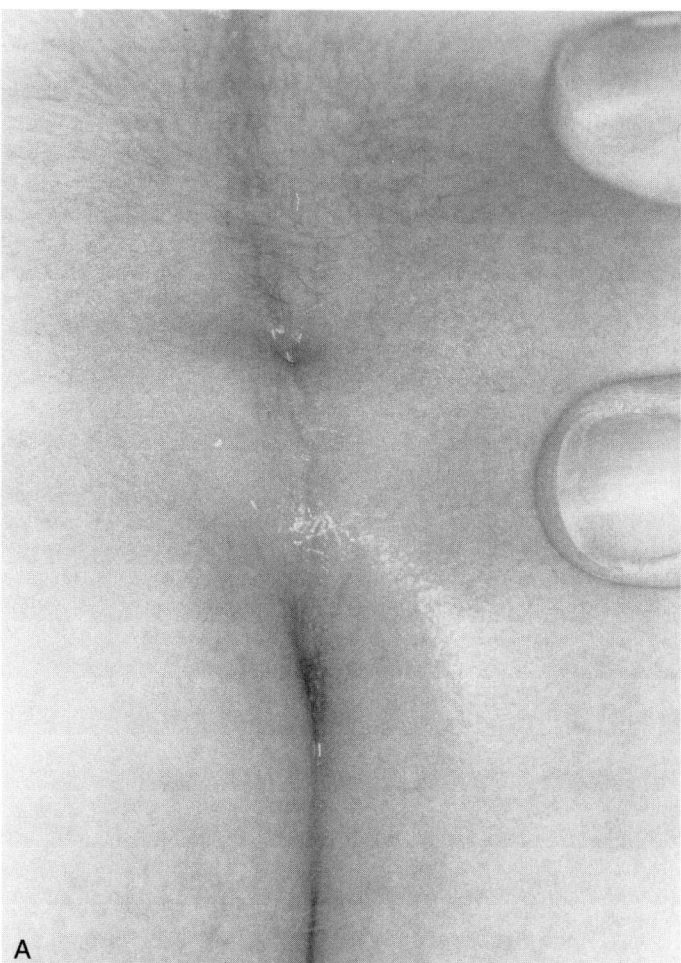

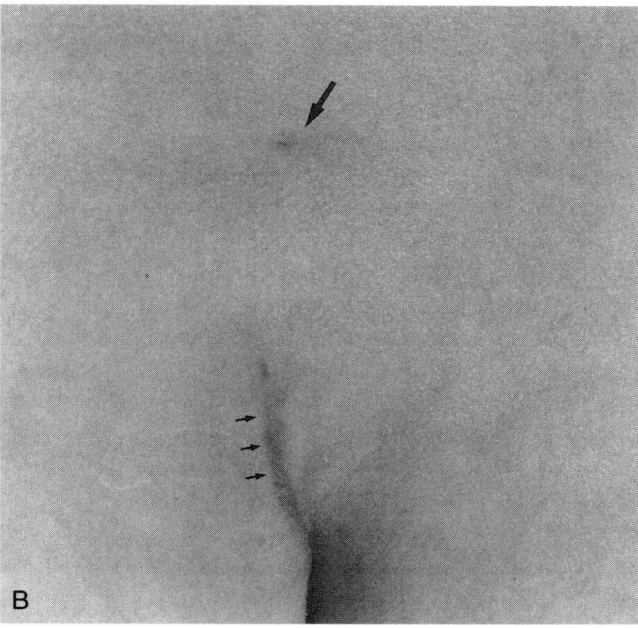

FIGURE 281–17. *A,* Innocent coccygeal dimple in a newborn infant. The gluteal folds have been pulled apart to reveal this small dimple within the folds of the gluteal cleft, overlying the coccyx. Note that the gluteal cleft is normally positioned in the midline. *B,* Pathologic sacral dermal sinus tract in another newborn infant. The tract *(large arrow)* is located well above the gluteal crease. The upper end of the gluteal crease is abnormally deflected toward the left *(small arrows).* (From McLone DG, Dias MS: Normal and abnormal embryology of the nervous system. In Cheek WR [ed]: Pediatric Neurosurgery: Surgery of the Developing Nervous System, 3rd ed. Philadelphia, WB Saunders, 1994, pp 3–39.)

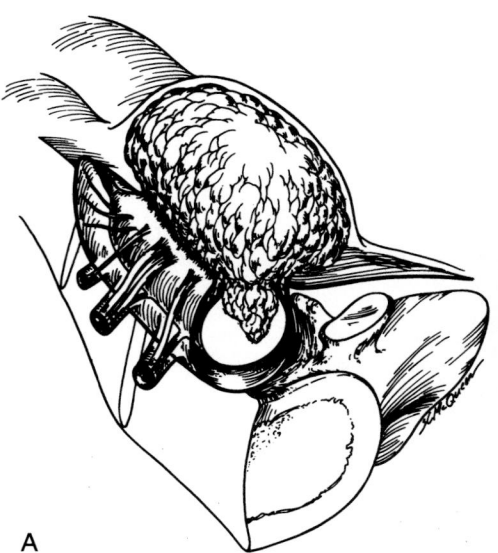

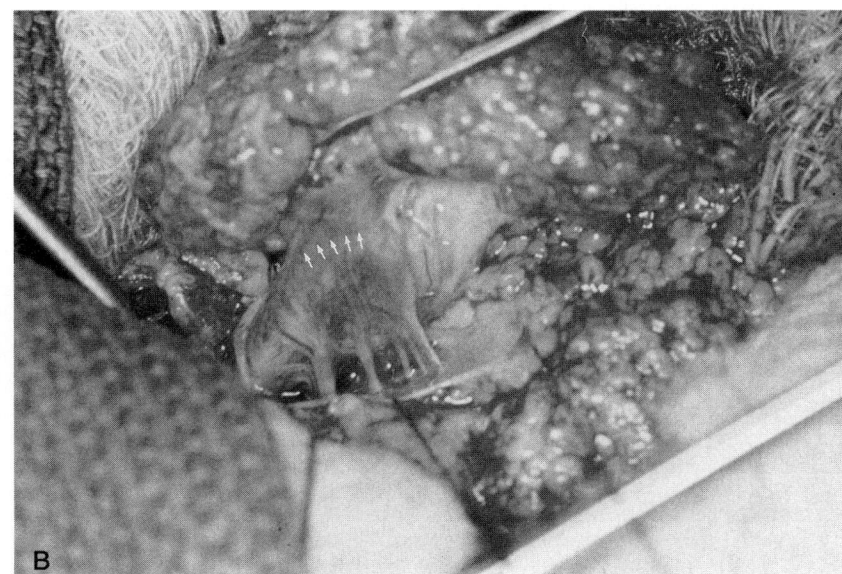

FIGURE 281–18. Spinal lipomas. *A,* Illustration of a spinal lipoma having both intra- and extramedullary components. *B,* Operative photograph of a lipoma. In both, the lipoma arises from the dorsal surface of the spinal cord, between the neural folds, and therefore medial to the dorsal root entry zones *(arrows).* (*A,* From Chapman PH: Congenital intraspinal lipomas: Anatomical considerations and surgical treatment. Childs Brain 9:37–47, 1982.)

dorsal, terminal, and transitional—depending on their relationship with the involved spinal cord segment.[229] All three extend in an exophytic fashion from the central canal of the spinal cord. The dorsal lipoma is exophytic dorsally with the spinal cord and sits atop the dorsal surface of the involved segment. The terminal lipoma is exophytic from the caudal end of the spinal cord and extends caudal to the tip of the conus medullaris (the fatty filum terminale is considered by many to be a form of terminal lipoma). The transitional lipoma represents a combination of the other types and is exophytic both dorsally and caudally from the conus medullaris.

The current theory of embryogenesis proposes that lipomas arise from premature dysjunction during primary neurulation.[230, 231] The cutaneous ectoderm prematurely separates from the neuroepithelium before neural fold fusion, allowing the surrounding mesenchymal cells to ingress between the neural tube and cutaneous ectoderm into the central canal of the developing neural tube (Fig. 281–19). When these mesenchymal cells are exposed to the outer surface of the neural tube, they are normally induced to form meninges; when they are instead exposed to the central canal of the spinal cord, they are thought to form fat.[231] When it is bilateral, premature dysjunction may produce a symmetrical midline fatty mass medial to the dorsal root entry zones. However, when premature dysjunction is unilateral, an eccentric mass may be produced. The spinal cord is rotated such that the dorsal root entry zone on the involved side lies most dorsal, nearest the fatty stalk, whereas the contralateral side is more ventral. Understanding these anatomic relationships is crucial to avoid injury to the spinal cord and roots during repair of the malformation.

Lipomas involving the neural tube caudal to S2 and the filum terminale must originate from the CCM and arise during secondary neurulation.[218, 231] In support of this concept, the histology of terminal lipomas differs from that of more rostral malformations; rostral lipomas usually contain only fat cells, whereas terminal lipomas more frequently contain striated muscle, mesenchyma, and other disparate tissue types derived from the CCM.[231] The nature of the underlying disorder

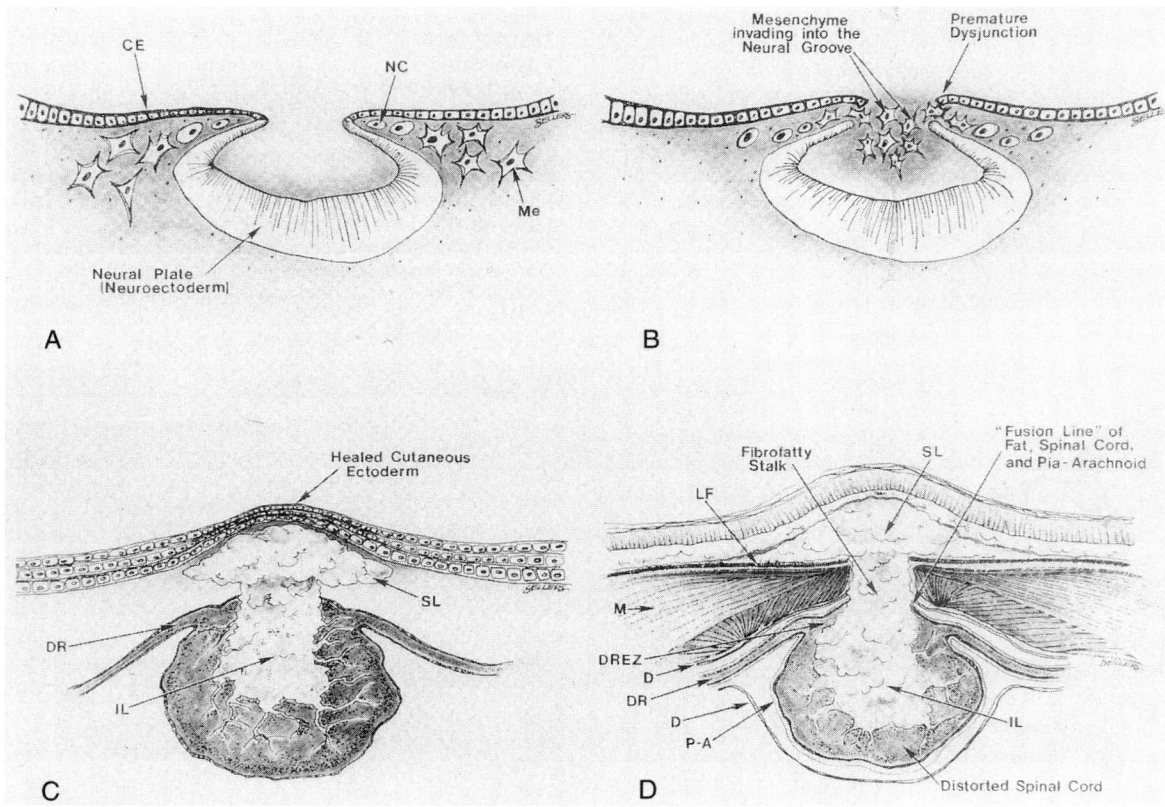

FIGURE 281–19. Embryogenesis of spinal lipomas. *A*, Neural plate during latter stages of neurulation. *B*, Premature dysjunction allows adjacent mesenchyma (Me) to ingress into the central canal of the neural tube. *C*, The ingressing mesenchymal cells are induced to form fibrofatty tissue, whereas extramedullary mesenchymal cells are induced to form pia-arachnoid (P-A). The cutaneous ectoderm is intact overlying the malformation. *D*, Dorsal roots (DR) and dorsal root ganglia arise from neural crest cells (derived from the neural folds) and are located immediately lateral to the fibrofatty mass. The pia-arachnoid surrounds the neural tube, except where the fatty mass fuses with the adjacent neural folds (the "fusion line"). CE, cutaneous ectoderm; D, dura; DREZ, dorsal root entry zone; IL, intramedullary lipoma; M, paraspinous muscles; NC, neural crest; SL, subcutaneous lipoma. (From Pang D: Tethered cord syndrome. In Neurosurgery: State of the Art Reviews, vol 1. Philadelphia, Hanley & Belfus, 1986, pp 45–79.)

of secondary neurulation that produces terminal lipomas is unknown.

Disorders of Gastrulation: Combined Spina Bifida, Split Cord Malformations, and Neurenteric Cysts

A number of seemingly unrelated disorders are thought to share a common embryogenesis. They include combined (anterior and posterior) spina bifida; split cord malformations (diastematomyelia); neurenteric cysts; intestinal malrotations, duplications, and fistulas; some cases of the Klippel-Feil malformation sequence; some cases of sacral agenesis; and a number of other unclassified complex dysraphic malformations, all of which manifest disorders involving all three primary germ layers. Variously described as the split notochord syndrome,[232] endodermal-ectodermal adhesion syndrome,[233] or accessory neurenteric canal syndrome,[234] the common element in most of these anomalies is a split cord malformation involving some portion of the neuraxis. The embryogenesis of these disorders is detailed by Dias and Walker[1] and is discussed here only briefly.

Split cord malformations may arise either in association with open neural tube defects or, more commonly, as occult malformations developing in isolation or in conjunction with other associated anomalies. Earlier classification schemes did little to foster our understanding about the embryogenesis of these lesions. The term *diastematomyelia* (from the Greek *diastema,* meaning "cleft," and *melos,* meaning "medulla") was used to describe malformations in which the spinal cord is split into two hemicords, each containing a single set of dorsal and ventral nerve roots. In contrast, the term *diplomyelia* was used to describe a complete duplication of the spinal cord, each side containing two sets of ventral and dorsal nerve roots.[235-237] In addition, it was widely believed that each of the two half cords in diastematomyelia was contained within its own separate dural sheath; an intervening osseous or fibrocartilaginous spur provided a point of tethering (Fig. 281–20A). In contrast, the duplicated cords in diplomyelia were both thought to lie within a single, common dural tube (see Fig. 281–20B), having no interposed tethering mesenchymal element.[235, 236] Diastematomyelia was commonly seen as a tethering malformation amenable to surgical treatment, whereas diplomyelia was regarded as an embryologic curiosity with no clinical relevance.

However, several observations suggest a common embryonic origin for these two malformations. The original description of diastematomyelia by James and Lassman[238] included 11 cases of single dural tube malformations, 8 of which contained midline tethering fibrous bands, analogous to the bony or fibrocartilaginous spurs of the double dural tube malformations.[238] These bands were also reported by Pang and colleagues[239] (Fig. 281–21A). The bands originated in the cleft between the two hemicords, traversed the subarachnoid space, and ended more caudally on the dura. They contained tough, fibrous connective tissue and prominent blood vessels, as well as dystrophic median nerve roots that originated from one or both of the hemicords (see later).[239] Just as the original description of diastematomyelia included cases of single dural tube malformations, the original descriptions of diplomyelia by Herren and Edwards[236] described both single and double dural tube malformations with approximately equal frequency, as well as many cases with intervening fibrous bands of tissue.

Moreover, dystrophic median nerve roots projecting

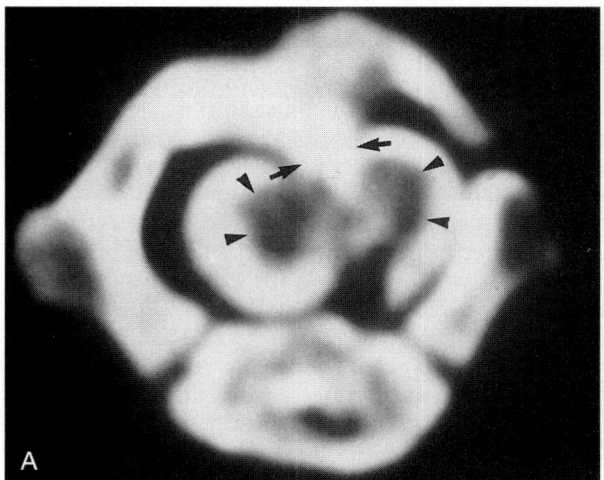
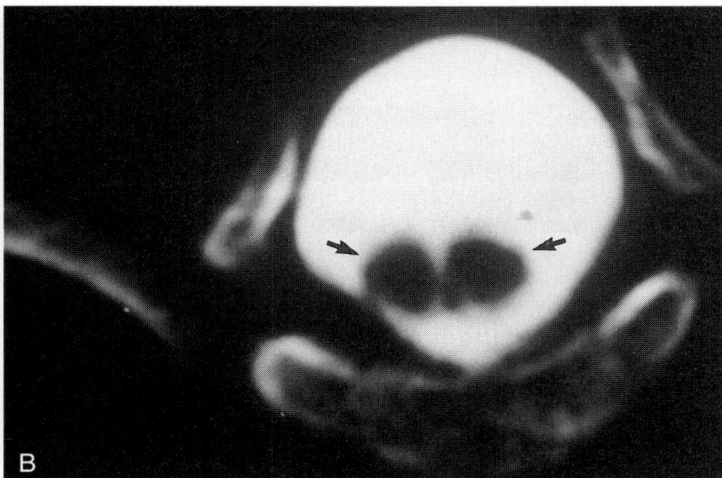

FIGURE 281–20. Split cord malformations. *A,* Axial view of a metrizamide computed tomographic myelogram shows a type I split cord malformation, with two hemicords separated by a thick, midline bony spur. Each hemicord is contained within its own separate dural sheath. *B,* Axial view of a metrizamide computed tomographic myelogram shows a type II split cord malformation, with two hemicords contained within a single dural sheath. No tethering elements are visible. (From Pang D, Dias MS, Ahab-Barmada M: Split cord malformation. Part I. A unified theory of embryogenesis for double spinal cord malformations. Neurosurgery 31:451–480, 1992.)

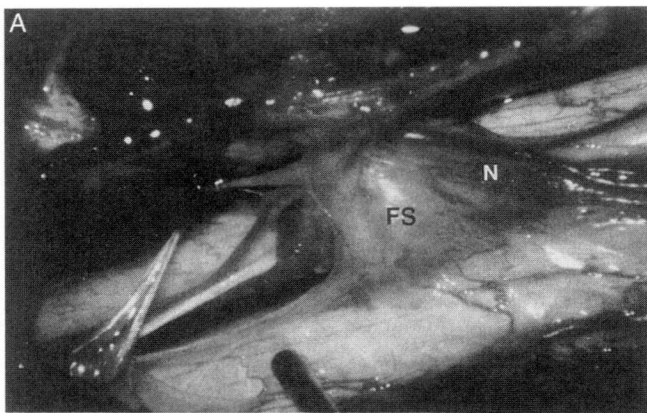

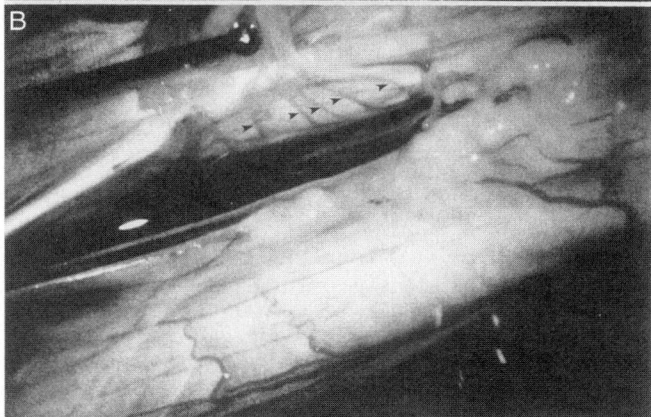

FIGURE 281–21. Operative photograph of a patient with a type II split cord malformation, with the dura open. *A,* A fibrous septum (FS) of tissue arises from between the two hemicords; immediately cranial to the stalk are small median nerve roots (N). *B,* After the stalk has been removed, the tiny median nerve roots are visible arising from the dorsal and ventral portions of the hemicord *(black arrows)* and crawling up to join the median fibrous septum. (From Pang D, Dias MS, Ahab-Barmada M: Split cord malformation. Part I. A unified theory of embryogenesis for double spinal cord malformations. Neurosurgery 31:451–480, 1992.)

from one or both hemicords and inserting onto the midline osseous spurs or fibrous bands have been described in both diastematomyelia and diplomyelia.[236, 238, 240–242] Although dorsal roots and ganglion cells are more frequent, ventral roots have been described as well (see Fig. 281–21B).[241, 242] The presence of both lateral and median sets of nerve roots arising from each hemicord strongly suggests the presence of at least a partial spinal cord duplication in both malformations. Pathologic descriptions of the hemicords from published examples of both diastematomyelia and diplomyelia demonstrate neither absolute splitting nor complete duplication of the cord. Rather, the hemicords are incomplete duplications, with relatively well-preserved lateral halves and dystrophic medial halves.[235, 236, 242–244]

These observations suggest that diastematomyelia and diplomyelia are different ends of a spectrum of split cord malformations that share a common embryonic origin and differ only in the subsequent fates of various tissue types (Fig. 281–22).[1, 239] Split cord

malformations are seen in association with a variety of anomalies, including combined (anterior and posterior) spina bifida; hemimyelomeningoceles; myelomeningoceles (occurring in up to one third of cases); cervical myelomeningoceles; neurenteric cysts; some examples of the Klippel-Feil anomaly, iniencephaly, and caudal agenesis; and certain intestinal duplications and diverticula (reviewed in Dias and Walker[1]). All these complex dysraphic malformations share common stereotypical anomalies involving tissues derived from all three primary germ layers, and they may share a common embryonic origin.[1, 190] Four theories have attempted to explain the underlying embryopathy.

Beardmore and Wigglesworth[245] proposed that an adhesion could develop between the epiblast and hypoblast and interfere with notochordal outgrowth. The elongating notochord, encountering this endodermal-ectodermal adhesion, could either deviate to one or the other side or split around the adhesion, producing two heminotochords, each inducing a neural hemicord. Associated remnants of the adhesion could give rise to endodermal remnants located anywhere between the gut and the cutaneous ectoderm. This mechanism works only if the notochord extends cranially from Hensen's node. If the notochord elongates by the addition of cells to its caudal end during Hensen's node regression (as it does in the chick), an adhesion of this type would not provide a barrier to notochordal outgrowth. Prop and colleagues[233] consequently modified this theory by postulating an adhesion within the primitive streak caudal to Hensen's node, around which the notochord might be split during node regression.

Bremer[234] studied patients with combined spina bifida (or split notochord syndrome), characterized by both anterior and posterior dysraphic malformations (Fig. 281–23). The involved vertebrae and spinal cord are split midsagittally to form two laterally displaced hemivertebral columns and a split cord malformation surrounding a central cleft (see Fig. 281–23). The cleft connects the dorsum with the peritoneal cavity; through the cleft passes a variable amount of endodermal tissue, from a simple neurenteric cyst to entire loops of bowel. Associated visceral malformations are exceedingly common and include intestinal malrotations, diverticula, or duplications.[245, 246]

Bremer[234] noted the similarities between the central cleft in combined spina bifida and the neurenteric canal of normal embryos, both seeming to bisect the embryo and connect the amniotic and yolk sacs. However, the dorsal opening of the neurenteric canal is the primitive pit, which ultimately comes to lie at the tip of the coccyx. In contrast, combined spina bifida and other split cord malformations involve more cranial levels of the neuraxis. Bremer therefore proposed the formation of an accessory neurenteric canal and suggested that a dorsal herniation of endoderm might split the notochord and neuroepithelium to form such a canal. However, the impetus for such a dorsal herniation is unknown. Moreover, it is difficult experimentally to split a normally formed notochord.[1]

McLetchie and associates[247] and Saunders[248] sug-

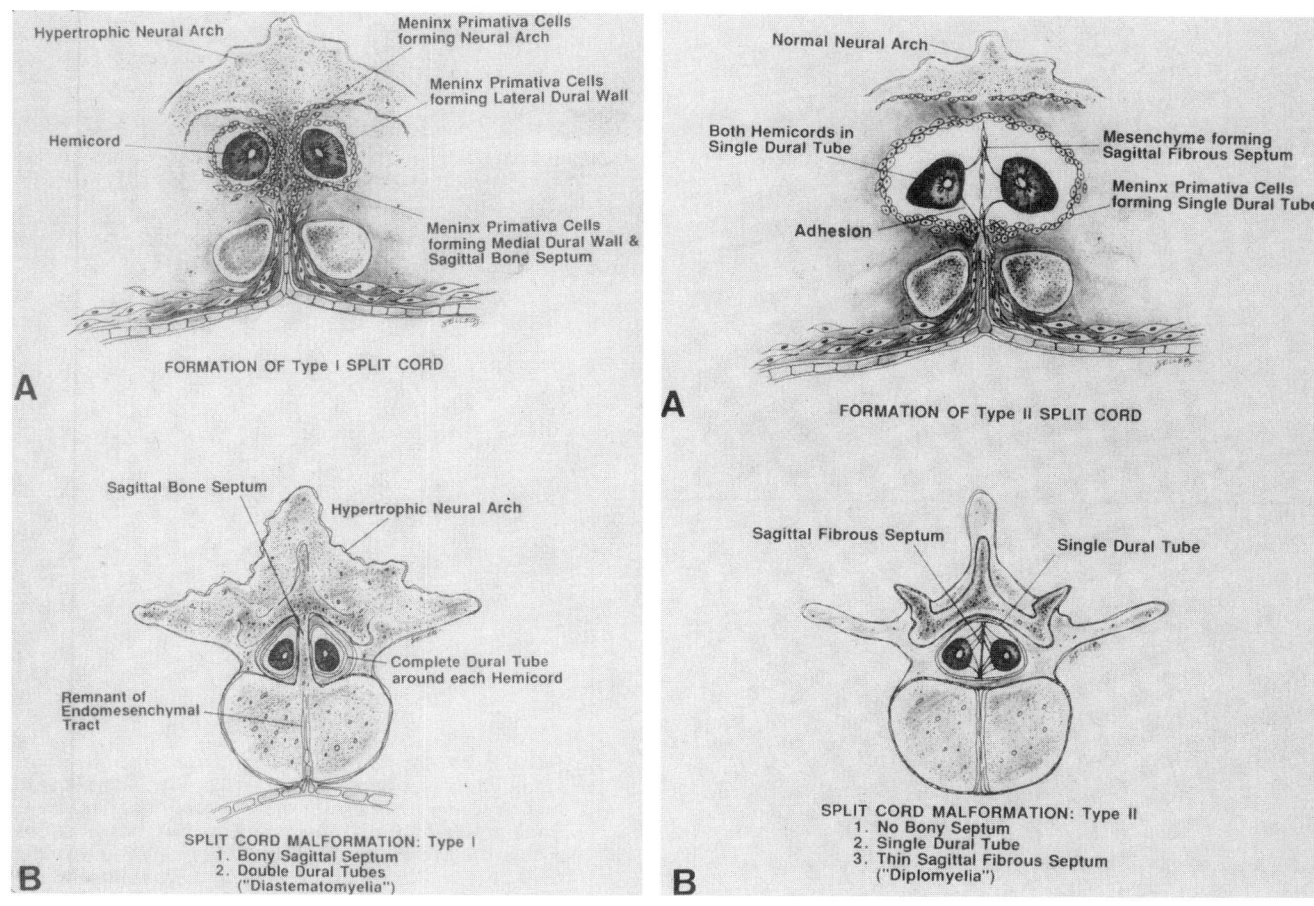

FIGURE 281–22. Embryogenesis of split cord malformations. *Left,* Type I malformation (diastematomyelia) in which the midline mesenchymal tract forms a median bony spur between the two hemicords; the surrounding meninx primitiva is induced to form two separate dural sheaths, each of which surrounds one of the two hemicords. *Right,* Type II malformation (diplomyelia) in which the mesenchymal tract is thinner and more delicate, forming only a fibrous midline septum that bisects and is frequently adherent to the medial aspect of the two hemicords. The meninx primitiva is induced to form a single dural sheath that contains both hemicords. (From Pang D, Dias MS, Ahab-Barmada M: Split cord malformation. Part I. A unified theory of embryogenesis for double spinal cord malformations. Neurosurgery 31:451–480, 1992.)

gested that the initial abnormality involves duplication of the notochord, followed by a secondary endodermal-ectodermal interaction between the duplicated notochords. Dodds[249] suggested that during normal embryogenesis, bilaterally paired prospective notochordal cell anlagen might be integrated into a single midline structure during regression of the primitive streak. Feller and Sternberg[250] proposed that abnormal rests of undifferentiated cells in Hensen's node might interfere with proper midline integration and result in paired notochords. Subsequent differentiation of these cell rests could give rise to a variety of midline anomalies composed of tissues derived from any of the three primary germ cell layers.

Dias and Walker[1] proposed that these malformations arise when prospective anlagen from all three germ layers are being laid down during gastrulation (Fig. 281–24). During normal development, paired notochordal anlagen are integrated to form a single notochordal process, and bilaterally paired prospective neu-

roepithelial cells flanking both sides of Hensen's node and the primitive streak are integrated to form a single midline neural plate. During the formation of complex dysraphic malformations, both the paired notochordal anlagen and adjacent prospective neuroepithelial regions remain separate, developing independently over a variable portion of their length to produce a split notochord and paired hemicords, respectively. Laterally displaced (and perhaps disrupted) somitic mesoderm forms abnormally widened spinal canals and numerous associated somitic malformations, including sagittally clefted (butterfly) vertebrae, fused vertebrae, hemivertebrae, absent vertebrae, or, if displaced widely enough, partially duplicated vertebral columns, as seen in combined spina bifida. The intervening space between the paired hemicords is composed of pluripotent primitive streak cells and could give rise to a variety of tissue types from any of the three primary germ layers (all having been described in association with split cord malformations): endodermal tissues (neu-

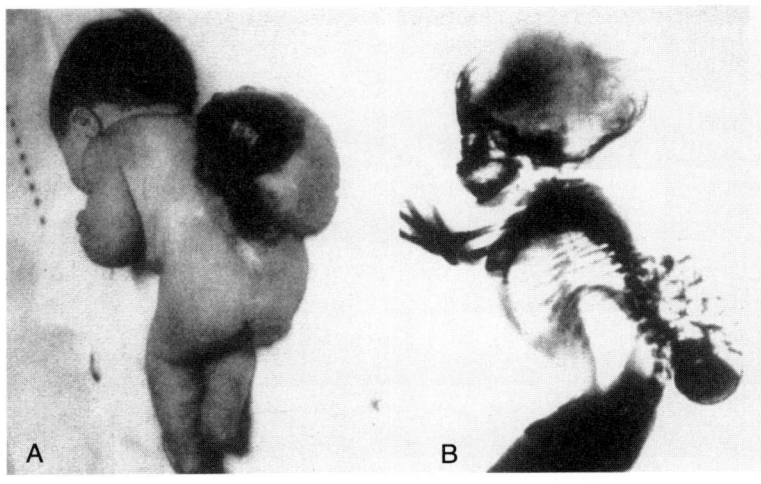

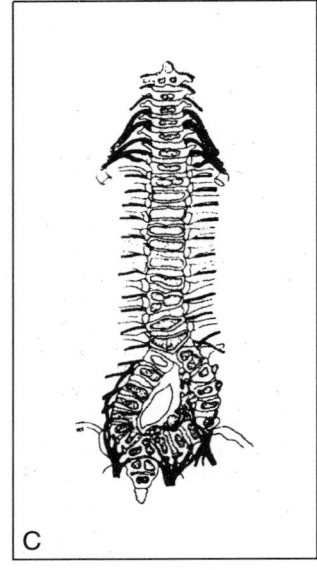

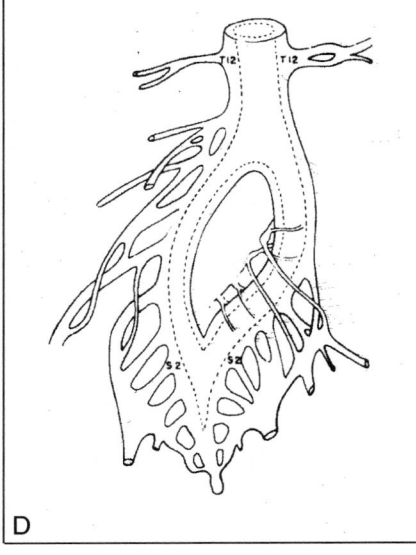

FIGURE 281–23. Combined (anterior and posterior) spina bifida (split notochord syndrome). *A,* Infant with a large mass arising from the thoracolumbar spine. *B,* Radiograph of the same infant shows bowel loops within the sac. *C* and *D,* Diagrams illustrating, respectively, the widely split bony vertebral elements and the spinal cord elements around a central cleft, through which the loops of bowel were extruded. (*A* and *B,* From Dénes J, Honti J, Léb J: Dorsal herniation of the gut: A rare manifestation of the split notochord syndrome. J Pediatr Surg 2:359–363, 1967. *C* and *D,* From Saunders RL: Combined anterior and posterior spinal bifida in a living neonatal human female. Anat Rec 87:255–278, 1943.)

renteric cysts, loops of bowel), mesodermal tissues (bony or fibrous midline structures, blood vessels, muscle, and fat encountered in split cord malformations; anomalous vertebrae; immature renal and müllerian tissues), ectodermal tissues (dermoid and epidermoid tumors), and even pathologic tissues such as teratomas and Wilms' tumors.[251–253]

The subsequent development of the two hemicords could also influence the type of resultant malformation. Successful neurulation of both hemicords would produce a split cord malformation. Failure of one hemicord to neurulate would produce a hemimyelomeningocele with an eccentric placode and asymmetrical neurological deficits.[254] A localized failure of both hemicords to neurulate would produce a myelomeningocele in association with an adjacent split cord malformation.

Similar malformations have been reproduced in chick embryos by splitting Hensen's node midsagittally into two heminodes during gastrulation.[1] Double neural tube malformations of variable extent are produced by these maneuvers and are associated with wide-spread open NTDs and multiple somitic abnormalities. Splitting the node during midgastrulation (when the primitive streak is at full extension) produces more cranial malformations. Manipulations performed slightly later during regression of the primitive streak cause more caudal malformations. Although preliminary, these data support the theory that complex dysraphic malformations are the result of disordered gastrulation.

Disorders of Secondary Neurulation: Thickened Filum Terminale, Myelocystocele, and Currarino's Triad

Abnormalities of secondary neurulation are thought to produce only skin-covered malformations because secondary neurulation occurs beneath an intact cutaneous ectoderm. The sacral spinal cord segments (below S2) and filum terminale are the only parts of the nervous system to develop from the caudal cell mass[27]; therefore, disorders of secondary neurulation produce malformations of these caudalmost structures. The

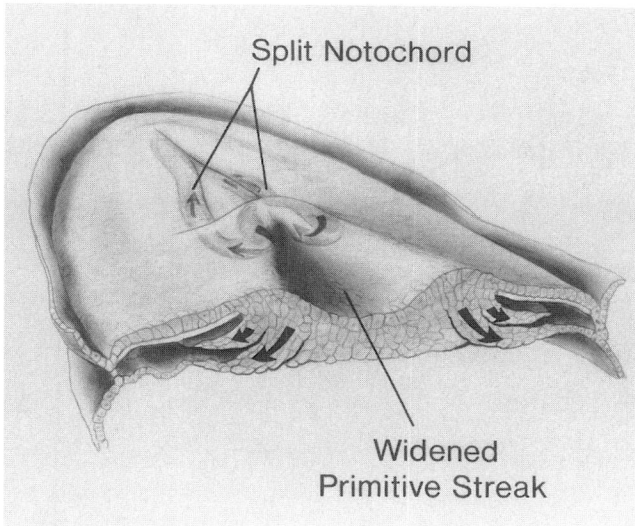

FIGURE 281–24. Proposed embryogenesis of split cord malformations and other complex dysraphic malformations. In normal human gastrulation, prospective notochordal cells located along the anterior margin of Hensen's node ingress through the primitive pit to become the notochordal process. The neuroectoderm flanking the node and primitive streak is integrated to form a single neural tube. Abnormal gastrulation results in a failure of midline axial integration (see Fig. 281–2B). The primitive streak is abnormally wide; prospective notochordal cells therefore begin ingressing more laterally than normal. As a result, two notochordal processes are formed. The caudal neuroepithelium flanking the primitive streak also fails to become integrated to form a single neuroepithelial sheet and instead forms two hemineural plates. (From Dias MS, Walker ML: The embryogenesis of complex dysraphic malformations: A disorder of gastrulation? Pediatr Neurosurg 18:229–253, 1992.)

more common malformations include shortened filum terminale, terminal myelocystocele, and Currarino's triad. The embryology of the shortened filum terminale is entirely unknown but may represent either an abnormal formation of the secondary neural tube from the caudal cell mass or an abnormality of retrogressive differentiation. The filum terminale is abnormally thickened and frequently infiltrated with adipose tissue; as mentioned earlier, this lesion is categorized by many as a terminal lipoma.

Terminal myelocystoceles (Fig. 281–25) are rare occult dysraphic lesions containing a cystic dilatation of the caudal spinal cord as a CSF-containing, glial or ependyma-lined terminal cyst (or myelocystocele).[255, 256] The dilated terminal cord is surrounded, in turn, by a dilated and ectatic dural sleeve. This produces a "double sac" in which the CSF within the dilated terminal cyst is contiguous with the central canal of the more cranial spinal cord, and the CSF in the outer, dural sac is contiguous with the more cranial subarachnoid space.[256] Ordinarily, there is no free communication between the inner and outer sacs.[256] An associated lipoma is almost universal and is contiguous with the caudal end of the dilated terminal cord. Malformations of other caudal organ systems (all derived from the CCM) are frequent[255–257] and include cloacal extrophy, imperforate anus, ambiguous genitalia, and multiple

caudal vertebral malformations, including segmentation anomalies and caudal agenesis. Myelocystoceles are one component of the OEIS (omphalocele, extrophy, imperforate anus, and spinal malformations) complex.[257]

Terminal myelocystoceles are thought to arise from the CCM during secondary neurulation.[255, 256, 258] The juxtaposition of cells in the CCM that give rise to multiple organ rudiments probably accounts for the frequent association of myelocystocele with other hindgut and cloacal anomalies.[256] One proposal is that CSF, unable to exit from the central canal, is vented into the terminal portion of the central canal during canalization of the secondary neural tube.[256] This proposal assumes that the central canals of the primary and secondary neural tubes are in continuity during canalization, as occurs in the mouse.[26] Alternatively, CSF could distend the terminal neural tube secondarily after it becomes integrated with the more cranial neural tube. Progressive accumulation of CSF would distend the central canal of the terminal spinal cord as well as the surrounding meningeal precursors, producing the double sac malformation. In addition, disruption of the surrounding mesenchyma (but not the cutaneous ectoderm) would result in a dorsal bony dysraphism and mesenchymal abnormality with intact overlying skin.[256] The nature of the underlying CSF disturbance is uncertain. The absence of hydrocephalus in most patients with terminal myelocystoceles suggests that the disturbance in CSF dynamics is probably regional rather than global.

Currarino's triad[259] is a caudal malformation involving the combination of anorectal stenosis, a presacral mass, and an anterior sacral bony defect or scimitar sacrum (Fig. 281–26). The most common enteric malformations include anal or anorectal stenosis, although anorectal agenesis, anorectal stenosis with rectovaginal fistula, and rectal ectopia have been described. An associated hemisacral, or scimitar sacral, defect is present; segmentation anomalies are less frequent. The presacral mass is most frequently a presacral teratoma or anterior meningocele; neurenteric cysts or dermoid tumors are unusual. At least 50% of cases are familial, and both X-linked and autosomal-dominant inheritance patterns have been described.[260–262]

These malformations were thought by Currarino to arise through an ectodermal-endodermal adhesion, either primarily or secondarily as a consequence of an abnormally split notochord, in a manner analogous to the split cord malformations and related complex dysraphic malformations described earlier.[232, 234, 247, 248] However, these mechanisms do not adequately fit our current understanding of caudal axial development. Whereas split cord malformations and their variants involve more cranial regions of the neuroectoderm formed from primary neurulation, Currarino's triad involves neuroectoderm and other embryonic tissues that normally form during development of the CCM through entirely different embryonic processes.[263]

The recent description of a child with both Currarino's triad and a caudal split cord malformation, in which one of the two hemicords was contiguous

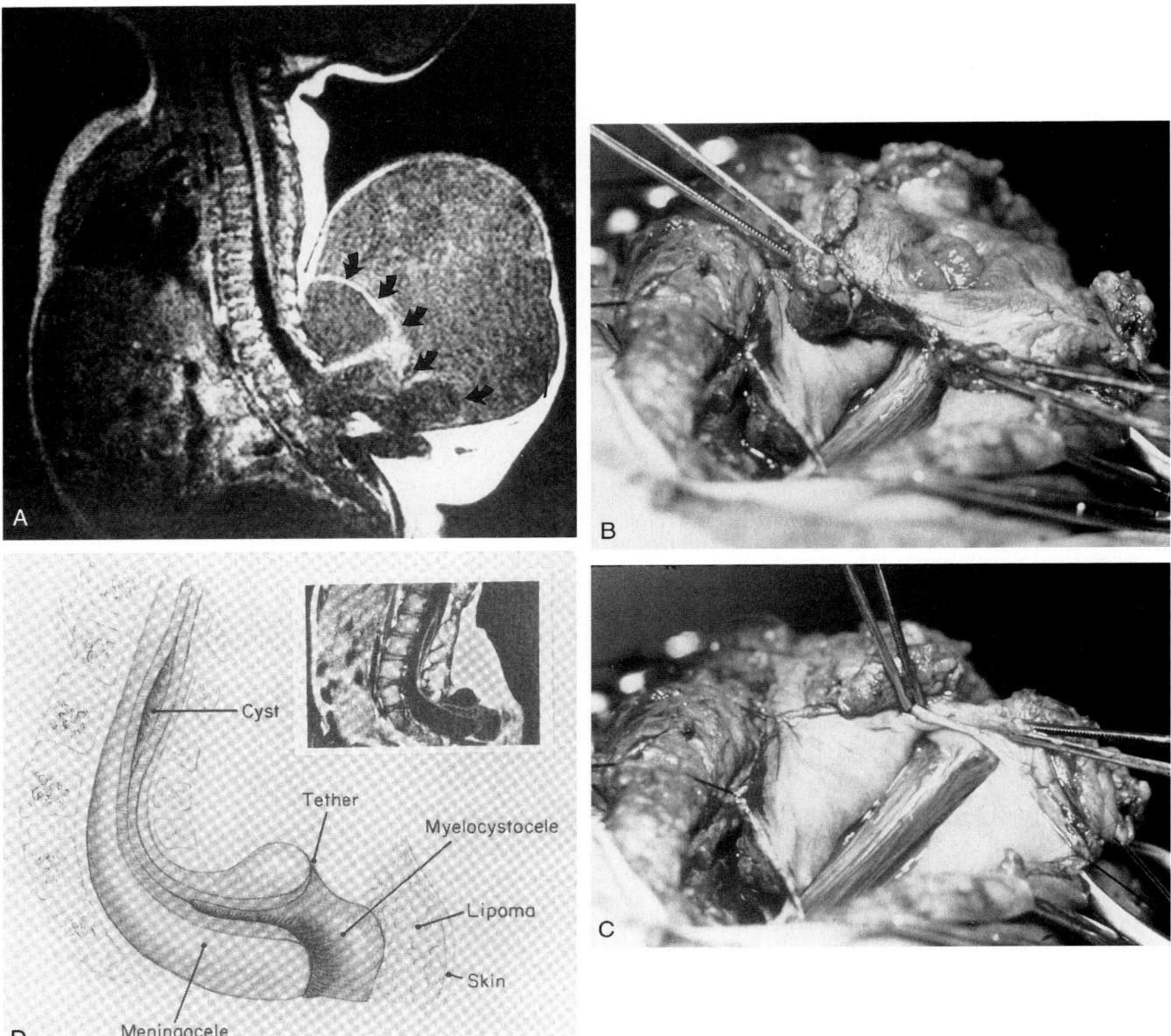

FIGURE 281–25. Terminal myelocystocele. *A,* Sagittal T1-weighted magnetic resonance imaging (MRI) scan shows a "sac within a sac" appearance, with the terminally dilated spinal cord *(curved arrows)* lying within a much larger dural sac containing cerebrospinal fluid. *B* and *C,* Operative photographs of a terminal myelocystocele. In *B,* the spinal cord ends caudally in a dilated sac representing the ballooned-out central canal. In *C,* the surrounding outer sac, composed of dura, is seen around the distal spinal cord. *D,* Diagram shows the distal spinal cord ending within a large sac of meninges (meningocele); the central canal of the spinal cord is grossly dilated to form a second sac (the myelocystocele) within the larger dural sac. An associated spinal lipoma is almost always present. *Inset,* Sagittal T1-weighted MRI scan demonstrating similar findings. (*B* and *C,* From McLone DG, Naidich TP: The tethered spinal cord. In McLaurin RL, Schut L, Venes JL, Epstein F [eds]: Pediatric Neurosurgery, 2nd ed. Philadelphia, WB Saunders, 1989. *D,* From Peacock WJ, Murovic JA: Magnetic resonance imaging in myelocystoceles: Report of two cases. J Neurosurg 70:804–807, 1989.)

through the sacral defect with a presacral teratoma and enteric duplication,[264] suggests a common embryogenetic pathway for caudal split cord malformations and Currarino's triad during the period of late gastrulation and development of the CCM. According to this theory, Currarino's triad represents a failure of a normal embryonic event: the dorsoventral separation of the CCM from the hindgut endoderm.[264] The subsequent disruption of secondary neurulation produces caudal neural tube occult dysraphic malformations in some cases. Cloacal maldevelopment produces anorectal stenosis, fistula, or other anorectal anomalies and also accounts

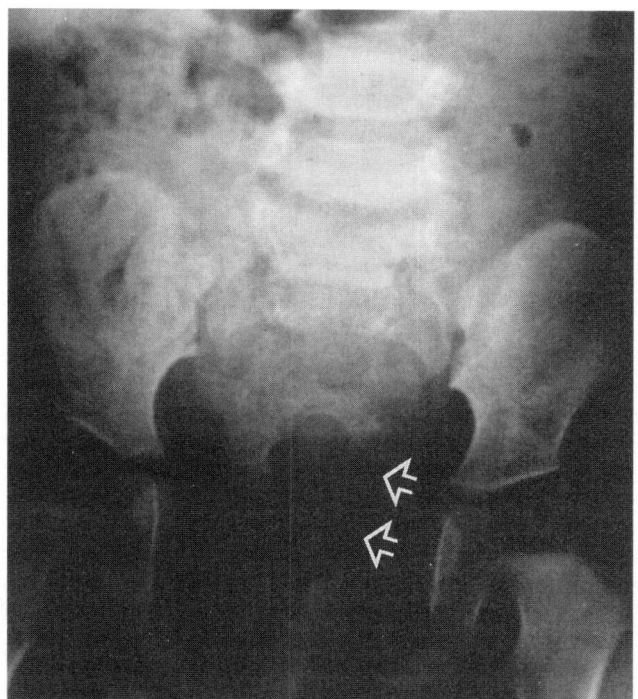

FIGURE 281–26. Caudal agenesis sequence. Anteroposterior radiograph shows absence of the coccyx and caudal portions of the sacrum *(open arrows)*.

tions.[267–274] The spinal canal is sometimes widened; in the extreme, combined spina bifida occurs.[190, 275–277]

The distal spinal cord is truncated (see Fig. 281–27), with the terminal spinal cord ending in a dysplastic glial nodule.[268, 278, 279] Motor deficits usually correspond to the level of the agenesis. In contrast, sensory sparing is characteristic,[269, 270, 272–274, 277, 280–283] suggesting a relative preservation of neural crest cells. Alternatively, migration of neural crest cells from more cranial spinal segments could conceivably occupy the territory rendered vacant by the agenesis. An associated myelomeningocele is present in as many as 50% of cases[272, 274, 281]; conversely, sacral agenesis is reported in as many as 24% of patients with myelomeningocele.[284] Split cord malformations (both single and double dural tube malformations) have been described in several reports.[272, 277, 285–287]

Associated limb anomalies are common and include flattened buttocks, gluteal atrophy, and equinovarus deformities. The legs are wasted distally, imparting an "inverted champagne bottle" appearance.[271] Histologic examination of involved muscles demonstrates a virtual absence of myocytes, with relative preservation of

for the rare associated genitourinary anomalies.[259, 261, 265, 266] Disruption of somitic and leptomeningeal mesenchymal condensation around the notochord and spinal cord produces both the scimitar sacrum and other sacral anomalies, as well as the anterior sacral meningocele. Finally, persistent multipotent stem cells of the caudal eminence produce the presacral teratoma.

Failure of Caudal Neuraxial Development: Caudal Agenesis

Caudal agenesis comprises a group of caudal malformations characterized by partial or complete absence of a variable number of sacral or lumbar vertebrae, together with corresponding regions of the caudal neural tube. The term *sacral agenesis* is not entirely accurate because the malformation is not always limited to the sacral spinal segments. In fact, lumbosacral agenesis and even suspended lumbar agenesis with sacral sparing have been described. Similarly, the term *caudal regression* is inaccurate because the malformation appears to involve a failure of the caudal segments to form, rather than a regression of previously formed spinal segments. These terms should therefore be discarded.

The vertebral anomalies are striking (Fig. 281–27). In addition to agenesis, other complex vertebral anomalies are often present cranial to the absent regions and include hemivertebrae, wedge-shaped vertebrae, fused vertebrae, sacralized lumbar vertebrae, posterior spina bifida, midline bony spurs, and abnormal rib articula-

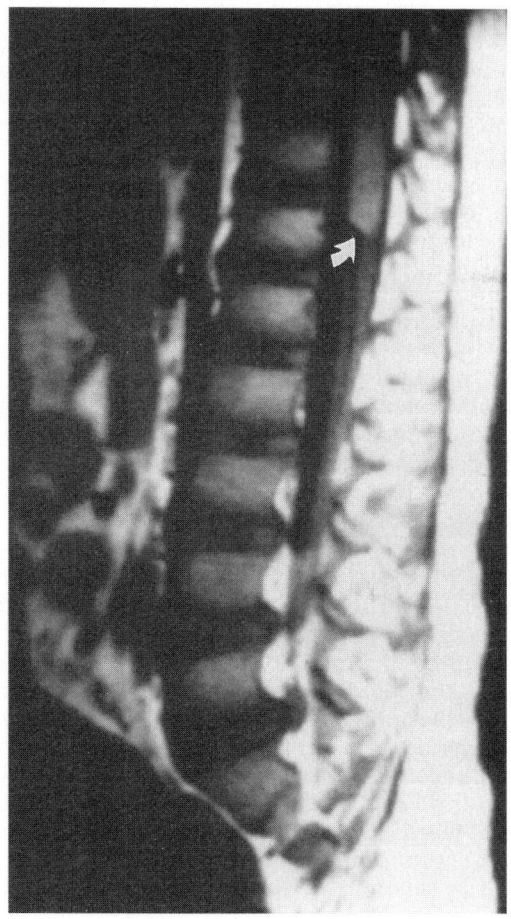

FIGURE 281–27. Caudal agenesis sequence. Sagittal T1-weighted magnetic resonance imaging scan shows an atrophic S2 vertebral body; the more caudal vertebrae are absent. The distal spinal cord ends abruptly *(curved arrow)*; the distal conus medullaris and the filum terminale are absent.

connective tissues.[268, 273, 278, 279] This pattern of findings suggests either denervation atrophy[271, 283] or a failure of somitic development to contribute myoblasts to prospective muscle masses.

Associated visceral malformations are present in 35% of patients with caudal agenesis[269] and most commonly include intestinal (tracheoesophageal fistula, Meckel's diverticulum, cloacal extrophy, omphalocele, intestinal malrotation) and urogenital (renal agenesis, horseshoe kidney, ureteral and bladder duplications, anomalies of external genitalia) malformations.[272, 273, 276, 279, 283, 288, 289] Some, but not all, of these malformations are derivatives of the CCM.

The cause of caudal agenesis is not completely known, although most authors agree that the malformation arises during early embryogenesis, probably before the 10th week.[271] The association of caudal agenesis with myelomeningoceles suggests a disorder that arises before or during closure of the caudal neural tube. The frequent occurrence of caudal agenesis in offspring of diabetic mothers is well described.[278, 280, 290, 291] "Rumpless" chickens exhibiting similar malformations have been produced by exposing embryos to insulin or other sulfur-containing compounds during early embryogenesis.[292–294] Similar malformations have also been produced by exposing mouse embryos to hyperglycemic medium or to β-hydroxybutyrate, a ketone body that is elevated during periods of ketoacidosis.[295] The optimal time for producing such anomalies is during late gastrulation, when caudal neuraxial structures are first being formed. Horton and Sadler[295] invoked an interference with the structure or function of glycoproteins known to be involved in early embryonic development.

Duhamel[296] proposed a common cause for a wide spectrum of malformations involving the caudal urogenital and gastrointestinal systems, including imperforate anus at one end and sirenomelia (caudal spinal agenesis, multiple visceral anomalies, and associated fusion of both hind limbs into a single appendage—the so-called mermaid syndrome) at the other extreme. Caudal agenesis is thought to be an intermediate form of these disorders. Sirenomelia has been produced in chickens by destroying the caudal axial mesoderm.[297] This finding has led to the suggestion that a disorder of an axial mesodermal "developmental field," responsible for orchestrating the migration and determination of prospective caudal mesodermal cells during gastrulation, might be responsible for caudal agenesis. According to this theory, malformations arise when epiblast cells migrating through the primitive streak "fail to make, at the proper time, the proper transition whereby they come to acquire mesodermal characteristics."[298] Failure of a caudal "organizer" has been implicated by others.[269, 272, 299] Such a developmental field or organizer is thought to act through cell-cell interactions mediated by cell surface morphogenesis proteins.[298, 300]

The association of caudal agenesis with the broader group of malformations collectively referred to earlier as complex dysraphic malformations suggests that caudal agenesis sometimes represents another expression of a disorder of midline axial integration during gastru-

lation.[1] In this case, gastrulation ceases altogether. Midline neuraxial structures (neural tube and notochord) are therefore deficient, and somitic development, which depends on proper notochordal development, is also severely impaired.

Secondarily Acquired Central Nervous System Anomalies: Chiari II Malformations

Although not strictly a spinal cord malformation, the Chiari II malformation is such an integral component of the myelomeningocele that we believe its embryology should be discussed. The Chiari II malformation is a complex disorder that, to a variable extent, encompasses anomalies of almost the entire neuraxis (Fig. 281–28). Most prominent among these are caudal displacement of the cerebellar vermis and tonsils into the cervical canal; elongation, kinking, and caudal displacement of the lower brainstem below the foramen magnum; and upward displacement of the superior cerebellum through a dysplastic, low-lying tentorial incisura. A small posterior fossa and lückenschädel of the skull, as well as many associated telencephalic and diencephalic anomalies (Table 281–2), suggest a pancerebral disorder involving much of the cranial neuraxis and chondrocranium.[301]

Theories regarding the embryology of Chiari malformations can generally be grouped into four types.[301] The first group, regarded as the dysgenesis–developmental arrest theories, presumed that the Chiari malformation was the result of a primary dysgene-

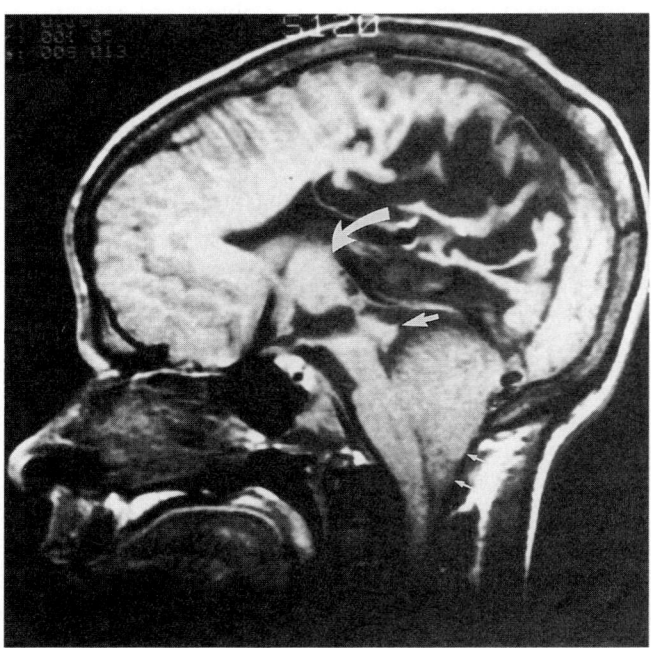

FIGURE 281–28. Chiari II malformation in a child with a myelomeningocele. The cerebellar vermis *(small white arrows)*, fourth ventricle, and caudal brainstem have all descended into the cervical canal. Additionally, the midbrain tectum is beaked *(large straight arrow)*, the massa intermedia of the thalamus is enlarged *(curved arrow)*, the corpus callosum is thin and misshapen, and several areas of cortical dysplasia (stenogyria) are present.

TABLE 281–2 ■ **Chiari-Associated Central Nervous System Malformations**

Disorders of the Skull

Lückenschädel of skull
Small posterior fossa
Low-lying tentorium cerebelli with large incisura
Scalloping of petrous bone
Shortening of clivus
Enlargement of foramen magnum

Disorders of the Posterior Fossa

Descent of cerebellar vermis through foramen magnum
Caudal displacement of pons and medulla
Rostral displacement of superior vermis through incisura
Kinking of brainstem
Loss of pontine flexure
Aqueductal stenosis or forking
Beaking of tectum

Disorders of the Cerebral Hemispheres

Stenogyria
Cortical heterotopias
Dysgenesis of the corpus callosum
Large massa intermedia of thalamus

sis of the neuraxis[302]; others suggested that a failure of pontine flexure might lead to a herniation of hindbrain contents.[303, 304] Neither of these theories can account for the frequent associated cerebral malformations.

The second group, referred to as the hydrocephalus-hydrodynamic theories, rely on the presence of fetal hydrocephalus that, because of a presumed imbalance (either static or dynamic) between supra- and infratentorial compartments, displaces the posterior fossa contents caudally. However, these theories ignore the small cranial volumes and absence of hydrocephalus in all early human fetuses with dysraphism and Chiari malformations.[305] Moreover, they fail to explain the small size of the posterior fossa, *upward* herniation of the superior cerebellar vermis, and associated cerebral anomalies.

The third group, referred to as the traction theories, suggests that traction on the caudal spinal cord by a myelomeningocele may pull the hindbrain caudally.[306, 307] However, experimental evidence suggests that the forces generated by spinal cord traction are dissipated within four spinal segments.[308] Moreover, these theories do not explain the upwardly herniated superior cerebellar vermis, the medullary kink and vermian peg, or associated cerebral anomalies.

The fourth group, referred to as the small posterior fossa–overgrowth theories, suggests that the Chiari malformation is caused by a primary disorder of paraxial mesoderm that causes a small posterior fossa that cannot adequately accommodate the burgeoning cerebellum and brainstem.[309] Padget and Lindenberg[310, 311] suggested that leakage of CSF from an open neural placode might result in acquired microcephaly with a small posterior fossa, leading to premature fusion of the cerebellar primordia and, with subsequent cerebellar growth, a Chiari malformation.

McLone and Knepper[301] proposed a unifying theory of embryogenesis for Chiari malformations that incorporates elements of each of the preceding theories.[305] According to this model, an open neural placode allows CSF to escape from the central canal of the caudal neural tube. In addition, spinal occlusion (which, in normal animals and in humans, precedes and is responsible for rapid brain enlargement) is incomplete in animal models of dysraphism and allows further leakage of CSF from the ventricles through the central canal. Finally, CSF leakage continues from the still open placode after spinal occlusion ends at stage 14 (POD 32). This persistent venting of CSF interferes with proper ventricular enlargement and eventually results in multiple central nervous system anomalies. For example, incomplete dilatation of the telencephalic ventricles results in disorganized migration of neurons from the ventricular zone, producing cortical heterotopias, gyral anomalies (stenogyria), and callosal dysgenesis. Inadequate distention of the third ventricle results in prolonged contact between the two thalami and an enlarged massa intermedia. Finally, inadequate enlargement of the rhombencephalic ventricle may similarly influence brainstem development and produce abnormalities of cranial nerve nuclei and their afferent and efferent connections.[301]

Most important, impaired ventricular enlargement affects the development of the chondrocranium, especially the posterior fossa. The growth and development of the chondrocranium are normally dependent on cues provided by the expansion of the underlying neural mass (the developing brain and ventricular system) during early embryogenesis.[312, 313] Incomplete distention of the rhombencephalic ventricle leaves the posterior fossa chondrocranium without an adequate inductive force. The posterior fossa is therefore smaller than normal, and the tentorium is low-set and deficient.[301, 305] This small posterior fossa is incapable of accommodating the later growth of the cerebellum. As a result, the posterior fossa contents are displaced both cranially through the tentorial incisura and caudally through the foramen magnum. Impaction of neural tissues at these levels impairs CSF flow through the foramina of Luschka and Magendie, as well as through the subarachnoid space at the foramen magnum and tentorial incisura, and results in hydrocephalus.

NORMAL DEVELOPMENT OF THE VERTEBRAL COLUMN

Gastrulation and the Formation of Somites

The normal development of the vertebral column begins during gastrulation, with formation of the notochord and somites (see earlier). During regression of the primitive streak, the prospective somitic mesoderm (the precursors of the vertebrae) migrate toward the cranial portion of the primitive streak, ingress through the primitive groove, and come to lie between the ectoderm and endoderm on either side of the developing notochord. Experimental evidence suggests that prospective somite cells from either side of the primitive streak are distributed bilaterally and contribute to somites on both sides of the embryo.[314] More caudal somites are formed during later embryogenesis from the caudal cell mass. As mentioned earlier, the posterior notochord is derived from the posterior notochordal center, located immediately cranial to the CCM.

Once in their final positions, the somite cells aggregate into discrete blocks of tissue, the somites. This process appears to be influenced by, but does not require, the presence of the adjacent notochord and neural tube, because somitic mesoderm, when cultured in isolation, is still capable of generating a discrete, metameric pattern.[315, 316] In humans, somites first become visible at stage 9 (PODs 19 to 21) in the future cervical region.[27] The formation of subsequent somites occurs in a rostral-to-caudal direction. Approximately five cranial somites are present at the time the neural folds first make contact during primary neurulation. The formation of succeeding caudal somites keeps pace with the caudal wave of neurulation.

As with the neural tube, the patterning of the somites is determined by the interaction of various homeobox genes and their gene products. The specification of a vertebra along the craniocaudal axis is thought to be due to its *Hox profile*—the degree of expression of various homeobox genes at that particular craniocaudal level. Misexpression of one or another homeobox gene can result in either anterior or posterior transformation of various vertebrae. For example, the overexpression of *Hoxa-7* in mice results in a posterior translocation of the cervical vertebrae, such that the last occipital somites, rather than contributing to the occiput, instead form an aberrant "pro-atlas." The true atlas, which normally would constitute only a ring and whose cells would ordinarily contribute to the formation of the dens, instead expresses a full vertebral body. In contrast, overexpression of the gene *Hoxc-6* results in anterior spinal translocation, creating a thoracic phenotype with an accompanying rib from the upper lumber vertebra.[317] The misexpression of homeobox genes in humans could similarly account for such malformations as occipitalized atlas, cervical ribs, and lumbarized or sacralized lumbosacral vertebrae.

The maximal number of somites in the human embryo is typically 42 to 44, although no more than 38 or 39 are required for the formation of the axial skeleton.[27] Most of the "excess" is due to coccygeal somitic segments that disappear during subsequent growth, although there also may be a rearrangement or loss of the cranialmost segments as well.[318] The number and size of the somites appear to be species specific and relatively constant within species.[319] If a number of somites are experimentally removed, the embryo is capable of compensating (regulating) to generate a normal number of somites of normal size.[320, 321] Regulation to produce normal numbers of vertebrae can occur even after removal of up to 90% of chick somites or after bilateral removal of a somitic pair. Reconstitution apparently occurs from the remaining somitic mesoderm with normal or only minimally malformed vertebrae.[321] Vertebral malformations of the type seen in

clinical practice are rare after experimental excision of somites, suggesting that such malformations may arise later in embryogenesis.

Formation of the Sclerotome and Dermomyotome

The developing somite is divided dorsoventrally into two elements: a more ventrally situated sclerotome, which will form the axial skeleton (the vertebrae and ribs), and a more dorsally situated dermomyotome, which will form the dermis and subcutaneous tissues of the back as well as the myocytes of the dorsal trunk musculature.[316] The sclerotome and dermomyotome are readily identified by the expression of various molecular markers. For example, the sclerotome is characterized by the expression of Pax1 and Pax9, whereas the dermomyotome is characterized by the expression of Pax3 and Pax7 as well as MyoD and other molecular species.[322]

The formation of the sclerotome and dermomyotome is regulated by the notochord or neural tube floor plate. A dorsally implanted notochord or floor plate represses the formation of the dermomyotome and instead induces an additional sclerotome, whereas excision of the notochord inhibits sclerotome formation ventrally.[316] The regulation of this dorsoventral polarity of the somites, as with the neural tube, is mediated by developmentally regulated proteins such as shh secreted from the developing notochord and floor-plate cells, Wnt and neurotrophin 3 (NT-3) from the adjacent dorsal neural tube, and BMP-4 from the lateral plate mesodermal precursors of the lateral body wall (Fig. 281–29).[153] Sonic hedgehog induces the sclerotome from the ventromedial region of the somite, whereas Wnt, NT-3, and BMP-4 all induce the dermomyotome from more dorsal regions. The dorsal misexpression of shh, like notochord transplantation, induces the formation of a dorsally situated accessory sclerotome. Antibodies that block the action of NT-3 prevent the formation of dermal elements from the dorsal somite.[153]

The subsequent development of the somites can be divided into three phases: the membranous phase during the fifth week of embryogenesis, the chondrification phase beginning at the sixth embryonic week, and the ossification phase beginning at around the ninth embryonic week.

MEMBRANOUS PHASE

During the membranous phase, sclerotomal cells migrate toward and surround both the notochord ventrally and the neural tube dorsally. The merging of cells from somites on either side of the notochord produces the vertebral centra, which first become visible in human embryos at stage 15 (POD 33). There is clear-cut experimental evidence that each sclerotome is divided into cranial and caudal halves, each expressing a different set of cellular and molecular markers.[316] This craniocaudal polarity begins during somite formation and is restricted to the sclerotomal portion of the somite.[322] The cranial portion of each sclerotome

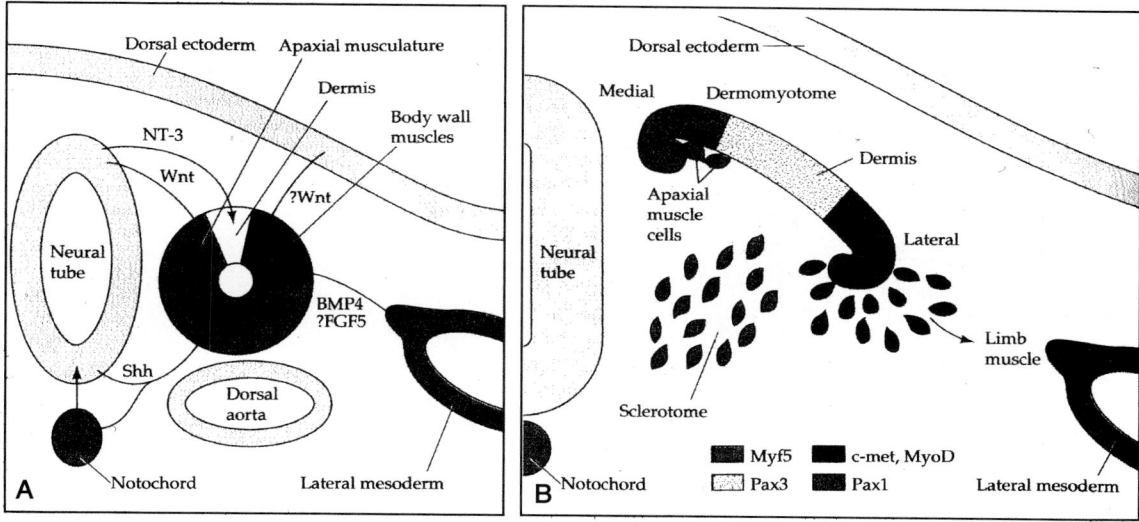

FIGURE 281–29. Formation of the somite. *A,* Postulated molecular interactions between the neural tube, dorsal (cutaneous) ectoderm, lateral plate mesoderm, and notochord in the formation of the somite. Sonic hedgehog from the notochord and floor-plate cells of the neural tube induces the sclerotome. Wnt from the dorsal neural tube induces the myotome precursors of the paraxial musculature; Wnt from the epidermis, together with BMP-4 from the lateral plate mesoderm, induces the myotomic precursors of the limb musculature. Neurotrophin 3 from the neural tube may induce the dermatomyotome. *B,* Expression of transcription factors from various regions of the somite. The sclerotomal cells express Pax1, and the medial dermatomyotomal cells express Myf5. Lateral dermatomyotomal cells express MyoD and c-met receptor for scatter factor. The central portion of the dermatomyotome expresses Pax3 and becomes dermis. (From Gilbert SF: Developmental Biology. Sunderland, MA, Sinauer Associates, 1997.)

contains more loosely packed cells, and the caudal portion contains more densely packed cells. Between the cranial and caudal portions lies a hypocellular cleft, called the fissure of von Ebner. The craniocaudal organization of the sclerotome is critical to axonal outgrowth, because the outgrowth of spinal nerves at each level of the neuraxis is restricted to the more loosely packed cranial portion of the sclerotome.[315, 322] The dorsal vertebral arch appears to be exclusively derived from the caudal, more densely packed half of the sclerotome.

There has been ongoing debate about whether each sclerotome forms a single vertebral centrum, or whether the caudal half (the dense-celled portion) of one sclerotome and the cranial half of the adjacent sclerotome combine to form a single vertebral body, with the hypocellular fissure of von Ebner contributing to the intervening intervertebral disk (a process called *resegmentation,* or *Neugliederung*). Resegmentation was originally proposed by Remak[323] in 1855 to account for the anatomic arrangement of the vertebral centra, dorsal vertebral arch, and spinal nerves. At each sclerotomal level, the spinal nerve passes through the cranial half-sclerotome, and the posterior vertebral arch is derived from the caudal half-sclerotome. Therefore, one would predict that the spinal nerve would exit cranial to the corresponding pedicle. The observed anatomic relationships of the pedicles to the anterior half of each vertebral body, with each spinal nerve passing *caudal* to the corresponding pedicle, can be accounted for only by resegmentation so that the cranial, loose-celled region of one sclerotome joins with the caudal, dense-celled region of the next more cranial sclerotome to form a single vertebral unit (Fig. 281–30).

The concept of resegmentation was opposed by Verbout,[324] Theiler,[325] and others, who suggested that each vertebra (including the vertebral centrum, posterior arch, transverse processes, ribs, and a single adjacent intervertebral disk) is derived exclusively from a single pair of somites. As a result, the concept of resegmentation fell into disfavor. However, much (but not all) subsequent experimental evidence has supported the concept of resegmentation.[326–331] For example, chick-quail chimeras (in which single chick somites are excised and replaced with quail vertebrae) and retroviral-mediated gene transfer paradigms (in which a recombinant retrovirus expressing a β-galactosidase marker is injected into single somites) have been used to follow the fate of the labeled somite over time. In these experiments, each somite contributes to two adjacent vertebral centra. The concept of resegmentation has therefore been resurrected, but it continues to be debated.

CHONDRIFICATION PHASE

Chondrification centers appear during the sixth embryonic week under the inductive control of secreted substances from the adjacent notochord and ventral neural tube. Ordinarily, three paired centers of chondrification appear (Fig. 281–31). The first pair surrounds the notochord ventral to the neural tube and forms the vertebral centrum. The second pair forms dorsolaterally and migrates medially, dorsal to the neural tube, to form the dorsal vertebral arches and spinous processes. The

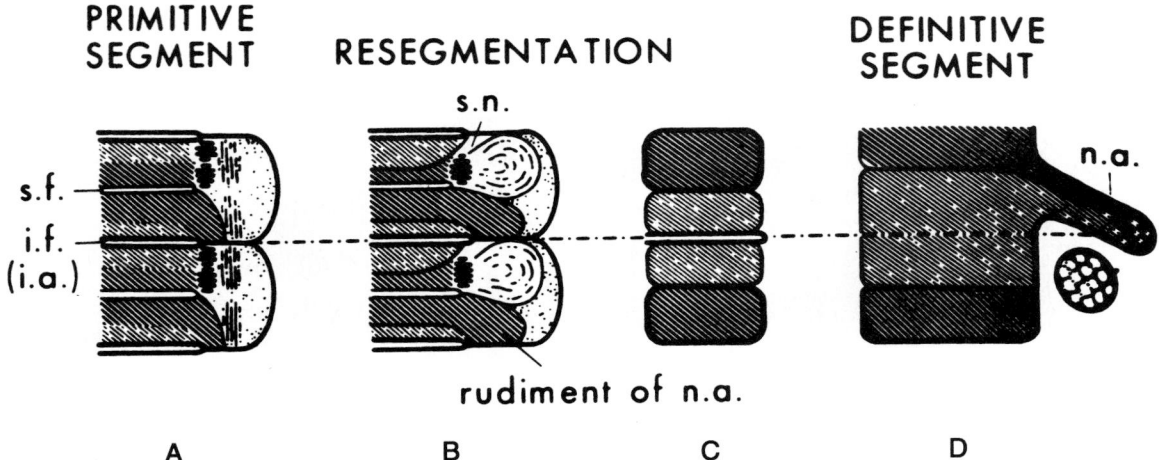

FIGURE 281–30. Resegmentation of the somites to form the definitive vertebrae. The densely hatched area is the dense-celled area; the lightly hatched area is the loose-celled area. ia, intersegmental artery; if, intersegmental fissure; sf, segmental fissure (of von Ebner). (From Tanaka T, Uhthoff HK: Significance of resegmentation in the pathogenesis of vertebral body malformations. Acta Orthop Scand 52:331–338, 1981.)

third pair develops between the dorsal and ventral pairs and forms the transverse processes and costal arches. The ventral centers appear earlier than the dorsal centers, resulting in chondrification of the vertebral centra before the dorsal arches. Chondrification initially begins at the cervicothoracic region and extends both cranially and caudally thereafter. During the chondrification phase, cells from perinotochordal tissues condense around the notochord to produce the annulus of the intervertebral disk, while phylosipharous cells of the notochord form the more centrally located nucleus pulposus.[332] The anterior and posterior

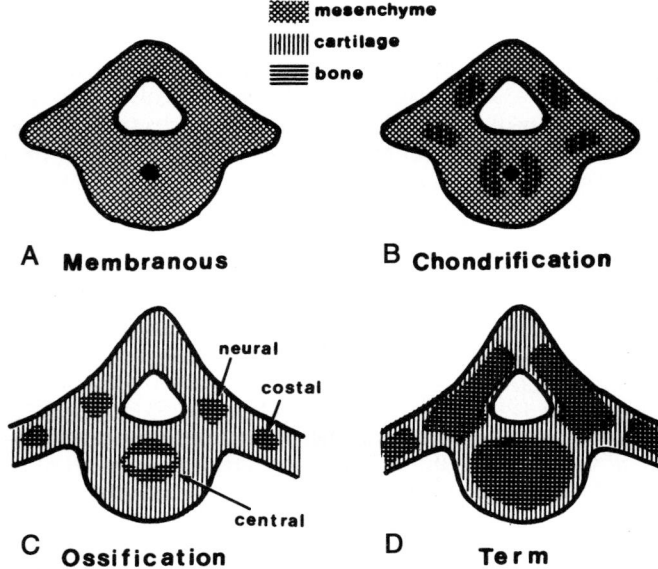

FIGURE 281–31. Chondrification and ossification of the vertebrae. (From Parke WW: Development of the spine. In Herkowitz HN, Garfin SR, Balderston RA, et al [eds]: Rothman-Simeone: The Spine, 4th ed. Philadelphia, WB Saunders, 1999, pp 3–27.)

longitudinal ligaments are formed during the chondrification phase from mesenchymal cells surrounding the cartilaginous vertebrae.

OSSIFICATION PHASE

Ossification of the vertebrae begins during the eighth embryonic week[333] and continues into postnatal life (see Fig. 281–31). Ossification is enhanced by the motion of the embryo.[332] The number of ossification centers that form within each vertebral segment is debated. Most authors suggest that there are three primary ossification centers—one for the vertebral centrum and one for each side of the dorsal vertebral arch. Within each side of the dorsal arch, the ossification centers extend to form three progressively independent zones of ossification—one each for the pedicles, lamina, and transverse processes. Others have proposed two independent ossification centers within each vertebral centrum—one forming dorsally and the other ventrally—with fusion of the two by the 20th to 24th embryonic week. Still others have suggested that as many as six primary ossification centers may be present: two forming the vertebral centrum; two forming the pedicles, lateral masses, and transverse processes; and two forming the laminae and spinous process (reviewed in reference 332).

Cartilaginous zones appear cranial and caudal to the ossification centers as the cartilaginous end plates. At the periphery of the cartilaginous end plates, between the developing intervertebral disk and the expanding ossification center of the vertebral centrum, lies the ring apophysis. Because of the ellipsoid growth of the ossification center, the ring apophysis is relatively deficient dorsally and more robust laterally and ventrally, forming a C shape. Eleven to 14 years postnatally, foci of ossification appear within the ring apophysis. They become confluent by 15 years of age and form the radiographic "ring" (the analog of the secondary ossification centers of long bones).[332] The ring eventually fuses with the vertebral centrum during mid to late adolescence. During childhood, the ring apophysis can fracture and its fragments can become displaced into the vertebral canal dorsolaterally, where they impinge on nerve roots in the lumbar foramina, simulating a herniated intervertebral disk. The junction of the paired posterior and the ventral ossification centers occurs at the neurocentral joint (of Luschka). It is important to recognize that the neurocentral joint lies *within* the vertebral body, not at the junction of the body and the pedicle. The vertebral body is therefore composed of elements derived from both the dorsal and the centrum ossification centers, and the terms *centrum* and *vertebral body* are therefore not strictly synonymous. Secondary ossification centers develop later in embryogenesis and are located in the apophysis (as described earlier) and at the tips of the spinous and transverse processes (see Fig. 281–31). The primary and secondary ossification centers fuse by 15 to 16 years of age.

Ossification of the vertebral centra slightly precedes that of the dorsal arch.[333, 334] Ossification of the vertebral centra begins at the thoracolumbar junction from T10 to L1 and rapidly spreads to involve the T2-L4 vertebrae. Thereafter, ossification proceeds in a bidirectional fashion to involve progressively more cranial and caudal vertebrae. In contrast, ossification of the dorsal arches begins simultaneously from C1 to L1 and proceeds monodirectionally in a craniocaudal direction. All ossification centers are visible by 14 weeks' gestation.[333, 334]

The notochord continues to contribute cells to the intervertebral disks during the fetal period and in the first few years of postnatal life. During the embryonic period, the notochord develops undulations, the first hint of segmentation. At the level of the intervertebral disks, the notochord assumes a more vacuolated appearance. The intervening portions are stretched into a "mucoid streak" that eventually begins to disappear as ossification centers appear in the adjacent centra. The remaining phylosipharous cells form the nucleus pulposus of the intervertebral disks; occasional microscopic rests may also be found within the vertebral bodies as well. By age 5 years, the proliferation of phylosipharous cells has largely ceased, and usually no viable cells remain in the disk. However, persistent notochordal cells have been found, particularly in incarcerated disks of the sacrum, and likely account for the sacral chordoma.[318]

Development of the Craniovertebral and Sacrococcygeal Regions

Development of the craniovertebral junction does not follow the pattern of the subaxial spine and is much more complex and embryologically unstable. Malformations of this region are therefore more common. The craniovertebral junction (encompassing the occiput, atlas, and axis) develops from the four occipital sclerotomes (formed from the somite pairs 1 to 4, respectively) and the first and second cervical sclerotomes (derived from somites 5 and 6, respectively) (Fig. 281–32). The basiocciput (occipital bone, lateral occipital

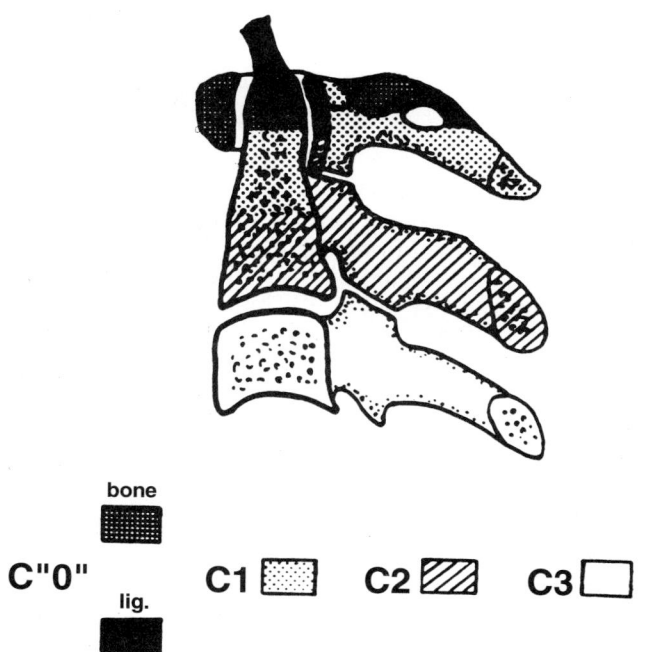

FIGURE 281–32. Development of the cervicomedullary junction from the fourth occipital and first three cervical somites. (From Parke WW: Development of the spine. In Herkowitz HN, Garfin SR, Balderston RA, et al [eds]: Rothman-Simeone: The Spine, 4th ed. Philadelphia, WB Saunders, 1999, pp 3–27.)

condyles, and clivus) is formed from the four occipital sclerotomes (somites 1 to 4). The anterior arch of the atlas is derived from a dense band of tissue, the hypochordal bow (an analog of the holocentrous vertebra in more primitive species), formed from the fourth occipital sclerotome (somite 4). The posterior arch of the atlas is derived from contributions from the fourth occipital and first cervical sclerotomes (somites 4 and 5, respectively). The anterior arch of the atlas is nonossified in 80% of newborns and usually ossifies between 6 and 24 months postnatally.[332]

The axis is derived from the fourth occipital sclerotome (somite 4) and the first and second cervical sclerotomes (somites 5 and 6). Rather than forming the centrum of the atlas, the ventral portion of the first cervical sclerotome (somite 5) forms the odontoid proper. Remnants of the notochord can be found within the odontoid at the level of the atlas arch, confirming its origin from the centrum.[318] The tip of the dens (the phylogenetic equivalent of the proatlas of reptile and avian embryos) is formed from the fourth occipital sclerotome (somite 4). The remainder of the axis (both the body and the dorsal vertebral arch) is derived from the second cervical sclerotome (somite 6). Ossification of the axis occurs from six ossification centers. The dens contains a bilaterally symmetrical pair of ossification centers that may not fuse until 3 months postnatally.[332] The tip of the dens (the portion derived from the fourth occipital sclerotome) contains an additional ossification center. Finally, the axis body contains three ossification centers—a ventral ossification center forming the centrum, and bilaterally paired dorsal ossification centers forming the dorsal arch. Fusion of the dens to the axis body at the dentocentral synchondrosis begins at about 4 years of age and is completed by 8 years; fusion of the apex of the dens to the dens proper occurs at around 12 years.

The sacrum and coccyx are also unique, and their development complex. In addition to the usual vertebral ossification centers already described, each sacral vertebra has one additional pair of ossification centers that provides ossification to the inferior and superior surfaces of each segment.[318] Three additional paired centers produce the sacral alae, forming anterolateral to the sacral foramina of the three upper sacral vertebrae.[318] The coccyx is formed from the caudalmost ventral sclerotomal segments; there are no corresponding dorsal ossification centers. The sacral segments are separated by intervertebral disks during early childhood, but fusion begins in late adolescence and is usually complete by the middle of the third decade. Coccygeal segments ossify postnatally—the first coccygeal segment before 5 years of age, and the remaining three more caudal segments at successive 5-year increments.[318]

ABNORMAL DEVELOPMENT OF THE VERTEBRAL COLUMN

There have been a number of attempts to classify vertebral malformations, the most recent and comprehensive by Tsou and colleagues[335] (Fig. 281–33), based on alleged embryogenetic mechanisms. Elements of this classification scheme have been modified by more recent embryonic data obtained by Tanaka and Uhthoff.[336] These schemes propose that most vertebral malformations arise during the membranous (resegmentation) or early chondrification phase of vertebral formation, although certain malformations may arise later during the ossification phase.[335, 336] Based on this classification scheme and subsequent modifications, we can divide vertebral malformations into several categories, according to reputed embryogenetic mechanisms (note that more than one mechanism may account for each malformation): (1) abnormalities of gastrulation (vertebral anomalies associated with split cord and other complex dysraphic malformations); (2) disordered alignment of sclerotomal rests, giving rise to hemimetameric shifts (hemivertebrae); (3) disordered formation of whole vertebrae (single or multiple) or of vertebral elements from sclerotomal precursors (vertebral wedging, hemivertebrae, caudal agenesis); (4) disordered segmentation of vertebrae, with or without associated vertebral formation defects (block vertebrae, Klippel-Feil syndrome); (5) disordered alignment of vertebrae (congenital vertebral dislocation); (6) disordered assimilation of sclerotomal cells across the midline (butterfly vertebrae); and (7) disordered ossification and fetal growth (isolated defects of vertebral centra). In this section, we give concrete examples to illustrate the various vertebral malformations and at-

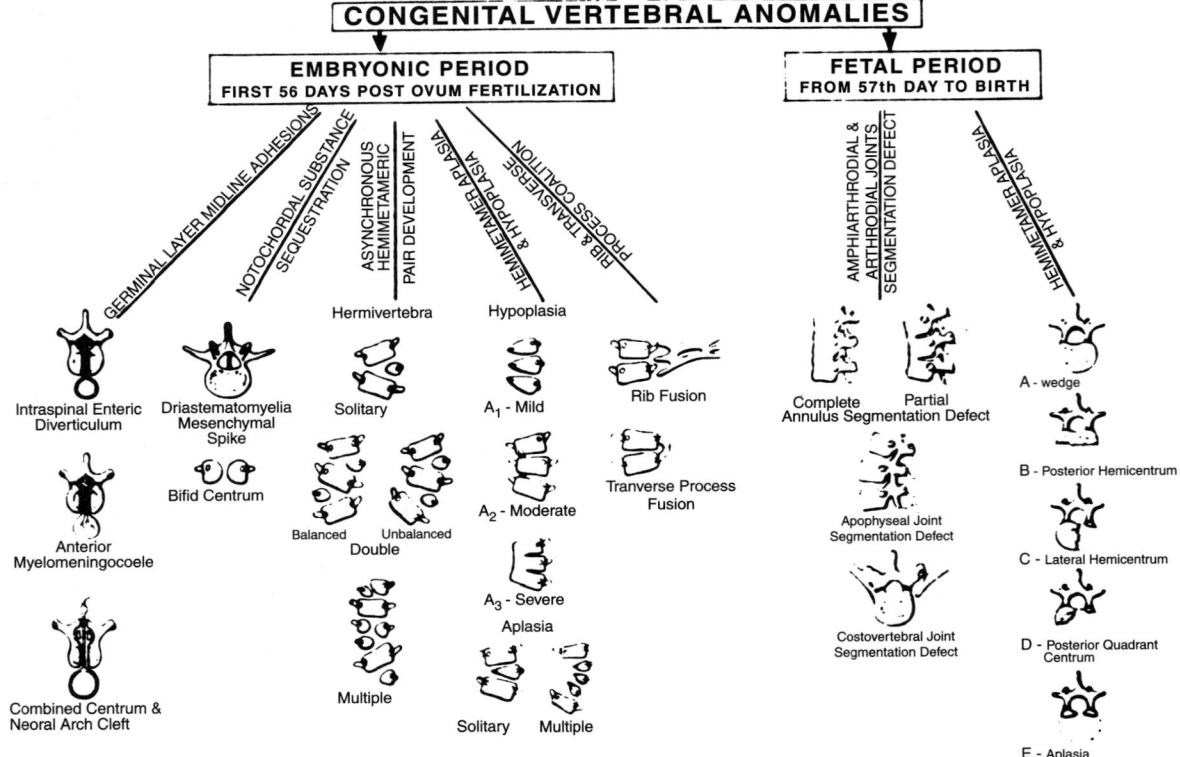

FIGURE 281–33. Proposed schematic of vertebral malformations. (From Tsou PM, Yau A, Hodgson AR: Embryogenesis and prenatal development of congenital vertebral anomalies and their classification. Clin Orthop 152:211–231, 1980.)

tempt to place them in the context of disordered embryogenesis. Neither the cellular nor the molecular mechanisms underlying these malformations are understood.

Disordered Gastrulation

This mechanism was thoroughly discussed earlier with regard to the dysraphic malformations. In addition to the multiple anomalies of the neural tube and other organ systems, a variety of vertebral malformations may arise from the secondary effects on the adjacent prospective somitic mesoderm in the proximal half of the primitive streak during gastrulation.[1] Hemivertebrae, sagittally clefted (butterfly) vertebrae, fused (block) vertebrae, midline osseous or fibrocartilaginous spurs or bands, some types of the Klippel-Feil anomaly, iniencephaly, and sacral agenesis have all been described (reviewed in Dias and Walker[1]). The association of these vertebral malformations with elements of the split cord malformation and its sequelae is the key to identifying this embryopathy.

Malalignment of Somitic Columns: Hemimetameric Shift

Lehman-Facius[337] first suggested in 1925 that hemivertebrae may arise as a result of a hemimetameric shift of the somitic column on one side of the embryo. Tsou and colleagues[335] argued that during the integration of the somitic mesoderm across the midline to form individual centra, the somites are normally at the same stage of development, and integration occurs between bilaterally juxtaposed pairs of somites. However, tardy development of a somite on one side might lead to a caudal metameric segmental shift of one somitic column with respect to the other, malalignment of the somites, and creation of an unpaired sclerotomic center, leading to a hemivertebra (Fig. 281–34). The key characteristic of this malformation is a hemivertebral seg-

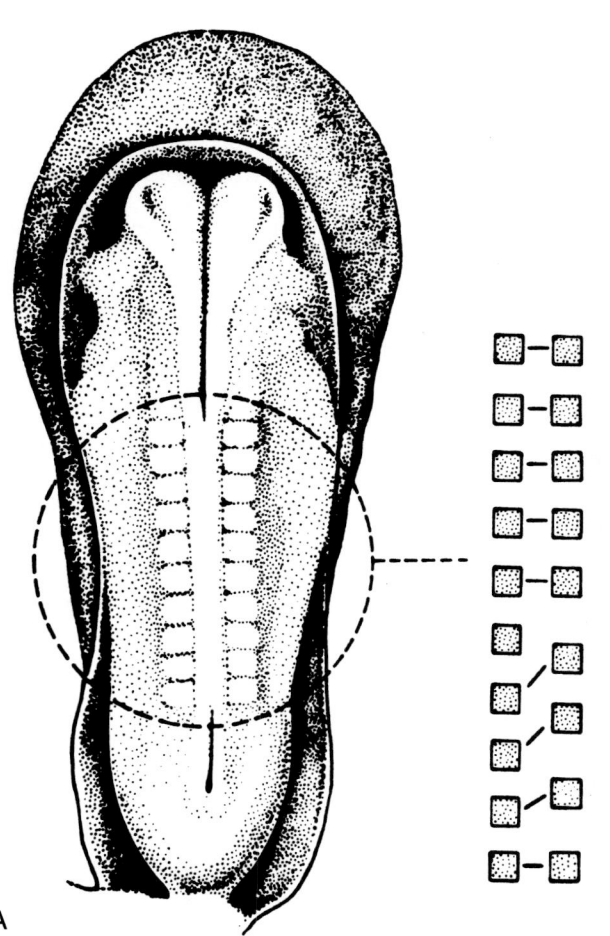
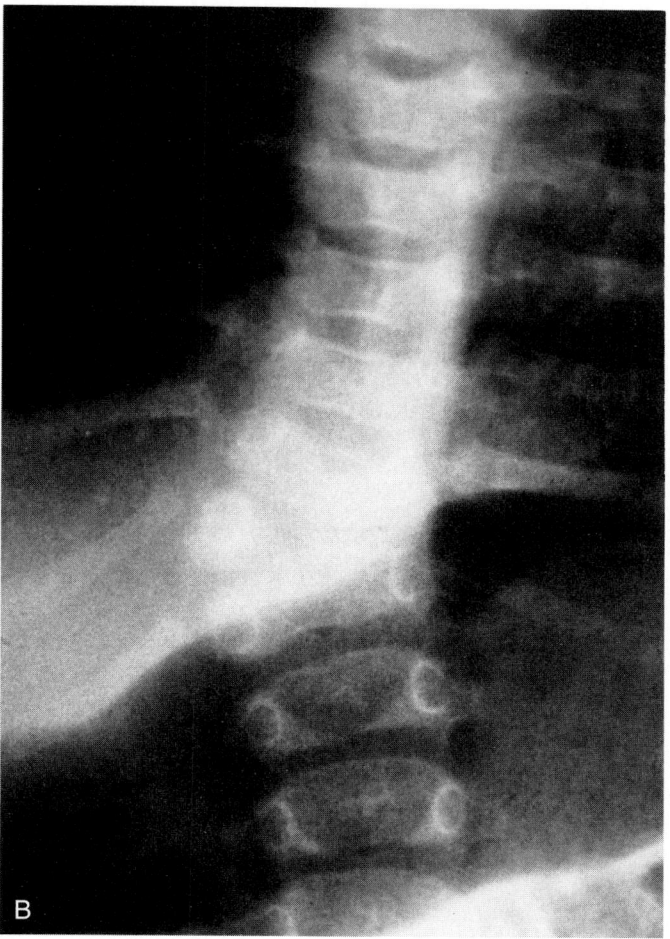

FIGURE 281–34. Hemivertebra. *A*, Illustration of hemimetameric somitic shift producing a hemivertebra. If paired somites are not at the same stage of maturation at the time of somitic midline fusion, the tardy side shifts one segment caudad, producing an isolated hemisomite that develops into a solitary hemivertebra. *B*, Anteroposterior radiograph of a hemivertebra. (*A*, From Tsou PM, Yau A, Hodgson AR: Embryogenesis and prenatal development of congenital vertebral anomalies and their classification. Clin Orthop 152:211–231, 1980.)

ment that has a rounded medial border and does not cross the midline. Both the portion of the vertebral centrum and the corresponding dorsal vertebral arch on the opposite side are congenitally absent. A fully formed posterior vertebral arch is present on the ipsilateral side but is often incorporated into the vertebral arch above or below the hemivertebra and may be difficult to see. The malformation may be uni- or multisegmental and may lead to balanced or imbalanced hemivertebrae. Tsou and colleagues[335] estimated that this mechanism accounts for most cases of hemivertebrae (58 of 63 cases in their series).

Disordered Vertebral Formation

Disruption or injury to either the somites or the sclerotomal precursors during the membranous phase could unilaterally decrease the ability of the sclerotome to contribute cells to the formation of the vertebra, resulting in unilateral vertebral hypoplasia or agenesis. Although a disorder of the ossification phase was originally proposed by Junghanns,[338] the presence of these malformations in embryos between 7 and 11.5 weeks of gestation[336, 339] clearly refutes such a mechanism. Ossification is likely affected only secondarily. Examples of partially disordered vertebral formation are wedge vertebrae and some cases of hemivertebrae. Tsou and colleagues[335] applied the term *hemimetamer hypoplasia or aplasia* to these malformations and identified three types related to the severity of the deficiency. A key component of these malformations is the involvement of both the vertebral centrum and the posterior vertebral arch.

In the mildest form, the quantity of chondrogenic precursors from the ipsilateral sclerotome is reduced, the height of the vertebral centrum is diminished unilaterally, and a wedge vertebra results (Fig. 281–35A). In the moderate form, the contributions to the posterior vertebral arch are deficient, and the laminae, apophyseal joints, and (in more severe forms) pedicles of adjacent segments fuse to form a dorsolateral unsegmented bar. In the thoracic region, multiple rib malformations are also formed (see Fig. 281–35B). In the most severe form, the vertebral centrum and dorsal arch are simultaneously affected, leading to a form of hemivertebra. In contrast to the hemivertebra formed by hemimetameric shift, however, the existing contralateral half-centrum in this instance is irregular and crosses the midline to a variable degree. A rudimentary rib may mark the site of the missing half-centrum. In the extreme, there is multisegmental failure, and the hemivertebral elements are replaced at multiple levels with poorly differentiated fibrocartilaginous tissue (see Fig. 281–35C).[335]

A number of dysraphic anomalies, most commonly split cord and related malformations, have been associated with hemivertebrae of this type. The combination of a single hemivertebra with a contralateral congenital dorsolateral unsegmented bar is most frequently (50% of cases) associated with an underlying spinal cord malformation.[340] Associated renal malformations are also common, particularly with lower thoracic and lumbar lesions. Embryologically, they are predicted by the close physical and temporal proximity of the embryonic intermediate mesoderm, which lies immedi-

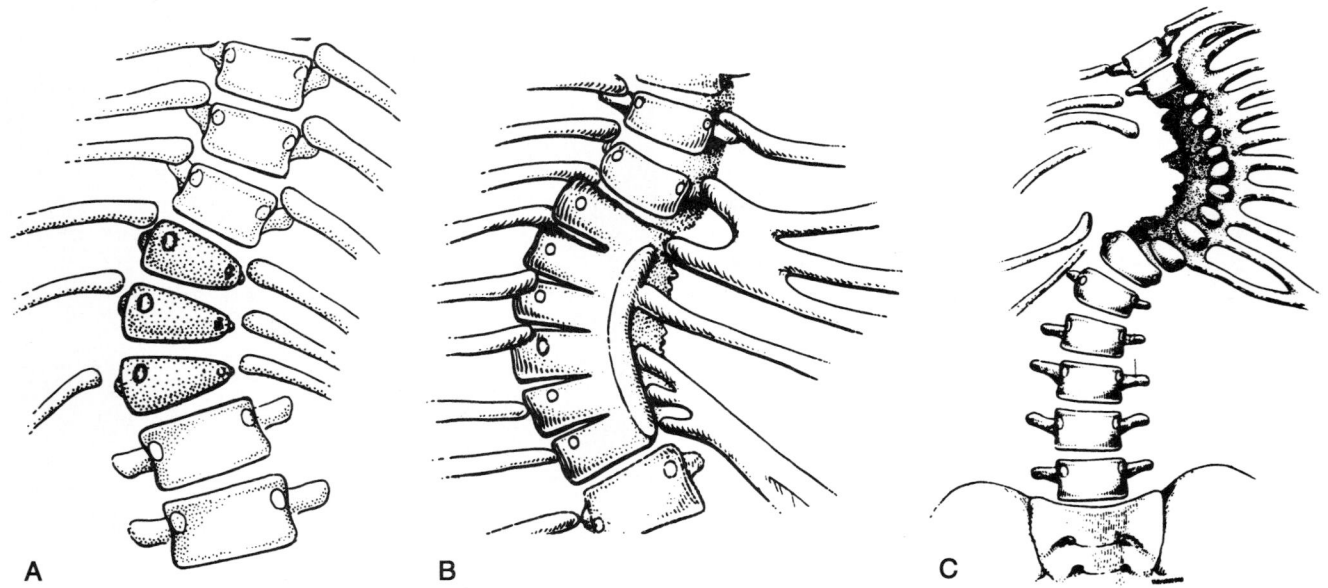

FIGURE 281–35. Hemimetamer hypoplasia producing hemivertebrae and segmental bars. *A,* Mild hypoplasia produces isolated lateral wedging of three adjacent vertebrae. *B,* More severe involvement produces a segmental bar formed from the vestiges of the ipsilateral neural arch elements and centra. Segmentation markings are lost on the involved side. *C,* Multiple hemimetamer aplasia produces multiple hemivertebrae. The involved side contains only undifferentiated fibrocartilaginous tissue. (From Tsou PM, Yau A, Hodgson AR: Embryogenesis and prenatal development of congenital vertebral anomalies and their classification. Clin Orthop 152:211–231, 1980.)

ately lateral to the somitic mesoderm and gives rise to the mesonephros of the kidney. When renal malformations coexist with hemivertebrae, they are always ipsilateral to the side of the missing half-vertebra.[341] The underlying cause of the injury or disruption of the sclerotome is unknown, although a vascular cause due to malformation or disruption of the intersegmental arteries during the membranous phase has been proposed by Tanaka and Uhthoff.[336] Those associated with dysraphic malformations likely arise before neural tube closure and involve a disorder of gastrulation, as discussed earlier.[1]

A number of craniocervical malformations may represent partial or complete failure of vertebral formation via similar mechanisms. There may be an absent anterior atlas arch (inadequate development of the hypochordal bow), a hypoplastic or absent posterior atlas arch or absent tip of the dens (inadequate development of the fourth occipital sclerotome [somite 4]), or a hypoplastic or absent dens (inadequate development of the first cervical sclerotome [somite 5]).

Disordered Vertebral Segmentation

A number of malformations can be ascribed to disorders of vertebral segmentation. The simplest example of isolated vertebral segmentation failure is the single block vertebra, in which two adjacent vertebrae are fused. These may be ventral (affecting only the vertebral body), dorsal (affecting only the dorsal vertebral arch), or both. An example of a more restricted dorsolateral failure is the unsegmented bar (discussed earlier). Multiple vertebral fusions may be involved in the Klippel-Feil syndrome (Fig. 281–36). Finally, at the craniocervical junction, atlas assimilation may represent a failure of segmentation of the fourth occipital sclerotome (somite 4) from the first cervical sclerotome (somite 5).

The simplest mechanistic explanation is a failure (within either the prospective somitic mesoderm or the somites themselves) to properly segment into discrete entities, perhaps because of disordered expression of homeobox genes or CAMs. Segmentation appears to be regulated by metameric segmentation genes of the homeobox class and others, and genetic mutations of these genes may be responsible for segmentation failure malformations. Keynes and Stern[315] described a number of segmentation-class gene mutations in mice that display a variety of fusions, deletions, and malformations. For example, in the mouse mutant pudgy, only rudimentary segmentation takes place, resulting in multiple segmentation anomalies and irregular, misshapen vertebrae.[317] Homologues of the *Drosophila* genes *Delta* and *Notch* appear to be particularly important in somite segmentation.[316] Mouse mutants lacking *Notch* expression exhibit severe defects of somitic segmentation and polarity, and microinjections of a dominant negative form of *X-Delta-2* into *Xenopus* embryos cause multiple disorders of segmentation and even abolish the segmental pattern. Whether the localized segmentation failures that produce, for example,

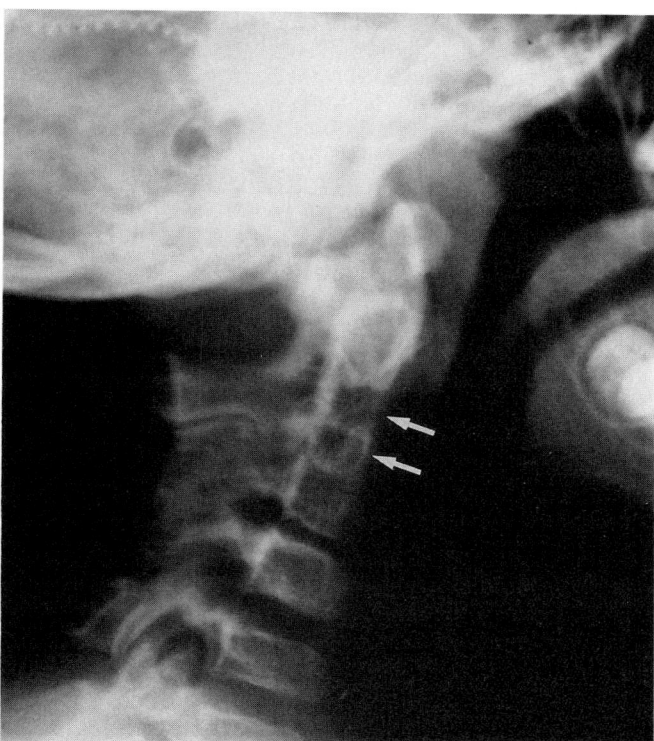

FIGURE 281–36. Failure of segmentation at C2-3 *(white arrows)* in a patient with Klippel-Feil syndrome.

block vertebrae are due to these or other mechanisms is unknown.

Alternatively, Tsou and colleagues[335] suggested that osseous metaplasia of the annulus ventrally or of the apophyseal or costovertebral joints dorsally during the ossification phase could account for vertebral fusions. However, descriptions of human embryos as early as 5 to 7.5 weeks with vertebral fusions suggest that these malformations occur much earlier, during or before the membranous phase, and reflect an earlier embryonic insult.[336, 339] Others have suggested that the cervical vertebral fusions seen in the Klippel-Feil syndrome may reflect a disruption in subclavian or vertebral artery blood supply to the involved structures at or soon before the sixth embryonic week. This disruption would give rise not only to the cervical vertebral fusions but also to Sprengel's deformity, hypoplastic pectoralis muscles, breast hypoplasia, and the terminal limb defects that are sometimes associated.[342, 343] However, it is difficult to explain the associated thoracolumbar or lumbar fusions (Klippel-Feil syndrome type III) that one occasionally sees in the disorder or the association with sacral agenesis (Klippel-Feil syndrome type IV).[344] Finally, the reported association of Klippel-Feil syndrome with split cord malformations[1, 345] raises the possibility, as reviewed earlier, that certain cases of Klippel-Feil syndrome may arise through disordered midline axial integration during gastrulation.

Disordered Vertebral Alignment

A condition referred to as *congenital vertebral dislocation* may represent an example of malalignment of verte-

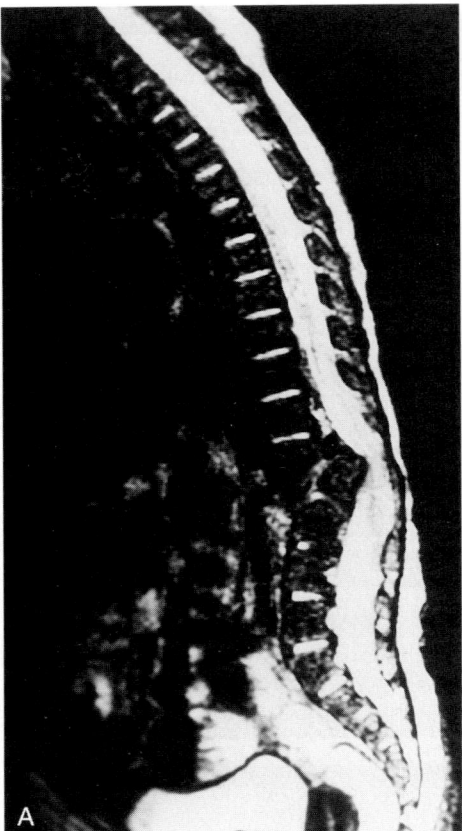

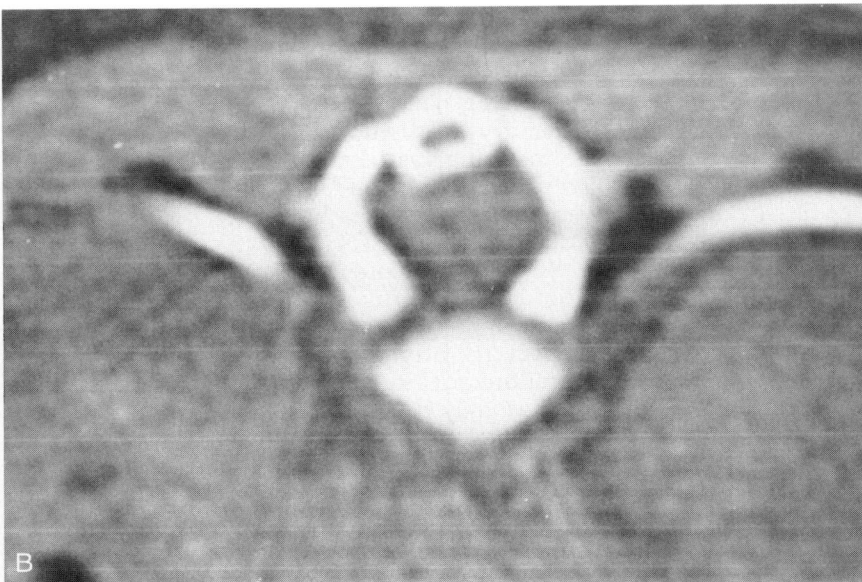

FIGURE 281–37. Congenital vertebral dislocation. *A,* Sagittal T2-weighted magnetic resonance imaging scan demonstrates a complete and abrupt spondyloptosis of T11 on T12. Note the alignment of the T12 body with the more caudal vertebral column. *B,* Axial computed tomographic myelogram in another case shows the spinal cord and thecal sac transposed dorsally to the extreme dorsal portion of the spinal canal *(arrows).* The pedicles are abnormally elongated, and the canal is extremely wide in the anteroposterior dimension. (From Dias MS, Li V, Landi M, et al: The embryogenesis of congenital vertebral dislocation: Early embryonic buckling? Pediatr Neurosurg 29:281–289, 1998.)

brae during early vertebral development. In this condition (Fig. 281–37), a complete vertebral spondyloptosis develops at a single vertebral level, usually at or near the thoracolumbar junction. The more inferior vertebrae are aligned one with another, as are the more superior vertebrae, suggesting that the entire vertebral column has been translocated at a single vertebral level. The spinal canal at the involved level is widened, the pedicles of the more superior vertebra are peculiarly elongated (see Fig. 281–37*B*), and the dorsal vertebral arch is often dysraphic as well. The spinal cord is intact across the lesion but is almost always lowlying (suggesting spinal cord tethering). Despite a severe translocation of the vertebral canal, these patients often have few, if any, neurological deficits. There are few associated malformations, but reported instances of tracheoesophageal fistula and unilateral renal agenesis suggest an early embryonic insult. This deformation has been postulated to arise as a result of simple mechanical buckling of the embryo between the fourth and sixth weeks of embryogenesis, after neurulation but before chondrification is complete.[346]

Failed Fusion of Sclerotome, Chondrification, and Ossification Centers

Various vertebral malformations may be due to disordered assimilation, or "fusion," of the various chondrification or ossification centers. For example, the sagittally clefted butterfly vertebra (Fig. 281–38) could arise from disordered integration of scleroderm pairs across the ventral midline and around the notochord, perhaps because of an abnormal perinotochordal sheath.[347] Butterfly vertebrae can be produced in rabbits by maternal oxygen deprivation at stages corresponding to stages 11 to 12 (PODs 23 to 27) in humans, and they have been described in Danforth's short-tail mice (reviewed in reference 348); in both, abnormalities of the notochord have been described. The timing of butterfly vertebrae in these models, as well as in the few described human fetal malformations,[348] supports the view that these defects arise during somatogenesis (stages 10 to 13; PODs 21 to 28). Alternatively, bilateral (left and right) chondrification centers could fail to become properly integrated as late as the sixth embryonic week.[348]

Localized failure of fusion of the ventral and dorsal ossification centers could result in malformations of the pedicles or facets, such as dysplastic spondylolysis. Moreover, a failure of fusion of the bilaterally paired dorsal chondrification or, later, ossification centers could result in spina bifida occulta, with a missing or malformed spinous process. Interestingly, a homeobox gene *Msx-2* (formerly known as *Hox-8*) is expressed in the spinous process and appears to be involved in the development of the dorsal vertebral arch during early embryogenesis. Mutations of the *Msx-2* gene produce mouse embryos that lack a spinous process.[317]

Finally, at the craniocervical junction, localized failure of fusion leads to well-known anomalies. Failure

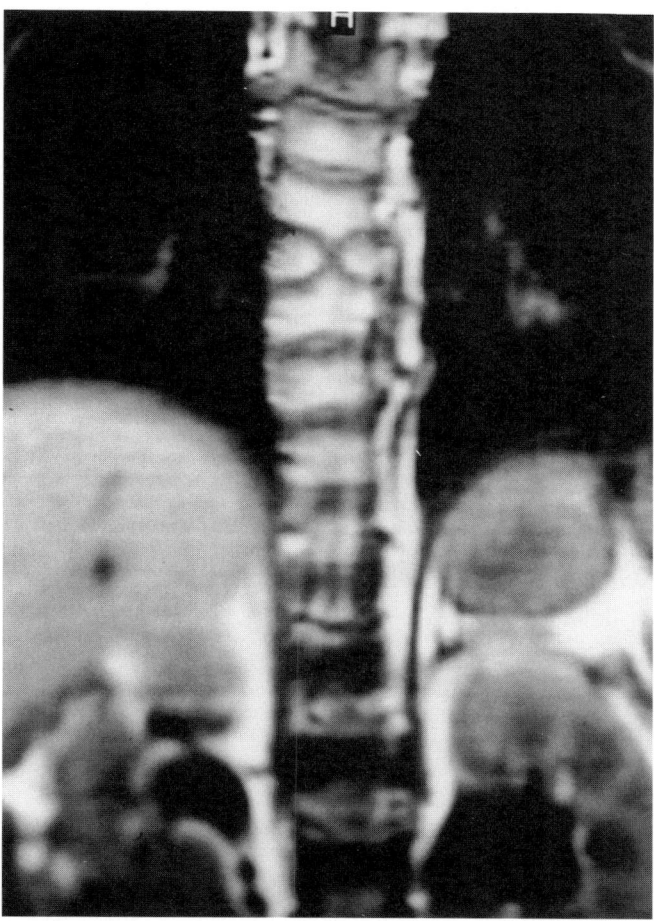

FIGURE 281–38. Coronal T1-weighted magnetic resonance imaging scan of a child with an isolated hemivertebra at T9.

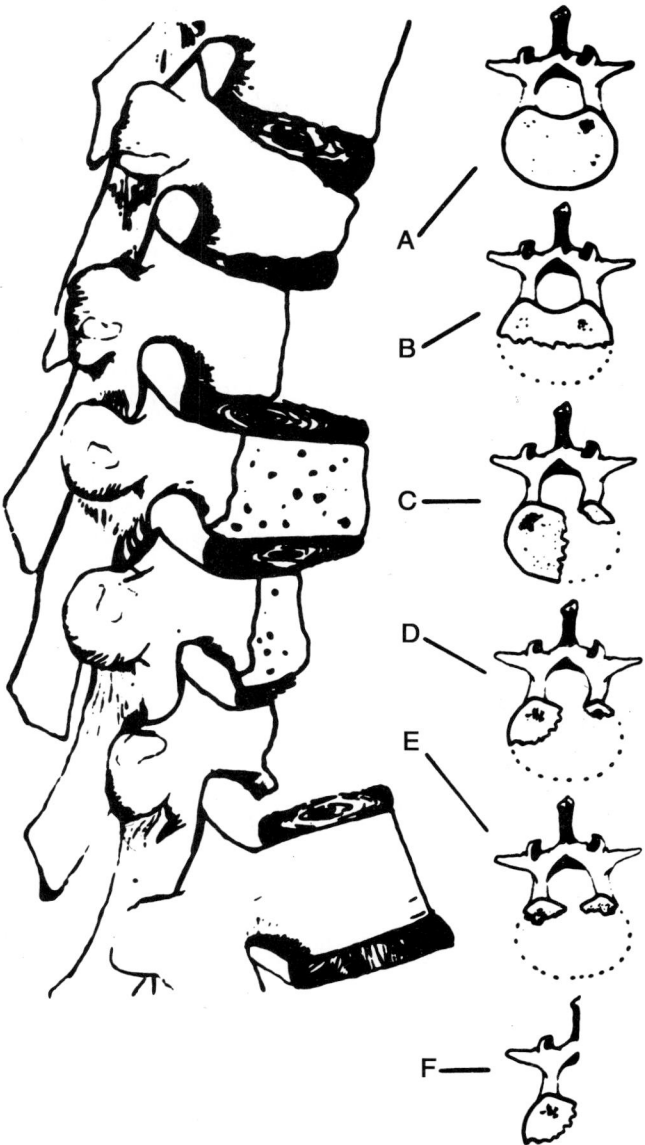

FIGURE 281–39. Centrum hypoplasia and aplasia. *A*, Wedge. *B*, Posterior hemicentrum. *C*, Lateral hemicentrum. *D*, Posterior quadrant centrum. *E*, Centrum aplasia. *F*, Asynchronous development of a hemimetamer pair. The lateral centrum of the unpaired hemivertebra suffers further anterior growth disturbance during the fetal period. The residue posterior quadrant centrum is accompanied by an ipsilateral hemiarch, in contrast to the intact neural arch of the posterior quadrant centrum in *D*. (From Tsou PM, Yau A, Hodgson AR: Embryogenesis and prenatal development of congenital vertebral anomalies and their classification. Clin Orthop 152:211–231, 1980.)

of the ossiculum terminale (fourth cervical sclerotome) to fuse with the odontoid proper (first cervical sclerotome) results in ossiculum terminale (or os avis), and failure of the odontoid proper to fuse with the axis body (second cervical sclerotome) results in os odontoideum.

Isolated Failure of Ossification and Growth

Isolated hypoplasia or aplasia of the vertebral centrum, without corresponding alterations in the dorsal vertebral arch, likely reflects a failure of centrum growth during later fetal stages.[335] All or part of the centrum is reduced or absent, but the pedicles, up to the neurocentral synchondrosis, remain (Fig. 281–39). In the absence of corresponding dorsal arch anomalies, a primary sclerotomal disorder is unlikely; disruption of the vascular supply has been proposed as a possible cause.[335] The posterior (dorsal) hemivertebra, in which there is isolated absence or wedging of the ventral portion of the centrum, may also occur during later vertebral development; growth of the centrum is most rapid ventrally, putting that area at the greatest risk for vascular compromise. Conversely, if there are indeed ventral and dorsal ossification centers within the cen-

trum, as some have described, an isolated failure of the ventral ossification center could also produce such a malformation.

SUMMARY

We have given a detailed and comprehensive description of normal early human development of the spinal cord and spine and have provided a mechanistic, or embryogenetic, classification scheme for many identified malformations based on a working knowledge of normal human embryogenesis. A variety of theories have been offered to explain the origin of these malformations; some have advanced our understanding of dysraphism, and others have fallen short of the mark. Although these theories are plausible, few have been rigorously tested experimentally, and none has been proved. Although the mechanisms may eventually be proved wrong, they provide a working framework on which we can begin to identify and classify human malformations, to understand their demographics and anatomy, and ultimately to guide their surgical management. A thorough understanding of normal anatomy and embryology provides a solid background for the accurate diagnosis and rational treatment of children with congenital spine and spinal cord malformations. Conversely, failing to understand these processes can lead to misidentification or mistreatment of these disorders.

REFERENCES

1. Dias MS, Walker ML: The embryogenesis of complex dysraphic malformations: A disorder of gastrulation? Pediatr Neurosurg 18:229–253, 1992.
2. Campbell LR, Dayton DH, Sohal GS: Neural tube defects: A review of human and animal studies on the etiology of neural tube defects. Teratology 34:171–187, 1986.
3. O'Rahilly R, Müller F: Developmental Stages in Human Embryos. Washington, DC, Carnegie Institution of Washington, 1987.
4. Vakaet L: Some new data concerning the formation of the definitive endoblast in the chick embryo. J Embryol Exp Morphol 10:38–57, 1962.
5. Modak SP: Experimental analysis of the origin of the embryonic endoblast in birds [French]. Rev Suisse Zool 73:877–908, 1966.
6. Fontaine J, Le Douarin NM: Analysis of endoderm formation in the avian blastoderm by the use of quail-chick chimaeras: The problem of the neurectodermal origin of the cells of the APUD series. J Embryol Exp Morphol 41:209–222, 1977.
7. Rosenquist GC: A radioautographic study of labeled grafts in the chick blastoderm: Development from primitive streak stages to stage 12. Contrib Embryol 38:73–110, 1966.
8. Nicolet G: Analyse autoradiographique de la localisation des différentes ébauches présomptives dans la ligne primitive de l'embryon de Poulet. J Embryol Exp Morphol 23:79–108, 1970.
9. Nicolet G: Avian gastrulation. Adv Morphog 9:231–262, 1971.
10. Schoenwolf GC, Sheard P: Fate mapping the avian epiblast with focal injections of a fluorescent-histochemical marker: Ectodermal derivatives. J Exp Zool 255:323–339, 1990.
11. Spratt NT: Regression and shortening of the primitive streak in the explanted chick blastoderm. J Exp Zool 104:69–100, 1947.
12. Schoenwolf GC, Smith JL: Gastrulation and early mesodermal patterning in vertebrates. In Tuan RS, Lo CW (eds): Methods in Molecular Biology: Developmental Biology Protocols, vol 1. Totowa, NJ, Humana Press, 1998.
13. Tam PPL, Behringer RR: Mouse gastrulation: The formation of a mammalian body plan. Mech Dev 68:3–25, 1997.
14. Hill JP, Florian J: A young human embryo (embryo Dobbin) with head-process and prochordal plate. Philos Trans R Soc Lond B 219:443–486, 1931.
15. Shaw W: Observations on two specimens of early human ova. BMJ 1:411–415, 1932.
16. Hendrickx AG: Description of stages IX, X, and XI. In Hendrickx AG (ed): Embryology of the Baboon. London, University of Chicago Press, 1971, pp 69–85.
17. O'Rahilly R, Müller F: The first appearance of the human nervous system at stage 8. Anat Embryol (Berl) 163:1–13, 1981.
18. Müller F, O'Rahilly R: The first appearance of the neural tube and optic primordium in the human embryo at stage 10. Anat Embryol (Berl) 172:157–169, 1985.
19. Müller F, O'Rahilly R: The first appearance of the major divisions of the human brain at stage 9. Anat Embryol (Berl) 168:419–432, 1983.
20. Müller F, O'Rahilly R: The development of the human brain and the closure of the rostral neuropore at stage 11. Anat Embryol (Berl) 175:205–222, 1986.
21. O'Rahilly R: Developmental Stages in Human Embryos, Including a Survey of the Carnegie Collection. Part A. Embryos of the First Three Weeks (Stages 1 to 9). Washington, DC, Carnegie Institution of Washington, 1973.
22. Golden JA, Chernoff GF: Multiple sites of anterior neural tube closure in humans: Evidence from anterior neural tube defects (anencephaly). Pediatrics 95:506–510, 1995.
23. Golden JA, Chernoff GF: Intermittent pattern of neural tube closure in two strains of mice. Teratology 47:73–80, 1993.
24. Van Allen MI, Kalousek DK, Chernoff GF, et al: Evidence for multi-site closure of the neural tube in humans. Am J Med Genet 47:723–743, 1993.
25. Urioste M, Rosa A: Anencephaly and faciocranioschisis: Evidence of complete failure of closure 3 of the neural tube in humans. Am J Med Genet 75:4–6, 1998.
26. Müller F, O'Rahilly R: The development of the human brain, the closure of the caudal neuropore, and the beginning of secondary neurulation at stage 12. Anat Embryol (Berl) 176:413–430, 1987.
27. Müller F, O'Rahilly R: Somitic-vertebral correlation and vertebral levels in the human embryo. Am J Anat 177:3–19, 1986.
28. Streeter GL: Developmental horizons in human embryos: Description of age group XI, 13 to 20 somites, and age group XII, 21 to 29 somites. Contrib Embryol 30:211–245, 1942.
29. Nichols DH: Formation and distribution of neural crest mesenchyme to the first pharyngeal arch region of the mouse embryo. Am J Anat 176:221–231, 1986.
30. Tan SS, Morris-Kay G: The development and distribution of the cranial neural crest in the rat embryo. Cell Tissue Res 240:403–416, 1985.
31. Müller F, O'Rahilly R: The first appearance of the future cerebral hemispheres in the human embryo at stage 14. Anat Embryol (Berl) 177:495–511, 1988.
32. Bronner-Fraser M: The neural crest: What can it tell us about cell migration and determination? Curr Top Dev Biol 15:1–25, 1980.
33. Perris R, Bronner-Fraser M: Recent advances in defining the role of the extracellular matrix in neural crest development. Comments Dev Neurobiol 1:61–83, 1989.
34. Bronner-Fraser M: Analysis of the early stages of trunk neural crest migration in avian embryos using monoclonal antibody HNK-1. Dev Biol 115:44–55, 1986.
35. Erickson CA: Morphogenesis of the neural crest. In Browder LW (ed): Developmental Biology, vol 2. New York, Plenum, 1986, pp 481–543.
36. Anderson DJ: The neural crest cell lineage problem: Neuropoiesis? Neuron 3:1–12, 1989.
37. Schoenwolf GC: Histological and ultrastructural observations of tail bud formation in the chick embryo. Anat Rec 193:131–147, 1979.
38. Schoenwolf GC: Tail (end) bud contributions to the posterior region of the chick embryo. J Exp Zool 201:227–246, 1977.
39. Schoenwolf GC, DeLongo J: Ultrastructure of secondary neurulation in the chick embryo. Am J Anat 158:43–63, 1980.
40. Schoenwolf GC: Histological and ultrastructural studies of secondary neurulation in mouse embryos. Am J Anat 169:361–376, 1984.
41. Lemire RJ: Secondary caudal neural tube formation. In: Lemire RJ, Loeser JD, Leech RW, et al (eds): Normal and Abnormal Development of the Human Nervous System. Hagerstown, MD, Harper & Row, 1975, pp 71–83.
42. Bolli P: Sekundäre Lumenbildungen im Neuralrohr und Rückenmark menschlicher Embryonen. Acta Anat 64:48–81, 1966.
43. Streeter GL: Factors involved in the formation of the filum terminale. Am J Anat 25:1–11, 1919.
44. Kunimoto K: The development and reduction of the tail and of the caudal end of the spinal cord. Contrib Embryol 8:161–198, 1918.

45. DiPietro MA: The conus medullaris: Normal US findings throughout childhood. Radiology 188:149–153, 1993.

46. Wilson DA, Prince JR: MR imaging determination of the location of the normal conus medullaris throughout childhood. AJR Am J Roentgenol 152:1029–1032, 1989.

47. Wolfe S, Schneble F, Tröger J: The conus medullaris: Time of ascendence to normal level. Pediatr Radiol 22:590–592, 1992.

48. Barson AJ: The vertebral level of termination of the spinal cord during normal and abnormal development. J Anat 106:489–497, 1970.

49. James CCM, Lassman LP: Spinal Dysraphism: Spina Bifida Occulta. London, Butterworths, 1972.

50. Jit I, Charnalia VM: The vertebral level of termination of the spinal cord during normal and abnormal development. J Anat Soc India 8:93–102, 1959.

51. Barson AJ: Spina bifida: The significance of the level and extent of the defect to the morphogenesis. Dev Med Child Neurol 12:129–144, 1970.

52. Reimann AF, Anson BJ: Vertebral level of termination of the spinal cord with report of a case of sacral cord. Anat Rec 88:127–138, 1944.

53. Schoenwolf GC, Smith JL: Mechanisms of neurulation: Traditional viewpoint and recent advances. Development 109:243–270, 1990.

54. Baker PC, Schroeder TE: Cytoplasmic filaments and morphogenetic movement in the amphibian neural tube. Dev Biol 15:432–450, 1967.

55. Burnside B: Microtubules and microfilaments in amphibian neurulation. Am Zool 13:989–1006, 1973.

56. Schroeder TE: Mechanisms of morphogenesis: The embryonic neural tube. Int J Neurosci 2:183–197, 1971.

57. Karfunkel P: The role of microtubules and microfilaments in neurulation in *Xenopus*. Dev Biol 25:30–56, 1971.

58. Handel MA, Roth LE: Cell shape and morphology of the neural tube: Implications for microtubule function. Dev Biol 25:78–95, 1971.

59. Messier P-E: Effects of β-mercaptoethanol on the fine structure of the neural plate cells of the chick embryo. J Embryol Exp Morphol 21:309–329, 1969.

60. Lyser KM: Early differentiation of motor neuroblasts in chick embryo as studied by electron microscopy. II. Microtubules and neurofilaments. Dev Biol 17:117–142, 1968.

61. Karfunkel P: The activity of microtubules and microfilaments in neurulation in the chick. J Exp Zool 181:289–301, 1972.

62. Nagele RG, Lee HY: Ultrastructural changes in cells associated with interkinetic nuclear migration in the developing chick neuroepithelium. J Exp Zool 210:89–106, 1979.

63. Schoenwolf GC, Powers ML: Shaping of the chick neuroepithelium during primary and secondary neurulation: Role of cell elongation. Anat Rec 218:182–195, 1987.

64. Herman L, Kauffman SL: The fine structure of the embryonic mouse neural tube with special reference to cytoplasmic microtubules. Dev Biol 13:145–162, 1966.

65. Wilson DB, Finta LA: Early development of the brain and spinal cord in dysraphic mice: A transmission electron microscopic study. J Comp Neurol 190:363–371, 1980.

66. Wilson DB, Finta LA: Fine structure of the lumbosacral neural folds in the mouse embryo. J Embryol Exp Morphol 55:279–290, 1980.

67. Löfberg J, Jacobson C-O: Effects of vinblastine sulphate, colchicine, and guanosine phosphate on cell morphogenesis during amphibian neurulation. Zoon 2:85–98, 1974.

68. Ferm VH: Colchicine teratogenesis in hamster embryos. Proc Soc Exp Biol Med 112:775–778, 1963.

69. O'Shea S: The cytoskeleton in neurulation: Role of cations. In Harrison RJ (ed): Progress in Anatomy. London, Cambridge University Press, 1981, pp 35–60.

70. Gustafson T, Wolpert L: Cellular mechanisms in the morphogenesis of the sea urchin larva: Change in shape of cell sheets. Exp Cell Res 27:260–279, 1962.

71. Gustafson T, Wolpert L: Cellular movement and contact in sea urchin morphogenesis. Biol Rev Camb Philos Soc 42:442–498, 1967.

72. Jacobson AG, Oster GF, Odell GM, et al: Neurulation and the cortical tractor model for epithelial folding. J Embryol Exp Morphol 96:19–49, 1986.

73. Schoenwolf GC, Alvarez IS: Roles of neuroepithelial cell rearrangement and division in shaping of the avian neural plate. Development 106:427–439, 1989.

74. Martins-Green M: Origin of the dorsal surface of the neural tube by progressive delamination of epidermal ectoderm and neuroepithelium: Implications for neurulation and neural tube defects. Development 103:687–706, 1988.

75. Roux W: Beiträge zur entwicklungsmechanik des embryo. Zeitschrift fuer Biologie 21:411–524, 1885.

76. Schoenwolf GC: Microsurgical analysis of avian neurulation: Separation of medial and lateral tissues. J Comp Neurol 276:498–507, 1988.

77. Marin-Padilla M, Ferm VH: Somite necrosis and developmental malformations induced by vitamin A in the golden hamster. J Embryol Exp Morphol 13:1–8, 1965.

78. Marin-Padilla M: Mesodermal alterations induced by hypervitaminosis A. J Embryol Exp Morphol 15:261–269, 1966.

79. Morriss GM, Solursh M: Regional differences in mesenchymal cell morphology and glycosaminoglycans in early neural-fold stage rat embryos. J Embryol Exp Morphol 46:37–52, 1978.

80. Morris-Kay GM, Crutch B: Culture of rat embryos with β-D-xyloside: Evidence of a role for proteoglycans in neurulation. J Anat 134:491–506, 1982.

81. Schoenwolf GC, Fisher M: Analysis of the effects of *Streptomyces* hyaluronidase on formation of the neural tube. J Embryol Exp Morphol 73:1–15, 1983.

82. Smits-van Prooije A, Poelmann R, Dubbeldam J, et al: The formation of the neural tube in rat embryos, cultured in vitro, studied with teratogens. Acta Histochem Suppl 32:41–45, 1986.

83. Anderson CB, Meier S: Effect of hyaluronidase treatment on the distribution of cranial neural crest cells in the chick embryo. J Exp Zool 221:329–335, 1982.

84. Tuckett F, Morriss-Kay GM: Heparitinase treatment of rat embryos during cranial neurulation. Anat Embryol (Berl) 180:393–400, 1989.

85. Morriss-Kay G, Tuckett F: Immunohistochemical localisation of chondroitin sulphate proteoglycans and the effects of chondroitinase ABC in 9- to 11-day rat embryos. Development 106:787–798, 1989.

86. Morriss-Kay GM, Tuckett F, Solursh M: The effects of *Streptomyces* hyaluronidase on tissue organization and cell cycle time in rat embryos. J Embryol Exp Morphol 98:59–70, 1986.

87. Jacobson AG: Morphogenesis of the neural plate and tube. In Connelly TG, Brinkeley LL, Carlson BM (eds): Morphogenesis and Pattern Formation. New York, Raven Press, 1981, pp 233–263.

88. Jacobson AG: Some forces that shape the nervous system. Zoon 6:13–21, 1978.

89. Jacobson AG, Gordon R: Changes in the shape of the developing vertebrate nervous system analyzed experimentally, mathematically and by computer simulation. J Exp Zool 197:191–246, 1976.

90. Gordon R: A review of the theories of vertebrate neurulation and their relationship to the mechanics of neural tube birth defects. J Embryol Exp Morphol 89(Suppl):229–255, 1985.

91. His W: Über mechanische Grundvorgänge thierischer Formbildung. Arch Anat Physiol u wiss Med: Anat Abthl 1:1–80, 1894.

92. Brun RB, Garson JA: Neurulation in the Mexican salamander (*Ambystoma mexicanum*): A drug study and cell shape analysis of the epidermis and the neural plate. J Embryol Exp Morphol 74:275–295, 1983.

93. Schroeder TE: Neurulation in *Xenopus laevis*: An analysis and model based upon light and electron microscopy. J Embryol Exp Morphol 23:427–462, 1970.

94. Schoenwolf GC, Franks MV: Quantitative analyses of changes in cell shapes during bending of the avian neural plate. Dev Biol 105:257–272, 1984.

95. Moore DC, Stanisstreet M, Evans GE: Morphometric analyses of changes in cell shape in the neuroepithelium of mammalian embryos. J Anat 155:87–99, 1987.

96. Youn BW, Malacinski GM: Axial structure development in ultraviolet-irradiated (notochord-defective) amphibian embryos. Dev Biol 83:339–352, 1981.

97. Malacinski GM, Youn BW: Neural plate morphogenesis and axial stretching in "notochord-defective" *Xenopus laevis* embryos. Dev Biol 88:352–357, 1981.

98. Smith JL, Schoenwolf GC: Notochordal induction of cell wedging in the chick neural plate and its role in neural tube formation. J Exp Zool 250:49–62, 1989.

99. Schoenwolf GC, Folsom D, Moe A: A reexamination of the role of microfilaments in neurulation in the chick embryo. Anat Rec 220:87–102, 1988.

100. Burnside B: Microtubules and microfilaments in newt neurulation. Dev Biol 26:416–441, 1971.

101. Schroeder TE: Cell constriction: Contractile role of microfilaments in division and development. Am Zool 13:949–960, 1973.

102. Nagale RG, Lee H: Studies on the mechanism of neurulation in the chick: Microfilament-mediated changes in cell shape during uplifting of neural folds. J Exp Zool 213:391–398, 1980.

103. Freeman BG: Surface modifications of neural epithelial cells during formation of the neural tube in the rat embryo. J Embryol Exp Morphol 28:437–448, 1972.

104. Morriss GM, New DAT: Effect of oxygen concentration on morphogenesis of cranial neural folds and neural crest in cultured rat embryos. J Embryol Exp Morphol 54:17–35, 1979.

105. Nagale RG, Lee H: Motility-related proteins in developing neuroepithelial cells in the chick. Am Zool 18:608, 1978.

106. Lee HY, Kosciuk MC, Nagele RG, et al: Studies on the mechanisms of neurulation in the chick: Possible involvement of myosin in elevation of neural folds. J Exp Zool 225:449–457, 1983.

107. Linville GP, Shephard TH: Neural tube closure defects caused by cytochalasin B. Nat New Biol 236:246–247, 1972.

108. Messier P-E, Auclair C: Effects of cytochalasin B on interkinetic nuclear migration in the chick embryo. Dev Biol 36:218–223, 1974.

109. Lee HY, Kalmus GW: Effects of cytochalasin B on the morphogenesis of explanted early chick embryos. Growth 40:153–162, 1976.

110. Wiley MJ: The effects of cytochalasins on the ultrastructure of neurulating hamster embryos in vivo. Teratology 22:59–69, 1980.

111. Morriss-Kay GM: Growth and development of pattern in the cranial neural epithelium of rat embryos during neurulation. J Embryol Exp Morphol 65(Suppl):225–241, 1981.

112. Greenaway JC, Shepard TH, Kuc J: Comparison of cytochalasins (A, B, D, and E) in chick explant teratogenicity and tissue culture systems. Proc Soc Exp Biol Med 155:239–242, 1977.

113. Lee H, Nagale RG: Neural tube defects caused by local anesthetics in early chick embryos. Teratology 31:119–127, 1985.

114. Shepard TH, Greenaway JC: Teratogenicity of cytochalasin D in the mouse. Teratology 16:131–136, 1977.

115. Webster W, Langman J: The effect of cytochalasin B on the neuroepithelial cells of the mouse embryo. Am J Anat 152:209–221, 1978.

116. Austin WL, Wind M, Brown KS: Differences in the toxicity and teratogenicity of cytochalasin D and E in various mouse strains. Teratology 25:11–18, 1982.

117. Morriss-Kay G, Tuckett F: The role of microfilaments in cranial neurulation in rat embryos: Effects of short-term exposure to cytochalasin D. J Embryol Exp Morphol 88:333–348, 1985.

118. Tuckett F, Morriss-Kay GM: The kinetic behaviour of the cranial neural epithelium during neurulation in the rat. J Embryol Exp Morphol 85:111–119, 1985.

119. Nagele RG, Pietrolungo JF, Lee H: Studies on the mechanisms of neurulation in the chick: The intracellular distribution of Ca⁺⁺. Experientia 37:304–306, 1981.

120. Moran DJ: A scanning electron microscopic and flame spectrometry study on the role of Ca²⁺ in amphibian neurulation using papaverine inhibition and ionophore induction of morphogenetic movement. J Exp Zool 198:409–416, 1976.

121. Moran D, Rice RW: Action of papaverine and ionophore A23187 on neurulation. Nature 261:497–499, 1976.

122. Lee H, Nagale R, Karasanyi N: Inhibition of neural tube closure by ionophore A23187 in chick embryos. Experientia 34:518–520, 1977.

123. Carter SB: Effects of cytochalasins on mammalian cells. Nature 213:261–264, 1967.

124. Carter SB: The cytochalasins as research tools in cytology. Endeavour 31:77–82, 1972.

125. Wessels NK, Spooner BS, Ash JF, et al: Microfilaments in cellular and developmental processes. Science 171:135–143, 1971.

126. Smith JL, Schoenwolf GC: Cell cycle and neuroepithelial cell shape during bending of the chick neural plate. Anat Rec 218:196–206, 1987.

127. Smith JL, Schoenwolf GC: Role of cell-cycle in regulating neuroepithelial cell shape during bending of the chick neural plate. Cell Tissue Res 252:491–500, 1988.

128. Sauer FC: The cellular structure of the neural tube. J Comp Neurol 63:13–23, 1935.

129. Martin A, Langman J: The development of the spinal cord examined by autoradiography. J Embryol Exp Morphol 14:25–35, 1965.

130. Langman J, Guerrant RL, Freeman BG: Behavior of neuro-epithelial cells during closure of the neural tube. J Comp Neurol 127:399–411, 1966.

131. van Straaten HWM, Hekking JWM, Wiertz-Hoessels EJLM, et al: Effect of the notochord on the differentiation of a floor plate area in the neural tube of the chick embryo. Anat Embryol (Berl) 177:317–324, 1988.

132. Edelman GM: Surface modulation in cell recognition and cell growth. Science 192:218–226, 1976.

133. McLone DG, Knepper PA: Role of complex carbohydrates and neurulation. Pediatr Neurosci 12:2–9, 1985.

134. Moran D, Rice RW: An ultrastructural examination of the role of cell membrane surface coat material during neurulation. J Cell Biol 64:172–181, 1975.

135. Lee H, Sheffield JB, Nagele RG Jr, et al: The role of extracellular material in chick neurulation. I. Effects of concanavalin A. J Exp Zool 198:261–266, 1976.

136. Sadler TW: Distribution of surface coat material on fusing neural folds of mouse embryos during neurulation. Anat Rec 191:345–349, 1978.

137. O'Shea KS, Kaufman MH: Phospholipase C–induced neural tube defects in the mouse embryo. Experientia 36:1217–1219, 1980.

138. Lee H, Nagale RG, Kalmus GW: Further studies on neural tube defects caused by concanavalin A in early chick embryos. Experientia 32:1050–1052, 1978.

139. Higbee RG, Fiacco JL, Vanden Hoek T, et al: Oligosaccharides and abnormal neurulation in the delayed splotch mutant [abstract]. Neuroscience 14:829, 1988.

140. Ersahin Y, Higbee RG, Vanden Hoek T, et al: Vitamin A–induced suppression/enhancement of protein glycosylation and neurulation. Pediatr Neurosci 13:293–303, 1987.

141. Fujimori T, Miyatani S, Takeichi M: Ectopic expression of N-cadherin perturbs histogenesis in *Xenopus* embryos. Development 110:97–104, 1990.

142. Detrick RJ, Dickey D, Kintner CR: The effects of N-cadherin misexpression on morphogenesis in *Xenopus* embryos. Neuron 4:493–506, 1990.

143. Mak LL: Ultrastructural studies of amphibian neural fold fusion. Dev Biol 65:435–446, 1978.

144. Revel JP: Scanning electron microscope studies of cell surface morphology and labelling, in situ and in vitro. Scanning Electron Microsc 1:542–548, 1974.

145. Bancroft M, Bellairs R: Differentiation of the neural plate and neural tube in the young chick embryo: A study by scanning and transmission electron microscopy. Anat Embryol (Berl) 147:309–335, 1975.

146. Gouda JG: Proceedings: Closure of the neural tube in relation to the developing somites in the chick embryo. J Anat 118:360–361, 1974.

147. Waterman RE: Topographical changes along the neural fold associated with neurulation in the hamster and mouse. Am J Anat 146:151–171, 1976.

148. Waterman RE: SEM observations of surface alterations associated with neural tube closure in the mouse and hamster. Anat Rec 183:95–98, 1975.

149. Schoenwolf GC: Observations on closure of the neuropores in the chick embryo. Am J Anat 155:445–465, 1979.

150. Gonzalez Santander R, Martinez Cuadrado G: Ultrastructure of the neural canal closure in the chicken embryo. Acta Anat (Basel) 95:368–383, 1976.

151. Geelen JAG, Langman J: Ultrastructural observations on closure of the neural tube in the mouse. Anat Embryol (Berl) 156:73–88, 1979.

152. Costanzo R, Watterson RL, Schoenwolf GC: Evidence that sec-

ondary neurulation occurs autonomously in the chick embryo. J Exp Zool 219:233–240, 1982.

153. Gilbert SF: Developmental Biology. Sunderland, MA, Sinauer Associates, 1997.

154. Hammerschmidt M, Brook A, McMahon AP: The world according to hedgehog. Trends Genet 13:14–21, 1997.

155. DeRobertis EM: Dismantling the organizer. Nature 374:407–408, 1995.

156. Spemann H, Mangold H: Über induktion von Embryonalanlagen durch Implantation artfremder Organisatoren. Roux Arch Entw Mech Org 100:599–638, 1924.

157. Dias MS, Schoenwolf GC: Formation of ectopic neurepithelium in chick blastoderms: Age-related capacities for induction and self-differentiation following transplantation of quail Hensen's nodes. Anat Rec 228:437–448, 1990.

158. Gallera J: Inductions cérébrales et médullaires chez les Oiseaux. Experientia 26:886–887, 1970.

159. Gallera J: Différence de réactivité à l'inducteur neurogène entre l'ectoblaste de l'aire opaque et celui de l'aire pellucide chez le Poulet. Experientia 26:1353–1354, 1970.

160. Lemaire L, Kessel M: Gastrulation and homeobox genes in chick embryos. Mech Dev 67:3–16, 1997.

161. Toivonen S, Wartiovaara J: Mechanisms of cell interaction during primary embryonic induction studied in transfilter experiments. Differentiation 5:61–66, 1976.

162. Toivonen S, Tarin D, Saxén L: The transmission of morphogenetic signals from amphibian mesoderm to ectoderm in primary induction. Differentiation 5:49–55, 1976.

163. Saxen L: Transfilter neural induction of amphibian ectoderm. Dev Biol 3:140–152, 1961.

164. Lemaire P, Kodjabachian L: The vertebrate organizer: Structure and molecules. Trends Genet 12:525–531, 1996.

165. Kelly OG, Melton DA: Induction and patterning of the vertebrate nervous system. Trends Genet 11:273–278, 1995.

166. Smith JL, Schoenwolf GC: Getting organized: New insights into the organizer of higher vertebrates. Curr Top Dev Biol 40:79–110, 1998.

167. Moon RT, Brown JD, Torres M: WNTs modulate cell fate and behavior during vertebrate development. Trends Genet 13:157–162, 1997.

168. Shawlot W, Behringer RR: Requirement for Lim1 in head-organizer function. Nature 374:425–430, 1995.

169. Lumsden A, Krumlauf R: Patterning the vertebrate neuraxis. Science 274:1109–1115, 1996.

170. Tanabe Y, Jessell TM: Diversity and pattern in the developing spinal cord. Science 274:1115–1123, 1996.

171. Ruiz i Altaba A, Jessell TM: Midline cells and the organization of the vertebrate neuraxis. Curr Opin Genet Dev 3:633–640, 1993.

172. George TM, McLone DG: Mechanisms of mutant genes in spina bifida: A review of implications from animal models. Pediatr Neurosurg 23:236–245, 1995.

173. Chatkupt S, Johnson WG: Waardenburg syndrome and myelomeningocele in a family. J Med Genet 30:83–84, 1993.

174. Anderson DJ: Cellular and molecular biology of neural crest cell lineage determination. Trends Genet 13:276–280, 1997.

175. Joyner AL, Guillemot F: Gene targeting and development of the nervous system. Curr Opin Neurobiol 4:37–42, 1994.

176. Grabowski CT: The effects of the excision of Hensen's node on the early development of the chick embryo. J Exp Zool 133:301–343, 1956.

177. Vakaet L: Résultats de la greffe de nœuds de Hensen d'âge différent sur le blastoderme de Poulet. C R Soc Biol 159:232–233, 1965.

178. Lumsden A: The cellular basis of segmentation in the developing hindbrain. Trends Neurosci 13:329–335, 1990.

179. Ang S-L: The brain organization. Nature 380:25–27, 1996.

180. Shimamura K, Martinez S, Puelles L, et al: Patterns of gene expression in the neural plate and neural tube subdivide the embryonic forebrain into transverse and longitudinal domains. Dev Neurosci 19:88–96, 1997.

181. Joyner AL: Engrailed, Wnt and Pax genes regulate midbrain-hindbrain development. Trends Genet 12:15–20, 1996.

182. Puelles L, Rubenstein JLR: Expression patterns of homeobox and other putative regulatory genes in the embryonic mouse forebrain suggest a neuromeric organization. Trends Neurosci 16:472–479, 1993.

183. Wilkinson DG, Krumlauf R: Molecular approaches to the segmentation of the hindbrain. Trends Neurosci 13:335–339, 1990.

184. Sperry RW: Chemoaffinity in the orderly growth of nerve fiber patterns and connections. Proc Natl Acad Sci U S A 50:703–710, 1963.

185. von Recklinghausen E: Untersuchungen über die Spina bifida. Arch Path Anat 105:243–373, 1886.

186. Morgagni JB: The Seats and Causes of Disease Investigated by Anatomy. London, A Millar & T Cadell, 1769.

187. Gardner WJ: Diastematomyelia and the Klippel-Feil syndrome: Relationship to hydrocephalus, syringomyelia, meningocele, meningomyelocele, and iniencephalus. Cleve Clin Q 31:19–44, 1964.

188. Gardner WJ: Embryologic origin of spinal malformations. Acta Radiol Diagn (Stockh) 5:1013–1023, 1966.

189. Gardner WJ: Hypothesis; overdistention of the neural tube may cause anomalies of non-neural organs. Teratology 22:229–238, 1980.

190. Gardner WJ: The Dysraphic States from Syringomyelia to Anencephaly. Amsterdam, Excerpta Medica, 1973.

191. Caldarelli M, McLone DG, Collins JA, et al: Vitamin A induced neural tube defects in a mouse. Concepts Pediatr Neurosurg 6:161–171, 1985.

192. Copp AJ, Brook FA, Estibeiro JP, et al: The embryonic development of mammalian neural tube defects. Prog Neurobiol 35:363–403, 1990.

193. Copp AJ: Genetic models of mammalian neural tube defects. In Bock G, Marsh J (eds): Neural Tube Defects. CIBA Foundation Symposium No. 181. Chichester, England, John Wiley & Sons, 1994, pp 118–143.

194. van Straaten HWM, Hekking JWM, Consten C, et al: Intrinsic and extrinsic factors in the mechanisms of neurulation: Effect of curvature of the body axis on closure of the posterior neuropore. Development 117:1163–1172, 1993.

195. Brook FA, Shum ASW, van Straaten HWM, et al: Curvature of the caudal region is responsible for failure of neural tube closure in the curly tail (ct) mouse embryo. Development 113:671–678, 1991.

196. Seller MJ, Embury S, Polani PE, et al: Neural tube defects in curly-tail mice. II. Effect of maternal administration of vitamin A. Proc R Soc Lond B Biol Sci 206:95–107, 1979.

197. Seller MJ: Maternal nutrition factors and neural tube defects in experimental animals. In Dobbing J (ed): Prevention of Spina Bifida and Other Neural Tube Defects. New York, Academic Press, 1983, pp 1–22.

198. Czeizel AE, Dudás I: Prevention of the first occurrence of neural-tube defects by periconceptional vitamin supplementation. N Engl J Med 327:1832–1835, 1992.

199. MRC Vitamin Study Research Group: Prevention of neural tube defects: Results of the Medical Research Council Vitamin Study. Lancet 338:131–137, 1991.

200. Wald NJ: Folic acid and neural tube defects: The current evidence and implications for prevention. In Bock G, Marsh J (eds): Neural Tube Defects. CIBA Foundation Symposium No. 181. Chichester, England, John Wiley & Sons, 1994, pp 192–211.

201. Seller MJ: Vitamins, folic acid and the cause and prevention of neural tube defects. In Bock G, Marsh J (eds): Neural Tube Defects. CIBA Foundation Symposium No. 181. Chichester, England, John Wiley & Sons, 1994, pp 161–179.

202. Fleming A, Copp AJ: Embryonic folate metabolism and mouse neural tube defeects. Science 280:2107–2109, 1998.

203. Scott JM, Wier DG, Molloy A, et al: Folic acid metabolism and mechanisms of neural tube defects. In Bock G, Marsh J (eds): Neural Tube Defects. CIBA Foundation Symposium No. 181. Chichester, England, John Wiley & Sons, 1994, pp 180–191.

204. Gordon N: Folate metabolism and neural tube defects. Brain Dev 17:307–311, 1995.

205. Buehler JW, Mulinare J: Preventing neural tube defects. Pediatr Ann 26:535–539, 1997.

206. Ubbink JB: Is an elevated circulating maternal homocysteine concentration a risk factor for neural tube defects? Nutr Rev 53:173–175, 1995.

207. Bower C: Folate and neural tube defects. Nutr Rev 53:S33–S38, 1995.

208. Rosenquist TH, Ratashak SA, Selhub J: Homocysteine induces congenital defects of the heart and neural tube: Effect of folic acid. Proc Natl Acad Sci U S A 93:15227–15232, 1996.

209. Whitehead AS, Gallagher P, Mills JL, et al: A genetic defect in 5,10 methylenetetrahydrofolate reductase in neural tube defects. QJM 88:763–766, 1995.

210. Steegers-Theunissen RPM, Boers GHJ, Trijbels FJM, et al: Neural-tube defects and derangement of homocysteine metabolism. N Engl J Med 324:199–200, 1991.

211. Steegers-Theunissen RP: Folate metabolism and neural tube defects: A review. Eur J Obstet Gynecol Reprod Biol 61:39–48, 1995.

212. Minns RA: Folic acid and neural tube defects. Spinal Cord 34:460–465, 1996.

213. Steegers-Theunissen RPM, Boers GHJ, Trijbels FJ, et al: Maternal hyperhomocysteinemia: A risk factor for neural tube defects? Metabolism 43:1475–1480, 1994.

214. Goyette P, Sumner JS, Milos R, et al: Human methlenetetrahydrofolate reductase: Isolation of cDNA, mapping and mutation identification. Nat Genet 7:195–200, 1994.

215. Nau H: Valproic acid-induced neural tube defects. In Bock G, Marsh J (eds): Neural Tube Defects. CIBA Foundation Symposium No. 181. Chichester, England, John Wiley & Sons, 1994, pp 144–152.

216. Finnell RH, Wlodarczyk BC, Craig JC, et al: Strain-dependent alterations in the expression of folate pathway genes following teratogenic exposure to valproic acid in a mouse model. Am J Med Genet 70:303–311, 1997.

217. Wlodarczyk BC, Craig J, Bennett GD, et al: Valproic acid–induced changes in gene expression during neurulation in a mouse model. Teratology 54:284–297, 1996.

218. French BN: Abnormal development of the central nervous system. In McLaurin RL, Venes JL, Schut L, et al (eds): Pediatric Neurosurgery: Surgery of the Developing Nervous System, 2nd ed. Philadelphia, WB Saunders, 1989, pp 9–34.

219. Humphreys RP: Spinal dysraphism. In Wilkins RH, Rengachary SS (eds): Neurosurgery, vol 3. New York, McGraw-Hill, 1985, pp 2041–2052.

220. Steinbok P, Cochrane DD: The nature of congenital posterior cervical or cervicothoracic midline cutaneous mass lesions: Report of eight cases. J Neurosurg 75:206–212, 1991.

221. Pang D, Dias MS: Cervical myelomeningoceles. Neurosurgery 33:363–373, 1993.

222. Boldrey EB, Elvidge AR: Dermoid cysts of the vertebral canal. Ann Surg 110:273, 1939.

223. Guidetti B, Gagliardi FM: Epidermoid and dermoid cysts: Clinical evaluation and late surgical results. J Neurosurg 47:12–18, 1977.

224. Walker AE, Bucy PC: Congenital dermal sinuses; a source of spinal meningeal infection and subdural abscesses. Brain 57:401–421, 1934.

225. Ehni G, Love JG: Intraspinal lipomas: Report of cases, review of the literature, and clinical and pathologic study. Arch Neurol Psychiatry 53:1–28, 1945.

226. Lassman LP, James CCM: Lumbosacral lipomas: Critical survey of 26 cases submitted to laminectomy. J Neurol Neurosurg Psychiatry 30:174–181, 1967.

227. McLone DG, Mutluer S, Naidich TP: Lipomeningoceles of the conus medullaris. In Raimondi AJ (ed): Concepts in Pediatric Neurosurgery, vol 3. Basel, S Karger, 1983, pp 170–177.

228. Walsh JW, Markesbery WR: Histological features of congenital lipomas of the lower spinal canal. J Neurosurg 52:564–569, 1980.

229. Chapman PH: Congenital intraspinal lipomas: Anatomic considerations and surgical treatment. Childs Brain 9:37–47, 1982.

230. Naidich TP, McLone DG, Mutluer S: A new understanding of dorsal dysraphism with lipoma (lipomyeloschisis): Radiologic evaluation and surgical correction. AJR Am J Roentgenol 140:1065–1078, 1983.

231. McLone DG, Naidich TP: Spinal dysraphism: Experimental and clinical. In Holtzman RN, Stein BM (eds): The Tethered Spinal Cord. New York, Thieme-Stratton, 1985, pp 14–28.

232. Bentley JFR, Smith JR: Developmental posterior enteric remnants and spinal malformations: The split notochord syndrome. Arch Dis Child 35:76–86, 1960.

233. Prop N, Frensdorf EL, van de Stadt FR: A postvertebral endodermal cyst associated with axial deformities: A case showing the "endodermal-ectodermal adhesion syndrome." Pediatrics 39:555–562, 1967.

234. Bremer JL: Dorsal intestinal fistula; accessory neurenteric canal; diastematomyelia. Arch Pathol 54:132–138, 1952.

235. Cohen J, Sledge CB: Diastematomyelia: An embryological interpretation with report of a case. AMA J Dis Child 100:257–263, 1960.

236. Herren RY, Edwards JE: Diplomyelia (duplication of the spinal cord). Arch Pathol 30:1203–1214, 1940.

237. Naidich TP, Harwood-Nash DC: Diastematomyelia: Hemicord and meningeal sheaths; single and double arachnoid and dural tubes. AJNR Am J Neuroradiol 4:633–636, 1983.

238. James CCM, Lassman LP: Diastematomyelia: A critical survey of 24 cases submitted to laminectomy. Arch Dis Child 39:125–130, 1964.

239. Pang D, Dias MS, Ahab-Barmada M: Split cord malformation. Part I. A unified theory of embryogenesis for double spinal cord malformations. Neurosurgery 31:451–480, 1992.

240. Pang D: Tethered cord syndrome. In Neurosurgery: State of the Art Reviews, vol 1. Philadelphia, Hanley & Belfus, 1986, pp 45–79.

241. Pang D: Split cord malformation. Part II. Clinical syndrome. Neurosurgery 31:481–500, 1992.

242. Ross GW, Swanson SA, Perentes E, et al: Ectopic midline spinal ganglion in diastematomyelia: A study of its connections. J Neurol Neurosurg Psychiatry 51:1231–1234, 1988.

243. Lichtenstein BW: "Spinal dysraphism": Spina bifida and myelodysplasia. Arch Neurol 44:792–810, 1940.

244. Rokos J: Pathogenesis of diastematomyelia and spina bifida. J Pathol 117:155–161, 1975.

245. Beardmore HE, Wigglesworth FW: Vertebral anomalies and alimentary duplications. Pediatr Clin North Am 5:457–474, 1958.

246. Burrows FGO, Sutcliffe J: The split notochord syndrome. Br J Radiol 41:844–847, 1968.

247. McLetchie NGB, Purves JK, Saunders RL: The genesis of gastric and certain intestinal diverticula and enterogenous cysts. Surg Gynecol Obstet 99:135–141, 1954.

248. Saunders RL: Combined anterior and posterior spina bifida in a living neonatal human female. Anat Rec 87:255–278, 1943.

249. Dodds GS: Anterior and posterior rhachischisis. Am J Pathol 17:861–872, 1941.

250. Feller A, Sternberg H: Zur Kenntnis der Fehlbildungen der Wirbelsäule. I. Die Wirbelkörperspalte und ihre formale Genese. Virchows Arch Pathol Anat 272:613–640, 1929.

251. Fernbach SK, Naidich TP, McLone DG, et al: Computed tomography of primary intrathecal Wilms tumor with diastematomyelia. J Comput Assist Tomogr 8:523–528, 1984.

252. Cameron AH: Malformations of the neuro-spinal axis, urogenital tract and foregut in spina bifida attributable to disturbances of the blastopore. J Pathol Bacteriol 73:213–221, 1957.

253. Ugarte N, Gonzalez-Crussi F, Sotelo-Avila C: Diastematomyelia associated with teratoma: Report of two cases. J Neurosurg 53:720–725, 1980.

254. Duckworth T, Sharrard WJ, Lister J, et al: Hemimyelocele. Dev Med Child Neurol 16:69–75, 1968.

255. Peacock WJ, Murovic JA: Magnetic resonance imaging in myelocystoceles: Report of two cases. J Neurosurg 70:804–807, 1989.

256. McLone DG, Naidich TP: Terminal myelocystocele. Neurosurgery 16:36–43, 1985.

257. Carey JC, Greenbaum B, Hall BD: The OEIS complex (omphalocele, exstrophy, imperforate anus, spinal defects). Birth Defects Orig Artic Ser 14(6B):253–263, 1978.

258. Lemire RJ, Beckwith JB: Pathogenesis of congenital tumors and malformations of the sacrococcygeal region. Teratology 25:201–213, 1982.

259. Currarino G, Coln D, Votteler T: Triad of anorectal, sacral, and presacral anomalies. AJR Am J Roentgenol 137:395–398, 1981.

260. Yates VD, Wilroy RS, Whitington GL, et al: Anterior sacral defects: An autosomal dominantly inherited condition. J Pediatr 102:239–242, 1983.

261. Cohn J, Bay-Nielsen E: Hereditary defect of the sacrum and coccyx with anterior sacral meningocele. Acta Paediatr Scand 58:268–274, 1969.

262. Ashcraft KW, Holder TM: Hereditary presacral teratoma. J Pediatr Surg 9:691–697, 1974.

263. Gaskill SJ, Marlin AE: The Currarino triad: Its importance in pediatric neurosurgery. Pediatr Neurosurg 25:143–146, 1997.

264. Dias MS, Azizkhan RG: A novel embryogenetic mechanism for Currarino's triad: Inadequate dorsoventral separation of the caudal eminence from hindgut endoderm. Pediatr Neurosurg 28:223–229, 1998.

265. Anderson FM, Burke BL: Anterior sacral meningocele: A presentation of three cases. JAMA 237:39–42, 1977.

266. Lee S-C, Chun Y-S, Jung S-E, et al: Currarino triad: Anorectal malformation, sacral bony abnormality, and presacral mass—a review of 11 cases. J Pediatr Surg 32:58–61, 1997.

267. Alexander E, Nashold BS: Agenesis of the sacrococcygeal region. J Neurosurg 13:507–513, 1956.

268. Frantz CH, Aitken GT: Complete absence of the lumbar spine and sacrum. J Bone Joint Surg Am 49:1531–1540, 1967.

269. Freedman B: Congenital absence of the sacrum and coccyx: Report of a case and review of the literature. Br J Surg 37:299–303, 1950.

270. Hamsa WR: Congenital absence of the sacrum. Arch Surg 30:657–666, 1935.

271. Pang D, Hoffman HJ: Sacral agenesis with progressive neurological deficit. Neurosurgery 7:118–126, 1980.

272. Renshaw TS: Sacral agenesis: A classification and review of twenty-three cases. J Bone Joint Surg Am 60:373–383, 1978.

273. Sarnat HB, Case ME, Graviss R: Sacral agenesis: Neurologic and neuropathologic features. Neurology 26:1124–1129, 1976.

274. Smith ED: Congenital sacral defects. In Stephens FD (ed): Congenital Malformations of the Rectum, Anus, and Genito-urinary Tracts. Edinburgh & London, E & S Livingstone, 1963, pp 82–105.

275. Rosselet P: A rare case of rachischisis with multiple malformations. AJR Am J Roentgenol 73:235–240, 1955.

276. Stewart SF: Absence of sacrum with report of a case, and a review of the literature. Arch Surg 9:647–652, 1924.

277. Williams DI, Nixon HH: Agenesis of the sacrum. Surg Gynecol Obstet 105:84–88, 1957.

278. Price DL, Dooling EC, Richardson EP Jr: Caudal dysplasia (caudal regression syndrome). Arch Neurol 23:212–220, 1970.

279. Rusnak SL, Driscoll SG: Congenital spinal anomalies in infants of diabetic mothers. Pediatrics 35:989–995, 1965.

280. Banta JV, Nichols O: Sacral agenesis. J Bone Joint Surg Am 51:693–703, 1969.

281. Blumel J, Butler MC, Evans EB, et al: Congenital anomaly of the sacrococcygeal spine: Report of eight cases of absence or malformation. Arch Surg 85:982–993, 1962.

282. Blumel J, Evans EB, Eggers GWN: Partial and complete agenesis or malformation of the sacrum with associated anomalies. J Bone Joint Surg Am 41:497–518, 1959.

283. Ignelzi RJ, Lehman RA: Lumbosacral agenesis: Management and embryological implications. J Neurol Neurosurg Psychiatry 37:1273–1276, 1974.

284. Naik DR, Lendon RG, Barson AJ: A radiological study of vertebral and rib malformations in children with myelomeningocele. Clin Radiol 29:427–430, 1978.

285. Lausecker H: Beitrag zu den misbildungen des Kreuzbeines. Virchows Arch Pathol Anat 322:119–129, 1952.

286. Lichtor A: Sacral agenesis: Report of a case. Arch Surg 54:430–433, 1947.

287. Sinclair JG, Duren N, Rude JC: Congenital lumbosacral defect. Arch Surg 43:473–478, 1941.

288. Girard PM: Congenital absence of the sacrum. J Bone Joint Surg 17:1062–1064, 1935.

289. Källén B, Winberg J: Caudal mesoderm pattern of anomalies: From renal agenesis to sirenomelia. Teratology 9:99–111, 1974.

290. Mills JL: Malformations in infants of diabetic mothers. Teratology 25:385–394, 1982.

291. Passarge E, Lenz W: Syndrome of caudal regression in infants of diabetic mothers: Observations of further cases. Pediatrics 37:672–675, 1966.

292. Duraiswami PK: Comparison of congenital defects induced in developing chickens by certain teratogenic agents with those caused by insulin. J Bone Joint Surg Am 37:277–294, 1955.

293. Landauer W: Rumplessness of chicken embryos produced by the injection of insulin and other chemicals. J Exp Zool 98:65–77, 1945.

294. Zwilling E: The effects of some hormones on development. Ann N Y Acad Sci 55:196–202, 1952.

295. Horton WE Jr, Sadler TW: Effects of maternal diabetes on early embryogenesis: Alterations in morphogenesis produced by the ketone body, β-hydroxybutyrate. Diabetes 32:610–616, 1983.

296. Duhamel B: From the mermaid to anal imperforation: The syndrome of caudal regression. Arch Dis Child 36:152–155, 1961.

297. Wolff E: La Science des Monstres. Paris, Gallimard, 1948.

298. Gardner RJM, Nelson MM: An association of caudal malformations arising from a defect in the "axial mesoderm" developmental field. Am J Med Genet Suppl 2:37–44, 1986.

299. Storm-Mathisen A: Myelodysplasia with absence of sacrum. Acta Psychiatr Neurol Scand 29:145–149, 1954.

300. Bennett D: The T-locus of the mouse. Cell 6:441–454, 1975.

301. McLone DG, Knepper PA: The cause of Chiari II malformation: A unified theory. Pediatr Neurosci 15:1–12, 1989.

302. Cleland J: Contribution to the study of spina bifida, encephalocele, and anencephalus. J Anat Physiol 17:257–292, 1883.

303. Daniel PM, Strich SJ: Some observations on the congenital deformity of the central nervous system known as the Arnold-Chiari malformation. J Neuropathol Exp Neurol 17:255–266, 1958.

304. Peach B: The Arnold-Chiari malformation: Morphogenesis. Arch Neurol 12:527–535, 1965.

305. McLone DG, Nakahara S, Knepper PA: Chiari II malformation: Pathogenesis and dynamics. Concepts Pediatr Neurosurg 11:1–17, 1991.

306. Penfield W, Coburn DF: Arnold-Chiari malformation and its operative treatment. Arch Neurol Psychiatry 40:328–366, 1938.

307. Lichtenstein BW: Distant neuroanatomic complications of spina bifida (spinal dysraphism): Hydrocephalus, Arnold-Chiari deformity, stenosis of the aqueduct of Sylvius, etc: Pathogenesis and pathology. Arch Neurol Psychiatry 47:195–214, 1942.

308. Goldstein F, Kepes JJ: The role of traction in the development of the Arnold-Chiari malformation: An experimental study. J Neuropathol Exp Neurol 25:654–666, 1966.

309. Marin-Padilla M, Marin-Padilla TM: Morphogenesis of experimentally induced Arnold-Chiari malformation. J Neurol Sci 50:29–55, 1981.

310. Padget DH: Development of so-called dysraphism; with embryologic evidence of clinical Arnold-Chiari and Dandy-Walker malformations. Johns Hopkins Med J 130:127–165, 1972.

311. Padget DH, Lindenberg R: Inverse cerebellum morphogenetically related to Dandy-Walker and Arnold-Chiari syndromes: Bizarre malformed brain with occipital encephalocele. Johns Hopkins Med J 131:228–246, 1972.

312. Jelinek R, Pexieder T: Pressure of the CSF and the morphogenesis of the CNS. I. Chick embryo. Folia Morphol (Praha) 18:102–110, 1970.

313. Coulombre AJ, Coulombre JL: The role of mechanical factors in brain morphogenesis. Anat Rec 130:289–290, 1958.

314. Schoenwolf GC, Garcia-Martinez V, Dias MS: Mesoderm movement and fate during avian gastrulation and neurulation. Dev Dyn 193:229–253, 1992.

315. Keynes RJ, Stern CD: Mechanisms of vertebrate segmentation. Development 103:413–429, 1988.

316. Gossler A, Hrabe de Angelis M: Somitogenesis. Curr Top Dev Biol 38:225–287, 1998.

317. Dietrich S, Kessel M: The vertebral column. In Thorogood P (ed): Embryos, Genes, and Birth Defects. Chichester, England, John Wiley & Sons, 1997, pp 281–302.

318. Parke WW: Development of the spine. In Herkowitz HN, Garfin SR, Balderston RA, et al (eds): Rothman-Simeone: The Spine, 4th ed. Philadelphia, WB Saunders, 1999, pp 3–27.

319. Flint OP, Ede DA, Wilby OK, et al: Control of somite number in normal and amputated mutant mouse embryos: An experimental and a theoretical analysis. J Embryol Exp Morphol 45:189–202, 1978.

320. Tam PPL: The control of somitogenesis in mouse embryos. J Embryol Exp Morphol 65(Suppl):103–128, 1981.

321. Bagnall KM, Sanders EJ, Higgins SJ, et al: The effects of somite removal on vertebral formation in the chick. Anat Embryol (Berl) 178:183–190, 1988.

322. Christ B, Schmidt C, Huang R, et al: Segmentation of the vertebrate body. Anat Embryol (Berl) 197:1–8, 1998.

323. Remak R: Untersuchungen über die Entwicklung der Wirbelthiere. Berlin, Reimer, 1855.

324. Verbout AJ: A critical review of the "neugliederung" concept in relation to the development of the vertebral column. Acta Biotheor 25:219–258, 1976.

325. Theiler K: Vertebral malformations. Adv Anat Embryol Cell Biol 112:1–99, 1988.

326. Ewan KBR, Everett AW: Evidence for resegmentation in the formation of the vertebral column using the novel approach of retroviral-mediated gene transfer. Exp Cell Res 198:315–320, 1992.

327. Bagnall KM: The migration and distribution of somite cells after labelling with the carbocyanine dye, Dil: The relationship of this distribution to segmentation in the vertebrate body. Anat Embryol (Berl) 185:317–324, 1992.

328. Bagnall KM, Higgins SJ, Sanders EJ: The contribution made by cells from a single somite to tissues within a body segment and assessment of their integration with similar cells from adjacent segments. Development 107:931–943, 1989.

329. Bagnall KM, Higgins SJ, Sanders EJ: The contribution made by a single somite to the vertebral column: Experimental evidence in support of resegmentation using the chick-quail chimaera model. Development 103:69–85, 1988.

330. Huang R, Zhi Q, Wilting J, et al: The fate of somitocoele cells in avian embryos. Anat Embryol (Berl) 190:243–250, 1994.

331. Huang R, Zhi Q, Neubüser A, et al: Function of simote and somitocoele cells in the formation of the vertebral motion segment in avian embryos. Acta Anat (Basel) 155:231–241, 1996.

332. Ogden JA, Ganey TM, Sasse J, et al: Development and maturation of the axial skeleton. In Weinstein SL (ed): The Pediatric Spine: Principles and Practice, vol 1. New York, Raven Press, 1994, pp 3–69.

333. Bareggi R, Grill V, Sandrucci MA, et al: Developmental pathways of vertebral centra and neural arches in human embryos and fetuses. Anat Embryol (Berl) 187:139–144, 1993.

334. Bareggi R, Grill V, Zweyer M, et al: A quantitative study on the spatial and temporal ossification patterns of vertebral centra and neural arches and their relationship to the fetal age. Anat Anz 176:311–317, 1994.

335. Tsou PM, Yau A, Hodgson AR: Embryogenesis and prenatal development of congenital vertebral anomalies and their classification. Clin Orthop 152:211–231, 1980.

336. Tanaka T, Uhthoff HK: The pathogenesis of congenital vertebral malformations: A study based on observations in 11 human embryos and fetuses. Acta Orthop Scand 52:413–425, 1981.

337. Lehman-Facius H: Die Keilwirbelbildung bei der Kongenitalen Skoliose. Frankfurter Pathol 31:389, 1925.

338. Junghanns H: Die Fehlbildungen der Wirbelkörper. Arch Orthop Unfallchir 38:1–24, 1937.

339. Tanaka T, Uhthoff HK: Significance of resegmentation in the pathogenesis of vertebral body malformation. Acta Orthop Scand 52:331–338, 1981.

340. McMaster MJ: Congenital scoliosis. In Weinstein SL (ed): The Pediatric Spine: Principles and Practice. New York, Raven Press, 1994, pp 227–244.

341. Tori JA, Dickson JH: Association of congenital anomalies of the spine and kidneys. Clin Orthop 148:259–262, 1980.

342. Bavinck JN, Weaver DD: Subclavian artery supply disruption sequence: Hypothesis of a vascular etiology for Poland, Klippel-Feil, and Möbius anomalies. Am J Med Genet 23:903–918, 1986.

343. Brill CB, Peyster RG, Keller MS, et al: Isolation of the right subclavian artery with subclavian steal in a child with Klippel-Feil anomaly: An example of the subclavian artery disruption sequence. Am J Med Genet 26:933–940, 1987.

344. Raas-Rothschild A, Goodman RM, Grunbaum M, et al: Klippel-Feil anomaly with sacral agenesis: An additional subtype, type IV. J Craniofac Genet Dev Biol 8:297–301, 1988.

345. David KM, Copp AJ, Stevens JM, et al: Split cervical spinal cord with Klippel-Feil syndrome: Seven cases. Brain 119:1859–1872, 1996.

346. Dias MS, Li V, Landi M, et al: The embryogenesis of congenital vertebral dislocation: Early embryonic buckling? Pediatr Neurosurg 29:281–289, 1998.

347. Ehrenhaft JL: Development of the vertebral column as related to certain congenital and pathological changes. Surg Gynecol Obstet 76:282–292, 1943.

348. Müller F, O'Rahilly R, Benson DR: The early origin of vertebral anomalies, as illustrated by a "butterfly vertebra." J Anat 149:157–169, 1986.

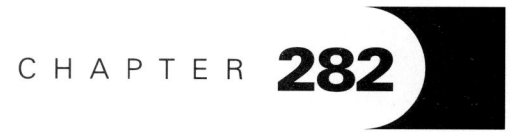

CHAPTER **282**

Approach to the Patient and Medical Management of Spinal Disorders

CHARLES KUNTZ IV ■ CHRISTOPHER I. SHAFFREY ■ W. PUTNAM WOLCOTT

A logical approach is essential to the evaluation and management of patients with suspected spinal disorders. As a fundamental guide to spinal pathology, an algorithm proposed by Borenstein and colleagues has been modified and expanded (Fig. 282–1). This algorithm classifies and organizes spinal pathology based on symptoms and signs at presentation. The following observations are used for categorization: (1) presence or absence of pain, (2) characteristics of the pain, (3) presence or absence of neurological deficit, (4) characteristics of the neurological deficit, and (5) presence or absence of systemic symptoms and signs. With this information, laboratory and radiologic evaluation can proceed, a diagnosis can be made, and appropriate surgical or medical management can be prescribed.[1, 2]

Our approach begins with characterization of the pain, evaluation for neurological deficit, and search for systemic symptoms and signs. Most patients with spinal disorders present with either pain or a neurological deficit. Most pathologic processes that involve primarily the musculoligamentous or bony spinal column manifest as progressive spinal or radicular pain, which may be followed by a progressive neurological deficit. Pathologic processes that involve primarily the spinal cord or nerve roots may manifest with either pain or neurological deficit.

The first section of this chapter deals with disorders that manifest predominantly with pain; the second section covers conditions that manifest predominantly with neurological deficits. Further subdivisions of these sections are based on the characteristics of the pain or neurological deficit and the presence of systemic symptoms or signs. Some overlap in presentation among groups is to be expected. The basic framework of the algorithm (see Fig. 282–1), however, should help clinicians classify spinal pathology based on clinical presentation, restrict the differential diagnoses, and proceed with the evaluation in a logical order. Other chapters discuss the evaluation and management of individual disease entities.[2–4]

PAIN

The most common reason for absenteeism from work is neck and lower back pain. Most patients with lower back or neck pain have some type of musculoligamentous strain that resolves with conservative therapy. Patients with persistent axial skeletal pain or radicular pain are much more likely to have a surgical lesion and to require more extensive diagnostic evaluation. Assessment of patients with persistent spinal or radicular pain begins with a history and physical examination, followed by laboratory investigation and diagnostic imaging.[3–7]

The history should focus on the onset, characteristics, location, aggravating and alleviating conditions, and similar episodes of pain. Systemic and associated symptoms must be sought. Medical history, family history, and social history elucidate conditions associated with spinal pathology. The physical examination should include a complete analysis of all systems. Anterior neck pathology, thoracic disease, and abdominal ailments can manifest with visceral pain referred to the neck or back, and systemic disease may first manifest in the spine. Evaluation of the spine should include inspection, palpation, and range-of-motion testing. A detailed neurological examination should look for brain, brainstem, spinal cord, peripheral nerve, and muscle involvement. When a neurological deficit is present after a long history of painful symptoms, the characteristics of the neurological deficit help establish the diagnosis.

Based on the clinical findings, appropriate laboratory and imaging studies are obtained. Standard laboratory studies include a complete blood count; electro-

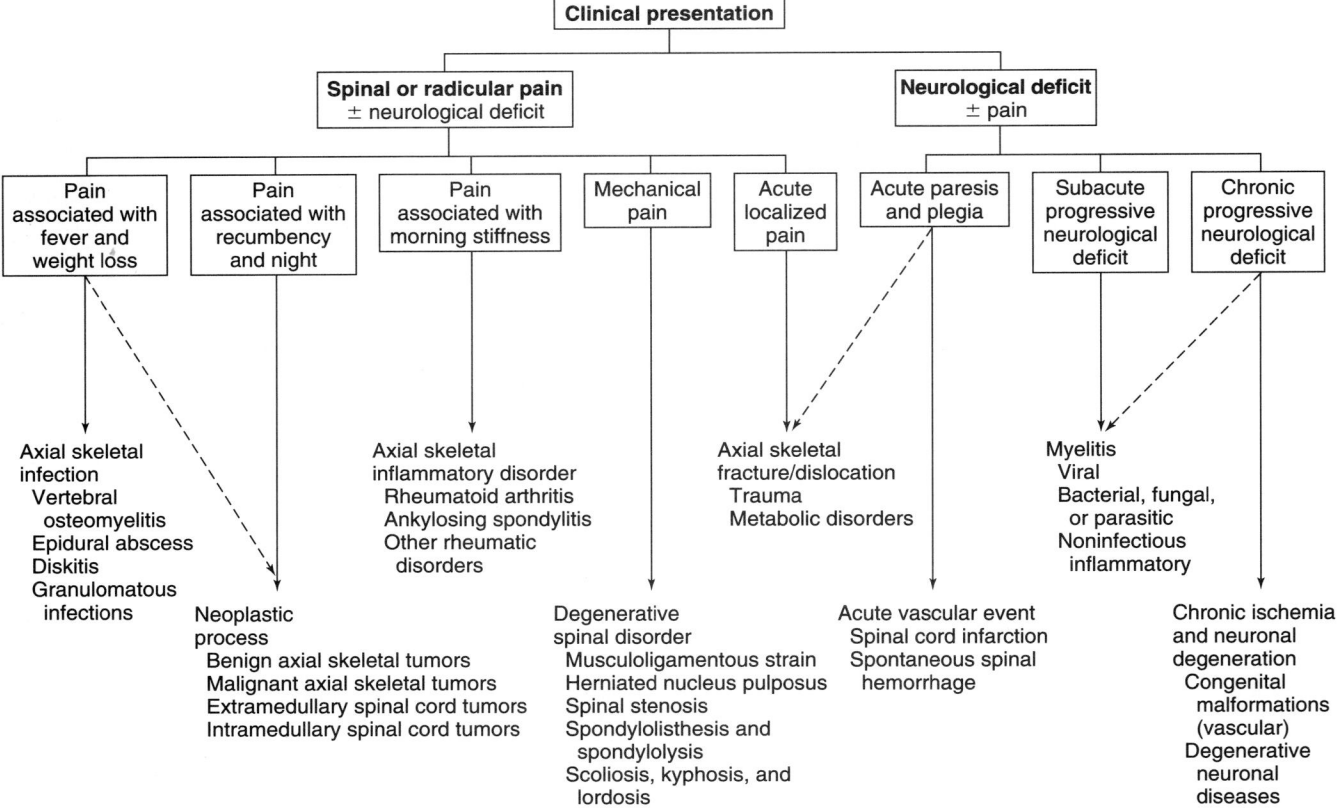

FIGURE 282–1. This algorithm classifies and organizes spinal pathology based on clinical presentation. The basic framework of the algorithm should help clinicians restrict the differential diagnoses, consider infrequently encountered conditions, and proceed with the workup in a logical manner.

lyte, blood urea nitrogen, creatinine, and glucose determinations; and a coagulation panel. Directed laboratory studies may include an erythrocyte sedimentation rate (ESR) and blood cultures to diagnose an infection, serum and urine studies to explore neoplasia, immunologic markers to diagnose inflammatory diseases, and endocrine and metabolic studies to investigate primary metabolic bone diseases.

Classically, imaging of the spine begins with plain radiographs, which should include anteroposterior, lateral, and flexion-extension views, as well as coned-down views of transitional areas. If the plain radiographs reveal evidence of pathologic disease or there is a high index of clinical suspicion despite normal radiographs, magnetic resonance imaging (MRI) or computed tomography (CT) of the spine should follow. As a general rule, MRI is better for imaging soft tissues and changes in tissue hydration, and CT is better for imaging bony detail. CT-myelography often improves delineation of the neural elements in relation to bony anatomy. Bone scans are highly sensitive for the detection of focal bony pathology but are relatively nonspecific. Various imaging techniques can be used to evaluate bone density. The laboratory studies and radiologic imaging may provide a definitive diagnosis, or pathologic evaluation of abnormal tissue may be required. When a definitive diagnosis has been obtained, medical or surgical treatment can proceed.[4–7]

Pain Associated with Fever and Weight Loss

Patients presenting with spinal or radicular pain associated with fever and weight loss are at increased risk of having an infectious process (Table 282–1). The presentation of neoplastic processes, specifically metastatic disease and lymphoma, can be similar. The presence of fever with spinal or radicular pain, however, should lead the physician to look for an axial skeletal infection first. Vertebral osteomyelitis, diskitis, epidural abscess, and granulomatous processes are the most common potential infectious conditions. Neurological deficits can occur, but they usually present weeks to months after the onset of pain and systemic symptoms.

VERTEBRAL OSTEOMYELITIS

Vertebral osteomyelitis typically results from a pyogenic infection of the vertebral column (Fig. 282–2). It is the most frequently encountered infection of the axial skeleton and accounts for 2% to 19% of all cases of osteomyelitis. Pyogenic infection of the vertebra may be the result of spinal trauma, extension from adjacent structures, or hematogenous spread. A definitive source of infection is found in less than 50% of cases. The most common foci are genitourinary, soft tissue, and respiratory, or the infection may be traced to intra-

TABLE 282-1 ■ Clinical Summary of Axial Skeletal Infections

INFECTION	INCIDENCE	CHARACTERISTICS	LOCATION
Vertebral osteomyelitis	Uncommon	Disease of the elderly and debilitated; males > females; gram-positive cocci most common	Lumbar > thoracic > cervical vertebral body
Spinal epidural abscess	Uncommon but clinically important	Most often spread hematogenously; gram-positive cocci most common	Thoracic > lumbar > cervical Posterior > anterior
Diskitis			
Adult	Uncommon	Postoperative infection after diskectomy; gram-positive cocci most common	Lumbar most common
Pediatric	Rare	Benign disease; either chronic inflammatory disorder or infection	Lumbar most common
Granulomatous infection	Uncommon in developed countries	Most common causative agent globally, *Mycobacterium tuberculosis*	Thoracic and lumbar most common
		Other rare causes: *Actinomyces israelii, Nocardia asteroides, Brucella, Cryptococcus neoformans,* candidiasis, aspergillosis, syphilis, *Echinococcus*	Vertebral body

venous drug abuse. The most common organisms isolated, the gram-positive cocci, constitute 60% to 70% of all cases. *Staphylococcus aureus* is the most prevalent, representing up to 60% of all positive cultures. Some series have reported a relative increase in gram-negative rods, which are found predominantly in parenteral drug abusers or immunocompromised patients. The lumbar spine is most often involved, followed by the thoracic and cervical spine. In more than 95% of cases, the vertebral body is involved. Less than 5% of cases involve the posterior elements.[8-12]

Vertebral osteomyelitis, a disease of the elderly and debilitated, has a male predominance. Advanced age, diabetes mellitus, steroid therapy, and intravenous drug abuse are predisposing factors. The most common symptom is insidious diffuse back pain, which occurs in about 90% of patients. Fever occurs in 50% to 70% of patients; weight loss, radicular symptoms, myelopathy, spinal deformity, and meningeal irritation are associated less frequently. Initially, the diagnosis can be missed because the presentation of the disease is relatively benign and nonspecific. Time from initial presentation to diagnosis ranges from 2 weeks to 5 months, with a mean of 6 to 8 weeks. Neurological compromise and decreased mobility are late complications. Diagnosis is based on pertinent laboratory findings, including an elevated ESR, blood and bone cultures, an elevated white blood cell count, and radiologic studies. The superior sensitivity and specificity of MRI make it the gold standard for detecting osteomyelitis. Bone scans are useful for diagnosis because of their high sensitivity, but they can be misleading because other inflammatory processes or neoplasia can mimic infection. CT reveals the extent of bony destruction.

Management is based on the results of biopsy. The preferred method is percutaneous aspiration and bone biopsy under computed tomographic or fluoroscopic guidance. Treatment entails bed rest and initiation of broad-spectrum antibiotics, followed by definitive antimicrobial therapy based on culture results. Anterior decompression with instrumentation and fusion may be required if there is evidence of extensive bony involvement or if neurological sequelae ensue from excessive bony destruction or abscess formation.[13-23]

SPINAL EPIDURAL ABSCESS

A spinal epidural abscess usually results from a pyogenic infection of the epidural space (Fig. 282-3). Although this is an uncommon clinical entity (reported incidence of 0.2 to 1.2 cases per 10,000 hospital admissions), its clinical importance overshadows its rarity. Approximately 50% of spinal epidural abscesses are the result of hematogenous spread to the epidural space. Other causes include direct extension of a preexisting osteomyelitis or diskitis and direct inoculation from surgical manipulation or trauma. The bacteria present in spinal epidural abscesses closely resemble the organisms found in vertebral osteomyelitis. Gram-positive cocci are the most prevalent, with *S. aureus* isolated in 60% to 65% of the positive cultures; other staphylococcal and streptococcal species are the next most common organisms isolated. In recent series, the frequency of gram-negative rods has increased. Thoracic involvement is commonly followed closely by lumbar involvement and then, much less frequently, by cervical involvement. A posterior location predominates in about two thirds of cases. An anterior abscess often results from direct extension of a ventrally located diskitis or vertebral osteomyelitis.[9-12]

Primarily adults are affected; occurrences in children are rare. There is no sex predominance. In most cases, axial skeletal pain is the initial clinical presentation. The pain may then develop a radicular component, with isolated sensory or motor dysfunction in the distribution of the nerve root. If untreated, paraplegia or quadriplegia ensues. The incidence of fever, leukocytosis, and neurological compromise is higher than in vertebral osteomyelitis. Laboratory investigations should include ESR and white blood cell count, which are elevated in most patients. MRI is the diagnostic procedure of choice. T1-weighted images reveal a hypointense epidural mass, which enhances with contrast. On T2-weighted images, the mass is hyperintense. Early diagnosis is important, because patients with spinal epidural abscess can deteriorate rapidly. Even on intravenous antibiotics, a patient's neurological condition can rapidly deteriorate to paraplegia or quadriplegia. The recommended treatment for a spinal

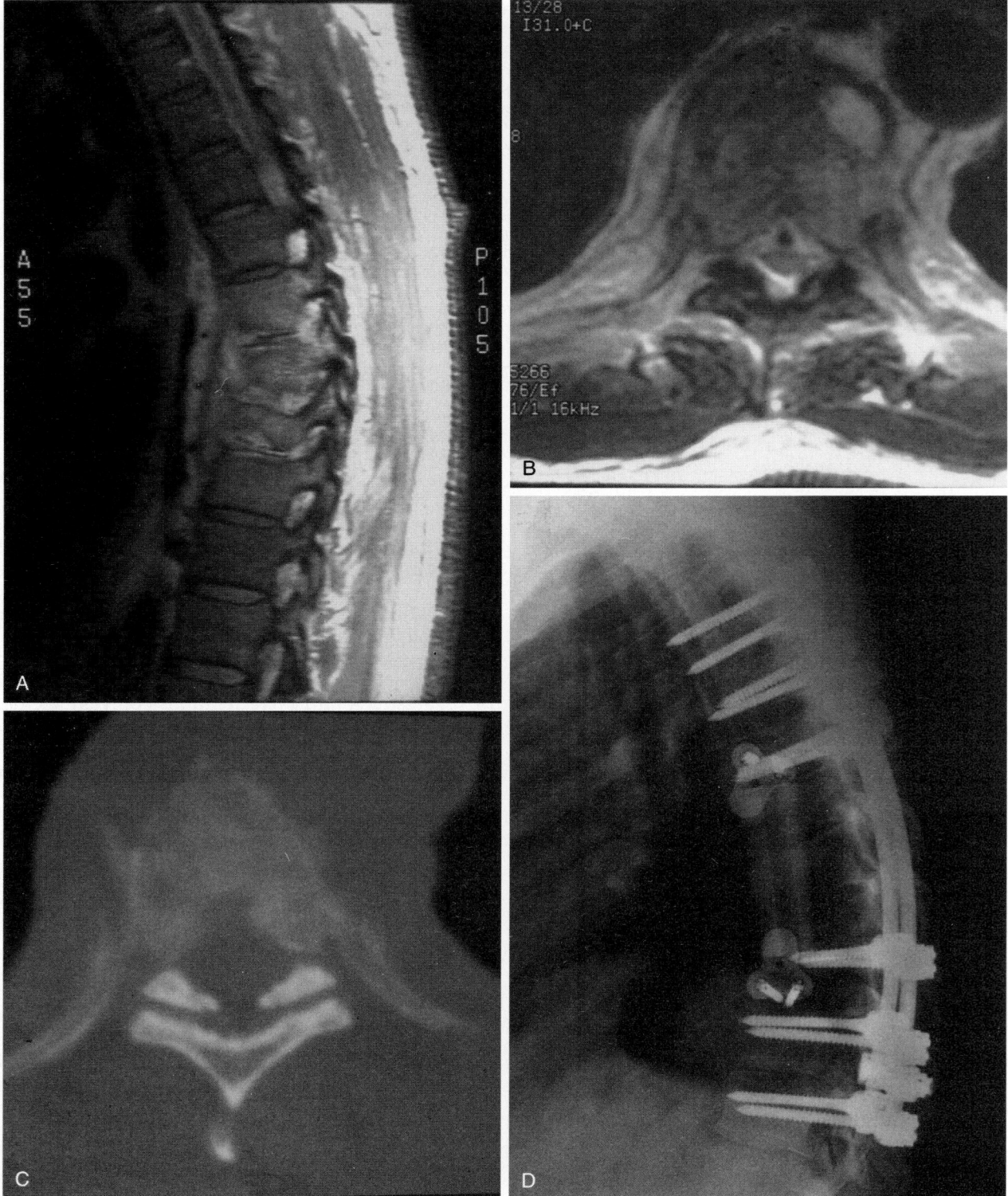

FIGURE 282–2. Vertebral osteomyelitis in a 51-year-old man with diabetes and a 5-month history of progressive midthoracic back pain, fever, and weight loss. *A,* Sagittal magnetic resonance proton density-weighted image. *B,* Axial T2-weighted contrast-enhanced magnetic resonance imaging scan of the thoracic spine. *A* and *B* show pyogenic thoracic osteomyelitis with progressive kyphosis and extension of the infection into the anterior epidural space. *C,* Axial computed tomographic scan through the T8 vertebral body shows extensive bony involvement. *D,* The patient underwent a two-level T7-8 anterior thoracic decompression and débridement, with placement of a T6-9 tibial allograft followed by a posterior segmental instrumentation and fusion from T4-11. Postoperatively, the patient was treated with culture-directed antibiotic therapy.

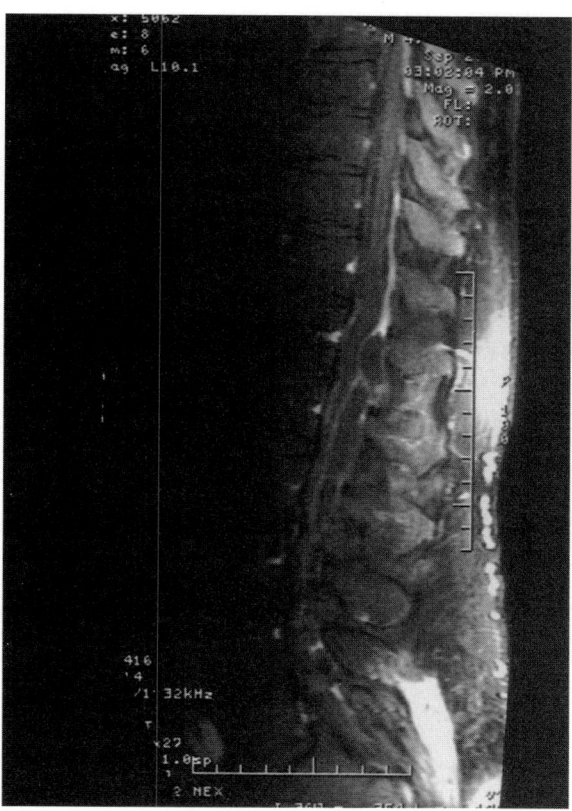

FIGURE 282–3. Spinal epidural abscess in a 47-year-old man with a history of intravenous drug abuse and a 4-month history of lower back pain and fever and new-onset mild lower extremity weakness. A sagittal T1-weighted, fat-suppressed, contrast-enhanced image of the thoracolumbar spine shows a posterior rim–enhancing spinal epidural abscess extending from T12 through L5. The pyogenic epidural infection was drained from a posterior approach through thoracolumbar laminectomies, and the patient was treated with culture-directed antibiotic therapy.

epidural abscess is surgical evacuation with administration of the appropriate antibiotics.[19, 24, 25]

DISKITIS

Diskitis represents two entirely different entities in adults and children. Classically, spontaneous diskitis is a disease of the pediatric population. In adults, diskitis is usually encountered in patients who have undergone diskectomy. Less often, adult diskitis is the result of hematogenous spread, often associated with intravenous drug abuse or debilitating disease. Early investigation and detection are important to prevent diskitis from progressing to vertebral osteomyelitis or epidural abscess.[25–29]

In children, diskitis has been described as a relatively benign disease that may be a chronic inflammatory disorder, a viral infection, or a low-grade bacterial infection. In adults, postoperative diskitis is usually a pyogenic infection that probably results from direct inoculation during surgical manipulation. Children are predisposed to diskitis because of the vascular anastomotic network around and through the cartilaginous

end plates and disk, which functions as a bacterial filter and end point (the vascular network disappears in late adolescence). Gram-positive cocci, specifically staphylococcal and streptococcal species, predominate in positive cultures (pediatric and adult). Biopsies and blood cultures are nondiagnostic in 20% to 50% of patients in most series. The lumbar spine is affected much more frequently than the thoracic or cervical spine in children and adults.[19, 30–32]

The clinical presentation of back pain and painful ambulation is related to the most common location—the lumbar spine. In adults, the onset of back pain 1 to 3 weeks after surgery at the operated level should alert physicians to the possibility of an infection. Typically, the ESR is elevated. Because of its ability to detect hydration changes in the disk, MRI is the most sensitive and specific modality both for detecting infection and for following efficacy of treatment. MRI scans show evidence of the infection sooner than does plain radiography. ESR is a sensitive laboratory test not only for detecting the infection but also for following the progression of treatment. Management consists of CT- or fluoroscopy-guided biopsy and culture, followed by bed rest and a brief course of intravenous antibiotics until symptoms attenuate. Oral antibiotic therapy is then initiated. The prognosis of uncomplicated cases is excellent.[10, 12, 30, 33–35]

GRANULOMATOUS INFECTIONS

Broadly, granulomatous infections include all processes that can initiate a chronic granulomatous response. Fungal, spirochetal, and uncommon bacterial organisms such as *Actinomyces, Nocardia,* and *Brucella,* as well as common *Mycobacterium tuberculosis* infections, can produce granulomatous disease of the axial skeleton.

Although rare in developed countries, globally, *tuberculous spondylitis* is the most common granulomatous infection affecting the axial skeleton (Fig. 282–4). Historically dubbed Pott's disease, tuberculous spondylitis is usually caused by *M. tuberculosis,* although another mycobacterium may be the culprit. Generally, tuberculous spondylitis results from the hematogenous spread of the pathogen via a pulmonary or genitourinary source. The granulomatous infection then spreads across the disk space along either the posterior or the anterior longitudinal ligament but tends to spare the disk space. The skeleton is involved in about 1% of all cases; of those, 50% to 60% have an infection of the axial skeleton. The thoracolumbar spine is affected most frequently; cervical and sacral involvement is rare.[19, 25, 36]

Historically, tuberculosis is a disease of the elderly in developed countries and predominates in children in developing countries. Currently, individuals infected with the human immunodeficiency virus (HIV) are responsible for most tubercular infections in the United States. Clinical presentation involves bone pain over the affected site—typically, the thoracolumbar spine—in conjunction with fever, malaise, and weight loss. Vertebral collapse, spinal deformity, epidural abscess, and subarachnoid seeding after dural erosion are

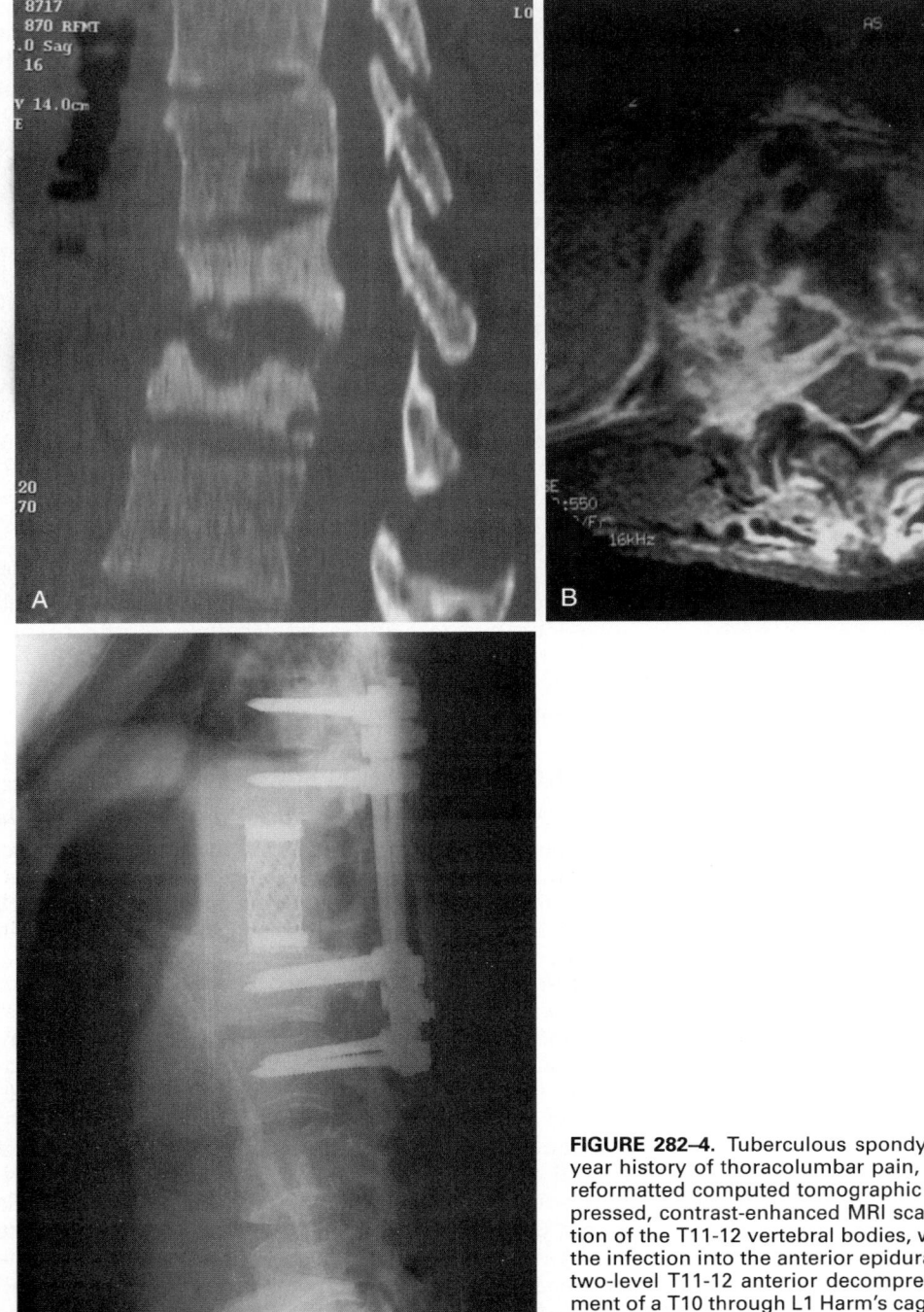

FIGURE 282–4. Tuberculous spondylitis in a 44-year-old man with a 2-year history of thoracolumbar pain, fever, and weight loss. *A*, Sagittally reformatted computed tomographic scan. *B*, Axial T1-weighted, fat-suppressed, contrast-enhanced MRI scan. *A* and *B* show extensive destruction of the T11-12 vertebral bodies, with early kyphosis and extension of the infection into the anterior epidural space. *C*, The patient underwent a two-level T11-12 anterior decompression and débridement, with placement of a T10 through L1 Harm's cage followed by a posterior segmental instrumentation and fusion from T9 through L2. Postoperatively, the patient continued to receive antituberculous treatment.

late sequelae. In the progressive stages of the disease, kyphosis and epidural abscesses are common. Neurological sequelae occur in 10% to 50% of patients with active disease. In 20% of cases, tuberculous spondylitis causes paraparesis.[37–41]

Plain radiography, MRI, and CT-myelography are the basis for evaluating treatment, disease progression, and surgical planning. MRI is superior for evaluating the involvement of soft tissue and the formation of abscesses. CT provides better bony detail. Treatment modalities are based on positive biopsy and culture results, degree of kyphosis, extent of neurological compromise, and disease refractory to medical management. Anterior decompression and débridement, combined with proper antibiotic therapy, are the accepted treatment modalities when a neurological deficit evolves. Prognosis and morbidity and mortality rates are related to the patient's age, extent of systemic involvement, and preoperative neurological status.[25, 42–45]

Actinomyces israelii is an anaerobic gram-positive bacterium. Infection leads to purulent abscesses, external draining sinuses, and characteristic sulfur granules on microscopic examination. Actinomycosis is found most often in the cervical spine, because most cases involve the mandible and supraclavicular areas, with direct extension to the adjacent vertebrae. *Nocardia asteroides*, a gram-positive bacterium, usually causes systemic illness but can represent a rare cause of back pain when the bony spinal column is involved. *Nocardia* usually spreads hematogenously from a pulmonary focus to the soft tissue organ systems, but osteomyelitis has occasionally been reported. *Brucella*, a gram-negative coccobacillus that is a pathogen of farm animals, is extremely uncommon in developed countries, primarily because milk is pasteurized and food sources are uncontaminated. Brucellosis is usually transmitted via digestion of contaminated food or inhalation of aerosols. The illness usually manifests systemically with indolent fever, lymphadenopathy, and generalized malaise. When the spine is involved, there is a lumbar predilection.[12, 25, 46, 47]

Fungal infections of the axial skeleton are rare even in endemic areas. Infection occurs by spore inhalation, with resultant pulmonary seeding and systemic spread. Fungal infections in patients with disseminated disease are associated with various degrees of spinal osseous involvement. Spinal osseous involvement with disseminated coccidioidomycotic and blastomycotic infection occurs in 10% to 50% of cases. *Cryptococcus neoformans* is a fungal infection more commonly known for central nervous system (CNS) involvement. Osseous involvement occurs in only 10% of cases, with minimal granuloma formation and cellular reaction. The incidence of axial skeletal involvement with candidiasis or aspergillosis is much lower. Both fungal infections tend to occur in immunocompromised hosts. Other rare granulomatous diseases of the axial skeleton include parasitic infections such as syphilis and echinococcosis.[12, 25, 48, 49]

Pain Associated with Recumbency and Nighttime

Pain is the most common presenting symptom for tumors involving the axial skeleton and spinal cord (extramedullary and intramedullary). The hallmark of neoplastic lesions of the axial skeleton is localized spinal pain associated with recumbency and nighttime (Table 282–2). Spinal cord tumors most often manifest with diffuse spinal or radicular pain that is not relieved by rest. Pain in the axial skeleton occurs in as many as 85% of patients in large series of vertebral column tumors. It usually begins well before any radicular pain or neurological deficit appears. Spinal cord tumors (extramedullary and intramedullary) manifest with pain; spinal cord tumors are associated with the insidious onset of diffuse spinal pain or spinal pain vaguely localized to the level of the tumor. Because of the insidious onset and diffuse nature of the pain associ-

ated with spinal cord tumors, radicular pain or neurological deficit is usually present by the time the tumor is diagnosed.

Age, location, incidence, and pathology exhibit a variety of correlations with axial skeletal lesions. Younger patients tend to have a greater incidence of benign bone tumors, whereas those older than 30 years are predisposed toward malignancy. Malignant lesions of the axial skeleton, whether metastatic or primary, are most often found in anterior locations; benign processes tend to favor posterior elements. The incidence of skeletal metastases outweighs the incidence of primary malignant bone tumors by a margin of 25:1 to 40:1.

Correlations for similar parameters can be deduced for spinal cord tumors. Approximately two thirds of spinal cord tumors are extramedullary, and one third are intramedullary. Extramedullary tumors involve the intradural space twice as frequently as the extradural space and are composed primarily of nerve sheath tumors and meningiomas. The origin of most intramedullary tumors, predominantly astrocytomas and ependymomas, is glial. The most common tumor to involve the meninges and spinal cord occurs in the epidural space as metastatic disease.

BENIGN TUMORS OF THE AXIAL SKELETON

Typically, benign tumors of the axial skeleton are found in a posterior location in individuals between 20 and 30 years old. In the axial skeleton, the more common types of benign lesions—osteochondromas, osteoid osteomas, and osteoblastomas—have a lower incidence of recurrence after resection overall than do malignant bone tumors. Other benign tumors include giant cell tumors, aneurysmal bone cysts, hemangiomas, and eosinophilic granulomas.[50–53]

An *osteochondroma* is a cartilage-capped bony protuberance that is thought to develop from an adjacent physis or a cartilaginous remnant of the physis. Osteochondromas are the most common of the benign bone tumors. More than 50% of symptomatic spinal lesions occur in the cervical region, and they almost always involve the posterior elements. Clinical presentation varies from a dull backache (small tumors) to decreased motion or deformity (large tumors). Neurological compromise is rare. When neurological compromise is present, the cervical spine, followed by the thoracic spine, is the most typical location, and myelopathic symptoms result. Plain radiographs usually demonstrate a protruding lesion with well-demarcated borders in the posterior elements. On rare occasions, pain, neurological deficit, or an accelerated growth pattern may necessitate surgical removal. Prognosis is usually excellent when the affected periosteum and surrounding cartilage are resected completely. Osteochondromas occasionally degenerate into malignant chondrosarcomas (usually in patients with multiple lesions).[50, 51, 53, 54]

Osteoid osteomas and *osteoblastomas* share a common pathologic origin, but their size and incidence of spinal involvement differ. These tumors are thought to be a

T A B L E 2 8 2 - 2 ■ **Clinical Summary of Neoplastic Processes**

NEOPLASTIC PROCESS	INCIDENCE	CHARACTERISTICS	LOCATION
Benign Tumors of the Axial Skeleton			
Osteochondroma	Uncommon	Age <30 yr	Symptomatic Cervical > thoracic Posterior elements
Osteoid osteoma	Common	Age <30 yr; males > females	Lumbar most common Posterior elements
Osteoblastoma	Uncommon	Age <30 yr	Distributed throughout spinal axis Posterior elements
Giant cell tumor	Rare	Third to fourth decades of life	Sacral most common
Aneurysmal bone cyst	Rare	Age <30 yr	Thoracic and lumbar most common Posterior elements
Hemangioma	Common	All ages	Thoracic and lumbar most common Vertebral body
Eosinophilic granuloma	Rare	Pediatric population	Vertebral body
Malignant Tumors of the Axial Skeleton			
Metastatic	25–40 times more common than primary tumors	Age >50 yr Breast, lung, and prostate	Thoracic and lumbar > cervical Vertebral body
Multiple myeloma and solitary plasmacytoma	Uncommon	Fifth to seventh decades of life Plasmacytoma, males > females	Thoracic > lumbar > cervical Vertebral body
Chordoma	Uncommon	Fifth to sixth decades of life	Lumbosacral > cervical Vertebral body
Chondrosarcoma	Rare	Primary or secondary	Evenly distributed throughout spinal axis
Osteogenic sarcoma	Rare	Primary or secondary	Evenly distributed throughout spinal axis Vertebral body
Ewing's sarcoma	Rare	Pediatric population	Sacral most common Vertebral
Extramedullary Spinal Cord Tumors			

Nerve sheath tumor
  Schwannoma
  Neurofibroma
	Rare	Fourth to fifth decades of life
		Neurofibromatosis
			Schwannoma > neurofibroma
			Dorsal root > ventral root

Meningioma	Rare	Fifth to seventh decades of life; females > males	Thoracic most common
Filum terminale ependymoma	Rare	Third to fifth decades of life	Proximal filum terminale

Other
  Dermoid
  Epidermoid
  Lipoma
  Teratoma
  Neuroenteric cyst
  Paraganglioma
  Hemangioblastoma
  Ganglioneuroma
  Arachnoiditis			

Intramedullary Spinal Cord Tumors			
Glial	Rare	Children: astrocytomas more common Adults: ependymomas more common	Cervical and thoracic

Astrocytoma
  Ependymoma
Other
  Ganglioglioma
  Oligodendroglioma
  Subependymoma
  Neurocytoma
  Hemiangioblastoma
  Metastasis			

chronic inflammatory reaction rather than true neoplasms. Osteoid osteomas account for 2.6% of all excised primary bone tumors and as many as 18% of axial skeletal primary tumors. By definition, osteoid osteomas are smaller than 2 cm; otherwise, the lesions are classified as osteoblastomas. Approximately 40% of spinal osteoid osteomas occur in the lumbar region, most in the posterior elements. Most patients with symptomatic lesions are young and male. Half of all symptomatic lesions appear in the second decade of life. On clinical presentation, patients report a dull ache that is exacerbated at night. This condition is believed to be the result of prostaglandin production by the tumor. Thus, classically, the pain is relieved by aspirin. Neurological deficits are rare, but osteoid osteomas are the most common lesions associated with painful scoliosis in adolescents. Radiologically, the lesion is characterized by a radiolucent area with a central nidus and an appropriate degree of surrounding sclerosis. Treatment is excision. Instrumentation and fusion may be required if scoliosis is severe. Minor deformities resolve with resection alone. Overall, the prognosis is excellent, and the rate of recurrence, which is related to inadequate excision of the nidus, is marginal.[50, 51, 53–56]

Osteoblastomas are larger than osteoid osteomas (>2 cm). Histologically, the two lesions cannot be differentiated. Less common than osteoid osteomas, osteoblastomas represent less than 2% of primary benign bone tumors but have a greater propensity for axial skeleton involvement. Approximately 30% to 40% of osteoblastomas involve the axial skeleton. The lesions are distributed throughout the longitudinal axis of the spine, most often involve the posterior elements, and have a propensity to produce a spinal deformity. In 90% of cases, osteoblastomas are found in patients 30 years or younger. Their male-to-female predominance is 2:1. Clinical presentation characteristically involves a higher incidence of neurological deficit related to the size of the lesion. Treatment is en bloc resection, which usually resolves the scoliotic deformity. With adequate removal, prognosis is favorable. Long-term recurrence rates approach 10%.[50, 51, 53–56]

Giant cell tumors are benign lesions, but their cellular origin is unknown. They are aggressive, carry some malignant potential, and are associated with a high incidence of local recurrence. They are responsible for 21% of all primary benign bone tumors and affect the spinal axis in 8% to 11% of all cases. When the spinal column is involved, the tumors typically occur in the sacral region. Unlike most primary bone tumors, giant cell tumors tend to be found in individuals in the third and fourth decades of life. Their frequency decreases in later years. Women are affected slightly more often than are men. Plain radiographs demonstrate cortical expansion with little reactive sclerosis or periosteal reaction. MRI scans reveal homogeneous signals; computed tomographic studies better delineate the degree of vertebral bone involvement and define surgical margins. Because the histologic characteristics of giant cell tumors are nondistinct, a thorough evaluation, including radiographic investigation coupled with histopathologic studies, is important to differentiate this condition from other primary bone tumors. Treatment is usually en bloc resection. Because of the high rate of recurrence (50%), the prognosis is relatively poor. These tumors have the potential for malignant transformation, especially after local radiation if surgical margins were inadequate.[50, 51, 53–57]

Aneurysmal bone cysts are benign, non-neoplastic, proliferative lesions. Although responsible for only 1% to 2% of all primary bone tumors, aneurysmal bone cysts affect the axial skeleton in 12% to 25% of reported cases. Their pathogenesis is unclear, but accepted theories include an underlying tumor or traumatic arteriovenous malformation (AVM) with subsequent development of a cyst. Histologically, aneurysmal bone cysts contain fluid-filled spaces separated by fibrous septa. Their incidence is greatest in the thoracolumbar region. As in most benign osseous lesions, 60% of spinal aneurysmal bone cysts occur in the posterior elements. Aneurysmal bone cysts typically occur in young patients in the second decade of life, with a slight predominance in women. MRI and CT demonstrate a multiloculated, expansile, highly vascular osteolytic lesion with a thin, well-demarcated, eggshell-like cortical rim. Multiple vertebral levels may be involved in as many as 40% of cases. Treatment involves preoperative embolization and surgical resection. Postoperative radiation may have a role if the margins obtained during surgical resection were inadequate. Recurrence rates vary from 6% to 70%, depending on the extent of surgical resection and the administration of postoperative radiation.[50, 51, 53–56, 58–62]

Hemangiomas are benign tumors of vascular origin and are probably the most common benign tumor of the spine. General autopsy studies have found hemangiomas of the axial skeleton in 10% to 12% of cases. Characterized by slow growth and a female predominance, vertebral hemangiomas most often occur in the thoracolumbar spine and have a predilection for the vertebral body. Symptomatic vertebral hemangiomas are exceedingly rare. When they do become symptomatic, however, the most common initial symptom is back pain with or without radiation into the lower extremities. The loose relationship between pregnancy and expansile vertebral hemangiomas that produce a neurological deficit is attributed to the physiologic increase in the volume of the circulatory system during pregnancy, which causes a previously asymptomatic lesion to expand. Symptomatic lesions are best diagnosed with MRI scans; asymptomatic lesions are discovered incidentally during other radiographic investigations. Treatment of symptomatic lesions involving the spine consists of a combination of embolization, surgical resection, and possibly radiotherapy.[50, 51, 53–56, 63–65]

Eosinophilic granulomas are the solitary osseous lesions in a continuum of disorders (histiocytosis X and Letterer-Siwe and Hand-Schüller-Christian diseases) characterized by an abnormal proliferation of Langerhans' cells. Eosinophilic granulomas are rare lesions of the axial skeleton and occur most frequently in the vertebral body. Most eosinophilic granulomas occur in children; the peak incidence is between ages 5 and 10. MRI and CT are the investigative procedures of choice, but the ultimate diagnosis requires biopsy. Treatment is somewhat controversial but commonly includes surgical curettage. Adjuvant radiotherapy or chemotherapy is reserved for disseminated versions of this uncommon disease of the axial skeleton.[50, 51, 53–56, 66–70]

MALIGNANT TUMORS OF THE AXIAL SKELETON

Malignant tumors of the axial skeleton can be either metastatic or primary. The most common metastatic spinal column tumors are breast, lung, and prostate malignancies; multiple myeloma, chordoma, chondrosarcoma, osteogenic sarcoma, and Ewing's sarcoma are the most common primary malignant neoplasms of the axial skeleton. Metastasis can result from direct extension or hematogenous spread. Primary malignant axial skeletal neoplasms and metastatic tumors most often involve the vertebral body. Malignant tumors of the axial skeleton are 25 to 40 times more likely to be metastatic than primary.[50, 51, 53–56]

Metastatic disease in the form of distant foci is evident at autopsy in 40% to 85% of cases of malignancy, and the spine is the most common site of skeletal metastasis. Breast, lung, and prostate malignancies account for most spinal metastatic lesions. Overall, metastatic lesions are spread equally throughout the thoracic and lumbosacral spine, but thoracic metastases tend to be symptomatic most often. Most series report that cervical lesions are symptomatic in only 6% to 8% of patients. The vertebral body is the structure most often involved. The axiom that acute neck or back pain in a patient with a known malignancy is metastatic disease until proved otherwise is a prudent guideline. Ultimate diagnosis relies on laboratory investigation, radiographic studies, and tumor biopsy results. MRI and CT-myelography help determine the extent of epidural compression and bone destruction, and they are used to screen for other areas of spinal involvement. Treatment options for metastatic disease of the spine include both radiation and surgical intervention. Operative intervention is palliative; pain control and maintenance of function and stability are the goals. Surgery is usually reserved for neurological compromise, radiation failure, spinal instability, or an uncertain diagnosis. Preoperative functional status and level of activity correlate directly with postoperative outcomes. Patients who suffer rapid progressive neurological deficits within a 24-hour period have a higher chance of developing permanent paraplegia than do those with slowly evolving deficits, who are more likely to regain ambulatory function. Overall, prognosis is directly related to neoplastic type, spinal location, and extent of systemic involvement.[50, 53, 56, 71–74]

Multiple myelomas and *solitary plasmacytomas* are two manifestations of B-cell lymphoproliferative disease. Multiple myelomas are the most common malignant neoplasms of bone in adults and affect the spine in 30% to 50% of reported cases. The thoracic spine is affected most commonly, followed by the lumbar spine and, rarely, the cervical spine (<10%). The vertebral body is usually the site of tumor involvement. Multiple myeloma is primarily a disease of the fifth, sixth, and

seventh decades of life and occurs equally among men and women. However, approximately 75% of solitary plasmacytomas occur in men. Unlike the classic presentation of pain with recumbency, the pain of multiple myeloma is sometimes relieved by rest and aggravated by mechanical agitation, mimicking other degenerative sources of pain. The diagnosis of multiple myeloma is based on characteristic serum protein abnormalities and radiologic imaging. Plain radiography and CT can be almost solely diagnostic because of the characteristic osteolytic picture, without sclerotic edges involving the vertebral body and sparing of the posterior elements. Treatment and prognosis depend on whether the diagnosis is solitary plasmacytoma or systemic multiple myeloma. Both conditions are exquisitely radiosensitive, but patients with solitary plasmacytomas have significantly longer survival rates.[50, 51, 53–56]

Chordomas, originally described by Virchow, are tumors that originate from the primitive notochord (Fig. 282–5). As tumors of the axial skeleton and skull base, chordomas constitute 1% to 2% of all skeletal sarcomas. Histologically, they are low-grade, locally invasive tumors, but metastases can occur in 5% to 43% of cases. More than 50% of these lesions are located in the lumbosacral region, 35% are in the clival and cervical area, and the remainder are spread throughout the vertebral column. Chordomas are the most common primary neoplasms of the sacrococcygeal region and occur predominantly in the fifth and sixth decades of life. Neurological deficits in the form of bowel and bladder dysfunction may be present at the time of diagnosis. MRI is the radiographic modality of choice for total tumor evaluation because of its ability to delineate soft tissue involvement. CT remains the modality of choice for imaging the extent of bony destruction. Diagnosis is based on CT- or fluoroscopy-guided biopsy. Treatment is en bloc resection when feasible. Radiation is usually reserved for local recurrences and surgically inaccessible disease. There is considerable debate on pathologic subtypes with respect to grade, recurrence, and outcome. Age at presentation is probably the best prognostic indicator for disease-free survival after surgery, with younger patients having better prognoses.[50, 51, 53–56, 75–79]

Chondrosarcomas are rare, malignant, cartilage-forming neoplasms that arise from cartilaginous elements. These tumors affect primarily the adult appendicular skeleton, and spinal involvement is rare (6% of cases). Chondrosarcomas arise either primarily or from preexisting solitary osteochondromas, hereditary multiple exostosis, or Paget's disease. There is an even distribution of tumor involvement among cervical, thoracic, and lumbosacral locations. Primary and secondary chondrosarcomas usually arise in middle-aged and older patients and show a predilection for men. Diagnostic characteristics on MRI and CT include bone destruction, associated soft tissue mass, and characteristic flocculent calcifications in the soft tissue mass. Definitive diagnosis is based on the results of tumor biopsy. Treatment is en bloc resection if feasible. Neither radiation therapy nor chemotherapy is of much benefit. Prognosis correlates with tumor extension and

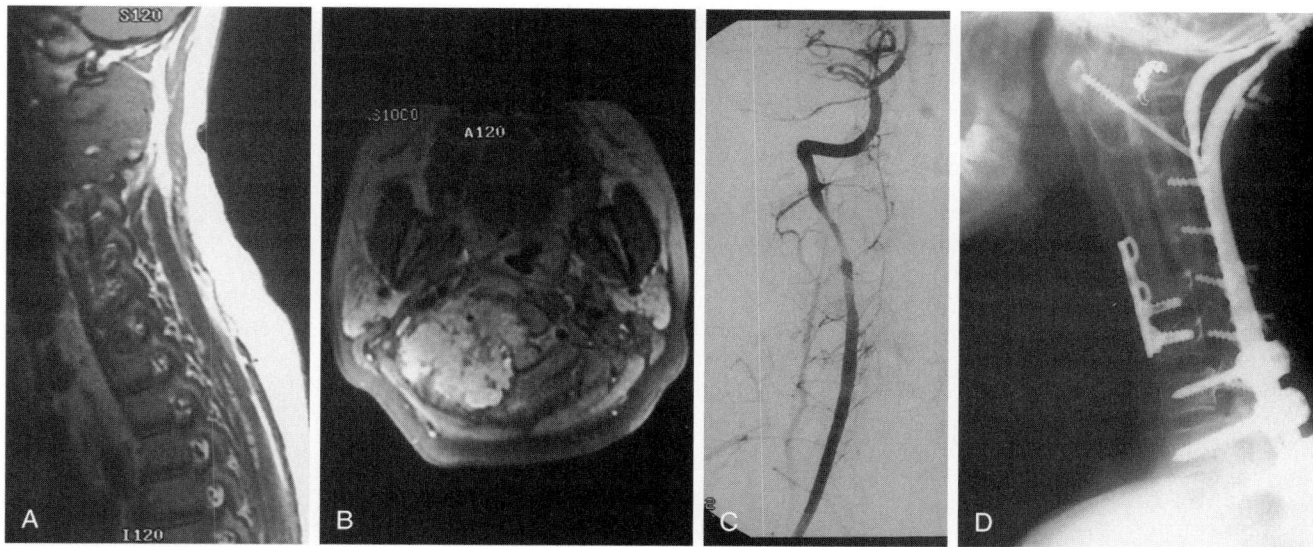

FIGURE 282–5. Chordoma in a 14-year-old boy with a 3-month history of progressively worsening neck pain that was exacerbated at night. *A,* Sagittal T1-weighted image of the cervical spine. *B,* Axial T2-weighted, fat-suppressed image of the cervical spine. *A* and *B* show a chordoma arising at C2 and extending inferiorly to C5. *C,* Angiogram shows stenosis and displacement of the right vertebral artery from the neoplastic lesion. *D,* The patient underwent preoperative embolization of the right vertebral artery, followed by en bloc tumor resection with anterior and posterior spinal reconstruction. Postoperatively, the patient was treated with proton radiation therapy.

grade. Patients with unresectable chondrosarcomas have a 5-year survival rate of only 20%.[50, 51, 53–56, 80–84]

Osteogenic sarcomas are malignant tumors of bone that are exceedingly rare in the axial skeleton. Only 2% of all osteogenic sarcomas arise in the spine. When they do involve the vertebral column, they are more likely to be metastatic than primary. The vertebral body is involved in more than 95% of cases, and the lesions are distributed evenly throughout the spine. Osteogenic sarcomas can arise primarily or secondarily. Most primary osteogenic sarcomas manifest in the first 20 years of life; secondary sarcomas arise in the fifth to sixth decades as a result of irradiated bone or preexisting Paget's disease. This neoplastic disease has a slight predilection for men. Radiologically, osteogenic sarcomas typically exhibit combined lytic and sclerotic lesions, with cortical destruction and ossification in the tumor mass. CT- or fluoroscopy-guided biopsy provides the diagnosis and guides preoperative adjuvant therapy. Preoperative embolization, chemotherapy, and surgical extirpation with adjuvant radiotherapy are the current treatment modalities. Overall, prognosis is poor, with a life expectancy of 10 months to 1.5 years; there are a few long-term survivors.[50, 51, 53–56]

Ewing's sarcoma is a small blue cell tumor of bone whose cell of origin remains unclear (Fig. 282–6). Only 3% to 4% of Ewing's sarcomas arise within the axial skeleton, and they constitute only 6% of all primary malignant bone tumors, making them rare primary neoplasms of the spinal column. The incidence of spinal column involvement decreases caudally to rostrally, with more than half of Ewing's sarcomas arising within the sacrum. The vertebral body is most often involved. Ewing's sarcoma is primarily a disease of children,

with more than 85% of cases occurring in the first 2 decades of life. Males are affected more often than are females, at a ratio of 2:1. MRI and CT usually reveal a lytic lesion, possibly with a blastic component. Diagnosis is based on biopsy of the tumor. Treatment involves a multidisciplinary approach that combines surgical extirpation, radiation, and chemotherapeutic protocols. Younger patients tend to have a better prognosis; survival at 5 years approaches 75%.[50, 51, 53–56, 85–87]

EXTRAMEDULLARY SPINAL CORD TUMORS

Extramedullary spinal cord tumors may be intradural or extradural, or both. Intradural extramedullary tumors account for 40% to 50% of all spinal cord tumors, and extradural tumors account for 30%. The most common extramedullary spinal cord tumors are nerve sheath tumors, meningiomas, and filum terminale ependymomas. Nerve sheath tumors and meningiomas constitute more than 70% to 80% of the extramedullary spinal cord tumors. Pain is an early symptom. Back pain is the most common initial complaint in adults harboring extramedullary spinal cord neoplasms. Children with extramedullary spinal cord tumors tend to present with neurological deficits in the form of motor or gait disturbances.[88–91]

Initially, the spinal pain in adults is diffuse and unrelated to mechanical activity, thus delaying diagnosis until the pain becomes radicular or symptoms caused by spinal cord compression ensue. Extradural lesions may be associated with more intense localized pain or a more rapid progression to radicular pain, leading to an earlier diagnosis. Symptoms can be nocturnal and are rarely relieved with rest or recumbency.

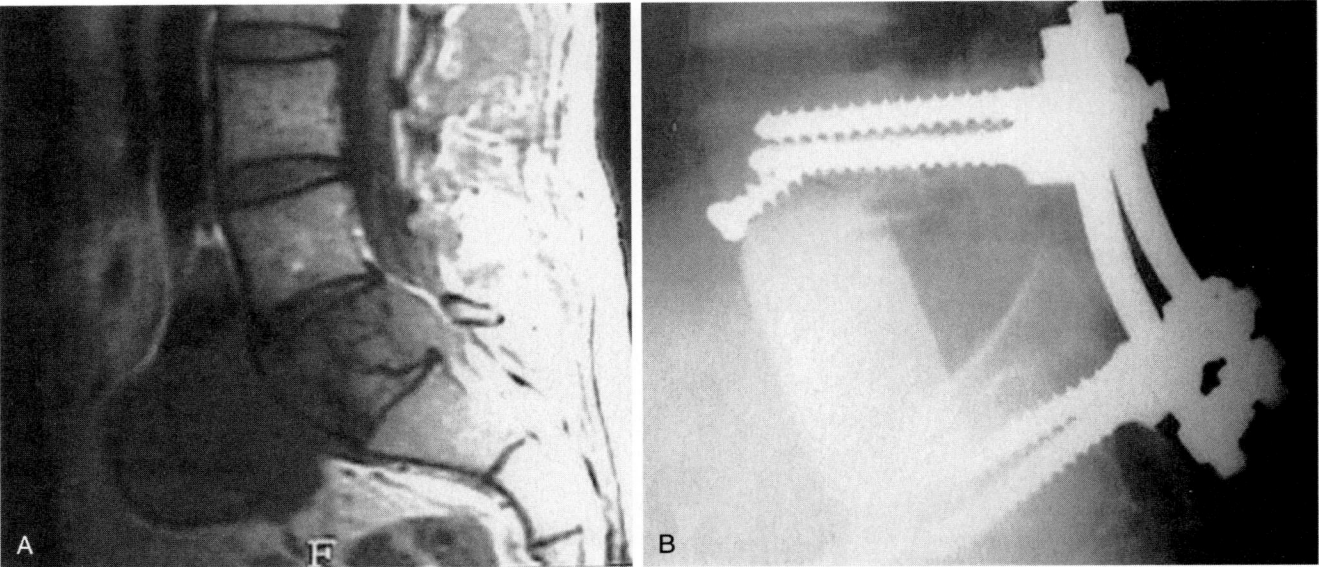

FIGURE 282–6. Ewing's sarcoma in a 15-year-old boy with progressive intractable lower back pain. *A,* Sagittal T1-weighted image of the lumbosacral spine shows a Ewing's sarcoma arising from the L5 vertebral body with anterior and posterior extension. *B,* The patient underwent gross total resection of the tumor, with placement of an anterior tibial allograft followed by posterior segmental instrumentation and fusion. Postoperatively, the patient underwent treatment with radiation and chemotherapy.

Early neurological compromise is uncommon because of the adaptive compressibility of the surrounding fat, cerebrospinal fluid (CSF), and adjacent vascular structures. Neurological compromise occurs when the compliance of surrounding structures is at its nadir and compression is transmitted directly to the spinal cord. The location of the neoplasm within the longitudinal spinal canal affects the evolution of the neurological deficit. Most extramedullary neoplasms produce local segmental deficits before a distant neurological deficit appears. Cervical lesions can produce weakness, fasciculation, and atrophy of hand muscles. Thoracic lesions can produce band paresthesias or Horner's syndrome, whereas lumbosacral or conus medullaris lesions can produce lower extremity weakness as well as bladder and bowel symptoms. Because of the anterolateral and posterolateral locations of many extramedullary spinal cord neoplasms, there is a higher incidence of Brown-Séquard syndrome with these tumors.[88–92]

Nerve sheath tumors are categorized as either schwannomas or neurofibromas (Fig. 282–7). Both are benign lesions of Schwann cell origin. Most nerve sheath tumors are schwannomas that occur proportionally throughout the spinal canal. Most are also entirely intradural. However, 10% to 15% extend through the dural root sleeve with both intradural and extradural components, and approximately 10% are entirely extradural. Most nerve sheath tumors arise from a dorsal nerve root; tumors arising from a ventral root are more likely to be neurofibromas. Although their malignant potential is low (2.5%), nerve sheath tumors can be locally destructive if allowed to progress. Caudally located nerve sheath tumors can displace adjacent nerve roots, with possible bone erosion of nearby foramina

as the neoplasm grows. Their peak incidence is in the fourth and fifth decades of life. On clinical presentation, patients with these tumors often exhibit vague localized spinal pain with radicular pain and evidence of nerve root or spinal cord impairment. Nerve sheath tumors occur commonly in patients with neurofibromatosis. MRI is the diagnostic procedure of choice and usually reveals a heterogeneously enhancing extramedullary anterolateral lesion, often with a widened neural foramen. Excision is recommended for symptomatic lesions. Recurrence is rare with complete removal.[88–95]

Spinal meningiomas tend to arise from the arachnoid cap cells embedded in the dura near the nerve root sleeve. Most tumors occur in the thoracic spine, although meningiomas are the most common benign tumor at the foramen magnum. Approximately 10% of meningiomas are either intradural and extradural or entirely extradural, but most are intradural. The majority present between the fifth and seventh decades of life, and more than 70% occur in women. Clinical presentation is similar to that of nerve sheath tumors, but radicular symptoms occur less frequently. MRI is the investigative modality of choice and reveals a homogeneously enhancing, posterolateral, dural-based lesion. Treatment is embolization followed by surgical excision. Ten years after gross total removal, the recurrence rate is 10% to 15%.[88–92, 96–98]

Filum terminale ependymomas are glial tumors that arise within the filum terminale and are almost always of the myxopapillary histologic type. These lesions account for approximately 15% of extramedullary spinal cord tumors. Approximately 40% of all spinal ependymomas arise within the proximal intradural filum. Most filum terminale ependymomas occur in the third

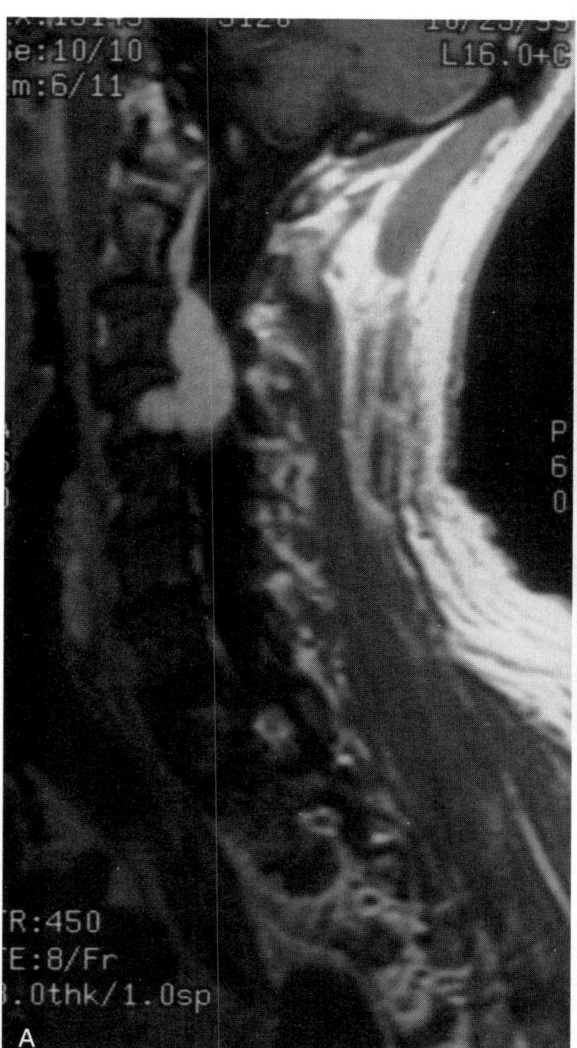
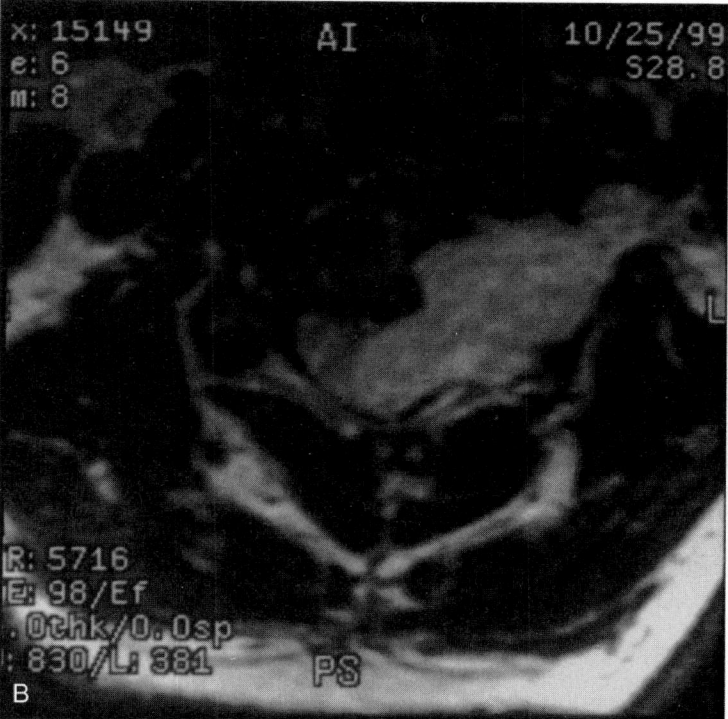

FIGURE 282–7. Nerve sheath tumor in a 48-year-old man with a long history of neck pain and a 4-month history of left upper extremity radicular pain. *A,* Sagittal T1-weighted contrast-enhanced image. *B,* Axial T2-weighted image. *A* and *B* show the cervical nerve sheath tumor arising at C4 on the left and extending through the neural foramen. The patient underwent combined posterior and anterior approaches to this lesion, with gross total resection.

to fifth decades of life. MRI is the diagnostic procedure of choice. Treatment is en bloc surgical resection, and recurrences are rare after gross total resection. Radiation is reserved for biologically aggressive tumors, which occur more frequently in the younger population.[88–92, 99–101]

The remaining extramedullary spinal cord tumors are rare and account for only 5% to 10% of such tumors. The majority of these lesions are intradural extramedullary tumors. Dermoids, epidermoids, lipomas, teratomas, and neuroenteric cysts are inclusion tumors and cysts that result from disordered embryogenesis. Occasionally, epidural lipomas are associated with Cushing's disease or exogenous steroid use and produce symptoms related to spinal cord compression. Paragangliomas are rare tumors that can arise from the filum terminale or cauda equina. Hemangioblastomas and ganglioneuromas can involve intradural nerve roots and present as extramedullary mass lesions. Arachnoiditis (though not strictly a tumor) can manifest with diffuse constant pain and is associated with paresthesias and sensory changes.[88–93]

INTRAMEDULLARY SPINAL CORD TUMORS

Intramedullary spinal cord tumors account for 2% to 4% of CNS neoplasms and are of neuroglial origin in 80% of cases. These lesions account for 20% to 25% of all spinal cord tumors, and most are astrocytomas and ependymomas. Gangliogliomas, oligodendrogliomas, subependymomas, hemangioblastomas, neurocytomas, and metastases occur much less frequently. Children are predisposed to astrocytic tumors. With age, however, ependymomas become more common than astrocytomas. Intramedullary spinal cord tumors manifest with insidious pain that localizes to the level of the tumor and is rarely radicular. Dysesthesias are more common than numbness. The pain associated with these lesions is usually unrelated to mechanical activity and is not relieved by recumbency or rest. An objective neurological deficit is usually present at diagnosis. Because of the insidious onset of symptoms, diagnosis can be delayed for as long as 2 years. The location of the intramedullary tumor within the longitudinal spinal canal dictates the evolution of the neurological deficit. Most intramedullary tumors produce local segmental and distant neurological deficits. Cervical segmental findings include weakness, fasciculation, and atrophy of the hand muscles. Upper thoracic tumors may produce Horner's syndrome, whereas lumbosacral or conus lesions may produce bladder or bowel symptoms. Because of their central location, intramedullary spinal cord tumors may produce a central cord-like syndrome, with relative sparing of the more radially located lumbosacral nerve tracts. Their central location renders Brown-Séquard syndrome unlikely.[89, 90, 92, 93]

Glial-derived tumors, astrocytomas and ependymomas, predominate in pediatric and adult intramedullary spinal cord tumors (Fig. 282–8). Astrocytomas can occur at any age but are most common in the first 3 decades of life. They constitute 90% of intramedullary tumors in patients younger than 10 years and 60% of intramedullary tumors in adolescents. Ependymomas are the most common intramedullary tumor in adults. Approximately 90% of pediatric astrocytic tumors are benign fibrillary astrocytomas or juvenile pilocytic astrocytomas; fibrillary astrocytomas prevail in adults. Only 10% of pediatric intramedullary astrocytomas are malignant, compared with 25% of adult astrocytic tumors. Histologically, almost all ependymomas are benign. Astrocytic tumors often infiltrate adjacent spinal cord tissue. Although unencapsulated, ependymomas are usually well circumscribed and do not infiltrate the adjacent spinal cord. MRI is the gold standard for evaluating intramedullary spinal cord tumors. Both astrocytomas and ependymomas produce fusiform dilatation of the spinal cord and are associated with low- to intermediate-intensity signals on T1-weighted images and a higher signal intensity on T2-weighted images; ependymomas tend to have more marked enhancement, better defined borders, and a more central location. With the advent of microneurosurgery, resection margins have improved, and morbidity and mortality rates have decreased. Adjuvant radiation therapy for glial tumors is controversial, and some investigators have found no significant benefit associated with this treatment.[92, 93, 102–111]

The remaining intramedullary spinal cord tumors are rare. Intramedullary hemangioblastomas most often occur in association with von Hippel–Lindau syndrome. These tumors usually have a pial attachment and are located dorsally or dorsolaterally. Gangliogliomas, oligodendrogliomas, and neurocytomas are rare intramedullary glial-derived tumors. Metastatic disease accounts for 1% to 2% of intramedullary spinal cord tumors.[89, 90, 92, 93, 107–109, 112]

Pain Associated with Morning Stiffness

Persistent axial pain that slowly tapers as mechanical activity increases is the hallmark of an inflammatory disorder affecting the spine (Table 282–3). Rheumatoid arthritis (RA) and ankylosing spondylitis are the two most common chronic inflammatory processes involving the axial skeleton. Although related, these diseases represent two vastly different pathologic conditions with regard to sex, age, axial location, associated clinical findings, immunologic characterization, and indications for surgical intervention. Neurological deficits are usually a late manifestation of these chronic disease processes. Other inflammatory disorders that may involve the axial skeleton include psoriatic arthritis, Reiter's syndrome, Behçet's disease, Whipple's disease, enteropathic arthritis, gout, and pseudogout.[113, 114]

RHEUMATOID ARTHRITIS

RA is a chronic systemic inflammatory disorder of unknown cause that involves primarily small blood vessels and synovium. The prevalence of RA is 1% for both genders by age 65. RA destroys joint articular surfaces, capsules, and supporting ligaments. The most common skeletal manifestation is involvement of the metatarsophalangeal joints, followed by involvement of the cervical spine. RA most often affects the cervical spine in one of three ways: atlantoaxial subluxation, basilar invagination, or subaxial subluxation. Craniocervical instability in the form of atlantoaxial subluxation is present in 19% to 70% of cases. Approximately 20% of patients with atlantoaxial subluxation have some degree of basilar invagination. Basilar invagination is less common than atlantoaxial subluxation but is more frequently associated with neurological

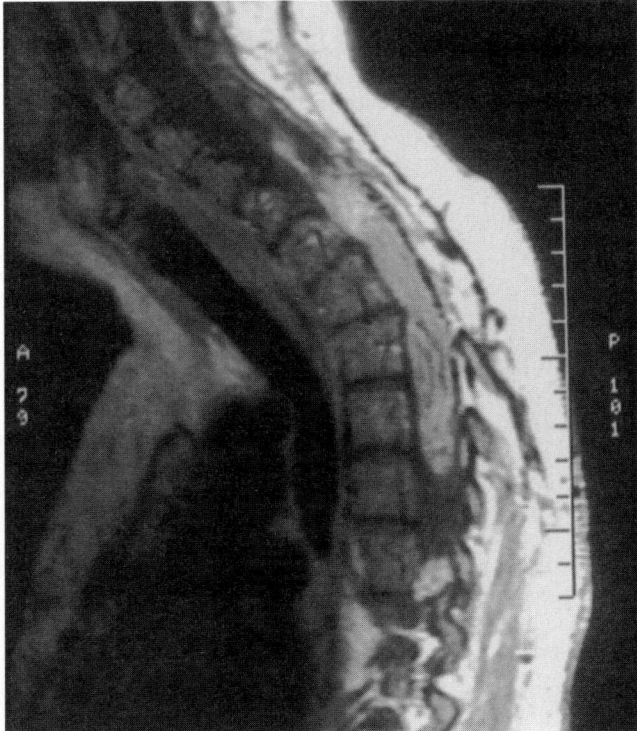

FIGURE 282–8. Spinal cord fibrillary astrocytoma in a 30-year-old woman who had previously undergone three resections and radiation therapy and presented with a history of progressive quadriparesis. Sagittal T1-weighted contrast-enhanced image of the cervicothoracic spine shows an enhancing intramedullary spinal cord tumor and associated syrinx. The patient underwent shunting of the progressively enlarging syrinx.

T A B L E 2 8 2 – 3 ■ **Clinical Summary of Axial Skeletal Inflammatory Disorders**

DISORDER	INCIDENCE	CHARACTERISTICS	LOCATION
Rheumatoid arthritis	Prevalence 1% by age 65	Elderly cervical spine, females > males Atlantoaxial subluxation Basilar invagination Subaxial subluxation	Cervical spine most common
Ankylosing spondylitis	2% incidence	Onset from puberty to 45 yr; males > females Spinal ankylosis Spinal deformity Pathologic fracture	Sacroiliac joints Lumbar spine most common

Other
  Psoriatic arthritis
  Reiter's syndrome
  Behçet's disease
  Whipple's disease
  Enteropathic arthritis
  Gout
  Pseudogout			

deficits. Subaxial subluxation most often occurs at C2-3 and C3-4, producing a "staircase" appearance on cervical radiographs.[113, 115, 116]

The peak onset of RA is in the fourth and fifth decades of life, and the disease has a female predominance. Diagnosis of RA is based on history, distribution of joint involvement, and positive rheumatoid factor. Neck pain warrants a thorough radiographic evaluation, including flexion-extension cervical spine radiographs and MRI scans to evaluate for neural compression. Radiographic sequelae include soft tissue swelling, narrowing of joint spaces, and ultimately bone erosion with deformity and instability. Surgical intervention with decompression or instrumentation with fusion, or both, is warranted for myelopathy, progressive subluxation, and severe pain.[117–120]

ANKYLOSING SPONDYLITIS

Ankylosing spondylitis is the most prevalent of the seronegative spondyloarthropathies, with an incidence of up to 2% in the white population (Fig. 282–9). The prototypical lesion is enthesopathic, affecting insertion sites of tendons and ligaments to bone, with inflammation, bony erosion, and ankylosis. The axial skeleton is affected most commonly, with a milder degree of peripheral involvement. Vertebral body osteoporosis, ankylosis of the apophyseal joints, intervertebral disk calcification, and ligamentous ossification are the characteristic pathologic changes. The pathogenesis is unclear, but there is a strong immunologic association with HLA-B27 positivity. The disease progresses in an ascending fashion from caudal to rostral, producing the characteristic "bamboo spine" and severe kyphotic deformity.[121–125]

Age at onset ranges from puberty to 45 years. Unlike RA, ankylosing spondylitis has a male predominance. The disease begins with insidious lower back pain in 80% to 90% of patients and peripheral joint pain in the hip or shoulder in 20% to 40% of patients. Sacroiliitis is usually one of the earliest manifestations of the disease. Clinical diagnosis is based on age younger than 45 years and a history of insidious onset of back pain with persistence for more than 3 months, morning stiffness, improvement with exercise, and limitation of chest expansion. HLA-B27 positivity is suggestive but not conclusive evidence of the disease. Radiographic studies reveal sacroiliitis followed by spinal ankylosis. It takes 3 to 7 years for the radiographic evidence of bilateral symmetrical sacroiliitis to become evident; therefore, back pain, morning stiffness, and loss of axial mobility are important symptoms and signs. Spinal ankylosis and associated kyphosis, fractures, stenosis, and rotary instability are the results of this chronic spondylitis. Prognosis and success of treatment relate directly to the time of diagnosis, initiation of physical therapy, and possibly phenotypic expression. Treatment options for severe kyphotic deformities include cervical or lumbar osteotomies with instrumentation and fusion. The disease course predicts its progression in the first 10 years, with the more aggressive subtypes causing greater deformity.[126–130]

OTHER RHEUMATIC DISORDERS

Other rheumatic disorders of the spine include the remainder of the spondyloarthropathies, such as psoriatic arthritis, Reiter's syndrome, Behçet's disease, Whipple's disease, enteropathic arthritis, gout, and pseudogout. These conditions represent other possible causes of back pain with or without deformity that may require either surgical intervention or, more commonly, conservative therapy for systemic symptoms. The clinical presentation and spinal involvement of the spondyloarthropathies obviously overlap. In general, these syndromes cause either instability or axial deformity.[113, 115, 123]

Mechanical Pain

Pain that is initiated and exacerbated by activity but without constitutional signs and symptoms is a large category that includes musculoligamentous strain, disk herniation, spinal stenosis, spondylolisthesis, spondy-

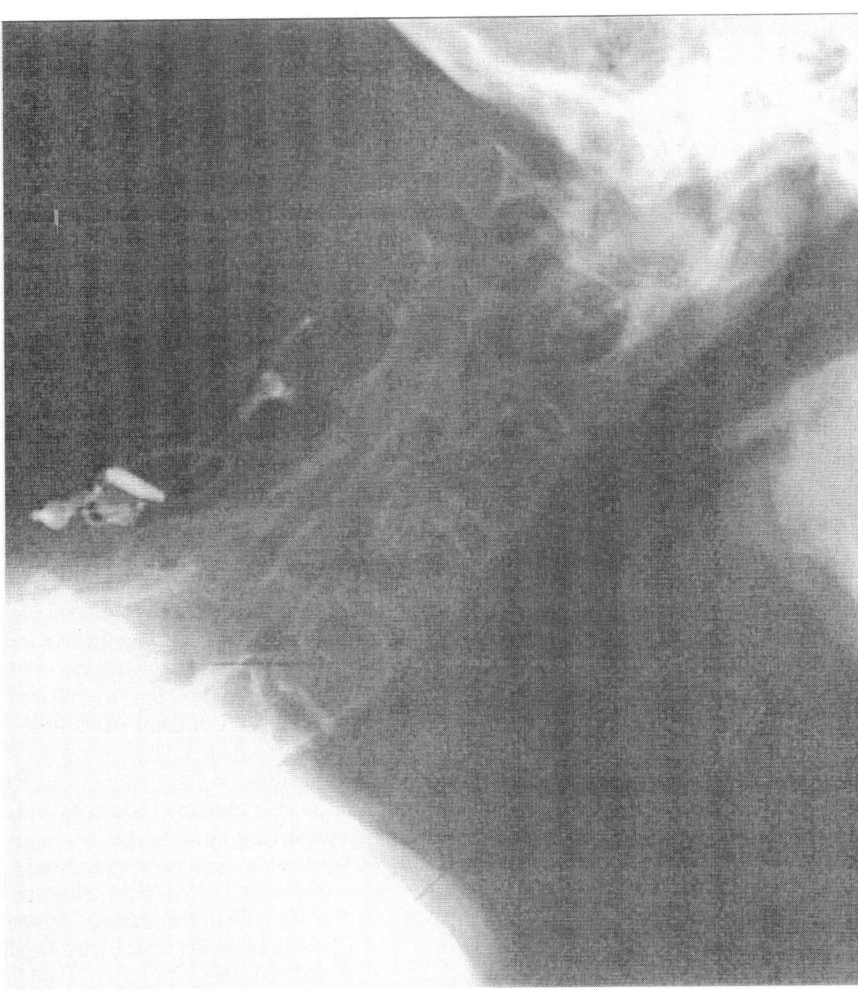

FIGURE 282–9. Ankylosing spondylitis in a 62-year-old man who presented with 90-degree cervical kyphosis and severe neck pain. A lateral cervical spine radiograph shows correction of the deformity with bony ankylosis after a cervical osteotomy was performed.

lolysis, and degenerative deformity (Table 282–4). Other entities such as sacroiliac joint dysfunction, facet syndrome, coccydynia, perineural cysts, dural ectasia, costovertebral syndromes, internal disk disruption, and soft tissue irritation disorders such as in piriformis syndrome are less well differentiated causes of lower back pain that are usually diagnosed clinically and managed conservatively. The differential diagnoses with respect to axial pain related to movement can be numerous, because most anatomic structures of the spine are reported to be pain generators.

The cause of spinal or radicular pain is mechanical in 90% of patients, and with conservative therapy, most patients improve. Treatment decisions for patients who fail conservative therapy can be difficult. Although the decision for surgical intervention is relatively straightforward in a patient suffering from acute disk herniation with progressive neurological deficit, treatment decisions for other degenerative disease such as spinal stenosis and spondylolisthesis are less clear. Evaluation of degenerative spinal disorders necessitates determining the character of pain and any associated neurological deficit. Age, history of onset, character and duration of symptoms, presence of a congenital disorder, and spinal deformity help differentiate among the more

common degenerative lesions. Plain radiography, MRI, and CT-myelography are most often used to evaluate degenerative spinal disorders.[131–136]

HERNIATED NUCLEUS PULPOSUS

Herniated disks can be classified as diffuse bulges of the annulus fibrosus, focal protrusions of the annulus fibrosus, extrusion of the nucleus pulposus through the annulus fibrosus, and extrusion of the nucleus pulposus with sequestration in the extradural space. Management of the different disk pathologic conditions depends on the characteristics of the pain—spinal or radicular—and associated signs of nerve root irritation. Typically, an acutely herniated nucleus pulposus manifests with the relatively acute onset of sharp radiating pain that follows a dermatomal pattern; occasionally, the pain is associated with significant radicular weakness, myelopathy, or cauda equina syndrome. Self-limited episodes of spinal pain can precede the acute symptoms. This condition is a common cause of cervical and lumbar radicular pain in adults and, less frequently, of thoracic symptoms. Diagnosis includes clinical findings consistent with the affected nerve root in the form of sensory, motor, and reflex deficits. Mechani-

TABLE 282-4 ■ Clinical Summary of Degenerative Spinal Disorders

DISORDER	INCIDENCE	CHARACTERISTICS	LOCATION
Musculoligamentous strain	Common at all ages	Local spinal pain and tenderness	Cervical and lumbar > thoracic
Herniated nucleus pulposus	Common; incidence increases with age	Radiculopathy ± myelopathy or cauda equina syndrome	Cervical and lumbar > thoracic
Spinal stenosis			
Central	Common; incidence increases with age	Cervical: radiculomyelopathy Lumbar: neurogenic claudication	Cervical and lumbar > thoracic
Foraminal	Common; incidence increases with age	Radiculopathy	Cervical and lumbar > thoracic
Spondylolisthesis	Common; incidence increases with age	Classification: Congenital Isthmic Degenerative Traumatic Pathologic	Lumbar most common
Spinal deformity	Common; incidence increases with age	Classification: Scoliosis Kyphosis Lordosis	Cervical, thoracic, and lumbar
Other Internal disk disruption Facet joint syndromes Sacroiliac joint dysfunction Coccydynia Costovertebral syndromes Perineural cysts Dural ectasia			

cal signs are important in the diagnosis of a herniated disk; the single most important mechanical sign is positive nerve root tension sign. MRI is the diagnostic procedure of choice. Most herniated disks respond to conservative therapy. Surgical intervention is reserved for severe pain, progressive neurological involvement, myelopathy, or cauda equina syndrome.[7, 133, 134, 137–147]

SPINAL STENOSIS

Spinal stenosis is a clinical diagnosis confirmed by radiographic imaging. The pathologic stenosis may involve the central spinal canal, the lateral spinal canal extending through the neural foramen, or a combination of the central and lateral canal. The classic presentation for cervical central spinal stenosis involves neck pain or radicular pain, with the subsequent development of progressive radiculopathy and myelopathy. Patients may present with any combination of these symptoms and a relatively indolent course or a more rapidly progressive course. Although rare, cervical spinal stenosis can manifest as a progressive myelopathy without pain.

The symptoms of lumbar central spinal stenosis are quite different, and the classic clinical presentation is the constellation of symptoms referred to as *neurogenic claudication*. Neurogenic claudication, characterized by the initial onset of pain followed by numbness, tingling, and weakness in the lower extremities, is typically induced by standing or walking and relieved by sitting. Obviously, neurogenic claudication must be differentiated from vascular claudication. The clinical picture of vascular claudication is progressive calf pain after ambulation with associated decreased peripheral pulses and chronic tissue changes in the cool, distal extremities.

Lateral spinal canal stenosis or neural foraminal stenosis involving the cervical or lumbar spine most often presents with neck or lower back pain associated with radicular pain and sensory or motor changes in the involved nerve root distribution.

The clinical diagnosis of central or lateral spinal canal stenosis is confirmed with MRI or CT-myelography. For both cervical and lumbar spinal stenosis, surgical intervention encompasses decompression with or without instrumentation and fusion.[3, 4, 147–158]

SPONDYLOLISTHESIS AND SPONDYLOLYSIS

Spondylolisthesis is anterior subluxation of one vertebral body on another (Fig. 282–10). A defect in the pars interarticularis is referred to as spondylolysis.

Spondylolisthesis can be classified according to cause: congenital, isthmic, degenerative, traumatic, or pathologic. Congenital spondylolisthesis is characterized by dysplasia of the facet joints on the upper sacrum, whereas isthmic spondylolisthesis is caused either by a lytic lesion from a stress fracture of the pars interarticularis or by an elongated pars interarticularis related to repeated fracture and healing. Degenerative spondylolisthesis is secondary to long-standing intersegmental instability and rarely progresses beyond 50% anterior vertebral body subluxation. Trauma or surgery is the pathogenesis in traumatic spondylolisthesis. Pathologic spondylolisthesis is the result of generalized bone disease. These conditions are common causes of back pain in both children and adults, and anterior subluxation of L5 on S1 is the most common site of

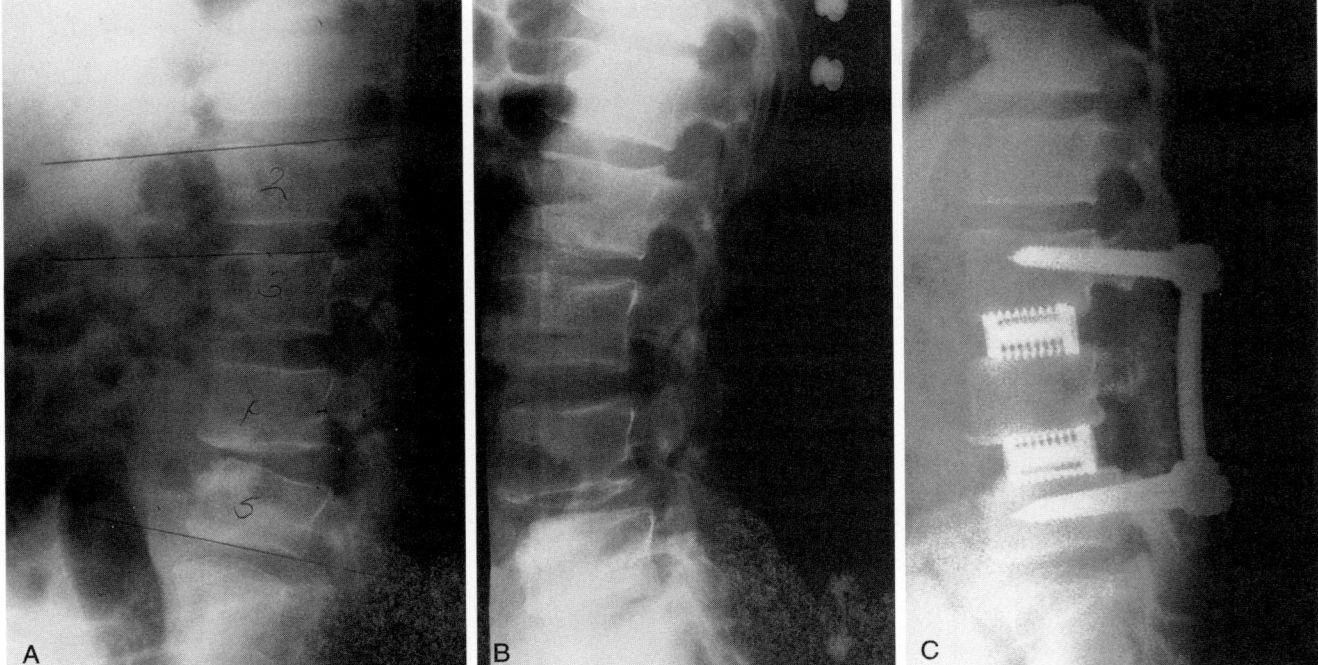

FIGURE 282–10. Spondylolysis in a 38-year-old man who presented with a transient cauda equina syndrome after a fall from a roof. *A,* Lateral flexion radiograph. *B,* Extension lumbar radiograph. *A* and *B* show old L3 and L4 pars interarticularis defects with segmental instability at L3-4 and L4-5. *C,* The patient underwent L3-4 and L4-5 lumbar interbody cage fusions, with an L3-5 posterior segmental instrumentation and fusion.

involvement. Spondylolisthesis is the most common cause of back pain in individuals younger than 30 years. Seitsalo and colleagues found that in the population younger than age 20 with spondylolisthesis, 50% to 86% had lower back pain, 82% had radicular pain, and 74% had both.[159, 160] Pain tended to correlate with the degree of lumbosacral kyphosis and not with the extent of slippage. Adults have a more vague and insidious presentation; back pain is the most common complaint, followed by claudication, radicular symptoms, and hamstring tightness. Treatment varies, depending on the type of pain, degree of slippage, and segmental instability. Surgical decompression with instrumentation and fusion is the mainstay for advanced disease.[150, 153, 161–165]

SCOLIOSIS, KYPHOSIS, AND LORDOSIS

There are three basic types of spinal deformity: scoliosis, kyphosis, and lordosis. Each disorder can occur alone or in combination. Deformities are classified according to cause, location, magnitude, and direction. Degenerative axial skeletal deformities represent another potential cause of spinal and radicular pain in adults. Adult lumbar scoliosis due to either idiopathic or degenerative causes (with a Cobb angle >10 degrees) is present in approximately 8% of adults with back pain. The prevalence of degenerative lumbar scoliosis increases with age. Although the exact cause of the pain is unclear, back pain was present in 86% of adult patients with lumbar scoliosis in one large series.

Most cases of minor (<20-degree Cobb angle) lumbar scoliosis are managed medically. Degenerative deformities in the sagittal plane are common in the elderly population and often remain asymptomatic or are associated with mild axial skeletal pain. Surgical intervention for degenerative scoliosis, kyphosis, and lordosis is reserved for progression of the deformity, severe spinal or radicular pain, segmental instability, and neurological deficits.[166–169]

Acute Localized Pain

The acute onset of localized pain can be related to the following causes (Table 282–5): (1) fractures, ligamentous injuries, or vertebral expansion caused by trauma or an underlying systemic condition or (2) acute hemorrhage involving the spinal column or cord. By far the most common cause of acute spinal or radicular pain is trauma, and the axiom that a patient complaining of spinal or radicular pain after trauma has a fracture or ligamentous injury until proved otherwise is an excellent guideline. Pathologic vertebral fractures can also produce severe localized axial skeletal pain and are often related to infections, tumors, inflammatory disorders, or metabolic diseases. These pathologic conditions can destroy or weaken the vertebral body, ultimately causing a fracture under normal physiologic loads. Infections, tumors, and inflammatory diseases are usually associated with a longer history of painful symptoms, as discussed previously. The most common metabolic diseases resulting in pathologic fractures or

TABLE 282–5 ■ **Clinical Summary of Axial Skeletal Fractures and Dislocations**

CAUSE	INCIDENCE	CHARACTERISTICS	LOCATION
Trauma	Common	Age <30 yr; males > females Penetrating Blunt	Focal

Metabolic disorders
Osteoporosis
	Common; incidence increases with age	Decreased normal-quality bone
		Causes:
		  Primary—idiopathic most common
		  Secondary—hyperthyroidism, hyperparathyroidism, Cushing's disease, steroid exposure, estrogen deficiency, prolonged bed rest
			Diffuse
			Thoracic-lumbar compression fractures most common

Osteomalacia	Uncommon	Inadequate mineralization of bone Cause: vitamin D deficiency most common globally	Diffuse
Paget's disease	Uncommon	? Slow viral infection Brittle bone matrix due to increased resorption and replacement	Focal
Other Ossification of posterior longitudinal ligament Diffuse idiopathic skeletal hyperostosis Calcium pyrophosphate arthropathy Dialysis-associated spondyloarthropathy Fibrous dysplasia Amyloidosis Acromegaly			

vertebral body expansion include osteoporosis (primary and secondary), osteomalacia, and Paget's disease. Acute disk herniation and spinal hemorrhage must also be included in the differential diagnosis of acute localized pain. An acute disk herniation is usually associated with mechanical pain and has already been discussed. The acute hemorrhage of a vertebral body tumor or the sudden rupture of a spinal AVM is a rare cause of acute neck or back pain and is usually associated with apoplectic neurological deficits.[2]

TRAUMA

Traumatic injury to the spinal column or cord may result from penetrating or blunt injury (Fig. 282–11). Penetrating trauma from a knife or gunshot injury seldom causes spinal column instability but may violate the dura and injure the spinal cord. Blunt trauma tends to cause spinal column instability with an intact dura. The mechanisms of blunt trauma—flexion, extension, rotation, compression, and distraction—can cause fracture-dislocations, pure fractures, or pure dislocations. Traumatic fracture-dislocations have the highest incidence of neurological deficits, followed by burst fractures. Traumatic fracture-dislocations of the cervical spine are the most common cause of quadriplegia. Compression fractures and flexion injuries are less likely to produce neurological deficits. Injuries at the level of the cauda equina are less likely to have an associated neurological deficit than are cervical or thoracic injuries.[170, 171]

Traumatic spinal injuries occur primarily in young men; more than half of the victims of spinal cord injury are between 15 and 30 years old. Patients who present with a history of trauma provide an obvious clue to the differential diagnosis of acute spinal or radicular pain. Any patient who presents acutely or subacutely with spinal or radicular pain after trauma should be evaluated rigorously for occult fractures or instability. An adequate history, including mechanism of injury, coupled with a detailed physical examination often pinpoints the site of injury (exquisite tenderness to palpation is common at the level of injury). After trauma, it is imperative to ascertain the absence of injury in the cervical spine. Appropriate methodology is disputed but usually includes a physical examination coupled with anteroposterior, lateral, and odontoid radiographs of the cervical spine. When a single spinal fracture has been identified, the entire spine needs to be radiographed, because 10% to 30% of these patients have concurrent spinal fractures. Most spinal fractures are evident on plain radiographs alone. MRI is the study of choice for suspected traumatic disk, spinal cord, and ligamentous injury; CT is considered superior for anatomic bony detail, especially to differentiate burst from compression fractures. Patients with vertebral fractures are emergently managed with immobilization and realignment of the spinal column. Individuals who sustain spinal cord injuries should receive methylprednisolone. Definitive treatment of spinal injuries may include cervical, thoracic, or lumbosacral orthosis, early or late decompression, and an anterior

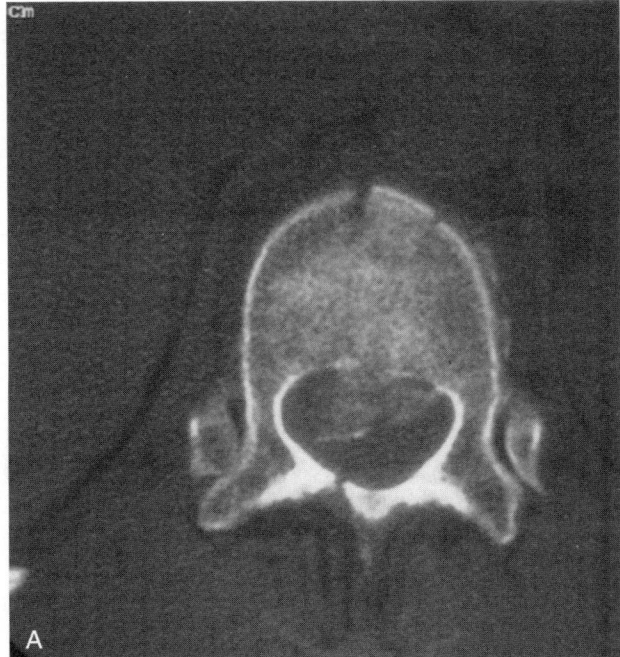
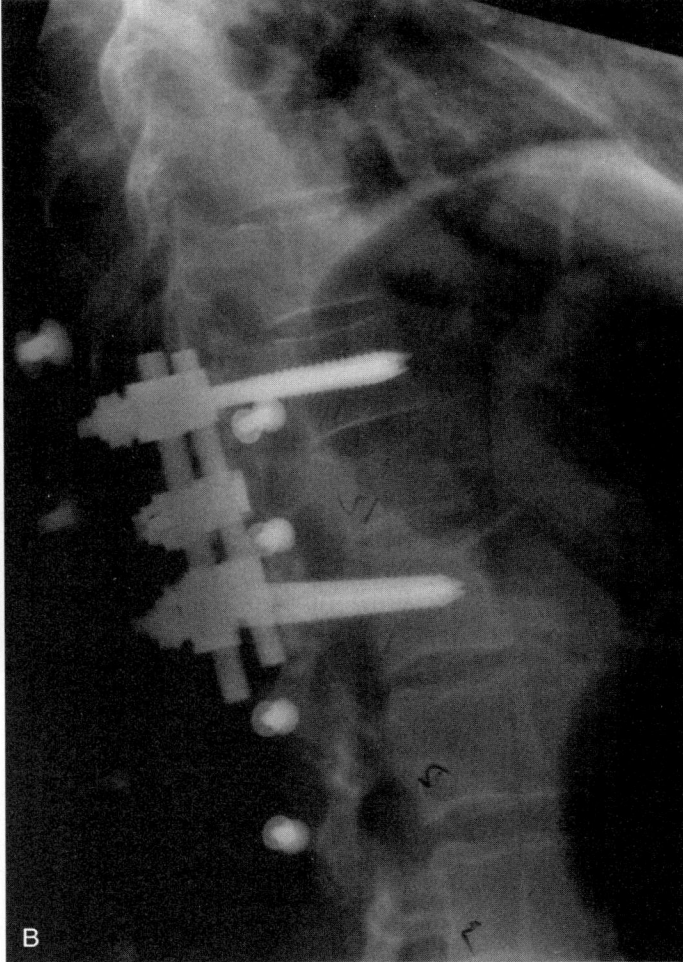

FIGURE 282–11. *A,* T12 burst fracture with an incomplete spinal cord injury in a 32-year-old woman involved in a motor vehicle accident. *B,* The patient underwent emergent posterior segmental instrumentation with correction of kyphosis, restoration of vertebral height, and reduction of fracture fragments through ligamentotaxis. Postoperatively, the patient was maintained in a thoracolumbosacral orthosis.

or posterior surgical approach with instrumentation and fusion.[170–178]

Post-traumatic syringomyelia should be included in the differential diagnosis of any patient who develops ascending deterioration of sensory or motor function after a traumatic spinal cord injury. Approximately 11% of all cases of syringomyelia are reported to be caused by trauma, and 3% of patients with severe cervical trauma with paraplegia or quadriplegia are said to develop post-traumatic syringomyelia. The time course to development ranges from 2 months to 36 years. Clinical presentation involves pain, an ascending sensory level, motor deficits, and loss of reflexes above the previous lesion. MRI is the radiologic procedure of choice to evaluate for post-traumatic syringomyelia. Surgical intervention may be required for pain, ascending deficits, or progressive spasticity.[179, 180]

METABOLIC DISORDERS

Most metabolic disorders that affect either bone mineralization or density are chronic processes. Although many of these disorders predispose patients to benign pathologic fractures, others, such as Paget's disease, can have malignant potential. Individuals with metabolic disorders first present with systemic symptoms and signs before reporting axial skeletal pain. The most common metabolic bone diseases are osteoporosis, osteomalacia, and Paget's disease. When these diseases involve the spine, the clinical presentation may include localized spinal pain secondary to the pathologic process, pathologic vertebral column fractures, or symptoms from bony entrapment of neural tissue (rarely). Most pathologic vertebral column fractures related to metabolic bone diseases cause acute localized spinal pain without neurological deficits. The formidable list of metabolic bone diseases is covered in other chapters. As a general rule, however, the metabolic bone diseases are managed medically. External support with an orthosis may help relieve pain in the acute phase of a vertebral fracture but should be discontinued when the symptoms resolve. Spinal surgery is reserved for fractures causing gross deformity, instability, or neurological impairment.[181]

Osteoporosis is characterized by decreased amounts of normal-quality bone, increasing the patient's susceptibility to fractures. Approximately 15 to 20 million individuals in the United States are afflicted, with a resultant 1 to 2 million pathologic skeletal fractures each year. Osteoporosis can be primary or secondary.

Primary osteoporosis is idiopathic, unrelated to any endocrinopathy or other disease state. Secondary osteoporosis can be the result of endocrinopathies, neoplastic diseases, hematologic disorders, mechanical disorders, biochemical collagen disturbances, or nutritional aberrations. Common causes of secondary osteoporosis include hyperthyroidism, hyperparathyroidism, Cushing's disease, hypothalamic hypogonadism, estrogen deficiency, diabetes mellitus, steroid exposure, multiple myeloma, leukemia, and prolonged bed rest.[181–185]

Osteomalacia and Paget's disease occur much less frequently than does osteoporosis, although Paget's disease is the second most common metabolic bone disturbance in the United States after osteoporosis. Osteomalacia is a metabolic bone disease characterized by inadequate mineralization of newly formed osteoid. It usually results from a deficiency of or resistance to vitamin D, intestinal malabsorption, acquired or hereditary renal disorders, intoxication with heavy metals (aluminum and iron), and other assorted causes. Paget's disease is characterized by an excess of hyperactive osteoclasts and osteoblasts, which increases bone resorption and marrow replacement by hypervascular fibrous tissue. The result is a brittle bone matrix that is susceptible to fracture. The annual occurrence rate of Paget's disease is 1 per 1000 persons. The vertebrae, pelvis, and femora are the most common bones involved with this disease. Malignant degeneration occurs in 1% to 10% of patients; the most frequently occurring malignant tumor in pagetic bone is osteogenic sarcoma. The clinical presentation of Paget's disease involving the spine can include local pain, vertebral fractures, or entrapment of nerve roots (radiculopathy or neurogenic claudication). Treatment is multidisciplinary, with surgery reserved for instability or progressive neurological deficits.[181, 186]

Other poorly understood metabolic diseases affecting the spine include ossification of the posterior longitudinal ligament, diffuse idiopathic skeletal hyperostosis, calcium pyrophosphate arthropathy, amyloidosis, acromegaly, fibrous dysplasia, and dialysis-associated spondyloarthropathy. The clinical presentation and treatment of these diseases are variable and are discussed in other chapters.[181, 187–189]

NEUROLOGICAL DEFICIT

Spinal cord and nerve root dysfunction can be manifested by a variety of pain, motor, sensory, bladder, and bowel disturbances. The time course of a neurological deficit, in conjunction with the pattern of pain and the presence of motor and sensory deficits, helps formulate the differential diagnosis. Obtaining a comprehensive history of symptom onset, characteristics, location, aggravating and alleviating conditions, and similar related episodes is the first step in evaluating a patient with neurological deficits. Antecedent infections and symptoms of systemic disease must be sought. Medical history, family history, and social history elucidate conditions associated with neuronal diseases. The physical examination should include a complete analysis of all systems. Occasionally, brain, brainstem, peripheral nerve, or muscular pathologic conditions masquerade as spinal cord disease. The skin should be inspected for cutaneous lesions overlying the spine, dermatomal rash, and evidence of phakomatosis. The spine should be evaluated during range-of-motion testing and palpation for step-off, focal tenderness, and subcutaneous mass lesions. Signs of nerve root tension should be elicited. A detailed neurological examination should be performed looking for brain, brainstem, spinal cord, peripheral nerve, and muscle involvement.

The anatomic location and distribution of a neurological deficit are extremely important and help determine the differential diagnosis and localization of the pathologic lesion. The single most important finding indicative of focal spinal cord pathology is a segmental spinal level below which the neurological deficit is present. This finding indicates a localized pathologic process affecting the ascending or descending spinal cord tracts. Focal neurological deficits in the anatomic distribution of a nerve root are also extremely accurate for localizing pathology to the spinal cord or segmental nerve roots. Based on the anatomic distribution of the sensory and motor deficits, the physical examination differentiates nerve root from central and peripheral neural disease, as well as from pure muscle pathology. In the absence of anatomic localization of a neurological deficit (diffuse disease), the pattern of sensory and motor involvement helps make the differential diagnosis but is less reliable for differentiating spinal cord pathology from central and peripheral neurological disease or from primary muscular pathology. Upper motor neuron pathology may be the result of spinal, brainstem, or brain pathologic processes. Diffuse muscular weakness and atrophy may be the result of spinal and peripheral nerve diseases or neuromuscular junction and muscular illnesses. Ataxia may be the result of cerebellar, brainstem, or spinal cord diseases. Sensory deficits may be the result of lesions anywhere along the neural axis. Localizing more diffuse neurological deficits to the spinal cord requires knowledge of the presentation of specific spinal diseases, combined with laboratory investigations, electrophysiologic studies, and radiographic imaging.[190]

Based on the patient's clinical history and neurological deficits, appropriate diagnostic investigation may begin. Standard laboratory studies include a complete blood count; electrolyte, blood urea nitrogen, creatinine, and glucose determinations; and a coagulation panel. Directed laboratory studies may include CSF analysis and culture, combined with immunologic studies for the investigation of myelitis, the level of serum cobalamin to diagnose subacute combined degeneration, and biochemical or genetic analysis to exclude hereditary spinal cord diseases. When the physical examination cannot localize a disease process precisely, electrophysiologic studies are the mainstay for identifying and characterizing the pathologic process. Electromyography, nerve conduction studies, and somatosensory evoked potentials are capable of differentiating among primary muscular, peripheral nerve, spinal, and brainstem pathology. Imaging of the spine should begin with plain radiography, followed by MRI. MRI is the study of choice because of its ability to detect subtle soft tissue changes indicative of a primary spinal cord pathologic condition. CT remains the superior imaging study to demonstrate acute hemorrhage and bony detail. Laboratory investigations, electrophysiologic evaluation, and radiologic imaging may be diagnostic, or the diagnosis may require biopsy of the pathologic lesion. Once a definitive diagnosis is made, medical or surgical treatment can begin.[191, 192]

Acute Paresis or Paralysis

The acute (minutes to hours) onset of paraparesis, quadriparesis, paraplegia, or quadriplegia is usually secondary to trauma or a vascular event involving the spinal cord (Table 282–6). Trauma is usually accompanied by severe spinal pain at the level of injury and was discussed in the setting of acute localized spinal pain. However, it is worth stressing that patients with a history of trauma and new-onset neurological deficits need to be evaluated rigorously for a spinal column or neural axis injury. When there is no history of trauma, the acute onset of paresis or paralysis involving the extremities is most likely related to either spinal cord infarction or spinal hemorrhage. A detailed neurological evaluation usually reveals motor and sensory deficits below the level of the vascular cord injury, thus allowing the clinician to localize the segmental level of the lesion rostrally to caudally. The pattern of the motor and sensory deficits localizes the lesion within the axial plane of the spinal cord. With the clinical history and the pattern of neurological deficit, a logical differential diagnosis can be deduced.

SPINAL CORD INFARCTION

Spinal cord infarction is rare. When there is an ischemic insult to the spinal cord, the vascular territory of the anterior spinal artery is typically involved. Spinal cord ischemia usually results from involvement of the segmental vessels rather than from direct involvement of the anterior spinal artery. Thromboembolic occlusion of spinal segmental arteries or dissection, clamping, or severe atheroma of the aorta is a common cause of spinal cord infarction. Anterior cord syndrome is the typical clinical presentation. The midthoracic level is the most common site of ischemia, as it lies in a vascular watershed zone. Less commonly, in cases of spinal cord infarction caused by systemic hypotension, the central gray matter of the lower thoracic and lumbosacral spinal cord may be involved. Occasionally, polyarteritis nodosa, syphilitic meningomyelitis, or emboli arising from a severely atherosclerotic aorta occlude a spinal medullary artery. Foix-Alajouanine disease produces a necrotizing myelopathy related to acute thrombosis of a spinal cord AVM. Occasionally, caisson disease and fibrocartilaginous embolism cause spinal cord infarction as a result of nitrogen bubbles after diving or fibrocartilage embolism after trauma, respectively.[192–198]

The most important vascular input to the cervical spinal cord comes from the vertebral arteries. The vertebral arteries provide the cephalic origin of the anterior median and the two posterior spinal arteries. Cervical radicular arteries may also provide segmental cervical arterial supply to the spinal cord. The thoracic and lumbar spinal cord is supplied by segmental branches of the aorta and branches of the internal iliac arteries. The most important segmental vessel is the artery of Adamkiewicz, which usually approaches the spinal cord on the left side between the T10 and L3 spinal segments. The border zone between these main

TABLE 282–6 ■ **Clinical Summary of Acute Vascular Events**

ACUTE VASCULAR EVENT	INCIDENCE	CAUSE	LOCATION
Spinal cord infarction*	Rare	Aortic dissection, clamping, or severe atheroma Hypotension Vasculitis Caisson disease Fibrocartilage embolism AVM thrombosis acutely	Thoracic > cervical
Spontaneous spinal hemorrhage Epidural-subdural	Rare	Apoplectic neurologic deficit Epidural venous plexus Bleeding diathesis Anticoagulation therapy Vascular malformation Neoplasm	Epidural > subdural > Subarachnoid > intramedullary
Subarachnoid-intramedullary		AVM Cavernous malformation Aneurysm Bleeding diathesis Anticoagulation therapy Neoplasm Syringomyelia	

*Anterior spinal cord syndrome most common.
AVM, arteriovenous malformation.

vascular systems is relatively vulnerable to ischemia, particularly in the midthoracic (T4-6) region of the spinal cord.[192]

Anterior spinal artery syndrome, also known as anterior cord syndrome, consists of motor paralysis, dissociated sensory loss, and paralysis of sphincteric function. It results from an infarction in the vascular territory of the anterior spinal artery, which supplies the anterior two thirds of the spinal cord. The posterior columns are usually spared, aiding in the diagnosis. Symptoms may develop instantaneously or over several hours. The prognosis for a functional recovery is poor.[192]

SPONTANEOUS SPINAL HEMORRHAGE

Spontaneous spinal hemorrhages are rare but may be epidural, subdural, subarachnoid, or intramedullary. Most are apoplectic, with rapidly developing neurological deficits. The most common causes of spontaneous epidural or subdural hematoma include bleeding diathesis, anticoagulant therapy, and vertebral body tumor; many cases are idiopathic. Spontaneous spinal epidural hematomas occur much more frequently than subdural hematomas, and their pathogenesis is thought to involve the epidural venous plexus. Spontaneous subarachnoid or intramedullary spinal hemorrhages are often the result of AVM, cavernous malformation, neoplasm, bleeding diathesis, anticoagulation therapy, and syringomyelia. The most common cause of spontaneous spinal subarachnoid hemorrhage is intradural type II spinal AVM. Spontaneous intramedullary spinal hemorrhage from any cause is exceedingly rare. MRI and CT are the diagnostic procedures of choice for spontaneous spinal hemorrhages. Treatment involves correction of an underlying hematologic disorder or coagulopathy and surgical evacuation of a compressive hematoma. Postoperative MRI, CT-myelography, and angiography help delineate the cause of the hemorrhage.[199–210]

Although the most common cause of spinal subarachnoid hemorrhage is intradural spinal AVM, most vascular malformations involving the spine become symptomatic with chronic, progressive neurological deterioration. The only spinal vascular malformations that tend to manifest as spinal hemorrhage are the rare type II (glomus) spinal AVMs. Spinal vascular malformations are discussed further in the context of chronic progressive neurological disorders.[199–210]

Subacute, Progressive Neurological Deficit

The clinical onset of a subacute (days to weeks), progressive neurological deficit indicates either an inflammatory disease involving the spinal cord or a more rapidly compressive spinal cord lesion (Table 282–7). The more rapidly compressive spinal cord lesions, vertebral infections, tumors, and large herniated disks are usually associated with a history of painful symptoms, as reviewed earlier. The myelitic disorders usually manifest with subacute progressive neurological deficits without a significant long-standing history of pain.

Myelitis is often, but not universally, associated with systemic symptoms and signs of infection. The absence of an infection or infectious prodrome does not preclude the diagnosis of myelitis.

The myelitic disorders include a relatively nonhomogeneous group of spinal cord inflammatory diseases. Myelitis may be related to viral, bacterial, fungal, and parasitic diseases and to noninfectious inflammatory lesions. The clinical spectrum of disease presentation can vary from days to weeks; rarely, the neurological symptoms evolve over hours or months. Clinical presentation may include the subacute onset of spinal pain at the level of the inflammatory damage. A detailed neurological evaluation reveals motor or sensory deficits, or both, at or below the level of the lesion. The pattern and progression of the motor and sensory deficits provide evidence about the possible cause of the inflammatory process. The inflammatory diseases of the spinal cord can be broadly classified by cause: (1) myelitis due to viruses; (2) myelitis due to bacterial, fungal, and parasitic diseases of the meninges and spinal cord; and (3) myelitis of the noninfectious inflammatory type. The diagnosis of myelitis is based on the patient's clinical history; physical examination; laboratory investigations, including CSF analysis; and MRI scans of the spinal cord to rule out a compressive spinal cord lesion.[192]

VIRAL MYELITIS

Viral myelitis can be caused by enteroviruses (poliovirus, coxsackievirus groups A and B, and echoviruses), herpesviruses (varicella-zoster virus, herpes simplex virus types 1 and 2, cytomegalovirus, and Epstein-Barr virus), rabies virus, herpesvirus B, human T-cell lymphotrophic virus type I (HTLV-I), and HIV. The enteroviruses, varicella-zoster virus, HIV, and HTLV-I are the important viral entities in this category. The enteroviruses have an affinity for neurons of the anterior horn of the spinal cord and the motor nuclei of the brainstem, whereas varicella-zoster virus has an affinity for the dorsal root ganglion. The pathologic characteristic of HIV myelitis is vacuolated spinal cord white matter, which is most severe in thoracic segments. As a general rule, viral infections of the spinal cord produce distinct clinical syndromes secondary to the affinity of the individual viruses for different neuronal cell populations. Viral infections of the spinal cord (with the exception of HTLV-I) usually do not produce transverse myelitis involving the entire cross-sectional area of the spinal cord with combined motor and sensory deficits. The cause of myelitis with significant sensory and motor deficits is seldom viral.[192, 211]

Poliovirus infections are rare in countries with successful vaccination programs. In the United States, there are approximately 15 cases of paralytic poliomyelitis each year. In countries with successful vaccination programs, other enteroviruses are now the most common causes of anterior poliomyelitis syndrome. The illnesses caused by these viruses are usually benign, and the paralysis is rarely significant. The pathogenesis of paralytic poliomyelitis is secondary to the destruc-

TABLE 282–7 ■ Clinical Summary of Myelitis

TYPE	INCIDENCE	CHARACTERISTICS	LOCATION
Viral			

Enteroviruses
  Poliovirus
  Coxsackievirus
	Rare	Motor paresis or paralysis secondary to virus affinity for motor neurons	Cervical and thoracic

Herpes zoster	Uncommon	Radicular pain or eruption secondary to virus affinity for sensory ganglia	Lower thoracic most common
HTLV-I	Rare	Tropical spastic paraparesis	Thoracic most common
HIV	Uncommon	White matter vacuolar myelopathy	Thoracic most common

Other
  Epstein-Barr virus
  Cytomegalovirus
  Herpes simplex viruses
  Rabies virus
  Herpesvirus B			

Bacterial, Fungal, and Parasitic			
Spinal epidural abscess	Uncommon but clinically important	Transverse spinal cord lesion—variable involvement	Thoracic > lumbar > cervical posterior > anterior
Neurosyphilis	Rare	Degeneration of posterior columns with lightning pains, ataxia, and urinary incontinence	Cervical and thoracic
Schistosomiasis	Rare	Conus medullaris syndrome	Conus most common

Other
  Spinal cord abscess
  Mycoplasma pneumoniae
  Lyme disease
  Tuberculosis
  Cysticercosis
  Sarcoid			

Noninfectious Inflammatory			
Postinfectious, postvaccinal Postinflammatory Multiple sclerosis Vasculitic disorders Paraneoplastic Encephalomyelitis	Rare	Transverse spinal cord lesion—variable involvement; severe forms cause necrosis over extended spinal segments	Thoracic > cervical

HIV, human immunodeficiency virus; HTLV-I, human T-cell lymphotropic virus type I.

tion of neurons in the anterior and intermediate horns of the gray matter of the spinal cord. The main reservoir for poliovirus is the human intestinal tract, and the main route of infection is fecal-oral. The distribution of spinal paralysis is variable. Most poliovirus infections are inapparent or are associated with only mild systemic symptoms. The remainder of poliovirus infections may be nonparalytic, preparalytic, or paralytic. The systemic symptoms of clinically apparent poliovirus infection include listlessness, headache, fever, stiffness, aching muscles, sore throat, anorexia, nausea, and vomiting. The manifestations of nervous system involvement include irritability, restlessness, and emotional lability, which are often followed by paralysis. Muscle weakness may develop rapidly over 48 hours or over a week or longer. Typically, the weakness does not progress after the patient's temperature has been normal for 48 hours. Patients may complain of paresthesias in the affected limbs, but objective sensory loss is rare. Urine may be retained acutely, but the problem seldom persists. Treatment of an acute poliovirus infection is supportive. Most patients with paralytic poliomyelitis improve over 3 to 4 months after the infection, but the mortality rate associated with acute infection is 5% to 10%.[211–214]

Herpes zoster represents reactivation of a varicella-zoster viral infection. After an infection with chickenpox, the virus becomes latent in neurons of the sensory ganglia. Herpes zoster is a common viral infection of the CNS, and its incidence increases with age. There are approximately 3 to 5 cases per 1000 persons each year. The pathologic changes include an acute inflammatory reaction involving isolated spinal or cranial sensory ganglia, the posterior gray matter of the spinal cord, and the adjacent leptomeninges. Clinically, herpes zoster is characterized by radicular pain, a vesicular cutaneous eruption and, less often, segmental motor or sensory loss. Almost any dermatome may be involved, but the thoracic dermatomes, particularly T5-10, are most often affected. Treatment includes acyclovir, which shortens the duration of acute pain and speeds healing but does not affect the incidence of postherpetic neuralgia. The prognosis in uncomplicated cases is excellent.[211, 215]

HIV and HTLV-I both may produce subacute to chronic myelitis. HIV infection of the spinal cord produces a white matter vacuolar myelopathy, most severely affecting the thoracic spinal cord segments. Clinical presentation is leg or leg and arm weakness developing over weeks. The clinical syndrome is often complicated by the other CNS disorders associated with HIV infection (patients with AIDS are prone to develop infectious encephalitis and cytomegalovirus radiculomyelopathy). Tropical spastic paraparesis is a chronic infective inflammatory disease of the spinal cord caused by the retrovirus HTLV-I. Its clinical presentation is a slowly progressive paraparesis with increased tendon reflexes and Babinski's sign. Disorder of sphincter control is usually an early sign, and sensory function in the lower extremities is variably affected. The cerebrum, brainstem, and upper extremities are usually spared. There are anecdotal reports of improvement after the intravenous administration of gamma globulin.[211, 216–220]

BACTERIAL, FUNGAL, AND PARASITIC MYELITIS

Included in this category of diseases is myelitis due to *Mycoplasma pneumoniae* and *Borrelia burgdorferi,* as well as pyogenic myelitis, tuberculous myelitis, and syphilitic myelitis. Both the spinal cord and meninges may be affected, or the spinal cord lesion may predominate. Analysis of the CSF often holds the clue to the causative mechanism. MRI and CT-myelography show the extent of spinal column and spinal cord involvement.[192]

Spinal epidural abscess is the most important clinical entity in this group of diseases. As discussed, almost any infection of the axial skeleton can produce an infection in the epidural space. Initially, symptoms are spinal pain and fever, followed by radicular symptoms. Pyogenic infections often have a more rapidly progressive clinical course. If the infection is allowed to progress untreated, patients develop paraplegia or quadriplegia. Granulomatous infections of the epidural space or meninges may become symptomatic with a more indolent clinical course, associated with a more subacute progressive neurological deficit. Rarely, the spinal subdural space may be infected. The clinical symptoms and signs are almost indistinguishable from those of an epidural infection. For further details, see the previous discussion of spinal epidural abscess.[9–12, 25]

Syphilis is caused by the spirochete *Treponema pallidum.* All forms of neurosyphilis begin as meningitis, and active meningeal inflammation invariably accompanies all forms of neurosyphilis. Neurosyphilis may affect the spinal cord and most commonly causes tabetic neurosyphilis (tabes dorsalis); however, it may also produce syphilitic meningomyelitis or spinal meningovascular syphilis. Tabetic neurosyphilis usually develops 15 to 20 years after the onset of the infection. The pathogenesis involves degeneration of the posterior columns of the spinal cord and the dorsal nerve roots. Other systemic signs of infection are usually present by the onset of tabes dorsalis and include papillary abnormalities in more than 90% of patients. The major symptoms of tabes dorsalis are lightning pains, ataxia, and urinary incontinence. The chief signs are absent lower extremity tendon reflexes, impaired vibratory and position sense in the feet and legs, and Romberg's sign. Muscular power is fully retained, and the ataxia is related to the sensory deficit. Approximately 1% to 10% of patients with tabes develop deafferented Charcot's joints, most commonly affecting the hips, knees, ankles and, occasionally, lumbar spine. In syphilitic meningomyelitis, there is a subpial loss of myelinated fibers and gliosis as a result of chronic fibrosing meningitis; gumma of the meninges or spinal cord is rare. Spinal meningovascular syphilis occasionally assumes the form of an anterior spinal artery syndrome. Diagnosis is confirmed with a positive CSF Venereal Disease Research Laboratories (VDRL) slide test. Treatment involves the administration of intravenous penicillin G, which improves or arrests the neurological disease process in most patients.[221, 222]

Rarely, a systemic infection with *M. pneumoniae* or *B. burgdorferi* (Lyme disease) may produce myelitis. The associated systemic symptoms and signs usually lead the clinician to the correct diagnosis. Other possible causes of inflammatory lesions of the spinal cord include tuberculous meningitis with spinal tuberculoma, schistosomiasis, spinal cord abscess, and sarcoid. Schistosomiasis is an important disease in developing countries. CNS involvement occurs in 3% of cases; spinal cord disease often involves the conus medullaris as an intramedullary or meningeal granuloma.[223–228]

NONINFECTIOUS INFLAMMATORY MYELITIS

Noninfectious inflammatory myelitis takes the form of a leukomyelitis with either demyelination or necrosis of the tracts of the spinal cord. Critical to the pathogenesis of this group of diseases is a disordered immune response rather than the direct effect of an infectious agent. Causes include postinfectious and postvaccinal myelitis, acute and chronic relapsing multiple sclerosis (MS), subacute necrotizing myelitis, myelopathy with lupus or other forms of angiitis, and paraneoplastic myelitis.[192, 229–231]

Postinfectious and postvaccinal myelitides are characterized by (1) a temporal relationship to a viral infection or vaccination, (2) the development of neurological signs and symptoms over several days, and (3) a monophasic temporal course (no recurrence). The usual clinical presentation involves progressive numbness and weakness of the feet and legs (less often, the hands and arms) over the course of a few days, with variable involvement of the sensory and motor spinal cord tracts. Headache or stiff neck may or may not be present. Differentiating the disease from Guillain-Barré syndrome involves the demonstration of a sensory level and upper motor neuron dysfunction. Sphincteric dysfunction and spinal pain are common during the evolution of the disease. The neurological dysfunction outweighs any painful symptoms. More often, there is incomplete spinal cord involvement that affects one side more than the other. T2-weighted MRI scans often show a signal abnormality in the spinal cord and slight gadolinium enhancement over two or three segments; the spinal cord may be swollen focally. Treatment is supportive. Although corticosteroids are often administered, there is no evidence that they alter the course of the disease. Prognosis is often better than the initial symptoms may suggest.[192, 231–236]

MS demyelinative myelitis shares many of the features of the postinfectious and postvaccinal myelitides. However, the clinical symptoms evolve more slowly over 1 to 3 weeks or longer. There is no antecedent infection or vaccination, and the condition is usually painless (Fig. 282–12). Only 0.6% of MS patients initially present with myelitis. In most cases, symptoms other than impairment of spinal cord function precede the myelopathy. Exercise or increased temperature (Uhthoff phenomenon) may worsen the symptoms and signs of MS. MRI, the modality of choice to confirm the diagnosis of myelitis, is positive in 85% to 95% of clinically defined MS patients. While investigating the possibility of MS plaque in the spinal cord, MRI scans of the brain should be performed to rule out much more common and usually recognizable changes in the brain. The clinical diagnosis is supported by laboratory studies, including CSF examination revealing oligoclonal bands and an immunoglobulin G index greater than 1.7. Evoked potentials detect CNS functional abnormalities that may be undetectable clinically. The multifocal nature of the disease may be supported by the discovery of a subclinical lesion in a site remote from the area of clinical dysfunction. Treatment with corticosteroids may lead to regression of symptoms, but the disease may relapse if the medication is tapered too quickly.[192, 237–241]

Acute necrotizing myelitis may be a variant of MS or other myelitic syndromes. The clinical manifestations of this necrotizing myelopathy that distinguish it from the more common types of myelitis include persistent and profound flaccidity of the legs or arms, areflexia, and atonicity of the bladder. These clinical findings reflect necrosis of the gray and white matter over a considerable vertical extent of the spinal cord. When both the optic nerves and spinal cord are involved, the disease is called *neuromyelitis optica*, or *Devic's disease*. Systemic lupus erythematosus, rare vasculitic disorders, and paraneoplastic myelitis also produce acute or subacute necrotizing myelopathies. Myelitis may also be one manifestation of a more diffuse disseminated encephalomyelitis.[192, 242–246]

Chronic, Progressive Neurological Deficit

The disorders discussed here usually manifest with chronic (weeks to months), progressive neurological deficits and minimal painful or systemic symptoms (Table 282–8). Almost any pathologic process that produces persistent spinal cord ischemia or slowly progressive spinal cord neuronal degeneration and dysfunction can cause a chronic, progressive neurological deficit. Differentiating the different disease entities is possible through a detailed clinical history and neurological evaluation, combined with laboratory investigation, electrophysiologic studies, and radiographic imaging.[2]

Chronic spinal cord ischemia may result from compression, traction (tethering), or blood-flow irregulari-

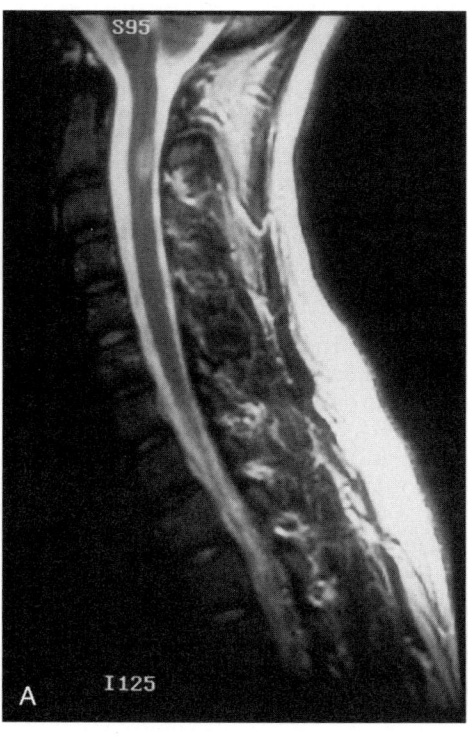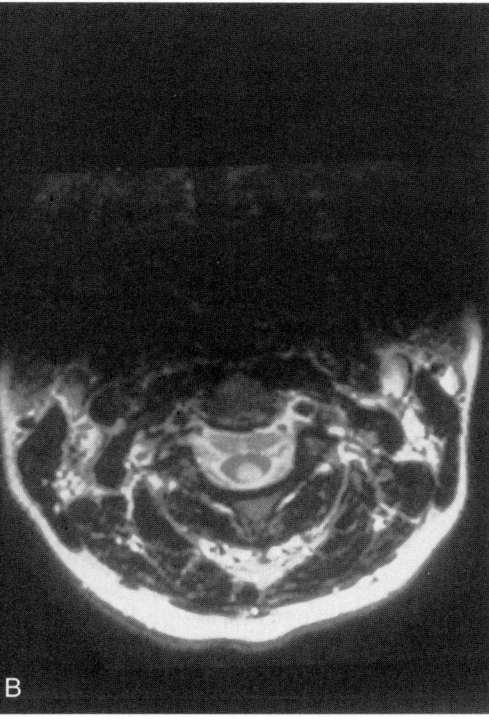

FIGURE 282–12. Multiple sclerosis in a 36-year-old woman who presented with the subacute onset of progressive ataxia with quadriparesis. Sagittal *(A)* and axial *(B)* T2-weighted images of the cervical spine show the classic intrinsic high-intensity signal from the spinal cord associated with lesions in multiple sclerosis. The patient was treated with corticosteroids, and her symptoms regressed.

TABLE 282–8 ■ Clinical Summary of Chronic Ischemia and Neuronal Degeneration

TYPE	CHARACTERISTICS	LOCATION
Congenital Malformations		

Open spinal dysraphism
  Meningocele
  Myelocele
  Myelomeningocele
	Open dysraphic defect at birth with high incidence of neurologic dysfunction	Lumbar > thoracic

Occult spinal dysraphism Incomplete vertebral arch (isolated)	Asymptomatic	L5-S1 most common
Tight filum terminale	Fatty filum, diameter >2 mm	Lumbar most common
Dorsal dermal sinus	Epithelial tract to dura or cord	Lumbar most common
Myelocystocele	Cystic dilatation of distal cord	Lumbar most common

Lipomyeloschisis
    Intradural lipoma
    Lipomyelocele
    Lipomyelomeningocele
	Intradural or extradural lipoma, or both; bony dysraphism; subcutaneous lipoma mass	Lumbar most common

Neoplasm
    Epidermoid
    Dermoid
    Neurenteric cyst and teratoma
	Inclusion tumors and cysts	Cervical, lumbar, and sacral

Split spinal cord malformations
    Diastematomyelia
    Diplomyelia
	Hemicord and duplicate cord malformations	Thoracic and lumbar

Caudal regression syndrome	Abnormal regressive differentiation	Sacral and coccygeal
Spinal Cord Cavitation Hydromyelia Syringomyelia	Central cavitation lined by ependyma or eccentric cavitation without ependyma	Cervical and thoracic
Axial Skeletal Deformities	Defects of segmentation and defects of formation	Thoracic and lumbar
Vascular Malformations		
Type I spinal AVM	Dural arteriovenous fistula; progressive neurological deficit; fourth to seventh decades of life; males > females	Thoracic most common
Type II spinal AVM	Intramedullary; compact nidus; subarachnoid hemorrhage, age <30	Cervical and thoracic
Type III spinal AVM	Intra- and extramedullary over multiple spinal segments; progressive neurologic deficit	Cervical most common
Type IV spinal AVM	Intradural extramedullary arteriovenous fistula; progressive neurologic deficit	
Cavernous Malformations	Fourth to fifth decades of life; females > males; progressive neurological deficit	Cervical and thoracic
Neuronal Degenerative Diseases		
Syndromes of muscular weakness and atrophy without sensory changes Upper motor neuron degeneration		
Primary lateral sclerosis	Fifth to sixth decades of life	Leg > arm
Hereditary spastic paraplegia	Age <35 yr	Leg > arm

Other
      Familial spastic paraplegias plus other neurological abnormalities
      Adrenoleukodystrophy
      Lathyrism
      Radiation myelopathy		

Lower motor neuron degeneration		
Progressive muscular atrophy	Adult onset	Arm > leg
Spinal muscular atrophy	Infancy to adolescence	Arm and leg

Other
      Fazio-Londe syndrome
      Kennedy's disease
      Postpolio syndrome		

Combined upper and lower motor neuron degeneration		
Amyotrophic lateral sclerosis	Age >50 yr	Leg > arm

Table continued on following page

TABLE 282-8 ■ **Clinical Summary of Chronic Ischemia and Neuronal Degeneration** *Continued*

TYPE	CHARACTERISTICS	LOCATION
Neuronal Degenerative Diseases		
Syndromes of progressive spinal ataxia		
Friedreich's ataxia	Age <25	Posterior column—DRG, corticospinal tract, and spinocerebellar degeneration
Non-Friedreich's ataxia	Age <25	Spinocerebellar and corticospinal tract degeneration
Combined System Disorders		
Subacute combined degeneration (SCD)	Vitamin B_{12} deficiency	Posterior and lateral column degeneration
SCD—nonpernicious anemia type	Idiopathic	Posterior and lateral column degeneration

AVM, arteriovenous malformation; DRG, dorsal root ganglion.

ties. Degenerative spondylosis, tumors, and the spondylitic disorders can produce chronic spinal cord compression, whereas the congenital malformations (including vascular malformations) often produce spinal cord tethering and blood flow abnormalities. The chronic spinal cord compressive disorders are usually associated with pain, as reviewed previously; the congenital malformations are seldom associated with painful symptoms, or the pain is minor compared with that of a progressive neurological deficit. When the patient's clinical history and neurological examination fail to differentiate compressive from congenital lesions, MRI, CT, and angiography help establish the diagnosis.

Chronic, progressive spinal cord neuronal degeneration and dysfunction may result from progressive neuronal degeneration, chronic myelitis, or intramedullary spinal cord tumors. Intramedullary tumors usually manifest with an insidious onset of pain, and chronic myelitis is usually associated with systemic symptoms and signs. In constrast, the neuronal degenerative diseases are seldom associated with pain or systemic symptoms and signs. Laboratory investigation, including CSF analysis, and MRI help exclude chronic myelitis and intramedullary tumors when diagnosing a neuronal degenerative disease.

CONGENITAL MALFORMATIONS

In most major developmental disorders of the neural tube, a physical examination at birth reveals a spinal defect with or without an associated neurological dysfunction. Other congenital malformations involving the spine may remain occult until symptoms develop as the spinal column grows.

Spinal dysraphism refers to a set of disorders arising from the incomplete formation of the dorsal midline structures during embryogenesis. The disordered embryogenesis may involve one or more of the embryonic layers, resulting in abnormalities of the skin, vertebral arch, neural tissue, or a combination thereof. Although a heterogeneous group of malformations, spinal dysraphism can be broadly categorized according to whether the malformation is open or is covered by a layer of skin.

Open spinal dysraphism (spina bifida aperta) refers to a defect in the vertebral arches with exposure of the meninges or neural tissue, or both. Before 1980, the incidence of spina bifida aperta with meningocele, myelocele, or myelomeningocele was reported to be 1 to 2 per 1000 live births. In many areas of the world, the incidence is now reported to be declining. More than 85% of meningoceles, myeloceles, and myelomeningoceles are found in the distal thoracic, lumbar, or sacral area. Myelomeningocele is associated almost universally with the Arnold-Chiari II malformation, as well as with syringomyelia, hydrocephalus, diastematomyelia, and cerebral malformations, including lobar agenesis, polymicrogyria, holoprosencephaly, cerebellar dysplasia, heterotopia, and schizencephaly. Neurological deficits associated with myelocele and myelomeningocele are almost universally present at birth as a result of the abnormal formation of the neural structures. Surgical intervention is directed at closing the defect and possibly decompressing the ventricles.[247, 248]

Occult spinal dysraphism refers to dorsal midline malformations covered by skin. The simplest form of occult spinal dysraphism is the absence of the spinous process and variable amounts of the vertebral arch, most often at L5 through S1. Bony dysraphism may be found in 20% to 30% of the general population. The CNS is seldom involved, and patients are usually asymptomatic. However, when a defect in the vertebral arch is associated with overlying cutaneous abnormalities, the incidence of occult intraspinal dysraphic lesions increases. Intraspinal abnormalities include tight filum terminale, dorsal dermal sinus tracts, myelocystoceles, intradural lipomas, lipomyeloceles, lipomyelomeningoceles, neoplasms, split-cord malformations, and caudal regression syndromes. A tight filum terminale is often associated with a low-lying spinal cord, fat in the filum, and a filum diameter greater than 2 mm. The dorsal dermal sinus represents a tract lined by epithelium that extends from the posterior midline surface of the skin to the underlying dura or spinal cord. A myelocystocele is a terminal dilatation of the central spinal canal associated with a meningocele and dorsal bony dysraphism. A simple intradural lipoma represents a collection of intradural fat with minimal vertebral arch malformation; the spinal cord may or may not be tethered. Lipomyelocele and lipomyelomeningocele consist of an intradural or extradural lipoma, dorsal bony dysraphism, spinal cord tethering, and prominent subcutaneous mass. Congenital dermoids and epidermoids may occur independently or in association with a dermal sinus tract and represent incomplete separation of the neural ectoderm from the epithelial ectoderm. Neurenteric cysts most often occur in the anterior cervical region and consist of a cyst of endodermal origin that may or may not have a fistulous tract. Intraspinal teratomas contain elements of all three germ layers. Diastematomyelia and diplomyelia are split spinal cord malformations that refer to the sagittal division of the spinal cord into two hemicords or two duplicated cords, respectively. In diastematomyelia, an associated fibrous or bony spur separates the two hemicords (Fig. 282–13). Caudal regression syndrome has been used to describe abnormal or absent coccygeal, sacral, and lumbar segments secondary to abnormal retrogressive differentiation. When occult spinal dysraphism becomes symptomatic, it is usually related to an intradural lesion with tethering of the spinal cord or, less frequently, with compression of the neural elements from the mass lesion. The neurological deficit usually progresses slowly over months and often coincides with the patient's growth. Symptoms include pain, structural deformities such as scoliosis, and gait or bladder dysfunction. It is important to identify occult intradural lesions early, because significant neurological deficits may not be reversible. Surgical intervention for occult spinal dysraphism is directed at untethering the spinal cord and resecting the mass lesion.[248–253]

Spinal cord cavitation is divided into hydromyelia and syringomyelia. Hydromyelia is a central cavitation of the spinal cord lined by ependyma; syringomyelia refers to an eccentric cavitation of the spinal cord *not* lined by ependyma. Syringomyelia tends to be more focal, but both conditions may involve the entire spinal cord. Hydromyelia has been described as "hydrocephalus of the spinal cord" and is often associated with inadequately treated hydrocephalus. Both conditions are associated with a multitude of primary problems, including Chiari malformation, posterior fossa cyst, platybasia, spinal cord tumor, diastematomyelia, tethered spinal cord, and trauma. The clinical presentation includes bilateral sensory loss, usually of the upper extremities; muscle weakness; spasticity; pain; incontinence; scoliosis; and kyphosis. MRI is the diagnostic procedure of choice to demonstrate the intramedullary fluid cavity and to exclude associated pathology. A posterior fossa decompression or shunting procedure is often required to prevent bulbar symptoms or spasticity or to relieve pain.[248, 253]

Congenital axial skeletal deformities are often secondary to anomalous vertebral development or spinal dysraphism. The two basic types of vertebral skeletal mal-

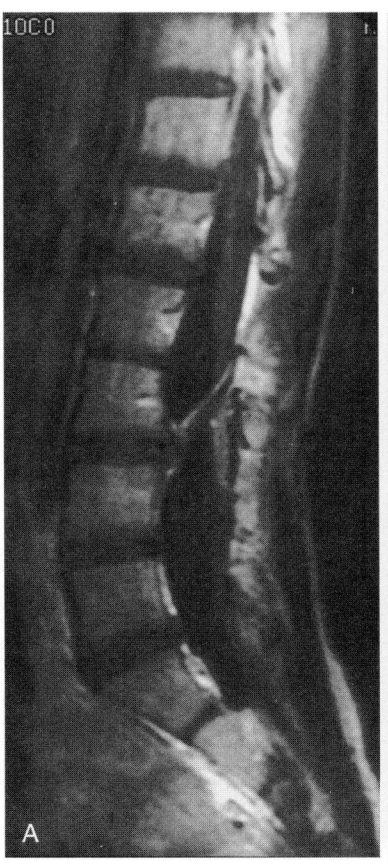
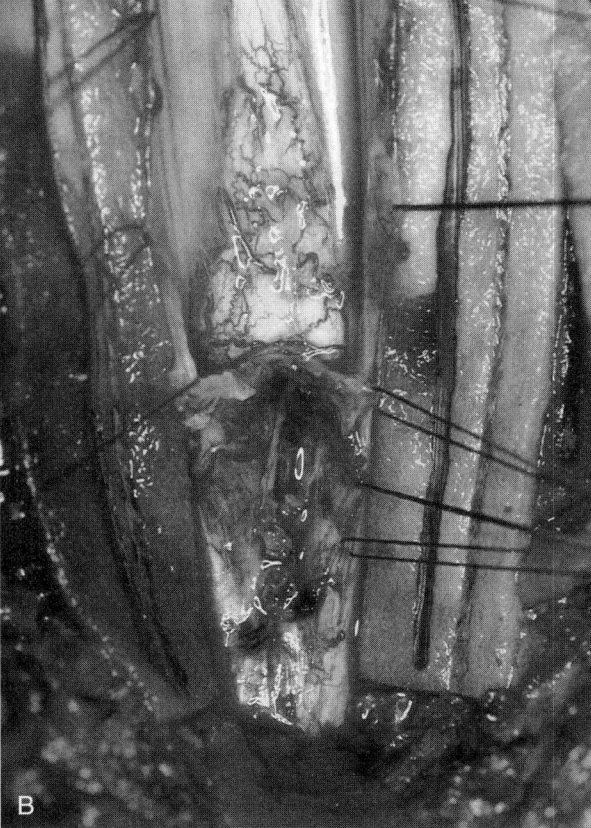

FIGURE 282–13. Diastematomyelia in a 14-year-old boy who presented with slowly progressive lower extremity dysfunction and the new onset of urinary incontinence. *A*, Sagittal T1-weighted image of the thoracolumbar spine shows diastematomyelia with tethering of the spinal cord. *B*, Intraoperative photograph shows the two hemicords after untethering with resection of the fibrous spur.

formations are defects of segmentation and defects of formation. The defects may result in scoliosis, kyphosis, or lordosis. The management of these deformities depends on the magnitude and progression of the deformity, associated pathology, and neurological deficit. Congenital scoliosis is often associated with spinal cord abnormalities: syringomyelia, diastematomyelia, neoplasm, tethered cord, and Arnold-Chiari malformation. Neurological symptoms in the form of sensory and motor dysfunction, spasticity, and bladder disturbances usually result from the underlying spinal cord disease. Treatment is directed at the underlying pathologic condition, correction of deformity, and prevention of further neurological deficits.[248, 254]

Spinal vascular malformations can be divided into three groups: dural arteriovenous fistulas (type I spinal AVMs), intradural AVMs (types II, III, and IV), and cavernous malformations. Type I spinal AVMs are typically dural arteriovenous fistulas with the nidus located within the dura mater of the proximal nerve root; these lesions constitute 80% to 85% of all spinal AVMs (Fig. 282–14). Type I spinal AVMs usually occur in the lower thoracic spinal cord and manifest between the ages of 40 and 70 in men. Neurological symptoms are caused by venous congestion and hypertension in these low-flow lesions. Their clinical presentation includes insidious onset of pain with progressive leg weakness, sensory changes, and disturbances of bladder and bowel function. Most patients have neurological dysfunction at the time of diagnosis. Type II spinal AVMs,

also known as glomus AVMs, are intramedullary AVMs with a true compact nidus. These high-flow malformations occur with equal frequency along the longitudinal axis of the spine and typically manifest in adolescence with a sudden hemorrhage (often a subarachnoid hemorrhage). Type III spinal AVMs, also known as juvenile AVMs, are larger, more extensive lesions that involve the intramedullary and extramedullary spaces over more than one spinal segment. They represent formidable high-flow lesions with a predilection for the cervicothoracic spine. Their typical clinical presentation is progressive neurological deficits that occur in adolescence or early adulthood. Type IV spinal AVMs are intradural extramedullary arteriovenous fistulas. These lesions are exceedingly rare and usually manifest with progressive neurological deficits rather than hemorrhage. Strenuous activity and postural changes can exacerbate the symptoms associated with type I and type III spinal AVMs. For types II, III, and IV lesions, both sexes are affected equally. MRI scans of dural arteriovenous fistulas may be normal or reveal nonspecific findings of increased signal intensity, or the signal intensity of the spinal cord may decrease with spinal cord expansion and evidence of venous congestion. In contrast to MRI, myelography is usually abnormal in dural arteriovenous fistulas and demonstrates the presence of the lesion. For intradural AVMs, MRI has replaced myelography as the initial diagnostic study of choice. Spinal angiography occasionally delineates arteriovenous lesions that cannot be identified on

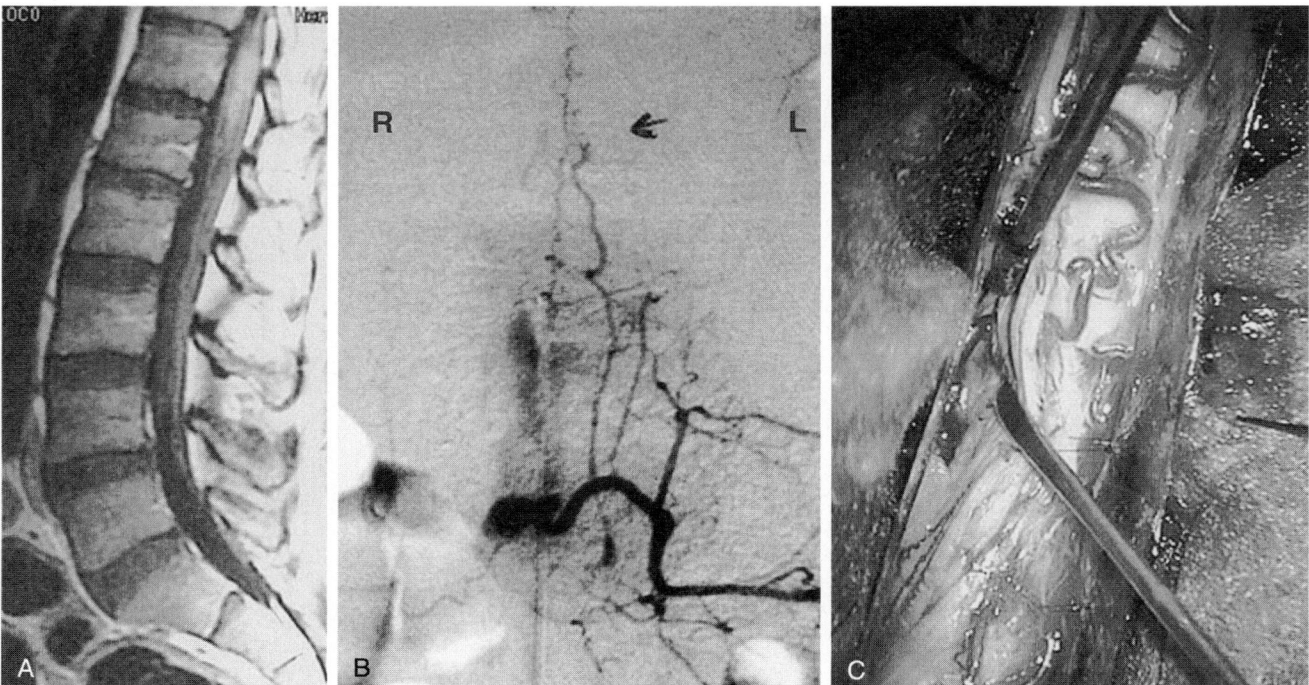

FIGURE 282–14. Type I spinal arteriovenous malformation in a 54-year-old man with vague lower back pain, progressive lower extremity weakness, and urinary incontinence. *A*, Sagittal T1-weighted image of the thoracolumbar spine shows dilatation and increased signal intensity from the conus medullaris. *B*, Spinal angiogram shows a T12 type I spinal arteriovenous malformation. R, right; L, left. *C*, Intraoperative photograph demonstrates the dural arteriovenous fistula before its obliteration.

MRI scans or myelography. The treatment of spinal AVMs is multidisciplinary, involving embolization and surgical resection.[255-258]

Histologically similar to their intracranial counterpart, *spinal cavernous malformations* are intramedullary lesions that represent 5% to 10% of all spinal vascular malformations. Cavernous malformations usually present in the fourth or fifth decade of life in women. The lesions occur with equal frequency along the neural axis. Their typical clinical presentation is progressive paraparesis and sensory loss with pain related to repetitive hemorrhages. MRI is the investigative procedure of choice, revealing mixed signal intensity on T1- and T2-weighted images with variable contrast enhancement. Microsurgical resection is the only therapeutic option.[256, 259, 260]

NEURONAL DEGENERATIVE DISEASES

The neuronal degenerative disorders encompass a broad spectrum of diseases that can affect the brain, spinal cord, or peripheral nerves. Those affecting the spinal cord can be divided broadly into syndromes of muscular weakness and atrophy without sensory changes, syndromes of progressive spinal ataxia, and combined system disorders. Despite this obvious oversimplification, most spinal cord neuronal degenerative diseases that must be distinguished from other pathologic entities (cervical spondylitic myelopathy, compressive neoplasm, and chronic myelitis) fall into one of these categories.[192]

The syndrome of muscular weakness and atrophy without sensory changes may be the result of degenerative diseases that affect upper motor neurons, lower motor neurons, or a combination of upper and lower motor neurons. The prognosis can vary greatly, depending on the clinical presentation and the motor neuron population involved.

The pure *upper motor neuron degenerative diseases* are primary lateral sclerosis and hereditary spastic paraplegia. Primary lateral sclerosis is a rare disease characterized by a slowly progressive degeneration of the corticospinal tracts. Pathologic studies have shown a decrease in the number of Betz's cells in the frontal cortex. Primary lateral sclerosis usually begins insidiously in the fifth or sixth decade of life with a slowly progressive spastic paraparesis that later involves the arms and oropharyngeal muscles. There are no lower motor neuron or sensory changes, and the clinical course is often prolonged. Clinically and genetically, hereditary spastic paraplegia is a heterogeneous disorder associated with progressive spasticity and mild weakness in the lower extremities. The pattern of inheritance is usually autosomal dominant. Onset of the more common form of the disease is before age 35 whereas onset of other forms is between the ages of 40 and 60 years. The clinical picture is that of a progressively worsening spastic gait with difficulty walking. Lower extremity spasticity, hyperreflexia, and extensor plantar responses are encountered on examination. In pure cases, lower motor neuron and sensory changes are lacking. The clinical course of hereditary spastic paraplegia is usually protracted. Treatment for these pure upper motor neuron degenerative diseases is symptomatic and directed at reducing spasticity.[261, 262]

Upper motor neuron degeneration may also be one manifestation of a more extensive neuronal degenerative process. Disorders involving other neural systems and the motor system in the form of upper motor neuron degeneration include the familial spastic paraplegias associated with other neurological abnormalities, adrenoleukodystrophy, lathyrism, and radiation myelopathy. The literature contains a number of reports of familial spastic paraplegias combined with other neurological abnormalities. Family history and associated neurological abnormalities almost always help determine the differential diagnosis. Adrenoleukodystrophy, an X-linked recessive disorder of males, most often manifests in children but may also present with spastic paraparesis in adolescence. Associated neurological abnormalities include dementia, optic atrophy, seizures, and adrenal insufficiency. Lathyrism, a disease of India and Africa, manifests as a subacute myelopathy caused by β-N-oxylylaminoalanine, a toxin in the grass pea *Lathyrus sativus*. Predominantly, the corticospinal and spinocerebellar tracts are affected. Another uncommon cause of slowly progressive subacute or chronic myelopathy may be radiation. Characteristically, radiation myelopathy is a complication of including the spinal cord in the field of radiation treatment and usually develops 6 months to 2 years after treatment. The corticospinal and spinothalamic pathways are involved early in the course of this disease. A rather stable, nonprogressive myelopathy may also be associated with cerebral spastic diplegia. Treatment for these neuronal disorders involves eliminating the causative agent when possible and supportive care directed at reducing spasticity.[192, 261-264]

The *lower motor neuron degenerative diseases* are a relatively nonhomogeneous group that includes progressive muscular atrophy and the spinal muscular atrophies (SMAs). Progressive muscular atrophy is an adult-onset disease characterized by pure lower motor neuron degeneration. Typically, progressive muscular atrophy presents in males as a symmetrical wasting of the hand muscles, slowly advancing to the more proximal arm musculature; less often, the atrophic weakness begins in the legs. Almost always, the distal extremities are involved before proximal weakness and atrophy appear. Progressive muscular atrophy progresses more slowly and its clinical course is more benign than that of amyotrophic lateral sclerosis (ALS). Some patients survive 15 years or longer. The SMAs are usually inherited as autosomal recessive traits and are linked to chromosome 5. SMA type I (Werdnig-Hoffman syndrome) is evident at birth or soon thereafter and is fatal in 85% of cases by age 2. SMA type II is similar to SMA type I, except that it appears between 6 and 12 months of age, and patients may survive beyond 2 years of age. The onset of SMA type III (Wohlfart-Kugelberg-Welander disease) is in late childhood or adolescence, and its clinical course is more benign. Included in this group of diseases are Fazio-Londe syndrome, Kennedy's disease, and postpolio syndrome. Fazio-Londe syndrome (childhood bulbar muscular atrophy) and Kennedy's disease (adult bulbar muscular atrophy) are degenerative diseases of the lower motor neurons with prominent bulbar signs; both diseases can progress to involve the spinal cord. The postpolio syndrome is defined as the new onset of muscle weakness, pain, and fatigue 30 to 40 years after a patient recovers from acute paralytic poliomyelitis. The disease is probably caused by premature aging affecting the chronically overworked surviving motor neurons. No evidence of reactivation of the old poliomyelitis has been found.[192, 261, 262, 265]

Combined upper and lower motor neuron degenerative diseases are the most common of the motor system diseases. ALS is the prototypical neurodegenerative disorder affecting upper and lower motor neurons. In most areas of the world, its overall incidence ranges between 1 and 2.5 cases per 100,000 population. Most cases of ALS are sporadic, but 10% are familial. Pathologically, ALS is distinguished by atrophy and death of motor neurons. The upper motor neurons in the brain (Betz's cells of the motor cortex) are affected, with secondary degeneration of the corticospinal tracts. The lower motor neurons involved include the anterior horn cells of the spinal cord and the brainstem nuclei for cranial nerves V, VII, IX, X, and XII. The extraocular muscle nuclei and Onuf's nucleus in the sacral spinal cord are relatively spared or affected late in the course of the disease. The incidence of ALS increases during each decade of life, with a mean age at onset of 55

years. The disease usually begins distally in one limb, most commonly the leg, and then spreads within the neural axis to involve contiguous groups of neurons. Approximately 50% of ALS patients die within 3 years of the onset of symptoms, although 20% live 5 years and 10% live 10 years. Progressive bulbar palsy is a condition in which the first and dominant symptoms are related to weakness of the muscles innervated by the lower brainstem. Progressive bulbar palsy almost always progresses to involve the spinal cord and is most likely a variant of ALS. Treatment of these diseases is supportive. Riluzole may prolong life 1 to 2 months.[262, 263, 266, 267]

The syndromes of progressive spinal ataxia include Friedreich's ataxia and non-Friedreich's ataxia. Friedreich's ataxia is characterized by degeneration of the posterior columns, dorsal root ganglia, corticospinal tracts, and spinocerebellar tracts. The disease onset almost always occurs before the 10th year of life, although a later onset (between 20 and 30 years) has been documented. Gait ataxia is usually the initial symptom, with both legs affected simultaneously. Difficulties in standing steadily and running are early symptoms. As the disease progresses, ataxia results from the sensory (secondary to posterior column degeneration) and cerebellar (secondary to spinocerebellar degeneration) deficits. Deep tendon reflexes are lost early in the course of the disease, and amyotrophy may be a late manifestation. Friedreich's ataxia is invariably progressive, and within 5 years, walking often is no longer

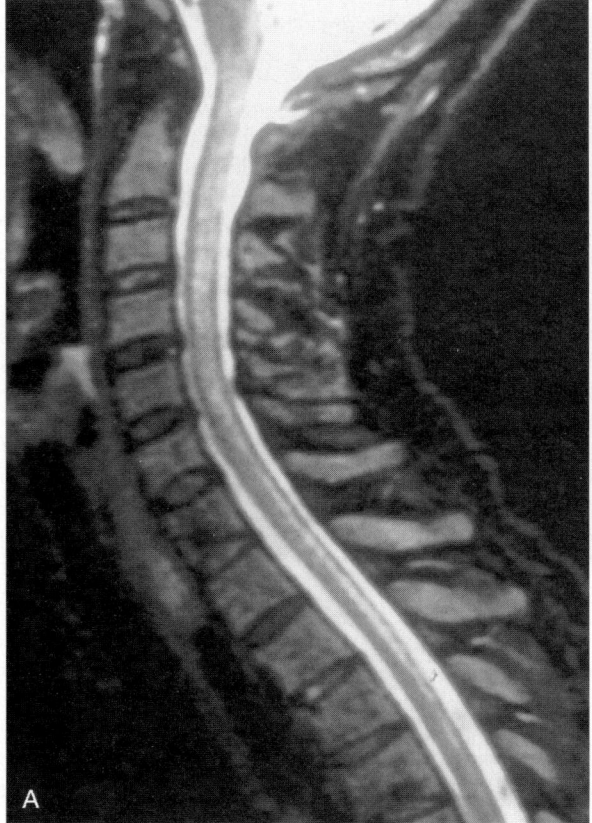

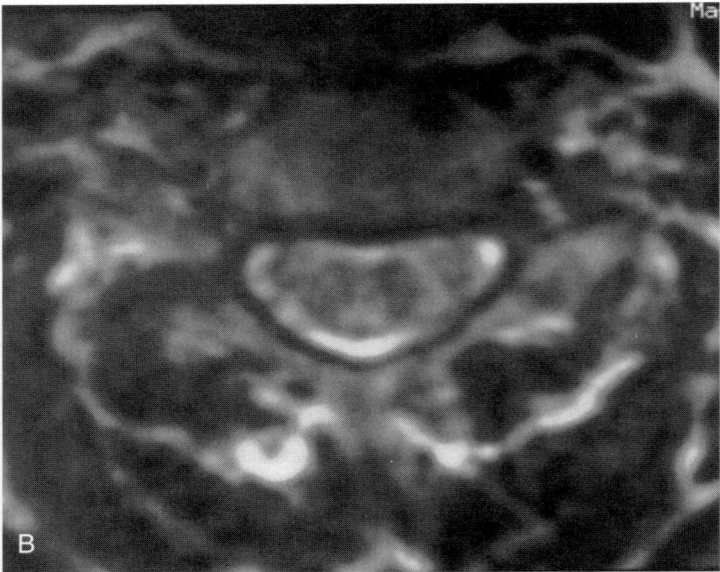

FIGURE 282–15. Subacute combined degeneration in a 52-year-old woman with constant paresthesias involving the hands and feet. She progressively lost proprioception, developed spastic paraparesis, and was diagnosed with subacute combined degeneration. Sagittal *(A)* and axial *(B)* T2-weighted images of the cervicothoracic spine show increased signal intensity from the posterior columns. The patient was treated with the administration of vitamin B$_{12}$ for life.

possible. Kyphoscoliosis and cardiomyopathy often contribute to death in patients with Friedreich's ataxia. Non-Friedreich's ataxia is the result of corticospinal and spinocerebellar degeneration. The clinical presentation of these two diseases is similar. In non-Friedreich's ataxia, however, the deep tendon reflexes are preserved, and there is no associated kyphoscoliosis or cardiomyopathy. Its prognosis is better than that of Friedreich's ataxia.[261, 268]

The combined system disorders are those diseases that affect the posterior and lateral spinal columns (Fig. 282–15). The diseases in this category are subacute combined degeneration and combined system disease of the nonpernicious anemia type. Subacute combined degeneration is due to a vitamin B_{12} (cobalamin) deficiency and may affect the brain, optic nerves, spinal cord, and peripheral nerves. The spinal cord is usually affected first and often solely. Pathologically, the disease is first characterized by degeneration of the posterior columns in the cervicothoracic region. Later, the disease progresses longitudinally and anterolaterally along the neural axis. The clinical presentation starts with constant and progressive paresthesias involving the hands and feet. As the illness advances, the gait becomes unsteady, and a spastic paraparesis develops. If untreated, spastic paraplegia ensues. Neurological examination reveals a disorder of the dorsal columns and corticospinal tracts. This disease is treatable, and the degree of reversibility is related to the duration of symptoms. Diagnosis is made in the appropriate clinical setting with laboratory studies that include a serum cobalamin level. Subacute combined degeneration may be present without anemia or an abnormal volume of red blood cells. MRI scans of the cervical and thoracic spine occasionally show pathologic increased signal intensity in the posterior columns. Treatment involves the immediate administration of vitamin B_{12} and its continuation for the remainder of the patient's life. Combined system disease of the nonpernicious anemia type is an idiopathic disease characterized by degeneration of the posterior and lateral columns. The signs of corticospinal tract disease dominate the clinical picture throughout the course of the illness. The cause is unknown, and the clinical course is slowly and chronically progressive. There is no known treatment for this disorder.[261, 269–273]

REFERENCES

1. Borenstein DG, Wiesel SW (eds): Low Back Pain: Medical Diagnosis and Comprehensive Management. Philadelphia, WB Saunders, 1989, pp 147–169.
2. Wolcott WP, Malik JM, Shaffrey CI, et al: Differential diagnosis of surgical disorders of the spine. In Benzel EC (ed): Spine Surgery: Techniques, Complication Avoidance, and Management. New York, Churchill Livingstone, 1999, pp 25–51.
3. Vukmir RB: Low back pain: Review of diagnosis and therapy. Am J Emerg Med 9:328–335, 1991.
4. Lindsley HB: Low back pain evaluation and management. Compr Ther 18:23–26, 1992.
5. Martinelli TA, Wiesel SW: Low back pain: The algorithmic approach. Compr Ther 17:22–27, 1991.
6. McCowin PR, Borenstein D, Wiesel SW: The current approach to the medical diagnosis of low back pain. Orthop Clin North Am 22:315–325, 1991.
7. Nachemson AL: Spinal disorders: Overall impact on society and the need for orthopedic resources. Acta Orthop Scand Suppl 241:17–22, 1991.
8. Bamberger DM: Osteomyelitis: A commonsense approach to antibiotic and surgical treatment. Postgrad Med 94:177–184, 1993.
9. Boden SD, Laws ER: Infections of the spine. In Boden SD (ed): The Aging Spine: Essentials of Pathophysiology, Diagnosis, and Treatment. Philadelphia, WB Saunders, 1991, pp 205–219.
10. Hitchon PW, Osenbach RK, Yuh WT, et al: Spinal infections. Clin Neurosurg 38:373–387, 1992.
11. Lifeso RM: Pyogenic spinal sepsis in adults. Spine 15:1265–1271, 1990.
12. Zeidman SM, Ducker TB: Infectious complications in spine surgery. In Benzel EC (ed): Spine Surgery: Techniques, Complication Avoidance, and Management. New York, Churchill Livingstone, 1999, pp 1445–1457.
13. Aliabadi P, Nikpoor N: Imaging osteomyelitis. Arthritis Rheum 37:617–622, 1994.
14. Anthony JP, Mathes SJ: Update on chronic osteomyelitis. Clin Plast Surg 18:515–523, 1991.
15. Cole WG: The management of chronic osteomyelitis. Clin Orthop 264:84–89, 1991.
16. Correa AG, Edwards MS, Baker CJ: Vertebral osteomyelitis in children. Pediatr Infect Dis J 12:228–233, 1993.
17. Crim JR, Seeger LL: Imaging evaluation of osteomyelitis. Crit Rev Diagn Imaging 35:201–256, 1994.
18. Dirschl DR, Almekinders LC: Osteomyelitis: Common causes and treatment recommendations. Drugs 45:29–43, 1993.
19. Keenan TL, Benson DR: Differential diagnosis and conservative treatment of infectious diseases. In Frymoyer JW (ed): The Adult Spine: Principles and Practice, 2nd ed. Philadelphia, Lippincott-Raven, 1997, pp 871–894.
20. Kramer J, Stiglbauer R, Wimberger D, et al: MRI of spondylitis. Bildgebung 59:147–151, 1992.
21. Krodel A, Sturz H, Siebert CH: Indications for and results of operative treatment of spondylitis and spondylodiscitis. Arch Orthop Trauma Surg 110:78–82, 1991.
22. Lafont A, Olive A, Gelman M, et al: *Candida albicans* spondylodiscitis and vertebral osteomyelitis in patients with intravenous heroin drug addiction: Report of 3 new cases. J Rheumatol 21:953–956, 1994.
23. Sapico FL, Montgomerie JZ: Vertebral osteomyelitis. Infect Dis Clin North Am 4:539–550, 1990.
24. Ansari A, Yock DH, Seymour JL, et al: Acute pyogenic spondylodiscitis with epidural phlegmon: Diagnosis and management by MRI and multidisciplinary approach. Minn Med 76:21–24, 1993.
25. Currier BL: Infections of the spine. In Rothman RH, Simeone FA: The Spine, 3rd ed. Philadelphia, WB Saunders, 1992, pp 1319–1380.
26. Connolly ES: Management of persistent or recurrent symptoms and signs in the postoperative lumbar disc patient. Neurosurg Clin N Am 4:161–166, 1993.
27. Crawford AH, Kucharzyk DW, Ruda R, et al: Diskitis in children. Clin Orthop 266:70–79, 1991.
28. Dendrinos GK, Polyzoides JA: Spondylodiscitis after percutaneous discectomy: A case diagnosed by MRI. Acta Orthop Scand 63:219–220, 1992.
29. Dirschl DR: Acute pyogenic osteomyelitis in children. Orthop Rev 23:305–312, 1994.
30. Petty RE: Septic arthritis and osteomyelitis in children. Curr Opin Rheumatol 2:616–621, 1990.
31. Ponte CD, McDonald M: Septic discitis resulting from *Escherichia coli* urosepsis. J Fam Pract 34:767–771, 1992.
32. du Lac P, Panuel M, Devred P, et al: MRI of disc space infection in infants and children: Report of 12 cases. Pediatr Radiol 20:175–178, 1990.
33. Garcia FF, Semba CP, Sartoris CC, et al: Diagnostic imaging of childhood spinal infection. Orthop Rev 22:321–327, 1993.
34. Morgenlander JC, Rozear MP: Disc space infection: A case report with MRI diagnosis. Am Fam Physician 42:983–986, 1990.
35. Torbiak R, Pugash R: Answer to case of the month #3. Pyogenic discitis: Staphylococcal discitis complicated by bilateral psoas abscesses. Can Assoc Radiol J 41:49–50, 1990.

36. Lifeso RM, Weaver P, Harder EH: Tuberculous spondylitis in adults. J Bone Joint Surg Am 67:1405–1413, 1985.

37. Bloch AB, Rieder HL, Kelly GD, et al: The epidemiology of tuberculosis in the United States. Semin Respir Infect 4:157–170, 1989.

38. Ellinas PA, Rosner F: Pott's disease in urban populations: A report of five cases and a review of the literature. N Y State J Med 90:588–591, 1990.

39. Fam AG, Rubenstein J: Another look at spinal tuberculosis. J Rheumatol 20:1731–1740, 1993.

40. Slater RR Jr, Beale RW, Bullitt E: Pott's disease of the cervical spine. South Med J 84:521–523, 1991.

41. Wurtz R, Quader Z, Simon D, et al: Cervical tuberculous vertebral osteomyelitis: Case report and discussion of the literature. Clin Infect Dis 16:806–808, 1993.

42. Freilich D, Swash M: Diagnosis and management of tuberculous paraplegia with special reference to tuberculous radiculomyelitis. J Neurol Neurosurg Psychiatry 42:12–18, 1979.

43. Gorse GJ, Pais MJ, Kusske JA, et al: Tuberculous spondylitis: A report of six cases and a review of the literature. Medicine (Baltimore) 62:178–193, 1983.

44. Janssens JP, de Haller R: Spinal tuberculosis in a developed country: A review of 26 cases with special emphasis on abscesses and neurological complications. Clin Orthop 257:67–75, 1990.

45. Upadhyay SS, Sell P, Saji MJ, et al: Surgical management of spinal tuberculosis in adults: Hong Kong operation compared with debridement surgery for short and long term outcome of deformity. Clin Orthop 302:173–182, 1994.

46. Laurin JM, Resnik CS, Wheeler D, et al: Vertebral osteomyelitis caused by *Nocardia asteroides*: Report and review of the literature. J Rheumatol 18:455–458, 1991.

47. Zaks N, Sukenik S, Alkan M, et al: Musculoskeletal manifestations of brucellosis: A study of 90 cases in Israel. Semin Arthritis Rheum 25:97–102, 1995.

48. D'Hoore K, Hoogmartens M: Vertebral aspergillosis: A case report and review of the literature. Acta Orthop Belg 59:306–314, 1993.

49. Lafont A, Olive A, Gelman M, et al: *Candida albicans* spondylodiscitis and vertebral osteomyelitis in patients with intravenous heroin drug addiction: Report of 3 new cases. J Rheumatol 21:953–956, 1994.

50. Boden SD, Laws ER: Tumors of the spine. In Boden SD (ed): The Aging Spine: Essentials of Pathophysiology, Diagnosis, and Treatment. Philadelphia, WB Saunders, 1991, pp 221–252.

51. Ebersold MJ, Hitchon PW, Duff JM, et al: Primary bony spinal lesions. In Benzel EC (ed): Spine Surgery: Techniques, Complication Avoidance, and Management. New York, Churchill Livingstone, 1999, pp 663–677.

52. Elghazawi AK: Clinical syndromes and differential diagnosis of spinal disorders. Radiol Clin North Am 29:651–663, 1991.

53. Masaryk TJ: Neoplastic disease of the spine. Radiol Clin North Am 29:829–845, 1991.

54. Boriani S, Weinstein JN: Differential diagnosis and surgical treatment of primary benign and malignant neoplasms. In Frymoyer JW (ed): The Adult Spine: Principles and Practice, 2nd ed. Philadelphia, Lippincott-Raven, 1997, pp 951–1014.

55. Dreghorn CR, Newman RJ, Hardy GJ, et al: Primary tumors of the axial skeleton: Experience of the Leeds Regional Bone Tumor Registry. Spine 15:137–140, 1990.

56. Weinstein JN: Tumors of the spine. In Rothman RH, Simeone FA (eds): The Spine, 3rd ed. Philadelphia, WB Saunders, 1992, pp 1279–1319.

57. Abdelwahab IF, Kenan S, Hermann G, et al: Case report 845: Fluid-filling giant cell tumor with an aneurysmal bone cyst component. Skeletal Radiol 23:317–319, 1994.

58. Chakravarty K, Brett F, Merry P: Aneurysmal bone cyst—an unusual presentation of neck pain in a young adult [letter]. Br J Rheumatol 33:597–598, 1994.

59. Gupta VK, Gupta SK, Khosla VK, et al: Aneurysmal bone cysts of the spine. Surg Neurol 42:428–432, 1994.

60. Lifeso RM, Younge D: Aneurysmal bone cysts of the spine. Int Orthop 8:281–285, 1985.

61. Scully SP, Temple HT, O'Keefe RJ, et al: Case report 830: Aneurysmal bone cyst. Skeletal Radiol 23:157–160, 1994.

62. Vandertop WP, Pruijs JE, Snoeck IN, et al: Aneurysmal bone cyst of the thoracic spine: Radical excision with use of the cavitron. A case report. J Bone Joint Surg Am 76:608–611, 1994.

63. Faria SL, Schlupp WR, Chiminazzo H: Radiotherapy in the treatment of vertebral hemangiomas. Int J Radiat Oncol Biol Phys 11:387–390, 1985.

64. Perrin RG, McBroom RJ: Thoracic spine tumors. Clin Neurosurg 38:353–372, 1992.

65. Tekkok IH, Acikgoz B, Saglam S, et al: Vertebral hemangioma symptomatic during pregnancy—report of a case and review of the literature. Neurosurgery 32:302–306, 1993.

66. Acciarri N, Paganini M, Fonda C, et al: Langerhans cell histiocytosis of the spine causing cord compression: Case report. Neurosurgery 31:965–968, 1992.

67. De Schepper AM, Ramon F, Van Marck E: MR imaging of eosinophilic granuloma: Report of 11 cases. Skeletal Radiol 22:163–166, 1993.

68. DeCandido P, Resnik CS, Aisner SC: Case report 792: Eosinophilic granuloma of bone. Skeletal Radiol 22:371–373, 1993.

69. Johnson S, Klostermeier T, Weinstein A: Case report 768: Eosinophilic granuloma of the cervical spine. Skeletal Radiol 22:63–65, 1993.

70. Sessa S, Sommelet D, Lascombes P, et al: Treatment of Langerhans-cell histiocytosis in children: Experience at the Children's Hospital of Nancy. J Bone Joint Surg Am 76:1513–1525, 1994.

71. Bednar DA, Brox WT, Viviani GR: Surgical palliation of spinal oncologic disease: A review and analysis of current approaches. Can J Surg 34:129–131, 1991.

72. Boogerd W, van der Sande JJ: Diagnosis and treatment of spinal cord compression in malignant disease. Cancer Treat Rev 19:129–150, 1993.

73. Gilbert RW, Kim JH, Posner JB: Epidural spinal cord compression from metastatic tumor: Diagnosis and treatment. Ann Neurol 3:40–51, 1978.

74. O'Connor MI, Currier BL: Metastatic disease of the spine. Orthopedics 15:611–620, 1992.

75. Bjornsson J, Wold LE, Ebersold MJ, et al: Chordoma of the mobile spine: A clinicopathologic analysis of 40 patients. Cancer 71:735–740, 1993.

76. Burger EL, Lindeque BG: Sacral and non-spinal tumors presenting as backache: A retrospective study of 17 patients. Acta Orthop Scand 65:344–346, 1994.

77. Caballero C, Fontaniere B: Sacrococcygeal chordoma: Fine needle aspiration cytological findings and differential diagnosis. Cytopathology 4:311–313, 1993.

78. O'Neill P, Bell BA, Miller JD, et al: Fifty years of experience with chordomas in southeast Scotland. Neurosurgery 16:166–170, 1985.

79. Samson IR, Springfield DS, Suit HD, et al: Operative treatment of sacrococcygeal chordoma: A review of twenty-one cases. J Bone Joint Surg Am 75:1476–1484, 1993.

80. Abdelwahab IF, Casden AM, Klein MJ, et al: Chondrosarcoma of a thoracic vertebra. Bull Hosp Jt Dis Orthop Inst 51:34–39, 1991.

81. Alpaslan AM, Acaroglu RE, Kis M: Three-stage excision of recurrent cervical chondrosarcoma: A case report. Arch Orthop Trauma Surg 112:245–246, 1993.

82. Kretzschmar HA, Eggert HR: Mesenchymal chondrosarcoma of the craniocervical junction. Clin Neurol Neurosurg 92:343–347, 1990.

83. Slater G, Huckstep RL: Management of chondrosarcoma. Aust N Z J Surg 63:587–589, 1993.

84. Young CL, Sim FH, Unni KK, et al: Chondrosarcoma of bone in children. Cancer 66:1641–1648, 1990.

85. Mameghan H, Fisher RJ, O'Gorman-Hughes D, et al: Ewing's sarcoma: Long-term follow-up in 49 patients treated from 1967 to 1989. Int J Radiat Oncol Biol Phys 25:431–438, 1993.

86. Sharafuddin MJ, Haddad FS, Hitchon PW, et al: Treatment options in primary Ewing's sarcoma of the spine: Report of seven cases and review of the literature. Neurosurgery 30:610–619, 1992.

87. Tekkok IH: Treatment options in primary Ewing's sarcoma of the spine: Report of seven cases and review of the literature [letter]. Neurosurgery 32:480, 1993.

88. Birch BD, McCormick PC: Intradural extramedullary spinal le-

sions. In Benzel EC (ed): Spine Surgery: Techniques, Complication Avoidance, and Management. New York, Churchill Livingstone, 1999, pp 623–634.

89. Cassidy JR, Ducker TB, Dienes EA: Intradural tumors. In Frymoyer JW (ed): The Adult Spine: Principles and Practice, 2nd ed. Philadelphia, Lippincott-Raven, 1997, pp 1015–1029.

90. Hughes JT: Neuropathology of the spinal cord. Neurol Clin 9: 551–571, 1991.

91. McCormick PC, Post KD, Stein BM: Intradural extramedullary tumors in adults. Neurosurg Clin N Am 1:591–608, 1990.

92. McCormick PC, Stein BM: Spinal cord tumors in adults. In Youmans JR (ed): Neurological Surgery: A Comprehensive Reference Guide to the Diagnosis and Management of Neurosurgical Problems, 4th ed. Philadelphia, WB Saunders, 1996, pp 3102–3133.

93. DeSousa AL, Kalsbeck JE, Mealey J Jr, et al: Intraspinal tumors in children: A review of 81 cases. J Neurosurg 51:437–445, 1979.

94. Levy WJ, Latchaw J, Hahn JF, et al: Spinal neurofibromas: A report of 66 cases and a comparison with meningiomas. Neurosurgery 18:331–334, 1986.

95. McCormick PC: Surgical management of dumbbell and paraspinal tumors of the thoracic and lumbar spine. Neurosurgery 38:67–75, 1996.

96. Honch GW: Spinal cord and foramen magnum tumors. Semin Neurol 13:337–342, 1993.

97. Levy WJ Jr, Bay J, Dohn D: Spinal cord meningioma. J Neurosurg 57:804–812, 1982.

98. Solero CL, Fornari M, Giombini S, et al: Spinal meningiomas: Review of 174 operated cases. Neurosurgery 25:153–160, 1989.

99. Conrad EU III, Olszewski AD, Berger M, et al: Pediatric spine tumors with spinal cord compromise. J Pediatr Orthop 12:454–460, 1992.

100. McCormick PC, Stein BM: Miscellaneous intradural pathology. Neurosurg Clin N Am 1:687–699, 1990.

101. Reyes MG, Torres H: Intrathecal paraganglioma of the cauda equina. Neurosurgery 15:578–582, 1984.

102. Cohen AR, Wisoff JH, Allen JC, et al: Malignant astrocytomas of the spinal cord. J Neurosurg 70:50–54, 1989.

103. Cooper PR: Outcome after operative treatment of intramedullary spinal cord tumors in adults: Intermediate and long-term results in 51 patients. Neurosurgery 25:855–859, 1989.

104. Cristante L, Herrmann HD: Surgical management of intramedullary spinal cord tumors: Functional outcome and sources of morbidity. Neurosurgery 35:69–76, 1994.

105. Epstein F, Epstein N: Surgical treatment of spinal cord astrocytomas of childhood: A series of 19 patients. J Neurosurg 57: 685–689, 1982.

106. Epstein FJ, Farmer JP, Freed D: Adult intramedullary astrocytomas of the spinal cord. J Neurosurg 77:355–359, 1992.

107. McCormick PC, Anson JA: Intramedullary spinal cord lesions. In Benzel EC (ed): Spine Surgery: Techniques, Complication Avoidance, and Management. New York, Churchill Livingstone, 1999, pp 615–622.

108. McCormick PC, Stein BM: Intramedullary tumors in adults. Neurosurg Clin N Am 1:609–630, 1990.

109. McCormick PC, Stein BM: Spinal intradural tumors. In Wilkins RH, Rengachary SS (ed): Neurosurgery, 2nd ed. New York, McGraw-Hill, 1996, pp 1769–1781.

110. McCormick PC, Torres R, Post KD, et al: Intramedullary ependymoma of the spinal cord. J Neurosurg 72:523–532, 1990.

111. Whitaker SJ, Bessell EM, Ashley SE, et al: Postoperative radiotherapy in the management of spinal cord ependymoma. J Neurosurg 74:720–728, 1991.

112. Costigan DA, Winkelman MD: Intramedullary spinal cord metastasis: A clinicopathological study of 13 cases. J Neurosurg 62:227–233, 1985.

113. Bessette L, Katz JN, Liang MH: Differential diagnosis and conservative treatment of rheumatic diseases. In Frymoyer JW (ed): The Adult Spine: Principles and Practice, 2nd ed. Philadelphia, Lippincott-Raven, 1997, pp 803–826.

114. Dougados M: Diagnosis and monitoring of spondylarthropathy. Compr Ther 16:52–56, 1990.

115. Clark CR: Rheumatoid arthritis: Surgical considerations. In Rothman RH, Simeone FA (eds): The Spine, 3rd ed. Philadelphia, WB Saunders, 1992, pp 1429–1445.

116. Delamarter RB, Bolesta MJ, Bohlman HH: Rheumatoid arthritis. In Frymoyer JW (ed): The Adult Spine: Principles and Practice, 2nd ed. Philadelphia, Lippincott-Raven, 1997, pp 827–843.

117. Heary RF, Simeone FA, Crockard HA: Rheumatoid arthritis. In Benzel EC (ed): Spine Surgery: Techniques, Complication Avoidance, and Management. New York, Churchill Livingstone, 1999, pp 463–481.

118. Kaplan JG, Rosenberg RS, DeSouza T, et al: Atlantoaxial subluxation in psoriatic arthropathy. Ann Neurol 23:522–524, 1988.

119. Kramer J, Jolesz F, Kleefield J: Rheumatoid arthritis of the cervical spine. Rheum Dis Clin North Am 17:757–772, 1991.

120. Nakano KK, Schoene WC, Baker RA, et al: The cervical myelopathy associated with rheumatoid arthritis: Analysis of patients, with 2 postmortem cases. Ann Neurol 3:144–151, 1978.

121. Bennett GJ: Ankylosing spondylitis. Clin Neurosurg 37:622–635, 1991.

122. Carbone LD, Cooper C, Michet CJ, et al: Ankylosing spondylitis in Rochester, Minnesota, 1935–1989: Is the epidemiology changing? Arthritis Rheum 35:1476–1482, 1992.

123. Eberson MJ, Jestus JA, Quast LM: Ankylosing spondylitis and related disorders. In Benzel EC (ed): Spine Surgery: Techniques, Complication Avoidance, and Management. New York, Churchill Livingstone, 1999, pp 483–488.

124. Gran JT, Husby G: The epidemiology of ankylosing spondylitis. Semin Arthritis Rheum 22:319–334, 1993.

125. Laurent-Haupt L, Westmark KD: Long-standing ankylosing spondylitis with back pain. Rheum Dis Clin North Am 17: 813–816, 1991.

126. Jaffray D, Becker V, Eisenstein S: Closing wedge osteotomy with transpedicular fixation in ankylosing spondylitis. Clin Orthop 279:122–126, 1992.

127. Kostuik JP: Ankylosing spondylitis: Surgical treatment. In Frymoyer JW (ed): The Adult Spine: Principles and Practice, 2nd ed. Philadelphia, Lippincott-Raven, 1997, pp 845–870.

128. Lin SY, Wu HJ, Chien SH: Correction osteotomy of flexion deformity of cervical spine in ankylosing spondylitis—a case report. Kao Hsiung I Hsueh Ko Hsueh Tsa Chih 6:454–460, 1990.

129. Simmons EH: Ankylosing spondylitis. In Rothman RH, Simeone FA (eds): The Spine, 3rd ed. Philadelphia, WB Saunders, 1992, pp 1447–1511.

130. Thiranont N, Netrawichien P: Transpedicular decancellation closed wedge vertebral osteotomy for treatment of fixed flexion deformity of spine in ankylosing spondylitis. Spine 18:2517–2522, 1993.

131. Avrahami E, Frishman E, Fridman Z, et al: Spina bifida occulta of S1 is not an innocent finding. Spine 19:12–15, 1994.

132. DonTigny RL: Anterior dysfunction of the sacroiliac joint as a major factor in the etiology of idiopathic low back pain syndrome. Phys Ther 70:250–265, 1990.

133. Fager CA: Identification and management of radiculopathy. Neurosurg Clin N Am 4:1–12, 1993.

134. Frymoyer JW: Radiculopathies: Lumbar disc herniation. In Frymoyer JW (ed): The Adult Spine: Principles and Practice, 2nd ed. Philadelphia, Lippincott-Raven, 1997, pp 1937–1946.

135. Heary RF, Stellar S, Fobben ES: Preoperative diagnosis of an extradural cyst arising from a spinal facet joint: Case report. Neurosurgery 30:415–418, 1992.

136. Jackson RP: The facet syndrome: Myth or reality? Clin Orthop 279:110–121, 1992.

137. Connolly ES: Management of persistent or recurrent symptoms and signs in the postoperative lumbar disc patient. Neurosurg Clin N Am 4:161–166, 1993.

138. Dubuisson A, Lenelle J, Stevenaert A: Soft cervical disc herniation: A retrospective study of 100 cases. Acta Neurochir (Wien) 125:115–119, 1993.

139. Frymoyer JW: Lumbar disk disease: Epidemiology. Instr Course Lect 41:217–223, 1992.

140. Garrido E: Lumbar disc herniation in the pediatric patient. Neurosurg Clin N Am 4:149–152, 1993.

141. Gokaslan ZL, Cooper PR: Treatment of disc and ligamentous diseases of the cervical spine by the anterior approach. In Youmans JR (ed): Neurological Surgery: A Comprehensive Reference Guide to the Diagnosis and Management of Neurosurgical Problems, 4th ed. Philadelphia, WB Saunders, 1996, pp 2253–2261.

142. Haid RW Jr, Dickman CA: Instrumentation and fusion for discogenic disease of the lumbosacral spine. Neurosurg Clin N Am 4:135–148, 1993.

143. Kelsey JL, Golden AL, Mundt DJ: Low back pain/prolapsed lumbar intervertebral disc. Rheum Dis Clin North Am 16:699–716, 1990.

144. Long DM: Decision making in lumbar disc disease. Clin Neurosurg 39:36–51, 1992.

145. Rogers MA, Crockard HA: Surgical treatment of the symptomatic herniated thoracic disk. Clin Orthop 300:70–78, 1994.

146. Singounas EG, Kypriades EM, Kellerman AJ, et al: Thoracic disc herniation: Analysis of 14 cases and review of the literature. Acta Neurochir (Wien) 116:49–52, 1992.

147. Williams RW: Lumbar disc disease: Microdiscectomy. Neurosurg Clin N Am 4:101–108, 1993.

148. Bernhardt M, Hynes RA, Blume HW, et al: Cervical spondylotic myelopathy. J Bone Joint Surg Am 75:119–128, 1993.

149. Boden SD, Laws ER: Metabolic bone disease and the spine. In Boden SD (ed): The Aging Spine: Essentials of Pathophysiology, Diagnosis, and Treatment. Philadelphia, WB Saunders, 1991, pp 253–259.

150. Caputy AJ, Luessenhop AJ: Long-term evaluation of decompressive surgery for degenerative lumbar stenosis. J Neurosurg 77:669–676, 1992.

151. Fisher WS III: Selection of patients for surgery. Neurosurg Clin N Am 4:35–44, 1993.

152. O'Duffy JD: Spinal stenosis: Development of the lesion, clinical classification, and presentation. In Frymoyer JW (ed): The Adult Spine: Principles and Practice, 2nd ed. Philadelphia, Lippincott-Raven, 1997, pp 769–779.

153. Herkowitz HN, Kurz LT: Degenerative lumbar spondylolisthesis with spinal stenosis: A prospective study comparing decompression with decompression and intertransverse process arthrodesis. J Bone Joint Surg Am 73:802–808, 1991.

154. Katz JN, Dalgas M, Stucki G, et al: Diagnosis of lumbar spinal stenosis. Rheum Dis Clin North Am 20:471–483, 1994.

155. Markwalder TM: Surgical management of neurogenic claudication in 100 patients with lumbar spinal stenosis due to degenerative spondylolisthesis. Acta Neurochir (Wien) 120:136–142, 1993.

156. Martinelli TA, Wiesel SW: Epidemiology of spinal stenosis. Instr Course Lect 41:179–181, 1992.

157. Newcombe DS: Intermittent spinal ischemia: A reversible cause of neurological dysfunction and back pain. Arthritis Rheum 37:142–144, 1994.

158. Porter RW: Central spinal stenosis: Classification and pathogenesis. Acta Orthop Scand Suppl 251:64–66, 1993.

159. Seitsalo S, Osterman K, Hyvarinen H, et al: Severe spondylolisthesis in children and adolescents: A long-term review of fusion in situ. J Bone Joint Surg Br 72:259–265, 1990.

160. Seitsalo S, Osterman K, Hyvarinen H, et al: Progression of spondylolisthesis in children and adolescents: A long-term follow-up of 272 patients. Spine 16:417–421, 1991.

161. Burkus JK, Lonstein JE, Winter RB, et al: Long-term evaluation of adolescents treated operatively for spondylolisthesis: A comparison of in situ arthrodesis only with in situ arthrodesis and reduction followed by immobilization in a cast. J Bone Joint Surg Am 74:693–704, 1992.

162. Grobler LJ, Wiltse LL: Classification, and nonoperative and operative treatment of spondylolisthesis. In Frymoyer JW (ed): The Adult Spine: Principles and Practice, 2nd ed. Philadelphia, Lippincott-Raven, 1997, pp 1865–1921.

163. Law MD Jr, Bernhardt M, White AA III: Cervical spondylotic myelopathy: A review of surgical indications and decision making. Yale J Biol Med 66:165–177, 1993.

164. Saraste H: Spondylolysis and spondylolisthesis. Acta Orthop Scand Suppl 251:84–86, 1993.

165. Satomi K, Hirabayashi K, Toyama Y, et al: A clinical study of degenerative spondylolisthesis: Radiographic analysis and choice of treatment. Spine 17:1329–1336, 1992.

166. Bilsky MH, Dimar JR, Shields CB, et al: Thoracic and lumbar deformities. In Benzel EC (ed): Spine Surgery: Techniques, Complication Avoidance, and Management. New York, Churchill Livingstone, 1999, pp 541–564.

167. Bradford DS: Adult scoliosis. In Lonstein JE, Bradford DS, Winter RB, Ogilvie JW (eds): Moe's Textbook of Scoliosis and Other Spinal Deformities, 3rd ed. Philadelphia, WB Saunders, 1995, pp 369–386.

168. Gundry CR, Heithoff KB: Imaging evaluation of patients with spinal deformity. Orthop Clin North Am 25:247–264, 1994.

169. Perennou D, Marcelli C, Herisson C, et al: Adult lumbar scoliosis: Epidemiologic aspects in a low-back pain population. Spine 19:123–128, 1994.

170. Chapman JR, Anderson PA: Cervical spine trauma. In Frymoyer JW (ed): The Adult Spine: Principles and Practice, 2nd ed. Philadelphia, Lippincott-Raven, 1997, pp 1245–1295.

171. Huler JH: Thoracolumbar spine fracture. In Frymoyer JW (ed): The Adult Spine: Principles and Practice, 2nd ed. Philadelphia, Lippincott-Raven, 1997, pp 1473–1511.

172. Aebi M, Mohler J, Zach GA, et al: Indication, surgical technique, and results of 100 surgically-treated fractures and fracture-dislocations of the cervical spine. Clin Orthop 203:244–257, 1986.

173. Bracken MB, Shepard MJ, Holford TR, et al: Methylprednisolone or tirilazad mesylate administration after acute spinal cord injury: 1-year follow up. Results of the third National Acute Spinal Cord Injury Randomized Controlled Trial. J Neurosurg 89:699–706, 1998.

174. Chapman JR, Anderson PA: Thoracolumbar spine fractures with neurological deficit. Orthop Clin North Am 25:595–612, 1994.

175. Fehlings MG, Tator CH: An evidence-based review of decompressive surgery in acute spinal cord injury: Rationale, indications, and timing based on experimental and clinical studies. J Neurosurg 91:1–11, 1999.

176. Gertzbein SD: Scoliosis Research Society: Multicenter spine fracture study. Spine 17:528–540, 1992.

177. Magerl F, Aebi M, Gertzbein SD, et al: A comprehensive classification of thoracic and lumbar injuries. Eur Spine J 3:184–201, 1994.

178. Maroon JC, Abla AA, Wilberger JI, et al: Central cord syndrome. Clin Neurosurg 37:612–621, 1991.

179. Sgouros S, Williams B: Management and outcome of posttraumatic syringomyelia. J Neurosurg 85:197–205, 1996.

180. Umbach I, Heilporn A: Post–spinal cord injury syringomyelia. Paraplegia 29:219–221, 1991.

181. Hall CH, Einhorn TA: Metabolic bone diseases of the adult spine. In Frymoyer JW (ed): The Adult Spine: Principles and Practice, 2nd ed. Philadelphia, Lippincott-Raven, 1997, pp 783–800.

182. Bostrom MP, Lane JM: Future directions: Augmentation of osteoporotic vertebral bodies. Spine 22:38S–42S, 1997; erratum in Spine 23:1922, 1998.

183. Lane JM, Nydick M: Osteoporosis: Current modes of prevention and treatment. J Am Acad Orthop Surg 7:19–31, 1999.

184. Meunier PJ, Delmas PD, Eastell R, et al: Diagnosis and management of osteoporosis in postmenopausal women: Clinical guidelines. International Committee for Osteoporosis Clinical Guidelines. Clin Ther 21:1025–1044, 1999.

185. Tamayo-Orozco J, Arzac-Palumbo P, Peon-Vidales H, et al: Vertebral fractures associated with osteoporosis: Patient management. Am J Med 103:44S–48S, 1997.

186. Ryan MD, Taylor TK: Spinal manifestations of Paget's disease. Aust N Z J Surg 62:33–38, 1992.

187. Cuffe MJ, Hadley MN, Herrera GA, et al: Dialysis-associated spondylarthropathy: Report of 10 cases. J Neurosurg 80:694–700, 1994.

188. Salcman M, Khan A, Symonds DA: Calcium pyrophosphate arthropathy of the spine: Case report and review of the literature. Neurosurgery 34:915–918, 1994.

189. Tsuyama N: Ossification of the posterior longitudinal ligament of the spine. Clin Orthop 184:71–84, 1984.

190. Adams RD, Victor M, Ropper AH: The clinical method of neurology. In Adams RD, Victor M, Ropper AH (ed): Principles of Neurology, 6th ed. New York, McGraw-Hill, 1997, pp 3–40.

191. Miller DW, Hahn JF: General methods of clinical examination. In Youmans JR (ed): Neurological Surgery: A Comprehensive Reference Guide to the Diagnosis and Management of Neurosurgical Problems, 4th ed. Philadelphia, WB Saunders, 1996, pp 3–43.

192. Adams RD, Victor M, Ropper AH: Diseases of the spinal cord. In Adams RD, Victor M, Ropper AH (eds): Principles of Neurology, 6th ed. New York, McGraw-Hill, 1997, pp 1227–1277.

193. Anderson NE, Willoughby EW: Infarction of the conus medullaris. Ann Neurol 21:470–474, 1987.

194. Blumbergs PC, Byrne E: Hypotensive central infarction of the spinal cord. J Neurol Neurosurg Psychiatry 43:751–753, 1980.

195. Mikulis DJ, Ogilvy CS, McKee A, et al: Spinal cord infarction and fibrocartilaginous emboli. AJNR Am J Neuroradiol 13:155–160, 1992.

196. Shenaq SA, Svensson LG: Paraplegia following aortic surgery. J Cardiothorac Vasc Anesth 7:81–94, 1993.

197. Thompson PD: Paraplegia and quadriplegia. In Bradley WG, Daroff RB, Fenichel GM, et al (eds): Neurology in Clinical Practice, 2nd ed. Boston, Butterworth-Heinemann, 1996, pp 261–273.

198. Yoong MF, Blumbergs PC, North JB: Primary (granulomatous) angiitis of the central nervous system with multiple aneurysms of spinal arteries: Case report. J Neurosurg 79:603–607, 1993.

199. Anagnostopoulos DI, Gortvai P: Spontaneous spinal subdural haematoma. BMJ 1:30, 1972.

200. Bernsen RA, Hoogenraad TU: A spinal haematoma occurring in the subarachnoid as well as in the subdural space in a patient treated with anticoagulants. Clin Neurol Neurosurg 94:35–37, 1992.

201. Brandt RA: Chronic spinal subdural haematoma. Surg Neurol 13:121–123, 1980.

202. Brandt M: Spontaneous intramedullary haematoma as a complication of anticoagulant therapy. Acta Neurochir (Wien) 52:73–77, 1980.

203. Calhoun JM, Boop F: Spontaneous spinal subdural hematoma: Case report and review of the literature. Neurosurgery 29:133–134, 1991.

204. Constantini S, Ashkenazi E, Shoshan Y, et al: Thoracic hematomyelia secondary to Coumadin anticoagulant therapy: A case report. Eur Neurol 32:109–111, 1992.

205. Groen RJ, Ponssen H: The spontaneous spinal epidural hematoma: A study of the etiology. J Neurol Sci 98:121–138, 1990.

206. Kulali A, von Wild K, Hobik HP: Subarachnoid haemorrhage with acute cauda symptom due to spinal tumour. Neurochirurgia (Stuttg) 32:87–90, 1989.

207. Lonjon MM, Paquis P, Chanalet S, et al: Nontraumatic spinal epidural hematoma: Report of four cases and review of the literature. Neurosurgery 41:483–487, 1997.

208. Mattle H, Sieb JP, Rohner M, et al: Nontraumatic spinal epidural and subdural hematomas. Neurology 37:1351–1356, 1987.

209. Wisoff HS: Spontaneous intraspinal hemorrhage. In Wilkins RH, Rengachary SS (eds): Neurosurgery, 2nd ed. New York, McGraw-Hill, 1996, pp 2559–2565.

210. Wisoff JH, Rovit RL, Ho V, et al: Spontaneous hematomyelia secondary to factor XI deficiency: Case report. J Neurosurg 63:293–295, 1985.

211. Adams RD, Victor M, Ropper AH: Viral infections of the nervous system. In Adams RD, Victor M, Ropper AH (eds): Principles of Neurology, 6th ed. New York, McGraw-Hill, 1997, pp 742–776.

212. Chumakov M, Voroshilova M, Shindarov L, et al: Enterovirus 71 isolated from cases of epidemic poliomyelitis-like disease in Bulgaria. Arch Virol 60:329–340, 1979.

213. Ross MA: Acquired motor neuron diseases. Neurol Clin 15:481–500, 1997.

214. Shindarov LM, Chumakov MP, Voroshilova MK, et al: Epidemiological, clinical, and pathomorphological characteristics of epidemic poliomyelitis-like disease caused by enterovirus 71. J Hyg Epidemiol Microbiol Immunol 23:284–295, 1979.

215. Devinsky O, Cho ES, Petito CK, et al: Herpes zoster myelitis. Brain 114:1181–1196, 1991.

216. Arimura K, Rosales R, Osame M, et al: Clinical electrophysiologic studies of HTLV-I–associated myelopathy. Arch Neurol 44:609–612, 1987.

217. Jordan BD, Navia BA, Petito C, et al: Neurological syndromes complicating AIDS. Front Radiat Ther Oncol 19:82–87, 1985.

218. Kaplan JE, Osame M, Kubota H, et al: The risk of development of HTLV-I–associated myelopathy/tropical spastic paraparesis among persons infected with HTLV-I. J Acquir Immune Defic Syndr 3:1096–1101, 1990.

219. Osame M, Matsumoto M, Usuku K, et al: Chronic progressive myelopathy associated with elevated antibodies to human T-lymphotropic virus type I and adult T-cell leukemialike cells. Ann Neurol 21:117–122, 1987.

220. Petito CK, Navia BA, Cho ES, et al: Vacuolar myelopathy pathologically resembling subacute combined degeneration in patients with the acquired immunodeficiency syndrome. N Engl J Med 312:874–879, 1985.

221. Adams RD, Victor M, Ropper AH: Infections of the nervous system (bacterial, fungal, and spirochetal, parasitic) and sarcoid. In Adams RD, Victor M, Ropper AH (eds): Principles of Neurology, 6th ed. New York, McGraw-Hill, 1997, pp 695–741.

222. Centers for Disease Control: Epidemic early syphilis—Escambia County, Florida, 1987 and July 1989–June 1990. JAMA 265:2782, 1991.

223. Berenguer J, Moreno S, Laguna F, et al: Tuberculous meningitis in patients infected with the human immunodeficiency virus. N Engl J Med 326:668–672, 1992.

224. Chen RC, McLeod JG: Neurological complications of sarcoidosis. Clin Exp Neurol 26:99–112, 1989.

225. Chen RC, McLeod JG: Neurological complications of sarcoidosis [letter]. Med J Aust 156:815, 1992.

226. Kelley RE, Bell L, Kelley SE, et al: Syphilis detection in cerebrovascular disease. Stroke 20:230–234, 1989.

227. Pitchenik AE, Fertel D, Bloch AB: Mycobacterial disease: Epidemiology, diagnosis, treatment, and prevention. Clin Chest Med 9:425–441, 1988.

228. Walsh TJ, Hier DB, Caplan LR: Fungal infections of the central nervous system: Comparative analysis of risk factors and clinical signs in 57 patients. Neurology 35:1654–1657, 1985.

229. Cumming WJ: Myelitis and toxic, inflammatory and infectious disorders. Curr Opin Neurol Neurosurg 5:549–553, 1992.

230. Dawson DM, Potts F: Acute nontraumatic myelopathies. Neurol Clin 9:585–603, 1991.

231. Thomas M, Thomas J Jr: Acute transverse myelitis. J La State Med Soc 149:75–77, 1997.

232. Black MJ, Motaghedi B, Robitaille Y: Transverse myelitis. Laryngoscope 90:847–852, 1980.

233. Fenichel GM: Neurological complications of immunization. Ann Neurol 12:119–128, 1982.

234. Huang TY, Sileo DR, Huang JT, et al: MR imaging of acute transverse myelitis. J Ky Med Assoc 97:165–167, 1999.

235. Isoda H, Ramsey RG: MR imaging of acute transverse myelitis (myelopathy). Radiat Med 16:179–186, 1998.

236. McCarthy JT, Amer J: Postvaricella acute transverse myelitis: A case presentation and review of the literature. Pediatrics 62:202–204, 1978.

237. DeLara F, Tartaglino L, Friedman D: Spinal cord multiple sclerosis and Devic neuromyelitis optica in children. AJNR Am J Neuroradiol 16:1557–1558, 1995.

238. Sorensen TL, Ransohoff RM: Etiology and pathogenesis of multiple sclerosis. Semin Neurol 18:287–294, 1998.

239. Tartaglino LM, Friedman DP, Flanders AE, et al: Multiple sclerosis in the spinal cord: MR appearance and correlation with clinical parameters. Radiology 195:725–732, 1995.

240. Weinshenker BG: Epidemiology of multiple sclerosis. Neurol Clin 14:291–308, 1996.

241. Weinshenker BG, Issa M, Baskerville J: Long-term and short-term outcome of multiple sclerosis: A 3-year follow-up study. Arch Neurol 53:353–358, 1996.

242. Aillievi A, Tangari N, Ferro H, et al: Transverse myelitis and systemic lupus erythematosus: A case report [in Spanish]. Medicina (B Aires) 51:351–354, 1991.

243. Boumpas DT, Patronas NJ, Dalakas MC, et al: Acute transverse myelitis in systemic lupus erythematosus: Magnetic resonance imaging and review of the literature. J Rheumatol 17:89–92, 1990.

244. Heller L, Keren O, Mendelson L, et al: Transverse myelitis associated with *Mycoplasma pneumoniae*: Case report. Paraplegia 28:522–525, 1990.

245. Lyu RK, Chen ST, Tang LM, et al: Acute transverse myelopathy and cutaneous vasculopathy in primary Sjogren's syndrome. Eur Neurol 35:359–362, 1995.

246. Propper DJ, Bucknall RC: Acute transverse myelopathy complicating systemic lupus erythematosus. Ann Rheum Dis 48:512–515, 1989.

247. Park TS: Myelomeningocele. In Albright AL, Pollack IF, Adelson

PD (eds): Principles and Practice of Pediatric Neurosurgery. New York, Thieme, 1999, pp 291–320.

248. Iskander BJ, Oakes WJ: Occult spinal dysraphism. In Albright AL, Pollack IF, Adelson PD (eds): Principles and Practice of Pediatric Neurosurgery. New York, Thieme, 1999, pp 321–351.

249. Castillo M, Hankins L, Kramer L, et al: MR imaging of diplomyelia. Magn Reson Imaging 10:699–703, 1992.

250. Davidoff AM, Thompson CV, Grimm JM, et al: Occult spinal dysraphism in patients with anal agenesis. J Pediatr Surg 26:1001–1005, 1991.

251. Miller A, Guille JT, Bowen JR: Evaluation and treatment of diastematomyelia. J Bone Joint Surg Am 75:1308–1317, 1993.

252. Petersen MC: Tethered cord syndrome in myelodysplasia: Correlation between level of lesion and height at time of presentation. Dev Med Child Neurol 34:604–610, 1992.

253. Reigel DH, Mclone DG: Tethered spinal cord. In Cheek WR (ed): Pediatric Neurosurgery: Surgery of the Developing Nervous System, 3rd ed. Philadelphia, WB Saunders, 1994, pp 77–95.

254. Bradford DS: Congenital scoliosis. In Lonstein JE, Bradford DS, Winter RB, Ogilvie JW (eds): Moe's Textbook of Scoliosis and Other Spinal Deformities, 3rd ed. Philadelphia, WB Saunders, 1995, pp 369–386.

255. Anson JA, Batjer HH, Spetzler RF: Spinal dural vascular malformations. In Benzel EC (ed): Spine Surgery: Techniques, Complication Avoidance, and Management. New York, Churchill Livingstone, 1999, pp 643–650.

256. Kopitnik TA, Batjer HH, Anson JA: Spinal intradural vascular malformations. In Benzel EC (ed): Spine Surgery: Techniques, Complication Avoidance, and Management. New York, Churchill Livingstone, 1999, pp 635–642.

257. Oldfield EH: Spinal vascular malformations. In Wilkins RH, Rengachary SS (eds): Neurosurgery, 2nd ed. New York, McGraw-Hill, 1996, pp 2541–2558.

258. Rosenblum B, Oldfield EH, Doppman JL, et al: Spinal arteriovenous malformations: A comparison of dural arteriovenous fistulas and intradural AVMs in 81 patients. J Neurosurg 67:795–802, 1987.

259. Ogilvy CS, Louis DN, Ojemann RG: Intramedullary cavernous angiomas of the spinal cord: Clinical presentation, pathological features, and surgical management. Neurosurgery 31:219–229, 1992.

260. Stein BM, McCormick PC: Intramedullary neoplasms and vascular malformations. Clin Neurosurg 39:361–387, 1992.

261. Adams RD, Victor M, Ropper AH: Degenerative diseases of the nervous system. In Adams RD, Victor M, Ropper AH (eds): Principles of Neurology, 6th ed. New York, McGraw-Hill, 1997, pp 1046–1107.

262. Tandan R: Disorders of the upper and lower motor neurons. In Bradley WG, Daroff RB, Fenichel GM (eds): Neurology in Clinical Practice, 2nd ed. Boston, Butterworth-Heinemann, 1996, pp 1687–1717.

263. Fitzgerald RH Jr, Marks RD Jr, Wallace KM: Chronic radiation myelitis. Radiology 144:609–612, 1982.

264. Goldwein JW: Radiation myelopathy: A review. Med Pediatr Oncol 15:89–95, 1987.

265. Dalakas MC: The post-polio syndrome as an evolved clinical entity: Definition and clinical description. Ann N Y Acad Sci 753:68–80, 1995.

266. Brown RH Jr: Amyotrophic lateral sclerosis: Insights from genetics. Arch Neurol 54:1246–1250, 1997.

267. Jackson CE, Bryan WW: Amyotrophic lateral sclerosis. Semin Neurol 18:27–39, 1998.

268. Gates PC, Paris D, Forrest SM, et al: Friedreich's ataxia presenting as an adult-onset paraparesis. Neurogenetics 1:297–299, 1998.

269. Katsaros VK, Glocker FX, Hemmer B, et al: MRI of spinal cord and brain lesions in subacute combined degeneration. Neuroradiology 40:716–719, 1998.

270. Mancall E: Subacute combined degeneration of the spinal cord. In Rowland LP (ed): Merritt's Textbook of Neurology, 9th ed. Baltimore, Williams & Wilkins, 1995, pp 691–694.

271. Timms SR, Cure JK, Kurent JE: Subacute combined degeneration of the spinal cord: MR findings. AJNR Am J Neuroradiol 14:1224–1227, 1993.

272. Waragai M, Shinotoh H, Hayashi M, et al: High signal intensity on T1 weighted MRI of the anterolateral column of the spinal cord in amyotrophic lateral sclerosis. J Neurol Neurosurg Psychiatry 62:88–91, 1997.

273. Waragai M: MRI and clinical features in amyotrophic lateral sclerosis. Neuroradiology 39:847–851, 1997.

Evaluation and Management of the Failed Back Syndrome

GEORGE W. SYPERT ■ E. JOY ARPIN-SYPERT

Chronic low back pain disorders, which include the so-called failed back syndrome, are significant health problems for our society.[1] Available evidence suggests that more than 75% of the population in a modern industrial society such as North America will suffer at least temporary disability from lumbago or sciatica.[2] The prevalence is approximately 20%, indicating that at any time, one fifth of the adult population will complain about low back pain if asked.[3] According to U.S. health statistics, low back pain is the most common specific complaint generating visits to primary care physicians, and it ranks sixth in terms of hospital bed-days per year. Further, it appears that low back pain disorders are the most expensive illnesses affecting adults in the United States, being responsible for the loss of more than 200 million person-days of work each year. It has been estimated that there are in excess of 7 million new low back pain sufferers each year in the United States, on whom more than 200,000 original surgical procedures are performed. In addition, the incidence of reoperation for low back disorders is greater than 20%. The economic impact of benign low back pain disorders is staggering. In 1990, it was estimated that it cost $24 billion to treat these disorders, including hospitalization, professional fees, diagnostic tests, medications, therapeutic appliances, compensation payments, and litigation settlements, but excluding lost productivity.[4]

Although lesions related to the intervertebral lumbar disk are the most common identifiable causes of acute and chronic low back pain disorders, the principal sources of low back pain syndromes are traumatic and degenerative diseases of the soft tissues, that is, myofascial syndromes.[5, 6] Although chronic degenerative lesions of the lumbar disks and the intervertebral facet joints and ligaments may account for many cases of chronic low back pain disorders, in many patients the exact cause of the chronic pain disorder cannot be identified.[7] The clinical problem is further complicated by the observation that, by age 40 years, 40% of asymptomatic adults with no history of low back pain or leg pain demonstrate one or more herniated lumbar disks on high-resolution magnetic resonance imaging (MRI).

Further, high-resolution MRI demonstrates significant lumbar spinal stenosis in 60% of asymptomatic adults by age 60 years. Such clinical and anatomic imaging data make the evaluation and management of chronic low back pain disorders exceedingly difficult. It is our opinion that the majority of patients with chronic low back pain or failed back syndrome suffer principally from a combination of myofascial "frozen back syndrome," psychosocioeconomic factors, and erroneous original diagnosis complicated by inappropriate treatment, both nonsurgical and surgical.[8] Such patients seldom have clinical syndromes that will respond to additional surgical therapy, which should be considered only as a last resort. Despite the importance of benign, chronic low back pain disorders as a major health and socioeconomic problem, their natural histories have not been adequately studied, nor have the various forms of therapy been rigorously evaluated using modern scientific methodology.

The evaluation and treatment of chronic low back pain disorders are complex topics. These patients often suffer from psychosocioeconomic disorders that may not be manageable using available health care techniques. To address this multifactorial disorder, the reader requires an understanding of the relevant anatomy, pathology, clinical syndromes, and available treatment modalities.

ANATOMY AND PHYSIOLOGY

The anatomy of the lower back includes the lumbar spine, sacrum, sacroiliac articulations, coccyx, and associated joints, muscles, tendons, ligaments, and neural elements (cauda equina, individual nerve roots, and peripheral nerves innervating the low back structures). All these structures are capable of contributing to chronic low back pain disorders.

The intervertebral disk is a fibrocartilaginous remnant of the embryonic notochord. It consists of an ovoid, paracentrally located, gelatinous nucleus pulposus contained within the firm, concentric, collagenous fibrous tissue rings of the annulus fibrosus and the cartilaginous end plates of the vertebral body above and below. In childhood, the nucleus is a semigelatinous, amorphous intercellular material (mainly water and proteoglycans) with bundles of collagenous fibers. The disk is an amphiarthrodial joint that appears to function as a cushion between the vertebral bodies, counteracting the axial compressive forces of weight bearing and redistributing these forces evenly in all directions. The nucleus pulposus alters its shape freely under pressure, transmitting the forces radially to the annulus fibrosus and the cartilaginous end plates. The basis of the shape-altering property is the semifluid nature of the nucleus pulposus, which renders it essentially incompressible. A normal nucleus pulposus, which occupies about half the disk surface, bears most of the vertical load, whereas the annulus fibrosus bears most of the tangential load. These biomechanical functions of the disk depend on the water content of the nucleus, which gradually diminishes with age, decreasing from 88% at birth to 66% at age 70 years.

Lumbar intervertebral disks normally have greater height anteriorly than posteriorly, resulting in a backward tilt that forms the normal lordotic curve of the lumbar spine. The thick, lamellated, fibrous annulus is anchored mainly to the bony, marginal ridges at the periphery of the adjacent vertebral bodies and to the margins of the hyaline cartilaginous end plates.

The nucleus pulposus is supplied with blood vessels via small perforations in the central cartilaginous end plates. These vessels undergo progressive obliteration during the first 3 decades of life, after which nutrition of the nucleus is supported only by lymphatic channels and extracellular fluid circulation. It is possible that this loss of nutrient supply during maturation may contribute to the progressive desiccation, degeneration, and collapse of the disk that accompanies the aging process (spondylosis).

This brief introduction to the lumbar intervertebral disk brings up the opportunity to address the ill-conceived concept of so-called diskogenic pain. A number of clinical investigators have hypothesized that the nucleus pulpolsus contains "toxic" pain-generating substances that, when released by traumatic or degenerative tears of the annulus, cause acute and chronic low back pain disorders. The only rationale for such a concept is that it permits these clinicians to perform a variety of unproven and ineffective interventional therapies on patients suffering low back pain disorders. Annular tears with leakage of disk material occur in all adults, but the majority do not suffer incapacitating low back pain that requires treatment. Individuals suffer herniated intervertebral disks, including free fragments within the spinal canal that may produce neurological deficits such as footdrop, without experiencing significant back or leg pain. The vast majority of private patients who undergo lumbar diskectomy for a free-fragment disk herniation awake from surgery with complete relief of their radicular pain and minimal low back pain, despite the presence of a substantial hole in the annulus fibrosus that would permit continuous long-term leakage of any hypothetical toxic material from the remaining nucleus. Therefore, we must conclude that such a concept has no scientific or clinical merit. Justification for surgical management based on such a concept appears to contribute substantially to the problem of the failed back syndrome, or more specifically, the failed back surgery syndrome.

The posterior primary ramus innervates the vertebral and paravertebral osseomusculoligamentous structures of the adjacent vertebral segment. A major branch of the posterior primary ramus is the recurrent nerve of Luschka (sinuvertebral nerve), which enters the dorsal root just distal to the ganglion outside the foramen and receives sensory branches from the dura, posterior longitudinal ligament, facet joint capsule, erector spinae muscles, and annulus, but not the nucleus pulposus. Pressure applied to the lumbar disk either by palpation at surgery under local anesthesia or during diskography produces poorly localized, aching low back pain with segmental nonradicular pain radiation into the ipsilateral leg. Radicular leg pain (sciatica) appears to require injury or inflammation of the nerve root, ganglion, or sciatic nerve.

The lumbar spine is largely responsible for flexion and extension movements of the lower spine. In fact, the vast majority of lumbar flexion-extension movement occurs at the L4-5 and L5-S1 motion segments. Given these stresses, as well as their increased vertical loading, it is not surprising that about 90% of lumbar disk herniations occur at these two levels.

Finally, it should be recognized that the lumbar spine is made up of a series of vertebrae, each of which is linked to its neighbor anteriorly by an intervertebral disk and posteriorly by two facet joints. Owing to the rigidity of the vertebrae, changes in any one component of this three-joint complex will result in changes in the other two components, as they function in concert. Therefore, any pathology that involves the disk will affect the facet joints, and vice versa.

PATHOLOGY

Intervertebral disk degeneration begins at an early age and is a normal part of the aging process. The nucleus progressively loses its hydration and proteoglycan content, with a resulting loss of disk height and increase in collagen content, which is fibrillated and disorganized. These biomechanical changes lead to loss of the fluid gel behavior of the nucleus and deterioration of the mechanical properties of the annulus. Physical stresses and trauma (either acute-severe or chronic-repetitive) certainly accelerate and contribute substantially to this degenerative process. Small circumferential tears develop in the annulus that eventually coalesce to form large circumferential tears and radial tears. Axial and tangential forces placed on the nucleus are unevenly distributed to a weakened and inelastic annulus, such that bulging, prolapse, or herniation of the nucleus through the annulus may occur. Low back pain may or may not accompany this degenerative process. If herniation of the nucleus occurs and significantly compresses a nerve root, radicular pain may develop, often associated with a reduction in the preexisting low back pain.

The pathogenetic process of disk degeneration can be divided into three stages: nuclear degeneration, nuclear prolapse, and fibrosis. It should be kept in mind that any pathology affecting any one part of the three-joint complex constituting a vertebral motion segment will result in pathologic alterations in the other joints. Therefore, dysfunction of the intervertebral disk will lead to changes in the posterior facet joints. The sequence of these changes is similar to that seen in any synovial joint: synovitis, synovial tags in the joint, capsular tears, capsular laxity, degeneration of the articular cartilage, and formation of osteophytes. Biomechanically, the pathologic processes involved in disk degeneration (spondylosis) can be divided into three stages[8]: dysfunctional stage (traumatic tears of the annulus and internal disruption of the nucleus), unstable stage (disk and facet degeneration and capsule laxity), and restabilization stage (disk collapse and fibrosis and osteophyte formation, producing a stiff motion segment). Interestingly, many individuals undergo this process and develop a severely degenerated spine without ever complaining of back pain or seeking medical attention. Moreover, in many patients with acute, severe low back pain disorders, symptoms frequently regress over time without any specific medical therapy.

Concurrent with the pathologic disk alterations, including loss of disk height and bulging of the annulus, there is progressive osteophyte formation (bone callus), degeneration and hypertrophy of the articular facets and ligaments, and overriding of the facets, all of which may contribute to nerve root compression syndromes (lateral and central spinal stenosis). Further, congenital anomalies such as a narrow spinal canal, malformed facet joints, or isthmic spondylolisthesis may contribute significantly to the development of neural compression or instability syndromes. Knowledge of the anatomy, physiology, and normal pathologic evolution, as well as their protean variations, is critical to an understanding of the wide spectrum of clinical syndromes causally related to benign acute and chronic low back pain disorders, including the role of interventional surgical management.

CLINICAL SYNDROMES

Lumbago (low back pain) and sciatica (radicular leg pain) are merely descriptions of symptom complexes. Low back pain of spinal origin may result from numerous pathologic conditions other than disease of the intervertebral disk. Similarly, sciatica may be caused by a variety of pathologic entities such as lumbar radiculopathy and radiculitis, lumbosacral plexopathy and plexitis, and sciatic entrapment syndromes. In addition to nerve root compression (e.g., herniated lumbar disk, spinal stenosis, vertebral fracture), lumbar radiculopathy may be caused by intraneural pathologic changes related to temporary or permanent neural injury from a neural compressive lesion or surgery, arachnoiditis, and perineural fibrosis, to mention only

a few. Finally, it must be recognized that a variety of pathologic conditions affecting low back structures can cause pain that is segmentally referred down the lower extremity. This form of pain is often misinterpreted by naive or inexperienced clinicians as radiculopathic pain. One of the most common sources of these symptoms in a failed back patient is the frozen back syndrome, which may occur with or without surgery due to soft tissue contractures related to protective immobilization of the injured lumbar spine's soft tissue structures (i.e., disks, facet joints and capsules, ligaments, muscles). Although lumbago and sciatica are frequently related to lumbar disk diseases, they are complex pain syndromes caused by a wide variety of pathologic conditions, some of which remain to be elucidated.

The clinical investigation of chronic low back pain disorders is usually complicated by psychological, social, and economic factors. Despite the development of numerous highly sophisticated diagnostic technologies (e.g., computed tomography [CT], myelography, MRI) that have contributed substantially to our understanding of low back pain disorders, it is often difficult even for experienced neurosurgeons to accurately diagnose the specific cause of low back or leg pain. Moreover, decision making regarding treatment is confounded by any prior surgical therapy. Consistent with our clinical observations of patients suffering from failed back surgery syndrome, review of the original records and neurodiagnostic imaging studies in the majority of such patients fails to demonstrate appropriate indications for the original surgical procedure.[10]

The preceding discussion suggests that decision making regarding the management of benign chronic low back pain disorders, particularly reoperative treatment, is difficult and will remain so until further knowledge of the pathogenetic factors involved and the natural history is obtained. At present, the indications for surgical treatment are limited to these five objectives: (1) decompression of compressed neural elements (i.e., cauda equina or nerve roots), (2) stabilization-arthrodesis of vertebral motion segments, (3) destruction of neural elements thought to be involved in the pathogenesis of pain, (4) electrical stimulation of neural structures to reduce the perception of pain, and (5) long-term intrathecal analgesia therapy. The generally accepted primary indication for surgical treatment of benign lumbar spine disorders is relief of persistent or recurrent neural compression. Therefore, lumbar spine surgery is most commonly directed toward the restoration of nerve root or cauda equina function or the relief of intractable nerve root compression pain (neural compression syndrome). A second major indication for lumbar spine surgery is the relief of carefully documented intractable and incapacitating "mechanical" low back pain disorders (instability syndrome) by way of a stabilization-arthrodesis procedure.[11, 12] It is our opinion that objectives (3), (4), and (5) are largely investigational at this time and should be reserved for patients suffering neuropathic pain syndromes related to irreversible neural injury.

To facilitate decision making regarding low back

TABLE 283–1 ■ **Classification of Spinal Pain Disorders**[9]

Myofascial syndrome
Neural compression syndrome
Mechanical (instability) syndrome
Inflammatory syndrome
Neuropathic syndrome
Psychosocioeconomic syndrome

pain disorders, we have found it useful to classify a patient's principal complaint of pain of lumbar spine origin into one or more of six general categories (Table 283–1). This presumes that the clinician has ruled out low back pain related to metabolic, nondegenerative, and extraspinal disease. Although such a classification scheme may appear simplistic, it is consistent with available knowledge regarding the pathogenesis of axial spinal pain and nerve root pain. In addition, this categorical scheme has proved helpful in educating patients, neurosurgical residents, fellows, colleagues, and referring physicians regarding diseases affecting the spine and their management, as well as in substantially reducing the application of unnecessary diagnostic and interventional therapy.

Myofascial Syndrome

The cause of low back and leg pain in the vast majority of patients is unknown. Some assume that the basic problem is degeneration of the lumbar disks, but this is an unproven and highly suspect hypothesis. The source of both low back and leg pain is most likely irritation or injury of musculoligamentous soft tissue structures innervated by the posterior primary ramus of the exiting spinal nerve, with pain being referred to the ipsilateral extremity. Most patients have a history of trauma or prior surgery and complain of low back pain with diffuse, nonspecific hip, groin, and leg pain radiation. Although the pain often follows the proximal course of the sciatic nerve, unlike with true sciatica, its termination and associated symptoms, such as appropriate sensory loss and paresthesias, are generally vague, histrionic, and nondermatomal. Moreover, objective neurological findings are typically absent unless there has been a prior nerve root injury.

The symptoms are usually worsened by activity and improved partially by rest, though in some patients this is reversed. Often these latter patients are worse in the morning and evening, with transient improvement during mild physical activity such as stretching and walking. Vigorous physical activity, particularly bending, twisting, and lifting, commonly aggravates the symptoms, whereas restriction of pain-producing activities results in improvement at least temporarily. Typical physical findings are nonspecific, including restricted range of motion of the spine, tight hamstring muscles, paravertebral muscle spasms, muscular trigger points, tenderness, and aggravation of symptoms on forward flexion and straight leg raising tests. In fact, the greater the restriction of range of motion,

the greater the complaints (frozen back syndrome). Objective reflex and neurologically appropriate motor and sensory alterations are usually not present.

Included in this category are patients who are subclassified by some specialists as having ill-defined lumbar facet and piriform syndromes. It is important that this group of patients be recognized and treated appropriately. Surgical therapy inflicts additional soft tissue injury, aggravating the primary condition. These patients, if compliant, do quite well with intensive rehabilitation programs directed at restoring full range of motion to the lumbar spine and hip regions. Such patients must accept the concept of "no pain, no gain." In other words, the patient will have to undergo pain-inducing reconditioning to achieve long-term functional pain reduction. In fact, as soon as full range of motion of the lumbar spine and hip soft tissues is restored, most symptoms resolve. These patients must be educated and treated with understanding and compassion. However, if the patient is noncompliant, further treatment should be limited, because it will only aggravate the disorder, particularly ineffectual surgical therapy.

Neural Compression Syndrome

Given the incidence and magnitude of complaints of chronic pain due to benign low back disorders, and the fact that neural compression syndromes are relatively infrequent, it is important that an accurate diagnosis be made and appropriate therapy applied, so that a serious problem does not go unrecognized. It is also important to understand that the vast majority of chronic low back pain disorders, including those following lumbar spine surgery, are benign and that they can generally be managed nonsurgically. The two most common benign lumbar spine disorders causing neural compression syndromes are herniated lumbar disk and lumbar spondylotic spinal stenosis.

An acute lumbar disk herniation with nerve root compression is usually a reasonably straightforward clinical syndrome and is not difficult to diagnose and treat appropriately. In patients suffering from chronic low back pain disorders, however, the situation is more complex. These patients usually complain of progressively worsening low back and leg pain, and they generally have a long history of back and leg pain following extensive therapy programs, often including multiple operations on the lumbar spine.[10, 12–15] Recurrent disk herniation or a secondary disk herniation at a different level is always possible. Sometimes the neural compression syndrome is clinically clear-cut, and the symptoms indicate the acute onset of a new syndrome. Because new symptoms are superimposed on old symptoms and signs, however, it is frequently difficult to separate them, especially in previously operated patients. Fortunately, modern high-resolution MRI with and without contrast enhancement is usually diagnostic, and appropriate microsurgical excision of the herniated disk fragment usually ameliorates the new symptoms.

Inadequately decompressed lateral spinal stenosis[16]

or acquired central and lateral spinal stenosis may contribute to the disability of patients with chronic low back pain disorders. The symptoms and signs are clinically much more difficult to differentiate in these patients than in those who present with lumbar spinal stenosis syndromes as the primary problem. Modern high-resolution MRI (with and without contrast enhancement in a previously operated patient) or high-resolution CT–myelography (in MRI-incompatible patients) is generally diagnostic of anatomic neural compression in these patients. Appropriate and adequate microsurgical decompression of the neural elements generally results in substantial relief of the symptoms caused by the neural compressive process, particularly when combined with a low back rehabilitation program.[8, 13]

Mechanical (Instability) Syndrome

Mechanical pain syndrome, due to instability of a lumbar spine motion segment, consists of low back pain or segmental leg pain generated by weight bearing and stress applied to the lumbar spine motion segments. In a failed back patient, prior decompressive surgery that severely disrupts the function of a lumbar motion segment may cause this syndrome. Typically, such patients complain of pain that is aggravated by weight bearing, bending, twisting, lifting, and other activities that mechanically stress the lumbar spine. These patients usually obtain nearly complete relief of symptoms from recumbency, when the spinal motion segments are not under stress. Unless there is a concomitant neural compressive lesion or previous neurological injury, objective neurological findings are absent. The diagnosis cannot reliably be made in patients with a limited range of motion of the lumbar spine, because all their symptoms could be due to a frozen back and myofascial disease. Therefore, these patients should undergo an intensive rehabilitation program with full restitution of range of motion, if possible, before entertaining the diagnosis of mechanical lumbar instability. It is our observation that when restitution of range of motion is achieved, most patients achieve relief of symptoms and do not experience a residual mechanical instability syndrome. A clinical trial in an appropriate lumbar orthosis used to reduce forces acting on the lumbar spine may play an adjunctive role in the symptomatic determination of mechanical pain.[11] It must be recognized that the only orthotic device that offers significant immobilization of the L4-5 and L5-S1 motion segments is a well-fitted "walking spica" that incorporates one thigh.[17] In fact, other orthotic devices designed for the lumbar spinal region may aggravate motion or stress of the lower lumbar region in certain circumstances.

The diagnosis of mechanical instability syndrome is solely clinical.[11, 12] Imaging studies have no role in the diagnosis except as an aid in localizing the lumbar motion segments that are producing the clinical symptoms. The neurodiagnostic imaging signs that can help localize the unstable motion segments and guide the neurosurgeon in deciding which levels to fuse include the following: spondylolisthesis, olisthesis, retrolisthesis, excessive motion on dynamic flexion-extension (rare), vacuum disk, disk arthropathy, vacuum facet, facet arthropathy, facet synovial cysts, and previously operated segments. In our opinion, diskography has no place in determining either the indications for stabilization or which segments to stabilize. However, like asymptomatic individuals with lumbar disk herniation and spinal stenosis on imaging studies, there are many individuals with imaging abnormalities consistent with instability of the lumbar spine who do not have clinical symptoms referable to those abnormalities. In patients with a true intractable and incapacitating clinical mechanical instability syndrome, including those with the failed back syndrome, appropriate surgical stabilization-arthrodesis can be gratifying.

Inflammatory Syndrome

Inflammatory syndromes are lumbar spine disorders related to inflammatory diseases such as diskitis, osteomyelitis, and ankylosing spondylitis, which are beyond the scope of this chapter. Generally, appropriate treatment of the primary diagnosis and adequate management of any associated neural compressive and mechanical instability syndrome will yield a satisfactory result.[18]

Neuropathic Syndrome

Neuropathic syndrome refers to pain of neural origin, that is, pain "wired" into the brain, spinal cord, nerve roots, or peripheral nerves, which generally follows permanent injury to these neural structures. Typically, such patients complain of constant burning, dysesthetic pain corresponding to an area of sensory loss. Unfortunately, with respect to the failed back syndrome patient, the principal cause of lumbar neuropathic syndrome appears to be iatrogenic—nerve root injury during surgery or other invasive interventional therapy. Additional causes include neural injury due to nerve root compression from herniated lumbar disk and spinal stenosis; adhesive arachnoiditis; lumbosacral plexus, femoral plexus, and sciatic nerve stretch injury; retroperitoneal or pelvic surgical injuries; and injection injuries. Recognition of this syndrome is essential if additional unsuccessful surgery is to be prevented, which in these patients carries a substantial risk of aggravating the clinical syndrome. The primary management is appropriate psychotropic, antidepressive, nonaddicting medications supplemented by psychological support under the direction of an experienced clinician familiar with the management of chronic benign pain syndromes. Based on personal experience and review of available clinical data, we believe that the neuroablative and so-called neuroaugmentative interventional therapies play a somewhat limited and investigational role in the management of neuropathic syndrome. Treating these unfortunate patients suffering intractable chronic pain syndromes with intraspinal narcotic infusion therapy is not rational and is ill advised.

Psychosocioeconomic Syndrome

Psychological, social, and economic factors operate in all patients who suffer intractable chronic pain. These factors are especially important in patients suffering from the failed back syndrome.[7, 10, 13–15, 19] Even the most stoic and highly motivated patient suffers some degree of psychological stress, fear, and depression related to the pain and associated impairment. These factors must be recognized early and addressed appropriately if one is to manage the problem successfully. Patient education regarding the cause of the pain and the role of psychosocioeconomic syndrome in the patient's disability and perception of pain is essential. Early on, the patient must be reassured and accept that permanent harm (i.e., irreversible loss of neurological function) is exceedingly rare and is not a significant consequence of an intensive low back rehabilitation program.

Among patients suffering from chronic low back pain disorders, those with myofascial syndromes tend to report higher levels of pain and are less likely to report periods of reduced pain than are those with structural neural compressive syndromes and instability syndromes.[14] In fact, most patients with chronic low back pain disorders should be categorized as myofascial when a pathoanatomic cause is not apparent.

Depression and somatization play a prominent role in chronic low back pain disorders and require appropriate therapy.[7, 10, 14] The most common psychological problem that seriously limits and complicates the successful management of these patients is personality dysfunction. More than 50% of the patients referred to a tertiary chronic pain treatment program suffered a significant personality dysfunction at some time.[10] Such patients have problems in virtually every sphere of living, making successful management very difficult even when these individuals have a pathoanatomically correctable problem.

Numerous studies have confirmed the observation that patients with chronic low back pain disorders who receive workers' compensation benefits or are involved in ongoing litigation tend to report more total pain, more severe disability, and more psychological distress than those who are not involved in such issues.[10, 14] Further, these socioeconomic issues negatively influence treatment outcome. In approaching such patients, the clinician must be aware of these problems and address them accordingly. When socioeconomic factors are important and are combined with a dysfunctional personality disorder, the likelihood of a successful management program is small.

CLINICAL EVALUATION

History and Physical Examination

A detailed history is essential in the evaluation of a patient suffering from a chronic low back pain disorder. Those patients who may benefit from surgical management usually have a history of neural compressive pain (clear-cut radicular pain, spinal claudication) or symptomatic mechanical instability pain.[5, 20, 21] Some aspects of the patient's history influence management decisions irrespective of the specific pathology or cause of pain. Many patients with chronic, intractable low back pain are incapacitated by personality dysfunction and psychosocioeconomic factors.[10, 13, 14] The patient's complaint of pain and pain behavior should correlate with demonstrated pathology and degree of physical impairment. Exaggerated and histrionic behavior is almost always related to psychosocioeconomic syndrome. A history of alcohol and substance abuse requires specific interventions and medications. Symptoms such as sleep disturbance, suicidal ideation, appetite disturbance, and irritability may indicate a significant depressive reaction that requires psychiatric therapy.

A complete general physical and neurological examination is requisite. During the musculoskeletal examination, particular attention should be given to range of motion of the lumbar spine, straight leg raising tests, and examination of the hips. Any neurological impairments must be documented, and an attempt should be made to determine when they occurred and whether such deficits are static or progressive, based on the patient's history and a review of medical records. During the history and physical examination, the clinician should carefully observe the patient for inconsistencies, exaggeration of impairment, histrionic behavior, and inappropriate signs. Waddell and colleagues[22] proposed five categories of inappropriate signs that correlated with psychosocioeconomic syndrome being a major contributor to a patient's low back pain disorder. These are (1) inappropriate tenderness that is superficial or widespread; (2) pain on simulated axial loading (performed by pressing on the top of the head) or simulated spine rotation (performed by holding the patient's arms to the side while rotating the hips, ensuring that the shoulders and hips rotate together); (3) distraction signs, such as inconsistent performance between straight leg raising in the seated position versus the supine position; (4) regional disturbances in strength and sensation that do not correspond to nerve root innervation patterns; and (5) overreaction during the physical examination. Positive findings in three of the five categories are indicative of substantial psychosocioeconomic syndrome.

All available medical records, operative reports, and neurodiagnostic imaging studies should be reviewed before ordering new diagnostic tests. If the original preoperative neurodiagnostic imaging studies failed to reveal a surgically treatable process, it is unlikely that surgery to correct the original inappropriate surgery will be beneficial. Further, the most recent neurodiagnostic imaging studies may be sufficient to complete the assessment and arrive at an accurate diagnosis and an appropriate treatment program.

After developing a working diagnosis based on a complete history, physical and neurological examinations, and review of preexisting medical records and neurodiagnostic studies, the clinician begins the secondary stage of diagnostic assessment to clarify the diagnosis. This is essential to developing an outline for an appropriate therapeutic regimen. In most cases, secondary assessment is straightforward, requiring specific high-quality neurodiagnostic spinal imaging tests.[23] Only in exceptional cases is it necessary to order additional tests, which generally yield little useful information and may further confound the problem.

Spinal Imaging

Conventional radiographic imaging is essential to an appropriate diagnosis. A lumbar spine radiographic series should include a weight-bearing anteroposterior view and lateral flexion-neutral-extension views (see Fig. 283–7). Oblique views have little diagnostic or therapeutic value and should not be routinely ordered. These images can exclude the presence of disease processes other than those related to the intervertebral disk, spondylosis, or trauma. The degree of disk degeneration or instability (vacuum disk, disk arthropathy), facet arthropathy, spondylolisthesis, olisthesis, retrolisthesis, scoliosis, transitional vertebra, and abnormal translational movement can be assessed on lumbar radiographs. It must be re-emphasized that such changes do not necessarily indicate the site of origin of the patient's symptoms.

High-quality, high-resolution MRI is the other essential imaging study. It permits excellent assessment of the lumbar disks, nerves, nerve roots, and all the soft tissues. With contrast enhancement, recurrent disk herniation can generally be differentiated from epidural fibrosis in a previously operated spine (Figs. 283–1 and 283–2). We have found that the bony anatomy and neural foramina can be examined in equal or greater detail with high-resolution MRI (Figs. 283–1 to 283–4) than can be achieved with high-resolution CT, including three-dimensional CT reconstruction. In addition, advanced MRI may be used to assess chronic microinstability of the lumbar motion segments. MRI evidence of segmental instability includes severe destruction of the intervertebral disks and associated end plates, reactive vertebral bone changes adjacent to the intervertebral disk (hypointense on T1 and hyperintense on T2), and marked facet arthropathy (Fig. 283–5). Myelography is seldom necessary unless combined with CT. CT–myelography is occasionally required for patients in whom satisfactory MRI cannot be accomplished. CT–myelography also allows excellent assessment of the cauda equina, the presence or absence of nerve root compression, and the relationship of the nerve roots to the lateral recesses, neural foramina, and disks. Both high-resolution MRI and CT–myelography can be used to image far-lateral disk herniations. However, CT–myelography has not proved useful in differentiating recurrent herniated lumbar disk and postoperative epidural or perineural fibrosis. Given the diagnostic accuracy of high-resolution MRI, the role of CT, CT–myelography, and bone scanning should be very limited, in an effort to reduce the substantial cost of diagnostic imaging in patients with persistent low back pain disorders.[24]

The patient's history, behavior, physical and neuro-

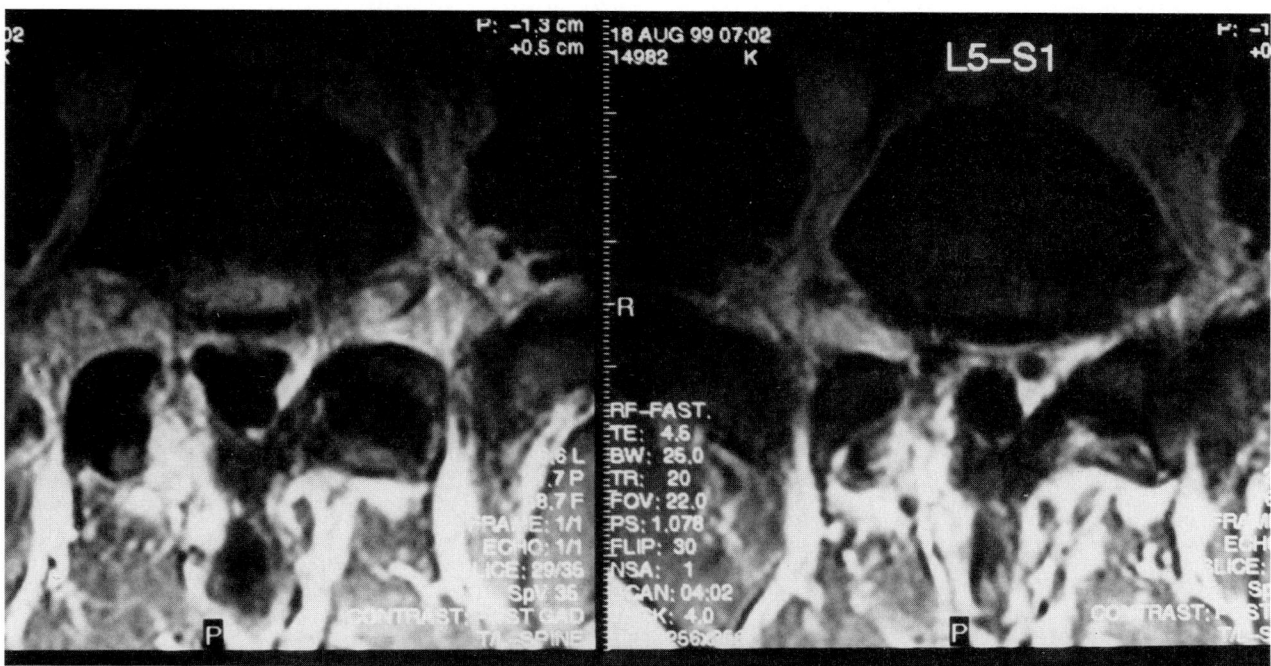

FIGURE 283–1. Magnetic resonance imaging (MRI) scan of a 36-year-old man—an unemployed construction worker receiving workers' compensation—who had two lumbar L5-S1 decompressive diskectomies with the persistent complaint of right low back and leg pain. The only objective finding on physical and neurological examination was exaggerated pain behavior. *Left,* Unenhanced axial MRI at L5-S1. *Right,* Enhanced axial MRI at L5-S1. Note the absence of neural compression and the presence of enhancing epidural fibrosis. Interestingly, the patient's pain resolved, and he returned to full-time work after settlement of the workers' compensation claim.

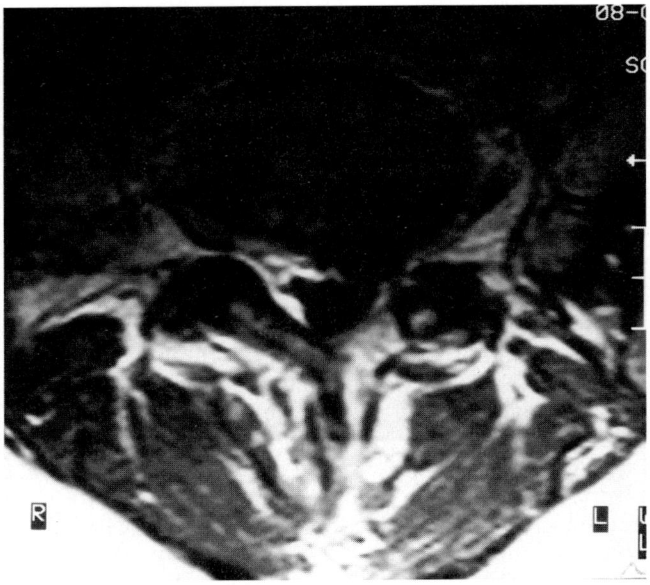

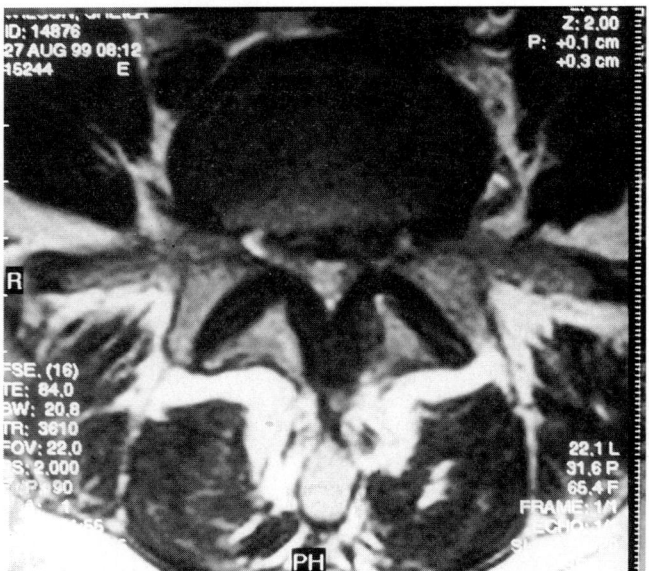

FIGURE 283–2. Magnetic resonance imaging scan of a 34-year-old female schoolteacher who suffered recurrent intractable left sciatica following three left L5-S1 decompressive diskectomies for free-fragment disk herniations. Physical and neurological examinations were consistent with a classic L5-S1 lumbar disk herniation syndrome, with pain behavior appropriate to her complaints and the clinical findings. On the contrast-enhanced T1-weighted scan, note the presence of a large, nonenhancing, ventral epidural mass lesion at L5-S1 on the left, consistent with a recurrent free-fragment disk herniation. Following microsurgical re-exploration and excision of the recurrent free-fragment herniated disk and arthrodesis, the patient's symptoms resolved, and she returned to work full-time.

FIGURE 283–3. Magnetic resonance imaging scan of a 77-year-old man with persistent intractable spinal claudication following lumbar decompression for spinal stenosis. Axial T2-weighted scan at L3-4 shows the rather severe, persistent neural compression from inadequate decompression of the patient's spondylotic spinal stenosis. Following bilateral microsurgical decompression at L3-4, the patient has been asymptomatic and has returned to playing golf 4 days a week.

logical examinations, and neurodiagnostic spinal imaging should all correlate. However, the weight given to anatomic imaging data requires careful assessment and excellent judgment. Clinicians must always keep in mind that they are treating patients, not images. The anatomic abnormalities found on these images may be asymptomatic and may not correlate with the clinical data, and their discovery does not necessarily constitute a rationale for a surgical or interventional procedure. Relevant anatomic abnormalities must be consistent with the patient's description of neural compressive or mechanical pain and the carefully observed impairments.

Neurodiagnostic Testing

Electrodiagnostic testing (electromyography, nerve conduction velocities, and spinal evoked potentials) and thermography have little role in the evaluation of spinal pain disorders. The use of electrodiagnostic testing should be limited to those few patients in whom the differential diagnosis is between a cauda equina syndrome and peripheral neuropathy and when it is necessary to elucidate a peripheral nerve entrapment syndrome. Thermography may occasionally be useful in the rare patient who develops a secondary reflex sympathetic dystrophy. Hence, these studies add little worthwhile information beyond that obtained by a thorough history and physical and neurological examinations and add substantially to the cost.

Physiologic Testing

Recently, there has been a strong resurgence of interest in provocative (diskography) and pain-relieving tests, largely by our colleagues performing orthopedic spinal surgery. Despite the fact that provocative lumbar diskography has been used for at least 3 decades, there is no scientifically credible evidence that this examination is diagnostic of the specific source of pain generation, reliable, or predictive of a response to therapy. Similarly, temporary local anesthetic blockade (e.g., zygopophyseal joint blockade, the so-called facet block) to assess the contribution of suspected spinal structures to low back pain disorders has not been demonstrated to have reliability, diagnostic specificity, or predictive value. Selective nerve root blocks and differential spinal anesthesia also remain unproved, unreliable adjuncts in the evaluation and management of patients with either acute or chronic low back pain disorders. Based on available studies, it is our opinion that these so-called physiologic tests generate unnecessary interventional procedures and add significantly to the economic impact of low back pain disorders.

Psychological, Social, and Economic Testing

Formal psychological testing such as the Minnesota Multiphasic Personality Inventory is impractical outside of an investigational setting. Moreover, there are

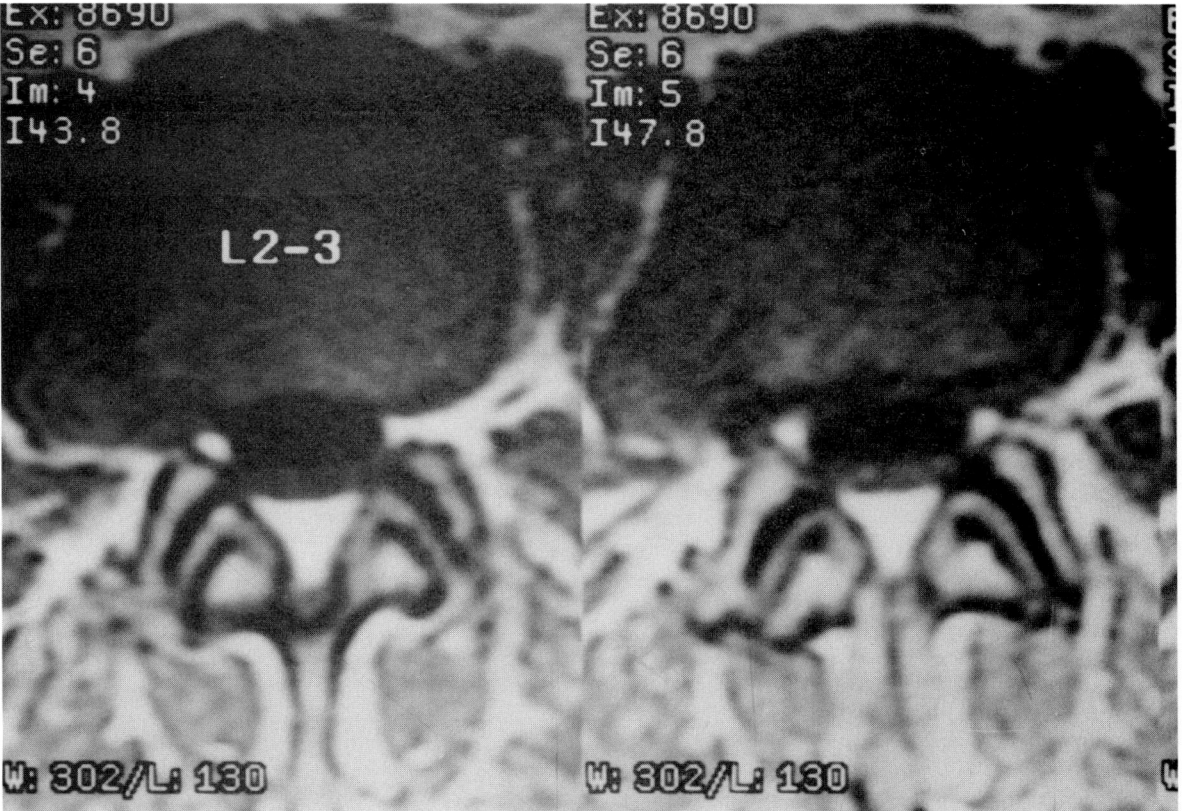

FIGURE 283–4. Adjacent axial T1-weighted magnetic resonance imaging scan at L2-3 in a 48-year-old man with persistent right anterior thigh radicular pain associated with weak quadriceps muscle and absent knee reflex following two right lumbar diskectomies at L4-5 performed for "bulging" disks. Note the large, right-sided far-lateral disk herniation. The patient became asymptomatic immediately after microsurgical excision of this far-lateral disk herniation.

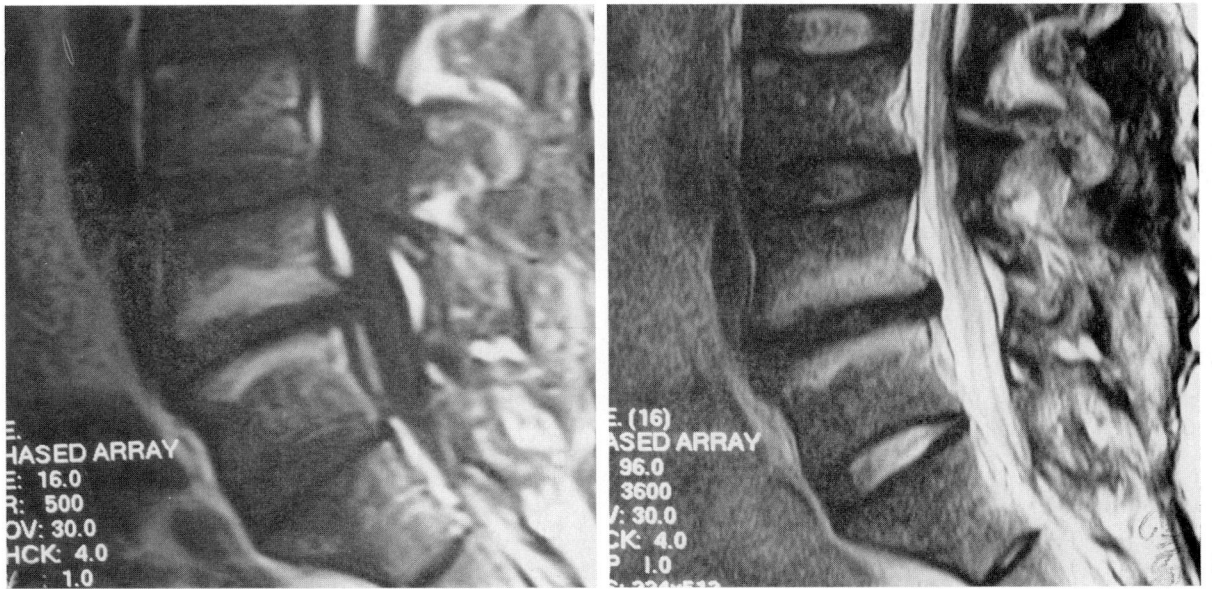

FIGURE 283–5. Sagittal T1-weighted *(A)* and T2-weighted *(B)* magnetic resonance imaging scans in a 38-year-old woman suffering 5 years of intractable and incapacitating "mechanical" low back pain despite extensive therapies. Note the hyperintense signal change adjacent to the L4-5 disk space, consistent with chronic microinstability. (Some patients demonstrate hypointensity on T1.)

no rigorous data indicating that these methods add any useful information beyond what an experienced clinician can obtain with an adequate history and physical and neurological examinations, supplemented by patient interaction after the initial visit. Therefore, we do not routinely use these examinations in the evaluation and management of chronic low back pain disorders. Patients who demonstrate significant psychosocial pathology are referred to a psychiatrist who is experienced in the evaluation and treatment of chronic benign pain syndromes complicated by psychosocioeconomic syndrome.

THERAPY

Having completed a comprehensive evaluation of the patient and arrived at a diagnosis of the cause of the patient's complaints, it should be possible to make rational decisions regarding appropriate management. Regardless of the specific diagnosis, all chronic low back pain patients require a rehabilitation program. If possible, the rehabilitation program should be the initial therapeutic approach in an attempt to avoid surgery. However, certain issues need to be addressed early if an appropriate and effective treatment program is to be developed. The treating neurosurgeon must determine whether there is a lumbar spine condition for which only surgical management will be effective. Obviously, the rare patient suffering loss of nerve root or cauda equina function due to a significant neural compressive process demands reasonably urgent microneurosurgical decompression to preserve function. The vast majority of these patients, however, are at essentially no risk of loss of neurological function.

There are only two clinical-anatomic conditions that demand early surgical intervention because a rehabilitative program would be ineffective without correction of the anatomic abnormality. The first is a neural compressive process such as severe spinal stenosis with intractable neurogenic claudication that cannot be effectively treated without adequate neural decompressive surgery. The second is overt, intractable, and incapacitating lumbar segmental instability. Although the use of an appropriate orthotic appliance may palliate symptoms temporarily, only surgical stabilization will correct the problem. In these circumstances, there is no benefit in delaying surgical management.

Rehabilitation

Ideally, the rehabilitation program should be initiated early in a vigorous attempt to avoid surgery. In fact, the principal diagnosis in the majority of these patients is a myofascial syndrome with a frozen back complicated by psychosocioeconomic syndrome. Under no circumstance would surgical therapy be appropriate for these patients; the only appropriate treatment in the majority is rehabilitation.

The rehabilitation program must be individualized to the patient. It must include a comprehensive approach that covers the major impairments that many of these patients develop, particularly psychosocioeconomic syndrome. Before initiating any program, it is essential that the patient be fully educated regarding the cause of his or her pain, including the role of any psychosocioeconomic issues; the rationale of appropriate therapy; and the importance of complying with and accepting personal responsibility for rehabilitation. Fundamental to the program is painful, intensive physical conditioning with restitution of muscle tone and full range of motion of the lumbar and hip regions.[25] In some patients, a progressive, professionally guided exercise program may be necessary.[13] Accompanying such a program must be a home program for which the patient is personally responsible. We believe that such a home program should be simple and should include uninterrupted walking for at least 2 miles per day and stretching exercises. The patient must be instructed that the personal home program is a lifetime commitment to prevent recurrence of the low back pain disorder.

Depression and anxiety must be treated, and drug abuse corrected. The use of all depressant, addictive medications must be curtailed. If drug-seeking behavior is serious, the patient should undergo a detoxification program before the rehabilitation program is initiated.

Pharmacologic Management

Pharmacologic management of the failed back syndrome poses a challenge. Although a number of different drug classes have been used, most have not been extensively evaluated in controlled clinical trials in patients with chronic low back pain disorders. Acetaminophen appears to be a reasonably safe analgesic for patients with mild chronic back pain. Nonsteroidal anti-inflammatory drugs (NSAIDs) are indicated for mild to moderate inflammatory pain, but there are significant toxicity concerns, especially in the elderly and in those with comorbid conditions. Although the role of inflammation in chronic low back pain remains undefined, NSAIDs are the most frequently prescribed medication for back pain. Tramadol hydrochloride (Ultram) is an effective analgesic for moderate to moderately severe chronic low back pain. It has a low abuse potential and a favorable safety profile. However, tramadol should not be used in patients who have a history of opioid dependence. Narcotic analgesics are indicated for severe acute pain, but their long-term use in chronic pain disorders such as the failed back syndrome is limited because of concerns about safety, depression, and abuse potential. Although narcotic analgesics have been reported to be effective in treating chronic low back pain disorders, their efficacy relative to other medications has not been evaluated in controlled clinical trials. Therefore, extended use of narcotic analgesics should be rigorously controlled and reserved for patients with severe pain that significantly compromises function and is resistant to other treatments.

Additional medications that have been used to treat chronic low back pain disorders include muscle relaxants, antidepressant medications, and anticonvulsants. Muscle relaxants have a limited role in the treatment of chronic low back pain disorders because spasm is an unlikely source of chronic pain. Moreover, these drugs produce undesirable effects, notably drowsiness and depression, which can aggravate the chronic pain syndrome. Tricyclic antidepressants are useful in patients with failed back syndrome who are clinically depressed. In such patients, amitriptyline, 150 mg daily, should reduce depressive symptoms and may decrease low back pain as well. The value of tricyclic antidepressants in nondepressed patients remains debatable. In some patients, low doses of tricyclic antidepressant agents may be effective as an adjunct to analgesic medications. Anticonvulsant medications such as gabapentin (Neurontin) may be useful in some patients suffering neuropathic pain syndromes.

Psychological, Social, and Economic Management

Psychiatric and psychosocioeconomic disorders require identification and treatment. Although most patients are very resistant to the concept that their psychological status may play a significant role in their perception of pain, they must be educated and their psychological dysfunction treated. Substantial psychological dysfunction severely limits the patient's ability to cope with and effectively participate in the rehabilitation process. Destructive pain behavior requires individualized psychotherapeutic management as part of the overall rehabilitation effort. In general, the so-called stereotypical pain program has proved to be ineffective in rehabilitating these patients. Most insurance carriers in the state of Florida, for example, will not approve treatment in these programs because they are not cost-effective. Nevertheless, the rather expensive, appropriately designed, comprehensive, multidisciplinary pain and rehabilitation program is an effective way to treat some patients with the failed back syndrome.[13]

Social and economic issues must also be addressed as part of the rehabilitative effort. In many patients, functional recovery cannot be accomplished without settlement of any ongoing compensation disputes or litigation.[14] Rehabilitative and appropriate surgical treatment in the face of substantial psychosocioeconomic dysfunction has a very high rate of failure when compared with motivated patients with minimal secondary dysfunction.[11, 13, 14]

Among patients suffering chronic low back pain disorders are many who have unmanageable psychosocial dysfunction, particularly those who have preexisting personality disorders. These patients are generally noncompliant with the rehabilitation program, despite valiant efforts by health care providers. In this instance, it is beneficial to all, including the patient, that the patient be placed at maximal medical improvement, health care delivery cease, an appropriate impairment rating be given, and the patient be discharged with appropriate functional restrictions based on objective anatomic, physical, and neurological abnormalities.[16, 26] The patient must become independent and take

personal responsibility for his or her own long-term management.

Surgical Management

The role of surgery in the management of intractable, incapacitating chronic low back pain disorders is limited to two specific goals: decompression of symptomatic neural compression syndromes, and stabilization-arthrodesis of symptomatic lumbar segmental instability. In both cases, the clinical complaints and physical and neurological examinations must be consistent with well-documented imaging abnormalities. In some patients, combined neural decompressive and stabilization-arthrodesis is required because they suffer simultaneous neural compressive and mechanical instability syndromes. So-called stereotypical salvage-type surgical procedures for persistent pain in a failed back syndrome patient without consideration of the consistency of the patient's symptoms and the physical, psychosocioeconomic, and anatomic components are guaranteed to fail and have a significant risk of further disabling the patient.

DECOMPRESSIVE SURGERY

Decompressive surgery is indicated when the patient's complaints of neural compressive pain are consistent with demonstrable neural compression on high-quality neurodiagnostic imaging studies. Typical diagnoses include recurrent disk herniation; retained disk fragment; persistent, recurrent, or delayed lateral stenosis (lateral recess foramina) (see Fig. 283–4); intraspinal or foraminal ganglionic cyst arising from an injured facet joint (see Fig. 283–5); and persistent, recurrent, or delayed central spinal stenosis. Unfortunately, in some patients it is impossible to differentiate neuropathic pain secondary to nerve root injury and neural compressive pain secondary to nerve root compression demonstrated by the imaging studies. Anatomically successful decompressive surgery generally fails to benefit a patient who suffers from a neuropathic pain disorder.

Postoperative epidural fibrosis is a common finding on high-resolution MRI in many asymptomatic patients. Such findings are also common in patients with failed back surgery syndrome. The presence of epidural fibrosis alone, despite the patient's complaints, is never an indication for surgical decompression. In our experience, these patients are rarely helped by surgical therapy and are often made worse.

Redo surgery for recurrent disk herniation, retained disk fragment, postoperative intraspinal ganglionic cyst, and persistent or recurrent lateral spinal stenosis is much more demanding than the initial interlaminar procedure and carries a substantially greater likelihood of failure owing to the possibility of preexisting neuropathic pain. In addition, there is a much greater risk of surgical neural injury and dural tear related to the perineural fibrotic process. A well-organized plan of attack by an experienced neurosurgeon is essential to avoid these pitfalls.

We strongly believe that the operating microscope is

essential to achieving the desired result. Its value is not the small size of the skin incision or even the reduced muscle dissection and retraction, but rather the outstanding lighting and magnification provided by this instrument. The latter is necessary to clearly delineate the tissue layers (e.g., bone, ligamenta flava, epidural scar, posterior longitudinal ligament, disk capsule) from the herniated disk, ganglionic cyst, hypertrophic osteophyte and ligament, and dura and nerve root sheaths. Therefore, complications such as dural tear or nerve root injury can be reduced using this device.

At the time of surgery, the relevant neurodiagnostic imaging studies must be on hand to ensure proper localization of the level of pathology. If, at the time of exposure of the interlaminar space, there is any doubt about the level, an intraoperative radiograph must be obtained.

Once satisfactory general endotracheal anesthesia has been induced, we prefer to position the patient prone on a spinal frame, with careful padding of all pressure points. If the patient is massively obese, the lateral position is used. In the prone position, care must be taken to eliminate lordosis by flexion and concurrently keeping the abdomen free to reduce venous congestion.

We do not permit the anesthetist to use paralyzing agents during any spinal operative procedures. A nonparalyzed patient exhibits motor movements whenever the nerve root or spinal cord is excessively manipulated during microdissection, giving immediate feedback to the surgeon and providing an additional margin of safety.[27] The disadvantage of not using paralytic agents is that muscle retraction is slightly more difficult, and the anesthesia techniques are somewhat more sophisticated. These minor difficulties are far outweighed by the reduced risk of neural injury.

The preferred posterior skin incision is midline, generally using the prior incisional scar. It is centered as nearly as possible over the involved intervertebral segments. The length of the incision should permit complete visualization of the entire hemilamina rostral and caudal to the appropriate interlaminar spaces, as well as the entire facet complex. The lumbodorsal fascia is incised with the electric knife just lateral to the spinous process and supraspinous ligament. Atraumatic dissection of the muscle off the spinous processes and laminae is accomplished with a periosteal elevator and the electric knife. After exposure of the appropriate interlaminar area and the entire rostral and caudal hemilamina, a self-retaining retractor is used to retract the musculofascial layers laterally, exposing the lateral portion of the facet joint. For massive disk herniations or central spinal stenosis with cauda equina compression, adequate bilateral exposure and bony and ligamentous decompression are required before attempting to dissect and retract the neural elements if a neurological catastrophe is to be avoided.

At this point, the operating microscope is brought into the field for microdissection. The initial goal is adequate exposure and dorsolateral decompression before neural manipulation and exploration. This is true for all spinal operative procedures. To accomplish this, adequate removal of bone is required. The bone removal is accomplished with a high-speed bur (AM-3, Midas Rex) and carried both rostrally and caudally well beyond the area of neural compressive pathology. The bony decompression must include a mesial facetectomy such that the lateral bone exposure is flush with the vertebral pedicle just caudal to the disk space. All residual ligamenta flava are gently microdissected from the dura and nerve root sheath and excised with either a 2- or 3-mm footplate modified Kerrison-type rongeurs. Exuberant epidural scar is then gently and sharply microdissected off the dura and nerve root sheath using microsurgical instrumentation, giving greater pliability to these delicate tissues. In general, all dissection should be carried out in the rostral-caudal plane, not the medial-lateral plane, to minimize the possibility of neural injury.

Once adequate dorsolateral decompression and exposure of the dural sac and involved nerve root have been accomplished, a generous foraminotomy is performed with the thin-plate Kerrison rongeurs and angled flat-back curets if lateral stenosis is contributing to the neural compression. If the neural compression is caused by an intraspinal ganglionic cyst arising from the facet joint, it is radically excised using microdissection, and the facet joint is cleaned of all residual synovial tissue. If the neural compressive lesion is a herniated disk fragment, the nerve root and dural sac are gently mobilized from the adherent fibrous tissue and herniated disk material. Once the dura and nerve root can be easily and gently retracted and a portion of the herniated disk exposed, a blunt nerve hook can be used to mobilize the disk fragment and tease it into the field for removal with a grasping pituitary rongeur. Upon removal of a significant extruded disk fragment, tension on the dura and nerve root is reduced, permitting further protection of the neural elements during the additional dissection required to fully expose the floor of the spinal canal and neural foramina to ensure complete excision of all herniated disk material and adequate neural decompression. After removal of all herniated disk material, the annulus is exposed, and the disk space is cleaned of all retained disk material using curets and pituitary rongeurs in an attempt to prevent recurrence. Finally, the neural retraction is discontinued, and the ventral epidural space and neural foramina are explored extensively with long, blunt, ball nerve hooks to ensure that there is no remaining neural compressive lesion. Although there is some controversy regarding the optimal material for covering the hemilaminectomy defect, we prefer to leave a thrombin-soaked Gelfoam pledget over the exposed dura when there is no residual normal epidural fat left for coverage.

Redo decompression of persistent or recurrent lumbar spinal stenosis is also a rather formidable procedure. In this case, the scar tissue is intimately associated with a considerable area of the dura compared with that encountered after prior lumbar hemilaminotomy, substantially increasing the possibility of a dural tear. The first step in the re-decompression of a complete laminectomy is a bilateral, subperiosteal dissection of the intact vertebrae immediately rostral and caudal to the levels of prior laminectomies. Once this has been accomplished, the electric knife is used to gradually incise the midline scar just superficial to the underlying dura. If there is a preexisting pseudomeningocele, great care must be taken to avoid entering the cerebrospinal fluid spaces, which increases the risk of nerve root or cauda equina injury. This portion of the dissection is greatly facilitated by the use of strong lateral retraction with self-retaining soft tissue retractors. In fact, strong lateral retraction often helps to perform the midline dissection and has not resulted in either dural or nerve root injury in our hands. Once the epidural scar has been thinned in the midline just superficial to the dura, the electric knife is used to expose the entire facet complexes bilaterally. The operating microscope is then brought into the field, and the bony decompression is accomplished using microdissection techniques. Using a high-speed bur (AM-3, Midas Rex) under microsurgical control, the laminectomy is widened bilaterally, and mesial facetectomies are performed vertically, flush with the pedicles. At all times, epidural scar and retained ligamenta flava are left intact to protect the dura during the bony decompression. Once bilateral, wide, dorsolateral bony decompression has been achieved, the epidural scar is microdissected free of the dura and excised. With the operating surgeon standing on the side opposite that to be laterally decompressed, dissection of the lateral dura and nerve roots from the hypertrophic bone, ligamenta flava, and scar is begun at one end, where normal, unscarred dura has been exposed and the plane of microdissection is readily established. We have found that various sizes of straight and angled flatback curets are ideal dissectors for developing the correct cleavage plane to separate the dura and nerve roots from the lateral scar, overlying hypertrophic bone, and ligamenta flava. Once this plane is fully developed, the lateral hypertrophic scar, ligamenta flava, and hypertrophic bone can be excised with various-sized angled, thin-plate, modified Kerrison rongeurs. Further undercutting of the neural foramina can then be accomplished with these rongeurs and various-sized angled curets so that extensive foraminal decompression is achieved. The microsurgical decompression is continued until large Murphy ball nerve hooks can be readily passed over each nerve root and out the neural foramina with ease, ensuring adequate neural decompression. The surgeon then switches to the opposite side of the operating table to microsurgically decompress the remaining side using identical techniques. Once adequate neural decompression has been accomplished bilaterally, the wound is carefully closed in layers.

Rigorous interpretation of the literature on lumbar spine reoperations for persistent or recurrent neural compression syndrome is difficult owing to a lack of adequate clinical and radiographic classification of the patient populations. Patient selection and differing preoperative clinical definitions further confound the variations in reported outcomes. For example, Greenwood and coworkers[28] reported 70% (47 cases) good or excellent results following reoperation for lumbar disk excision in 67 patients. They further reported 100% (17 cases) good results in those patients in whom a recurrent herniated disk fragment was identified. However, only 13 of 24 patients (54%) in whom epidural fibrosis was the primary pathology had a good result. Similarly, Schlarb and Wenker[29] performed one or more decompressive reoperations on 132 patients, representing 10.4% of the total operations for lumbar disk disease. When a recurrent disk herniation was found, the failure rate was 32%; it rose to 76% if epidural fibrosis was discovered. Finnegan and associates[30] and Schuler and colleagues[31] also reported an overall rate of about 80% satisfied patients after carefully selected decompressive reoperations for presumed recurrent herniated lumbar disks. Law and coworkers[32] reported a successful outcome in only 16 of 53 patients (26%) undergoing reoperations for failed lumbar disk surgery. Essentially all the successful results were in patients with recurrent herniated disk fragments.

Certainly, third and fourth reoperations carry an even greater risk of failure. With each recurrent neural compressive syndrome and each reoperation, the risk of permanent neural injury and irreversible neuropathic pain increases. On those rare occasions when we have treated a third or fourth recurrence of free-fragment disk herniation at the same level, a stabilization-arthrodesis procedure was performed along with neural decompression in selected patients, with the goal of preventing any further extrusion of residual disk material. The literature regarding reoperations for persistent or recurrent lumbar stenosis is lacking. However, we have observed that good or excellent results can be achieved in more than 80% of patients undergoing repeat microsurgical decompressive procedures for neural compression syndromes. To achieve such results, rigorous patient selection is required, aided by careful clinical analysis and modern high-resolution imaging, and appropriate surgical procedures must be carefully and meticulously executed to ensure satisfactory neural decompression.[33] If significant psychosocioeconomic factors are involved, the success rate is only about 50%, despite rigorous patient selection and adequate microsurgical decompression.

The complications after decompressive reoperations are no different from those encountered during or after a primary decompressive procedure. However, certain complications are more likely to occur owing to the inherent technical difficulties related to the epidural fibrotic process. Among these are nerve root and root sleeve damage, pseudomeningocele, cerebrospinal fluid leakage, arachnoiditis, and postoperative instability related to additional facet complex damage. Fortunately, in our experience, complications are rare, with minor postoperative neurological dysfunction occurring in less than 0.5% of patients. We have had no cases of lumbar cerebrospinal fluid leakage or pseudomeningocele formation.

STABILIZATION-ARTHRODESIS SURGERY

Stabilization-arthrodesis surgery is indicated when the patient's complaints of intractable and incapacitating mechanical low back or segmental leg pain (clinical instability syndrome) are consistent with demonstrated segmental instability on neurodiagnostic imaging studies. Typical imaging findings include spondylolisthesis, olisthesis, retrolisthesis, focal rotoscoliosis, excessive translational movement on dynamic flexion-extension radiographs, disk arthropathy (vacuum disk), traction spurs, disk destruction on MRI, adjacent vertebral body reactive changes on MRI (hypo- or hyperintensity on T1 and hyperintensity on T2), severe facet arthropathy (vacuum facet, hypertrophic changes, synovial cyst formation), facet subluxation, facet fracture, prior facet surgical destruction, pseudarthrosis, and evidence of prior surgery. Unfortunately, there is no preoperative diagnostic test that can reliably determine that these abnormal segments are the cause of the patient's mechanical pain syndrome. Therefore, the neurosurgeon must use his or her best judgment in deciding on the appropriate levels to be stabilized. When it is reasonable, we prefer to perform arthrodesis at all levels that may be involved in the instability process.

Once a final decision to perform lumbar spine stabilization-arthrodesis has been made, the technique must be considered. At present, there are three generally accepted techniques for arthrodesis of the lumbosacral spine for intractable, benign, mechanical pain syndromes: posterolateral (intertransverse process) fusion, posterior lumbar interbody fusion (PLIF), and anterior lumbar interbody fusion (ALIF). It must always be kept in mind that long-term stability is dependent solely on successful bony fusion. The role of spinal segmental instrumentation is limited to correcting spinal deformity and temporarily stabilizing the spine to improve the probability of a successful long-term arthrodesis (motion segment bony fusion).[8, 11, 12]

PLIF was introduced by Cloward in 1945.[34] Its initial acceptance was less than enthusiastic due to its technical difficulty, the potential complications, and the understandable controversy about the role of lumbosacral arthrodesis in the management of low back pain disorders. However, the technique has improved over the years, and interest in this technique has increased.[35–38] Its advantages include distraction-decompression of the spinal canal and foramina; total diskectomy, preventing recurrent disk herniation; immediate mechanical stability; the ability to use allograft bone; the presence of contact compressive forces, which favors bone fusion; and the fact that the skin and muscle dissection required is essentially equivalent to that needed in an ordinary bilateral posterior lumbar decompression. The disadvantages include technical difficulty; substantial excision of dorsolateral spine structures for exposure, which reduces some of the support and stability achieved by the grafts; high pseudarthrosis rate (15% to 30%); excessive retraction of neural elements, with risk of neurological injury, arachnoiditis, and dural tear; substantial epidural fibrosis following the considerable epidural exposure; graft migration (6% to 15%), with risk of neural injury; and risk of great vessel and intra-abdominal injury.

Given these disadvantages, PLIF failed to gain significant popularity among spinal surgeons. However,

the recent development of lumbar interbody threaded fusion cage implants and techniques has resulted in a resurgence of interest in lumbar interbody fusion as a potentially superior technique for lumbar segmental fixation and arthrodesis.[39] Adequate prospective clinical trials have been completed using these implants, and the U.S. Food and Drug Administration has approved their use for lumbar interbody fusion. The threaded fusion cages may be used for the treatment of lumbar segmental instability at one or two levels from L2 to S1 (Fig. 283–6). Contraindications to the threaded fusion cage technique include grade II or greater spondylolisthesis, three or more levels of fusion, osteoporosis, pregnancy, skeletal immaturity, previous attempted PLIF, and active infection. In the multicenter prospective studies of these techniques, successful interbody fusion was reported to have occurred in 96% to 98% of patients at 12 months, with a reasonably low neurological complication rate of less than 3%.[40, 41] Although long-term follow-up studies are not available at this time, no unusual delayed complications have been encountered in 4 years. Despite the lack of long-term follow-up, available data indicate that the threaded fusion cage technique for PLIF will play an important role in the treatment of lumbar instability when it is limited to one or two motion segments and a wide decompression is necessary.

ALIF is also used by some surgeons in the management of low back pain disorders. Despite improvements over the years, ALIF continues to have a high rate of pseudarthrosis and complications.[42–45] The advantages of this approach include no need to work in an area of previous spinal surgery, avoidance of intraspinal injury and scarring, distraction-decompression of the spinal canal and foramina, immediate mechanical stability, ability to use allograft bone, and presence of contact compressive forces. The disadvantages include inability to surgically decompress neural elements; lack of familiarity with anterior approaches; high pseudarthrosis rate (13% to 44%); risk of gastrointestinal, genitourinary, and great vessel injury; high incidence of thromboembolic disease (5% to 8%); and impotence and sterility from retrograde ejaculation. With the advent of lumbar threaded interbody fusion technology, there has been an explosion of interest in using these implants for ALIFs during the past few years. Both open and endoscopic anterior lumbar transabdominal approaches, with application of threaded interbody fusion techniques, are rapidly gaining popularity. The cage technique provides a comparatively simple method of performing a lumbar interbody fusion and has a substantially higher rate of fusion than the original ALIF procedure; however, the role of ALIF in the failed back syndrome requires further definition with long-term follow-up, which is not available at this time.

Although complete fusion of the anterior and posterior spinal elements would be biomechanically ideal, the so-called 360-degree or two-staged posterior-anterior operative procedure for low back pain disorders has no scientific merit or redeeming value. It merely

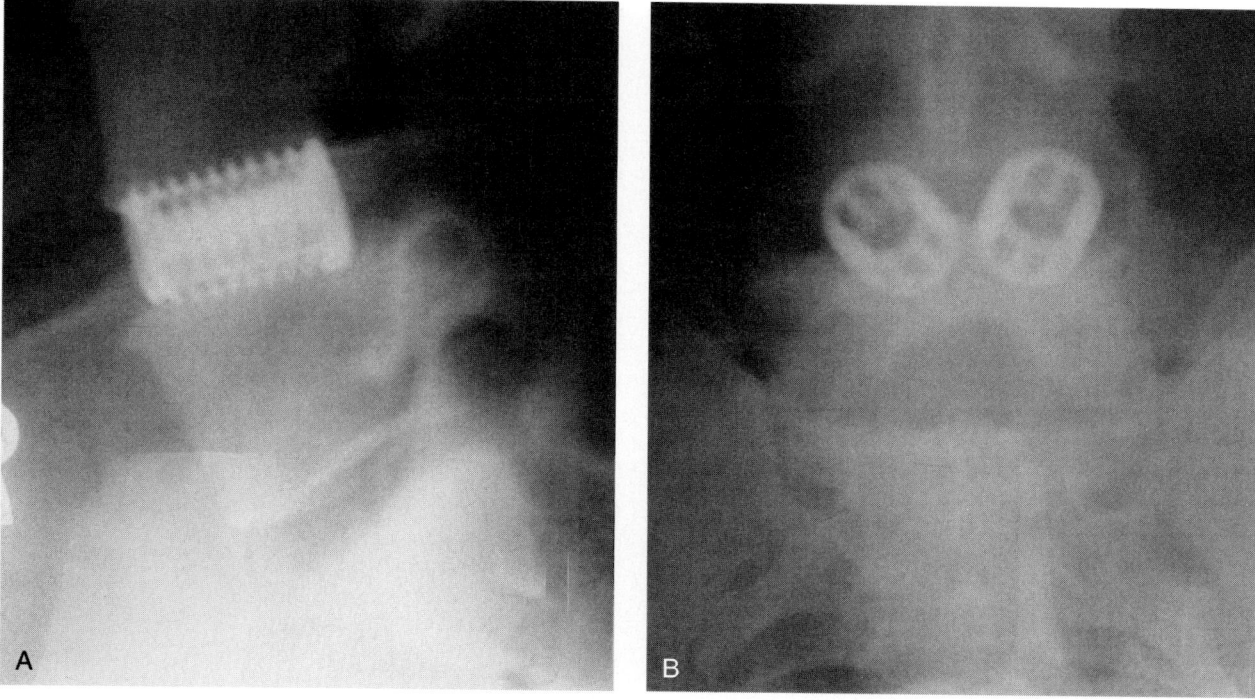

FIGURE 283–6. Postoperative lumbar spine radiographs of the patient from Figure 283–5. Three years after segmental stabilization with Ray threaded fusion cages and interbody autogenous arthrodesis, the patient is asymptomatic, works full-time, jogs 4 days a week, and enjoys golf on the weekends.

adds significantly to the complication rate in the surgical management of benign low back pain disorders.

Another major advance in lumbosacral arthrodesis occurred with the evolution of fusion of the posterolateral spinal elements, so-called posterolateral intertransverse process fusion. The first clinical series was published by Cleveland and associates in 1948.[46] Autogenous matchstick grafts were shown to be the optimal material for the induction of fusion.[7, 11, 46–49] Moreover, bilateral posterolateral fusion produces fewer adverse effects in the unfused motion segments while yielding good stabilization of the fused motion segments in comparison with direct posterior fusion and anterior interbody fusion.[50] The advantages of this technique include a high fusion rate (90% for one level, 80% for two levels, 90% for multiple levels with segmental instrumentation)[8, 11, 12]; no need to expose neural elements; no bone overgrowth leading to spinal stenosis; no risk of neural injury from graft extrusion; and excellent biomechanical support for resistance to torsional forces, which appear to be highly detrimental to degenerating intervertebral disks.[29] The disadvantages include blood loss from donor site and recipient bone, absence of contact compressive forces, lack of any immediate stability, absence of distraction-decompression of the spinal canal and foramina, and substantial traumatic injury to and denervation of the lumbar paravertebral muscles. To overcome some of these disadvantages, a segmental distraction-stabilization instrumentation system may be used for single and multiple motion segment fusions to give immediate stability, increase the probability of successful fusion,[8,

[11, 12, 51] and further decompress the neural elements in the foramina.[8, 11, 12]

The role of lumbar spine segmental instrumentation in the surgical management of the failed back syndrome does not differ substantially from the role of such implants in the management of patients suffering from mechanical instability syndromes who have not had prior surgery. Fundamentally, the principal role of these devices is to improve the probability of successful floating or multilevel, long-term bony arthrodesis. A second virtue of the fixation system is instant stability. An additional theoretical benefit from a distraction system is the possibility of achieving additional neural decompression by opening the neural foramina. Correction of deformity or olisthesis by these systems probably has little or no relationship to clinical outcome, other than producing elegant postoperative images. Clinical success is dependent on three factors: (1) a correct preoperative clinical diagnosis of mechanical instability pain; (2) achievement of a stable, solid bony arthrodesis (fusion); and (3) absence of surgical complications.[8, 11, 12] All spinal segmental instrumentation must be considered temporary, as there is a race between the achievement of bony arthrodesis and implant failure. If bony fusion is not achieved, the spinal implant will loosen or break over time, necessitating a second operation for repair or removal.

A wide variety of posterior segmental fixation systems has been used in the surgical management of presumed lumbar segmental instability syndromes. These systems include dual rod distraction systems with or without wire (cable) fixation, modified Luque rectangle sublaminar wire fixation systems, and pedicle screw fixation systems. Each system has its proponents, but there are no rigorous scientific data indicating that one system is better than another. At present, the choice among these various systems is based on surgeon preference. In an early study of the role of segmental stabilization-arthrodesis for lumbar instability pain in more than 200 consecutive patients with the failed back syndrome, a simple dual distraction rod segmental stabilization system supplemented with sublaminar cable fixation was used to achieve a 96% fusion rate without any neurological complications.[8, 12] However, the lumbar pedicle screw fixation systems have been shown to be superior to other posterior systems, based on biomechanical properties, involvement of fewer motion segments, high rate of osseous union, and versatility.[52] Despite the excellent biomechanical characteristics of pedicle screw fixation systems, the technique is associated with significant surgical risks, particularly neurological injury and deep lumbar infections. One report indicates that pedicle screw fixation systems are an effective and reasonably safe procedure for internal fixation of the lumbar spine when meticulous surgical techniques are used, with a fusion rate approximating 97%.[52] Therefore, pedicle screw fixation systems are the procedure of choice among most spinal surgeons when the threaded fusion cage technique is contraindicated (Fig. 283–7).

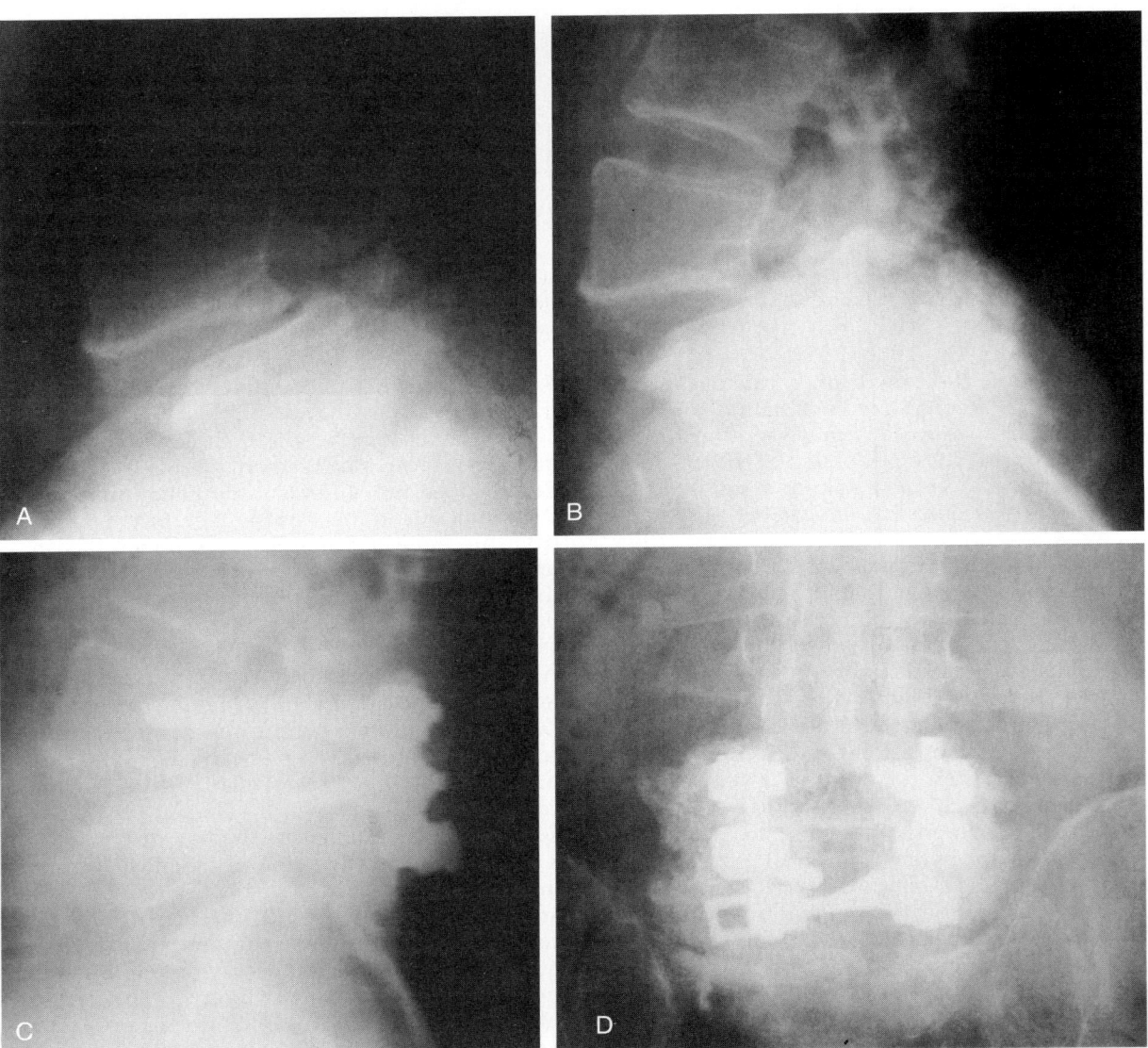

FIGURE 283–7. Preoperative lateral flexion-extension (*A* and *B*) and postoperative anteroposterior and lateral (*C* and *D*) lumbar spine radiographs in a 55-year-old retired professional football player with intractable and incapacitating "mechanical" low back pain following two L4-5 decompressions and lateral fusions for failed lytic spondylolisthesis. Note the translation and opening of the anterior disk space on the preoperative images, consistent with gross segmental instability. Five years after pedicle screw segmental stabilization and posterior-lateral autogenous arthrodesis, the patient is asymptomatic and enjoys golf and tennis.

The literature regarding the outcome from surgical stabilization-arthrodesis in patients with persistent or recurrent symptoms after lumbar surgery is even more difficult to interpret. In 125 posterolateral fusions performed at the Mayo Clinic during the period 1960 to 1967 as so-called salvage procedures following failed lumbar disk surgery, Stauffer and Coventry[53] reported a satisfactory outcome in 81% of their patients. In 1985, Jackson and colleagues[54] reported a prospective study of 144 consecutive bilateral posterolateral fusions, with improvement noted in 80% and solid fusion in 87%. In a more recent series of 67 patients selected using the clinical definitions of lumbar instability as developed in this chapter, we reported that 54% excellent results (asymptomatic) and 32% good results (normal life, employed, occasional non-narcotic analgesics for minor low back pain) can be achieved with adequate neural decompression and stabilization in patients with failed back syndrome.[8, 12] The complications in the latter series consisted of two cases of pseudarthrosis and implant dislodgment (3%, both osteoporotic) and one deep wound infection (1%). More recently, Masferrer and coworkers[52] reported a retrospective study of lumbar instability treated by a posterior surgical approach with pedicle screw fixation and posterolateral arthrodesis. Lumbar pain improved in 84% of patients with failed back syndrome, but 7% suffered a substantial worsening of pain after surgery. There were no significant neurological complications. However, 5.2% of patients developed deep lumbar wound infection. Therefore, lumbar stabilization-arthrodesis appears to have a definite, albeit infrequent, role in the surgical management of highly selected cases of failed low back pain disorders. However, stereotypical procedures applied to the complaint of pain without an understanding of the type of pain syndrome or the physical and psychosocioeconomic components of chronic pain syndrome are generally guaranteed to fail to benefit the patient.

NEUROPATHIC PAIN SURGERY

In our experience, the use of interventional surgical therapy for lumbar neuropathic pain syndromes is limited. We have never examined a patient with failed back syndrome suffering from neuropathic pain who functionally benefited from any of the various pain-relieving procedures. The current surgical approaches to neuropathic pain include neuroablative procedures (dorsal rhizotomies, dorsal root ganglionectomies, anterolateral cordotomies), neuroaugmentative procedures (implanted dorsal column stimulators, deep brain stimulation), and implanted intraspinal drug infusion therapies.

Although some clinical investigators have reported some success with dorsal rhizotomy and dorsal root ganglionectomy in the management of selected failed back syndrome patients,[55] careful analysis of the clinical data by unbiased investigators indicates that the overall results of these neuroablative procedures are poor and fail to justify their performance.[56, 57] Percutaneous or open anterolateral cordotomy has no role in

the management of benign chronic pain syndromes; the resultant pain relief is limited to 1 to 2 years, and the original pain is frequently replaced by severe dysesthetic pain of central origin. Other cerebral ablative procedures such as stereotactic cingulotomy appear to be rather radical, with limited results.

In our experience, the use of transcutaneous nerve stimulation has a limited role in the management of lumbar neuropathic pain syndromes. But because it is without significant risk, it is certainly worth a try, along with appropriate psychotherapeutic management. In contrast, implantable spinal cord stimulation (SCS) systems have been used to treat failed back syndrome patients, with some modest success. The SCS systems have gradually improved over their 30-year evolution. In rigorously selected patients suffering from end-stage failed back syndrome and treated with SCS, approximately 50% reported greater than 50% pain relief at long-term follow-up, with substantial improvement in their quality of life.[58] This technique is effective only in relieving leg pain; it has little effect on axial back pain. A more recent study indicated that despite the considerable expense associated with SCS treatment of the failed back syndrome, the technique can lower overall medical costs for these difficult-to-treat patients.[59]

Deep brain stimulation is available in only a few specialized centers, which have reported varying success in controlling pain in failed back syndrome patients. Given its limited success, as well as the serious complications that can occur, the role of deep brain stimulation in the treatment of the failed back syndrome remains problematic.

Finally, we are greatly concerned about the proliferation of implantable intraspinal drug infusion systems, particularly those that use habituating and addicting substances. Owing to the limitations and risks associated with this technology, there appears to be little rational basis for their use in the management of long-term chronic pain syndromes, particularly the failed back syndrome. Because of the cost, labor intensity, high probability of failure, and complications, their use in benign chronic pain syndromes is not warranted.[60]

SUMMARY

The failed back syndrome may be defined as "the failure of lumbar spine therapy to relieve pain and incapacitation." The term *failed back syndrome* is often used synonymously with *failed back surgery syndrome*. Unfortunately, this syndrome is a common phenomenon in our society and a difficult therapeutic challenge. It is a multifactorial disease process with organic, psychological, and socioeconomic factors interacting in complex ways.

Because the major symptom of the failed back syndrome is pain, an understanding of this complex symptom is requisite not only to the evaluation and treatment of the failed back syndrome but also to the initial evaluation and treatment of an individual first presenting with an intractable low back pain disorder. In this regard, it is important to recognize that pain is a subjective behavior to the clinician. Although acute pain usually closely approximates the stimulus (nociception), pain behavior in patients complaining of chronic pain often has little correlation with objective physical evidence of active tissue irritation or damage. In fact, exhaustive studies of patients with chronic, intractable low back pain (>6 months) frequently fail to detect any evidence of peripheral nociceptive activity. Therefore, it is likely that operant mechanisms (non-nociceptive factors) may play a principal role in the persistence of symptoms. Learned operant responses (psychosocioeconomic pain) include primary gains (reduction of conflict or stress, such as avoidance of unpleasant tasks), secondary gains (environmental gains, such as compensation, litigation, sympathy), and tertiary gains (gains achieved by persons other than the patient, such as the spouse and health care professional). These important factors must always be kept in mind when treating a patient with an intractable chronic low back pain disorder. In general, the evaluation of failed back syndrome patients does not differ substantially from that of other patients suffering recent onset low back pain. It is important to obtain complete background information, such as the patient's original presentation, the details of previous examinations, the actual prior neurodiagnostic imaging studies, and reports of prior interventional therapies.

Treatment of the failed back syndrome requires that certain general principles be followed in all cases, irrespective of the pathologic process present or prospects for interventional therapy. Initially, intercurrent psychological, social, and economic issues must be addressed. In some cases, hospitalization in a pain management program may be necessary. Abuse of medications, particularly narcotics and benzodiazepines, must be curtailed. All patients require intensive physical reconditioning programs to relieve their myofascial pain related to the frozen back syndrome and careful instructions in body biomechanics to prevent further insults.

The primary concept regarding the failed back syndrome is that prevention is more important than treatment. Prevention requires an understanding of the natural history of low back pain disorders and the operant psychosocioeconomic factors involved. It is essential that an accurate diagnosis be established and a simple, rational, and appropriate treatment-rehabilitation program be instituted without delay. If the pain is allowed to become "fixed," no form of treatment is likely to rehabilitate the patient and return him or her to a satisfactory, productive life.

Finally, the limitations and benefits of interventional surgical therapy must be recognized. Surgical management can achieve only two objectives: neural decompression and spinal stabilization. If the patient's principal problem is not a neural compression or mechanical instability pain syndrome, interventional therapy will only contribute to the devastating failed back surgery syndrome. It is now recognized that the most common reason for the failed back surgery syndrome is misdiagnosis and inappropriate patient selection for surgical therapy. However, making an accurate diagnosis and rendering appropriate therapy can substantially benefit some patients suffering from the failed back syndrome.

REFERENCES

1. Frymoyer JW, Gordon SL: Research perspectives in low back pain: Report of a 1988 workshop. Spine 14:1384–1390, 1989.
2. Kelsey TL, White A: Epidemiology and impact of low back pain. Spine 5:133, 1980.
3. Nagi SZ, Riley LE, Newby LG: A social epidemiology of back pain in a general population. J Chron Dis 26:769, 1973.
4. Loeser JD, Volinn E: Epidemiology of low back pain. Neurosurg Clin N Am 2:713, 1991.
5. Sypert GW: Lumbar disk disease. Part 1. Natural history and diagnosis. Neurol Neurosurg Update Ser 7(11):1, 1987.
6. Sypert GW: Lumbar disk disease. Part 2. Therapy. Neurol Neurosurg Update Ser 7(12):1, 1987.
7. Loeser JD: Low back pain. In Bonica JJ (ed): Pain. New York, Raven Press, 1980, pp 363–377.
8. Sypert GW, Arpin-Sypert EJ: Non-neoplastic lumbar spinal disorders. In Little JR, Awad IA (eds): Reoperative Neurosurgery. Baltimore, Williams & Wilkins, 1992, pp 155–182.
9. Kirkaldy-Willis WH: The pathology and pathogenesis of low back pain. In Kirkaldy-Willis WH (ed): Managing Low Back Pain. New York, Churchill Livingstone, 1983, pp 23–44.
10. Long DM, Filtzer DL, DenDebba M, Hendler MH: Clinical features of the failed-back syndrome. J Neurosurg 69:61, 1988.
11. Sypert GW: Low back pain disorders: Lumbar fusion? Clin Neurosurg 33:457, 1986.
12. Sypert GW, Arpin-Sypert EJ: The role of spinal instrumentation in the failed back. In Hardy RW Jr (ed): Lumbar Disc Disease. New York, Raven Press, 1993, pp 201–208.
13. Cassissi JE, Sypert GW, Salamon A, Kapel L: Independent evaluation of a multidisciplinary rehabilitation program for chronic low back pain. Neurosurgery 25:877, 1989.
14. Cassissi JE, Sypert GW, Lagana L, et al: Pain, disability, and psychological functioning in chronic low back pain subgroups: Myofascial versus herniated disc syndrome. Neurosurgery 33:1, 1993.
15. Hoon PW, Feuerstein M, Papciak AS: Evaluation of the chronic low back pain patient: Conceptual and clinical considerations. Clin Pychol Rev 5:377, 1985.
16. Burton CV, Kirkaldy-Willis WH, Yong-Hing K, Heithoff KB: Causes of failure of surgery on the lumbar spine. Clin Orthop 157:191, 1981.
17. Sypert GW: External spinal orthotics. Neurosurgery 20:642, 1987.
18. Arpin-Sypert EJ, Sypert GW: Septic complications of spinal surgery. In Tarlov EC (ed): Neurosurgical Topic: Complications of Spinal Surgery. Park Ridge, Ill, American Association of Neurological Surgeons, 1991, pp 29–40.
19. Korbon GA, DeGood DE, Schroeder ME, et al: The development of a somatic amplification rating scale for low-back pain. Spine 12:787, 1987.
20. Sypert GW: Failed back syndrome. In Long DM (ed): Current Therapy in Neurological Surgery 2. Philadelphia, BC Decker, 1989, pp 286–289.
21. Deyo RA, Rainville J, Kent DL: What can the history and physical examination tell us about low back pain? JAMA 268:760, 1992.
22. Waddell G, McCullouch JA, Kummel E, Vernner RM: Nonorganic physical signs in low back pain. Spine 5:117, 1980.
23. Ackerman SJ, Steinber EP, Bryan RN, et al: Persistent low back pain in patients suspected of having herniated nucleus pulposus: Radiologic predictors of functional outcome—implications for treatment selection. Radiology 203:815, 1997.
24. Ackerman SJ, Steinberg EP, Bryan RN, et al: Trends in diagnostic imaging for low back pain: Has MR imaging been a substitute or add-on? Radiology 203:535, 1997.
25. Adams MS, Sypert GW, Benzel EL: The nonoperative management of neck and back pain. In Benzel EC (ed): Spine Surgery. Philadelphia, Churchill Livingstone, 1999, pp 1393–1397.
26. Waddell G, Kummel EG, Lotto WN, et al: Failed lumbar disc surgery and repeat surgery following industrial injuries. J Bone Joint Surg Am 61:201, 1979.

27. Sypert GW, Saunders RL, Benzel EC: Intraoperative nonparalytic monitoring. In Benzel EC (ed): Spine Surgery. Philadelphia, Churchill Livingstone, 1999, pp 1267–1269.
28. Greenwood J Jr, McGuire TH, Kimbell F: A study of the causes of failure in the herniated intervertebral disc operation: An analysis of 67 reoperated cases. J Neurosurg 9:15, 1952.
29. Schlarb H, Wenker H: Re-operation performed on patients suffering from an intervertebral disc prolapse in the lumbar region. Adv Neurosurg 4:32, 1977.
30. Finnegan WJ, Fenlin JM, Marvel JP, et al: Results of surgical intervention in the symptomatic multiply-operated back patient. J Bone Joint Surg Am 61:1077, 1979.
31. Schuler P, Clemens D, Rossak K: Nachuntersuchungs-ergebnisse nach lumbalen. Z Orthop 121:33, 1983.
32. Law JD, Ralph RAW, Kirsch WM: Reoperations after lumbar intervertebral disc surgery. J Neurosurg 48:259, 1978.
33. North RB, Campbell JN, James CS, et al: Failed back surgery syndrome: 5 year follow-up in 102 patients undergoing repeated operation. Neurosurgery 28:685, 1991.
34. Cloward RB: The treatment of ruptured intervertebral discs by vertebral body fusion. J Neurosurg 10:151, 1953.
35. Cloward RB: Posterior lumbar interbody fusion updated. Clin Orthop 193:16, 1985.
36. Collis JS: Total disc replacement: A modified posterior lumbar interbody fusion. Clin Orthop 193:64, 1985.
37. Hutter CG: Posterior intervertebral body fusion: A 25-year study. Clin Orthop 179:86, 1983.
38. Lin PM: Posterior lumbar interbody fusion technique: Complications and pitfalls. Clin Orthop 193:90, 1983.
39. Onesti ST, Ashkenazi E: The Ray threaded fusion cage for posterior lumbar interbody fusion. Neurosurgery 42:200, 1998.
40. Ray CD: Threaded titanium cages for lumbar interbody fusion. Spine 22:667, 1997.
41. Yuan HA, Kushlich SD, Dowdle JA, et al: Prospective Multi-Center Clinical Trial of the BAK Interbody Fusion System. Minneapolis, Minn, Spine Tech, 1977.
42. Hodgson AR, Wong SK: A description of a technic and evaluation of results in anterior spinal fusion for deranged intervertebral disk and spondylolisthesis. Clin Orthop 56:133, 1968.
43. Stauffer RN, Coventry MB: Anterior interbody lumbar spine fusion. J Bone Joint Surg Am 54:756, 1972.
44. Chow SP, Leong JCY, Yau ACMC: Anterior spinal fusion for deranged lumbar intervertebral disc. Spine 9:686, 1984.
45. Leong JCY, Chun SY, Grange WJ, Fang D: Long-term results of lumbar intervertebral disc prolapse. Spine 8:793, 1983.
46. Cleveland M, Bosworth DM, Thompson FR: Pseudoarthrosis in the lumbosacral spine. J Bone Joint Surg Am 30:302, 1948.
47. Young HH, Love JG, Svien HJ, et al: Low back and sciatic pain: Long-term results after removal of protruded intervertebral disk with or without fusion. Clin Orthop 5:128, 1955.
48. Truchly G, Thompson WAL: Posterolateral fusion of the lumbosacral spine. J Bone Joint Surg Am 44:505, 1962.
49. Wiltse LL, Bateman JG, Duey R: Experiences with transverse process fusions in the lumbar spine. J Bone Joint Surg Am 44:1013, 1962.
50. Lee CK, Langrana NA: Lumbosacral spine fusion: A biomechanical study. Spine 9:429, 1984.
51. Flatley TJ, Derderian H: Closed loop instrumentation of the lumbar spine. Clin Orthop 196:273, 1985.
52. Masferrer R, Gomez CH, Karahalios DG, et al: Efficacy of pedicle screw fixation in the treatment of spinal instability and failed back surgery: A 5-year review. J Neurosurg 89:371, 1998.
53. Stauffer RN, Coventry MB: Posterolateral lumbar spine fusion. J Bone Joint Surg Am 54:1195, 1972.
54. Jackson RK, Boston DA, Edge AJ: Lateral mass fusion: A prospective study of a consecutive series with long-term follow-up. Spine 10:828, 1985.
55. Hoppenstein R: A new approach to the failed back syndrome. Spine 5:13, 1982.
56. Onofrio BM, Campa HK: Evaluation of rhizotomy: A review of 12 years' experience. J Neurosurg 36:751, 1972.
57. Loeser JD: Dorsal rhizotomy for the relief of chronic pain. J Neurosurg 36:745, 1972.
58. North RB, Kidd DH, Zahuak M: Spinal cord stimulation for chronic intractable pain: Experience over two decades. Neurosurgery 32:384, 1993.
59. Bell GK, Kidd DH, North RB: Cost effective analysis of spinal cord stimulation in treatment of failed back syndrome. Pain Symptom Manage 13:286, 1997.
60. Anderson VC, Burchiel KJ: A prospective study of long-term intrathecal morphine in the management of chronic nonmalignant pain. Neurosurgery 44:289, 1999.

CHAPTER 284

Metabolic and Other Nondegenerative Causes of Low Back Pain

EDWARD S. CONNOLLY ■ H. BRUCE HAMILTON

Low back pain is one of the most common afflictions of humans, with up to 80% of the population experiencing low back pain in their lifetimes.[1-3] Most patients improve within the first month, and 90% are symptom free by 3 months. Low back pain is a symptom and not in itself an illness.

Degenerative and mechanical disorders of the lower back afflict most patients presenting with low back pain. Fewer patients have nondegenerative low back pain from metabolic, inflammatory, infectious, neoplastic, hematologic, and vascular diseases and from visceral referred pain syndromes. Those presenting with back pain and fever, weight loss, continuous stiffness, acute bone pain, and pain at rest should be evaluated for these nondegenerative disorders.

METABOLIC BONE DISEASE

The endocrine system maintains bone homeostasis through the interplay of parathyroid hormone, calcitonin, and 1,25-dihydroxycholecalciferol, a major metabolite of vitamin D. Parathyroid hormone prevents serum calcium from falling by increasing resorption of calcium and phosphate from bone, increasing reabsorption of calcium from the renal tubules, and decreasing absorption of phosphate from the kidney. Calcitonin prevents abnormal increases in renal calcium and phosphate by decreasing absorption of calcium and phosphate from bone and decreasing reabsorption of calcium and phosphate from the renal tubules. Vitamin D maintains the ionized calcium transport system in bone, increases absorption of calcium and phosphate from the digestive tract, and decreases reabsorption of calcium from the kidneys.[4] Two thirds of bone weight is from mineral sources, and the remainder is from collagen and water. Bone mineral is present as hydroxyapatite crystals and amorphous calcium phosphate.[5] Bone is continuously being formed and resorbed by the actions of osteoblasts and osteoclasts. Osteoblasts form new bone on the surfaces of bone and are actively involved in the synthesis of bone matrix—primarily collagen—and facilitate the movement of mineral ions between the extracellular fluid and the bones. After the osteoblasts are embedded in the bone matrix, they become osteocytes and act as a cellular syncytium for the transport of mineral in and out of bone, deep to the bone surface. The osteoclasts are responsible for bone reabsorption and are capable of solubilizing bone matrix and releasing calcium and phosphate and of transporting them into the extracellular fluids.

If the metabolic system becomes unbalanced, bone disease occurs. The two major metabolic diseases affecting the vertebral column are osteomalacia and osteoporosis.

Osteomalacia

Osteomalacia is the failure of the bone matrix to mineralize normally.[5, 6] The most frequent causes of this failure to mineralize are a decrease in the concentration of calcium and phosphate in the extracellular fluid, abnormal functioning of osteoblasts, abnormal defective collagen production, and a low pH at the sites of mineralization. Osteomalacia can result from vitamin D deficiency caused by inadequate exposure to sunlight without vitamin D supplements, gastrointestinal disease that interrupts normal absorption of vitamin D, and impaired synthesis of 1,25-dihydroxycholecalciferol.[7, 8] Osteomalacia also can be caused by phosphate deficiency from low dietary intake, failure of intestinal absorption of phosphates, or impaired renal tubular phosphate reabsorption. Other causes include systemic acidosis,[9] drug side effects,[10, 11] tumor toxins,[12] and primary mineralization defects.

The most common cause of osteomalacia is malabsorption of calcium and vitamin D from the intestinal tract. The biologically active metabolites of vitamin D are secreted in the bile, and conditions such as biliary fistula, chronic steatorrhea, sprue, or surgical resections of a large portion of the distal jejunum and ileum may also produce osteomalacia.[8] Another cause of osteomalacia is chronic renal disease with impaired synthesis of 1,25-dihydroxycholecalciferol and the loss of calcium resorption. Phosphate-deficient diets, such as in those of vegetarians who do not eat diary products and of patients who take large doses of aluminum hydroxide,[12] which blocks the absorption of phosphate the intestines, also cause osteomalacia. Severe phosphate wasting is associated with certain tumors such as sclerosing hemangiomas, angiosarcomas, hemangiopericytomas, and nonossifying fibromas.[12]

Osteomalacia frequently is asymptomatic, but as the condition advances, diffuse skeletal pain and muscle weakness develop. Kyphosis is seen as a result of vertebral collapse and deformities of the ribs and long bones. An osteomalacia patient has a characteristic waddling gait due to proximal muscle weakness and low back pain on leg motion.

Initially, there is a mild hypercalcemia and increased serum parathyroid hormone level, a normal or slightly decreased serum phosphate concentration, and a decreased serum 2,5-dihydroxycholecalciferol level. As osteomalacia progresses, hypocalcemia occurs with a further decline in the concentration of 2,5-dihydroxycholecalciferol and an increase in the serum parathyroid hormone level.

There is initially some decrease in bone density that is indistinguishable from osteoporosis. The most pathognomonic radiologic finding in osteomalacia is the pseudofracture in long bones—a radiolucent band running perpendicular to the bone surface.[13] Pseudofractures are sometimes called Fraser's zones or milkman's fractures. As the disease progresses, compression fractures of the vertebrae may occur with little or no trauma.

Patients with vitamin D deficiency are treated with oral doses of ergocalciferol 0.05 μg (2000 IU) and regular periods of exposure to artificial or natural ultraviolet light. However, patients with malabsorption from the intestine do not respond well to vitamin D and require 5 μg (200,000 IU) of oral ergocalciferol per day or 40,000 to 80,000 IU intravenously.[14] Renal tubular acidosis is corrected with sodium bicarbonate. Tumor-induced osteomalacia responds to surgical removal of the tumor.

Osteoporosis

Osteoporosis, a generalized bone disorder characterized by loss of bone mass that causes bone fragility, is the most common metabolic bone disease. It occurs most commonly in postmenopausal women and the very old of both sexes. An estimated 20% of women suffer an osteoporotic fracture by the age of 65 years, and 40% of women have an osteoporotic fracture sometime during their lives.[14] Vertebral and hip fractures are the most common. The major etiologic factors in osteoporosis are deficiency in sex hormones and a deficiency of calcium intake in the elderly.[14–19] Research has identified genes that predispose the individual to osteoporosis.[20] Other risk factors include alcohol abuse, smoking, immobilization and lack of exercise,[21] and excessive exercise with weight loss and amenorrhea.[22, 23] Drug-induced osteoporosis is seen with the use of corticosteroids, thyroid hormone, and anticonvulsant drugs.[10, 11, 24]

Osteoporosis is also seen in genetic disorders such as Turner's syndrome and Klinefelter's syndrome. Two more forms of osteoporosis of unknown origin are juvenile osteoporosis, which occurs in late childhood and is self-limiting, and a malignant young-adult form, which may progress rapidly to a complete collapse of the axial skeleton and death from respiratory failure.[14]

The first symptom of osteoporosis is a vertebral compression fracture with localized pain in the back that is sometimes associated with radicular radiation. Weight bearing aggravates the pain, and bed rest improves the pain. Healing of the fracture and continued pain may last 4 to 8 weeks. Subsequent vertebral fractures may occur, producing chronic back pain (Fig. 284–1). Common findings are a dorsal kyphosis (i.e., window's hump) and loss of height.

In senile osteoporosis, serum calcium, alkaline phosphatase, and intact parathyroid hormone levels are within normal range. Quantitative computed tomography (CT) shows direct measurements of decreased bone mass in the central portion of the vertebral body.

Senile or postmenopausal osteoporosis is treated with oral calcium supplements (1 to 2 g of elemental calcium per day) plus estrogen (0.625 μg/day for 3 of 4 weeks). Progesterone (5 to 10 μg) is given during the last 10 days of the estrogen cycle.[14, 25] In elderly men, combined androgen and estrogen therapy is given. Decreasing intake of alcohol and tobacco and increasing

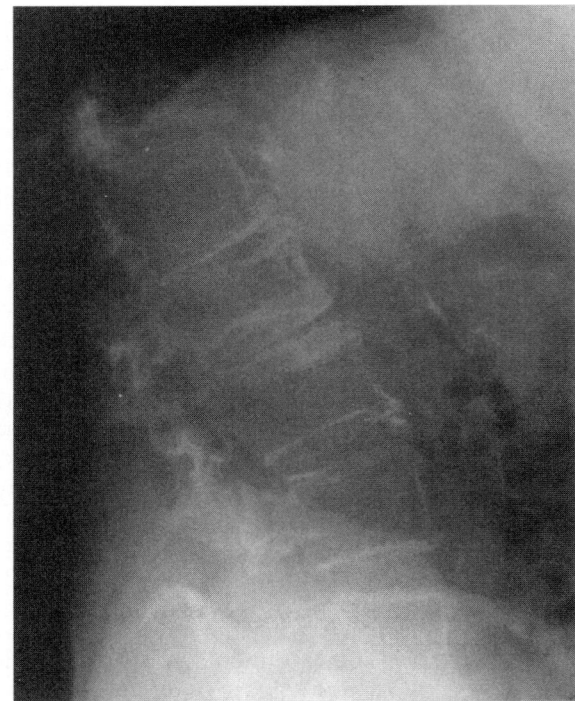

FIGURE 284–1. Osteopenia with severe compression of T12 and moderate compression of L1 is characteristic of osteoporosis associated with back pain.

exercise are also helpful. Thoracolumbosacral orthosis and Jewett braces are helpful in preventing further vertebral compressions. Sodium fluoride (50 μg/day) has been shown to aid the healing of vertebral compression fractures but has significant untoward side effects.[26] Kyphoplasty or vertebral plasty, which consists of injecting methyl acrylic into compression fracture, frequently relieves pain.

Paget's Disease (Osteitis Deformans)

Paget's disease is a focal disorder of bone metabolism characterized by uncontrolled bone reabsorption and formation by excessive numbers of osteoblasts and osteoclasts, leading to the formation of thick but soft bone. Paget's disease has a predilection for the lumbosacral spine. Paget's disease is unevenly distributed geographically, with a much higher incidence in England and Germany and a rare incidence in Scandinavia, Africa, the Mid-East, and Asia. Nuclear inclusions resembling virus particles have been seen in osteoclasts, suggesting a slow virus as a possible cause of Paget's disease.[27, 28]

Paget's disease may produce back pain from compression fracture or by causing nerve root compression from stenosis of the spinal canal and foramen. Severe focal bone pain may also occur with sarcomatous degeneration.

Serum calcium, phosphate, magnesium, and parathyroid hormone levels are normal. There are marked increases in the concentrations of alkaline phosphatase and acid phosphatase.

Radiologic abnormalities range from purely osteolytic lesions to combined osteolytic and sclerotic lesions. Thickening of the vertebrae, compression fracture, and disappearing vertebrae can be identified.[29]

Only symptomatic patients are treated. Decompressive laminectomies are indicated for severe spinal stenosis. Calcitonin (100 U/day given subcutaneously or intramuscularly) is the most common medical treatment, with bisphosphonates and mithramycin used for severe resistant cases.[29–31]

INFLAMMATORY DISORDERS

Spondyloarthropathies are a category of related diseases characterized by systemic involvement of bone, joints, ligaments, tendons, and muscles. These diseases are characterized by inflammation of the joints of the axial skeleton, the sacroiliac joints, and large peripheral joints. When spinal involvement occurs, it is usually diffuse. In most of these diseases, the rheumatoid factor is absent, and the diseases in which this factor is absent comprise the seronegative spondyloarthropathies.

Patients with spondyloarthropathies present with pain on arising in the morning that improves with activity. This pain and tenderness is most noticeable over the spine and sacroiliac joints, and motion is restricted. Laboratory tests reveal a nonspecific systemic inflammatory response.

Ankylosing Spondylitis

Inflammation, erosions, and ankylosis of joints and the point of attachment of ligaments, tendons, and joint capsules to bone constitute the classic pathologic pattern of ankylosing spondylitis. The sacroiliac, apophyseal, and costovertebral joints and the annulus and vertebral end plates are involved in the inflammation and ankylosis of the axial skeleton, whereas involvement with the appendicular skeleton is similar to rheumatoid arthritis.

The system for immune recognition, the major histocompatibility complex, appears to be a factor in the pathogenesis of ankylosing spondylitis. Human leukocyte antigen B27 (HLA-B27) is found in 8% of American whites but in at least 87.5% of American whites with ankylosing spondylitis.[32] The prevalence of HLA-B27 among blacks in the United States is about 2%, and ankylosing spondylitis is rare in blacks.

Extra-articular manifestations occur in the ocular, cardiovascular, and pulmonary systems. Uveitis occurs in 20% to 25% of those with ankylosing spondylitis, whereas aortitis, valvular dysfunction, and cardiomegaly occur in 3% to 10%. Pulmonary apical disease and fibrosis appear in just over 1% of patients affected with ankylosis spondylitis. Approximately 0.1% to 0.2% of the white population is affected by ankylosing spondylitis, and the disease seems to be three to nine times more prevalent in men. Ankylosing spondylitis is milder and less rapidly progressive in women. Typically, the disease begins in people 15 to 40 years of age.[32, 33]

An insidious onset of low back pain and stiffness in the second and third decade is the usual manifestation. This pain may extend from the thoracic spine to the buttocks, radiating into the legs above the knee, and it is usually worse in the morning but improves with exercise. Peripheral joint complaints and the nonspecific systemic manifestations of fatigue, anemia, low-grade fevers, and weight loss are often present.

The earliest and most specific radiographic abnormalities for ankylosing spondylitis are erosions and sclerosis of subchondral bone in the lower portion of the sacroiliac joint that are usually bilateral and symmetrical. As the disease progresses, ankylosis of this joint predominates. Anterior ossification of the longitudinal ligaments of the vertebrae, causing squaring of the vertebrae, calcifications of the intraspinous and supraspinous ligaments, and apophyseal joint fusion, is common and develops sequentially in a caudal-to-rostral manner, producing the characteristic bamboo-spine appearance (Fig. 284–2).

Treatment of ankylosing spondylitis is directed at maintaining normal posture and mobility through physical therapy and medications. Irradiation was used in the past but is now limited to those intolerant of medical therapy and with very focal disease. Nonsteroidal anti-inflammatory drugs are effective in controlling the pain and stiffness of ankylosing spondylitis but do not alter progression of the disease. Corticosteroids, gold therapy, d-penicillamine, and antimalarial drugs have no treatment benefits in these patients.

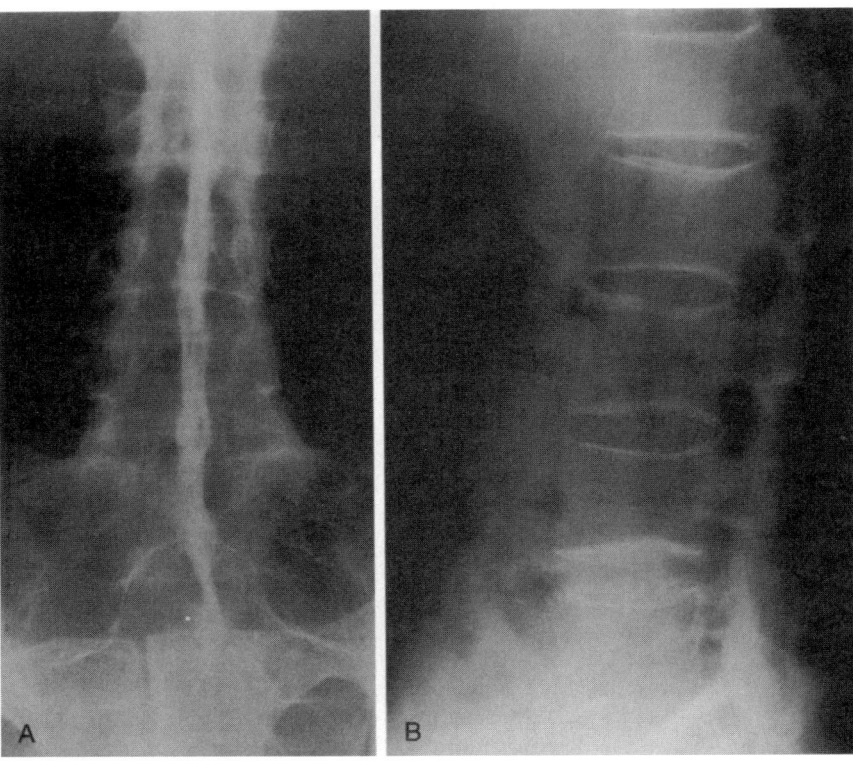

FIGURE 284–2. Early changes in a bamboo spine include fusion of the sacroiliac joints. *A,* Anterior-posterior view. *B,* Lateral view.

Reiter's Syndrome

The triad of urethritis, conjunctivitis, and arthritis is the classic description of Reiter's syndrome, with some authorities adding keratodermia blennorrhagia and circinate balanitis. This syndrome is associated with nongonococcal urethritis and enteral infections with *Shigella, Salmonella, Campylobacter,* and *Yersinia,* and it usually occurs during or shortly after these infections. The HLA-B27 antigen is present in 80% of these patients.[32, 33] The arthritic component of Reiter's syndrome typically includes a periarterial arthropathy that is acute, involves a few joints (often asymmetrically), and most commonly involves the lower extremities. Axial involvement includes sacroiliitis that occurs in more than one third of these patients and arthropathy of the lumbosacral spine. The sacroiliitis in Reiter's syndrome may be unilateral and asymmetrical, unlike ankylosing spondylitis and inflammatory bowel disease, but it is otherwise indistinguishable. Spinal involvement, including ossification and syndesmophyte formation, occurs less often and in a more random fashion than in ankylosing spondylitis.

Genitourinary symptoms occur in 93% of patients. Iritis and conjunctivitis with pain and photophobia occur in 20%.[32] One third experience fever, anorexia, and fatigue. Mucocutaneous lesions are also common.

The arthritis occurs 1 to 3 weeks after the initial infection, most commonly with asymmetrical pain in the knees, ankles, feet, and sacroiliac joint. The sacroiliac joint is involved in 30% to 90% of these patients and accounts for most back pain.[32, 33]

Psoriatic Arthropathy

Psoriatic arthritis occurs in 7% of the patients with psoriasis and is primarily located in the hands, feet, and axial skeleton. This arthritis most commonly manifests asymmetrically in a few joints of the peripheral skeleton but may occur symmetrically, and in 20% of patients, it involves the axial skeleton. Arthritis mutilans, a severe form of the disease, occurs in 5% of patients with psoriatic arthritis and causes extensive joint destruction of the hands and feet.

The uric acid concentration is elevated in 20% of patients who may develop gout, whereas 35% to 60% of those with axial skeletal involvement have elevated expression of HLA-B27.[32, 33]

Radiographically, osteolysis of the proximal phalanx, widening of the distal interphalangeal joint, and long-bone periosteal reaction are seen in the extremities, but the axial findings are indistinguishable from those in Reiter's syndrome. Sacroiliitis usually occurs in an asymmetrical fashion and may be unilateral, but ossification and syndesmophyte formation of the joint are asymmetrical.

Psoriasis occurs equally in men and women, with most cases occurring in temperate climates. Among all patients with psoriasis, 5% develop psoriatic arthritis, usually after the onset of skin changes. Severity of skin and nail changes increase the risk of developing psoriatic arthritis but do not correlate with the arthritis symptoms. Spinal involvement occurs in 20% of psoriatic arthritic patients and tends to predominate in male patients and have an onset later in life.[32, 33]

The pain of psoriatic arthritis occurs most commonly in the fingers and toes. Asymptomatic decreased motion of the spine and joints can occur, as well as tenderness at the sacroiliac joints and spine.

Enteropathic Arthritis

The association of inflammatory bowel disease and spondyloarthropathy of the axial skeleton is called enteropathic arthritis. Division of these patients into three groups is based on the temporal relationship of the bowel disease and onset of the spondyloarthropathy—whether the spondyloarthropathy preceded, followed, or was concurrent with the inflammatory bowel disease.

Peripheral arthritis occurs concurrently with exacerbations of bowel disease, whereas the spinal disease progresses independently of the bowel disease. Of all patients with enteropathic arthropathy, 5% are HLA-B27 positive, but among patients with axial skeletal involvement, this percentage increases to 50% to 75%.[32]

Peripheral joints exhibit soft tissue swelling and effusions without the presence of joint space narrowing and destruction on radiographic examination, but the axial skeletal changes are identical to those in ankylosing spondylitis: bilateral, symmetrical sacroiliitis; ossification; and progressive syndesmophyte formation in a symmetrical fashion.

Spondyloarthropathy occurs in about 2% to 12% of cases of ulcerative colitis and Crohn's disease.[32] Pain and stiffness of peripheral and axial joints that improve with ambulation are common, along with the symptoms and signs associated with the bowel disease. Ulcerations of the gastrointestinal tract, iritis, erythema nodosum, and pyoderma gangrenosum are common.

Myofascial Pain Syndrome (Fibromyositis of Fibromyalgia)

Myofascial syndrome may occur as a generalized or focal problem. The focal myofascial syndromes are common, estimated to occur in 6% to 15% of the population, and constitute one of the most common causes of musculoskeletal pain.[34] This syndrome frequently affects the low back and neck, usually occurring in middle-aged patients, with a marked female preponderance. Approximately one half of patients with this syndrome admit to sleep disturbance. It is frequently initiated by injury or overuse. Diagnosis depends on the presence of a trigger point. The treatment consists of injecting the trigger points with local analgesics, followed by stretching exercises of the involved muscle groups. Strengthening exercises should be avoided. Heat and massage may be beneficial.

Rheumatoid Arthritis

Rheumatoid arthritis is a chronic inflammatory disease affecting many joints, including those of the spine. Joint involvement is usually symmetrical, and the disease affects multiple joints, most commonly the metacarpal phalangeal, proximal interphalangeal, wrist, and knee joints. Multiple other joints are commonly involved. When spinal involvement occurs, it is almost exclusively in the cervical spine, conspicuously sparing the thoracolumbar spine. Back pain is not a usual symptom in rheumatoid arthritis.

INFECTIONS

Infectious processes involving the lumbar spine are common sources of back pain. These infections may affect the intervertebral disk, the vertebral body, the pedicles and laminae, and other soft tissues immediately surrounding the spine.

Infections of the disk space should be divided into two separate categories: pediatric and adult. Pediatric infectious diskitis is almost always bacterial, although viral causes can be found. These cases of diskitis are believed to be from a hematogenous source. Immobilization and antibiotics are curative in most cases. The adult disk space infection is usually a complication of spinal surgery, although hematogenous spread from distant areas does occur and is usually related to a genitourinary tract infection. Blood cultures and tuberculin tests should be performed on all patients. Antibiotic treatment is usually effective in treating the infection, and immobilization alleviates pain. In resistant cases and in those associated with epidural abscess, surgical débridement and drainage may be necessary.

Osteomyelitis of the spine develops when the infectious organism enters the bone. The involved bone is usually the body of the vertebra and only rarely the posterior element of the spine. The most frequent site of infection is the lumbar spine, followed by the thoracic spine and the cervical and sacral bones. The source of the infectious agent is usually through hematogenous spread from a distant infection. Immunosuppressed patients and diabetics are more susceptible, as are intravenous drug users. *Staphylococcus aureus* remains the most common organism causing pyogenic osteomyelitis of the spine. Infections with gram-negative rod organisms are closely associated with genitourinary infections. Osteomyelitis may occur from urinary and genital tract manipulations that cause phlebitis of Batson's plexus and after spinal surgery or from adjacent local infections. Bacterial, viral, fungal, and parasitic organisms can cause osteomyelitis of the spine. The incidence increases with age.

Paraspinal abscesses usually arise next to an area of osteomyelitis. They infrequently occur independently of other spinal infections or in association with previous spinal surgery.

Pyogenic Infections

Pyogenic infections of the spine almost exclusively involve the vertebral body, occurring most commonly in the lumbar spine and occasionally the thoracic spine. They usually arise from hematogenous spread of an infectious process elsewhere in the body, although genitourinary manipulations, spinal surgery, and adjacent infections may be causative. These infections may manifest acutely, subacutely, or chronically, depending on the virulence of the organism and on the host response to the infection.

The patient's history may indicate an increased likelihood of pyogenic spinal infections. Patients with sickle cell anemia may be infected with *Salmonella*, intravenous drug users with *Pseudomonas aeruginosa*, and those who have had urinary tract procedures with *Escherichia coli* and *Proteus*. Diabetes, prior spinal surgeries, and trauma also predispose patients to pyogenic vertebral infections.

Pain and tenderness exacerbated by motion and palpation are the most common symptoms. Motion may be severely limited, and a hip flexion deformity may result from psoas muscle irritation. Most patients do not appear septic, although they may have fever, chills, and malaise. Only a few patients have an increased temperature.

The erythrocyte segmentation rate is usually elevated, and the white blood cell count is frequently normal, although the differential count is usually abnormal, showing a left shift. Blood cultures for infectious agents are positive in 50% of cases.

Radiographic examination is normal within the first few days of the infection. A paravertebral shadow and disk space loss are often the initial signs of infection and do not occur before 2 or 3 weeks. Vertebral end plates show an increased density at approximately 12 weeks, and lytic changes in these end plates develop later, leading to vertebral destruction and collapse in the worst cases (Fig. 284–3). CT reveals bone erosion and vertebral destruction quite early and delineates the soft tissue abnormalities at the infection site. Magnetic

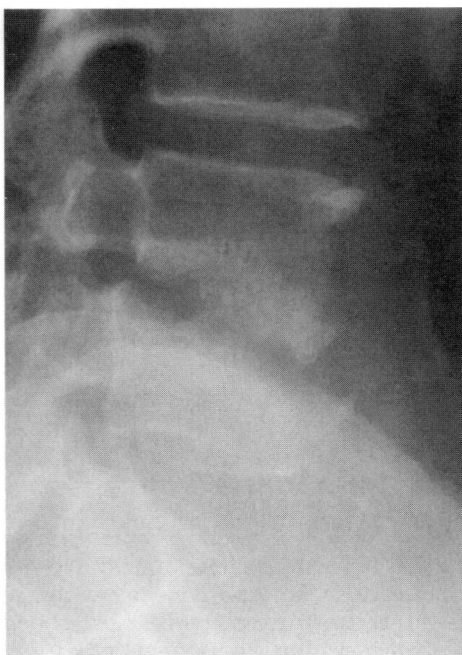

FIGURE 284–3. Loss of the disk space and lytic changes of the vertebral end plates are characteristic of pyogenic infection of the vertebrae.

resonance imaging (MRI) is becoming the most sensitive and specific method of diagnosing pyogenic infections of the spine because it has a sensitivity of 96%, specificity of 92%, and accuracy of 94%.[35] A bone scan may localize the area before radiographic evidence exists and is extremely sensitive to inflammatory changes quite early. The earliest positive diagnostic test is MRI, showing gadolinium enhancement of the disk space (Figs. 284–4).

Treatment includes rest, immobilization if pain is severe, and appropriate antibiotics after cultures are obtained. A 6-week course of intravenous antibiotics is a general guideline. If the clinical response is not seen within the first 3 weeks, if neurological compromise exists or progresses, or if evidence of a chronic infection exists (i.e., draining sinus tract), surgical débridement should be considered. If bone destruction is sufficient to produce instability, reconstruction and fusion are indicated.

Granulomatous Disease

Granulomatous infections are caused by organisms that elicit a granulomatous immune response. When granulomatous bony infection occurs, the spine is a frequent site of involvement, with the vertebral body being most commonly involved. The source of the infecting organism is usually pulmonary with hematogenous spread to the spine.

Patients with granulomatous disease present with localized back pain that is aggravated by movement. As destruction of the vertebral bodies, intervertebral disks, and ligaments progresses, angulation of the spine, spinal collapse, and inflammatory material compressing the neural elements may occur.

Radiographic appearance is similar in all granulomatous spinal infections. Vertebral end plates are subject to lytic destruction, and as the disease progresses, vertebral collapse and spinal angulation occur.

Laboratory evaluation and medical treatments are specific for each disease. Otherwise, conservative and surgical management are similar for all granulomatous spinal infections.

The most common granulomatous infection is tuberculosis. Fungal infections caused by *Blastomyces dermatitidis*, *Cryptococcus neoformans*, *Coccidioides immitis*, *Aspergillus*, and *Histoplasma capsulatum*, as well as bacteria of the genus *Brucella*, *Actinomyces bovis*, and *Actinomyces israelii*, give rise to granulomatous disease of the spine.

NEOPLASTIC DISEASE

Neoplasia of the lumbar spine is an uncommon cause of low back pain, but when neoplastic disease involves the spine, pain is the most prominent and common symptom. The differential diagnosis of low back pain should include neoplastic disorders because of the associated morbidity and mortality and the likelihood that the prognosis can be significantly improved with early diagnosis and treatment.

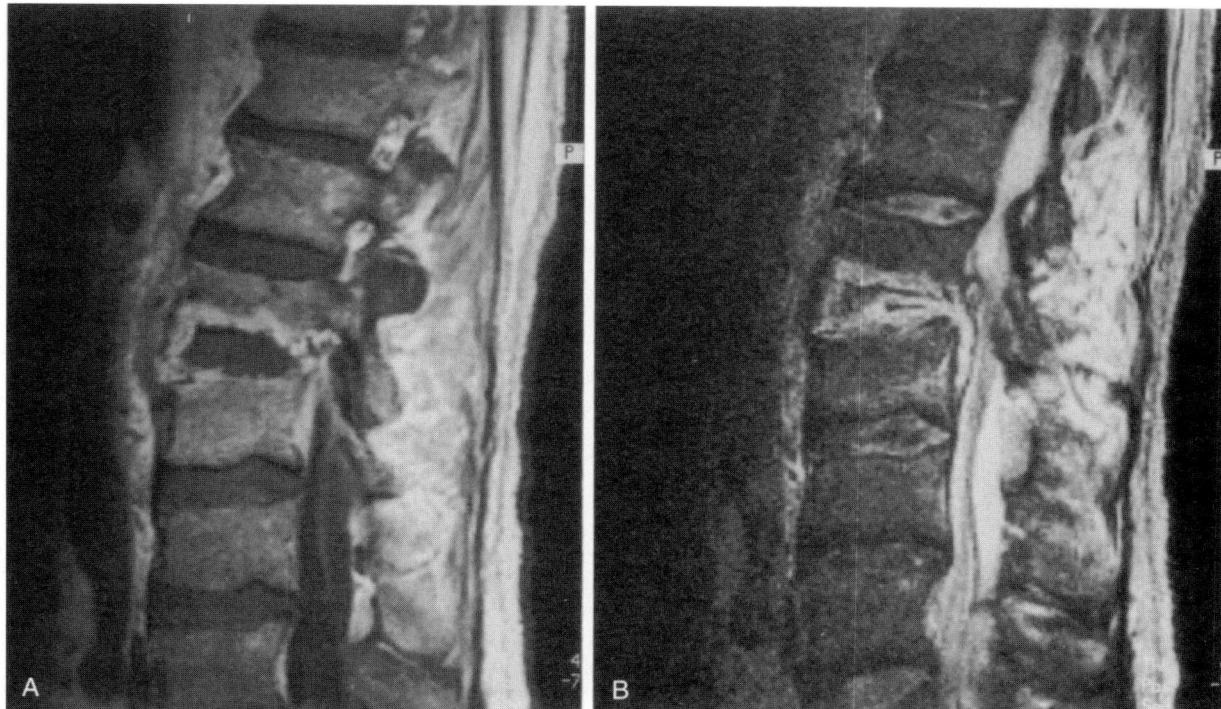

FIGURE 284–4. *A,* Gadolinium enhancement of the infected disk joint is seen on magnetic resonance imaging. *B,* The T2-weighted image shows an epidural mass compressing the thecal sac.

Neoplastic spinal lesions may arise from local lesions within or adjacent to the spinal column or from the metastatic spread of distant malignancies. Local lesions consist of primary tumors of bone, the spinal cord, nerve roots, meninges, and adjacent soft tissues. Metastatic lesions may arise from almost all malignancies; however, breast carcinoma, pulmonary carcinoma, lymphoreticular malignancies, and genitourinary tract cancers are the most common primary tumor types, accounting for more than one half of these lesions.

Primary bony tumors and metastases can be found throughout all regions of the spine and in all age groups. However, the metastatic lesions are far more common. Metastases involve the skeleton 40 times more frequently than all other tumors involving the bones, and the vertebral column is the most common site. Primary tumors are rare, accounting for a very small percentage of all spinal tumors. A variety of extradural and intradural soft tissue tumors may give rise to low back pain. Focal pain is the most common symptom in spinal neoplasia. This pain is progressive, unremitting, and may worsen with recumbency at night. Radicular symptoms may also be present. Spine deformation may occur initially from pain and paraspinous spasm and later from bony destruction and instability. Weakness and neurological deficits exist in nearly one half of these patients.

The rate of symptom progression, the patient's age, and tumor location are of diagnostic and prognostic significance. Rapid progression of symptoms and neurological compromise are associated with the more malignant tumors, whereas slow, symptomatic progression is associated with the more benign tumors. Metastatic disease is most common in the fifth and sixth decades because of the peak incidence of carcinoma and lymphoreticular disease in this period. Primary tumors occurring after the age of 21 are usually malignant, and those occurring before 21 years are most likely benign. Most malignant disease manifests as tumors involving the vertebral body and the pedicles. Posterior element tumors tend to be benign.

Benign Primary Tumors

OSTEOID OSTEOMA AND OSTEOBLASTOMA

Osteoid osteoma and osteoblastoma are pathologically similar diseases that are differentiated by size. Osteoid osteomas are less than 1.5 cm in diameter, and osteoblastomas are larger than or equal to 1.5 cm.[36] These lesions are solitary, painful, and osteoblastic, and they are most commonly seen in the bones of the lower extremities, with a propensity for spinal involvement by 10% to 41% of these lesions.[37, 38]

When they occur in the spine, the posterior elements are almost always the site of origin. They are rarely found in the vertebral body. The lumbar spine is most frequently involved. These lesions occur most frequently in the second and third decades, and they are more common in men.

Pain is the characteristic complaint; it is persistent but more severe at night. Less than 50% of cases show dramatic improvement of the pain with aspirin.[37–39] A few lesions are painless, and some patients have associated radicular involvement.

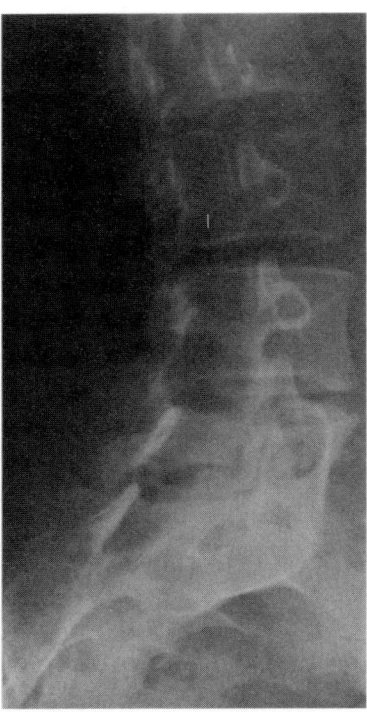

FIGURE 284–5. Osteoblastoma involves the pedicle.

Radiographic films show an expansion of cortical bone that has a dense sclerotic edge with a central radiolucent nidus involving the posterior elements of the spine (Fig. 284–5). Radioisotope bone scans and CT are the diagnostic tests of choice when plain radiography is unrevealing.

Excision of the lesions is the treatment of choice, but curettage is effective when excision is not feasible. With complete excision, pain is eliminated in 92% of patients.[38]

OSTEOCHONDROMA

Osteochondromas are common, benign bone lesions, with vertebral involvement occurring in roughly 7% of all cases. Hyaline cartilage–capped bony growths extend from the growth plate as solitary or multiple lesions that usually grow quite slowly.

These lesions are usually asymptomatic, but although rare, symptoms of cord and root compression may occur. Radiographic examination reveals the bony portion of the lesion, but the cartilaginous cap is rarely visualized on plain radiography. CT, MRI, and myelography may be required for complete visualization.

Surgical excision is the treatment of choice. Recurrence is uncommon and is usually delayed if it does occur.

ANEURYSMAL BONE CYST

Aneurysmal bone cysts are benign neoplastic lesions of bone consisting of anastomosis of cavernous spaces. Spine involvement is rare, but when the spine is in-

volved, the lumbar spine is the most frequent site, with cysts typically involving the posterior elements. Most lesions appear in the second and third decades of life and are more common in women.

Pain, tenderness, and local swelling are the most common symptoms at initial presentation. As the lesion expands, spinal cord and root compression may occur.

Radiographically, these lesions often extend between multiple adjacent vertebrae. The expansive osteolytic capita with their thin cortexes have a bubbly appearance that gives the lesion its name (Fig. 284–6).

The treatment of choice is excision when feasible, but curettage seems to be similarly efficacious. Cysts recur in approximately 10% to 15% of cases, but a second resection or curettage is quite effective.

HEMANGIOMA

Hemangioma, the most common primary tumor of the spine, usually develops in the thoracic spine. These benign tumors of vascular origin occur most commonly around the fifth decade of life and affect women slightly more frequently than men.

Hemangiomas are rarely symptomatic, but if present, they usually cause focal pain and spinal deformity. Neurological symptoms may be produced by pathologic fracture and focal swelling or by soft tissue extension and compression of neurological structures.

Radiographically, the vertebral body appears to have decreased density with prominent vertical striations throughout the body. CT shows a classic starburst appearance (Fig. 284–7).

These radiosensitive tumors may sometimes be cured by selective irradiation.[40] Surgical resection should be considered in symptomatic cases when irradiation is not feasible or when neurological compres-

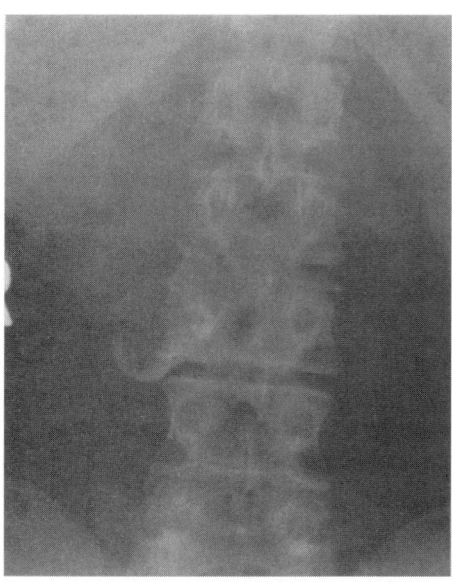

FIGURE 284–6. The osteolytic lesion with a bubbly appearance is an aneurysmal bone cyst.

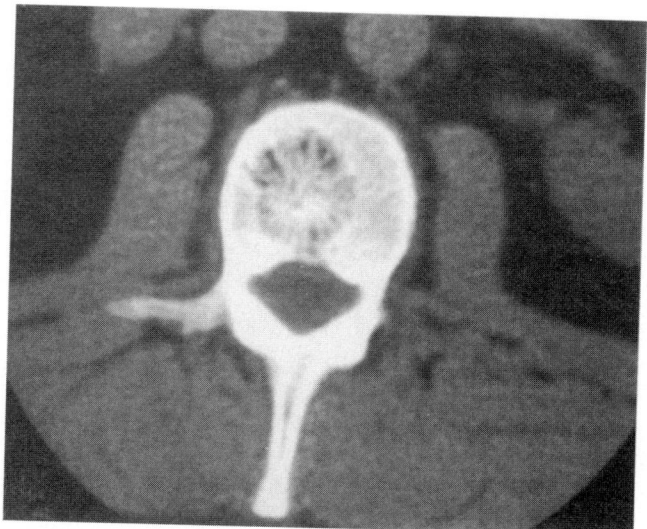

FIGURE 284–7. Classic starburst appearance is characteristic of a hemangioma of the vertebral body.

sion occurs. Angiography is frequently performed before surgical excision to evaluate the vertebral vascularity and to embolize the lesion, limiting severe blood loss.[41, 42]

EOSINOPHILIC GRANULOMA

Eosinophilic granuloma is a benign lesion that is a member of the reticuloendothelial proliferative diseases. Called Langerhans' histiocytosis or histiocytosis X, eosinophilic granuloma has an uncertain origin. When spinal involvement occurs, a single vertebra is usually involved, most commonly a cervical vertebra and least commonly a lumbar vertebra. The vertebral body is generally involved. Eosinophilic granuloma can occur in all age groups.[43]

Pain, focal spasm, and vertebral deformity are common at presentation. As the lesion expands, bony destruction may lead to partial vertebral collapse. More complete collapse leads to the classic vertebra plana. This bony destruction is believed to be the cause of the initial signs and symptoms and the source of later neurological compression and malfunction.

Radiographically, a central lytic lesion with poorly defined margins and a periosteal reaction is revealed early in the disease, with vertebral collapse into the vertebra plana appearing with disease progression. The disk is spared.

Because the disease is self-limited, many patients do not require treatment. When neurological compromise occurs, steroids and low-dose radiation therapy with immobilization is a widely accepted treatment.

GIANT CELL TUMOR (OSTEOCLASTOMA)

Giant cell tumors of bone are locally aggressive, benign lesions made up of mononuclear cells interposed with multinucleated osteoclast-like giant cells. Spinal involvement occurs in 2% to 3% of patients with these lesions, but there is no preference for any spinal level.[44, 45] Almost all lesions involve the vertebral body, but the posterior elements also may be involved. Women are affected slightly more frequently than men, with a peak incidence in the third decade.

Paraspinous muscular spasm is the most common presenting symptom. Pain and radicular changes are less common.

A lytic lesion that is well circumscribed or expansive, depending on the aggressiveness of the lesion, can be seen on plain radiography. A well-defined pseudocapsular margin is visible on CT, which allows complete tumor delineation and evaluation of tumor expansion beyond anatomic borders (Fig. 284–8).

Because of the locally aggressive nature of these lesions, complete excision is the treatment of choice. When complete removal is not possible, phenol, cement, cryosurgery, curettage, and radiotherapy should be employed as adjunctive therapy.

Malignant Primary Tumors

PLASMACYTOMA

Plasmacytomas are tumors composed of malignant plasma cells. They may occur as a part of systemic bone marrow disease, forming multiple myelomas, or they may exist as a lesion that is outside of bone marrow (i.e., extramedullary plasmacytoma) or a solitary lesion of bone (i.e., solitary plasmacytoma). The prognosis for patients with extramedullary plasmacytomas appears to be better than that for the multiple myelomas or solitary bone plasmacytomas.[46] The spine is the initial site at presentation in 25% to 50% of cases of solitary plasmacytomas. These tumors usually appear after the fifth decade of life and are three times more common in men than women. The thoracic spine is the most common site of involvement, but the lum-

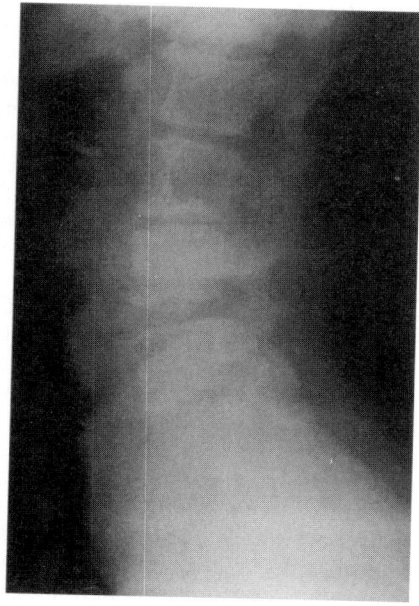

FIGURE 284–8. A giant cell tumor involves the vertebral body.

bar spine is frequently involved. Some plasmacytomas may be secretory.

The initial presenting symptom of patients with solitary plasmacytomas is deep and persistent focal pain. Neurological involvement may result from tumor impingement on neural structures or from compression fractures. Associated paraprotein secretion, which is generally much less than in multiple myeloma, can lead to a variety of syndromes, including hyperviscosity, coagulation abnormalities, renal disease, and amyloidosis. Radiographically, these lesions are lytic and usually sharply demarcated in the spine. Bone scanning results may be normal or show decreased radionuclide uptake. CT and MRI are useful in delineating spinal lesions.

In minimally involved vertebrae, irradiation is the treatment of choice. With extensive bony destruction, surgical excision and anterior reconstruction and fusion should be undertaken.

MULTIPLE MYELOMA

Multiple myeloma is a systemic disease in which malignant plasma cells begin to proliferate within the marrow and spread throughout the body. Spinal involvement occurs in all cases of multiple myeloma. Multiple myeloma is rare, occurring in 4.7 of 100,000 white men and in 3.2 of 100,000 white women, with twice that frequency among blacks. In most cases, the disease appears after the sixth decade, with a male preponderance in both races.[47]

The symptoms are similar to those of isolated plasmacytoma but appear more widespread. Bone pain, anemia, neurological changes from compression, and compression fractures are common. Paraprotein syndromes such as coagulation disorders, renal disease, amyloidosis, and a decreased ability to fight infection are common in patients with multiple myeloma.

Radiographically, the lytic lesions of multiple myeloma are identical to those of isolated plasmacytomas but are more widespread and have a salt-and-pepper appearance (Fig. 284–9).

Corticosteroids, antineoplastic agents, and selective radiation therapy are used in the treatment of this systemic disease. When neurological compromise occurs, surgical decompression may be also indicated.

The prognosis is considerably worse in multiple myeloma compared with solitary plasmacytomas. Disease-free survival is possible for patients with solitary lesions, but for those with systemic multiple myeloma, median survival is 28 months, with a 25% to 29.3% 5-year survival rate.[47] When spinal cord involvement exists, the prognosis is worse in both diseases.

OSTEOSARCOMA

Osteosarcoma is the most common primary malignant tumor of bone after myeloma, accounting for nearly 20% of osseous tumors. These osteoblastic tumors develop most commonly in the rapidly growing bones of the extremities as primary osteosarcoma and occur in a variety of other conditions, such as Paget's disease,

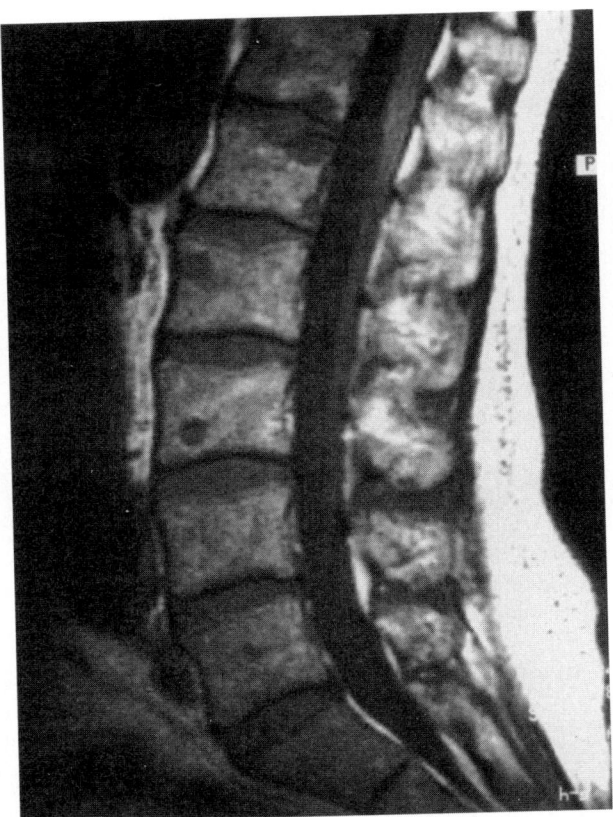

FIGURE 284–9. Multiple lytic lesions of the vertebrae are seen in patients with multiple myeloma.

fibrous dysplasia, and some benign tumors, and after irradiation. Spinal involvement exists in 1% to 3% of patients with these tumors, with 95% of the lesions arising from anterior elements of the spine. Osteogenic sarcomas are most common between the ages of 10 and 20 years, but spinal involvement is most common in adults. Secondary lesions occur later in life. Men are affected slightly more often than women.[48]

Pain at the tumor site is the most common presenting symptom, but two thirds of patients with osteosarcomas present with a neurological deficit. Tumor extension is responsible for these symptoms.

Radiographically, these lesions are classified as osteolytic, sclerotic, and mixed. Most lesions in the spine show a mixed picture of lytic and sclerotic areas, with cortical erosion and a marked periosteal reaction producing the typical sunburst pattern. CT and MRI delineate the soft tissue extension, canal involvement, and the presence of metastases.

Treatment with chemotherapy followed by excision and irradiation has been advocated. The prognosis for patients with this disease is dismal; the median survival is 6 months, with occasional long-term survivors.

EWING'S SARCOMA

Ewing's sarcoma makes up 0.5% of primary malignant bone tumors of the spine. These small, round-cell tumors of unknown origin arise predominantly in the sacrum and lumbar spine and demonstrate male predominance. They appear most commonly in the second decade of life, at an average age of 16.5 years.[49]

At presentation, localized pain is the most common symptom; radicular symptoms and urinary and bowel problems are frequently identified. One fourth of patients are febrile.

Plain radiographic examination reveals lytic, moth-eaten destruction of bone with a sclerotic rim. Vertebral collapse may develop in severe disease.

Surgical excision is the treatment of choice. Multiagent chemotherapy and high-dose radiotherapy are required, because surgical excision is seldom complete. The 5-year survival rate of 40% is increasing as therapies improve.

CHORDOMA

Chordoma is a rare, primary malignant tumor that arises from remnants of the primitive notochord of the sacrococcygeal and basioccipital regions and occasionally from notochordal rests in the vertebrae. These lesions account for about 20% of malignant tumors of the axial skeleton, one half in the sacrococcygeal region and 15% in the vertebrae above the sacrum.[50] Men develop sacral chordomas three times more often than women, and most of these tumors appear in the fifth through seventh decades of life. There is no sexual preference in clival or vertebral chordomas.[50-53]

Pain in the low back and sacrum is the most common presenting symptom. Radicular changes, bladder and bowel difficulties, and a palpable mass are frequently encountered.

Typical radiographic findings include bony destruction, associated with a large soft tissue mass, calcifications in the sacrum, and lytic destruction of the vertebrae with a sclerotic rim in the lumbar spine. The vertebral disk is spared. CT and MRI are useful for delineating tumor extent (Fig. 284–10).

Complete surgical resection with wide margins is the treatment of choice. High-dose radiation therapy may serve a palliating role in the control of pain and neurological deficit. Chemotherapy is generally ineffective. The median 5-year survival is 66% for sacral chordomas and 50% for vertebral chordomas.[52]

CHONDROSARCOMA

Chondrosarcoma, a rare malignant tumor of cartilaginous origin, may arise as a primary malignancy or develop from benign cartilaginous tumors after irradiation. Approximately 10% of these tumors arise in the spine, with a uniform distribution through all segments. Men are affected more commonly than women, and the mean age at presentation is in the fourth decade.[43]

Pain is the most common presenting symptom, with neurological compromise taking place as the tumor progresses. Swelling can occur.

Radiographically, these lesions appear as areas of bone destruction and an associated soft tissue mass

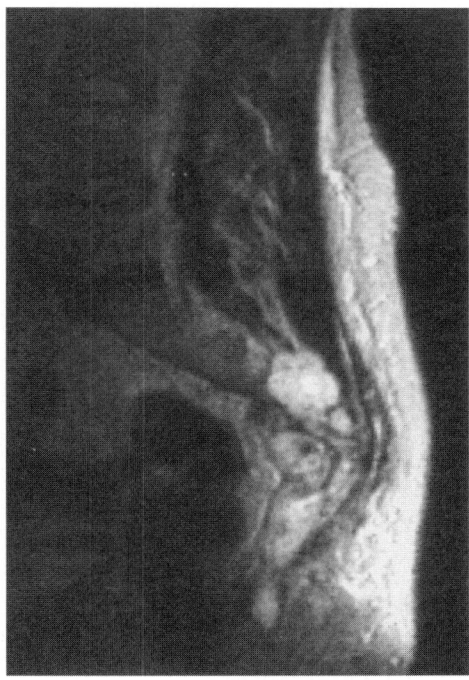

FIGURE 284–10. A chordoma of the sacrococcygeal joints is identified on magnetic resonance imaging.

that is frequently calcified. CT and MRI can delineate tumor extent.

Complete surgical excision is the treatment of choice. Radiotherapy is seldom indicated; it is useful only in those with residual tumor and only for palliative treatment. Chemotherapy has no role in the treatment of these tumors. The median survival rate at 5 years is 50%.

Malignant Secondary Tumors

The axial skeleton is the third most common site of metastases after lung and liver. Metastases are by far the most common skeletal tumors, and the spine is the most common site of involvement. Metastases account for 70% of all tumors of the spine, and the lumbar spine is most frequently involved.[1] The most common primary tumor types are carcinoma of the breast, carcinoma of the lung, lymphoma, and carcinoma of the prostate.

Involvement of the spine may occur through marrow replacement by tumor cells, through hematogenous spread, or by direct extension from an adjacent lesion. Tumor-bone interaction is both destructive and proliferative. Destruction of bone may occur by direct tumor lysis or indirectly through vascular derangement and the release of diffusible substances that increase osteoclastic activity. The osteoblastic response to bony destruction accounts for the proliferative phase.

Despite the wide variety of spinal neoplasia, a common syndrome of pain, neurological compression, and segmental destruction and instability is typical. In metastasis, the first and most common symptom is pain,

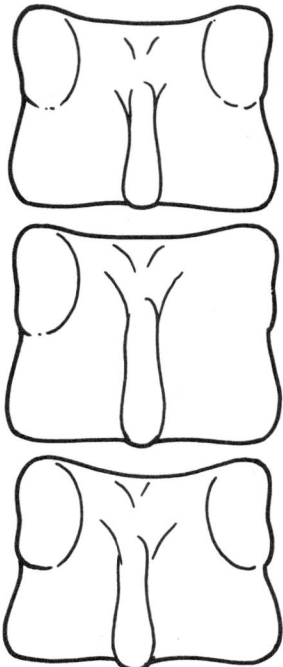

FIGURE 284–11. Loss of the outline of one pedicle of the vertebra, which is usually the first sign of metastatic involvement, is seen as the winking owl sign on an anteroposterior view of a plain radiograph.

which is progressive, persistent, localized, and worse at night.

Radiographically, these lesions are classified as osteolytic, osteoblastic, or mixed; most are osteolytic. The osteoblastic reaction is most common in prostate carcinoma and Hodgkin's disease; occasionally, cervical, gastric, and breast carcinomas produce "ivory vertebrae." The first radiographic involvement is seen in the pedicle, producing the winking owl sign (Fig. 284–11). MRI, the most helpful diagnostic test for metastatic tumors of the spine, shows lesions before they are visible on plain radiography and reveals their soft tissue extension and neural components (Fig. 284–12).

For most patients, radiotherapy has been the treatment of choice for spinal metastases. Tumors of the prostate and lymphoreticular system are very radiosensitive. Most breast carcinomas are sensitive, but gastrointestinal and renal tumors are quite resistant. Surgery is indicated when the diagnosis is in doubt. Surgical treatment is indicated for patients with radioresistant lesions and for healthy individuals who have an isolated lesion that is producing a neurological deficit or severe pain. Laminectomy is seldom indicated, and surgical treatment requires resection of the vertebral body involvement, followed by reconstruction and fusion.

NONVERTEBRAL SPINAL TUMORS

A variety of intradural and extradural soft tissue tumors arising about the spinal column give rise to low back pain.

Intramedullary Tumors of the Spine

One fifth of the intradural tumors are intramedullary tumors of the spinal cord, and more than one half of these intramedullary tumors are ependymomas. Astrocytomas make up approximately 40%, with the remainder being hemangioblastomas, lipomas, and dermoids.[54] One half of these lesions arise in the lumbar region, with slightly more than one third arising in the thoracic spine. There is no age or sexual preference for these tumors.

The most common presenting symptom is back pain that is not radicular but that may be associated with a band of hypoesthesia. Myelopathic changes usually follow as the disease progresses.

Complete excision of these tumors, if technically possible, is the treatment of choice. Ependymomas offer the best chance at total surgical resection and cure. Astrocytomas are usually unresectable and have a high recurrence rate; those with a higher pathologic grade should be irradiated.

Extramedullary Intradural Tumors of the Spine

Two thirds of the intradural spinal tumors are extramedullary and are usually benign. Neurofibromas and meningiomas account for nearly 70% of extramedullary tumors and occur equally frequently. Sarcomas account for 10%; epidermoids and dermoids occur less frequently. For the three most common tumors (i.e., neu-

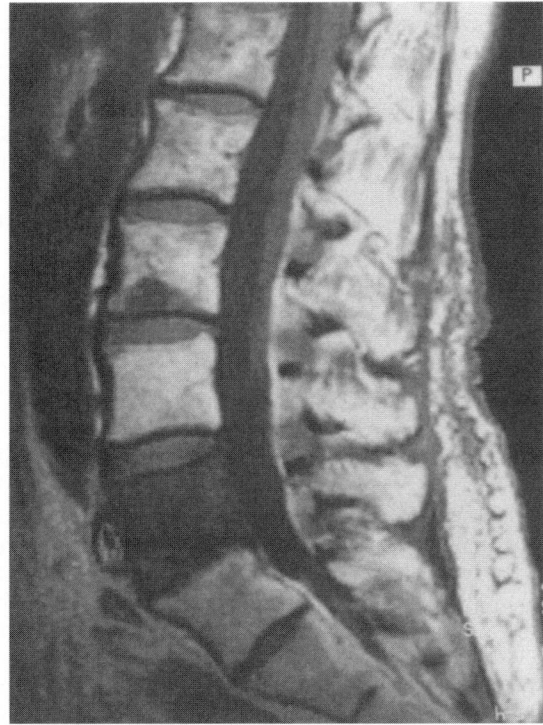

FIGURE 284–12. Magnetic resonance imaging shows metastatic carcinomatous involvement of L4 with a narrow compression and an associated lesion at L2.

rofibromas, meningiomas, and sarcomas), the frequency increases with increasing age. Neurofibromas and sarcomas affect men and women equally, but 80% of meningiomas occur in women.[54]

Radicular pain is the most common symptom at presentation, but back pain, with a tendency to worsen at night, also occurs. Radiculopathy and myelopathy occur as the disease progresses.

The recommended treatment is complete excision, which often is curative for patients with neurofibromas, meningiomas, dermoids, and epidermoids. Sarcomas in these sites require adjuvant therapy as in other locations.

RETROPERITONEAL AND PELVIC DISORDERS

Disease processes in the retroperitoneal space or pelvis may manifest as back pain. Periodic low back pain may occur in persons with endometriosis and may even be associated with leg pain if the lumbosacral plexus is involved. The back pain usually begins just before the menses. The usual treatment is hormone manipulation. Retroperitoneal inflammatory processes, such as perforation of a retroperitoneal appendix, sigmoid diverticulitis, and posterior wall duodenal ulcer, may manifest as low back pain. Tumors in the retroperitoneal space involving the pancreas, kidney, or rectum are associated with back pain. Aortic aneurysms with dissection produce severe, acute back pain. All of these processes are characterized by nonfocal pain, unlike the very focal pain characteristic of vertebral involvement.

REFERENCES

1. Posner JB: Back pain and epidural spinal cord compression. Med Clin North Am 71:185–205, 1987.
2. Martinelli TA, Wiesel SW: Low back pain: The algorithmic approach. Compr Ther 17:22–27, 1991.
3. McCowin PR, Borenstein D, Wiesel SW: The current approach to the medical diagnosis of low back pain. Orthop Clin North Am 22:315–325, 1991.
4. Neer RM: Calcium and inorganic phosphate homeostasis. In DeGroot LJ, Besser GM, Cahill GF Jr, et al (eds): Endocrinology, 2nd ed. Philadelphia, WB Saunders, 1989, pp 927–953.
5. Frame B, Parfitt MA: Osteomalacia: Current concepts. Ann Intern Med 89:966–982, 1978.
6. Goldring SR, Krane SM: Disorders of calcification: Osteomalacia and rickets. In DeGroot LJ, Besser GM, Cahill GF Jr, et al (eds): Endocrinology, 2nd ed. Philadelphia, WB Saunders, 1989, pp 1165–1187.
7. Fraser D, Kooh SW, Kind HP, et al: Pathogenesis of hereditary vitamin-D–dependent rickets: An inborn error of vitamin D metabolism involving defective conversion of 25-hydroxyvitamin D to 1α,25-dyhydroxy-vitamin D. N Engl J Med 289:817–822, 1973.
8. Morgan DB, Hunt G, Paterson CR: The osteomalacia syndrome after stomach operations. Q J Med 39:395–410, 1970.
9. Morris RC Jr, Sebastian A, McSherry E: Symposium on acid-base homeostasis: Renal acidosis. Kidney Int 1:322–340, 1972.
10. Hahn TJ, Hendin BA, Scharp CR, et al: Serum 25-hydroxycalciferol levels and bone mass in children on chronic anticonvulsant therapy. N Engl J Med 292:550, 1975.
11. Maclaren N, Lifshitz F: Vitamin D–dependency rickets in institutionalized, mentally retarded children on long term anticonvulsant therapy. II. The response to 25-hydroxycholecalciferol and to vitamin D₂. Pediatr Res 7:914–922, 1973.
12. Ryan EA, Reiss E: Oncogenous osteomalacia: Review of the world literature of 42 cases and report of two new cases. Am J Med 77:501–512, 1984.
13. Steinbach HL, Noetzli M: Roentgen appearance of the skeleton in osteomalacia and rickets. Am J Roentgenol Radium Ther Nucl Med 91:955–972, 1964.
14. Riggs BL: Osteoporosis. In DeGroot LJ, Besser GM, Cahill GF Jr, et al (eds): Endocrinology, 2nd ed. Philadelphia, WB Saunders, 1989, pp 1188–1207.
15. Cann CE, Martin MC, Genant HK, et al: Decreased spinal mineral content in amenorrheic women. JAMA 251:626–629, 1984.
16. Ettinger B, Genant HK, Cann CE: Long-term estrogen replacement therapy prevents bone loss and fractures. Ann Intern Med 102:319–324, 1985.
17. Lindsay R, Hart DM, Aitken JM, et al: Long-term prevention of postmenopausal osteoporosis by oestrogen: Evidence for an increased bone mass after delayed onset of oestrogen treatment. Lancet 1:1038–1041, 1976.
18. Consensus Conference Development Panel (Peck WA, Barrett-Connor E, Buckwalter JA, et al): Osteoporosis. JAMA 252:799–802, 1984.
19. Riggs BL, Melton LJ III: Involutional osteoporosis. N Engl J Med 314:1676–1686, 1986.
20. Mundy GR, Gregory R: Osteoporosis: Boning up on genes. Nature 367:216–217, 1994.
21. Aloia JF, Cohn SH, Ostuni JA, et al: Prevention of involutional bone loss by exercise. Ann Intern Med 89:356–358, 1978.
22. Drinkwater BL, Nilson K, Chestnut CH III, et al: Bone mineral content of amenorrheic and eumenorrheic athletes. N Engl J Med 311:277–281, 1984.
23. Marcus R, Cann C, Madvig P, et al: Menstrual function and bone mass in elite women distance runners: Endocrine and metabolic features. Ann Intern Med 102:158–163, 1985.
24. Paul TL, Kerrigan J, Kelly AM, et al: Long-term l-thyroxine therapy is associated with decreased hip bone density in premenopausal women. JAMA 259:3137–3141, 1988.
25. Riis B, Thomsen K, Christiansen C: Does calcium supplementation prevent postmenopausal bone loss? A double-blind, controlled clinical study. N Engl J Med 316:173–177, 1987.
26. Riggs BL, Seeman E, Hodgson SF, et al: Effect of the fluoride/calcium regimen on vertebral fracture occurrence in postmenopausal osteoporosis: Comparison with conventional therapy. N Engl J Med 306:446–450, 1982.
27. Arnold A: Paget's disease of bone: Pathophysiology and diagnosis. In DeGroot LJ, Besser GM, Cahill GF Jr, et al (eds): Endocrinology, 2nd ed. Philadelphia, WB Saunders, 1989, pp 1208–1244.
28. Singer FR, Mills BG: Evidence for a viral etiology of Paget's disease of bone. Clin Orthop 178:245–251, 1983.
29. Freeman DA: Paget's disease of bone. Am J Med Sci 295:144–158, 1988.
30. Strewler GE: Paget's disease of bone. Medical Staff Conference, University of California, San Francisco. West J Med 140:763–768, 1984.
31. Wallach S: Treatment of Paget's disease. In Stollerman GH (ed): Advances in Internal Medicine, vol 27. Chicago: Year Book Medical Publishers, 1982, pp 1–43.
32. Kahn MA, van der Linden SM: Ankylosing spondylitis and other spondyloarthropathies. Rheum Dis Clin North Am 16:551–579, 1990.
33. Wollheim FA: Ankylosing spondylitis. In Kelly WN, Harris ED Jr, Ruddy S, et al (eds): Textbook of Rheumatology, 4th ed. Philadelphia, WB Saunders, 1993, pp 943–960.
34. Yunus M, Masi AT, Calabro JJ, et al: Primary fibromyalgia (fibrositis): Clinical study of 50 patients with matched normal controls. Semin Arthritis Rheum 11:151–171, 1981.
35. Modic MT, Feiglin DH, Piraino DW, et al: Vertebral osteomyelitis: Assessment using MR. Radiology 157:157–166, 1985.
36. Nemoto O, Moser RP Jr, Van Dam BE, et al: Osteoblastoma of the spine: A review of 75 cases. Spine 15:1272–1280, 1990.
37. Byers PD: Solitary benign osteoblastic lesions of bone. Osteoid osteoma and benign osteoblastoma. Cancer 22:43–57, 1968.
38. Kirwan EO, Hutton PA, Pozo JL, et al: Osteoid osteoma and benign osteoblastoma of the spine: Clinical presentation and treatment. J Bone Joint Surg Br 66:21–26, 1984.
39. Janin Y, Epstein JA, Carras R, et al: Osteoid osteomas and osteoblastomas of the spine. Neurosurgery 8:31–38, 1981.

40. Yang ZY, Zhang LJ, Chen ZX, Hu HY: Hemangioma of the vertebral column: A report on twenty-three patients with special reference to functional recovery after radiation therapy. Acta Radiol Oncol 24:129–132, 1985.

41. Graham JJ, Yang WC: Vertebral hemangioma with compression fracture and paraparesis treated with preoperative embolization and vertebral resection. Spine 9:97–101, 1984.

42. Hemmy DC, McGee DM, Armbrust FH, et al: Resection of a vertebral hemangioma after preoperative embolization. J Neurosurg 47:282–285, 1977.

43. Berry DH, Becton DL: Natural history of histiocytosis-X. Hematol Oncol Clin North Am 1:23–34, 1987.

44. Dahlin DC: Giant-cell tumor of vertebrae above the sacrum: A review of 31 cases. Cancer 39:1350–1356, 1977.

45. Savini R, Gherlinzoni F, Morandi M, et al: Surgical treatment of giant-cell tumor of the spine: The experience at the Instituto Ortopedico Rizzoli. J Bone Joint Surg Am 65:1283–1289, 1983.

46. Knowling MA, Harwood AR, Bergsagel DE: Comparison of extramedullary plasmacytomas with solitary and multiple plasma cell tumors of bone. J Clin Oncol 1:255–262, 1983.

47. Riedel DA, Pottern LM: The epidemiology of multiple myeloma. Hematol Oncol Clin North Am 6:225–247, 1992.

48. Sundaresan N, Schiller AL, Rosenthal: Osteosarcoma of the spine. In Sundaresan N, Schmidek HH, Schiller AL, et al (eds): Tumors of the Spine. Philadelphia, WB Saunders, 1990, pp 128–145.

49. Bradway JK, Pritchard DJ: Ewing's tumor of the spine. In Sundaresan N, Schmidek HH, Schiller AL, et al (eds): Tumors of the Spine. Philadelphia, WB Saunders Company, 1990, pp 235–239.

50. Healey JH, Lane JM: Chordoma: A critical review of diagnosis and treatment. Orthop Clin North Am 20:417–426, 1989.

51. O'Neill P, Bell BA, Miller JD, et al: Fifty years of experience with chordomas in Southeast Scotland. Neurosurgery 16:166–170, 1985.

52. Sundaresan N, Galicich JH, Chu FC, Huvos AG: Spinal chordomas. J Neurosurg 50:312–319, 1979.

53. Paavolainen P, Teppo L: Chordoma in Finland. Acta Orthop Scand 47:46–51, 1976.

54. Connolly ES: Spinal cord tumors in adults. In Youmans JR (ed): Neurological Surgery, 2nd ed. Philadelphia, WB Saunders, 1982, pp 3196–3215.

BIBLIOGRAPHY

Altman RD, Collins-Yudiskas B: Synthetic human calcitonin in refractory Paget's disease of bone. Arch Intern Med 147:1305, 1987.

Amendola BE, Amendola MA, Oliver E, et al: Chordoma: Role of radiation therapy. Radiology 158:839, 1986.

Anderson M: Management of cerebral infection. J Neurol Neurosurg Psychiatry 56:1243, 1993.

Andrews WC: What's new in preventing and treating osteoporosis? Postgrad Med 104:89, 1998.

Angtuaco EJC, McConnell JR, Chadduck WM, et al: MR imaging of spinal epidural sepsis. AJR Am J Roentgenol 149:1249, 1987.

Arnaud CD: Calcium homeostasis: Regulatory elements and their integration. Fed Proc 37:2557, 1978.

Auwerx J, Bouillon R: Mineral and bone metabolism in thyroid disease: A review. Q J Med 60:737, 1986.

Baker ND, Greenspan A, Neuwirth M: Symptomatic vertebral hemangiomas: A report of four cases. Skeletal Radiol 15:458, 1986.

Belza MG, Urich H: Chordoma and malignant fibrous histiocytoma: Evidence for transformation. Cancer 58:1082, 1986.

Bennett RM: The fibromyalgia syndrome: Myofascial pain and the chronic fatigue syndrome. In Kelley WN, Harris ED Jr, Ruddy S, et al (eds): Textbook of Rheumatology, 4th ed. Philadelphia, WB Saunders, 1993, pp 471–483.

Bogduk N: The causes of low back pain. Med J Aust 156:151, 1992.

Boulware DW, Schmid LD, Baron M: The fibromyalgia syndrome: Could you recognize and treat it? Postgrad Med 87:211, 1990.

Bremnes RM, Hauge HN, Sagsveen R: Radiotherapy in the treatment of symptomatic vertebral hemangiomas: Technical case report. Neurosurgery 39:1054, 1996.

Bringhurst FR: Calcium and phosphate distribution, turnover, and metabolic actions. In DeGroot LJ, Besser GM, Cahill GF Jr, et al (eds): Endocrinology, 2nd ed. Philadelphia, WB Saunders, 1989, pp 805–843.

Buskila D: Fibromyalgia, chronic fatigue syndrome, and myofascial pain syndrome. Curr Opin Rheumatol 11:119, 1999.

Calderone RR, Larsen JM: Overview and classification of spinal infections. Orthop Clin North Am 27:1, 1996.

Campbell SM, Clark S, Tindall EA, et al: Clinical characteristics of fibrositis: I. A "blinded," controlled study of symptoms and tender points. Arthritis Rheum 26:817, 1983.

Cecil M, Dimar JR II: Paraspinal pyomyositis, a rare cause of severe back pain: Case report and review of the literature. Am J Orthop 26:785, 1997.

Congdon CC: Benign and malignant chordomas: A clinico-anatomical study of twenty-two cases. Am J Pathol 28:793, 1952.

Constans JP, de Divitiis E, Donzelli R, et al: Spinal metastases with neurological manifestations: Review of 600 cases. J Neurosurg 59:111, 1983.

Corwin J, Lindberg RD: Solitary plasmacytoma of bone vs. extramedullary plasmacytoma and their relationship to multiple myeloma. Cancer 43:1007, 1979.

Cummings BJ, Hodson DI, Bush RS: Chordoma: The results of megavoltage radiation therapy. Int J Radiat Oncol Biol Phys 9:633, 1983.

Currier BL, Eismont FJ: Infections of the spine. In Rothman RH, Simeone FA (eds): The Spine, 3rd ed. Philadelphia, WB Saunders, 1992, pp 1319–1380.

Dagi TF, Schmidek HH: Vascular tumors of the spine. In Sundaresan N, Schmidek HH, Schiller AL, et al (eds): Tumors of the Spine: Diagnosis and Clinical Management. Philadelphia, WB Saunders, 1990, pp 181–191.

Danner RL, Hartman BJ: Update of spinal epidural abscess: 35 cases and review of the literature. Rev Infect Dis 9:265, 1987.

Delmas PD, Chapuy M-C, Edouard C, et al: Beneficial effects of aminohexane diphosphonate in patients with Paget's disease of bone resistant to sodium etidronate. Am J Med 83:276, 1987.

Devogelaer J-P, Maldague B, Malghem J, et al: Appendicular and vertebral bone mass in ankylosing spondylitis. A comparison of plain radiographs with single- and dual-photon absorptiometry and with quantitative computed tomography. Arthritis Rheum 35:1062, 1992.

Edgar MA, Ghadially JA: Innervation of the lumbar spine. Clin Orthop 115:35, 1976.

Eismont FJ, Bohlm HH, Soni PL, et al: Pyogenic and fungal vertebral osteomyelitis with paralysis. J Bone Joint Surg Am 65:19, 1983.

Emery SE, Chan DPK, Woodward HR: Treatment of hematogenous pyogenic vertebral osteomyelitis with anterior débridement and primary bone grafting. Spine 14:284, 1989.

Ergan M, Macro M, Benhamou CL, et al: Septic arthritis of lumbar facet joints: A review of six cases. Rev Rhum Engl Ed 64:386, 1997.

Eriksson B, Gunterberg B, Kindblom LG: Chordoma: A clinicopathologic and prognostic study of a Swedish national series. Acta Orthop Scand 52:49, 1981.

Feldenzer JA, McKeever PE, Schaberg DR, et al: The pathogenesis of spinal epidural abscess: Microangiographic studies in an experimental model. J Neurosurg 69:110, 1988.

Floman Y, Bar-On E, Mosheiff R, et al: Eosinophilic granuloma of the spine. J Pediatr Orthop B 6:260, 1997.

Fox MW, Onofrio BM, Kilgore JE: Neurological complications of ankylosing spondylitis. J Neurosurg 78:871, 1993.

Fraser RD, Osti OL, Vernon-Roberts B: Iatrogenic discitis: The role of intravenous antibiotics in prevention and treatment: An experimental study. Spine 14:1025, 1989.

Frymoyer JW, Cats-Baril WL: An overview of the incidences and costs of low back pain. Orthop Clin North Am 22:263, 1991.

Frymoyer JW, Newberg A, Pope MH, et al: Spine radiographs in patients with low-back pain: An epidemiological study in men. J Bone Joint Surg Am 66:1048, 1984.

Frymoyer JW, Pope MH, Clements JH, et al: Risk factors in low back pain. J Bone Joint Surg Am 65:213, 1983.

Glorieux FH, Scriver CR, Reade TM, et al: Use of phosphate and vitamin D to prevent dwarfism and rickets in X-linked hypophosphatemia. N Engl J Med 287:481, 1972.

Goldenberg DL: Fibromyalgia syndrome: An emerging but controversial condition. JAMA 257:2782, 1987.

Gordan GS, Picchi J, Roof BS: Antifracture efficacy of long-term estrogens for osteoporosis. Trans Assoc Am Physicians 86:326, 1973.

Gruber HE, Ivey JL, Baylink DJ, et al: Long-term calcitonin therapy in postmenopausal osteoporosis. Metabolism 33:295, 1984.

Hehne H-J, Zielke K, Böhm H: Polysegmental lumbar osteotomies and transpedicle fixation for correction of long-curved kyphotic deformities in ankylosing spondylitis: Report on 177 cases. Clin Orthop 258:49, 1990.

Helliwell PS, Zebouni LNP, Porter G, et al: A clinical and radiological study of back pain in rheumatoid arthritis. Br J Rheumatol 32: 216, 1993.

Hirsch C, Ingelmark B-E, Miller M: The anatomical basis for low back pain. Acta Orthop 33:1, 1963.

Ho EKW, Chan FL, Leong JCY: Postsurgical recurrent stress fracture in the spine affected by ankylosing spondylitis. Clin Orthop 247: 87, 1989.

Horenstein S: Chronic low back pain and the failed low back syndrome. Neurol Clin 7:361, 1989.

Hosrman A, Jones M, Francis R, et al: The effect of estrogen dose on postmenopausal bone loss. N Engl J Med 309:1405, 1983.

Hudson TM, Galceran M: Radiology of sacrococcygeal chordoma: Difficulties in detecting soft tissue extension. Clin Orthop 175: 237, 1983.

Hutter RVP, Worcester JN Jr, Francis KC, et al: Benign and malignant giant cell tumors of bone. Cancer 15:653, 1962.

Huvos AG, Butler A, Bretsky SS: Osteogenic sarcoma associated with Paget's disease of bone: A clinicopathologic study of 65 patients. Cancer 52:1489, 1983.

Ireland P, Fordtran JS: Effect of dietary calcium and age on jejunal calcium absorption in humans studied by intestinal perfusion. J Clin Invest 52:2672, 1973.

Kellgren JH: On the distribution of pain arising from deep somatic structures with charts of segmental pain areas. Clin Sci 4:35, 1939.

Kenny JB, Hughes PL, Whitehouse GH: Discovertebral destruction in ankylosing spondylitis: The role of computed tomography and magnetic resonance imaging. Br J Radiol 63:448, 1990.

Kirkaldy-Willis WH, Hill RJ: A more precise diagnosis for low-back pain. Spine 4:102, 1979.

Kirwan EOG: Back pain. In Wall PD, Melzack R (eds): Textbook of Pain, 2nd ed. New York, Churchill Livingstone, 1989, pp 335–340.

Kirwan J, Edwards A, Huitfeldt B, et al: The course of established ankylosing spondylitis and the effects if sulphasalazine over 3 years. Br J Rheumatol 32:729, 1993.

Koppel BS, Tuchman AJ, Mangiardi JR, et al: Epidural spinal infection in intravenous drug abusers. Arch Neurol 45:1331, 1988.

Krol G, Sundaresan N, Deck M: Computed tomography of axial chordomas. J Comput Assist Tomogr 7:286, 1983.

Lane JM: Osteoporosis: Medical prevention and treatment. Spine 22(Suppl):32S, 1997.

Lane JM, Nydick M: Osteoporosis: Current modes of prevention and treatment. J Am Acad Orthop Surg 7:19, 1999.

Larsson S-E, Lorentzon R, Boquist L: Giant-cell tumors of the spine and sacrum causing neurological symptoms. Clin Orthop 111: 201, 1975.

Lau CS, Burgos-Vargas R, Louthrenoo W, et al: Features of spondyloarthritis around the world. Rheum Dis Clin North Am 24: 753, 1998.

Leithner A, Windhager R, Lang S, et al: Aneurysmal bone cyst: A population based epidemiologic study and literature review. Clin Orthop 363:176, 1999.

Lichtenstein L: Benign osteoblastoma: A category of osteoid- and bone-forming tumors other than classical osteoid osteoma, which may be mistaken for giant-cell or osteogenic sarcoma. Cancer 9: 1044, 1956.

Liebergall M, Chaimsky G, Lowe J, et al: Pyogenic vertebral osteomyelitis with paralysis. 289:142, 1991.

MacLaughlin J, Holick MF: Aging decreases the capacity of human skin to produce Vitamin D₃. J Clin Invest 76:1536, 1985.

Macnab I, McCulloch J: Backache, 2nd ed. Baltimore, Williams & Wilkins, 1990, pp 22–25.

McCain GA, Harth M, Bell DA, et al: Septic discitis. J Rheumatol 8: 100, 1981.

Meyers SP, Wiener SN: Diagnosis of hematogenous pyogenic vertebral osteomyelitis by magnetic resonance imaging. Arch Intern Med 151:683, 1991.

Miettinen M, Lehto V-P, Virtanen I: Malignant fibrous histiocytoma within a recurrent chordoma: A light microscopic, electron microscopic, and immunohistochemical study. Am J Clin Pathol 82: 738, 1984.

Miller PD, Brown JP, Siris ES, et al: A randomized, double-blind comparison of risedronate and etidronate in the treatment of Paget's disease of bone. Paget's Risedronate/Etidronate Study Group. Am J Med 106:513, 1999.

Mitchell MJ, Sartoris DJ, Moody D, et al: Cauda equina syndrome complicating ankylosing spondylitis. Radiology 175:521, 1990.

Mooney V: The classification of low back pain. Ann Med 21:321, 1989.

Mooney V: The syndromes of low back disease. Orthop Clin North Am 14:505, 1983.

Mooney V: Where is the lumbar pain coming from? Ann Med 21: 373, 1989.

Nachemson AL: Newest knowledge of low back pain: A critical look. Clin Orthop 279:8, 1992.

Nassim JR, Saville PD, Cook PB, et al: The effects of vitamin D and gluten-free diet in idiopathic steatorrhoea. Q J Med 28:141, 1959.

Nilas L, Christiansen C: Bone mass and its relationship to age and the menopause. J Clin Endocrinol Metab 65:697, 1987.

Nittner K: Spinal meningiomas, neurinomas and neurofibromas and hourglass tumours. In Vinken PJ, Bruyn GW (eds): Handbook of Clinical Neurology. New York, American Elsevier, 1976, pp 177–322.

Odell WD, Swerdloff RS: Male hypogonadism. West J Med 124: 446, 1976.

Ozuna RM, Delamarter RB: Pyogenic vertebral osteomyelitis and postsurgical disc space infections. Orthop Clin North Am 27: 87, 1996.

Padovani R, Poppi M, Pozzati E, et al: Spinal epidural hemangiomas. Spine 6:336, 1981.

Paillas J-E, Alliez B, Pellet W: Primary and secondary tumours of the spine. In Vinken PJ, Bruyn GW (eds): Handbook of Clinical Neurology. New York, American Elsevier, 1976, pp 19–54.

Papagelopoulos PJ, Galanis EC, Sim FH, et al: Clinicopathologic features, diagnosis, and treatment of osteoblastoma. Orthopedics 22:244, quiz 248, 1999.

Pardo-Mindan FJ, Guillen FJ, Villas C, et al: A comparative ultrastructural study of chondrosarcoma, chordoid sarcoma, and chordoma. Cancer 47:2611, 1981.

Parfitt AM, Gallagher JC Heaney RP, et al: Vitamin D and bone health in the elderly. Am J Clin Nutr 36:1014, 1982.

Paris SV: Anatomy as related to function and pain. Orthop Clin North Am 14:475, 1983.

Porter RW: Mechanical disorders of the lumbar spine. Ann Med 21: 361, 1989.

Ralston SH, Urquhart GDK, Brzeski M, et al: Prevalence of vertebral compression fractures due to osteoporosis in ankylosing spondylitis. BMJ 300:563, 1990.

Ratliff JK, Connolly ES: Intramedullary tuberculoma of the spinal cord: Case report and brief review of the literature. J Neurosurg 90:125, 1999.

Rich TA, Schiller A, Suit HD, et al: Clinical and pathologic review of 48 cases of chordoma. Cancer 56:182, 1985.

Riggs BL, Gallagher JC, DeLuca HF, et al: A syndrome of osteoporosis, increased serum immunoreactive parathyroid hormone, and inappropriately low serum 1,25-dyhydroxyvitamin D. Mayo Clin Proc 53:701, 1978.

Riggs BL, Melton LJ III: Evidence for two distinct syndromes of involutional osteoporosis. Am J Med 75:899, 1983.

Rigotti NA, Nussbaum SR, Herzog DB, et al: Osteoporosis in women with anorexia nervosa. N Engl J Med 311:1601, 1984.

Rowed DW: Management of cervical spinal cord injury in ankylosing spondylitis: The intervertebral disc as a cause of cord compression. J Neurosurg 77:241, 1992.

Saifuddin A, White J, Sherazi Z, et al: Osteoid osteoma and osteoblastoma of the spine. Factors associated with the presence of scoliosis. Spine 23:47, 1998.

Salisbury JR, Isaacson PG: Demonstration of cytokeratins and an epithelial membrane antigen in chordomas and human fetal notochord. Am J Surg Pathol 9:791, 1985.

Schofferman L, Schofferman J, Zucherman J, et al: Occult infections causing persistent low-back pain. Spine 14:417, 1989.

Scoles PV, Quinn TP: Intervertebral discitis in children and adolescents. Clin Orthop 162:31, 1982.

Seeman E, Melton LJ, O'Fallon WM, et al: Risk factors for spinal osteoporosis in men. Am J Med 75:977, 1983.

Selecki BR, Sewell M: Neurosurgical management of spinal condition—an overview. Aust N Z J Surg 54:37, 1984.

Silver JJ, Einhorn TA: Osteoporosis and aging: Current update. Clin Orthop 316:10, 1995.

Singh M, Riggs BL, Beabout JW, et al: Femoral trabecular-pattern index for evaluation of spinal osteoporosis. Ann Intern Med 77: 63, 1972.

Slooff JL, Kernahera JW, MacCarty CS: Primary Intramedullary Tumors of the Spinal Cord and Filum Terminale. Philadelphia, WB Saunders, 1964.

Stamp TCB, Round JM: Seasonal changes in human plasma levels of 25-hydroxyvitamin D. Nature 247:563, 1974.

Stone DB, Bonfiglio M: Pyogenic vertebral osteomyelitis. Arch Intern Med 112:491, 1963.

Tsai KS, Heath H III, Kumar R, et al: Impaired vitamin D metabolism with aging in women: Possible role in pathogenesis of senile osteoporosis. J Clin Invest 73:1668, 1984.

van der Linden S, van der Heijde D: Ankylosing spondylitis: Clinical features. Rheum Dis Clin North Am 24:663, vii, 1998.

Vecht CJ: Effect of age on treatment decisions of low-grade glioma. J Neurol Neurosurg Psychiatry 56:1259, 1993.

Villas C, López R, Zubieta JL: Case report. Osteoid osteoma in the lumbar and sacral regions: Two cases of difficult diagnosis. J Spinal Disord 3:418, 1990.

Vukmir RB: Low back pain: Review of diagnosis and therapy. Am J Emerg Med 9:328, 1991.

Waldvogel FA, Medoff G, Swartz MN: Medical progress. Osteomyelitis: A review of clinical features, therapeutic considerations and unusual aspects (first of three parts). N Engl J Med 282:198, 1970.

Waldvogel FA, Medoff G, Swartz MN: Medical progress. Osteomyelitis: A review of clinical features, therapeutic considerations and unusual aspects (second of three parts). N Engl J Med 282:260, 1970.

Waldvogel FA, Medoff G, Swartz MN: Medical progress. Osteomyelitis: A review of clinical features, therapeutic considerations and unusual aspects (third of three parts). N Engl J Med 282:316, 1970.

Waldvogel FA, Vasey H: Medical progress. Osteomyelitis: The past decade. N Engl J Med 303:360, 1980.

Weinstein J: Neurogenic and nonneurogenic pain and inflammatory mediators. Orthop Clin North Am 22:235, 1991.

Weinstein JN, McLain RF: Tumors of the spine. In Rothman RH, Simeone FA (eds): The Spine, 3rd ed. Philadelphia, WB Saunders, 1992, pp 1279–1318.

Whalen JL, Brown ML, McLeod R, et al: Limitations of indium leukocyte imaging for the diagnosis of spine infections. Spine 16: 193, 1991.

Wiley AM, Trueta J: The vascular anatomy of the spine and its relationship to pyogenic vertebral osteomyelitis. J Bone J Surg Br 41:796, 1959.

Will R, Edmunds L, Elswood J, et al: Is there sexual inequality in ankylosing spondylitis? A study of 498 women and 1202 men. J Rheumatol 17:1649, 1990.

Yonemoto T, Tatezaki S, Takenouchi T, et al: The surgical management of sacrococcygeal chordoma. Cancer 85:878, 1999.

York JE, Kaczaraj A, Abi-Said D, et al: Sacral chordoma: 40-year experience at a major cancer center. Neurosurgery 44:74, discussion 79, 1999.

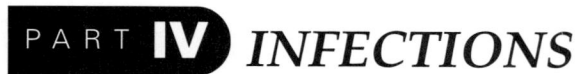
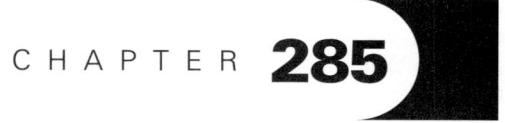

CHAPTER **285**

Infections of the Spine and Spinal Cord

NITIN TANDON ■ DENNIS G. VOLLMER

Infections of the spinal axis have afflicted humans throughout history. Evidence of tubercular disease of the spine has been found in Egyptian and South American mummies.[1, 2] Sociologic changes and advances in medical technology have changed the spectrum of causative organisms and the characteristics of patients who acquire these infections. However, the uneven nature of these socioeconomic changes around the globe has led to regional variability in the epidemiology of spinal infections. The growth of medical technologies has enhanced the ease of detection and the options for definitive management of spinal infections. Ironically, technologic advances have also promoted the occurrence of spinal infections by increasing the number of patients with iatrogenic immunosuppression, enhancing the life expectancy of patients with chronic medical illnesses, and increasing the complexity of spinal procedures and therefore the potential for infectious complications.[3]

From a neurosurgical perspective, infections can be subdivided into three broad categories: spontaneous pyogenic infections, iatrogenic infections, and infections caused by mycobacteria, fungi, unusual bacteria, and parasites. We use the term *pyogenic* to refer only to bacterial infections that produce a predominantly neutrophilic infiltrate and purulence. Although mycobacterial, actinomycetic, nocardial, and certain fungal infections can produce purulence, this is a lymphocyte-predominant immune response—the so-called cold pus. The clinical behavior and management of such infections differ enough from that of pyogenic infections to merit discussion in a separate section.

SPONTANEOUS PYOGENIC SPINAL INFECTIONS

Traditionally, spinal infections have been categorized based on their anatomic locus. The terminology used—osteomyelitis, diskitis, and epidural abscess—relied solely on whether the vertebral body, disk space, or epidural space was primarily affected. The widespread availability of magnetic resonance imaging (MRI) for the diagnosis of these conditions has made it clear that such terminology may not accurately reflect the nature of the infection. Most spinal infections spread to involve more than one of these regions, and it is not uncommon for all three to be affected.[4–10] Further, a classification based on these anatomic boundaries does not contribute much to determining the optimal management for an individual patient. Although a somewhat longer duration of antibiotic therapy is needed to cure an osteomyelitis compared with an infection of the disk or the epidural space, the role of surgical intervention, the incidence of neurological deficits, and the chances of failure with maximal medical management are poorly predicted by these traditional anatomy-based descriptors. In addition, all three subcategories of infection share similar epidemiology, risk factors, and clinical presentations and are diagnosed using the same laboratory tests and imaging studies.

We find it more useful to categorize these infections by the neurological condition of the patient (presence or absence of deficits) and by the vertebral level affected. A classification based on these descriptors is concordant with the biology of these infections and facilitates decisions based on the patient's clinical condition and the radiographic findings rather than on an arbitrary anatomic label.

Epidemiology

The incidence and demographics of pyogenic spinal infections (PSIs) have been significantly influenced by changes in social behavior, advances in medical technology, and the acquired immunodeficiency syndrome (AIDS) pandemic. The incidence of spinal infections appears to be on the rise.[11, 12] In years past, the incidence of epidural abscess was estimated to be around

0.2 to 2 per 10,000 hospital admissions[4, 7]; recent authors cite higher rates.[13–16] The annual incidence of all PSIs is now probably about 1 per 100,000 individuals.[11] Older series[17, 18] described two age-related spikes—one during the first decade of life, and the second around the fifth or sixth decade, reflecting the proclivity of very young and older individuals to acquire such infections. Infections still occur in these demographic groups, perhaps with no change in frequency,[19] but they are overshadowed in number by infections that occur in adults with frequent bacteremia, significantly impaired host defenses, or both.[13, 21–23] Intravenous drug abuse and AIDS—the most common risk factors for PSIs[9, 16, 24–29]—have reached epidemic proportions.[30, 31] Medical advances have also led to an increased prevalence of individuals who are susceptible to spinal infection. Patients with diabetes, end-stage renal disease, and cirrhosis now live longer.[32] Immunosuppression of transplant recipients,[33] long-term steroid therapy for autoimmune diseases, chemotherapy, chronic indwelling catheters for venous access,[34] splenectomy, genitourinary instrumentation, and other medical interventions also enhance a patients' risk for contracting an infection of the spine.[3, 20, 23, 25, 35–37]

In susceptible patients, remote pyogenic infections (e.g., skin, genitourinary tract, lungs, gastrointestinal tract) can result in bacterial seeding of the spine. Spontaneous bacteremia with the potential to inoculate the spine is probably a relatively common event, rendered inconsequential by competent immune mechanisms. A Danish database of all patients with staphylococcal bacteremia in that country suggested that hematogenous vertebral osteomyelitis developed in 145 patients—roughly 1% of all those who had clinically apparent bacteremia.[13] In some patients with predisposing conditions for PSI, no overt source of primary infection is found; in others, infection occurs in the absence of any particular risk factors. Greater awareness of spinal infections as a cause of fevers of unknown origin and the widespread availability of MRI may have contributed to an increase in the diagnosis of this condition.

Pathogenic Mechanisms

Infective organisms can be carried to the spine by four routes: via the arterial blood supply, retrograde by the vertebral venous plexus,[38, 39] by direct inoculation (e.g., a contaminated surgical instrument or needle or a penetrating injury), or direct extension from an adjacent nidus of infection (e.g., pulmonary abscess or sacral decubitus ulcer). Most infections probably occur by the first of these routes. In adults, the nutrient artery of the metaphyseal end plate is an endartery, derived from the periosteal arteries. Infected thrombi that lodge in this metaphyseal artery produce avascular necrosis in a portion of the metaphysis, which creates a sizable nidus for infection.[40] Small anastomotic arteries that branch off from metaphyseal arteries are unable to supplant the blood flow to an ischemic metaphysis. These connect the metaphyseal plates at opposite ends of a vertebra and are the likely pathway for the spread of infection to transequatorial metaphyses, while sparing the intervening equatorial region of the vertebra.[41] The equatorial region of the vertebra is supplied by multiple branches from the main segmental artery, making it very vascular and relatively resistant to the phenomenology that results in infarction of the metaphysis. In addition to the devitalization of the metaphyseal bone, thrombosis of the metaphyseal artery results in ischemia of the intervertebral disk, resulting in an infection of the disk as well as chronic aseptic necrosis. This results in gradual loss of disk height and, occasionally, in the production of frank pus in the disk space. Purulence in the disk or the bone can result in septic thrombosis of draining veins, which relay the infection to the epidural venous plexus, resulting in the formation of an epidural abscess.

The presence of infection in all three areas—vertebral body, disk, and epidural space—is common but not constant, and the relative predominance of infection in a single region was the basis for the traditional categorization of these lesions (discussed earlier). The microvascular anatomy of the vertebrae and disk is slightly different in children than in adults; thus, infection in children tends to be limited to the disk space (see the section on pediatric spinal infections).

Not all infections arrive in the spine through an arterial route. Transvenous dissemination may also occur, somewhat akin to the metastasis of genitourinary and gastrointestinal malignancies to the spine. Infections involving the left kidney may be more likely to spread to the spine, because the left renal vein often communicates with Batson's plexus.[37] Occasionally, infection may be restricted to the epidural veins, which act as a portal to the spine, resulting in the production of contiguous or heterotopic epidural abscesses over multiple spinal segments without significant involvement of bony or cartilaginous components of the spine.[6] Similar mechanisms may be involved in the infrequent occurrence of infections arising within the posterior elements of the spine.[42, 102, 103] Less than 5% of spinal infections are isolated to the posterior spinal elements[6, 43, 44] (Fig. 285–1; see also Fig. 285–15).

Bacteria can also reach the spine through contaminated needles or other instruments used during diskography, epidural anesthesia, or surgery; by contiguous spread from surrounding infected tissues; and by penetrating injuries or following cutaneous breakdown (especially over the sacrum and the lower lumbar region). The presentation and management of such infections are addressed later.

Neurological deficits develop as a result of compression or ischemia of the spinal cord or cauda equina in 5% to 50% of all cases of PSI.[24, 25, 43, 45–47] Such compression and ischemia can occur either by an expanding epidural abscess or, more commonly, by kyphosis of the spine due to the loss of bony integrity, resulting in bony compression and distortion of neural elements. The lumbar spinal canal is relatively capacious relative to the size of the cauda equina that needs to be accommodated. Thus, sizable epidural collections and retropulsed bony fragments are tolerated in the lumbar

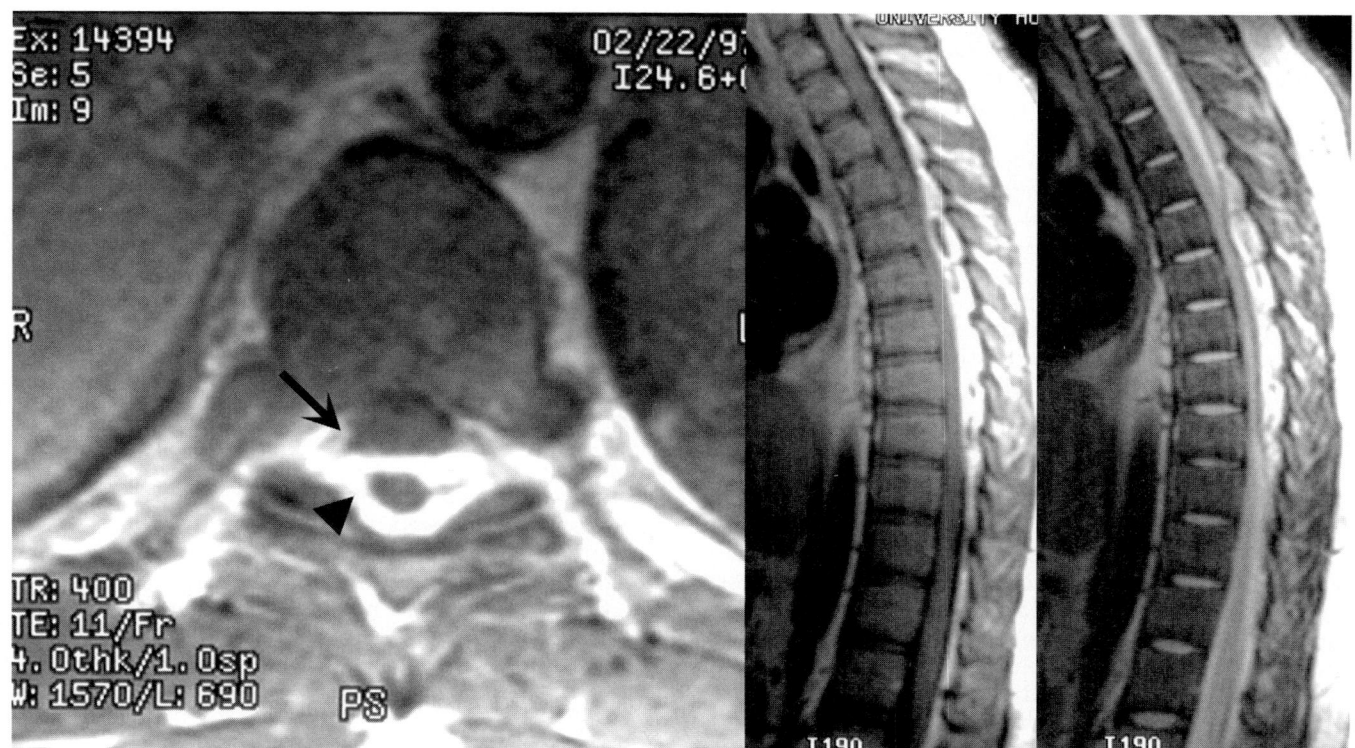

FIGURE 285–1. Magnetic resonance imaging scans of a 24-year-old man without any obvious risk factors for infection who presented with a sensory level at T7 and paraparesis of about 12 hours' duration. The spinal cord is displaced anteriorly by a dorsally situated epidural abscess that enhances peripherally and has a central liquid component. He underwent an emergent laminectomy from T4 to T10 and had an excellent neurological outcome.

spinal canal; in contrast, there is very little "spare" room around the cord in the cervical and thoracic spinal canals. For this reason, even though PSI affecting the lumbar region is relatively common,[24, 48, 53] neurological deficits are seen predominantly with infections of the cervical and thoracic regions.[6, 46, 49] In addition, immunocompromised patients are more likely than others to develop neurological deficits as a consequence of a spinal infection.[24]

Microbiology

The most common causative organism of PSI is *Staphylococcus aureus*.* *S. aureus* and other gram-positive organisms such as *Staphylococcus epidermidis*, *Streptococcus viridans*, *Streptococcus pneumoniae*, *Streptococcus faecalis* (enterococcus), *Propionibacterium* species, and diphtheroids account for the vast majority of PSIs. Gram-negative organisms such as *Escherichia coli*, *Pseudomonas*, *Salmonella*, *Enterobacter*, *Klebsiella*, *Haemophilus*, and *Proteus* are less frequent and may be associated with gastrointestinal or genitourinary sources of infection.[15, 45, 55, 56] Infections in intravenous drug abusers are most likely to be caused by staphylococcal species as well,[14, 54, 57, 58] but *Pseudomonas* infection may be relatively more common in this patient group.[24, 26, 49, 57, 59] Rarely, anaer-

obes such as *Peptostreptococcus* and *Bacteroides* may cause spinal infections,[4, 60] also with relatively greater frequency in intravenous drug abusers. Anaerobic infections are more likely than aerobic infections to be polymicrobial. Care should be taken to process all materials submitted for culture both aerobically and anaerobically.[61]

Clinical Presentation

The diagnosis of PSI is easy to miss unless a high index of suspicion is maintained.* Given the large number of visits to emergency rooms for complaints of back pain, recognizing this comparatively rare, sometimes subtle, but treatable condition is challenging. Additionally, patients with a history of substance abuse, who are especially prone to such infections, can be poor historians and manifest drug-seeking behavior, confounding matters further.[57]

Early in the course of their disease, patients typically present with isolated back pain that they may relate to strenuous activity or a minor injury.[24, 48] Systemic signs of infection such as fever or an elevated leukocyte count may be absent. Such patients may be discharged from emergency departments or physicians' offices

---

*See references 4, 6, 8, 9, 22, 27, 28, 47, 50–55.

* See references 3, 4, 15, 17, 19, 23, 25, 27, 46, 53, 56.

without a definitive diagnosis, only to return later with progressive symptoms or neurological deficits.

Heusner described the clinical evolution of epidural abscess in four stages: pain, radiculopathy, weakness, and paralysis.[7] In practice, however, such a distinct progression of the infection is rarely seen. Patients can present anywhere along a spectrum of predominantly local manifestations of focal spinal or radicular pain at one end to systemic manifestations of infection (e.g., fevers, chills, malaise, night sweats) at the other end. The presence of systemic manifestations may herald a bacteremia, and this is an opportune time to obtain blood cultures. Unusual characteristics of the back pain, such as a midline location over the thoracic or upper lumbar spine, worsening with recumbency (especially at night), and associated thoracic radiculopathy, should prompt consideration of a nondegenerative cause of the pain. Careful screening for risk factors such as intravenous drug abuse, AIDS, diabetes, recent steroid therapy, or the presence of other immunocompromised states helps detect those patients who merit further evaluation. Neurological symptoms are more common with infections of the cervical and thoracic spine, compared with the lumbar region. The rate of progression of infection and of the neurological deficits is variable—some infections are relatively indolent, while others can progress rapidly, resulting in profound neurological deficits in a matter of hours.

On examination, there is usually exquisite tenderness to percussion of the affected spinal segment. When there is a prominent bony component to the infection, a gibbous deformity may be clinically obvious. A dermatomal level of sensory, motor, or combined deficits is common in patients presenting with deficits. Examination is usually consistent with an acute spinal cord injury with bladder and bowel involvement. The measurement of postvoid bladder residual followed by bladder catheterization provides an objective measure of urologic dysfunction at presentation and prevents secondary injury of the detrusor muscle. Rarely, with relatively indolent infections, chronic compression of the spinal cord may occur, and long-tract signs may be seen at presentation.[62]

Occasionally, patients may present in florid sepsis,[63] with an altered level of consciousness and an inability to provide any history. This is somewhat more common in immunocompromised patients, in those who have delayed seeking medial attention, and in patients with previous, more rostral spinal cord injuries who are insensate to pain and have no neurological function below the infected level.[64] In such cases, the diagnosis of PSI may be delayed for hours or days until the patient is stable enough to undergo MRI.

Diagnosis

LABORATORY MARKERS

The diagnosis of PSI is suggested by the clinical features described earlier. Laboratory markers of acute inflammation—leukocyte count, erythrocyte sedimentation rate (ESR), and C-reactive protein (CRP)—are helpful in screening patients for further evaluation and in establishing the diagnosis when the imaging changes are nondiagnostic. Of these, the leukocyte count is least commonly affected[11, 24, 48, 65]; the ESR is usually affected, often in a dramatic fashion.[6, 16, 17, 45, 48, 50, 66] Measurement of the The ESR is an inexpensive test and reasonably sensitive, though nonspecific. It is an excellent parameter to follow in determining the response to therapy and should be measured at the time of presentation even if the diagnosis is already clear. Given its lack of specificity, the ESR should always be interpreted in the context of the patient's overall condition. This lack of specificity is especially important in the management of patients with PSI and a preexisting elevated baseline ESR, such as those with cirrhosis. In such cases, the elevated ESR is refractory to treatment of the infection, and it is hard to determine whether the infection is responding. The diagnosis is also strongly suggested by a persistently elevated CRP. Measurement of CRP may be useful in detecting early infections, but given the individual variability in normal CRP values, it is most useful when a baseline measurement of the CRP is also available.

RADIOGRAPHIC DIAGNOSIS

The diagnosis of a PSI requires that the physician first establish the presence of an infection and then arrive at a bacteriologic diagnosis. The first of these goals is dependent on adequate radiographic data. The radiographic diagnosis is usually established by MRI. Plain radiographs and computed tomographic scans can also play a role in the diagnosis. Occasionally, MRI scans are either not feasible or nondiagnostic. In such cases, the diagnosis needs to be made by an overall interpretation of the patient's clinical picture, laboratory parameters, and radiographic findings. Additional imaging data such as radionuclide scans may be useful in such cases.

Plain radiographs and computed tomographic scans typically show few if any changes during the early stages of infection.[23] These imaging modalities are valuable in the evaluation of more advanced infections, when bony changes are manifest, and in the evaluation of vertebral bony integrity and spinal stability in patients in whom surgical management is being considered. Changes seen on plain radiographs several weeks after the onset of infection include increasing prevertebral and paravertebral soft tissue volume, loss of disk height, trabecular erosion, and eventually destruction of the entire vertebral end plate on either side of the disk. Vertebral collapse, loss of normal lordosis around the affected level, and development of a kyphotic deformity occur with advanced infection[67, 68] (see Figs. 285–3*A* and 285–8*A*).

Computed tomographic scans are generally more sensitive and specific than plain radiographs. Contrast-enhanced scans reveal inflammation of the prevertebral and paravertebral soft tissues, visible as stranding and the loss of normal tissue planes, in infections that have been present for several days. Enhancing epidural collections may also be visible on a high-quality, contrast-

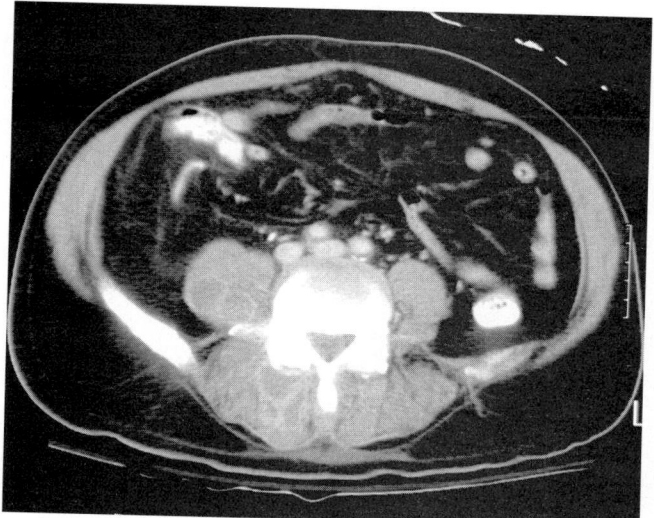

FIGURE 285–2. Paraspinous muscle involvement in a patient with a pyogenic spinal infection as seen on an abdominal computed tomographic scan obtained after contrast administration.

enhanced computed tomographic scan of the spine. Computed tomography (CT) is an appropriate modality for the detection and percutaneous management of psoas abscesses and paravertebral abscesses that result from the unchecked progression of the prevertebral and paravertebral components of a PSI. CT guidance is useful for the percutaneous aspiration of disk spaces, paravertebral fluid collections, and necrotic bone to provide specimens for a bacteriologic diagnosis (Fig. 285–2). Myelography with postmyelographic CT is another way of visualizing spinal cord or cauda equina compression when MRI cannot be performed.

MRI is the diagnostic test of choice for the detection of PSI and should be obtained in all patients unless contraindicated. Imaging should be carried out without and with the administration of paramagnetic contrast agents. Unenhanced T1-weighted images reveal a hypointense signal in the vertebral body, especially at the end plates; the normal hyperintense fat signal in the vertebral bone marrow is lost. Disk height is reduced and may be markedly diminished. T2-weighted images reveal high signal (edema) in the disk space and occasionally in the bone and the paravertebral soft tissues.[8, 51, 69] Gadolinium-enhanced T1-weighted imaging is perhaps the most diagnostic sequence; enhancement of the vertebral end plates, vertebral body, prevertebral and paravertebral soft tissues, and epidural space can be seen[68] (Fig. 285–3). The entire spine should be imaged if an infection is detected because, much like metastatic tumors, spinal infections can occasionally be multifocal[70, 71] (see Fig. 285–15).

Occasionally, it is not feasible to evaluate a patient using MRI. The presence of incompatible devices such as cardiac pacemakers, ferromagnetic aneurysm clips, or shrapnel is an absolute contraindication. Other problems such as patient size, claustrophobia, and ongoing mechanical ventilation or other monitoring may render the performance of a high-quality MRI scan difficult or

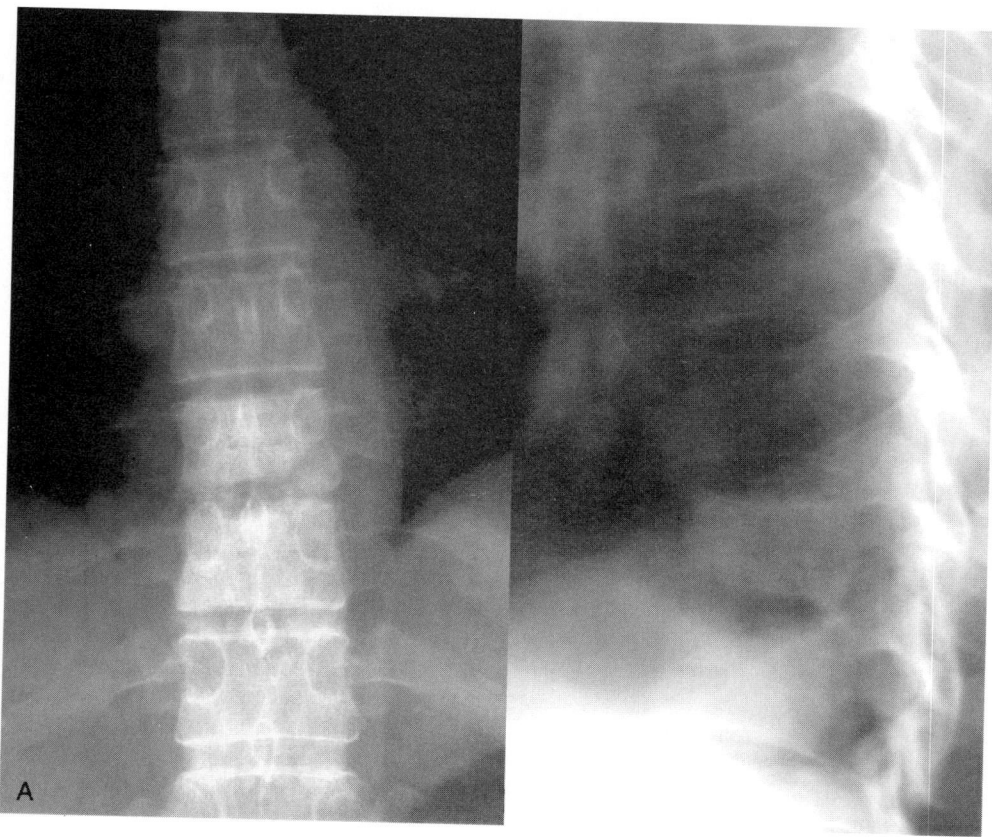

FIGURE 285–3. *A,* Plain radiographic changes suggestive of a pyogenic spinal infection. Increased paravertebral soft tissue shadow, loss of disk height, and loss of normal trabecular pattern at T10 are seen.

Illustration continued on following page

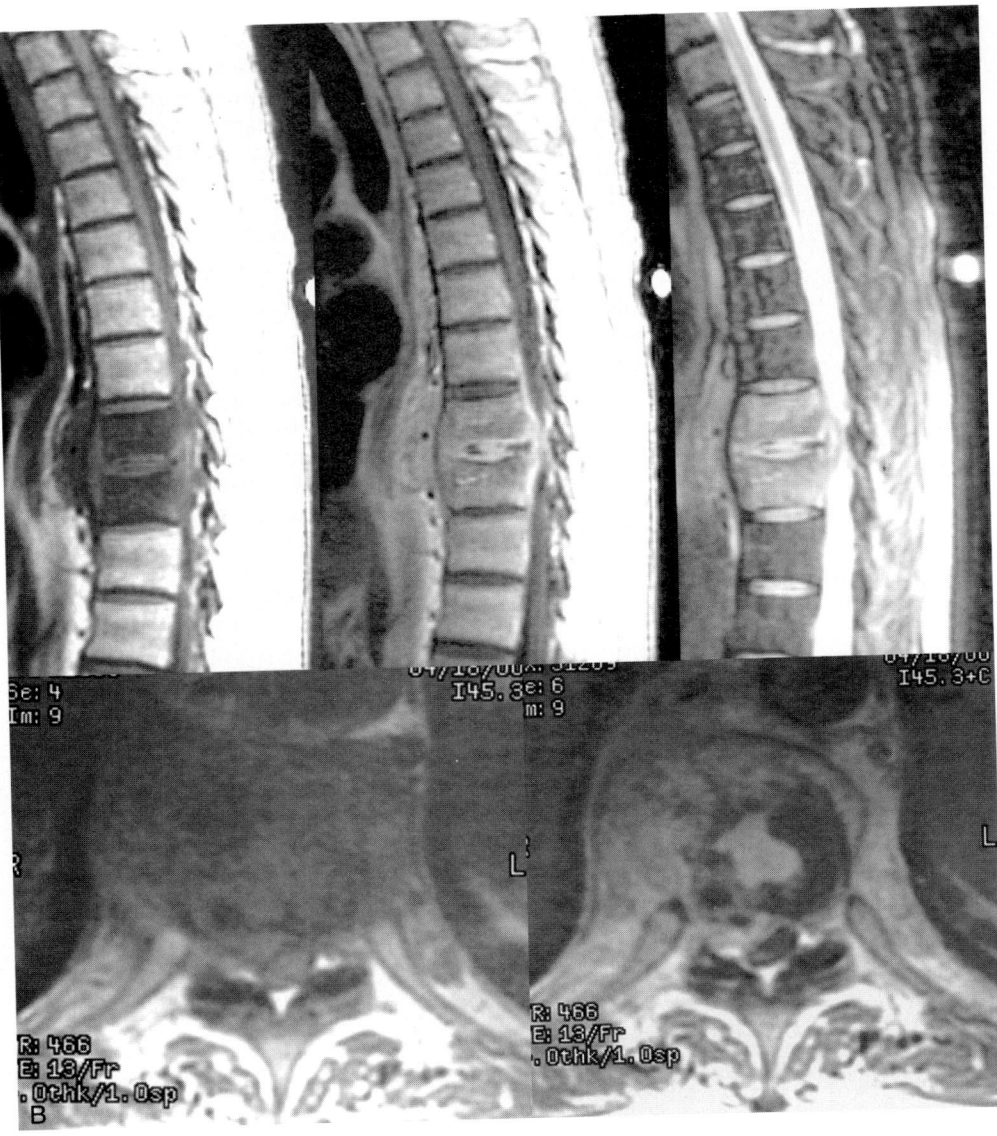

FIGURE 285–3. *Continued. B,* Magnetic resonance imaging changes typical of a spinal infection. There is hypointense signal in the vertebral body on T1-weighted images, with enhancement of the vertebral end plates, vertebral body, prevertebral and paravertebral soft tissues, and epidural space after contrast administration. The T2-weighted image reveals high signal (edema) in the disk space, bone, and paravertebral soft tissues.

too time-consuming. Further, MRI scans may be less specific in patients with extensive or pronounced spondylosis or those who have suffered recent trauma. Finally, the scans of some patients with MRI-compatible metallic implants are affected by sufficient artifact to render them nondiagnostic. In all cases in which MRI is either not possible or not diagnostic, CT–myelography and nuclear medicine scans should be considered (Fig. 285–4).

Gallium 67 and technetium 99 both have reasonable sensitivity for the detection of PSI. Gallium binds to iron-binding proteins at the site of inflammation, and technetium reflects blood flow to the bone. Gallium scans are therefore more specific for PSI than technetium scans are, but neither method is very specific.[72] Focal uptake can be seen in spondylosis, following trauma, and in tumors. In comparison, scans using white cells tagged with radionuclide are more specific for the detection of infection. Leukocytes from the buffy layer of the patient's blood are tagged with in-

dium 111 and reinjected into the patient. These labeled cells localize to sites of ongoing inflammation; focal uptake in the spine strongly suggests the diagnosis of a PSI, although false-positive results can be seen in the case of tumors, especially hematogenous malignancies involving the spine (Figs. 285–4 and 285–5). Chronic infections can occasionally lead to false-negative results with indium scanning.

BACTERIOLOGIC DIAGNOSIS

The second component of the diagnostic evaluation is the bacteriologic characterization of the infection. The causative organism may be isolated from either blood or spinal tissue. Blood cultures should be obtained in all cases, and if possible, multiple sets should be collected, coinciding with spikes in the patient's temperature. If the blood cultures are positive, appropriate therapy can be started without performing further, more invasive testing. Unfortunately, blood cultures

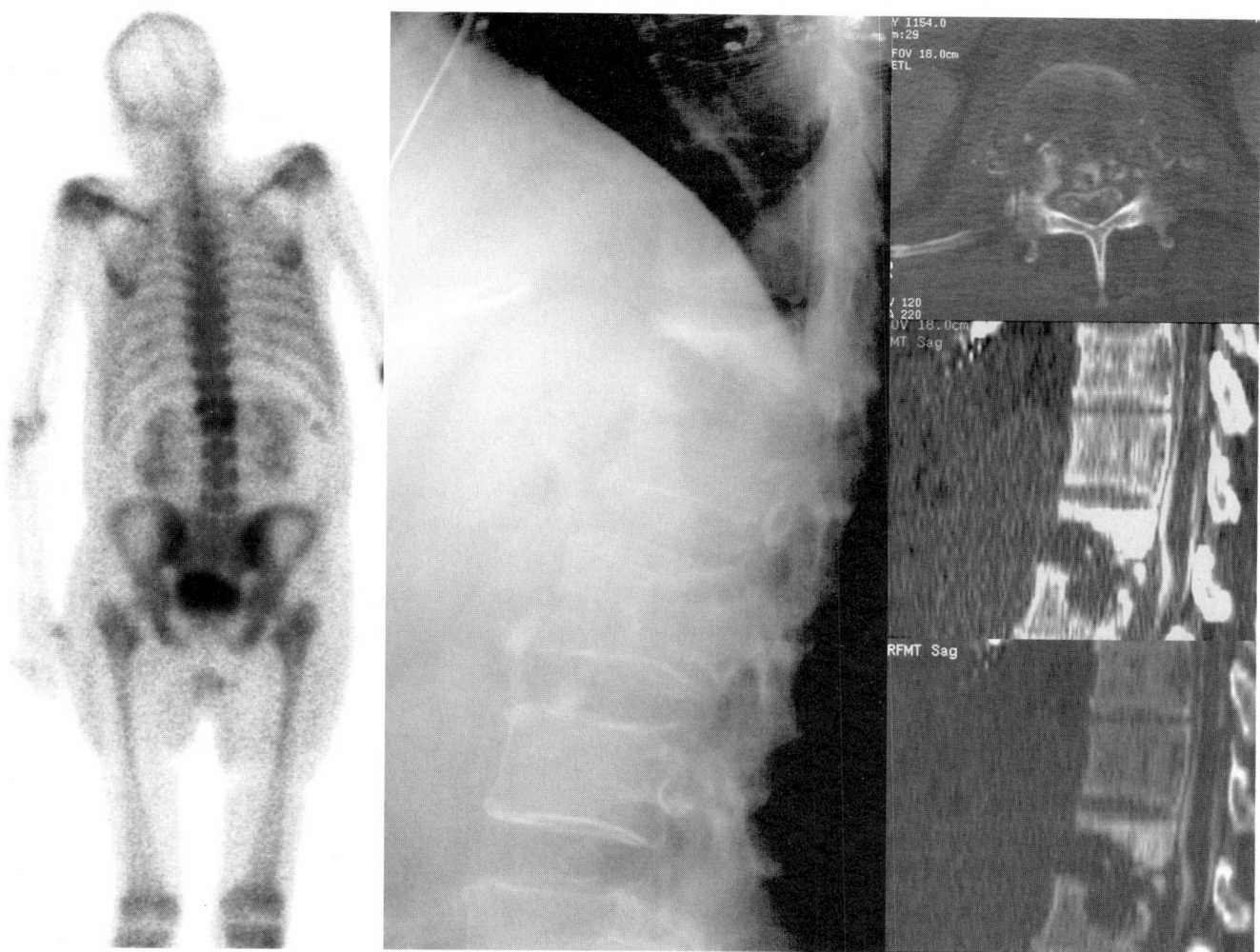

FIGURE 285–4. Technetium-99 bone scan and computed tomography–myelogram performed by cisternal puncture on a 54-year-old man with diabetes. The plain myelogram films reveal a "block" at T11-12. Compression of the thecal sac is seen on the axial computed tomographic scan. The radionuclide scan reveals increased uptake at the thoracolumbar junction.

are positive in only about 30% to 60% of cases, possibly because some infections are indolent and some patients receive antibiotics before cultures are obtained. In such cases, a biopsy of the vertebra or the disk space using CT or fluoroscopic guidance has a higher rate of success in culturing the organism (Fig. 285–6).[73] The biopsy may need to be repeated if no growth results from culturing the aspirate. A larger-bore needle that obtains a core of tissue may yield superior microbiologic results compared with aspirates of fluid from bone. The use of a nucleotome for percutaneous suction aspiration of the infected disk space has also been described.[74] Biopsies of a core of tissue can also be submitted for histopathologic analysis to confirm the diagnosis. If these measures fail and the imaging diagnosis is reasonably definitive for a PSI, an open biopsy may be necessary. This is best done in an operating suite under fluoroscopic guidance.

The bacteriologic diagnosis is difficult to establish if empirical antibiotic therapy is begun before obtaining cultures. It is important to withhold antibiotics until it is clear that an organism has been cultured, unless the patient is septic or has major systemic manifestations, in which case delaying therapy may be inappropriate.[56] Even a single dose of a broad-spectrum intravenous antibiotic may significantly decrease the probability of culturing an organism. In patients with neurological deficits, antibiotics should be withheld until specimens are collected intraoperatively. If antibiotic treatment is initiated before a bacteriologic diagnosis is established in patients who are neurologically intact, it may be reasonable to terminate this empirical therapy and obtain fresh cultures with the patient off the antimicrobials. In a small number of cases, no organism can be cultured despite multiple attempts.[6, 74] Mycobacterial or fungal infections should be considered in such cases. Once this possibility is reasonably excluded, empirical antibiotic therapy is the only option. Patients treated empirically with antibiotics need to be followed closely to confirm a response to the treatment.

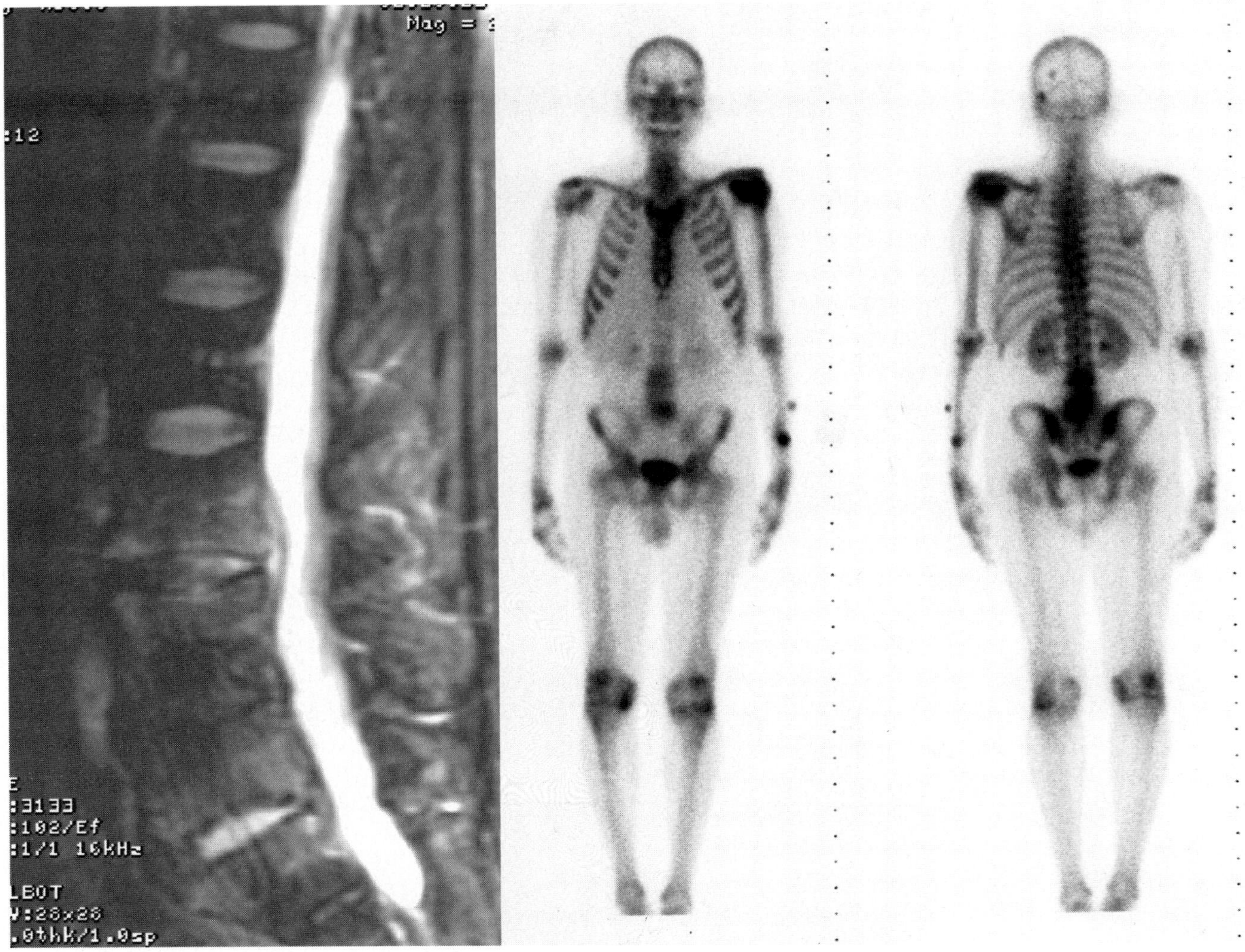

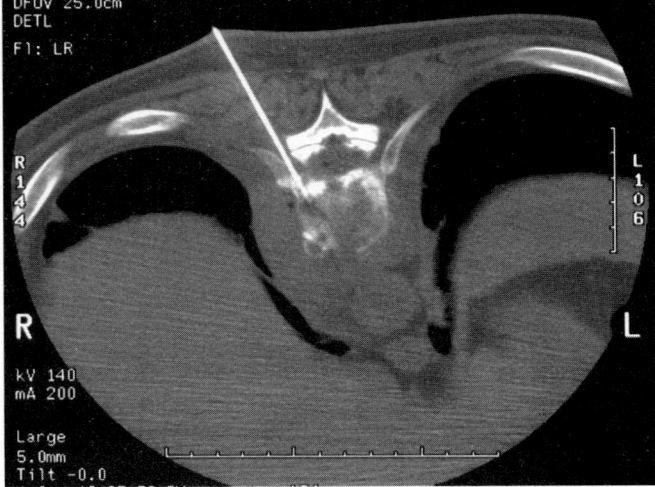

FIGURE 285–5. Magnetic resonance imaging scans in a patient with cirrhosis were nondiagnostic for a pyogenic spinal infection. The diagnosis was made using an indium-111 tagged white cell scan that reveals focal uptake.

FIGURE 285–6. Computed tomography–guided biopsy for bacterial diagnosis of a pyogenic spinal infection.

DIAGNOSIS OF ASSOCIATED CONDITIONS

Patients with PSIs are at risk for concomitant pyogenic infections elsewhere in the body. The risk of bacterial endocarditis is especially high, and patients should be examined for cardiac murmurs and evidence of embolization to the retina and the skin. If endocarditis is suspected, echocardiography, preferably by a transesophageal route, should be performed to look for valvular vegetations.

Often, a cutaneous pyogenic lesion that represents the index location of the infection is still present when the patient is evaluated by a neurosurgeon.[75] Such lesions can often be used to obtain cultures for a bacteriologic diagnosis. Patients should also undergo an assessment of risk factors responsible for the infection. Certain risk factors may be obvious; others may be discovered only after careful evaluation. For instance, patients may be reluctant to admit to intravenous drug abuse. In some cases of indolent infection, the drug abuse may have occurred several months previously. It is reasonable to offer intravenous drug abusers testing for human immunodeficiency virus (HIV) and for viral hepatitis types B and C, along with appropriate counseling.

It should be emphasized that the evaluation of a PSI is incomplete unless the patient is assessed for extraspinal manifestations of the infection. Infections can track along fascial planes adjacent to the infected vertebrae, resulting in psoas abscesses, paraspinous muscle abscesses, empyemas, sympathetic pleural effusions, and retropharyngeal abscesses[76] (see Fig. 285–2). Infections can breach the dura spontaneously or with the unintended assistance of a biopsy or lumbar puncture needle. Mental status changes, nuchal rigidity, or emesis in a patient with a known or suspected PSI should lead to the consideration of meningitis or parameningeal inflammation as a diagnostic possibility (Fig. 285–7). The diagnosis of meningitis is best confirmed by obtaining cerebrospinal fluid from a cisternal rather than a lumbar puncture—unless the locus of infection is clearly remote from the site of the puncture.[57]

Differential Diagnosis

Occasionally, patients with severe back pain and laboratory studies consistent with acute inflammation have spinal MRI scans that fail to reveal changes diagnostic of a PSI. In such cases, it is prudent to wait for definitive imaging changes to develop or to obtain radionuclide scans if the diagnosis of a PSI is strongly suspected. It is also essential to consider alternative diagnoses that can mimic PSI.

Conditions with similar clinical presentations to PSI, but that can be differentiated based on imaging, include pyogenic arthritis of the hip, septic or autoimmune sacroiliitis, pyelonephritis, primary psoas abscess, autoimmune spondylitis, spinal trauma, osteoporotic compression fractures, spinal epidural hematoma, spontaneous spinal subarachnoid hemorrhage, and leptomeningeal metastatic disease. Certain conditions may be harder to distinguish based on imaging alone. Nonpyogenic (tubercular or fungal) spinal infection can occasionally mimic PSI rather closely, as can tumors metastatic to adjacent vertebral levels. Greater involvement of the vertebral body than the disk space and the development of paravertebral abscesses early in the course of the infection suggest a tubercular rather than a pyogenic cause.[65] A definitive diagnosis can usually be established by a needle biopsy in such cases. Tubercular infection and lymphomas should always be considered in the differential diagnosis in patients with AIDS.[77] Degenerative changes[78] seen in advanced spondylosis can sometimes be confused with infections, because both are preferentially localized to the vertebral end plates. Degeneration can usually be differentiated from infection, because a degenerated disk is usually dehydrated and therefore hypointense, whereas an infected disk is hyperintense on T2-weighted images. Enhancement of the disk itself is also indicative of PSI, whereas enhancement of vertebral bone can be seen with either entity. The presence of gas within the disk, the vacuum disk phenomenon, is much more suggestive of degeneration than infection.[68] A rare entity that may mimic PSI is avascular

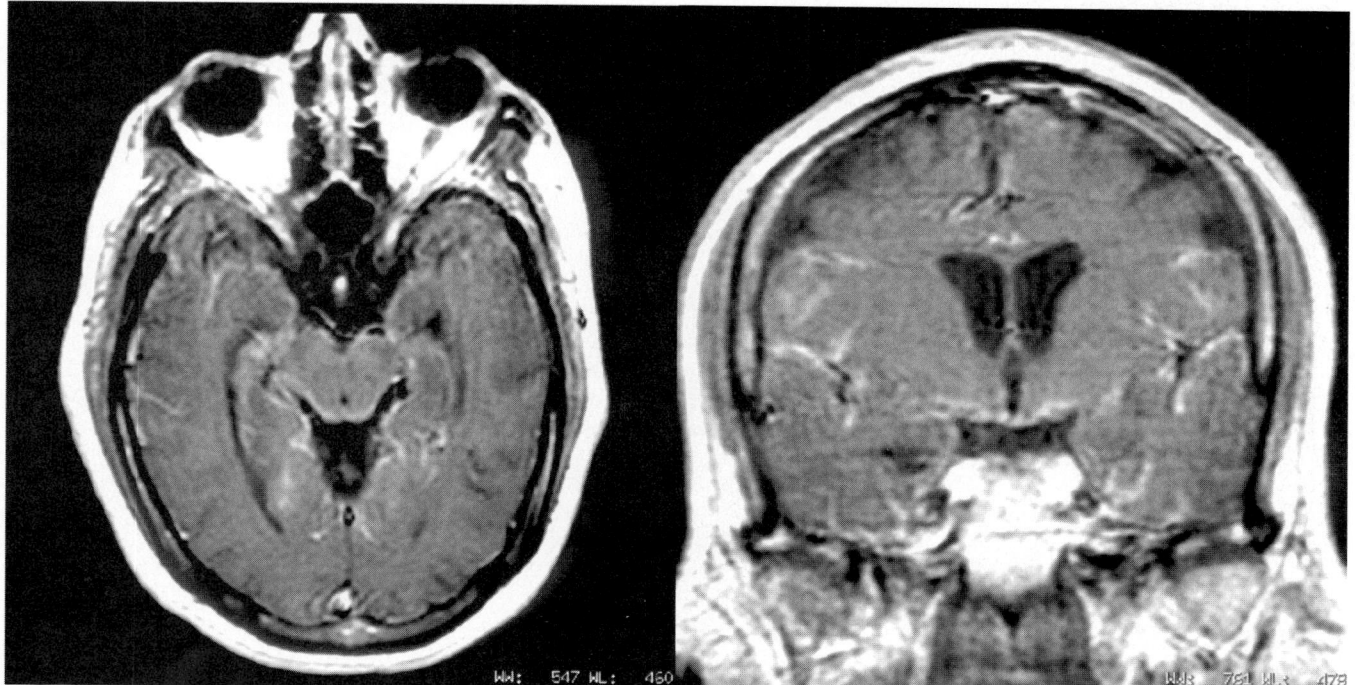

FIGURE 285–7. Contrast-enhanced magnetic resonance imaging scan in a patient with a pyogenic spinal infection and markedly altered mentation reveals leptomeningeal enhancement, indicative of meningitis.

necrosis of the vertebral body. This is usually associated with a significant collapse of the vertebral body and intravertebral vacuum clefts. Changes in the intravertebral vacuum clefts are seen as a consequence of spinal loading and unloading. A T2-weighted image obtained immediately after the patient lies supine on the scanner reveals a hypointense signal due to the presence of air, but as fluid enters the cleft, this signal becomes hyperintense.[79, 80]

Management

Once a diagnosis of PSI has been made, an important decision is whether operative intervention is indicated. Although all patients need antibiotic therapy, the term *medical management* in the present context refers to the use of antibiotics without planned surgical débride-

ment at the site of infection. *Surgical management*, in contrast, implies operative intervention with débridement of necrotic tissue, decompression of neural elements, correction of deformity, fusion, and instrumentation as indicated by the clinical situation, coupled with appropriate antimicrobials.

SURGICAL MANAGEMENT

The decision to perform surgery should be made after consideration of the patient's neurological status, vertebral level of involvement, extent of vertebral destruction, and MRI findings. In the past, the decision to proceed with emergent surgery was often made solely on the basis of an enhancing epidural component. The guiding principle has been that an epidural abscess constitutes a neurosurgical emergency. It has become

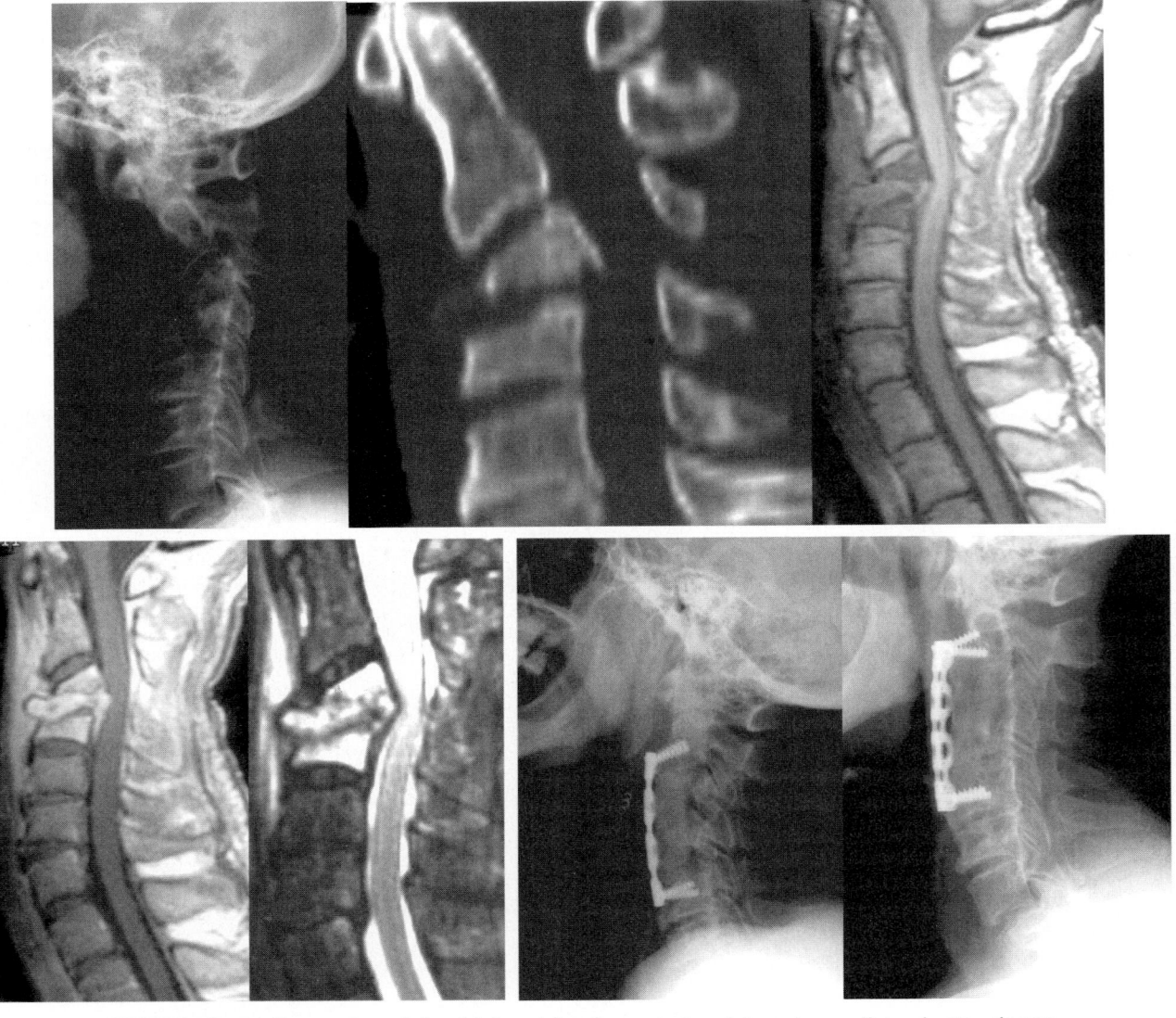

FIGURE 285–8. Destruction of the third and fourth cervical vertebrae by an *Enterobacter cloacae* infection in a 50-year-old intravenous drug abuser. The spine was grossly unstable, and a C3-4 corpectomy was performed, followed by fusion using iliac crest autograft and an anterior cervical plate. The second cervical radiograph was obtained 2 years after the initial operation and reveals incorporation of the bone graft.

increasingly clear, however, that there is heterogeneity in the composition of epidural collections. Entirely liquid "abscesses" are rare, and in most cases, a phlegmon with minimal if any liquid abscess is seen. This heterogeneity also applies to the clinical manifestations of epidural collections—some produce rapidly progressive neurological deficits, and others produce no deficits. Further, neurological deficits occur more often from spinal instability or deformity than from compression of the cord or cauda equina by an abscess component. Thus, there is often a poor correlation between

an imaging diagnosis of "epidural abscess" and the development of neurological deficits. This lends further credence to the notion that management decisions in PSI are best made by using multiple clinical and radiographic criteria rather than a simple anatomic classification of the infection.

The presence of neurological deficits is the most important of these criteria. Emergent surgical intervention should be considered in all patients with neurological deficits, regardless of the duration of weakness, unless the deficits are minimal (e.g., radiculopathy)

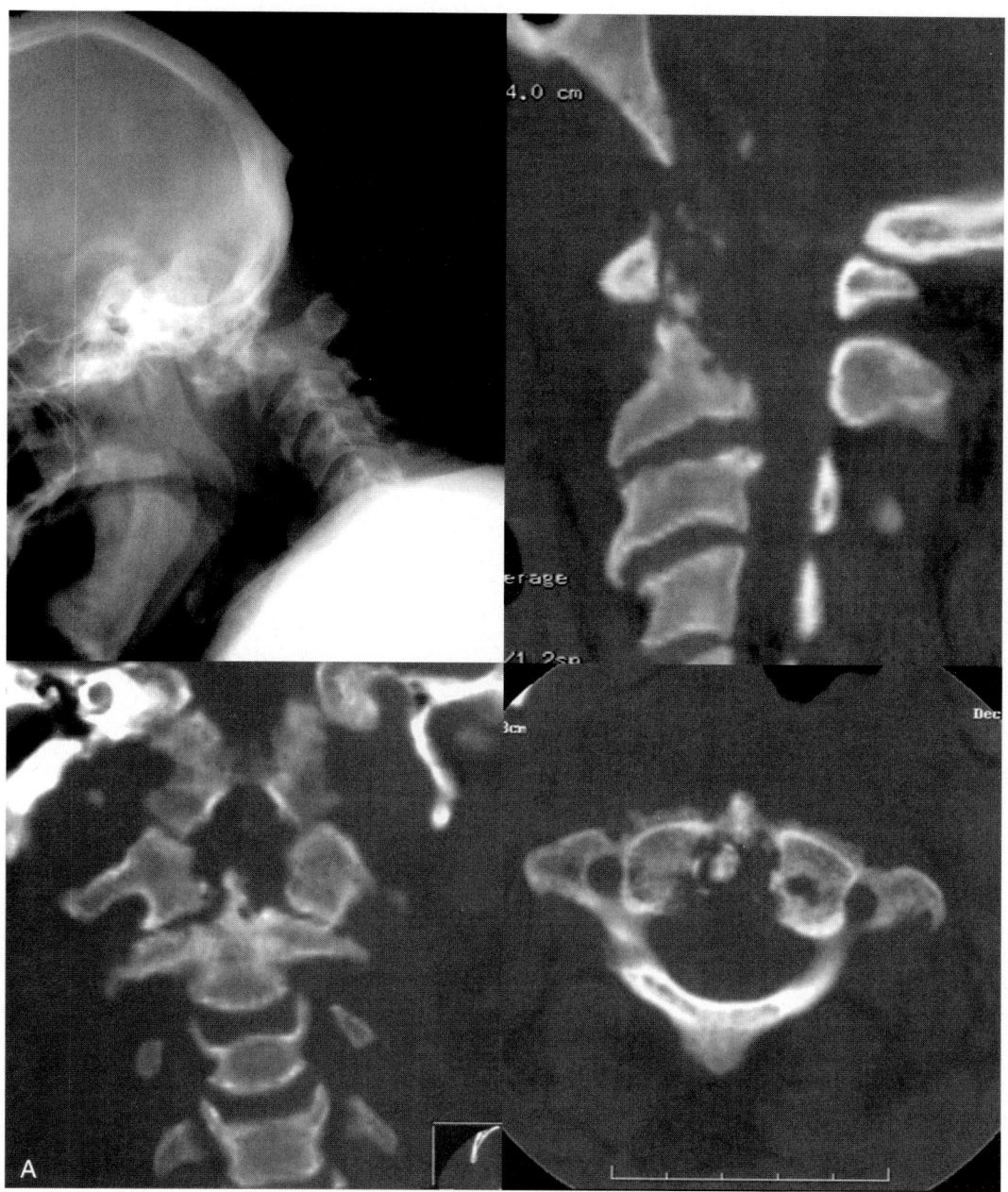

FIGURE 285–9. *A,* Pyogenic spine infection of the odontoid with C1-2 instability. The odontoid is eroded and the transverse ligament is likely disrupted, leading to the widening of the atlanto-dental interval on the lateral flexion roentgenogram.

Illustration continued on following page

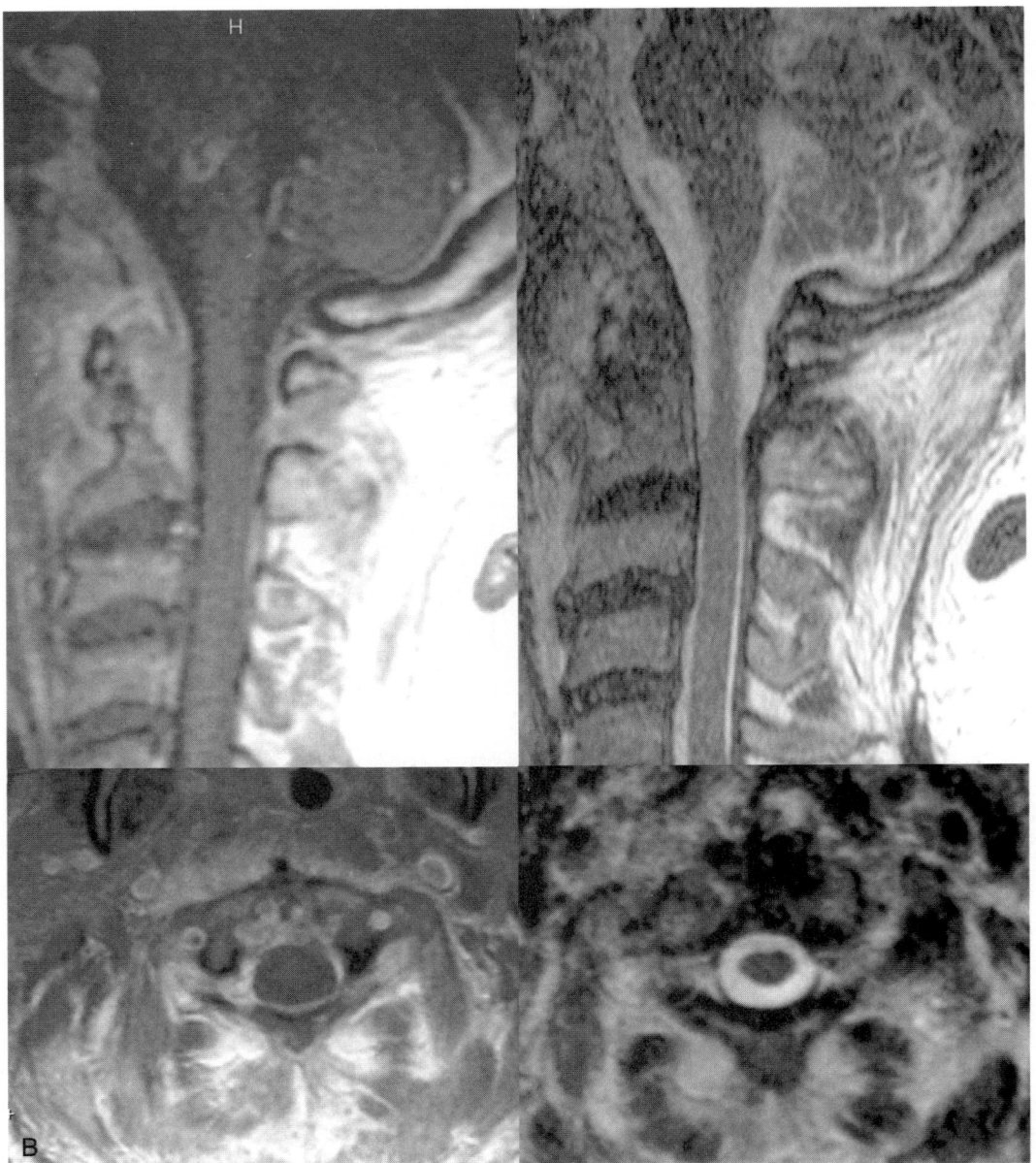

FIGURE 285–9. *Continued. B,* MRI scans reveal an enhancing mass that has replaced most of the odontoid. No obvious compromise of the spinal canal is seen in the neutral position.

or the patient's medical comorbidities (coagulopathy, sepsis) preclude rapid surgical intervention. If the decision is made to treat a patient with minimal neurological deficits nonsurgically, the patient must be carefully monitored to detect any progression early. Deficits can sometimes progress rapidly, in just a few hours.

Surgical intervention for neurological deficits needs to address the location of the compressive lesion (e.g., ventral or dorsal to the spinal cord or cauda equina). Although this sounds simplistic, ignoring this principle may result in destabilization of an already compromised spine, with worsening deficits.[36, 44, 46, 81] The nature of the compressive lesion—liquid pus versus a mass of granulation tissue or retropulsed bone—is also an important consideration in determining the optimal

surgical approach. Whereas pus can be accessed and drained by various routes, a simple laminectomy does not afford adequate decompression of a solid, ventrally situated extradural lesion and can exacerbate the deficits produced by a kyphotic deformity. Finally, the various anatomic regions of the spine dictate the potential approaches available and the likelihood of postoperative instability.

In the cervical spine, the surgical approach usually coincides with the location of the compressive lesion—an anterior approach for ventral compression, and a posterior approach for dorsal compression[9, 49] (Fig. 285–8). An exception may be ventral abscesses without major bony involvement extending over more than two or three levels. In these cases, pus can usually

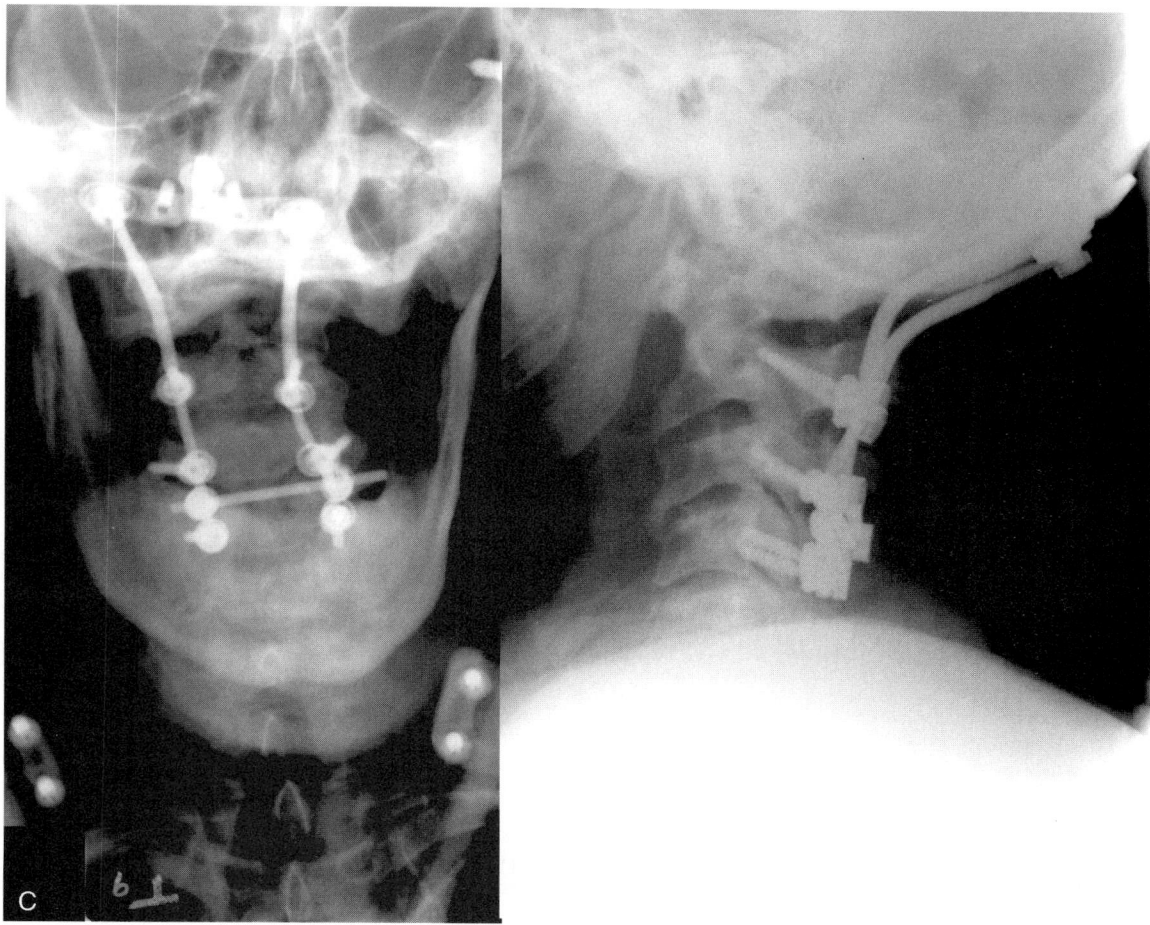

FIGURE 285–9. *Continued. C,* Given the absence of neurological deficits despite the gross spinal instability, the patient was managed with a transoral biopsy followed by an occipitocervical fusion (occiput to C4).

be drained from a posterior approach without the morbidity of multilevel corpectomy and fusion. Infections of the odontoid, though rare, have been reported. If such an infection has produced instability, it is best managed by occipitocervical fusion and a transoral biopsy or decompression of the thecal sac (Fig. 285–9). Stable lesions at this level can be managed medically.[82, 83] At the cervicothoracic junction and in the upper thoracic spine, anterior lesions may be difficult to access from a ventral approach because of the presence of the great vessels. Partial sternotomy or manubrial resection may provide adequate access in such cases, but technical challenges remain in the débridement and reconstruction of the anterior column. Further, a kyphotic deformity produced by the infection can make access to the apex of the deformity via an anterior approach more difficult. Transpedicular, lateral extracavitary,[84–86] or periscapular[87, 88] approaches may be used in these cases. These approaches can be used to decompress the ventral aspect of the spinal cord, and potential or apparent segmental instability can be addressed by concurrent posterior thoracic fusion with instrumentation.[36, 44, 81] Recent technologic advancements have in-

creased the options available for fixation over the cervicothoracic junction.

Surgical approaches for PSI of the midthoracic spine are best tailored to the site of compression. Thoracotomy approaches offer excellent visualization of the ventral and ventrolateral aspects of the spinal canal. Anterior reconstruction following a vertebrectomy is readily performed by this exposure (Fig. 285–10). Alternatively, the lateral extracavitary approach[84–86] or the retropleural approach[88] can be used. The temptation to perform a laminectomy for ventral disease in the thoracic spine, other than for liquid pus, should be resisted, as it can result in the cord being draped over the compressive lesion, with concomitant loss of the stability offered by the posterior tension band.[44, 46, 81] The extent of spinal instrumentation required to restore stability is a function of the number of segments involved, the degree of kyphotic deformity, the patient's bone stock, and the integrity of the posterior tension band.

In the lower thoracic spine and upper lumbar spine, anterior débridement via a thoracoabdominal approach affords excellent exposure for resection of the involved

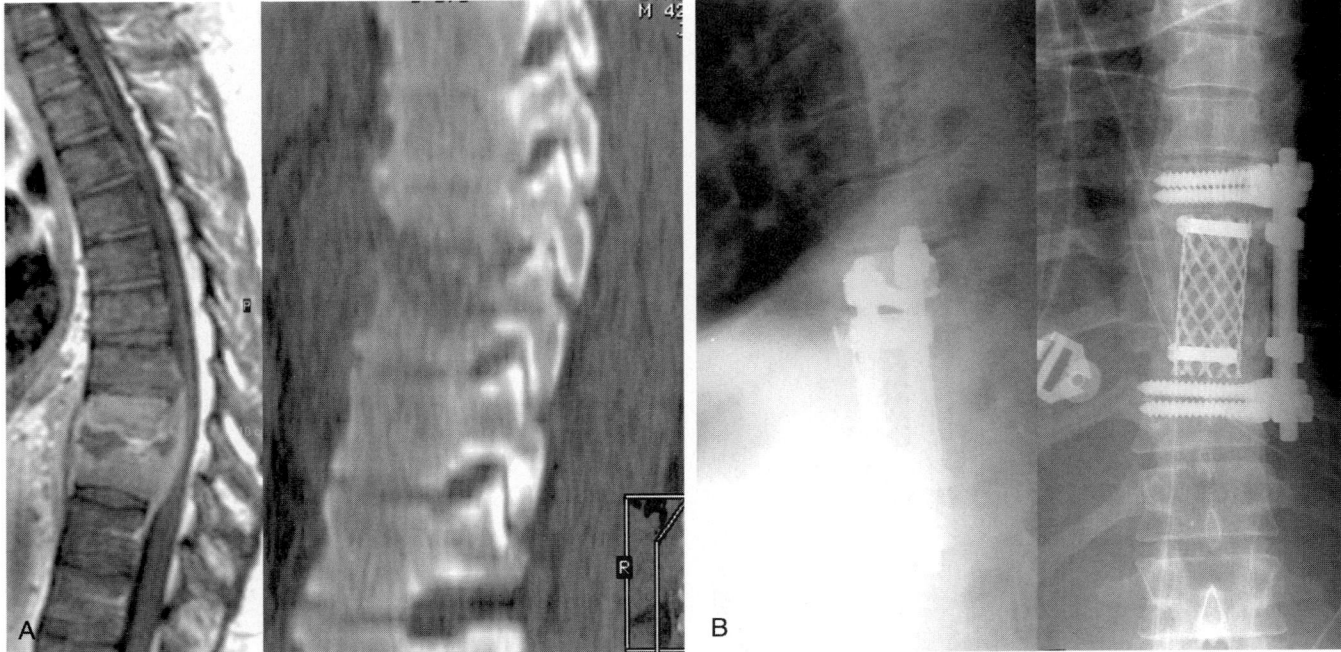

FIGURE 285–10. Pyogenic infection caused by *Staphylococcus aureus* at T9-10 in a 38-year-old man who presented with paraparesis. Management consisted of anterior débridement and reconstruction with a Harms cage, autograft, and Kaneda-type construct.

vertebral bodies and reconstruction of the anterior and middle columns.[19, 24, 50] When the posterior elements are intact, an anterior approach alone may suffice. Anterior débridement and fusion followed by posterior instrumentation and posterolateral fusion[89, 90] may be an option in selected cases when there is concern about the appropriate placement of instrumentation via the anterior approach used for decompression (Fig. 285–11).

Infections of the middle and lower lumbar spine may be approached by either a retroperitoneal or a transperitoneal approach for débridement and anterior reconstruction (Fig. 285–12). Below the conus, a posterior approach can be used to decompress the neural elements; however, reconstruction of the anterior and middle columns is difficult by this approach. Transpedicular instrumentation can provide a measure of stability in such cases, but it may occasionally fail if an anterior column reconstruction is not performed.

Following fusion and instrumentation for spinal infections, an external orthotic device appropriate for the level in question should be prescribed for approximately 3 months.

In addition to patients presenting with neurological deficits, surgical intervention is indicated in patients who have failed medical therapy, in those with chronic pain following medical management, and in patients with a prominent deformity or overt instability.[6, 29, 91] Relapses of infection can be treated with either a second course of antibiotics or surgery, depending on the clinical scenario and the patient's preference. It has been postulated that relapses occur owing to the presence of necrotic bone (sequestrum) within the vertebral body that lacks a blood supply and provides a nidus for persistent infection. Surgical treatment in these cases includes débridement of the infected vertebral body (i.e., corpectomy), followed by reconstruction.

Some surgeons have a bias toward the surgical management of patients with prominent bony components to their infection, because they believe that the bacteriologic cure rates are higher and a cure is achieved earlier. This bias remains unvalidated by clinical trials; however, the fact that an aggressive débridement eliminates a sizable portion of infected and necrotic bone lends credence to this viewpoint.

Timing of Surgery

Surgery needs to be performed emergently in patients with rapidly progressive neurological deficits.[52] In cases in which the deficits are slowly progressive or the patient has significant medical comorbidities (e.g., septicemia, coagulopathy, endocarditis with cardiac failure), the timing of surgical intervention should be more carefully considered. Surgery can be carried out on an elective basis in patients with no deficits when the goal is to stabilize the spine or débride a necrotic focus of infection.

The role of steroids, at doses used for the acute management of spinal cord injury,[92, 93] is questionable, in that there are no prospectively collected data addressing this issue, nor are there likely to be any, given the relatively small number of cases seen at any one institution. Our experience, though anecdotal, suggests that the use of steroids at high doses in patients with significant neurological deficits in the perioperative period is safe and may be effective as a neuroprotectant.

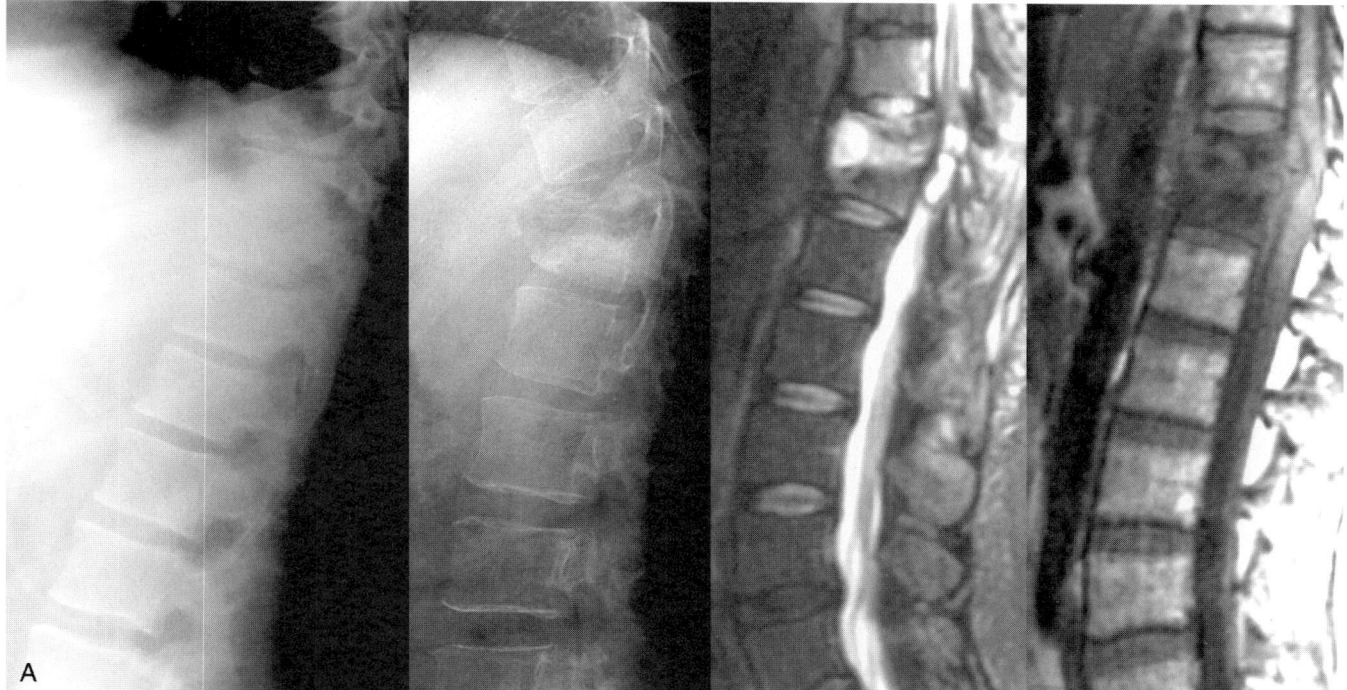

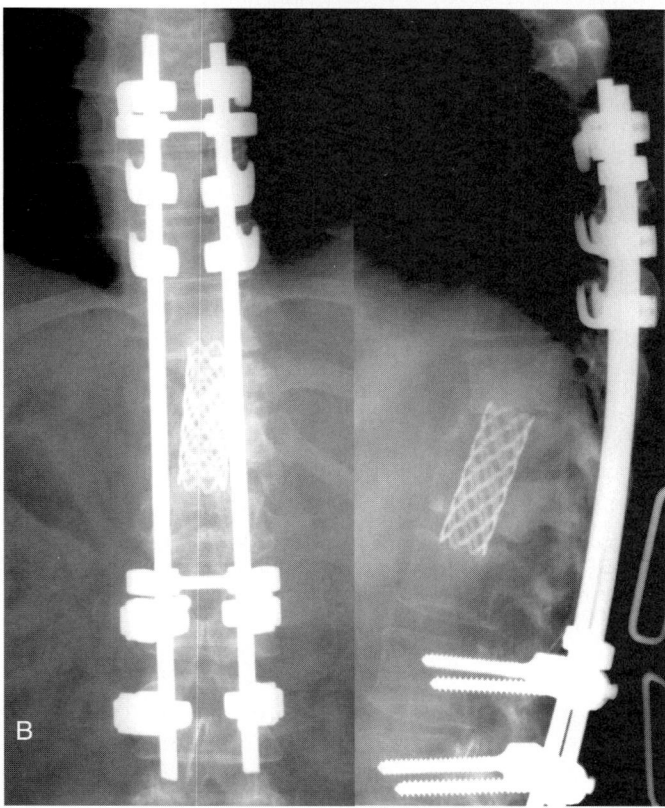

FIGURE 285–11. Pyogenic infection at T11-12 with a 4-day history of dense paraplegia in a 49-year-old intravenous drug abuser *(A)*, managed by T11-12 corpectomy and fusion with a Harms cage and autograft, followed by T7-L3 posterior fusion *(B)*. The patient is now ambulatory.

Implantation of Bone Grafts and Hardware

The surgical wound created during the operative management of a PSI is heavily contaminated by the organisms responsible for the infection. Yet the spine in such cases is often unstable, and some method of spinal reconstruction is essential. In the past, the implantation of devitalized bone or metal into such a field was considered contraindicated. Recent clinical experience by multiple groups has tended to refute this viewpoint. Many studies have shown that if the necrotic bone is adequately débrided, implantation of a

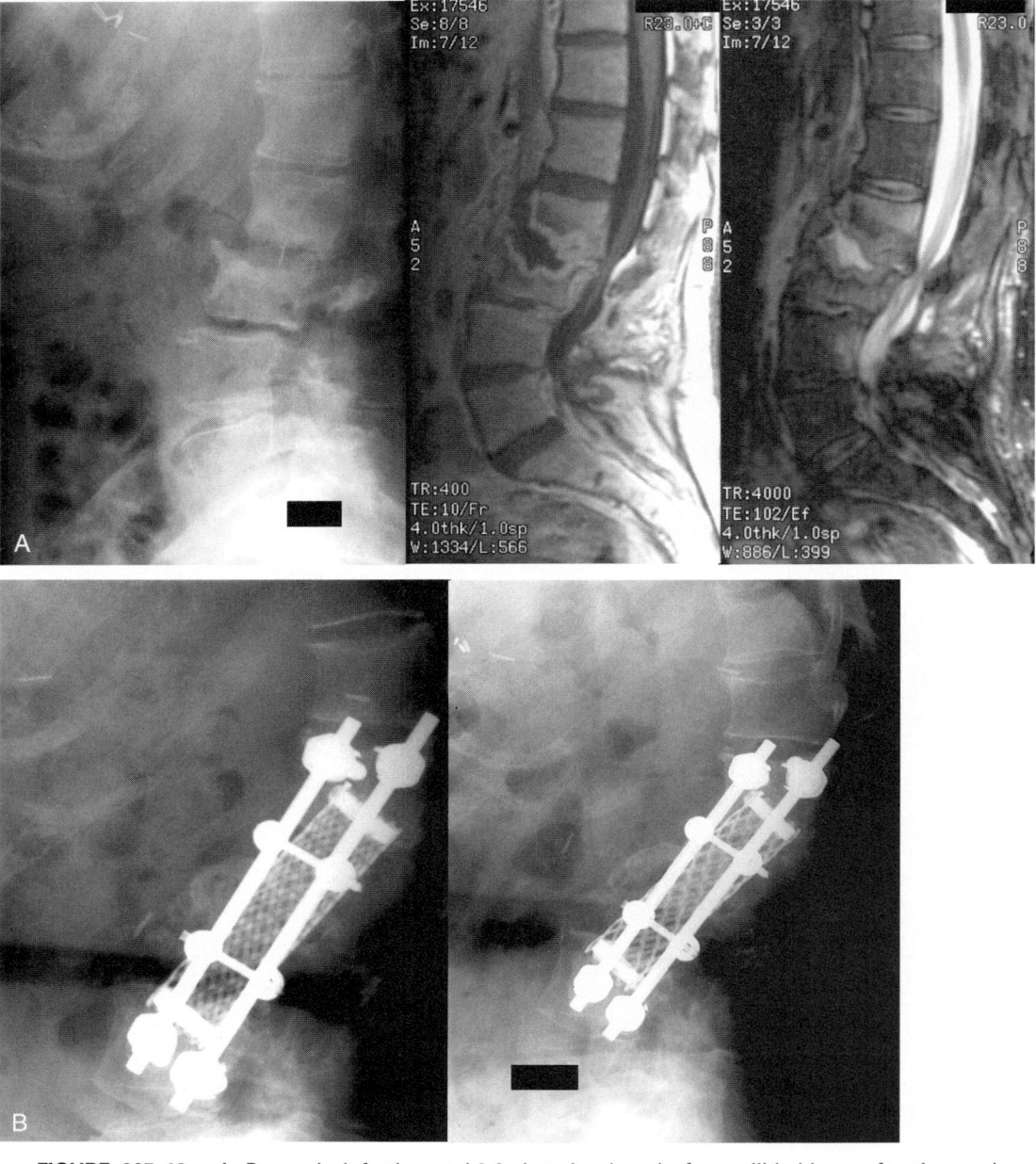

FIGURE 285–12. *A,* Pyogenic infection at L2-3 that developed after gallbladder perforation and *Salmonella* sepsis in a 58-year-old woman. *B,* She undewent L2-3 corpectomy, fusion with a Harms cage and autograft, and stabilization with a Kaneda-type construct. The angulation of the hardware was stable on images obtained 2 years postoperatively, indicating a solid bony union.

bone graft (allograft or autograft) and instrumentation is safe and effective in patients who receive an appropriate course of postoperative antibiotics.[6, 27, 29, 36, 49, 63, 75, 81, 94] Follow-up over time reveals that the implantation of hardware and bone grafts is remarkably effective in producing a bony union at the site of infection. This may be partly due to the enhanced vascularity of the region with the infection. Implanted hardware and bone grafts seldom get secondarily infected as long as the necrotic bone is well débrided and the patient receives an appropriate course of antibiotics (Fig. 285–13). Given that inadequate débridement is often the

cause of recrudescence of infection, and that the placement of hardware is safe if the débridement is adequate, thorough débridement is an important goal of surgical intervention in PSI.

MANAGEMENT OF EPIDURAL ABSCESSES

The management of epidural abscesses merits a separate discussion, given the controversies that surround it. There are no prospectively collected data addressing the surgical versus medical management of these lesions. Because patients with true "abscesses are at some

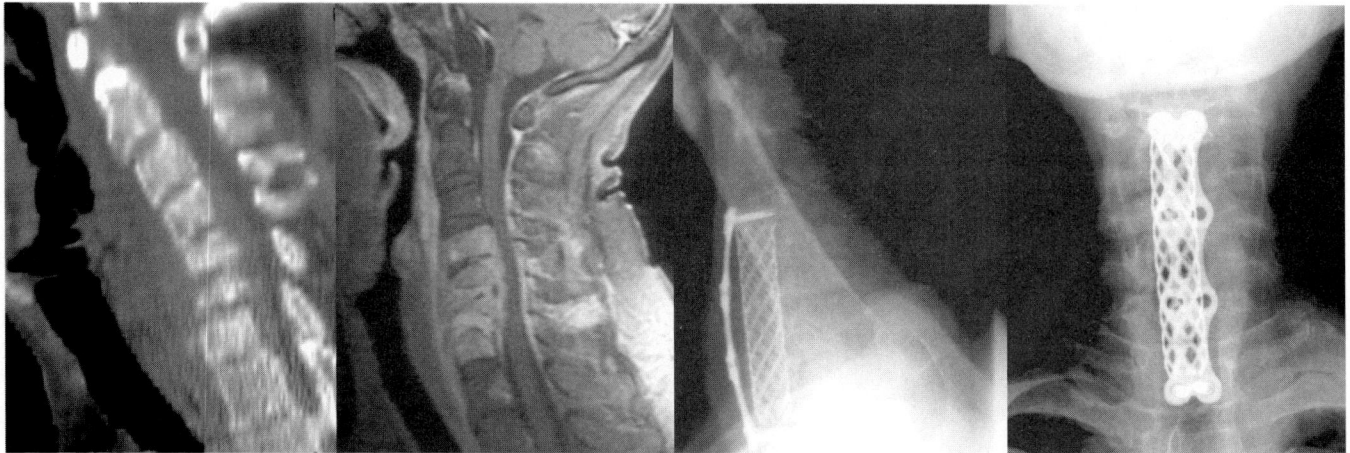

FIGURE 285–13. Pyogenic infection of C4-7 caused by *Pseudomonas aeruginosa*. The patient underwent C4-7 corpectomy, fusion with a Harms cage and autograft, and stabilization with an anterior cervical plate and halo. The infection was treated, and the patient' s mild preoperative paraparesis improved gradually.

risk for acute neurological deterioration and fatality," an observation that dates back to Dandy,[95] the prevailing recommendation has been to treat all abscesses surgically[7, 14, 32, 96]—"*ubi pus, ibi evacua.*" However, a review of the existing literature, as well as our own experience in dealing with such lesions, suggests that carefully selected patients can have an excellent outcome with medical management alone.[16, 22, 26, 28, 44, 52, 54, 97, 98]

The clinical condition of the patient and the imaging characteristics of the epidural collection are the determining factors in making a management decision. Careful evaluation of the MRI characteristics of epidural lesions can determine their fluid versus formed nature and prevent unnecessary, potentially harmful intervention. A collection that enhances only peripherally, has a central nonenhancing portion, and is hyperintense on T2-weighted images likely consists of fluid that can be easily drained. Lesions that are homogeneously enhancing and isointense or hypointense on T2-weighted images likely represent phlegmons—collections of granulation tissue. Such collections need to be addressed surgically only if they produce neurological deficits (Fig. 285–14).

A questionable situation arises in the case of a patient with a fluid abscess but no detectable deficits. If an organism is identified and the patient can be monitored closely, medical management is an option. If a bacteriologic diagnosis is not forthcoming, the patient's symptoms persist or worsen despite medical therapy, or there is difficulty obtaining reliable serial neurological assessments, surgical intervention is desirable.[91] Epidural abscesses of the cervical and thoracic spine are at higher risk for the sudden onset of neurological deficits than are similar lesions below the conus; they therefore have a lower threshold for surgical intervention. The presence of an epidural abscess over several segments or of paralysis of more than 3 days' duration does not present a contraindication for surgical intervention[22, 98] (Fig. 285–15). Good outcomes can be obtained by decompressions over discontinuous segments, and patients with relatively long-standing deficits may, occasionally, improve neurologically with surgical intervention.

It cannot be overemphasized that patients with epidural abscesses who are managed conservatively need to be carefully and serially monitored with regard to their neurological status.

MEDICAL MANAGEMENT

The management strategy in patients without neurological deficits or sepsis involves immobilization of the affected vertebral levels and administration of the appropriate intravenous antibiotics.[19] Medical management should be initiated as soon as an organism has been isolated, or after cultures have been obtained in patients who present in septic extremis. The goal of therapy is to sterilize the infected vertebral levels, prevent the occurrence of a neurological deficit, and prevent the formation of a painful deformity as the infection clears. The duration of therapy may be dependent on the extent of bony involvement seen on MRI. In patients with a minimal amount of bony infection and a competent immune system, the duration of therapy can be restricted to 6 weeks. If there is a prominent osteomyelitis component extending over multiple segments or the patient is immunocompromised (e.g., AIDS, cirrhosis, poorly controlled diabetes), an 8-week course of antibiotic therapy may be more effective in preventing the relapse of infection.[23] The efficacy of medical management can be gauged by diminishing pain, malaise, and fever and a decrease in the ESR. In all cases in which there are no coexisting reasons for its persistent elevation, the ESR should be followed closely to measure the effect of treatment. The response of the ESR to appropriate treatment is, unfortunately, unpredictable. Although a significant decrease in the ESR within a few weeks of treatment usually augurs a good prognosis, sustained elevations do not in them-

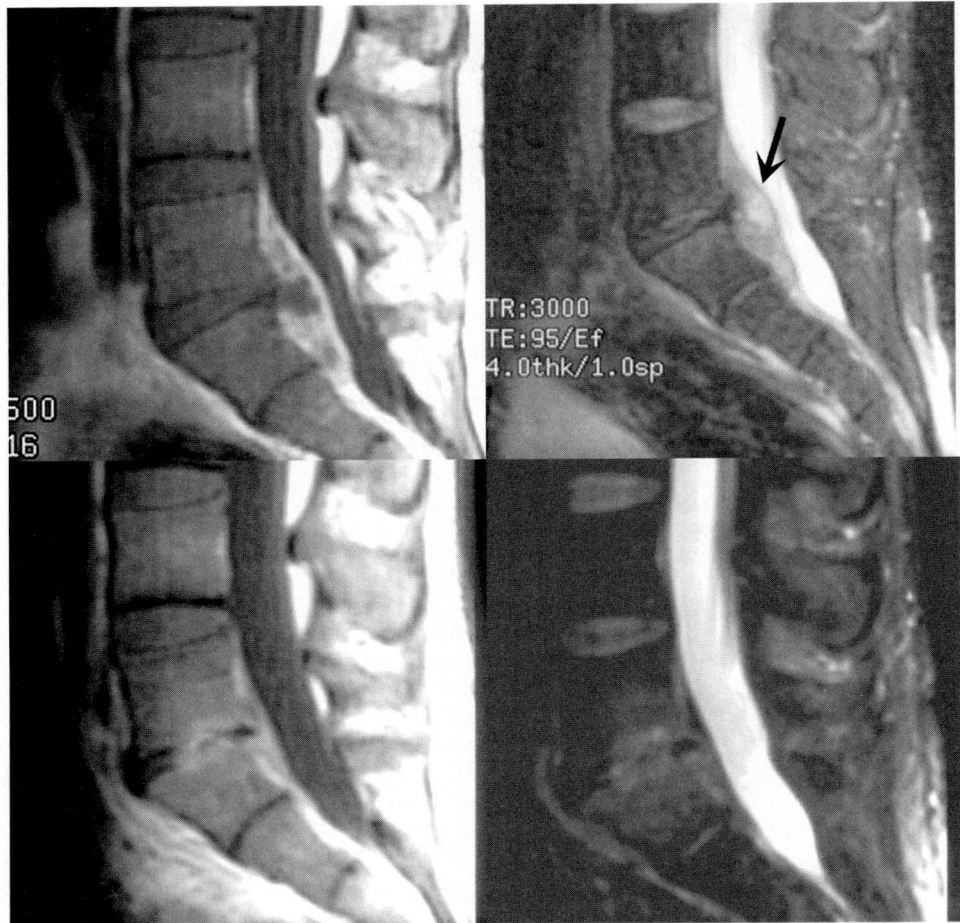

FIGURE 285–14. Pyogenic spinal infection with a prominent epidural abscess component from L4 to S2 managed with intravenous penicillin for 6 weeks. Resolution is apparent on a follow-up scan obtained at the end of medical therapy. The arrow points to a "fluid" component of epidural abscess.

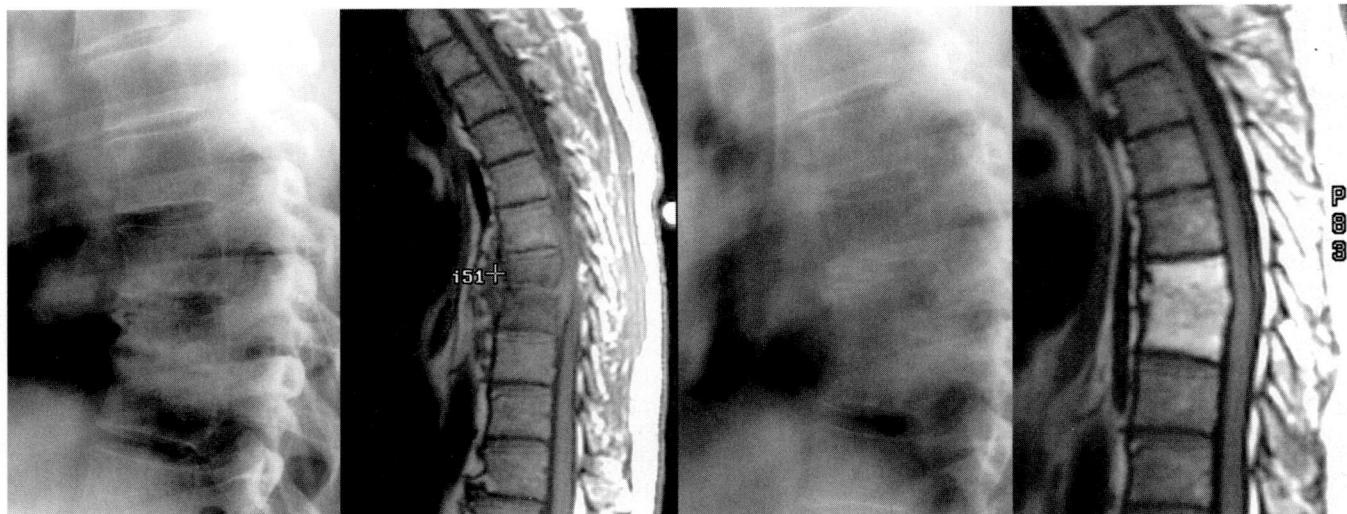

FIGURE 285–15. Pyogenic infection at T7-8 without neurological deficits or significant kyphosis, managed with antibiotic therapy alone. Radiographs and magnetic resonance imaging scan reveal spontaneous fusion across the infected disk space and increased signal intensity of the affected vertebral level on T1-weighted images, suggesting replacement of the marrow with fat.

selves imply therapy failure.[65] The ESR should be viewed in context of the patient's overall clinical picture. If the decrement in the ESR takes far longer than expected, consideration should be given to extending the duration of antibiotic therapy. If, after several weeks of therapy, there is no significant alteration in the ESR and the patient continues to be symptomatic, consideration should be given to reestablishing the radiographic and bacteriologic diagnosis.[17, 99]

Antibiotic therapy is guided by the in vitro sensitivity of the isolated organism. Given that staphylococcal and streptococcal species account for the vast majority of PSIs, the beta-lactams (penicillin, oxacillin, methicillin, nafcillin), ureidopenicillins (ticarcillin and piperacillin), cephalosporins, and vancomycin are the most commonly prescribed antibiotics. The addition of an aminoglycoside, trimethoprim-sulfa, a fluoroquinolone, or rifampin as a second agent may have a synergistic effect in vivo and should be considered in cases with extensive bony involvement, because vancomycin and certain cephalosporins may penetrate poorly into devascularized bone and the disk.[100] The addition of fusidic acid to a treatment regimen of penicillinase-stable penicillins appears to decrease the chance of failure of medical therapy.[23]

If no causative organism is isolated after multiple attempts or empirical treatment was started before a full microbiologic workup, the patient needs to be followed especially closely. Recommendations for empirical antibiotics vary somewhat with the epidemiologic factors of the case. Intravenous drug abusers may have a relatively greater proportion of infections caused by *Pseudomonas*.[24, 26, 49, 57] Failure of empirical therapy should prompt consideration of unusual pathogens—fungi and mycobacteria (see later). Patients also need to be monitored for adverse effects of the drugs used, appropriate antibiotic levels, and management of predisposing factors and associated complications.

In addition to antibiotics, patients are prescribed about 2 weeks of bed rest and are fitted with an orthosis appropriate to the spinal level of infection to prevent deformity or to help correct a mild deformity present at the time of diagnosis.

The role of oral antibiotics in PSIs is poorly defined. The practice of placing patients on oral agents after a prolonged course of intravenous antibiotics is widespread for osteomyelitis in various locations,[54, 96, 101] yet there is little evidence of their efficacy in treating spinal infections.[11] It is unlikely that residual infection after an appropriate course of intravenous antibiotics would be cleared by oral antibiotics, which may simply suppress recrudescence of the infection rather than sterilize the nidus of infection.

Infections isolated to the facet joints are rare.[102, 103] They are usually well managed by medical treatment, with surgery being reserved for patients with neurological compromise. A dorsal approach for débridement is usually adequate in these cases, and disruption of a single facet does not usually compromise spinal stability.

Outcomes

Patients with PSIs who present with incomplete neurological deficits of recent onset can have surprisingly good neurological recoveries, provided that timely, aggressive surgical therapy is instituted.[16, 36, 46, 49, 63, 75] The prognosis is more guarded in patients with profound deficits and in those whose diagnosis or treatment is delayed. Nonetheless, some of these patients may show substantial improvement in neurological function over time, justifying an aggressive therapeutic stance even when severe deficits are encountered.

It is our experience that the neurological outcome for patients with deficits secondary to PSI is better than that for patients with other acute causes of myelopathy, such as traumatic spinal cord injury. This is probably because the compressive forces acting on the spinal cord in PSI develop slowly, are gradually progressive, and are likely smaller in magnitude than those accompanying traumatic spinal cord injury. In some cases, however, deficits associated with PSI are the result of related vascular events such as venous or arterial thrombosis with infarction. Under these circumstances, recovery is less dramatic.

An analysis of outcome in patients with epidural abscesses suggests that older patients and patients presenting in sepsis, with neurological deficits of more than 72 hours' duration, or with significant compression of the spinal cord by imaging studies were more likely to have a poor outcome than were patients without these characteristics.[52, 104]

In patients who are managed medically, prognosis depends to some extent on the patient's age, the rate of decrease in ESR, and whether the patient is substantially immunocompromised. An immunocompromised state and infections caused by virulent organisms such as *S. aureus* (as opposed to *S. epidermidis* or *Propionibacterium*) may be associated with higher mortaliy rates.[24] Old age itself may be an independent indicator of a bad outcome; studies have suggested that the elderly have a poor outcome,[24, 52] but with aggressive surgical management, they may fare rather well.[19, 20]

Serial plain radiographs may be considered in patients with a prominent bony component to the infection for the early detection of vertebral body collapse or the development of a deformity. Successful treatment of the infection is seen radiographically as incorporation of the bone graft (if the patient was managed surgically) or sclerosis of the vertebral end plates on plain radiographs and CT. In cases of prominent disk space or bone infection, a spontaneous fusion at the affected level may occur. MRI scans show resolution of the typical changes, with the vertebral body tending to have a fatlike signal quality. Serial MRI scanning is not indicated unless a relapse of infection is suspected on clinical grounds. Radiographic findings respond very slowly to successful treatment compared with the clinical response and are therefore not immediately useful in assessing the response to therapy[51] (Fig. 285–16).

Pyogenic Spinal Infections in Children

PSIs in young children are common. Those affected usually have no risk factors for infection other than

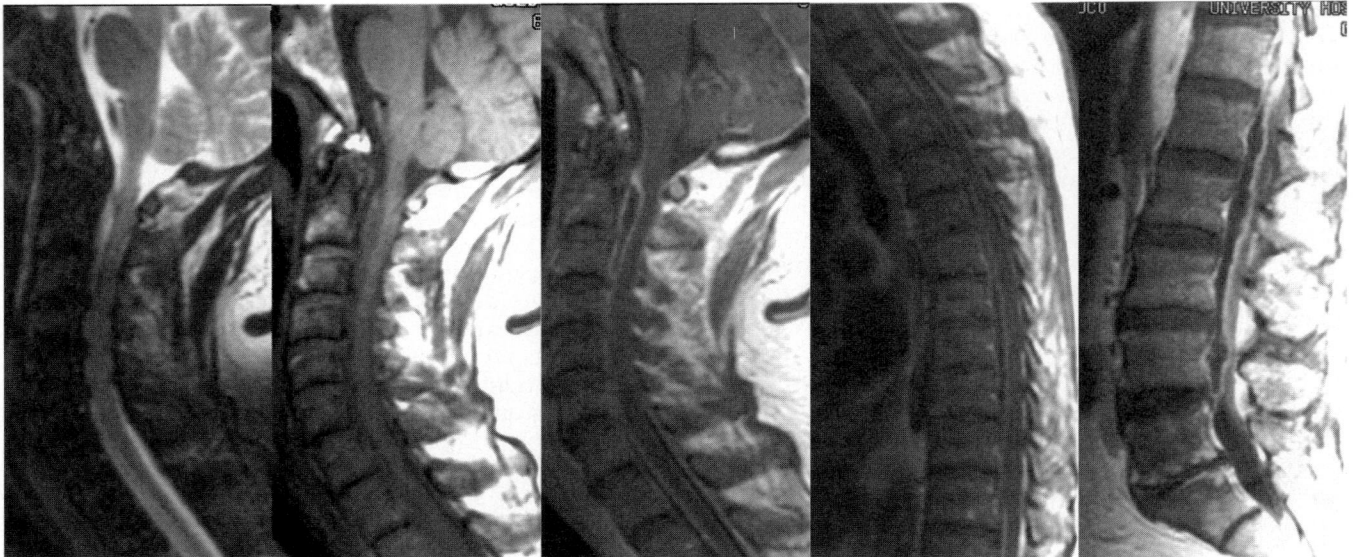

FIGURE 285–16. Epidural abscess involving the entire spine in a 65-year-old man with multiple gingival abscesses who presented with a sensory level at T5 and mild paraparesis. He was managed with laminectomies at C1-2, T5, and L2-4, which revealed infection by *Streptococcus viridans*.

their age. Infections have been reported in neonates[105] and infants[106, 107] and occur throughout childhood into early adolescence. The predilection for these infections appears to be a result of the frequent bacteremia that occurs in childhood. The distinct pattern of infection is thought to result from the peculiarities of pediatric spinal vascular anatomy.

Until about 7 years of age, profuse anastomoses exist between the intraosseous spinal arteries, preventing devascularization and infarction of large portions of the metaphysis when septic emboli occlude a metaphyseal artery. This tends to limit the extent of metaphyseal and osseous infection to the cartilaginous end plate at either end of the vertebra. Hence, hematogenous spread to the pediatric spine tends to be limited to the disk space. Additionally, the pediatric disk retains vascularity, unlike the situation in adults, and occasionally blood-borne pathogens may lodge directly in the disk space in children, without any involvement of the metaphyseal end plates.[108]

There is controversy regarding whether pediatric diskitis can exist without the presence of infection. It has been postulated that some cases may occur secondary to a partial dislocation of the epiphysis due to a hyperflexion injury.[109] Indeed, the rate of successful culturing of organisms from the disk in young children with radiographic changes consistent with infection is lower than that in adults.[67, 110, 111] Other studies, however, support the notion that these are true infections and are best treated by intravenous antibiotic therapy.[10]

Young children may be unable to provide an accurate history or accurately describe their symptoms, so the diagnosis should be considered whenever a child with fever refuses to bear weight or assumes a posture that avoids bending of the spine. The differential diagnosis includes conditions that mimic PSI in adults, but idiopathic intervertebral disk calcification, urinary tract infection, and appendicitis must also be considered in the pediatric population. The clinical and radiographic disease in children is often milder than that seen in adults. If no organisms are isolated, management with immobilization alone may be reasonable, but patients managed in this way should be followed closely for clinical and radiographic evidence of deterioration. In all cases in which infection is suspected or confirmed, appropriate antibiotic therapy, based on the culture results, should be initiated. Surgical intervention is only rarely indicated, usually if there is a significant epidural extension of the infection leading to neural compromise.[97, 112] Patients appear to do well with relatively short courses of antibiotic therapy and immobilization. In the long term, these patients may be at high risk for the development of block vertebra and vertebra magnum.[106, 113]

IATROGENIC INFECTIONS

Infections of the spine can occur after a variety of invasive diagnostic and therapeutic procedures, notably surgical procedures on the spine. The true scope of the term *iatrogenic* also includes infections resulting from hematogenous inoculation of the spine precipitated by the manipulation of a remotely contaminated or infected site (e.g., dental manipulation, urologic instrumentation, or drainage of a noncontiguous abscess). Infections resulting from such iatrogenic bacteremia are similar in most aspects to spontaneous pyogenic infections.

This section deals specifically with infections that result from direct spinal interventions. These procedures can render the spine susceptible to infection due to implanted instrumentation, devascularized bone graft, suture, and hematoma and by the production of ischemic or necrotic tissue through dissection and retraction.

Postoperative Spinal Infections

Postoperative spinal infections can occasionally be catastrophic, resulting in prolonged (and expensive) hospital stays and significant long-term disability.[114, 115] In the preantibiotic era, the rate of infection for spinal operations was about 0.9% to 4.6%. In series reported after the advent of Harrington instrumentation, the infection rate rose to between 1% and 12%, with an average of 6%.[116] Today, however, postoperative infection rates have decreased substantially in spite of the increased complexity of surgical procedures.

Currently, the average rate of infection following spinal procedures is around 2%. Of course, rates vary by procedure and are impacted by many variables. Contamination of the surgical wound by skin commensals occurs in as many as half of all surgical cases.[117] The host response to this contamination plays a significant role in determining whether an infection develops. Patient factors that predispose to infection include prior surgery, prior irradiation, preexisting neoplasm, chronic steroid therapy, diabetes, malnutrition, paraplegia, smoking, rheumatoid arthritis, poor nutritional state, and intercurrent infection.[118–120] In addition, there are numerous technical factors that influence the infection risk, including the duration of surgery, length of the wound, duration and force of retraction used, presence of a cerebrospinal fluid leak, use of antibiotic irrigation solutions, and implantation of instrumentation. Prophylactic antibiotics in the perioperative period are probably useful in preventing colonization of the wound and, if used for appropriate durations, are not associated with the development of infection by resistant organisms.[121–124] Double gloving is another practice that may reduce infection risk. The use of Bovie monopolar cauterization has been implicated in the increased risk of postoperative infection.[125] Interestingly, a lack of experience by the surgeon (e.g., residents and fellows in training) does not seem to increase the risk of infection.[126] For diskectomy procedures, the risk of postoperative spondylodiskitis may be reduced by placing a gentamicin-impregnated collagen sponge into the disk space[127, 128] and adding bacitracin to the irrigation fluid used during surgery.[129] This seeming efficacy of locally delivered antibiotics finds support from studies that show unreliable and poorly sustained levels of antibiotics in the disk space following systemic administration.[130, 131] Microneurosurgical approaches for diskectomy may also be associated with a lower infection risk than traditional laminectomy and diskectomy.[132]

Potential infections that can occur following spinal surgery include superficial wound infections, deep infections (below the fascia), spondylodiskitis, epidural abscess, and meningitis. The occurrence and management of most of these infections are affected significantly by whether instrumentation and bone grafting were carried out.

SURGERY WITHOUT INSTRUMENTATION OR BONE GRAFT

The incidence of infection after lumbar laminectomy or diskectomy is approximately 1%.[133] Postoperative diskitis occurs in about 0.1% to 5% of patients following lumbar diskectomy.[127, 134] The incidence is similar for posterior cervical operations but may be slightly lower when an anterior approach to the cervical spine is used. Infection usually occurs after intraoperative contamination,[129] and the typical causative organisms are skin flora—commonly *S. aureus* and *S. epidermidis*. Rarely, however, gram-negative organisms and anaerobes may produce fulminant infections in the surgical bed.[135] The typical scenario is the recurrence of symptoms in a patient who initially experienced good relief of preoperative symptoms (e.g., radiculopathy) immediately after surgery. The surgical incision may appear to be healing uneventfully. A history of a small amount of drainage soon after surgery is occasionally obtained. The diagnosis is strongly suggested by a persistently elevated ESR[127, 136] or CRP and by typical changes on MRI. However, both the acute-phase reactants and the radiographic changes need to be distinguished from expected postoperative changes. The ESR usually returns to normal within 2 weeks after uncomplicated surgery. Measurement of CRP levels, which return to normal sooner, may be useful in detecting early infections, but given the individual variability in CRP values, this is most useful when a baseline value is available. Measurement of a specific acute-phase reactant, such as elastase-α_1 proteinase inhibitor, may allow the earlier detection of infection, but it has not been shown to be relevant outside of a research setting.[137] MRI with contrast almost always reveals changes suggestive of a postoperative spondylodiskitis, but it may yield false-positive results[134, 138] and should be evaluated in the context of the patient's clinical picture and laboratory data.

Depending on the number of levels operated on and the size of the postoperative fluid collection, the infection can be managed either with antibiotics alone or with surgical débridement in addition.[139] Because there is little devascularized tissue or foreign material in such wounds, antibiotic penetration is usually excellent, and these infections can often be eradicated by a few weeks of intravenous therapy alone.

SURGERY WITH INSTRUMENTATION AND BONE GRAFT

The modern management of spinal disorders often includes the use of instrumentation to facilitate fusion. Instrumentation provides immediate spinal stabilization, early mobilization of the patient, and a higher rate of bony fusion. However, the use of instrumentation clearly increases the risk of postoperative infectious complications. Data demonstrating the effect of instrumentation on the risk of postoperative infection first became available in a series involving Harrington rod instrumentation.[140] Recent estimates of infection risk in instrumented cases range from 2% to 8.5%.[118, 119,]

[141, 142] Infections associated with spinal instrumentation are far more common after posterior or posterolateral approaches to the spine; a lower rate of infection is observed after anterior cervical or anterior thoracolumbar instrumentation.[118] This is presumably related to an increase in necrosis of the paraspinous muscles and other soft tissues due to devascularization that results from dissection and ischemia from prolonged retraction. Prolonged retraction is known to cause disruption of normal muscle physiology and compromise of perfusion; thus the duration and extent of retraction should be minimized.[143, 144] In addition to frank tissue necrosis, ischemia can promote the formation of a large seroma in the wound, a fertile ground for colonization by multiple organisms.[115]

Infections following spinal instrumentation can manifest in either an acute or a delayed fashion. Patients with acute infections usually present between 2 and 8 weeks after the initial surgery with erythema of the wound, partial wound dehiscence, and drainage of seropurulent fluid.[118] Fever and leukocytosis may or may not be present, although the ESR is usually elevated. The causative organism can usually be cultured from the wound if cultures are obtained before starting antibiotic therapy.

A distinction needs to be made between early infections that are limited to the skin and subcutaneous tissues and those that extend below the fascia. Superficial infections usually occur in obese patients with large amounts of subcutaneous fat and in those with impaired wound healing. These infections can be closed after thorough débridement and irrigation, if there is minimal necrosis, or they can be managed with sterile dressing changes and delayed secondary closure, if there is more substantial soft tissue loss. Early infections following instrumentation are usually caused by *S. aureus*—sometimes by a strain resistant to the antibiotic administered perioperatively. Such infections necessitate thorough débridement of the wound, removal of suture material and necrotic tissue, and intravenous antibiotic therapy. They can usually be managed without removal of the implants.[115, 118] A concern in the management of deep infections following instrumentation has been the ability to deliver bactericidal concentrations of antibiotics to potentially devascularized regions. To accomplish this, some surgeons advocate the use of continuous suction-irrigation systems to deliver antibiotics to the wound.[115, 118, 145] Others prefer to augment local bacterial control at the surgical graft site by implanting materials that release antibiotics locally over an extended period.[146] However, Rath has stated that if the delivery vehicle is an acrylic implant, it may allow the infective foci to persist.[36] Many other surgeons, including us, prefer multiple débridements or serial open packing of the wound until all necrotic tissue is removed and a delayed secondary closure can be performed. Occasionally, catastrophic mixed infections by organisms that can cause a synergistic necrotizing fasciitis or gangrene can complicate débridements, but fortunately, they are rare.[147]

Delayed infections manifest several months after the initial operation. Such infections are almost always attributable to indolent organisms such as *Propionibacterium acnes*, *S. epidermidis*, or *Corynebacterium*. If enough time has elapsed since bone grafting and a rigid bony fusion is found at surgery, a case can be made for removal of the infected hardware.[142, 148] Dubousset has argued that these delayed infections are not true infections but may reflect a fretting corrosion of the metal implant that results in a seemingly sterile chronic inflammation surrounding the instrumentation.[149] It has been shown, however, that if the intraoperative tissue cultures are maintained in the laboratory for at least 7 days, slow-growing organisms such as the ones mentioned can be isolated.[142, 150] These infections likely result from intraoperative contamination of the instrumentation by organisms that multiply slowly.[148] The instrumentation is coated by an avascular exopolysaccharide—the glycocalyx—produced by these bacteria, which prevents the body's immune mechanisms and antibiotics from eradicating them. Additionally, the glycocalyx prevents truly representative organisms from detaching in sufficient numbers to be detected by a simple aspiration and culture. Because such infections usually present late, removal of the instrumentation may not compromise the bony fusion. Hardware removal is the most effective way of eradicating the glycocalyx and thereby the nidus of the infection. This forms the basis of some authors' recommendation for hardware removal.[142, 148] Following hardware removal, adequate débridement, and intravenous antibiotics for about 4 weeks, these infections are usually eliminated.

Postdiskography Infections

Infections develop after diskography in about 0.16% to 3% of disks injected.[151–154] Although the most common infectious complication is diskitis, an epidural abscess[151, 155] or even a subdural abscess can result following diskography. Patients usually present with severe local pain a few days after the diskogram. The hematologic markers of acute inflammation[156] are significantly elevated. The diagnosis is made by obtaining an MRI scan without and with contrast. Management is chiefly medical, with antibiotics tailored to staphylococcal species—the most common causative organisms—or to culture results if an organism can be aspirated from the disk. The risk of spinal infection from diskography can be minimized by the administration of a broad-spectrum antibiotic either intravenously or mixed with the contrast dye.[157] The use of styletted needles and a double-needle technique, as recommended by Fraser, may also aid in the prevention of iatrogenic contamination of the disk space.[152]

Infections Following Epidural Catheter Placement

Epidural catheters used for pain control can occasionally provide a tract for the entry of infection into the epidural space. The usual pathogenic organisms are *S. epidermidis* and *S. aureus*, which likely reflect contamination of the catheter by skin flora.[158] The reported incidence of such infections is widely variable—from approximately 1 infection per 2000 catheter placements[159] to a 12% infection rate. Much of this variability can be explained by differences in the duration of epidural catheterization use, with a rise in infection risk as the duration of catheterization increases. When the incidence is expressed as the number of infections per catheter-days, there is much more homogeneity in the infection risk. The incidence stated in this way is between 0.2 and 0.77 per 1000 catheter-days.[160–162] Long-term epidural anesthesia is used in the management of cancer pain, and the "per-patient" risk of infection is higher in this population.[162] Given the wide use of epidural anesthesia during parturition, a large majority of reports of infection of these catheters comes from the obstetric literature.

Factors that appear to correlate with the occurrence of catheter infection include prolonged time of catheter insertion, immunocompromised patient, and recent trauma.[160, 163, 164] Early warning signs of the presence of infection include focal pain around the site of catheter insertion, superficial infection of the catheter entry site, and catheter dysfunction.[162] These early signs can progress to the rapid development of neurological deficits.[162] MRI scanning with contrast provides a reliable diagnosis in most cases.[162, 165] Management depends on the condition of the patient at the time of presentation. If the infection is detected early, it can be managed by removing the catheter and treating the patient with appropriate antibiotics. Patients who have developed deficits should be evaluated for urgent surgical intervention.[163, 165] Surgical intervention can improve the chances of neurological recovery in patients who develop deficits, but many patients may not improve despite aggressive intervention.[164] Culture of the catheter after its removal usually identifies the causative organism, and antimicrobial therapy can be tailored accordingly. Patients with chronic pain who are debilitated may develop sepsis following the development of an epidural abscess and may succumb to this.[162] Tunneling the catheter for a distance before exiting the skin may help reduce the risk of infection.[166]

The use of 0.5% chlorhexidine in 80% ethanol instead of 10% povidone-iodine to prepare the skin before placement of an epidural catheter has been promoted by some as a method of preventing catheter infection.[167] It finds support in the scientific literature, where chlorhexidine solutions have been shown to be more effective than povidone-iodine in decreasing the number of bacterial colonies cultured from the skin[168–170] and in preventing vascular catheter-related infection.[171–174] Some consider the latter set of studies to be analogous to epidural space catheterization, due to similarities in the risk factors for catheter colonization. However, two prospective, randomized studies comparing the use of chlorhexidine versus povidone-iodine for skin preparation before the placement of epidural catheters failed to agree with each other; one study showed a beneficial effect of using chlorhexidine in a pediatric population, and the other study showed no difference in an adult population.[175, 176]

Other Iatrogenic Infections

Spinal infections may develop after minimally invasive procedures on the spine. The risk of infections devel-

oping after kyphoplasty,[177] the placement of epidural spinal cord stimulators,[178] and intradiskal electrothermy[179] is extremely low. The use of careful sterile technique and periprocedural antibiotics minimizes these risks. Early detection and aggressive medical therapy are usually adequate in the management of infections in this setting, with surgical intervention reserved for cases of neurological deficits or the presence of infected nonbiologic material.

UNUSUAL BACTERIAL PATHOGENS

As noted previously, the vast majority of spinal infections are caused by gram-positive organisms, with staphylococcal species predominating. Other pathogens that are relatively common infectious agents, such as enterococci, *E. coli*, *Pseudomonas* species, and *Proteus* species, make up most of the remainder. Infections due to uncommon organisms such as *Nocardia* species and *Actinomyces* have been described sporadically.

Actinomycosis and Nocardiosis

Actinomyces species are gram-positive, filamentous bacteria that are most commonly associated with chronic draining infections. The presence in the drainage of "sulfur granules," discrete yellow particulate material consisting of clumps of the organism itself, is pathognomonic of *Actinomyces* infection. Common sites of infection include the oral cavity and paranasal sinuses, with extension into the soft tissues of the face or neck. Spinal involvement is rare and generally the result of contiguous spread from adjacent sites of infection, especially the lungs and sinuses.[180, 181] Vertebral destruction with deformity is uncommon with *Actinomyces* infection. Neurological compromise is usually due to extensive spread of the infection to the epidural space. The first-line treatment of *Actinomyces* osteomyelitis is intravenous penicillin G. Ciprofloxacin and rifampicin are also effective for eradicating vertebral infections.[182] Surgical intervention is rarely indicated and should generally be reserved for cases of neurological compromise.[183, 184]

Nocardia are filamentous, branching, gram-positive aerobic bacteria. They are normally found in the soil and are associated primarily with pulmonary infection in immunocompromised patients. Spinal involvement is rare—there are only about a dozen cases reported in the literature[185–187]—and occurs both by direct extension of intrathoracic infections and through hematogenous spread. Most reported infections have been caused by the *asteroides* species. Treatment is with sulfonamides, cephalosporins, aminoglycosides, or synthetic penicillins. Although a prolonged course of antibiotics may be required to cure osteomyelitis, elimination of the infection occurs in most patients. Surgery is generally reserved for stabilization and the correction of deformity.

Brucellosis

Infections with *Brucella* species in humans are uncommon in the United States and northern and central

Europe. This group of pathogens continues to pose a significant problem in many underdeveloped regions of the world, however. Endemic areas include the Mediterranean region, the Middle East, and Central and South America. Most human infections are associated with contact with livestock or products related to livestock, such as untanned hides or unpasteurized milk.

Osteoarticular complications of infection with *Brucella* species are common, occurring in about 25% of cases.[188] Spinal involvement is perhaps the most common bony infection, accounting for about half the cases of osteoarticular extension. Vertebral infection occurs in about 6% to 12% of cases of brucellosis.[189, 190] The presenting signs and symptoms of spinal brucellosis are nonspecific and similar to those associated with other forms of spinal osteomyelitis.[191] The symptom onset of spinal brucellosis tends to be subacute, and the radiologic manifestations are nonspecific, with some similarity to cases of tuberculosis (TB). However, the proliferative changes associated with bony repair in brucellosis are not seen in tuberculous infection, and deformities of the spine, which are common in TB, are rarely seen with brucellosis. Radionuclide bone scans are highly sensitive in demonstrating areas of involvement in patients with *Brucella* infections who have musculoskeletal complaints.[192]

Antimicrobial therapy is effective in most cases, with a cure possible in approximately 90% of cases of skeletal brucellosis; there is some evidence, however, that spinal infections may be more refractory. A number of antibiotics in various combinations have been used to treat *Brucella* osteomyelitis, including tetracyclines, trimethoprim-sulfa, and aminoglycosides. Surgical intervention in these cases is infrequent and is typically reserved for cases in which a bacteriologic diagnosis is not possible by other means; for decompression of the neural elements, when necessary; and, occasionally, for correction of deformity.

Tuberculosis

TB is perhaps the most lethal infectious disease worldwide, accounting for nearly 3 million deaths per year.[193] More than 1.5 billion people either are presently infected or have had tuberculous infection in the past. The AIDS pandemic has been cited as the cause of the recent resurgence in reported cases of TB, especially in eastern and central Africa, where the incidence of HIV infection is especially high. In the Western world as well, there is evidence of an increase in tuberculous infections in high-risk groups, especially those with immunosuppression or immunodeficiency syndromes, with substandard nutrition and living conditions, and at the extremes of age.

Osseous and articular involvement is a common manifestation of well-established mycobacterial disease and occurs in approximately 3% to 5% of cases. Interestingly, the incidence of skeletal involvement in patients with concurrent HIV infection rises to 60%. The most common site of skeletal involvement is the spine, with nearly half of all cases of osseous TB being spinal. Spinal infections typically have the most serious consequences, with severe deformity and paraplegia being

the most significant. Although tuberculous involvement can be seen at any spinal level, the frequency of involvement varies widely, with a peak occurrence at the thoracolumbar junction and decreasing frequencies at more rostral and caudal levels. Overall, the cervical spine accounts for about 10% of cases of tuberculous spondylitis, the thoracic spine for 50%, and the lumbar spine 40%.[188] Although spinal involvement may result from direct extension from adjacent structures (e.g., lung and pleural cavity), spread to the vertebral column is more common through a vascular route. Work by Hodgson in the 1960s and 1970s suggested that a major mechanism for the spread of infection is via Batson's venous plexus. The strong association of spinal involvement with intra-abdominal infection, such as renal TB, is consistent with this hypothesis.

The nature of tuberculous spinal infection is somewhat different from that of the pyogenic infections described earlier. TB tends to manifest in a more indolent fashion. It commonly exhibits concurrent involvement of the posterior elements and is therefore more likely to induce deformity. Because of the slow rate of development, these deformities are often observed without severe neurological compromise. The disks are often relatively preserved, but associated paraspinous masses of inflammatory tissue or abscess are common. The appearance of tuberculous infection on imaging may be more difficult to distinguish from neoplastic processes as a result. The actual nature of the pathology is dependent on the stage of the disease process. Initial inflammatory changes are followed by abscess formation. Occasionally, a large amount of liquid pus is present and may cause mass effect on the neural elements with deficit. As the infection evolves, caseous material forms. Necrosis of bone with erosion and loss of ligamentous integrity contributes to the development of angulation and deformity. Retropulsion of sequestered bone into the spinal canal may cause acute deficits. With resolution of the acute infectious process, a more chronic situation may develop that includes the formation of fibrous scarring, which acts to restore relative stability. Calcification and ultimately ossification may occur, which in some cases produce cord compression as a chronic process.

DIAGNOSIS

The diagnosis of spinal TB requires a high level of suspicion. In the absence of a history of active pulmonary or renal TB, the initial symptoms overlap with a variety of spinal disorders, depending on the level of involvement. The course of symptoms may be more suggestive of neoplasm than infection, and the systemic complaints of a patient with active TB may be mistaken for signs of disseminated cancer. Patients with concurrent AIDS and pediatric patients may present with greater acuity. The initial evaluation usually consists of plain radiographs, MRI scanning with and without contrast, blood culture, urine culture, and percutaneous biopsy or aspiration. CT may supplement the other imaging modalities by better defining the degree of bony destruction and the likelihood of segmental instability. Open biopsy is infrequently necessary to obtain satisfactory diagnostic material. Surgical intervention is reserved primarily for therapeutic purposes, as discussed later.

TREATMENT

Chemotherapy

The mainstay of treatment for spinal TB, as with other sites of infection, is effective antituberculous chemotherapy. Modern methods of characterizing TB strains using the polymerase chain reaction have provided clues in the prospective determination of possible drug resistance. Standard antituberculous therapy involves multiple agents administered for protracted periods. Triple-drug therapy with isoniazid, rifampin, and pyrazinamide is a frequently used regimen. Duration of therapy is often debated, but the incidence of relapse of bony infection may be unacceptable with less than 12 months of triple-drug therapy. Longer durations may be required in patients who are slow to respond.

Adjunctive Treatment

The role of bed rest or orthoses in the management of spinal TB is not well defined. Some authors advocate an early period of recumbency at the beginning of drug treatment, with the rationale of decreasing the development of deformity. Others use orthoses and maintain the patient's ambulatory status. Many larger studies of therapy for tuberculous spondylitis are derived from underdeveloped countries, where the difficulty of providing for prolonged recumbency or problems in fitting and maintaining appropriate orthoses may have made positive results from these measures unlikely. Nonetheless, the presence of significant instability or deformity is probably best treated with surgical means, if other patient factors allow.

Surgery

Surgical treatment is considered in the presence of spinal instability or progressive neurological symptoms with evidence of cord compression or deformation. In the past, surgical drainage of large paraspinal "cold" abscesses was advocated on the grounds that this maneuver accelerated the patient's improvement. More recently, the experience in centers treating a large volume of spinal TB cases suggests that routine drainage of these extraspinal collections may have little or no impact on outcome. Similarly, it has been held that surgical débridement of involved bone and soft tissue may have utility in clearing the infection. There is good evidence, however, that simple débridement of the infected focus adds little to effective chemotherapy. When deformity, neurological deficit, or instability exists, however, the role of decompression, débridement of affected tissue, reconstruction, and stabilization seems clear.

As with other types of spinal infection, most of the involvement centers in the vertebral bodies. As a result, decompression, débridement, and reconstruction of the affected anterior and middle columns require anterior or anterolateral approaches. For cervical lesions, the standard approaches for multilevel anterior disease are applicable. In patients with considerable deformity that cannot be completely corrected from the front, an additional posterior fixation may need to be considered.

Thoracic levels are generally accessed through a thoracotomy approach, which is sufficient to allow anterior débridement, anterior reconstruction with allograft strut or cylindrical cage and autograft, and placement of an anterior internal fixation device. If the posterior elements are intact and kyphosis is not marked, this is usually sufficient. Alternatively, if there is more pronounced kyphosis with cord compression in the thoracic region (T4-L1), a lateral extracavitary approach[85] may be quite effective in affording visualization of spinal cord decompression and allowing a long posterior construct for deformity correction through a single operative field. Anterior reconstruction using autologous rib or allograft strut or cage can generally be performed with this approach. Finally, planned anterior and posterior surgery carried out sequentially in a single session may be required to produce optimal débridement, deformity correction, and long-term stability.

FUNGAL INFECTIONS

Fungal infections of the spine are infrequent and tend to occur in patients with predisposing conditions or, rarely, as the consequence of iatrogenic interventions. Examples of comorbid conditions usually seen in patients with fungal spinal infections include prolonged corticosteroid administration, immunosuppression after organ transplantation, severe systemic illness associated with malnutrition and multiple antibiotic use, HIV infection, diabetes, alcohol or intravenous drug abuse, and parenteral nutrition.

Candida species have become some of the most common nosocomial pathogens in critically ill patients. Osteoarticular involvement can be expected to increase as the overall incidence of disseminated candidiasis increases. Certain endemic respiratory pathogens such as *Coccidioides* and *Blastomyces* involve the spine as a consequence of dissemination. Recognition of the possibility of these infections in their various endemic regions is the key to diagnosis. Because bacterial infection is much more prevalent, a high degree of clinical suspicion, especially in patients with the previously mentioned risk factors, is critical to making the appropriate diagnosis and initiating effective antifungal therapy. *Aspergillus, Blastomyces,* and *Coccidioides* infections of the spine closely mimic mycobacterial infections and should be considered in the differential diagnosis of Pott's disease.

Aspergillosis

Aspergillus, a ubiquitous species of fungus, is usually pathogenic only in patients with impaired immune defenses. Spinal infection with *Aspergillus* species is rare in immunocompetent patients. Predisposing factors that have been described in clinical reports include systemic corticosteroid therapy, uncontrolled diabetes, immunosuppression following organ transplantation, AIDS, chronic granulomatous disease, chemotherapy, hematologic malignancy, and prolonged neutropenia.[205-207] Aspergillus typically invades the spine from a contiguous site of infection (usually pulmonary), but can also be spread hematogenously. Though rare, *Aspergillus* vertebral infections have been reported in immunocompetent hosts as well.[208, 209] Differentiation must be made from tuberculosis, which can closely

mimic aspergillosis of the spine, using serologic testing. Cases diagnosed early can usually be managed medically. Intravenous amphotericin B is the primary therapeutic agent although one of the growing group of azole antifungal agents may also be effective. Once an *Aspergillus* infection is established in the spine, rapid destruction of the intervertebral disk and vertebral bodies can occur, causing deformity and neurological deficits. Surgical débridement is indicated in cases with abscess formation, significant vertebral destruction or neurological deficit. (Fig. 285–17). Spinal instrumenta-

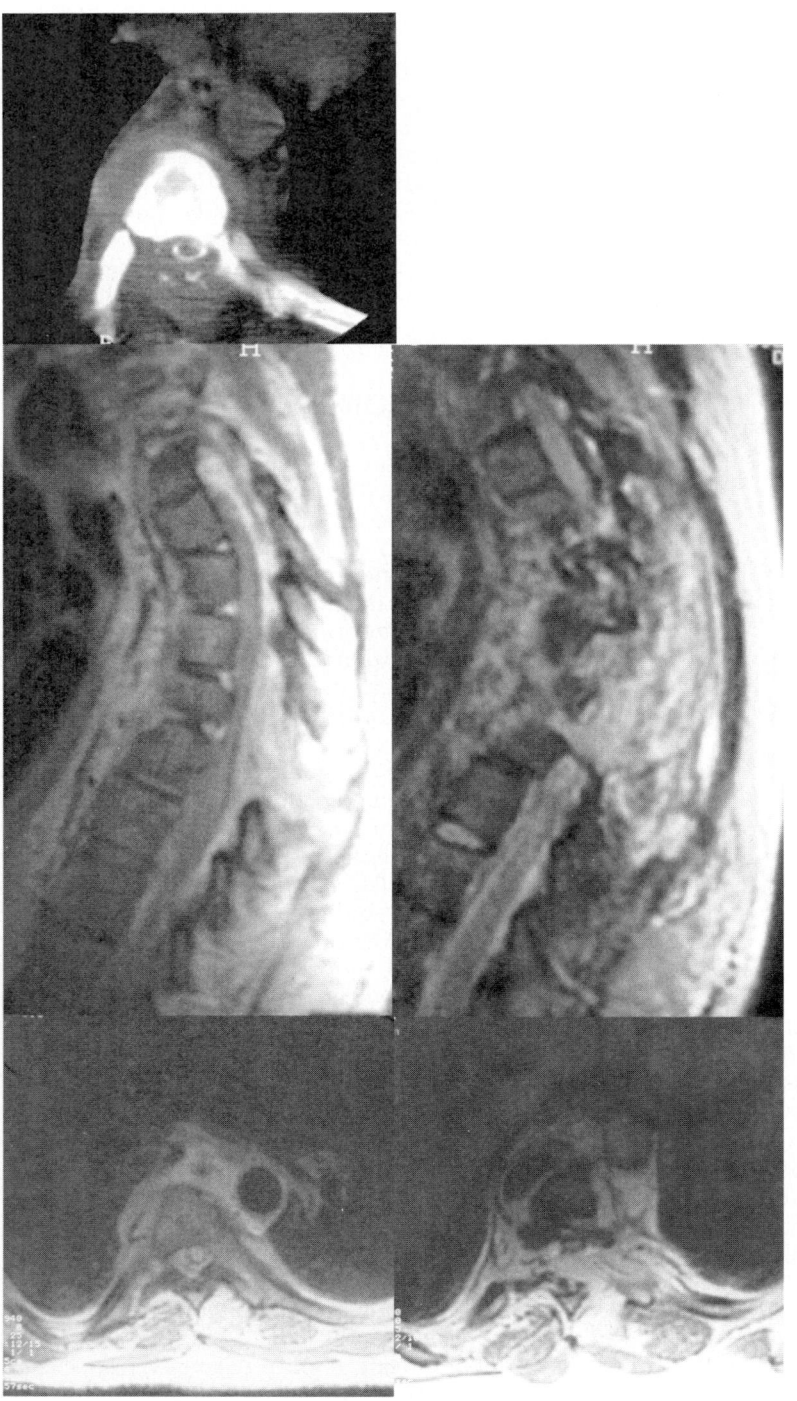

FIGURE 285–17. Thirty-six-year-old woman with blastomycosis of the spine.

tion is usually necessary to restore spinal stability and maintain alignment.[208, 210, 211]

Blastomycosis

North American blastomycosis is predominantly a granulomatous cutaneous or respiratory infection. It is caused by *Blastomyces dermatitides,* a dimorphic fungus endemic to regions along the Mississippi and Ohio river valleys and the southern and eastern United States. Males are more susceptible to infection than females, and blacks are more commonly affected than whites. All ages can be affected, but the disease appears to have a predilection for those in the second through fifth decades of life. The infection may be self-limited or may progress to dissemination. Disseminated disease produces generalized symptoms of fever, malaise, anorexia, and night sweats. Secondary osseous involvement is common, with the spine being a prime target. Vertebral involvement produces a destructive lesion often associated with a large paraspinous mass. The lower thoracic and lumbar spine is most often the site of the infection. Fever and skin lesions typical of blastomycosis may be seen.[213] Blastomycosis of the spine must be distinguished from tuberculosis and coccidioidomycosis. In tuberculosis the posterior elements of the vertebral body are not infected, whereas in coccidioidomycosis and blastomycosis all bony elements of the spine may be involved. Additionally, blastomy-

cosis has a greater tendency to produce cutaneous fistulae.[212] The definitive diagnosis is typically made through positive cytology or histologic examination of biopsy specimens. A high index of suspicion is justified in endemic areas and in immunocompromised or otherwise susceptible hosts. Like most fungal osteomyelitis, standard treatment is with amphotericin B, although newer azole antifungals (e.g., itraconazole) may be effective, with surgery reserved for spinal instability or neurological deterioration (Fig. 285–18).

Candidiasis

Candida species are common opportunistic infections in patients with various forms of immunocompromise, including diabetes, systemic malignancy, HIV infection, prolonged antibiotic administration, or bone marrow or organ transplantation.[25] The presence of a central venous catheter, the use of broad-spectrum antibiotics, and intravenous drug abuse are other factors that increase the risk of candidal osteomyelitis.[214] Approximately one-half to two-thirds of all patients who are ultimately diagnosed with candida osteomyelitis have had at least one episode of candidemia in the past, usually within a year of presentation.[215, 216] Non-*albicans* species such as *C. glabrata, C. tropicalis,* and *C. dublinensis* are assuming greater importance as opportunistic pathogens. This is significant as there is an increase in resistance to antifungal chemotherapy in

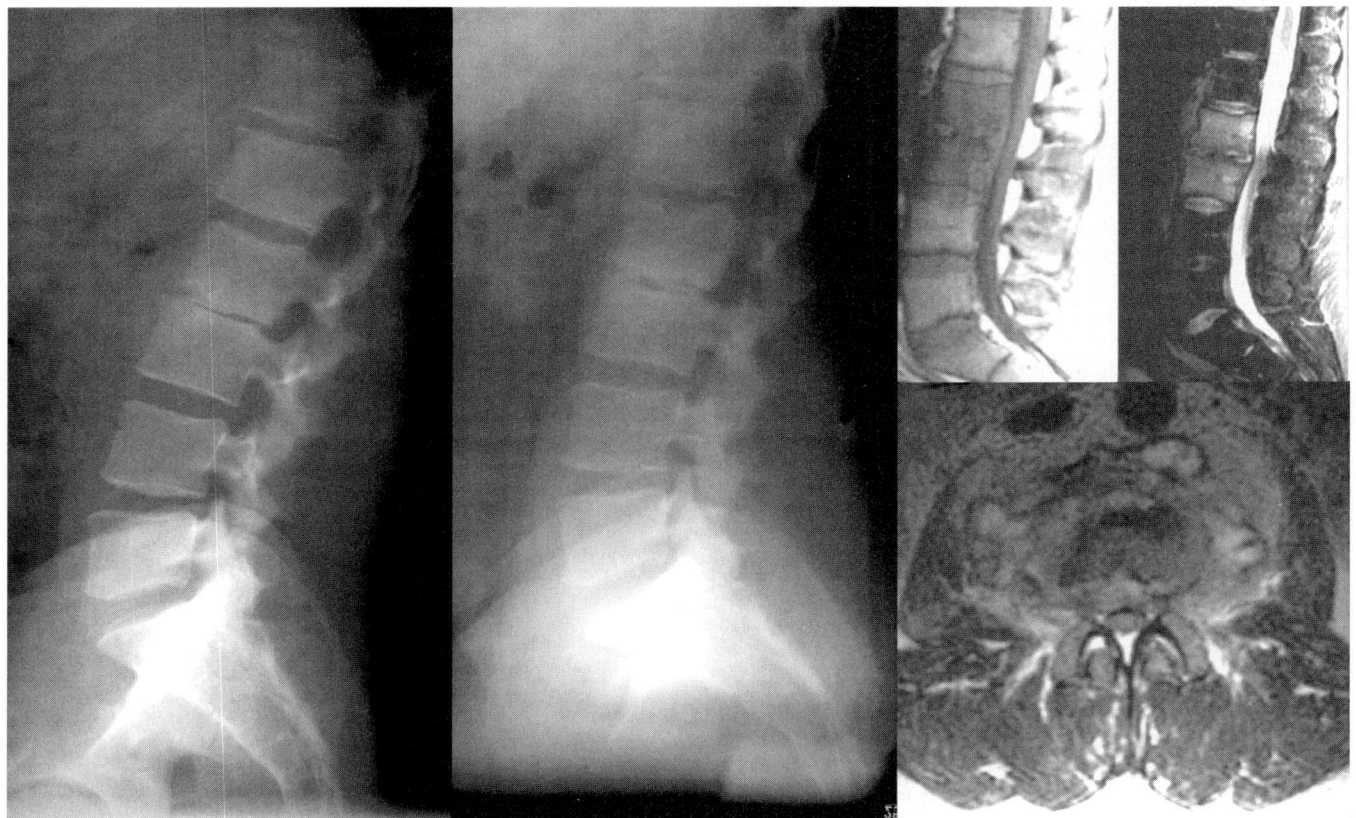

FIGURE 285–18. Thirty-year-old man with mucormycosis of the spine.

many of these "nontraditional" species. Most patients have an elevated ESR, positive blood cultures are obtained in about 50% of patients,[214] and the organism can usually be isolated by percutaneous CT-guided biopsy,[216] although with a lower success rate as compared to pyogenic infections.[73] Both culture and histology of biopsy specimens have utility in confirming the correct diagnosis. MRI characteristics of Candida spondylitis (akin to aspergillus spondylitis) that are distinct from pyogenic osteomyelitis are the absence of disk hyperintensity and the relative preservation of the intranuclear cleft on T2-weighted images.[217]

Amphotericin B is the standard form of medical therapy, though newer triazole derivatives may be successful with lower rates of toxicity but need to be administered on a continuous basis for prolonged periods.[216] Variations in drug sensitivity must be considered when planning therapy. The ESR can be useful in assessing the response to treatment. As with other forms of infection, surgical debridement, fusion, and instrumentation are required for cases of advanced deformity, neurological compromise, and instability and in cases where there is no response to appropriate antifungal therapy.[215] Overall, between 67% and 85% of patients will respond to treatment with cure of the osteomyelitis.[214, 216] Because of the significance of comorbid conditions, however, mortality rates in Candida spinal osteomyelitis remain high.

Coccidioidomycosis

Coccidioidomycosis is endemic to the southwestern United States, Mexico, and Central and South America. Infection with *Coccidioides immitis* occurs after inhalation of the arthroconidia in the dust in endemic areas. It is usually a benign infection that is asymptomatic or generates mild symptoms referable to the respiratory tract. Extrapulmonary disease occurs in perhaps 5% of all cases of infection, affects the musculoskeletal system and the central nervous system, and is most likely in patients with disordered cell-mediated immunity, as in Hodgkin's disease, uremia, collagen-vascular disorders, AIDS, and patients on immunosuppressant drugs.[222] Epidemiologic observations seem to suggest that Filipino, African-American, and Asian individuals are intrinsically more susceptible to contracting the infection than are Caucasians.[218, 219] Spinal infections usually involve the vertebral body, are destructive, and, like other granulomatous infections, relatively spare the disk.[220, 221] Differention from tuberculosis can be made by the presence of skull lesions, which, although common in coccidioidomycosis, are rare in tuberculosis; the presence of nodular skin lesions is highly suggestive[223]; a serum anticoccidioidal IgG CFA titer above 1:32 indicates a diagnosis of disseminated coccidioidomycosis, particularly if the coccidioidal skin test fails to show delayed-type hypersensitivity.[222] Multifocal spinal involvement while common in this disease is rare in tuberculosis. Treatment is initially medical with intravenous antifungal agents such as amphotericin B. This is usually successful if there is not much paravertebral infection. Operative débridement is often neces-

sary in cases with multilevel disease, significant paravertebral involvement, disease at junctional levels, cases with significant deformity, or those with neurological deficits.

PARASITIC INFECTIONS

Parasitic infections of the spine are rare except in areas where parasitic infestation is endemic and a significant proportion of the population is infected. In these regions, a relatively greater incidence of parasitic involvement of the spine is seen. *Echinococcus granulosus* (hydatid disease), *Schistosoma haematobium, Schistosoma mansoni, Schistosoma japonicum* (bilharziosis), *Taenia solium* (cysticercosis), and *Dracunculus medinensis* (guinea worm infection) have been implicated with some regularity as causes of spinal infection. Of these, echinococcal[224–226] and dracuncular infections[227, 228] occasionally result in truly extra-axial lesions that compress the neural elements. Cysticercosis[229–231] and schistosomiasis[232, 233] of the spine are usually parenchymal diseases of the spinal cord or subarachnoid. Readers interested in further information on these highly unusual infections are referred to the literature cited, most of which reflects the experience in endemic areas.

REFERENCES

1. Lyons AS, Pertucelli RJ: Medicine: An Illustrated History. New York, Harry N. Abrams, 1987.
2. Gerszten PC, Gerszten E, Allison MJ: Diseases of the spine in South American mummies. Neurosurgery 48:208–213, 2001.
3. Sapico FL, Montgomerie JZ: Pyogenic vertebral osteomyelitis: Report of 9 cases and review of the literature. Rev Infect Dis 1:754, 1979.
4. Baker AS, Ojemann RG, Swartz MN, Richardson EP Jr: Spinal epidural abscess. N Engl J Med 293:463, 1975.
5. Darouiche RO, Hamill RJ, Greenberg SB, et al: Bacterial spinal epidural abscess: Review of 43 cases and literature survey. Medicine 71:369–385, 1992.
6. Hadjipavlou AG, Mader J, Necessary JT, Muffoletto AJ: Hematogenous pyogenic spinal infections and their surgical management. Spine 25:1668–1679, 2000.
7. Heusner AP: Nontuberculous spinal epidural infections. N Engl J Med 239:845–847, 1948.
8. Kuker W, Mull M, Mayfrank L, et al: Epidural spinal infection—variability of clinical and magnetic resonance imaging findings. Spine 22:544–551, 1997.
9. Messer HD, Litvinoff J: Pyogenic cervical osteomyelitis. Arch Neurol 33:571–576, 1976.
10. Ring D, Wenger DR: Pyogenic infectious spondylitis in children: The evolution to current thought. Am J Orthop 25:342–348, 1996.
11. Chelsom J, Solberg CO: Vertebral osteomyelitis at a Norwegian university hospital 1987–97: Clinical features, laboratory findings and outcome. Scand J Infect Dis 30:147–151, 1998.
12. Jensen AG, Espersen F, Skinhoj P, et al: Increasing frequency of vertebral osteomyelitis following Staphylococcus aureus bacteraemia in Denmark 1980–1990. J Infect 34:113–118, 1997.
13. Espersen F, Frimodt-Moller N, Thamdrup Rosdahl V, et al: Changing pattern of bone and joint infection due to Staphylococcus aureus: Study of cases of bacteremia in Denmark 1959–1988. Rev Infect Dis 13:347–358, 1991.
14. Hlavin ML, Kaminski HJ, Ross JS, Ganz E: Spinal epidural abscess: A ten-year perspective. Neurosurgery 27:177–184, 1990.
15. Jones NS, Anderson DJ, Stiles PJ: A five year study showing an increase in subacute osteomyelitis. J Bone Joint Surg Br 69:779–783, 1987.
16. Rigamonti D, Liem L, Sampath P, et al: Spinal epidural abscess: Contemporary trends in etiology, evaluation, and management. Surg Neurol 52:189–196, 1999.

17. Digby JM, Kersley JB: Pyogenic non-tuberculous spinal infection: An analysis of thirty cases. J Bone Joint Surg Br 61:47, 1979.
18. Waldvogel FA, Medoff G, Swartz NM: Osteomyelitis: A review of clinical features, therapeutic considerations and unusual aspects. N Engl J Med 282:316–322, 1970.
19. Cahill DW, Love LC, Rechtine GR: Pyogenic osteomyelitis of the spine in the elderly. J Neurosurg 74:878, 1991.
20. Belzunegui J, Intxausti JJ, De Dios JR, et al: Haematogenous vertebral osteomyelitis in the elderly. Clin Rheumatol 19:344–347, 2000.
21. Broner FA, Garland DE, Zigler JE: Spinal infections in the immunocompromised host. Orthop Clin North Am 27:37–46, 1996.
22. Grieve JP, Ashwood N, O'Neill KS, Moore AJ: A retrospective study of surgical and conservative treatment for spinal extradural abscess. Eur Spine J 9:67–71, 2000.
23. Jensen AG, Espersen F, Skinhoj P, Frimodt-Moller N: Bacteremic *Staphylococcus aureus* spondylitis. Arch Intern Med 158:509–517, 1998.
24. Carragee EJ: Pyogenic vertebral osteomyelitis. J Bone Joint Surg Am 79:874–880, 1997.
25. Colmenero JD, Jimenez-Mejias ME, Sanchez-Lora FJ, et al: Pyogenic, tuberculous and brucellar vertebral osteomyelitis: A descriptive and comparative study of 219 cases. Ann Rheum Dis 56:709–715, 1997.
26. Patzakis MJ, Rao S, Wilkins J, et al: Analysis of 61 cases of vertebral osteomyelitis. Clin Orthop 264:178, 1991.
27. Przybylski GJ, Sharan AD: Single-stage autogenous bone grafting and internal fixation in the surgical management of pyogenic discitis and vertebral osteomyelitis. J Neurosurg (Spine) 94:1–7, 2001.
28. Reihsaus E, Waldbaur H, Seeling W: Spinal epidural abscess: A meta-analysis of 915 patients. Neurosurg Rev 23:175–204, 2000.
29. Schuster JM, Avellino AM, Mann FA, et al: Use of structural allografts in spinal osteomyelitis: A review of 47 cases. J Neurosurg 93(1 Suppl):8–14, 2000.
30. Adler MW: ABC of AIDS: Development of an epidemic. BMJ 322:226–229, 2001.
31. Centers for Disease Control and Prevention: Trends in injection drug use among persons entering addiction treatment—New Jersey, 1992–1999. JAMA 285:2706–2707, 2001.
32. Del Curling O Jr, Gower DJ, McWhorter JM: Changing concepts in spinal epidural abscess: A report of 29 cases. Neurosurgery 27:185, 1990.
33. Datta S, Hussain IR, Madden B: Spinal osteomyelitis and diskitis: A rare complication following orthotopic heart transplantation. J Heart Lung Transplant 20:1213–1216, 2001.
34. Obrador GT, Levenson DJ: Spinal epidural abscess in hemodialysis patients: Report of three cases and review of the literature. Am J Kidney Dis 27:75–83, 1996.
35. Hanley EN, Phillips ED: Profiles of patients who get spine infections and the type of infections that have a predilection for the spine. Semin Spine Surg 2:257–267, 1990.
36. Rath SA, Neff U, Schneider O, Richter HP: Neurosurgical management of thoracic and lumbar vertebral osteomyelitis and discitis in adults: A review of 43 consecutive surgically treated patients. Neurosurgery 38: 933–938, 1996.
37. Siroky MB, Movlan RA, Austen G, et al: Metastatic infection secondary to genito-urinary tract sepsis. Am J Med 61:351–360, 1976.
38. Anderson R: Diodrast studies of the vertebral and cranial venous systems to show their possible role in cerebral metastases. J Neurosurg 8:411, 1951.
39. Batson OV: The function of vertebral veins and their role in the spread of metastases. Ann Surg 112:138, 1940.
40. Wiley AM, Trueta J: The vascular anatomy of the spine and its relationship to pyogenic vertebral osteomyelitis. J Bone Joint Surg Br 41:796, 1959.
41. Ratcliffe JF: Anatomic basis for the pathogenesis and radiologic features of vertebral osteomyelitis and its differentiation from childhood discitis. Acta Radiol Diagn 26:137, 1985.
42. Babinchak TJ, Riley DK, Rotheram EB: Pyogenic vertebral osteomyelitis of the posterior elements. Clin Infect Dis 25:221–224, 1997.
43. Griffiths HED, Jones DM: Pyogenic infection of the spine: A review of 28 cases. J Bone Joint Surg Br 53:383, 1971.
44. Kemp HBS, Jackson JW, Jeremiah JD, et al: Anterior fusion of the spine for infective lesions in adults. J Bone Joint Surg Br 55: 715, 1973.

45. Collert S: Osteomyelitis of the spine. Acta Orthop Scand 48: 283, 1977.
46. Eismont FJ, Bohlman HH, Soni PL, et al: Pyogenic and fungal vertebral osteomyelitis with paralysis. J Bone Joint Surg Am 65: 19, 1983.
47. Silverthorn KG, Gillespie WJ: Pyogenic spinal osteomyelitis: A review of 61 cases. N Z Med J 99:62, 1986.
48. Hitchon PW, Osenbach RK, Yuh WTC, et al: Spinal infections. Clin Neurosurg 38:373, 1992.
49. Stone JL, Cybulski GR, Rodroguez J, et al: Anterior cervical débridement and strut grafting for osteomyelitis of the cervical spine. J Neurosurg 70:879–883, 1989.
50. Carragee EJ: Instrumentation of the infected and unstable spine: A review of 17 cases from the thoracic and lumbar spine with pyogenic infections. J Spinal Disord 10:317–324, 1997.
51. Carragee EJ: The clinical use of magnetic resonance imaging in pyogenic vertebral osteomyelitis. Spine 22:780–785, 1997.
52. Khanna RK, Malik GM, Rock JP: Spinal epidural abscess: Evaluation of factors influencing outcome. Neurosurgery 39:958–964, 1996.
53. Malawski SK, Lukawski S: Pyogenic infection of the spine. Clin Orthop Rel Res 272:58–66, 1991.
54. Mampalam TJ, Rosegay H, Andrew BT, et al: Nonoperative treatment of spinal epidural infections. J Neurosurg 71:208, 1989.
55. Waldvogel FA, Vasev H: Osteomyelitis: The past decade. N Engl J Med 303:360–370, 1980.
56. Frederickson B, Yuan H, Olans R: Management and outcome of pyogenic vertebral osteomyelitis. Clin Orthop 131:160, 1978.
57. Koppel BS, Tuchman AJ, Mangiardi JR: Epidural spinal infection in intravenous drug abusers. Arch Neurol 45:1331–1337, 1988.
58. Sapico FL: Microbiology and antimicrobial therapy of spinal infections. Orthop Clin North Am 27:9–13, 1996.
59. Lewis R, Gorbach D, Halpern M: Spinal pseudomonas chondroosteomyelitis in heroin users. N Engl J Med 286:1303, 1973.
60. Brook I: Two cases of diskitis attributable to anaerobic bacteria in children. Pediatrics 107:E26, 2001.
61. Hall BB, Fitzgerald RH, Rosenblatt JE, et al: Anaerobic osteomyelitis. J Bone Joint Surg 65:30–35, 1983.
62. Yin KS, Wang C, Lucero Y: Myelopathy secondary to spinal epidural abscess: Case reports and a review. J Spinal Cord Med 21:348–354, 1998.
63. Lifeso RM: Pyogenic spinal sepsis in adults. Spine 15:1265–1271, 1990.
64. Frisbie JH, Gore RL, Strymish JM, Garshick E: Vertebral osteomyelitis in paraplegia: Incidence, risk factors, clinical picture. J Spinal Cord Med 23(1):15–22, 2000.
65. Carragee EJ, Kim D, van der Vlugt T, Vittum D: The clinical use of erythrocyte sedimentation rate in pyogenic vertebral osteomyelitis. Spine 22:2089–2093, 1997.
66. Garcia A Jr, Grantham SA: Hematogenous pyogenic vertebral osteomyelitis. J Bone Joint Surg Am 42:429, 1960.
67. Crawford AH, Kucharyzk DW, Ruda R, et al: Diskitis in children. Clin Orthop 266:70–79, 1991.
68. Rothman SL: The diagnosis of infections of the spine by modern imaging techniques. Orthop Clin North Am 27:15–31, 1996.
69. Dagirmanjian A, Schils J, McHenry M, Modic MT: MR imaging of vertebral osteomyelitis revisited. AJR Am J Roentgenol 167: 1539–1543, 1996.
70. Chow GH, Gebhard JS, Brown CW: Multifocal metachronous epidural abscesses of the spine: A case report. Spine 21:1094–1097, 1996.
71. Pfister HW, von Rosen F, Yousry T: MRI detection of epidural spinal abscesses at noncontiguous sites. J Neurol 243:315–317, 1996.
72. Nolla-Solé JM, Lourdes MS, Rozadilla-Sacanell A, et al: Role of technetium-99m diphosphonate and gallium-67 citrate bone scanning in the early diagnosis of infectious spondylodiscitis: A comparative study. Ann Rheum Dis 51:665–667, 1992.
73. Chew FS, Kline MJ: Diagnostic yield of CT-guided percutaneous aspiration procedures in suspected spontaneous infectious diskitis. Radiology 218(1):211–214, 2001.
74. Yu WY, Siu C, Wing PC, et al: Percutaneous suction aspiration for osteomyelitis. Spine 16:198–202, 1991.
75. Liebergall M, Chaimsky G, Lowe J, et al: Pyogenic vertebral osteomyelitis with paralysis: Prognosis and treatment. Clin Orthop 269:142, 1991.
76. Bass SN, Ailani RK, Shekar R, Gerblich AA: Pyogenic vertebral osteomyelitis presenting as exudative pleural effusion: A series of five cases. Chest 114:642–647, 1998.

77. Thurnher MM, Post MJD, Jinkins JR: MRI of infections and neoplasms of the spine and spinal cord in 55 patients with AIDS. Neuroradiology 42:551–563, 2000.

78. Modic MT, Steinberg PM, Ross JS: Degenerative disc disease: Assessment of changes in vertebral body marrow with MR imaging. Radiology 166:193–199, 1988.

79. Malghem J, Maldague B, Labaisse M, et al: Intravertebral vacuum cleft: Changes in content after supine positioning. Radiology 187:483–487, 1993.

80. Naul LG, Peet GJ, Maupin WB: Avascular necrosis of the vertebral body: MR imaging. Radiology 172:219–222, 1989.

81. Arnold PM, Baek PN, Bernardi RJ, et al: Surgical management of nontuberculous thoracic and lumbar vertebral osteomyelitis. Surg Neurol 47:551–561, 1997.

82. Young WF, Weaver M: Isolated pyogenic osteomyelitis of the odontoid process. Scand J Infect Dis 31:512–515, 1999.

83. Wiedau-Pazos M, Curio G, Grusser C: Epidural abscess of the cervical spine with osteomyelitis of the odontoid process. Spine 24:133–136, 1999.

84. Benzel EC: The lateral extracavitary approach to the spine using the three-quarter prone position. J Neurosurg 71:837–841, 1989.

85. Larson SJ, Holst RA, Hemmy DC, Sances A Jr: Lateral extracavitary approach to traumatic lesions of the thoracic and lumbar spine. J Neurosurg 45:628–637, 1976.

86. McCormick PC: Surgical management of dumbbell and paraspinal tumors of the thoracic and lumbar spine. Neurosurgery 38:67–74, discussion 74–75, 1996.

87. Fessler RG, Dietze DD Jr, Millan MM, Peace D: Lateral parascapular extrapleural approach to the upper thoracic spine. J Neurosurg 75:349–355, 1991.

88. McCormick PC: Retropleural approach to the thoracic and thoracolumbar spine. Neurosurgery 37:908–914, 1995.

89. Krodel A, Kruger A, Lohscheidt K, et al: Anterior débridement, fusion and extrafocal stabilization in treatment of osteomyelitis of the spine. J Spinal Disord 12:17–26, 1999.

90. Safran O, Rand N, Kaplan L, et al: Sequential or simultaneous, same-day anterior decompression and posterior stabilization in the management of vertebral osteomyelitis of the lumbar spine. Spine 23:1885–1890, 1998.

91. Harrington P, Millner PA, Veale D: Inappropriate medical management of spinal epidural abscess. Ann Rheum Dis 60:218–222, 2001.

92. Bracken MB, Shepard MJ, Collins WF, et al: A randomized, controlled trial of methylprednisolone or naloxone in the treatment of acute spinal-cord injury: Results of the second national acute spinal cord injury study. N Engl J Med 322:1405–1411, 1990.

93. Bracken MB, Shepard MJ, Holford TR, et al: Methylprednisolone or tirilazad mesylate administration after acute spinal cord injury: 1-year follow up. Results of the third national acute spinal cord injury randomized controlled trial. J Neurosurg 89:699–706, 1998.

94. Dietze DD, Fessler RG, Jacob RP: Primary reconstruction for spinal infections. J Neurosurg 86:981–989, 1997.

95. Dandy WE: Abscesses and inflammatory tumors in the spinal epidural space (so called pachymeningitis externa). Arch Surg 13:477–494, 1926.

96. McGee-Collett M, Johnson IH: Spinal epidural abscess: Presentation and treatment. A report of 21 cases. Med J Aust 155:14, 1991.

97. Bair-Merritt MH, Chung C, Collier A: Spinal epidural abscess in a young child. Pediatrics 106:E39, 2000.

98. Leys D, Lesoin F, Viaud C, et al: Decreased morbidity from acute bacterial spinal epidural abscess using computed tomography and nonsurgical treatment in selected patients. Ann Neurol 17:350–355, 1985.

99. McCain GA, Harth M, Bell DA: Septic discitis. J Rheumatol 8:100–109, 1981.

100. Eismont FJ, Wiesel SW, Brighton CT, Rothman RH: Antibiotic penetration into rabbit nucleus pulposus. Spine 12(3):254–256, 1987.

101. Mader JT, Cantrell JS, Calhoun J: Oral ciprofloxacin compared with standard parenteral antibiotic therapy for chronic osteomyelitis in adults. J Bone Joint Surg Am 72:104, 1990.

102. Roberts WA: Pyogenic vertebral osteomyelitis of a lumbar facet joint with associated epidural abscess. A case report with a review of the literature. Spine 13:948–952, 1988.

103. Muffoletto AJ, Nader R, Westmark RM, et al: Hematogenous pyogenic facet joint infection of the subaxial cervical spine. A report of two cases and review of the literature. Neurosurg 95(1 Suppl):135–138, 2001.

104. Mackenzie AR, Laing RB, Smith CC: Spinal epidural abscess: The importance of early diagnosis and treatment. J Neurol Neurosurg Psychiatry 65:209–212, 1998.

105. van Dalen IV, Heeg M: Neonatal infectious spondylitis of the cervical spine presenting with quadriplegia: A case report. Spine 25:1450–1452, 2000.

106. Eismont FJ, Bohlman HH, Soni PL, et al: Vertebral osteomyelitis in infants. J Bone Joint Surg Br 64:32–35, 1982.

107. Lee J, Kim J, Kim S, et al: Anterior cervical spinal epidural abscess in an infant. Childs Nerv Syst 15:137–139, 1999.

108. Rudert M, Tillmann B: Lymph and blood supply of the human intervertebral disc: Cadaver study of correlations to discitis. Acta Orthop Scand 64:37–40, 1993.

109. Alexander CJ: The etiology of juvenile spondyloarthritis (discitis). Clin Radiol 21:178–187, 1970.

110. Brown R, Hussain M, McHugh K, et al: Discitis in young children. J Bone Joint Surg Br 83:1, 106–111, 2001.

111. Ryoppy S, Jaaskelainen J, Rapola J, Alberty A: Nonspecific discitis in children: A non-microbial disease? Clin Orthop 297:95–99, 1993.

112. Fischer EG, Green CS, Winston KR: Spinal epidural abscess in children. Neurosurgery 9:257, 1981.

113. Jansen BRH, Hart W, Schreuder O: Diskitis in childhood: 12–35 year follow up of 35 patients. Acta Orthop Scand 64:33, 1993.

114. Kirkland KB, Briggs JP, Trivette SL, et al: The impact of surgical-site infections in the 1990s: Attributable mortality, excess length of hospitalization, and extra costs. Infect Control Hosp Epidemiol 20:725–730, 1999.

115. Thalgott JS, Cotler HB, Sasso RC, et al: Post-operative infections in spinal implants: Classification and analysis—a multi-center study. Spine 16:981–984, 1991.

116. Theiss SM, Lonstein JE, Winter RB: Wound infections in reconstructive spine surgery. Orthop Clin North Am 27:105–110, 1996.

117. Dietz FR, Koontz FP, Found EM, et al: The importance of positive bacterial cultures of specimens obtained during clean orthopedic procedures. J Bone Joint Surg Am 73:1200–1207, 1991.

118. Levi AD, Dickman CA, Sonntag VK: Management of postoperative infections after spinal instrumentation. J Neurosurg 86:975–980, 1997.

119. Massie JB, Heller JG, Abitbol JJ, et al: Postoperative posterior spinal wound infections. Clin Orthop 284:99–108, 1992.

120. Stambough JL, Beringer D: Postoperative wound infections complicating adult spine surgery. J Spinal Disord 5:277–285, 1992.

121. Fraser RD, Osti OL, Vernon-Roberts B: Iatrogenic discitis: The role of intravenous antibiotics in prevention and treatment. An experimental study. Spine 14:1025–1032, 1989.

122. Mader JT, Cierny G: The principles of the use of preventative antibiotics. Clin Orthop 190:72–75, 1984.

123. Ozuna RM, Delamarter RB: Pyogenic vertebral osteomyelitis and postsurgical disc space infections. Orthop Clin North Am 27:87–94, 1996.

124. Savitz M, Savitz S, Malis L: Ethical issues in the history of prophylactic antibiotic use in neurosurgery. Br J Neurosurg 13:306–311, 1999.

125. Kumar K, Crawford AH: Role of "Bovie" in spinal surgery: Historical and analytical perspective. Spine 27:1000–1006, 2002.

126. Banco SP, Vaccaro AR, Blam O, et al: Spine infections: Variations in incidence during the academic year. Spine 27:962–965, 2002.

127. Rohde V, Meyer B, Schaller C, Hassler WE: Spondylodiscitis after lumbar discectomy: Incidence and a proposal for prophylaxis. Spine 23:615–620, 1999.

128. Zink PM, Frank MA, Trappe AE: Prophylaxis of postoperative lumbar spondylodiscitis. Neurosurg Rev 12:297–303, 1989.

129. Tronnier V, Schneider R, Kunz U, et al: Postoperative spondylodiscitis: Results of a prospective study about aetiology of spondylodiscitis after operation for lumbar disc herniation. Acta Neurochir 117:149–152, 1992.

130. Rhoten RLP, Murphy MA, Kalfas IH, et al: Antibiotic penetration into cervical discs. Neurosurgery 37:418–421, 1995.

131. Luer MS, Hatton J: Appropriateness of antibiotic selection and use in laminectomy amd microdiskectomy. Am J Hosp Pharm 50:667–670, 1993.

132. Dauch WA: Infection of the intervertebral space following conventional and microsurgical operation on the herniated lumbar intervertebral disc: A controlled clinical trial. Acta Neurochir (Wien) 82:43–49, 1986.
133. Horwitz NH, Curtin JA: Prophylactic antibiotics and wound infections following laminectomy for lumber disc herniation. J Neurosurg 43:727–731, 1975.
134. Grane P: The postoperative lumbar spine: A radiological investigation of the lumbar spine after discectomy using MR imaging and CT. Acta Radiol Suppl 414:1–23, 1998.
135. Kristopaitis T, Jensen R, Gujrati M: *Clostridium perfringens*: A rare cause of postoperative spinal surgery meningitis. Surg Neurol 51:448–450, 1999.
136. Puranen J, Makela J, Lahde S: Postoperative intervertebral discitis. Acta Orthop Scand 55:461–465, 1984.
137. Huber A, Kainz C, Witzmann A, et al: Peri-operative elastase-alpha-1 proteinase inhibitor in patients with postoperative intervertebral discitis. Acta Neurochir (Wien) 120:150–154, 1993.
138. Kylanpaa-Back ML, Suominen RA, Salo SA, et al: Postoperative discitis: Outcome and late magnetic resonance image evaluation of ten patients. Ann Chir Gynaecol 88:61–64, 1999.
139. Schultz KP, Assheuer J: Discitis after procedures on the intervertebral disc. Spine 19:1172–1177, 1994.
140. Lonstein J, Winter R, Moe J: Wound infection with Harrington instrumentation and spine fusion for scoliosis. Clin Orthop 96:222–233, 1973.
141. Abbey DM, Turner DM, Warson JS, et al: Treatment of postoperative wound infections following spinal fusion with instrumentation. J Spinal Disord 8:278–283, 1995.
142. Richards BR, Emara KM: Delayed infections after posterior TSRH spinal instrumentation for idiopathic scoliosis: Revisited. Spine 26:1990–1996, 2001.
143. Lu K, Liang C, Cho C, et al: Oxidative stress and heat shock protein response in human paraspinal muscles during retraction. J Neurosurg (Spine 1) 97:75–81, 2002.
144. Kawaguchi Y, Matsui H, Tsuji H: Back muscle injury after posterior lumbar spine surgery. Part 2. Histologic and histochemical analysis in humans. Spine 19:2598–2602, 1994.
145. Garrido E, Rosenwasser RH: Experience with the suction-irrigation technique in the management of spinal epidural infection. Neurosurgery 12:678–679, 1983.
146. Dietze DD, Haid RW: Antibiotic impregnated methylmethacrylate in treatment of infections with spinal instrumentation. Spine 17:981–986, 1992.
147. Kauffman CP, Bono CM, Vessa PP, Swan KG: Postoperative synergistic gangrene after spinal fusion. Spine 25:1729–1732, 2000.
148. Viola RW, King HA, Adler SM, Wilson CB: Delayed infection after elective spinal instrumentation and fusion: A retrospective review of eight cases. Spine 22:2444–2450, 1997.
149. Dubousset J, Shufflebarger H, Wenger D: Late "infection" with CD instrumentation. Orthop Trans 18:121, 1994.
150. Clark CE, Shufflebarger HL: Late developing infection in instrumented idiopathic scoliosis. Spine 24:1909–1912, 1999.
151. Connor PM, Darden BV II: Cervical discography complications and clinical efficacy. Spine 18(14): 2035–2038, 1993.
152. Fraser RD, Osti OL, Vernon-Roberts B: Discitis after discography. J Bone Joint Surg Br 68:26–35, 1987.
153. Guyer RD, Ohnmeiss DD, Mason SL, Shelokov AP: Complications of cervical discography: Findings in a large series. J Spinal Disord 10(2):95–101, 1997.
154. Zeidman SM, Thompson K, Ducker TB: Complications of cervical discography: Analysis of 4400 diagnostic disc injections. Neurosurgery 37(3):414–417, 1995.
155. Junila J, Niinimaki T, Tervonen O: Epidural adscess after lumbar discography: A case report. Spine 22(18):2191–2193, 1997.
156. Guyer RD, Collier R, Stith WJ, et al: Discitis after discography. Spine, 13(12):1352–1354, 1988.
157. Osti OL, Fraser RD, Vernon-Roberts B: Discitis after discography. The role of prophylactic antibiotics. J Bone Joint Surg Br 72(2):271–274, 1990.
158. Sakuragi T, Yasunaka K, Hirata K, et al: The source of epidural infection following epidural analgesia identified by pulsed-field gel electrophoresis. Anesthesiology 89(5): 1254–1256, 1998.
159. Wang Lars P, Hauerberg J, Schmidt JF: Incidence of spinal epidural abscess after epidural analgesia: A national 1-year survey. Anesthesiology 91:1928, 1999.
160. Byers K, Axelrod P, Michael S, Rosen S: Infections complicating tunneled intraspinal catheter systems used to treat chronic pain. Clin Infect Dis 21:403–408. 1995.
161. Du Pen L, Peterson DG, Williams A, Bogosian AJ: Infection during chronic epidural catheterization: Diagnosis and treatment. Anesthesiology 73:905–909, 1990.
162. Sillevis Smitt P, Tsafka A, van den Bent M, et al: Spinal epidural abscess complicating chronic epidural analgesia in 11 cancer patients: Clinical findings and magnetic resonance imaging. J Neurol 246:815–820, 1999.
163. Bulow PM, Biering-Sorensen F: Paraplegia, a severe complication to epidural analgesia. Acta Aneaesthesiol Scand 43:233–235, 1999.
164. Wang LP, Hauerberg J Schmidt JF: Long-term outcome after neurosurgically treated spinal epidural abscess following epidural analgesia. Acta Anaesthesiol Scand 45(2):233–239, 2001.
165. Royakkers AA, Willigers H, van der Ven AJ, et al: Catheter-related epidural abscesses—don't wait for neurological deficits. Acta Anaesthesiol Scand 46(5):611–615, 2002.
166. Aram L, Krane EJ, Kozloski LJ, Yaster M: Tunneled epidural catheters for prolonged analgesia in pediatric patients. Anesth Anal 92(6):1432–1438, 2001.
167. Sato S, Sakuragi T, Dan K: Human skin flora as a potential source of epidural abscess. Anesthesiology 85(6):1276–1282, 1996.
168. Mimoz O, Karim A, Mercat A, et al: Chlorhexidine compared with povidone-iodine as skin preparation before blood culture. A randomized, controlled trial. Ann Intern Med 131(11):834–837, 1999.
169. Pereira LJ, Lee GM, Wade KJ: An evaluation of five protocols for surgical handwashing in relation to skin condition and microbial counts. J Hosp Infect 36(1):49–65, 1997.
170. Peterson AF, Rosenberg A, Alatary SD: Comparative evaluation of surgical scrub preparations. Surg Gynecol Obstet 146(1):63–65, 1978.
171. Chaiyakunapruk N, Veenstra DL, Lipsky BA, Saint S: Chlorhexidine compared with povidone-iodine solution for vascular catheter-site care: A meta-analysis. Ann Intern Med 136(11):792–801, 2002.
172. Goldblum SE, Ulrich JA, Goldman RS, et al: Comparison of 4% chlorhexidine gluconate in a detergent base (Hibiclens) and povidone-iodine (Betadine) for the skin preparation of hemodialysis patients and personnel. Am J Kidney Dis 2(5):548–552, 1983.
173. Maki DG, Ringer M, Alvarado CJ: Prospective randomised trial of povidone-iodine, alcohol, and chlorhexidine for prevention of infection associated with central venous and arterial catheters. Lancet 338(8763):339–343, 1991.
174. Mimoz O, Karim A, Mercat A, et al: Chlorhexidine compared with povidone-iodine as skin preparation before blood culture. A randomized, controlled trial. Ann Intern Med 131(11):834–837, 1999.
175. Kasuda H, Fukuda H, Togashi H, et al: Skin disinfection before epidural catheterization: Comparative study of povidone-iodine versus chlorhexidine ethanol. Dermatology 204(Suppl 1):42–46, 2002.
176. Kinirons B, Mimoz O, Lafendi L, et al: Chlorhexidine versus povidine iodine in preventing colonization of continuous epidural catheters in children: A randomized, controlled trial. Anesthesiology 94(2):239–244, 2001.
177. Amar AP, Larsen DW, Esnaashari N, et al: Percutaneous transpedicular polymethylmethacrylate vertebroplasty for the treatment of spinal compression fractures. Neurosurgery 49(5): 1105–1114; discussion 1114–1115, 2001.
178. Spincemaille GH, Klomp HM, Steyerberg EW, et al: ESES study group. Technical data and complications of spinal cord stimulation: Data from a randomized trial on critical limb ischemia. Stereotact Funct Neurosurg 74(2):63–72, 2000.
179. Saal JA, Saal JS: Intradiscal electrothermal treatment for chronic discogenic low back pain. Prospective outcome study with a minimum 2-year follow-up. Spine 27(9):966–973; discussion 973–974, 2002.
180. Oruckaptan HH, Senmevsim O, Soylemezoglu F, Ozgen T: Cervical actinomycosis causing spinal cord compression and multisegmental root failure: Case report and review of the literature. Neurosurgery 43:937–940, 1998.
181. Yung BC, Cheng JC, Chan TT, et al: Aggressive thoracic actinomycosis complicated by vertebral osteomyelitis and epidural abscess leading to spinal cord compression. Spine 25:745–748, 2000.

182. Voisin L, Vittecoq O, Mejjad O, et al: Spinal abscess and spondylitis due to actinomycosis. Spine 23:487–490, 1998.

183. Houman MH, Ben Ghorbel I, Ben Achour NR, et al: Vertebral actinomycosis with spinal cord compression: A case report. Rev Med Interne 22:567–570, 2001.

184. Eftekhar B, Ketabchi E, Ghodsi M, Ahmadi A: Cervical epidural actinomycosis: Case report. J Neurosurg 95(1 Suppl):132–134, 2001.

185. Graat HC, Van Ooij A, Day GA, McPhee IB: *Nocardia farcinica* spinal osteomyelitis. Spine 27:E253–E257, 2002.

186. Harvey AL, Myslinski J, Ortiz L: A case of *Nocardia* epidural abscess. J Emerg Med 16:579–581, 1998.

187. Laurin JM, Resnik CS, Wheeler D, Needleman BW: Vertebral osteomyelitis caused by *Nocardia asteroides*: Report and review of the literature. J Rheumatol 18:455–458, 1991.

188. Colmenero JD, Reguera JM, Fernandez-Nebro A, Cabrera-Franquelo F: Osteoarticular complications of brucellosis. Ann Rheum Dis 50(1):23–26, 1991.

189. Ariza J, Gudiol F, Valverde F, et al: Brucellar spondylitis: A detailed analysis based on current findings. Rev Infect Dis 7:656–664, 1985.

190. Lifeso RM, Harder E, McCorkell SJ: Spinal brucellosis. J Bone Joint Surg Br 67:345–351, 1985.

191. Tekkok IH, Berker M, Ozcan OE, et al: Brucellosis of the spine. Neurosurgery 33:834–844, 1993.

192. Madkour MM, Sharif HS, Abed MY, Al-Fayez MA: Osteoarticular brucellosis: Results of bone scintigraphy in 140 patients. AJR Am J Roentgenol 150:1101–1105, 1988.

193. Adams JC: Technique, dangers, and safeguards in osteotomy of the spine. J Bone Joint Surg Br 334:225–232, 1952.

194. Chen WJ, Chen CH, Shih CH: Surgical treatment of tuberculosis spondylitis. Acta Orthop Scand 66;137–142. 1995.

195. Griffith DLI: Short-course chemotherapy in the treatment of spinal tuberculosis. J Bone Joint Surg Br 68:158, 1986.

196. Medical Research Council Working Party on Tuberculosis of Spine: A 10-year assessment of controlled trials of inpatient and outpatient treatment and of plaster of Paris jackets for tuberculosis of the spine in children on standard chemotherapy: Studies in Massan and Pusan, Korea. J Bone Joint Surg Br 67:103–110, 1985.

197. Medical Research Counsel Working Party on Tuberculosis of Spine: A controlled trial of ambulant outpatient and inpatient rest in bed in the management of tuberculosis of the spine in young Korean patients on standard chemotherapy. Studies in Massan and Pusan, Korea. J Bone Joint Surg Br 55:678–697, 1973.

198. Moon MS, Ha KY, Sun DH, et al: Pott's paraplegias—67 cases. Clin Orthop 323:122–128, 1996.

199. Moon MS, Yoo YK, Lee KS, et al: Posterior instrumentation and anterior interbody fusion for tuberculosis kyphosis of dorsal and lumbar spine. Spine 20:1910–1916, 1995.

200. Moon MS: Combined posterior instrumentation and anterior interbody fusion for active tuberculosis kyphosis of the thoracolumbar spine. Current Orthopedics 5:177–179, 1991.

201. Pattison PRM: Pott's paraplegia: An account of the treatment of 89 consecutive patients. Paraplegia 24:77–91, 1986.

202. Rajasekaran S, Soundarapandian S: Progression of kyphosis in tuberculosis of the spine treated by anterior arthrodesis. J Bone Joint Surg Am 71:1314–1323, 1989.

203. Upadhyay SS, Saji MJ, Yau CMC: Duration of antituberculous chemotherapy in conjunction with radical surgery in the management of spinal tuberculosis. Spine 21:1898–1903, 1996.

204. Upadhyay SS, Sell P, Saji MJ, et al: Seventeen year prospective study of surgical management of spinal tuberculosis in children: Hong Kong operation compared with debridement surgery for short- and long-term outcome of deformity. Spine 18:1704–1711, 1993.

205. Cortet B, Richard R, Deprez X, et al: Aspergillus spondylodiscitis: Successful conservative treatment in 9 cases. J Rheumatol 21(7):1287–1291, 1994.

206. Vinas FC, King PK, Diaz FG: Spinal aspergillus osteomyelitis. Clin Infect Dis 28(6):1223–1229, 1999.

207. Martinez M, Lee AS, Hellinger WC, Kaplan J: Vertebral Aspergillus osteomyelitis and acute diskitis in patients with chronic obstructive pulmonary disease. Mayo Clin Proc 74(6):579–583, 1999.

208. Govender S, Kumar KP: Aspergillus spondylitis in immunocompetent patients. Int Orthop 25(2): 74–76, 2001.

209. Schubert M, Schar G, Curt A, Dietz V: Aspergillus spondylodiscitis in an immunocompetent paraplegic patient. Spinal Cord 36(11):800–803, 1998.

210. Bridwell KH, Campbell JW, Barenkamp SJ: Surgical treatment of hematogenous vertebral Aspergillus osteomyelitis. Spine 15(4):281–285, 1990.

211. van Ooij A, Beckers JM, Herpers MJ, Walenkamp GH: Surgical treatment of aspergillus spondylodiscitis. Eur Spine J 9(1):75–79, 2000.

212. Hadjipavlou AG, Mader JT, Nauta HJ, et al: Blastomycosis of the lumbar spine: Case report and review of the literature, with emphasis on diagnostic laboratory tools and management. Eur Spine J 7(5):416–421, 1998.

213. Saccente M, Abernathy RS, Pappas PG, et al: Vertebral blastomycosis with paravertebral abscess: Report of eight cases and review of the literature. Clin Infect Dis 26(2):413–418, 1998.

214. Miller DJ, Mejicano GC: Vertebral osteomyelitis due to Candida species: Case report and literature review. Clin Infect Dis 33(4):523–530, 2001.

215. Hendrickx L, Van Wijngaerden E, Samson I, Peetermans WE: Candidal vertebral osteomyelitis: Report of 6 patients, and a review. Clin Infect Dis 32(4):527–533, 2001.

216. Hennequin C, Bouree P, Hiesse C, et al: Spondylodiskitis due to *Candida albicans*: Report of two patients who were successfully treated with fluconazole and review of the literature. Clin Infect Dis 23(1):176–178, 1996.

217. Williams RL, Fukui MB, Meltzer CC, et al: Fungal spinal osteomyelitis in the immunocompromised patient: MR findings in three cases. AJNR Am J Neuroradiol 20(3):381–385, 1999.

218. Pappagianis D, Lindsay S, Beall S, et al: Ethnic background and the clinical course of coccidioidomycosis [letter]. Am Rev Respir Dis 120:959–961, 1979.

219. Williams PL, Sable DL, Mendez P, et al: Symptomatic coccidioidomycosis following a severe natural dust storm. An outbreak at the Naval Air Station, Lenmoore, California. Chest 76:566–570, 1979.

220. Zeppa MA, Laorr A, Greenspan A, et al: Skeletal coccidioidomycosis: Imaging findings in 19 patients. Skeletal Radiol 25:337–343, 1996.

221. Olson EM, Duberg AC, Herron LD, et al: Coccidioidal spondylitis: MR findings in 15 patients. AJR Am J Roentgenol 171(3):785–789, 1998.

222. Wrobel CJ, Chappell ET, Taylor W: Clinical presentation, radiological findings, and treatment results of coccidioidomycosis involving the spine: Report on 23 cases. J Neurosurg 95(1):33–39, 2001.

223. Dalinka MK, Greendyke WH: The spinal manifestations of coccidioidomycosis. J Can Assoc Radiol 22:93–99, 1971.

224. Pamir MN, Ozduman K, Elmaci I: Spinal hydatid disease. Spinal Cord 40:153–160, 2002.

225. Govender TS, Aslam M, Parbhoo A, Corr P: Hydatid disease of the spine: A long-term followup after surgical treatment. Clin Orthop 378:143–147, 2000.

226. Islekel S, Ersahin Y, Zileli M, et al: Spinal hydatid disease. Spinal Cord 36:166–170, 1998.

227. Legmann P, Chiras J, Launay M, et al: Epidural dracunculiasis: A rare cause of spinal cord compression. Neuroradiology 20:43–45, 1980.

228. Dinakar I, Seetharam W, Leelanaidu PS, et al: Spinal compression due to an extradural guinea worm abscess: A case report. Neurol India 25:191–192, 1977.

229. Mohanty A, Das S, Kolluri VR, Das BS: Spinal extradural cysticercosis: A case report. Spinal Cord 36:285–287, 1998.

230. Bandres JC, White AC Jr, Samo T, et al: Extraparenchymal neurocysticercosis: Report of five cases and review of management. Clin Infect Dis 15:799–811, 1992.

231. McDonald JB, Turner PT, Miller AH: Cysticercosis and spinal cord compression [letter]. Ann Neurol 6:367–368, 1979.

232. Pittella JE: The relation between involvement of the central nervous system in schistosomiasis mansoni and the clinical forms of the parasitosis: A review. J Trop Med Hygiene 94:15–21, 1991.

233. Scrimgeour EM, Gajdusek DC: Involvement of the central nervous system in *Schistosoma mansoni* and *S. haematobium* infection: A review. Brain 108:1023–1038, 1985.

Treatment of Disk and Ligamentous Diseases of the Cervical Spine

ROBERT J. JACKSON ■ ZIYA L. GOKASLAN

Degenerative disk and ligamentous diseases of the cervical spine are thought to represent anatomic adaptations to the continuous wear and tear of the involved structures. This process leads to structural changes in the involved joints, with thickening and calcification of the ligaments and appositional bone formation. *Cervical spondylosis* is a commonly used term to describe these degenerative changes and has been defined as "vertebral osteophytosis secondary to degenerative disease."[1] Degenerative disease of the cervical spine is extremely common in adults. Radiographic evidence of cervical spondylosis is present in 25% to 50% of the population by age 50 and increases to 75% to 85% by age 65.[2–4] Successful treatment of degenerative disk and ligamentous disease of the cervical spine requires an understanding of the degenerative process and a careful analysis of the patient's clinical history, physical findings, and imaging studies. Many patients can be treated nonoperatively; however, when surgical treatment is indicated, the procedure should be directed to the particular pathologic condition responsible for the symptoms without producing additional morbidity.

HISTORICAL BACKGROUND

In the early 1900s, the routine surgical approach to the cervical spine was through a midline posterior incision. In 1943, Semmes and Murphy described unilateral rupture of the sixth cervical disk causing compression of the seventh cervical root at the neural foramen.[5] In the 1940s, Spurling and Scoville[6] and Frykholm[7] described the technique of posterior foraminal decompression. In 1955, Robinson and Smith described their operative technique for anterior cervical diskectomy and interbody fusion using a horseshoe-shaped autograft.[8] Three years later, Cloward reported his technique of anterior disk excision, removal of compressive structures, and fusion with a bone dowel.[9] The Cloward

technique emphasized direct visualization and removal of compressive structures, whereas Robinson and Smith[8] thought that offending posterior osteophytes would resorb once fusion had occurred, making their removal unnecessary. In 1960, Bailey and Badgley published their method of onlay strut grafting for cervical stabilization.[10] Numerous modifications have been made in the anterior approach to the cervical spine for the treatment of cervical spondylosis. The introduction of operative magnification allowed better visualization of the neural elements so that compressive structures could be removed safely. There have also been numerous variations in the source and configuration of the interbody graft.[11] Multilevel anterior cervical corpectomy and stabilization with strut grafting and instrumentation have been successfully used to decompress the anterior cervical cord for the treatment of spondylotic myelopathy.[12–18]

Advances in the posterior approach and treatment of cervical spondylosis have been made as well. Cervical laminoplasty was developed by surgeons in Japan after a high incidence of postlaminectomy kyphosis was encountered. Oyama and associates[19] described an expansive Z-shaped laminoplasty that was subsequently modified by Hirabayashi and colleagues[20] to an open-door expansive laminoplasty. Several variations of the cervical laminoplasty were subsequently developed in an effort to maintain spinal stability and to prevent late neurologic deterioration.[21] Others have achieved good results after dorsal decompression followed by posterior fusion with instrumentation.[22, 23] The ability to use anterior and posterior instrumentation now allows spinal surgeons to perform more extensive decompressive procedures safely, which might otherwise carry the risk of instability.

PATHOPHYSIOLOGY

With aging, there is a qualitative and quantitative change in the proteins that compose the nucleus pulposus of the intervertebral disk; in addition, water content in the disk drops from approximately 88% at infancy to approximately 70% at age 72.[24] The disk therefore loses height, the annulus fibrosis begins to bulge, and the facets override each other.[25] This degenerative process may lead to increased motion at that spinal segment, which may further damage the intervertebral disk. In addition, increased stress across the uncovertebral and facet joints leads to capsular thickening and osteophyte formation within these joints. The annulus may weaken and rupture, allowing acute disk herniation. Eventually, the bulging annulus elevates the adjacent periosteum of the vertebral body in the region of Sharpey's fibers. The elevation leads to subperiosteal bone formation, creating an osteophyte or a spondylotic ridge.

As the disk space loses height and the annulus bulges, the cross-sectional area of the spinal canal diminishes. Infolding, thickening, and calcification of the ligamentum flavum, along with hypertrophy of the facet joints, may further diminish the cross-sectional area of the spinal canal. Ossification of the posterior longitudinal ligament also contributes to stenosis of the spinal canal.

Excess segmental spinal motion contributes to the degenerative process and hastens the development of symptomatic cervical spondylosis.[2, 26] This process can be seen in the level adjacent to a fused segment of congenital, degenerative, or surgical origin.[27, 28] Patients with conditions that cause an increase in cervical motion (such as torticollis, athetosis) or those with ligamentous laxity (as seen in Down syndrome) are more severely affected by spondylosis.[29, 30] The osteophytic changes of spondylosis are thought to be a mechanism to increase both the weight-bearing surface of the vertebral body and to limit excessive motion, thereby stabilizing the spine.[31]

CLINICAL PRESENTATION

The common clinical manifestations of degenerative disk and ligamentous diseases of the cervical spine include neck pain, radiculopathy, and myelopathy. These symptoms may occur alone or in combination. The sudden herniation of an intervertebral disk is typically associated with acute symptoms, whereas cervical spondylosis causes a more insidious clinical picture. Less common symptoms include dysphagia secondary to the presence of large anterior osteophytes or vertebrobasilar insufficiency.[32, 33]

Cervical Pain

The neck pain associated with cervical degenerative disease tends to be posterior, located in the paraspinous muscular region. Patients may have associated occipital headaches as well as interscapular pain. This pain is frequently exacerbated by motion and may be due to facet joint disease, disk disease, ligamentous stretching, segmental instability, or a combination of these factors. The posterior annulus, dura, and poste-

rior longitudinal ligament are innervated by the sinuvertebral nerve, which emerges from the primary ventral ramus and gray ramus communicans. The anterior portion of the disk and anterior longitudinal ligament are innervated by branches from the gray ramus.[34] Irritation of any of these structures may result in cervical pain.

Cervical Radiculopathy

Soft disk herniations or the osteophytic changes of spondylosis may cause cervical radicular pain (i.e., pain in the distribution of a nerve root). Regardless of the cause of nerve root compression, the symptoms and signs tend to be similar. In both conditions, neck pain and arm pain in a radicular distribution are the hallmarks of the clinical picture. These symptoms typically develop suddenly in acute cervical disk herniation. Although trauma may precipitate an acute clinical picture, spondylotic radiculopathy usually develops episodically and chronically.

Usually, sensation to pinprick and touch is lost in the appropriate dermatomal distribution. Weakness and decrease or loss of the deep tendon reflex in the corresponding myotome are typical. Although sensory and motor changes most often occur simultaneously, one may be present without the other. Wasting and fasciculations are unusual unless the nerve root compression is chronic. Because spondylosis may involve more than one segment, symptoms may be more diffuse than those associated with an isolated disk herniation.

The C5-6 interspace and the C6-7 interspace are the most commonly degenerated levels in the cervical spine. The cervical nerve roots exit above the correspondingly numbered vertebral body. For example, a disk herniation at the C5-6 level will usually compress the C6 nerve root, causing a C6 radiculopathy. A classic C6 radiculopathy may be characterized by pain along the posterior neck, radiating down the biceps, the lateral aspect of the forearm, and into the dorsum of the hand, thumb, and index fingers. Radicular pain may be exacerbated by simultaneous lateral flexion, slight rotation, and vertex compression (Spurling's sign) and may be diminished with shoulder abduction.[6, 35] Elbow flexor and wrist extensor weakness can often be detected on examination before the patient is aware of this loss of strength. Diminution or loss of the biceps reflex is an objective test that supports the diagnosis of C6 radiculopathy. Sensory changes are variable but usually occur in the dorsum of the hand and over the thumb and index fingers.

Disk degeneration with herniation or spondylosis at the C6-7 interspace may cause a C7 radiculopathy. A C7 radiculopathy can be characterized by pain radiating across the back of the shoulder and neck, across the triceps, and down the posterolateral aspect of the forearm into the middle finger. Pain radiating to the index and ring fingers is not uncommon. The triceps reflex may be diminished or absent, and the elbow extensors, wrist flexors, and finger extensors at the metacarpophalangeal joint may be weakened. Again, sensory loss is variable, but the C7 dermatome includes the middle portion of the hand and the middle finger.

A C8 radiculopathy is characterized by pain radiating down the medial aspect of the forearm to the ring and small finger with associated numbness of the medial forearm, medial ring finger, and small finger and weakness of the hand intrinsic muscles. Radiculopathy in the C5 distribution is less common and is characterized by pain radiating from the side of the neck to the top of the shoulder. Weakness of the deltoid and sensory changes over the region of the deltoid may occur. Radiculopathy of the C3 or C4 root is rare and is associated with pain and numbness in the mastoid region (C3) and posterior neck (C4). There is no readily detectable weakness with compression of these roots.

These patterns of pain, weakness, and sensory changes are classically described and are intended as guidelines for clinicians. Overlapping distributions of nerve roots, anatomic variations, multilevel disease, chronic disease, and comorbidities may significantly complicate the diagnostic picture.

Cervical Myelopathy

Cervical disk disease and spondylosis may be associated with a variety of spinal cord syndromes. Complete spinal cord injury with loss of all motor and sensory modalities below the level of functional transection, although rare, may occur as a result of acute central soft disk herniation or minor cervical trauma in a patient with spondylosis and preexisting canal compromise. Incomplete spinal cord injury and related syndromes occur more frequently, however. These acute syndromes include the central spinal cord syndrome, the Brown-Séquard syndrome, and the anterior cord syndrome.

The central spinal cord syndrome is characterized by a disproportionately greater loss of motor strength in the upper extremities than in the lower extremities with varying degrees of sensory loss.[36] Classically, this pattern of deficits was attributed to a central cord injury that damaged medial arm and hand fibers in the presumed lamination of the corticospinal tract.[37] However, evidence in humans and primates suggests that the hand, arm, and leg fibers in the corticospinal tract are intermingled and that the corticospinal tract is critical for hand function but not for lower extremity function.[38–41] The Brown-Séquard syndrome is characterized by ipsilateral hemiparesis, ipsilateral loss of joint position and vibratory sense, and contralateral loss of pain and temperature sensation.[42] The initial description of anterior cord syndrome was based on two patients with acute spinal cord injuries that resulted in immediate and complete paralysis with some sparing of touch and vibration sense. Both patients reportedly recovered substantially after operative decompression.[43] The preceding syndromes of incomplete acute spinal cord injury may occur with some variation or in combination.

Cervical spondylotic myelopathy (CSM) is defined as spinal cord compromise arising from degenerative changes in the cervical spine. It is the most serious consequence of degenerative disk and ligamentous disease of the cervical spine, and it is the leading cause of spinal cord dysfunction in patients older than 55 years.[44] Although earlier descriptions of CSM reported that the course of neurologic deterioration tended to stabilize, more recent studies report relentlessly progressive neurologic decline, with a few patients experiencing brief periods of stability.[14, 45–47] CSM typically manifests with subtle gait deterioration and clumsiness of the hands.[14] Lower extremity spasticity is thought to have a greater effect on gait than the associated proximal muscular weakness.[14] The gait disturbance is usually insidious and slowly progressive. As spasticity and weakness worsen, gait difficulties become more obvious. The result is a broad-based, stooped, and spastic gait that often progresses until a wheelchair is necessary for locomotion.[48] Sensory loss and weakness contribute to the loss of fine motor skills in the hands. Activities of daily living, such as buttoning a shirt or writing, are often impaired.

A neurologic examination of the patient with CSM characteristically reveals upper extremity and hand weakness, proximal lower extremity weakness, hyperreflexia, and patchy sensory loss. The Babinski upgoing plantar reflex and the Hoffman thumb and finger flexion reflex indicate disruption of normal upper motor neuron inhibition and are frequently elicited in patients with CSM. Approximately 25% of patients with CSM experience a generalized electric shock or paresthesia sensation with voluntary flexion of the neck, which is known as *Lhermitte's sign*.[49]

Bladder, bowel, and sexual dysfunction occur in cases of severe cervical myelopathy. These symptoms were present in 5% to 10% of the patients who presented with CSM in a 1999 study.[14]

DIAGNOSTIC STUDIES

The importance of the clinical history and the neurologic examination in the diagnostic evaluation cannot be overemphasized. The majority of middle-aged and elderly patients will have some degree of degenerative change in their cervical spine on imaging studies, but few will have symptoms of spinal cord or root compression. In two studies, more than 50% of asymptomatic individuals were found to have radiographic evidence of cervical degeneration or cervical protrusion on magnetic resonance imaging (MRI), with frank spinal cord compression in 26%.[50, 51] A careful history and meticulous neurologic examination are essential to correlate imaging abnormalities accurately with the patient's clinical picture.

Plain Radiography

Initial imaging studies should include roentgenographic images with anteroposterior, lateral, and oblique views. An open-mouth view is useful to evaluate the atlantoaxial region. Lateral views are useful to assess disk degeneration, disk space height, osteophytes, spinal canal size, alignment, and the curvature of the cervical spine. Oblique views are useful to assess the neural foramina. Flexion and extension views of the cervical spine are useful to assess the presence of instability. Roentgenographic images are also important in demonstrating other causes of myelopathy such as tumor, infection, trauma, and congenital abnormalities.

Osteophytic intrusions into the spinal canal must be assessed in relation to the size of the canal. A relatively small bone spur may cause significant spinal cord compression in a congenitally narrow canal, whereas a spacious canal can tolerate much larger intrusions. On a standard lateral cervical radiograph, an anteroposterior diameter of 12 mm is considered to be the lower limit of normal for the spinal canal. Any spinal canal less than 12 mm in diameter is said to be congenitally narrow. Because plain radiographic images are often magnified, it is often helpful to measure the ratio of the sagittal diameter of the spinal canal to the anteroposterior width of the vertebral body, with a ratio of less than 0.8 being considered significantly stenotic.[52, 53]

Myelography

Injection of water-soluble contrast material into the subarachnoid space allows visualization of the nerve roots and spinal cord. In assessing spinal cord compression, the lateral view is most helpful. Anteroposterior films are useful for the assessment of cervical root sleeve dye-filling defects, which may represent compression of a nerve root by an osteophyte or vertebral disk. Postmyelography computed tomography (CT) greatly enhances the utility of myelography.

Computed Tomography

With its cross-sectional views, CT provides significantly more information regarding the size and shape of the spinal canal than do plain radiographs. The size and shape of osteophytic ridges are also clearly demonstrated. Although plain CT is an excellent diagnostic tool in assessing bony anatomy, the spinal cord, nerve roots, and other soft tissue abnormalities are not visualized satisfactorily. CT–myelography may be the "gold standard" for imaging cervical spondylosis. It provides an excellent definition of herniated disks and spondylotic ridges and demonstrates their relationship to the nerve roots and the spinal cord.

Magnetic Resonance Imaging

MRI provides a means of examining the cervical spine for disk and spondylotic disease without the use of ionizing radiation or invasive myelography and is the preferred initial screening study for patients who present with cervical myelopathy or radiculopathy. Many surgeons do not consider MRI to be the definitive preoperative imaging modality in patients with cervical spondylosis. Although the details of bony anatomy can be inferred from the MRI study, CT–myelography is still the study of choice in assessing the extent of spondylotic disease. Nevertheless, MRI provides excellent details of the spinal cord, nerve roots, subarachnoid space, and soft tissue abnormalities, such as disk herniation, and is the preferred examination in assessing the presence of an intramedullary process and intra- or extradural neoplastic processes. The quality of MRI continues to improve and, in certain cases, may offer sufficient preoperative information for surgical planning. Preoperatively, MRI and plain CT are frequently used to complement each other to define specific anatomy of the bone and soft tissue structures and their relationship to neural structures.

NONOPERATIVE MANAGEMENT

Although patients with progressive neurologic deficits secondary to nerve root or spinal cord compression typically require surgical intervention, a trial of nonoperative management is usually indicated for patients who have only neck or arm pain. The majority of patients with cervical pain, arm pain, or both, can be effectively managed nonoperatively. Cervical radiculopathy will often respond to conservative management with rest, nonsteroidal anti-inflammatory drugs, physical therapy, and time, whereas CSM tends to be progressive with conservative care.[54–57]

As suggested for the treatment of lumbar radiculopathy, we usually recommend a 2-day course of bed rest along with nonsteroidal anti-inflammatory medications, or a tapering dose pack of corticosteroids after an initial episode or exacerbation of cervical pain, radiculopathy, or both. In the treatment of lumbar radiculopathy, a short course of bed rest has been found to be as effective as a longer course, without the deleterious effects of deconditioning, loss of bone density, and diminished muscular strength.[58–60] A 1-week course with a soft cervical collar may help decrease cervical pain and spasm, despite the collar's inability to limit cervical motion significantly. This improvement may occur through a proprioceptive mechanism or through a local heat trapping effect of the cervical collar on the skin.[61] Immobilization should not be continued indefinitely to prevent the patient from becoming dependent on the brace.[62]

Daily isometric cervical exercises are soon initiated to prevent loss of muscle tone and atrophy in this early period of decreased mobility and pain.[62] This process involves exercising the shoulder and neck muscles against fixed resistance without any accompanying spinal motion. Home cervical traction therapy was retrospectively found to provide relief in 81% of patients with mild to moderately severe symptoms of cervical spondylosis.[63] Aerobic conditioning, flexibility exercises and, finally, progressive resistive exercises of the upper trunk, shoulder girdle, and cervical spine musculature are initiated to strengthen support of the cervical spine. Selective lifestyle modifications, including weight loss, smoking cessation, stress management, postural training, and workplace ergonomic evaluation, may play a role in the treatment of certain patients.

OPERATIVE TREATMENT

Cervical Pain

Disabling cervical pain that is unresponsive to conservative treatment should be considered for surgical treatment. Anatomic correlation between the pain and a defined structural abnormality must be unequivocal in these cases. Surgical fusion should be considered as a last therapeutic means to resolve the painful condition only in patients whose clinical findings correlate with the changes observed radiologically.[64]

It is often difficult to define the source of pain in these patients. Facet joints and intervertebral disks and their surrounding joint capsules, collagenous envelopes, and ligaments may be a source of pain. Pain secondary to cervical instability from degenerative, traumatic, iatrogenic, or neoplastic processes responds well to surgical stabilization.[64–67] Identifying a source of cervical pain in a patient without gross instability may be more difficult. Facet joint pain can sometimes be identified by palpation. Fluoroscopically directed selective facet blocks with local anesthesia and steroid medication may help confirm the diagnosis.[68–70] Dorsal cervical fusion at the symptomatic level should be considered when there are no neurologic symptoms or signs.[71] Alternatively, one may consider percutaneous radiofrequency neurotomy for chronic cervical facet joint pain.[72]

The concept of diskogenic pain and the validity of diskography are more controversial. Patients characteristically complain of axial neck pain and stiffness, often with referred pain to the interscapular region, shoulders, and posterior cervical region, and are without neurologic deficit. This pain may be reproduced by injecting a small amount of fluid into the disk space. Injection of a small amount of local anesthetic should relieve the pain. The pain-producing disk is then removed, and the space is fused. Good to excellent results with regard to pain relief have been achieved in 70% to 93% of patients in selected series.[48, 73–75] Diskometry may help identify patients who have cervical pain and no neurologic deficit (and have failed conservative therapy) who might benefit from surgery. Patients with normal plain radiographs and normal MRI results or those with diffuse multilevel arthritic changes should not undergo diskometry.[76] Surgical intervention for neck pain without neurologic symptoms should be contemplated only after conservative treatment is unsuccessful. In addition, surgical stabilization should be considered only in cases in which the clinical pain pattern is thought to arise from specific radiographic changes of the cervical spine.

Radiculopathy

Surgical intervention is typically indicated for patients with degenerative disease of the cervical spine and radiculopathy who have disabling pain that is refractory to conservative measures, progressive muscular weakness, or sensory impairment. Again, precise correlation between clinical and imaging studies is necessary before successful surgical intervention.

The operative approach must be tailored to the patient's particular anatomy, pathologic condition, and symptoms. When nerve root compression and radiculopathy are due to a posterolateral disk herniation or osteophyte at one or more levels (Fig. 286–1), we usually prefer a posterior approach and a keyhole foraminotomy more than an anterior interbody approach.[6, 8, 9, 77] The foraminotomy has the advantage of sparing the motion segment and associated adjacent level disease, which is important in the spondylotic patient. In selected patients, posterior cervical foraminotomy can be performed safely on an outpatient basis, with good to excellent results in 91% of patients and with minimal complications and recurrences.[27, 77] With a keyhole foraminotomy, which is approximately 1 cm in diameter and centered on the medial third of the facet, postoperative instability is rare.

The posterior foraminotomy is an elegant operation with excellent results and minimal morbidity in selected patients with cervical radiculopathy. A review of eight series that were published between 1953 and 1997, providing a cumulative evaluation of 1364 patients who underwent posterior foraminotomy for radiculopathy, revealed a range of "excellent/good" outcomes in 86% to 100% (mean, 92%) of patients.[6, 57, 77–82] The morbidity rate ranged from 0% to 1.5% (mean, 1%), with only one death reported in all the series combined. The recurrence rate, when reported, ranged from 0% to 6%.

In patients with radiculopathy related to the presence of ventral osteophytes or to a slightly more centrally located herniated disk or in those with evidence of spinal cord compression or mechanically produced

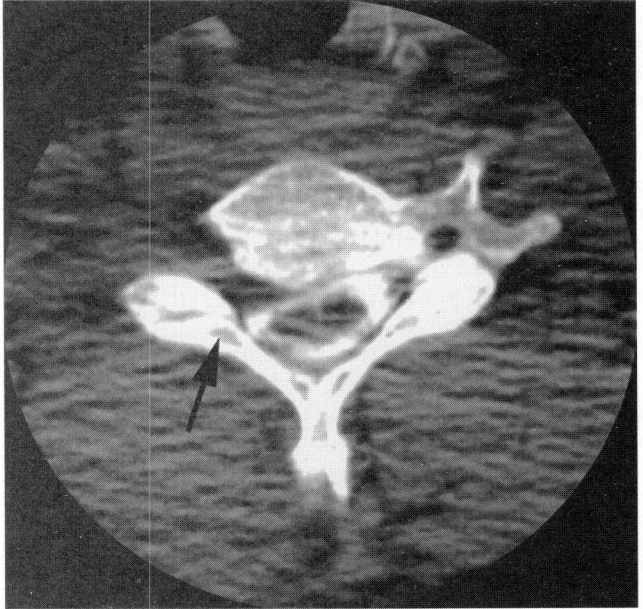

FIGURE 286–1. Postmyelography computed tomographic scan reveals lateral C6-7 disk herniation in a patient with persistent C7 radiculopathy refractory to conservative treatment. This patient's symptoms were relieved after a posterior keyhole foraminotomy was performed and the disk fragment was removed. *Arrow* indicates site of compression and approach to decompression.

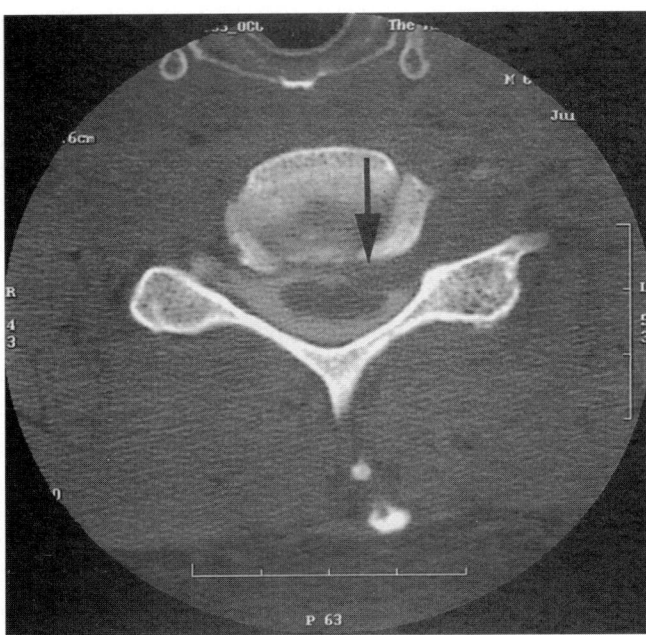

FIGURE 286–2. Postmyelography computed tomographic scan reveals lateral C5-6 paramedian disc herniation in a patient with C6 radiculopathy. This patient's symptoms were relieved after anterior cervical discectomy, foraminotomy, and fusion. *Arrow* indicates site of compression and approach to decompression.

neck pain (Fig. 286–2), we prefer the anterior interbody approach with fusion. This approach allows complete decompression of the neural elements and anterior foraminotomy under direct view, usually with the assistance of the operating microscope. Although excellent results have been achieved without placement of an interbody graft, we prefer to use either allograft fibula or tricortical iliac crest autograft, depending on the patient's and surgeon's preference, to maintain the foraminal opening, to prevent possible kyphosis, and to reduce postoperative pain.[83, 84] Anterior cervical plating is used selectively in patients with single-level disease and is almost always used with multilevel diskectomies or corpectomies. Although others have achieved good results without anterior cervical plating, the addition of anterior cervical instrumentation provides immediate spinal stabilization, limits graft displacement and collapse, increases fusion rates, and minimizes the need for postoperative immobilization.[85–87]

It is difficult to compare results directly among series of anterior cervical diskectomies (with or without fusion) performed for cervical radiculopathy; it is even more difficult to compare these results with those from posterior foraminotomy series. A review of 12 series published between 1989 and 1998 with a cumulative review of 998 patients revealed a range of "excellent/good" outcomes in 49% to 95% (mean, 89%), with a morbidity rate of 3% to 34% (mean, 14%) and only one postoperative death in all the series combined.[50, 83, 88–97] Complications, or the lack thereof, were not reported in certain series. These more recent results appear to be better than historical results. A review of 15 series published between 1962 and 1992 by Whitecloud and

Werner revealed that an "excellent/good" outcome was achieved in 51% to 97% (mean, 76%) of 1782 patients undergoing anterior cervical diskectomy, with or without fusion, for cervical radiculopathy.[98]

The preceding series on the treatment of cervical radiculopathy were mostly retrospective and without third-party independent review. A more recent prospective study with an independent review compared the surgical treatment (51 patients) with the medical treatment (104 patients) of cervical radiculopathy and revealed a 75% "cure" rate with surgery, an 80% patient satisfaction rate with surgery, and a 60% satisfaction rate with medical treatment.[54] Surgical treatment was mixed and included anterior cervical diskectomy with or without fusion, fusion with or without instrumentation, posterior foraminotomy, and even laminectomy.

Potentially serious complications associated particularly with the anterior approach include injury to the carotid artery, vertebral artery, trachea or esophagus, sympathetic chain, and the superior or recurrent laryngeal nerve.[99–106] A delayed postoperative wound hematoma with subsequent compromise of the airway is a potentially fatal complication. Injuries to the spinal cord or nerve roots, which may occur with either the anterior or posterior approach, are potentially devastating complications.

Graft site complications have been reported to occur in as many as 20% of patients.[107] Donor site complications can be eliminated with the use of allograft or biomechanical spacers or by diskectomy without fusion.[11] However, diskectomy without fusion may lead to greater cervical pain in the postoperative period, new radiculopathy on the opposite side of the decompression, or angular deformation.[104] Accelerated spondylosis at the levels adjacent to the fusion can be a problem. Hilibrand and associates[27] found a 2.9% per year rate of symptomatic, adjacent-level disease after anterior cervical arthrodesis. Surprisingly, the rate of symptomatic adjacent-level disease was significantly lower for multilevel anterior arthrodesis. With the anterior approach, there may be a need for postoperative immobilization and greater restriction against participating in contact sports and similar activities while awaiting fusion.

When surgical management is indicated for the treatment of cervical radiculopathy, the procedure should address the particular pathologic condition and symptoms of the individual patient. Both anterior and posterior surgical approaches have specific roles in the management of cervical radiculopathy. Both approaches have been shown to be effective in carefully selected patients. Surgeons should be familiar with the indications, technique, and associated complications of both the anterior and posterior surgical approaches for the management of cervical radiculopathy.

Myelopathy

Surgical decompression is almost always indicated in cases of acute myelopathy due to compressive lesions. Acute cervical myelopathy may occur after a central soft disk herniation or after minor cervical trauma in a patient with spondylosis and preexisting compromise of the spinal canal. Again, precise correlation between the clinical and imaging studies is necessary before surgical intervention. The operative approach must be tailored to a particular patient's anatomy and pathologic condition. In the majority of patients with acute myelopathy secondary to compression from a soft disk or a spondylotic ridge, the lesion is located ventrally; consequently, the surgical procedure of choice is usually an anterior decompression. The anterior approach allows direct visualization and safe removal of the offending lesion. In patients with acute myelopathy secondary to cervical disk herniation, the outcome is related to the duration and severity of neurologic dysfunction before decompression and the level of neurologic function in the first few days after treatment.[108]

Surgical planning and the operative treatment for CSM are significantly more complex than for an acute herniated disk. Successful treatment of CSM requires an understanding of the anatomic, mechanical, and physiologic factors that lead to this progressive disease. The pathophysiology of CSM, which involves a combination of a sagittally narrowed spinal canal, progressive spondylosis with further circumferential narrowing, dynamic mechanical factors that cause additional spinal cord compression with flexion and extension, and progressive ischemic changes, was well described in a review by Fehlings and Skaf.[109] Surgical treatment should address the pathologic condition responsible for the static and dynamic compressive factors without creating additional iatrogenic morbidity. To do so may involve an anterior, posterior, or combined approach depending on the site of compression, the curvature of the cervical spine, and the stability of the spine before and after surgical decompression.

Laminectomy was traditionally the procedure of choice for multilevel spondylosis, but delayed neurologic deterioration and the failure to address certain static and dynamic compressive factors of CSM have led to the popularity of alternative procedures.[44, 110–112] Current strategies in the treatment of CSM include the anterior approaches, corpectomy and strut grafting or multilevel diskectomy and grafting, and the posterior approaches, which include laminectomy with or without fusion and canal-expansive laminoplasty. Several technical variations for each procedure are discussed in detail in subsequent chapters. Additional procedures described for the treatment of CSM include multilevel oblique corpectomies without fusion and the dorsolateral decompressive procedure.[113, 114] The large number and variety of procedures to treat a single disease attest to the complexity and difficulty of treating CSM.

The optimal surgical approach varies among individual patients. Patient age, general medical condition, spinal stability, spinal curvature, and the location and extent of compression are factors that must be considered. The very elderly or debilitated patient may have difficulty tolerating a lengthy and complex procedure and a solid fusion may be less likely to develop in these patients, thus making an anterior procedure or a fusion procedure less desirable. Older patients may also have greater intrinsic spinal stability related to the

spondylotic process, which may decrease the need for fusion after posterior decompression. In those in whom a hypermobile or unstable spine is thought to contribute to the myelopathy, a stabilization and fusion procedure should be considered. Spinal curvature (kyphotic, straight, or lordotic) and location of compression (anterior or posterior) are probably the two most important factors in the decision-making process about the surgical approach.

Batzdorf and Batzdorff[115] and Benzel[116] eloquently described the importance of spinal geometry in guiding the approach for decompression in patients with CSM. The cervical curvature is measured according to the relationship of the dorsal aspects of the C3-7 vertebral bodies to a line drawn from the dorsocaudal aspect of C2 to the dorsocaudal aspect of C7. An "effective" kyphosis has been defined as a configuration of the cervical spine in which any aspect of the dorsal portions of the C3-7 vertebral bodies crosses a line drawn from the dorsocaudal aspect of the C2 vertebral body down to the dorsocaudal aspect of the C7 vertebral body. When no aspect of the C3-7 vertebral bodies crosses this line, the patient is said to have an "effective" cervical lordosis. This line from the dorsocaudal aspect of C2 to the dorsocaudal aspect of C7 is associated with a few millimeters of a gray zone of uncertainty, in which the surgeon's bias and clinical judgment play a role in determining the predominant spinal configuration (Fig. 286–3).

An anterior approach is most effective for removing anterior compressive pathology and is the procedure of choice in the kyphotic spine.[47, 64, 71, 112, 115, 116] Laminectomy in this situation is unlikely to relieve anterior compression adequately and may lead to further kyphosis, compression, and neurologic deterioration.[44, 110–112, 117] Anterior or posterior decompression may be effective in the straightened cervical spine; the surgeon's preference and individual patient factors may influence the choice of approach in these cases. In patients with congenital spinal canal stenosis with minimal anterior spondylosis and in those with lordosis or hyperlordosis, a posterior decompression may be the procedure of choice.[22, 71] Just as a laminectomy may be ineffective in the treatment of compression caused by anterior osteophytes, an anterior procedure may not relieve compression in the hyperlordotic spine.

It is difficult to compare the results from anterior and posterior approaches for the treatment of CSM. Indications for surgery, preoperative condition, patient assessment, and follow-up vary. No prospective randomized trials have compared one approach to the other, and it is unlikely that one will ever be conducted because the indications for each approach differ. Historical results for laminectomy in the treatment of CSM reveal neurologic improvement in 31% to 85% of patients treated, with an average of 64% of patients improving. These findings are clearly better than the natural history of CSM.[18, 21, 44, 46, 49, 114, 117–121] The greatest neurologic improvement after laminectomy has occurred in patients with normal cervical lordosis.[115, 117] Late deterioration after laminectomy may be limited by appropriate patient selection with respect to spinal

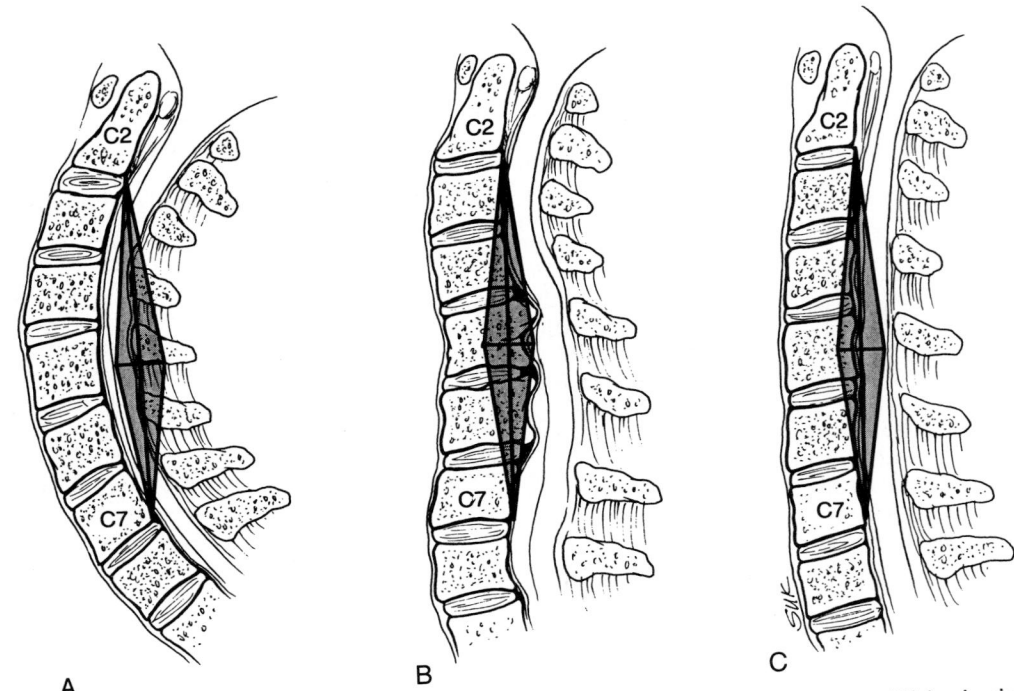

FIGURE 286–3. An illustration of a midsagittal cervical spine with preserved lordosis *(A)*, kyphosis *(B)*, or straightened configuration *(C)*. A line has been drawn from the dorsocaudal portion of the C2 vertebral body to the dorsocaudal aspect of the C7 vertebral body. If any portion of the dorsal aspect of the C3-7 vertebral bodies crosses this line, the cervical spine is said to have an "effective" kyphosis, and an anterior decompressive approach is generally indicated. Conversely, if no portion of the dorsal C3-7 vertebral body crosses this line, the cervical spine is considered to have a lordotic configuration, and a posterior decompressive approach is generally preferred. This imaginary line from C2-7 is associated with a few millimeter "gray zone" (demarcated by the shaded diamond) within which the surgeon's bias and clinical judgment play a role in the determination of the predominant spinal configuration and approach for decompression. (Adapted from Benzel E: Cervical spondylotic myelopathy: Posterior surgical approaches. In Cooper P [ed]: Degenerative Disease of the Cervical Spine. Park Ridge, Ill, American Association of Neurological Surgeons, 1993, pp 91–104.)

stability, spinal curvature, and the location and extent of compression.[44, 110–112] Additional reasons for poor outcome after laminectomy include intraoperative spinal cord trauma, intraoperative hypotension, inappropriate length of decompression (laminectomy of too few segments may cause the spinal cord to kink, whereas laminectomy over too many levels may lead to kyphosis, especially when crossing the cervicothoracic junction), and inappropriate width of the laminectomy (too narrow may not adequately decompress; too wide may destabilize).

Canal-expansive laminoplasty may decompress the cervical spinal cord effectively and may prevent further spinal cord compression by postlaminectomy scarring (Fig. 286–4). Although laminoplasty may reduce the incidence of postoperative cervical kyphosis, neurologic outcome after laminoplasty does not appear to differ from that of laminectomy.[76] Laminoplasty may not fully address the dynamic factors involved in CSM and may be associated with significant postoperative neck and shoulder pain.[22, 114, 122, 123] In cases of preoperative instability or if a particularly wide laminectomy or multiple foraminotomies are performed, surgical fusion should be considered after posterior decompression to prevent progressive instability and kyphosis

(Fig. 286–5). In the adult population, the true incidence of kyphosis after simple posterior decompression remains unclear.[124] Successful stabilization and fusion should eliminate the dynamic compressive factors and prevent abnormal angulation of the spine and subsequent late deterioration. It may also arrest the progression of spondylosis in the fused levels. Some have achieved excellent results with no evidence of late deterioration using laminectomy and posterior fusion for the treatment of CSM, although routine fusion after cervical laminectomy remains controversial.[22, 23]

It is difficult to compare directly the results among series of posterior and anterior decompression in the treatment of CSM because of differences in patient selection, indications, severity of disease, follow-up, and outcome assessment. The amount of neurologic improvement after anterior corpectomy and fusion is variable and has been reported to occur in 47% to 100% of patients.[12–15, 18, 44, 107, 125–127] The most recent studies by well-respected groups have shown significant neurologic improvement in 80% to 87% of patients after anterior corpectomy and fusion, with a complication rate of approximately 20%.[12–14] Complications are similar to those previously described for anterior cervical diskectomy and fusion and are mostly related to the

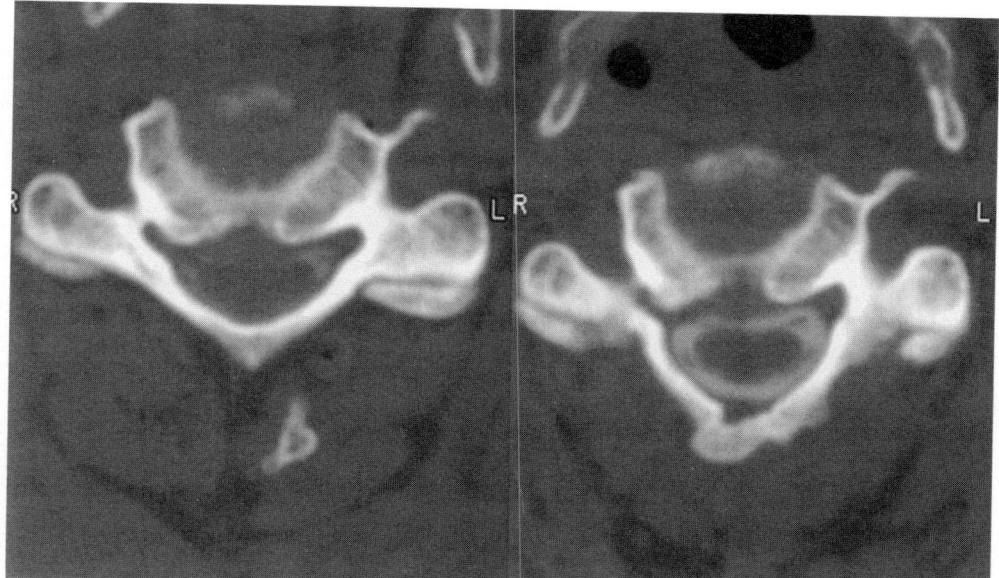

FIGURE 286–4. *Left,* Preoperative postmyelography computed tomographic scan reveals narrowed spinal canal. *Right,* Postmyelography CT 1 year after canal-expansive laminoplasty.

exposure of the spine and the bone graft. Typically, complications are increased with multilevel decompression and grafting relative to a single-level diskectomy and fusion because of the increased exposure needed and the decreased fusion rate seen when attempting to fuse across a greater distance or at multiple levels.

For patients with CSM and "effective" kyphosis or (in certain cases) a straightened spine, we favor anterior decompression and strut grafting with fibular allo-

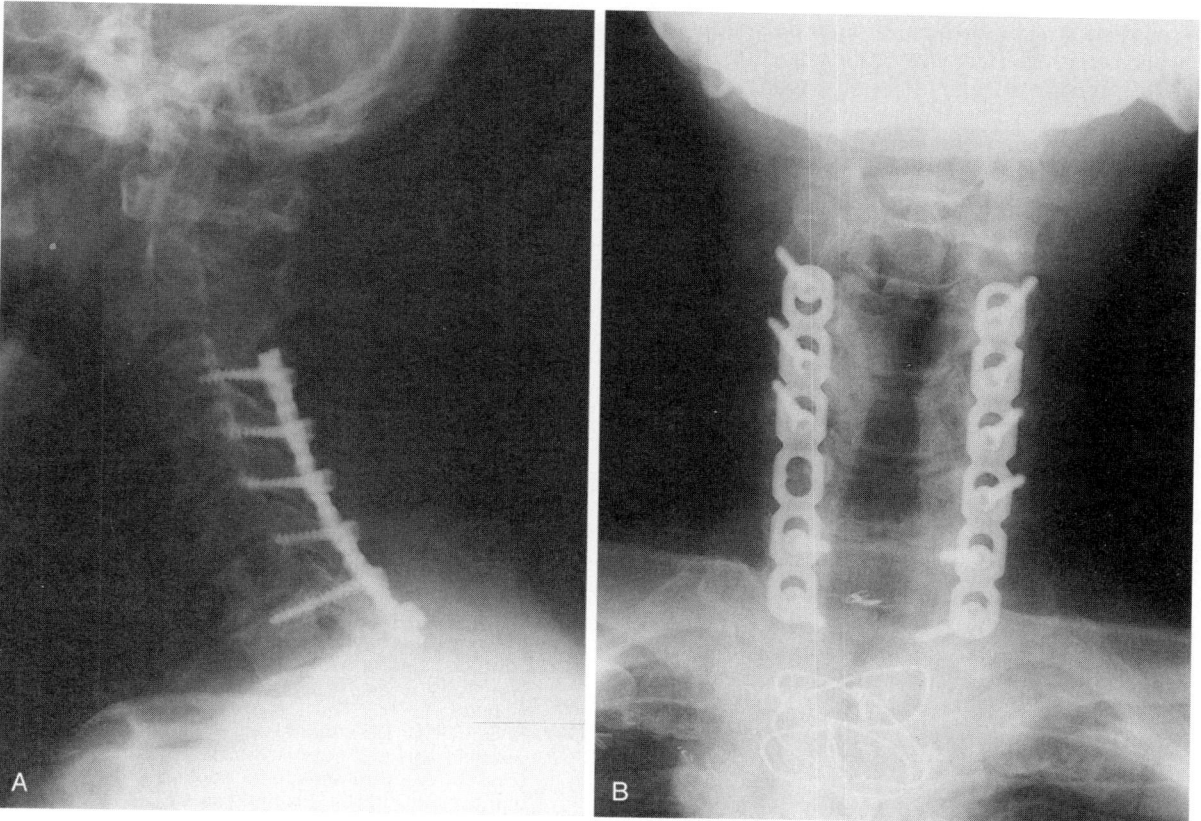

FIGURE 286–5. Lateral *(A)* and anteroposterior *(B)* radiographs demonstrating posterior fusion and bilateral plate fixation in a patient who had a wide laminectomy and multiple foraminotomies.

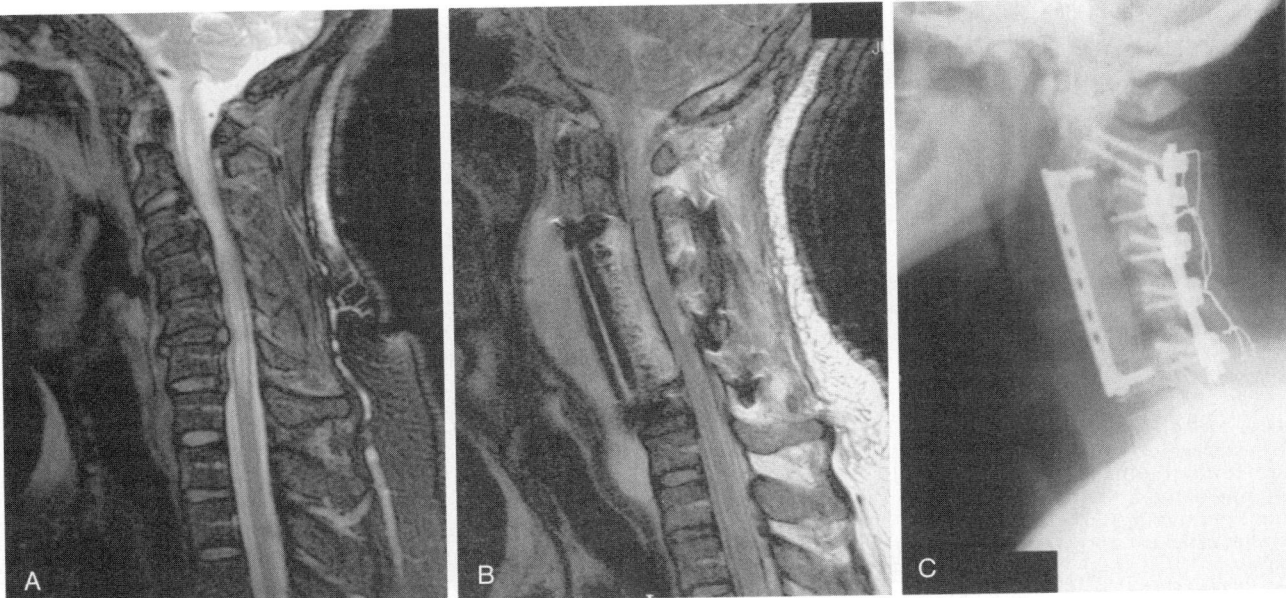

FIGURE 286–6. *A,* Midsagittal magnetic resonance imaging (MRI) reveals multilevel cervical spondylosis, spinal cord compression, and "effective" cervical kyphosis in this patient with progressive cervical myelopathy. *B,* Postoperative midsagittal MRI after multilevel anterior corpectomy, fibular allograft fusion, and anteroposterior stabilization. *C,* Postoperative lateral radiograph demonstrating strut graft and anteroposterior fixation.

graft or autologous iliac crest supplemented by anterior plate instrumentation. Posterior fusion and instrumentation with lateral mass plates, spinous process wiring, or both, are used in selected patients undergoing multilevel corpectomies to increase stability and fusion rates (Fig. 286–6). This strategy may represent overtreatment; three- and four-level anterior corpectomies have been performed with only anterior instrumentation[13] or without instrumentation,[128] although a few of these patients have experienced acute graft failure or required an external halo orthosis. While adding only a slightly increased risk of potential operative morbidity, 360-degree stabilization provides immediate spinal stability and almost a 100% fusion rate, thereby reducing postoperative graft complications, neurologic deterioration, and the need for external halo orthosis.

We prefer cervical laminectomy for those with hyperlordosis or normal lordosis without anterior compression. A posterior fusion and stabilization procedure is performed if instability is suspected either preoperatively (radiographically or in patients with significant axial spinal pain) or after the decompression, such as in multilevel foraminotomies or laminectomy across the cervicothoracic junction. Posterior fusion and instrumentation may also be indicated in cases in which posterior decompression is preferred despite relative straightening of the cervical spine.

CONCLUSIONS

Successful treatment of degenerative disk and ligamentous disease of the cervical spine requires an understanding of the degenerative process and a careful analysis of the patient's clinical history, physical findings, and imaging studies. Many patients can and should be treated nonoperatively; however, when surgical treatment is indicated, the procedure should be directed to the particular pathologic condition responsible for the symptoms without producing additional morbidity. Surgeons must be familiar with the indications and techniques for both the anterior and posterior approaches to the cervical spine for performing both decompression and arthrodesis in order to provide optimal care for the patient suffering from degenerative disk and ligamentous diseases of the cervical spine.

REFERENCES

1. Weinstein P, Ehni G, Wilson C: Lumbar Spondylosis: Diagnosis, Management and Surgical Treatment. Chicago, Year Book Medical, 1977.
2. Adams CB, Logue V: Studies in cervical spondylotic myelopathy. I. Movement of the cervical roots, dura and cord, and their relation to the course of the extrathecal roots. Brain 94: 557–568, 1971.
3. Bohlman HH, Emery SE: The pathophysiology of cervical spondylosis and myelopathy. Spine 13:843–846, 1988.
4. Connell MD, Wiesel SW: Natural history and pathogenesis of cervical disk disease. Orthop Clin N Am 23:369–380, 1992.
5. Semmes R, Murphy F: The syndrome of unilateral rupture of the sixth cervical intervertebral disc. JAMA 121:1209–1214, 1943.
6. Spurling R, Scoville W: Lateral rupture of the cervical intervertebral discs: A common cause of shoulder and arm pain. Surg Gynecol Obstet 78:350–358, 1944.
7. Frykholm R: Deformities of dural pouches and strictures of dural sheaths in the cervical region producing nerve-root compression: A contribution to the etiology and operative treatment of brachial neuralgia. J Neurosurg 4:403–413, 1947.
8. Robinson R, Smith G: Anterolateral cervical disc removal and interbody fusion for cervical disc syndrome. Bull Johns Hopkins Hosp 96:223–224, 1955.

9. Cloward R: Anterior approach for removal of ruptured cervical discs. J Neurosurg 15:602–617, 1958.
10. Bailey RW, Badgley CE: Stabilization of the cervical spine by anterior fusion. J Bone Joint Surg Am 42:565–594, 1960.
11. Whitecloud TS 3rd: Modern alternatives and techniques for one-level discectomy and fusion. Clin Orthop 359:67–76, 1999.
12. Fessler RG, Steck JC, Giovanini MA: Anterior cervical corpectomy for cervical spondylotic myelopathy. Neurosurgery 43:257–657, 1998.
13. Eleraky MA, Llanos C, Sonntag VK: Cervical corpectomy: Report of 185 cases and review of the literature. J Neurosurg 90(1 Suppl):35–41, 1999.
14. Chiles BW 3rd, Leonard MA, Choudhri HF, Cooper PR: Cervical spondylotic myelopathy: Patterns of neurological deficit and recovery after anterior cervical decompression. Neurosurgery 44:762–770, 1999.
15. Saunders RL, Bernini PM, Shirreffs TG Jr, Reeves AG: Central corpectomy for cervical spondylotic myelopathy: A consecutive series with long-term follow-up evaluation. J Neurosurg 74:163–170, 1991.
16. Bernard TN Jr, Whitecloud TS 3rd: Cervical spondylotic myelopathy and myeloradiculopathy: Anterior decompression and stabilization with autogenous fibula strut graft. Clin Orthop 221:149–160, 1987.
17. Hanai K, Fujiyoshi F, Kamei K: Subtotal vertebrectomy and spinal fusion for cervical spondylotic myelopathy. Spine 11:310–315, 1986.
18. Boni M, Cherubino P, Denaro V, Benazzo F: Multiple subtotal somatectomy: Technique and evaluation of a series of 39 cases. Spine 9:358–362, 1984.
19. Oyama M, Hattori S, Moriwaki N: A new method of posterior decompression. Cent Jpn J Orthop Traumatol Surg 16:792–794, 1973.
20. Hirabayashi K, Miyakawa J, Satomi K, et al: Operative results and postoperative progression of ossification among patients with ossification of cervical posterior longitudinal ligament. Spine 6:354–364, 1981.
21. Ducker T, Ziedman S: Cervical radiculopathies and myelopathies: Posterior approaches. In Frymoyer J (ed): The Adult Spine: Principles and Practice, 2nd ed. Philadelphia, Lippincott-Raven, 1997, pp 1381–1400.
22. Kumar VG, Rea GL, Mervis LJ, McGregor JM: Cervical spondylotic myelopathy: Functional and radiographic long-term outcome after laminectomy and posterior fusion. Neurosurgery 44:771–778, 1999.
23. Maurer PK, Ellenbogen RG, Ecklund J, et al: Cervical spondylotic myelopathy: Treatment with posterior decompression and Luque rectangle bone fusion. Neurosurgery 28:680–684, 1991.
24. Keyes D, Compere E: The normal and pathological physiology of the nucleus pulposus of the intervertebral disc: An anatomical, clinical, and experimental study. J Bone Joint Surg 14:897–938, 1932.
25. Dunsker S: Cervical spondylotic myelopathy: Pathogenesis and pathophysiology. In Dunsker S (ed): Cervical Spondylosis. New York, Raven Press, 1981, pp 119–133.
26. Barnes MP, Saunders M: The effect of cervical mobility on the natural history of cervical spondylotic myelopathy. J Neurol Neurosurg Psychiatry 47:17–20, 1984.
27. Hilibrand AS, Carlson GD, Palumbo MA, et al: Radiculopathy and myelopathy at segments adjacent to the site of a previous anterior cervical arthrodesis. J Bone Joint Surg Am 81:519–528, 1999.
28. Ehni G: Cervical Arthosis: Diseases of Cervical Motion Segments. Chicago, Year Book Medical, 1984, pp 197–233.
29. Ebara E, Yamazaki Y, Harada T, et al: Motion analysis of the cervical spine in athetoid cerebral palsy. Spine 15:1097–1103, 1990.
30. Olive PM, Whitecloud TS 3rd, Bennett JT: Lower cervical spondylosis and myelopathy in adults with Down's syndrome. Spine 13:781–784, 1988.
31. Hoff JT, Wilson CB: The pathophysiology of cervical spondylotic radiculopathy and myelopathy. Clin Neurosurg 24:474–487, 1977.
32. Lambert JR, Tepperman PS, Jimenez J, Newman A: Cervical spine disease and dysphagia: Four new cases and a review of the literature. Am J Gastroenterol 76:35–40, 1981.
33. Giroux JC: Vertebral artery compression by cervical osteophytes. Adv Otorhinolaryngol 28:111–117, 1982.
34. Ball P, Benzel E: Pathology of disc degeneration. In Menezes A, Sonntag V (eds): Principles of Spinal Surgery. New York, McGraw-Hill, 1986, pp 507–516.
35. Davidson RI, Dunn EJ, Metzmaker JN: The shoulder abduction test in the diagnosis of radicular pain in cervical extradural compressive monoradiculopathies. Spine 6:441–446, 1981.
36. Schneider R, Cherry G, Patnek H: The syndrome of acute central spinal cord injury. J Neurosurg 11:546–577, 1954.
37. Schneider RC, Crosby EC, Russo RH, Gosch HH: Traumatic spinal cord syndromes and their management. Clin Neurosurg 20:424–492, 1973.
38. Phillips C, Porter R: Cortical Spinal Neurones: Their Role in Movement. London, Academic Press, 1977.
39. Eidelberg E: Consequences of spinal cord lesions upon motor function, with special reference to locomotor activity. Prog Neurobiol 17:185–202, 1981.
40. Nathan P, Smith M: Long descending tracts in man: Review of present knowledge. Brain 78:248–304, 1956.
41. Levi AD, Tator CH, Bunge RP: Clinical syndromes associated with disproportionate weakness of the upper versus the lower extremities after cervical spinal cord injury. Neurosurgery 38:179–185, 1996.
42. Brown-Séquard C: Course of Lectures on the Physiology and Pathology of the Central Nervous System. Philadelphia, Collins, 1860.
43. Schneider RC: A syndrome in acute cervical spine injuries for which early operation is indicated. J Neurosurg 8:360–367, 1951.
44. Ebersold MJ, Pare MC, Quast LM: Surgical treatment for cervical spondylitic myelopathy [see comments]. J Neurosurg 82:745–751, 1995.
45. Brain W, Northfield D, Wilkinson M: Neurological manifestations of cervical spondylosis. Brain 75:187–225, 1952.
46. Nurick S: The natural history and the results of surgical treatment of the spinal cord disorder associated with cervical spondylosis. Brain 95:101–108, 1972.
47. Orr RD, Zdeblick TA: Cervical spondylotic myelopathy: Approaches to surgical treatment. Clin Orthop 359:58–66, 1999.
48. Montgomery DM, Brower RS: Cervical spondylotic myelopathy: Clinical syndrome and natural history. Orthop Clin N Am 23:487–493, 1992.
49. Crandall PH, Batzdorf U: Cervical spondylotic myelopathy. J Neurosurg 25:57–66, 1966.
50. Gore DR, Sepic SB, Gardner GM: Roentgenographic findings of the cervical spine in asymptomatic people. Spine 11:521–524, 1986.
51. Teresi LM, Lufkin RB, Reicher MA, et al: Asymptomatic degenerative disk disease and spondylosis of the cervical spine: MR imaging. Radiology; 164:83–88, 1987.
52. Torg JS, Pavlov H, Genuario S, et al: Neuropraxia of the cervical spinal cord with transient quadriplegia. J Bone Joint Surg Am 68:1354–1370, 1986.
53. Ehni G: Developmental variations, including shallowness of the cervical spinal canal. In Post M (ed): Radiographic Evaluation of the Cervical Spine. New York, Mason, 1980, pp 469–474.
54. Sampath P, Bendebba M, Davis JD, Ducker T: Outcome in patients with cervical radiculopathy: Prospective, multicenter study with independent clinical review. Spine 24:591–597, 1999.
55. Beck D: Cervical spondylosis: Clinical findings and treatment. Contemp Neurosurg 13:1–6, 1991.
56. Persson LC, Carlsson CA, Carlsson JY: Long-lasting cervical radicular pain managed with surgery, physiotherapy, or a cervical collar: A prospective, randomized study. Spine 22:751–758, 1997.
57. Spurling R, Scoville W: Lateral intervertebral disc lesions in the lower cervical region. JAMA 151:354–359, 1953.
58. Deyo RA, Diehl AK, Rosenthal M: How many days of bed rest for acute low back pain? A randomized clinical trial. N Engl J Med 315:1064–1070, 1986.
59. Krolner B, Toft B: Vertebral bone loss: An unheeded side effect of therapeutic bed rest. Clin Sci 64:537–540, 1983.
60. Muller EA: Influence of training and of inactivity on muscle strength. Arch Phys Med Rehabil 51:449–462, 1970.
61. Kurz LT: Nonoperative treatment of degenerative disorders of

the cervical spine. In The Cervical Spine Research Society Editorial Committee (ed): The Cervical Spine, 3rd ed. Philadelphia, Lippincott-Raven, 1998, pp 779–783.

62. Tan JC, Nordin M: Role of physical therapy in the treatment of cervical disk disease. Orthop Clin N Am 23:435–449, 1992.

63. Swezey RL, Swezey AM, Warner K: Efficacy of home cervical traction therapy. Am J Phys Med Rehabil 78:30–32, 1999.

64. Grob D: Surgery in the degenerative cervical spine. Spine 23: 2674–2683, 1998.

65. Herman JM, Sonntag VKH: Cervical corpectomy and plate fixation for postlaminectomy kyphosis. J Neurosurg 80:963–970, 1994.

66. Caspar W, Pitzen T, Papavero L, et al: Anterior cervical plating for the treatment of neoplasms in the cervical vertebrae. J Neurosurg 90(1 Suppl):27–34, 1999.

67. Jackson RJ, Gokaslan ZL: Occipitocervicothoracic fixation for spinal instability in patients with neoplastic processes. J Neurosurg 91(1 Suppl):81–89, 1999.

68. Hove B, Gyldensted C: Cervical analgesic facet joint arthrography. Neuroradiology 32:456–459, 1990.

69. Roy DF, Fleury J, Fontaine SB, Dussault RG: Clinical evaluation of cervical facet joint infiltration. Can Assoc Radiol J 39:118–120, 1988.

70. Ehni G, Benner B: Occipital neuralgia and the C1–C2 arthrosis syndrome. J Neurosurg 61:961–965, 1984.

71. Batzdorf U, Sauders R, Benzel E: Cervical spondylosis. In Benzel E (ed): Spine Surgery: Techniques, Complication Avoidance, and Management. New York, Churchill Livingstone, 1999, pp 411–419.

72. Lord SM, Barnsley L, Wallis BJ, et al: Percutaneous radio-frequency neurotomy for chronic cervical zygapophyseal-joint pain [see comments]. N Engl J Med 335:1721–1726, 1996.

73. Roth DA: Cervical analgesic discography: A new test for the definitive diagnosis of the painful-disk syndrome. JAMA 235: 1713–1714, 1976.

74. Siebenrock KA, Aebi M: Cervical discography in discogenic pain syndrome and its predictive value for cervical fusion. Arch Orthop Trauma Surg 113:199–203, 1994.

75. Whitecloud TS 3rd, Seago RA: Cervical discogenic syndrome: Results of operative intervention in patients with positive discography. Spine 12:313–316, 1987.

76. Zeidman SM, Ducker TB: Evaluation of patients with cervical spine lesions. In The Cervical Spine Research Society Editorial Committee (ed): The Cervical Spine, 3rd ed. Philadelphia, Lippincott-Raven, 1998, pp 143–161.

77. Tomaras CR, Blacklock JB, Parker WD, Harper RL: Outpatient surgical treatment of cervical radiculopathy [see comments]. J Neurosurg 87:41–43, 1997.

78. Henderson CM, Hennessy RG, Shuey HM Jr, Shackelford EG: Posterior-lateral foraminotomy as an exclusive operative technique for cervical radiculopathy: A review of 846 consecutively operated cases. Neurosurgery 13:504–512, 1983.

79. Zeidman SM, Ducker TB: Posterior cervical laminoforaminotomy for radiculopathy: Review of 172 cases. Neurosurgery 33: 356–362, 1993.

80. Epstein JA, Lavine LS, Aronson HA, Epstein BS: Cervical spondylotic radiculopathy: The syndrome of foraminal constriction treated by foraminotomy and the removal of osteophytes. Clin Orthop 40:113–122, 1965.

81. Aldrich F: Posterolateral microdiscectomy for cervical monoradiculopathy caused by posterolateral soft cervical disc sequestration [see comments]. J Neurosurg 72:370–377, 1990.

82. Davis RA: A long-term outcome study of 170 surgically treated patients with compressive cervical radiculopathy. Surg Neurol 46:523–533, 1996.

83. Savolainen S, Rinne J, Hernesniemi J: A prospective randomized study of anterior single-level cervical disc operations with long-term follow-up: Surgical fusion is unnecessary. Neurosurgery 43:51–55, 1998.

84. Sonntag VKH, Klara P: Controversy in spine care: Is fusion necessary after anterior cervical discectomy? Spine 21:1111–1113, 1996.

85. Tippets RH, Apfelbaum RI: Anterior cervical fusion with the Caspar instrumentation system. Neurosurgery 22(6 Pt 1):1008–1013, 1988.

86. Connolly PJ, Esses SI, Kostuik JP: Anterior cervical fusion: Outcome analysis of patients fused with and without anterior cervical plates. J Spinal Disord 9:202–206, 1996.

87. Caspar W, Geisler FH, Pitzen T, Johnson TA: Anterior cervical plate stabilization in one- and two-level degenerative disease: Overtreatment or benefit? J Spinal Disord 11:1–11, 1998.

88. Brodke DS, Zdeblick TA: Modified Smith-Robinson procedure for anterior cervical discectomy and fusion. Spine 17(Suppl): S427–S430, 1992.

89. Tegos S, Rizos K, Papathanasiu A, Kyriakopulos K: Results of anterior discectomy without fusion for treatment of cervical radiculopathy and myelopathy. Eur Spine J 3:62–65, 1994.

90. Gaetani P, Tancioni F, Spanu G, Rodriguez y Baena R: Anterior cervical discectomy: An analysis on clinical long-term results in 153 cases. J Neurosurg Sci 39:211–218, 1995.

91. Pointillart V, Cernier A, Vital JM, Senegas J: Anterior discectomy without interbody fusion for cervical disc herniation. Eur Spine J 4:45–51, 1995.

92. Brigham CD, Tsahakis PJ: Anterior cervical foraminotomy and fusion: Surgical technique and results. Spine 20:766–770, 1995.

93. Bucciero A, Vizioli L, Cerillo A: Soft cervical disc herniation: An analysis of 187 cases. J Neurosurg Sci 42:125–130, 1998.

94. Bohlman HH, Emery SE, Goodfellow DB, Jones PK: Robinson anterior cervical discectomy and arthrodesis for cervical radiculopathy: Long-term follow-up of one hundred and twenty-two patients. J Bone Joint Surg Am 75:1298–1307, 1993.

95. Kozak JA, Hanson GW, Rose JR, et al: Anterior discectomy, microscopic decompression, and fusion: A treatment for cervical spondylotic radiculopathy. J Spinal Disord 2:43–46, 1989.

96. Bhandari M, Louw D, Reddy K: Predictors of return to work after anterior cervical discectomy. J Spinal Disord 12:94–98, 1999.

97. Watters WC 3rd, Levinthal R: Anterior cervical discectomy with and without fusion: Results, complications, and long-term follow-up. Spine 19:2343–2347, 1994.

98. Whitecloud TS 3rd, Werner J: Cervical spondylosis and disc herniation: The anterior approach. In Frymoyer J, (ed): The Adult Spine: Principles and Practice, 2nd ed. Philadelphia, Lippincott-Raven, 1997, pp 1357–1379.

99. Whitecloud TS 3rd: Complications of anterior cervical fusion: Instructional Course Lecture, American Academy of Orthopedic Surgeons, vol 27. St. Louis, CV Mosby, 1978, pp 223–227.

100. Cosgrove GR, Theron J: Vertebral arteriovenous fistula following anterior cervical spine surgery: Report of two cases. J Neurosurg 66:297–299, 1987.

101. Tew JM Jr, Mayfield FH: Complications of surgery of the anterior cervical spine. Clin Neurosurg 23:424–434, 1976.

102. Flynn TB: Neurological complications of anterior cervical interbody fusion. Spine 7:536–539, 1982.

103. Graham JJ: Complications of cervical spine surgery. In The Cervical Spine Research Society Editorial Committee (ed): The Cervical Spine, 2nd ed. Philadelphia, JB Lippincott, 1989, pp 831–837.

104. Bertalanffy H, Eggert HR: Complications of anterior cervical discectomy without fusion in 450 consecutive patients. Acta Neurochir (Wien) 99(1–2):41–50, 1989.

105. Bulger RF, Rejowski JE, Beatty RA: Vocal cord paralysis associated with anterior cervical fusion: Considerations for prevention and treatment. J Neurosurg 62:657–661, 1985.

106. Cloward RB: Complications of anterior cervical disc operation and their treatment. Surgery 69:175–182, 1971.

107. Whitecloud TS 3rd, LaRocca H: Fibular strut graft in reconstructive surgery of the cervical spine. Spine 1:33–43, 1976.

108. Jackson R, Baskin D: Spinal cord injury. In Evans R, Baskin D, Yatsu F (eds): Prognosis of Neurological Disorders, vol 2. New York, Oxford University Press, 2000, pp 381–393.

109. Fehlings MG, Skaf G: A review of the pathophysiology of cervical spondylotic myelopathy with insights for potential novel mechanisms drawn from traumatic spinal cord injury. Spine 23:2730–2737, 1998.

110. Yonenobu K, Okada K, Fuji T, et al: Causes of neurologic deterioration following surgical treatment of cervical myelopathy. Spine; 11:818–823, 1986.

111. Sim FH, Svien HJ, Bickel WH, Janes JM: Swan-neck deformity following extensive cervical laminectomy: A review of twenty-one cases. J Bone Joint Surg Am 56:564–580, 1974.

112. Butler JC, Whitecloud TS 3rd: Postlaminectomy kyphosis: Causes and surgical management. Orthop Clin N Am 23:505–511, 1992.

113. George B, Gauthier N, Lot G: Multisegmental cervical spondylotic myelopathy and radiculopathy treated by multilevel oblique corpectomies without fusion. Neurosurgery 44:81–90, 1999.

114. Hidai Y, Ebara S, Kamimura M, et al: Treatment of cervical compressive myelopathy with a new dorsolateral decompressive procedure. J Neurosurg 90(4 Suppl):178–185, 1999.

115. Batzdorf U, Batzdorff A: Analysis of cervical spine curvature in patients with cervical spondylosis. Neurosurgery 22:827–836, 1988.

116. Benzel E: Cervical spondylotic myelopathy: Posterior surgical approaches. In Cooper P (ed): Degenerative Disease of the Cervical Spine. Park Ridge, Ill, American Association of Neurological Surgeons, 1993, pp 91–104.

117. Naderi S, Ozgen S, Pamir MN, et al: Cervical spondylotic myelopathy: Surgical results and factors affecting prognosis. Neurosurgery 43:43–50 1998.

118. Carol MP, Ducker TB: Cervical spondylitic myelopathies: Surgical treatment. J Spinal Disord 1:59–65, 1988.

119. Epstein JA, Carras R, Lavine LS, Epstein BS: The importance of removing osteophytes as part of the surgical treatment of myeloradiculopathy in cervical spondylosis. J Neurosurg 30:219–226, 1969.

120. Fager CA: Results of adequate posterior decompression in the relief of spondylotic cervical myelopathy. J Neurosurg 38:684–692, 1973.

121. Guidetti B, Fortuna A: Long-term results of surgical treatment of myelopathy due to cervical spondylosis. J Neurosurg 30:714–721, 1969.

122. Matsunaga S, Sakou T, Nakanisi K: Analysis of the cervical spine alignment following laminoplasty and laminectomy. Spinal Cord 37:20–24, 1999.

123. Hosono N, Yonenobu K, Ono K: Neck and shoulder pain after laminoplasty: A noticeable complication [see comments]. Spine 21:1969–1973, 1996.

124. Albert TJ, Vacarro A: Postlaminectomy kyphosis. Spine 23:2738–2745, 1998.

125. Banerji D, Acharya R, Behari S, et al: Corpectomy for multilevel cervical spondylosis and ossification of the posterior longitudinal ligament. Neurosurg Rev 20:25–31, 1997.

126. Macdonald RL, Fehlings MG, Tator CH, et al: Multilevel anterior cervical corpectomy and fibular allograft fusion for cervical myelopathy. J Neurosurg 86:990–997, 1997.

127. Seifert V: Anterior decompressive microsurgery and osteosynthesis for the treatment of multi-segmental cervical spondylosis: Pathophysiological considerations, surgical indication, results and complications: A survey. Acta Neurochir (Wien) 135(3–4):105–121, 1995.

128. Saunders RL, Pikus HJ, Ball P: Four-level cervical corpectomy. Spine 23:2455–2461, 1998.

Posterior Approach to Cervical Degenerative Disease

GREGORY C. WIGGINS ■ CHRISTOPHER I. SHAFFREY

There are many surgical approaches to the management of degenerative disorders of the cervical spine. Deciding which is the best method for a patient requires the surgeon to be aware of the advantages as well as the complications and limitations of each approach. Laminectomy was developed early in the 19th century and initially received little support because the mortality rate was nearly 100%. The first successful laminectomy was performed in 1828, by Alban G. Smith, a little-known surgeon in Danville, Kentucky.[1] The patient's paraplegia improved after Smith performed a three-level laminectomy. Posterior approaches dominated cervical operations until the 1950s, when anterior approaches were developed.

Dorsal exposures have several advantages. They generally require less surgical effort in exposing multiple levels, and they frequently do not require stabilization, fusion, or instrumentation as part of the procedure. The procedure does not necessitate stiffening the spine and therefore does not accelerate spondylotic degeneration at adjacent levels. The nerve roots are decompressed under direct visualization, and there is little risk to major vessels, the esophagus, or recurrent laryngeal nerve. Posterior surgical approaches to the cervical spine are familiar and have been established as safe and efficacious.[2–9] Some disadvantages of posterior techniques include postoperative neck pain, the potential for spinal instability, and an inability to access ventral canal osteophytes, which may be the major cause of neurological deficits. Conceptually, posterior cervical approaches are simple and straightforward operations that offer direct thecal sac and nerve root decompression. The complications are predictable and usually can be avoided with attention to detail and proper patient selection.

Because spinal deformities can occur as a result of inappropriate patient selection or inadequate attention to anatomic detail, it is imperative to determine which patients are going to most benefit from a posterior cervical approach compared with an anterior decompression. A range of posterior surgical procedures exists, including laminectomy, laminoplasty, and posterior spinal instrumentation with or without laminectomy. The most important factors in patient selection for a particular procedure are the clinical signs and symptoms and the radiographic alignment of the spine. To treat the patient optimally, the surgeon must consider the location of the pathology, the type of pathology, the patient's general condition, and the static and dynamic sagittal spine balance. Appropriate patient selection maximizes the chance of optimal neurological outcomes and minimizes complications. In this chapter, we look at posterior cervical approaches for radiculopathy (i.e., laminoforaminotomy), myelopathy and myeloradiculopathy (i.e., laminectomy or laminoplasty), and posterior stabilization techniques that may be necessary after a posterior decompression.

PATHOLOGY OF DEGENERATIVE CERVICAL DISEASE

The essential feature of degenerative cervical disk disease is desiccation of the disk material. The dehydration and fragmentation of the nuclear material of the disk is a natural process. With aging, some of the vertical height provided by the disk is lost as the disk loses elasticity. With disk degeneration, the articular cartilage and vertebral end plates are subjected to greater stress. Osteophytic spurs develop at the margins of the end plates and project into the spinal canal posteriorly and into the prevertebral space anteriorly. The facet joints are subjected to the development of osteophytic spurs that impinge on the posterolateral spinal canal and neural foramen. These osteophytic spurs attempt to stabilize the adjacent vertebrae by increasing the area of the weight-bearing surface of the vertebral end plates and facets. The ligamentum flavum also becomes inelastic with age. With disk degeneration, the ligamentum flavum is required to perform more of a stabilizing role. It therefore hypertrophies and can lead to significant canal compromise, especially in extension. The changes in the disk, facets, and ligamentum flavum can lead to significant spinal canal compromise, neural compression, and myelopathy.

Disk degeneration along with the formation of annular fissures is the central feature leading to the sequestered disk syndrome. Acute hyperflexion or rotation, or both, can precede rupture of a disk. The annulus and often the posterior longitudinal ligament tear and allow the nucleus material to herniate into the spinal canal. There, the nuclear material can compress the spinal cord, causing myelopathy, or compress the adjacent roots as they exit into the neural foramen, which can lead to radiculopathy. Most often, acute disk rupture occurs laterally in the spinal canal because of the relative deficiency of the posterior longitudinal ligament in this location.

CLINICAL EVALUATION

The most important aspect of preoperative planning is the clinical evaluation of the patient, which includes a history, physical examination, and radiographic evaluation. The clinical syndrome caused by degenerative cervical disease depends on the location of neural compression in addition to the overall size of the spinal canal.

Soft disk herniations frequently are found laterally in the spinal canal. Consequently, the nucleus herniation causes root compression and radiculopathy more often than cord compression and myelopathy. The lower cervical segments (C4-7) are usually involved. Patients present with classic radicular arm and neck pain. Turning and extending the neck can reproduce the radicular pain, and elevating the affected arm above the head may relieve the pain.[10–12] Weakness in the myotome with loss of the corresponding stretch reflex is typical. Paresthesias may accompany the pain in the appropriate dermatome. Atrophy and fasciculations are unusual.

A central disk herniation into the spinal canal causes variable amounts of compression on the spinal cord, depending on the degree of preexisting spinal canal stenosis. Relatively mild spinal trauma can cause the development of a variety of spinal cord syndromes. Most commonly, patients present with signs and symptoms of myelopathy, but incomplete spinal cord syndromes such as central cord syndrome, the Brown-Sequard syndrome, and anterior spinal artery syndrome can occur.

Cervical spondylosis usually does not manifest with an acute disk herniation, but rather as a slow, insidious nerve root or cord compression with resultant radiculopathy or myelopathy. Although trauma may occasionally precipitate radiculopathy, spondylotic radiculopathy usually develops episodically and chronically. Because spondylosis may affect more than one cervical segment, symptoms may be more diffuse than those seen with a unilateral soft disk herniation.

Cervical spondylotic myelopathy (CSM) is slowly progressive with episodes of acute decline. A complete history is useful to rule out other causes of spinal cord dysfunction such as amyotrophic lateral sclerosis, cerebrovascular disease, demyelinating disease, intracranial lesions, hydrocephalus, syringomyelia, tabes dorsalis, myopathy, peripheral neuropathy, and metabolic or alcoholic encephalopathy.[13] Patients with CSM have neck pain, difficulty walking, and unsteadiness on their feet. Pain, numbness, paresthesias, weakness, and loss of dexterity of the upper extremities are common findings. Patients also may have radicular symptoms. Bowel or bladder dysfunction is unusual and should prompt further workup in search of another cause. Patients with CSM may have coexisting lumbar stenosis.[14]

Patients with CSM have upper motoneuron findings that can occur in the lower extremities and lower motoneuron findings that can occur in the upper extremities at the level of the compressive lesion. Upper motoneuron findings may be present in the upper extremities caudal to the lesion; the deep tendon reflexes may be hyperactive in the upper and lower extremities. Patients may have myelopathy indicated by the Hoffmann reflex, the inverted radial reflex[15] (i.e., spontaneous flexion of the digits with the brachioradialis reflex), the Lhermitte sign, or clonus. The inverted radial reflex is virtually pathognomonic of CSM.[15] The Babinski sign usually is not present until late in the disease. Sensory examination may reveal changes to light touch, but changes in position sense and vibratory sense are more specific. Dysdiadochokinesia is one of the earliest findings in CSM. Patients may also have a myelopathic gait, characterized by circumduction, scissoring, and decreased stride length.

RADIOGRAPHIC ANATOMY AND BIODYNAMICS

In choosing the best operation for a patient with cervical disease, it is necessary to identify the major sites of pathology and coexistent spinal stenosis or spinal instability. Generally, patients undergoing evaluation for cervical spondylosis should have anteroposterior and lateral cervical spine radiographs. If there is a suspicion that instability exists, lateral flexion and extension radiographs should be performed.

A developmentally narrow spinal canal can be ruled out if the anteroposterior spinal canal diameter is 13 mm or more on a standard lateral cervical radiograph.[16] This definition is based on studies that documented the anteroposterior dimensions of the normal spinal canal from C3 to C7 to be 16 to 18 mm.[17] Patients with CSM had an average canal diameter of 11.8 mm; patients with canal diameters of less than 10 mm are more likely to have myelopathy.[18–23] These absolute measurements can be affected by the radiographic technique. The Pavlov ratio,[24] which is anteroposterior diameter of the spinal canal divided by the anteroposterior diameter of the vertebral body at the same level (Fig. 287–1), is not affected by radiographic technique or magnification and therefore is a better guide to diagnosing cervical canal stenosis. A ratio of 1.0 is normal; a ratio less than 0.8 indicates a developmentally narrow canal.

The lateral radiograph shows the overall sagittal balance. Figure 287–2 illustrates the importance of sagittal balance in determining the optimal approach for

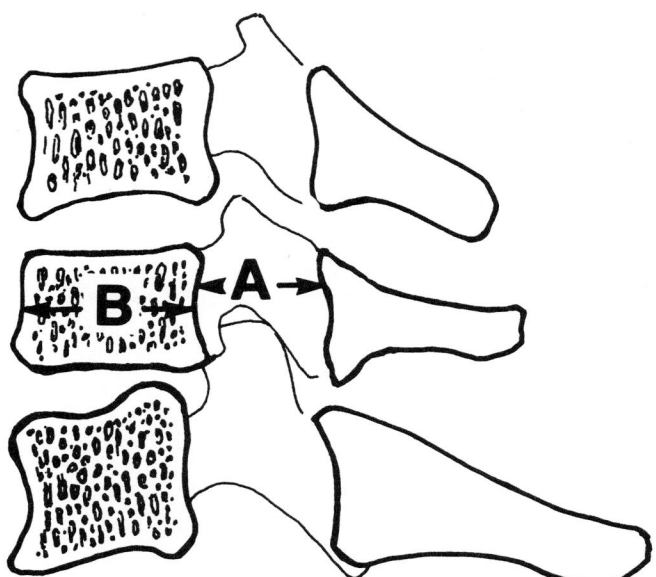

FIGURE 287–1. The Pavlov ratio is the anteroposterior diameter of the spinal canal *(A)* divided by the anteroposterior diameter of the vertebral body at the same level *(B),* as measured on a lateral radiograph. It is normally about 1.0. A ratio of less than 0.8 indicates a developmentally narrow cervical spinal canal. (From Wiggins GC, Shaffrey CI: Laminectomy in the cervical spine: Indications, surgical techniques, and avoidance of complications. Contemp Neurosurg 21:2, 1999.)

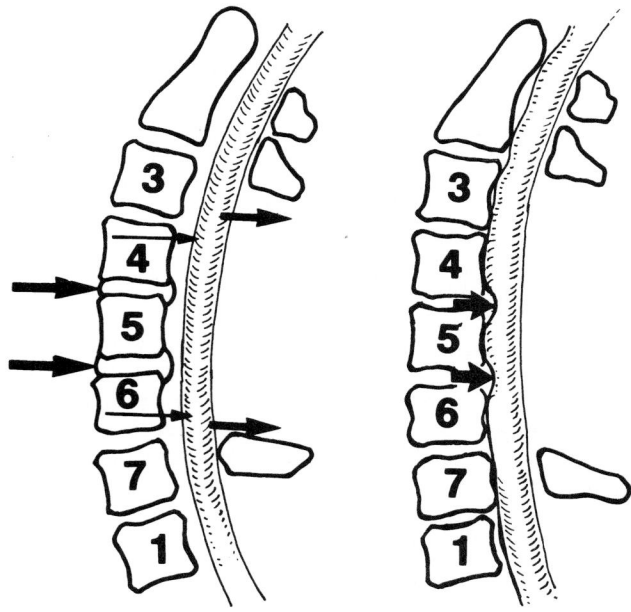

FIGURE 287–2. *Left,* Normal lordotic curve of the cervical vertebral column permits posterior migration of the spinal cord after laminectomy. *Right,* Cervical vertebral column with loss of normal lordotic curvature prevents reduction of anterior spinal cord compression by laminectomy. (From Wiggins GC, Shaffrey CI: Laminectomy in the cervical spine: Indications, surgical techniques, and avoidance of complications. Contemp Neurosurg 21: 2, 1999.)

treating cervical pathology. Cervical spinal cord decompression after laminectomy cannot be obtained in patients with reversal of lordosis of the cervical spine, because the spinal cord is draped over anterior pathology despite a satisfactory posterior decompression. Preservation of lordosis is needed to allow adequate room for the spinal cord to migrate dorsally off any ventral compression. The cervical spine usually has 14.4 degrees of lordosis from C2 to C7.[25] If the patient has a straight or kyphotic cervical spine, an anterior approach or a laminectomy combined with posterior segmental instrumentation is needed because of the risk of postoperative kyphosis, especially in children. If instability is present even in the lordotic cervical spine, posterior instrumentation and arthrodesis at the time of cervical laminectomy should be considered.

Neurodiagnostic studies must include the entire cervical spine to avoid missing a significant pathology at other levels. Magnetic resonance imaging (MRI) is excellent for evaluating the soft tissues of the cervical spine and specifically for assessing the intrinsic spinal cord pathology.[26–28] Figure 287–3 provides the preoperative and postoperative magnetic resonance images of a 71-year-old patient after laminectomy that reveals the extent of canal decompression and maintenance of cervical lordosis. The T2-weighted, gradient-echo image may reveal increased signal, indicating injury to the spinal cord. Dynamic (e.g., flexion, extension) MRI may reveal compression of the spinal cord with motion that was not evident on the static imaging.

The compression ratio (Fig. 287–4) is a useful measurement that can be made on axial MRI or on postmyelographic axial computed tomography (CT).[29] The compression ratio is measured by dividing the smallest anteroposterior dimension of the spinal cord (i.e., sagittal diameter) by the broadest transverse diameter at the same level. A compression ratio of 0.4, especially after decompression, is associated with a poor recovery.[29] Conversely, a compression ratio of more than 0.4 or greater than 40 mm² in the transverse area of the spinal cord correlates with improved clinical recovery.[25, 30] Measurement of the transverse area of the spinal cord at the affected level has been the most accurate predictor of neurological recovery.

Some patients have the clinical picture of CSM but do not show severe compression on neuroimaging. These patients may have intermittent compression that is revealed only by dynamic imaging studies. Brieg and colleagues[31] and Reed[8] studied the effects of flexion and extension maneuvers in cadaver specimens. In flexion, although the canal enlarges, axial tension on the spinal cord narrows the anteroposterior diameter. This deforms the lateral columns and anterior horns and simultaneously compromises circulation. Hyperextension narrows the spinal canal and improves the perfusion of the cord as axial tension is released. However, the spinal cord thickens and reduces the space available. It is important to maintain neutral alignment while positioning a patient.

Dynamic MRI can reveal compression of the spinal cord by the ligamentum flavum and dynamic annular bulging.[8, 32, 33] This repetitive compression may cause

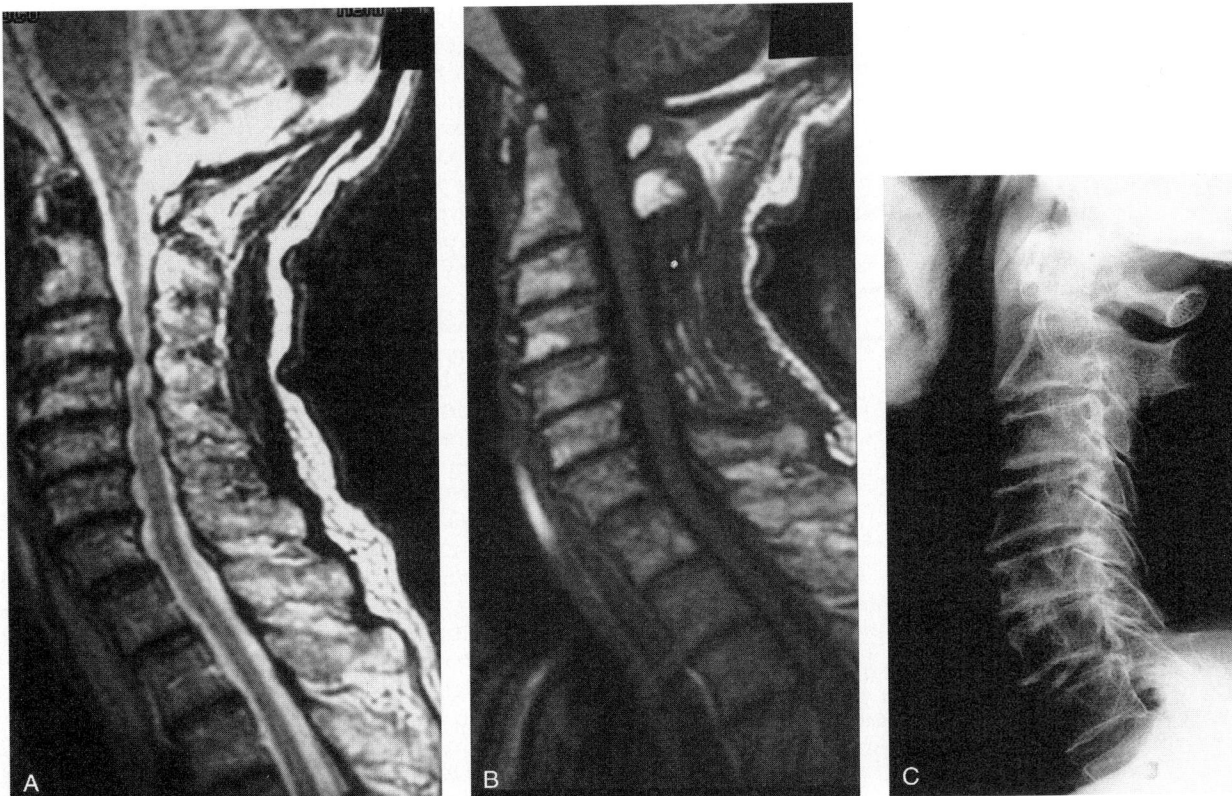

FIGURE 287–3. *A,* Sagittal, preoperative magnetic resonance imaging (MRI) of a 71-year-old patient with progressive myelopathy. *B,* Postoperative MRI of the same patient. *C,* Postoperative cervical spine radiograph demonstrates maintenance of cervical lordosis. (From Wiggins GC, Shaffrey CI: Laminectomy in the cervical spine: Indications, surgical techniques, and avoidance of complications. Contemp Neurosurg 21:3, 1999.)

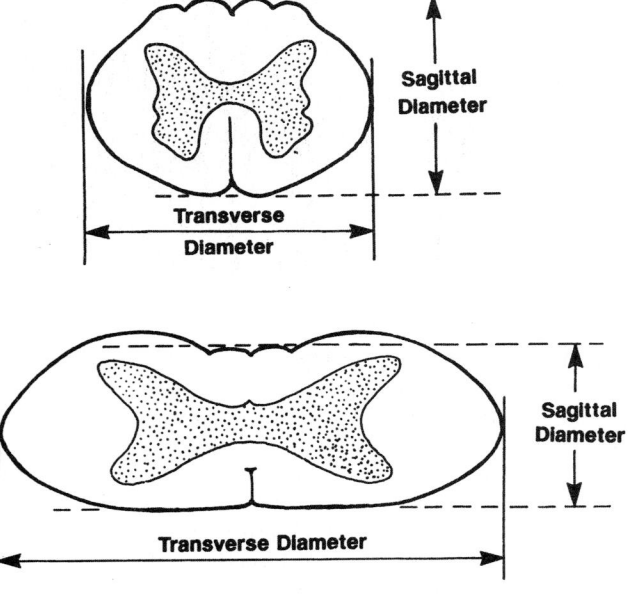

FIGURE 287–4. The compression ratio is the smallest antero-posterior diameter (i.e., sagittal diameter) of the spinal cord divided by the broadest transverse diameter at the same level. (From Wiggins GC, Shaffrey CI: Laminectomy in the cervical spine: Indications, surgical techniques, and avoidance of complications. Contemp Neurosurg 21:3, 1999.)

microtrauma to the spinal cord and result in a slow evolution of symptoms and signs. Myelography and postmyelographic CT are excellent modalities for showing dynamic compression and bony compression or ossification of the posterior longitudinal ligament.

TREATMENT OF CERVICAL SPONDYLOTIC MYELOPATHY

Cervical radiculopathy, even when severe, frequently improves without operative intervention. In some patients, pain may persist, despite a variety of nonoperative treatments. In other patients the pain regresses, but the motor deficit can worsen, indicating continued nerve damage. Lees and Turner[34] reported a long-term study of 95 patients in which 44 with cervical radiculopathy were followed for 3 to 40 years. Most of their patients had bouts of increased symptoms followed by quiescent periods or periods of mild improvement. Repeated episodes generally left the patient worse than before.

Therapy for cervical radiculopathy includes rest, cervical traction, and nonsteroidal anti-inflammatory drugs (NSAIDs). NSAIDs are effective for acute radiculopathy, but chronic use can lead to gastric irritation or renal dysfunction in some patients. Generally, conservative therapy should be continued as long as the patient is improving.

Many factors are important in the timing of surgery for radiculopathy. Significant and profound motor weakness is an indication for a more urgent operation. If the problem is a progressive neurological deficit, it requires a rapid radiologic evaluation to make an accurate diagnosis. If the development of symptoms and neurological deficits is more chronic, several examinations spaced over different office visits can allow the surgeon to attain a full appreciation of the disease. It is important that the radiologic studies correlate with the clinical examination to achieve the best surgical results. Comorbidities such as diabetes mellitus can influence the diagnosis and outcome in the treatment of cervical radiculopathy.

Profound neurological deficits resulting from untreated radiculopathy are rare. The primary goal of surgical treatment is to improve the patient's quality of life. Patients who need operative care generally fall into two categories: younger patients with a soft herniated disk and older patients with osteophytic nerve root compression (i.e., hard disk), and the specific procedure selected should take into consideration the anticipated pathology.[10, 11, 35, 36]

Nonoperative Therapy

Understanding the natural history of CSM is important in selecting patients for surgery. Although the natural history of CSM has been investigated, it is difficult to accurately predict the clinical course for a single patient. In 1956, Clark and Robinson[37] published a review of 120 patients with CSM in which they commented that spontaneous regression was clinically observed in two patients, but no patient ever returned to a normal state. They found that 75% of their patients had recurring episodes and 66% had new symptoms of myelopathy and neurological deterioration. Of their 120 patients, 5% had rapid onset of symptoms followed by a long period of neurological plateau. Other studies have reported clinical improvement rates as high as 36% to 50% for patients managed with nonoperative treatments.[4, 34] This statistic must be compared with improvement rates of 68% to 95% and cure rates of 33% reported for surgically treated patients.[4, 21, 38] The prognosis for the recovery of spinal cord function postoperatively is variable and depends on the duration and severity of symptoms. The best results have been obtained for patients who were decompressed within 6 months to 1 year after onset of symptoms; those who had early, mild myelopathy[30, 39]; and those in whom the transverse area of the spinal cord increased to more than 40 mm² postoperatively.[29, 30]

Conservative therapy is indicated for patients who have mild neurological complaints without ongoing progression of symptoms and for patients with advanced CSM and fixed deficits whose advanced age and medical comorbidity pose a significant risk for operative intervention. Nonoperative therapy includes temporary cervical immobilization with a firm orthosis, the use of NSAIDs, physical therapy, and cervical trac-

tion. Patients can perform cervical traction at home three times each day for about 15 minutes each time. Care should be taken not to extend the neck while in cervical traction, because this can lead to neurological decline.[40] Manipulation of the neck is discouraged because extension of the neck leads to narrowing of the spinal canal.[8, 18, 32, 33, 41] Patients who are poor surgical candidates may benefit from an epidural steroid injection to help control symptoms.[42]

Indications for Surgical Treatment

The primary consideration in selecting patients for surgical therapy is the extent to which a patient's symptoms affect his or her lifestyle and the surgeon's confidence that the symptoms are caused by cervical compression. Failures of operative therapy may result from poor patient selection or poor operation selection for the patient.

Surgery for CSM is almost always performed on an elective basis. A variety of factors affect the timing of surgical intervention. Indications for more expedient intervention include progressive muscle weakness due to a coexisting radiculopathy, severe disabling sensory impairment, and significant spinal cord compression causing myelopathy. Relative indications for operative intervention on a less urgent basis include pain, weakness, or sensory deficit that is not disabling but can cause unacceptable lifestyle changes because of a need for medication or restriction of activities.

Absolute contraindications to surgery are rare. There are few situations in which appropriate decompressive surgery cannot be undertaken, especially when spinal cord compression is the issue. There are some relative contraindications, including advanced age with osteoporosis, severe pulmonary disease making it difficult to wean a patient from mechanical ventilation, and severe cardiac disease. Surgery can be performed in all but the sickest patients if attention is paid to minimizing blood loss and operative time, maintaining blood pressure to prevent cardiac and spinal cord ischemia, and in some cases, keeping patients intubated until they no longer need large doses of narcotics for pain control. Generally, multilevel posterior decompressions can be performed more rapidly and with less morbidity than multilevel anterior procedures; however, multilevel posterior laminectomies are contraindicated in patients with cervical kyphosis because of a high rate of surgical failure due to persistent anterior compression or progression of the kyphosis (Fig. 287–5). Similarly, patients with preoperative instability or anterior column incompetence should not undergo isolated posterior cervical decompression because of the risk of kyphosis. Some patients with focal, flexible kyphosis or limited instability can undergo laminectomy with the use of posterior instrumentation such as lateral mass plates to help maintain or create some lordosis. Table 287–1 gives some indications for selecting laminectomy in treating a patient with cervical spine pathology. It is important to select the operation that best addresses the pathology and maximizes the chance of

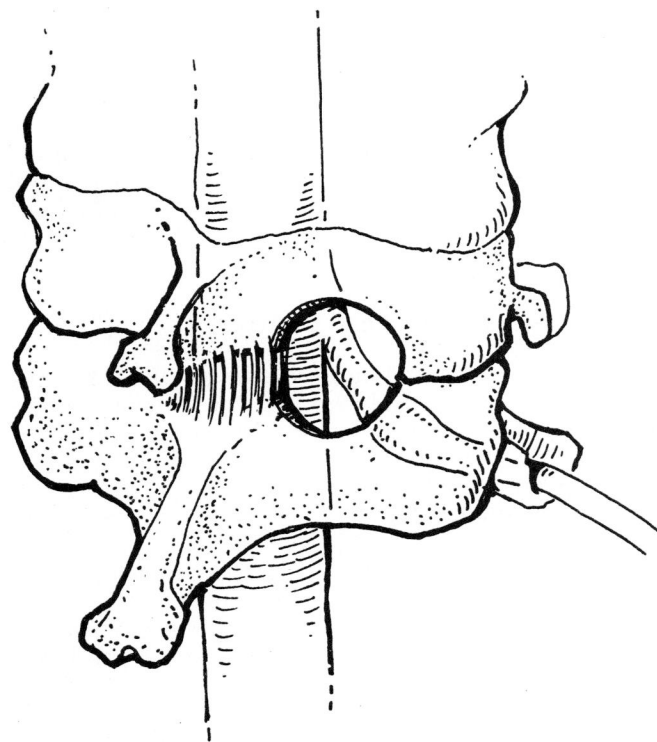

FIGURE 287–5. Operative exposure for laminoforaminotomy. A high-speed drill is used to create a small laminotomy. The drawing shows the relationship of the nerve root to the bony opening.

patient improvement but at the same time minimizes morbidity.

Preoperative Evaluation

Before an elective operation is performed, the patient's medical status must be thoroughly evaluated. Any cardiac risk factors must be identified and medical therapy optimized. Some patients require stress testing and

TABLE 287–1 ■ **Indications for Cervical Laminectomy**

Single or multilevel disease
Congenital stenosis—developmental changes
To access intradural pathology (extramedullar and intramedullar)
Difficulty in performing anterior procedure
   Failure of previous surgery
   Mechanical difficulties: obesity, short neck, barrel chest, difficulty positioning
Operative factors (decreasing risk)
   Less operative time and anesthesia
   Better tolerated than anterior approach by elderly patients
   Limited blood loss; rarely requires transfusion
   Superior visualization of nerve roots
Combined supplementary procedure in anterior and posterior approach
Need to perform posterior instrumentation
Tracheostomy: open procedure
Extensive anterior cervical soft tissue pathology preventing anterior approach

cardiac revascularization before surgical treatment of cervical myelopathy. All NSAIDs should be discontinued an adequate time before surgery. Aspirin derivatives should be stopped 1 week before surgery and ibuprofen 3 days before surgery to prevent platelet dysfunction. The patient's prothrombin time, partial thromboplastin time, routine electrolyte levels, and complete blood cell count should be checked preoperatively.

Anesthesia and Positioning

In most instances, general anesthesia is preferred to local or regional anesthesia. General anesthesia facilitates positioning, airway control, and hemodynamic monitoring. Neuromuscular junction blocking agents can be used during induction of general anesthesia. After positioning and initial dissection, the neuromuscular junction blockade can be reversed, especially if cervical foraminotomies are anticipated. This allows detection of excessive nerve root manipulation or trauma to be viewed as arm movement.

Fiberoptic intubation with the patient awake is advisable to avoid passive extension of the neck and the resultant neural compression. A urinary catheter and pneumatic compression stockings are placed, and the patient is given antibiotics before the incision is made. We use 1 g of cefazolin or vancomycin if the patient is allergic to penicillin. Although controversial, in cases of significant spinal cord compression, we administer 1 g of methylprednisolone, which theoretically protects the spinal cord from intraoperative insult such as hypotension or mechanical trauma, or both. When positioning the patient, care is taken to ensure all bony prominences are padded to prevent pressure on the ulnar or peroneal nerves.

Positioning the cervical spine of the patient is critical in preventing worsening neurological deficit. The neck must be kept in neutral alignment. The prone position is preferred for most dorsal approaches to the spine. In the prone position, the patient's head is most predictably held with three-point fixation, avoiding pressure on the face or eyes. Some surgeons advocate the sitting position despite its risks, which include the potential for postural hypotension and air embolism.[43, 44] Although significant morbidity associated with the sitting position is uncommon, air has been detected entering the venous system in nearly 7% of cervical laminectomies performed with the patient in the sitting position.[35] If the sitting position is selected despite these drawbacks, monitoring includes precordial Doppler ultrasonography, an end-tidal CO_2 monitor, a central venous catheter placed in the right atrium, and an arterial line. If air embolism occurs, the wound must be packed with wet sponges, and venous bleeding sites must be sequentially identified and coagulated, with the anesthesiologist applying jugular compression to increase venous backflow. Rarely is it necessary to bring the patient's head down and turn the table left side down to lock the air in the right atrium. Because of these potential complications with the sitting position, we use the prone position almost exclusively.

Electrical monitoring for somatosensory evoked potentials and nerve root function (i.e., electromyography) may be considered in cases that involve extensive surgery, long operative times, use of segmental instrumentation, tumor removal, or significant risk of neurological injury due to positioning. Epstein[45] reported 270 cervical spine procedures, including posterior and anterior approaches, between 1989 and 1994. This series had no operative cord injuries, and there were only seven nerve root injuries. Despite these results and because of the extremely low likelihood of nerve root or spinal cord injury with cervical decompression, it is doubtful whether such monitoring is cost effective for routine posterior cervical decompressions.

Laminoforaminotomy

Spurling and Scoville[12] in 1944 and Frykholm[46] in 1947 described the technique of posterolateral decompression of the cervical nerve root as it enters the neural foramen. This procedure is designed to decompress the nerve root and has little effect if there is spinal cord compression or canal stenosis. This technique is used for the relief of cervical radiculopathy due to disk herniation or osteophyte encroachment. The medial portion of the cervical facet can be approached from a midline or paramedian muscle-splitting approach. The simpler midline approach is more common. In cases of soft disk herniation without spinal stenosis or spinal cord compression, flexion of the cervical spine during positioning reduces the bony removal required to provide exposure.

After the patient is positioned and monitored appropriately, the skin is prepared and the patient draped. The incision infiltrated with 0.25% Marcaine with a 1:100,000 solution of epinephrine to help with hemostasis and postoperative pain. The level is localized with an intraoperative lateral radiograph. A vertical midline incision is made to expose only the dorsal elements that need to be addressed during the surgical procedure. Electrocautery is used to incise the ligamentum nuchae only on the affected side, followed by subperiosteal dissection and retraction of the paracervical muscles, with care taken to preserve the facet capsules. Unnecessary dissection can increase postoperative discomfort and cause facet joint damage, unnecessary postoperative scarring, and soft tissue injury that can result in additional morbidity. The paracervical muscles are then held with self-retaining retractors, which are released every 20 minutes to allow adequate perfusion, avoiding necrosis of the muscles and denervation.

Advocates of the alternative muscle-splitting approach claim that it produces less postoperative pain.[47] A skin incision is made diagonally to the spinous process, parallel to the fibers of the trapezius muscle. The trapezius is split longitudinally along its fibers, which exposes the fascia of the serratus posterior. This fascia is divided, exposing the fibers of the splenius capitis that run perpendicular to the fibers of the trapezius. These fibers are split longitudinally, exposing the multifidi and semispinatus muscles. These muscles are subperiosteally dissected off the lamina and facet, gain-

ing exposure similar to that using the midline approach. With improvement in instrumentation for minimally invasive spinal surgery techniques, muscle-sparing paramedian approaches will probably gain popularity in the near future.

After the exposure is completed, the remainder of the procedure is performed with loupe or microscope magnification. The keyhole laminoforaminotomy is then performed. A curet is used to identify the edge of the superior lamina and the articular process. A high-speed air drill is used for bone removal. Dissection begins on the superior lamina at the junction with the articular process and carried out superiorly about 5 mm and then medially about 5 mm. A similar amount of bone is removed from the inferior lamina, starting at the junction of the lamina and the articular facet and progressing medially and inferiorly (Fig. 287-5). The ligamentum flavum lies medially, and a plexus of veins and connective tissue covers the nerve root sleeve laterally. The ligamentum flavum is sharply divided and removed. A nerve hook is then used to identify the medial edge of the superior and inferior pedicles. The inferior pedicle marks the axilla of the nerve and the principal location of a sequestered disk or osteophyte compressing the nerve root. Bone removal is then carried laterally over the nerve root sleeve into the facet. No more than 50% of the facet complex should be removed.

Epidural bleeding can be troubling during the medial facetectomy. Hemostasis is obtained with thrombin-soaked Gelfoam. After decompression is completed, a nerve hook is used to identify the medial edge of the venous plexus. This is coagulated along

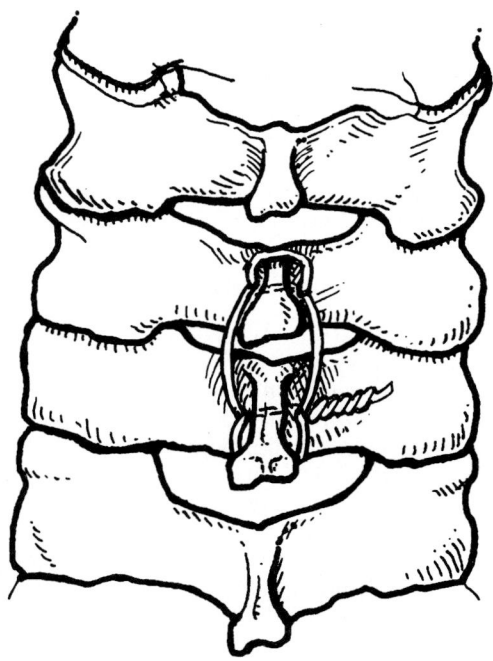

FIGURE 287-6. Triple wire technique. A single wire is passed through the superior spinous process and then wrapped around the superior spinous process and back through the spinous process. This process is repeated with the inferior spinous process, and the free ends of the wire are tightened.

the course of the nerve root with bipolar cautery at a low setting to prevent thermal injury to the nerve root. The coagulated plexus is sharply transected along the axis of the nerve root, fully exposing the nerve root. At this point, the nerve root should be completely freed dorsally. Any remaining tissue on top of the root should be sharply divided.

The nerve root is explored with a blunt nerve hook. The nerve root axilla is the most critical location to explore, because this is the common location for sequestered disk material or osteophytes. Care is taken to not mistake a separate motor nerve root sleeve for a sequestered disk. It may be necessary to incise the annulus fibrosis near the axilla to allow extrusion of disk material retained by the ligament. This process can be encouraged by applying gentle pressure with the nerve hook on the annulus fibrosis. Free disk material is removed with a rongeur. To avoid injuring anterior structures, the disk space should not be entered too deeply. If an osteophyte is identified, removal is optional, because the nerve root has been dorsally decompressed. If desired, the osteophyte can be removed with a diamond-bit drill. Next, a nerve hook or Woodson elevator is used to assess the adequacy of the lateral nerve root decompression.

Hemostasis of epidural bleeding is obtained with Gelfoam soaked in thrombin. The wound is copiously irrigated with antibiotic solution. The muscles and fascia are closed with Vicryl suture. The subcutaneous layer is closed with 2–0 Vicryl suture and the subcuticular layer with 3–0 Vicryl suture. The skin is reapproximated with staples to prevent postoperative wound dehiscence.

Prophylactic antibiotics are continued for the first 24 hours. The patient is transferred to the regular unit, and early ambulation is encouraged. Rehabilitation therapy is started early to encourage strengthening of the cervical musculature and to maintain cervical lordosis. Because stability has not been compromised, an orthosis is unnecessary. However, the patient sometimes benefits from a soft collar for comfort. The patient is usually discharged in 24 to 48 hours.

Laminoforaminotomy with Posterior Spinal Fusion

Posterior spinal instrumentation and fusion should be considered when preexisting instability exists, a complete facetectomy is performed, bilateral facetectomies (>50%) are performed, significant anterior column deficiency is present, or when revising failed anterior procedures. In approximately 5% of anterior cervical diskectomies, a nonunion occurs, and 2% to 3% of these patients develop painful radiculopathy.[48] Some of these patients require a second operation to address the radiculopathy caused by the disk space collapse and nonunion. Posterior cervical laminoforaminotomy with stabilization can decompress the cervical roots, and the fusion performed can help relieve pain.[48] After successful posterior fusion, the previous anterior pseudarthrosis usually goes on to solid arthrodesis.

The posterior fusion can be performed using the

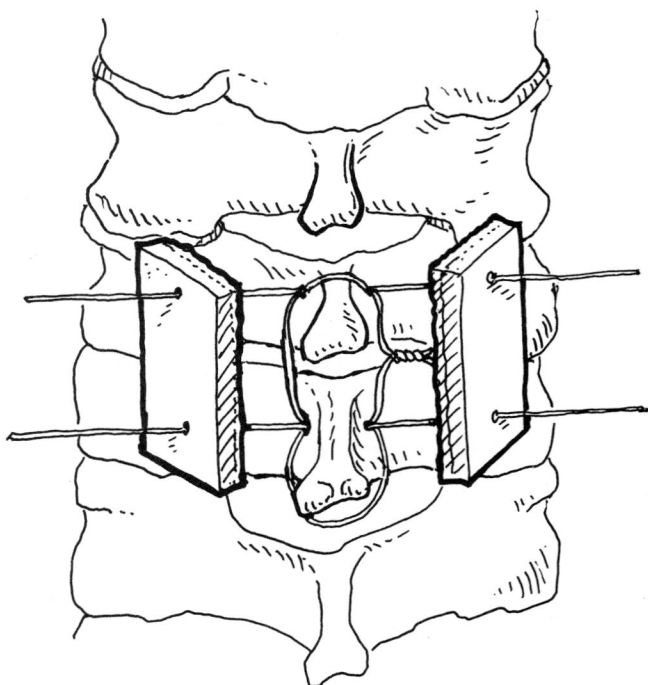

FIGURE 287–7. The triple wire technique is completed by taking separate wires through the spinous process and through the bone graft on each side. The free ends of the wires are tightened, bringing the bone in contact with the previously decorticated lamina.

standard triple wire technique (Fig. 287–6). A single wire is placed through the spinous process of the superior vertebra and wrapped above and below it. The wire is then passed beneath the inferior vertebral spinous process and secured to itself. Separate wires are passed through holes at the base of each spinous process and then through a hole in the iliac crest bone graft. The wires are then tightened, placing the bone grafts under compression against the lamina and base of the spinous process at each level (Fig. 287–7). Lateral mass plating is another effective method of achieving spinal arthrodesis and is discussed later in this chapter.

Laminectomy and Laminoplasty

Positioning for laminectomy or laminoplasty is the same as for a patient undergoing laminoforaminotomy, except that the exposure is bilateral at the affected lamina. If the patient is to undergo a multilevel laminectomy that includes C3, it is possible to identify the spinous process of C2 and count from there; otherwise, an intraoperative radiograph is obtained to identify the level.

The actual technique used for laminectomy probably does not affect patient outcome, but it is advisable to avoid placing any instrument under the lamina in an area of severe spinal cord compression because of the risk of worsening any neurological injury. A Kerrison punch with a low-profile footplate can be used safely to begin the laminectomy working along the lateral aspect of the lamina. We prefer to use a high-speed

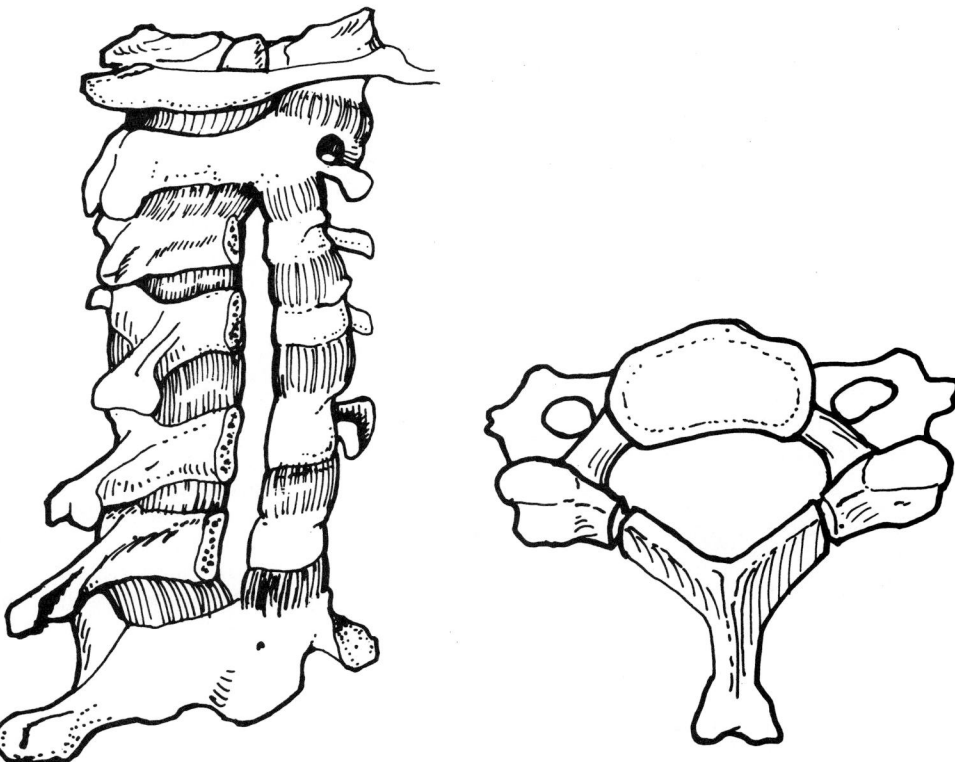

FIGURE 287–8. Operative technique for cervical laminectomy. Bilateral gutters are created using a high-speed bur as shown in the posterolateral (left) and axial (right) drawings. (Adapted from Wiggins GC, Shaffrey CI: Laminectomy in the cervical spine: Indications, surgical techniques, and avoidance of complications. Contemp Neurosurg 21:6, 1999.)

drill. The supraspinous and interspinous ligaments at the top and bottom extent of the laminectomy are transected. A high-speed bur drill is used to create a gutter at the junction of the lamina and medial aspect of the lateral mass through the outer cortical bone and cancellous bone bilaterally (Fig. 287–8). The inner cortical bone also is thinned. Using a 1-mm Kerrison rongeur, transection of the lamina and ligamentum

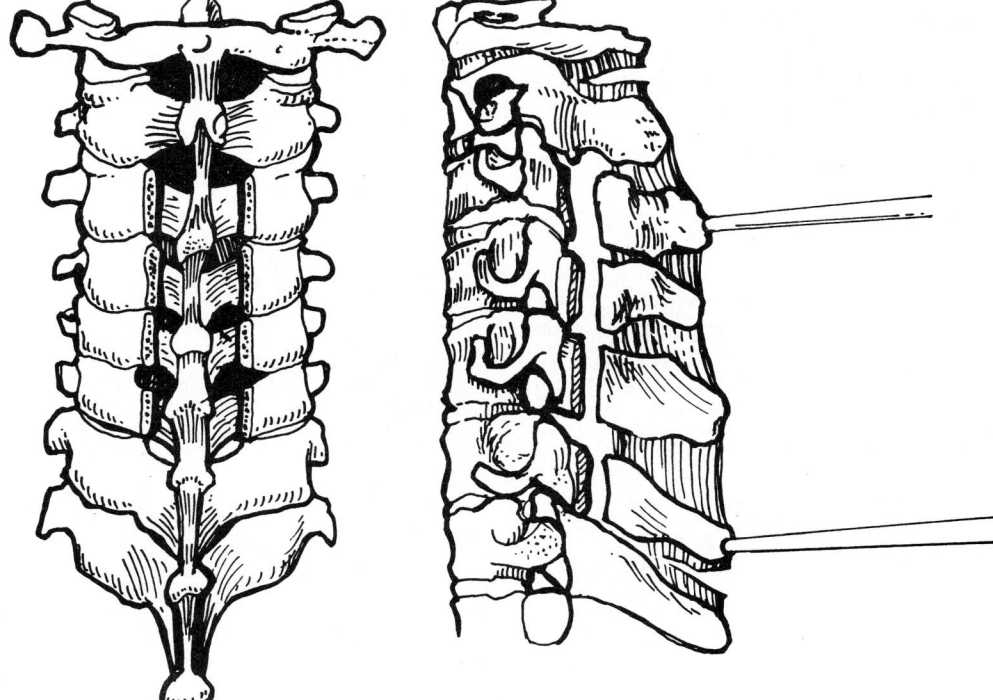

FIGURE 287–9. Operative technique for cervical laminectomy. The lamina are removed en bloc with Kocher clamps as shown in the posterior *(A and C)* and lateral *B and D)* drawings. Care is taken not to lever the lamina into the thecal sac. (Adapted from Wiggins GC, Shaffrey CI: J Neurosurg [Spine 2] 90:170, 1999.)

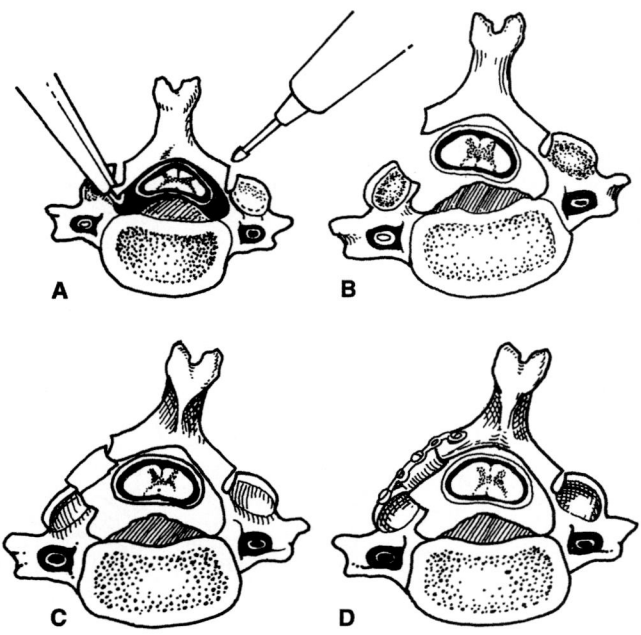

FIGURE 287–10. Operative technique for a modified open-door laminoplasty. *A,* Bilateral gutters are created using a high-speed bur. The lamina and ligamentum flavum are transected with a Kerrison rongeur. *B,* Greenstick osteotomy. *C,* Placement of a bone graft with notching to lock it into place. *D,* Stabilization of the level with a titanium miniplate. (Adapted from Wiggins GC, Shaffrey CI: J Neurosurg [Spine 2] 90:170, 1999.)

flavum is performed bilaterally. Two Kocher clamps are used to lift the dorsal elements by the spinous processes en bloc while the remaining attachments are transected (Fig. 287–9). Care is taken not to rock or tilt the lamina and create impingement on the cord.

Adequate laminectomy length typically requires the removal of one lamina above and one below the maximal cord compression to prevent recurrent stenosis or spinal cord "kinking" on the edge of the lamina. If necessary, C2 and T1 can be undercut, but to reduce

the risk of postoperative kyphosis, we avoid removing C2 or T1. The width of the laminectomy should be to the lateral aspect of the dural sac. Care is taken to remove no more than 25% of the facet complexes. If necessary, a foraminotomy can be performed. If more than 50% of the facet is removed or bilateral foraminotomies are performed, instrumentation and fusion should be considered.

Historically, laminectomy was supplemented by opening the dura and sectioning the dentate ligaments to allow the cord to migrate dorsally. Reid[8] determined that the normal function of the dentate ligaments was to transmit cephalocaudal axial stresses between the spinal cord and the dura. The dentate ligaments should not be sectioned, and complications from opening the dura should be avoided.

In some patients, the canal is reconstructed using a laminoplasty. A prospective study comparing surgical management of CSM found laminoplasty plus anterior decompression to be superior to laminectomy.[49] A variety of laminoplasty techniques exists, but most are modifications of the "open-door" technique. We use a high-speed bur drill to create a gutter at the junction of the lamina and medial aspect of the lateral mass through the outer cancellous bone (Fig. 287–10A). The cancellous bone on the opening side of the laminoplasty is removed and the inner cortex thinned. Using a 1- or 2-mm Kerrison rongeur, transection of the lamina and ligamentum flavum is performed. On the closing side, the gutter also is formed at the junction of the lamina and the lateral mass. This gutter must be sufficiently wide to permit a closing wedge osteotomy with eventual approximation of the lamina against the lateral mass. Generally, approximately 4 mm of bone is resected. Most of the cancellous bone is removed, as well as the outer cortex, but the inner cortex is left intact.

A greenstick osteotomy is performed by carefully displacing the spinous processes toward the closing osteotomy side while elevating the opening side of the lamina with a nerve hook (see Fig. 287–10B). The lam-

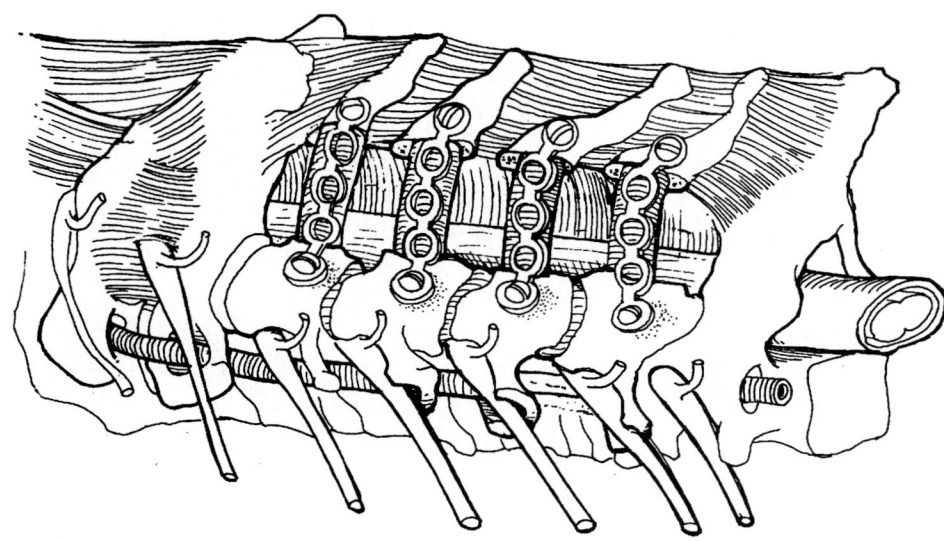

FIGURE 287–11. The schematic drawing shows the orientation of the bone grafts and titanium miniplates for a C3-6 laminoplasty. (From Wiggins GC, Shaffrey CI: J Neurosurg [Spine 2] 90:170, 1999.)

ina is opened en bloc on the side with greatest radiographic compression or with the most prominent signs and symptoms of myeloradiculopathy. Fibular or iliac crest allograft is soaked in antibiotic solution and then cut into strips 1.1 to 1.5 cm high, 0.5 to 0.7 cm wide, and 0.5 to 0.7 cm deep. Allograft tricortical iliac crest is used to generate bicortical bone graft segments. A notch is burred into the superior and inferior aspects of the graft, which firmly lock it into place in the open-door portion of the laminoplasty between the opened lamina and lateral mass (see Fig. 287–10C). Stabilization of each level is then performed using a 2-mm titanium miniplate. An appropriate segment (four or five holes) of straight plate is bent into an open Z shape (see Fig. 287–10D). The plate is secured using a 2 × 6 mm screw at the superior aspect of the lamina and a 2 × 8 mm screw at the corresponding lateral mass (Fig. 287–11). Figure 287–12 shows preoperative, sagittal, T2-weighted MRI and postoperative, T2-weighted MRI of a 58-year-old patient with progressive myelopathy who underwent a laminoplasty. Figure 287–13 shows the postoperative anteroposterior and lateral radiographs of the same patient and demonstrate the miniplate reconstruction and maintenance of cervical lordosis.

Hemostasis of epidural bleeding is obtained with Gelfoam soaked in thrombin. The wound is copiously irrigated with antibiotic solution. A 10 Fr suction drain is placed if there is significant oozing. The muscles and fascia are closed with Vicryl suture. The subcutaneous layer is closed with 2–0 Vicryl suture and the subcuticular layer with 3–0 Vicryl suture. The skin is reapproximated with staples to prevent postoperative wound dehiscence.

Prophylactic antibiotics are continued for the first 24 hours or until the drain is removed. The patient is transferred to the regular unit, and early ambulation is encouraged. Rehabilitation therapy is started early to encourage strengthening of the cervical musculature and maintain cervical lordosis. The patient wears a soft collar for comfort and usually is discharged after a hospital stay of 3 to 4 days.

Posterior Cervical Segmental Instrumentation and Laminectomy

Occasionally, during cervical laminectomy, bilateral nerve root decompression with more than 50% facet resection is needed to obtain complete nerve root and thecal sac decompression. This can lead to cervical instability and deformity. Proper instrumentation at the time of an initial decompression in patients with abnormal segmental motion or absent lordosis markedly decreases their risk for developing postlaminectomy kyphosis, can help maintain sagittal alignment,

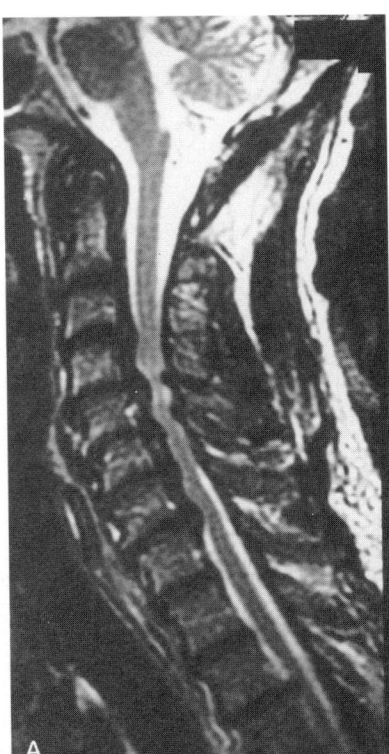
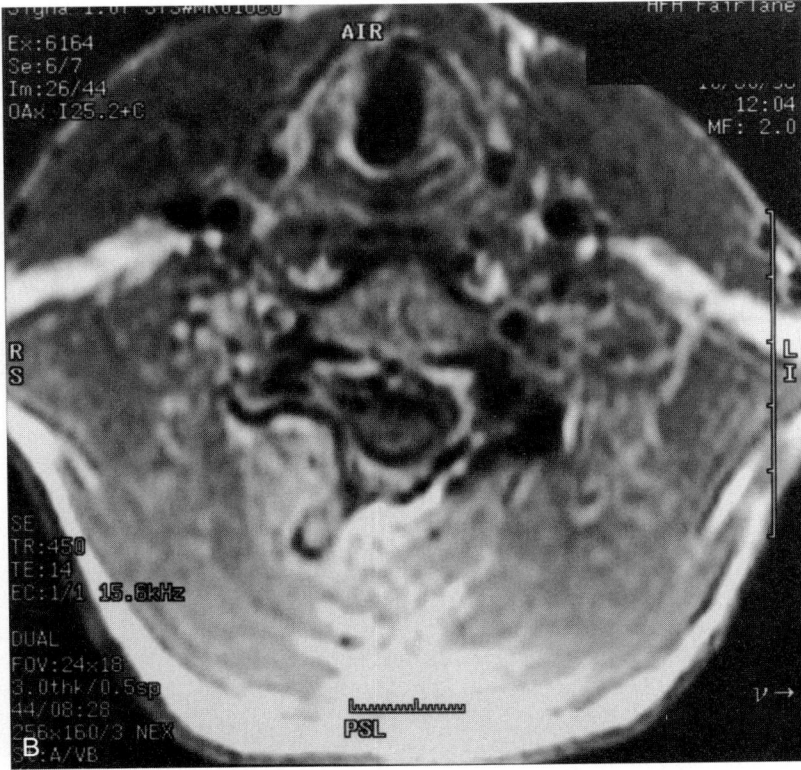

FIGURE 287–12. *A,* Preoperative, sagittal, T2-weighted magnetic resonance imaging (MRI) of a 58-year-old patient with progressive myelopathy. *B,* Postoperative, axial, T2-weighted MRI of the same patient after cervical laminoplasty. Notice the deviated spinous process and enlarged canal area. (Adapted from Wiggins GC, Shaffrey CI: Laminectomy in the cervical spine: Indications, surgical techniques, and avoidance of complications. Contemp Neurosurg 21:7, 1999.)

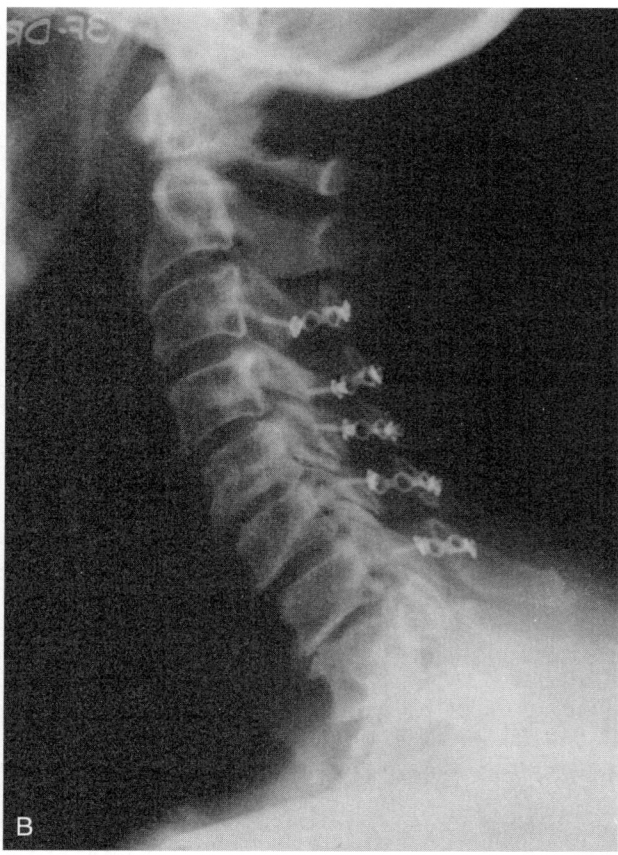

FIGURE 287–13. In the anteroposterior *(A)* and lateral *(B)* postoperative radiographs of the patient in Figure 287–12, notice the titanium miniplate reconstruction and the maintenance of cervical lordosis. (Adapted from Wiggins GC, Shaffrey CI: Laminectomy in the cervical spine: Indications, surgical techniques, and avoidance of complications. Contemp Neurosurg 21:7, 1999.)

and can prevent future neurological decline or delayed pain (Fig. 287–14). Similarly, in cases of instability and kyphosis, instrumentation is usually required. In selected cases of circumferential spinal decompression, gross instability resulting from three-column compromise, or after multilevel anterior decompressions, a combined anterior and posterior fusion procedure may be indicated (Fig. 287–15).

The goal of any fixation system is to provide structural stability until a solid bone fusion forms. Several techniques of posterior cervical stabilization have been described. Many wiring techniques have been developed, but most require the presence of intact posterior elements for fixation. These techniques are not useful in a patient after laminectomy. Cervical spine stabilization techniques available after laminectomy include interfacet wiring, facet wiring, and lateral mass plates.

INTERFACET WIRING

Fixation may be obtained by interfacet wiring, as described by Johnson[50] in the 1970s. The advantage of this technique is that it is effective in achieving stability against rotational and shear forces. The disadvantage is that it requires violation of an intact and unfused facet, which can lead to postoperative pain. The inferior facet at the level of injury and one below the level of injury are exposed. A drill hole is made through each inferior facet at a 90-degree angle to the plane of the facet joint, with a Freer elevator placed in the interarticular surface to prevent overpenetration during drilling (Fig. 287–16). A wire is passed from posterior to anterior through the inferior facet at the uninjured level and the injured level. The wire is twisted over the surface of the facet (Fig. 287–17).

FACET WIRING

Facet fusion can be used to prevent postlaminectomy instability. The exposure should include all the levels to be fused and their facets. The soft tissue and facet capsules are stripped. The articular cartilage of the facet joint is removed using a fine curet. Holes are drilled in the inferior facets as described previously. Separate braided, 22-gauge wires are then passed through the inferior facet holes at each level from superior to inferior and exiting the facet joint medially. A posterior iliac bone graft large enough to span the affected levels is harvested. Holes are placed in the bone graft slightly medially to allow maximal graft

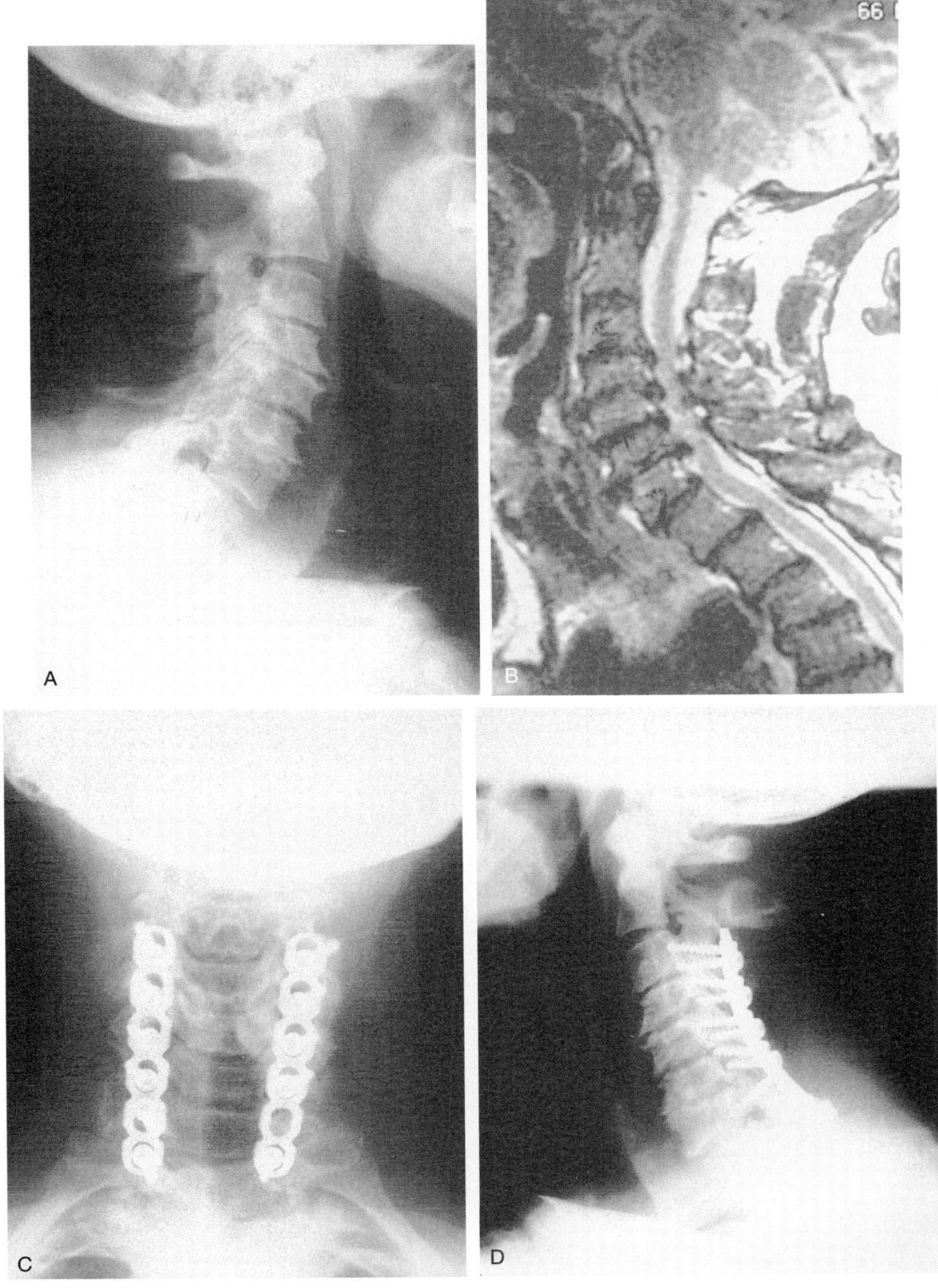

FIGURE 287–14. The lateral radiograph *(A)* showing C7-T1 instability in a 68-year-old patient with neck pain, hand atrophy, C8 radiculopathy, and myelopathy was obtained preoperatively, as was the T2-weighted magnetic resonance image *(B)*. Anteroposterior *(C)* and lateral *(D)* radiographs after a C3-T1 laminectomy with lateral mass plating and arthrodesis. Notice the C7 and T1 transpedicular fixation without a left C7 pedicle screw because of excessive bone resection during the decompression.

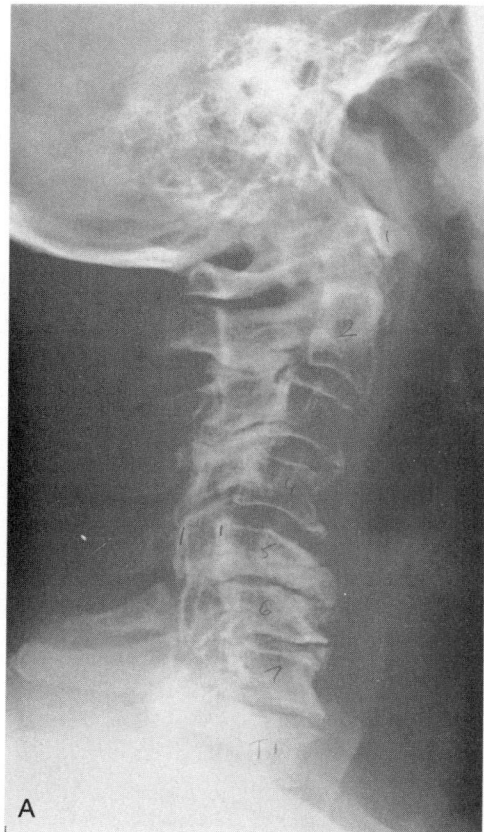

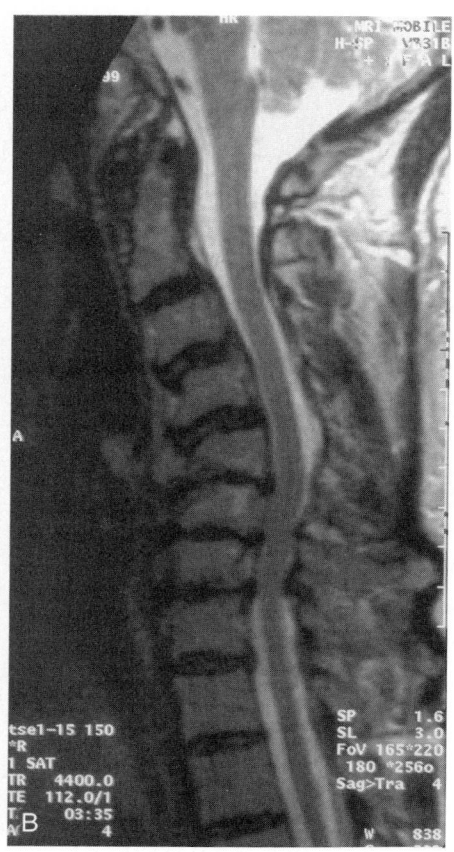

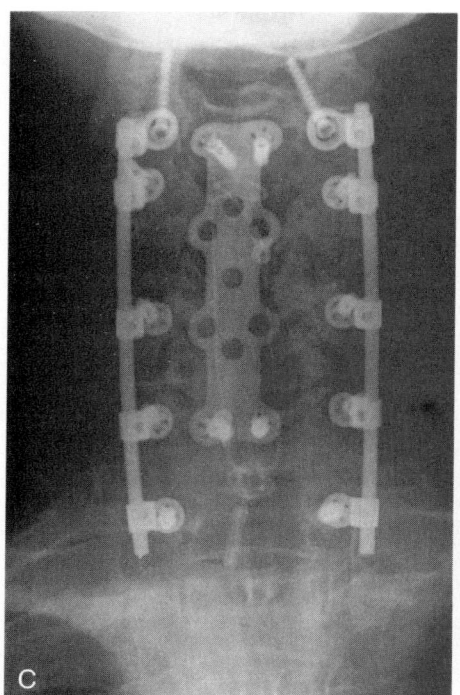

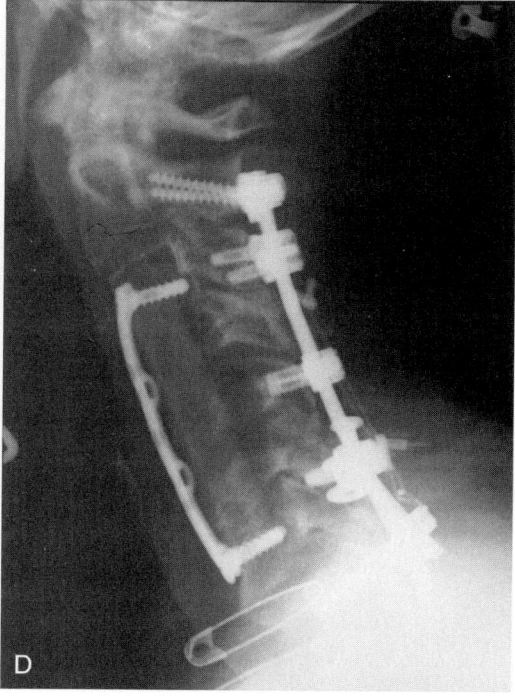

FIGURE 287–15. The lateral radiograph *(A)* of a 47-year-old patient with neck pain and myelopathy with a significant, fixed, midcervical kyphosis was obtained before surgery, as was the T2-weighted magnetic resonance image *(B)*. Anteroposterior *(C)* and lateral *(D)* radiographs 12 weeks after multilevel corpectomy and anterior reconstruction followed by posterior segmental instrumentation.

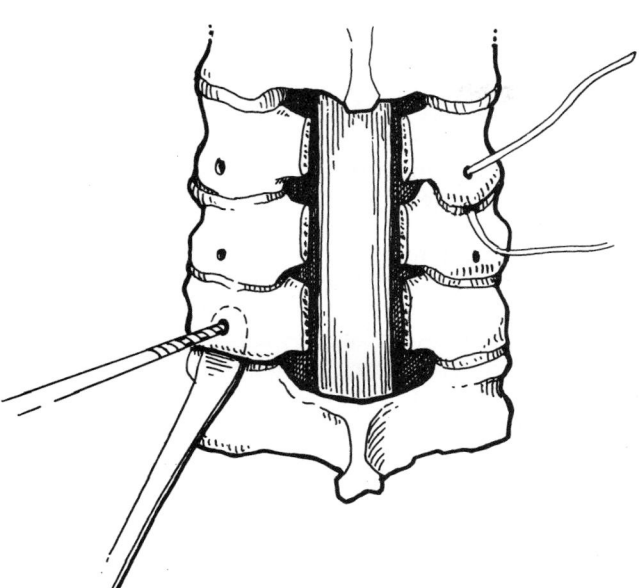

FIGURE 287–16. Placement of a drill hole in the inferior facet. A Freer elevator is placed in the interarticular surface to prevent overpenetrating during drilling. A wire is then passed posterior to anterior through the drill hole.

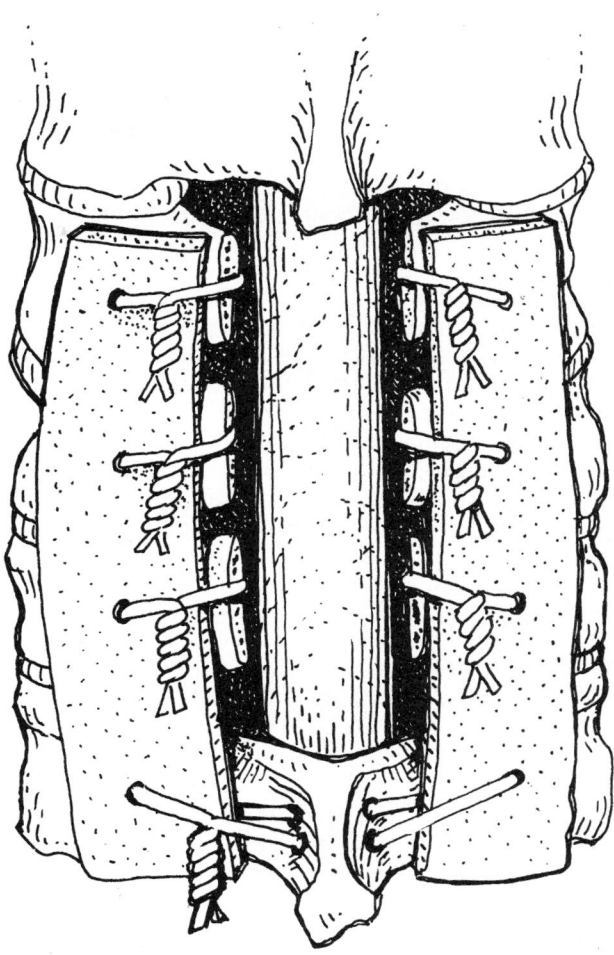

FIGURE 287–18. Facet wiring is achieved with facet wires passed up through an iliac graft. Notice that the inferior wire is passed through the spinous process to avoid injuring an unfused level.

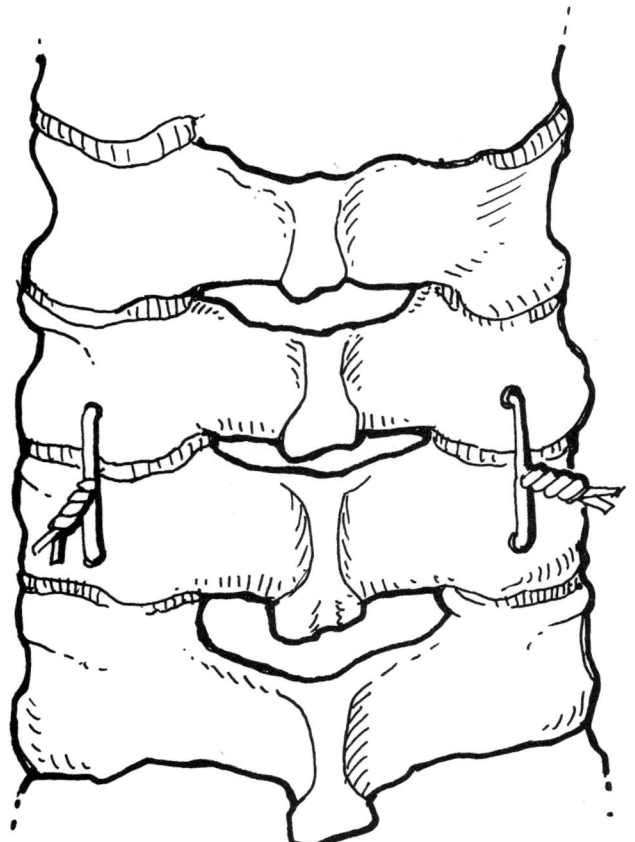

FIGURE 287–17. Interfacet wiring is completed with a single wire passed through two adjacent inferior facets.

contact with the facet. Each facet wire is passed through the corresponding hole in the bone plate. The other end of the wire is brought around the medial aspect of the bone graft. After the facet surfaces have been slightly decorticated, the graft is placed in contact with the facets, and the wires are sequentially tightened (Fig. 287–18).

The graft should be secured to the first stable facet above the laminectomy. The inferior wire should be secured to the first spinous process below the laminectomy rather than traversing an unaffected facet level. Cancellous autograft can then be packed into the facet joints and laid laterally along the grafts to promote arthrodesis.

LATERAL MASS PLATES

Several surgeons[51–56] have described the technique of using cervical lateral mass plates. The technique involves fixation of a small plate into the lateral masses with screws. These devices provide superb flexural stability and resist torsion and extension significantly better than spinous process wiring.[54] Lateral mass plate fusion requires significantly less operative time than segmental facet fixation with wire. The enhanced stability can decrease or eliminate the need for postoperative orthosis. Disadvantages of lateral mass plates include cost and potential injury to the exiting nerve root and vertebral artery.

Several screw placement techniques have been described. The technique developed by Roy-Camille[54] places the screw halfway between the articular surfaces of the facets and halfway between the lamina facet line and the lateral margin of the lateral mass. The screw is placed at the midpoint of the lateral mass and angled 10 degrees laterally. Magerl and coworkers[53] described another technique. The entry point is 1 mm medial and 1 to 2 mm cephalad to the center of the lateral mass. The screw angles 25 degrees laterally and 30 degrees cephalad. In an anatomic and biomechanical study, the Magerl technique was observed to avoid the neurovascular structures better than the Roy-Camille technique.[57] Because the Magerl technique parallels the facet, longer screws could be placed (20 versus 14 mm) and were able to accommodate a greater load before failing.[58] It appears that the Magerl technique provides greater immediate stability and lower risk to neurovascular structures.

This screw technique is used for C3-6 segments. A C2 screw can be placed, but it is usually placed into the C2 pars. The starting point is 3 mm superior and lateral to the most medial aspect of the C2-3 facet, with 10- to 15-degree medial and 35-degree cephalad trajectories. The C7 and T1 levels can be incorporated into the fusion by placing pedicle screws. A small laminotomy can be performed to identify the medial pedicle during screw placement. The entry point is 1 mm below the facet joint and at the intersection of the lamina and transverse process. The angle is 25 to 30 degrees medially and perpendicular to bone in the superior-inferior plane. Lateral fluoroscopy can be helpful in identifying the pedicles during pedicle screw placement in the upper thoracic spine.

The technique of placing lateral mass plates involves a standard midline exposure extended laterally to expose the lateral aspect of the lateral masses bilaterally. The facet capsules are removed, and the articular cartilages and surfaces are roughened. Cancellous bone or bone from the spinous processes is packed into the facet joint space. The holes are drilled before plate insertion to obtain the ideal screw position in the lateral mass. There is no compromise in the hole position to help fit the plate's hole spacing. The midpoint of the lateral mass is identified, and the entry point 1 mm medial and 1 to 2 mm cephalad is identified. The dorsal cortex of the lateral mass is pierced perpendicularly with an awl. The hole is drilled using the Magerl technique and a drill with a depth stop of about 15 to 16 mm. Although bicortical purchase is considered superior to unicortical fixation, it is not mandatory because of the increased risk of neurovascular injury with bicortical screw fixation. Care is taken not to fracture the lateral mass, which can happen if the drilling angle is too steep. The dorsal cortex is tapped before screw insertion.

After all the holes are drilled, an appropriate plate is selected and contoured to the cervical lordosis. The screws are placed to secure the plate to the lateral masses. Generally, 14-mm screws are used for most female and small male patients, and 16-mm screws are used in larger male patients. When one plate is secured, the contralateral side is drilled, the plate placed, and final screws tightened. Although it is generally recommended to place lateral mass plates in situ, lateral mass plates occasionally can be used to correct a kyphosis.

Complications with lateral mass plates include neural injury, vertebral artery injury, and hardware failure leading to pseudarthrosis. Heller and colleagues[59] performed the most complete analysis of complications after lateral mass plating. They found a 0.69% incidence of nerve root injury per screw placed. There was a 1.17% incidence of screw loosening, which had no effect on their 98.6% fusion rate. Infections occurred in 1.3% of patients. They observed 3.8% adjacent segment degeneration with neck pain. No vertebral artery injuries or spinal cord injuries have been reported.

Complications and Complication Avoidance

A variety of complications associated with posterior cervical approaches have been reported (Table 287–2),[4, 60–75] but most can be prevented by paying strict attention to detail and operative technique. The complications can be grouped into three categories: general, neurological, and biomechanical.

The general category includes air embolism, infection,[67] epidural hematoma,[74] cerebellar hemorrhage,[62] deep venous thrombosis, dural tear,[64] and adhesive arachnoiditis.[70] For most surgeons, avoiding the use of the sitting position for surgery is emphasized[24] to lessen the operation preparation time, risk of hypotension, risk of positional and pressure-related peripheral nerve injury, and air embolism.

Neurological complications generally are caused by

**T A B L E   2 8 7 – 2 ■ Complications of Cervical
Laminectomy**

Neurologic worsening: quadriparesis, quadriplegia, mononeuropathy
   Impaired perfusion: hypotension, hypervolemia, microcirculation
   Iatrogenic trauma
   Abnormal clotting factors
   Postoperative hematoma
Kyphotic deformity: loss of facets, denervation of erector spinae muscles
Air embolus: venous, paradoxical, pins in head holder
Laceration of dura, nerve roots, cerebrospinal fluid fistula, meningocele
   Operative manipulation, scarring
   Air drill injury
Brachial plexus injury: positioning
Central retinal artery thrombosis in the prone position, horseshoe facial support

failure of technique or conceptual failure in planning. These failures often are preventable. Complications include injury to the spinal cord during the operation,[74, 75] residual compression of the neural elements,[4, 65, 66] delayed central spinal cord syndrome,[68] and syringomyelia.[69] Unacceptable results may occur because of inappropriate selection of operation, intraoperative spinal cord or nerve root trauma, inappropriate width of laminectomy, or inappropriate length of laminectomy. The risks of inappropriate operation selection cannot be overemphasized. If the patient has preoperative kyphosis or focal anterior pathology, a dorsal approach is unlikely to help the patient improve.

The incidence of intraoperative neural trauma is low during routine laminectomy,[5] but the procedure can lead to unacceptable operative results. It is completely avoidable. Injury can potentially occur by placing too large of a Kerrison punch below the lamina. Thinning the lamina with a high-speed drill can reduce the risk of this complication.

The width of the laminectomy is critical. A laminectomy that is not wide enough cannot decompress the neural elements and may lead to continued neurological symptoms. Conversely, a laminectomy that is too wide may lead to instability. If the laminectomy is taken to the lateral extent of the dural sac, the neural elements can be decompressed without risk of instability.

The length of the laminectomy is also important. If it is too long, spinal deformity and instability are encouraged unnecessarily. These complications are most commonly encountered with the removal of the first thoracic lamina, leading to kyphosis.[76] Pal and Routal[77] used 40 dry adult cervical spines to assess the relative weight bearing of the cervical lamina. They concluded that the lamina of C2 and C7 are heavily loaded, whereas the others are not. Laminectomy at C2 and C7 would tend to lead to instability, whereas between C3 and C6, instability would be less likely. All attempts are made to preserve the lamina and spinous process of C2, where the insertion of the erector spinae muscles maintains stability. If the laminectomy is too short, it does not adequately decompress the spinal cord and can lead to the spinal cord kinking as it migrates posteriorly into the laminectomy defect.

The extent of decompression after cervical laminectomy may also contribute to the rate of C5 nerve root paresis. Yonenobu and coworkers[74] reviewed anterior and posterior cervical approaches. They found 13 instances of C5 nerve root paresis or plegia without sensory involvement in a group of 384 patients. Paresis of the deltoid was the most common weakness. They believed the weakness was caused by tethering of the nerve root by fibrosis or by spondylotic changes at the foramen and root canal. Dorsal shift of the spinal cord could exert traction on the nerve root that resulted in loss of motor function.[71, 74, 78] The C5 nerve root seems to be the most affected nerve because it is usually at the midpoint in a cervical laminectomy and would be at the point of maximum displacement of the cord. In a review of 287 patients with cervical laminectomy Dai and coworkers[63] identified 37 patients (12.9%) with postoperative radiculopathy. Although C5 radiculopathy was the most common type, they felt that this could be predicted preoperatively with electrophysiologic studies. Local trauma to the nerve root is another possible explanation for postoperative paresis. No matter what the cause, postoperative C5 paresis usually resolves with time.

Postoperative spinal deformity is frequently an iatrogenic disease. In most instances, it can be prevented or predicted preoperatively and treated with stabilization at the time of decompression. To prevent postoperative instability, the surgeon must identify the factors that place a patient at higher risk. Intimate knowledge of the biomechanics that lead to postoperative instability can help guide the surgeon away from procedures that leave the patient unstable. Postcervical laminectomy instability can be one of two types. Postoperative kyphosis is the most common, but hyperlordosis and segmental instability also can occur.

Laminoplasty is one method of preventing postoperative instability after laminectomy. Some reports[79, 80] suggest that laminoplasty provides greater stability and greater range of motion compared with laminectomy, which may protect against postoperative instability.[81] Open-door laminoplasty reduces cervical spinal motion from 50% to 62%,[82–84] and reduced motion may help to prevent the progression of cervical spondylotic disease. A prospective study by Herkowitz[49] compared anterior cervical decompression and fusion (ACDF), laminoplasty, and laminectomy. ACDF and laminoplasty provided superior results with no statistical difference between them. Laminoplasty did retain some cervical motion.

The mechanism for postoperative instability lies in the amount of facet resection, age of the patient, and the length of laminectomy. A cervical kyphotic deformity refers to a reversal of 5 degrees or more of the natural cervical lordosis. During cervical laminectomy, the erector spinae muscles are partially denervated and weakened. The spinous processes, lamina, and ligamentum flavum are removed. The head's center of gravity usually is slightly anterior to the cervical spine. Weakening of the posterior tension band favors a kyphotic deformity (Fig. 287–19). The risk of postoperative kyphotic deformity is greater in children because they have a relatively more flexible cervical spine. The epiphyses in the growing spine respond to asymmetric forces by causing a ventral wedging of the vertebral bodies. The orientation of the facet joints in the immature spine is more horizontal than the 45-degree angle in the mature spine, leading to less resistive force to flexion.[85]

The exact incidence of postoperative kyphosis after cervical laminectomy is unknown. It appears to occur more often in children than in adults.[61, 62, 72, 73] Studies vary with respect to the type and significance of deformity. The overall incidence of adult postlaminectomy (without facetectomy) deformity is between 6% and 52%.[49, 62, 70, 75, 86–88] Rarely (0% to 3%) do these patients develop symptoms directly related to their deformity. The extent of laminectomy seems to be one factor in determining postoperative kyphosis. Cusick and asso-

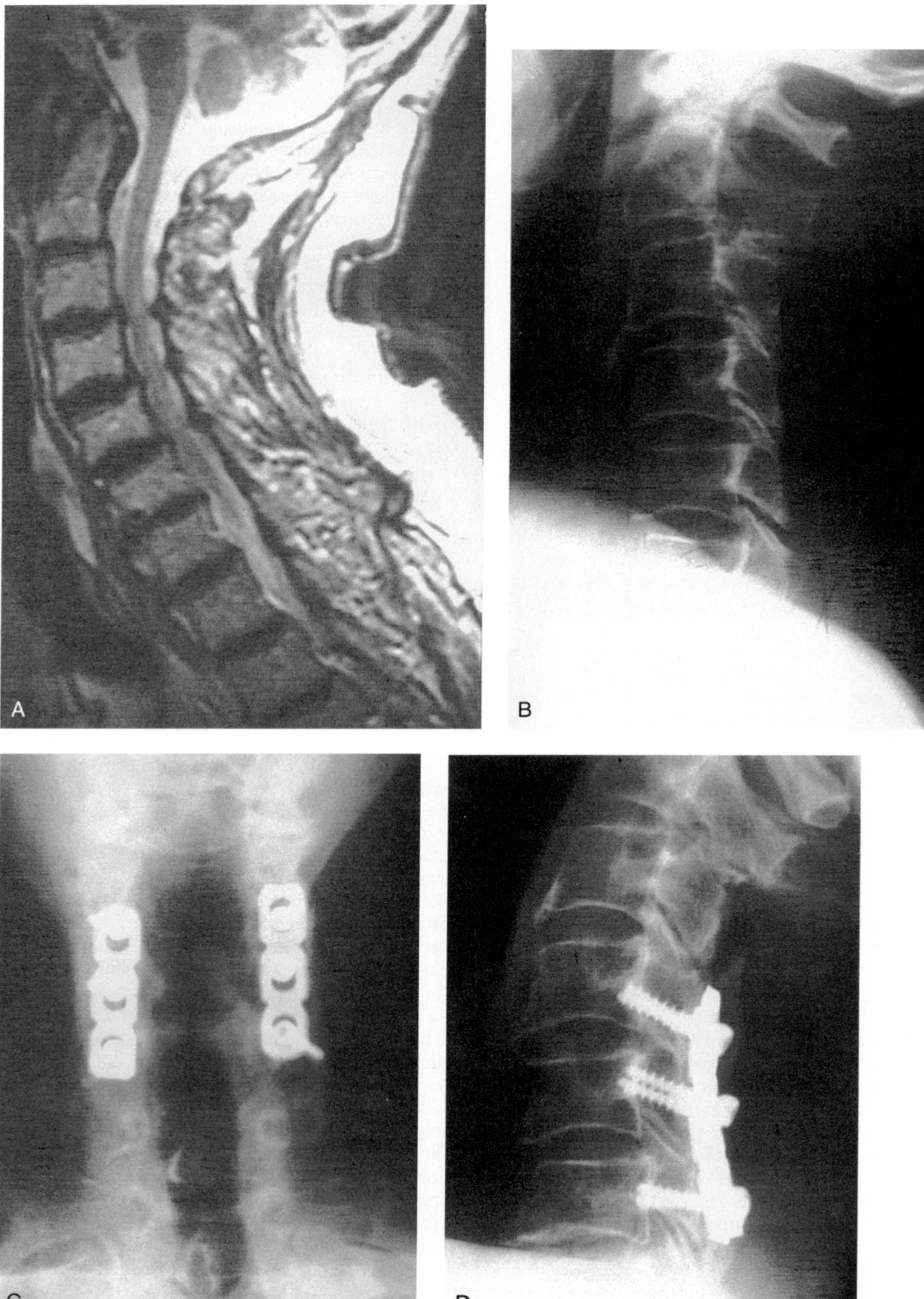

FIGURE 287–19. *A,* Preoperative, T2-weighted magnetic resonance image shows slight C5 on C6 anterolisthesis and kyphosis. *B,* A postoperative, lateral-view radiograph shows C5 on C6 instability and bilateral C6 radiculopathies. Anteroposterior *(C)* and lateral *(D)* radiographs were obtained after lateral mass plate fixation with resolution of all symptoms.

ciates[89] looked at the biomechanics of cervical laminectomy without facetectomy and concluded that laminectomy alone induces significant increases in total cervical spine flexibility. If the C2 or C7 lamina or spinous process is removed, the risk seems to be increased.[62, 86, 90] Removal of the C2 lamina damages most of the musculus semispinalis cervicis and musculi suboccipitales, which are attached to the spinous process of C2. Because they are damaged, the posterior tension band is weakened.

The width of the laminectomy and, more importantly, the width of the facetectomy are critical in determining the risk of postoperative kyphosis. Several studies in vitro have shown that the extent of facet resection can destabilize the cervical spine and can potentially contribute to accelerated degenerative changes.[25, 89, 91] In a study in which a multilevel cervical laminectomy model was used, Nowinski and associates[92] concluded that concurrent arthrodesis should be performed if bilateral facetectomy of more than 25% is performed in conjunction with a multilevel laminectomy. In a study of cervical spine mechanics, Panjabi and colleagues[93] demonstrated a progressively increasing degree of cervical instability to flexion loads with sequential removal of posterior supporting elements of the spine. Zdeblick and associates[25] studied the effect of progressive facet resection after laminectomy in human specimens. Facetectomy of more than 50% caused a statistically significant loss of stability in flexion and torsion. In a similar study, Zdeblick and coworkers[91] found a significant loss of stability after 55% capsular resection. Two finite element studies looked at the effect of graded facetectomies.[94, 95] Their mathematical models suggest that the greatest change in stability occurred between 50% and 75% facet resection bilaterally. Resection of more than 50% of the bilateral facet complexes can lead to pronounced increases in angular rotation and intervertebral disk stresses.

Munechica[96] studied the relative contribution of the facets and the lamina to spinal stability in monkeys. Laminectomy alone did not lead to deformity, but a gibbus developed when laminectomy was combined with resection of one facet. In a clinical study, Epstein[97] emphasized the importance of the facet joint contribution to stability and advocated that not more than one fourth to one third of the facets should be removed during foraminal decompression. In a comparison of treatment modalities for multilevel spondylotic radiculopathy, Herkowitz[49] found a 25% incidence of postoperative kyphotic deformities within 2 years after cervical laminectomy with partial bilateral facetectomies. The facetectomy should be limited to 25% to 50% to limit the risk of postoperative instability; otherwise, stabilization must be considered.

A variety of complications associated with posterior cervical decompression have been discussed. Complication avoidance involves taking care in each step: preoperative evaluation of patients, evaluation of preoperative radiographs, the operation itself, and postoperative follow-up. Proper patient selection can avoid operations on patients unlikely to benefit from surgery. Choosing the appropriate operation to address the spe-

cific pathology helps to avoid missing or incompletely treating the pathology. Close inspection of the radiographs identifies the nature of the pathology, location of pathology, and the levels that need to be addressed. During the operation, care is taken to avoid iatrogenic injury from the laminectomy or the degree of facetectomy. Postoperatively, patients must be followed, and care must be taken to identify postoperative instability or neurological deterioration. Ultimately, the success of any operative approach depends on the correct selection of the surgical candidate and on the skill, judgment, and experience of the surgeon.

Outcomes

In patients with radiculopathy, the most common operation is a posterior cervical laminoforaminotomy. In several series, more than 90% of patients undergoing laminoforaminotomy have shown good or excellent results.[10, 11, 35, 36, 98–100] Scoville and coworkers[11] reported excellent or good results for 95% of the patients who underwent posterior surgery. Krupp and colleagues[36] reviewed 230 patients undergoing laminoforaminotomy for lateral disk herniation with radiculopathy. These patients had the soft disk material removed if present, but no attempt was made to remove anterior osteophytes after the posterior root decompression was completed. One hundred sixty-one patients were available, with an average follow-up period of 3.5 years. They reported excellent or good results for 98% of patients with a soft disk, 84% of patients with a hard disk, and 91% of patients with combined pathology. Overall, 93% of patients had complete improvement of paresis, and 82% had improvement of sensory deficits. Ninety-two percent of patients were able to return to their previous occupations. Other surgeons have advocated removing any offending osteophyte, if present. In 1990, Aldrich[98] evaluated 36 patients with posterolateral disk herniations. In this selected population, 100% had improvement of preoperative motor complaints, and 100% had significant pain relief. Of the 21 patients with sensory deficits, 7 had improvement immediately after the operation, and 16 of 18 with long-term follow-up had a reduction in their sensory complaints.

A review of the literature regarding the efficacy of cervical laminectomy indicates a 40% to 78% rate of resolution of the myelopathy associated with cervical spondylosis or stenosis.[5, 41, 60, 66, 87, 101–106] Improvement rates of 68% to 95% and cure rates of 33% have been reported in some surgically treated patients.[4, 21, 38] Although a few series suggest that prelaminectomy malalignment of the cervical column is not associated with subsequent clinical improvement, most reviews indicate that alterations of spinal curvature may be an important determinant of a poor clinical outcome.[2, 41, 70, 88, 102] Attention to maintaining lordosis and anatomic alignment is indicated to improve patient outcomes. Some patients develop immediate or delayed impairment of neural function after laminectomy.[107, 108] Brain and associates[109] found impairment of neural function in 19% of patients who had been treated with laminectomy. Crandall and Gregorius,[107] after long-term follow-up, reported that 9 of 15 patients treated by laminectomy were worse postoperatively. Failure may be caused by loss of neural function with cervical laminectomy from intraoperative manipulation of the spinal cord, failure to treat the causes of anterior compression, and loss of stability of the spine.

Many of the studies of laminectomy were performed in the late 1970s. Since then, attention has been placed on atraumatic cervical spine surgery. A long-term study by Kato and coworkers[110] of laminectomy for cervical myelopathy caused by ossification of the posterior longitudinal ligament revealed that the neurological recovery rate was 44.2% after 1 year and 42.9% after 5 years. The surgical outcome was maintained after 5 years but worsened between 5 and 10 years after surgery. Most patients' neurological decline was caused by falls. In the appropriately selected patient, neurological recovery is expected, with maintenance of this recovery over 5 years.

CONCLUSIONS

Posterior cervical approaches for the treatment of degenerative disk disease are successful and have been performed since the 1950s. As with any operation, it is important to select the appropriate operation and tailor it to the individual patient. It is critical to evaluate a patient's pathology (i.e., location and type) in addition to the static and dynamic sagittal spine balance. Complications can be avoided with careful attention to detail. The success of the operation ultimately depends on the surgeon's judgment and experience and on patient selection.

REFERENCES

1. Smith AG: Account of a case in which portions of three dorsal vertebrae were removed for the relief of paralysis from fracture, with partial success. North Am Med Surg J 8:94–97, 1829.
2. Batzdorf U, Batzdorff A: Analysis of cervical spine curvature in patients with cervical spondylosis. Neurosurgery 22:827–836, 1988.
3. Benzel EC, Lancon J, Kesterson L, et al: Cervical laminectomy and dentate ligament section for cervical spondylotic myelopathy. J Spinal Disord 4:286–295, 1991.
4. Carol MP, Ducker TB: Cervical spondylitic myelopathies: Surgical treatment. J Spinal Disord 1:59–65, 1988.
5. Fager CA: Results of adequate posterior decompression in the relief of spondylotic cervical myelopathy. J Neurosurg 38:684–692, 1973.
6. Fager CA: Reversal of cervical myelopathy by adequate posterior decompression. Lahey Clin Found Bull 18:99–108, 1969.
7. Morgan TH, Wharton GW, Austin GN: The results of laminectomy in patients with incomplete spinal cord injuries. Paraplegia 9:14–23, 1971.
8. Reid JD: Effects of flexion-extension movements of the head and spine upon the spinal cord and nerve roots. J Neurol Neurosurg Psychiatry 23:214–221, 1960.
9. Rogers L: The surgical treatment of cervical spondylitic myelopathy. Mobilisation of the complete cervical cord into an enlarged canal. J Bone Joint Surg Br 43:3–6, 1961.
10. Murphey F, Simmons JCH, Brunson B: Surgical treatment of laterally ruptured cervical disc: Review of 648 cases, 1939 to 1972. J Neurosurg 38:679–683, 1973.
11. Scoville WB, Dohrmann GJ, Corkill G: Late results of cervical disc surgery. J Neurosurg 45:203–210, 1976.
12. Spurling RG, Scoville WB: Lateral rupture of the cervical intervertebral discs. Surg Gynecol Obstet 78:350–358, 1944.
13. Bernhardt M, Hynes RA, Blume HW, et al: Current concepts review: Cervical spondylotic myelopathy. J Bone Joint Surg Am 75:119–128, 1993.
14. Epstein NE, Epstein JA, Carras R, et al: Coexisting cervical and lumbar spinal stenosis: Diagnosis and management. Neurosurgery 15:489–496, 1984.
15. Simeone FA, Rothman RH: Cervical disc disease. In Rothman RH, Simeone FA (eds): The Spine, 2nd ed. Philadelphia, WB Saunders, 1982, pp 440–496.
16. Parke W: Correlative anatomy of cervical spondylotic myelopathy. Spine 13:831–837, 1988.
17. Arnold JG Jr: The clinical manifestations of spondylochondrosis (spondylosis) of the cervical spine. Ann Surg 141:872–889, 1955.
18. Adams CB, Logue V: Studies in cervical spondylotic myelopathy. II. The movement and contour of the spine in relation to the neural complications of cervical spondylosis. Brain 94:568–586, 1971 .
19. Burrows EH: The sagittal diameter of the spinal canal in cervical spondylosis. Clin Radiol 14:77–86, 1963.
20. Edwards WC, LaRocca H: The developmental segmental sagittal diameter of the cervical spinal canal in patients with cervical spondylosis. Spine 8:20–27, 1983.
21. Epstein BS, Epstein JA, Jones MD: Cervical spinal stenosis. Radiol Clin North Am 15:215–226, 1977.
22. Epstein JA, Carras R, Hyman RA, et al: Cervical myelopathy caused by developmental stenosis of the spinal canal. J Neurosurg 51:362–367, 1979.
23. Hayashi H, Okada K, Hamada M, et al: Etiologic factors of myelopathy: A radiographic evaluation of the aging changes in the cervical spine. Clin Orthop 214:200–209, 1987.
24. Pavlov H, Torg JS, Robie B, et al: Cervical spinal stenosis: Determination with vertebral body ratio method. Radiology 164:771–775, 1987.
25. Zdeblick TA, Zou D, Warden KE, et al: Cervical stability after foraminotomy: A biomechanical in vitro analysis. J Bone Joint Surg Am 74:22–27, 1992.
26. Al-Mefty O, Harkey LH, Middleton TH, et al: Myelopathic cervical spondylotic lesions demonstrated by magnetic resonance imaging. J Neurosurg 68:217–222, 1988.
27. Matsuda Y, Miyazaki K, Tada K, et al: Increased MR signal intensity due to cervical myelopathy: Analysis of 29 surgical cases. J Neurosurg 74:887–892, 1991.
28. Okada Y, Ikata T, Yamada H, et al: Magnetic resonance imaging study on the results of surgery for cervical compressive myelopathy. Spine 18:2024–2029, 1993.
29. Fujiwara K, Yonenobu K, Ebara S, et al: The prognosis of surgery for cervical compression myelopathy: An analysis of the factors involved. J Bone Joint Surg Br 71:393–398, 1989.
30. Koyanagi T, Hirabayashi K, Satomi K, et al: Predictability of surgical results of cervical compression myelopathy based on presurgical computed tomographic myelography. Spine 18:1958–1963, 1993.
31. Breig A, Turnbull I, Hassler O: Effects of mechanical stresses on the spinal cord in cervical spondylosis: A study of fresh cadaver material. J Neurosurg 25:45–56, 1966.
32. Gruninger W, Gruss P: Stenosis and movement of the cervical spine in cervical myelopathy. Paraplegia 20:121–130, 1982.
33. Penning L: Some aspects of plain radiography of the cervical spine in chronic myelopathy. Neurology 12:513–519, 1962.
34. Lees F, Turner J: Natural history and prognosis of cervical spondylosis. Br Med J 2:1607–1610, 1963.
35. Henderson CM, Hennessy RG, Shuey HJ, et al: Posterior-lateral foraminotomy as an exclusive operative technique for cervical radiculopathy: A review of 846 consecutive operated cases. Neurosurgery 504–512, 1983.
36. Krupp W, Schattke H, Muke R: Clinical results of the foraminotomy as described by Frykholm for the treatment of lateral cervical disc herniation. Acta Neurochir 107:22–29, 1990.
37. Clarke E, Robinson PK: Cervical myelopathy: A complication of cervical spondylosis. Brain 79:483–510, 1956.
38. Epstein JA, Carras R, Epstein BS, et al: Myelopathy in cervical

spondylosis with vertebral subluxation and hyperlordosis. J Neurosurg 32:421–426, 1970.

39. Lesoin F, Bouasakao N, Clarisse J, et al: Results of surgical treatment of radiculomyelopathy caused by cervical arthrosis based on 1000 operations. Surg Neurol 23:350–355, 1985.

40. Cusick JF: Pathophysiology and treatment of cervical spondylotic myelopathy. Clin Neurosurg 37:661–681, 1991.

41. Adams CB, Logue V: Studies in cervical spondylotic myelopathy. III. Some functional effects of operations for cervical spondylotic myelopathy. Brain 94:587–594, 1971.

42. Murphy MJ, Lieponis JV: Nonsurgical treatment of cervical spine pain. In the Cervical Spine Research Society Editorial Committee (eds): The Cervical Spine, 2nd ed. Philadelphia, JB Lippincott, 1989, pp 670–677.

43. Matjasko J, Petrozza P, Cohen M, et al: Anesthesia and surgery in the seated position: Analysis of 554 cases. Neurosurgery 17:695–702, 1985.

44. Standefer M, Bay JW, Trusso R: The sitting position in neurosurgery: A retrospective analysis of 488 cases. Neurosurgery 14:649–658, 1984.

45. Epstein NE, Danto J, Nardi D: Somatosensory evoked potential monitoring during 100 cervical operations. Spine 18:737–747, 1993.

46. Frykholm R: Deformities of dural pouches and strictures of dural sheaths in the cervical region producing nerve-root compression: A contribution to the etiology and operative treatment of brachial neuralgia. J Neurosurg 4:403–413, 1947.

47. Ducker TB, Zeidman SM: The posterior operative approach for cervical radiculopathy. Neurosurg Clin N Am 4:61–74, 1993.

48. Farey ID, McAfee PC, David RF, et al: Pseudoarthrosis of the cervical spine after anterior arthrodesis: Treatment by posterior nerve-root decompression, stabilization, and arthrodesis. J Bone Joint Surg Am 72:1171–1177, 1990.

49. Herkowitz HN: A comparison of anterior cervical fusion, cervical laminectomy, and cervical laminoplasty for the surgical management of multiple level spondylotic radiculopathy. Spine 13:774–780, 1988.

50. Johnson R: Surgical approaches to the spine. In Rothman R, Simeone F (eds): The Spine. Philadelphia, WB Saunders, 1982, pp 140.

51. Cherny WB, Sonntag VKH, Douglas RA: Lateral mass posterior plating and facet fusion for cervical spine instability. Barrow Neurol Inst Q 7:2–11, 1991.

52. Cooper PR, Cohen A, Rosiello A, et al: Posterior stabilization of cervical spine fractures and subluxations using plates and screws. Neurosurgery 23:300–306, 1988.

53. Magerl F, Grob D, Seemann P: Stable dorsal fusion of the cervical spine (C2-Th1) using hook plates. In Kehr P, Weidner A (eds): Cervical Spine, vol 1. New York, Springer-Verlag, 1987, pp 217–221.

54. Roy-Camille R, Saillant G, Mazel C: Internal fixation of the unstable cervical spine by a posterior osteosynthesis with plates and screws. In the Cervical Spine Research Society Editorial Committee (eds): The Cervical Spine, 2nd ed. Philadelphia, JB Lippincott, 1989, pp 390–403.

55. Weidner A: Internal fixation with metal plates and screws. In the Cervical Spine Research Society Editorial Committee (eds): The Cervical Spine, 2nd ed. Philadelphia, JB Lippincott, 1989, pp 404–421.

56. An HS, Gordin R, Renner K: Anatomic considerations for plate-screw fixation of the cervical spine. Spine 16(Suppl):S548–S451, 1991.

57. Montesano PX, Jauch E, Jonsson H: Anatomic and biomechanical study of posterior cervical spine plate arthrodesis: An evaluation of two different techniques of screw placement. J Spinal Disord 5:301–305, 1992.

58. Heller JG, Carlson GD, Abitbol JJ, et al: Anatomic comparison of the Roy-Camille and Magerl techniques for screw placement in the lower cervical spine. Spine 16(Suppl):S552–S557, 1991.

59. Heller JG, Estes BT, Zaouali M, et al: Biomechanical study of screws in the lateral masses: Variables affecting pullout resistance. J Bone Joint Surg Am 78:1315–132, 1996.

60. Callahan RA, Johnson RM, Margolis RN, et al: Cervical facet fusion for control of instability following laminectomy. J Bone Joint Surg Am 59:991–1002, 1977.

61. Cattell HS, Clark GL Jr: Cervical kyphosis and instability following multiple laminectomies in children. J Bone Joint Surg Am 49:713–720, 1967.

62. Chadduck WM: Cerebellar hemorrhage complicating cervical laminectomy. Neurosurgery 9:185–189, 1981.

63. Dai L, Ni B, Yuan W, et al: Radiculopathy after laminectomy for cervical compression myelopathy. J Bone Joint Surg Br 80:846–849, 1998.

64. Eismont FJ, Weisel SW, Rothman RH: Treatment of dural tears associated with surgery. J Bone Joint Surg Am 63:1132–1136, 1981.

65. Epstein NE, Epstein JA, Benjamin V, et al: Traumatic myelopathy in patients with cervical spinal stenosis without fracture or dislocation: Methods of diagnosis management, and prognosis. Spine 5:489–496, 1980.

66. Guidetti B, Fortuna A: Long-term results of surgical treatment of myelopathy due to cervical spondylosis. J Neurosurg 30:714–721, 1969.

67. Haines SJ: Systematic antibiotic prophylaxis in neurological surgery. Neurosurgery 6:355–361, 1980.

68. Levy WJ, Dohn DF, Hardy RW: Central cord syndrome as a delayed postoperative complication of decompressive laminectomy. Neurosurgery 11:491–495, 1982.

69. Middleton TH, Al-Mefty O, Harkey LH, et al: Syringomyelia after decompressive laminectomy for cervical spondylosis. Surg Neurol 28:458–462, 1987.

70. Mikawa Y, Shikata J, Yamamuro T: Spinal deformity and instability after multilevel cervical laminectomy. Spine 12:6–11, 1987.

71. Tsuzuki N, Abe R, Saiki K, et al: Extradural tethering effect as one mechanism of radiculopathy complicating posterior decompression of the cervical spinal cord. Spine 21:203–211, 1996.

72. Yasuoka S, Peterson HA, Laws ER Jr, et al: Pathogenesis and prophylaxis of postlaminectomy deformity of the spine after multiple level laminectomy: Difference between children and adults. Neurosurgery 9:145–152, 1981.

73. Yasuoka S, Peterson HA, MacCarty CS: Incidence of spinal column deformity after multilevel laminectomy in children and adults. J Neurosurg 57:441–445, 1982.

74. Yonenobu K, Hosono N, Iwasaki M, et al: Neurologic complications of surgery for cervical compression myelopathy. Spine 16:1277–1282, 1991.

75. Yonenobu K, Okada K, Fuji T, et al: Causes of neurologic deterioration following surgical treatment of cervical myelopathy. Spine 11:818–823, 1986.

76. Kurz LT, Herkowitz HN: Modified anterior approach to the cervicothoracic junction. Paper presented at the Cervical Spine Research Society Annual Meeting, November 29, 1990, San Antonio, TX.

77. Pal GP, Routal RV: The role of the vertebral laminae in the stability of the cervical spine. J Anat 188:485–489, 1996.

78. Stoops WL, King RB: Neural complications of cervical spondylosis: Their response to laminectomy and foraminotomy. J Neurosurg 16:986–999, 1962.

79. Itoh T, Tsuji H: Technical improvements and results of laminoplasty for compressive myelopathy in the cervical spine. Spine 10:729–736, 1985.

80. Sato T: Radiological follow-up of motion in the cervical spine after surgery. J Jpn Orthop Assoc 66:607–620, 1992.

81. Kamioka Y, Yamamoto H, Tani T, et al: Postoperative instability of cervical OPLL and cervical radiculopathy. Spine 14:1177–1183, 1989.

82. Hirabayashi K, Wananabe K, Wakano K, et al: Expansive open-door laminoplasty for cervical spinal stenotic myelopathy. Spine 8:693–699, 1983.

83. Kimura I, Shingu H, Nasu Y: Long-term follow-up of cervical spondylotic myelopathy treated by canal-expansive laminoplasty. J Bone Joint Surg Br 77-B:956–961, 1995.

84. Kohno K, Kumon Y, Oka Y, et al: Evaluation of prognostic factors following expansive laminoplasty for cervical spinal stenotic myelopathy. Surg Neurol 48:237–245, 1997.

85. White AA III, Panjabi MM: Clinical Biomechanics of the Spine, 2nd ed. Philadelphia, Lippincott-Raven, 1990.

86. Ishida Y, Suzuki K, Ohmori K, et al: Critical analysis of extensive cervical laminectomy. Neurosurgery 24:215–222, 1989.

87. Jenkins DH: Extensive cervical laminectomy: Long-term results. Br J Surg 60:852–854, 1973.

88. Miyazaki K, Kirita Y: Extensive simultaneous multisegment laminectomy for myelopathy due to the ossification of the posterior longitudinal ligament in the cervical region. Spine 11: 531–542, 1986.

89. Cusick JF, Yoganandan N, Pintar FA, et al: Biomechanics of cervical spine facetectomy and fixation techniques. Spine 13: 808–812, 1988.

90. Guigui P, Benoist M, Deburge A: Spinal deformity and instability after multilevel cervical laminectomy for spondylotic myelopathy. Spine 23:440–447, 1998.

91. Zdeblick TA, Abitbol JJ, Kunz DN, et al: Cervical stability after sequential capsule resection. Spine 18:2005–2008, 1993.

92. Nowinski GP, Visarius H, Nolte LP, et al: A biomechanical comparison of cervical laminaplasty and cervical laminectomy with progressive facetectomy. Spine 18:1995–2004, 1993.

93. Panjabi MM, White AA, Johnson RM: Cervical spine biomechanics as a function of transection of components. J Biomech 8: 327–336, 1975.

94. Kumaresan S, Yoganandan N, Pintar FA, et al: Finite element modeling of cervical laminectomy with graded facetectomy. J Spinal Disord 10:40–46, 1997.

95. Voo LM, Kumaresan S, Yoganandan N, et al: Finite element analysis of cervical facetectomy. Spine 22:964–969, 1997.

96. Munechica Y: Influence of laminectomy on the stability of the spine: An experimental study with special reference to the extent of laminectomy and the resection of the intervertebral joint. J Jpn Orthop Assoc 47:111–126, 1973.

97. Epstein JA: The surgical management of cervical spinal stenosis, spondylosis and myeloradiculopathy by means of the posterior approach. Spine 13:864–869, 1988.

98. Aldrich F: Posterolateral microdiscectomy for cervical monoradiculopathy caused by posterolateral soft cervical disc sequestration. J Neurosurg 72:370–77, 1990.

99. Williams RW: Microcervical foraminotomy: A surgical alternative for intractable radicular pain. Spine 8:708–716, 1983.

100. Zeidman SM, Ducker TB: Posterior cervical laminoforaminotomy for radiculopathy: Review of 172 cases. Neurosurgery 33: 356–362, 1993.

101. Bishara SN: The posterior operation in treatment of cervical spondylosis with myelopathy: A long-term follow-up study. J Neurol Neurosurg Psychiatry 34:393–398, 1971.

102. Epstein JA, Janin Y, Carras R, et al: A comparative study of the treatment of cervical spondylotic myeloradiculopathy: Experience with 50 cases treated by means of extensive laminectomy, foraminotomy, and excision of osteophytes during the past 10 years. Acta Neurochir (Wien) 61:89–104, 1982.

103. Gonzalez FL, Peraita PP: Cervical spondylotic myelopathy: A cooperative study. Clin Neurol Neurosurg 78:19–33, 1975.

104. Gorter K: Influence of laminectomy on the course of cervical myelopathy. Acta Neurochir (Wien) 33:265–281, 1976.

105. Kurz LT, Herkowitz HN: Surgical management of myelopathy. Orthop Clin North Am 23:495–504, 1992.

106. Nurick S: The natural history and the results of surgical treatment of the spinal cord disorder associated with cervical spondylosis. Brain 95:101–108, 1972.

107. Crandall PH, Gregorius FK: Long-term follow-up of surgical treatment of cervical spondylotic myelopathy. Spine 2:139–146, 1977.

108. Gregorius FK, Estrin T, Crandall PH: Cervical spondylotic radiculopathy and myelopathy: A long-term follow-up study. Arch Neurol 33:618–625, 1976.

109. Brain WR, Northfield D, Wilkinson M: The neurological manifestations of cervical spondylosis. Brain 75:187–225, 1952.

110. Kato Y, Iwasaki M, Fuji T, et al: Long-term follow-up results of laminectomy for cervical myelopathy caused by ossification of the posterior longitudinal ligament. J Neurosurg 89:217–223, 1998.

Anterior Approach including Cervical Corpectomy

JUAN BARTOLOMEI ■ VOLKER K. H. SONNTAG

The progression of cervical spondylosis can be insidious. Patients may be relatively asymptomatic or have symptoms ranging from minor findings to significant spinal cord compression with associated myelopathic findings. Symptoms result from degenerated cervical intervertebral disks, herniated disks, bulging disks, or disk-osteophyte complexes. The radiographic incidence of cervical spondylosis has been cited as 20% to 25% for the population 50 years of age or younger and 70% to 95% for the 65-year-old age group.[1, 2] Despite radiographic findings suggesting degenerative cervical disk disease, relatively few patients are symptomatic, and most have transient episodes that respond to conservative measures.

Progress in diagnostic imaging, surgical techniques, and spinal instrumentation has changed the management of degenerative cervical spondylosis and intervertebral disk disease, but the most appropriate surgical approach and management strategy for this condition continue to be debated. This chapter addresses the pathophysiology of degenerative cervical disk disease, associated clinical symptoms, diagnostic imaging modalities, and anterior operative treatment of cervical disease and spondylosis.

HISTORICAL PERSPECTIVE

In the early 20th century, Elliot[3] first reported how arthritis in the cervical spine appeared to be responsible for compression at the neural foramina and development of radicular symptoms. Stookey[4] later identified pathologic syndromes caused by cervical disk herniations that previously were incorrectly attributed to chondromas. Stookey divided the compression of these extradural chondromas into three regions: those compressing one half of the ventral aspect of the spinal cord, those compressing both halves of the spinal cord, and those laterally compressing the nerve roots. Elsberg[5] classified these chondroma-like lesions as ecchondrosis and local hyperplasia of the cartilage. Stookey and Elsberg were the first surgeons to address the surgical removal of chronic degenerated cervical

disks. The classic paper by Mixter and Barr[6] first correlated radicular symptoms with the lateral herniation of lumbar disks. This observation generated an intense interest in the role of cervical disk degeneration and herniation in the development of cervical radiculopathy and myelopathy.

The surgical approach for the treatment of cervical disk disease has been refined in past decades. In 1955, Robinson and Smith[7] described their anterior approach for removing the disk and performing an arthrodesis with a horseshoe-shaped bone graft and later expanded the success of this technique.[8, 9] In 1958, Cloward[10] presented his technique for removing the disk and performing an interbody fusion with a cylindrical bone graft. In 1960, Bailey and Badgley[11] introduced interbody fusion through a keystone technique. In the late 1960s, Verbiest[12] expanded the anterior approach to incorporate a more anterolateral exposure for resecting the foramen transversarium and controlling the vertebral artery. These procedures have enjoyed tremendous success for the treatment of cervical spondylosis and degenerative disk disease. The advent of newer imaging modalities further improved our understanding of the natural history of cervical spondylosis, and innovative spinal instrumentation permits safe and extensive decompression with excellent clinical outcomes.

ANATOMY AND PHYSIOLOGY OF THE CERVICAL SPINE

Anatomy

The cervical segment of the spine consists of seven vertebrae. Within the cervical spine are three distinct anatomic, physiologic, and biomechanical regions. Because the cervical vertebrae bear the least weight of any spinal region, the vertebral bodies are small in relation to their respective arch and transverse foramina. The transverse diameter is greater than the anteroposterior diameter. Except for the upper two cervical vertebrae, each vertebra articulates with adjoining vertebrae at the intervertebral disk interspace and at the facet joints posteriorly. The disks are wider anteriorly than posteriorly, and this configuration creates a natural lordotic posture. Within the intervertebral space, the superior surfaces of the vertebrae turn sharply upward in a superolateral direction to form the uncinate processes.

A unique feature of cervical vertebrae is the transverse foramen, which perforates the transverse processes. The anterior aspect of the transverse process represents a fused costal joint that arises from the vertebral body. The lateral portion of the transverse process contains two projections referred to as the anterior and posterior tubercles. The anterior tubercle serves as the origin of the anterior cervical musculature, and the posterior tubercle serves as the origin and insertion of the posterior musculature. The spinal nerves exit through a deep groove within the tubercles. As it traverses from C6 to the skull base, the vertebral artery is located anterior to the spinal nerve roots.

The articulation between vertebral bodies is formed by the disks. Intervertebral disks consist of a semifluid gelatinous matrix, the nucleus pulposus, surrounded by the annulus fibrosus. The intervertebral disk adheres firmly to the vertebral bodies by the cartilaginous end plate. More posteriorly, the position of the nucleus pulposus is slightly eccentric. In younger age groups, the nucleus pulposus has a high water content. With time, however, it dehydrates, leading to degeneration. The annulus fibrosus consists of well-defined fibrous lamellae that adhere strongly to the vertebral end plate. In addition to containing the nucleus pulposus, the annulus fibrosus withstands considerable shearing and tensile forces from all directions. The annulus fibrosus is innervated by the sinuvertebral nerve, which may play a role in the origin of diskogenic pain.[13]

The intervertebral disk is supported by the anterior longitudinal ligament (ALL) and posterior longitudinal ligament (PLL). The ALL is stronger than the PLL. The PLL is formed by two bands of fibers. The superficial fibers extend through several vertebral bodies and are attached to their posterior midline. A deeper band extends no more than two vertebral segments and attaches itself firmly into the disks. Laterally, the PLL becomes thinner and does not extend completely to the lateral margins of the disk. These features make this region more susceptible to disk herniations. Lateral disk herniations can compress exiting nerve roots and cause radiculopathy. Central compression of the spinal cord can occur with central disk herniation and the concomitant development of osteophytes from adjacent vertebral bodies. In some instances, multisegmental ossification of the PLL can also cause severe spinal cord compression.

Biomechanics

Within the cervical spine, several functional regions are responsible for motion. Approximately 40% of axial rotation occurs at the atlantoaxial joints. The anatomic configuration of the atlantoaxial joint, which is stabilized by the transverse and alar ligaments, permits

only rotation. The remaining axial rotation is evenly distributed among the subaxial vertebrae, but the middle and lower (C4-7) segments provide the most motion, in part because of the orientation of their facets. Almost 30% to 50% of flexion occurs at the occipital-C2 region; the remaining force is distributed unevenly throughout the spine, with the lower cervical segments being mostly responsible for flexion.[14]

The height of the intervertebral disk accounts for about one fourth of the total height of the cervical spine. The lenticular shape of the disk in the sagittal dimension permits the disk to slide forward. The superior vertebral body overrides the inferior one to increase flexion. Cervical lateral flexion is partially limited by the large pars articularis, intertransverse ligaments, and orientation of the facets. During lateral flexion, considerable coupling related to the horizontal orientation of the facets provides lateral support and increases lateral rigidity. The anatomic configuration of the facet in conjunction with large lateral masses makes hyperextension injuries associated with slight head rotation devastating.

Pathophysiology

Most reports on the natural history of cervical spondylosis were published before the advent of contemporary imaging techniques and do not accurately represent the natural history of cervical spondylosis.[15–21] Newer imaging techniques, however, are improving our understanding of the natural history and progression of symptomatic cervical spondylosis and cervical pathophysiology. Gore and colleagues[1] reported that the radiographic incidence of cervical spondylosis in asymptomatic patients was about 95% for men and 70% for women in the seventh decade of life.

The onset of symptoms usually occurs in the sixth decade, and men are affected more than women. C5-6 and C6-7 are the levels most involved because of their relatively extensive range of motion. The onset of symptoms is usually insidious, with long periods of stabilization and intermittent episodes of decline. The outcome of symptomatic cervical spondylosis depends on the severity of radiculopathy and myelopathic signs and on the age of patients when they seek treatment.[15, 16, 19, 21]

Development of cervical spondylosis is a consequence of disk degeneration and dynamic processes. The vertebra of the cervical spine contains five joints: two zygapophyseal (facets) joints, two neurocentral (Luschka) joints, and the intervertebral disk. The anatomic configuration of the facet joints allows a significant degree of motion in flexion and extension and permits some lateral bending. Moreover, the shape of the intervertebral disk in conjunction with its interface with the end plates of the adjacent vertebra permits flexion, extension, lateral bending, and shearing motion. The neurocentral joints are located laterally. They confine the intervertebral disk and closely abut the superior end plate of the adjacent vertebral body with little cushioning. Progressive degeneration of these joints leads to compression of the exiting nerve root and clinical symptoms of radiculopathy.

The anatomy of the cervical spine and its relationship to the neural elements are unique compared with other regions of the spine. The cross-sectional area of the cervical spinal canal is almost entirely occupied by the spinal cord and exiting nerve roots. In contrast, the lumbar region is mostly occupied by nerve roots. This anatomic relationship, coupled with increasing cervical motion, makes the cervical spine vulnerable to small degenerative changes that may manifest clinically.[22, 23]

Degeneration of any disk is a dynamic process that begins with the loss of absorptive and viscoelastic properties due to dehydration and changes in proteoglycans. Events that increase motion, chronic heavy use, and smoking can accelerate these degenerative changes. Disk dehydration alters the biomechanical properties. The resulting loss of height and annular bulging make the disk and end plates more vulnerable to injury. Altered physical demands on the disk produce gradual fibrocartilaginous changes that blur the boundaries between the nucleus pulposus and the annulus fibrosus until they are indistinguishable. These biomechanical changes can increase segmental motion, thereby accelerating degeneration.

As degeneration ensues, fissures in the annulus make the disk more susceptible to herniation and narrow its height. As the disk narrows, the facet joints override each other, and the neurocentral joints rub against the superior end plates. Reparative efforts between adjacent end plates and the joints cause sclerosis of subchondral bone and the formation of osteophytes. As the extent of contact surfaces and the transfer of force to equilibrate the new biomechanical demands increase, the surfaces expand and form disk-osteophyte complexes that constrict the neural foramen and spinal canal.[19, 23–25]

Unlike lumbar nerve roots that exit the foramen after a long, oblique course, cervical nerve roots exit through the neural foramen in a more direct, short, transverse route. Moreover, the cervical neural foramen is mostly filled by the nerve root. These features make it difficult for nerve roots to accommodate a decrease in the surface area of their foraminal exit. Consequently, clinical radiculopathy can be associated with an insignificantly small to moderately sized bone spur. Another potential cause of a disk-osteophyte complex is calcified, herniated disk material.[26] Overt trauma may exacerbate symptoms of cervical spondylosis, but its association with the development of cervical spondylosis has not been clearly established.[27]

As a degenerating disk fails biomechanically, load shared by the facets increases. Together with the ligamentum flavum, these structures become hypertrophied, further compromising the spinal canal posteriorly and the neural foramen.[28] As the facet joints degenerate, this region becomes incompetent in response to shear stresses, leading to spondylolisthesis or retrolisthesis. Posterior disk-osteophyte complexes form from the inferior articular joint and may further constrict the dimensions of the intervertebral foramen, leading to clinical symptoms.[29] Occasionally, disk-osteophyte complexes become quite large but remain clinically silent. However, in individuals with congeni-tal cervical stenosis, relatively small osteophytes can compromise a large percentage of the spinal canal, producing significant clinical findings. Patients with spinal canals larger than 13 mm in the anteroposterior dimension rarely develop symptomatic cervical myelopathy.[30, 31]

In addition to anatomic constraints, the area of the cervical canal changes during flexion and extension.[28, 32] During flexion, the spinal cord lengthens and bows anteriorly, abutting the posterior surfaces of the vertebral column.[33] In the presence of a posteriorly displaced osteophytic complex, the spinal cord stretches over these bars. As documented in autopsy studies, chronic changes develop.[28, 33] Local changes in areas of significant compression may affect the physiologic state of local neurons or axons through compressive forces or vascular compromise (venous or arterial).[28, 30, 34]

During extension, the posterior elements become a critical factor in the development of cervical stenosis. Extension of the cervical spine allows the ligamentum flavum to buckle inward, and it shortens the cross-sectional area available for the spinal cord. The spinal cord also shortens during extension, increasing its cross-sectional area and further compromising the cervical canal.[30, 35] In patients with degenerated disks, loss of height, disk-osteophyte complexes, and hypertrophied joints occur, as seen in the elderly population, and extension injuries can be neurologically devastating.[36]

The overriding hypertrophied facets narrow the foramen, impaling the exiting nerve roots. The size of the foramen can be further compromised by lateral bending and flexion, which cause radicular symptoms.[30]

The critical size of the spinal canal and foramen responsible for clinical symptoms is difficult to characterize with current imaging modalities. The anatomic and local biomechanical factors that are responsible for the development of these symptoms must be evaluated carefully on an individual basis.[28, 37] Excessive motion can cause ligamentous laxity and segmental instability, contributing to myelopathic symptoms. The ligaments become incompetent and hypertrophied, and this condition is usually seen adjacent to surgically or degenerated fused levels. Excessive segmental loading results in degenerative subluxations that further compromise the spinal canal.[38, 39]

CLINICAL MANIFESTATIONS

Clinical symptoms of cervical spondylosis can develop in an insidious fashion and may include axial neck pain, occipital pain, shoulder pain, radiculopathy, and myelopathy. Axial neck pain can result from segmental instability caused by disk degeneration and from direct nerve root compression. Myofascial syndromes have also been implicated in the development of axial neck pain.[40] Occipital pain has been attributed to arthritic changes or instability at the C1 and C2 junction, resulting in compression of the exiting C2 nerve root.[41] Shoulder pain may be related to cervical disk degeneration, brachial neuritis, or nerve root compression at C3, C4, or C5.[42–45]

The symptoms of cervical radiculopathy follow a specific dermatomal pattern corresponding to the involved nerve root. These features can include the loss of motor strength, decreased reflexes, loss of sensation, and well-delineated pain along the dermatome of the nerve root. The most common radiculopathies involve the C5, C6, and C7 nerve roots.[22, 46] C5 nerve root compression manifests as pain or loss of sensation along the shoulder region and proximal aspect of the arm laterally. Patients usually complain of an inability to abduct their arm and difficulty placing objects overhead. Examination usually reveals deltoid weakness, and the biceps occasionally may be involved by weakness in the external rotators of the shoulder.

C6 nerve root compression usually manifests with radiating symptoms from the neck into the biceps and extends into the thumb and index finger. Weakness of the biceps and wrist extensor and a depressed biceps and brachioradialis reflex may also be present. C7 nerve root compression is common because of the excessive motion possible at C6-7. Patients with C7 radiculopathy often complain of radiating pain down the posterior and posterolateral aspects of their arm, shoulder, and scapular region and distally along the triceps into the middle finger. Patients experience weakness of the triceps, pronator, and pectoralis muscles and a depressed triceps reflex. Wrist flexion and finger extension also may be weak.

C8 radiculopathies typically are associated with radiating symptoms along the ulnar distribution into the small finger. Because the C8 nerve root supplies many of the hand muscles, particularly the interossei, hand grasp is usually weak and patients often report an inability to hold objects. Because the C8 nerve has more motor fibers than sensory fibers, weakness is more common than pain.

T1 radicular symptoms usually follow a distribution similar to that of C8. However, the sensory symptoms do not extend into the hands, except for a subtle weakness of the intrinsic hand musculature.

In all cases of radiculopathy, the clinician can attempt to elicit radiating symptoms through provocative maneuvers. Spurling's maneuver, performed by slight extension with lateral bending toward the symptomatic side and axial compression, can exacerbate and elicit radicular symptoms along a compromised nerve root.

Cervical disk disease and spondylosis may be associated with myelopathy. Patients typically exhibit subtle changes in their gait, which tends to be broad based, stumbling, spastic, and ataxic. Patients report difficulties going up an incline, buckling of their legs, and sensory disturbances in their extremities proximally. They also may report profound weakness and clumsiness of their hands, difficulty with writing and joint position sensing, fine tremor, chronic and ill-defined numbness, and intrinsic musculature dysfunction. Persons with cervical disk disease may have bowel or bladder dysfunction characterized by urinary incontinence or retention. During flexion and extension, pa-

tients often report electrical shock sensations up and down the spine, known as Lhermitte's sign. This sign usually indicates severe spinal cord compression and a dynamic component, possibly with incompetent structural support.

Physical findings in myelopathic patients include lower motor neuron disease at the level of the lesion and upper motor neuron disease below the level of the lesion. Hoffman's sign may be elicited by flicking the middle finger and observing flexion contractions of the thumb and index finger. Reflex abnormalities may include hyporeflexia at the level of the compromised nerve root and hyperreflexia distally. Other findings may include altered suspended sensory disturbances, diffuse spasticity, diffuse hand weakness, proximal lower extremity weakness, clonus, and Babinski's sign. The differential diagnosis of patients with symptoms of cervical spondylosis who may have myelopathy can include intrinsic medullary tumors, syringomyelia, multiple sclerosis, extramedullary tumors in the cervical or thoracic spine, subacute combined degeneration, hereditary spastic paraplegia, amyotrophic lateral sclerosis (ALS), normal-pressure hydrocephalus, and arteriovenous malformations.[2, 20, 27, 47–49]

Unusual presentations of cervical spondylosis can include Brown-Séquard syndrome with ipsilateral hemiparesis, contralateral sensory loss to pain and temperature, and ipsilateral loss of joint perception.[50] Although rare, an anterior spinal artery syndrome can result from thrombosis caused by compression of this vessel. This syndrome is associated with complete loss of motor and sensation below the lesion with preserved joint and vibratory sensation. Vertebrobasilar insufficiency, manifested by nausea, vertigo, dizziness, and visual disturbances, also has resulted from osteophytic overgrowth in the transverse foramen.[51, 52] Anterior osteophytic spurs can grow quite large and cause dysphagia. This condition, however, is rare because osteophytes grow slowly and the esophagus is flexible and mobile.[53, 54]

DIAGNOSTIC STUDIES

The diagnosis of cervical spondylotic myelopathy and radiculopathy includes the use of radiologic or electrophysiologic studies. Radiographic evaluation of cervical disease begins with comprehensive plain radiographic studies that include anteroposterior, lateral, and oblique views. Swimmer's views are used to assess the cervicothoracic junction. Flexion and extension views can be helpful in patients with a history of trauma, evidence of spondylolisthesis, and prior surgical fusions. Plain radiographs must be evaluated carefully for the presence of congenital stenosis, misalignment, degenerative changes, and instability. A spinal canal less than 12 mm in diameter is considered to be abnormally narrow. One difficulty in relying on plain radiographs is the almost ubiquitous findings of cervical spondylosis in the aging population and the presence of degenerative changes in asymptomatic patients.[1, 32, 55, 56] Moreover, plain radiographs are inadequate for the assessment of soft tissue compression, such as ligamentous and disk herniations.

Magnetic resonance imaging (MRI) has become the mainstay for assessing cervical degenerative changes. It is rapid and accurate without the use of ionizing radiation. It has become the preferred method for screening patients with suspected radiculopathy or myelopathy (Fig. 288–1).[57–59] MRI clearly visualizes neural elements and the ligamentous and soft tissue structures. High-intensity signals within the spinal cord occur in areas of severe compression and suggest intrinsic neural damage, which has implications for postoperative prognosis.[34, 60–62] MRI can provide excellent visualization of ligamentous disruption caused by trauma.[63] MRI demonstrates the cervical spine in a multiplanar fashion, facilitating visualization and ana-

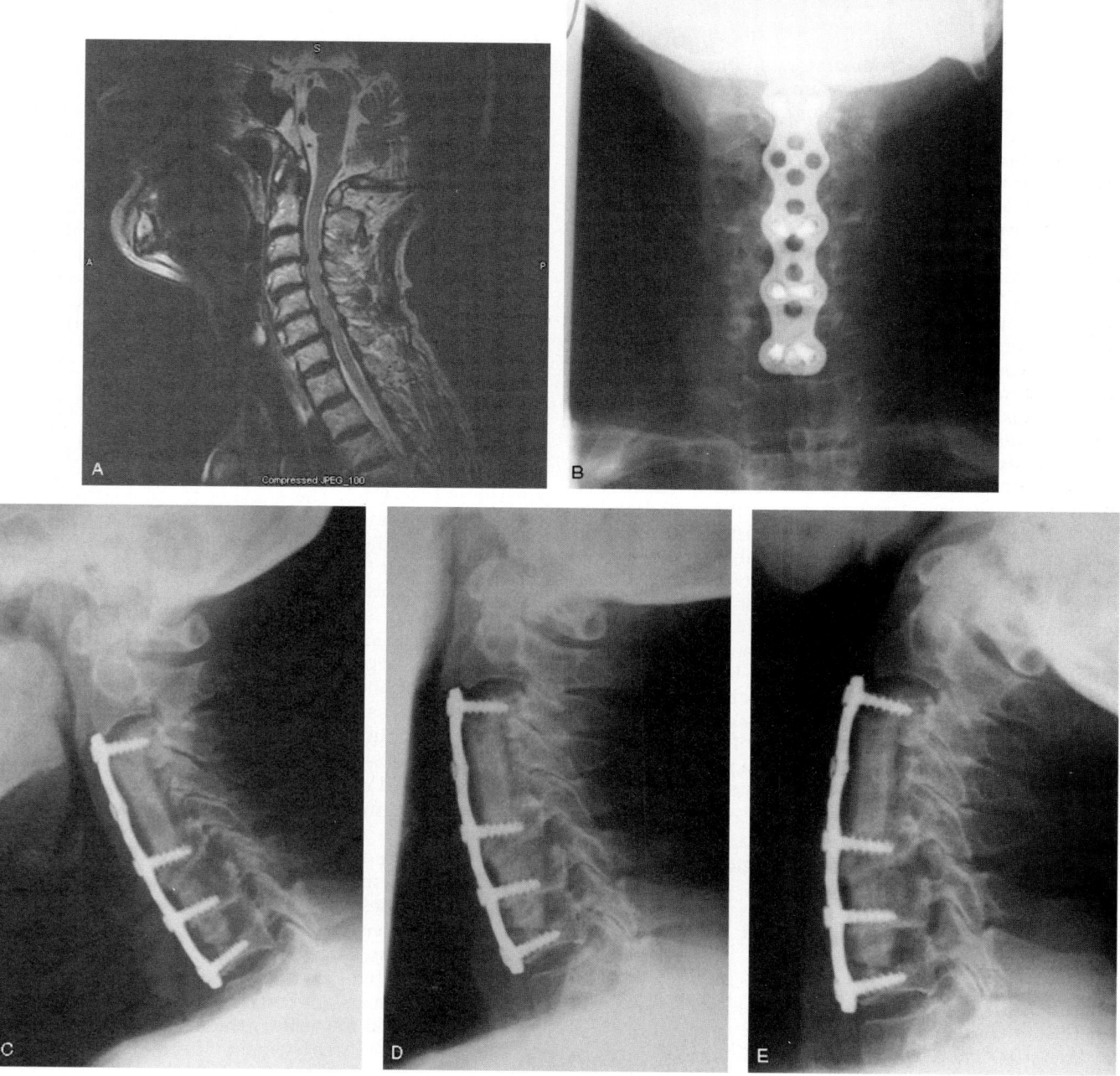

FIGURE 288–1. A 65-year-old woman with a 2-month history of gait ataxia, hand numbness, and urinary incontinence was found to have multilevel cervical stenosis on T2-weighted sagittal magnetic resonance imaging *(A).* She underwent a C4 corpectomy with C5-6 and C6-7 diskectomies with allograft fusion and plating *(B).* Postoperatively, she had a short course of physical therapy, and her symptoms resolved completely. Lateral radiographs at 6 months show the incorporation of the allograft with no evidence of motion in flexion *(C),* neutral *(D),* and extension *(E)* views.

tomic definition of disks, neural foramina, and their compression of exiting nerve roots. MRI can visualize bone marrow changes that suggest neoplastic, degenerative, inflammatory, or infectious processes, and it is a valuable tool for postoperative evaluation. However, MRI cannot adequately assess bony or osseous features, which should be imaged with computed tomography (CT).

CT provides cross-sectional views of the cervical spine, allowing clear visualization of disk-osteophyte complexes and calcified ridges. Myelography with injection of water-soluble contrast into the subarachnoid space delineates the spinal cord and segmental nerve roots. Lateral and anteroposterior radiographs provide limited definition of compressive lesions. However, the combination of cervical myelography with postmyelography CT provides excellent definition of osteophytic ridges, herniated disks, and their relationships to the nerve roots and spinal cord. In cases of severe compression, CT–myelography allows visualization distal to myelographic blocks.[64] CT–myelography is complementary to MRI for patients suffering from an ossified PLL and for those with prior instrumented fusions. In some instances, CT–myelography has provided enough definition to avoid vertebrectomy, thereby providing another point of fixation for the instrumentation and enhancing stability.

Electrodiagnostic studies can also be used to evaluate patients with radiculopathy or myelopathy. These tests include electromyography (EMG), nerve conduction velocity (NCV), and somatosensory evoked potentials (SSEP). These studies are usually performed when there are discrepancies between clinical and radiographic findings or when other underlying conditions, such as ALS, multiple sclerosis, or peripheral neuropathy, are suspected. EMG and NCV are performed concomitantly and can differentiate among radiculopathy, peripheral nerve pathology, and brachial plexus pathology. All of these electrodiagnostic tools suffer from a lack of specificity and sensitivity to localize or grade the extent of compression. In selected cases, SSEP changes may serve as an objective measurement of the progression of cervical spondylosis.[65] In their model of chronic spinal cord compression, Al-Mefty and coworkers[34] found that changes in SSEP existed almost immediately before or at the time of neurological presentation. Preoperative diagnostic images must be evaluated carefully to ensure proper surgical planning.

OPERATIVE TECHNIQUE FOR THE ANTERIOR APPROACH

On the morning of surgery, informed consent is obtained, and unless contraindicated (e.g., history of trauma), the patient is asked to extend and flex his or her neck voluntarily to assess for any clinical symptoms. In this way, the surgeon and anesthesiologist can limit their manipulations and not exceed the patient's own range of motion. The anesthesiologist can also determine if flexible fiberoptic intubation is necessary.

After the patient is placed on the operating table, the anesthesiologist secures the airway through orotracheal access. When fiberoptic intubation is used, the patient is intubated while awake but under conscious sedation and local anesthesia. After the patient is anesthetized, SSEP leads are placed so that functional feedback can be obtained during surgery. Appropriate venous access is obtained, and the patient is secured to the bed in a supine position.

After the leads are placed, the patient's neck is extended slightly. A small towel roll may be placed in the interscapular space, or the patient can be placed in a Caspar head holder (Aesculap, San Francisco, CA) (Fig. 288–2). Five- to 10-pound traction may be placed with the use of Gardner-Well tongs or an occipitomental traction device.

The shoulders are taped to the foot of the bed or hands wrapped with a Kerlix bandage. Securing the shoulders provides traction if the lower spine needs to be visualized radiographically. The Kerlix bandage allows the hands to be pulled to help visualize the lower cervical spine. Care is exerted to avoid overstretching the shoulder to prevent a brachial plexus injury. Neurovascular structures at risk for compression are padded carefully. One dose of prophylactic, intravenous antibiotics is administered before the skin incision is made.

Surface landmarks do not correspond to exact levels of the cervical spine but do provide general reference points. The cricothyroid membrane identifies the C6 vertebral level. The thyroid cartilage corresponds to C3-4, and the space halfway between these two points corresponds to C4-5. The angle of the jaw corresponds to C2-3. For skin incisions, a distance of two fingerbreadths above the clavicle usually corresponds to C6-7, and a distance of three fingerbreadths corresponds to C4-5. The C6 anterior tubercle can be palpated in thin patients. C-arm fluoroscopy can also be used to determine where the skin incision should be made.

The side of approach depends on the surgeon's preference. Right-handed surgeons prefer operating from the right. A possible disadvantage of operating from the right is a recurrent laryngeal nerve with an aberrant course. On the left side, the thoracic duct may be in the surgical field in the lower spine. Patients with vocal cord paralysis must be approached from the side of paralysis.

For simple one- or two-level diskectomies, a transverse incision is made along a skin crease. When multilevel diskectomies or corpectomies are considered, the border of the sternocleidomastoid is incised obliquely (Fig. 288–3). The transverse incision should be 5 or 6 cm long and extend medially near the anatomic midline. After the incision is delineated, the area is prepared and draped in sterile fashion. If an autograft will be harvested, the area (usually the left iliac crest) is also prepared for surgical access.

The platysma muscle is divided sharply along its fibers or along the axis of the transverse incision. The platysma muscle is undermined with sharp dissection to permit adequate access to the deeper surgical field. Undermining also minimizes superficial tension that

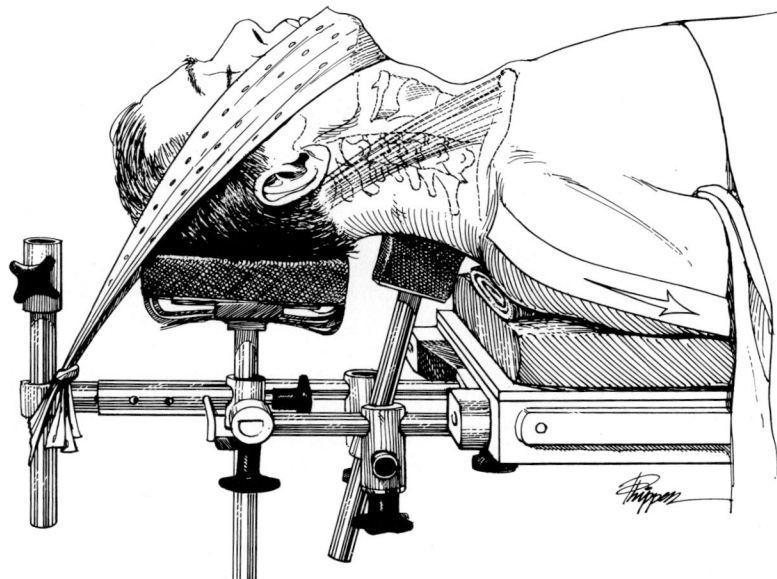

FIGURE 288–2. The patient is positioned using the Caspar head holder. The patient's head is maintained in a neutral position and secured by an elastic band around the chin and attached to the frame. Cervical lordosis can be recreated by positioning the mobile neck holder in the middle or lower cervical region and by providing slight pressure to the posterior aspect of the neck. The shoulder can be taped to the frame or pulled down from the bottom of the table to improve visualization of the lower cervical region. (Courtesy of the Barrow Neurological Institute, Phoenix, AZ.)

can rotate retractors. Reapproximation of this layer during closure is important for cosmesis.

Deep to the platysma muscle lies the anterior jugular plexus. The veins can be ligated or mobilized. The medial border of the sternocleidomastoid is identified under the platysma muscle. The muscle may be mobilized with blunt dissection and retracted laterally. The laryngeal strap muscles are also identified and carefully mobilized medially. In an extended exposure of the lower cervical spine, the omohyoid muscle may be in the surgical field. This muscle can be divided to help the exposure.

After the sternocleidomastoid muscle is mobilized using digital palpation, the surgeon can feel the pulsations of the carotid artery. The carotid sheath is re-

tracted laterally with Cloward retractors, and the trachea and esophagus are retracted medially (Fig. 288–4A). The pretracheal and prevertebral facial layers are identified and easily dissected to expose the spine. The longus colli muscles are identified laterally, and the ALLs overlie the anterior aspect of the cervical spine. At this point, a bayonetted spinal needle is placed in the disk space, and lateral radiographs are obtained to identify the level of interest (Fig. 288–5A).

After the correct level is identified, the longus colli muscle is dissected laterally off the anterior vertebral body with bipolar cauterization and periosteal elevators. The muscle is mobilized from its medial insertion in a rostrocaudal direction to provide about 20 mm of exposure of the anterior aspect of the vertebral body

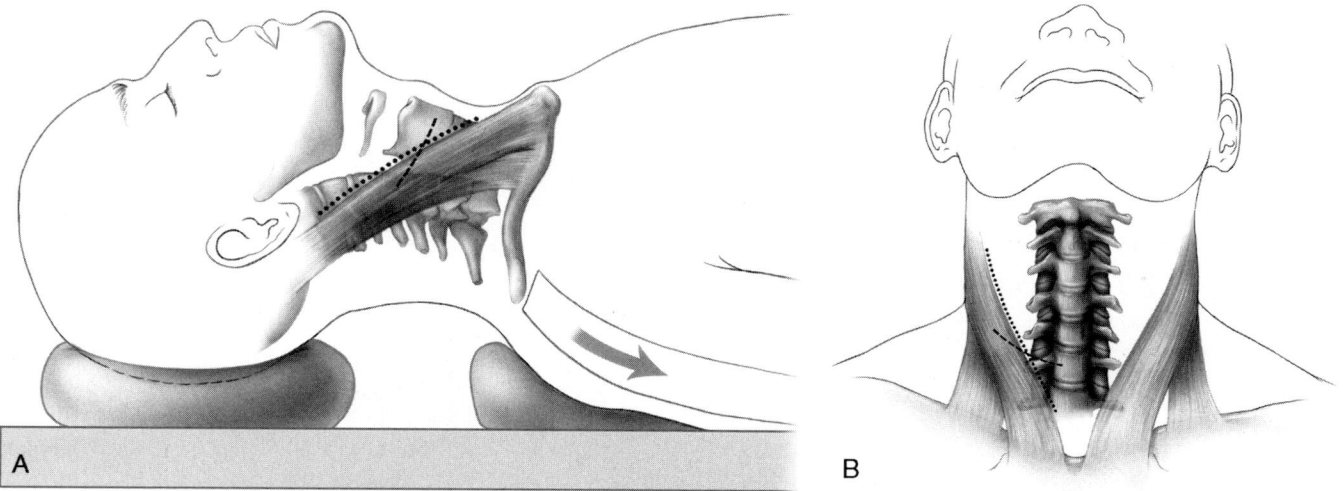

FIGURE 288–3. Lateral *(A)* and anterior *(B)* views of the patient's position and planned skin incisions for single- or two-level diskectomies *(dashed line)* and multilevel diskectomies or corpectomies *(dotted line)*. (Courtesy of the Barrow Neurological Institute, Phoenix, AZ.)

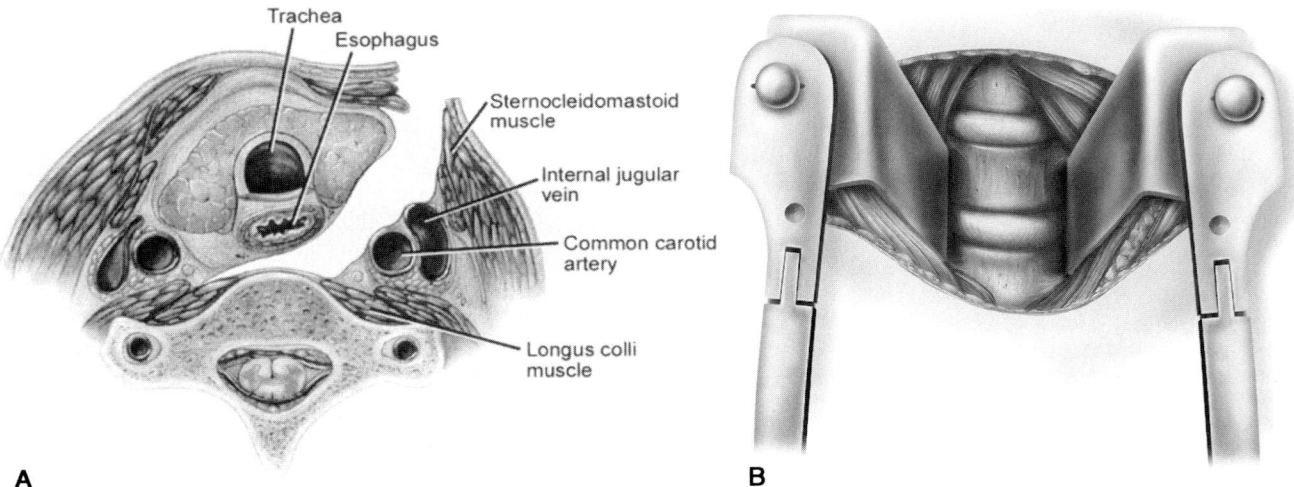

FIGURE 288–4. *A,* Axial views of the surgically relevant anatomic structures and plane of dissection. The carotid sheath and jugular vein are gently retracted laterally while the esophagus and trachea are mobilized medially. *B,* The longus colli muscles are mobilized laterally, and self-retaining retractors are placed under their medial border to obtain a full view of the anterior cervical spine. (Courtesy of the Barrow Neurological Institute, Phoenix, AZ.)

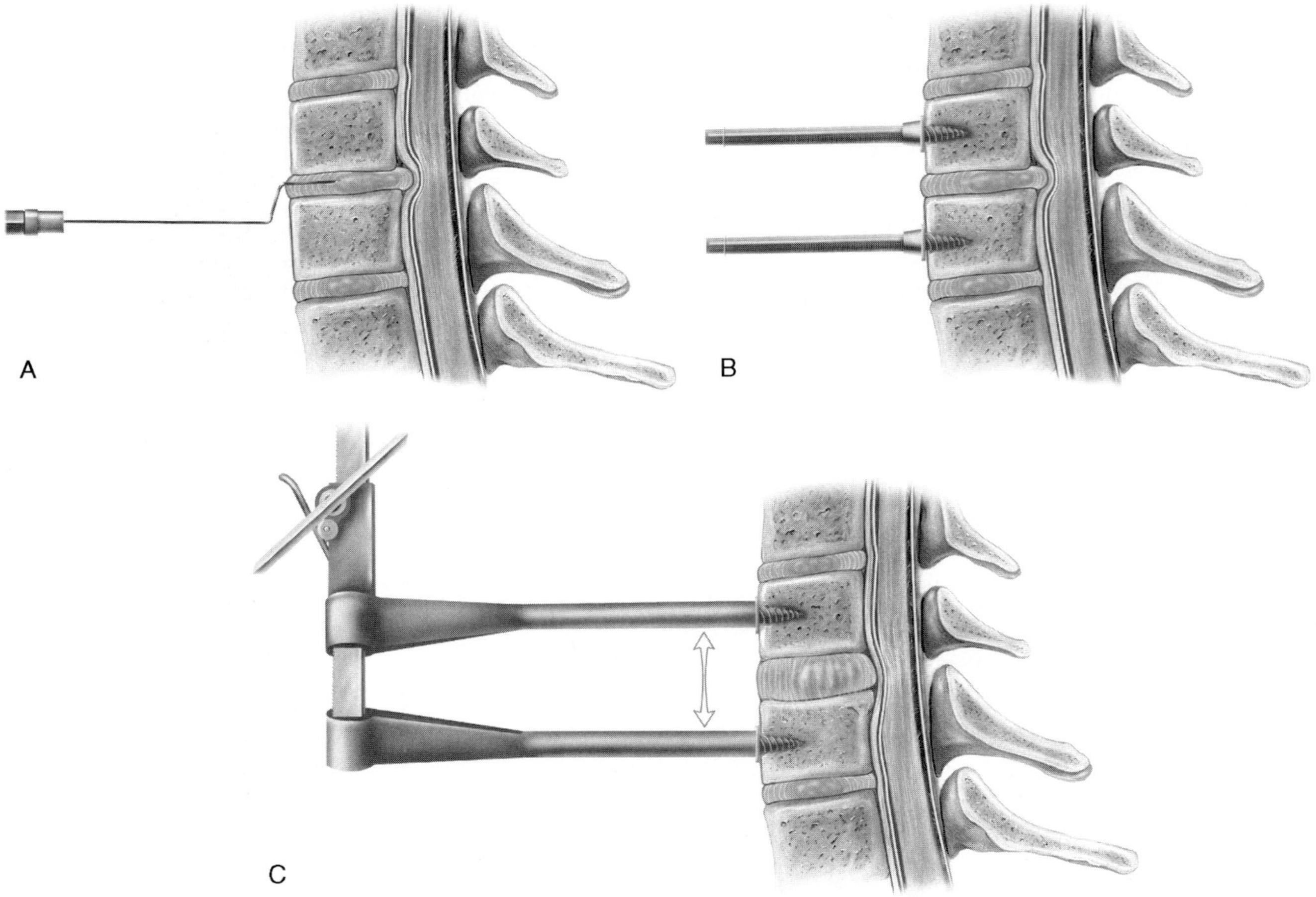

FIGURE 288–5. *A,* A bayonetted spinal needle is placed at the desired level, and a radiograph is obtained to confirm the level. *B,* A Caspar pin retractor is placed in the middle of the vertebral body. *C,* An interbody spreader helps distract the collapsed disk space. (Courtesy of the Barrow Neurological Institute, Phoenix, AZ.)

or disk, or both. Aggressive dissection of the muscle can disrupt the sympathetic fibers that course along its medial edge or inadvertently injure the vertebral artery.[66, 67]

After the muscle is mobilized, self-retaining retractors are placed with the teeth of the retractor under the muscle (see Fig. 288–4B). Placing the retractors incorrectly can cause excessive retraction on the esophagus and carotid artery. A second set of retractors can be placed in a rostrocaudal direction to gain full exposure of the area of interest. Alternatively, Caspar distracting pins can be placed at the midlevel of the vertebral body to obtain adequate exposure and to provide distraction that facilitates identification of the intervertebral space (see Fig. 288–5B and C).

Diskectomy and Corpectomy

After the anterior aspect of the spine is exposed, the microscope is brought into the surgical field for the diskectomy. The diskectomy begins by removing the anterior aspect of the annulus fibrosis circumferentially with a sharp knife (Fig. 288–6). The superficial disk is resected with curets and pituitary rongeurs. When significant osteophytic ridges are present, a high-speed, small-diameter bur is used to approach the PLL cautiously. A mental picture of the midline is necessary to avoid wandering too far laterally. The Luschka joints are excellent anatomic landmarks that help the surgeon to avoid inadvertent injury to the vertebral artery, which lies immediately lateral to the joint.

The PLL is identified and removed to determine whether any subligamentous disk material is present. The safest way to elevate the PLL is by placing a blunt hook in the lateralmost aspect of the canal near the exit of the nerve root, where the PLL is weakest and thinnest. Sometimes, resection and drilling of the Luschka joint must be extended laterally. After the PLL is elevated, it can be resected safely with up-biting curets or small Kerrison punches that do not compromise the spinal canal during their insertion.

Central disk-osteophyte complexes can be removed safely by using 1- to 2-mm Kerrison punches and minimizing their protrusion into the spinal canal. Alternatively, osteophytes can be thinned, elevated, and removed with up-biting curets. In patients with radiculopathy, decompression of the foramen must be ample; drilling the foramen and resecting the Luschka joints may be required to visualize the exiting nerve root clearly (Fig. 288–7). Nerve root decompression can also be confirmed by palpating the pedicle of the lower cervical vertebrae with a blunt hook. Bleeding from epidural veins is controlled with low-powered bipolar coagulation devices or Avitene (MecChem, Woburn, MA).

When a corpectomy is performed, diskectomies are performed above and below the corpectomy sites to obtain a visual gauge of where the spinal canal lies (Fig. 288–8). The longus colli muscle is dissected laterally until the body begins to curve laterally and posterolaterally. The vertebrectomy can begin by using a narrow Leksell rongeur spanning from one disk to

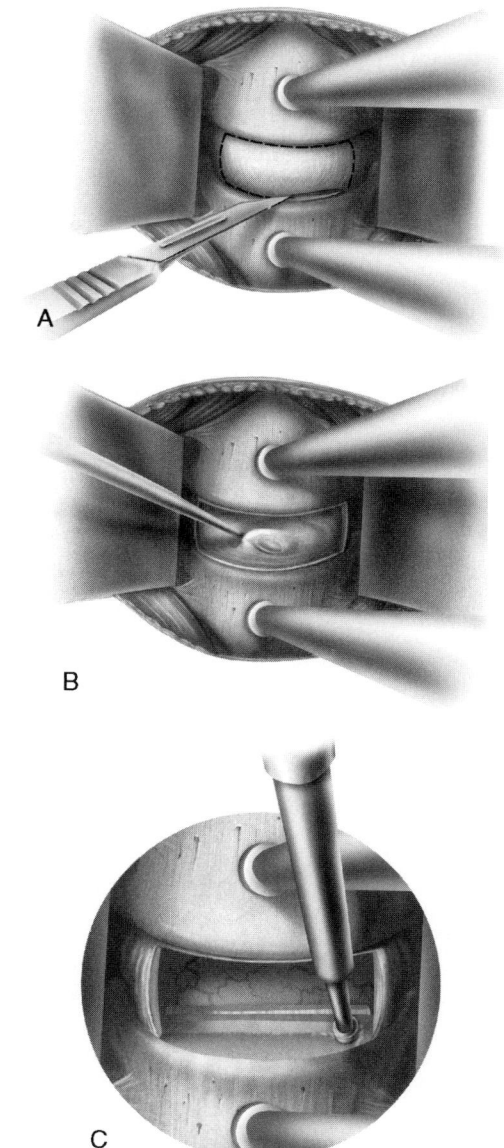

FIGURE 288–6. *A,* After the area of interest is identified, the diskectomy begins with dissection of the annulus with a no. 11 blade. *B,* The disk material is removed with curets or pituitary rongeurs. Distraction is applied, and the posterior longitudinal ligament is resected with curets or thin-plated Kerrison rongeurs. *C,* The end plates are prepared by removing the cartilaginous surface with curets or a high-speed drill. A small posterior shelf is created to prevent retromigration of the graft into the spinal canal. (Courtesy of the Barrow Neurological Institute, Phoenix, AZ.)

another. The remaining corpectomy can be performed by using a high-speed drill and drilling deep into the posterior cortex. At this point, the cortex is elevated by using up-biting curets, and the PLL is identified posteriorly. Large emissary and epidural veins are carefully controlled by bipolar coagulation. At levels of severe compression, osteophytic ridges that may be adherent to the underlying dura are dissected carefully.

After the central decompression is completed, 1- to

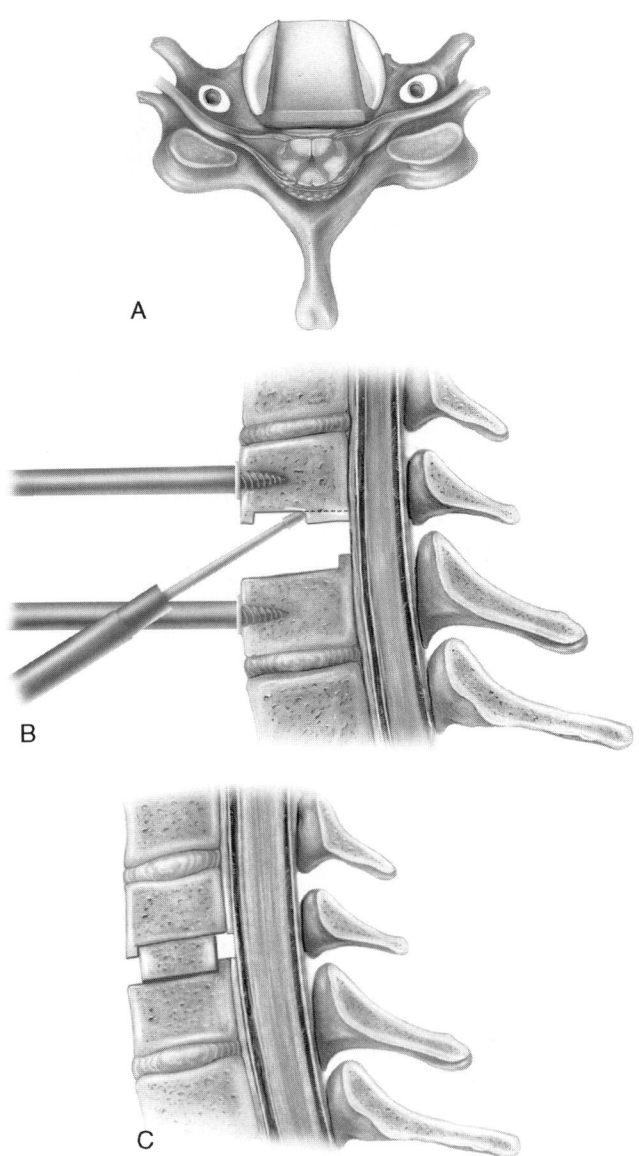

FIGURE 288–7. *A,* Axial view of the final appearance of the operative site after diskectomy. The posterior longitudinal ligament has been removed, decompressing the spinal canal. The foramen is also removed after an osteophytectomy. *B,* Sagittal view of the operative site. The end plates are prepared with a high-speed drill to avoid retrograde and anterograde migration of the graft. *C,* The graft is placed under compression. (Courtesy of the Barrow Neurological Institute, Phoenix, AZ.)

2-mm Kerrison punches are used to widen the canal from pedicle to pedicle. A decompression spanning 15 to 20 mm typically provides ample space. At the level of the vertebral body, extensive lateral dissection is unnecessary because myelopathy is a central phenomenon and because radiculopathy, a more lateral phenomenon, is addressed during the diskectomy portion of the decompression.

Fusion

After the diskectomy or corpectomy is performed, the end plates are prepared to enhance bony fusion. Three types of fusion techniques, which have been modified over the past decades, can be used after diskectomy. The Cloward technique uses a cylindrical bone dowel from the iliac crest or a specially prepared iliac allograft.[10] The surgeon prepares the diskectomy site by drilling a circular hole 10 to 14 mm deep and 12 to 16 mm in diameter. The bone graft mostly sits on soft cancellous bone, predisposing it to a slight degree of collapse compared with the other techniques. Despite this minor disadvantage, the Cloward technique effectively deals with cervical disk disease.

Another technique, popularized by Simmons and Bhalla,[68] uses a keystone-shaped graft. The graft is seated in a triangularly shaped notch located at each end plate and oriented posteriorly. With the use of intraoperative traction, the graft is fitted and locked into place preventing its migration posteriorly or anteriorly. Similar to Cloward's technique, a substantial portion of the graft sits on soft cancellous bone, which predisposes the graft to settling and potential kyphosis.

The most commonly used procedure is the Smith and Robinson technique with various modifications. This technique uses a horseshoe-shaped graft seated on stronger subchondral bone that resists settling to some degree. The height of the graft is 6 to 10 mm. Initially, end plates were prepared by perforating them with curets to enhance fusion across the graft. New modifications use a drill to create bleeding surfaces without complete resection of the end plates. A 1- to 2-mm posterior shelf of bone is created in the superior aspect of the inferior vertebral body to prevent migration of the graft into the spinal canal. A lip is left in the inferior end plate of the superior vertebral body to prevent anterior dislodgment of the graft. For corpectomy sites, the end plates are prepared in a similar fashion as for diskectomy.

The use of allograft or autograft from the iliac crest or fibula depends on the surgeon's preferences and experience. Careful preparation of the end plate ensures successful incorporation of the graft and prevents it from being dislodged.[69, 70] Meticulous attention is needed to measure the height of the graft accurately and to modify it to preserve normal cervical lordosis.

In diskectomy and corpectomy, the grafts are placed while the end plates are distracted. After the graft is placed, the distraction is removed slowly to provide compression along the graft site to enhance fusion according to Wolfe's law. Lateral radiographs are obtained to assess for evidence of overdistraction that could cause postoperative pain and to confirm good bone-to-graft surface contact.

Plating

A variety of plates are available for the cervical spine. The intention of this chapter is not to promote one or discuss in detail any particular plating system. The basic principles of anterior instrumentation and plating are discussed. Some of the advantages of cervical plating include increased segmental stiffness, prevention of graft-related complications, and restoration of cervical lordosis. Fusion success rates with anterior cervical plat-

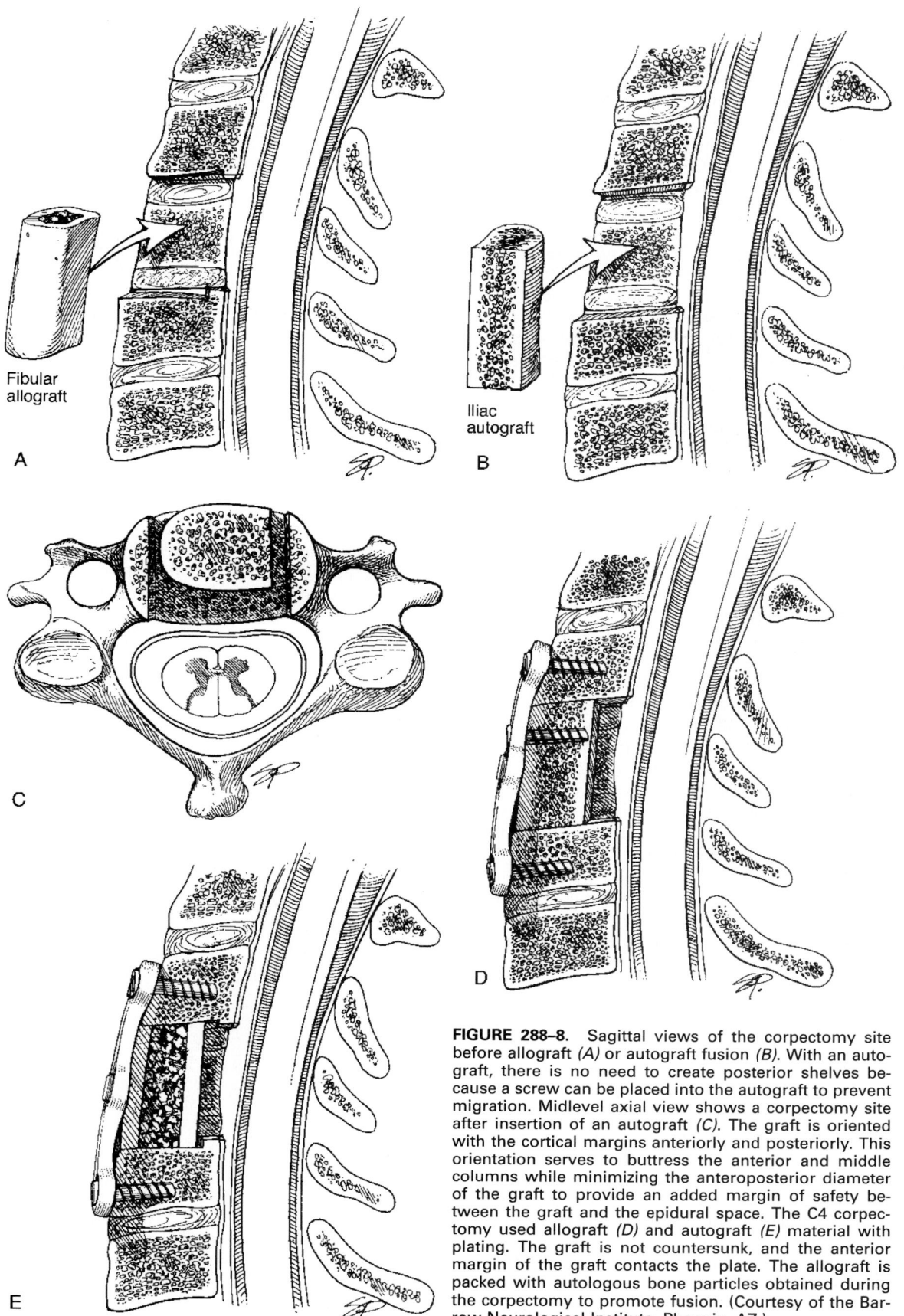

FIGURE 288–8. Sagittal views of the corpectomy site before allograft *(A)* or autograft fusion *(B)*. With an autograft, there is no need to create posterior shelves because a screw can be placed into the autograft to prevent migration. Midlevel axial view shows a corpectomy site after insertion of an autograft *(C)*. The graft is oriented with the cortical margins anteriorly and posteriorly. This orientation serves to buttress the anterior and middle columns while minimizing the anteroposterior diameter of the graft to provide an added margin of safety between the graft and the epidural space. The C4 corpectomy used allograft *(D)* and autograft *(E)* material with plating. The graft is not countersunk, and the anterior margin of the graft contacts the plate. The allograft is packed with autologous bone particles obtained during the corpectomy to promote fusion. (Courtesy of the Barrow Neurological Institute, Phoenix, AZ.)

ing for one-level fusion have been questioned in the literature.[71, 72] However, more compelling data support the use of anterior plating for multilevel fusions.[73, 74] After the interbody graft is placed and plating is considered, the surgeon has to remove the anteriorly located osteophytes to allow flush contact of the plate with the vertebral body. This can be performed with a high-speed drill or with a Leksell or pituitary rongeur. Careful attention is needed to not remove the anterior cortex of the vertebral body, because it provides a significant amount of screw pullout resistance. The interbody graft is not countersunk, and it is placed flushed with the anterior vertebral body margin to maximize the contact surface with the fusion construct. When using a corpectomy autograft, the graft can be secured to the plate using a bicortical screw. This cannot be performed with fibular allograft because it is too brittle to accept any screw without affecting its structural integrity.[75, 76]

Depending on the plating system used, the surgeon has the option of using fixed or variable angle screws, and most of the new systems have locking mechanisms to resist screw pullout. Real-time fluoroscopy aids in monitoring screw placement. The screw should be placed in the dense bone tissue in the subchondral region without violating the end plate. Violation of the end plate by the screw results in a poor biomechanical construct and physiomechanical alteration of a normal adjacent segment. The ideal torque is to finger tightness to avoid stripping the screw. If stripping occurs, the construct can be secured by a rescue screw of a larger diameter or by moving the entire plate and redirecting new screw trajectories. Methyl methacrylate can be infused into the initial hole to bolster the screw purchase. The cervical plates can also be contoured to maximize surface contact, but manipulation can cause plate fatigue and should be minimized. When multilevel diskectomies or corpectomies are being performed, multiple fixation points can provide a more biomechanically sound construct. This is particularly important at the caudal levels, where most of the stress is placed on the construct.[75, 76]

Direct inspection and fluoroscopy are used to assess placement of the instrumented construct and the final position of the intervertebral graft. Self-retaining retractors are removed, and meticulous hemostasis is obtained with bipolar cautery. The esophagus and carotid artery are inspected with hand-held retractors for evidence of injury. The wound is irrigated with an antibiotic-containing solution, and the platysma layer is closed with interrupted absorbable suture. The dermis is approximated with a subcuticular closure.

Postoperative orthosis is dictated by the underlying condition and bone integrity of the patient. One-level diskectomies generally do not require a hard cervical collar postoperatively. We recommend a soft cervical collar when patients develop some neck pain, and we encourage disuse when they are comfortable. Multilevel diskectomies, corpectomies, or trauma-associated injuries are generally maintained with a hard collar for approximately 6 weeks. At that time, cervical radiographs are obtained with flexion-extension views to assess incorporation of the graft. In the absence of complicating features, patients are asked to wean themselves from using the collar over several weeks and to start isometric exercises to strengthen cervical neck musculature. Patients with metabolic derangements or with poor bone integrity (e.g., those with rheumatoid arthritis) are sometimes managed with a longer course of a hard collar and or halo vest, depending on the extent of their construct.

Complications

Several complications have been reported after anterior spinal surgery. The most common complications are transient vocal cord paralysis, breathing difficulties, dysphagia, and odynophagia.[75, 76] Permanent vocal cord paralysis is rare, with an estimated incidence of 0.5% to 1%.[77, 78] Postoperative hoarseness usually resolves within weeks to months. Breathing difficulties may result from soft tissue swelling after prolonged and excessive retraction or from postoperative hematomas. Large hematomas compromising the airway should be addressed surgically and can be prevented by placement of a drain. During anterior spinal procedures, the carotid artery, jugular veins, trachea, and esophagus are at risk for injury (Fig. 288–9). Careful dissection and meticulous attention to retractor placement should prevent injuries to these vital structures. The retractors should be placed bilaterally under direct vision under

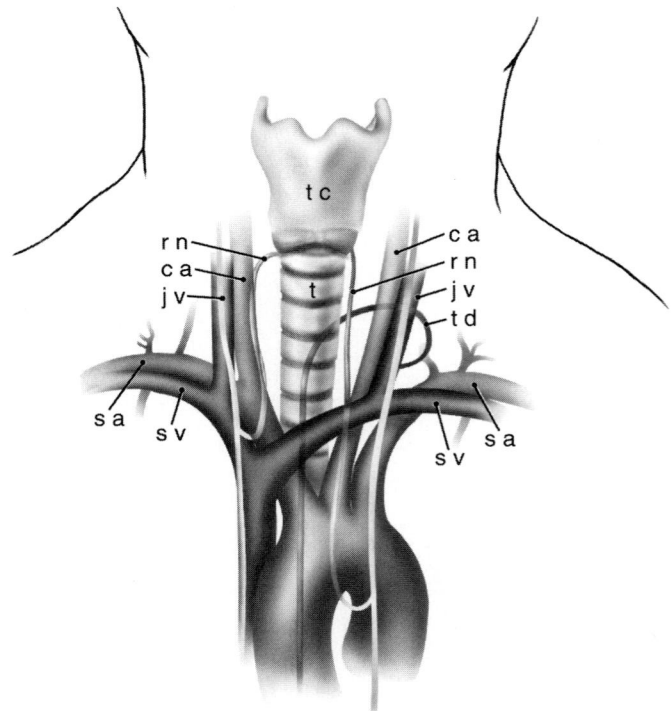

FIGURE 288–9. Surgical anatomy relevant to the anterior cervical approaches. The subclavian artery (sa), subclavian vein (sv), carotid artery (ca), jugular vein (jv), recurrent laryngeal nerve (rn), thoracic duct (td), trachea (t), and thyroid cartilage (tc) are indicated. (Courtesy of the Barrow Neurological Institute, Phoenix, AZ.)

the longus colli muscle to avoid inadvertent injury to the esophagus. Although rare, esophageal injuries carry a significant morbidity, with possible development of mediastinitis and lethal abscesses. After completion of surgery, the esophagus needs to be thoroughly inspected along its length to check for rents. Methylene blue dye can be instilled in the pharynx, and any suspicious areas are carefully inspected for dye extravasation. If a rent is identified, it needs to be repaired primarily. Treatment of an infected esophageal repair requires surgical revision, drainage, nasogastric aspiration, intravenous or local antibiotics, and in some instances, esophageal diversion.[79, 80]

Severe neurological injuries are rare after anterior cervical procedures.[81] They can result from surgical trauma, overdistraction with cord impingement, or retropulsion of interbody grafts. If postoperative neurological deterioration is encountered, an epidural hematoma should be suspected and addressed emergently. Vertebral artery injuries are also rare and result from loss of midline orientation, screw placement, or aggressive resection of laterally placed disk osteophytes.[82] Cerebrospinal fluid fistulas are uncommon. They are usually seen in patients with ossified posterior longitudinal ligament (OPLL) with extensive adhesion to the dura. Most defects are small and can be handled by local application of a Gelfoam pledget and fibrin glue and by postoperative elevation of the head of the bed. Direct closure is technically difficult in these instances, and if there is any concern, lumbar drainage can be implemented with good results. Other rare complications include Horner's syndrome (i.e., anhydrosis, miosis, and ptosis) from interruption of the sympathetic chain located on the anterior surface of the longus colli; pneumothorax when addressing pathology at the cervicothoracic junction; and thoracic duct disruption when approaching the lower cervical region through the left side.

Complications from iliac crest harvest can include localized pain, meralgia paresthetica from disruption of the lateral femoral cutaneous nerve, wound infection, and hip fractures. The use of oscillating saws rather than osteotomes may reduce the incidence of hip fractures.[83] Graft displacement and angulation have been reported in 2% to 8% of cases.[68, 84] A well-fitted graft under compression may reduce the incidence of this problem. Depending on the symptoms, extruded grafts may require surgical intervention. The risk of pseudarthrosis has been reported in most series addressing anterior cervical diskectomy and fusion.[68, 71, 72, 74, 84–92] The rate of pseudarthrosis for one-, two-, and three-level fusion has been reported to be as high as 20%, 50%, and 56%, respectively.[93–100] Reports on the use of cervical plating have shown significant improvement in fusion rates for two- and three-level fusions.[73, 101] Development of pseudarthrosis does not necessarily result in a poor surgical outcome. However, patients who have symptomatic pseudarthrosis have resolution of their symptoms after posterior fusion at the involved levels. Other potential complications with the use of instrumentation include esophageal erosion and hardware failure. Use of a nonconstraining screw plate may allow graft settling and prevent plate and screw breakage.

CONCLUSIONS

A patient with cervical spondylosis requires a thorough evaluation by the clinician. Potential sources for pain and neurological deficits must be ruled out by appropriate diagnostic imaging or electromyographic studies, or both. After the diagnosis has been narrowed to pathology of the cervical spine, an appropriate treatment plan should be formulated for the patient. The degree and extent of neurological injury determine the need for conservative or surgical management. Patients with radicular symptoms may be treated conservatively, whereas patients with myelopathic symptoms need careful and expeditious management, usually requiring surgery.

The anterior cervical approach to the spine has undergone a tremendous evolution over the last 5 decades and is well accepted by surgeons. This approach is extremely versatile, allowing the surgeon full access to all the pathologic components responsible for clinical symptoms. Foraminal distraction, spinal cord decompression, and lordotic curvature can be performed by placement of a graft and subsequent stabilization, if required. Fusion can be enhanced through meticulous preparation of the end plate, maximizing bone-to-graft contact at the interface and compression. Excellent results are usually achieved with little or acceptable morbidity.

REFERENCES

1. Gore DR, Sepic SB, Gardner GM: Roentgenographic findings of the cervical spine in asymptomatic people. Spine 11:521–524, 1986.
2. Montgomery DM, Brower RS: Cervical spondylotic myelopathy. Clinical syndrome and natural history. Orthop Clin North Am 23:487–493, 1992.
3. Elliott GR: A contribution to spinal osteoarthritis involving the cervical region. J Bone Joint Surg Am 8:42–52, 1926.
4. Stookey B: Compression of the spinal cord due to ventral extradural chordomas: Diagnosis and surgical treatment. Arch Neurol Psychiatry 20:275–291, 1928.
5. Elsberg CA: Extradural spinal tumors—primary, secondary, metastatic. Surg Gynecol Obstet 46:10–20, 1928.
6. Mixter WJ, Barr JS: Rupture of the intervertebral disc with involvement of the spinal canal. N Engl J Med 211:210–214, 1934.
7. Robinson RA, Smith GW: Anterolateral cervical disc removal and interbody fusion for cervical disc syndrome. Bull Johns Hopkins 96:223–224, 1955.
8. Robinson RA, Walker AE, Ferlic DC, et al: The results of an anterior interbody fusion of the cervical spine. J Bone Joint Surg Am 44:1587, 1962.
9. Smith GW, Robinson RA: The treatment of certain spine disorders by anterior removal of the intervertebral disc and interbody fusion. J Bone Joint Surg Am 40:607–624, 1958.
10. Cloward RB: The anterior approach for removal of ruptured cervical disks. Neurosurgery 15:602–617, 1958.
11. Bailey RW, Badgley CE: Stabilization of the cervical spine by anterior fusion. J Bone Joint Surg Am 42:565–594, 1960.
12. Verbiest H: A lateral approach to the cervical spine: Technique and indications. J Neurosurg 28:191–203, 1968.
13. Bogduk N, Windsor M, Inglis A: The innervation of the cervical intervertebral discs. Spine 13:2–8, 1988.

14. Panjabi M, White AA 3rd: Biomechanics of nonacute cervical spinal cord trauma. Spine 13:838–842, 1988.

15. Campbell AMG, Phillips DG: Cervical disc lesions with neurological disorder. Br Med J 2:481–485, 1960.

16. Clarke E, Robinson PK: Cervical myelopathy: A complication of cervical spondylosis. Brain 79:483–510, 1956.

17. Gregorius FK, Estrin T, Crandall PH: Cervical spondylotic radiculopathy and myelopathy: A long-term follow-up study. Arch Neurol 33:618–625, 1976.

18. Lees F, Turner JWA: Natural history and prognosis of cervical spondylosis. Br Med J 2:1607–1610, 1963.

19. Nurick S: The pathogenesis of the spinal cord disorder associated with cervical spondylosis. Brain 95:87–100, 1972.

20. Rowland LP: Surgical treatment of cervical spondylotic myelopathy: Time for a controlled trial. Neurology 42:5–13, 1992.

21. Phillips DG: Upper limb involvement in cervical spondylosis. J Neurol Neurosurg Psychiatry 38:386–390, 1975.

22. Friedenberg ZB, Miller WT: Degenerative disc disease of the cervical spine: A comparative study of asymptomatic and symptomatic patients. J Bone Joint Surg Am 45:1171–1178, 1963.

23. Vernon-Roberts B, Pirie CJ: Degenerative changes in the intervertebral discs of the lumbar spine and their sequelae. Rheumatol Rehabil 16:13–21, 1977.

24. Payne EE, Spillane JD: The cervical spine: An anatomico-pathological study of 70 specimens (using a special technique) with particular reference to the problem of cervical spondylosis. Brain 80:571–596, 1957.

25. Raynor RB, Koplik B: Cervical cord trauma: The relationship between clinical syndromes and force of injury. Spine 10:193–197, 1985.

26. Wilkinson M: The morbid anatomy of cervical spondylosis and myelopathy. Brain 83:589–616, 1960.

27. Brain WR, Northfield D, Wilkinson M: The neurologic manifestations of cervical spondylosis. Brain 75:187–225, 1952.

28. White AA 3rd, Panjabi MM: Biomechanical considerations in the surgical management of cervical spondylotic myelopathy. Spine 13:856–860, 1988.

29. Kelsey JL, White AA 3rd, Astides H, et al: The impact of musculoskeletal disorders on the population of the United States. J Bone Joint Surg Am 61:959–964, 1979.

30. Parke WW: Correlative anatomy of cervical spondylotic myelopathy. Spine 13:831–837, 1988.

31. Zeidman SM, Ducker TB: Cervical disk disease: Part I. Treatment options and outcomes. Neurosurg Q 2:116–143, 1992.

32. Alexander J, Natural history and nonoperative management of cervical spondylosis. In Menezes AH, Sonntag VKH (eds): Principles of Spinal Surgery. New York, McGraw-Hill, 1996, pp 547–557.

33. Breig A, Turnbull I, Hassler O: Effects of mechanical stresses on the spinal cord in cervical spondylosis: A study on fresh cadaver material. J Neurosurg 25:45–56, 1996.

34. al-Mefty O, Harkey HL, Marawi I, et al: Experimental chronic compressive cervical myelopathy. J Neurosurg 79:550–561, 1993.

35. Epstein JA, Carras R, Lavine LS, et al: The importance of removing osteophytes as part of the surgical treatment of myeloradiculopathy in cervical spondylosis. J Neurosurg 30:219–226, 1969.

36. Symonds C: The interrelation of trauma and cervical spondylosis in impression of the cervical cord. Lancet 1:451–454, 1953.

37. Mann KS, Khosla VK, Gulati DR: Cervical spondylotic myelopathy treated by single-stage multilevel anterior decompression: A prospective study. J Neurosurg 60:81–87, 1984.

38. Barnes MP, Saunders M: The effect of cervical mobility on the natural history of cervical spondylotic myelopathy. J Neurol Neurosurg Psychiatry 47:17–20, 1984.

39. Cusick JF, Steiner RE, Berns T: Total stabilization of the cervical spine in patients with cervical spondylotic myelopathy. Neurosurgery 18:491–495, 1986.

40. Travell JG, Simons DG: Myofascial Pain Syndromes and Dysfunction. The Trigger Point Manual. Baltimore, Williams & Wilkins, 1983.

41. Ehni G, Benner B: Occipital neuralgia and the C1-2 arthrosis syndrome. J Neurosurg 61:961–965, 1984.

42. Ahlgren BD, Garfin SR: Cervical radiculopathy. Orthop Clin North Am 27:253–263, 1996.

43. McCarty EC, Tsairis P, Warren RF: Brachial neuritis. Clin Orthop 368:37–43, 1999.

44. Poletti CE: Third cervical nerve root and ganglion compression: Clinical syndrome, surgical anatomy, and pathological findings. Neurosurgery 39:941–949, 1996.

45. Ruggieri PM: Cervical radiculopathy. Neuroimaging Clin N Am 5:349–366, 1995.

46. Henderson CM, Hennessy RG, Shuey HM Jr, et al: Posterior-lateral foraminotomy as an exclusive operative technique for cervical radiculopathy: A review of 846 consecutively operated cases. Neurosurgery 13:504–512, 1983.

47. Clark CR: Cervical spondylotic myelopathy: History and physical findings. Spine 13:847–849, 1988.

48. Clifton AG, Stevens JM, Whitear P, et al: Identifiable causes for poor outcome in surgery for cervical spondylosis: Postoperative computed myelography and MR imaging. Neuroradiology 32:450–455, 1990.

49. Li TM, Day SJ, Alberman E, et al: Differential diagnosis of motor neurone disease from other neurological conditions. Lancet 2:731–733, 1986.

50. Jabbari B, Pierce JF, Boston S, et al: Brown-Sequard syndrome and cervical spondylosis. J Neurosurg 47:556–560, 1977.

51. Bakay L, Leslie EV: Surgical treatment of vertebral artery insufficiency caused by cervical spondylosis. J Neurosurg 23:596–602, 1965.

52. Smith DR, Vanderark GD, Kempe LG: Cervical spondylosis causing vertebrobasilar insufficiency: A surgical treatment. J Neurol Neurosurg Psychiatry 34:388–392, 1971.

53. Gamache FW Jr, Voorhies RM: Hypertrophic cervical osteophytes causing dysphagia: A review. J Neurosurg 53:338–344, 1980.

54. Ladenheim SE, Marlowe FI: Dysphagia secondary to cervical osteophytes. Am J Otolaryngol 20:184–189, 1999.

55. Irvine DH, Foster JB, Newell DJ, et al: Prevalence of cervical spondylosis in a general practice. Lancet 1:1089–1092, 1965.

56. Wilkinson HA, LeMay ML, Ferris EJ: Clinical-radiographic correlations in cervical spondylosis. J Neurosurg 30:213–218, 1969.

57. Brown BM, Schwartz RH, Frank E, et al: Preoperative evaluation of cervical radiculopathy and myelopathy by surface-coil MR imaging. AJR Am J Roentgenol 151:1205–1212, 1988.

58. Larsson EM, Holtas S, Cronqvist S, et al: Comparison of myelography, CT myelography and magnetic resonance imaging in cervical spondylosis and disk herniation: Pre- and postoperative findings. Acta Radiol 30:233–239, 1989.

59. Vanderburgh DF, Kelly WM: Radiographic assessment of discogenic disease of the spine. Neurosurg Clin N Am 4:13–33, 1993.

60. al-Mefty O, Harkey HL, Middleton TH, et al: Myelopathic cervical spondylotic lesions demonstrated by magnetic resonance imaging. J Neurosurg 68:217–222, 1988.

61. Wada E, Ohmura M, Yonenobu K: Intramedullary changes of the spinal cord in cervical spondylotic myelopathy. Spine 20:2226–2232, 1995.

62. Takahashi M, Yamashita Y, Sakamoto Y, et al: Chronic cervical cord compression: Clinical significance of increased signal intensity on MR images. Radiology 173:219–224, 1989.

63. Vaccaro AR, Madigan L, Schweitzer ME, et al: Magnetic resonance imaging analysis of soft tissue disruption after flexion-distraction injuries of the subaxial cervical spine. Spine 26:1866–1872, 2001.

64. Litt AW: Imaging and diagnosis of degenerative disease of the cervical spine. In Cooper PR (eds): Degenerative Diseases of the Cervical Spine. Park Ridge, IL, American Association of Neurological Surgeons, 1992, pp 73–90.

65. Restuccia D, Di Lazzaro V, Lo Monaco M, et al: Somatosensory evoked potentials in the diagnosis of cervical spondylotic myelopathy. Electromyogr Clin Neurophysiol 32:389–395, 1992.

66. Ebraheim NA, Lu J, Yang H, et al: Vulnerability of the sympathetic trunk during the anterior approach to the lower cervical spine. Spine 25:1603–1606, 2000.

67. Lu J, Ebraheim NA, Nadim Y, et al: Anterior approach to the cervical spine: Surgical anatomy. Orthopedics 23:841–845, 2000.

68. Simmons EH, Bhalla SK: Anterior cervical discectomy and fusion. A clinical and biomechanical study with eight-year follow-up. J Bone Joint Surg Br 51:225–237, 1969.

69. Saunders RL, Bernini PM, Shirreffs TG Jr, et al: Central corpec-

tomy for cervical spondylotic myelopathy: A consecutive series with long-term follow-up evaluation. J Neurosurg 74:163–170, 1991.

70. Saunders RL: Corpectomy for cervical spondylotic myelopathy. In Menezes AH, Sonntag VKH (eds): Principles of Spinal Surgery. New York, McGraw-Hill, 1996, pp 559–569.

71. Connolly PJ, Esses SI, Kostuik JP: Anterior cervical fusion: Outcome analysis of patients fused with and without anterior cervical plates. J Spinal Disord 9:202–206, 1996.

72. Want JC, McDonough PW, Endow K, et al: The effect of cervical plating on single-level anterior cervical discectomy and fusion. J Spinal Disord 12:467–471, 1999.

73. Kaiser MG, Haid RW Jr, Subach BR, et al: Anterior cervical plating enhances arthrodesis after discectomy and fusion with cortical allograft. Neurosurgery 50:229–238, 2002.

74. Want JC, McDonough PW, Endow K, et al: Increased fusion rates with cervical plating for two-level anterior cervical discectomy and fusion. Spine 25:41–45, 2000.

75. Vishteh AG, Baskin JJ, Sonntag VKH: Techniques of cervical discectomy with and without fusion. Oper Tech Neurosurg 1:85–89, 1998.

76. Baskin JJ, Vishteh AG, Dickman CA, et al: Techniques of anterior cervical plating. Oper Tech Neurosurg 1:90–102, 1998.

77. Bertalanffy H, Eggert HR: Complications of anterior cervical discectomy without fusion in 450 consecutive patients. Acta Neurochir (Wien) 99:41–50, 1989.

78. Bulger RF, Rejowski JE, Beatty RA: Vocal cord paralysis associated with anterior cervical fusion: Considerations for prevention and treatment. J Neurosurg 62:661–661, 1985.

79. Gaudinez RF, English GM, Gebhard JS, et al: Esophageal perforations after anterior cervical surgery. J Spinal Disord 13:77–84, 2000.

80. Smith MD, Bolesta MJ: Esophageal perforation after anterior cervical plate fixation: A report of two cases. J Spinal Disord 5:357–362, 1992.

81. Flynn TB: Neurologic complications of anterior cervical interbody fusion. Spine 7:536–539, 1982.

82. Golfinos JG, Dickman CA, Zabramski JM, et al: Repair of vertebral artery injury during anterior cervical decompression. Spine 19:2552–2556, 1994.

83. Porchet F, Jacques B: Unusual complications at iliac crest bone graft donor site: Experience with two cases. Neurosurgery 39:856–859, 1996.

84. Gore DR, Sepic SB: Anterior cervical fusion for degenerated or protruded discs. A review of one hundred forty-six patients. Spine 9:667–671, 1984.

85. Aronson N, Filtzer DL, Bagan M: Anterior cervical fusion by the Smith-Robinson approach. J Neurosurg 29:396–404, 1968.

86. Brodke DS, Zdeblick TA: Modified Smith-Robinson procedure for anterior cervical discectomy and fusion. Spine 17(Suppl):S427–S430, 1992.

87. Clements DH, O'Leary PF: Anterior cervical discectomy and fusion. Spine 15:1023–1025, 1990.

88. Cloward RB: Complications of anterior cervical disc operation and their treatment. Surgery 69:175–182, 1971.

89. Herkowitz HN, Kurz LT, Overhold DP: Surgical management of cervical soft disc herniation: A comparison between the anterior and posterior approach. Spine 15:1026–1030, 1990.

90. Kozak JA, Hanson GW, Rose JR, et al: Anterior discectomy, microscopic decompression, and fusion: A treatment for cervical spondylotic radiculopathy. J Spinal Disord 2:43–46, 1989.

91. Riley LH Jr, Robinson RA, Johnson KA, et al: The results of anterior interbody fusion of the cervical spine: Review of ninety-three consecutive cases. J Neurosurg 30:127–133, 1969.

92. Schneeberger AG, Boos N, Schwarzenbach O, et al: Anterior cervical interbody fusion with plate fixation for chronic spondylotic radiculopathy: A 2- to 8-year follow-up. J Spinal Disord 12:215–221, 1999.

93. Brown MD, Malinin TI, Davis PB: A roentgenographic evaluation of frozen allografts versus autografts in anterior cervical spine fusions. Clin Orthop 119:231–236, 1976.

94. Cloward RB: Gas-sterilized cadaver bone grafts for spinal fusion operations: A simplified bone hook. Spine 5:4–10, 1980.

95. Emery SE, Fisher JR, Bohlman HH: Three-level anterior cervical discectomy and fusion: Radiographic and clinical results. Spine 22:2622–2625, 1997.

96. Grossman W, Peppelman WC, Baum JA, et al: The use of freeze-dried fibular allograft in anterior cervical fusion. Spine 17:565–569, 1992.

97. Malinin TI, Rosomoff HL, Sutton CH: Human cadaver femoral head homografts for anterior cervical spine fusions. Surg Neurol 7:249–251, 1977.

98. Rish BL, McFadden JT, Penix JO: Anterior cervical fusion using homologous bone grafts: A comparative study. Surg Neurol 5:119–121, 1976.

99. Young WF, Rosenwasser RH: An early comparative analysis of the use of fibular allograft versus autologous iliac crest graft for interbody fusion after anterior cervical discectomy. Spine 18:1123–1124, 1993.

100. Zdeblick TA, Ducker TB: The use of freeze-dried allograft bone for anterior cervical fusions. Spine 16:726–729, 1991.

101. Bolesta MJ, Rechtine GR 2nd, Chrin AM: Three- and four-level anterior cervical discectomy and fusion with plate fixation: A prospective study. Spine 25:2040–2046, 2000.

Cervical Spondylotic Myelopathy

V.G.R. KUMAR ■ CHRISTOPHER MADDEN ■ GARY L. REA

Cervical spondylosis is ankylosis of the vertebral joints in the neck and probably represents normal, age-related degenerative changes in the cervical spine. Cervical stenosis is vertebral canal narrowing seen on radiographic images. Either of these conditions may be symptomatic or asymptomatic.[1-3] In some individuals, spondylosis progresses to such severe stenosis that the cervical spinal cord is injured and the patient becomes myelopathic. Although there are a number of causes of canal stenosis and cord compromise, the most common is related to the degenerative process called cervical spondylotic myelopathy (CSM).

Case reports in the 19th and early 20th centuries noted the existence of degenerative, compressive spinal cord lesions. Key[4] provided what was probably the first description of a spondylotic bar causing paraplegia (though this was not in the cervical region). Gowers[5] described "vertebral exostosis," which may cause cord compression, but he considered this to be an exceedingly rare lesion. Stookey[6] noted cervical cord compression by what he described as ventral extradural chondromas and described the different clinical syndromes that could occur with this compression. Recognition that chondromas represented disk material came in the 1930s with the articles of Mixter and Barr[7] and Peet and Echols.[8]

Brain[9] is credited with developing the first cogent clinical description of CSM in 1948. His insight lay in recognizing the difference between an acute disk herniation, which was likely to produce radicular symptoms, and a chronic osteophytic disease process, which was more apt to produce myelopathic symptoms. This theme was developed in subsequent years by Brain and others, but half a century after the description of this condition, many controversies remain regarding its pathophysiology, clinical course, and treatment. Some of this difficulty has arisen from inconsistencies in reporting (e.g., inclusion of mixed patient populations having cervical root symptoms and not myelopathy, or asymptomatic patients with cervical spondylosis) and a general failure to apply standard preoperative and postoperative criteria when assessing outcomes.[10, 11]

PATHOPHYSIOLOGY

The exact circumstances or combination of circumstances that leads to CSM has not been completely elucidated. Stenosis normally occurs secondary to the formation of osteophytic bars at the level of the disk space. Cord injury likely occurs as the result of several interrelated factors: direct compression of the cord, microtrauma associated with neck flexion and extension, and vascular injury.

Spinal canal diameter between C3 and C7 in a normal adult is about 17 to 18 mm. This number varies slightly between the sexes but has been confirmed in a number of studies. Adams and Logue[12] found that in patients with CSM, the average canal diameter was 11.8 mm, with a range of 9 to 15 mm. Osteophytic bars progressively encroach on the canal, decreasing its diameter, as the degenerative condition worsens. Persons with congenitally small canals characterized by low laminar arches and short pedicles may become symptomatic at an earlier stage of degeneration.

Spondylotic changes seem to begin with disk degeneration at one level. The cervical disk is thicker anteriorly to maintain the cervical lordosis, and as it collapses, a segmental flexion deformity occurs at that level. The degenerated disk allows for abnormal motion at that level. The uncinate processes override, and the proximity of the vertebral bodies allows for reactive spur formation at that level. Abnormal movement may also contribute to ligamenta flava and facet hypertrophy, leading to posterior encroachment on the canal. The flexion at the degenerated disk space can lead to hyperextension at the superior levels.

Hayashi and coworkers[13] demonstrated that the hyperostosis and spondylotic bars appear radiographically first at the lower levels (C5-6 and C6-7). As the joint space becomes fused, there is less motion at these levels and more stress and movement associated with the higher levels. At the upper levels of C3-4 and C4-5, more retro- or anterolisthesis develops later with relative increased motion. This seems to indicate that the spondylotic process is progressive: degenerative changes in the lower cervical spine are followed by osteophytes and decreased motion at that level, leading to abnormal movement at the disk segments above and degeneration at those levels.

Regarding the production of myelopathy, several mechanisms have been proposed, including direct compression of neural elements, ischemic injury secondary to vascular compromise, and repetitive spinal cord microtrauma associated with normal neck movements. Experimental studies in dogs have shown that mechanical compression of the spinal cord leads to irreversible large motoneuron loss, necrosis, and cavitation in the cord parenchyma when normal movements impinge on an already compromised spinal cord.[14, 15] Extension of the neck with subsequent buckling of the ligamenta flava diminishes the size of the canal. In flexion, the cord may be draped over the osteophytic spurs anteriorly. It is postulated that when this compression exists, the normal movements of the spine cause repetitive injury to the cervical cord. Although no one has demonstrated anterior artery occlusion, there is a wealth of experimental and pathologic data suggesting that compression can occlude the sulcal and terminal branches of the anterior artery, causing ischemic injury to the cord.[15]

NATURAL HISTORY

Studies of the natural history of CSM have resulted in varied opinions regarding its clinical course. Clarke and Robinson's[16] study of 120 patients in 1956 noted that after the patient had become symptomatic, neurological examinations did not return to normal. Motor changes tended to persist; sensory and sphincter changes tended to be transient. Seventy-five percent of patients presented with a series of episodes during which they experienced new signs and symptoms. In two thirds of these patients (i.e., 50% of the series), there was a slow, steady progression punctuated by new episodes; in one third (25% of the series), the condition stabilized between episodes. In 20% of patients, the clinical course was a slow, steady progression after initial presentation. The remaining 5% of patients presented with rapid onset of symptoms followed by a lengthy period of stability. With conservative treatment, approximately 50% of patients experienced some improvement in both the radicular and the gait components of their symptoms.

In 1963, Lees and Turner[17] looked at two groups of patients with cervical stenosis: one group of 44 patients who had myelopathy with stenosis, and one group of 51 patients who had evidence of stenosis without myelopathy. In the myelopathic group, the initial development of symptoms was followed by a period of neurological stability or improvement. In those who had disease longer than 10 years, some had episodes of deterioration that led to progressive neurological deficit. These further episodes, however, also tended to be followed by periods of stabilization or improvement. The patients rarely deteriorated in a steadily progressive fashion. Those patients who had cervical stenosis without evidence of myelopathy did not develop symptoms. Nurick's[18] review of 37 conservatively treated patients echoed Lees and Turner's assessment. He thought that it was a "generally benign disorder" in which "disability develops in an initial phase" and "later remains static except in older patients, in whom it may progress."[19]

In 1967, Symon and Lavender[20] reviewed the data of Lees and Turner and noted that although 55% of patients had shown some improvement, only 18% improved in terms of their disability category. In their own patients, they noted that 67% had a steadily progressive course, challenging the notion that the disease was episodic in nature with a relatively benevolent course. In 1973, Phillips[21] looked at patients treated only with a collar and noted that there was improvement in one third; that improvement was related to the duration of symptoms before treatment. Fifty percent of patients who had been symptomatic for less than 1 year improved, but only 40% of those who had been symptomatic for 1 to 2 years improved. There was no improvement in those who had been symptomatic for more than 2 years. Roberts[22] reviewed 24 patients treated with collar immobilization and found that, with regard to motor disability, 29% were improved, 38% were unchanged, and 33% had deteriorated at follow-up, which ranged from 4 months to 6.5 years. Sadasivan and colleagues[23] reported on 22 patients admitted for surgery in whom the natural history appeared to be progressive deterioration without regression of symptoms. Epstein and associates[24] evaluated four series of patients and found that in the combined group of 114 patients, 36% were improved, 38% were unchanged, and 26% were worse.

Rowland[11] criticized the lack of knowledge about the natural history of CSM. Although most clinicians do not consider it a benign condition, further studies are needed to accurately characterize its natural history.

CLINICAL PRESENTATION

CSM can present with a protean range of symptoms, depending on the level and degree of compression and the number of levels involved. Typically, the patient is middle-aged or elderly with a broad-based, stooped, hesitant gait and complaints of loss of dexterity in the hands, particularly in fine movements. Gait abnormalities may predate upper extremity symptoms,[25] but the hand symptoms often lead the patient to seek medical attention. Patients often complain of difficulty writing, buttoning buttons, or fastening a brassiere. East Asians often complain of difficulty using chopsticks. The hands may have paresthesias and numbness, and patients occasionally complain of arm pain. Leg symptoms include weakness and stiffness. Bladder symptoms (usually urgency) are not uncommon, but bowel incontinence is relatively rare. Neck pain may or may not be present, and the symptoms in the extremities are usually painless. The onset of symptoms is usually insidious, although acute and subacute presentations are possible.

On examination, the patient commonly exhibits lower motoneuron findings at the level of the lesion (these may be unilateral) and upper motoneuron findings below the level of the lesion. If the spondylosis affects the nerve root foramen and the exiting nerve root, there may be weakness, atrophy, or fasciculations in the distribution of that nerve root. Reflexes associated with the nerve root may be diminished, and there may be sensory loss referable to that nerve root. Pathologic reflexes indicating upper motoneuron disease (Babinski's, Hoffmann's, inverted radial reflex, and clonus) may be present. Lhermitte's sign may be present in some cases with flexion of the neck. Hyperreflexia is generally noted in the lower extremities. Sensory findings in the lower extremities tend to reflect dorsal column involvement. Occasionally, there is loss of superficial sensation, but it is usually asymmetrical and can be patchy. The motor examination is remarkable for slow, stiff opening and closing of the hands, and there may be weakness and atrophy of the hands if the lesion is severe and long standing. In the lower extremities, frank weakness is not appreciable, although spasticity can be prominent. The presence of an abnormal jaw jerk reflex, tongue fasciculations, or cranial nerve findings suggests another cause for the symptoms, as does the complete absence of sensory findings.

Several authors have commented on various aspects of the hand findings in cervical myelopathy. Ono and coworkers[26] describe a "myelopathy hand," in which spastic dysfunction and deficient pain sensation are associated with gait disturbance. Ebara and colleagues[27] describe an amytrophic myelopathy hand, in which there is diffuse or localized wasting of the intrinsic or extrinsic muscles, mild or no sensory disturbances, and weakness, often appearing as a deficiency in extension of the fingers. Involvement is mostly unilateral, but if it is bilateral, it favors one side. High cervical lesions (C3-5) may present with a syndrome of "numb, clumsy hands." The hands are noted to have diminished proprioception and vibration sense, with little associated sensory deficit and minimal motor findings.[28]

Attempts at grading disease severity have focused on the degree of associated neurological disability. Nurick[18, 19] provided a system based on the degree of gait abnormality ranging from grade 0 (radiculopathy without myelopathy, or no disability) to grade 5 (chair bound or bedridden). The Japanese Orthopedic Association score evaluates upper and lower extremity motor and sensory function, trunk sensation, and bladder function, providing a more comprehensive clinical picture for purposes of pre- and postoperative assessment and comparison.[29]

In some cases (5% to 13%), the patient suffers from stenosis in both the cervical and the lumbar regions. Such patients often present with intermittent neurogenic claudication, a progressive gait disturbance, and a mixed pattern of upper and lower motoneuron signs in both the upper and lower extremities, like that found in amyotrophic lateral sclerosis. It is important to recognize these patients, because the condition is usually amenable to treatment. In these instances, the more symptomatic region is typically treated first.[24, 30, 31]

Ferguson and Caplan[32] described four clinical syndromes related to cervical spondylosis: (1) primarily radicular (lateral), (2) myelopathic (medial), (3) combined radicular and myelopathic, and (4) a vascular pattern with sudden onset that is not amenable to surgical reversal. In this last case, radiographic images do not usually demonstrate a degree of stenosis commensurate with the symptoms, and the time course suggests an apoplectic event.

Crandall and Batzdorf[33] delineated five clinical syndromes seen in association with cervical spondylosis. The transverse lesion syndrome involves the corticospinal and spinothalamic tracts and dorsal columns, and patients exhibit severe spasticity with frequent sphincter involvement. This was the most frequent type encountered, and the authors believed that it might represent the end stage of the disease process, because patients with this type had had symptoms for the longest time. The motor system syndrome involves the corticospinal tract and anterior horn cells, with insignificant or no sensory impairment. Severe spasticity was present in 75% of patients. In the central cord syndrome, upper extremity motor and sensory involvement is greater than lower extremity involvement. These patients have useless hands, painful paresthetic dysesthesias, and Lhermitte's sign in 50%. Brown-Séquard syndrome involves a unilateral cord lesion with ipsilateral corticospinal deficit and contralateral analgesia below the level of the lesion. Painful paresthetic sensations were present in 50% of patients. The brachialgia and cord syndrome consists of upper limb pain and associated long-tract involvement, either motor or sensory or both.

Given that the symptoms and physical findings in CSM are shared with many other disease processes, and that asymptomatic cervical spondylosis is so common, it is important that the clinical examination be carefully correlated with the radiographic images. Important differential diagnostic considerations include multiple sclerosis, amyotrophic lateral sclerosis, subacute combined degeneration, syringomyelia, Chiari malformation, vertebrobasilar insufficiency, Guillain-Barré syndrome, poliomyelitis, peripheral neuropathy, and cerebral hemisphere disease. Other space-occupying lesions, including tumor, arteriovenous malformation, acute disk herniation, epidural abscess, and hematoma, may be excluded with magnetic resonance imaging (MRI).

RADIOGRAPHIC FINDINGS

A cervical spinal canal with an anteroposterior diameter less than 11 to 13 mm represents stenosis, and a canal that is 10 mm or less represents absolute stenosis, because the cord in that region measures approximately 1 cm in diameter. This can be measured on a lateral cervical spine film as the distance from the posterior vertebral body to the edge of the lamina, though this measurement may be unreliable if a lateral spur creates the impression of central canal stenosis. Oblique views may demonstrate foraminal stenosis at the involved level, and flexion-extension views can assess gross instability. Computed tomography shows cross-sectional bony anatomy and allows for direct measurement of the canal diameter. When used in conjunction with myelography, it provides information

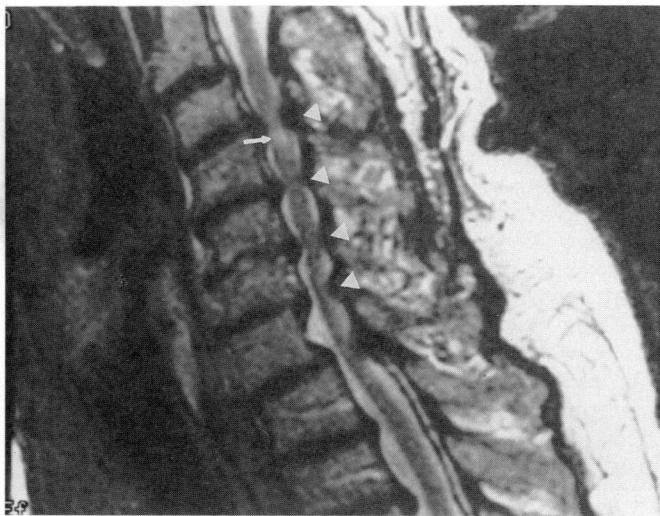

FIGURE 289–1. Sagittal magnetic resonance imaging scan of a patient with progressing myelopathy shows multilevel compression by posterior ligamentous hypertrophy *(arrowheads)*, anterior disk protrusion, and an area of hyperintensity at C3-4 *(arrow)*.

about foramina, nerve root impingement, and compression of the thecal sac.

MRI can also assess canal diameter and provides superior soft tissue imaging (Fig. 289–1). It can be used to exclude other causes of the myelopathy, such as tumor or syrinx. In some patients with CSM, preoperative MRI scans demonstrate an area of increased T2 signal in the spinal cord at the area of greatest compression. The exact cause of the increased signal is unknown, but it is believed to represent an area of edema, inflammation, gliosis, vascular ischemia, or myelomalacia. Several studies have suggested that surgical outcome is not as good in patients who exhibit this area of T2 hyperintensity, and the surgical outcome may be better in those patients in whom the cord lesion disappears postoperatively,[15, 34, 35] though this correlation is not invariable.[36]

TREATMENT

The management of CSM is controversial. The confounding variables are the often slow, variable natural history and the absence of randomized, controlled studies to allow evidence-based treatment choices. Surgical treatment of significant cord compression should be considered once the diagnosis of CSM has been made and alternative diagnoses excluded. However, a subgroup of patients with myelopathy and stenosis may not be surgical candidates either because they refuse surgery or because they are so medically frail that surgery is not an option.

Nonsurgical

The mainstay of nonoperative treatment of stenosis has been immobilization in a hard collar to prevent further

neurological deterioration secondary to motion. Various results have been reported,[16–18, 22, 37–39] but there are no large prospective trials. It is not clear that the results with collar immobilization are different from the natural history of the disease. One of the difficulties with the collar is noncompliance, which has been documented by a number of authors.[40] It has been suggested that more extensive immobilization (e.g., a Minerva collar) may be more effective in preventing neurological deterioration.[31]

Surgical

Successful surgical treatment depends on understanding the pathophysiology of CSM. It seems logical that surgical treatment should address both static and dynamic components of the disorder.[13, 14, 41] CSM is usually treated with either anterior or posterior decompression with or without fusion. Each has its merits and disadvantages, and the choice is often determined by the surgeon's preference.

SELECTION OF PATIENTS

Surgical outcome could be improved if there were preoperative indicators allowing the selection of patients who are likely to improve. Factors that may be associated with poor outcomes in patients with CSM are poor initial clinical condition,[42] long duration of symptoms,[43–45] presence on MRI of high-intensity lesions or cord atrophy,[34–36] presence of other serious medical or emotional conditions,[42, 46] and operative complications.[34] Monro[47] noted that although younger patients with a shorter duration of symptoms did better in some reports, there was considerable uncertainty about other variables.

The preoperative evaluation of evoked potentials or the use of other electrophysiologic tests, including cortical magnetic stimulation, has not been predictive of outcome.[48–54] However, the technology is continually evolving, and Chang and Lin[55] reported a measure of prediction based on a grading of motor conduction velocity in the thoracolumbar cord.

Fundamental to patient selection for surgery are the severity of the patient's symptoms and their impact on the patient's lifestyle; however, prophylactic surgery for possible sudden catastrophic neurological deterioration may be indicated in some patients with mild symptomatic disease and significant neural encroachment.[56–58] This factor and the possibility that patients with better initial clinical status will have better outcomes must be weighed against the risk of surgery for the individual patient.[42, 59]

SURGICAL APPROACHES

An open-minded approach toward selection of the operation is necessary, and consideration of spinal geometry is an important determinant of the surgical approach.[60–62]

Benzel[62] emphasized the high probability of failure associated with posterior decompression alone in patients with an effective cervical kyphosis. Such a kyphosis has been defined as a configuration of the cervical spine in which any part of the dorsal aspect of the C3-7 vertebral bodies crosses a line drawn in the midsagittal plane (on a lateral cervical radiograph or MRI scan) from the dorsocaudal aspect of the vertebral body of C2 to the dorsocaudal aspect of the vertebral body of C7. An effective cervical lordosis has been defined as a configuration of the cervical spine in which no part of the dorsal aspect of any of the C3-7 vertebral bodies crosses this line. The definition of this imaginary line has also been associated with a zone of uncertainty ("gray zone") within which the surgeon's clinical judgment determines whether the predominant configuration is lordosis or kyphosis. Patients whose spinal configuration falls within the gray zone have been defined as having a straightened spine.

It is suggested that patients with an effective cervical kyphosis receive an anterior surgical approach and that patients with an effective lordosis undergo a posterior surgical approach. Patients with a straight spine may be approached from either front or back, and other factors may be considered. Another issue in planning the surgical approach is the patient's age. An older patient with a lordotic spine compressed at three levels is less likely to become kyphotic, so laminectomy without fusion can be considered.

Anterior Approaches

The most common procedure used to treat myelopathy secondary to cervical spondylosis is an anterior cervical decompression, ranging from a simple diskectomy at one or more levels to multiple-level vertebrectomies. Single-level diskectomies can be performed with or without bone graft or fixation, and vertebrectomies have been done with or without fixation.

Anterior cervical disk decompression has traditionally been supplemented with fusion,[63, 64] but as long ago as 1960, Hirsch[65] questioned this. More than 40 years later, the question still remains unanswered.[66–70] The theoretical advantages of interbody graft include improvement in achieving bony fusion, preservation of the size of the neural foramen at the operated level, and prevention of segmental collapse with kyphotic deformity. The potential disadvantages are the complications of graft extrusion, donor site complications, and accelerated disease at adjacent levels. There have been at least four prospective, randomized studies of diskectomy with and without bone grafting, none of which has demonstrated any significant difference in outcome.[66, 71–73] The rate of bony fusion at the operated level is higher in the grafted group, 97% versus 70%. Patients having diskectomy alone had shorter hospital stays, needed less postoperative analgesia, and returned to work sooner,[71, 73] but patient satisfaction and return to preoperative activity level were similar in both groups.

For more widespread anterior compression, the results of anterior cervical corpectomy have been reported by a number of authors.[74–78] Common indications are the presence of osteophytes, an ossified posterior longitudinal ligament, disk material posterior to the vertebral body, or a narrow canal posterior to the vertebral body. The anterior column is then reconstituted with autograft or allograft bone. There have been reports of corpectomies with and without internal fixation. Saunders and colleagues[76] reported a long-term cure rate of almost 60% with multiple-level corpectomies with autograft and no internal fixation. They reported an overall complication rate of 47.5%, but long-term sequelae and regression of improvement were low. Similarly, Fessler and associates[79] reported significant improvement in myelopathic patients after corpectomies. In 93 patients, there was one permanent quadriparesis, two permanent vocal cord paralyses, six graft displacements, and reoperations for screw pullout. The plating decreased the need for surgical revision from 13% in patients using a collar to 7.4% (two screw pullouts) (Fig. 289–2).

Specific Considerations in the Anterior Approach

1. If the patient has severe pain or numbness in the arms or legs with extension while awake, or there is evidence of instability, an awake fiber-optic intubation should be strongly considered. The neck must be in a flexed or neutral position during surgery in cases of severe cord compression anteriorly.

2. Perioperative steroids may be beneficial.

3. A carefully placed transverse incision can expose one or two vertebral levels, but for more than two disk spaces, the less cosmetically appealing longitudinal incision can be used.

4. A left-sided approach decreases the incidence of recurrent laryngeal nerve palsy, but in the lower levels of the cervical spine, this may increase the risk of injury to the thoracic duct.

5. Releasing the self-retaining retractors for 5 minutes every 45 to 60 minutes may decrease the risk of recurrent laryngeal nerve injury.

6. A trough 15 mm wide with a corpectomy will adequately decompress the cord and may not increase the risk of C5 radiculopathy.

7. Anesthesia without paralytic agents allows the surgeon to note irritation of nerve roots or cord during decompression or bipolar electrocautery.

8. The microscope adds light, improves vision, and facilitates the participation of an assistant during actual decompression.

9. In plating, the anterior osteophytes are removed so that the plate sits flush against the bone.

10. With or without plating, the graft and vertebral surfaces must be prepared meticulously.

11. Plates must be of appropriate length, and the screws must be placed accurately.

12. Screws placed into allograft bone may weaken or shatter it.

Posterior Approaches

The traditional surgical treatment for CSM has been cervical laminectomy. The simplicity of the procedure, the familiarity of the technique, its ability to address all affected levels, and its relative safety have contrib-

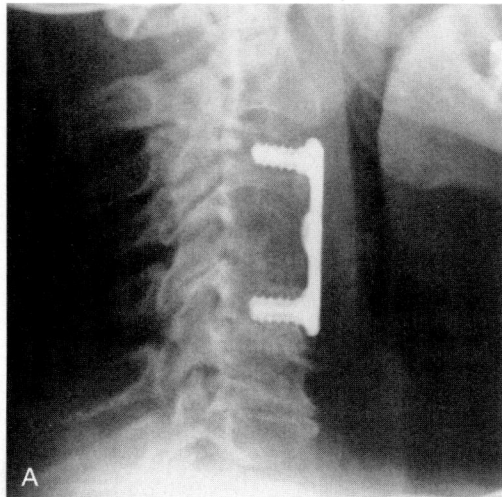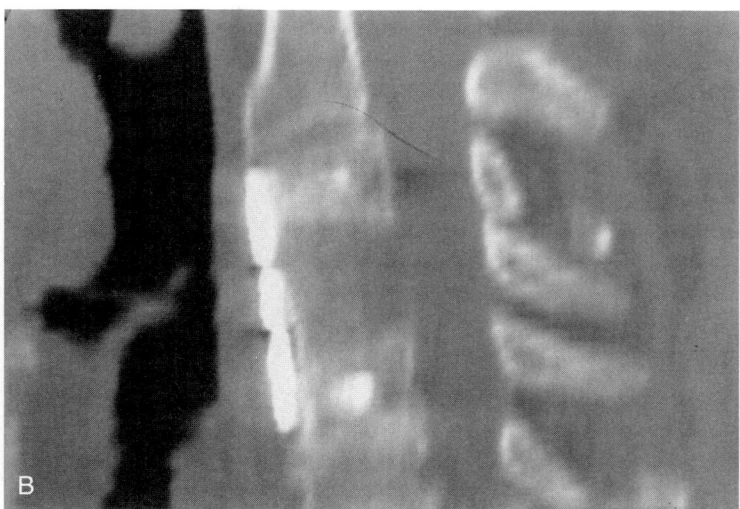

FIGURE 289–2. *A*, Postoperative film after C4 corpectomy with allograft and plate fixation. The patient had myelopathy from osteophyte formation at C3-4 and C4-5 and a canal that was narrow at the C4 body. *B*, Postoperative computed tomographic reconstruction of the same patient shows allograft and no posterior osteophytes.

uted to its popularity. The main criticisms of the procedure have been that late instability with progressive kyphotic or swan-neck deformity can develop[80–84] and that it does not directly address the ventral compression or correct the dynamic component.

Surgical modifications to address these shortcomings include dentate ligament section to permit the spinal cord to move dorsally[85, 86] and excision of osteophytes after laminectomy.[87–89] To achieve stability and address the dynamic component, various techniques to fuse the spine after laminectomy have been proposed.[42, 44, 90–92] Cervical laminaplasty has also been advocated as an alternative to laminectomy to address some of these issues. Since the first description of the procedure by Hirabayashi,[95] a number of technical modifications have been reported.[93, 94, 96]

Specific Considerations in the Posterior Approach

1. If the patient has severe pain or numbness in the arms or legs with extension while awake, or there is evidence of instability, an awake fiber-optic intubation is indicated. The neck must be in a flexed or neutral position during surgery.

2. Perioperative steroids may be beneficial.

3. If the patient has a lordotic spine, is older than 70 years, has compression at three disk levels, and has no listhesis at C3-4 or C4-5, a laminectomy alone is reasonable.

4. If a laminectomy alone is performed, the muscle should be stripped only to the medial edge of the facet to decrease the risk of denervation and instability.

5. If performing a stabilization with the laminectomy, the lateral mass plates should be placed before removing the lamina.

6. Arthrodesis with removal of synovial tissue is required, but placement of bone graft between the facets is not necessary when doing a posterior fusion-fixation.

7. Ultrasonography confirms the posterior movement and good pulsations of the cord with adequate decompression.

8. Many patients take nonsteroidal anti-inflammatory drugs, which may cause oozing after surgery, so a drain may be placed.

9. A posterior decompression-fixation tends to cause more postoperative pain than the anterior approach for about the first 2 to 3 months.

10. Cervical laminaplasty is more technically demanding than a laminectomy and fusion, is more difficult to revise, and does not have clearly superior clinical results.

OUTCOME

The clinical course of CSM is slow and variable. Because of this, any study looking at either the natural history or the outcome after surgical intervention must have reasonably long-term follow-up and evaluation using objective, validated measurements (Table 289–1). Greater standardization of outcome measurements would allow meaningful comparison of results among studies. Because CSM is rarely fatal or completely cured, clear end points for outcome assessment do not exist, which makes it even more important to record other indices that contribute to overall outcome, such as pain, general well-being, coexisting disease, emotional state, and satisfaction with care.

Generic measures of general health, such as the short-form health survey (SF-36) or the Euroqol instrument,[97, 98] can be used to measure outcome in patients who have undergone spinal procedures. Objective measurement of function in CSM can be accomplished using a number of scales, including the Japanese Orthopedic Association's scale, the Myelopathy Disability Index, or the European Myelopathy Scale.[29, 99] This review concentrates on studies that had follow-up longer

TABLE 289-1 ■ Surgical Outcomes of Cervical Spondylotic Myelopathy

SERIES	TOTAL	BETTER (%)	UNCHANGED (%)	WORSE (%)	COMPLICATIONS	FOLLOW-UP	COMMENTS
Anterior							
Boni et al[74]	29	51	47 (less better)	2	10 of 39 cases, 2 requiring reoperations	0.5–13 yr	No criteria for diagnosis; imaging not specified; results rated as good, moderate, & poor; x-ray follow-up good. 7 of 16 cases (47%) developed degeneration in levels above and below
Lunsford et al[25]	37	50		50	Mortality 3%; morbidity 23%	1–7 yr	Good evaluation criteria; myelography only. 2 patients later diagnosed with MS & ALS
Seifert & Stolke[77]	22	77	23 (improved)	0	3 (14%), 1 needing reoperation	21 mo/12 patients	CTM or MRI; patients with myelopathy, no objective criteria for FU
Emery et al[101]	108 87 motor	92	7	1	Mortality (2%); quadriplegia 1%; morbidity 19% (20 patients), of whom 5 (5%) needed reoperations	>2 yr	Imaging not stated specifically; patients date back from 1974; objective assessment; only myelopathy; OPLL excluded. Further operation (13%) long term; pseudarthrosis (15%)
Saunders et al[76]	40	57.5 (cure)		15	Mortality 2.5%; morbidity 47.5%	2–5 yr	Myelo, CTM, MRI; objective evaluation
Chiles et al[59]	76	80	14	7	Mortality 1.3%; morbidity 9%, 2 patients requiring reoperations	Mean, 31 mo	MRI/CTM; objective initial assessment. Only 21 (28%) examined at 1 yr after surgery, the rest at mean 3.6 mo; no follow-up imaging; later deterioration in 5 more requiring operation at adjacent levels
Fessler et al[79]	93	86	13	1	18%; 1 neurological deterioration; 2 reoperations	2–137 mo (mean, 39 mo)	Myelo, CTM, MRI; objective evaluation; 55% have 1-yr FU
Laminectomy							
Epstein et al[88]	50	86	6	8	No mention	1–7 yr	Myelo, CTM; included patients with myelopathy & myeloradiculopathy; excision of osteophytes
Fager[109]	35	68.5	26	5.5	5 (14%) transient deficit; 1 (3%) wound infection	1–7 yr	Laminectomy + dentate section; myelopathy only. Postop myelo in 13 (37%)
Gorter[110]	75	51 67	23 13	26 20	No mention	Mean, 2–6 yr	Older series with myelo only
Bishara[111]	59	61	25	14	Mortality 5%; no other mention of early complications	5–20 yr	Older series with myelo only. 3 patients on FU had MS; 1 parasagittal meningitis; at 10 yr FU, 51% remained better

Table continued on following page

TABLE 289-1 ■ **Surgical Outcomes of Cervical Spondylotic Myelopathy** *Continued*

SERIES	TOTAL	BETTER (%)	UNCHANGED (%)	WORSE (%)	COMPLICATIONS	FOLLOW-UP		COMMENTS
Snow & Weiner[102]	90	77	13	10	Mortality 2%; morbidity 2%	6 mo–4 yr	CTM & MRI	Telephone; FU mostly; no objective evaluation
Laminectomy & Fusion								
Maurer et al[92]	10	90	10	0	20% wound infection; 30% wound seroma	10 mo	CTM & MRI; objective evaluation	
Kumar et al[42]	25	80	20	0	Morbidity 8%	>2 yr (mean, 4 yr)	CTM & MRI; objective evaluation; FU MRI	
Anterior or Posterior								
Ebersold et al[43]	33 A / 51 P	55 / 37	27 / 26	18 / 37	2 (6%) in anterior; not mentioned for posterior	3–9.5 yr (mean, 7.35 yr)	Objective evaluation & FU CTM & MRI	
Carol & Decker[112]	81 A / 125 P	73 / 68	25 / 30	2 / 2	7% graft failure—reoperation; 2% mortality		CT/CTM	
Laminaplasty								
Ohmori et al[96]						6–69 mo (mean, 29 mo)		Mixed cases, including lumbar & thoracic + OPLL
Hase et al[94]	30					2–7 yr (mean 4 yr)		Includes OPLL & CSM
Satomi et al[107]	18					5–13 yr (mean, 8 yr)		Includes OPLL & CSM
Kimura et al[105]						5–14 yr (mean, 7 yr)		Includes OPLL & CSM
Inoue et al[104]	50	76		24	Not specifically mentioned	5–13 yr (mean, 8 yr)	Myelo, pre & post surgery; long, meticulous FU; compared with OPLL	Kyphosis in 3 (6%), straightening in 2 (4%), worse kyphosis in 3 (6%); the 24% deterioration is at late FU
Kohno et al[106]	12					3–8 yr (mean, 5 yr)		Includes OPLL & CSM
Fornari et al[93]	7					<1 yr		

A, anterior; ALS, amyotrophic lateral sclerosis; CSM, cervical spondylotic myelopathy; CT, computed tomography; CTM, CT–myelography; FU, follow-up; MRI, magnetic resonance imaging; MS, multiple sclerosis; myelo, myelogram; OPLL, ossification of the posterior longitudinal ligament; P, posterior.

than 1 year and that used objective outcome measurements.

In 1957, Bradshaw[38] observed that among his patients with CSM treated by laminectomy, 17% were worse at 1-year follow-up, and 50% were worse at 2-year follow-up. Adams and Logue[12] noted that 6 of the 24 patients who deteriorated neurologically, as measured by myelopathy grades, did so at an average postoperative period of 2.3 years. On long-term follow-up, they reported improvement in only 25%, with 50% remaining neurologically stable and 25% deteriorating.

Epstein and Epstein,[100] in a comprehensive review in 1989, noted that 73% of 353 patients improved after anterior surgery, 68% of 444 patients improved after laminectomy, and 85% of 116 patients improved after laminectomy and removal of osteophytes.

Rowland,[11] in a literature review of the results of treatment for CSM, reported that after laminectomy, 60% of 261 patients improved, 34% remained unchanged, and 6% worsened. After anterior surgery, 52% of 385 patients improved, 24% remained unchanged, and 23% worsened. After conservative treatment, 44% of 136 patients improved, 33% remained unchanged, and 23% worsened.

Analysis of the results of surgical therapy reported in the literature, especially in the early literature, is particularly difficult. Interpretation is confounded by dissimilarities in treatment protocols. Very few studies used objective criteria to evaluate patients preoperatively or considered a period of conservative treatment before surgery, other possible diagnoses such as multiple sclerosis or amyotrophic lateral sclerosis were excluded, and consistent criteria for surgery were not identified. Also, pre- or postoperative changes were not recorded in a standard way, and there were no uniform criteria for evaluation of outcome.

If one restricts the analysis to more contemporary studies (reflecting the improved diagnostic ability of computed tomography–myelography and MRI) that included only patients with myelopathy, had a follow-up of at least 1 year, and attempted to evaluate objective outcome measures, a pattern of results emerges.

After anterior surgery, rates of improvement ranged from 77% to 92%; 14% of patients were stable neurologically, without deterioration; and 0% to 15% worsened on follow-up.[59, 76, 77, 79, 101] The surgical mortality ranged from 0% to 3%, and morbidity from 13% to 47.5%.

One of the two contemporary series detailing the results after laminectomy alone reported that 77% of patients improved, 13% remained unchanged, and 10% worsened. The mortality (2%) and morbidity (2%) in this series are well within reported limits in other series. Seventy-eight percent of these patients were followed for more than 1 year.[102] Ebersold and coworkers[43] evaluated the outcomes in 51 patients who had undergone cervical laminectomies. Of the 19 patients (37.3%) who were worse, 14 (74%) showed late deterioration at an average follow-up of 7.6 years.

The main criticism of laminectomy for the treatment of CSM has been the development of delayed instability with progressive kyphosis or S-shaped deformity. The other criticism of the procedure is that it does not address the motion-related forces in the spinal canal.[12, 40] Campbell and Phillips[37] and Cusick and colleagues[103] have emphasized the possible importance of immobilization.

The surgical procedures that have been used to allay these two criticisms are cervical laminaplasty and cervical laminectomy with posterior fusion. Since its first description by Hirabayashi[95] in 1978, laminaplasty has become well established as a technique for posterior cervical decompression. A number of studies detailing the results at relatively long-term follow-up (4 to 8 years) after various techniques of laminaplasty have been encouraging.[94, 96, 104–107] All these studies, however, looked at a mixed population of patients with cervical myelopathy, including patients with ossified posterior longitudinal ligament. Inoue and colleagues[104] described 50 patients with CSM followed for 5 to 13 years (mean, 8 years) and compared them with 26 similar

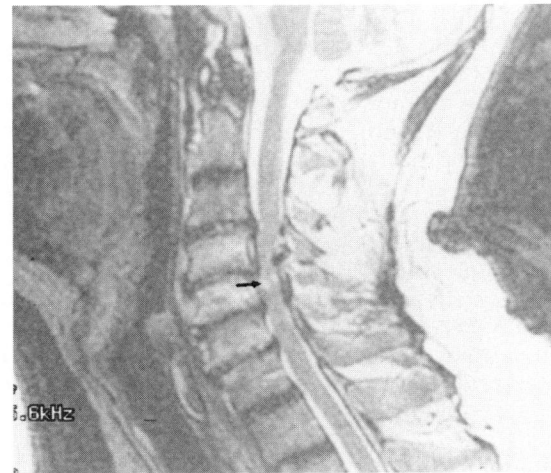

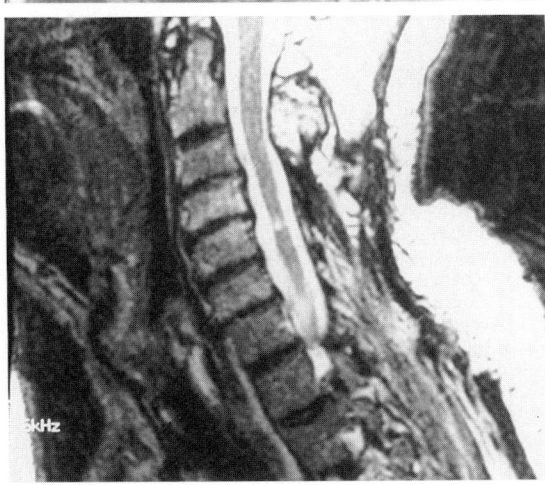

FIGURE 289-3. *A,* Preoperative sagittal magnetic resonance imaging (MRI) scan shows multilevel compression that is greatest at C4-5 and C5-6 and less at C3-4 and C6-7 in an elderly patient with myelopathy. There is a hyperintense lesion in the cord at C4-5 *(arrow). B,* Postoperative MRI scan after laminectomy and fusion-fixation of C3-7. The cord is away from any anterior osteophytes, without the need for dentate sectioning, and the area of hyperintensity can still be seen. The patient made a full recovery and is functioning normally.

patients with ossified posterior longitudinal ligament. Good recovery was noted, with no neurological deterioration, at initial follow-up and at 1 year. However, at later follow-up, deterioration was noted in 12 (24%) patients; in 4 (8%), reconstriction with cord compression was found, but in 8 (16%), there was no obvious radiologic explanation. This study underscores the need for long-term evaluation and imaging.

Cervical laminectomy with simultaneous posterior fusion by bone graft, metal rectangles, or lateral mass plates has been described to address the criticisms of laminectomy alone.[42, 44, 92] The most recent of these studies reported improvement of myelopathy scores in 76% of patients. There was no neurological deterioration or instability at a mean follow-up of almost 4 years, and follow-up MRI scans showed continued decompression (Fig. 289–3).[42]

CONCLUSION

Patients with CSM are not a homogeneous group. Studies of the natural history of the condition are dated (before the current era of modern neuroimaging). Published data do not reveal the superiority of any one surgical approach. Dissatisfaction with the standard procedures is implied in the reports of new ones.

There have been many calls for a prospective, randomized trial, which would, of necessity, have to be multicenter and possibly multinational.[11, 108] In the absence of such a trial, all centers that deal with patients with CSM should gather data in a prospective manner, with a clear protocol defining the surgical rationale and technique. Objective pre- and postoperative evaluations should be done using a standardized generic scale, with the aim of achieving long-term clinical and radiologic follow-up.

REFERENCES

1. Teresi L, Lufkin R, Reicher M, et al: Asymptomatic degenerative disk disease and spondylosis of the cervical spine: MR imaging. Radiology 164:83–88, 1987.
2. Hitselberger W, Witten R: Abnormal myelograms in asymptomatic patients. J Neurosurg 28:204–208, 1968.
3. Friedenberg Z, Miller W: Degenerative disc disease of the cervical spine: A comparative study of asymptomatic and symptomatic patients. J Bone Joint Surg Am 45:1171–1178, 1963.
4. Key C: Guy's Hosp Rep 3:17, 1838.
5. Gowers W: Diseases of the Nervous System, vol 1, 2nd ed. London, Churchill, 1892, p 260.
6. Stookey B: Compression of the spinal cord due to ventral extradural cervical chondromas. Arch Neurol Psychiatry 20:275–291, 1928.
7. Mixter W, Barr J: Rupture of the intervertebral disc with involvement of the spinal canal. N Engl J Med 211:210, 1934.
8. Peet M, Echols D: Herniation of nucleus pulposus: Cause of compression of the spinal cord. Arch Neurol Psychiatry 32:924, 1934.
9. Brain WR: Discussion on rupture of the intervertebral disc in the cervical region. Proc R Soc Med 41:509, 1948.
10. Alexander J: Natural history and nonoperative management of cervical spondylosis.
11. Rowland LP: Surgical treatment of cervical spondylotic myelopathy: Time for a controlled trial. Neurology 42:5–13, 1992.
12. Adams CBT, Logue V: Studies in cervical spondylotic myelopa-

13. Hayashi H, Okada K, Hashimoto J, et al: Cervical spondylotic myelopathy in the aged patient: A radiological evaluation of the aging changes in the cervical spine and etiologic factors of myelopathy. Spine 13:618–625, 1988.
14. Harkey HL, Al-Mefty O, Marawi I, et al: Experimental chronic compressive cervical myelopathy: Effects of decompression. J Neurosurg 83:336–341, 1995.
15. Al-Mefty O, Harkey L, Middleton T, et al: Myelopathic cervical spondylitic lesions demonstrated by magnetic resonance imaging. J Neurosurg 68:217–222, 1988.
16. Clarke E, Robinson P: Cervical myelopathy: A complication of cervical spondylosis. Brain 79:483–510, 1956.
17. Lees F, Aldren Turner JW: Natural history and prognosis of cervical spondylosis. BMJ 2:1607–1610, 1963.
18. Nurick S: The pathogenesis of the spinal cord disorder associated with cervical spondylosis. Brain 95:87–100, 1972.
19. Nurick S: The natural history and the results of surgical treatment of the spinal cord disorder associated with cervical spondylosis. Brain 95:101–108, 1972.
20. Symon L, Lavender P: The surgical treatment of cervical spondylotic myelopathy. Neurology 17:117–127, 1967.
21. Phillips D: Surgical treatment of myelopathy with cervical stenosis. J Neurol Neurosurg Psychiatry 36:879–884, 1973.
22. Roberts A: Myelopathy due to cervical spondylosis treated by collar immobilization. Neurology 16:951–954, 1966.
23. Sadasivan K, Reddy R, Albright J: The natural history of cervical spondylotic myelopathy. Yale J Biol Med 66:235–242, 1993.
24. Epstein N, Epstein J, Carras R, et al: Coexisting cervical and lumbar stenosis: Diagnosis and management. Neurosurgery 15:489–496, 1984.
25. Lunsford LD, Bissonette DJ, Zorub DS: Anterior surgery for cervical disc disease. Part 2. Treatment of cervical spondylotic myelopathy in 32 cases. J Neurosurg 53:12–19, 1980.
26. Ono K, Ebara S, Fuji T, et al: Myelopathy hand: New clinical signs of cervical cord damage. J Bone Joint Surg Br 69:215–219, 1987.
27. Ebara S, Yonenobu K, Fujiwara K, et al: Myelopathy hand characterized by muscle wasting, a different type of myelopathy hand in patients with cervical stenosis. Spine 13:785–791, 1988.
28. Good D, Couch J, Wacaser L: Numb, clumsy hands and high cervical spondylosis. Surg Neurol 22:285–291, 1984.
29. Hukuda S, Mochizuki T, Ogata M, et al: Operations for cervical spondylotic myelopathy: A comparison of the results of anterior and posterior procedures. J Bone Joint Surg Br 67:609–615, 1985.
30. Dagi T, Tarkington MA, Leech J: Tandem lumbar and cervical stenosis, natural history, prognostic indices, and results after surgical decompression. J Neurosurg 66:842–849, 1987.
31. Teng P, Papatheodorou C: Combined cervical and lumbar stenosis. Arch Neurol 10:298–308, 1964.
32. Ferguson R, Caplan L: Cervical spondylitic myelopathy. Neurol Clin 3:373–382, 1985.
33. Crandall P, Batzdorf U: Cervical spondylotic myelopathy. J Neurosurg 25:57–66, 1966.
34. Mehalic TF, Pezzuti RT, Applebaum BI: Magnetic resonance imaging and cervical spondylotic myelopathy. Neurosurgery 26:217–227, 1990.
35. Matsuda Y, Miyazaki K, Tada K, et al: Increased MR signal intensity due to cervical myelopathy. J Neurosurg 74:887–894, 1991.
36. Yone K, Sakou T, Yanase M, Ijiri K: Preoperative and postoperative magnetic resonance image evaluations of the spinal cord in cervical myelopathy. Spine 17(Suppl 10):S388–S392, 1992.
37. Campbell AMG, Phillips DG: Cervical disk lesions with neurological disorder. BMJ 2:481–485, 1960.
38. Bradshaw P: Some aspects of cervical spondylosis. Q J Med 26:177–208, 1957.
39. Balla J, Walton J, Hankinson J: Newcastle Med J 28:191–203, 1964.
40. Barnes MP, Saunders M: The effect of cervical mobility on the natural history of cervical spondylotic myelopathy. J Neurol Neurosurg Psychiatry 47:17–20, 1984.
41. Al-Mefty O, Harkey HL, Marawi I, et al: Experimental chronic compressive cervical myelopathy. J Neurosurg 79:550–561, 1993.

42. Kumar VGR, Rea GL, Mervis LJ, McGregor JM: Cervical spondylotic myelopathy: Functional and radiographic long-term outcome after laminectomy and posterior fusion. Neurosurgery 44: 771–778, 1999.

43. Ebersold MJ, Pare MC, Quast LM: Surgical treatment for cervical spondylotic myelopathy. J Neurosurg 82:745–751, 1995.

44. Gonzalez-Feria L: The effect of surgical immobilization after laminectomy in the treatment of advanced cases of cervical spondylotic myelopathy. Acta Neurochir (Wien) 31:185–193, 1975.

45. Guidetti B, Fortuna A: Long-term results of surgical treatment of myelopathy due to cervical spondylosis. J Neurosurg 30: 714–721, 1969.

46. Thomas NW, Rea GL, Pikul BK, et al: Quantitative outcome and radiographic comparisons between laminectomy and laminotomy in the treatment of acquired lumbar stenosis. Neurosurgery 41:567–575, 1997.

47. Monro P: What has surgery to offer in cervical spondylosis? In Warlow C, Garfield J (eds): Dilemmas in the Management of the Neurosurgical Patient. Edinburgh, Churchill Livingstone, 1984, pp 168–187.

48. Jaskolski DJ, Jarratt JA, Jakubowski J: Clinical evaluation of magnetic stimulation in cervical spondylosis. Br J Neurosurg 3: 541–548, 1989.

49. Leblhuber F, Reisecker F, Boehm-Jurkovic H, et al: Diagnostic value of different electrophysiologic tests in cervical disc prolapse. Neurology 38:1879–1881, 1988.

50. Maertens de Noordhout A, Remacle JM, Pepin JL, et al: Magnetic stimulation of the motor cortex in cervical spondylosis. Neurology 41:75–80, 1991.

51. Peioglou-Harmoussi S, Fawcett PRW, Howell D, Barwick DD: F-response frequency in motor neurone disease and cervical spondylosis. J Neurol Neurosurg Psychiatry 50:593–599, 1987.

52. Thacker AK, Misra S, Katiyar BC: Nerve conduction studies in upper limbs of patients with cervical spondylosis and motor neurone disease. Acta Neurol Scand 78:45–48, 1988.

53. Ueta E, Tani T, Shinichirou T, et al: Diagnostic value of cervical somatosensory evoked potentials recorded from the intervertebral discs after median and ulnar nerve stimulation in cervical spondylotic myelopathy. J Spinal Disord 11:514–520, 1998.

54. Yiannikas C, Shahani BT, Young RR: Short latency somatosensory evoked potentials from radial, median, ulnar, and peroneal nerve stimulation in the assessment of cervical spondylosis. Arch Neurol 43:1264–1271, 1986.

55. Chang C, Lin S: Measurement of motor conduction in the thoracolumbar cord: A possible predictor of surgical outcome in cervical spondylotic myelopathy. Spine 21:485–491, 1996.

56. Epstein JA, Carras R, Hyman RA, Crockard HA: Cervical myelopathy caused by developmental stenosis of the spinal canal. J Neurosurg 51:363–367, 1979.

57. Foo D: Spinal cord injury in 44 patients with cervical spondylosis. Paraplegia 26:301–306, 1986.

58. Regenbogen VS, Rogers LF, Atlas SW, Kim KS: Cervical spinal cord injuries in patients with cervical spondylosis. AJR Am J Roentgenol 146:277–284, 1986.

59. Chiles BW, Leonard MA, Choudhri HF, Cooper PR: Cervical spondylotic myelopathy: Patterns of neurological deficit and recovery after anterior cervical decompression. Neurosurgery 44:762–770, 1999.

60. Batzdorf U, Batzdorff A: Analysis of cervical spine curvature in patients with cervical spondylosis. Neurosurgery 22:827–836, 1988.

61. Benzel EC: Cervical spondylotic myelopathy. In Cooper PR (ed): Degenerative Disease of the Cervical Spine. Park Ridge, Ill, American Association of Neurological Surgeons, 1993, pp 91–104.

62. Benzel EC: Cervical spondylotic myelopathy: Posterior surgical approaches. In Menezes AH, Sonntag VKH (eds): Principles of Spinal Surgery. New York, McGraw-Hill, 1996, pp 571–580.

63. Cloward RB: The anterior approach for removal of ruptured cervical disks. J Neurosurg 15:602–617, 1958.

64. Smith GW, Robinson RA: The treatment of certain cervical-spine disorders by anterior removal of the intervertebral disc and interbody fusion. J Bone Joint Surg Am 40:607–624, 1958.

65. Hirsch C: Cervical disc rupture: Diagnosis and therapy. Acta Orthop Scand 30:172–186, 1960.

66. Savolainen S, Rinne J, Hernesniemi J: A prospective randomized study of anterior single-level cervical disc operations with long-term follow-up: Surgical fusion is unnecessary. Neurosurgery 43:51–55, 1998.

67. Murphy MA, Trimble MB, Piedmonte MR, Kalfas IH: Changes in the cervical foraminal area after anterior discectomy with and without a graft. Neurosurgery 34:93–96, 1994.

68. Bertalanffy H, Eggert H: Clinical long-term results of anterior discectomy without fusion for the treatment of cervical radiculopathy and myelopathy. Acta Neurochir (Wien) 90:122–135, 1988.

69. Klaiber R, von Ammon K, Sarioglu A: Anterior microsurgical approach for degenerative cervical disc disease. Acta Neurochir (Wien) 114:36–42, 1992.

70. Thorell W, Cooper J, Hellbusch L, Leibrock L: The long-term clinical outcome of patients undergoing anterior cervical discectomy with and without intervertebral bone graft placement. Neurosurgery 43:268–274, 1998.

71. Dowd GC, Wirth FP: Anterior cervical discectomy: Is fusion necessary? J Neurosurg (Spine 1) 90:8–12, 1999.

72. Martins AN: Anterior cervical discectomy with and without interbody bone graft. J Neurosurg 44:290–295, 1976.

73. Rosenorn J, Hansen EB, Rosenorn M: Anterior cervical discectomy with and without fusion: A prospective study. J Neurosurg 59:252–255, 1983.

74. Boni M, Cherubino P, Denaro V, Benazzo F: Multiple subtotal somatectomy: Technique and evaluation of a series of 39 cases. Spine 9:358–362, 1984.

75. Harsh GR, Sypert GW, Weinstein PR, et al: Cervical spine stenosis secondary to ossification of the posterior longitudinal ligament. J Neurosurg 67:349–357, 1987.

76. Saunders RL, Bernini PM, Shirreffs TG, Reeves AG: Central corpectomy for cervical spondylotic myelopathy: A consecutive series with long-term follow-up evaluation. J Neurosurg 74: 163–170, 1991.

77. Seifert V, Stolke D: Multisegmental cervical spondylosis: Treatment by spondylectomy, microsurgical decompression, and osteosynthesis. Neurosurgery 29:498–503, 1991.

78. Zdeblick TA, Bohlman HH: Cervical kyphosis and myelopathy: Treatment by anterior corpectomy and strut-grafting. J Bone Joint Surg Am 71:170–182, 1989.

79. Fessler RG, Steck JC, Giovanini MA: Anterior cervical corpectomy for cervical spondylotic myelopathy. Neurosurgery 43: 257–267, 1998.

80. Mikawa Y, Shikata J, Yamamuro T: Spinal deformity and instability after multilevel cervical laminectomy. Spine 12:6–11, 1987.

81. Miyazaki K, Tada K, Matsuda Y, et al: Posterior extensive simultaneous multisegment decompression with posterolateral fusion for cervical myelopathy with cervical instability and kyphotic and/or S-shaped deformities. Spine 14:1160–1170, 1989.

82. Sim FH, Svien HJ, Bickel WH, Janes JM: Swan-neck deformity following extensive cervical laminectomy. J Bone Joint Surg Am 56:564–580, 1974.

83. Yasuoka S, Peterson HA, Laws ER, MacCarty CS: Pathogenesis and prophylaxis of postlaminectomy deformity of the spine after multiple level laminectomy: Difference between children and adults. Neurosurgery 9:145–152, 1981.

84. Yasuoka S, Peterson HA, MacCarty CS: Incidence of spinal column deformity after multilevel laminectomy in children and adults. J Neurosurg 57:441–445, 1982.

85. Brieg A, Turnbull I, Hassler O: Effects of mechanical stresses on the spinal cord in cervical spondylosis. J Neurosurg 25: 45–56, 1966.

86. Kahn EA: The role of the dentate ligaments in spinal cord compression and the syndrome of lateral sclerosis. J Neurosurg 4:191–199, 1947.

87. Epstein JA, Carras R, Lavine LS, Epstein BS: The importance of removing osteophytes as part of the surgical treatment of myeloradiculopathy in cervical spondylosis. J Neurosurg 30: 219–226, 1969.

88. Epstein JA, Janin Y, Carras R, Lavine LS: A comparative study of the treatment of cervical spondylotic myeloradiculopathy: Experience with 50 cases treated by means of extensive laminectomy, foraminotomy, and excision of osteophytes during the past 10 years. Acta Neurochir (Wien) 61:89–104, 1982.

89. Mayfield FH: New instrument. J Neurosurg 14:469, 1957.

90. Callahan RA, Johnson RM, Margolis RN, et al: Cervical facet fusion for control of instability following laminectomy. J Bone Joint Surg Am 59:991–1002, 1977.

91. Fehlings MG, Cooper PR, Errico TJ: Posterior plates in the management of cervical instability: Long-term results in 44 patients. J Neurosurg 81:341–349, 1994.

92. Maurer PK, Ellenbogen RG, Ecklund J, et al: Cervical spondylotic myelopathy: Treatment with posterior decompression and Luque rectangle bone fusion. Neurosurgery 28:680–684, 1991.

93. Fornari M, Luccarelli G, Giombini S, Chiapparini L: Artificial lamina-assisted laminoplasty performed in seven cases. J Neurosurg (Spine 1) 91:43–49, 1999.

94. Hase H, Watanabe T, Hirasawa Y, et al: Bilateral open laminoplasty using ceramic laminas for cervical myelopathy. Spine 16:1269–1276, 1991.

95. Hirabayashi K: Expansive open-door laminoplasty for cervical spondylotic myelopathy. Operation (Jpn) 32:1159–1163, 1978.

96. Ohmori K, Ishida Y, Suzuki K: Suspension laminotomy: A new surgical technique for compression myelopathy. Neurosurgery 21:950–957, 1987.

97. Brazier J, Jones N, Kind P: Testing the validity of the Euroquol and comparing it with the SF-36 health survey questionnaire. Qual Life Res 2:169–180, 1993.

98. McHorney CA, Ware JE, Lu JFR, Sherbourne CD: The MOS 36-item short-form health survey (SF-36). III. Tests of data quality, scaling assumptions, and reliability across diverse patient groups. Med Care 32:40–66, 1994.

99. Casey ATH, Bland JM, Crockard HA: Development of a functional scoring system for rheumatoid arthritis patients with cervical myelopathy. Ann Rheum Dis 55:901–906, 1996.

100. Epstein JA, Epstein NE: The surgical management of cervical spinal stenosis, spondylosis, and myeloradiculopathy by means of the posterior approach. In Cervical Spine Research Society (ed): The Cervical Spine. Philadelphia, Lippincott, 1989, pp 625–669.

101. Emery SE, Bohlman HH, Bolesta MJ, Jones PK: Anterior cervical decompression and arthrodesis for the treatment of cervical spondylotic myelopathy. J Bone Joint Surg Am 80:941–951, 1998.

102. Snow RB, Weiner H: Cervical laminectomy and foraminotomy as surgical treatment of cervical spondylosis: A follow-up study with analysis of failures. J Spinal Disord 6:245–251, 1993.

103. Cusick JF, Steiner RE, Berns T: Total stabilization of the cervical spine in patients with cervical spondylotic myelopathy. Neurosurgery 18:491–495, 1986.

104. Inoue H, Ohmori K, Ishida Y, et al: Long-term follow-up review of suspension laminotomy for cervical compression myelopathy. J Neurosurg 85:817–823, 1996.

105. Kimura I, Shingu H, Nasu Y: Long-term follow-up of cervical spondylotic myelopathy treated by canal-expansive laminoplasty. J Bone Joint Surg Br 77:956–961, 1995.

106. Kohno K, Kumon Y, Oka Y, et al: Evaluation of prognostic factors following expansive laminoplasty for cervical spinal stenotic myelopathy. Surg Neurol 48:237–245, 1997.

107. Satomi K, Nishu Y, Kohno T, Hirabayashi K: Long-term follow-up studies of open-door expansive laminoplasty for cervical stenotic myelopathy. Spine 19:507–510, 1994.

108. Braakman R: Management of cervical spondylotic myelopathy and radiculopathy. J Neurol Neurosurg Psychiatry 57:257–263, 1994.

109. Fager CA: Results of adequate posterior decompression in the relief of spondylotic cervical myelopathy. J Neurosurg 30:684–692, 1973.

110. Gorter K: Influence of laminectomy on the course of cervical myelopathy. Acta Neurochir (Wien) 33:265–268, 1976.

111. Bishara SN: The posterior operation in treatment of cervical spondylosis with myelopathy. J Neurol Neurosurg Psychiatry 34:393–398, 1971.

112. Carol MP, Decker TB: Cervical spondylotic myelopathies: Surgical treatment. J Spinal Disord 1:59–65, 1988.

CHAPTER 290

Spondyloarthropathies, including Ankylosing Spondylitis

MICHAEL R. GALLAGHER ■ REGIS W. HAID

The spondyloarthropathies are a group of related arthritic disorders of uncertain cause characterized by peripheral inflammatory arthritis, sacroiliitis, and a tendency toward extensive spinal involvement. Additionally, extra-articular features such as uveitis, conjunctivitis, and cardiac and pulmonary dysfunction may be observed. The spondyloarthropathies are all associated with the genetic marker HLA-B27. Rheumatoid factor is usually absent.[1, 2]

Ankylosing spondylitis is generally considered the prototype of the spondyloarthropathies. Other commonly recognized types include Reiter's syndrome (reactive arthritis), psoriatic arthritis, and enteropathic arthritis. Many patients share certain features of spondyloarthropathies but do not fulfill diagnostic criteria for any of the currently established categories of spondyloarthropathies. These conditions have been referred to as *undifferentiated spondyloarthropathies.*

This chapter focuses on features of the spondyloarthropathies of clinical interest to neurosurgeons, with an emphasis on ankylosing spondylitis. The clinical presentations and distinguishing features of the other spondyloarthropathies are summarized. As a whole, this diverse group of rheumatic disorders presents a significant challenge to neurosurgeons because of their complex effects on the spine and their potential neurological and functional sequelae. Recognition and treatment of these conditions require a thorough understanding of their epidemiology, pathogenesis, clinical features, and natural history. These areas, along with the basic principles of surgical and nonsurgical management, are also addressed.

ANKYLOSING SPONDYLITIS

Epidemiology

The prevalence of ankylosing spondylitis varies widely, depending on the population studied, the methods of study, and the diagnostic criteria employed. A long-term U.S. population–based study yielded an adjusted incidence rate of 7.3 per 100,000 patient-years.[3] In general, the prevalence of ankylosing spondylitis closely parallels the frequency of HLA-B27 in most populations.[4] However, a direct correlation is lacking in some populations.[5] Relative disease risk in HLA-B27–positive patients appears to be 1% to 2%.[6] In HLA-B27–positive first-degree relatives of patients with ankylosing spondylitis, this risk is increased to 20% to 30%.[6] More recent studies have demonstrated a link between HLA-B60 in both HLA-B27–positive and –negative patients.[3, 7] This link suggests that B60 (or a tightly linked gene) can increase susceptibility to ankylosing spondylitis independent of B27. Clinically, the disease is seen more commonly in males than in females, with a male-female ratio of 2:1 to 3:1.[8]

Cause

The cause of ankylosing spondylitis and the other spondyloarthropathies has yet to be determined. A genetically determined host response to a ubiquitous environmental factor or factors appears to be responsible.[2, 9–11] Among environmental factors, infectious causes have long been suspected. The number of recognized microbial triggering agents for reactive arthritis continues to grow, and they include bacterial agents with an established HLA-B27 relationship: *Campylobacter, Chlamydia, Clostridium, Salmonella, Shigella,* and *Yersinia.*[12] Multiple additional bacteria, as well as some viruses and parasites, may also be associated with reactive arthritis, but without an established link to HLA-B27.[12] However, the potential relationship between infection or exposure to such agents and the development of ankylosing spondylitis remains undetermined. Statistical analysis from more recent studies of twins with ankylosing spondylitis suggests that environmental triggers play only a small role and that genetic factors are largely responsible for susceptibility.[11,13]

The strong epidemiologic association between HLA-B27 and ankylosing spondylitis has led to detailed study of its role. Several mechanisms of association have been proposed.[11, 14–17] Whatever the mechanism, multiple factors and considerable heterogeneity are likely involved. Indeed, most persons positive for B27 do not have the disease, despite the proposed ubiquitous nature of the environmental trigger or triggers.[5] Further, the disease may occur in B27-negative individuals, although its clinical form may differ.[18]

The spondyloarthropathies characteristically involve variable combinations of synovitis, spinal inflammation (spondylitis), dactylitis (sausage digits), and, importantly, enthesitis (inflammation at the site where a ligament, tendon, or capsule inserts into bone) and bone formation.[19,20] Enthesitis is a major feature of spondyloarthropathy associated with spinal disease and peripheral tendinitis. Imaging studies of early synovitis suggest that the first abnormality to appear in these swollen joints is enthesitis.[19] This observation has led to a hypothesis that the synovitis seen in spondyloarthropathy occurs secondary to the release of proinflammatory mediators (e.g., cytokines and growth factors) from the enthesis.[19] If this hypothesis holds true, arthritis could be classified as either primary synovial (rheumatoid like) or enthesial (spondyloarthropathy like).[19] However, details of this pathogenesis remain unclear. Studies suggest that growth factors (such as bone morphogenetic proteins and transforming growth factor-β) play an essential role in the development of the vertebral ossification seen in ankylosing spondylitis.[21–23]

Pathology

Ankylosing spondylitis involves inflammation, bone erosion, and ankylosis. The target tissues are diarthrodial joints and entheses that represent the attachment sites of ligaments, tendons, and joint capsules to bone. In the axial skeleton, the sacroiliac, apophyseal, and costovertebral joints typically are affected and may become ankylosed. Enthesopathy is manifested in the axial skeleton at the junction of the annulus fibrosus and vertebral end plates. The inflammation usually is chronic and involves lymphocytes, plasma cells, and histiocytes.[24] These inflammatory and fibrotic changes subsequently lead to ossification, with much of the disk eventually replaced by bone after destruction of the cartilage and subchondral plate.[24] Such ossification

of the disk accounts for the characteristic radiographic appearance.[24] Syndesmophytes typically occur at the disk margins (marginal syndesmophytes) and predominate on the anterior and lateral aspects of the spine.[21, 25, 26] This relative anterior predominance may be attributable to a higher number of mesenchymal cells potentially responsive to cytokines and various growth factors in the anterior ligamentous structures.[27]

Clinical Features

SPINAL

Ankylosing spondylitis typically presents in the second or third decade of life with the insidious onset of chronic, persistent lower back pain. Women and children are more likely than men to have pain in the hips, knees, and other peripheral joints.[28] The pain generally is dull and centered in the lumbar and sacroiliac or gluteal regions, but it may be referred locally. Unlike pain from sciatica, however, pain from ankylosing spondylitis seldom radiates below the knee.[28, 29] The pain may be exacerbated by coughing or straining. The pain of sacroiliitis initially may be unilateral and intermittent, but eventually it becomes bilateral and persistent.

Back stiffness represents another common feature. Although stiffness is usually located in the lumbosacral region, it may be felt anywhere in the spine.[6] Typically, back stiffness worsens after prolonged rest and improves with mild activity or exercise. Several features differentiate the pain and stiffness of ankylosing spondylitis from that associated with other causes of back pain (Table 290–1).[30, 31] Eventually, some patients may develop diffuse ankylosis of the lumbar, thoracic, and cervical regions of the spine. Typically, fusion begins in the lumbar area and ascends. Classically, patients assume a posture of lumbar flexion, transferring weight away from the inflamed apophyseal joints.[29,32] Eventually, thoracic kyphosis and cervical extension develop, resulting in a progressively stooped posture that may become extreme (Fig. 290–1). The costovertebral joints are often involved; their involvement results in decreased chest expansion, which is often further reduced by a stooped posture.

TABLE 290–1 ■ **Classification of Back Pain**

FACTORS	MECHANICAL	INFLAMMATORY	INFECTIOUS	NEOPLASTIC
Age	15–19 yr	<40 yr	5–90 yr	>40 yr
Family history	Absent	Present	Absent	Absent
Onset	Acute	Insidious	Acute	Subacute
Nocturnal pain	Rare	Common	Common	Common
Morning stiffness	Rare	Common	Absent	Absent
Improvement with rest	Yes	No	No	No
Improvement with exercise	No	Yes	No	No
Radiation	Radicular	Diffuse	Diffuse	Localized
Neurological signs	Common	None	Uncommon	Common
Extraspinal involvement	None	Common	Uncommon	Common
Fever	Absent	Rare	Common	Uncommon
Erythrocyte sedimentation rate	Normal	High	High	Variable

Adapted from Calin A: Ankylosing spondylitis. In Kelley WN, Harris ED Jr, Ruddy S, et al (eds): Textbook of Rheumatology. Philadelphia, WB Saunders, 1985, pp 993–1006.

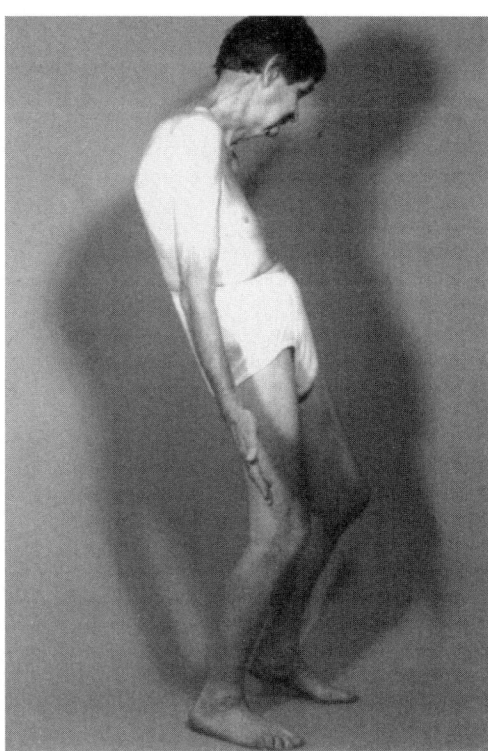

FIGURE 290–1. Adult male with advanced ankylosing spondylitis. The severely stooped posture is the result of lumbar flexion, thoracic kyphosis, and cervical extension.

Multiple complications can arise from spinal involvement in ankylosing spondylitis, including fracture, pseudarthrosis, spinal deformity, upper cervical instability, spondylodiskitis, spinal stenosis, and, rarely, cauda equina syndrome.

Spinal fractures represent a serious potential complication and may occur after relatively minor trauma, frequently falls. The lack of mobile segments, combined with secondary osteoporosis, predisposes the ankylosed spine to fracture. Patients with total spinal involvement are at greatest risk.[33–35] These fractures resemble the transverse shear pattern seen with fractures of osteoporotic tubular bone.[36] Such fractures may occur at any level but are most common (75%) in the cervical spine.[37] The lower cervical spine and cervicothoracic junction are the most frequently injured levels, followed by the thoracolumbar junction.[36–41] The ossified disk space represents the weakest area of the fixed spinal column and thus is prone to fracture.[33, 42] Such fractures may also involve adjacent portions of the vertebral body.[37] Fractures may be associated with epidural hematoma or, rarely, with herniated disks.[33, 43, 44] These injuries tend to be highly unstable and are associated with a significant risk of neurological deficit.[33, 45, 46] Not uncommonly, a pattern of secondary neurological deterioration may occur with a free interval between trauma and the onset of deficits, or further neurological deterioration may occur in a patient with an established spinal cord injury.[45, 46] In either case, repeat imaging is imperative to evaluate for the presence of an epidural hematoma or an interval change in spinal alignment.[45]

Spondylodiskitis is an erosive and sclerotic process that involves the intervertebral disk and adjacent vertebral bodies. Its cause is not completely understood. One view is that it represents an inflammatory process affecting the intervertebral disk and surrounding bone. Biopsy data support this view.[47, 48] Another belief is that it occurs after trauma, with excessive forces localized at one intervertebral segment causing mechanical destruction and pseudarthrosis. Both mechanisms may result in similar destructive disk lesions, and the term *spondylodiskopathy* has been suggested.[49, 50] The radiographic appearance is fairly typical, characterized by widening of the erosive disk space, breakdown of subchondral bone, and sclerosis of the surrounding bone. The radiologic appearances of spondylodiskitis, pseudarthrosis, and infectious diskitis are similar.[29] Spondylodiskitis has a reported incidence of approximately 5% in patients with ankylosing spondylitis.[48, 51, 52] Slightly more than 50% of patients are asymptomatic, and approximately 50% of afflicted patients present with back pain of mechanical character.[48, 49, 51] Most of the lesions develop in the lower thoracic spine.

Other spinal complications are encountered even less frequently. Spinal stenosis rarely occurs due to ankylosis of the posterior longitudinal ligament.[29, 33] As the only remaining area with mobile joints, the upper cervical spine may become unstable as the enthesopathic process reaches it.[33] Cauda equina syndrome is also rarely encountered. Its pathogenesis is unclear. Radiographically, arachnoid diverticula with posterior element erosion are noted.[49] It may involve chronic nerve root injury related to gravitational traction by arachnoid diverticula.[53] A varied picture of cauda equina damage as a result of fibrosis, demyelination, and atrophy has been noted.[54] Its natural history tends to be slowly progressive.[53]

EXTRASPINAL

Peripheral arthritis occurs in ankylosing spondylitis and may be chronic in up to 25% of patients.[28] Occasionally, it is the presenting manifestation, particularly with early onset.[6]

Acute iritis (acute anterior uveitis) is the most common extra-articular manifestation of ankylosing spondylitis.[6] It is more common in HLA-B27–positive than HLA-B27–negative patients, and its precise relationship to the disease is poorly defined.[55]

Other systemic manifestations are relatively uncommon and are observed mainly in patients with long-standing disease. Cardiovascular complications include aortitis, valvular dysfunction, and conduction disturbances. Apical pulmonary fibrosis may occur, with males at higher risk than females.[29, 56] Lung cavities may develop and subsequently become infected. Secondary amyloidosis may lead to renal dysfunction. Inflammatory bowel disease may be an associated disorder, although its relationship to ankylosing spondylitis is uncertain.[28, 57] Study of muscles in affected patients suggests that they are secondarily affected by pain-related inhibition and disuse.[58]

OTHER SPONDYLOARTHROPATHIES

Other spondyloarthropathies include psoriatic and enteric arthritis, undifferentiated spondyloarthropathies, and the reactive arthritic disorders, including Reiter's syndrome. These conditions constitute a wide spectrum of disease with some overlap, and "incomplete" forms are observed. Two sets of diagnostic criteria have been developed: the European Spondyloarthropathy Study Group and the Amor criteria (Tables 290–2 and 290–3).[59, 60] The specificity and sensitivity of both are similar.[61] Classification of these disorders into subtypes may be helpful in understanding prognosis and guiding therapy.[62]

Psoriatic Arthritis

Psoriatic arthritis is an inflammatory arthritis associated with psoriasis.[63] It affects men and women equally, and its peak onset is in the fourth decade.[30] The presentation is quite variable, and multiple patterns are possible: distal joint disease, asymmetrical oligoarthritis, polyarthritis (often asymmetrical), and arthritis mutilans. The most common extra-articular feature is a skin lesion, usually psoriasis vulgaris. Spine involvement occurs in approximately 20% of patients.[64, 65] The spondyloarthropathy of psoriatic arthritis has a different pattern than that of ankylosing spondylitis. Sacroiliitis tends to be asymmetrical, whereas in ankylosing spondylitis, it is symmetrical.[30] In ankylosing spondylitis, syndesmophytes tend to occur at the disk margins with a symmetrical distribution.[30] In psoriatic arthritis, marginal and nonmarginal syndesmophytes occur, often skipping vertebrae.[30] Typically, ligamentous calcification is relatively absent, and the apophyseal joints are spared.[64, 66] A relative lack of progression with relative preservation of spinal mobility has been observed, but involvement can be severe.[64, 66] HLA-B27 occurs less frequently in psoriatic arthritis than in ankylosing spondylitis.[30]

T A B L E 2 9 0 – 2 ■ **European Spondylarthropathy Study Group Preliminary Criteria for the Classification of Spondylarthropathy**

Inflammatory spinal pain or synovitis—asymmetrical, predominantly in the lower limbs and one or more of the following:
Positive family history
Inflammatory bowel disease
Urethritis, cervicitis, or acute diarrhea within 1 mo before arthritis
Buttock pain alternating between right and left gluteal areas
Enthesopathy
Sacroiliitis

Adapted from Schumacher H, Bardin T: The spondyloarthropathies classification and diagnosis: Do we need new terminologies? Baillieres Clin Rheumatol 12:551–565, 1998.

T A B L E 2 9 0 – 3 ■ **Amor Criteria for the Classification of Spondyloarthropathies**

FEATURE	POINTS*
Past or Current Clinical Manifestations	
Back pain at night, back stiffness in the morning, or both	1
Asymmetrical oligoarthritis	2
Gluteal path without other details or	1 or
Alternating gluteal pain	2
Sausage-like digit or toe	2
Heel pain or other enthesopathy	2
Iritis	2
Nongonococcal urethritis or cervicitis within 1 mo before the onset of arthritis	1
Diarrhea within 1 mo before the onset of arthritis	1
Past or current psoriasis, balantidiasis, or inflammatory bowel disease	2
Roentgenographic Changes	
Sacroiliitis (stage 2 or more if bilateral, stage 3 or more if unilateral)	3
Predisposing Genetic Factors	
Presence of the HLA-B27 antigen or positive family history for ankylosing spondylitis, Reiter's syndrome, psoriasis, uveitis, or chronic bowel disease	2
Responsiveness to Treatment	
Improvement within 48 hrs after initiation of a nonsteroidal anti-inflammatory drug	1

*Patients with a total score of 6 points or more are classified as having a spondyloarthropathy.
Adapted from Schumacher H, Bardin T: The spondyloarthropathies classification and diagnosis: Do we need new terminologies? Baillieres Clin Rheumatol 12:551–565, 1998.

Reactive Arthritis

Reactive arthritis refers to a group of aseptic arthritic disorders that develop during or soon after an enteric or genitourinary tract infection. Its overall prevalence is uncertain, but it is most common in young men.[2] Classic Reiter's syndrome consists of the triad of nongonococcal urethritis, conjunctivitis, and asymmetrical oligoarthritis. However, an incomplete form, which is more common than the classic form, is recognized.[1, 67] The peripheral arthritis may be accompanied by other extra-articular features, including iritis and mucocutaneous lesions.[29] Typically, the peripheral arthritis is acute and oligoarticular, with preferential lower extremity involvement.[29] Sacroiliitis occurs in more than a third of patients with Reiter's syndrome.[68] However, when it does occur, disability is mainly due to calcaneal disease rather than to spinal involvement.[68]

Many potential triggering microorganisms have been mentioned. The prevalence of HLA-B27 among whites is approximately 75%.[2] The patterns of spinal involvement in Reiter's syndrome and psoriatic arthritis are quite similar and distinct from those associated with enteric arthritis and ankylosing spondylitis. Patients with Reiter's syndrome tend to have a better functional status than those with enteric arthritis and ankylosing spondylitis, even when the extent of radiographic involvement is taken into account.[29] Reactive arthritis usually has a self-limited course of 3 to 12 months.[69] However, some patients develop chronic, indolent arthritis.[30]

Enteropathic Arthropathy

Inflammatory bowel disease may be associated with spondyloarthropathy that has a pattern identical to that of ankylosing spondylitis. Arthritis occurs in as many as 20% of patients with inflammatory bowel disease.[70] Some patients may actually present with arthritis before the inflammatory bowel disease is recognized.[30] It may occur at any age but is seen most often in young adults and affects males and females equally.

The pattern of arthritis is variable. It is commonly asymmetrical and affects primarily the lower extremity joints.[30] In ulcerative colitis, unlike in Crohn's disease, the arthritic activity parallels the course of bowel inflammation.[30]

The spondyloarthropathy of inflammatory bowel disease constitutes a minority of the arthropathy and clinically is very similar to idiopathic ankylosing spondylitis.[30] Spinal involvement is more common in men than women and is not affected by the bowel inflammation.[30] Table 290–4 summarizes some comparative features of the spondyloarthropathies.

Undifferentiated Spondyloarthropathies

Patients with undifferentiated spondyloarthropathies have clinical and radiographic features of spondyloarthropathies but do not fulfill the diagnostic criteria for any of the currently established disease categories.[71] This definition implies a wide spectrum of disease manifestations with highly variable presentations and courses.[71] Such a definition encompasses patients who present with an early stage of a definite spondyloarthropathy, an abortive form of a definite spondyloarthropathy, an overlap syndrome, or an unknown and etiologically undefined subcategory of spondyloarthropathy.[71]

The features of undifferentiated spondyloarthropathies include arthritis (asymmetrical, mainly mono-oligoarticular, and preferentially involving the lower extremities), enthesitis, sacroiliitis, spondylitis, and systemic manifestations (including uveitis, conjunctivitis, and mucocutaneous lesions).[71] Patients with such features have been ignored in previous epidemiologic studies, resulting in an underestimation of the prevalence of spondyloarthropathies.[2, 72]

PATIENT EVALUATION

Indications for Surgery

Operative indications for patients with ankylosing spondylitis are difficult to define categorically. As with other surgical decisions, an individualized approach is necessary. Broadly stated, multiple categories of patients requiring surgical intervention exist. One category would be selected patients with acute fractures, particularly highly unstable fractures, or fractures with a significant associated deformity or neurological deficit. (Fracture management in patients with ankylosing spondylitis is somewhat controversial; see "Complications of Surgical Management.") An additional subgroup would be patients with acute fractures and associated compressive lesions (e.g., epidural hematoma or diskogenic lesion). A second general category of patients requiring operative intervention would be those with severe, fixed deformities resulting in significant functional impairment. Less common indications would include patients with bony, compressive lesions and resultant neural compromise, selected patients with spondylodiskitis (or pseudarthrosis), and patients with extensive cervical spinal involvement and upper cervical instability.

As with any spinal surgery, an appropriate preoper-

T A B L E 2 9 0 – 4 ■ **Comparison of the Spondyloarthropathies**

FEATURE	PSORIATIC ARTHRITIS	ANKYLOSING SPONDYLITIS	REITER'S SYNDROME	ENTEROPATHIC ARTHROPATHY
Gender (M:F)	1:1	9:1	8:1	1:1
Age of onset (yr)	35–45	20–29	20–29	Any age
Peripheral arthritis	96%	25%	90%	Common
Distribution	Any joint	Axial, lower limbs	Lower limbs	Lower limbs
Dactylitis	35%	Uncommon	Common	Uncommon
Enthesitis	Common	Common	Common	Less common
Sacroiliitis	40%	100%	80%	20%
Skin lesions	100%	Rare	Common	Occasional
Type	Psoriasis vulgaris, guttate, nail lesions	Nil specific	Keratoderma blennorrhagicum, nail	Pyoderma gangrenosum, erythema nodosum
Mucous membrane	Uncommon	Uncommon	Common	Uncommon
Conjunctivitis	Occasional	Rare	Common	Rare
Uveitis	Occasional	Occasional	Common	Occasional
Urethritis	Occasional	Rare	Common	Rare
Aortic regurgitation	Rare	Occasional	Common	Occasional
Familial aggregation	Common	Common	Occasional	Occasional
HLA-B27	40%	90%	80%	Common 30%

Adapted from Gladman D: Clinical aspects of the spondyloarthropathies. Am J Med Sci 316:234–238, 1998.

ative evaluation is crucial for a successful outcome. In addition to customary laboratory and systemic evaluations, several specific problems should be addressed. Because the spondyloarthropathies may be associated with enteropathies, nutritional status and general bone density should be evaluated.[47] Respiratory function may be compromised by thoracolumbar kyphosis and ankylosis of costovertebral articulations. Less commonly, intrinsic pulmonary disease can occur. The hip joints should also be evaluated clinically and radiographically. A total hip replacement should be performed, if indicated, before any spinal deformity is corrected surgically.[47] Atlantoaxial instability and subaxial subluxation are rare but, if present, are managed in a fashion similar to that for rheumatoid arthritis.[47] The preoperative examination should also include cardiac evaluation because of the increased incidence of aortic stenosis.

Radiologic evaluation should include standing views in the neutral position, with additional flexion-extension studies to assess potential instability. The chin-brow–to–vertical angle should be measured clinically with the patient's neck in a neutral position, and the measurements should be transposed to a lateral view of the spine.[47] The amount of bone resection required at each level can then be measured. Anteroposterior and lateral standing views are needed. Overall truncal balance, including the degree of hip flexion and sacral position, should be analyzed.[73]

Diagnostic Evaluation

A complete clinical history is essential to diagnose ankylosing spondylitis and may serve to distinguish it from other causes of mechanical back pain. A high degree of suspicion is required for clinical diagnosis, particularly when patients are in the early stages of the disease. Ankylosing spondylitis should always be considered in the differential diagnosis of lower back pain, particularly in young men. Clinical features that differentiate inflammatory lower back pain from other causes include the presence of a family history, insidious onset with persistent course, classic morning stiffness, and improvement with exercise (see Table 290–1).[74]

Physical examination should include analysis of habitus, posture, and flexibility of the spine. Flexibility is decreased in almost all patients with ankylosing spondylitis and can be measured with multiple techniques, including Schober's flexion test, Moll's lateral flexion test, and measurement of fingertip-to-floor distance. In Schober's flexion test, the top of the sacrum is identified, and points 10 cm above and 5 cm below it are marked. The patient is then asked to flex forward, and the distance between the two points is measured. In 95% of normal individuals, this distance increases by at least 5 cm.[75] Of course, none of these tests is specific, and they may yield abnormal results in patients with mechanical back pain or hip disease.[29] Chest expansion has a high degree of specificity, although it may be negative early in the disease.[29, 76, 77] These clinical measurements may be useful for regular follow-up of disease progression and severity.[78]

Laboratory analysis is of limited usefulness for diagnosis. Determination of the erythrocyte sedimentation rate, although nonspecific, is inexpensive and easy, and it may differentiate ankylosing spondylitis (elevated values) from mechanical back pain (normal values). The erythrocyte sedimentation rate and C-reactive protein may not be particularly useful for assessing disease activity.[79]

Radiography is the most specific testing modality for diagnosing ankylosing spondylitis.[29] The presence of sacroiliitis is required for a definitive diagnosis.[2, 28]

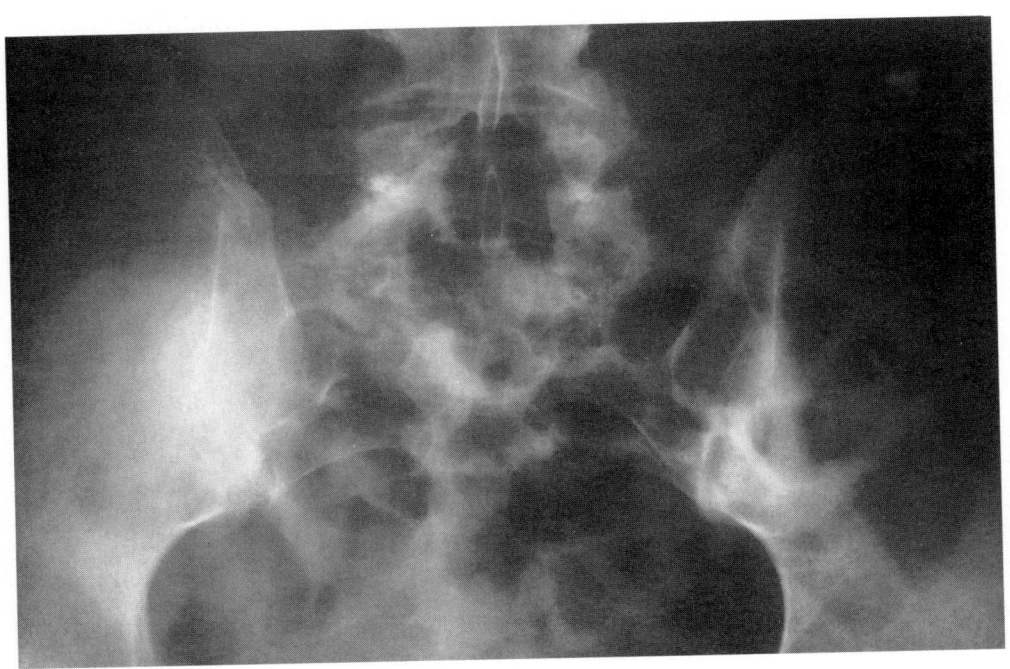

FIGURE 290–2. This anteroposterior radiograph from a patient with ankylosing spondylitis demonstrates advanced sacroiliitis with diffuse, symmetrical bilateral sclerosis and ankylosis. (Courtesy of Glenn Strome, MD.)

A plain anteroposterior view of the pelvis is usually adequate. However, radiographic assessment may be difficult, particularly early in the disease's course.[2, 28] Early changes consist of small, localized areas of erosion or sclerosis but with preservation of joint width. Subsequent progression is manifested by erosion, sclerosis, widening, or narrowing with ankylosis. Eventually, total ankylosis may occur (Fig. 290–2). If early ankylosing spondylitis is suspected, radiographic studies can be repeated in 6 months and routine medical measures initiated.[80] Alternatively, computed tomography or magnetic resonance imaging may be helpful. Computed tomography may be more sensitive than magnetic resonance imaging for demonstrating narrowing of the joint space, sclerosis, and erosion.[28, 81] Dynamic contrast-enhanced magnetic resonance imaging is also useful for detecting sacroiliitis in its early stages (when conventional radiography may still be negative).[82] Typical changes on magnetic resonance imaging include contrast enhancement of inner joint spaces, joint erosions, and juxta-articular osteitis.[82] Bone abnormalities have been demonstrated by single photon emission computed tomography in the lower thoracic and lumbar spines of patients with established symptomatic ankylosing spondylitis, but the role of this modality in daily practice remains unclear.[83]

Radiographic evaluation of bone density in patients with ankylosing spondylitis has yielded mixed results.[84,85] In mild disease, the reduction of bone mineral density is significant.[84] In advanced disease, increased lumbar bone mineral density has been reported.[84] This finding conflicts with clinical experience and the general appearance of plain radiographs, which demonstrate osteopenia and trabecular bone loss. The reason for these seemingly paradoxical findings is probably that osteoporosis persists in the advanced stage as trabecular osteopenia, but the advanced enthesopathy is followed by new bone formation in peripheral layers of the vertebral column, resulting in increased lumbar bone mineral density measurements.[84] This theory is supported by quantitative computed tomography, which has revealed decreased trabecular density in such patients.[86] A bone configuration of this nature may also explain the fracture patterns observed in advanced disease: the segmental spinal form is changed into a curved tubular structure with compression and tension surfaces and resultant transvertebral and transdiskal stress fractures.[86, 87]

The changes that occur in the vertebral bodies on plain radiographs are well known. "Squaring" results from bone erosion at the sites of disk attachment to the end plates. "Shiny corners" occur secondary to sclerosis at the disk. Bony bridging between the adjacent vertebrae is due to syndesmophyte formation and calcification of interspinous and supraspinous ligaments at sites of enthesopathy (Fig. 290–3).[29] Long-term involvement may eventually lead to diffuse radiographic fusion, resulting in the classic "bamboo spine" (Fig. 290–4). Typically, spinal changes develop sequentially from the sacrum to the cervical spine. A scoring system (the Stoke ankylosing spondylitis spine score) has been developed that uses a lateral lumbar radio-

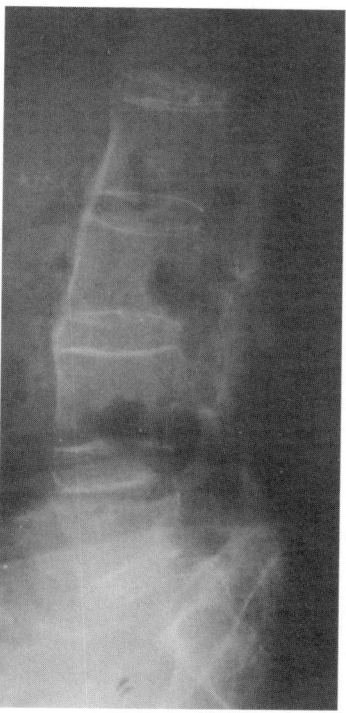

FIGURE 290–3. This lateral radiograph of the lumbosacral spine in a patient with long-standing ankylosing spondylitis illustrates typical "squaring," "shiny corner," syndesmophyte formation and ligamentous calcification.

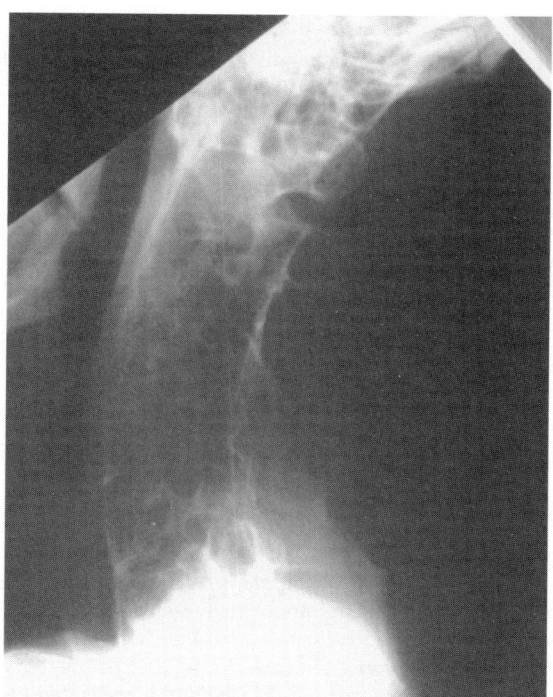

FIGURE 290–4. This lateral cervical radiograph demonstrates diffuse cervical involvement with the classic "bamboo spine" appearance.

TABLE 290–5 ■ **Criteria for Ankylosing Spondylitis**

ROME, 1961	NEW YORK, 1966	MODIFIED NEW YORK, 1984
Clinical 1. Low back pain and stiffness for more than 3 mo not relieved by rest 2. Pain and stiffness in the thoracic region 3. Limited motion in the lumbar spine 4. Limited chest expansion 5. History or evidence of iritis or its sequelae	**Clinical** 1. Limitation of motion of the lumbar spine in all three planes: anterior flexion, lateral flexion, and extension 2. Pain at the dorsolumbar junction or in the lumbar spine 3. Limitation of chest expansion to 2.5 cm or less measured at the level of the fourth intercostal space	**Clinical** 1. Low back pain of at least 3 mo duration improved by exercise and not relieved by rest 2. Limitation of motion of the lumbar spine in sagittal and frontal planes 3. Chest expansion decreased relative to normal values for age and sex 4. Bilateral sacroiliitis grade 2–4 5. Unilateral sacroiliitis grade 3–4
Radiologic Roentgenogram showing bilateral sacroiliac changes characteristic of ankylosing spondylitis (this would exclude osteoarthritis of the sacroiliac joints)	**Definite** 1. Grade 3–4 bilateral sacroiliitis with at least one clinical criterion 2. Grade 3–4 unilateral or grade 2 bilateral sacroiliitis with clinical criterion 1 or with both clinical criteria 2 and 3	**Definite** Unilateral grade 3 or 4 or bilateral grade 2–4 sacroiliitis and at least one of the three other clinical criteria
Definite 1. Grade 3–4 bilateral sacroiliitis with at least one clinical criterion 2. At least four clinical criteria	**Probable** Grade 3–4 bilateral sacroiliitis with no clinical criteria	

0, normal; 1, suspicious; 2, minimal sacroiliitis; 3, moderate sacroiliitis; 4, ankylosis.
Adapted from Kahn MA, van der Linden SM: Ankylosing spondylitis and other spondyloarthropathies. Rheum Dis Clin North Am 16:551, 1990.

graph and correlates with clinical features.[88] It may prove useful as an outcome measure.

Because back pain is a common symptom in the general population, numerous attempts at standardizing diagnostic criteria have been made. Currently, however, there are no validated diagnostic criteria for ankylosing spondylitis. The modified New York criteria (Table 290–5) remain the current standard. Criteria for all spondyloarthropathies have been discussed (see Tables 290–2 and 290–3). All these criteria, however, represent classification criteria rather than diagnostic criteria. As such, they are designed for application to groups of affected patients for epidemiologic purposes rather than to individual patients.[8] As noted, many patients with early disease (or formes frustes) may not fulfill the requirements for a particular classification. Of course, treatment decisions should be based on clinical signs and symptoms and need not depend on the formal fulfillment of criteria.[8] Nonetheless, such criteria are necessary for categorization and comparative study of these patients and for outcome assessments.

MANAGEMENT

Nonsurgical

The primary goals of management are (1) the optimization of functional status through the maintenance of proper upright posture and joint mobility and (2) the minimization of pain and stiffness, which promotes increased activity and exercise. The former objective is achieved through physical therapy and the latter through pharmacologic management.

Three main groups of drugs are used to treat ankylosing spondylitis.[89] The first group includes the main drugs used for pain control, the nonsteroidal anti-inflammatory drugs (NSAIDs), which do not influence the disease process itself but control the inflammatory process. The second group is composed of adjuvant drugs to control pain if the NSAIDs fail or are poorly tolerated. The third group includes drugs with theoretical or potential disease-modifying activity as observed in rheumatoid arthritis. This group is considered second-line treatment and includes sulfasalazine, which may be the only such drug used to treat ankylosing spondylitis.

NSAIDs constitute a cornerstone in the pharmacologic therapy of ankylosing spondylitis because they control inflammatory symptoms. In addition, these drugs have analgesic, antipyretic, and platelet-inhibiting activity.[90, 91] For reasons that are unclear, these drugs are more effective than aspirin and other salicylate compounds.[28] Despite extensive study, no NSAID has documented superiority in terms of efficacy and safety.[61] Individual patients respond to NSAIDs differently, and the choice of drug should be based on the patient's response.

Phenylbutazone, the first drug of this type to become available, has been used with some success. However, concerns about toxicity (i.e., its potential for producing agranulocytosis and aplastic anemia) have limited its use. The efficacy of indomethacin is well supported, and it remains the drug of choice of many rheumatologists.[28, 92] Naproxen is a widely used alternative with proven efficacy.[6] Many other alternatives, such as sulindac, tolmetin, piroxicam, diclofenac, and ibuprofen, exist.[49]

The most prominent side effects of NSAIDs are gastrointestinal disturbances. Indeed, these side effects represent the single most important factor limiting the drugs' usefulness.[91] The more recently introduced selective COX-2 inhibitors (e.g., celecoxib) may be useful in these patients.[89] Other significant side effects include renal impairment, hematologic reactions, adverse effects on the central nervous system, and mucocutaneous reactions.[89]

NSAIDs relieve musculoskeletal pain and stiffness and reduce peripheral joint swelling. In the spine, increased mobility may favorably influence a patient's functional status. Some authorities recommend an "on-and-off" regimen in which the drug is administered selectively during periods of high disease activity and withdrawn during quiescent periods.[91] No studies have demonstrated any benefit to the continuous administration of NSAIDs, and potential side effects may be reduced or avoided with their intermittent use.[91] To avoid unnecessary or inappropriate shifting between drugs, appropriate dosages must be used for a sufficient duration (generally at least 6 weeks) before a particular drug is abandoned.[91] The timing of drug administration is also important. For example, because pain and stiffness are frequently most severe at night and early in the morning, it may be helpful to schedule a relatively large dose near bedtime and a second dose on awakening.[91] Alternatively, agents with a long half-life (e.g., the oxicams) may be effective in a single daily dose.[89]

There has been significant interest in treating ankylosing spondylitis with disease-modifying antirheumatic drugs. Unfortunately, no drug has yet been found that consistently improves systemic disease activity and prevents progression. Sulfasalazine is the only drug with demonstrated efficacy in suppressing disease activity. However, some data are equivocal.[8] Sulfasalazine may help reduce synovitis in patients with polyarticular involvement without significant effect on axial involvement.[93, 94] Its use may be considered in patients with long-standing disease, a high level of disease activity (as measured by laboratory variables such as erythrocyte sedimentation rate), and active peripheral arthritis.[91] Gastrointestinal discomfort and central nervous system symptoms represent the major limiting side effects of this drug; fever, skin rash, hepatotoxicity, and leukopenia are less prominent. Most adverse reactions tend to develop within the first 3 months of sulfasalazine use.

Despite substantial interest, effective remittance therapy for ankylosing spondylitis is lacking. Oral or parenteral gold, azathioprine, the antimalarial drugs, and penicillamine have no demonstrated efficacy in the treatment of ankylosing spondylitis.[28, 89, 91] Methotrexate has rarely been used and has not been studied in a controlled fashion.[89] Despite some anecdotal reports, it has no proven efficacy.[89, 95, 96]

The anti-inflammatory effects of glucocorticoids are less marked in patients with ankylosing spondylitis than in patients with rheumatoid arthritis or systemic lupus erythematosus. This observation underscores the difference between pure inflammation and inflammation leading to bony ankylosis. Thus, administration of oral corticosteroids rarely produces any significant, lasting benefit.[91, 97] However, use of intra-articular corti-

costeroids can be quite helpful in selected patients with peripheral arthritis, enthesitis, and sacroiliitis.[25, 61, 89, 91, 98]

Physical therapy is essential for the successful management of patients with ankylosing spondylitis. Regular therapeutic exercise for the prevention of deformity and disability is one of the most important adjuncts to medical management.[6] Spinal ossification cannot be prevented by currently available medications. In patients with incomplete spinal ossification, an erect position can be achieved and maintained with the help of extension exercises.

Exercise programs are designed to strengthen back extensor muscles and to maintain motion in the spine, hips, shoulders, and thoracic cage.[29] The beneficial effects of exercise, including improved lumbar flexion, chest expansion, and mobility, have been well demonstrated.[99–102] Swimming is a particularly valuable exercise in these patients. Extension exercises should be performed once or twice a day.

Patient education should stress appropriate postural habits and strict compliance with regular exercise. Patients should walk as erect as possible and sleep on a firm mattress with minimal use of pillows. Patients should sleep while extended in the supine or prone position and should avoid sleeping on the side in flexion.[6] Compliance with exercise regimens tends to be poor, and continuous encouragement and regular follow-up by a physician and therapist are useful.[29, 103] Support groups for these patients may also help enhance compliance.[104]

Surgical

Most patients with ankylosing spondylitis do not require surgical therapy. General categories of patients for whom surgery is indicated, as well as basic considerations for preoperative assessment, were addressed under "Indications for surgery." General contraindications to surgery include poor general health and advanced age; these patients may be unable to tolerate the demands of surgery, immobilization, and rehabilitation.[105] Significant abdominal scarring or advanced atherosclerosis may preclude anterior correction or extension osteotomy of the lumbar spine.[105] Finally, the patient and family must have an appropriate understanding of the nature of the procedure and the potential associated morbidity.

In the correction of fixed flexion deformities, the site of the primary deformity should be determined clinically and radiographically. Ideally, primary correction is performed at this level; however, the patient's overall status, relative benefits and risks, and goals of postoperative function should be considered.[47] Flexion or kyphotic deformities involve different considerations, depending on the segment of the spine involved.

A primary flexion deformity may occur in the cervical region or, frequently, at the cervicothoracic junction. Simmons stressed the importance of recognizing an underlying fracture, particularly in patients who present with new or acute axial pain.[106] Patients with such acute fractures are typically managed with halo traction, followed by immobilization with radiographic follow-up or by posterior stabilization. If such fractures go unrecognized, they eventually heal, leaving the patient with a fixed, often severe, flexion deformity. At this stage, osteotomy is required for correction.

The goals of cervical osteotomy include correction of "chin-on-chest" deformity (facilitating forward view), prevention of atlantoaxial dislocation, relief of tracheal and esophageal kinking, and relief of myelopathy and radiculopathy caused by traction or kinking.[47] The first cervical osteotomy was reported by Urist in 1958.[80] In 1962, Law published a report of cervical osteotomies. His technique employed general anesthesia, frequently with correction at C3-4 or C5-6, and included grafting with wire or plate fixation and postoperative immobilization with a Minerva or halo vest.[107] Owing to potential difficulties with intubation and neurological deterioration with correction, Simmons advocated the use of local anesthesia, with good results.[48, 106, 108] This technique involves cervical osteotomy between C7 and T1 with the patient in a sitting position. Multiple anatomic advantages are associated with this level: relatively wide spinal canal, mobility, relatively diminished morbidity from compromise of the C8 root, and relatively reduced risk to the vertebral arteries.[48]

Kostuik employed a similar technique with some modifications (Figs. 290–5 and 290–6).[109] A halo is applied preoperatively to assist with reduction. If the osteotomy can be closed operatively, internal fixation is used. If pain or neurological difficulties (significant symptoms or monitoring changes) prohibit full surgical correction, additional postoperative closed correction is achieved with halo traction, followed by halo cast application.[109] McMaster reported 15 patients managed with a similar C7-T1 extension osteotomy technique using halo traction with general anesthesia and monitoring. A mean correction of 54 degrees was obtained.[110]

Some amount of thoracic kyphosis is commonly associated with ankylosing spondylitis; however, it is relatively rare for such a deformity to be the only or the primary deformity that requires correction in this area.[48] Patients with thoracolumbar kyphosis may be broadly grouped into two categories.[105] The first group includes patients with significant thoracic kyphosis and

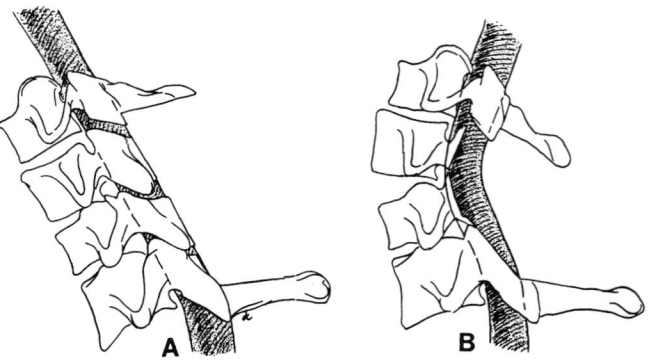

FIGURE 290–6. Kostuik cervical osteotomy technique. This lateral view of the cervical spine reveals the contour after osteotomy *(A)* and following the correction of kyphosis *(B).* (From Kostuik JP: The surgical treatment of ankylosing spondylitis. Semin Spine Surg 5:243, 1993.)

relatively normal cervical and lumbar lordosis. This group requires correction at the site of major deformity—the thoracic spine. In patients with rigid thoracic kyphosis, multiple anterior diskectomies and grafting via a transthoracic approach are performed, followed by postoperative halo traction and a delayed second-stage posterior correction involving multilevel V-shaped osteotomies and closure with compressive instrumentation.[48] Less commonly, in patients with relatively mobile thoracic kyphosis, preoperative halo traction is used, followed by a similar posterior procedure and then a second-stage anterior procedure with resection and grafting of areas of spondylodiskitis.[48] In this manner, significant correction can be obtained, but it is spread over multiple levels, thereby avoiding a single major angular correction that would pose an undue risk. In addition, some correction is obtained in the interval between stages by traction in an awake patient, thereby further reducing the potential risk.[48]

The second group includes patients with generalized kyphosis of the entire thoracolumbar spine with loss of lumbar lordosis.[105] This group is corrected with lumbar extension osteotomy. Multiple variations, including opening or closing osteotomies and single or multilevel procedures, exist. Theoretically, neurological risk is reduced at the lumbar level. The most important goal is restoration of the physiologic sagittal vertical axis.[105] Overcorrection must be avoided because of the lack of compensatory cervical motion and possible secondary effects on the pelvis, hips, and lower extremities.[73,105] In the event of severe overall deformity that requires multiregion correction, the cervical osteotomy should be performed first (because correction here is more limited), followed by the lumbar osteotomy (where realignment can be finally adjusted).[105]

In 1945, Smith-Petersen and colleagues described a posterior V-shaped extension osteotomy technique.[111] Since then, multiple alternatives have been described.[73, 106, 109–112] Figure 290–7 illustrates the general principles involved. Law reported a series of 120 patients using the Smith-Petersen technique with the addition of internal fixation to maintain correction and permit early

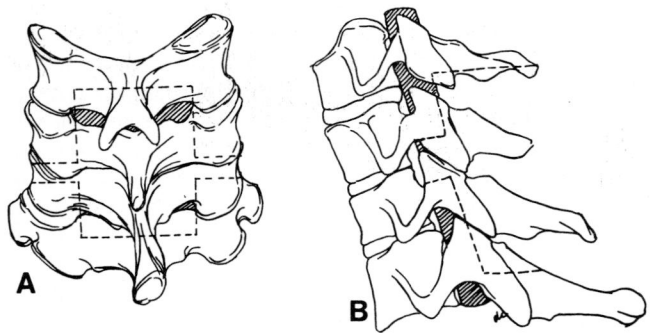

FIGURE 290–5. Posterior *(A)* and lateral *(B)* views of the Kostuik method for cervical osteotomy. The bone block to be resected is outlined. (From Kostuik JP: The surgical treatment of ankylosing spondylitis. Semin Spine Surg 5:243, 1993.)

A   B   C

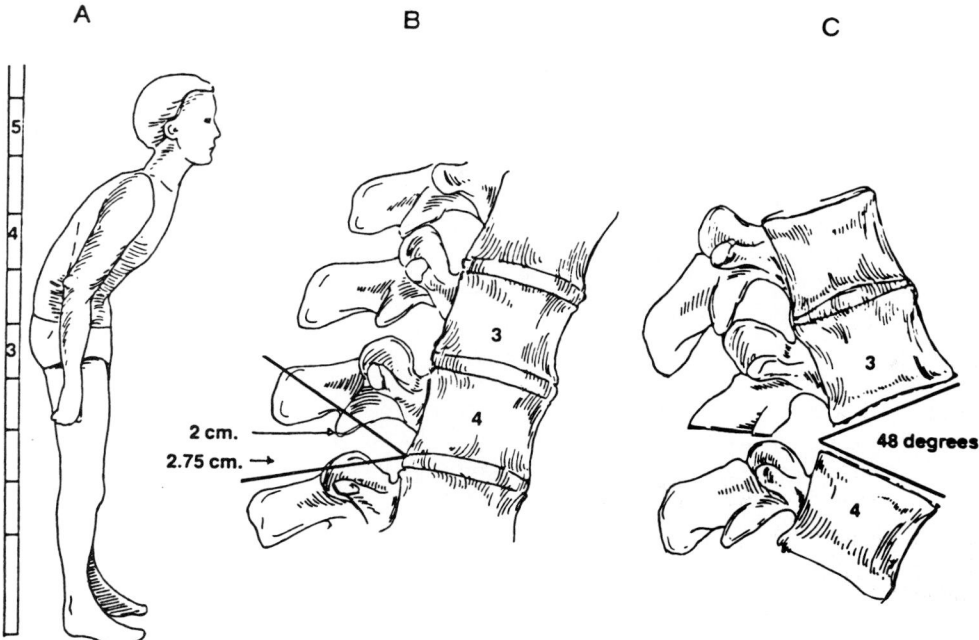

FIGURE 290–7. *A–C,* Lateral view of an ankylosing spondylitis patient standing with the hips and knees extended. The chin-brow–to–vertical angle has been measured and transposed to a lateral view of the lumbar spine with its apex at L3-4 so that the amount of bone resection required for correction can be determined. (From Kostuik JP: Ankylosing spondylitis. In Frymoyer JW (ed): The Adult Spine: Principles and Practice. New York, Raven Press, 1991, pp 719–743.)

mobilization.[113] Many other series support this benefit.[73, 109, 112, 114] Kostuik,[109] Thomasen,[115] and McMaster[69] successfully employed posterior monosegmental techniques caudal to the conus with supplemental instrumentation. Puschel and Zielke advocated multilevel (three or more) wedge osteotomies to reproduce lumbar lordosis (supplemented by pedicle screws and Zielke rods).[116] However, other authors have pointed out that the correction obtained is no greater than that achieved with monosegmental osteotomy and that the main correction with such techniques tends to occur at one level.[112, 114] Posterior techniques have potentially reduced the risk of vascular compromise, radicular compression or traction, and instability in comparison with anterior opening techniques.[73] Lazennec and coworkers reported their experience with 31 lumbar osteotomy patients using modern techniques.[73] These authors progressively changed to posterior monosegmental closing osteotomies with osteoclasty and supplemental monobloc fixation, with good results and correction up to 75 degrees.[73] They believed that monosegmental correction was faster and easier and resulted in less blood loss.[73]

COMPLICATIONS OF SURGICAL MANAGEMENT

Complication rates of surgery in patients with ankylosing spondylitis, particularly deformity correction, can be significant, even in experienced hands. Mortality rates ranging from 2.3% to 10% have been reported.[69, 117, 118] When spinal fractures are present, mortality rates as high as 13% to 50% (the latter number in older series) have been reported.[47, 119] Neurological complication rates are also significant. In a series of lumbar osteotomy patients, Lazennec and coworkers reported neurological complications in 6 of 19 patients undergoing anterior osteotomies and in 2 of 12 patients undergoing posterior procedures.[73] Fractures in patients with ankylosing spondylitis (which tend to be unstable three-column injuries) are associated with an incidence of neurological injury as high as 87%.[120] Additional potential complications include recurrent deformity and nonunion (which tend to occur concomitantly), loss of fixation, dural tears, vascular injury, and medical complications. This significant potential morbidity must be considered before undertaking these major procedures. As noted, appropriate patient selection and thorough preoperative evaluation and planning are crucial. Neurological injuries appear to be less frequent in recent series, possibly reflecting improved monitoring and earlier intervention.[105] The incidence of fixation loss and recurrent deformity may be reduced with transpedicular fixation compared with older techniques.[114] Restoration of sagittal balance can diminish the likelihood of recurrent deformity above or below instrumented levels.[105]

Fractures represent a frequent complication of ankylosing spondylitis, and they often remain undiagnosed. A high index of suspicion is therefore required. Spinal fractures may occur after even mild trauma. In general, patients with total spinal involvement are at greatest risk for injury.[33, 34] New or exacerbated back or neck pain in these patients warrants a thorough search for fractures. Fractures may be multiple and are most commonly associated with hyperextension injuries.[33, 34, 121, 122] Consequently, radiographic evaluation in such patients should be of the entire spine rather than just the symptomatic region.[33, 123] The majority of fractures occur in the lower cervical spine, followed by the thoracolumbar junction. As noted, these fractures tend to be extremely unstable and carry a high risk of neurological deficit (Fig. 290–8).

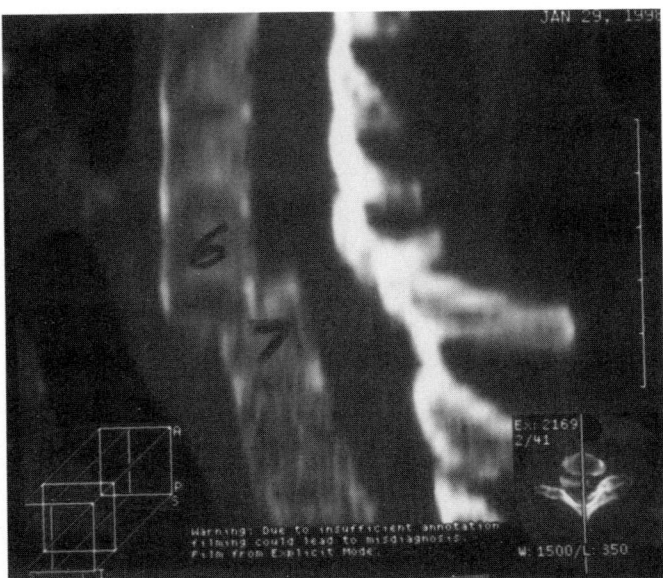

FIGURE 290–8. Midline sagittal computed tomographic reconstruction from spondyloarthropathy patient demonstrating typical cervical fracture pattern. This patient presented with new cervicothoracic axial pain and myeloradiculopathy. This injury required closed reduction via halo traction with subsequent posterior fixation and arthrodesis.

The optimal management of these fractures remains controversial.[124] Grisolia, Weinstein, and others have advocated conservative management for patients without neurological deficits, persistent vertebral dislocation, or fracture fragments within the canal because of the high surgical morbidity rate.[33, 42, 125, 126] However, other authorities have advocated primary surgical management using decompression (if needed), fixation, and external immobilization.[33, 35, 47] In separate series by Detwiler and Fox and their colleagues, primary operative management for cervical fractures was used successfully, including initial axial traction for realignment, followed by early posterior stabilization and postoperative halo vest (or cervicothoracic orthosis) immobilization.[33, 35] In a more recent series by Olerud and associates, similar primary operative management, but generally using anterior and posterior fixation, was advocated.[120]

Thoracolumbar fractures involve similar considerations. Minimally displaced fractures with a normal sagittal contour may be managed with a posterior compression construct and fusion.[105] However, fractures with significant anterior displacement or concomitant anterior kyphosis may be managed optimally with posterior and anterior surgery.[105] Supplemental rigid postoperative immobilization also may be helpful in these fractures.[105]

Management of symptomatic spondylodiskitis involves surgical considerations similar to those for acute thoracolumbar fractures.[105] As noted, these lesions most commonly occur in the lower thoracic spine. They may be managed with a posterior compression construct to shift the weight-bearing line posteriorly.[105, 118] A second-stage anterior grafting procedure can address residual kyphosis and anterior column deficits.[105]

Patients with ankylosing spondylitis with cervical involvement may develop associated C1-2 instability. This area should be screened intensely in such patients before intubation or surgery and should be followed clinically and radiographically in patients with known cervical involvement.[127] In a study of the natural history of atlantoaxial instability in patients with ankylosing spondylitis, 5 of 22 patients underwent posterior fusion over a 2-year period; surgery was necessitated by the development of myelopathy in 2 patients and by radiographic progression in 3.[128] Management considerations are similar to those for rheumatoid involvement, with C1-2 posterior arthrodesis used for atlantoaxial instability and occipital-cervical fusion used for vertical subluxation or extensive atlanto-occipital joint involvement (which is often the last joint affected).[129]

Rarely, a cauda equina syndrome develops in the late stage of ankylosing spondylitis. Lumboperitoneal shunt placement has been reported as a potentially effective option, although its efficacy and mechanism of benefit remain unclear.[130]

OUTCOMES AND CONCLUSIONS

Analysis of the natural history and prognosis of ankylosing spondylitis is complicated by the clinical heterogeneity of the disease. Despite this diversity, certain generalizations can be made. In 1988, Little summarized the natural history of ankylosing spondylitis on the basis of older studies. Since then, these generalizations have undergone many refinements and alterations but still remain applicable:[131]

1. The onset is insidious.
2. Exacerbations and remissions of the disease occur.
3. Spinal limitation and deformity are progressive.
4. Peripheral joint involvement, if present, occurs early.
5. Iritis tends to be early and recurrent.
6. The course is more severe if a patient's symptoms begin before age 16 years.
7. The course in women tends to be milder.

Early onset of disease is generally associated with slightly increased rates of morbidity and mortality; however, this mortality risk probably does not apply to the entire population with the disease. Khan and associates observed that the survival of patients with mild disease (the majority of patients) is comparable to that of the general population, although treatment and disease-related complications may contribute to premature death.[132]

In 1994, Amor and colleagues reported a long-term outcome study of ankylosing spondylitis with at least 10 years of follow-up.[133] Seven variables correlated with disease and outcome: hip arthritis, erythrocyte sedimentation rate over 30, poor efficacy of NSAIDs, limitation of lumbar spine, sausage-like fingers or toes, oligoarthritis, and onset before or at age 16 years.[133] If none of these factors was present at presentation, the patient could be expected to have a mild outcome. Conversely, if hip involvement or more than three factors were present, a severe outcome could be predicted.[133]

In 1997, Gran and Skomsvoll reported an outcome study of 100 patients with ankylosing spondylitis.[134] After a mean disease duration of 16.5 years, 51.5% of the patients remained in full-time work. Work cessation occurred at a mean disease duration of 15.6 years and was significantly associated with female gender, low educational level, acute anterior uveitis, "bamboo spine," and coexistence of nonrheumatic disease. Most of the functional loss occurred in the first 10 years of the disease and correlated with the occurrence of peripheral arthritis, spinal radiographic changes of ankylosing spondylitis, and the development of "bamboo spine." After more than 20 years of disease, more than 80% of the patients complained of daily pain and stiffness, and more than 60% used medications daily.[134] Such knowledge of the natural history of ankylosing spondylitis is an essential factor in guiding management decisions involving these patients. Future prospective studies of both surgically and nonsurgically treated patients would also be useful.

ACKNOWLEDGMENTS

The authors gratefully acknowledge the significant contributions of Eileen M. Sheehan, MS, CNRN, and Debbie Kilgore in the preparation of this chapter.

REFERENCES

1. Arnett FC: Seronegative spondyloarthropathies. Rheumatol Dis 37:1–12, 1987.
2. Khan MA, van der Linden SM: Ankylosing spondylitis and other spondyloarthropathies. Rheum Dis Clin North Am 16:551–579, 1990.
3. Carbone LD, Cooper C, Michet CJ, et al: Ankylosing spondylitis in Rochester, Minnesota 1935–1989: Is the epidemiology changing? Arthritis Rheum 35:1476–1482, 1992.
4. Gran JT, Husby G: The epidemiology of ankylosing spondylitis. Semin Arthritis Rheum 22:319–334, 1993.
5. Gran JT, Husby G: Clinical, epidemiologic and therapeutic aspects of ankylosing spondylitis. Curr Opin Rheumatol 10:292–298, 1998.
6. Shah BC, Khan MA: Review of ankylosing spondylitis. Compr Ther 13:52–59, 1987.
7. Brown MA, Pike KD, Kennedy LG, et al: HLA class I associations of ankylosing spondylitis in the white population in the United Kingdom. Ann Rheum Dis 55:268–270, 1996.
8. van der Linden S, van der Heijde D: Ankylosing spondylitis. Rheum Dis Clin North Am 24:663–676, 1998.
9. Ahearn JM, Hochberg MC: Epidemiology and genetics of ankylosing spondylitis. J Rheumatol 15:22–28, 1988.
10. Amor B: Suspected infectious agent and host environment interactions in spondyloarthropathies. Clin Exp Rheumatol 5:19–24, 1987.
11. Brown M, Wordsworth P: Predisposing factors to spondyloarthropathies. Curr Opin Rheumatol 9:308–314, 1997.
12. Toivanen A, Toivanen P: Epidemiologic aspects, clinical features, and management of ankylosing spondylitis and reactive arthritis. Curr Opin Rheumatol 6:354–359, 1994.
13. Brown MA, Duncan E, Shatford JL, et al: Susceptibility to ankylosing spondylitis in twins. Arthritis Rheum 40:1823–1828, 1997.
14. Archer JR, Whelan MA, Badakere SS, et al: Effect of a free sulphydryl group on expression of HLA-B27 specificity. Scand J Rheumatol 87:44–50, 1990.
15. Woodrow JC: Genetic aspects of the spondyloarthropathies. Clin Rheumatol 11:1–24, 1985.
16. Nickerson CL, Luthra HS, Savarirayan S, et al: Susceptibility of HLA-B27 transgenic mice to *Yersinia enterocolitica* infection. Hum Immunol 28:382–396, 1990.
17. Davenport MP: The promiscuous B27 hypothesis [letter]. Lancet 346:500–501, 1995.
18. Khan MA: Ankylosing spondylitis and heterogeneity of HLA-B27. Semin Arthritis Rheum 18:134–141, 1988.
19. McGonagle D, Gibbon W, Emery P: Classification of inflammatory arthritis by enthesitis. Lancet 352:1137–1140, 1998.
20. Resnick D, Niwayama G: Entheses and enthesopathy: Anatomical, pathological and radiological correlation. Radiology 146:1–9, 1983.
21. Ono K, Yonenobu K, Miyamoto S, et al: Pathology of ossification of the posterior longitudinal ligament and ligamentum flavum. Clin Orthop 359:18–26, 1999.
22. Forestier J, Rotes-Querol J: Senile ankylosing hyperostosis of the spine. Ann Rheum Dis 9:321–330, 1950.
23. Resnick D, Niwayama G: Radiographic and pathologic features of spinal involvement in diffuse idiopathic skeletal hyperostosis (DISH). Radiology 119:559–566, 1976.
24. Cruickshank B: Pathology of ankylosing spondylitis. Clin Orthop 74:43–58, 1971.
25. Cunnane G, Brophy DP, Gipney RG, et al: Diagnosis and treatment of heel pain in chronic inflammatory arthritis using ultrasound. Semin Arthritis Rheum 25:383–389, 1996.
26. Hammoudeh M, Siam AR, Khanjar I: Spinal stenosis due to posterior syndesmophytes in a patient with seronegative spondyloarthropathy. Clin Rheumatol 14:464–466, 1995.
27. Miyamoto S, Kuratsu S, Yonenobu K, et al: Evaluation of cell proliferating potentials in ossification of the spinal ligaments by argyrophilic nucleolar organizer region (AgNOR) staining. In Kurokawa T (ed): Annual Report of the Investigation Committee for Ossification of the Spinal Ligaments under the Auspices of Japanese Ministry of Health and Welfare. Tokyo, Department of Orthopedics, University of Tokyo, 1992, pp 160–165.
28. Escalante A: Ankylosing spondylitis: A common cause of low back pain. Postgrad Med 94:153–166, 1993.
29. Katz JN, Liang MH: Differential diagnosis and conservative treatment of rheumatic disorders. In Frymoyer JW (ed): The Adult Spine. New York, Raven Press, 1991, pp 669–718.
30. Gladman D: Clinical aspects of the spondyloarthropathies. Am J Med Sci 316:234–238, 1998.
31. Calin A: Ankylosing spondylitis. In Kelley WN, Harris ED, Ruddy S, et al (eds): Textbook of Rheumatology. Philadelphia, WB Saunders, 1985, pp 993–1006.
32. Simkin PA, Downey DJ, Kilcoyne RF: Apophyseal arthritis limits lumbar motion in patients with ankylosing spondylitis. Arthritis Rheum 31:798–802, 1988.
33. Fox MW, Onofrio BM, Kilgore JE: Neurological complications of ankylosing spondylitis. J Neurosurg 78:871–878, 1993.
34. Murray GC, Persellin RH: Cervical fracture complicating ankylosing spondylitis: A report of eight cases and review of the literature. Am J Med 70:1033–1041, 1981.
35. Detwiler KN, Loftus CM, Godersky JC, et al: Management of cervical spine injuries in patients with ankylosing spondylitis. J Neurosurg 72:210–215, 1990.
36. Harding JR, McCall IW, Park WM, et al: Fracture of the cervical spine in ankylosing spondylitis. Br J Radiol 58:3–7, 1985.
37. Karasick D, Schweitzer M, Abidi N, et al: Fractures of the vertebrae with spinal cord injuries in patients with ankylosing spondylitis: Imaging findings. Am J Radiol 165:1205–1208, 1995.
38. Fox MW, Onofrio BM, Kilgore JE: Neurological complications of ankylosing spondylitis. J Neurosurg 78:871–878, 1993.
39. Weinstein PR, Karpman RR, Gall EP, et al: Spinal cord injury, spinal fracture, and spinal stenosis in ankylosing spondylitis. J Neurosurg 57:609–616, 1982.
40. Goldberg AL, Keaton NL, Rothfus WE, et al: Ankylosing spondylitis complicated by trauma: MR findings correlated with plain radiographs and CT. Skeletal Radiol 22:333–336, 1993.
41. Simmons EH, Bernstein AJ: Fractures of the spine in ankylosing spondylitis. In Floman Y, Farcy J, Argenson C (eds): Thoraco-

lumbar Spine Fracture. New York, Raven Press, 1993, pp 385–408.

42. Weinstein PR, Karpman RR, Gal EP, et al: Spinal cord injury, spinal fracture, and spinal stenosis in ankylosing spondylitis. J Neurosurg 57:609–616, 1982.

43. Hunter T, Dubo HI: Spinal fractures complicating ankylosing spondylitis: A long-term follow-up study. Arthritis Rheum 26:751–759, 1983.

44. Rowed DW: Management of cervical spinal cord injury in ankylosing spondylitis: The intervertebral disc as a cause of cord compression. J Neurosurg 77:241–246, 1992.

45. Tico N, Ramon S, Garcia-Ortun F, et al: Traumatic spinal cord injury complicating ankylosing spondylitis. Spinal Cord 36:349–352, 1998.

46. Colterjohn N, Bednar D: Identifiable risk factors for secondary neurologic deterioration in the cervical spine-injured patient. Spine 20:2293–2297, 1995.

47. Kostiuk JP: Ankylosing spondylitis. In Frymoyer JW (ed): The Adult Spine: Principles and Practice. New York, Raven Press, 1991, pp 719–743.

48. Simmons EH: Surgery of the spine in ankylosing spondylitis and rheumatoid arthritis. In Chapman MW (ed): The Spine. Philadelphia, JB Lippincott, 1993, pp 2815–2850.

49. Rasker J, Prevo R, Lanting P: Spondylodiscitis in ankylosing spondylitis; inflammation or trauma? Scand J Rheumatol 25:52–57, 1996.

50. Hunter T: The spinal complications of ankylosing spondylitis. Semin Arthritis Rheum 19:172–182, 1989.

51. Little H, Urowitz MD, Smythe HA, et al: Asymptomatic spondylodiscitis: An unusual feature of ankylosing spondylitis. Arthritis Rheum 17:487–492, 1974.

52. Rosen PS, Graham DC: Ankylosing spondylitis: A clinical review of 128 cases. Arch Int Rheumatol 5:158–211, 1962.

53. Sant S, O'Connell D: Cauda equina syndrome in ankylosing spondylitis: A case report and review of the literature. Clin Rheumatol 14:224–226, 1995.

54. Tyrrell P, Davies A, Evans N: Neurological disturbances in ankylosing spondylitis. Ann Rheum Dis 53:714–717, 1994.

55. Edmunds L, Elswood J, Calin A: New light on uveitis in ankylosing spondylitis. J Rheumatol 18:50–52, 1991.

56. Rosenow E, Strimlan CV, Muhm JR, et al: Pleuropulmonary manifestations of ankylosing spondylitis. Mayo Clin Proc 52:641–649, 1977.

57. Mielants H, Veys EM, Goemaere S, et al: Gut inflammation in the spondyloarthropathies: Clinical radiologic, biologic and genetic features in relation to the type of histology: A prospective study. J Rheumatol 18:1542–1551, 1991.

58. Faus-Riera S, Martinez-Pardo S, Blanch-Rubio J, et al: Muscle pathology in ankylosing spondylitis: Clinical, enzymatic, electromyographic and histologic correlation. J Rheumatol 18:1368–1371, 1991.

59. Amor B, Dougados M, Mijiyawa M: Criteres de classification des spondylarthropathies. Rev Rheumatol 57:85–89, 1990.

60. Dougados M, van der Linden SS, Juhlin R, et al: The European Spondylarthropathy Study Group preliminary criteria for the classification of spondylarthropathy. Arthritis Rheum 34:1218–1227, 1991.

61. Olivieri I, Cantini F, Salvarani C: Diagnostic and classification criteria, clinical and functional assessment, and therapeutic advances for spondyloarthropathies. Curr Opin Rheumatol 9:284–290, 1997.

62. Schumacher H, Bardin T: The spondylarthropathies classification and diagnosis: Do we need new terminologies? Bailliers Clin Rheumatol 12:551–565, 1998.

63. Gladman DD: Psoriatic arthritis. In Kelley WN, Harris ED, Ruddy S, Sledge CB (eds): Textbook of Rheumatology, 5th ed. Philadelphia, WB Saunders, 1997, pp 999–1005.

64. Hanly JG, Russell ML, Gladman DD: Psoriatic spondyloarthropathy: A long term prospective study. Ann Rheum Dis 47:386–393, 1988.

65. Vasey FB: Psoriatic arthritis. In Schumacher HR (ed): Primer in the Rheumatic Diseases, 9th ed. Atlanta, Arthritis Foundation, 1988, pp 151–153.

66. McEwen C, DiTata D, Lingg C, et al: Ankylosing spondylitis and spondylitis accompanying ulcerative colitis, regional enteritis, psoriasis and Reiter's disease: A comparative study. Arthritis Rheum 14:291–318, 1971.

67. Arnett FC, McClusky OE, Schacter BZ, et al: Incomplete Reiter's syndrome: Discriminating features and HL-A W27 in diagnosis. Ann Intern Med 84:8–12, 1976.

68. Fox R, Calin A, Gerber RC, et al: The chronicity of symptoms and disability in Reiter's syndrome: An analysis of 131 consecutive patients. Ann Intern Med 91:190–193, 1979.

69. McMaster MJ: A technique for lumbar spinal osteotomy in ankylosing spondylitis. J Bone Joint Surg Br 67:198–210, 1985.

70. Gravallese EM, Kantrowitz G: Arthritic manifestations of inflammatory bowel disease: Clinical review. Am J Gastroenterol 83:703–709, 1988.

71. Zeidler H, Mau W, Khan MA: Undifferentiated spondyloarthropathies. Rheum Dis Clin North Am 18:187–202, 1992.

72. Khan MA, van der Linden SM: A wider spectrum of spondyloarthropathies. Semin Arthritis Rheum 20:107–113, 1990.

73. Lazennec JY, Saillant G, Saidi K, et al: Surgery of the deformities in ankylosing spondylitis: Our experience of lumbar osteotomies in 31 patients. Eur Spine J 6:222–232, 1997.

74. Calin A, Porta J, Fries JF, et al: Clinical history as a screening test for ankylosing spondylitis. JAMA 237:2613–2614, 1977.

75. Merritt JL, McLean TJ, Erickson RP, et al: Measurement of trunk flexibility in normal subjects: Reproducibility of three clinical methods. Mayo Clin Proc 61:192–197, 1991.

76. Khan MA: Ankylosing spondylitis. In Calin A (ed): Spondyloarthropathies. Orlando, Fla, Grune & Stratton, 1984, pp 1–17.

77. Rigby AS, Wood PHN: Observations on diagnostic criteria for ankylosing spondylitis. Clin Exp Rheumatol 11:5–12, 1993.

78. Viitanen JV, Kokko M-L, Lehtinen K, et al: Correlation between mobility restrictions and radiologic changes in ankylosing spondylitis. Spine 20:492–496, 1995.

79. Spoorenberg A, van der Heijde D, de Klerk E, et al: Relative value of erythrocyte sedimentation rate and C-reactive protein in assessment of disease activity in ankylosing spondylitis. J Rheumatol 26:980–984, 1999.

80. Urist MR: Osteotomy of the cervical spine: Report of a case of ankylosing rheumatoid arthritis spondylitis. J Bone Joint Surg 40:833–843, 1958.

81. Kozin F, Carrera GF, Ryan LM, et al: Computed tomography in the diagnosis of sacroiliitis. Arthritis Rheum 24:228–233, 1981.

82. Bollow M, Braun J, Hamm B, et al: Early sacroiliitis in patients with spondyloarthropathy: Evaluation with dynamic gadolinium-enhanced MR imaging. Radiology 194:529–536, 1995.

83. Ryan P, Gibson T, Fogelman I: Spinal bone SPECT in chronic symptomatic ankylosing spondylitis. Clin Nucl Med 22:821–824, 1997.

84. Mullaji AB, Upadhyay SS, Ho EK: Bone mineral density in ankylosing spondylitis. J Bone Joint Surg Br 76:660–665, 1994.

85. Lee YS, Schlotzhauer T, Ott SM, et al: Skeletal status of men with early and late ankylosing spondylitis. Am J Med 103:233–241, 1997.

86. Devogelaer JP, Maldague B, Malghem J, et al: Appendicular and vertebral bone mass in ankylosing spondylitis: A comparison of plain radiographs with single- and dual-photon absorptiometry and with quantitative computed tomography. Arthritis Rheum 35:1062–1067, 1992.

87. Thorngren KG, Liedberg E, Aspelin P: Fractures of the thoracic and lumbar spine in ankylosing spondylitis. Arch Orthop Trauma Surg 98:101–107, 1981.

88. Dawes PT: Stoke ankylosing spondylitis spine score. J Rheumatol Br 26:993–996, 1999.

89. Toussirot E, Wendling D: Current guidelines for the drug treatment of ankylosing spondylitis. Drugs 56:225–240, 1998.

90. Brooks PM, Day RO: Nonsteroidal anti-inflammatory drugs: Differences and similarities. N Engl J Med 324:1716–1725, 1991.

91. Gran JT, Husby G: Ankylosing spondylitis: Current drug treatment. Drugs 44:585–603, 1992.

92. Calin A, Elswood J: Prospective nationwide cross-sectional study of NSAID usage in 1331 patients with ankylosing spondylitis. J Rheumatol 17:801–803, 1990.

93. Clegg DO, Reda DJ, Weisman MH, et al: Comparison of sulfasalazine and placebo in the treatment of ankylosing spondylitis: A Department of Veterans Affairs cooperative study. Arthritis Rheum 39:2004–2012, 1996.

94. Dougados M, van der Linden S, Leirisalo-Repo M, et al: Sulphasalazine in the treatment of spondylarthropathy: A randomized, multicenter double-blind, placebo-controlled study. Arthritis Rheum 38:618–627, 1995.

95. Yamane K, Saito C, Natsuda H, et al: Ankylosing spondylitis successfully treated with methotrexate. Intern Med 32:53–56, 1993.

96. Ostendorf B, Specker C, Schneider M: Ankylosing spondylitis: Clinical and serological response to methotrexate therapy compared with rheumatoid arthritis [abstract]. Arthritis Rheum 38: S203, 1995.

97. Richter MB, Woo P, Panayi GS: The effects of intravenous pulse methylprednisolone on immunological and inflammatory processes in ankylosing spondylitis. Clin Exp Rheumatol 53:51–59, 1983.

98. Maugars Y, Mathis C, Vilon P, et al: Corticosteroid injection of the sacroiliac joint in sero-negative spondylarthropathies: First report of our experience. Arthritis Rheum 35:564–568, 1992.

99. Khan MD, Yue CC: Molecular basis for HLA association of rheumatic diseases. Autoimmunity Forum Rheumatol 1:2–4, 1989.

100. Kraag G, Stokes B, Groh J, et al: The effects of comprehensive home physiotherapy and supervision on patients with ankylosing spondylitis: A randomized controlled trial. J Rheumatol 17: 228–233, 1990.

101. Russell P, Unsworth A, Haslock I: The effect of exercise on ankylosing spondylitis: A preliminary study. J Rheumatol Br 32: 498–506, 1993.

102. Viitanen JW, Suni J, Kautiainen H, et al: Effect of physiotherapy on spinal mobility in ankylosing spondylitis. Scand J Rheumatol 21:38–43, 1992.

103. Gross M, Brandt KD: Educational support groups for patients with ankylosing spondylitis: A preliminary report. Pat Counsel Health Educ 3:6–12, 1981.

104. Barlow JH, Macey SJ, Struthers G: Psychosocial factors and self-help in ankylosing spondylitis patients. Clin Rheumatol 11: 220–225, 1992.

105. Hammerberg KW: Ankylosing spondylitis. In Bridwell KH, De-Wald RL (eds): The Textbook of Spinal Surgery, 2nd ed. Philadelphia, Lippincott-Raven, 1997, pp 1109–1127.

106. Simmons EH: The surgical correction of flexion deformity of the cervical spine in ankylosing spondylitis. Clin Orthop 86: 132–143, 1972.

107. Law WA: Osteotomy of the spine. J Bone Joint Surg 44:1199–1206, 1962.

108. Simmons EH, Duncan CP: Fracture of the cervical spine in ankylosing spondylitis: An analysis of its influence on severe deformity presenting for spinal osteotomy. Clin Orthop 133: 277, 1978.

109. Kostuik JP: The surgical treatment of ankylosing spondylitis. Semin Spine Surg 5:243–255, 1993.

110. McMaster MJ: Osteotomy of the cervical spine in ankylosing spondylitis. J Bone Joint Surg Br 79:197–203, 1997.

111. Smith-Petersen MN, Lawson CB, Aufranc OE: Osteotomy of the spine for correction of flexion deformity in rheumatoid arthritis. J Bone Joint Surg 27:1–11, 1945.

112. van Royen BJ, Slot GH: Closing-wedge posterior osteotomy for ankylosing spondylitis. J Bone Joint Surg Br 77:117–121, 1995.

113. Law WA: Osteotomy of the spine. Clin Orthop 66:70–76, 1969.

114. Weale AE, Marsh CH, Yeoman PM: Secure fixation of lumbar osteotomy. Clin Orthop 321:216–222, 1995.

115. Thomasen E: Vertebral osteotomy for correction of kyphosis in ankylosing spondylitis. Clin Orthop 194:142–152, 1985.

116. Puschel J, Zielke K: Korrekturoperation bei Bechterew-Kyphose: Indikation, Technik, Ergebnisse. Z Orthop 120:338–342, 1982.

117. Hehne HJ, Zielke K, Bohm H: Polysegmental lumbar osteotomies and transpedicular fixation for correction of long curved kyphotic deformities in ankylosing spondylitis: Report on 177 cases. Clin Orthop 258:49–55, 1990.

118. Simmons EH: Surgery of the spine in rheumatoid arthritis and ankylosing spondylitis. In Evarts CM (ed): Surgery of the Musculoskeletal System. New York, Churchill Livingston, 1983, p 4.

119. Graham B, Van Peteghem K: Fracture of the spine in ankylosing spondylitis: Diagnosis, treatment and complications. Spine 14: 803–807, 1989.

120. Olerud C, Frost A, Bring J: Spinal fractures in patients with ankylosing spondylitis. Eur Spine J 5:51–55, 1996.

121. Osgood CP, Abbasy M, Mathews T: Multiple spine fractures in ankylosing spondylitis. J Trauma 15:163–166, 1975.

122. Young JS, Chesire DJE, Pierce JA, et al: Cervical ankylosing with acute spinal cord injury. Paraplegia 15:133–146, 1977.

123. Kiwerki J, Wieclawek H, Garwacka I: Fractures of the cervical spine in ankylosing spondylitis. Int Orthop 8:243–246, 1985.

124. Exner G, Botel U, Kluger P, et al: Treatment of fracture and complication of cervical spine with ankylosing spondylitis. Spinal Cord 36:377–379, 1998.

125. Broom MJ, Raycroft JF: Complications of fractures of the cervical spine in ankylosing spondylitis. Spine 13:763–766, 1988.

126. Grisolia A, Bell RL, Peltier LF: Fractures and dislocations of the spine complicating ankylosing spondylitis: A report of six cases. J Bone Joint Surg Am 49:339–344, 1967.

127. Simmons EH: The cervical spine in ankylosing spondylitis. In Bridwell KH, DeWald RL (eds): The Textbook of Spinal Surgery, 2nd ed. Philadelphia, Lippincott-Raven, 1997, pp 1129–1158.

128. Ramos-Remus C, Gomez-Vargas A, Hernandez-Chavez A, et al: Two year follow-up of anterior and vertical atlantoaxial subluxation in ankylosing spondylitis. J Rheumatol Am 24: 507–510, 1997.

129. Garfin SR, Bradley D, Ahlgren BD: Current management of cervical spine instability. Curr Opin Rheumatol 7:114–119, 1995.

130. Kawasaki T, Hukuda S, Katsuura A, et al: Lumboperitoneal shunt for cauda equina syndrome in ankylosing spondylitis. J Spinal Disord 9:72–75, 1996.

131. Little H: The natural history of ankylosing spondylitis [editorial]. J Rheumatol Am 15:1179–1180, 1988.

132. Khan MA, Khan MK, Kushner I: Survival among patients with ankylosing spondylitis: A life table analysis. J Rheumatol Am 8:86–90, 1981.

133. Amor B, Santos RS, Nahal R, et al: Predictive factors for the long term outcome of spondyloarthropathies. J Rheumatol Am 21:1883–1887, 1994.

134. Gran JT, Skomsvoll JF: The outcome of ankylosing spondylitis: A study of 100 patients. J Rheumatol Br 36:766–771, 1997.

Ossification of the Posterior Longitudinal Ligament and Other Enthesopathies

PHILIP V. THEODOSOPOULOS ■ PHILIP R. WEINSTEIN

Enthesopathies are disorders caused by inflammation of tendinous and ligamentous attachments to bone. The most common and neurologically important of these disorders is ossification of the posterior longitudinal ligament (OPLL), which lines the posterior surface of the spinal vertebral bodies (anterior surface of the neural canal) from the foramen magnum to the sacrum.[1] The dysplastic process leading to ossification is associated with growth of a hyperplastic mass within the posterior longitudinal ligament, which causes spinal cord compression due to formation of a progressively enlarging mass of ligament and bone in the floor of the spinal canal.

Other enthesopathies, such as diffuse idiopathic skeletal hyperostosis, are systemic disorders that involve both the appendicular and axial skeleton and may accompany OPLL.[2] Spinal enthesopathies, including degenerative spondylosis, ossification of the anterior longitudinal ligament, and ankylosing spondylitis, may occur alone or in conjunction with OPLL.

Advances in diagnosis using computed tomography and magnetic resonance imaging (MRI) have led to more frequent identification of OPLL as a surgically treatable cause of myelopathy.[3, 4] Originally thought to occur only in persons of Japanese descent, OPLL affects other Asians and whites as well.[5, 6] Although the indications for surgical treatment have been defined, selection of the most effective operation remains controversial.[7–9]

PATHOGENETIC FACTORS

Hereditary Prevalence

An increased incidence of OPLL has been reported in families of Japanese patients with the disease.[10] A 30% incidence was found radiographically in first-degree relatives.[11] In one study, the prevalence of cervical OPLL detected radiographically among asymptomatic Japanese adults was 2% (143 of 6994), compared with 0.95% among Koreans, 0.17% to 0.2% among whites, and 0.1% to 0.14% among African Americans.[12] More recent studies suggest a higher prevalence among whites in the United States (0.7%) and Italy (1.7%).[13, 14] Prevalence also depends on age and sex. In Japan, 4.3% of asymptomatic 60-year-old men and 2.4% of 60-year-old women had OPLL in the cervical spine; among patients older than 60 years, the prevalence was greater than 10% in both men and women.[15] Most patients with radiographic evidence of OPLL are asymptomatic. No familial patterns of inheritance have been described for diffuse idiopathic skeletal hyperostosis or ankylosing spondylitis.

Hormonal and Metabolic Factors

The possibility that hormonal and metabolic factors are involved in pathologic ligamentous ossification has been investigated. The incidence of diabetes is higher in patients with OPLL and in those with diffuse idiopathic skeletal hyperostosis.[16, 17] In another study, however, insulin, which may stimulate bone growth, was found at higher levels in patients with diffuse idiopathic skeletal hyperostosis than in controls.[18]

The serum level of growth hormone–binding protein, which reflects the density of growth hormone receptors, was significantly higher in 26 Japanese patients with OPLL than in normal controls.[19] However, levels of growth hormone and insulin-like growth factor were not increased. In another study, the serum growth hormone response to insulin tolerance testing was much greater in patients with diffuse idiopathic skeletal hyperostosis than in controls.[20] Growth hormone stimulates new bone growth in patients with acromegaly and also stimulates precursor cells for cartilage and bone formation; therefore, it could play a synergistic role with insulin and bone growth factors in the pathogenesis of ligamentous ossification. A more recent study of 28 patients with diffuse idiopathic skeletal hyperostosis and controls matched for age, sex, and body mass index showed a positive correlation between the presence of the disease and increases in the serum insulin level; there was no correlation with serum retinol, glucose, uric acid, or cholesterol levels.[21]

Hypoparathyroidism, which may cause ectopic calcification and ossification, is not more common in patients with OPLL or diffuse idiopathic skeletal hyperostosis.[22, 23] Japanese patients with OPLL were found to have decreased calcium clearance, as determined by the calciuric response to an oral tolerance test, compared with patients without radiographic evidence of ligamentous ossification.[24] Plasma fibronectin levels were higher in patients with OPLL or ossification of the ligamenta flava than in age- and sex-matched controls.[25] Because this glycoprotein is an essential factor for endochondral ossification, it could mediate pathologic ligamentous ossification. An unexplained association of extraspinal ligament and tendon calcification has been reported after prolonged treatment of skin disorders such as psoriasis and rheumatoid arthritis with isotretinoin, a vitamin A–like retinoid.[26] Patients with diffuse idiopathic skeletal hyperostosis but not OPLL have increased retinoid levels.[27]

Bone Growth Factors

Tissue culture studies of the phenotypic characteristics of posterior longitudinal ligament osteoblasts obtained from nonossified sites in surgical patients with OPLL show many more cells with osteoblastic activity than in specimens obtained from patients with disk herniation or spondylosis.[28] High alkaline phosphatase activity and the metabolic response pattern to parathyroid hormone, calcitonin, prostaglandin E_2, and bone-seeking cytokines observed in those studies suggest that regulation of the proliferation and differentiation of ligament cells is altered in patients with OPLL.[29]

Immunohistochemical staining of ossified and adjacent normal specimens of ligament from a single surgical patient with OPLL demonstrated bone morphogenetic protein (BMP)-2 in both areas.[30] Transforming growth factor-β was also present in ossified matrix and adjacent cartilaginous areas but not in mesenchymal fibroblastic cells in uninvolved tissue. In a study of five specimens from patients with OPLL and two similar specimens from control patients with cervical spondylosis, several BMP and activin receptors were found to be preferentially elevated in the OPLL specimens.[31] Activins are multifunction proteins that also modulate induction of ectopic bone formation by BMP. BMP-2 stimulates mesenchymal progenitor cells to differentiate into osteoblasts; subsequently, transforming growth factor-β may stimulate ectopic ossification. In a study of the effect of BMP-2 on spinal ligament cells from patients with OPLL compared with controls from patients without OPLL, Kon and associates found that BMP-2 induces an increase in DNA synthesis, in procollagen type I carboxyl-terminal peptide synthesis, and in alkaline phosphatase activity in OPLL cells versus non-OPLL cells.[32]

Radiologic studies of mineral density in the distal radius of patients with OPLL suggest that during a mean follow-up of 3.9 years, trabecular bone mass decreased and cortical bone mass remained constant in patients whose disease progressed compared with those who did not have progression.[33] Other studies suggest that although bone mineral content was, in general, increased in cases of OPLL, those patients with the most severe myelopathy had a relative decrease.[34] These results suggest that the dysregulation of bone growth in OPLL is due to a complex, multifactorial systemic disturbance that remains poorly understood.

Genetic Markers

Genetic factors that might promote ligamentous ossification have also been evaluated. Recent work by Okawa and colleagues has shed some light on the genetics of OPLL. In a study of the ttw/twy (tiptoe-walking) mouse, a naturally occurring mutant that exhibits ossification of the spinal ligaments, especially the posterior longitudinal ligament, they determined that a nonsense mutation in the Npps gene, which encodes nucleotide pyrophosphatase, causes the phenotype.[35, 36] The Npps gene lies on chromosome 10 in the mouse genome. In humans, several studies have localized the genetic locus associated with OPLL to chromosome 6p, very close to the HLA gene.[37–39] Koga and coworkers reported marker D6S276 to be very closely linked to OPLL in 91 affected sibling pairs in Japan.[38] Numasawa and colleagues demonstrated a genetic link between the OPLL phenotype and the HLA complex on chromosome 6 by showing that molecular variants of the intergenic region between the retinoic X receptor b and collagen 11A2 are associated with OPLL in a statistically significant fashion.[39]

Initial studies showed that human leukocyte antigen (HLA) B27, which has been associated with hyperostotic conditions, is not more prevalent in patients with diffuse idiopathic skeletal hyperostosis.[40] Yet in a study by Ramos-Remus and associates of the prevalence of OPLL in patients with ankylosing spondylitis, 15% to 30% of those with ankylosing spondylitis and other spondyloarthropathies also had OPLL, a number higher than expected based on the relatively low frequency of HLA B27 among patients with OPLL.[41] HLA BW40 and SA5, but not B27, were found more frequently in Japanese patients with OPLL than in the normal population.[17] In a familial study of 33 patients with OPLL, the disease was present radiographically in 10 of 18 siblings (56%) who shared two rare HLA haplotype clusters with the patients.[42] In another review of HLA haplotypes in 24 patients and their siblings, 53% of the siblings with two identical haplotypes had OPLL, 24% of the ones with one identical haplotype had OPLL, and only 1 of the 24 patients without any identical HLA haplotypes had OPLL.[43] Inheriting related HLA genes from both parents is thought to establish a genetic predisposition for the interaction of additional factors that contribute to spinal ligament ossification, including aging, biomechanical stress, trauma, and degenerative processes.

The mode of inheritance for OPLL is still obscure. In a radiographic study of 129 relatives of 62 patients with OPLL, a simple dominant mode of inheritance was suggested.[10] Yet in a report of four family members with OPLL, an autosomal-recessive genetic trait was described by Hamanishi and colleagues.[44] Results of the analysis of blood groups, serum groups, and erythrocyte isoenzyme groups were inconclusive in identifying additional genetic markers. Familial studies of non-Japanese Asians or other racial groups have not been reported.

ANATOMY AND PHYSIOLOGY

Ossification of the Posterior Longitudinal Ligament

The posterior longitudinal ligament restrains and reverses flexion of the vertebral column. It attaches to the annulus of each intervertebral disk and to the adjacent posterior cortical surface of the vertebral bodies. In adults, this ligament is normally 1 to 2 mm thick; it is wider at the disk level and narrows at each midbody level. It contains longitudinally oriented collagen and elastin fibers that are most dense centrally and are thinner at the site of the most lateral attachment to the annulus.

Hypertrophy, calcification, and ossification of the ligament occur segmentally in association with degenerative disk disease or after traumatic herniation as spondylosis develops. Such changes can represent a benign degenerative process of aging, but in some cases, intermittent episodes of spinal pain, presumably due to inflammation, may occur. OPLL, however, is diagnosed when ossification originates within or spans the space between adjacent disks to involve the ligament overlying the centrum of the vertebral body. The ossified mass may replace or arise from the ligament, causing progressive occlusion of the spinal canal.

The clinical manifestations are more severe and occur at an earlier age in patients with developmental spinal stenosis. In such cases, the reserve space normally found in the neural canal has already been diminished by the inadequate length and horizontal orientation of the pedicle. No hereditary link has been established between developmental spinal stenosis and OPLL. However, personal observations suggest that cases of OPLL that are identified because of symptoms or signs of radiculomyelopathy rather than by incidental radiographic studies are more likely to be associated with a developmentally small neural canal. A high percentage of clinically symptomatic patients with OPLL also have degenerative cervical spondylosis.[45]

OPLL involves the cervical spine in 90% of patients. C5 is most commonly affected, followed by C4 and C6. The disease may also occur in the upper cervical levels; we have treated two patients with myelopathy due to ligamentous ossification restricted to C1 to C3. In our original series of patients with cervical OPLL diagnosed and treated in the United States, the mean number of vertebral bodies involved was 2.25.[46] However, 3 of 20 patients required surgical decompression from C3 to C7. In our subsequent series, three or more levels

were typically involved, perhaps reflecting referral of more complex cases to a neurospinal surgery center. Several patients have had upper thoracic as well as cervical lesions. Yonenobu and colleagues reported that involvement of the thoracic spine with myelopathy due to OPLL occurs in only 9% of cases; ossification of the ligamenta flava was also found in 12 of 15 patients in that series, and 6 patients had thoracic lesions associated with cervical lesions that were not contiguous.[47] The lumbar spine is rarely involved. Lumbar lesions are also commonly associated with ossification of the lumbar ligamenta flava and with cervical lesions.[48]

OPLL is classified anatomically into four types of lesions.[49] Segmental lesions are discrete sites of ossification adjacent to a single vertebral body centrum; adjacent disks are unaffected. Segmental lesions may skip one or more normal vertebral bodies between levels of involvement. Continuous lesions span two or more disks. Localized lesions span a single disk but involve two adjacent vertebral bodies. Mixed lesions combine two of the preceding types. In Japanese patients, the mean area of ossification, measured radiographically, was 0.36 cm² for segmental lesions, 2.36 cm² for continuous lesions, and 2.6 cm² for mixed lesions.[49] In the cervical spine, 32% of lesions were segmental, 35% were continuous, 30% were mixed, and 3% were localized. Thoracic spinal involvement was continuous in 87% of cases and localized in 13%; lumbar lesions were continuous in 42% and localized in 58%.

Progressive enlargement of the ossified mass lesion in the anteroposterior, lateral, and longitudinal directions has been documented radiographically. Although growth rates are variable, serial radiographic studies in 13 Japanese patients revealed a mean annual increase in lesion size of 4.07 mm longitudinally and 0.67 mm anteroposteriorly; clinical correlation with lesion growth was not provided.[50] Most patients with a radiographic diagnosis of OPLL do not have neurological signs or symptoms, perhaps because neural canal stenosis is not present or because displacement or compression of the spinal cord and nerve root is chronic and gradual in onset (Fig. 291–1). Ossification within the posterior longitudinal ligament eventually proceeds beyond its posterior margin.[51] The enlarging mass may be round, cuboidal, triangular, or polypoid. Its base of attachment may be flat and broad or narrow and pedunculated.[52] Radiographically, the mass appears to arise from the posterior vertebral body cortex, displacing the ventral dura, indenting the spinal cord, and stretching the overlying nerve roots. In advanced cases, the spinal cord is deformed into a thin, crescent-shaped structure that is concave anteriorly.

Spinal cord compression may be further exacerbated not only by developmental stenosis but also by diskogenic osteophytes or ligamenta flava hypertrophy.[50] A spinal canal narrowing ratio, calculated as the anteroposterior diameter of the mass divided by the diameter of the entire canal, has been proposed as a quantitative radiographic parameter to assess the extent of cord entrapment and to predict the risk of neurological complications. In asymptomatic patients, the ratio between

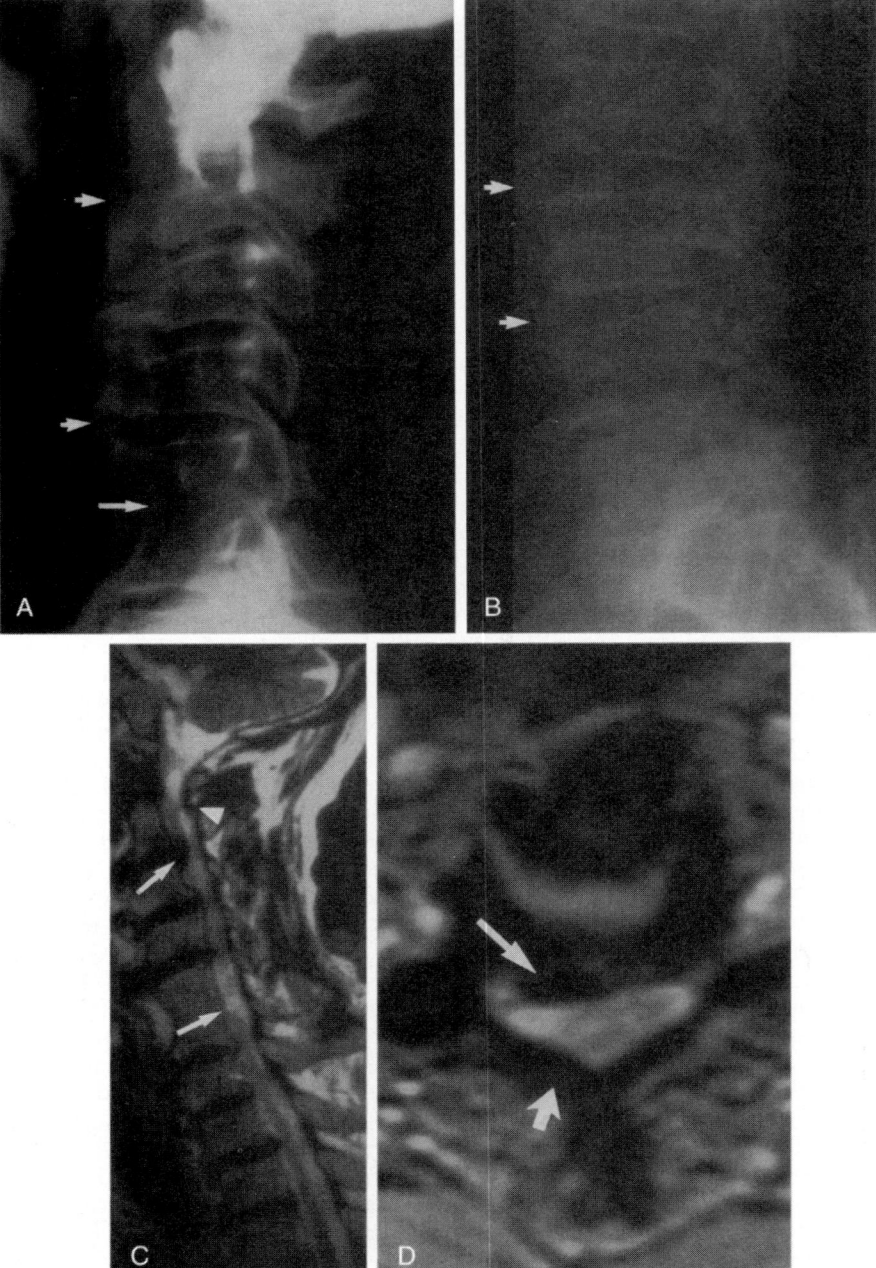

FIGURE 291–1. *A,* Lateral radiograph of the cervical spine in a 57-year-old man with slowly progressive cervical myelopathy shows large osteophytes *(small arrows),* the typical manifestation of diffuse idiopathic skeletal hyperostosis, in an ossified anterior longitudinal ligament extending from C2 to C5. Anterior cervical diskectomy and fusion *(large arrow)* at C5-6 had been performed previously to treat neck and arm pain. *B,* Lateral radiograph of the lumbar spine in the same patient demonstrates large anterior osteophytes at L2-3 and L3-4 *(arrows). C,* Sagittal T2-weighted magnetic resonance image shows severe developmental spinal stenosis and cord compression; note cord edema at C5-6 *(lower large arrow).* Multilevel diskogenic *(upper large arrow)* and ligamentous *(arrowhead)* osteophytes are present, most prominently at C2-3. Ossification of the ligamenta flava causes dorsal cord compression at C1-2. *D,* Axial gradient echo magnetic resonance image at C2-3 demonstrates segmental ossification of the posterior longitudinal ligament *(long arrow)* with severe stenosis, also due to ossification of the ligamenta flava *(short arrow).* C2 to C7 laminaplasty was performed, and the previous occurrence of spontaneous fusion was verified intraoperatively.

C3 and C5 was 0.2 or less, whereas in patients with radiculopathy only, the ratio was 0.2 to 0.3, and in those with myelopathy, it was greater than 0.3.[53] The important variable is, of course, the residual canal diameter, or the minimal distance between the ventral mass and the rostral edge of the dorsal lamina, which determines the size of the subarachnoid space and the space available to the spinal cord. Myelopathy is expected to develop when the residual anteroposterior canal diameter is less than 9 mm.[30] The area of the neural canal in the axial plane has also been correlated with the outcome after surgical decompression.[54] In another study, the axial cord area, the presence of increased intramedullary signal on T2-weighted MRI scans, and the duration of the neurological deficit were used to predict the postoperative outcome.[55] Nakamura and Fujimura studied the correlation between T2 hyperintensity in the cord and outcome in patients with OPLL and showed that high T2 signal correlates with poor outcome only in patients with a history of trauma.[56]

Post-traumatic or degenerative vertebral column deformities due to kyphosis or spondylolisthesis may exacerbate stretching or compression of the spinal cord and nerve roots due to OPLL. Diskogenic osteophytes and ossified ligaments also restrict or prevent normal intervertebral joint movement, which results in loss of flexibility of the vertebral column. The spinal cord may be further stretched over a large ventral osteophyte during flexion, when motion occurs at uninvolved levels above and below a site of segmental or localized ligament ossification. Asymptomatic patients may experience the acute onset of myelopathy after an episode of relatively trivial trauma or sudden neck flexion. In a study of the role of MRI in the diagnosis and treatment of OPLL, Koyanagi and coworkers showed that the presence of disk protrusion is an important predictor for the development of myelopathy, and it is present in 81% of patients with the segmental type of OPLL.[57] Cervical extension is less likely to be associated with spinal cord concussion or contusion if no movement occurs at the affected segments, because spontaneous arthrodesis has occurred over multiple levels. However, if intervertebral joint mobility persists at sites of severe stenosis, a paralytic spinal cord injury may occur during forced neck extension. Repetitive minor trauma may also occur, especially where the cord crosses the caudal edge of the ossified lesion. Delayed conduction of spinal cord somatosensory evoked potentials is most common at the most inferior pole of the lesion.[58]

Other Enthesopathies

OPLL is occasionally found as part of the diathesis for ligamentous ossification in patients with ankylosing spondylitis and in up to 50% of patients with diffuse idiopathic skeletal hyperostosis. Other systemic manifestations of diffuse idiopathic skeletal hyperostosis occur in more than half of patients with OPLL. Ossification of intraspinal ligaments is more severe in patients with diffuse idiopathic skeletal hyperostoses than in those with OPLL alone.[2, 59] The prevalence of diffuse idiopathic skeletal hyperostosis is 3% in adults older than 40 years and 12% to 15% in those older than 65 years.[2, 60] In these patients, hyperostosis develops along with calcification of ligaments and tendons at their insertion sites. The anterior and posterior longitudinal ligaments, as well as the ligamenta flava and interspinous ligaments, may be involved. Lumbar spinal stenosis may result.[61] Appendicular joints most commonly affected include the knee, ankle, and elbow. It is tempting to consider the possibility that OPLL represents a genetically or pathophysiologically related disorder that presents as an anatomically limited manifestation of diffuse idiopathic skeletal hyperostosis. However, neither condition has been correlated with abnormalities of calcium or phosphorus metabolism, endocrine abnormalities, histocompatibility locus antigens, or the presence of rheumatoid factor.

Ankylosing spondylitis is another systemic skeletal disorder that causes calcification and ossification of the intervertebral disks and ligamentous attachments. Apophyseal joints fuse, and the annulus fibrosus and anterior longitudinal ligament ossify; the posterior longitudinal ligament is rarely involved.[62] Interspinous ligaments and ligamenta flava routinely ossify, which causes spontaneous arthrodesis of the anterior, middle, and posterior components of the vertebral column, resulting in a rigid "bamboo" or "poker" spine. This disorder may be associated with severe, progressive thoracic kyphosis and stress or traumatic fractures across fragile osteoporotic vertebra or ossified disks. Ankylosing spondylitis has also been reported in association with lumbar spinal stenosis.[63] Manubrosternal and costovertebral joint involvement may restrict thoracic mobility and limit respiratory function. The occurrence of inflammatory synovial proliferation and hypervascularity that erodes adjacent cartilage and bone, and the association with atlantoaxial joint instability and basilar invagination, link ankylosing spondylitis pathologically with rheumatoid arthritis. OPLL may be radiographically evident in patients with ankylosing spondylitis, but it is rarely, if ever, associated with progressively enlarging mass lesions or neurological deficit.[64]

Ossification of both the posterior longitudinal ligament and the ligamenta flava, causing severe paraparesis due to cauda equina compression (hyperostotic lumbar spinal stenosis), has been reported in Japan.[48] A review of 2403 lumbosacral spine radiographs found ossification of the ligamenta flava in 206 cases (8.6%). Symptomatic multilevel ossification of the ligamenta flava without OPLL has also been reported. Treatment of this condition by simple laminectomy and foraminotomy relieves the radiculopathy.

Spinal stenosis and myelopathy due to intraspinal ligamentous hypertrophy and calcification have been reported in patients with mucopolysaccharidoses.[65] Patients with Hunter-Hurler and Scheie's syndromes may develop acquired spinal stenosis due to thickening of the ligamenta flava and posterior longitudinal ligament in adult life without the anatomic stigmata of dwarfism seen in achondroplasia or spondyloepiphyseal dysplasia (Morquio's syndrome). Ankylosing spondylitis has been reported in cases of diffuse idiopathic skeletal hyperostosis; some radiologic features such as anterior spinal syndesmophytes may be similar.[66] Ankylosing spondylitis is also associated with combined cervical and lumbar spinal stenosis without OPLL or ossification of the ligamenta flava.[67]

PATHOLOGY

As in other types of compressive myelopathy, pathologic changes in the spinal cord have been observed only in patients with advanced, untreated OPLL. In such cases, it is difficult to distinguish the effect of biomechanical stresses and tissue compression from the effects of ischemic necrosis due to vascular compromise. Autopsy studies have shown distortion and compression of the cord into a thin crescent of residual tissue over the ossified anterior ligamentous mass.[68] Extensive damage to gray and white matter is observed. The extent of gray matter changes and the degree of spinal cord compression correlate with anterior horn deformity and with the severity of myelopathy.[69] There is histologic evidence of venous stasis, edema, ischemic neuronal necrosis, and infarction. Cavitation and gliosis occur in gray matter; spongiform atrophy, demyelination, and axon loss occur in white matter.[70]

Central gray matter and adjacent dorsal and lateral column fibers are most severely damaged. Terminal arteriolar degeneration of central perforating branches of the anterior spinal artery is seen and may represent the mechanism of progressive quadriplegia.[71] Demyelination, axon loss, and atrophy occur in nerve roots that have been stretched or compressed. The pathologic alterations described, including retrograde and anterograde degeneration of long tracts, are similar to those seen at compression sites in advanced cases of cervical spondylosis.[72]

OPLL occurs by the process of endochondral bone formation, beginning with the most superficial layer.[49, 73] The histologic findings in surgical specimens are indistinguishable from those of heterotopic bone formation seen in spondylosis or in response to mechanical stress and trauma in other ligaments.[74] Fibroblast hyperplasia and increased collagen deposition are followed by mineralization of the thickened ligament.[75] Cartilage cells and bone matrix proliferate in the vertebral body periosteum, annulus fibrosus, and, in some cases, dura mater, as well as in the posterior longitudinal ligament.[73]

As the ossified mass enlarges and extends longitudinally, lamellar bone eventually matures with well-developed haversian canals and few marrow cavities. The ossified ligament is not always continuous with the vertebral body cortex, being separated by connective tissue at some levels.[71] Even when the ossified ligament merges with the adjacent vertebral cortex, the calcified ligamentous structure is preserved within the lamellar bone of the lesion. Similarly, the annulus fibrosus remains separate and uninvolved with ossification at certain levels. As with the formation of osteophytes in patients with spondylosis and of syndesmophytes in those with spinal ankylosis, the hyperostosis does not affect the posterior vertebral cortex.

The vertebral and osseous pathology of ankylosing spondylitis is characterized by chondroid metaplasia followed by calcification and ossification.[62] Apophyseal joint involvement begins with rheumatoid-like erosive changes that progress to cartilaginous destruction, joint space narrowing, and ankylosis. Inflammatory synovial proliferation and vascularization occur. Annulus fibrosus or posterior longitudinal ligament ossification follows. Ankylosing spondylosis is not associated with proliferative osteoneogenesis producing growth of intraspinal osteophytes.[76]

Diffuse idiopathic skeletal hyperostosis is characterized pathologically as a selective, multiarticular, ligamentous hypertrophy with adjacent subperiosteal new bone formation.[61] The anterior longitudinal ligament is characteristically involved, with the formation of bony outgrowth from the anterolateral surfaces of the vertebral bodies. However, no specific histologic characteristics of this disorder have been identified.[77]

CLINICAL PRESENTATION AND NATURAL HISTORY

The clinical syndromes of OPLL and related disorders are ones of slowly progressing compressive myelopathy with or without radiculopathy. They are localized neurologically to the levels of spinal involvement, unless both cervical and thoracic lesions are present. In rare cases, cervical pain syndromes without radicular radiation or neurological deficit may occur. No differences in the history or physical findings between Asian and non-Asian patients have been reported.[8, 45, 78] Yet Wang and colleagues showed a statistically significant difference in diet, with OPLL patients having higher salt intake and lower meat intake than patients with cervical spondylosis.[79]

Symptoms described in addition to neck pain (42%) and arm pain or dysesthesia (48%) include arm weakness (19%), leg weakness (15%), and urinary incontinence (10%).[17] In our series, arm and leg clumsiness or weakness, arm numbness or paresthesias, and gait difficulties each occurred in at least 80% of patients.[46] Limited cervical spinal motion, hyperreflexia, extensor-plantar response, and arm or leg weakness were found in 65% of our patients. Hypalgesia below segmental levels on the torso were present in 60%, and radicular sensory loss was found in 55%.

The acute onset of symptoms or signs of neurological involvement may also occur after trivial trauma. Existing neurological syndromes were exacerbated by cervical injury in 6 of our initial 20 patients.[46] Acute episodes that precipitated symptoms were described as a remote part of the history in an additional five cases.

The median duration of symptoms before diagnosis was 7.5 months (range, 0 to 36 months) in our series. Acceleration of neurological deterioration often led to diagnosis and treatment. Difficulty in diagnosis can result in delay of treatment or inappropriate treatment. In the Japanese cooperative study, 19% of patients were physically incapable of self-care, and 23% required assistance with walking.[17] In another series, previous surgery had been unsuccessful because of misdiagnosis in 6 of 14 patients.[59] Two of our 20 patients failed to improve or worsened neurologically after a previous cervical laminectomy, and 4 did not respond to a previous anterior cervical diskectomy.

The natural history of OPLL is one of progressive enlargement of the lesion posteriorly and laterally as well as longitudinally, depending on the type of ligamentous involvement, hereditary factors, and spinal stress.[49] Neurological symptoms and signs can be expected to develop when the lesion occupies more than 65% of the neural canal.[71] Analysis of sequential spinal radiographs confirmed this observation in untreated patients.[17, 50, 51] However, lesion growth has not been measured over time on axial spine scans or in non-Asian patients without hereditary risk factors or an associated systemic enthesopathy. Therefore, there is no firm rationale for treating asymptomatic patients surgically or advising prophylactic total excision of all ossified ligamentous tissue. Prospective long-term follow-up studies are needed, especially in patients with spontaneous fusion of affected vertebral motion segments.

DIAGNOSIS

OPLL and other enthesopathies are diagnosed radiographically. Diffuse idiopathic skeletal hyperostosis and ankylosing spondylitis are easily detected on spinal radiographs (see Fig. 291–1). OPLL is visible as retrovertebral calcification on plain films in approximately one third of cases (Fig. 291–2).[6, 80] MRI should be the initial diagnostic imaging procedure in any patient with nontraumatic myeloradiculopathy. On T1- and T2-weighted images, ligamentous calcification or ossification appears as a region of low signal intensity (Fig. 291–3).[81] Sagittal images demonstrate the longitudinal extent of anterior epidural lesions and their anatomic type.[82] Axial images can demonstrate the extent of neural canal stenosis, including developmental and acquired anterior and posterior components. Disk herniation and spondylosis can easily be identified. Infection and neoplasm can be detected on contrast-enhanced images. Spinal deformity due to trauma or congenital disorders can be diagnosed on sagittal images. Spinal cord compression, hemorrhage, edema, and atrophy can be demonstrated on both axial and sagittal images.[83] Such information is critical for making an accurate anatomic diagnosis, for selecting the most effective surgical treatment, and for estimating the prognosis.

Clinical correlation with the findings on MRI has been excellent in our experience (see Fig. 291–2). In some cases, however, MRI tends to exaggerate the severity of stenosis and the extent of obliteration of the subarachnoid cerebrospinal fluid space. When the level of involvement is difficult to determine neurologically

in complex cases, computed tomographic scanning after intrathecal administration of contrast material is recommended, especially when previous surgery has been performed (Fig. 291–4). Computed tomography provides better resolution of osseous detail than MRI and may demonstrate the severity and extent of calcification and ossification more clearly. The information derived may show that fewer levels require surgical decompression and can be used to determine whether the anterior or posterior approach should be used.

Flexion-extension radiographs are useful for assessing vertebral hypermobility or instability. In cases of borderline stenosis, MRI during spinal flexion or extension may demonstrate compression and show where it is most severe.[59] Somatosensory evoked potentials may be used as an adjunct to the neurological examination to localize the level of maximal spinal cord compression and to predict the response to surgical decompression.[58]

TREATMENT

The treatment of spinal stenosis due to OPLL and other enthesopathies is based on standard principles of managing neurospinal disease. Acute episodes of pain and the onset or increase of neurological deficit are treated with rest, external spinal immobilization with a collar or brace, and analgesics, including anti-inflammatory or antispasmodic medications when indicated. Acute cervical or thoracic spinal cord contusion can be treated with high-dose steroids.

Surgery is indicated for patients with acute or chronic progression of neurological deficits or recurrent temporary disability from reversible neurological deficits, including impairment of manual dexterity and leg coordination. In some cases, intermittent postural paresthesias, such as occur in Lhermitte's syndrome, are incapacitating. In others, lower extremity spasticity and impairment of bladder control become intolerable. Because the natural history of enthesopathies is variable and the occurrence of spontaneous arthrodesis may be protective, surgery is not routinely advised for asymptomatic patients. However, some high-risk patients with mild or transient deficits and anteroposterior neural canal diameters of 9 mm or less may choose prophylactic surgery to avoid restrictions of precarious forms of work and recreational activity. Further, projection of a large bone mass directly into the anterior surface of a chronically constricted spinal cord, causing ventral indentation and anterior spinal artery displacement, is likely to lead to future neurological deficits that could be irreversible. Preventive surgery should be offered to patients wishing to avoid such risks.

Selection of Surgical Procedure

The choice of operation depends on the anatomy of the lesion causing spinal cord and nerve root compression.[84] Spinal stenosis due to ossification of the ligamenta flava is best treated by posterior decompression

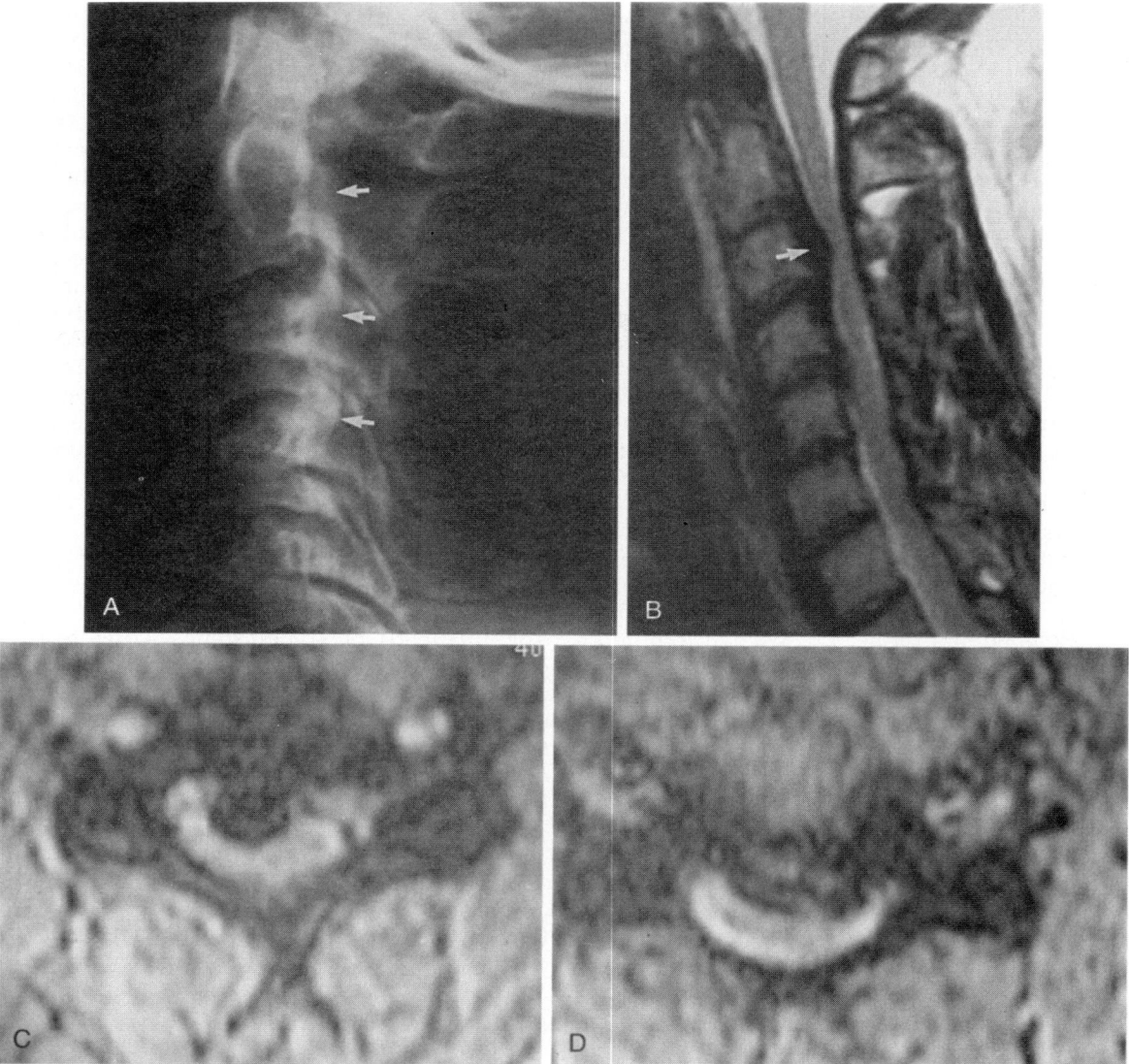

FIGURE 291–2. Radiographic studies of the cervical spine of a 40-year-old Japanese American man with recurrent myelopathy localized to C4 who had undergone two unsuccessful thoracic laminectomies for ossification of the thoracic posterior longitudinal ligament. Eventually, he was treated successfully with transthoracic T4 corpectomy and fusion. *A,* Lateral radiograph demonstrates an ossified mass *(arrows)* extending along the posterior surface of the vertebral bodies from C2 to C5. *B,* Sagittal T2-weighted magnetic resonance image 2 mm to the right of the midline demonstrates diffuse spinal cord compression that extends down to T2 and is most severe at the midbody C3 level *(arrow). C,* Axial image at that level shows a pedunculated osteophyte that projects 9 mm into the stenotic neural canal, causing severe spinal cord compression. *D,* Axial image at the midbody C5 level demonstrates a broad-based ligamentous osteophyte that measures 20 mm in the transverse dimension and reduces the midline anteroposterior diameter of the neural canal from 12 to 6 mm. This lesion has features of the continuous type of ligamentous ossification (see text). Because of the patient's short, thick neck and systemic medical illness, the lesion was treated by laminectomy from C2 to T2 and posterior fusion from C4 to C7, which were the only segments that demonstrated mobility intraoperatively. Ossification of the ligamenta flava was also present.

and laminectomy. Complex cases of thoracic ligamentous ossification involving both the ligamenta flava and the posterior longitudinal ligament may require both posterolateral extracavitary thoracotomy for lateral decompression or transthoracic anterior corpectomy and fusion, and posterior decompression and fusion by laminectomy and instrumentation for inter-

nal fixation.[85] Based on the natural curvature of the spine, Kurosa and colleagues advocate anterior decompression for midthoracic lesions centered at the apical vertebrae of the thoracic S curve, anterior or posterior decompression for the upper thoracic spine, and "anterior decompression through a posterior approach" for the lower thoracic spine.[86] Because of the flexibility of

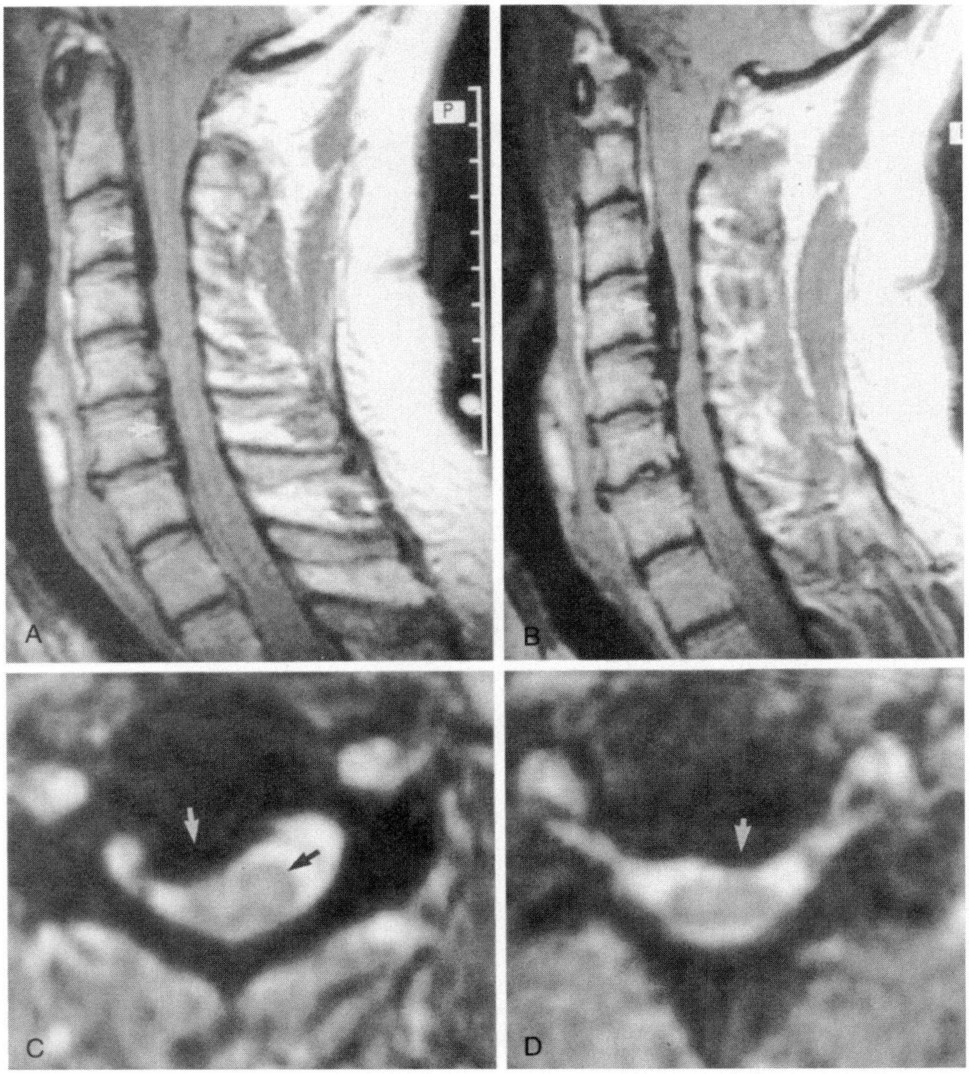

FIGURE 291–3. Magnetic resonance images of the cervical spine of a 50-year-old Hawaiian man with a 2-year history of persistent neck pain after being rear-ended in a motor vehicle accident; there were no neurological deficits or radicular symptoms. *A,* Midline sagittal T1-weighted magnetic resonance image demonstrates osseous hypertrophy of the posterior longitudinal ligament *(arrows)* that extends from C2 to C7 but skips the midbody portion of C4. This case represents the mixed type of lesion in a patient without developmental stenosis. The lesion at C3 reduces the anteroposterior neural canal diameter from 14 to 10 mm on this image. *B,* Sagittal image 4 mm to the right of the midline demonstrates a large ventral mass *(arrow)* that extends from C3 to C5, crossing the C3-4 and C4-5 disks. On this image, the lesion reduces the anteroposterior canal diameter from 14 to 5 mm. *C,* Axial T2-weighted magnetic resonance image at the C4 midbody level demonstrates a large focal osteophyte *(white arrow)* arising from the posterior longitudinal ligament and projecting into the floor of the neural canal. The spinal cord *(dark arrow)* is compressed and rotated, but no intramedullary focus of increased signal was seen to suggest edema. *D,* Axial T2-weighted magnetic resonance image at C6-7 demonstrates a relatively low-profile lesion consistent with a broad-based diskogenic osteophyte *(arrow)* that is not associated with spinal cord or nerve root compression or displacement. Here the neural canal diameter is reduced from 16 to 11 mm by the lesion. There is no developmental stenosis. Surgical treatment was not advised but will probably be necessary in the future. Follow-up magnetic resonance images will be obtained in 1 year.

the cauda equina and its capacity to elongate, anterior decompression is rarely necessary in the lumbar spine.[48] Further, lesions of the lumbar posterior longitudinal ligament tend to be relatively smaller with respect to the anteroposterior canal diameter than are cervical and thoracic lesions. They are more likely to be segmental than continuous.

In most cases of cervical and thoracic myelopathy due to OPLL, anterior decompression and arthrodesis are indicated.[87] Only in the rare case of focal segmental lesions that do not extend above or below the disk does a simple interbody diskectomy and fusion suffice.[88] Moreover, complete resection of the lesion requires microsurgical removal of the involved posterior longitu-

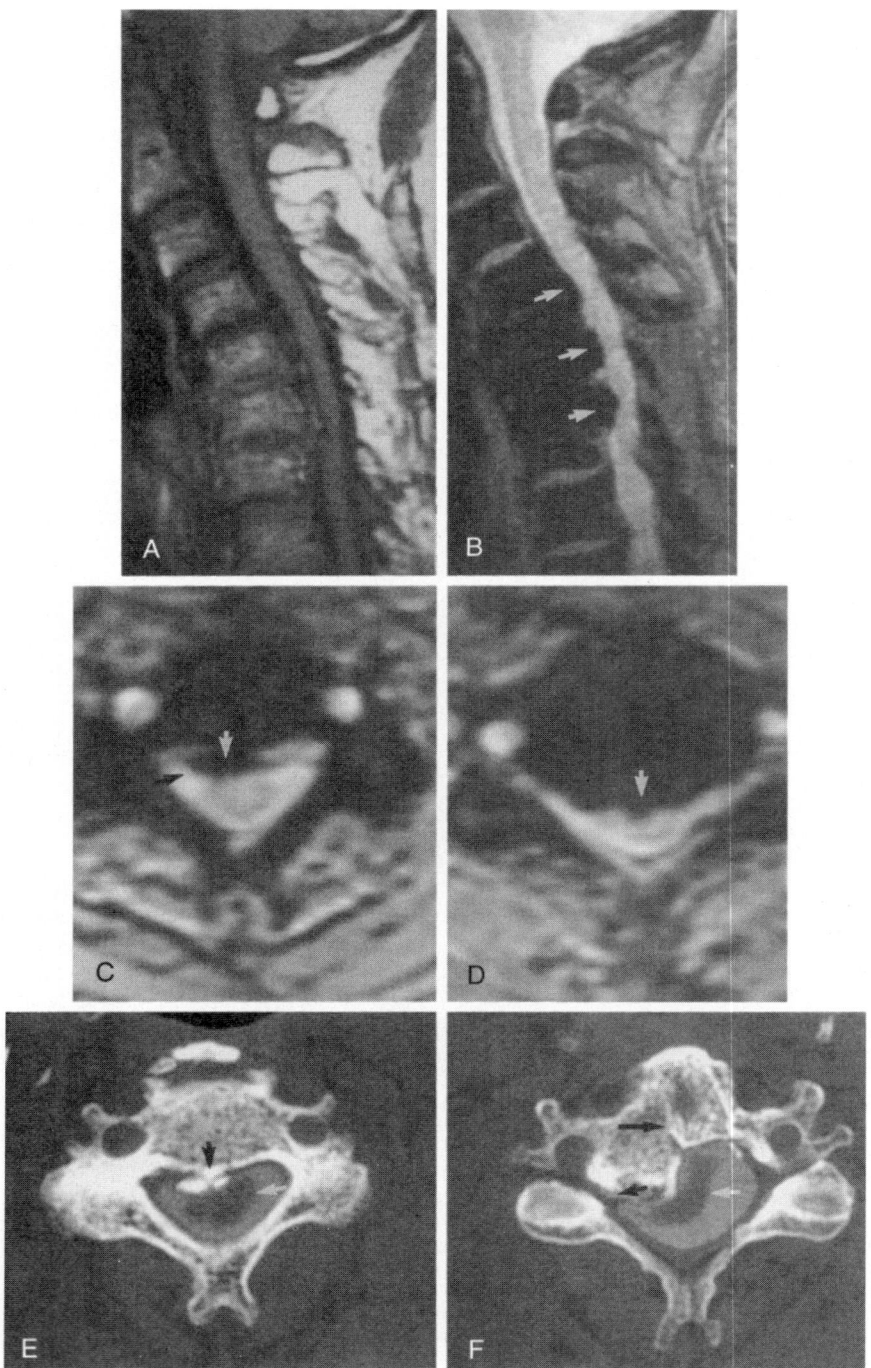

FIGURE 291–4. Images of the cervical spine in a 71-year-old Iranian man with spastic quadriparesis that worsened acutely and progressed chronically after anterior diskectomy without fusion at C5-6 and C6-7. Anterior median corpectomy and fusion 4 years later resulted in dramatic and unexpected recovery, with restoration of ambulation and manual dexterity. One year after the second operation, left arm pain and right C7 numbness without myelopathy recurred. *A,* Before corpectomy, a midline sagittal T1-weighted magnetic resonance image demonstrates severe developmental stenosis from C5 to C7 and a kyphotic deformity centered at the C5-6 level. *B,* T2-weighted image shows ossification of the posterior longitudinal ligament with multiple segmental lesions adjacent to both the C4-5 (previously unoperated) level and the previously operated C5-6 and C6-7 disks *(arrows). C,* Axial T2-weighted image at C4 demonstrates ossification concentrated in the central portion of the ligament *(white arrow)* and mild compression of the subarachnoid space *(dark arrow). D,* Axial magnetic resonance image at the C6-7 disk level shows more severe developmental and acquired neural canal stenosis due to recurrent hypertrophic ossification of the disk and ligament *(arrow). E,* One year after corpectomy, axial computed tomographic scan obtained after intrathecal administration of contrast material demonstrates rostral extension of ligamentous ossification *(dark arrow)* without compression of the rotated cord *(white arrow)* above the level of previous surgery at C4. *F,* Scan at C5-6 demonstrates residual osteophyte causing neural foramen *(small dark arrow)* but not canal stenosis at C5-6. Note the right-to-left slant of the corpectomy trench and iliac crest bone graft *(large dark arrow),* which has fused satisfactorily. The atrophic spinal cord *(white arrow)* is rotated but not compressed. This is an example of the most frequently encountered cause of recurrent or residual radiculomyelopathy after anterior decompression. Symptoms resolved without reoperation.

dinal ligament and adjacent osteophytes, which may be technically difficult and dangerous when surgical exposure is limited to the intervertebral space. Anterior diskectomy and corpectomy without resection of the posterior longitudinal ligament failed to relieve spinal cord compression in almost half the cases reported.[89] Theoretically, the incompletely resected but diseased ligament may reattach to vertebral body resection margins and ultimately resume growth.

Anterior diskectomy, median corpectomy (somatectomy), and fusion are now considered the optimal operation for spinal cord and nerve root decompression and vertebral stabilization in most patients with OPLL.[90] The ossified ligament and all attached intraspinal osteophytes can be totally excised. Spinal stabilization is accomplished by placement of an iliac crest (one to three levels) or fibular strut (three to five levels) bone graft. This approach relieves the major source of spinal cord compression and prevents its recurrence; it also prevents postoperative kyphotic spinal deformity or instability.

Circumferential surgery is an important addition to the treatment of cervical OPLL. Epstein performed anterior corpectomies with posterior wiring and fusion in 22 patients with cervical OPLL and reported good outcomes, with an average operative time of less than 10 hours and low complication rates.[91]

Although laminectomy has been used for decompression in patients with cervical OPLL,[92] the risks of spinal cord injury during decompression, recurrence or progression of myelopathy due to persistence or further growth of the lesion, and development of a swan-neck kyphotic deformity are substantial. In a retrospective study of 52 patients who underwent cervical laminectomy for OPLL, progressive kyphosis developed in 47%, and further spread of OPLL was noted in 70% of the patients.[93] Because the posterior vertebral column bone and ligamentous structures have already been resected, anterior corpectomy after a failed laminectomy carries a greater risk of complications due to postoperative instability. In patients with diffuse idiopathic skeletal hyperostosis or ankylosing spondylitis who develop spontaneous arthrodesis of the disk and facet joints, laminectomy without fusion may be an acceptable means of decompressing severe multilevel developmental stenosis and OPLL (see Fig. 291–1).

Single-stage resection of four or five vertebral central and adjacent disks is feasible in patients with favorable anatomy. However, sufficient surgical exposure to allow bone graft placement may be difficult to achieve at C2 or T1. Although additional exposure can be provided by a mandibulotomy above or a sternotomy below, some patients can also be managed with anterior resection of the most extensive lesions at the accessible midcervical levels and posterior laminectomy for decompression at the C1-2 and C7-T1 or T2 levels, where the anterior lesion is often relatively flat and the neural canal is larger. Staged or combined anterior and posterior decompression may be necessary in patients with mixed or continuous OPLL.[94] Posterior decompression alone is a suboptimal but palliative treatment for OPLL; it may be appropriate when the lesion extends across five or more vertebrae and in certain elderly or debilitated patients or in those with systemic illness who may not tolerate a more lengthy and extensive anterior decompression and fusion.

Osteoplastic laminaplasty has been used as an alternative posterior operation for enlarging the cervical or thoracic neural canal with less theoretical risk of postoperative instability or kyphosis. However, the theoretical rationale for establishing spinal stability without bone grafting and for preventing further enlargement of the ossified posterior longitudinal ligament remains to be established by prospective studies.[84] Osteoplastic laminaplasty consists of an en bloc laminectomy that leaves the laminar arch and spinous process attached to the ligamenta flava unilaterally but disconnected from both pedicles.[95] Sutures to overlying fascia or interposed bone struts and wires or screw plates are used to elevate the detached arch and separate it from its previous site of attachment on the side of transection of the ligamenta flava. The goal is to decompress the spinal cord dorsally while reconstructing the posterior elements, so as to prevent spinal instability by allowing reattachment of the paraspinal muscles and the nuchal ligament. This goal can also be achieved by simple laminectomy and posterior facet fusion with internal fixation by placing lateral mass screw plates and using laminectomy bone or iliac crest autograft for arthrodesis.

Surgical Technique

Anterior cervical median corpectomy is performed through a standard surgical exposure of the anterior vertebral column. Endotracheal intubation is performed under topical anesthesia with the patient awake to avoid cervical spinal cord injury due to spinal hyperextension. The tube remains in place to protect the airway for 24 to 72 hours after surgery. During this time, respiratory insufficiency is a risk owing to excessive secretions, laryngeal and tracheal edema, vocal cord paralysis, cervical spinal cord edema at C3-4, and phrenic nerve–mediated diaphragm motor dysfunction. Steroids are administered perioperatively to prevent these complications. Somatosensory and motor evoked potentials are monitored intraoperatively to detect compromise in dorsal or lateral column function due to surgical manipulation.

An oblique incision parallel to the medial border of the sternocleidomastoid muscle may be needed for multilevel exposure. The anterior longitudinal ligament is exposed by retracting the carotid sheath laterally and the tracheoesophageal complex medially. A lateral localizing radiograph is obtained with an intradiskal needle in place to identify the level of exposure. The longus colli muscles are elevated. Transverse and longitudinal anterior cervical retractors are placed and secured. Using a headlight and magnifying loupes, the surgeon initiates a diskectomy at each level. If the vertebral body is deformed, it may be necessary to verify the location of the midline radiographically by reference to the axial MRI or computed tomographic images. A 12- to 16-mm-wide median corpectomy trench is created with the high-speed drill and a 5-mm cutting bur. To avoid interfering with arthrodesis, thrombin-soaked Gelfoam powder rather than bone wax is used for osseous hemostasis. As the trench approaches the posterior vertebral body cortex, it is widened by undercutting with a 3-mm bur to extend the decompression across the entire transverse interpedicular canal diameter of 18 to 22 mm.

The diskectomies and corpectomies are completed under the operating microscope. Diskogenic osteophytes are removed, and the posterior vertebral cortex is resected with a diamond bur to expose the ossified posterior longitudinal ligament. Bone is débrided from the ligament by drilling until flexible ligament or dura is exposed. To avoid prematurely detaching and mobilizing a large central osseous mass before internal reduction has been safely accomplished, ligamentous bone is resected by working from the midline laterally rather than in the reverse direction. Bilateral foraminotomies are performed at each level with the drill and microcurets. The rostral and caudal edges of the corpectomy are further extended by undercutting the margins of the remaining vertebral bodies to completely decompress the stenosis. The posterior longitudinal ligament is then perforated if necessary and elevated over a blunt hook or angled dissector inserted into the epidural space. Transverse and longitudinal incisions are made, and the ligament is totally resected with angled curets and a 2-mm punch. Dura involved with the ossified lesion is resected as well; the dural defect is covered with Gelfoam or bovine collagen tissue adhesive and sealed with fibrin glue. If cerebrospinal fluid drainage results from an opening in the arachnoid, a lumbar subarachnoid drain is placed after closure.

During completion of the median corpectomy, a mortise step is cut into the rostral and caudal surfaces of the lower and upper vertebral body end plates to secure and lock in the fusion graft. After the corpectomy dimensions have been measured, the bone graft is harvested from the donor iliac crest or fibular site or is prepared from allograft bone bank material. Cylindrical mesh titanium cages that can be filled with cancellous autograft bone obtained from the corpectomy or iliac crest are also available for implant as a vertebral body prosthesis. To allow sufficient space for anterior expansion of the decompressed thecal sac, the graft or implant should not be more than 10 to 12 mm deep in the anteroposterior plane. The bone graft is trimmed transversely so that it will be slightly wider than the trench to ensure a snug fit. To maintain adequate foramen circumference, a moderate amount of distraction is applied with a vertebral distractor during the final longitudinal trimming and impaction of the bone graft. After a single-level corpectomy, external immobilization with a hard collar is adequate. After two- to three-level corpectomy, internal screw plate fixation or external immobilization with a halo brace is used. After four- or five-level corpectomy, separate screw plates may be placed at the upper and lower ends of the graft, although placement of a long single plate is preferable, if feasible.

Pitfalls and Complications

The most common technical error leading to inadequate decompression is right-to-left slanting of the corpectomy trench, leaving residual ossification and stenosis on the patient's right (see Fig. 291–4). These residua are easily seen on postoperative scans, which are usually obtained because of persistent or recurrent neurological deficit. This error can be avoided by obtaining an intraoperative fluoroscopic or radiographic image with a metallic marker in place to demonstrate the transverse diameter and lateral extent of decompression at each level. Intraoperative ultrasound scanning may also be used to detect this error and to verify that a complete decompression has been achieved. When available, computer-based image-guided surgery systems can be used to direct and monitor adequate decompression. Intraoperative computed tomographic scanning can also be used for visualization and verification of the neural canal and foraminal decompression. For a right-handed surgeon operating from the patient's right, changing position to the left side of the operating table makes it easier to decompress the lateral recesses and foramina on the right. Alternatively, use of a surgical diploscope or optical bridge attachment allows the assistant to complete the decompression on the right side.

In our experience with 100 anterior corpectomy cases, surgical complications have been infrequent. They include temporary paraparesis due to epidural hematoma requiring evacuation in one case; new cervical radiculopathy due to residual foramen stenosis, despite the use of distraction during placement of the bone graft, in one case (subsequently treated by posterior foraminotomy); temporary recurrent laryngeal nerve and superior laryngeal nerve palsy due to retraction injury in two cases; anterior bone graft displacement not requiring reoperation in two cases; and halo pin site infection in one case. Delayed onset of progressive myelopathy due to cord edema occurred 3 to 5 days postoperatively in two patients; this responded well to posterior decompression by laminectomy to relieve relative stenosis above or below the corpectomy site. Such patients would be best treated with circumferential surgery initially. Respiratory insufficiency due to upper airway obstruction after premature tracheal extubation required reintubation in two cases. One patient died of esophageal perforation, retropharyngeal abscess, sepsis, and liver failure due to preexisting cirrhosis. Late removal of an anterior screw plate was required in one patient because of persistent dysphagia and esophageal compression at C3. To date, one patient required reoperation 6 years after corpectomy by laminectomy and fusion at additional vertebral levels because of OPLL extension and degenerative spondylosis above and below the previous fusion at C3-4 and C7-T1.

RESULTS

In our initial series of 18 cases of OPLL treated by anterior corpectomy and fusion with 2- to 5-year follow-up, outcome was assessed with a spinal function scale (0% to 100%).[96] Functional recovery was good to excellent (60% to 100%) in 8 of 18 patients (44%); it was fair (40% to 60%) in 3 others. Seven patients had little or no improvement in neurological function. No subsequent delayed deterioration was observed. The mean recovery score was 55%, indicating that the overall outcome was fair.

All patients who do not recover satisfactorily undergo neuroimaging studies to assess the adequacy of decompression (Fig. 291–5). Flexion-extension radiographs are obtained to verify the stability of the fusion. There have been no cases of pseudarthrosis identified. Reoperation is recommended only for treatment of progressive postoperative neurological deterioration.

In a recent review of 44 non-Japanese patients with OPLL, 34 improved neurologically, 4 were stable, and 3 deteriorated.[45] Epstein reviewed the neurological outcome in six published series of surgically treated patients for comparison with preoperative neurological grades.[8] Although substantial neurological improvement was documented in each series, this analysis did not demonstrate an outcome advantage for anterior or posterior decompression. However, experience in some of these series suggests that the incidence of new postoperative neurological deficit is lower after anterior surgery.[8, 87] In the most recent report of a single surgical series of 51 cases treated in the United States, better results were obtained after anterior decompression than after posterior decompression.[8] There were no neurological complications in that series; however, new postoperative quadriplegia has been described in 2% to 10% of cases in the past. Fujimura and coworkers reported on 33 patients who underwent anterior decompression and fusion for thoracic OPLL with myelopathy, with 53% good recovery and a mean follow-up of 8 years and 2 months.[97] Delayed deterioration in neurological function commonly occurs between 5 and 10 years postoperatively and is usually a slow, insidious process.[93, 97] To date, no prospective study comparing the results of anterior and posterior operations has been reported.

In the future, it is likely that selection of the safest, anatomically most appropriate operation and the use of meticulous microsurgical technique, intraoperative neurophysiologic monitoring, and internal fixation to enhance fusion will result in further improvement in the surgical outcome. Circumferential surgery combining both anterior and posterior operations may be necessary in selected patients.

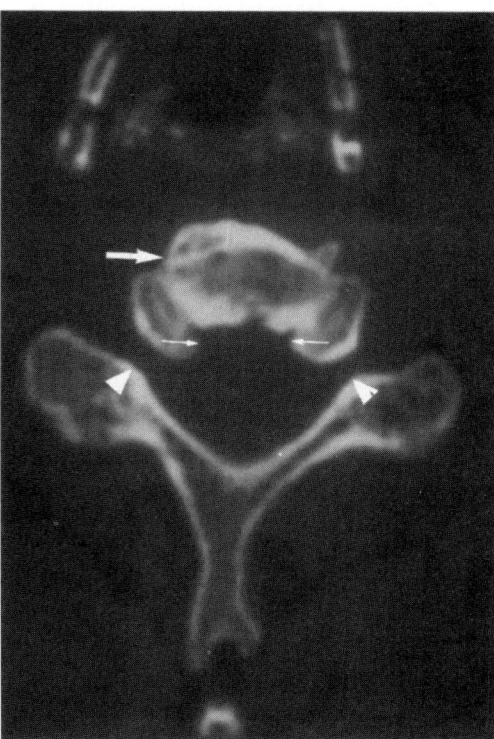

FIGURE 291–5. Axial computed tomographic scan at C4-5 1 year after C5-6 corpectomy for decompression of stenosis and ossification of the posterior longitudinal ligament demonstrates adequate neural canal diameter, patent foramina *(arrowheads)*, midline position of the corpectomy trench *(small arrows)*, and satisfactory incorporation of the iliac crest bone graft *(large arrow)*.

REFERENCES

1. Shaibani A, Workman R, Rothschild BM: The significance of enthesopathy as a skeletal phenomenon. Clin Exp Rheumatol 11: 399–403, 1993.
2. Resnick D, Niwayama G: Radiographic and pathologic features of spinal involvement in diffuse idiopathic skeletal hyperostosis (DISH). Radiology 119:559–568, 1976.
3. Otake S, Matsuo M, Nishizawa S, et al: Ossification of the posterior longitudinal ligament: MR evaluation. AJNR Am J Neuroradiol 13:1059–1067, 1992.
4. Klara PM, McDonnell DE: Ossification of the posterior longitudinal ligament in Caucasians: Diagnosis and surgical intervention. Neurosurgery 19:212–217, 1986.
5. Del Conte L, Tassinari T, Trucco M, et al: Ossification of the posterior longitudinal ligament (OPLL) in the cervical spine: Clinical, neuroradiological and neurophysiological study on 9 cases. Ital J Neurol Sci 13:767–780, 1992.
6. Dietemann JL, Dirheimer Y, Babin E, et al: Ossification of the posterior longitudinal ligament (Japanese disease): A radiological study in 12 cases. J Neuroradiol 12:212–222, 1985.
7. Cheng WC, Chang CN, Lui TN, et al: Surgical treatment for ossification of the posterior longitudinal ligament of the cervical spine. Surg Neurol 41:90–97, 1994.
8. Epstein N: The surgical management of ossification of the posterior longitudinal ligament in 51 patients. J Spinal Disord 6:432–454, discussion 454–455, 1993.
9. Yang DY, Wang YC, Lee CS, Chou DY: Ossification of the posterior cervical longitudinal ligament. Acta Neurochir (Wien) 115: 15–19, 1992; erratum in 115:165, 1992.
10. Wada K: [Genetic studies on the ossification of the posterior longitudinal ligament.] Nippon Seikeigeka Gakkai Zasshi 61: 171–183, 1987.
11. Ohtsuka K, Terayama K, Yanagihara M, et al: A radiological population study on the ossification of the posterior longitudinal ligament in the spine. Arch Orthop Trauma Surg 106:89–93, 1987.
12. Izawa K: [Comparative roentgenographical study on the incidence of ossification of the posterior longitudinal ligament and other degenerative changes of the cervical spine among Japanese, Koreans, Americans and Germans.] Nippon Seikeigeka Gakkai Zasshi 54:461–474, 1980.
13. Albisinni U, Merlini L, Terayama K, et al: [X-ray epidemiology of ligament ossification and disc degeneration of the cervical spine.] Chir Organi Mov 70:15–22, 1985.
14. Firooznia H, Benjamin VM, Pinto RS, et al: Calcification and ossification of posterior longitudinal ligament of spine: Its role

in secondary narrowing of spinal canal and cord compression. N Y State J Med 82:1193–1198, 1982.

15. Nakanishi T, Mannen T, Toyokura Y: Asymptomatic ossification of the posterior longitudinal ligament of the cervical spine: Incidence and roentgenographic findings. J Neurol Sci 19:375–381, 1973.

16. Littlejohn GO: Insulin and new bone formation in diffuse idiopathic skeletal hyperostosis. Clin Rheumatol 4:294–300, 1985.

17. Tsuyama N: Ossification of the posterior longitudinal ligament of the spine. Clin Orthop 47:71–84, 1984.

18. Smythe HA: Osteoarthritis, insulin and bone density. J Rheumatol 14:91–93, 1987.

19. Ikegawa S, Kurokawa T, Hizuka N, et al: Increase of serum growth hormone–binding protein in patients with ossification of the posterior longitudinal ligament of the spine. Spine 18:1757–1760, 1993.

20. Altomonte L, Zoli A, Mirone L, et al: Growth hormone secretion in diffuse idiopathic skeletal hyperostosis. Ann Ital Med Int 7:30–33, 1992.

21. Troillet N, Gerster JC: [Forestier disease and metabolism disorders: A prospective controlled study of 25 cases.] Rev Rhum 60:274–279, 1993.

22. Lambert RG, Becker EJ: Diffuse skeletal hyperostosis in idiopathic hypoparathyroidism. Clin Radiol 40:212–215, 1989.

23. Okazaki T, Takuwa Y, Yamamoto M, et al: Ossification of the paravertebral ligaments: A frequent complication of hypoparathyroidism. Metabolism 33:710–713, 1984.

24. Seichi A, Hoshino Y, Ohnishi I, Kurokawa T: The role of calcium metabolism abnormalities in the development of ossification of the posterior longitudinal ligament of the cervical spine. Spine 17(3 Suppl):S30–S32, 1992.

25. Miyamoto S, Yonenobu K, Ono K: Elevated plasma fibronectin concentrations in patients with ossification of the posterior longitudinal ligament and ossification of the ligamentum flavum. Spine 18:2267–2270, 1993.

26. DiGiovanna JJ, Helfgott RK, Gerber LH, Peck GL: Extraspinal tendon and ligament calcification associated with long-term therapy with etretinate. N Engl J Med 315:1177–1182, 1986.

27. Lussier A, Esdaile J, Trojan D, et al: Ossification of the posterior spinal ligaments: A different disease than DISH [abstract]. Rev Mex Rheumatol 5(Suppl 1):134, 1990.

28. Ishida Y, Kawai S: Characterization of cultured cells derived from ossification of the posterior longitudinal ligament of the spine. Bone 14:85–91, 1993.

29. Ishida Y, Kawai S: Effects of bone-seeking hormones on DNA synthesis, cyclic AMP level, and alkaline phosphatase activity in cultured cells from human posterior longitudinal ligament of the spine. J Bone Miner Res 8:1291–1300, 1993.

30. Kawaguchi H, Kurokawa T, Hoshino Y, et al: Immunohistochemical demonstration of bone morphogenetic protein-2 and transforming growth factor-beta in the ossification of the posterior longitudinal ligament of the cervical spine. Spine 17(3 Suppl):S33–S36, 1992.

31. Yonemori K, Imamura T, Ishidou Y, et al: Bone morphogenetic protein receptors and activin receptors are highly expressed in ossified ligament tissues of patients with ossification of the posterior longitudinal ligament. Am J Pathol 150:1335–1347, 1997.

32. Kon T, Yamazaki M, Tagawa M, et al: Bone morphogenetic protein-2 stimulates differentiation of cultured spinal ligament cells from patients with ossification of the posterior longitudinal ligament. Calcif Tissue Int 60:291–296, 1997.

33. Morio Y, Yamamoto K, Kishimoto H, et al: Bone mineral density of the radius in patients with ossification of the cervical posterior longitudinal ligament: A longitudinal study. Spine 18:2513–2516, 1993.

34. Maezumi H: [Bone mineral analysis in patients with ossification of the posterior longitudinal ligament of the spine.] Nippon Seikeigeka Gakkai Zasshi 64:534–545, 1990.

35. Okawa A, Nakamura I, Goto S, et al: Mutation in Npps in a mouse model of ossification of the posterior longitudinal ligament of the spine. Nat Genet 19:271–273, 1998.

36. Okawa A, Ikegawa S, Nakamura I, et al: Mapping of a gene responsible for twy (tip-toe walking Yoshimura), a mouse model of ossification of the posterior longitudinal ligament of the spine (OPLL). Mamm Genome 9:155–156, 1998.

37. Koga H, Hayashi K, Taketomi E, et al: Restriction fragment length polymorphism of genes of the alpha 2(XI) collagen, bone morphogenetic protein-2, alkaline phosphatase, and tumor necrosis factor-alpha among patients with ossification of posterior longitudinal ligament and controls from the Japanese population. Spine 21:469–473, 1996.

38. Koga H, Sakou T, Taketomi E, et al: Genetic mapping of ossification of the posterior longitudinal ligament of the spine. Am J Hum Genet 62:1460–1467, 1998.

39. Numasawa T, Koga H, Ueyama K, et al: Human retinoic X receptor beta: Complete genomic sequence and mutation search for ossification of posterior longitudinal ligament of the spine. J Bone Miner Res 14:500–508, 1999.

40. Perry JD, Wolf H, Festenstein H, Storey GO: Ankylosing hyperostosis: A study of HLA A, B, and C antigens. Ann Rheum Dis 38:72–73, 1979.

41. Ramos-Remus C, Russell AS, Gomez-Vargas A, et al: Ossification of the posterior longitudinal ligament in three geographically and genetically different populations of ankylosing spondylitis and other spondyloarthropathies. Ann Rheum Dis 57:429–433, 1998.

42. Sakou T, Taketomi E, Matsunaga S, et al: Genetic study of ossification of the posterior longitudinal ligament in the cervical spine with human leukocyte antigen haplotype. Spine 16:1249–1252, 1991.

43. Matsunaga S, Yamaguchi M, Hayashi K, Sakou T: Genetic analysis of ossification of the posterior longitudinal ligament. Spine 24:937–938, discussion 939, 1999.

44. Hamanishi C, Tan A, Yamane T, et al: Ossification of the posterior longitudinal ligament: Autosomal recessive trait. Spine 20:205–207, 1995.

45. Trojan DA, Pouchot J, Pokrupa R, et al: Diagnosis and treatment of ossification of the posterior longitudinal ligament of the spine: Report of eight cases and literature review. Am J Med 92:296–306, 1992.

46. Harsh G, Weinstein P: Cevical myeloradiculopathy secondary to ossification of the posterior longitudinal ligament. In Saunders R, Bernini P (eds): Cervical Spondylotic Myelopathy. Cambridge, Mass., Blackwell Scientific, 1992, pp 186–202.

47. Yonenobu K, Ebara S, Fujiwara K, et al: Thoracic myelopathy secondary to ossification of the spinal ligament. J Neurosurg 66:511–518, 1987.

48. Kurihara A, Tanaka Y, Tsumura N, Iwasaki Y: Hyperostotic lumbar spinal stenosis: A review of 12 surgically treated cases with roentgenographic survey of ossification of the yellow ligament at the lumbar spine. Spine 13:1308–1316, 1988.

49. Saika M: [A morphological study of the etiology and growth of ossification of the posterior longitudinal ligament of the spine.] Nippon Seikeigeka Gakkai Zasshi 61:1059–1072, 1987.

50. Sato M, Turu M, Yada K: [The anteroposterior diameter of the cervical spinal canal in ossification of the posterior longitudinal ligament.] No Shinkei Geka 5:511–517, 1977.

51. Takahashi M, Kawanami H, Tomonaga M, Kitamura K: Ossification of the posterior longitudinal ligament—a roentgenologic and clinical investigation. Acta Radiol Diagn 13:25–36, 1972.

52. Kadoya S, Nakamura T, Tada A: Neuroradiology of ossification of the posterior longitudinal spinal ligament: Comparative studies with computer tomography. Neuroradiology 16:357–358, 1978.

53. Nose T, Egashira T, Enomoto T, Maki Y: Ossification of the posterior longitudinal ligament: A clinico-radiological study of 74 cases. J Neurol Neurosurg Psychiatry 50:321–326, 1987.

54. Koyanagi T, Hirabayashi K, Satomi K, et al: Predictability of operative results of cervical compression myelopathy based on preoperative computed tomographic myelography. Spine 18:1958–1963, 1993.

55. Okada Y, Ikata T, Yamada H, et al: Magnetic resonance imaging study on the results of surgery for cervical compression myelopathy. Spine 18:2024–2029, 1993.

56. Nakamura M, Fujimura Y: Magnetic resonance imaging of the spinal cord in cervical ossification of the posterior longitudinal ligament: Can it predict surgical outcome? Spine 23:38–40, 1998.

57. Koyanagi I, Iwasaki Y, Hida K, et al: Magnetic resonance imaging findings in ossification of the posterior longitudinal ligament of the cervical spine. J Neurosurg 88:247–254, 1998.

58. Shinomiya K, Furuya K, Sato R, et al: Electrophysiologic diagnosis of cervical OPLL myelopathy using evoked spinal cord potentials. Spine 13:1225–1233, 1988.
59. McAfee PC, Regan JJ, Bohlman HH: Cervical cord compression from ossification of the posterior longitudinal ligament in non-Orientals. J Bone Joint Surg Br 69:569–575, 1987.
60. Julkunen H, Heinonen OP, Knekt P, Maatela J: The epidemiology of hyperostosis of the spine together with its symptoms and related mortality in a general population. Scand J Rheumatol 4: 23–27, 1975.
61. Karpman RR, Weinstein PR, Gall EP, Johnson PC: Lumbar spinal stenosis in a patient with diffuse idiopathic skeletal hypertrophy syndrome. Spine 7:598–603, 1982.
62. Cruickshank B: Pathology of ankylosing spondylitis. Clin Orthop 74:43–58, 1971.
63. Leroux JL, Legeron P, Moulinier L, et al: Stenosis of the lumbar spinal canal in vertebral ankylosing hyperostosis. Spine 17:1213–1218, 1992; see comments.
64. Forestier J, Rotes-Querol J: Senile ankylosing hyperostosis of the spine. Ann Rheum Dis 9:321–330, 1950.
65. Kulkarni MV, Williams JC, Yeakley JW, et al: Magnetic resonance imaging in the diagnosis of the cranio-cervical manifestations of the mucopolysaccharidoses. Magn Reson Imaging 5:317–323, 1987.
66. Ramos-Remus C, Gomez-Vargas A, LeClercq S, Russell AS: Radiologic features of DISH may mimic ankylosing spondylitis. Clin Exp Rheumatol 11:603–608, 1993.
67. Laroche M, Moulinier L, Arlet J, et al: Lumbar and cervical stenosis: Frequency of the association, role of the ankylosing hyperostosis. Clin Rheumatol 11:533–535, 1992.
68. Hashizume Y, Iijima S, Kishimoto H, Yanagi T: Pathology of spinal cord lesions caused by ossification of the posterior longitudinal ligament. Acta Neuropathol (Berl) 63:123–130, 1984.
69. Mizuno J, Nakagawa H, Iwata K, Hashizume Y: Pathology of spinal cord lesions caused by ossification of the posterior longitudinal ligament, with special reference to reversibility of the spinal cord lesion. Neurol Res 14:312–314, 1992.
70. Murakami N, Muroga T, Sobue I: Cervical myelopathy due to ossification of the posterior longitudinal ligament: A clinicopathologic study. Arch Neurol 35:33–36, 1978.
71. Ono K, Ota H, Tada K: Cervical myelopathy secondary to multiple spondylotic protrusions: A clinicopathologic study. Spine 2: 109–127, 1977.
72. Ono K, Ota H, Tada K, et al: Ossified posterior longitudinal ligament: A clinicopathologic study. Spine 2:126–138, 1977.
73. Tsuzuki N, Imai T, Hotta Y: [Histopathologic findings of ossification of the posterior longitudinal ligament of the cervical spine and their significance.] Nippon Seikeigeka Gakkai Zasshi 55: 387–397, 1981.
74. Goto S: [Studies of ossification of the posterior longitudinal ligament in the cervical spine using microradiography and histochemistry.] Nippon Seikeigeka Gakkai Zasshi 55:451–466, 1981.
75. Yasui N, Ono K, Yamaura I, et al: Immunohistochemical localization of types I, II, and III collagens in the ossified posterior longitudinal ligament of the human cervical spine. Calcif Tissue Int 35:159–163, 1983.
76. Weinstein PR, Karpman RR, Gall EP, Pitt M: Spinal cord injury, spinal fracture, and spinal stenosis in ankylosing spondylitis. J Neurosurg 57:609–616, 1982.
77. Resnick D, Guerra J Jr, Robinson CA, Vint VC: Association of diffuse idiopathic skeletal hyperostosis (DISH) and calcification and ossification of the posterior longitudinal ligament. AJR Am J Roentgenol 131:1049–1053, 1978.
78. Lee T, Chacha PB, Khoo J: Ossification of posterior longitudinal ligament of the cervical spine in non-Japanese Asians. Surg Neurol 35:40–44, 1991.
79. Wang PN, Chen SS, Liu HC, et al: Ossification of the posterior longitudinal ligament of the spine: A case-control risk factor study. Spine 24:142–144, discussion 145, 1999.
80. Gui L, Merlini L, Savini R, Davidovits P: Cervical myelopathy due to ossification of the posterior longitudinal ligament. Ital J Orthop Traumatol 9:269–280, 1983.
81. Yoshino MT, Seeger JF, Carmody RF: MRI diagnosis of thoracic ossification of posterior longitudinal ligament with concomitant disc herniation. Neuroradiology 33:455–457, 1991.
82. Hirai T, Korogi Y, Yamashita Y, et al: Ossification of posterior longitudinal ligaments: Evaluation with MRI. J Magn Reson Imaging 8:398–405, 1998.
83. Takahashi M, Sakamoto Y, Miyawaki M, Bussaka H: Increased MR signal intensity secondary to chronic cervical cord compression. Neuroradiology 29:550–556, 1987.
84. Yonenobu K, Fuji T, Ono K, et al: Choice of surgical treatment for multisegmental cervical spondylotic myelopathy. Spine 10: 710–716, 1985.
85. Tomita K, Kawahara N, Baba H, et al: Circumspinal decompression for thoracic myelopathy due to combined ossification of the posterior longitudinal ligament and ligamentum flavum. Spine 15:1114–1120, 1990.
86. Kurosa Y, Yamaura I, Nakai O, Shinomiya K: Selecting a surgical method for thoracic myelopathy caused by ossification of the posterior longitudinal ligament. Spine 21:1458–1466, 1996.
87. Abe H, Tsuru M, Ito T, et al: Anterior decompression for ossification of the posterior longitudinal ligament of the cervical spine. J Neurosurg 55:108–116, 1981.
88. Tominaga S: The effects of intervertebral fusion in patients with myelopathy due to ossification of the posterior longitudinal ligament of the cervical spine. Int Orthop 4:183–191, 1980.
89. Hanai K, Inouye Y, Kawai K, et al: Anterior decompression for myelopathy resulting from ossification of the posterior longitudinal ligament. J Bone Joint Surg Br 64:561–564, 1982.
90. Kojima T, Waga S, Kubo Y, et al: Anterior cervical vertebrectomy and interbody fusion for multi-level spondylosis and ossification of the posterior longitudinal ligament. Neurosurgery 24:864–872, 1989.
91. Epstein NE: Circumferential surgery for the management of cervical ossification of the posterior longitudinal ligament. J Spinal Disord 11:200–207, 1998.
92. Rozario RA, Levine H, Stein BM: Cervical myelopathy and radiculopathy secondary to ossification of the posterior longitudinal ligament. Surg Neurol 10:17–20, 1978.
93. Kato Y, Iwasaki M, Fuji T, et al: Long-term follow-up results of laminectomy for cervical myelopathy caused by ossification of the posterior longitudinal ligament. J Neurosurg 89:217–223, 1998.
94. Hirabayashi K, Miyakawa J, Satomi K, et al: Operative results and postoperative progression of ossification among patients with ossification of cervical posterior longitudinal ligament. Spine 6:354–364, 1981.
95. Nakano N, Nakano T, Nakano K: Comparison of the results of laminectomy and open-door laminoplasty for cervical spondylotic myeloradiculopathy and ossification of the posterior longitudinal ligament. Spine 13:792–794, 1988.
96. Harsh GRT, Sypert GW, Weinstein PR, et al: Cervical spine stenosis secondary to ossification of the posterior longitudinal ligament. J Neurosurg 67:349–357, 1987.
97. Fujimura Y, Nishi Y, Nakamura M, et al: Long-term follow-up study of anterior decompression and fusion for thoracic myelopathy resulting from ossification of the posterior longitudinal ligament. Spine 22:305–311, 1997.

CHAPTER 292

Benign Extradural Lesions of the Dorsal Spine

PAUL SANTIAGO ■ ANDREW D. FINE ■ DAVID SHAFRON ■ RICHARD G. FESSLER

The diagnosis and treatment of thoracic disk herniation have evolved considerably during the last century. Significant changes have been brought about by new surgical techniques and improved technology, such as the recent development of endoscopic techniques. Diagnostic imaging techniques have contributed to earlier diagnosis and treatment. Before the era of magnetic resonance imaging (MRI) and computed tomography (CT), thoracic disk herniation was diagnosed by myelography and plain film roentgenography. These methods yielded false-negative results in 8% of cases and provided a correct diagnosis in only 56% of symptomatic thoracic disk herniations.[1, 2] These imaging studies, coupled with the protean manifestations of this disorder, often resulted in delayed diagnosis or even misdiagnosis.

Intervertebral disk herniation in the cervical and lumbar spine is relatively common. The diagnosis and management of cervical and lumbar disk herniation, though not without controversy, have been well described. This is not the case with thoracic disk herniation. With the routine availability of MRI over the past 2 decades, thoracic disk protrusions are being diagnosed with increasing frequency. Autopsy series suggest that the incidence of thoracic disk herniation is between 7% and 15%.[3] Clinically, however, thoracic disk herniations represent only approximately 1% of symptomatic intervertebral disk herniations. The estimated prevalence, therefore, ranges from 1/1000 to 1/ 1 million in the general population.[2-8] Loss of motor, sensory, bowel, bladder, and sexual function has been associated with thoracic disk herniation. The potential for devastating neurological sequelae makes rapid diagnosis and appropriate treatment of paramount importance. This chapter reviews the essentials of diagnosing and managing this challenging disease process.

HISTORY AND EPIDEMIOLOGY

The study and treatment of thoracic disk herniation began in the 20th century, with the notable exception of Key's 1838 report of thoracic disk herniation as a cause of spinal cord injury.[9] Most early reports classified these disk herniations as cartilaginous tumors. They were called enchondroms, chondromas, and ecchondromas.[10-12] Middleton and Treacher[13] and then Dandy[14] described post-traumatic thoracic disk herniations. In 1934, Mixter and Barr retrospectively reviewed a series of 25 thoracic spinal cord tumors from Massachusetts General Hospital and reclassified nearly 80% of them as disk herniations.[15] Surgical intervention for this disease was first described by Adson in 1922.[16]

Although no large series or epidemiologic data exist, review of the available literature suggests that there is a slight male predominance. Thoracic disk herniation most commonly occurs in the fourth through sixth decades, with a mean age of 50 years.[6, 11, 17-21] A history of trauma is reported in only 22% to 50% of symptomatic patients.[4, 6, 21, 22] When such a history is present, it frequently is related to a fall, with the patient describing landing on the feet or buttocks, combined with an axial spinal rotation. The lower incidence of thoracic disk herniations compared with cervical and lumbar disk herniations has been attributed to the limited motion of the thoracic spine and the relatively small size of the thoracic intervertebral disk.[23]

CLINICAL PRESENTATION AND DIFFERENTIAL DIAGNOSIS

The most frequent history elicited is one of prolonged dorsal spine pain, with or without radiation or sensory changes, and progressive long-tract signs.[4, 22] Radiculopathy from thoracic disk disease is classically unilateral, lancinating, and dermatomal but may be bilateral. Because adjacent levels overlap to a sufficient degree, dermatomal sensory loss is absent. Patients often complain of progressive gait difficulty, characterized by increasing stiffness, cramping, and weakness of the lower extremities. Common complaints reported in several series are summarized in Table 292–1. When

T A B L E   2 9 2 – 1 ■ **Presenting Complaints of Thoracic Disk Herniation**

COMPLAINT	STILLERMAN & WEISS[40]	MAIMAN ET AL[7]	ARCE & DOHRMANN[4,22]	OTANI ET AL[21]	FESSLER[20]
Weakness	59%	43%	50%	100%	41%
Local pain	59%	78%	57%		88%
Sensory loss	39%	87%	56%	100%	88%
Bowel/bladder dysfunction	18%	43%	31%	78%	47%
Radicular pain	16%	35%	9%		65%
Spinal cord syndrome			9% Brown-Séquard	100%, 7 complete myelographic blocks	41%, spasticity ± Babinski's reflex

associated with acute trauma, patients tend to present within 1 to 30 days with spinal cord or radicular symptoms. Commonly, pain is rated as moderate, aggravated by movement, and relieved with rest. Occasionally, pain may be absent. Bladder dysfunction (i.e., urgency, dribbling) is a common complaint.

Several authors have described syndromes that correspond to disk herniations at particular thoracic levels. Horner's syndrome, presumably resulting from preganglionic sympathetic fiber injury from a lateral disk herniation at the C7-T1 or T1-2 level, has been reported in the literature.[24–27] Dysesthesias of the medial arm may be misdiagnosed as a sign of cardiovascular disease (myocardial infarction, angina, thoracic aortic dissection) or of apical bronchogenic carcinoma (Pancoast's tumor). In the mid to lower thoracic spine, disk herniations can present as Brown-Sequard or anterior spinal artery syndromes, and at the thoracolumbar junction, a disk herniation may manifest itself as a conus medullaris syndrome.[2, 4, 22] Certainly, the identification of a spinal cord syndrome focuses the physician's attention on the spine and spinal cord. Delayed diagnosis can occur when symptomatic exacerbations alternate with remissions, suggesting the presence of a demyelinating disease, or when pain is not a component of the initial presentation, suggesting a primary motoneuron disease, neuromuscular disease, myopathy, muscular dystrophy, or motor neuropathy. Radicular dysesthesias may be misdiagnosed as visceral referred pain (e.g., renal colic, gallbladder colic, colitis), intercostal neuritis, or costochondritis.

RADIOLOGIC EVALUATION

Plain Radiographs

Plain films of the spine are commonly the first studies ordered in the evaluation of back pain. They are useful screening tools for the presence of diskitis, osteomyelitis, and destructive lesions such as primary or metastatic tumors. In addition, they are invaluable in identifying pathologic fractures or traumatic instability. The findings on plain radiographs that suggest possible thoracic disk herniation are degenerative disk space disease, calcifications (within the disk space itself or within the canal), vertebral body end plate osteophytes,

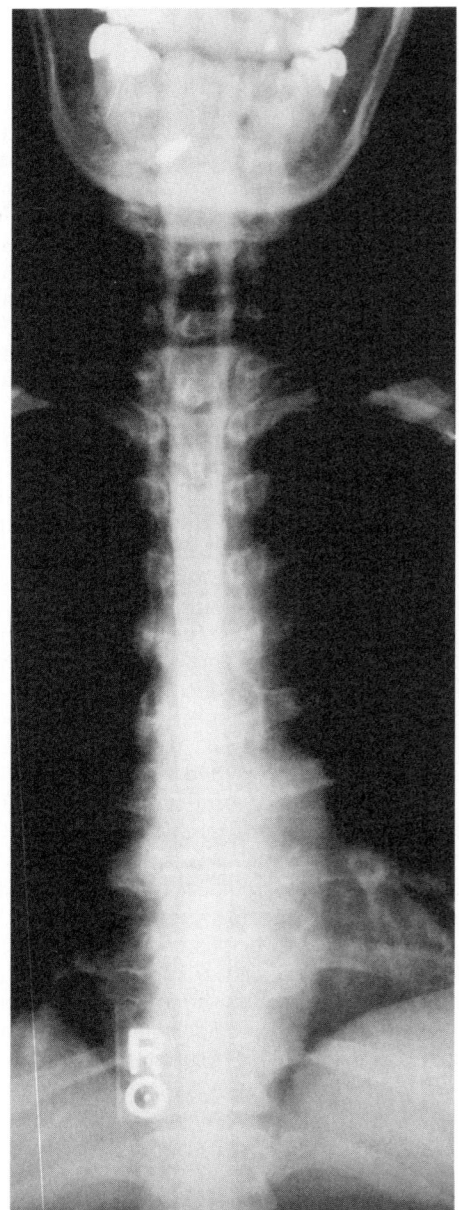

FIGURE 292–1. Anteroposterior thoracic myelogram demonstrating a two-level nerve root cutoff due to a centrolaterally herniated disk.

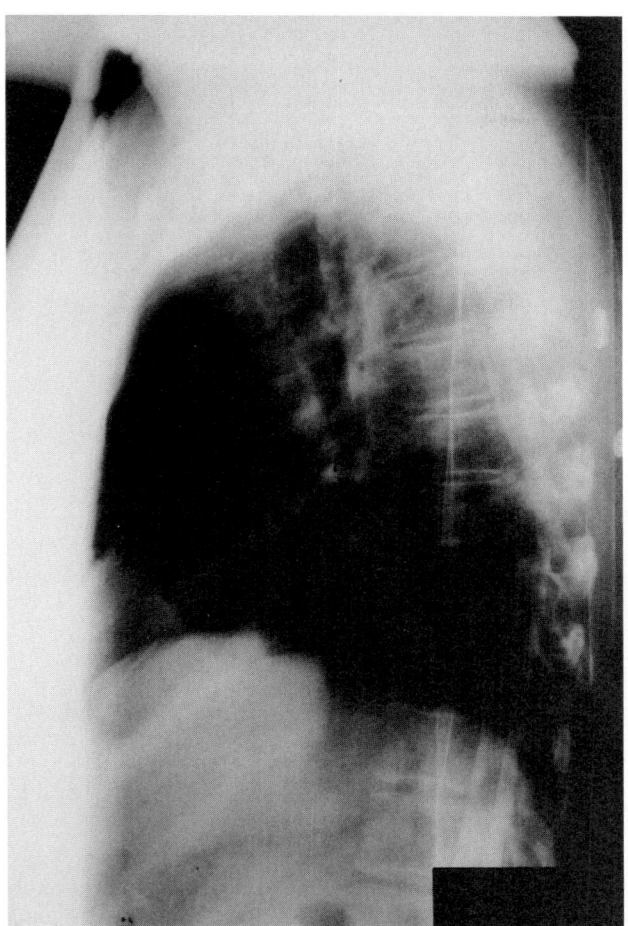

FIGURE 292–2. Lateral thoracic myelogram in the same patient as in Figure 292–1.

and localized kyphosis. Although the significance of disk space calcification is questionable, calcification within the spinal canal is highly suggestive of thoracic disk herniation and may be associated with intradural extension of the disk.

Myelography and Postmyelography Computed Tomography

The combination of thoracic myelography and postmyelography CT is the gold standard in the diagnosis of thoracic disk herniation. Although the myelogram shows a typical extradural defect consistent with many disease processes, its localization at the disk space is typical (Figs. 292–1 and 292–2). The postmyelogram CT image often reveals a mixed soft tissue density with calcium in association with end plate osteophytes (Figs. 292–3 and 292–4). Thoracic disk herniations are central or paracentral in 70% to 90% of cases causing spinal cord or nerve root compression.[25, 28–30] Twelve percent of thoracic disk herniations are associated with calcification within the spinal canal. In our experience, and in the experience of others, this suggests the possibility of intradural extension.[25, 28–30]

Magnetic Resonance Imaging

MRI of the thoracic spine has several advantages. It is a noninvasive procedure that provides detailed information about the thoracic vertebrae, disk spaces, spinal cord, and surrounding soft tissues in multiple planes (Figs. 292–5 and 292–6). MRI is very sensitive for the identification of thoracic disk protrusion but has a relatively high false-positive rate (14.5%), making clinical correlation critical.[31, 32] Exaggeration of the magnitude of disk protrusion, especially on sagittal MRI, is not unique to the thoracic spine and is partly a conse-

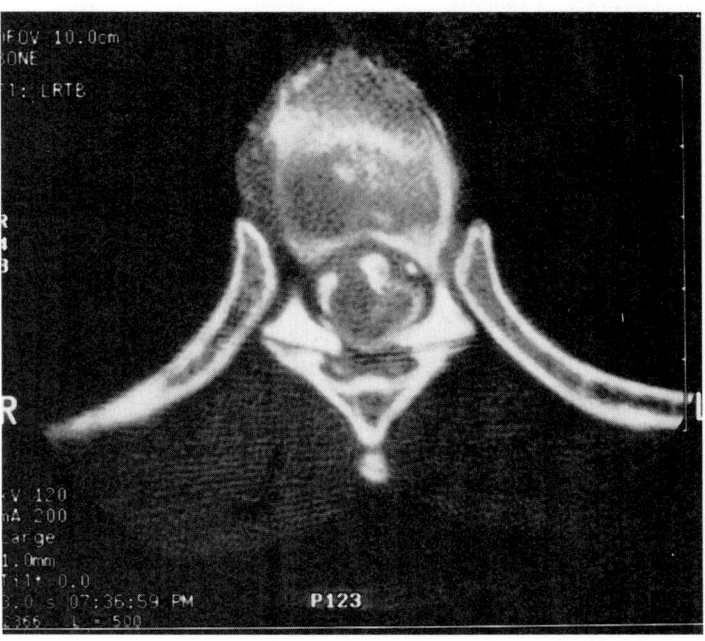

FIGURE 292–3. Axial postmyelogram computed tomographic scan demonstrating a massive centrally herniated disk filling the majority of the spinal canal.

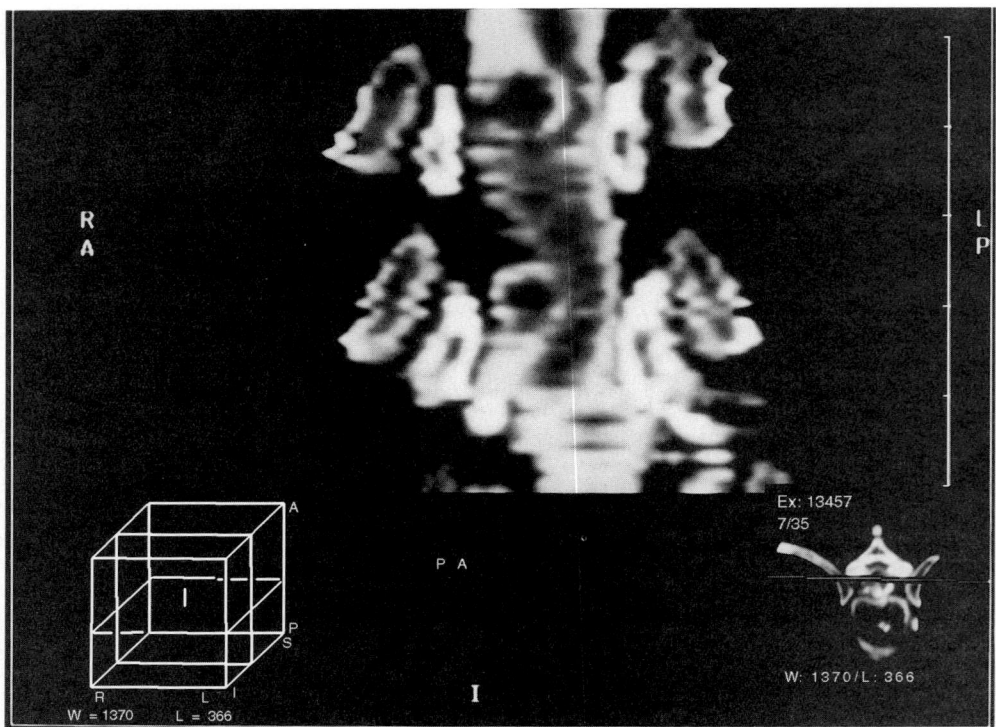

FIGURE 292–4. Coronal reconstruction of a postmyelogram computed tomographic scan in the same patient as in Figure 292–3. It demonstrates significant deviation of the spinal cord to the left and a massive right-sided disk herniation spanning two levels.

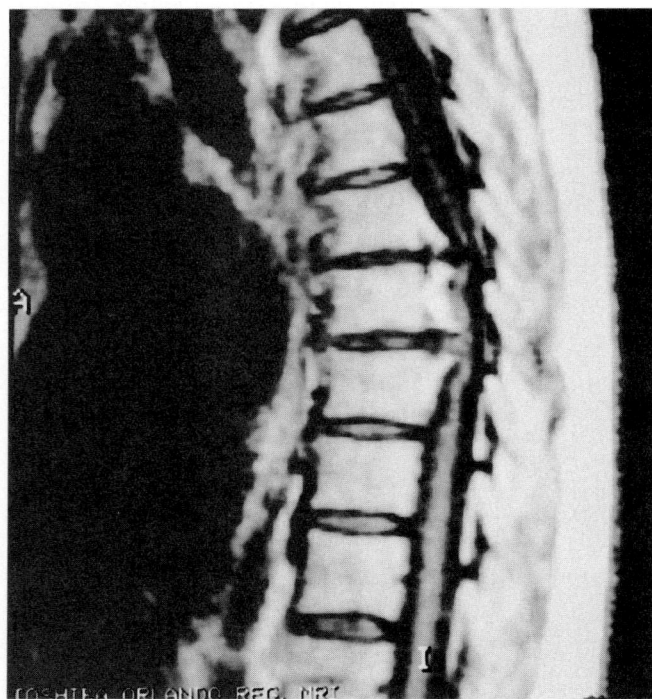

FIGURE 292–5. Sagittal T1-weighted magnetic resonance imaging sequence demonstrating large disk herniations at two adjacent levels, causing severe cord compression.

quence of an "edge effect" that occurs when two substances of different proton densities lie adjacent to each other. In this case, the "edge" occurs between the disk herniation and the adjacent cerebrospinal fluid, creating a distortion in the magnetic field that is especially noticeable on T2-weighted images. Enlarging the field of view and refocusing the magnetic field are techniques that can decrease this distortion, but they also result in some loss of detail in resolution. MRI of the thoracic spine should be used as a screening study for potential thoracic disk herniation and to rule out other pathology of the thoracic spine or spinal cord. We recommend performing a follow-up thoracic myelogram and postmyelogram CT to specifically identify the extent and level of thoracic disk herniation.[29, 33]

Owing to improved imaging technology, the identification of thoracic disk herniation has increased. Clinical experience and a detailed neurological examination, however, must be used to determine the clinical significance of radiographic findings. The incidence of asymptomatic thoracic disk herniations identified by myelogram and postmyelogram CT approximately equals the false-positive rate of MRI as reported in the radiology literature.[5] Awwad and colleagues reported a 13.5% false-positive rate when diagnosing thoracic disk herniation with postmyelogram CT.[5] Although these investigators attempted to identify radiographic criteria to differentiate asymptomatic from symptomatic thoracic disk herniations, they concluded that there was no reliable method. They found that spinal cord distortion and flattening could be present to a marked

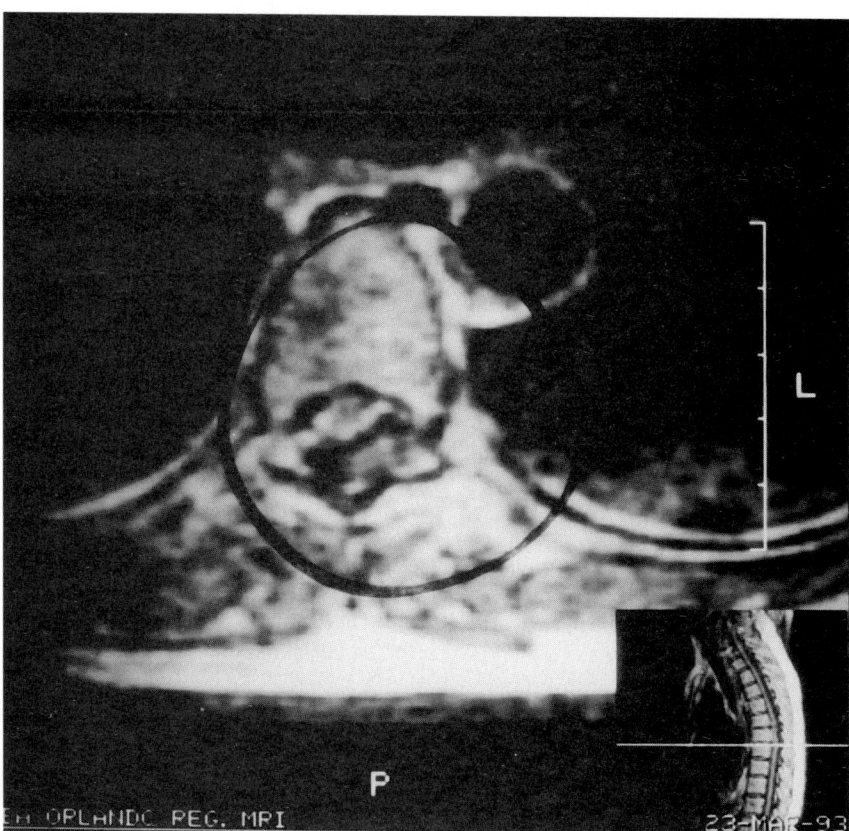

FIGURE 292–6. Axial magnetic resonance imaging scan of the same patient as in Figure 292–5, showing deviation of the spinal cord to the left.

degree even in asymptomatic patients. Spinal angiography is mentioned only to state that it has no role in the routine diagnosis and management of thoracic disk herniation.

MANAGEMENT

The treatment of thoracic disk herniation is dictated by the clinical presentation.[34] Myelopathy due to thoracic disk herniation is an absolute indication for surgery. Without surgery, these patients tend to follow a progressive course of neurological deterioration.[4, 22] Severe radicular pain may be disabling, and when it is refractory to a 3- to 6-month course of conservative therapy, surgery should be considered. Conservative measures may include restricted activity, nonsteroidal anti-inflammatory drugs, a hyperextension brace, oral steroids, and epidural steroids.[20, 29, 30, 35] With increased awareness of thoracic disk herniation and improved neurodiagnostic imaging, neurosurgeons are being called on to evaluate patients with thoracic disk herniation more frequently. If the clinical presentation is one of localized back pain and radiculopathy, plain films are recommended. If these films are normal, conservative management is the initial recommendation. If plain radiography is positive for intradiskal or intraspinal calcification, large osteophytes, or localized spondylosis, or if the patient presents with myelopathic findings on physical examination, MRI is also indi-

cated. Before surgery, a thoracic myelogram and postmyelogram CT should be performed to further delineate the relation of the disk to the spinal cord and nerve roots and to absolutely identify the level of disk protrusion. Figure 292–7 is a diagnostic and therapeutic algorithm we have found useful in the management of thoracic disk herniation.

Surgical approaches to thoracic disk disease are determined by numerous anatomic factors, including the bony rib cage, scapula and periscapular shoulder musculature, mediastinal contents, lungs, diaphragm, level and laterality of the disk herniation, and extent of calcification of the disk fragment. Specific approaches may be more or less appropriate for disk herniations at various levels of the thoracic spine because of the unique anatomy of each region. In general, the thoracic spine can be divided into three divisions based on anatomic and biomechanical characteristics: T1-4, or upper thoracic spine; T5-9, or midthoracic spine; and T10-12, or thoracolumbar spine. Thoracic disk herniations of the upper thoracic spine are rare and require unique surgical approaches because of the anatomy of the thoracic outlet and superior mediastinum.[20, 29, 36, 37] The midthoracic spine has the added stabilizing influences of the rib cage, and the thoracolumbar spine is a transition zone of vertebral configuration and facet orientation, predisposing it to failure under stress.[32, 38, 39] Independent of the specific division of the thoracic spine involved, other factors can also influence the choice of surgical approach. For example, the patient's

PRESENTATION

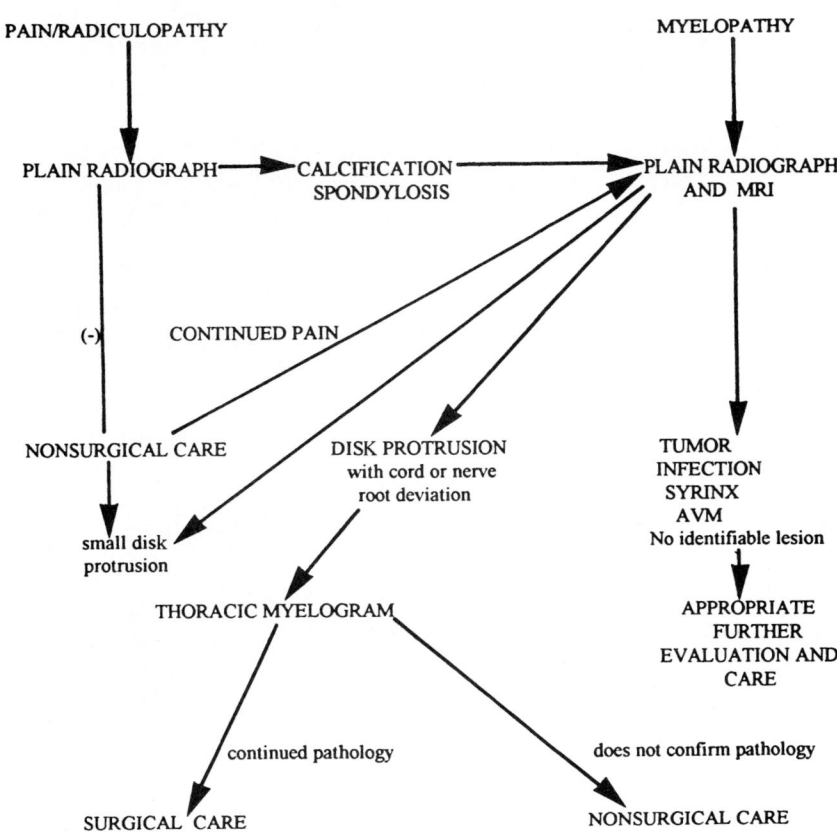

FIGURE 292–7. Diagnostic and therapeutic algorithm for thoracic disk herniation. (Modified from Dietze DD Jr, Fessler RG: Thoracic disc herniations. Neurosurg Clin N Am 4:75–90, 1993.)

age and general medical condition and the surgeon's experience with a particular approach are important factors that can influence outcome.[40] Thus, if the herniated disk is soft, the disk of origin is without significant degenerative change, and the disk is positioned lateral to the spinal cord, a posterior transpedicular approach may be considered.[3, 41, 42] The advantage of the posterior approaches is that they do not require transpleural or transmediastinal dissection, violation of the rib cage, or ligation of the neurovascular bundle. Moreover, they

TABLE 292–2 ■ **Advantages and Disadvantages of Surgical Approaches to Thoracic Disk Herniation**

SURGICAL APPROACH	ADVANTAGES	DISADVANTAGES
Laminectomy	Technical ease	Poor results Thecal sac retraction
Transpedicular	Technical ease Adequate for soft lateral disk	Limited exposure
Costotransversectomy	Posterolateral approach, extrapleural Visualization to midline Adequate for soft/hard lateral disk	Difficult to see across midline
Lateral extracavitary	Lateral approach, extrapleural Excellent exposure across midline Access to multiple levels Access for fusion Access for intradural exploration	Lung retraction (extrapleural)
Transthoracic	Anterolateral approach Excellent exposure across midline Access to multiple levels Access for fusion	Transpleural dissection Difficult intradural access

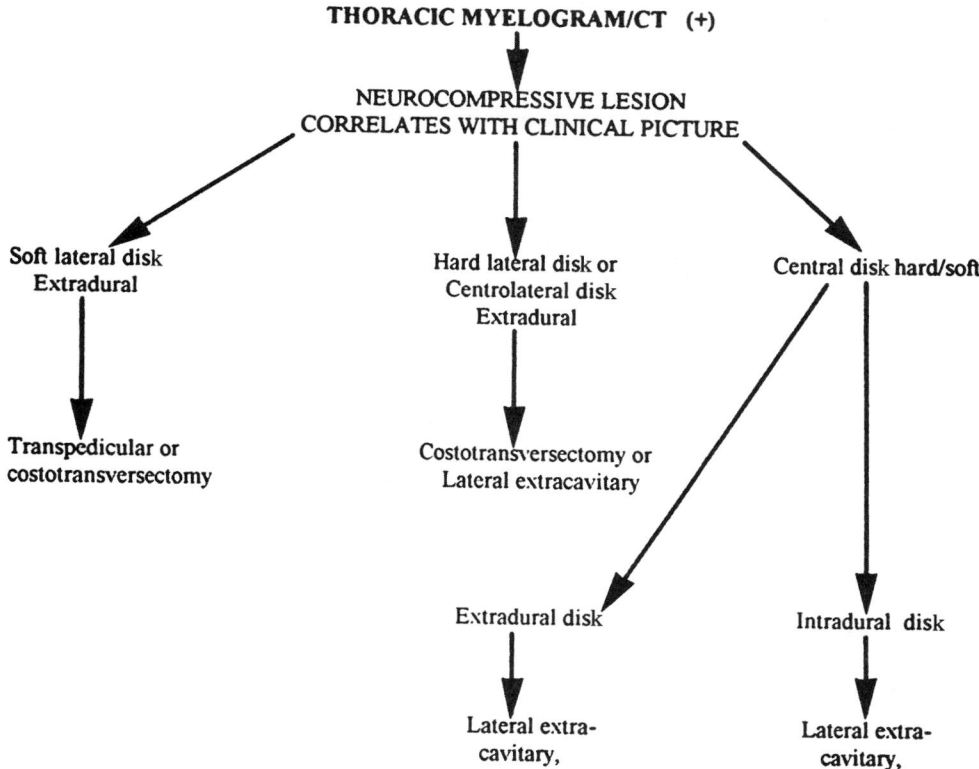

THORACIC MYELOGRAM/CT (+)

**NEUROCOMPRESSIVE LESION
CORRELATES WITH CLINICAL PICTURE**

Soft lateral disk
Extradural

Hard lateral disk or
Centrolateral disk
Extradural

Central disk hard/soft

Transpedicular or
costotransversectomy

Costotransversectomy or
Lateral extracavitary

Extradural disk

Intradural disk

Lateral extra-
cavitary,
transthoracic

Lateral extra-
cavitary,
transthoracic

FIGURE 292–8. Therapeutic algorithm for determining the best surgical approach for resection of a thoracic disk herniation. (Modified from Dietze DD Jr, Fessler RG: Thoracic disc herniations. Neurosurg Clin N Am 4:75–90, 1993.)

may be associated with less operative time and bleeding and are familiar to all neurosurgeons. When done from a posterior approach, a portion of the disk resection can be performed without direct visualization of the disk and ventral aspect of the dural sac. If a calcified herniated disk is positioned central or centrolateral with respect to the spinal cord and is associated with degenerative changes or has the potential for dural adhesions, posterior approaches have been associated with increased surgical risk and poorer outcomes compared with anterior or lateral approaches. In experienced hands, thoracoscopy has all the advantages of the anterior approaches and fewer complications than thoracotomy. Table 292–2 summarizes the advantages and disadvantages of the surgical approaches used in the treatment of thoracic disk herniation. Figure 292–8 presents a therapeutic algorithm for the choice of a surgical approach.

SURGICAL APPROACHES

Posterior Approaches: Laminectomy and Transpedicular

Laminectomy for removal of lesions positioned anterior to the spinal cord is associated with a 45% risk of either no benefit or neurological deterioration.[43–45] Therefore, laminectomy alone has no role in the treatment of thoracic disk disease. The transpedicular approach allows access anterolateral to the thecal sac

and involves removal of the facet joint and pedicle ipsilateral to the lesion. By drilling a small trough in the posterior vertebral body, the disk or osteophyte can be fractured away from the dura (Fig. 292–9). Patterson and Arbit,[41] Epstein,[46] and Le Roux and coworkers[47] reported success with this approach for resection of lateral disk herniations. The advantage of this approach is that it is less extensive than other approaches; the primary disadvantage is limited visibility of the ventral aspect of the spinal canal. Attempted decompression of a centrally herniated disk via this approach would be performed blindly. Fusion is generally not required with this approach because the integrity of the rib cage, the anterior longitudinal ligament, and the majority of the posterior ligaments are maintained. However, there is one report of a delayed compression fracture after a transpedicular approach.[48]

Anterior Approach: Transthoracic and Thoracoscopic

Transthoracic approaches are appropriate for lesions below T4 that are positioned central or centrolateral to the spinal cord. Perot and Munro[42] and Ransohoff and colleagues[49] simultaneously pioneered the use of the transthoracic approach for thoracic disk herniations. This approach provides direct access to the anterior and anterolateral spinal column and requires a transpleural dissection after removal of one or more ribs (including the rib head and neck) to expose the disk space and intervertebral foramen (Fig. 292–10).[38, 40] The

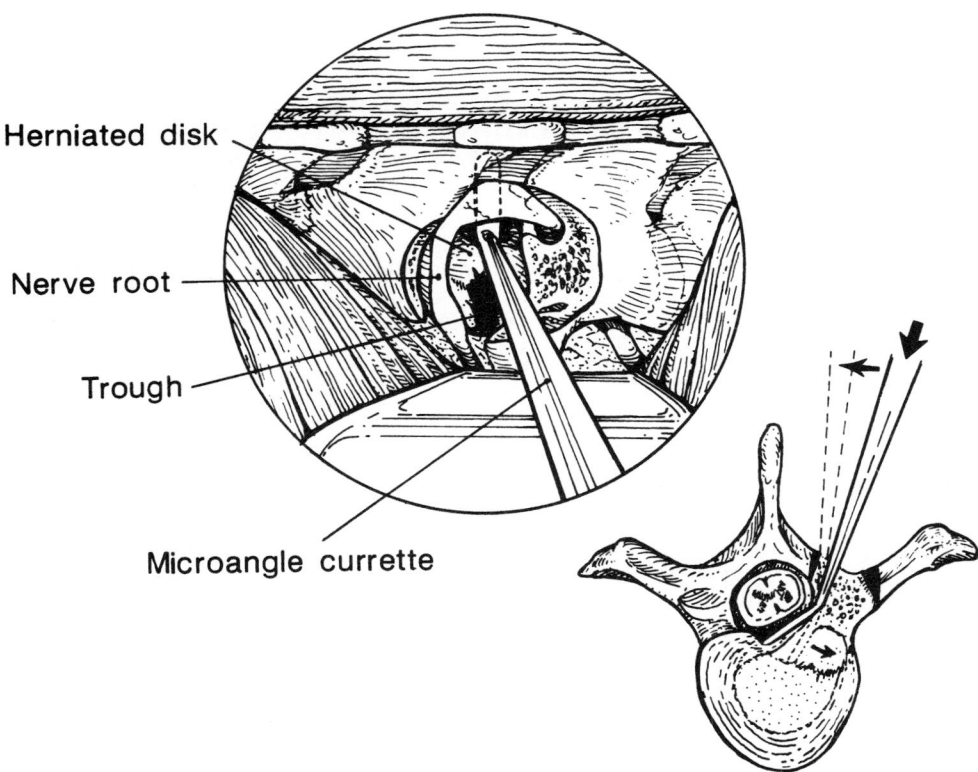

Herniated disk

Nerve root

Trough

Microangle currette

FIGURE 292–9. Transpedicular approach to thoracic disk resection. A complete laminectomy has been performed, with a subtotal unilateral facetectomy and total pediculectomy. The disk has been incised, and a partial diskectomy has been performed to allow evacuation of the herniated disk into the disk space.

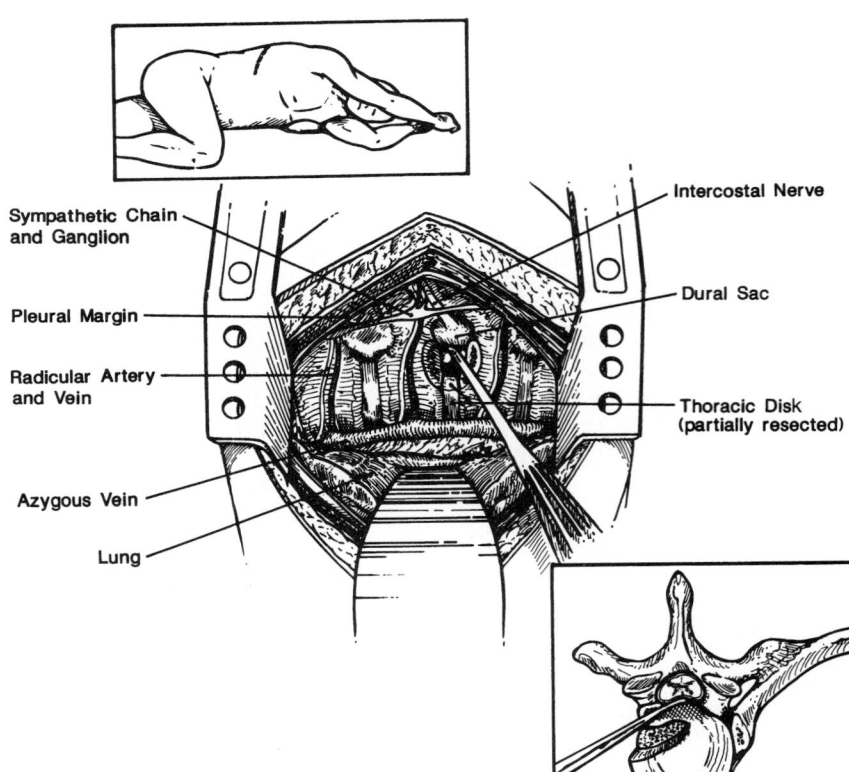

Sympathetic Chain and Ganglion

Pleural Margin

Radicular Artery and Vein

Azygous Vein

Lung

Intercostal Nerve

Dural Sac

Thoracic Disk (partially resected)

FIGURE 292–10. Transthoracic approach for thoracic disk resection. A transpleural dissection reveals the disk space. Resection of the rib head and adjacent vertebral end plates must also be performed. A partial diskectomy exposes the dural sac and nerve root. Insets demonstrate the positioning, incision, and axial view of the diskectomy.

transthoracic approach provides excellent exposure of anterior midline lesions, while preserving the pedicle and providing exposure for anterior interbody bone graft fusion. In addition, it provides exposure over multiple levels. There are several disadvantages to this approach. First, the neural elements are approached blindly during decompression. Because up to 18% of thoracic disk herniations dissect intradurally, this is a potentially significant limitation.[40, 50] Other disadvantages include (1) the diaphragm must be partially taken down at the thoracolumbar junction; (2) exposure of thoracic viscera is associated with several potential complications, including pneumonia, pleural effusion, and cerebrospinal fluid pleural fistula; (3) mediastinal structures are at risk for injury; (4) closed chest drainage is required postoperatively; and (5) patients are at risk for post-thoracotomy pain syndrome.

Fusion is generally not required with this approach after resection of extradural herniations.[51] Removal of one or two ribs, however, has been shown not to disrupt the biomechanical integrity of the spine–rib cage complex unless the sternum is also disrupted.[7, 52] Nevertheless, some surgeons perform anterior interbody fusions because of the removal of one or more rib insertions. The transthoracic approach preserves the integrity of the anterior longitudinal ligament, pedicles, facet complexes, and posterior ligaments. The posterior longitudinal ligament, posterior annulus fibrosus, and posterior vertebral body are disrupted. Thus, one could argue that there is increased potential for delayed kyphosis. Using Denis's three-column model for the thoracic spine, however, only the middle column is disrupted. With completely intact anterior and posterior columns, the thoracic spine should be stable. Anterior interbody fusion is usually required after resection of a herniated thoracic disk with intradural extension because of the extent of vertebral body resection required to adequately expose the dura. Transition of the facet complexes and pedicle orientation at the thoracolumbar junction increases susceptibility to translational and rotational forces; therefore, care should be taken to verify the integrity of the anterior and posterior columns preoperatively (e.g., recognition of advanced degenerative changes in the vertebral bodies and facet complexes, evidence of listhesis or kyphosis, dynamic translational movement). Failure to do so may lead to progressive postoperative instability.

Thoracoscopy was first performed on humans by Jacobeus and reported in 1910.[53] It was used to lyse tuberculous pleural adhesions in 1921.[54] This technology was improved with the addition of fiber-optics and optical lens systems. In the 1970s, a video camera was mounted to the endoscope.[55–58] This was a major advance, allowing the surgeon to maintain a sterile field without the need to look directly into the objective lens. In the 1990s, Rosenthal and associates performed the first thoracoscopic spine procedure—removal of a thoracic disk.[59–61] Surgical dissecting tools for use with the endoscope have also been developed specifically for neurosurgical applications.

For thoracoscopy, the patient is turned and prepared in the lateral decubitus position.[62–64] A double-lumen endotracheal tube is used for single lung ventilation. The patient must be secured to the table to allow for 30 to 40 degrees of rotation. This causes the atelectatic lung to fall away from the spine, with minimal need for retraction. Three or four small intercostal portals are placed to allow adequate visualization and assistance. The viewing portal should be directly lateral to the level of interest, as determined by fluoroscopy, and in the zone between the midaxillary and posterior axillary lines. The surgeon is positioned facing the patient's chest to allow the most appropriate angle of attack to the spine. The working portals are placed in the zone beween the midaxillary and anterior axillary lines.

After entering the chest, the level of interest is identified by counting the ribs from within the thoracic cavity. The pleura is incised at the level of the corresponding proximal rib, and the segmental vessels are identified and ligated. The proximal 2 cm of rib and pedicle are resected, and the lateral aspect of the dura is visualized. The rib should be saved in the event fusion is required. Early visualization of the dura is critical to performing the diskectomy safely. Next, a cavity must be created in the dorsal disk space. This allows instruments to approach the herniated disk without entering the already compromised spinal canal. If the disk is large, ossified, or intradural, a corpectomy can be performed to increase the working space. If the disk herniation is intradural, the dura is repaired with endoscopic sutures, dural graft, and fibrin glue after removal of the disk. A lumbar drain is placed. A chest tube is inserted and placed to water seal rather than the usual suction. Epidural hemostasis is obtained with the use of Gelfoam or bipolar cautery. If Surgicel is used, it should be limited to a single layer to prevent mass effect. Postoperatively, the chest tubes are removed when the output is less than 100 mL/day. In the absence of an obvious cerebrospinal fluid leak, lumbar drainage should be continued for a minimum of 72 hours.

Lateral Approach

Early lateral approaches to the thoracic spine were designed for the treatment of Pott's tuberculous disease of the spine.[65–67] Hulme reported good results using the costotransversectomy approach for thoracic disk herniation.[68] The lateral extracavitary and lateral parascapular extrapleural approaches are far-lateral approaches that maximize exposure of the anterolateral spinal column for metastatic, infectious, and traumatic pathology.[29, 38, 50] Maiman and coworkers[7] used the lateral extracavitary approach for thoracic disk herniation with good results and low morbidity. Their approach involved resection of approximately 8 cm of dorsal rib and rib head and ligation of the intercostal nerve approximately 3 cm distal to the dorsal root ganglion. The segmental neurovasculature was divided, and partial pediculectomies were performed to widen the intervertebral foramen. A posterior vertebral body trough was then created, into which calcified disk and osteophytes were fractured, decompressing the dura.

The advantage of this approach is direct visualization of neural elements before and during decompression. In addition, the "extrapleural" dissection eliminates the need for closed chest drainage and the need to take down the diaphragm at the thoracolumbar junction. If necessary, anterior interbody fusion and posterior spinal fusion and fixation with posterior instrumentation can be performed simultaneously. Multilevel disease can also be treated using this approach. The disadvantage is the potential intercostal neuralgia or anesthesia dolorsa from intercostal nerve resection. We have modified the lateral extracavitary approach to preserve the neurovascular bundle; minimize muscle, bone, and ligament disruption; and decrease blood loss, operative time, and hospital stay.

SURGICAL PROCEDURE

Positioning. Intubation is performed using a single-lumen endotracheal tube. A jet ventilator is used to allow for continuous ventilation with minimal lung excursion into the operative field. The patient is positioned prone on chest rolls on a radiolucent operating table. Intraoperative fluoroscopy is used to mark the appropriate levels and draw out the skin incision. A curved hockey-stick incision is made extending from two disk space levels above to two disk space levels below the pathologic level (generally about 6 inches long in the midline and curved for a length of about 4 inches).

Exposure of the Thoracic Cage and Removal of the Rib. The skin is incised down to the dorsal thoracolumbar fascia, and a musculocutaneous flap is reflected incorporating the trapezius and rhomboid muscles (if above T6) (Fig. 292–11*A*). The transverse processes and dorsal ribs are palpated, and intraoperative fluoroscopy is used to verify the appropriate rib for resection (i.e., the rib that articulates with the inferior vertebra of the disk level to be treated). The spinalis and longissimus muscles of the paraspinous musculature are subperiosteally dissected off the transverse processes and costotransverse articulations, and the iliocostalis muscles are dissected off the dorsal ribs. Muscular attachments to the laminae and spinous processes are left intact. The intercostal musculature and neurovasculature are dissected subperiosteally off the appropriate rib, and the costotransverse and costovertebral joints are disarticulated. The appropriate rib is removed, and the neurovascular bundles are dissected and preserved.

Exposure of the Anterolateral Thecal Sac and Lateral Vertebral Column. The intercostal nerve is traced to the intervertebral foramen, and a dorsal foraminectomy (involving partial facetectomy with preservation of the pedicles) allows exposure of the lateral thecal sac and dorsal root ganglion (see Fig. 292–11*B*). The epidural venous plexus is coagulated, and bleeding is controlled with Gelfoam. The posterior longitudinal ligament and vertebral bodies are identified.

Thecal Sac Decompression. The annulus fibrosus is opened laterally. The thoracic disk space is generally narrow and thus is widened by drilling the posterior end plates of the adjacent vertebral bodies. This creates room for curettage and allows the posterior vertebral osteophytes to be fractured away from the dura. The posterior longitudinal ligament is removed at the disk space to ensure complete thecal sac decompression and to evaluate for possible intradural extension.

Intradural Exploration and Spinal Fusion. If there is intradural extension, removal of the inferior vertebral transverse process and pedicle with a hemilaminectomy allows exposure of the lateral thecal sac from the posterior longitudinal ligament to the spinolaminar line dorsally. The dura is incised along the long axis of the spinal canal and flapped anteriorly by transverse incisions at each end (suture tags on the corners keep the dura stretched and retracted; see Fig. 292–11*C*). Microsurgical technique is used to remove the intradural pathology with minimal manipulation of the spinal cord. Primary dural closure is performed, and the wound is covered with Gelfoam. If dural resection was required, dural reconstruction is accomplished with thoracolumbar fascial autograft, allograft, or dural substitute. Fibrin glue may be used to seal the closure. If the pedicle is removed, an intertransverse rib graft is secured with wire across the operative defect for added stability.

Wound Closure and Postoperative Care. Before wound closure, the operative field is filled with saline and observed for an air leak. If a pleural tear is identified, a pediatric chest tube is placed through the operative field and brought out dorsolaterally behind the musculocutaneous flap. A layered wound closure is performed, and a Jackson-Pratt drain is placed deep in the operative field and brought out through a separate stab incision inferior to the musculocutaneous flap. The operative procedure takes 4 hours, and the average blood loss is 300 mL. The patient is observed in the intensive care or intermediate care unit for 8 to 12 hours and monitored for respiratory distress. The drain is removed on postoperative day 1. Mobilization in a clamshell orthosis begins on postoperative day 1. The average hospital stay is 5 days, and a clamshell orthosis is worn for 6 to 12 weeks if a fusion was required.

RESULTS

The results of operative treatment for thoracic disk herniation should be considered in the context of the indication for which the procedure was performed: myelopathy versus back or radicular pain. This rationale is based, in part, on the extensive nature of the surgical approaches, which can induce substantial pain themselves. Some reports indicate that back and radicular symptoms respond favorably to surgery in 94% of patients.[39, 40] In our experience, patients with back and radicular symptoms who failed conservative therapy experienced clinical relief of their symptoms only 67% of the time; complete resolution of back pain was even less frequent.[29] In various series, myelopathic symp-

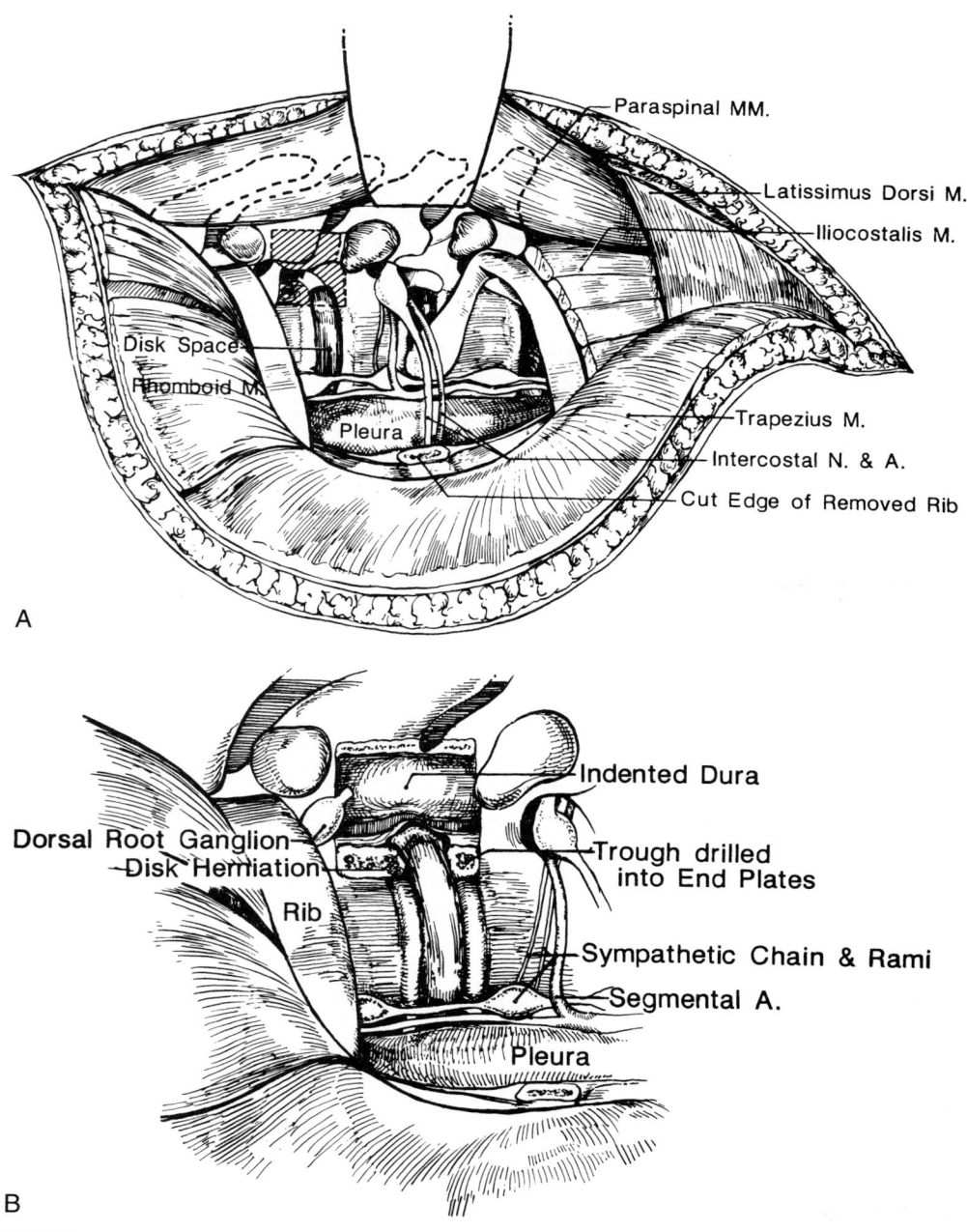

FIGURE 292–11. Steps of the modified lateral extracavitary approach to thoracic disk herniations. *A,* Operative view after reflection of the musculocutaneous flap, dissection and retraction of the paraspinous musculature, and removal of the selected rib. Identifiable are the pleura, sympathetic chain along the anterolateral vertebral body, intervertebral foramina, and dissected intercostal neurovascular bundle. Important concepts are as follows: (1) The neurovascular bundle is preserved; the segmental vasculature crosses over the lateral mid–vertebral body to reach the intervertebral foramen. (2) The dissected neurovascular bundle from the resected rib enters the intervertebral foramen at the level inferior to the pathologic process; the rib head articulates over the disk space of the interspace above (i.e., the sixth rib head articulates over the T5-6 disk space). (3) The paraspinous muscles need not be completely mobilized off the spinous processes; only the attachments to the lamina and transverse processes need be dissected to allow elevation of the muscle belly, exposing the facet complex of the pathologic level. The hatched box overlies the facet complex at the pathologic level, which is removed along with a trough in the posterior vertebral end plates to expose the anterolateral thecal sac. *B,* The operative field after removal of the facet complex and drilling of the troughs in the posterior vertebral end plates. Important concepts are as follows: (1) The facet complex is removed to allow identification of the thecal sac before approaching the pathology. (2) Drilling the troughs in the posterior vertebral end plates allows the disk protrusion to be fractured away from the thecal sac without manipulation of the thecal sac. (3) The lateral exposure gives excellent visualization across the midline without the added morbidity of a transpleural exposure. (There is a relative blind spot on the opposite anterolateral surface of the thecal sac.) (4) If the posterior longitudinal ligament (PLL) is not removed, an eroded disk herniation through the PLL can be missed.

Illustration contiunued on following page

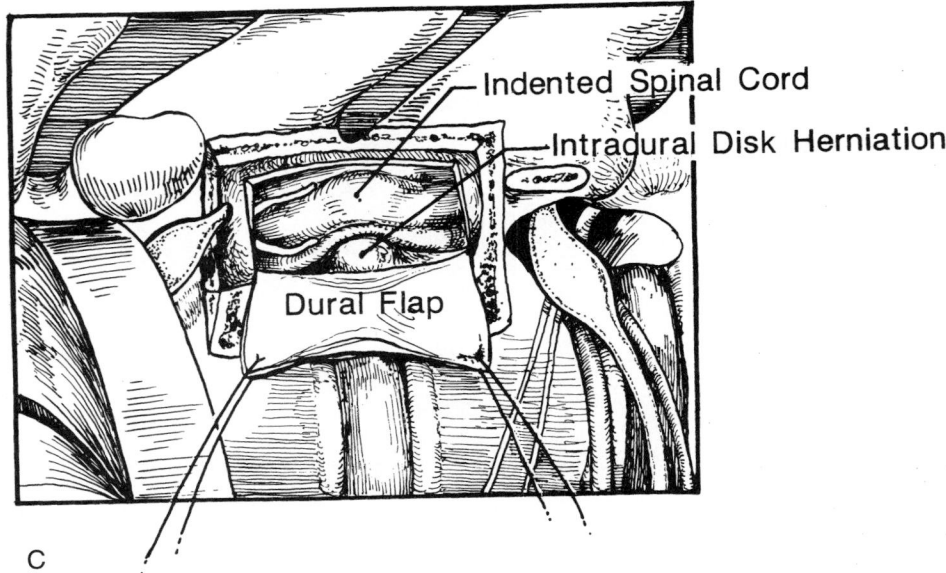

C

FIGURE 292–11. *Continued. C*, The operative field after a dural opening has been made to extract an intradural disk herniation. When intradural exploration is required, the inferior vertebral pedicle and transverse process are removed to enlarge the exposure of the thecal sac. The dura is opened along its posterolateral margin and flapped anteriorly by two vertical incisions at each end of the longitudinal opening. Excellent visualization of the anterior, lateral, and posterior subarachnoid spaces around the spinal cord is obtained. Microsurgical technique is used to excise adhesions to the spinal cord, and the disk material is fractured away from the spinal cord, minimizing manipulation of the spinal cord. The dura can be closed with suture; if there is a large dural defect from the disk erosion, reconstruction is performed and sealed with fibrin glue. (Modified from Dietze DD Jr, Fessler RG: Thoracic disc herniations. Neurosurg Clin N Am 4:75–90, 1993.)

toms showed clinical improvement in 71% to 97% of cases.[20, 21, 29, 43] A summary of the results in three recent surgical series is presented in Table 292–3. In experienced hands, the results of thoracoscopy are equal to those of open surgery, and the complications may be fewer.

COMPLICATIONS OF THORACIC DISK RESECTION

Among the numerous reports available in the literature, few provide adequate detail or sufficient numbers of patients for the assessment of surgical and postoperative complications. Seventeen reports that had at least some discussion of complications were summarized to determine morbidity and mortality rates associated with specific surgical approaches (Table 292–4). In general, before 1960, most procedures for the management of thoracic disk herniation used laminectomy. Since 1960, the transpedicular, costotransversectomy, lateral extracavitary, and transthoracic procedures have all been used. The majority of patients since 1960 have undergone lateral extracavitary or transthoracic approaches. In the early literature, little information on morbidity was available beyond reports of increased paresis, paralysis, or death. Mixter and Barr,[15] Hawk,[23] Mueller,[16] Love and Keifer,[2] Loque,[45] and Tovi and Strang[69] have all reported poor results using laminectomy. These series reported increased neurological deficits in 18% to 66% of cases and mortality ranging from 14% to 50%. Based on these poor results, the treatment of thoracic disk herniation with laminectomy was abandoned.

T A B L E 2 9 2 – 3 ■ **Results of Three Surgical Series**

RESULTS	STILLERMAN & WEISS[40]	MAIMAN ET AL[7]	FESSLER
No. of patients	51	23	17
Surgical approach	Transthoracic (3 lateral extracavitary)	Lateral extracavitary	Lateral extracavitary
Pain	33/35 (94%) improved or resolution	17/18 (94%) improved or resolution	10/15 (67%) improved or resolution
Myelopathy	7/9 (97%) improved	19/22 (86%) improved	5/7 (71%) improved
Bowel/bladder dysfunction	7/9 (78%)	6/10 (60%)	7/7 (100%)
Neurological deterioration	None	None	None

T A B L E 2 9 2 – 4 ■ **Morbidity and Mortality of Specific Surgical Approaches**

APPROACH	NO. OF PATIENTS	TOTAL MORBIDITY: NO. (%)	TOTAL MORTALITY: NO. (%)
Laminectomy	63	33 (59)	8 (13)
Transpedicular	11	1 (9)	0 (0)
Costotransversectomy	17	2 (12)	0 (0)
Lateral extracavitary	76	10 (12)	0 (0)
Transthoracic	88	10 (12)	0 (0)

With the lateral extracavitary, transthoracic, thoracoscopic, and transpedicular approaches, mortality has been virtually eliminated. Increased paresis or paralysis has become the exception, rather than the rule, in the surgical treatment of thoracic disk herniation. Having minimized these major complications, several authors in the past decade have evaluated the less devastating morbidities associated with surgical treatment of thoracic disk herniation. Maiman and coworkers,[7] Stillerman and Weiss,[40] Fessler and coauthors,[20, 50, 70] Rosenthal and colleagues,[59–61] and Dickman and associates[63] reported no mortalities in a total of 180 cases using the lateral extracavitary, transthoracic, or thoracoscopic approach. Maiman and coworkers[7] and Fessler and colleagues[20, 50, 70] reported no increase in neurological deficits using the lateral extracavitary approach in 40 patients. Stillerman and Weiss[40] reported increased neurological deficits in 2% of 51 patients undergoing the transthoracic approach. Rosenthal's and Dickman's groups[59–61, 63] reported no permanent increase in neurological deficits in 55 patients. Other complications included infections, either deep or superficial, reported in 2% to 12% of cases[7, 20, 21, 29, 71]; pleural tears, reported as a complication in 13% of cases during lateral extracavitary approaches by Maiman's group[7] (this complication is not reported as a morbidity in the transthoracic or thoracoscopic approaches because transpleural dissection is a component of these approaches); and a 4% incidence of anesthesia dolorosa.[7, 20, 50, 70] A summary of these complications can be found in Table 292–5.

SUMMARY

Surgeons should maintain a high level of suspicion for thoracic disk herniation in patients with unexplained localized back pain or sensorimotor deficits. These patients should have MRI as a screening test, and if a disk is identified, confirmatory myelogram and postmyelogram CT should be performed. Although the natural history is anecdotal, there appears to be a tendency for myelopathic symptoms and signs to be progressive, warranting surgical intervention. For radicular dysfunction or localized back pain, a conservative therapeutic plan is recommended. If intractable radicular pain is demonstrated and the diagnosis is certain, surgical intervention should be considered.

Appropriate surgical decision making depends on an understanding of the variety of surgical options available, their advantages and disadvantages, and spinal biomechanics. When selecting an approach, consideration must be given to the specific anatomic location of the disk herniation, the patient's overall health, and the surgeon's experience. To ensure safe and effective thoracic disk surgery, the surgeon must minimize spinal cord manipulation, preserve the neurovascular supply whenever possible, minimize manipulation of the intercostal nerve, and preserve bony and ligamentous attachments.

REFERENCES

1. Baker HL, Love JG, Uihlein A: Roentgenologic features of protruded thoracic and intervertebral discs. Radiology 84:1059–1065, 1965.
2. Love JG, Kiefer EJ: Root pain and paraplegia due to protrusions of thoracic intervertebral discs. J Neurosurg 7:62–69, 1950.
3. Carson J, Grumpert J, Jefferson A: Diagnosis and treatment of thoracic intervertebral disc protrusions. J Neurol Neurosurg Psychiatry 34:68–77, 1971.
4. Arce CA, Dohrmann GJ: Thoracic disc herniation: Improved diagnosis with computed tomographic scanning and a review of the literature. Surg Neurol 23:356–361, 1985.
5. Awwad EE, Martin DS, Smith KR, Baker BK: Asymptomatic versus symptomatic herniated thoracic discs: Their frequency and characteristics as detected by computed tomography after myelography. Neurosurgery 28:180–186, 1991.
6. Benson MKD, Bynes DP: The clinical syndromes and surgical treatment of thoracic intervertebral disc prolapse. J Bone Joint Surg Br 57:471–477, 1975.

T A B L E 2 9 2 – 5 ■ **Complications of Surgical Treatment of Thoracic Disk Herniation**

COMPLICATION	STILLERMAN & WEISS[40]	MAIMAN ET AL[7]	FESSLER[50]
Mortality	0/51	0/23	0/17
Superficial wound infection	1/51 (2%)	2/23 (8.6%)	0/17
Urinary tract infection	0/51	1/23 (4%)	0/17
Atelectasis	2/51 (4%)	2/23 (8.6%)	
Transient paraparesis (48 hr)	1/51 (2%)	0/23	0/17
Postoperative seizure	1/51 (2%)	0/23	0/17
Anesthesia dolorosa	0/51	1/23 (4%) (resolved after dorsal root ganglionectomy)	1/17 (6%) (incomplete resolution)
Compression fracture	1/51 (2%)	0/23	0/17
Pleural tears		3/23 (13%)	0/17
Pneumonia			1/17 (6%)

7. Maiman DJ, Larson SJ, Luck E, El-Ghatit A: Lateral extracavitary approach to the spine for thoracic disc herniation: Report of 23 cases. Neurosurgery 14:178–182, 1984.
8. Sekhar LN, Jannetta PJ: Thoracic disc herniation: Operative approaches and results. Neurosurgery 12:303–305, 1983.
9. Key CA: On paraplegia depending on disease of the ligaments of the spine. Guys Hosp Rep 3:17–34, 1838.
10. Bucy PC: Chondroma of intervertebral disk. JAMA 94:1552–1554, 1930.
11. Elsberg CA: Extradural spinal tumors—primary, secondary metastatic. Surg Gynecol Obstet 46:1–20, 1928.
12. Stookey B: Compression of the spinal cord due to ventral extradural cervical chondromas. Arch Neurol Psychiatry 20:275–291, 1928.
13. Middleton GS, Teacher JH: Injury of the spinal cord due to rupture of an intervertebral disc during muscular effort. Glasgow Med J 1:16, 1911.
14. Dandy WE: Loose cartilage from intervertebral disk simulating tumor of the spinal cord. Arch Surg 19:660–672, 1929.
15. Mixter WJ, Barr JS: Rupture of the intervertebral disc with involvement of the spinal canal. N Engl Surg Soc 211:210–215, 1934.
16. Muller R: Protrusion of thoracic intervertebral discs with compression of the spinal cord. Acta Med Scand 139:99–104, 1951.
17. Abbot KH, Retter RH: Protrusions of thoracic intervertebral disks. Neurology 6:1–10, 1956.
18. Arseni C, Marisius M: Thoracic disc hernia (clinical-therapeutic considerations on 42 operated cases). Neurol Psychiatr Neurochir 15:331–338, 1970.
19. Arseni C, Nash F: Thoracic intervertebral disc protrusion: A clinical study. J Neurosurg 17:418–430, 1960.
20. Fessler RG, Dietze DD, MacMillan M, et al: Lateral parascapular extrapleural approach to the upper thoracic spine. J Neurosurg 75:349–355, 1991.
21. Otani K, Yoshida M, Fujii E: Thoracic disc herniation: Surgical treatment in 23 patients. Spine 13:1262–1267, 1988.
22. Arce CA, Dohrmann GJ: Herniated thoracic disks. Neurol Clin 3:383–392, 1985.
23. Hawk WA: Spinal compression caused by ecchondrosis of the intervertebral fibrocartilage: With a review of the recent literature. Brain 59:204–224, 1936.
24. Gelch MM: Herniated thoracic disc at T1-2 level associated with Horners syndrome: Case report. J Neurosurg 48:128, 1978.
25. Hann EC: Experience with ruptured T1-T2 discs. J Indiana State Med Assoc 73:598–599, 1980.
26. Kumar R, Nuckley T: First thoracic disc protrusion. Spine 11:449, 1986.
27. Lloyd TV, Johnson JC, Paul DJ: Horner's syndrome secondary to herniated disc at T1-T2. Am J Radiol 134:184–185, 1980.
28. Chowdhary UM: Intradural thoracic disc protrusions. Spine 12:718–719, 1987.
29. Dietze DD, Fessler RG: Thoracic disc herniations. Neurosurg Clin N Am 4:75–90, 1993.
30. Hamilton MG, Thomas HG: Intradural herniation of a thoracic disc presenting as flaccid paraplegia: Case report. Neurosurgery 27:482–484, 1990.
31. Williams MP, Cherryman GR, Husband JE: Significance of thoracic disc herniation demonstrated by MR imaging. J Comput Assist Tomogr 13:211, 1989.
32. Williams MP, Cherryman GR: Thoracic disk herniation: MR imaging. Radiology 167:874–875, 1988.
33. Blumenkopf B: Thoracic intervertebral disc herniations: Diagnostic value of magnetic resonance imaging. Neurosurgery 23:36–40, 1988.
34. Wood KB, Blair JM, Aepple DM, et al: The natural history of asymptomatic thoracic disc herniations. Spine 22:525–530, 1997.
35. Ogilivie JW: Thoracic disc herniation. In Bridwell KH, DeWold RL (eds): Textbook of Spinal Surgery. Philadelphia, JB Lippincott, 1991, pp 711–718.
36. Nanson EM: The anterior approach to upper dorsal sympathectomy. Surg Gynecol Obstet 104:118–120, 1957.
37. Sundaresan N, Shah J, Foley KM, Rosen G: An anterior surgical approach to the upper thoracic vertebrae. J Neurosurg 61:686–690, 1984.

38. Larson SJ, Holst RA, Hemmy DC, Sances A: Lateral extracavitary approach to traumatic lesions of the thoracic and lumbar spine. J Neurosurg 45:628–637, 1976.
39. Maiman DJ, Pintar FA: Anatomy and clinical biomechanics of the thoracic spine. Clin Neurosurg 38:296–324, 1991.
40. Stillerman CB, Weiss MH: Management of thoracic disc disease. Clin Neurosurg 38:325–352, 1991.
41. Patterson RH, Arbit E: A surgical approach through the pedicle to protruded thoracic discs. J Neurosurg 48:768–772, 1978.
42. Perot PL, Munro DD: Transthoracic removal of midline thoracic disc protrusions causing spinal cord compression. J Neurosurg 31:452–458, 1969.
43. Bennett MH, McCallum JE: Experimental decompression of spinal cord. Surg Neurol 8:63–67, 1977.
44. Doppman JL, Girton M: Angiographic study of the effect of laminectomy in the presence of acute anterior epidural masses. J Neurosurg 45:195–202, 1976.
45. Loque V: Thoracic intervertebral disc prolapse with spinal cord compression. J Neurol Neurosurg Psychiatry 15:227–241, 1952.
46. Epstein JA: Commentary on Sekhar LN, Jannetta PA: Thoracic disc herniation: Operative approaches and results. Neurosurgery 12:305, 1983.
47. Le Roux PD, Haglund MM, Harris AB: Thoracic disc disease: Experience with the transpedicular approach in twenty consecutive patients. Neurosurgery 33:58–66, 1993.
48. Singounas EG, Karvounis P: Thoracic disc protrusion. Acta Neurochir (Wien) 49:245–254, 1979.
49. Ransohoff J, Spencer F, Siew F: Transthoracic removal of thoracic disc: Report of three cases. J Neurosurg 31:459–461, 1969.
50. Fessler RG, Sturgill M: Review: Complications of surgery for thoracic disc disease. Surg Neurol 49:609–618, 1998.
51. Broc GG, Crawford NR, Sonntag VKH, et al: Biomechanical effects of transthoracic microdiscectomy. Spine 22:605–612, 1997.
52. Patrick L, Kroell C, Mertz H: Forces on the human body in simulated crashes. In Proceedings of the Ninth Annual Stapp Car Crash Conference, Society of Automotive Engineers, 1965.
53. Jacobeus HC: Possibility of the use of the cystoscope for investigation of serious cavities. Munich Med Wochenschr 57:2090–2092, 1910.
54. Jacobeus HC: The practical importance of thoracoscopy in surgery of the chest. Surg Gynecol Obstet 32:493–500, 1921.
55. Das K, Rothberg M: Thoracoscopic surgery: Historical perspectives. Neurosurg Focus 9:1–3, 2000.
56. Horovitz MB, Moossy JJ, Julian T, et al: Thoracic discectomy using video assisted thoracoscopy. Spine 19:1082–1086, 1994.
57. Regan JJ, Mack MJ, Picetti GD III: A technical report on video-assisted thoracoscopy in thoracic spinal surgery: Preliminary description. Spine 20:831–837, 1995.
58. Rosenthal DJ, Dickman CA: The history of thoracoscopic spine surgery. In Dickman CA, Rosenthal DJ, Perin NI (eds): Thoracoscopic Spine Surgery. New York, Thieme, 1999, pp 1–5.
59. Rosenthal DJ, Dickman CA: Thoracoscopic microsurgical excision of herniated thoracic discs. J Neurosurg 89:224–235, 1998.
60. Rosenthal D, Dickman C, Lornez R, et al: Thoracic disc herniation: Early results after surgical treatment using microsurgical endoscopy [abstract]. J Neurosurg 84:334A, 1996.
61. Rosenthal D, Rosenthal R, de Simone A: Removal of a protruded thoracic disc using microsurgical endoscopy: A new technique. Spine 19:1087–1091, 1994.
62. Dickman CA, Rosenthal DJ: Thoracoscopic access strategies: Portal placement techniques and portal selection. In Dickman CA, Rosenthal DJ, Perin NI (eds): Thoracoscopic Spine Surgery. New York, Thieme, 1999, pp 107–124.
63. Dickman CA, Rosenthal DJ, Perin NI: Thoracoscopic microsurgical discectomy. In Dickman CA, Rosenthal DJ, Perin NI (eds): Thoracoscopic Spine Surgery. New York, Thieme, 1999, pp 221–244.
64. Rosenthal DJ, Dickman CA: Operating room setup and patient positioning. In Dickman CA, Rosenthal DJ, Perin NI (eds): Thoracoscopic Spine Surgery. New York, Thieme, 1999, pp 95–106.
65. Alexander GL: Neurological complications of spinal tuberculosis. Proc R Soc Med 39:730–734, 1946.
66. Capener N: The evolution of lateral rachotomy. J Bone Joint Surg 36:173–179, 1954.
67. Menard V: Cause de la paraplegie dans la maladie de Patt, son

traiement chirurgical par l'ouverutre direct du foyer tuberculeaux des vertebras. Rev Orthop 5:47–64, 1984.

68. Hulme A: The surgical approach to thoracic intervertebral disc protrusions. J Neurol Neurosurg Psychiatry 23:133–137, 1960.

69. Tovi D, Strang RR: Thoracic intervertebral disc protrusions. Acta Chir Scand 267:3–41, 1960.

70. Fessler RG, Dietze DD: Lateral parascapular approach to the upper thoracic spine. Perspect Neurol Surg 3:85–105, 1992.

71. McAfee PC, Regan JR, Zdeblick T, et al: The incidence of complications in endoscopic anterior thoracolumbar spinal reconstructive surgery: A prospective multicenter study comprising the first 100 consecutive cases. Spine 20:1624–1632, 1995.

Treatment of Disk Disease of the Lumbar Spine

RUSSELL W. HARDY, JR. ■ PERRY A. BALL

HISTORY

The symptoms of sciatica, pain beginning in the back and radiating into the buttock and leg, were mentioned in ancient Greek and Roman texts but were often grouped with pain originating from the hip joint. In 1764, Cotugno clearly associated the symptoms with the sciatic nerve. He believed that the condition was due to irritation of the nerve by "acrid humours" derived from the blood.[1]

The intervertebral disk was described by Vesalius in 1555, and in 1858, Luschka observed at autopsy the degenerative processes of the disk. The connection between the disk and the syndrome of sciatica, however, remained elusive. In the first part of the 20th century "enchondromas" were noted in the lumbar spine but were thought to be of neoplastic origin. In 1929, Dandy described two cases of cauda equina syndrome that he thought were due to material derived from the intervertebral disk.[2] The breakthrough in establishing the association between the intervertebral disk and the syndrome of sciatica came in 1934, when Mixter and Barr described 34 patients whose symptoms they believed were caused by degenerative changes in the disk that were amenable to surgical treatment.[3] The idea was quite controversial at the time,[4] but lumbar disk excision is now a commonly performed procedure. Refinements have occurred in diagnosis, imaging, and surgical technique; however, some uncertainties remain in patient selection and outcome.

ANATOMY

Each lumbar vertebra consists of a vertebral body and a neural arch. The neural arch consists of two pedicles, the transverse processes, the superior and inferior articular facets, the laminae, and the spinous process. Each vertebra is attached to its neighbors by the intervertebral disk, the facet joints, and the spinal ligaments.

The strongest of these ligaments, the anterior longitudinal ligament, attaches to the anterior surface of the vertebral bodies and serves to resist extension. The

posterior longitudinal ligament runs along the posterior aspect of the vertebral bodies, but it is attached primarily to the disks. The fibers of this ligament are thickest in the midline and thin out laterally (Fig. 293–1). The ligamenta flava are attached to the undersurface of adjacent laminae; they are thinnest in the midline and widen laterally. The intertransverse ligament joins the transverse processes, and the interspinous ligament connects the spinous processes.

The facet joints are synovia-lined joints composed of the articular processes of adjacent vertebrae; they are surrounded by the capsular ligaments. These joints bear a significant amount of weight only when the spine is in extension.

The intervertebral disk also acts as a joint between adjacent vertebrae and bears the axial load of upright posture. The disk consists of three parts: (1) the cartilaginous end plate, a structure covering the bone of adjacent vertebrae and acting as a barrier between the nucleus pulposus and the adjacent vertebral bodies; (2) the nucleus pulposus, the semigelatinous center of the

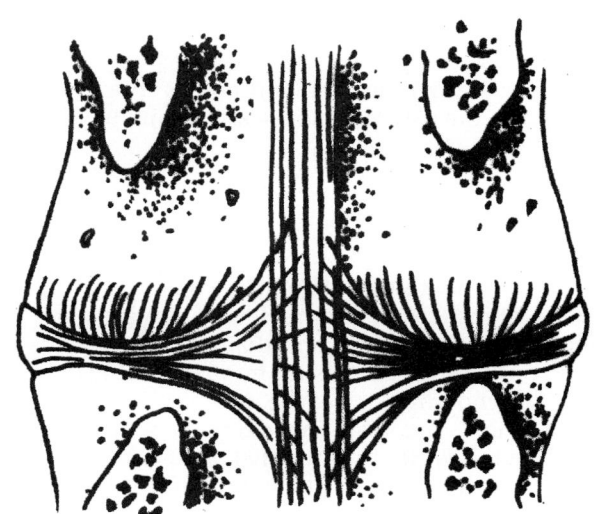

FIGURE 293–1. The fibers of the posterior longitudinal ligament, showing the thickest portion in the midline.

disk that serves as a physiologic shock absorber; and (3) the annulus fibrosus, a circular fibrous structure composed largely of collagen that restrains the lateral forces produced by the compressed nucleus. The disk is able to support weight because it contains a variety of proteoglycans, which results in a substantial osmotic gradient between the disk and the plasma. The resulting force favoring the flow of water into the disk is opposed by the compressive force of upright posture. These two opposing forces reach a balance point based on position, so that water flows into the disk in the supine position and is forced out in the upright position.

The spinal canal is formed by the neural arch dorsally and the vertebral bodies and disks ventrally. In most individuals, the spinal cord ends at the lower end of L1; the cauda equina, composed of motor and sensory nerve roots, occupies the dural sac below that level. Nerve roots leave the canal at each level of the lumbar spine. Each root leaves the dural sac, crosses the disk space, and enters the lateral recess. This space is formed by the posterior aspect of the vertebral body, adjacent disk, medial wall of the pedicle, and superior articular facet. The root then passes around the pedicle and into the neural foramen, where it leaves the spine.

Each spinal segment is innervated by the recurrent nerve of Luschka, which arises from the posterior ramus of each nerve root and supplies sensory branches to the dura, the posterior longitudinal ligament, and the fibers of the annulus fibrosus. No pain fibers are present within the nucleus pulposus.

The arterial supply to the disks and vertebrae comes from the lumbar arteries, which arise from the aorta. These vessels supply each vertebra in a segmental fashion in which radicular branches enter the dura with each nerve root. A major radicular branch, the artery of Adamkiewicz, supplies the spinal cord and may enter as low as the L3 nerve root. The disk itself is avascular but contains chondrocytes, which are mesenchymal cells that produce and maintain the collagen and proteoglycans of the disk. In adults, these cells derive nutrients through diffusion from the plasma. The venous drainage is derived from the internal venous plexus located on the floor of the canal. The plexus also drains the vertebral bodies in a segmental fashion into the external plexus and ultimately into the vena cava.

PATHOPHYSIOLOGY

The process of disk degeneration occurs in both the annulus fibrosus and the nucleus pulposus. The mechanical strength of the annulus decreases with age, which results in an increasing frequency of tears in the fibers. The chondrocytes of the disk also produce fewer glycoproteins. The resulting decrease in the osmotic force drawing water into the disk results in a decrease in both the total water content of the disk and the ability of the disk to expand.

These degenerative changes progress with increasing age; however, strikingly, the incidence of disk her-

niation does not: it peaks in the fourth decade. The explanation for this has been delineated by Kramer[5] and is depicted in Figure 293–2. The disk's ability to expand appears to be important in the development of disk herniation. At younger ages, the disk has a substantial ability to expand, but the annulus is strong enough to contain these forces. In the sixth and seventh decades, despite a weakened annulus, the disk has lost much of its ability to expand, and disk herniations are less common. It is in the third through the fifth decades, when the disk still has the ability to expand and the annulus is becoming weaker, that disk herniations are most common.

The most common direction for lumbar disk herniations to occur is posterolateral, which corresponds to the region of the spinal canal between the midline and the neural foramen (Fig. 293–3). As mentioned previously, this is the region where the fibers of the posterior longitudinal ligament are thin and thus less effective in constraining the disk. Disk herniations that occur at or lateral to the foramen were not clearly

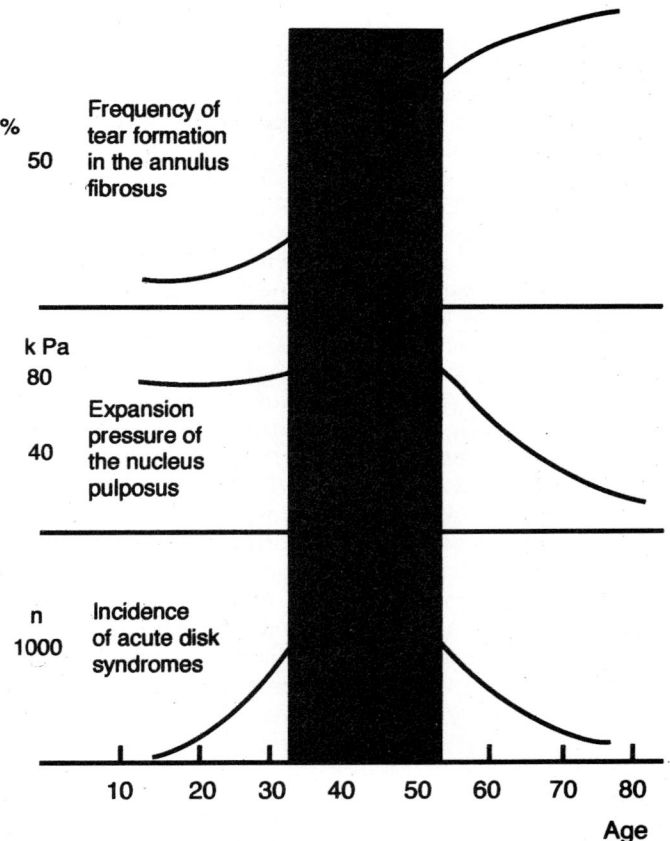

FIGURE 293–2. Explanation for the age incidence of lumbar disk herniations. There is an increase in the number or annular tears with increasing age; however, the disk's ability to expand also decreases with age. Disk herniations are uncommon early in life because of the ability of the annulus to constrain the disk. In later life, although the ability of the annulus to constrain the disk is diminished, the ability of the disk to expand has decreased, and disk herniations again become less common. (Adapted from Kramer J: Intervertebral Disc Diseases: Causes, Diagnosis, Treatment and Prophylaxis, 2nd ed. New York, Thieme Medical, 1990.)

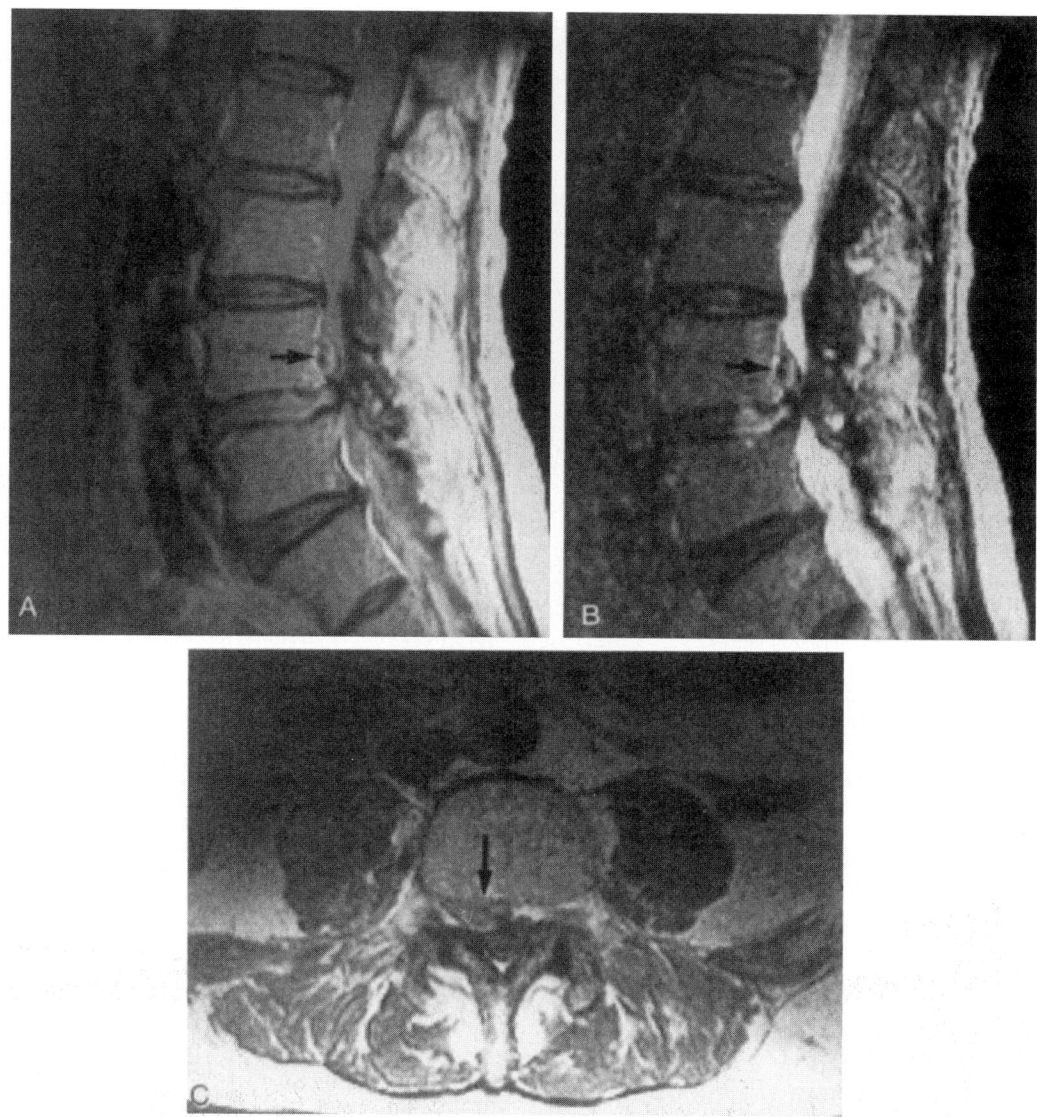

FIGURE 293–3. Sagittal spin-density *(A)*, sagittal T2-weighted *(B)*, and axial spin-density *(C)* magnetic resonance images demonstrate an extruded disk fragment *(arrow)*.

described until 1974,[6] because they often were not visualized by myelography. With modern imaging techniques, it has been recognized that they constitute about 10% of lumbar disk herniations.[7, 8] A number of terms (extraforaminal, extreme lateral, far lateral) have been used to refer to these herniations; far lateral is probably the most commonly used term (Fig. 293–4). Central disk herniations are rare but important, because they are usually the cause of cauda equina syndrome (Fig. 293–5).

A posterolateral disk herniation usually affects the nerve root exiting under the pedicle of the lower vertebral body. For instance, a disk herniation between the L4 and L5 vertebral bodies most commonly affects the L5 root. However, a lateral disk herniation often affects the nerve root exiting under the pedicle of the upper vertebral body. This is illustrated in Figure 293–6.

The pathophysiology of the radicular pain of sciatica

has been the subject of considerable investigation but is incompletely understood. Certainly, disk herniation that results in sciatica involves some degree of mechanical pressure on the nerve root. Experimental studies using animal models have demonstrated edema, alteration in nutrient transport, and inhibition of axonal conduction with mechanical pressure on the nerve root.[9] Although it is likely that mechanical compression plays a role, there are reasons to believe that it is not the sole factor in the generation of sciatica. Nerve compression is not always accompanied by sciatica; imaging studies of the lumbar spine in asymptomatic subjects typically show that about 20% have disk herniation.[10] Further, sciatica can resolve spontaneously, and when imaging is repeated after the resolution of symptoms, the degree of nerve root compression is often unchanged.[11]

Investigators have examined the role of inflamma-

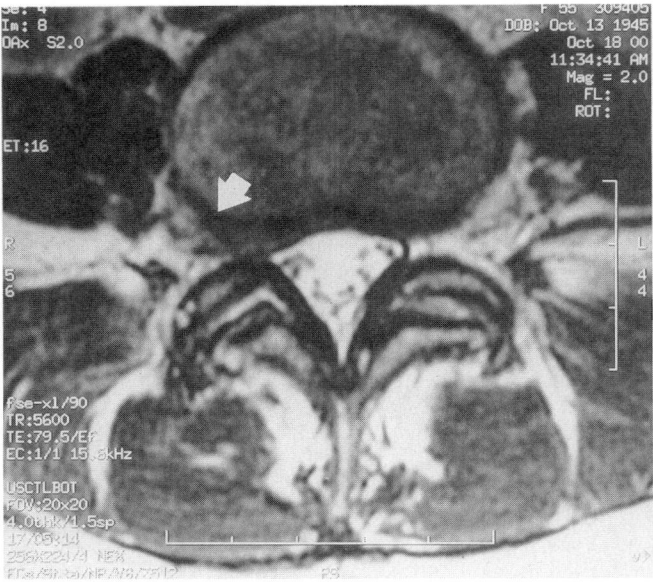

FIGURE 293–4. Arrow points to far-lateral disk herniation.

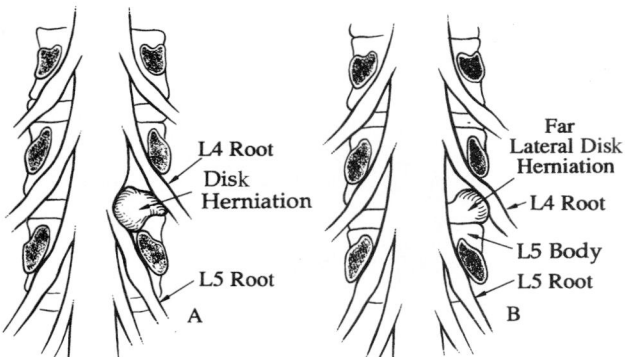

FIGURE 293–6. The lumbar spine with the dorsal elements removed. Note the relationship of the nerve roots to the disk spaces. In most cases, a herniated disk compresses the highest numbered root as it crosses the disk space rather than the root that exists in the corresponding foramen. Thus, an L4 disk protrusion usually causes L5 radiculopathy. Far-lateral disk ruptures or fragments *(A)* that migrate superiorly *(B)* may compress the root corresponding to the number of the space (in this illustration, a far-lateral L4 disk herniation would cause an L4 radiculopathy). Rarely, a disk fragment that migrates distally might compress a more distal nerve root instead of, or in addition to, the expected root. In this instance, a large distal fragment might cause L5 and S1 root signs.

tion in the generation of sciatica. Some studies have found evidence of inflammatory cells in disk specimens removed at surgery. Phospholipase A_2, an inflammatory mediator involved in the liberation of arachidonic acid and leukotrienes, has also been found in surgically resected disk specimens.[12] Another line of investigation has demonstrated that the experimental application of nucleus pulposus without compression to nerve roots results in alterations in blood flow and nerve conduction velocity.[13, 14]

CLINICAL PRESENTATION

Symptoms

The initial symptom of a herniated lumbar disk is usually back pain. There may be a history of recent

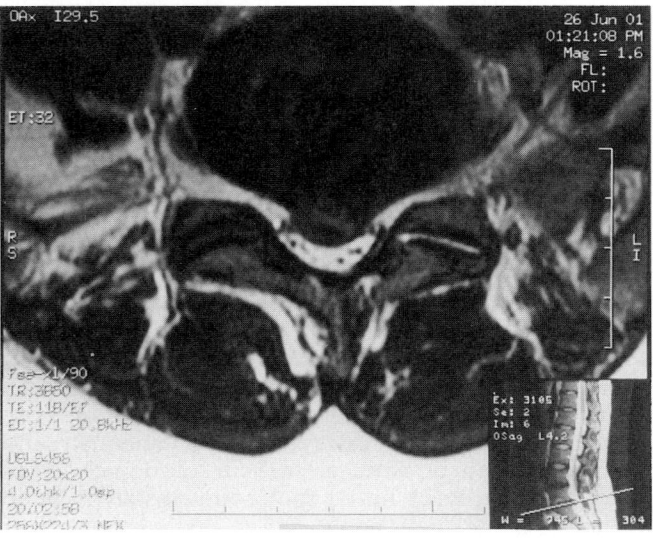

FIGURE 293–5. Central disk herniation.

trauma, but frequently the pain begins insidiously. This is often followed days to weeks later by radiation of pain into the leg, numbness, and paresthesias. The back pain often improves as the leg pain becomes more prominent. The pain may be aggravated by sitting, standing, and walking, as well as by coughing, sneezing, or straining. The patient is usually able to trace the distribution of the pain along the dermatome of the affected nerve root (Fig. 293–7). For an L4 radiculopathy, this extends down the anterior thigh, anterior shin, and medial ankle. An L5 radiculopathy characteristically radiates from the posterior hip along the posterolateral thigh and leg, with numbness of the great toe. The distribution of S1 symptoms is usually in the posterior thigh and calf, with numbness of the lateral surface of the foot.

A midline disk herniation may produce back pain and vague leg pain that radiates from side to side. A large central protrusion can result in cauda equina syndrome, characterized by perineal numbness, loss of bladder and bowel control, and some degree of motor weakness in the legs.

Differential Diagnosis

Numerous conditions can cause pain and weakness that mimic radiculopathy, and these should be considered in the differential diagnosis.

Tumors. Tumors of the conus or cauda equina, such as ependymomas, neurofibromas, and schwannomas, can present with back pain with radiation into the extremity. The back pain has often been present for some time—even years—and the extremity discomfort is often diffuse. The pain is typically more pronounced at night or when first waking rather than being more

	L4	L5	S1
Sensory	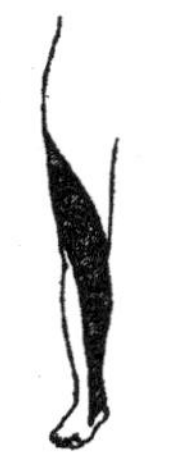	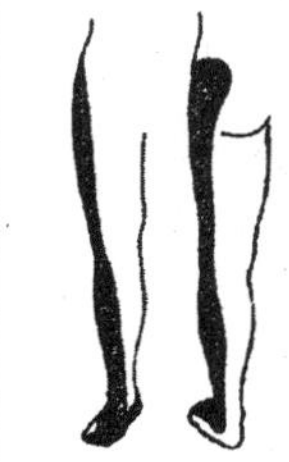	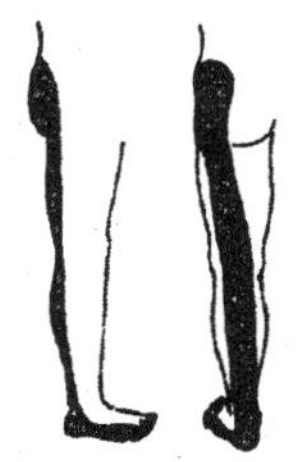
Motor	Quadriceps	EHL Tibialis Anterior	Gastrocnemius
Reflex	Patellar	None	Achilles

FIGURE 293–7. The sensory, motor, and reflex abnormalities expected with L4, L5, and S1 radiculopathies.

pronounced with activity. Metastatic disease to the lumbar vertebrae often involves the pedicle, so root irritation may accompany the onset of back pain. In a patient with a known malignancy, this should be a consideration.

Peripheral Nerve Lesions. Diabetic amyotrophy (Bruns-Garland syndrome) is characterized by the sudden onset of pain in the back and hip, often initially on one side with progression to bilateral symptoms. The pain abates spontaneously and is followed by profound quadriceps weakness and atrophy that may progress over several months. There is eventually incomplete improvement in strength. Although most patients with the syndrome have a known history of diabetes, the diagnosis of diabetes is occasionally made at the time of pain onset.[15, 16] A hematoma in the psoas muscle can produce sudden weakness in the femoral nerve. Peroneal nerve palsy due to trauma or peripheral neuropathy can produce footdrop, which can be confused with an L5 radiculopathy; the distinction can be difficult on clinical grounds alone. Peroneal nerve palsy is usually painless, and foot inversion is often preserved, as this is performed mostly by muscles supplied by the tibial nerve. The sciatic nerve can be involved in the pelvis with neoplasms and endometriosis. The piriformis syndrome is a controversial entity purported to be caused by irritation of the sciatic nerve as it exits under the piriformis muscle in the sciatic notch. Physical examination may demonstrate tenderness to palpation of the sciatic notch, pain on internal rotation of the hip in the neutral position, and pain on abduction and external rotation of the hip in the flexed position. The controversy surrounding this entity stems largely from the fact that this is essentially a diagnosis of exclusion, and imaging studies are often normal. Injection of local anesthetic directly into the piriformis muscle may provide relief, and decompression of the sciatic nerve through sectioning of the piriformis muscle can be considered.[17]

Rheumatologic Conditions. Osteoarthritis of the hip can produce buttock and leg pain. There is often radiation of pain into the groin, and pain can be reproduced by internal and external rotation of the hip (Patrick's sign). Trochanteric bursitis produces pain that radiates along the lateral side of the leg; the pain can be reproduced by pressure over the greater trochanter.

Cysts. Synovial cysts arising from the lumbar facet joints can irritate the underlying nerve root and produce radiculopathy. The appearance of these lesions on magnetic resonance imaging (MRI) is characteristic (Fig. 293–8). Surgical resection usually produces gratifying results.[18] Tarlov cysts, which are collections of cerebrospinal fluid within the nerve sheath of the sacral roots, are a relatively common incidental finding but may cause radiculopathy. Various approaches to their management, including percutaneous drainage and open cyst fenestration, have been proposed; however, it can be challenging to determine definitively that the cyst is the cause of the patient's symptoms.[19]

Examination

The examination of a patient with suspected lumbar disk herniation begins with testing the range of motion of the lumbar spine. Flexion and extension are often limited due to muscle splinting. Passive lateral bending

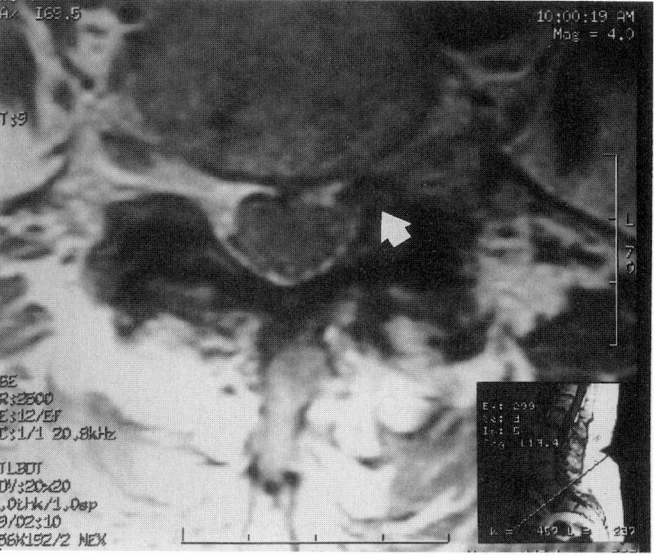

FIGURE 293–8. Arrow points to a synovial cyst arising from the facet joint.

of the spine may reproduce the patient's pain. When the protrusion is at the shoulder of the nerve root, movement toward that side may stretch the nerve root and cause leg pain; conversely, if the fragment is in the axilla of the root, movement away from the affected side may produce root stretch and radicular pain. This is illustrated in Figure 293–9.

The test of Lesègue, often referred to as the straight leg raising test, is an important part of the examination. With the patient in the supine position, the affected leg is passively flexed at the hip with the knee kept in extension. It should be possible to raise the leg to nearly 90 degrees without provoking symptoms other than hamstring tightness. At about 30 degrees, the nerve root moves in the foramen, and in the presence of root irritation, this stretch reproduces the patient's sciatic pain. This reproduction of pain is considered a positive test; back pain is not. In some patients, raising the contralateral, unaffected leg reproduces the pain in the affected leg. This is the crossed straight leg raising test, in which the affected nerve root is drawn medially by the movement of the contralateral root. This is illustrated in Figure 293–10. A meta-analysis of studies assessing the accuracy of these tests in diagnosing disk

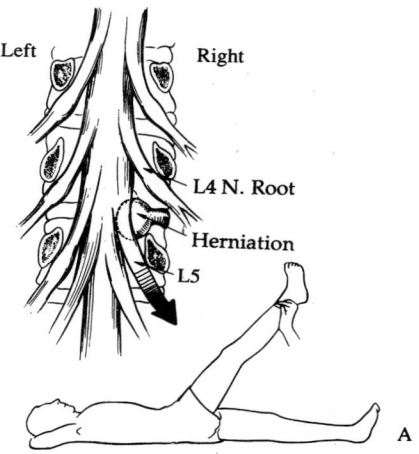

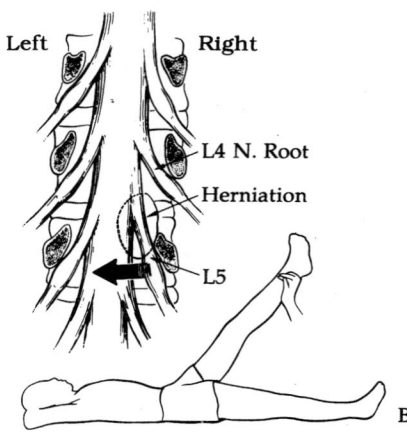

FIGURE 293–10. Straight leg raising test. *A,* Usually, extension of the leg stretches the nerve root that is compressed by the herniated disk and reproduces ipsilateral pain. *B,* Rarely, when a large fragment is present (or when a fragment is in the axilla at the root), extension of the contralateral leg pulls the root medially; when this occurs, the root is stretched and pain is reproduced in the leg ipsilateral to the herniated disk.

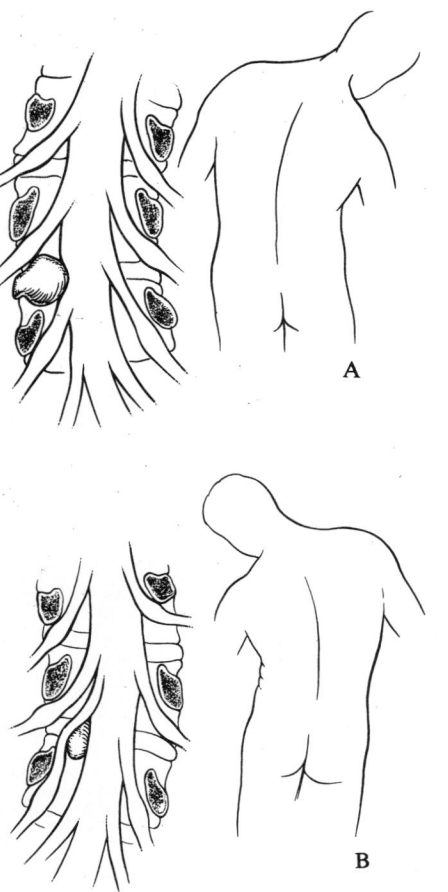

FIGURE 293–9. A lateral herniated disk most often displaces the root medially. *A,* Pain is reduced on bending away from the affected side, and it is increased on bending toward it. *B,* When a disk fragment is in the axilla of the root, the converse is true.

herniation suggests that the straight leg raising test has high sensitivity but low specificity, whereas the opposite is true of the crossed straight leg raising test, which has low sensitivity but high specificity.[20]

Patients with upper lumbar disk herniations may not have a positive straight leg raising test but may have reproduction of pain with the femoral nerve traction test. This is performed by placing the patient in the lateral decubitus position with the unaffected side down and the head flexed. The leg is extended at the hip joint with the knee in extension initially and then in flexion. The test is considered positive if these maneuvers reproduce the patient's radicular pain.[21]

Imaging

Magnetic Resonance Imaging. MRI is the preferred imaging study for demonstrating lumbar disk herniation. Axial images demonstrate the relationship of the disk herniation to the midline and the neural foramen. These images also allow the identification of any component of facet hypertrophy and lateral recess stenosis. Sagittal images can demonstrate whether there has been extension of the disk in the cephalad or caudad direction (Fig. 293–11), as well as the alignment of the vertebrae. A great advantage of MRI is that it allows visualization of the conus and cauda equina to exclude the possibility of neoplasm. Some patients, however, are unable to undergo MRI, including those with retained metallic fragments and cardiac pacemakers. Patients who have severe claustrophobia may need sedation before undergoing imaging.

Computed Tomography. Many lumbar disk herniations can be visualized on computed tomographic scanning, and this is a reasonable means of diagnosing patients who cannot tolerate MRI or when MRI is not available (Fig. 293–12). A significant drawback of computed tomography is that intradural abnormalities, including tumors, can be missed unless myelography is added.

Myelography. The use of myelography and postmyelographic computed tomographic scanning can be helpful in certain instances. In patients with equivocal

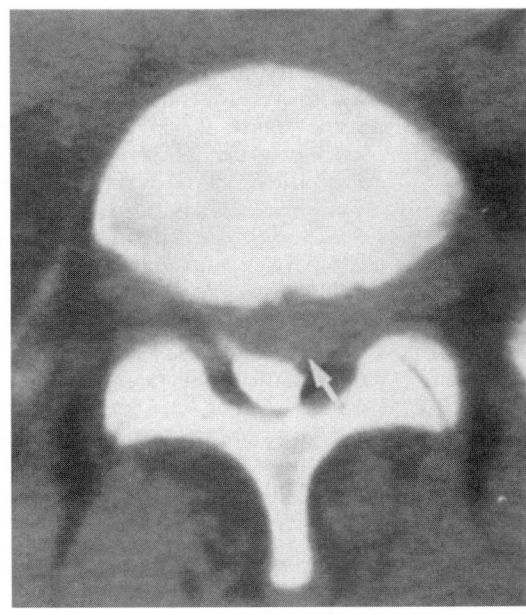

FIGURE 293–12. Computed tomography after myelography demonstrates a large disk herniation *(arrow).*

findings on MRI or in whom there may be a significant element of lateral recess stenosis, myelography may be able to better define the anatomy.

Diskography. Diskography has been a source of controversy for decades. It is clear that diskography does not provide better information than MRI in cases of nerve root compromise.[22] The current controversy surrounds provocative diskography. Advocates of this technique argue that if a patient's back pain is reproduced during injection of dye into the disk space, this is evidence that the disk is the source of pain, and treatments such as fusion may be beneficial.[23] Others argue that this test is unreliable, and the results of treatments based on diskography have been disappointing.[24]

SURGERY

Indications

Surgery for lumbar disk herniation has a high success rate and a low complication rate. In a retrospective study of more than 900 patients who underwent lumbar diskectomy with a mean follow-up of 10 years, good results were noted in 89%, with a 4% complication rate.[25] Similarly, a prospective study of 100 patients who underwent lumbar diskectomy showed that at 1-year follow-up, 96% were pleased with the result and 93% had returned to work.[26] Conversely, many patients with sciatica improve without surgical intervention. A study of nonoperative management of 64 patients with lumbar radiculopathy due to disk herniation reported good outcomes in 90%.[27] Selection bias in these studies makes it difficult to know which treatment is superior. There has been one randomized, controlled, pro-

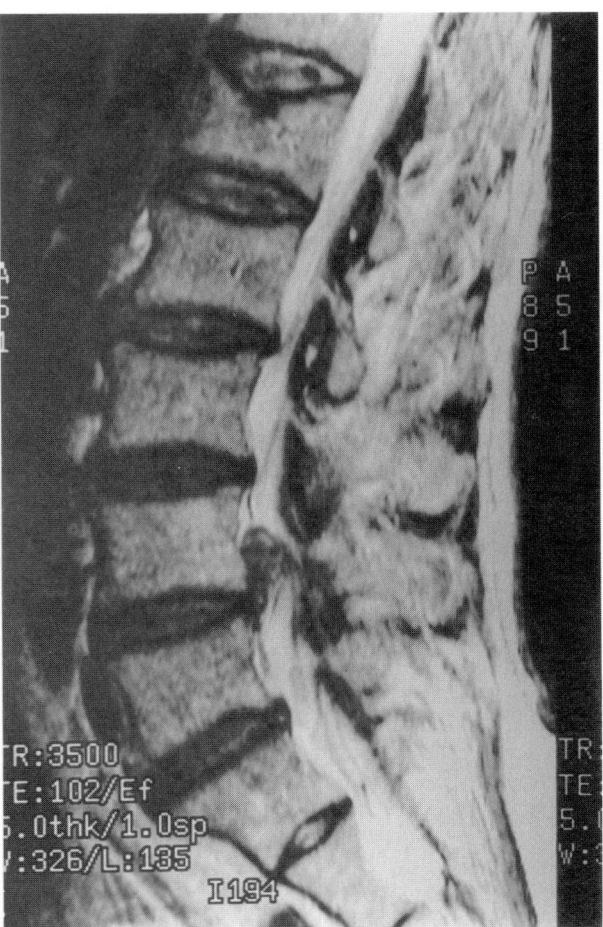

FIGURE 293–11. Sagittal magnetic resonance imaging scan demonstrating cephalad migration of disk herniation.

spective study of surgical versus nonoperative management of lumbar disk herniation reported by Weber in 1983.[28] One hundred twenty-six patients who presented with sciatica were randomized to surgery or a program on nonoperative management. At 1 year, the surgical group had better outcomes, but at 10-year follow-up, there was essentially no difference between the groups. This widely cited and influential paper has been used to argue that there is no long-term difference between operative and nonoperative management. These results, however, must be viewed with caution. Sixty-seven patients were excluded from the study because their symptoms at presentation were so severe that they underwent surgery. In addition, 20% of the patients initially randomized to nonsurgical treatment crossed over and had surgery, introducing a possible bias toward more favorable outcomes from nonsurgical management.

The dilemma in selecting treatment for patients with lumbar disk herniations is to not operate too hastily on patients who may improve without surgery but not withhold surgery for prolonged periods if patients do not respond to nonoperative measures. It is here that some individualization is necessary based on the severity of the symptoms, the examination, and the imaging study results.

Patients who present with cauda equina syndrome should be considered for urgent surgery. Shapiro reviewed 44 patients who presented with cauda equina syndrome secondary to lumbar disk herniation and found a significantly higher likelihood of recovery of bladder function and resolution of pain and motor deficits in patients undergoing operation within 48 hours of symptom onset.[29] It should be noted, however, that the severity of the initial neurological deficit probably influences the ultimate outcome, and others have not reported such a clear association between the timing of surgery and the recovery of bladder function.[30]

Patients with profound motor weakness should be considered for early surgery. Although in Weber's series the recovery of motor strength was equal in patients randomized to surgical and nonsurgical treatment, the degree of weakness was not specified. Motor weakness that progresses or a Medical Research Council grade[31] of less than 4 in quadriceps or foot dorsiflexion strength is a reasonable indication to proceed with decompression. Some degree of extensor hallucis longus weakness is common with L5 radiculopathy and usually improves with improvement in other symptoms.

In patients with pain but without significant motor deficit or sphincter disturbance, there is often some improvement within the first 4 weeks, so an initial attempt at nonoperative management is reasonable. Analgesics, either nonsteroidal anti-inflammatory or mild narcotic medications, are an important part of initial management. A short course of oral steroid medication is occasionally beneficial. Because symptoms are often exacerbated by activity, some limitation of activity is reasonable. Epidural injection of corticosteroids may lead to significant improvement. The patient's response to these nonoperative measures should be monitored; if there is no improvement, it is reasonable to proceed with diskectomy.

Lumbar disk herniation in children and adolescents is uncommon, but the symptoms of back and radicular pain are similar to those in adults. Some studies have demonstrated a high incidence of associated spinal structural abnormalities such as scoliosis, spina bifida occulta, and spondylolisthesis; thus, it is reasonable to obtain plain radiographs before considering surgery.[32, 33] At operation, the disk material is often less firm than in adults.

Although the initial results of surgery in pediatric patients are good, an understandable concern is the long-term outcome in terms of reoperation and back pain. In studies with sufficiently long follow-up, rates of reoperation appear to be about 20%.[34, 35] Despite this, the long-term functional outcome is quite good. Durham and colleagues studied a group of patients who underwent lumbar diskectomy when younger than 17 years old, with a mean follow-up of 8.5 years. These authors did not find a high incidence of chronic back pain, and the Short Form Health Survey questionnaire (SF-36) scores were similar to those of age-matched controls.[35]

Technique

The surgical procedure should be preceded by a review of the imaging studies to reconfirm the side and level of disk herniation. In most situations, general endotracheal anesthesia is preferable; however, in selected cases, spinal or local anesthesia can be used. The use of short-acting muscle relaxants on induction allows the blockade to wear off before the portion of the procedure in which the nerve is manipulated. This affords an extra margin of safety, because excessive heat or retraction on the root often produces a muscular response.

Positioning of the patient should be directed at avoiding pressure on the abdomen, to minimize pressure in the lumbar epidural veins. For most patients, this can be accomplished with use of the knee-chest position. Alternatively, the prone position can be used, with rolls placed under the patient to support the weight on the rib cage and iliac crests. Several positioning frames are also available. Morbidly obese patients can be difficult to adequately ventilate in the prone position; in these patients, the lateral decubitus position with the symptomatic side up can be used. In all positions, the anesthesiologist should confirm that there is no direct pressure on the eye, to avoid optic ischemia.

The incision is made sharply in the midline and carried to the level of the lumbodorsal fascia. This is opened using electrocautery, and the paraspinal muscles are dissected off the spinous processes of the vertebrae above and below the involved disk. Further dissection of the muscles off the laminae can be accomplished using periosteal elevators. The level of the dissection should be confirmed by lateral radiograph. A towel clamp can be placed on one of the spinous processes for reference. At this point, the procedure is made easier with the use of visual magnification. This can be achieved with either loupes or the operating microscope. The operating microscope has the advantages of providing brilliant focused illumination and allowing the surgeon and the assistant to share the same field of view.

The inferior edge of the superior lamina is dissected using a curet; then, using a Kerrison punch, a laminotomy is performed. It is necessary to remove about half the lamina, and the dissection is then extended laterally to the medial facet (Fig. 293–13). The ligamenta flava are now visible and are incised sharply (Fig. 293–14). The underlying dura or epidural fat should be visible. A Penfield no. 4 dissector is then placed into the opening in the ligamenta flava to ensure that there are no adhesions between the ligament and the dura. The remaining ligament is then removed with a Kerrison punch. The dura is inspected, and the nerve root is identified. It may be necessary at this point to use the Kerrison punch to remove additional bone and ligament laterally to the medial edge of the facet joint. To avoid injuring the nerve root, it is helpful to probe under the ligament first with the Penfield no. 4 dissector, because the ligament becomes thinner laterally, and the nerve root may be pressed up against it by the underlying disk herniation. At this point, the nerve root should be visible and can be retracted medially with the Penfield dissector, and the underlying disk herniation can be visualized (Fig. 293–15). If the posterior longitudinal ligament is intact, it is incised with a no. 11 blade. The underlying herniated disk material usually extrudes through the opening. This material is removed with a pituitary rongeur. The rongeur is advanced into the disk space, and additional disk material is removed. It is probably necessary to remove only enough disk material to adequately decompress

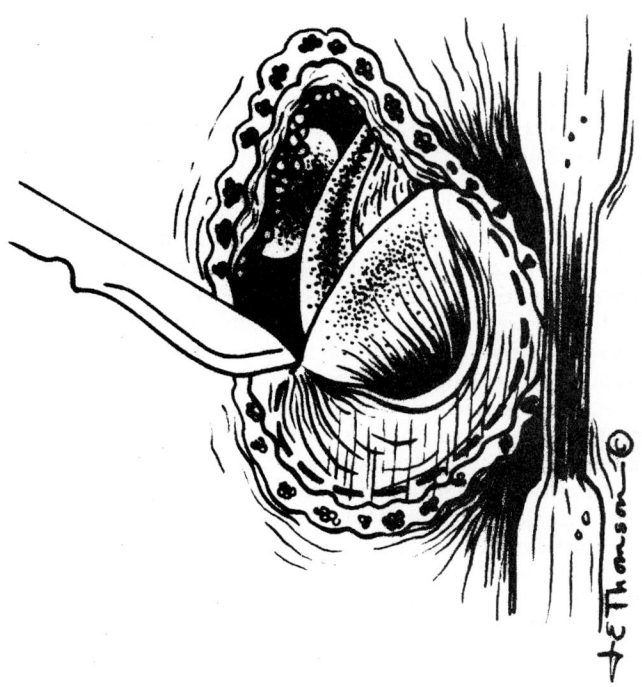

FIGURE 293–14. Incising the ligamenta flava.

the nerve root. Care must be exercised not to advance the rongeur too deeply within the disk space to avoid injuring structures in the retroperitoneum on the opposite side of the disk space, such as the bowel or vessels.

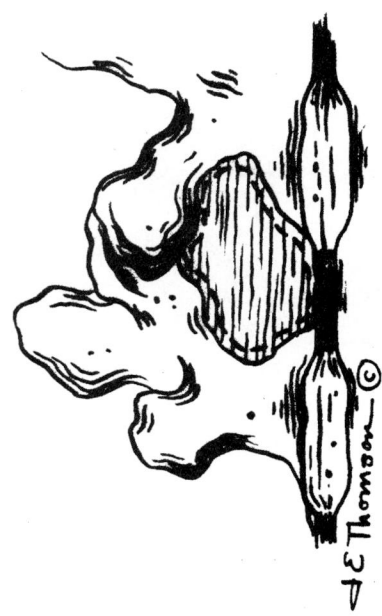

FIGURE 293–13. The approximate extent of the laminotomy and underlying ligamenta flava.

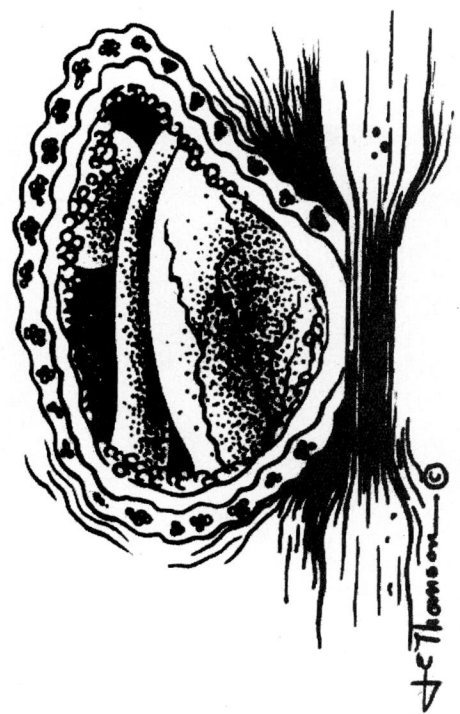

FIGURE 293–15. The dura and root sleeve with the disk herniation at the shoulder of the root.

If the posterior longitudinal ligament is not intact when first inspected, it is possible that a disk fragment has been extruded and has migrated cephalad, caudad, or into the axilla of the root. At the conclusion of the procedure, if the root is well decompressed, it should be pulsatile. The wound is irrigated and closed in layers.

In the case of a large central disk herniation, and especially in the presence of cauda equina syndrome, it is best to perform a bilateral laminectomy for exposure. This allows the dura to be retracted medially on each side without further compromising the roots. The herniated disk material can then be removed from each side using a pituitary rongeur.

As mentioned previously, about 10% of disk herniations occur at or lateral to the neural foramen. The surgeon's view of this region is obscured by the facet joint, and a variety of approaches have been described to address disk herniations in this location. The most straightforward of these involves a medial facetectomy. The standard diskectomy approach is extended laterally into the medial portion of the facet joint, and the disk fragment can be removed by angling the rongeur laterally. Abdullah and associates reported excellent results with this technique.[7] This approach is most useful if a component of the herniation is within the canal.

When the fragment lies farther laterally in the extraforaminal space, it can be reached from the extraforaminal approach first described by Frankhauser and de Tribolet.[36] A paramedian incision is made, and the intermuscular septum between the multifidus and longissimus muscles is identified (Fig. 293–16). Dissection in this plane leads down to the facet joint. The intertransverse muscle is dissected off the lateral edge of the facet. Bone removal is accomplished with either a Kerrison punch or a drill, starting at the isthmus of the

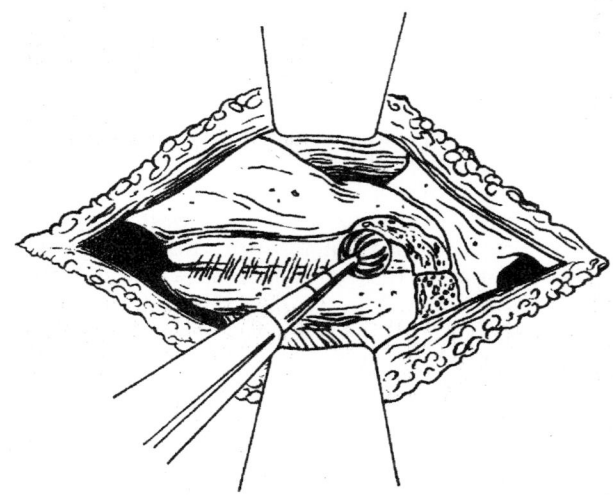

FIGURE 293–17. Bone removal along the isthmus of the lamina. (Adapted from Porchet F, Chollet-Bornand A, de Tribolet N: Long-term follow up of patients surgically treated by the far-lateral approach for foraminal and extraforaminal lumbar disc herniations. J Neurosurg [Spine 1] 90:59–66, 1999.)

superior lamina and proceeding cephalad to the level of the pedicle (Fig. 293–17). The lateral edge of the ligamenta flava should be visible, and once this is removed, the underlying nerve and dorsal root ganglion will be visible. The disk herniation lies under the root and can be removed using a pituitary rongeur (Fig. 293–18). Good results have been reported using this technique,[37] but the principal limitation is the difficulty of removing any portion of the fragment that lies medial to the foramen within the spinal canal. An alternative in this situation is to combine a standard

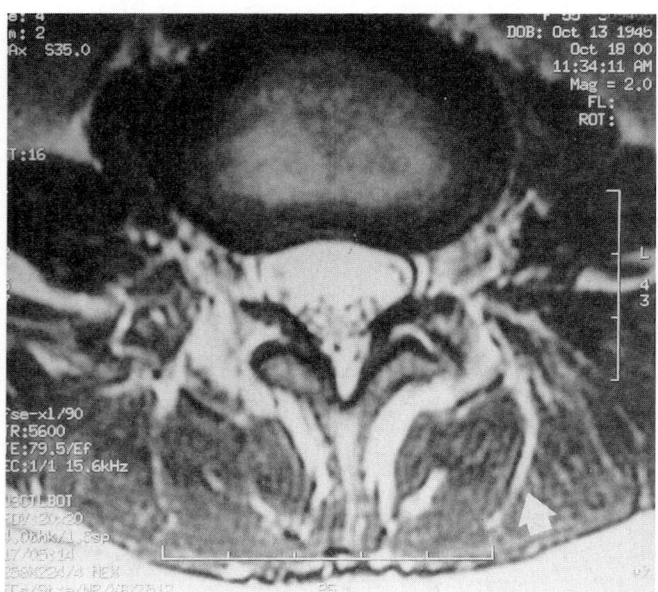

FIGURE 293–16. Arrow points to the intermuscular septum, which leads to the facet joint.

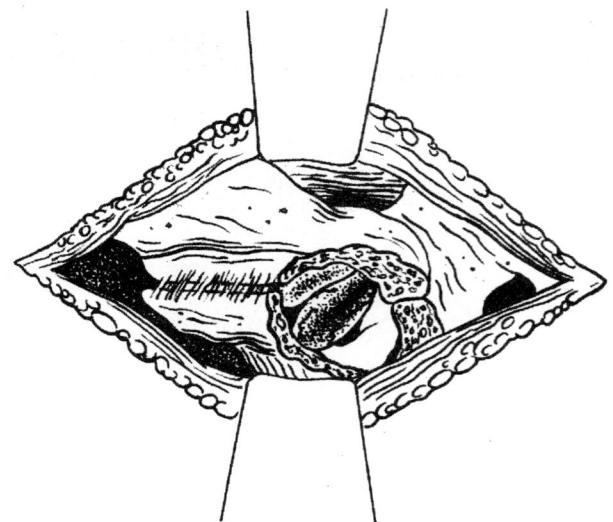

FIGURE 293–18. After removal of ligament, the nerve root and underlying disk herniation will be visible. (Adapted from Porchet F, Chollet-Bornand A, de Tribolet N: Long-term follow up of patients surgically treated by the far-lateral approach for foraminal and extraforaminal lumbar disc herniations. J Neurosurg [Spine 1] 90:59–66, 1999.)

hemilaminotomy with an extraforaminal approach as described by Jane and colleagues.[38] This provides visualization of the root from within the canal and into the extraforaminal space.

Far-lateral disk herniations at the L5-S1 interspace can be problematic. The pedicles are quite far apart at this level, and access to the extraforaminal space can be restricted by the sacrum. In this situation, drilling of the costal process of the sacrum can provide visualization of the extraforaminal space.[39]

Occasionally, none of these approaches provides satisfactory exposure. One option is to perform a unilateral complete facetectomy. This provides excellent visualization of the root but raises concerns about postoperative instability. This complication is not as common as might be expected, however. Garrido and Connaughton performed unilateral complete facetectomies in 41 patients and, with a mean follow-up of nearly 2 years, noted instability requiring fusion in only one patient.[8]

Intraoperative Complications

Negative Exploration. If the findings at the explored disk space do not correspond to what was expected based on the imaging studies, it should be confirmed that the side of the exposure corresponds to the side of the patient's symptoms. Next, it is reasonable to repeat the intraoperative radiograph to ensure that the dissection has not inadvertently proceeded a level cephalad or caudad of the intended level. If the correct side and level are confirmed, one should consider the possibility of an intradural herniation of the fragment.[40]

Durotomy. The dura can be opened inadvertently, resulting in the appearance of cerebrospinal fluid in the wound. If the rent can be directly visualized, any exposed nerve roots should be reduced with the aid of a cottonoid patty, and the opening should be sutured. It is not always possible to suture or even directly view the opening, however, especially if it is anterior or in the axilla of the root. In this case, the wound is closed and the patient is kept on flat bed rest for 24 hours and then mobilized. If cerebrospinal fluid leaks from the wound, the patient is returned to bed rest, and the would is oversewn. If this fails to stop the leakage, a lumbar drain is inserted percutaneously and left in place for 3 to 5 days.

Retroperitoneal Injury. Injury to the structures in the retroperitoneum, including the great vessels and the bowel, can occur if there is penetration of the anterior longitudinal ligament, usually by a pituitary rongeur, during removal of disk material from a posterior approach. Measurements of the diameter of the lower three lumbar vertebrae demonstrate that although the anteroposterior dimension is quite variable, it is consistently greater than 3 cm.[41] The risk of anterior penetration can therefore be reduced if penetration of instruments into the disk space is limited to less than 3 cm.

The aorta and vena cava and their branches lie di-

rectly in front of the anterior longitudinal ligament of the lumbar spine. Injuries to these structures are rare but carry a high mortality. The injury can be arterial or venous, or it can result in the development of an arteriovenous fistula. The first indication of a vascular injury may be brisk bleeding from the disk space; however, this is present in only about half the cases.[42, 43] The development of unexplained signs of volume depletion, such as hypotension and tachycardia, should raise suspicion of a vascular injury. If a vascular injury is strongly suspected, the wound should be packed, the patient rolled into the supine position, the abdomen prepped, and a laparotomy commenced while awaiting the assistance of a general or vascular surgeon.

Injury to the bowel is also a rare complication. Most reported cases involved injury to the ileum during surgery at the L5-S1 disk space. The injury is often not apparent at the time of surgery but presents as increasing abdominal pain in the first few days after surgery, but reports have been that of chronic wound infection.[44] Treatment involves consultation with a general surgeon.

Postoperative Complications

Failure of Pain Relief. Most patients undergoing lumbar diskectomy experience prompt improvement of their preoperative radicular pain, despite the presence of incisional pain. If there is no improvement in the patient's radicular pain in the early postoperative period, imaging studies should be performed to rule out the possibility that the procedure was performed at the wrong level or that residual retained disk material is present. If these are found, re-exploration is indicated.

Recurrence of Pain. The return of radicular pain after a period of improvement suggests either recurrent disk herniation or epidural scar formation. The symptoms in either situation are often similar to the original

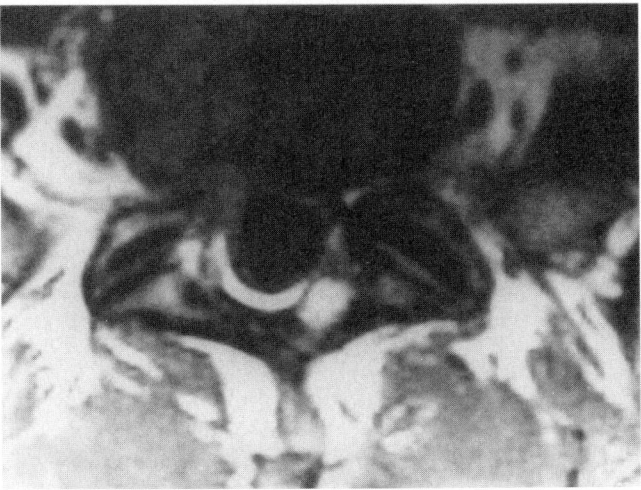

FIGURE 293–19. Magnetic resonance imaging without gadolinium enhancement.

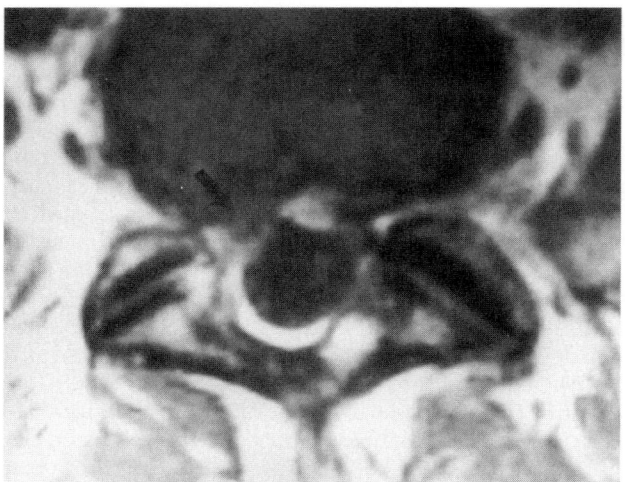

FIGURE 293–20. Magnetic resonance imaging with gadolinium enhancement. Note the lack of enhancement of the recurrent disk fragment *(arrow)*.

sciatica. MRI with and without gadolinium enhancement can provide valuable information. Areas of epidural scarring enhance brightly after the administration of gadolinium, whereas recurrent disk herniation does not. This is illustrated in Figures 293–19 and 293–20.

Epidural scarring occurs to some extent following any procedure in the epidural space. The pathogenesis of the pain is thought to be related to tethering of the nerve root in the foramen by scar tissue. Most patients present with recurrent pain within the first year following surgery.[45] It is not clear why a small minority of patients become symptomatic from the epidural scar-

ring that is inevitably present following lumbar diskectomy, while the majority of patients do not. A prospective study of patients undergoing lumbar diskectomy found a correlation between the extent of scarring and the presence of recurrent pain, but even among patients with the most extensive scar formation, pain was present in less than 20%.[46] Surgery is ineffective in this situation.[47] The use of a barrier gel has shown some promise in reducing the occurrence of scar formation.[48]

Recurrent disk herniation can occur at the same level as the initial surgery or at a different level. The overall rate of recurrent disk herniation appears to be about 8%,[49] with an average pain-free interval of about 8 years.[45] The indications for repeat diskectomy are similar to those for initial diskectomy, and the overall outcomes appear to be similar as well.[50] It should be noted, however, that surgery for recurrent disk herniation is a more challenging procedure than initial diskectomy, and the risk of durotomy or injury to the nerve root is higher owing to the presence of scarring. The procedure involves opening the previous incision and identifying the superior and inferior laminae. Scar tissue usually obscures the prior laminotomy site and is adherent to the dura. Using a curet, the edge of the previous laminotomy site is identified, and using a Kerrison rongeur, additional bone is removed circumferentially from around the previous opening in the bone. This allows the identification of dura that is not invested in scar. Exploration is then carried to the level of the disk space, and any recurrent disk material is removed.

Infection. The development of infection within the disk space is a rare occurrence following lumbar diskectomy, with an estimated frequency of about 0.5%. The most common presenting symptom of disk space

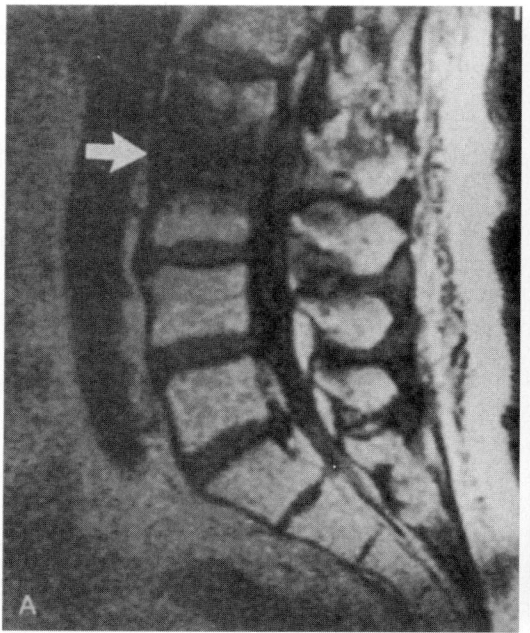
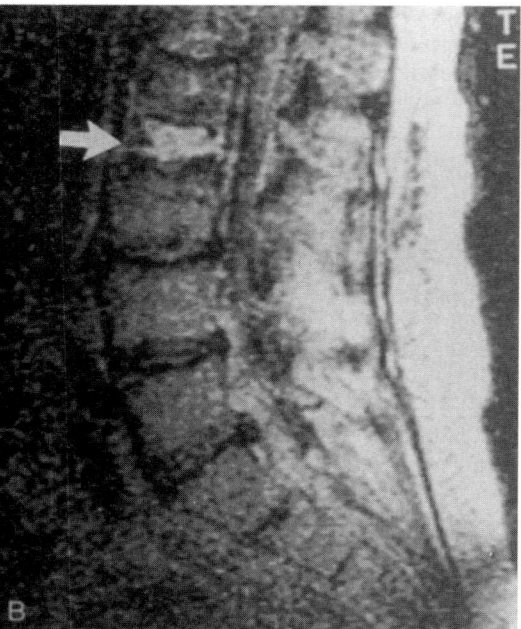

FIGURE 293–21. Sagittal T1-weighted *(A)* and T2-weighted *(B)* magnetic resonance imaging demonstrates a disk space infection at L2-3 *(arrows)*.

infection is the onset of worsening back pain, often accompanied by paravertebral muscle spasm. This usually begins 1 to 4 weeks postoperatively but has been reported as long as 8 months following surgery.[51] Fever and marked leukocytosis may be absent; however, the erythrocyte sedimentation rate is reliably elevated.[51] The difficulty with using the erythrocyte sedimentation rate as a screening test for diskitis is that it increases after uncomplicated lumbar diskectomy and does not return to normal for several weeks. The C-reactive protein level, however, increases postoperatively but returns to normal within 5 to 14 days following uncomplicated surgery.[52] The C-reactive protein level may be at least as sensitive as the erythrocyte sedimentation rate for the detection of postoperative diskitis, and it is more specific.[53, 54] MRI can identify changes in the disk space quite early in the course of the disease (Fig. 293–21).

If the imaging and laboratory findings are suspicious for diskitis, percutaneous biopsy of the disk space for culture and histology can be useful in guiding therapy. *Staphylococcus aureus* is the most common organism isolated.[51, 54] If organisms are detected on biopsy, appropriate antibiotics based on sensitivities should be started. The usual recommendation is for 6 weeks of therapy. If no organisms are detected on biopsy, the appropriate therapy is somewhat controversial. Some argue that antibiotics directed against the most common organisms should be used if the imaging and laboratory findings are consistent with a disk space infection.[54] Others argue that if the cultures are negative and the histology of the sampled tissue is not suggestive of active infection, this represents a "mechanical" diskitis that can be treated with only rest.[55] In either case, serial measurements of the erythrocyte sedimentation rate should be made, with an expectation that levels will start to decrease within 3 weeks of treatment.

REFERENCES

1. Viets H: Dominico Cotugno: His description of the cerebral spinal fluid, with a translation of part of his De Ischiade Nervosa Commentarius (1764) and a bibliography of his important works. Bull Inst Hist Med 3:701–738, 1935.
2. Dandy WE: Loose cartilage from intervertebral disc simulating tumor of the spinal cord. Arch Surg 19:660–672, 1929.
3. Mixter WJ, Barr JS: Rupture of the intervertebral disc with involvement of the spinal canal. N Engl J Med 211:210–214, 1934.
4. Parisien R, Ball P: Historical perspective: William Jason Mixter (1880–1958): Ushering in the "dynasty of the disc." Spine 23: 2363–2366, 1998.
5. Kramer J: Intervertebral Disc Diseases: Causes, Diagnosis, Treatment and Prophylaxis, 2nd ed. New York, Thieme Medical, 1990.
6. Abdullah AF, Ditto EW III, Byrd EB, Williams R: Extreme-lateral lumbar disc herniations. J Neurosurg 41:229–234, 1974.
7. Abdullah AF, Wolber PG, Warfield JR, Gunadi IK: Surgical management of extreme lateral lumbar disc herniations: Review of 138 cases. Neurosurgery 22:648–653, 1988.
8. Garrido E, Connaughton PN: Unilateral facetectomy approach for lateral lumbar disc herniation. J Neurosurg 74:754–756, 1991.
9. Olmarker K, Holm S, Rosenqvist AL, Rydevik B: Experimental nerve root compression. A model of acute, graded compression of the porcine cauda equina and an analysis of neural and vascular anatomy. Spine 16:61–69, 1991.
10. Boden SD, Davis DO, Dina TS, et al: Abnormal magnetic resonance scans of the lumbar spine in asymptomatic subjects: A prospective investigation. J Bone Joint Surg Am 72:403–408, 1990.
11. Bozzao A, Galluci M, Masciocchi C: Lumbar disc herniation: MR imaging assessment of natural history in patients treated without surgery. Radiology 185:135–141, 1992.
12. Saal JS, Franson RC, Dobrow R, et al: High levels of inflammatory phospholipase A_2 activity in lumbar disc herniations. Spine 15:674–678, 1990.
13. Olmarker K, Rydevik B, Nordborg C: Autologous nucleus pulposus induces neurophysiologic and histologic changes in porcine cauda equina nerve roots. Spine 18:1425–1432, 1993.
14. Otani K, Arai I, Mao GP, et al: Nucleus pulposus–induced nerve root injury: Relationship between blood flow and motor nerve conduction velocity. Neurosurgery 45:614–619, 1999.
15. Barohn R, Sahenk Z, Warmolts JR, Mendell JR: The Bruns-Garland syndrome (diabetic amyotrophy). Arch Neurol 48:1130–1135, 1991.
16. Garland H: Diabetic amyotrophy. BMJ 2:1287–1290, 1955.
17. Rodrigue T, Hardy RW: Diagnosis and treatment of the piriformis syndrome. Neurosurg Clin N Am 12:311–319, 2001.
18. Howington JU, Connolly ES, Voorhies RM: Intraspinal synovial cysts: 10 year experience at the Ochsner Clinic. J Neurosurg (Spine 2) 91:193–199, 1999.
19. Mummaneni PV, Pitts LH, McCormack BM, et al: Microsurgical treatment of symptomatic sacral Tarlov cysts. Neurosurgery 47: 74–79, 2000.
20. Devillé WLJM, et al: The test of Lesègue: Systematic accuracy in diagnosing herniated discs. Spine 25:1140–1147, 2000.
21. Dyck P: The femoral nerve traction test with lumbar disc protrusions. Surg Neurol 6:163–166, 1976.
22. Gibson MJ, Buckley J, Mawhinney R, et al: Magnetic resonance imaging and discography in the diagnosis of disc degeneration. J Bone Joint Surg Br 68:369–373, 1986.
23. Calhoun E, et al: Provocation discography as a guide to planning operations on the spine. J Bone Joint Surg Br 70:267–271, 1988.
24. Pallatroni HF, Ball PA: Argument against lumbar fusion for low back pain. Semin Neurosurg 11:177–181, 2000.
25. Davis RA: A long-term outcome analysis of 984 surgically treated herniated lumbar discs. J Neurosurg 80:415–421, 1994.
26. Lewis PJ, Weir BK, Broad RW, Grace MG: Long-term prospective study of lumbosacral discectomy. J Neurosurg 67:49–53, 1987.
27. Saal JA, Saal JS: Nonoperative treatment of herniated lumbar intervertebral disc with radiculopathy: An outcome study. Spine 14:431–437, 1989.
28. Weber H: Lumbar disc herniation: A controlled, prospective study with ten years observation. Spine 8:131–140, 1983.
29. Shapiro S: Medical realities of cauda equina syndrome secondary to lumbar disc herniation. Spine 25:348–352, 2000.
30. Gleave J, Macfarlane R: Prognosis for recovery of bladder function following lumbar central disc prolapse. Br J Neurosurg 4: 205–210, 1990.
31. Brain GO: Aids to the Examination of the Peripheral Nervous System. London, Ballière Tindall, 1986.
32. DeOrio JK, Bianco AJ: Lumbar disc excision in children and adolescents. J Bone Joint Surg Am 64:991–996, 1982.
33. Shilito J: Pediatric lumbar disc surgery: 20 patients under 15 years of age. Surg Neurol 46:14–18, 1996.
34. Ebersold MJ, Quast LM, Bianco AJ: Results of lumbar discectomy in the pediatric population. J Neurosurg 67:643–647, 1987.
35. Durham SR, Sun PP, Sutton LN: Surgically treated lumbar disc disease in the pediatric population: An outcome study. J Neurosurg (Spine 1) 92:1–6, 2000.
36. Frankhauser H, de Tribolet N: Extreme lateral lumbar disc herniation. Br J Neurosurg 1:111–129, 1987.
37. Porchet F, Chollet-Bornand A, de Tribolet N: Long-term follow up of patients surgically treated by the far-lateral approach for foraminal and extraforaminal lumbar disc herniations. J Neurosurg (Spine 1) 90:59–66, 1999.
38. Jane JA, Haworth CS, Broaddus WC, Lee JH: A neurosurgical approach to far-lateral disc herniation. J Neurosurg 72:143–144, 1990.
39. Muller A, Reulen HJ: A paramedian tangential approach to lumbosacral extraforaminal disc herniations. Neurosurgery 43:854–861, 1998.
40. Schisano G, Franco A, Nina P: Intraradicular and intradural

lumbar disc herniation: Experiences with nine cases. Surg Neurol 44:536–543, 1995.

41. Anda S, Aakhus S, Skaanes KO, et al: Anterior perforations in lumbar discectomies: A report of four cases of vascular complications and a CT study of the prevertebral lumbar anatomy. Spine 16:54–60, 1991.

42. Montorsi W, Ghiringhelli C: Genesis, diagnosis and treatment of vascular complications after intervertebral disk surgery. Int Surg 58:233–235, 1973.

43. DeSaussure RL: Vascular injury coincident to disc surgery. J Neurosurg 16:222–229, 1959.

44. Smith EB, DeBord JR, Hanigan WC: Intestinal injury after lumbar discectomy. Surg Gynecol Obstet 173:22–24, 1991.

45. Jönsson B, Strömqvist B: Clinical characteristics of recurrent sciatica after lumbar discectomy. Spine 21:500–505, 1996.

46. Ross JS, Robertson JT, Frederickson RC, et al: Association between peridural scar and recurrent radicular pain after lumbar discectomy: Magnetic resonance evaluation. ADCON-L European Study Group. Neurosurgery 38:855–863, 1996.

47. Fiume D, Sherkat S, Callovini GM, et al: Treatment of the failed back surgery syndrome due to lumbro-sacral epidural fibrosis. Acta Neurochir Suppl (Wien) 64:116–118, 1995.

48. de Tribolet N, Porchet F, Lutz TW, et al: Clinical assessment of a novel antiadhesion barrier gel: Prospective, randomized, multicenter clinical trial of ADCON-L to inhibit postoperative peridural fibrosis and related symptoms after lumbar discectomy. Am J Orthop 27:111–120, 1998.

49. Connolly ES: Surgery for recurrent lumbar disc herniation. Clin Neurosurg 39:211–216, 1992.

50. Suk K, Lee H, Moon S: Recurrent disc herniation: Results of operative management. Spine 26:672–676, 2001.

51. Rawlings CE, Wilkins RH, Gallis HA, et al: Postoperative intervertebral disc space infection. Neurosurgery 13:371–376, 1983.

52. Thelander U, Larsson S: Quantitation of C-reactive protein levels and erythrocyte sedimentation rate after spinal surgery. Spine 17:400–404, 1992.

53. Meyer B, Schaller K, Hassler W: The C-reactive protein for detection of early infections after lumbar microdiscectomy. Acta Neurochir (Wien) 136:145–150, 1995.

54. Bilsky MH, SCB: Complications of lumbar disc surgery. Contemp Neurosurg 17:1–6, 1995.

55. Fouquet B, Goupille P, Jattiot F, et al: Discitis after lumbar disc surgery: Features of "aseptic" and "septic" forms. Spine 17:356–358, 1992.

Lumbar Spinal Stenosis

NANCY E. EPSTEIN

Verbiest first described the syndrome of lumbar spinal stenosis in the early 1950s after observing that laminectomy relieved radiculopathic symptoms in four patients with narrowed spinal canals.[1-4] He described two types of lumbar stenosis. The first, congenital stenosis, is characterized by vertebrae with short pedicles and shallow sagittal canal diameters of 10 mm or less. Patients with achondroplasia have the purest form of congenital lumbar stenosis.[5] In these individuals, the vertebrae are trapezoidal with short, thick pedicles, hypertrophied lamina, and thickened vertebral end plates that contribute to further narrowing of the spinal canal. Periosteal bone formation adds to circumferential compression of the normal-sized cauda equina and nerve roots.

The second type, relative or acquired stenosis, indicates that the canal is between 10 and 12 mm in anteroposterior diameter but originally had normal dimensions. Here, progressive narrowing is attributed to acquired degenerative changes such as thickened laminae, medially impinging arthrotic facets, hyperlordosis with laminar shingling, infolding of hypertrophied yellow ligament, and ossification of the posterior longitudinal ligament. Endocrinopathies such as Paget's disease, acromegaly, and fluorosis also contribute to canal compromise.

Lateral recess and subarticular stenosis, as defined by Epstein and colleagues and Getty,[6-8] also contributes to lateral thecal sac and nerve root entrapment beneath the superior articular facets. With significant lateral recess stenosis, more acute radicular deficits arise from relatively small intrusions. This is due to the lack of available "reserve" space within a spinal canal with a trefoil configuration and a normal central canal diameter. Central and lateral recess stenosis may coexist.

Primary and acquired developmental stenosis may arise focally over one or two segments, or it may be found diffusely throughout the lumbar spinal canal. The most frequent site of stenosis is the L4-5 level, followed in descending order of frequency by L3-4, L2-3, L5-S1, and, rarely, L1-2.

ANATOMY AND PATHOPHYSIOLOGY OF STENOSIS

The epidural compartment is multisegmented, with large patches of dura in immediate contact with the canal wall.[9] Dorsally, the ligamentum flavum is angled inward and fused in the midline, where it is covered by an underlying fat pad. Ventrally and centrally, disk, spurs, and dilated veins are found; anterolaterally, disk, spur (osteophyte), and hypertrophic changes in the posterior longitudinal ligament further compromise available space. Congenital anomalies, such as benign Tarlov cysts, may balloon into neural foramina, sometimes reaching extremely large proportions in the distal lumbar spinal canal.[10]

Animal models simulate the pathophysiologic changes occurring with progressive lumbar stenosis. In Delamarter and coworkers' canine model, progressive cauda equina compression contributed to increased neurological deterioration and a loss of evoked potentials attributed to venous congestion adding to atrophy, neural demyelination caused by obstruction of axoplasmic flow, and wallerian degeneration.[11]

Radiculopathy and neurogenic claudication associated with spinal stenosis are attributed to either direct mechanical compression or indirect vascular insufficiency leading to lack of adequate blood flow and oxygenation of the lumbar nerve roots or cauda equina. Standing and walking transiently increase lordosis, accentuating stenosis by exaggerating the infolding of the ligamentum flavum into the central canal or lateral recesses, thus exacerbating symptoms. In contrast, sitting and recumbency typically reverse the lordosis, open the canal, improve blood flow, and relieve complaints. Watanabe and Park observed that the direct vascular compromise that occurs with ambulation is mostly arterial, resulting in "demyelinization, pia-arachnoidal adhesions, interstitial fibrosis, and thick-walled congested veins."[12] Complaints of neurogenic claudication were attributed to "ectopic neural impulses" that fluctuated with the adequacy of the vascular supply to the cauda equina.

CLINICAL PICTURE

Symptoms

Patients with congenital lumbar stenosis become symptomatic earlier, often in their 30s and 40s, while those with acquired stenosis develop radicular or claudicatory complaints in their 50s to 60s. Radiculopathy often starts unilaterally, then slowly becomes bilateral. Neurogenic claudication typically begins as a bilateral complaint characterized by leg pain, numbness, tingling, and weakness that are increased with standing and walking and relieved with rest, especially by sitting, lying down, or assuming any posture that reverses the lordotic curve. Although these patients usually cannot walk, they are comfortable driving long distances. When Jonsson and Stromqvist looked at 100 consecutive patients with disk disease, 100 with lateral recess stenosis, and 100 with central stenosis, they found that all three groups showed comparable degrees of pain at rest, pain at night, and pain on coughing.[13] In Louis and Nazarian's lumbar stenosis series (350 patients), 57% showed unilateral radiculopathy, and 67% exhibited neurogenic claudication.[14] Lemaire and associates demonstrated that 87% of their patients with stenosis complained of low back pain, 82% had radiculopathy, and 58% presented with claudication.[15]

Many patients who have not yet developed significant neurological deficits can be managed successfully without surgery, using rehabilitation or multidisciplinary pain centers. Surgery is usually reserved for those with intractable pain and progressive disability or evolving radicular or cauda equina syndromes.[16] On occasion, patients with stenosis complicated by acute disk herniation may demonstrate the rapid onset of mono- or paraplegia with sphincteric dysfunction.

Signs

Mechanical findings of entrapment, including the Lasègue and reversed Lasègue signs, may be seen in 60% of patients with absolute stenosis and 43% of patients with mixed stenosis.[2, 17] Mechanical, motor, reflex, and sensory signs most frequently reflect the level or levels of involvement. In descending order, the L5 root syndromes are correlated with L4-5 disease, L4 root syndromes with L3-4 pathology, L3 root syndromes with L2-3 disease, and S1 root pathology with L5-S1 compression.[18] Many patients, however, present with minimal or no neurological deficits early in the course of this disorder. Lemaire and associates determined that in patients with spinal stenosis exhibiting a complete myelographic block, 37% showed significant motor, reflex, sensory, and sphincteric deficits.[15] Postoperative improvement in back pain occurred in 60% of patients, radicular pain improved in 89%, and neurogenic claudication in 90%.

Chronic bladder dysfunction is often subclinically present in patients with lumbar stenosis. Deen and colleagues found that all patients (average age, 71 years) undergoing two- to four-level laminectomies for severe lumbar stenosis exhibited some degree of preoperative bladder compromise.[19] They documented that 6 months after laminectomy, although only 45% of patients showed objective (cystoscopy or urodynamic testing) improvement in urinary function (i.e., decrease in postvoiding residual volume), subjectively, 60% thought that their urinary dysfunction had improved.

Diagnostic Studies

A complete preoperative evaluation of lumbar stenosis includes plain radiographs, magnetic resonance imaging (MRI) and computed tomography (CT) examinations, and optimally a three-dimensional CT or CT–myelography evaluation. Plain anteroposterior and lateral radiographs provide an immediate overview of the vertebrae and the lumbar spine; additionally, they show the curvature in two views and the presence of olisthy on dynamic studies. They may also demonstrate a lumbosacral anomaly 7% of the time.[20] For example, a lumbosacral transitional vertebra may contribute to increased stress above the level of the anomaly, with early disk degeneration increasing the incidence of spondyloarthrosis and contributing ninefold to disk herniation at the immediate cephalad interspace. Flexion-extension radiographs may further document hypermobility and instability manifested by greater than 4 mm of translation and greater than 10 to 12 degrees of angulation at the level of olisthy.[21–24]

MRI scans are the first noninvasive study performed in most patients presenting with symptoms of lumbar stenosis (Figs. 294–1 and 294–2).[25] MRI studies, whether static or dynamic, better demonstrate soft tissue changes laterally, foraminally, and far laterally, and they show longitudinal pathology in three dimensions, extending to the thoracolumbar junction. CT studies, however, are better at showing bony abnormalities. Three-dimensional MRI with gadolinium DTPA affords a near "myelographic" view of the entire subarachnoid space, especially in postoperative patients, providing an 82.6% correlation between operative and MRI findings.[26, 27] Further, enhanced MRI scans accurately differ-

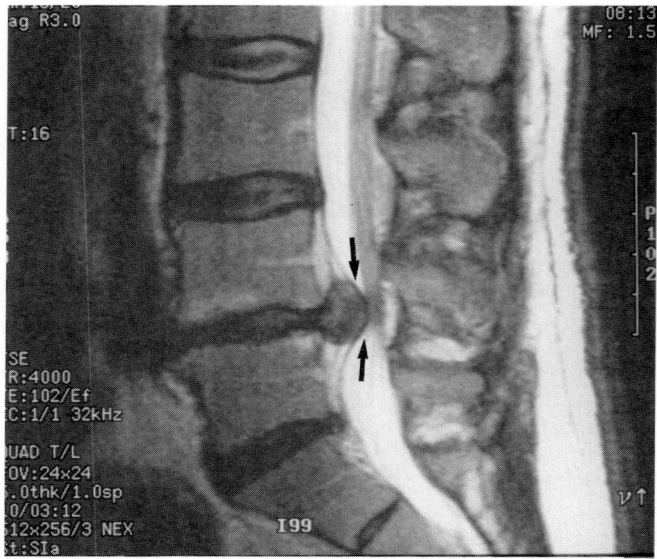

FIGURE 294–1. Midline sagittal T2-weighted magnetic resonance imaging scan of an L4-5 type IV limbus vertebral fracture resulting in a cauda equina syndrome (Case 1). There is a large, central, hypointense mass protruding from the L4-5 interspace, resulting in marked cauda equina compression *(arrows)*. Note how the limbus vertebral fracture elevates the posterior longitudinal ligament cephalad and caudad to the interspace.

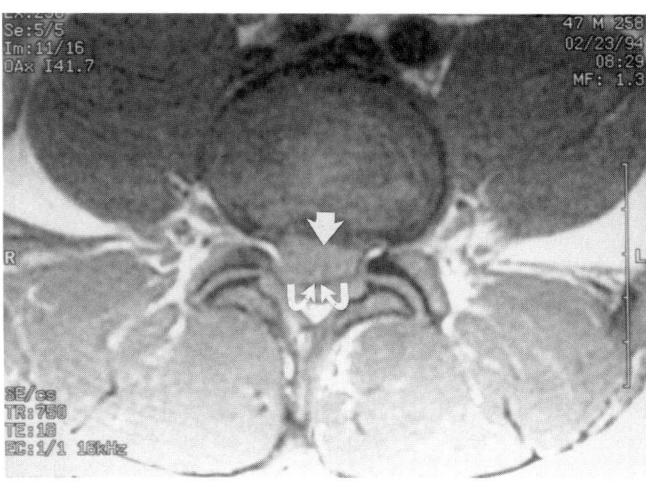

FIGURE 294–2. Transaxial T1-weighted magnetic resonance imaging scan demonstrates a massive type IV limbus fracture compressing the thecal sac and contributing to secondary spinal stenosis at the L4-5 level (Case 1). The large, ventral, somewhat hyperintense limbus vertebral fracture nearly obliterates the canal *(white arrows).*

entiate scar from disk 96% of the time. MRI may also screen for more cephalad cervical and thoracic disease, while also identifying tumors, demyelinating syndromes, adhesive arachnoiditis, and infections.[28] Nevertheless, one must recognize the high frequency of asymptomatic lesions found on MRI studies. For example, in Boden and coworkers' experience, among patients older than 60 years, 36% had herniated disks and 21% had spinal stenosis, yet only 33% were symptomatic.[25]

The noncontrast CT examination, supplemented with two- and three-dimensional reconstructed images, provides excellent structural definition of lumbar stenosis and accompanying pathology: recurrent stenosis, disk herniation, limbus fracture, olisthy, ossification of the posterior longitudinal ligament (OPLL), ossification of the yellow ligament (OYL), and changes in a fusion mass (Figs. 294–3 to 294–8). For instance, Laasonen and Soini found 157 CT abnormalities in 48 patients who remained symptomatic after lumbar fusions: 12 of 27 major lesions included fusion mass fractures, hairline pseudarthroses, and unrelieved spinal stenosis, all confirmed at surgery.[29]

Three-dimensional CT or CT–myelography evaluations provide sagittal, coronal, and transaxial images

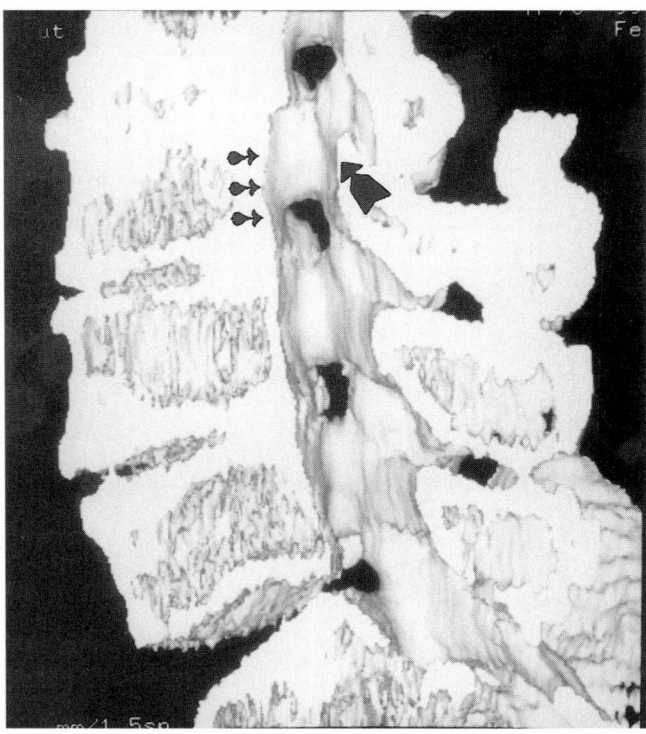

FIGURE 294–3. Midline sagittal three-dimensional computed tomographic scan demonstrates L3-S1 lumbar spinal stenosis that is most marked at the L3-4 level (Case 2). Dorsal laminar shingling is typical of lumbar stenosis *(small arrows)* and is most severe at the L3-4 level.

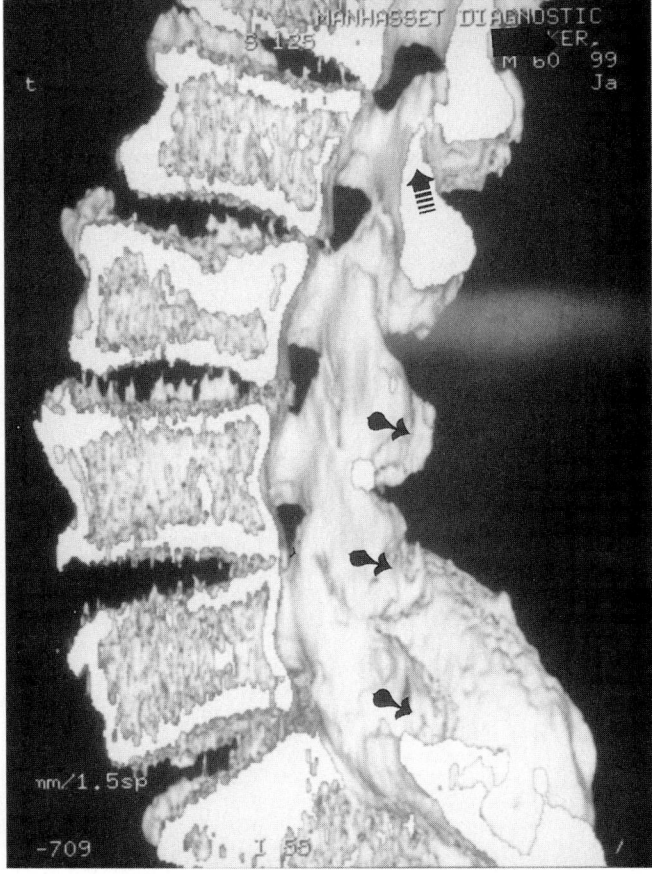

FIGURE 294–4. Two years after surgery, this midline sagittal three-dimensional computed tomographic scan shows new L2-3 stenosis *(larger interrupted arrow)* cephalad to the prior L3-S1 laminectomy defect *(single rounded arrows)* (Case 2).

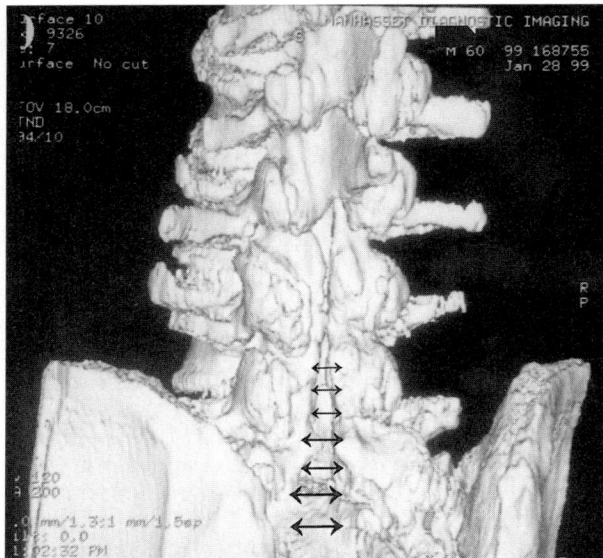

FIGURE 294–5. Two years after surgery, this dorsal three-dimensional computed tomographic scan demonstrates recurrent stenosis at the previously decompressed L3-S1 levels (Case 2). The recurrent lumbar stenosis is nearly obliterating the prior laminectomy defect *(arrows).*

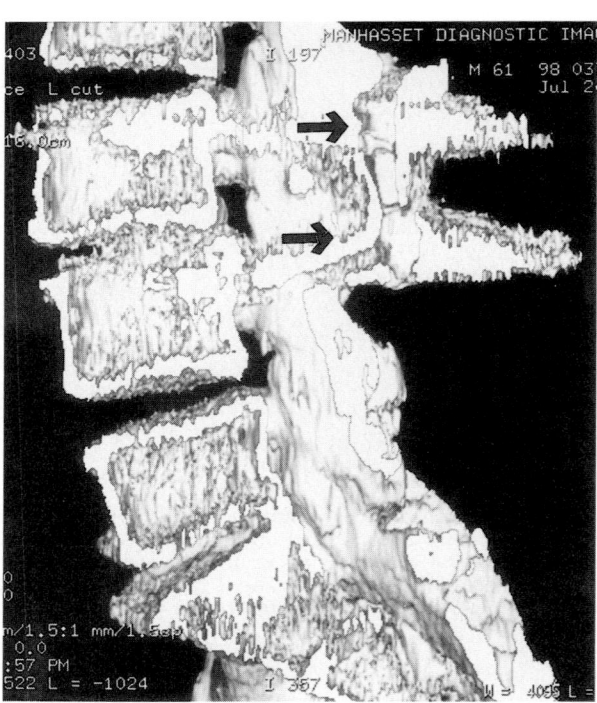

FIGURE 294–7. Midline sagittal three-dimensional computed tomographic scan shows a dorsal fusion mass at the L3-4 level *(arrows)* 4 months after a Texas Scottish Rite Hospital instrumented fusion (Case 3). This 61-year-old man originally had an L3-S1 laminectomy for spinal stenosis. Five years later, he developed recurrent stenosis and instability at the L3-4 level and underwent the second procedure.

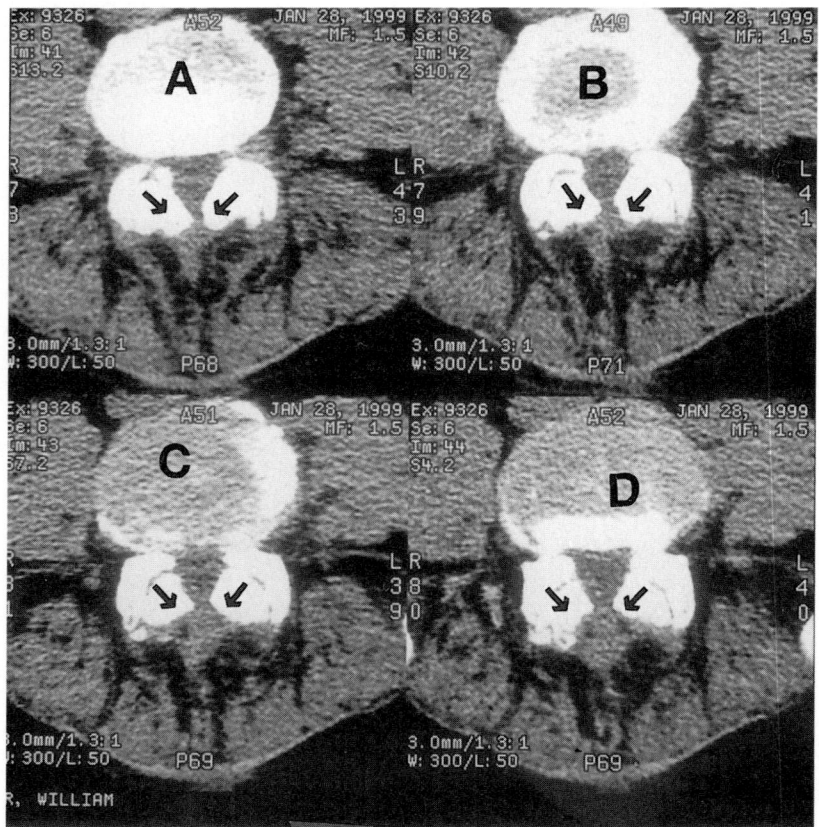

FIGURE 294–6. Two years after surgery, this transaxial noncontrast computed tomographic scan confirms recurrent stenosis at the L3-4 level (Case 2) (A–D). There is near complete obliteration of the prior laminectomy defect *(arrows)* due to further hypertrophic changes of the facet joints.

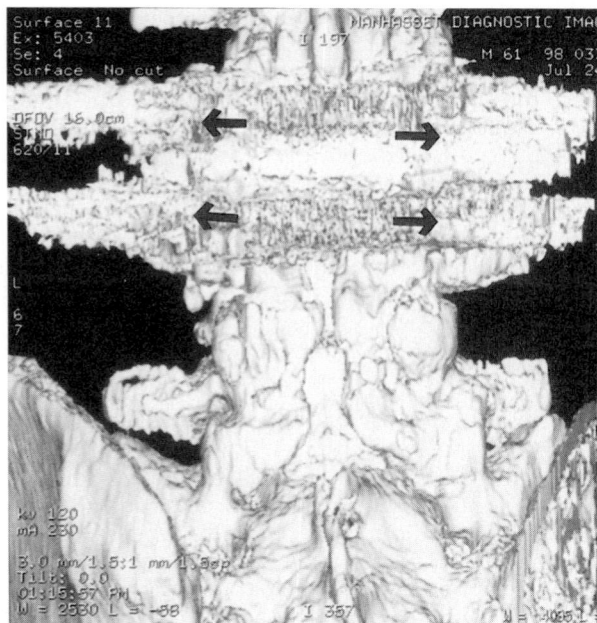

FIGURE 294–8. Dorsal three-dimensional computed tomographic scan shows a large lateral fusion mass at the L3-4 level *(arrows)* 4 months after a Texas Scottish Rite Hospital fusion (Case 3). Additionally, the prior inferior laminectomy defect extending to the sacrum can be visualized.

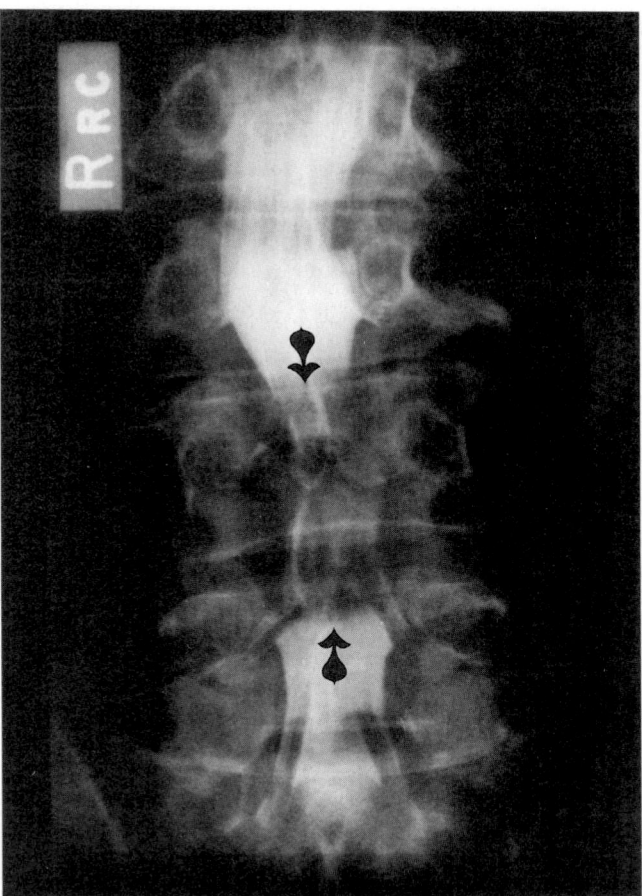

FIGURE 294–10. Anteroposterior myelogram of L3-5 *(arrows)* shows the classic bilateral, waistlike deformity of lumbar stenosis (Case 4).

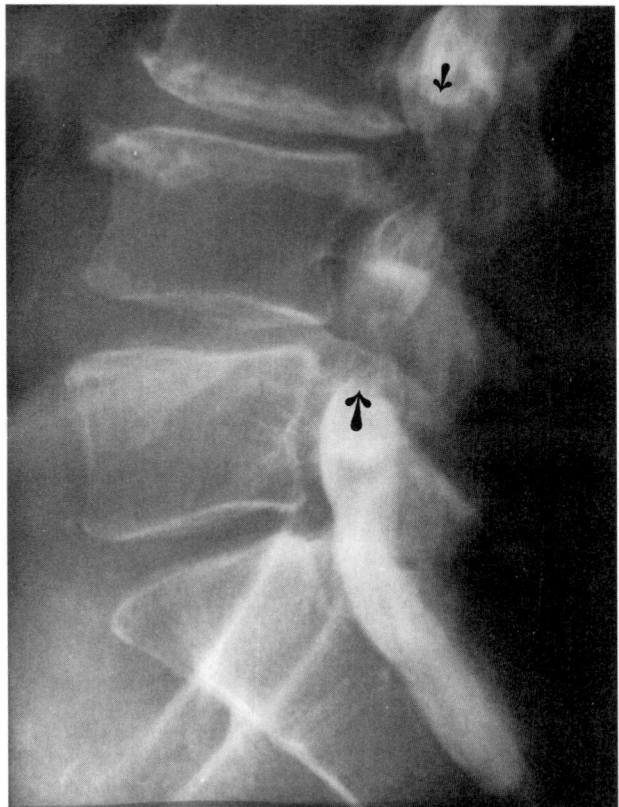

FIGURE 294–9. This 63-year-old man with neurogenic claudication and partial footdrop bilaterally had a lateral myelogram demonstrating diffuse central lumbar stenosis at L3-5 *(arrows)* (Case 4). Observe the multilevel circumferential narrowing of the thecal sac at the L3-4 and L4-5 levels.

of the spinal canal, allowing an overview of the lateral foraminal and far lateral compartments (Figs. 294–9 to 294–12). Ventral pathology identified by these studies includes disk disease, spurs or spondylosis, limbus fracture, and OPLL. Posteriorly, ossification of the yellow or capsular ligaments and arthrotic changes of the facet joints may also be identified. Two- and three-dimensional reconstructions best illustrate olisthy, lysis, scoliosis, and foraminal changes.[30, 31]

Such diagnostic studies may also be used for prognostic purposes. In Herno and colleagues' studies, the severity of the preoperative myelographic block helped predict the quality of outcome in 251 patients managed with laminectomy and followed for an average of 4.2 years postoperatively.[32–34] Although 76% of patients with complete myelographic block had good to excellent outcomes, only 56% with absolute stenosis and 61% with relative stenosis and a trefoil canal had comparable good to excellent results.[34]

Somatosensory Evoked Potential and Electromyographic Monitoring

Preoperative, intraoperative, and postoperative somatosensory evoked potentials may be used to deter-

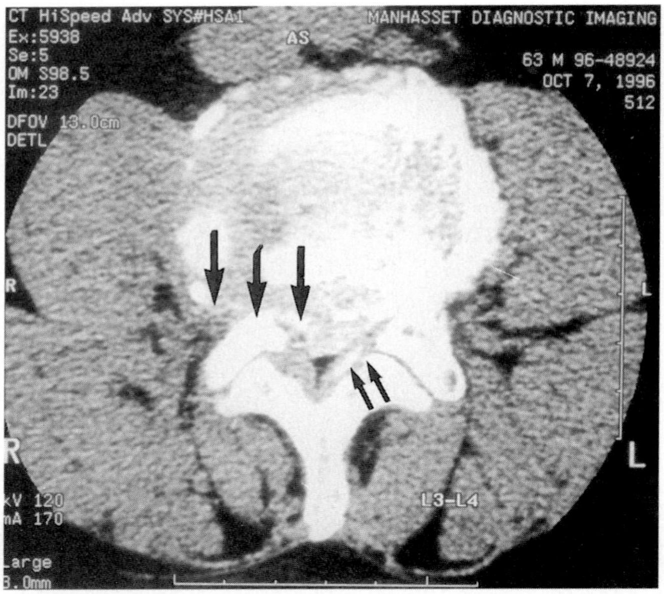

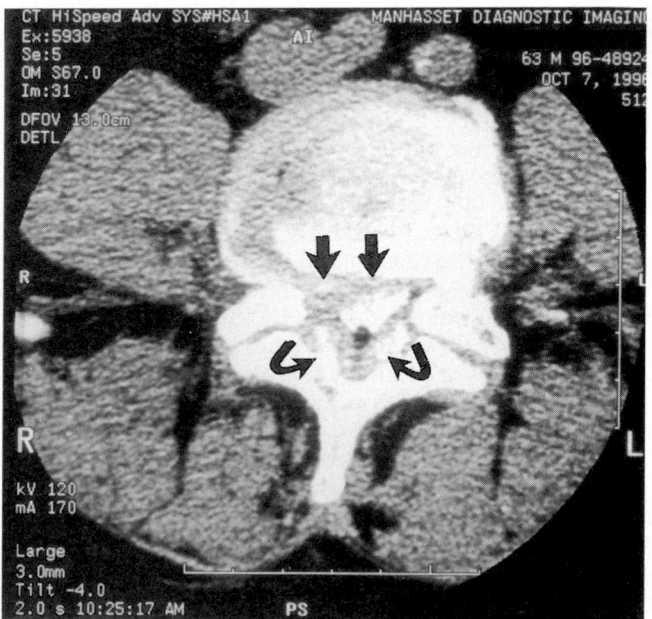

FIGURE 294–11. Transaxial computed tomography–myelography at the L3-4 level demonstrates right-sided lateral, foraminal, and far lateral stenosis, spondyloarthrosis, and disk herniation *(triple large arrows)*, along with dorsolateral ossification of the yellow ligament *(small double arrows)* (Case 4).

FIGURE 294–12. Transaxial computed tomography–myelography at the L4-5 level shows marked diffuse stenosis, a right-sided anterolateral disk herniation *(double arrows)*, and bilateral dorsolateral ossification of the yellow ligament *(curved arrows)* (Case 4). This resulted in marked compression of the thecal sac, the right L4 nerve root as it exits far laterally, and the L5 nerve roots bilaterally (right greater than left).

mine whether nerve roots have been adequately decompressed. In Gepstein and Brown's series, successive improvement in somatosensory evoked potentials recorded intraoperatively and 3 weeks and 3 months postoperatively predicted ample nerve root release in 27 patients with herniated disks and in 14 with spinal stenosis.[35] Intraoperative electromyography may also be used to provide immediate feedback regarding the adequacy of decompression, as well as to indicate when excessive manipulation and retraction are being used.

Differential Diagnosis

Accompanying Cervical and Thoracic Stenosis. Patients presenting with diffuse lower back or leg pain may actually suffer from cervical or thoracic stenosis. Therefore, particularly when stenosis is found in older patients, an examination of the entire neuraxis may be warranted to ensure that symptoms are not arising from more cephalad disease. Up to one third of patients undergoing cervical decompression for stenosis experience improvement in their lumbar symptoms, even when significant lumbar pathology is present.[36] Similarly, those with thoracic stenosis respond favorably to thoracic decompression.[37–41] Other entities mimicking lumbar disease include thoracic disk herniation, achondroplasia, ankylosing spondylitis, osteochondrodystrophy, diabetic peripheral neuropathy, acromegaly, familial hypophosphatemic vitamin D–refractory rickets, Scheuermann's disease, OPLL, OYL, Paget's disease, and arthritis of the hips.

Ossification of the Yellow and Posterior Longitudinal Ligaments. OYL may significantly contribute to lumbar stenosis. Postacchini and associates found that the ligamenta flava from 10 stenotic patients showed unique degenerative changes not found in others having surgery for lumbar disk herniations or trauma.[42] OYL originates as an ingrowth of fibrocartilage due to proliferation of type II collagen. Next, ligamentous hypertrophy and calcium crystal deposition lead to progressive ossification, which begins laterally at the enthesis and extends medially.[43] Crystals consist of calcium pyrophosphate dihydrate with occasional hydroxyapatite and calcium orthophosphate. Ten percent of OPLL is located in the proximal lumbar canal, 10% in the proximal thoracic spine (T1-4), and 80% in the distal cervical canal.[44, 45]

OPLL and OYL may both contribute to thoracic or lumbar stenosis.[37, 38, 44, 45] Twenty-six of 1100 patients (2.3%) operated on for spinal stenosis from 1986 to 1997 had OYL or OPLL: 11 patients had OPLL, 12 had OYL, and 3 had both.[44] This group of patients averaged 64 years of age (range, 26 to 77 years), was half male and half female, and was followed an average of 3.7 years. The patients presented with thoracic myelopathy (4 patients), radiculopathy and neurogenic claudication (20 patients), and cauda equina syndromes (2 patients). Laminectomy, completed in 24 patients, addressed OPLL (average of 3.7 levels) or OYL (average of 4.4 levels). Two patients with both thoracic OPLL and

OYL required simultaneous anterior transthoracic and posterior decompressions. Using Odom's criteria, good to excellent outcomes were achieved in 73% of OPLL patients and 83% of OYL patients.

Amyloidosis. Amyloidosis may also contribute to lumbar stenosis. Using light and electron microscopy, D'Agostino and coworkers found that 12 of 97 patients having lumbar surgery for stenosis had a thickened ligamentum flavum that contained amyloid crystals.[46]

Ankylosing Hyperostosis. Ankylosing hyperostosis also contributes to lumbar stenosis. Leroux and colleagues studied the radiographs and computed tomographic scans of 46 patients with ankylosing hyperostosis and compared these examinations with those of 54 normal subjects.[47] They found that the diagnosis could be confirmed when four of the following six criteria were met: somatic osseous proliferation at the (1) anterior or (2) posterior lateral margin, or proliferation of the nonarticular portion of the (3) posterior facet joints, (4) articular capsule, (5) yellow ligament, or (6) supraspinal ligament.

Diabetes: Neuropathy, Angiopathy, and Other Comorbidities. Patients with diabetic peripheral neuropathy, femoral amyotrophy, or angiopathy may be misdiagnosed as having lumbar radiculopathy or neurogenic claudication. Cinotti and associates prospectively diagnosed lumbar stenosis and performed successful lumbar laminectomies in 25 diabetic and 25 nondiabetic patients averaging 71 years of age and followed an average of 3.4 years.[48] Outcomes for diabetic and nondiabetic patients were comparable, although one patient with diabetes was misdiagnosed and had a peripheral neuropathy, and another had angiopathy. Additionally, preoperative nerve conduction studies demonstrated slowing in 80% of diabetics but in only 25% of controls; peripheral vascular disease was confirmed in 20% of diabetics but in only 4% of nondiabetics. Clinical symptoms signaling diabetes rather than stenosis as the underlying pathology included the abrupt onset of pain accompanied by night pain, burning dysesthesia, and the lack of posture-related pain relief.

Even when the diagnosis of lumbar stenosis was correct, Simpson and coworkers noted that diabetics undergoing lumbar laminectomy had poorer outcomes than nondiabetics.[49] Long-term assessment showed significantly higher postoperative infection rates and longer hospital stays, with good to excellent results in only 39% of their 44 diabetic patients (followed a mean of 5 years) versus good to excellent results in 95% of their 55 nondiabetic patients (followed a mean of 7 years).

Neurogenic versus Vascular Claudication. Patients with vascular claudication, unlike those with neurogenic claudication, experience cramping calf or leg pain brought on by ambulation and relieved by rest alone. They do not have to alter their posture (bend forward or sit down) to get relief. Lower extremity arterial pulses, arterial Doppler studies of the lower extremities, ultrasonography of the abdominal aorta, and angi-

ography contribute to the diagnosis of aortofemoral or peripheral vascular insufficiency. When vascular and neurogenic claudication coexist, vascular surgery should precede lumbar intervention.

Tumors. Tumors of the cervical, thoracic, or lumbar spine (especially the cauda equina or conus), including ependymomas, neurofibromas, meningiomas, metastatic carcinomas, and others, may mimic the symptoms of spinal stenosis. Here, extensive preoperative evaluation should be performed using MRI studies enhanced with gadolinium DTPA.

NONSURGICAL MANAGEMENT OF LUMBAR STENOSIS

Most patients with mild radiologic evidence of spinal stenosis can be successfully managed with conservative therapy. Rosomoff and Rosomoff believe that many patients with MRI- and CT-documented moderate to severe stenosis, even with significant neurological deficits, may improve when treated at multimodality pain centers.[16] Onel and coauthors showed that 145 patients demonstrating preoperative positive mechanical findings (100%), neurogenic claudication (100%), sensory deficits (47%), and motor deficits (29%) were adequately managed without surgery.[50] Conservative management included infrared heat treatments, ultrasonic diathermy, and active lumbar flexion exercises. The duration of relief is often compromised with the passage of time.

Herno and colleagues completed several studies focusing on the surgical results in lumbar stenosis patients with and without prior surgery.[51-53] In particular, they compared the outcomes (Oswestry questionnaire and surgeon's clinical assessment) in 54 similar matched pairs with lumbar stenosis who were treated conservatively (nonoperatively) or with laminectomy.[52, 53] The sample included 440 surgical patients (1974 to 1987) followed an average of 4.1 years and 54 nonsurgical patients (1980 to 1987) followed an average of 4.3 years. Although the overall data showed no statistically significant difference in outcome between matched pair groups, the men undergoing surgical decompression demonstrated significantly improved outcomes when compared with the nonoperated group.

SURGICAL MANAGEMENT OF LUMBAR STENOSIS

Laminectomy

Older patients are prophylactically immobilized in hard cervical collars with gel pads under the chin at the time of intubation or are placed in three-pin head holders. Those with significant cervical spondylostenosis but no evidence of myelopathy require awake intubation and positioning under somatosensory evoked potential monitoring. Foley catheters are routinely placed in older patients. Intraoperative monitoring devices include end-tidal carbon dioxide analysis, pulse oximetry, electrocardiogram assessment, arterial lines, and central lines; Swan-Ganz catheters are reserved for those with significant cardiopulmonary problems. Prophylactic antibiotics and 10 mg of intravenous dexamethasone are also given. Whereas the fenestration technique may be used for more focal stenosis in younger patients with less evident spondylostenosis, laminectomy is preferred to address more severe changes.[54-56] Shorter procedures may be completed with the patient in the knee-chest position if there is no attendant hip, knee, or peripheral vascular pathology or massive obesity. For longer operations with the attendant comorbidities mentioned earlier, the Cloward saddle or Wilson frame is preferred.

The wound is infiltrated with 30 mL of 0.5% bupivacaine with 1:200,000 dilution of epinephrine. This diminishes the blood loss and immediate postoperative pain and reduces anesthetic requirements, allowing for earlier reversal at the end of surgery. Subperiosteal dissection of the paraspinal muscles from the spinous processes is accomplished using coagulation cautery, a periosteal elevator, and 2-inch vaginal packing. Retraction is then achieved with multiple Taylor or Collis retractors; Addson suboccipital retractors are routinely placed at either end. Next, an intraoperative radiograph is taken either with a clamp on a spinous process or interspinous ligament or with a Penfield elevator in the spinal canal or disk space. This helps avoid decompressing the wrong surgical levels—one of the most common reasons for failure in stenosis surgery.

The spinous processes may be removed with a rib cutter or Leksell rongeur. Next, an en face laminectomy is completed with a combination of a rongeur and a high-speed air drill using a coarse diamond bur (no. 6), which facilitates shaving down hypertrophied laminae and medially impinging facet joints. Once the laminae have been shaved down, a small curet can be used to dissect the ligamentum flavum away from the most caudal lamina. Because stenosis is typically most severe at the L4-5 level, it is safer to enter the canal at L5-S1 and thereby define the dural-ligamentous plane and progressively remove the laminae cranially. Central stenosis is decompressed first, a maneuver that involves removal of the midline and paramedian laminae and secondarily the ligamentum flavum. Next, lateral recess stenosis and foraminal compromise are addressed using angled 2- to 4-mm Kerrison rongeurs with their filed-down footplates. Medial facetectomy and foraminotomy are completed, paying careful attention to preserving the lateral two thirds of the facet joints using an undercutting technique. At this point, the canal, once it is decompressed bilaterally, is inspected for disk herniations, limbus fractures, or other pathology that may warrant the use of the operating microscope (use of surgical telescopes is routine). At this point, some surgeons evaluate the wound with intraoperative ultrasonography. Using this technique in 104 patients, Montalvo and coworkers discovered residual disk material 41% of the time and additional stenosis 23% of the time, requiring resection before closing.[57]

Damage to the cauda equina or nerve roots or pro-

duction of a cerebrospinal fluid fistula can best be avoided by dissecting as indicated from the normal to the abnormal, maintaining close contact between the lateral bony margins and the tip of any cutting instrument. After performing lateral bony contours with an up-biting curet and carefully dissecting soft tissues with either a Penfield elevator or a dental tool, variously sized Kerrison punches can be introduced. If a cerebrospinal fluid leak has occurred during the dissection (as it does in 5% of first and 10% of second lumbar decompressions), the leakage site should be sutured using 7–0 Gore-Tex under the operating microscope or closed with a dural titanium stapler (1.4 mm); this should be supplemented with fibrin sealant. In the absence of a leak, a medium Hemovac drain is frequently inserted and brought out through a cephalad stab incision. The wound is closed using 0 and 2–0 absorbable suture (Vicryl), followed by subcuticular or staple closure of the skin. As soon as the last suture is in place, the anesthetic is reversed, and the patient is examined awake on the stretcher while still in the operating room. If the patient is neurologically intact, he or she is transferred to the recovery room.

EXTENT

The number of levels included in a laminectomy should be based on a combination of clinical and radiographic (MRI and CT) findings. It is generally accepted that all stenosis levels should be decompressed at the first surgery, because one of the most common reasons for failure is an insufficient original decompression.[54-56, 58, 59] However, Sato and Kikuchi, evaluating 81 patients with either L4-5 or L3-4–L4-5 stenosis followed an average of 4.6 years, found that only the critical, symptomatic level had to be decompressed; the other levels rarely become symptomatic.[60] This issue remains controversial.

SUCCESS

Performing a meta-analysis of 74 papers in the literature encompassing multiple surgeon-based outcome measures (e.g., Odom's criteria and Prolo and coauthors' scheme),[61] Turner and colleagues found that patients achieve good to excellent outcomes 64% to 85% of the time irrespective of the mode of lumbar decompression used (i.e., with or without fusion).[62] Deyo and coworkers also studied clinical outcomes, including morbidity, mortality, and resource utilization, in patients undergoing laminectomy with or without fusion for the management of lumbar stenosis.[63, 64] They discovered that outcomes were comparable for decompression versus decompression with fusion, but mortality was increased twofold in the geriatric population by fusion, along with an increase in morbidity (20%), blood transfusion requirements (5.4 times greater), nursing home referrals, and so forth.

Herron and Mangelsdorf performed a surgeon-based outcome study involving 140 patients averaging 63 years of age and followed an average of 42 months postoperatively. They found that leg pain improved in

82% of patients, and back pain improved in 71%.[65] Poor prognoses were observed in females, those involved in compensation claims or litigation, those with prior "failed" surgery, and those exhibiting new postoperative sensory deficits.

In Tuite and coauthors' study, the results of long-term outcome questionnaires versus the results of physical examinations by physicians were compared for 119 laminectomy patients followed an average of 4.6 years.[66] Patients rated themselves as much improved (37%), somewhat improved (29%), unchanged (17%), somewhat worse (5%), or much worse (12%). The patient-based outcomes were considerably worse than those based on physicians' assessments.

Second Operations

Operative success rates of 80% to 85% following initial decompression of lumbar stenosis (with or without fusion) deteriorate to less than 50% when secondary procedures are performed.[54-56, 63-65, 67-71] In Herno and colleagues' retrospective study of outcomes using the Oswestry questionnaire, outcomes were excellent to good in 67% of patients undergoing a single procedure, but only 46% showed comparable results after repeated procedures.[51] Poorer outcomes correlated not only with multiple procedures but also with an interval of less than 18 months between operations and the presence of significant comorbidities. Of note, the presence of severe myelographic block in multiply operated patients did not positively correlate with a better postoperative result. When Herno and colleagues next reported on 41 similarly matched pairs of patients (averaging 51 years of age and followed 4.4 to 4.6 years), results of subjective disability questionnaires confirmed that patients undergoing one operation had significantly better outcomes than those undergoing two procedures, especially when the interval between procedures was short.[53]

FREQUENCY

The frequency of secondary decompression or fusion to address recurrent stenosis or instability ranges from 9.3% to 28%.[51-53, 72-74] Among Caputy and Luessenhop's 100 patients (averaging 67 years old and followed more than 5 years), 16 demonstrated recurrent stenosis at or above previously decompressed levels.[74] Herno and colleagues found that 10 of 108 patients (9.3%) required second operations for recurrent stenosis (average 6.8-year follow-up).[32] In McCullen and coworkers' assessment of 118 patients having lumbar decompression without fusion for stenosis, 50 were examined at follow-up to determine the incidence of reoperation.[75] Only 6% of men but 28% of women required additional surgery to address recurrent stenosis with or without slip. Five of the 290 patients in my series of patients undergoing initial laminectomy for degenerative spondylolisthesis required secondary fusions because of progressive olisthy with symptomatic instability.[76]

The longer the follow-up after original decompressive laminectomy for degenerative lumbar stenosis, the higher the reoperation rate. When Katz and associates evaluated 88 consecutive patients, 6% warranted repeat surgery to address instability or recurrent stenosis within 1 year, and 15% at 3 years.[72] Comorbidities correlating with poorer long-term outcome included osteoarthritis, cardiac or pulmonary disease, rheumatoid arthritis, or previous inadequate decompression (i.e., single rather than multilevel laminectomy).

PATHOLOGY

The pathology addressed at secondary procedures for lumbar stenosis also significantly affects outcome. Jonsson and Stromqvist performed a prospective evaluation of 93 patients who had prior lumbar surgery for disk herniations (65 patients) or lumbar stenosis (28 patients).[13] The 19 patients having surgery for recurrent disk herniation and the 19 undergoing single-nerve root decompression for focal recurrent stenosis did well, while the 20 with recurrent central stenosis and the 35 with additional perineural involvement and stenosis at more cephalad or caudad levels did poorly. To determine the reasons for recurrent pain in these patients and to define the indications for additional surgery, accurate radiographic assessment with enhanced MRI studies and CT-based examinations (i.e., three-dimensional CT, CT–myelography) is critical.

Laminotomy

Unilateral Laminotomy. Unilateral laminotomy is an alternative approach to decompressing ipsilateral lumbar stenosis. Single-level stenosis can occasionally be successfully addressed using a unilateral laminotomy with bilateral ligamentectomy as described by Poletti for the management of OYL.[77] In a human cadaver model, Spetzger and coworkers performed microsurgical unilateral laminotomies to resect even diffuse stenosis, which included partial removal of the medial facet joints bilaterally and excision of the medial laminar arch and the entire ligamentum flavum.[78] Although these more restricted approaches may minimize the risk of instability, the cadaver model might not be applicable in vivo, where one would risk significant damage to the contralateral nerve root and cauda equina.

Bilateral Laminotomy (Fenestration Procedures) for Central Stenosis. In younger patients and in selected older individuals, moderate central lumbar stenosis can be managed using wide bilateral fenestration approaches over single or multiple levels.[79-84] The microsurgical fenestration technique preserves the spinous processes, interspinous ligaments, medial yellow ligaments, and lateral two thirds (weight-bearing portions) of the facet joints. Decompression of the nerve roots and cauda equina, however, extends centrally, laterally, and foraminally. In Nakai and associates' series of 34 patients with stenosis followed an average of 5.5 years after such fenestration approaches, patients demonstrated lasting symptomatic relief and new bone deposition contributing to stability but not to recurrent stenosis.[79] In Caspar and colleagues' 58 consecutive patients, the fenestration procedure provided adequate nerve root decompression while maximally preserving the overlying bone and stability.[80] Good to excellent results were achieved in 71% of patients using surgeon-based outcome measures, compared with 76% using patient-based outcome questionnaires.

Bilateral Laminotomy (Fenestration Procedures) for Lateral Recess Stenosis. Single or multilevel bilateral fenestration procedures may also be used to treat single or multilevel lateral recess stenosis.[8, 85, 86] Lateral recess compromise can be attributed to congenital stenosis, acquired spondylostenosis, OYL, disk herniation, limbus fracture, scoliosis, or degenerative slip. High-speed air drills using diamond bits (coarse or smooth) may facilitate decompression of nerve roots tethered in tight lateral recesses. In Aryanpur and Ducker's series of 32 patients with lateral recess stenosis undergoing fenestration procedures, 90% demonstrated excellent postoperative results as determined by the operating surgeon 5 years later.[85]

Trumpet Laminectomy

Routine laminectomy with bilateral medial facetectomy and foraminotomy is the primary procedure of choice in severe stenosis.[54–56] However, the trumpet laminectomy or coronal hemilaminectomy is an alternative to both the more restricted fenestration approach and the less restricted laminectomy for the management of single-level stenosis. This procedure includes removal of two thirds of the cephalad lamina and spinous process and one third to one half of the caudad lamina and spinous process. When Kanamori and coworkers compared the results of trumpet laminectomy with those of routine laminectomy (35 patients), a lower incidence of postoperative scoliosis and instability was reported over an average follow-up of 5.2 years.[87]

Expansive Laminaplasty

The expansive laminaplasty, frequently performed to decompress cervical spondylostenosis, can also be used in the lumbar spine. Tsuji and associates determined that lumbar laminaplasty provides adequate enlargement of the spinal canal, ensuring stability, and Matsui and colleagues showed that enlargement of the canal was maintained for 3 years postoperatively.[88, 89] In the latter study, noncontrast CT in 10 patients showed 119% rectangular enlargement of the spinal canal, and 73% of patients had good to excellent long-term outcomes.

DISK HERNIATION

Disk herniation accompanied lumbar stenosis in 15% of Hall's patients, 33% of Heath's patients, and 45% of my series of 857 individuals.[54–56, 58, 59] Disk herniation similarly accompanied degenerative spondylolisthesis in 4.3% of patients in Tsou and Hopp's series and in up to 20% of patients in Alexander and coauthors' study.[69, 90]

Far Lateral Pathology

The far lateral compartment, located beyond the neural foramen, is bordered superiorly by the pedicle, anteriorly by the disk, medially by the vertebral body and leading edge of the superior articular facet, and laterally by fat.[91–95] Far lateral disk herniations, constituting 7% to 12% of all disk herniations, typically migrate cranially as they extend laterally, foraminally, and far laterally. Far lateral stenosis similarly compromises the superiorly exiting nerve root in the far lateral compartment; compression may also be attributed to spondylostenosis, arthrosis, limbus vertebral fracture, olisthy with or without lysis, and scoliosis.[91–93] Far lateral disease affects the cephalad rather than caudad nerve root, most often impinging on the L4 root at the L4-5 level, followed in descending order of frequency by the L3 root at L3-4, the L5 root at L5-S1, and the L2 root at L2-3.[93] Because the majority of the far lateral compartment is located beyond the dural sleeve, MRI and CT studies often do not provide data on the far lateral pathology itself. However, CT myelography in older patients has been found to identify significant attendant stenosis warranting further decompression up to 72% of the time.[91]

Three techniques—medial facetectomy, intertransverse procedure, and full facetectomy—can be used to approach far lateral pathology.[92, 93] The medial facetectomy and foraminotomy may adequately expose the lateral neural foramen at the least stenotic level, such as L5-Sl, as long as a foraminal tail of the disk fragment is identified. The most critical limitation of this approach is the greater potential for retained far lateral sequestered fragments. The intertransverse approach requires a combined medial and far lateral exposure. Here, an interlaminar laminotomy with medial facetectomy and foraminotomy is completed first, followed by the far lateral exposure, consisting of the removal of the superolateral aspect of the facet joint while preserving the pars interarticularis. An obvious advantage of this technique is preservation of pars interarticularis stability while providing direct access to far lateral disease and avoiding retained fragments medially in the foramen. Finally, the full facetectomy allows one to handle the most stenotic or spondyloarthrotic canal, greatly simplifying the anatomy and limiting the risk of inadvertent damage to the nerve root within a stenotic neural foramen. However, this increases the risk of instability.[92, 93, 95]

Author's Series of Far Lateral Disk Surgery

Between 1984 and 1994, surgery was performed on 170 of my patients with far lateral disk herniations or stenosis.[93] Patients averaged 55 years old and included 112 males and 58 females. Neurological findings included ipsilateral knee contracture (143 patients), positive Lasègue's maneuvers (159 patients), positive femoral stretch tests (145 patients), and focal motor deficits (126 patients). MRI and CT studies confirmed 68 far lateral disk herniations at L4-5, 63 at L3-4, 33 at L5-S1, 4 at L2-3, and 2 at L1-2. Diffuse stenosis was demonstrated in 36 patients, and lateral recess stenosis in 134. Far lateral stenosis complicated the surgery for far lateral disk herniations in 30 cases, and another 23 individuals demonstrated degenerative spondylolisthesis. Patients with more severe stenosis typically required full facetectomy, whereas those with less severe stenosis could be managed with the intertransverse or medial facetectomy procedures.[92, 93]

The surgeon's assessment of outcome, using Odom's criteria, revealed excellent results in 73 patients, good results in 51, fair results in 26, and poor results in 20.[94] Of greatest interest was the notation that the type and extent of facet resection did not significantly impact outcome: good to excellent results were achieved in 79% of patients having intertransverse approaches, 70% having full facetectomy, and 68% undergoing medial facetectomy. Similar outcomes were encountered following routine disk surgery in An and coworkers' study of routine disk herniations, as well as in other far lateral disk series.[96–98]

Fusion Requirements in Far Lateral Disk Surgery

Few patients undergoing far lateral disk surgery, even those having a full facetectomy, warrant secondary fusion. Only 4 of the 170 patients (2.4%) undergoing far lateral disk surgery in my series required secondary fusion.[93] Of note, all 4 patients became unstable following L4-5 laminectomy for decompression of stenosis accompanied by grade I olisthy and unilateral L4-5 full facetectomy for excision of foraminal and far lateral disk herniations with stenosis. Instrumented fusions using pedicle screws and rods successfully managed the resultant spinal instability. In Garrido and Connaughton's series of 41 full facetectomies in patients having far lateral disk surgery, only 1 patient (2.4%) required subsequent fusion.[95]

Outcome of Far Lateral Disk Surgery

A long-term surgeon and patient-based outcome study involved 76 of my original 170 patients (45%) having far lateral disk surgery from 1984 to 1994. Outcomes were assessed by the surgeon using Odom's criteria, and the patients filled out the Medical Outcomes Trust SF-36 questionnaire. When the follow-up interval between surgery and the surgeon's last assessment was less than 4.5 years, surgeon and SF-36 outcomes were most closely correlated, especially on Physical Function, Role Physical, and Bodily Pain scales. Such outcome-based studies may significantly contribute to future medical and surgical policy-making decisions and should be integrated into future studies.

LIMBUS VERTEBRAL FRACTURE

Four types of limbus vertebral fractures may accompany lumbar stenosis.[99–102] Type I fractures include a curvilinear posterior shelf of cortical bone. The remaining three types include both cortical and cancellous bone, with type II fractures occurring centrally; type III fractures occurring laterally, foraminally, and far laterally; and type IV fractures extending from one interspace to the next. Type I, II, and IV fractures contribute to cauda equina compression, and types I, III, and IV produce radiculopathy.

These lesions should be identified with a combination of MRI and CT-based examinations.[99–102] Whereas MRI delineates soft tissue compression and occasionally the marrow associated with the cancellous element of the limbus fracture, the CT evaluation, particularly on 1-mm cuts, directly defines the full extent of the calcific pathology.

Limbus fractures typically require extensive decompression to facilitate resection and avoid contributing to a postoperative cauda equina syndrome. Laminectomy or coronal hemilaminectomy can address type I, II, and IV lesions contributing to cauda equina compression, thus facilitating exposure of the thecal sac and bilaterally exiting nerve roots. Alternatively, ipsilateral hemilaminectomies are required for lateral type III lesions involving the cephalad or caudad vertebral limbus, which brings pathology to the superior or inferior midpedicular level. Once exposed, limbus fractures can be excised in a piecemeal fashion, avoiding undue retraction, with a down-biting curet, tamp, and mallet technique.

DEGENERATIVE SPONDYLOLISTHESIS WITH AN INTACT NEURAL ARCH

Cause. The lumbar spine, particularly the L4-5 level, is uniquely predisposed to olisthy when the facet joints are congenitally oriented sagittally rather than coronally. Progressive arthrosis of these facets leads to a typical 25% olisthy; the ultimate locking mechanism resisting further slip is the hugely hypertrophied posterior facet joints. In contrast, L5-S1 remains stable, rarely demonstrating olisthy, because it is typically below the intercrestal line, where greater support is afforded by longer transverse processes and the iliotransverse ligaments.

Mechanism of Stenosis. The progressive scissoring, leading to both cauda equina and nerve root compression, that occurs with grade I olisthy is further complicated by the intrusion of markedly hypertrophied facet joints. The slip itself leads to ventral compression, and the enlarged facet joints contribute to dorsolateral intrusion on the thecal sac and superiorly exiting nerve root as it extends foraminally and far laterally. Simultaneously, the inferiorly exiting root may be compromised by a hypertrophied yellow ligament, congenitally or developmentally narrowed lateral recess, and additional arthrotic spurs. Disk herniations, reported in up to 20% to 45% of patients with olisthy, add to nerve root compromise.

Clinical Presentation. Most patients presenting with

degenerative spondylolisthesis with an intact neural arch are women in their 50s to 80s.[54–56, 76, 103–108] The female-to-male ratio varies from 2:1 to 10:1, and patients average 67 years old (range, 38 to 82 years). Although symptoms may evolve over several months to decades, patients initially present with neurogenic claudication followed by radiculopathy, with only half exhibiting minor, late neurological signs. Later in the course of the disease, motor and sensory complaints become more prominent, in the relative absence of mechanical findings.

Levels of Olisthy. Degenerative spondylolisthesis is an acquired variant of lumbar stenosis typically found at the L4-5 level, followed in descending order of frequency at the L3-4, L2-3, and L5-S1 interspaces.[54–56, 76, 103–108]

In my 1983 series of 60 patients with degenerative spondylolisthesis, 56 had disease at L4-5, 2 at L3-4, and 2 at L5-S1.[107] As noted in my 1998 series of 290 patients with degenerative spondylolisthesis, 86% of patients had olisthy at one level: 214 had a slip at L4-5, 20 at L3-4, and 16 at L5-S1.[76] Two-level olisthy was found in the remaining 14% of patients: 34 at both the L3-4 and L4-5 levels, 5 at L4-5 and L5-S1, and 1 at L2-3 and L4-5.

Surgery for Olisthy. For patients with "stable" degenerative spondylolisthesis without an active slip of greater than 4 mm or greater than 10 to 12 degrees of angulation, laminectomy alone is appropriate; the secondary fusion rate for instability is less than 10%.[76, 103–108]

Younger patients with moderate focal stenosis may be managed with fenestration procedures, such as Getty and associates' partial undercutting facetectomy or diPierro and colleagues' procedure consisting of unilateral decompression and contralateral fusion.[86, 109] Of my 290 patients with olisthy, 41 were managed with the fenestration technique, addressing an average of 1.7 levels of olisthy and 3.2 levels of stenosis.[76] Successful long-term outcomes (average 5-year follow-up) have been reported with fenestration procedures, and new bone deposition fails to contribute to significant recurrent stenosis.

Older patients with olisthy and more severe spondylostenosis are more safely managed with laminectomy or coronal hemilaminectomy.[110] In my 1983 study of 60 patients with olisthy and stenosis, 40 had multilevel laminectomies, 14 had coronal hemilaminectomies, and only 6 had fenestration procedures.[107] In my more recent study, 249 of the 290 patients with stenosis and olisthy were treated with laminectomy over an average of 3.4 levels.[76]

Disk Herniation in Conjunction with Olisthy. Disk herniations accompany olisthy 4.3% to 20% of the time, compared with a 15% to 45% frequency seen with routine spinal stenosis.[54–56, 76, 103–108] Twenty percent of my 290 patients with olisthy demonstrated disk herniation; 47 patients had routine extruded or sequestered disks, and in 12 patients the herniated disk was located foraminally or far laterally.[76]

Unique Surgical Considerations Associated with Olisthy. Removal of the diving lamina at the olisthetic level is greatly facilitated by a diamond bur, which avoids placing a Kerrison punch under a stenosing lamina. Great attention is paid to preserving the facet joints at the level of maximal slip. More extensive foraminal stenosis magnified by the slip warrants decompression using an undercutting technique. Portions of the leading edge of the inferior vertebral body may have to be tamped down or resected along with the most inferior aspect of the pedicle to facilitate nerve root and thecal sac decompression. Instability may be minimized by limiting contralateral foraminal decompression or by the presence of preexisting intervertebral fusion.

New and Increased Olisthy Following Laminectomy. Following laminectomy for stenosis with olisthy, further progression of olisthy is not necessarily symptomatic and often does not warrant a second surgery.[65, 76, 111–114] Shenkin and Nash observed that among 59 patients with stenosis managed with laminectomy and full bilateral facetectomy, 10% demonstrated slip progression, but only 3.3% warranted secondary fusion.[111] Herron and Mangelsdorf observed that 83% of patients undergoing laminectomy for stenosis and olisthy did well without fusion, despite the mild progression of slip over 1.5 years.[65] Similarly, Johnsson and colleagues' patients with preoperative stenosis and olisthy showed an increase in postoperative slip but remained symptom free.[113, 114] In my series of 290 patients with stenosis and a degenerative slip, only 4 (2.4%) warranted secondary fusion for gross instability following L4-5 laminectomy with full unilateral facetectomy for far lateral disk excision.[76]

Fusion Requirements for Degenerative Spondylolisthesis

Criteria for Instability. Lumbar instability measured on flexion and extension lateral radiographs is defined by greater than 4 mm of translation (8%) or greater than 10 to 12 degrees of angular displacement.[21, 22, 115] The determination of instability using these criteria may well lead to fusion. Nevertheless, in Turner and coauthors' meta-analysis of the stenosis literature, including olisthy, 64% of patients showed excellent results irrespective of whether fusion accompanied laminectomy.[62]

Fusion Required to Address Secondary Unstable Olisthy. Only 8 (2.8%) of my 290 patients with degenerative spondylolisthesis presenting without instability and treated originally with laminectomy later required secondary fusion. Five with instability associated with increased olisthy (new in four patients, old in one) and three others exhibiting new disk herniations and more cephalad stenosis (two patients) or recurrent stenosis (one patient) warranted secondary fusion.[76]

Outcome of Laminectomy without Fusion. Between 69% and 85% of patients undergoing initial laminectomy for stenosis with olisthy do well.[54–56, 62–64, 76, 103–108, 115–117] Among Nasca's 80 patients, 71% with degenerative spondylolisthesis showed excellent results up to 5 years after laminectomy.[116] Silvers and coworkers noted that 75% of 258 patients undergoing decompression for stenosis with or without a degenerative slip had achieved good to excellent results after an average of 4.7 years.[117] When Prolo's outcome scale was applied to the 290 patients with olisthy in my series, 69% of patients showed excellent, 13% good, 12% fair, and 6% poor postoperative results over an average 10-year follow-up period.[61, 76]

Fusion Required to Address Original Unstable Olisthy. Carefully selected patients demonstrating significant instability before surgery for olisthy may warrant primary laminectomy with fusion. In all 28 of my patients with spinal stenosis and unstable olisthy, laminectomy was accompanied by instrumented fusion.[115] Patients averaged 64 years of age and included 13 males and 15 females followed for an average of 38 months. Grade I slips were observed in 25 patients, and grade II olisthy in 3. Patients had an average of four levels of stenosis. Disk herniations were encountered in 16 patients—at the level of olisthy in 11, far laterally in 4, and foraminal in 1. In this series, all levels decompressed were simultaneously fused using the Texas Scottish Rite Hospital pedicle rod system, supplemented with autologous iliac crest bone graft to avoid instability adjacent to a prior fusion. Outcomes rated using Prolo's economic and functional scale were categorized as excellent in 71%, good in 14%, fair in 11%, and poor in 4% of patients. Note that these results are comparable to those observed for patients with olisthy who were managed with laminectomy alone.

Advocating more universal fusion for patients with degenerative spondylolisthesis with or without demonstrated motion, Bolesta and Bohlman presumptively and primarily performed decompression and posterolateral fusion, believing that the slip would progress without stabilization.[106] Further evaluating the role of primary fusion for the management of olisthy, Herkowitz and Kurz prospectively studied 50 patients with olisthy treated with laminectomy alone (25 patients) or laminectomy with fusion (25 patients).[118] They too concluded that fused patients were less symptomatic an average of 3 years after surgery.

Outcome of Laminectomy with Fusion. Some have determined that patients with lumbar stenosis and "unstable" olisthy do best when simultaneous fusion is performed.[106, 118, 119] Postacchini and Cinotti's 10 patients undergoing decompression with fusion for olisthy exhibited less bony regrowth and better outcomes over 8.6 postoperative years compared with 6 patients having decompression alone.[82] Colemont and colleagues observed an initial 84% rate of good to excellent results 6 months after laminectomy with fusion but saw this rate decline to 56% due to further slip progression.[120]

Careful patient selection for laminectomy with fusion for unstable olisthy is critical in the geriatric population. In Deyo and coworkers' series, 43% of patients warranting fusion were older than 65 years, placing them at greater risk for peri- and postoperative compli-

cations, including double the mortality rate for fusion than for laminectomy alone.[63, 64]

SPONDYLOLISTHESIS WITH LYSIS

Posterior or anterior fusion or both may be warranted for the management of isthmic spondylolisthesis. Markwalder and colleagues employed microsurgical decompression and Louis plate fixation for grade I olisthy and the Cotrel-Dubousset pedicle screw system for grade II lesions in 72 patients; excellent results were achieved in 82% of patients, good results in 14%, and poor results in 4%.[121] Boos and associates, treating a similar population with the Cotrel-Dubousset pedicle screw-rod system and following those patients for 25 months, observed a 76% rate of good to excellent clinical response and a 96% rate of solid fusion.[122] Kim and Kim noted that 87% of patients undergoing anterior interbody fusion showed good to excellent outcomes 1 year after surgery.[123]

Although younger, unstable patients with spondylolisthesis and lysis typically warrant laminectomy with fusion, older individuals with spinal stenosis, listhesis, and lysis may not necessarily require fusion.[54–56] Many of these older individuals can be adequately managed with laminectomy alone, showing no significant postoperative progression of listhesis accompanying their lytic defects.

DEGENERATIVE SCOLIOSIS

Degenerative scoliosis is characterized by a rotational and conformational narrowing of the spinal canal attributed to degenerative changes.[54–56] This results in the progressive loss of alignment and may lead to laminectomy with facetectomy or foraminotomy, particularly on the concave side of the curve, where profuse spondyloarthrotic changes extensively narrow the foramina and exiting nerve roots. Many older patients with severe multilevel stenosis and scoliosis can be managed with laminectomy alone. However, Simmons and Simmons and others believe in performing simultaneous instrumented fusions, achieving postoperative pain relief in 93% of patients over an average follow-up of 44 months.[124–126]

FUSION FOR SPINAL STENOSIS

Age-Related Risk Factors. Younger patients with preoperative instability typically warrant simultaneous fusion. However, fusion for geriatric patients carries higher morbidity and mortality rates.[63, 64] Most important, reoperation and failure rates were unchanged by the performance of these high-risk fusions.[62, 127]

Low Incidence of Postlaminectomy Instability. Postlaminectomy instability rarely warrants secondary fusion; the frequency varies from 0.8% to 4.6%.[69, 76, 111, 117] Further, the more levels decompressed, the greater the frequency of olisthy. Decompression of two or fewer levels is associated with a 6% incidence of slip, increasing to 15% for three or more levels.[111]

Arguments for and against Primary Fusion for Stenosis. Some authors report a high (13% to 43%) frequency of biomechanical postlaminectomy instability warranting secondary fusion, as well as the poor clinical outcome observed in nonfused patients.[103–106, 128–131] Nevertheless, fusion failures must also be considered, including a 27.3% rate of pseudarthrosis and a 13% to 18% frequency of slip progression.[129] CT abnormalities found in Laasonen and Soini's 48 patients with recurrent symptoms following lumbar fusion for stenosis included 16 fusion mass fractures, 9 hairline pseudarthroses, and 8 instances of recurrrent stenosis, all of which contributed to a 42% reoperation rate.[29]

Fusion Techniques

Determinants of Fusion. Many studies fail to identify any real indications for the performance of lumbar fusion following laminectomy for stenosis.[62, 72, 73, 117] Therefore, Katz and colleagues designed a prospective multicenter study to identify how the decision to fuse is made.[73] In their study, 272 patients having surgery (laminectomy versus laminectomy and fusion) by eight surgeons in four centers were examined using satisfaction questionnaires obtained 6 and 24 months postoperatively. Of these patients, 37 had noninstrumented fusion and 41 had instrumented fusion. The major predictor of whether a fusion was performed was the individual surgeon ($P = 0.0001$). Noninstrumented fusion was associated with better relief of low back pain at 6 and 24 months but showed borderline significance. There were no other significant differences across management groups.

Bilateral Intertransverse Process Fusions. Bilateral intertransverse process fusion was the most commonly performed fusion before the availability of instrumentation techniques. In Brodsky's 32-year review of 184 patients treated with L4-5 floating fusions for disk disease and instability, 83.7% showed excellent to good outcomes, 79% demonstrated fusion, and only 2.7% developed new L5-S1 disk herniations mandating excision and fusion to the sacrum.[70]

Posterior Lumbar Interbody Fusion without Supplemental Instrumentation. Posterior lumbar interbody fusion (PLIF), a less common alternative to posterolateral fusion, requires a complete diskectomy with intracanalicular fusion. Cloward,[71] among others, advocated noninstrumented PLIF for the treatment of disk herniation or single-level instability.[132, 133] Mitsunaga and coworkers similarly used microscopically assisted PLIF to achieve successful fusion in patients with spondylolisthesis or chronic low back pain.[132] However, complications included graft expulsion and cauda equina or nerve root compression, particularly with noninstrumented PLIF. In Wetzel and LaRocca's series, 37 procedures were completed in 12 patients; "failure" of PLIF was attributed to marked epidural fibrosis in 11 cases, pseudarthrosis in 9, and instability at nearby levels in 4.[133]

INSTRUMENTATION TECHNIQUES

Pedicle Screw-Rod Fixation

Markwalder prospectively compared the results of translaminar screw, pedicle screw-plates, and pedicle screw-rod fusion techniques in 100 patients undergoing lumbar decompression and fusion for stenosis with degenerative spondylolisthesis.[134] The best surgical results were achieved with the pedicle screw-rod system, with patients demonstrating overall excellent (91%), good (4%), fair (2%), and poor (1%) results over an average follow-up of 2.9 years.

Pedicle rod fixation is indicated for the management of lumbar stenosis, as well as for fractures, failed fusions, spondylolisthesis, and failed back syndrome. It offers the advantage of immediate stabilization, along with higher rates of fusion, easy contouring, and more available space for bone graft compared with pedicle screw-plate systems in particular.[135–137] Marchesi and colleagues cited an 88% rate of good to excellent results for these fusions, plus a low 6% pseudarthrosis rate.[138] Whitecloud and associates observed a somewhat lower 62.5% rate of good to excellent results; a 29% complication rate was seen in de novo cases, but this rose to 63% for reoperations.[135]

Pedicle screw placement carries its own risks and complications.[136–140] Weinstein and coworkers reported a 21% incidence of inaccurate screw placement in cadavers.[139] In vivo, Matsuzaki and colleagues documented that 11% of patients exhibited new postoperative motor deficits and 3.5% had new sensory deficits; screw breakage occurred 5.7% of the time in 21% of patients.[140] McAfee and coauthors similarly observed a 4.18% screw complication rate.[136]

Other complications associated with rigid internal fixation using pedicle screw-rod systems include an increased incidence of adjacent disease. Etebar and Cahill followed 125 consecutive patients undergoing instrumented fusion for degenerative instability and found that 18 (14.4%) developed next-segment degeneration at previously asymptomatic levels over an interval of 44.8 months.[141] Adjacent segment disease included spondylolisthesis (39%), spinal stenosis with or without disk herniation (33%), stress fracture of adjacent vertebrae (28%), and scoliosis (17%).

Another consideration is whether the addition of instrumentation to these fusions improves postoperative outcome. Mullin and associates observed a 54% rate of postlaminectomy instability in patients undergoing decompression for stenosis alone: 62% of these patients required aid in walking.[142] According to Katz and colleagues' findings, patients undergoing noninstrumented fusion demonstrated better symptomatic relief 6 and 24 months postoperatively compared with those having laminectomy alone or instrumented fusion.[73] Additionally, a laminectomy alone cost $12,615, a laminectomy with noninstrumented fusion cost $18,495, and laminectomy with instrumented fusion cost $25,914. McCulloch, evaluating 21 patients undergoing microsurgical decompression and single-level noninstrumented fusion for spinal canal stenosis with degenerative spondylolisthesis, found that 86% of patients were satisfied.[143] Nork and coworkers used an SF-36 survey and functional questionnaire to retrospectively analyze 30 patients with degenerative spondylolisthesis who had undergone instrumented fusion. They found a 90% satisfaction rate with 93% successful fusion; only three patients required secondary surgery for pseudarthrosis (two patients) and a deep infection (one patient).[144]

Anterior Fusion

Anterior interbody fusion is an alternative to the posterior management of instability in patients with spinal stenosis.[125, 145] In 75 patients with grade I to III spondylolisthesis (involving the L5 body in 55% of cases), Kim and Kim observed a 77% frequency of successful anterior fusion and an 87% frequency of excellent or good clinical outcome.[123] Similarly, Kostuik and Matsusaki successfully treated patients with late post-traumatic thoracic or thoracolumbar kyphosis using anterior fusion techniques; pain relief was seen in nearly 100% of those with spinal stenosis.[145] BAK cages, Z-plates, and other instrumentation devices are alternatives to supplement anterior lumbar fusion.

SUCCESS WITH AND WITHOUT FUSION

Success without Fusion

Success rates following decompressions for lumbar stenosis without fusion vary from 80% to 96%. Alexander and colleagues quoted a 91% rate of good to excellent results at 3 years and an 87% rate at 6 years for 50 patients with degenerative spondylolisthesis treated with laminectomy and facetectomy.[90] Hall and associates noted an 84% success rate following decompression for stenosis in 68 patients after 4 years.[58] Similarly, in Mauersberger and Nietgen's series, 80% of those with lumbar stenosis improved with laminectomy alone.[146]

When patient outcome measures are added to surgeon-based assessments, the quality of outcomes is more variable. Using the Oswestry disability questionnaire in 438 patients who had undergone laminectomy for lumbar stenosis 4.3 years earlier, Airaksinen and coworkers found that only 62% of women and 57% of men reported good to excellent results; poor prognostic factors included diabetes, hip joint arthrodesis, and preoperative spinal fracture.[147] Guigui and associates found that among 50 patients having laminectomy for stenosis and followed for an average of 38 months, 42 had good to excellent results and 8 had fair results; here, favorable prognostic factors for motor recovery included the presence of a herniated disk, stenosis at one level, preoperative weakness of less than 6 weeks' duration, age younger than 65 years, and monoradicular deficit.[148] When examining outcomes following 50 microscopic laminotomies for degenerative spinal stenosis, Tsai and coauthors observed a close correlation

between surgeon and patient-based outcome measures: the surgeon reported 34 good to excellent, 8 fair, and 8 poor outcomes, whereas 30 patients were very satisfied, 10 were somewhat satisfied, and 10 were very dissatisfied.[149]

However, success rates following laminectomy alone deteriorated with time. In Katz and associates' series, 6% of patients required second operations within the first postoperative year, and within 3 years, 15% of patients required secondary surgery for combinations of instability and stenosis.[72] Poor prognostic factors positively correlated with an increased reoperation rate included osteoarthritis, cardiovascular or pulmonary disease, rheumatoid arthritis, and initial procedures restricted to only one interspace.

Success with Fusion

Some authors advocate primary fusion for lumbar stenosis, particularly degenerative spondylolisthesis.[105, 106, 115, 118, 121, 122, 128, 129] Lombardi and colleagues noted a 90% rate of good to excellent results following intertransverse process fusion without instrumentation, compared with an 80% rate of good results following laminectomy and a 33% rate of good results after laminectomy with complete facetectomy.[105] In Louis and Nazarian's series of 350 patients with spinal stenosis, 65% of those having decompressions alone did well, but 85% who were simultaneously fused enjoyed the best outcomes.[14]

Prophylactic extension of decompression to adjacent levels of stenosis and primary fusion in selected patients, especially those with spondylolisthesis, are recommended by some. Caputy and Luessenhop's 5-year evaluation of patients undergoing decompressive laminectomies alone revealed an initial 27% failure rate, which, if projected over a lifetime, could approach 50%.[74] Half the failures were associated with recurrent stenosis observed at previously operated sites, and the other half were associated with new neurological deficits attributed to adjacent stenosis.

SURGICAL COMPLICATIONS

Age-Related Complications without and with Fusion. Geriatric patients (older than 70 to 75 years) with lumbar stenosis and no significant comorbidities who are managed with laminectomy alone do not experience significantly increased morbidity and mortality compared with their younger counterparts. Quigley and coworkers found that the surgical outcome of laminectomy alone was not uniquely impacted by age: at the end of nearly 3 years, 66.6% of patients had no or minimal symptoms, and 77.3% enjoyed good postoperative outcomes.[150] However, laminectomy with fusion in this same geriatric population—often for identical preoperative indications—resulted in a twofold greater mortality rate and an 18% higher morbidity rate.[63, 64]

Patient Selection. Poor outcomes are most clearly correlated with poor patient selection and inadequate decompression for lumbar spinal stenosis. Criteria that should be met include documentation of significant neurogenic claudication, clear-cut radiographic evidence of severe lumbar stenosis, and performance of an adequately extensive lumbar laminectomy. Patients with vague complaints of back pain without clear neurological deficits or neurodiagnostic abnormalities, or those involved in compensation cases or litigation, do not make good surgical candidates.[112] Morbidity also significantly increases with the number of major medical comorbidities, particularly cardiovascular or pulmonary disease, diabetes, and hypertension.

Cerebrospinal Fluid Fistulas. Cerebrospinal fluid fistulas occur during 5% of primary and 10% of secondary decompressions, with or without fusion, for lumbar spinal stenosis.[54-56] Other sources of cerebrospinal fluid may include a prior lumbar puncture (i.e., myelogram) or a dural defect due to OYL or a prior fusion. Direct watertight dural repair is critical to avoiding future wound breakdown. Dural repairs are greatly facilitated by use of the operating microscope, particularly in larger patients with deeper wounds. One may use 7–0 Gore-Tex suture or the microdural titanium stapler (1.4-mm staples). The Gore-Tex suture, which is larger than the needle and therefore not a nidus of increased leakage, may be applied in an interrupted fashion. Next, sutures are used to elevate and evert the dural edges, allowing for staple placement. More complex dural defects require bovine pericardial grafts or rotation muscle flaps. Supplementing dural repairs with fibrin sealant (not fibrin glue) is critical to increase the strength of the closure.

REFERENCES

1. Verbiest H: A radicular syndrome from developmental narrowing of the lumbar vertebral canal. J Bone Joint Surg Br 36:230–237, 1954.
2. Verbiest H: Neurogenic intermittent claudication in cases with absolute and relative stenosis of the lumbar vertebral canal (ASLC, RSLC) in cases with narrow lumbar intervertebral foramina, and in cases with both entities. Clin Neurosurg 20:204–210, 1972.
3. Verbiest H: Results of surgical treatment of idiopathic developmental stenosis of the lumbar vertebral canal: A review of 27 years experience. J Bone Joint Surg Br 59:181–188, 1977.
4. Verbiest H: Introduction: Spinal stenosis. In Hopp E (ed): Spine: State of the Art Reviews. Philadelphia, Hanley & Belfus, 1987, pp 361–368.
5. Epstein JA, Malis LI: Compression of spinal cord and cauda equina in achondroplastic dwarfs. Neurology 5:875–881, 1955.
6. Epstein JA, Epstein BS, Rosenthal AD, et al: Sciatica caused by nerve root entrapment in the lateral recess: The superior facet syndrome. J Neurosurg 36:584–589, 1972.
7. Epstein JA, Epstein BS, Lavine LS, et al: Lumbar nerve root compression at the intervertebral foramina caused by arthritis of the posterior facets. J Neurosurg 39:362–369, 1973.
8. Getty CJM: Lumbar spinal stenosis: The clinical spectrum and the results of operation. J Bone Joint Surg Br 62:481–485, 1980.
9. Hogan QH: Lumbar epidural anatomy: A new look by cryomicrotome section. Anesthesiology 75:767–775, 1991.
10. Tarlov IM: Spinal perineurial and meningeal cysts. J Neurol Neurosurg Psychiatry 33:833–843, 1970.
11. Delamarter RB, Bohlman HH, Dodge LD, et al: Experimental lumbar spinal stenosis: Analysis of the cortical evoked potentials, microvasculature, and histopathology. J Bone Joint Surg Am 72:110–120, 1990.
12. Watanabe R, Park WW: Vascular and neural pathology of lumbosacral spinal stenosis. J Neurosurg 64:64–70, 1986.
13. Jonsson B, Stromqvist B: Symptoms and signs in degeneration of the lumbar spine: A prospective, consecutive study of 300 operated patients. J Bone Joint Surg Br 75:381–385, 1993.
14. Louis R, Nazarian SL: Lumbar stenosis surgery: The experience of the orthopaedic surgeon. Chir Organi Mov 77:23–29, 1992.
15. Lemaire JJ, Sautreaux JL, Chabannes J, et al: Lumbar canal stenosis: Retrospective study of 158 operated cases. Neurochirurgie 41:89–97, 1995.
16. Rosomoff H, Rosomoff RS: Nonsurgical aggressive treatment of lumbar spinal stenosis. In Hopp E (ed): Spine: State of the Art Reviews. Philadelphia, Hanley & Belfus, 1987, pp 583–600.
17. Verbiest H: Stenosis of the lumbar vertebral canal and sciatica. Neurosurg Rev 3:75–89, 1980.
18. Epstein JA, Epstein BS, Lavine L: Nerve root compression associated with narrowing of the lumbar spinal canal. J Neurol Neurosurg Psychiatry 25:165–170, 1962.
19. Deen HG Jr, Zimmerman BS, Swanson SK, et al: Assessment of bladder function after lumbar decompressive laminectomy for spinal stenosis: A prospective study. J Neurosurg 80:971–974, 1994.
20. Elster AD: Bertolotti's syndrome revisited: Transitional vertebrae of the lumbar spine. Spine 14:1373–1377, 1989.
21. Amundsen T, Seber H, Lileas F, et al: Lumbar spinal stenosis: Clinical and radiographic features. Spine 20:1178–1186, 1995.
22. Wood KB, Popp CA, Transfeldt EE, et al: Radiographic evaluation of instability in spondylolisthesis. Spine 19:1697–1703, 1994.
23. Dvorak J, Panjabi MM, Novotny JE, et al: Clinical validation of functional flexion-extension roentgenograms of the lumbar spine. Spine 16:943–950, 1991.
24. Sano S, Yukukura S, Nagata Y, et al: Unstable lumbar spine without hypermobility in postlaminectomy cases: Mechanism of symptoms and effect of spinal fusion with and without spinal instrumentation. Spine 15:1190–1197, 1990.
25. Boden SD, Davis DO, Dina TS, et al: Abnormal magnetic-resonance scans of the lumbar spine in asymptomatic subjects: A prospective investigation. J Bone Joint Surg Am 72:403–408, 1990.
26. Jia LS, Shi ZR: MRI and myelography in the diagnosis of lumbar canal stenosis and disc herniation: A comparative study. Chin Med J 104:303–306, 1991.
27. Ross JS, Modic MI: Current assessment of spinal degenerative disease with magnetic resonance imaging. Clin Orthop 279:68–81, 1992.
28. Djukic S, Lang P, Morris J, et al: The postoperative spine: Magnetic resonance imaging. Orthop Clin North Am 21:603–624, 1990.
29. Laasonen EM, Soini J: Low-back pain after lumbar fusion: Surgical and computed tomographic analysis. Spine 14:210–213, 1989.
30. Annertz M, Holtas S, Cronqvist S, et al: Isthmic lumbar spondylolisthesis with sciatica: MR imaging vs. myelography. Acta Radiol 31:449–453, 1990.
31. Giles LG, Kaveri MJ: Some osseous and soft tissue causes of human intervertebral canal (foramen) stenosis. J Rheumatol 17:1474–1481, 1990.
32. Herno A, Airaksinen O, Saari T: Long-term results of surgical treatment of lumbar spinal stenosis. Spine 18:1471–1474, 1993.
33. Herno A, Airaksinen O, Saari T: Computed tomography after laminectomy for lumbar spinal stenosis: Patients' pain patterns, walking capacity, and subjective disability had no correlation with computed tomographic findings. Spine 19:1975–1978, 1994.
34. Herno A, Airaksinen O, Saari T, et al: The predictive value of preoperative myelography in lumbar spinal stenosis. Spine 19:1335–1338, 1994.
35. Gepstein R, Brown MD: Somatosensory evoked potentials in lumbar nerve root decompression. Clin Orthop 245:69–71, 1989.
36. Epstein NE, Epstein JA, Carras R, et al: Coexisting cervical and lumbar spinal stenosis: Diagnosis and management. Neurosurgery 15:489–496, 1984.
37. Epstein N, Schwall G: Thoracic spinal stenosis: Diagnostic treatment challenges. J Spinal Disord 7:259–269, 1994.
38. Epstein N: Clinical opinion: Thoracic ossification of the posterior longitudinal ligament, ossification of the yellow ligament from T9-T12 with superimposed acute T10-T11 disc herniation:

Controversies in surgical management. J Spinal Disord 9:446–450, 1996.

39. Barnett GH, Hardy RW, Little JR, et al: Thoracic spinal canal stenosis. J Neurosurg 66:338–344, 1987.

40. Marzluff JM, Hunderford GH, Kempe LG: Thoracic myelopathy caused by osteophytes of the articular processes. J Neurosurg 50:779–783, 1979.

41. Okada K, Oka S, Tohge K, et al: Thoracic myelopathy caused by ossification of the ligamentum flavum: Clinicopathologic study and surgical treatment. Spine 16:280–287, 1991.

42. Postacchini F, Gumina S, Cinotti G, et al: Ligamenta flava in lumbar disc herniation and spinal stenosis: Light and electron microscopic morphology. Spine 19:917–922, 1994.

43. Baba H, Maezawa Y, Furusawa N, et al: The role of calcium deposition in the ligamentum flavum causing a cauda equina syndrome and lumbar radiculopathy. Paraplegia 33:219–223, 1995.

44. Epstein NE: Ossification of the yellow ligament and spondylosis and/or ossification of the posterior longitudinal ligament of the thoracic and lumbar spine. J Spinal Disord 12:250–256, 1999.

45. Epstein N, Hollingsworth R, Carras R: Acute paraplegia due to ossification of the yellow ligament (OYL) in the thoracic spine: A case report. Neuro-Orthopedics 16:93–101, 1994.

46. D'Agostino AN, Mason MS, Quinn SF: Lumbar spinal stenosis and spondylosis associated with amyloid deposition in the ligamentum flavum. Clin Neuropathol 11:146–150, 1992.

47. Leroux JL, Legeron P, Moulinier L, et al: Stenosis of the lumbar spinal canal in vertebral ankylosing hyperostosis. Spine 18:2368–2369, 1993.

48. Cinotti G, Postacchini F, Weinstein JN: Lumbar spinal stenosis and diabetes: Outcome of surgical decompression. J Bone Joint Surg Br 76:215–219, 1994.

49. Simpson JM, Silveri CP, Balderston RA, et al: The results of operations on the lumbar spine in patients who have diabetes mellitus. J Bone Joint Surg Am 75:1823–1829, 1993.

50. Onel D, Sari H, Donmez C: Lumbar spinal stenosis: Clinical/radiologic therapeutic evaluation in 145 patients. Conservative treatment or surgical intervention? Spine 18:291–298, 1993.

51. Herno A, Airaksinen O, Saari T, et al: Surgical results of lumbar spinal stenosis: A comparison of patients with or without previous back surgery. Spine 20:964–969, 1995.

52. Herno A, Airaksinen O, Saari T, et al: Lumbar spinal stenosis: A matched-pair study of operated and non-operated patients. Br J Neurosurg 10:461–465, 1996.

53. Herno A, Airaksinen O, Saari T, et al: The effect of prior back surgery on surgical outcome in patients operated on for lumbar spinal stenosis: A matched-pair study. Acta Neurochir (Wien) 138:357–363, 1996.

54. Epstein NE, Epstein JA: Surgery for spinal stenosis. In Wiesel SW, Weinstein JN, Herkowitz H, et al (eds): The Lumbar Spine, vol 2, 2nd ed. Philadelphia, WB Saunders, 1995, pp 737–756.

55. Epstein NE, Epstein JA: Lumbar spinal stenosis. In Julian R (ed): Neurological Surgery, vol 3, 4th ed. Philadelphia WB Saunders, 1996, pp 2390–2415.

56. Epstein NE, Epstein JA: Lumbar decompression for spinal stenosis: Surgical indications and techniques with and without fusion. In Frymoyer JW (ed): The Adult Spine: Principles and Practice, vol 2, 2nd ed. New York, Lippincott-Raven, 1997, pp 2055–2088.

57. Montalvo BM, Quencer RM, Brown MD, et al: Lumbar disk herniation and canal stenosis: Value of intraoperative sonography in diagnosis and surgical management. AJR Am J Roentgenol 154:821–830, 1990.

58. Hall S, Bartelson JD, Onofrio BM, et al: Spinal stenosis: Clinical features, diagnostic procedures, and results of surgical treatment in 68 patients. Ann Intern Med 103:271–275, 1985.

59. Heath JM: The clinical presentation of lumbar spinal stenosis. Ohio Med 85:484–487, 1989.

60. Sato K, Kikuchi S: Clinical analysis of two-level compression of the cauda equina and the nerve roots in lumbar spinal canal stenosis. Spine 22:1998–1903, 1997.

61. Prolo DJ, Oklund SA, Butcher M: Toward uniformity in evaluating the results of lumbar spine operations: A paradigm applied to posterior lumbar interbody fusions. Spine 11:601–606, 1986.

62. Turner JA, Ersek M, Herron L, et al: Surgery for lumbar spinal stenosis: Attempted meta-analysis of the literature. Spine 17:1–8, 1992.

63. Deyo RA, Cherkin DC, Loeser JD, et al: Morbidity and mortality in association with operations on the lumbar spine: The influence of age, diagnosis, and procedure. J Bone Joint Surg Am 74:536–543, 1992.

64. Deyo RA, Ciol MA, Cherkin DC, et al: Lumbar spinal fusion: A cohort study of complications and resource use in the Medicare population. Spine 18:1463–1470, 1993.

65. Herron LD, Mangelsdorf C: Lumbar spinal stenosis: Results of surgical treatment. J Spinal Disord 4:26–33, 1991.

66. Tuite GF, Stern JD, Doran SE, et al: Outcome after laminectomy for lumbar stenosis. Part I. Clinical correlations. J Neurosurg 82:912–918, 1995.

67. Wilste LL: Salvage of failed lumbar spinal stenosis surgery. In Hopp E (ed): Spine: State of the Art Reviews. Philadelphia, Hanley & Belfus, 1987, pp 421–450.

68. Vanden Berghe L, Maes G, Fabry G, et al: In situ posterolateral fusion for spondylolisthesis. Acta Orthop Belg 57(Suppl 1):214–218, 1991.

69. Tsou PM, Hopp E: Postsurgical instability in spinal stenosis. In Hopp E (ed): Spine: Sate of the Art Reviews. Philadelphia, Hanley & Belfus, 1987, pp 533–550.

70. Brodsky AE: Post-laminectomy and post-fusion stenosis of the lumbar sine. Clin Orthop Rel Res 115:130–139, 1976.

71. Cloward RB: Spinal stenosis: Treatment by posterior lumbar interbody fusion. In Hopp E (ed): Spine: State of the Art Reviews. Philadelphia, Hanley & Belfus, 1987, pp 457–516.

72. Katz JN, Lipson SJ, Larson MG, et al: The outcome of decompressive laminectomy for degenerative lumbar stenosis. J Bone Joint Surg Am 73:809–816, 1991.

73. Katz JN, Lipson SJ, Lew RA, et al: Lumbar laminectomy alone or with instrumented or noninstrumented arthrodesis in degenerative lumbar spinal stenosis: Patient selection, costs, and surgical outcomes. Spine 22:1123–1131, 1997.

74. Caputy AJ, Luessenhop AJ: Long-term evaluation of decompressive surgery for degenerative lumbar stenosis. J Neurosurg 77:669–676, 1992.

75. McCullen GM, Bernini PM, Bernstein SH, et al: Clinical and roentgenographic results of decompression for lumbar spinal stenosis. J Spinal Disord 7:380–387, 1994.

76. Epstein NE: Decompression in the surgical management of degenerative spondylolisthesis: Advantages of a conservative approach in 290 patients. J Spinal Disord 11:116–122, 1998.

77. Poletti CE: Central lumbar stenosis caused by ligamentum flavum: Unilateral laminotomy for bilateral ligamentectomy: Preliminary report of two cases. Neurosurgery 37:343–347, 1995.

78. Spetzger U, Bertalanffy H, Naujokat C, et al: Unilateral laminotomy for bilateral decompression of lumbar spinal stenosis. Part I. Anatomical and surgical considerations. Acta Neurochir (Wien) 139:392–396, 1997.

79. Nakai O, Okawa A, Yamaura I: Long-term roentgenographic and functional changes in patients who were treated with wide fenestration for central lumbar stenosis. J Bone Joint Surg Am 73:1184–1191, 1991.

80. Caspar W, Papavero L, Sayler MK, et al: Precise and limited decompression for lumbar spinal stenosis. Acta Neurochir (Wien) 131:130–136, 1994.

81. Young S, Veerapen R, O'Laoire S: Relief of lumbar canal stenosis using multilevel subarticular fenestrations as alternative to wide laminectomy: Preliminary report. Neurosurgery 23:628–633, 1988.

82. Postacchini F, Cinotti G: Bone regrowth after surgical decompression for lumbar spinal stenosis. J Bone Joint Surg Br 74:862–869, 1992.

83. Lin PM: Internal decompression for multiple levels of lumbar spinal stenosis: A technical note. Neurosurgery 11:546–549, 1982.

84. Sanderson P, Wood PL: Surgery for lumbar spinal stenosis in old people. J Bone Joint Surg Br 75:393–397, 1993.

85. Aryanpur J, Ducker T: Multilevel lumbar laminotomies: An alternative to laminectomy in the treatment of lumbar stenosis. Neurosurgery 26:429–433, 1990.

86. Getty CJM, Johnson JR, Kirwan EO, Sullivan MF: Partial undercutting facetectomy for bony entrapment of the lumbar nerve root. J Bone Joint Surg Br 63:330–335, 1981.

87. Kanamori M, Matsui H, Hirano N, et al: Trumpet laminectomy for lumbar degenerative spinal stenosis. J Spinal Disord 6:232–237, 1993.

88. Tsuji H, Itho T, Sekido H, et al: Expansive laminoplasty for lumbar spinal stenosis. Int Orthop 14:308–314, 1990.

89. Matsui H, Tsuji H, Sekido H, et al: Results of expansive laminoplasty for lumbar spinal stenosis in active manual workers. Spine 17(Suppl):S37–S40, 1992.

90. Alexander E, Kelly DL, Davis CH, et al: Intact arch spondylolisthesis: A review of 50 cases and description of surgical treatment. J Neurosurg 63:840–844, 1985.

91. Epstein NE: Review article: Different surgical approaches to far lateral lumbar disc herniations. J Spinal Disord 8:383–394, 1995.

92. Epstein NE, Epstein JA, Carras R, et al: Far lateral lumbar disc herniations and associated structural abnormalities: An evaluation in 60 patients of the comparative value of CT, MR, and myelo-CT in diagnosis and management. Spine 15:534–539, 1990.

93. Epstein NE: An evaluation of varied surgical approaches employed in the management of 170 far lateral lumbar disc herniations. J Neuosurg 83:648–656, 1995.

94. Epstein NE, Hood DC: A comparison of surgeon's assessment to patient's self analysis (Short Form 36) after far lateral lumbar disc surgery: An outcome study. Spine 22:2422–2428, 1997.

95. Garrido E, Connaughton PN: Unilateral facetectomy approach for lateral lumbar disc herniation. J Neurosurg 76:342–343, 1992.

96. An HS, Vaccaro A, Simeone FA, et al: Herniated lumbar disc in patients over the age of fifty. J Spinal Disord 3:143–146, 1990.

97. Faust SE, Ducker TB, Van Hassent JA: Lateral lumbar disc herniations. J Spinal Disord 5:97–103, 1992.

98. Hood RS: Far lateral lumbar disc herniations. Neurosurg Clin N Am 4:117–124, 1993.

99. Epstein NE, Epstein JA, Mauri T: Treatment of fractures of the vertebral limbus and spinal stenosis in 5 adolescents and 5 adults. Neuorsurgery 24:596–604, 1989.

100. Epstein NE, Epstein JA: Limbus vertebral fractures of the lumbar spine and spinal stenosis in five adolescents with further evaluation of type III fractures. Neuro-Orthopedics 9:33–52, 1990.

101. Epstein NE, Epstein JA: Limbus lumbar vertebral fractures in 27 adolescents and adults. Spine 16:962–966, 1991.

102. Epstein NE: Lumbar surgery for 56 limbus fractures emphasizing non-calcified type III lesions. Spine 17:1489–1496, 1992.

103. Schlegel JD, Smith JA, Schleusener RL: Lumbar motion segment pathology adjacent to thoracolumbar, lumbar, and lumbosacral fusions. Spine 21:970–981, 1996.

104. Cauchoix J, Benoist M, Chassaing V: Degenerative spondylolisthesis. Clin Orthop 115:122–129, 1976.

105. Lombardi JS, Wilste LL, Reynolds J, et al: Treatment of degenerative spondylolisthesis. Spine 10:821–827, 1985.

106. Bolesta MJ, Bohlman HH: Degenerative spondylolisthesis. Instr Course Lect 38:157–168, 1989.

107. Epstein NE, Epstein JA, Carras R, et al: Degenerative spondylolisthesis with an intact neural arch: A review of 60 cases with an analysis of clinical findings and the development of surgical management. Neurosurgery 13:555–561, 1983.

108. Epstein JA, Epstein BS, Lavine LS, et al: Degenerative lumbar spondylolisthesis with an intact neural arch (pseudospondylolisthesis). J Neurosurg 44:139–147, 1976.

109. diPierro CG, Helm GA, Shaffrey CI, et al: Treatment of lumbar stenosis by extensive unilateral decompression and contralateral autologous bone fusion: Operative technique and results. J Neurosurg 84:166–173, 1996.

110. Jonsson B, Annertz M, Sjoberg C, et al: A prospective and consecutive study of surgically treated lumbar spinal stenosis. Part I. Clinical features related to radiographic findings. Spine 22:2932–2937, 1997.

111. Shenkin HA, Nash CJ: Spondylolisthesis after multiple bilateral laminectomies and facetectomies for lumbar spondylosis: Follow-up review. J Neurosurg 50:45–47, 1979.

112. Epstein NE: Surgical management of lumbar stenosis: Decompression and indications for fusion. Neurosurg Focus 3:1–14, 1997.

113. Johnsson KE, Willner S, Jonsson K: Postoperative instability after decompression for lumbar spinal stenosis. Spine 11:107–110, 1986.

114. Johnsson KE, Redlund-Johnell I, Uden A, et al: Preoperative and postoperative instability in lumbar spinal stenosis. Spine 14:591–593, 1989.

115. Epstein NE: Primary fusion for the management of "unstable" degenerative spondylolisthesis. Neuro-Orthopedics 23:45–52, 1998.

116. Nasca RJ: Rationale for spinal fusion in lumbar spinal stenosis. Spine 14:451–454, 1989.

117. Silvers HR, Lewis PJ, Asch HL: Decompressive lumbar laminectomy for spinal stenosis. J Neurosurg 78:695–701, 1993.

118. Herkowitz HN, Kurz LT: Degenerative lumbar spondylolisthesis with spinal stenosis: A prospective study comparing decompression with decompression and intertransverse process arthrodesis. J Bone Joint Surg Am 73:802–808, 1991.

119. Yone K, Sakou T, Kawauchi Y, et al: Indication of fusion of lumbar spinal stenosis in elderly patients and its significance. Spine 21:242–248, 1996.

120. Colemont J, Heinrich E, Giehl JP, et al: Stabilization of the lumbosacral spine in postlaminectomy syndromes: Technique and 2-year results. Acta Orthop Belg 57(Suppl 1):247–254, 1991.

121. Markwalder TM, Saager C, Reulen HJ: Isthmic spondylolisthesis—an analysis of the clinical and radiological presentation in relation to intraoperative findings and surgical results in 72 consecutive cases. Acta Neurochir (Wien) 110:154–159, 1991.

122. Boos N, Marchesi D, Aebi M: Treatment of spondylolysis and spondylolisthesis with Cotrel-Dubousset instrumentation: A preliminary report. J Spinal Disord 4:472–479, 1991.

123. Kim NH, Kim DFJ: Anterior interbody fusion for spondylolisthesis. Orthopedics 14:1069–1076, 1991.

124. Roy-Camille R, Saillant G, Mazel C: Internal fixation of the lumbar spine with pedicle screw plating. Clin Orthop Rel Res 203:7–17, 1986.

125. West JL, Bradford DS, Ogilvie JW: Results of spinal arthrodesis with pedicle screw-plate fixators. J Bone Joint Surg Am 73:1179–1184, 1991.

126. Simmons ED Jr, Simmons EH: Spinal stenosis with scoliosis. Spine 17(Suppl):S117–S120, 1992.

127. Grob D, Humke T, Dvorak J: Degenerative lumbar spinal stenosis: Decompression with and without arthrodesis. J Bone Joint Surg Am 77:1036–1041, 1995.

128. Harrison, MJ, Sundaresan N: Spinal instrumentation for degenerative disease of the lumbar spine. Mt Sinai J Med 58:169–176, 1991.

129. Lee CK: Lumbar spinal instability (olisthesis) after extensive posterior spinal decompression. Spine 8:429–433, 1983.

130. White AA, Panjabi MM: Biomechanical considerations in the surgical measurement of the spine. In Clinical Biomechanics of the Spine, 2nd ed. Philadelphia, JB Lippincott, 1990, pp 511–631.

131. Wilste LL, Kirkaldy-Willis WH, McIvor GW: The treatment of spinal stenosis. Clin Orthop 115:83–91, 1976.

132. Mitsunaga MM, Chong G, Maes KE: Microscopically assisted posterior lumbar interbody fusion. Clin Orthop 263:121–127, 1991.

133. Wetzel FT, LaRocca H: The failed posterior lumbar interbody fusion. Spine 16:839–845, 1991.

134. Markwalder TM: Surgical management of neurogenic claudication in 100 patients with lumbar spinal stenosis due to degenerative spondylolisthesis. Acta Neurochir (Wien) 120:136–142, 1993.

135. Whitecloud TS 3rd, Butler JC, Cohen JL, et al: Complications with the variable spinal plating system. Spine 14:472–476, 1989.

136. McAfee PC, Weiland DJ, Carlow JJ: Survivorship analysis of pedicle spinal instrumentation. Spine 16(Suppl):S422–S427, 1991.

137. Puno RM, Bechtold JE, Byrd JA 3rd, et al: Biomechanical analysis of transpedicular rod systems: A preliminary report. Spine 16:973–980, 1991.

138. Marchesi DG, Thalgott JA, Aebi M: Application and results of the AO internal fixation system in nontraumatic indications. Spine 16:S162–S169, 1991.

139. Weinstein JN, Spratt KF, Spendler D, et al: Spinal pedicle fixation: Reliability and validity of roentgenogram-based assessment and surgical factors on successful screw placement. Spine 13:1012–1018, 1988.

140. Matsuzaki H, Tokuhashi Y, Matsumoto F, et al: Problems and solutions of pedicle screw plate fixation of the lumbar spine. Spine 15:1159–1165, 1990.

141. Etebar S, Cahill DW: Risk factors for adjacent-segment failure following lumbar fixation with rigid instrumentation for degenerative instability. J Neurosurg 90:163–169, 1999.

142. Mullin BB, Rea GL, Irsik R, et al: The effect of postlaminectomy spinal instability on the outcome of lumbar spinal stenosis patients. J Spinal Disord 9:107–116, 1996.

143. McCulloch JA: Microdecompression and uninstrumented single-level fusion for spinal canal stenosis with degenerative spondylolisthesis. Spine 23:2243–2252, 1998.

144. Nork SE, Hu SS, Workman KL, et al: Patient outcomes after decompression and instrumented posterior spinal fusion for degenerative spondylolisthesis. Spine 24:561–569, 1999.

145. Kostuik JP, Matsusaki H: Anterior stabilization, instrumentation, and decompression for post-traumatic kyphosis. Spine 14:379–386, 1989.

146. Mauersberger W, Nietgen T: Surgical treatment of lumbar stenosis: Long-term results. Neurosurg Rev 12:291–295, 1989.

147. Airaksinen O, Herno A, Turunen V, et al: Surgical outcome in 438 patients treated surgically for lumbar spinal stenosis. Spine 22:2278–2282, 1997.

148. Guigui P, Benoist M, Delecourt C, et al: Motor deficit in lumbar spinal stenosis: A retrospective study of a series of 50 patients. J Spinal Disord 11:283–288, 1998.

149. Tsai RY, Yang R, Bray RS: Microscopic laminotomies for degenerative lumbar spinal stenosis. J Spinal Disord 11:389–394, 1998.

150. Quigley MR, Kortyna R, Goodwin C, et al: Lumbar surgery in the elderly. Neurosurgery 30:672–674, 1992.

CHAPTER 295

Spondylolysis and Spondylolisthesis

GREGORY J. BENNETT

Since 1782, spondylolisthesis has been recognized as a disorder characterized by a visible lumbosacral deformity, slipped vertebrae, and fractures or other deformities of the pars interarticularis.[1] Several classifications that vary in their descriptions of the deformed but intact pars interarticularis and facet joint anatomy have been proposed. Degenerative spondylolisthesis with an intact pars interarticularis has been included in these classifications, whereas other segmental instability syndromes such as retrolisthesis have been excluded. Most classifications include six types of spondylolisthesis:

Type I: Congenital
Type II: Isthmic
Type III: Degenerative
Type IV: Traumatic
Type V: Pathologic
Type VI: Postsurgical

CLINICAL AND RADIOLOGIC FINDINGS

Congenital spondylolisthesis is seen most often in adolescents and is associated with congenital deformities of the sacrum, including spina bifida; a dorsal displacement of the sacrum, which may be at the posterior apex of the iliac crest; and deformities of the superior articular process of the sacrum, which lacks the coronal-plane surface needed to resist a forward slip. An elongated but intact pars interarticularis has been described in this syndrome but has also been classified with type II. Congenital spondylolisthesis is rare in general neurosurgical practice. An example is shown in Figure 295–1.

The isthmic type of spondylolisthesis is familiar to most neurosurgeons and has been studied extensively. A stress fracture of the pars interarticularis detaches the stabilizing posterior elements from the motion segment and results in biomechanically inappropriate translational and shear forces on the disk annulus. The annulus gradually fails as the vertebral bodies become displaced. Fibrocartilage proliferates at the fracture site, resulting in compression of the nerve exiting the foramen at that level, typically the L5 nerve in a patient with an L5-S1 spondylolisthesis. The disk may herniate posteriorly and compress the lateral nerve (L5 at L5-S1) and, occasionally, the medial nerve (S1 at L5-S1). The forward slip of the upper vertebrae may be accompanied by an angular sagittal-plane deformity, which creates a localized kyphosis. A compensatory hyperlordosis can occur above the spondylolisthesis with an associated retrolisthesis (retrodisplacement) and symptomatic disk herniation. Axial and sagittal views of a typical L5-S1 isthmic spondylolisthesis are shown on magnetic resonance imaging (MRI) (Fig. 295–2A) and computed tomography (CT) (see Fig. 295-2B), and are also depicted graphically (Fig. 295-3).

Degenerative spondylolisthesis is most common at L4-5 in women but may occasionally be seen at L3-4 and, rarely, at L5-S1. The facet joints at these levels normally have synovial surfaces with biomechanical significance in the coronal and sagittal planes. The sagittal-plane portion resists rotation in the y-axis (i.e., axial plane rotation), whereas the coronal plane portion resists translation in the z-axis (i.e., forward slippage) (Fig. 295-4). If the coronal plane portion is anatomically deficient or damaged by degenerative disease, the upper vertebra at that motion segment can slip forward. Because the neural arch is intact, forward slippage frequently causes spinal stenosis with neurogenic claudication. Variations in facet and laminar shape and dimensions have been commonly observed in degenerative spondylolisthesis and may be causally related.

Traumatic spondylolysis is rare in neurosurgical practice. Some physicians have restricted this diagnosis to cases of major trauma involving fractures of the pedicle but not of the pars interarticularis. Radiographs obtained after minor injury and showing a spondylolysis usually reveal sclerotic changes, indicating that the fracture is old. This is frequently an issue in personal injury liability and workers' compensation cases. Spontaneous healing of acute traumatic fractures can occur and can be seen as hyperostotic or densely sclerotic deformities of the pars interarticularis. However, most healed pars interarticularis fractures result from cumulative trauma, not from the acute trauma in question in liability cases.

Pathologic spondylolisthesis is occasionally seen by neurosurgeons and is usually caused by infection or tumor, which damages the facets and pedicles bilaterally.

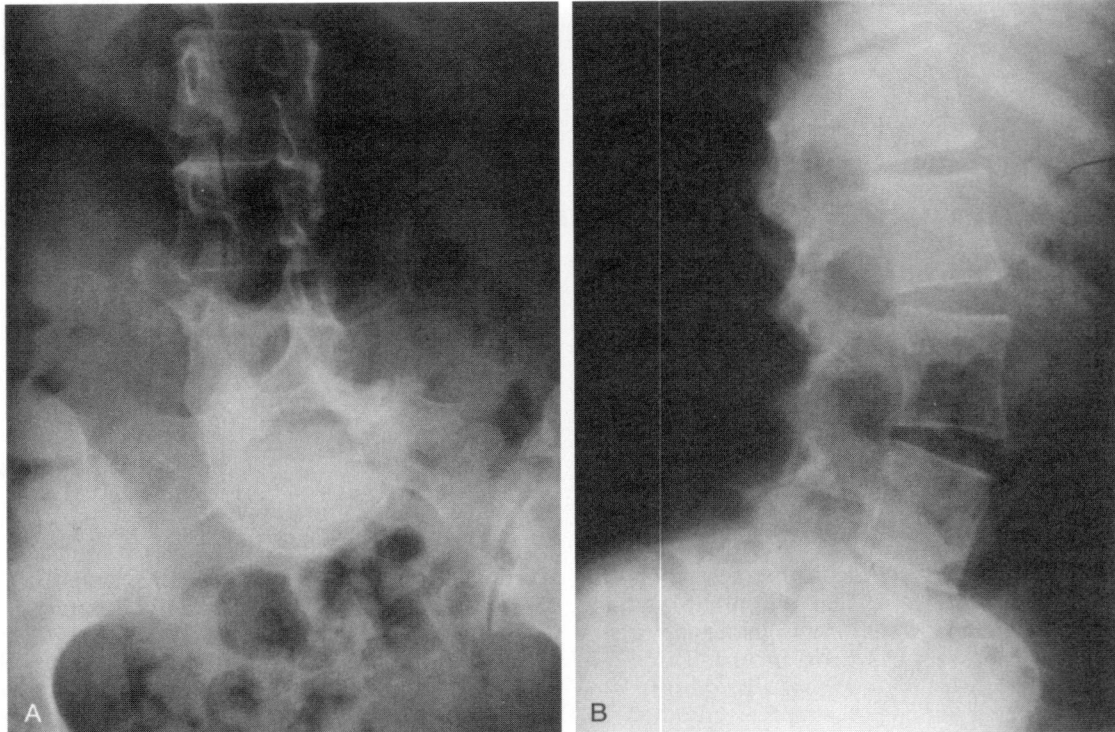

FIGURE 295–1. Congenital spondylolisthesis is demonstrated on the anteroposterior and lateral radiographs of a 19-year-old woman with hamstring tightness and back and leg pain. Notice the intact facet joints of S1 on the anteroposterior view *(A)* and the elongated but intact pars interacticularis of L5-S1 on the lateral view *(B)*.

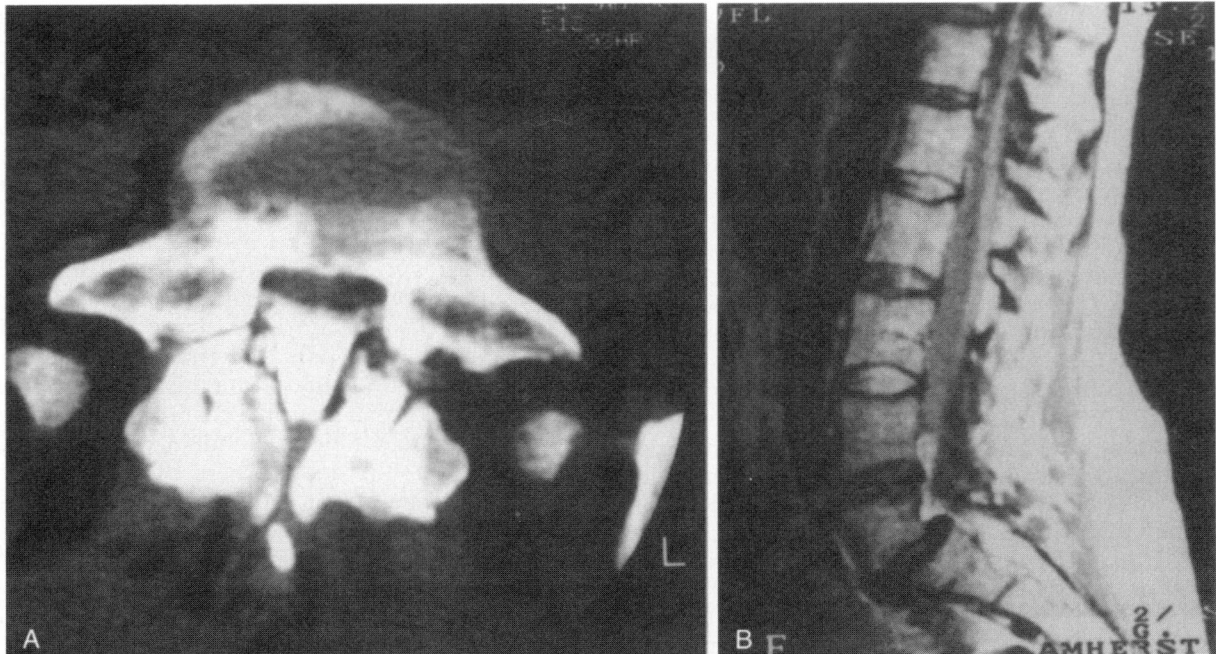

FIGURE 295–2. Isthmic spondylolisthesis is shown on axial computed tomography *(A)* and lateral magnetic resonance imaging *(B)* in a 32-year-old woman. The pars interarticularis defect is best seen on axial computed tomography, and the slip percentage and disk changes are best viewed on lateral magnetic resonance imaging. The L4-5 disk is degenerated but not herniated.

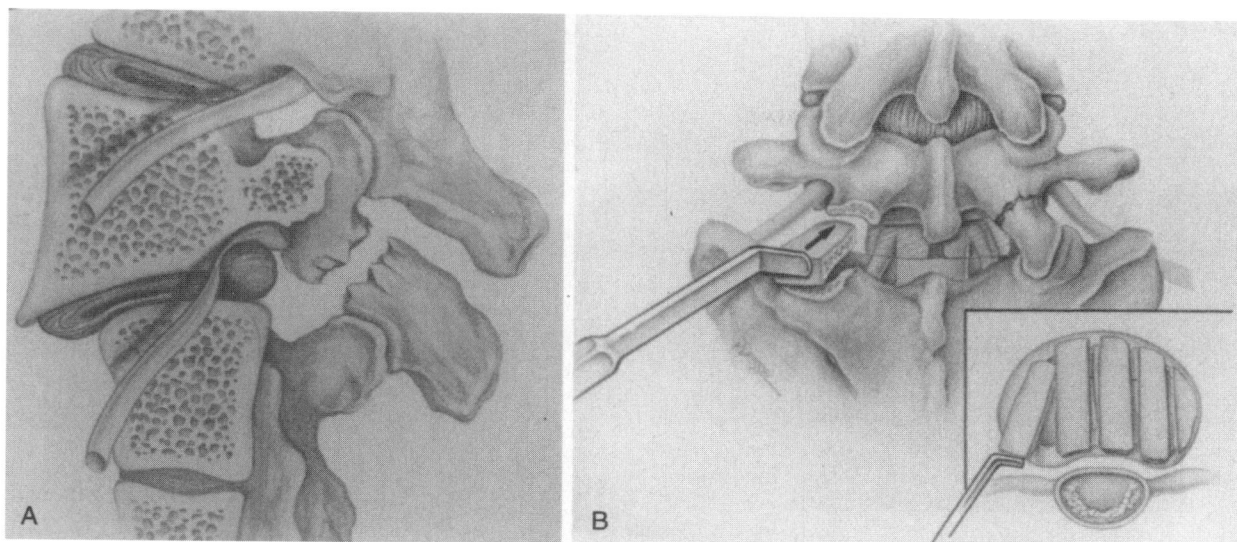

FIGURE 295–3. Nerve compression and radicular symptoms are usually caused by reactive fibrocartilage at the pars interarticularis defect, with the nerve immediately ventral to the cartilage *(A).* After removal of the lamina and pars interarticularis, a disk herniation occasionally contributes to the compression of the L5 nerve. After diskectomy, the space between the L5 and S1 nerves is carefully developed to permit the insertion of bone grafts with a minimum of nerve retraction *(B).*

Postlaminectomy spondylolisthesis is caused by surgical damage to the facet joint, disk, or pars interarticularis. The slip is usually low grade and very symptomatic, but it can progress to about 50% of the anterior-posterior diameter of the vertebral body (Fig. 295–5). A related disorder, known as *spondylolysis acquisita,* is seen in patients with prior diskectomy at the adjacent caudal level or fusion at an adjacent level. The patient with spondylolisthesis after laminectomy has back and leg pain with obvious radiologic findings that typically develop months after surgery. The patient with spondylolysis after prior diskectomy usually has an associated disk herniation, and the lysis frequently is not seen on CT before reoperation.

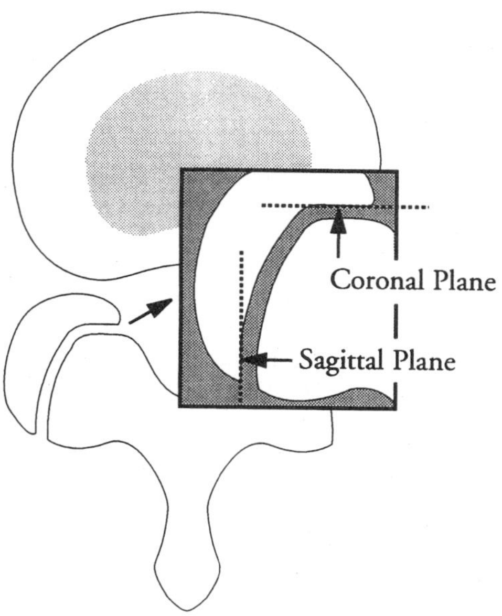

BIOMECHANICS AND PATHOGENESIS

Type I: Congenital

The vertebral weakness that causes spondylolisthesis is considered to begin in the posterior elements. Congenital spondylolisthesis as described by Wiltse and Rothman[2] is a facet dysplasia characterized by a predominantly axial or sagittal plane orientation rather than by the normal coronal orientation at L5-S1. Elongation of the pars interarticularis is considered to be secondary, caused by vertebral slippage and by the developmental plasticity of juvenile bone. Wiltse and Rothman[2] have further classified patients with an elongated but intact pars interarticularis, facet dysplasia, and in 32%, an associated spina bifida as having a variant of isthmic spondylolisthesis. Other observers have described patients with congenital disease as having an elongated pars interarticularis with or without a defect; spina bifida of the sacrum, which is rotated and displaced dorsally; a high-grade slip with angulation; and facet dysplasias.[3] These same investigators also found an increased incidence of isthmic spondylolisthesis and congenital spondylolisthesis in first-degree relatives of both types of patients, suggesting that an underlying genetic predisposition exists in both disorders, most prominently in the congenital variety.

The age of onset is usually younger than 20 years. Overlap cases occur, and the distinction is probably

FIGURE 295–4. Normally, facets at L4-5 have significant coronal and sagittal configurations. However, in degenerative spondylolisthesis, the facets lack the coronal portion, and the L4 lamina is narrow; this permits the lamina to move anteriorly.

Coronal Plane

Sagittal Plane

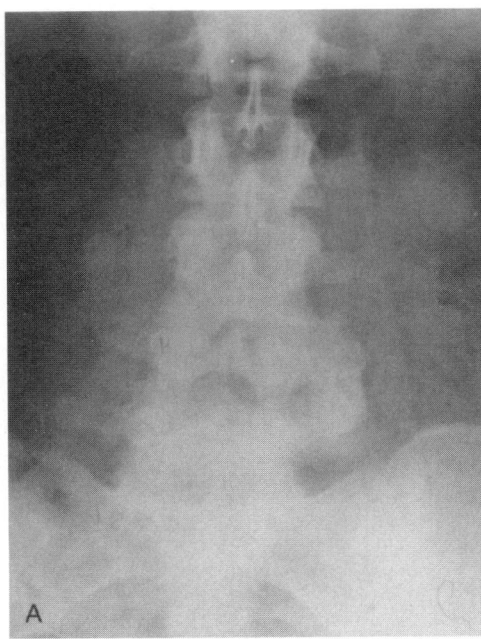 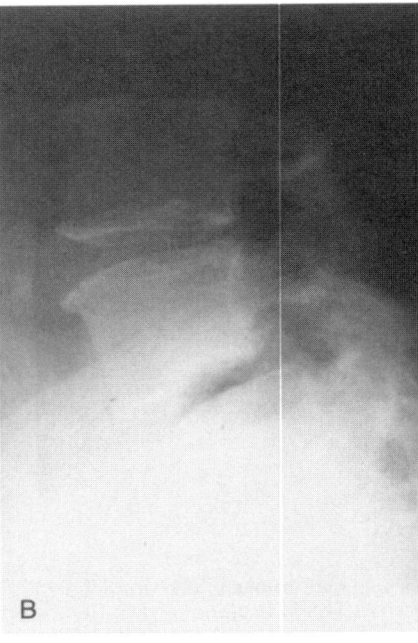

FIGURE 295–5. Spondylolisthesis developing after diskectomy in a 48-year-old woman is evident on anteroposterior *(A)* and lateral *(B)* radiography. An intertransverse fusion was performed in situ without pedicle fixation. The slip progressed despite the presence of a visible fusion mass. At surgery, a pseudarthrosis was found between the fusion mass and the L4 transverse process. This case demonstrates the limitations of radiologic evaluation of intertransverse fusion.

unimportant to prognosis and treatment. Regardless of the type, if the pars interarticularis is infact and not elongated and if spina bifida is absent, high-grade slippage can occur, causing severe spinal stenosis and neurological deficit such as that occasionally seen in degenerative spondylolisthesis. Patients should be considered for decompression at the time of their initial surgery. Symptomatic patients with significant deformities and no neural compression can be treated with an in situ fusion with a low risk of neurological deficit.[4] A variety of related disorders and very detailed clinical and radiologic reports have been summarized by Hensinger[5]; however, for clinicians, the most significant associated disorder is scoliosis.

Thoracolumbar or lumbar scoliosis is seen in up to 48% of young patients with spondylolisthesis, whereas a 6.2% incidence of pars interarticularis defects is seen among patients with scoliosis.[6, 7] In patients with mild lumbar curves of less than 20 degrees, the scoliosis results from back pain and muscle spasm. Surgical treatment of the spondylolisthesis alone results in significant improvements in the curves. Thoracolumbar curves are usually more advanced than such curves and are structural in origin. For a variety of reasons, the patient may require surgery for scoliosis in addition to lumbosacral fusion. A minor but progressive lumbar or thoracolumbar curve may indicate the need for lumbosacral fusion for spondylolisthesis to prevent the development of a fixed structural curve requiring subsequent surgery for scoliosis.

Type II: Isthmic

Isthmic spondylolisthesis is thought to result from a stress fracture in the pars interarticularis, which is associated with a variety of biomechanical stresses. A congenital predisposition exists in as many as one third of patients.[8] Spina bifida of the sacrum or the L5 lamina; hypoplasia of the superior articular facet of the sacrum; occasionally, a significant disk herniation; and bilateral or, rarely, unilateral pars interarticularis defects are seen in patients with the congenital variety of isthmic spondylolisthesis.[9] Pars interarticularis defects have been reported in children as young as 4 months of age, and their prevalence increases until the age of 16 years. Strenuous athletic activities, such as gymnastics and blocking in football, are associated with pars interarticularis fractures. The stresses in these activities are diverse, but hyperextension has been identified as the one most likely to cause a pars interarticularis fracture. Failure of the L4 pars interarticularis during extension at L4-5 has been reported at loads of up to 5800 N (approximately 1400 lb) under biomechanical testing conditions.[10, 11] This observation is inconsistent with the occurrence of most pars interarticularis defects and suggests that fatigue fracture mechanisms are the cause in most patients. After a fracture, the pars interarticularis may heal unilaterally or bilaterally; however, the usual response is formation of fibrocartilage, which can proliferate and compress the exiting nerve root. Consequently, the disk, posterior ligaments, and intersegmental muscles must sustain all of the load across the motion segment. The segmental vertebral deformity is predominantly a forward slip. The reason for this is not clear, but it is probably related to the normal lordotic angle, which places a dependent anterior load on the spine in an upright position. Occasionally, a localized kyphotic angulation that is highly unstable and likely to progress can occur. Surgical decompression and stabilization employing a variety of procedures have been used for symptomatic patients, although the goals and rationale for surgery are largely empirical and not based on a defined biomechanical correction of the disorder in all patients.

Type III: Degenerative

Degenerative spondylolisthesis was first described in 1930 as pseudospondylolisthesis by Junghanns[12] during an examination of the extensive Schmorl collection of vertebrae. Hallgrimson[13] described 22 cases in 1941. In 1950, MacNab,[14] who called the disorder *spondylolisthesis with an intact neural arch* and described its pathologic anatomy, demonstrated its instability radiographically and discussed treatment options. Newman and Stone[15] proposed the current term *degenerative spondylolisthesis,* and Epstein and coworkers[16] and Kirkaldy-Willis[17] emphasized the occurrence of spinal stenosis in patients with the disorder. The clinical recognition of the relationship between spinal stenosis and facet pathology by Verbiest[18] has contributed directly to the gradual understanding of degenerative spondylolisthesis.

A variety of anatomic and biomechanical changes in the facets have been described and characterized in patients with degenerative spondylolisthesis. The disorder is most commonly seen in women at the L4-5 level but may also be seen at the L3-4 level. The apparent cause is a progressive degeneration of the facet joints. Because this occurs in association with sacralization of L5 in many patients, the facet degeneration could be explained as a hypermobility syndrome.[19] As in isthmic spondylolisthesis, the adjacent levels may develop a compensatory hyperlordosis with retrolisthesis and contribute to symptoms. However, the primary causes of symptoms are lateral recess stenosis, which results from the forward slippage of the inferior articular process, and disk herniation, which contributes to the central stenosis created by the intact neural arch (Fig. 295–6). Historically, the primary objective in treatment has been lateral recess decompression, which involves removal of the lamina and partial removal of the anteriorly displaced inferior articular facet and adjacent superior facet.

In the past, clinical examination of these patients has focused on the extent of decompression (i.e., partial versus total facetectomy) and has attempted to anticipate the occurrence of instability syndromes after decompression. These questions underscore the dilemma faced by the surgeon in selecting which patients should undergo fusion and which should be observed after decompression. In an attempt to rationalize the timing of surgery, observations of the natural history of the disorder and spontaneous restabilization mechanisms have been made. Fitzgerald and Newman[20] found that patients who do not demonstrate radiologic features such as narrowing of the disk space, subcartilaginous sclerosis, ossification of the ligaments, and spur formation are at increased risk for progression of the slip. Generalized ligamentous laxity has been recognized by these and other investigators as a possible cause of the slip.[21]

Using nonaxial CT and findings from postmortem dissections of 19 lumbar spines, Farfan[22] identified two types of degenerative slip: rotation with obliquity suggesting listhesis, and rotation with true listhesis. After further observations, Farfan concluded that medial displacement of the pedicle causes symptoms and myelographically observable defects. Other clinicians were more impressed with the importance of a narrow lamina and a narrow inferior articular process.

Wiltse and colleagues[23] found that, of the patients presenting with degenerative spondylolisthesis who had narrow laminae at L4, one third also had narrow laminae and sagittal facets at the other lumbar levels,

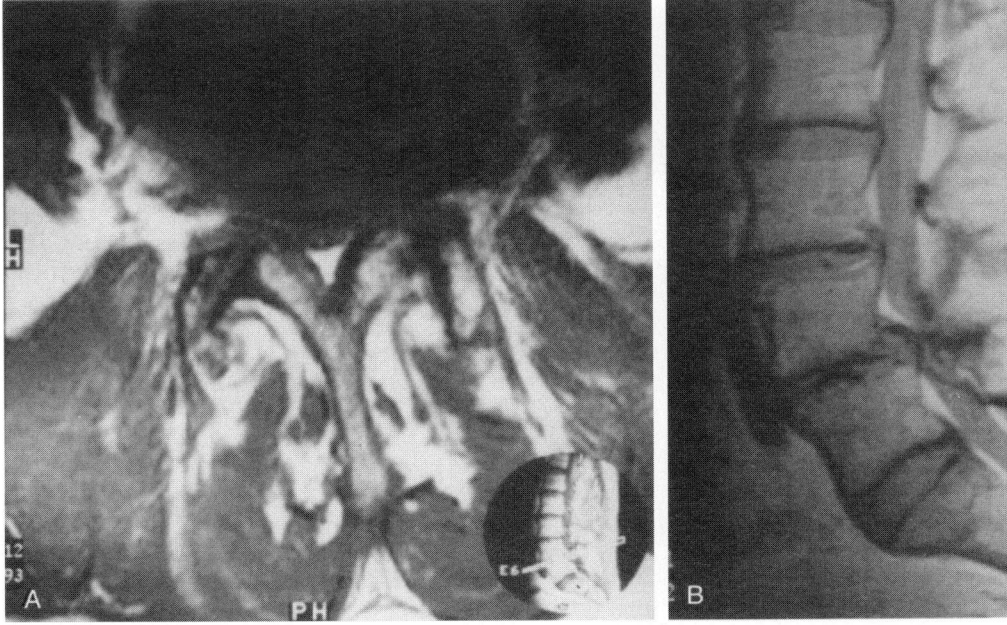

FIGURE 295–6. Degenerative spondylolisthesis and spinal stenosis in a 68-year-old man are visualized on anteroposterior *(A)* and lateral *(B)* magnetic resonance imaging. Notice the predominantly sagittal orientation of the facets and central disk herniation, best seen on the anteroposterior view *(A).*

suggesting a developmental origin of disease in this group of patients. Later, Sato and associates[24] used CT to classify the configuration of laminae in the lumbar spine. In an investigation of 98 patients with L4-5 degenerative spondylolisthesis and 257 controls that focused on the axial-plane orientation of facet joints and on the coronal-plane width of the lamina and inferior articular processes, the occurrence of degenerative spondylolisthesis was found to correlate with the presence of a narrow lamina in the coronal plane (Fig. 295–7A). A sagittal-plane orientation of the facets permitted the facet joints to be seen on plain anteroposterior radiographs, as well as the trefoil shape of the spinal canal in these patients. Axial-plane facet angles of less than 40 degrees correlated with the presence of degenerative spondylolisthesis (see Fig. 295–7B). Narrow laminae at L4 also correlated with the severity of symptoms and a myelographic block. Another distinct group of patients with degenerative spondylolisthesis had a frontal facet orientation, a shallow triangular canal, low-grade slips of 6 to 8 mm, and anterior defects consistent with disk herniation, as observed on myelography (see Fig. 295–7C). Their instability problem was predominantly diskogenic, and the spinal stenosis was caused by a combination of pedicle shortness and central disk herniation.

In summary, the cause of degenerative spondylolisthesis is multifactorial. Probable pathogenetic mechanisms include localized hypermobility, variations in facet orientation and dimensions, variations in laminar dimensions, disk degeneration, and restabilization changes. Decisions regarding the timing and extent of surgery for this disorder continue to be made on the basis of clinical and empirical findings.

Type IV: Traumatic

Acute traumatic spondylolysis with spondylolisthesis is usually associated with major trauma and is probably caused by hyperextension. Lumbar fractures at L2-5 that are associated with vertebral subluxation are usually much more extensive than with the other types, involving severe disruption of the facets, disk, and vertebral body.[25] Although the occasional patient seen with a new fracture of the pars interarticularis usually does not have a slip present at the time of the injury, the slip presumably could occur months to years later as the disk degenerates under shear loads that it cannot sustain. However, this manner of occurrence has not been documented, and a causal relationship cannot be inferred in an individual patient for liability purposes.

Type V: Pathologic

Pathologic spondylolysis with spondylolisthesis is usually caused by damage to the pars interarticularis or, more commonly, to the pedicle in patients with infection or tumor in the vertebral body. In my experience, pathologic spondylolisthesis is also frequently associated with a prior laminectomy. Rare generalized bone diseases, such as syphilis, arthrogryposis, and Albers-Schönberg disease (i.e., osteopetrosis), have been associated with spondylolisthesis.

Type VI: Postsurgical

Postsurgical spondylolisthesis occurs in a small percentage of patients who undergo decompressive laminectomy for spinal stenosis. It sometimes occurs after dis-

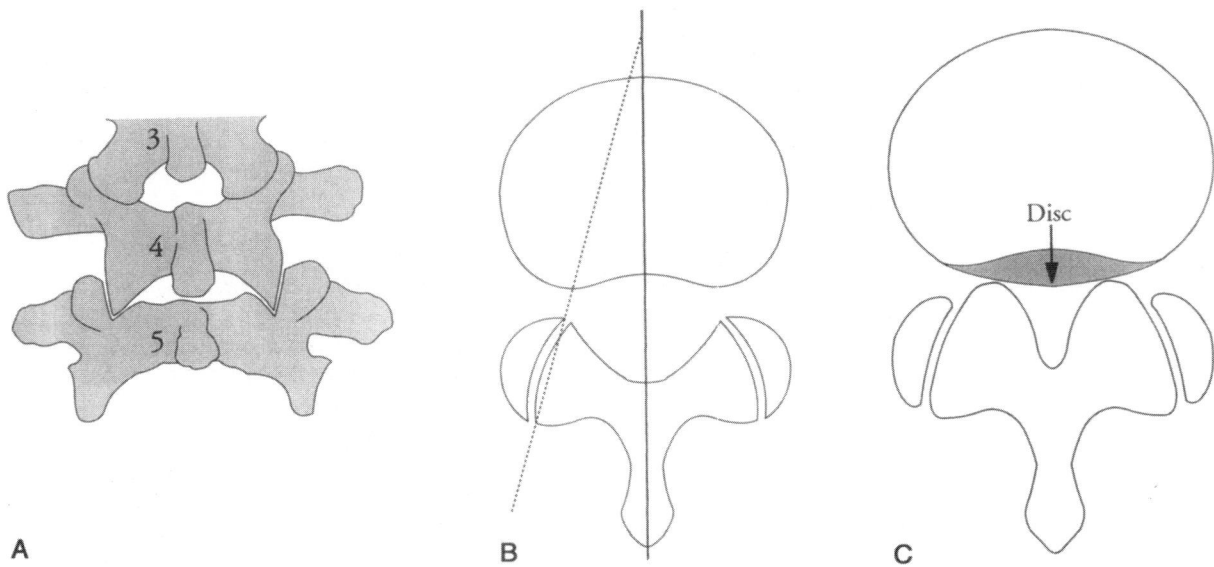

A   **B**   **C**

FIGURE 295–7. The lamina in degenerative spondylolisthesis is frequently narrow, and the inferior articular processes do not overlap the facet joint in the coronal plane *(A)*. This permits anteroposterior radiography to demonstrate the joint space. The transverse facet angle created by the joint plane and a line perpendicular to the coronal plane *(B)* is less than 40 degrees in patients with degenerative spondylolisthesis. The disk is frequently herniated centrally, and in patients with short pedicles, the clinical presentation is neurogenic claudication with instability *(C)*.

kectomy or fusion. Four general categories of postsurgical spondylolisthesis and spondylolysis can be described:

1. Spondylolisthesis after laminectomy with partial or complete facetectomy for spinal stenosis
2. Spondylolisthesis after diskectomy and partial facetectomy
3. Spondylolysis and recurrent disk herniation after diskectomy
4. Spondylolysis after fusion at an adjacent level or coextensive with a previous fusion as part of a pseudarthrosis

The occurrence of spondylolisthesis after laminectomy has long been recognized, and most investigators have concentrated on identifying the preoperative risk factors so that a decision regarding whether to fuse the spine at the time of initial decompression can be made. A study of such risk factors determined that, if displacement as demonstrated on standing flexion-extension radiographs averages 1.2 mm (compared with 0.2 mm in normal patients), the risk of progressive postsurgical slippage is increased.[26] Complete facetectomy, especially in women, was found to be associated with a greater rate of postsurgical slippage and poor clinical outcome. A 3-year follow-up study of 59 patients who underwent laminectomy and facetectomy at two or more levels for the treatment of spinal stenosis revealed that 6 patients (9.8%) developed spondylolisthesis, and two of these had instability symptoms sufficient to warrant fusion.[27] A two-level radical decompression resulted in a rate of instability of 6%, whereas a decompression of three or more levels resulted in a rate of 15%. All slips occurred in patients younger than 70 years of age.

Diskectomy alone presents a very low risk for the postoperative development of spondylolysis and spondylolisthesis. Nevertheless, one woman in my fusion series developed a symptomatic L4-5 spondylolisthesis after prior diskectomy and partial facetectomy and subsequently underwent lumbar fusion (see Fig. 295–5). No predisposing risk factors such as a history of trauma, were present. Two other patients, one man and one woman, developed symptomatic, unilateral spondylolysis after prior diskectomy and responded to lumbar fusion.

I treated spondylolysis with recurrent disk herniation after prior diskectomy with fusion surgery in four patients (fusion at L4-5 in three and fusion at L3-4 in one). Presumably, prior diskectomy and partial facetectomy reduced the failure strength of the motion segment in axial and extension loading. In all cases, the pars interarticularis defect was ipsilateral to the prior posterior decompression and diskectomy. Lumbar disk degeneration displaces caudad the instantaneous axis of rotation and increases translational and rotational movements in the sagittal plane, which increases the strain on the posterior stabilizing ligaments. After diskectomy, similar changes may be caused by early loss of height at the disk space and an increase in disk space range of motion before settling of the facet joints and vertebral bodies. Axial loads on the facet joints also increase with diskectomy, and this factor may contribute to joint failure and to translational or rotational deformities.

The occurrence of spondylolysis after lumbar fusion (i.e., spondylolysis acquisita) is well recognized. Degenerative spondylolisthesis can also occur at adjacent segments. Lee[28] reported 18 cases with the condition, including 3 cases of spondylolysis and 2 of degenerative spondylolisthesis. Lee and Langrana's[29] biomechanical experiments and mathematical models have shown that posterior fusions result in the most significant adverse effects on adjacent segments, especially at the facet joints, compared with other fusion procedures. Intertransverse fusions cause a slight increase in stress at adjacent facet joints, whereas anterior fusions increase shear stress and compressive stress on adjacent disks. Postsurgical spondylolisthesis after an incomplete fusion for an L4 burst fracture in a 13-year-old girl is shown in Figure 295–8. The girl was treated surgically with a lateral extracavitary approach for removal of the bone fragments from L4 and with placement of Cotrel-Dubousset rods and hooks at L2-5. The anterior graft did not extend through the L4-5 disk space to L5. Additional surgery at L4-5 involved posterior lumbar interbody fusion and revision of the implant to include pedicle screws in L5, resulting in a stable fusion of L2-5. The superior lamina hooks on L5 permitted a rotational deformity of the surgical construct and development of L4-5 spondylolisthesis with a failed posterior fusion at L4-5.

In neurosurgical practice, the most common clinical situation in which the issue of spondylolysis acquisita must be considered is before elective lumbar fusion. Patients should be advised before surgery that increased stress on adjacent motion segments will necessitate occupational and other lifestyle changes if the risk of symptom recurrence is to be reduced. Unfortunately, very little is known about the exact risk for these patients under specific loading conditions, such as riding in motor vehicles or repetitive lifting. As a result, patients must frequently make occupational and lifestyle decisions that entail significant economic consequences without the benefit of having detailed clinical follow-up information on recurrent herniation and instability syndromes related to such activities.

RADIOLOGIC ANALYSIS

Several radiologic findings describe the severity of a spondylolisthesis deformity as defined by Wiltse and Winter[30]:

1. Percentage of anterior displacement
2. Sacral inclination
3. Sagittal rotation
4. Sacral rounding
5. Wedging of the olisthetic vertebra
6. Lumbosacral angles

Anterior displacement is reported as a percentage (Fig. 295–9). Sacral inclination is the angle between vertical and the posterior margin of the S1 segment of the sacrum (Fig. 295–10). Sagittal rotation is described

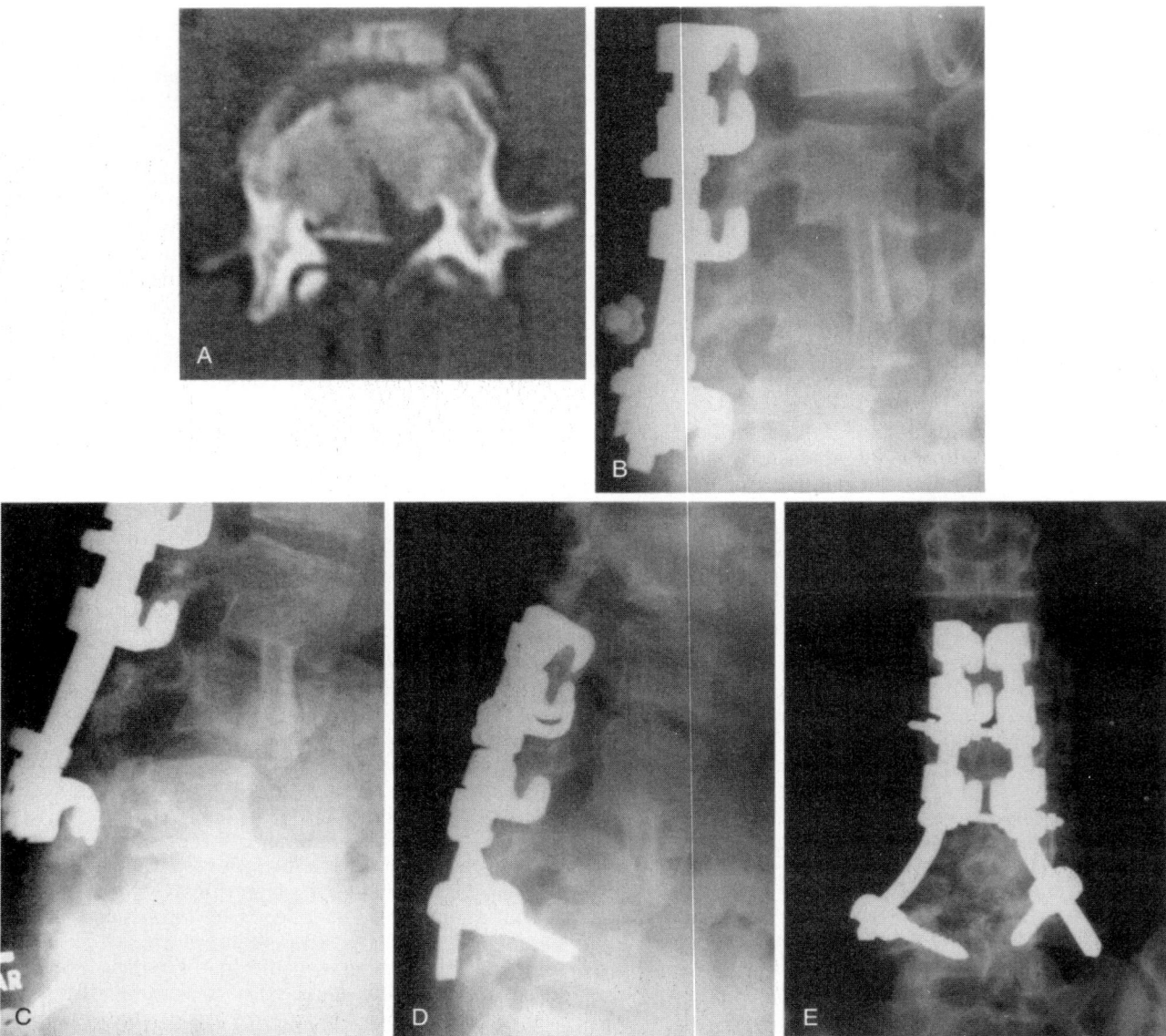

FIGURE 295–8. A 13-year-old girl with an L4 burst fracture, as seen on axial computed tomography *(A)*, was treated surgically with the removal of retropulsed bone and with interbody grafting that did not cross the L4-5 disk space, as shown on the lateral radiograph *(B)*. The posterior fixation device with clawed hooks on the L5 lamina did not provide stability sufficient to prevent the development of spondylolisthesis 18 months later *(C)*. Revision of the implant with the use of pedicle screws in L5 and posterior lumbar interbody fusion at L4-5 resulted in fusion (*D* and *E*).

as the angle between the anterior margin of L5 and the posterior margin of the S1 segment of the sacrum (Fig. 295–11). Sacral rounding is calculated as the percentage of the superior end plate of the sacrum that is deformed inferiorly, usually at the anterior margin of the sacrum (Fig. 295–12). Wedging of the olisthetic vertebra is expressed as the percentage reduction in the height of the slipped vertebrae (Fig. 295–13). A variety of lumbosacral angles have been defined to quantify the sagittal plane orientation of lumbar vertebrae and the sacrum (Fig. 295–14).

This terminology enables precise comparison of disease severity and the results of surgical correction of the deformity. The most frequently used descriptions

are the slip percentage and the angle of sagittal rotation. Severity of disease, biomechanical instability, and the risk of progressive deformity are greater in patients with increased sacral rounding and angles of sagittal rotation. Slip percentages in the moderate range (10% to 50%) are not associated with a significant risk of progressive deformity. Compensatory hypertrophic changes in the sacrum can restabilize the motion segment if the rotational deformity is not great. Wedging of the slipped vertebra may be surgically significant, because greater anterior height presents a relative barrier to reduction and requires distraction or superior sacral end-plate resection with partial removal of the anterior L5 vertebra to create the space needed to re-

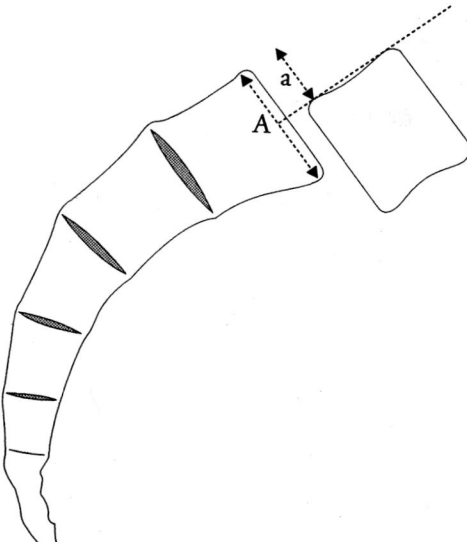

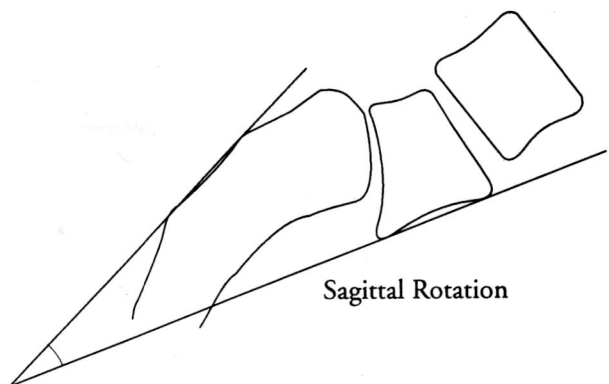

FIGURE 295–11. *Sagittal rotation* is the angle between the posterior margin of S1 and the anterior margin of L5. Increased sagittal rotation angles are a sign of instability in spondylolisthesis and are associated with an increased risk of slip progression.

FIGURE 295–9. The ratio of vertebral displacement to maximal sacral width (a/A) can be easily calculated and reported as *slip percentage.* The posterior osteophytes of L5 are excluded from line a, whereas line A is defined as parallel to the superior end plate of the sacrum. Slip percentage = a/A × 100.

duce the L5 vertebra. Knowledge of the lumbosacral angles is helpful when sagittal plane alignment is considered, but these measurements are largely related to secondary or compensatory phenomena that return to normal after lumbar fusion.

Radiographic findings in spondylolisthesis can be enhanced through comparison of recumbent projec-

tions with standing projections, especially for young adults. In one report on military personnel, 13 (26%) of 50 patients developed increased displacement of greater than 2 mm on standing, whereas standing flexion-extension projections showed only a small additional displacement.[31] The radiographic technique did not include use of the method of Wiltse and Winter[30] for defining the posterior margin of the L5 vertebral body to exclude marginal osteophytes, and it is possible that significant variations in the measurements (approximately 2 mm) were permitted. This illustrates the need for the standardization of radiographic analysis.

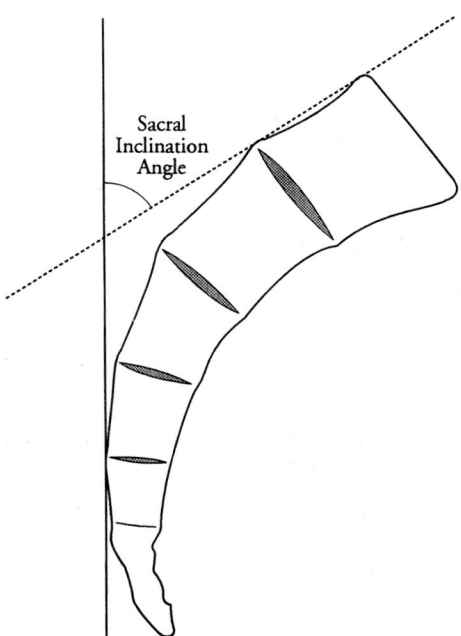

FIGURE 295–10. *Sacral inclination* is the sagittal plane orientation of the sacrum as measured by the intersection of a line extended from the posterior S1 vertebral body to the y axis with the caudal sacrum parallel to the y axis.

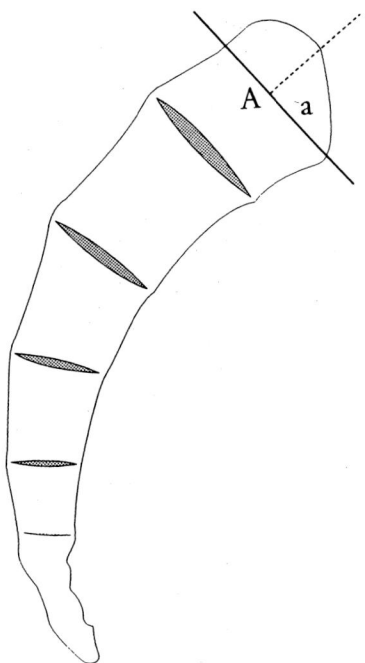

FIGURE 295–12. *Sacral rounding* is the percentage of the sacral end plate that is deformed caudad, usually at the anterior border of the sacrum. Sacral rounding is a sign of instability and represents a barrier to reduction of the slipped vertebra. Percentage of sacral rounding = a/A × 100.

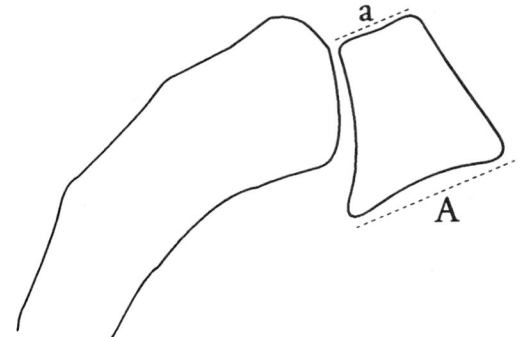

FIGURE 295–13. Wedging of the olisthetic vertebra is the ratio of the posterior margin to the anterior margin of L5. Wedging is surgically significant because it represents a barrier to reduction of the slipped vertebra. % wedging = a/A × 100.

SURGICAL TREATMENT

Congenital and Isthmic Spondylolisthesis in Children

Surgery for children with congenital and isthmic spondylolisthesis is indicated for intractable symptoms of back and leg pain, hamstring tightness, and disabling deformity. Deformities in patients with moderate degrees of slippage (<30%) can usually be stabilized with a posterolateral fusion. More severe deformities may

be better treated with a combination of interbody and intertransverse fusion and pedicle fixation. Decompression for patients with severe leg pain involves removal of the detached laminar arch of L5, fibrocartilage, disk, and residual bone adjacent to the L5 nerve root. Surgeons who prefer to avoid decompression in patients without neurological deficit generally report relief of leg pain and occasionally recovery of footdrop after fusion in situ.[32, 33] The fusion is extended to L4 or L3 in cases of spondyloptosis treated with fusion in situ. Other surgeons have reported satisfactory long-term results with fusion in situ.[34]

Persistence of deformities resulting in cosmetic changes and the occasional progressive slippage with elongation of the posterior bone mass despite an intact fusion have prompted attempts at performing closed and open reduction.[35] Closed reduction is generally safe, with cast techniques being the most effective methods for correction of sagittal rotation.[36] Numerous surgeons have reported successful open reduction and fusion of spondylolisthesis with the use of pedicle fixation techniques.[37–39] Some risk of neurological damage is associated with these procedures because of distraction of the L5 spinal nerve when the L5 vertebral body is retracted from the pelvis into anatomic alignment or the L1-3 spinal nerves, which are stretched by elongation of the entire lumbar segment in relation to the pelvis.[40] Intraoperative evoked potential monitoring of tibial nerve stimulation and wake-up testing may re-

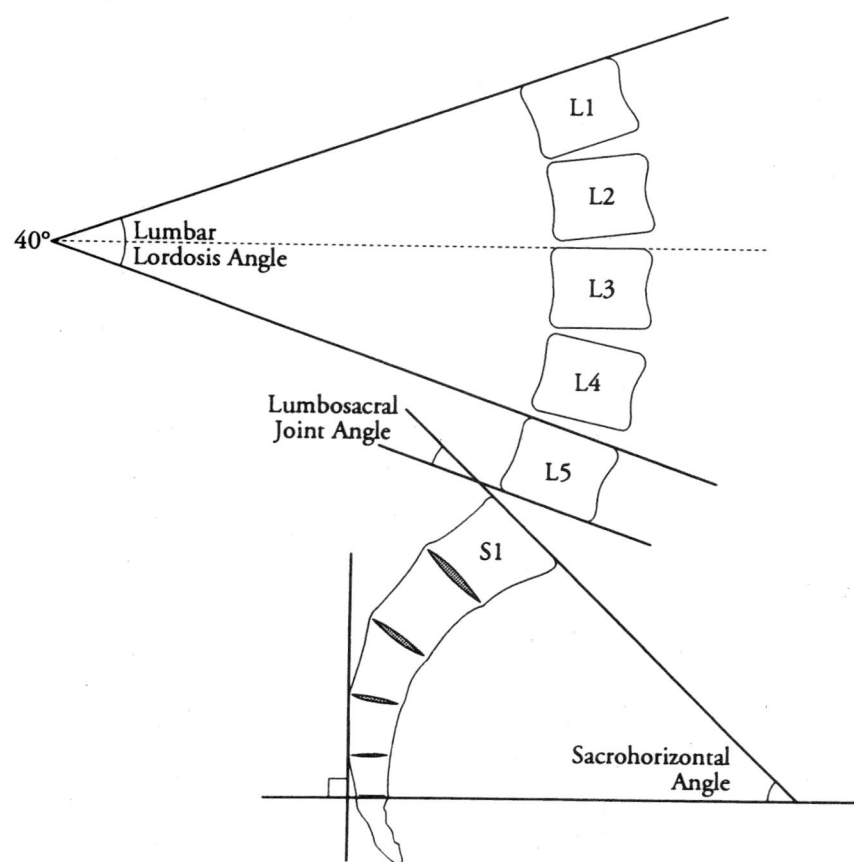

FIGURE 295–14. *Sagittal plane orientation at the lumbosacral junction can be defined by a variety of angles, including the sacrohorizontal angle, the angle of lumbar lordosis, and the lumbosacral joint angle.*

duce the risk of severe damage, but significant limitations still remain and include problems with interpretation of test results and the possibility of delayed development of neurological deficit. Resection of the deformed superior end plate of the sacrum and the anterior wedge of L5 combined with a thorough diskectomy reduces the elongation sufficiently to correct the deformity and may reduce the risk associated with these procedures. Some surgeons have used combined anterior transperitoneal and posterior approaches to stabilize and fuse severe spondylolisthesis, with minimal deformation of the spinal nerves and no neurological morbidity and with adequate success.[41] The L5 vertebral body can be resected using a retroperitoneal or transperitoneal approach to permit a staged reduction of the deformity in cases of spondyloptosis without excessive elongation of the spine.[42]

In summary, the surgical techniques for decompression and stabilization of spondylolisthesis in children include posterior intertransverse fusions with minimal decompression for all patients; a variety of posterior procedures involving decompression, fusion, and stabilizing implants; and combined anterior and posterior procedures. Neurological morbidity is unacceptable with any procedure, because safe alternatives exist for every patient. The challenge is to obtain relief of symptoms and satisfactory spinal alignment with minimal morbidity. Based on the reported findings discussed earlier, certain conclusions appear warranted:

1. Pedicle fixation permits laminectomy and posterior decompression in all patients with radicular leg symptoms without increasing the risk of failed fusion.

2. Excessive elongation of the spine and distraction of individual nerve roots can be difficult to diagnose during open reduction and should be avoided in patients with an initial slippage of 10% to 25%. Surgical shortening of the spine should be undertaken from a posterior approach in patients with slippage of 30% to 90% and from an anterior approach in those with slippage of greater than 90%.

3. Interbody fusion procedures have immediate mechanical and biologic advantages over intertransverse fusion procedures and should be considered in patients with failed posterior fusion, in those considered at risk for a failed fusion, or in those for whom axial loads may exceed the bending strength of the spinal implant.

Isthmic Spondylolisthesis in Adults

The objective of surgery for isthmic spondylolisthesis in adults is the treatment of patients with symptoms of back and leg pain who are unresponsive to conservative measures. The relatively benign course of the disorder in those patients treated without surgery has been noted by several observers.[43, 44] Nevertheless, significant numbers of patients continue to seek treatment for these symptoms, which historically has involved excision of the loose lamina and decompression of the nerve roots.[45] Late follow-up reports revealed significant numbers of patients with recurrent symptoms due to instability.[46, 47] With the use of decompression and

primary fusion, treatment failures persist, and the risk factors predicting poor results have been analyzed. Symptoms have occurred in a high percentage of men who have work-related injuries and who smoke, and slippage of more than 25% has been associated with pseudarthrosis and persistent radicular pain.[48] Cloward[49] reported the use of posterior lumbar interbody fusions without pedicle fixation in 122 patients, with a 3% rate of fusion failure in adults. Others have confirmed that fusion rates are greater for combined anterior and posterior procedures performed in adults.[50]

I have surgically treated 34 adult patients for isthmic spondylolisthesis between 1987 and 1993. The results of treatment are as follows:

L5-S1 spondylolisthesis, L4-5 disk: normal, fusion at L5-S1 (24 patients)
1. L5 laminectomy, L5-S1 intertransverse fusion with pedicle fixation (18 patients)
   Outcome: 17 good; 1 poor with failed fusion
2. L5 laminectomy, L5-S1 posterior lumbar interbody fusion with allografting and autografting and use of Steffee plates (5 patients)
   Outcome: all good
3. L5 laminectomy, L5-S1 posterior lumbar interbody fusion with autografting only (1 patient)
   Outcome: fair, with bone donor site pain

This group demonstrates that decompression and one-level fusion with instrumentation is a well-tolerated procedure with favorable overall results. The one patient with a poor outcome had fusion failure. No advantage is seen with posterior lumbar interbody fusions compared with intertransverse fusions.

L5-S1 spondylolisthesis, L4-5 disk herniation, fusion at L4-S1 (10 patients)
1. L5 laminectomy, L4-5 diskectomy, L5-S1 diskectomy, two-level posterior lumbar interbody fusion with use of Steffee plates (5 patients)
   Outcome: 3 good, 1 fair, and 1 poor
2. L5 laminectomy, L4-5 diskectomy, L4-S1 intertransverse fusion with use of Steffee plates (4 patients)
   Outcome: 1 good, 2 fair, and 1 poor
3. L5 laminectomy, L4-5 diskectomy, L4-S1 fusion with autografting, no implant (1 patient)
   Outcome: poor

This group had significantly worse outcomes than did the patients who underwent one-level surgery. Two diabetic patients had poor results. One developed diskitis and osteomyelitis in the interbody bone at a posterior lumbar interbody fusion site, and the other experienced fusion failure after a preoperative course of prednisone therapy ordered by a rheumatologist. The third poor result (in a man who was obese and who smoked) was also a fusion failure. Stabilization with pedicle fixation appears to be essential, and an improved result with posterior lumbar interbody fusion is suggested.

Degenerative Spondylolisthesis

Surgery for degenerative spondylolisthesis has consisted of laminectomy with partial preservation of the facets, laminectomy with complete facetectomy, and laminectomy with facetectomy and fusion. Numerous observers have noticed slip progression after facetectomy without fusion. This procedure is not recommended unless very extensive stabilizing changes exist at the disk space, including the presence of large marginal osteophytes, significant disk narrowing with advanced sclerosis, and no disk herniation requiring diskectomy as part of the decompression. Research intended to answer the question of whether laminectomy with partial facetectomy is the best procedure for all patients is limited by a failure to take into account these anatomic and other behavioral and biomechanical risk factors for slip progression. Nevertheless, many patients can benefit from a decompressive procedure with relief of neurogenic claudication symptoms. Several investigators have reported series in which patients with healthy lifestyles and signs of stability at

the disk for whom the loads on the motion segment after decompression without fusion are not anticipated to be excessive frequently do quite well.[51, 52] However, these investigators listed about 12% of their patients as having experienced treatment failure (i.e., they had symptoms that suggested an instability disorder). Some investigators have found slightly higher rates of good outcomes (approximately 10%) for patients with fusion; these rates seemed to increase at 1 and 3 years of follow-up.[53] Others have noted higher fusion rates with the use of pedicle fixation in a group of patients who underwent intertransverse fusion.[54]

In summary, it appears that patients who are at risk for the development of a postdecompression instability disorder can derive some benefit from a primary fusion. General risk factors for instability remain somewhat obscure but include female sex, obesity, mobility on preoperative radiography, a relatively young age

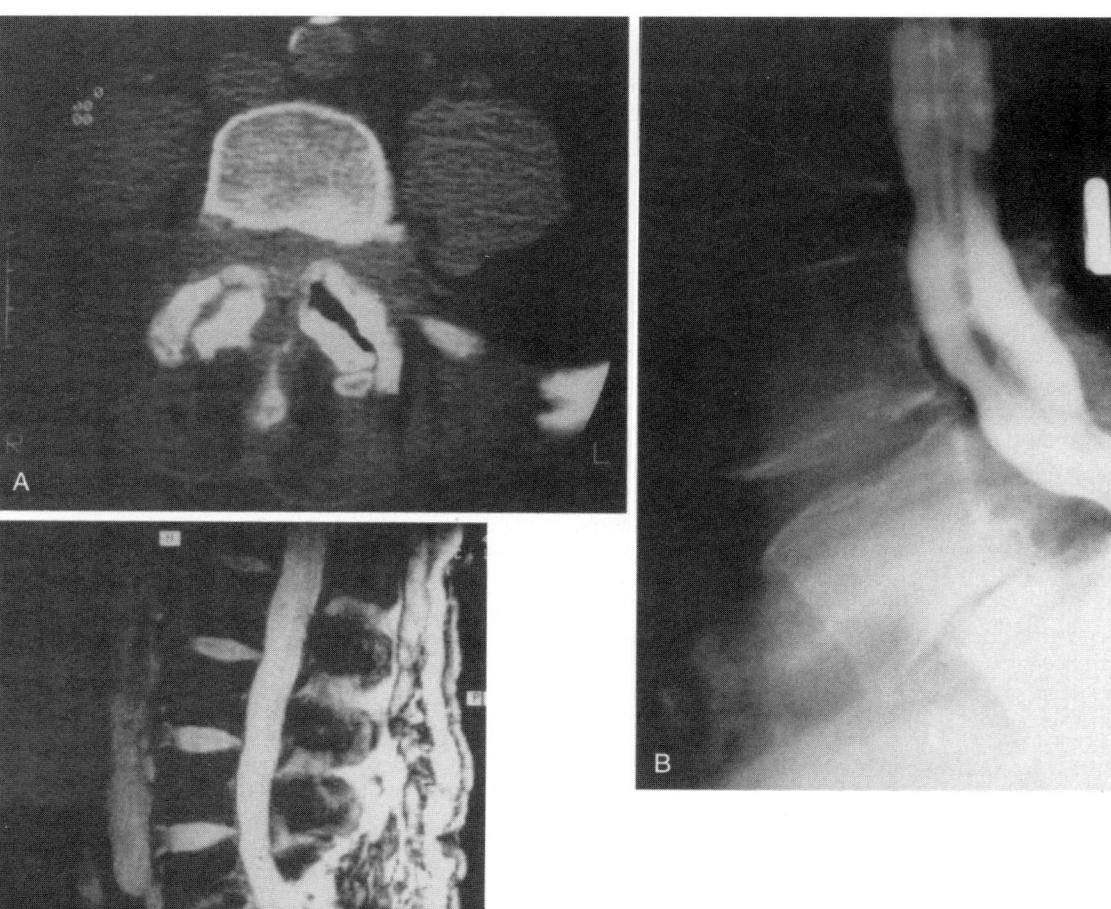

FIGURE 295–15. Degenerative spondylolisthesis and spinal stenosis at L4-5 in a 57-year-old woman whose leg pain was initially relieved by laminectomy but who subsequently developed a progressive slip (*A* and *B*). Notice the severe degeneration of the facets and sagittal configuration *(A)*, which are risk factors for the occurrence of degenerative spondylolisthesis. Notice also the absence of stabilizing changes in the disk, which is severely degenerated but not narrowed. Progressive slippage can also be seen (*B* and *C*).

and greater level of activity, and a large disk space with herniation and without marginal osteophytes. More specific risk factors, such as measured ligamentous laxity and facet dimensions and orientation, have been proposed and are under investigation.

The best guides for the surgeon making a preoperative decision are a patient's general risk factors, the status of the disk, and the facet dimensions and orientation. Patients who are obese and in poor physical condition are at risk for persistent back pain after decompression. When these patients also have narrow lamina, a herniated disk at the same level, and a sagittal orientation of the facets, primary fusion is advisable.

I treated 15 patients with degenerative spondylolisthesis for back and leg pain between 1987 and 1993. Nine women and five men (mean age, 58 years) underwent lumbar fusion procedures with instrumentation (two of these were intertransverse procedures, and the remainder were posterior lumbar interbody fusion procedures). One of the patients, an obese woman, had a previous laminectomy performed by me and developed a progressive symptomatic slip (Fig. 295–15). Surgical treatments and their results are as follows:

1. L4-5 posterior lumbar interbody fusion with pedicle fixation (4 patients)
   Outcome: 4 good
2. L4-5, L5-S1 posterior lumbar interbody fusion (4 patients), intertransverse fusion (1 patient), all with pedicle fixation
   Outcome: all good
3. L3-4, L4-5 posterior lumbar interbody fusion (3 patients), intertransverse fusion (1 patient), all with pedicle fixation
   Outcome: 2 good, 1 fair, 1 poor
4. L3-4 posterior lumbar interbody fusion with use of Steffee plates (1 patient)
   Outcome: good
5. L5-S1 posterior lumbar interbody fusion with use of Steffee plates (1 patient)
   Outcome: good

As reported, this surgical series included fusion patients exclusively, and therefore its results cannot be used to address the issues of instability after laminectomy (with the exception of the one laminectomy failure) (Fig. 295–16). The patient with a poor outcome developed localized instability at L2-3 at 1 year postoperatively and had a lateral and anterior slip that may require future surgery. The fair result was obtained in an obese and deconditioned woman with chronic back pain. Fusion surgery at L3-4 and above entails somewhat higher risk for nerve damage because of the reduced space available for introducing graft material into the interspace and of the narrowed transverse diameter of the pedicle, which increases the risk of screw insertion.

Postsurgical Spondylolysis and Spondylolisthesis

From 1987 to 1993, I treated 14 patients with postsurgical instability syndromes by means of reoperation and fusion. The results were as follows:

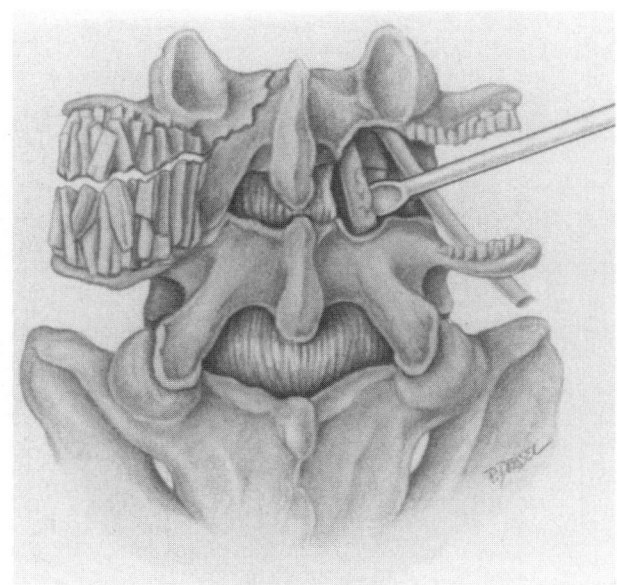

FIGURE 295–16. The surgical approach to decompression and fusion after prior failed fusion begins with a careful exploration and removal of the fusion bone mass. The transverse process and pedicle at each level must be identified. Then, the facets can be removed with osteotomes and rongeurs for identification of the medial and lateral nerves, the disk space, and fresh dural margins. Diskectomy is followed by careful introduction of contoured bone grafts, which are secured by compression across pedicle screws.

1. Spondylolisthesis after laminectomy for spinal stenosis (2 patients) and for degenerative spondylolisthesis (1 patient); all underwent fusion with pedicle fixation
   Outcomes: 2 good, 1 fair
2. Spondylolysis after diskectomy (2 patients), spondylolisthesis after diskectomy (1 patient); all fusions with pedicle fixation
   Outcomes: 2 good, 1 fair
3. Spondylolysis and ipsilateral recurrent disk herniation (4 patients); all underwent posterior lumbar interbody fusion with a variety of pedicle fixation devices
   Outcomes: 3 good, 1 poor (did not recover preoperative footdrop)
4. Spondylolysis adjacent to failed fusion (3 patients), and spondylolisthesis coextensive with failed fusion (1 patient); fusions revised with pedicle fixations and posterior lumbar interbody fusion
   Outcomes: 3 good, 1 fair

Surgery for these patients restored useful function and provided relief of symptoms. During reoperations, complete facetectomy exposed previously nonoperated tissues without scar, which made identification of dural margins easier and safer.

With this approach, diskectomy and posterior lumbar interbody fusion are achieved with a minimum of nerve retraction. Pedicle fixation is essential for stabilization of the spine. Accordingly, the pedicles should

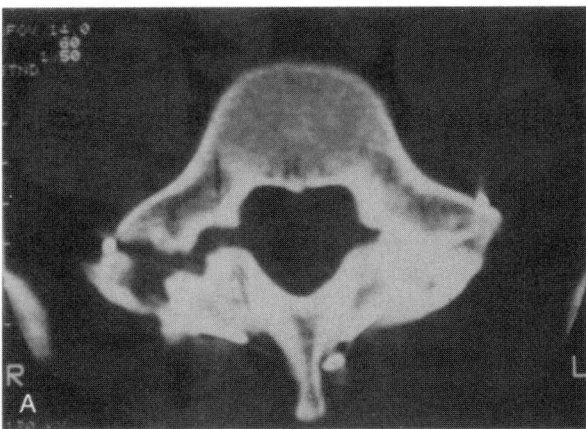

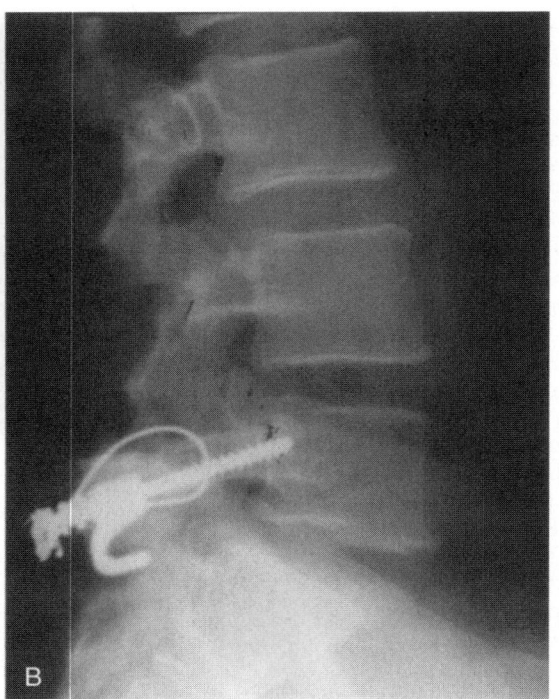

FIGURE 295–17. A 32-year-old man with back and leg pain from spondylolysis underwent removal of the pars interarticularis and fusion with autografting, which was supplemented by allografting on the right side and by placement of wires between the transverse process and spinous process bilaterally. The side with allografting failed to fuse *(A)*. After revision of the fusion with autografting alone and placement of a screw and hook implant *(B)*, fusion and relief of symptoms occurred.

be defined and preserved carefully during removal of bone from previous fusion surgeries. Before bone removal, the pars interarticularis and area of prior fusion (when present) should be carefully examined for defects. This approach is illustrated in Figure 295–16.

Fusion Techniques for Spondylolysis without Spondylolisthesis

Direct repair of the pars interarticularis defect in patients without spondylolisthesis has been performed since 1970.[55] The rationale for this treatment is to preserve movement at the disk caudal to the defect, which would be eliminated by fusion. Placement of wire under tension between the transverse process and spinous process had been the primary stabilizing technique until pedicle screws with hooks or wire on the lamina came into use.[56–58] The procedure is most effective in patients younger than 30 years of age and requires autografting. My experience with this procedure is limited to three patients, two of whom were treated with wire and posterior bone fusion, and the third was treated with a construct of Steffee screws and Isola hooks with posterior bone fusion. The operation involves removal of the fractured pars interarticularis and reactive fibrocartilage, which compresses the L5 spinal nerve and nerve root, and is followed by the placement of overlay bone grafts. These grafts cross the defect and extend from the transverse process of L5 to the lamina and spinous process of L5 and, in effect, create a new pars interarticularis. Both patients in whom wire was used had failed fusions, one unilateral failure (Fig. 295–17) and one bilateral failure. In the unilateral case, failure occurred on the side on which allografting was used in combination with auto-

grafting to limit damage to the iliac crest donor site. Both patients with failed fusions underwent reoperation; the reoperation for the unilateral failure employed the screw and hook construct, and that for the bilateral failure involved the use of a Luque rectangle and posterior intertransverse fusion L4-5. The patient treated with Steffee screws and Isola hooks improved but finds the bulky hooks uncomfortable because of their relatively posterior location at the caudal margin of the L5 lamina.

This procedure is most appropriate for young adults with intractable back and leg pain and a normal disk caudal to the pars interarticularis defect. In the future, a low-profile screw and hook construct will probably be available and will represent the optimal implant. Autografting is essential for direct repair of the pars interarticularis.

REFERENCES

1. Herbiniaux G: Traité sur divers accouchaments Laborieux, et sur les Polypes de la Matrice. Brussels, De Boubers, 1782.
2. Wiltse LL, Rothman SLG: Spondylolisthesis: Classification, diagnosis, and natural history. Semin Spinal Surg 1:78, 1989.
3. Wynne-Davies R, Scott JH: Inheritance and spondylolisthesis: A radiographic family survey. J Bone Joint Surg Br 61:301–305, 1979.
4. Maurice HD, Morley TR: Cauda equina lesions following fusion in situ and decompressive laminectomy for severe spondylolisthesis: Four case reports. Spine 14:214–216, 1989.
5. Hensinger RN: Current concepts review: Spondylolysis and spondylolisthesis in children and adolescents. J Bone Joint Surg Am 71:1098–1107, 1989.
6. Goldstein LA, Haake PW, Devanny JR, et al: Guidelines for the management of lumbosacral spondylolisthesis associated with scoliosis. Clin Orthop 117:135–148, 1976.
7. Seitsalo S, Osterman K, Poussa M: Scoliosis associated with lumbar spondylolisthesis: A clinical survey of 190 young patients. Spine 13:899–904, 1988.

8. Farfan HF, Osterial V, Lamy C: The mechanical etiology of spondylolysis and spondylolisthesis. Clin Orthop 117:40–55, 1976.
9. Scoville WB, Corkill G: Lumbar spondylolisthesis with ruptured disc. Neurosurgery 40:529–534, 1974.
10. Lamy C, Bazergui A, Kraus H, et al: The strength of the neural arch and the etiology of spondylosis. Orthop Clin North Am 6:215–231, 1975.
11. Troup JDG: Mechanical factors in spondylolisthesis and spondylolysis. Clin Orthop 117:59–67, 1976.
12. Junghanns HI: Spondylolisthesis ohne Spalt im Zwischengelenkstück. Arch Orthop Unfallchir (München) 29:118, 1930.
13. Hallgrimson S: A case of pseudospondylolisthesis with affection of spinal roots. Acta Orthop Scand 12:309, 1941.
14. MacNab I: Spondylolisthesis with an intact neural arch: The so-called pseudo-spondylolisthesis. J Bone Joint Surg Br 32:325, 1950.
15. Newman H, Stone KH: The etiology of spondylolisthesis. J Bone Joint Surg Br 45:39, 1963.
16. Epstein JA, Epstein BS, Lavine LS, et al: Degenerative lumbar spondylolisthesis with an intact neural arch (pseudospondylolisthesis). Neurosurgery 44:139–147, 1976.
17. Kirkaldy-Willis WH: Radiologic diagnosis of degenerative lumbar spinal instability. Spine 10:262–276, 1985.
18. Verbiest H: Neurogenic intermittent claudication in cases with absolute and relative stenosis of the lumbar vertebral canal (ASLC and RSLC), in cases with narrow lumbar intervertebral foramina, and in cases with both entities. Clin Neurosurg 20:204, 1972.
19. Rosenberg N: Degenerative spondylolisthesis, predisposing factors. J Bone Joint Surg Am 57:467–474, 1975.
20. Fitzgerald JA, Newman PH: Degenerative spondylolisthesis. J Bone Joint Surg Br 58:184–192, 1976.
21. Matsunaga S, Sakou T Morizono Y et al: Natural history of degenerative spondylolisthesis: Pathogenesis and natural course of the slippage. Spine 15:1204–1210, 1990.
22. Farfan HF: The pathological anatomy of degenerative spondylolisthesis: A cadaver study. Spine 5:412–418, 1980.
23. Wiltse LI, Newman PH, Macnab I: Classification of spondylolysis and spondylolisthesis. Clin Orthop 117:23–29, 1976.
24. Sato K, Wakamatsu K, Yoshimuzi A, et al: The configuration of the laminas and facet joints in degenerative spondylolisthesis. Spine 14:1265–1271, 1989.
25. Levine AM, Bosse M, Edwards CC: Bilateral facet dislocations in the thoracolumbar spine. Spine 13:630–640, 1988.
26. Johnsson KE, Redlund-Johnell I, Uden A, et al: Preoperative and postoperative instability in lumbar spine stenosis. Spine 13:591–593, 1989.
27. Shenkin HA, Hash CJ: Spondylolisthesis after multiple bilateral laminectomies and facetectomies for lumbar spondylosis. J Neurosurg 50:45–47, 1979.
28. Lee CK: Accelerated degeneration of the segment adjacent to a lumbar fusion. Spine 13:375–377, 1988.
29. Lee CK: Langrana NA: Lumbosacral spinal fusion: A biomechanical study. Spine 9:574–581, 1984.
30. Wiltse LL, Winter RB: Terminology and measurement of spondylolisthesis. J Bone Joint Surg Am 65:768–772, 1983.
31. Lowe RW, Hayes TD, Kaye Jr, et al: Standing roentgenograms in spondylolisthesis. Clin Orthop 117:80–84, 1976.
32. Laurent LE, Osterman K: Operative treatment of spondylolisthesis in young patients. Clin Orthop 117:85–91, 1976.
33. Wiltse LL, Jackson DW: Treatment of spondylolisthesis and spondylolysis in children. Clin Orthop 117:92–100, 1976.
34. Johnson JR, Kirwan EO: The long-term results of fusion in situ for severe spondylolisthesis. J Bone Joint Surg Br 65:43–46, 1983.
35. Boxall D, Bradford DS, Winter RB, et al: Management of severe spondylolisthesis in children and adolescents. J Bone Joint Surg Am 61:479–495, 1979.
36. Bradford DS: Closed reduction of spondylolisthesis. Spine 13:580–587, 1988.
37. Louis R: Fusion of the lumbar and sacral spine by internal fixation with screw plates. Clin Orthop 203:18–33, 1986.
38. Sijbrandij S: Reduction and stabilization of severe spondylolisthesis. J Bone Joint Surg Br 65:40–42, 1983.
39. Steffee AD, Sitkowski DJ: Reduction and stabilization of grade IV spondylolisthesis. Clin Orthop 227:82–89, 1988.
40. Transfeldt EE, Dendrinos GK, Bradford DS: Paresis of proximal lumbar roots after reduction of L5-S1 spondylolisthesis. Spine 14:884–887, 1989.
41. Lindholm TS, Ragni P, Ylikoski M et al.: Lumbar isthmic spondylolisthesis in children and adolescents. Spine 15:1350–1355, 1990.
42. Gaines RW, Nichols WK: Treatment of spondyloptosis by two-stage 15 vertebrectomy and reduction of L4 onto S1. Spine 10:680–686, 1985.
43. Apel DM, Lorenz MA, Zindrick MR: Symptomatic spondylolisthesis in adults: Four decades later. Spine 14:348–348, 1989.
44. Harris IE, Weinstein SI: Long-term follow-up of patients with spondylolisthesis. J Bone Joint Surg Am 69:960–969, 1987.
45. Amuso SJ, Neff RS, Coulson DB, et al: The surgical treatment of spondylolisthesis by posterior element resection. J Bone Joint Surg Am 52:529–536, 1970.
46. Hanley EN Jr, Levy JA: Surgical treatment of isthmic lumbosacral spondylolisthesis. Spine 14:48–50, 1989.
47. Osterman K, Lindholm TS, Laurent LS: Late results of removal of the loose posterior element (Gill's operation in the treatment of lytic lumbar spondylolisthesis). Clin Orthop 117:121–128, 1976.
48. Gill GG, Manning JG, White HL: Surgical treatment of spondylolisthesis without spine fusion. J Bone Joint Surg Am 37:493, 1955.
49. Cloward RB: Spondylolisthesis: Treatment by laminectomy and posterior interbody fusion. Clin Orthop 154:74–82, 1981.
50. Kim SS, Denis F, Lonstein JE, et al: Factors affecting fusion rate in adult spondylolisthesis. Spine 15:979–984, 1990.
51. Epstein NE, Epstein JA, Carras R, et al: Degenerative spondylolisthesis with an intact neural arch: A review of 60 cases with an analysis of clinical findings and the development of surgical management. Neurosurgery 13:555–561, 1983.
52. Herron LD, Trippi AC: L4-5 degenerative spondylolisthesis. Spine 14:534–538, 1989.
53. Lombardi JS, Wiltse LL, Reynolds JD, et al: Treatment of degenerative spondylolisthesis. Spine 10:821–827, 1985.
54. Bridwell KH, Sedgewick TA, O'Brien MF, et al: The role of fusion and instrumentation in the treatment of degenerative spondylolisthesis with spinal stenosis. J Spinal Disord 6:461–472, 1993.
55. Nachemson A: Repair of the spondylolisthetic defect and intertransverse fusion for young patients. Clin Orthop 117:101–105, 1976.
56. Bradford DS, Iza J: Repair of the defect in spondylolysis or minimal degrees of spondylolisthesis by segmental wire fixation and bone grafting. Spine 10:673–679, 1985.
57. Buck JE: Direct repair of the defect in spondylolisthesis. J Bone Joint Surg Br 52:432–437, 1970.
58. Hambly M, Lee CK, Gutteling E, et al: Tension band wiring—bone grafting for spondylolysis and spondylolisthesis. Spine 14:455–460, 1989.

Adult Thoracolumbar Scoliosis

SEAN A. SALEHI ■ STEPHEN L. ONDRA

Traditionally, neurosurgery has dealt with diseases of the spine that produced neurological compression. With improved understanding of the pathophysiology and biomechanics of spine disease, there has been steady expansion of our ability to treat patients with complex disorders of the spine, including problems of neurologic compression and disorders that result in axial back pain or mechanical imbalance. New surgical techniques and instrumentation systems allow us to apply powerful stabilizing and corrective forces to the spine. This ability to change the biomechanics of the spine requires us to develop a deeper understanding of the pathophysiology of spinal disease and the biomechanical forces at work. The long-term implications of spinal disease and treatment are important considerations for the neurosurgeon treating adult thoracolumbar scoliosis. The principles of evaluation and management of adult spinal deformity are discussed in this chapter.

Scoliosis is defined as a coronal-plane deformity of the spine that is greater than 10 degrees when measured by the Cobb angle method. It typically has structural rotation at the apical motion segment[1] (Fig. 296–1). Adult degenerative scoliosis is the presentation of a spinal deformity greater than 10 degrees in the coronal plane after the age of 20 years or after having reached skeletal maturity. This deformity typically is exacerbated by degenerative changes in the spinal elements.[2] The degenerative changes that result in deformity progression frequently cause back pain and neurological compression. To adequately treat the resulting pain syndromes, the surgeon must consider the biomechanical changes that are being created by the deformity and by the planned treatment. By understanding the interplay of these two biomechanical forces, an optimal long-term result can be obtained for the patient.

DEMOGRAPHICS AND NATURAL HISTORY

Adolescent idiopathic scoliosis is believed to be an inherited disease process that follows an autosomal-dominant pattern with incomplete penetrance. It is more prevalent in women, with a female-to-male inci-

dence of approximately 7:1. This increased incidence in adolescents leads to an increased incidence of degenerative scoliosis due to late progression of idiopathic curves in women. This process is further accelerated by the higher incidence of osteoporosis in women. Presentations of de novo degenerative scoliotic curves are equal for men and women.[3] There appears to be no exacerbation in either group due to pregnancy.[4]

Degenerative curves of all types typically present after the age of 40 years. It is estimated that degenerative thoracolumbar scoliosis occurs in 1.9% to 3.9% of the population older than 40 years.[5, 6] Other studies have found up to a 30% incidence in scoliosis in patients between the ages of 50 and 84 years.[7] These figures incorporate all patients with adult scoliosis regardless of classification and demonstrate the age-related increase in deformity due to degeneration of the vertebral column metabolic bone disease, degenerative disk disease, and degenerative joint disease.[7–9] It is believed that the population with adult spinal deformity will increase because of the relative aging of the population and the increasing incidence of degenerative spinal disease and osteoporosis. It is estimated that the average degenerative scoliotic curve will progress at a rate of 1 to 2 degrees per year. Because a standard measurement error of 3 degrees is allowed, no curve should be considered progressive until it has increased at least 5 degrees.

Thoracolumbar curves greater than 50 degrees are at highest risk for progression.[10] In the study by Collins,[11] it was estimated that 65% of all curves would progress by 5 degrees or more during the follow-up period. In addition to the coronal curve measurement, the degree of axial rotation also has an effect. The greater is the axial rotation, the greater the degeneration and higher rate of curve progression.

SYMPTOMS OF SCOLIOSIS

Back, buttock, and leg pain are the overwhelming presenting symptoms of patients with adult degenerative scoliosis. It is estimated that 48% to 79% of adult patients complain of pain as their primary symptoms.[5, 8, 12] Lower extremity paresthesias, radiculopathy, sacroiliac

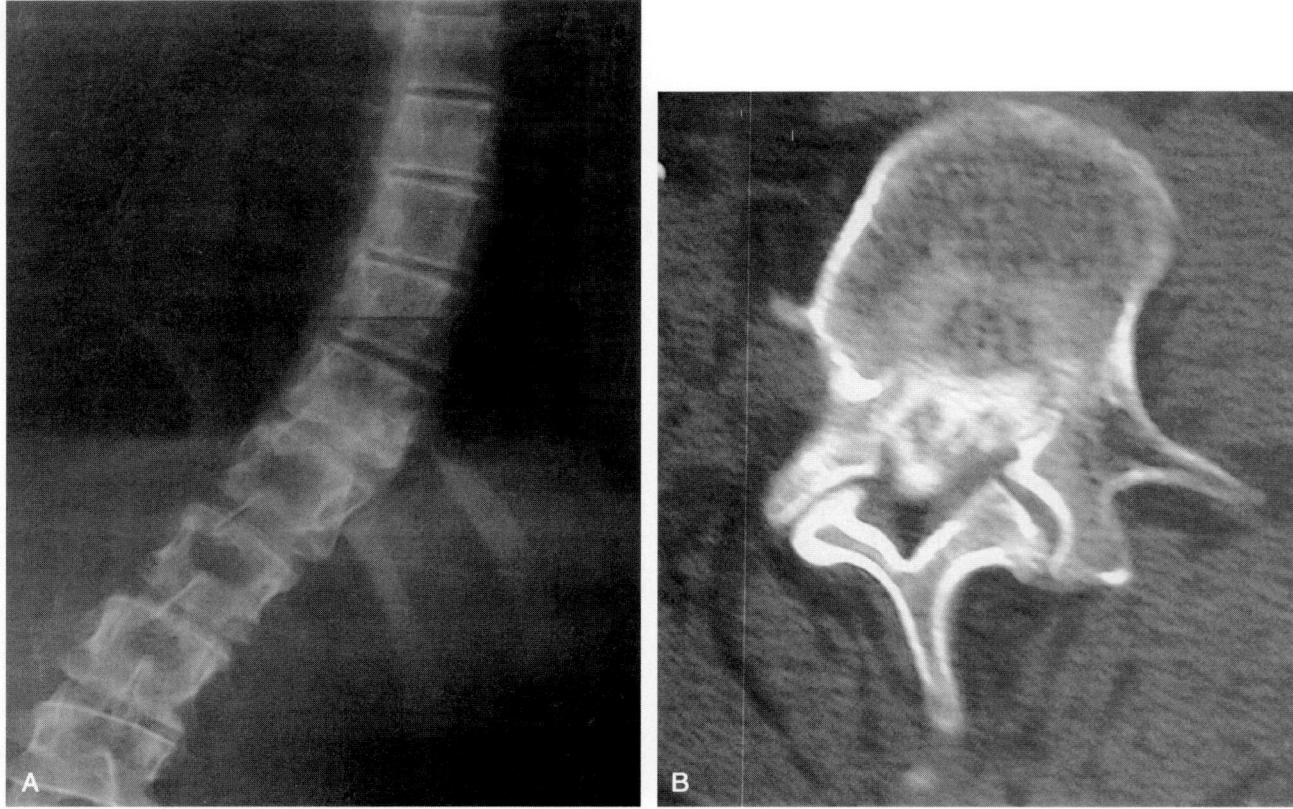

FIGURE 296–1. *A,* Anteroposterior view of the thoracolumbar spine shows rotation of the vertebrae in the axial plane. Notice the rotation of the pedicles. *B,* Computed tomography shows rotation of the vertebrae in the apex of the curve. This rotation is thought to be the primary driving force for the progression of the curve.

joint pain, and muscle spasms are also common manifestations. Complaints of pain in the thigh muscles from hip flexion is common in patients with a sagittal-plane imbalance and is characteristic of flat back. Patients may complain of gait disturbance caused by sagittal-plane imbalance. Some adults also notice progressing deformity of their backs.

Because back and lower extremity radiating pain is common in the general population, it is essential that a careful history and physical examination be conducted. Eliciting factors such as location and duration of the pain, activities that increase or decrease pain, character and location of pain radiation, paresthesias, and urinary symptoms should be carefully reviewed. Areas of muscle spasm and tightness should also be defined. Winter and colleagues[13] describe a characteristic pain pattern in scoliotic patients. Pain over the concavity of the scoliosis curve is thought to be caused by facet degeneration, whereas pain over the convexity is thought to be caused by muscle spasm. Pain in the midscapular and trapezius region typically results from cervical rather than thoracolumbar pathology.[13] Posture and the possible coexistence of sacroiliac joint pathology should be evaluated. In this way, confusion about the cause of the pain can be avoided.[14] By understanding the true cause of the pain, the risk of overtreating the problem can be minimized.

The importance of this careful evaluation is best demonstrated in a study by Nachemson.[15] In his 30-year follow-up, he found that patients with adult scoliosis did not have a greater incidence of spine pain than in the general population.[15] He also concluded that low back pain in patients with scoliosis should undergo the same conservative management as patients with nonscoliotic degenerative disease. Weinstein and co-workers[10] echoed Nachemson's finding when they reported that there was no relation between the severity of pain and the amount of scoliotic curve.[10] These investigators demonstrated the importance of remembering that not all pain in patients with scoliosis is caused by the curve. This is important because the biomechanical requirements of surgery in scoliosis patients often preclude routine procedures and demand extensive reconstruction. The history, physical examination, and diagnostic testing can direct the physician in treating the proper source of the patient's symptoms to obtain maximal effectiveness and minimal morbidity.

CLASSIFICATION

The Scoliosis Research Society has divided idiopathic spinal deformity into a variety of basic categories. Although idiopathic scoliosis is primarily diagnosed and treated in adolescence, adult degenerative scoliosis can result from a late progression of preexisting idiopathic curve. It may also develop de novo from degenerative disease of the spine or traumatic changes after skeletal maturity has occurred. Degenerative scoliosis is a separate classification of spinal deformity and cannot be categorized in the King system.[16] Late progression of a preexisting idiopathic curve is typically classified as one of the categories defined by King. The King classification defines five distinct curve patterns (Table 296–1). These patterns specifically apply to patients with preexisting idiopathic curves. Problems of pain and deformity are accelerated in all groups by degenerative disk disease, degenerative facet joint disease, and osteoporosis.

All spinal deformity curves have two potential components. The structural portion of the curve is a rigid deformity that is not correctable by the patient's bending when observed on physical examination or in radiographic studies. The compensatory portion of the curve is a physiologic curve that assists the patient in establishing better spinal balance for the rigid (structural) portion of the spinal deformity. It can be brought into normal alignment with the remainder of the spine by having the patient bend and adjust position. Traditionally, the King classification system defines the structural or rigid part of the deformity. In adolescence, correction of this single portion of the curve allows the sacral plumb line to come into alignment. This allows for shorter segment fusion than might be initially expected by a static standing film.

In adults, a portion of the curve that was previously physiologic as an adolescent often becomes structural from long-standing, uncorrected deformity and the progression of degenerative disease. This degenerative progression increasingly stiffens the spine, making most adult curves true thoracolumbar rigid deformities. The sagittal-plane portion of the deformity becomes an increasing problem for adults with degenerative scoliosis when compared with children and adolescents.[8] Kyphosis at the thoracolumbar junction is the rule in adult degenerative scoliosis. This results in a sagittal-plane imbalance characterized by a loss of lumbar lordosis and thoracolumbar junction kyphosis. The imbalance throws the C7 plumb line anterior to the sacrum and requires the patient to increasingly flex at the hips to regain spinal-pelvic balance, which can result in hip flexor contraction and a characteristic posture and gait of flat back syndrome from the loss of lumbar lordosis.

T A B L E   2 9 6 – 1 ■ **Curve Patterns in Idiopathic Scoliosis according to the King Classification**

CLASS	CURVE PATTERN
King 1	Major lumbar, minor thoracic
King 2	Major thoracic, minor lumbar
King 3	Single thoracic curve
King 4	Thoracolumbar curve
King 5	Double thoracic curve

As in all types of spinal deformity, adult degenerative scoliosis should be characterized based only on the structural portion of the curve. If the adult curve does not fit easily into the King system, it should be characterized by stating the degree of curve measured by the method of Cobb and the apical and caudal vertebrae used in that measurement for each rigid portion of the curve. The sagittal portions of the curve should also be stated. In this way, all adult curves can be classified by their component levels. Equally important is the ability provided by such measurements to assess progression of the curve on sequential films.

EVALUATION

Any patient being considered for reconstructive spinal surgery should undergo a careful assessment for the presence of associated adult degenerative scoliosis. The initial evaluation begins with a careful clinical examination. In addition to the standard neurological examination performed on patients with spinal disease, careful assessment of the spine, posture, and extremities should be performed. Patients should be dressed in a gown, and ideally, a standing examination is performed. The overall posture should be assessed from anterior, posterior, and lateral perspectives. From the anterior and posterior perspectives, the shoulders and pelvis should be examined to see if there is any tilt (i.e., discrepancy in height from right to left) that may indicate an underlying coronal scoliotic curve. The spine itself should also be examined and palpated to assess for any evidence of curvature. From the lateral perspective, assessment of overall posture and the sagittal plane should occur. This includes evaluation about whether the head, shoulders, and pelvis fall into alignment and whether the cervical and lumbar lordosis and the thoracic kyphosis are of normal contour. The hip posture should be evaluated to assess if there is rotation of the hips to compensate for an imbalance of the spine in the sagittal plane. Assessment of the knee and hips should be done. Hip flexion may indicate compensation for a sagittal-plane imbalance of the spine. The leg length should be assessed. A leg length discrepancy may indicate long-standing spinal imbalance. Gait should be assessed to evaluate the patient for a neurological change and for an abnormal gait caused by a structural change.

Having completed the surface examination of the patient's skeletal structure and balance, a general neurological and medical evaluation should be performed. The neurological examination should look for evidence of radiculopathy or myelopathy. This includes careful motor, reflex, and sensory examinations. Evidence for a primary neuromuscular disease or neurocutaneous syndrome should also be sought. The general medical examination should pay particular attention to the pulmonary and cardiovascular systems. Any patient with a significant thoracic kyphosis, coronal curve greater than 70 degrees, or the clinical suggestion of pulmonary disease should undergo formal pulmonary function tests.

After physical examination of the patient is completed, diagnostic imaging studies are done. The most important diagnostic imaging method for patients who are thought to have adult degenerative scoliosis is plain radiography.[14] All patients being considered for reconstructive surgery of the thoracolumbar spine should have standard anteroposterior, lateral, and lateral flexion and extension films of the spine. If there is any suggestion on physical examination or on x-ray films of a coronal- or sagittal-plane imbalance, standard 36-inch, upright, anteroposterior and lateral scoliosis films should be obtained. In this way, the coronal- and sagittal-plane balance of the patient can be carefully assessed. If the patient has a spinal imbalance, right- and left-side bending films should be obtained in addition to the flexion-extension films. Areas of the curve that correct with bending reflect simple compensatory curves and may not need to be included fully in the fusion. Areas of the deformity curve that do not change with bending are structural and require reconstruction and correction. Follow-up plain x-ray films give a wealth of information about progression of the curve.[1]

The lateral scoliosis film allows detailed assessment of sagittal-plane balance. A plumb line dropped from C7 should fall through the body of L1 and the body of S1. This is normal spinal balance in the sagittal plane.

In general, the normal thoracic kyphosis is 35 to 45 degrees, with an average of 40 degrees. The normal lumbar lordosis has higher variability and may be 30 to 60 degrees, with a mean of 45 to 50 degrees. Any loss of lumbar lordosis (i.e., flat back) or thoracic kyphosis results in the spine's plumb line being shifted anterior to the sacrum. This is typically compensated for by rotation of the pelvis and flexion of the hips, and the spine is returned to balance over the pelvis. This causes difficulty in ambulation and a tired, aching feeling in the thighs. Increase in thoracic kyphosis or lumbar hyperlordosis results in the plumb line falling posterior to the sacrum. In these cases, the patient leans forward to try to restore spinal-pelvic balance. In both cases, correction of the abnormal curve is required to restore normal spinal balance. When abnormalities have been long-standing, often both thoracic and lumbar curves are abnormal. Correction of one leaves the patient out of balance or can possibly worsen the spinal balance. Correction of both curves is necessary for restoration of spinal balance. Imbalance in the sagittal plane is much more debilitating to patients than coronal imbalance, and particular attention should be paid to understanding and correcting sagittal balance.

The anteroposterior scoliosis film provides significant information regarding the scoliotic curve of a patient with adult degenerative scoliosis. The coronal curve is established in the same way as sagittal curves. The angle of deformity is typically measured with the method described by Cobb. A line is drawn parallel with the superior end plate of the apical vertebra of the curve. An additional line is drawn parallel to the inferior end plate of the caudal vertebra of the curve. Perpendicular lines are drawn to each of the end-plate

lines. The angle of the curve is measured by assessing the angle defined by the intersection of these two lines (Fig. 296–2). Angles should always be given, with the apical and caudal vertebrae used to establish the angle given within parentheses next to the absolute number. In this way, intraobserver variability is minimized, and accurate comparison with old films is enhanced.

The anteroposterior scoliosis films allows the examiner to establish whether the patient is in coronal balance. A line drawn from C7 should fall through L1 and the middle of the sacrum. Any deviation from the sacral midline indicates a coronal imbalance. The stable vertebra of the curve is the vertebra bisected by the central sacral line (Fig. 296–3). Rotation is typically measured using the Nash method. The neutral vertebra is the one that has both pedicles without rotation. The apical vertebra is the segment at the maximal deformity of the coronal curve.

Typically, patients with evidence of neurological progression have magnetic resonance imaging (MRI) performed. MRI is essential in evaluating the patient

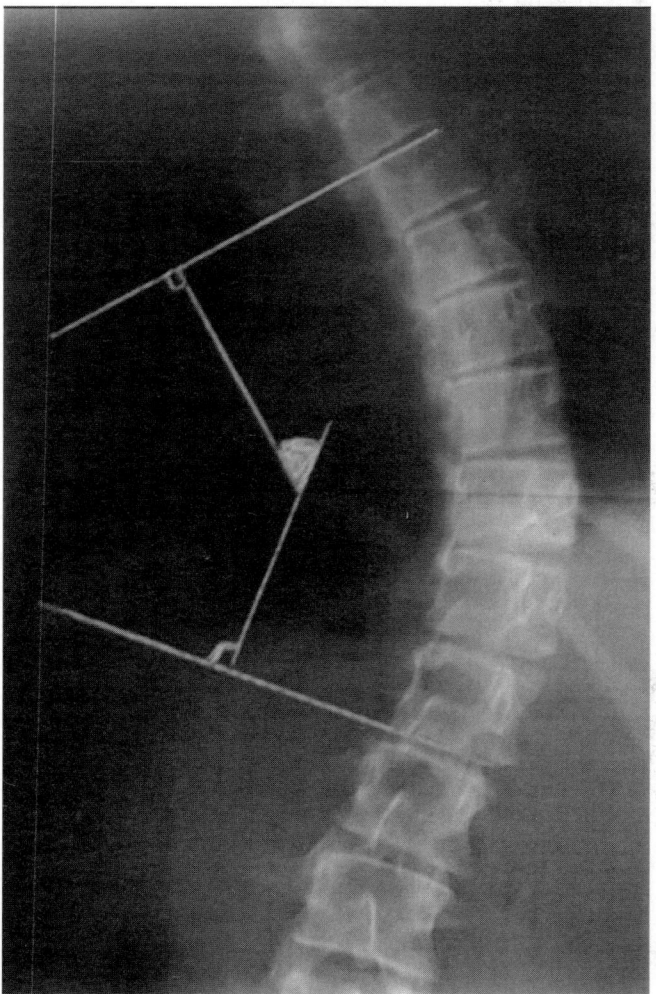

FIGURE 296–2. The method of Cobb is used to measure the degree of curvature in the coronal plane. Perpendicular lines are drawn to two lines drawn along the superior end plate of the top vertebra and the inferior end plate of the bottom vertebra.

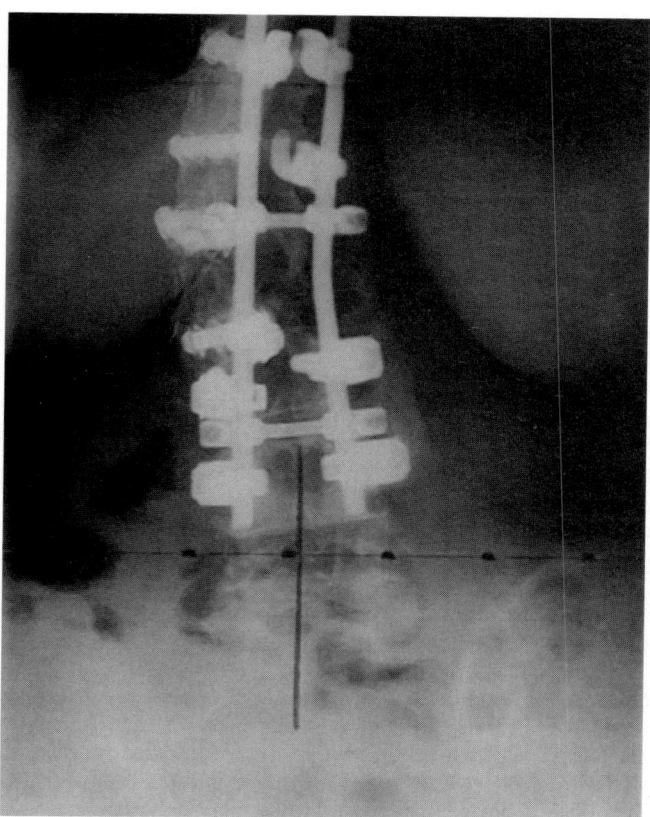

FIGURE 296–3. A stable vertebra is defined as the vertebra bisected by the center sacral line (i.e., perpendicular line drawn from the middle of sacrum). Here, L4 is the stable vertebra.

for areas of spinal canal or foraminal compression. Disk hydration and degeneration can also be assessed, in addition to herniation and neurological compression. The physician may also get a rough assessment of the scoliosis on the sagittal and coronal reconstructions. Axial reconstructions may indicate evidence of rotation associated with a scoliotic curve. The most important aspect of the MRI is evaluation of disk hydration and degeneration. In general, a spinal reconstructive procedure should not be ended at the level of a severely degenerated or dehydrated disk.

MRI of patients with severe scoliosis may be difficult to assess. Because of the rotation and angulation present, the amount of nerve root compression may be deceiving. In these cases, myelography and postmyelogram computed tomography (CT) can provide important and additional information to help identify areas of neurological compression.

Myelography and postmyelogram CT are often helpful in assessing areas of neurological compression. The myelogram is sometimes easier to interpret than axial images in cases of deformity. Nerves can be evaluated for compression without the confusion of axial images that are distorted by the curve.

Diskography has been used by some[17] to assess the disk status at the caudal or cephalad end of a reconstructive fusion. A negative diskogram result indicates that it is safe to conclude the fusion at this disk level, whereas a positive diskogram result suggests that the fusion should be extended.

Bone density evaluation by dual-energy x-ray absorptiometry (DEXA) often provides important information regarding the quality of the bone and its ability to hold instrumentation and withstand the forces needed for deformity correction and stabilization. Patients with poor bone mineral density may only be able to have fusion in situ, because it is unlikely they can withstand the forces needed for correction. Patients with extremely poor bone mineral density may not be candidates for fusion at all. In these cases, alternative treatment measures may need to be considered.

Electromyography (EMG) can be very useful in assessing patients with degenerative scoliosis. A positive finding may indicate which of the multiple abnormal foramina in patients with this disorder result in neurological compression, which is often difficult to assess clinically or radiographically. Some investigators[18] have suggested that simple correction of the deformity may obviate the need for decompression. This is a minority view, but decompression only in areas with a positive EMG result may limit the amount of decompression performed, preserving additional bone surface for fusion. Bone density evaluation is also important in patients who have evidence of osteoporosis on plain x-ray films. A patient with degenerative scoliosis who suffers from thoracic hyperkyphosis should undergo pulmonary function testing (PFT) whether surgery is contemplated or not.[11] We routinely recommend patients with curves of more than 70 degrees, because the rate of pulmonary compromise in this group is high. For patients who complain of pulmonary symptoms and do not plan to undergo surgery, PFT at regular intervals may pick up subtle worsening of pulmonary function. Preoperative PFT can help the surgeon in better postoperative care planning, such as using a longer postoperative intubation period as a safety factor. PFT is also important for asymptomatic patients who have comorbid conditions such as asthma, emphysema, lung cancer, or cardiac disease.

The acquisition of these data gives clear definition of the scoliotic deformity in the sagittal and coronal planes. It also defines areas of spinal stability and instability. These are critical measures when assessing potential correction and reconstruction. Without this careful assessment, suboptimal long-term results of spinal stabilization are achieved, and a new imbalance can be introduced into the spine, worsening the patient's condition.

MEDICAL MANAGEMENT

Patients who present with back pain, no clinical evidence of neurological compression, and a curve less than 45 degrees should initially undergo a course of medical management.[19] This includes nonsteroidal anti-inflammatory agents and limited use of oral narcotics. In general, narcotics should only be used for finite periods during episodes of severe pain. Physical therapy is also useful in treating associated muscle spasm, improving body mechanics, and strengthening the supporting musculature of the spine. In general, bracing is of no use in deformity stabilization or correction in adults.[20] Some patients may benefit from a short course of brace stabilization until an exacerbation of acute pain resolves. A program of weight loss combined with physical therapy can significantly reduce the stress on the deformed, degenerative spine. Patients with osteoporosis should be considered for medications that may slow or reverse ongoing bone loss.

Minimally invasive management options consist primarily of injections. These include injections of painful, degenerative facets; trigger point injections for muscle spasm; and epidural steroid injections.[19]

These are many of the measures used in the management of nonscoliotic degenerative spine pain. Nachemson's study[15] found that the incidence of back pain in patients with degenerative adult scoliosis did not significantly differ from the incidence of pain in age-matched populations. In view of this, all medical treatment for pain in adult scoliosis patients should be exhausted before surgical intervention is contemplated or the patient falls into the curve parameters that predict scoliotic decompensation.[15]

SURGICAL MANAGEMENT

Surgical indications for patients with adult scoliosis include severe and disabling back pain that fails to respond to maximal medical management; severe, nonresponsive radiculopathy; and progression of physiologic disturbances such as pulmonary dysfunction. Patients whose pain may or may not be manageable can also become surgical candidates based on mechanical evaluation and prediction of decompensation. Mechanical indications for surgery include the progression of sagittal- or coronal-plane imbalance of more than 5 to 10 degrees per year.[2] A curve larger than 50 degrees is also at high risk for decompensation. Progressively unacceptable gait imbalance and cosmetic issues may also enter into the decision to operate.

Decompression Alone

In a patient with severe radiculopathy and well-controlled back pain, consideration can be given to decompression alone[15] after carefully assessing the patient's curve and stability. The surgeon must also consider how destabilizing the decompression will be and where in the curve the mechanics will be altered.[21]

Curve decompensation and progression are more likely if decompression is being done at the apex of the curve. Full laminectomies are also more destabilizing than hemilaminectomies because of the loss of muscle attachment and ligamentous support. When a foramenotomy is being performed, it should not remove more than one third of the facet. High-degree curves with significant rotation also have a higher risk of decompensation when decompression alone is carried out.

Other considerations include bone density and quality and the physical demand that the patient will place on the spine. In general, a very stiff spine identified on bending radiographs in a low-demand patient is at lower risk for decompensation than a more mobile spine in an active patient. If these factors are considered, decompression for radiculopathy or neurogenic claudication may be appropriate.

Posterior Segmental Correction

In deformity of the spine, instrumentation provides the corrective forces to reestablish spinal balance and internal fixation until fusion occurs. Many systems have been designed for the correction of scoliotic deformity.[22-24] Initially, the Harrington rod system allowed some correction and stabilization of curves. The corrective force for this system was primarily provided by distraction, which resulted in frequent loss of sagittal-plane balance, flat back syndrome, and a high rate of pseudoarthrosis. Luque rods were another early system for deformity correction. It required multiple sublaminar wires and had a higher rate of postoperative correction loss.[25]

The introduction of posterior segmental instrumentation and correction by Cotrel and Dubousset revolutionized deformity correction. By controlling the spine across multiple segments with a combination of hooks, pedicle screws, and cables, powerful correction and immobilization forces could be applied to the spine.[26] Cotrel and Dubousset's concept is to control each critical segment of the spine with a bone fixation device (i.e., hook or pedicle screw). A rod is then bent to the desired sagittal and coronal contours. The spine is brought to the rod segment by segment in a three-plane correction. This involves derotation and translation of the bone fixators to the rod and then affixing them to the rod with a connector. The concept of segmental three-dimensional correction of the spine is the basis of all current deformity correction systems. It has resulted in improved rates of fusion and better maintenance of correction.

The most important step in spinal deformity correction is preoperative planning. Realistic goals should be set to achieve spinal balance, not simply straighten a portion of the spine. In patients who are relatively balanced and have no major cosmetic or pulmonary issue, an instrumented in situ posterior stabilization and fusion is a reasonable consideration. When deformity correction is needed to achieve balance, additional planning is required.

In general, a 50% correction of any segment is realistic in an adult. To achieve this, the typically rigid adult spine needs to be made mobile for correction. After the areas for release have been decided, the pattern of corrective forces should be drawn out to consider all three planes of desired correction. This provides a template for surgery that allows spinal balance and stabilization.

Before corrective forces can be applied, the spine must be mobilized by release of partially fused, ankylosed segments. This is done by performing osteotomies where corrective forces will be applied. In simple corrections in patients with preserved disks, posterior osteotomies alone may suffice. These are done in a wedge shape, with the larger part of the wedge on the convex side that is to be closed. Simple linear osteotomies can be done for sagittal-plane correction. When large corrections are needed or the spine is very rigid, an anterior diskectomy and osteotomy may need to precede the posterior release and instrumentation. This is typically done by a thoracoabdominal approach on the convex side of the curve with a diskectomy and concave osteotomy. We typically use disk replacement cages placed eccentrically to the concave side to maintain sagittal-plane correction.

There are general guidelines for posterior segmental instrumentation constructs. In thoracolumbar correction, the construct should not end near the apex of a coronal or sagittal curve. This can result in a junctional deformity due to mechanical stress. The construct should not end at a spinal junction such as the thoracolumbar junction. If the construct is planned to T12, it should be extended to L1 or L2 to avoid a junctional decompensation. If the construct ends at L5, consideration should be given to extending it to the sacrum, although some feel that, if the L5-S1 disk is competent, the morbidity of extending the fusion to the sacrum exceeds the morbidity of lumbar-sacral decompensation and the need for revision.

Fusions at L5-S1 have a variety of problems. There is a higher rate of instrumentation loosening and pseudoarthrosis at L5-S1.[27] This risk can be reduced by obtaining rigid lumbar-sacral junction fixation. When possible, interbody fusion devices placed at L5-S1 can decrease the stress on the caudal screws. Bicortical fixation of the S1 screws should also be obtained. Additional screw placement at S2 or the use of an intrasacral rod technique can be considered. Ilial fixation can be accomplished by the Galveston technique or its modification. Although such techniques do improve stability, they alter pelvic motion and gait. They can also cause late pain due to rod loosening in the ilium from residual motion at the sacroiliac joint. We do not recommend their use in patients who are ambulatory, but we have found them quite helpful in nonambulatory patients with paralytic scoliosis.

The rod should end at a stable vertebra at each end. In adults, the disk below the fusion should be assessed to ensure that it is not degenerative. Ending a long deformity construct on a degenerative disk can lead to early failure of the segment adjacent to the fusion.

If possible, the thoracolumbar or lumbar sacral junctions should be left out of the fusion. This allows patients a residual area of spinal motion that they can use to correct themselves over any residual or new imbalance in the reconstructed spine. If both junctions must be included, as is often the case, extraordinary care should be taken to optimize the patient's reconstruction balance in the sagittal and coronal planes. With both junctions included in the reconstruction, the patient's only remaining compensating mechanisms for balance are pelvic. Further spinal compensation is not possible. A patient with significant hip disease has no compensatory mechanisms.

After the extent of the fusion has been determined, the pattern of segmental correction should be planned. In general, we prefer pedicle screws when possible because of their greater strength. Pedicle diameter in cases of deformity can be highly variable, even within the same spinal segment. Assessment of pedicle size is mandatory to ensure that safe screw placement is possible. This can done with conventional CT, MRI, or three-dimensional CT obtained for image guidance. Segments that cannot accept pedicle screws can be controlled with hooks. Hook patterns should end in a claw construct (i.e., down-going hook at the top of the construct facing an up-going hook) at the ends of the rod. The intervening pattern should allow forces to be applied at the segments that are to be corrected. Typically, this includes the segments one or two levels above and below the apical vertebra, the stable vertebra, and a neutral vertebra at each end. A combination of transverse process, pedicle, and lamina hooks can be used. The hooks and screws can be supplemented with sublaminar cables at intervening levels.

In thoracolumbar curves, the hooks are placed to allow compression across the convex apex of the lumbar curve. This helps to derotate the spine and correct the coronal plane. Because the compression is posterior to the instantaneous axis of rotation, it also allows restoration or lordosis of the lumbar spine, which invariably is hypolordotic. The thoracic hooks are set up to allow distraction and derotation along the concave aspect of the thoracic curve. This helps to correct the coronal deformity, derotate the spine, and restore thoracic kyphosis.

The typical hook-rod pattern is then set up to accept the first rod along the thoracic concave curve and the lumbar convex curve. The desired sagittal contour initially fits into the coronal curves at 60 to 90 degrees from its desired end point. After the rod is seated and loosely captured by the hooks and screws, it is turned back to its desired position and then fixed in place. This is the classic derotation maneuver, which restores balance in the sagittal and coronal planes. Equivalent results can be obtained by slowly translating the spine to the rod segmentally (Fig. 296–4).

Anterior Segmental Correction

The concept of single-stage anterior correction has gained popularity for treating the adolescent and adult populations. Anterior correction allows single-stage stabilization and correction with less blood loss and two or three fewer segments of fusion. The mechanical evaluation and principles of correction applied to the preoperative planning are similar to those for posterior correction.

This technique is possible if the posterior elements are not ankylosed, the correction can be accomplished within the limits of T8 to L4, and the curve does not exceed 60 degrees. Patients who do not fit these criteria should not be considered for single-stage anterior correction. An anterior release is performed, and disk replacement cages are placed in a fashion similar to the anterior release done for posterior correction. Bicortical

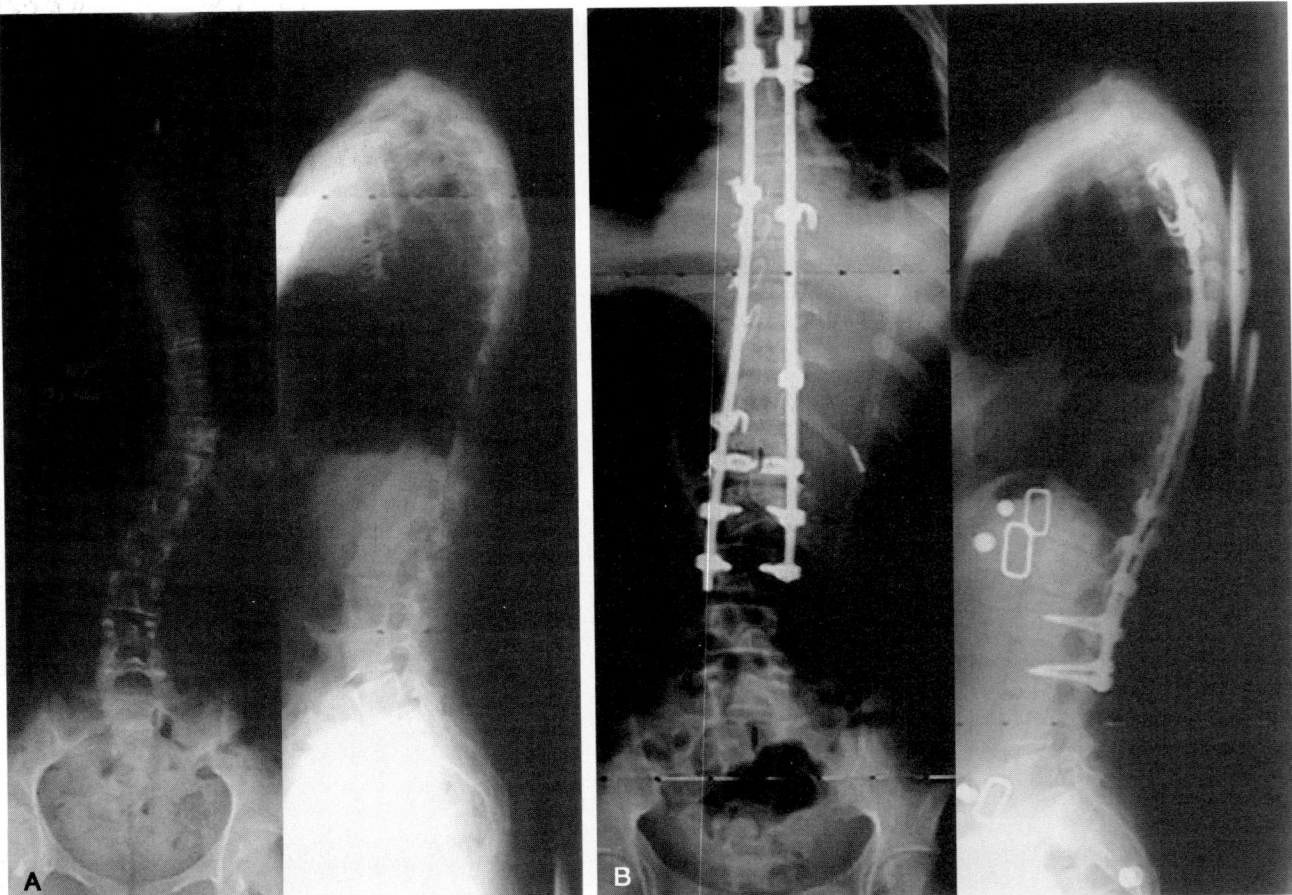

FIGURE 296–4. Preoperative *(A)* and postoperative *(B)* plain radiographs of the spine. T3 and L3 are the stable vertebrae, and the fusion has been extended between these two vertebrae. The Cobb angle has been reduced from 45 to 5 degrees. Maintenance of the normal sagittal-plane balance is achieved.

vertebral body screws are then placed, and the rod is contoured to the desired correction. The rod is then placed and derotated. Final compression and distraction are performed with the knowledge that the rod is anterior to the axis of rotation. As such, compression causes a mild loss of lordosis. If space permits, a second rod can be placed and cross-linked (Fig. 296–5).

RESULTS

Several studies have found good to excellent results in terms of pain relief in 70% to 90% of patients.[3, 28–30]

Although these results compare favorably with the surgical treatment for radicular and back pain from other causes, the magnitude of adult deformity surgery carries significant risk of complications. The rates of major and minor complications from adult deformity surgery range from 20% to 53%[12, 29, 31, 32] (Table 296–2 and Table 296–3). Most complications can be minimized by careful attention to nutrition, wound care, activity, venous thrombosis prophylaxis, and preoperative planning.

Most complications are relatively minor and transient and of limited long-term consequence. Major complications with serious sequelae occur often

T A B L E   2 9 6 – 2 ■ **Studies Evaluating Complication Rates for Scoliosis Surgery**

STUDY	NO. OF PATIENTS	COMPLICATION (%)	NEUROLOGICAL DEFICIT (%)	PSEUDOARTHROSIS (%)	INFECTION (%)	INSTRUMENTATION FAILURE (%)	DEATHS
Byrd[28]	26	85	7.7	0	0	11.5	0
Kostuik[31]	107	47	0.7	10	10	10	1
Ondra*	42	42	0	5	2	15	1
Simmons[29]	49	41	0	0	0	12.2	0
Swank[32]	222	53	0.5	11	8	12	3
Van Dam	91	33	1.1	15	1	5	0

* Unpublished data.

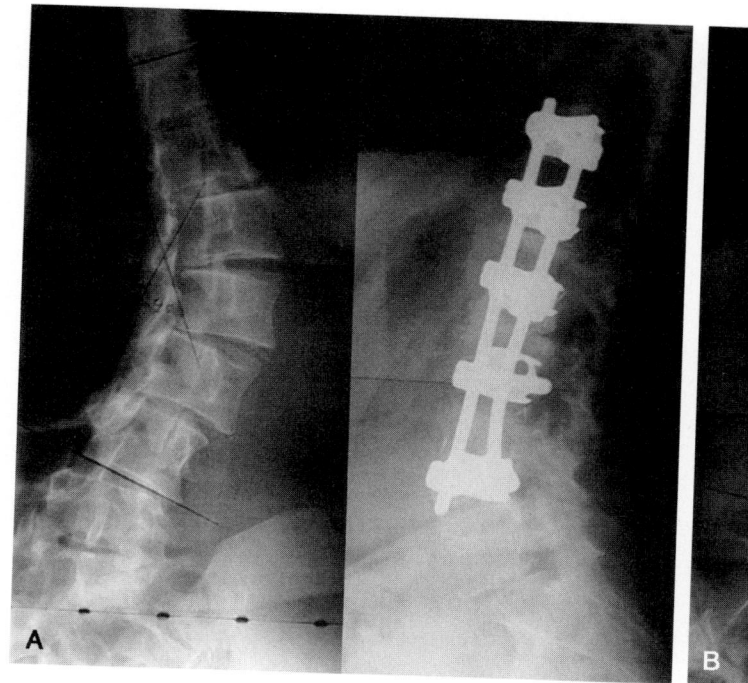
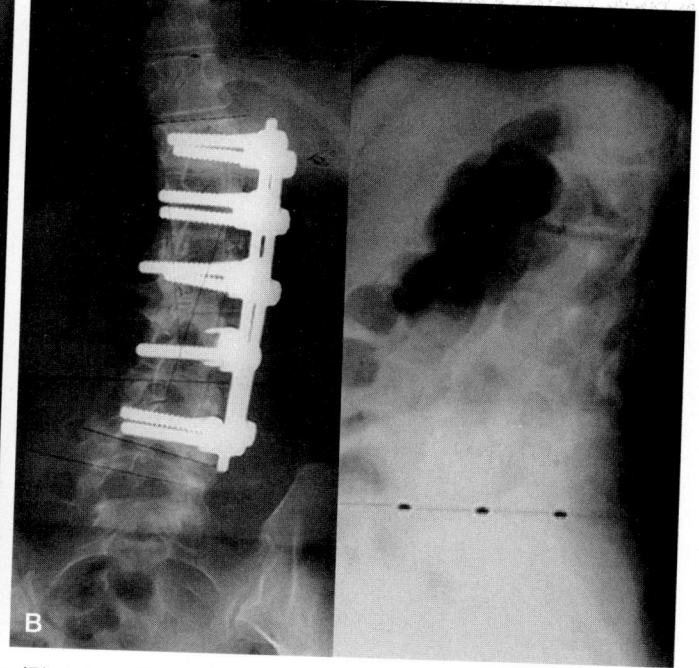

FIGURE 296–5. Preoperative *(A)* and postoperative *(B)* plain radiographs of the spine. Anterior rods have been placed between T12 and L4. The Cobb angle has been reduced from 45 to 21 degrees. Notice that derotation of the spine is achieved with instrumentation.

enough that caution and experience should be employed when considering adult deformity correction.

Technical Considerations

CAUDAL EXTENSION OF FUSION

The distal end of the fusion should include the stable vertebra and the neutral vertebrae, and it should be in the stable Harrington zone. The construct should not be extended below L4 so bending is not compromised. Hayes and colleagues,[23] in a biomechanical study of the lumbar spine after scoliosis correction, showed that patients fused down to L3-4 have an increased incidence of retrolisthesis, increased translational motion,

TABLE 296–3 ■ **Complications Associated with Scoliosis Correction**

Neurologic Complications
  Paralysis
  Paraparesis
  Dural tear
  Pseudomeningocele
  Blindness
Non-neurologic Complications
  Pulmonary embolus
  Myocardial infarction
  Pneumonia
  Wound infection
  Ileus
  Abdominal hernias
  Instrumentation failure
  Pseudoarthrosis
  Hip pain

and low back pain compared with higher levels of fusion. Such observations were not made when correction was done at a higher level than L3. The fusion should not extend to the sacrum to minimize limitation of ambulation. This means that fusion for King 2, 3, and 5 curves is carried down to the stable vertebrae. In King 1 and 4 curves, in which the lumbar curve is part of the major curve, it is routinely necessary to extend the fusion down to L4. The T2 vertebra should be included in the fusion of King 5 curves to neutralize shoulder asymmetry.

In the case of a patient with degenerative scoliosis who is not ambulatory for any reason or the neutrality of L4-5 is in question, fusion down to the sacrum is recommended to assist with sitting and structural support to the spine. When fusion down to the sacrum is contemplated, we recommend simultaneous fusion of L4-5 and L5-S1 disk spaces when possible through a posterior lumbar interbody fusion or an anterior approach for diskectomy and placement of structural interbody cages. This step is added because fusion at the lumbosacral junction has a high rate of failure if only a posterior approach is used. Kostuik's[27] earlier results with Harrington rods had shown a pseudoarthrosis rate of up to 50% at the lumbar-sacral junction.

DEGENERATION BEYOND FUSION

Even though the caudal extent of fusion is determined as described previously, the surgeon should also include findings from the diskogram and MRI to extend the fusion beyond the disk space where degeneration and symptoms may develop.[2] Fusion should never stop at the thoracolumbar junction, because the chances of kyphosis progression increase tremendously. For example, although the stable vertebra may be T12 in a King type 2 curve, fusion should be extended down to at least L2 to include the junctional zone.

PSEUDOARTHROSIS

In adult degenerative scoliosis, especially in an osteoporotic patient who has a poor instrument-bone interface, a high rate of pseudoarthrosis can be expected. In a study by Nuber and Schafer,[12] a 16.7% pseudoarthrosis rate was quoted for a patient population of 19 patients using a Harrington rod instrumentation system. However, in a study by Marchesi and Aebi[18] a 4% pseudoarthrosis rate was observed in a patient population of 27 using a Cotrel-Dubousset system or AO internal fixator.[18] This high rate of fusion compared with older studies using the Harrington rod is caused by the biomechanical properties of such newer systems.

A major risk factor for pseudoarthrosis is fusion to the sacrum. Saer and colleagues[34] had 2 of 17 pseudoarthrosis patients who were fused down to the sacrum. Grubb and coworkers[8] reported a 17.5% pseudoarthrosis rate after surgery for patients fused to the sacrum. This rate can be reduced by combining the S1 pedicle screw fixation with a technique such as Jackson intrasacral rod fixation. Placement of cages through an anterior approach or a posterior approach should also reduce this high rate of pseudoarthrosis.

A combined anterior and posterior approach to scoliosis surgery may decrease the rate of pseudoarthrosis further.[12, 35] Byrd and associates,[28] in a series of 26 patients with adult scoliosis, reported no cases of pseudoarthrosis. Meticulous surgical principles, such as resection of the soft tissue as much as possible and arthrodesis of the bony surface, are paramount. In our institutional experience, using an external orthosis for a period of 3 months is recommended to further decrease the rate of pseudoarthrosis.

LOSS OF CORRECTION

Nuber and Schafer,[12] in their series of 62 adults with degenerative scoliosis, corrected by a Harrington, Luque, or an anterior-posterior procedure, showed that the rate of curve correction loss can be as high as 6.7 degrees in patients with Harrington rod instrumentation at 27 months' follow-up, 4.2 degrees with the Luque rod instrumentation at 18 months' follow-up, and 4.1 degrees with combined anterior-posterior procedures at 27 months. Using an anterior and posterior approach, Van Dam[36] reported only a 6% loss of curve, compared with 8% to 14% loss for a posterior approach by other surgeons in the mid-1970s to mid-1980s.

These results show that a segmental fusion technique or a combined procedure reduces the rate of curve correction loss. With better instrumentation, such as the Cotrel-Dubousset system, better rates of fusion can be expected.

Thoracoplasty

Although thoracoplasty puts the patient at risk for declining pulmonary function, especially the patient with poor preoperative pulmonary function, it has many advantages.[36, 37] The rib hump created from the spinal rotation in the axial plain does not completely resolve after fusion. This leaves the patient with an unacceptable rib hump which may be cosmetically unacceptable to the patient or may cause symptoms such as pain when lying flat. In our institution, we routinely perform thoracoplasty in a patient with acceptable pulmonary function who desires better cosmesis or symptomatic relief from the rib hump. We use the same midline incision and perform a subfascial dissection down to the ribs in the apex of the curve. At least two ribs above and two ribs below the apex of the curve are identified. The ribs are resected to the apical angle of the hump, typically 7 to 10 cm. This releases the hump, and an immediate result is observed. Some surgeons may extend the rib resection more anteriorly, but in our experience, this is not necessary because it requires a separate incision and does not accomplish much more in terms of cosmesis. The only time to consider going more distally is when the surgeon desires more autogeneous bone graft. To prevent creating a ridge postoperatively, we routinely shave off the transverse processes of the involved vertebrae on the convex side.

If the pleura is opened, the surgeon may attempt closing it primarily and then obtain a chest x-ray film before closure of the incision. If the opening is large enough, a chest tube is necessary until the pleura heals.

Postoperative Management

In our institution, we place our patients into a thoracolumbosacral orthosis for 3 months to reduce strain on the implant-bone interface. After the 3-month period, we place the patients in a lumbosacral corset to transition them while they strengthen their muscles in therapy for an additional 6 weeks. For patients who have had fusion down to the sacrum or pelvis, a leg extension can be used to limit the motion along the sacroiliac joint.

Because of the magnitude of the procedure, all patients older than 40 years of age are excluded if myocardial infarction is a factor, and careful fluid management is performed. Patients are sedated until they are ready to be extubated, typically in less than 24 hours.

Postoperative anteroposterior and lateral plain radiographs of the spine are performed to ensure the stability of the construct. Regular postoperative laboratory values, such as hemoglobin, electrolytes, creatinine, and coagulation factors, are checked daily and adjusted as required.

Perioperative myocardial infarction is always a consideration, and we always rule out patients at risk for this condition as determined by enzymes. Increased requirement for transfusion and massive fluid shifts during the surgery in an adult with low myocardial reserve predispose the patient to some cardiac events.

Pulmonary embolus is unfortunately a common

complication of deformity correction. The length of the procedure and possible coagulopathy intraoperatively predispose the patient to having a pulmonary embolus. We routinely use venous compression devices perioperatively and place patients on mini-dose heparin 24 hours after surgery. In patients at high risk for pulmonary embolus (i.e., obese or a history of coagulopathy), a prophylactic caval filter is placed preoperatively. Routine lower extremity venous duplex sonography is performed on a weekly basis while patients are still in the hospital.

Ileus is a complication of spinal surgery of long duration, especially if a retroperitoneal approach is used for anterior fixation. In patients with ileus, we routinely use a nasogastric tube with wall suction to decompress the gastrointestinal system and rest it.

Wound infection is minimized by meticulous surgical techniques and use of perioperative antibiotics. In patients who develop wound infections postoperatively that are superficial to the fascial plain, local wound care is performed. For infections that extend beyond the fascial plain, a surgical débridment is performed. If necessary, a flap can be placed over the instrumentation. We do not remove the hardware, even in cases of deep infection. In our experience, débridment of the devitalized tissue as described previously, followed by long-term intravenous and oral antibiotics, controls the infection.

Nutritional support is of paramount importance in patients postoperatively. In patients who for any reason cannot have any adequate enteral feeding, hyperalimenation is used 24 hours after surgery because of the high metabolic demands of the body. Physical therapy and occupational therapy are used postoperatively to mobilize the patients as soon as possible.

CONCLUSIONS

Changes in surgical techniques and instrumentation have given us unparalleled ability to stabilize and correct the spine. When such power is applied correctly, we are able to treat many conditions that in the past had few options and often left patients debilitated with a deteriorating quality of life. When such power is applied incorrectly or poorly thought out, it can leave a patient in worse condition than before treatment.

This increased technical ability demands an equal increase in understanding of the pathophysiology and biomechanics of adult spinal disease in general and scoliosis in particular. As newer techniques are developed that allow manipulation of the biologic environment of the spine and provide less invasive techniques for correction, it will even be more important to understand the underlying forces and disease processes.

REFERENCES

1. Ogilvie JW: Adult scoliosis: Evaluation and nonsurgical treatment [review]. Instr Course Lect 41:251–255, 1992.

2. Kostuik JP: Adult scoliosis: The lumbar spine. In Bridwell KH, DeWald RL (eds): The Textbook of Spinal Surgery, 2nd ed. Philadelphia, Lippincott-Raven, 1997.
3. Grubb SA, Lipscomb HJ, Suh PB: Results of surgical treatment of painful adult scoliosis. Spine 19:1619–1627, 1994.
4. Betz R, Bunnell W, Lambrecht-Mulier E, et al: Scoliosis and pregnancy. J Bone Joint Surg Am 69:90, 1987.
5. Kostuik JP, Bentivoglio J: The incidence of low-back pain in adult scoliosis. Spine 6:268–273, 1981.
6. Shands AR, Eisenberg HV: The incidence of scoliosis in the state of Delaware. J Bone Joint Surg Am 37:1243, 1955.
7. Robin GC, Span Y, Steinberg R, et al: Scoliosis in the elderly: A follow-up study. Spine 7:355–359, 1982.
8. Grubb SA, Lipscomb HJ, Coonrad RW: Degenerative adult onset scoliosis. Spine 13:241–245, 1988.
9. Vanderpool DW, James JIP, Wynne-Davis R: Scoliosis in the elderly. J Bone Joint Surg Am 51:446–455, 1969.
10. Weinstein SL, Zavala DC, Ponsetti I: Idiopathic scoliosis: Long-term follow-up and prognosis in the untreated patients. J Bone Joint Surg Am 63:702–712, 1983.
11. Collins DK, Ponsetti IV: Long-term follow-up of patients with idiopathic scoliosis not treated surgically. J Bone Joint Surg Am 51:425–445, 1969.
12. Nuber GW, Schafer MF: Surgical management of adult scoliosis. Clin Orthop 208:228–237, 1986.
13. Winter RB, Lonstein JE, Denis F: Pain patterns in adult scoliosis. Orthop Clin North Am 19:339–345, 1988.
14. Epstein JA, Epstein BS, Jones MD: Symptomatic lumbar scoliosis with degenerative changes in the elderly. Spine 4:542–547, 1979.
15. Nachemson A: Adult scoliosis and back pain. Spine 4:513–517, 1979.
16. King H, Moe JH, Bradford DS, Winter RB: Selection of fusion levels in thoracic idiopathic scoliosis. J Bone Joint Surg Am 65: 1302–1313, 1983.
17. Kostuik JP: Recent advances in the treatment of painful adult scoliosis. Clin Orthop 147:238–252, 1980.
18. Marchesi DG, Aebi M: Pedicle fixation devices in the treatment of adult lumbar scoliosis. Spine 17(Supp 8):S304–S309, 1992.
19. Van Dam BE: Nonoperative treatment of adult scoliosis [review]. Orthop Clin North Am 19:347–351, 1988.
20. Ascani E, Bartolozzi P, Logroscino CA, et al: Natural history of untreated idiopathic scoliosis after skeletal maturity. Spine 11: 784–789, 1986.
21. Bener B, Ehni G: Degenerative lumbar scoliosis. Spine 4:548–552, 1979.
22. Dwyer AF, Newton NC, Sherwood AA: An anterior approach to scoliosis: A preliminary report. Clin Orthop 62:192–202, 1969.
23. Luque ER: Segmental spinal instrumentation for correction of scoliosis. Orthopedics 163:192–198, 1982.
24. Moe JH, Prucell GA, Bradford DS: Zielke instrumentation (VDS) for correction of spinal curvature. Clin Orthop 180: 133–153, 1983.
25. Wegner DR, Carollo JJ, Wilkerson JA: Biomechanics of scoliosis correction by segmental spinal instrumentation. Spine 7:260–264, 1982.
26. Cotrel Y, Dubousset J, Guillaumat M: New universal instrumentation in spinal surgery. Clin Orthop 227:10–23, 1988.
27. Kostuik JP, Gleason TF, Errico TJ: The surgical correction of flat back syndrome (iatrogenic lumbar kyphosis). Orthop Trans 9: 131, 1985.
28. Byrd A, Scoles PV, Winter RB, et al: Adult idiopathic scoliosis treated by anterior and posterior spinal fusion. J Bone Joint Surg Am 69:843–850, 1987.
29. Simmons ED Jr, Kowalski JM, Simmons EH: The results of surgical treatment for adult scoliosis. Spine 18:718–724, 1993.
30. Van Dam BE, Bradford DS, Lonstein JE, et al: Adult idiopathic scoliosis treated by posterior spinal fusion and Harrington instrumentation. Spine 12:32–36, 1987.
31. Kostuik JP, Israel J, Hall JE: Scoliosis surgery in adults. Clin Orthop 226:225, 1973.
32. Swank S, Lonstein JE, Moe JH, et al: Surgical treatment of adult scoliosis: A review of two hundred and twenty-two cases. J Bone Joint Surg Am 63:268–287, 1981.
33. Hayes MA, Tompkins SF, Herndon WA, et al: Clinical and radio-

logical evaluation of lumbosacral motion below fusion levels in idiopathic scoliosis. Spine 13:1161–1167, 1988.

34. Saer EH, Winter RB, Lonstein JE: Long scoliosis fusion to the sacrum in adults with nonparalytic scoliosis: An improved method. Spine 15:650–653, 1990.

35. Johnson J, Holt R: Combined use of anterior and posterior sur-gery for adult scoliosis. Orthop Clin North Am 19:361–366, 1988.

36. Van Dam BE: Operative treatment of adult scoliosis with poste-rior fusion and instrumentation [review]. Orthop Clin North Am 19:353–359, 1988.

37. Steel H: Rib resection and spine fusion in correction of convex deformity in scoliosis. J Bone Joint Surg Am 65:920–925, 1983.

PART VI ADULT CONGENITAL ABNORMALITIES

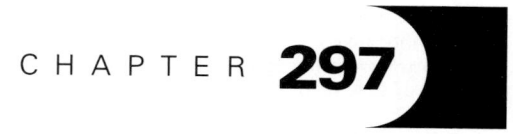

CHAPTER 297

Acquired Abnormalities of the Craniocervical Junction

ARNOLD H. MENEZES

The craniocervical junction is the most complex region of the axial skeleton. The geometry of the articular surfaces provides mobility at the cost of stability. The latter is provided by the ligamentous structures as well as by the development of cervical musculature.[1] The synovial lining of the craniocervical joints is affected early in rheumatoid disease and plays a significant role in the subsequent destructive changes that occur in this region.[2, 3] Other nonrheumatoid entities that affect the craniocervical junction are inflammation (e.g., ankylosing spondylitis, juvenile rheumatoid arthritis [RA], psoriasis, regional ileitis, Reiter's syndrome), degeneration (e.g., osteoarthritis, calcium pyrophosphate "pseudogout"), and infection (e.g., pyogenesis, Grisel's syndrome).[4]

RHEUMATOID ARTHRITIS

Rheumatoid arthritis is one of the most common disabling diseases. The overall prevalence in Europe for proven RA is 0.8% among adults older than 15 years.[5] The prevalence in Sudbury, Massachusetts, was similar at 0.9%,[6] and it was 1% in a national sample of the white population in United States.[7, 8] The number of patients with RA totals 2 million to 2.4 million in the United States and 630,000 to 650,000 in the United Kingdom. Based on available studies, a significant number will develop involvement of the cervical spine that requires attention.

In 1890 Garrod first described RA of the cervical spine as a clinical entity.[9] In that series of 500 patients, 178 had involvement of the cervical spine. According to Conlon and coworkers, if lateral cervical radiographs were made of the general population, cervical spine involvement compatible with RA would be detected in about 6%.[10] However, cases with clinical involvement are only a fraction of this percentage. In the initial studies by Conlon and coworkers, it was believed that involvement of the cervical spine did not cause neurological deficits. Unfortunately, this conclusion led to the common but erroneous belief that rheumatoid involvement of the craniocervical junction should be treated conservatively. In 1974, however, Mathews pointed out that progressive atlantoaxial subluxation occurred in as many as 25% of patients with RA and that rheumatoid cranial settling occurred in 6% to 18% of individuals.[11]

RA is a chronic, relapsing, inflammatory arthritis that usually affects multiple diarthrodial joints with a varying degree of systemic involvement.[12–14] RA occurs worldwide in all racial groups and affects females two to four times more frequently than males. It causes substantial morbidity and attendant economic burden. Approximately 50% of patients are unable to work within 10 years of onset, and the lifetime costs of the disease rival those of coronary artery disease or stroke.[14] Joints, articular tissue, serosa, and the eyes are commonly affected, but the spectrum of organ damage can be vast, especially when vasculitis develops in the course of the disease.[15]

Immunologic Features

The immunologic features of RA include rheumatoid factors, antinuclear antibodies, immune complexes, and the characteristic complement levels.[16]

Rheumatoid factors are antibodies with specificity for the Fe fragment of IgG.[15, 17] The latex agglutination test is positive in 80% of patients meeting the American Rheumatism Association criteria for RA[18] (Table 297–1). High titers are associated with the presence of subcutaneous nodules, extra-articular manifestations, and vasculitis. A negative rheumatoid factor test by routine laboratory procedures does not exclude the diagnosis of RA because 20% of patients who meet the American

T A B L E   2 9 7 – 1 ■ **American Rheumatism Association Criteria for Rheumatoid Arthritis (RA)**

Morning stiffness
Pain on motion or tenderness in at least one joint
Swelling of at least one joint
Swelling of at least one other joint
Symmetrical swelling of the same joint, right and left
Subcutaneous nodules
Radiographic changes typical of RA
Positive serum test for rheumatoid factors
Poor mucin clotting of synovial fluid
Characteristic histologic changes of RA

Rheumatism Association criteria test negative for RA. These patients may have IgG or 7 IgM rheumatoid factor that is not detectable by routine test techniques.[16]

Antinuclear antibodies have been found in 14% to 28% of patients with RA. The tests that use monoclonal rheumatoid factors in the CLq binding assay are more frequently positive in patients with RA than are all the various assays for detecting immune complexes.[13] However, the assays correlate poorly with the indices of disease activity. A positive test, however, is usually associated with an increased incidence of extra-articular manifestations, particularly vasculitis.

Although the cause of RA is unknown, it is postulated that the disease is triggered either directly or indirectly (e.g., by molecular mimicry) by an infectious agent or agents in a genetically predisposed individual.[14] The ensuing pathogenetic events are believed to be driven by T-cell (and B-cell) responses to the inciting agents or self-antigens, or both, in the synovium, with elaboration of proinflammatory cytokines that induce the up-regulation of endothelial adhesion molecules, the influx of chronic inflammatory cells, protease expression, and subsequent tissue destruction.[19] Non–T-cell–dependent mechanisms may contribute to disease perpetuation, including aberrantly regulated cytokine cascades, impaired regulation of growth and programmed death among synovial cells, and cell-to-cell and cell-matrix interactions that autonomously drive inflammatory mechanisms.[20, 21]

Genetic susceptibility to RA is strongly attributable to the inheritance of a specific human leukocyte antigen (DRB-1) that encodes a common five–amino acid sequence ("shared epitope") in the antigen-binding groove of the DR molecule.[22] Homozygosity for the epitope confers risk for the most severe expression of the disease. The synovial membrane is infiltrated predominantly by CD4 T cells, an expressed activation marker that originates predominantly in macrophages and fibroblasts. The proinflammatory cytokine tumor necrosis factor (TNF-α) plays a central role in the pathogenesis of inflammation and tissue injury in RA.[23] Clinical advances include more aggressive treatment of early RA facilitated by the availability of increasingly effective therapeutic agents, including methotrexate, leflunomide, and biologic agents directed against TNF-α.[21, 24, 25] The latter agents appear to be more active in retarding tissue destruction. Combination therapy, including concomitant use of methotrexate and anti–

TNF-α agents, is more efficacious than monotherapy and causes less toxicity.[24, 26–28]

Synovial lymphocytes produce an altered immunoglobulin G that subsequently stimulates a local immune response in the synovial fluid. This response activates the complement system in joints, resulting in histamine release, production of chemotactic factors, and a marked influx of neutrophils into the joint fluid. The polymorphonuclear cells release lysosomal enzymes, oxygen radicals, and arachidonic acid metabolites that produce inflammation and cause tissue damage. There are perivascular collections of small lymphocytes, lymphoblasts, plasma cells, mast cells, and macrophages within the synovium. Further tissue damage within the joint is induced by mediators of the inflammation released by these cells.[20, 22]

Rheumatoid pannus forms in the inflamed joints from proliferating fibroblasts and inflammatory cells, leading to granulation tissue.[29] The pannus itself produces collagenase and proteolytic enzymes capable of destroying adjacent cartilage, tendons, and bones.[19] The result is loss of cartilage, ligamentous laxity, rupture of tendons, and bone erosion. In general, the joints deteriorate and become symptomatic within the first year of disease onset.

Clinical manifestations of RA include constitutional symptoms; arthritis involving large, medium, and small joints; and extra-articular manifestations that include subcutaneous nodules, nail bed thrombi, pleurisy, pulmonary fibrosis, pericarditis, nerve entrapment syndromes, scleritis, and vasculitis. The most common vascular complications are peripheral cutaneous ulcers and neuropathy.[30–34]

The earliest changes in the cervical spine most likely occur at the superficial joints and lateral margins of the disks. Neurocentral synovitis results in granulation tissue with fibroblasts and capillaries that erode and replace the disk annulus and neighboring disk-bone border. There is no active bone formation.[35] Therefore, osteophytic formation around disks and apophyseal joints is inconspicuous and enhances the possibility of dislocation.[11, 36, 37]

Fibrosis and ankylosis of apophyseal joints are common in untreated cases, and the disease tends to terminate in segmental immobilization with loss of the disk. Stepwise subluxations are seen in the subaxial cervical region. The active inflammatory lesions with fibrinoid changes are similar to those in the tendons of the hand and are thus seen in the apical ligaments, in the transverse ligament of the craniocervical junction, and in biopsy specimens of the interspinous ligaments.[38] The transverse ligament becomes insufficient because of inflammatory erosion of the posterior surface of the odontoid process by granulation tissue arising in the synovial joints between the transverse ligament and the posterior surface of the odontoid process. Osteoporosis is a frequent finding in the rheumatoid cervical spine and may contribute to weakening of the bone beneath the ligamentous attachments.[38, 39]

Rheumatoid Involvement of the Spine

Winfield and colleagues evaluated 100 rheumatoid patients diagnosed within a year of disease onset.[40] At a

5-year follow-up, 12 patients had atlantoaxial subluxation of more than 7 mm, and subaxial subluxation had occurred in 20. In three individuals, the odontoid process had migrated vertically. Similarly, Pellicci and coworkers studied RA patients over a 5-year period.[41] The mortality rate in their patients was 17%, compared with a 9% mortality rate for the same age group without rheumatoid disease. Subluxations worsened in 80%, and new subluxations occurred in 27%. From a postmortem study of 104 patients with RA, Mikulowski and associates found that the cause of death in 11 was atlantoaxial dislocation with cervicomedullary compression.[42] This finding had not been suspected ante mortem. Two had myelomalacia, and three had vascular complications of the cervical vertebral artery related to dislocation. In 1981 Marks and Sharp reported 31 patients with RA and upper cervical spine involvement with dislocations.[36] Fifteen died within 6 months of presentation. All who were untreated died, as did 50% of those treated with a soft cervical collar alone. Only fusion provided a reasonable chance of survival. Delamarter and Bohlman performed a postmortem analysis of patients with paralysis related to RA of the cervical spine.[3] Cervical cord compression was the main cause of death in 10 patients. Once cervical myelopathy sets in, the natural history is grave without surgical intervention.[34, 43–45]

Because of the large number of synovial joints, the cervical spine is the most common site affected by RA. The most common lesion is atlantoaxial dislocation, followed by cranial settling and then rheumatoid granulation tissue. Subaxial subluxation occurs in 12% to 22% of individuals, predominantly at C4 and C5.[46]

Atlantoaxial subluxation is initiated by loss of tensile strength and stretching of the transverse ligament. Similar changes occur in the synovial joints around the odontoid process as occur in the joints of the lateral atlantoaxial and occipitoatlantal regions: erosive changes in the adjacent bone, formation of granulation tissue in the synovial joints, loss of bone volume, osteoporosis, angulation of the softened bone, and occasional fractures. The laxity of the ligaments and the changes in the bone lead to horizontal or anteroposterior translation, as well as to rotary luxation of the atlas and axis vertebrae (Fig. 297–1).[42, 47–53]

Vertical penetration of the odontoid process into the foramen magnum has been termed *rheumatoid basilar invagination, odontoid vertical migration, rheumatoid translation,* and *cranial settling.*[7, 11] The condition results from bone loss from the lateral mass of the atlas vertebra, with rostral migration of the axis vertebra. In severe cases with lateral displacement, the lateral atlantal masses can fracture.[29] The odontoid then penetrates farther through the foramen magnum. The destructive changes can be severe enough that the occipital condyles rest on the lateral masses of the axis vertebrae, separating and displacing the anterior and posterior arches of the atlas and their respective directions (Fig. 297–2).[54] The anterior arch of the atlas settles downward, telescoping onto the axis body, and the odontoid process invaginates superiorly. This condition is not basilar invagination or basilar impression but rather cranial settling.[7, 29, 31, 55–57]

Excessive proliferation of granulation tissue can lead to complete destruction of the odontoid process, with the granulation mass and pannus emanating from the rest of the synovial joints.[34] This mass causes ventral and lateral cervicomedullary compression with gross dislocation in all directions (Fig. 297–3). At times the bony spicule of the odontoid process is left as a "ghost" and can penetrate the tectorial membrane. Subsequently, it embeds in the ventral aspect of the pons

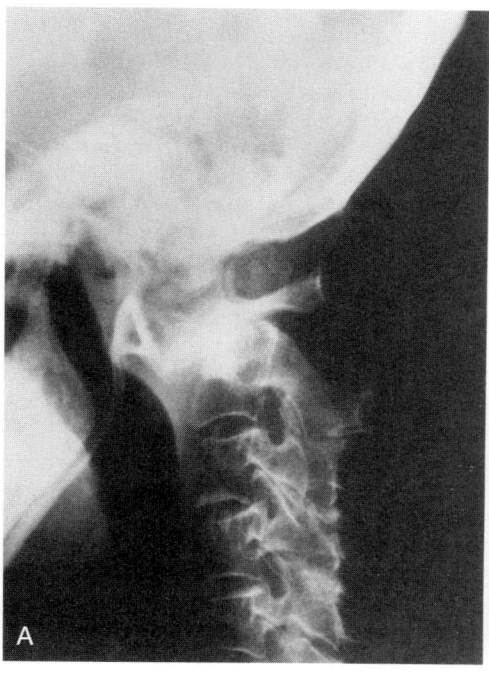
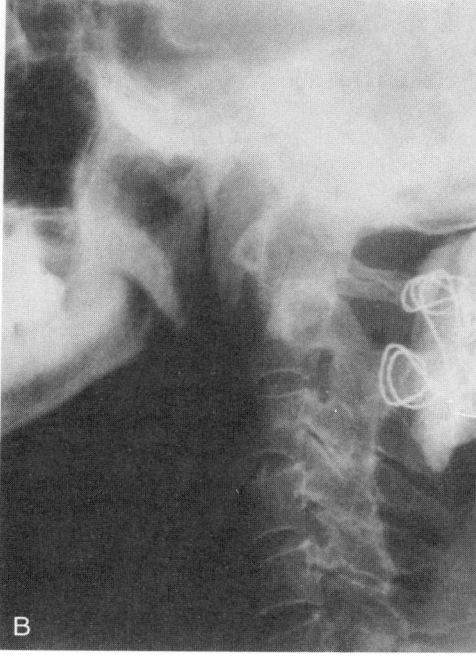

FIGURE 297–1. Composite of preoperative *(left)* and postoperative *(right)* cervical spine radiographs in a 68-year-old individual with Felty's syndrome. Preoperative atlantoaxial dislocation is evident and was easily reduced with cervical traction and maintained with interlaminar fusion.

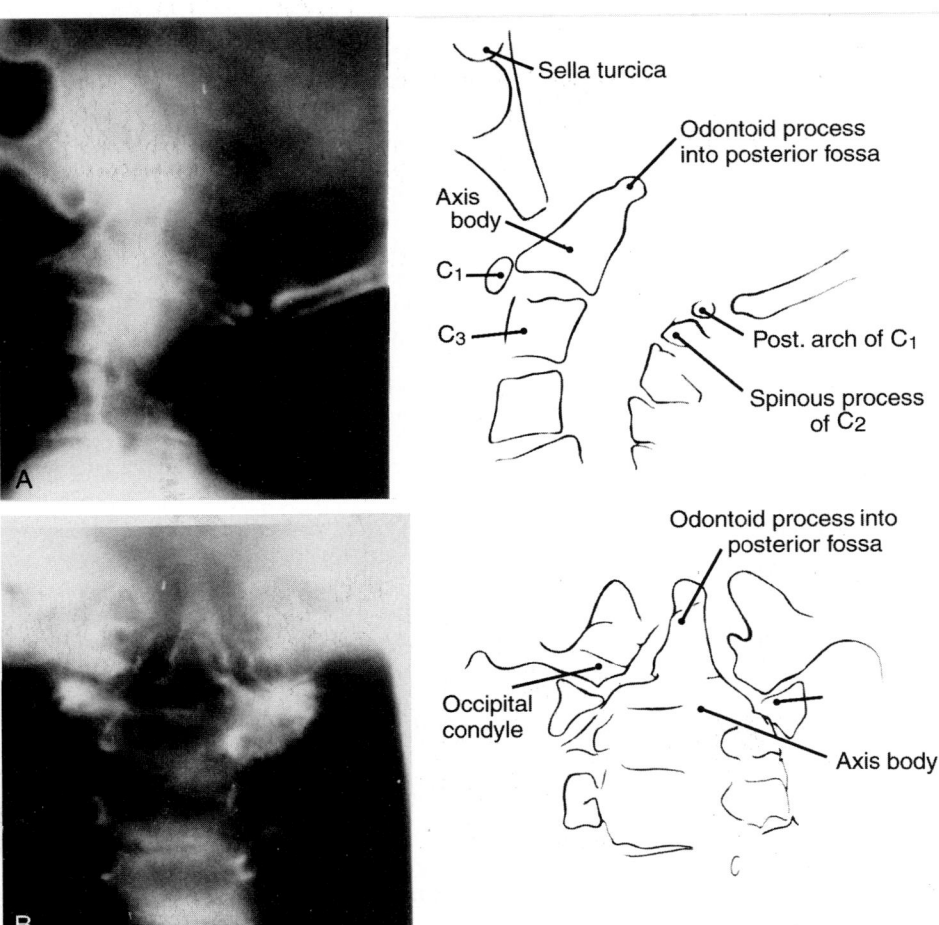

FIGURE 297-2. *A,* Midline polytomogram of the craniocervical junction and line drawing illustrate penetration of the odontoid process into the posterior fossa. The anterior atlas arch is at the C2-3 disk interspace. *B,* Frontal tomogram and line drawing through the plane of the odontoid process with cranial settling in the same patient. The lateral atlantal masses are widely separated. The occipital condyles appear to rest on the slopes of the axis.

and medulla and attaches itself to the vertebrobasilar arterial tree. Occasionally, rheumatoid dural nodules and pachymeningitis follow the rheumatoid process. The rheumatoid pannus can be associated with granulation tissue and can be tough and fibrotic.[34] It seldom recedes with immobilization. In contrast, active pannus that resembles the active disease in other joints recedes with cervical immobilization.[57-60]

Subluxations below the second cervical vertebra occur in 17% to 29% of patients with RA, typically at C4-5. Serial cervical subluxations producing a "staircase" appearance are common.[10, 61]

Autopsy analysis of spinal cords from rheumatoid patients suffering from paralysis related to atlantoaxial dislocation, cranial settling, or both has shown abnormal histology within the spinal cord at the site of compression.[3] Common to all patients were gliosis and axonal degeneration. Nuclear damage within the ganglion cells often appeared in different stages of progression. No parenchymal hemorrhage was seen. Delamarter and Bohlman identified three histologic types of spinal cord compression.[3] In the first type, distortion with flattening and destruction of the spinal cord and secondary wallerian degeneration of the ascending and descending tracts without anoxic or ischemic neural changes suggested that the damage was related to

chronic mechanical compression. In the intermediate stage of compression, called type II, vascular compression was associated with ischemic damage to the spinal cord, with necrosis of the lateral columns and the ischemic watershed regions supplied by the anterior and posterior spinal arteries. Type III was mild mechanical compression, which manifested only as focal gliosis at the site of compression, without ascending or descending tract injury. Nakano and colleagues analyzed two autopsy cases and found maximal changes in the central gray matter and adjacent posterior and lateral columns.[49] The changes were attributed to direct intermittent compression and narrowing of the transverse branches of the anterior spinal artery. These findings have been confirmed by Bland[2] and by Casey and colleagues.[44] Thus, the space available for the spinal cord at the craniocervical junction is of great prognostic significance.[4, 44, 45]

Extra-articular Manifestations

Extra-articular manifestations are myriad in patients with severe RA and high titers of rheumatoid factor. Pericarditis, myocarditis, and coronary vasculitis are common.[16, 32, 33, 62] RA can present in the lungs as pleural effusions and pleuritis, intraparenchymal rheumatoid

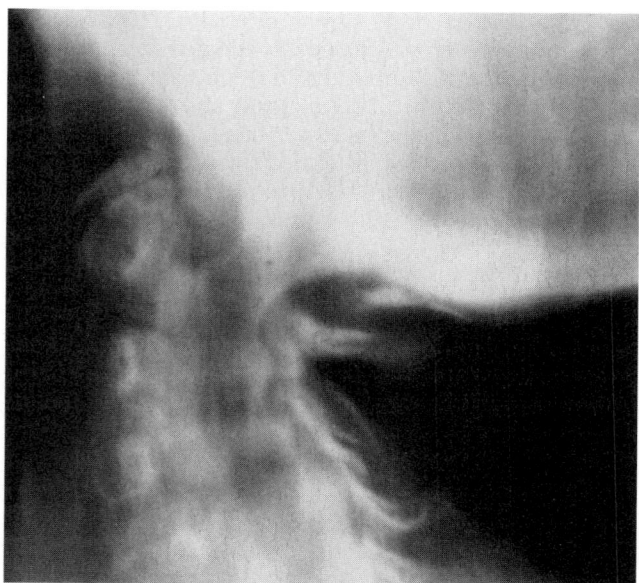

FIGURE 297–3. Midline sagittal polytomogram with iohexol contrast outlining the subarachnoid space and spinal cord. The odontoid process is atrophic. A large ventral mass behind the axis body and odontoid process represents tough pannus markedly compressing the ventral cervicomedullary junction. The patient underwent ventral decompression and a dorsal occipitocervical fusion.

nodules, and Caplan's syndrome (rheumatoid nodules with pneumoconiosis, diffuse pulmonary fibrosis, bronchiolitis, and pulmonary hypertension disproportionate to coexistent lung disease).[17, 32, 63–65] Pleuritis is the most common thoracic manifestation (5% to 15%), and rheumatoid effusions occur in 50% of patients in the first 5 years after the onset of arthritis.[66] Pulmonary fibrosis was found in 10 of 18 patients with RA who underwent thin-section computed tomography of the chest. The plain radiographs were reported as normal.[67] Thus, it is important that pulmonary function tests be performed in patients with RA before they undergo an operative procedure and general anesthesia.

Pharyngeal dysfunction may be a manifestation of neurological involvement or floppy arytenoid cartilages with an abnormal swallowing mechanism as a result of the disease process.

General Treatment

The ideal management of patients with RA requires an interdisciplinary approach involving the primary care physician, rheumatologic consultant, occupational therapist, physical therapist, and various surgical specialists. In the past, drugs such as sulfasalazine, gold, and penicillin were used. Methotrexate in combination with cyclophosphamide has been tolerated well and provides good control of the active disease and of pain.[14] For patients with RA, a new era in treatment has begun.[25] This optimistic view, which is widely shared by rheumatologists, reflects the recent introduction of novel agents to treat this painful and debilitating condition. These agents include the TNF blockers,

which limit the inflammation and retard the destruction of cartilage and bone.[22–25]

Clinical Presentation

Atlantoaxial subluxation may manifest within 2 years of disease onset, but it is unusual for myelopathy to develop early.[41, 54, 68] The most frequent symptom of rheumatoid abnormalities of the craniocervical junction is occipital headaches.[34] Typically the headaches are described as occipital pain radiating to the skull vertex and aggravated by an upright posture. They are present in 60% of patients with atlantoaxial subluxation and in 90% of individuals with cranial settling. Between 1977 and 1994, the author evaluated 780 symptomatic patients with RA affecting the craniocervical region.[34] The three main categories of radiographic abnormalities were atlantoaxial instability, cranial settling, and primary granulation tissue masses.

Cervical myelopathy is insidious, and disability may be mistaken for progression of rheumatoid disease, rheumatoid joint dysfunction, hypothyroidism, and poor nutritional status.[11, 29, 43, 69, 70] The clearest indications of cervical myelopathies are progressive physical disability and the inability to perform daily tasks.[43, 49] It is difficult to detect abnormal neurological signs of myelopathy in rheumatoid patients with deforming painful arthritis and associated neuropathy. The peripheral neuropathy itself can cause areflexia. Thus, the presence of normal reflexes in patients with advanced RA should raise suspicion of myelopathy. The author has found neurophysiologic testing with somatosensory evoked potentials to be of no use in this situation, despite reports to the contrary.[7]

Limb paresthesias, numbness, weakness, and sphincter disturbance can herald myelopathy. Dizziness, vertigo, and syncope can be associated with vertebrobasilar ischemia, and nystagmus can be evident. Among individuals with cranial settling, 55% complained of transient blackout spells.[29] Gradual, progressive difficulty with ambulation was a chief complaint in 76% of individuals with cervical myelopathy. An acute onset of quadriparesis was experienced by 15%.[34]

In the author's experience, abnormal neurological signs include brainstem evidence of internuclear ophthalmoplegia, facial diplegia, nystagmus, spastic quadriparesis, and sleep apnea, especially in patients with cranial settling. These signs, either alone or in combination, were present in 20% of individuals. An additional 20% lost pain and touch sensation in the distribution of the trigeminal nerve, and each patient had more than 10 mm of invagination of the odontoid process above the foramen magnum.[34] The cranial nerves most affected by cranial settling were the glossopharyngeal and vagus, followed by the hypoglossal. Among individuals with cranial settling, 20% had evidence of dysfunction of one or more cranial nerves.[71] Nine individuals with cranial settling had undergone previous tracheostomy for the diagnosis of rheumatoid pharyngeal dysfunction.

Radiologic Features of Cervical Spine Involvement

The radiographic changes reflect the pathologic processes described. Plain lateral cervical spine radiographs, as well as anteroposterior and open-mouth views, are usually obtained. At times, dynamic flexion-extension views are obtained, with the patient assuming the extended and flexed position without forced extremes of head position. Neurological deficits, a 7- to 8-mm predental space, and abnormal radiographic pathology such as cranial settling, atrophy of the odontoid process, and subaxial subluxation justify magnetic resonance imaging (MRI). This modality shows the relationship of the cervical spine to the contained cervicomedullary junction and cervical spinal cord.

Both T1- and T2-weighted MRI scans must be obtained in the sagittal and axial planes. Dynamic views in the flexed and extended positions identify the instability as well as the manner of potential compression (Fig. 297–4).[59–61, 72, 73] Active synovitis with ligamentous involvement is best identified with spin-echo imaging. Contrast-enhanced, T1-weighted spin-echo MRI can discriminate between joint effusion and various forms of pannus in patients with RA of the craniocervical junction. Stiskal and coworkers found that joint effusions appeared as low signal intensity on unenhanced T1-weighted images and as high signal intensity on enhanced T1-weighted images. All lesions had a rim-like zone at the periphery that was redistributed with delayed images (Fig. 297–5).[60] On T2-weighted graded images with and without contrast, hypervascular pan-

nus appeared as high signal intensity. However, the signal intensity of the fibrous pannus was reduced on T2-weighted, gradient-recalled echo images and on pre- and postcontrast T1-weighted spin-echo images.[73] From a surgical perspective, these findings are important. Craniocervical immobilization with fusion will not cause the ventral mass of fibrous hypovascular pannus to disappear (see Fig. 297–3). However, dorsal stabilization resolves active pannus and synovitis associated with hypervascular tissue.

Thin-section computed tomography and three-dimensional computed tomography of the affected area provide further information about the osseous integrity, the anatomic relationships, and the extent of osteoporosis and osteopenia (Fig. 297–6).[34]

Cranial settling is reducible in 77% to 80% of individuals with the use of positioning or cervical traction as high as 9 to 10 pounds for 4 to 5 days (Fig. 297–7). Cranial settling is irreducible in individuals who exhibit more than 15 mm of odontoid penetration through the foramen magnum, in those with large pannus or a fractured odontoid process, or if cranial settling is complicated by lateral or rotational dislocation in addition to the primary phenomenon (Fig. 297–8).[34, 71] Complex cranial settling with posterior dislocation is considered potentially lethal at any time from distraction of the vertebral artery complex. Such individuals should undergo a fusion procedure immediately.

Operative Indications

The results of natural history studies vary. Failure to identify and appreciate cranial settling makes it diffi-

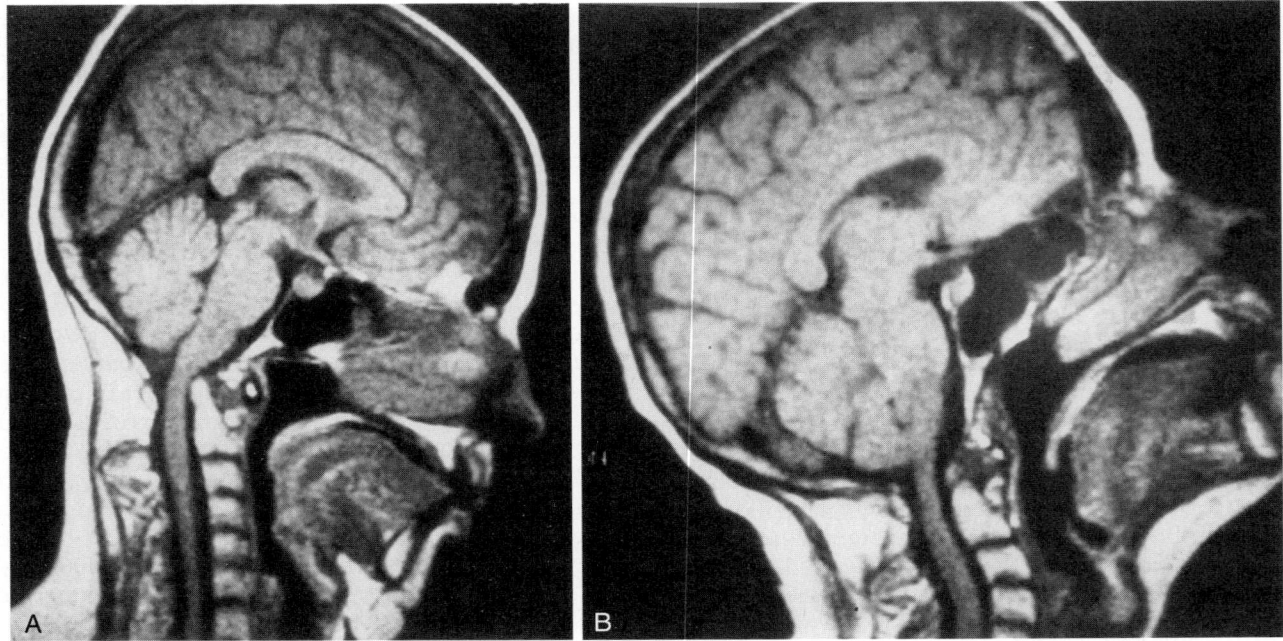

FIGURE 297–4. *A,* Midsagittal T1-weighted magnetic resonance imaging (MRI) scan of the brain and cervical spinal cord in the flexed position shows atlantoaxial dislocation with ventral compression on the cervicomedullary junction in this 42-year-old individual with rheumatoid arthritis. *B,* Midsagittal T1-weighted MRI scan in extension shows reduction of the atlantoaxial dislocation.

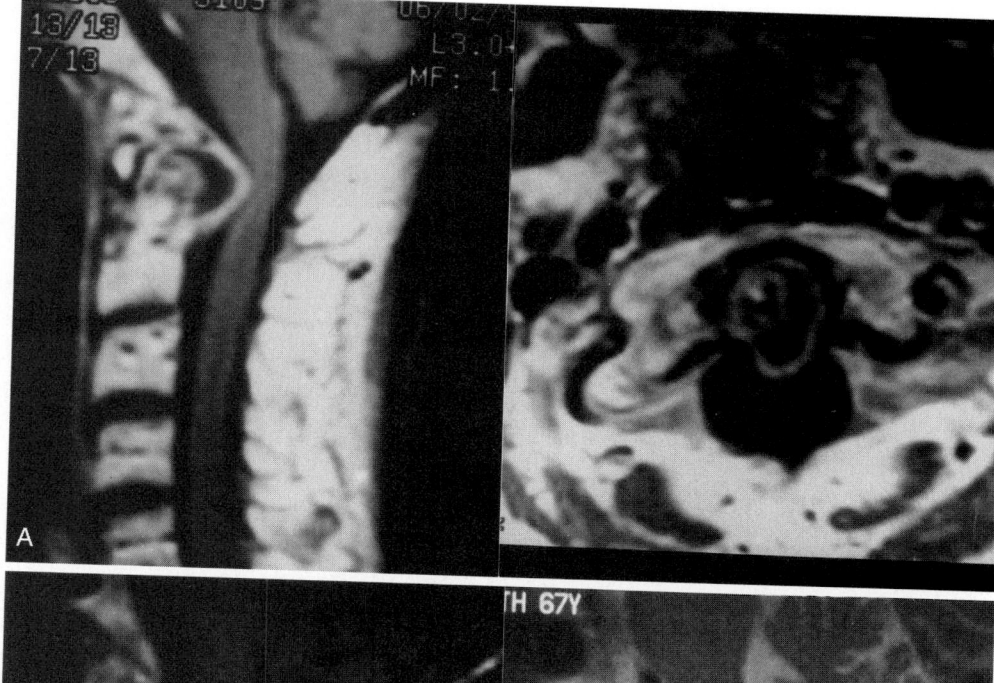

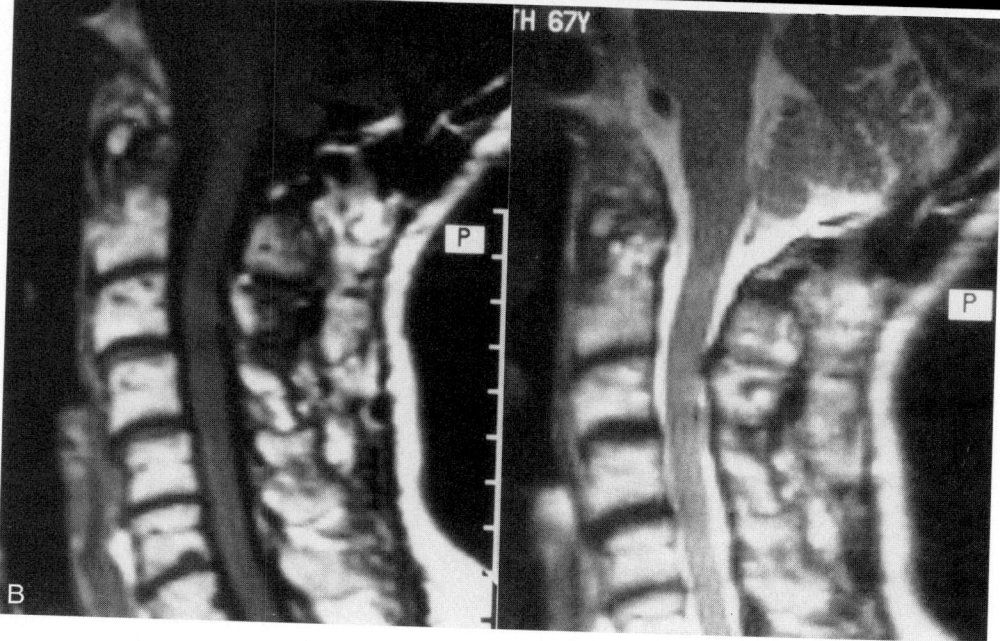

FIGURE 297–5. *A,* Composite midsagittal *(left)* and axial *(right)* magnetic resonance imaging (MRI) scan through the plane of the odontoid in a 67-year-old individual with rheumatoid arthritis. On the gadolinium-enhanced T1-weighted image, the rimlike zone at the periphery of the lesion with ventral cervicomedullary compression is active pannus. *B,* Composite midsagittal MRI scan of the craniocervical junction with T1-weighted *(left)* and T2-weighted *(right)* modes 3 months after dorsal occipitocervical fusion with titanium loop instrumentation and rib grafts. The pannus has regressed completely.

cult to draw conclusions about the efficacy of surgical intervention.[29] An example is the increased incidence of transoral decompression and dorsal occipitocervical fusion procedures in the presence of potentially reducible (80%) cranial settling. However, there is consensus that surgical intervention must be advocated for progressive neurological dysfunction, cranial settling, and intractable pain.[4, 38, 39, 49, 53, 54, 68, 74] Cervical myelopathy and instability, especially after decompressive laminectomy, are urgent indications for operative intervention.

Atlantoaxial dislocation of more than 8 to 9 mm must be examined carefully on MRI. In 1994 Boden showed that a posterior atlantal dental interval (PADI) greater than 14 mm (on plain radiographs) is safe,[45] not including the presence of pannus or other tissues that reduce the effective diameter of the subarachnoid space. However, if the PADI was greater than 14 mm, there was a 94% chance that the patient would experience paralysis. Depending on the thickness of pannus, a patient with a PADI of 13 mm could have much less space available for the spinal cord.

The Ranawat classification of neurological deficit in rheumatoid patients does not differentiate severity in class IIIB (Table 297–2).[75] Reporting on Crockard's series, Casey and associates recognized high rates of postoperative morbidity and mortality in patients categorized as Ranawat class IIIB.[44] The detailed investigation of a cohort of 55 such patients was quoted. The early postoperative mortality rate was 12.7%, and 25% of the patients were dead within 6 months. When the spinal cord area was less than 44 mm², a poor outcome was more likely than when it was larger. This finding

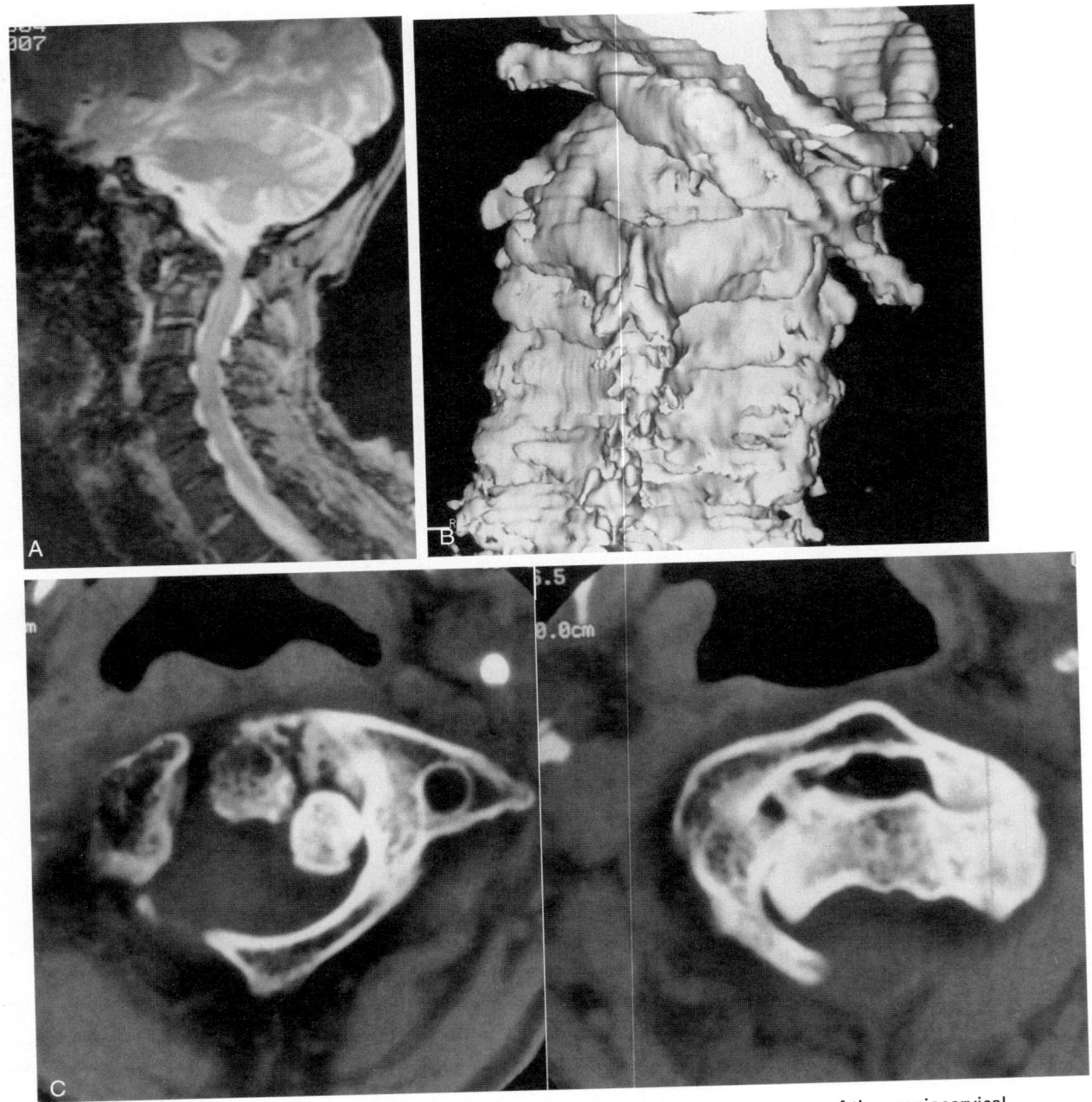

FIGURE 297–6. *A*, Midsagittal T2-weighted magnetic resonance imaging scan of the craniocervical junction in a 68-year-old individual with advanced rheumatoid arthritis. The patient was quadriparetic with a marked head tilt to the right. Note the hourglass constriction of the subarachnoid sac at C1. *B*, Three-dimensional reconstruction of the skull and cervical spine of same patient shows lateral dislocation of C1 and C2 with a 35-degree angulation. *C*, Composite axial computed tomographic scan through the upper *(left)* and lower *(right)* rims of the atlas arch shows an odontoid fracture with the superior segment adjacent to the odontoid stub. Note the fixed atlantoaxial dislocation.

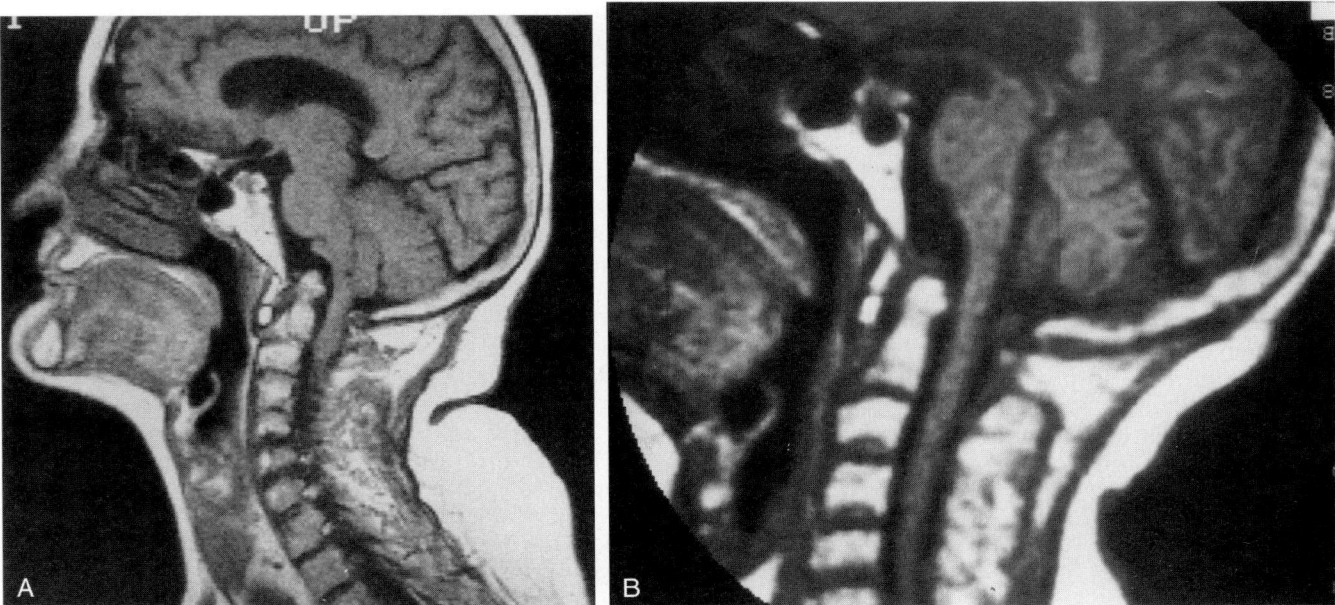

FIGURE 297–7. *A,* Midsagittal T1-weighted magnetic resonance imaging (MRI) scan of the brain and cervical spinal cord in a patient with cranial settling and vertical odontoid penetration into the posterior fossa. *B,* Midsagittal T1-weighted MRI scan of the craniocervical junction in the same patient 48 hours after halo traction. The vertical odontoid penetration into the foramen magnum is reduced, and the cervicomedullary compression is relieved.

FIGURE 297–8. *A,* Composite midline sagittal computed tomographic scan of the craniocervical junction and line drawing show the odontoid penetration into the foramen magnum and the fractured odontoid process. *B,* Composite axial computed tomographic scans 1 cm *(left)* and 3 cm *(right)* above the plane of the foramen magnum. The subarachnoid space is opacified with iohexol. The tip of the odontoid process is anchored in the ventral medulla at the level of the formation of the basilar artery by the two vertebral arteries.

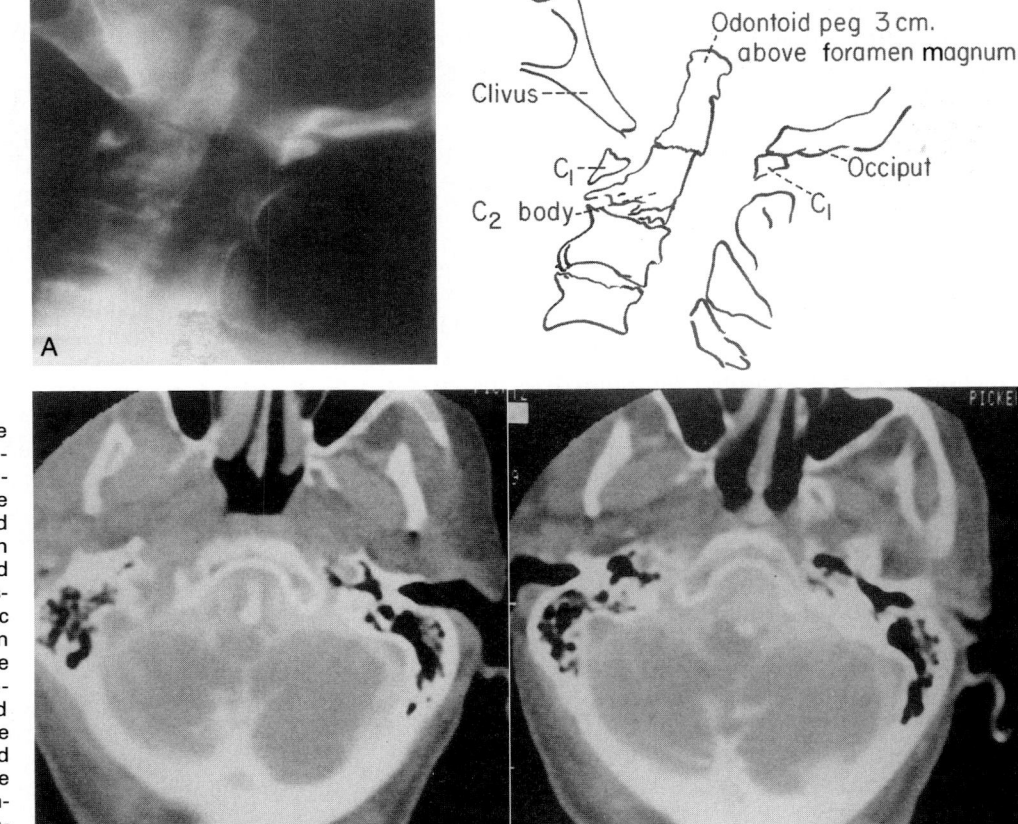

TABLE 297-2 ■ **Ranawat Classification of Neurological Deficit**

Class I	Pain, no neurological deficit
Class II	Subjective weakness, hyperreflexia, dysesthesias
Class IIIA	Ambulatory
Class IIIB	Nonambulatory

correlated with patients who had an increased degree of "vertical translocation." Before the era of MRI, Weissman and colleagues actually proposed the same relationships without providing a true statistical analysis.[76] Boden likewise recognized that when the preoperative PADI was less than 10 mm, the prognosis for return of motor function was poor.[45] In contrast, significant postoperative motor recovery could be appreciated in patients who had preoperative PADIs of 14 mm or greater.

Treatment of Rheumatoid Involvement of the Craniocervical Junction

The primary treatment goals for patients with RA at the craniocervical junction are relief of neuraxial compression and elimination of instability.[29] Achieving these goals depends on the precise identification of pathology and motion mechanics. For treatment purposes, these lesions are divided into reducible and irreducible lesions.[4] A reducible lesion is defined as one in which compression of the cervicomedullary neural structures can be relieved by restoring the craniocervical junction to a more anatomic relationship. Positioning or cervical traction can be used. A stabilization procedure then becomes paramount. In irreducible lesions, the basic tenet is decompression in the manner in which encroachment has occurred, followed by dorsal fixation.

All patients who require surgical attention must first be evaluated for articular and extra-articular involvement of the rheumatoid process. Nutritional status is best evaluated with a total lymphocyte count and liver function tests.[34] A lymphocyte count less than 1000/mm^3 is indicative of protein deficiency. All salicylate and nonsteroidal anti-inflammatory agents must be discontinued for a week before surgery. During this time, drugs such as methotrexate and steroids must be used for symptomatic relief of pain. Cardiac status and pulmonary function should always be evaluated.

Before surgical treatment, patients with rheumatoid involvement of the craniocervical junction should undergo an attempt to align the osseous anatomy and relieve the neural compression. Traction is contraindicated only for complex rotary luxations and posterior occipitoatlantoaxial dislocations.[34] These individuals require immediate stabilization. All patients undergoing cervical traction should be observed in a monitored nursing setting with pulse oximetry and the capacity to monitor respiratory function. Traction is applied via

a crown halo ring started at 5 to 7 pounds and gradually increased to a maximum of 11 to 12 pounds. Maximal weight is obtained at 36 hours. Periodic radiographic evaluation is essential to identify the degree of reduction, as well as to make changes in the force vectors for distraction. Mild extension to a neutral position is necessary in most individuals. If reduction is not achieved within 4 to 5 days, the patient's lesion should be considered irreducible, especially in the conditions described previously. Dorsal fusion of an irreducible ventral pathologic condition can be associated with adverse outcomes (Fig. 297-9).

Irreducible pathologic conditions causing ventral cervicomedullary neural compression (e.g., cranial settling with odontoid invagination into the medulla) require ventral removal of the offending pathology first.[34, 71] The transoral-transpharyngeal route provides a rapid, safe, and effective approach to the ventral craniocervical junction. This procedure must be accompanied by dorsal fixation. Cranial settling mandates occipitocervical arthrodesis.[29]

Reducible atlantoaxial dislocation is best managed with transarticular screw fixation if the lateral atlantal masses are intact and the quality of bone is satisfactory, as in younger individuals (Fig. 297-10).[7, 30, 34, 77-79] All fusions, however, must be supplemented with bone. Dorsal interlaminar fixation can be performed with rib graft.[71] The fusion rate has been reported at 98.2%.[79] The Halifax clamp for atlantoaxial dorsal fixation is associated with a failure rate of 17% to 20%.[71] Placement of a large rectangle of iliac crest between the posterior arch of C1 and C2 with cable retention is associated with a high rate of failure (Fig. 297-11). Internal fixation obviates the need for postoperative halo immobilization or the like.

Dorsal occipitocervical fusion is necessary in all individuals with rheumatoid cranial settling and in those who have had rheumatoid pannus resected. In a few individuals with active pannus, dorsal fixation stabilizes and reduces the ventral soft tissue mass because the active process immediately abates with stabilization (as with active effusion in other joints). Dorsal occipitocervical stabilization necessitates the placement of bone to anchor the cervical spine to the occiput as far laterally as possible to prevent lateral rotation as well as flexion and extension; it also provides for axial loading.[71, 80-82]

Instrumentation is essential in most rheumatoid individuals undergoing dorsal occipitocervical fusion. The procedure includes a custom-contoured threaded titanium loop fixed to the skull and upper cervical spine[34, 83] to allow bone supplementation for long-term osseous integration. Whether the use of calvarial bone in disabled patients with RA increases morbidity or mortality rates has been questioned.[7, 54] The success rate of occipital bone is well documented.[83-85] In the author's experience, a modified custom-built occipitocervical shell brace has proved satisfactory for occipitocervical stabilization. This custom-molded orthosis is similar to a modified Minerva brace and enjoys a high degree of patient acceptance and compliance.

Although methyl methacrylate has been used to

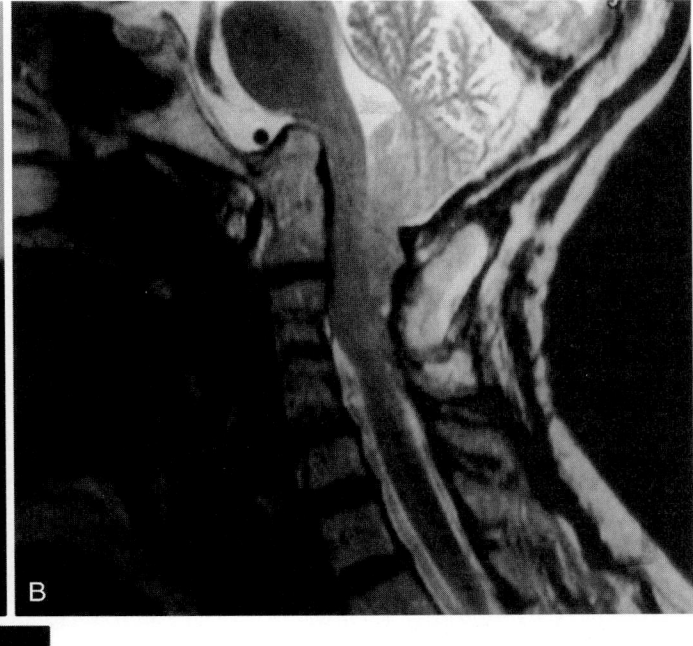

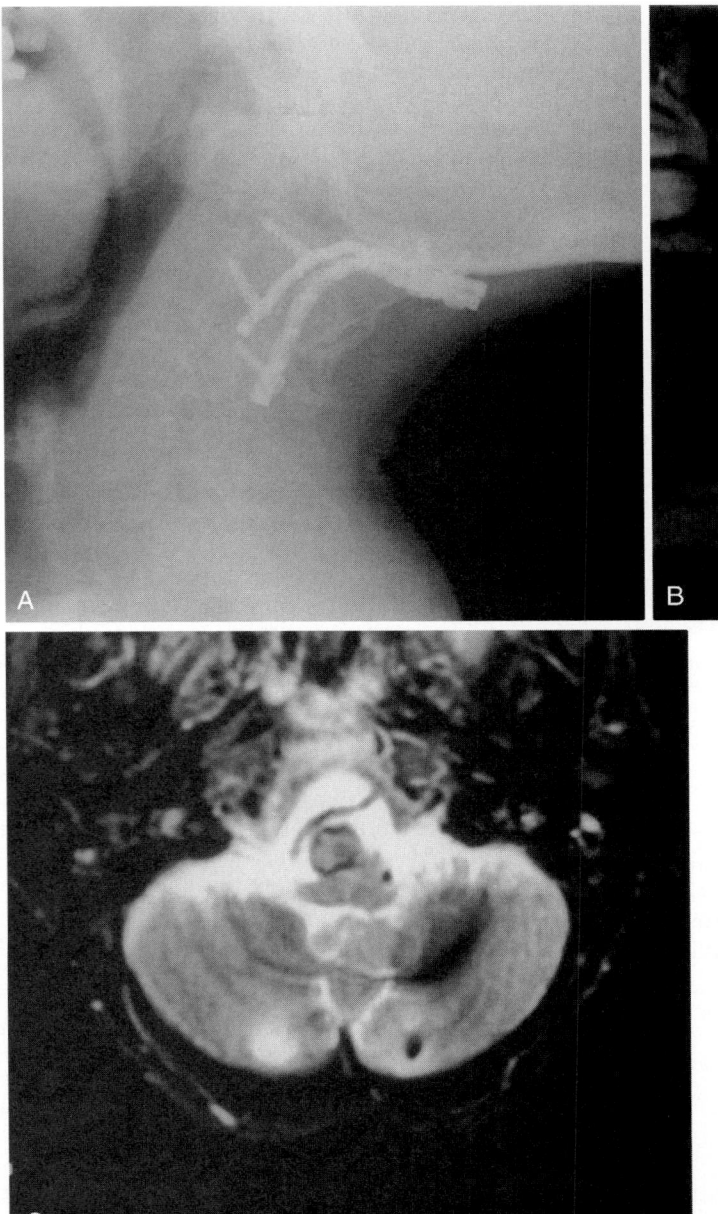

FIGURE 297–9. *A*, Lateral cervical radiograph in a 54-year-old individual with rheumatoid arthritis who had difficulty swallowing, diplopia, and quadriparesis. A previous dorsal occipitocervical fusion with plate and screws and iliac crest bone graft had been performed to treat ventral pontomedullary compression with cranial settling, without addressing the ventral pathology. *B*, T2-weighted magnetic resonance imaging (MRI) scan in the midsagittal plane of the craniocervical junction reveals odontoid penetration into the foramen magnum, compressing the ventral pontomedullary junction. Note the position of the vertebrobasilar arterial tree and the acquired hindbrain herniation. *C*, Axial T2-weighted MRI scan 1 cm above the plane of the foramen magnum shows the odontoid process posterior to the vertebrobasilar system, compressing the ventral and right lateral medulla.

supplement a bone construct to provide rigid internal immobilization, the occipitocervical contoured loop has definite advantages in achieving intraoperative reduction and in maintaining the reduction.

Transarticular screw fixation between C2 and C1 requires that the width of the pars interarticularis at C2 be satisfactory. The integrity of the lateral mass of C1 cannot be compromised by atrophy, compression, or significant osteoporosis, so that purchase for screw fixation can be gained.[30] Unfortunately, in 25% to 30% of individuals who fulfill these criteria for transarticular screw fixation, the vertebral artery groove may encroach on the pars interarticularis and may be injured even in the most experienced hands.[78] This situation can be identified as a potential problem on preoperative computed tomographic scans of the area of screw placement.

Several difficult situations arise in RA patients with debilitating symptoms. For instance, the ideal treatment (e.g., transoral odontoid resection) for bedridden patients who will never be mobile must be weighed against practical issues. Such an individual would have a poor outcome; hence, the operative procedure should be tailored to individual needs. Pain can be handled with fusion. However, the basic tenet of decompression with significant ventral pathology must be addressed first. The quality of bone and the patient's nutritional status also play a large role in the decision. Likewise,

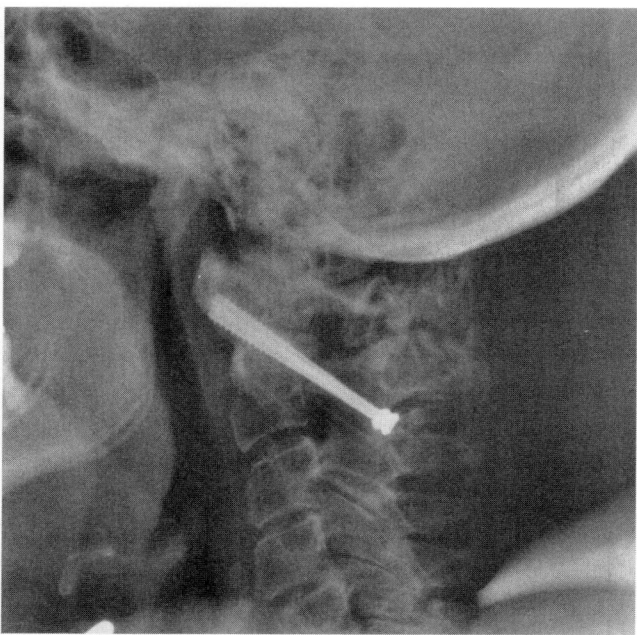

FIGURE 297–10. Lateral cervical spine radiograph of a 72-year-old individual with severe atlantoaxial dislocation that was reduced by traction. Note the transarticular screw fixation and bone obtained from the calvaria for dorsal occipitocervical fusion. The dislocation has been reduced.

fusion could fail due to the quality of the recipient bone, tissue vascular changes, and the inability to achieve satisfactory postoperative immobilization. These difficulties are just a few of those encountered in the management of patients with this affliction.

SPONDYLOARTHRITIDES OR NONRHEUMATOID INVOLVEMENT OF THE CRANIOCERVICAL JUNCTION

The term *seronegative spondyloarthritides* refers to conditions that cause inflammatory states of the spine and sacroiliac joints with an absence of rheumatoid factor.[86, 87] These conditions include ankylosing spondylitis, Reiter's syndrome, some forms of psoriatic arthritis, infectious arthritis, and arthritis associated with inflammatory bowel disease. In these conditions, the anatomic site of involvement in the ligament is the tendinous insertion into bone; hence the term *enthesis*.[85–97] This metabolically active transition in the region between two collagenous surfaces is particularly susceptible to torsion-related injury and can be the site of chronic inflammation. Conditions that result from inflammation of the enthesis are referred to as enthesopathies and overlap with the seronegative spondyloarthritides. In contrast, the central structure involved in rheumatic conditions is a synovial membrane. Although synovial involvement can occur in the seronegative arthritides, it tends to be less severe and is believed to be secondary to the primary area of injury.

Atlantoaxial instability, although common in cases of RA, is rare in seronegative spondyloarthritides.

Ankylosing spondylitis, or "bamboo spine," usually affects the axial skeleton, sparing the atlantoaxial region.[93] The fusion in the subaxial spine leads to an excessive dynamic load at the atlantoaxial level, with subsequent dislocation and further progression. It also may lead to secondary basilar invagination.[96] The fused mid and lower cervical and thoracic portions of the spine act as a single segment, transmitting load to the craniocervical region (Fig. 297–12). Suarez-Almazor and Russell observed a substantial increase in atlantoaxial instability in patients with ankylosing spondylitis who had associated psoriasis, Reiter's syndrome, or inflammatory bowel disease.[98] Of 39 patients, one third had peripheral disease involving psoriasis or an inflammatory bowel.

Juvenile RA occurs in children and adolescents and is not a single disease but a group of disorders classified by mode of onset.[16, 99] This entity includes Still's disease, polyarticular onset, pauciarticular onset, and RA. It is believed to be more than one disease. Therefore, multiple origins are expected and include factors such as infection, autoimmunity, and trauma. Viruses have been considered because they are associated with arthritis in children, and the rubella virus has been isolated from phytohemagglutinin-stimulated lymphoblasts.[34, 88] Illness that simulates juvenile RA is common in patients with immunoglobulin A deficiency and agammaglobulinemia or C2 complement deficiency. Seventy percent of patients experience a spontaneous and prominent remission by adulthood. Children with positive latex fixation tests have the worst prognosis.[34, 48] The major complications are impaired growth and irreversible developmental retardation due to early apophyseal closure. Ten percent of children develop amyloidosis.

Psoriatic arthropathy occurs in 7% of patients with psoriasis.[95, 100–102] The skin change tends to precede the onset of arthritis. Spinal involvement develops in 20% of patients with psoriatic arthritis and affects the craniocervical junction much the same way as ankylosing spondylitis.[102–104] Blau and Kaufman reviewed the clinical histories of 28 patients with both psoriasis and inflammatory arthritis between 1971 and 1984.[94] The cervical spine was involved in 75% of the group; 13 of 21 had ankylosing, and 8 of 21 had inflammatory characteristics. Three patients developed cervical myelopathy.

The relationship between inflammatory bowel disease and craniocervical disease has seldom been addressed. In 1986 Jordan and coworkers reported the first case in which inflammatory bowel disease was associated with atlantoaxial instability.[89] The patient presented with C1-2 instability and was diagnosed as having Crohn's disease. The triad of arthritis, urethritis, and ocular disease, referred to as Reiter's syndrome, seldom manifests simultaneously. The arthropathy may be acute and at times associated with reactive arthritis. As a result of the synovitis, atlantoaxial subluxation can occur. The treatment of these conditions is as previously outlined for RA.

Calcium pyrophosphate dehydrate deposition

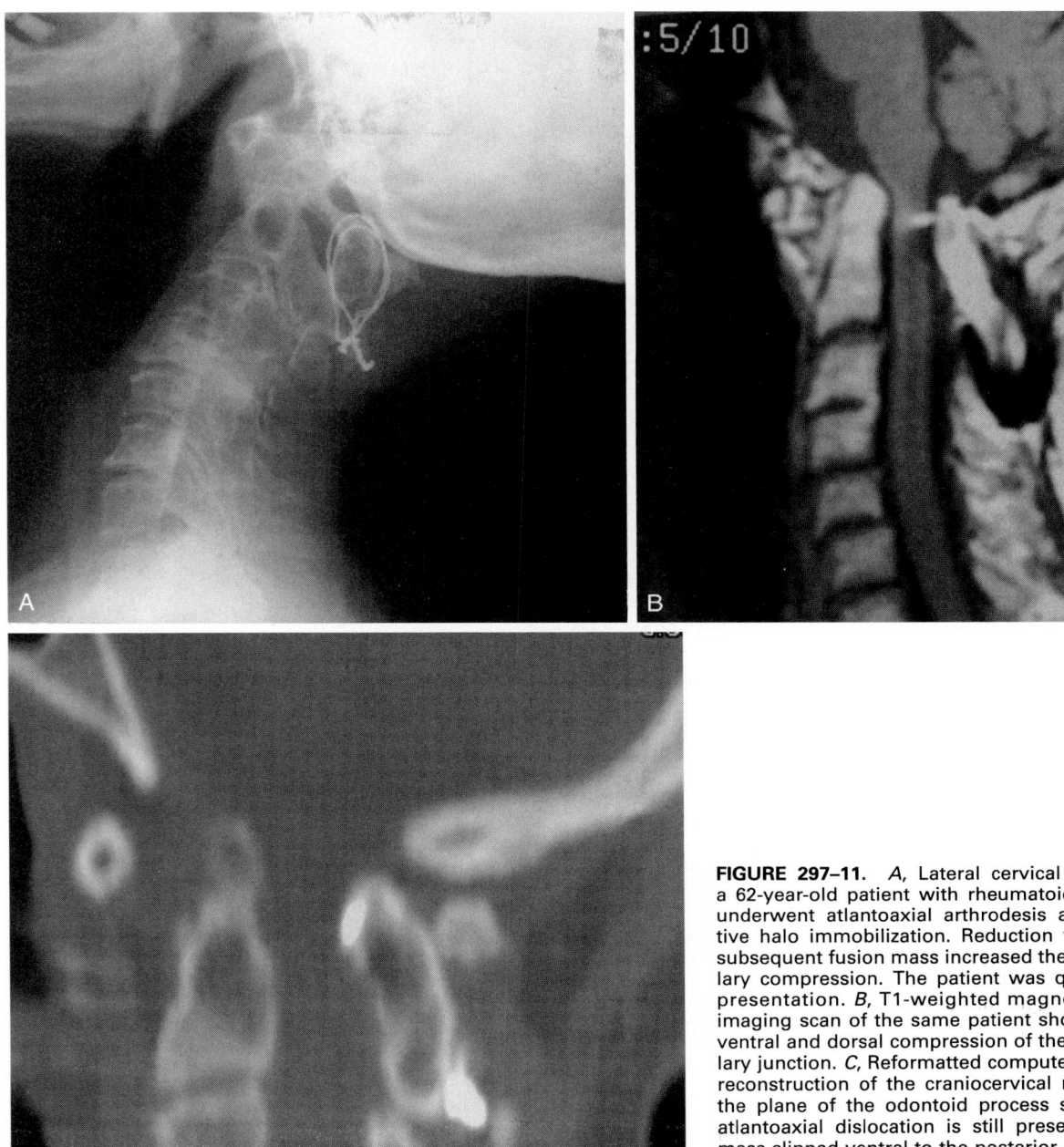

FIGURE 297–11. *A*, Lateral cervical radiograph of a 62-year-old patient with rheumatoid arthritis who underwent atlantoaxial arthrodesis and postoperative halo immobilization. Reduction failed, and the subsequent fusion mass increased the cervicomedullary compression. The patient was quadriparetic at presentation. *B*, T1-weighted magnetic resonance imaging scan of the same patient shows irreducible ventral and dorsal compression of the cervicomedullary junction. *C*, Reformatted computed tomographic reconstruction of the craniocervical region through the plane of the odontoid process shows that the atlantoaxial dislocation is still present. The fusion mass slipped ventral to the posterior arch of C1, and the inferior aspect of the graft incorporated with the posterior arch of C2. The patient required ventral odontoid resection, dorsal bony decompression, and fusion.

(CPDD) is considered one of the most common forms of crystal-induced arthritis.[105] The disease has not been recognized in individuals younger than 70 years and is more common in individuals older than 85 years. CPDD can act as a retro-odontoid mass, causing ventral cervicomedullary compression. The diagnostic features are small areas of calcification within the mass on computed tomographic scans; a mostly isointense mass on T1-weighted MRI scans; mixed density, with the signal changing from hypo- to hyperintense, on T2-weighted MRI scans; and peripheral enhancement of the mass on postgadolinium MRI scans (Fig. 297–13).[34, 106] Based on these findings, retro-odontoid CPDD-induced masses can be diagnosed with a high degree of certainty before surgery. CPDD can be approached via the transoral route to halt or reverse the progression of neurological deterioration. The surgical pathologist must be alerted to the possibility of this diagnosis so that the surgical specimen is handled appropriately to reveal the diagnostic birefringent rhomboid CPDD crystals.

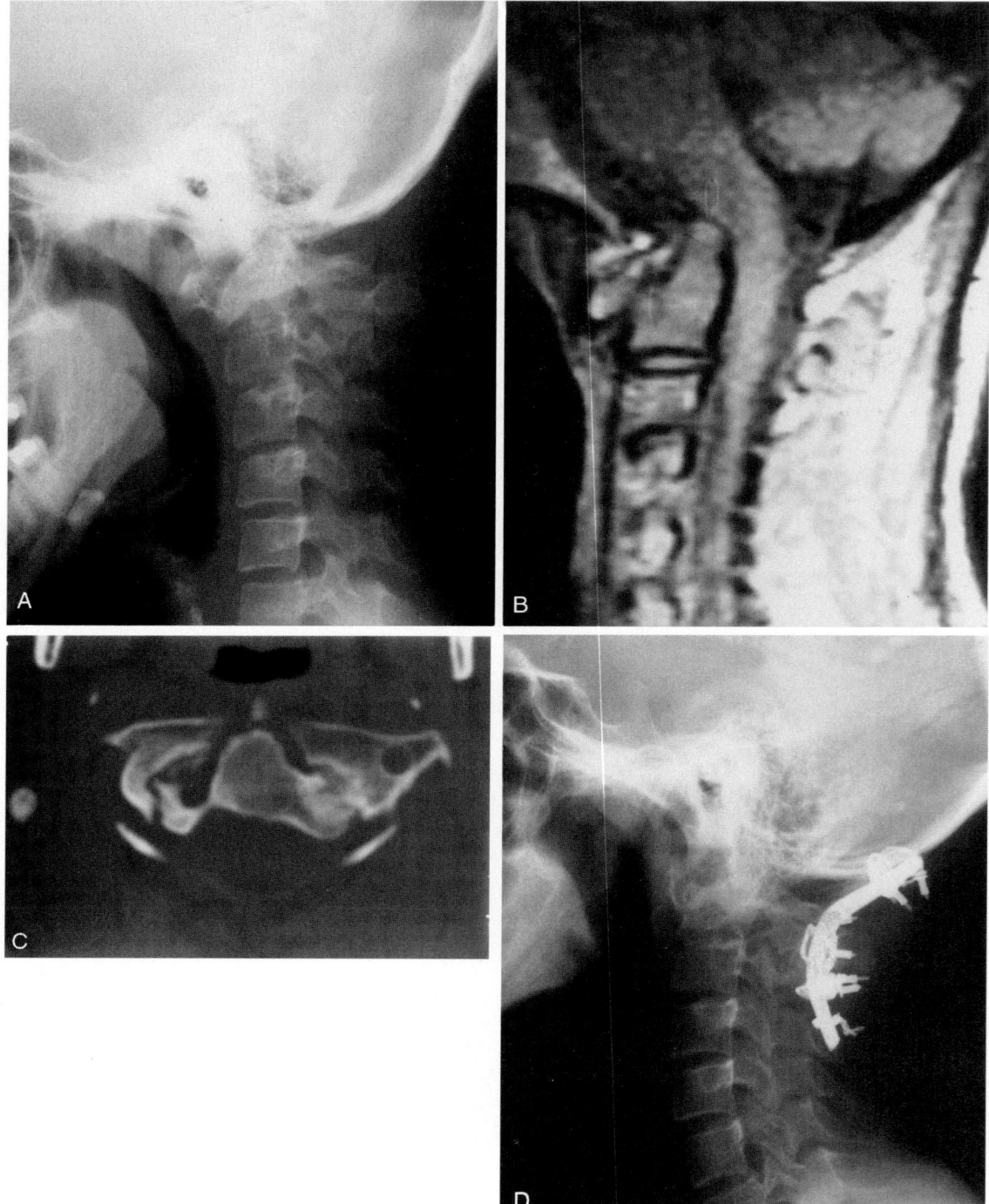

FIGURE 297–12. *A,* Lateral craniocervical radiograph of a 22-year-old man with severe ankylosing spondylitis shows atlantoaxial dislocation. He presented with a 6-month history of severe neck pain and quadriparesis that was worse in the legs than in the arms. The anterior arch of the atlas is displaced inferiorly; the posterior arch of the atlas is displaced ventrally. *B,* Midsagittal T1-weighted magnetic resonance imaging scan shows odontoid migration into the posterior fossa, with compression of the inferior ventral medulla. *C,* Axial computed tomographic scan through the plane of the atlas shows atlantoaxial dislocation, with fusion between the superior surface of the axis body and the lateral atlantal mass. *D,* Lateral craniocervical radiograph obtained 6 months after transoral ventral decompression of the atlas and odontoid process shows a dorsal occipitocervical fixation with loop instrumentation and rib graft. The patient recovered neurologically.

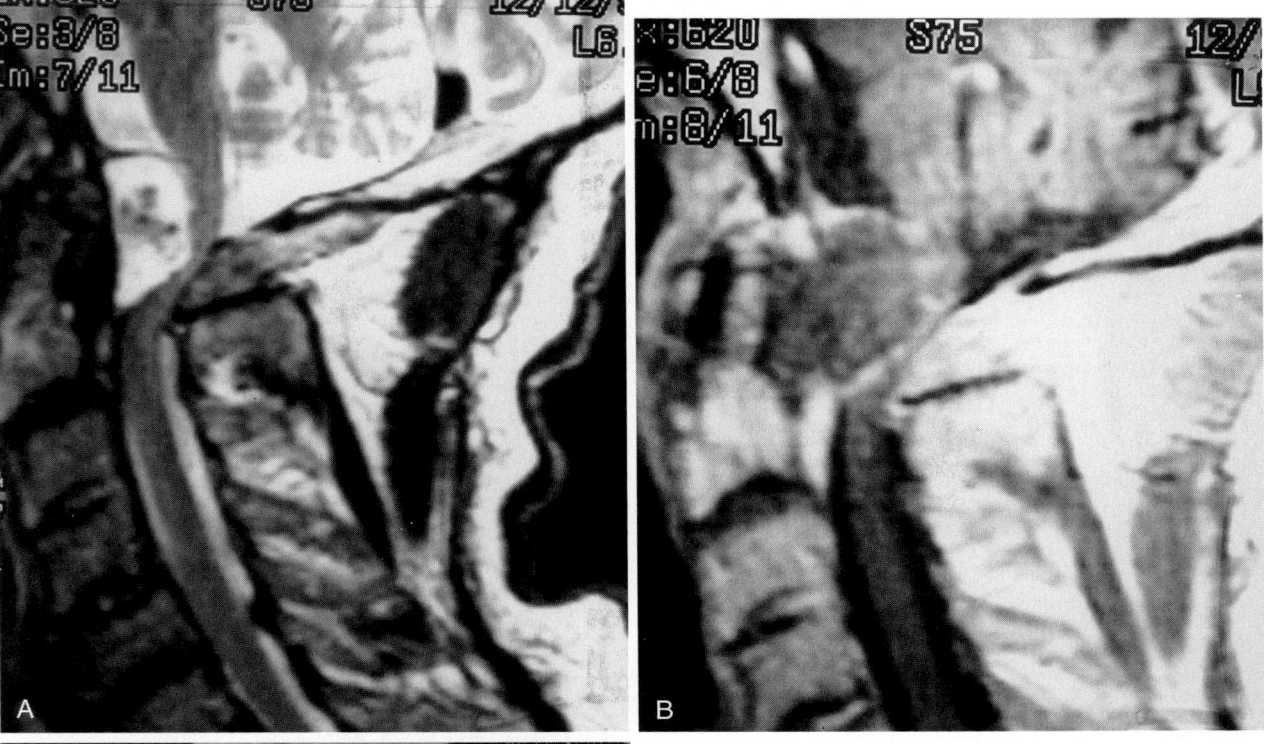

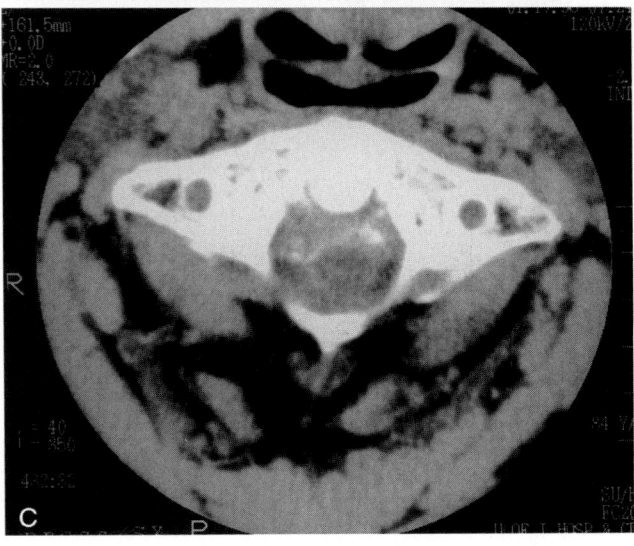

FIGURE 297–13. *A,* T2-weighted magnetic resonance imaging (MRI) scan in an 82-year-old individual with calcium pyrophosphate mass (pseudogout) shows a mass ventral to the cervicomedullary junction in the retro-odontoid region. The patient presented with lower cranial nerve disturbance and quadriparesis. *B,* Midsagittal T1-weighted MRI scan with gadolinium enhancement shows the rimlike enhancement of the retro-odontoid mass. *C,* Axial computed tomographic scan through the plane of the odontoid process and atlas shows calcifications in the retro-odontoid mass.

REFERENCES

1. Goel VK, Clark CR, Gallaes K, et al: Movement-rotation relationships of the ligamentous occipito-atlanto-axial complex. J Biomech 21:673–680, 1988.
2. Bland JH: Rheumatoid arthritis of the cervical spine: Review. J Rheumatol 1:319–342, 1974.
3. Delamarter RB, Bohlman HH: Postmortem osseous and neuropathologic analysis of the rheumatoid cervical spine. Spine 19:2267–2274, 1994.
4. Menezes AH, VanGilder JC: Anomalies of the craniovertebral junction. In Youmans J (ed): Neurological Surgery, vol 2, 3rd ed. Philadelphia, WB Saunders, 1990, pp 1359–1420.
5. Engel A: Rheumatoid arthritis in US adults 1960–1962. In Bennett PH, Wood PHN (eds): Population Studies of the Rheumatic Diseases. Amsterdam, Exerta Medica, 1968, pp 83–89.
6. Cathcart E, O'Sullivan JB: Rheumatoid arthritis in a New England town: A prevalence study in Sudbury, Massachusetts. N Engl J Med 282:421–442, 1970.
7. Casey ATH, Crockard HA: Rheumatoid arthritis. In Dickman CA, Spetzler RF, Sonntag VKH (eds): Surgery of the Craniovertebral Junction. New York, Thieme, 1998, pp 151–174.
8. Kauppi M, Hakala M: Prevalence of cervical spine subluxations and dislocations in a community-based rheumatoid arthritis population. Scand J Rheumatol 23:133–136, 1994.
9. Garrod AE: A Treatise on Rheumatism and Rheumatoid Arthritis. London, 1890, pp 1–342.
10. Conlon PW, Isdale IC, Rose BS: Rheumatoid arthritis of the cervical spine: An analysis of 333 cases. Ann Rheum Dis 25:120–126, 1966.
11. Mathews JA: Atlanto-axial subluxation in rheumatoid arthritis: A 5-year followup study. Ann Rheum Dis 33:526–531, 1974.

12. Vasey FB: Psoriatic arthritis. In Schumacher HR (ed): Primer in the Rheumatic Diseases, 9th ed. Atlanta, Arthritis Foundation, 1988, pp 151–153.

13. Silman AJ: Rheumatoid arthritis and infection: A population approach. Ann Rheum Dis 48:707–710, 1989.

14. Koopman WJ: Prospects for autoimmune disease: Research advances in rheumatoid arthritis. JAMA 285:648–650, 2001.

15. Zvaifler NJ: Rheumatoid arthritis: Epidemiology, etiology, rheumatoid factor, pathology, pathogenesis. In Schumacher HR (ed): Primer on the Rheumatic Diseases, 9th ed. Atlanta, Arthritis Foundation, 1988, pp 83–87.

16. Condemi JJ: The autoimmune diseases. JAMA 268:2882–2892, 1992.

17. Young ID, Ford SE, Ford PM: The association of pulmonary hypertension with rheumatoid arthritis. J Rheumatol 16:1266–1269, 1989.

18. Arnett FC, Edworthy SM, Bloch DA, et al: The American Rheumatism Association 1987 revised criteria for the classification of rheumatoid arthritis. Arthritis Rheum 31:315–324, 1988.

19. Cush JJ, Lipsky PE: The immunopathogenesis of rheumatoid arthritis: The role of cytokines in chronic inflammation. Clin Aspects Autoimmune 1:2–13, 1987.

20. Deleuran BW: Cytokines in rheumatoid arthritis: Localization in arthritic joint tissue and regulation in vitro. Scand J Rheumatol Suppl 104:1–34, 1996.

21. Feldmann M, Brennan FM, Maini RN: Role of cytokines in rheumatoid arthritis. Ann Rev Immunol 14:397–440, 1996.

22. Moreland LW, Koopman WJ: Biologic response modifiers for treating musculoskeletal disorders. In Koopman WJ (ed): Arthritis and Allied Conditions, 14th ed. Philadelphia, Lippincott Williams & Wilkins, 2001, pp 877–930.

23. Weinblatt ME, Kremer JM, Bankhurst AD, et al: A trial of etanercept, a recombinant tumor necrosis factor receptor:Fc fusion protein, in patients with rheumatoid arthritis receiving methotrexate. N Engl J Med 340:253–259, 1999.

24. Lovell DJ, Giannini EH, Reiff A, et al: Etanercept in children with polyarticular juvenile rheumatoid arthritis: Pediatric Rheumatology Collaborative Study Group. N Engl J Med 342:763–769, 2000.

25. Pisetsky DS: Tumor necrosis factor blockers in rheumatoid arthritis. N Engl J Med 342:810–811, 2000.

26. Tugwell P, Pincus T, Yocum D, et al: Combination therapy with cyclosporine and methotrexate in severe rheumatoid arthritis: The Methotrexate-Cyclosporine Combination Study Group. N Engl J Med 333:137–146, 1995.

27. Wallace CA: The use of methotrexate in childhood rheumatic diseases. Arthritis Rheum 41:381–391, 1998.

28. Bertolini DR, Nedwin GE, Bringman TS, et al: Stimulation of bone resorption and inhibition of bone formation in vitro by human tumour necrosis factors. Nature 319:516–518, 1986.

29. Menezes AH, VanGilder JC, Clark CR, et al: Odontoid upward migration in rheumatoid arthritis: An analysis of 45 patients with "cranial settling." J Neurosurg 63:500–509, 1985.

30. Clark CR, Menezes AH: Rheumatoid arthritis: Surgical considerations. In Herkowitz HN, Garfin SR, Balderston RA, et al (eds): The Spine, vol 2, 4th ed. Philadelphia, WB Saunders, 1999, pp 1281–1301.

31. Delamarter RB, Bolesta MJ, Bohlman HH: Rheumatoid arthritis. In Frymoyer J (ed): The Adult Spine: Principles and Practice, vol 1. New York, Raven Press, 1991, pp 745–762.

32. Helmers R, Galvin J, Hunninghake GH: Pulmonary manifestations associated with rheumatoid arthritis. Chest 100:235–238, 1991.

33. Hurd ER: Extraarticular manifestations of rheumatoid arthritis. Semin Arthritis Rheum 8:151–176, 1979.

34. Menezes AH: Rheumatological disorders. In Menezes AH, Sonntag VKH (eds): Principles of Spinal Surgery, vol 1. New York, McGraw-Hill, 1996, pp 705–722.

35. Sharp J, Purser DW, Lawrence JS: Rheumatoid arthritis of the cervical spine in the adult. Ann Rheum Dis 17:303–313, 1958.

36. Marks JS, Sharp J: Rheumatoid cervical myelopathy. Q J Med 50:307–319, 1981.

37. Ball J, Sharp J: Rheumatoid arthritis of the cervical spine. In Hill AGS (ed): Modern Trends in Rheumatology, 2nd ed. London, Butterworth, 1971, pp 117–138.

38. Lorber A, Pearson CM, Rene RM: Osteolytic vertebral lesions as a manifestation of rheumatoid arthritis and related disorders. Arthritis Rheum 4:514–532, 1961.

39. VonTorklus D, Gehle W: The upper cervical spine: Regional anatomy, pathology and traumatology. In Verlag GT (ed): A Systemic Radiological Atlas and Textbook. New York, Grune & Stratton, 1972, pp 1–99.

40. Winfield J, Cooke D, Brook AS, et al: A prospective study of the radiological changes in the cervical spine in early rheumatoid disease. Ann Rheum Dis 40:109–114, 1981.

41. Pellicci PM, Ranawat CS, Tsairis P, et al: A prospective study of the progression of rheumatoid arthritis of the cervical spine. J Bone Joint Surg Am 63:342–350, 1981.

42. Mikulowski P, Wollheim FA, Rotmil P, et al: Sudden death in rheumatoid arthritis with atlanto-axial dislocation. Acta Med Scand 198:445–451, 1975.

43. Crockard HA, Essigman WK, Stevens JM, et al: Surgical treatment of cervical cord compression in rheumatoid arthritis. Ann Rheum Dis 44:809–816, 1985.

44. Casey AT, Crockard HA, Bland JM, et al: Predictors of outcome in the quadriparetic nonambulatory myelopathic patient with rheumatoid arthritis: A prospective study of 55 surgically treated Ranawat class IIIb patients. J Neurosurg 85:574–581, 1996.

45. Boden SD: Rheumatoid arthritis of the cervical spine: Surgical decision making based on predictors of paralysis and recovery. Spine 19:2275–2280, 1994.

46. Hernandez LA, Buchanan WW, Sturrock RD: C4 and C5 body vertebral erosions in early rheumatoid disease. Clin Rheumatol 7:331–334, 1988.

47. Dodge LD, Bohlman HH, Rechtine GR: Paralysis secondary to rheumatoid arthritis—pathogenesis and results of treatment. Orthop Trans 11:473, 1987.

48. Martel W: The occipito-atlanto-axial joints in rheumatoid arthritis and ankylosing spondylitis. AJR Am J Roentgenol 86:223–240, 1961.

49. Nakano KK, Schoene WC, Baker RA, et al: The cervical myelopathy associated with rheumatoid arthritis: Analysis of 32 patients with two postmortem cases. Ann Neurol 3:144–151, 1978.

50. O'Leary P, Ranawat CS, Pellicci PM: The cervical spine in rheumatoid arthritis. Contemp Surg 7:13–17, 1975.

51. Redlund-Johnell I, Pettersson H: Radiographic measurements of the cranio-vertebral region: Designed for evaluation of abnormalities in rheumatoid arthritis. Acta Radiol Diagn 25:23–28, 1984.

52. Sambrook PN, Eisman JA, Champion GD, et al: Determinants of axial bone loss in rheumatoid arthritis. Arthritis Rheum 30:721–728, 1987.

53. Santavirta S, Slatis P, Kankaanpaa U, et al: Treatment of the cervical spine in rheumatoid arthritis. J Bone Joint Surg Am 70:658–667, 1988.

54. Crockard HA: Surgical management of cervical rheumatoid problems. Spine 20:2584–2590, 1995.

55. Macedo TF, Gow PJ, Heap SW, et al: Bilateral hypoglossal nerve palsy due to vertical subluxation of the odontoid process in rheumatoid arthritis. Br J Rheumatol 27:317–320, 1988.

56. Sherk HH: Atlantoaxial instability and acquired basilar invagination in rheumatoid arthritis. Orthop Clin North Am 9:1053–1063, 1978.

57. Zygmunt S, Saveland H, Brattstrom H, et al: Reduction of rheumatoid periodontoid pannus following posterior occipitocervical fusion visualised by magnetic resonance imaging. Br J Neurosurg 2:315–320, 1988.

58. Zoma A, Sturrock RD, Fisher WD, et al: Surgical stabilisation of the rheumatoid cervical spine: A review of indications and results. J Bone Joint Surg Br 69:8–12, 1987.

59. Larsson EM, Holtas S, Zygmunt S: Pre- and postoperative MR imaging of the craniocervical junction in rheumatoid arthritis. AJR Am J Roentgenol 152:561–566, 1989.

60. Stiskal MA, Neuhold A, Szolar DH, et al: Rheumatoid arthritis of the craniocervical region by MR imaging: Detection and characterization. AJR Am J Roentgenol 165:585–592, 1995.

61. Bundschuh C, Modic MT, Kearney F, et al: Rheumatoid arthritis of the cervical spine: Surface-coil MR imaging. AJR Am J Roentgenol 151:181–187, 1988.

62. Case records of the Massachusetts General Hospital: Weekly clinicopathological exercises. Case 37-1992: A 68-year-old woman with rheumatoid arthritis and pulmonary hypertension. N Engl J Med 327:873–880, 1992.

63. Eaton AM, Serota H, Kernodle GH Jr, et al: Pulmonary hypertension secondary to serum hyperviscosity in a patient with rheumatoid arthritis. Am J Med 82:1039–1045, 1987.

64. Price TML, Skelton MO: Rheumatoid arthritis with lung lesions. Thorax 11:234–240, 1956.

65. Wiedemann HP, Matthay RA: Pulmonary manifestations of the collagen vascular diseases. Clin Chest Med 10:677–722, 1989.

66. Epler GR, McLoud TC, Gaensler EA, et al: Normal chest roentgenograms in chronic diffuse infiltrative lung disease. N Engl J Med 298:934–939, 1978.

67. Fewins HE, McGowan I, Whitehouse GH, et al: High definition computed tomography in rheumatoid arthritis associated pulmonary disease. Br J Rheumatol 30:214–216, 1991.

68. Boden SD, Dodge LD, Bohlman HH, et al: Rheumatoid arthritis of the cervical spine: A long-term analysis with predictors of paralysis and recovery. J Bone Joint Surg Am 75:1282–1297, 1993.

69. Christophidis N, Huskisson EC: Misleading symptoms and signs of cervical spine subluxation in rheumatoid arthritis. BMJ 285:364–365, 1982.

70. Saway PA, Blackburn WD, Halla JT, et al: Clinical characteristics affecting survival in patients with rheumatoid arthritis undergoing cervical spine surgery: A controlled study. J Rheumatol 16:890–896, 1989.

71. Menezes AH: Surgical approaches to the craniocervical junction. In Frymoyer J (ed): The Adult Spine: Principles and Practice, vol 2. New York, Raven Press, 1991, pp 967–986.

72. Semble EL, Elster AD, Loeser RF, et al: Magnetic resonance imaging of the craniovertebral junction in rheumatoid arthritis. J Rheumatol 15:1367–1375, 1988.

73. Winalski CS, Aliabadi P, Wright RJ, et al: Enhancement of joint fluid with intravenously administered gadopentetate dimeglumine: Technique, rationale, and implications. Radiology 187:179–185, 1993.

74. Grob D, Wursch R, Grauer W, et al: Atlantoaxial fusion and retrodental pannus in rheumatoid arthritis. Spine 22:1580–1584, 1997.

75. Ranawat CS, O'Leary P, Pellicci PM, et al: Cervical spine fusion in rheumatoid arthritis. J Bone Joint Surg Am 61:1003–1010, 1979.

76. Weissman BN, Aliabadi P, Weinfeld MS, et al: Prognostic features of atlantoaxial subluxation in rheumatoid arthritis patients. Radiology 144:745–751, 1982.

77. Dickman CA, Crawford NR, Paramore CG: Biomechanical characteristics of C1-2 cable fixations. J Neurosurg 85:316–322, 1996.

78. Paramore CG, Dickman CA, Sonntag VKH: The anatomical suitability of the C1-2 complex for transarticular screw fixation. J Neurosurg 85:221–224, 1996.

79. Sawin PD, Traynelis VC, Menezes AH: A comparative analysis of fusion rates and donor-site morbidity for autogeneic rib and iliac crest bone grafts in posterior cervical fusions. J Neurosurg 88:255–265, 1998.

80. Newman P, Sweetnam R: Occipito-cervical fusion: An operative technique and its indications. J Bone Joint Surg Br 51:423–431, 1969.

81. Sakou T, Kawaida H, Morizono Y, et al: Occipitoatlantoaxial fusion utilizing a rectangular rod. Clin Orthop 239:136–144, 1989.

82. MacKenzie AI, Uttley D, Marsh HT, et al: Craniocervical stabilization using Luque/Hartshill rectangles. Neurosurgery 26:32–36, 1990.

83. Robertson SC, Menezes AH: Occipital calvarial bone graft in posterior occipitocervical fusion. Spine 23:249–255, 1998.

84. Walters BC: Cranial bone grafts for use in posterior fixation of the cervical spine: Technical note. J Neurosurg 79:286–288, 1993.

85. Sagher O, Malik JM, Lee JH, et al: Fusion with occipital bone for atlantoaxial instability: Technical note. Neurosurgery 33:926–929, 1993.

86. Fries JF: The reactive enthesopathies. Dis Mon 31:1–46, 1985.

87. Ryken TC, Menezes AH: Inflammatory bowel disease and the craniocervical junction [article 10]. Neurosurg Focus, vol 6, 1999.

88. Helliwell PS, Hickling P, Wright V: Do the radiological changes of classic ankylosing spondylitis differ from the changes found in the spondylitis associated with inflammatory bowel disease, psoriasis, and reactive arthritis? Ann Rheum Dis 57:135–140, 1998.

89. Jordan JM, Obeid LM, Allen NB: Isolated atlantoaxial subluxation as the presenting manifestation of inflammatory bowel disease. Am J Med 80:517–520, 1986.

90. Kerr R, Resnick D: Radiology of the seronegative spondyloarthropathies. Clin Rheum Dis 11:113–146, 1985.

91. Lee ST, Lui TN: Psoriatic arthritis with C-1–C-2 subluxation as a neurosurgical complication. Surg Neurol 26:428–430, 1986.

92. Yulish BS, Lieberman JM, Newman AJ, et al: Juvenile rheumatoid arthritis: Assessment with MR imaging. Radiology 165:149–152, 1987.

93. Sharp J, Purser DW: Spontaneous atlanto-axial dislocation in ankylosing spondylitis and rheumatoid arthritis. Ann Rheum Dis 20:47–77, 1961.

94. Blau RH, Kaufman RL: Erosive and subluxing cervical spine disease in patients with psoriatic arthritis. J Rheumatol 14:111–117, 1987.

95. Fam AG, Cruickshank B: Subaxial cervical subluxation and cord compression in psoriatic spondylitis. Arthritis Rheum 25:101–106, 1982.

96. McEwen C, DiTata D, Lingg C, et al: Ankylosing spondylitis and spondylitis accompanying ulcerative colitis, regional enteritis, psoriasis and Reiter's disease: A comparative study. Arthritis Rheum 14:291–318, 1971.

97. Kransdorf MJ, Wehrle PA, Moser RP Jr: Atlantoaxial subluxation in Reiter's syndrome: A report of three cases and review of the literature. Spine 13:12–14, 1988.

98. Suarez-Almazor ME, Russell AS: Anterior atlantoaxial subluxation in patients with spondyloarthropathies: Association with peripheral disease. J Rheumatol 15:973–975, 1988.

99. Ball J: Enthesopathy of rheumatoid and ankylosing spondylitis. Ann Rheum Dis 30:213–223, 1971.

100. Dzioba RB, Benjamin J: Spontaneous atlantoaxial fusion in psoriatic arthritis: A case report. Spine 10:102–103, 1985.

101. Hanly JG, Russell ML, Gladman DD: Psoriatic spondyloarthropathy: A long-term prospective study. Ann Rheum Dis 47:386–393, 1988.

102. Killebrew K, Gold RH, Sholkoff SD: Psoriatic spondylitis. Radiology 108:9–16, 1973.

103. Paimela L, Laasonen L, Kankaanpaa E, et al: Progression of cervical spine changes in patients with early rheumatoid arthritis. J Rheumatol 24:1280–1284, 1997.

104. Reynolds MD, Rankin TJ: Diagnosis of "rheumatoid variants," ankylosing spondylitis, the arthritides of gastrointestinal diseases and psoriasis, and Reiter's syndrome. West J Med 120:441–447, 1974.

105. Chuzhin Y, Panush RS: CPPDDD: What it is and why it is underrecognized. Bull Rheum Dis 44:3–5, 1995.

106. Zunkeler B, Schelper R, Menezes AH: Periodontoid calcium pyrophosphate dihydrate deposition disease: "Pseudogout" mass lesions of the craniocervical junction. J Neurosurg 85:803–809, 1996.

Basic Principles of Spinal Internal Fixation

GEOFFREY ZUBAY ■ CURTIS A. DICKMAN
VOLKER K. H. SONNTAG ■ NEIL R. CRAWFORD

The spine is composed of 28 vertebrae: 7 cervical vertebrae, 12 thoracic vertebrae, 5 lumbar vertebrae, and 4 sacral vertebrae that typically exist as a single fused unit. Each vertebra (except for C1, C2, and the sacral vertebrae) is composed of a body, pedicle, facet, lamina, and spinous process. As one proceeds down the spinal column rostrally to caudally, the size of the vertebrae increases, and the orientation of the facets changes gradually from parallel sloping to upright blocking. The normal spine has a cervical lordosis, a thoracic kyphosis, and a lumbar lordosis.

The spinal column is supported by numerous ligamentous and soft tissue elements. Spinal stability is provided by the facet joints, intervertebral disks, posterior spinous ligaments, and numerous accessory elements adjacent to the spine. After retrospectively reviewing the radiographic images of 412 thoracolumbar fractures, Denis[1] devised the three-column theory of spinal stability. The anterior column consists of the anterior half of the vertebral body, the anterior half of the annulus fibrosus, and the anterior longitudinal ligament. The middle column consists of the dorsal half of the vertebral body, the dorsal half of the annulus fibrosus, and the posterior longitudinal ligament. The posterior column consists of the pedicles, facets, lamina, pars interarticularis, and posterior ligamentous complex. Denis proposed that an injury that compromises two of the three columns leads to pathologic instability at the affected level (Fig. 298–1).

The spinal motion segment is the fundamental biomechanical unit on which all principles of internal fixation are based. It is composed of two adjacent vertebrae and all the surrounding supportive connective tissue and ligaments. Pathologic instability of a spinal motion segment can compromise the spinal canal, spinal cord, and nerve root foramina. Abnormal movement or instability can lead to clinical symptoms of myelopathy when the spinal cord is compromised, to radicular symptoms when the nerve root foramen or cauda equina is compromised, and to back pain when abnormal motion occurs.

The goal of surgical treatment is to correct pathologic instability by promoting bony fusion at the affected level. Orthotic immobilization after spinal fusion has been the standard of care for decades. Mechanical hardware as an adjunct has become more popular because it allows early mobilization of the patient.

The goal of spinal internal fixation is to reconstruct the compromised columns *within* a spinal motion segment with nonbiologic materials to afford temporary immobilization and stabilization until bony fusion can develop. Fixation is successful when a construct can withstand the wear and tear of mechanical stresses and strains until fusion occurs. Successful application of the available hardware and instrumentation techniques begins with a sound and fundamental understanding of the origin of these stresses and strains and how they are modified by different instrumentation techniques.

BASIC BIOMECHANICS

The spine is subjected to numerous forces, typically from gravitational loads, muscular and ligamentous loads, and acceleration and deceleration loads. Forces applied to the spine can be directed to induce compression, tension, shear, bending, or torsion. Forces applied to the spine can be envisioned as vectors (Fig. 298–2). A force vector has magnitude and direction in three-dimensional space. Force causes displacement or distortion of an object if it is, respectively, unopposed or opposed.

The effect of a force depends on its orientation to a body's axis of rotation or neutral axis. The axis of

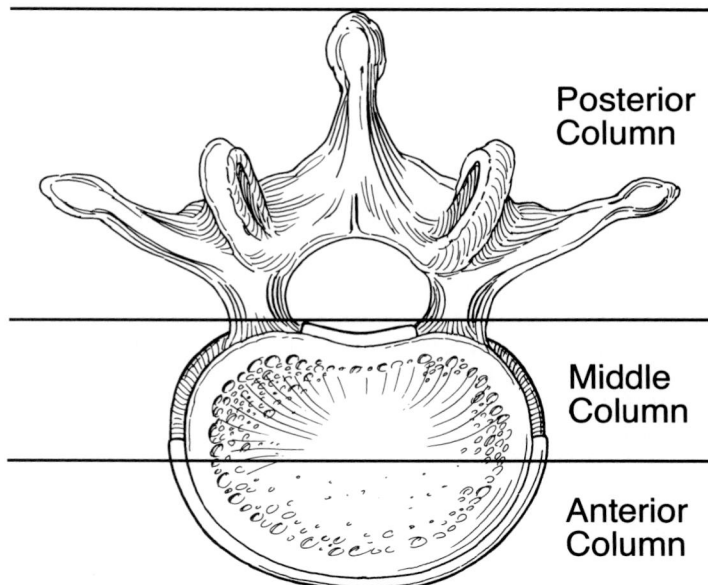

FIGURE 298–1. Illustration of a vertebral body showing the columns of spinal stability as originally described by Denis.[1] (Courtesy of Barrow Neurological Institute, Phoenix, AZ.)

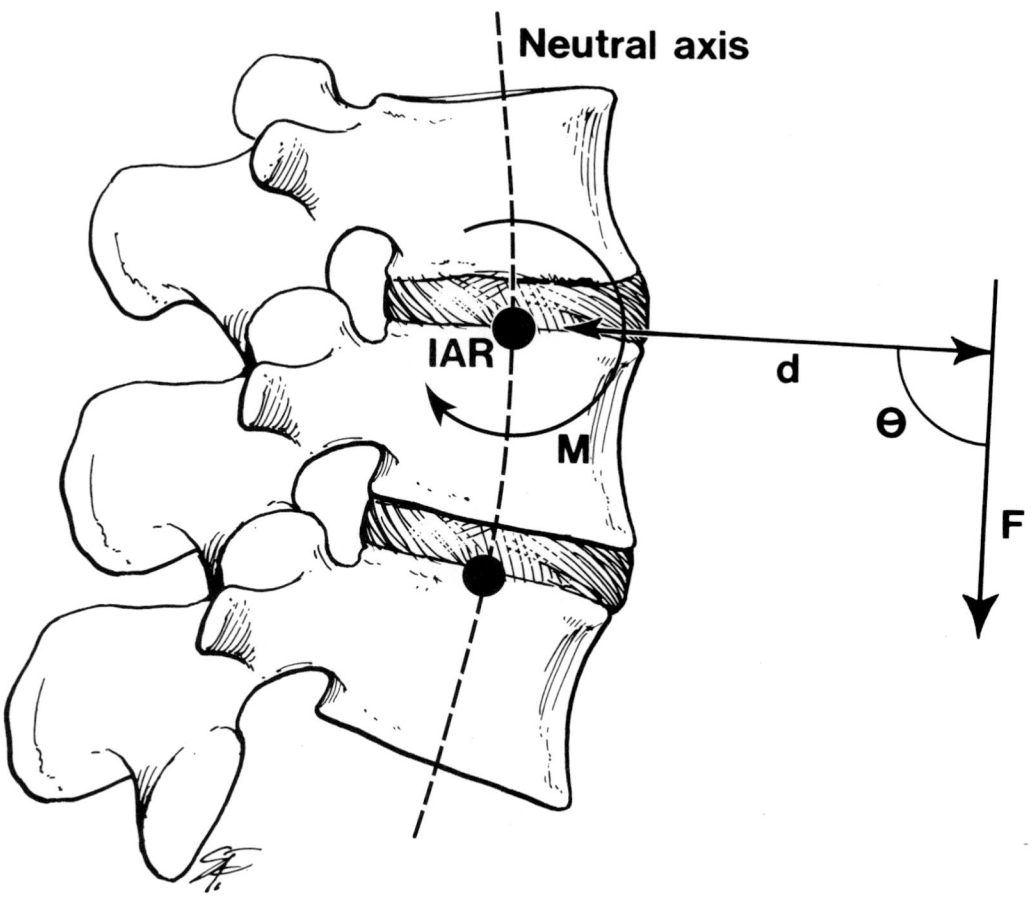

FIGURE 298–2. Lateral illustration of a spinal motion segment showing the instantaneous axis of rotation (IAR) and the spinal column's neutral axis *(dashed line)* during flexion. A force vector (F) is depicted applied at an angle (θ) and distance (d) relative to the IAR. The moment (M) occurring at the IAR is depicted by the curved arrow. The magnitude of the moment is represented by the equation M = Fdsinθ. (Courtesy of Barrow Neurological Institute, Phoenix, AZ.)

rotation is the axis about which a structure bends or rotates. For example, when a door swings open, a line through its hinges would be the axis of rotation. In the spine, it is frequently referred to as the *instantaneous axis of rotation* (IAR) because its location shifts as the spine moves through its normal range of motion in response to forces. Therefore, instantaneous measurement at one time point provides one "snapshot" of the location of the axis of rotation during that particular phase of the movement. In the normal spine, the IAR for a given bending or twisting motion usually remains in or near the disk space because the disk material is more flexible and deforms more easily than the rigid vertebral bodies. The location of the IAR can often be predicted from the curvature of the facet joints and disk.[2]

The *neutral axis* is the longitudinal axis along which no axial stresses or strains occur during bending or twisting. For example, when the lumbar spine bends in flexion, the anterior disk fibers compress axially while the posterior fibers stretch axially. The fibers in between, through which the neutral axis runs, neither compress nor stretch (although they may shear anteroposteriorly if the axis of rotation is below the disk space, as is often the case). The neutral axis intersects at right angles the IARs of each spinal motion segment along the entire spine (see Fig. 298–2). The neutral axis is a term that applies only during bending or twisting of the spine. No neutral axis exists during pure distraction, compression, or shear because the entire spine is under unidirectional loading in these cases.

Forces applied to the spine are often interpreted in terms of the moments they create at locations of interest, such as at the axis of rotation, along the neutral axis, or at the site of fixation. The moment, M, created by a force, F, is described by the formula

$$M = Fd \sin\theta$$

where d is any measured distance between the line of action of the force and the location where the moment is assessed, and θ is the angle between the line along which distance is measured and the force vector. The magnitude of the moment increases as the distance from the line of force to the location where moment is measured (i.e., the moment arm) increases.

Newton's third law states that each force is opposed by an equal and opposite force. When an internal force from the muscles or an external force from gravity, acceleration, or contact is applied to the spinal motion segment, the ligaments, disk, and joint surfaces react as the primary sources of this equal and opposing force. The mechanical properties of these supporting tissues dictate how the force will be dissipated by the system.

When normalized, the loads and displacements that occur within a system are defined as *stress* and *strain*. Stress is defined as the force, F, applied over an initial cross-sectional area, A

$$Stress = F/A$$

Strain is defined as the change in length of a material over the original length of the material, as defined in the formula

$$Strain = (L_n - L_i)/L_i$$

where L_n is the new length and L_i is the initial length. Stress and strain are directly proportional to each other: as stress increases, strain increases. The amount of stress needed to produce a given strain (i.e., the ratio of stress over strain) is Young's modulus, or the stiffness of a material.

Most biologic materials are much less stiff than the materials used in spinal fixation. However, most biologic materials have both viscous and elastic (viscoelastic) properties, whereas implant materials act primarily as elastic elements. The viscous properties present in the spine permit long-term and rate-dependent responses to loads. With the application of stress to a material with viscoelastic properties, elastic strain is apparent immediately, whereas viscous strain becomes apparent over time as the stress in the system declines exponentially. Strains applied to viscoelastic materials at a high rate, such as during a car accident, cause higher stresses in the tissues resisting the strains than do the same strains applied at a lower rate, such as during a lifting accident.

Physiologic *range of motion* is the range through which the spine can move without injury and is dictated by the viscoelastic properties of the spinal motion segment (Fig. 298–3). For small deformations, ligaments and other soft tissues are lax, and consequently, the stiffness of the system is low. The portion of the

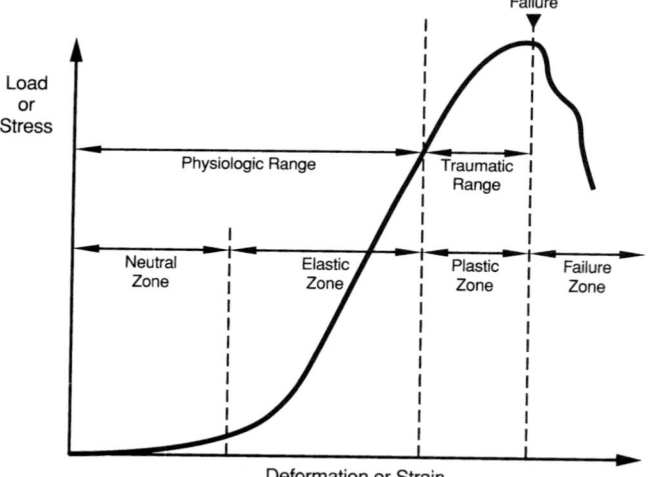

FIGURE 298–3. Graph illustrating range of motion (ROM) and other parameters in a spinal motion segment as they relate to stress and strain. The neutral zone is the range of spinal movement in which large deformations occur in response to small amounts of applied stress. The elastic zone is the range in which exceedingly larger forces are required to produce small incremental changes in the ROM. The physiologic range is the ROM and includes both the neutral and elastic zones. Once the elastic zone is exceeded, the system sustains injury, which can lead to further deformation and eventual failure of the spinal motion segment. (Adapted from White AA, Punjabi MM: Clinical Biomechanics of the Spine, 2nd ed. Philadelphia, Lippincott Williams & Wilkins, 1990, p 21.)

range of motion at which little stress is required to produce large deformations of the spinal motion segment is known as the *neutral zone*. In contrast, in the *elastic zone*, exceedingly larger forces are required to produce small incremental changes in deformation. In the elastic zone, the ligaments and other soft tissues are stretching, whereas in the neutral zone, they have not yet begun to stretch.[3]

When the elastic zone and range of motion are exceeded, the elastic limits of the tissues are surpassed, and permanent (plastic) deformation occurs. In a biologic system, the source of plastic deformation is the tearing of individual tissue fibers. In a nonbiologic system, the source of plastic deformation is the sliding of atoms past one another into a new lattice location, or microfractures of the material's structure. In both systems, larger scale tears and fractures represent failure of the system.

Different materials, biologic and nonbiologic, display different behaviors when they reach the traumatic and failure zones. Some materials fail gradually, and others fail instantaneously. Materials such as methyl methacrylate, ceramic, and some alloys may be strong, but they are brittle and fail completely with small deformations. Other materials are better at tolerating strain. Steel, for example, gradually bends instead of snapping when its elastic limits are exceeded. The behavior of a material in terms of the extent of stresses and strains it must endure is an important consideration when designing or choosing a construct for stabilizing a spinal motion segment.

When a normal spinal motion segment fails, the elastic limit of the ligaments, disk, or bone is exceeded. When a spinal fusion construct fails, the elastic limit of either the fixation hardware or the remaining biologic tissues is exceeded. In either fused or normal motion segments, stability is afforded when the elastic limits of the tissues or mechanical hardware are obeyed. Failure of the system leads to the dissipation of the unopposed force or moment applied to the system. Translation of this load to the neural elements of the spine can result in mechanical compression or injury of the spinal cord.

PHYSIOLOGIC SPINAL LOADING

When the normal spine assumes a physiologic upright position, the center of gravity is far anterior to the spine's IAR and neutral axis. The anterior location of the body's center of gravity imposes a flexion bending moment on the spine, which is counteracted by extensor muscle forces in the dorsal elements of the spine posterior to the IAR. The total compressive load, P, caused by body weight plus muscle contraction to counteract the bending moment imposed by gravity in a spinal motion segment, is estimated as

$$P = w + w(L_g/L_d)$$

where w is the weight of the body above the spinal motion segment, L_g is the distance from the IAR to the center of gravity, and L_d is the distance from the IAR

to the dorsal muscles of the spine. Because L_g is always larger than L_d when standing upright, the actual compression experienced by the spinal motion segment is often two to four times that due to simple gravitational loading. When the orientation of the IAR or center of gravity changes, the load that must be exerted by the posterior muscles changes. When holding an object in one's arms in front of the torso, for example, the center of gravity is displaced anteriorly from the IAR, and the compressive load increases. This point is important, because when the posterior muscle tissues are compromised by surgery or trauma, or when the IAR is shifted by surgery, degeneration, or trauma, spinal biomechanics change significantly.

BASICS OF SPINAL INSTRUMENTATION

Historical anecdotes cite the use of screws, rods, and wires to correct and stabilize spinal deformities as early as the mid to late 1800s. However, the rapid advances that have led to contemporary spinal instrumentation and fixation techniques began in 1962, when Harrington introduced his spinal instrumentation system. To appreciate the intrinsic shortcomings and strengths of different fixation techniques, one must be familiar with the mechanical and metallurgic qualities of the components in any given instrumentation system.

Screws

Screws are used in a variety of applications in the spine. Each application requires different biomechanical considerations. Regardless of the specific application, all screws share common features. Each screw has a head, a shaft, and a threaded portion. The minor diameter of the screw is the width of the shaft beneath the threads; the major diameter is the width of the shaft with the threads.

The mechanical bending strength of a screw is a function of the diameter of the shaft. Changes in the minor diameter significantly increase or decrease the bending strength of a screw.[4] A twofold change in the minor diameter increases the screw's bending strength eightfold because the highest stress, S, applied to a screw during three-point bending is a function of the equation

$$S = F(16L/\pi d^3)$$

where F is the force applied at either end of the screw, L is the length of the screw, and d is its minor diameter (Fig. 298–4). Often, the bending moment or shear force at the proximal aspect of the screw shaft is large because of the orientation of forces at the screw head–plate junction, which can mimic the claw of a hammer prying the head of a nail. Because the transition from the threaded to the nonthreaded portion of the shaft is accompanied by an abrupt increase in the minor diameter of the screw, this area can function as the weak point in the screw and is often the site of screw failure.[5, 6]

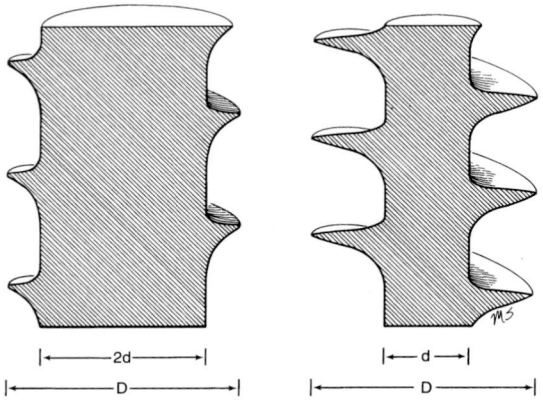

Pullout strength ($^D/_b$)^2 = 1

Bending strength ($^{2d}/_d$)^3 = 8

FIGURE 298–4. The theoretical bending strength of a screw is directly proportional to the third power of the minor screw diameter (d). The pullout strength of a screw is proportional to the square of the major diameter (D) and is affected by the density of the bone beneath the screw threads. Theoretically, a twofold increase in the minor screw diameter with no change in the major diameter increases the bending strength eightfold without affecting the pullout strength. (Courtesy of Barrow Neurological Institute, Phoenix, AZ.)

The pullout strength of a screw depends on numerous variables. Most important are the screw-bone interface and the quality of the bone.[4] Cortical bone provides a more secure purchase than does trabecular bone. Diseased osteopenic bone provides poor structural support. During screw insertion, trauma related to poor drilling techniques or overheating can impair the screw's purchase or lead to the pathologic resorption of bone around the screw.[7] Rescue screws used in cervical plating systems and thoracolumbar pedicle screws have a wider diameter to recover purchase in a stripped or enlarged screw hole. The pullout strength of a screw depends on the depth at which the screw is placed and the screw's major diameter.[8] Note that unlike a screw's bending strength, the pullout strength is affected little by the screw's minor diameter (except when the dimensions of the major and minor diameters are too close to create bite, or when the bone surrounding the hole is not uniform). Hence, a twofold increase in minor diameter that causes an eightfold increase in bending strength should have little or no effect on pullout strength (see Fig. 298–4).

Screws can be categorized as self-tapping, non–self-tapping, cortical, cancellous, lag, cannulated, locking, and nonlocking.[9, 10] Self-tapping and non–self-tapping screws differ by the design of the threads (Fig. 298–5). Self-tapping screws typically have sharp threads, whereas non–self-tapping screws are less sharp.

Cancellous screws are usually self-tapping. They tend to have a small minor diameter and a large major diameter to allow the threads to bite across a larger portion of the porous, weak trabeculae and increase their holding power in trabecular bone. When cancel-lous screws obtain a purchase in the distal bone cortex, their pullout strength increases significantly.

Cortical screws are traditionally non–self-tapping and usually are threaded along the entire shaft. Typically, they are placed using a drill bit the size of the screw's minor diameter and a tap the size of the screw's major diameter. In early instrumentation systems, non–self-tapping screws were used instead of self-tapping screws because there was concern about cracking the bone under the expansive force of screw insertion. Modern manufacturers are shifting more toward self-tapping cortical systems as screw designs improve.

Lag screws place bone fragments under compression. The shaft of a lag screw has both threaded and nonthreaded portions. The threaded portion of the shaft, which is the distal portion, is used to engage a distal bone fragment. As the screw is tightened, the distal fragment is compressed toward the proximal fragment as long as the threaded portion of the shaft does not cross the fracture line. A lag effect in a fully threaded screw can be obtained by drilling the proximal portion of the screw hole to the screw's major diameter so that the screw obtains no purchase proximally. A lag effect can also be obtained by using a screw with a threaded shaft divided into two portions, based on a difference in the pitch and depth of the thread. This difference causes the distal portion of the screw to advance more rapidly than the proximal portion, which consequently compresses the bone fragments.[10]

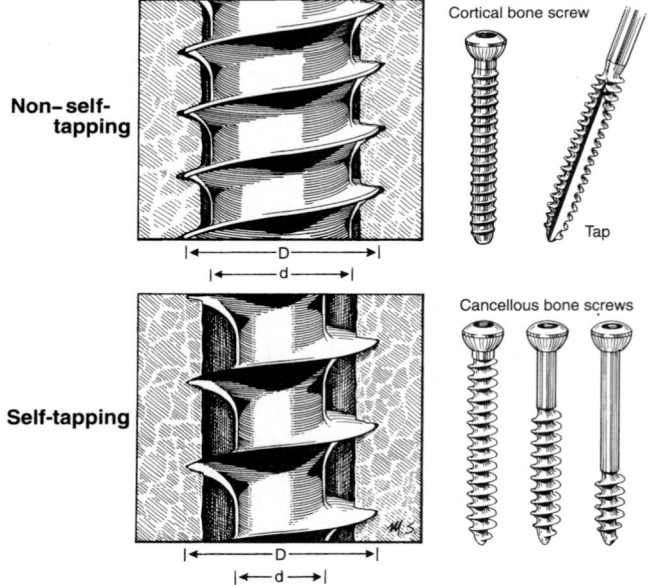

FIGURE 298–5. Non–self-tapping screws have a larger minor diameter and require the use of an appropriately sized tap. Typically, cortical bone screws are non–self-tapping and threaded along the entire shaft. Self-tapping screws have a small minor diameter and large threads that bite deeply into the bone. This feature increases their holding strength in trabecular bone. Cancellous bone screws tend to be self-tapping and may not be threaded along the entire shaft. (Courtesy of Barrow Neurological Institute, Phoenix, AZ.)

Cannulated screws have a hollow shaft that allows the screw to be placed over a thin surgical guide wire. These screws are used when precise placement is needed, as in transarticular screw placement. The hollow aspect of the screw's shaft slightly reduces its bending strength but does not affect its pullout strength.[11] Because the outer region of metal in a screw shaft is more important in resisting bending than the core is, substantial bending strength can still be maintained with cannulation. For example, a 2.5-mm minor diameter screw with a 1.5-mm diameter cannula is theoretically 87% as strong in bending as a solid 2.5-mm diameter screw; a 3-mm minor diameter screw with a 1.5-mm diameter cannula is theoretically 94% as strong in bending as its solid counterpart.

Screws also differ based on their relationship to the overlying plate or rod (Fig. 298–6). When the screw head's interface with the overlying apparatus is rigid, the system is described as constrained. When the screw head's interface is nonrigid, the system is described as nonconstrained. The design of the hardware determines whether a constrained screw can have a variable trajectory during placement. For example, in most cervical plating systems, screws placed with a fixed trajectory are, by definition, constrained screws because of how the screw head–plate interface is designed. In contrast, in most pedicle screw systems, the trajectory of the screw does not affect the screw's ability to rigidly fixate to the overlying rod, so these screws can be described as variable-trajectory screws in a constrained system.

Constrained screws provide more rigid immobilization and are generally more desirable when treating traumatic instability. Nonconstrained screws are desirable when treating degenerative instability because they allow settling at the screw-plate interface while the adjacent fusion mass subsides over time.

Rods and Plates

Typically, rods are used for posterior fixation of the thoracolumbar spine. Plates are used in the cervical spine for anterior or posterior fixation techniques and in the thoracolumbar spine for ventrolateral fixation. Rods and plates are made from stainless steel, titanium alloys, or pure titanium. The most commonly used steel alloy is type 316L stainless steel (17% chromium, 13% nickel, and 2.25% molybdenum). Stainless steel alloys are the standard with regard to strength and workability properties. The ferromagnetic quality of steel alloys interferes with magnetic resonance imaging, and their nickel content can contraindicate their use in patients with cutaneous nickel allergies.

Titanium alloys are also used, the most common of which is Ti-64, a mixture of titanium, aluminum, and vanadium. The tensile strength of titanium alloys is almost equivalent to that of stainless steel alloys, but they tend to be brittle. Titanium is available in different grades, based on its purity (grades 1 to 4). Less pure grades of titanium tend to be less brittle than higher-purity grades, but all grades of unalloyed titanium are more brittle than the commonly used titanium alloys.

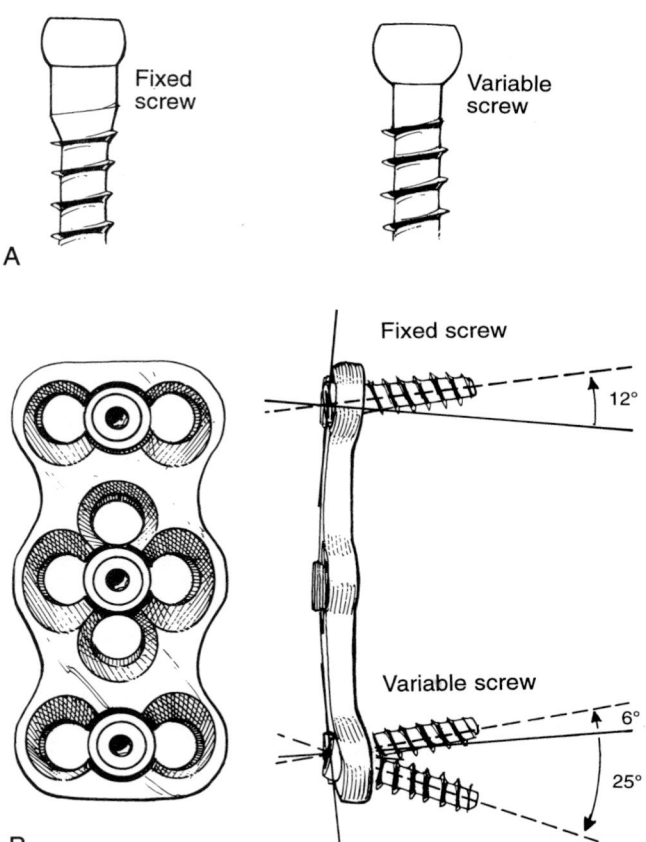

FIGURE 298–6. *A,* Fixed- and variable-trajectory screws differ, based on their interface with the overlying implant. Shown are the screws in the Atlantis cervical plating system (Medtronic Sofamor Danek, Memphis, TN). The fixed screw head is shaped so that it locks at its interface with the overlying plate to prevent toggling. The variable screw is shaped so that it can toggle. *B,* Fixed-trajectory screws function like a fixed moment arm cantilever beam fixation device. This rigid fixation device provides optimal biomechanical stability. It is preferred when fixation is needed to correct instability caused by trauma. In contrast, variable-trajectory screws function like a tension band or nonfixed moment arm cantilever, because the angle of fixation has the ability to change as depicted. This feature may allow the implant to dissipate the stress and strain introduced as a graft subsides over time. (Courtesy of Barrow Neurological Institute, Phoenix, AZ.)

Titanium is also more resistant to corrosion than are steel alloys and permits osteointegration, which should theoretically increase the rate of fusion.[4, 7]

Manipulating rods and plates before their application can affect their integrity. Stress risers result from contouring rods and plates, so excessive contouring should be avoided. Notching, which also occurs from contouring techniques, results when the structural integrity of the rod or plate is compromised. Titanium is especially susceptible to both stress risers and notching-related phenomena. A notch as small as 1% can reduce the fatigue resistance of 316L stainless steel wire by 63%.[12] Notching also increases the corrosion rate of the implant.

All instrumentation should be made of the same

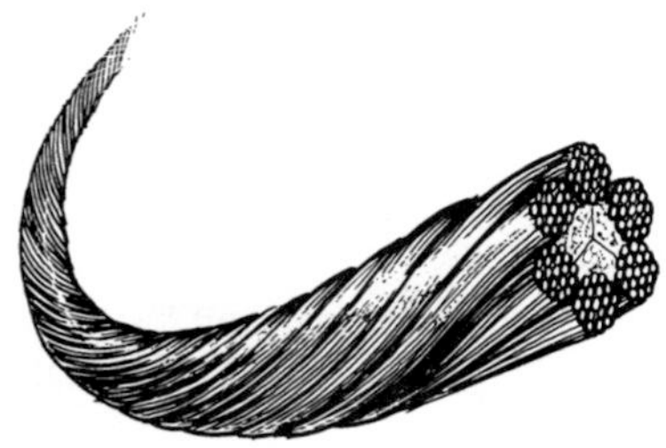

FIGURE 298–7. Cross-sectional view of a braided cable commonly used in tension band fixation techniques. (Courtesy of Barrow Neurological Institute, Phoenix, AZ.)

material. Mixing different alloy components could generate a galvanic current that could facilitate corrosion.

Wires

Wires are used in a variety of posterior fixation techniques. Sublaminar wiring and spinous process wiring are some of the oldest techniques used in posterior spinal fixation. There are single-stranded wires, twisted wires, and braided cables. Braided cables tend to be the strongest and distribute tension most evenly.[13] Braided cable is available in both titanium and stainless steel alloys, with stainless steel cables generally providing better strength and resistance to fatigue (Fig. 298–7).[13] Although cables and wires are commonly used, there is growing evidence that screw systems are more rigid and less susceptible to loosening than are wired alternatives.[14]

BIOMECHANICS OF FIXATION TECHNIQUES

Simple Distraction Techniques

Simple distraction is used to reestablish the height loss associated with chronic degenerative changes (foraminal stenosis, osteodegeneration of the spine, insufficiency fractures) or traumatic changes (compressive fractures of the spine). Distractive forces are usually applied alone only when they can be centered along the neutral axis of the spine. Otherwise, the distractive devices can serve as fulcrums that can lead to bending moments and promote deformity. Distractive forces can be applied ventrally or dorsally.

The dorsal application of distractive forces with dorsal sublaminar hooks was once commonly used to treat foraminal stenosis. Dorsally applied distractive techniques are now used only within a larger construct to facilitate the application of complex reduction forces and techniques (e.g., a universal spine instrumentation system). When distractive forces are applied posteriorly, the disk fibers posterior to the IAR are in tension to resist the distraction. Hardware that appeared rigid at the time of surgery may loosen because of viscous dissipation, causing exaggeration of kyphotic abnormalities, loosening of the hardware, and eventual hard-

ware failure (Fig. 298–8). The hardware also compromises the biomechanical behavior during normal bending. The hooks serve as a new pivot point for the motion segment in extension, shifting the IAR far posterior from its normal position. The fulcrum created by the hardware causes loads to be distributed abnormally during extension: all disk fibers are placed in tension.

Ventral application of distractive forces is used in interbody fusion techniques. Synthetic cages or bone grafts can be placed as interbody struts. These techniques distract the spine near its normal IAR and therefore do not change the normal loading of the spine as much as posterior distraction does. However, depending on the shape and location of the interbody graft, the graft can create unusual pivot points that can lead to damage to the remaining disk and instability.

Three-Point Fixation Techniques

Three-point fixation techniques are used to correct abnormal curvatures. The Harrington rod system is an example of a three-point fixation technique. Such a construct applies dorsally directed forces at the termini and a ventrally directed force at the fulcrum, which should be the site of the abnormal curvature. This construct is fundamentally different from the distraction model discussed earlier because the rod connecting the termini contacts the spine in the midpoint of the construct to permit a ventrally applied force vector (Fig. 298–9).[12] In a three-point fixation construct, the magnitude of the moment generated at the fulcrum of the construct is proportional to the length of the construct.[15] Therefore, there is a mechanical advantage to using longer constructs for reduction.

How the system is assembled affects the mechanical advantage of the construct. Bends in the rods or strategically placed sleeves at the fulcrum that increase the diameter of the rod can increase the mechanical advantage at the fulcrum to facilitate reduction.[16] Bends placed in rod constructs are less efficacious than sleeves placed at the fulcrum, because the former are susceptible to rotational changes, which may occur as the construct fatigues. Lamina, pedicle, or transverse process hooks are designed to resist chiefly either flexion or extension, depending on the direction in which the hook is oriented and whether it is placed on the rostral or caudal margin of the bony process. Placing several hooks in opposing directions on adjacent vertebrae gives the construct the ability to resist both flexion and extension, and unseating of the hooks during normal activity is avoided.

Tension Band Techniques

Tension band techniques are used both ventrally and dorsally. Dorsal applications include posterior wiring techniques, posterior clamps, and rods and screws. When a tension band is in place, the moment that would be required at the IAR to cause the motion segment to bend away from the band depends on the distance between the tension band and the IAR.[12] When

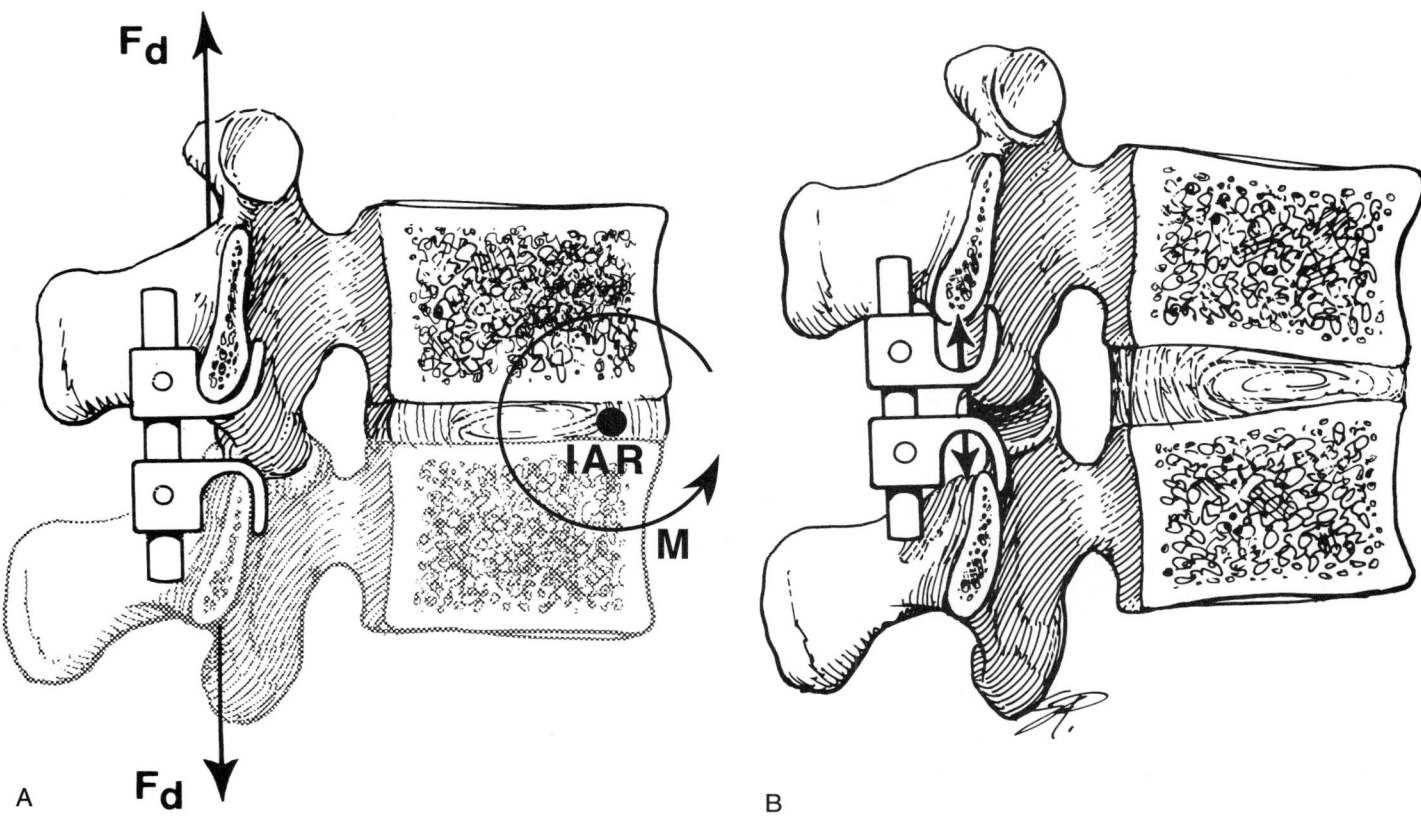

FIGURE 298–8. *A,* Illustration of a spinal motion segment showing a pure distraction model of fixation. Sublaminar hooks are interconnected by a vertical rod that does not contact the spine. The distracting force (F_d) is depicted by the solid arrows, and the moment (M) that would be necessary at the former location of the axis of rotation to resist these forces is depicted by the solid curved arrow. *B,* The system fails when the interanchor distance increases. The hardware then loses its points of contact with the spine, leading to loss of immobilization. IAR, instantaneous axis of rotation. (Courtesy of Barrow Neurological Institute, Phoenix, AZ.)

a tension band is applied posteriorly, it can resist a large bending moment, because the IAR is located ventrally. When a tension band is applied anteriorly, the proximity of the IAR reduces the magnitude of the bending moment that it can resist.

Tension band techniques are applied most successfully over short segments. In a long segment, the mobility of the vertebrae between the termini leads to questionable stability—imagine trying to hold a tall stack of blocks together with two fingers, versus holding just two blocks together. As their name suggests, tension bands work only in tension, not in compression. Most tension band implants are rigid constructs that do not respond to decreases in interanchor distances (Fig. 298–10A). For example, initially a compressive force is associated with posterior interspinous wiring. However, if the disk degenerates, the interanchor distance of the wire fixation decreases, but the wire fixation device does not change in size because it is inelastic. The compressive force disappears, and the slack introduced to the system causes loss of rigidity of the construct, which becomes more susceptible to fatigue failure from repetitive loading and unloading during normal movement (see Fig. 298–10B). Because of this tendency, tension band techniques are usually accompanied by application of an adjacent distraction

technique such as an interbody strut or interspinous process strut, as used in anterior cervical plating and C1-2 interspinous fusions, respectively.

Cantilever Beam Fixation

Cantilever beam fixation has been widely applied to instrumentation of the spine and is used to treat both degenerative and traumatic instability. It is most popular as a short-segment fixation technique and is usually confined to a level above and below the pathology. There are several forms of cantilever beam fixation: fixed moment arm, nonfixed moment arm, and applied moment arm.[4] Typically, the cantilever beam construct consists of screws placed either ventrally or dorsally into a vertebral body and connected longitudinally with a system of rods or plates. The classic model is the pedicle screw system (Fig. 298–11A), which is a fixed moment arm cantilever.

The fixed moment arm cantilever beam fixation system resists both bending and axial loading. The magnitude of the loads that a cantilever device must be capable of resisting depends on the extent of interaction of the biologic and nonbiologic components of the construct. The presence or absence of ventral load sharing can significantly alter the magnitude of the

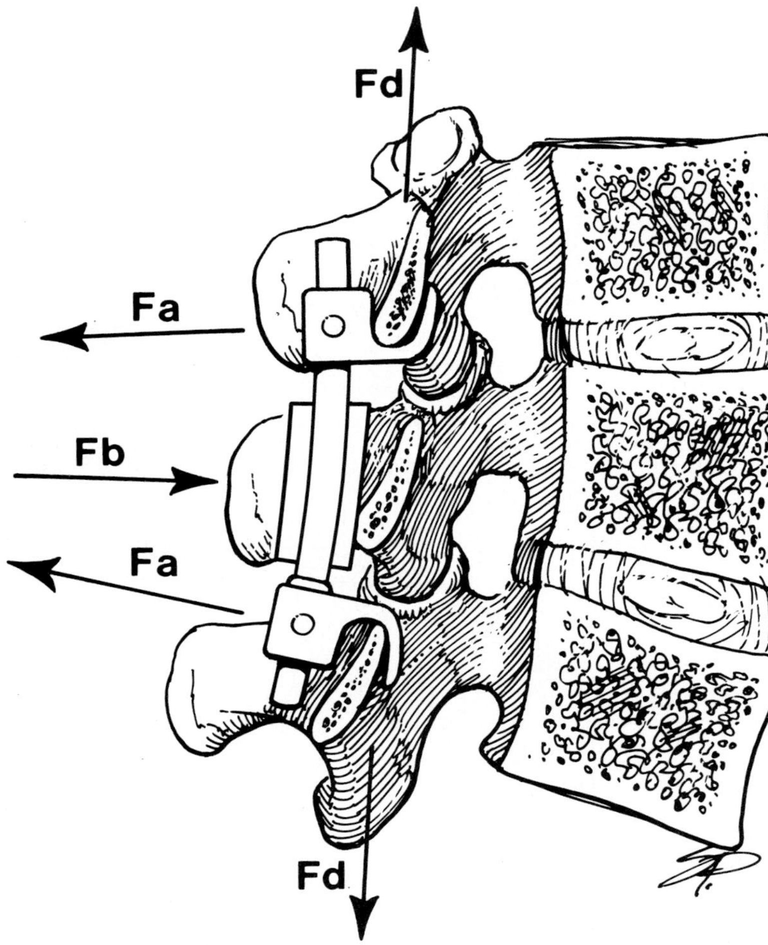

FIGURE 298–9. Illustration of a segment of the spine showing a three-point bending system. The terminal hooks are depicted with their distracting force vectors (F_d). The intervening rod has a sleeve that contacts the lamina, allowing a ventrally directed force vector (F_b) to be applied. At the termini, dorsally directed force vectors (F_a) are produced. (Courtesy of Barrow Neurological Institute, Phoenix, AZ.)

loads at the screw head or proximal shaft. The magnitude of stress that different portions of the hardware experience also depends on the intrinsic features of the system, such as screw design, screw placement, and hardware assembly.

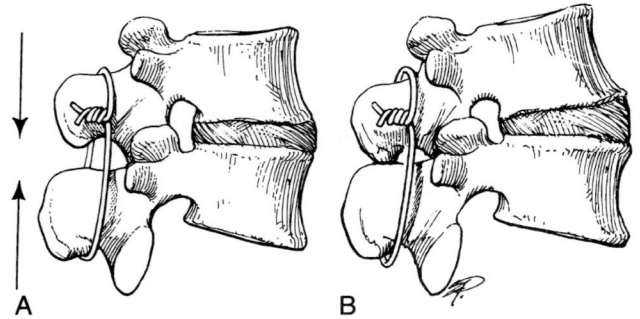

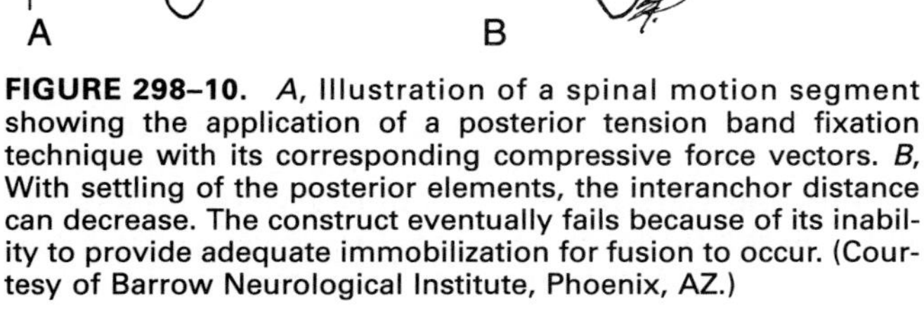

FIGURE 298–10. *A,* Illustration of a spinal motion segment showing the application of a posterior tension band fixation technique with its corresponding compressive force vectors. *B,* With settling of the posterior elements, the interanchor distance can decrease. The construct eventually fails because of its inability to provide adequate immobilization for fusion to occur. (Courtesy of Barrow Neurological Institute, Phoenix, AZ.)

Typically, the screw in a thoracolumbar pedicle screw construct is rigidly fixed to the longitudinally connecting rods. Older pedicle screw systems were nonfixed moment arm cantilever beam systems. These systems allowed screws to toggle, which led to high rates of screw pullout. They are now rarely used in the thoracolumbar spine but are still common in the cervical spine, where less load bearing is required. Some anterior cervical spine plating systems are fixed moment arm cantilever beams. Typically, these cervical plating systems are used to fixate traumatic fractures when a rigid fixation technique is needed to treat pathologic instability. Other cervical plating systems are nonfixed moment arm cantilever beam systems that make allowances for changes caused by subsidence in the spinal motion segment. In these cases, the biomechanical model of the nonconstrained cervical plate can be interpreted as either an anterior tension band technique (during extension) or an anterior nonfixed moment arm cantilever beam technique (during flexion or extension).

Applied moment arm cantilever beam fixation techniques are used when significant moments must be applied to reduce an angulation deformity or to provide active compression or distraction. In this tech-

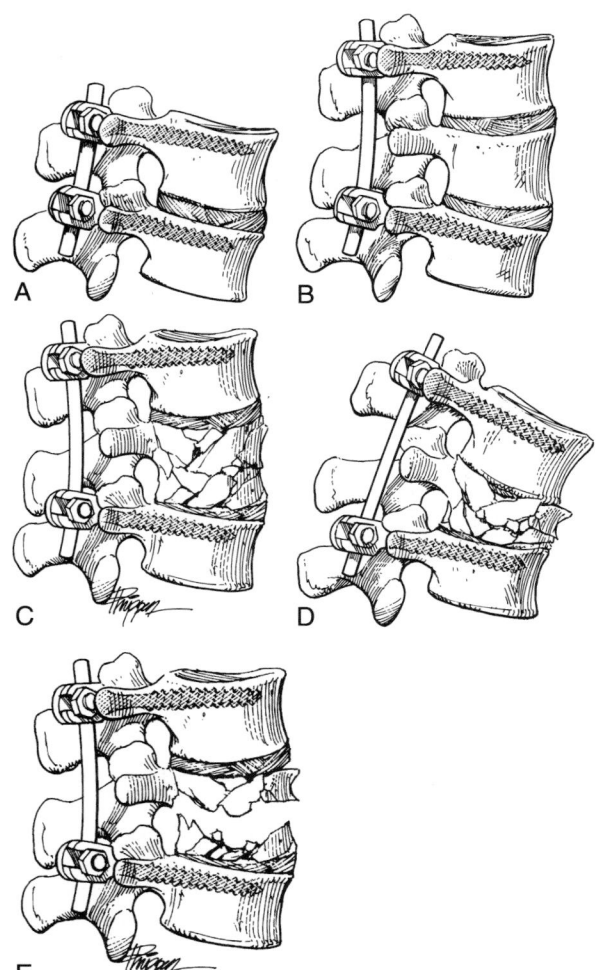

FIGURE 298–11. *A,* Illustration of a segment of the spine showing a fixed moment arm cantilever beam fixation system. The healthy intervening disk space allows ventral load sharing and prevents the hardware from supporting all loads on the motion segment. *B,* A healthy intervening vertebral body can also participate in ventral load sharing. *C,* A fractured body is depicted with no loss of height, demonstrating that it is still able to participate in anterior loading sharing. *D,* A deformed vertebral body is associated with loss of height and an abnormal kyphotic angulation. However, the intervening vertebral body is still able to participate in some load sharing because the system is assembled in situ, with no reduction of the abnormal angulation or height. *E,* A fractured vertebral body with associated loss of height is depicted after correction of a kyphotic angulation, demonstrating how it is unable to participate effectively in load sharing and translates compression and flexion loads to the hardware posteriorly. (Courtesy of Barrow Neurological Institute, Phoenix, AZ.)

nique, the plate or rod is rigidly attached to the screw head while the plate or rod is under a residual "spring-loaded" torque. Because such fixation techniques require the surgeon to apply significant forces before rigid fixation, they have significant failure rates. More levels can be incorporated above and below the deformity to reduce stress on the hardware by load sharing.

The simplest application of the pedicle screw system is its use to treat degenerative disk disease associated with instability (see Fig. 298–11*A*). In this situation, the pedicle screw construct spans one disk space. Pedicle screws are placed in adjacent vertebrae. Load in the pedicle screw system is distributed between the vertebral bodies and posteriorly through the instrumentation. Because the disk space is usually small or collapsed from the degenerative pathology, the vertebral bodies participate in load sharing by acting as a contiguous support column. This feature greatly reduces the stress on the system. When the disk space is large, interbody strut grafts can be used to facilitate fusion as well as to participate in load sharing.

A more complex application of the pedicle screw system is its use to treat traumatic instability. When a destabilizing injury spares the vertebral body, a pedicle screw construct can be assembled to extend from the vertebra above the fracture to the one below it (see Fig. 298–11*B*). When the vertebral body is fractured but no height is lost, the load-bearing capacity is probably reduced. The extent of the reduction, however, depends on the severity and pattern of the fracture. Many investigators have reported good fusion rates and low failure rates with constructs that span a fractured vertebral body when the loss of height or kyphotic angulation is minor.[17–19]

In contrast, when the vertebral body is significantly compromised and associated with a considerable loss of height or abnormal angulation, the biomechanics of the system are altered significantly. The changes in interbody height and angle cause the neutral axis and IAR to be shifted posteriorly away from the injury. Load distribution changes and probably contributes to the abnormal kyphotic angulation that develops. A cantilever beam fixation system can be used to halt the progression of this deformity by fusing the spine without correcting any deformity, or it can be used to correct a height and angulation deformity (see Fig. 298–11*C* and *D*). Pedicle screws are typically placed above and below the level of the pathology. When the deformity is fixated in situ with no attempt to reduce the kyphotic angulation, the intervening vertebral body may still share some load, at least in compression-flexion. When the angulation and loss of height at the affected level are reduced during the application of the pedicle screw construct, however, the intervening vertebral body is unable to share the load effectively (see Fig. 298–11*E*). All compressive, bending, and torsional stresses are borne by the hardware, making the system more prone to failure. To reduce the magnitude of the stress supported by individual linkages of the system, healthy vertebrae above and below can be incorporated into the construct to help share the load.

Based on experimental models, the bending moment at the screw-plate interface in a fixed moment arm cantilever system appears to increase more than five-fold when no intervening vertebral body participates in the load sharing.[15] Ventral constructs can be applied to provide load sharing to reduce the magnitude of the bending moment experienced by the hardware in flexion-compression.[4, 15, 20, 21] Ventral constructs are typically interbody struts. These struts need a sufficient cross-sectional area to resist subsidence into the vertebral body when gravitational loads are applied.[22] This goal is readily achieved with allograft from the femur or humerus. Multiple rib constructs also provide a sufficient cross-sectional area to resist subsidence. The resistance of titanium mesh cages to subsidence is comparable.[22] Some manufacturers provide cages with end caps to reduce the rate of cage subsidence associated with axial loading.

Optimizing Hardware

Surgeons can apply numerous techniques to existing constructs of all types to reduce the failure rate. Using the largest diameter screw possible reduces the stress applied to the screw.[23] Setting screws deeply into the pedicle lowers the profile of the hardware and decreases the moment arm at the screw head, lowering the susceptibility of the proximal shaft to failure from gravitational loads.[7] Placing longer screws deeper into the vertebral body reduces the propensity for screw pullout.[19, 24] When the cancellous bone–screw interface is poor, a bicortical screw purchase may be desirable to increase the pullout strength of the screw. Incorporating additional vertebral levels above and below the construct leads to load sharing and reduces the bending moment experienced at each level. Placing patients in external orthotic devices after surgery reduces the propensity for mechanical bending, which is usually well in excess of any gravitational load applied to the system.

Preventing rods from being placed in a parallel orientation can reduce complications related to rotational or torsional strain (the parallelogram effect).[20, 25, 26] Placing rods in a convergent orientation or using transverse connectors can reduce the propensity for failure due to this problem.

PRACTICAL APPLICATIONS OF THE BIOMECHANICS OF SPINAL FIXATION

White and Panjabi[27] cited four basic indications for spinal stabilization: (1) restoration of stability when stability is compromised by trauma or degenerative changes, (2) maintenance of alignment after alignment correction, (3) prevention of further alignment deformities, and (4) alleviation of pain related to instability or pathologic movement. Fixation techniques are used to provide the spine with temporary rigid or semirigid fixation until osseous fusion can occur. The basis of almost all internal fixation techniques is successful bone fusion. With continued repetitive loading in the absence of osseous fusion, all fixation methods eventually fatigue and fail. In fact, some surgeons advocate—and certain clinical situations require—the eventual removal of nonbiologic hardware after osseous fusion has developed.

The following sections broadly review the specific fixation techniques used in treating different pathologic conditions of the spine. The basic biomechanical principles applied with each technique are elucidated to help readers understand when an application is appropriate.

Cervical Spine

Odontoid fractures are treated with either odontoid screw or C1-2 fusion techniques. Odontoid screw fixation techniques use a lag screw, which stabilizes the fracture temporarily and approximates fragments until osseous fusion develops. When odontoid screw techniques cannot be applied because of a soft tissue injury or an ill-suited fracture pattern, a C1-2 fusion is performed. Traditional C1-2 fusion techniques use a posterior wiring technique (tension band) and an interspinous bone strut (simple distraction). The presence of an interspinous bone strut counteracts the tendency for the posterior wiring technique to fail from narrowing of the interanchor distance. The interspinous bone strut also permits osseous fusion. The Gallie and Sonntag fusion techniques are examples (Fig. 298–12). The additional application of transarticular screws helps form a rigid construct that promotes osseous fusion by counteracting the system's tendency to fail because of its susceptibility to rotational stresses (Fig. 298–13). Either transarticular screws or a halo vest is required to stabilize C1-2 adequately for most types of injuries.[28]

Ventral cervical bone grafts are used to treat both trauma and degenerative conditions. A ventral bone graft functions as a simple distractive force. Although not shown clinically to be a necessary adjunct in most cases, ventral plating functions as a fixed or nonfixed cantilever beam system that provides axial load sharing and immobilization to promote fusion. It also reconstructs the ventral tension band.

Both posterior sublaminar wiring and interspinous wiring function as tension band constructs. Their benefit is greatest in stabilizing flexion forces and weakest with respect to extension. By itself, wire probably does not provide a stable construct, because the interanchor space tends to narrow. The consequent lack of immobilization can lead to nonunion and eventual hardware failure. The use of Luque rods and rectangles with

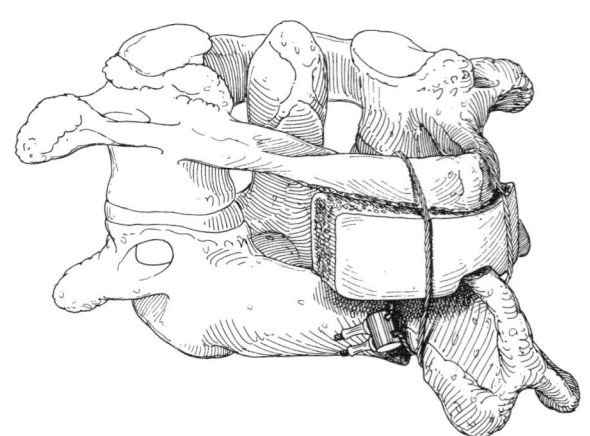

FIGURE 298–12. Interspinous wiring of C1 and C2. Braided cable is used to secure the posterior tension band. An intervening bone graft promotes fusion and prevents hardware failure by fixing the interanchor distance between C1 and C2. (Courtesy of Barrow Neurological Institute, Phoenix, AZ.)

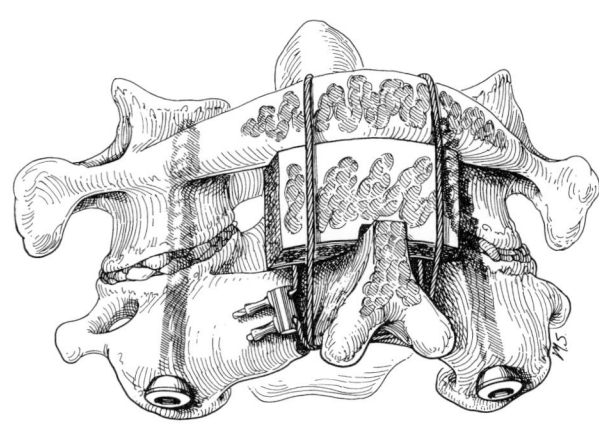

FIGURE 298–13. A C1-2 fusion with transarticular screw fixation. The transarticular screws enhance immobilization, promoting fusion of the bone graft. (From Marcotte P, Dickman CA, Sonntag VKH, et al: Posterior atlantoaxial facet screw fixation. J Neurosurg 79:234–237, 1993.)

wiring techniques provides a three-point bending fixation that can help correct pathologic deformities.

In less active patients, lateral mass plates are sometimes used as motion limiters instead of as load bearers to allow close to normal rotation but prevent hyperrotation. In this hardware application, fusion is not necessarily the desired outcome. In such cases, the lateral mass plates limit flexion by acting as tension bands. Because low loads and infrequent testing of limits are expected in the cervical region in these patients, these implants can survive for many years without failure.

Thoracolumbar Spine

The Harrington rod system is a classic three-point bending system. It is a long segment–short fusion system used to correct angulation deformities of the spine. Most Harrington rod systems incorporate simple distractive forces and tension band forces at the termini of the construct to augment their stability and decrease rates of failure.

Universal spinal systems consist of hooks, screws, and rods. Typically, they are long segment–long fusion systems that incorporate principles of three-point bending, simple distraction, and tension band reconstruction. These systems permit the correction of long-segment spinal deformities and allow early mobilization of patients; they also increase fusion rates.

Pedicle screw systems are short segment–short fusion fixed moment arm cantilever beam systems. Alone, they are used to treat glacial instability from acquired or degenerative spondylolisthesis. When used to treat angulation deformities caused by traumatic or osteodegenerative fractures, they usually require the application of a ventral strut (simple distraction) to reduce gravitational load bearing by the hardware. The ventral strut may be a bone graft or a titanium mesh cage when a corpectomy is performed. When the pathology is confined to the disk space, the ventral strut may be an anterior lumbar interbody fusion device or a posterior lumbar interbody fusion device (e.g., BAK cage, Sulzer Spine-Tech, Inc., Minneapolis, MN).

Ventrolateral thoracolumbar plating techniques include the Z-plate (Medtronic Sofamor Danek, Memphis, TN) and the Kaneda system (DePuy AcroMed, Inc., Raynham, MA). Typically, they are used to treat pathologic fractures of the spine. They apply fixed moment arm or applied moment arm cantilever beam fixation with a ventral strut (simple distraction) to facilitate compressive load sharing, reconstruction of the anterior tension band, and osseous fusion.

Interbody fusion in the lumbar spine incorporating interbody grafts such as the BAK cage is used to treat diskogenic disease. The grafts apply a simple distractive force. When the grafts are applied anteriorly, the surgical approach compromises the anterior tension band (anterior longitudinal ligament). When interbody grafts are applied posteriorly, the surgical approach compromises the facets and the posterior tension band. In the absence of additional hardware such as a fixed moment arm cantilever beam system to reconstruct the missing tension band, interbody cages may be unstable constructs. To date, however, no long-term clinical outcome results have been compiled to support or disprove this notion.

CONCLUSION

The basic principles of spinal internal fixation are founded on fundamental principles of spinal biomechanics. Appropriate treatment of degenerative or traumatic instability begins with an understanding of what constitutes clinical instability. When the unstable component of the spine is identified, spinal fixation can be targeted at reestablishing the continuity of the compromised column to provide temporary stabilization until bony fusion can occur.

When applied anteriorly, laterally, or posteriorly, plate, rod, and wire techniques provide different types of biomechanical stabilization. Hardware failure is an eventual certainty. The failure of hardware before bone fusion occurs often reflects a failure to recognize the summary stresses and strains being applied to a construct. The stresses and strains applied to a system are often a function of the extent that the spine is compromised by degenerative changes or traumatic injury. A sound biomechanical understanding of the limits of each fixation technique and the degree of instability associated with a given condition is required to choose the appropriate technique, hardware, and fusion modality.

Ongoing biomechanical research constantly improves our ability to understand clinical instability and how it can be interpreted based on radiographic and clinical findings. Furthermore, new and improved fixation techniques are constantly being developed. Knowledge of the fundamentals on which these principles are built is the key to understanding not only how currently available techniques work but also the advantages and disadvantages of new fixation techniques as they are introduced.

REFERENCES

1. Denis F: The three column spine and its significance in the classification of acute thoracolumbar spinal injuries. Spine 8:817–831, 1983.
2. Penning L, Wilmink JT: Rotation of the cervical spine: A CT study in normal subjects. Spine 12:732–738, 1987.
3. Panjabi MM: The stabilizing system of the spine. Part II. Neutral zone and instability hypothesis. J Spinal Disord 5:390–396, 1992.
4. Benzel EC: Biomechanics of Spinal Stabilization: Principles and Practice. New York, McGraw-Hill, 1995.
5. Cunningham BW, Sefter JC, Shono Y, et al: Static and cyclical biomechanical analysis of pedicle screw spinal constructs. Spine 18:1677–1688, 1993.
6. Yoganandan N, Larson SJ, Pintar F, et al: Biomechanics of lumbar pedicle screw/plate fixation in trauma. Neurosurgery 27:873–880, 1990.
7. Bennett GL: Materials and materials testing. In Benzel EC (ed): Neurosurgical Topics: Spinal Instrumentation. Park Ridge, Ill, American Association of Neurological Surgeons, 1994, pp 31–46.
8. Skinner R, Maybee J, Transfeldt E, et al: Experimental pullout testing and comparison of variables in transpedicular screw fixation: A biomechanical study. Spine 15:195–201, 1990.
9. Baskin JJ, Vishteh AG, Dickman CA, et al: Techniques of anterior cervical plating. Operative Tech Neurosurg 1:90–92, 1998.
10. Dickman CA, Sonntag VKH: General principles of spinal screw fixation. In Dickman CA, Sonntag VKH, Spetzler RF (eds): Surgery of the Craniovertebral Junction. New York, Thieme Medical, 1998, pp 711–718.
11. Collinge CA, Stern S, Cordes S, et al: Mechanical properties of small fragment screws. Clin Orthop 373:277–284, 2000.
12. Weiser MW, Luevano CA, Goel VK, et al: Spinal implant attributes: Distraction, compression, and three-point bending. In Benzel EC (ed): Spine Surgery. Philadelphia, Churchill Livingstone, 1999, pp 979–990.
13. Dickman CA, Papadopoulos SM, Crawford NR, et al: Comparative mechanical properties of spinal cable and wire fixation systems. Spine 22:596–604, 1997.
14. Hurlbert RJ, Crawford NR, Choi WG, et al: A biomechanical evaluation of occipitocervical instrumentation: Screw compared with wire fixation. J Neurosurg 90:84–90, 1999.
15. Duffield RC, Carson WL, Chen LY, et al: Longitudinal element size effect on load sharing, internal loads, and fatigue life of tri-level spinal implant constructs. Spine 18:1695–1703, 1993.
16. Edwards CC, Levine AM: Early rod-sleeve stabilization of the injured thoracic and lumbar spine. Orthop Clin North Am 17:121–145, 1986.
17. Daniaux H, Seykora P, Genelin A, et al: Application of posterior plating and modifications in thoracolumbar spine injuries: Indication, techniques, and results. Spine 16:S125–S133, 1991.
18. Esses SI, Botsford DJ, Wright T, et al: Operative treatment of spinal fractures with the AO internal fixator. Spine 16:S146–S150, 1991.
19. Lindsey RW, Dick W: The fixateur interne in the reduction and stabilization of thoracolumbar spine fractures in patients with neurological deficit. Spine 16:S140–S145, 1991.
20. Gaines RW Jr, Carson WL, Satterlee CC, et al: Experimental evaluation of seven different spinal fracture internal fixation devices using nonfailure stability testing: The load-sharing and unstable-mechanism concepts. Spine 16:902–909, 1991.
21. Maiman DJ, Pintar F, Yoganandan N, et al: Effects of anterior vertebral grafting on the traumatized lumbar spine after pedicle screw-plate fixation. Spine 18:2423–2430, 1993.
22. Hollowell JP, Vollmer DG, Wilson CR, et al: Biomechanical analysis of thoracolumbar interbody constructs: How important is the endplate? Spine 21:1032–1036, 1996.
23. Misenhimer GR, Peek RD, Wiltse LL, et al: Anatomic analysis of pedicle cortical and cancellous diameter as related to screw size. Spine 14:367–372, 1989.
24. Krag MH, Beynnon BD, Pope MH, et al: Depth of insertion of transpedicular vertebral screws into human vertebrae: Effect upon screw-vertebra interface strength. J Spinal Disord 1:287–294, 1988.
25. Gurr KR, McAfee PC, Shih CM: Biomechanical analysis of anterior and posterior instrumentation systems after corpectomy: A calf-spine model. J Bone Joint Surg Am 70:1182–1191, 1988.
26. Carson WL, Duffield RC, Arendt M, et al: Internal forces and moments in transpedicular spine instrumentation: The effect of pedicle screw angle and transfixation—the 4R-4bar linkage concept. Spine 15:893–901, 1990.
27. White AA 3rd, Panjabi MM: Clinical Biomechanics of the Spine. Philadelphia, Lippincott-Raven, 1990.
28. Crawford NR, Hurlbert RJ, Choi WG, et al: Differential biomechanical effects of injury and wiring at C1-C2. Spine 24:1894–1902, 1999.

Technical Aspects of Bone Graft Harvest and Spinal Fusion

LAWRENCE S. LIU ■ PAUL J. MARCOTTE

More than a quarter of a million spinal fusions are performed in the United States each year.[1] A similar number of other arthrodeses are performed in all the other areas of the body. Of these, the majority require bone as part of the fusion process. Recent developments in technique and technology have not obviated the need for bone graft materials to achieve a successful spinal arthrodesis. A large variety of materials is available for bone grafting, including autograft, cadaveric allograft, demineralized bone matrix, and other novel synthetic biomaterials. Nonautograft sources of bone have been sought to eliminate the complications of bone graft harvest, to extend the volume of graft available, and to increase the efficiency and effectiveness of the fusion process. This chapter discusses the techniques and complications of bone graft harvest and describes the various alternatives to autograft as they apply to spinal fusions.

HISTORY

Bone grafting originated in the 19th century with autograft and allograft implantation by Walther in 1820 and Macewen in 1878.[2] In 1911, Albee[2a] reported the transplantation of bone from the tibia into the spine for tuberculosis, showing that an autologous bone graft could induce a spinal fusion. That same year, Hibbs[2b] published his technique of using autologous laminar bone for dorsal fusion in scoliotic patients. The ensuing half century was marked by attempts at improving spinal stabilization and allowing graft material to fuse in situ. These techniques improved the rate of fusion. Advances in material sciences and biomechanics have produced better metal alloys (Vitallium, titanium, and titanium alloys), bone allograft material, and instrumentation design. Today, bone grafting and the goal of achieving fusion are often wed to the use of appropriate instrumentation.

Advances in the understanding of bone physiology and the identification of cytokine signaling systems have added a new frontier and expanded the potential for improving fusion rates. In 1965, Urist, an orthopedist, discovered the first of a group of compounds now termed bone morphogenetic proteins (BMPs).[3, 4] Their properties led to an influx and activation of osteoprogenitor and mesenchymal cells, which trigger subsequent bone growth and remodeling at an injured or grafted site. Current research is focused on the incorporation of recombinant BMP and other compounds into implants to induce bone growth and fusion. The science of bone morphogenesis is progressing. Clinical applications are now gaining approval for selected indications. Further research and development will likely revolutionize the techniques of bone grafting and spinal fusion.

PRINCIPLES OF FUSION

Knowledge of the basic physiology of bone growth aids in understanding the complexities of bone fusion. Basic bone physiology can be broken down into three components: cellular, humoral, and matrix related. The three cell types found in bone are osteoblasts, osteoclasts, and osteocytes. Osteoblasts are the bone matrix–producing cells, derived from mesenchymal progenitor cells. They lay down the precursor matrix of collagen that later becomes mineralized to form bone. Osteocytes, or mature bone cells, are similar in function and are derived from osteoblasts. They are the most abundant cells in bone and are responsible for recruiting other cells to form and resorb bone. Osteoclasts reside in Howship's lacunae and are involved in resorbing and remodeling the bony matrix. The extracellular matrix is composed of approximately 70% inorganic hydroxyapatite, 5% water, and 25% organic matrix. The organic matrix is composed of collagen, predominantly proteoglycans, and other matrix proteins. Complex cell-matrix and cell-cell interactions create a dynamic pattern of growth and resorption that underlies the process of bone graft incorporation at the host site during fusion. The cellular components function within a bony or collagen matrix, creating a constant turnover of bone. The human body's skeletal mass is replaced, on average, once every 10 years.[5]

To augment the process of bone fusion, a source of bone graft is typically required to bridge appropriately prepared host surfaces to induce fusion.[6] The process of bone healing and fusion includes the phases of osteogenesis, osteoinduction, and osteoconduction. *Osteogenesis* refers to the cellular component of fusion. Within the freshly harvested autograft is a variety of cells, including precursor cells and osteoblasts, which are recruited and stimulated to produce bone.[7] Implant and graft materials without a cellular component do not have osteogenic potential. *Osteoinduction* is the process by which molecular signaling agents stimulate undifferentiated mesenchymal cells to form osteoblasts.[8] The ability to induce bone growth was initially attributed to the discovery of BMPs by Urist, as mentioned earlier. Other compounds with osteoinductive properties have since been discovered, including 15 forms of BMP. An osteoinductive compound has the capacity to produce bone formation after introduction into a heterotopic (nonbony) site. These agents have tremendous potential to assist in promoting fusion and are the subject of extensive research. *Osteoconduction* involves the progress of bone growth across the site of the intended fusion. It occurs on the scaffold provided by the bone graft matrix. This conduction process requires bony proliferation associated with neovascularization. The process of osteoconduction is most efficient when the graft substrate is cancellous autograft. Allograft and cortical bone are less efficient conductors of osteogenesis. Osteoconduction is not limited to bone grafts; metal implants can also exhibit bone growth on their surfaces.

The ideal bone graft material would have properties of osteogenesis, osteoinduction, and osteoconduction. Autograft is the only graft substance that possesses all three qualities. The matrix of the corticocancellous bone graft provides the osteoconductive properties of the bone graft. The bone marrow cells, matrix, and serum in the bone graft provide a source of factors for osteogenesis and osteoinduction. BMPs and cells in the bone graft are present in limited concentrations. Recombinant molecular biologic techniques are now being used to manufacture analogous morphogenetic proteins to augment the osteogenetic and osteoinductive processes.

A number of other bone graft substitutes have been used,[9] including allograft, xenograft, hydroxyapatite crystals,[10] and demineralized bone matrix.[11] Although these autograft substitutes have been successful for specific indications, none of these substances is as efficacious as autograft in all clinical applications.[12]

The achievement of bone healing and fusion is a complex metabolic process.[13] However, once it is induced, either by a fracture or by the environment across which fusion is desired, factors stimulating osteoblast differentiation, activation, and mesenchymal cell recruitment occur. This stimulation of osteogenesis requires a complex array of BMPs and related factors to initiate and sustain the repair process. BMPs stimulate cellular migration, proliferation, and differentiation. As the cells are converted to osteoblasts and induce bone formation, they gradually extend across the defect between the two bones being fused. Neovascularization of the area also occurs and progresses with the migration of the osteoblasts. The osteoconductive properties of the marrow and bone elements provide a scaffolding across which the osteoblasts migrate and the vasculature proliferates. The deposition of hydroxyapatite by the cells produces ossification of the callus. With time, the fusion mass is remodeled to fortify the strength of the fusion. The stress placed across the fusion site orients the remodeling process to optimize the strength of the newly formed bone (Wolff's law).[14, 15]

A number of factors are thought to promote the fusion process. A sufficient volume of bone graft probably augments the process.[6] It provides the framework on which osteoconduction can occur and, in the presence of fresh autograft, provides a source of osteoinductive, osteogenic, and osteoconductive factors. Lengthy strips that bridge directly across the site of fusion, without interruption, may also enable a more efficient migration of osteoblasts and blood vessels through the marrow channels, as opposed to multiple bone fragments, which would require migrating osteogenic tissue to bridge gaps between the graft fragments. Bone graft placed under compression seems to be an optimal configuration for graft incorporation and successful fusion.[14] This phenomenon may also relate to the presence of graft in continuity between the host surfaces being fused. Interbody grafting and packing of the facet joints are situations in which the bone graft can be placed under compression. Intertransverse and posterior onlay grafts are typically not under compression. Fusion is also promoted by immobilization of the vertebrae along the fused segment. External and internal devices have been developed for fixation. Other chapters of this textbook describe the various instrumentation systems in detail.

Factors that inhibit the fusion process include the presence of chronic disease, infection, and osteoporosis. Also, steroids and smoking are thought to impair fusion. Recent research in rabbits to determine the effects of steroids on a posterolateral fusion model indicated that steroids have a negative effect at multiple steps in the fusion process.[16] Clinical and animal studies have revealed a decrease in trabecular bone volume and fusion mass with exposure to nicotine.[17] Physiologic alterations occur with cellular abnormalities, including decreased osteoblast differentiation. Calcitonin resistance is thought to develop in elderly smokers. Impairment of vascularization also occurs due to increased platelet aggregation and vasoconstriction.

GRAFT SUBSTRATES

There are two types of bone sources available for fusion: cancellous bone and cortical bone. Cortical, cancellous, or a combination of corticocancellous bone sources can be obtained as autograft or are available as allograft. Fresh autologous cancellous bone has all three characteristics conducive to fusion: osteoinduction, osteogenesis, and osteoconduction. Cancellous allograft has osteoconductive and limited osteoinductive properties. Cancellous bone does not have good weight-bearing capacity and usually fails under compression. It can be used as an onlay graft over the posterior elements, packed into the facet joints, or used in conjunction with cortical bone. If it is placed in the interspace, a load-sharing device must be inserted. Carbon fiber or titanium cages or a cortical graft can be used in the interspace to provide weight-bearing resistance. The cancellous graft acts as a nidus for bone formation. Cortical bone shares all the same characteristics as cancellous bone, although its osteoinductive and osteogenetic characteristics are less effective. The main advantage of a cortical bone graft is its ability to resist compression. Hence, it is useful as an interbody graft. Combining a cortical graft with a source of cancellous bone (see Fig. 299–5C) augments the osteogenetic and osteoinductive properties of the cortical graft material.

Allograft bone is devoid of cellular activity and retains a relatively small fraction of its osteoinductive potential. It acts mainly as an osteoconductive material and a load-bearing device when cortical bone is a component of the graft. The method by which the allograft is processed and stored determines its immunogenicity and consistency. Two common techniques for processing and storing allograft are fresh-freezing and freeze-drying.[18, 19]

Allograft bone graft harvesting usually takes place under aseptic conditions. Depending on the technique of preservation, immunogenic soft tissue, blood, and marrow contents and cellular debris can be removed during processing.[20] A freeze-dried allograft contains no more than 6% moisture. It can be stored at room temperature in this manner for approximately 5 years.[21, 22] The freeze-drying technique decreases the immunogenicity of the bone and alters its strength and quality.[6, 22] Bone tends to be more brittle when freeze-dried. Gamma radiation also adversely affects bone quality. The use of ethylene oxide decreases the biologic activity of bone.[19, 21, 23, 24]

Demineralized bone matrix is derived from allograft bone by exposing the bone to acid, which extracts the minerals. The precise technique used to demineralize and treat the bone can affect the osteoinductive potential of the bone graft. Exposure to heat, ethylene oxide, and gamma radiation and multiple freezing and thawing cycles adversely affect the osteoinductive qualities of demineralized bone matrix.[14] Exposure to antibiotics apparently does not alter the osteoinductive capacity. Demineralized bone matrix is supplied in different forms, including gel, putty, and flexible sheets. Currently, it is used as a graft extender or is combined with allograft rings as an osteoinductive agent.

Originally collected from amputated limbs, most allograft material currently used for spinal surgery is derived from cadaveric sources. Collection and storage of allograft material were first undertaken in the 1950s during the Korean War. The navy created a tissue bank, where it saved bone in anticipation of mass casualties. The use of cadaveric sources has grown significantly in the United States, with up to 150,000 allografts implanted per year.[25, 26]

Disease transmission is an ongoing concern when using allograft. Human immunodeficiency virus (HIV), prion diseases, and hepatitis are the greatest concerns. The Centers for Disease Control and Prevention documented two cases of HIV transmission through bone allograft. One patient was the recipient of a femoral head in 1984; mass screening for HIV became available in 1985. The donor had a history of lymphadenopathy and drug abuse. In 1991, a 22-year-old organ and tissue donor transmitted HIV to four organ recipients and three bone graft recipients. He had had two negative HIV tests in 1985.[27–29]

Donor screening, by history and antibody testing, is an effective means of avoiding HIV transmission. By questionnaire screening alone, 90% of inappropriate donors can be identified and eliminated. The use of polymerase chain reaction and amino assays reduces the likelihood of disease transmission by five- to six-log-fold.

Processing allograft with alcohol, bleach, and other sterilizing agents significantly diminishes its infectivity.[30] Recent advances in viral deactivation by Osteotec (Shrewsbury, NJ) have shown a decrease in viral loads of 6- to 12-log-fold for cytomegalovirus, hepatitis B and C, HIV, and polio.[31]

Coralline hydroxyapatite (CH) has been used as a graft substitute for a number of indications.[32, 33] The material is sea coral treated by a hydrothermal process whereby the calcium carbonate is converted to hydroxyapatite. However, it does contain some nonapatitic calcium phosphate. In a study by Boden and colleagues, the use of CH in posterolateral fusions was examined.[32] Forty-eight rabbits were placed into three study groups using hydroxyapatite with bone marrow, CH with autogenous iliac crest bone graft, and CH with 500 μg of bovine-derived osteoinductive bone protein extract. The fusion rates were 0%, 50%, and 100%, respectively. Based on this result, CH was not considered an adequate substitute or extender for posterolateral fusion bone. CH was also used at one time as an interbody graft for cervical fusions. It was somewhat brittle, however, and its use has been abandoned.

Xenograft implants were used in the 1980s as a cervical interbody graft substitute.[9] Graft collapse and a lack of incorporation were frequent complications. A significant immune response causing graft sequestration occurred, which prevented osteoconduction.[14] Xenograft is no longer used as an autograft substitute.

HARVESTING TECHNIQUES AND COMPLICATIONS

Spinal fusion is a process by which bone is induced to bridge across a motion segment and join the adjacent vertebrae. The placement of bone graft is required to stimulate the process. Bone can be placed under compression across the interspace or placed over the posterior elements as an onlay graft.[34] Depending on the location of the graft, the segment of spine involved, and the nature of the instrumentation used in conjunction with the graft, cancellous or corticocancellous graft can be used.[35, 36] The major source of autogenous bone graft for spinal fusion is the iliac crest. Graft can be harvested both anteriorly and posteriorly. The fibula and the rib are also potential sources of autograft.

Fibular autograft has been used in the past as a strut graft to reconstruct the spine after a vertebrectomy. More recently, microvascular anastomosis has been used to provide a vascularized fibular strut graft.[37, 38] This technique has not gained widespread acceptance because the success rate of cervical fusion is quite high using nonvascularized fibular autograft or allograft with appropriate stabilization.

Rib grafts can also be harvested for vertebral reconstruction.[39–41] Again, the success rate with other sources of allograft and autograft struts has made it unnecessary to harvest rib grafts through a separate incision. However, the rib can be a convenient source of bone graft for limited thoracic reconstruction, because the graft can be harvested during the thoracotomy.

The iliac crest is an abundant source of both cancellous and corticocancellous bone. Weight-bearing and non–weight-bearing graft can be harvested from the iliac crest for spinal fusion. The anterior and posterior aspects of the crest are potential sources of bone harvest. The site of the harvest is determined by the type of graft required (cancellous versus corticocancellous), the volume of bone needed, the nature of the surgery, and the approach undertaken to treat the spinal pathol-ogy. The harvest of bone graft from the iliac crest is associated with risk,[14, 42–44] including localized pain and injury to surrounding neurovascular or soft tissues. Although technique and experience may reduce the frequency of complications, anatomic variability of the bony pelvis and surrounding structures and other patient factors will prevent the total elimination of graft harvest complications.[43]

Anterior Iliac Crest Harvest

The anterior iliac crest region is a frequent site for bone graft harvest. Bi- and tricortical segments of bone can be harvested from the ridge of the crest. The iliac crest acts as an insertion point for various muscles of the lower extremity and abdominal wall. Along the lateral aspect of the crest, the quadriceps and gluteal muscles insert on the iliac crest. The iliacus muscle inserts along the medial aspect of the iliac crest. The most anterior point of the iliac crest is the insertion site of the inguinal ligament and sartorious muscle at the anterior superior iliac spine. The abdominal muscles also insert along the superior aspect of the crest. Both the abdominal wall and the gluteal muscle fascia cover these muscles. Sensory nerves are present in the subcutaneous fat in the region of the anterior iliac spine. In particular, the lateral femoral cutaneous nerve is in proximity to the anterior spine (Fig. 299–1). Typically, it is medial to

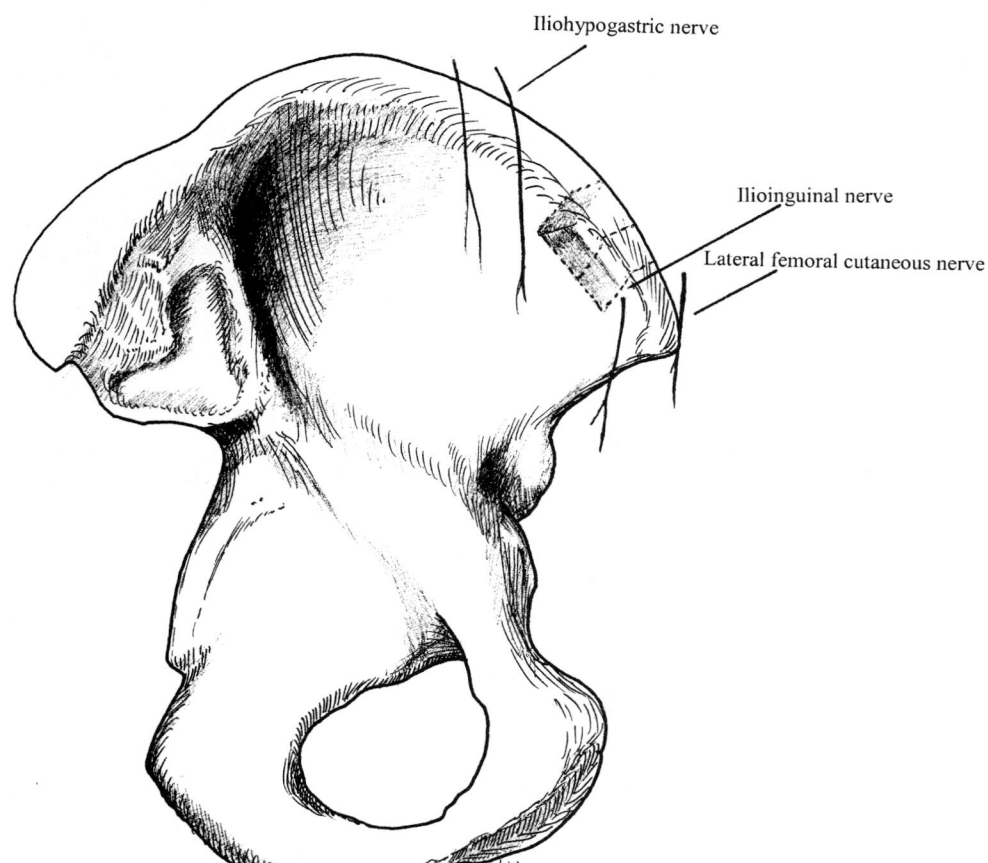

Iliohypogastric nerve

Ilioinguinal nerve

Lateral femoral cutaneous nerve

FIGURE 299–1. Anterior iliac crest harvest. The iliohypogastric nerve lies along the iliac crest, and the lateral femoral cutaneous nerve runs medial to the anterior superior iliac spine. Graft harvest can be initiated safely 1 inch posterior to the anterior superior iliac spine.

the anterior superior iliac spine and exits from the pelvis below the inguinal ligament. It provides sensation to the anterolateral aspect of the thigh. This nerve can have an anomalous course, exiting the pelvis posterior to the anterior superior iliac spine, over the crest of the iliac bone.[43] In this position, it is more vulnerable to injury during the harvest of a tricortical piece of bone. Branches of the iliohypogastric nerve extend over the lateral aspect of the iliac crest (see Fig. 299–1) to provide sensation to this region.[42, 43]

To harvest a segment of the anterior iliac crest bone, the ridge of the crest must be exposed. The skin incision should be started approximately 1 inch posterior to the anterior superior iliac spine region to reduce the likelihood of damaging the lateral femoral cutaneous nerve,[42, 43] which exits in this region, and also to maintain some anterior iliac crest bone at the level of the anterior spine to reduce the likelihood of fracture. The incision is typically made over the ridge of the iliac crest. However, some surgeons advocate making an incision inferior to the ridge to avoid an incision over a bony prominence,[42] which might reduce the likelihood of postoperative pain. Regardless of the site of the incision, the subcutaneous dissection should be carried down to the ridge of the iliac crest. Fascia and muscle cover the ridge of the crest. Often a plane between the insertion of the abdominal fascia and muscles and the lower extremity fascia and muscles can be identified. At this junction, the fascia is directly applied to the bone without intervening muscle. If this junction can be identified, dissection of the fascia and muscle can commence at this point, limiting the amount of muscle trauma required to expose the crest. Coagulating current and elevators can be used to dissect the fascia and muscle off the iliac crest. If cancellous graft is required, exposure can be limited to the ridge or the lateral aspect of the crest. If a tricortical segment of bone is harvested, the muscles along the medial and lateral aspects of the crest must be mobilized to obtain the graft. Once the iliac crest bone is exposed, drills, osteotomes, or curets can be used to harvest the bone graft (see Fig. 299–1).

After the bone graft harvest, hemostasis of the raw bony surface can be achieved by bone wax or Gelfoam packing. Gelfoam is preferred, because the use of bone wax prevents reuse of the donor site in the future. The fascia and muscle should be reapproximated over the site of the bony defect.[43]

COMPLICATIONS

A variety of complications can result from the harvest of bone graft.[14, 21, 42–49] Besides the general complications of surgery, including infection and wound breakdown, complications can result from the manipulation of bone and surrounding structures during the harvest, resulting in symptoms. The most common complications of bone graft harvest are pain and sensory nerve dysfunction. Although these complications are often transient, permanent sequelae can occur; however, they are rarely severe or functionally limiting.[42–44]

There are many potential sources of donor site pain

following graft harvest, yet the origin of some pain syndromes is uncertain. Some patients, despite an uncomplicated harvest of a small amount of graft, have tenderness over the graft site. The origin of this pain is uncertain, and the characteristics of the pain are nonspecific, except for localized tenderness to contact or manipulation of the area. The sources of pain may be the overlying soft tissue, neural structures, or bone. In the absence of a clear cause, it is difficult to determine how to avoid or treat such pain syndromes. Empirically, prominent bony edges should be avoided at the harvest site by resecting such prominences when present. Some advocate filling the iliac crest defect with allograft or demineralized bone matrix before the soft tissue closure. A firm reapproximation of the fascia and muscle over the bony defect may reduce the likelihood of tenderness at the surgical site.

The history, physical examination, and ancillary tests can help determine the cause of pain syndromes. Injury to a superficial nerve in the region of the bone graft harvest can result in pain. The nature of this pain is quite characteristic of sensory nerve injury; it can be dysesthetic and associated with numbness. The distribution of the pain is typically not confined to the incision site but is limited to an area surrounding the harvest site, extending inferiorly. Branches of the iliohypogastric nerve may be the injured nerve element. Expectant treatment should be considered.

A more severe pain syndrome can result if the iliac crest fractures (Fig. 299–2).[50, 51] Such a fracture is usually located at the anterior aspect of the iliac wing and incorporates the anterior superior iliac spine. A fracture is more likely to result if the graft is harvested very close to the anterior superior iliac spine or extends deep into the iliac crest, thereby isolating the anterior superior iliac spine from the rest of the iliac bone. Aggressive use of the osteotome, or use of a dull osteotome, can transmit the force from the hammer to an area remote from the harvest site, weakening the surrounding structures and predisposing to a fracture.[52] Osteoporosis may be a risk factor for fracture. A frac-

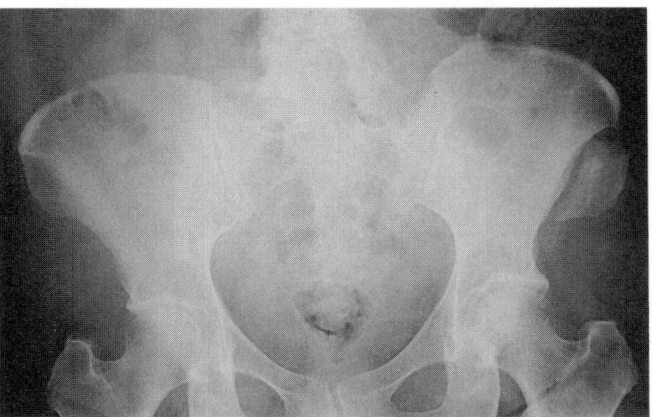

FIGURE 299–2. Avulsion fracture of the left anterior superior iliac spine. The fracture fragment has migrated inferiorly. The patient was treated expectantly, and the localized pain resolved without neurological deficits.

ture of the iliac crest is typically diagnosed with plain pelvic radiographs (see Fig. 299–2). A computed tomographic scan may more clearly define the extent and displacement of the fracture.

Although a fracture can happen at the time of surgery, fractures may also occur in a delayed manner, weeks after the harvest. In our experience, increasing the load on the ipsilateral leg, such as stepping off a curb or stairs, can cause a fracture. Often, patients complain of acute, severe localized pain. A lateral femoral cutaneous nerve injury can occur in association with a fracture, depending on the location of the nerve and the size and displacement of the fracture. The subacute fracture results from an avulsion of the bone by the attached quadriceps and sartorius muscles. Expectant treatment should be considered, because the fragment usually stabilizes spontaneously, and the associated pain gradually dissipates. Exploration of the area risks injury to the lateral femoral cutaneous nerve during the attempt to mobilize and reduce the fragment. Stabilizing the fragment can be problematic.

A wound hematoma can cause localized graft site pain (Fig. 299–3). This pain typically occurs in the immediate postoperative period, although a subacute onset following surgery is also possible. The presence of significant swelling with or without bloody leakage from the wound is highly suggestive of a hematoma. Bleeding or swelling may be seen only if there is an associated dehiscence of the fascial closure. Wound hematomas below the deep fascia occur on the medial or lateral aspects of the iliac wing. A hematoma deep to the iliac crest is probably more common, because bleeding may be more difficult to see along this aspect

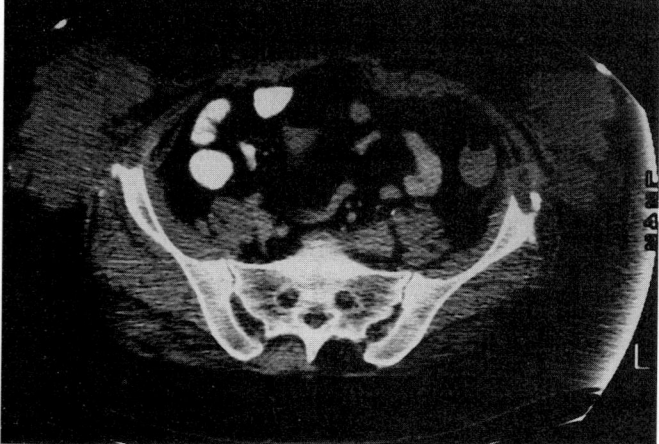

FIGURE 299–3. Computed tomographic scan of the pelvis. The patient is obese and has had bilateral cancellous bone graft harvest for interbody fusions with titanium cages. The anterior aspects are comminuted due to the graft harvest. She has bilateral superficial hematomas (right greater than left) above the muscle fascia. She had evacuation of the right hematoma, which was producing localized pain and swelling. The study was performed with oral contrast medium, which outlines the small intestine. No defect in the abdominal wall is seen, and there is no herniation of abdominal contents. Also, the proximity of the sacroiliac (SI) joints to the posterior superior iliac spine (PSIS) is demonstrated. The SI joint is medial and deep to the PSIS.

of the iliac crest at the time of surgery. The blood vessels can retract into the muscle, and the bleeding can be occult and track away from the site of surgery. The patient feels localized pain and pressure in the area. In the days or weeks after the bleeding, the patient may experience some radiating pain and swelling in the inguinal region or, in a male, to the ipsilateral testicle. The radiating pain results from anteromedial tracking of the hematoma or dependent migration of the blood as it metabolizes. It is uncommon to have internal organ dysfunction or neurological sequelae accompanying the pain from a hematoma. Computed tomography or magnetic resonance imaging of the pelvis can demonstrate the presence and extent of the hematoma (see Fig. 299–3). Most hematomas resolve spontaneously. A patient with a larger hematoma or more extreme symptoms may benefit from operative evacuation of the hematoma. This expedites resolution of the hematoma and the associated symptoms.[53]

Other potential causes of localized graft site pain include infection or an incisional hernia. A superficial wound infection, involving the skin or subcutaneous fat, is readily diagnosed and treated with oral antibiotics. A more problematic situation is a deep infection extending to the bone surface. An obvious concern is osteomyelitis, and eradicating the infection and achieving secondary healing of an abscess cavity at the harvest site can be difficult when it extends below the fascia to the bone. A more aggressive approach to treating these infections should be considered. Exploration of the area for débridement, adequate drainage, and an attempt to close the muscle layers and deep fascia over the bony defect are preferable. In more recalcitrant cases, a muscle flap inserted by plastic surgery may be required to achieve wound closure.

Although exceedingly rare, an incisional hernia can result if the iliacus or abdominal muscles are traumatized or not closed during the graft harvest.[43] Herniation through the abdominal wall and the presence of bowel at the graft site can produce pain. Uncommonly, a hernia can extend from the iliac crest incision inferiorly through the femoral canal to the upper leg. A computed tomographic scan of the pelvis may assist in identifying the abdominal wall defect and the presence of bowel at the site (see Fig. 299–3). Caution should be taken when re-exploring the graft site for pain, because a hernia may be present. A general surgeon should be consulted for primary closure or mesh repair of an incisional hernia.

Sensory nerve injury can result from damage to a localized distal sensory nerve branch or to the lateral femoral cutaneous nerve.[54] The presence of a nerve injury is typically manifested by a patch of numbness that extends beyond the immediate incision site.[42, 43] Dysesthetic pain, as mentioned earlier, can be a manifestation of a sensory nerve injury. For a sensory nerve branch injury in the region of the incision, no specific treatment is required. The symptoms should resolve spontaneously, or at least the patch of numbness should significantly diminish in size. Typically, the patient becomes accustomed to such numbness and is not disabled by the abnormal sensation.

A lateral femoral cutaneous nerve injury causes a large patch of sensory deficit involving the anterolateral thigh. This may be accompanied by dysesthetic pain. The nerve injury can result from direct trauma or transection of the nerve, a wound hematoma, or fracturing of the anterior superior iliac spine. In the absence of an aberrant course, the lateral femoral cutaneous nerve can be directly traumatized during surgery if the dissection extends through the iliacus muscle medially or medial to the anterior superior iliac spine. If the patient has retained tactile sensation over the distribution of the nerve, the injury is likely in continuity. The principles of peripheral nerve repair should be used when deciding how to treat such injuries. Many lateral femoral cutaneous neuropathies are reversible, so expectant treatment is prudent initially.

Despite the broad spectrum of potential complications associated with anterior iliac crest bone graft harvest, the likelihood of a significant complication is small.[42, 44, 48, 55] The incidence of significant complications requiring further surgery or resulting in a permanent symptom or deficit appears to be low (2.8%).[44] Other authors have found a similar complication rate.[42]

INDICATIONS

The anterior iliac crest is the usual source of tricortical structural bone graft for cervical or upper thoracic surgery. Its use in the mid and lower thoracic spine is limited owing to the small cross-sectional area of the iliac crest relative to the surface area of the vertebral bodies in these segments. Tricortical graft can be used for an interbody graft following diskectomy or for vertebral reconstruction after vertebrectomy. Depending on the size and configuration of the patient's iliac crest, grafts from a few millimeters up to 50 or 55 mm long can be harvested for cervical reconstruction. With sufficient exposure, an unlimited segment of the iliac crest can be harvested. However, as the crest courses posterior across the upper rim of the pelvis, the curvature of the edge limits the useful length of crest available for vertebral reconstruction.

The absolute cross-sectional diameter of graft available for harvest depends on the size of the patient's crest. Typically, the width of the crest varies along its course. The iliac crest ridge is relatively narrow in the anterior superior iliac spine region. At a point 2 to 3 inches posterior to the anterior superior iliac spine, which is typically over the most lateral aspect of the iliac crest, the crest is frequently much wider than along the more anterior segment.

Cancellous bone can also be harvested from the marrow space of the iliac wing. Only the ridge of the iliac crest has to be exposed; there is no need to dissect muscle off the medial or lateral aspects of the crest. Once the cortical surface of the ridge is removed, a curet can be used to enter the marrow space and resect cancellous bone. The harvest can be extended anterior, posterior, and deep to the entry point to obtain larger volumes of graft. A cancellous harvest should be taken over the widest part of the iliac crest, typically at its lateral margin. In this location, the volume of the cancellous space is greatest. Also, dissection in this area avoids the anterior superior iliac spine region, thereby reducing the likelihood of fracture.

Posterior Iliac Crest Harvest

The posterior iliac crest region is a source of abundant cancellous or corticocancellous bone. The bone is usually harvested deep in the region of the posterior superior iliac spine. If a tricortical piece of bone is required during a posterior approach, one can open or extend an incision laterally along the posterior aspect of the ridge of the iliac crest.

The landmark for harvesting bone posteriorly from the iliac crest is the posterior superior iliac spine (Fig. 299–4). Unless the patient is quite obese, this site is usually palpable as a prominence approximately 2 to 3 inches off the midline, adjacent to the L5-S1 spinous process interspace. In a lean person, it can be identified visually as dimpling of the skin in this region. Access to this area is gained either by a direct incision overlying the posterior superior iliac spine or by dissection lateral from the midline lumbar spine incision in a plane between the fascia and the subcutaneous fat. Once the deep fascia overlying the posterior superior iliac spine is reached, dissection is carried through the soft tissue with elevators or the coagulating current to expose the bone in this area. Depending on the volume and configuration of the cancellous graft required, the ridge of the posterior spine alone can be exposed to gain access to the marrow space for cancellous fragments, or the gluteus muscles can be dissected off the lateral aspect of the crest to gain access for cancellous and corticocancellous strips. If one stays within the confines of the marrow cavity, bone dissection can be extended in all four directions to obtain bone graft. As the dissection is carried laterally and deep along the iliac wing, the marrow space narrows. Deep and medial dissection extends toward the sacroiliac joint (see Figs. 299–3 and 299–4).

COMPLICATIONS

The complications associated with bone graft harvest from the posterior superior iliac spine region are similar to those associated with anterior crest harvest. Injury to the surrounding soft tissue or the iliac bone itself can result in a pain syndrome or neurovascular complications. Graft site pain without an associated injury can result from iliac crest harvest. The specific cause of this pain is unknown. Avoidance of bony prominences and adequate soft tissue coverage of the site during closure may reduce the likelihood of such a pain syndrome.[42, 56, 57]

The superior cluneal nerves provide sensation over the lateral aspect of the buttock. These nerves perforate the fascia superior to the iliac crest and course inferiorly and laterally over the buttock.[58] Injury to these sensory nerves can result during the harvest of bone graft from the posterior iliac crest and the posterior superior iliac spine region. Injury is more likely from harvest along the posterior iliac crest, because these

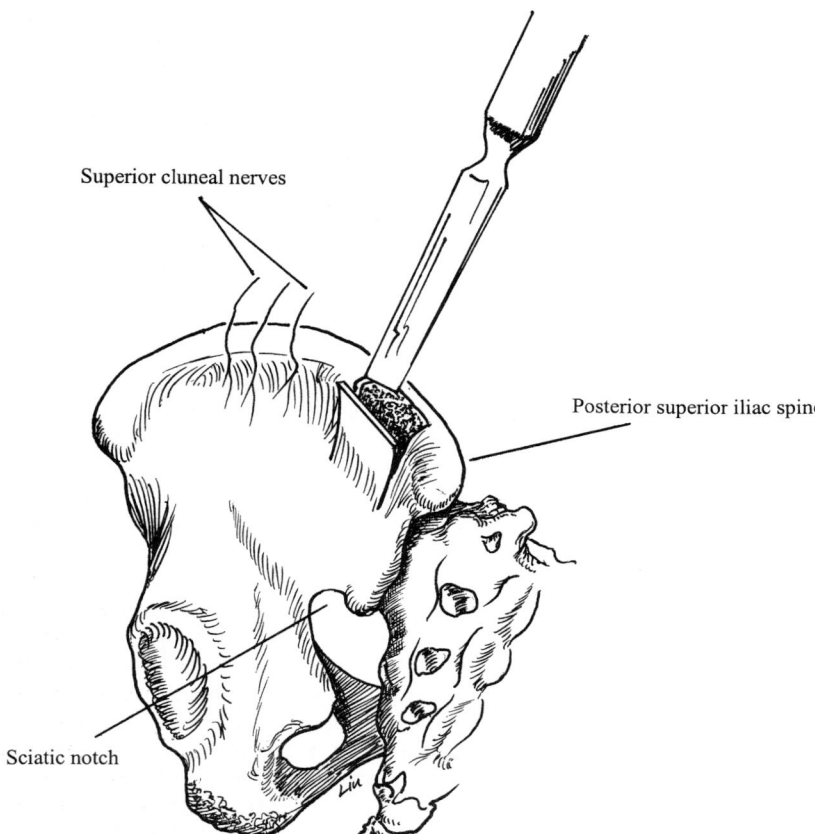

Superior cluneal nerves

Posterior superior iliac spine

Sciatic notch

FIGURE 299–4. Posterior iliac crest harvest. Bone graft is removed from the posterior superior iliac crest region. The skin incision and soft tissue incision should be within 8 cm of the midline to avoid injuring the superior cluneal nerves. The depth of the dissection should be limited to prevent encroachment on the sciatic notch and its neurovascular structures.

nerves do not originate in the midline and they extend laterally in their superficial course. To minimize the likelihood of a cluneal nerve injury during a posterior iliac crest harvest, the skin incision should be kept within 7 to 8 cm of the midline.[42, 43, 58] Incisions more laterally placed are more likely to injure a cluneal nerve over the posterior iliac crest.[42, 43, 58] The undermining technique to approach the posterior superior iliac spine and crest is also intended to reduce the risk of injuring the cluneal nerves.[42] Anomalies in the course of the cluneal nerve can predispose to injury. The medial cluneal nerves perforate the deep fascia paramedian in the low sacral region.[42, 43] They have not been characterized as a source of neuropathy or pain associated with posterior iliac crest harvest.

As one extends deep along the iliac bone at the level of the posterior superior iliac spine, eventually the sciatic notch is encountered (see Fig. 299–4). The sciatic nerve and vascular branches feeding the gluteal muscles exit the pelvis through this sciatic notch.[43, 53] Major neurological or vascular morbidity can result if the dissection, retraction, or bone resection is carried deep into this region. Published guidelines regarding a safe depth for this dissection have not been established. In our experience, for the average adult, dissection down 3 inches should avoid the foramen and the neurovascular structures. To optimize the safety of the graft harvest, the muscle dissection and bone removal should be performed under direct visualization.

As mentioned earlier, the sacroiliac joint is in proximity to the posterior superior iliac spine marrow space (see Figs. 299–3 and 299–4). One should avoid violating the medial cortex of the iliac bone in this region. Theoretically, trauma to the sacroiliac joint can lead to a pain syndrome,[43] although confirmation of this following a graft harvest is difficult.

As for anterior crest harvest (described earlier), infection at the graft site is a potential risk of posterior crest harvest. The previously mentioned considerations regarding superficial versus deep infection are applicable to this segment of the iliac crest as well.

CLINICAL APPLICATIONS

Allograft versus Autograft

Many factors are involved in the decision to use autograft versus allograft for a spinal fusion. The nature of the underlying pathology, the fusion procedure contemplated, the segment of the spine involved, and patient factors all influence the choice of a graft substrate. To determine which type of graft to use in the procedure, the surgeon must weigh the risks and benefits of each one and the prevailing clinical circumstances.[59, 60]

As outlined earlier, from a fusion perspective, autograft is considered the optimal graft substrate. It is immune compatible, and disease transmission is not a consideration. However, there are attendant morbidities during graft harvest,[22] including pain syndromes, neurovascular damage, blood loss, and infection. Also, the volume of bone graft available is limited,[22] especially in children, the elderly, osteoporotic patients, and those who have had previous graft harvests. The immunology and osteogenic properties of allograft are less favorable compared with autograft. However, the use of allograft eliminates harvest complications,[43] and an unlimited supply of cortical and cancellous bone, of all varieties and sizes, is available.

In general, autograft is recommended when there is a paucity of healthy cancellous surfaces, the blood supply is poor, and tensile strain predominates. Allograft is preferable when a large volume of graft is required or as part of a mixture with autograft as a graft extender. Allograft is useful when a lengthy weight-bearing graft is required, such as in multilevel cervical vertebrectomies, and in the low thoracic and lumbar regions.[61]

Fusion Procedures

CERVICAL

As discussed earlier, bone graft is required as a substrate for spinal fusion. The graft can be applied to the anterior or posterior aspects of the spine. In general, anteriorly placed bone graft is under compression, because it usually replaces the vertebral body or disk, which are the main load-bearing components of the spinal complex (Fig. 299–5). Unless instrumentation or an interbody device can provide the weight-bearing function of a fused segment, a component of cortical bone is required to maintain the vertical height of the grafted segment. Anteriorly placed cancellous bone functions to stimulate the fusion process. Posterior fusions typically incorporate cancellous bone alone as an onlay substrate. The choice between allograft and autograft depends on the segment of the spine involved and the indication for fusion.[62]

Anterior interbody fusions and vertebral reconstructions following corpectomy require a weight-bearing graft for spinal reconstruction. Optimally, a source of cancellous bone should also be incorporated into the fusion,[63] although cortical graft alone has been used successfully for anterior cervical fusions. Regardless of the substrate, high fusion rates have been documented in the literature with either autograft or allograft.[44, 55, 64] Cervical reconstruction failure appears to correlate most closely with reconstruction extending over multiple levels. The failure likely results from biomechanical instability and graft displacement.[6] Supplementation of the graft by instrumentation has a positive effect by reducing the likelihood of graft displacement and permitting load sharing with the graft to reduce subsidence.[65]

To optimize the chance of incorporation of the graft after a diskectomy or vertebrectomy, the end plates at the ends of the host site should be adequately prepared.[6, 14] The end plates should be denuded of disk material and cartilage. Exposure of the bone graft to the cancellous portion of the vertebral bodies would optimize graft incorporation; however, complete resection of the cortical end plate and placement of the bone graft on the decorticated cancellous bone surface significantly increase the likelihood of the bone graft subsiding into the vertebral body. Subsidence can result in loss of the cervical lordotic curve and predispose to nonunion by increasing the translational instability of the motion segment, because the tension on the bridging ligaments is lost.

The use of anterior plating to supplement a reconstruction or interbody fusion has become common.[6] Debate exists regarding the need to plate, particularly for short-segment reconstructions. The function of plating is to load-share with the graft and increase the

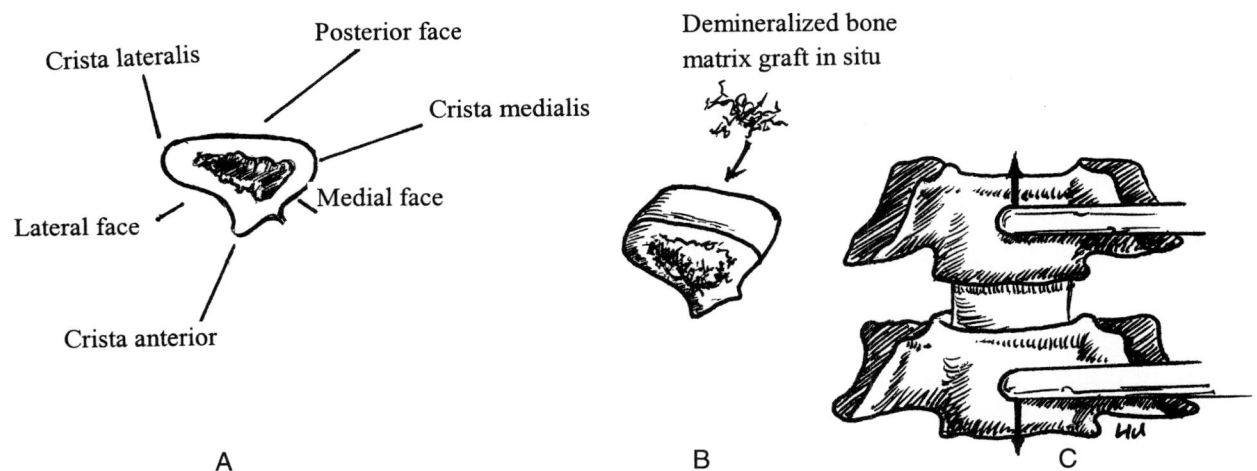

FIGURE 299–5. Cross-sectional anatomy of the fibula *(A)*. To augment the osteoinductive properties of a fibular allograft, the fibula marrow cavity can be packed with cancellous graft or demineralized bone matrix *(B)*. An anterior cervical interbody graft is placed between the two cervical vertebrae *(C)*. Typically, the interspace is distracted open with a retractor or interbody distraction pins to enable the graft to be interposed in the space under compression.

translational stability of the involved spinal segment. The biomechanics of plating and its advantages and disadvantages have been studied over the past 2 decades, during which the frequency of cervical plating has significantly increased. Further discussion of cervical plating can be found in other chapters of this textbook.

Synthetic interbody cages, both cylindrical and ring shaped, have been developed to substitute for interbody autografts and allografts.[66, 67] Initial studies suggest that fusion rates comparable to those of existing interbody substrate techniques can be achieved without the use of harvested bone graft.[66] It is still early in their use, and the true benefits of these devices remain uncertain.

Posterior cervical fusion typically incorporates cancellous bone that is laid on the posterior elements or in the facet joint spaces of the cervical vertebrae. Cancellous grafts from a remote site or allograft chips can be used for this purpose. However, the small amount of graft required for cervical fusion enables local harvest from the spinous processes of the cervical spine.

Cortical strips can also be incorporated as part of a posterior cervical fusion.[39, 68–70] The cortical strips are typically used as a vertical member that is secured to adjacent vertebrae by wiring as a form of segmental fixation. The cortical strips can be fixed to the lateral masses or to the spinous processes, the latter as part of the Bowman triple-wire fusion technique.[68]

THORACOLUMBAR

Thoracolumbar fusion can be performed by anterior and posterior techniques. The major components of the spine and the available bone graft substrates are similar for cervical and thoracolumbar fusions; however, there are many differences between these two segments of the spine that affect fusion rates and graft sources.[71]

The vertebrae at the cervicothoracic junction and uppermost aspect of the thoracic spine are similar in size to the lower cervical vertebrae. Hence, the use of iliac crest graft as an interbody fusion substrate or for vertebral reconstructions in short segments is feasible. The biomechanics of this segment of the spine, however, are different from those in the midcervical spine. Thus, fixation techniques used in conjunction with grafting must be carefully thought out to optimize the success of the fusion and reconstruction.[72]

In the mid and lower thoracic and lumbar spinal segments, the cross-sectional diameter of the vertebral bodies and the compressive force exerted on these segments make it difficult to use iliac crest autograft as a source of corticocancellous bone for reconstruction or interbody fusion. The allograft ring, or a synthetic load-sharing device (titanium, carbon fiber, or acrylic), can be used as a weight-bearing component of the spinal reconstruction.[73–75] Except for palliative reconstructions for cancer, the synthetic devices are supplemented with a source of bone to promote fusion across the motion segment.[69] The bone graft is placed in or around the

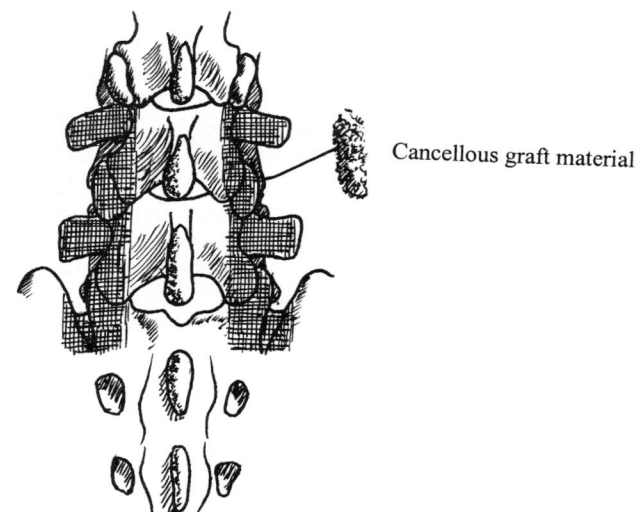

Cancellous graft material

FIGURE 299–6. Lumbar posterolateral fusion. The transverse processes and facets are prepared for fusion by denuding them of soft tissue and then decorticating the bone surfaces. Strips of cancellous graft are placed between the transverse processes, and bone can be packed into the facet joints.

synthetic device in the vertebral body space, or it is placed posteriorly.

Posterior lumbar fusion, like its cervical counterpart, includes onlay graft placement (Fig. 299–6). The distances required to bridge the mid and upper thoracic vertebrae are limited, and fixation techniques are quite effective for this component of the spine. Therefore, both allograft and autograft are potential sources of bone graft for posterior fusion of this spinal segment. Achieving a successful fusion at the thoracolumbar junction and in the lumbar spine is more difficult than in the cervical or thoracic spine, for a variety of reasons. These segments of the spine incur the most stress, the distance between adjacent posterior elements is great, and fixation of the lumbar spine is more difficult than in the upper segments of the spine. With few exceptions,[28] cancellous allograft is not recommended as a source of bone graft for posterior lumbar fusion.[14, 21, 22]

FUTURE DIRECTIONS

Although a great deal has been elucidated about the physiology of spinal fusion and bone grafting, there is still a significant failure rate for fusion, and bone graft harvest morbidity still exists. Current and future research has been directed to help optimize the success rate of spinal fusion and reduce or eliminate bone graft harvest morbidity or the need for bone grafting altogether. By defining the molecular and cellular processes involved in bone healing and growth,[76] more effective means of improving fusion rates may be found. Much emphasis is now being placed on identifying and synthetically producing the factors that induce and sustain bone growth. A number of factors involved in the process of osteogenesis have been iden-

TABLE 299-1 ■ Factors Related to Bone Growth

SUBSTANCE	PROPERTIES
TGF-β	Growth and differentiation factor released by platelets and osteoprogenitor cells; synergizes with BMPs
BMPs	TGF-β–related glycoproteins that induce extracellular and skeletal organogenesis and bone growth
OP-1	BMP-7; has shown osteoinductive characteristics in animal and human studies
FGF	Angiogenic growth factor that stimulates the vascularization of grafts
GDF-5	Member of the TGF-β family involved in normal skeletal development
LMP-1	Increases the synthesis of BMPs; involved in osteoblast differentiation and both endochondral and membranous ossification

BMP, bone morphogenetic protein; FGF, fibroblast growth factor; GDF-5, growth and differentiation factor-5; LMP-1, LIM mineralization protein-1; OP-1, osteogenic protein-1; TGF-β, transforming growth factor-β.

tified (Table 299–1). Their interaction and regulation are incompletely understood.

Transforming Growth Factor-β

Transforming growth factor-β is a member of a larger family of transforming growth factors. These components are related to mesenchymal cell division and differentiation. The bone morphogenetic proteins are a subset of the transforming growth factor-β superfamily.

Bone Morphogenetic Proteins

Bone morphogenetic proteins (BMPs) are a family of glycoproteins that share sequence homology and protein structure similarities with the transforming growth factor-β superfamily. The initial protein was discovered from bone extracts and was first described by Urist in 1965.[3, 4] Over the past several decades, 15 unique members of the BMP family have been identified. Their myriad functions stimulate and guide the differentiation of mesenchymal cells into osteoblasts, generating a cascade of cytokines leading to bone growth via endochondral or membranous ossification. The pattern of the BMP-cytokine profile over time shows a highly regulated process that promotes cellular migration and differentiation leading to bone growth, remodeling, and fusion. Their varied interactions and their ability to form heterodimeric and active compounds reveal a complex interplay in an autocrine and paracrine fashion.[8, 77]

BMPs were incorporated into ceramic sponges to assess the potential for improving fusion rates in implants. Previous models demonstrated a significant enhancement of fusion.[11, 67, 78–85]

LIM Mineralization Protein-1

LIM mineralization protein-1 (LMP-1) is named after the originally described homeodomain proteins of

Caenorhabditis elegans: lin-11, isl-1, and mec-3.[84, 86, 87] This protein was revealed during differential gene expression analysis for glucocorticoid-induced BMP-6–modulated osteoblast differentiation.[88, 89] LMP-1 modulated downstream and BMP-cytokine expression and subsequent osteoblast differentiation and bone formation. LMP-1 is expressed intracellularly as an osteoinductive agent and assists in modulating BMP-cytokine expression, which provokes osteoblast differentiation and bone formation.[90]

Other Substances

A host of other factors are involved in bone regeneration, bone homeostasis, revascularization, and growth. Insulin-like growth factor-1, platelet-derived growth factor, osteoinductive factor-1, and fibroblast growth factors have all been implicated.[91]

These morphogenetic factors act in concert to produce bone by inducing localized cells to become osteoblasts, without the need for a bone graft substrate. The hope is to isolate the various factors and produce them using bioengineering and genetic techniques. Early forms of recombinant BMP have been developed[78, 92] and have received approval for clinical use by the Food and Drug Administration for specific indications. A BMP-impregnated sponge (recombinant human BMP-2) has been approved as a bone graft substitute for use in titanium interbody cages for lumbar fusion.

SUMMARY

Much has been learned about the basic science and technical aspects of bone graft harvest and fusion in the decades since the pioneers in spinal surgery developed their early techniques. Autograft remains the optimal form of graft substrate because it is osteoinductive, osteogenic, and osteoconductive. However, the advantages of autograft must be weighed against the potential morbidity of the graft harvest. Pain, injury to surrounding neurovascular and soft tissue structures, fracture, hematoma, and poor cosmesis are all potential complications of graft harvest from the iliac crest. Although a clear understanding of the anatomy of the iliac crest and surrounding structures and meticulous operating technique can minimize these complications, they cannot be eliminated. Severe, permanent complications are rare, however.

Allograft has comparable osteoconductive properties to autograft but is less effective as an osteoinductive agent and has no osteogenic capacity because there are no viable mesenchyma or osteoblasts in these processed specimens. An unlimited supply of cancellous and corticocancellous graft material is available. Coralline and xenografts have clearly defined limitations as autograft substitutes.

Discovery of the morphogenetic protein subclasses and bioengineering technology should optimize the efficiency of the fusion process. The future of bone fusion will likely involve the addition of bioengineered

BMP to autograft or allograft or its use as a single agent without the need for bone graft.

REFERENCES

1. Health Care Research—Spinal Implants Market. Bank America Research Division, San Francisco, Nov 24, 1997.
2. Chase SW, Herndon CH: The fate of autogenous and homogenous bone graft: A historical review. J Bone Joint Surg Am 37: 809, 1955.
2a. Albee FH: Transplantation of a portion of the tibia into the spine for Pott's disease. JAMA 57:885–886, 1911.
2b. Hibbs RA: An operation for progressive spinal deformities. NY State J Med 93:1013, 1911.
3. Peltier LF: The classic: Bone: Formation by autoinduction. Clin Orthop 395:4–10, 2002.
4. Urist MR: Bone: Formation by autoinduction. Science 150:890–899, 1965.
5. Frost HM: Tetracycline-based histologic analysis of bone remodeling. Calcif Tissue Res 3:211–237, 1969.
6. Nasca RJ, Whelchel JD: Use of cryopreserved bone in spinal surgery. Spine 12:222–227, 1987.
7. Ludwig SC, Boden SD: Osteoinductive bone graft substitutes for spinal surgery: A basic science summary. Orthop Clin North Am 30:635–645, 1999.
8. Yoon ST, Boden SD: Osteoinductive molecules in orthopedics: Basic science and preclinical studies. Clin Orthop 395:33–43, 2002.
9. Greenwald S, Boden SD, Goldberg VM, et al: Bone graft substitutes: Facts, fictions and applications. J Bone Joint Surg Am 83(Suppl 2):98–103, 2001.
10. Pintar FA, Maiman DJ, Hollowell JP, et al: Fusion rate and biomechanical stiffness of hydroxylapatite versus autogenous bone grafts for anterior discectomy—an in vivo study. Spine 19:2524–2528, 1994.
11. Iwata H, Sakano S, Itoh T, Bauer TW: Demineralized bone matrix and native bone morphogenetic protein in orthopedic surgery. Clin Orthop 395:99–109, 2002.
12. LeGeros RZ: Properties of osteoconductive biomaterials: Calcium phosphates. Clin Orthop 395:81–98, 2002.
13. Stevenson S: Biology of bone grafts. Orthop Clin North Am 30: 543–552, 1999.
14. Prolo DJ, Rodrigo JJ: Contemporary bone graft physiology and surgery. Clin Orthop 200:322–342, 1985.
15. Wolff J: Die Lehre von den functionellen Knochengestalt. Virchows Arch 155:256, 1899.
16. Sawin PD, Dickman CA, Crawford NR, et al: The effects of dexamethasone on bone fusion in an experimental model of posterolateral lumbar spinal arthrodesis. J Neurosurg (Spine 1) 94:76–81, 2001.
17. Riebel GD, Boden SD, Whitesides TE, Hutton WC: The effect of nicotine on incorporation of cancellous bone graft in an animal model. Spine 20:2198–2002, 1995.
18. Boyce T, Edwards J, Scarborough N: Allograft bone: The influence of processing on safety and performance. Orthop Clin North Am 30:571–598, 1999.
19. Butterman GR, Glazer PA, Bradford DS: The use of bone allografts in the spine. Clin Orthop 324:75–85, 1996.
20. Sedlin ED, Hirsch C: Factors affecting the determination of the physical properties of femoral cortical bone. Acta Orthop Scand 37:29–48, 1966.
21. Herron LD, Newman MH: The failure of ethylene oxide gas-sterilized freeze-dried bone graft for thoracic and lumbar spinal fusion. Spine 14:496–500, 1989.
22. Malinin TI, Brown MD: Bone allografts in spinal surgery. Clin Orthop 154:68–73, 1981.
23. Currey JD, Foreman J, Laketic I, et al: Effects of ionizing radiation on the mechanical properties of human bone. J Orthop Res 15: 111–117, 1997.
24. Thoren K, Aspenberg P: Ethylene oxide sterilization impairs allograft incorporation in a conduction chamber. Clin Orthop 318:259–264, 1995.
25. Kagan RJ (ed): Standards for Tissue Banking. McLean, VA, American Association of Tissue Banks, 1998.
26. Tomford WW, Mankin HJ: Bone banking: Update on methods and materials. Orthop Clin North Am 30:565–570, 1999.
27. Centers for Disease Control: Transmission of HIV through bone transplantation: Case report and public health recommendations. MMWR Morb Mortal Wkly Rep 39:597–599, 1988.
28. Knapp DR, Jones ET: Use of cortical cancellous allograft for posterior spinal fusion. Clinical Orthop 229:99–106, 1988.
29. Simmonds RJ, Holmberg SD, Hurwitz RL: Transmission of human immunodeficiency virus type 1 from a seronegative organ and tissue donor. N Engl J Med 326:726–732, 1992.
30. Tomford WW: Transmission of disease through transplantation of musculoskeletal allografts: Current concepts review. J Bone Joint Surg Am 77:1742–1754, 1995.
31. Scarborough NL, White EM, Hughes JV, et al: Allograft Safety: Viral Inactivation with Bone Demineralization. Shrewsbury, NJ, Osteotech, 2002.
32. Boden SD, Martin GJ, Morone MA, et al: The use of coralline hydroxyapatite with bone marrow, autogenous bone graft, or osteoinductive bone protein extract for posterolateral lumbar spine fusion. Spine 24:320–327, 1999.
33. Bucholz RW: Nonallograft osteoconductive bone graft substitutes. Clin Orthop 395:44–52, 2002.
34. Davy DT: Biomechanical issues in bone transplantation. Orthop Clin North Am 30:553–563, 1999.
35. Hitchon PW, Traynelis VC, Rengechary S: Techniques in Spinal Fusion and Stabilization. New York, Thieme, 1995.
36. Sandhu HS, Grewal HS, Parvataneni H: Bone grafting for spinal fusion. Orthop Clin North Am 30:685–699, 1999.
37. Bradford DS: Anterior vascular pedicle bone grafting for the treatment of kyphosis. Spine 5:318–323, 1980.
38. Taylor GI: Microvascular free bone transfer, a clinical technique. Orthop Clin North Am 8:425, 1977.
39. Cohen MW, Drummond DS, Flynn JM, et al: A technique of occipitocervical arthrodesis in children using autologous rib grafts. Spine 26:825–829, 2001.
40. Govender S, Suresh Kumar KP, Med PCM: Long term follow-up assessment of vascularized rib pedicle graft for tuberculosis kyphosis. J Pediatr Orthop 21:281–284, 2001.
41. Nakamura H, Yamano Y, Seki M, et al: Use of folded vascularized rib graft in anterior fusion after treatment of thoracic and upper lumbar lesions. J Neurosurg (Spine 2) 94:323–327, 2001.
42. Banwart JC, Asher MA, Hassanein RS: Iliac crest bone graft harvest donor site morbidity. Spine 20:1055–1060, 1994.
43. Kurz LT, Garfin SR, Booth RF: Harvesting autogenous iliac bone grafts: A review of complications and techniques. Spine 14:1324–1331, 1989.
44. Schnee CL, Freese A, Weil RJ, Marcotte PJ: Analysis of harvest morbidity and radiographic outcome using autograft for anterior cervical fusion. Spine 22:2222–2227, 1997.
45. Arrington ED, Smith WJ, Chambers HG, et al: Complications of iliac bone graft harvesting. Clin Orthop 329:300–309, 1996.
46. Brown CA, Eismont FJ: Complications in spinal fusion. Orthop Clin North Am 29:679–699, 1998.
47. Fujita T, Kostuik JP, Huckell CB, et al: Complications of spinal fusion in adult patients more than 60 years of age. Orthop Clin North Am 29:669–678, 1998.
48. Goulet JA, Senunas LE, DeSilva GL, Greenfield ML: Autogenous iliac crest bone graft—complications and functional assessment. Clin Orthop 339:76–81, 1997.
49. Robertson PA, Wray AC: Natural history of posterior iliac crest bone graft donation for spinal surgery—a prospective analysis of morbidity. Spine 26:1473–1476, 2001.
50. Hu RW, Bohlman HH: Fracture at the iliac bone graft harvest site after fusion of the spine. Clin Orthop 309:208–213, 1994.
51. Porchet F, Jaques B: Unusual complications at iliac crest bone graft donor site: Experience with two cases. Neurosurgery 39: 856–859, 1996.
52. Jones AAM, Dougherty PJ, Sharkey NA, Benson DR: Iliac crest bone graft—osteotome versus saw. Spine 18:2048–2052, 1993.
53. Shin AY, Moran ME, Wenger DR: Superior gluteal artery injury secondary to posterior iliac crest bone graft harvesting—a surgical technique to control hemorrhage. Spine 21:1371–1374, 1996.
54. Ghent WR: Further studies on meralgia paresthetica. Can Med Assoc J 85:871–875, 1961.
55. Riley LH, Robinson RA, Johnson KA, Walker AE: The results of anterior interbody fusion of the cervical spine. J Neurosurg 30: 127–133, 1969.

56. Behairy YM, Al-Sebai W: A modified technique for harvesting full-thickness iliac crest bone graft. Spine 26:695–697, 2001.

57. Hutchinson MR, Dall BE: Midline fascial splitting approach to the iliac crest for bone graft—a new approach. Spine 19:62–66, 1994.

58. Lu J, Ebraheim NA, Huntoon M, et al: Anatomic considerations of superior cluneal nerve at posterior iliac crest region. Clin Orthop 347:224–228, 1998.

59. Malloy KM, Hilibrand AS: Autograft versus allograft in degenerative cervical disease. Clin Orthop 394:27–38, 2002.

60. Young WF, Rosenwasser RH: An early comparative analysis of the use of fibular allograft versus autologous iliac crest graft for interbody fusion after anterior cervical discectomy. Spine 18:1123–1124, 1993.

61. Singh K, DeWald CJ, Hammerberg KW, Dewald RL: Long structural allografts in the treatment of anterior spinal column defects. Clin Orthop 394:121–129, 2002.

62. Grossman W, Peppelman WC, Baum JA, Kraus DR: The use of freeze-dried fibular allograft in anterior cervical fusion. Spine 62:565–569, 1991.

63. Zdeblick TA, Ducker TB: The use of freeze-dried allograft bone for anterior cervical fusions. Spine 16:726–729, 1991.

64. Bishop RC, Moore KA, Hadley MN: Anterior cervical interbody fusion using autogeneic and allogeneic bone graft substrate: A prospective comparative analysis. J Neurosurg 85:206–210, 1996.

65. Macdonald RL, Fehlings MG, Tator CH, et al: Multilevel anterior cervical corpectomy and fibular allograft fusion for cervical myelopathy. J Neurosurg 86:990–997, 1997.

66. Hacker RJ, Cauthen JC, Gilbert TJ, Griffith SL: A prospective randomized multicenter clinical evaluation of an anterior cervical fusion cage. Spine 25:2646–2654, 2000.

67. Vaccaro AR, Cirello J: The use of allograft bone and cages in fractures of the cervical, thoracic, and lumbar spine. Clin Orthop 394:19–26, 2002.

68. Bohlman HH: Acute fractures and dislocations of the cervical spine: An analysis of three hundred hospitalized patients and review of the literature. J Bone Joint Surg Am 61:1119–1142, 1979.

69. Elia M, Mazzara JT, Fielding JW: Onlay technique for occipitocervical fusion. Clin Orthop 280:170–174, 1992.

70. Sawin PD, Traynelis VC, Menezes AH: A comparative analysis of fusion rates and donor-site morbidity for autogeneic rib and iliac crest bone grafts in posterior cervical fusions. J Neurosurg 88:255–265, 1988.

71. Yuan HA, Garfin SR, Dickman CA: A historical and cohort study of pedicle screw fixation in thoracic, lumbar, and sacral spinal fusions. Spine 19(Suppl 20):2279s–2296s, 1994.

72. Bookvar JA, Philips MF, Telfeian AE, et al: Results and risk factors for anterior cervicothoracic junction surgery. J Neurosurg 94(1 Suppl):12–17, 2001.

73. Finkelstein JA, Chapman JR, Mirza S: Anterior cortical allograft in thoracolumbar fractures. J Spinal Disord 125:424–429, 1999.

74. Hellman EW, Glassman SD, Dimar JR II: Clinical outcome after fusion of the thoracic or lumbar spine in the adult patient. Orthop Clin North Am 29:859–869, 1998.

75. Kleinstueck FS, Hu SS, Bradford DS: Use of allograft femoral rings for spinal deformity in adults. Clin Orthop 394:84–91, 2002.

76. Urist MR: Bone transplants and implants. In Urist MR (ed): Fundamental and Clinical Physiology of Bone. Philadelphia, JB Lippincott, 1980, p 331.

77. Boden SD, Martin GJ, Morone MA, et al: Posterolateral lumbar intertransverse process spine arthrodesis with recombinant human bone morphogenetic protein 2/hydroxyapatite-tricalcium phosphate after laminectomy in the nonhuman primate. Spine 24:1179–1185, 1999.

78. Boden SD, Zdeblick TA, Sandhu HS, et al: The use of rhBMP-2 in interbody fusion cages: Definitive evidence of osteoinduction in humans: A preliminary report. Spine 25:376–381, 2000.

79. Boden SD: Editorial: Evaluation of carriers of bone morphogenetic protein for spinal fusion. Spine 26:850, 2001.

80. Commentary. J Bone Joint Surg Am 83(Suppl 1):S159–S164, 2001.

81. Morone AA, Boden SD, Martin G, et al: Gene expression during autograft lumbar spine fusion and the effect of bone morphogenetic protein-2. Clin Orthop 351:252–265, 1998.

82. Ripamonti U, Ramoshebi LN, Matsaba T, et al: Bone induction by BMPs/OPs and related family members in primates. J Bone Joint Surg Am 83(Suppl 1):S116–127, 2001.

83. Valentin-Opran A, Wozney J, Csimma C, et al: Clinical evaluation of recombinant human bone morphogenetic protein-2. Clin Orthop 395:110–120, 2002.

84. Way JC, Chalfie M: Mec-3, a homeobox-containing gene that specifies the differentiation of the touch receptor neurons in *C. elegans.* Cell 54:5–16, 1988.

85. Wang EA, Rosen V, D'Alessandro JS, et al: Recombinant human bone morphogenetic protein induces bone formation. Proc Natl Acad Sci USA 87:2220–2224, 1990.

86. Freyd G, Kim SK, Horvitz HR: Novel cysteine-rich motif and homeodomain in the product of the *Caenorhabditis elegans* cell lineage gene lin-11. Nature 344:876–879, 1990.

87. Karlsson O, Thor S, Norberg T, et al: Insulin gene enhancer binding protein Isl-1 is a member of a novel class of proteins containing both a homeodomain and a Cys-His domain. Nature 344:879–882, 1990.

88. Boden SD, Liu Y, Hair GA, et al: LMP-1, a LIM-domain protein, mediates BMP-6 effects on bone formation. Endocrine 139:5125–5134, 1998.

89. Boden SD, Titus L, Hair G, et al: Lumbar spine fusion by local gene therapy with a cDNA encoding a novel osteoinductive protein (LMP-1). Spine 23:2486–2492, 1998.

90. Viggeswarapu M, Boden SD, Liu Y, et al: Adenoviral delivery of LIM mineralization protein-1 induces new-bone formation in vitro and in vivo. J Bone Joint Surg Am 83:364–376, 2001.

91. Bauer TW, Smith ST: Bioactive materials in orthopaedic surgery: Overview and regulatory considerations. Clin Orthop 395:11–22, 2002.

92. Boden SD, Kang J, Sandhu H, Heller JG: Use of recombinant human bone morphogenetic protein-2 to achieve posterolateral lumbar spine fusion in humans. Spine 27:2662–2673, 2002.

Biology of Bone Grafting and Healing in Spinal Surgery

PAUL D. SAWIN

The 1990s witnessed a revolution in the field of spinal fusion surgery. New devices to facilitate internal spinal fixation are being developed at an unprecedented pace. These devices allow surgeons to approach complex spinal disorders in a manner previously deemed impossible with more traditional techniques. Despite the sophistication of today's hardware, internal fixation is an adjunct to spinal fusion and is not intended to confer long-term spinal stability. Hardware, by its nature, is susceptible to loosening, fatigue, and breakage. Ultimately, the success of any spinal stabilization construct relies on the biologic process of bone fusion. Without solid bone fusion, all constructs (regardless of design) will eventually fail.

This chapter reviews the following concepts: bone anatomy, biochemistry, and physiology; types of bone grafts available for spinal surgery; bone healing, as it pertains to fracture repair and bone grafting; and factors promoting and inhibiting bone fusion.

ANATOMY OF BONE

Bone is the distinguishing characteristic of vertebrate species. This tissue possesses the capacity for continuous differentiation, internal remodeling, and flawless regeneration, the only such tissue in the human organism.[1] In addition to its vital role in supporting locomotion and protecting delicate soft tissue structures (e.g., brain, spinal cord), the human endoskeleton serves as a vast reservoir for the regulation of calcium and phosphorus metabolism.

Embryologically, bone forms by either intramembranous ossification or endochondral ossification. Intramembranous ossification forms bone without an intermediate cartilaginous phase. Mesenchymal cells aggregate in sheets and, under the influence of osteoinductive proteins, differentiate into osteoblasts that deposit collagen and osteoid. With ossification, the primitive woven bone is remodeled into inner and outer plates of cortical bone surrounding a middle cancellous layer. Membranous bones include the facial bones, clavicles, and cranial vault.

Endochondral ossification occurs through a transitional stage of cartilage formation. In this process, mesenchymal cells differentiate into primitive hyaline cartilage that calcifies. As the calcified cartilage is resorbed by osteoclasts, osteoblasts deposit new bone. Bones of the appendicular skeleton, the vertebrae, and the skull base form through endochondral ossification.

In adults, bone is found in one of three states: (1) woven bone, (2) cancellous bone, and (3) cortical bone. Woven bone is found during periods of rapid bone turnover, including fracture repair and certain disease states such as Paget's disease and hyperparathyroidism. Woven bone is relatively weak owing to its loose and disorderly architecture of collagen fibers and vascular spaces lined with osteoblasts. In most cases, woven bone is remodeled to a more mature cortical or cancellous form.[2]

Cortical bone constitutes the external surfaces of the long bones and the outer and inner tables of the flat bones. Cortical bone is dense and structurally sound, accounting for most of the load-bearing capacity of the skeleton. The fundamental structural unit of cortical bone is the osteon. Osteons are tubes or cylinders of compact lamellar bone surrounding a central vascular channel, the haversian canal. Osteocytes, the terminally differentiated form of bone-producing osteoblasts, reside within lacunae in the lamellar bone. They extend cytoplasmic processes via canaliculi to the capillaries of the haversian canal and to adjacent lacunae. Adjacent osteons are connected via Volkmann's canals, which are oriented at right angles to the haversian canals.

Cancellous (or trabecular) bone is situated between cortical bone surfaces. Hematopoietic cells reside within the vascular-rich stroma of the bone marrow, situated between bony trabeculae. To augment structural support, most trabeculae are oriented perpendicular to external force vectors created by muscle tension and weight bearing. The density, size, and distribution of trabeculae within cancellous bone are determined by the weight-bearing requirements of a particular bone. As such, the cancellous bone of the femur is stronger than that of the iliac crest.[3] The trabeculae of cancellous bone also house osteocytes, which are interconnected by gap junctions. A thin layer, the endosteum, lines the trabecular spaces, insulating the hematopoietic elements, undifferentiated mesenchymal cells, and capillaries.

Surrounding the cortical bone surfaces is the double-layered periosteum. The outer fibrous layer is detachable; the inner cambial layer is nondetachable and contains osteoblasts capable of surviving transplantation and of forming callus.[3] The periosteum serves as the attachment site for skeletal muscles via tendinous fibrils called Sharpey's fibers. This layer also contains small unmyelinated pain fibers and postganglionic sympathetic neurons that cover the cortical bone surfaces and penetrate the haversian canals.

Cellular elements of bone include osteoblasts, osteoclasts, osteogenic precursor cells (including undifferentiated mesenchymal cells), and hematopoietic cells. Osteoblasts are primary bone-producing cells that secrete the nonmineralized organic components of the bone matrix, collectively called osteoid. These metabolically active cells, which contain receptors for parathyroid hormone and calcitonin, also participate in initiating mineralization of osteoid.[3] As the osteoid mineralizes, some osteoblasts become entrapped within the bone substance and form osteocytes. Within their lacunae, osteocytes are surrounded by a loose matrix that permits diffusion of bone fluid. Osteocytes communicate with one another and with the blood vessels of the haversian canals via cytoplasmic processes transmitted through canaliculi.

Osteoclasts are responsible for bone resorption. These multinucleated cells, derived from monocyte precursors, exhibit a "homing action," traveling through the bloodstream to sites of bone resorption in remodeling bone and grafts.[3] Groups of osteoclasts called *cutting cones* work in concert to enzymatically dissolve the matrix of mature bone and calcified cartilage.

BONE BIOCHEMISTRY AND MOLECULAR BIOLOGY

Bone tissue is a composite of organic and inorganic elements. Whole cortical bone is about 70% inorganic mineral, 20% organic matrix, and 10% water.[4] The inorganic constituents, referred to as bone ash, include mainly calcium phosphate and calcium carbonate, with lesser amounts of magnesium, sodium, and fluoride. These mineral elements crystallize to form hydroxyapatite, $Ca_{10}(PO_4)_6(OH)_2$, which is deposited among the collagen fibers of the osteoid matrix. Osteoblasts, secretors of osteoid, also secrete mediators that regulate the formation and maturation of hydroxyapatite crystals.[3]

The organic matrix of bone is 90% type I collagen and 10% noncollagenous "ground substance." Type I collagen molecules are composed of two α_1 chains and one α_2 chain arranged in a triple helix. These fibers are extensively cross-linked and insoluble in physiologic fluids.[3] The noncollagenous matrix proteins are a mixture of glycoproteins, proteoglycans, glycosaminogly-

TABLE 300–1 ■ **Regulatory Proteins Involved in Bone Growth and Development**

PROTEIN	FUNCTION
BMP	Initiates and regulates osteoinduction
Epidermal growth factor	Promotes osteoblast proliferation
Fibronectin	Binds osteoinductive proteins to mesenchymal cells
FGF	Promotes osteoblast proliferation, angiogenesis
IGFs	Stimulate osteoblast proliferation, collagen synthesis
Osteocalcin	Binds calcium, regulates matrix calcification
OIF	Stimulates osteoblast differentiation, inhibits osteoclasts
Osteonectin	Promotes collagen and hydroxyapatite deposition
Osteopontin	Mediates cell adhesion in bone matrix
PDGF	Promotes osteoinduction, osteoblast proliferation
PGE₁, PGE₂	Mediates bone remodeling
SGF	Identical to IGF; stimulates osteoblast proliferation
TGF-β	Regulates osteoblast proliferation, differentiation; inhibits osteoclasts

BMP, bone morphogenetic protein; FGF, fibroblast growth factor; IGF, insulin-like growth factor; OIF, osteoinductive factor; PDGF, platelet-derived growth factor; PGE, prostaglandin E; SGF, skeletal growth factor, TGF-β, transforming growth factor-β.

cans, sialoproteins, phosphoproteins, and albumin (Table 300–1). Several of these noncollagenous proteins exert specific effects on bone growth and development.

Bone Growth Factors

Bone is both a reservoir and the target organ of a host of polypeptide growth factors that regulate bone formation, maturation, and remodeling. Growth factors are also released from platelets, fibroblasts, and macrophages after injury (e.g., fracture or bone grafting). These proteins stimulate mesenchymal cells such as monocytes and fibroblasts to migrate to the site of injury (chemotaxis), where they proliferate and differentiate. Similar to soft tissue wound healing, growth factors regulate the orderly repair of injured bone through a well-established sequence of events.

When bone is injured or grafted, platelets migrate to the site of injury. Platelets liberate transforming growth factor-β (TGF-β) and platelet-derived growth factor into the extracellular space; both growth factors are chemoattractive to macrophages. The arriving macrophages are stimulated to secrete their own TGF-β and platelet-derived growth factor, which in turn are chemotactic for fibroblasts. Once lured to the site of injury, the fibroblasts proliferate and join with platelets and macrophages in liberating bone growth factors.[3] Osteoblasts and chondrocytes also synthesize and secrete TGF-β under certain conditions, including fracture repair and endochondral ossification.[5] These cells also secrete basic fibroblast growth factor, a potent stimulus for endothelial cell migration and proliferation.[6]

The resultant milieu is rich in growth factors promoting bone repair. Platelet-derived growth factor stimulates chemotaxis in macrophages and fibroblasts, induces mesenchymal cell proliferation, and enhances type I collagen production. TGF-β is also chemoattractive for macrophages and fibroblasts and stimulates the production of collagen, fibronectin, osteonectin, osteopontin, and prostaglandin E.[3] In addition, TGF-β mediates chondrocyte and osteoblast proliferation and regulates the maturation of cartilage to bone in endochondral ossification.[5] Basic fibroblast growth factor promotes angiogenesis in healing bone, essential for neovascularization of grafts and fracture sequestrum.

Osteoinduction and the Bone Morphogenetic Proteins

Bone growth factors exert their activity on differentiated cells of chondro-osseous lineage. In contrast, bone morphogenetic proteins (BMPs) are responsible for osteoinduction, a process of genetic conversion by which undifferentiated mesenchymal cells are transformed into competent bone-producing cells.[1, 7] Urist isolated a substance from demineralized, lyophilized bone matrix that had the capacity to induce new bone formation in the extraskeletal tissues of a rat.[1, 7] He termed this osteoinductive substance *bone morphogenetic protein*. Subsequent investigation has demonstrated that BMP is actually a family of highly conserved polypeptides with various degrees of osteoinductive activity in vivo.[8, 9] BMP is found in quantities of less than 1 μg/kg in cortical bone; cancellous bone contains only picogram amounts of BMP per kilogram.[3]

The target cell for BMP-mediated osteoinduction is the pluripotential mesenchymal-derived pericyte.[3, 7] During the morphogenetic phase of new bone formation, which lasts 2 to 3 days, BMP alters gene expression in undifferentiated perivascular cells, such that these cells disaggregate, migrate, reaggregate, and proliferate along an osteogenic lineage.[1, 3, 7] By day 5, cartilage has formed. By day 10, woven bone is present and is remodeled to lamellar bone by day 20. Bone marrow is evident by day 30.[1, 3, 7] By controlling osteoinduction, BMP regulates bone remodeling, fracture repair, and bone graft incorporation.[7]

Initially, BMP could be obtained only by processing several kilograms of cortical bone to yield a few milligrams of partially purified BMP product. Recombinant DNA technology has allowed the identification and mass production of a series of pure osteoinductive polypeptides that have been named BMP-1, -2, -3, -4, -5, -6, and -7. All but BMP-1 are members of the TGF-β family of proteins; BMP-3 is identical to osteogenin.[2, 3] Recombinant human BMP-2, a potent osteoinductive agent, is being produced commercially and is currently the subject of numerous clinical trials. At the time of this writing, none of the BMPs have been approved for clinical use by the Food and Drug Administration.

BONE GRAFTS AND GRAFTING

Bone grafts are used to augment bone healing when reconstructing or replacing skeletal defects.[10] Bone grafts strengthen and supplement arthrodesis, reinforce fracture repair, and fill skeletal defects created by tumor or infection. The ideal bone graft provides four elements critical for successful bone healing: (1) an osteoconductive matrix, (2) osteoinductive factors, (3) viable osteogenic cells, and (4) structural support.[10]

Osteoconduction is the process by which new capillaries, perivascular tissue, and osteogenic precursor cells from the recipient bed invade the structural framework of an implant or bone graft.[7] An osteoconductive matrix facilitates new bone ingrowth by providing a scaffolding conducive to this process. Osteoconductive activity is dictated by the structural properties of this scaffold that promote cell adhesion, cell migration, cell differentiation, and vascular ingrowth.[2] The osteoconductive matrix can be biologic (e.g., autograft bone, allograft bone) or nonbiologic (e.g., ceramics, plastics). When a biologic matrix is used, osteoconduction is coupled with resorption and replacement (remodeling) of the implant; with a nonbiologic scaffold, remodeling of the implant does not occur. As such, biologic implants are more rapidly and completely incorporated than are nonbiologic materials.[7]

Osteoinduction, the process of transforming pluripotential mesenchymal perivascular cells into competent bone-producing cells, is initiated and regulated by BMP. Consequently, the osteoinductive capacity of a given graft depends on its concentration of BMP. Some graft materials, such as ceramics or processed allograft bone, contain essentially no active BMP and thus have no osteoinductive capability. Others, such as demineralized bone matrix (DBM), function almost entirely as osteoinductive agents.

A relatively small percentage of viable osteogenic cells survives transplantation, even in freshly harvested autografts, owing to anoxia and the trauma of surgery. Most mature osteocytes perish soon after transplantation, leaving empty lacunae. Less differentiated cells of osteogenic lineage fare better, particularly those within cancellous bone, and may survive to produce new bone at the implant-host interface.[7] Most bone-producing cells at the graft site, however, are derived from the tissues of the recipient bed. Only fresh autografts contribute viable osteogenic cells to the developing fusion. Processed allografts contain no living cellular elements.

In addition to osteoconduction, osteoinduction, and osteogenic cells, the ideal graft contributes structural support to the fusion construct. In some instances, such as a noninstrumented anterior cervical fusion, the interbody graft is entirely responsible for load bearing. When instrumentation is placed, the graft may participate in load sharing with the hardware, but the extent of support conferred by the graft varies from construct to construct. For example, a cortical strut graft used in conjunction with plate-screw instrumentation in an anterior thoracolumbar reconstruction is responsible for most of the axial load bearing. In contrast, the morcellized corticocancellous bone graft used in an instrumented posterolateral lumbar fusion provides almost no structural support.

Cortical bone grafts are compact, resist compressive and tensile loads, and provide immediate load sharing and structural support to a fusion construct.[11] The structural integrity of a cortical graft, however, degrades over time as remodeling ensues. After an initial phase of osteointegration at the ends of the graft, non-viable bone is removed by osteoclast-mediated resorption. The resorptive phase may last 6 to 18 months; during this time, the graft may lose as much as one third of its mechanical strength.[12] Even years after implantation, a cortical graft retains islands of nonviable bone that have not been remodeled.

Cancellous grafts behave quite differently after implantation. Initially, cancellous grafts confer very little mechanical strength to the fusion construct.[11] This situation, however, changes rapidly as the porous, osteoconductive matrix of cancellous bone undergoes osteointegration. Graft strength continues to increase during remodeling, as bone mass accumulates along lines of stress. The ideal graft contains both cortical bone (for initial structural support) and cancellous bone (for rapid, complete osteointegration).

Types of Grafts

A variety of materials is currently available for bone grafting (Table 300–2). Bone grafts can be classified as autografts, allografts, syngrafts, and xenografts.[2] Autografts are harvested from one site and transplanted to another in the same individual. Allografts are harvested from one individual and transplanted to another individual of the same species. Syngrafts are tissues transplanted between genetically identical members of the same species. Xenografts are transplanted between members of different species. In addition, various nonbiologic materials can be used as fusion substrates in lieu of bone.

No single graft material is ideal for all situations. Consequently, the selection of a graft substrate must be individualized to each clinical situation.

AUTOGRAFT BONE

Autograft bone remains the standard against which all graft materials are measured. For 2 centuries, autogenous bone has been used routinely to repair skeletal defects; its use is documented in the oldest medical records.[13] Autografts may be cancellous, cortical, or corticocancellous. Cancellous autografts are maximally osteoconductive, osteoinductive, and osteogenic but provide little immediate structural support. Consequently, they must be supplemented with rigid internal fixation. Cortical autografts confer far greater mechanical strength, at least initially, and can participate in load sharing with hardware to enhance the structural integrity of a construct. The dense structure of cortical bone, however, possesses less surface area per unit weight for osteoconduction and creates a barrier to vascular ingrowth and remodeling. Grafts with both cortical and cancellous components, such as the tricortical iliac crest wedge or strut graft, combine the desirable attributes of both.

Many skeletal sites, including the calvaria, iliac crest (anterior and posterior), rib, fibula, and scapula, have been used to procure autograft bone. Typically, autologous bone can be harvested from any site that is both accessible and expendable. Accessibility is dictated by proximity of the donor site to the skin surface and the primary surgical site and by the nature and importance of the overlying tissues. Expendable bone is that which plays no major role in weight bearing or organ protection.

The prototypical donor site that fulfills these criteria is the iliac crest. For spinal surgery, the iliac crest is readily accessible regardless of the patient's position (supine, prone, or lateral decubitus). It is expendable because it is not primarily involved in weight bearing, muscle attachment, or protection of vital organs. In addition, the iliac crest is a versatile source of graft material. Tricortical wedge and corticocancellous strut grafts can be procured in a variety of shapes and sizes for reconstruction of the anterior spinal column. Abundant cancellous bone can be harvested for posterior spinal onlay fusions. Although other sites may be used (and even preferred) for certain applications,[14] no other site offers more versatility than the iliac crest for spinal procedures.

Most autogenous grafts are nonvascularized bone, transplanted orthotopically between noncontiguous sites. Fully vascularized grafts from the fibula, rib,

TABLE 300–2 ■ Properties of Common Graft Materials

GRAFT MATERIAL	OSTEOCONDUCTION	OSTEOINDUCTION	OSTEOGENESIS	IMMUNOGENICITY	STRUCTURAL SUPPORT
Cortical autograft	+	++	+	−	++
Cancellous autograft	++	+	++	−	±
Freeze-dried cortical allograft	+	+	−	+	++
Freeze-dried cancellous allograft	++	±	−	+	±
Demineralized bone matrix	+	+	−	±	−
Ceramics	++	−	−	−	±
Bone morphogenetic protein	−	++	−	−	±

++, strong effect or property; +, weak effect or property; − no effect or property; ±, equivocal.

and iliac crest are occasionally used and offer some advantages in select cases. A vascularized graft, either transposed locally on a vascular pedicle or reanastomosed via microsurgical techniques, remains viable throughout and does not suffer as much cell necrosis as does devascularized bone.[10] Vascularized grafts therefore promote rapid osseous incorporation and provide superior mechanical strength, without the initial phase of resorption and weakening common to devascularized grafts.[2] Vascularized bone grafts also have the ability to hypertrophy in response to mechanical stress.[10] Although not applicable for routine procedures, vascularized grafts are most useful when the recipient bed is scarred or irradiated (or if radiation therapy is anticipated) or when the defect that must be bridged is extremely long.[2, 10] Shortcomings of vascularized autografts include difficulty maintaining vascular patency, limited donor sites, and prolonged operative time.

Autograft bone offers several advantages over other fusion substrates. It is histocompatible, does not transfer disease, and retains viable osteogenic cells that participate in new bone formation. Unfortunately, the disadvantages of autograft bone are substantial. The quantity of graft available may be insufficient, particularly for long-segment fusions and in children. Moreover, the quality of the graft material can be a concern in patients with osteoporosis, metabolic disorders of bone (e.g., renal insufficiency, hyperparathyroidism, rickets), or neoplasia.

The primary disadvantage of autograft bone is morbidity at the donor site.[14–16] General harvest-related complications include chronic pain at the donor site, scarring and contour abnormalities, infection, nerve injury, blood loss, and increased anesthesia time. Other site-specific complications include meralgia paresthetica, abdominal wall hernia, buttock anesthesia, femoral neuropathy, iliac fracture (with iliac crest harvest), pneumothorax, intercostal neuralgia (with rib harvest), and gait disturbance (with fibula harvest). Although donor site morbidity amounts to no more than an annoyance for most patients, it can be severe and debilitating in as many as 25% of cases.[14, 16]

ALLOGRAFT BONE

Efforts to eliminate the donor site morbidity associated with autograft bone harvest have led to the development of alternative graft materials to promote bone fusion. The one most commonly used is allograft bone. Allograft bone provides structural support and an osteoconductive matrix, but it is neither osteogenic nor significantly osteoinductive. The latter accounts for the generally inferior outcomes obtained when allograft rather than autograft is used for spinal fusion.[17–20]

Allograft bone is available in fresh, frozen, or freeze-dried preparations. Owing to its inherent antigenicity, fresh allograft evokes an intense immunologic response and thus is inappropriate for most spinal applications. Frozen allografts are less immunogenic and are biomechanically sound, but they are somewhat cumbersome to transport and store because the temperature must be maintained below −60°C before implantation. Consequently, most allograft bone used in spinal surgery is freeze-dried (lyophilized).

Freeze-dried allograft is processed to remove water from the frozen bone tissue, after which it may be vacuum-packed and stored at room temperature. In addition to facilitating transport and storage, freeze-drying reduces the antigenicity of allograft bone while maintaining its limited osteoinductive properties. In the process, however, freeze-dried bone is altered biomechanically, losing some of its compressive and tensile strength.[10] All processing techniques currently used destroy all viable osteoprogenitor cells within the graft.

Allograft bone is available in myriad shapes, sizes, and configurations. Bi- and tricortical iliac crest struts and strips, fibula struts and wedges, and patella wedges can be used for anterior cervical applications. Larger pieces, such as humerus, tibia, and femoral rings and shafts, are useful for anterior thoracolumbar reconstructions. For posterior spinal surgery, iliac crest, rib strips, and morcellized cancellous chips are frequently used. Allograft bone can be used alone or in combination with autograft as a "graft extender" when the quantity or quality of autogenous bone is limited.[2]

The principal advantage of allograft bone is elimination of the donor site morbidity associated with autograft harvest. Also, the supply of allograft bone is almost limitless—a particularly important issue in children or those with diseased bone stock. The disadvantages of allograft bone include delayed vascular penetration, slow osteogenesis, graft resorption, fibrous encapsulation, delayed or incomplete incorporation, and graft rejection.[2, 3, 17, 21–23] Regardless of the processing technique, allograft bone elicits an immunologic reaction to proteins retained in the transplanted tissue.[21–23]

A final important consideration for both patients and clinicians is the potential for transmitting disease with allograft bone transplantation. Of greatest concern is the transmissibility of the hepatitis viruses and human immunodeficiency virus (HIV). Established in 1976, the American Association of Tissue Banks regulates and certifies member institutions that comply with stringent harvesting and processing standards. Since December 1993, the Food and Drug Administration has made compliance with these standards mandatory, thus regulating the practices of all tissue banks and requiring comprehensive donor screening, tissue testing, long-term graft tracking, and regular inspections of facilities.[10] When such stringent requirements are followed, the risk of transmitting HIV is less than 1 in 1 million.[24] Preimplantation testing is critical, however, because freezing and freeze-drying provide no protection from disease transmission.[2, 24]

Additional steps can be incorporated into the processing of allograft bone to reduce the risk of infection even further. Ethylene oxide gas sterilization, in addition to reducing immunogenicity, eradicates viruses and bacteria in tissue while maintaining the structural integrity of the graft.[25–27] Although effective as a sterilizing agent, irradiation may disrupt the matrix proteins of bone and weaken its structure.[2, 3] Like heating or autoclaving, irradiation should be considered inferior to ethylene oxide as a means of sterilization.

DEMINERALIZED BONE MATRIX

DBM is prepared by acid extraction of allograft cortical and corticocancellous bone. This process preserves noncollagenous bone proteins, collagen, and bone growth factors (including BMP) in the bone matrix while reducing antigenicity.[7, 10] Many bone banks process DBM in house; several proprietary DBM formulations, such as Grafton (Osteotech, Shrewsbury, NJ) and Osteofil (Medtronic Sofamor Danek, Memphis, Tenn), are marketed commercially. DBM is available freeze-dried as powder, crushed granules, chips, gel, or putty.

DBM is osteoinductive and osteoconductive. It is not osteogenic and serves no structural or mechanical function. DBM is most effective when used in conjunction with internal fixation and as an adjunct to other graft materials. To date, the role of DBM in spinal fusions has not been clearly established.

CERAMICS

The term *ceramic* has been used to describe both natural calcium carbonate and synthetic calcium phosphate preparations used as bone graft substitutes. Most ceramics are composed of hydroxyapatite, tricalcium phosphate, or a combination of the two.[10] Natural replamineform ceramics are primarily hydroxyapatite, derived from the calcium carbonate skeletons of sea coral. Synthetic calcium phosphate ceramics are created by a high-temperature process called sintering, combined with high-pressure compaction.[10]

Ceramics provide only an osteoconductive matrix for bone ingrowth. These materials have no osteoinductive or osteogenic properties. Ceramics tend to be brittle and possess little tensile strength. However, the biomechanical properties of ceramics vary widely, depending on their chemical composition. Tricalcium phosphate is porous and is remodeled more quickly than hydroxyapatite is, but it is mechanically weaker because of its rapid resorption. Hydroxyapatite is considerably stronger, particularly in compression, but is remodeled slowly and incompletely.[10] In clinical situations, a composite of hydroxyapatite and tricalcium phosphate is often used to take advantage of these complementary properties. In most cases, however, ceramics must be shielded from loads by rigid internal fixation until bony remodeling occurs.

Pore size influences the osteoconductive properties of ceramics and can vary significantly in both natural and synthetic preparations. The optimal pore size for osteoconduction in ceramics appears to be from 150 to 500 μm, mimicking that of cortical and cancellous bone. Commercially, corallin hydroxyapatite ceramics are available as Pro Osteon (Interpore Orthopaedics, Irvine, Calif) in a variety of pore sizes within this range.

Ceramics are biocompatible and osteoconductive and evoke almost no inflammatory foreign body response. Unfortunately, they have no inherent osteoinductivity and provide little structural support. At present, ceramics are most effective when used as bone graft expanders, particularly when incorporated in compressive applications.[10] Improvements in composite strength and supplementation with bone growth factors such as BMP may increase the utility of ceramics for spinal surgery in the future.

RECOMBINANT HUMAN BONE MORPHOGENETIC PROTEIN

Although they are not technically graft materials, recombinant human BMP and other soluble bone growth factors may soon revolutionize the way bone grafts and spinal fusions are performed. BMP is a potent inducer of bone cell differentiation but is a weak mitogen.[1, 3, 7] Although low-molecular-weight bone growth factors have little inherent osteoinductive capacity, they are powerful mitogens for differentiated cells of osseous lineage.[3] The synergistic activity of BMP and bone growth factors can dramatically augment the healing of fractures, skeletal defects, and fusions.

Human BMP is already available in a purified, recombinant form; bone growth factors may be synthesized in similar fashion. In the near future, it is conceivable that spinal fusions will be performed with no bone graft at all. Instead, only a carrier substance may be used to deliver BMP and growth factors to the appropriate site and then release them along optimal concentration gradients. Likely, the design of a suitable carrier substance will be site and application specific. That is, depending on the demands of the construct, a synthetic carrier would need to satisfy some (or all) of the following criteria: (1) mechanical support to augment skeletal integrity, (2) protection of neural elements, (3) osteoconductivity, (4) biodegradability, (5) histocompatibility, and (6) controlled, sustained release of BMP or growth factors.[3]

PHYSIOLOGY OF GRAFT HEALING

Stages in Bone Graft Incorporation

Over the 20th century, several investigators have delineated with great uniformity the histologic events that transpire during graft incorporation.[13] The following generic description outlines the fundamental stages of repair for a nonvascularized, autogenous bone graft. As mentioned previously, the incorporation of cortical and cancellous bone, as well as that of autografts and allografts, differs. Also, the stages of repair and healing are modified somewhat with vascularized grafts. It is important to realize that graft healing and incorporation involve an interaction between the graft and the recipient site, with each playing vital roles.

Much of what is known about bone graft incorporation has been extrapolated from observations of fracture healing, a remarkably similar process.[2] Bone graft healing takes place in three distinct phases: inflammation, repair, and remodeling.[2, 28, 29]

Immediately after transplantation, a hematoma is

formed around the implanted bone graft. Most osteogenic cells within the graft perish from ischemia; only those on the periphery of the graft, near the trabecular and cortical surfaces, survive by diffusion.[13] As necrosis of the nonvascularized graft ensues, a local inflammatory reaction is incited. Within days, host-derived macrophages, monocytes, lymphocytes, granulocytes, and fibroblasts invade the graft, obeying chemical messengers liberated by the necrotic bone tissue. This invasion creates a fibrovascular stroma, or "granulation tissue," that encapsulates the graft, forming a bridge between the recipient bed and the graft. From this fibrovascular stroma, new blood vessels penetrate the graft, carrying the pluripotential mesenchymal cells that will differentiate into new osteogenic cells. If the inflammatory response is inhibited (e.g., with corticosteroids, cytotoxic agents, or nonsteroidal anti-inflammatory drugs) during this crucial period, bone healing may not occur.

Cancellous bone offers little resistance to vascular ingrowth; in fact, its porosity is conducive to rapid revascularization without significant resorption of the graft. As a consequence, cancellous bone incorporates rapidly and completely, and bone mass, density, and mechanical strength increase progressively. Cortical bone grafts behave differently. Invading vascular buds follow preexisting haversian or Volkmann's canals to establish a foothold in the dense cortical bone. These channels are widened by osteoclastic resorption, substantially increasing porosity and decreasing overall mass.[13] After this osteoclastic phase, which may last months, new bone formation replaces bone resorption, and bone mass and structural integrity are restored. With dense cortical grafts, however, this process is only partially accomplished. Even years after apparently successful incorporation of cortical grafts, substantial amounts of nonviable, nonremodeled bone persist.

Revascularization coincides with the recruitment of recipient-derived mesenchymal cells into the graft. Through the process of osteoinduction, these pluripotential cells differentiate along osteogenic lines to become competent bone-producing cells. As new bone is formed, the old necrotic bone of the graft is replaced with a continuous bone mass. This process, which begins at the ends of the graft and proceeds to its center, is termed *creeping substitution.*[2, 3, 29]

Repair of nonvascularized bone grafts through creeping substitution requires weeks to months to complete. Thereafter, the incorporated bone is remodeled over months to years. The process of remodeling is slow, occurring in response to the mechanical stresses placed on the graft. Through this process, the incorporated graft assumes its final configuration and strength.

Factors Influencing Graft Healing

Both endogenous and exogenous factors may substantially influence the incorporation of bone grafts. Proper preparation of the recipient bed, which includes thoroughly decorticating and exposing the cancellous bone and maximizing the contact area of the graft-recipient bed, enhances the likelihood of successful graft incorporation. Mechanical stability, frequently provided by internal fixation, also promotes bone healing. Ideally, however, stress shielding of the graft is avoided because mechanical loading is also a strong stimulus for graft incorporation and remodeling. Biochemical factors in the local milieu that promote bone healing include the various bone growth proteins and BMP. Systemic hormonal influences, such as anabolic steroids, estrogen, testosterone, calcitonin, growth hormone, somatomedin, parathyroid hormone, thyroxine, and vitamins A and D, also enhance the probability of successful graft incorporation.[2]

Special mention should be made of the impact of electromagnetic stimulation on bone healing. A half-century ago, continuous electric current was shown to stimulate new bone growth in rabbit femora.[3] Subsequently, direct-current electrodes were demonstrated to induce osteogenesis around the negative electrode and bone resorption around the positive electrode.[3] Since these pioneering efforts, many laboratory and clinical investigations have been undertaken to establish the efficacy of electromagnetic fields for this application.

Electromagnetic stimulation promotes rapid angiogenesis, inhibits osteoclastic resorption, and stimulates osteogenesis in bone, leading to more rapid bone graft incorporation. No hazardous side effects have been identified. Electrical fields can be delivered via implantable stimulators, with a cathode placed at the site of bone repair and an anode in nearby subcutaneous tissues. Electrical fields can also be delivered by external collars or belts that place skin electrodes on opposite sides of the bone to be stimulated. Several studies have demonstrated the efficacy of electromagnetic stimulation in enhancing spinal fusion, whereas others have shown little or no effect from these devices.[30–33] At present, the role of electromagnetic stimulation for spinal fusion remains poorly defined. Given the cost of these devices, their routine use in uncomplicated cases is probably unwarranted. However, for patients who are at high risk of pseudarthrosis or those with documented fusion failure, the use of electromagnetic stimulation may be justified.

Several factors exert an inhibitory effect on bone graft incorporation. Inadequate preparation of the recipient bed, poor graft carpentry, excessive mechanical motion, and stress shielding increase the likelihood of fusion failure. Systemic conditions such as malnutrition, obesity, anemia, diabetes mellitus, infection, malignancy, alcoholism, Paget's disease, osteoporosis, and rheumatoid arthritis all inhibit bone healing.[2, 13] Medications, including corticosteroids, nonsteroidal anti-inflammatory drugs, chemotherapeutic agents, myelosuppressants, and antimetabolites, exert a profound negative effect on graft healing, presumably through their anti-inflammatory and cytotoxic effects.[2, 13, 34]

Cigarette smoking (and nicotine use in general) has long been established as a potent inhibitor of spinal fusion.[35, 36] Smoking diminishes the vertebral blood supply and promotes osteoporosis and intervertebral disk degeneration.[3] Nicotine is a potent inhibitor of angiogenesis and neovascularization, which, when coupled with the hypoxia found in smokers, probably accounts for the substantial incidence of pseudarthrosis in smokers.

Irradiation of the fusion bed inhibits bone graft incorporation via both acute and chronic mechanisms. Acutely, radiation inhibits cellular proliferation and incites acute vasculitis. Chronic radiation-induced changes include osteonecrosis and scar formation, which create a poorly vascularized environment for bone growth and repair.[2]

CONCLUSIONS

Despite the current emphasis on techniques of internal fixation in spinal surgery, the long-term success of any fusion construct depends on the integrity of the bone fusion. A basic understanding of bone anatomy, biochemistry, and physiology enhances the surgeon's ability to manipulate these factors to enhance bone healing, thereby increasing the probability of attaining a solid arthrodesis.

REFERENCES

1. Urist MR, DeLange RJ, Finerman GAM: Bone cell differentiation and growth factors. Science 220:680–686, 1983.
2. Dickman CA: The biology of spinal fusion. In Dickman CA, Spetzler RF, Sonntag VKH (eds): Surgery of the Craniovertebral Junction. New York, Thieme, 1998, pp 685–698.
3. Prolo DJ: Biology of bone. In Menezes AH, Sonntag VKH (eds): Principles of Spinal Surgery. New York, McGraw-Hill, 1996, pp 141–149.
4. Triffitt JT: The organic matrix of bone tissue. In Urist MR (ed): Fundamental and Clinical Bone Physiology. Philadelphia, JB Lippincott, 1980, pp 45–82.
5. Joyce ME, Bolander ME: Role of transforming growth factor-β. In Habal MB, Reddi AH (eds): Bone Grafts and Bone Substitutes. Philadelphia, WB Saunders, 1992, pp 99–111.
6. Folkman J, Klagsbrun M: Angiogenic factors. Science 235:442–447, 1987.
7. Urist MR: Bone morphogenetic protein, bone regeneration, heterotopic ossification and the bone–bone marrow consortium. Bone Mineral Res 6:57–112, 1989.
8. Wang EA, Rosen V, Cordes P, et al: Purification and characterization of other distinct bone-inducing factors. Proc Natl Acad Sci U S A 85:9484–9488, 1988.
9. Wozney JM, Rosen V, Celeste AL, et al: Novel regulators of bone formation: Molecular clones and activities. Science 242:1528–1534, 1989.
10. Gazdag AR, Lane JM, Glaser D, et al: Alternatives to autogenous bone graft: Efficacy and indications. J Am Acad Orthop Surg 3:1–8, 1995.
11. Hayes WC: Biomechanics of cortical and trabecular bone: Implications for assessment of fracture risk. In Mow VC, Hayes WC (eds): Basic Orthopaedic Biomechanics. New York, Raven Press, 1991, pp 93–142.
12. Enneking WF, Burchardt H, Puhl JJ, et al: Physical and biological aspects of repair in dog cortical-bone transplants. J Bone Joint Surg Am 57:237–252, 1975.
13. Friedlaender GE: Bone grafts: The basic science rationale for clinical application. J Bone Joint Surg Am 69:786–790, 1987.
14. Sawin PD, Traynelis VC, Menezes AH: A comparative analysis of fusion rates and donor-site morbidity for autogenous rib and iliac crest bone grafts in posterior cervical fusions. J Neurosurg 88:255–265, 1998.
15. Laurie SWS, Kaban LB, Mulliken JB, et al: Donor-site morbidity after harvesting rib and iliac bone. Plast Reconstr Surg 73:933–938, 1984.
16. Summers BN, Eisenstein SM: Donor site pain from the ilium: A complication of lumbar spine fusion. J Bone Joint Surg Br 71:677–680, 1989.
17. Aurori BF, Weierman RJ, Lowell HA, et al: Pseudarthrosis after spinal fusion for scoliosis: A comparison of autogeneic and allogeneic bone grafts. Clin Orthop 199:153–158, 1985.
18. Ferneyhough JC, White JI, LaRocca H: Fusion rates in multilevel cervical spondylosis comparing allograft fibula with autograft fibula in 126 patients. Spine 16:S561–S564, 1992.
19. Stabler CL, Eismont FJ, Brown MD, et al: Failure of posterior cervical fusions using cadaveric bone graft in children. J Bone Joint Surg Am 67:370–375, 1985.
20. Zdeblick TA, Ducker TB: The use of freeze-dried allograft bone for anterior cervical fusions. Spine 16:726–729, 1991.
21. Bos GD, Goldberg VM, Powell AE, et al: The effects of histocompatibility matching on canine frozen bone allografts. J Bone Joint Surg Am 65:89–96, 1983.
22. Brooks DB, Heiple KG, Herndon CH, et al: Immunological factors in homogenous bone transplantation. IV. The effect of various methods of preparation and irradiation on antigenicity. J Bone Joint Surg Am 45:1617–1626, 1963.
23. Friedlaender GE, Strong DM, Sell KW: Studies on the antigenicity of bone. II. Donor specific anti-HLA antibodies in human recipients of freeze-dried allografts. J Bone Joint Surg Am 66:107–112, 1984.
24. Buck BE, Malinin TI, Brown MD: Bone transplantation and human immunodeficiency virus: An estimate of risk of acquired immunodeficiency syndrome (AIDS). Clin Orthop 240:129–136, 1989.
25. Herron LD, Newman MH: The failure of ethylene oxide gas-sterilized freeze-dried bone graft for thoracic and lumbar spinal fusion. Spine 14:496–500, 1989.
26. Pelker RR, Friedlaender GE: Biomechanical aspects of bone autografts and allografts. Orthop Clin North Am 18:235–239, 1987.
27. Prolo DJ, Pedrotti PW, White DH: Ethylene oxide sterilization of bone, dura mater, and fascia lata for human transplantation. Neurosurgery 6:529–539, 1980.
28. Burchardt H: Biology of bone transplantation. Orthop Clin North Am 18:187–196, 1987.
29. Kaufman HH, Jones E: The principles of bony spinal fusion. Neurosurgery 24:264–270, 1989.
30. Kane WJ: Direct current electrical bone growth stimulation for spinal fusion. Spine 13:363–365, 1988.
31. Kahanovitz N, Arnoczky SP, Hulse D, et al: The effect of postoperative electromagnetic pulsing on canine posterior spinal fusion. Spine 9:273–279, 1984.
32. Lindsey RW, Grobman J, Leggon RE, et al: Effects of bone graft and electrical stimulation on the strength of healing bony defects in dogs. Clin Orthop 222:275–280, 1987.
33. Mooney V: A randomized double-blind prospective study of the efficacy of pulsed electromagnetic fields for interbody lumbar fusions. Spine 15:708–712, 1990.
34. Sawin PD, Dickman CA, Crawford NR, et al: Dexamethasone inhibits bone fusion in an experimental model of posterolateral lumbar spinal arthrodesis. J Neurosurg 94:76–81, 2001.
35. Blumental SL, Baker J, Dossett A, et al: The role of anterior lumbar fusion for internal disc disruption. Spine 13:566–569, 1988.
36. Brown CW, Orme TJ, Richardson HD: The rate of pseudarthrosis (surgical nonunion) in patients who are smokers and patients who are nonsmokers: A comparison study. Spine 11:942–943, 1986.

PART VIII *Instrumentation*

CHAPTER **301**

Anterior Cervical Instrumentation

JONATHAN J. BASKIN ■ A. GIANCARLO VISHTEH ■ CURTIS A. DICKMAN ■
VOLKER K. H. SONNTAG

Pathologic processes that compromise the biomechanical integrity of the cervical spine ultimately require management that incorporates rigid internal fixation of the vertebral column. The application of anteriorly based screw-plate systems to facilitate reconstruction of the cervical spine is a relatively recent innovation in the history of spinal surgery. This instrumentation confers immediate segmental stability along the vertebral column and ensures patient compliance by locating the "orthosis" internally. Its use has been associated with improved fusion and postoperative comfort; those who receive the implants tend to return to work more rapidly than patients who do not.[1-7] Consequently, anterior cervical screw-plate systems have become an integral part of the surgical armamentarium for achieving vertebral interbody arthrodesis within the subatlantal (C2-7) cervical spine after procedures involving diskectomy or corpectomy. Since the early 1990s, an intense evolution within this domain of instrumentation has taken place, and several anterior cervical screw-plate systems are commercially available. In pursuing the "clinical ideal" of product versatility, enhanced fusion rates, and ease of application, each new generation of anterior plating system has built on the growing body of biomechanical research and clinical experience. Aggressive advertising espouses the relative benefits of these individual systems, whose aggregate market was projected at more than $100 million in 1999.[8]

This chapter details the indications, techniques, and potential complications intrinsic to anterior screw-plate fixation of the cervical spine. In comparing the features of several different commercially available systems, we attempt to trace their development rather than endorse any particular one. The information presented here should be considered only one facet of a thoughtful approach to managing patients who present with cervical spine instability or who are at risk for developing instability after an anterior cervical procedure. Treat-ment plans must be individualized based on each patient's underlying pathologic condition and associated medical condition.

INDICATIONS FOR ANTERIOR CERVICAL SCREW-PLATE FIXATION

Anteriorly directed decompressive procedures for the subaxial cervical spine can be performed without grafting material (simple diskectomy), with grafting material (fusion procedure), and with graft material augmented by screw-plate instrumentation (fusion and internal fixation). Even without the placement of grafting material (simple diskectomy), spontaneous interbody arthrodesis is frequently observed. Clinical results reported by the senior author (VKHS) attest to the efficacy of the simple diskectomy procedure in younger patients characterized preoperatively by normal cervical lordosis, stable flexion and extension plain radiographs, absence of significant axial (neck) pain, and degenerative disease limited to one or two levels.[9]

The rationale for performing internal fixation and fusion of the subaxial cervical spine can be distilled as follows: to restore stability to the structurally compromised spine, to maintain alignment after correction of a deformity, to prevent progression of a deformity, and to alleviate pain.[10] Degenerative, neoplastic, infectious or inflammatory, traumatic, and iatrogenic (postsurgical) causes of vertebral column instability, with or without concomitant neural compression, are well suited for treatment with rigid internal fixation from an anterior surgical approach. Anterior cervical plates function to optimize the environment for osseous union by providing immediate rigid fixation across the span of desired arthrodesis. Internal fixation with screw-plate systems is performed solely in conjunction with a grafting procedure. The proximity of this instrumentation to the fusion substrate functions to resist graft displacement or disruptive micromotion at the graft-vertebral body interface and frequently obviates the need for postoperative bracing with an external orthosis.

At our institution, absolute criteria for cervical plate instrumentation include procedures that involve any extent of formal corpectomy or patients with post-traumatic spinal instability. In the event of a particularly severe ("three-column") injury,[11] an isolated anterior construct might not impart sufficient stabilization. In this circumstance, the addition of a posterior fixation procedure (circumferential fusion) to reconstruct the posterior tension band or the use of a rigid external orthosis would be necessary.[12–15] Diskectomy and fusion procedures that involve three or more adjacent levels are now routinely performed in conjunction with anterior instrumentation.[16]

In general, degenerative disease that is limited to one or two motion segments and does not involve disruption of the posterior ligamentous elements can be managed without internal fixation. Individual patient characteristics, however, can adversely affect the anticipated success of bone healing and provide relative indications for incorporating internal fixation in the operative strategy. Malnutrition, the active use of tobacco, the presence of significant osteoporosis or other disorders that result in poor bone quality, the need for exogenous steroids, or a history of previously unsuccessful fusion efforts (at the same or different vertebral levels) often leads to the patient being managed with an anterior cervical plate.[17, 18]

The presence of gross infection at the operative site and metal sensitivity are the primary contraindications to screw-plate insertion.

OPERATIVE TECHNIQUE

Preoperative Preparation and Positioning

After informed consent for the surgical procedure has been obtained, patients are brought to the operating room wearing antiembolic stockings. Intravenous and intra-arterial access is secured, and a single prophylactic dose of antibiotic is administered 30 minutes before the skin is incised. In patients with evidence of myelopathy or significant compromise of the vertebral canal, baseline evoked potentials (somatosensory and motor) are measured before the patient is intubated or positioned. Muscle paralytics are avoided during surgery to provide an immediate indication of neural irritation and to avoid exacerbating spinal instability. Patients with post-traumatic cervical instability or preexisting myelopathy undergo fiberoptic or awake intubation with the surgeon in attendance. Patients with preexisting myelopathy receive methylprednisolone in accordance with the National Acute Spinal Cord Injury Study (NASCIS) III protocol immediately before the procedure begins.[19] Drug infusion is continued throughout the procedure and is discontinued after surgery when the patient's neurologic examination is seen to be stable. A urinary catheter is placed after general anesthesia is induced if the procedure is antici-

pated to exceed 3 hours. When patients are positioned, bony and soft tissue prominences are carefully padded to avoid pressure sores or peripheral neuropathies.

Before surgery, patients are counseled regarding the choice of autograft or allograft for their fusion substrate. Given the slightly lower but comparable rate of anterior cervical fusion using fibular allograft instead of autograft (particularly for single-level procedures) and the opportunity to avoid the complications associated with harvesting a tricortical segment of autologous iliac crest, most of our patients choose an allograft fusion procedure.[18, 20] Among the choices for allograft sources, we prefer fibular allograft given its greater compressive strength compared with tricortical iliac crest allograft.[5, 18, 21, 22]

Reported donor site complications after autologous iliac crest harvest include acute and chronic pain, infection, arterial hemorrhage, peripheral nerve injury, pelvic instability, cosmetic deformity, hernia formation, and postoperative hematoma.[23] The risk of transplanting human immunodeficiency virus (HIV)-infected bone has been estimated at less than 1 in 1 million when stringent screening criteria are used.[5, 22, 24] If an autograft is to be harvested from the iliac crest, the appropriate hip is elevated with a towel roll. Patient preference determines the side from which the autograft is removed. An intrascapular roll, tape along the lateral aspect of the arms, and soft wrist ties that can be manipulated by the circulating nurse are helpful adjuncts that facilitate intraoperative radiographic visualization of the distal vertebral column.

We prefer the Caspar headholder (Aesculap, San Francisco, California) to support the patient's head and cervical spine (Fig. 301–1), even if the patient is already wearing a halo orthosis. The head is maintained in a neutral position, and the neck is maintained neutrally or is extended minimally with the assistance of a chin strap. The evoked potentials should be observed carefully for any changes, and intraoperative fluoroscopy should be available to confirm the maintenance of cervical alignment (anatomic or best attainable) after positioning is completed. At our institution, the convenience and cost-effectiveness of using cross-table fluoroscopy from the beginning of the procedure are well established compared with the relative expense and delays associated with obtaining intraoperative plain film radiographs. The importance of fluoroscopy in confirming the operative level, selecting an appropriately sized cervical plate, directing screw trajectories, assessing final screw positions, and evaluating plate alignment relative to the vertebral column cannot be overstated.

Skin Incision

The operative approach is directed from the side that is most comfortable for the surgeon and usually corresponds to the patient's right side in a right-handed surgeon. On the right side, however, the recurrent laryngeal nerve is more susceptible to injury given its relatively anterolateral course outside the tracheo-esophageal groove when compared with the left side.[25]

Consequently, some surgeons may prefer an approach directed from the patient's left side. However, injury to the thoracic duct has been reported as a complication of approaching the caudal cervical spine from the left side.[26] If the patient has already undergone a cervical procedure, we pursue operative access from the ipsilateral side. Although this strategy requires contending with scar tissue and altered anatomic planes, it avoids the more daunting possibility of incurring bilateral injury to vagal nerve branches, the unilateral manifestations of which may be subtle and otherwise undetected unless specifically looked for after the previous procedure.

A general orientation along the cervical spine can be estimated by external anatomic landmarks (Fig. 301–2), but intraoperative fluoroscopy ensures a more precise placement of the skin incision and limits the amount of soft tissue dissection necessary to obtain adequate visualization of the targeted segment of the vertebral column. Preoperative use of the fluoroscope to define the most rostral and caudal levels of exposure necessary for decompression and stabilization also assists in selecting the optimal orientation for the incision. We have found that a transverse incision located within a skin crease is cosmetically superior to a longitudinal incision that follows the medial border of the sternocleidomastoid muscle. When extended adequately (beyond the midline and laterally across the sternocleidomastoid muscle) and accompanied by gen-

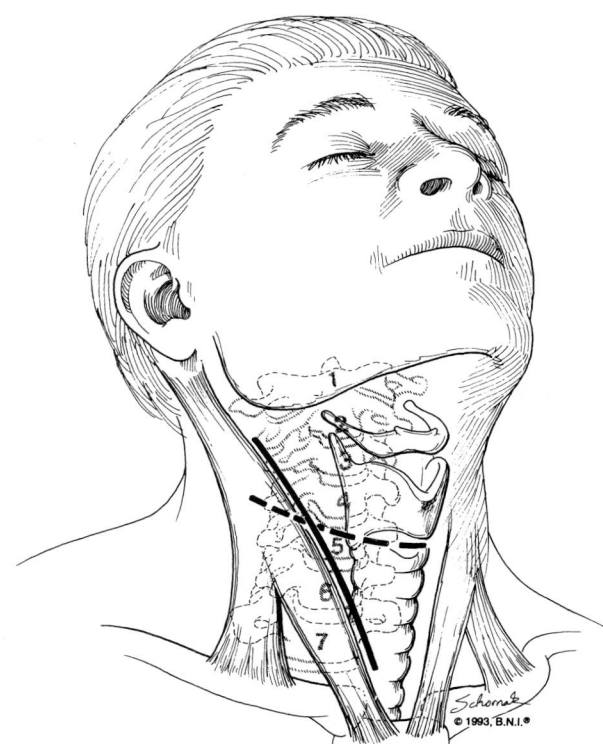

FIGURE 301–2. Orientation to the vertebral column may be estimated by palpating superficial anatomic structures. The hyoid bone sits roughly at the level of the C2-3 disk space. The top of the thyroid cartilage can be estimated as the C3-4 disk space. The inferior border of the thyroid cartilage can be estimated as the C4-5 level. The cricoid ring approximates the level of the C5-6 disk space. The C7-T1 disk space sits approximately one finger's breadth above the clavicle. Our preference is to expose the vertebral column through a transversely oriented skin incision. (Courtesy of Barrow Neurological Institute, St. Joseph's Hospital and Medical Center, Phoenix, AZ.)

erous undermining of the platysma muscle, a transverse incision rarely fails to provide sufficient access and visualization to enable multiple corpectomies to be performed with an accompanying fusion and plating procedure. However, the longitudinal incision may be more functional in patients with difficult anatomy or in whom a particularly long fusion construct is required.

Soft Tissue Dissection and Exposure of the Vertebral Column

After the patient has been prepared and draped, the skin is sharply incised to the level of the platysma muscle. Hemostasis is obtained with electrocauterization, and the platysma layer is traversed. Early attention to broad undermining of this subcutaneous muscle is greatly rewarded by the rostral and caudal extents of surgical exposure that can be attained. The underlying sternocleidomastoid muscle and tracheoesophageal bundle are identified, and the avascular plane between these structures is developed with careful, blunt dissection. A trajectory medial to the carotid sheath is followed, and the underlying vertebral column is palpated (Fig. 301–3). Comparing the osteophytic

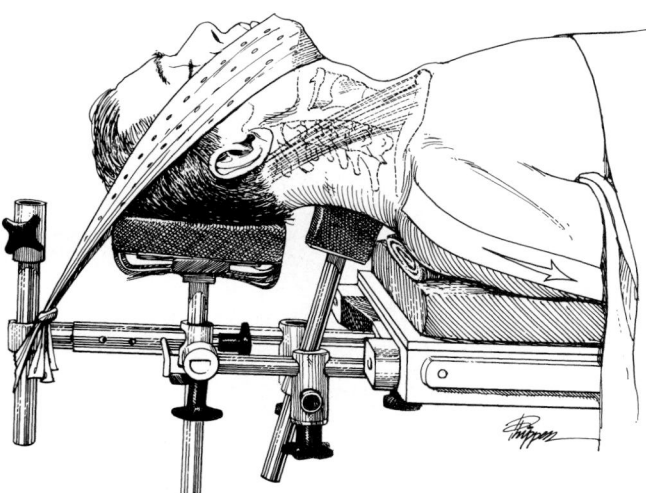

FIGURE 301–1. Patient positioning with the Caspar headholder. The patient's head is maintained in a neutral position by means of an elastic chin strap. The cervical spine is carefully maintained in either a neutral or minimally extended posture to recreate cervical lordosis. Adhesive tape is run along the lateral margin of the shoulder joint and arm and affixed to the foot of the bed to assist with intraoperative fluoroscopic visualization of the distal cervical spine. The tape should not be run directly over the clavicle to avoid a pressure injury to the brachial plexus. An intrascapular roll facilitates operative access by allowing the shoulders to fall below the coronal plane of the cervical spine. Both the scalp leads for evoked potential monitoring and the endotracheal tube (not shown) would be rostral in the operative field. (Courtesy of Barrow Neurological Institute, St. Joseph's Hospital and Medical Center, Phoenix, AZ.)

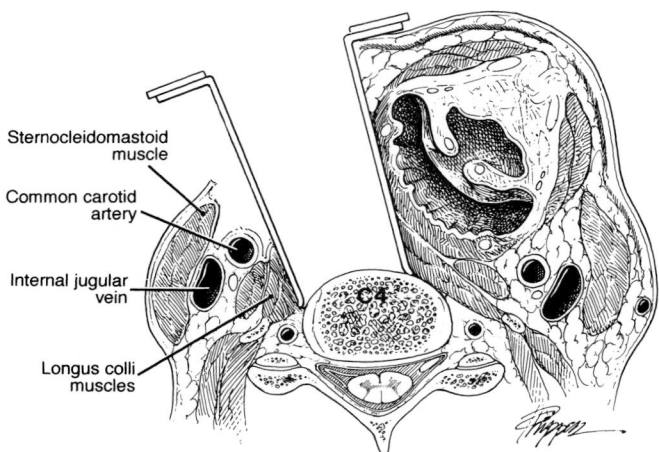

FIGURE 301–3. The relative anatomy and trajectory for an anterior transcervical retropharyngeal approach to the cervical vertebral column. A plane of dissection is maintained lateral to the tracheoesophageal bundle and medial to the carotid sheath. Bilaterally, the longus colli muscles are dissected subperiosteally to provide a submuscular pocket for seating the toothed retractor blades. Failure to seat these blades beneath the longus colli muscles properly places the esophagus and adjacent vascular structures at risk for perforation. When the vertebral column is approached anterolaterally, the tendency is to direct decompression eccentric to the contralateral side. Thus, regardless of whether the operative approach is conducted from the patient's left or right side, it is important to ensure that the ipsilateral neural foramen receives adequate attention and decompression. When anterior cervical plates are applied, the tendency is to place the plates slightly eccentric to the side from which dissection is directed. Ideally, the plates should be applied in as midline a position as possible to minimize the risk of injuring the vertebral artery and to provide as optimal a biomechanical construct as possible. (Courtesy of Barrow Neurological Institute, St. Joseph's Hospital and Medical Center, Phoenix, AZ.)

topography to preoperative or intraoperative radiographs can often help orient the surgeon along the cervical column, but fluoroscopy is used for definitive localization along the cervical spine. The prevertebral fascia is opened, and the ventral aspect of the anterior longitudinal ligament is cleaned of overlying soft tissue. The medial insertions of the longus colli muscles are elevated bilaterally from the vertebral column.

Several self-retaining retractor systems are available for enhancing exposure of the anterior vertebral column. Fundamental to all these retractors is the requirement that their laterally directed blades be seated deep to the longus colli musculature to avoid injury to the adjacent tracheoesophageal bundle or carotid artery. Injury to the vagal innervation of the larynx can result in silent aspiration (superior laryngeal branch) or hoarseness (recurrent laryngeal nerve). Apfelbaum and Kriskovich[7] reported that injury to the recurrent laryngeal nerve during anterior cervical surgery is most likely due to compression of the endolaryngeal segment of this nerve against the shaft of the endotracheal tube after the retractor is placed rather than to direct injury from dissection. To protect against this neuropraxia, they describe transiently deflating the cuff of the endotracheal tube after placing the self-retaining retractors and then reinflating the cuff to "just seal"

pressure. This allows the endotracheal tube to recenter within the larynx and remove pressure from the laryngeal wall. This technique improved the incidence of injury to the recurrent laryngeal nerve, which decreased from 6.4% in 250 patients undergoing anterior cervical plating without this maneuver to 1.7% of the next 650 consecutive patients in whom it was used.

Rostral-caudal exposure can be improved by placing a second retractor perpendicular to the first (Fig. 301–4). We avoid placing distraction posts within the vertebral bodies destined for screw placement to avoid compromising their bony integrity and adversely affecting the quality of screw purchase. Use of the high-speed drill to remove obstructing osteophytes, in conjunction with the superior illumination and magnification offered by the surgical microscope, has significantly diminished the amount of active cervical distraction necessary to confirm adequate neural decompression during a diskectomy procedure. However, if ultimately deemed necessary, distraction posts can be inserted one level rostral and one level caudal to the vertebrae targeted for screw insertion to improve exposure without potentially compromising screw purchase. Alternatively, some surgeons maintain vertebral distraction by placing patients in axial traction using Gardner-Wells tongs at the start of the procedure[27] or through gentle, even traction applied by the anesthesiologist during graft impaction. If the patient is maintained in tongs during the procedure, it is crucial to remember to release this distraction after the grafting material has been inserted and before the fixation hardware is placed.

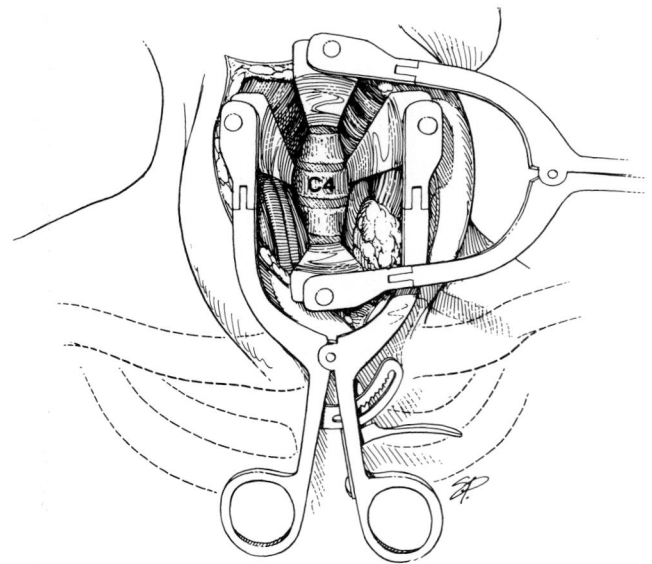

FIGURE 301–4. A second, perpendicularly oriented Caspar retractor system assists with rostral-caudal exposure of the vertebral column. These longitudinally oriented retractor blades are without teeth. Alternatively, the Caspar vertebral body distraction posts can be used to help retract soft tissue in this plane. If the latter system is used, the posts are preferentially placed in the vertebral bodies rostral and caudal to those intended for screw placement. (Courtesy of Barrow Neurological Institute, St. Joseph's Hospital and Medical Center, Phoenix, AZ.)

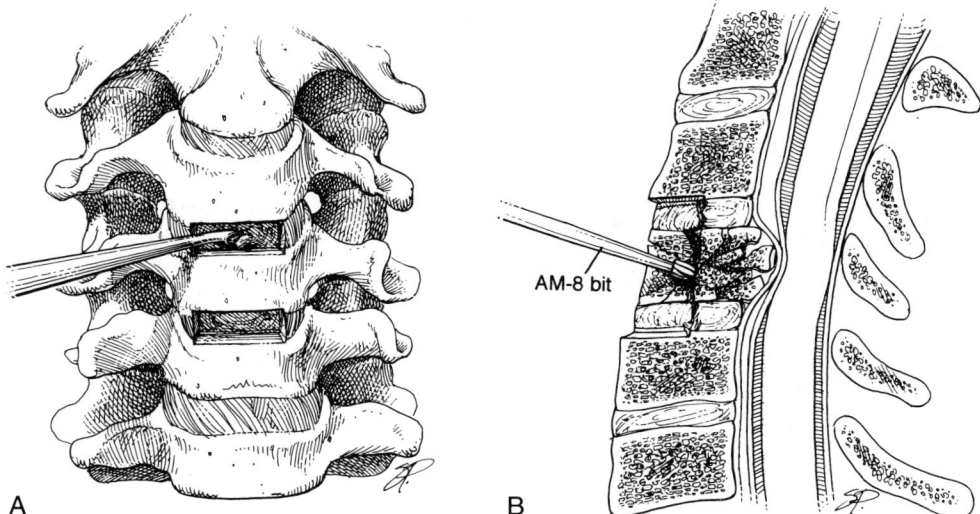

FIGURE 301–5. *A,* Anterior view of partially completed C3-4 and C4-5 diskectomies. The lateral extent of disk removal is the uncovertebral joints bilaterally. If a corpectomy is planned, the adjacent disk spaces are similarly first defined, and superficial diskectomies are performed before the vertebral body is resected. The superficial aspect of the corpectomy can then be performed easily with either a bone rongeur or a Midas Rex (Midas Rex Pneumatic Tools, Inc., Fort Worth, Tex.) drill. Typically, we prefer to use the AM-8 Midas bit to perform the corpectomy. *B,* Sagittal view of a C4 corpectomy. The deeper aspects of the diskectomies and corpectomy are performed under the operating microscope to ensure the safe exposure and decompression of the epidural space. Once the epidural space has been identified at the level of the rostral and caudal disk spaces, the remaining posterior cortex of the interval vertebral body is removed with bone punches. (Courtesy of Barrow Neurological Institute, St. Joseph's Hospital and Medical Center, Phoenix, AZ.)

Diskectomy with or without Corpectomy

Once orientation at the level of pathology has been confirmed, annulotomies are performed and superficial diskectomies are initiated with straight and angled curettes (Fig. 301–5A). If an interval corpectomy is necessary, a bone rongeur can be used to resect the anterior half of the vertebral body and the Midas Rex drill (Midas Rex Pneumatic Tools, Inc., Fort Worth, TX) used to complete the deeper aspect of bone removal (see Fig. 301–5B). If placement of an allograft strut (fibular) is planned, autologous bone from the vertebrectomy site is saved for packing the hollow center of the allograft shaft. The operative microscope is routinely used to assist with the removal of deeper bone and soft tissues to facilitate safe exposure of the dura. The epidural space is inspected, and posteriorly based osteophytes are removed from the vertebral bodies and foramen to ensure adequate decompression of the spinal cord and nerve roots. When possible, "generous diskectomies" are substituted for a corpectomy if adequate neural decompression can be achieved through wide and deep undercutting of the offending posterior vertebral body surfaces. The benefits of avoiding a complete corpectomy include preserving additional sites for screw fixation along the plate and circumventing the higher risk of nonunion or hardware failure that accompanies fusion constructs involving multiple segments.[28, 29] This latter point is particularly relevant for patients who require multilevel decompressions.

When completed, the typical lateral extent of tissue removed for diskectomies or corpectomies spans up to 20 mm. Reliable identification of the vertebral midline is crucial to ensure adequate decompression of neural tissue and to avoid vascular complications related to injury of the vertebral artery.[30–32] Frequently, severe degenerative disease, traumatic disruption, or scarring from previous surgical procedures results in the loss of the otherwise apparent anatomic midline. Typically, however, several anatomic cues remain and can be used to provide orientation to the midline for both decompressive maneuvers and plate positioning (Table 301–1). Marking the midline of the vertebral bodies with monopolar cauterization before the longus colli muscles are elevated can also provide helpful reference as the procedure progresses. It is also worthwhile to

TABLE 301–1 ■ Anatomic Cues Available for Maintaining Midline Orientation

Location of longus colli muscle
Location of uncovertebral joints
Curvature of vertebral body (lateral margin, waist)
Location of epidural veins and fat
Curvature of dural tube
Visualization of nerve roots
Palpation of pedicles
Location of sternomanubrial notch (angle of Louis)
Use of anteroposterior fluoroscopy (pedicle, spinous process location)

From Baskin JJ, Vishteh AG, Dickman CA, Sonntag VKH: Techniques of anterior cervical plating. Operative Tech Neurosurg 1:90–102, 1998.

confirm with the anesthesiologist that the patient's head has not deviated from the midline position established at the beginning of the procedure.

Bone Grafting and Plate Fixation

Screw-plate application provides immediate rigid fixation of the cervical spine and functions analogously to an "internal" halo brace. By ideally imparting some combination of load-bearing to the vertebral column and load-sharing properties through the graft site, plating systems protect the neural elements from trauma while facilitating the development of a fusion response, respectively. Bone and instrumentation deform and reform as stress is applied.[33] Over time, even the most rigid constructs permit some segmental motion across the site of fixation. In the absence of an osseous union, repetitive loading will fatigue an implant to the point of failure through loosening or breakage. Consequently, perhaps the most fundamental principle related to performing rigid internal fixation is that the presence of instrumentation does not substitute for a carefully conceived and meticulously prepared fusion site.[34, 35] In the absence of an associated arthrodesis, hardware failure is a time-dependent certainty (Fig. 301–6).

We typically use the Robinson-Smith technique for interbody fusion after a cervical diskectomy.[36] Techniques to optimize the chances for successful arthrodesis (Table 301–2) at the operative site can be subdivided into (1) those that enhance the natural capacity for bone healing to occur, (2) those that minimize the extent of iatrogenically induced impediments to bone graft incorporation, and (3) those that maximize the biomechanical advantage of the hardware construct.

TABLE 301–2 ■ **Techniques to Optimize Fusion Hardware Contrast**

MANEUVER	BENEFIT
Insert graft under compression	Improves graft incorporation
Maximize surface of implant-bone interface	Improves graft incorporation
Remove soft tissue from fusion interface	Avoids fibrous healing
Maintain integrity of cortical end plate	Prevents telescoping of graft
Irrigate while drilling	Prevents thermal injury with impaired bone healing and resorption
Avoid contouring plate	Avoids fatiguing of implant
Avoid overtightening screws	Prevents stripping screw hole and diminishing bone purchase
Insert angulated screws	Improves pull-out strength
Use longest screws possible	Improves pull-out strength

From Baskin JJ, Vishteh AG, Dickman CA, Sonntag VKH: Techniques of anterior cervical plating. Operative Tech Neurosurg 1:90–102, 1998.

Enhancing the Natural Capacity for Bone Healing

Bone grafts are incorporated with the greatest success when the fusion construct is maintained under a compressive load (Wolff's law).[37] Consequently, the vertical dimension of the graft material being used is typically sized a few millimeters longer than the measured diskectomy or corpectomy defect to ensure mechanical compression of the graft within the recipient bed. At the time the graft is placed, the adjacent vertebral bodies can be distracted mildly through several techniques (disk space spreader, vertebral body distraction

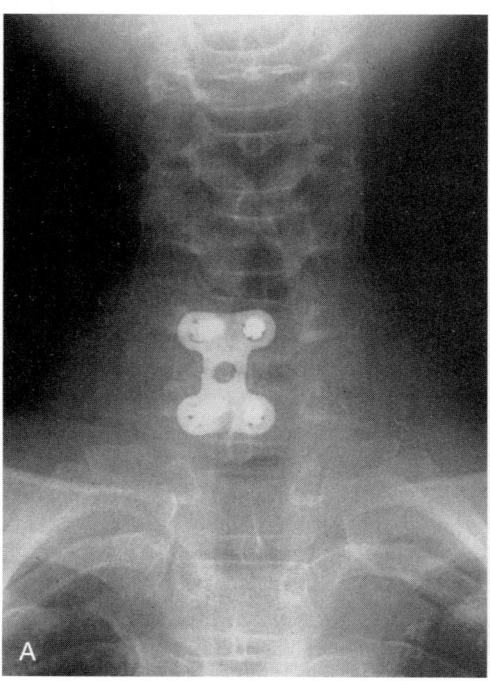
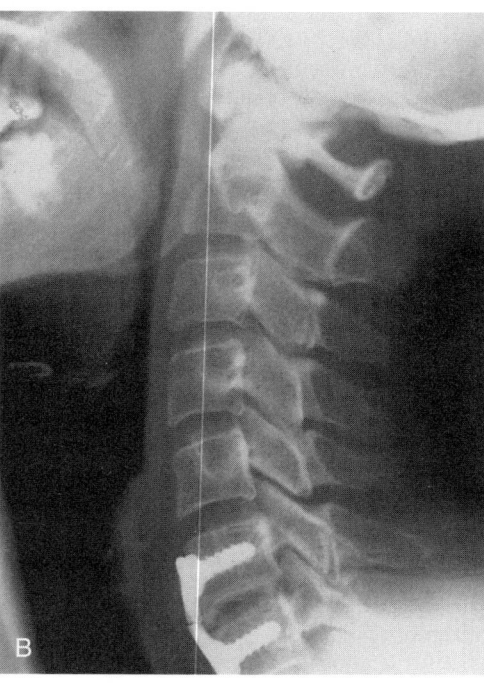

FIGURE 301–6. *A,* Anteroposterior *(A)* and lateral *(B)* views of a patient treated at an outside facility with a failed anterior cervical plate. Note the transversely oriented fracture at the plate's midline. The rostral and caudal screw sets maintain good position. There is no evidence of arthrodesis spanning the discectomy site.

posts, axial traction, or gentle vertical distraction by the anesthesiologist) to ensure that the graft ultimately experiences a compressive load. After the posterior half of the graft has been tamped into place, the vertebral body distraction is released and the remainder of the graft advanced. These maneuvers promote seating and avoid excessive impaction of the graft. When relying on axial traction applied with cranial tongs to achieve vertebral distraction during the decompressive portion of the procedure, it is important not to overlook requesting its release before proceeding to internal fixation.

After final positioning, graft security and an appropriate epidural margin are confirmed by palpating posterior to the graft with a nerve hook and visualizing the posterior border of the graft with fluoroscopy. Before the graft is inserted, all soft tissues are removed from the graft material and fusion interfaces (end plate articular cartilage) to prevent the delayed differentiation of fibrous tissue that might hinder bone formation. The creation of smooth, apposing surfaces along the bone graft and vertebral bodies serves to improve the environment for fusion by maximizing the area of surface contact at the bony interfaces.

Iatrogenic Impediments to Fusion Biology

High-speed drills are convenient for denuding articular surfaces within the fusion bed and for shaping the fusion surfaces of the vertebral bodies and graft. During all drilling, consistent irrigation is needed to avoid thermal injury that can incite subsequent bone resorption and interfere with the fusion response. Similarly, the excessive use of monopolar cauterization to expose the vertebral column can impede healing as a result of direct thermal injury and bone devascularization. The recipient bed (vertebral surfaces) is the source of almost all the osteogenic components critical to the fusion response. Even when using an autologous bone graft, few of the "transplanted" osteoblasts and osteocytes actually survive to contribute to healing.[18] As such, the surface area of healthy vascularized bone in the fusion bed should be maximized. Using monopolar cauterization for deep tissue dissection also places adjacent soft tissues (e.g., esophagus, recurrent laryngeal nerve) at greater risk. Bone bleeding within the recipient site can be controlled with thrombin-soaked Gelfoam sponge (Upjohn, Kalamazoo, MI), Avitene powder (MecChem, Woburn, MA) or, if particularly intractable, bone wax. These substances hinder the fusion response and should be used sparingly at the graft-vertebral body interface.

Optimizing the Fusion and Hardware Construct

Most available cervical plates are machined with an established lordotic curve to conform to the contour of the cervical spine. Although most of these plates can be further shaped using special devices at their time of insertion, this action weakens the plate and should be avoided if possible. Ventral osteophytes should be removed to allow a flush application of the plate to the midline of the spinal column. Its position can be confirmed fluoroscopically and by the absence of "seesawing" when the sides or the rostral and caudal ends of the plate are alternately compressed against the vertebral column. When osteophytes are removed, as much of the cortical bone layer as possible should be retained because it contributes substantially to an individual screw's resistance to pulling out. This point is particularly important when screw-plate systems that rely only on unicortical bone purchase are implanted.

In contrast to cervical fusion procedures that do not include instrumentation, the graft material is not countersunk away from the ventral margin of the disk space. Instead, the anterior border of the bone plug or strut is left in line with the anterior margin of the adjacent vertebral bodies to maximize the contact surface between the plate and the entire fusion construct. For a single-level procedure using autograft or allograft, a trough along the posterior aspect of one of the vertebral bodies protects against graft retropulsion and epidural compression. Autograft struts that span more than one level are secured to the plate with a bicortically anchored screw to prevent graft retropulsion. Typically, fibular allograft is too brittle to accept a bone screw, and posterior troughs are created at the upper and lower vertebral levels to protect against its displacement (Fig. 301–7).

When the recipient site is prepared for graft placement, the cortical end plates are thinned sufficiently to expose bleeding bone but are left intact to minimize "telescoping" of the graft material through the adjacent vertebral bodies. This step is particularly important when allograft material is implanted, because its rigidity makes this complication more likely than when autograft is used, especially in patients with osteopenic or otherwise soft bone. Loss of graft height, due to either settling or resorption, adds further mechanical stress to the screw-plate construct and increases the risk for implant failure and pseudarthrosis. Proper attention to graft harvesting (autograft) or preparation (allograft) optimizes the load-bearing capabilities of these materials. We prefer to harvest autologous iliac crest bone using an oscillating saw to avoid osteotome-related microfractures, which can reduce the compressive strength of the graft.[38] Failure to reconstitute the freeze-dried allograft appropriately in saline (minimum of 30 minutes) before it is shaped or implanted compromises its structural integrity.[18]

"Two-finger tightness" is the desired final torque when inserting bone screws. Overtightening screws can "strip" the threads of the screw hole and diminish their resistance to pulling out. If the tapped threads are stripped, there are several options for securing the construct. A larger diameter "rescue" screw (if available) can be substituted for the initially placed fixation screw. A new screw path can be drilled within the same plate-hole site if the screw trajectory can be varied. The entire plate can be moved so that a new hole for a fixed trajectory screw can be drilled. Finally, the initial screw's purchase can be bolstered with methylmethac-

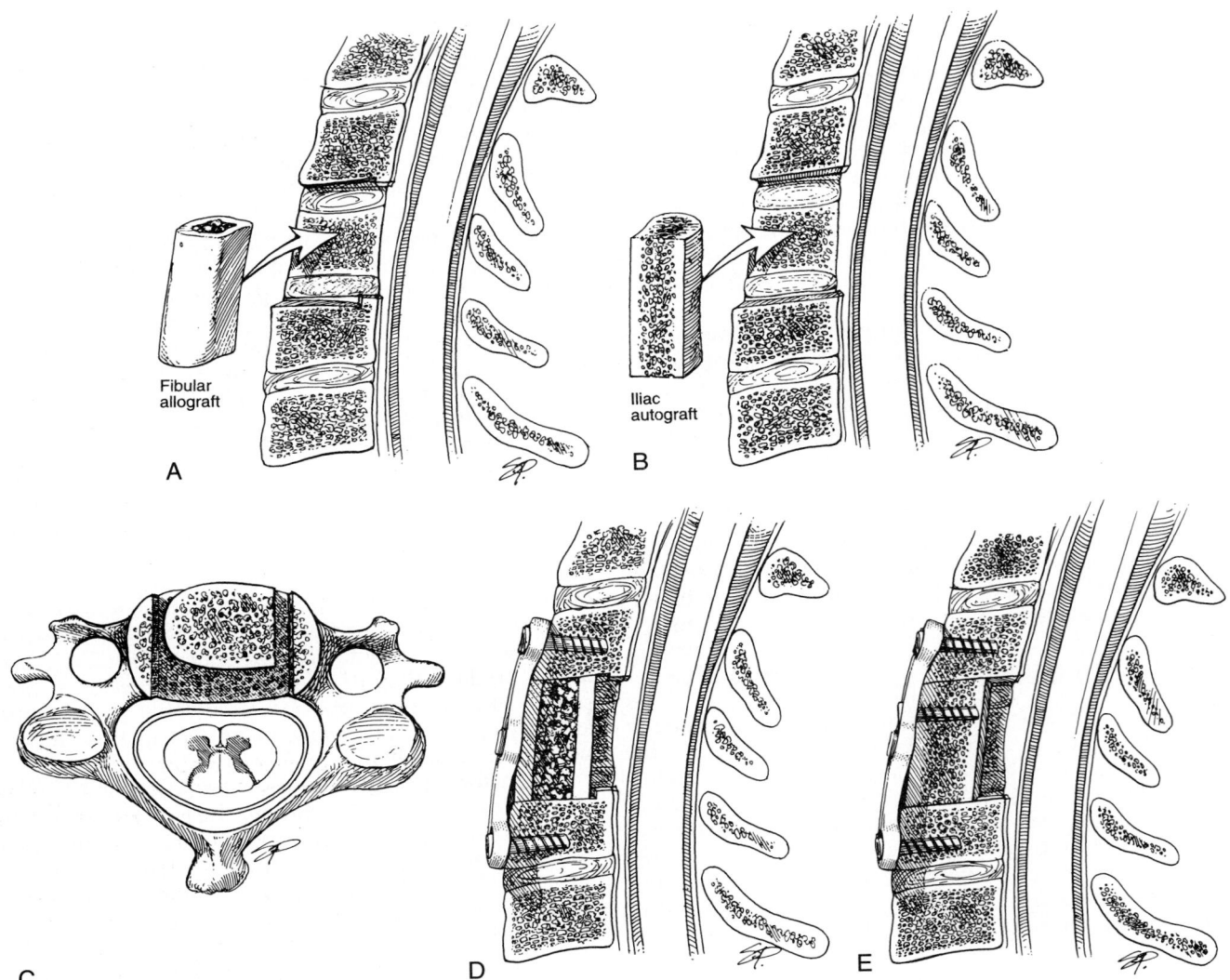

FIGURE 301–7. Sagittal views of corpectomy defects before allograft (A) and autograft (B) fusion procedures. Because a screw can be used to secure the autograft to the anterior cervical plate, posterior troughs are unnecessary to prevent graft retropulsion. Conversely, the allograft material is usually too brittle to accept a screw, and rostral and caudal troughs are created within the respective vertebral bodies to protect the epidural space. The height of the troughs is 1 to 2 mm, and a concerted effort is made to maintain the integrity of the adjacent vertebral end plates to minimize the risk of the graft telescoping through the adjacent vertebral bodies. C, Midlevel axial view through a corpectomy defect after insertion of an autologous bone graft illustrates the preference for orienting autologous graft material. As placed, the cortical margins serve to buttress the anterior and middle columns while minimizing the anteroposterior diameter of the graft. C4 corpectomy site after allograft (D) and autograft (E) fusion with plating procedures. In both cases, the graft material has not been countersunk; the anterior margin of the graft material is flush with the undersurface of the plate. The allograft material is packed with autologous bone from the corpectomy site to promote fusion. A bicortical screw fixes the autograft to the cervical plates. (Courtesy of Barrow Neurological Institute, St. Joseph's Hospital and Medical Center, Phoenix, AZ.)

rylate. Pilot-hole drilling and screw placement should always be monitored with real-time fluoroscopy, irrespective of the surgeon's experience with screw-plate fixation.

If possible, the screw trajectory should capture the denser bone tissue in the subchondral region of the vertebral body while respecting the end plate of the vertebral body. Crossing the distal vertebral end plate results in a suboptimal screw purchase that can further loosen over time because of motion across the violated disk space. Alternatively, this misplacement risks incorporating a normal motion segment within the fusion construct. If unicortical screw placement is pursued, the longest screws that can be accepted by an individual patient's anatomy are used for plate fixation because they resist pulling out better than their shorter counterparts. When fixation involves multiple segments, the plate should be secured at as many points as possible. This step is particularly important at the caudal aspect of the plate given the greater failure stresses transmitted to that location.[28, 29] Because additional sites for fixation are preserved, partial corpectomies or "generous diskectomies" are desirable substitutes for a completed corpectomy. Obviously, minimizing bone removal presupposes satisfying the goal of adequate neural decompression. Midsagittal application of the plate fosters optimal load sharing among the fixation points and is facilitated by fluoroscopic guidance, as noted further on.

Closure

Final inspection of the operative site includes assessing the alignment of the vertebral column after fixation, the position of the graft with respect to the epidural space, and the length of the plate and position of the screws with respect to the rostral and caudal disk spaces. Midline location and vertical orientation of the plate can be assessed fluoroscopically by observing the parallel overlap of plate holes and screw trajectories on "true lateral" cross-table views. An anteroposterior view can be obtained as the fluoroscope is removed from the operative field. Location of the plate midway between the vertebral pedicles and in line with the superimposed spinous processes confirms placement in the vertebral midline. The asymmetrical application of a plate most often is a consequence of the caudal aspect of the plate being shifted toward the side of surgical approach (see Fig. 301–6*A*).

Bacitracin-containing saline is used to irrigate the wound, and hemostasis is obtained with bipolar cauterization. Self-retaining retractors are removed, and the trachea, esophagus, and carotid sheath are inspected for evidence of injury with a hand-held retractor. The presence of a carotid pulse above and below the level of self-retaining retractors is confirmed. The platysma muscle and dermis are closed as separate layers using interrupted absorbable sutures, and the skin is further reapproximated with a running subcuticular suture and sterile adhesive strips. We have found no need to maintain a surgical drain within the operative site, and current evidence does not support the routine use of prophylactic postoperative antibiotics in otherwise immunocompetent patients.

ORTHOSES AND POSTOPERATIVE FOLLOW-UP

The nature of the patient's preoperative pathologic condition, the extent of the underlying mechanical instability, and the length of the fusion construct dictate the type of postoperative cervical orthosis prescribed. In patients who have a three-column traumatic disruption of their spinal column or who suffer from an underlying metabolic impediment to healing (e.g., rheumatoid arthritis), a halo brace should be considered for additional postoperative stabilization. Multilevel plate constructs are more prone to failure than their shorter counterparts.[28, 29] A patient whose procedure involves three or more corpectomies should be managed in a halo brace or undergo augmentation with posterior

fusion.[28] When screw purchase is good in patients undergoing a single-level fusion and plating procedure for spondylotic disease, they likely can be maintained without a collar after surgery.

Baseline radiographic (fluoroscopic or plain film) documentation of the fusion and instrumentation construct is obtained at the completion of the surgical procedure. Plain films are repeated 4 to 6 weeks after surgery and are expanded to include dynamic views (flexion and extension) if there is evidence of graft incorporation and stable hardware position. When evidence of a fusion response (bridging trabeculated bone across the graft-vertebral interface) is obtained, patients are instructed in neck-strengthening exercises. Those who have been wearing a cervical collar are instructed to taper its use and to initiate flexion exercises. Dynamic views are obtained 6 to 8 weeks after surgery in patients managed in a halo brace with the halo ring disconnected from the vest but still attached to the skull. The halo ring is removed only after mechanical stability is demonstrated. Such patients are then placed in a hard cervical collar, the use of which is tapered while they perform cervical strengthening exercises.

EVOLUTION OF SCREW-PLATE SYSTEMS

The first reported use of screw-plate fixation in the anterior cervical spine occurred in 1964 and is attributed to Bohler and Gaudernak.[39] They relied on the available hardware of the time, which was intended for long bone (extremity) fixation. In 1982, Caspar described a novel technique and instrumentation system (retractors, distractors, and screw-plates) that popularized the practice of anterior cervical plate application.[40] From this beginning, several anterior cervical screw-plate systems have emerged. Some of the more frequently used systems are listed in Table 301–3. Each system has its own advocates and detractors, and the relative merits of one product compared with another largely remain subject to an individual surgeon's preference rather than to an objectively demonstrated superiority of one system over another. Our institutional experience with anterior cervical plates has been derived primarily from the use of five different systems (Caspar, Aesculap, San Francisco, CA; Synthes, Synthes Spine, Paoli, PA; Orion, Medtronic Sofamor Danek, Memphis, TN; Codman, Codman and Shurtleff Inc., Johnson & Johnson, Raynham, MA; and Atlantis, Medtronic Sofamor Danek, Memphis, TN) whose specifications are detailed further on. The ABC system (Aesculap, San Francisco, CA) is included in this comparison, although we have no clinical experience with it.

From biomechanical and biologic perspectives, the ideal plating system would offer a combination of "static" and "dynamic" elements. These seemingly contradictory but complementary characteristics promote arthrodesis by minimizing disruptive motion within the fusion bed and by facilitating remodeling through load sharing, respectively. The earlier plating systems offered one or the other of these qualities in

TABLE 301–3 ■ Comparison of Anterior Screw-Plate Systems

PLATE SYSTEM	YEAR COMMERCIALLY AVAILABLE	PRE-CONTOURED LORDOSIS	REQUIRED SCREW PURCHASE	SCREW LOCKING MECHANISM	SCREW TRAJECTORY	BIOMECHANICAL CHARACTER	AVAILABLE PLATE LENGTHS (END-TO-END) (mm)	AVAILABLE SCREW TYPES DIAMETER (LENGTH) (mm)	SAMPLE 2000 CATALOGUE PRICE		
									Plate Length (28 mm)	Individual Screw in mm	Minimum Construct Cost*
Caspar	1980	No	Bicortical	None	Variable	Dynamic, nonconstrained	26–90	3.5 (10–28) 4.5 (17–24)	$464.50	All screws $34.60 each	$ 602.90
Synthes	1991	Yes	Unicortical	Separate anchor screw (all sites)	Fixed	Static, constrained	22–92	4.0 (12, 14, or 16) 4.35 (12, 14, or 16) (all available in standard or self-tapping) Locking screw	$525 standard $620 small stature	Standard 4.0 $110† Standard 4.35 $154† Self-tapping 4.0 $133† Self-tapping 4.35 $187† Locking (anchor) $22.75	$1056.00
Orion	1993	Yes	Unicortical	Separate locking screw (limited to rostral and caudal ends)	Fixed	Static, constrained	21.5–110	4.0 (10–24) 4.35 (11, 13, or 15) 4.50 (11, 13, or 15) (available in only self-tapping) Locking screw	$618	4.0 $132† 4.35 $141† 4.5 $168† Locking screw $61	$1268.00
Codman	1996	Yes	Unicortical	Integrated cam (all sites)	Variable	Dynamic, nonconstrained	24–110	4.5 (10–26) (standard) 4.5 (12–16) (self-tapping)	$697	Standard 12 or 15 $109 Standard other lengths $130 Self-tapping 12 or 15 $135 Self-tapping 13, 14, or 16 $155	$1133.00
Atlantis	1998	Yes	Unicortical	Integrated locking screw (all sites)	Both	Static, constrained or dynamic, nonconstrained (depending on screw selection)	19–110	4.0 (10–20)‡ 4.5 (13, 15, or 17)‡ (standard or self-tapping)	$813	All 4.0 standard $153§ All 4.0 self-tapping $176 All 4.5 standard $195 All 4.5 self-tapping $225§	$1425.00
ABC	1999	Yes	Unicortical	Internal screw mechanism (all sites)	Variable	Dynamic, constrained	20–103	4.0 (10–18) self-tapping 4.0 (10–28) bicortical flat tip 4.5 (13, 15, or 17)	$424.50	All screws $278	$1536.50

*28-mm plate and all necessary screws (least expensive available).
†No price difference related to length.
‡Fixed or variable trajectory screw type.
§No price difference based on screw length or fixed or variable trajectory.
Adapted from Baskin JJ, Vishteh AG, Dickman CA, Sonntag VKH: Techniques of anterior cervical plating. Operative Tech Neurosurg 1:90–102, 1998.

isolation; they were either solely dynamic (Caspar) or static (Synthes and Orion). Thus, the selection of a plating system at that time had to be based on prioritizing the relative merits of a load-bearing (constrained or static) or load-sharing (nonconstrained or dynamic) construct.

Historically, the coupling between the screw head and plate has determined whether these instrumentation systems were classified as constrained (static) or nonconstrained (dynamic). The variable trajectory screws of the Codman and Atlantis systems are nonrigidly locked to their plates. Although the screw is unable to back away from the plate, its angulation within the plate hole can change over time (dynamic quality) and allows limited vertical subsidence. In contrast, fixed trajectory screws are rigidly secured to their plate so that their angulation relative to the plate surface cannot change (Synthes, Orion, or Atlantis [fixed trajectory screw]). A unique aspect of the newly introduced ABC system is that a variable trajectory screw can be rigidly secured to its plate (constrained or static feature) and concomitantly offer limited stress shielding through vertical migration of the screws within their respective slots (dynamic feature).

The current manufacture of all screw-plate systems in titanium or one of its alloys has combined material strength (90% strength of steel) with magnetic resonance imaging compatibility. The introduction of a "locking plate" design (screw head secured to the plate) significantly simplified implantation of these systems by replacing the requirement for a bicortical screw (Caspar) with the technically easier option of placing a unicortical screw (Synthes, Orion, Codman, Atlantis, and ABC). Later generations of "unicortical" systems have become successively easier to use because of the trend of incorporating the locking mechanism within the plate (Codman, Atlantis) or screw itself (ABC) instead of the locking mechanism existing as a separate component (Synthes, Orion).

Most systems now offer an expanded selection of screw lengths and the option of "standard" or "self-tapping" screws. However, there is often a substantial disparity in cost between the standard screws and their self-tapping counterparts and between screw lengths considered to be "regular" and those that are "expanded" (see Table 301-3). A common inclusion within most of the recent generations of systems is a temporary "holding pin" that stabilizes the plate during screw-hole drilling and screw placement. These pins prove to be useful during multilevel plate fixation and are placed either through designated holes along the plate midline or within one of the plate's screw holes.

Although fixed trajectory screws are associated with less error in screw placement, they offer little opportunity for the surgeon to compensate for a patient's abnormal anatomy or to correct for suboptimal screw tracks or stripped tap holes. Similarly, the ability to contour plates using fixed trajectory screws is limited by the effect that bending would have on the final screw position. Fixed trajectory systems can also be difficult to use at the extremes of cervical placement, where bony structures (mandible or clavicle) can pro-

hibit the necessary angulation of instruments for drilling and inserting screws along a predetermined path. Variable screws are attractive because they offer greater diversity in screw placement and allow surgeons to optimize screw purchase. However, they also carry a greater risk for complications related to screw malposition than do fixed trajectory systems.

Individual Plating Systems

CASPAR SYSTEM

Introduced commercially in 1982, the Caspar "osteosynthetic plate"(Aesculap, San Francisco, CA) is the only system that requires bicortical screw purchase (Fig. 301-8). The screw trajectory is variable, and no locking mechanism secures the screw head to the plate (nonconstrained-dynamic system). The requirement for bicortical screw purchase makes this the most technically challenging system to use because the depth of posterior cortical penetration must be determined precisely to avoid compromising the epidural space. The plates are machined without contour in the sagittal plane but can be curved as desired. The slotted configuration allows screws to be positioned and redirected as necessary. The recommended screw trajectory is directed 15 degrees medially and parallel to the adjacent vertebral end plate. The appropriate plate length should measure 2 mm from the rostral and caudal end plates of the respective rostral and caudal vertebral bodies that are incorporated in the fusion construct.[29, 41] The posterior longitudinal ligament sufficiently shields the dura as long as the blunt-tipped bicortically placed screw does not extend further than the width of one screw thread beyond the posterior cortex.

Although bicortical screw placement poses a greater potential risk for dural violation and spinal cord injury

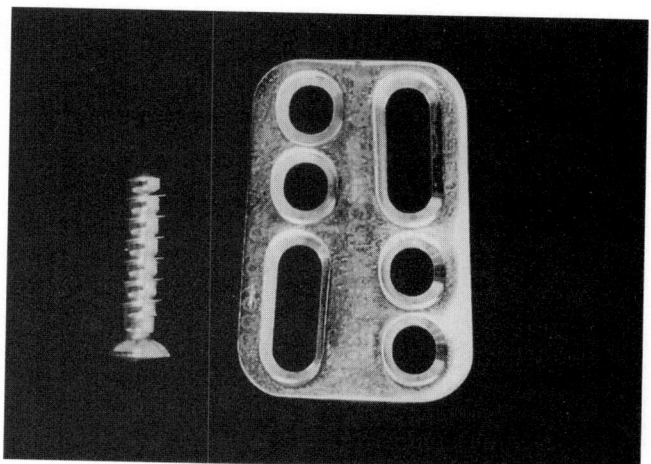

FIGURE 301-8. Early-generation Caspar plate (28 mm) and screw. Bicortical screw purchase prevents the need to fixate the screw head rigidly to the plate. Newer generation Caspar plates are titanium and have midline holes for "holding-pin" placement. (From Baskin JJ, Vishteh AG, Dickman CA, Sonntag VKH: Techniques of anterior cervical plating. Operative Tech Neurosurg 1: 90–102, 1998.)

than does a unicortically positioned screw, the Caspar system has been in clinical use longer than any of the available screw-plate systems. It remains popular, with a very low reported rate of complication.[41] The newer generation Caspar titanium plate has been modified to include midline holes for "holding-pin" placement and is marked to orient surgeons to its rostral and caudal ends. It is the least expensive of the available screw-plate systems (see Table 301–3).

SYNTHES

Introduced in 1986, the Synthes unicortical system (Cervical Spine Locking Plate; Synthes Spine, Paoli, PA) uses fixation screws that accommodate a separate internal 1.8-mm expansion locking screw (Fig. 301–9). This combination rigidly secures the screw head to the plate (constrained-static system). The rostral and caudal fixation screws are directed in a fixed, medially convergent trajectory that increases the resistance to pulling out. The upper screws are angled 12 degrees cephalad to approximate the cervical lordosis, and the lower screws are directed perpendicular to the plate in the sagittal plane.[22, 42] Initially available in only a 4-mm diameter and 14-mm length, the fixation screws are now produced in 12-, 14-, and 16-mm lengths in both standard and self-tapping varieties. The working screw diameter for the set is 4 mm, and a 4.35-mm "rescue" screw is available in standard and self-tapping forms. As is the case with all the plating systems, self-tapping screws are significantly more expensive than the standard variety (see Table 301–3).

The plate has an established lordotic curve as well as a fixed rostral and caudal orientation (indicated by an arrow at the plate's rostral end). Bending, which further weakens the plate's structure, should be performed away from the screw holes to avoid altering the integrity of the locking mechanism. Bending also

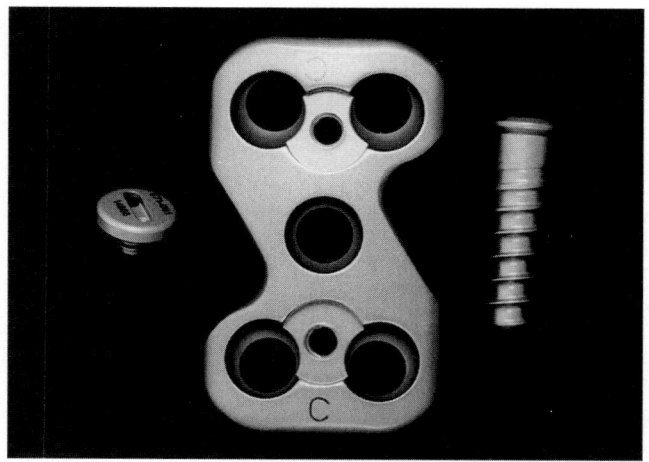

alters the fixed screw trajectory and can compromise the final screw position. The Synthes plates are available in "small stature" dimensions, but they cost more than the standard sizes.

ORION

The Orion (Sofamor Danek, Memphis, Tennessee) is a contoured system that uses a fixed trajectory screw (constrained-static system) that is medially convergent (6 degrees) with 15 degrees of angulation at the rostral and caudal ends (divergent) (Fig. 301–10). As with the Synthes system, further plate bending alters the cephalad and caudal angulations of screw placement. In contrast to every other "locking plate" system, the Orion plate accommodates locking screws (separate components) only at its rostral and caudal ends. The head of each locking screw overlaps the tops of the paired 4-mm-diameter fixation screws at the respective ends of the plate. Additional anchoring screws can be placed through a variable interval slot (4.35-mm diameter screws recommended) that is present within the longer plates. However, screws in this location cannot be secured to the plate with a locking screw and preferably are placed with a bicortical purchase. A 4.5-mm "rescue" screw is available within this system. The 4-, 4.35-, and 4.5-mm screws are currently produced only in a self-tapping form.

Insertion of the locking screw requires an orientation that is truly perpendicular to the plate surface. Failure to achieve this angle, which may be particularly difficult in the vicinity of the mandible or clavicle, can prevent successful placement of the locking screw. A self-limiting torque mechanism causes the driver for the locking screw to twist free from the screw head when it is secured appropriately. Plate sizing must allow for the fixed screw angulation of 15 degrees. Because of the vertical angle of the screws, the plate length should span just beyond the margins of the

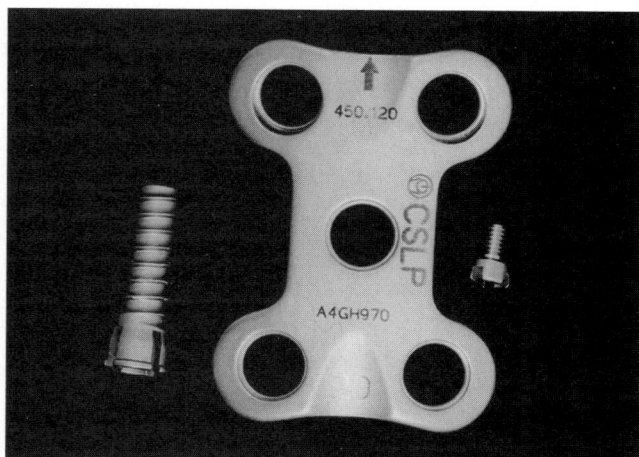

graft site to ensure that the screws do not violate the adjacent end plates.[43]

CODMAN ANTERIOR CERVICAL PLATE

The Codman anterior cervical plate (Codman and Shurtleff Inc., Raynham, MA) is a contoured titanium plate (Fig. 301–11) that offers variable trajectories for screw insertion and has no specific rostral or caudal end. A locking cam mechanism integrated into the plate resists screw "back-out" and allows unicortical screw fixation. However, the screw head is not rigidly fixed within its plate hole and can change its angulation relative to the plate (nonconstrained). This "dynamic" aspect of the system allows some load sharing and affords the system some tolerance for delayed vertebral settling that might occur from graft resorption or "telescoping."

When the locking cam engages the screw head appropriately, the cam driver "clicks." Extremes in screw angulation (>16 degrees) can prevent the cam system from formally engaging the screw head and cause the cam to continue to rotate as directed by the cam driver. In this case, the cam can be left in its "lock zone" between 240 and 270 degrees of rotation to offer some resistance to the screw backing out. This incomplete contact between the locking cam and screw head further influences the degree of delayed angulation that can occur between the screw head and plate. If the plate is bent to optimize contact with the vertebral column, its curvature should be distributed evenly throughout its length and limited to the thinner, designated "bend zones" to prevent the locking cam mechanism from failing.

The more commonly used 12- and 15-mm drill bits, taps, and screws are color coded (blue and gold, re-

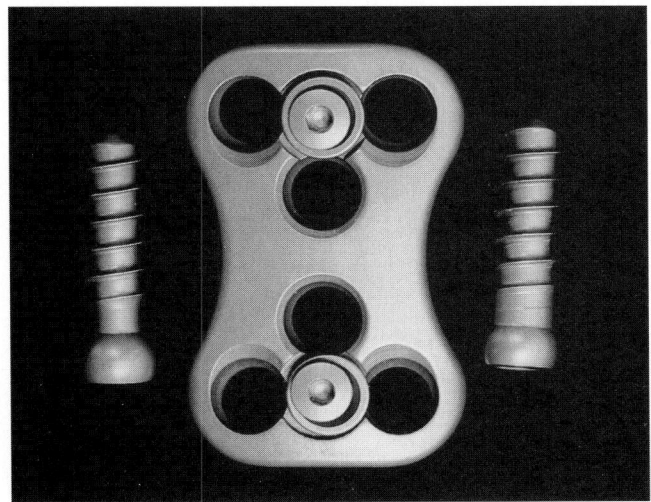

FIGURE 301–12. Atlantis plate (27.5 mm) with variable *(left)* and fixed *(right)* trajectory fixation screws. Fixation screw heads at any location on the plate are within access of one of the integrated locking screws. (From Baskin JJ, Vishteh AG, Dickman CA, Sonntag VKH: Techniques of anterior cervical plating. Operative Tech Neurosurg 1:90–102, 1998.)

spectively) to simplify use of the system. However, a wide range of screw lengths is available, and they can be inserted using the available variable-depth drill guide and taps. All screws in this system are 4.5 mm in diameter, the size typically reserved for "rescue" screws in other systems. The recommended screw placement is 10 degrees medially and parallel to the orientation of the adjacent disk space in the sagittal plane. The recommended plate length is from the rostral subchondral region of the most rostral vertebral body to the caudal subchondral region of the most caudal vertebral body included in the fusion construct.[44]

ATLANTIS SYSTEM

With the Atlantis system (Sofamor Danek, Memphis, TN), fixed or variable screw trajectories are available for any plate level or screw site (Figs. 301–12 and 301–13). The system includes specific drill guides that

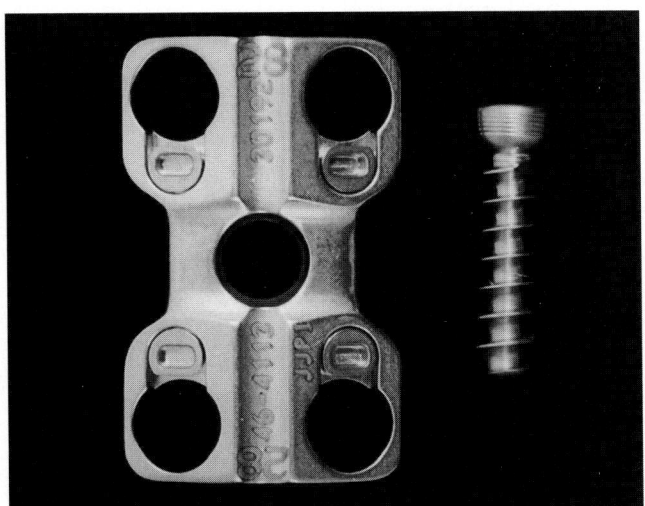

FIGURE 301–11. Codman plate (28 mm) with fixation screw. Note the integrated locking cam mechanism. Each fixation screw site has its own individual corresponding locking cam site. (From Baskin JJ, Vishteh AG, Dickman CA, Sonntag VKH: Techniques of anterior cervical plating. Operative Tech Neurosurg 1:90–102, 1998.)

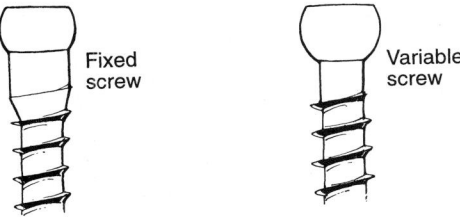

FIGURE 301–13. The fixed and variable trajectory screws of the Atlantis system. The configuration of the head and proximal shaft of the fixed screw results in a rigid or constrained interface with the Atlantis plate in contrast to the nonconstrained interface between the variable screw and the Atlantis plate. (Courtesy of Barrow Neurological Institute, St. Joseph's Hospital and Medical Center, Phoenix, AZ.)

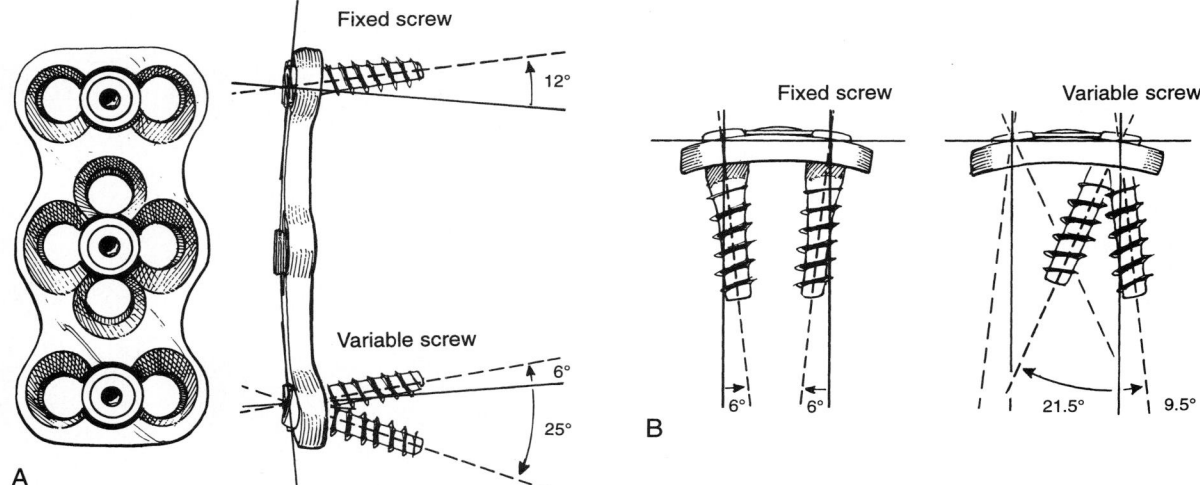

FIGURE 301–14. *A,* Anterior and sagittal views of the Atlantis plate. The sagittal view shows the fixed screw trajectory angled 12 degrees rostral to a line that is perpendicular to the plate at the rostral screw site and the range of angulation available with the variable screw at the caudal screw site. Because the screw hole is eccentric on the plate, the arc of rotation possible in the sagittal plane is 6 degrees toward the plate relative to a line perpendicular to the plate, or 25 degrees from this line. *B,* Axial view of the Atlantis plate showing the fixed medial (convergent) trajectory of 6 degrees relative to a line drawn perpendicular to the plate and the angulation available with the variable screw (4-mm diameter) relative to the same perpendicular line. The degree of angulation possible in the axial and sagittal planes is less with the larger diameter 4.5-mm screw. (Courtesy of Barrow Neurological Institute, St. Joseph's Hospital and Medical Center, Phoenix, AZ.)

either lock in a fixed position in the plate screw hole (12 degrees divergent in sagittal plane, 6 degrees medially convergent) or allow variable angulation through an arc of approximately 31 degrees relative to the axis of the screw hole (Fig. 301–14). The diameter of the holding pin available for "hands-off" stabilization of the plate during drilling is small enough that an anchoring screw can ultimately be passed along its track (Fig. 301–15). The option of fixed or variable screw trajectories within any one plate-hole site enables the produc-

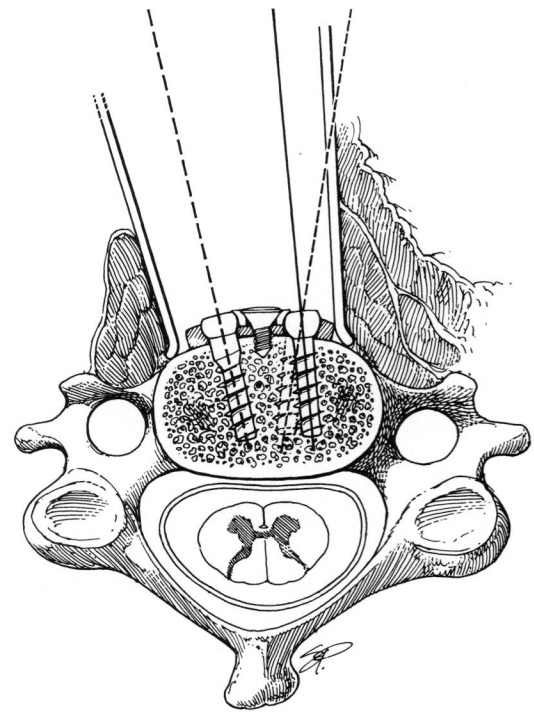

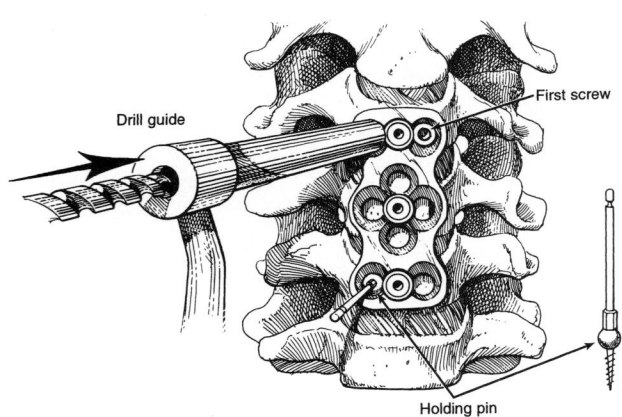

FIGURE 301–15. A holding pin is available to stabilize the plate while other screw sites are drilled and tapped. The individual plate holes in the Atlantis system can accommodate either a fixed or variable trajectory drill guide or screw. A locking screw is available for all plate-hole sites. (Courtesy of Barrow Neurological Institute, St. Joseph's Hospital and Medical Center, Phoenix, AZ.)

FIGURE 301–16. Atlantis plate system with a fixed trajectory screw (medially directed) used at one position and a variable trajectory screw at the neighboring site. This flexibility allows the surgeon to compensate for a patient's aberrant anatomy or for suboptimal screw positions or purchases. Consequently, the biomechanical stability of the fixation construct can be optimized. (Courtesy of Barrow Neurological Institute, St. Joseph's Hospital and Medical Center, Phoenix, AZ.)

tion of constrained, nonconstrained, or hybrid biomechanical constructs based on the underlying pathologic condition of the vertebral column (Fig. 301–16).

The locking mechanism of the Atlantis plate consists of a locking screw and washer, which compress and cover the fixation screw heads in pairs (Fig. 301–17). Similar to the Codman system, extremes in screw angulation can result in an incomplete interface between the anchor screw and locking mechanism. At the time of screw insertion, it is important to make certain that the locking washer remains above the level of the fixation screw head. Because of its mobility while in an "unlocked" position, the locking washer can be caught under the head of the anchor screw as the latter is advanced into the vertebral body. The anchor screw would then be prevented from fully seating within its plate hole, and locking the pair of anchor screws to the plate would be precluded. The Atlantis plate is manufactured with all the locking screws in the open, elevated position. Before the wound is closed, *all* locking screws should be recessed to minimize the profile of the fixation construct.

ABC SYSTEM

Released for use in 1999, the ABC system (Aesculap, San Francisco, CA) is composed of precontoured, slotted, trapezoidal plates and a variable trajectory screw (Fig. 301–18). The screw head consists of five compressible "petals" that snap into the plate slot and prevent the screw from backing out (Fig. 301–19). The screws also have a self-contained locking mechanism: An internal pin, engaged by a locking tool, can be pulled up into the screw head and functions to "block" the petals in their respective positions and to secure the screw head rigidly to the plate (Fig. 301–20). Although the

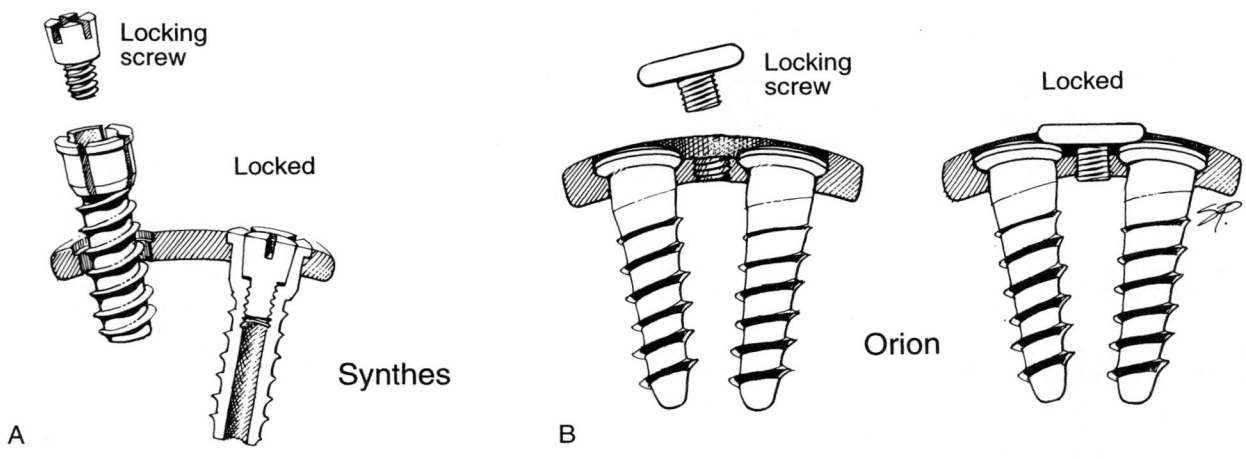

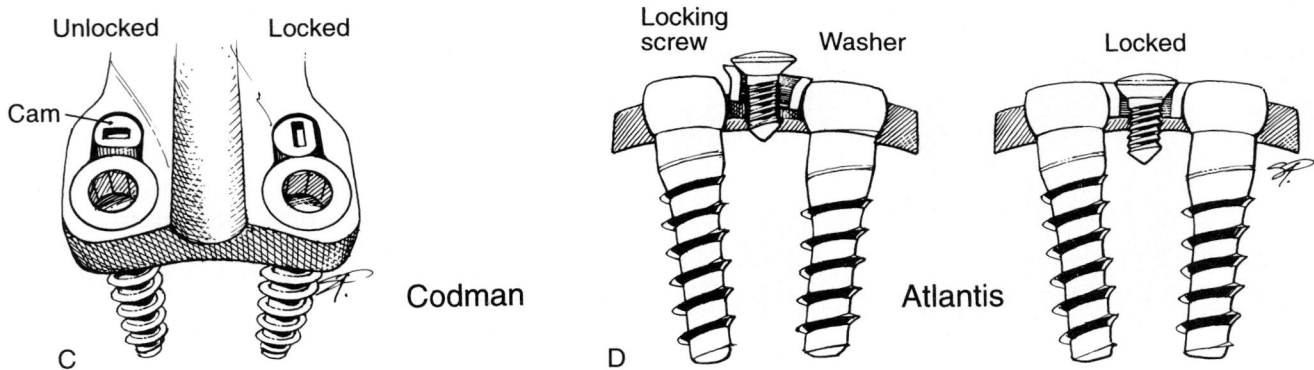

FIGURE 301–17. Comparison of the screw-locking mechanisms offered by the Synthes *(A)*, Orion *(B)*, Codman *(C)*, and Atlantis *(D)*, cervical plating systems. (Courtesy of Barrow Neurological Institute, St. Joseph's Hospital and Medical Center, Phoenix, AZ.)

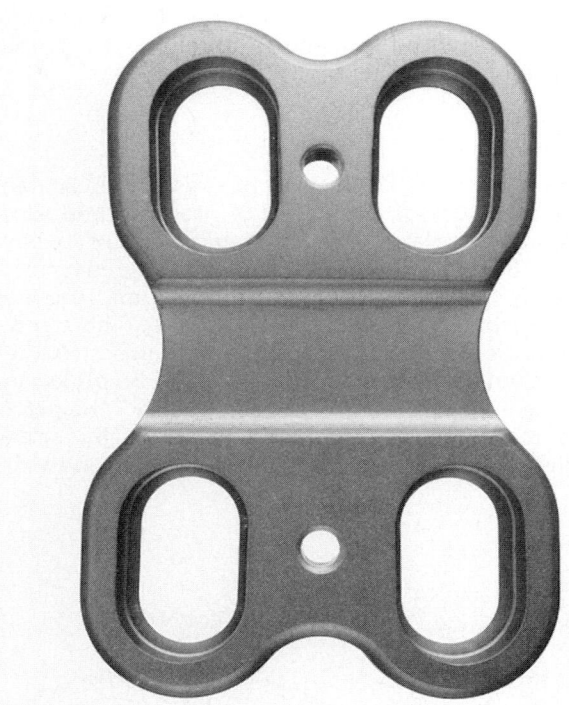

FIGURE 301–18. ABC trapezoidal plate. The slotted configuration promotes load sharing by allowing vertical settling of the fixation construct. Midline holes are for the holding pins. (Courtesy of Aesculap Anterior Plating System, South San Francisco, CA.)

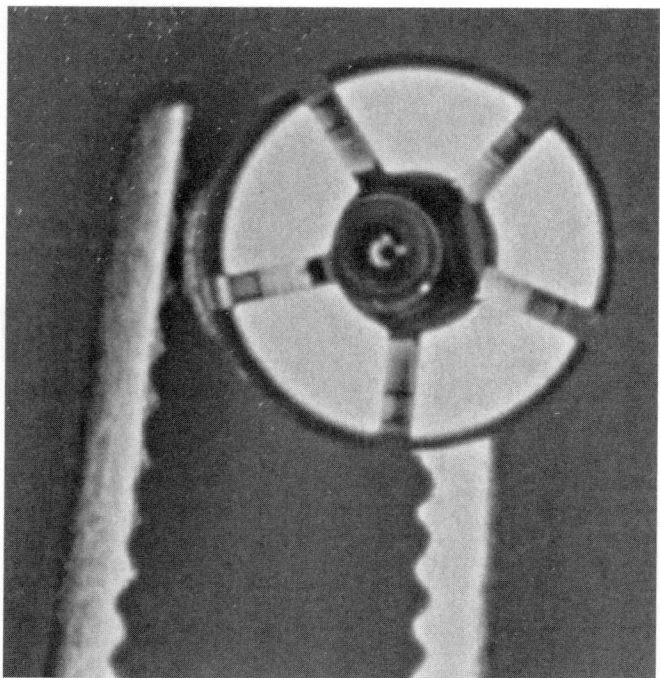

FIGURE 301–19. Axial view of the ABC screw head. The head is composed of five compressible "petals" that snap into the ABC plate slot. The top of the internal "blocking pin" is recessed within the screw shaft (unlocked position). (Courtesy of Aesculap Anterior Plating System, South San Francisco, CA.)

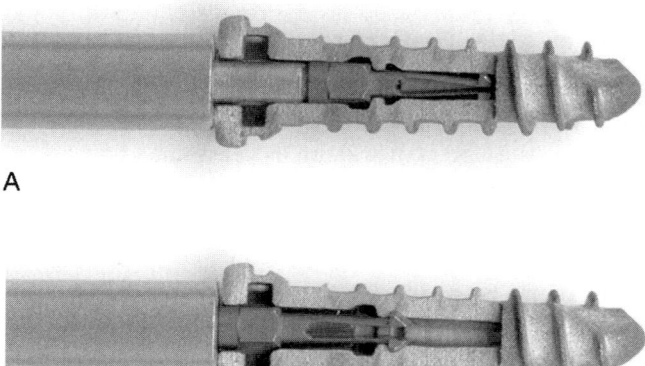

FIGURE 301–20. Longitudinal view of the ABC screw with internal blocking pin in the unlocked *(A)* and locked *(B)* positions. When engaged, the blocking pin prevents compression of the screw head's petals, thus rigidly locking the screw head to the plate (fixed pitch). (Courtesy of Aesculap Anterior Plating System, South San Francisco, CA.)

angle between the screw head and plate is fixed (constrained), the screws can migrate vertically within their slots. This capacity to maintain axial loading despite graft subsidence permits load sharing by minimizing the presence of "stress shielding" and promotes fusion.[45]

The screws are available in self-tapping unicortical and nontapping flat-tipped bicortical versions. The system design allows angulation of plus or minus 30 degrees in the vertical axis and plus or minus 8 degrees medially and laterally in the coronal axis. The optimal ABC plate length is one in which the midpoints of the uppermost and lowermost screw slots overlie the adjacent graft–vertebral body interface. Stated in other terms, 50% of the screw slot should overlap the graft and 50% should overlap the adjacent vertebral body. To further accommodate settling, the individual screws should be positioned at the most distal aspect of their respective slots. These positions should correspond to an entry site at the most caudal end of the rostral vertebral body and the rostral end of the most caudal vertebral body. Temporary fixation pins can be placed through designated holes along the plate's midline axis to stabilize it during insertion.

COMPLICATIONS

The risks related to screw-plate stabilization of the cervical spine include all risks intrinsic to a routine anterior cervical diskectomy and fusion procedure[46, 47]: injury to branches of the vagus nerve (recurrent or superior laryngeal nerves), dysphagia, radicular or myelopathic injury, cerebrospinal fluid leakage, infection, graft migration, postoperative hematoma, stroke and, if autologous graft is used, donor-site morbidity. The development of pseudarthrosis (fibrous union) and instrumentation failure are intimately related. The primary occurrence of either can result directly in the other and necessitate revision of the entire fusion and fixation construct. Alternatively, successful arthrodesis can develop in the presence of failed instrumentation,[48, 49] thus illustrating the "race" between bony healing and implant fatigue. In this circumstance, the need to remove the hardware is not absolute and would have to be considered in the context of the patient's symptoms (if any) and the risk for tracheoesophageal or neurovascular injury.

CONCLUSIONS

Anterior cervical plating has dramatically changed the treatment of the structurally compromised vertebral column. For patients in whom cervical immobilization with a halo orthosis would have historically been considered (those recovering after fusion for trauma, tumor, infectious processes, or severe degeneration), internal fixation with a screw-plate system may obviate this requirement. Several anterior cervical plating systems are available for stabilizing and reconstructing a structurally compromised vertebral column. Regardless of what accompanying instrumentation is used, the basis for a successful arthrodesis remains meticulous preparation of the graft and recipient bed.

A socioeconomic argument for using screw-plate systems after anterior cervical diskectomy and fusion is that patients who receive these implants may require briefer hospitalizations, may have less or no need for an external cervical orthosis, and may return to work earlier than those who undergo cervical fusion procedures without plating. The cost of plates and screws varies greatly among systems. Individual hospital contracts with manufacturers can dramatically influence the cost of using one instrumentation construct compared with another. The figures listed in Table 301–3 reflect the manufacturers' catalog citations for the year 2000. Additional surgeons' fees for performing internal fixation, the extra operating time needed, the expense and radiation exposure associated with the fluoroscopy necessary to perform this procedure safely, and postoperative radiography are other variables that should be considered when calculating the cost-to-benefit ratio of screw-plate insertion.

As experience with anterior cervical plating systems has increased, the differences in operative time between procedures that incorporate plating and those that do not continue to narrow. Later generations of screw-plate systems have become progressively easier to insert, offering the convenience of unicortical bone screw purchase, an integrated locking mechanism to prevent retropulsion of the anchoring screws, and self-tapping screws. Anterior cervical plates are an integral method of treatment for the diseased cervical spine.

REFERENCES

1. Caspar W: Anterior stabilization with the trapezial osteosynthetic plate technique in cervical spine injuries. In Kehr P, Weidner A (eds): Cervical Spine I. New York, Springer-Verlag, 1987, pp 198–204.

2. Caspar W, Barbier DD, Klara PM: Anterior cervical fusion and Caspar plate stabilization for cervical trauma. Neurosurgery 25:491–502, 1989.
3. Suh PB, Kostuik JP, Esses SI: Anterior cervical plate fixation with the titanium hollow screw plate system: A preliminary report. Spine 15:1079–1081, 1990.
4. Tippets RH, Apfelbaum RI: Anterior cervical fusion with the Caspar instrumentation system. Neurosurgery 22:1008–1013, 1988.
5. Shapiro S: Banked fibula and the locking anterior cervical plate in anterior cervical fusions following cervical discectomy. J Neurosurg 84:161–165, 1996.
6. Aebi M, Zuber K, Marchesi D: Treatment of cervical spine injuries with anterior plating: Indications, techniques, and results. Spine 16:S38–S45, 1991.
7. Apfelbaum RI, Kriskovich MD: On the incidence, cause, and prevention of recurrent laryngeal nerve palsies during anterior cervical spine surgery [abstract]. Paper presented at the 27th Annual Meeting of the Cervical Spine Research Society, Salt Lake City, Utah, 1999.
8. Mendenhall Associates: 1999 Spinal Surgery Update. Orthopedic Network News 10:1–20, 1999.
9. Hadley MN, Sonntag VKH: Cervical disc herniations: The anterior approach to symptomatic interspace pathology. Neurosurg Clin N Am 4:45–52, 1993.
10. White AA, Panjabi MM: Biomechanical considerations in the surgical management of the spine. In White AA, Panjabi MM (eds): Clinical Biomechanics of the Spine. Philadelphia, Lippincott-Raven, 1990, pp 511–634.
11. Denis F: The three column spine and its significance in the classification of acute thoracolumbar spinal injuries. Spine 8:817–831, 1983.
12. McAfee PC, Bohlman HH: One-stage anterior cervical decompression and posterior stabilization with circumferential arthrodesis: A study of twenty-four patients who had a traumatic or a neoplastic lesion. J Bone Joint Surg Am 71:78–88, 1989.
13. McNamara MJ, Devito DP, Spengler DM: Circumferential fusion for the management of acute cervical spine trauma. J Spinal Disord 4:467–471, 1991.
14. Stauffer ES, Kelly EG: Fracture-dislocations of the cervical spine: Instability and recurrent deformity following treatment by anterior interbody fusion. J Bone Joint Surg Am 59:45–48, 1977.
15. Van Peteghem PK, Schweigel JF: The fractured cervical spine rendered unstable by anterior cervical fusion. J Trauma 19:110–114, 1979.
16. Sonntag VKH: Point of view. Spine 22:2625, 1997.
17. Bishop RC, Moore KA, Hadley MN: Anterior cervical interbody fusion using autogeneic and allogeneic bone graft substrate: A prospective comparative analysis. J Neurosurg 85:206–210, 1996.
18. Dickman CA, Maric Z: The biology of bone healing and techniques of spinal fusion. BNI Q 10:2–12, 1994.
19. Bracken MB, Shepard MJ, Holford TR, et al: Administration of methylprednisolone for 24 or 48 hours or tirilazad mesylate for 48 hours in the treatment of acute spinal cord injury: Results of the Third National Acute Spinal Cord Injury Randomized Controlled Trial. JAMA 277:1597–1604, 1997.
20. Vishteh AG, Harrington T, Theodore N, et al: Cervical spine fusion: Allograft versus autograft [abstract]. Presented at the Rocky Mountain Neurosurgical Society, Telluride, Colorado, June 16–20, 1996.
21. Sachs B, Brennan W: Comparison of freeze-dried allograft versus autograft in anterior cervical spine fusions [abstract]. Cervical Spine Research Society meeting report, 140–142, 1992.
22. Shapiro S: Banked fibula, the locking anterior cervical plate, and allogeneic bone matrix in anterior cervical fusions following cervical discectomy. In Rengachary SS, Wilkins RH (eds): Neurosurgical Operative Atlas. Park Ridge, IL, American Association of Neurological Surgeons, 1996, pp 233–239.
23. Kurz LT, Garfin SR, Booth RE Jr: Harvesting autogenous iliac bone grafts: A review of complications and techniques. Spine 14:1324–1331, 1989.
24. Buck BE, Malinin TI, Brown MD: Bone transplantation and human immunodeficiency virus: An estimate of risk of acquired immunodeficiency syndrome (AIDS). Clin Orthop 240:129–136, 1989.

25. Ebraheim NA, Lu J, Skie M, et al: Vulnerability of the recurrent laryngeal nerve in the anterior approach to the lower cervical spine. Spine 22:2664–2667, 1997.

26. Hart AK, Greinwald JH Jr, Shaffrey CI, et al: Thoracic duct injury during anterior cervical discectomy: A rare complication: Case report. J Neurosurg 88:151–154, 1998.

27. McAllister P, Pait TG: Unicortical anterior cervical plate fixation. Techniques Neurosurg 1:117–122, 1995.

28. Paramore CG, Dickman CA, Sonntag VKH: Radiographic and clinical follow-up review of Caspar plates in 49 patients. J Neurosurg 84:957–961, 1996.

29. Harkey HL, Caspar W, Tarassoli Y: Caspar plating of the cervical spine. In Rengachary SS, Wilkins RH (eds): Neurosurgical Operative Atlas. Park Ridge, IL, American Association of Neurological Surgeons, 1992, pp 261–271.

30. Xu R, Ebraheim NA: Essential bony anatomy of the cervical spine relative to instrumentation. Neurosurg Q 8:172–179, 1998.

31. Pait TG, Killefer JA, Arnautovic KI: Surgical anatomy of the anterior cervical spine: The disc space, vertebral artery, and associated bony structures. Neurosurgery 39:769–776, 1996.

32. Golfinos JG, Dickman CA, Zabramski JM, et al: Repair of vertebral artery injury during anterior cervical decompression. Spine 19:2552–2556, 1994.

33. Benzel EC: Qualitative attributes of spinal implants. In Benzel EC (ed): Biomechanics of Spine Stabilization: Principles and Clinical Practice. New York, McGraw-Hill, 1995, pp 135–150.

34. Prolo DJ: Biology of bone fusion. Clin Neurosurg 36:135–146, 1990.

35. Kaufman HH, Jones E: The principles of bony spinal fusion. Neurosurgery 24:264–270, 1989.

36. Robinson RA, Smith GW: Anterolateral cervical disc removal and interbody fusion for cervical disc syndrome. Bull Johns Hopkins Hosp 96:223–224, 1955.

37. Wolff J, Maquet P, Furlong R: The Law of Bone Remodeling. Berlin, Springer-Verlag, 1986.

38. Dougherty PJ, Jones AAM, Sharkey N, et al: Iliac crest bone graft: Osteotome versus saw [abstract]. Cervical Spine Research Society meeting report, 1992.

39. Bohler J, Gaudernak T: Anterior plate stabilization for fracture-dislocations of the lower cervical spine. J Trauma 20:203–205, 1980.

40. Caspar W: Advances in cervical spine surgery: First experiences with trapezoidal osteosynthetic plate and a new surgical instrumentation for anterior interbody stabilization. Orthop News 4: 7–8, 1982.

41. Harkey HL: Bicortical anterior cervical plate fixation. Techniques Neurosurg 1:108–116, 1995.

42. Rengachary SS: Anterior stabilization of the cervical spine using a locking plate system. In Rengachary SS, Wilkins RH (eds): Neurosurgical Operative Atlas. Park Ridge, IL, American Association of Neurological Surgeons, 1993, pp 423–434.

43. Lowery KL: Stabilization of the cervical spine with the Orion anterior cervical plate system. In Rengachary SS, Wilkins RH (eds): Neurosurgical Operative Atlas. Park Ridge, IL, American Association of Neurological Surgeons, 1996, pp 101–108.

44. Hurlbert RJ, Sonntag VKH: Anterior cervical spine stabilization with the Codman locking plate system. In Rengachary SS (ed): Neurosurgical Operative Atlas. Park Ridge, IL, American Association of Neurological Surgeons, 1997, pp 157–165.

45. Apfelbaum RI, Dailey AT, Barbera J: Clinical experience with a new load-sharing anterior cervical plate. Paper presented at the 27th Annual Meeting of the Cervical Spine Research Society, 1999.

46. Bulger RF, Rejowski JE, Beatty RA: Vocal cord paralysis associated with anterior cervical fusion: Considerations for prevention and treatment. J Neurosurg 62:657–661, 1985.

47. Flynn TB: Neurological complications of anterior cervical interbody fusion. Spine 7:536–539, 1982.

48. Dickman CA, Fessler RG, MacMillan M, et al: Transpedicular screw-rod fixation of the lumbar spine: Operative technique and outcome in 104 cases. J Neurosurg 77:860–870, 1992.

49. McAfee PC, Farey ID, Sutterlin CE, et al: 1989 Volvo Award in basic science: Device-related osteoporosis with spinal instrumentation. Spine 14:919–926, 1989.

CHAPTER 302

Posterior Cervical Stabilization and Fusion Techniques

PAUL D. SAWIN

HISTORICAL PERSPECTIVE

The past century has witnessed major advances in the treatment of cervical spine instability. Early surgical pioneers used autogenous bone grafts applied to the posterior elements in onlay fashion to stimulate fusion. Because this technique conferred little inherent stability, lengthy periods of bed rest, traction, bracing, or all three were required to maintain proper alignment while awaiting bone healing. In 1891 Hadra[1] used a wire to secure adjacent cervical vertebrae rendered unstable by Pott's disease and trauma, and the era of internal spinal fixation was born.

Hadra's seminal work represented a quantum leap in the treatment of spinal instability by using nonbiologic materials to restore and maintain stability before bone healing. Similar reports followed, describing a variety of surgical techniques that incorporated wire to secure the posterior elements of the cervical spine. Many of these methods remain viable options for managing cervical instability in contemporary neurosurgical practice.

Although inexpensive and typically easy to perform, posterior wiring techniques do not provide rigid fixation and thus may be unsuitable for complex instability problems. To deal with these more challenging scenarios, osteosynthetic screw-rod and screw-plate systems, hook-rod fixators, and interlaminar clamps have been developed and refined in the past decade. These devices impart immediate internal stability to a cervical construct, thereby protecting the neural elements and preventing pain and deformity until the bone fusion matures and can assume this role. Thus, the need for cumbersome bracing is reduced or eliminated, patient comfort is enhanced, compliance is assured, and early mobilization and rehabilitation are facilitated. More rigid fixation also allows "shorter" fusion constructs (i.e., fewer segments incorporated) by imparting intrinsic strength, rigidity, and load-sharing properties to the construct. As a result, residual cervical motion is maximized while the motion arm created by the fusion mass is minimized.

This chapter reviews standard posterior subaxial cervical fusion techniques, emphasizing surgical indications, operative techniques, potential complications, and outcomes. More complex instability may mandate more rigid fixation strategies using screw-plate or screw-rod devices, but the options for treating less demanding pathology are wide and varied. In general terms, the choice of construct should be dictated by the surgeon's familiarity, the nature and extent of instability, and (to a lesser extent) cost.

SURGICAL INDICATIONS

Indications for spinal stabilization encompass the following: (1) to restore structural stability to the unstable spine, thereby protecting the neural elements; (2) to correct deformity; (3) to maintain reduction after a deformity is corrected; and (4) to alleviate pain.[2] Most posterior cervical fusions are undertaken to treat existing instability or to prevent instability from developing over time. In global terms, spinal instability, deformity, or both may arise from congenital-developmental anomalies, trauma, degenerative disease, inflammatory spondyloarthropathy, or neoplasia, or they may be iatrogenic as a consequence of surgical destabilization (Table 302–1). Regardless of cause, the surgeon must gauge both the nature and the extent of the existing instability and must appreciate the future demands created by progression of the underlying disease process.[3-5] The *nature* of instability refers to the loss of integrity of the specific anatomic structures that normally confer stability to the intact spine. Is the injury purely ligamentous, as with cervical facet dislocation, or is a bony injury present as well? What about the integrity of the intervertebral disk? The *extent* of instability is determined by which spinal columns (i.e., anterior, middle, posterior) are affected, as well as by the number of motion segments involved.[3, 4, 6] Establishing the nature and extent of instability before surgery allows the surgeon to judge whether surgical intervention is required and, if so, what type of construct would be optimal.

TABLE 302-1 ■ **Indications for Posterior Cervical Stabilization**

CAUSE	TYPE
Fracture	Articular facet fracture
	Pedicle or lamina fracture
	Vertebral body fracture
Ligamentous injury	Facet dislocation, capsular ligaments
	Supra- or infraspinous ligaments
	Anterior or posterior longitudinal ligaments*
Congenital	Klippel-Feil syndrome
	Segmentation anomalies
	Hemi- or block vertebrae
Spondylosis	Facet arthropathy
	Stenosis
	Intervertebral disk degeneration
Iatrogenic destabilization	Postlaminectomy, lordosis maintained
	Postlaminectomy, lordosis absent
	Postlaminectomy, established kyphosis*
	Diskectomy or corpectomy*
Infection	Diskitis
	Osteomyelitis
	Granulomatous disease
Chronic inflammation	Rheumatoid arthritis
	Ankylosing spondylitis
	Gout or pseudogout
	Other inflammatory spondyloarthropathy
Neoplasia	Primary osseous (benign, malignant)
	Metastatic osseous
	Neurogenic

*Consider anterior stabilization.

Traumatic Instability

Instability arising from trauma is the most common indication for posterior cervical stabilization and fusion.[7-11] Cervical spine injuries are identified in as many as 4% of all trauma patients, affecting about 5 persons per 100,000 population annually.[12] Flexion-type injuries are most common, constituting almost 80% of all cervical injuries.[13] The subaxial cervical segments are particularly susceptible to injury from high-energy flexion and distraction forces owing to the inherent hypermobility of the cervical spine and its relatively small and flat articular processes. Traumatic disk protrusion, vertebral body fracture, facet capsule ligament disruption, vertebral subluxation, facet dislocation, and spinal cord contusion may result from high-energy deceleration injuries.

Many patients with cervical spine injuries do not require surgery. In almost all cases, initial management consists of spinal realignment (when necessary), neural decompression (if required), and stabilization. Often, external immobilization is adequate to protect the neural elements while healing occurs if spinal alignment is acceptable and neural compression is absent. Nonoperative management is most effective when the injury is primarily osseous; ligamentous disruption is poorly responsive to conservative measures.[14, 15]

Operative intervention for open reduction and internal fixation is undertaken when conservative management is inappropriate or ineffectual. Posterior stabilization is most effective when the injury involves primarily the posterior or posterolateral elements. Facet capsule ligament disruption, facet dislocation, and fracture of the posterior elements are well suited for posterior fixation. In most cases, stabilization across the injured motion segment alone is sufficient to reestablish stability. When the instability is more severe or when less rigid fixation techniques are used, multiple levels may need to be incorporated. Posterior element fractures typically require fixation of at least one intact level above and below the level of injury to achieve a stable construct. Many of the posterior wiring techniques require intact posterior elements to be effective. Consequently, such injuries may preclude the use of these methods and favor others.

Injuries of the anterior load-bearing columns of the cervical spine or their supporting ligamentous structures are often difficult to stabilize with posterior constructs. Anterior ligamentous disruption, vertebral body fracture, and intervertebral disk injury are most effectively addressed via an anterior approach, particularly when the ventral spinal canal is compromised. In these cases, the ventral approach provides optimal neural decompression and spinal stabilization.[16] Primarily anterior column injuries have been treated effectively with posterior stabilization, but this procedure should be attempted only if the articular facets at the level of injury are intact, because these structures contribute substantially to axial load bearing under these conditions.[9, 17] If a posterior approach is chosen, multiple adjacent segments above and below the level of injury must be incorporated to minimize the risk of progressive kyphosis.[7, 8, 10]

Posterior cervical stabilization may be used to complement anterior fixation when instability is severe or when the anticipated load-bearing requirements of the ventral construct are deemed excessive. A 360-degree or circumferential fusion procedure is reserved for cases of severe three-column instability, for which a single approach would not adequately restore structural competence.[18, 19] Such an approach restores the stability in almost all motion planes and prevents the complications, such as progressive kyphosis and graft dislodgment, that may accompany ventral fixation alone.[20, 21] If an anterior-posterior arthrodesis is required, I prefer to perform both under a single anesthetic. If desired, however, each may be staged separately.

Nontraumatic Instability

Posterior cervical fixation techniques are also frequently used to address instability unrelated to trauma. Neoplastic disease, whether primary or metastatic, may create spinal instability by destroying the load-bearing elements. Additional destabilization may occur with attempts at surgical resection. Typically, instability created by malignant tumors mandates multilevel fixation, and frequently a circumferential or 360-degree approach is required. In all cases, the construct must incorporate disease-free segments, both rostral and caudal to the involved levels.[3] The surgeon also must anticipate the likelihood of disease recurrence or progression and its impact on future stability. External beam radiotherapy, when required as adjunctive treatment, creates a hostile environment for bone healing by devascularizing and destroying osteogenic precursor cells at the site. In such cases, more rigid and extensive stabilization should be considered.

Spondylotic or degenerative disease is a frequent indication for posterior cervical fixation. Segmental instability arising from degenerative disease may be encountered de novo or may be the result of surgical destabilization. For patients with cervical stenosis who undergo posterior cervical decompression, internal fixation can reduce the incidence of progressive post-laminectomy kyphotic deformities, particularly if the normal cervical lordosis has been lost. Posterior stabilization, however, is much less effective when treating established kyphosis. Such deformities are best managed with anterior reconstruction.[22]

Often, spinal stabilization is undertaken to prevent instability that may arise as a consequence of disease progression. The loss of structural integrity associated with spinal neoplasia, infection, chronic inflammatory conditions, or degenerative disease may be progressive. An accurate assessment of the underlying disease process and sound preoperative planning are required to address not only the existing instability but also the instability that will occur over time. The surgeon must attempt to gauge the demands that will be placed on a particular construct by the disease process, anticipating both the amount of support required from the implant and the duration of that requirement. In some settings, an implant must fulfill 100% of the load-bearing requirements for the remainder of the patient's life. These issues profoundly influence the selection of the appropriate construct. Consequently, solutions for most instability problems must be formulated on a case-by-case basis.

CONSTRUCT SELECTION AND DESIGN

Frequently, several stabilization alternatives may be acceptable to treat a given problem. If there is no clear advantage among stabilization options, the technique selected should be determined by the following: the surgeon's familiarity, the patient's bone quality, the patient's general medical and neurological condition, postoperative bracing requirements, imaging compatibility, the patient's comfort and compliance, and cost.

General Considerations

In assessing the structural ramifications of cervical disease, three questions must be answered: Is the spine stable or unstable? If it is unstable, how severe is the structural embarrassment? Is surgical intervention the best way to restore stability? In theory, spinal instability is a difficult concept to define. White and Panjabi offered perhaps the most widely accepted definition of

TABLE 302–2 ■ **Grading Scale for Instability in Cervical Spine Injuries**

CRITERION	POINT VALUE*
Anterior elements incompetent	2
Posterior elements incompetent	2
Translation (sagittal plane) >3.5 mm	2
Angulation (sagittal plane) >11 degrees	2
Positive stretch test	2
Spinal cord injury	2
Nerve root injury	1
Disk space narrowing	1
"Dangerous" loading anticipated	1

*Cervical instability if total >5 points.
Data from White AA, Panjabi MM: Biomechanical considerations in the surgical management of the spine. In White AA, Panjabi MM (eds): Clinical Biomechanics of the Spine. Philadelphia, JB Lippincott, 1990, pp 511–634.

clinical spinal instability: "loss of the ability of the spine under physiologic loads to maintain its pattern of displacement so that there is no initial or additional neurological deficit, no major deformity, and no incapacitating pain."[2] Even this definition, however, is unwieldy in the clinical setting, because the terminology is overly qualitative and not readily quantifiable.

Fortunately, determining instability in practice is usually more straightforward. Instability of the cervical spine is suggested by static radiographs and, if necessary, confirmed by dynamic studies. Static studies include plain radiography, computed tomography, myelography, and magnetic resonance imaging. Frequently, cervical instability can be predicted on the basis of these studies alone. Occasionally, dynamic studies, consisting primarily of flexion-extension radiographs and, less frequently, pluridirectional tomography, are required to identify occult instability. Dynamic radiographs are particularly useful for identifying an isolated ligamentous injury, such as capsular disruption without associated bony fracture. Of course, dynamic radiographs should be avoided when static films demonstrate significant structural compromise and in unconscious patients.

Several grading schemes have been established to identify and quantify cervical instability. White and colleagues proposed a point system predicated on the radiographic appearance of the injury and the presence or absence of neurological deficit (Table 302–2).[23] An extrapolation of Denis's three-column thoracolumbar fracture classification scheme is often applied to cervical spine injuries (Table 302–3).[6] Although often useful in gauging the degree of structural compromise and the resultant instability, these grading strategies have their limitations. They were developed to assess acute traumatic injury and thus may not apply to instability arising from tumors, infections, or degenerative diseases. Further, none has been subjected to stringent evaluation in clinical outcome studies. Consequently, they should be considered only as guidelines that can be used in the context of each clinical scenario.

Nonoperative Treatment

Once the presence of cervical instability has been established, a treatment strategy must be developed and

TABLE 302-3 ■ **Denis's Three-Column Classification Scheme for Acute Spinal Injuries**

LOAD-BEARING COLUMN*	ANATOMIC CONSTITUENTS
Anterior	Anterior longitudinal ligament
	Anterior annulus fibrosus
	Anterior vertebral body
Middle	Posterior longitudinal ligament
	Posterior annulus fibrosus
	Posterior vertebral body
Posterior	Posterior neural arch
	Articular facets
	Supraspinous and infraspinous ligaments

*Instability with injury to two or more columns.

Data from Denis F: The three column spine and its significance in the classification of acute thoracolumbar spinal injuries. Spine 8:817–831, 1983.

instituted. Treatment options are surgical (internal fixation) or nonsurgical (external orthoses for immobilization). In select cases with minimal instability, a simple cervical collar may be all that is required to restore stability and promote healing.

Frequently, however, nonoperative stabilization of more significant cervical injuries requires the use of a halo vest. This device is the most effective means of immobilizing the cervical spine externally.[24] Despite its substantial encumbrances, however, the halo vest allows considerable segmental motion through a process of paradoxical spinal motion described as "snaking."[25] Segmental motion is restricted but not abolished. The average residual of normal flexion and extension across each subaxial segment is 31%.[26] In highly unstable cervical injuries, the residual motion allowed by the halo vest may be clinically significant, permitting progressive deformity and neurological injury.

Nonoperative stabilization with external immobilization is most effective for treating primarily bony injuries in which bone healing contributes significantly to restoring spinal stability.[27] Purely ligamentous injuries, such as cervical facet dislocations, heal poorly with bracing alone and often fail nonoperative treatment.[14, 15, 27, 28] Hadley and coworkers reported a 23% incidence of persistent instability despite prolonged halo vest immobilization in patients with cervical facet dislocations.[27] Of those who failed nonoperative treatment, most had ligamentous disruption alone without an associated facet fracture. If an injury is primarily ligamentous, surgical treatment for internal fixation should be considered strongly.

Operative Stabilization

Internal fixation is the most reliable means of restoring structural integrity to an unstable spinal motion segment. The procedure may involve simple maneuvers such as intraspinous wiring or more complicated techniques requiring screw fixation of the cervical lateral masses or pedicles. To select the appropriate technique

for a given instability problem, the surgeon must appreciate the structural demands created by the injury. If the degree of instability is mild and the demands on the construct are relatively small, a simple wiring technique may suffice. More severe instability necessitates a more aggressive surgical approach. Optimal construct design requires matching the implant with the instability on a case-by-case basis.[3, 4]

As a general rule, posterior stabilization techniques are most effective when used to treat pathology involving the dorsal, rather than ventral, spinal elements. Nonetheless, some authors have reported successful stabilization of vertebral body fractures and anterior ligamentous injuries with posterior constructs.[7, 10, 17] In most cases, however, it is unreasonable to expect any implant to function optimally when placed in a biomechanically disadvantageous position.

All posterior instrumentation provides a measure of immediate internal stability to the injured cervical spine. None, however, confers long-term structural integrity, which requires bony fusion. Bone, as well as other dynamic fixators such as wire or braided cables, exhibits "plastic" properties at the implant-bone interface, deforming and reforming as stress is applied.[29] With repetitive loading, even the most rigid construct permits some segmental motion across the sites of fixation. Unless bone fusion ensues, the implant will fail. Consequently, the long-term stability of any spinal fixation construct depends on the quality of the bone fusion.

With few exceptions, cervical implants are applied in the neutral mode. In contrast, thoracolumbar fixation devices can be applied in distraction, compression, neutral, flexion, extension, or lateral bending modes. Therefore, cervical deformity must be reduced and anatomic spinal alignment restored before internal fixation. Generally, posterior cervical implants are used to maintain alignment, not to accomplish reduction. Even with the most rigid devices, the reductive forces that can be applied are small and usually insufficient to achieve anatomic spinal alignment.

Posterior cervical instrumentation restores stability through several mechanisms of load bearing. Almost all function involves tension-band fixators that reestablish the integrity of the posterior tension band to resist flexion. Some techniques, such as interspinous wiring, afford little else, conferring almost no resistance to extension, lateral bending, or axial rotation.[30] Other more rigid devices such as articular mass plates or plate-screw or rod-screw constructs provide three-point bending and fixed or nonfixed cantilever beam fixation in addition to their tension-band function. These more complex load-bearing mechanisms confer pluridirectional stability, resisting flexion, extension, lateral bending, axial rotation, and axial loading.

In practice, selecting the most appropriate posterior fixation construct for a given clinical scenario requires understanding the characteristics of these implants as they relate to the structural demands created by the pathology. Successful outcomes depend on sound preoperative planning and construct design. The implant must match the instability.

OPERATIVE TECHNIQUES

Anesthesia and Spinal Cord Monitoring

In almost all cases, posterior cervical stabilization is facilitated by general anesthesia. For patients with cervical instability or severe stenosis, laryngoscopy and endotracheal intubation must be approached with extreme caution. Awake fiber-optic laryngoscopy may be performed with little or no neck manipulation and thus affords maximal protection from iatrogenic spinal cord injury as the airway is secured. The awake patient is then positioned, and neurological function is assessed before general anesthesia is induced. This technique should be considered in all patients with known cervical instability.[7, 31] Awake laryngoscopy requires patient compliance, however, and should be avoided in patients who are unwilling or unable to cooperate. Under these circumstances, direct laryngoscopy under general anesthesia may be undertaken with great care, provided the head and neck are stabilized adequately during the intubation sequence.[31]

Patients with spinal cord injuries and resultant autonomic instability represent a particular challenge for neurosurgeons and anesthesiologists. Neurogenic shock, manifest by profound arteriohypotension and bradycardia, frequently accompanies complete cervical spinal cord injury because sympathetic tone is abolished.[27] Most anesthetic agents exacerbate arteriohypotension, and agents should be selected carefully to minimize this effect. Intraoperative hypotension must be treated aggressively with volume repletion and sympathomimetic vasopressor agents to restore intervascular volume, vascular tone, and cardiac contractility. Inadequate resuscitation can lead to additional neurological deficits as a consequence of spinal cord ischemia.[27]

Pharmacologic paralysis with neuromuscular blocking agents should be used judiciously in patients with cervical instability. The posterior cervical paraspinous musculature, which can maintain some resting tone even under profound general anesthesia, may function as a "physiologic splint" that helps maintain alignment. Neuromuscular blockade eliminates the support conferred by the cervical musculature and thus may exacerbate instability. Intraoperatively, spinal cord function can be monitored by recording somatosensory or motor evoked potentials. Spinal cord monitoring is particularly useful as an adjunct to decompressive surgery or open reduction in patients with at least partial preservation of neurological function in whom inadvertent spinal cord manipulation might be detected by a change in the amplitude, latency, or general morphology of the waveform. Although it is widely used, electrophysiologic spinal cord monitoring for trauma or degenerative disease remains controversial. If spinal cord function is monitored, baseline studies should be obtained before surgery to aid in interpretation.

Patient Positioning

Patients with cervical instability must be positioned on the operating table with great care. Inadvertent cervical manipulation could have devastating consequences. The surgeon should directly supervise all aspects of positioning and is responsible for maintaining the proper cervical alignment throughout this process. This oversight is imperative when anesthetized patients who are incapable of assisting with this task are positioned. Fluoroscopic imaging can be an invaluable tool to assess cervical alignment in real time during the positioning process.

With the exception of the occasional sitting procedure, most posterior cervical stabilization procedures are performed with the patient prone. The neck is maintained in a neutral posture or, at most, in slight extension.[4, 8, 10, 32] During exposure, alignment is maintained by axial in-line cervical traction or by rigid fixation with a pin head-holder system. Once positioning is finalized, alignment is assessed with plain radiography or cervical fluoroscopy to ensure that reduction has been maintained and alignment is optimal. For patients who are intubated while awake, positioning can be undertaken before general anesthesia is induced, affording the opportunity to assess neurological function throughout the positioning process. Any change in neurological function mandates a prompt reappraisal of cervical alignment. For patients intubated under general anesthesia, a postpositioning neurological assessment is not possible, and radiographic confirmation of alignment and evoked potential wave morphology must suffice.

Exposure

Once the patient has been positioned, general anesthesia induced, and appropriate cervical alignment verified, the surgical procedure can begin. The posterior aspect of the cervical spine is exposed via a dorsal midline approach. The operative site is prepared with antiseptic solution and draped in the usual sterile manner. Infiltration of the dermis and subcutaneous tissues with a dilute epinephrine solution provides vasoconstriction and facilitates hemostasis. The midline incision is carried sharply to the ligamentum nuchae, and self-retaining retractors are placed gently. Dissection proceeds through the superficial and deep layers of the ligamentum nuchae with cutting monopolar electrocauterization until the spinous processes are encountered. The paraspinous musculature is dissected from the spinous processes and lamina in a subperiosteal manner and retracted laterally. Sharp tissue dissection techniques are preferable to avoid inadvertent cervical manipulation. Caution must be exercised during subperiosteal dissection, particularly when the posterior elements are fractured. When feasible, supporting soft tissue elements (intraspinous or supraspinous ligaments, facet capsules) should be preserved.

The extent of surgical exposure in the rostrocaudal and mediolateral dimensions is dictated by the extent of the pathology and the method of fixation. Some techniques, such as simple interspinous wiring, require minimal exposure of the dorsal elements. Lateral mass and pedicular fixation mandates extensive lateral dissection to fully expose the lateral masses at all instrumented levels. Care should be taken to avoid trauma to the facet capsule ligaments above and below the levels to be instrumented to limit the risk of junctional instability.

Once the exposure is adequate, the primary pathology can be addressed. Persistent spinal deformity or malalignment should be corrected promptly. Despite aggressive attempts at closed reduction before surgery, some dislocations will not reduce adequately. Irreducible injuries necessitate open reduction, either with cautious intraoperative manipulation or with partial facetectomy. If spinal cord or nerve root compression persists despite restoration of anatomic spinal alignment, a decompressive procedure is undertaken. Key load-bearing elements may need to be sacrificed, which can exacerbate segmental instability. The surgeon must be prepared to reassess the degree and extent of instability continually during the decompressive procedure and to alter the stabilization strategy when necessary.

SUBAXIAL CERVICAL FIXATION TECHNIQUES

Posterior subaxial cervical fixation can be divided into four general categories: wire and cable techniques, interlaminar clamps, articular mass plates, and articular mass pedicle screw-rod or hook-rod constructs.

Wire and Cable

Many wire and cable techniques for fixation of the posterior cervical spine have been described. Each technique has its own nuances, but all posterior wiring techniques can be divided into three general subcategories: spinous process wiring, facet wiring, and sublaminar wiring. Although it is still useful for atlantoaxial and occipitocervical stabilization, sublaminar wiring has almost been abandoned as a means of securing the subaxial cervical spine, because passage of the wire is associated with a risk of neurological injury.[33, 34] Other techniques provide stability that is equivalent or superior to that associated with sublaminar wiring. Consequently, the risks of wiring are rarely justified.[34] I do not advocate the routine use of sublaminar wiring in the subaxial cervical spine, and these techniques are not discussed.

Posterior wire and cable techniques are simple to perform, require no special equipment, and use inexpensive materials. Biomechanically, these methods reconstitute the posterior tension band and so are most effective in resisting flexion.[30] Typically, wiring alone provides insufficient multiplanar stability to be used as a stand-alone construct. This type of fixation must be supplemented with bone graft, methyl methacrylate, or external bracing to augment stability until bone fusion occurs.

Wire techniques may use single-strand wire, twisted wire, or braided cables. For most of the methods described here, surgeons initially used a single-strand, small-gauge, stainless steel wire. Many surgeons now prefer to use larger-gauge wire (16 or 18 gauge) for additional strength. These thicker wires, however, are less flexible and more difficult to manipulate. Smaller braided or twisted wires afford a compromise between strength and malleability. Two strands of 22-gauge wire braided together are not only stronger but also easier to handle than a single-strand 18-gauge wire.[35] When twisted wire is passed, care must be taken to avoid "sawing" through bone.

Braided multistrand cables have replaced wire for most applications. Cables offer the advantages of higher tensile strength, more uniform distribution of applied tension, and ease of handling. Braided cables are available in stainless steel and titanium; the latter are preferable to facilitate postoperative imaging. These cables are substantially more expensive than wire, but their inherent advantages tend to offset this cost differential. Unlike wire, which deforms and "stays put," multistrand cable exhibits a property referred to as "memory." This property is probably insignificant biomechanically, but it alters the handling characteristics when applied to traditional wiring methods.

SPINOUS PROCESS WIRING TECHNIQUES

Simple Interspinous Wiring

Rogers initially described interspinous wiring in 1942 as a means to stabilize the cervical spine rendered unstable by trauma.[36] Multiple modifications have been proposed since, but the fundamental technique remains unaltered. The basic Rogers method is designed to stabilize a single subaxial cervical motion segment. Additional segments can be incorporated by repeating the maneuver at adjacent levels. The spinous processes and laminae at the levels to be stabilized are exposed as described earlier, again taking care to avoid trauma to the facet capsule and ligaments rostral and caudal, respectively. A right-angle dental drill is used to create a single hole through the base of the spinous process just dorsal to the spinal laminar junction at each level. A single wire or cable is looped in opposite directions through the hole in the superior spinous process. The cable is then double-passed through the inferior spinous process, creating a loop that encircles the caudal portion of the process. The free ends of the wire or cable are tightened as desired (Fig. 302–1). Surfaces are prepared for bone fusion by thoroughly decorticating the spinous processes and laminae and the onlay of bone graft. Graft material also may be packed medial to the wires' parasagittal limbs or within the articular spaces.

The Rogers interspinous wiring method is a simple, quick, inexpensive, and biomechanically sound treatment option for some cervical injuries if the instability is not too extensive or severe. Successful interspinous wiring requires intact posterior elements at the levels to be stabilized. If the posterior elements are competent, wiring across a single motion segment usually suffices. If the posterior elements are unsound, an intact level rostral or caudal to the unstable motion segment must be incorporated. Overtensioning of the cables or wires, which can induce cervical hyperextension and exacer-

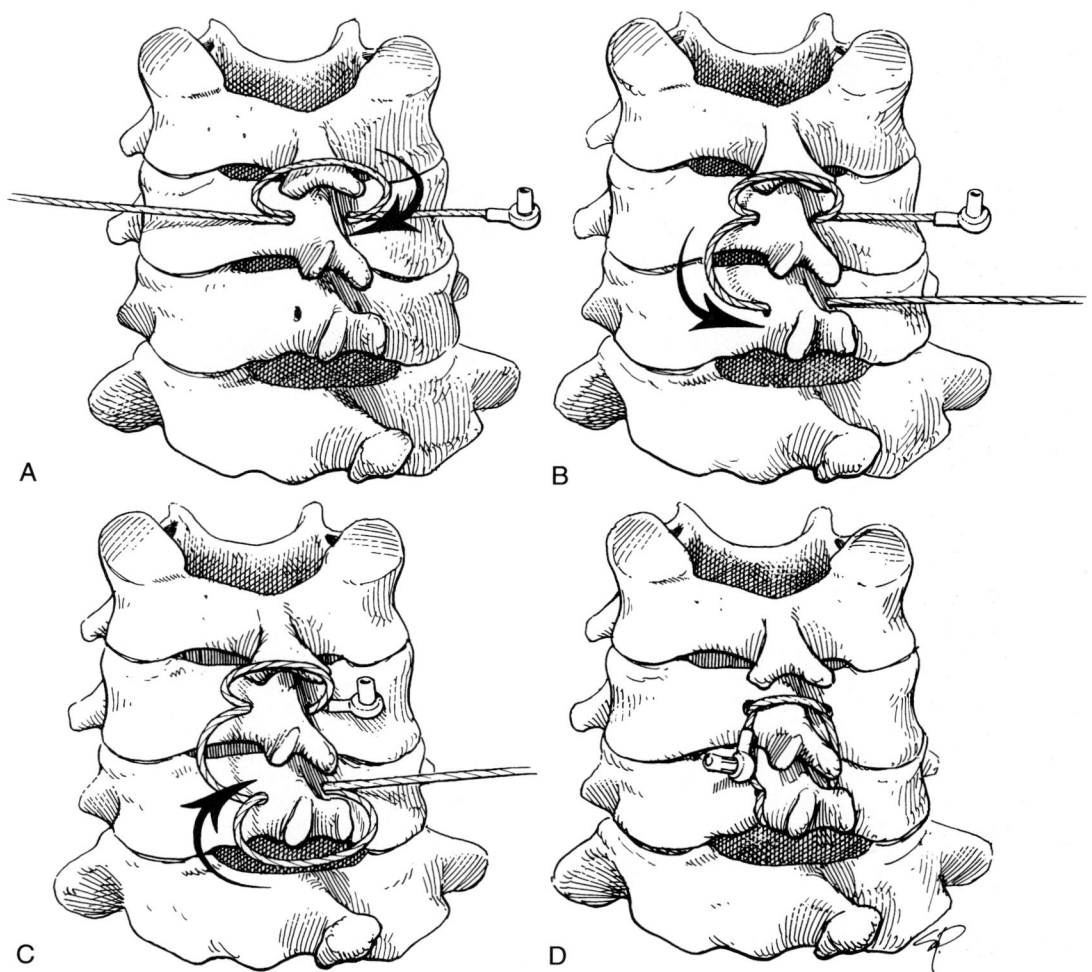

FIGURE 302–1. Rogers interspinous wiring technique. *A*, A single cable is looped through a hole in the base of the superior spinous process, with the loop passing above its respective process. *B*, The free end of the cable is passed through the inferior spinous process. *C*, The inferior loop encircles the inferior spinous process. *D*, The cable is tightened as desired. (Courtesy Barrow Neurological Institute.)

bate central canal or neural foraminal stenosis, must be avoided. A rigid external cervical brace should be worn while the bone fusion matures, because simple interspinous wiring confers insufficient immediate internal stability in most cases.

Several modifications of Rogers's original technique have been propagated. Perhaps the simplest is Whitehill's method (Fig. 302–2).[37] All simple interspinous wiring variations reestablish the integrity of the posterior tension band but serve no other function. They perform best when treating flexion-type injuries in which the anterior and middle load-bearing columns remain intact. Patients with more complex injuries, particularly those with concomitant vertebral body, intervertebral disk, or anterior ligamentous injury or those with extensive posterior element fractures, are best treated with other methods.

Interspinous Wiring with Integral Bone Grafts

Some modifications of Rogers's basic interspinous wiring technique incorporate bone graft as an integral

part of the stabilization construct. Benzel and Kesterson modified Whitehill's method by incorporating a second "compression wire" passed through the interspinous space beneath the cerclage wire.[38] This wire secures two matched corticocancellous bone grafts against the decorticated spinous processes and laminae, pressing the custom-contoured grafts against the posterior elements, cortical sides out (Fig. 302–3).

Bohlman and McAfee devised perhaps the best-known and most biomechanically sound modification of simple interspinous wiring.[39-41] The triple-wire technique uses three separate wires to stabilize each motion segment. Holes are created in the base of each spinous process as described earlier. The first wire secures the two adjacent spinous processes in the manner of Rogers. Single wires are then passed separately through each spinous process so that the horizontally oriented wires parallel one another. The bone graft is split longitudinally into two matching corticocancellous halves. The horizontal wires are passed through holes in the grafts and tightened, thereby securing the grafts

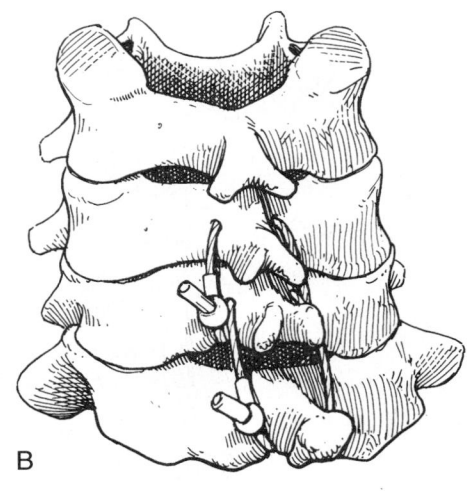

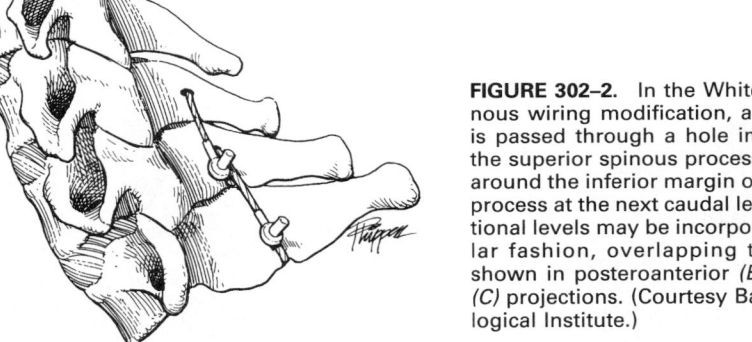

FIGURE 302–2. In the Whitehill interspinous wiring modification, a single cable is passed through a hole in the base of the superior spinous process and looped around the inferior margin of the spinous process at the next caudal level *(A)*. Additional levels may be incorporated in similar fashion, overlapping the wires as shown in posteroanterior *(B)* and lateral *(C)* projections. (Courtesy Barrow Neurological Institute.)

against the decorticated spinous processes and laminae on either side (Fig. 302–4).

These techniques offer several advantages over simple interspinous wiring. Bone grafts are incorporated as an integral part of the construct, acting as buttresses to augment torsional stability. Compression wires load the grafts, optimizing conditions for bone fusion.

FACET WIRING TECHNIQUES

The following techniques use the inferior articular facet as the primary point of attachment rather than the spinous process. Consequently, these techniques are slightly more technically demanding than interspinous wiring, although they are still fairly quick and easy to perform.

Oblique Facet Wiring

Cahill and colleagues described a technique of wiring the facet to the spinous process in an oblique fashion to treat traumatic cervical instability.[42] As originally described, this method was developed to address the unique requirements of facet fracture-dislocations because the rotational stability provided by simple interspinous wiring techniques can be inadequate to maintain reduction in this setting. This technique is also useful when the lamina or spinous process of the adjacent rostral motion segment is missing. Oblique

facet wiring stabilizes the injured motion segment without extending to an adjacent level.

The spinous processes, laminae, and articular masses of the involved motion segment are exposed in routine fashion. The inferior articular facets of the rostral vertebra are isolated, and the facet capsules are removed. The joint spaces are opened with a small elevator, and the articular cartilage is removed with a drill or fine curet. Holes are drilled through the midportion of the inferior articular processes bilaterally, perforating the bone perpendicular to the articular surfaces (Fig. 302–5A). A small dissector placed in the joint space protects the underlying nerve root and vertebral artery during drilling. A cable is passed through the articular process and looped beneath the intact spinous process of the vertebra below (see Fig. 302–5B). The maneuver is repeated on the contralateral side (see Fig. 302–5C). The spinous processes and laminae are decorticated, and bone graft is placed in onlay fashion and packed into the facet joint spaces. Fixation must be undertaken bilaterally, even in the context of unilateral facet injury. Unilateral facet–to–spinous process wiring is unsound biomechanically and can allow redislocation as a result of persistent rotatory instability.

Facet Wiring

In certain cases, the spinous processes, laminae, or both are unavailable owing to fracture or previous

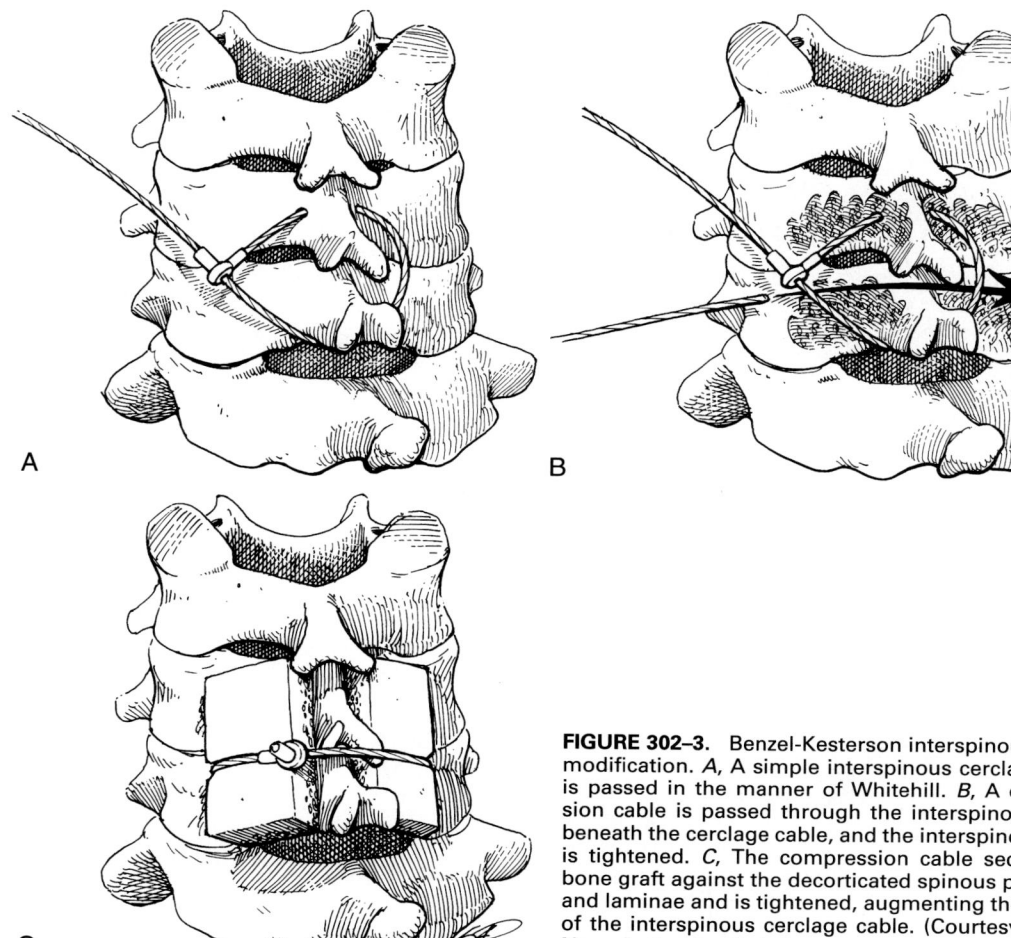

FIGURE 302–3. Benzel-Kesterson interspinous wiring modification. *A,* A simple interspinous cerclage cable is passed in the manner of Whitehill. *B,* A compression cable is passed through the interspinous space beneath the cerclage cable, and the interspinous cable is tightened. *C,* The compression cable secures the bone graft against the decorticated spinous processes and laminae and is tightened, augmenting the tension of the interspinous cerclage cable. (Courtesy Barrow Neurological Institute.)

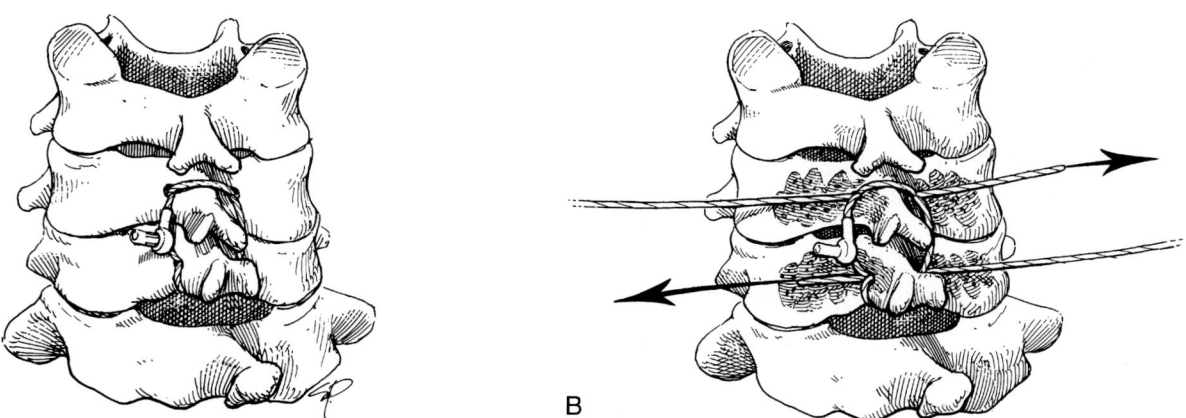

FIGURE 302–4. Bohlman triple-wire technique. *A,* The first cable creates an interspinous loop after the manner of Rogers. *B,* Two separate cables are passed through holes in the superior and inferior spinous processes.

Illustration continued on following page

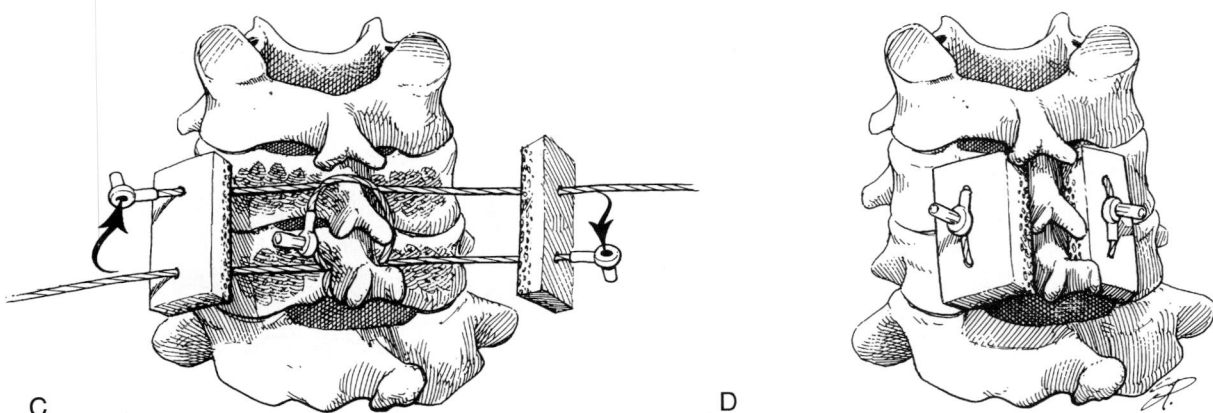

FIGURE 302–4. *Continued. C*, The ends of these cables are passed through holes in the two autologous bone grafts. *D*, The cables are tightened, securing the grafts against the decorticated spinous processes and laminae. (Courtesy Barrow Neurological Institute.)

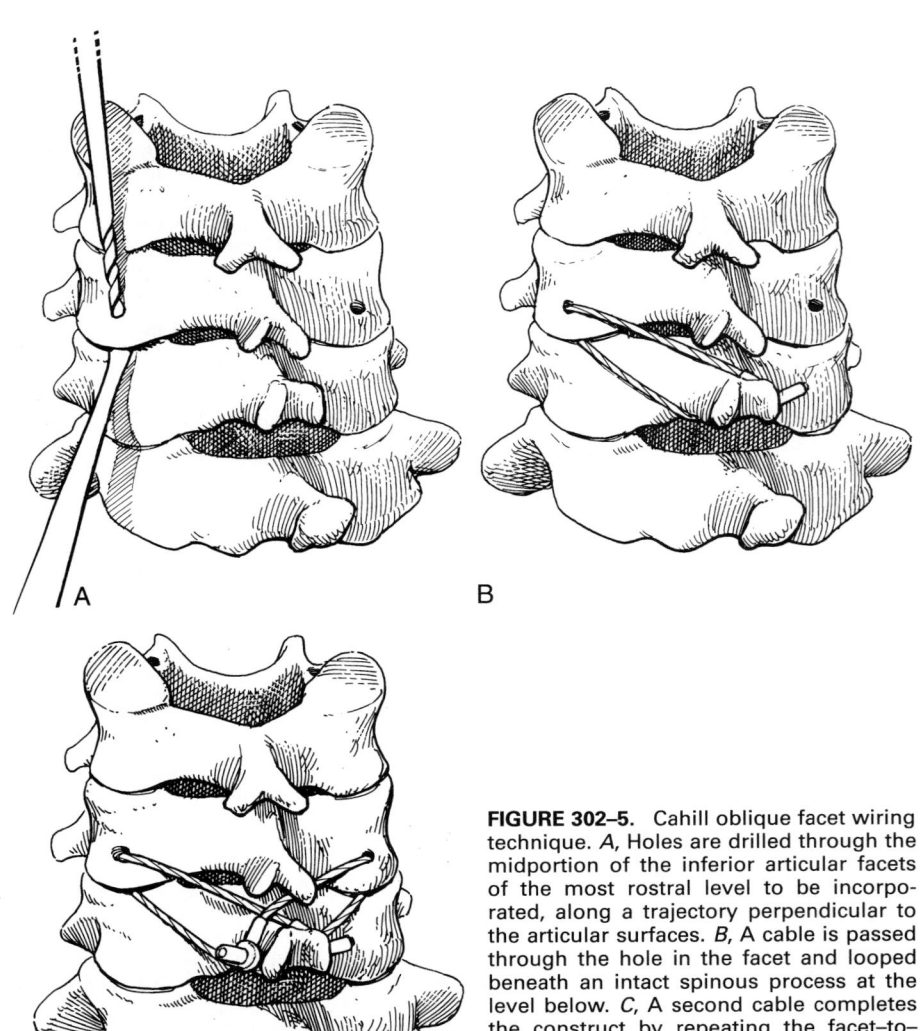

FIGURE 302–5. Cahill oblique facet wiring technique. *A*, Holes are drilled through the midportion of the inferior articular facets of the most rostral level to be incorporated, along a trajectory perpendicular to the articular surfaces. *B*, A cable is passed through the hole in the facet and looped beneath an intact spinous process at the level below. *C*, A second cable completes the construct by repeating the facet–to–spinous process wiring maneuver on the contralateral side. (Courtesy Barrow Neurological Institute.)

surgical removal. Under these conditions, the articular processes can be used for segmental fixation. Callahan and associates devised a method of facet wiring to prevent kyphosis after laminectomy.[43] This method is equally effective in the setting of trauma, where posterior element fracture can render interspinous wiring techniques infeasible. Facet wiring is relatively simple and provides multiplanar stability, resisting flexion-extension, axial rotation, and translation. Conceptually, facet wiring most closely resembles articular mass plate or rod stabilization. Both involve segmental fixation of the articular masses to a longitudinal member.

The articular masses and facet joint spaces are exposed as previously described. Holes are drilled through the inferior articular processes at each level, oriented perpendicular to the articular surfaces (Fig. 302–6A). A wire or cable is passed through each hole, rostrally to caudally, exiting through the joint space.

Two strut grafts of sufficient length to span the entire construct are procured, from either a rib or the posterior iliac crest. A rib may be preferable because its natural curvature conforms to the cervical lordosis, circumferential cortex, and length.[32] Holes are placed through the graft at intervals corresponding to the spacing of each inferior articular process. The lateral masses are decorticated, and the facet wires are passed through the graft (see Fig. 302–6B). Wires should always be passed around the medial aspect of the graft to prevent the strut from being displaced into the spinal canal. The struts are advanced over the wires and segmentally transfixed against the articular masses (see Fig. 302–6C). In lieu of bone struts, small contoured metal rods or a Luque rectangle can be used.[44] Additional bone graft may be packed into the joint spaces or placed in onlay fashion alongside the longitudinal components. The caudal end of the graft can be secured

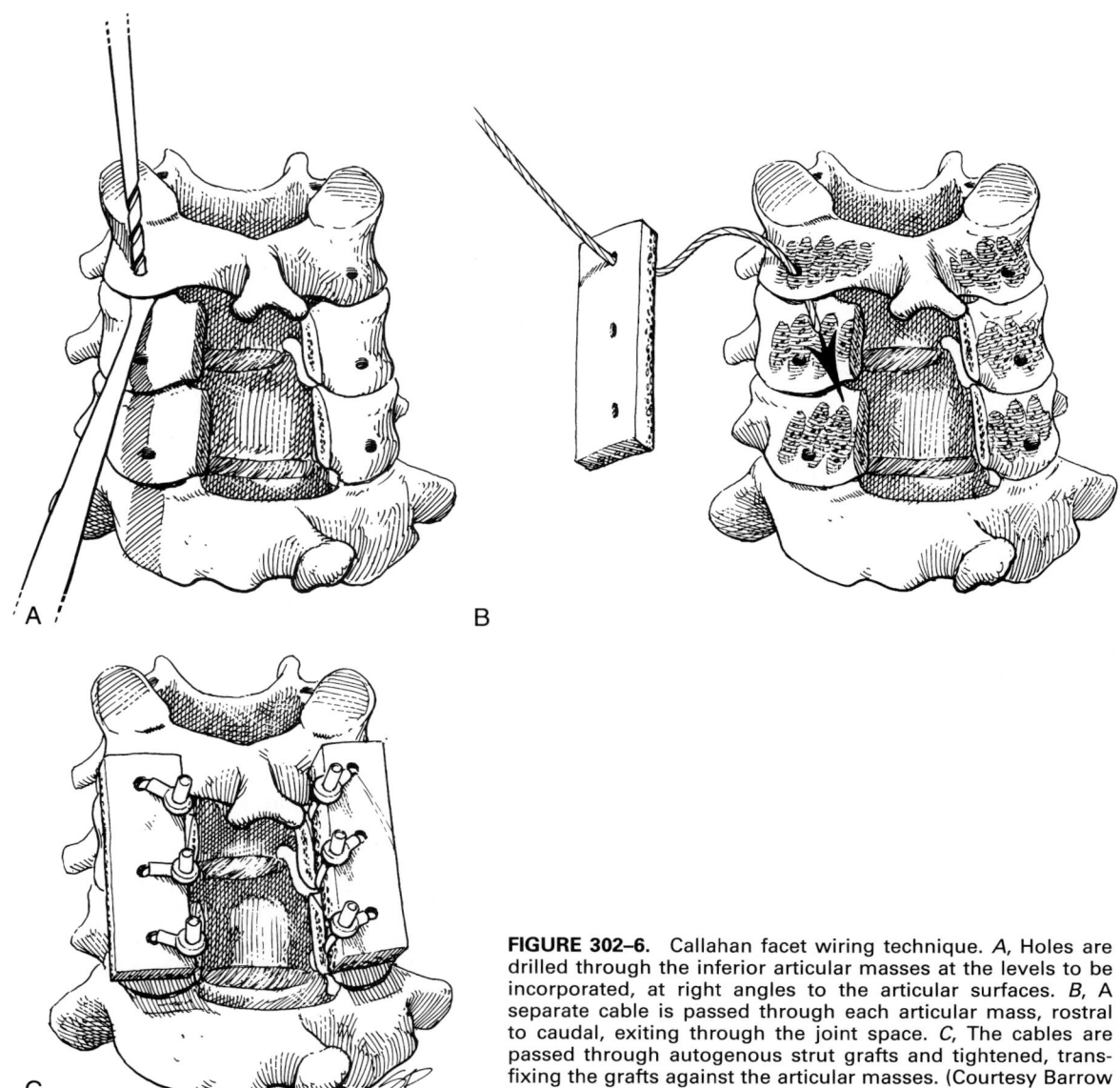

FIGURE 302–6. Callahan facet wiring technique. *A*, Holes are drilled through the inferior articular masses at the levels to be incorporated, at right angles to the articular surfaces. *B*, A separate cable is passed through each articular mass, rostral to caudal, exiting through the joint space. *C*, The cables are passed through autogenous strut grafts and tightened, transfixing the grafts against the articular masses. (Courtesy Barrow Neurological Institute.)

to the spinous process rather than to the inferior articular facet to avoid the chronic pain that occasionally results from violating an unfused facet joint.

Interlaminar Clamps

Stabilization of the subaxial cervical spine with interlaminar clamps was first described in 1975.[45] These devices are most effective for treating isolated posterior flexion injuries, because they reestablish the integrity of the posterior tension band. Although multisegmental fixation is technically possible, interlaminar clamps perform optimally when used to stabilize a single motion segment. The implants are available in a variety of sizes and configurations in both stainless steel and titanium alloy.

Interlaminar clamps are relatively easy to apply. The leading edge of the superior lamina above and the trailing edge of the inferior lamina below must be thinned bilaterally to enlarge the interlaminar spaces rostral and caudal to the unstable motion segment. Appropriately sized clamps are selected and separated into their two principal components—fitted laminar hooks. The threaded upper half of the clamp is hooked over the leading edge of the most rostral lamina, and the unthreaded lower half of the clamp is placed under the trailing edge of the most caudal lamina. A machine screw secures the two hooks. As the screw is tightened, the two laminae are apposed by drawing the hooks together (Fig. 302–7). The dorsal and dorsolateral elements are prepared for bone fusion, and the graft is applied.[46]

Although some have had acceptable results with unilateral interlaminar clamp fixation, most surgeons advocate bilateral placement to optimize fixation and augment multiplanar stability.[46–48] Multilevel fixation with these devices, which is associated with excessive construct failure, should be avoided.[46, 48] Other disadvantages of this method are the requirement for intact lamina at the levels to be instrumented and the risk of neurological deficit created by metal stenosis from the sublaminar hooks.[48]

Articular Mass Screw-Plate and Screw-Rod Fixation

Posterior stabilization of the subaxial cervical spine has been revolutionized by articular mass screw fixation. Screw-plate and screw-rod devices confer immediate internal stability, are equally effective for single and multilevel fixation, and do not require intact posterior elements for use (Fig. 302–8). Several screw-plate and three screw-rod systems are available for clinical use in the United States (Table 302–4). Curiously, none of them have been approved by the Food and Drug Administration for application in the subaxial cervical spine.

The general operative technique for articular mass screw fixation is similar for both screw-plate and screw-rod systems. There are four fundamental steps: drilling the articular masses, sizing and contouring the longitudinal component (e.g., plate or rod), selecting and placing the screw, and securing the longitudinal component.

DRILLING THE ARTICULAR MASSES

The articular masses to be instrumented are exposed fully to both their rostrocaudal and mediolateral margins. Again, care should be taken to preserve the facet capsules at the rostral and caudal limits of the construct to minimize the risk of junctional instability. Once the lateral mass has been exposed, its midpoint is identified. In most cases, drilling is initiated at a point 1 to 2 mm medial to the center of the lateral mass.

Various screw trajectories have been described. Roy-Camille and others have advocated entering the lateral mass in its center and drilling perpendicular to the sagittal plane while angling laterally 10 degrees.[10, 30] The widely used Magerl technique engages the lateral mass 1 mm medial and rostral to the center of the lateral mass, and the trajectory is drilled 25 degrees lateral and 40 degrees cephalad.[49] The cephalad angulation orients the screw parallel to the facet joint. Several variations of the Magerl technique have been described.[3, 7, 50] A lateral and cephalad screw trajectory is usually advisable to avoid injuring the nerve root and vertebral artery.

I advocate a slight variant of the Magerl technique, the so-called 25/25 trajectory.[3, 4] The lateral mass is engaged at a point 1 mm medial to its midportion. Drilling proceeds along a course 25 degrees cephalad

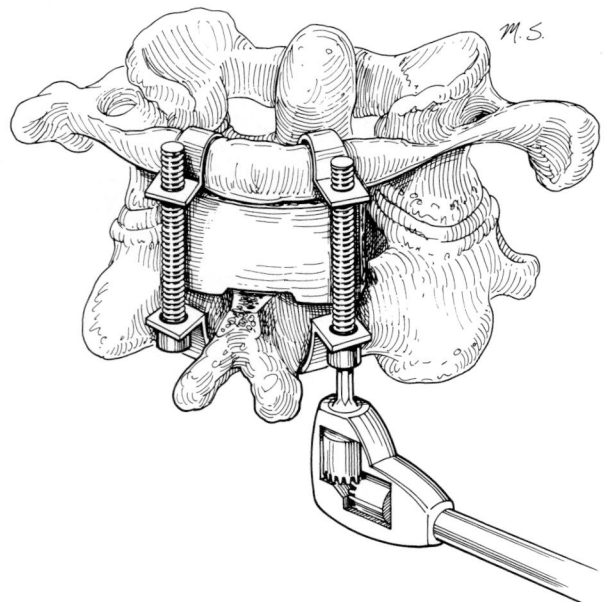

FIGURE 302–7.   Interlaminar clamps. The leading edge of the lamina above and the trailing edge of the lamina below are thinned bilaterally to increase the interlaminar spaces above and below the segment to be fused. The upper (threaded) half-clamp is hooked over the rostral lamina, and the lower (unthreaded) half-clamp is hooked under the caudal lamina. A machine screw transfixes the clamp halves and is tightened, apposing the laminae by drawing the two hooks together. (Courtesy Barrow Neurological Institute.)

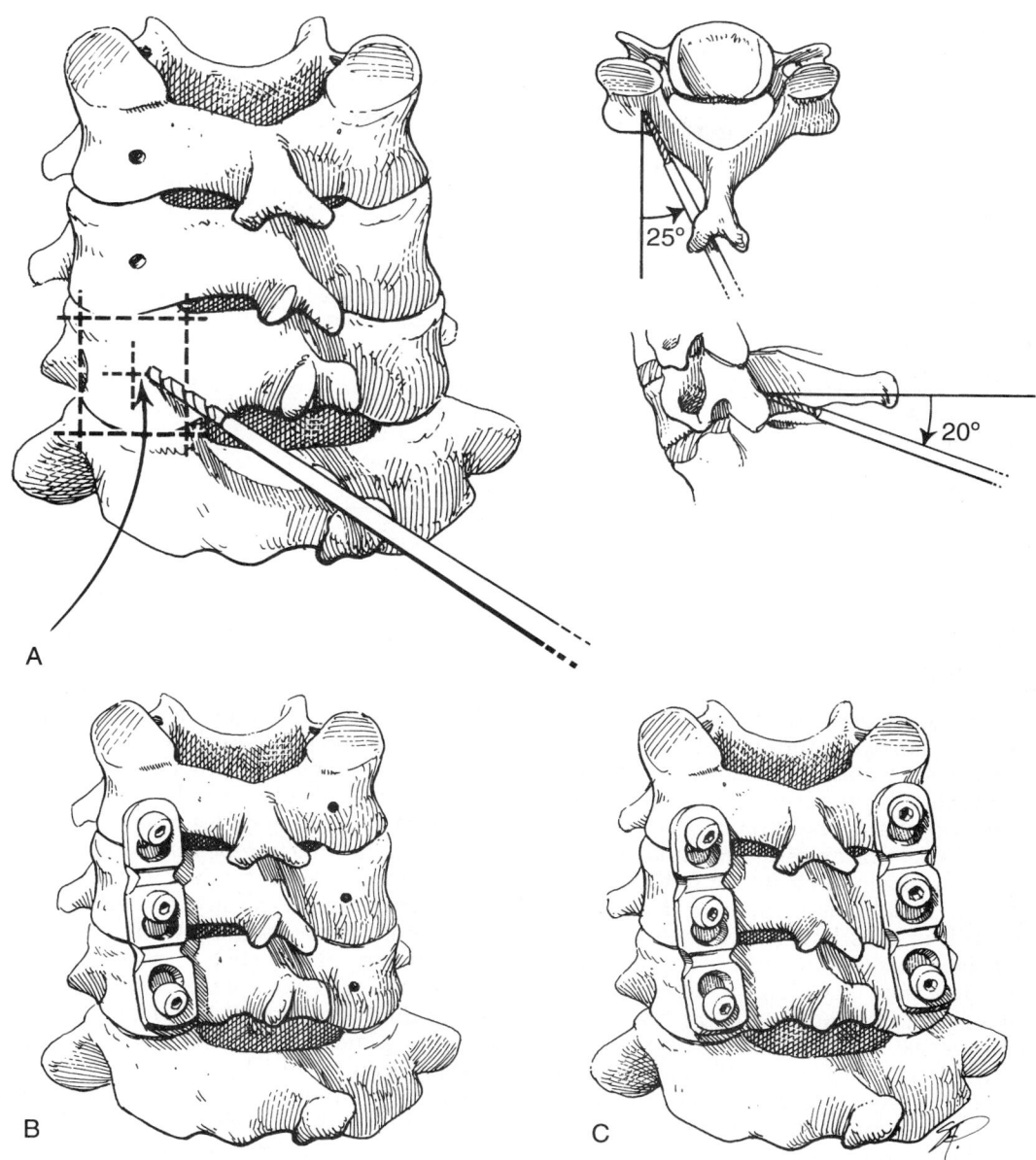

FIGURE 302–8. Articular mass plates. *A,* Holes are drilled in the inferior articular masses at each level to be incorporated, along a trajectory 15 degrees cephalad and 20 to 30 degrees lateral. *B,* The plate is sized, contoured, and secured against the lateral masses with bicortical screws at each level. *C,* The process is then repeated on the contralateral side. (Courtesy Barrow Neurological Institute.)

and 25 degrees lateral. This trajectory can be approximated by visualizing the articular mass intraoperatively as a box or cube. The drill is aimed from its entry point in the center of the dorsal surface to the superolateral corner of the ventral surface. This trajectory affords both reasonable protection from neurovascular injury and solid bicortical purchase. It can be used reliably at C3, C4, C5, and C6.

The screw trajectory is often altered somewhat due to the relatively small size of the C7 lateral mass. A slightly more lateral and cephalad trajectory often accommodates this anatomic constraint. Because fixation in the small lateral mass of C1 can be suboptimal, it is often preferable to obtain transpedicular fixation at C7 and T1. This strategy is particularly useful when the construct ends at C7 or T1, because pedicular fixation provides a solid base for the caudal end of the construct. The C7 and T1 pedicles tend to be large and may be entered 1 mm caudal to the facet joint along a trajectory medialized 25 to 30 degrees.[3, 4] A small laminotomy allows direct visualization and palpation of the pedicle to assist in accurate screw placement. Alternatively, image guidance with frameless stereotaxy can be used to help place transpedicular screws.

Each screw hole should be positioned optimally in its respective lateral mass. Therefore, holes are oriented with reference to the patient's anatomy, not placed

T A B L E 3 0 2 – 4 ■ **Features of Posterior Cervical Screw-Rod Systems**

	ROD-SCREW SYSTEM		
FEATURE	**Cervifix Starlock**	**Summit**	**Vertex**
Material	Titanium	Titanium alloy	Titanium alloy
Screw diameter (mm)	3.5/4.0	3.5/4.5	3.5/4.0
Screw length (mm)	8–54	8–30	10–52
Self-tapping	Yes	Yes	No
Hooks	Yes	No	Yes
Rod diameter (mm)	3.5	3.0	3.2
Connectors	Lateral offset	Polyaxial screw, lateral offset	Polyaxial screw, lateral offset
Sagittal angulation (degrees)	0–50	0–60	0–60
Screw-rod interface	0–50	0–60	0–60
Crosslink	Yes	Yes	Yes
Profile (mm)	8	10	11
Approved for cervical use	Yes*	No	Yes*

*Hooks only; screws approved for occipital and thoracic use only.

according to the "lie" of the hardware. This issue is of greater concern with screw-plate instrumentation than with screw-rod devices because of the decreased rostrocaudal and mediolateral variability inherent in posterior cervical plate constructs. To minimize this tendency, drilling screw holes through the plate should be avoided. The fixation system should be sufficiently versatile to accommodate properly positioned screws.

Once the entry point and the screw trajectory have been selected, the outer cortex of the articular mass is pierced with an awl or small cutting bur to facilitate initial drilling. The lateral masses may be drilled with an unprotected drill or Kirschner wire. To avoid overpenetration, however, a drill bit with a depth stop at 14 to 16 mm is preferable. Toggling, which may yield an irregular or oversized hole, should be minimized. Toggling is of greatest concern when a high-speed power drill is used. Drilling by hand reduces these concerns. Bicortical screw purchase is desirable, and typically the drill bit can be felt penetrating the anterolateral cortex of the lateral mass. If penetration occurs before the predetermined depth set by the drill stop is reached, drilling should cease immediately. In most cases, a fractured facet is unsuitable for fixation, and the construct must be extended to incorporate the next intact lateral mass.

SIZING AND CONTOURING THE LONGITUDINAL COMPONENT

In almost all cases, articular mass fixation should be bilateral and symmetrical. If a plate is chosen as the longitudinal component, the shortest plate that allows screw purchase in each articular mass should be selected.[51] The posterior elements have been approximated with an interspinous wire, enabling the use of a plate that initially appeared to be too short.[4, 51] This maneuver may confer a biomechanical advantage by preloading the construct and compression loading the facet joint to enhance the probability of successful fusion.[51]

The ideal alignment of the instrumented cervical spine should approximate normal lordotic posture. However, articular mass devices should be considered in situ fixators. Consequently, they should not be relied on to alter cervical alignment through the application of reductive forces. If lordosis cannot be achieved by preoperative traction, intraoperative manipulation, or both, the cervical spine may be instrumented in neutral alignment. It is more appropriate to modify the contour of the longitudinal component to fit the patient rather than attempt to alter the patient's anatomy to conform to the hardware. Typically, posterior cervical devices should not be applied if kyphosis is present, because the curvature places such a construct at a substantial biomechanical disadvantage. Sizing and contouring the longitudinal component are far more tedious processes for screw-plate systems. Screw-rod devices allow infinite rostrocaudal variability and enhanced mediolateral tolerances via the use of polyaxial screw heads, lateral offset connectors, or both. The added variability inherent in screw-rod fixators is useful when instrumenting the transition zones at the cervicothoracic and occipitocervical junctions.

SELECTING AND PLACING THE SCREW

Most posterior cervical fixation systems are replete with primary screws that are 3.5 mm in diameter in a multitude of lengths. Larger-diameter screws are available for "rescue" applications. Safe bicortical purchase is usually obtained with 14- to 16-mm screws. Bicortical fixation is preferable, particularly for devices using a nonconstrained screw-plate or screw-rod interface. Fully constrained, rigid screw-rod systems accommodate unicortical screw purchase, but these systems should be considered less than optimal. Cancellous screws provide better purchase in the articular masses than those with cortical threads. Depending on the system, the screws may or may not be self-tapping. If the screw is not self-tapping, at least the posterior cortex of the articular mass should be tapped before the screw is inserted. Most screw-rod devices allow final screw placement before the longitudinal component is secured.

Caution must be exercised to avoid overtightening the screws, which can strip the screw bed. Unacceptable screw purchase may result from osteoporotic bone, irregular or oversized drill holes, or improper trajectory. When purchase is inadequate, a salvage technique must be used. The primary screw is removed and may be replaced by a rescue screw with a larger diameter to improve purchase. Rescue screws are not placed without peril, however, because the articular mass can fracture. This risk is greater when the articular mass is small or when the entry site is lateral to the facet midline.

SECURING THE LONGITUDINAL COMPONENT

Before placing the plate or rod, provisions are made for bony arthrodesis. The facet joint spaces are thoroughly decorticated and packed with bone graft. Additional graft material can be placed in onlay fashion over the lateral masses themselves. For screw-plate fixation, the appropriately sized and contoured plate is applied flush to the lateral masses and secured by the articular mass screws. For the constrained screw-rod devices, the rod is secured to the preplaced screws via polyaxial screw heads, lateral offset connectors, or both, and locking or set screws are engaged.

Articular mass screw fixation provides unsurpassed immediate multiplanar stability to the posterior subaxial cervical spine, often eliminating the need for cumbersome postoperative bracing. With this technique, successful arthrodesis has been reported in 98% of cases, with extremely low rates of operative morbidity.[52] In a meta-analysis of almost 500 cases, the incidence of neurovascular injury was substantially less than 1%.[52]

WOUND CLOSURE AND POSTOPERATIVE CARE

Once internal fixation has been accomplished, intraoperative radiographs should be obtained to confirm appropriate spinal alignment and hardware position before the wound is closed. If indicated, the neck may be flexed gently and extended under direct vision, fluoroscopy, or both to ensure that stability has been reestablished. The wound is then reapproximated in anatomic layers. In most cases, absorbable suture is used. If postoperative external beam radiotherapy is anticipated, nonresorbable suture may be preferable.

The patient is turned supine, and typically general anesthesia is reversed. A detailed neurological examination is mandatory at this point. New deficits must be investigated promptly with imaging studies, surgical re-exploration, or both. Postoperative imaging is facilitated by the use of titanium implants, and this factor should be considered when selecting an instrumentation system.

The need for postoperative orthotic immobilization is dictated by the nature and extent of the patient's preoperative instability, the patient's general medical and neurological status, and the integrity of the internal fixation. The more rigid constructs seldom require supplementation with external bracing. A less rigid construct may necessitate a more aggressive bracing strategy. Patients are followed with serial clinical and radiographic examinations until a solid bone fusion is confirmed.

CONCLUSIONS

Internal fixation of the injured or diseased cervical spine restores segmental spinal stability, relieves pain, minimizes deformity, and protects the neural elements from further trauma. The need for external bracing is often eliminated, thereby enhancing the patient's comfort and ensuring compliance. This advantage results in rapid, safe mobilization and facilitates aggressive rehabilitation strategies.

REFERENCES

1. Hadra BE: Wiring the vertebrae as a means of immobilization in fractures and Pott's disease. Trans Am Orthop Assoc 4:206, 1891.
2. White AA, Panjabi MM: Biomechanical considerations in the surgical management of the spine. In White AA, Panjabi MM, (eds): Clinical Biomechanics of the Spine. Philadelphia, JB Lippincott, 1990, pp 511–634.
3. Sawin PD, Sonntag VKH: Techniques of posterior subaxial cervical fusion. Tech Neurosurg 1:72–83, 1998.
4. Sawin PD, Traynelis VC: Posterior articular mass plate fixation of the subaxial cervical spine. In Menezes AH, Sonntag VKH (eds): Principles of Spinal Surgery. New York, McGraw-Hill, 1996, pp 1081–1104.
5. Sawin PD, Traynelis VC: Cervical construct design. In Benzel EC (ed): Spine Surgery: Techniques, Complication Avoidance, and Management. New York, Churchill Livingstone, 1999, pp 1129–1140.
6. Denis F: The three column spine and its significance in the classification of acute thoracolumbar spinal injuries. Spine 8:817–831, 1983.
7. Anderson PA, Henley MB, Grady MS, et al: Posterior cervical arthrodesis with AO reconstruction plates and bone graft. Spine 16(Suppl):S72–S79, 1991.
8. Cherny WB, Sonntag VKH: Lateral mass posterior plating and facet fusion for cervical spine instability. BNI Q 7:2–11, 1991.
9. Cooper PR: Stabilization of fractures and subluxations of the lower cervical spine. In Cooper PR (ed): Management of Posttraumatic Spinal Instability. Park Ridge, Ill, American Association of Neurological Surgeon, 1990, pp 111–133.
10. Cooper PR, Cohen A, Rosiello A, et al: Posterior stabilization of cervical spine fractures and subluxations using plates and screws. Neurosurgery 23:300–306, 1988.
11. Savini R, Parisini P, Cervellati S: The surgical treatment of late instability of flexion-rotation injuries in the lower cervical spine. Spine 12:178–182, 1987.
12. Bracken MB, Freeman DH Jr, Hellenbrand K: Incidence of acute traumatic hospitalized spinal cord injury in the United States, 1970–1977. Am J Epidemiol 113:615–622, 1981.
13. Daffner RH: Evaluation of cervical vertebral injuries. Semin Roentgenol 27:239–253, 1992.
14. Bucholz RD, Cheung KC: Halo vest versus spinal fusion for cervical injury: Evidence from an outcome study. J Neurosurg 70:884–892, 1989.
15. Sonntag VK, Hadley MN: Nonoperative management of cervical spine injuries. Clin Neurosurg 34:630–649, 1988.
16. Bohlman HH, Anderson PA: Anterior decompression and arthro-

desis of the cervical spine: Long-term motor improvement. Part I. Improvement in incomplete traumatic quadriparesis. J Bone Joint Surg Am 74:671–682, 1992.

17. Capen DA, Nelson RW, Zigler J, et al: Surgical stabilization of the cervical spine: A comparative analysis of anterior and posterior spine fusions. Paraplegia 25:111–119, 1987.

18. McAfee PC, Bohlman HH: One-stage anterior cervical decompression and posterior stabilization with circumferential arthrodesis: A study of twenty-four patients who had a traumatic or a neoplastic lesion. J Bone Joint Surg Am 71:78–88, 1989.

19. McNamara MJ, Devito DP, Spengler DM: Circumferential fusion for the management of acute cervical spine trauma. J Spinal Disord 4:467–471, 1991.

20. Stauffer ES, Kelly EG: Fracture-dislocations of the cervical spine: Instability and recurrent deformity following treatment by anterior interbody fusion. J Bone Joint Surg Am 59:45–48, 1977.

21. Van Peteghem PK, Schweigel JF: The fractured cervical spine rendered unstable by anterior cervical fusion. J Trauma 19:110–114, 1979.

22. Herman JM, Sonntag VK: Cervical corpectomy and plate fixation for postlaminectomy kyphosis. J Neurosurg 80:963–970, 1994.

23. White AA III, Johnson RM, Panjabi MM, et al: Biomechanical analysis of clinical stability in the cervical spine. Clin Orthop 109:85–96, 1975.

24. Krag MH: Biomechanics of the cervical spine: Orthoses. In Frymoyer JW (ed): The Adult Spine: Principles and Practice. Philadelphia, Lippincott-Raven, 1997, pp 1110–1117.

25. Benzel EC: Spinal orthotics. In Menezes AH, Sonntag VKH (eds): Principles of Spinal Surgery. New York, McGraw-Hill, 1996, pp 181–190.

26. Koch RA, Nickel VL: The halo vest: An evaluation of motion and forces across the neck. Spine 3:103–107, 1978.

27. Hadley MN, Fitzpatrick BC, Sonntag VK, et al: Facet fracture-dislocation injuries of the cervical spine. Neurosurgery 30:661–666, 1992.

28. Morone MA, Ball PA: Spinal traction. In Benzel EC (ed): Spine Surgery: Techniques, Complication Avoidance, and Management. New York, Churchill Livingstone, 1999, pp 1353–1362.

29. Benzel EC: Qualitative attributes of spinal implants. In Benzel EC (ed): Biomechanics of Spine Stabilization: Principles and Clinical Practice. New York, McGraw-Hill, 1995, pp 135–150.

30. Roy-Camille R, Saillant G, Mazel C: Internal fixation of the unstable cervical spine by posterior osteosynthesis with plates and screws. In Cervical Spine Research Society Editorial Committee (ed): The Cervical Spine. Philadelphia, JB Lippincott, 1989, pp 390–404.

31. Sawin PD, Todd MM, Traynelis VC, et al: Cervical spine motion with direct laryngoscopy and orotracheal intubation: An in vivo cinefluoroscopic study of subjects without cervical abnormality. Anesthesiology 85:26–36, 1996.

32. Sawin PD, Traynelis VC, Menezes AH: A comparative analysis of fusion rates and donor-site morbidity for autogeneic rib and iliac crest bone grafts in posterior cervical fusions. J Neurosurg 88:255–265, 1998.

33. Geremia GK, Kim KS, Cerullo L, et al: Complications of sublaminar wiring. Surg Neurol 23:629–635, 1985.

34. Sutterlin CE III, McAfee PC, Warden KE, et al: A biomechanical evaluation of cervical spinal stabilization methods in a bovine model: Static and cyclical loading. Spine 13:795–802, 1988.

35. Osenbach RK, Moores LE: Subaxial wire and cable techniques in the cervical spine. Tech Neurosurg 1:128–138, 1995.

36. Rogers WA: Treatment of fracture dislocations of the cervical spine. J Bone Joint Surg 24A:245–258, 1942.

37. Whitehill R, Reger SI, Fox E, et al: The use of methylmethacrylate cement as an instantaneous fusion mass in posterior cervical fusions: A canine in vivo experimental model. Spine 9:246–252, 1984.

38. Benzel EC, Kesterson L: Posterior cervical interspinous compression wiring and fusion for mid to low cervical spinal injuries. J Neurosurg 70:893–899, 1989.

39. Bohlman HH: Acute fractures and dislocations of the cervical spine: An analysis of three hundred hospitalized patients and review of the literature. J Bone Joint Surg Am 61:1119–1142, 1979.

40. Weiland DJ, McAfee PC: Posterior cervical fusion with triple-wire strut graft technique: One hundred consecutive patients. J Spinal Disord 4:15–21, 1991.

41. McAfee PC, Bohlman HH: The triple wire fixation technique for stabilization of acute cervical fracture-dislocations. Orthop Trans 9:142, 1985.

42. Cahill DW, Bellegarrigue R, Ducker TB: Bilateral facet to spinous process fusion: A new technique for posterior spinal fusion after trauma. Neurosurgery 13:1–4, 1983.

43. Callahan RA, Johnson RM, Margolis RN, et al: Cervical facet fusion for control of instability following laminectomy. J Bone Joint Surg Am 59:991–1002, 1977.

44. Garfin SR, Moore MR, Marshall LF: A modified technique for cervical facet fusions. Clin Orthop 230:149–153, 1988.

45. Tucker HH: Technical report: Method of fixation of subluxed or dislocated cervical spine below C1-C2. Can J Neurol Sci 2:381–382, 1975.

46. Aldrich EF, Weber PB, Crow WN: Halifax interlaminar clamp for posterior cervical fusion: A long-term follow-up review. J Neurosurg 78:702–708, 1993.

47. Holness RO, Huestis WS, Howes WJ, et al: Posterior stabilization with an interlaminar clamp in cervical injuries: Technical note and review of the long term experience with the method. Neurosurgery 14:318–322, 1984.

48. Schulder M: Interlaminar clamps: Indications, techniques, and results. In Menezes AH, Sonntag VKH (eds): Principles of Spinal Surgery. New York, McGraw-Hill, 1996, pp 1121–1132.

49. Heller JG, Carlson GD, Abitbol JJ, et al: Anatomic comparison of the Roy-Camille and Magerl techniques for screw placement in the lower cervical spine. Spine 16(Suppl):S552–S557, 1991.

50. An HS, Gordin R, Renner K: Anatomic considerations for plate-screw fixation of the cervical spine. Spine 16(Suppl):S548–S551, 1991.

51. Gill K, Paschal S, Corin J, et al: Posterior plating of the cervical spine: A biomechanical comparison of different posterior fusion techniques. Spine 13:813–816, 1988.

52. Traynelis VC: Anterior and posterior plate stabilization of the cervical spine. Neurosurg Q 2:59–76, 1992.

Occipitocervical Fusion

JONATHAN J. BASKIN ■ CURTIS A. DICKMAN ■ VOLKER K. H. SONNTAG

The craniovertebral junction (CVJ) is comprised of the occipital bone, the first two cervical vertebrae (atlas and axis), and their soft tissue attachments. In their role as a stable but functionally mobile transition zone between the axial skeleton and skull, the occipitoatlantoaxial joints compose the most anatomically and kinematically complex articulations of the spinal axis.[1-4] A variety of pathologic processes can compromise the structural integrity of these osseous elements, their tethering ligaments, or both, creating instability in this region as a consequence.

In the acute setting of a traumatically disrupted CVJ, the clinical outcome is frequently fatal. Immediate survivors of occipitoatlantal dislocation (OAD) are predisposed to repeated subluxations and sudden death. Immediate and aggressive efforts at internal fixation are therefore integral to their survival,[5-9] particularly with the vertically and posteriorly displaced forms of OAD.[3] Alternatively, several disease entities (degenerative, inflammatory, metabolic, infectious, congenital, or neoplastic) predispose patients to an insidiously worsening mechanical incompetence of the CVJ that manifests as progressively worsening symptoms of cervicomedullary irritation, vertebrobasilar or anterior spinal artery insufficiency, altered cerebrospinal fluid (CSF) dynamics, or radicular pain (C1-2).[3, 10-19] Regardless of the cause, the surgical management of pathology involving the occipitocervical junction must satisfy the fundamental goals of reducing subluxations, ensuring neural decompression, and achieving structural stabilization.

An extreme range of motion is normally available at the CVJ. The occipitoatlantal joint allows 13 degrees of flexion and extension and 8 degrees of lateral bending, but no rotation.[4] The atlantoaxial complex provides 10 degrees of flexion and extension, no lateral bending, and a 94-degree range of rotation.[4] Historically, the mobility inherent to the CVJ has hindered efforts to attain arthrodesis in this region. From the initial description by Pilcher in 1910 of an inadvertent occipitocervical fusion after open reduction of an atlantoaxial dislocation[20] and onlay grafting with fibula by Foerster in 1927 to treat an unstable odontoid fracture,[21] operative techniques for stabilization of the CVJ have evolved to promote osseous union through increas-

ingly rigid internal multisegmental fixation constructs. The earliest surgical efforts that relied on subperiosteal dissection with onlay grafting were accompanied by a significant incidence of failure and pseudarthrosis and entailed prolonged periods of bed rest.[22-25] The practice of fixing autologous bone struts to the occiput and cervical spine with wire (in conjunction with rigid external bracing) improved outcomes but still failed in 5% to 30% of patients.[22, 23, 26-33] The subsequent introduction and continued refinement of metallic implants (multistranded cables, pins, frames, screws, and plates) have provided the most effective means of conferring immediate rigid internal fixation across the unstable occipitocervical junction and have significantly improved the frequency of arthrodesis in this region.[29, 32-53]

Most contemporary spine surgeons rely on titanium-based fixtures because they combine strength and compatibility with magnetic resonance imaging.[54] Despite the superior biomechanical properties of the currently available instrumentation constructs, hardware fatigue and failure are time-dependent certainties if a solid arthrodesis is not achieved (Fig. 303–1). Therefore, meticulous attention to the time-honored biologic and mechanical principles that affect the fusion response is crucial to attaining a successful osseous integration.[55-57] Although several factors determine both the choice of postoperative orthosis prescribed after an occipitocervical fusion procedure and the duration of its use, the development of superior rigid internal fixation has reduced reliance on rigid external bracing.[3, 46, 58, 59] Consequently, convalescence is more comfortable, and the exposure of this frequently frail population to the potential complications associated with a constrictive orthosis is limited.[60-62]

Several internal fixation systems are available to facilitate occipitocervical fusion. Clinical success has been reported with constructs that rely on contoured pins, malleable rods, and frames that are fixated with sublaminar and suboccipital cables, plate and rod-plate combinations that are secured with lateral mass, transarticular and occipital bone screws, and hybrid constructs that use calvarial screws and sublaminar wires.[29, 32–50, 52, 53] This chapter focuses on our (VKHS and CAD) preferred technique for stabilizing the occipitocervical junction using a contoured and grooved

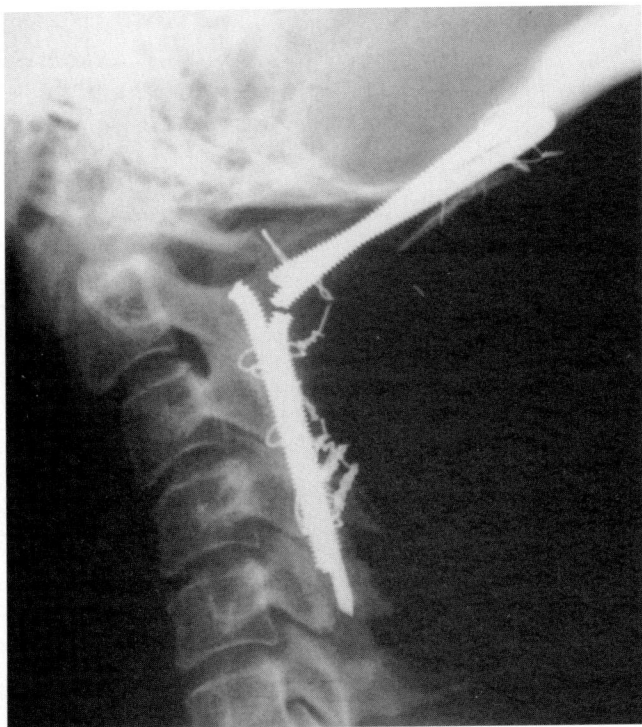

FIGURE 303–1. Fractured fixation rod in a patient with rheumatoid arthritis. Fortuitously, the instrument breakage was asymptomatic and associated with a solid fusion. The rod failed 16 months after surgery (before development of the BendMeister, Sofamor-Danek; Memphis, TN), and the patient remained stable without sequelae through 37 months of follow-up. (From Apostolides PJ, Dickman CA, Golfinos JG, et al: Threaded Steinmann pin fusion of the craniovertebral junction. Spine 21:1630–1637, 1996.)

titanium rod that is anchored with suboccipital and sublaminar cables. This technique has been used extensively and its efficacy documented.[46] Alternative methods of stabilizing the CVJ are also described.

INDICATIONS FOR OCCIPITOCERVICAL FUSION

Occipitocervical fusion is indicated for patients with occipitocervical instability: rheumatoid settling, primary or secondary basilar impression, OAD, neoplastic disease (primary or metastatic), or congenital anomalies that involve the CVJ. In patients with brain stem compression related to rheumatoid settling or basilar impression, preoperative in-line axial traction is attempted to reduce odontoid impaction and to optimize craniocervical alignment for fusion in situ. Weight is added continuously and cautiously over a period of days while the patient is observed in the intensive care unit (initiate at 3 pounds, increase to a maximum of 12 to 15 pounds).[3, 15] If the odontoid migration is irreducible, a ventrally directed decompressive procedure (transoral odontoidectomy) is necessary and should precede the posterior stabilization procedure. Indicators of irreducibility include an odontoid migration

greater than 15 mm above the foramen magnum, an intra-arachnoid location, or the presence of a sequestrum.[3] Approximately 70% to 80% of patients undergoing a transpalatopharyngeal (transoral) decompression will require subsequent occipitocervical fixation.[3, 37, 63–65] Patients who do not undergo fusion immediately after the transoral decompression require careful long-term monitoring to detect incipient instability.[3, 63] Occipitocervical fusion can also be required as a "salvage" procedure in patients who have atlantoaxial instability if a previous effort at C1-2 internal fixation has failed or in patients with complex atlantoaxial fractures for which C1-2 wiring or transarticular screw placement is infeasible or contraindicated.

OPERATIVE TECHNIQUES

In devising an occipitocervical fusion construct, the surgeon must balance the seemingly contrary goals of achieving adequate rigidity while minimizing the number of cervical motion segments sacrificed for that purpose (as long as necessary, as short as possible). The inclusion of each additional subaxial motion segment in the fusion construct forfeits approximately 10 degrees of flexion-extension, lateral bending, and axial rotation.[66] This loss must be considered in the context of an occipitoatlantoaxial fixation that is already anticipated to eliminate 25 to 30 degrees of flexion-extension and the first 35 to 40 degrees of lateral rotation that occurs at the atlantoaxial joint.[3]

The degree of preoperative CVJ instability obviously influences the number of levels that should be incorporated within a particular occipitocervical fusion. For patients with occipitocervical instability with intact posterior laminar elements who have not undergone basilar invagination or destabilizing anterior decompressive surgery, we perform the fusion procedure through the axial level (occiput–C1-2). Patients who have undergone an anteriorly directed decompressive procedure require additional points of fixation to stabilize their CVJ sufficiently, as do patients with evidence of basilar invagination. We immobilize these patients with a construct that incorporates C3 and possibly C4. In patients who require anterior decompressive and posterior stabilization procedures, we preferentially stage these interventions as sessions separated by 1 to 2 days. Patients are maintained in a halo orthosis in the interim and remain intubated given the associated postoperative pharyngeal and lingual edema that follows the transpalatopharyngeal approach. For patients with incompetent posterior elements, either resulting from trauma or after a posteriorly directed decompression of the vertebral canal, we extend the occipitocervical fusion caudally enough to incorporate at least two levels with normal laminar anatomy.

Preoperative Preparation and Positioning

Patients with occipitocervical instability arrive in the operating room wearing some form of protective external cervical immobilization. Patients with rheumatoid settling or basilar invagination typically undergo in-line axial traction preoperatively. In patients with OAD, the profound extent of instability produced by ligamentous disruption mandates the use of a halo orthosis and specifically contraindicates the mechanically distracting effects of in-line traction or a hard cervical collar.[5] These patients should be maintained in a flat position. Their craniospinal alignment is precarious despite the presence of the halo brace. Patients with milder degrees of CVJ instability can be maintained preoperatively in a hard cervical collar.

Intravascular access is secured, and a prophylactic dose of antibiotic (cefazolin) is administered within 30 minutes of making the skin incision. The patient is intubated, often using an awake or fiberoptic technique to minimize the risk of neurologic injury from inadvertent occipitocervical or atlantoaxial dislocation. Paralytic medications are avoided so as not to exacerbate CVJ instability and to allow clinical recognition of inadvertent spinal cord or nerve root irritation during the surgical procedure. A urinary catheter and antiembolic stockings are placed after general anesthesia is induced.

Intraoperatively, somatosensory and brain stem auditory evoked potentials are monitored continuously to assess the physiologic status of the spinal cord and brain stem during the procedure. Baseline waveforms are obtained before the patient is rotated to the prone position. If the waveform alters significantly after prone positioning, the patient is returned to the supine position and reexamined. After confirming that the baseline neurologic examination remains intact, we have found it helpful to reposition these patients in the prone orientation while they are awake and during continued evoked potential monitoring. General anesthesia is then resumed after confirming that the patient's baseline motor examination remains stable in the prone position. If preoperative evidence of myelopathy is present, methylprednisolone is administered in accordance with the North American Spinal Cord Injury Study (NASCIS III) guidelines.[67] Postoperatively, this steroid infusion is discontinued if the patient's neurologic examination is stable.

The Mayfield head holder (Codman, Inc., Raynham, MA) secures the cranium during the procedure and is applied while the patient is supine. Maintaining a hard cervical collar in place until prone positioning is completed helps guard against undesirable cervical movement during patient rotation (Fig. 303–2A). If the patient is wearing a halo brace, the Mayfield head holder adaptor (Durr-Fillauer Medical, Inc., Chattanooga, TN) is connected to the halo ring to fix the patient to the operating table (see Fig. 303–2B). The posterior aspect of the halo vest is then removed to allow access to

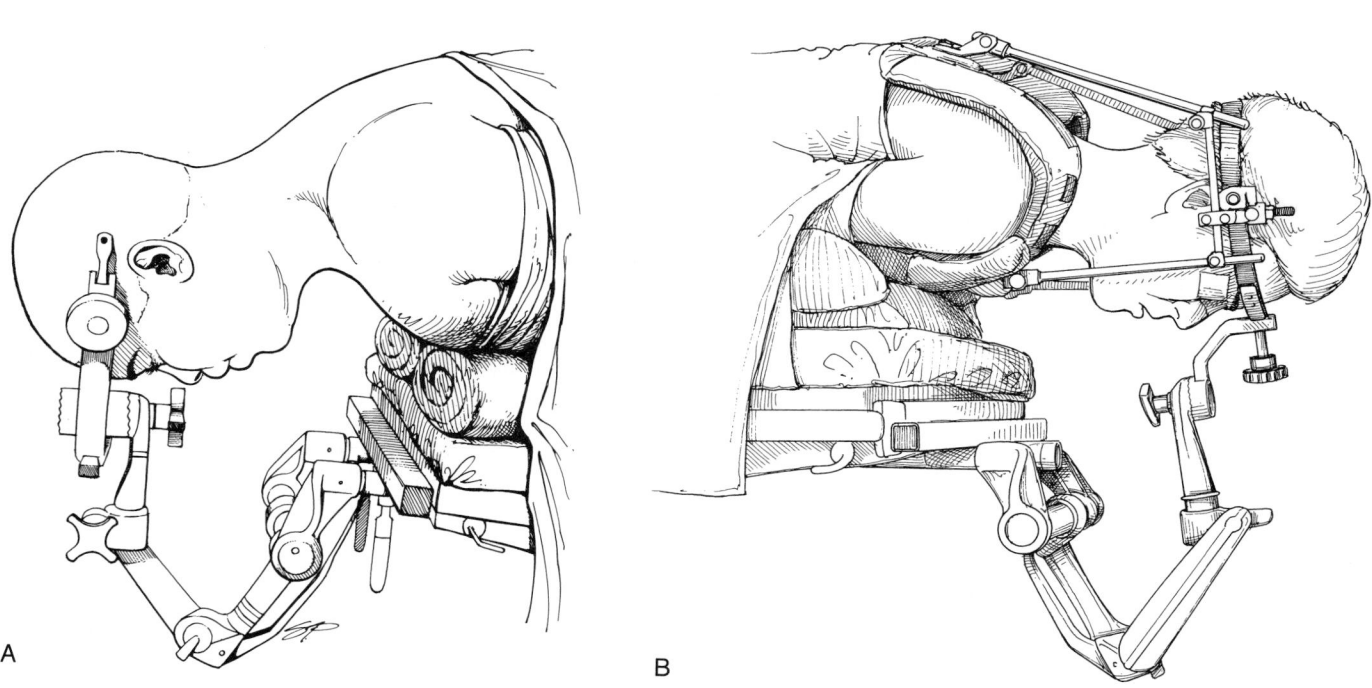

A   B

FIGURE 303–2. *A,* Prone positioning with use of the Mayfield head holder (Codman, Inc., Raynham, MA). The head holder is applied while the patient is supine. The patient is rotated into the prone position while wearing a hard cervical collar (not shown) to guard against occipitocervical or atlantoaxial dislocation. Baseline evoked potentials are measured before positioning as well as throughout the remainder of the procedure. *B,* The Mayfield halo adapter (Durr-Fillauer Medical, Inc., Chattanooga, TN) is used to secure patients wearing a halo brace. The posterior aspect of the halo apparatus is removed to allow access to autologous graft sites. Atraumatic positioning of extremities and joints is particularly crucial in patients whose craniovertebral junction pathology is related to arthritic or bone-softening diseases. (Courtesy of Barrow Neurological Institute, St. Joseph's Hospital and Medical Center, Phoenix, AZ.)

the cervical region and autologous graft site. Menezes advocates the use of dynamic axial traction during the operation and reserves fixing the halo ring to the operating table only for patients with grossly unstable CVJ pathology.[3, 58]

A lateral cervical radiograph is obtained after the patient is positioned to assess craniovertebral alignment. Intraoperative fluoroscopy is used for closed manipulation of the CVJ before the procedure begins, for performing open reduction before instrumentation is placed, or for monitoring alignment in patients with particularly unstable injuries (OAD). The absence of rotation at the occipitoatlantal joint means that a "true" lateral view of the skull also provides a "true" lateral view of C1. This point is helpful when confirming anatomic alignment of the CVJ or atlantoaxial complex before internal fixation. Attention is directed toward appropriately padding soft tissues and bony prominences and to atraumatic positioning of the particularly fragile joints or extremities of patients with rheumatoid arthritis, osteogenesis imperfecta, or other bone-softening disorders that manifest with a CVJ deformity.[15, 19, 68]

Skin Incision and Soft Tissue Dissection

The rostral aspect of the surgical exposure is the external occipital protuberance. The minimal extent of caudal dissection includes complete exposure of the dorsal elements of the first three cervical vertebrae. Further caudal dissection may be necessary if additional fixation points are warranted to maximize the stability of the construct. Soft tissue dissection is limited to the levels of craniovertebral instability to avoid further (iatrogenic) destabilization or, particularly in children, the inadvertent fusion of normal motion segments.

The patient's hair is shaved in the occipitocervical midline from the inion to over the spinous process of C5. After a standard sterile preparation, the inscribed midline incision is infiltrated with 0.5% lidocaine with epinephrine for hemostasis. The skin and subcutaneous tissues are incised down to the dorsal cervical fascia, and this plane is developed laterally to allow placement of hemostatic clips and to facilitate a multilayered closure when the procedure is completed. The avascular midline plane between the cervical paraspinal muscles is developed, ideally using sharp dissection and periosteal elevators. An effort is made to avoid devascularizing the adjacent musculature and to spare the bony tissue of the graft bed from the potentially injurious effects of monopolar cauterization. As the depth of soft tissue dissection progresses, care must be taken to avoid dislocation of unstable vertebral segments. Menezes notes the utility of stabilizing the operative exposure by placing angled retractors perpendicular to each other to prevent motion at the craniocervical joint and also by securing the C2 spinous process with a towel clip while elevating the paraspinous musculature.[3]

Soft tissue dissection is adequate when the occipital squama, foramen magnum, and posterior elements of the upper three cervical vertebrae are clearly visible. The vertebral exposure should extend to the lateral

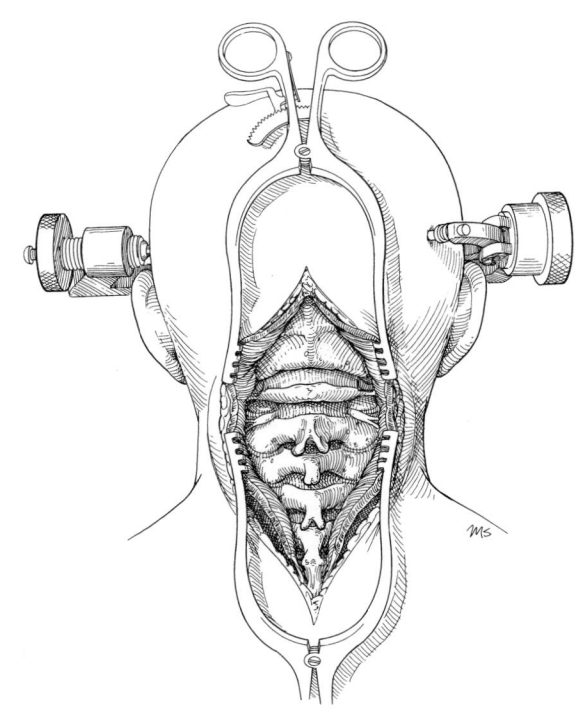

FIGURE 303–3. Posterior midline surgical incision used for occipitocervical fusion. The minimal exposure required demonstrates the dorsal elements of the first three cervical vertebrae out to the lateral margins of their facet joints (bilaterally) and the occipital squama. The cosurgeon can stand across the table from the primary surgeon or assist while positioned at the cranial vertex. (Courtesy of Barrow Neurological Institute, St. Joseph's Hospital and Medical Center, Phoenix, AZ.)

margin of the facet joints bilaterally. The available occipital surface must be able to accommodate the fixation construct (Fig. 303–3). All soft tissue in the region of the proposed fusion bed should be removed, including the occipitoatlantal membrane and posterior spinal ligaments (interspinous and ligamentum flavum). After the surgical site has been irrigated generously with an antibiotic-containing solution, the graft bed is further prepared using a high-speed air drill to decorticate the relevant facet joints and adjacent occipital and laminar surfaces. This step maximizes the available surface area for fusion and is most easily and thoroughly performed before the occipitocervical instrumentation is placed.

OCCIPITOCERVICAL INSTRUMENTATION

A variety of metallic fixtures is available for stabilizing the occipitocervical junction. The fixtures can primarily be subdivided into wire (cable)-based and screw-based systems. Common to all these devices are the prefixation steps and precautions already described. As is the case with any implant, the individual components should be composed of the same metal to avoid a potentially corrosive (redox) reaction that increases the risk of hardware fatigue and failure.[44, 45, 52]

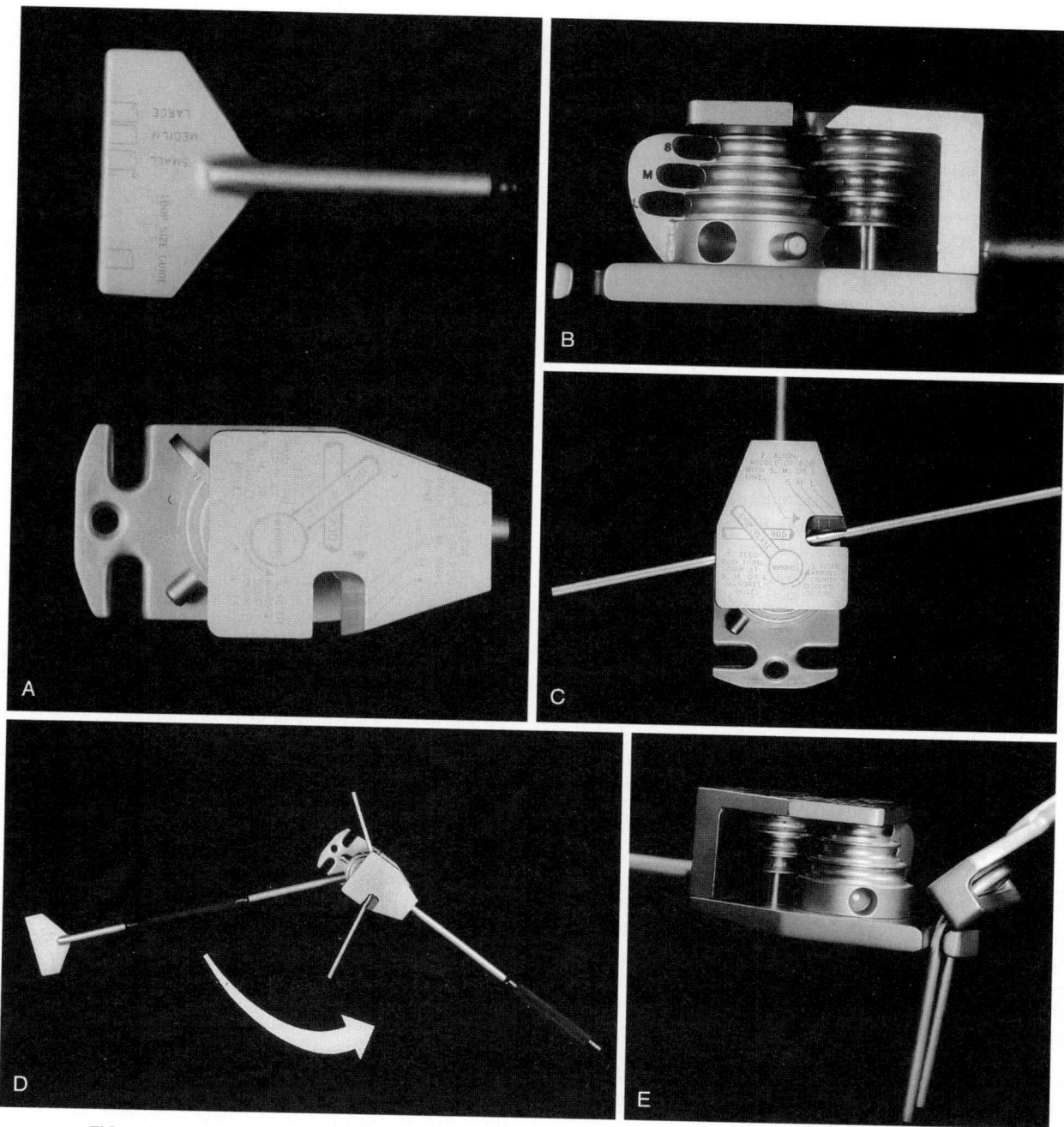

FIGURE 303–4. *A*, The BendMeister rod bender (Sofamor-Danek, Memphis, TN) is composed of a rod bender handle (*top*) and the rod bender proper (*bottom*). The manufacturer's price is $3567 (U.S.). The device provides the mechanical advantage necessary to create precise, uniform curvatures within metallic rods while minimizing the risk of producing nicks, cracks, or stress risers. *B*, Lateral view of the rod bender bending mandrel with choice of small (S), medium (M), and large (L) radii of curvature for producing circular bends (primary loop). Selection of the optimal radius of curvature is facilitated by using a malleable endotracheal tube stylet to model the unique topography of an individual patient's craniovertebral junction. *C*, Lateral surface of the rod bender with instructions for use. Note the attached lever arm (12 o'clock position) and the bending anvil for producing angular (secondary) curves (6 o'clock position). *D*, The straight end of the rod bender handle is inserted into the mandrel and rotated counterclockwise to produce the primary bend. Before the fixation pin is shaped, the rod grip plate is rotated to its starting position as far clockwise as possible. The pin is inserted through the appropriate hole (based on the desired radius of curvature), and its midpoint is aligned with the appropriate etching on the lateral surface of the rod bender. *E*, The "legs" of the preliminarily contoured loop are held in the slotted anvil. The primary curve is passed through the paddle end of the rod bender handle, and the secondary curve is produced. Again, reference to the malleable endotracheal tube stylet optimizes the pin's final contour. Unilateral bends can be made in the fixation rod using the "bending hole" within the anvil. (*A–C* from Apostolides PJ, Karahalios DG, Yapp RA, Sonntag VKH: Use of the BendMeister rod bender for occipitocervical fusion: Technical note. Neurosurgery 43: 389–391, 1998; *D* and *E* from Dickman CA, Apostolides PJ, Karahalios DG: Surgical techniques for upper cervical spine decompression and stabilization. Clin Neurosurg 44:137–160, 1997.)

Occipitocervical Wiring Techniques

The grooved titanium fixation rod (Stromer/Southwest Medical Inc., Scottsdale, AZ) is our preferred means of cable-based fixation of the CVJ. The threaded character of the pin helps resist settling, "telescoping," or vertical translation of the fusion construct.[44, 46] The wide diameter of the rod (5/32 inch) minimizes the risk of implant breakage. The fixation rod is most easily contoured to the CVJ before the anchoring suboccipital and sublaminar cables are placed. A sterile, malleable endotracheal tube stylet can be used to model the shape of the fusion bed and to serve as a template for contouring the pin outside the surgical wound. The pin must be shaped precisely to maximize the area of metal-bone interface. Gaps between the pin and bone surfaces suboptimally fixate the unstable segments and can allow detrimental motion that fosters instrument failure and nonunion. The ends of the pin are cut so that they do not extend beyond the lowest segment to be fused. Failure to do so can result in destabilizing leverage on the fixation construct or the unintentional incorporation of an additional motion segment within the fusion mass.

We use a unique rod bender developed by the senior author (VKHS) (BendMeister, Sofamor-Danek, Memphis, TN) that permits easily reproducible contouring of the pins with smooth primary and secondary curves.[69] Other methods of rod shaping (table vises, bending irons, French benders) can produce mechanically disadvantageous sharp angles and notches that predispose these implants to failure. Smooth curves distribute forces more uniformly along the rod and help to increase resistance to breaking. The rod bender further simplifies an occipitocervical fusion procedure because only a single-length titanium pin is needed in the operating room at the time of custom sizing (Fig. 303–4). In contrast, reliance on precontoured loops or frames requires an inventory of implant sizes and shapes (degrees of curvature) to be available for any one patient. Contouring the implant to fit the architecture of the CVJ, rather than the reverse, is crucial to achieving a biomechanically sound and clinically tolerated fixation construct.[70]

The sublaminar wires are passed as medially as possible given the more generous dimensions of the epidural space in this region. Notching the rostral and caudal aspects of the laminae at this medial point further facilitates safe passage of the cable by reducing the epidural distance that the wire must traverse and by improving direct visualization of the dura during passage of the wire. The posterior rim of the foramen magnum can be enlarged with a high-speed air drill to facilitate suboccipital epidural wire passage for anchoring the titanium rod to the skull base. Three bur holes are placed within the occipital bone approximately 1 cm away from the margin of the enlarged foramen magnum and off the midline (Fig. 303–5). The dura is dissected away from the inner table of the skull toward the foramen magnum, and the epidural space is defined under the laminae of interest. If the foramen magnum is relatively inaccessible because of anoma-

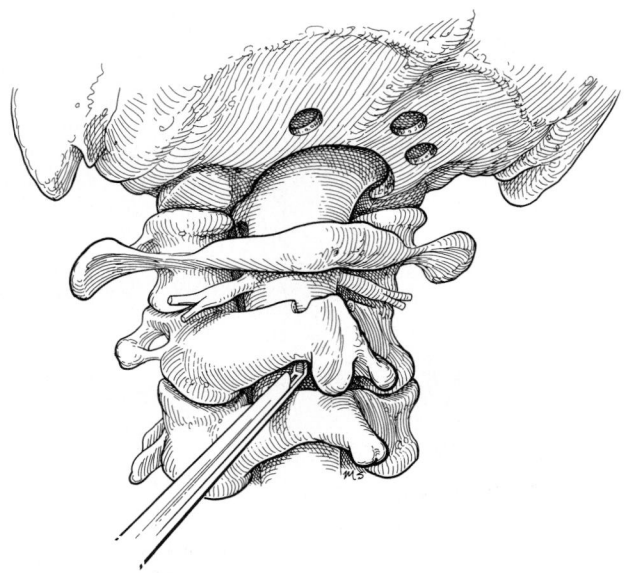

FIGURE 303–5. Preparation for placement of suboccipital and sublaminar cable. Wire passage is simplified by using a high-speed drill to resect the thickened posterior rim of the foramen magnum. The contoured rod is secured to the occipital bone with three points of fixation. Sublaminar cables are passed as medially as possible because of the generous epidural space in this region. Notching the rostral and caudal aspects of the laminae shortens the sublaminar distance that must be traversed and allows monitoring for potentially injurious dural distortion. (From Barrow Neurological Institute, St. Joseph's Hospital and Medical Center, Phoenix, AZ.)

lous anatomy (occipitalized atlas) or if cervical flexion is otherwise limited, an alternative means of obtaining occipital fixation is to place three sets of bur holes around the periphery of the foramen magnum and to pass a cable between each set.

Multistranded cables are used because of their greater resistance to stress fatigue compared with their single-stranded counterparts.[71] The cable (Sofamor-Danek, Memphis, TN) is passed under the laminae by first passing the blunt end of a large needle attached to a 2–0 Vicryl suture through the epidural space underlying the lamina of interest (Fig. 303–6). The Vicryl suture is pulled through the epidural space using a blunt nerve hook and tied to a cable pair that is connected by a single rigid leader. As a single unit, the cables are advanced carefully through the epidural space using a two-handed technique in which simultaneous "pulling and feeding" allow the wire to "hug" the undersurface of the bone (Fig. 303–7). Once passed, the leader that joins the doubled cables is halved with a wire cutter and a cable pulled to each side. Single cables are similarly passed under the occipital squama between sets of bur holes or between single bur holes and the enlarged foramen magnum. The leader of the single cable can be looped back on itself to allow tying to it the suture and to create a blunt surface for epidural transit.

Complications associated with suboccipital or sublaminar wire passage are related to dural violation by the cable or ventral bowing of the cable with com-

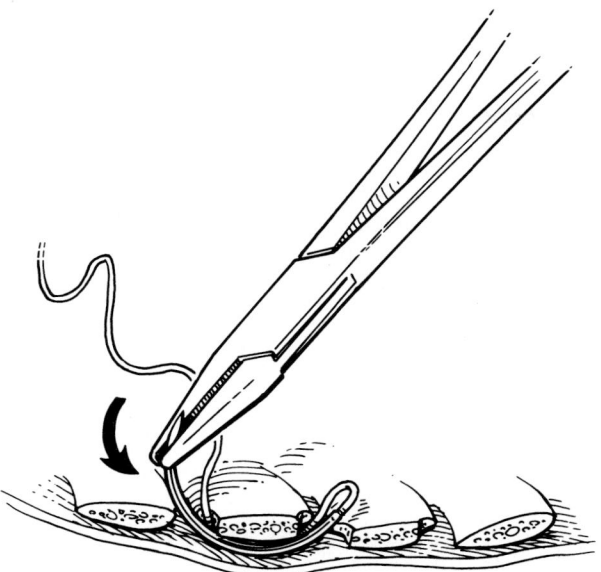

FIGURE 303–6. The technique for sublaminar cable placement begins with the sublaminar passage of a thick (00) Vicryl suture. The suture is attached to a needle that is passed in a retrograde fashion through the epidural space. The "loop" of suture that appears within the adjacent interlaminar space is pulled through with a nerve hook. (From Barrow Neurological Institute, St. Joseph's Hospital and Medical Center, Phoenix, AZ.)

pression of the underlying cerebellum or spinal cord, respectively. These maneuvers can cause cerebrospinal fluid leaks, subdural hemorrhages, and parenchymal injuries.[72, 73] Every effort is therefore expended to define the planned epidural path cleanly and to ensure that the cable maintains as low a profile as possible within the epidural space. If the lamina of a particular level is incompetent, facet wires have been used to anchor the titanium rod.[44, 45, 74] Sublaminar wires are preferred over facet wires because more rigid immobilization is attain-

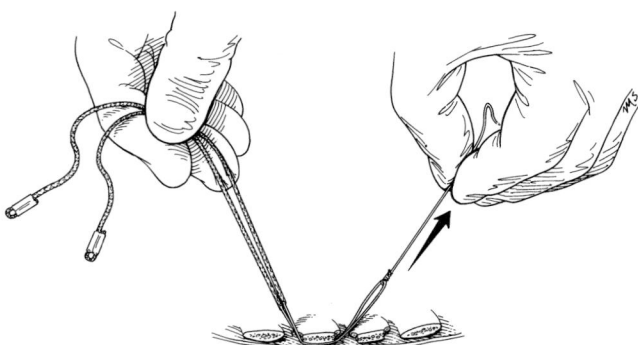

FIGURE 303–7. The Vicryl suture is tied to the doubled cable (two multistranded cables connected by a single leader) and simultaneously pulled and advanced with a two-handed technique through the epidural space (atlas cable [Sofamor-Danek, Memphis, Tenn]; double cable, $422; single cable, $331). Cable redundancy is avoided to avert dural compression. (From Barrow Neurological Institute, St. Joseph's Hospital and Medical Center, Phoenix, AZ.)

able, and their resistance to pulling out is comparatively greater.[75]

The pin is cinched against the occiput and cervical laminae or facets. The sublaminar wires are positioned at the most lateral extent of their respective laminae. The cables are tightened and crimped in a sequential manner that carefully maintains the position of the pin against the previously decorticated surfaces of the fusion bed (Fig. 303–8). The individual cables are maintained under tension before their final tightening to prevent ventral buckling and secondary dural compression. Individual cable sites must be inspected to ensure that all slack has been removed before crimping and to guard against overtightening the cable, which can cause it to cut through the fixation point. Generous amounts of autologous cancellous bone graft are placed in the regions to be fused. If a suboccipital craniectomy or cervical laminectomy is required to decompress the neural elements, a unicortical plate of iliac crest bone can be sutured or wired to the central portion of the pin to act as a template for the fusion mass and to preserve the dural decompression (Fig. 303–9). Self-retaining retractors are removed and hemostasis is obtained. No further irrigation is performed after the cancellous autograft is placed. A routine, multilayered wound closure is performed. No surgical drain is used.

The operative techniques for occipitocervical fixation using other cable-based contoured loops or frames are identical to those described for the threaded rod.[38–43] The smooth surfaces of several of the alternative implants may predispose these constructs to settling, telescoping, or vertical translocation, particularly in patients whose dorsal stabilization was preceded by traction-induced reduction of a ventrally based compressive deformity (Fig. 303–10).[45, 76] The Cotrel-Dubousset screw-plate rod is a hybrid implant that requires sublaminar wires and occipital bone screws. A transverse cross-link at the caudal end of the construct provides additional rotational stability (Fig. 303–11).

Occipitocervical Screw-Based Techniques

The various occipitocervical screw-based constructs provide an option for fixation that does not require sublaminar passage of wires. These implants are therefore especially useful if the cervical laminae are incompetent or absent, or if the risk of sublaminar wire passage is considered too high for a particular patient. Biomechanical evaluation of occipitocervical instrumentation further suggests that screw-based fixation better resists fatigue and vertical settling, provides superior immobilization of the CVJ, and requires the incorporation of fewer vertebral segments compared with cable-based methods.[76, 77]

Screw-based methods of fixation are technically demanding and require anatomic precision. Subaxial anchoring of implants with lateral mass (articular pillar) screws and fixation to the atlantoaxial complex with transarticular screws place the cervical nerve roots and vertebral arteries at risk of injury. Historically, the relative thinness of the occipital bone has limited the quality of screw purchase attainable in this region. The

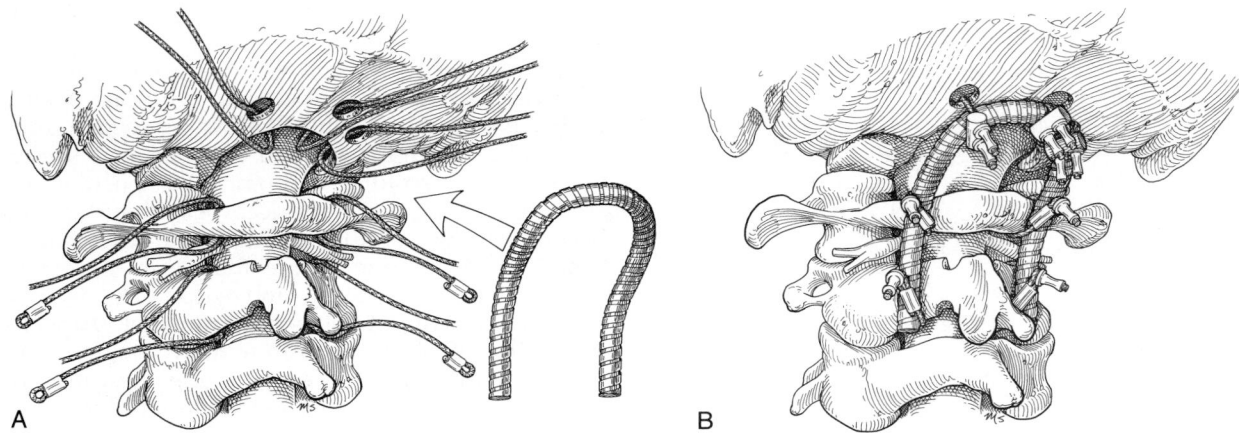

FIGURE 303–8. *A*, The individual sublaminar cables are pulled to the lateral extent of their respective laminae. All cables are maintained in tension to avoid buckling in the cranial or spinal epidural space. The previously contoured rod is inserted through the cable loops and is seated against the occipitocervical junction (CVJ; Titanium Fixation Rod, $675 [U.S.], 10 inch, $700 12 inch, Stromer Southwest, Scottsdale, AZ). *B*, The rod is fixed against the CVJ. The cable tension that can be expected before crimping is diminished compared with normal as a result of the soft bone that frequently characterizes patients with CVJ instability. Attention must be directed to ensure that the cables do not cut through their anchoring bone sites. Furthermore, vigilance is required to prevent displacement of the rod during sequential tightening of the cables. Use of multiple "provisional crimp" attachments with the tensionometer device (Sofamor-Danek, Memphis, Tenn) allows cable tensions or positions to be sampled at multiple sites and readjusted as necessary before final tightening. (From Barrow Neurological Institute, St. Joseph's Hospital and Medical Center, Phoenix, AZ.)

occipital bone rapidly thins as it progresses laterally from its fuller midline crest, the average thickness of which is 14 mm at the nuchal line.[35] Heywood and coworkers reported that the thickness of lateral suboc-

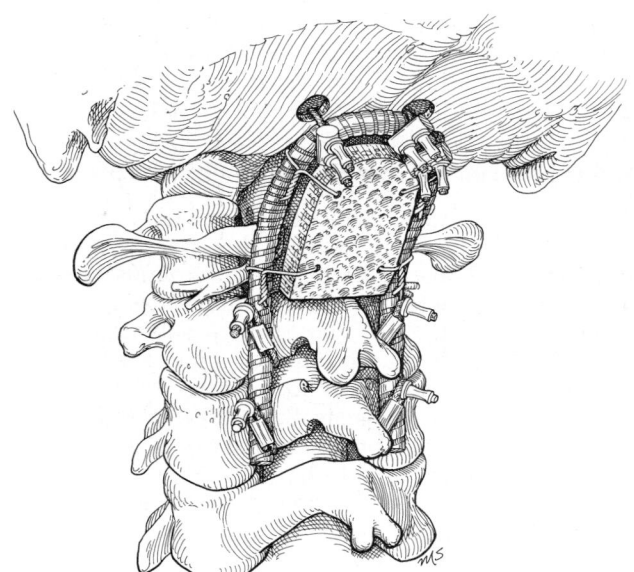

FIGURE 303–9. When a C1 laminar defect is present, a unicortical piece of iliac crest is wired or sutured to the rod to function as a template for fusion and to preserve decompression of the CVJ. The fixation construct has been extended to C3 in the interest of recruiting two normal laminar segments to anchor the construct. (From Barrow Neurological Institute, St. Joseph's Hospital and Medical Center, Phoenix, AZ.)

cipital bone ranged from 3 to 9 mm.[49] Careful preoperative measurement of the thickness of the occipital bone has therefore been fundamental to calculating the depth of screw insertion and to avoiding complications related to dural penetration. Pait and colleagues have addressed this difficulty with an innovative modification in occipital screw placement (Fig. 303–12; see color section in this volume). Their so-called inside-out technique allows an atraumatic, broad-based surface to purchase the occipital squama and renders the thickness of the occipital bone irrelevant.[51]

Lateral mass, pars interarticularis, and transarticular screws should be placed under direct fluoroscopic visualization. Although screw-based fixation typically limits the fusion procedure to unstable motion segments, poor bone quality may preclude adequate screw purchase and require additional fixation points to optimize the stability of the construct. In this setting, sublaminar wiring may offer biomechanical superiority.

PLACEMENT OF PARS INTERARTICULARIS AND TRANSARTICULAR SCREWS

Prospective analysis has demonstrated that the regional anatomy (location of vertebral artery and width of pars interarticularis) of almost 20% of patients contraindicates placement of a transarticular screw on at least one side.[78] Thus, if transarticular screw fixation is contemplated, the preoperative radiographic evaluation should include fine-cut computed tomographic images in the plane of the transarticular screw with sagittal reconstructions.[78] When bilateral screw placement is contraindicated, unilateral posterior transartic-

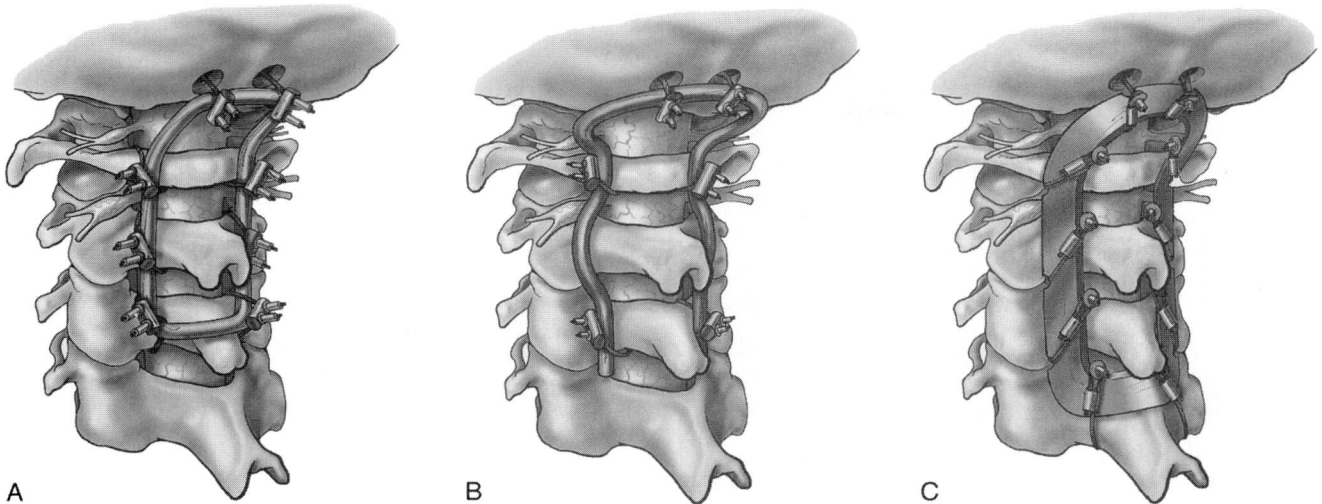

FIGURE 303–10. Metal implants available for occipitocervical fixation. *A,* Hartshill rectangle (Surgicraft, Redditch, Worcestershire, UK). *B,* Ransford loop (Surgicraft, Redditch, Worcestershire, UK). *C,* Titanium (Ti) frame (Codman, Raynham, MA). (From Barrow Neurological Institute, St. Joseph's Hospital and Medical Center, Phoenix, AZ.)

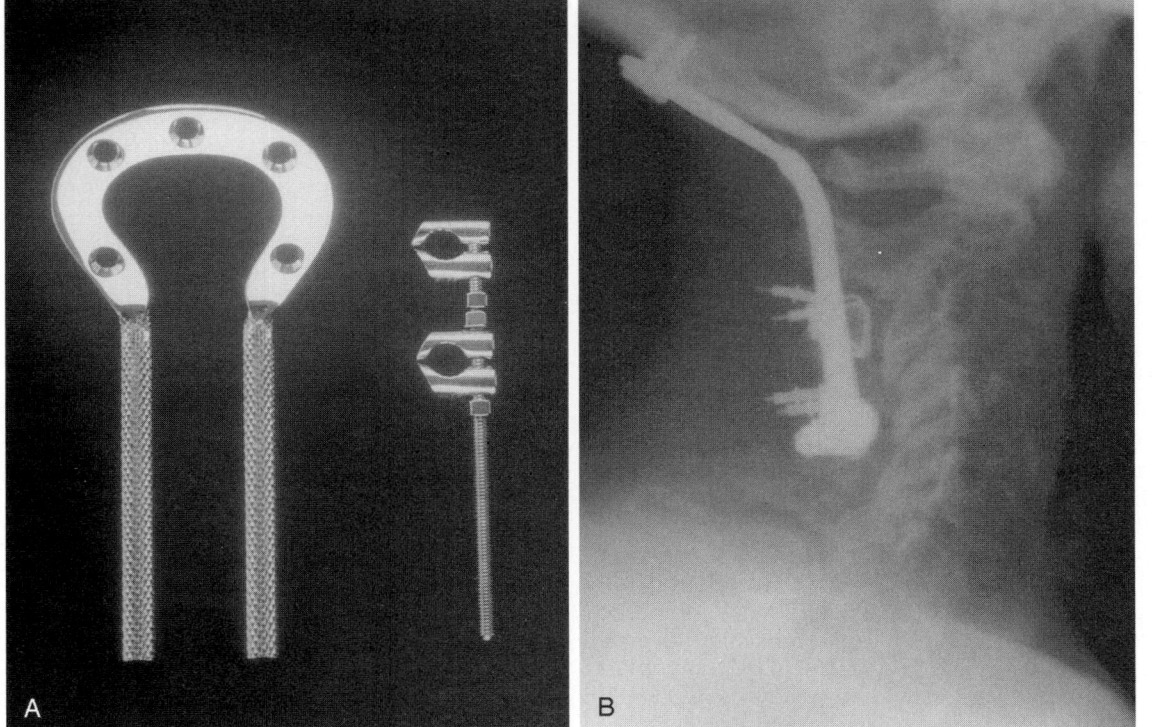

FIGURE 303–11. *A,* The Cotrel-Dubousset rod-screw plate and cross-link. The limbs are knurled to combat settling or vertical displacement. *B,* Postoperative plain radiograph illustrating occipitocervical fixation that extends to C4. Occipital bone screws must be measured carefully to prevent violation of the dura. Sublaminar cables are evident at C3 and C4; atlantoaxial fixation is precluded by incompetent posterior bony elements at C1 and C2. (From Apostolides PJ, Spetzler RF, Sonntag VKH: Occipitocervical wiring techniques. In Dickman CA, Spetzler RF, Sonntag VKH [eds]. Surgery of the Craniovertebral Junction. New York, Thieme, 1998, pp 795–808.)

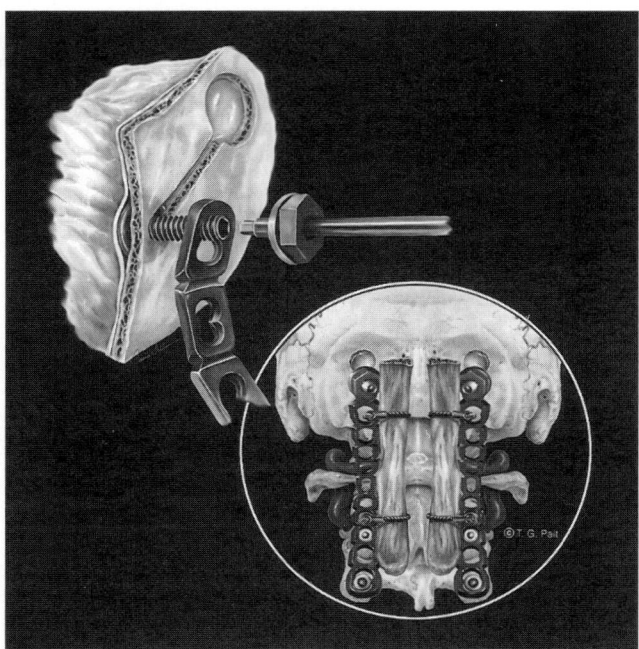

FIGURE 303–12. Illustration of the "inside-out" technique for occipital bone screw placement as described by Pait and associates.[15] (From Pait TG, Al-Mefty O, Boop FA, et al: Inside-outside technique for posterior occipitocervical spine instrumentation and stabilization: Preliminary results. J Neurosurg 90:1–7, 1999 [cover illustration].)

ular screw placement can provide valuable fixation for the treatment of atlantoaxial instability.[79] An incompletely reduced atlantoaxial dislocation precludes transarticular screw placement because it is associated with a higher risk of vertebral artery injury.[80] When transarticular screw placement is impossible, limiting the position of the screw to the pars interarticularis provides a "next best" fixation point for the occipitocervical fusion construct.

The C1-2 facet can be directly visualized by using a dissector to gently retract the C2 nerve root and its associated venous plexus rostrally. The medial border of the pars interarticularis is also visualized directly to ensure that screw placement does not violate its medial border (Fig. 303–13). The screw entry point is 2 to 3 mm above the caudal edge of the C2 inferior facet and an equal distance lateral to the medial border of the facet (Fig. 303–14). Percutaneous delivery is often necessary to achieve the desired screw trajectory through the atlantoaxial complex (Fig. 303–15). Ultimately, a cannulated screw is directed over a K wire along the central axis of the pars interarticularis (0- to 10-degree medial angulation) and proceeds across the atlantoaxial joint to purchase the lateral mass of C1 (Fig. 303–16). An absent anterior C1 tubercle has been associated with screw malposition.[80] Thus, we attempt to preserve as much of this landmark as possible during anterior decompressive procedures. Transarticular screw placement begins on the side of the nondominant vertebral artery. Suspicion of a vertebral artery injury contraindicates placement of the contralateral transarticular

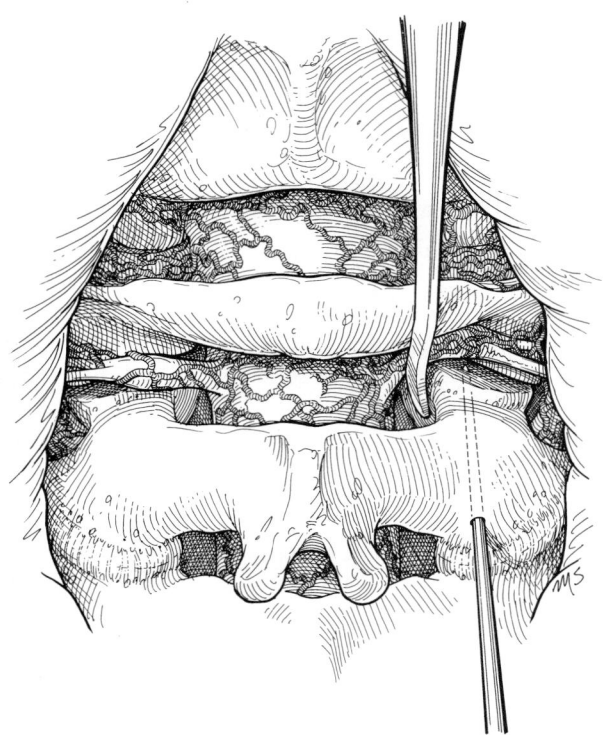

FIGURE 303–13. Anatomic landmarks for placement of transarticular or pars interarticularis screws. The rostral aspect of the pars interarticularis is followed ventrally to the atlantoaxial joint. The C2 nerve root and its associated venous plexus are gently retracted rostrally to facilitate exposure of the pars. The proposed mediolateral screw trajectory should not violate the medial cortex of the pars as indicated by the positioned Penfield dissector. A sagittal screw trajectory is planned using intraoperative fluoroscopy as detailed in Figure 303–16*B*. (From Barrow Neurological Institute, St. Joseph's Hospital and Medical Center; Phoenix, AZ.)

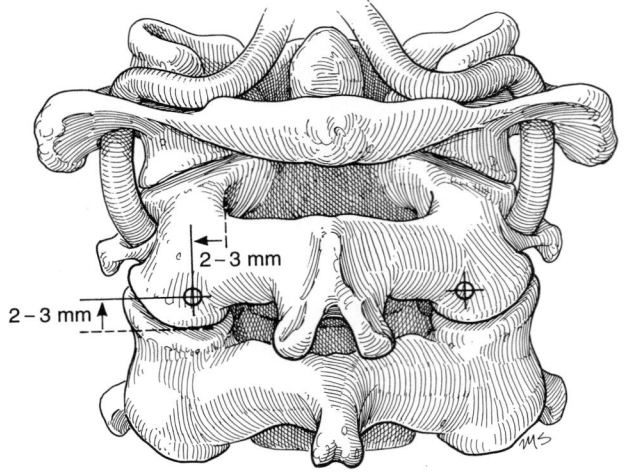

FIGURE 303–14. Entry site for placement of transarticular or pars interarticularis screws. The C2–3 facet joint is followed to its medial extent. An entry point 2 to 3 mm lateral to the medial border of the joint and 2 to 3 mm rostral to the joint is marked and decorticated with a drill bit or bone awl. The illustration demonstrates an anatomically favorable circumstance for bilateral transarticular screw placement. (From Barrow Neurological Institute, St. Joseph's Hospital and Medical Center, Phoenix, AZ.)

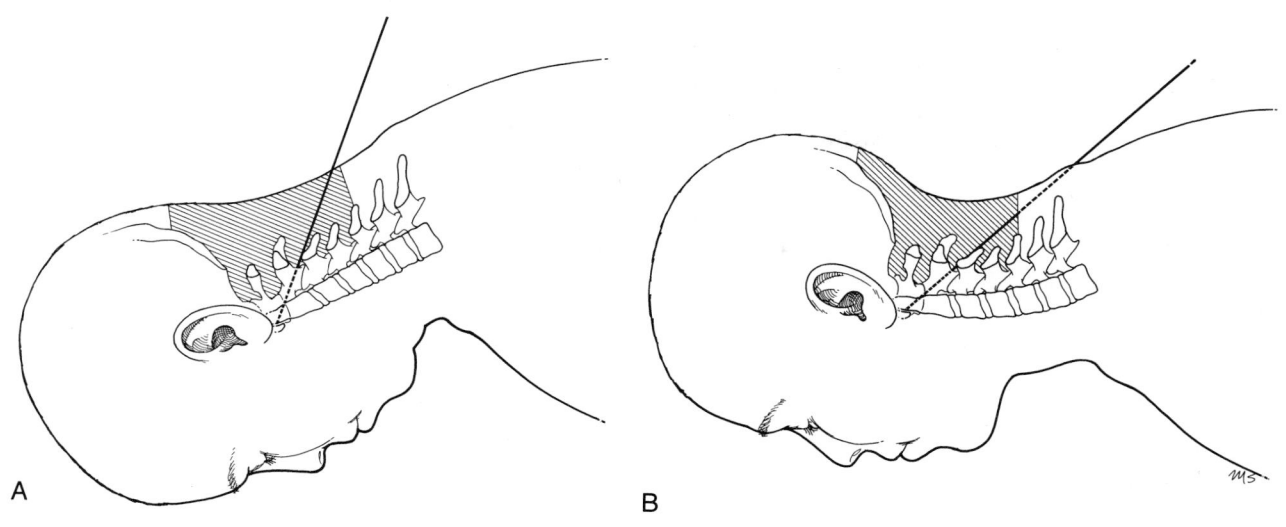

FIGURE 303–15. Transincisional (*A*) or percutaneous (*B*) delivery of transarticular or C2 pars interarticularis screws. The shaded area indicates the extent of incision and in both cases spans from the inion to the spinous process of C5. The ability to flex the cervical spine sufficiently directs the appropriate method. Cervical manipulation is performed under direct fluoroscopic visualization. The location of the paired percutaneous entry sites can be extrapolated using a long instrument that is juxtaposed over the spine along the necessary screw trajectory (sagittal) during fluoroscopy. Percutaneous entry sites are included within the sterile field and must be calculated at the start of the procedure. Percutaneous placement is always performed in conjunction with open dissection of the atlantoaxial complex to permit sufficient monitoring of the mediolateral screw trajectory. (From Barrow Neurological Institute, St. Joseph's Hospital and Medical Center, Phoenix, AZ.)

screw, but the alternative of a pars interarticularis screw remains an option. All screws are placed using imaging guidance (direct fluoroscopy or frameless stereotactic navigation).

PLACEMENT OF LATERAL MASS SCREWS

The placement of lateral mass screws for posteriorly directed stabilization of the subaxial cervical spine is

well described.[36, 81–86] The articular pillars of the C3-6 vertebrae can be used as caudal fixation points for occipitocervical fusion procedures. The center of the lateral mass is identified as the midpoint between the superior and inferior facets rostrocaudally and the lateral edge of the lamina and lateral border of the facet mediolaterally.[83] The screw entry point, 1 mm medial to this midpoint, is marked with a bone awl (Fig.

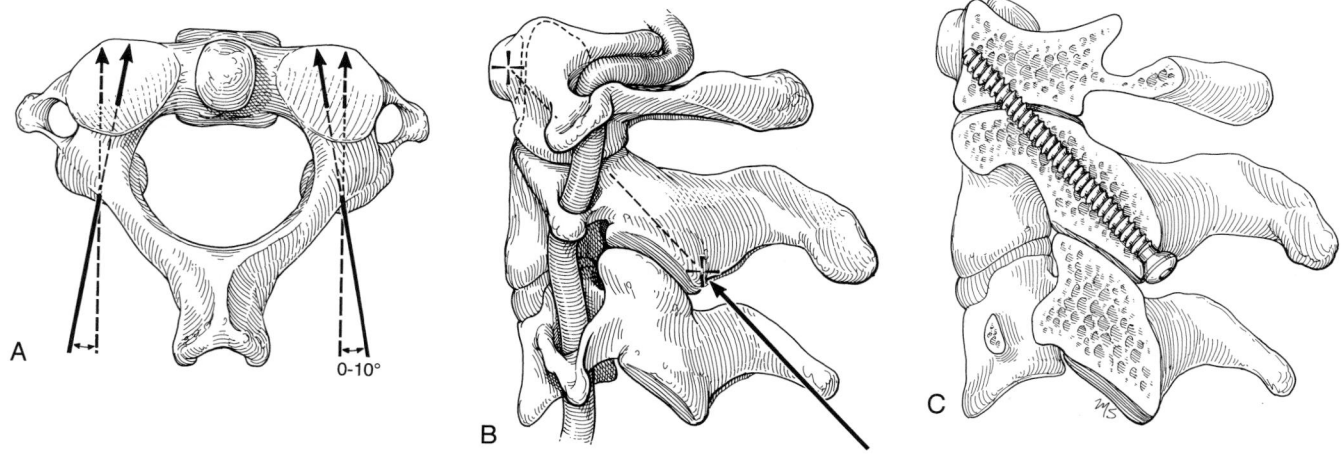

FIGURE 303–16. Axial (*A*) and sagittal (*B*) trajectories for transarticular screw placement. The screw is passed down the central axis of the pars interarticularis (0 to 10 degrees medially) and is targeted in the sagittal plane toward the posterior cortex of the anterior arch of C1. Failure to reduce anterior atlantoaxial displacement and the absence of the anterior C1 tubercle are associated with an elevated incidence of suboptimally positioned screws and injured vertebral arteries. *C,* Final position of a fully threaded, cannulated transarticular screw. A pars interarticularis screw would be placed using similar landmarks and trajectories, but with only limited passage along the pars interarticularis. (From Barrow Neurological Institute, St. Joseph's Hospital and Medical Center, Phoenix, AZ.)

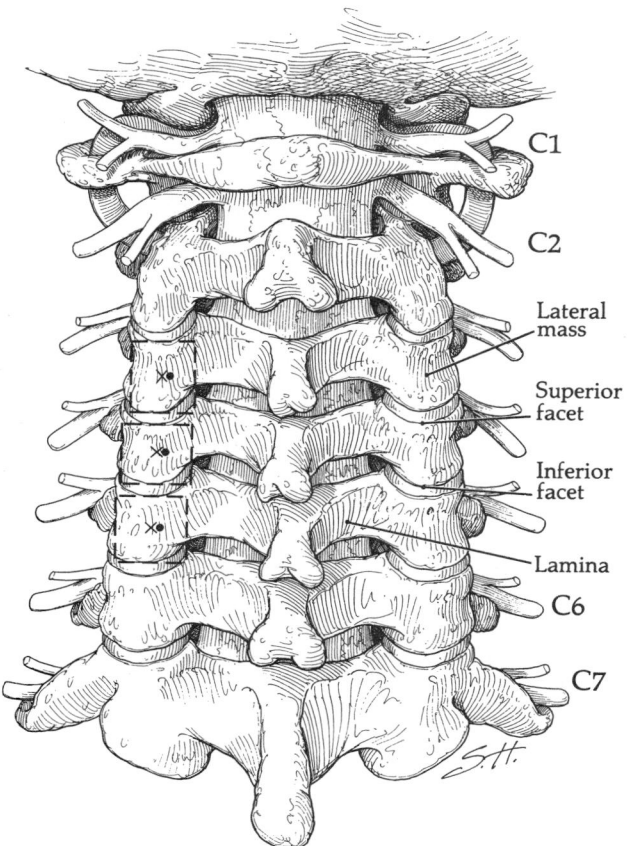

FIGURE 303–17. Entry point (*dot*) for lateral mass screw placement. The rostral, caudal, medial, and lateral borders of the articular pillar are defined, and the midpoint is identified (*X*). Our (VKHS and CAD) preferred entry site for lateral mass screws is 1 mm medial to this point. (From Barrow Neurological Institute, St. Joseph's Hospital and Medical Center, Phoenix, AZ.)

303–17). In most adults, the vertebral artery lies more than 16 mm from this site of screw entry.[83] Pilot holes are drilled and screws are directed 20 to 30 degrees rostrally (parallel to the facet joint orientation) and 20 to 30 degrees laterally (Fig. 303–18). Bicortical purchase of the articular pillar is sought with the screw tip residing in the ventral extent of the superolateral aspect of the lateral mass. This region has been designated as the "safe quadrant," under which there are no neurovascular structures.[84] Facet joints within the fixation construct are decorticated with a curette or drill to facilitate their fusion. This maneuver is most easily performed before the hardware is inserted.

PLACEMENT OF FIXATION PLATES

Given the tight anatomic constraints inherent to positioning posterior cervical screws, entry sites and screw trajectories for transarticular and lateral mass screws are drilled before the implant is shaped or placed. Only after these relatively immutable anchoring points are defined and the patient's craniovertebral alignment considered is the fixation hardware contoured (Fig. 303–19). In the event that cervical screw purchase is

compromised at a particular site because of a suboptimal placement that cannot be corrected or poor bone quality that cannot be compensated for with a larger diameter screw, a sublaminar or facet cable may be connected to the plate to salvage that fixation point. Tenuous screw sites can also be reinforced with methyl methacrylate, but this option is undesirable because it diminishes the surface area available for the fusion response to occur.[44] The addition of autologous bone to the decorticated surgical bed remains paramount to promoting long-term stability of the mechanically compromised CVJ.

BONE GRAFTS

Autologous bone is the preferred fusion substrate for posterior cervical fusion procedures.[87, 88] The use of autogeneic bone from the iliac crest was first described for occipitocervical fusion in 1935[89] and has essentially served as the senior authors' exclusive source of corticocancellous bone for occipitocervical fusion. The techniques for harvesting autologous iliac crest bone are well described.[90, 91] The side of autologous graft harvest is directed by the patient's preference and may be influenced by preexisting difficulties with arthritis or gait. Although the ilium offers relatively easy access to an ample amount of excellent quality grafting substrate, a considerable morbidity rate is associated with iliac crest bone harvest and is likely even underreported.[92] In particular, donor site pain (acute and chronic) can impede a patient's convalescence. In one series, it affected 49% of 290 patients who underwent harvest of autologous iliac crest bone.[93]

In a retrospective analysis that compared fusion rates and donor site morbidity associated with autogeneic rib and iliac crest bone grafts in cervical fusion procedures, Sawin and colleagues demonstrated the benefits of rib autograft as a fusion material.[92] In their series of 600 patients, 300 underwent posterior cervical spine fusion procedures with autologous rib. The rib graft was successfully incorporated in 296 (98.8%) of these patients. Included in this cohort were 196 patients who underwent an occipitocervical fusion procedure. Graft-related morbidity occurred in 11 (3.7%) patients who underwent rib harvest, with pneumonia being the most common complication. No cases of pneumothorax, intercostal neuralgia, or chronic chest wall pain were noted. In contrast, the incidence of graft-associated morbidity associated with iliac crest harvest exceeded 25%. In this subgroup, debilitating pain (17%) was the most prevalent complication.

ORTHOSES AND POSTOPERATIVE FOLLOW-UP

Supplemental external orthoses help control motion and reduce loads on the fixation instrumentation while the fusion response matures. A Philadelphia collar or sterno-occipitomandibular immobilizer (SOMI brace) is appropriate when the patient's bone quality is good,

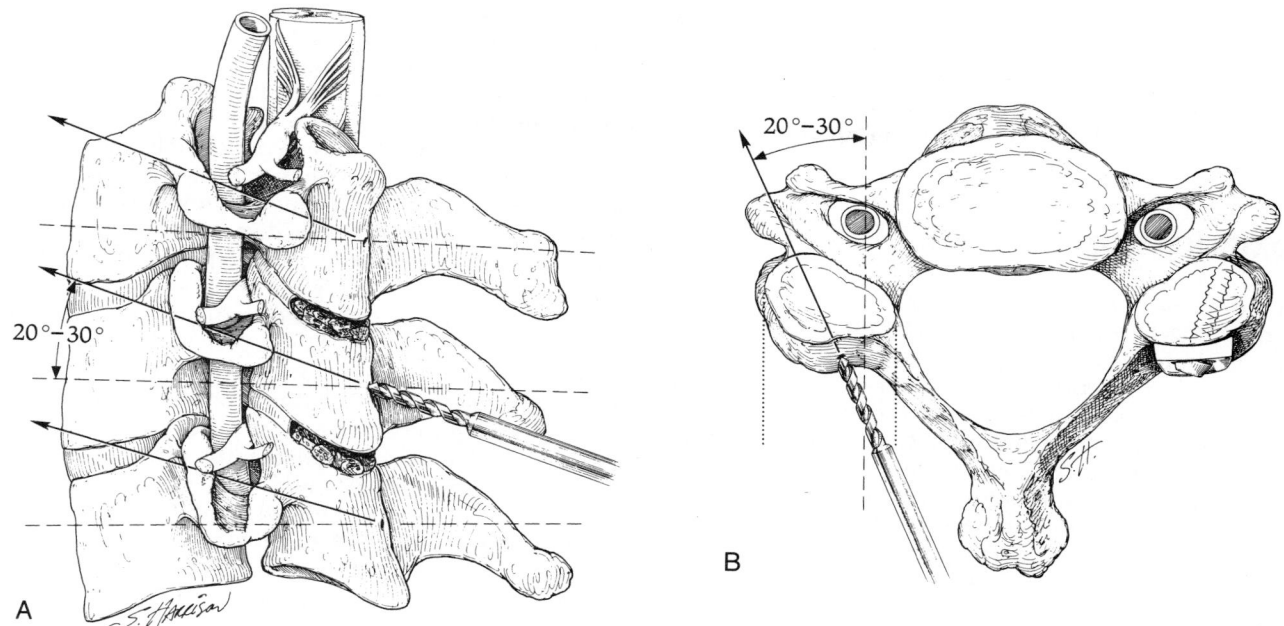

FIGURE 303–18. Sagittal (*A*) and axial (*B*) depictions of lateral mass screw trajectories. Sagittal orientation is parallel to the facet joint, and screws are placed fluoroscopically with the intention of gaining bicortical purchase. Note the decorticated facet joints. The screw track is angled 20 to 30 degrees laterally in the axial plane and can be approximated by seating the instrument at the entry site and angling the shaft of the drill guide or screwdriver to contact the adjacent spinous process. (From Barrow Neurological Institute, St. Joseph's Hospital and Medical Center, Phoenix, AZ.)

the fixation is strong, and deforming forces are minimal. A more rigid orthosis (halo or Minerva brace) is needed for poor fixation (soft bone), extensive instability (OAD), excessive loading of the vertebrae, widespread bony destruction, or individual patient characteristics that portend a diminished fusion response (e.g., malnutrition, tobacco use, osteoporosis or metabolic disorders associated with poor bone quality, and exogenous steroid or drug requirements that limit bone healing).[52]

In the senior authors' experience with occipitocervical cable-based fixation, no significant differences in fusion response were associated with the type of postoperative immobilization (Philadelphia collar or halo brace) in patients treated for comparable CVJ pathologic conditions.[46] Although patients were previously maintained in a halo brace for 12 to 16 weeks, rigid postoperative external bracing is now avoided. Patients wear a hard collar and are evaluated at 2- to 4-week intervals to assess clinical progress and monitor

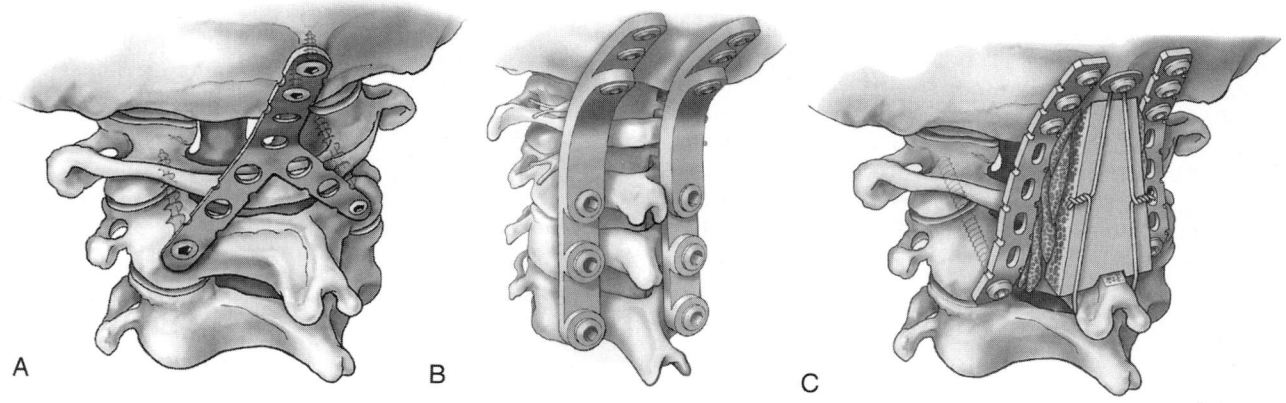

FIGURE 303–19. Occipitocervical screw-plate constructs. *A*, Grob "Y" screw plate with transarticular screw fixation of the atlantoaxial complex. *B*, Roy-Camille occipitocervical reinforced plate. *C*, Magerl technique with transarticular screw and wire fixation of the autologous graft. (From Barrow Neurological Institute, St. Joseph's Hospital and Medical Center, Phoenix, AZ.)

radiographic alignment. After 12 weeks, evidence of fusion prompts dynamic radiographs (cervical flexion and extension) to assess stability of the construct. In the case of a stable arthrodesis, patients are weaned from their hard collar and begin cervical strengthening exercises.

COMPLICATIONS

The potential risks associated with cranioverterbral stabilization techniques include infection, bleeding that requires transfusion with the associated possibilities of transfusion reactions or infection (e.g., hepatitis or human immunodeficiency virus [HIV]), medical complications (e.g., myocardial infarction, stroke, pneumonia, urinary tract infections, or deep venous thrombosis), high cervical myelopathy with the associated need for tracheostomy and gastrostomy, lower cranial neuropathy, intracranial hemorrhage related to suboccipital wire passage or screw placement, dural tears associated with a cerebrospinal fluid leak, suboccipital numbness, inadequate bone healing (fibrous union or pseudarthrosis), or hardware failure with displacement of instrumentation. The risks of surgery also include complications at the donor site (e.g., infection, hematomas, cosmetic deformities, and prolonged pain or numbness).

Recognition of the medical frailty of many patients who make up this population is a key point to minimizing postoperative rates of morbidity. Efforts to optimize nutrition can avert difficulties with wound healing and pulmonary and laryngeal edema.[3] The metabolic derangements inherent to certain causes of CVJ pathology should be corrected as best as possible before surgery with the assistance of a multidisciplinary team. The rate of operative morbidity in patients with bone-softening diseases is higher than that of age-matched controls and has been reported to exceed 40%.[15] The justifiably feared risk of myelopathy related to cervical sublaminar wire placement can be minimized by carefully passing cables in the "pull-push" method described earlier and by exposing the dura sufficiently so that distortion can be recognized as the cable is passed. Anteriorly based compressive pathology is most safely addressed before pursuing posterior stabilization with a sublaminar cable. Attention to radiographic and anatomic detail when placing posterior cervical screws is crucial, both because of the proximity of vulnerable neurovascular structures and the inferior bone purchase frequently associated with attempts to correct a suboptimally positioned screw (measure twice, screw once).

CONCLUSIONS

Increasing success in securing arthrodesis at the occipitocervical junction is a direct result of the evolution of progressively more effective and aggressive methods of achieving rigid internal fixation along this region. Various metallic implants are available through which immediate rigid internal fixation can be achieved in patients with occipitocervical instability. Their development has enabled a transition away from rigid external bracing during the postoperative management of patients who have undergone CVJ stabilization procedures, thus providing a more comfortable and "maintenance-free" convalescence. Patients with CVJ deformities often have chronic systemic disorders (e.g., rheumatoid settling, Paget's disease, osteogenesis imperfecta, rickets, osteomalacia, hyperparathyroidism), which can contribute to higher rates of morbidity. Optimization of primary metabolic or medical ailments should not be overlooked as a pre- and postoperative requirement for a successful outcome. Absolute familiarity with the regional anatomy is mandatory for surgeons planning to perform these procedures, and attention to detail is crucial when intubating, positioning, and operating on patients with CVJ pathology. Surgical planning must remain faithful to the goals of neural decompression and mechanical stabilization.

Our clinical experience in surgically managing the unstable CVJ is primarily derived from the application of a contoured, grooved pin fixed with braided cables to the occiput and cervical laminae. Screw-based systems offer the opportunity to avoid complications related to sublaminar wire placement but introduce the potential of injuring the cervical or hypoglossal nerve roots or vertebral arteries. Long-term clinical success is a function of osseous integration, but diseased bone tissue heals slowly and tolerates hardware poorly. Increasingly sophisticated instrumentation does not supplant the fundamental requirement for a carefully conceived and meticulously performed fusion procedure.

REFERENCES

1. White AA 3rd, Panjabi MM: The clinical biomechanics of the occipitoatlantoaxial complex. Orthop Clin North Am 9:867–878, 1978.
2. Menezes AH, VanGilder JC: Anomalies of the craniovertebral junction. In Youmans JR (ed): Neurological Surgery. Philadelphia, WB Saunders, 1990, pp 1359–1420.
3. Menezes AH: Posterior occipitocervical fixation. Tech Neurosurg 1:72–81, 1995.
4. White AA 3rd, Panjabi MM: Clinical Biomechanics of the Spine. Philadelphia, JB Lippincott, 1978.
5. Dickman CA, Papadopoulos SM, Sonntag VKH, et al: Traumatic occipitoatlantal dislocations. J Spinal Disord 6:300–313, 1993.
6. Papadopoulos SM, Dickman CA, Sonntag VKH, et al: Traumatic atlantooccipital dislocation with survival. Neurosurgery 28:574–579, 1991.
7. Traynelis VC, Marano GD, Dunker RO, et al: Traumatic atlanto-occipital dislocation. Case report. J Neurosurg 65:863–870, 1986.
8. Bucholz RW, Burkhead WZ: The pathological anatomy of fatal atlanto-occipital dislocations. J Bone Joint Surg Am 61:248–250, 1979.
9. Pang D, Wilberger JE Jr: Traumatic atlanto-occipital dislocation with survival: Case report and review. Neurosurgery 7:503–508, 1980.
10. Crockard HA, Essigman WK, Stevens JM, et al: Surgical treatment of cervical cord compression in rheumatoid arthritis. Ann Rheum Dis 44:809–816, 1985.
11. Menezes AH, VanGilder JC: Transoral-transpharyngeal approach to the anterior craniocervical junction. Ten-year experience with 72 patients. J Neurosurg 69:895–903, 1988.
12. Zeidman SM, Ducker TB: Rheumatoid arthritis. Neuroanatomy, compression, and grading of deficits. Spine 19:2259–2266, 1994.

13. McWhorter JM, Alexander E, Davis CH, et al: Posterior cervical fusion in children. J Neurosurg 45:211–215, 1976.
14. Walpin LA, Singer FR: Paget's disease. Reversal of severe paraparesis using calcitonin. Spine 4:213–219, 1979.
15. Shiau JSC, Arginteanu MS, Perin NI: Arthritic and bone-softening diseases of the craniocervical junction. Neurosurg Q 8:180–190, 1998.
16. Sharp J, Purser DW: Spontaneous atlanto-axial dislocation in ankylosing spondylitis and rheumatoid arthritis. Ann Rheum Dis 20:47–77, 1961.
17. Taylor AR, Chakrovorty BC: Clinical syndromes associated with basilar impression. Arch Neurol 10:475–484, 1964.
18. Hakuba A, Komiyama M, Tsujimoto T, et al: Transuncodiscal approach to dumbbell tumors of the cervical spinal canal. J Neurosurg 61:1100–1106, 1984.
19. Harkey HL, Capel WT: Bone softening diseases and disorders of bone metabolism. In Dickman CA, Spetzler RF, Sonntag VK (eds): Surgery of the Craniovertebral Junction. New York, Thieme, 1998, pp 197–208.
20. Pilcher LS: Atlo-axoid fracture-dislocation. Ann Surg 51:208–211, 1910.
21. Foerster O: Die Leitungsbahnen des Schmerzgefühls und die chirurgische Behandlung der Schmerzzustände. Berlin, Urban and Schwarzenberg, 1927.
22. Murphy MJ, Southwick WO: Posterior approaches and fusions. In Cervical Spine Research Society (ed): The Cervical Spine. Philadelphia, JB Lippincott, 1989, pp 775–791.
23. Newman P, Sweetnam R: Occipito-cervical fusion. An operative technique and its indications. J Bone Joint Surg Br 51:423–431, 1969.
24. Elia M, Mazzara JT, Fielding JW: Onlay technique for occipitocervical fusion. Clin Orthop 280:170–174, 1992.
25. Fielding JW, Hawkins RJ, Ratzan SA: Spine fusion for atlanto-axial instability. J Bone Joint Surg Am 58:400–407, 1976.
26. Sherk HH, Snyder B: Posterior fusions of the upper cervical spine: Indications, techniques, and prognosis. Orthop Clin N Am 9:1091–1099, 1978.
27. Grantham SA, Dick HM, Thompson RC Jr, et al: Occipitocervical arthrodesis. Indications, technic and results. Clin Orthop 65:118–129, 1969.
28. Hamblen DL: Occipito-cervical fusion. Indications, technique and results. J Bone Joint Surg Br 49:33–45, 1967.
29. Menezes AH, VanGilder JC, Graf CJ, et al: Craniocervical abnormalities. A comprehensive surgical approach. J Neurosurg 53:444–455, 1980.
30. Wertheim SB, Bohlman HH: Occipitocervical fusion. Indications, technique, and long-term results in thirteen patients. J Bone Joint Surg Am 69:833–836, 1987.
31. Yashon D: Surgical management of trauma to the spine. In Schmidek HH, Sweet WH (eds): Operative Neurosurgical Techniques. Indications, Methods and Results. Orlando, Grune & Stratton, 1988, pp 1449–1469.
32. Robinson RA, Southwick WO: Surgical approaches to the cervical spine. In American Academy of Orthopedic Surgeons (ed): Instructional Course Lectures. St. Louis, CV Mosby, 1960, pp 299–330.
33. Fehlings MG, Errico T, Cooper P, et al: Occipitocervical fusion with a five-millimeter malleable rod and segmental fixation. Neurosurgery 32:198–207, 1993.
34. Dickman CA, Douglas RA, Sonntag VKH: Occipitocervical fusion: Posterior stabilization of the craniovertebral junction and upper cervical spine. BNI Q 6:2–14, 1990.
35. Grob D, Dvorak J, Panjabi M, et al: Posterior occipitocervical fusion. A preliminary report of a new technique. Spine 16:S17–S24, 1991.
36. Roy-Camille R, Saillant G, Mazel C: Internal fixation of the unstable cervical spine by a posterior osteosynthesis with plates and screws. In Cervical Spine Research Society (ed): The Cervical Spine. Philadelphia, JB Lippincott, 1989, pp 390–403.
37. Crockard HA, Pozo JL, Ransford AO, et al: Transoral decompression and posterior fusion for rheumatoid atlanto-axial subluxation. J Bone Joint Surg Br 68:350–356, 1986.
38. MacKenzie AI, Uttley D, Marsh HT, et al: Craniocervical stabilization using Luque/Hartshill rectangles. Neurosurgery 26:32–36, 1990.
39. Ransford AO, Crockard HA, Pozo JL, et al: Craniocervical instability treated by contoured loop fixation. J Bone Joint Surg Br 68:173–177, 1986.
40. Sakou T, Kawaida H, Morizono Y, et al: Occipitoatlantoaxial fusion utilizing a rectangular rod. Clin Orthop 239:136–144, 1989.
41. Ellis PM, Findlay JM: Craniocervical fusion with contoured Luque rod and autogeneic bone graft. Can J Surg 37:50–54, 1994.
42. Itoh T, Tsuji H, Katoh Y, et al: Occipito-cervical fusion reinforced by Luque's segmental spinal instrumentation for rheumatoid diseases. Spine 13:1234–1238, 1988.
43. Smith MD, Anderson P, Grady MS: Occipitocervical arthrodesis using contoured plate fixation. An early report on a versatile fixation technique. Spine 18:1984–1990, 1993.
44. Sonntag VKH, Dickman CA: Craniocervical stabilization. Clin Neurosurg 40:243–272, 1993.
45. Sonntag VKH, Dickman CA: Occipitocervical instrumentation. In Hitchon PW, Traynelis VC, Rengachary SS (eds): Techniques in Spinal Fusion and Stabilization. New York, Thieme, 1995, pp 107–121.
46. Apostolides PJ, Dickman CA, Golfinos JG, et al: Threaded Steinmann pin fusion of the craniovertebral junction. Spine 21:1630–1637, 1996.
47. Songer MN, Spencer DL, Meyer PR Jr, et al: The use of sublaminar cables to replace Luque wires. Spine 16:S418–S421, 1991.
48. Dickman CA, Sonntag VKH, Marcotte PJ: Techniques of screw fixation of the cervical spine. BNI Q 8:9–26, 1992.
49. Heywood AW, Learmonth ID, Thomas M: Internal fixation for occipito-cervical fusion. J Bone Joint Surg Br 70:708–711, 1988.
50. Malcolm GP, Ransford AO, Crockard HA: Treatment of non-rheumatoid occipitocervical instability. Internal fixation with the Hartshill-Ransford loop. J Bone Joint Surg Br 76:357–366, 1994.
51. Pait TG, Al-Mefty O, Boop FA, et al: Inside-outside technique for posterior occipitocervical spine instrumentation and stabilization: Preliminary results. J Neurosurg 90:1–7, 1999.
52. Apostolides PJ, Sonntag VKH, Dickman CA: Occipitocervical wiring techniques. In Dickman CA, Spetzler RF, Sonntag VKH (eds): Surgery of the Craniovertebral Junction. New York, Thieme, 1998, pp 795–808.
53. Grob D, Dvorak J, Panjabi MM, et al: The role of plate and screw fixation in occipitocervical fusion in rheumatoid arthritis. Spine 19:2545–2551, 1994.
54. Rupp R, Ebraheim NA, Savolaine ER, et al: Magnetic resonance imaging evaluation of the spine with metal implants. General safety and superior imaging with titanium. Spine 18:379–385, 1993.
55. Dickman CA, Maric Z: The biology of bone healing and techniques of spinal fusion. BNI Q 10:2–12, 1994.
56. Prolo DJ: Biology of bone fusion. Clin Neurosurg 36:135–146, 1990.
57. Kaufman HH, Jones E: The principles of bony spinal fusion. Neurosurgery 24:264–270, 1989.
58. Menezes AH: Posterior occipital C1–C2 fusion. In Menezes AH, Sonntag VK (eds): Principles of Spinal Surgery. New York, McGraw-Hill, 1996, pp 1051–1065.
59. Sonntag VK, Dickman CA: Posterior occipital C1–C2 instrumentation. In Menezes AH, Sonntag VK (eds): Principles of Spinal Surgery. New York, McGraw-Hill, 1996, pp 1067–1079.
60. Glaser JA, Whitehill R, Stamp WG, et al: Complications associated with the halo-vest. A review of 245 cases. J Neurosurg 65:762–769, 1986.
61. Lind B, Nordwall A, Sihlbom H: Odontoid fractures treated with halo-vest. Spine 12:173–177, 1987.
62. Polin RS, Szabo T, Bogaev CA, et al: Nonoperative management of Types II and III odontoid fractures: The Philadelphia collar versus the halo vest. Neurosurgery 38:350–357, 1996.
63. Dickman CA, Locantro J, Fessler RG: The influence of transoral odontoid resection on stability of the craniovertebral junction. J Neurosurg 77:525–530, 1992.
64. Hadley MN, Spetzler RF, Sonntag VKH: The transoral approach to the superior cervical spine. A review of 53 cases of extradural cervicomedullary compression. J Neurosurg 71:16–23, 1989.
65. Menezes AH, VanGilder JC, Clark CR, et al: Odontoid upward migration in rheumatoid arthritis. An analysis of 45 patients with "cranial settling." J Neurosurg 63:500–509, 1985.
66. Krag MH: Biomechanics of the cervical spine including bracing,

surgical constructs, and orthosis. In Frymoyer JW, Ducker TB, Hadler NM, et al (eds): The Adult Spine: Principles and Practice. New York, Raven, 1991, pp 929–965.

67. Bracken MB, Shepard MJ, Holford TR, et al: Administration of methylprednisolone for 24 or 48 hours or tirilazad mesylate for 48 hours in the treatment of acute spinal cord injury. Results of the Third National Acute Spinal Cord Injury Randomized Controlled Trial. National Acute Spinal Cord Injury Study. JAMA 277:1597–1604, 1997.

68. Sawin PD, Menezes AH: Basilar invagination in osteogenesis imperfecta and related osteochondrodysplasias: Medical and surgical management. J Neurosurg 86:950–960, 1997.

69. Apostolides PJ, Karahalios DG, Yapp RA, et al: Use of the Bend-Meister rod bender for occipitocervical fusion: Technical note. Neurosurgery 43:389–391, 1998.

70. McCormick PC: Use of the BendMeister rod bender for occipitocervical fusion [commentary]. Neurosurgery 43:391, 1998.

71. Dickman CA, Papadopoulos SM, Crawford NR, et al: Comparative mechanical properties of spinal cable and wire fixation systems. Spine 22:596–604, 1997.

72. Clark CR, Goetz DD, Menezes AH: Arthrodesis of the cervical spine in rheumatoid arthritis. J Bone Joint Surg Am 71:381–392, 1989.

73. Geremia GK, Kim KS, Cerullo L, et al: Complications of sublaminar wiring. Surg Neurol 23:629–635, 1985.

74. Sonntag VKH, Dickman CA: Occipitocervical and high cervical stabilization. In Rengachary S, Wilkins R (eds): Neurosurgical Operative Atlas. Baltimore, Williams & Wilkins, 1991, pp 327–339.

75. Pelker RR, Duranceau JS, Panjabi MM: Cervical spine stabilization. A three-dimensional, biomechanical evaluation of rotational stability, strength, and failure mechanisms. Spine 16:117–122, 1991.

76. Hurlbert RJ, Crawford NR, Choi WG, et al: A biomechanical evaluation of occipitocervical instrumentation: Screw compared with wire fixation. J Neurosurg 90:84–90, 1999.

77. Montesano PX, Juach EC, Anderson PA, et al: Biomechanics of cervical spine internal fixation. Spine 16:S10–S16, 1991.

78. Paramore CG, Dickman CA, Sonntag VKH: The anatomical suitability of the C1–2 complex for transarticular screw fixation. J Neurosurg 85:221–224, 1996.

79. Song GS, Theodore N, Dickman CA, et al: Unilateral posterior atlantoaxial transarticular screw fixation. J Neurosurg 87:851–855, 1997.

80. Madawi AA, Casey AT, Solanki GA, et al: Radiological and anatomical evaluation of the atlantoaxial transarticular screw fixation technique. J Neurosurg 86:961–968, 1997.

81. Weidner A: Internal fixation with metal plates and screw. In Cervical Spine Research Society (ed): The Cervical Spine. Philadelphia, JB Lippincott, 1989, pp 404–421.

82. An HS, Gordin R, Renner K: Anatomic considerations for plate-screw fixation of the cervical spine. Spine 16:548–551, 1991.

83. Cherny WB, Sonntag VKH, Douglas RA: Lateral mass posterior plating and facet fusion for cervical spine instability. BNI Q 7:2–11, 1991.

84. Pait TG, McAllister PV, Kaufman HH: Quadrant anatomy of the articular pillars (lateral cervical mass) of the cervical spine. J Neurosurg 82:1011–1014, 1995.

85. Sawin PD, Traynelis VC: Posterior articular mass plate fixation of the subaxial cervical spine. In Menezes AH, Sonntag VKH (eds): Principles of Spinal Surgery. New York, McGraw-Hill, 1996, pp 1081–1104.

86. Heller JG, Carlson GD, Abitbol JJ, et al: Anatomic comparison of the Roy-Camille and Magerl techniques for screw placement in the lower cervical spine. Spine 16:S552–S557, 1991.

87. Koop SE, Winter RB, Lonstein JE: The surgical treatment of instability of the upper part of the cervical spine in children and adolescents. J Bone Joint Surg Am 66:403–411, 1984.

88. Stabler CL, Eismont FJ, Brown MD, et al: Failure of posterior cervical fusions using cadaveric bone graft in children. J Bone Joint Surg Am 67:371–375, 1985.

89. Kahn EA, Yglesias L: Progressive atlanto-axial dislocation. JAMA 105:348–352, 1935.

90. Kurz LT, Garfin SR, Booth RE, Jr: Harvesting autogenous iliac bone grafts. A review of complications and techniques. Spine 14:1324–1331, 1989.

91. Yonemura KS: Bone grafts: Types of harvesting and their complications. In Menezes AH, Sonntag VKH (eds): Principles of Spinal Surgery. New York, McGraw-Hill, 1996, pp 151–156.

92. Sawin PD, Traynelis VC, Menezes AH: A comparative analysis of fusion rates and donor-site morbidity for autogeneic rib and iliac crest bone grafts in posterior cervical fusions. J Neurosurg 88:255–265, 1998.

93. Summers BN, Eisenstein SM: Donor site pain from the ilium. A complication of lumbar spine fusion. J Bone Joint Surg Br 71:677–680, 1989.

CHAPTER 304

Anterior Thoracic Instrumentation

MICHAEL G. KAISER ■ ANDREW T. PARSA ■
BARRY D. BIRCH ■ PAUL C. McCORMICK

Operative techniques for anterior reconstruction of the thoracic spine have changed significantly in the last several decades. The early efforts of surgical pioneers to stabilize the spine after the destruction of the anterior spinal elements were often met with high rates of morbidity and construct failure. Currently, effective anterior stabilization of the thoracic spine can be achieved with an evolving array of spinal instrumentation. Although surgical intervention for ventral thoracic pathology is practiced regularly, it is by no means routine. Surgical success is predicated on the practitioner's understanding of the appropriate operative indications, thoracic surgical anatomy, and spinal biomechanics. Up-to-date knowledge of available implants is also essential.

This chapter describes the background and surgical practice of anterior instrumentation of the thoracic spine. Constructs for anterior thoracic spinal fixation are designed primarily to stabilize from the midthoracic through thoracolumbar regions. Lesions of the upper thoracic spine, especially traumatic lesions, are less common and do not produce the same degree of instability.

HISTORICAL BACKGROUND

The impetus for developing thoracic instrumentation can be found in the literature as far back as 1928. In that year, Royle[1] described anterior decompression of the spine for scoliotic deformities, without subsequent spinal reconstruction. Hodgson and Stock[2] later described similar decompressive procedures for Pott's disease. These efforts did not include spinal reconstruction; as a result, their patients suffered from postoperative instability and progressive deformity. In 1958, Humphries and Hawk[3] published one of the first reports on ventral instrumentation developed for stabilization following transperitoneal decompression of patients with Pott's disease. Their ventral plate and screw construct provided little biomechanical support and was later abandoned. In the 1970s, advances in construct design were applied surgically by Dwyer and coworkers[4, 5] and Zielke and colleagues.[6] The screw-

cable construct of Dwyer and the screw-rod construct of Zielke successfully corrected scoliotic deformities. However, these constructs were not rigid enough to provide structural support. In the late 1970s, Dunn developed a double-rod, double-screw construct that provided adequate stability for anterior thoracolumbar reconstruction.[7, 8] In 1986, however, the Dunn device was removed from clinical use after reports of great vessel erosion.[9] The material properties of newer-generation titanium constructs, such as the Kaneda device (Acromed, Cleveland, OH) and the ZPlate II (Sofamor-Danek, Memphis, TN), have improved, and their profiles are lower than those of earlier devices. They are also compatible with magnetic resonance imaging.

INDICATIONS FOR OPERATIVE INTERVENTION

Neoplasm

Most neoplastic disorders affecting the spinal column are malignant. Between 20% and 70% of patients with metastatic disease have some form of spinal involvement, with approximately 80% to 90% of these metastases involving the vertebral bodies.[10–13] The incidence of patients with spinal metastases has increased over the years, reflecting improvements in adjuvant therapy and longer survival times.

Metastatic involvement of the spine can manifest with pain, progressive deformity, or neurological deficits. Operative intervention is appropriate for tissue diagnosis, neurological decompression, and spinal stabilization. Other indications include resection of radioresistant neoplasms, resection of isolated recurrences, and neurological deterioration after adjuvant treatment. Posterior decompression for anterior metastatic disease has been ineffective and sometimes detrimental.[14] Resection of the posterior elements removes the posterior tension band and decreases the ability of the spine to resist flexion forces if the anterior elements are compromised. Neurological deficits can follow extrusion of bone fragments into the spinal cord or anterior tethering of the spinal cord as a kyphotic deformity develops. Historically, clinical outcomes associated with posterior surgical intervention were so poor that radiotherapy became the treatment of choice.[10, 14–16] Advances in surgical technique led to the development of ventral spinal approaches without excessive complications. An anterior approach provides a direct means to address ventral pathology and to reconstruct the spine at the origin of instability. Currently, clinical outcomes for patients with metastatic spinal disease after anterior decompression are superior to those associated with posterior decompression with or without adjuvant radiotherapy.[12, 17–23] However, selection of appropriate patients for surgical intervention remains a challenge.

Several considerations determine whether patients with neoplastic disease of the spine are operative candidates. A poor baseline medical condition increases the risk of surgical complications. Age and preoperative functional status are independent predictors of postoperative survival. The Karnofsky performance scale has been used as an assessment of functional status and quality of life, and survival rates are higher in patients with a score of 70 or higher.[24–26] Typically, surgical intervention is reserved for patients with a life expectancy of at least 12 months. The cost of subjecting patients with a limited life expectancy to a prolonged course of hospitalization and rehabilitation must be considered, but surgical intervention should not be withheld if it will significantly improve quality of life. The value of restoring neurological function, such as ambulation or sphincter control, must be judged on an individual basis.

Other considerations in selecting patients for operative intervention include type of tumor, compromise of spinal canal, degree of neurological deficit, and level of pain. Neurological deficits associated with tumor invasion of the spinal canal are not always a clear indication for operative intervention.[10, 11, 27] Certain tumors, such as prostate neoplasms, lymphoma, and myeloma, are sensitive to adjuvant treatments. A trial of radiation, chemotherapy, or hormonal therapy should be considered before operative intervention. Radiotherapy has been associated with favorable outcomes when the spinal canal is compromised by soft tissue alone.[14] In contrast, surgical decompression is indicated if retropulsed bone fragments from a pathologic fracture compromise the spinal canal. Emergent surgical decompression is appropriate for patients with progressive neurological deficits caused by a tumor known to be unresponsive to adjuvant therapies. After a complete spinal cord injury of at least 24 hours' duration, recovery from a neurological deficit is extremely rare, even after successful decompression. In such cases, surgical intervention is seldom effective unless a significant degree of instability will interfere with the patient's care.

Nonoperative intervention is also appropriate for patients with stable myelopathy and spinal cord compression. Close observation is required whenever radiation is applied to a lesion within the spinal canal. Radiation-induced cell death can cause edema to form, and the resultant spinal cord compression is responsive to treatment with steroids. However, persistent deterioration after radiotherapy is more likely the result of

tumor progression and warrants surgical decompression. Surgical intervention may be the only recourse for patients who have received maximal levels of adjuvant therapy. Intractable pain can result from several factors, including direct neurological compression, invasion of the periosteum, and spinal instability. If overt instability is absent, as many as 85% of patients can achieve pain control with radiation or analgesics.[11]

Neurological deterioration is rare after operative intervention for metastatic spinal disease. Perioperative mortality rates range from 6% to 8%, and overall complication rates range from 8% to 11%. In these reports, some patients were not initially treated with an anterior approach, and it is possible that an anterior approach alone would decrease the combined rate of morbidity and mortality.[12]

Trauma

Most thoracic spine fractures occur at the thoracolumbar junction; about 50% to 80% occur between T10 and L2.[28, 29] The thoracolumbar region is particularly susceptible to traumatic injury for several reasons: instability associated with transition from the stable thoracic spine to the mobile lumbar region, loss of rigidity provided by the intact rib cage, instability associated with transition from kyphosis to lordosis, and change in orientation of the facet.[30, 31] Based on the three-column model of stability, Denis[32] categorized these fractures into four classes: compression fractures, burst fractures, seat-belt-type fractures, and fracture-dislocations. The most common types of fractures are compression and burst fractures.[32]

Neurological injury results from direct compression of the spinal cord by retropulsed bone fragments or tethering of the spinal cord over a kyphotic deformity. Conservative management of thoracic fractures with external bracing is associated with excellent outcomes, with no gross destruction of the anterior spinal elements, no significant compromise of the spinal canal or neurological deficits, and an intact posterior column.[29, 33, 34] Typically, fractures that produce a 40% loss in the height of the vertebral body, a 50% compromise of the spinal canal without neurological deficits, a kyphotic deformity of 30 degrees, or neurological deficits require operative intervention.[35, 36]

The choice of surgical procedure remains controversial. Posterior fusion and fixation may be appropriate if there is no significant ventral deformity or spinal canal compromise. This approach, however, is inadequate for lesions that cause ventral neuronal compression or a significant deformity. Ligamentotaxis is an unreliable means of decompressing the ventral spinal canal. Outcomes after posterior decompression, reduction, and stabilization are comparable to the results obtained with conservative management of lesions producing ventral compression.[37–41] Lesions producing ventral compression or significant biomechanical compromise of the anterior and middle columns are indications for an anterior approach. Previous reports have documented better outcomes with an anterior approach compared with isolated posterior stabilization.[35, 38, 42, 43] If the posterior elements have been injured significantly, an anterior construct may be insufficient to resist flexion forces. Loss of the posterior tension band may require supplementation with posterior stabilization. Patients with a complete injury may still benefit from spinal stabilization. Surgical stabilization optimizes the rehabilitation process and possibly decreases the length of hospitalization.

Infection

Hodgson and Stock[2] were among the first to describe successful anterior decompression in patient's with Pott's disease. With advances in diagnosis and antibiotics, most cases of vertebral osteomyelitis and diskitis can now be treated effectively without surgical intervention. As many as 90% of patients respond to intravenous antibiotics and immobilization.[44] Failed medical management may require surgical débridement and stabilization. Evidence of antibiotic failure includes an elevated erythrocyte sedimentation rate and white blood cell count, persistent or worsening pain, radiographic evidence of progression, and continued bacteremia. Infections rarely spread to the ventral epidural space; less than 20% of spinal epidural abscesses occur anterior to the spinal cord.[45] Neurological deficits can result from medullary or radicular vessel inflammation and is not always an indication to proceed with surgery. Surgical débridement is necessary to obtain a diagnostic culture and in the case of failed medical treatment, neurological deficits related to a ventral collection, and severe vertebral body destruction that causes a significant deformity. Despite the presence of an active infection, insertion of an interbody strut graft and instrumentation construct does not appear to increase the incidence of postoperative infection.[46, 47]

Deformity and Degenerative Conditions

A symptomatic deformity of the thoracic spine can occur as a late complication of trauma, infection, or neoplasm. Iatrogenic deformities can follow laminectomy or repair of a developmental anomaly. Anatomic indications for surgical intervention include kyphosis greater than 30 degrees as well as progressive scoliotic deformity. Clinical indications for operative intervention include intractable axial or radicular pain and progressive neurological deficits.

Unfavorable results obtained with posterior fusion and fixation have made the anterior approach the treatment of choice. Anterior fusion without instrumentation has been unsuccessful in stabilizing the spine for deformity correction, particularly at the thoracolumbar junction.[48] Instrumentation is necessary to resist the dynamic biomechanical forces encountered at this level.[49, 50] Without the added stability of instrumentation, most patients require prolonged bed rest to facilitate fusion. Success has been reported with either posterior or anterior constructs.[48-51] However, the higher failure rate with posterior constructs makes anterior instrumentation, alone or in combination with a posterior construct, preferable.

In the spine, the overwhelming majority of degenerative disease is encountered rostral or caudal to the thoracic region. Disk herniations are the most common type of degeneration at the thoracic level. Most of these rare lesions can be resected successfully through a posterolateral approach without the addition of fusion and fixation.[52]

SURGICAL APPROACHES TO THE ANTERIOR THORACIC SPINE

The anterior thoracic spine can be exposed through a variety of approaches. The spinal level and the surgeon's preference often determine the approach. The availability of a general or thoracic surgeon may also play a role in the decision-making process. Exposure of the upper thoracic spine is confounded by the complex anatomy of the superior mediastinum, depth of the exposure, and kyphotic angulation of the vertebral bodies away from the surgeon. Pathology affecting the middle to lower thoracic spine (T5-10) can be exposed with either a posterolateral (lateral extracavitary) or an anterolateral (thoracotomy-retropleural) approach. If a transcavitary approach is chosen, the assistance of a thoracic surgeon is recommended. For the thoracolumbar region (T10-L2) a thoracoabdominal approach, combining one of the approaches for the lower thoracic spine with a retroperitoneal approach, is used.

Surgical Anatomy

A clear understanding of the regional anatomy is essential for any anterior approach to the thoracic spine. Exposure of the upper thoracic spine requires entrance into the upper mediastinum through the thoracic inlet. This oval passage at the cervicothoracic junction has a mean sagittal diameter of about 5 cm and a mean coronal diameter of 10 cm. The approach is initiated from the left to avoid injury to the recurrent laryngeal nerve. The left recurrent laryngeal nerve reverses its course at the aorta, whereas the right recurrent laryngeal nerve reverses its course at the innominate artery. A disadvantage of the left exposure is the presence of the thoracic duct, which empties into the jugulosubclavian junction within the thoracic inlet. The extent of this exposure is limited caudally by the aortic arch and the innominate vessels. Other major vessels encountered include the common carotid artery, subclavian artery, and internal jugular vein.

Transcavitary approaches to the middle and lower thoracic spine project through the pleural and peritoneal spaces, whereas the anterolateral approaches avoid these compartments. All three approaches require the identification and division of several important structures along the posterior and lateral thoracoabdominal walls. The posterior back muscles are divided into three layers. The superficial layer consists of the trapezius, latissimus dorsi, and rhomboid muscles. The intermediate layer contains the serratus posterior superior and inferior muscle groups. The deep muscle layer is composed of the erector spinae group, including the spinalis, longissimus, and iliocostalis muscles, and the underlying intrinsic muscles of the back. The erector spinae bundle is oriented longitudinally along the length of the spine, dorsolateral to the paraspinal transversospinalis group. The fascial investment of the erector spinae muscles is continuous laterally with the transversus aponeurosis of the abdominal wall, providing a dissection plane to the lateral spinal compartment. Toward the thoracolumbar junction, this fascial investment separates these muscles from the quadratus lumborum and intertransversarii muscles.

The external, internal, and innermost intercostal muscles occupy the intercostal space and are continuous with the anterior abdominal musculature. The intercostal nerve and blood vessels run in the inferior costal groove, between the internal and innermost intercostal muscles. The course is continued medially, where the internal intercostal muscle is continuous with the superior costotransverse ligament. Deep to the intercostal musculature lies the endothoracic fascia (also known as Sibson's fascia in the upper thorax), which is loosely opposed to the parietal pleura. Transection of this fascial layer allows the surgeon to gain access to the retropleural space. A left-sided exposure is favored because the aorta is easily mobilized once the segmental vessels are ligated. The hemiazygos and accessory hemiazygos veins also lie along the left anterolateral aspect of the spine and join the azygos vein anterior to the spine. The thoracic duct lies along the left anterolateral spine as it passes rostrally to empty into the left brachiocephalic vein. A meshwork of splanchnic nerves courses with the aorta through the diaphragmatic hiatus. Prominent vascular structures encountered on the right are the inferior vena cava and azygos vein. The esophagus and associated splanchnic nerves also deviate toward the right. Inferiorly, the parietal pleura forms a costodiaphragmatic sinus on each side. The most inferior aspect of the lung ends approximately 5 cm above this sinus, forming a pleural sac known as Fontan's space.

The aponeurosis of the transversus abdominis runs posteromedially from the tip of the 12th rib to join the thoracolumbar fascia. Deep to the transversus abdominis is the transversalis fascia, the abdominal equivalent of the endothoracic fascia. Division of the transversus abdominis aponeurosis allows entrance into the retroperitoneal space, which contains the kidneys, ureters, adrenals, and perinephric fat. Different structures are encountered within the retroperitoneal space, depending on the side of approach. The right retroperitoneal space is occupied by the right hemidiaphragm, right lobe of the liver, hepatic flexure of the colon, duodenopancreatic junction, inferior vena cava, and renal vessels. On the left side are the spleen, stomach fundus, splenic colon flexure, pancreatic tail, and aorta and its major branches, including the celiac trunk, superior mesenteric artery, and renal artery.

The thoracic spine is composed of 12 vertebrae whose size increases rostrally to caudally. The anterior height of the thoracic vertebral bodies is several millimeters shorter than the posterior height, creating a natural kyphosis. The kyphotic nature of the upper thoracic spine makes ventral exposure difficult because the spine courses away from the surgeon when the patient is supine. Overall, the vertebral bodies are cylindrical; however, the dorsal aspect of the vertebral body is concave. An understanding of the configuration of the posterior wall is necessary to avoid violation of the spinal canal during insertion of a vertebral body screw. Underestimating this concavity can lead to neural injury by passing a screw into the spinal canal. At the upper thoracic levels, each rib articulates with the disk space above and the respective transverse process. The costovertebral articulation is secured by a series of ligaments; the most important of these are the radiate and costotransverse ligaments, which attach the rib head to the lateral surface of the disk space and the ventral surface of the transverse process (Fig. 304–1). The 11th and 12th ribs articulate with the superior aspect of the corresponding vertebral body and lack a costotransverse articulation.

Understanding the anatomy of the diaphragm is mandatory for approaches to the thoracolumbar junction (Fig. 304–2). The diaphragm is a dome-shaped muscle with anterior attachments to the tips of the lower six costal cartilages, the lower four ribs, and the xiphoid process. Posteriorly, the diaphragm originates from the anterior surface of the upper lumbar vertebrae and the 12th rib. The right hemidiaphragm extends along the posterior thoracic wall to the T8-9 intercostal space, where it is penetrated by the inferior vena cava.

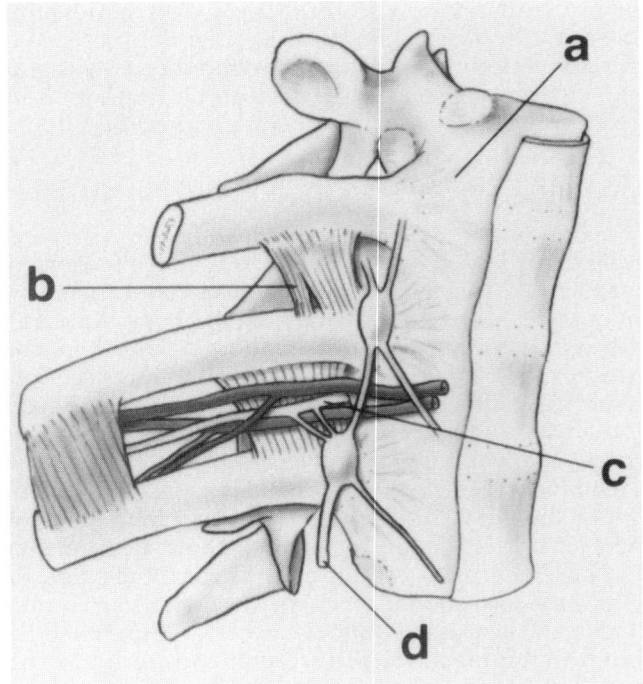

FIGURE 304–1. Ligamentous attachments and surrounding anatomy of the costovertebral joint: radiate ligament (a), costotransverse ligament (b), intercostal neurovascular bundle (c), sympathetic chain (d). (From Desai RD, McCormick PC: Anterior fusion techniques for thoracolumbar junction pathology. In Menezes AH, Sonntag VKH [eds]: Principles of Spinal Surgery. New York, McGraw-Hill, 1996, p 1189.)

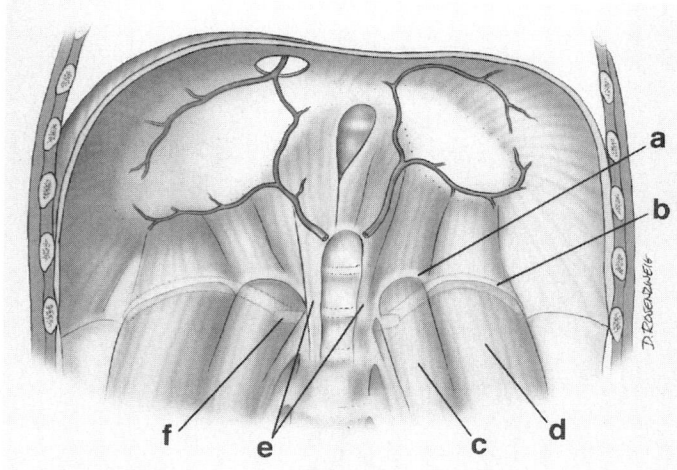

FIGURE 304–2. Inferior view of the diaphragmatic dome: medial arcuate ligament (a), lateral arcuate ligament (b), psoas muscle (c), quadratus lumborum muscle (d), diaphragmatic crura (e), transverse process of L1 (f). (From Desai RD, McCormick PC: Anterior fusion techniques for thoracolumbar junction pathology. In Menezes AH, Sonntag VKH [eds]: Principles of Spinal Surgery. New York, McGraw-Hill, 1996, p 1189.)

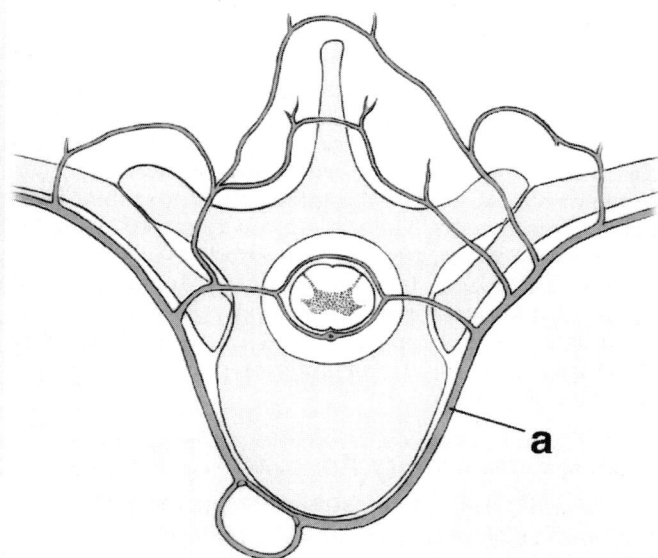

FIGURE 304–3. Collateral blood supply to the spine and spinal cord. Division of the segmental vessels midway between the aortic origin and intervertebral foramen maintains the collateral flow (a). (From Desai RD, McCormick PC: Anterior fusion techniques for thoracolumbar junction pathology. In Menezes AH, Sonntag VKH [eds]: Principles of Spinal Surgery. New York, McGraw-Hill, 1996, p 1190.)

The esophageal hiatus is opposite the vertebral body of T10, and the aortic hiatus lies at the level of T12. The diaphragmatic crura attach medially to the lumbar spine, with the right crus extending from L1 through L3 and the left from L2 to L3. The medial arcuate ligament crosses the psoas muscle from the vertebral body of L1 to the lateral tip of the transverse process. The lateral arcuate ligament extends over the quadratus lumborum muscle from the tip of the transverse process of L1 to the ventral surface of the 12th rib. The phrenic nerves, originating from C3 through C5, innervate the diaphragmatic domes in a central-to-peripheral configuration. Along the superior surface of the diaphragm, the pleura is tightly adherent, providing an additional layer of strength for suturing the muscle if it is transected.

The segmental vessels of the upper thoracic cord originate from the vertebral, thyrocervical, and costo-cervical arteries and are seldom encountered in a ventral exposure. In the middle and lower thoracic spine, the radicular arteries exit the lateral aspect of the aorta and course toward the vertebral foramen. Before entering the foramen, numerous anastomotic branches are sent to the spine and spinal cord (Fig. 304–3). Transection of radicular arteries distal to the neuronal foramen, particularly the radiculomedullary artery of Adamkiewicz, should be avoided so as not to disrupt collateral blood flow to the spinal cord. Sacrificing the artery of Adamkiewicz places the spinal cord at significant risk for infarction. Although the artery of Adamkiewicz is located on the left 80% of the time, spinal angiography may be warranted with a lower thoracic approach to verify its location. Preoperative identification of a significant radiculomedullary artery within the planned exposure can necessitate an alternative anterolateral approach from the opposite side or a transcavitary approach.

Approach to the Upper Thoracic Spine

In 1957, Cauchoix and Binet[53] were among the first to describe an anterior approach to the upper thoracic spine. Subsequently, variations of this approach, differing in the degree of bone resection at the sternoclavicular joint and use of a thoracotomy, have been reported.[54–57] These approaches allow more lateral exposure than earlier approaches did. All, however, are limited caudally by the great vessels of the superior mediastinum, usually at T3-4. For lesions within the paraspinal region, a ventral approach may fail to offer adequate exposure. In this situation, a posterolateral approach such as the lateral extracavitary exposure may be more appropriate.

OPERATIVE TECHNIQUE

The patient is positioned supine with the neck in slight extension. The incision starts along the medial border of the sternocleidomastoid muscle and extends inferiorly through the midline of the sternum up to the xiphoid process. The dissection along the superior portion of the incision is conducted in a manner similar to the traditional anterior cervical exposure. The contents of the carotid sheath are retracted laterally, and the trachea and esophagus are retracted medially. The attachments of the sternohyoid muscle to the medial sternum and clavicle are identified and detached. The soft tissue and vascular structures, especially the brachiocephalic trunk, are cleared from the deep surface of the sternum into the mediastinum with blunt dissection. If the superior thyroid artery is identified, it should be ligated. Using an oscillating saw, a median sternotomy is performed up to the xiphoid process, and the mediastinum is opened with a crank retractor. The pleural surfaces are identified, carefully dissected, and retracted. The esophagus is bluntly dissected off the prevertebral fascia. Because the longus colli muscles at the thoracic level are unable to accommodate retractor blades, a table-mounted retractor system facilitates visualization. The viscera are retracted from the prevertebral space, revealing the underlying vertebral bodies. The fascia is cleared of any remaining soft tissue, and an intraoperative radiograph is obtained to document the appropriate level. Decompression and stabilization similar to an anterior cervical procedure can then be performed.

Lateral Extracavitary Approach

The lateral extracavitary approach introduced by Larson and colleagues[58] in 1976 is a derivative of the lateral costotransversectomy. It is ideally suited for lesions with a significant anterior paraspinal extension, with or without a substantial intraspinal component. This approach provides a familiar exposure and orientation for neurosurgeons and extensive access to all three spinal compartments.[59] The lateral extracavitary approach is entirely extrapleural and avoids the perioperative complications associated with the transthoracic exposure. In addition, circumferential stabilization of the spine is possible through a single incision. The lateral extracavitary approach is versatile and can be modified based on a tumor's size, level of involvement, relationship to neural structures, and need for spinal stabilization.

OPERATIVE TECHNIQUE

Once anesthesia is induced, the patient is placed in a three-quarter prone position. For the initial exposure, the operative table is tilted toward the side of pathology so the patient is in a true prone position. An intraoperative anteroposterior radiograph is obtained to identify the appropriate level, and a wide area of skin over the back is prepared and draped. The drapes are positioned in a rectangular fashion with at least 15 cm of lateral exposure on the surgical side.

A hockey-stick incision is centered over the level of pathology (Fig. 304–4). Adequate caudal exposure is needed before the incision is extended laterally, or the caudal extent of the exposure will be limited, particularly when posterior instrumentation or laminectomy is planned. The lateral limb of the incision is curved gently toward the side of the pathology, extending 8 to 10 cm from the midline. The midline incision proceeds through the subcutaneous tissue to the level of the spinous processes and thoracodorsal fascia. A routine subperiosteal dissection of the paraspinal muscles is performed with a Cobb dissector and monopolar cauterization. The takedown is performed bilaterally if a posterior exposure is required for laminectomy or instrumentation; otherwise, a unilateral exposure is sufficient. The lateral limb of the incision is opened by

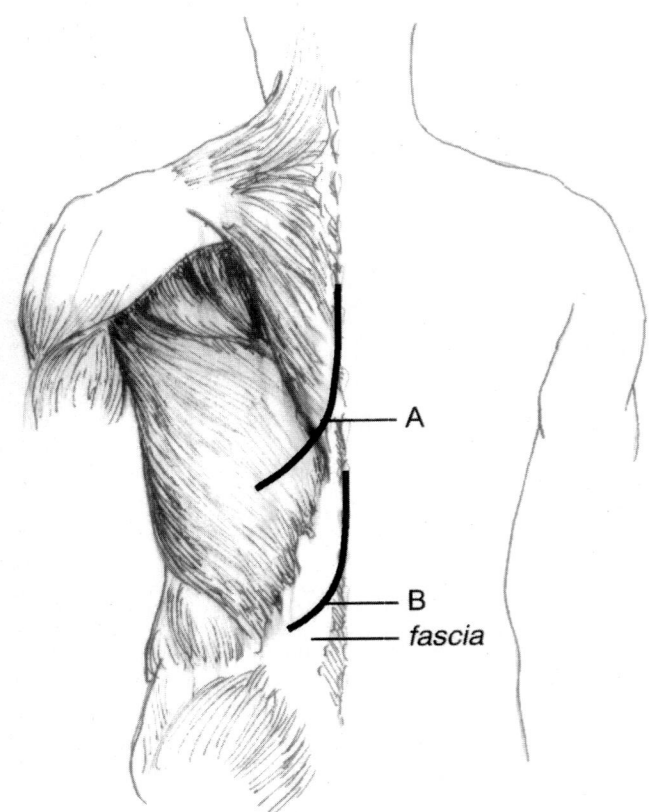

FIGURE 304–4. Typical incisions used for the lateral extracavitary approach of the midthoracic *(A)* and thoracolumbar *(B)* regions of the spine. Thoracolumbar fascia is identified. (From McCormick PC: Surgical management of dumbbell and paraspinal tumors of the thoracic and lumbar spine. Neurosurgery 38:67–74, 1996.)

transecting the transversely oriented thoracic muscles (i.e., latissimus dorsi, trapezius, rhomboid) in line with the skin incision. The myocutaneous flap is elevated, exposing the longitudinally oriented erector spinae musculature (Fig. 304–5).

The paraspinal musculature runs in the trough created by the ribs, transverse process, facet joint, and pedicle. The lateral margin of the erector spinae is identified and dissected medially to expose the underlying ribs. This dissection is then carried further over the facet joint, eventually communicating with the posterior dissection. The mobilization of the erector spinae muscle allows access to the lateral spinal compartment (Fig. 304–6). The longitudinal muscle mass is wrapped in a moist sponge to avoid desiccation and positioned medially or laterally, allowing the surgeon to work on either side.

Complete dissection of the vertebral elements above and below the pathologic level ensures adequate ventral exposure. The dorsal and lateral rib surfaces are exposed with a Cobb elevator up to the vertebral body articulation. The ventral soft tissue is dissected free in a subperiosteal fashion with a Doyne rib dissector. The exposed transverse process at the level of pathology, along with 6 to 8 cm of the corresponding rib, is then

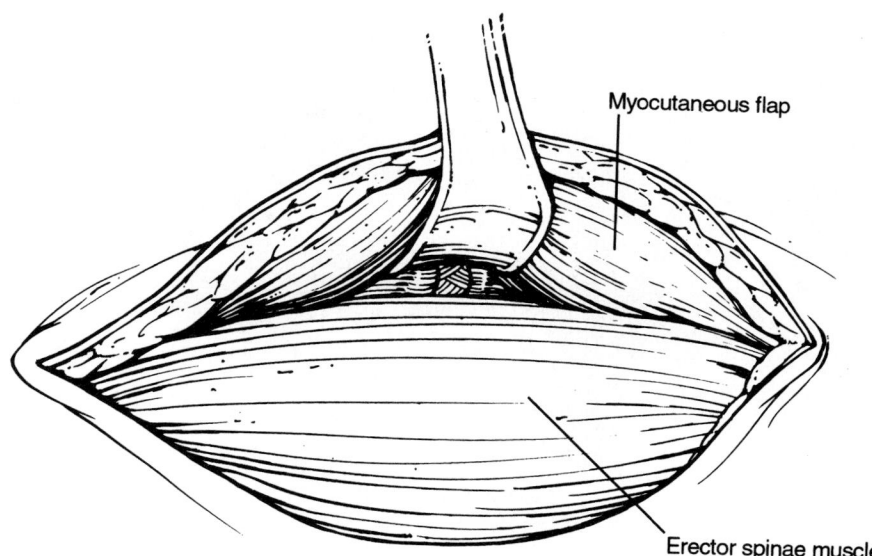

FIGURE 304–5. Medial retraction of the myocutaneous flap exposes the erector spinae muscles.

resected with a rib cutter and rongeur. The costotransverse and costovertebral joints are disarticulated and transected sharply. Resection of the rib head exposes the anterolateral surface of the spine, including the pedicle and intervertebral foramen. At the levels above and below, a portion of rib is also resected to enhance the ventral exposure. Only 3 to 4 cm of rib is resected at these levels to avoid a flail chest deformity.

Once the rib and transverse processes are removed, the neurovascular bundle is identified within the endothoracic fascia, deep to the intercostal musculature. The segmental nerves above and at the level of pathology are dissected free and divided, with the proximal stump elevated medially toward the intervertebral foramen. Unlike at lumbar levels, the nerves at thoracic levels can be sacrificed without a detectable deficit. Once the nerve is free, the parietal pleura is displaced ventrally to provide access to the anterior spinal com-

partment. The parietal pleura is kept out of the operative field with a table-mounted retractor system. A padded, wide retractor blade helps avoid a pleural tear. At this point, the operative table is returned to a true prone position, enhancing the ventral visualization. The parietal pleura, diaphragm, or both are bluntly dissected free from the ventrolateral aspect of the vertebral bodies with a Cobb elevator. Sharp dissection may be required at the level of the disk space if more adherent connective tissue is present. The sympathetic chain is identified along the ventrolateral aspect of the vertebral bodies. The rami communicantes are transected at the involved spinal segments, and the sympathetic chain is mobilized through a subperiosteal dissection. Dorsal and foraminal vessels are identified, cauterized, and transected. The previously elevated nerve stump facilitates dissection to the foramen and pedicle. Resection of the pedicle allows identification

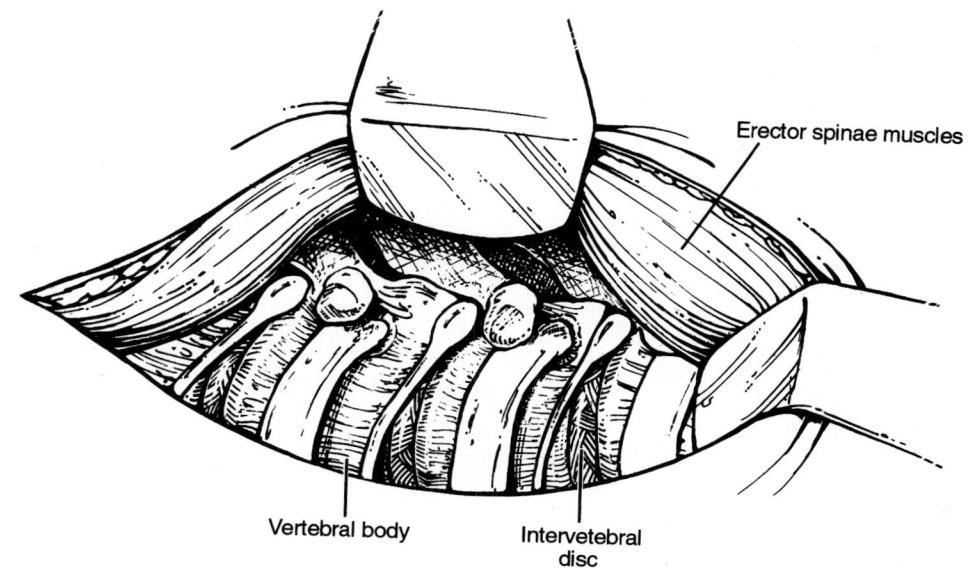

FIGURE 304–6. Mobilization of the erector spinae muscles exposes the lateral spinal compartment and dorsal surface of the ribs.

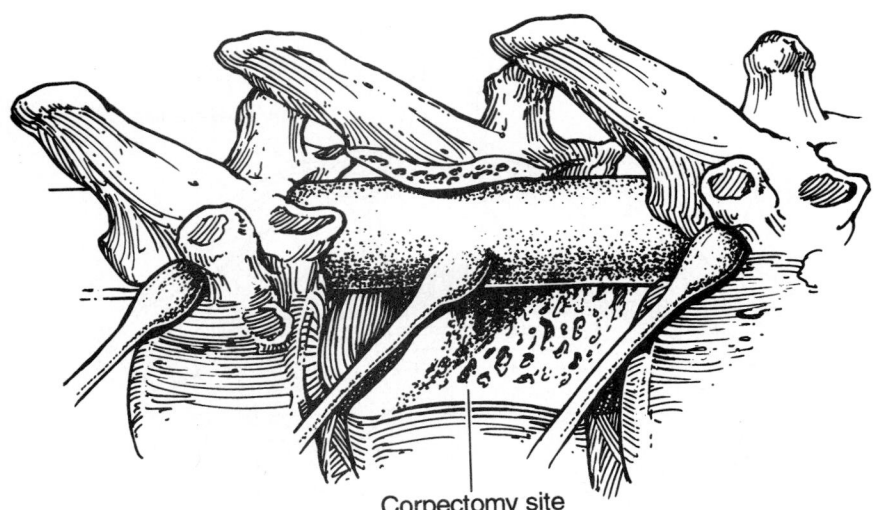

Corpectomy site

FIGURE 304–7. Access to the spinal canal can be obtained through both the posterior and the anterolateral compartments with the lateral extracavitary approach. Resection of the lamina, pedicle, facet joint, and ventral vertebral body provides a wide exposure of the spinal canal.

of the ventral spinal canal. A distinct advantage of the lateral extracavitary approach is the simultaneous access provided to both the anterolateral and the posterior spinal compartments. The spinal canal can be exposed through resection of either or both of the posterior and anterior elements (Fig. 304–7). Depending on the degree of pathologic involvement, a corpectomy is then performed in the standard fashion.

Once the pathology has been resected, a spinal stabilization procedure may be required. The sectioned rib provides an excellent source of graft material. Positioning the rib with the concave side directed dorsally assumes the natural kyphotic curvature of the thoracic spine. Ventral plating followed by dorsal instrumentation may be inserted as deemed appropriate. The parietal pleura is inspected for air leaks. Minor leaks can be repaired primarily. A significant leak mandates placing a chest tube for the immediate postoperative period. Once the pleura has been inspected and repaired, the remainder of the wound is closed in layers.

Retropleural Thoracotomy

Contemporary techniques for anterolateral approaches to the thoracic spine were based, in part, on Hodgson and Stock's[2] operative treatment of Pott's disease. The

retropleural thoracotomy is appropriate for pathology extending up to two spinal segments. A left-sided approach is preferred because the aorta is easier to mobilize than the vena cava, and the liver will not obstruct views of the lower thoracic spine. A double-lumen endotracheal tube is used for procedures of the upper thoracic spine but is not required for pathology located below T6. Unlike the lateral extracavitary approach, the retropleural and transpleural approaches provide a greater degree of ventral exposure at the expense of access to the posterior compartment.

OPERATIVE TECHNIQUE

The patient is placed in a lateral position with an axillary roll and appropriate padding to prevent pressure neuropathies. The correct level for the approach is determined with an intraoperative radiograph obtained after the patient has been positioned. Because of the caudal rib angulation, the incision for an anterolateral approach should be made two levels above the pathology. For example, a lesion at T8 would be approached through an incision over the sixth rib. The incision for a retropleural approach starts approximately 4 cm from the midline over the rib of interest and extends to the midaxillary line (Fig. 304–8). The

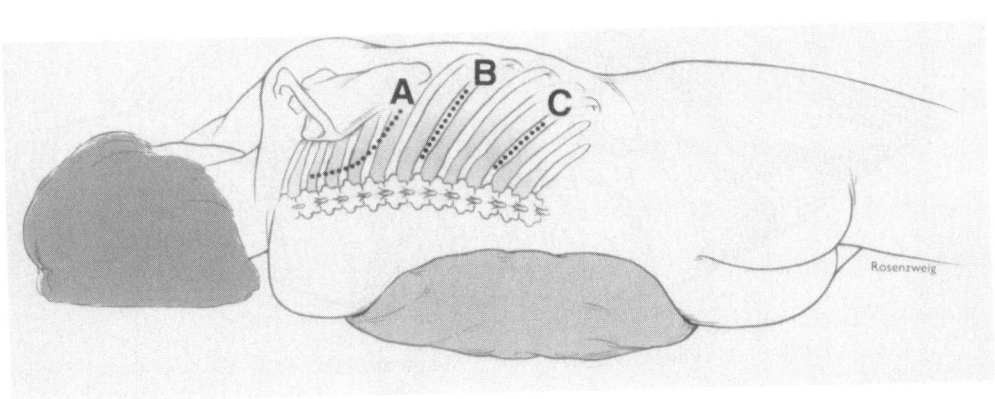

Rosenzweig

FIGURE 304–8. Relationship of a retropleural skin incision to the underlying spine and rib cage for the upper thoracic (A), midthoracic (B), and thoracolumbar (C) levels.

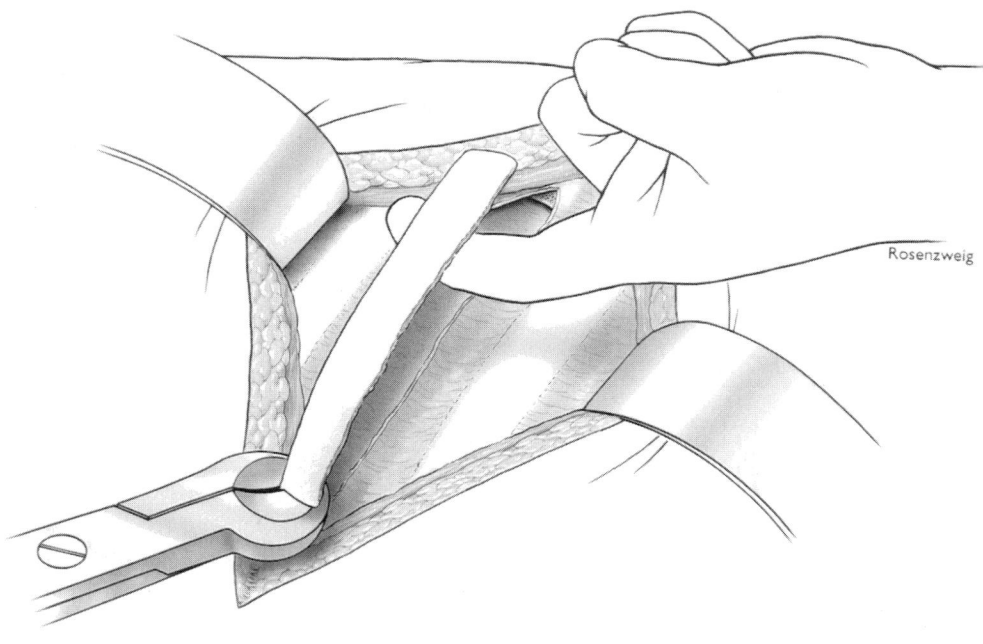

FIGURE 304–9. Resection of the rib reveals the underlying periosteum and endothoracic fascia. The resected rib may be used for grafting at the time of fusion. (From Desai RD, McCormick PC: Anterior fusion techniques for thoracolumbar junction pathology. In Menezes AH, Sonntag VKH [eds]: Principles of Spinal Surgery. New York, McGraw-Hill, 1996, p 1191.)

subcutaneous tissue and underlying muscles are transected with monopolar cauterization to expose the periosteum of the rib. The surrounding soft tissue is detached from the dorsal aspect of the rib using an Addison dissector, preserving the intercostal neurovascular bundle. A Doyne dissector is used to free the ventral periosteum along the length of the rib. This dissection continues as far medially as possible, usually 1 to 2 cm lateral to the costotransverse joint. The section of rib is resected and saved for possible grafting (Fig. 304–9).

The endothoracic fascia is identified as the shiny tissue layer deep to the rib periosteum but superficial to the parietal pleura. This fascial layer is sharply incised in line with the skin incision (Fig. 304–10). The underlying parietal pleura is freed in all directions using blunt dissection with a finger or sponge dissector (Fig. 304–11). This maneuver exposes the costotransverse joint and anterolateral aspect of the vertebral bodies. For exposure of the lower thoracic region and thoracolumbar junction, the lateral attachments of the diaphragm must be divided so that the retropleural and retroperitoneal spaces are in communication. Instead of incising the diaphragm circumferentially from the anterior chest wall, the 11th and 12th rib attachments to the diaphragm are dissected subperiosteally through a smaller, more caudal diaphragmatic opening. This dissection continues medially to elevate the lateral and medial arcuate ligaments from the underlying muscles. At the transverse process of L1, a cuff of muscle is left intact to help reapproximate the diaphragm. Finally, the left crus is divided to complete the communication of the retropleural and retroperitoneal cavities. The peritoneum is gently swept from the posterior abdominal wall, with special attention paid to the area near the central tendon, where the peritoneum

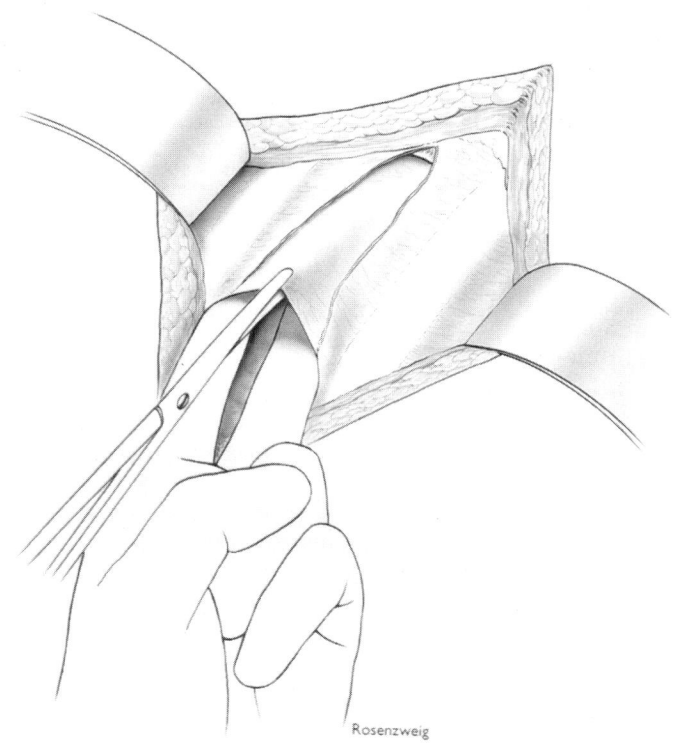

FIGURE 304–10. The endothoracic fascia is incised in line with the skin incision to gain access to the retropleural space. (From Desai RD, McCormick PC: Anterior fusion techniques for thoracolumbar junction pathology. In Menezes AH, Sonntag VKH [eds]: Principles of Spinal Surgery. New York, McGraw-Hill, 1996, p 1192.)

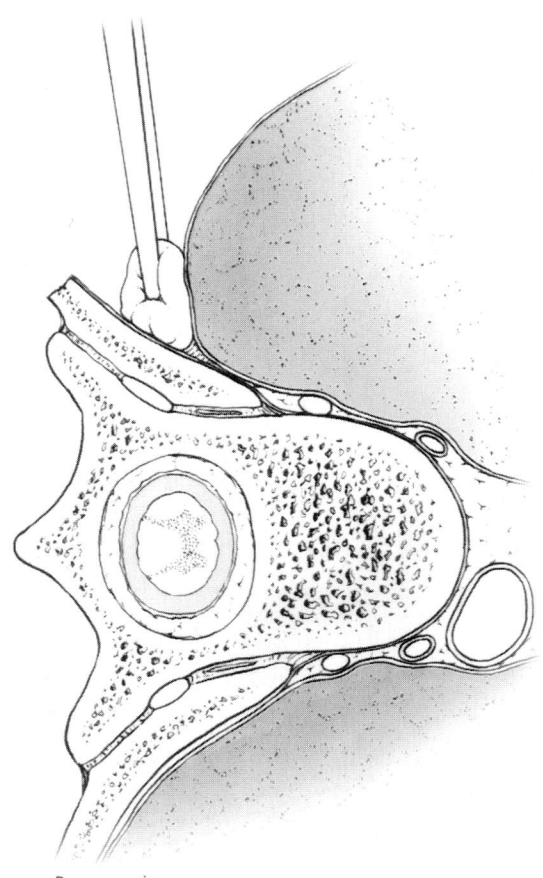

Rosenzweig

FIGURE 304–11. The pleura is bluntly dissected from the antero-lateral aspect of the spine using a cotton sponge or finger. A wide separation of the pleura in a rostral-caudal direction helps prevent pleural tears when the lung is retracted. (From Desai RD, McCormick PC: Anterior fusion techniques for thoracolumbar junction pathology. In Menezes AH, Sonntag VKH [eds]: Principles of Spinal Surgery. New York, McGraw-Hill, 1996, p 1192.)

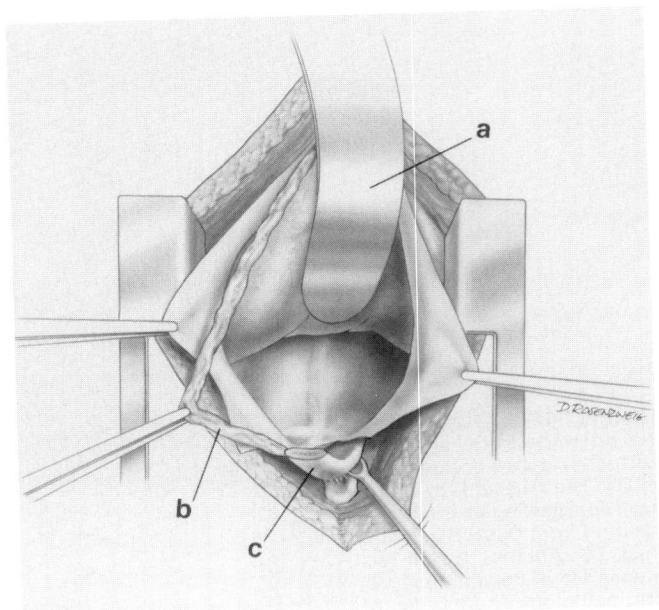

FIGURE 304–12. The proximal rib head (c) is resected using sharp dissection with a curet. The neurovascular bundle (b) and lung are retracted with a smooth, wide retractor blade (a), revealing the anterolateral surface of the spine. (From Desai RD, McCormick PC: Anterior fusion techniques for thoracolumbar junction pathology. In Menezes AH, Sonntag VKH [eds]: Principles of Spinal Surgery. New York, McGraw-Hill, 1996, p 1193.)

is thinner. The hemiazygos and accessory azygos veins should be identified and may require cauterization or clipping. The proximal rib head is resected sharply, exposing the lateral aspect of the vertebral body (Fig. 304–12). A table-mounted retractor is positioned and used to retract the lung and peritoneal contents. Using a well-padded retractor blade avoids injury to the underlying structures.

Details of the stabilization procedure are discussed in subsequent sections. Once the fusion and fixation are complete, the surgical site is irrigated and inspected. If the diaphragm was incised, its edges are reapproximated with an absorbable stitch and reattached to the psoas, transverse process of L1, quadratus, and intercostal cuff. Primary repair is required for any pleural tear, and a chest tube should be inserted if significant air leaks are evident. The primary incision is closed in layers, taking care to avoid injuring the intercostal nerves.

Transpleural Thoracotomy

The transpleural approach is similar to the previously described retropleural approach. The patient is placed in the lateral position, and the skin incision is made over the rib two levels above the area of interest. Unlike the retropleural approach, the parietal pleura is incised in line with the endothoracic fascia after the rib is resected, allowing access to the pleural cavity. The lung is deflated and retracted with a well-padded blade from a table-mounted retractor. If the diaphragm is to be incised, a 1-cm cuff is left intact for reapproximation at the end of the procedure. The rest of the approach to the anterolateral spine is identical to the retropleural approach. Unlike the retropleural approach, however, a chest tube is always required at closure.

FUSION TECHNIQUES OF THE ANTERIOR THORACIC SPINE

Anterior Interbody Graft Materials

Various graft materials have been used for interbody fusion of the anterior thoracic spine. The decision regarding which material to use is based on the type of lesion, the patient's life expectancy, and the surgeon's and patient's preferences. A solid fusion is the goal for patients with a traumatic injury, benign tumor, developmental deformity, or degenerative disease or those with an extended life expectancy. Under these circumstances, acceptable graft materials include bone autograft or allograft and titanium cages packed with bone. For patients with malignant neoplasms and a life expectancy less than 2 years, a synthetic graft such as acrylic or polymethyl methacrylate (PMMA) or a titanium cage provides the necessary structural support. Each type of graft has clear advantages and disadvantages. Long-term results with titanium cages are not yet available. No strong clinical evidence supports the application of one graft type over another.

The most commonly used material for interbody grafting is bone, either autograft or allograft. Autogenous bone is the most successful material for forming a solid fusion and is considered the gold standard.[60–62] Fusion rates are higher with autograft bone because of its superior osteoconductive, osteoinductive, and osteogenic properties.[62] Autograft bone can be harvested from a number of sites, including the iliac crest, rib, humerus, tibia, and fibula. The risk of a complication associated with harvesting autologous bone ranges from 9.4% to 49%.[63–67] Severe complications are rare but can occur as a result of injury to the lateral femoral cutaneous nerve, damage to the peritoneum, hip fracture, donor site pain, hematoma formation, and infection. Bone harvesting also increases the operative time and blood loss. All soft tissue must be stripped meticulously from the graft to maximize the potential for fusion. Inserting a vascularized graft is technically demanding but may be warranted for conditions associated with a poor fusion rate, such as previously irradiated graft sites.[68–70]

The use of allogeneic bone has increased because processing techniques have improved and because it is desirable to avoid the complications associated with harvesting autologous bone. The supply and diversity of allograft bone are greater than those of autologous bone, offering an important advantage to surgeons attempting to fill a corpectomy defect. However, the rate of interbody fusion is slightly less than that associated with autologous bone.[69, 71, 72] Fusion rates may be enhanced with the application of demineralized bone matrix and bone morphogenetic proteins; the osteoinductive properties of these two substances are well established experimentally.[62, 73–77] A disadvantage of allograft bone is the relatively increased time required for fusion formation. The longer fusion time increases the chance of pseudarthrosis and the formation of stress fractures. Allograft bone tends to have a higher degree of stiffness, which increases its axial load tolerance but also increases the chance of the graft's telescoping into adjacent vertebral bodies. Although the risk is low, viral transmission is still possible with allograft bone and may cause unnecessary anxiety for certain patients.[78, 79] Under normal circumstances, the difference in fusion rates obtained with autograft and allograft is irrelevant clinically. In some patients at increased risk for pseudarthrosis, however, the use of autologous bone may be warranted. Patients with a history of smoking, diabetes, a previously failed fusion, or cancer who receive adjuvant therapy may fall into this category.

For patients with malignant disease, using bone as an interbody graft has several disadvantages. If life expectancy is limited, there may not be enough time or the need for a solid fusion to occur. Adjuvant therapies, such as radiation and chemotherapy, affect fusion negatively.[62] Maintaining structural integrity is the most important consideration, and tumor infiltration or adjuvant therapies typically weaken a bone graft. Diffuse metastatic disease can limit the available supply of autogenous bone and increase the risk of complications related to bone harvesting. Consequently, patients with malignant disease are more likely to receive synthetic graft materials. The traditional material used for patients with metastatic disease of the spine has been PMMA. Acrylic provides the structural support to resist axial loads, is easy to shape, and attains its strength in a short time. No osteointegration occurs between the surfaces of the acrylic and bone. Over time, the acrylic-bone interface is likely to loosen; therefore, grafting with PMMA is often supplemented with Steinmann pins.[80, 81] Other synthetic implants now available include titanium cages, carbon-fiber cages, hydroxyapatite blocks, and ceramic implants.[62, 81]

Fusion Technique

Once the anterolateral surface of the spine is exposed adequately, the corpectomy is performed. Before the vertebral body is resected, the intervertebral disks above and below the involved levels are removed. The lateral surface of the disk is incised, and the disk material is extracted with pituitary rongeurs and curets (Fig. 304–13). These lateral elements are resected to gain access to the lateral dural margin and thereby improve exposure of the ventral spinal canal. The pedicle and facet joint are removed with either a high-speed drill

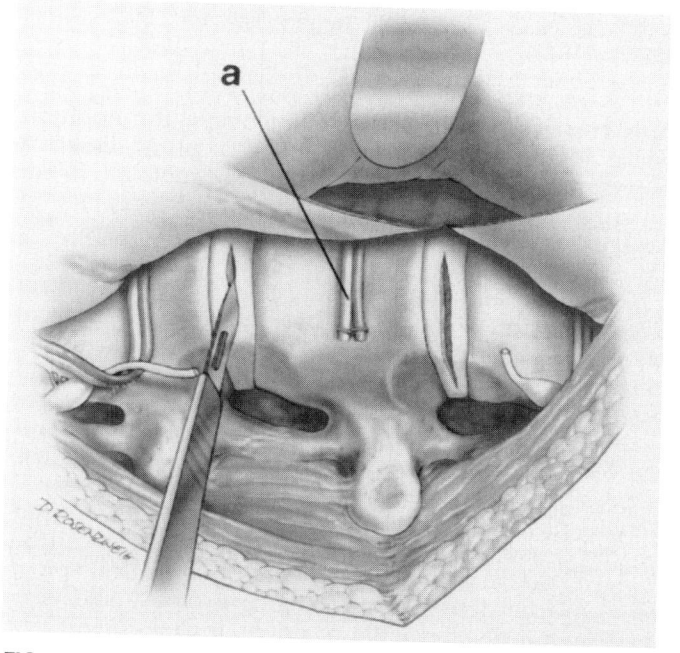

FIGURE 304–13. The disks above and below the corpectomy site are incised and then resected before any bone removal. Ligation of the segmental vessels along the anterolateral surface of the vertebral body preserves collateral blood supply to the spinal cord (a). (From Desai RD, McCormick PC: Anterior fusion techniques for thoracolumbar junction pathology. In Menezes AH, Sonntag VKH [eds]: Principles of Spinal Surgery. New York, McGraw-Hill, 1996, p 1193.)

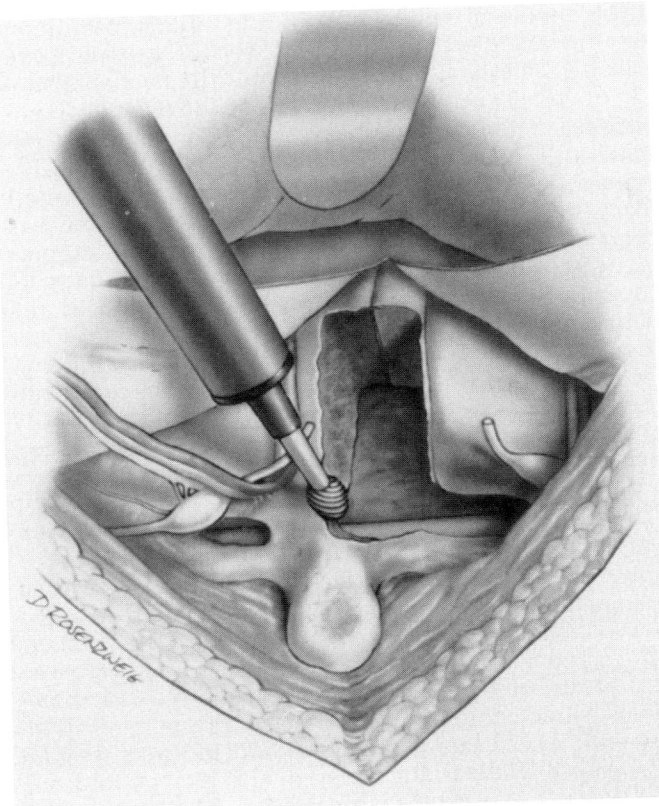

FIGURE 304–14. High-speed drill and rongeurs are used to perform the corpectomy and prepare the end plates for graft insertion. (From Desai RD, McCormick PC: Anterior fusion techniques for thoracolumbar junction pathology. In Menezes AH, Sonntag VKH [eds]: Principles of Spinal Surgery. New York, McGraw-Hill, 1996, p 1194.)

or a rongeur. During these maneuvers, the epidural space is probed with a nerve hook or blunt dissector to ensure that the thecal sac and nerve roots are freed. During drilling, adequate irrigation is necessary to keep excess heat from accumulating and damaging the underlying dura.

Once the lateral dural margin is exposed, ventral decompression is achieved by drilling the vertebral body (Fig. 304–14). Initially, a trough is drilled in the vertebral body, leaving a thin shelf of dorsal cortical bone in place. With a reverse-angle curet, this remaining bone is delivered into the created trough, and the corpectomy is completed. Considerable blood loss is possible because of the proximity of the perineural venous plexus. The anesthesiologist should be advised of this possibility so that excessive blood loss can be replaced adequately. A lesion within the ventral spinal canal can be delivered into the corpectomy site with the use of a reverse-angle or down-angled curet. Contralateral visualization of the spinal canal can be obtained with an angled dental mirror.

Insertion of an interbody strut graft begins with preparation of the end plates within the corpectomy site. The cartilaginous end plates are excised with a high-speed drill, curet, or osteotome. The cortical end plate is removed until bleeding cancellous bone is en-

countered at several points. Removal of the entire cortical portion of end plate compromises the axial load-resisting capabilities of the vertebral bodies. If the entire end plate is removed, the graft will telescope into the vertebral body because the underlying cancellous bone is too weak to support axial loads. Settling of the graft into the vertebral bodies increases the risk of kyphotic deformity and posterior graft displacement into the spinal cord. A small shelf of end plate is left intact at the posterior border of the vertebral body to help prevent this posterior displacement. The rostral and caudal end plates should lie parallel to each other when preparation is complete. Slanting the end plates predisposes the graft to loosening and dislodgment.

The corpectomy site is measured to determine the size of the interbody graft. The graft is cut to the appropriate size, and a trial insertion is performed. Final adjustments are made using a high-speed drill or rongeur. Ideally, the graft is slightly longer than the relaxed corpectomy site. Excessive drilling of an autologous graft and the corpectomy site should be avoided, because thermal injury can destroy viable osteogenic cells. The vertebral bodies are distracted, and the graft is inserted with a mallet and impactor. The graft should fit tightly within the corpectomy site, requiring some force for insertion. The graft is mortised into the end plates to help prevent its dislodgment (Fig. 304–15). After placement, the graft should lie flush with or slightly recessed from the ventral edges of the vertebral

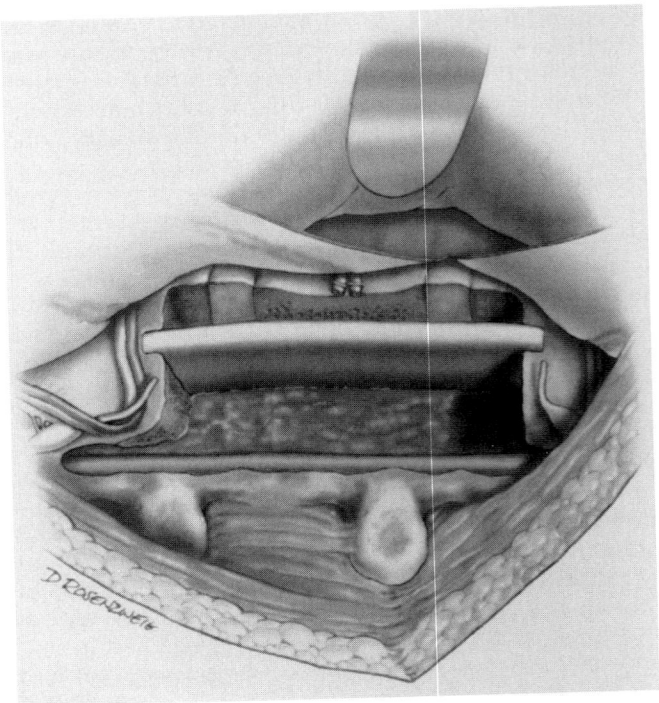

FIGURE 304–15. The graft is mortised into the vertebral body above and below the corpectomy site to help prevent migration. The space ventral to the graft can be packed with corticocancellous bone chips to enhance fusion potential. (From Desai RD, McCormick PC: Anterior fusion techniques for thoracolumbar junction pathology. In Menezes AH, Sonntag VKH [eds]: Principles of Spinal Surgery. New York, McGraw-Hill, 1996, p 1194.)

bodies. Corticocancellous bone chips are placed ventral to the graft to enhance the potential for fusion. The posterior border is checked with a nerve hook to ensure that the graft does not impinge on the spinal cord.

INSTRUMENTATION OF THE ANTERIOR THORACIC SPINE

Biomechanical Considerations

A detailed discussion of spinal biomechanics is beyond the scope of this chapter. However, some basic concepts apply to the most rudimentary exercise in anterior thoracic stabilization. Spinal instability, as defined by White and Panjabi,[82] is the inability of the spine to resist normal physiologic stresses, with resultant abnormal motion causing pain, deformity, or neurological irritation. Denis[32] has defined three columns of stability in the spine. The anterior column consists of the anterior longitudinal ligament and the anterior halves of the vertebral body and intervertebral disks; the middle column consists of the posterior halves of the vertebral body and disk and the posterior longitudinal ligament. These two columns contribute the majority of the axial load-bearing support for the spine. In the thoracic spine, axial loads are often translated into a bending moment because of the thoracic spine's kyphotic posture and ventrally displaced instantaneous axis of rotation. Destruction of the anterior or middle column leads to spinal instability and a progressive kyphotic deformity. Subsequently, the spinal cord can be injured by ventrally extruded bone fragments or tethering of the spinal cord over the kyphotic deformity.

A ventral approach is optimal for reconstruction of the anterior and middle columns. The interbody strut replaces the anterior and middle columns in resisting axial loads but requires an intact posterior column to resist excessive flexion, extension, or rotational forces. The optimal position of the interbody graft depends on the nature of the posterior elements, the degree of kyphotic deformity, and the locations of the instantaneous axis of rotation and neutral axis. The kyphotic angulation or curvature radius can indicate the severity of deformity and help determine the appropriate position for the graft. The neutral axis, the region where flexion and extension do not produce significant compression or distraction, lies at the junction of the anterior and middle columns. In this position, axial load-resisting capabilities are maximal; however, the ability of the graft to resist flexion forces may be compromised. Positioning within the neutral axis is best suited for patients with minimal deformity over a short segment and with intact posterior elements. A more ventrally placed graft allows axial loads to be shared by the posterior elements and increases the ability of the graft to resist flexion forces. The more ventrally the graft is placed from the neutral axis, the greater is its ability to resist the forces contributing to a kyphotic deformity.[83, 84] Another important step in avoiding complications involving a construct is an accurate preoperative biomechanical assessment. Compromise of the

posterior column suggests that a ventral construct alone may be insufficient to provide adequate stability. If a considerable portion of the posterior elements is destroyed in conjunction with anterior instability, a circumferential approach is required to achieve adequate stabilization.[85]

Ventral instrumentation constructs are divided into two categories termed *rigid* or *dynamic*, depending on the amount of motion allowed between components of the construct.[86] Implants that allow no motion between components are considered rigid and function through a fixed or applied moment arm. This type of instrumentation is designed to immobilize the spine completely and to maximize stabilization. Rigid constructs are stiffer than dynamic constructs and promote fusion by decreasing the amount of motion across the fusion interface. The increased stiffness of the construct also eliminates the need for bicortical screw purchase. Because of the construct's rigidity, most forces applied are absorbed by the construct and produce the phenomenon known as *stress shielding*. Stress shielding can interfere with the development of a solid fusion because the fusion-enhancing forces that promote bone healing are absorbed by the construct. Continued stress shielding can also lead to stress-reduction osteoporosis. Rigid constructs are associated with an increased risk of implant failure because the forces are primarily absorbed by the construct and not shared with the spine. Over time, the material properties of the construct and the connections between the individual elements are weakened. Rigid constructs also require a static condition during implantation. No compression or distraction forces can be applied to the inserted screws once the plate is positioned, because the screw passes through a fixed hole within the plate.

Constructs that allow some motion between elements are known as dynamic constructs and function through a nonfixed cantilever beam. The dynamic nature of these implants distributes the load among the construct, graft, and intrinsic spinal elements. Force is distributed because the screw is allowed to toggle at its interface with either the plate or the rod, decreasing the stresses supported by the implant. The movement between the implant components diffuses the applied stresses. Theoretically, this motion reduces the chance of construct failure and failure at the bone-implant interface. To increase construct stiffness, however, it is typically recommended that the inserted screws achieve bicortical purchase. Distribution of the stress across the segments also creates load sharing between the implant and the graft. These load-sharing properties promote bony fusion owing to the compressive forces encountered by the graft. It is believed that the forces applied to the bone stimulate vascular growth and the proliferation of osteoblasts from the host bone. Another advantage of a dynamic system is the ability to apply compressive or distractive forces across the graft during insertion.

Bone undergoes deformation when a force is applied; therefore, no construct can be completely rigid. Over time, the motion that occurs at the bone-implant interface causes even a rigid construct to become dynamic. Therefore, designating one construct as rigid and one as dynamic may be a matter of semantics. Clinical outcomes associated with dynamic or rigid constructs have not been shown to differ.

Types of Constructs

Initial anterior instrumentation constructs, such as the Dwyer and Zielke devices, were used to correct scoliotic deformities. These constructs lacked the mechanical integrity to restore load-bearing capabilities. Instead, these construct were intended to treat chronic instability leading to a slowly progressive deformity. The constructs applied forces to the spine, "persuading" it to assume a more physiologic configuration.

Kaneda and associates,[87] Dunn,[7] and Kostuik[43] subsequently developed more rigid systems to restore mechanical stability. Dunn's construct was among the more stable, but it was later removed from clinical use owing to reports of great vessel erosion.[9] The continued development of anterior instrumentation has led to both screw-rod and screw-plate constructs that are easier to implant and have a lower profile, which allows fixation of shorter segments. They are also compatible with magnetic resonance imaging. Examples of screw-rod constructs include the Zielke device, the Kostuik-Harrington device, the Kaneda SR Anterior Spinal System (Acromed, Cleveland, OH), and the Ventrofix system (Synthes, Paoli, PA). Plating systems include the Anterior Thoracolumbar Locking Plate (Synthes, Paoli, PA), and the ZPlate II (Sofamor-Danek, Memphis, TN).

The Zielke technique, introduced in 1976, was a modification of the Dwyer procedure and offered the ability to correct the rotational and coronal deformities associated with scoliosis.[6] This technique has been given the generic designation *ventral derotation spondylodesis* (VDS). The vertebral body screws are placed laterally and connected to a threaded rod. Compressive forces are applied to the convex curve of the deformity. The Zielke VDS is associated with an excellent fusion rate and good correction of deformities, and it decreases the number of levels that require fusion. The primary indication for the Zielke VDS is correction of a scoliotic deformity in the thoracolumbar or lumbar region. Contraindications for the use of a Zielke device include a rigid deformity related to degenerative ankylosis, a rigid compensatory thoracic curve greater than 30 degrees, and a significant rib cage deformity.[88] There is little value in using a Zielke VDS after corpectomy, because more rigid constructs that are easier to insert and that allow fixation over fewer motion segments are available.

The Kostuik-Harrington device was developed to improve on the poor results obtained with posterior Harrington distraction rods.[89] Unlike plate systems, the Kostuik-Harrington system allows the application of distractive forces in addition to fixation. This system provides adequate stabilization as long as it is constructed in a rectangular or parallelogram fashion. The construct consists of a standard Harrington distraction system along with a compression rod. Two types of collar-ended screws are crimped over the compression rod and ratcheted to fit onto the distraction rod. With no toggle at the screw-rod interface, this system is classified as a rigid distraction construct. Clinical success has been reported with the Kostuik-Harrington device,[49, 88–90] but newer constructs tend to be less cumbersome and easier to implant.

The Kaneda SR Anterior Spinal System was developed in 1984 for the treatment of thoracolumbar fractures[87] (Fig. 304–16A). This device consists of spiked vertebral plates, cancellous screws, a smooth rod, and transverse couplers. The vertebral plate has four spikes on its undersurface and is impacted into the ventrolateral surface of the vertebral body. These plates serve as templates for screw placement, prevent screw migration, and help resist axial loads. After the rod is inserted, both compressive and distractive forces can be applied to the construct before final tightening of the screw. The transverse coupler increases the stability of the construct against both rotational and flexion-extension forces. The Kaneda device also allows multisegmental fixation, with intervening vertebral bodies fastened to the construct through separate screws. The indications for this construct are identical to those for the Kostuik-Harrington construct and include correction of scoliotic deformities. The fusion rate is greater than 95%.[91]

The Ventrofix device is a newer-generation rigid anterior screw-rod construct intended to stabilize the lower thoracic and lumbar spines (see Fig. 304–16B). Direct axial compression can be applied across the graft site through a sliding mechanism between the rods and vertebral body clamps. The system can be implanted as a double- or single-rod construct, depending on the space limitations of the anatomy. The rod is secured to a clamp rather than to individual screws, increasing the stability of the system. This additional stability eliminates the need for a transverse coupler when a single level is stabilized. For longer constructs, a parallel connector is used to maintain rod alignment. The construct is assembled outside the operative field by inserting the free end of each rod into the open hole of the opposing clamp. Because the system is rigid, the trajectory of the screws is critical to properly engage the machine threads of the screw head to the clamp hole. The rods are allowed to pass through the opposite clamp during compression and are secured using two pairs of setscrews. This system has multiple configurations for stabilizing either complete or partial corpectomies.[92]

The Anterior Thoracolumbar Locking Plate is designed to stabilize the spine across the thoracolumbar junction and lumbar spine (see Fig. 304–16C). Despite the construct's rigidity, the graft can be compressed during plate insertion using a separate set of screws. Two cancellous bone screws are inserted into the angled dynamic compression plate holes and sequentially tightened to produce temporary compression. This places compressive forces on the vertebral body before insertion of the locking screws. Once the temporary fixation is complete, the locking screws are inserted and permanently maintain the compression placed across the graft. The plate hole is threaded so

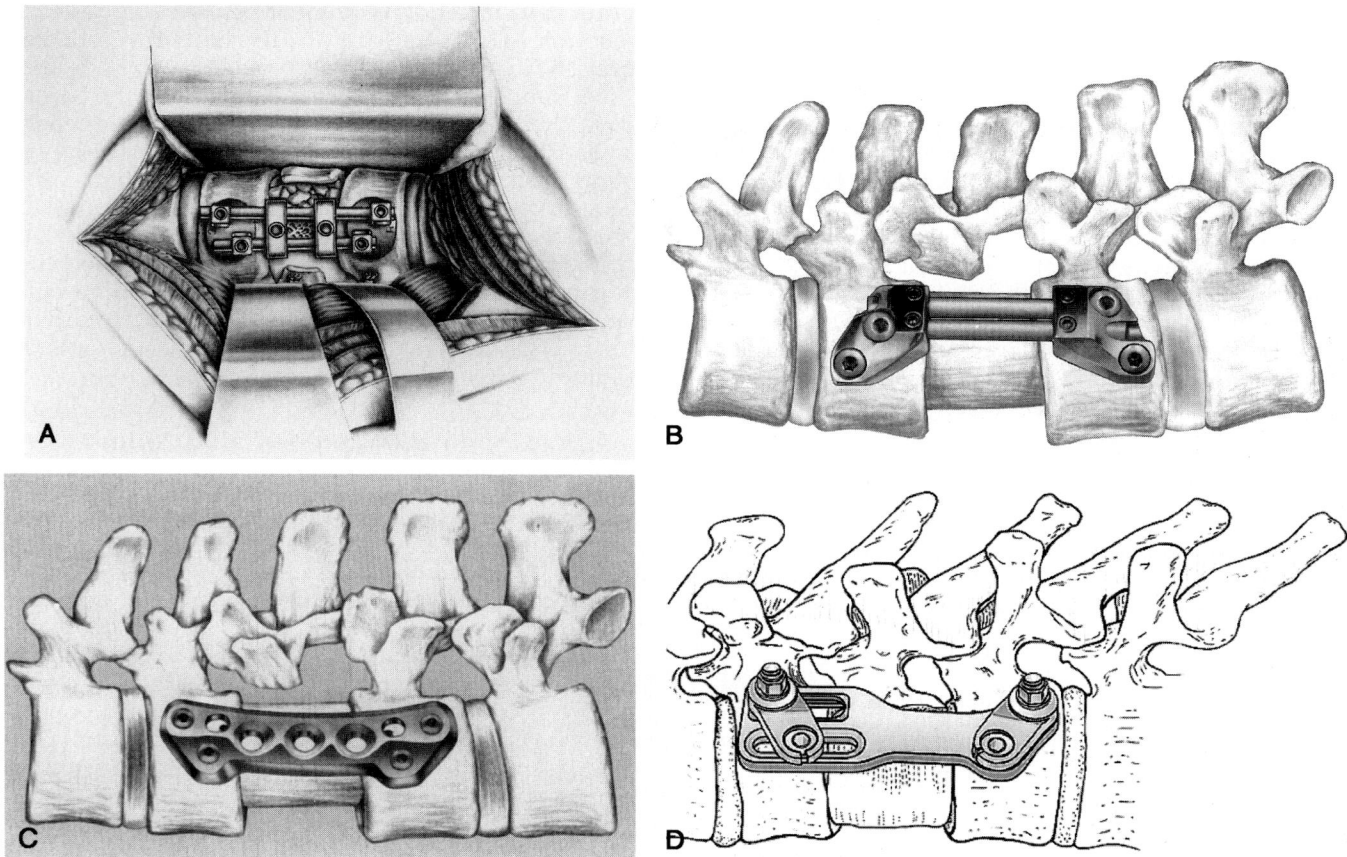

FIGURE 304–16. *A*, The Kaneda SR construct (Acromed, Cleveland, OH). *B*, The Ventrofix system (Synthes, Paoli, PA). *C*, The Anterior Thoracolumbar Locking Plate (Synthes, Paoli, PA). *D*, The ZPlate II (Sofamor-Danek, Memphis, TN).

the locking screw trajectory is perpendicular to the plate to ensure proper insertion. Therefore, this system is rigid.[93] Clinical results with this system have been favorable and support its use as a safe and effective anterior fixation construct.[94]

The ZPlate II is an advanced system that uses a combination of screws and bolts (see Fig. 304–16D). Unlike the original ZPlate designed primarily for the thoracolumbar junction, the ZPlate II has two categories of plates: the ZPlate II—ATL (anterior thoracolumbar) and the ZPlate II—Thoracic. The goal of the developers of the ZPlate II was to create an anterior fixation system that would permit anterior load sharing as well as distraction and compression across the graft, maintain a low profile, be compatible with computed tomography and magnetic resonance imaging, and be relatively easy to implant. The ZPlate II is classified as a dynamic implant because the multiaxial design of the bolts and screws allows movement between the components and promotes load sharing with the graft. The posteriorly placed bolts act as anchors for distraction of the corpectomy site to reduce the deformity. After the plate is positioned for precise seating of the graft, the slotted design of the ZPlate II allows compression across the corpectomy site. Adjustments made to create the ZPlate II—Thoracic include an intrinsic

kyphotic curvature, a narrower plate, a smaller curvature on the plate underside, and smaller bolts and screws. The bolts are inserted at predetermined coordinates based on the anatomy of the vertebral body. There are no specific clinical studies of the ZPlate II; however, clinical trials with the original ZPlate produced stable fixation, maintained deformity correction, and produced solid bony fusion comparable to other instrumentation techniques.[95, 96] Its ease of use makes it one of the preferred anterior thoracic instrumentation devices at our institution.

General Principles of Implantation

Several general principles should be followed during the implantation of ventral thoracic instrumentation. Despite specifics for both rod and plate constructs, the basic principles for insertion are the same. The systems available today are implanted primarily along the ventrolateral aspect of the vertebral bodies. The goals are to provide the greatest degree of stability with the lowest profile and to maximize implant-bone contact. Unequal stresses at the various bone-implant surfaces should be avoided by contouring the implant as closely as possible to the vertebral body surface and completely removing the costovertebral articulation and any protruding osteophytes.

Owing to the lateral insertion of the screws into the vertebral body, a clear understanding of the anatomy is essential to avoid compromising the spinal canal. The concave surface of the posterior vertebral body wall may lead to canal compromise if the posterior screws are not angled anteriorly.[97] Ideally, the posterior screw or bolt is inserted at a point 4 to 5 mm anterior to the posterior margin of the vertebral body and angled slightly ventrally to avoid the spinal canal. The anterior screws are placed either perpendicular to the posterior wall or slightly dorsally (Fig. 304–17). This placement triangulates the screws, increasing the resistance to screw pullout and parallelogram deformity. Some newer-generation rigid constructs, such as the Anterior Thoracolumbar Locking Plate and the Ventrofix, allow unicortical screw purchase. Implant insertion is easier, and the possible complications of impinging on contralateral structures are avoided. Patients with poor bone quality, such as osteoporotic patients, still need bicortical purchase to maximize stability.

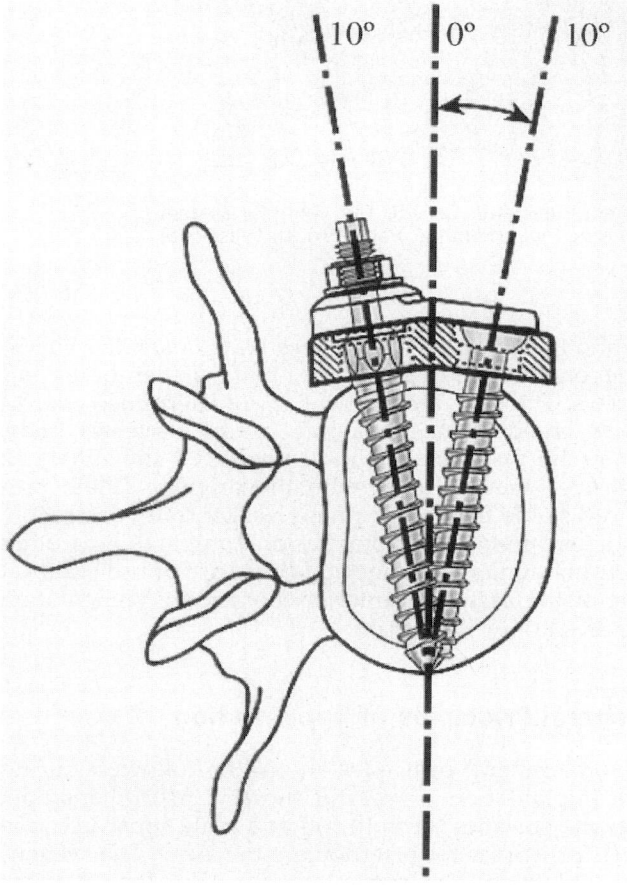

FIGURE 304–17. Axial section through a vertebral body demonstrating the appropriate trajectories of the vertebral body screws. The concave configuration of the posterior vertebral body wall necessitates a ventral trajectory of the dorsal screw to avoid the spinal canal. (From Zdeblick TA: ZPlate II Anterior Fixation System—Surgical Technique. Memphis, TN, Medtronic/Sofamor Danek, 1999, p 23.)

An intrinsic bending moment between the rods can cause a translational deformity with the rod constructs.[98] This problem can be avoided by cross-fixation of the parallel rods and triangulation of the screws within the vertebral body. Some of the newer-generation constructs avoid a parallelogram construct by offsetting the screws in a rostral-caudal orientation within a single vertebral body. Distraction and compression forces are applied to the screws before and after the graft is inserted. Excessive distraction across the defect can cause spinal cord injury from stretch and vascular compromise. Distraction is therefore limited, especially if distraction-resisting ligaments, such as the anterior longitudinal ligament, are incompetent.

Implantation of the Kaneda SR Anterior Spinal System

The unique feature of the Kaneda device is the tetraspiked spinal plates that serve as templates for insertion of the vertebral body screws. The plates are available in three sizes: small, medium, and large. The plate should maximally cover the lateral aspect of the vertebral body, with all four spikes located within the confines of the vertebral cortex. The plates are designed in pairs with a specific rostral and caudal component. Each plate is clearly marked to assist in this distinction. The plate must be orientated correctly to ensure that the anterior screws are inserted at the rostral and caudal limits of the construct. To ensure maximal contact with the bone, the lateral surface of the vertebra should be cleared of any soft tissue and protruding osteophytes. The plate is then driven into the lateral vertebral surface with the plate impactor (Fig. 304–18A).

The Kaneda screws serve to anchor the longitudinal rod to the vertebral body and are available in an open or closed design. The screw-rod interface is secured with a V-groove hollow ground connection and a setscrew. This contact site must be tightened to a minimum of 60 inch-pounds to obtain an acceptable connection. Screws are 6.25 mm in diameter and available in various lengths in 5-mm increments. The correct screw length can be determined either with preoperative images or by measuring the corpectomy defect directly. Bicortical screw purchase is optimal for maximal stability and is checked with intraoperative imaging or direct palpation. The posterior screw is inserted parallel to a vertebral end plate and angled about 10 degrees ventrally. The anterior screws are inserted parallel to the same vertebral end plate and perpendicular to the lateral aspect of the vertebral body. The same vertebral end plate should be used as a reference to achieve a perpendicular orientation between the screws and rods. The screws are inserted until the heads are recessed within the vertebral plate and aligned for rod placement (see Fig. 304–18B). Two open screws will not fit into the same vertebral plate.

The corpectomy site is reduced to as near an anatomic alignment as possible by distracting the rostral and caudal screws with a vertebral body spreader. The corpectomy site is measured, and an appropriately sized interbody strut is impacted into position (see Fig.

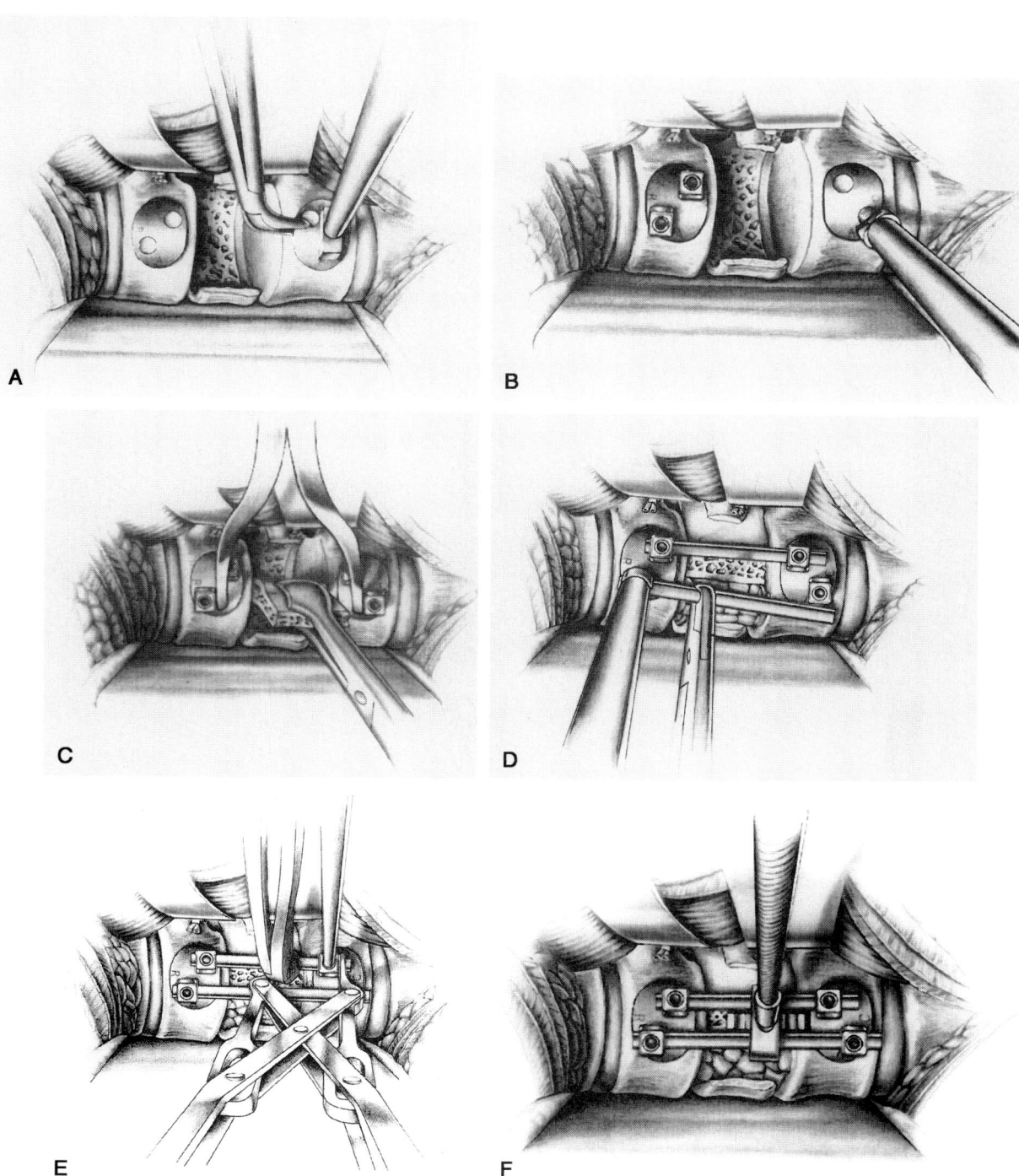

FIGURE 304–18. *A,* The tetra-spiked Kaneda SR spinal plate acts as a template for the placement of vertebral body screws. Each plate is marked with letters for correct orientation during placement. Once the correct size plate is selected, it is positioned on the lateral surface of the vertebral body and impacted. *B,* The screws are driven until the heads are recessed into the surface of the plate and aligned to allow rod passage. *C,* The vertebral body spreader is placed between the rostral and caudal screws, and distraction is applied. An appropriately sized graft is impacted into the corpectomy site. Morselized bone can be packed anterior to the graft to fill the defect. *D,* To aid in rod insertion, one screw is rotated away from the longitudinal axis of the construct, and the rod is inserted. The screw is rotated back to its original position, and the rod is passed through the second screw. *E,* The rod is correctly positioned in relation to either the rostral or caudal screw, and the setscrew is tightened. A rod holder is clamped onto a rod approximately 2 cm from the unsecured screw and acts as a compression anchor. Compression is applied across the rod holder and unsecured screw, and the setscrew is tightened. *F,* The upper and lower portions of the coupler are positioned perpendicular to each other, and the lower portion is passed between the longitudinal rods. The lower portion of the coupler is then rotated into position and engaged into the rod with upward traction. The bolt is tightened with a ⅛-inch wrench. (From Kaneda K, Gaines RW: Surgical Technique for Anterior Thoracolumbar Corpectomy, Graft Placement, and Stabilization Using the Kaneda SR Anterior Spinal System. Cleveland, OH, Acromed, 1996, pp 5–10.)

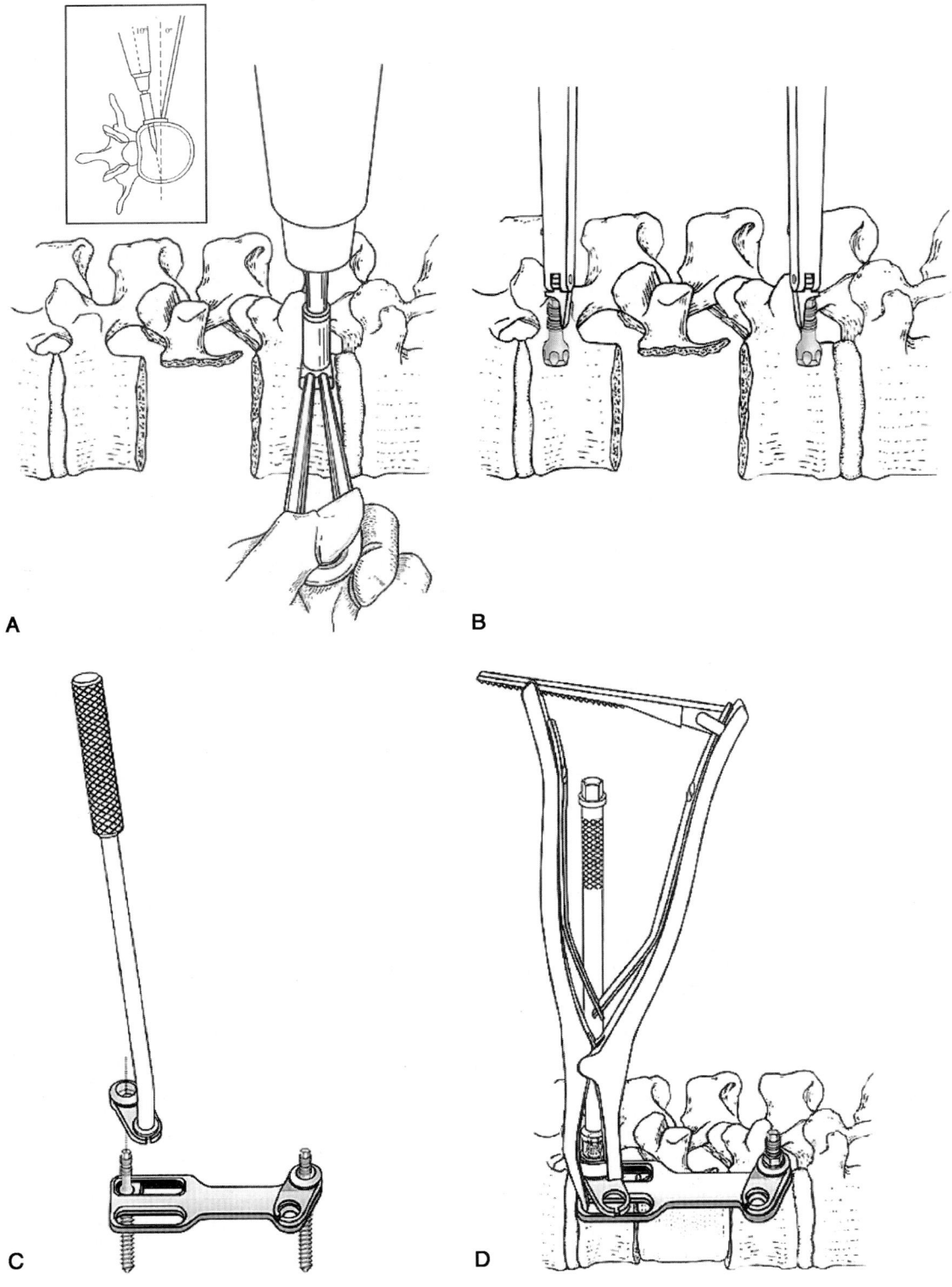

FIGURE 304–19. *A*, The bolt position guide is used to prepare the insertion point for the posteriorly placed bolts. Inset: The guide is placed parallel to the edge of the posterior cortex, and the awl is driven into the vertebral body with a 10-degree dorsal inclination. *B*, Placing the rack distracter over the machine-thread portion of the posteriorly placed bolts allows final distraction of the corpectomy site. *C*, Using a washer holder, the variable and slot washers are placed over the bolt posts and aligned with the anterior plate hole or slot. The bolt nuts are then tightened only to finger pressure. *D*, The shoe of the compressor is slipped around the base of the superior nut driver. Gentle compression is applied by squeezing the compressor, making sure that its tip remains within the plate slot and the shoe cradles the nut driver.

Illustration continued on following page

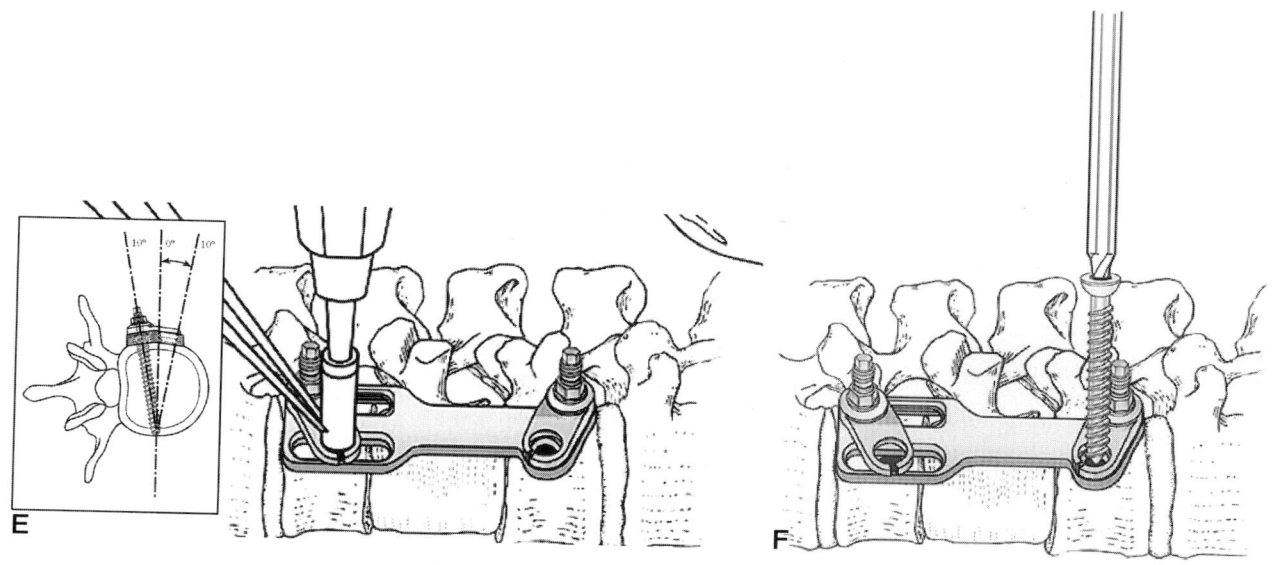

FIGURE 304–19. *Continued. E,* Using the screw position guide and awl, the holes for the anterior screws are prepared. Inset: The holes are directed through the retaining ring hole in the variable and slot washers and directed between 0 and 10 degrees posteriorly. *F,* The anterior screws are inserted into the previously prepared holes. The screw is tightened until the head is seated beneath the retaining ring of the washer. (From Zdeblick TA: ZPlate II Anterior Fixation System—Surgical Technique. Memphis, TN, Medtronic/Sofamor Danek, 1999, pp 9–24.)

304–18*C*). The distance between posterior screws is measured, and length is added so that the rod extends about 2 mm from either screw edge. An appropriately sized rod is inserted into the screws. The anterior rod is measured and inserted in an identical fashion (see Fig. 304–18*D*). The setscrews for the four V-groove hollow ground connections are inserted but not tightened. The posterior rod is placed in the final position relative to either the superior or inferior screw, and the respective setscrew is tightened. A rod clamp is attached to the posterior rod several centimeters from the unsecured screw to act as an anchor. Compression is applied across the rod clamp and unsecured screw (see Fig. 304–18*E*). Once an adequate amount of compression is achieved, the final setscrew is tightened. The anterior rod is placed under compression in an identical manner.

To maximize stability, the manufacturer recommends placing a transverse coupler at the rostral and caudal ends of the implant. The correct size of the coupler is determined with a transverse coupler template. The coupler is loaded onto a self-retaining ⅛-inch wrench, and the upper and lower portions of the coupler are oriented perpendicular to each other. The lower portion is passed between the rods and rotated into its final position, parallel to the upper portion (see Fig. 304–18*F*). The coupler bolt is tightened, approximating the lower and upper portions. Final tightening is achieved with the modular ⅛-inch wrench. Once the construct is complete, all setscrews and transverse coupler bolts are tightened to at least 60 inch-pounds.

Implantation of the ZPlate II

Zdeblick[99] describes the technique for surgical implantation of the ZPlate II anterior fixation system. Measurement of the coronal diameter of the vertebral body is the initial step. This measurement is used to determine the appropriate size bolts and screws and is obtained intraoperatively with a depth gauge or from preoperative imaging. The length of the bolts and screws chosen should be slightly longer than the coronal diameter to ensure bicortical purchase. Bolts are placed into the posterosuperior corner of the rostral vertebra and the posteroinferior corner of the caudal vertebra. The insertion point is 4 to 5 mm away from the adjacent disk space and 4 to 5 mm anterior to the posterior cortical wall. A high-speed drill is used to clear the lateral surface of the vertebral body of osteophytes, especially at the end plate. The bolt position guide is placed parallel to the edge of the inferior vertebral body, and the bone awl is used to prepare the initial insertion site (Fig. 304–19*A*). The first bolt is inserted at an anterior angle of 10 degrees, until the bolt driver is flush with the vertebral body. The second bolt is inserted into the superior vertebral body in an identical manner.

Distracting the end plates with a lamina spreader and manually compressing the posterior spine initially reduce the deformity. The rack distracter is fitted to the machine-threaded portion of the exposed bolts, and final distraction is applied (see Fig. 304–19*B*). The corpectomy site is measured with a set of calipers, and the appropriate size interbody graft is inserted. The rack distracter is not within the corpectomy site, allowing easy access to both end plates. Once it is inserted, the distraction is released, and the thoracic template is placed over the bolts to determine the appropriate size plate. When using the ZPlate II–Thoracic, the kyphosis present in the plate must be aligned with the natural kyphosis of the thoracic spine. For a left-sided approach, the plate is placed so that the slots are oriented at the superior end of the plate. The appropriate size plate is placed over the bolts. The shortest plate possible is chosen to maximize compression and minimize impingement on the superior disk space. The variable and slot washers are assembled over the bolts and aligned with the plate slot or hole. The nuts are threaded onto the bolts and tightened with the nut driver using finger pressure (see Fig. 304–19C). Once the superior nut is provisionally tightened, the shoe of the compressor is placed around the base of the nut driver. Gentle compression is applied while ascertaining that the tip of the compressor rests within the plate slot and the cradle is secured around the base of the nut driver on the superior bolt (see Fig. 304–19D). The superior nut is tightened with a deflection torque wrench to 80 to 100 inch-pounds while the compression is maintained. Countertorque should be applied during final tightening with a rod pusher. The inferior nut is then tightened to the same torque using the torque wrench.

The anterior body screws should measure 5 mm longer than the posterior bolts, ensuring bicortical screw purchase. Using the screw positioning guide and awl, the pilot hole is created for the screws through the retaining ring hole of the variable and slot washers (see Fig. 304–19E). The anterior screws are offset in a superior-inferior orientation from the posterior bolts and directed 10 degrees posterior to achieve triangulation between the screw and bolt. The screws are tightened with a hex driver until the screw head is seated beneath the retaining ring of the washers (see Fig. 304–19F). The bolt extensions are removed with the post-breakoff wrench in a clockwise fashion. Countertorque should be applied during this maneuver. Once the screws are inserted, an intraoperative fluoroscopic image or radiograph is obtained to document the correct position of the screws. The surgical site is irrigated copiously, and the wound is closed in routine fashion.

COMPLICATIONS RELATED TO OPERATIVE INTERVENTION

The key to avoiding complications related to ventral instrumentation of the thoracic spine is appropriate preoperative planning. Appropriate imaging studies indicate the extent of pathology and identify its association with the surrounding anatomy. All patients require a comprehensive preoperative medical evaluation. Pulmonary status is important to assess, because approaches to the thoracic spine involve the pleural cavity to a certain extent. Trauma patients should undergo a thorough assessment of all organ systems to rule out any additional life-threatening injuries before surgery.

Complications related to the implantation of ventral thoracic instrumentation can occur at any point during the procedure or afterward. Rare injuries to internal organs (lungs, diaphragm, kidneys, ureters) or major vessels (aorta, vena cava) have been reported.[100] During a transcavitary exposure, the assistance of a thoracic or general surgeon can significantly reduce the incidence of such injuries. Damage to the neural elements is more likely to occur during decompression and reconstruction. Excessive distraction of the deformity can lead to a stretch injury or vascular compromise and should be avoided. If the dura is violated, every attempt should be made to obtain a watertight closure. Persistent tears in the dura significantly increase the risk of infection and interfere with wound healing, particularly if a chest tube must be inserted. In such a scenario, the chest tube should never be placed on more than 20 cm water suction and should be turned to water seal as soon as possible to prevent formation of a cerebrospinal fluid fistula.

Possible early complications include pulmonary problems (pneumothorax, atelectasis, pneumonia), deep venous thrombosis, and minor infection. Proper closure of the incision avoids wound dehiscence and decreases the incidence of superficial infection. Complications related to the instrumentation or fusion usually occur during the postoperative period or after recovery. Instrumentation failures, including fracture, loosening, or pullout, can be reduced by appropriate selection of constructs and insertion techniques. Despite these precautions, instrumentation fails in as many as 15% of cases. The more catastrophic complications, such as large vessel erosion, have not been reported since the newer, low-profile constructs were introduced. Deep infections related to anterior instrumentation are rare.

CONCLUSION

A wide variety of pathologies can affect the anterior thoracic spine. These lesions may reach the attention of spine surgeons for a number of reasons, including pain, neurological deficits, or worsening structural deformities. One of the most important steps in managing these lesions is learning the appropriate indications for surgical intervention. Advances in surgical techniques and the development of instrumentation constructs allow spine surgeons to treat this category of spinal pathology effectively. The specific approach and the instrumentation construct used depend on the nature of the pathology and the surgeon's preference. No randomized, prospective studies have compared the outcomes associated with the various constructs, and the utility of such studies remains questionable because the biomechanical properties of most constructs are now comparable.

REFERENCES

1. Royle ND: The operative removal of an accessory vertebra. Med J Aust 1:467, 1928.
2. Hodgson A, Stock F: Anterior spinal fusion: A preliminary communication on radical treatment of Pott's disease and Pott's paraplegia. Br J Surg 44:266–275, 1956.
3. Humphries AW, Hawk WA: Anterior fusion of the lumbar spine using an internal fixative device. Surg Forum 9:770–773, 1958.
4. Dwyer AF, Newton NC, Sherwood AA: Anterior approach to scoliosis: A preliminary report. Clin Orthop 62:192–202, 1969.

5. Dwyer AF, Schafer MF: Anterior approach to scoliosis: Results of treatment in fifty-one cases. J Bone Joint Surg Br 56:218–224, 1974.

6. Zielke K, Stunkat R, Beaujean F: Ventrale derotations-spondy-lodesis [German]. Arch Orthop Unfallchir 85:257–277, 1976.

7. Dunn HK: Anterior stabilization of thoracolumbar injuries. Clin Orthop 189:116–124, 1984.

8. Dunn HK: Anterior spine stabilization and decompression for thoracolumbar injuries. Orthop Clin North Am 17:113–119, 1986.

9. Brown LP, Bridwell KH, Holt RJ, et al: Aortic erosions and lacerations associated with the Dunn anterior spinal instrumentation. Paper presented at the Scoliosis Research Society, 1985.

10. Gilbert RW, Kim JH, Posner JB: Epidural spinal cord compression from metastatic tumor: Diagnosis and treatment. Ann Neurol 3:40–51, 1978.

11. Greenberg HS, Kim JH, Posner JB: Epidural spinal cord compression from metastatic tumor: Results with a new treatment protocol. Ann Neurol 8:361–366, 1980.

12. Sundaresan N, Digiacinto GV, Hughes JE: Surgical treatment of spinal metastases. Clin Neurosurg 33:503–522, 1986.

13. Wong DA, Fornasier VL, MacNab I: Spinal metastasis: The obvious, the occult, and the impostors. Spine 15:1–4, 1990.

14. Findlay GF: Adverse effects of the management of malignant spinal cord compression. J Neurol Neurosurg Psychiatry 47:761–768, 1984.

15. Black P: Spinal metastasis: Current status and recommended guidelines for management. Neurosurgery 5:726–746, 1979.

16. Young RF, Post EM, King GA: Treatment of spinal epidural metastases: Randomized prospective comparison of laminectomy and radiotherapy. J Neurosurg 53:741–748, 1980.

17. Johnson JR, Leatherman KD, Holt RT: Anterior decompression of the spinal cord for neurological deficit. Spine 8:396–405, 1983.

18. Siegal T, Tiqua P, Siegal T: Vertebral body resection for epidural compression by malignant tumors: Results of forty-seven consecutive operative procedures. J Bone Joint Surg Am 67:375–382, 1985.

19. Harrington KD: Anterior decompression and stabilization of the spine as a treatment for vertebral collapse and spinal cord compression from metastatic malignancy. Clin Orthop 233:177–197, 1988.

20. Sundaresan N, Digiacinto VG, Hughes JE, et al: Treatment of neoplastic spinal cord compression: Results of a prospective study. Neurosurgery 29:645–650, 1991.

21. Cooper PR, Errico TJ, Martin R, et al: A systematic approach to spinal reconstruction after anterior decompression for neoplastic disease of the thoracic and lumbar spine. Neurosurgery 32:1–8, 1993.

22. Sonntag VKH, Marcotte P: Comment on Cooper PR, et al: A systematic approach to spinal reconstruction after anterior decompression for neoplastic disease of the thoracic and lumbar spine. Neurosurgery 32:1–8, 1993.

23. Sundaresan N, Krol G, Steinberger AA, Moore F: Management of tumors of the thoracolumbar spine. Neurosurg Clin N Am 8:541–553, 1997.

24. Karnofsky DA, Abelmann WH, Craver LF, et al: The use of nitrogen mustards in the palliative treatment of carcinoma: With particular reference to bronchogenic carcinoma. Cancer 1:634–656, 1948.

25. Mahaley MS, Mettlin C, Natarajan N, et al: National survey of patterns of care for brain-tumor patients. J Neurosurg 71:826–836, 1989.

26. Tokuhashi R, Matsuzaki H, Toriyama S, et al: Scoring system for the preoperative evaluation of metastatic spine tumor prognosis. Spine 15:1110–1113, 1990.

27. Boland PJ, Lane JM, Sundaresan N: Metastatic disease of the spine. Clin Orthop 169:95–102, 1982.

28. Keene JS: Radiographic evaluation of thoracolumbar fractures. Clin Orthop 189:58–64, 1984.

29. Mumford J, Weinstein JN, Spratt KF, et al: Thoracolumbar burst fractures: The clinical efficacy and outcome of nonoperative management. Spine 18:955–970, 1993.

30. Errico T, Bauer R, Waugh T (eds): Spinal Trauma. Philadelphia, JB Lippincott, 1990, pp 195–336.

31. Berg EE: The sternal-rib complex: A possible fourth column in thoracic spine fractures. Spine 18:1916–1929, 1993.

32. Denis F: The three column spine and its significance in the classification of acute thoracolumbar spinal injuries. Spine 8:817–831, 1983.

33. Davies WE, Morris JH, Hill V: An analysis of conservative (non-surgical) management of thoracolumbar fractures and fracture-dislocations with neural damage. J Bone Joint Surg Am 62:1324–1328, 1980.

34. Weinstein JN, Collalto P, Lehmann TR: Thoracolumbar "burst" fractures treated conservatively: A long-term follow-up. Spine 13:33–38, 1988.

35. Bohlman HH: Treatment of fractures and dislocations of the thoracic and lumbar spine. J Bone Joint Surg Am 67:165–169, 1985.

36. Willen J, Lindahl S, Nordwall A: Unstable thoracolumbar fractures: A comparative clinical study of conservative treatment and Harrington instrumentation. Spine 10:111–122, 1985.

37. Gertzbein SD, Macmichael D, Tile M: Harrington instrumentation as a method of fixation in fractures of the spine. J Bone Joint Surg Br 64:526–529, 1982.

38. Esses SI, Botsford DJ, Kostuik JP: Evaluation of surgical treatment for burst fractures. Spine 15:667–673, 1990.

39. Moreland DB, Egnatchik JG, Bennett GJ: Cotrel-Dubousset instrumentation for treatment of thoracolumbar fractures. Neurosurgery 27:69–73, 1990.

40. Zou D, Yoo JU, Edwards WT, et al: Mechanics of anatomic reduction of thoracolumbar burst fractures: Comparison of distraction versus distraction plus lordosis, in the anatomic reduction of thoracolumbar burst fractures. Spine 18:195–203, 1993.

41. Dekutoski MB, Conlan ES, Salciccioli GG: Spinal mobility and deformity after Harrington rod stabilization and limited arthrodesis of thoracolumbar fractures. J Bone Joint Surg Am 75:168–176, 1993.

42. Bohlman HH, Freehafer A, Dejak J: The results of treatment of acute injuries of the upper thoracic spine with paralysis. J Bone Joint Surg Am 67:360–369, 1985.

43. Kostuik JP: Anterior fixation for burst fractures of the thoracic and lumbar spine with or without neurological involvement. Spine 13:286–293, 1988.

44. Cahill D: Infections of the spine. Contemp Neurosurg 15:1–8, 1993.

45. Baker AS, Ojemann RG, Swartz MN, et al: Spinal epidural abscess. N Engl J Med 293:463–468, 1975.

46. Kostuik JP: Anterior spinal cord decompression for lesions of the thoracic and lumbar spine, techniques, new methods of internal fixation results. Spine 8:512–531, 1983.

47. Oga M, Arizono T, Takasita M, et al: Evaluation of the risk of instrumentation as a foreign body in spinal tuberculosis: Clinical and biologic study. Spine 18:1890–1894, 1993.

48. Malcolm BW, Bradford DS, Winter RB, et al: Post-traumatic kyphosis: A review of forty-eight surgically treated patients. J Bone Joint Surg Am 63:891–899, 1981.

49. Roberson JR, Whitesides TE Jr: Surgical reconstruction of late post-traumatic thoracolumbar kyphosis. Spine 10:307–312, 1985.

50. Kostuik JP, Matsusaki H: Anterior stabilization, instrumentation, and decompression for post-traumatic kyphosis. Spine 14:379–386, 1989.

51. Chang KW: Oligosegmental correction of post-traumatic thoracolumbar angular kyphosis. Spine 18:1909–1915, 1993.

52. Le Roux PD, Haglund MM, Harris AB: Thoracic disc disease: Experience with the transpedicular approach in twenty consecutive patients. Neurosurgery 33:58–66, 1993.

53. Cauchoix J, Binet J: Anterior surgical approaches to the spine. Ann R Coll Surg Engl 21:234–243, 1957.

54. Standefer M, Hardy RW Jr, Marks K, et al: Chondromyxoid fibroma of the cervical spine: A case report with review of the literature and a description of an operative approach to the lower anterior cervical spine. Neurosurgery 11:288–292, 1982.

55. Micheli LJ, Hood RW: Anterior exposure of the cervicothoracic spine using a combined cervical and thoracic approach. J Bone Joint Surg Am 65:992–997, 1983.

56. Kurz LT, Pursel SE, Herkowitz HN: Modified anterior approach to the cervicothoracic junction. Spine 16(10 Suppl):S542–S547, 1991.

57. Nazzaro JM, Arbit E, Burt M: "Trap door" exposure of the cervicothoracic junction: Technical note. J Neurosurg 80:338–341, 1994.

58. Larson SJ, Holst RA, Hemmy DC, et al: Lateral extracavitary approach to traumatic lesions of the thoracic and lumbar spine. J Neurosurg 45:628–637, 1976.

59. McCormick P: The lateral extracavitary approach to the thoracic and lumbar spine. In Holtzman R, Stein B, Farcy J, et al (eds): Spinal Instability. New York, Raven Press, 1993, pp 335–348.

60. Heiple KG, Chase SW, Herndon CH: A comparative study of healing process following different types of bone transplantation. J Bone Joint Surg Am 45:1593–1616, 1963.

61. Prolo DJ, Rodrigo JJ: Contemporary bone graft physiology and surgery. Clin Orthop 200:322–342, 1985.

62. Boden SD, Schimandle JH: Biologic enhancement of spinal fusion. Spine 20(24 Suppl):113S–123S, 1995.

63. Laurie SW, Kaban LB, Mulliken JB, et al: Donor-site morbidity after harvesting rib and iliac bone. Plast Reconstr Surg 73:933–938, 1984.

64. Keller EE, Triplett WW: Iliac bone graft: Review of 160 consecutive cases. J Oral Maxillofac Surg 45:11–14, 1987.

65. Summers BN, Eisenstein SM: Donor site pain from the ilium: A complication of lumbar spine fusion. J Bone Joint Surg Br 71:677–680, 1989.

66. Younger EM, Chapman MW: Morbidity at bone graft donor sites. J Orthop Trauma 3:192–195, 1989.

67. Banwart JC, Asher MA, Hassanein RS: Iliac crest bone graft harvest donor site morbidity: A statistical evaluation. Spine 20:1055–1060, 1995.

68. Bradford DS: Anterior vascular pedicle bone grafting for the treatment of kyphosis. Spine 5:318–323, 1980.

69. McBride GG, Bradford DS: Vertebral body replacement with femoral neck allograft and vascularized rib strut graft: A technique for treating post-traumatic kyphosis with neurologic deficit. Spine 8:406–415, 1983.

70. Shaffer JW, Field GA, Goldberg VM, et al: Fate of vascularized and nonvascularized autografts. Clin Orthop 197:32–43, 1985.

71. Blumenthal SL, Baker J, Dossett A, et al: The role of anterior lumbar fusion for internal disc disruption. Spine 13:566–569, 1988.

72. Hanley EJ, Harvell J, Shapiro D, et al: Use of allograft bone in cervical spine surgery. Semin Spine Surg 1:262–270, 1989.

73. Urist MR, Dowell TA, Hay PH, et al: Inductive substrates for bone formation. Clin Orthop 59:59–96, 1968.

74. Einhorn TA, Lane JM, Burstein AH, et al: The healing of segmental bone defects induced by demineralized bone matrix: A radiographic and biomechanical study. J Bone Joint Surg Am 66:274–279, 1984.

75. Dahners LE, Jacobs RR: Long bone defects treated with demineralized bone. South Med J 78:933–934, 1985.

76. Gepstein R, Weiss RE, Hallel T: Bridging large defects in bone by demineralized bone matrix in the form of a powder: A radiographic, histological, and radioisotope-uptake study in rats. J Bone Joint Surg Am 69:984–992, 1987.

77. Hulth A, Johnell O, Henricson A: The implantation of demineralized fracture matrix yields more new bone formation than does intact matrix. Clin Orthop 234:235–249, 1988.

78. Leads from the MMWR: Transmission of HIV through bone transplantation: Case report and public health recommendations. JAMA 260:2487–2488, 1988.

79. Buck BE, Malinin TI, Brown MD: Bone transplantation and human immunodeficiency virus: An estimate of risk of acquired immunodeficiency syndrome (AIDS). Clin Orthop 240:129–136, 1989.

80. Arbit E, Galicich J: Vertebral body reconstruction with a modified Harrington rod distraction system for stabilization of the spine affected with metastatic disease. J Neurosurg 83:617–620, 1995.

81. Johnson J, Pare L, Torres R: Thoracolumbar vertebral body replacement: Materials and techniques. Contemp Neurosurg 20:1–8, 1998.

82. White AA III, Panjabi MM: Clinical Biomechanics of the Spine. Philadelphia, JB Lippincott, 1990.

83. Benzel EC: Spinal deformities. In Benzel EC (ed): Biomechanics of Spine Stabilization: Principles and Clinical Practice. New York, McGraw-Hill, 1995, pp 76–77.

84. Benzel EC: Spinal fusion. In Benzel EC (ed): Biomechanics of Spine Stabilization: Principles and Clinical Practice. New York, McGraw-Hill, 1995, pp 103–105.

85. Kanayama M, Ng JT, Cunningham BW, et al: Biomechanical analysis of anterior versus circumferential spinal reconstruction for various anatomic stages of tumor lesions. Spine 24:445–450, 1999.

86. Benzel EC: Qualitative attributes of spinal implants. In Benzel EC (ed): Biomechanics of Spine Stabilization: Principles and Clinical Practice. New York, McGraw-Hill, 1995, pp 42–45, 47–49, 135–136.

87. Kaneda K, Abumi K, Fujiya M: Burst fractures with neurologic deficits of the thoracolumbar-lumbar spine: Results of anterior decompression and stabilization with anterior instrumentation. Spine 9:788–795, 1984.

88. Oglivie J: Zielke instrumentation of the spine. In An H, Cotler J (eds): Spinal Instrumentation. Baltimore, Williams & Wilkins, 1992, pp 353–358.

89. Kostuik JP: Anterior Kostuik-Harrington distraction systems. In An H, Cotler J (eds): Spinal Instrumentation. Baltimore, Williams & Wilkins, 1992, pp 359–377.

90. Kostuik JP: Anterior fixation for fractures of the thoracic and lumbar spine with or without neurologic involvement. Clin Orthop 189:103–115, 1984.

91. Kaneda K: Kaneda anterior spinal instrumentation for the thoracic and lumbar spine. In An H, Cotler J (eds): Spinal Instrumentation. Baltimore, Williams & Wilkins, 1992, pp 413–433.

92. Aebi M, Thalgott J, Webb J: Stabilization techniques: Thoracolumbar spine. In Aebi M, Thalgott J, Webb J (eds): AO ASIF Principles in Spine Surgery. Berlin, Springer, 1998, pp 94–100.

93. Aebi M, Thalgott J, Webb J: Stabilization techniques: Thoracolumbar spine. In Aebi M, Thalgott J, Webb J (eds): AO ASIF Principles in Spine Surgery. Berlin, Springer, 1998, pp 85–88.

94. Thalgott JS, Kabins MB, Timlin M, et al: Four year experience with the AO anterior thoracolumbar locking plate. Spinal Cord 35:286–291, 1997.

95. Ghanayem AJ, Zdeblick TA: Anterior instrumentation in the management of thoracolumbar burst fractures. Clin Orthop 335:89–100, 1997.

96. Aydin E, Solak AS, Tuzuner MM, et al: Z-plate instrumentation in thoracolumbar spinal fractures. Bull Hosp Jt Dis 58:92–97, 1999.

97. Ebraheim NA, Xu R, Ahmad M, et al: Anatomic considerations of anterior instrumentation of the thoracic spine. Am J Orthop 26:419–424, 1997.

98. Benzel EC: Anterior cantilever beam fixation and related techniques. In Benzel EC (ed): Biomechanics of Spine Stabilization: Principles and Clinical Practice. New York, McGraw-Hill, 1995, pp 187–189.

99. Zdeblick TA: ZPlate II Anterior Fixation System—Surgical Technique. Memphis, TN, Medtronic/Sofamor Danek, 1999, pp 9–24.

100. Matsuzaki H, Tokuhashi Y, Wakabayashi K, et al: Penetration of a screw into the thoracic aorta in anterior spinal instrumentation: A case report. Spine 18:2327–2331, 1993.

CHAPTER 305

Posterior Thoracic Instrumentation

SCOTT L. SIMON ■ JAMES M. SCHUSTER

The safe and effective insertion of posterior instrumentation in the thoracic spine is one of the more challenging tasks in spinal surgery. This is due in part to the anatomic constraints and the proximity to neural and vascular structures, allowing for a very small margin of error. Therefore, a thorough understanding of the anatomy and biomechanics of the thoracic spine in general, and of the patient's specific anatomy and pathology through preoperative radiographic evaluation, is essential in achieving a good outcome. Decision making regarding the use of posterior instrumentation in the thoracic spine requires the consideration of multiple factors, including surgical experience, indications and limitations of various instrumentation methods, level of pathology, nature of the pathologic process, surgical anatomy above and below the level of involvement, bone quality, biomechanical requirements for stabilization, desired surgical result (e.g., kyphosis correction, distraction), patient's medical condition (which may limit blood loss or length of surgery), patient life expectancy, and requirements for postoperative magnetic resonance imaging. The following discussion is more pertinent to traumatic, oncologic, and degenerative processes than to scoliosis and deformity, which are discussed elsewhere in this book.

ANATOMY

The use of posterior instrumentation to treat disorders of the thoracic spine mandates a thorough understanding of the anatomy of this region. The three-dimensional bony anatomy in this region is relatively small in comparison to that of the lumbar spine, allowing little margin for error, especially in the mid and upper thoracic spine. This three-dimensional anatomy also changes throughout the thoracic spine and varies from patient to patient, requiring careful preoperative evaluation. Determining the quality and size of the pedicles and lamina that will be incorporated into a construct should be done before choosing the type of fixation to be used. A fractured lamina does not provide a viable point of fixation for a sublaminar wire or a sublaminar hook. Pedicle size determines the practicality of using pedicle screw fixation and the screw size required,

especially in the upper thoracic spine and across the cervicothoracic junction. The presence of significant osteoporosis further influences the type of fixation chosen. Poor bone quality limits the effectiveness of screw fixation and diminishes screws' mechanical advantage over hooks and sublaminar wires.[1–3] However, there have been recent reports of augmenting pedicle screw pullout strength with cements such as methyl methacrylate[4] and hydroxyapatite.[5–8]

The musculature overlying the dorsal surface of the thoracic spine contributes to the maintenance of sagittal balance and aids in controlling rotation. The trapezius muscle lies in the superficial muscular group and extends from the occipital protuberance and the C7 spinous process to the T12 spinous process. The deep musculature is composed of the erector spinae group, which lies in the vertebrocostal groove, and extends from the posterior inferior sacrum and iliac crest throughout the length of the spine. This group of muscles acts primarily as an extensor but can cause bending when acting unilaterally. Deep to the erector spinae muscles are the paravertebral muscles, which have their origins in the transverse processes and insert on the spinous processes. Proper exposure for placement of thoracic instrumentation requires visualization of the facets and transverse processes, requiring extensive, careful muscle dissection. Using fascial planes and subperiosteal dissection reduces blood loss, postoperative pain, and wound complications.

In the lumbar spine, the transverse processes are often used as an external landmark for the location of the pedicle. However, there is more anatomic variability in the thoracic spine. A cadaver study by McCormack and colleagues[9] found that the midline of the transverse process is cephalad to the pedicle in the upper thoracic spine, in line with the pedicle in the middle thoracic spine, and caudal to the pedicle in the lower thoracic spine. In addition, considerable individual variability exists with regard to the dimensions of the thoracic pedicle, which mandates a thorough preoperative evaluation with computed tomography before attempting transpedicular fixation.[10]

In general, the pedicular dimensions are larger in men.[11] The width of the pedicle decreases from T1 to T4 and then gradually increases to T12, whereas the pedicle height and length tend to increase from T1 to T12.[11] The transverse angle of the pedicle, however, decreases from T1 to T12, such that the pedicles become less medially aligned the closer they are to the thoracolumbar junction. At T1 and T2, the pedicles have a medial projection of 30 to 40 degrees; at T3 to T11, this transverse angle is 20 to 25 degrees; and at T12, the transverse angle has been measured at 10 degrees.[11] Conversely, the pedicular sagittal angle remains relatively consistent throughout the thoracic spine.[11] The majority of the pedicle is composed of cancellous bone, which is encased in a shell of cortical bone that is significantly thicker medially than laterally. This may account for the finding that most screw-related pedicle fractures occur laterally.[12]

The thecal sac abuts the medial wall of the pedicle, and the nerve roots exit under the inferior wall of the pedicle. The nerve roots tend to have a more cephalad angulation and a closer relationship to the pedicle in the upper thoracic spine and a more caudal angulation and more distant relationship in the lower thoracic spine.[13] Attached to the superior and inferior surfaces of the pedicles are the facets, which are oriented in the coronal plane throughout most of the thoracic region (T1-10). This orientation provides stability against anteroposterior translation. In the lower thoracic spine, the facets take on a more sagittal orientation, which provides greater stability against rotation. The lateral portion of the facet joints plays an important role in providing spinal stability and should be preserved to minimize postoperative kyphotic deformity and segmental instability when performing a wide decompressive laminectomy, especially in adjacent segments not incorporated in a fusion. The spinous processes project inferiorly in the upper and middle thoracic spine but have a more horizontal configuration in the lower thoracic spine.

The spinal ligaments and joint capsules preserve the articulated nature of the spine, allowing a requisite but restrained amount of movement. The anterior longitudinal ligament contains a relatively higher proportion of collagen and acts to prevent hyperextension and overdistraction. Testing has found that the strength of the anterior longitudinal ligament increases as it descends toward the thoracolumbar junction.[14] The posterior longitudinal ligament functions to limit hyperflexion of the spine. Its tensile strength is about half that of the anterior longitudinal ligament. The integrity of the posterior longitudinal ligament is essential when attempting to perform indirect reductions of fractures through ligamentotaxis with posterior instrumentation.

BIOMECHANICS

The inherent stability of the thoracic spine is provided by the rib cage; therefore, considerable force or disruption is required to cause instability, especially in the upper thoracic spine. Whitesides[15] defined a stable spine as one that can withstand stress without further neurological damage or progressive deformity. The degree of spinal stability and classifications for clinical management are often based on spinal columns in trauma. The three-column model proposed by White and Panjabi[14] was the basis for the fracture classification systems of Denis[16, 17] and McAfee and associates.[18] Gertzbein and others[19, 20] have proposed a more extensively descriptive system using pathomorphologic characteristics and based on a two-column model.[15] Several authors have proposed similar methods for characterizing spinal stability in primary and metastatic tumors, with an emphasis on degree of anterior column involvement.[21, 22] Although no system can account for all possible diagnostic and therapeutic permutations, these systems provide a rough framework within which rational decision making can be initiated.

Regardless of the method used to determine clinical instability, a careful evaluation must be made of the thoracic spine's ability to protect the spinal cord from initial or subsequent damage and prevent the development of incapacitating deformity or severe pain under physiologic loads. Several contributing factors make the thoracic spine susceptible to this descriptive definition of instability. In this region of the spine, there is relatively less free space surrounding the spinal cord, as well as a more tenuous blood supply, making the spinal cord more susceptible to canal compromise.[14] In addition, the normal thoracic spine possesses a kyphosis, which predisposes it to instability in flexion.[14] This kyphosis is formed in utero and is maintained by the differences in the anterior and posterior vertebral body and disk dimensions. The height of the ventral surface of the thoracic vertebral body is approximately 1 to 2 mm less than that of the dorsal surface.[23] This slight height difference is also seen in the thoracic intervertebral disks. Further, the thoracic spine is less mobile and more rigid than the cervical or lumbar spine owing to the steep orientation of the facets as well as its relationship to the rib cage. The rib cage restricts motion in the sagittal, coronal, and transverse planes and adds stiffness to the spine, giving additional support to the thoracic spine.[24, 25] Rib articulations exist on the thoracic vertebral bodies, pedicles, and, except for T1, T11, and T12, transverse processes and give the thoracic spine its most identifiable feature. This transition between relative mobility and immobility that exists at the cervicothoracic and thoracolumbar junctions produces a stress riser, making these junctions more susceptible to traumatic injury and destabilization.[26, 27] Therefore, treating junctional instability often requires relatively longer constructs with multiple points of fixation, as well as consideration of supplementing the posterior construct with anterior instrumentation.[28, 29]

Spinal instrumentation is designed to maximize the preservation of neurological function, maintain alignment or reduce deformity, provide mechanical stability to allow early return of function, and provide security until fusion.[30] Without anterior column integrity (i.e., a weight-bearing graft), the posterior instrumentation bears a majority of the load (however, the ribs provide some support in the thoracic spine). In the long term, posterior fusion alone cannot compensate for a defect in the anterior column. In the case of trauma, posterior fusion as a bridge fixation technique for thoracolumbar burst fractures assumes eventual healing of the anterior column. More points of fixation in the bridge are required for more complex and extensive fractures to increase stress transfer and reduce failure, especially at transition levels such as the cervicothoracic and thoracolumbar junctions. If there is no chance that the anterior column will eventually contribute to load sharing, some type of anterior column support will be required to avoid posterior failure. Placement of an anterior column support substantially reduces the fraction of the load supported by the posterior implant, which then serves as more of a tension band system. Additionally, posterolateral arthrodesis has been shown to decrease the strain on posterior instrumentation; however, it takes several weeks for this process to occur.[31] Posterior reconstructions with pedicle screws in tumor cases often require extension of the construct for more levels above and below the lesion than with trauma, especially at the thoracolumbar junction, to increase the load sharing of the screws.[32]

TECHNIQUES OF POSTERIOR INTERNAL FIXATION

An educated evaluation of the biomechanical stability of the spine is necessary when determining the best course of treatment for a disease process that affects the thoracic spine. Such information determines whether surgery is indicated or whether bracing or bed rest alone will suffice. If surgery is needed, the decision regarding whether anterior fixation, posterior fixation, or combined anterior and posterior fixation is required is based on the mechanics of the region, how these mechanics are compromised by pathology, and what the goals of the operation are. This information may ultimately be tempered by patient factors, such as the patient's wishes, general health, and prognosis. As stated previously, circumferential stabilization is often required in extensive fractures in which the anterior column is unlikely to ever contribute to the structural stability. In tumor cases, circumferential stabilization is usually required when there is extensive anterior and posterior decompression; resection of more than two levels; or lesions at the thoracolumbar junction, where there is increased transitional stress.[32] In patients who cannot tolerate anterior procedures, or in patients with primarily posterior disease or localized anterior disease accessible from a posterolateral approach, an exclusively posterior approach is a reasonable option.[33] The anterior column can be decompressed through a posterolateral approach.[34-38] Nerve roots in the thoracic spine can be sacrificed, which often aids exposure. The anterior column can then be reconstituted with methacrylate or a structural graft, such as an allograft or cage.[33] Subsequently, a posterior instrumented fusion can be undertaken without the morbidity associated with a transthoracic or transabdominal approach. This posterior approach to the thoracic spine can be less morbid and far more straightforward than the anterior approaches, especially when treating lesions at the upper thoracic spine and cervicothoracic junc-

tion.[28, 34] In these cases, it is often beneficial to place the pedicle screws before decompression, because decompression can introduce significant instability. Additionally, when there is the potential for significant blood loss, such as in patients with metastatic renal cell carcinoma, placement of the spinal hardware before decompression allows for rapid completion of stabilization at the end of the decompression or if the patient becomes hemodynamically unstable.

Despite the increased level of technical difficulty associated with placement, pedicle screws provide several distinct advantages over other fixation techniques. Pedicle screws can be placed at levels where there have been wide laminectomies, lamina fractures, or even partial pedicle removal.[32] Additionally, pedicle screws do not require placement of implants in the spinal canal, as is the case with hooks and sublaminar wires.

Pedicle screw constructs are more rigid compared with sublaminar wire and hook constructs, thus increasing the potential for successful fusion.[14] Pedicle screw fusion also decreases the number of adjacent segments that need to be incorporated to obtain stability compared with wire and hook systems.[14, 39, 40] Finally, pedicle screws provide the most versatility with regard to intraoperative manipulation for correction of deformity (Fig. 305-1).

Fixation devices using screws are more at risk of failing at the bone-metal interface when force is applied in the direction of screw pullout. Further, bone quality and the diameter of the screw determine the magnitude of the resistance to pullout.[41, 42] For thoracic pedicle screws, pullout is therefore due to either failure of the screw to anchor in the bone or fracture of the pedicle.[43] If a screw diameter is too small, the flanges are less able to capture cortical bone. If the screw diameter is too large, the risk of pedicle fracture is increased. By providing three-column fixation, thoracic pedicle screws provide a biomechanically more rigid construct than fixation using hooks or wires, provided that screw placement, screw diameter, and bone quality are optimal.

Properly inserting thoracic pedicle screws demands a thorough knowledge of the anatomy of the thoracic pedicles and the surrounding structures, as well as the specific anatomy of the individual patient, because there is considerable variability in pedicle size and orientation. The placement of pedicle screws can be especially difficult in the upper thoracic spine, where the pedicles may be only slightly larger than the diameter of the screw. Proper insertion may be further impeded by the presence of a rotational or translational deformity. This again emphasizes the necessity of preoperative bone imaging to assess the diameter of the pedicles and to identify anatomic abnormalities and alignment irregularities.

Several descriptions of the proper starting point for pedicle screw fixation exist. Roy-Camille[44] and associates first described the starting point for thoracic pedicle screw insertion as the intersection of the middle of the transverse process and the middle of the facet joint. This description was modified by Magerl,[45] who suggested that the starting point for pedicle screw in-

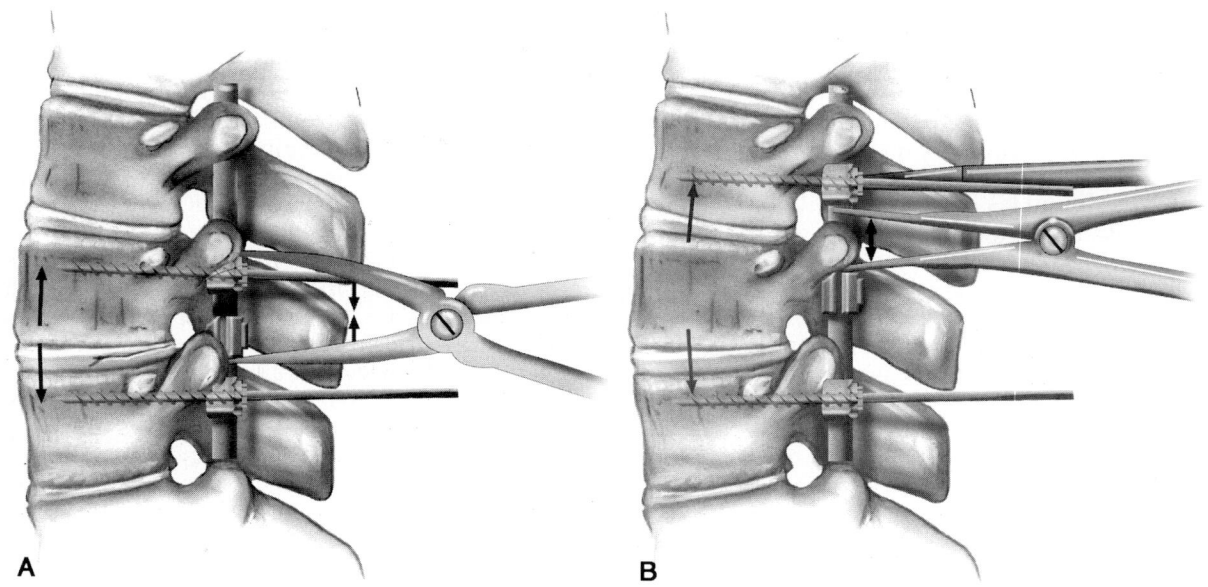

FIGURE 305–1. *A*, The construct acts as a posterior tension band as a compression forceps is used to approximate the screws and correct the kyphosis. *B*, Restoration of vertebral body height without risking displacement of fracture fragments into the spinal canal is accomplished by distraction.

sertion at the lower thoracic spine lies at the junction of the midline of the transverse process and the lateral margin of the facet joint. Cadaver studies by An and colleagues[46] and Ebraheim[11] attempted to locate the starting point for thoracic pedicle screw insertion more exactly. An and colleagues suggested that the starting point for pedicle screw insertion in the upper thoracic spine is 1 mm below the midportion of the facet joint.[46] Ebraheim and coworkers located the starting point for T1 and T2 at approximately 7 to 8 mm medial to the lateral edge of the superior facet and 3 to 4 mm superior to the midline of the transverse process; the starting point for T3 to T12 lies 4 to 5 mm medial to the lateral margin of the facet and 5 to 8 mm superior to the midline of the transverse process.[11]

To avoid spinal cord, nerve root, or vascular injury from improper insertion of a thoracic pedicle screw, pedicle screw angulation must be correct. The screws should be angled downward 10 to 20 degrees, such that their sagittal orientation is approximately parallel to the superior end plates. However, because the pedicle height is greater than its width, with the exception of the T1 and T2 pedicles, the insertion point is less forgiving in the medial-lateral plane. Roy-Camille and associates recommended that the screw be placed perpendicular to the posterior plane of the facet.[44] An and colleagues and Magerl advocated a medial insertion angle of 10 to 20 degrees, and Ebraheim and coworkers recommended a medially oriented 30- to 40-degree angle of insertion at T1 and T2, 20 to 25 degrees at T3 to T11, and 10 degrees at T12[11] (Fig. 305–2). The differences in the insertion angles advocated by various individuals reflect the differences in the pedicle starting points they use.

Because of individual variability and pathology, lo-

cating starting points and trajectory angles based on published techniques can lead to inaccuracy. They can be used as general guidelines but must be modified by radiographic examination and intraoperative observation. Morphometric studies have revealed significant individual variation in the size and orientation of the thoracic pedicles.[47] In this regard, intraoperative fluoroscopy is helpful in determining the starting point and the sagittal plane trajectory. Use of a completely radiolucent table with end supports that allow free movement of the fluoroscope under the table is very beneficial.

From T4 to T11, we use an entry point just below the rim of the upper facet and approximately 3 mm lateral to the center of the joint (near the base of the transverse process).[30] The entry point is verified by lateral fluoroscopy, which also aids in sagittal trajectory. The medial angulation is gauged from preoperative computed tomography and by knowledge of the pedicle's medial inclination in the each region of the thoracic spine. T12 is often a transitional segment with regard to facet configuration. Fluoroscopy is again useful in determining the entrance point. Anteroposterior views allow verification of entry point and trajectory. In general, if a thoracic pedicle screw crosses the midline in an anteroposterior view, there is a high risk of violation of the spinal canal. Lateral wall violation can also be determined with an anteroposterior view. We use a similar entry point for the upper thoracic levels (T1-3), but because of the difficulty with intraoperative imaging, we rely more heavily on laminotomies and palpation of the pedicle. Additionally, drilling the pilot hole with a 2-mm K-wire and an adjustable drill guide improves control and accuracy.[48]

The type and size of the pedicle screw are deter-

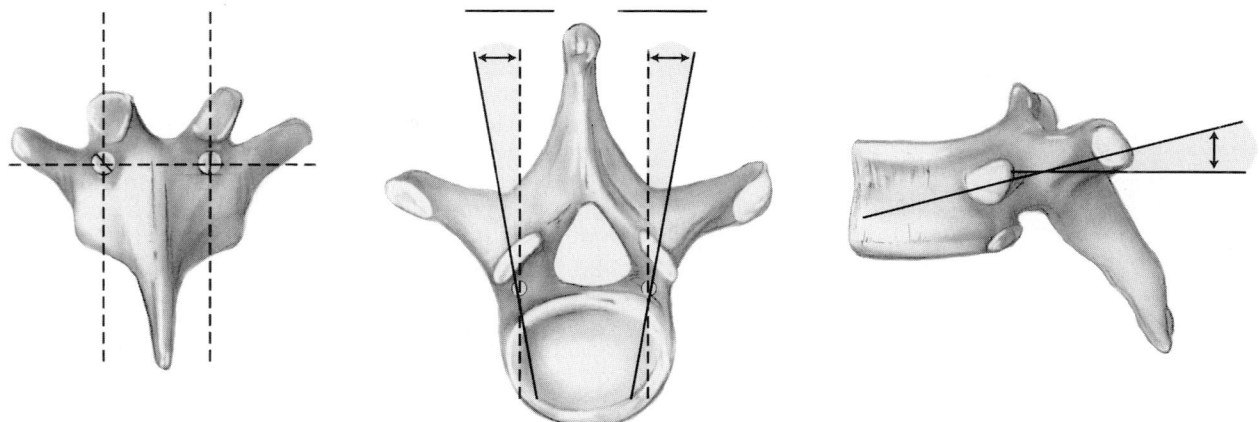

FIGURE 305–2. From T4 to T11, we use a pedicle screw starting point that lies just below the rim of the upper facet and approximately 3 mm lateral to the center of the joint (near the base of the transverse process). The sagittal trajectory can be verified by fluoroscopy. The screws should be angled more medially in the upper thoracic spine than in the middle and lower thoracic spine, where the pedicles take on a more perpendicular orientation.

mined by where the surgeon wishes to place the screw and why. Titanium screws greatly reduce artifacts on computed tomography and magnetic resonance imaging compared with steel implants.[49] The ability to obtain meaningful images of the spinal canal postoperatively is especially important when treating benign and malignant tumors of the spine. One other theoretic advantage is that titanium better approximates the elasticity of bone compared with stainless steel.[30]

Complications associated with thoracic pedicle screw insertion include nerve root, spinal cord, and vascular injury. An improperly placed screw in the sagittal plane may injure a nerve root. Esses and co-workers' series of 617 cases of pedicle screw fixation contained 169 complications, 29 of which were nerve root injuries.[50] Matsuzaki and colleagues' series of 57 cases had 6 patients with postoperative radiculopathies.[51] Even in the face of a spinal deformity, thoracic transpedicular fixation may be used safely. In Suk and associates'[52] series of 462 patients with spinal deformity, only one patient suffered a transient neurological paraparesis from a delayed epidural hematoma.

Good intraoperative radiographic evaluation of the thoracic spine can be difficult, especially in the upper thoracic spine and at the cervicothoracic junction. This can affect the ability to localize the levels of interest, often requiring the surgeon to count up or down from better-visualized levels. Use of fluoroscopy for intraoperative guidance in the placement of instrumentation is often limited in the upper thoracic spine, requiring more reliance on direct visualization through a laminotomy or perhaps through frameless stereotaxy.

Several methods have been used to increase the safety of pedicle screw placement, including fluoroscopy, frameless stereotaxy, direct palpation of the pedicles through laminotomies,[53, 54] and electrophysiologic monitoring. Electrophysiologic monitoring has been used with some success to assess the placement of lumbar pedicle screws.[55] A screw placed completely within the pedicle requires a higher-voltage stimulation

to achieve an electromyographic limb response than does a screw placed with a breach in the pedicle wall.[55] However, a threshold value has not been determined to identify a misplaced pedicle screw in the thoracic spine.[55]

Frameless stereotactic techniques are being used more frequently for the placement of pedicle screws in an attempt to improve accuracy.[54, 56, 57] Although their full utility has yet to be realized, there are several potential drawbacks. These systems are not foolproof, and as with intracranial frameless stereotaxy, they can provide misinformation. Also, if a surgeon's experience involves placement only with image guidance, he or she may not recognize an aberrant trajectory. Because the spine is multiarticulated, there is the potential for varying alignment between preoperative images and operative positioning, requiring adjustments with intraoperative registration. Finally, frameless stereotaxy often adds significant time to the case.

Variations in pedicle anatomy sometimes require the combined use of screws and hooks, further increasing versatility (Fig. 305–3). This is especially true at the cervicothoracic junction, where the pathology can be very challenging. Combining cervical lateral mass and possibly C7 pedicle screws with upper thoracic pedicle screws or hooks provides excellent stability and versatility at the cervicothoracic junction[48, 58, 59] (Fig. 305–4) compared with other techniques such as the Luque rectangle and sublaminar wires.

The use of laminar, transverse process, and pedicle hooks provides constructs that can better control axial loading in comparison to sublaminar wires. However, hooks require intact lamina, pedicles, and transverse processes and have significantly less pullout strength than pedicle screws, except in cases of osteoporosis. When treating patients with osteoporosis, hooks may provide rigidity comparable to that of pedicle screw constructs.[1, 60] First used in the correction of scoliotic deformities, laminar hooks can be placed around either the superior or inferior portion of the lamina, de-

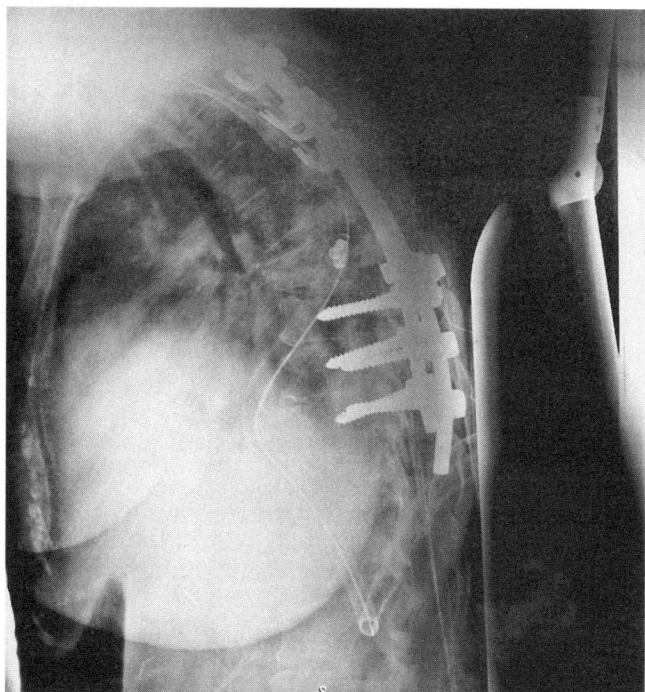

FIGURE 305–3. Lateral radiograph depicting the use of pedicle screws at the lower end of the construct and hooks at its upper end.

pending on the configuration needed. Distraction or compression can therefore be achieved to correct deformity and provide stability. The insertion of laminar, transverse process, and pedicle hooks is technically less demanding and carries less of a risk of iatrogenic injury than does pedicle screw insertion, especially in the upper thoracic spine, where the pedicles are relatively smaller. However, hooks do require the placement of instrumentation in the spinal canal. Again, hooks can serve as cephalad points of attachment of a construct that uses pedicle screws at its more caudal end. Offset laminar hooks may also be used in conjunction with pedicle screws to augment the stiffness of the construct.[61] Fixation using hooks relies on relatively long constructs, which provide a greater lever arm for better deformity correction. Complications of hooks include instrumentation failure, fracture of the posterior elements, and encroachment of the hook into the spinal canal, leading to a neurological deficit. In addition, the use of hooks has been shown to apply additional stresses to the vertebral body, further increasing the risk of failure.[43]

When an extended thoracic fixation is needed, rods secured by sublaminar wires can be an effective and relatively simple option. Using sublaminar wires allows for multiple points of fixation that can readily span the cervicothoracic and thoracolumbar junctions (Fig. 305–5). This technique provides stability in flexion, extension, and lateral rotation and is able to restore 50% of the rotational stiffness of the intact spine. The stability of the construct is directly dependent on the number of points of fixation it incorporates.

Panjabi and coworkers,[62] using a cadaver injury model, studied the three-dimensional stability provided by eight spinal fixation devices spanning the thoracolumbar junction. The Luque rectangle secured using sublaminar wires spanning five vertebrae was found to provide the most stability in flexion, extension, and lateral bending; the Luque rectangle spanning three vertebrae was the least stable. However, sublaminar wiring cannot provide and maintain corrective distraction or compression forces, because the position of the wires is not fixed as they wrap around the rod. Therefore, this construct cannot support axial loads or restore vertebral body height.[40, 62, 63] Before passing the wires, the lamina should be cleared of soft tissue and undermined using an up-going curet. Care most be taken not to compress the thecal sac when passing the wires. Severe neurological complications resulting from the passage of sublaminar wires have been reported.[64, 65] Several parameters have been identified to limit encroachment of the wire into the spinal canal.[66] A lateral passage should be avoided, and the spinous process should be removed to facilitate a midline passage of the wire. In addition, the radial curvature of the wire should at least equal the width of the lamina, and the bend of the wire tip should be no greater than 45 degrees. The wires should be restrained after passing

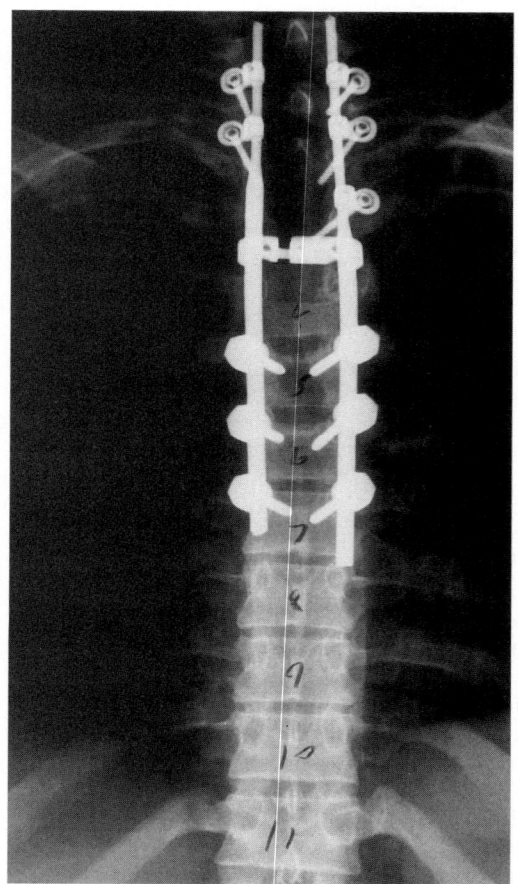

FIGURE 305–4. Anteroposterior radiograph depicting a construct with tapered rods to allow the use of smaller-diameter pedicle screws at the cervicothoracic junction.

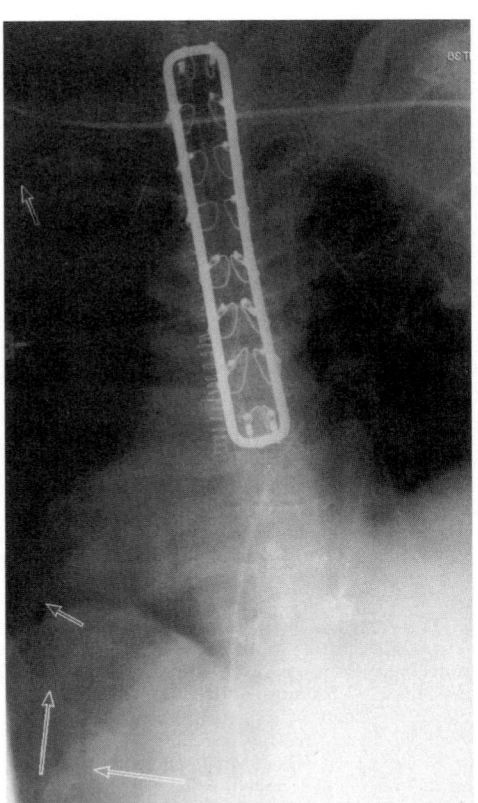

FIGURE 305–5. Anteroposterior radiograph of a Luque rectangle secured by sublaminar wires crossing the cervicothoracic junction.

them under the lamina to avoid any inadvertent canal encroachment. Correction of a deformity can be accomplished through the use of the segmental wiring and cantilever bending technique. The application of sublaminar wires is less technically demanding than transpedicular fixation, and in experienced hands, the procedure carries a low risk of morbidity.[67-69] Use of double-ended braided cables (such as a Songer cable) at each level facilitates passage, reduces the number of passes per level, and allows easy tensioning and securing of the wire.[65]

SUMMARY

The use of internal thoracic fixation to achieve stabilization demands a thorough knowledge of the anatomy and biomechanics of the thoracic spine preoperatively. Computed tomography and magnetic resonance imaging are complementary imaging modalities that provide valuable information about the patient's specific anatomy and clearly define the pathology. This information, along with other patient factors such as bone quality and general health, enables the surgeon to choose the optimal type of instrumentation to provide stability and correct any deformity. The location of the pathology and the presence of deformity dictate the length of the construct. The significant curvatures

across the cervicothoracic and thoracolumbar junctions place an increased amount of translational force and stress on fixation devices and make it technically more difficult to gain good screw purchase in the vertebral bodies during the procedure. Fixation supplementation with an anterior construct or extension of the fixation over multiple levels must be considered when attempting to stabilize the thoracic spine, especially when the construct crosses the cervicothoracic or thoracolumbar junction. Pedicle screw fixation provides the most rigid anchor and the greatest versatility if placed correctly in bone of adequate quality. However, correctly inserting thoracic pedicle screws is technically challenging, especially in the upper thoracic spine, and carries some risk of iatrogenic neurovascular injury. Therefore, the surgeon's familiarity with the instrumentation, as well as the adjuncts available, such as fluoroscopy and possibly frameless stereotaxy, should also guide the choice of a fixation technique.

REFERENCES

1. Butler TE Jr, Asher MA, Jayaraman G, et al: The strength and stiffness of thoracic implant anchors in osteoporotic spines. Spine 19:1956–1962, 1994.
2. Coe JD, Warden KE, Herzig MA, McAfee PC: Influence of bone mineral density on the fixation of thoracolumbar implants: A comparative study of transpedicular screws, laminar hooks, and spinous process wires. Spine 15:902–907, 1990.
3. Skinner R, Maybee J, Transfeldt E, et al: Experimental pullout testing and comparison of variables in transpedicular screw fixation: A biomechanical study. Spine 15:195–201, 1990.
4. Sarzier JS, Evans AJ, Cahill DW: Increased pedicle screw pullout strength with vertebroplasty augmentation in osteoporotic spines. J Neurosurg 96:309–312, 2002.
5. Sanden B, Olerud C, Johansson C, Larsson S: Improved bone-screw interface with hydroxyapatite coating: An in vivo study of loaded pedicle screws in sheep. Spine 26:2673–2678, 2001.
6. Sanden B, Olerud C, Larsson S: Hydroxyapatite coating enhances fixation of loaded pedicle screws: A mechanical in vivo study in sheep. Eur Spine J 10:334–339, 2001.
7. Sanden B, Olerud C, Petren-Mallmin M, Larsson S: Hydroxyapatite coating improves fixation of pedicle screws: A clinical study. J Bone Joint Surg Br 84:387–391, 2002.
8. Yerby SA, Toh E, McLain RF: Revision of failed pedicle screws using hydroxyapatite cement: A biomechanical analysis. Spine 23:1657–1661, 1998.
9. McCormack BM, Benzel EC, Adams MS, et al: Anatomy of the thoracic pedicle. Neurosurgery 37:303–308, 1995.
10. Panjabi MM, O'Holleran JD, Crisco JJ 3rd, Kothe R: Complexity of the thoracic spine pedicle anatomy. Eur Spine J 6:19–24, 1997.
11. Ebraheim NA, Xu R, Ahmad M, Yeasting RA: Projection of the thoracic pedicle and its morphometric analysis. Spine 22:233–238, 1997.
12. Kothe R, O'Holleran JD, Liu W, Panjabi MM: Internal architecture of the thoracic pedicle: An anatomic study. Spine 21:264–270, 1996.
13. Ebraheim NA, Jabaly G, Xu R, Yeasting RA: Anatomic relations of the thoracic pedicle to the adjacent neural structures. Spine 22:1553–1557, 1997.
14. White AA 3rd, Panjabi MM: Clinical Biomechanics of the Spine. Philadelphia, JB Lippincott, 1990.
15. Whitesides TE Jr: Traumatic kyphosis of the thoracolumbar spine. Clin Orthop 128:78–92, 1977.
16. Denis F: The three column spine and its significance in the classification of acute thoracolumbar spinal injuries. Spine 8:817–831, 1983.
17. Denis F: Spinal instability as defined by the three-column spine concept in acute spinal trauma. Clin Orthop 189:65–76, 1984.
18. McAfee PC, Yuan HA, Fredrickson BE, Lubicky JP: The value of computed tomography in thoracolumbar fractures: An analysis

of one hundred consecutive cases and a new classification. J Bone Joint Surg Am 65:461–473, 1983.

19. Gertzbein SD: Spine update: Classification of thoracic and lumbar fractures. Spine 19:626–628, 1994.

20. Magerl F, Aebi M, Gertzbein SD, et al: A comprehensive classification of thoracic and lumbar injuries. Eur Spine J 3:184–201, 1994.

21. Kostuik JP, Errico TJ, Gleason TF, Errico CC: Spinal stabilization of vertebral column tumors. Spine 13:250–256, 1988.

22. Weinstein JN: Surgical approach to spine tumors. Orthopedics 12:897–905, 1989.

23. Maiman D, Pintar F: Anatomy and clinical biomechanics of the thoracic spine. Clin Neurosurg 38:296–324, 1992.

24. Oda I, Abumi K, Cunningham BW, et al: An in vitro human cadaveric study investigating the biomechanical properties of the thoracic spine. Spine 27:E64–E70, 2002.

25. Oda I, Abumi K, Lu D, et al: Biomechanical role of the posterior elements, costovertebral joints, and rib cage in the stability of the thoracic spine. Spine 21:1423–1429, 1996.

26. Goldberg W, Mueller C, Panacek E, et al: Distribution and patterns of blunt traumatic cervical spine injury. Ann Emerg Med 38:17–21, 2001.

27. Holmes JF, Miller PQ, Panacek EA, et al: Epidemiology of thoracolumbar spine injury in blunt trauma. Acad Emerg Med 8:866–872, 2001.

28. Boockvar JA, Philips MF, Telfeian AE, et al: Results and risk factors for anterior cervicothoracic junction surgery. J Neurosurg 94:12–17, 2001.

29. Oxland TR, Lin RM, Panjabi MM: Three-dimensional mechanical properties of the thoracolumbar junction. J Orthop Res 10:573–580, 1992.

30. Aebi M, Thalgott J, Webb J: AO ASIF Principles in Spine Surgery. Berlin, Springer, 1998.

31. Kanayama M, Cunningham BW, Weis JC, et al: Maturation of the posterolateral spinal fusion and its effect on load-sharing of spinal instrumentation: An in vivo sheep model. J Bone Joint Surg Am 79:1710–1720, 1997.

32. Fourney DR, Abi-Said D, Lang FF, et al: Use of pedicle screw fixation in the management of malignant spinal disease: Experience in 100 consecutive procedures. J Neurosurg 94:25–37, 2001.

33. Cahill DW, Kumar R: Palliative subtotal vertebrectomy with anterior and posterior reconstruction via a single posterior approach. J Neurosurg 90:42–47, 1999.

34. Bilsky MH, Boland P, Lis E, et al: Single-stage posterolateral transpedicle approach for spondylectomy, epidural decompression, and circumferential fusion of spinal metastases. Spine 25:2240–2249, discussion 2250, 2000.

35. Graham AW 3rd, MacMillan M, Fessler RG: Lateral extracavitary approach to the thoracic and thoracolumbar spine. Orthopedics 20:605–610, 1997.

36. Steck JC, Dietze DD, Fessler RG: Posterolateral approach to intradural extramedullary thoracic tumors. J Neurosurg 81:202–205, 1994.

37. Tomita K, Kawahara N, Baba H, et al: Total en bloc spondylectomy for solitary spinal metastases. Int Orthop 18:291–298, 1994.

38. Tomita K, Kawahara N, Kobayashi T, et al: Surgical strategy for spinal metastases. Spine 26:298–306, 2001.

39. Ferguson RL, Tencer AF, Woodard P, Allen BL Jr: Biomechanical comparisons of spinal fracture models and the stabilizing effects of posterior instrumentations. Spine 13:453–460, 1988.

40. Gurr KR, McAfee PC, Shih CM: Biomechanical analysis of posterior instrumentation systems after decompressive laminectomy: An unstable calf-spine model. J Bone Joint Surg Am 70:680–691, 1988.

41. Hackenberg L, Link T, Liljenqvist U: Axial and tangential fixation strength of pedicle screws versus hooks in the thoracic spine in relation to bone mineral density. Spine 27:937–942, 2002.

42. Liljenqvist U, Hackenberg L, Link T, Halm H: Pullout strength of pedicle screws versus pedicle and laminar hooks in the thoracic spine. Acta Orthop Belg 67:157–163, 2001.

43. Gayet L, Pries P, Hamcha H, et al: Biomechanical study and digital modeling of traction resistance in posterior thoracic implants. Spine 27:707–714, 2002.

44. Roy-Camille R, Saillant G, Mazel C: Plating of the thoracic, thoracolumbar, and lumbar injuries with pedicle screw plates. Orthop Clin North Am 17:147–159, 1986.

45. Dick W, Kluger P, Magerl F, et al: A new device for internal fixation of thoracolumbar and lumbar spine fractures: The fixateur interne. Paraplegia 23:225–232, 1985.

46. An HS, Gordin R, Renner K: Anatomic considerations for plate-screw fixation of the cervical spine. Spine 16:5548–5551, 1991.

47. Vaccaro A, Rizzolo S, Allardyce T, et al: Placement of pedicle screws in the thoracic spine. Part I. A morphometric analysis of the thoracic vertebrae. J Bone Joint Surg Am 77:1193–1199, 1995.

48. Chapman JR, Anderson PA, Pepin C, et al: Posterior instrumentation of the unstable cervicothoracic spine. J Neurosurg 84:552–558, 1996.

49. Ebraheim NA, Rupp RE, Savolaine ER, Reinke D: Use of titanium implants in pedicular screw fixation. J Spinal Disord 7:478–486, 1994.

50. Esses SI, Sachs BL, Dreyzin V: Complications associated with the technique of pedicle screw fixation. A selected survey of ABS members. Spine 18:2231–2238, 1993.

51. Matsuzaki H, Tokuhashi Y, Matsumoto F, et al: Problems and solutions of pedicle screw plate fixation of lumbar spine. Spine 15:1159–1165, 1990.

52. Suk SI, Kim WJ, Lee SM, et al: Thoracic pedicle screw fixation in spinal deformities. Spine 26:2049–2057, 2001.

53. Xu R, Ebraheim NA, Ou Y, Yeasting RA: Anatomic considerations of pedicle screw placement in the thoracic spine: Roy-Camille technique versus open-lamina technique. Spine 23:1065–1068, 1998.

54. Youkilis AS, Quint DJ, McGillicuddy JE, Papadopoulos SM: Stereotactic navigation for placement of pedicle screws in the thoracic spine. Neurosurgery 48:771–778, discussion 778–779, 2001.

55. Lewis SJ, Lenke LG, Raynor B, et al: Triggered electromyographic threshold for accuracy of thoracic pedicle screw placement in a porcine model. Spine 26:2485–2490, 2001.

56. Assaker R, Reyns N, Vinchon M, et al: Transpedicular screw placement: Image-guided versus lateral-view fluoroscopy: In vitro simulation. Spine 26:2160–2164, 2001.

57. Jang JS, Lee WB, Yuan HA: Use of a guide device to place pedicle screws in the thoracic spine: A cadaveric study: Technical note. J Neurosurg 94:328–333, 2001.

58. Albert TJ, Klein GR, Joffe D, Vaccaro AR: Use of cervicothoracic junction pedicle screws for reconstruction of complex cervical spine pathology. Spine 23:1596–1599, 1998.

59. Vaccaro R, Conant RF, Hilibrand AS, Albert TJ: A plate-rod device for treatment of cervicothoracic disorders: Comparison of mechanical testing with established cervical spine in vitro load testing data. J Spinal Disord 13:350–355, 2000.

60. Hackenberg L, Link T, Liljenqvist U: Axial and tangential fixation strength of pedicle screws versus hooks in the thoracic spine in relation to bony mineral density. Spine 27:937–942, 2002.

61. Chiba M, McLain RF, Yerby SA, et al: Short-segment pedicle instrumentation: Biomechanical analysis of supplemental hook fixation. Spine 21:288–294, 1996.

62. Panjabi MM, Abumi K, Duranceau J, Crisco JJ: Biomechanical evaluation of spinal fixation devices. II. Stability provided by eight internal fixation devices. Spine 13:1135–1140, 1988.

63. Gurr KR, McAfee PC, Shih CM: Biomechanical analysis of anterior and posterior instrumentation systems after corpectomy: A calf-spine model. J Bone Joint Surg Am 70:1182–1191, 1988.

64. Pampliega T, Beguiristain JL, Artieda J: Neurologic complications after sublaminar wiring: An experimental study in lambs. Spine 17:441–445, 1992.

65. Parsons JR, Chokshi BV, Lee CK, et al: The biomechanical analysis of sublaminar wires and cables using Luque segmental spinal instrumentation. Spine 22:267–273, 1997.

66. Goll SR, Balderston RA, Stambough JL, et al: Depth of intraspinal wire penetration during passage of sublaminar wires. Spine 13:503–509, 1988.

67. Benson ER, Thomson JD, Smith BG, Banta JV: Results and morbidity in a consecutive series of patients undergoing spinal fusion for neuromuscular scoliosis. Spine 23:2308–2317, discussion 2318, 1998.

68. Girardi FP, Boachie-Adjei O, Rawlins BA: Safety of sublaminar wires with Isola instrumentation for the treatment of idiopathic scoliosis. Spine 25:691–695, 2000.

69. Segal LS, Schwentker EP: Wire-holding frame for sublaminar segmental spinal instrumentation. Spine 19:1190–1192, 1994.

CHAPTER 306

Anterior Lumbar Instrumentation

MICHAEL G. KAISER ■ ANDREW T. PARSA ■
PETER ANGEVINE ■ PAUL C. MCCORMICK

Ventral instability of the lumbar spine is a common clinical problem encountered by spinal surgeons. Effective management requires a comprehensive understanding of spinal biomechanics, anterior spinal anatomy, ventral surgical approaches, and evolving techniques for spinal stabilization. Ventral instability can be caused by pathologic destruction of the vertebral body, or it can occur as an iatrogenic consequence of surgical decompression. Neoplastic, traumatic, infectious, and degenerative processes all may lead to ventral instability. Anterior stabilization strategies are aimed at fortifying biomechanical elements that have been compromised by these pathologic processes. The development of anterior fixation constructs has enabled contemporary spinal surgeons to immobilize the lumbar spine to promote bony fusion. During the last 20 years, surgical techniques and methods of internal fixation have progressed rapidly, providing effective tools for managing anterior lumbar instability while minimizing the associated risks.

HISTORICAL PERSPECTIVE

In 1916, Elsberg[1] established posterior decompression as the treatment of choice for most compressive lesions involving the spine. Posterior fusion procedures, developed in the early 1900s by such pioneers as Albee[2] and Hibbs,[3] were also used to treat ventral lumbar disease. The development of anterior approaches to the spine was delayed, primarily because of inadequate antiseptic and anesthetic techniques. In 1906, Müller[4] described the first successful ventral approach to the lumbar spine for the treatment of Pott's disease. He later abandoned this approach after subsequent failures. In 1933, Burns,[5] recognizing that dorsal fusion procedures treated ventral instability inefficiently, performed a successful transabdominal approach for an interbody fusion of a traumatic L5-S1 spondylolisthesis. Ito and coworkers[6] subsequently modified the approach to treat Pott's disease with a lumbosacral sympathetic ganglionectomy through an extraperitoneal exposure. Despite their important contributions, credit for the ventral approach is attributed to Hodgson and Stock,[7] who developed a transthoracic approach to treat Pott's disease. They demonstrated that ventral decompression, stabilization, and correction of deformities could all be performed through a single incision.

After the ventral fusion procedures were introduced, the development of anterior fixation constructs to enhance spinal immobilization soon followed. In 1961, Humphries and coworkers[8] reported the use of an anterior lumbar compression plate but observed a fusion failure rate of 30%. Recognizing the deficiencies of dorsal fixation for the treatment of ventral scoliotic deformities, in 1969, Dwyer and associates[9] introduced a ventral screw-cable construct that applied an even compressive force across the convex surface of a scoliotic deformity. Since then, the number of anterior spinal instrumentation constructs has increased dramatically. Current construct designs include screw-rod implants, screw-plate implants, and interbody fixation devices. The continued development of these constructs has improved insertion techniques and enhanced bony fusion formation while decreasing radiographic artifacts.

INDICATIONS

The goals of surgical intervention are to decompress the neural elements, reduce the existing spinal deformity, and restore the load-bearing capabilities of the spine. A clear understanding of surgical indications based on the origin of instability is essential to achieve favorable outcomes.

Neoplasm

Advances in surgical techniques have made ventral decompression and stabilization viable options for the treatment of primary and metastatic neoplastic disease of the lumbar spine. Primary tumors of the spine are extremely rare; less than 10% of reported bone tumors and soft tissue sarcomas involve the spine.[10, 11] Most primary lesions are malignant. In a review from the Mayo Clinic, 510 of 655 primary spinal lesions were malignant. Plasma cell tumors, including multiple myelomas and plasmacytomas, were the most common malignant lesions encountered.[11]

Metastatic disease is a frequent feature of many solid tumors,[12-14] and the spinal column is the most common site of bony metastases.[15] As many as 66% of spinal malignancies originate from breast, lung, prostate, and hematopoietic cancers.[14, 16-19] It is estimated that 90% of prostate cancers, 75% of breast carcinomas, and 45% of lung carcinomas involve the spine to various degrees.[20-22] Metastatic lesions are distributed in relation to the amount of bone marrow available. Consequently, the thoracic spine is the most common site of infiltration, followed by the lumbar region.[23] The location of a lesion can help formulate the differential diagnosis. Primary benign tumors, such as osteoblastomas and aneurysmal bone cysts, tend to involve the posterior elements, whereas primary malignant and metastatic tumors involve the medullary spaces of the vertebral body.[11, 24-26]

Neoplastic infiltration of the lumbar spine occurs through several mechanisms. In most cases, the tumor disseminates to the vertebral body through hematogenous channels, possibly through the basivertebral plexus.[27, 28] Additional mechanisms of infiltration include lymphatic spread and direct local extension from the paraspinal region.[29]

Clinical manifestations result from expansion of the periosteum or cortex, pathologic compression fractures, spinal instability, deformity progression, and direct neural element compression. By far the most common symptom produced by either primary or metastatic lesions is pain.[12, 30-33] Unfortunately, this pain is often difficult to distinguish from lower back pain caused by more common disorders. Some classic features suggestive of tumor involvement include constant pain that rest fails to relieve and that intensifies at night. Progression of the tumor beyond the confines of the vertebral body produces various degrees of myeloradiculopathy as a result of both direct compression of neural elements and vascular compromise.

The presence and extent of neurological involvement depend on the type of tumor, its location along the spine, and the degree of spinal canal compromise. The existence of objective neurological deficits at the time of presentation can correlate with 20% to 55% compromise of the spinal canal, depending on the spinal region.[11, 16, 34-38] Prognosis after complete loss of function is poor, irrespective of the tumor's location. Studies that have shown improved neurological function after treatment in patients with partial loss of function provide the impetus for aggressive surgical intervention.[39, 40]

The role of surgery for the treatment of ventral and ventrolateral lumbar neoplastic disease continues to evolve. Early reports from the 1970s demonstrated no difference in neurological outcome when patients were treated with a posterior approach and radiation compared with radiation alone.[30, 41] Based on this early experience, many surgeons played an ancillary role in the treatment of patients with neoplastic spinal disease. With the development of ventral surgical approaches and spinal instrumentation and improved comprehen-

sion of tumor biology, spinal surgeons now have a more active role in the initial management of spinal metastatic disease.[21, 42] Although indications for surgical intervention continue to be updated, spinal instability and the presence of neural compression from retropulsed bone fragments will remain important indications for operative intervention. Several schemes have been proposed for classifying spinal instability due to neoplastic disease.[21, 43-45] Prognostic factors, including tumor type and location, preoperative neurological status, and overall medical condition, correlate with surgical outcome.[46, 47]

Numerous series have reported the successful treatment of spinal neoplastic disease with a ventral or ventrolateral approach.[19, 40, 42, 48-57] Sundaresan and colleagues[42] reported a prospective series of 54 patients with various spinal malignancies. A ventral or ventrolateral decompression was performed in 83% of the patients. Forty-four percent were nonambulatory before treatment, and 13% demonstrated severe paresis or cauda equina compression. After surgery, all patients were ambulatory, and the overall complication rate was 20%. Cooper and colleagues[40] reported 33 patients who underwent ventral decompression for thoracic and lumbar neoplastic disease. The percentage of patients who were ambulatory improved from 75% before surgery to 88% afterward. Their overall complication rate was 22%, and the average length of survival was 10 months for patients with metastatic disease. Unfortunately, it is difficult to compare these studies owing to a number of variables, including patient selection, operative techniques, timing of intervention, outcome assessment, region of spinal involvement, definition of complications, and length of follow-up. Despite limitations in methodology, these reports demonstrate that the surgical management of ventral neoplastic disease has improved. The decision to pursue surgery should be individualized for each patient.

Open procedures for diagnostic purposes are being done less frequently as image-guided needle biopsy techniques have improved.[58] Some specialists reserve surgery as an option if medical measures fail[13, 36, 59]; however, many adjuvant therapies increase the risk of surgical morbidity. In addition, neurological deficits are less likely to improve the longer they have been present.[60, 61]

Trauma

Compared with fractures of the thoracolumbar junction, fractures of the lumbar spine are relatively uncommon. Less than 4% of all fractures involve L3 through L5.[62, 63] The inherent stability of the lumbar spine reduces the incidence of traumatic fracture. The increased mass of the individual vertebral bodies, their lordotic posture, and the surrounding soft tissues are major factors that increase the load-bearing capabilities of the lumbar spine. As a result of the lordotic curvature and coupled motions, fractures of the lumbar spine often assume familiar patterns.

Various classification schemes have been proposed for spinal fractures, many of which are based on Denis's three-column model of spinal stability and mechanism of spinal injury.[64-67] McCormack and coworkers[68] introduced a load-sharing classification system that focuses on the ability of the fracture to heal without further deformity. This scheme considers the degree of fragment displacement and the ability to bear an applied stress. The amount of comminution, the apposition of fragments, and the degree of deformity are graded on a scale of 1 to 3. Unlike other classification systems that consider soft tissue injury, this approach is unable to assess overall stability. Its value lies in helping surgeons to choose an appropriate approach and instrumentation construct once the decision to operate has been made.

The diagnosis of a lumbar fracture must be entertained in any patient involved in a high-energy trauma. Certain mechanisms of injury tend to be associated with lumbar fractures. Falls from a significant height that produce substantial axial loads are associated with both thoracolumbar and lumbar fractures. Passengers wearing lower abdominal seat belts during motor vehicle accidents often sustain flexion or flexion-distraction injuries to the lumbar spine, with the seat belt acting as a fulcrum. Other clinical sequelae associated with lumbar fractures include calcaneal fractures, abdominal trauma, lower back pain, and spinal fractures outside the lumbar region. In some studies, certain patterns of noncontiguous fractures involved the lumbar spine in about 5% of cases of spinal trauma.[69, 70] Initially, additional fractures were missed in about 50% of these cases, and the mean delay to diagnosis was 52 days. A careful evaluation of the entire spine is therefore warranted whenever a spinal fracture is identified.

The decision to pursue operative or nonoperative treatment of a spinal fracture is based on a multitude of factors. The ultimate goal of any intervention is to restore normal anatomy and to prevent future deformities that could lead to functional compromise. Several authors have designed guidelines to determine whether operative intervention is indicated.[71-82] In addition to the presence of a neurological deficit, the extent of spinal canal encroachment, loss of vertebral body height, degree of kyphosis, and fracture pattern have all been used as operative criteria. Bohlman[71] and Brown[72] recommend surgery for fractures producing more than a 40% loss in height of a vertebral body and more than 1 cm of retropulsed fragments. Denis and coworkers[76] suggest operative treatment for destruction of the middle column associated with severe compromise of the spinal canal. Willen and colleagues[73] believe that operative intervention is needed for a 50% loss of vertebral height and 50% compromise of the spinal canal. These guidelines are by no means absolute, but they do provide a reference for formulating treatment plans for patients with lumbar fractures.

The presence or progression of a neurological deficit is key in determining the timing of treatment. Individuals who are neurologically intact do not require emergent surgical decompression. The decision to operate on this patient population depends on the stability of the spine and the presence of a deformity and its potential to progress. The three-column model of Denis

has been validated as a useful tool for defining spinal stability.[83] Typically, a fracture that compromises the middle column is considered unstable, but more recent evidence points to the posterior column as a significant contributor to stability.[84]

The degree of kyphosis and the presence of comminuted fracture fragments are also important considerations when choosing between operative and conservative management. A significant kyphosis can result in a progressive deformity that eventually leads to neurological deterioration. More chronic problems caused by a stable kyphosis include back pain and fatigue, consequences of the "flat back syndrome."[62, 85, 86] The extent of fracture-fragment displacement determines the load-bearing capacity and potential for a worsening deformity. Fragments within the spinal canal produce not only acute neural compression but also long-standing stenotic changes that lead to significant disability. A spinal canal already compromised with fracture fragments may potentiate later degenerative changes at the injured segment. However, the presence of fracture fragments within the spinal canal is not an absolute indication for surgical intervention, because spontaneous resorption has been described.[86]

The decision to operate on a patient with a partial neurological deficit is based on the fracture pattern and the potential for restoring neurological function. If neural elements are compressed, immediate steps should be taken to relieve the compression. Although postural reduction has been reported, it is not recommended for a neurologically compromised patient with an unstable spine. Surgical decompression is the treatment of choice in a patient whose deficit is caused by external compression. Emergent decompression is recommended for a progressive neurological deficit and a grossly unstable spine.

The indications for operative treatment of patients with fixed neurological deficits are less clear. Advocates who favor delaying surgery believe that the elements of an acute injury, such as edema and induration, subside over time, thus reducing the risk of neural injury and decreasing intraoperative blood loss.[86, 87] Delaying intervention also facilitates a comprehensive evaluation and the organization of an experienced operating room staff. Proponents believe that early surgery provides the best opportunity for neurological recovery. Patients are mobilized quickly and therefore avoid the complications associated with prolonged bed rest. Delaying surgery may make the fracture more difficult to reduce or decompress, increasing the risk of injury to both the dura mater and neural elements. Finally, early mobilization provides both patient and family with a psychological advantage.[88]

When a patient with a spinal cord injury is evaluated, it is important to rule out spinal shock in the acute period, before a complete injury can be diagnosed. The bulbocavernosus reflex is the lowest reflex mediated by the spinal cord and returns first (within 48 hours of injury) in 99% of patients with an incomplete injury.[89] The prognosis of a patient with a complete deficit after this period is significantly worse, with little chance of neurological recovery.[90] In such circumstances, spinal stabilization can help mobilize patients and maximize their rehabilitation potential.

Any decision to operate on a lumbar fracture must be tailored to the patient's clinical presentation and radiographic data. The criteria described in the literature should serve only as a guide. Other important factors to consider include age, general medical condition, and presence of associated injuries. If additional injuries are severe enough to increase the risk of surgery significantly, a conservative course may be indicated.

Degenerative Disease

Degenerative disease is a common affliction of the lumbar spine. Aging, congenital abnormalities, and iatrogenic destabilization all contribute to the degenerative process. Unlike the acute instability produced by traumatic injury, degenerative disease typically produces a chronic and progressive instability, often classified as "glacial instability" or "dysfunctional segmental motion."[91] The degenerative process most commonly affects the intervertebral disk, facet joints, and posterior ligamentous structures. Selection of appropriate patients for surgical treatment, whether from a posterior or an anterior approach, is not a straightforward process. In addition to the difficulty with patient selection based on clinical and radiographic data, it has been shown that low socioeconomic status, psychological disturbances, cigarette smoking, litigation, and workers' compensation are all negative prognostic indicators.[92–96] The decision-making process is further confounded by the lack of uniform selection criteria among neurosurgeons, resulting from the lack of properly controlled outcome analyses.

Most degenerative processes are treated either conservatively or with a standard posterior approach. As our understanding of spinal biomechanics has improved, anterior lumbar interbody fusion (ALIF) techniques have become increasingly popular. The biomechanical advantages of an ALIF procedure include reconstruction of the anterior column, improved sagittal balance, restoration of the lumbar lordotic curvature, and enlargement of the neural foramina.[97, 98] Various devices are available for ALIF in a wide range of materials, including titanium alloy, tantalum, carbon fiber, and allograft bone. Threaded metallic cages have become a popular interbody graft for use in ALIF procedures.[99–101]

Primary indications for ALIF include a wide range of degenerative processes such as disk disease, lumbar instability, iatrogenic instability from a previous posterior procedure, pseudarthrosis of a previous posterior fusion, or grade I or II spondylolisthesis.[98, 102–109] An incapacitating radiculopathy associated with lower back pain caused by a diffuse degenerative disk is a common indication for ALIF. Symptoms should be unresponsive to aggressive conservative measures for a prolonged period before an ALIF procedure is considered.[106, 110, 111] Negative psychosocial prognostic factors warrant consideration in patients undergoing ALIF

procedures because the primary indication, chronic pain, is more subjective than objective.

There are absolute and relative contraindications for the insertion of a threaded interbody fusion cage.[98, 102, 112–115] These devices should not be used when the ligamentous structures of the spine are disrupted extensively. The interbody fixation devices depend on the annulus and ligaments to stabilize the spine when placed in distraction. Severe osteoporosis is another absolute contraindication because the graft can telescope into the weakened vertebral bodies. Other absolute contraindications include grades III to V spondylolisthesis and extensive vertebral body destruction. Relative contraindications include an active disk space infection, posterior compressive pathology, concern (among young males) about retrograde ejaculation, disseminated malignancy, history of multiple abdominal operations, anomalous genitourinary anatomy, and severe atherosclerotic vascular disease.

Infection

Early reports asserted that epidural abscesses and vertebral osteomyelitis occur in isolation of each other.[116–118] The advent of magnetic resonance imaging has revealed just the opposite scenario. Most cases of osteomyelitis form an epidural abscess if untreated, and an epidural abscess in the absence of an associated osteomyelitis is rare unless the epidural space has been violated directly.[119] Bacterial organisms, most often *Staphylococcus aureus*, are the most common causes of spinal infections. However, as the incidence of fungal and parasitic infections has increased, the number of immunocompromised patients has grown.[119, 120]

Historically, Pott's disease was a common indication for an anterior fusion and stabilization procedure.[4, 6, 7] Today, however, an infectious involvement of the lumbar spine that requires anterior instrumentation is rare. Most spinal infections are treated with intravenous antibiotics and immobilization before the onset of a neurological deficit and spinal deformity.[119–121] Unfortunately, the diagnosis can be delayed owing to the nonspecific nature of the complaints. Under such circumstances, surgical intervention may be warranted.

Operative indications include severe infections leading to a significant spinal deformity and neurological deficit or, rarely, to a lack of response to appropriate antibiotic therapy. Because infections of the vertebral body affect the anterior and middle columns, any surgical approach must provide access to the ventral spine. Débridement of the active infection often involves removal of the disk and a corpectomy of the involved vertebral body, followed by a fusion procedure. To avoid the complications associated with prolonged bed rest and external immobilization, many patients are offered the option of internal fixation with anterior instrumentation. The use of ventral instrumentation in the setting of an acute infection remains controversial. Recent experience, however, suggests that the rate of postoperative infection does not increase if débridement has been adequate, particularly in the case of tuberculous spondylitis.[119, 122]

SURGICAL ANATOMY

A clear understanding of the regional anatomy is required to approach pathology of the ventral lumbar spine effectively. Preoperative evaluation with computed tomography and multiplanar magnetic resonance imaging is invaluable for developing an operative plan. Failure to recognize the relationships among various anatomic structures can lead to an inadequate exposure, increase the risk of surgical complications, and prevent the successful implantation of a fusion-fixation construct.

Lumbar Spine

In terms of width, depth, and height, the vertebral bodies in the lumbar spine are more massive than in other regions.[123, 124] Their increased size translates into an increased ability of the lumbar spine to resist loads. The vertebral bodies are cylindrical with a concave posterior cortical wall (Fig. 306–1). This configuration must be understood to avoid violating the ventral spinal canal when vertebral body screws are placed. Defining the pedicle, which arises just inferior to the intervertebral disk, is key when decompressing the

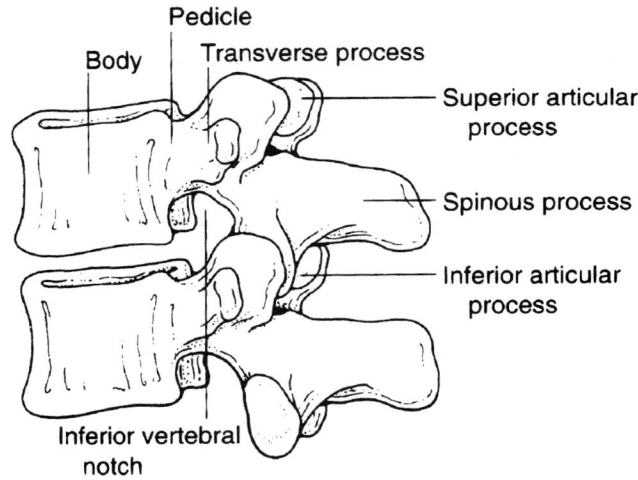

FIGURE 306–2. Two lumbar vertebrae. The neural foramen is defined by pedicles superiorly and inferiorly, the facet joint posteriorly, and the intervertebral disk space anteriorly. (From Benzel EC: Spine Surgery: Techniques, Complication Avoidance, and Management. Philadelphia, Churchill Livingstone, 1999.)

ventral spinal canal. The boundaries of the neural foramen, through which the nerve root and radicular vessels pass, are defined rostrally and caudally by the pedicles, anteriorly by the intervertebral disk space, and posteriorly by the facet joint (Fig. 306–2). Exposure of the superior lumbar spines requires manipulation of the 11th and 12th ribs. Unlike other ribs, the 11th and 12th ribs lack a neck and tubercle and do not articulate at the intervertebral disk space or with a transverse process.

Ventral Lumbar Musculature

The psoas and quadratus lumborum muscles lie deep and lateral to the erector spinae muscle and compose the posterior abdominal wall. The psoas major and minor muscles, flexors of the hip and lumbar spine, originate along the ventrolateral aspect of T12-L5 and insert on the femur and anterior pelvic rim (Fig. 306–3). The quadratus lumborum originates from the iliolumbar ligament and medial iliac crest and inserts onto the transverse processes of L1 through L4 and the medial surface of the 12th rib. This is a muscle of inspiration, increasing the vertical thoracic diameter.

The diaphragm and its attachments are important anatomic obstacles when the upper lumbar spine must be exposed. The lumbar portion of the diaphragm is composed of the right and left crura and three arcuate ligaments (Fig. 306–4). The right crus originates from the ventrolateral surface of the superior three lumbar vertebrae, and the left crus originates from the surface of L1 and L2. Both crura blend into the anterior longitudinal ligament inferiorly. The median arcuate ligament unites the medial surfaces of the two crura. The medial arcuate ligament crosses over the psoas between the crus and the transverse process of L1. The lateral arcuate ligament extends over the quadratus lumborum muscle from the transverse process of L1 to

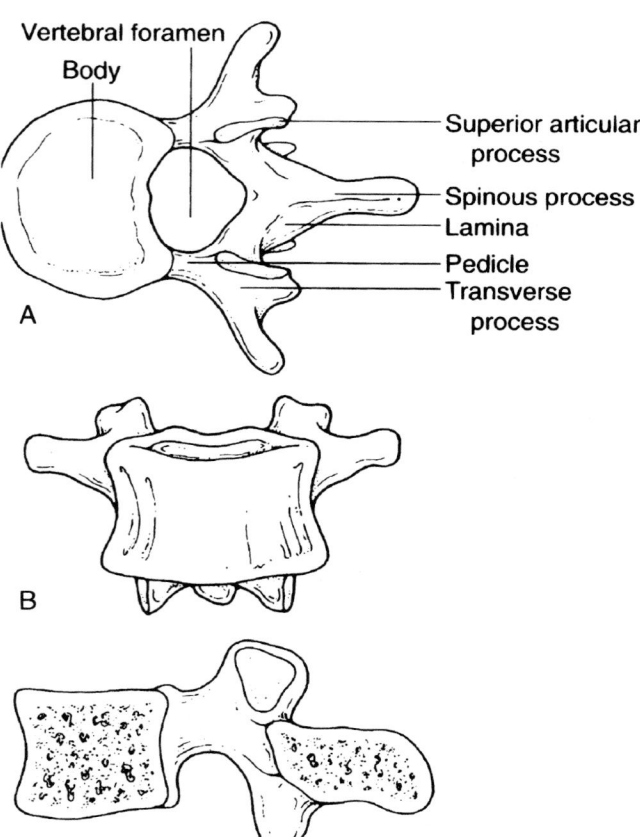

FIGURE 306–1. Superior *(A)*, anterior *(B)*, and midsagittal *(C)* views of a lumbar vertebra. (From Benzel EC: Spine Surgery: Techniques, Complication Avoidance, and Management. Philadelphia, Churchill Livingstone, 1999.)

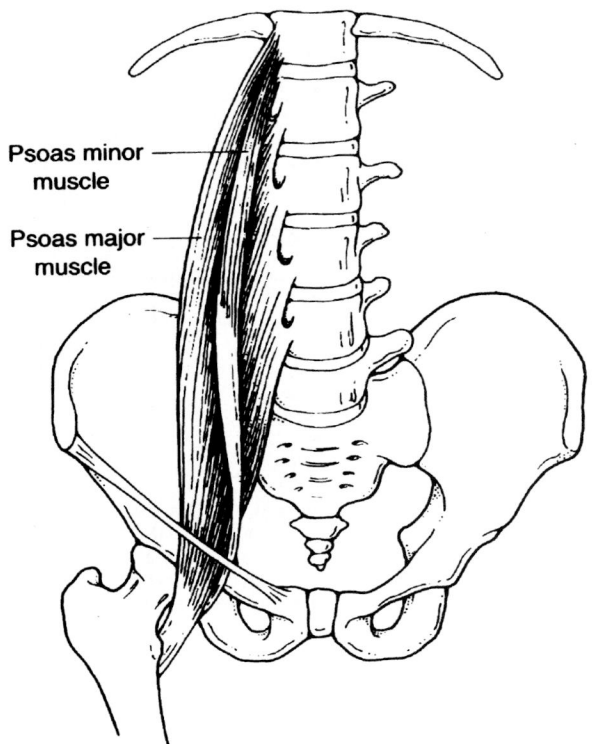

FIGURE 306–3. The psoas muscles originate along T12 to L5 and insert on the femur. (From Benzel EC: Spine Surgery: Techniques, Complication Avoidance, and Management. Philadelphia, Churchill Livingstone, 1999.)

the caudal margin of the 12th rib. The phrenic nerve descends onto the central diaphragm and sends radial fibers to the periphery of the diaphragmatic dome. The configuration of the phrenic nerve must be considered during dissection of the diaphragmatic dome for exposure of the superior lumbar spine (Fig. 306–5).

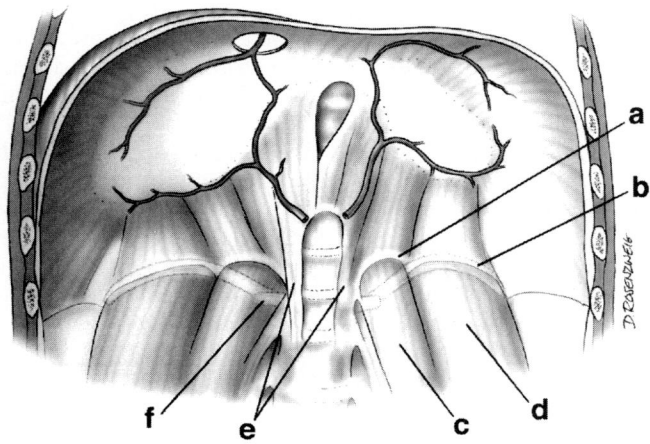

FIGURE 306–4. The diaphragm viewed inferiorly. a, medial arcuate ligament; b, lateral arcuate ligament; c, psoas; d, quadratus lumborum; e, crura of the diaphragm; f, transverse process of L1.

Great Vessels

The abdominal aorta extends from the T12-L1 disk space, at the diaphragmatic hiatus, to its bifurcation into the iliac arteries, at the L4 vertebral body. The paired lumbar arteries arise from the dorsolateral surface of the aorta and divide into dorsal and ventral branches. The ventral branch passes deep to the quadratus lumborum muscle and merges with the epigastric plexus. The dorsal branch courses dorsolaterally to the articular processes and gives rise to the radicular arteries and the anastomotic network of vessels supplying the spine and spinal cord (Fig. 306–6). Depending on where the interruption is located, violation of these vessels can lead to spinal cord ischemia. Transection of the radicular vessel at the neural foramen places the spinal cord at significant risk of an ischemic insult because these terminal arteries arise distal to anastomotic branches. Ischemia is particularly likely if the radiculomedullary artery of Adamkiewicz is disrupted. Although this vessel usually occurs in the mid to lower thoracic region, it has been reported in the upper lumbar region as well. A more proximal interruption of the vessels before the anastomotic network, as typically occurs with a ventrolateral approach, is desired.

The inferior vena cava begins at the right ventrolateral surface of the fifth lumbar vertebrae by the union of the common iliac veins. It ascends along the right side of the posterior abdominal wall, directly on the L3-5 vertebral bodies, and exits through the foramen of the vena cava in the central tendon of the diaphragm. The inferior vena cava receives many branches, not all of which have arterial counterparts. Tributaries to the inferior vena cava include the iliac veins, third and fourth lumbar veins, right testicular or ovarian veins, azygos vein, renal veins, right suprarenal vein, inferior phrenic vein, and hepatic veins. The superior lumbar veins unite to form the ascending lumbar vein that lies posterior to the psoas muscle. The azygos vein is formed on the right, and the hemiazygos vein is formed on the left.

Neuronal Structures

Both somatic and autonomic nerves are associated with the ventral surface of the lumbar spine. The lumbar plexus originates within the psoas muscle from the roots of L2 through L4 and gives rise to the obturator and femoral branches. The ilioinguinal and iliohypogastric nerves are derived from the L1 nerve root and enter the abdominal cavity dorsal to the medial arcuate ligament. Both pass along the ventral surface of the quadratus lumborum muscle. The genitofemoral nerve arises from the L1 and L2 nerve roots and courses along the psoas muscle, dividing into genital and femoral branches lateral to the iliac vessels. The nerve roots of L4 and L5 give rise to the lumbosacral trunk that descends over the ala of the sacrum into the pelvis. The sympathetic and parasympathetic nerves originate from plexuses of nerves located along the ventral surface of the aorta. The major components associated with the ventral lumbar spine are the celiac ganglia,

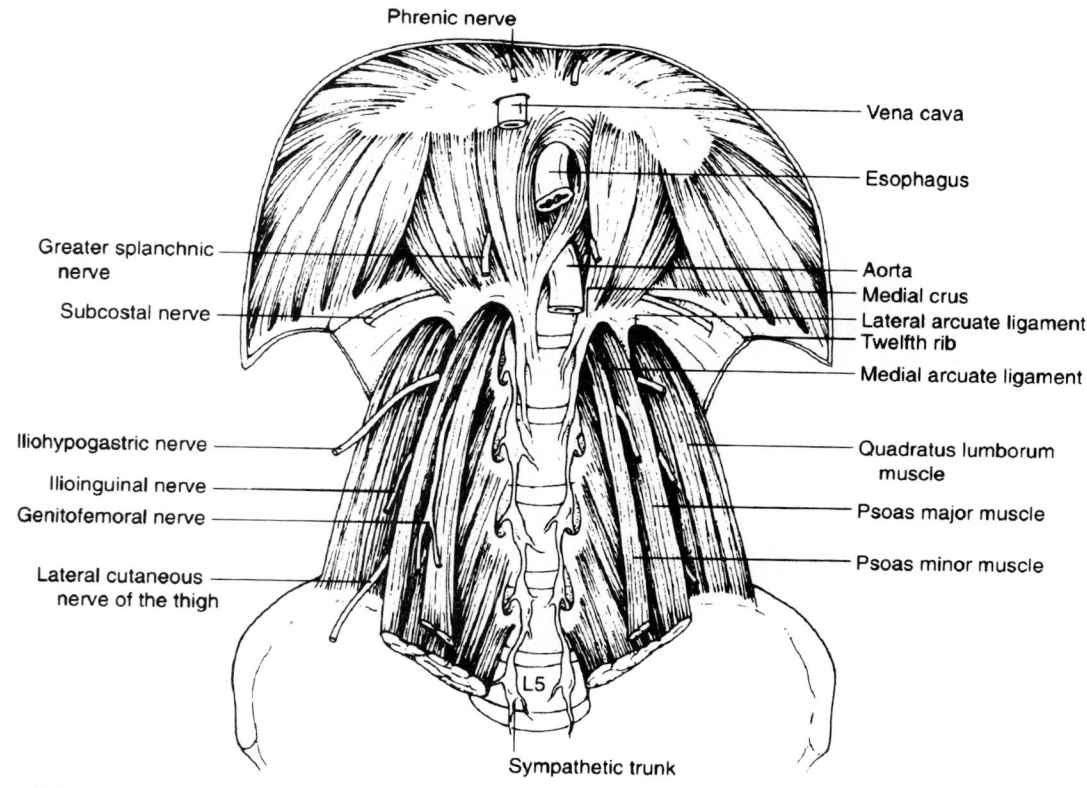

FIGURE 306–5. The diaphragm and its anatomic relationships with neural structures. (From Benzel EC: Spine Surgery: Techniques, Complication Avoidance, and Management. Philadelphia, Churchill Livingstone, 1999.)

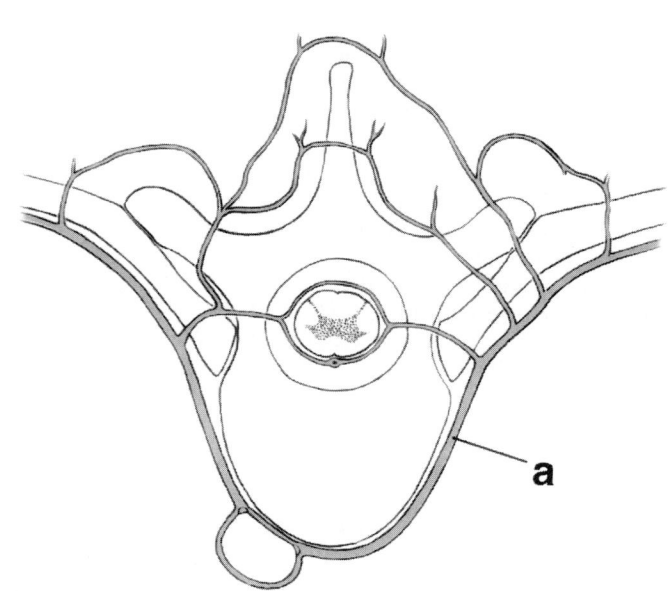

FIGURE 306–6. Segmental spinal cord blood supply. Proximally, dividing segmental vessels (a) preserve the spinal cord supply via anastomotic vessels. (From Benzel EC: Spine Surgery: Techniques, Complication Avoidance, and Management. Philadelphia, Churchill Livingstone, 1999.)

the splanchnic nerves, and the hypogastric plexus. The hypogastric plexus is particularly important because it innervates the bladder and internal vesicular sphincter and the vas deferens and seminal vesicles in males (Fig. 306–7). These structures all contribute to the neurophysiology of ejaculation. Injury to the hypogastric plexus can lead to retrograde ejaculation.

Visceral Structures

The cisterna chyli lies along the right ventrolateral surface of the first two lumbar vertebrae and marks the origin of the thoracic duct. This structure lies between the abdominal aorta and azygos vein, dorsal to the right crus of the diaphragm.

Each kidney lies within the retroperitoneal space, lateral to the lumbar spine against the psoas muscle. The ureter runs almost vertically through the retroperitoneum, along the psoas major muscle. On the right, it is adjacent to the vena cava. Bilaterally, the ureters cross the pelvic brim and external iliac arteries just beyond the bifurcation of the common iliac arteries. The ureter is adherent to the peritoneum and is often retracted with the peritoneum during the approach.

SURGICAL APPROACHES

The decision of which ventral approach to use is influenced by the lumbar level involved and the type of

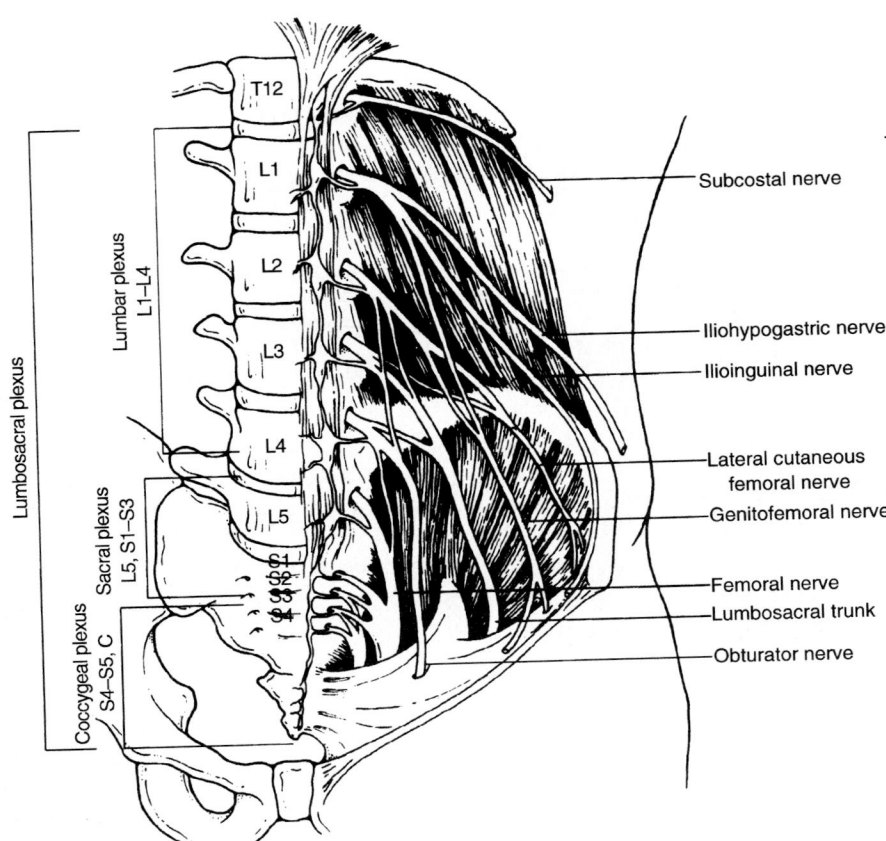

FIGURE 306–7. The lumbosacral plexus. (From Benzel EC: Spine Surgery: Techniques, Complication Avoidance, and Management. Philadelphia, Churchill Livingstone, 1999.)

pathology. Over the years, ventral approaches have been developed for a variety of pathologic processes.[108, 109, 125–128] The approach selected should maximize visualization of the lesion and regional anatomy. An insufficient exposure makes decompression and internal fixation more difficult and increases the risk of complications. Exposure of the thoracolumbar junction for visualization of L1 requires a thoracoabdominal approach and release of the diaphragm. Lesions located from L2 to L5 can be addressed through the flank with a retroperitoneal approach. If bilateral exposure of L2 to L5 is required, a transperitoneal approach may be more appropriate. The side of exposure is ultimately determined by the pathology, but a left-sided approach is preferred, owing to the anatomic constraints encountered on the right side. The vena cava is more difficult to mobilize than the aorta because its walls are thinner and more friable. The liver blocks a right-sided exposure more so than the spleen, but either organ can be injured if retraction is excessive. The assistance of a general or vascular surgeon often facilitates adequate exposure, and an appropriate preoperative evaluation and clear surgical plan enable neurosurgeons to avoid mishaps.

Retroperitoneal Approach

The retroperitoneal approach was developed from the standard flank incision that had been used for lumbar

sympathectomies. In the 1950s, Harmon popularized its application to spinal surgery, using this exposure to fuse the lumbar spine in the treatment of degenerative disk disease.[129] Compared with the transperitoneal route, the retroperitoneal approach provides the necessary exposure of the vertebral bodies at a decreased risk of visceral and vascular injury. Unlike the lateral extracavitary approach, this exposure requires no manipulation of nerve roots and avoids the destabilizing effects of dissecting the posterior musculature. Its disadvantages include unilateral exposure and the anatomic obstacles encountered if a right-sided approach is required. Despite these limitations, the retroperitoneal approach provides excellent visualization, allowing surgeons to identify the neural elements and thecal sac to gain access from L2 through L5. Either a midline or a lateral exposure can be used to enter the retroperitoneal space; the primary distinction is the position of the skin incision and the degree of muscle transection.

Ventrolateral Retroperitoneal Approach

A flank incision is used to start the ventrolateral retroperitoneal approach. The patient is placed in a lateral decubitus position with appropriate padding to avoid pressure ulcerations and neuropathies. The patient is positioned so that flexion of the operating table opens the space between the iliac crest and costal margin.

The incision begins in the midaxillary line between the ribs and iliac crest and follows an inferior oblique course to the lateral edge of the rectus sheath. The level of the incision depends on the desired level of exposure (Fig. 306–8). For lesions of the upper lumbar spine, the incision should be made above the umbilicus along the 11th or 12th rib. The rib can be resected to improve exposure and to provide a substrate for a fusion. For lesions in the midlumbar spine, the incision starts at the level of the umbilicus. The lower lumbar spine is accessed through an incision superior to the midpoint, between the umbilicus and symphysis pubis. Exposure of the lumbosacral junction is obtained through an incision inferior to this point.

The underlying musculature, including the latissimus dorsi, serratus posterior inferior, external oblique, and internal oblique muscles, is transected in line with the skin incision. The transversalis fascia is identified and transected to enter the retroperitoneal space. The underlying peritoneum is identified as a semitranslucent layer and carefully separated from the abdominal wall using digital dissection or a sponge stick. Adhesions, particularly toward the midline at the rectus sheath, may require sharp dissection. A plane between the quadratus lumborum muscle and retroperitoneal organs is developed, and the viscera, including the kidney, perirenal fat, and ureter, are retracted medially

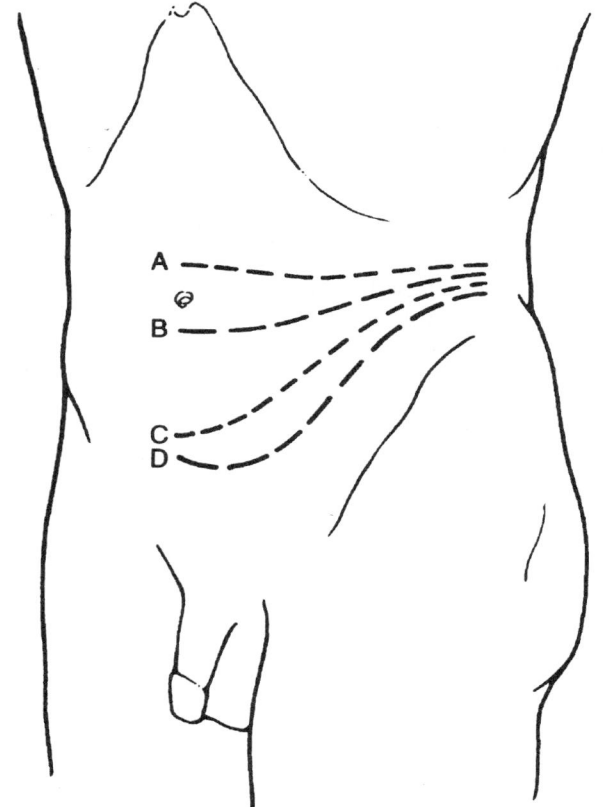

FIGURE 306–8. Transverse incisions for the retroperitoneal approach: L2-3 *(A)*, L3-4 *(B)*, L4-5 *(C)*, and L5-S1 *(D)*. (From Benzel EC: Spine Surgery: Techniques, Complication Avoidance, and Management. Philadelphia, Churchill Livingstone, 1999.)

(Fig. 306–9). Dissection of the fat plane posterior to the psoas muscle ends in a blind pouch. The dissection is continued inferiorly, mobilizing the peritoneum off the posterior abdominal wall to the level of the sacrum. The retroperitoneal organs and peritoneal contents are retracted medially and positioned outside the operative field with a well-padded, table-mounted retractor system. The dissection continues medially to identify the psoas muscle and genitofemoral nerve. This nerve lies along the ventral surface of the psoas and should not be injured. The psoas muscle may require dorsal mobilization with either a Cobb elevator or monopolar coagulation to expose the spine. If the psoas cannot be mobilized adequately, it is transected with monopolar cauterization. Aggressive retraction or transection of the psoas should be avoided to prevent injury to the lumbosacral plexus located within this muscle. The sympathetic trunk, which lies just medial to the psoas along the ventrolateral surface of the vertebral bodies, should be preserved. The ganglia at L1 and L2 provide fibers to the hypogastric plexus and are essential for ejaculatory function. At the lower lumbar regions, the common iliac vessels lie along the lateral aspect of the vertebral bodies and may require medial mobilization to increase exposure.

The lateral surface of the lumbar vertebrae is concave, and the surface of the intervertebral disk is convex. The lateral vertebral elements, including the pedicle and transverse process, are cleared of soft tissue with curets to identify the intervertebral foramen and neurovascular bundle. Unlike in the thoracic region, the nerve roots of the lumbar spine should not be sacrificed. The segmental vessels are ligated midway between the aorta and foramen with either a suture or metal ligature to preserve blood flow to the neural elements. Ligation of the segmental vessels allows easier mobilization of the aorta and iliac vessels to expose the anterolateral surface of the vertebral bodies.

Exposure of the upper lumbar region requires detachment of the left diaphragmatic crus from the anterior longitudinal ligament at the level of L2. A cuff of tissue is left to permit the crus to be reapproximated at closure. Mobilization of the ureter, necessary to allow medial retraction of the kidney, requires delicate manipulation. A generous cuff of tissue is left to preserve the microcirculation of the ureter. At the lumbosacral junction, the exposure is directed between the iliac vessels. The dissection continues over the left common iliac artery to expose the anterior longitudinal ligament. The plane between the anterior longitudinal ligament and vertebral body is defined just medial to the iliac artery. All the prevertebral tissues, including the hypogastric plexus, are then swept together toward the contralateral side. Steinmann pins are inserted into the lateral surface of the vertebral body to retract the iliac vessels away from the midline. Alternatively, the iliac vessels can be mobilized and retracted toward the contralateral side to provide a lateral oblique exposure of the lumbosacral region. Once the vertebral elements are cleared of soft tissue, decompression, fusion, and internal fixation are performed. After the procedure, the retroperitoneal and peritoneal contents are returned

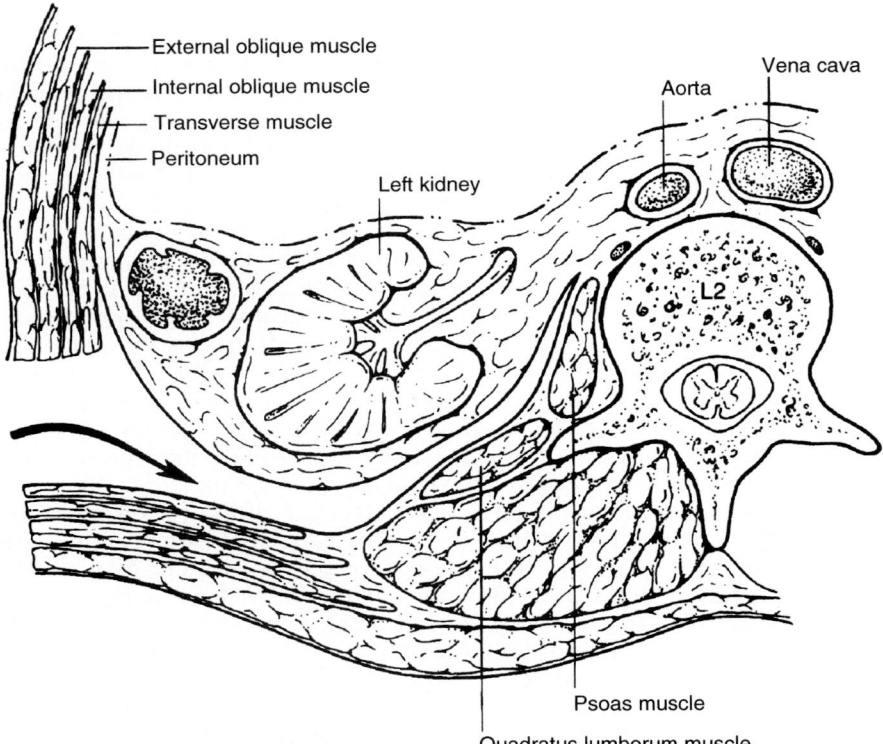

External oblique muscle
Internal oblique muscle
Transverse muscle
Peritoneum

Left kidney

Aorta

Vena cava

L2

Psoas muscle

Quadratus lumborum muscle

FIGURE 306–9. Axial view of ventrolateral retroperitoneal approach. (From Benzel EC: Spine Surgery: Techniques, Complication Avoidance, and Management. Philadelphia, Churchill Livingstone, 1999.)

to their normal anatomic positions. The muscle layers are reapproximated individually and sutured with a heavy, absorbable suture. The skin is closed with either staples or a subcuticular stitch. Postoperatively, the patient is placed in an external orthosis such as a thoracolumbar spinal orthosis, and imaging is obtained to assess the alignment and position of the fixation construct. The patient is mobilized after the position of the construct is confirmed.

Paramedian Retroperitoneal Approach

Direct anterior exposure of the lower lumbar and lumbosacral levels can also be obtained through a paramedian retroperitoneal route. Compared with the ventrolateral retroperitoneal approach, the paramedian approach provides a more direct anterior exposure, avoids transecting the muscles of the anterior abdominal wall, and can easily be converted to a transperitoneal approach if necessary. The paramedian approach is particularly useful for inserting an interbody graft when decompression of the spinal canal is not required and exposure of the anterior surface of the vertebral bodies is necessary.

The patient is positioned supine with a bolster placed below the lower back to elevate the sacrum and facilitate the exposure. A variety of skin incisions, including a vertical midline, paramedian, or traditional Pfannenstiel's incision, can be used (Fig. 306–10). The incisions are located below the level of the umbilicus several centimeters rostral to the symphysis pubis. Exposure of lumbar levels above L4 requires a vertical

incision that extends rostral to the umbilicus. The rectus sheath is opened along the medial or lateral border, depending on the location of the incision, and the muscles are retracted to expose the posterior rectus sheath and transversalis fascia (Fig. 306–11). The transversalis fascia and arcuate line are incised in a vertical orientation to expose the underlying preperitoneal fat and peritoneum.

The plane between the transversalis fascia and peritoneum is developed with blunt dissection, and the parietal peritoneum is freed from the lateral abdominal wall (Fig. 306–12). The abdominal contents and freed peritoneum are reflected medially and upward to expose the ventral lumbar spine (Fig. 306–13). The remainder of the dissection is similar to the ventrolateral retroperitoneal approach. The prevertebral tissues are dissected toward the contralateral side, and the iliac vessels are retracted laterally with Steinmann pins (Fig. 306–14). As in the ventrolateral retroperitoneal approach, extreme care is required when the hypogastric plexus is manipulated, especially in males. Once the procedure is completed, the abdominal contents are returned to their normal anatomic position, and the skin incision is closed in routine fashion. Postoperative care is identical to that for the ventrolateral approach.

Transperitoneal Approach

The transperitoneal approach provides the most direct route to the anterior lumbar spine and is ideal for visualizing L4-5 and the lumbosacral junction. Higher lumbar levels can be exposed, but considerable vessel

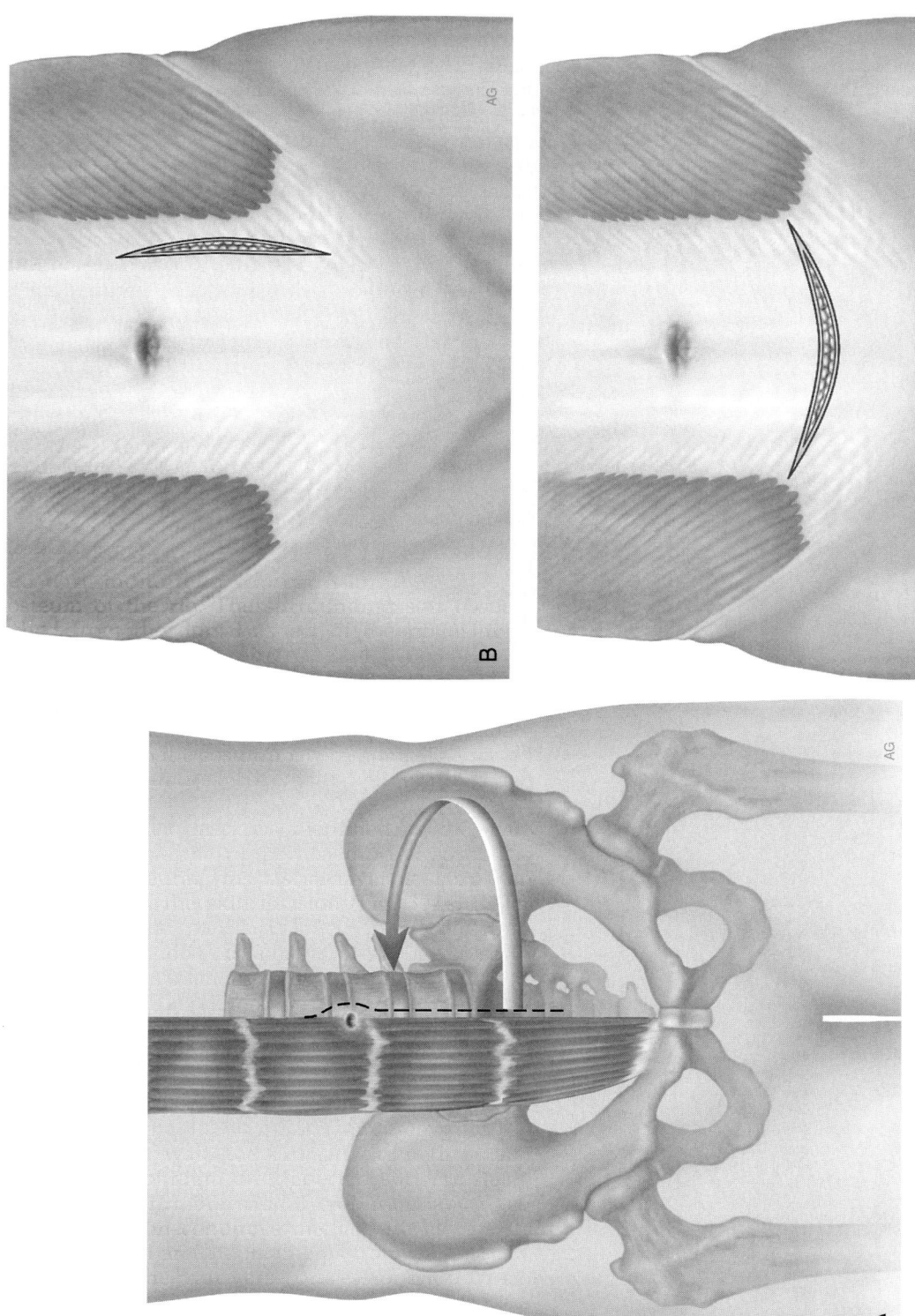

FIGURE 306–10. The midline incision *(A)* for the paramedian retroperitoneal approach. Paramedian *(B)* and Pfannenstiel's *(C)* incisions may also be used.

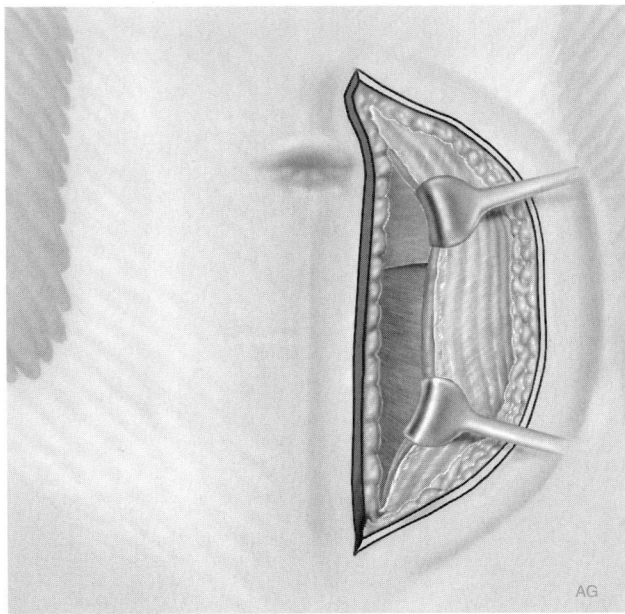

FIGURE 306–11. Exposure of the posterior rectus sheath and transversalis fascia.

retraction is required. Owing to the increased risk of vessel injury, lumbar levels above L4 are more appropriately exposed through a retroperitoneal exposure.

The assistance of a general or vascular surgeon is essential for a transperitoneal approach. Preoperatively, the patient must receive a bowel cathartic to cleanse the intestines. Broad-spectrum antibiotics are administered in case the bowel is perforated. The patient is positioned in a similar fashion as used with the paramedian retroperitoneal approach. A midline, paramedian, or Pfannenstiel's incision, identical to that for the paramedian retroperitoneal approach, can be used. The umbilicus serves as an indication of the level. An incision caudal to the umbilicus, several centimeters rostral to the pubis, exposes L5-S1. The underlying fascia, subcutaneous tissue, and peritoneum are incised in line with the incision to enter the abdominal cavity.

The abdominal contents are packed in a moist sponge and retracted into the upper abdomen to expose the posterior peritoneum. The peritoneum is incised in the midline over the aorta. The incision continues caudally over the right common iliac vessels to enter the retroperitoneal space. At the level of the iliac vessels, the incision proceeds medially to avoid the ureter. The peritoneal flaps are retracted laterally over the iliac vessels. The retroperitoneal portions of the large bowel are mobilized and retracted to the left to expose the aortic bifurcation and sacral promontory. Adjacent to the aorta, the ureters and hypogastric plexus are also visualized and treated with caution. Typically, the aortic bifurcation lies at L4 and the inferior vena cava origin starts at L5, but variations are common. The surgeon must be aware of these anatomic variants and adjust the operative plan as needed. Ante-

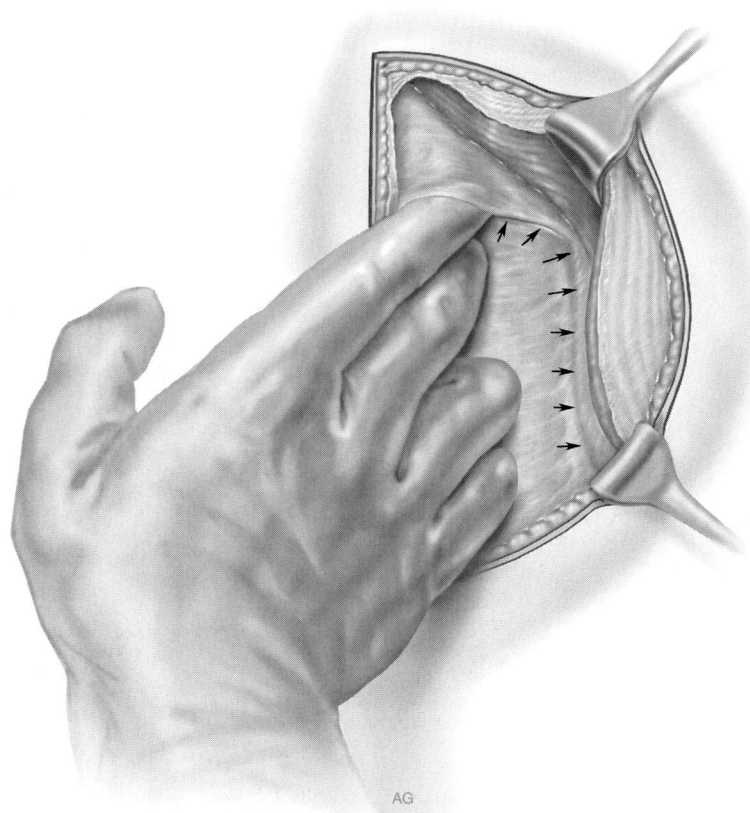

FIGURE 306–12. Blunt dissection is used to develop the plane between the peritoneum and the transversalis fascia.

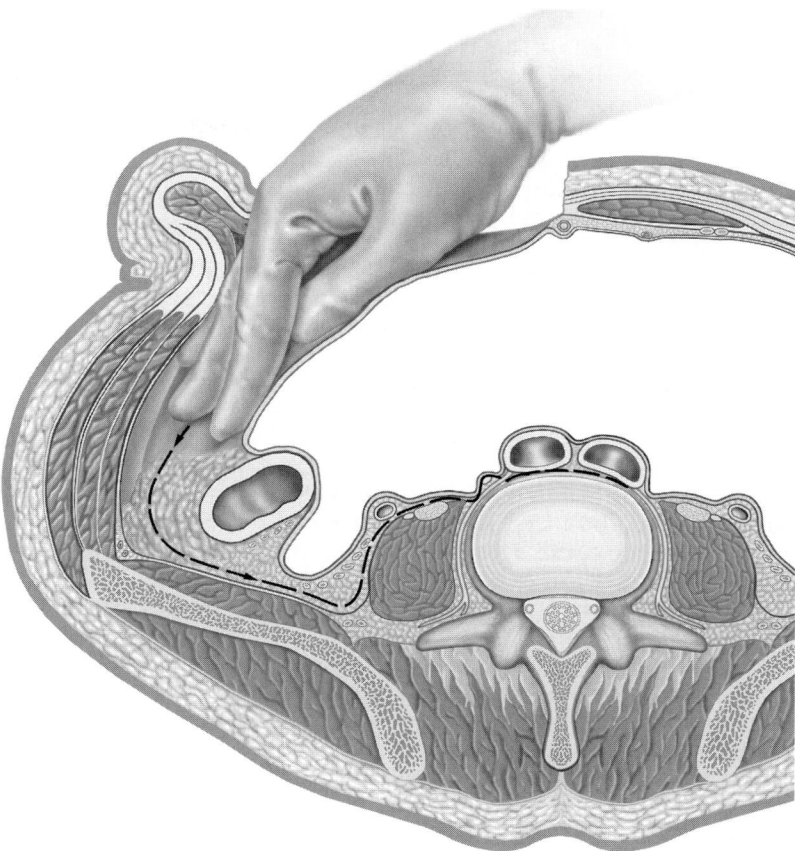

FIGURE 306–13. The plane between the transversalis fascia and the peritoneum is developed laterally. The abdominal contents are mobilized medially.

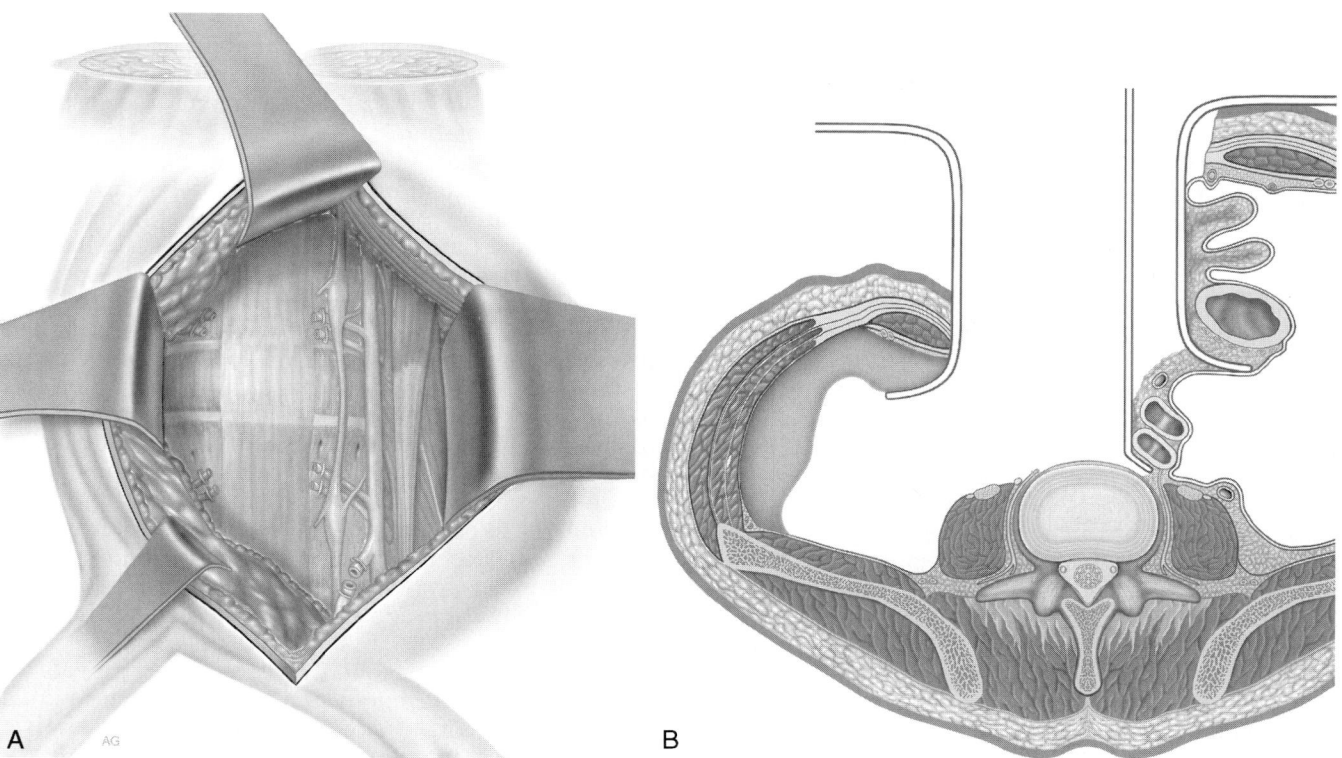

A

B

FIGURE 306–14. Anterior *(A)* and cross-sectional *(B)* views of the final exposure. Segmental vessels are divided proximally to preserve the anastomotic supply to neural structures.

rior branches of the aorta, including the inferior mesenteric artery, the middle sacral artery, and the segmental lumbar arteries, are also encountered with the transperitoneal approach.

For exposure of L5-S1, the dissection proceeds just medial to the left common iliac artery. The plane between the anterior longitudinal ligament and vertebral body is developed, and all the prevertebral tissues, including the hypogastric plexus, are swept toward the right. Dissection deep to the anterior longitudinal ligament avoids injury to the hypogastric plexus. The middle sacral artery and vein are identified inferior to the aortic bifurcation and ligated with either a suture or a metal clip. The middle sacral vein follows a variable course and may empty into one of the common iliac veins instead of into the origin of the inferior vena cava. The iliac vessels are mobilized, retracted laterally, and held in position with Steinmann pins driven into the vertebral bodies. L4-5 is best approached through a left lateral aortic route because the vena cava typically originates ventral to L5. If the origin of the vena cava is abnormally high, an interiliac approach may be attempted. The lateral aortic route also decreases the chance of injury to the hypogastric plexus. The aorta and iliac artery are mobilized and retracted toward the right. Retraction is facilitated by ligation of segmental lumbar vessels. The segmental vessels should be divided midway between their origin and the intervertebral foramen to preserve collateral blood flow to the spinal canal.

When the spinal procedure is completed, the posterior peritoneum is closed with an absorbable suture. Drainage of the retroperitoneal space is seldom required. The abdominal contents are then returned to their anatomic position to avoid intestinal torsion and obstruction. The individual layers are reapproximated with absorbable sutures. After the procedure, bowel function should be assessed before the patient's diet is advanced. The patient is placed in an external orthosis, imaged to document the position of the graft and construct, and mobilized as tolerated.

BIOMECHANICS OF ANTERIOR LUMBAR INSTRUMENTATION

A detailed discussion of biomechanics is beyond the scope of this chapter, but several basic concepts require review. The response of the spine to applied stress is mediated by the intrinsic biologic properties of the individual elements, as well as by their spatial relationships. Clinical instability, as defined by White and Panjabi,[130] is the inability of the spine to prevent abnormal motions that produce pain, deformity, or neurological deficits under physiologic loads. Spinal instability should not be considered an all-or-none phenomenon; rather, it is a point along a continuum.

Instability can be divided into acute and chronic forms. Benzel[91] subcategorized each of these two forms into two separate types. Acute instability can be divided into overt instability, or the inability of the spine to support the torso under normal loads, and limited instability, which is a lesser injury in which the spine provides some support with normal activity. Overt instability implies disruption of all three columns as described by Denis,[64] and limited instability is the loss of either ventral or dorsal stabilizing elements, but not both. Overt instability requires immediate operative intervention. Limited instability may be treated conservatively, with an understanding that progression to either overt or chronic instability is possible. Overt instability is often the result of a traumatic injury and is less common in the lumbar spine than is limited instability.

Chronic instability is divided into glacial instability, in which the deformity progresses slowly with no realistic chance of rapid deterioration, and dysfunctional motion segments, an instability in which degenerative changes of the disk and vertebral body increase the potential for spinal pain.[91] Glacial instability results from a number of causes, including degeneration, trauma, tumor, congenital deformity, and infection. This form of instability is common in the lumbar spine owing to the increased loads that it supports and the propensity for degenerative changes.

A number of "column" concepts of spinal integrity have been described in the literature.[64, 131–134] The three-column model of Denis has gained the most widespread acceptance. This model divides the spine into three columns. The vertebral bodies, disks, anterior longitudinal ligaments, and posterior longitudinal ligaments are separated into the anterior and middle columns; the posterior bony arch and ligaments compose the posterior column.[64] The recognition of a middle column incorporating the neutral axis separates the Denis model from other models of spinal stability.[91] The neutral axis undergoes minimal compression or distraction during flexion and extension, supports the majority of an axial load, and contains the instantaneous axis of rotation.

White and Panjabi[130] developed a point system to determine the extent of acute instability, incorporating the three-column concept and radiographic, clinical, and historical data. The validity of this scale has not yet been verified with a well-controlled, prospective study. On the scale, a score of 5 points implies overt instability, and 2 to 4 points correlates with limited instability. No scale has been created to assess chronic instability, so the diagnosis depends primarily on imaging, including dynamic radiographs; the clinical examination; and the clinician's bias. The lack of objective data, particularly in the diagnosis of a dysfunctional motion segment, creates considerable variability and controversy in diagnosing and treating chronic instability. Yet any attempt to treat instability on a purely arbitrary point system, without the use of common sense and clinical judgment, is sure to lead to diagnostic errors.

Anterior instrumentation constructs can be categorized based on the interaction among the individual spinal components.[135] A construct is classified as *rigid* if no motion is intended at the interface between adjoining elements. These constructs immobilize the spine and provide immediate stability. However, the rigid construct shields the graft from fusion-promoting forces, a phenomenon known as *stress shielding*. Fusion occurs only if the construct remains intact over a sufficient period. Eventually, the fusion assumes the stress-bearing work of the construct, or the construct fails. Constructs that intentionally allow variable degrees of movement between the individual components are termed *dynamic* constructs. The permissive movement of dynamic constructs is designed to expose the graft to fusion-enhancing forces, a phenomenon known as *load sharing*. The movement allowed between the components decreases the risk of failure at the bone-construct interface. A dynamic construct, however, may not provide enough support for a grossly unstable spine, in which progression of deformity is a serious risk.

Anterior constructs, whether rigid or dynamic, impart complex forces to the spine.[135] For the sake of simplicity, an anterior implant can be placed in either a distraction or a compression mode. There are two fundamental types of anterior distraction implants, an interbody strut and a cantilever beam construct. The interbody strut acts as a simple distraction buttress when placed in the neutral axis. Intrinsic or surgically created resistance to distraction is required for an interbody strut to provide support effectively. A cantilever beam construct, using screws or staples, provides stabilization in a nonfixed, fixed, or applied moment arm configuration. A rigid construct produces a fixed or applied and acts as a buttress when encompassing the neutral axis. A deformity can be corrected with a rigid cantilever construct by producing an intrinsic bending moment between the longitudinal members of the implant. The bending moment is produced within the construct by applying opposite forces to the individual longitudinal members. Cross-linking of the longitudinal members increases the stability of the construct. A nonfixed moment arm is produced with a dynamic construct. When placed in distraction, this construct produces extension and enhances load sharing. If a fulcrum exists between the terminal ends of the construct, a three-point bending force limits the degree of extension.[135–138]

An anterior cantilever beam construct that resists distraction is considered an anterior compression, or tension-band, fixation device.[135, 137–139] Unlike the distraction devices described earlier, an interbody strut graft does not provide the desired forces to the spine. The compression produced by the construct increases the degree of load supported by the spine or interbody strut and decreases the stress placed on the bone-implant interface. This force distribution decreases the risk of implant failure, increases load sharing, and increases the fusion-forming forces applied to the graft. This concept applies only if intrinsic or inserted spinal elements can accept the axial load applied by the construct. Tension-band fixation devices resist bending opposite the side of insertion; therefore, an anterior compression construct is designed to resist extension. As with distraction constructs, the anterior compression construct fails under excessive flexion forces if a posterior tension band is absent. The anterior constructs are unable to compensate for an incompetent posterior tension band during flexion, most often causing the implant to fail at the bone-construct interface.

INSTRUMENTATION CONSTRUCTS

During the past 2 decades, various constructs have become available. The different designs include screw-rod implants, such as the Kaneda SR Anterior Spinal System (AcroMed Corp., Cleveland, OH) and the VentroFix system (Synthes, West Chester, PA); screw-plate implants, such as the Anterior Thoracolumbar Locking Plate (ATLP; Synthes, West Chester, PA) and Z-plate II (Sofamor-Danek, Memphis, TN); and interbody fusion implants, such as the BAK Interbody Fusion System (Sulzer Spine-Tech, Minneapolis, MN) and the Ray Threaded Fusion Cage (Surgical Dynamics, Norwalk, CT). The use of these devices requires a commitment from surgeons to learn the insertion technique of each construct in detail. Manufacturer-sponsored training sessions can be invaluable in developing the necessary surgical skills. The continued development of these devices has led to constructs with a low profile, advanced biomechanics, reduced radiographic artifact, and improved insertion techniques. Although randomized, prospective trials are lacking, the clinical effectiveness of several constructs has been demonstrated.[140–145]

Screw-Rod Constructs

The Kaneda SR Anterior Spinal System was first developed in 1984 for the treatment of thoracolumbar fractures.[146] This device consists of vertebral body plates, cancellous screws, paired rods, and transverse couplers (Fig. 306–15*A*). The spiked vertebral body plate, unique to the Kaneda system, is impacted into the ventrolateral surface of the vertebra. It serves as a template for screw placement to prevent screw migration and to provide mechanical support. Each plate anchors two vertebral body screws. The ventral screws provide an anchor for distraction across the defect during insertion of an interbody strut graft. The rods are secured to the screw with a patented V-Groove Hollow Ground junction using a circumferential grip connector. Once the rods are in position, compression across the construct is applied before final tightening of the lock screws. The transverse coupler increases the stability of the construct against both rotatory and flexion-extension forces. This device allows multisegmental fixation to a maximum of four motion segments.

The VentroFix system is one of the newer generation implants, a hybrid between the screw-plate and screw-rod designs (see Fig. 306–15*B*). It consists of a pair of clamps secured to the vertebral bodies that anchor the intervening rods. Unlike in the standard screw-rod design, the rods are secured to the clamps rather than to individual vertebral body screws. The trajectory of the screws is critical, because the heads of the vertebral body screws are threaded and engage the clamp (Fig. 306–16). No motion is allowed between the screw and

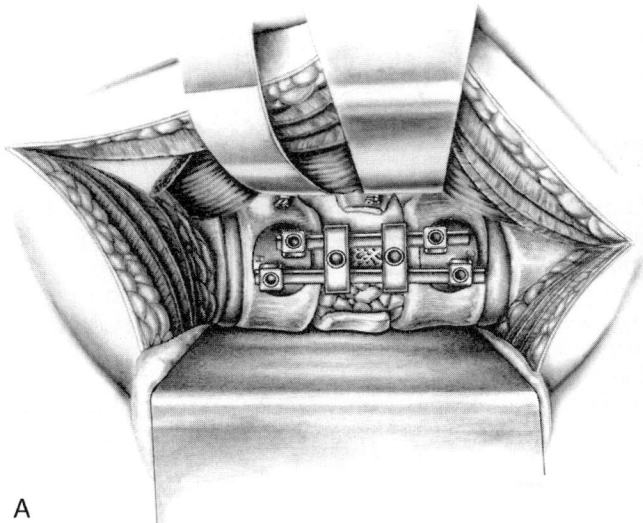

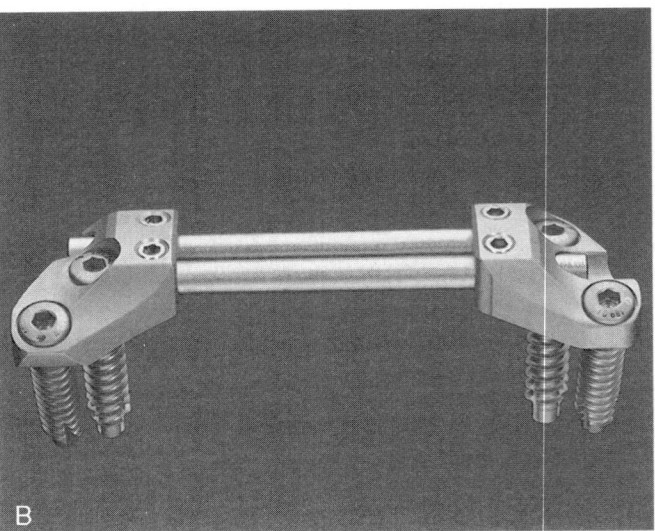

A

B

FIGURE 306–15. *A*, Kaneda SR Anterior Spinal System. *B*, VentroFix fixation system. (*A*, From Kaneda K, Gaines RW: Surgical Technique for Anterior Thoracolumbar Corpectomy, Graft Placement, and Stabilization Using the Kaneda SR Anterior Spinal System. Cleveland, OH, Acromed, 1996. *B*, From VentroFix and Anterior Thoracolumbar Locking Plate technique guides. West Chester, PA, Synthes, 1998. Used with permission of Synthes.)

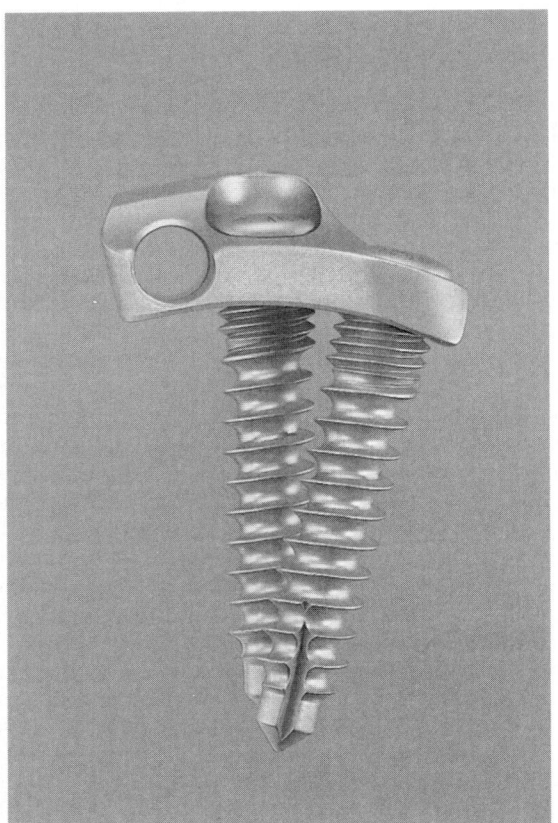

FIGURE 306–16. VentroFix screws engage bone and clamp with separate threads. (From VentroFix and Anterior Thoracolumbar Locking Plate technique guides. West Chester, PA, Synthes, 1998. Used with permission of Synthes.)

vertebral clamp, creating a rigid construct. The increased stability eliminates the need for a transverse coupler when stabilizing a single level. For longer constructs, a parallel connector is used to maintain alignment of the rod. Compressive forces can be applied across the construct because the clamps are open-ended and allow the rods to slide through. The VentroFix system is extremely versatile, with a variety of vertebral body clamps available for partial or multilevel corpectomies.[147]

Screw-Plate Constructs

The ATLP is a rigid construct consisting of a precontoured titanium locking plate, cancellous vertebral body screws, and compression screws (Fig. 306–17*A*). A machine-threaded head on the vertebral body screws, similar to the VentroFix system, locks the screw to the plate. Distraction across the corpectomy site is obtained with a separate instrument, because the plate provides no anchor for distraction. Once the graft is in place, compression is applied through a separate set of screws inserted into the angled dynamic compression plate (DCP) holes. These screws can cause up to 3 mm of compression when driven into the bone. The vertebral body screws have a wide cancellous pitch that allows unicortical purchase. For proper insertion, the trajectory of the locking screw must be perpendicular to the plate to facilitate the interface of threads from the screw and plate. Once the locking screws are set, the compression is maintained and the DCP screws are removed. This simple design is one advantage of the ATLP system; however, only a limited degree of compression can be applied.[147]

The Z-plate II is one of the most dynamic plating systems currently available (see Fig. 306–17*B*). There

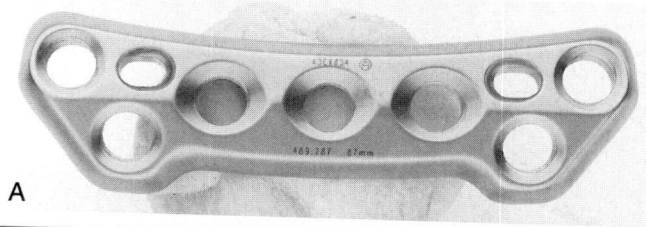

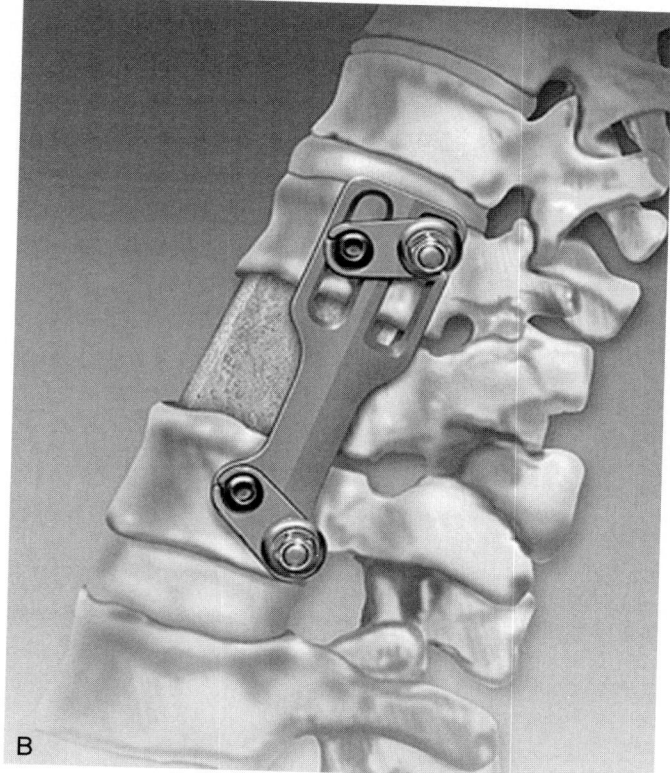

FIGURE 306–17. *A*, Anterior Thoracolumbar Locking Plate (ATLP) system. *B*, Z-plate system. (*A*, From VentroFix and Anterior Thoracolumbar Locking Plate technique guides. West Chester, PA, Synthes, 1998. Used with permission of Synthes. *B*, Courtesy of Medtronic/Sofamor Danek, Memphis, TN.)

are two categories of plates: the Z-plate II—ATL (anterior thoracolumbar) and the Z-plate II—thoracic. The implant consists of the slotted plate, multiaxial bolts and screws, a slot and variable washer, and tightening nuts. The Z-plate II is classified as a dynamic implant because the multiaxial design of the bolts and screws allows movement between the components and promotes load sharing with the graft. The posteriorly placed bolts act as anchors for distraction across the corpectomy defect, facilitating insertion of the graft and correction of a deformity. The slotted design of the Z-plate II allows compression across the corpectomy site after the plate is positioned for precise seating of the graft.

Interbody Fusion Devices

Compared with more traditional posterior fusion constructs, anterior interbody fusion devices have several surgical and biomechanical advantages.[148–152] Anterior approaches for the insertion of these devices tend to be less invasive than the standard posterior approach.[153–156] Successful techniques for delivering these devices include laparoscopic intraperitoneal surgery and the "mini" open laparotomy.[157–159] These approaches restore disk height and lumbar lordosis, distract the intervertebral foramen, provide a favorable graft environment, and do not disturb the posterior tension band. They also decrease intraoperative blood loss, eliminate the need for nerve root manipulation, and decrease operative time and length of hospitalization.[157, 160, 161] The device is positioned within the neutral axis because the interbody cage is an extremely rigid construct and because of the location of the instantaneous axis of rotation. It eliminates motion efficiently and enhances the possibility of fusion formation.[150] The risk of settling with the cage is increased because the threads breach the end plate and expose cancellous bone. Revision is also difficult once the cage is inserted.

A number of different metallic cages, including the Interfix (Sofamor-Danek, Memphis, TN), the BAK Interbody Fusion System, and the Ray Threaded Fusion Cage, are now available (Fig. 306–18). Ideally, the metallic cage is packed with autograft bone and threaded into the distracted disk space. The cage is fenestrated along the rostral and caudal faces to allow the ingrowth of fusion bone. The threads of the cage prevent migration, resist shear stresses, and expose the cancellous bone to promote fusion. Continued development has produced a variety of cages composed of different materials (titanium, carbon fiber, and allograft cortical bone) and available in a number of shapes. Biomechanical data indicate that most of these devices increase stability beyond that of the normal intact spine, but no conclusive studies have demonstrated the superiority of one device over another.

IMPLANTATION TECHNIQUES

Technique guides are available from the manufacturers for all the constructs described in this chapter. For the sake of completeness, the insertion technique for each design category is detailed based on the manufacturer's guide to surgical techniques.

General Principles

A number of general principles are followed when instrumentation is to be inserted into the ventrolateral lumbar spine, regardless of the type of construct chosen. The main surgical goal is to achieve stability with the lowest profile and maximal implant-to-bone contact. Maximal surface contact between the bone and implant is desirable to distribute the application of forces evenly. "Gardening" the spine refers to the removal of osteophytes and other bony protrusions before the construct and implant are placed to allow an implant to lie flush against the vertebral surface.

Typically, vertebral body screws are inserted at fixed coordinates based on the concave configuration of the

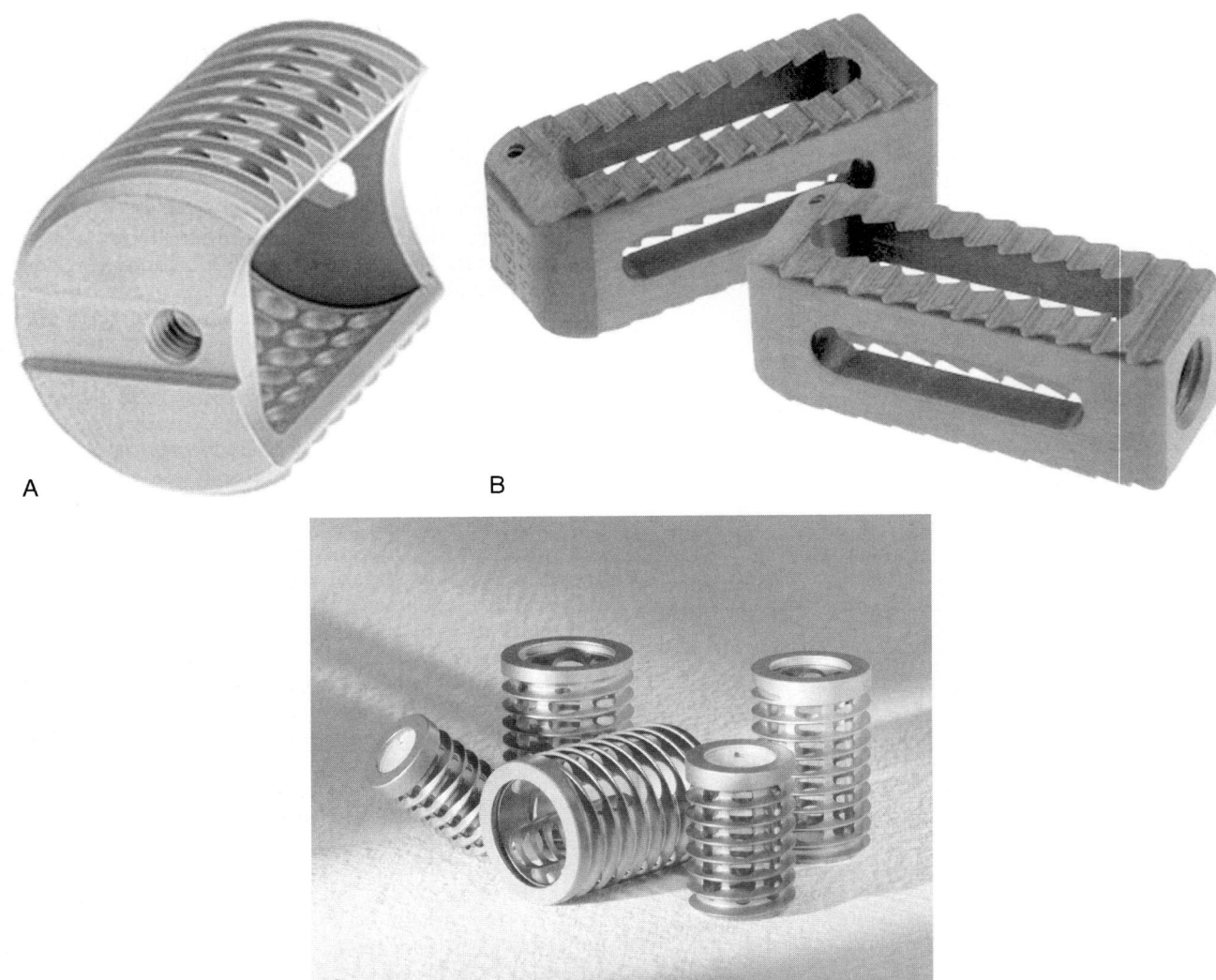

FIGURE 306–18. Representative cages. *A*, InterFix system. *B*, BAK system. *C*, Ray Threaded Fusion Cages. (*A*, Courtesy of Medtronic/Sofamor Danek, Memphis, TN. *B*, Courtesy of Sulzer Spine-Tech, Minneapolis, MN. *C*, Courtesy of Surgical Dynamics, Norwalk, CT.)

posterior cortical wall. The dorsal screws are placed 8 to 10 mm ventral to the posterior cortical surface and 8 to 10 mm either caudal or rostral from the end plates (Fig. 306–19). These coordinates, along with a trajectory inclined 10 degrees ventrally, ensure that the screw does not enter the spinal canal. Ventral screws are inserted either parallel or with a slight dorsal inclination to triangulate the screws and decrease the risk of pullout. All screws should be countersunk within the construct to obtain a low profile. Several systems require only unicortical screw purchase, but bicortical purchase increases the stability of any construct. Penetrating the contralateral cortex more than 2 to 3 mm should be avoided. In general, an awl should be used to start any screw hole before drilling to avoid slippage and catastrophic injury. Additional technical guidelines are specific for the construct chosen.

A translational deformity can occur with rod constructs due to an intrinsic bending moment between the rods.[137] It can be avoided by cross-fixation of parallel rods and triangulating the screws within the vertebral body. Some of the newer constructs avoid a parallelogram configuration by offsetting the screws in the sagittal and coronal planes within a single vertebral body. Distraction and compression are applied to the screws before and after the graft is inserted. Excessive distraction across the defect can cause spinal cord injury from stretch and vascular compromise, especially if distraction-resisting ligaments, such as the anterior longitudinal ligament, are incompetent.

VentroFix System

The VentroFix system is intended to stabilize the ventrolateral spine from T8 through L5. The appropriate screw length can be selected from preoperative imaging or thorough intraoperative measurements. After the corpectomy, the coronal width of the superior and

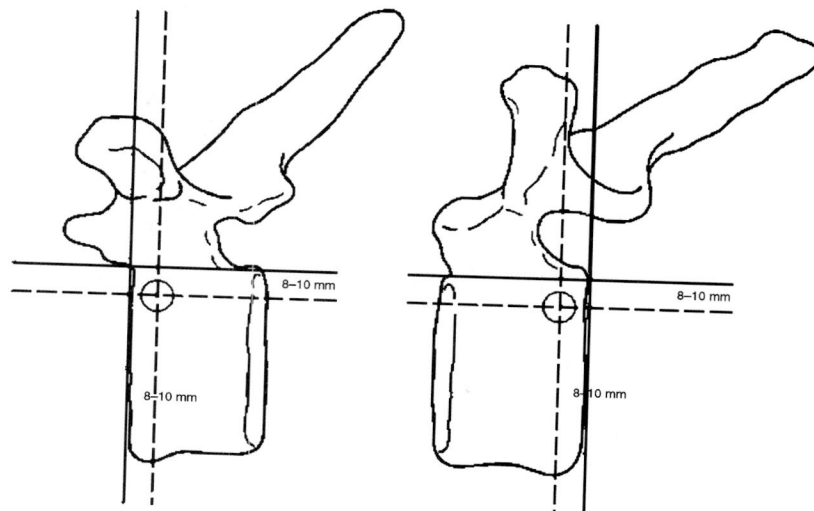

FIGURE 306–19. The screw insertion sites are 8 to 10 mm inferior or superior to the superior or inferior end plate, respectively, and 8 to 10 mm anterior to the posterior margin of the vertebral body. (Courtesy of Medtronic/Sofamor Danek, Memphis, TN.)

inferior end plates is measured with a depth gauge. The manufacturer recommends a screw length 5 mm shorter than the coronal width of the end plate. Unicortical purchase is sufficient secondary to the rigid nature of the construct. Once the interbody graft is inserted, the ventrolateral surfaces of the vertebral bodies are cleared of protruding osteophytes. The distance across the corpectomy is measured with a rod template to determine the length of the construct. The appropriate rods are chosen and cut to the desired length with a rod cutter if necessary. The vertebral body clamps have a specific orientation, with both upper and lower clamps based on a left lateral approach. Although the manufacturer has designated a rostral-caudal orientation for the clamps, this placement is not absolute, and the clamps are interchangeable when an alternative construct is preferred. When only a portion of the vertebral body is resected, a "fracture clamp" that is smaller than the standard clamp can be used (Fig. 306–20A).

The construct is assembled before implantation. A 6-mm rod is inserted in the closed hole of each clamp and secured by tightening the setscrew. The free end of each rod is inserted into the open hole of the opposite clamp (see Fig. 306–20B). The construct is adjusted to the desired length, and the setscrew is tightened to maintain the appropriate length. If the rod protrudes more than 5 mm from the open hole, it should be removed and cut to the appropriate length. A threaded drill guide is inserted into the posterior holes of each clamp (see Fig. 306–20C). The construct holder is seated on both rods and attached to the straight threaded drill-guide applicator. For constructs that span several levels, a VentroFix parallel connector is used to maintain parallel rod alignment. This connector must be preloaded onto the rods before the clamp is inserted. The connector is not intended for end-to-end rod coupling.

The construct is placed on the ventrolateral aspect of the vertebral bodies and held in position with the construct holder. A posterior hole is drilled into the vertebral bodies through one of the threaded drill guides using a 5-mm flexible drill bit equipped with a permanent stop (see Fig. 306–20D). The drill guide is removed, and a 7.5-mm self-tapping screw of the appropriate length is inserted into the hole. A flexible or straight hexagonal screwdriver is used to insert the screw. The construct must be held firmly in position to ensure that the screw is inserted perpendicular to the clamp and engages the self-locking threads. The sequence is repeated for the other posterior hole. The straight threaded drill guide is removed from the construct holder, leaving the construct holder in place to provide an anchor for compression across the construct. Two 5-mm threaded drill guides are inserted into the anterior holes with the straight threaded drill guide. The anterior screws are inserted in a similar fashion as the posterior screws. If compression is desired, the setscrews for the open clamp holes can be loosened to allow the rods to slide through. Compression must be applied along the rod opposite the one with the construct holder. The compression forceps are placed against the construct holder and the countersink of the clamp (see Fig. 306–20E). Once compression is applied, the setscrews on the open clamp holes are tightened to lock the rods in place (see Fig. 306–20F). The compression forceps and construct holder are removed, and the closure is performed in standard fashion.

Anterior Thoracolumbar Locking Plate System

The ATLP system is designed to stabilize the anterior spine from T10 through L5. The proper plate size is selected, making sure that all screw holes, vertebral body screws, and DCP screws are placed over the vertebral body. As with the VentroFix system, drill guides are threaded onto the plate to ensure a proper trajectory for the screw holes. A threaded drill guide is secured to the center hole of the plate and attached to the threaded drill-guide applicator. The plate is posi-

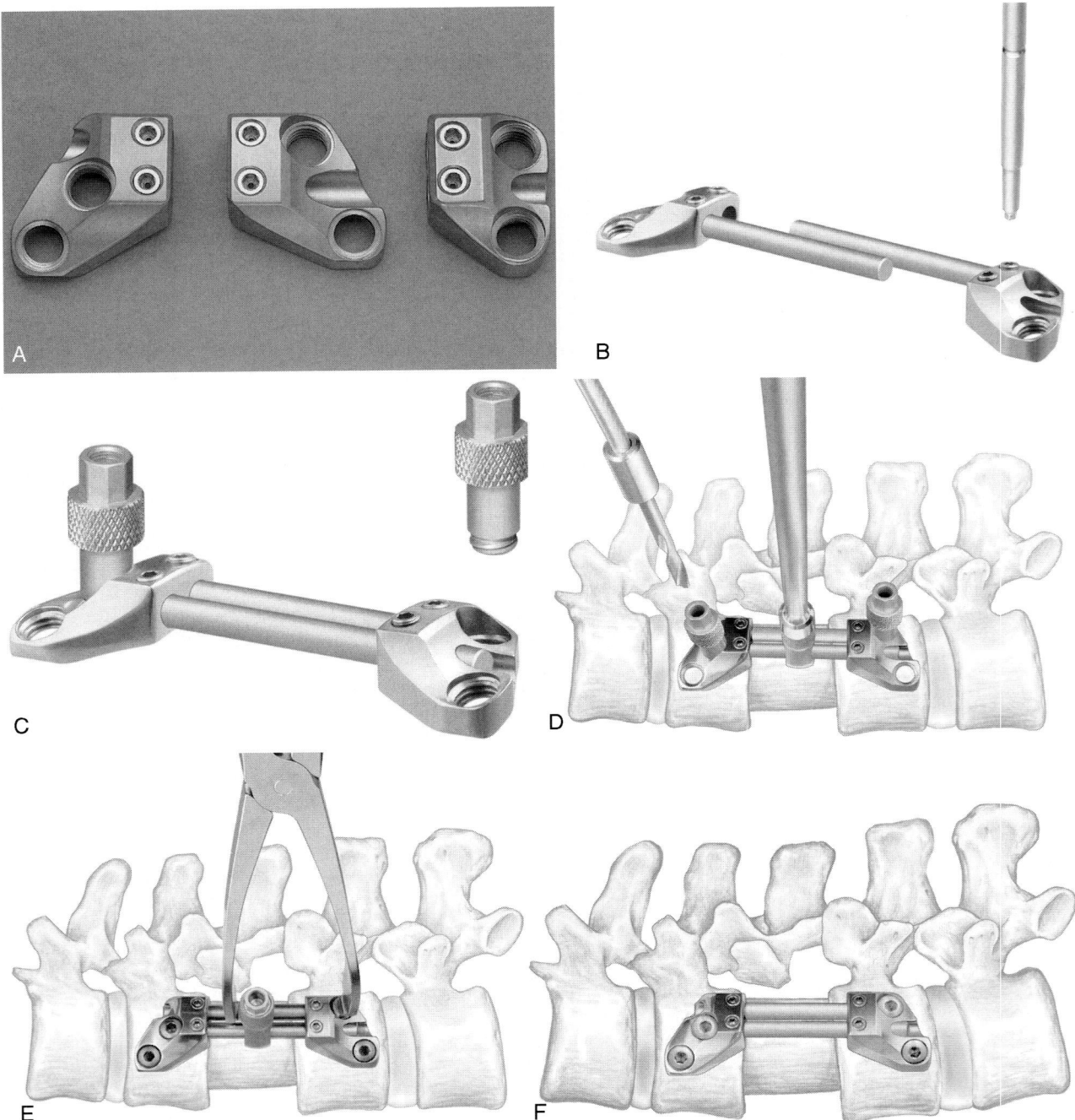

FIGURE 306–20. *A,* VentroFix titanium clamps. *From left to right,* upper, lower, and fracture clamps. *B,* Preimplantation assembly of VentroFix construct. *C,* Threaded drill guides are inserted into the posterior hole of each clamp. *D,* The construct holder is mounted on the straight threaded drill-guide applicator and attached to either rod of the construct. The construct is then held firmly in the desired position, and a posterior hole is drilled with a 5-mm flexible drill bit with a permanent stop. *E,* Compression can be applied to the construct. The setscrews on the open hole of each clamp are loosened. Compression is applied along the rod that does not have the construct holder. Compression must be maintained while the setscrews are tightened. *F,* The completed VentroFix construct. (From VentroFix and Anterior Thoracolumbar Locking Plate technique guides. West Chester, PA, Synthes, 1998. Used with permission of Synthes.)

tioned onto the ventrolateral surface of the vertebral bodies and held in position with the drill-guide applicator (Fig. 306–21*A*). A 2.5-mm-long DCP drill guide is positioned in one of the DCP holes, and the hole is drilled with the 2.5-mm three-fluted drill bit equipped with an intrinsic 30-mm stop. Pointing the arrow on

the drill guide at the graft site ensures proper orientation of the DCP hole (see Fig. 306–21*B*). A 4-mm cancellous screw is inserted into the DCP hole but not tightened completely. A second screw is inserted into the opposite DCP site. Each screw is then sequentially tightened to place the graft under compression.

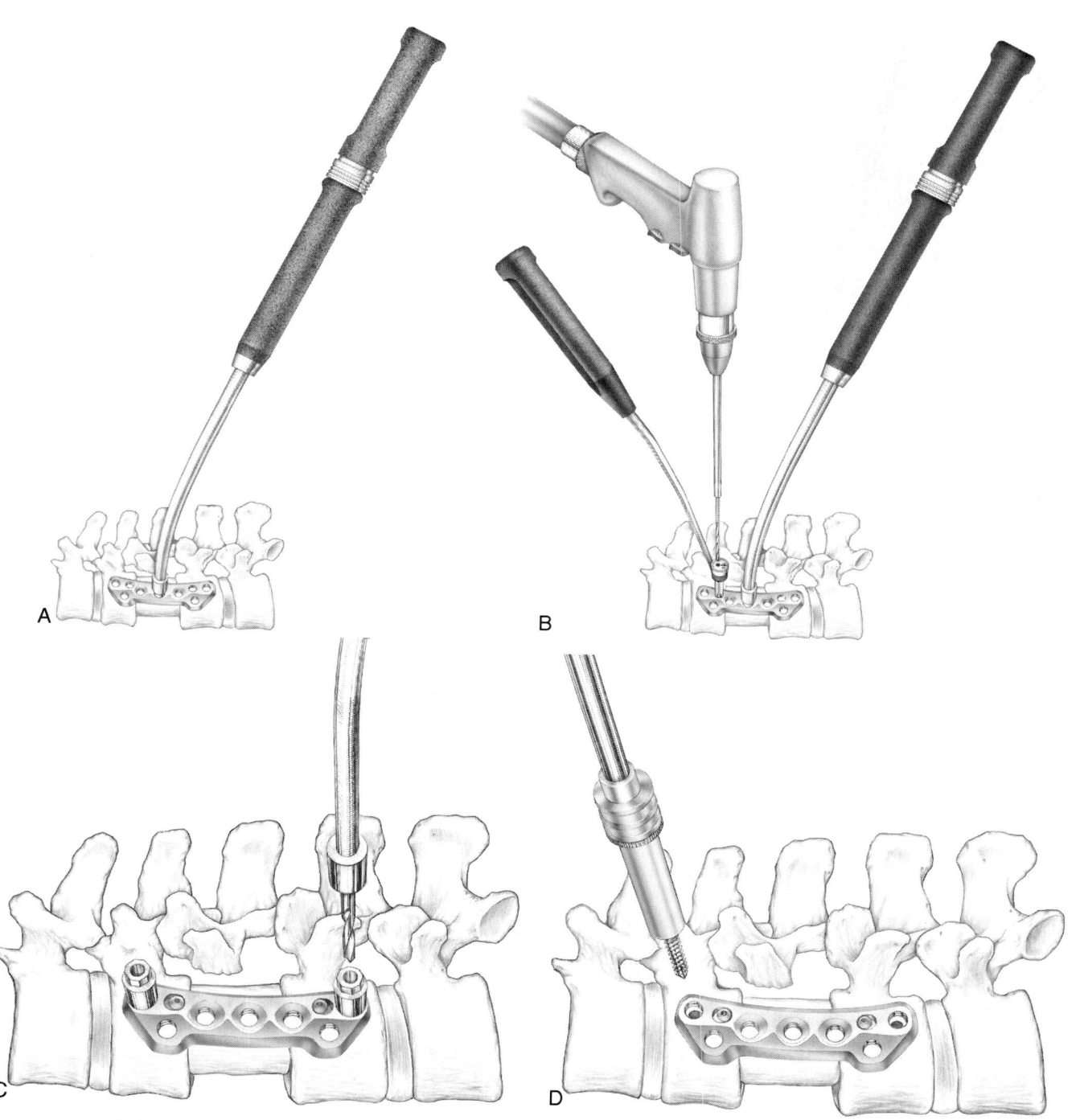

FIGURE 306–21. *A*, The threaded drill-guide applicator is used to hold the Anterior Thoracolumbar Locking Plate (ATLP) on the ventrolateral surface of the vertebral bodies. *B*, Temporary fixation holes are drilled using the drill guide and a 2.5-mm bit with a 30-mm stop. The arrow on the drill guide must point toward the graft site to achieve compression. *C*, The posterior holes are drilled first. *D*, 7.5-mm screws are inserted into the holes. (From VentroFix and Anterior Thoracolumbar Locking Plate technique guides. West Chester, PA, Synthes, 1998. Used with permission of Synthes.)

The threaded drill guide is removed from the center hole and placed into one of the posterior holes. A second drill guide is placed in the opposite posterior hole. A hole is drilled using the 5-mm flexible drill bit with an automatic stop at 30 mm (see Fig. 306–21C). The drill guide is removed, and a 7.5-mm self-tapping anterior spinal locking screw is inserted (see Fig. 306–21D). The screw must be inserted perpendicular to the plate to engage its locking mechanism. The opposite posterior screw is inserted in an identical manner. Once the posterior vertebral body screws are in position, the 4-mm cancellous screws are removed from the DCP holes to allow insertion of the anterior screws. Threaded drill guides are placed into the anterior plate holes. The same sequence used for the posterior screws is used for the anterior screws.

Spine-Tech BAK Interbody Fusion Device

When an interbody fusion cage is to be placed, selection of the correct size implant is critical to obtain optimal results. Radiographic templating helps select the appropriately sized distraction plug and implant to maximize implant–end plate contact, distract the disk space, and place the annulus under tension. Radiographic templates are available from the manufacturer for use with plain radiography, computed tomography, or magnetic resonance imaging. The template provides information on implant and distraction plug size, a magnification and reduction scale, and anteroposterior and lateral representations of the implant and distraction plug. Lateral plain radiographs are used to determine the proper implant length by overlying the lateral implant representations. The reaming depth and implant that can be safely contained within the boundaries of the disk space are chosen. An adjacent normal disk space on the lateral radiograph is used to determine the appropriate distraction plug size (Fig. 306–22A). The sizes of the implant and the distraction plug are then compared using the range chart provided. As a general rule, the implant should be at least 3 mm larger than the distraction plug to obtain proper purchase of the end plates. The final measurement is made with the anteroposterior representations of the implant and an anteroposterior radiograph (see Fig. 306–22B). The largest implant representation contained in the lateral margins is selected. Axial implant images are available for size selection based on either computed tomography or magnetic resonance imaging.

The first step in inserting the fusion implant is to ensure proper alignment with the disk space, which is achieved with the alignment guide (see Fig. 306–22C). A pilot hole is drilled through the alignment guide using an 8-mm drill, and the disk material is removed with pituitary rongeurs or curets (see Fig. 306–22D). The distraction plugs are impacted within the drill holes to distract the vertebral bodies and to tense the annulus (see Fig. 306–22E). The size of the plug and annular tensing are appropriate when significant resistance is encountered while trying to remove the plug. The drill tube is placed over the distraction plug obturator, and the tube's teeth are allowed to engage the superior and inferior end plates. The tube must be perpendicular to the coronal plane of the disk space to achieve the appropriate implant trajectory. Additional disk material is loosened with the reamer and removed with pituitary rongeurs (see Fig. 306–22F). A trial implant is inserted into the disk space, and its position is assessed with a lateral radiograph. The implant is removed, and the hole is tapped with the bone tap (see Fig. 306–22G).

The leading chamber of the selected implant is packed with morcellized bone graft, and the opposite end is attached to the implant driver (see Fig. 306–22H). The orientation of the implant is correct when the driver T-handle is parallel to the disk space. Once inserted, the implant should lie between 3 and 4 mm below the anterior margin of the disk space. The trailing chamber is then packed with bone graft (see Fig. 306–22I). An end cap can be placed over the anterior face of the implant to prevent expulsion of the bone graft. Proper depth is determined through ruled etchings on the sides of the instruments and with intraoperative lateral radiographs.

Under certain circumstances, the insertion technique may be modified. If a spondylolisthesis cannot be reduced, the drill tube and sheath will not sit evenly over the anterior margins of the disk space, and the implant will not lie parallel in the disk space. The anterior margin of the slipped vertebral body must be removed before the drill tube is impacted. If mobilization of the great vessels appears inadequate, a BAK proximity cage can be used to facilitate bilateral implantation. Alternatively, a single implant can be used. If the bone thread is stripped, the next larger sized cage should be implemented to achieve the appropriate purchase. If stripping occurs with the largest available cage (19 mm), a 22-mm bone dowel is available to fill the defect. Finally, any large marginal osteophytes at the location of the drill should be removed.

COMPLICATIONS

Potential complications related to anterior lumbar instrumentation can be divided into major and minor and are classified as visceral, vascular, neurological, and construct related. Complications related to the graft and instrumentation include pseudarthrosis, graft or construct dislodgment, and fracture of individual construct elements. Overall complication rates for anterior spinal fusion have been reported as high as 40%.[162, 163] Major catastrophic complications occur less often.

Vascular injuries have been reported to follow anterior lumbar fusion in about 15% of cases.[164, 165] Such injuries are more common with a rectus incision than with a flank incision.[164] The aorta, inferior vena cava, common iliac vessels, and their associated branches are all at risk. The left-sided approach is favored not only because arterial structures are easier to mobilize than venous structures but also because hemorrhage from an arterial vessel is usually easier to control. Bleeding from either type of vessel should be managed directly and expeditiously. Digital pressure is often the initial

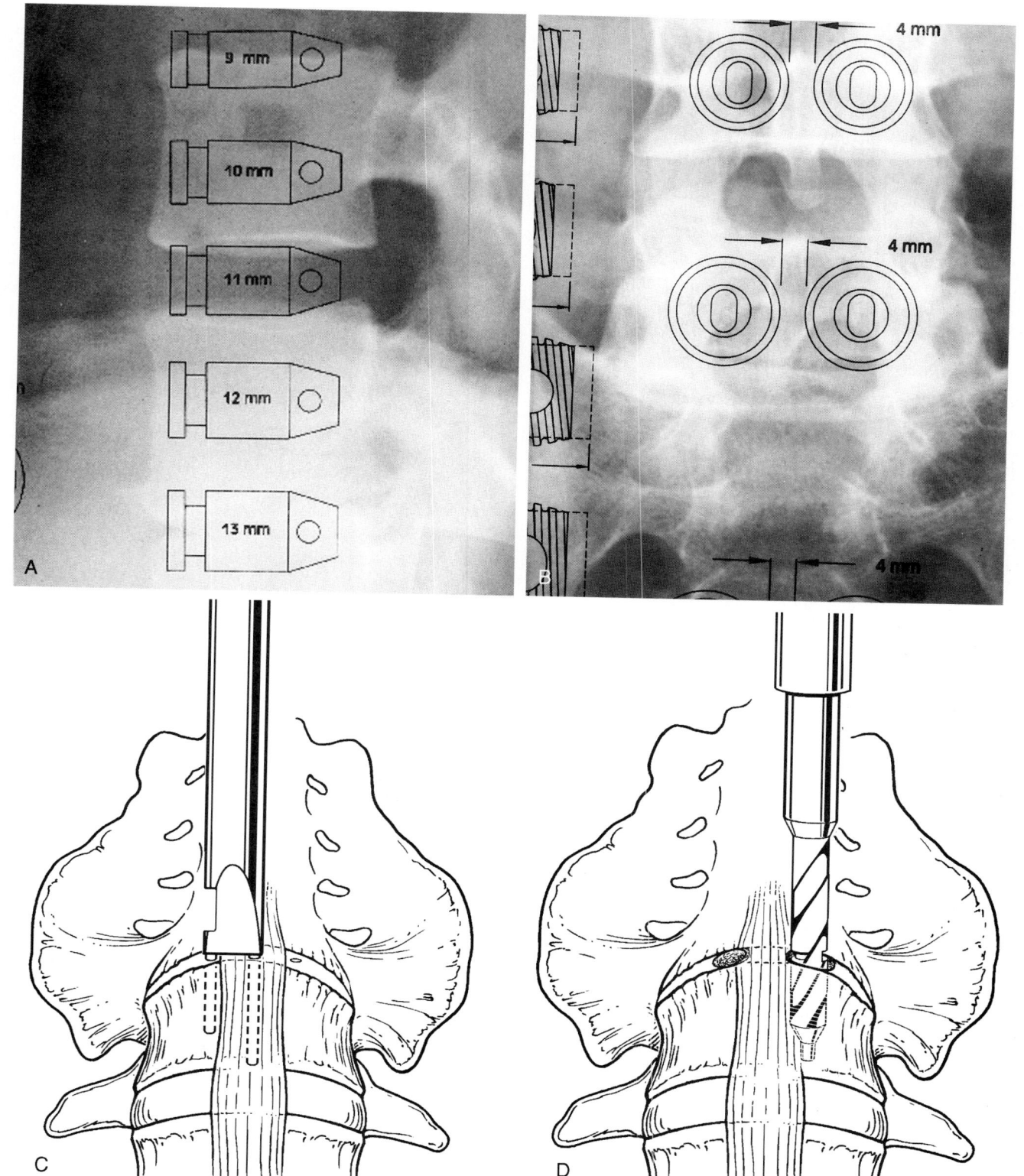

FIGURE 306–22. *A,* The distraction plug overlay is used with a lateral radiograph to determine the proper plug size. *B,* The proper implant diameter is confirmed on an anteroposterior radiograph. *C,* The alignment guide is used to create landmarks for the proper placement of two BAK implants. The longer tip is placed in a midline pilot hole, and the lateral cutting tip is lightly impacted on each side. *D,* The 8-mm drill is used to drill each hole created by the alignment guide. The proper depth is achieved when the groove in the bit is even with the anterior cortex of the spine. A pituitary rongeur or small curet is used to clean each hole.

Illustration continued on following page

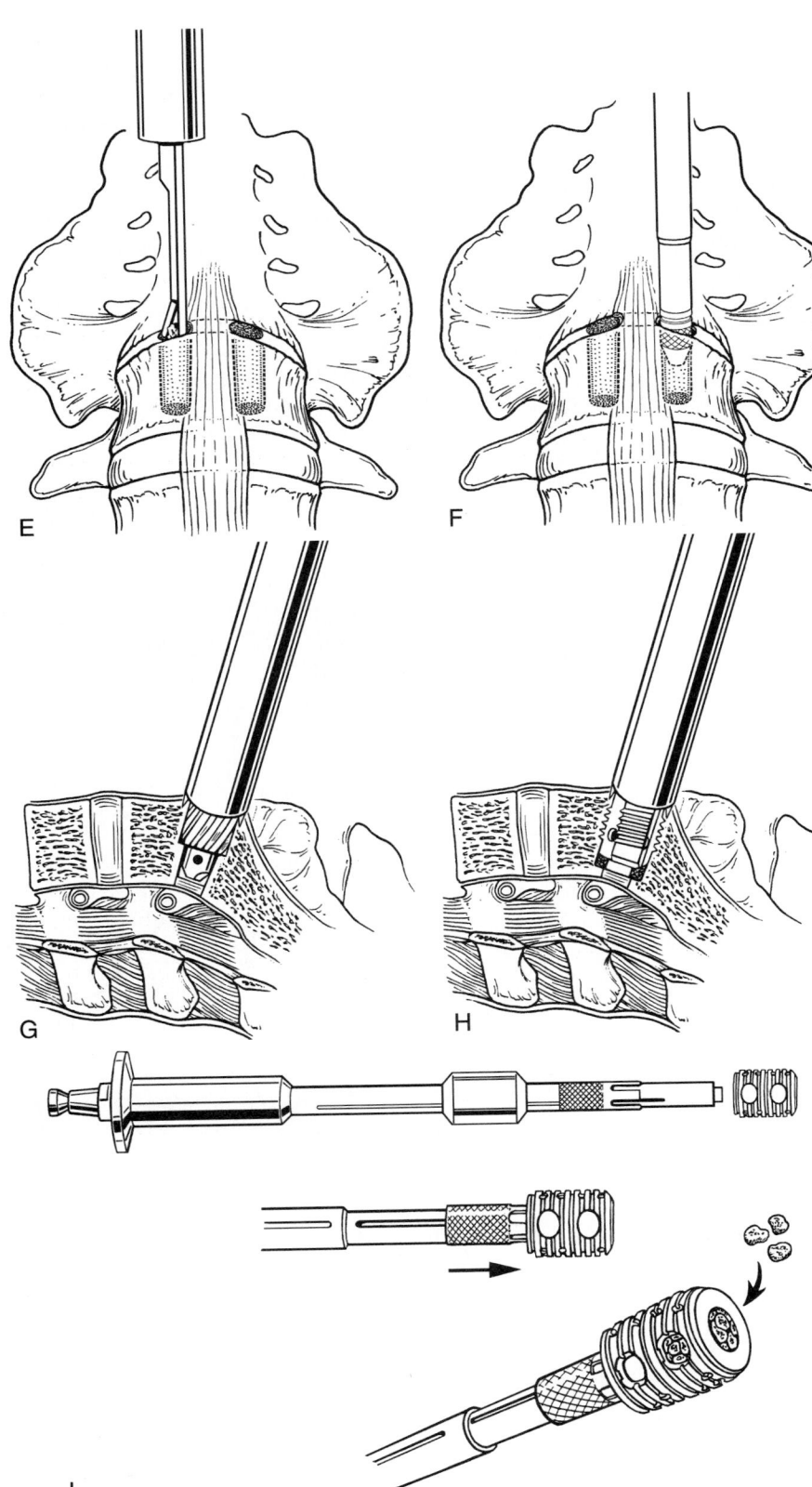

FIGURE 306–22. *Continued. E,* A distraction plug is impacted into one hole. A proper-sized plug gives significant resistance when removal is attempted. *F,* A reamer is used to clean the drilled hole. *G,* The bone tap is used to thread each hole. *H,* The leading chamber and large holes are packed with morcellized autograft bone. *I,* The implant is inserted, with care taken to maintain the same angle as used for drilling and tapping. (Courtesy of Sulzer Spine-Tech, Minneapolis, MN.)

step in controlling a vessel laceration. Temporary hemostatic clamps can also be placed to control bleeding and to allow repair of the defect. Inflammatory, neoplastic, or degenerative processes or adjuvant therapy for neoplastic disease, such as radiation or chemotherapy, may increase scarring around the vessels, making dissection more difficult. Hemorrhage associated with the resection of a vascular neoplasm may be palliated with the use of preoperative embolization. Excessive lateral retraction of the iliac vessels can lead to spasm or thrombosis. If a thrombus occurs, the assistance of a vascular surgeon may be required to perform a thrombectomy.

Most visceral complications consist of bowel and ureter injuries. Bowel perforations, common with a transperitoneal approach, should be repaired by a general surgeon. Inadequate closure can lead to peritonitis, sepsis, or abscess formation. A functional ileus is common after intra-abdominal surgery and typically resolves spontaneously within 2 to 3 days.[166] A mechanical ileus may result if the bowels are not returned to their normal anatomic location. Failure to recognize a mechanical obstruction can compromise blood flow and lead to the devastating consequences of bowel ischemia. The ureter is frequently manipulated during a retroperitoneal approach but is usually lateral to the transperitoneal exposure. Excessive mobilization or traction can lead to injury or fibrosis. If mobilization is required, particularly with a rostral lumbar exposure, a generous cuff of soft tissue should be left surrounding the ureter to preserve blood flow.

Various neurological injuries are associated with an anterior lumbar approach. Sympathetic fibers originating from the L1 and L2 ganglia supply the fibers to the hypogastric plexus, innervating the internal vesicular sphincter. Deinnervation of this sphincter results in retrograde ejaculation, a significant complication in men. The reported incidence of this complication ranges from 5% to 22%.[163, 167, 168] Within 1 to 2 years, function returns completely or partially in as many as a third of these patients. Penile erection is mediated through the parasympathetic plexus and should not be injured when standard anterior approaches are used.[169] If erectile dysfunction is associated with an anterior lumbar procedure, it is usually nonorganic. Injury to the lumbosacral plexus and to the femoral and genitofemoral nerves is possible during dissection or retraction of the psoas muscle; ipsilateral leg weakness or paresthesias result. Decompression and graft insertion can injure the exiting nerve roots and cauda equina, producing lower extremity or bowel and bladder deficits. Careful technique and planning can help avoid such injuries.

FUTURE AND CURRENT INNOVATIONS

Surgical adjuncts such as frameless stereotactic and laparoscopic modalities are now providing advantages over more traditional surgical approaches. These evolving adjuncts should be integrated cautiously into the technical repertoire of practicing neurosurgeons, however. In particular, laparoscopic procedures are associated with a treacherous learning curve that may preclude application of this technique outside spine centers that treat large numbers of patients. Recently, Rodts and colleagues[170] described their experience with 32 patients over a 2-year period who underwent single-level laparoscopic ALIF at the L4-5 or L5-S1 interspace. Patients were treated for degenerative disk disease, degenerative lumbar instability, less than grade II spondylolisthesis, postoperative spinal instability, or pseudarthrosis after attempted posterior fusion. Postoperative complications included one disk space infection that was treated successfully with antibiotics, one nerve root contusion, two iliac vein thromboses that required anticoagulation, and three cases of retrograde ejaculation. In addition, two procedures were converted to open procedures owing to adhesions, and one was converted to an open procedure to facilitate visualization of a spinal deformity. Additional reports in the literature have described success with laparoscopic techniques using anterior approaches.[171–176] As with all innovations, the formal evaluation of these techniques will require multicenter, randomized, prospective trials in a specifically selected group of patients followed by diligent outcome analysis.

CONCLUSION

Ventral instrumentation of the lumbar spine has become a necessary tool for the effective treatment of anterior lumbar pathology. With advances in construct design, contemporary spinal surgeons have an array of instrumentation constructs from which to choose. The decision to use instrumentation and the choice of construct should not be approached in a cavalier manner. A thorough understanding of the appropriate indications, biomechanics, and surgical techniques is required before these implants are used. Practicing surgeons should always consider several questions when contemplating the use of instrumentation constructs: (1) What is the indication for a spinal implant? (2) How has the pathology affected the biomechanics of the spine? (3) What is the appropriate type of construct to restore the integrity of the spine? (4) What is the goal of placing an implant? Surgeons should avoid formulating generalized treatment plans for all pathology of the anterior lumbar spine. Instead, each case should be treated individually. Any attempt at generalizing a treatment plan in this complex arena is sure to result in poor clinical outcomes.

REFERENCES

1. Elsberg C: Diagnosis and Treatment of Surgical Diseases of the Spinal Cord and Its Membranes. Philadelphia, WB Saunders, 1916.
2. Albee F: Transplantation of a portion of the tibia into the spine for Pott's disease: A preliminary report. JAMA 57:885–886, 1911.
3. Hibbs R: An operation for progressive spinal deformities. N Y Med J 93:1013–1016, 1911.
4. Muller W: Transperitoneale Freilegung der Wirbelsaule bei Tuberkuloser Spondylitis. Dtsch Z Chir 85:128–135, 1906.

5. Burns BH: An operation for spondylolisthesis. Lancet 1:1233, 1933.

6. Ito H, Tsuchiya J, Asami G: A new radical operation for Pott's disease: Report of ten cases. J Bone Joint Surg 16:499–515, 1934.

7. Hodgson A, Stock F: A preliminary communication on the radical treatment of Pott's paraplegia. Br J Surg 44:266–275, 1956.

8. Humphries A, Hawk W, Berndt A: Anterior interbody fusion of lumbar vertebrae: A surgical technique. Surg Clin North Am 41:1685–1700, 1961.

9. Dwyer AF, Newton NC, Sherwood AA: An anterior approach to scoliosis: A preliminary report. Clin Orthop 62:192–202, 1969.

10. Boring C, Squires T, Tong T: Cancer statistics 1993. CA Cancer J Clin 43:7–26, 1993.

11. Ebersold M, Hitchon P, Duff J, et al: Primary bony spinal lesions. In Benzel E (ed): Spine Surgery: Techniques, Complication Avoidance, and Management. Philadelphia, Churchill Livingstone, 1999, pp 663–677.

12. Bach F, Larsen BH, Rohde K, et al: Metastatic spinal cord compression: Occurrence, symptoms, clinical presentations and prognosis in 398 patients with spinal cord compression. Acta Neurochir (Wien) 107:37–43, 1990.

13. Byrne TN: Spinal cord compression from epidural metastases. N Engl J Med 327:614–619, 1992.

14. Constans JP, de Divitiis E, Donzelli R, et al: Spinal metastases with neurological manifestations: Review of 600 cases. J Neurosurg 59:111–118, 1983.

15. Malawer M, Delaney T: Treatment of metastatic cancer to bone. In De Vita V, Hellman S, Rosenberg S (eds): Cancer: Principles and Practice of Oncology. Philadelphia, Lippincott-Raven, 1993, pp 2225–2246.

16. Boland PJ, Lane JM, Sundaresan N: Metastatic disease of the spine. Clin Orthop 169:95–102, 1982.

17. Sundaresan N, Digiacinto GV, Hughes JE: Surgical treatment of spinal metastases. Clin Neurosurg 33:503–522, 1986.

18. Sundaresan N, Galicich JH, Bains MS, et al: Vertebral body resection in the treatment of cancer involving the spine. Cancer 53:1393–1396, 1984.

19. Sundaresan N, Galicich JH, Lane JM, et al: Treatment of neoplastic epidural cord compression by vertebral body resection and stabilization. J Neurosurg 63:676–684, 1985.

20. Wong DA, Fornasier VL, MacNab I: Spinal metastases: The obvious, the occult, and the imposters. Spine 15:1–4, 1990.

21. Sundaresan N, Krol G, Digiacinto GV, et al: Metastatic tumor of the spine. In Sundaresan N, Schmiedek H, Schiller A, et al (eds): Tumors of the Spine: Diagnosis and Clinical Management. Philadelphia, WB Saunders, 1990, pp 279–304.

22. Algra PR, Bloem JL, Tissing H, et al: Detection of vertebral metastases: Comparison between MR imaging and bone scintigraphy. Radiographics 11:219–232, 1991.

23. Algra PR, Heimans J, Valk J, et al: Do metastases in vertebrae begin in the body or the pedicles? Imaging study in 45 patients. AJR Am J Roentgenol 158:1275–1279, 1992.

24. Sundaresan N, Krol G, Hughes JE, et al: Tumors of the spine: Diagnosis and management. In Tindall G, Cooper P, Barrow D (eds): The Practice of Neurosurgery. Philadelphia, Williams & Wilkins, 1996, pp 1303–1322.

25. Tillotson C, Rosenthal D: Radiology of spine tumors: General considerations. In Sundaresan N, Schmiedek H, Schiller A, et al (eds): Tumors of the Spine: Diagnosis and Clinical Management. Philadelphia, WB Saunders, 1990, pp 34–45.

26. Boriani S, Campanna R, Donati D, et al: Osteoblastoma of the spine. Clin Orthop 278:37–45, 1992.

27. Arguello F, Baggs RB, Duerst RE, et al: Pathogenesis of vertebral metastasis and epidural spinal cord compression. Cancer 65:98–106, 1990.

28. Batson O: The role of the vertebral veins in metastatic processes. Ann Intern Med 16:38–45, 1942.

29. Berrettoni BA, Carter JR: Mechanisms of cancer metastasis to bone. J Bone Joint Surg Am 68:308–312, 1986.

30. Gilbert RW, Kim JH, Posner JB: Epidural spinal cord compression from metastatic tumor: Diagnosis and treatment. Ann Neurol 3:40–51, 1978.

31. Jaeckle KA, Young DF, Foley KM: The natural history of lumbosacral plexopathy in cancer. Neurology 35:8–15, 1985.

32. Weinstein JN, McLain RF: Primary tumors of the spine. Spine 12:843–851, 1987.

33. Delaney T, Oldfield E, Spinal cord compression. In Devita V, Hellman S, Rosenberg S (eds): Cancer: Principles and Practice of Oncology. Philadelphia, Lippincott-Raven, 1993, pp 2118–2128.

34. Siegal T: Current considerations in the management of neoplastic spinal cord compression. Spine 14:223–228, 1989.

35. Fornasier VL, Horne JG: Metastases to the vertebral column. Cancer 36:590–594, 1975.

36. Grant R, Papadopoulos SM, Greenberg HS: Metastatic epidural spinal cord compression. Neurol Clin 9:825–841, 1991.

37. Sorensen S, Borgesen SE, Rohde K, et al: Metastatic epidural spinal cord compression: Results of treatment and survival. Cancer 65:1502–1508, 1990.

38. Maranzano E, Latini P, Checcaglini F, et al: Radiation therapy in metastatic spinal cord compression: A prospective analysis of 105 consecutive patients. Cancer 67:1311–1317, 1991.

39. Solini A, Paschero B, Orsini G, et al: The surgical treatment of metastatic tumours of the lumbar spine. Ital J Orthop Traumatol 11:427–442, 1985.

40. Cooper PR, Errico TJ, Martin R, et al: A systematic approach to spinal reconstruction after anterior decompression for neoplastic disease of the thoracic and lumbar spine. Neurosurgery 32:1–8, 1993.

41. Black P: Spinal metastasis: Current status and recommended guidelines for management. Neurosurgery 5:726–746, 1979.

42. Sundaresan N, Digiacinto GV, Hughes JE, et al: Treatment of neoplastic spinal cord compression: Results of a prospective study. Neurosurgery 29:645–650, 1991.

43. Cybulski GR: Methods of surgical stabilization for metastatic disease of the spine. Neurosurgery 25:240–252, 1989.

44. Kostuik J, Weinstein JN: Differential diagnosis and surgical treatment of metastatic spine tumors. In Frymoyer J (ed): The Adult Spine: Principles and Practice. Philadelphia, Raven, 1991, pp 861–888.

45. DeWald RL, Bridwell KH, Prodromas C, et al: Reconstructive spinal surgery as palliation for metastatic malignancies of the spine. Spine 10:21–26, 1985.

46. Barcena A, Lobato RD, Rivas JJ, et al: Spinal metastatic disease: Analysis of factors determining functional prognosis and the choice of treatment. Neurosurgery 15:820–827, 1984.

47. Tokuhashi Y, Matsuzaki H, Toriyama S, et al: Scoring system for the preoperative evaluation of metastatic spine tumor prognosis. Spine 15:1110–1113, 1990.

48. Fidler MW: Anterior decompression and stabilisation of metastatic spinal fractures. J Bone Joint Surg Br 68:83–90, 1986.

49. Kostuik JP: Anterior spinal cord decompression for lesions of the thoracic and lumbar spine: Techniques, new methods of internal fixation, results. Spine 8:512–531, 1983.

50. Loquet E, Thibaut R, Thibaut H, et al: Surgical treatment of spinal metastases. Acta Orthop Belg 59:79–82, 1993.

51. Onimus M, Schraub S, Bertin D, et al: Surgical treatment of vertebral metastasis. Spine 11:883–891, 1986.

52. Overby MC, Rothman AS: Anterolateral decompression for metastatic epidural spinal cord tumors: Results of a modified costotransversectomy approach. J Neurosurg 62:344–348, 1985.

53. Siegal T: Surgical decompression of anterior and posterior malignant epidural tumors compressing the spinal cord: A prospective study. Neurosurgery 17:424–432, 1985.

54. Siegal T, Tiqva P: Vertebral body resection for epidural compression by malignant tumors: Results of forty-seven consecutive operative procedures. J Bone Joint Surg Am 67:375–382, 1985.

55. Arbit E, Galicich JH: Vertebral body reconstruction with a modified Harrington rod distraction system for stabilization of the spine affected with metastatic disease. J Neurosurg 83:617–620, 1995.

56. Muhlbauer M, Pfisterer W, Eyb R, et al: Minimally invasive retroperitoneal approach for lumbar corpectomy and anterior reconstruction: Technical note. J Neurosurg 93:161–167, 2000.

57. McAfee PC, Zdeblick TA: Tumors of the thoracic and lumbar spine: Surgical treatment via the anterior approach. J Spinal Disord 2:145–154, 1989.

58. Kattapuram S, Rosenthal D: Percutaneous needle biopsy of the spine. In Sundaresan N, Schmiedek H (eds): Tumors of the Spine: Diagnosis and Clinical Management. Philadelphia, WB Saunders, 1990, pp 46–51.

59. Bridwell KH: Treatment of metastatic prostate cancer of the spine. Urol Clin North Am 18:153–159, 1991.
60. Martenson JA Jr, Evans RG, Lie MR, et al: Treatment outcome and complications in patients treated for malignant epidural spinal cord compression (SCC). J Neurooncol 3:77–84, 1985.
61. Sundaresan N, Bains M, McCormack P: Surgical treatment of spinal cord compression in patients with lung cancer. Neurosurgery 16:350–356, 1985.
62. An HS, Simpson JM, Ebraheim NA, et al: Low lumbar burst fractures: Comparison between conservative and surgical treatments. Orthopedics 15:367–373, 1992.
63. Levine AM, Edwards CC: Low lumbar burst fractures: Reduction and stabilization using the modular spine fixation system. Orthopedics 11:1427–1432, 1988.
64. Denis F: Spinal instability as defined by the three-column spine concept in acute spinal trauma. Clin Orthop 189:65–76, 1984.
65. Levine A: Classification of spinal injury. In Levine A, Eismont F, Garfin S, et al (eds): Spine Trauma. Philadelphia, WB Saunders, 1998, pp 123–132.
66. McAfee PC, Yuan HA, Fredrickson BE, et al: The value of computed tomography in thoracolumbar fractures: An analysis of one hundred consecutive cases and a new classification. J Bone Joint Surg Am 65:461–473, 1983.
67. Magerl F, Aebi M, Gertzbein SD, et al: A comprehensive classification of thoracic and lumbar injuries. Eur Spine J 3:184–201, 1994.
68. McCormack T, Karaikovic E, Gaines RW: The load sharing classification of spine fractures. Spine 19:1741–1744, 1994.
69. Keenen TL, Antony J, Benson DR: Non-contiguous spinal fractures. J Trauma 30:489–491, 1990.
70. Calenoff L, Chessare JW, Rogers LF, et al: Multiple level spinal injuries: Importance of early recognition. AJR Am J Roentgenol 130:665–669, 1978.
71. Bohlman HH: Treatment of fractures and dislocations of the thoracic and lumbar spine. J Bone Joint Surg Am 67:165–169, 1985.
72. Brown G: Bone resorption in the canal following a thoracolumbar fracture with a displaced diaphyseal fragment. Iowa Orthop 9:69–71, 1989.
73. Willen J, Lindahl S, Nordwall A: Unstable thoracolumbar fractures: A comparative clinical study of conservative treatment and Harrington instrumentation. Spine 10:111–122, 1985.
74. Dunn HK: Anterior spine stabilization and decompression for thoracolumbar injuries. Orthop Clin North Am 17:113–119, 1986.
75. Jacobs RR, Casey MP: Surgical management of thoracolumbar spinal injuries: General principles and controversial considerations. Clin Orthop 189:22–35, 1984.
76. Denis F, Armstrong GW, Searls K, et al: Acute thoracolumbar burst fractures in the absence of neurologic deficit: A comparison between operative and nonoperative treatment. Clin Orthop 189:142–149, 1984.
77. Ferguson RL, Allen BL Jr: An algorithm for the treatment of unstable thoracolumbar fractures. Orthop Clin North Am 17:105–112, 1986.
78. Kostuik JP: Anterior fixation for fractures of the thoracic and lumbar spine with or without neurologic involvement. Clin Orthop 189:103–115, 1984.
79. Krompinger WJ, Frederickson BE, Mino DE, et al: Conservative treatment of fractures of the thoracic and lumbar spine. Orthop Clin North Am 17:161–170, 1986.
80. DeWald RL: Burst fractures of the thoracic and lumbar spine. Clin Orthop 189:150–161, 1984.
81. Weitzman G: Treatment of stable thoracolumbar spine compression fractures by early ambulation. Clin Orthop 76:116–122, 1971.
82. Roy-Camille R, Saillant G, Mazel C: Plating of thoracic, thoracolumbar, and lumbar injuries with pedicle screw plates. Orthop Clin North Am 17:147–159, 1986.
83. Panjabi MM, Oxland TR, Kifune M, et al: Validity of the three-column theory of thoracolumbar fractures: A biomechanic investigation. Spine 20:1122–1127, 1995.
84. James KS, Wenger KH, Schlegel JD, et al: Biomechanical evaluation of the stability of thoracolumbar burst fractures. Spine 19:1731–1740, 1994.
85. Fredrickson BE, Yuan HA, Miller H: Burst fractures of the fifth lumbar vertebra: A report of four cases. J Bone Joint Surg Am 64:1088–1094, 1982.
86. Stauffer E: Thoracolumbar spine fractures without neurological deficit. Monograph series, American Academy of Orthopedic Surgeons, 1993.
87. Holdsworth F: Fractures, dislocations, and fracture-dislocations of the spine. J Bone Joint Surg Am 52:1534–1551, 1970.
88. Wang J, Delamarter R: Lumbar fractures of the spine. In Capen D, Haye W (eds): Comprehensive Management of Spine Trauma. Philadelphia, CV Mosby, 1998, pp 214–234.
89. Spivak JM, Vaccaro AR, Cotler JM: Thoracolumbar spine trauma. I. Evaluation and classification. J Am Acad Orthop Surg 3:345–352, 1995.
90. Wagner FC Jr, Chehrazi B: Early decompression and neurological outcome in acute cervical spinal cord injuries. J Neurosurg 56:699–705, 1982.
91. Benzel E: Stability and instability of the spine. In Benzel E (ed): Biomechanics of Spine Stabilization: Principles and Clinical Practice. New York, McGraw-Hill, 1995, pp 25–38.
92. Brown HA, Pont ME: Disease of lumbar discs: Ten years of surgical treatment. J Neurosurg 20:410–417, 1963.
93. Fager CA, Freidberg SR: Analysis of failures and poor results of lumbar spine surgery. Spine S:87–94, 1980.
94. Long DM, Filtzer DL, BenDebba M, et al: Clinical features of the failed-back syndrome. J Neurosurg 69:61–71, 1988.
95. Long DM: Failed back surgery syndrome. Neurosurg Clin N Am 2:899–919, 1991.
96. Spengler DM, Freeman C, Westbrook R, et al: Low-back pain following multiple lumbar spine procedures: Failure of initial selection? Spine 5:356–360, 1980.
97. Oxland T, Kuslich S, Kohrs D, et al: The BAK interbody fusion system: Biomechanical rationale and early clinical results. In Margulies J, et al (eds): Lumbosacral and Spinopelvic Fixation. Philadelphia, Lippincott-Raven, 1996, pp 545–561.
98. Dickman CA: Internal fixation and fusion of the lumbar spine using threaded interbody cages. BNI Q 13:4–25, 1997.
99. Leong JC, Chow SP, Yau AC: Titanium-mesh block replacement of the intervertebral disk. Clin Orthop 300:52–63, 1994.
100. Enker P, Steffee AD: Interbody fusion and instrumentation. Clin Orthop 300:90–101, 1994.
101. Brantigan JW, Steffee AD: A carbon fiber implant to aid interbody lumbar fusion: Two-year clinical results in the first 26 patients. Spine 18:2106–2107, 1993.
102. Watkins R: Assessment of results and complications of anterior lumbar fusion. In Lin P, Gill K (eds): Lumbar Interbody Fusion. Rockville, MD, Aspen, 1989, pp 153–169.
103. Stauffer RN, Coventry MB: Anterior interbody lumbar spine fusion: Analysis of Mayo Clinic series. J Bone Joint Surg Am 54:756–768, 1972.
104. Sacks S: Anterior interbody fusion of the lumbar spine: Indications and results in 200 cases. Clin Orthop 44:163–170, 1966.
105. Sacks S: Anterior interbody fusion of the lumbar spine. J Bone Joint Surg Br 47:211–223, 1965.
106. Leong J: Anterior interbody fusion. In Lin P, Gill K (eds): Lumbar Interbody Fusion. Rockville, MD, Aspen, 1989, pp 133–148.
107. Flynn JC, Hoque MA: Anterior fusion of the lumbar spine: End-result study with long-term follow-up. J Bone Joint Surg Am 61:1143–1150, 1979.
108. Freebody D, Bendall R, Taylor RD: Anterior transperitoneal lumbar fusion. J Bone Joint Surg Br 53:617–627, 1971.
109. Crock HV: Anterior lumbar interbody fusion: Indications for its use and notes on surgical technique. Clin Orthop 165:157–163, 1982.
110. Loguidice VA, Johnson RG, Guyer RD, et al: Anterior lumbar interbody fusion. Spine 13:366–369, 1988.
111. Chow SP, Leong JC, Ma A, et al: Anterior spinal fusion or deranged lumbar intervertebral disc. Spine 5:452–458, 1980.
112. Oxland TR, Lund T, Jost B, et al: The relative importance of vertebral bone density and disc degeneration in spinal flexibility and interbody implant performance: An in vitro study. Spine 21:2558–2569, 1996.
113. Collis J, Rojas C, Janack M: Anterior total disc replacement: A modified anterior lumbar interbody fusion. In Lin P, Gill K (eds): Lumbar Interbody Fusion. Rockville, MD, Aspen, 1989, pp 149–152.

114. Gill K: Technique and complications of anterior lumbar interbody fusion. In Lin P, Gill K (eds): Lumbar Interbody Fusion. Rockville, MD, Aspen, 1989, pp 95–106.

115. Watkins R: Anterior approaches to the lumbar spine. In Torres M, Dickson R (eds): Operative Spinal Surgery. New York, Churchill Livingstone, 1991, pp 161–171.

116. Hitchon PW, Osenbach RK, Yuh WT, et al: Spinal infections. Clin Neurosurg 38:373–387, 1992.

117. Hulme A, Dott M: Spinal epidural abscess. BJM 1:64–68, 1958.

118. Baker AS, Ojemann RJ, Swartz MN, et al: Spinal epidural abscess. N Engl J Med 293:463–468, 1975.

119. Cahill DW: Pyogenic infections of the spine. In Menezes AH, Sonntag VKH (eds): Principles of Spinal Surgery. New York, McGraw-Hill, 1996, pp 1453–1465.

120. Vincent K, Benson DR: Differential diagnosis and conservative treatment of infectious disease. In Frymoyer J (ed): The Adult Spine: Principles and Practice. New York, Raven, 1991, pp 763–785.

121. Zeidman S, Ducker T: Infectious complications of spine surgery. In Benzel E (ed): Spine Surgery: Techniques, Complication Avoidance, and Management. New York, Churchill Livingstone, 1999, pp 1445–1457.

122. Sridhar K, Ramamurthi B: Granulomatous fungal and parasitic infections of the spine. In Menezes AH, Sonntag VKH (eds): Principles of Spinal Surgery. New York, McGraw-Hill, 1996, pp 1467–1495.

123. Berry JL, Moran JM, Berg WS, et al: A morphometric study of human lumbar and selected thoracic vertebrae. Spine 12:362–367, 1987.

124. Benzel EH: Biomechanically relevant anatomy and material properties of the spine and associated elements. In Benzel EH (ed): Biomechanics of Spine Stabilization: Principles and Clinical Practice. New York, McGraw-Hill, 1995, pp 3–16.

125. McCormack B, Maher D, Fessler RG: Anterior approaches to the lumbar spine. In Menezes AH, Sonntag VKH (eds): Principles of Spinal Surgery. New York, McGraw-Hill, 1996, pp 1293–1306.

126. Kirkaldy-Willis WH, Thomas TG: Anterior approaches in the diagnosis and treatment of infections of the vertebral bodies. J Bone Joint Surg Am 47:87–110, 1965.

127. Blumenthal SL, Baker J, Dossett A, et al: The role of anterior lumbar fusion for internal disc disruption. Spine 13:566–569, 1988.

128. Sturgill M, Fessler RG, Woodard E: The lumbar and sacral spine. In Benzel EH (ed): Spine Surgery: Techniques, Complication Avoidance, and Management. Philadelphia, Churchill Livingstone, 1999, pp 169–191.

129. Harmon P: Anterior extraperitoneal lumbar disk excision and vertebral body fusion. Clin Orthop 18:169–184, 1960.

130. White AA, Panjabi M: Clinical Biomechanics of the Spine. Philadelphia, Lippincott Williams & Wilkins, 1990.

131. Louis R: Spinal stability as defined by the three-column spine concept. Anat Clin 7:33–42, 1985.

132. Kelly RP, Whitesides TE Jr: Treatment of lumbodorsal fracture-dislocations. Ann Surg 167:705–717, 1968.

133. Holdsworth F: Fractures, dislocations, and fracture dislocations of the spine. J Bone Joint Surg Br 45:6–20, 1963.

134. Bailey RW: Fractures and dislocations of the cervical spine: Orthopedic and neurosurgical aspects. Postgrad Med 35:588–599, 1964.

135. Benzel EH: Qualitative attributes of spinal implants. In Benzel EH (ed): Biomechanics of Spine Stabilization: Principles and Clinical Practice. New York, McGraw-Hill, 1995, pp 135–150.

136. Benzel EH: Anterior spinal neutral and distraction fixation. In Benzel EH (ed): Biomechanics of Spine Stabilization: Principles and Clinical Practice. New York, McGraw-Hill, 1995, pp 177–181.

137. Benzel EH: Anterior cantilever beam fixation and related techniques. In Benzel EH (ed): Biomechanics of Spine Stabilization: Principles and Clinical Practice. New York, McGraw-Hill, 1995, pp 187–189.

138. Benzel EH: Mechanical quantitative attributes of spinal implants: Construct types. In Benzel EH (ed): Biomechanics of Spine Stabilization: Principles and Clinical Practice. New York, McGraw-Hill, 1995, pp 151–162.

139. Benzel EH: Anterior spinal compression (tension-band) fixation. In Benzel EH (ed): Biomechanics of Spine Stabilization: Principles and Clinical Practice. New York, McGraw-Hill, 1995, pp 183–186.

140. Aydin E, Solak AS, Tuzuner MM, et al: Z-plate instrumentation in thoracolumbar spinal fractures. Bull Hosp Jt Dis 58:92–97, 1999.

141. Ghanayem AJ, Zdeblick TA: Anterior instrumentation in the management of thoracolumbar burst fractures. Clin Orthop 335:89–100, 1997.

142. Kaneda K: Kaneda anterior spinal instrumentation for the thoracic and lumbar spine. In An HS, Cotler JM (eds): Spinal Instrumentation. Baltimore, Williams & Wilkins, 1992, pp 413–433.

143. Thalgott JS, Kabins MB, Timlin M, et al: Four year experience with the AO anterior thoracolumbar locking plate. Spinal Cord 35:286–291, 1997.

144. Ray CD: Threaded titanium cages for lumbar interbody fusions. Spine 22:667–680, 1997.

145. Kuslich SD, Danielson G, Dowdle JD, et al: Four-year follow-up results of lumbar spine arthrodesis using the Bagby and Kuslich lumbar fusion. Spine 25:2656–2662, 2000.

146. Kaneda K, Abumi K, Fujiya M: Burst fractures with neurologic deficits of the thoracolumbar-lumbar spine: Results of anterior decompression and stabilization with anterior instrumentation. Spine 9:788–795, 1984.

147. Aebi M, Thalgott JS, Webb J: AO ASIF Principles in Spine Surgery. Berlin, Springer-Verlag, 1998.

148. Evans JH: Biomechanics of lumbar fusion. Clin Orthop 193:38–46, 1985.

149. Dickman CA, Maric Z: The biology of bone healing and techniques of spinal fusion. BNI Q 10:2–12, 1994.

150. Ray CD: Spinal interbody fusions: A review, featuring new generation techniques. Neurosurg Q 7:135–156, 1997.

151. Benzel EH: Spinal fusion. In Benzel EH (ed): Biomechanics of Spine Stabilization: Principles and Clinical Practice. New York, McGraw-Hill, 1995, pp 103–108.

152. Goel VK, Kim YE, Lim TH, et al: An analytical investigation of the mechanics of spinal instrumentation. Spine 13:1003–1011, 1988.

153. Chen T, Maiman D: Anterior lumbar fusions. Tech Neurosurg 4:256–264, 1998.

154. Lazennec JY, Pouzet B, Ramare S, et al: Possibilities of anterior approach to the lumbar spine by minimal retroperitoneal access: Anatomical bases. Technical principles and initial results [French]. Chirurgie 122:468–477, 1997.

155. Ogon M, Maurer H, Wimmer C, et al: Minimally invasive approach and surgical procedures in the lumbar spine [German]. Orthopade 26:553–561, 1997.

156. Newman MH, Grinstead GL: Anterior lumbar interbody fusion for internal disc disruption. Spine 17:831–833, 1992.

157. Dickman CA, Sonntag VKH, Russell JC: The laparoscopic approach for instrumentation and fusion of the lumbar spine. BNI Q 13:26–36, 1997.

158. Mahvi DM, Zdeblick TA: A prospective study of laparoscopic spinal fusion: Technique and operative complications. Ann Surg 224:85–90, 1996.

159. Mayer HM: A new microsurgical technique for minimally invasive anterior lumbar interbody fusion. Spine 22:698–700, 1997.

160. Regan JJ, Yuan H, McAfee PC: Laparoscopic fusion of the lumbar spine: Minimally invasive spine surgery. A prospective multicenter study evaluating open and laparoscopic lumbar fusion. Spine 24:402–411, 1999.

161. Zdeblick TA, Ulschmid S, Dick J: The surgical treatment of L5-S1 degenerative disc disease: A prospective randomized study. Paper presented at the 10th Annual Meeting of the North American Spine Society, Oct 18–21, 1995, Washington, DC, p 168.

162. Faciszewski T, Winter RB, Lonstein JE, et al: The surgical and medical perioperative complications of anterior spinal fusion surgery in the thoracic and lumbar spine in adults: A review of 1223 procedures. Spine 20:1592–1599, 1995.

163. Rajaraman V, Vingan R, Roth P, et al: Visceral and vascular complications resulting from anterior lumbar interbody fusion. J Neurosurg 91:60–64, 1999.

164. Westfall SH, Akbarnia BA, Merenda JT, et al: Exposure of the anterior spine: Technique, complications, and results in 85 patients. Am J Surg 154:700–704, 1987.

165. Baker JK, Reardon PR, Reardon MJ, et al: Vascular injury in anterior lumbar surgery. Spine 18:2227–2230, 1993.

166. Sicard GA, Reilly JM, Rubin BG, et al: Transabdominal versus retroperitoneal incision for abdominal aortic surgery: Report of a prospective randomized trial. J Vasc Surg 21:174–181, 1995.

167. Inoue S, Watanabe T, Hirose A, et al: Anterior discectomy and interbody fusion for lumbar disc herniation: A review of 350 cases. Clin Orthop 183:22–31, 1984.

168. Tiusanen H, Seitsalo S, Osterman K, et al: Retrograde ejaculation after anterior interbody lumbar fusion. Eur Spine J 4:339–342, 1995.

169. Johnson RM, McGuire EJ: Urogenital complications of anterior approaches to the lumbar spine. Clin Orthop 154:114–118, 1981.

170. Rodts G, McLaughlin M, Zhang J, et al: Laparoscopic anterior lumbar interbody fusion. Proc Cong Neurol Surgeons 47:541–556, 1999.

171. Hannon JK, Faircloth WB, Lane DR, et al: Comparison of insufflation versus retractional technique for laparoscopic-assisted intervertebral fusion of the lumbar spine. Surg Endosc 14:300–304, 2000.

172. Bhatnagar MK, Mathur SK, Mess CF: Laparoscopic spinal fusion. Md Med J 48:161–164, 1999.

173. Hawasli A, Thusay M, Elskens DP, et al: Laparoscopic anterior lumbar fusion. J Laparoendosc Adv Surg Tech A 10:21–25, 2000.

174. Lieberman IH, Willsher PC, Litwin DE, et al: Transperitoneal laparoscopic exposure for lumbar interbody fusion. Spine 25:509–515, 2000.

175. Zdeblick TA, David SM: A prospective comparison of surgical approach for anterior L4-L5 fusion: Laparoscopic versus mini anterior lumbar interbody fusion. Spine 25:2682–2687, 2000.

176. Cowles RA, Taheri PA, Sweeney JF, et al: Efficacy of the laparoscopic approach for anterior lumbar spinal fusion. Surgery 128:589–596, 2000.

CHAPTER 307

Posterior Lumbar Instrumentation

PAUL TOLENTINO ■ RICHARD G. FESSLER

Lumbar spinal fusion provides stabilization of a mobile and unstable lumbar spinal level, increasing the load that the fused spinal level can bear and improving the quality of life of the patient. Instability can be caused by degenerative, traumatic, infectious, or malignant diseases affecting the vertebral bodies, intervertebral disks, facet joints, or ligamentous structures. Instrumentation to augment spinal fusion of the lumbar spine has been used for decades. The techniques have evolved over time, and the indications continue to be a topic of considerable study and debate. The goal of this chapter is to review the indications for lumbar spinal instrumentation, discuss the outcomes for different clinical diseases, and review techniques of decompression, fusion, and stabilization.

INDICATIONS FOR INSTRUMENTATION

Instrumentation of the lumbar spine has neurologic and orthopedic goals. Neurologic goals include minimization of ongoing injury, spinal cord decompression, and functional recovery. Orthopedic goals include mechanical spinal stability, correction of malalignment and deformity, and remedy or prevention of pseudoarthrosis. The surgeon must also consider the length of hospitalization, patient rehabilitation, and pain relief associated with the procedure.[1]

Trauma

Lumbar spine trauma often manifests with indications for spinal stabilization. Denis[2] and McAfee and colleagues[3] devised models for describing different types of spine injuries and their impact on spine stability. Trauma that results in two- or three-column injury or injury to the posterior ligamentous complex is sufficiently unstable to require surgical stabilization (Table 307–1).[2, 3]

Degenerative Disease

Frymoyer and Selby[4] developed a classification scheme for defining the different degenerative processes (i.e., primary degenerative disease and fixed deformity) and provided criteria for fusion. Primary degenerative disease is divided into translational instability, retrolisthetic instability, torsional instability, disk disruption, and scoliosis. Indications for surgery vary for different conditions:

1. Translational instability: forward displacement seen on a plain, standing radiograph; persistent or recurrent low back pain or lumbar claudication; relatively preserved disk space; minimal bridging osteophytes; and more than 8 degrees of motion on flexion-extension
2. Retrolisthetic instability: posterior displacement seen on a standing radiograph, increased and decreased deformity during flexion and extension seen on radiographs, and lateral recess symptoms
3. Torsional instability: criteria similar to those for translational instability, but including spinous process malalignment and myelographic *pedicle-to-pedicle defect*
4. Disk degeneration: recurrent disk herniation and diskographic disk disruption with reproduction of symptoms
5. Degenerative scoliosis: progression of the scoliotic curve; increased symptoms of stenosis; translation seen on a lateral, standing radiograph; rotational deformity; and potentially destabilizing surgery

Hanley[5] further reviewed the indications for lumbar spinal fusion and instrumentation, including the role of fusion for isthmic spondylolisthesis. Indications for fusion of isthmic spondylolisthesis include persistence of painful mechanical or neurological symptoms in children after an appropriate course of nonoperative management, progression and symptoms in children with more than 33% slippage, initial presentation of a symptomatic slip of more than 50%, and persistent symptoms of back pain or neurological symptoms in adults not associated with psychosocial or work-related issues.

Osteomyelitis

Spinal stabilization may be necessary when osteomyelitis erodes more than 50% of the vertebral body or when aggressive débridement would result in an unstable spine. Traditionally, débridement and stabilization

TABLE 307-1 ■ **Characteristics of Spinal Fracture Models**

FRACTURE TYPES		SPINAL COLUMN FAILURE			STABILITY	
Denis	McAfee	Anterior	Middle	Posterior	Denis	McAfee
Wedge compression		F			Stable	Stable
Seat belt	Chance		F	F	Unstable	Stable
	Flexion-distraction	F	F	F		Unstable
Burst	Stable burst	F	F		Unstable	Stable
	Unstable burst	F	F	F		Unstable
Fracture-dislocation	Transitional injury	F	F	F	Unstable	Unstable

F, fracture. Data from Denis F: The three column spine and its significance in the classification of acute thoracolumbar spine injuries. Spine 8:817–831, 1983, and from McAfee PC, Yuan HA, Fredrickson BE, et al: The value of computed tomography in thoracolumbar fractures: An analysis of one hundred consecutive cases and a new classification. J Bone Joint Surg Am 65:461–473, 1983.

were performed as separate procedures. Later, anterior débridement with autograft fusion was performed with good results. However, in a prospective study, Krodel and associates[6] demonstrated that dorsal extrafocal stabilization could be performed in conjunction with anterior débridement and fusion. After an average follow-up period of 22 months, solid bony fusion was achieved in all 33 patients, with only 2 patients showing failure of screw-rod connections. This allowed rehabilitation and earlier ambulation without a brace, improving recovery.

Similar findings supporting same-day sequential or simultaneous anterior decompression and posterior stabilization using transpedicular screw fixation were described by Safran and coworkers.[7] In their study, 10 patients underwent sequential or simultaneous anterior decompression with posterior stabilization for vertebral osteomyelitis. One patient required a second surgical procedure because of expulsion of the bone graft and instrumentation pullout. Thirty months after surgery, all patients regained motor function, and all had correction of their kyphotic deformity.

Tumor

Primary and metastatic spinal tumors can cause instability, pain, deformity, and neurologic deficits. The goal of surgery is to alleviate pain, provide stability, and achieve decompression of neural elements. An anterior, posterior, or combined approach may be chosen. The decision is largely based on the location of the disease and the patient's medical condition.[8, 9]

A study using a calf spine corpectomy model compared different techniques of spinal instrumentation in restoring stability after destruction of the anterior and middle columns.[10] The goal of surgical treatment is to restore spinal stability while decompressing the neural elements. This study concluded that a cross-linked, rectangular, anterior Texas Scottish Rite Hospital (TSRH) construct and a combined construct of posterior segmental Luque rods with a cross-linked anterior TSRH construct were able to restore axial, sagittal, and torsional stiffness approaching control levels.

RADIOGRAPHIC STUDIES

Initial radiographic evaluation of the lumbar spine usually includes anteroposterior and lateral lumbosacral spine films. Radiographs may show evidence of degenerative disk changes and abnormalities of the posterior facet joints, end plates, or vertebral bodies that suggest congenital, neoplastic, infectious, metabolic, spondylolisthetic, or traumatic lesions.[11] If spondylolysis is suspected, oblique views may be obtained. However, if the oblique views are difficult to interpret, a bone scan may be useful in establishing a diagnosis of acute spondylolysis.[12] A bone scan may also aid in the diagnosis of infection or malignancy. To evaluate spondylolisthesis and monitor progression of disease, standing, lateral-view radiographs and flexion-extension films may prove useful.[11]

Myelography is useful in characterizing disease of the lumbar spine, especially for the diagnosis of lumbar stenosis and herniated nucleus propulsus.[13] Myelography can identify the effects of extradural, intradural, and intramedullary lesions on the thecal sac and exiting nerve roots. Advantages of myelography include the ability to visualize the entire lumbar spine and the ability to obtain dynamic studies. However, myelography is an invasive study that involves administration of contrast. The dye may cause symptoms, including nausea, vomiting, headache, seizures, and arachnoiditis. The usefulness of myelography is enhanced by postmyelography computed tomography (CT). Postmyelography CT can better identify the nature of the spinal disease, especially in cases of foraminal stenosis, facet hypertrophy, and lateral disk herniations.

Magnetic resonance imaging (MRI) provides a noninvasive method of visualizing lumbar spinal disease in multiple planes. MRI is superior to the previously mentioned studies in identification of soft tissue abnormalities associated with lumbar spinal disease, and the use of MRI contrast has been helpful in differentiating recurrent disk disease from postsurgical epidural fibrosis. However, bony pathology is better visualized on postmyelography CT than on MRI; these studies may complement each other, depending on the clinical situation.

Diskography is another radiographic study that can be used in diagnosing disk disease. In 1948, Lindblom[14] injected radiopaque dye into a disk as a method of diagnosing herniated disk disease. The appearance of the disk on diskography provides detailed information on internal structure. Adams and colleagues[15] defined six stages of disk degeneration based on diskograms.

Perhaps more important than the appearance of the disks is the reproduction of the patient's back or leg pain on disk injection. However, the use of diskography remains controversial because of the high false-positive rate and low specificity.[16–18]

Although any of the studies previously described may identify a structural abnormality, the surgeon must consider whether such findings warrant surgical intervention. Any structural finding characterized on radiographic studies should have a functional significance or be symptomatic. In 1994, Jensen and associates[19] found that 28% of asymptomatic subjects had evidence of disk protrusion or extrusion on lumbar MRI. In 1988, Hayes and coworkers[20] showed that there were 7 to 14 degrees of angulation and 2 to 3 mm of translation motion in the lumbar spines of asymptomatic individuals undergoing routine flexion-extension films, thereby questioning the value of this study as a primary determinant of lumbar segmental instability. Although radiographic studies are an integral part of the evaluation of lumbar spinal disease and are critical to surgical decision making, the clinical picture and natural history of the disease must also be considered before final surgical planning.

SURGICAL MANAGEMENT

Overview of Instrumentation Systems

Posterior fusion of the lumbar spine was described in 1953 by Watkins.[21] The original study described posterior intertransverse process fusion for pseudoarthrosis, postlaminectomy instability, and complications from tuberculosis. The technique required significant paraspinal muscle retraction and autologous bone graft. The technique did not provide increased stiffness, deformity correction, or alignment maintenance. However, 9 of the 10 patients who underwent the procedure experienced clinical improvement.

POSTERIOR ROD-HOOK

The Harrington system, using a distraction-compression rod system, was used as early as 1947 for the correction of scoliosis (Fig. 307–1). Fixation points above and below the segment of interest are required if posterior elements are removed for decompression.[22] Inclusion of these fixation points above and below the level of disease results in immobilization of the adjacent, normal-motion segments. These systems are not rigid; rather, they require distraction and ligamentotaxis to achieve a rigid construct. There is usually a loss of lumbar lordosis. Complications include overdistraction, "flat back syndrome," neural compression by the laminar hooks, and hook failure.

The use of Harrington rods as an adjunct for lumbosacral spinal fusion has been reviewed. For indications such as spinal stenosis, scoliosis, spondylolisthesis, and multioperated backs, decompression followed by lumbosacral fusion with Harrington rods and intersegmental wiring was shown to improve clinical outcome.[23] In

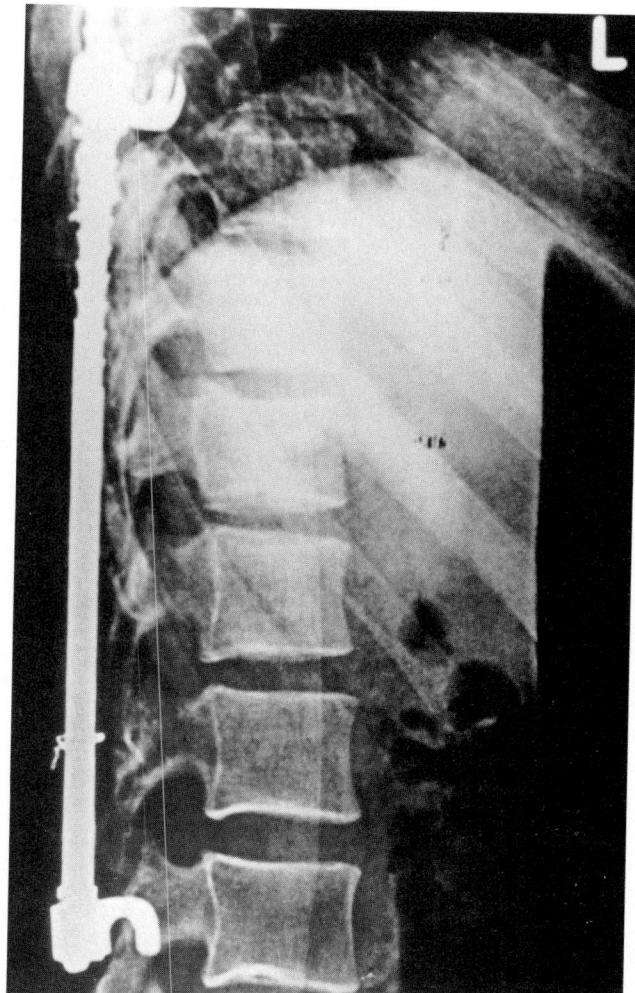

FIGURE 307–1. The Harrington system is a distraction-compression rod system.

1958, Harrington first used posterior instrumentation and fusion for stabilization of a fracture-dislocation, and Harrington rods have since been used successfully in the stabilization of lumbar spine fractures.[24]

POSTERIOR WIRE-ROD CONSTRUCTS

The Luque rod segmental spinal instrumentation system using sublaminar wires and rods was first described for use in patients with postpoliomyelitis and idiopathic scoliosis, and the system was developed as an alternative to Harrington rod instrumentation in soft, postpoliomyelitic bone (Fig. 307–2). Like the Harrington rod system, it also requires fixation points above and below the diseased segment.[25] Complications from this system include neurologic deficits after passage of sublaminar wires and migration of Luque rods through a laminectomy defect, leading spinal cord or cauda equina compression.[26] This system does not provide support against axial loads, and it provides limited support in cases such as burst fracture and vertebrectomy for tumor or osteomyelitis, in which

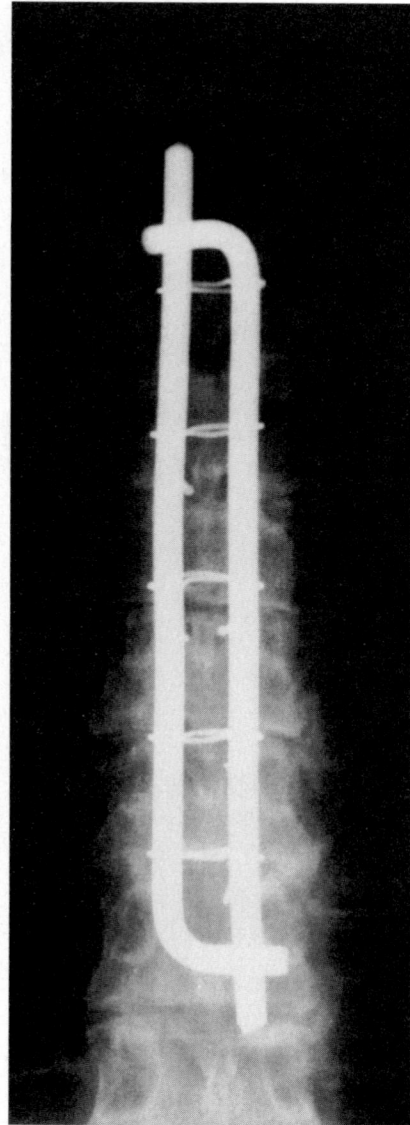

FIGURE 307–2. Luque rod segmental spinal instrumentation system.

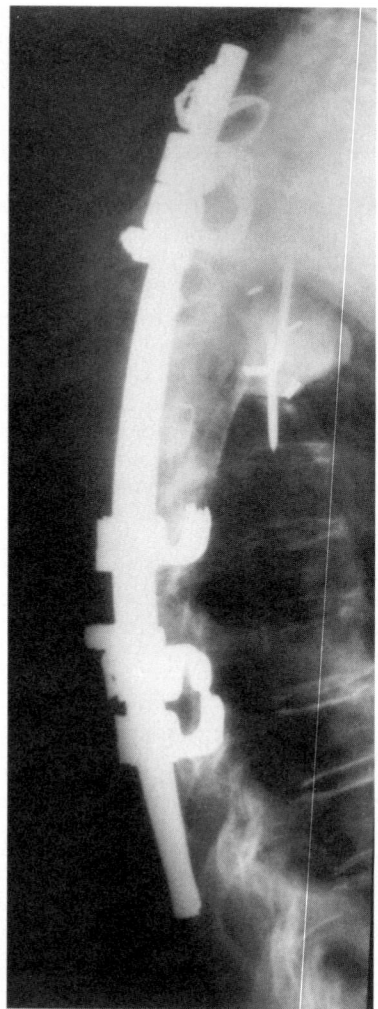

FIGURE 307–3. Cotrel-Dubousset instrumentation system using multiple laminar hooks.

axial load on the posterior instrumentation is significant.

POSTERIOR ROD–MULTIPLE HOOK CONSTRUCTS

In 1988, the Cotrel-Dubousset instrumentation system using multiple laminar hoods was described for use in adults with scoliosis, kyphosis, pseudoarthrosis, spondylolisthesis, traumatic fracture, and tumor (Fig. 307–3).[27] Notably, pedicle screws were used as alternatives to the hook construct in cases requiring laminectomy. The Cotrel-Dubousset system had an advantage over Luque and Harrington systems in requiring fewer segments above and below the diseased level for adequate fixation.

TRANSPEDICULAR SCREWS

The use of pedicle screw plates for spinal fixation began in 1963 (Fig. 307–4). Roy-Camille and associates[28] described the use of pedicle screw fixation for lumbar fracture, malunion, lumbar metastases, primary spine tumor, lumbosacral fusion, and high-grade spondylolisthesis. This technique has the advantage of requiring the least amount of normal anatomy to be involved in the fusion, but care must be taken in placing the pedicle screw to prevent injury to the nerve root. Pedicle screw devices can be used to provide distraction, compression, and translation. Pedicle screw fixation is discussed more extensively later in this chapter.

Outcomes

TRAUMA

Traumatic injury leading to clinical instability is a common indication for lumbar fusion with instrumentation. The addition of internal fixation to lumbar fusion

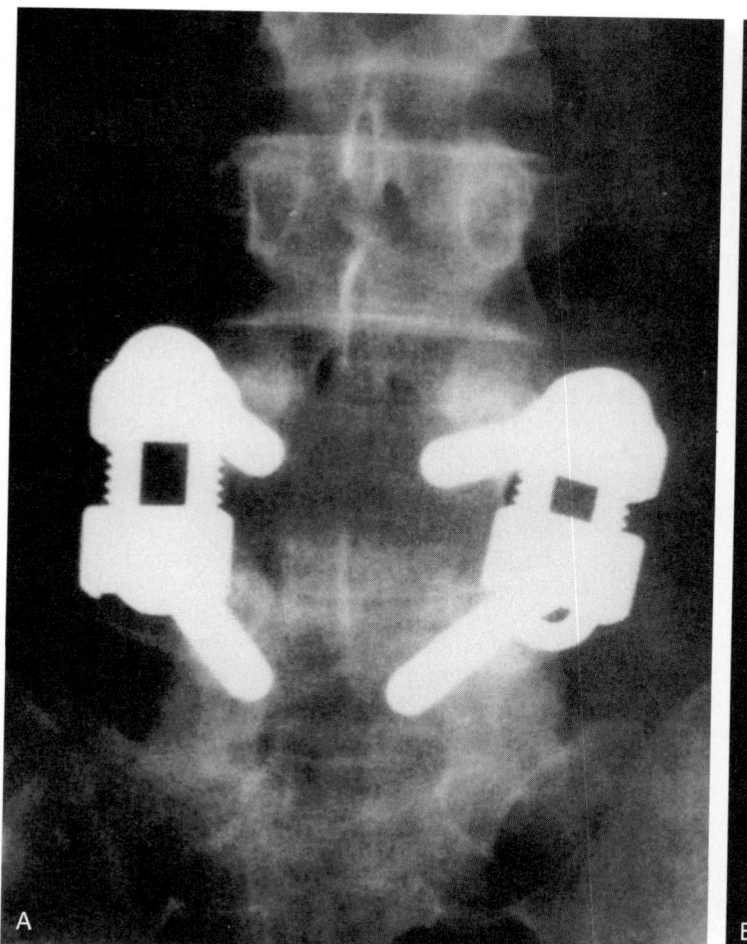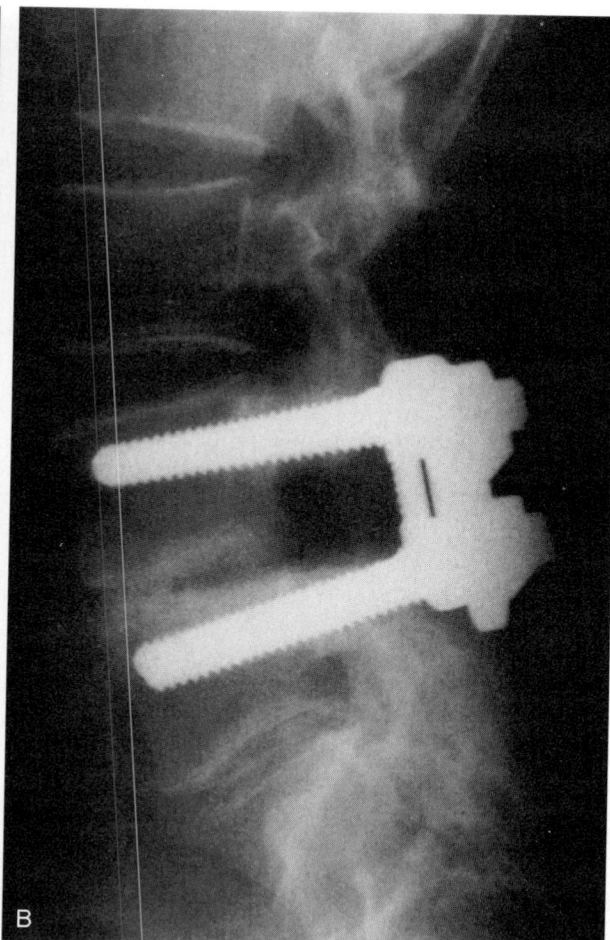

FIGURE 307–4. *A* and *B,* Pedicle screw–plate system.

has the advantages of deformity reduction, restoration of normal alignment, enhancement of fusion rates by providing decreased mobility, and earlier patient mobilization. The outcomes from alternative fixation techniques were compared in a meta-analysis by Dickman and colleagues[29] in 1994. In their review covering cases published from January 1975 to December 1993, the fusion rate using pedicle screw devices (99.4%) was significantly higher than the fusion rates using various hook-rod systems (96.9%) and anterior devices (94.8%). There was no significant difference between the treatment groups in overall complication rates. However, the hook-rod devices did have an increased incidence of loss of fixation compared with the pedicle screw devices, and the Luque instrumentation group had a greater incidence of wound complications compared with all other groups.

The superiority of pedicle screw fixation in supporting lumbar fusion may result from its ability to provide a nonmobile environment in which fusion can occur. Biomechanical data generated from cadaveric spine models described by Ferguson and coworkers[30] suggest that pedicle screw constructs provide increased stiffness compared with other models. In their in vitro model, a pedicle screw construct was found to provide the greatest degree of stiffness in iatrogenically destabilized spine models. By providing decreased mobility, the pedicle screw construct could provide the best environment for a solid fusion to occur.

The use of pedicle fixation allows rigid short-segment fixation of the anterior and posterior spinal columns, minimizing the number of motion segments required for fusion. Pedicle screw systems can also be used to provide distractive forces to restore vertebral body height, reestablish lumbar lordosis, and prevent translational and rotational instability. However, pedicle screw systems are not ideal in all settings. For example, axial loading of the anterior columns may be better treated with an anterior reconstruction or with combined anterior and posterior fixation. The nature of the trauma-induced instability and the biomechanical advantages and disadvantages of each type of instrumentation must be considered when deciding on a fusion technique.[31]

IATROGENIC INSTABILITY

Postsurgical iatrogenic instability may arise from a subclinical instability in a pathologic segment that does not cause symptoms or have radiographic findings until that segment is further destabilized by surgical intervention. The occurrence of iatrogenic instability is probably related to the degree of underlying instability and the amount of surgical intervention. Using a biomechanical model with a human cadaveric lumbar spine, Abumi and colleagues[32] demonstrated that bilateral medial facetectomy of more than 50% or unilateral total facetectomy resulted in instability. Postlaminectomy instability is a recognized phenomenon, especially in cases of preexisting spondylolisthesis and multiple laminectomies.[33-36]

Lee[37] demonstrated that pedicle screw fixation was an effective treatment for postlaminectomy lumbar instability. Eighty-two percent of patients with symptomatic, postlaminectomy lumbar instability received near-complete to complete relief of their preoperative symptoms. Comorbidities that contributed to treatment failures included osteoporosis, concomitant disk herniation, and persistent spinal stenosis.

DEGENERATIVE SPONDYLOLISTHESIS

Degenerative spondylolisthesis occurs when disk and facet joint disease allow the rostral vertebrae to slip forward. This condition occurs predominantly at L4-5 and is more common in women. Most patients with degenerative spondylolisthesis are asymptomatic and do not require surgical intervention. Most patients respond to conservative management with physical therapy and nonsteroidal anti-inflammatory medications. The indications for surgery and fusion are persistent pain unresponsive to conservative management and progressive subluxation.

Mardjetko and associates[38] reviewed the results of surgical decompression, fusion, and instrumentation in a meta-analysis of 11 studies published from January 1970 to December 1993. Their analysis revealed that 69% of all patients who underwent decompression alone had satisfactory outcomes. The combination of lumbar fusion with decompression increased the percentage of patients who had a satisfactory outcome to 90%, with a fusion rate of 86%. This difference in percentage of patients with satisfactory outcomes with decompression and fusion was statistically significant when compared with decompression alone. The addition of spinal instrumentation improved the fusion rate but did not improve the percentage of satisfactory outcomes.

The results of the retrospective meta-analysis are comparable to the prospective data reviewed by Bridwell and coworkers.[39] Forty-four patients with degenerative spondylolisthesis were randomized to three groups. Group I had decompression alone; group II had decompression with posterolateral fusion; and group III had decompression with fusion and instrumentation with pedicle fixation. If a patient had evidence of excessive motion (i.e., more than 10 degrees of angular motion or 3 mm of translational motion) at the slip location, he or she was not randomized, but was instead assigned to group III. In this study, only 33% of the patients who underwent decompression alone experienced a satisfactory outcome. The addition of transverse process fusion to decompression did not change the percentage of patients who had satisfactory outcomes (30%), and the fusion rate was also 30%. Pedicle fixation instrumentation with fusion and decompression increased the fusion rate to 87%, and the percentage of patients with satisfactory outcomes increased to 83%. The addition of instrumentation increased the fusion rate and increased the number of patients who had a functional improvement.

Another prospective, randomized study examining the role of fusion and instrumentation in degenerative spondylolisthesis was performed by Zdeblick.[40] In this series, 124 patients underwent lumbar and lumbosacral fusion for degenerative disease, including 56 patients with degenerative spondylolisthesis. The study had three groups. Group I had posterolateral fusion alone; group II had posterolateral fusion with a semi-rigid, pedicle screw–plate fixation system (i.e., Luque II system); and group III had posterolateral fusion with a rigid, pedicle screw–rod fixation system (i.e., TSRH system). When fusion alone was compared with fusion plus rigid instrumentation, the percentage of patients with a good clinical outcome increased (71% to 95%), and the fusion rate increased (65% to 95%). The use of semi-rigid fixation resulted in more modest differences when compared with noninstrumented cases, with a good clinical outcome rate of 89% and fusion rate of 77%. Instrumentation increased good clinical outcome and fusion rates, and the effect was more pronounced using rigid fixation.

Despite these positive study results, there is conflicting evidence that instrumentation does not necessarily improve the clinical outcome of patients. A randomized, prospective study by Fischgrund and colleagues[41] compared the results of 67 patients with degenerative lumbar spondylolisthesis who underwent decompression and posterolateral intertransverse process arthrodesis with and without transpedicular instrumentation using a screw-plate fixation system. The fusion rate for patients who received instrumentation was 82%, in contrast to the 45% fusion rate for patients who received no instrumentation. Despite this large difference in fusion rates, good clinical outcome was achieved in 76% of patients who received instrumentation and in 85% of patients who did not receive instrumentation. The difference was not statistically significant. Although the fusion rate improved with instrumentation, outcome did not. In another randomized, prospective study, Thomsen and associates[42] compared outcomes and fusion rates for patients with degenerative spondylolisthesis who underwent decompression and posterolateral fusion with and without Cotrel-Dubousset pedicle screw instrumentation. The investigators found no statistically significant difference in fusion rate or clinical outcome.

When performing a decompression and posterolateral intertransverse process fusion for degenerative spondylolisthesis, the decision about whether to place posterior instrumentation must take into account the risks and benefits. From the previously described clinical studies, it appears that rigid fixation with pedicle screw constructs improves the fusion rate. In many studies, rigid fixation also improves the clinical outcome. Instrumentation provides the ability to correct deformity, allowing improved alignment. However, these benefits must be balanced by the disadvantages of instrumentation, including factors such as increased surgical trauma, possible nerve root injury from misplaced pedicle screws, placement of additional foreign body into the surgical wound, and cost.

DEGENERATIVE DISK DISEASE

Lumbar disk disease is the most common cause of back and leg pain. The clinical presentation ranges from isolated low back pain to radicular pain to neurogenic claudication. The earliest manifestation is usually low back pain. The anatomic cause of the patient's symptoms is difficult to identify at this stage, and routine radiographic studies fail to reveal any abnormalities. As disk degeneration progresses, disk protrusion and herniation occur from mechanical stress of forward flexion and axial rotation combined with degenerative changes. The usual treatment for disk disease is diskectomy, although lumbar fusion may be indicated if abnormal or excessive translational motion is identified on dynamic imaging studies.

The role of vertebral body fusion for treating lumbar disk disease was described as early as 1953 by Cloward.[43] He described posterolateral interbody fusion (PLIF) after diskectomy, with an 85% response rate. In 1987, White and associates[44] compared the outcomes of diskectomy with and without lumbar fusion supplemented by posterior instrumentation. This study found no benefit from fusion with instrumentation. In 1992, Grubb and Lipscomb[45] identified disk disease with diskography and performed lumbosacral fusion with and without instrumentation. The postoperative pseudoarthrosis rate without instrumentation was 35%, compared with 6% using instrumentation. Fusion rate correlated with decreased pain, decreased disabled time, and increased rates of return to work. Poor outcomes were associated with prolonged preoperative disability and long-term disability claims, illustrating the importance of nonorganic factors in determining the outcome of surgical interventions. Similar findings were described by Parker and colleagues,[46] who examined the outcomes of posterolateral fusion in patients with diskogenic low back pain. In their study, poor outcomes were identified in patients receiving worker's compensation for more than 3 months.

From the previous discussion, it would appear that routine lumbar fusion for degenerative disk disease is not indicated. Because 28% of asymptomatic individuals have evidence of lumbar disk disease on MRI,[19] it is likely that such incidental findings would also be identified in patients with low back pain. The diagnostic reliability of diskography is controversial and does not clearly identify surgical lesions amenable to fusion. Organic and nonorganic factors influence the outcome of surgical intervention even in the face of a successful fusion. Lumbar fusion should be reserved for cases of lumbar disk disease in which the radiographic and clinical presentations suggest symptoms caused by instability.

LUMBAR STENOSIS

This discussion of surgical management of lumbar stenosis focuses on acquired lumbar spinal stenosis from degenerative disease. Acquired lumbar stenosis is a common condition caused by many factors, including a bulging degenerative disk, enlarged lamina, ligamentum flavum hypertrophy, facet hypertrophy, and osteophyte formation. Surgical intervention is indicated for patients with lumbar stenosis who have intractable leg pain, neurogenic claudication, or progressive lower extremity weakness. The principal surgery involves bilateral laminectomies with medial facetectomies to achieve wide decompression of the central canal and lateral recesses to adequately decompress the nerve roots. In most cases, bilateral laminectomies with medial facetectomies maintain spinal stability.

Although decompression is the primary surgical therapy for lumbar stenosis, lumbar fusion is occasionally indicated concomitantly with decompression. Indications for lumbar fusion include preoperative instability or the creation of iatrogenic instability. Johnsson and coworkers[35] showed that preoperative instability confers a poor prognosis for patients undergoing decompression for stenosis and that the patients with postoperative instability were more often radically decompressed that the stable group. Caputy and Luessenhop[47] showed that the prevalence of spondylolisthesis was higher among patients who failed surgical decompression for lumbar stenosis, and they suggested that stabilization be performed at levels of spondylolisthetic stenosis. In patients with preoperative instability and in patients who will undergo radical decompression, lumbar fusion may be indicated to improve outcomes. Fusion is also indicated for patients with concomitant degenerative spondylolisthesis and for patients with degenerative scoliosis.[48] Lumbar fusion is seldom required in cases of simple degenerative lumbar stenosis.

Technical Considerations

CHOICE OF INSTRUMENTATION

Lumbar instrumentation involves the placement of longitudinal plates or rods anchored to the spine using hooks, screws, or wires. Using these techniques, immediate and rigid spinal immobilization is achieved, providing an improved environment for bone graft fusion and allowing earlier patient mobilization. Lumbar instrumentation can be used to correct deformity and maintain proper alignment while the bone graft incorporates. The nature of the disease may dictate the type of instrumentation used. In a biomechanical analysis comparing Harrington distraction instrumentation with Luque segmental spinal instrumentation, it was shown that Harrington instrumentation is superior against axial loads and is better suited than Luque instrumentation for unstable burst fractures, whereas Luque instrumentation is superior in achieving rotational stability in translational injuries and is better suited than Harrington instrumentation for fracture-dislocations.[49]

The choice of instrumentation depends on the clinical disease being addressed and on patient factors that affect the success of particular construct. For example, the nature of a traumatic spinal fracture or morphometric considerations may prevent the placement of a single type of construct for stable instrumentation. In these cases, the instrumentation must be extended beyond the region of the diseased segment, with subsequent loss of the adjacent motion segment. However, different techniques of fixation may be combined in these cases. For example, in cases of osteoporosis or pedicle fracture, one biomechanical analysis suggested that a hook-claw construct may be used to replace one pedicle screw in a posterior construct.[50]

Osteoporosis is another major consideration in choosing the type of instrumentation. In one biomechanical study studying pedicle screws, osteoporosis was shown to correlate with pedicle fracture during placement.[51] Another group suggested that preoperative measurement of bone mineral density be performed before transpedicular screw placement in osteoporotic bone.[52] In a study using human cadaveric spines, Coe and associates[53] compared measures of bone mineral density with failure of different fixation devices. They showed that laminar hooks were superior to spinous process wires and transpedicular screws in situations of decreased bone mineral density such as osteoporosis.

TRANSPEDICULAR FIXATION

For lumbar fixation, transpedicular screw fixation systems are used more commonly than other systems. Since the 1970s, Roy-Camille and colleagues[54] and Louis[55] have used transpedicular screws to fix plates to the spine. In the 1980s, Steffee and associates[56] and Luque[57] used slotted plates in an attempt to alleviate the problem of screw breakage in screw and plate systems. Steffee's[58] variable screw placement system provided rigid fixation and excellent fusion rates, but screw breakage continued to be a problem. A tendency for intertransverse bone graft to resorb caused some concern that the rigid fixation and stress shielding achieved with transpedicular screw fixation might result in excessive stresses on adjacent motion segments. This led some surgeons to consider removing the implants after successful arthrodesis.[58]

The pedicle screw–rod system, which was first introduced by Magerl[59] and modified by others, was a further advancement, providing improved three-dimensional adjustments, increased versatility at the screw-rod interface, and a larger surface area on which to place bone graft.[60] The screw-rod system allows axial, angular, and rotational adjustability, permitting instrumented segments of the spine to be held in distraction, compression, or derotation.

Operative Technique

POSITIONING AND EXPOSURE

General endotracheal anesthesia is administered with the patient supine on the bed or table, and pneumatic

compression stockings are applied to the legs. Unless contraindicated, the patient is connected to a blood product recycling unit. Prophylactic antibiotics are administered preoperatively and continued 48 hours postoperatively. If possible, arrangements are made for autologous blood donation.

Intraoperative anteroposterior, oblique, and lateral fluoroscopy is performed using a radiolucent operating table with an adjustable fluoroscopic C-arm image intensifier and a patient frame or chest rolls. The patient is placed in the prone position on the operating table, with the thorax supported laterally to avoid epidural venous distention from abdominal compression. Alternatively, the patient is placed on a Jackson table, specifically designed for patient rotation to facilitate cases that require combined anterior and posterior approaches. A midline lumbar incision is extended 2 to 3 inches above and below the segments for instrumentation. Subperiosteal muscle dissection of the segments to be fused is performed with a wide exposure to the lateral tips of the transverse processes. Neural decompression and vertebral body reconstruction are performed, as indicated, before posterior instrumentation.

PEDICLE PREPARATION

After the lumbar spine segments are exposed and decompressed, the external landmarks are localized. Fluoroscopic confirmation is obtained for pedicle identification, hole preparation, and screw placement.

In the lumbar spine, the external landmarks for the pedicles are at the intersection of the axial plane through the middle of the transverse processes and the sagittal plane through the superior facet (Fig. 307–5). Identification of the facet complex is facilitated by mov-

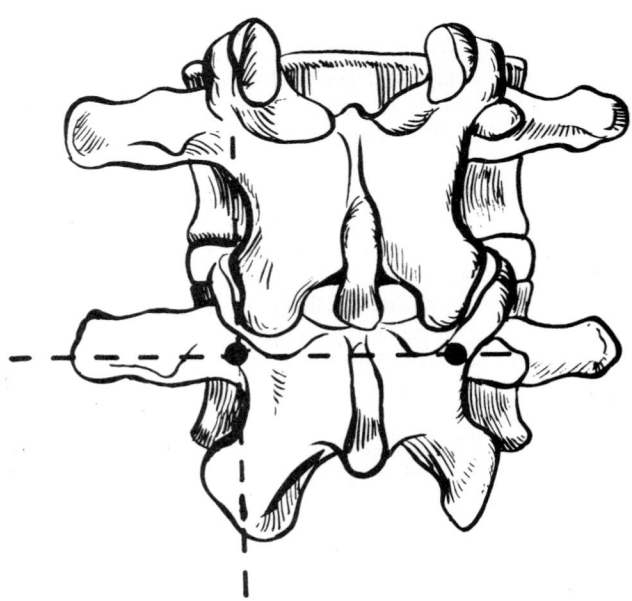

FIGURE 307–5. Pedicle landmarks for placement of transpedicular screws into lumbar vertebral segments. A line is drawn at the intersection of the axial plane through the middle of the transverse process and the sagittal plane through the superior facet.

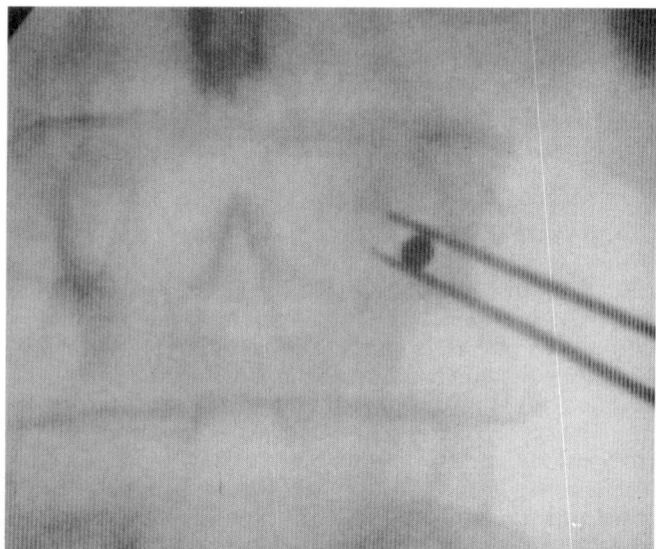

FIGURE 307–6. Fluoroscopic image shows the alignment of the pedicle and Steinmann pin.

ing the spinous process with a Kocher clamp and removing the soft tissue from the surface of the superior facet. A Steinmann pin is placed over the external landmark, and the correct entry position is verified with fluoroscopy (Fig. 307–6). The pin is oriented along the long axis through the center of the pedicle. On the anteroposterior or slightly oblique fluoroscopic images, the pedicle and Steinmann pin appeared as an oval structure with a central dot.

Sacral screw sites are prepared in the same manner as lumbar pedicle screw sites. The external anatomic landmarks differ, because there is no sacral transverse process (Fig. 307–7). Manipulation of the L5 spinous process helps to identify the L5-S1 facets. Soft tissue is cleared from the sacrum to delineate the first dorsal sacral foramina and the osseous recession caudal to the L5-S1 facets. The external landmark for the first sacral

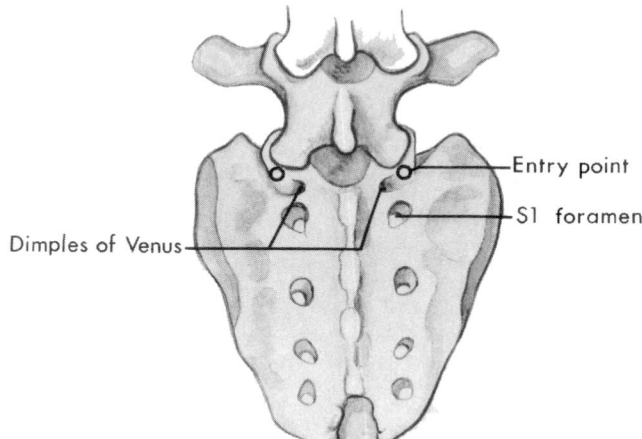

FIGURE 307–7. Pedicle landmarks for placement of the transpedicular screws into sacral vertebral segments.

pedicle is located at the inferolateral portion of the superior S1 facet. Fluoroscopy is used to confirm correct entry sites.

Screw holes are prepared by penetrating through the posterior cortex, deepening the hole past the narrow midportion of the pedicle, and completing the hole to the desired depth. Preparation of the hole and insertion of the screw require proper orientation relative to the pedicle's central axis. Under fluoroscopic monitoring, a hole is made in the pedicle with a Steinmann pin with a diameter corresponding the minor diameter of the screw. The pin is affixed to a Jacobs chuck on a T-handle and manually driven through the center of the pedicle with a firm twisting motion. This procedure is repeated at each pedicle. The progress of pin and screw penetration into the vertebral body is monitored using lateral imaging. Each pin is driven until positioned into the end plate of the vertebrae, avoiding penetration into the disk space. This requires a vertical orientation for the lumbar spine and a 30-degree caudal angle for the sacrum. The medial trajectory corresponds to the angle of the pedicles at each level. Biomechanical studies have shown that the sagittal insertion angle can affect the bending moments forced on the pedicle screws and that cephalad-angled screws experience significantly greater bending moments and are therefore more likely to fail.[61]

After all pins are placed into the vertebral bodies to create paths for the pedicle screws, the Steinmann pins are removed, and the superficial 5- to 10-mm area of each track is enlarged with a drill. This allows the screw threads to gain purchase into the bone. Pedicle screw sizes are preselected on the basis of the computed tomographic characteristics of the particular vertebra. The screws are placed into the prepared holes with the same trajectory as that of the Steinmann pins. Screw purchase is obtained by advancing the screw with a screwdriver to a depth of 70% to 80% of the vertebral body. The anterior portion of the vertebral body is not penetrated to avoid injury to vascular and visceral structures in the retroperitoneum.

ROD SYSTEM ASSEMBLY

A malleable template is used to approximate the desired rod curvature. The rods are selected, cut to proper length, and bent to match the template contours. For contour, an S-shaped curve is used for thoracolumbar rods, and a lordotic curve is used for lumbar or lumbosacral rods. The rods are connected bilaterally to the pedicle screws by threading the rods through the screws (i.e., Cotrel-Dubousset system) or attaching the eyebolts to the rods (i.e., TSRH system). The nut assemblies are then tightened, securing the rods.

Final adjustments in rod contour are achieved with in situ rod benders. Spinal reductions are performed, and instruments are placed under compression, distraction, or in neutral position, as indicated by the particular case. A transverse traction device (i.e., Cotrel-Dubousset system) or cross-linking rods (i.e., TSRH system) connect the longitudinal rods. All connections are securely tightened for final fixation.

FUSION SITE PREPARATION

The vertebrae beneath the full length of the instrument system are fused using the technique originally described by Watkins.[21] The fusion sites are prepared before rod placement, providing more working space for bone preparation. After all soft tissue is removed from the surface of the fusion bed, a high-speed drill is used to decorticate the transverse processes, facet joints, and other bone fusion surfaces. The articular surfaces of the facet joints are curetted or drilled to remove cartilage. Cancellous bone grafts are packed into the facets. After rod placement and wound irrigation with antibiotic-containing solution, cancellous bone and cortical matchstick grafts are placed for a posterolateral fusion. Autogenous iliac crest bone is the preferred bone graft. Closed suction drainage systems are placed into the wound, and multilayer wound closure is completed.

POSTOPERATIVE CARE

All wound drains are removed 24 to 48 hours after surgery. Patients with lumbar fusions wear a thoracolumbosacral orthosis for 3 to 6 months. Patients with lumbosacral fusions wear an orthotic device with one thigh immobilized. Patients are ambulatory within the first few postoperative days. Physical therapy for rehabilitation is then provided.

Results with Transpedicular Screw Fixation

Yahiro[62] reviewed the outcomes for pedicle screw technique by meta-analysis of published studies from 1984 through 1993. He reported an overall fusion rate of 95%, with complication rates of 7.1% for broken pedicle screws, 2.5% for malpositioned pedicle screws, 1.7% for neural deficits, 1.1% for dural tears, and 0.2% for broken rods. In a prospective study by Simmons and colleagues,[63] the results from 342 patients undergoing transpedicular fixation were reviewed with a 24-month follow-up. Clinical indications included degenerative disk disease, multioperated back, and vertebral fractures. They reported a 92% fusion rate with a statistically significant improvement in pain scores. The intraoperative complication rate was 22%, with a 7% rate of dural tears, 3.6% rate of difficulty or inability to instrument the pedicle, and 1.1% rate of excessive hemorrhage. A retrospective study by Stambough[64] reported a rate of 92% for arthrodesis with transpedicular screw instrumentation; with salvage of nonunion and delayed union cases, the fusion rate increased to 98%. Stambough[64] reported that the learning curve influenced operative time but not pedicle screw placement.

Given the rigidity of transpedicular fixation systems, one concern for a potential postoperative complication is increased degenerative disease at the transition zone between the instrumented and noninstrumented spine. Wiltse and colleagues[65] reviewed the incidence and severity of transition zone degeneration in patients who underwent transpedicular fixation over more than two vertebrae between L3 and S1. The average follow-up period was 7 years. Their study showed that transpedicular screw fixation did not increase the incidence or severity of transitional zone degeneration; rather, 65% of the control group and only 38% of the instrumented group developed new transitional zone changes.

CONCLUSIONS

Although lumbar sacral instrumentation can provide a powerful adjunct to spinal fusion, increasing the fusion rate, allowing earlier patient mobilization, and improving patient satisfaction, the indications for instrumentation are still a matter of considerable debate and investigation. Current studies suggest that fusion with instrumentation may prove beneficial in cases of spondylolisthesis, deformity, instability leading to chronic pain, and traumatic injury. However, each case must be considered individually before deciding on a particular surgical intervention.

REFERENCES

1. Fessler RG: Decision making in spinal instrumentation. Clin Neurosurg 40:227–242, 1993.
2. Denis F: The three column spine and its significance in the classification of acute thoracolumbar spine injuries. Spine 8:817–831, 1983.
3. McAfee PC, Yuan HA, Fredrickson BE, et al: The value of computed tomography in thoracolumbar fractures: An analysis of one hundred consecutive cases and a new classification. J Bone Joint Surg Am 65:461–473, 1983.
4. Frymoyer JW, Selby DK: Segmental instability: Rational for treatment. Spine 10:280–286, 1985.
5. Hanley EN: The indications for lumbar fusion with and without instrumentation. Spine 20(Suppl):143S–153S, 1985.
6. Krodel A, Kruger A, Lohscheidt K, et al: Anterior debridement, fusion, and extrafocal stabilization in the treatment of osteomyelitis of the spine. J Spinal Disord 12:17–26, 1999.
7. Safran O, Rand N, Kaplan L, et al: Sequential or simultaneous, same-day anterior decompression and posterior stabilization in the management of vertebral osteomyelitis of the lumbar spine. Spine 23:1885–1890, 1998.
8. Harrington KD: Current concepts review: Metastatic disease of the spine. J Bone Joint Surg Am 68:1110–1115, 1986.
9. Kostuik JP, Errico TJ, Gleason TF, Errico CC: Spinal stabilization of vertebral column tumors. Spine 13:250–256, 1988.
10. Heller JG, Zdeblick TA, Kunz R, et al: Spinal instrumentation for metastatic disease: In vitro biomechanical analysis. J Spinal Disord 6:17–22, 1993.
11. Ramsey RG: Disorders of the spine and myelography. In Neuroradiology. Philadelphia, WB Saunders, 1987, pp 669–795.
12. Amundson G, Edwards CC, Garfin SR: Spondylolisthesis: Radiographic studies. In Rothman RH, Simeone FA (eds): The Spine. Philadelphia, WB Saunders, 1992, pp 926–935.
13. Bell GR, Rothman RH, Booth RE, et al: A study of computer assisted tomography: Comparison of metrizamide myelography and computed tomography in the diagnosis of herniated lumbar disc and spinal stenosis. Spine 9:552–556, 1984.
14. Lindblom K: Diagnostic puncture of intervertebral disks in sciatica. Acta Orthop Scand 17:231–239, 1948.
15. Adams MA, Dovan P, Hutton WC: The stages of disc degeneration as revealed by discograms. J Bone Joint Surg 68:36–41, 1986.
16. Grubb SA, Lipscomb HJ, Guilford WB: The relative value of lumbar roentgenograms, metrizamide myelography and discography in the assessment of patients with chronic low back syndrome. Spine 12:282–286, 1987.
17. Holt EP: The question of lumbar discography. J Bone Joint Surg Am 50:720–726, 1968.

18. Simmons JW, April CN, Dwyer AP, et al: A reassessment on Holt's data on: "The question of lumbar discography." Clin Orthop 237:120, 1988.

19. Jensen MC, Brant-Zawadzki MN, Obuchowski N, et al: Magnetic resonance imaging of the lumbar spine in people without back pain. N Engl J Med 331:69–73, 1994.

20. Hayes MA, Tompkins SF, Herndon WA, et al: Clinical and radiological evaluation of lumbosacral motion below fusion levels in idiopathic scoliosis. Spine 13:1161–1167, 1988.

21. Watkins MB: Posterolateral fusion of the lumbar and lumbosacral spine. J Bone Joint Surg 35:1014–1018, 1953.

22. Harrington PR: Treatment of scoliosis: Correction and internal fixation by spinal instrumentation. J Bone Joint Surg Am 44: 591, 1962.

23. White AH, Zucherman JF, Hsu K: Lumbosacral fusions with Harrington rods and intersegmental wiring. Clin Orthop 203: 185–190, 1986.

24. Cotler JM, Vernace JV, Michalski JA: The use of Harrington rods in thoracolumbar fractures. Orthop Clin North Am 17: 87–103, 1986.

25. Luque ER: The anatomic basis and development of segmental spinal instrumentation. Spine 7:256–259, 1982.

26. Quint DJ, Salton G: Migration of Luque rods through a laminectomy defect causing spinal cord compression. Am J Neuroradiol 14:395–398, 1993.

27. Gurr KR, McAfee PC: Cotrel-Dubousset instrumentation in adults, a preliminary report. Spine 13:510–520, 1988.

28. Roy-Camille R, Saillant G, Mazel C: Internal fixation of the lumbar spine with pedicle screw plating. Clin Orthop 203:7–17, 1986.

29. Dickman CA, Yahiro MA, Lu HT, Melkerson MN: Surgical treatment alternatives for fixation of unstable fractures of the thoracic and lumbar spine: A meta-analysis. Spine 19(Suppl):2266S–2273S, 1994.

30. Ferguson RL, Tencer AF, Woodard P, et al: Biomechanical comparisons of spinal fracture models and the stabilizing effects of posterior instrumentations. Spine 13:453–460, 1988.

31. Stambough JL: Posterior instrumentation for thoracolumbar trauma. Clin Orthop 335:73–88, 1997.

32. Abumi K, Panjabi MM, Kramer KM, et al: Biomechanical evaluation of lumbar spinal stability after graded facetectomies. Spine 15:1142–1147, 1990.

33. Shenkin HA, Hash CJ: Spondylolisthesis after multiple bilateral laminectomies and facetectomies for lumbar spondylosis: Follow-up review. J Neurosurg 50:45–47, 1979.

34. Johnsson KE, Willner S, Johnsson K: Postoperative instability after decompression for lumbar spinal stenosis. Spine 11:107–110, 1986.

35. Johnsson KE, Redlund-Johnell I, Uden A, Willner S: Preoperative and postoperative instability in lumbar spinal stenosis. Spine 14: 591–593, 1989.

36. Sienkiewicz PJ, Flatley TJ: Postoperative spondylolisthesis. Clin Orthop 221:172–180, 1987.

37. Lee TC: Transpedicular reduction and stabilization for postlaminectomy lumbar instability. Acta Neurochir 138:139–145, 1996.

38. Mardjetko SM, Connolly PJ, Shott S: Degenerative lumbar spondylolisthesis: A meta-analysis of literature 1970–1993. Spine 19: 2256S–2265S, 1994.

39. Bridwell KH, Sedgewick TA, O'Brien MF, et al: The role of fusion and instrumentation in the treatment of degenerative spondylolisthesis with spinal stenosis. J Spinal Disord 6:461—472, 1993.

40. Zdeblick TA: A prospective, randomized study of lumbar fusion: Preliminary results. Spine 18:938–991, 1993.

41. Fischgrund JS, Mackay M, Herkowitz HN, et al. Degenerative lumbar spondylolisthesis with spinal stenosis: A prospective, randomized study comparing decompressive laminectomy and arthrodesis with and without spinal instrumentation. Spine 22: 2807–2812, 1997.

42. Thomsen K, Christensen FB, Eiskjaer SP, et al: The effect of pedicle screw instrumentation on functional outcome and fusion rates in posterolateral lumbar spinal fusion: A prospective randomized clinical study. Spine 22:2813–2822, 1997.

43. Cloward RB: The treatment of ruptured lumbar intervertebral discs by vertebral body fusion. J Neurosurg 10:154–168, 1953.

44. White AH, von Rogov P, Zucherman J, Heiden D: Lumbar laminectomy for herniated disc: A prospective controlled comparison with internal fixation fusion. Spine 12:305–307, 1987.

45. Grubb SA, Lispcomb HJ: Results of lumbosacral fusion for degenerative disc disease with and without instrumentation: Two and five year follow-up. Spine 17:349–355, 1992.

46. Parker LM, Murrell SE, Boden SD, et al: The outcome of posterolateral fusion in highly selected patients with discogenic low back pain. Spine 21:1909–1917, 1996.

47. Caputy AJ, Luessenhop AJ: Long term evaluation of decompressive surgery for degenerative lumbar stenosis. J Neurosurg 77:669–676, 1992.

48. Esses SI, Huler RJ: Indications for lumbar fusion in the adult. Clin Orthop 279:87–100, 1992.

49. McAfee PC, Werner FW, Glisson RR: A biomechanical analysis of spinal instrumentation system in thoracolumbar fractures: Comparison of traditional Harrington distraction instrumentation with segmental spinal instrumentation. Spine 10:204–217, 1985.

50. Margulies JY, Caruso SA, Chattar-Cora D, et al: Substitution of transpedicular screws by hook claws in a vertebrectomy model. J Spinal Disord 11:36–40, 1998.

51. Hirano T, Hasegawa K, Washio T, et al: Fracture risk during pedicle screw insertion in osteoporotic spine. J Spinal Disord 11: 493–497, 1998.

52. Okuyama K, Sato K, Abe E, et al: Stability of transpedicle screwing for the osteoporotic spine, an in vitro study of mechanical stability. Spine 18:2240–2245, 1993.

53. Coe JD, Warden KE, Herzig MA, et al: Influence of bone mineral density on the fixation of thoracolumbar implants. Spine 15: 902–907, 1990.

54. Roy-Camille R, Saillant G, Berteaux D, et al: Vertebral osteosynthesis using metal plates: Its different uses. Chirurgie 105:597–603, 1979.

55. Louis R: Fusion of the lumbar and sacral spine by internal fixation with screw plates. Clin Orthop 203:18–33, 1986.

56. Steffee A, Biscup R, Sitkowski D: Segmental spine plates with pedicle screw fixation: A new internal fixation device for disorders of the lumbar and thoracic spine. Clin Orthop 203:43–54, 1986.

57. Luque E: Interpeduncular segmental fixation. Clin Orthop 203: 54–57, 1986.

58. Whitecloud TS, Butler JC, Cohen JL, et al: Complications with the variable spinal plating system. Spine 14:471–476, 1989.

59. Magerl F, Dick W, Kluger P, et al: A new device for internal fixation of thoraco lumbar and lumbar spine fractures: The "fixateur interne." Paraplegia 23:225–232, 1981.

60. Haid RW, Dickman CA: Instrumentation and fusion for discogenic disease of the lumbosacral spine. Neurosurg Clin N Am 4: 135–148, 1993.

61. Youssef JA, McKinley TO, Yerby SA, et al: Characteristics of pedicle screw loading: Effects of sagittal insertion angle on intrapedicular bending moments. Spine 24:1077–1081, 1999.

62. Yahiro MA: Comprehensive literature review: Pedicle screw fixation devices. Spine 20(Suppl):2274S–2278S, 1994.

63. Simmons JW, Anderson GBJ, Russell GS, et al: A prospective study of 342 patients using transpedicular fixation instrumentation for lumbosacral spine arthrodesis. J Spinal Disord 11:367–374, 1998.

64. Stambough JL: Lumbosacral instrumented fusion: Analysis of 124 consecutive cases. J Spinal Disord 12:1–9, 1999.

65. Wiltse LL, Radecki SE, Biel HM, et al: Comparative study of the incidence and severity of degenerative change in the transition zones after instrumented versus noninstrumented fusions of the lumbar spine. J Spinal Disord 12:27–33, 1999.

CHAPTER 308

Image-Guided Spinal Navigation

IAIN H. KALFAS

Image-guided spinal navigation is a computer-based surgical technology that was developed to improve intraoperative orientation to the unexposed anatomy during complex spinal procedures.[1, 2] It evolved from the principles of stereotaxy, which have been used by neurosurgeons for several decades to help localize intracranial lesions. *Stereotaxy* is defined as the localization of a specific point in space using three-dimensional coordinates. The application of stereotaxy to intracranial surgery initially involved the use of an external frame attached to the patient's head. However, computer-based technologies have eliminated the need for this frame and have allowed the expansion of stereotactic technology into other surgical fields, in particular, spinal surgery.

The management of complex spinal disorders has been influenced by the acceptance and use of spinal instrumentation devices, as well as the development of complex operative exposures. Many of these techniques place a greater demand on the spinal surgeon by requiring a precise orientation to spinal anatomy that is not exposed in the surgical field. In particular, the various fixation techniques that involve the placement of bone screws into the pedicles of the thoracic, lumbar, and sacral spine; into the lateral masses of the cervical spine; and across joint spaces in the upper cervical spine require "visualization" of the unexposed spinal anatomy. Although conventional intraoperative imaging techniques such as fluoroscopy have proved useful, they are limited because they provide only two-dimensional imaging of a complex three-dimensional structure. Consequently, the surgeon must extrapolate the third dimension based on an interpretation of the images and a knowledge of the pertinent anatomy. This so-called dead reckoning of the anatomy can result in varying degrees of inaccuracy when placing screws into the unexposed spinal column.

Several studies have shown the unreliability of routine radiography in assessing pedicle screw placement in the lumbosacral spine. The rate of penetration of the pedicle cortex by an inserted screw ranges from 21% to 31% in these studies.[3–5] The disadvantage of these conventional radiographic techniques is that they display, at most, only two planar images. Although the lateral view can be relatively easy to assess, the antero-posterior or oblique view can be difficult to interpret. In the majority of screw fixation procedures, the position of the screw in the axial plane is the most important, because this plane best demonstrates the position of the screw relative to the neural canal. Conventional intraoperative imaging cannot provide this view. To assess the potential advantage of axial imaging for screw placement, Steinmann and colleagues used an image-based technique for pedicle screw placement that combined computed tomographic axial images of cadaver spine specimens and fluoroscopy.[6] This study demonstrated an improvement in pedicle screw insertion accuracy, with an error rate of only 5.5%.

Image-guided spinal navigation minimizes much of the guesswork associated with complex spinal surgery. It allows for the intraoperative manipulation of multiplanar computed tomographic images that can be oriented to any point in the surgical field. Although it is not an intraoperative imaging device, it provides the spinal surgeon with superior image data compared with conventional intraoperative imaging technology (i.e., fluoroscopy). It improves the speed, accuracy, and precision of complex spinal surgery and, in most cases, eliminates the need for cumbersome intraoperative fluoroscopy.

PRINCIPLES

The use of an image-guided navigational system for localizing intracranial lesions has been described elsewhere.[7, 8] Image-guided navigation establishes a spatial relationship between preoperative computed tomographic image data and the corresponding intraoperative anatomy. Both the image data and the anatomy can be viewed as three-dimensional coordinate systems, with each point having a specific x, y, and z Cartesian coordinate. Using defined mathematical algorithms, a specific point in the image data set can be "matched" to its corresponding point in the surgical field. This process is called *registration*, and it represents the critical step of image-guided navigation. A minimum of three points must be matched, or registered, to allow for accurate navigation.

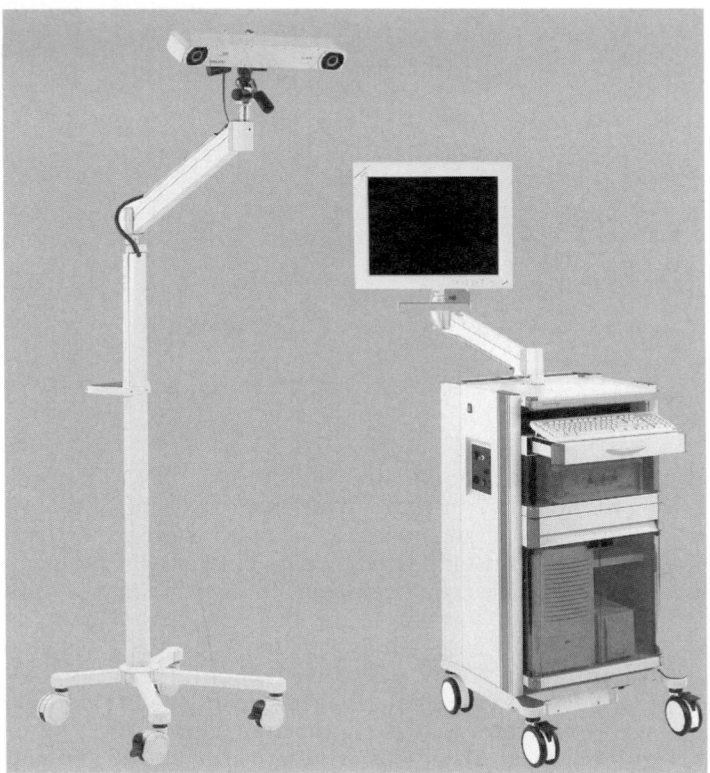

FIGURE 308–1. Image-guided navigational workstation with infrared camera localizer system.

A number of navigational systems have evolved over the past decade. The common components of most of these systems include an image-processing computer workstation interfaced with a two-camera optical localizer (Fig. 308–1). When positioned during surgery, the optical localizer emits infrared light toward the operative field. A hand-held navigational probe mounted with a fixed array of passive reflective spheres serves as the link between the surgeon and the computer workstation (Fig. 308–2). Alternatively, passive reflectors can be attached to standard surgical instruments. The spacing and positioning of the pas-

sive reflectors on each navigational probe or customized trackable surgical instrument are "known" by the computer workstation. The infrared light transmitted toward the operative field is reflected back to the optical localizer by the passive reflectors. This information is then relayed to the computer workstation, which calculates the precise location of the instrument tip in the surgical field, as well as the location of the anatomic point on which the instrument tip is resting.

The initial application of navigational principles to spinal surgery was not intuitive. The early application of navigational technology to intracranial surgery in-

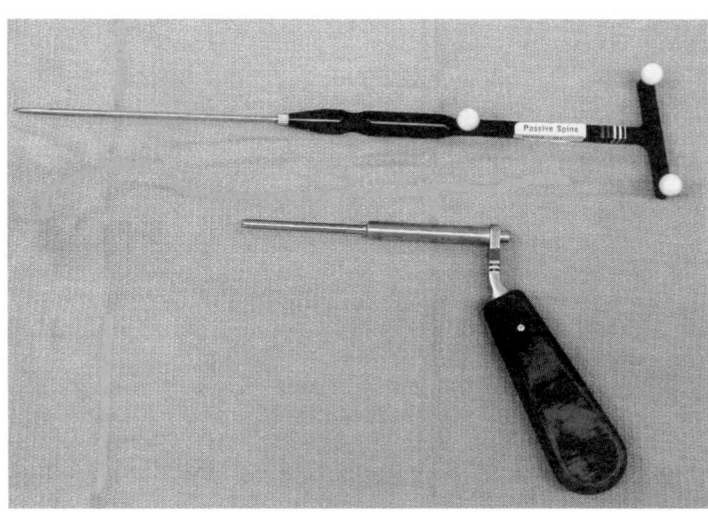

FIGURE 308–2. Navigation probe and drill guide for spinal surgery.

volved an external frame mounted on the patient's head to provide a point of reference to link preoperative image data to intracranial anatomy. This was not practical for spinal surgery. The current generation of intracranial navigational technology uses reference markers or fiducials that are attached to the patient's scalp before imaging. However, the use of these surface-mounted fiducials for spinal navigation is not practical because of accuracy problems related to the greater degree of skin movement over the spinal column.[9, 10] This is less of a problem with intracranial applications because of the relatively fixed position of the overlying scalp to the attached fiducials.

The application of navigational technology to spinal surgery involves using the rigid spinal anatomy itself as a frame of reference. Bony landmarks on the exposed surface of the spinal column provide the points of reference necessary for image-guided navigation. Specifically, any anatomic landmark that can be identified both intraoperatively and in the preoperative image data set can be used as a reference point. The tip of a spinous or transverse process, a facet joint, and a prominent osteophyte can all be reference points (Fig. 308–3). Because each vertebra is a fixed, rigid body, the spatial relationship between the selected registration points and the vertebral anatomy at a single spinal level is not affected by changes in body position.

Two different registration techniques can be used for spinal navigation: paired point registration and surface matching. Paired point registration involves selecting a series of corresponding points in a computed tomographic or magnetic resonance imaging data set and in the exposed spinal anatomy. The registration process is performed immediately after surgical exposure and before any planned decompressive procedure. This allows the spinous processes to be used as registration points.

A specific registration point in the computed tomo-graphic image data set is selected by highlighting it with the computer cursor. The tip of the probe is then placed on the corresponding point in the surgical field, and the reflective spheres on the probe handle are aimed toward the camera. Infrared light from the camera is reflected back, allowing the spatial position of the probe's tip to be identified. This initial step of the registration process effectively links the point selected in the image data with the point selected in the surgical field. When a minimum of three such points have been registered, the probe can be placed on any other point in the surgical field, and the corresponding point in the image data set will be identified on the computer.

Alternatively, registration can be accomplished with surface matching. This technique involves selecting multiple nondiscrete points on the exposed and débrided surface of the spine in the surgical field. It does not require the preselection of points in the image set, although several discrete points in both the image data set and the surgical field are frequently required to improve the accuracy of surface mapping. Positional information about these points is transferred to the workstation, and a topographic map of the selected anatomy is created and "matched" to the patient's image set.[11]

Typically, paired point registration can be done more quickly than surface mapping. The average time needed for paired point registration is 10 to 15 seconds, whereas in difficult cases, the time needed for surface mapping can be as much as 10 to 15 minutes. Because several registration processes must be performed during each surgery, this time difference can significantly affect the length of the navigational procedure and the surgery itself.[12]

The purpose of the registration process is to establish a precise spatial relationship between the image space of the data and the physical space of the patient's corresponding surgical anatomy. If the patient is

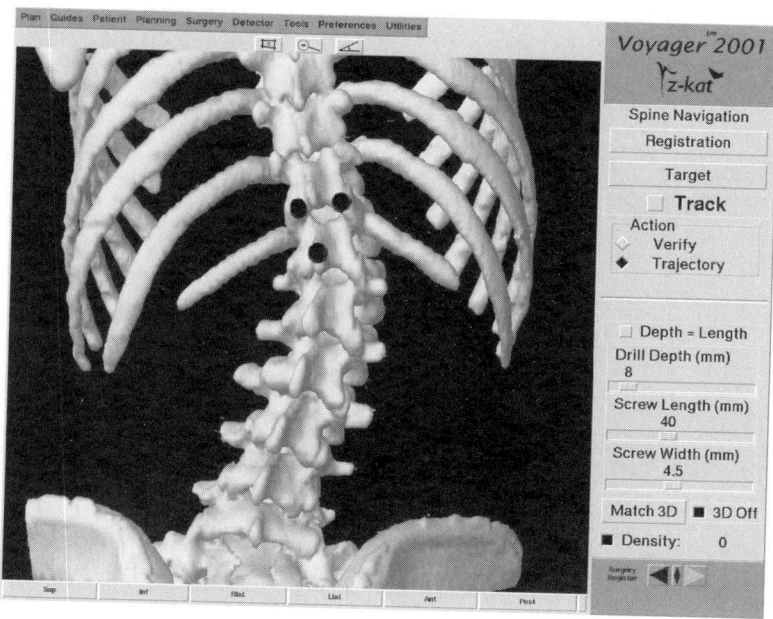

FIGURE 308–3. Navigational workstation screen demonstrating a paired point registration plan for the insertion of T12 pedicle screws. Three discrete bony landmarks are selected at the T12 level. In this case, the lateral margins of the two T12 transverse processes and the tip of the T12 spinous process have been selected.

moved after registration, this spatial relationship is distorted, making the navigational information inaccurate. This problem can be minimized by the optional use of a spinal tracking device that consists of a separate set of passive reflectors mounted on an instrument that can be attached to the exposed spinal anatomy (Fig. 308–4). The position of the reference frame can be tracked by the camera system. Movement of the frame alerts the navigational system to any inadvertent movement of the spine. The system can then make corrections to keep the registration process accurate and eliminate the need to repeat it. The disadvantage of using a tracking device is the extra time needed to attach it to the spine, the need to maintain a line of sight between it and the camera, and the inconvenience of having to perform the procedure with the device in the surgical field. It is particularly cumbersome when image-guided navigation is used during cervical procedures.

Alternatively, image-guided spinal navigation can be performed without a tracking device.[1, 12] This involves acknowledging the effect of patient movement on the accuracy of image-guided navigation and maintaining a reasonably stable patient position during the relatively short time needed (10 to 20 seconds) for the selection of each appropriate screw trajectory. Patient movement can occur with respiration, from the surgical team leaning on the table, or from a change of table position. Movement associated with patient respiration is negligible and does not require tracking, even in the thoracic spine. Although movement associated with

leaning on the table or repositioning the table or the patient can affect registration accuracy, this is easily avoided during the short navigational procedure. If inadvertent patient movement does occur, the registration process can be repeated. Repeating the registration process is easier when using the paired point technique as opposed to the more time-consuming surface mapping technique.

When the registration process has been completed, the probe can be positioned on any surface point in the surgical field, and three separate, reformatted computed tomographic images centered on the corresponding point in the image data set will immediately be presented on the workstation monitor. Each reformatted image is referenced to the long axis of the probe. If the probe is placed on the spinal anatomy directly perpendicular to its long axis, the three images will be in the sagittal, coronal, and axial planes. A trajectory line representing the orientation of the long axis of the probe will overlie the sagittal and axial planes. A cursor representing a cross section through the selected trajectory will overlie the coronal plane. The insertional "depth" of the trajectory can be adjusted to correspond to selected screw lengths. As the depth is adjusted, the specific coronal plane will adjust accordingly, with the position of the cursor demonstrating the final position of the tip of a screw placed at that depth along the selected trajectory. As the probe is moved to another point in the surgical field, the reformatted images as well as the position of the cursor and trajectory line will change. The planar orientation of the three re-

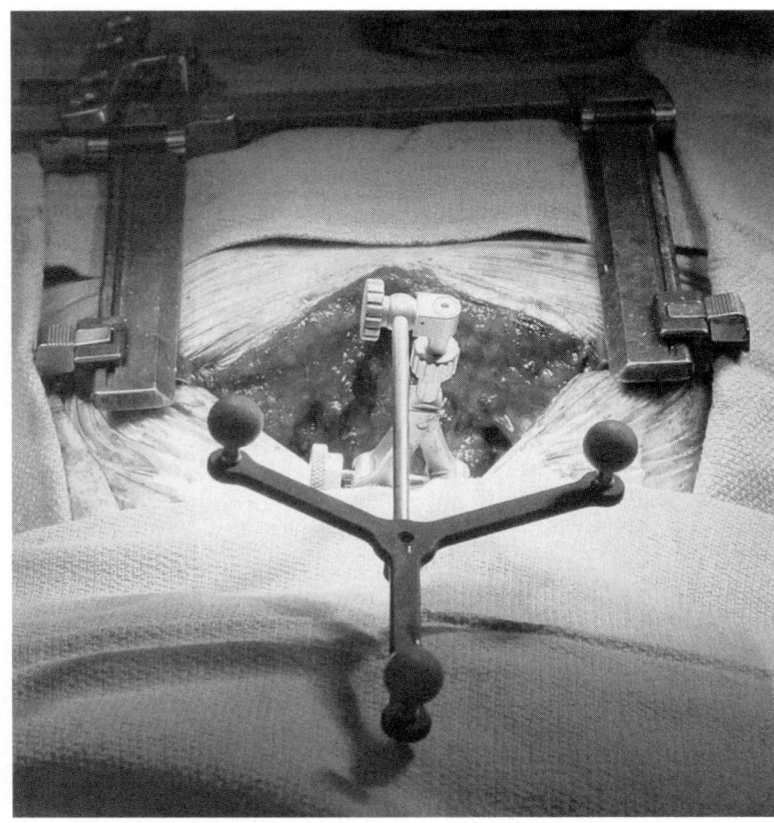

FIGURE 308–4. Reference frame attached to a spinous process in the surgical field. The reference frame monitors inadvertent movement of the spinal anatomy that may affect navigational accuracy.

formatted images will also change as the probe's angle relative to the spinal axis changes. When the probe's orientation is not perpendicular to the long axis of the spine, the images displayed will be in oblique or orthogonal planes. Regardless of the probe's orientation, the navigational workstation provides the surgeon with a greater degree of anatomic information than can be provided by any intraoperative imaging technique.

CLINICAL APPLICATIONS

Image-guided spinal navigation was initially evaluated for the insertion of pedicle screws in the thoracic and lumbosacral spines of cadaver specimens. The accuracy of screw insertion was documented by plain film radiography and thin-section computed tomographic imaging of the instrumented levels. All inserted pedicle screws were satisfactorily placed.[2] The clinical application of image-guided spinal navigation began with its use in lumbosacral pedicle fixation.[1, 13, 14] Other spinal applications gradually evolved, including transoral decompression, cervical screw fixation, thoracic pedicle fixation, anterior thoracolumbar decompression and fixation procedures, and treatment of spinal metastasis.[12, 15–20]

The application of image-guided navigation to spinal surgery is directed by the complexity of the procedure and, specifically, by the need to "visualize" the unexposed spinal anatomy. Image-guided navigation can be used with or without standard intraoperative imaging techniques such as fluoroscopy. In either case, image-guided navigation provides the surgeon with an improved orientation to the pertinent spinal anatomy, which facilitates the accuracy and effectiveness of the procedure.

Pedicle Fixation

Pedicle fixation has gained acceptance as an effective and reliable method of spinal stabilization. However, because of individual variations in pedicle anatomy, the safe and precise placement of pedicle screws can be difficult. Suboptimal screw placement can result in varying degrees of neural injury and fixation failure. These complications can be minimized if the surgeon is provided with an accurate spatial orientation to each pedicle to be instrumented before screw insertion.

Image-guided spinal navigation can now be used routinely in place of fluoroscopy for the insertion of pedicle screws in both the thoracic and lumbosacral spine. Although fluoroscopy provides real-time imaging of spinal anatomy, the views generated are two-dimensional images of a complex three-dimensional structure. Manipulation of the fluoroscopic unit can reduce this problem, but these maneuvers can be cumbersome and time-consuming. Other disadvantages include radiation exposure and the need to wear lead aprons during the procedure. Most important, fluoroscopy cannot provide a view of the spinal anatomy in the axial plane. The axial view obtained by image-

guided navigation makes it superior to fluoroscopy for spinal screw fixation procedures.

The application of image-guided navigation to the spine involves obtaining a preoperative computed tomographic scan through the spinal segments to be instrumented. The images consist of a three-dimensional volume data set of contiguous axial images. Alternatively, magnetic resonance imaging data can be used. The image data are then transferred to the computer workstation via an optical disk or a high-speed data link. If paired point registration is used, three to five reference points for each spinal segment to be instrumented are selected and stored in the image data set.

Intraoperatively, a standard exposure of the spinal levels to be instrumented is performed. A lateral radiograph can be obtained to confirm the appropriate level. The computer workstation and camera localizer are then positioned. The infrared camera detector is mounted at the foot of the table and aimed rostrally for thoracic and lumbosacral procedures.

Image-guided navigation is typically used before any planned decompression so that the intact posterior elements can act as registration points. The first spinal segment to be instrumented is registered using either the paired point or surface mapping technique. When the registration process has been completed, the navigational workstation calculates and displays a registration error (expressed in millimeters) that is directly dependent on the surgeon's registration technique. This error does not represent a linear error but rather a volumetric calculation comparing the spacing of registration points in the surgical field with the spacing of the corresponding points in the image data set. This figure is, at best, a relative indicator of accuracy.

A better method of ensuring registration accuracy is the verification step, which is typically performed immediately after completing the registration process. The surgeon places the navigational probe on a discrete landmark in the surgical field, and the navigational system tracks the movement and position of the probe. If accurate registration has been achieved, the trajectory line and cursor on the workstation screen will move to the corresponding point in the image data set. If registration accuracy has not been achieved, the cursor and trajectory line may rest on a point other than that selected in the surgical field. If this occurs to a significant degree, the registration process must be repeated. This step is an absolute indicator of registration accuracy and should be performed before proceeding with navigation.

When an accurate registration of the first spinal level to be instrumented has been verified, standard bony landmarks for pedicle localization are used to approximate the screw entry point. A drill guide is placed on this entry point, and the navigation probe is passed through the guide. The navigational system is activated, permitting tracking of the probe in the surgical field. Three separate reformatted views are displayed on the workstation screen. Each view represents a separate plane passing through the selected point in the surgical field. For most pedicle fixation cases, these views typically consist of a sagittal, axial, and coronal reconstruction. A trajectory line referenced to the long axis of the probe is superimposed on the sagittal and axial views. A round cursor, representing a cross section through the selected trajectory, is superimposed on the coronal view. As the probe is moved through the surgical field, the position of the trajectory line and cursor changes accordingly. Both the width of the trajectory line and the diameter of the cursor can be adjusted to match the relative diameter of the pedicle screws. The length of the trajectory line can also be adjusted (Fig. 308–5).

As the probe is placed on each pedicle entry point, the images on the workstation screen are presented in real time. As the angle of the probe is adjusted in both the axial and sagittal planes, the images update to show the corresponding trajectories. The depth of the coronal view can be adjusted to show the cross-sectional anatomy at any point along the selected trajectory. The orientation of each pedicle to be instrumented can be assessed rapidly and accurately. Any errors in trajectory or entry point selection can be determined and corrected by adjusting the position of the probe and the drill guide through which it passes.

When a satisfactory screw entry point and trajectory have been selected, the current images on the workstation screen are frozen, the probe is removed from the drill guide, and a drill (3-mm diameter) is positioned through the guide. The purpose of the drill guide is to preserve the physical trajectory and entry point information acquired through the navigation of that pedicle. If a drill guide is not used, it may be difficult to precisely position a drill or pedicle probe on the same point and with the same trajectory as the removed navigational probe. The drill guide also permits the use of a hand-held drill to place the small pilot hole, as opposed to trying to re-create the navigational information with a blunt and awkward pedicle probe. When the pilot hole is placed, a sound can be passed down

the hole to ensure adequate positioning. Navigation is then performed for the contralateral pedicle.

For each additional vertebra to be instrumented, a new set of registration points at that level is selected. This method, termed *segmental registration*, eliminates any potential discrepancy in anatomic orientation related to a change in patient position between the preoperative computed tomographic scan and the surgery. Because each vertebra is a fixed, rigid body, the spatial relationship of the selected registration points to the vertebral anatomy at a single spinal level is not affected by changes in body position.

After all pilot holes have been drilled, they are tapped, and appropriate-size screws are inserted. C-arm fluoroscopy or serial radiographs are not required. Typically, the average time for registration, navigation, and insertion of four pedicle screws is approximately 8 to 10 minutes when using a paired point registration technique. This time is considerably longer when using a surface mapping technique.

In addition to screw placement in the large pedicles of the lumbosacral spine, image-guided navigation can facilitate screw placement into the smaller pedicles of the thoracic spine (Fig. 308–6). The added precision of screw placement into thoracic pedicles greatly expands the fixation options for managing the unstable thoracic spine and cervicothoracic junction.

Image-guided navigation can also be used in place of fluoroscopy for the placement of interbody cages in the lumbosacral spine. During removal of the intervertebral disk, the navigational probe can be inserted into the evacuated disk space. With the trajectory length set at zero, the three reformatted images displayed provide optimal spatial orientation to the disk space, allowing precise placement of the cages (Fig. 308–7).

C1-2 Transarticular Screw Fixation

This procedure involves passing a screw through the pars interarticularis of C2, across the facet joint, and

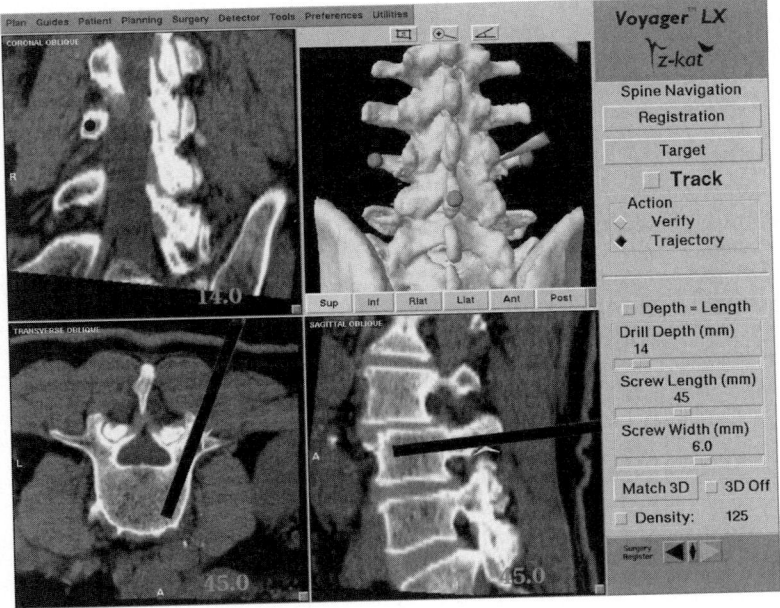

FIGURE 308–5. Workstation screen demonstrating navigation for an L3 pedicle screw.

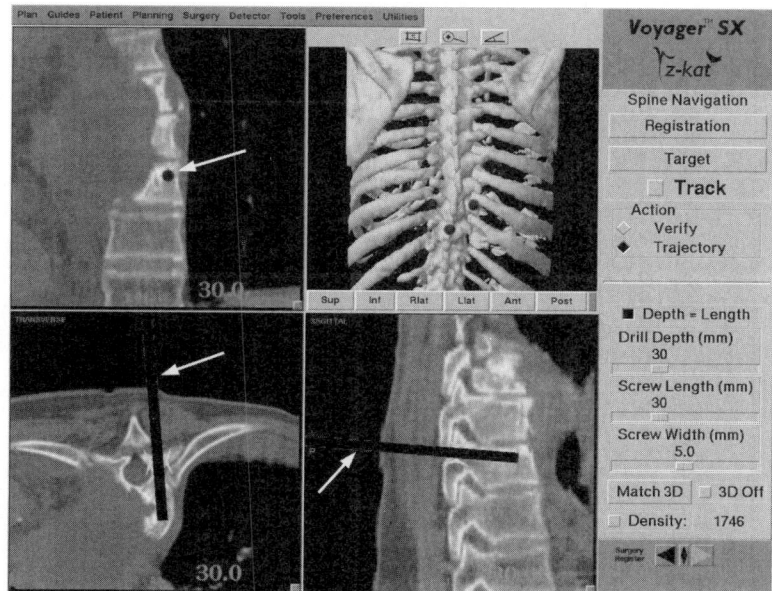

FIGURE 308–6. Workstation screen demonstrating navigation for a T8 pedicle screw in a patient with a mycotic aneurysm of the aorta.

into the lateral mass of C1. The risks of screw insertion include injury to the vertebral artery if the screw is placed too laterally or ventrally, injury to the spinal cord if the screw is placed too medially, and failure to engage the lateral mass of C1 if the screw trajectory is too ventral. The insertion of a screw on either side may be contraindicated if the pars interarticularis of C2 is too narrow. The procedure is typically performed bilaterally using fluoroscopic guidance.

Selection of the appropriate screw entry site and trajectory requires a thorough understanding of the atlantoaxial anatomy. Although fluoroscopy provides real-time imaging of the relevant spinal anatomy, the disadvantages discussed earlier for pedicle fixation also apply here. The application of image-guided navigation to this procedure adds a significant degree of accuracy in screw placement.

To apply image-guided navigation to posterior C1-2 screw fixation, a preoperative computed tomographic scan is required that extends from the lower occipital region to C3. The image data are transferred to the computer workstation and can be used to create a preoperative screw trajectory plan. A proposed entry point and target can be selected at the C2 and C1 levels, respectively. The image data set can then be manipulated in multiple planes between these two points to demonstrate the position of a screw placed along the selected trajectory. In addition to a sagittal image that demonstrates the same information provided by lateral fluoroscopy, two other images are presented. One of these images lies perpendicular to the sagittal image along the selected trajectory. It represents an orthogonal view that lies approximately midway between the coronal and axial planes through the spine, demonstrating a second view of the selected trajectory.

An additional view demonstrates an image oriented perpendicular to the long axis of the probe and, there-fore, the selected trajectory. A cursor superimposed on this image shows the position of the screw tip along the selected trajectory in increments of millimeters. By scrolling through this image, the proposed position of the screw along the selected trajectory can be assessed for its entire path. Although this planning technique does not ensure safe screw placement intraoperatively, it can alert the surgeon to avoid screw placement in patients with insufficient anatomy and to select an alternative approach.

Intraoperatively, the patient is positioned, and the posterior C1-2 complex is exposed. A wire (cable) and bone graft stabilization procedure at the C1-2 level is performed before navigation and screw insertion. Performing this step first minimizes any independent motion between C1 and C2 during navigation and makes tap and screw insertion easier. If a reference frame is used, it is typically attached to the spinous process of C2.

Following placement of the graft and cable, three to five registration points are selected at the C2 level. It is not necessary to include registration points at C1. Although the spatial relationship of C1 and C2 may change between the preoperative scanned position and the intraoperative position, the ability of image-guided navigation to facilitate accurate screw placement is not significantly affected. The most technically difficult part of this procedure is accurate passage of the screw through the narrow pars interarticularis of C2. The lateral mass of C1 is a relatively large target that can be easily reached, provided there is acceptable realignment of C1 and C2, as well as optimal positioning of the screw within the appropriate C2 anatomy. Although the relative position of C1 and C2 in both the preoperative image set and the surgical field is important, it is not critical enough to interfere with the process of image-guided navigation.

Two separate stab incisions are made on either side

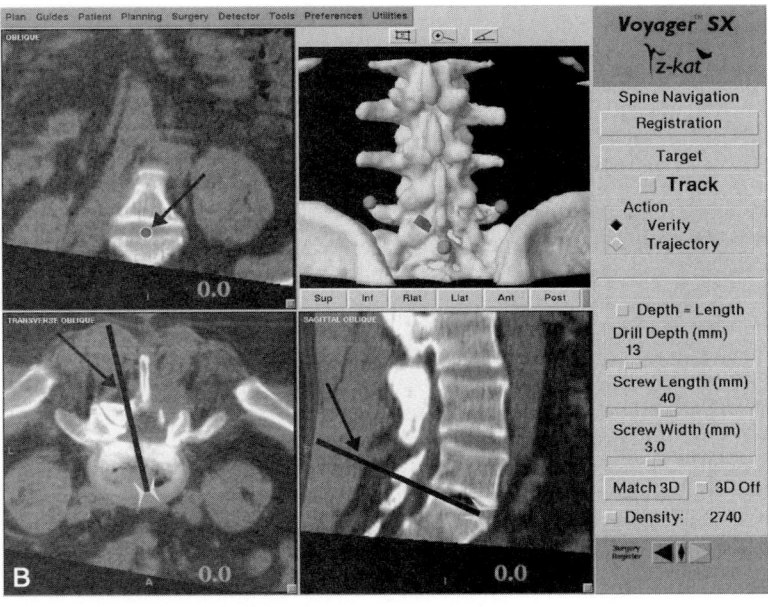

FIGURE 308–7. *A,* Workstation screen before L5-S1 disk excision for a posterior interbody fusion. (Probe tip location and trajectory highlighted by arrows.) *B,* Workstation screen after L5-S1 disk excision. The depth within the disk space and the extent of disk removal can be determined before cage or bone graft insertion. Fluoroscopy is not needed. (Probe tip location and trajectory highlighted by arrows.)

of the midline at the C7-T1 level. A drill guide is placed through one of the stab incisions and passed through the paravertebral musculature and into the operative field. A small divot is drilled at the proposed entry site to provide for secure placement of the drill guide. The registration process is performed at the C2 level, and its accuracy is confirmed using the verification step. The probe is passed through the drill guide, and as its position is adjusted in the surgical field, the images on the workstation screen adjust accordingly to show the corresponding trajectory in two separate planes and the projected location of the screw tip in the third plane. Orientation to the correct screw position can be assessed rapidly and accurately (Fig. 308–8). Any errors in trajectory or entry point selection can be determined and corrected by adjusting the position of the probe

and the drill guide through which it passes. When the correct screw insertion parameters have been selected, the probe is removed from the drill guide, and a drill is inserted. A hole is drilled along the selected trajectory and tapped, and the appropriate-length screw is inserted. The process is repeated on the opposite side.

The purpose of the drill guide is to preserve the physical trajectory and entry point information just acquired through the navigation of that pedicle. If a drill guide is not used, it may be difficult to precisely position a drill or pedicle probe on the same point and with the same trajectory previously conveyed by the navigational probe after probe removal.

Although image-guided navigation does not guarantee accurate screw placement, it does provide the surgeon with a greater degree of anatomic information

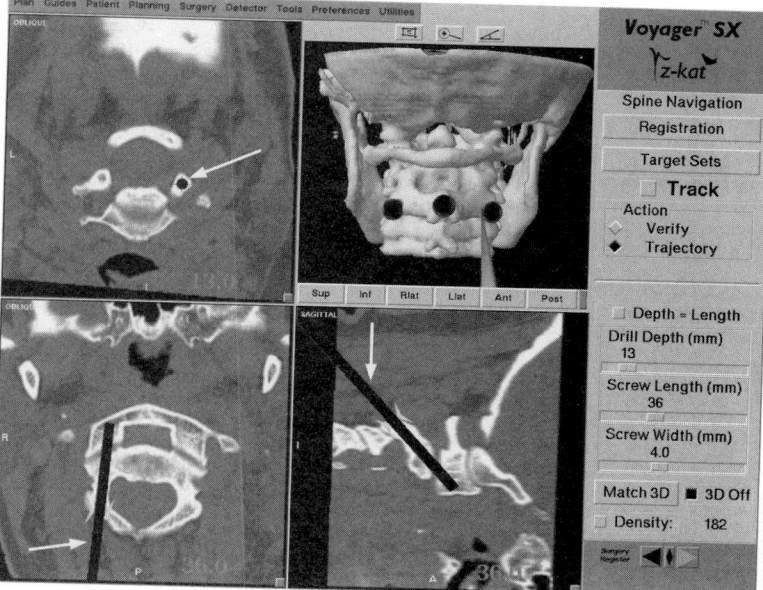

FIGURE 308–8. Workstation screen demonstrating a trajectory for insertion of a C1-2 transarticular screw. The lower right screen shows the trajectory in the sagittal plane. The lower left screen represents an orthogonal plane lying between the axial and coronal planes. It conveys the medial-lateral trajectory. The upper left screen represents a plane that is perpendicular to the two other images. It demonstrates the location of the screw tip inserted along the selected trajectory at the indicated depth. (Screw trajectory and tip location highlighted by arrows.)

than fluoroscopy alone. The addition of fluoroscopy to this navigational technique provides the greatest degree of precision. In this case, however, navigational technology significantly reduces the time required for intraoperative fluoroscopy, which is typically used only to help position the patient preoperatively and as a final check of the selected trajectory in the sagittal plane immediately following the navigational step.

Segmental C1-2 Screw Fixation

As an alternative to transarticular screw fixation, segmental fixation of C1-2 can be used to manage atlantoaxial instability.[21] The procedure involves placing a screw into each of the two lateral masses of C1 and two screws down the pedicles of C2. The polyaxial screw heads on each side are then connected with rods. Although this approach potentially reduces the risk of injury to the vertebral artery during screw insertion, it does not eliminate the risk altogether. As with the transarticular technique, precise anatomic orientation is required to avoid arterial or neural injury. Image guidance can supplement intraoperative fluoroscopy to provide the necessary orientation for accurate screw insertion.

As with the transarticular screw fixation technique, a preoperative computed tomographic scan is obtained. The posterior C1-2 spine is exposed, and a wire and cable fixation procedure is carried out. Registration is first performed at C1 for placement of the C1 lateral mass screws. The three registration points typically used at C1 are the midline posterior tubercle and the bilateral points marked by the junction of the small pedicle of C1 and its lateral mass (immediately above the two exiting C2 nerve roots). Once registration is complete, the correct trajectory into the lateral mass is displayed on the workstation screen, and the screws can be inserted (Fig. 308–9).

To use image guidance for inserting C2 pedicle screws, the same registration points are used as for transarticular fixation (the C2 spinous process and the two lateral margins of the C2-3 facet). The entry point for the screw is more lateral, and the trajectory is more medially oriented, than for a transarticular screw. The navigation probe is placed through a drill guide onto this entry point, and the selected trajectory is displayed on the workstation screen. When the correct entry point and trajectory have been selected, the probe is removed, a drill is inserted, and the pilot hole is drilled. The process is then repeated on the other side, and the heads of the screws are connected with two short rods.

Transoral Surgery

Transoral decompression of the upper cervical spine typically requires intraoperative fluoroscopy to help maintain proper anatomic orientation during the procedure. Although orientation in the sagittal plane is easy to obtain with fluoroscopy, depth and medial-lateral orientation are more difficult to assess. Image-guided technology can be used to orient the surgeon in multiple planes during transoral surgery.[12, 22]

Unlike in other spinal applications of image guidance, discrete registration points are not readily available during transoral surgery. In this setting, surface-mounted markers (fiducials) are applied to the patient before obtaining the preoperative computed tomographic scan. Typically, two fiducials are applied to the mastoid processes, and two are applied to the lateral orbital margins or to both malar eminences. The nasal septum can also be used as an inherent registration point.

The patient is positioned in a three-point head holder. The registration process is performed, using the surface-mounted fiducials, before draping the patient. Because the registration points will not be accessible

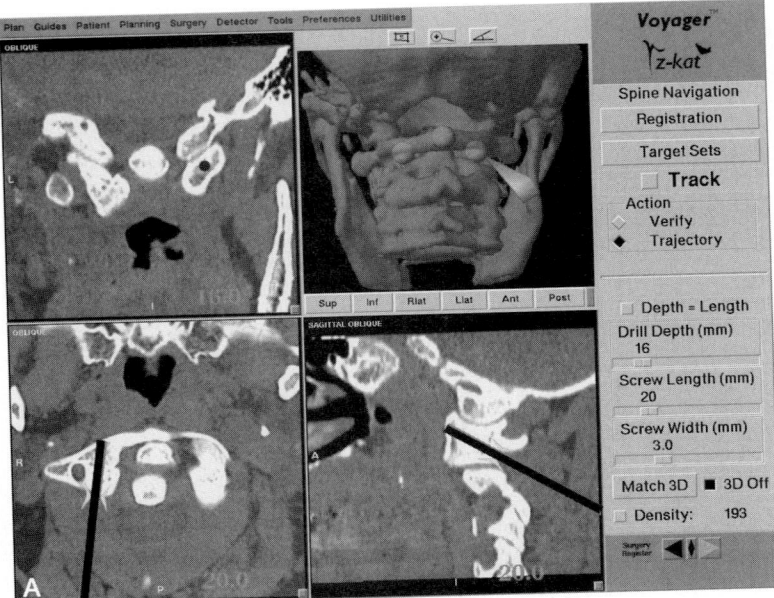

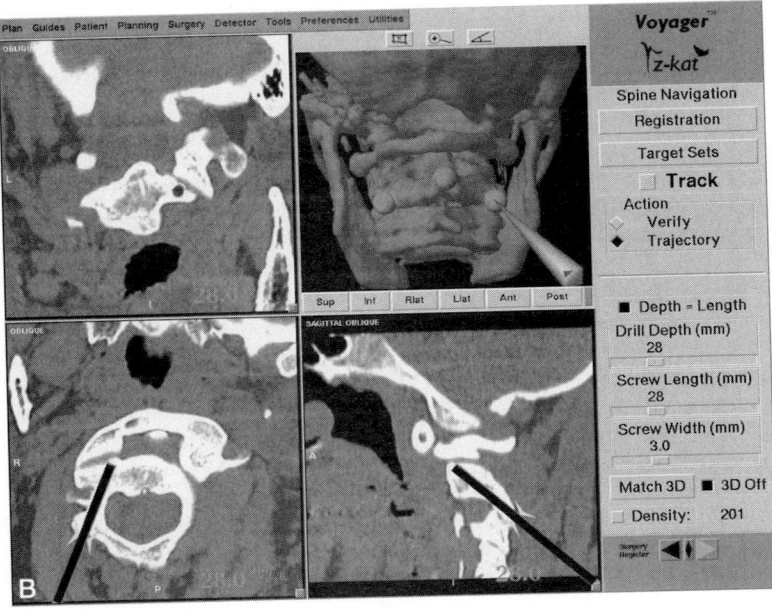

FIGURE 308–9. *A*, Workstation screen demonstrating navigational information for placement of a screw into the lateral mass of C1. *B*, Workstation screen demonstrating navigational information for placement of a screw into the pedicle of C2.

during the procedure, a reference frame is used for transoral navigation. This allows for changes in patient positioning during surgery without the need to reregister. The reference frame can be attached to the three-point head holder.

During the procedure, the probe can be placed into the site of the decompression. Reformatted sagittal, axial, and coronal computed tomographic images are immediately generated, providing the surgeon with a precise orientation to the pertinent surgical anatomy. In particular, orientation in the axial plane minimizes the risk of lateral deviation toward the vertebral artery during the decompression (Fig. 308–10). If posterior fixation is indicated following transoral decompression, the same computed tomographic image data set can be used for C1-2 screw placement

Anterior Thoracolumbar Surgery

Image-guided spinal navigation can be applied to anterior thoracolumbar surgery to help orient the surgeon to the extent of anterior decompression and to facilitate the precise placement of fixation screws. Although the selection of reference points for anterior spinal surgery is limited by the relative lack of prominent bony landmarks on the anterior aspect of the spinal column, the degree of accuracy required is less than that needed for most posterior screw fixation procedures. This degree of accuracy, termed *clinically relevant accuracy*, varies according to the procedure being performed. It represents the degree of accuracy needed to achieve a particular surgical task. For example, insertion of a C1-2 transarticular screw demands a higher clinically

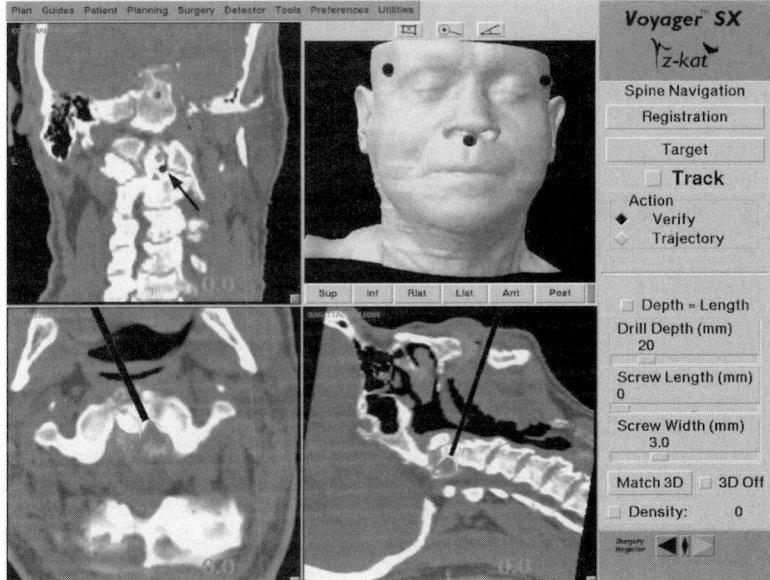

FIGURE 308–10. Workstation screen demonstrating navigational information during transoral decompression. (Probe tip location and trajectory highlighted by arrows.)

relevant accuracy than does placing an anterior fixation screw across a large thoracic or lumbar vertebral body. In both cases, image-guided navigation provides clinically relevant accuracy more consistently than does fluoroscopy alone.

Potential registration points for the use of image-guided navigation in anterior thoracolumbar surgery include selected landmarks on the vertebral end plates, pedicles, head of the rib, and prominent ventral osteophytes. In general, higher registration errors can be tolerated because of the lower accuracy requirements for most anterior thoracolumbar procedures compared with posterior screw fixation procedures. Performing the accuracy verification step immediately after registration can confirm the achievement of clinically relevant accuracy before proceeding with navigation.

During anterior decompression, the probe can be placed into the partially decompressed site to orient the surgeon to the contralateral margin of the spinal column and, more important, to the location of the epidural space (Fig. 308–11*A*). Orientation to tumor margins can also be obtained by placing the probe into the partially decompressed tumor bed. Following decompression, image guidance can be used to guide anterior fixation screws across the vertebrae at either end of the corpectomy site (see Fig. 308–11*B*).

Other Spinal Applications

Image-guided technology has several other applications in the management of complex spinal disorders. Any procedure in which intraoperative imaging is required to improve a surgeon's orientation to nonexposed spinal anatomy can benefit from image guidance. Other procedures to which image guidance has been applied include anterior screw fixation for nondisplaced odontoid fractures, cervical lateral mass screw fixation, cervical corpectomy, and the removal of para-

spinal neoplasms. The navigational workstation also provides superior image manipulation capabilities. This allows the surgeon to scroll through reformatted computed tomographic images in multiple planes, providing for optimal preoperative planning as well as improved intraoperative anatomic assessment.

PITFALLS

Although image-guided spinal navigation has proved to be a versatile and effective tool for facilitating complex surgical procedures, several problems can occur. In general, these pitfalls and errors are related to issues of accuracy, technique, and overall ease of use of the technology during surgery. A thorough understanding of these potential problems is required to ensure the efficient and effective use of image-guided navigation for spinal surgery.

Like any other computer-based technology, image-guided navigation is highly dependent on the quality of the information imported into the system. Although obtaining the properly formatted computed tomographic images and having them correctly transferred to the navigational workstation are important, the critical step of image guidance is the registration process. If the surgeon takes too casual an approach to registration, inaccurate information will be displayed during intraoperative navigation.

Another important principle of image guidance is the understanding that the navigational information provided must be correlated with the surgeon's own knowledge of the surgical anatomy and the appropriate screw trajectories through that anatomy. Image-guided navigation cannot replace the surgeon's understanding of the pertinent spinal anatomy and surgical technique. It merely helps confirm the surgeon's estimation of the nonexposed anatomy by providing im-

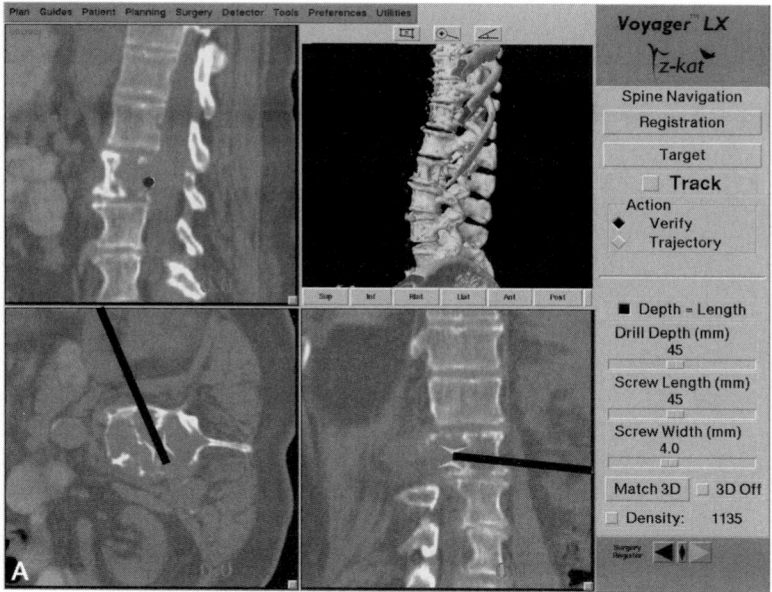

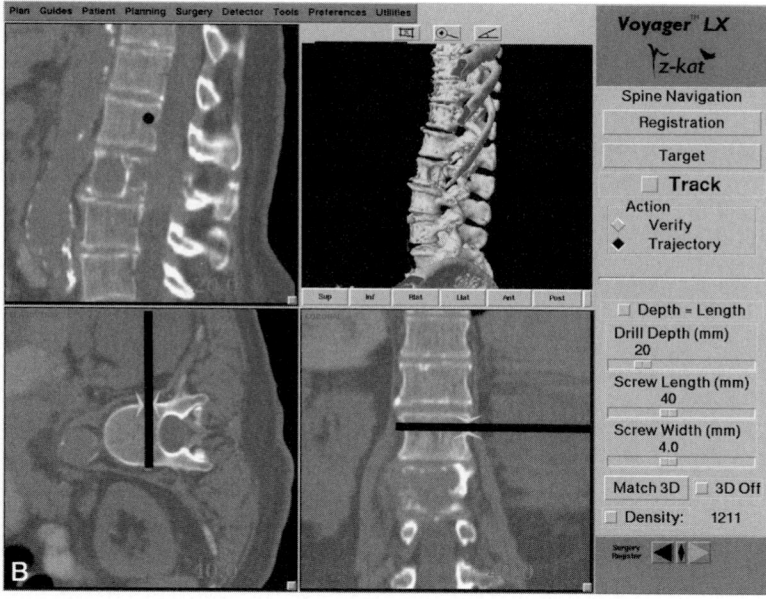

FIGURE 308–11. *A,* Workstation screen demonstrating navigation during removal of an L2 metastasis. Orientation to the contralateral side as well as the epidural space can be obtained. *B,* Workstation screen demonstrating a selected trajectory for an anterior lumbar fixation screw.

age information that exceeds that provided by intraoperative fluoroscopy.

Image-guided technology also has varying degrees of intraoperative functionality, depending on the features of the navigational system used. This translates into an ease-of-use factor that can either simplify or complicate the overall procedure. Typically, using surface mapping registration and a reference frame adds time to the navigational procedure, frequently making it longer and more complicated than using fluoroscopy alone. Using the paired point registration technique without a reference frame simplifies the spinal navigation process. With this approach, the insertion of four pedicle screws typically takes no more than 8 to 10 minutes. By optimizing the ease of use of navigational technology, standard fluoroscopy becomes unnecessary for most spinal screw fixation procedures.

FLUOROSCOPIC NAVIGATION

Fluoroscopic navigation is the combination of standard fluoroscopy and image-guided navigational technology. It was developed to counter the user difficulties of some earlier image-guided systems that typically took much longer to use than standard fluoroscopy did.[23] Its advantage is that it allows a reduction in fluoroscopic time during the procedure. Before surgery, but with the patient in position, anteroposterior and lateral fluoroscopic views of the pertinent spinal anatomy are obtained. This is done with a customized reference frame attached to the C-arm or to the patient. This frame serves to superimpose a specific grid on the two images obtained. The navigational workstation then takes the two images and relates the spatial position of the imaged anatomy to a navigational probe. A

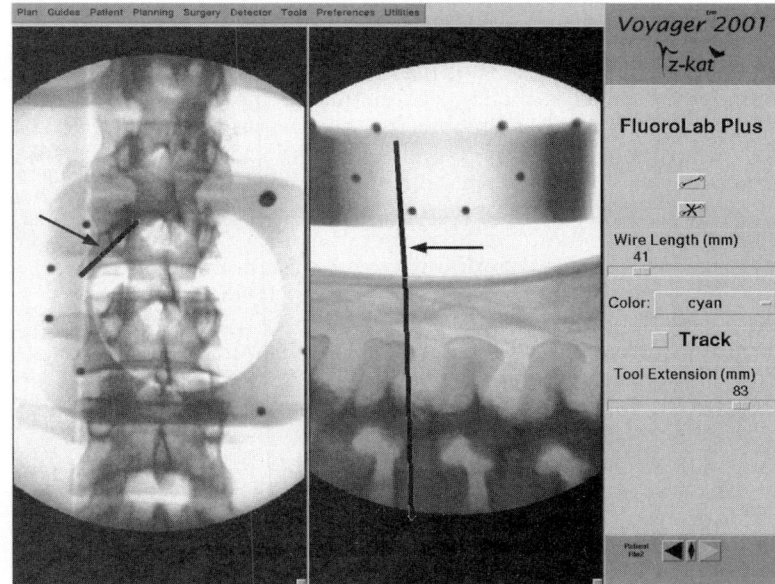

FIGURE 308–12. Workstation screen of a fluoroscopic navigational system. Only the standard anteroposterior and lateral views are provided. Unlike computed tomography–based image-guided navigation, fluoroscopic navigation does not provide the critical axial plane view.

navigational trajectory line and cursor can then be superimposed on the lateral and anteroposterior images, respectively. As the probe is moved over the exposed spinal anatomy during surgery, the trajectory line and cursor adjust their position on the stationary fluoroscopic images (Fig. 308–12).

The disadvantage of fluoroscopic navigation is that it is still only fluoroscopy. The same difficulties experienced with standard fluoroscopy are present with fluoroscopic navigation. Difficulties with anatomic visualization can occur in the upper thoracic region and in the lumbosacral region in obese individuals. More important, conventional fluoroscopy provides only anteroposterior and lateral images, whereas the critical plane for most spinal screw fixation procedures is the axial plane. This is the only plane that can definitively demonstrate violation of the spinal canal by a medially displaced screw. Computed tomography–based image-guided navigation provides images in the axial plane. Conventional fluoroscopy cannot provide this image.

A variation of conventional fluoroscopy called isocentric fluoroscopy may provide some solutions. With this technology, the fluoroscopic C-arm is swept in a 190-degree arc around the patient positioned on the operating table. Much like conventional computed tomographic imaging, the acquired images can then be reconstructed into multiplanar images, including images in the axial plane. Although the images are not of the same quality as standard computed tomographic imaging, they can be used for spinal navigation. This technology also offers the advantage of being able to acquire additional images during the course of the procedure.

CONCLUSION

The early goals of image-guided spinal navigation were to improve the surgeon's orientation to the intra-operative spinal anatomy in a time- and cost-efficient manner and to ultimately replace fluoroscopy. Although earlier image-guided systems were difficult to use intraoperatively, several advances have made some systems much easier to use. Several years of clinical experience have helped modify and improve navigational techniques. Paired point registration and the optional use of a reference frame both significantly reduce the difficulties of using image-guided technology for spinal procedures. Advances in computer and localizer technology have also contributed to the improved functionality of these systems. The greater ease of use of current image-guided systems, coupled with superior accuracy, image manipulation, and orientation capabilities, gives image-guided technology a clear advantage over any fluoroscopic-based technology.

Image-guided navigational technology has been successfully applied to spinal surgery. By linking digitized image data to spinal surface anatomy, image-guided spinal navigation facilitates the surgeon's orientation to unexposed spinal structures, improving the precision and accuracy of the surgery. It is typically used to optimize the placement of spinal fixation screws and to monitor the extent of complex decompressive procedures. It can also be used as a preoperative planning tool.

Although image-guided spinal navigation is a versatile and effective technology, it cannot replace the surgeon's thorough knowledge of the pertinent spinal anatomy and the correct surgical techniques. It is merely an additional source of information used by the surgeon to make intraoperative decisions. In this way, it is similar to more conventional intraoperative imaging techniques (e.g., fluoroscopy), except that it provides much more information to the surgeon.

Despite the advantages of image guidance, the surgeon must ultimately assess the information provided by these systems and determine whether it correlates with his or her estimation of the nonexposed anatomy and the proposed surgical plan. If good correlation exists between the two, the surgical step can be carried out. However, if sufficient correlation is lacking, the surgeon needs to reassess both the spinal anatomy and the accuracy of the image-guided registration before proceeding.

Ideally, the clinical application of this technology to spinal surgery should reduce operative time, morbidity, and costs. It should minimize or eliminate the need for conventional intraoperative imaging. It should be fast, easy to use, reliable, and capable of providing accurate intraoperative information while minimizing any disruption in the routine of the surgical procedure. Ultimately, beyond each individual surgical application, image-guided navigation technology needs to be clinically versatile. The routine use of this technology by multiple surgical specialties will drive its continued evolution and development, as well as establishing it as a cost-effective surgical tool.

REFERENCES

1. Kalfas IH, Kormos DW, Murphy MA, et al: Application of frameless stereotaxy to pedicle screw fixation of the spine. J Neurosurg 83:641–647, 1995.
2. Murphy MA, McKenzie RL, Kormos DW, Kalfas IH: Frameless stereotaxis for the insertion of lumbar pedicle screws: A technical note. J Clin Neurosci 1:257–260, 1994.
3. George DC, Krag MH, Johnson CC, et al: Hole preparation technique for transpedicle screws: Effect on pull-out strength from human cadaveric vertebrae. Spine 16:181–184, 1991.
4. Gertzbein SD, Robbins SE: Accuracy of pedicle screw placement in vivo. Spine 15:11–14, 1990.
5. Weinstein JN, Spratt KF, Spengler D, et al: Spinal pedicle fixation: Reliability and validity of roentgenogram-based assessment and surgical factors on successful screw placement. Spine 13:1012–1018, 1988.
6. Steinmann JC, Herkowitz HO, El-Kommos H, Wesolowski DP: Spinal pedicle fixation: Confirmation of an image-based technique for screw placement. Spine 18:1856–1861, 1993.
7. Barnett GH, Kormos DW, Steiner CP, Weisenberger J: Use of a frameless, armless stereotactic wand for brain tumor localization with two-dimensional and three-dimensional neuroimaging. Neurosurgery 33:674–678, 1993.
8. Barnett GH, Kormos DW, Steiner CP, Weisenberger J: Intraoperative localization using an armless, frameless stereotactic wand: Technical note. J Neurosurg 78:510–514, 1993.
9. Brodwater BK, Roberts DW, Nakajima T, et al: Extracranial application of the frameless stereotactic operating microscope: Experience with lumbar spine. Neurosurgery 32:209–213, 1993.
10. Bryant JT, Reid JG, Smith BL, Stevenson JM: A method for determining vertebral body positions in the sagittal plane using skin markers. Spine 14:258–265, 1989.
11. Pellizzari CA, Levin DN, Chen GTY, Chen CT: Image registration based on anatomic surface matching. In Maciunas RJ (ed): Interactive Image-Guided Neurosurgery. Park Ridge, IL, American Association of Neurological Surgeons, 1993, pp 47–62.
12. Kalfas IH: Image-guided spinal navigation. Clin Neurosurg 46:70–88, 1999.
13. Foley KT, Smith MM: Image-guided spine surgery. Neurosurg Clin N Am 7:171–186, 1996.
14. Glossop ND, Hu RW, Randle JA: Computer-aided pedicle screw placement using frameless sterotaxis. Spine 21:2026–2034, 1996.
15. Assaker R, Reyns N, Vinchon M, et al: Transpedicular screw placement: Image-guided versus lateral-view fluoroscopy: In vitro simulation. Spine 26:2160–2164, 2001.
16. Kalfas IH: Image-guided spinal navigation: Application to spinal metastasis. In Maciunas RJ (ed): Advanced Techniques in Central Nervous System Metastasis. Rolling Meadows, IL, AANS Publications, 1998, pp 245–254.
17. Kalfas IH: Frameless stereotaxy assisted spinal surgery. In Renganchary SS (ed): Neurosurgery Operative Color Atlas. Rolling Meadows, IL, AANS Publications, 2000, pp 123–134.
18. Laine T, Lund T, Ylikoski M, et al: Accuracy of pedicle screw insertion with and without computer assistance: A randomised controlled clinical study in 100 consecutive patients. Eur Spine J 9:235–240, 2000.
19. Welch WC, Subach BR, Pollack IF, Jacobs GB: Frameless sterotactic guidance for surgery of the upper cervical spine. Neurosurgery 40:958–964, 1997.
20. Youkilis AS, Quint DJ, McGillicuddy JE, Papadopoulos SM: Stereotactic navigation for placement of pedicle screws in the thoracic spine. Neurosurgery 48:771–778, 2001.
21. Harms J, Melcher R: Posterior C1-C2 fusion with polyaxial screw and rod fixation. Spine 26:2467–2471, 2001.
22. Welch WC, Subach BR, Pollack IF, Jacobs GB: Frameless sterotactic guidance for surgery of the upper cervical spine. Neurosurgery 40:958–964, 1997.
23. Foley KT, Simon DA, Rampersaud YR: Virtual fluoroscopy: Computer-assisted fluoroscopic navigation. Spine 26:347–351, 2001.

Thoracoscopic Approaches to the Spine

NICHOLAS THEODORE ■ CURTIS A. DICKMAN

Minimal incisional surgery has become a major goal across surgical subspecialties. Issues as diverse as cost containment, wound aesthetics, and decreased pain have all served as an impetus to refine these techniques. Technologic advances have helped make these procedures safe, viable options for a wide variety of pathologic conditions.

Advances in endoscopic imaging devices have played an important role in the development of minimally invasive surgery. Endoscopic image resolution now far surpasses that previously obtained because of improved technology such as computer interfacing, optical chips, fiberoptic cables, video endoscopy, and three-dimensional imaging. Endoscopes provide illumination, visualization, magnification, and a conduit to access areas of the human nervous system as diverse as the ventricular system and spine.

Endoscopic techniques in spinal surgery are now common for a variety of pathologic conditions: posterolateral percutaneous approaches to the lumbar disk spaces and neural foramina, anterior laparoscopic and anterolateral retroperitoneal endoscopic approaches to the lumbar spine, and thoracoscopic approaches to the thoracic spine.[1–14] Typically, rigid rod-lens endoscopes are used to visualize the anatomy and pathology; however, flexible fiberoptic endoscopes have also been used to inspect small spaces such as the neural foramina and syringomyelia cavities.[7–10, 13, 15] The resolution and image quality of flexible fiberoptic endoscopes are poorer than that of rigid endoscopes.

Endoscopes have found a valuable place in the treatment of thoracic spine disorders. Thoracoscopy was first widely used by cardiothoracic surgeons, and the techniques for thoracoscopic spinal surgery are adapted from their methods.[16–19] Today, thoracoscopic surgical techniques are used to perform sympathectomies, diskectomies, and vertebrectomies; to correct deformities; to stabilize the spine, and to biopsy and resect tumors.

HISTORICAL OVERVIEW

Beginning in the early 1900s, thoracoscopy was used as a diagnostic tool to evaluate pleural disease.[20–23]

During the late 1980s, techniques and instrumentation for endoscopic surgical procedures improved dramatically. In the early 1990s, thoracoscopic techniques were refined and applied to a broad spectrum of pathologic conditions involving the thorax.[16–19]

Today, many thoracic procedures previously performed via a thoracotomy are routinely performed thoracoscopically. These procedures include biopsy or resection of pleural or lung lesions, lymph node biopsy, biopsy and resection of mediastinal masses, lobectomy, pneumonectomy, pleural sclerotherapy, treatment of blebs, esophageal procedures, and sympathectomy, among others.[16–19, 24] For the treatment of thoracic pathology, thoracoscopy seems to have significant advantages compared with thoracotomy.[24–26] In the resection of pulmonary lesions, for example,[24–26] small thoracoscopic incisions have minimized dissection and retraction of the chest wall, reduced postoperative pain, decreased blood loss, shortened intensive care unit and overall hospital stays, improved postoperative pulmonary and shoulder function, hastened recovery times, and decreased complications.[16–19, 24–26]

The techniques of thoracoscopic spine surgery were independently developed by John Regan and coworkers[3, 6] in the United States and Daniel Rosenthal and colleagues[5, 27] in Germany. The first report of thoracoscopy for spinal diseases was published by Mack and associates[28] who described 10 patients with diverse spinal pathology effectively treated thoracoscopically without major complications. Rosenthal and colleagues[5] and Horowitz and coworkers[4] published separate reports that described the techniques for performing thoracic microdiskectomy thoracoscopically. Since then, numerous reports have demonstrated the effectiveness of thoracoscopic spinal surgery for the treatment of a wide variety of spinal disorders.[16, 29–31]

INDICATIONS

Thoracoscopy can be used to access the sympathetic chain, disks, vertebral bodies, and the ipsilateral pedicle; however, it cannot be used to access the posterior elements of the spine. Thoracoscopic approaches have been used to treat herniated thoracic disks,[2–6, 28] to drain

TABLE 309–1 ■ **Potential Indications for Thoracoscopic Spinal Surgery**

Sympathectomy
Diskectomy
Corpectomy with reconstruction
Biopsy of vertebral body or disk
Drainage of vertebral or perivertebral abscess
Resection of neurogenic tumor
Anterior release to correct a kyphotic deformity
Scoliosis to correct a deformity

TABLE 309–3 ■ **Contraindications for Thoracoscopic Procedures**

Previous ipsilateral thoracotomy or thoracoscopy (relative)
History of previous pleural inflammatory disease (relative)
Cardiac or pulmonary disease precluding unilateral ventilation (absolute)
Dense pleural adhesions (absolute)
Medical reasons prohibiting surgery (absolute)

vertebral epidural abscesses, to débride vertebral osteomyelitis and diskitis, to decompress fractures, to biopsy and resect neoplasms,[1–3, 28] and to perform vertebrectomies and interbody fusions, vertebral body reconstructions and instrumentation,[1–3, 28, 30] sympathectomies,[32–34] and anterior releases for the treatment of kyphosis and scoliosis (Table 309–1).[2, 3, 6, 28, 30]

Costotransversectomy, thoracotomy, and thoracoscopy are the three major techniques available to address thoracic vertebral and disk pathologic conditions. Each technique has distinct advantages and disadvantages (Table 309–2). When the ventral aspect of the dura must be visualized well, an anterior approach (thoracotomy or thoracoscopy) is necessary. Most spinal surgeons use thoracotomy reluctantly because of the complications and pain associated with the procedure and the need for a cardiothoracic surgeon to perform the exposure and closure.[29, 35–44] A transthoracic approach, however, significantly improves visualization of the ventral surfaces of the spine and spinal cord to facilitate decompression, reconstruction, and internal fixation compared with posterolateral approaches. Thoracoscopy can be used for almost any procedure that is suitable for thoracotomy and provides a more direct, complete view of the ventral aspect of the thoracic spine and dura than does costotransversectomy. This being said, costotransversectomy and other posterolateral approaches, such as the transpedicular approach, still have a place for lateral pathologic conditions.

CONTRAINDICATIONS

Contraindications to a thoracoscopic approach are similar to those for open approaches and include medical reasons that would prohibit surgery (uncontrollable coagulopathy, terminal illness, or severe cardiac or pulmonary disease). Requirements specific to thoracoscopic approaches include the ability to tolerate prolonged single-lung ventilation and the absence of significant pleural adhesions or advanced pulmonary disease. Patients with conditions such as chest trauma, emphysema, or hemothorax, or those who have undergone a prior thoracotomy may have extensive adhesions that prohibit thoracoscopic access. Extensive scar tissue from an earlier operation at the site of spinal pathology also precludes thoracoscopy. Consequently, most patients should be evaluated before surgery by a pulmonologist or internist as well as by a cardiothoracic surgeon when indicated. The preoperative assessment can include spirometry, blood gas determinations, and pulmonary function studies as needed (Table 309–3).

EDUCATIONAL ISSUES

Thoracoscopy represents a technique that is fundamentally unfamiliar to most spinal surgeons. Because of

TABLE 309–2 ■ **Comparison of Operative Approaches to the Thoracic Spine**

CHARACTERISTIC	THORACOSCOPY	THORACOTOMY	COSTOTRANSVERSECTOMY
Direction of approach	Anterolateral	Anterolateral	Posterolateral
View of ventral surface of spinal cord	Full, direct	Full, direct	Oblique, indirect
Size of incisions	0.5–1 inch (× 3–4 inches)	6 to 15 inches	4 to 12 inches
Muscle transection	Minimal	Extensive	Moderate or extensive
Relationship to pleura	Intrapleural	Intrapleural	Extrapleural
Postoperative chest tube	Yes	Yes	No
Access to posterior spinal elements for decompression or fixation	No	No	Yes
Access to vertebral bodies for screw-plate fixation	Yes	Yes	No
Extent of rib resection or rib retraction	1 inch of rib head and proximal rib removed, no retraction	6 to 12 inches of rib removed, extensive retraction	3 to 7 inches of rib removed, moderate retraction
Incidence of postoperative intercostal neuralgia	Rare, usually transient	Common, often prolonged	Uncommon, often transient

From Dickman CA, Karahalios DG: Thoracoscopic spinal surgery. Clin Neurosurg 43:392–422, 1996.

the restricted portals of entry, thoracoscopic techniques require new psychomotor skills for navigating and manipulating instruments from a distance while watching the procedure in real time on a video monitor. The clinical application of thoracoscopic techniques should only follow a comprehensive training program that includes didactic and practical components. Extensive practice in a surgical skills laboratory in either animal or human models is mandatory. Because of the rather steep "learning curve," surgeons should observe or assist individuals with significant thoracoscopic experience. Procedures also should be performed with the assistance of a cardiothoracic surgeon so that open exposure can be performed immediately if needed. Although there are no specific "guidelines" for the practice of thoracoscopic spinal surgery, the cardiothoracic surgery community has outlined the ethical and educational issues relating to the use of this technique by their practitioners.[15, 45]

THORACOSCOPIC TECHNIQUE

General Considerations

Thoracoscopic spinal surgery requires a thorough familiarity with the anatomy of the thoracic spine, spinal cord, thorax, and mediastinum. The decision to approach from the left or right side depends on the location, lateralization, and extent of the pathology. The position of the great vessels is also important to consider and may be evaluated on preoperative computed tomography or magnetic resonance imaging studies. Midline lesions are most often approached on the right side because more spinal surface area is usually available behind the azygos vein than behind the aorta. If a lesion is on the left side, a left-sided approach is more appropriate. A left-sided approach is also preferred for lesions below T9 because the diaphragm rides high on the right side at this level. In general, an exposure from T1 to the T11-12 interspace is possible via the thoracoscopic approach.

Thoracoscopic Imaging

In thoracoscopy the endoscope is used for illumination, visualization, and magnification. Unlike other endoscopic techniques, working channels within the scope are rarely used. Several separate portals are inserted in the chest wall for the endoscope and various instruments. A standard 5-mm- or 1-cm-diameter rigid-rod lens endoscope with a 0- to 30-degree angle of view is connected to a two-dimensional or three-dimensional camera, which transmits the image to a video monitor. High-resolution three-dimensional endoscopes can vividly represent complex regional anatomy and enhance the surgeon's ability to use instruments in this region. Xenon or halogen light sources are primarily used and delivered via fiberoptic cables. The endoscope is usually affixed to a table-mounted endoscopic holder with or without voice-activated robotic control to free the surgeon's and assistant's hands.

A clear endoscopic image is essential, and the lens must remain free of debris. The lens can be cleaned manually or by using the irrigating and automated wiper mechanisms on the tips of some endoscopes. Fogging is avoided by prewarming the endoscope, using warmed irrigation solution, and periodically wiping the lens with an antifogging agent. Frequent irrigation and suctioning eliminate blood from pooling in the thoracic cavity. Otherwise, blood absorbs a significant amount of light and darkens the operative field.

Instruments

The actual working distance in thoracoscopic surgery is much longer than in "open" procedures. Depending on the patient's size and the position of the portals, this distance ranges from 14 to 30 cm. Most of the long tools developed for thoracoscopic spine surgery require two hands for precise control during dissection and decompression of the nerves and spinal cord. These long tools also amplify motions differently than do shorter tools. Techniques to master the use of long endoscopic spine tools and avoid unnecessary movements should be practiced in the laboratory before clinical application.

Commercially available instruments for use in thoracoscopic spinal surgery include soft tissue dissectors, microscissors, fine tissue forceps, Babcock clamps, Allis clamps, right-angled forceps, suction-irrigation tools, mono- and bipolar cautery devices, and peanut dissectors. Bone and disk instruments include various straight and curved curettes, Kerrison and Leksell rongeurs, Penfield instruments, nerve hooks, periosteal elevators, rib dissectors, disk space rongeurs, osteotomes, and bone graft impactors. High-speed drills with a pistol grip and long drill bits are also available commercially (Midas Rex Pneumatic Tools, Inc., Fort Worth, Tex).

During all thoracoscopic cases, a complete thoracotomy tray should be opened onto the sterile field in the operating room in the unlikely event that a major vessel is damaged or immediate conversion to an open thoracotomy is needed for another reason.

Hemostatic Agents

The techniques used to obtain hemostasis are identical to the methods used in open surgery. A number of tools and methods can be used for hemostasis in thoracoscopic spinal surgery, including vascular clips and monopolar and bipolar cauterization devices. As in "open" procedures, monopolar cauterization should be used with caution in the region of the spinal cord and nerve roots. Cotton-tipped peanut dissectors can be used to apply bone wax. Gelatin sponges, microfibrillar collagen, and oxidized regenerated cellulose absorbable hemostatic agents can also be used to tamponade epidural venous bleeding gently. Cotton surgical patties with long strings can be used, but the end of the string must be anchored outside the chest wall to prevent loss of the pattie within the thoracic cavity. In the event of massive hemorrhage resulting from injury to the great vessels, a tightly rolled 4 × 4 sponge on a long clamp (sponge stick) can be used to provide gentle tamponade until the chest is opened.

Operating Room Setup and Patient Positioning

Because of the extensive equipment and large number of personnel needed for most thoracoscopic cases, a large operating room is preferred. In addition to the patient, there are typically two or three surgeons (spinal surgeon, assistant, and cardiothoracic surgeon), the scrub and circulating nurses, a clinical neurophysiology monitoring technician, and an anesthesiologist. A radiographic technician and videographer–medical photographer may also be present.

A radiolucent operating table is used so that fluoroscopic images can be obtained intraoperatively. Initially, the patient is placed supine on the operating room table while a double-lumen endotracheal tube is placed. Fiberoptic bronchoscopic equipment should be kept in the room should the endotracheal tube need to be repositioned or the patient suctioned during the procedure. Typically, the anesthesiologist is positioned at the head of the operating table (Fig. 309–1). An arterial line, central venous and urinary catheters, and pneumatic compression stockings are placed. Somatosensory or motor evoked potential leads, or both, are connected and baseline recordings are obtained before the patient is positioned.

The patient is then turned and placed in a lateral decubitus position with the side to be operated on facing up. The anesthesiologist reassesses the position

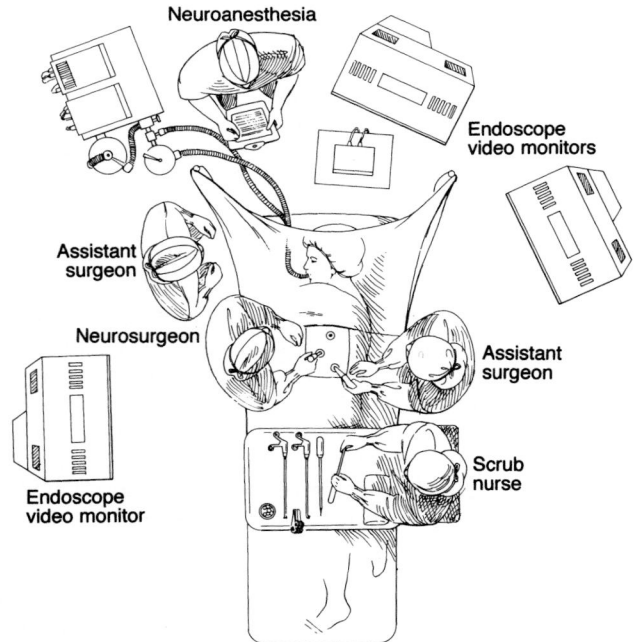

FIGURE 309–1. Position of the patient, surgeon, assistant, scrub nurse, video monitors, and anesthesiologist during a thoracoscopic procedure. (Courtesy of Barrow Neurological Institute, St. Joseph's Hospital and Medical Center, Phoenix, AZ.)

of the double-lumen endotracheal tube to ensure that it has not migrated. During a thoracoscopic procedure, the deflated lung is allowed to re-expand several minutes each hour to decrease the chance of the patient developing symptomatic atelectasis after surgery.

A foam axillary roll is used to pad the dependent axilla. The legs are flexed at the knees, and all bony prominences are meticulously padded with pillows and foam padding. The hips and shoulder are firmly secured to the operating table so that the patient can be tilted safely during surgery. The tilting allows the nonventilated lung to fall away from the spine and sometimes reduces the need to retract the lung mechanically. The patient's dependent arm is placed on a padded arm board, and the upper arm is elevated on a pillow or secured via a sling or ether screen. Abduction of the upper arm moves the scapula dorsally and increases exposure of the chest wall.

Intraoperative image-intensification (C-arm) is positioned to obtain a clear anteroposterior view of the thoracic spine to verify the appropriate level before the skin is marked with indelible ink. Preoperative markings on the skin include the position of the portals, scapula, and potential thoracotomy incision. The patient's entire chest, axillary region, proximal arm, back, and abdomen are then sterilely scrubbed, prepared, and draped.

During the procedure the surgeon and assistant stand anterior to the patient facing the anterior thorax. The scrub nurse can stand on the same side as the surgeon or across the operating table next to a Mayo stand. Ideally, two video monitors are used. The first is placed across the operating table for viewing by the surgeons. The second is positioned for the scrub nurse. A backup system should be available. Before surgery, the endoscope lens is prewarmed in irrigation solution, dried, and treated with a lens defogging solution.

Portal Insertion

Depending on the procedure, two to four portals are inserted to gain access to the thoracic cavity (Fig. 309–2). The portals should be spread far enough apart so that the surgeon's hands are neither too close together nor too close to the endoscope. The working portals (for instruments) are best positioned anterolaterally between the anterior and middle axillary lines. The endoscope portal is best positioned posterolaterally between the middle and posterior axillary line. This technique allows the surgeon's hands to rest comfortably during the procedure. The axilla and first and second interspaces are never entered to avoid injury to the brachial plexus and great vessels, respectively. Exposure from T9 through T12 requires caudal retraction of the diaphragm to expose the costophrenic recess. This exposure can be enhanced by a reverse Trendelenburg position and a fan retractor.

When a 0 degree–angled endoscope is used, the portal is placed directly over the spinal segment of interest. When a 30 degree–angled endoscope is used, the portal position must be offset above or below the level of pathology and the scope angled obliquely.

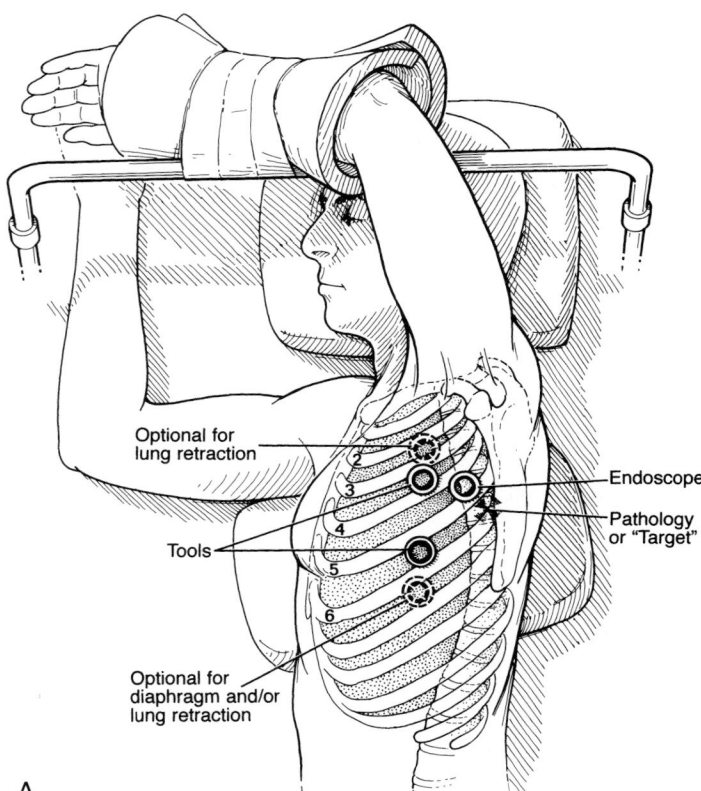

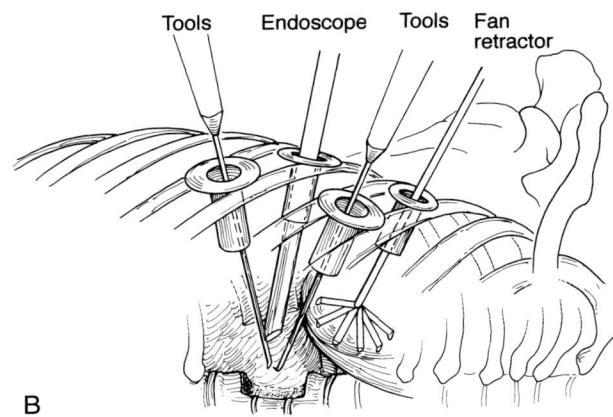

FIGURE 309–2. *A,* Patient in the right lateral decubitus position. The endoscopic port is placed posteriorly between the middle and posterior axillary lines situated over the level of interest. Working portals for instruments and retractors are placed anterolaterally between the anterior and middle axillary lines effectively "triangulating" the level of pathology. An optional superior (lung retraction) or inferior (diaphragm or lung retraction, or both) portal can be placed as needed. *B,* Close-up view of the principle of "triangulating" the endoscope and instruments around the level of pathology. The portals should be placed far enough apart to avoid "fencing." (*A* Courtesy of Barrow Neurological Institute, St. Joseph's Hospital and Medical Center, Phoenix, Ariz. *B* from Dickman CA, Rosenthal DJ: Thoracoscopic access strategies: Portal placement techniques and portal selection. In Dickman CA, Rosenthal DJ, Perin NI [eds]: Thoracoscopic Spine Surgery. New York, Thieme, 1999, pp 107–124.)

The positions of the portals are triangulated over the region of pathology and ideally evenly spaced rostral and caudal to the surgical target. The configuration is much like a baseball diamond: The surgeon is positioned at home plate, the target (and endoscope) is positioned at second base, and the working portals are at first base and third base. If needed, a fan retractor can be placed between the anterior and middle axillary lines, rostral or caudal to the working portals.

Flexible portals are used in thoracoscopic spinal procedures to avoid injury to the intercostal nerves. Portals serve to keep blood and debris off the endoscope and instruments. An 11- or 15-mm portal is adequate for most purposes. A smaller portal can be used for a suction-irrigation tool (7 mm). A larger portal is needed when bone grafts or instrumentation is to be placed.

Before the portals are placed, the skin is infiltrated and an intercostal nerve block is administered with a local anesthetic (1% bupivicaine and epinephrine [Marcaine with epinephrine]). The skin is incised parallel to the superior surface of the rib to avoid injury to the neurovascular bundle. A hemostat is passed through the intercostal muscles and parietal pleura directly adjacent to the superior surface of the rib. A finger can be inserted to check for lung adhesions that would preclude the introduction of a portal at that site. Portals are placed over a rigid trocar, which is removed immediately after the portals have been placed (Fig. 309–3). The proximal end of the portal is stapled or sutured to the skin to anchor it to the chest wall during surgery.

The endoscope is placed after the first portal is in-

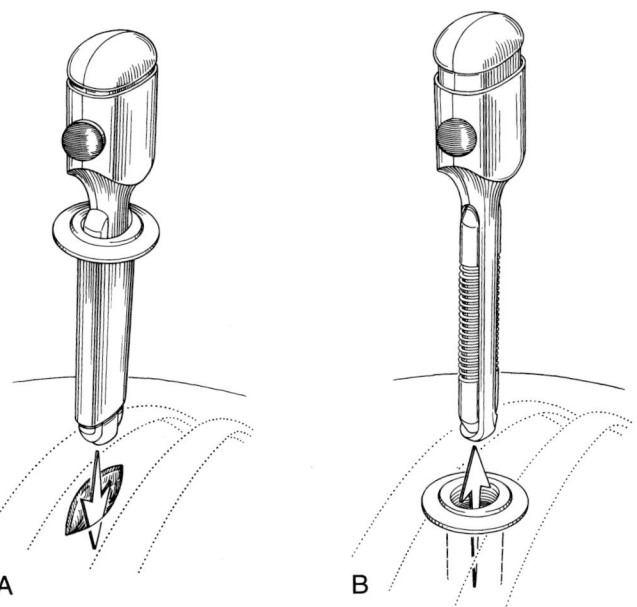

FIGURE 309–3. *A,* Technique of portal insertion. After a small incision is made parallel to the superior surface of the rib and access to the thoracic cavity with a hemostat has been obtained, a flexible portal is inserted with a trocar. *B,* The trocar is removed, leaving the portal in place. Portals can be secured with suture or surgical staples. Subsequent portals are placed under direct endoscopic vision. (Courtesy of Barrow Neurological Institute, St. Joseph's Hospital and Medical Center, Phoenix, AZ.)

serted. Additional portals are placed under direct endoscopic visualization. Small adhesions can be addressed with sharp or blunt dissection techniques; however, dense, diffuse adhesions usually preclude thoracoscopic access and require conversion to a thoracotomy.

Initial Spinal Exposure

As the lung is deflated, the thoracoscope is inserted to visualize the thoracic cavity. If necessary, the operating room table is rotated 30 to 40 degrees anteriorly to allow the lung to fall away from the spine and minimize the need for retraction. An endoscopic fan retractor can be inserted through another portal for gentle lung retraction. This instrument, however, must be opened and closed under visualization to avoid lacerating the lung. When present, pleural adhesions can be detached with cauterization and scissors to mobilize the lung.

Wound Closure and Postoperative Management

At the conclusion of the procedure after hemostasis has been obtained, the contents of the thoracic cavity are inspected carefully with the thoracoscope. All tissue debris and blood are thoroughly irrigated from the thoracic cavity. The fan retractors are removed, and the surface of the lung is inspected for air leaks or contusions as it is inflated. One or two chest tubes are placed through separate, preexisting portal incisions under direct thoracoscopic visualization to ensure proper positioning. The chest tube is secured with a heavy-gauge silk or nylon suture. The apical chest tube is used to reinflate the lung, and the posteroinferior tube is used to drain fluid and blood from the thorax after surgery.

The wounds are closed with a subcuticular skin closure. The chest tubes are placed to 20 cm H_2O of suction. The skin entry sites for the chest tubes are sealed with an occlusive dressing and nylon suture material. Postoperative chest and spine radiographs are obtained.

THORACIC ENDOSCOPIC SYMPATHECTOMY

Several clinical syndromes that result from pathologically elevated sympathetic tone can be treated surgically by thoracic sympathectomy. These entities include palmar or axillary hyperhidrosis, pain syndromes involving the upper extremities such as reflex sympathetic dystrophy (RSD), ischemic syndromes of the hand such as Raynaud's disease, and malignant tachyarrhythmias that are refractory to medical management. Physiologically, these disease processes are mediated primarily through the second, third, and sometimes fourth sympathetic ganglia. Thoracic endoscopic sympathectomy, a technique first described in 1951,[46] provides an appealing alternative for patients

with conditions that are treatable by sympathetic denervation.

Surgical Indications

Several major groups of disorders can be treated by thoracoscopic sympathectomy (Table 309–4), and contraindications for the procedure are few. Idiopathic (essential) palmar hyperhidrosis is the most common indication for thoracoscopic sympathectomy. Most patients who receive a neurosurgical referral for this condition have been evaluated for metabolic (hyperthyroidism) or neoplastic causes and have failed efforts at medical management with topical and anticholinergic agents.

In clinical series, the success rate of sympathectomy for permanent relief of palmar hyperhidrosis ranges from 90% to 100%.[33, 34, 47–55] Axillary hyperhidrosis and bromhidrosis (axillary malodor) can also be addressed through a sympathectomy that targets the T3 and T4 ganglia.[48] Associated plantar hyperhidrosis often (50%) resolves when hyperhidrosis of the upper extremities is relieved and is referred to as a "dividend benefit" of the procedure because it is not an expected effect of transecting the upper thoracic sympathetic chain.

Reflex sympathetic dystrophy (also known as *complex regional pain syndrome type I*)[56] is one of a number of pain syndromes that typically follow trauma. Current evidence suggests that an upregulated sensitivity of α-adrenoreceptors for catecholamines in the injured limb reduces reflex sympathetic dystrophy. Medical therapy tends to be ineffective in terms of both the degree and duration of relief. Patients who experience symptomatic relief after percutaneous blocks of the stellate ganglion with local anesthetic agents are considered candidates for surgical sympathectomy.[33, 49, 54] Long-term clinical benefits have been reported for this indication in more than 50% of patients.[57, 58]

Patients with severe upper extremity ischemia due to Raynaud's disease or related disorders may also benefit from sympathectomy.[33, 49, 54] Although the ischemic process is typically progressive, sympathectomy can be used to avoid limb amputation and to improve the associated complaints of pains.

Sympathectomy can also effectively relieve pain re-

TABLE 309–4 ■ **Indications for Sympathectomy**

Hyperhidrosis
    Palmar
    Axillary
    Plantar
Pain syndromes
    Post-traumatic (complex regional pain syndrome)
    Reflex sympathetic dystrophy
    Phantom pain
    Cancer pain
    Pancreatic
Ischemic syndromes
    Raynaud's disease
Tachyarrhythmia

From Dickman CA, Baskin JJ, Theodore N: Thoracic endoscopic sympathectomy. In Fessler RG, Sekhar LN (eds): Atlas of Neurosurgical Techniques. New York, Thieme, in press.

lated to pancreatic carcinoma.[59] This procedure entails lesioning the sympathetic ganglia on the left side from T5 through T9 to denervate the greater splanchnic nerve and lesioning the T10 and T11 ganglia to denervate the lesser splanchnic nerve.

Relative hyperactivity of left-sided sympathetic tone increases the QT interval on electrocardiography.[32, 57, 60] Conversely, stimulation on the right side from the T1 through T4 ganglia decreases the QT interval. Lesioning the ganglia on the left side from T1 through T4 shortens the QT interval and reduces the risk of a malignant arrhythmia developing in conjunction with a prolonged QT interval.[61]

Surgical Goals

Sympathetic denervation can be achieved through several actions. The autonomic tissue can be resected or the connections between the ganglia and the autonomic chain can be disrupted using sharp transection or thermal methods. Our practice has shifted from en bloc excision of these neural structures (ganglia with the interval sympathetic chain) to sharp transection of the ganglia and sympathetic chain with cauterization and scissors.

While this procedure is performed, the accessory innervations to the sympathetic chain must be addressed. The accessory nerve of Kuntz, if present, arises from the sympathetic trunk at the level of T1, T2, or T3. It must be transected to optimize the chances of the sympathectomy being effective.[62] Preserving the rostral half of the stellate ganglion in its position overlying the first rib head avoids incurring Horner's syndrome during the sympathectomy.

Patient Positioning

Although the supine position has been used, we prefer to place the patient in a lateral decubitus position.[51] This position permits dependent retraction of the lung and rapid conversion to an open procedure if necessary.

If a bilateral sympathectomy is necessary, the procedures are performed sequentially under the same anesthetic with the patient being repositioned and redraped between procedures. Palmar temperature is monitored bilaterally to document vasodilatation related to the sympathectomy.

The patient is rotated approximately 40 degrees toward the surgeon, which allows gravity to retract the lung and brings the thoracic vertebral column within view. A mild reverse Trendelenburg position allows the lung to fall away from the apex of the pleural cavity. The procedure is performed through two incisions (5 mm each) in the chest wall. The first 5-mm-diameter portal is placed in the middle or posterior axillary line within the fourth or fifth intercostal space (Fig. 309–4). Care is exerted to avoid the intercostal bundle along the caudal aspect of the rostral rib. The 5-mm-diameter rigid rod-lens thoracoscope is passed through this portal. A second 5-mm portal incision is placed in the anterior axillary line within the *third* intercostal space,

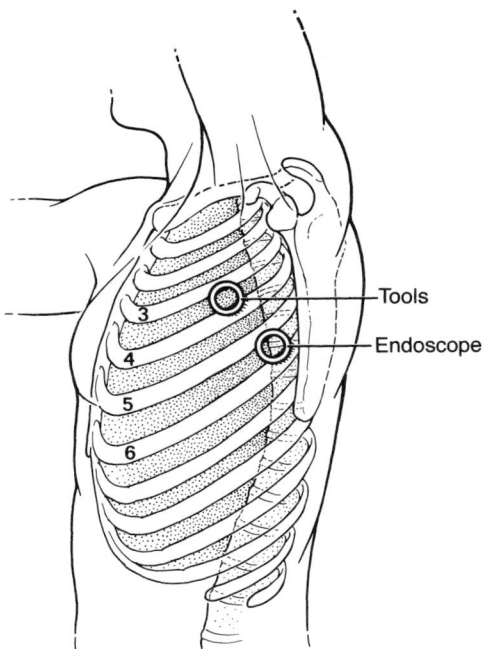

FIGURE 309–4. Patient positioning and portal insertion sites for a left-sided thoracoscopic sympathectomy. For a right-sided approach, the patient is similarly positioned on the opposite side. (Courtesy of Barrow Neurological Institute, St. Joseph's Hospital and Medical Center, Phoenix, AZ.)

and a hemostat is used to perforate the parietal pleura under direct visualization with the thoracoscope. Care is taken to avoid the subclavian vessels near the first and second intercostal spaces. The 5-mm-diameter endoscopic monopolar scissors are passed into the thoracic cavity. Gently patting the deflated lung with an endoscopic dissection tool produces further atelectasis and improves the visualization of the spinal column. If the lung continues to obscure exposure, a third incision can be made so that a lung (fan) retractor can be placed.

Anatomic Orientation

Typically, the stellate ganglion, sympathetic chain, and accessory sympathetic innervation can be visualized beneath the parietal pleura. The sympathetic chain is recognized as it crosses over the rib heads (Fig. 309–5). The first rib can be palpated, and the second through fourth ribs can be visualized directly. The stellate ganglion is located directly over the head of the first rib and typically is surrounded by a fat pad within the thoracic outlet, adjacent to the subclavian vasculature.

Care must be taken to avoid injuring the several large regional vessels. On the right side, tributaries of the second, third, and fourth intercostal veins merge to form the superior intercostal vein, which then empties into the azygos vein. The first intercostal vein drains directly into the brachiocephalic vein. On the left side, the subclavian artery and intercostal vessels are adjacent to the region of dissection. Because the sympathetic chain is positioned superficial to the segmental

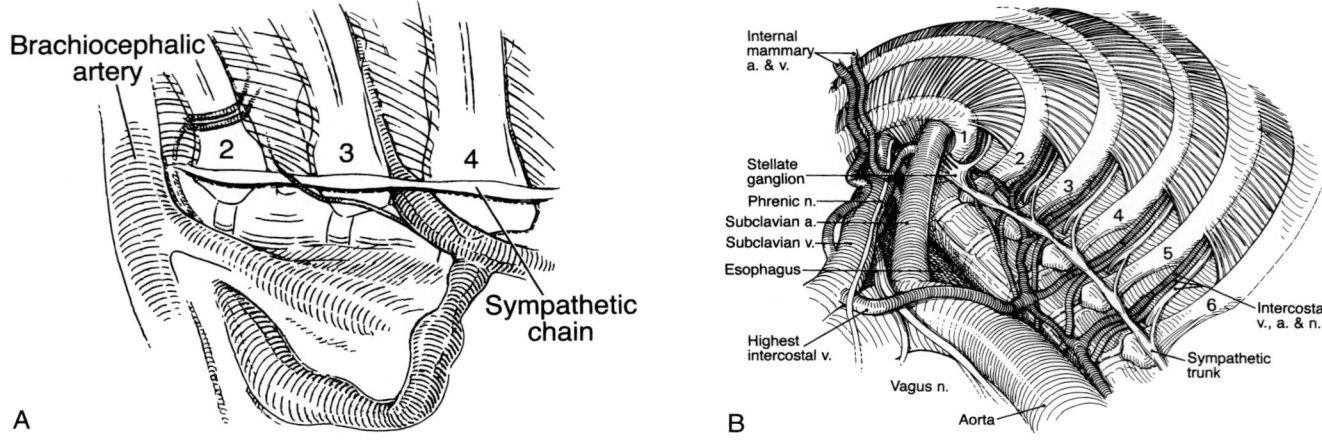

Brachiocephalic artery

2 3 4

Sympathetic chain

A

Internal mammary a. & v.

Stellate ganglion
Phrenic n.
Subclavian a.
Subclavian v.
Esophagus

Highest intercostal v.

Vagus n.

Aorta

1 2 3 4 5 6

Intercostal v., a. & n.

Sympathetic trunk

B

FIGURE 309–5. *A,* Regional anatomy for a right-sided thoracoscopic sympathectomy. The sympathetic chain lies over the rib head and is easily identified. *B,* Similar anatomic overview of the left thoracic cavity. The first rib and overlying stellate ganglion can be palpated; they are rarely visualized. (Courtesy of Barrow Neurological Institute, St. Joseph's Hospital and Medical Center, Phoenix, AZ.)

and intercostal vessels, it can be transected without sacrificing any of these vessels.

Sympathectomy

At the levels of interest, the sympathetic chain is transected using the monopolar cauterization scissors (Fig. 309–6). We routinely isolate the T2 ganglia for palmar hyperhidrosis by transecting the sympathetic chain over the second and third rib heads and include the T3 and T4 ganglia for axillary hyperhidrosis. In our experience, outcomes with this technique are comparable to those obtained after an en bloc resection of the sympathetic chain. Because the sympathetic chain does not have to be dissected away from the vertebral column, this modified procedure is safer and faster to perform. The scissors are used to "hook" and elevate the sympathetic ganglia away from the rib head. The

tissue is swept laterally (away from the segmental vessels) and coagulated. When the monopolar scissors are used, the lung parenchyma must be protected from thermal injury. Centering the dissection directly over the rib head protects the intercostal nerve.

The effectiveness of the sympathectomy is judged intraoperatively by monitoring palmar skin temperature. A unilateral increase of 1°C to 3°C occurs when an adequate sympathectomy has been performed.[5,17,48,53,55] This increase in temperature typically occurs over 10 to 20 minutes. If palmar skin temperature fails to increase, the presence of an aberrant accessory sympathetic supply that is still functional must be sought. Another possibility is that the inferior third of the stellate ganglion is contributing sympathetic input that needs to be addressed.

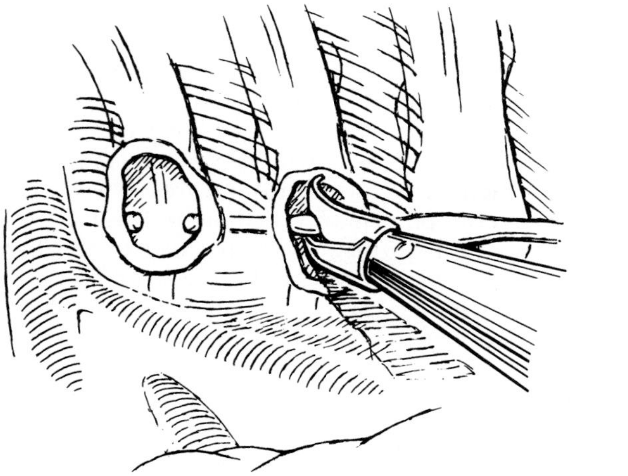

Closure

After lesioning is completed, a small-diameter (22F) apical chest tube is inserted through the same incision used to insert the monopolar scissors. The lung is reinflated by the anesthesiologist under direct thoracoscopic visualization. The chest tube is connected to suction to evacuate intrapleural air. If a contralateral sympathectomy is to be performed, the chest tube is left in place with an occlusive dressing. This strategy protects against difficulties with oxygenation or ventilation related to the deflation of both lungs. After the contralateral sympathectomy has been completed, the lung is reinflated and the chest tubes are removed bilaterally. Incisions are closed using subcuticular sutures and sterile adhesive strips (Steristrips, 3M Healthcare, St. Paul, Minn). A chest radiograph (upright, anteroposterior view at end expiration) is obtained in the recovery room to confirm the absence of persistent pneumothoraces. Patients are observed on a regular hospital floor and typically discharged within 24 hours of the procedure.

FIGURE 309–6. Transection of the right T2 and T3 ganglia using monopolar cauterization scissors during a right-sided thoracoscopic sympathectomy. (Courtesy of Barrow Neurological Institute, St. Joseph's Hospital and Medical Center, Phoenix, AZ.)

Surgical Outcomes

The success rate of endoscopic sympathectomy is highest for treating palmar hyperhidrosis. Several series, which reflect the prevalence of this disease in Asian populations, have reported success rates between 95% and 100%.[1-6, 17, 28, 33, 34, 47-50, 52-55, 63] Lesioning the sympathetic chain with a subsequent increase in the intraoperative palmar temperature of at least 3°C has provided the best immediate and long-term clinical outcomes. Sympathectomy for palmar hyperhidrosis relieves plantar hyperhidrosis in one half to two thirds of cases.[48] Axillary hyperhidrosis and bromhidrosis improve in 80% of patients who undergo lesioning of the T3 and T4 ganglia.[48]

Complications

In a significant number of patients, sympathectomy for hyperhidrosis can cause a postoperative compensatory hyperhidrosis syndrome (CHS), which involves increased sweating of the chest, abdomen, legs, back, or a combination of these sites (nondenervated areas).[47, 48, 53, 62] CHS symptoms typically improve or resolve within 6 months of surgery.[53] The incidence of CHS after sympathectomy ranges between 40% and 75%.[51] Most patients who develop CHS have mild or moderate sweating and are satisfied with the relief of their palmar sweating. Only 5% to 10% of patients who develop CHS have severe sweating that drenches their clothing and bedsheets and creates a disabling problem. CHS reflects the important thermoregulatory need for sweating to dissipate heat and ongoing generalized sympathetic hyperreactivity.

Horner's syndrome is avoided by sparing the rostral stellate ganglia and usually resolves spontaneously even if it does occur. Electrical or mechanical stimulation of this structure causes pupillary dilatation that can be observed by the anesthesiologist. It has been reported as a useful test for this structure.[58] Gustatory sweating, the result of aberrant synapses developing between sympathetic fibers and the vagus nerve, has been reported in 1% to 2% of patients.

THORACIC ENDOSCOPIC DISKECTOMY, VERTEBRECTOMY, AND RECONSTRUCTION

Indications

The indications for thoracoscopic microdiskectomies and vertebrectomies are the same as for open posterolateral and anterior approaches. The indications include symptomatic calcified or noncalcified central or centrolateral disk herniations and all types of infectious, traumatic, degenerative, or neoplastic processes of the ventral thoracic spine.

The thoracoscopic approach provides access to the anterior and anterolateral vertebrae (the vertebral bodies, ipsilateral pedicles, and ipsilateral transverse processes), disk spaces, and ventral aspect of the dura.

This exposure cannot access posterior spinal elements (laminae, spinous processes, facets), the contralateral pedicle, or the contralateral transverse process. The extent of exposure and visualization ventrally is identical to the exposure achieved with thoracotomy. Unequivocally, this anterior approach provides full visualization of the anterior spine and spinal cord, a view that cannot be achieved with posterolateral approaches. When thoracoscopy is not feasible, other operative options include thoracotomy, transsternal approaches, or costotransversectomy, depending on the location of the pathology.

Thoracic Spine Anatomy

The middle of the thoracic vertebral body has a slightly concave surface (Fig. 309–7). The segmental arteries and veins course over the middle of the vertebral bodies. The disk spaces and end plates form a convex surface. Intraoperatively, the surface contours are important clues for determining anatomic relationships.

The pedicles are dense oval cylinders of bone with a cancellous center. They connect the vertebral bodies with the remainder of the posterior arch (i.e., transverse processes, pars interarticularis, facets, laminae, and spinous processes). The pedicles are adjacent to the upper third of the vertebral body. The relationship of the pedicle to the disk space, vertebral body, and spinal canal is critical for intraoperative anatomic orientation. The neural foramen is formed by the boundaries of the pedicles of two adjacent vertebrae. Within the neural foramen, the nerve roots are surrounded by a large amount of epidural fat, a rich epidural venous plexus, and radicular arteries. The dura is therefore best exposed by removing the thoracic pedicles rather than by entering the neural foramen. The upper surface of the pedicle is contiguous with the superior surface of the vertebral end plates. Tracing the upper surface of the pedicle anteriorly leads to the disk space.

The rib heads provide essential landmarks for localization. The sympathetic ganglia and sympathetic chain are located just lateral to the rib heads beneath the parietal pleura. The ribs articulate with the transverse processes and the pedicles by strong ligamentous attachments. The costotransverse and costovertebral ligaments are dense, thick, and relatively inelastic. A triangular space is formed by the rib overlying the transverse process, pedicle, and vertebral body. The rib head, which articulates with the base of the pedicle and the vertebral body just caudal to or at the level of the disk space, serves to orient the surgeon to the relative position of the disk space and pedicles. The T9 rib, for example, leads to the T8-9 disk space. The costovertebral joint is a shallow ball-and-socket type of joint with a glistening surface that is a helpful anatomic feature for verifying that the rib head has been resected completely.

The costovertebral triangle is the key to unlocking the spinal canal and visualizing the nerve roots, dura, and spinal cord. It is defined by the space between the point at which the rib joins the transverse process and the vertebral body. The surface of the pedicle is ex-

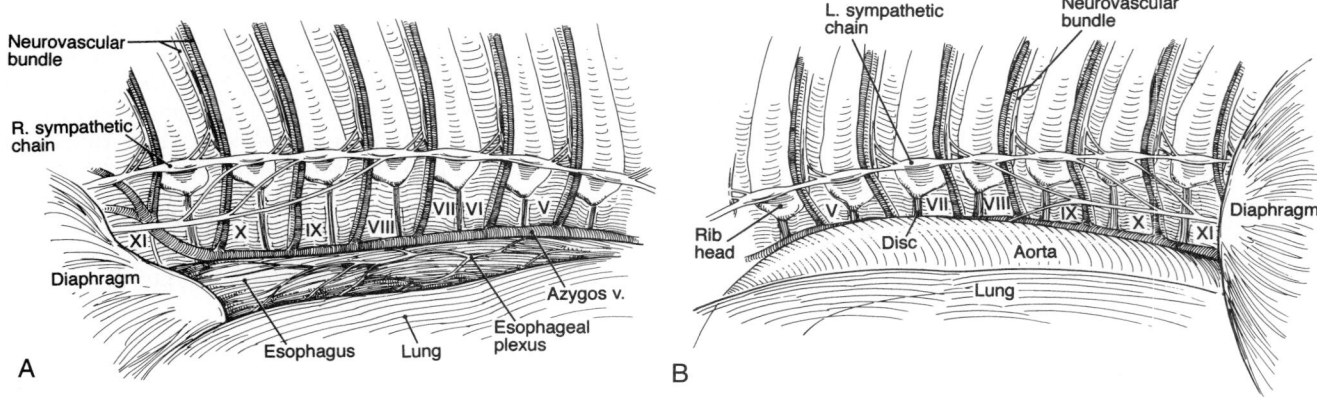

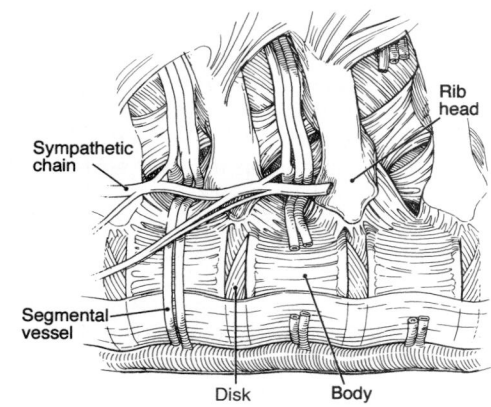

FIGURE 309–7. *A*, Overview of thoracoscopic anatomy and key landmarks for a right-sided approach. A lower thoracic pathology may require the placement of a retractor to keep the diaphragm out of the surgical field. *B*, Thoracoscopic anatomy and landmarks for a left-sided approach. *C*, Close-up of thoracic vertebral anatomy. The ribs are attached to the vertebrae via the costotransverse and costovertebral ligaments. The head of the rib articulates with the base of the pedicle and the vertebral body just below or at the disk space. The segmental vessels cross the middle of the concave surface of the vertebral bodies. (Courtesy of Barrow Neurological Institute, St. Joseph's Hospital and Medical Center, Phoenix, AZ.)

posed by removing the proximal 2 to 3 cm of rib en bloc. The pedicle is then removed to unlock the lateral aspect of the thecal sac. Removing the pedicle early in the dissection allows the dura to be visualized clearly so that the surgeon can remain oriented to the position of the spinal cord during dissection.

A predictable anatomic relationship exists among the intercostal vein, artery, and nerve. The segmental artery and vein course over the middle of the concave surface of the vertebral body. At the neural foramen, the segmental nerve joins the segmental vessels. As the neurovascular bundle extends laterally, from a cephalad to caudal direction, the vein, artery, and nerve run in the groove on the undersurface of each rib (see Fig. 309–7C).

Thoracic Microdiskectomy

After the pathologic disk space is exposed and confirmed by intraoperative radiography, the pleura over the medial surface of each rib is incised. Cobb periosteal elevators are used to expose a 2- to 3-cm segment of the proximal rib and rib head. The neurovascular bundle and muscular attachments are detached from the rib margins using subperiosteal dissection with periosteal elevators and large curved curettes. The neurovascular bundle is detached from the undersurface of the rib with careful dissection using curved curettes. Bleeding from the intercostal artery or vein encoun-

tered during rib dissection is controlled with bipolar cauterization. The intercostal nerve is identified and preserved.

A Cobb periosteal elevator and curved curettes are used to divide the costotransverse and costovertebral ligaments sharply. The rib head is detached from its articulation with the vertebral body, and all soft tissues are removed (Fig. 309–8A). A rib cutting tool or the Midas Rex (Midas Rex Pneumatic Tools, Inc., Fort Worth, TX) drill with an R-8 bit or footplate attachment (R-1) is used to create an osteotomy to transect the rib. The rib head and the proximal rib are removed en bloc. Enough of the proximal rib should be removed to ensure that the disk space, pedicle, and foramen are exposed satisfactorily. At this point, the pedicle is identified and fully exposed using a periosteal elevator and curved curettes. The nerve root and adjacent epidural fat are then identified within the neural foramen.

The amount of the pedicle that needs to be resected depends on the extent and location of herniated disk material. If the herniation is confined to the level of the disk space, only the superior half of the pedicle of the caudal vertebrae is removed. If the disk is broadbased or situated caudally, the entire pedicle must be resected. By removing the pedicle, the lateral aspect of the thecal sac is exposed. This visualization is critical because it enables the surgeon to protect the dura and spinal cord. Typically, the pedicle of the caudal vertebrae adjacent to the disk space must be removed.

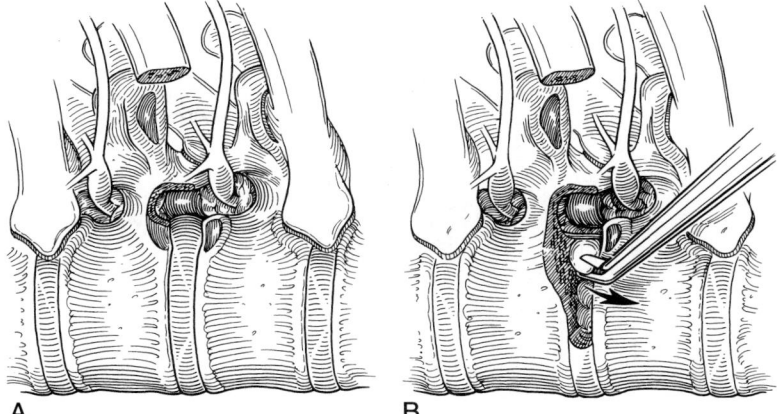

FIGURE 309–8. *A,* The disk space of interest after disarticulation and resection of the rib and upper half of the caudal pedicle to visualize the dura adjacent to the disk space. The nerve root in the foramen is surrounded by epidural fat, a venous plexus, and arterial branches. *B,* A 1- to 2-cm cavity is made in the dorsal vertebral bodies adjacent to the disk space to create a working space. The spinal cord can then be decompressed by dissecting the herniated disk away from the dura. (Courtesy of Barrow Neurological Institute, St. Joseph's Hospital and Medical Center, Phoenix, AZ.)

If the T9-10 disk is being removed, the T10 pedicle is resected. The pedicle is removed with a combination of drills and Kerrison rongeurs.

After the dura has been identified, the diskectomy is performed. The annulus fibrosus of the involved disk space is incised first. The thoracic disk spaces are narrow, and the annulus is best incised with a Cobb periosteal elevator. A drill with a cutting bur is used to create a cavity 1 to 2 cm wide in the dorsal vertebral bodies adjacent to the disk space (see Fig. 309–8*B*). Herniated disk material can then be curetted into the cavity and away from the spinal cord. Creating the cavity within the disk space and along the dorsal vertebrae minimizes the entry of tools into the compromised epidural space. Microsurgical tools and small curettes are used to move the herniated disk material away from the spinal canal into the cavity. Calcified disk material or osteophytes can be removed with a fine-tipped drill. The depth of the decompression is assessed by direct visualization and can be verified with intraoperative radiographs or fluoroscopic images. The decompression can be extended completely across the ventral aspect of the dura to the contralateral pedicle. Although interbody fusion is usually unnecessary after a routine thoracoscopic diskectomy, the proximal rib harvested during the spinal exposure can be used for this purpose if needed.

Thoracic Corpectomy

The exposure for thoracic corpectomy is similar to that for thoracic microdiskectomy. First, the pleura is dissected widely from the surface of the involved vertebrae and the adjacent ribs. The segmental vessels are mobilized, occluded with hemoclips, and cut between the clips. A circumferential subperiosteal dissection of the proximal 2 to 3 cm of the adjacent ribs is performed. The neurovascular bundle is dissected from the undersurface of the proximal ribs. The ligamentous attachments of the ribs are sectioned, osteotomies are performed, and the ribs are removed (Fig. 309–9*A*). The pedicles of the involved vertebrae are removed with a Kerrison rongeur, carefully exposing the lateral aspect of the dura and nerve roots. Diskectomies are

performed to define the cephalad and caudal boundaries of the bone dissection (see Fig. 309–9*B*). A large cavity is created within the center of the involved vertebral body with a high-speed drill, osteotomies, curettes, and rongeurs. The posterior longitudinal ligament and any elements compressing the spinal cord can be clearly visualized and safely removed by curetting the material away from the spinal cord into the cavity created within the vertebrae (see Fig. 309–9*C*). This sequence of dissection enables the dura to be visualized throughout the procedure and maximizes its safety. A strut graft can be placed within the corpectomy defect as detailed further on.

Vertebral Reconstruction

After thoracic corpectomy, various options exist for stabilization. Osseous defects from a corpectomy can be reconstructed using autologous iliac crest struts, allograft bone shafts (Fig. 309–10*A*), or methylmethacrylate. Autologous rib or a whole-diameter (allograft) humerus shaft usually fits well within the thoracic vertebrectomy site. The length, width, and depth of the bone graft and the vertebrectomy defect are measured precisely. Before the defect is measured and the graft is inserted, the spinous processes are pushed forward externally at the apex of the patient's kyphosis to optimize spinal alignment. The bone graft is sized to the exact length of the vertebrectomy defect. One end of the graft is cut with a slightly beveled surface to allow the graft to be wedged into position. The bone graft is inserted "end-on," through a 20-mm flexible portal into the thoracic cavity. The bone graft is grasped with an endoscopic clamp and positioned in the vertebrectomy defect. Bone-graft impactors and mallets are used to compress the bone grafts precisely into the vertebrectomy bed. The relationship of the graft to the dura must be observed throughout the insertion of the graft. This relationship can be confirmed with intraoperative radiography.

Another method of spinal stabilization that can be used for neoplastic disease is methylmethacrylate reconstruction (see Fig. 309–10*B* and *C*). After the dimensions of the resection defect have been measured, a

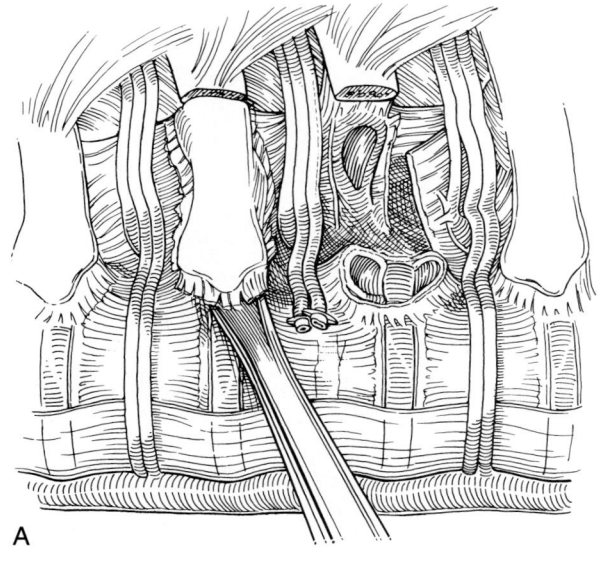

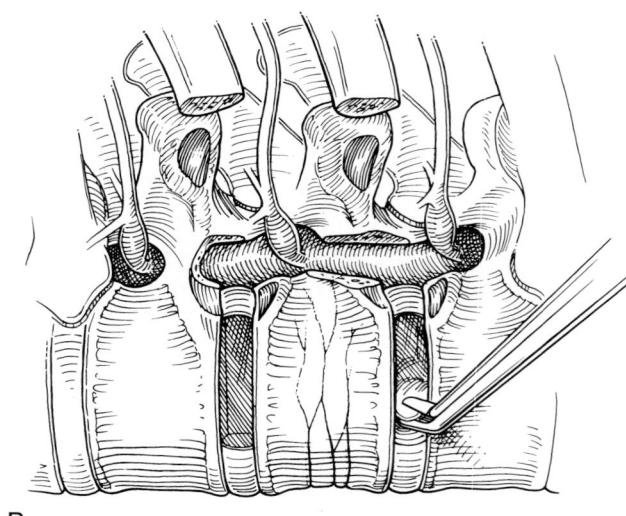

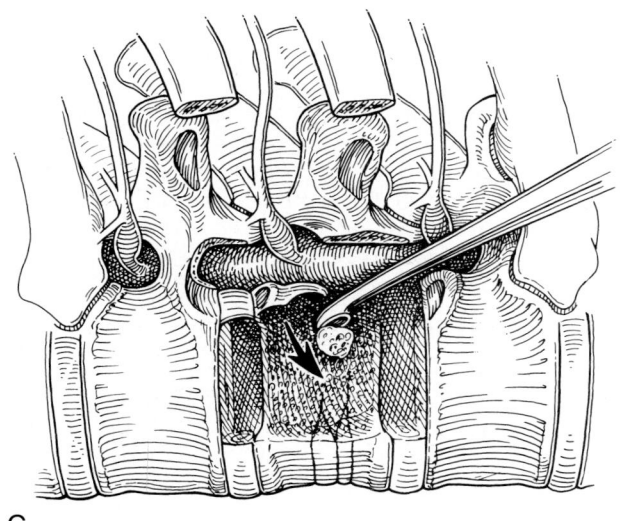

FIGURE 309–9. Technique of thoracoscopic corpectomy. *A*, Resection of the rib at the inferior level overlying the vertebral body of interest. *B*, Completion of the superior diskectomy. *C*, Decompression of the spinal canal by removing the vertebral body away from the ventral dura. (Courtesy of Barrow Neurological Institute, St. Joseph's Hospital and Medical Center, Phoenix, AZ.)

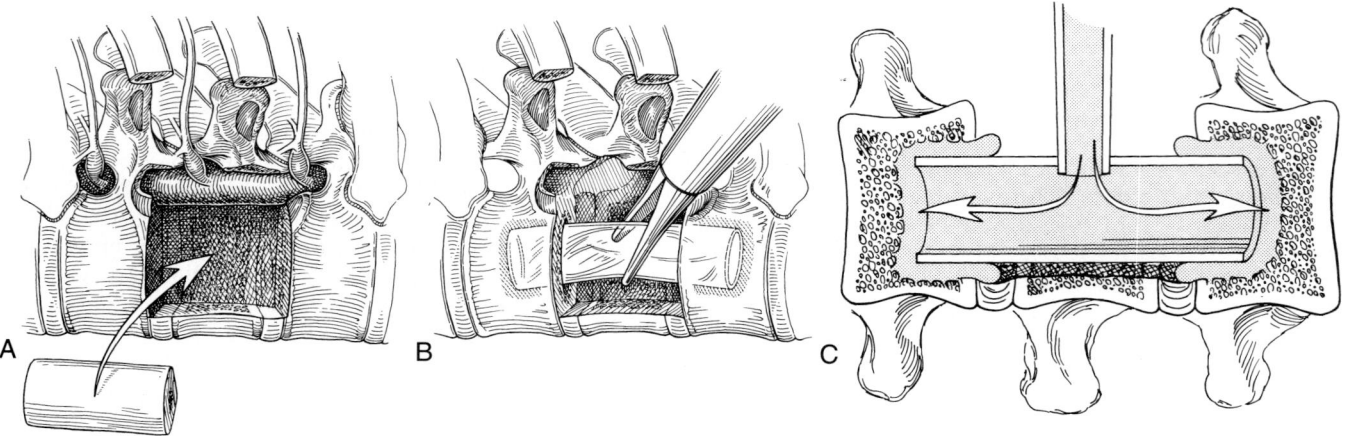

FIGURE 309–10. Technique of vertebral body reconstruction. *A*, Placement of humeral allograft into corpectomy defect. *B*, Placement of silicone tubing into corpectomy defect. *C*, Subsequent injection of methylmethacrylate to anchor it to surrounding bone. (Courtesy of Barrow Neurological Institute, St. Joseph's Hospital and Medical Center, Phoenix, AZ.)

sterile polymeric silicone (Silastic) tube is cut 5 to 6 mm longer than the end plates at the margin of the vertebrectomy defect. Holes are made in the adjacent vertebral end plates with drills and curettes to fit the tube diameter. The silicone tube, which serves as a template for the methylmethacrylate until it sets, is telescoped into the bodies of the adjacent vertebrae. A hole is cut in the middle of the tube to allow injection of methylmethacrylate. A long, wide-bore needle with a pressure syringe is used to inject the methylmethacrylate. Slow-setting cranioplasty methylmethacrylate is preferred to rapid-setting methacrylate, because it allows the polymer to be injected and produces much less heat as it sets, minimizing the risk of injury to the spinal cord. The methylmethacrylate is injected until it completely fills the silicone tubing and seeps through the ends into the adjacent vertebrae. The silicone tube acts like a mold while the methylmethacrylate hardens. Extrusion of the methacrylate into the adjacent bone is mandatory to provide an anchor that will prevent the polymer from loosening or becoming displaced. Additional methacrylate can be added ventral and lateral to the tube; however, care should be taken to ensure that the dura and spinal cord are not compressed by the polymer.

These reconstructive techniques can be augmented with screw-plate devices applied thoracoscopically or with posterior instrumentation constructs.

COMPLICATIONS

The potential complications of thoracoscopic spinal surgery include pneumothorax, hemothorax, chylothorax, atelectasis, pneumonia, neurologic injury, intercostal neuralgia, infection, spinal instability, hardware- or fixation-related complications, or injury to the great vessels or contents of the mediastinum. Postoperative atelectasis and pneumonia can be minimized by temporarily reinflating the lung intraoperatively. We recommend ventilating the lung 10 minutes for every 2 hours of surgical time. Postoperatively, patients are routinely placed on aggressive pulmonary physiotherapy regimens. If no intraoperative pulmonary complications occur and there is no air leak or excessive drainage through the thoracostomy tube, it can usually be removed either immediately after surgery or within 24 hours.

Vascular injury requiring conversion to an open procedure is rare and can be minimized by defining the regional anatomy with the endoscope before the instruments are placed. Pneumothorax requiring replacement of a chest tube is rare as long as the visceral pleura of the lung is not violated. Intercostal neuralgia is avoided by minimizing dissection and traction against the neurovascular bundle.

Cardiac arrhythmias are prevented by avoiding monopolar cauterization near the heart, and pulmonary lacerations are avoided by minimizing or avoiding lung retraction and by using blunt fan retractors carefully. The fan retractors should only be opened or closed when visualized directly with the endoscope and after they have been removed from the surface of the lung. Radicular and spinal cord injuries are prevented by meticulous dissection techniques under direct visualization.

CONCLUSIONS

The advantage of thoracoscopic techniques for extensive spinal decompression and reconstruction procedures is that they minimize the disruption of the superficial thoracic soft tissues. Previously, operative procedures for anterior thoracic spinal pathology have been performed exclusively with thoracotomy or costotransversectomy through large incisions. Although the basic anatomy and the dissection techniques of open thoracic surgery are familiar to most spinal surgeons, distinct technical challenges accompany thoracoscopic surgery. These challenges include significant adaptations of conventional surgical techniques: longer tools, restricted access to the surgical site, and new methods of visualizing and magnifying the operative site. Technologic improvements in endoscopic optical resolution and in the development of new tools have facilitated the application of endoscopic surgical approaches to the treatment of a broad spectrum of spinal disorders.

Thoracoscopy is more appropriately termed *surgery with minimal incisions* rather than *minimally invasive surgery* because the same extensive amount of spinal dissection is performed as with open surgery. It is, however, achieved through smaller incisions and without extensive retraction. Neural decompression, interbody fusion, vertebral body reconstruction, and internal fixation can be performed with these thoracoscopic techniques using minimal incisions. Thoracoscopic spinal surgery has tremendous potential for improving patients' comfort and cosmetic outcomes and for shortening recovery times.

REFERENCES

1. Dickman CA, Rosenthal D, Karahalios DG, et al: Thoracic vertebrectomy and reconstruction using a microsurgical thoracoscopic approach. Neurosurgery 38:279–293, 1996.
2. McAfee PC, Regan JR, Zdeblick T, et al: The incidence of complications in endoscopic anterior thoracolumbar spinal reconstructive surgery. A prospective multicenter study comprising the first 100 consecutive cases. Spine 20:1624–1632, 1995.
3. Regan JJ, Mack MJ, Picetti GD III, et al: A comparison of video-assisted thoracoscopic surgery (VATS) with open thoracotomy in thoracic spinal surgery. Today Ther Trend 11:203–218, 1994.
4. Horowitz MB, Moossy JJ, Julian T, et al: Thoracic discectomy using video assisted thoracoscopy. Spine 19:1082–1086, 1994.
5. Rosenthal D, Rosenthal R, de Simone A: Removal of a protruded thoracic disc using microsurgical endoscopy. A new technique. Spine 19:1087–1091, 1994.
6. Regan JJ, Mack MJ, Picetti GD III: A technical report on video-assisted thoracoscopy in thoracic spinal surgery. Preliminary description. Spine 20:831–837, 1995.
7. Burman MS: Myeloscopy or the direct visualization of the spinal canal and its contents. J Bone Joint Surg 13:695–696, 1931.
8. Pool JL: Direct visualization of dorsal nerve roots of the cauda equina by means of the myeloscope. Arch Neurol Psychol 39:1308–1312, 1938.
9. Pool JL: Myeloscopy: Diagnostic inspection of the cauda equina by means of the endoscope. Bull Neurol Inst NY 7:178–189, 1938.

10. Pool JL: Myeloscopy: Intrathecal endoscopy. Surgery 11:169–182, 1942.
11. Onik G, Helms CA, Ginsburg L, et al: Percutaneous lumbar discectomy using a new aspiration probe. AJR Am J Roentgenol 144:1137–1140, 1985.
12. Kambin P, Schaffer JL: Percutaneous lumbar discectomy. Review of 100 patients and current practice. Clin Orthop 238:24–34, 1989.
13. Ooi Y, Satoh Y, Morisaki N: Myeloscopy: The possibility of observing the lumbar intrathecal space by use of an endoscope. Endoscopy 5:901–906, 1973.
14. Mathews H: Paper presented at the First International Symposium on Lasers in Orthopaedics, 1991, San Francisco, Calif.
15. McKneally MF: Video-assisted thoracic surgery: Standards and guidelines. Chest Surg Clin N Am 3:345–351, 1993.
16. Kaiser LR: Video-assisted thoracic surgery: Current state of the art. Ann Surg 220:720–734, 1994.
17. Landreneau RJ, Mack MJ, Hazelrigg SR, et al: Video-assisted thoracic surgery. Basic technical concepts and intercostal approach strategies. Ann Thorac Surg 54:800–807, 1992.
18. Coltharp WH, Arnold JH, Alford WC Jr, et al: Videothoracoscopy: Improved technique and expanded indications. Ann Thorac Surg 53:776–779, 1992.
19. Mack MJ, Aronoff RJ, Acuff TE, et al: Present role of thoracoscopy in the diagnosis and treatment of diseases of the chest. Ann Thorac Surg 54:403–409, 1992.
20. Jacobaeus HC: Possibility of the use of the cystoscope for investigation of serious cavities. Munch Med Wochenschr 57:2090–2092, 1910.
21. Jacobaeus HC: The practical importance of thoracoscopy in surgery of the chest. Surg Gynecol Obstet 34:289–296, 1922.
22. Jacobaeus HC: The cauterization of adhesions in pneumothorax treatment of tuberculosis. Surg Gynecol Obstet 32:493–500, 1921.
23. Jacobaeus HC: Endopleural operations by means of a thoracoscope. Beitr Klin Tuberk 35:1, 1915.
24. Landreneau RJ, Hazelrigg SR, Mack MJ, et al: Postoperative pain-related morbidity: Video-assisted thoracic surgery versus thoracotomy. Ann Thorac Surg 56:1285–1289, 1993.
25. Hazelrigg SR, Landreneau RJ, Boley TM, et al: The effect of muscle-sparing versus standard posterolateral thoracotomy on pulmonary function, muscle strength, and postoperative pain. J Thorac Cardiovasc Surg 101:394–401, 1991.
26. Ferson PF, Landreneau RJ, Dowling RD, et al: Comparison of open versus thoracoscopic lung biopsy for diffuse infiltrative pulmonary disease. J Thorac Cardiovasc Surg 106:194–199, 1993.
27. Rosenthal D, Lorenz R: The use of the microsurgical endoscopic technique for treating affections of the dorsal spine: Indications and early results. J Neurosurg 82:342A, 1995.
28. Mack MJ, Regan JJ, Bobechko WP, et al: Application of thoracoscopy for diseases of the spine. Ann Thorac Surg 56:736–738, 1993.
29. Yuan HA, Mann KA, Found EM, et al: Early clinical experience with the Syracuse I-plate: An anterior spinal fixation device. Spine 13:278–285, 1988.
30. Dickman CA, Mican CA: Multilevel anterior thoracic discectomies and anterior interbody fusion using a microsurgical thoracoscopic approach. Case report. J Neurosurg 84:104–109, 1996.
31. Dickman CA, Karahalios DG: Thoracoscopic spinal surgery. Clin Neurosurg 43:392–422, 1996.
32. Krasna MJ, Mack MJ: Sympathectomy. In Krasna MJ, Mack MJ, (eds): Atlas of Thoracoscopic Surgery. St. Louis, Quality Medical, 1994, pp 139–149.
33. Robertson DP, Simpson RK, Rose JE, et al: Video-assisted endoscopic thoracic ganglionectomy. J Neurosurg 79:238–240, 1993.
34. Kao M-C, Tsai J-C, Lai D-M, et al: Autonomic activities in hyperhidrosis patients before, during, and after endoscopic laser sympathectomy. Neurosurgery 34:262–268, 1994.
35. Bohlman HH, Zdeblick TA: Anterior excision of herniated thoracic discs. J Bone Joint Surg Am 70:1038–1047, 1988.
36. Benjamin V: Diagnosis and management of thoracic disc disease. Clin Neurosurg 30:577–606, 1983.
37. Crafoord C, Hiertonn T, Lindblom K, et al: Spinal cord compression caused by a protruded thoracic disc: Report of a case treated with antero-lateral fenestration of the disc. Acta Orthop Scand 28:103–107, 1958.
38. Fidler MW, Goedhart ZD: Excision of prolapse of thoracic intervertebral disc. A transthoracic technique. J Bone Joint Surg Br 66:518–522, 1984.
39. Kaneda K, Abumi K, Fujiya M: Burst fractures with neurologic deficits of the thoraco-lumbar spine. Results of anterior decompression and stabilization with anterior instrumentation. Spine 9:788–795, 1984.
40. Kostuik JP: Anterior spinal cord decompression for lesions of the thoracic and lumbar spine, techniques, new methods of internal fixation results. Spine 8:512–531, 1983.
41. Kostuik JP: Anterior fixation for fractures of the thoracic and lumbar spine with or without neurologic involvement. Clin Orthop 189:103–115, 1984.
42. Perot PL Jr, Munro DD: Transthoracic removal of midline thoracic disc protrusions causing spinal cord compression. J Neurosurg 31:452–458, 1969.
43. Ransahoff J, Spencer F, Siew F, et al: Transthoracic removal of thoracic disc. Report of three cases. J Neurosurg 31:459–461, 1969.
44. Otani K, Nakai S, Fujimura Y, et al: Surgical treatment of thoracic disc herniation using the anterior approach. J Bone Joint Surg Br 64:340–343, 1982.
45. Statement of the AATS/STS Joint Committee on Thoracoscopy and Video Assisted Thoracic Surgery. Ann Thorac Surg 54:1, 1992.
46. Kux E: The endoscopic approach to the vegetative nervous system and its therapeutic possibilities. Dis Chest 20:139–147, 1951.
47. Cloward RB: Hyperhydrosis. J Neurosurg 30:545–551, 1969.
48. Kao MC: Video endoscopic sympathectomy using a fiberoptic CO_2 laser to treat palmar hyperhidrosis. Neurosurgery 30:131–135, 1992.
49. Kuntz A: Distribution of the sympathetic rami to the brachial plexus: Its relation to sympathectomy affecting the upper extremity. Arch Surg 15:871–877, 1927.
50. Kux M: Thoracic endoscopic sympathectomy in palmar and axillary hyperhidrosis. Arch Surg 113:264–266, 1978.
51. Lai Y-T, Yang L-H, Chio C-C, et al: Complications in patients with palmar hyperhidrosis treated with transthoracic endoscopic sympathectomy. Neurosurgery 41:110–115, 1997.
52. Lin CC: A new method of thoracoscopic sympathectomy in hyperhidrosis palmaris. Surg Endosc 4:224–226, 1990.
53. Ray B: Sympathectomy of the upper extremity: Evaluation of surgical methods. J Neurosurg 10:624–633, 1953.
54. Shih CJ, Wang YC: Thoracic sympathectomy for palmar hyperhidrosis: Report of 457 cases. Surg Neurol 10:291–296, 1978.
55. Stolman LP: Treatment of excess sweating of the palms by iontophoresis. Arch Dermatol 123:893–896, 1987.
56. Stanton-Hicks M, Jänig W, Hassenbusch S, et al: Reflex sympathetic dystrophy: Changing concepts and taxonomy. Pain 63:127–133, 1995.
57. Johnson JP, Ahn SS: Thoracoscopic sympathectomy. Tech Neurosurg 3:308–314, 1997.
58. Segal R, Ferson PM, Nemoto E, et al: Blood flow–monitored transthoracic endoscopic sympathectomy. In Rengachary SS, Wilkins RH (eds): Neurosurgical Operative Atlas. Park Ridge, Ill, American Association of Neurological Surgeons, 1998, pp 163–171.
59. Lee KH, Hwang PYK: Video endoscopic sympathectomy for palmar hyperhidrosis. J Neurosurg 84:484–486, 1996.
60. Schwartz PJ, Locati E, Priori SG, et al: The idiopathic long QT syndrome. In Zipes DP, Jalife J (eds): Cardiac Electrophysiology: From Cell to Bedside. Philadelphia, WB Saunders, 1990, pp 589–605.
61. Ouriel K, Moss AJ: Long QT syndrome: An indication for cervicothoracic sympathectomy. Cardiovasc Surg 3:475–478, 1995.
62. Johnson JP, Obasi C, Hahn MS, et al: Endoscopic thoracic sympathectomy. J Neurosurg 91:90–97, 1999.
63. Dickman CA, Mican C: Thoracoscopic approaches for the treatment of anterior thoracic spinal pathology. BNI Q 12:4–19, 1996.

Intradiskal and Percutaneous Treatment of Lumbar Disk Disease

THOMAS C. CHEN ■ LAWRENCE T. KHOO ■ CHARLES B. STILLERMAN

This chapter introduces the concept of intradiskal and percutaneous treatment of lumbar disk disease. Because lumbar disk disease includes such a large variety of disorders, ranging from diskogenic pain to herniated disks, the topic is immense. Its socioeconomic impact is obvious; lumbar disk disease is a tremendous source of lost productivity for patients and society. This chapter is especially pertinent in this era of minimally invasive approaches for surgical treatment. Managed care and the need to rein in health care costs also place an increased emphasis on cost-effective treatment.

This chapter is divided into three main sections. The first deals with posterior percutaneous and intradiskal approaches to the lumbar spine. Some of the techniques described have been used in the past with mixed results, including chemonucleolysis, automated percutaneous lumbar diskectomy, and laser-assisted percutaneous diskectomy.[1] Newer approaches such as endoscopic diskectomy are beginning to be used with more frequency as the instrumentation improves. The second section covers anterior approaches to the lumbar disk. In anterior approaches, the goal is to treat lumbar disk disease by disk removal and fusion. These procedures include laparascopic anterior lumbar interbody fusion and retroperitoneal endoscopic approaches to the lumbar spine. New technologies with only preliminary clinical experience are discussed in the third section. These new technologies offer tremendous potential for future development and growth. Procedures such as intradiskal electrothermal annuloplasty (IDET), use of bone morphogenetic protein (BMP) to accelerate fusion, and gene therapy are discussed as future technologies that may have promise.

POSTERIOR PROCEDURES

Chemonucleolysis

Chemonucleolysis by means of enzymatic digestion of the intervertebral nucleus pulposus has been used as an alternative to surgical treatment of lumbar disk herniation for nearly half a century. Diskolysis with either chymopapain or collagenase is accomplished via cleavage of disk matrix proteoglycans, with the resultant shrinkage of the central nuclear volume and pressure. With this reduction in the nucleus pulposus, indirect compression of the lumbar nerve roots by herniation is reduced. Injection with chymopapain has generally been limited to the same population of patients who would benefit from an open surgical excision of a proven herniated fragment. Despite Food and Drug Administration (FDA) approval and more than 40 years of overall successful findings from well-designed, carefully controlled clinical trials, the indications, efficacy, and safety of chemonucleolysis continue to be hotly debated. As MacNab observed on its use: "Arguments regarding its efficacy changed chemonucleolysis into a cause rather than scientific grounds. The mere mention of chemonucleolysis could rapidly change a friend into an acquaintance!"[2]

HISTORICAL PERSPECTIVE AND BACKGROUND

Working with crude papain extracted in bulk from a homogenate of proteolytic enzymes, Jansen and colleagues isolated chymopapain from papayas in 1941.[3] In 1956 Thomas reported the first use of this proteolytic enzyme on rabbits. After intravenous injection, it was observed that chymopapain had a selective affinity for the ground substance of cartilage, without any obvious effect on cartilage or nervous tissue. Only the microcirculation was digested, as capillary vessels are bound together by proteoglycans; large-caliber vessels did not collapse, as they contain collagen in their walls.[4] In 1959 Hirsch[5] suggested the possible use of this proteolytic enzyme in the disk space to accelerate degeneration to the point where the offending disk would become stable and asymptomatic. The possible therapeutic advantages of chymopapain in the treatment of disk herniations were then extensively investigated in the intervertebral spaces of hundreds of cats, rabbits, and dogs at the Baxter Laboratories in Chicago. The drug was injected directly into the nucleus pulposus of the disk space to achieve selective enzymatic digestion of the proteoglycans. The enzyme was also injected into the intrathecal, intradural, intravascular, and perivertebral spaces to examine its local effects. The long-term results of this work demonstrated consistent disk reduction even at minimal doses, with delayed reconstruction seen in the disks on necropsy after 2 years.[6] Additionally, these tests established the safety and toxicity of chymopapain, leading to its approval by the FDA for human investigation. Smith[7] administered the first injection of chymopapain (Discase) in a patient for the treatment of lumbar disk herniation on July 13, 1963. The clinical practice of chemonucleolysis had thus been established.

From its inception, chemonucleolysis has been saddled with controversy and debate. Although Smith achieved excellent results in the first 10 patients treated with chymopapain, two of his next 20 patients suffered catastrophic complications. The first patient demonstrated a postinjection Brown-Séquard syndrome, and the second developed acute paraplegia. Although a subsequent investigation could not establish the enzyme as the cause of these complications, chymopapain became widely known in 1964 as "a dangerous drug, and one which should not have been used in the first place."[8] Proceeding alone, Smith went on to perform chemonucleolysis in 100 patients, with excellent results and a minimum of complications. After presenting his experience in 1966 to the Clinical Orthopedic Society in Chicago, Wiltse, Day, Brown, and Ford agreed to participate in a prospective clinical investigation on chemonucleolysis. The following decade thus saw a renaissance of the procedure, with more than 14,000 patients treated by 55 different orthopedic and neurological surgeons.[9, 10] This period ended when the initial results of the first double-blind study comparing Discase and placebo were published. Patients injected with chymopapain did not have a statistically significant improvement of their symptoms compared with those injected with placebo (saline). As such, the manufacturer (Baxter Travenol, Chicago) withdrew its application for Discase's approval as a "new" investigational drug in 1976.[11] Although clinical use of chymopapain was thus halted in the United States, it continued to be widely used in Canada over the ensuing decade, with favorable results.

Spurred by these positive clinical findings, Smith's nephew formed Smith Laboratories in 1979 and developed a more selective formulation of chymopapain known as Chymodiactin. With strict adherence to a rigid protocol, this new formulation was used in 1498 patients, with good results achieved in 82% overall and a less than 2% incidence of complications.[12] Based on these results and those from another prospective trial, Chymodiactin was released for clinical use in the United States in 1984. As a result, chemonucleolysis underwent a resurgence, with more than 100,000 patients treated over the next few years. Despite an overall excellent clinical response, public attention became focused on the 55 adverse outcomes that were seen in this cohort. Adverse publicity and attention to this very low (0.055%) complication rate was enough to cause a marked decrease in chymopapain use. Since that time, chemonucleolysis has been performed at a fairly steady rate of 3000 patients per year in the United States and at least three times that number internationally.[10]

INDICATIONS

Overall, the patient indications for chemonucleolysis are similar, if not identical, to those for open surgical diskectomy.[13, 14] The converse, however, is not necessarily correct.[15] The typical patient is one with a symptomatic lumbar disk herniation proved on magnetic resonance imaging (MRI), computed tomography (CT), or myelography and the absence of any other major spinal disease (i.e., tumor or fracture). These patients should be unresponsive to at least a 6-week course of conservative management. Patients without secondary gain issues are also more likely to benefit from chemonucleolysis. Whereas radicular signs such as pain on straight leg raising are a good indication for treatment, several authors have suggested that patients with severe neurological signs such as focal weakness or incontinence should be taken to surgery for open decompression.[16] Therefore, adequate imaging to fully understand the nature and extent of the disk herniation is highly recommended before treatment. If the annulus has been breached, with leaking of nuclear material (i.e., sequestered fragments), the majority of experienced surgeons believe it is unacceptably risky to perform the procedure. Partially contained or extruded fragments are still considered acceptable for injection.[10] Retrospective analysis has found that neither the size of the herniated fragment nor the shape of the spinal canal seems to adversely affect the outcome of chemonucleolysis.[11, 17]

Relative contraindications to the use of chymopapain include a history of previous laminectomy or chemonucleolysis, a rapidly progressing neurological deficit, evidence of a cauda equina or conus compression syndrome, recurrent disk herniation at the same level, spinal tumor, severe spinal stenosis, spondylolisthesis or severe deformity, multiple levels of disk herniation, sequestered disk fragments, cerebrospinal fluid leak or fistula, open or closed neural tube defect, severe allergy, diabetes, or pregnancy.[18, 19] A general rule of thumb is that chemonucleolysis should not be performed in a patient with a history of previous treatment (i.e., diskectomy, laminectomy, injection) at the same level because of the presumed risk of chymopapain leaking through the adhesions between the disk and the dura mater into the subarachnoid space, resulting in potentially devastating hemorrhage.[20] For this reason, chemonucleolysis at a previously operated level is not approved by the FDA.

Allergic reactions to chymopapain and collagenase continue to be a concern. Preoperative skin testing with ChymoFAST (Biowhitaker, Inc., Palo Alto, CA) or similar systems is advocated as a screening tool to prevent anaphylaxis resulting from chymopapain exposure. Patients with any evidence of immunoglobulin E antibody reaction to the enzyme should be excluded from treatment.[21]

TECHNIQUE

Chemonucleolysis has generally been performed as an ambulatory procedure with a short recovery time. Appropriate routine screening for medical conditions should be completed in all patients, and adequate preoperative planning with radiographs is wise to ensure that an appropriate needle trajectory can be achieved. The chemonucleolysis technique itself is similar to the standard technique of posterolateral diskogram injection commonly used by radiologists, anesthetists, and orthopedic surgeons (Fig. 310–1A).

Before the procedure, many authors advocate a 24-hour period of medication with H_1 and H_2 blockers to blunt the potentially violent histamine reaction to chymopapain in sensitized patients.[22] Experimental studies examining histamine and catecholamine levels with and without premedication with hydroxyzine and tranexamic acid did not demonstrate any effect on the incidence of systemic clinical signs of anaphylaxis. Additionally, the study concluded that the use of local rather than general anesthesia was essential to allow for early detection of an allergic response.[23] Nevertheless, preoperative testing with ChymoFAST or similar tests is the mainstay of avoiding allergic complications.[21] Early recognition and immediate treatment with 0.1 to 0.3 mL of subcutaneous epinephrine (1:1000, 1 mg/mL) are effective in minimizing sequelae from established reactions.

It is important to emphasize that the use of local anesthesia with supplemental intravenous sedation is crucial for the safety of the procedure. General anesthetic techniques increase the risk of complications; they can blunt systemic responses and mask anaphylactic reactions, thereby delaying proper treatment. Agents used during general anesthesia may also have an additive effect on histamine release.[9] Further, accidental nerve injury and improper needle placement can be avoided by having ready feedback from an awake patient. Inadvertent injection or penetration of a nerve root can occur in up to 7% of patients under general anesthesia. This unacceptably high complication rate falls precipitously when the patient is able to report any radicular numbness or pain radiating below the knee. Additionally, more dangerous complications such as transverse myelitis and systemic collapse due to anaphylaxis are significantly more common in patients undergoing general anesthesia.[24]

After induction of local anesthesia and placement of one or two large-bore intravenous catheters, proper patient positioning on the operative table or fluoroscopy gantry is crucial to ensure optimal needle placement. The patient is typically secured in a left-lateral decubitus position, such that the target disk space is easily accessible. Some authors routinely use a prone position with success. A good fluoroscopy unit that can acquire real-time images in all three orthogonal planes is essential. Before initiation of the procedure, the end plates of the disk space to be injected must be visualized in at least two planes. A permanent marker is used to identify the needle entry site on the skin. Although numerous techniques have been described, a mark is usually made 6 to 12 cm lateral of the midline (as defined by the spinous processes) on the superior (i.e., right) side of the patient's back. The surgeon should also remain cognizant of anatomic considerations and variants that are unique to each patient. After reconfirmation of the target, the patient and fluoroscopy tube are prepped and draped. Proper planning is also needed to allow for the full range of motion of the fluoroscopy unit without compromising the sterility of the procedure. Then 1 to 2 mL of 0.5% lidocaine solution is infused subcutaneously under the previous skin marks. A 15- to 20-cm 18-gauge needle is passed at a 45-degree angle from the sagittal plane down to the level of the disk annulus (see Fig. 310–1A). Depending on the exact level, the angle of insertion is usually 30 to 60 degrees caudally. The passage of this needle should be done under careful fluoroscopic guidance. Once the needle has been seated at the disk annulus, repositioning the fluoroscope to a second orthogonal plane 90 degrees from the first is prudent for reconfirmation.

At this point, several authors advocate the use of a two-needle technique to decrease the incidence of infection. The stylus is removed from the 18-gauge needle, and a 20-cm 22-gauge needle is passed through the larger needle to the disk space itself. Fraser[12] and others believe that because the 22-gauge needle has not penetrated the skin, the chance of introducing skin flora into the disk space is greatly reduced. Many clinicians inject 1 to 3 mL of contrast medium to perform a confirmatory diskogram to ensure placement of the needle at the correct level (see Fig. 310–1B and C). Dangerous annular tears and fistulas between the annulus and intrathecal space can often be visualized as well. Potential leakage of the enzyme into the epidural or subarachnoid space can occur in such cases. Some authors have reported an increased incidence of complications with the use of concomitant contrast and enzyme injection. Experimental data from primate studies suggest that there may be a synergistic harmful effect of chymopapain when combined with contrast material in the intrathecal space.[6, 25] Several of the more severe complications after chemonucleolysis have involved the use of simultaneous diskograms as well.[10]

Once the needle is seated within the annulus of the desired disk level, approximately 1 to 2 mL of chymopapain-type enzyme is gently injected into the space until some resistance is encountered (see Fig. 310–1D and E). If strong resistance is met or the patient complains of severe pain during injection, further forceful enzyme infusion is best deferred or abandoned. This cautious use of a slow, gradual injection may help prevent hydraulic extrusion of free disk fragments by reducing the fluid pressure and by allowing for feedback from the patient as an early warning sign of potential neural injury.[9]

For most patients, the postprocedural course is typically short and uncomplicated, with the majority being able to leave after 2 to 4 hours of observation. Among the possible immediate side effects, back pain and muscle spasm are the most common and limiting. Recent

Chymopapain

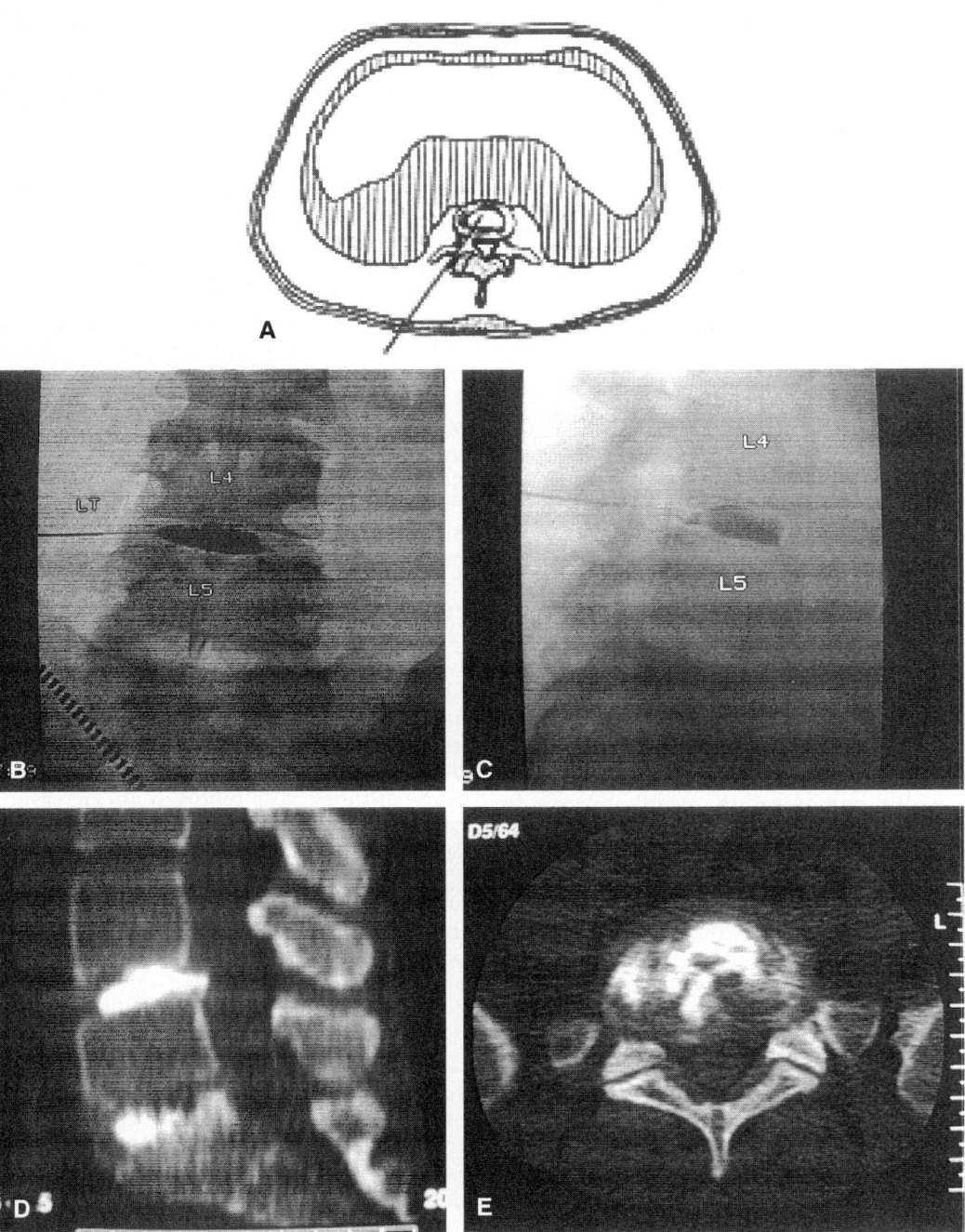

FIGURE 310–1. Chemonucleolysis using chymopapain is performed in an outpatient setting for a herniated L4-5 disk. A standard posterolateral approach, similar to that for a posterolateral diskogram, is used. *A,* A 15- to 20-cm 18-gauge needle is passed at a 45-degree angle from the sagittal plane down to the level of the disk annulus. Depending on the exact level, the angle of insertion is usually 30 to 60 degrees caudally. *B* and *C,* Once the needle is confirmed to be at the correct location by fluoroscopy, a diskogram is performed using 1 to 3 mL of contrast medium, allowing for visualization of dangerous annular tears or fistulas. Once the disk is demonstrated to be contained, 1 to 3 mL of chymopapain can be injected into the L4-5 disk space. Typically, if little or no backpressure is felt, up to 3 mL can be injected. *D,* Lateral view after injection. *E,* Confirmation by computed tomographic scan.

studies suggest that lowering the dose of Chymodiactin to as little as 25% (1000 U) of the standard dosage (4000 U) can help alleviate these uncomfortable sequelae. A prospective, double-blind trial comparing the use of 2000 U versus 4000 U of enzyme could not, however, demonstrate any significant decrease in post-injection back pain.[26] Injection of bupivacaine at the periphery of the disk annulus has also been described to reduce iatrogenic chemonucleolysis discomfort. A study using such a technique found back pain in only 3.8% of 80 patients at 3 weeks after the procedure. Compared with the typical 30% to 40% reported incidence of pain in most series, this was a significant reduction.[27]

RESULTS AND COMPLICATIONS

Because the clinical experience with chemonucleolysis spans almost 5 decades, a large body of clinical retrospective and prospective data is available for review.[22] Retrospective review of 7335 injected patients from 45 cohorts spanning 1985 to 1993 found an average success rate of 76%.[10] A subsequent meta-analysis of more than 130,000 patients treated between 1975 and 1994 revealed an average success rate of 88%.[28] Three large prospective, randomized, double-blind studies have been conducted comparing injection of chymopapain with placebo. In an open-label, double-blind, multicenter study of Chymodiactin conducted in 1498 patients, success rates ranging from 80% to 90% were reported. Patient selection in this series was especially strict regarding radicular symptoms, radiographic criteria, and patient demographics.[12] The most definitive U.S. prospective clinical trial was conducted in 105 patients.[15] At 6 weeks after injection, 75% of patients injected with the enzyme were significantly improved, compared with 45% of placebo patients ($P = 0.003$). At 6 months, the placebo success rate had fallen to 38%, with no change in the enzyme-injected group ($P > 0.001$). Placebo patients were then injected with chymopapain as well, with 91% achieving relief at 1-year follow-up. Another double-blind study conducted in Australia found that 80% of patients injected with chymopapain still considered the procedure efficacious after 10 years, compared with only 34% of patients injected with saline. Both patients and physicians were blinded to whether saline or enzyme was used during the course of the study.[29] An overall efficacy rate of 50% to 80% for chemonucleolysis was agreed on by several experienced authors who participated in a diagnostic and therapeutic technology assessment conducted by the American Medical Association.[16]

Because chymopapain use has been closely monitored by the FDA for its safety and toxicity since 1982, outcomes from 135,000 patients are available from postmarketing surveillance.[30] These data revealed 7 fatalities from anaphylaxis, 24 infections, 32 hemorrhagic complications, 32 neurological complications, and 16 miscellaneous other problems. An overall mortality rate of 0.019% and a complication rate of 0.090% were calculated. A subset analysis of 77,181 patients revealed that 385 had some degree of reaction to chymopapain

(0.5%). Most cases occurred within the first few years after Chymodiactin's approval in 1982, with an allergy rate of only 0.2% in the last 5 years of the study. A decreased standard enzyme dosage, routine screening with the ChymoFAST test, avoidance of general anesthetics, and pretreatment with antihistamines are thought to account for this decreased incidence.

For series with concomitant diskography, up to 25% of chemonucleolysis procedures may result in some amount of enzyme leakage into the epidural space.[16] However, numerous animal studies have consistently demonstrated that leakage of chymopapain and Chymodiactin into the epidural space at concentrations 100 times that used in humans has no harmful effect.[6] Intrathecal injection, in contrast, can be quite dangerous, causing subarachnoid hemorrhage, paralysis, and other catastrophic consequences. All experienced authors emphasize the need for correct needle placement with biplanar fluoroscopic confirmation to avoid such devastating complications. Widespread media publicity of such disastrous sequelae has greatly decreased the popularity of chemonucleolysis in the United States over the last decade.[6, 7]

An objective assessment of the available data, however, reveals a much lower incidence of serious sequelae. From the FDA data, only 17 (21%) of the 80 hemorrhagic, neurological, and other serious miscellaneous events could be directly related to chymopapain or the manner in which it was administered. Thus, the serious complication rate was only 0.0125% among the 135,000 tracked cases. Similarly, in another cohort of 80,000 patients treated with chemonucleolysis, there were only 46 cases of serious central nervous system complications, for a rate of 1 in 2000 (0.05%).[24] Indeed, when compared with open surgical diskectomy or laminectomy, chemonucleolysis has an objectively smaller procedural risk to the patient. A meta-analysis of 43,662 patients treated with chymopapain versus 2051 patients treated surgically revealed an overall complication rate of 3.7% and 26%, respectively.[31] There were three surgically related deaths and no mortality from chemonucleolysis. When Nordby and Wright[28] compared the results of their extensive analysis with standard surgical outcome data, they found that surgery had a 3 times higher mortality rate, a 15 times higher incidence of infection, and a 40 times higher rate of neurological or hemorrhagic sequelae. Although the efficacy of chemonucleolysis continues to be a point of controversy, it seems that the procedure itself is relatively safe and carries little unwarranted risk to the patient.

CONCLUSION

Chemonucleolysis by means of injecting chymopapain into the intradiskal space represents the first step toward a minimally invasive treatment for herniated intervertebral disks. In comparison to many other contemporary minimally invasive intradiskal techniques, the outcomes and complications of chemonucleolysis are well established in a large body of literature spanning more than 40 years. The enzyme appears to be safe in the epidural space but can cause serious consequences if injected intrathecally. Although disastrous complications were encountered early during the clinical use of this technique, analysis of the recent literature reveals that such sequelae have become extremely rare. Based on a review of the worldwide literature, chemonucleolysis seems to have a reproducible success rate of 60% to 80%, a morbidity rate of around 3% to 4%, and a mortality rate of less than 0.1%. Although chymopapain injection is clearly not as efficacious as open surgical diskectomy, it represents an alternative treatment for patients who are either unable or unwilling to undergo general anesthesia, and it carries a significantly lower overall risk to the patient. Further, the waxing and waning of chemonucleolysis's popularity may have been due, in large part, to nonscientific influences.

Automated Percutaneous Lumbar Diskectomy

As a result of the controversies surrounding chemonucleolysis, alternative mechanical means of decompressing the intervertebral disk space have been aggressively investigated and developed. Although varied in their exact technique, these procedures typically share two common goals. Like traditional open surgery, their first aim is to either directly or indirectly reduce a herniated disk fragment and alleviate the patient's low back and radicular symptoms. Second, they seek to achieve this decompression through a minimally invasive percutaneous technique with little or no bony or soft tissue manipulation. A review of the literature reveals a flowering of these minimally invasive spinal techniques over the last 2 decades.[32] These include automated percutaneous lumbar diskectomy (APLD), posterior and posterolateral arthroscopic and endoscopic diskectomy, and laser diskectomy. Aside from chemonucleolysis, APLD was, until recently, the most widely used alternative means of intradiskal decompression worldwide. There have been more than 120,000 cases published in the literature since the early 1980s, and the technical ease and safety of the procedure have been well established. Like chemonucleolysis, however, the indications and efficacy of APLD continue to be heavily debated in the clinical realm.

HISTORICAL PERSPECTIVE AND BACKGROUND

Hijikata[33] reported the first successful use in 1975 of "percutaneous nucleotomy" to accomplish a partial decompression and removal of the nucleus pulposus via a small posterolateral skin incision. Typically, a 4- to 8-mm working cannula is passed from the skin down to the desired intervertebral level. Some combination of pituitary forceps, curets, suction, and irrigation is then passed through this cannula to remove a variable quantity of intradiskal material. In the initial experience with 100 patients, Hijikata reported a 70% success rate, with one case of infection and one case of vascular injury. Concurrently, Kambin and Schaffer[34] achieved a

success rate of 85% in their 100 patients treated by a similar percutaneous posterolateral approach. Hoppenfeld[35] also claimed to be a pioneer of the technique and reported a nearly identical 86% of patients with good outcomes and no significant complications at 10-year follow-up. Since these initial reports, numerous modifications of this procedure have been adopted worldwide.[36] For instance, Schreiber and coworkers[37] reported the addition of a fiber-optic endoscope or arthroscope to directly visualize the material being removed, with a success rate of 72% in 109 patients.

From a theoretical standpoint, both chemonucleolysis and percutaneous diskectomy techniques work on a similar hypothesis. APLD centrally decompresses the nucleus pulposus, thereby decreasing the transmitted pressure through the annular tear into the herniated fragment. Although most of these techniques do not remove the herniation itself, it is thought that the indirect or secondary reduction in intradiskal pressure results in decreased pressure on the affected nerve root. It follows that the clinical success rate of any percutaneous procedure would be highly dependent on the selection of patients who have this picture of an extruded or protruding disk.[38–40]

The large size of the surgical instruments and the working cannula used during the early studies was often associated with a significant risk of muscular trauma, nerve root injury, and major vessel damage. Onik and his group[41] developed an APLD technique using a reciprocating suction cutting device for removal of the disk material. This device is contained in an outer cannula with a 2.8-mm diameter and uses a guillotine-like blade that reciprocates across a side port enclosed in the blunt-tipped outer sheath at a rate of approximately 180 Hz. Much like with chemonucleolysis, proper placement of the cannula and nucleotome is achieved by adequate anatomic planning and biplanar fluoroscopic visualization. Owing to the device's small size, the incidence of associated soft tissue injury is much smaller compared with previous manual percutaneous techniques. Because the outer cannula is passed first, the nucleotome itself does not encounter skin, which is associated with a lower infection rate. From their subsequent body of clinical experience in 200 consecutive patients, the authors reported an overall success rate of 77.5% at a mean follow-up of 6 months.[41] Subsequent modifications of both the device and the technique occurred over the next 15 years. Whereas Onik's original device was disposable, permanent versions of the nucleotome were created overseas and used with similar success rates.[42] As experience with the procedure grew, difficulties unique to the L5-S1 disk space were increasingly encountered, due to anatomic limitations. To ameliorate these targeting problems, Onik later developed a special set of curved cannulas and nucleotomes to enter the L5-S1 space through a standard posterolateral approach.[41] After a lag of many years, more than 50,000 procedures were eventually performed in the United States. An extremely low morbidity rate of 0.2% was reported, with the most common complication being diskitis.[43] From his review of 120,000 procedures performed worldwide, Onik could find no case of death attributable to the procedure itself.[44]

Despite the many reports of early success with manual and automated percutaneous lumbar diskectomy, these methods did not gain widespread popularity initially. A historical analysis may help explain this seeming lack of interest. First, the medical instrumentation industry was still in its infancy at this time and nowhere near the burgeoning enterprise it is today. Because there was little business interest behind APLD, no standardized commercial instrumentation sets were readily available. Additionally, owing to this lack of commercial backing, there was no concerted effort to widely publicize APLD and educate surgeons in its use. The absence of uniform criteria for patient selection and for the technique itself led to a heterogeneous initial clinical experience with the procedure. Many surgeons simply abandoned the procedure after a few attempts because of its steep learning curve and the lack of a good clinical support structure.[43] Subsequently, success rates as low as 40% to 50% were reported during this period.[45] Concurrently, a renaissance of chemonucleolysis occurred both in the United States and abroad. In many instances, interest in percutaneous diskectomy techniques was simply overshadowed by the wave of excitement generated by chymopapain injection.[7, 46] Last, a lack of financial incentive may have played a significant role in stifling the use of APLD. The procedure was deemed experimental by the National Blue Cross Blue Shield Technology Assessment Committee. As a result, Blue Cross and many other insurance carriers did not reimburse for APLD procedures for many years after their introduction.[47]

For these and other reasons, well-controlled, prospective, randomized clinical series were simply lacking during the development of APLD. Despite increasing enthusiasm on the part of the few clinical centers using APLD, skepticism regarding its efficacy continues to prevail among the community of seasoned spinal surgeons. As Mayer wrote in his critical analysis of the subject, "The large gap between the empirical data and scientific studies, the hazard of overuse and abuse, the poor definition of selection criteria, the lack of scientific validity proven in prospective controlled studies, and the tremendous commercial impact of percutaneous diskectomy is feeding a still ongoing controversial discussion about its value."[47]

INDICATIONS

As with all surgical procedures, success with APLD is directly correlated with selecting patients whose pathology is amenable to the postulated mechanism of indirect decompression. As such, APLD is most effective in treating patients with small to moderate, contained disk herniations with both clinical and radiographic findings suggesting radicular nerve root irritation and compression.[48] These patients should have sciatica, with leg pain greater than back pain, and some constellation of the classic findings of atrophy, paresis, sensory and reflex changes, and positive tension signs (e.g., straight leg raising or femoral nerve

stretch). Most authors believe that patients with severe or rapidly progressive weakness and bowel or bladder dysfunction should not be considered for APLD and may require timely open surgical decompression. Because disk herniations are thought to represent a spectrum of pathologic changes from the normal to the sequestered fragment, candidates for APLD ideally should have either MRI or CT evidence consistent with a herniated fragment that is still confined by the annulus and posterior longitudinal ligament. The presence of a sequestered or free disk fragment should be regarded as a strong contraindication for the procedure.[49] Other radiographic or clinical pictures that should exclude patients from APLD are diffuse or circumferential disk bulges without herniation, isolated "black-disk" disease, severe lateral recess or central spinal stenosis, calcified disk herniation, spondylolisthesis, evidence of instability, tumor, infection, or adjacent trauma. Patients with severe degenerative disease are more likely to have persistent or possibly worsened back pain after the procedure.[50] In short, APLD patients should meet the same criteria used for chemonucleolysis.

The most significant difficulty in patient selection lies in the ability to radiographically distinguish which disk herniations are contained and which are sequestered. Use of clinical criteria to identify patients with free or extruded fragments has been uniformly ineffective.[51] In a careful study correlating radiographic and surgical findings, Freis and coworkers[52] demonstrated that herniations occupying greater than half the spinal canal diameter on CT had a more than 90% likelihood of being sequestered at surgery. Similarly, the most definitive radiographic finding of a sequestered disk was the presence of a disk fragment superior or inferior to the actual disk space. Herniations with an acute angle and irregular shape on sagittal MRI were more likely to be extruded than were fragments with an obtuse angle and smooth margins.

Although the use of diskography is controversial among spinal surgeons, it may be helpful in identifying patients likely to have extruded fragments. If the herniation is well outlined by contrast material injected into the disk space and is contained within the posterior longitudinal ligament line, a contained fragment is likely. If there is extravasation of contrast within the spinal canal, an extruded disk is likely, and APLD should not be considered.[44] Use of concomitant CT with diskography can provide additional information on the size of the annular tear. Clinical studies have demonstrated an overall success rate of 80% for patients with wide communications, whereas those with narrow necks are associated with only a 50% success rate.[53]

Based on the available literature, certain subgroups of patients with lumbar disk disease have been identified that are most likely to benefit from APLD. These include patients who are young, those with far-lateral herniations, and those with a history of previous surgery. Young patients with well-hydrated disks on MRI are thought to have an overall better communication between the central nuclear material and the disk fragment. As such, the chance of reducing the herniation is better in these patients.[45] In cases of far-lateral disk herniations, standard posterior microsurgery often involves more bony removal from the facet to obtain adequate visualization. APLD is thought to be an ideal procedure for such cases, as the nucleotome and cannula often pass very near this area and may often directly traverse it.[54] For the approximately 5% to 10% of patients with reherniation after open surgery, APLD may provide a good salvage option, because the procedure avoids the epidural space, distortion, and prior scarring. For patients with reherniation and evidence of a connection to the central disk space, success rates as high as 80% to 90% have been reported.[47]

TECHNIQUE

Like all minimally invasive posterolateral techniques, the key to APLD lies in guiding the nucleotome apparatus into the center of the target disk space under precise fluoroscopically guided control.[55] Preoperative imaging with plain radiographs and CT is essential to define the anatomic variants unique to each patient. For example, some patients have a portion of the colon in a retroperitoneal position behind the psoas, and such preoperative assessment can avoid complications. Further, anatomic variations of the vascular tree are not uncommon and should be looked for specifically. Anteroposterior images alone are not adequate in this regard.

Similar to chemonucleolysis, the patient is placed in the lateral decubitus position, which allows for flexion and extension as needed during the procedure. Maximal access and exposure of the posterolateral aspect of the disk space are achieved by minimizing lordosis and maintaining a very straight, unrotated lateral decubitus position.[42] Like chymopapain injection, APLD is best performed with the patient under local anesthesia to allow for patient feedback and avoid accidental neural violation. Biplanar fluoroscopy is used to count up from the sacrum to ensure the proper level. Recent experience with intraoperative MRI, ultrasonography, and image guidance may help refine these techniques further.[56, 57]

Identifying the ideal entry point for APLD is similar to the technique already discussed in the section on chemonucleolysis. A small 22- or 25-gauge spinal needle is used initially to numb the skin, muscle, and outer fascial layers. The outer 18-gauge trocar is then inserted 8 to 14 cm off midline at the level of the target disk space (although this varies greatly with the patient's frame). The trocar is gradually advanced under real-time fluoroscopic guidance down to the level of the disk annulus. The main benefit of having an awake patient is the ability to withdraw and redirect the trocar should there be any radicular pain reported. On a true anteroposterior projection, the trocar should be lateral to a line formed by the medial border of the pedicles to ensure that it lies outside of the spinal canal.[47] Before advancement, many authors advocate swinging the fluoroscope to reconfirm positioning in the lateral view. The trocar is then advanced into the

center of the nucleus pulposus and again reconfirmed with biplanar imaging. Some authors advocate use of a two-trocar technique to reduce the incidence of diskitis, which is the most common complication. Strict adherence to sterile technique during APLD is mandatory.

Approach to the L5-S1 disk space can be especially problematic, owing to the position of the iliac crest and the difficulty in obtaining an adequate posterolateral trajectory.[57] A far-oblique trajectory must often be used, with fluoroscopy used to determine the entry point. The intersection of the iliac crest and a line tangential to the outside of the sacroiliac joint extending superiorly usually demarcates the insertion point for the procedure.[44] Teng and associates[42] described the use of preoperative CT to achieve such a trajectory in the majority of their 430 patients treated at this level. Beginning with the small-gauge local anesthetic needle, it is placed in the intended oblique trajectory toward the disk. Under lateral fluoroscopy, the angle of the needle with respect to the disk space is assessed. If the needle is in the plane of the disk, the entry point is moved about 2 cm laterally and then rechecked. If the needle is still in the plane of the disk, the entry point is again moved laterally such that the most lateral entry point that permits entrance into the disk space is achieved. Use of a specialized curved cannula and nucleotome is often necessary when such a straight oblique trajectory cannot be achieved. With this curved apparatus, the L5-S1 disk space can be successfully approached in more than 90% of cases.[41]

After final positioning of the trocar, a tissue dilator and cannula are passed over it down to the outer annulus. The dilator is removed, and the cannula is advanced slightly farther until it rests firmly against the annular fibers. The fluoroscope is again swung 90 degrees to make sure that the cannula is indeed flush against the disk annulus. A sharp trephine is passed through the cannula and over the trocar, such that an incision is made into the annulus. The trocar and trephine are then withdrawn, leaving the cannula in place. Moderate use of irrigation at this point helps to clear some of the blood, debris, and contaminants that may have accumulated in the cannula. Also, copious irrigation may help decrease the incidence of diskitis from skin flora introduced during the initial puncture. The nucleotome is then passed through the cannula into the center of the disk space. Performing biplanar fluoroscopy and acquiring permanent images for record keeping are prudent at this point to document correct placement of the instrument.

Activation of the foot pedal–controlled suction cutting device begins the diskectomy. The inner cutter of the Onik device reciprocates at 180 Hz, with an average aspiration pressure of 600 mm Hg.[58] The procedure should be carefully monitored throughout its course by watching the material that accumulates in the aspiration trap. Irrigation solution that contains an antibiotic (e.g., bacitracin or gentamicin) is infused by the device and returns with the disk material suspended within it. There should be little or no blood, as the nuclear material is avascular. Through rotation, elevation, and depression of the nucleotome's tip at different depths, significant amounts of disk material can be removed.[44] The procedure is terminated when no more disk fragments can be aspirated. On average, approximately 5 to 7 g of nuclear material is removed.[49] The nucleotome is removed, and irrigation solution is passed through the cannula. Typically, the actual diskectomy takes approximately 15 to 45 minutes. The puncture site is cleaned and bandaged. For most patients, observation in the postanesthesia recovery area for 3 to 4 hours is adequate, with same-day discharge being the rule. It is extremely important to monitor these patients for any evidence of acute or subacute blood loss. Also, careful monitoring of vital signs and the puncture site and for evidence of retroperitoneal-type pain can help circumvent potentially life-threatening problems.[57] Owing to the mechanical effects of central nucleotomy, many authors advocate an aggressive physical therapy and trunk stabilization program early on for patients undergoing APLD.

COMPLICATIONS

Although controversy persists over the efficacy and indications for the procedure, it is evident from the literature that APLD is one of the safest minimally invasive means of treating the intervertebral disk. Based on a review of more than 50 series comprising well over 5000 patients, there have been remarkably few complications, with no severe sequelae noted.[44] Postprocedural back pain and muscle spasms were far less common (<10%) for patients undergoing APLD than for those undergoing chemonucleolysis and were typically self-limited.[45] The most common long-term complication was diskitis, with an incidence of approximately 0.2% in the literature. In comparison to the previous literature on manual percutaneous diskectomy, with the use of larger cannulas and pituitary-type rongeurs, the incidence of soft tissue injury and hematoma is almost negligible for APLD[57]; compared with open diskectomy, this rate is three to five times lower. Importantly, there is still no clear case of mortality being associated with APLD among the more than 130,000 procedures performed worldwide.[38]

RESULTS

Questions regarding the overall efficacy of APLD are difficult to answer, as there is a lack of well-controlled, prospective, double-blind data on the subject. Onik and Helms[59] conducted a prospective, multi-institutional study of more than 500 patients, with careful selection of only patients with the "classic" criteria for disk herniation. With such stringent patient indications, these workers were able to achieve a 75% success rate at 6 months, with failures being attributed primarily to unrecognized free fragments. Interestingly, only 15% of these failures required open diskectomy. There was a very low incidence of diskitis (<0.2%), and no other serious complications were reported. Within this study, many APLD procedures were also performed on patients who did not meet the classic selection criteria. For this subset of patients, who often had compensa-

tion and social issues as well, the success rate of the procedure decreased to 50%. Although the value of APLD over placebo in these patients is questionable, some authors believe that its low morbidity makes it a possible salvage procedure for patients who have exhausted all conservative means of management.[60] Nevertheless, Onik[44] has emphasized that the ideal patients for APLD are those with the classic picture of disk herniation, as opposed to the "black" bulging disks seen in patients with diskogenic pain. Bocchi and colleagues[61] conducted a similar prospective, multicenter evaluation of APLD in 600 patients and found a similar 72% success rate. Nonrandomized, prospective long-term follow-up has also been published on APLD. Two separate series of 146 and 45 patients with 2-year follow-up found an overall success rate of 77% and 70%, respectively.[62, 63] In a much longer study of 62 patients, Gill and Blumenthal[64] found an overall success rate of 78% at 4.5 years and a much higher 93% rate of good outcomes for patients without compensation issues. Although most failures are due to retained free fragments or other factors, a reherniation rate of 3% to 5% within the first 6 months has been demonstrated in several series of APLD.[50, 65, 66]

This optimistic set of outcomes must be viewed cautiously, however, in light of other data on APLD. Mayer,[43] in his recent objective analysis of APLD outcome data, found significant errors and biases in many of the clinical series used to support APLD use. Applying the same criteria presently used for publication in the journal *Spine*, he could not demonstrate a single report that completely met all selection criteria. Further, he found an unacceptably high incidence of two- and three-level procedures that were based primarily on multilevel diskograms. Among the few controlled, prospective trials left after screening the papers, the clinical success rates were quite varied. From a prospective, controlled, multicenter trial of 327 patients, a clinical success rate of 75.2% was observed at 1 year. However, a smaller controlled, multi-institutional trial of 38 patients examined the actual pain and functional outcomes of patients after APLD and found that only 55% could return to work after 1-year follow-up.[55] Another prospective, randomized, multicenter trial comparing APLD and chemonucleolysis in 141 patients reported dismal 37% and 66% respective success rates at 1-year follow-up.[45] This study, however, has been appropriately criticized for its poor inclusion criteria, which allowed many patients with disk herniations greater than 30% to 50% of the canal. From this global review of the APLD literature, Mayer concluded, "There is no scientifically proven validity of automated percutaneous lumbar diskectomy compared with standard surgical methods and chemonucleolysis. The majority of articles analyzed did not fulfill the selection criteria of *Spine*. Additional prospective, randomized and controlled studies are needed to define the eventual role of percutaneous lumbar diskectomy on a scientific basis."[43]

CONCLUSION

APLD is a logical extension of the push toward minimally invasive treatment of herniated intervertebral disks. Like chemonucleolysis, APLD aims to reduce compression of the affected nerve root by indirectly reducing pressure in the central intradiskal space. As such, it is logical that only a limited subset of patients can benefit from such an indirect reduction of disk herniation. From the available data, APLD appears to be helpful in approximately 70% of properly selected patients. The primary difficulty is how to identify the characteristics of the ideal APLD patient. Because significant well-controlled, prospective, randomized trials of APLD are lacking, these criteria remain uncertain at the present. As a clinical procedure, however, APLD is a reasonable alternative to open surgical decompression and carries extremely low morbidity and mortality rates.

Laser-Assisted Percutaneous Diskectomy

With the advent and subsequent refinement of percutaneous diskectomy techniques, it was simply a matter of time before alternative techniques of disk ablation were explored. In parallel with recent advances in technology, innovations in fiber-optics and miniaturization have brought laser technology into the realm of medical therapeutics. Laser energy is formed from focused light emitted from a medium that has been excited by an external power supply. This energy must be absorbed by biologic tissue to have an effective surgical result. This effect is primarily one of ablation, necrosis, and cautery.[67] The delivery of laser energy to the disk through a small percutaneous portal thus represents a logical union of the fields of minimally invasive surgery and laser technology. Attractive aspects of percutaneous laser diskectomy include (1) single-step insertion of a very small working cannula, as laser fibers are thin; (2) resultant easier access to the L5-S1 disk space; (3) more aggressive nucleotomy, as ablation can extend well beyond the reach of a standard manual nucleotome by increasing the power and pulse time of the laser; and (4) shortened treatment time. Lasers are further defined by the characteristics of their emitted energy, which is monochromatic, coherent (i.e., nondivergent), and collimated within the same phase. Adjustments of these properties allow for alterations of the power level, pulse mode, and wavelength of each individual laser. Currently, lasers of the infrared, visible-light, and ultraviolet spectrum have been used clinically in surgical procedures.

The first surgical use of a laser for disk removal occurred in 1984 when a carbon dioxide (CO_2) laser was used as an adjunct during standard open anterior cervical diskectomy.[68] Choy and colleagues[69] reported the first clinical use in humans of a neodymium:yttrium-aluminum-garnet (Nd:YAG) laser (1.32-μm wavelength) for nonendoscopic percutaneous laser disk decompression and nucleotomy in 1987. Remarkably, this first report preceded any experimental studies in animals. Since that time, numerous centers have adopted the use of laser energy for intradiskal ablation. Because it is one of the newest means of nucleotomy, controlled, prospective data are lacking. As such, the clinical indications for and limitations of percutaneous laser diskectomy are in a state of evolution and refinement.

HISTORICAL PERSPECTIVE AND BACKGROUND

A full grasp of percutaneous laser diskectomy requires a solid understanding of intervertebral disk histology. The annulus is composed primarily of type I collagen at the periphery, whereas type II fibers predominate near the central portion. The nucleus pulposus has a gel-like consistency that results from a matrix of highly hydrated proteoglycans. The matrix contains approximately 60% to 70% water, but this varies with age and use. Experimental studies have found a water content of 90% in infants, 80% in young adults, and 70% in elderly patients.[70] Thus, the most effective laser energy for nuclear ablation is one that is well absorbed by water.

Lane and colleagues[71] examined the ablative properties of CO_2 (10.6 μm), argon Nd:YAG (1.32 μm), and holmium:YAG (2.1 μm) lasers and their effect on thawed fresh-frozen human intervertebral disks. Similarly, Cummings[72] examined the Nd:YAG laser in canine models. They both observed that the effectiveness of disk ablation was directly a function of the laser energy's water absorption characteristics. Lasers with the highest water absorption had the highest amount of ablation and the lowest amount of surrounding thermal necrosis from heat transmission to the end plates or posterior longitudinal ligament. This is defined as a low ablation threshold. Further, lasers that were not delivered by fiber-optic fibers (e.g., CO_2 laser) were associated with a higher index of heat transmission and adjacent thermal tissue injury (high ablation threshold). This phenomenon was underscored by Mayer and associates,[73] who compared energy transmission of Nd:YAG versus erbium (Er):YAG (2.94 μm) lasers and found that Er:YAG ablation had improved vaporization and less unnecessary disk heating. Clinical use of Er:YAG lasers was not feasible in 1994, however, as no fiber-optic fibers were available to deliver 2.94-μm wavelength energy.

The majority of lasers used for intradiskal ablation are in the infrared spectrum. CO_2 lasers exist in the far-infrared spectrum and are highly absorbed by water, with excellent ablative qualities and a low ablation threshold. Their clinical use, however, is severely limited by the lack of fiber-optic delivery capability.[74] Most clinical lasers used today occupy the mid-infrared range (1 to 4 μm) and can be delivered via flexible fiber-optic catheters through small working cannulas and needles. Near-infrared lasers are poorly absorbed by water and by the white avascular tissue of the nucleus pulposus. Their effectiveness can be improved by the addition of chromophores to tissue for better absorption of the laser energy. The fiber can be modified to absorb the laser energy, creating a contact ablation mode. Visible-light lasers, like near-infrared beams, are poorly absorbed by water. These lasers also tend to diffuse heavily into white avascular tissue such as the disk, with significant heat diffusion, boiling, and vaporization, leading to a typically char-lined crater.[74]

Ultraviolet lasers are more powerful than either infrared or visible-light lasers and have lower ablation thresholds per quantum of energy expended. As such, they cause far less surrounding thermal injury. Ablation with ultraviolet light, however, requires photochemical decomposition of peptide bonds within collagen molecules. Clinical use of ultraviolet lasers is thus ineffective at present owing to the slow rate of ablation. Whereas the majority of percutaneous laser diskectomies are done with mid-infrared lasers (i.e., Nd:YAG, Ho:YAG), the first laser to be approved by the FDA for laser diskectomy was the KTP/532 system (0.532-μm wavelength). As it is in the near infrared–visible light range, this laser is generally used in conjunction with the chromophore indigo carmine (indigotindisulfinate sodium) to stain the disk material, enhance energy absorption, and lower the ablation threshold.

Concerns regarding iatrogenic thermal energy to adjacent structures led Yunezawa and colleagues[75] to complete a systematic study of percutaneous laser diskectomy with the Nd:YAG laser in living rabbit and goat models. Using standard parameters and settings (400-μm fiber thickness, 18-gauge trocar needle) as defined by Choy and colleagues,[76] they discovered a significant amount of end plate destruction, along with burns to the trocar needle and laser fiber itself. This high amount of heat transmission was thought to result primarily from a "burn-back" phenomenon of tissue as it was vaporized by the laser's thermal energy. They then developed a double-lumen 18-gauge outer, 23-gauge inner needle system to allow for simultaneous aspiration of vaporized disk material during the procedure, which greatly minimized this phenomenon.[75, 77] Follow-up histologic analysis of rabbit disks 8 weeks after percutaneous laser disketomy found changes comparable to those described after conventional surgical diskectomy.

In addition to their thermal work, Yunezawa's group[75] completed biomechanical testing of the disks both before and after laser ablation. The animal specimens undergoing percutaneous laser diskectomy had significant changes in their response to vertical load, which were equivalent to the changes in animals treated by aggressive mechanical nucleotomy with microcurets. Choy and Altman[78] introduced 1000 J of Nd:YAG energy into the L5-S1 interspaces of cadaveric human spines and observed a 55.6% decrease in intradiskal pressures on axial loading after ablation. Similar findings were documented by Prodoehl and colleagues[79] for the Ho:YAG laser and for L4-5 human cadaveric disks treated by percutaneous laser diskectomy. For lasers with a higher ablation index and more thermal effect, there may also be a delayed mechanical and structural benefit. In light of recent work with radiofrequency electrothermocautery of the central nucleus, some authors have hypothesized that the thermal injury may induce shortening of collagen fibers and cause a delayed reorganization of the fiber structure during the healing process. Such data have been studied more extensively in work on restoration of shoulder and hip capsular integrity with thermal cautery probes.

From a historical perspective, all the studies cited earlier were published well after the first clinical use of percutaneous laser diskectomy in humans in 1987. Choy and his group[76] did, however, complete a preclinical feasibility study of percutaneous laser diskectomy in the intervertebral disks of 13 dogs before this. They could demonstrate no deleterious effects in the canines who were sacrificed 2 to 3 weeks after treatment. Despite this lack of significant experimental studies, laser diskectomy became increasingly popular at several institutions worldwide. It has been widely used in the treatment of both lumbar and thoracic disk herniations. In light of subsequent animal studies and modifications of the technical aspects of the procedure, percutaneous laser diskectomy has been fortunate in having very low morbidity and mortality rates associated with it.

INDICATIONS

Most clinicians working with percutaneous laser diskectomy agree that it is, in essence, a variation on the concept of manual and automated percutaneous diskectomy techniques. Ultimately, all three techniques derive their benefit from volumetric decompression of the central nucleus pulposus without removing the disk herniation itself. As such, most senior authors have stated that the patient selection criteria and indications for percutaneous laser diskectomy are the same as those used for microdiskectomy, chemonucleolysis, and mechanical percutaneous diskectomy, as discussed earlier. Although clinical experience with laser diskectomy is not as extensive as with other nucleotomy techniques, the consensus is that the ideal patient is one who meets all the classic radiographic and clinical criteria for a herniated disk.[80] Additionally, it is recommended that patients should have had at least 6 weeks of unsuccessful conservative therapy. Some concerns have been raised, however, in cases with suspected severe scarring from previous surgery, inflammation, or arachnoiditis. Whereas the nucleotomy of APLD is limited by the mechanical device and can easily be contained within the annulus by the operator, laser diskectomy carries the potential for inadvertent local diffusion of the laser energy, as well as distal thermal propagation. In cases in which severe distortion of the normal anatomy has occurred, scarred neural and vascular structures may be much closer than anticipated. Laser diskectomy may carry increased risk in such redo procedures, owing to the increased chance of inadvertent thermal transmission to these adherent vital structures.[81]

TECHNIQUE

Like APLD and chemonucleolysis, laser diskectomy is done with the patient in either a prone or lateral decubitus position, with the painful side placed superiorly. Biplanar image intensification via fluoroscopy is essential, as with all percutaneous intradiskal procedures. For reasons already discussed, general anesthesia should be avoided if possible to prevent inadvertent neurovascular compromise. With good intravenous access and local sedation, the procedure can be safely performed in either a radiology or operating suite. Strict sterile technique should be maintained, regardless of the venue of treatment. A point of entry is chosen and accessed before initiating the procedure. For a patient in the lateral decubitus position, a mark is usually made 7 to 8 cm off midline on the symptomatic side. In the prone position, this point is slightly more lateral, at around 10 cm.[82] An adequate subcutaneous infusion of lidocaine (0.5% or 1%) is made at a 45-degree angle to the coronal plane down to the level of the annulus with a large-bore needle (16 to 18 gauge). This anesthetic needle should be advanced slowly and withdrawn or repositioned should radicular pain be encountered. Continuous real-time visualization of the needle location with the image intensifier is crucial. Once the disk has been encountered, reconfirmation in a second orthogonal plane of view is generally prudent. After the trocar needle has definitely punctured the outer portion of the disk annulus, the inner stylet is withdrawn. Like with chemonucleolysis, some authors advocate a two-needle technique to enter the disk space (see earlier) to decrease the incidence of diskitis. A two-needle system can also be used to simultaneously aspirate and irrigate during the procedure to decrease "back-burn" thermal injury.[76] The laser fiber (usually 400 μm thick) is advanced through the trocar into the center of the nucleus pulposus. Biplanar fluoroscopic confirmation of the central placement of the radiopaque laser fiber tip is mandatory both for the patient's safety and for documentation purposes. Variations of this technique for a dorsolateral approach to the thoracic disks and a right ventrolateral approach to the cervical disks have been described.[80]

The laser probe is then activated, with the exact settings and duration dependent on the type of energy used. For Nd:YAG lasers (1.32-μm wavelength), typical settings are a 20- to 23-W output at the tip with 1-second pulses and 1-second pauses used to deliver 1000 to 1850 J to the disk space.[83] KTP/532 laser diskectomy is similar but uses a 1.8-mm "SpineStat" probe that optically diverts the laser energy 70 degrees, resulting in a vaporization zone 60 to 80 degrees from the fiber axis due to the 20-degree beam divergence. Usually 1250 to 1875 J of energy is delivered circumferentially.[81] For the Ho:YAG laser, a 400-μm fiber is advanced into the center of the disk space and activated using 1.5-J pulses at a rate of 10 Hz for 15-J bursts separated by 5-second pauses. Up to a total of 1200 J is thus delivered to the nucleus.[82] After treatment, the patient is allowed to recover from anesthesia for 2 to 4 hours under observation. Typically, only mild nonsteroidal anti-inflammatory drugs or weak narcotics are needed for pain control. Most patients are discharged several hours after the procedure.

Laser diskectomy through a working endoscope with real-time visualization has also been described. After initial placement of the trocar needle, the stylet is removed, and a guide wire is advanced over it. The needle is removed, and a 2-mm cannula with an inner trephine is introduced into the central portion of the disk space. The trephine and guide wire are removed after fluoroscopic confirmation of their location, leaving only the working cannula. A 1.7-mm endoscope with channels for the laser fiber, illumination fiber, image fiber, and flush lumen is then advanced through the cannula into the disk space. Models with a flexible tip are also available to allow up to 90 degrees of deflection. As described, ablation is begun and directly visualized during the pauses between cycles of the Ho:YAG laser. Irrigation through the endoscope offers the advantage of decreasing "burn-back" thermal injury and overheating, as well as decreasing the risk of sequestra and diskitis. However, irrigation also increases the amount of laser energy required for ablation to approximately 10,000 to 15,000 J.[84]

RESULTS AND COMPLICATIONS

Clinical experience with laser diskectomy has been limited by its relatively recent introduction. From the available data, percutaneous laser diskectomy may be as effective as other types of percutaneous nucleotomy. Choy and associates[83] performed 333 percutaneous laser diskectomies with the Nd:YAG laser and performed up to 1-year follow-ups using MacNab's criteria.[2] In this prospective, uncontrolled study, the authors found that 261 patients (78.4%) had a fair to good response, and 72 (21.6%) had a poor response. Eleven patients underwent a second laser diskectomy, with seven (64%) deriving subsequent benefit. There was a less than 1% overall complication rate, with diskitis being most common (<0.2%).

Using the KTP/532 laser after its FDA approval, Yeung[85] completed another prospective, uncontrolled study of 1000 patients undergoing percutaneous laser diskectomy. The average dose was 1250 J of laser energy. Strict patient selection criteria were used to include only those with contained disk herniations on MRI or CT, no evidence of dye leak on diskography, clinical findings consistent with sciatica, and failure to respond to conservative therapy. Based on these indications, they reported good to excellent outcomes in 840 (84%) of their patients. They reported no mortality and a less than 1% incidence of complications. In a similar study by Bosacco and coworkers[86] of KTP/532 laser diskectomies on 63 patients, 72% achieved relief of radicular pain, 54% had relief of lumbago, and 59% were able to return to work an average of 4 weeks after treatment.

Rhodes and colleagues[87] used the Ho:YAG laser for percutaneous lumbar laser nucleotomy and delivered 1200 J of energy to 25 consecutive patients in a prospective but uncontrolled trial. Using quite stringent selection criteria and a Dallas Pain Questionnaire for follow-up assessment, they found that 20 patients (80%) reported significant improvement of their symptoms. Twenty-three (92%) had resolution of abnormal physical findings, and 21 (84%) were able to return to work.

One of the largest studies of laser diskectomy patients was by Hellinger,[80] who retrospectively analyzed more than 2535 patients treated between 1989 and 1993. He found that 80% of lumbar patients and 86% of cervical patients reported some degree of symptomatic improvement. Thoracic cases seemed to do especially well. This subjective improvement rate lagged behind a reported 90% rate of improved physical findings. Like other published reports, this series quoted a low rate of complications (<1%), but it provided details of the few complications that were encountered. There was one case of diskitis requiring open débridement, one case of transient sympathectomy syndrome, one case of thermally induced paresis of the foot dorsiflexors, and one case of acute paraplegia after cervical laser diskectomy. Despite the low complication rate, these sequelae serve as a reminder that laser diskectomies are by no means risk free.

In one of the few prospective, controlled trials of laser diskectomy, Sherk[84] studied 68 patients who met classic radiographic and clinical criteria for herniated lumbar disks. Of these patients, 47 underwent laser diskectomy, and the other 21 were observed. Although the intention was to perform randomization, the patients generally refused random assignment. Assignment to either the laser diskectomy or control group was thus based solely on the patient's informed decision. Using a Dallas Pain Questionnaire for follow-up, no significant difference could be observed between the two groups ($P > 0.7$). There was, however, significant improvement of physical findings in the laser diskectomy group.

CONCLUSION

Percutaneous nucleotomy with the use of laser fibers represents an interesting technologic advancement in the field of minimally invasive treatment of herniated lumbar disks. Like any new tool, however, statements regarding its utility, efficacy, and safety must be qualified until prospective, controlled, randomized trials are conducted to compare its treatment outcomes with those of standard procedures. Laser diskectomy is attractive in its ability to achieve larger volumes of disk ablation through smaller working channels than even automated percutaneous diskectomy. The long-term effects of laser energy within the intervertebral disks, however, are poorly understood. Additionally, there may be thermally induced permanent alterations in the actual architecture of the disk itself. Although some of the available clinical data suggest that laser fibers may be as effective as the nucleotome in decompressing the nucleus pulposus, controlled series have yet to validate the benefit of laser diskectomy over more conservative therapy. Lack of such data should not discount laser diskectomy as a useful alternative to open microdiskectomy for patients unsuitable for surgery. Like chymopapain and the nucleotome were at one time, the laser fiber is simply the newest tool available for percutaneous diskectomy and requires further study to better delineate its indications and outcomes.

Endoscopic Diskectomy

Endoscopic diskectomy affords real-time direct visualization of the disk being removed. It represents an improvement over the "blind" percutaneous diskectomy that was previously used. It was not developed until sufficient experience had been obtained with the percutaneous paramedian approach to the lumbar spine under fluoroscopic control and small, rigid endoscopes or arthroscopes had been developed. Since then, instrumentation for endoscopic diskectomy has progressed from modified arthroscopes used for visualization to endoscopes that afford direct visualization with the ability to insert instruments for bone and disk removal. This section discusses three techniques used for endoscopic diskectomy: arthroscopic diskectomy, transforaminal diskectomy, and microendoscopic diskectomy (MED).

HISTORICAL PERSPECTIVE AND BACKGROUND

Initial experience with the posterolateral approach to the lumbar disk identified a triangular working zone defined inferiorly by the proximal vertebral plate, posteriorly by the superior facet of the inferior body, and anteriorly by the exiting nerve root. Once this triangular working space was defined as a safe area to introduce instrumentation, small-caliber rigid endoscopes or arthroscopes were developed to visualize this region.[88] Arthroscopes were first used as a means of visualizing this triangular working space. In 1983 Hausmann and Forst described a nucleoscope that could be used during open diskectomy to ensure that loose intradiskal fragments were adequately extracted.[89] Schreiber and associates used dual portals for arthroscopic nucelotomy.[89] Subsequently, Kambin developed a biportal access for the introduction of arthroscopes, with various angles through one portal and the ability to insert articulating instruments through the opposite port for uninterrupted visualization and removal of contained or nonmigrated posterior extraligamentous herniations.[89] To eliminate the biportal entry with arthroscopes, Mayer[43] popularized the use of a percutaneous endoscope angled to 70 degrees, coupled with a television and video unit for visualization. Rigid straight, angled, and flexible forceps with automated high-power suction shaver and cutter systems can then be introduced to remove "contained" lumbar disk herniations and small "noncontained" lumbar disk herniations.

Both the arthroscopic and the percutaneous endoscopic techniques use a posterolateral approach to the disk space. As a result, the procedure was largely confined to intradiskal work and was not suitable for patients with free fragments. Ditsworth[90] designed an endoscope that can bend up to 90 degrees and pass completely through the foramen into the spinal canal (transforaminal) to directly remove free fragments and reconfigure the disk, allowing for root and dural decompression at all lumbar levels. This technique expanded percutaneous endoscopy to include noncontained disk herniations and even migrated free fragments. More recently, Foley and Smith[91, 92] developed MED, which allows introduction of the endoscope, direct removal of bone using drills or Kerrison rongeurs, and removal of the disk. MED now allows the surgeon to perform a direct microdiskectomy, without the limitations of a contained disk or a foraminal free fragment.

INDICATIONS

The arthroscopic and percutaneous endoscopic techniques are especially suited for patients with contained disk herniations (outer border of the annulus fibrosus intact) and those with small, noncontained disk herniation (extrusion at the level of the disk space and occupying no more than one third of the sagittal diameter of the spinal canal). Mayer and coworkers[73] perform a diskogram on patients to confirm these criteria. The procedure is aborted if there is evidence of contrast leak into the epidural space or a subligamentous prolapse occupying more than one third of the sagittal diameter of the spinal canal. These strict selection criteria have led some surgeons to question the overall utility of the endoscopic procedure. Kleinpeter and associates[93] found that only 13 of 326 patients (4%) were candidates for an endoscopic procedure. Of these 13 patients, only 8 were wholly suitable and were operated on percutaneously. Patients should have clinical symptoms secondary to nerve root compression, such as positive straight leg raising test, sciatica, sensory disturbances, or mild motor weakness. These patients have posterolateral disk herniations that may be accessible using the posterolateral approach to the disk space. Patients with large, noncontained disk herniations extending cranially or caudally to the level of the disk space are not suitable, because the endoscope and the arthroscope are not designed to work at the level of the spinal canal. Patients with sequestered disk, spinal stenosis, or spondylolisthesis are not good candidates for this technique. Instead, they should be considered for open diskectomy or fusion.

Noncontained disk herniations may be removed using the transforaminal technique or MED. The ideal lesion for the transforaminal technique is a unilateral, one-level extruded disk and free fragments—preferably, free fragments in the spinal canal that are readily accessible to the foramen and soft and compressible enough to be delivered via the foramen using a small scope.[90] MED theoretically can be applied to all disk fragments (contained or noncontained) and can also be used in patients with symptomatic lateral stenosis secondary to bony hypertrophy. It is especially well suited for patients with far-lateral disk herniations, because a lateral incision is used for MED to begin with.[92]

TECHNIQUE

Both the arthroscopic and the percutaneous endoscopic techniques employ a posterolateral trajectory to the herniated disk.[94] In the arthroscopic technique popularized by Kambin, a biportal approach is used for the removal of large central or paramedian subligamentous and extraligamentous herniations; the uniportal approach is used for the removal of extraforaminal, foraminal, and smaller paramedian herniations.[89] In the arthroscopic technique, biportal access is used for introduction of the arthroscopes, with various angles through one portal and articulating instruments through the opposite port. Typically, an 18-gauge spinal needle is introduced into the disk space of choice under fluoroscopic visualization. Repeated puncturing of the spinal disk is performed to ensure that the disk space is indeed there. A guide wire is inserted into the spinal needle, and a trocar is passed into the disk space via the guide wire. The trocar then serves as the conduit for a rigid, 6.4-mm-outside-diameter working cannula. Instruments such as a straight forceps and up-biting forceps can then be introduced through the working portal into the disk to be removed. At the same time, another portal is established for visualization of the disk and the equipment used. Savitz[95] modified the arthroscopic approach by using the laser to help with the diskectomy.

In Mayer's technique, an endoscope is introduced percutaneously using the same posterolateral trajectory. The disk is approached from the symptomatic side. The skin is entered between 9 and 11 cm lateral to the midline, and the disk space is entered with a cannula. Before inserting the endoscope, a diskogram is performed. If contrast medium leaks into the epidural space or reveals a subligamentous prolapse occupying more than one third of the sagittal diameter of the spinal canal, the procedure is aborted. A guide wire is inserted via the cannula and serves as the conduit for a trocar, which is inserted into the disk space. The trocar then serves as the guide for the working cannula, from which rigid forceps may be introduced to remove a small amount of nucleus pulposus from the center of the disk. The endoscope can then be inserted to visualize the degree of disk removal. If the disk is midline, another endoscope is inserted to visualize the disk removal, much like Kambin's biportal arthroscope.[43, 73]

The transforaminal diskectomy was proposed by Ditsworth as an attempt to remove freely herniated disks via the neural foramen. Because of the small size of the working space and the 90-degree angle, the endoscope had to be small and flexible so that it could bend up to 90 degrees and pass completely through the foramen and into the spinal canal to directly remove free fragments and configure the disk. Unlike Kambin's 6.4-mm straight working cannula, the outer cannula is only 4.2 mm, and a flexible 2.8-mm endoscope can be passed through it and into the foramen. The procedure is done in two steps. First, an annulotomy and disk decompression are performed through the standard posterolateral appproach using a straight cannula. After the decompression, a curved cannula is inserted, and the flexibe endoscope is passed through the foramen. A combination of instruments may be passed through the endoscope, including a hook, a grasper, and a curet to remove a free disk fragment.[90, 96]

MED was developed by Foley and Smith[91] and allows for direct removal of herniated disks using a combination of endoscopic and standard open microsurgical techniques, with the goal of minimizing paraspinous muscle trauma. The procedure is performed in an outpatient setting, using epidural anesthesia. The patient is positioned prone on a Wilson frame, and the appropriate level is identified with a spinal needle using a fluoroscope. A paramedian incision (4.5 to 5 cm lateral to midline, ipsilateral to the side of herniation) is made and carried only to the subcutaneous tissues. The lumbodorsal fascia is identified, and a K-wire is directed through the incision, through the fascia, and toward the junction of the transverse process and the pars articularis. A cannulated dilator is placed over the K-wire, and the wire is removed (Fig. 310–2*A* and *B*). The position of the dilator, at the junction of the transverse process and the pars articularis, is verified using a combination of bony landmark palpation and fluoroscopy. The second and third dilators are placed, and a 16-mm-diameter tubular retractor is held in place by an articulated arm. These dilators establish an operative corridor between the fibers of the lumbar paraspinous muscles, leaving the normal paraspinous muscle attachments intact. A 25-degree rod-lens endoscope is then placed down the tubular retractor and connected to the coupler and camera, the light source, and the suction tube (see Fig. 310–2*C*). The endoscopic image is oriented to the patient's position. Under direct endoscopic visualization, a hemilaminotomy, medial facetectomy, resection of ligamenta flava, retraction of nerve root, and removal of disk are performed (see Fig. 310–2*D* to *F*). For removal of far-lateral herniated disks, the transverse process–pars articularis junction is exposed. Typically, the pars artery is identified, coagulated, and divided early in the exposure. The pars artery can be quite vascular if it is inadvertently violated, leading to difficulty in visualization with the endoscope. The lateral edge of the pars is identified. An angled curet is used to dissect the undersurface of the inferomedial aspect of the transverse process and pars, thereby releasing the medial aspect of the intertransverse ligament (Fig. 310–3*A*). A small portion of the inferomedial transverse process and the most lateral aspect of the pars is removed using an angled Kerrison rongeur (see Fig. 310–3*B*). This exposure allows for identification of the lateral aspect of the neural foramen and identification of the exiting nerve root adjacent to the pedicle. The nerve root is then followed toward the disk (see Fig. 310–3*C*). If necessary, the lateral margin of the superior articular process is identified and resected using a Kerrison rongeur. The nerve root is clearly exposed, and the sequestered disk fragments can be removed (see Fig. 310–3*D* and *E*). Once the nerve root has been deemed to be decompressed, the wound is irrigated, and the tubular retractor is removed. The muscle is minimally traumatized, the subcutaneous tissue is reapproximated, and the skin is sewn with subcuticular stitches.

Although MED allows the most direct approach to the disk space of all the endoscopic procedures, it still enables only two-dimensional visualization of the herniated disk. Moreover, it requires a steep initial learning curve to recognize the anatomy through the limited view of the endoscope and to work using the heads-up display of the endoscope. Additional disadvantages are the need to work through unfamiliar anat-

omy (as viewed through the endoscope) and the expense of buying the MED kit. However, it is especially useful for patients with far-lateral disks.[97] In these cases, MED has the advantage of a paramedian incision, ideal placement, and minimal trauma to the paraspinous muscles. Foley and Smith[91] reported the use of MED in 41 patients, with a follow-up of 7 to 18 months. All patients had substantial relief of their radiculopathy. The only complication was one patient with a cerebrospinal fluid leak. Foley and colleagues[92] also reported a small series of 11 consecutive patients with far-lateral disks operated on with MED. The operative time in their hands ranged from 90 to 120 minutes. All patients were discharged home less than 6 hours after the procedure. No patients required parenteral analgesic medication. After discharge, no patient required readmission to the hospital or the emergency room. The follow-up period ranged from 12 to 27 months. All patients improved using the modified MacNab criteria to qualify outcome. Of the nine patients with preoperative sensory abnormalities, four had residual decreased sensation. No patient experienced any residual motor deficits. One patient experienced some degree of nonradicular pain. Eight patients returned to work 3 weeks after surgery.

RESULTS

The results for endoscopic procedures are excellent if patient selection is done properly. Kambin and associates[98] reported their results with arthroscopic microdiskectomy. Between 1988 and 1998, they operated on a total of 175 patients for herniated lumbar disks; 169 patients were available for follow-up. Fifty-nine patients with a central herniated disk or a nonmigrated sequestered fragment were treated with bilateral biportal posterolateral approaches; 116 patients with radiographic evidence of a paramedian, foraminal, or extraforaminal herniation were treated using the unilateral uniportal approach. All patients were followed for a minimum of 24 months postoperatively. Outcome analysis demonstrated that 149 procedures were successful; 20 procedures (11.8%) were failures, with persistent radiculopathy that required open laminotomy in some cases. Complications were relatively few, including one disk space infection, one transient peroneal neurapraxia, and four index extremity hypersensitivity. All complications resolved without further sequelae. In a separate analysis, Kambin and Zhou[89] reported that patients with sequestered migrated herniations and large central herniations at L5-S1 and individuals with elevated iliac crests may be better served by open surgery instead of a percutaneous arthroscopic procedure.

Mayer also performed percutaneous lumbar disk procedures, but using an endoscope instead of an arthroscope, bypassing the need for biportal entry in selected cases. In an initial study of 40 patients with "contained" lumbar disk herniations (outer border of the annulus fibrosus intact) and small, "noncontained" lumbar disk herniations (at the level of the disk space, occupying less than one third the sagittal diameter of

MED 1

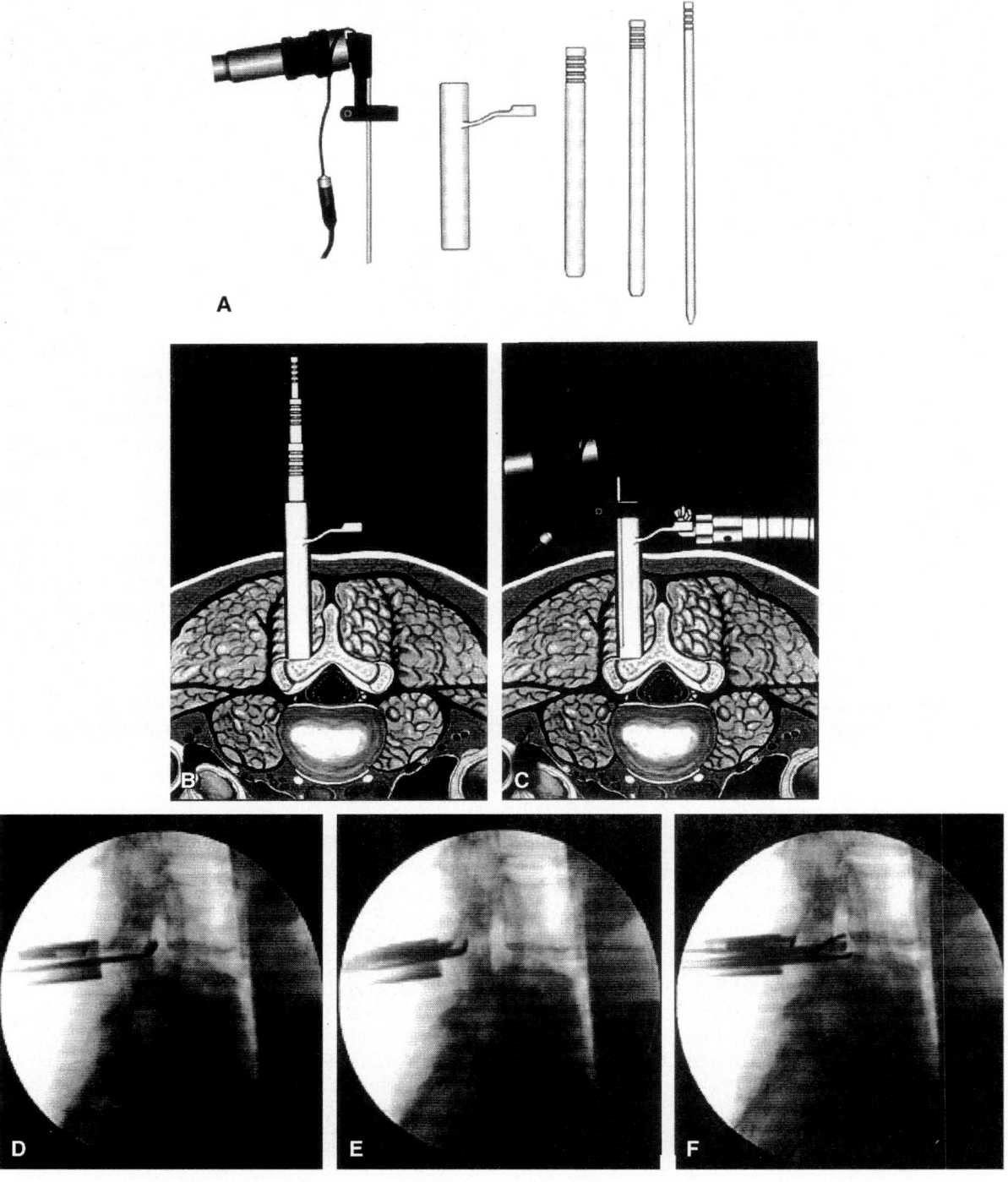

FIGURE 310–2. *A*, Microendoscopic diskectomy allows the direct removal of herniated disks using a series of dilated cannulas, a tubular retractor, and a 25-degree rod-lens endoscope. A paramedian incision is made, and a K-wire is directed through the incision, through the fascia, and toward the junction of the pars articularis and the transverse process. *B*, Three dilators are placed, establishing an operative corridor between the fibers of the lumbar paraspinous muscles, leaving the normal paraspinous muscle attachments intact. *C*, A 25-degree rod-lens endoscope is placed down the tubular retractor, and its position is verified using fluoroscopy. Serial fluoroscopic images are obtained during the microdiskectomy, demonstrating placement of the angle curet *(D)*, Kerrison rongeur *(E)*, and pituitary rongeurs to remove the disk *(F)*.

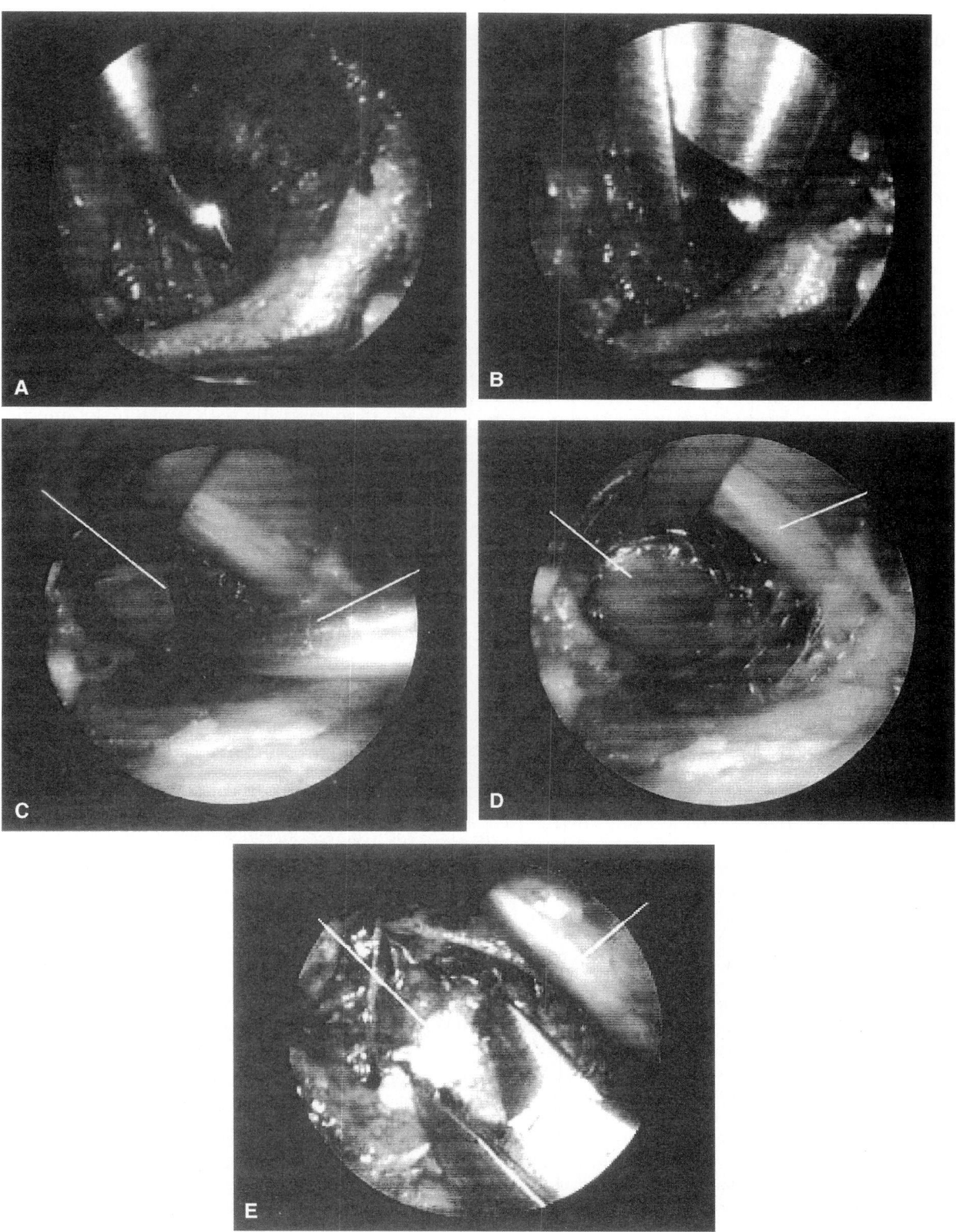

FIGURE 310–3. A laterally herniated disk is removed quite readily using the microendoscopic technique. The laterally placed incision allows for easy identification of the transverse process–pars articularis junction. The pars artery is identified and coagulated early in the procedure. *A,* An angled curet is used to dissect the undersurface of the inferomedial aspect of the transverse process and the pars, releasing the medial aspect of the intertransverse ligament. *B,* The lateral margin of the superior articular process is identified and resected using a Kerrison rongeur. *C,* The nerve root is now clearly exposed and can be gently retracted. *D,* The disk is clearly visualized. *E,* The disk is removed using pituitary rongeurs.

spinal canal), Mayer and Brock compared the results of percutaneous endoscopic diskectomy and microdiskectomy. The results from the standpoint of disappearance of sciatica, low back pain, and motor and sensory deficits between the two groups after 2 years of follow-up were similar. However, the number of patients who had returned to their previous occupations was 72.2% for the microdiskectomy group versus 95% for the percutaneous endoscopic diskectomy group.[43] A recent review article examined published papers in which a percutaneous technique was performed in 40 or more patients, with a minimum follow-up of 2 years. Of the six studies considered, five were retrospective, uncontrolled investigations. A compilation of the results demonstrated that over a follow-up period ranging from 3 months to 7.75 years (mean, 2.75 years), the results were very good, good, or fair in 72.5% of the patients. In 26.6% of the patients, a second operation was needed, usually because of residual or recurrent disk herniaiton. In eight patients (7.3%), spondylodiskitis developed at the operative level, and another two patients developed transient lumbar plexus injury. The sigmoid artery was injured in one patient, who had a full recovery after vascular surgery.[43]

Ditsworth has been the primary proponent of the endoscopic transforaminal lumbar diskectomy. Over a 6-year period, he reported 110 patients who had endoscopic transforaminal procedures, with a success rate of 95% (good or excellent) in 75 patients with disks presenting lateral to the dura and a success rate of 83% in 35 patients with "non-lateral presenting" disks, for an overall success rate of 91%. There was only one complication in a patient who developed diskitis.[90]

The MED procedure has been popularized by industry. The overall success rate is difficult to quantify because of the broad range of people using the device. However, in the hands of Foley and Smith, who popularized and designed the instrumentation used in this procedure, the success rates have been very good. They reported a series of 41 patients with disk levels ranging from L2-3 to L5-S1; 5 of 41 cases had far-lateral disk herniations, and the rest were within the spinal canal. Twenty-five of the 41 patients had free fragment pathology. Surgery was performed under epidural anesthesia on an outpatient basis. They reported good to excellent results in all patients using the modified MacNab criteria. All patients were discharged home within 6 hours of surgery, except for the first patient, who suffered a cerebrospinal fluid leak and was admitted for 48 hours. Return to work ranged from 2 to 40 days in the non–workers' compensation group and 14 to 107 days in the workers' compensation group.[91] Foley and coworkers[92] also used the MED technique in 11 patients with unilateral, single-level radiculopathy secondary to far-lateral disk herniations. There were four contained and seven sequestered disk herniations. Ten results were excellent, and one good result was obtained.

CONCLUSION

Endoscopic microdiskectomy is still evolving. Its indications have expanded from decompression of contained disks to direct attack on herniated disks or performance of foraminal decompression. The next area of development will come in the form of three-dimensional visualization. Currently, all techniques use two-dimensional screen visualization; three-dimensional visualization provided by the operating microscope is not available.

ANTERIOR PROCEDURES

Laparoscopic Anterior Interbody Fusion

Anterior lumbar interbody fusion may be performed using an "open" or laparoscopic approach.

HISTORICAL PERSPECTIVE AND BACKGROUND

Cloward pioneered the work on lumbar interbody fusion. In 1943 he advocated the use of posterior lumbar interbody fusion (PLIF) to treat the degenerative lumbar motion segment. He cited the importance of opening the disk space to increase neural foraminal diameter and creating a fusion across the unstable motion segment. PLIF, however, fell out of favor because Cloward's initial results could not be duplicated, and retropulsion of the bone graft sometimes occurred. With the development of modern posterior instrumentation, however, PLIF has again come into favor.

Anterior lumbar interbody fusion for disk disease has become increasingly common with better understanding of anterior approaches to the spine and the development of various interbody fusion devices.[99, 100] Compared with posterior lumbar fusion, anterior fusion tends to have less blood loss and does not require nerve root retraction. The original concept of a fusion cage was developed by Bagby for use in horses with cervical spondylosis and published in 1988.[101] It was later manufactured into the BAK cage. Subsequently, other cages have been developed and used in large clinical series, such as the Ray cage.[102] The first reported laparoscopic lumbar diskectomy was performed in 1991; the first two human cases of laparoscopic anterior lumbar fusion were performed at the L5-S1 junction in 1993. Since then, anterior laparoscopic spinal fusion has become increasingly popular.[103]

INDICATIONS

Anterior interbody fusion is used for patients with diskogenic back pain. It is performed for patients with mechanical back pain and instability secondary to degenerative disk disease of the lumbar spine. Patients with degenerative disk disease report low back pain that may radiate to the paraspinal regions or the buttocks. The pain is aggravated by standing and becomes particularly severe when attempting to bend the lumbar spine; lying down with the hips and knees flexed lessens the pain. Frequently, there is a referred component to the pain, with radiation down the sacroiliac joint, buttocks, or proximal thigh. Patients may also have radicular symptoms such as paresthesias or signs such as diminished reflexes corresponding to the unstable segment.

Radiographic confirmation is obtained by plain x-ray films, which may demonstrate narrowing at the appropriate level. Flexion-extension views may show evidence of degenerative instability, with motion defined as sagittal rotation in excess of 20 degrees or listhesis greater than 20% of body width. T2-weighted MRI demonstrates the so-called black disk, which is thought to be secondary to desiccation and changes in the collagen content of the disk. Significant disk protrusion, herniation, or nerve root compression is usually not present. In patients in whom radiographic confirmation by plain x-rays or MRI is not possible, diskograms are performed. Provocative diskography is performed under fluoroscopic guidance by experienced physicians (neuroradiologists at our institution). The diskogram is performed under the standard posterolateral approach, and Isovue contrast is injected into the disk space. Concordant (corresponding to the suspected disk space) or discordant (not corresponding to the suspected disk space) pain is recorded. A fluoroscopic image after contrast injection and a computed tomographic scan after the diskogram confirm extravasation of contrast from the suspected disk. Patients fitting the clinical syndrome of diskogenic back pain are therefore candidates for anterior interbody fusion.

TECHNIQUE

Laparoscopic anterior diskectomy and fusion are performed with the patient in a supine, steep Trendelenburg position with the knees flexed and a lumbar roll placed to maintain lumbar lordosis during surgery, allowing gravity to pull the intestines rostrally out of the operating field.[104] Although the laparoscopic procedure may be used for both L4-5 and L5-S1 disks, it is much easier and safer for L5-S1 disks.[105–107] An insufflator needle is placed at the umbilicus, and CO_2 is insufflated into the peritoneal cavity to a pressure of approximately 15 mm Hg. A 10-mm trocar and a 30-degree endoscope are then placed through the opening. Three other 5-mm working ports are placed—two on one side, one on the other side. The working port on the left has retractor fans used to retract the sigmoid colon laterally and superiorly; the other ports are used for suction-irrigation and dissection instruments. At the proposed interspace site, a fifth port for passage of the instruments and the screw cage is placed. A Steinmann pin is passed into the peritoneum under endoscopic visualization just above the symphysis pubis in the midline. The Steinmann pin is verified to be in the exact midline using anteroposterior and lateral fluoroscopy. A special punch is used to mark the insertion points for each of the two planned implants. A number of implants have been used with similar degrees of efficacy, including the BAK cage, bone dowels, Ray cage, or Harms cage. The drill is then used to make a pilot hole (Fig. 310–4A), and the disk space is expanded by placing dilators into the disk space (see Fig. 310–4B). The largest fitting dilator is left in place, and the other pilot hole is expanded. The instrumenta-

tion cannula is passed over the dilator; its teeth are used to engage the interspace. Reamers are used to remove disk material (see Fig. 310–4C), and a tap is used to prepare the vertebral end plate for the cage (see Fig. 310–4D). The cage is filled with cancellous bone that was previously harvested from the iliac crest, and it is inserted into the disk space (Fig. 310–4E). The implant is recessed below the level of the vertebral body so that it does not rub against the overlying soft tissues. The second implant is placed in a similar fashion. The fan retractor is then removed, and the great vessels are inspected for iatrogenic injury. The cage allows for permanent distraction and fusion of the degenerated disk space.[108]

RESULTS

Published results of laparoscopic anterior interbody fusion have generally been favorable. Riley and colleagues[109] performed a biomechanical and histologic analysis in a pig model to determine the effectiveness of an open versus a laparoscopic procedure. They found that pigs operated on with the laparoscopic technique had a less extensive diskectomy, less end plate decortication, and less resultant bone growth compared with pigs that had an open interbody fusion. In patients, results from selected centers with wide experience in laparoscopic technique have been uniformly good, albeit with limited long-term follow-up. Zucherman and coworkers[110] published results on 17 patients, with an average follow-up of 8 months (range, 6 to 12 months), who underwent this procedure. There were 14 single-level fusions and 3 two-level fusions, all involving L4-S1 levels. Only two patients required conversion to open procedures, without sequelae; two patients had remote donor site wound infections eradicated with incision and drainage and antibiotics, and one patient required subsequent posterior spinal decompression because of a displaced end plate fracture. The average hospital stay was 2 days, excluding the two patients with infections and prolonged hospital stays. Mahvi and Zdeblick[111] reported on 20 consecutive patients with diskogenic back pain who were prospectively treated with laparoscopic anterior lumbar instrumentation and fusion. Three technical complications occurred, all in the first four patients, necessitating two conversions to open transperitoneal fusion. Hospital stay for patients treated by laparoscopic instrumentation and fusion averaged 1.7 days. Twelve of 20 patients reported excellent pain relief; no motion was identified by flexion-extension films in 16 patients. Harkey and associates[112] reported results of laparosopic anterior interbody fusion using composite cages in seven patients. In two of the seven patients, the laparoscopic approach was converted to an open anterior lumbar interbody fusion because of iliac vein injury or poor visualization. Mean operative time was 120 minutes, mean blood loss was 75 mL, and mean hospital stay was 3.2 days. All patients achieved radiographic fusion. Retrograde ejaculation did occur in one patient. Martin and Yuan[113] similarly reported excellent results using laparoscopically placed BAK cages. In

ALIF

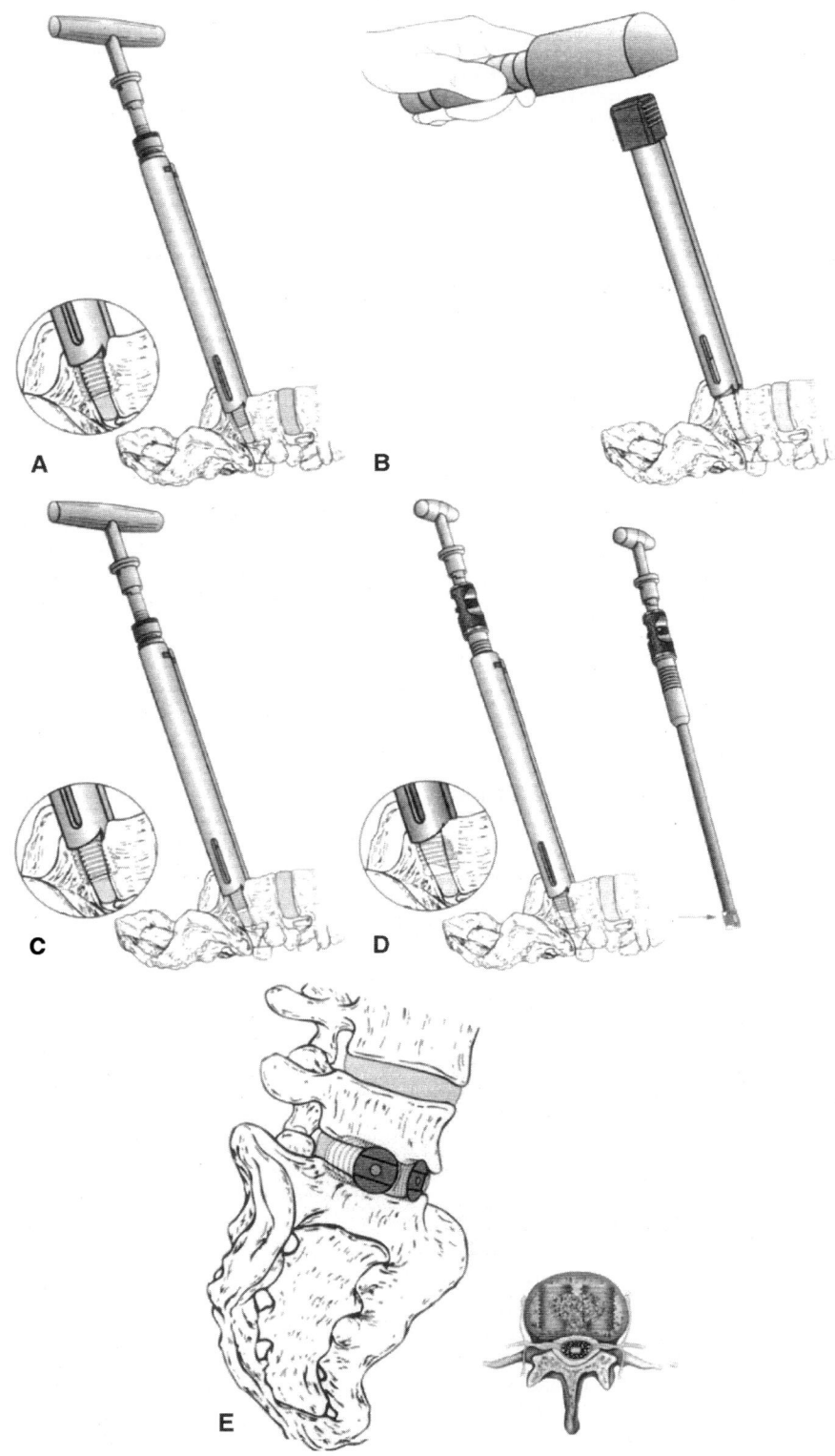

FIGURE 310–4. Schematic of an anterior lumbar fusion performed for the placement of cages at L5-S1. The Steinmann pin is passed under direct endoscopic visualization into the L5-S1 disk space. *A,* A drill is used to make a pilot hole. *B,* Progressive dilators are placed into the disk space, expanding it, and the largest fitting dilator is left in place. *C,* A reamer is used to remove the disk material, and loose disk fragments are removed using a pituitary rongeur. *D,* A tap is used to prepare the vertebral end plate for the cage. *E,* Once the cages are placed, previously harvested cancellous bone from the iliac crest is inserted into the cages.

IDET

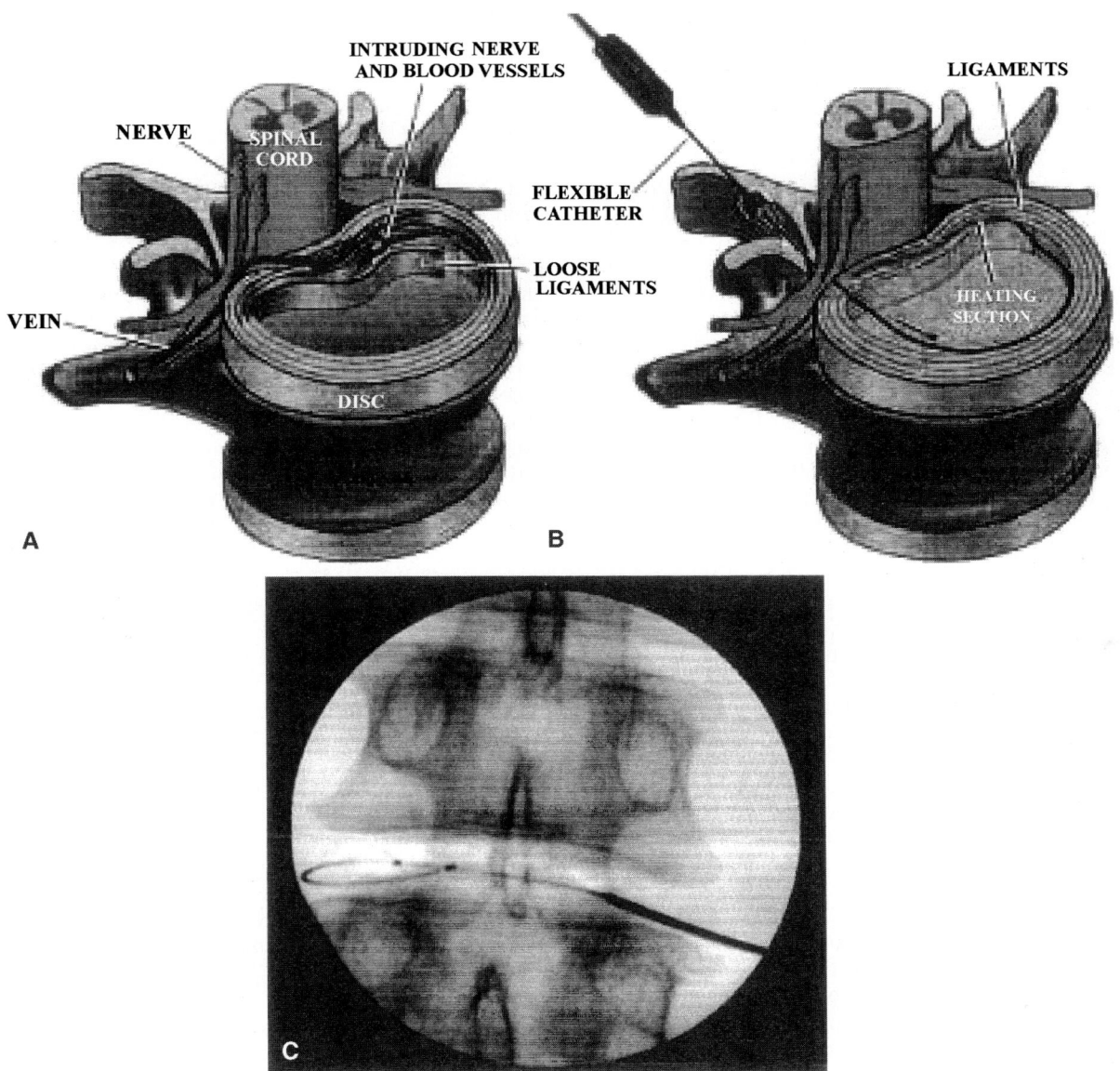

FIGURE 310–5. Schematic of the intradiskal electrothermal annuloplasty procedure. *A,* The degenerated disk has loose ligaments. Targeted thermal delivery to the degenerated disk will shrink collagen fibrils and thermocoagulate nervous tissue. *B,* A steerable SpineCATH intradiskal catheter is fed from the introducer into the posterior wall of the disk. *C,* Thermal treatment is applied over 17 minutes at a maximal tissue temperature of approximately 75°C after verification of the appropriate position of the catheter.

of rhBMP-2 in inducing fusion in the presence of various carrier agents has been tested in a number of papers.[129] Helm and coworkers[130] tested both demineralized bone matrix and type I collagen gel in 40 female beagles undergoing posterolateral fusion. They found that type I collagen served as a good osteoinductive agent, whereas demineralized bone matrix actually had an inhibitory effect on solid bone fusion in the spine. The rhBMP-2 strongly enhanced the amount of bone

formation at the fusion site and increased the number of intervertebral levels that were solidly fused. Similar results were found by David and associates,[131] who demonstrated in a posterolateral adult beagle fusion model that rhBMP-2 in the presence of type I collagen provided 100% fusion without adverse events. Boden and colleagues[132] used hydroxyapatite–tricalcium phosphate (HA-TCP) as a carrier block for rhBMP-2 for posterolateral fusions in rhesus monkeys. They examined HA-TCP blocks loaded with a solution containing 0, 6, 9, or 12 mg rhBMP-2 and demonstrated that all the monkeys treated with HA-TCP blocks and all dosages of rhBMP-2 underwent fusion. The monkeys that were not treated with rhBMP-2 showed bone ingrowth, but not through the ceramic block. When the ceramic blocks were loaded with rhBMP-2, there was a dose-dependent increase in the amount and quality of bone fused. Minamide and coworkers[133] examined the use of sintered bovine bone coated with type I collagen and rhBMP-2. Their rationale for the use of sintered bone was that it provided a natural trabecular structure and an organized crystal of bone mineral. Using a rabbit posterolateral fusion model, they demonstrated that the sintered bovine bone coated with type I collagen and rhBMP-2 had a superior fusion rate compared with autograft bone alone.

To determine the dose of rhBMP-2 that is effective for spinal fusion, Itoh and associates[134] examined a rabbit L4-5 transverse process fusion model using various dosages of rhBMP-2 and collagen. They found that the optimal rhBMP-2 dose for achieving posterolateral spinal fusion was approximately 50 μg per segment in rabbits. Martin and colleagues[114] performed the same experiments in a monkey model for L4-5 fusion and found that rhBMP-2 was extremely effective in promoting fusions in nonhuman primate spines; the presence of a laminectomy defect with exposed dura did not preclude the use of rhBMP-2. Meyer and associates[135] carried the question one step further by opening up the dura, leading to an egress of cerebrospinal fluid. They found that cerebrospinal fluid does not have a deleterious effect on spinal fusion.

The effectiveness of rhBMP-2 in inducing fusion was tested by Sandhu and coworkers,[136] who demonstrated that rhBMP-2 induced posterolateral fusion in dogs that did not receive traditional decortication of posterior elements. Martin and colleagues[114] showed that rhBMP-2 was able to overcome the detrimental effects of ketorolac, a nonsteroidal anti-inflammatory drug, on posterolateral fusion in a rabbit model. Boden and coworkers[137] demonstrated that a video-assisted lateral intertransverse process arthrodesis could be obtained by making a lateral incision in the paraspinal muscles. The use of rhBMP-2 was sufficient to ensure fusion using this technique alone.

The effectiveness of rhBMP-2 on anterior fusion has also been evaluated in animal models. Hecht and associates[138] demonstrated that rhBMP-2 was able to induce an anterior interbody fusion in rhesus monkeys undergoing L7-S1 interbody fusion using rhBMP-2–soaked collagen sponges placed in a cortical dowel allograft. Radiographic evidence of fusion was seen as early as 8 weeks in the animals receiving rhBMP-2; the control animals had evidence of pseudarthrosis in two of three monkeys. A similar study was performed by Boden and coworkers,[139] who demonstrated that titanium interbody threaded cages filled with collagen sponge containing 0 to 1.5 mg/mL of rhBMP-2 could be implanted into adult rhesus monkey models laparoscopically. They demonstrated excellent fusion in the animals that received rhBMP-2 versus the control animals.

Alden and colleagues[140] looked at the possibility of delivering the *BMP-2* gene via an adenovirus vector for a percutaneous spinal fusion. The adenovirus construct consisted of the CMV promoter and the *BMP-2* gene (Ad-BMP-2). They injected Ad-BMP-2 into the paraspinal muscle adjacent to the transverse process and demonstrated that an intertransverse process fusion occurred.

Besides rhBMP-2, other members of the BMP family may be used to induce fusion. Morone and coworkers[141] pointed out that although most of the in vitro and in vivo work has been performed with rhBMP-2, other BMPs, especially BMP-6, may actually be more important in the fusion process. In their study, looking at L4-5 posterolateral fusion in New Zealand rabbits, they divided the fusion mass into central and lateral zones of fusion and demonstrated that most nonunions occurred at the central zone. This central nonunion may be secondary to the fact that the central zone is compromised geographically. Eventually, the fusion process extends centrally, but in some cases, it is too late; the bone graft resorbs before fusion has occurred, and a nonunion results. BMP-6, not BMP-2, was found to be the important protein for central zone fusion, raising the question of whether rhBMP-6 should be the one studied. Another BMP family member, osteogenic protein-1 (OP-1; BMP-7), has also been demonstrated to be useful in initiating spinal fusion. Paramore and associates[142] demonstrated that OP-1 induced a strong fusion in 30 posterolateral fusions in dogs. In some of the animals, the dura was open, but OP-1 still induced an effective fusion. However, the authors found that bone growth can occur over exposed, decompressed dura, and it can form in the subdural and subarachnoid spaces, leading to spinal cord compression. Last, the cDNA for LIM mineralization protein (LMP-1) has been shown by Boden and colleagues[143] to be capable of being transfected into bone marrow cells. These cells were then placed into bone matrix and placed onto a single-level posterior lumbar and thoracic arthrodesis in athymic rats. Good fusion was obtained in all circumstances.

Gene Therapy

The use of gene therapy for lumbar disk disease may present a viable option in the near future. Wehling and coworkers[144] demonstrated that chondrocytic cells from bovine intervertebral end plates may be infected in vitro with retroviruses containing the bacterial β-galactosidase (*LacZ*) gene and the complementary DNA of the interleukin-1 receptor antagonist gene. However, the transduction rate was low (only about 1% of the transduced chondrocytes were β-galactosidase positive), secondary to the fact that retroviruses require actively dividing cells to transduce effectively. In an effort to improve transduction, Nishida and colleagues[145] used adenovirus vectors, which may transduce both replicating and nonreplicating cells. They demonstrated that cell cultures established from nucleus pulposus tissue can be infected with an adenovirus containing the *LacZ* gene (Ad-LacZ). Moreover, Ad-

LacZ can be injected directly into the disk space of rabbits in vivo, resulting in the efficient transduction of a considerable number of cells. Marker gene expression was seen in vivo at an apparently undiminished level for at least 12 weeks. Although Nishida's group did not demonstrate direct transfer of an adenovirus capable of secreting proteins (i.e., proteoglycans) necessary to prevent further disk degeneration, it did demonstrate transduction and expression of the β-galactosidase gene to the nucleus pulposus cells. More recently, Nishida and colleagues[146] demonstrated that the same adenovirus strategy can be used for transducing the nucleus pulposus of New Zealand white rabbits with the gene for human transforming growth factor-β1 (TGF-β1). TGF-β1 was chosen because it is known to stimulate the formation of extracellular matrix (i.e., proteoglycans). Injection of adenovirus TGF-β1 resulted in the nucleus pulposus tissues demonstrating a 30-fold increase in active TGF-β1 production and a 5-fold increase in total (active and latent) TGF-β1 production compared with control disks. More important, the increase in TGF-β1 expression was functionally significant, as these tissues exhibited a 100% increase in proteoglycan synthesis compared with control tissue. Recently, Helm and coworkers[147] showed that adenovirus containing BMP-13 can be injected into the thigh musculature of athymic rats, leading to the migration of progenitor cells between the transduced muscle fibers. These cells were able to proliferate, differentiate, and secrete large amounts of collagenous extracellular matrix. By 100 days after injection, the induced tissue had histologic and ultrastructural appearance of neotendon or ligament. These findings led to the proposal that the *BMP* gene may be an effective therapy for the healing of damaged spinal ligaments and the fibrocartilaginous nucleus pulposus. Using a similar approach, Riew and associates[148] demonstrated that good bony fusion can be induced by an adenovirus containing rhBMP-2.

Gene therapy is a powerful investigational tool for determining the importance of different factors in the induction of bony fusion. Elucidation of this mechanism will become more apparent with our increasing knowledge of its biology. Moreover, gene therapy as a therapeutic tool will become a real possibility in the future as our understanding of gene transduction and in vivo transfer improves.

REFERENCES

1. Quigley MR, Maroon JC: Intradiscal treatment of lumbar disc disease. In Youmans JR (ed): Neurological Surgery, 4th ed. Philadelphia, WB Saunders, 1996, pp 2382–2389.
2. MacNab I: Chemonucleolysis. Can J Surg 14:280, 1971.
3. Martin GJ, Boden SD, Titus L: Recombinant human bone morphogenetic protein-2 overcomes the inhibitory effect of ketorolac, a nonsteroidal anti-inflammatory drug (NSAID), on posterolateral lumbar intertransverse process spine fusion. Spine 24:2188–2196, 1999.
4. Thomas L: Reversible collapse of rabbit ears after intravenous papain. J Exp Med 104:245, 1956.
5. Hirsch C: Studies on the pathology of low back pain. J Bone J Surg Br 41:237–243, 1959.
6. Garvin P, Jennings RB, Smith L, Gessler RM: Chymopapain: A pharmacologic and toxicologic evaluation in experimental animals. Clin Orthop 41:204, 1965.
7. Smith L: Chemonucleolysis—personal history, trials, and tribulations. Clin Orthop 287:117–124, 1993.
8. Smith L: Enzyme dissolution of nucleous pulposus in humans. JAMA 1:97–137, 1964.
9. Brown MD: Intradiscal Therapy: Chymopapain or Collagenase. Chicago, Yearbook Medical Publishers, 1983, p 173.
10. Brown MD: Update on chemonucleolysis. Spine 21:62S–68S, 1996.
11. Schwetschenau PR, Ramirez A, Johnston J, et al: Double-blind evaluations of intradiscal chymopapain for herniated lumbar disc: Early results. J Neurosurg 45:622–628, 1976.
12. Fraser RD: Chymopapain for the treatment of intervertebral disc herniations: The final report of a double-blind study. Spine 9:815–818, 1984.
13. Apostolides PJ, Jacobwitz R, Sonntag VK: Lumbar discectomy microdiscectomy: The gold standard. Clin Neurosurg 43:228–237, 1996.
14. Ebni BL, Benzel EC: Lumbar discectomy. pp 389–399.
15. Javid MJ: Efficacy of chymopapain chemonucleolysis: A long-term review of 105 patients. J Neurosurg 62:662–666, 1985.
16. Cole H: Diagnostic and therapeutic technology assessment (DATTA). JAMA 262:953–956, 1989.
17. Wapner KL, Vaccaro AR, Albert TJ, et al: The results of chemonucleolysis as a function of three dimensional volumetric analysis of disc herniations. J Spinal Disord 6:324–332, 1993.
18. Diaz JH, Connolly ES: Anesthetic management of chemonucleolysis with chymopapain. South Med J 79:1554–1561, 1986.
19. Nachemson A, Zdeblick TA, O'Brien JP: Lumbar disc disease with discogenic pain—what surgical treatment is most effective? Spine 21:1835–1838, 1996.
20. McCulloch JA: Chemonucleolysis: Experience with 2000 cases. Clin Orthop 146:128–135, 1980.
21. Grammer LC, Schafer M, Bernstein D, et al: Prevention of chymopapain anaphylaxis by screening chemonucleolysis candidates with cutaneous chymopapain testing. Clin Orthop 234:12–15, 1988.
22. Kitchel SH, Brown MD: Complications of chemonucleolysis [review]. Clin Orthop 284:63–74, 1992.
23. Occelli G, Rauccoules M, Philip F, et al: [Changes in plasma histamine and catecholamine levels after injection of chymopapain in chemonucleolysis] [review]. Ann Fr Anesth Reanim 10:516–521, 1991.
24. Agre K, Wilson RR, Brim M, McDermott DJ: Chymodiactin post-marketing surveillance. Spine 9:479–485, 1984.
25. Agre K: Serious neurological adverse events associated with administration of Chymodiactin. In Brown JE (ed): Chemonucleolysis. Thorofare, NJ, Slack, 1985, pp 203–215.
26. Benoist M, Bonneville JF, Lassale B, et al: [Foraminal and neuroforaminal hernia: Mid-term results of percutaneous techniques nucleolysis-nucleotomy.] Neurochirurgie 39:110–115, 1993.
27. Abdel-Salam A, Eyres KS, Cleary J: A new paradiscal injection technique for the relief of back spasm after chemonucleolysis. Br J Rheumatol 31:491–493, 1992.
28. Nordby EJ, Wright PH: Efficacy of chymopapain in chemonucleolysis. Spine 19:2578–2583, 1994.
29. Gogan WJ, Fraser RD: Chymopapain: A 10-year, double-blind study. Spine 17:388–394, 1992.
30. Nordby EJ, Wright PH, Schofield SR: Safety of chemonucleolysis: Adverse effects reported in the USA 1982 to 1989. Clin Orthop 293:122–134, 1993.
31. Bouillet R: Treatment of sciatica: A comparative survey of complications of surgical treatment and nucleolysis with chymopapain. Clin Orthop 251:144–152, 1990.
32. Weber H: Spine update—the natural history of disc herniation and the influence of intervention. Spine 19:2234–2238, 1994.
33. Hijikata S: Percutaneous nucleotomy: A new concept. Technique and 12 years' experience. Clin Orthop 238:9–23, 1989.
34. Kambin P, Schaffer JL: Percutaneous lumbar discectomy: Review of 100 patients and current practice. Clin Orthop 238:24–34, 1989.
35. Hoppenfeld S: Percutaneous removal of herniated lumbar discs:

50 cases with ten-year follow-up periods. Clin Orthop 238: 92–97, 1989.

36. Friedman WA: Percutaneous discectomy: An alternative to chemonucleolysis? Neurosurgery 13:542–547, 1983.

37. Schreiber A, Suezawa MD, Leu H: Does percutaneous nucleotomy with discoscopy replace conventional discectomy? Eight years of experience and results in treatment of herniated lumbar disc. Clin Orthop 238:35, 1989.

38. Gobin P: Percutaneous automated lumbar nucleotomy. J Radiol 71:401, 1990.

39. Onik G, Helms CA, Ginsburg L, et al: Percutaneous lumbar discectomy using a new aspiration probe. AJR Am J Roentgenol 144:1137–1140, 1985.

40. Smith MM, Watson JC, Maroon JC: Percutaneous approaches to lumbar discectomy. pp 401–407.

41. Onik G, Maroon JC, Davis GW: Automated percutaneous discectomy at the L5-S1 level: Use of a curved cannula. Clin Orthop 238:71–76, 1988.

42. Teng GJ, Jeffrey RF, Guo JH, et al: Automated percutaneous lumbar discectomy: A prospective multi-institutional study. J Vasc Interv Radiol 8:457–463, 1997.

43. Mayer HM: Spine update: Percutaneous lumbar disc surgery. Spine 23:2719–2723, 1994.

44. Onik GM: Automated percutaneous lumbar discectomy. In White AH, Schofferman JA (eds): Spine Care. St Louis, Mosby, 1995, pp 1018–1027.

45. Revel M, Payan C, Vallee C, et al: Automated percutaneous lumbar discectomy versus chemonucleolysis in the treatment of sciatica, a randomized multicenter trial. Spine 18:1–7, 1992.

46. Gunzburg R, Fraser RD, Moore R, Vernon-Roberts B: An experimental study comparing percutaneous discectomy with chemonucleolysis. Spine 18:218–226, 1993.

47. Davis GW, Onik GM, Helms CA: Automated percutaneous discectomy. Spine 16:359–367, 1991.

48. Onik GM, Helms C: Nuances in percutaneous discectomy. Radiol Clin North Am 36:523–533, 1998.

49. Maroon JC, Quigley MR, Gleason PL: Is there a future for percutaneous intradiscal therapy? Clin Neurosurg 239–251, 1990.

50. Luft C: Automated percutaneous lumbar discectomy (APLD)—method and 1-year follow-up. Eur Radiol 2:292, 1992.

51. Wilson LF, Mulholland RC: Automated percutaneous discectomy versus surgery: A prospective randomized study of treatment for lumbar disc protrusion. Paper presented at the Third Annual Meeting of the European Spine Society, Sept 3, 1992, Cambridge.

52. Freis J, Abodely D, Vijungo J, et al: Computed tomography of herniated and extruded nucleus pulposus. J Comput Assist Tomogr 6:874, 1982.

53. Castro WH, Jerosch J, Hepp R, Schulitz KP: Restriction of indication for automated percutaneous lumbar discectomy based on computed tomographic discography. Spine 17:1239, 1992.

54. Vanneroy F: A new deal with far lateral lumbar disk herniations (FLHD): Automated percutaneous discectomy. Eur Radiol 1(Suppl):S163–S167, 1992.

55. Kahanovitz N: Percutaneous discectomy. Clin Orthop 284:75–82, 1992.

56. Onik G, Richardson D, Amaral J, et al: Percutaneous anterior discectomy under ultrasound guidance. Minim Invasive Neurosurg 38:90–95, 1995.

57. Schenk JF, Jolesz FA, Roemer PB, et al: Superconducting open-configuration MR imaging system for image-guided therapy. Radiology 195:805–814, 1995.

58. Davis GW, Onik G: Clinical experience with automated percutaneous lumbar discectomy. Clin Orthop 238:98–103, 1989.

59. Onik GM, Helms CA: Automated percutaneous lumbar discectomy. AJR Am J Roentgenol 156:531–540, 1991.

60. Bonaldi G, Belloni G, Prosetti D, Moschini L: Percutaneous discectomy using Onik's methods: Three years' experience. Neuroradiology 33:516–521, 1991.

61. Bocchi L, Ferrata P, Passarello F: The Onik method of automated percutaneous lumbar discectomy (APLD): Criteria of selection, technique, and evaluation of results. Ital J Orthop Traumatol 17: 5–14, 1991.

62. Schweigel J: Automated percutaneous discectomy: Comparison with chymopapain. In Automated Percutaneous Discectomy. San Francisco, Radiology Research and Education Foundation, 1988.

63. Ulrich HW: Automated percutaneous discectomy: Indication, technique, and results after 2 years. Z Orthop 130:45, 1992.

64. Gill K, Blumenthal SL: Clinical experience with automated percutaneous discectomy: The nucleotome system. Orthopedics 14: 757–762, 1991.

65. Phelip X, Troussier B, Chirossel JP: La nucleotomie percutanee automatisee dans le traitement des hernies discales lombaires. Presse Med 21:1604–1613, 1992.

66. Stern MB: Early experience with percutaneous lateral discectomy. Clin Orthop Jan:233:50–55.

67. Quigley MR, Maroon JC: Laser discectomy: A review. Spine 19: 53–56, 1994.

68. Gropper GR, Robertson JH, McClellan G: Comparative histologic and radiographic effects of CO_2 laser versus surgical anterior cervical discectomy in the dog. Neurosurgery 14:42–47, 1984.

69. Choy DSJ, Case RB, Ascher PW: Percutaneous laser ablation of the lumbar disc. Annu Meet Orthop Res Soc 1:19, 1987.

70. Oegema RT: Biochemistry of the intervertebral disc. Clin Sports Med 12:419–424, 1993.

71. Lane GT, et al: An experimental comparison of CO_2, argon, Nd: YAG, and Ho:YAG laser ablation of intervertebral discs. Spine State Art Rev 7:1–7, 1993.

72. Cummings RS: Laser ablation of intervertebral discs using the Nd:YAG 1.44 μm laser. Spine State Art Rev 7:37, 1993.

73. Mayer HM, Brock M, Stern E, Muller G: Percutaneous endoscopic laser discectomy: Experimental results. In Mayer HM, Brock M (eds): Percutaneous Lumbar Discectomy, 1st ed. Heidelberg, Germany, Springer Verlag, 1989, pp 187–196.

74. Choy DSJ, Altman PA, Case RB, et al: Interaction of laser radiation with human intervertebral discs at wavelengths of 193 nm, 488 nm, 514 nm, 1064 nm, 1318 nm, 2150 nm, 2940 nm, 10600 nm. Clin Orthop 267:245–250, 1990.

75. Yunezawa T, Tanaku S, Watanabe H, et al: Percutaneous intradiscal laser discectomy. In Mayer HM, Brock M (eds): Percutaneous Lumbar Discectomy, 1st ed. Heidelberg, Germany, Springer Verlag, 1989, pp 197–204.

76. Choy DSJ, Case R, Fielding W: Percutaneous laser ablation of lumbar discs: A preliminary report of in vitro and in vivo experience in animals and four human patients [abstract 323]. Paper presented at the 33rd Annual Meeting of the Orthopaedic Research Society, Jan 1987, San Francisco.

77. Yunezawa T, Ononmura J, Kosaky R, et al: System and procedure of percutaneous intradiscal laser nucleotomy. Spine 15: 1175–1185, 1990.

78. Choy DSJ, Altman PA: Fall of intradiscal pressure with laser ablation. Spine State Art Rev 7:11–16, 1993.

79. Prodoehl JA, et al: The effects of lasers on intervertebral disc pressures. Spine State Art Rev 7:17–21, 1993.

80. Hellinger J: Technical aspects of the percutaneous cervical and lumbar laser disc decompression and nucleotomy. Neurol Res 21:99–102,1999.

81. Liebler WA: Percutaneous laser disc nucleotomy. Clin Orthop 310:58–66, 1995.

82. Quigley MR, Shih T, Elrifai A, et al: Percutaneous laser discectomy with the Ho:YAG laser. Laser Surg Med 12:621–624, 1992.

83. Choy DSJ, et al: Percutaneous laser decompression: A new therapeutic modality. Spine 17:949–956, 1992.

84. Sherk HH: Results of percutaneous laser discectomy with lasers. Spine State Art Rev 7:141, 1993.

85. Yeung AT: Considerations for use of the KTP laser for disc decompression and ablation. Spine State Art Rev 7:67–70, 1993.

86. Bosacco SJ, Bosacco DN, Berman AT, et al: Am J Orthop 25: 825–828, 1996.

87. Rhodes A: Clinical use of the 2.1 micron holmium:YAG laser and percutaneous discectomy. Spine State Art Rev 7:49–54, 1993.

88. Guyer RD, Kambin P: Arthroscopic microdiscectomy: Posterolateral approach. Surg Tech 257–273.

89. Kambin P, Zhou L: History and current status of percutaneous arthroscopic disc surgery. Spine 21:57S–61S, 1996.

90. Ditsworth DA: Endoscopic transforaminal lumbar discectomy

and reconfiguration: A posterior lateral approach into the spinal canal. Surg Neurol 49:588–598, 1998.

91. Foley KT, Smith MM: Microendoscopic discectomy. Tech Neurosurg 3:301–307, 1997.

92. Foley KT, Smith MM, Rampersaud YR: Microendoscopic approach to far-lateral lumbar disc herniation. Neurosurg Focus 7, 1999.

93. Kleinpeter G, Markowitsch MM, Böck F: Percutaneous endoscopic lumbar discectomy: Minimally invasive, but perhaps only minimally useful? Surg Neurol 43:534–541, 1995.

94. Roh SW, Kim DH, Cardoso AC, Fessler RG: Endoscopic foraminotomy using a microendoscopic discectomy system in cadaveric specimens. Neurosurg Focus 4, 1998.

95. Savitz MH: Same-day microsurgical arthroscopic lateral-approach laser-assisted (SMALL) fluoroscopic discectomy. J Neurosurg 80:1039–1045, 1994.

96. Ondra SL, Smith MM: Lumbar foramenoscopic microdiscectomy. Tech Neurosurg 3:280–288, 1997.

97. Perin NI: Endoscopic lumbar microdiscectomy for far-lateral discs. Tech Neurosurg 3:275–279, 1997.

98. Kambin P, O'Brien E, Zhou L, Schaffer JL: Arthroscopic microdiscectomy and selective fragmentectomy. Clin Orthop 347:150–167, 1998.

99. Heary RF, Benzel EC, Vaicys C: Anterior lumbar interbody. pp 333–346.

100. Penta M, Frasier RD: Anterior lumbar interbody fusion. Spine 22:2429–2434, 1997.

101. Bagby GW: Arthrodesis by the distraction-compression method using a stainless steel implant. Orthopedics 11:931–934, 1988.

102. Ray CD: Threaded fusion cages for lumbar interbody fusions. Spine 22:681–685, 1997.

103. Detwiler PW, Porter RW, Sonntag VKH, Dickman CA: Laparoscopic anterior lumbar interbody fusion. Contemp Spine Surg 1:35–39.

104. Heini PF, Krahenbuhl L, Schwarazenbach O, Lottenbach M: Laparoscopic assisted spine surgery. Dig Surg 15:185–186, 1998.

105. Katkhouda N, Campos G, Mavor E, et al: Is laparoscopic approach to lumbar spine fusion worthwhile? Am J Surg 178:458–461, 1999.

106. Regan JJ, Aronoff RJ, Ohnmeiss DD, Sengupta DK: Laparoscopic approach to L4-L5 for interbody fusion using BAK cages: Experience in the first 58 cases. Spine 24:2171–2175, 1999.

107. Regan JJ, Yuan H, McAfee PC: Laproscopic fusion of the lumbar spine: Minimally invasive spine surgery. Spine 24:402–411, 1999.

108. Sandhu HS, Turner S, Kabo JM, et al: Distractive properties of a threaded interbody fusion device. Spine 21:1201–1210, 1996.

109. Riley LH, Eck JC, Hiroyu Y, et al: Laparoscopic assisted fusion of the lumbosacral spine. Spine 22:1407–1412, 1997.

110. Zucherman JF, Zdeblck TA, Bailey SA, et al: Instrumented laparoscopic spinal fusion. Spine 20:2029–2035, 1995.

111. Mahvi DM, Zdeblick TA: A prospective study of laparoscopic spinal fusion. Ann Surg 224:85–90, 1996.

112. Harkey HL, McGuire RA, Poole GV: Laparoscopic anterior interbody fusion of the lumbar spine. Tech Neurosurg 3:330–335, 1997.

113. Martin RJ, Yuan HA: Laparascopic anterior interbody fusion of the lumbar spine. Tech Neurosurg 3:322–329, 1997.

114. Martin GJ, Boden SD, Morone MA, Moskovitz PA: Posterolateral intertransverse process spinal arthrodesis with BMP-2 in a nonhuman primate: Important lessons learned regarding dose, carrier, and safety. J Spinal Disord 12:179–186, 1999.

115. Pineda S, Bauerle W, Goldstein J, et al: Laparoscopic lumbar spinal fusion using the BAK interbody fusion device. Tech Neurosurg 4:246–255, 1998.

116. Onimus M, Papin P, Gangioff S: Extraperitoneal approach to the lumbar spine with video assistance. Spine 21:2491–2494, 1996.

117. Rosenthal D, Paolucci V, Yahya H, et al: Microsurgical endoscopic-assisted retroperitoneal approaches to the thoraco-lumbar and lumbar spine. Tech Neurosurg 3:315–321, 1997.

118. Palmgren T, Grönblad M, Virri J, et al: An immunohistochemical study of nerve structures in the anulus fibrosus of human normal lumbar intervertebral discs. Spine 24:2075–2079, 1999.

119. Habtemariam A, Gronblad M, Virri J, et al: Immunocytochemical localization of immunoglobulins in disc herniations. Spine 21:1864–1869, 1996.

120. Olmarker K, Larsson K: Tumor necrosis factor α and nucleus-pulposus-induced nerve root injury. Spine 23:2538–2544, 1998.

121. Özaktay AC, Kallakuri S, Cavanaugh JM: Phospholipase A$_2$ sensitivity of the dorsal root and dorsal root ganglion. Spine 23:1297–1306, 1996.

122. Saal JS, Saal JA: A novel approach to painful internal disc derangement: Collagen modulation with a thermal percutaneous navigable intradiscal catheter: A prospective trial. Paper presented at the 13th Annual Meeting of the North American Spine Society, Oct 28–31, 1998, San Francisco.

123. Troussier B, Lebas JF, Chirossell JP, et al: Percutaneous intradiscal radio-frequency thermocoagulation. Spine 20:1713–1718, 1995.

124. Saal JA, Saal JS: Intradiscal electrothermal annuloplasty (IDET) treatment for chronic multi-level discogenic pain: Prospective one year follow up outcome study. Paper presented at the 14th Annual Meeting of the North American Spine Society, Oct 20–23, 1999, Chicago.

125. Karasek M, Karasek D, Bogduk NA: A controlled trial of the efficacy of intradiscal electrothermal treatment for internal disc disruption. Paper presented at the 14th Annual Meeting of the North American Spine Society, Oct 20–23, 1999, Chicago.

126. Chen TC: Recombinant human morphogenetic protein: Its future role in spinal fusions. Neurosurg Focus 4, article 11, 1998.

127. Urist MR, Huo YR, Brownell AG, et al: Purification of bovine bone morphogenetic protein by hydroxyapatite chromatography. Proc Natl Acad Sci U S A 81:371–375, 1984.

128. Wang EA, Rosen V, D'Alessandro JS, et al: Recombinant human bone morphogenetic protein induces bone formation. Proc Natl Acad Sci U S A 87:2220–2224, 1990.

129. Boden SD, Zdeblick TA, Sandhu HS, Heim SE: The use of rhBMP-2 interbody fusion cages. Spine 25:376–381, 2000.

130. Helm GA, Sheehan JM, Sheehan J, et al: Utilization of type I collagen gel, demineralized bone matrix, and bone morphogenetic protein-2 to enhance autologous bone lumbar spinal fusion. J Neurosurg 86:93–100, 1997.

131. David SM, Gruber HE, Meyer RA, et al: Lumbar spinal fusion using recombinant human bone morphogenetic protein in the canine: A comparison of three dosages and two carriers. Spine 24:1973–1979, 1999.

132. Boden SD, Martin GJ, Morone MA, et al: Posterolateral lumbar intertransverse process spine arthrodesis with recombinant human bone morphogenetic protein 2/hydroxyapatite-tricalcium phosphate after laminectomy in the nonhuman primate. Spine 24:1179–1185, 1999.

133. Minamide A, Tamaki T, Kawakakami M, et al: Experimental spinal fusion using sintered bovine bone coated with type I collagen and recombinant human bone morphogenetic protein-2. Spine 24:1863–1872, 1999.

134. Itoh H, Ebara S, Kamimura M, et al: Experimental spinal fusion with use of recombinant human bone morphogenetic protein 2. Spine 24:1402–1405, 1999.

135. Meyer RA, Gruber HE, Howard BA, et al: Safety of recombinant human bone morphogenetic protein-2 after spinal laminectomy in the dog. Spine 24:747–754, 1999.

136. Sandhu H, Kanim L, Toth J, et al: Experimental spinal fusion with recombinant human bone morphogenetic protein-2 without decortication of osseous elements. Spine 22:1171–1180, 1997.

137. Boden S, Moskovitz P, Morone M, Toribitake Y: Video-assisted lateral intertransverse process arthrodesis. Spine 21:2689–2697, 1996.

138. Hecht BP, Fischgrund JS, Herkowitz HN, et al: The use of recombinant human bone morphogenetic protein 2 (rhBMP-2) to promote spinal fusion in a nonhuman primate anterior interbody fusion model. Spine 24:629–636, 1999.

139. Boden S, Martin GJ, Horton W, et al: Laparoscopic anterior spinal arthrodesis with rhBMP-2 in a titanium interbody threaded cage. J Spinal Disord 11:95–101, 1998.

140. Alden TD, Pittman DD, Beres EJ, et al: Percutaneous spinal fusion using bone morphogentic protein-2 gene therapy. J Neurosurg (Spine 1) 90:109–114, 1999.

141. Morone M, Boden S, Hair G, et al: Gene expression during autograft lumbar spine fusion and the effect of bone morphogenetic protein 2. Clin Orthop 351:252–265, 1998.

142. Paramore C, Lauryssen C, Rauzzino J, et al: The safety of OP-1

for lumbar fusion with decompression—a canine study. Neurosurgery 44:1151–1156, 1999.

143. Boden S, Titus L, Hair G, et al: Lumbar spine fusion by local gene therapy with a cDNA encoding a novel osteoinductive protein (LMP-1). Spine 23:2486–2492, 1998.

144. Wehling P, Schulitz KP, Robbins PD, et al: Transfer of genes to chondrocytic cells of the lumbar spine. Spine 22:1090–1097, 1997.

145. Nishida K, Kang JD, Suh JK, et al: Adenovirus-mediated gene transfer to nucleus pulposus cells. Spine 23:2437–2443, 1998.

146. Nishida K, Kang JD, Gilbertson LG, et al: Modulation of the biologic activity of the rabbit intervertebral disc by gene ther-

apy: An in vivo study of adenovirus-mediated transfer of the human transforming growth factor B1 encoding gene. Spine 24:2419–2427, 1999.

147. Helm G, Zhong J, Alden T, et al: A light and electron microscopic study of ectopic tendon and ligament formation induced by bone morphogenetic protein-13 adenoviral gene therapy. Neurosurg Focus 8, article 6, 2000.

148. Riew KD, Wright NM, Cheng S-L, et al: Induction of bone formation using a recombinant adenoviral vector carrying the human BMP-2 gene in a rabbit spinal fusion model. Calcif Tissue Int 63:357–360, 1998.

CHAPTER **311**

Tumors of the Craniovertebral Junction

ARNOLD H. MENEZES ■ VINCENT C. TRAYNELIS ■ JASON HETH

The craniovertebral junction is a biomechanical and anatomic unit that comprises the clivus, foramen magnum, and upper two cervical vertebrae. The neoplasms that arise within the structures are osseous or extensions from the soft tissues that surround the craniovertebral junction, or they are neoplasms that arise from the neural structures contained within the bony anatomy.[1, 2] The diagnosis of such lesions has been greatly facilitated by modern neurodiagnostic imaging.

There is no single symptom or neurological finding that is pathognomonic for a lesion in this location.[3, 4] Because of the generous size of the subarachnoid spaces at the cervicomedullary junction, symptoms arise only after a lesion has achieved large proportions. These patients have a fluctuating neurological course, and an erroneous diagnosis is common owing to the anatomic complexities of the decussation of the sensory and motor tracts.

The first systematic evaluation of foramen magnum tumors was performed by Elsberg and Strauss.[5] Several authors have since reported extra-axial lesions affecting the region, such as meningiomas and neurinomas. Osseous neoplastic involvement of the craniovertebral junction may be due to chordoma, chondrosarcoma, plasmacytoma, osteoblastoma, fibrous dysplasia, metastatic tumor, and giant cell tumor. Table 311–1 summarizes the senior author's (AHM) experience.

COMMON CLINICAL MANIFESTATIONS OF CRANIOVERTEBRAL JUNCTION TUMORS

Tumors of the craniovertebral junction, whether extracranial with secondary involvement of the intracranial and intraspinal structures or primarily intracranial with secondary extension into the spinal canal, have characteristics that reflect compression of neighboring structures or traction. They also may have distal effects such as hydrocephalus, syringohydromyelia, and vas-cular compromise.[6–10] Chordoma often involves the cranial base and upper cervical spine extensively and may be associated with only minimal complaints of headache and neck pain for several years. Unfortunately, this hiatus is followed by a rapid progression of brainstem and cervical spinal cord dysfunction that brings the lesion to light. In the report of Meyer and coworkers, the time from the onset of symptoms to the diagnosis of extramedullary tumor at the foramen magnum was 2.5 years.[2]

The clinical presentation of craniovertebral junction tumors can be divided into intracranial lesions, "straddle lesions," and those affecting the high cervical spinal cord.[5] The effects of vascular compromise and alterations of cerebrospinal fluid (CSF) circulation add to the constellation of symptoms and signs.

Patients with intracranial lesions present with involvement of the lower cranial nerves, brainstem dysfunction, and occasionally cerebellar symptoms. Patients with straddle lesions have a paucity of cranial nerve dysfunction and a predominance of high cervical myelopathy. High cervical lesions do not produce cranial nerve and cerebellar signs, except for involvement of the spinal accessory nerves and sometimes the descending tracts of the trigeminal nerve and the lower decussations of the motor and sensory tracts.

The most common presentation is pain referred to the second cervical dermatome.[1] The head is held flexed, and the condition may resemble torticollis. The pain is described as an aching sensation that is aggravated by neck and head motion and referred to the suboccipital region. Unfortunately, the symptom of pain alone may predate other clinical findings for many years. Paresthesias or dysesthesias of the face, hands, and limbs are frequently reported. An abnormal cold sensation of the lower extremities was described by Elsberg and Strauss[5] and by Beatty[8] as being pathognomonic of lesions of the high cervical cord. Most frequently, pain and temperature sensation is affected, followed by loss of joint sensation. This finding is

T A B L E 3 1 1 – 1 ■ **Disease at the Craniovertebral Junction Requiring Surgical Treatment**

LOCATION	CONGENITAL	ACQUIRED	PRIMARY NEOPLASTIC	SECONDARY NEOPLASTIC	EXTRA–INTRADURAL
Clivus	Pro-atlas segmentation failure Neurenteric cyst	Basilar invagination Basilar impression Rickets Paget's disease Osteogenesis imperfecta	Eosinophilic granuloma Fibrous dysplasia Chordoma Chondroma Chondrosarcoma Plasmacytoma	Metastasis Nasopharyngeal malignancy Ectopic pituitary tumor Craniopharyngioma	Meningioma Neurofibroma Chordoma Glomus tumor Rhabdomyosarcoma
Atlas	Assimilation with segmentation failure	Stenosis in achondroplasia Morquio's syndrome Chronic dislocation	Chordoma Chondroma Osteoblastoma Giant cell tumor Osteoid osteoma	Metastasis Plasmacytoma Extension of local malignancy	Neurofibroma Meningioma
Axis	Dystopic os Axis segmentation failure Neurenteric cyst	Basilar invagination Basilar impression (e.g., osteogenesis, Paget's disease, acro-osteolysis, skeletal dysplasia, rheumatoid arthritis, psoriasis, ileitis) Chronic dislocation Osteomyelitis	Chordoma Plasmacytoma Osteoblastoma Giant cell tumor	Metastasis Extension of local malignancy	Meningioma Neurofibroma

seen in the upper extremities and may then proceed clockwise around the limbs. A suspended sensory loss with patches of preservation of sensation in the upper extremities may confuse the presentation. "Dissociated" sensory loss has been described in about one fourth of extracranial lesions of the cervicomedullary junction, even though this finding has been considered to reflect an intramedullary process.[2]

Spastic weakness of the extremities is a prominent feature in patients with tumors in this region. The weakness may begin in the ipsilateral limb and progress to the lower limb of the same side, followed by weakness of the contralateral lower limb; finally, weakness becomes apparent in the contralateral upper limb. This distinct progression of motor symptoms is an important characteristic of lesions of the cervicomedullary junction.[9] Localized wasting of the intrinsic muscles of the hand may develop ipsilateral to the lesion. Taylor and Byrnes postulate venous stagnation of the anterior horn cells and the lower cervical cord as a result of decreased venous drainage, which typically occurs rostral to the lower portion of the cervical spinal cord.[11] Other proposed mechanisms include anterior spinal artery compression, hydromyelia secondary to CSF obstruction, venous obstruction with spinal cord edema, and spinal cord rotation with contralateral traction.

A tumor at the foramen magnum may produce a mixture of upper motor neuron findings in the upper and lower extremities. This pattern reflects the pyramidal decussation that begins just below the obex and ends near the uppermost cervical spinal cord. The more medial fibers of the pyramidal tract carry impulses to the upper extremities and cross superior to the lateral fibers that serve the lower extremities. Similarly, the

sensory decussation of the medial lemniscus may produce a varied pattern of sensory abnormalities.[12] Thus, a tumor situated at the ventral aspect of the cervicomedullary junction can cause sensory aberrations in the lower extremities first. The syndrome of cruciate paralysis has been associated with trauma as well as with tumors with basilar invagination.[13]

Transient symptoms may be due to both vascular changes and instability at the craniovertebral junction. Such symptoms can manifest as paralysis, paresthesias, drop attacks, and vertebrobasilar syndromes such as migraine and visual loss in the homonymous visual fields. Cranial nerve palsies may be the result of nuclear involvement in the brainstem, traction, compression of the subarachnoid segments, or interosseous disease.[1] The most common cranial nerves affected are the vagus, glossopharyngeal, and hypoglossal. Their involvement leads to dysphagia, slurred speech, and repeated episodes of aspiration into the tracheobronchial tree, resulting in pneumonia and weight loss. Tumors of the upper cervical canal can present with involvement of the spinal root of the accessory nerve, manifesting as torticollis and weakness of the trapezius and sternocleidomastoid muscles. About 15% to 20% of patients develop tinnitus, vertigo, and hearing loss related to involvement of the vestibulocochlear nerve.[9]

The differential diagnoses considered most often by Meyer and coworkers in their initial evaluation of 102 documented cases of benign extramedullary tumors of the foramen magnum included cervical spondylosis (25%), multiple sclerosis (18%), syringomyelia (17%), intramedullary tumor (15%), Chiari malformation (5.5%), and carpal tunnel syndrome (5.5%).[2] Other erroneous diagnoses in patients with lesions at the craniovertebral junction are intramedullary tumors of the brainstem and upper cervical cord, amyotrophic lateral sclerosis, and subacute combined degeneration. Cervical spondylosis may be difficult to differentiate when it coexists. The presentation of restless legs syndrome in patients with craniovertebral compressive pathology has been well documented by Glasauer and Egnatchick.[14]

NEURODIAGNOSTIC IMAGING

The complex anatomy and pathology of tumors in this region demand precise definition and depiction of the tumor's extent and its relationship to the vital structures of the brainstem and spinal cord, lower cranial nerves, and vascular structures. Thus, complementary multimodality imaging includes plain radiography, magnetic resonance imaging (MRI), magnetic resonance angiography, computed tomography (CT), and three-dimensional CT-angiography. The sensitivity of MRI is greatly enhanced by the addition of intravenous gadolinium and by performing separate magnetic resonance venography and angiography.

Cerebral angiography is useful in understanding the dynamics of collateral circulation and tumor vascularity. Temporary balloon occlusion is a means of assessing a patient's tolerance of vascular occlusion of the carotid or vertebral circulation before surgery.[9, 15] Such information is especially useful when lesions are encased by tumor. These two tests provide information about the resectability of difficult lesions.

ELECTROPHYSIOLOGIC TESTS

Intraoperatively, we monitor somatosensory brainstem evoked potentials and perform facial electromyography when lesions extend to the cerebellopontine angle and when using the preauricular infratemporal fossa approach.[16–19] The intraoperative evaluation of cranial nerve IX and cranial nerve X function is accomplished by placing electrodes in the soft palate and against the true vocal cords, incorporating these latter electrodes in the endotracheal tube for the anesthetic. Hypoglossal nerve electromyography supplements the evaluation with an electrode placed directly into the tongue. Brainstem monitoring still yields a significant number of false negatives and false positives, but improved techniques make these adjuncts useful in the intraoperative assessment of the function of the cervicomedullary junction.

SURGICAL APPROACHES AND DECISION MAKING

The goal of treating benign osseous pathology differs from that of treating malignant disease, where complete excision is the objective. Benign lesions create a space among the neurovascular structures, thereby allowing surgical debulking and resection "from within." Malignant disease, however, requires a much more radical resection with clean margins. In most instances, benign lesions such as chordomas are radioresistant; hence, gross total resection should be the aim. Craniovertebral stability, both before and after operative intervention, must be considered in the development of approaches.[17, 20] Thus, the factors that influence the specific treatment of tumors arising in this region are (1) mechanism of compression and direction of encroachment, (2) whether the lesion is benign or malignant, (3) whether the lesion has an associated vascular or intramedullary component (e.g., syringomyelia), (4) craniospinal stability, and (5) patient age.

Lesions of the craniovertebral junction do affect the pediatric population, although to a lesser extent than they affect adults.[21–25] In children, the potential for growth, concerns about stability, and the patient's size are critical. From this perspective, midface growth centers are the nasal septum and the pterygoid plates. Hence, in a child, a transpalatal approach to the clivus and the sella would be considered before a sublabial transsphenoidal or a maxillary drop-down procedure, with the goal of avoiding damage to the growth centers.[26]

Advances in neurodiagnostic imaging and microsurgical instrumentation have allowed the development of extensive surgical approaches based on an understanding of the complex anatomy, craniovertebral dynamics, and site of encroachment. Consequently, the entire circumference of the foramen magnum is within the neurosurgeon's reach (Fig. 311–1) . However, several surgical limitations and considerations must be appreciated when designing an approach to the craniovertebral junction (Table 311–2). The most frequently used anterior route is the transoral-transpalatopharyngeal approach.[9, 27–29] Laterally, this approach is limited by the pterygoid plates, the hypoglossal canal, the eustachian tubes, and the width between the vertebral arteries. The limitation imposed by the pterygoid plates can be overcome by using a transmaxillary route with down-fracture of the maxilla and an extended maxillotomy if needed.[1, 30] A combined exposure with mandibulotomy and midline glossotomy lowers the midline exposure to C5.[9, 31–34] The disadvantages of the ventral approaches are overshadowed by their easy access, ability to cross the midline, and vertical extensions. The ventral and dorsal midline approaches permit the anterior and posterior 90 degrees of the craniovertebral junction to be scanned, respectively.

As a general rule, midline extra-axial tumors are best approached in an extra-axial fashion without retracting the brain or violating the dura. A lateral avenue should be used for tumors that are situated laterally. The transsphenoidal-transsphenoethmoidal approach provides a shallow operative depth and is well tolerated as a route to the upper two thirds of the clivus.[28, 35, 36] This exposure provides better access to the contralateral side; hence, at times, a bilateral approach may be necessary. The transfacial routes provide wide access to the anterior and midline skull base and include the ventral aspect of the clivus.[37, 38] This

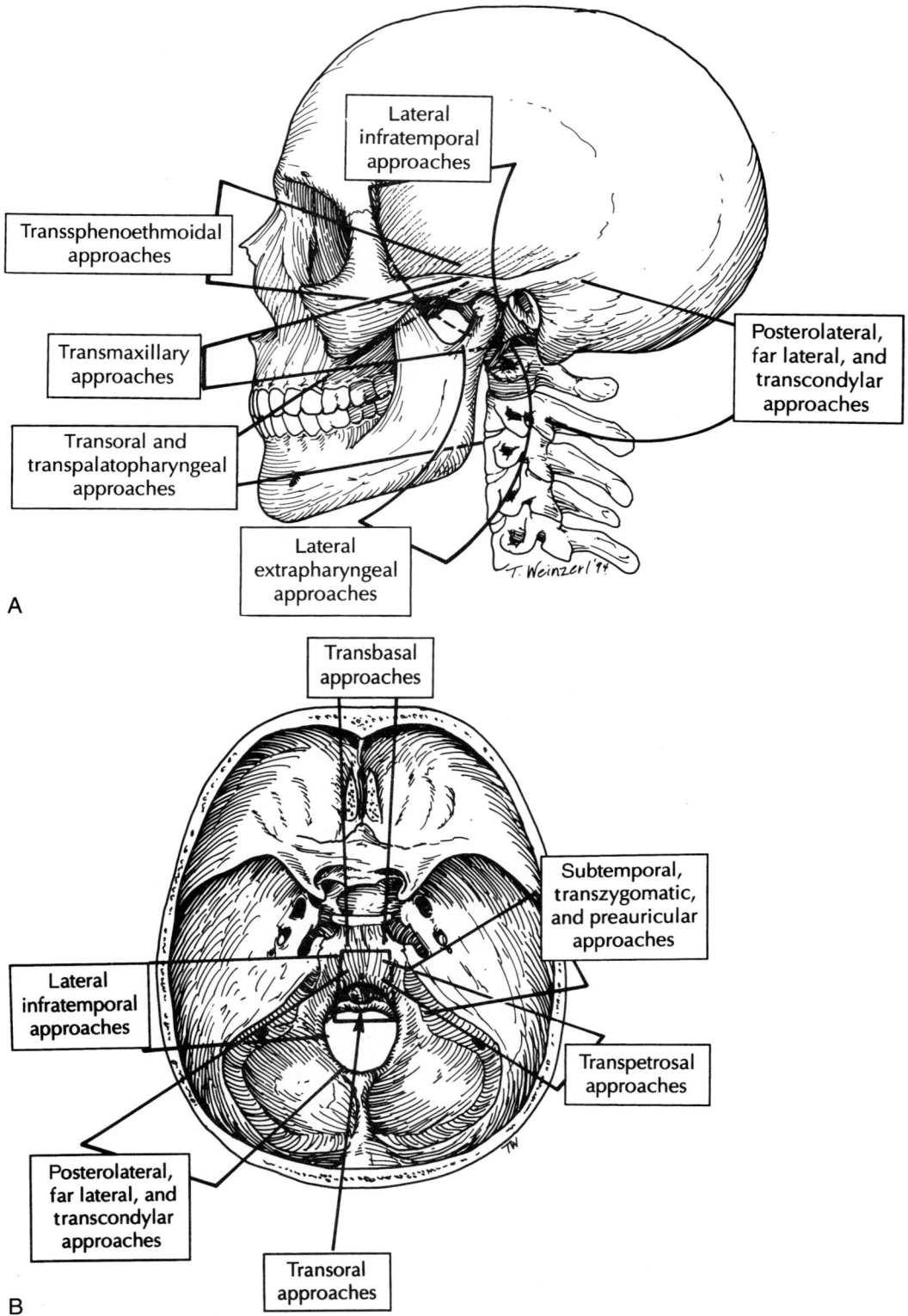

FIGURE 311–1. *A*, Illustration of exposure available via various approaches to the craniovertebral region in a lateral perspective. *B*, Illustration of exposure via various approaches to the clivus, foramen magnum, and upper cervical spine, as viewed from above the skull base.

TABLE 311–2 ■ Surgical Approaches to the Craniovertebral Junction

PROCEDURE	EXTENT OF EXPOSURE	COMMON PATHOLOGY	ADVANTAGES	LIMITATIONS	RISKS AND LONG-TERM SIDE EFFECTS
Transoral-transpalatopharyngeal	20–30 mm width of ventral midline, lower clivus, atlas, axis	Congenital development and degenerative diseases; extradural tumors	Simple, direct; may be combined with palatal split, mandibular split	Pterygoid plate, hypoglossal nerves, eustachian tubes, vertebral arteries	CSF leakage, inability to achieve clival closure, and possible instability; hence, intradural surgery to be avoided Injury to optic nerves and cavernous sinus
Transsphenoethmoidal	Good exposure of clivus and opposite side if ethmoid approach used; transsphenoid route is midline only	Extradural clival and sellar disease	Well-tolerated midline approach to clivus only; shortened operative depth	Lower clivus poorly accessible and no access below; cavernous sinus limits exposure	Limited exposure of clivus; careful reconstruction of base with bone, fascia, and pericranium
Transbasal	Anterior skull base; exposure of clivus is limited by two optic nerves going below sella	Lesions of sphenoethmoid bones and anterior skull base (e. g., meningioma, fibrous dysplasia, chordoma)	May be combined with pterional approach to access middle fossa; exposure of anterior fossa, clivus, C1 Wide exposure	Optic nerves, sella, cavernous carotid artery	Tracheostomy required; facial incision; closure and coverage of dura and pharynx poor
Transfacial	Uses Le Fort osteotomies of maxilla exposure from anterior fossae to sphenoid and entire clivus; lateral extent is into sphenomaxillary spaces and sinuses	Extradural disease; chordoma, angiofibroma, fibrous dysplasia		Poor dural coverage for CSF leak; miniplates needed to secure maxilla	
Lateral extrapharyngeal transcervical	Retropharyngeal midline CVJ and C1-2; laterally to carotid canal and inferior petrosal sinus; exposure widened by facial nerve dissection and removal of submandibular salivary gland	Chordoma, metastasis, plasmacytoma, basilar invagination	No communication with oral cavity; may be able to stabilize with bone or methyl methacrylate	Deep field with refraction of cranial nerves IX and XII and pharynx; midline and contralateral exposure better	Pharyngeal dysfunction and palsies of cranial nerves IX and XII; lower facial nerve palsies
Lateral transcondylar	Lower clivus and jugular bulb area below internal auditory canal; retrosigmoid craniectomy made	Extradural and intradural disease; meningioma, neurinoma, chordoma	No oral penetration; can be combined with infratemporal fossa procedures and may descend to expose vertebral artery for control; lateral brainstem easily visualized Control of carotid; no brain retraction	Sigmoid sinus and condyle with hypoglossal nerve	CSF leakage versus plexus bleeding; stabilization may be needed if more than half of condyle removed
Lateral basal with infratemporal fossa exposure	Petrous bone, upper clivus, ventrolateral brainstem middle cranial fossa	Intradural tumors; meningioma, epidermoid, aneurysm, neurinoma		Combined approach needed to access lower clivus and foramen magnum; visibility across midline inadequate	Hearing loss; cuts across external ear canal and temporomandibular joint; facial nerve palsy; trismus
Dorsolateral far-lateral lateral cerebellar	Midline posterior fossa to mastoid air cells, lateral half of condyle, lateral atlantal masses; posterolateral spinal canal; inferior clivus, CP angle, lateral CVJ and cervical canal	Extradural and intradural disease at lower clivus and CVJ; aneurysms of proximal basilar artery	Rapid exposure, familiar field; good control of vertebral artery, CP angle, ventral brainstem, cord, may be combined with fusion; no brainstem retraction	May be combined with presigmoid posterior fossa exposure; basilar artery, anterior inferior cerebellar artery, occiput-C1 joints are limits	CSF leakage; communicating hydrocephalus; cranial nerves XI and XII at risk
C1-2 Posterior midline suboccipital laminectomy	Covers 120 degrees of CVJ dorsal circumference; access to both sides of midline	Dorsolateral and dorsal tumors; bony decompression of foramen magnum	May be combined with dorsal fusion	Cannot be used for lateral or ventral lesions	Very few disadvantages when approach is indicated

CP, cerebellopontine; CSF, cerebrospinal fluid; CVJ, craniovertebral junction.

4803

approach is ideal for treating extradural lesions such as chordomas, angiofibromas, and fibrous dysplasias. Dural coverage must be provided by vascularized muscle flaps obtained from the temporalis muscle.

The transbasal approach provides access to the anterior skull base. Unless combined with removal of the supraorbital bar, this approach is limited by the distance between the two optic nerves and the need to work beneath the sella turcica.[20] Nonetheless, we have used this approach in several patients and have achieved good reconstruction of the floor.

A lateral extrapharyngeal route is effective and safe for reaching the upper cervical spine.[39–41] At the clivus, however, access becomes difficult because of the pyramidal narrowing of the exposure at the depths of the wound. In an effort to correct this problem, we reroute the facial nerve with upward displacement of the angle of the mandible,[26] thereby exposing the lower clivus. We believe that this approach should be limited to metastases, chordomas, and plasmacytomas that affect the axis and atlas vertebrae. Its use for the treatment of basilar invagination and intradural pathology is limited.

The true lateral transcondylar approach to the ventral aspect of the lower brainstem and clivus, as well as the upper cervical cord, demands resection of a portion of the lateral atlantal mass and the occipital condyle. Exposure of the lower clivus and the ventral brainstem is enhanced when combined with a retrosigmoid craniectomy. It is useful in the treatment of both extradural and intradural lesions such as chordomas, meningiomas, and neurofibromas.[3, 7, 9, 42–44] When combined with infratemporal procedures, it allows both anterior and posterior extensions that overcome the limitations of the sigmoid sinus and the hypoglossal nerve.[26, 45–47] The risk of CSF leakage and the possibility of destabilization are high. Troublesome bleeding is routinely encountered from the paravertebral venous plexuses.

The posterolateral route has been recognized for many years. It enables scanning of the foramen magnum to the 90 degrees available with the posterior midline approach as well as to the 90 degrees available with the lateral transcondylar approach.[1] The latter uses a standard midline posterior exposure with a lateral cerebellar approach and includes partial resection of the mastoid process and the posterior third to half of the occipital condyle to provide exposure of the jugular bulb and the medial aspect of the lateral atlantal mass. This provides access to the vertebral artery, which can be rerouted and displaced from the foramen transversarium, thus allowing for control from the C2 level upward. The ability to create a fusion makes this an ideal approach for posterior, lateral, and ventrolateral lesions. Thus, the entire circumference of the foramen magnum is accessible.

EXTRADURAL TUMORS OF THE CRANIOVERTEBRAL JUNCTION

Neoplasms that affect the craniovertebral junction are extradural or intradural in location. Glomus jugulare tumors and congenital and acquired abnormalities of the craniovertebral junction are discussed elsewhere.

Clival and Craniovertebral Junction Chordomas

Chordomas are rare, aggressive, locally destructive tumors of presumed notochordal origin that arise along the vertebral axis and show a proclivity for the spheno-occipital and sacral regions.[1, 6, 36, 48] Chordomas of the clivus and craniovertebral junction are the most common extradural neoplasms in this region. The overall incidence of chordomas is 0.2 to 0.5 per 100,000 persons per year, and they account for about 0.15% of all intracranial tumors.[49] About 25% of chordomas occur at the base of the skull arising from the clivus. Although usually midline, the notochord may have distal projections that extend to the clinoid processes of the petrous bones. Most patients experience symptoms referable to the tumor for more than a year before diagnosis.[1]

PATHOLOGY

Chordomas have been divided into classic chordomas, chondroid chordomas, and atypical chordomas.[50] Classic chordomas are lobulated, pinkish gray, gelatinous tumors that infiltrate bone but may appear grossly as somewhat demarcated; they account for 80% to 85% of all chordomas. Histologically, they exhibit a variable mix of sheets and cords or clusters of small polygonal cells with eosinophilic cytoplasm and hyperchromatic nuclei. A myxoid matrix is present. Cytologic atypia is absent or minimal.

A subpopulation, the chondroid chordoma, arises in the spheno-occiput and exhibits cartilaginous differentiation. Some authors dispute the existence of chondroid chordomas, preferring to regard these cartilage-containing neoplasms as chondrosarcomas. Chondroid chordomas have a more indolent clinical course; the survival rate is 15.8 years, compared with 4.1 years for typical classic chordomas.[48, 50] Chondroid chordomas account for 5% to 15% of all chordomas.

Atypical chordomas have a sarcomatoid appearance, with round cells and epithelial or spindle cells present with large areas of necrosis. These solid tumors are aggressive and account for 1.3% to 8% of all chordomas. In the series by Heffelfinger and coworkers, only one patient with an atypical chordoma survived more than 10 years, whereas almost 50% of those with chondroid chordomas survived more than 10 years.[50] The frequency of mitotic figures, nuclear pleomorphology, and hyperchromatism does not seem to affect the ultimate outcome.[51, 52] In rare circumstances, chordomas may dedifferentiate into malignant chondrosarcomas, fibrosarcomas, and even osteosarcomas.

The immunohistochemical profile of reactivity with antibodies to vimentin, cytokeratin, epithelial membrane antigen, and S-100 protein tend to distinguish chordomas from other sarcomatoid round cell or myxoid neoplasms.[51, 52] Chondrosarcomas are negative for cytokeratin, epithelial membrane antigen, and carcinoembryonic antigen. Vimentin and S-100 protein are present in both chondrosarcomas and chordomas. Immunostaining from keratin has no prognostic value regarding the aggressiveness of the tumor. Chondrosarcomas have been lumped with chordomas because of supposed parallel lines of occurrence, location, and aggressive behavior.

IMAGING CHARACTERISTICS

Cranial-based chordomas are clearly defined by the use of high-resolution CT, on which they appear as solitary or multiple areas of decreased attenuation within the clivus. T2-weighted MRI reveals a bright signal from the marrow in the skull base, signifying replacement of bone by tumor.[6, 26] At times, calcification is noted in the abnormal areas in the retropharyngeal space, representing sequestered bone fragments in tumor. Chordomas enhance with intravenous contrast and are well visualized by MRI. Chordomas are isointense on T1-weighted MRI (Fig. 311–2).

PRESENTATION

Chordomas usually occur in adults, with a peak incidence in the fourth decade of life.[6, 48, 53] Less than 5% of these tumors arise in children, and they have a predilection for the spheno-occipital region.[23, 26, 54] Headaches are often occipitocervical in location and aggravated by changes in craniovertebral positioning. In the senior author's series, 55% of patients benefited from craniovertebral stabilization in addition to tumor

resection, owing to involvement of the occipital condyles.[26] Lateral extensions of these tumors can give rise to unilateral symptoms, such as hypoglossal nerve palsy. Larger tumors have the potential to cause both upper and lower cranial nerve palsies and a variety of problems related to brainstem compression. Chordomas often cause symptoms from local growth into the nasal cavity, pharynx, and paranasal sinuses.

SURGICAL SERIES

Although the number of reported cases of untreated intracranial chordoma is small, only brief survival after diagnosis is a consistent finding. Several series of aggressive surgical extirpation followed by conventional radiation and proton beam therapy are discussed here.

Forsyth and colleagues[53] reviewed 51 intracranial chordomas treated surgically between 1960 and 1984 at the Mayo Clinic. The median age at presentation was 46 years, and 19 tumors were classified as chondroid chordomas. Eleven patients (22%) underwent biopsy, and 40 patients (78%) had subtotal resection. The survival rates for patients who underwent biopsy were 36% and 0% at 5 and 10 years, respectively, whereas survival rates in those with subtotal resections were 55% and 45% at 5 and 10 years, respectively. Patients who underwent postoperative radiation therapy tended to have longer disease-free survival times. Disease-free survival was the same for patients with chondroid chordomas as for those with typical chordomas.

Watkins and associates[55] described 38 patients

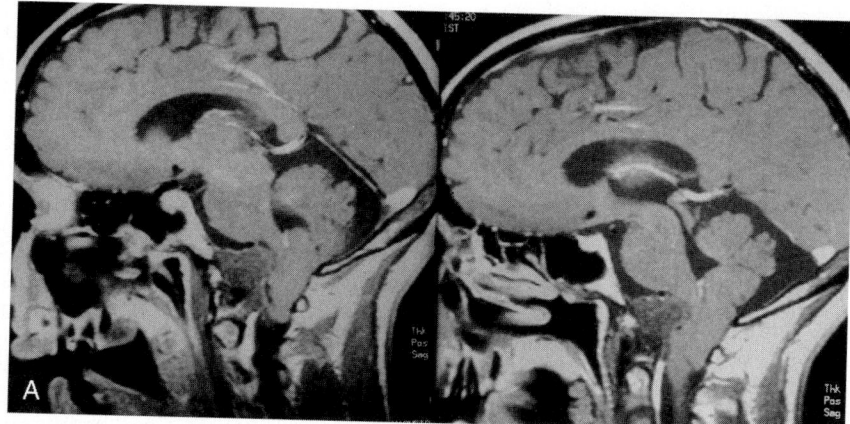

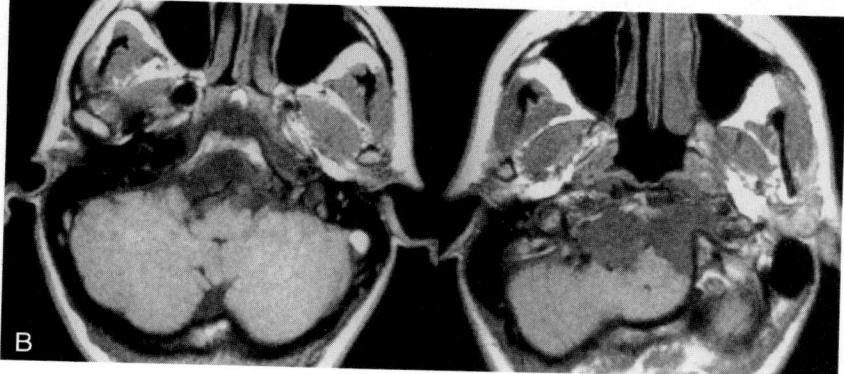

FIGURE 311–2. *A,* Composite of parasagittal and midsagittal gadolinium-enhanced magnetic resonance imaging (MRI) scans of the head and upper spinal canal in a 42-year-old woman with a craniovertebral chordoma. She presented with dysphagia, nasal regurgitation, unsteady gait, headaches, and tongue atrophy. Note the hindbrain herniation as a result of the tumor mass. *B,* Composite of T1-weighted gadolinium-enhanced MRI scans in the axial plane through the fourth ventricle *(left)* and the foramen magnum *(right).* Retropharyngeal as well as extradural and intradural tumor engulfs the left vertebral artery.

Illustration continued on following page

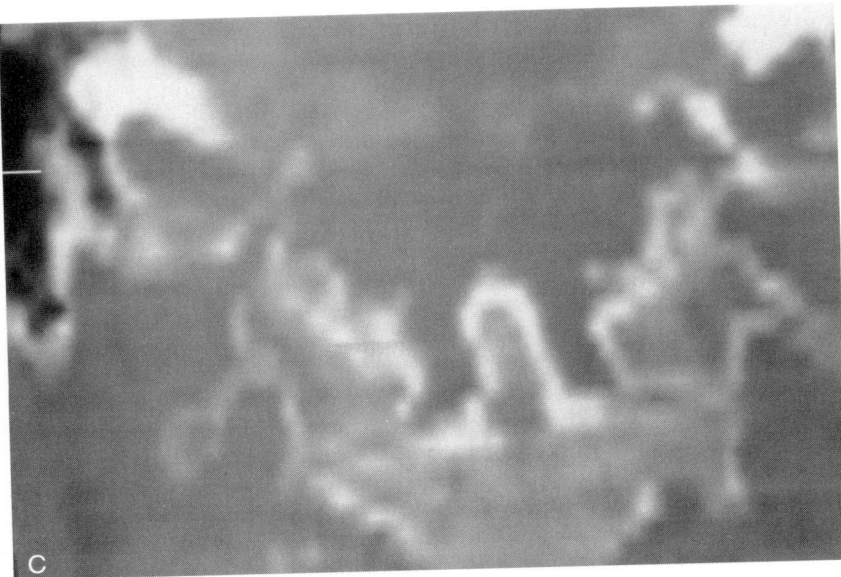

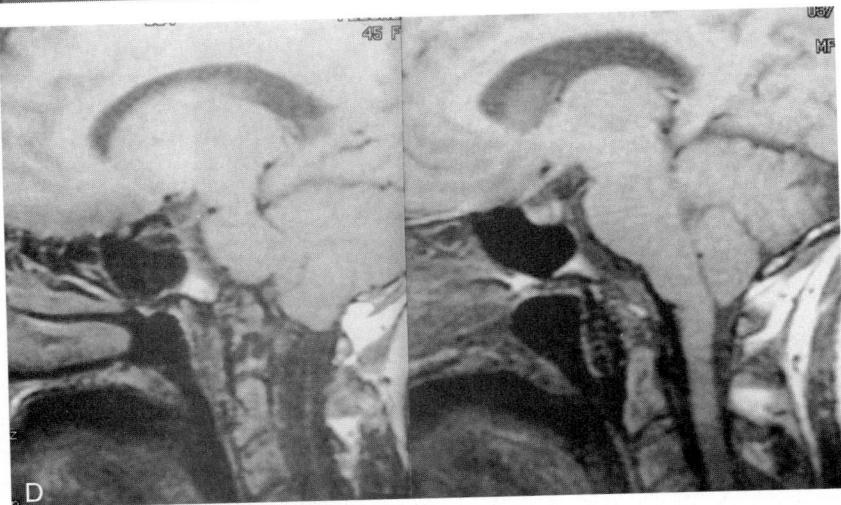

FIGURE 311–2. *Continued. C,* Reformatted computed tomographic scan of the craniovertebral junction in the frontal projection through the plane of the odontoid process. The occipital condyles are eroded bilaterally. *D,* Composite of postoperative T1-weighted MRI scans in the parasagittal and midsagittal planes at the craniovertebral junction. The hindbrain herniation has receded significantly, and there is no evidence of tumor visible. Eleven years have elapsed since this patient's transpalatopharyngeal resection of the clivus and craniovertebral junction chordoma.

treated at the National Hospital of Neurology and Neurosurgery in London between 1958 and 1988. Craniotomies were used in 28 patients, and transoral or transmaxillary routes were used in 10 others. All patients underwent postoperative external beam radiotherapy of 50 to 60 Gy. Recurrence developed in 23 patients, and 13 died within 5 years. Twelve patients were lost to follow-up. The authors concluded that two groups existed: one with indolent disease and another with aggressive growth and poor outcomes.

Gay and colleagues[48] reviewed the management of 46 chordomas and 14 chondrosarcomas involving the cranial base between 1984 and 1993 at the University of Pittsburgh. They recommended an aggressive approach to achieve long-term recurrence-free survival. Fifty percent of patients had undergone previous surgery before referral, and 22% had undergone previous external beam radiation therapy. The surgical approach was a subtemporal-infratemporal fossa approach, sometimes combined with a transpetrous approach. In other instances, an extended subfrontal approach was used, and in a few cases, the lateral transcondylar approach was used. There was a high tendency to stay between the subtemporal-infratemporal fossa approach and the extended subfrontal approach. Using this technique, the rate of total or near-total resection was 67%. Eighteen patients had died by the 5-year follow-up. Postoperatively, 20% of the patients underwent external beam, proton beam, or gamma radiation therapy. In patients who had total resection, the overall 5-year recurrence-free survival rate was 84%, compared with 64% in those with partial resection. However, the rate of morbidity was high. Thirty percent developed CSF leaks, 10% experienced meningitis, and 80% had an immediate new cranial nerve deficit. Using the Karnofsky performance score, 40% of patients had permanent functional deterioration. Based on this experience, the authors advocated aggressive initial surgical resection, with the sparing application of radiation therapy.

In 1997, Al-Mefty and Borba[6] reported their results with an aggressive surgical approach combined with postoperative proton beam therapy in 25 patients treated between 1990 and 1996. Radical or subtotal (>90%) removal was achieved in 84% of patients undergoing multiple procedures, when necessary, and extensive drilling of bone beyond the limits of tumor involvement. Postoperatively, 68% of the patients received a mean of 68 cGy–equivalent proton beam radiotherapy. The postoperative mortality rate was 4%. The postoperative rate of morbidity, however, was 48%, although only 8% suffered permanent neurological deficits. Eighteen percent of the patients treated with proton beam therapy developed radiation necrosis. The mean follow-up was only 25 months, however, making conclusions about outcome and survival difficult.

Maira and coworkers[36] achieved total tumor removal in 7 of 10 patients undergoing repeated transsphenoidal procedures for chordomas. They reported no evidence of disease in these patients at a mean of 38 months after surgery and encountered a cranial nerve complication in only one.

During the past 15 years, cranial-based exposures of the clivus and upper cervical–craniovertebral chordomas have become accepted. Thus, it is important to compare recent series with at least a 5- to 10-year follow-up. Since 1985, 25 males and 18 females with cranial-base chordomas have been treated at the University of Iowa Hospitals and Clinics.[26] Fourteen (34%) had undergone previous surgery; 11 (25%) had undergone previous radiation therapy, 5 of whom had proton beam therapy. The 43 patients underwent 49 skull base procedures, and 9 required stabilization. Fifteen patients underwent a transoral-transpalatopharyngeal approach, eight underwent a transmaxillary approach, six underwent a transsphenoethmoidal approach, four underwent an infratemporal fossa primary approach, four underwent a lateral extrapharyngeal approach, six underwent a transcondylar approach, five underwent a transfacial approach, and one underwent a transbasal approach. Gross total resection was possible in 12 of the 43 individuals (Fig. 311–3). Subtotal resection (>90%), which was documented on postoperative MRI, was achieved in 14 individuals. Seven patients died during the 15-year follow-up period. All patients had typical chordomas and underwent detailed histologic and immunohistochemical analysis of the tumor. Of the 15 individuals who underwent a transpalatopharyngeal approach, 5 died, 3 within 2 years of the transoral procedure at our institution. Each of these three patients had previously undergone more than four operative approaches to the tumor and had also undergone proton beam therapy. The time from proton beam radiation to the recurrence presenting at our institution was less than 3 years. There were no cases of postoperative CSF leakage, meningitis, or new cranial nerve deficits.

Chordomas in children are rare; only 30 cases have been reported. Classic chordoma is seen in 28%, and atypical chordoma in 72%. Thus, the prognosis reflects atypical lesions. All children with atypical lesions died within a mean of 6 months. Patients with classic chordomas treated within the last 10 years have survived a mean of 17 months. Metastasis occurs in approximately 60% of children younger than 5 years.

RADIATION THERAPY

The role of radiation therapy in the management of skull base chordomas is now fairly well established. Amendola and colleagues concluded that conventional radiation therapy provided better local control when administered postoperatively than when delivered for a recurrence following surgical resection.[56] Patients receiving more than 80 Gy had an 80% local control rate, whereas patients receiving 40 to 60 Gy had a 20% success rate. There has been a consistent movement toward achieving a higher dosage with conventional external beam radiotherapy. Radiation therapy itself has severe risks, including tumor recurrence, brain radiation necrosis, and radiation vasculitis.

In 1993, Forsyth and coworkers[53] reported the results of 39 patients treated with surgery and conventional radiation therapy. The overall survival rate was 51% at 5 years and 35% at 10 years. Fractionated proton beam therapy exploits favorable dose-localization characteristics and can deliver between 70 and 80 Gy to the tumor, whereas nearby nervous structures receive much lower doses. Researchers at both Harvard and the Berkeley Laboratory have published results with this modality.[57–61] Their patients had an impressive actuarial control rate of 82% at 5 years and 58% at 10 years. Of the relapses, 95% were local recurrences, and 20% had distant metastases. A poor prognosis was associated with tumors with a volume greater than 75 mL, more than 10% tumor necrosis, and involvement of the cervical spine. There was no histologic correlation with poor prognosis. Under this same protocol, 18 children, ranging in age from 4 to 18 years, were treated with proton beam therapy. The median tumor dose was 69 Gy, with a 72-month median follow-up. Over a 5-year period, the actuarial survival was 68%, and the 5-year disease-free survival rate was 63%.

In summary, the data strongly support the view that radiation therapy, particularly proton beam therapy combined with surgery, represents a substantial improvement over the natural history of chordoma (see Fig. 311–3C and D). Gamma radiation therapy may deliver the benefits of proton therapy with fewer complications, but this remains to be demonstrated.[62]

SURGICAL INTERVENTION

It is difficult to cure a patient with chordoma by surgical resection alone. No single operative approach can be used for all craniovertebral chordomas.[6, 26, 48] We believe that most cases are best approached with the initial intent to resect rather than just biopsy the tumor. Location of the tumor is the single most important factor in determining the approach. In some cases, several different approaches are necessary for adequate resection. We strongly believe that gross surgical resection or near-total resection should be the goal. The overall rate of morbidity associated with management must be weighed against the rate of recurrence and the extent of tumor resection. A close follow-up with postoperative imaging is essential and may be needed every 3 months for the first year, especially for aggres-

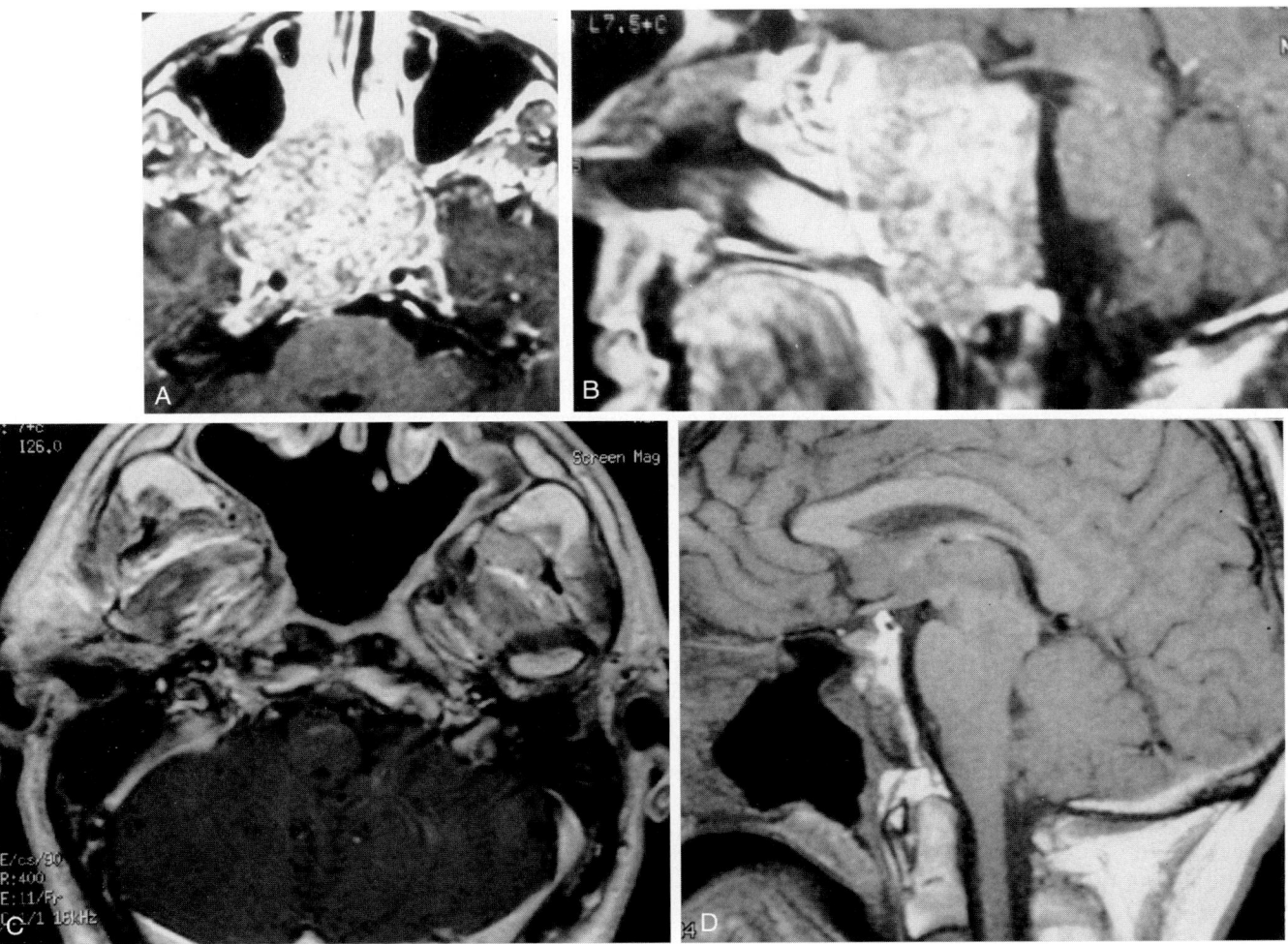

FIGURE 311–3. *A*, Axial gadolinium-enhanced magnetic resonance imaging (MRI) scan through the skull base in a patient with a chordoma of the clivus and anterior midline skull base. He presented with difficulty breathing, palsy of left cranial nerve VI, and pain in the left trigeminal distribution. The tumor extends between the two pterygoid plates and occupies the anterior midline skull base, with clival erosion. The carotid arteries are encased. *B*, Midsagittal gadolinium-enhanced MRI scan of the skull base revealing extensive tumor in the anterior midline skull base from the cribriform plate, including the dorsum sellae, to the anterior atlantal arch. *C*, Postoperative axial MRI scan through the plane of the lower brainstem and the anterior cranial base. The patient underwent a Le Fort I drop-down, swing-door maxillotomy with tumor resection, followed by proton beam therapy. Nine years have elapsed since his surgery. *D*, Postoperative gadolinium-enhanced midsagittal MRI scan of the head and face showing enhancement of the dural graft and tectorial membrane.

sive lesions. We reoperate on patients with gross tumor recurrence before subjecting them to radiation therapy. In subtotal resections, atypical lesions, and children, proton beam therapy has been offered after immediate reduction of the tumor's volume.

Plasmacytomas

Solitary plasmacytomas are clinical entities distinct from multiple myelomas, even though both are manifestations of a continuum of B-cell lymphoproliferative diseases.[40, 63, 64] The clinical distinction between the two is in the long-term prognosis. In a review of 84 patients with solitary plasmacytomas of the spine, McLain and Weinstein found that 44% of patients had developed disseminated disease at the end of 5 years, and the 5-

year survival rate was 60%.[65] In contrast, the 5-year mortality rate of disseminated myeloma (multiple myeloma) of the spinal column is 82%. Despite this improved outlook for solitary plasmacytomas, once a solitary plasmacytoma disseminates, the disease behaves much like multiple myeloma.[64]

The primary abnormality in multiple myeloma is slow, uncontrolled proliferation of immature and mature plasma cells in the bone marrow.[63, 66] This monoclonal population of cells produces a homogeneous immunoglobulin composed of a single class of heavy chain and one type of light chain, referred to as the M protein. Multiple myeloma is associated with plasmacytosis of the bone marrow and the presence of IgA-X monoclonal immunoglobulin in the cytoplasm of the tumor cell as well as in the serum. These serum and bone marrow findings are diagnostic. In contrast, plasmacytoma does not appear in the bone marrow and is localized to the tissue involved. We have seen plasmacytomas in the craniovertebral junction involving the occipital bone, the axis, and the atlas vertebrae.[1, 40, 67]

On gross examination, plasmacytomas are soft, grayish, moderately vascular lesions. They often reside within the diploic bone and only initially respect the cortices. When they expand, the cortex is destroyed. The tumor invades the vertebral bodies of the skull base and engulfs the vertebral vessels. When such tumors are present in the spinal canal, 20% involve the pedicles. The treatment of plasmacytoma involves diagnostic biopsy and stabilization. Because surgical attempts at resection can be fairly bloody, we advocate preoperative tumor embolization (Fig. 311–4).[40] In our experience, surgery requires internal and external fixation with instrumentation, followed by radiation therapy. Occasionally, decompression of the cervicomedullary junction is essential and may be performed from a transoral-transpalatopharyngeal route or from a lateral extrapharyngeal-transcervical approach. Careful follow-up, including evaluation of serum, urine, and bone marrow, is essential.

Eosinophilic Granulomas

Eosinophilic granuloma affecting the spine is a childhood disease. The age of symptomatic involvement is 11 to 12 years. The most common area of occurrence is the thoracic and lumbar spine, although the upper cervical spine and clivus can be involved. The incidence of solitary eosinophilic granuloma of the spine is 8%. In children, multiple lesions occur in 38% of cases.[24, 68–70]

The presenting complaint is local segmental spinal pain and paravertebral muscle spasm. Neurological symptoms may develop as a result of vertebral collapse, which produces focal spasm and torticollis at the craniovertebral junction. The pathologic findings on plain radiographs are an osteolytic defect with an occasional sclerotic rim and various grades of vertebral collapse with flattening of the vertebral body. The latter feature has led to the term *vertebra plana*. Mild to moderate kyphosis may be present as a result of collapse or segmental paravertebral muscle spasm.

When treating patients with eosinophilic granuloma of the craniovertebral junction, the senior author prefers to obtain a bone scan to identify lesions that may be present elsewhere. In some cases, an easily excised frontal bone or parietal bone lesion can lead to the diagnosis. The aim of treatment is to obtain an accurate diagnosis of a solitary lytic lesion. The differential diagnosis includes tuberculosis, pyogenic osteomyelitis, and osteochondritis. Percutaneous needle biopsy is an option, but the senior author believes that the risk of hemorrhage and the frequently nondiagnostic nature of percutaneous specimens make open biopsy preferable. Posterior resection of bony elements should be avoided, because the granuloma involves the vertebral body rather than the lamina and pedicles. Should the lesion require resection of the craniovertebral junction,

it is extremely important to have bony reconstitution anteriorly and posteriorly when stabilization is performed.

Treatment of eosinophilic granuloma with low-dose radiation has been advocated and reported to be effective.[71, 72] Simple biopsy and immobilization usually lead to reconstitution of the vertebral height,[25] because eosinophilic granulomas spare the endochondral ossifications within the vertebral bodies. Multiple lesions with systemic conditions such as Letterer-Siwe and Hand-Schüller-Christian diseases are the progressive form of this entity and require chemotherapy. Chemotherapy is not indicated for solid vertebral body lesions.

Osteoid Osteomas and Osteoblastomas

These lesions are osteoblastic, with a propensity to involve the posterior elements of the cervical spine.[40] Osteoblastomas and osteoid osteomas are differentiated from each other primarily on the basis of their size.[1] Osteoid osteomas are more common in males and are usually less than 1 to 1.5 cm. They are limited to the cortical framework and have no paraspinal extension. Patients with osteoid osteomas usually present in the second or third decade of life. They commonly complain of neck pain that worsens at night and is relieved by salicylates. Radiographically, these lesions have a central circular nidus that appears within a radiolucent area surrounded by a sclerotic border. The lesion is well outlined on CT, and the bone scan is invariably positive.[73, 74]

In contrast, osteoblastomas have been called *giant osteoids* or *osteofibromas*. These highly vascular lesions are predominantly lytic; they expand into the spinal canal and creep into the paravertebral space. Osteoblastomas tend to involve the pedicles and laminae as well as the spinous processes.[68] The neoplasms expand the medullary bone and appear on radiographs as lytic lesions with expansion of the cortical margin. Less peripheral sclerosis is seen than with osteoid osteomas. Like osteoid osteomas, osteoblastomas are well localized on isotope bone scans.

The treatment of both osteoblastoma and osteoid osteoma is resection. Curettage and bone grafting of vertebral osteoblastomas have provided good long-term results. Complete excision is desirable but may not be possible at the craniovertebral junction. Radiation therapy may be considered in individuals who have undergone subtotal resection and bone grafting. Radiation alone may provide reconstitution of bone and preserve spinal stability if immobilization is adequate. A very small number of such lesions may undergo malignant transformation. Long-term follow-up of treated patients is mandatory.

INTRADURAL TUMORS

Foramen Magnum Meningiomas

Meningiomas are common at the foramen magnum and account for 2% to 3% of all meningiomas.[2, 7, 21]

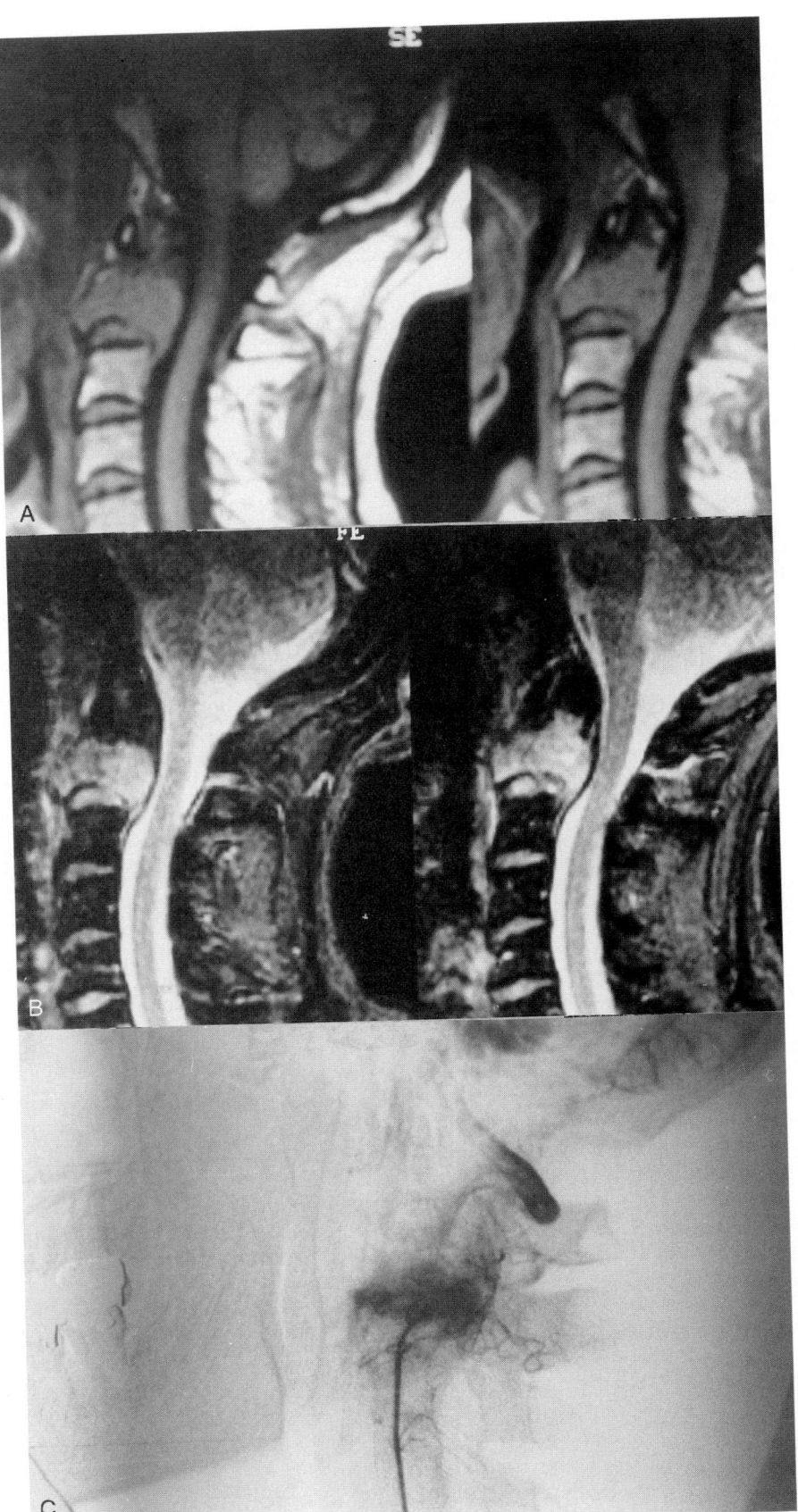

FIGURE 311–4. *A,* Composite of midsagittal and parasagittal T1-weighted magnetic resonance imaging (MRI) scans of the cervical spine in a 48-year-old man with plasmacytoma of the axis. He presented with severe occipital headaches and neck pain. The entire axis body has been replaced by the mass, which expands dorsally into the cervical canal. *B,* Composite of midsagittal and parasagittal T2-weighted MRI scans of the craniovertebral junction showing the high signal intensity of the plasmacytoma in the axis body, which has expanded and compressed the ventral cervical spinal cord. *C,* Selective lateral vertebral angiogram demonstrating tumor blush in the axis body. The tumor was embolized successfully. The patient then underwent a transoral resection of the plasmacytoma and dorsal occipitocervical fusion.

Females represent between 66% and 73% of cases.[3, 4, 46] Typically, patients become symptomatic between 35 and 60 years old, although meningiomas occasionally occur at the foramen magnum in children.[1, 22] Foramen magnum meningiomas may occur in the setting of neurofibromatosis.[75, 76]

Typically, the lesions are attached to the anterior rim of the foramen magnum and frequently invade the region of the entrance around the vertebral artery and the exit of the cervical nerve roots.[7, 46] These globoid and often fibrous lesions usually extend above and below the foramen magnum equally (Fig. 311–5). Occasionally, they show a marked predilection for either intracranial or intraspinal development. Many subtypes of meningioma have been identified at the foramen magnum, including meningothelial, transitional, fibrous, xanthomatous, clear cell, and lymphoplasmacytic-rich meningiomas.[22, 77, 78]

Plain radiographs may show evidence of increased pressure, such as erosion or calcification around the foramen magnum and widening of the interpedicular spaces of the upper cervical vertebrae. The concomitant finding of cervical spondylosis frequently results in an erroneous primary diagnosis of spondylosis as the cause of myelopathy.

MRI provides excellent high-resolution information about the tumor, vascular encasement, its relationship to the brainstem, and CSF spaces. Typically, meningiomas are isointense on T1-weighted images and iso- to hypointense on T2-weighted images and enhance intensely after gadolinium administration. Magnetic resonance angiography provides critical arterial detail, including vertebral artery patency. It is used routinely as an alternative to conventional angiography.[7] Magnetic resonance venography can be used to evaluate the vein of Labbé, sigmoid sinus, and dominance of the transverse sinus; thus it can help plan the surgical approach in some patients.

TREATMENT

The mainstay of treatment for foramen magnum meningioma is surgical resection. Samii and colleagues[46] reported complete removal in 63% of cases and subtotal removal in 30%, and their patients' mean Karnofsky performance scores increased from 63 to 73. George and associates[3] reported complete removal in 86% and subtotal removal in 11% of their patients. Clinical grade improved in 90% of patients, stabilized in 2.5%, and worsened in 7.5%—the latter corresponding to the three deaths in their series.

Meningiomas located at the ventral foramen magnum are more difficult to resect than are those at the posterior foramen magnum. Two major reasons account for this difference. First, the posterolateral approaches required to expose the ventral foramen magnum are larger and more complex than are the posterior approaches. Second, several critical structures, including the vertebral artery, occipital condyle, brainstem, and lower cranial nerves, impede exposure of the ventral foramen magnum. During a posterolateral approach, any of these structures can be subjected to injury, causing significant morbidity and mortality.

Despite these difficulties, Arnautovic and colleagues[7] reported 67% gross total resections, 11% near-total resections, and 22% subtotal resections in patients harboring ventral foramen magnum meningiomas. These results are similar to the surgical results for all foramen magnum meningiomas. Furthermore, Karnofsky performance scores increased postoperatively in 15 patients. Statistical analysis demonstrated that gross or near-total resection and a higher preoperative Karnof-

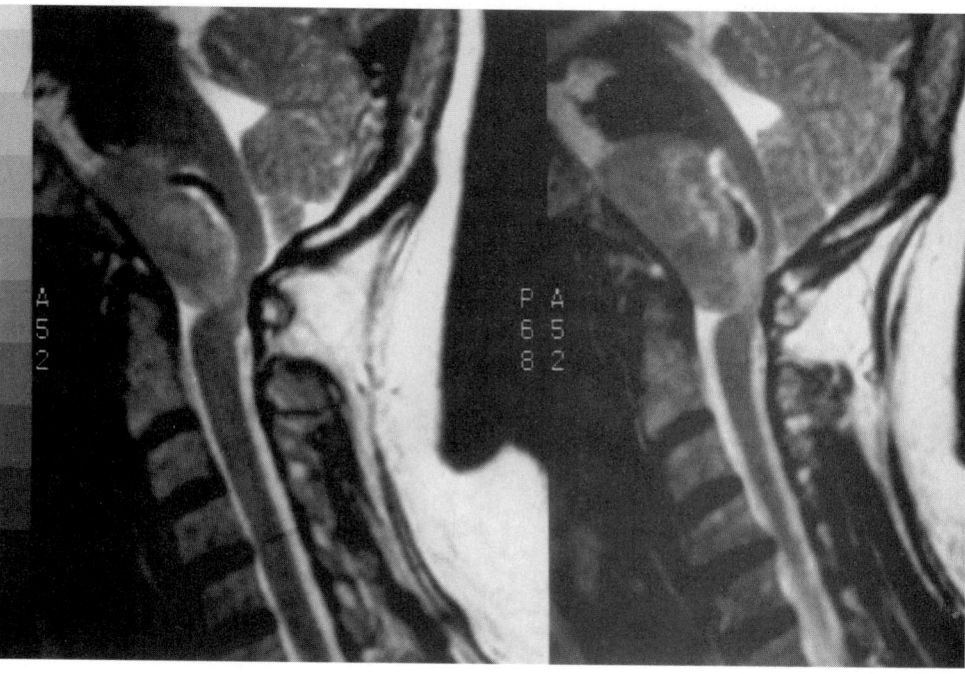

FIGURE 311–5. Composite of T2-weighted magnetic resonance imaging scans in the midsagittal and parasagittal planes of the craniovertebral junction. This 54-year-old woman was quadriparetic, with paralysis of the right glossopharyngeal, vagus, spinal accessory, and hypoglossal nerves. The encasement of the vertebral artery was controlled at surgery. She underwent a posterolateral far-lateral transcondylar approach to the cerebellopontine angle and the ventral aspect of C1, with rerouting of the vertebral artery at the foramen transversarium.

sky score indicated a significantly improved outcome. These series demonstrate that complete resection of foramen magnum meningiomas can be obtained in most cases, particularly during the first resection, and that resection can improve patients' postoperative performance scores.

Postoperative lower cranial palsies are the most frequent surgical complication. These palsies are significant because they are associated with longer periods of hospitalization.[7, 46] Lower cranial nerve palsies resulting in aspiration pneumonia and death accounted for the mortality rates in several series. Multiple regression analysis indicated that recurrent tumor, arachnoid scarring, craniovertebral meningioma, and no preoperative cranial nerve deficits were predictors of postoperative aspiration. Aggressive, comprehensive treatment is recommended once these deficits are discovered, including speech therapy, possible vocal cord medialization or injection, tracheostomy, or gastric tube placement.

Severe preoperative deficits and poor Karnofsky performance scores are also predictors of postoperative morbidity and mortality. Weakness and poor mobility predispose patients to pneumonia, deep venous thrombosis, and pulmonary embolism, which may account for up to 50% of postoperative mortality.[3, 7, 46]

Other postoperative complications include CSF leaks, meningitis, and hydrocephalus that may require insertion of a ventriculoperitoneal shunt. Other cranial nerve palsies can occur, but most resolve. Occipitocervical instability can occur, but this complication can be eliminated with judicious resection of no more than a third to a half of the occipital condyle. In recent series, the overall morbidity rate has been about 30%, and perioperative mortality rates have ranged from 0% to 7.5%. Incomplete tumor removal and aggressive recurrence of invasive meningioma have responded to conventional radiation.[79–82]

Muthukumar and colleagues[83] reported their experience treating five foramen magnum meningiomas using stereotactic radiosurgery. Patients with tumors less than 35 mm in diameter and with a reasonable performance status were selected for treatment. At a median follow-up of 36 months, no tumor growth had occurred and cranial nerve deficits had not worsened, but the series was small and the follow-up data were limited. Furthermore, their population represented ideal surgical candidates, whose results were likely to be more favorable than those of nonideal patients for whom nonsurgical treatment would be preferable. Much more experience in patient selection is required before stereotactic radiosurgery can be considered a primary treatment for foramen magnum meningiomas. Others have performed surgical resection with low thresholds for leaving adherent tumor and used postoperative gamma knife radiosurgery to treat the residual tumor.[84] Therefore, stereotactic radiosurgery may represent a valuable adjunctive therapy.

Intradural Extramedullary Tumors at C1 and C2

The most common extramedullary intradural spinal tumors are meningiomas, neurofibromas, and schwannomas. Together, these tumors represent about 55% of spinal tumors.[2, 3, 7, 9, 43, 76, 85, 86] Other intradural tumors, such as hemangioblastomas, dermoids, epidermoids, neurenteric cysts, and mixed tumors, are uncommon.[1, 87–90] Many of these lesions are benign and resectable, and the outlook after surgical therapy is excellent.

Overall, the clinical presentation and examination of patients with intradural extra-axial tumors in the region of the atlas and axis are similar to those of patients with foramen magnum meningiomas. This is true for two reasons: Tumors attached to the foramen magnum often expand caudally into the upper cervical canal, and tumors arising in the upper cervical canal expand rostrally through the foramen magnum. The radiographic evaluation is also similar in both groups of patients.

Neurofibromas produce symptoms in patients be-

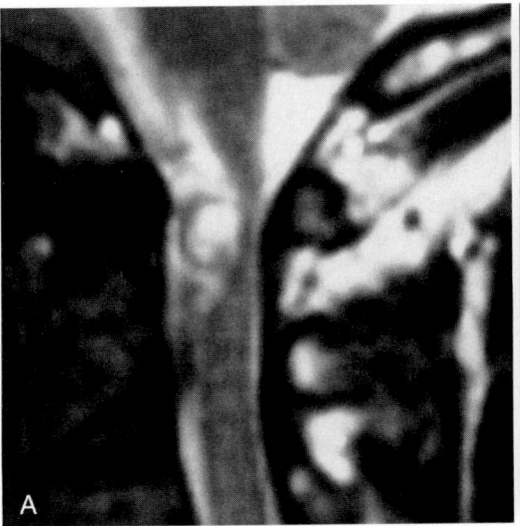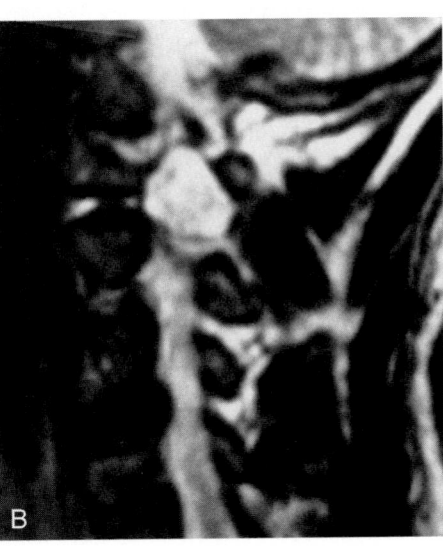

FIGURE 311–6. *A,* Midsagittal T2-weighted magnetic resonance imaging (MRI) scan of the cervicomedullary junction in a 55-year-old man. The patient presented with severe right-sided occipital pain and quadriparesis that was more pronounced in the right arm and leg than on the contralateral side. The area of high signal intensity represents a discrete ventral neurofibroma in the subarachnoid space at C1. The cervicomedullary junction is compressed dorsally. *B,* Parasagittal T2-weighted MRI scan through the neural foramen on the right side of the cervical canal demonstrates the high-signal-intensity tumor in the C1-2 neural foramen.

tween 20 and 60 years old.[1, 2] Patients with neurofibromatosis type 1 tend to become symptomatic at younger ages[10] and have multiple or bilateral tumors.[43] Neurinomas occur more frequently at C2 than at C1. The median time from onset of symptoms to diagnosis is 24 months. Although neurinomas are associated with nerve roots, symptoms tend to manifest distally with weakness and poor coordination or, less commonly, in a radicular pattern.[43, 85] Clinical signs also mirror those of foramen magnum meningiomas; however, hypesthe-

sia in the second cervical division is an important localizing sign.[91]

Although findings on plain radiographs may be normal or demonstrate cervical spondylosis, the pressure of an enlarged intervertebral foramen is highly suggestive of a nerve root tumor. Neurinomas are usually iso- to hypointense on T1-weighted MRI and hyperintense on T2-weighted MRI (Fig. 311–6).[86] Intratumoral hemorrhage and cyst formation can affect the postcontrast appearance of neurinomas (homogeneous, heteroge-

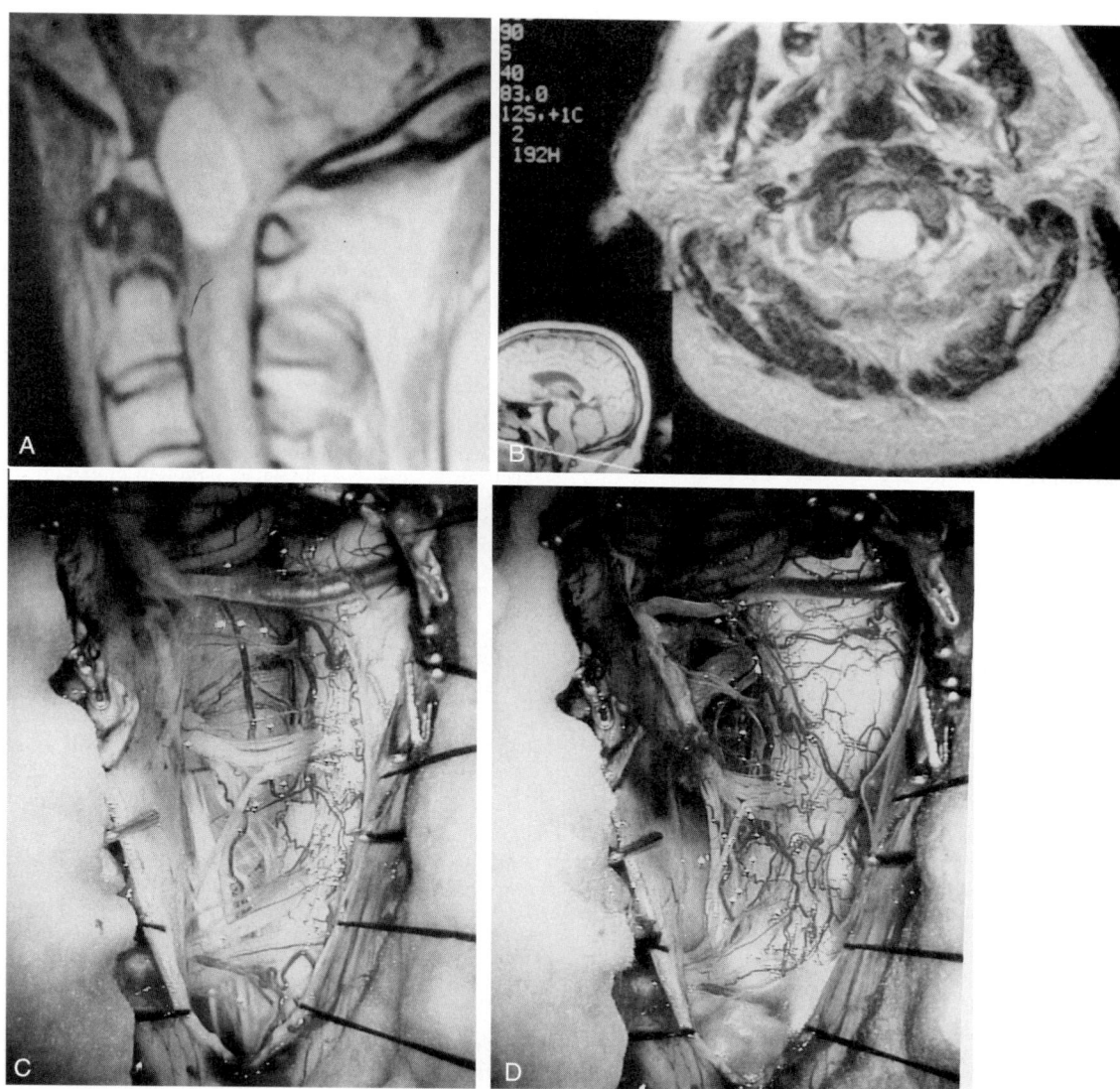

FIGURE 311–7. *A,* T1-weighted midsagittal magnetic resonance imaging (MRI) scan through the craniovertebral junction in a 24-year-old man with a neurenteric cyst ventral to the cervicomedullary junction. Note the high signal intensity caused by the proteinaceous material within the cystic mass. *B,* Axial T1-weighted MRI scan just below the plane of the foramen magnum. Dorsally, the ventral extra-axial mass displaces the cervicomedullary junction. *C,* Operative photograph through the microscope after a posterolateral transcondylar exposure of the ventral cerebellopontine angle and cervicomedullary junction. An intra-arachnoid mass is ventral to the cerebellum, medulla, and cervicomedullary junction. The dorsal branches of the posterior inferior cerebellar artery are at the top of the field; the upper cervical nerves are visualized, together with the spinal accessory nerve, in the most lateral portion of the ventral subarachnoid space. *D,* Operative photograph through the microscope after resection of the neurenteric cyst ventral to the medulla and cervicomedullary junction. The lower cranial nerves, as well as the upper cervical nerve roots and the posterior inferior cerebellar branches, are preserved.

neous, and even ring enhancement).[92] If necessary, magnetic resonance angiography can evaluate the vertebrobasilar arterial tree. CT provides detailed bony definition. If MRI is contraindicated, CT-myelography may improve intradural visualization of the tumor.

Neurenteric cysts are a developmental abnormality resulting in a cystic endodermal structure that can impinge on the spinal cord. Although most common in the cervical and thoracic regions, neurenteric cysts rarely appear in the region of the foramen magnum, typically in an anterior location. Their clinical presentation is similar to that of other foramen magnum lesions, with the exception that the cysts can lead to repeated episodes of meningitis.[90] Plain radiographs can demonstrate vertebral segmentation failure. CT is useful for fully delineating bony abnormalities. MRI demonstrates a cystic structure with T1- and T2-weighted imaging characteristics similar to those of proteinaceous CSF (Fig. 311–7).[88, 90]

TREATMENT

The aim of the surgical approach is to maximize exposure of the tumor affecting the spinal cord or brainstem while minimizing bone removal to maintain the stability of the craniovertebral junction. Early diagnosis, when neurological deficits are minor and the tumor is small, tends to lead to better surgical outcomes and prognoses. Thus, neurologically devastated individuals are less likely to attain gainful resolution of their neurological deficits.

Preoperative cardiopulmonary assessment is essential, as is discussion with the patient and family about the possibility of prolonged postoperative tracheal intubation or tracheostomy. Patients with large lesions within the spinal canal require preoperative evaluation of cervical motion to assess stability and determine whether neurological deficits develop during flexion due to compression of the brainstem by the tumor.[1, 91] This evaluation allows appropriate positioning under general anesthesia.

In most benign lesions, surgical exposure is obtained via a posterior midline or posterolateral approach. Surgical principles employed to remove benign tumors include the compulsory use of an operating microscope, tumor debulking early during the exposure, and gentle traction maintained away from the neural structures. In many cases, the use of an ultrasonic aspirator is beneficial. Electrophysiologic monitoring using motor and sensory evoked responses or bipolar recording rostral to the lesion has been used by the authors but is not mandatory for such surgical procedures.

Although posterior approaches are most commonly used to resect neurinomas, use of the anterolateral[3] and transoral exposures has been reported.[27] In rare instances, schwannomas of the craniovertebral junction may be ventral to the dentate ligament; in such cases, section of the ligament or even of the spinal accessory nerve may be required. Dumbbell neurofibromas can cause craniovertebral instability, and this possibility must be kept in mind at the time of reconstruction. The surgical outcome of neurinoma resection is excellent.

Patients with myelopathy and quadriparesis typically improve significantly, or their symptoms resolve completely. Resection rarely causes new radicular symptoms and usually improves existing radicular symptoms.

Neurenteric cysts have been resected through several approaches: posterior midline, posterolateral, far lateral, and transoral. Complete resection is mandatory, because cyst aspiration results in reaccumulation of the cyst contents and symptomatic recurrence.[90] Resection is typically associated with significant improvement or resolution of symptoms.

REFERENCES

1. Menezes AH, Traynelis VC: Tumors of the craniovertebral junction. In Youmans J (ed): Neurological Surgery. Philadelphia, WB Saunders, 1995, pp 3041–3072.
2. Meyer FB, Ebersold MJ, Reese DF: Benign tumors of the foramen magnum. J Neurosurg 61:136–142, 1984.
3. George B, Lot G, Boissonnet H: Meningioma of the foramen magnum: A series of 40 cases. Surg Neurol 47:371–379, 1997.
4. Howe JR, Taren JA: Foramen magnum tumors: Pitfalls in diagnosis. JAMA 225:1061–1066, 1973.
5. Elsberg CA, Strauss I: Tumors of the spinal cord which project into the posterior cranial fossa. Arch Neurol Psychiatry 21:261–273, 1929.
6. Al-Mefty O, Borba LAB: Skull base chordomas: A management challenge. J Neurosurg 86:182–189, 1997.
7. Arnautovic KI, Al-Mefty O, Husain M: Ventral foramen magnum meningiomas. J Neurosurg 92:71–80, 2000.
8. Beatty RA: Cold dysesthesia: A symptom of extramedullary tumors of the spinal cord. J Neurosurg 33:75–78, 1970.
9. Menezes AH: Tumors of the craniocervical junction. In Menezes AH, Sonntag VKH (eds): Principles of Spinal Surgery. New York, McGraw-Hill, 1996, pp 1335–1353.
10. Yasuoka S, Okazaki H, Daube JR, et al: Foramen magnum tumors: Analysis of 57 cases of benign extramedullary tumors. J Neurosurg 49:828–838, 1978.
11. Taylor AR, Byrnes DP: Foramen magnum and high cervical cord compression. Brain 97:473–480, 1974.
12. Cohen L, McCrae D: Tumors in the region of the foramen magnum. J Neurosurg 19:462–469, 1962.
13. Bell HS: Paralysis of both arms from injury of the upper portion of the pyramidal decussation: "Cruciate paralysis." J Neurosurg 33:376–380, 1970.
14. Glasauer FE, Egnatchick JE: Restless legs syndrome: An unusual cause for a perplexing syndrome. Spinal Cord 37:862–865, 1999.
15. Choi IS, Berenstein A: Surgical neuroangiography of the spine and spinal cord. Radiol Clin North Am 26:1131–1141, 1988.
16. Forbes HJ, Allen PW, Waller CS, et al: Spinal cord monitoring in scoliosis surgery: Experience with 1168 cases. J Bone Joint Surg Br 73:487–491, 1991.
17. Menezes AH: Surgical approaches to the craniocervical junction. In Frymoyer JW (ed): The Adult Spine: Principles and Practice, New York, Raven Press, 1991, pp 967–985.
18. May DM, Jones SJ, Crockard HA: Somatosensory evoked potential monitoring in cervical surgery: Identification of pre- and intraoperative risk factors associated with neurological deterioration. J Neurosurg 85:566–573, 1996.
19. Smith NJ, Beer D, Clark SA, et al: Monitoring cortical evoked potentials (EP) in operations on the cervical spine. In Jones SJ, Boyd S, Hetreed M, et al (eds): Handbook of Spinal Cord Monitoring: Proceedings of the Fifth International Symposium on Spinal Cord Monitoring. Dordrecht, Netherlands, Kluwer Academic, 1994, pp 216–221.
20. Derome PJ: Surgical management of tumours invading the skull base. Can J Neurol Sci 12:345–347, 1985.
21. Akalan N, Seckin H, Kilic C, Ozgen T: Benign extramedullary tumors in the foramen magnum region. Clin Neurol Neurosurg 96:284–289, 1994.
22. Germano A, Galatioto S, La Rosa G, et al: Xanthomatous poste-

rior pyramid meningioma in a 2-year-old girl. Childs Nerv Syst 13:406–411, 1997.

23. Handa J, Suzuki F, Nioka H, et al: Clivus chordoma in childhood. Surg Neurol 28:58–62, 1987.

24. Osenbach RK, Youngblood LA, Menezes AH: Atlanto-axial instability secondary to solitary eosinophilic granuloma of C2 in a 12-year-old girl. J Spinal Disord 3:408–412, 1990.

25. Sherk HH, Nicholson JT, Nixon JE: Vertebra plana and eosinophilic granuloma of the cervical spine in children. Spine 3:116–121, 1978.

26. Menezes AH, Gantz BJ, Traynelis VC, et al: Cranial base chordomas. Clin Neurosurg 44:491–509, 1997.

27. Crockard HA, Bradford R: Transoral transclival removal of a schwannoma anterior to the craniocervical junction: Case report. J Neurosurg 62:293–295, 1985.

28. Kobayashi S, Takemae T, Sugita K: Combined transsphenoidal and transoral approach for the clivus chordoma. No Shinkei Geka 12:1339–1346, 1984.

29. Seifert V, Laszig R: Transoral transpalatal removal of a giant premesencephalic clivus chordoma. Acta Neurochir (Wien) 112:141–146, 1991.

30. Cocke EW Jr, Robertson JH, Robertson JT, et al: The extended maxillotomy and subtotal maxillectomy for excision of skull base tumors. Arch Otolaryngol Head Neck Surg 116:92–104, 1990.

31. Arbit E, Patterson RH Jr: Combined transoral and median labio-mandibular glossotomy approach to the upper cervical spine. Neurosurgery 8:672–674, 1981.

32. Hall JE, Denis F, Murray J: Exposure of the upper cervical spine for spinal decompression by a mandible and tongue splitting approach: Case report. J Bone Joint Surg Am 59:121–123, 1977.

33. Honma A, Murota K, Shiba R, et al: Mandible and tongue-splitting approach for giant cell tumor of axis. Spine 14:1204–1210, 1989.

34. Moore LJ, Schwartz HC: Median labiomandibular glossotomy for access to the cervical spine. J Oral Maxillofac Surg 43:909–912, 1985.

35. Lalwani AK, Kaplan MJ, Gutin PH: The transsphenoethmoid approach to the sphenoid sinus and clivus. Neurosurgery 31:1008–1014, 1992.

36. Maira G, Pallini R, Anile C, et al: Surgical treatment of clival chordomas: The transsphenoidal approach revisited. J Neurosurg 85:784–792, 1996.

37. Janecka IP, Sen CN, Sekhar LN, et al: Facial translocation: A new approach to the cranial base. Otolaryngol Head Neck Surg 103:413–419, 1990.

38. Uttley D, Moore A, Archer DJ: Surgical management of midline skull base tumors: A new approach. J Neurosurg 71:705–710, 1989.

39. McAfee PC, Bohlman HH, Riley LH Jr, et al: The anterior retropharyngeal approach to the upper part of the cervical spine. J Bone Joint Surg Am 69:1371–1383, 1987.

40. Piper JG, Menezes AH: Management strategies for tumors of the axis vertebra. J Neurosurg 84:543–551, 1996.

41. Stevenson GC, Stoney RJ, Perkins RK, et al: A transcervical transclival approach to the ventral surface of the brain stem for removal of a clivus chordoma. J Neurosurg 24:544–551, 1966.

42. Dowd GC, Zeiller S, Awasthi D: Far lateral transcondylar approach: Dimensional anatomy. Neurosurgery 45:95–100, 1999.

43. Lot G, George B: Cervical neuromas with extradural components: Surgical management in a series of 57 patients. Neurosurgery 41:813–822, 1997.

44. Sen CN, Sekhar LN: An extreme lateral approach to intradural lesions of the cervical spine and foramen magnum. Neurosurgery 27:197–206, 1990.

45. Hakuba A, Nishimura S, Jang BJ: A combined retroauricular and preauricular transpetrosal-transtentorial approach to clivus meningiomas. Surg Neurol 30:108–116, 1988.

46. Samii M, Klekamp J, Carvalho G: Surgical results for meningiomas of the craniocervical junction. Neurosurgery 39:1086–1095, 1996.

47. Sen CN, Sekhar LN: The subtemporal and preauricular infratemporal approach to intradural structures ventral to the brain stem. J Neurosurg 73:345–354, 1990.

48. Gay E, Sekhar LN, Rubinstein E, et al: Chordomas and chondrosarcomas of the cranial base: Results and follow-up of 60 patients. Neurosurgery 36:887–897, 1995.

49. Raffel C, Wright DC, Gutin PH, et al: Cranial chordomas: Clinical presentation and results of operative and radiation therapy in twenty-six patients. Neurosurgery 17:703–710, 1985.

50. Heffelfinger MJ, Dahlin DC, MacCarty CS, et al: Chordomas and cartilaginous tumors at the skull base. Cancer 32:410–420, 1973.

51. Bottles K, Beckstead JH: Enzyme histochemical characterization of chordomas. Am J Surg Pathol 8:443–447, 1984.

52. Rich TA, Schiller A, Suit HD, et al: Clinical and pathologic review of 48 cases of chordoma. Cancer 56:182–187, 1985.

53. Forsyth PA, Cascino TL, Shaw EG, et al: Intracranial chordomas: A clinicopathological and prognostic study of 51 cases. J Neurosurg 78:741–747, 1993.

54. Plese JPP, Borges JM, Nudelman M, et al: Unusual subarachnoid metastasis of an intracranial chordoma in infancy. Childs Brain 4:251–256, 1978.

55. Watkins L, Khudodas ES, Kaleoglu M, et al: Skull base chordomas: A review of 38 patients, 1958–1988. Br J Neurosurg 7:241–248, 1993.

56. Amendola BE, Amendola MA, Oliver E, et al: Chordoma: Role of radiation therapy. Radiology 158:839–843, 1986.

57. Austin JP, Urie MM, Cardenosa G, et al: Probable causes of recurrence in patients with chordoma and chondrosarcoma of the base of skull and cervical spine. Int J Radiat Oncol Biol Phys 25:439–444, 1993.

58. Austin-Seymour M, Munzenrider J, Goitein M, et al: Fractionated proton radiation therapy of chordoma and low-grade chondrosarcoma of the base of the skull. J Neurosurg 70:13–17, 1989.

59. Berson AM, Castro JR, Petti P, et al: Charged particle irradiation of chordoma and chondrosarcoma of the base of the skull and cervical spine: The Lawrence Berkeley Laboratory experience. Int J Radiat Oncol Biol Phys 15:559–565, 1988.

60. Castro JR, Lindstadt DE, Bahary JP, et al: Experience in charged particle irradiation of tumors of the skull base: 1977–1992. Int J Radiat Oncol Biol Phys 29:647–655, 1994.

61. Suit HD, Griffin T, Almond P, et al: Particle radiation therapy. Cancer Treat Symp 1:147–160, 1984.

62. Kondziolka D, Lunsford LD, Flickinger JC: The role of radiosurgery in the management of chordoma and chondrosarcoma of the cranial base. Neurosurgery 29:38–46, 1991.

63. Corwin J, Lindberg RD: Solitary plasmacytoma of bone vs. extramedullary plasmacytoma and their relationship to multiple myeloma. Cancer 43:1007–1013, 1979.

64. Dimopoulos MA, Goldstein J, Fuller L, et al: Curability of solitary bone plasmacytoma. J Clin Oncol 10:587–590, 1992.

65. McLain RF, Weinstein JN: Solitary plasmacytoma of the spine: A review of 84 cases. J Spinal Disord 2:69–74, 1989.

66. Alexanian R, Dimopoulos M: The treatment of multiple myeloma. N Engl J Med 330:448–489, 1994.

67. Miyachi S, Negoro M, Sato K, et al: Myeloma manifesting as a large jugular tumor: Case report. Neurosurgery 27:971–977, 1990.

68. Bohlman HH, Sachs BL, Carter JR, et al: Primary neoplasms of the cervical spine: Diagnosis and treatment of twenty-three patients. J Bone Joint Surg Am 68:483–494, 1986.

69. Green NE, Robertson WW Jr, Kilroy AW: Eosinophilic granuloma of the spine with associated neural deficit: Report of three cases. J Bone Joint Surg Am 62:1198–1202, 1980.

70. Sanchez RL, Llovet J, Morena A: Symptomatic eosinophilic granuloma of the spine: Report of two cases and review of the literature. Orthopaedics 7:1721–1726, 1984.

71. Vera CL, Kempe LA, Powers JM: Plasmacytoma of the clivus presenting with an unusual combination of symptoms: Case report. J Neurosurg 52:857–861, 1980.

72. Ferguson L, Shapiro LM: Eosinophilic granuloma of the second cervical vertebra. Surg Neurol 11:435–437, 1979.

73. Di Lorenzo N, Palatinsky E, Bardella L, et al: Benign osteoblastoma of the clivus removed by a transoral approach: Case report. Neurosurgery 20:52–55, 1987.

74. Marsh BW, Bonfiglio M, Brady LP, et al: Benign osteoblastoma: Range of manifestations. J Bone Joint Surg Am 57:1–9, 1975.

75. Harada H, Kumon Y, Hatta N, et al: Neurofibromatosis type 2 with multiple primary brain tumors in monozygotic twins. Surg Neurol 51:528–535, 1999.

76. Barber DB, Quattrone BE, Lomba ME, Able AC: Neurofibromatosis: An unusual cause of cervical myopathy. J Spinal Cord Med 21:148–150, 1998.

77. Castellano F, Ruggiero G: Meningiomas of the posterior fossa. Acta Radiol Suppl (Stockh) 104:1–177, 1953.

78. Yamaki T, Ikeda T, Sakamoto Y, et al: Lymphoplasmacyte-rich meningioma with clinical resemblance to inflammatory pseudotumor: Report of two cases. J Neurosurg 86:898–904, 1997.

79. Carella RJ, Ransohoff J, Newall J: Role of radiation therapy in the management of meningioma. Neurosurgery 10:332–339, 1982.

80. Forbes AR, Goldberg ID: Radiation therapy in the treatment of meningioma: The Joint Center of Radiation Therapy experience 1970 to 1982. J Clin Oncol 2:1139–1143, 1984.

81. Mirimanoff RO, Dosoretz DE, Linggood RM, et al: Meningioma: Analysis of recurrence and progression following neurosurgical resection. J Neurosurg 62:18–24, 1985.

82. Petty AM, Kun LE, Meyer GA: Radiation therapy for incompletely resected meningiomas. J Neurosurg 62:502–507, 1985.

83. Muthukumar N, Kondziolka D, Lunsford LD, Flickinger JC: Stereotactic radiosurgery for anterior foramen magnum meningiomas. Surg Neurol 51:268–273, 1999.

84. Lin C, Node Y, Teramoto A: Treatment of posterior skull base tumors. Nippon Ika Daigaku Zasshi 65:316–319, 1998.

85. Bucci MN, McGillicuddy JE, Taren JA, Hoff JT: Management of anteriorly located C1-C2 neurofibromata. Surg Neurol 33:15–18, 1990.

86. Hu HP, Huang QL: Signal intensity correlation of MRI with pathological findings in spinal neurinomas. Neuroradiology 34:98–102, 1992.

87. Breeze RE, Nichols P, Segal JT, et al: Intradural epithelial cyst at the craniovertebral junction: Case report. J Neurosurg 73:788–791, 1990.

88. Koksel T, Revesz T, Crockard HA: Craniospinal neurenteric cyst. Br J Neurosurg 4:425–428, 1990.

89. Lee WY, Tseng HM, Lin MC, Chuang SM: Neurenteric cyst at craniocervical junction: Report of a case. J Formos Med Assoc 91:722–724, 1992.

90. Menezes AH, Ryken TC: Craniocervical intradural neurenteric cysts. Pediatr Neurosurg 22:88–95, 1995.

91. Stein BM: Spinal intradural tumors. In Wilkins RE, Rengachary S (eds): Neurosurgery. New York, McGraw-Hill, 1985, pp 1048–1061.

92. Friedman DP, Tartaglino LM, Flanders AE: Intradural schwannomas of the spine: MR findings with emphasis on contrast-enhancement characteristics. AJR Am J Roentgenol 158:1347–1350, 1992.

CHAPTER 312

Spinal Cord Tumors in Adults

THEODORE H. SCHWARTZ ■ PAUL C. MCCORMICK

Spinal cord tumors account for about 15% of central nervous system (CNS) neoplasms.[1] Most intradural tumors arise from the cellular constituents of the spinal cord and filum terminale, nerve roots, or meninges. Metastatic involvement of the spinal intradural compartment rarely manifests as a mass lesion. Intradural spinal cord tumors are broadly categorized according to their relationship to the spinal cord. Intramedullary tumors arise within the substance of the spinal cord, whereas extramedullary tumors are extrinsic to the spinal cord. A small number of neoplasms may have both intramedullary and extramedullary components that usually communicate either through a nerve root entry zone or the conus medullaris–filum terminale transition. Similarly, some intradural tumors may extend through the nerve root sleeve into the extradural compartment.

EXTRAMEDULLARY TUMORS

About two thirds of spinal cord tumors in adults are extramedullary (Table 312–1). Nerve sheath tumors, meningiomas, and filum terminale ependymomas account for most extramedullary neoplasms.[2] Metastases, inclusion tumors and cysts, paragangliomas, and melanocytic neoplasms are rare. With few exceptions, extramedullary tumors are histologically benign and amenable to complete surgical resection.

TABLE 312–1 ■ **Incidence of Tumors in Adults**

EXTRAMEDULLARY (Two Thirds of Cases)	%	INTRAMEDULLARY (One Third of Cases)	%
Nerve sheath tumor	40	Ependymoma	45
Meningioma	40	Astrocytoma*	40
Filum ependymoma	15	Hemangioblastoma	5
Miscellaneous**	5	Miscellaneous†	10

*Includes oligodendroglioma, ganglioglioma, neurocytoma, and subependymoma.
**Includes paraganglioma, drop metastases, granuloma.
†Includes metastatic tumor, inclusion tumor (e.g., lipoma), inflammation (e.g., abscess, tuberculosis, sarcoid), vascular condition (e.g., cavernous malformation, aneurysm).

Incidence and Etiology

Nerve Sheath Tumors. Nerve sheath tumors are categorized as schwannomas or neurofibromas. Although evidence from tissue culture, electron microscopy, and immunohistochemistry supports a common Schwann cell origin for neurofibromas and schwannomas, the morphologic heterogeneity of neurofibromas suggests participation of additional cell types such as perineural cells and fibroblasts. Neurofibromas and schwannomas merit separate consideration because of their distinct demographic, histologic, and biologic characteristics.

The histologic appearance of neurofibromas consists of an abundance of fibrous tissue and the conspicuous presence of nerve fibers within the tumor stroma.[3] Grossly, the tumor produces fusiform (plexiform) enlargement of the involved nerve, which makes it impossible to distinguish between tumor and nerve tissue. Multiple neurofibromas establish the diagnosis of neurofibromatosis (NF), but this syndrome should be considered even in patients with apparent solitary involvement. Both NF1 and NF2 are associated with nerve sheath tumors. Although neurofibromas predominate in NF1, schwannomas are more common in NF2.[4]

Schwannomas appear grossly as smooth globoid masses, which do not enlarge the nerve but are suspended eccentrically from it with a discrete attachment. Their histologic appearance consists of elongated bipolar cells with fusiform, darkly staining nuclei arranged in compact interlacing fascicles with a tendency toward palisade formation (Antoni-A). A loosely arranged pattern of stellate-shaped cells (Antoni-B) is less common.[5] Multiple schwannomas or "schwannomatosis" can occur in patients without NF, and these currently have no known genetic basis.[6, 7]

Nerve sheath tumors account for about 25% of intradural spinal cord tumors in adults,[2, 8] with an annual incidence of 0.3 to 0.4 per 100,000.[7] Most are solitary schwannomas that occur proportionally throughout the spinal canal (Fig. 312–1). The fourth through sixth decades of life represent the peak incidence of occurrence. Men and women are affected equally.

Most nerve sheath tumors arise from a dorsal nerve root. Neurofibromas represent a higher proportion of

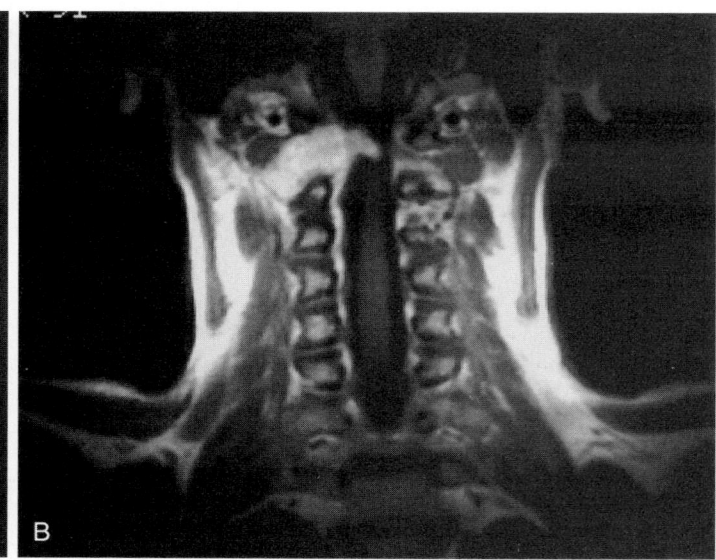

FIGURE 312–1. *A,* Axial T1-weighted magnetic resonance imaging (MRI) scan with contrast showing a dumbbell cervical schwannoma impinging on the spinal cord. *B,* Coronal MRI scan showing an extraforaminal component. *C,* Intraoperative photograph of the schwannoma showing extradural portion of the tumor *(arrows)*.

ventral root tumors and often exhibit dumbbell growth.[9] Most nerve sheath tumors are entirely intradural, but 30% extend through the dural root sleeve as a dumbbell tumor with both intradural and extradural components (see Fig. 312–1).[7] About 10% of nerve sheath tumors are epidural or paraspinal in location. Transdural growth is common in cervical tumors because the intradural root segment is short.[7] One percent of nerve sheath tumors are intramedullary and are thought to arise from the perivascular nerve sheaths that accompany penetrating spinal cord vessels.[7] Centripetal growth of a nerve sheath tumor may also result in subpial extension, most often with plexiform neuro-fibromas. In these cases, both intra- and extramedullary tumor components are apparent. Brachial or lumbar plexus neurofibromas may extend centrally into the intradural space along multiple nerve roots. Conversely, retrograde intraspinal extension of a paraspinal schwannoma usually remains epidural.

About 2.5% of intradural spinal nerve sheath tumors are malignant.[10] At least half occur in patients with NF. Malignant nerve sheath tumors carry a poor prognosis; survival rarely extends beyond 1 year. These tumors must be distinguished from the rare cellular schwannoma that displays aggressive histologic features but is associated with a favorable prognosis.

Meningiomas. Meningiomas and nerve sheath tumors occur with about equal frequency in adults. They usually arise from the arachnoid cap cells embedded in the dura near the root sleeve, accounting for their predominantly lateral location. Meningiomas may also arise from pia or dural fibroblasts, reflecting their probable mesodermal origin.[3]

Meningiomas arise in any age group, but the majority occur in individuals between the fifth and seventh decades of life. Seventy-five to 85% occur in women and about 80% are thoracic (Fig. 312–2).[2, 11–13] These demographics have led some to propose that a large fraction of spinal meningiomas is associated with microfractures in the osteoporotic spine.[14] The upper cervical spine and foramen magnum are also common sites.[15] Here, meningiomas often occupy a ventral or ventrolateral position and may adhere to the vertebral artery near its intradural entry and initial intracranial course (Fig. 312–3). Low cervical and lumbar meningiomas are rare. Most spinal meningiomas are entirely intradural, but about 10% may be both intradural and extradural or entirely extradural.[2]

Their gross characteristics range from smooth and fibrous to the more frequent variegated, fleshy, and friable appearance. Microscopic calcification may occur. The dural attachment is often broader than expected. *En plaque* examples are unusual but have been described.[16] The well-defined epidural space of the spine precludes bony involvement. Unlike intracranial meningiomas, spinal meningiomas do not penetrate the pia. This feature simplifies surgical resection and has been attributed to the presence of an "intermediate leptomeningeal layer" between the pia and arachnoid.[17] Another explanation is that spinal meningiomas manifest with signs of spinal cord compression early in their course and therefore are treated surgically before they have a chance to penetrate the pia.[17]

Filum Terminale Ependymomas. About 40% of spinal canal ependymomas arise within the filum terminale,[1] most in its proximal intradural portion. Astrocytomas, oligodendrogliomas, and paragangliomas can also originate in the filum terminale but are rare. Filum terminale ependymomas occur throughout life but are most common in the third to fifth decades. They occur in men slightly more often than in women. Filum ependymomas and cauda equina nerve sheath tumors occur with about equal frequency.

Myxopapillary ependymomas are by far the most common histologic type encountered in the filum terminale. Their histologic appearance consists of a papillary arrangement of cuboidal or columnar tumor cells surrounding a vascularized core of hyalinized and poorly cellular connective tissue.[5] Almost all are histologically benign.[18] These tumors, however, tend to be more biologically aggressive in younger age groups.[19]

Miscellaneous Pathologic Processes. Numerous neoplastic and non-neoplastic processes occasionally present as an extramedullary mass lesion. Dermoids, epidermoids, lipomas, teratomas, and neurenteric cysts

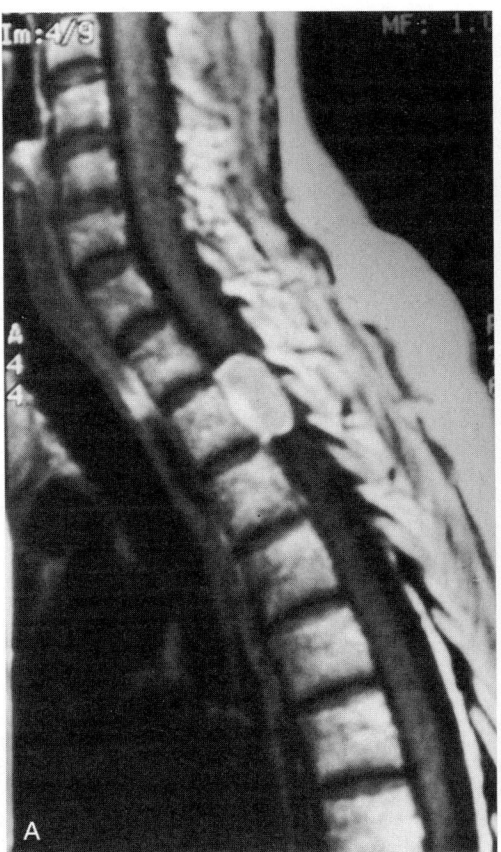
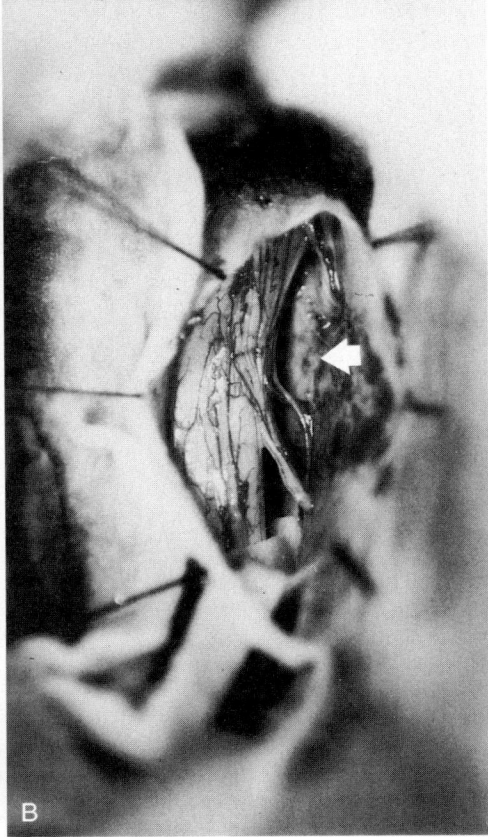

FIGURE 312–2. *A,* Sagittal gadolinium-enhanced MRI scan showing a ventral thoracic meningioma. *B,* Intraoperative photograph showing the resection cavity *(arrow)* anterior to the spinal cord after surgery.

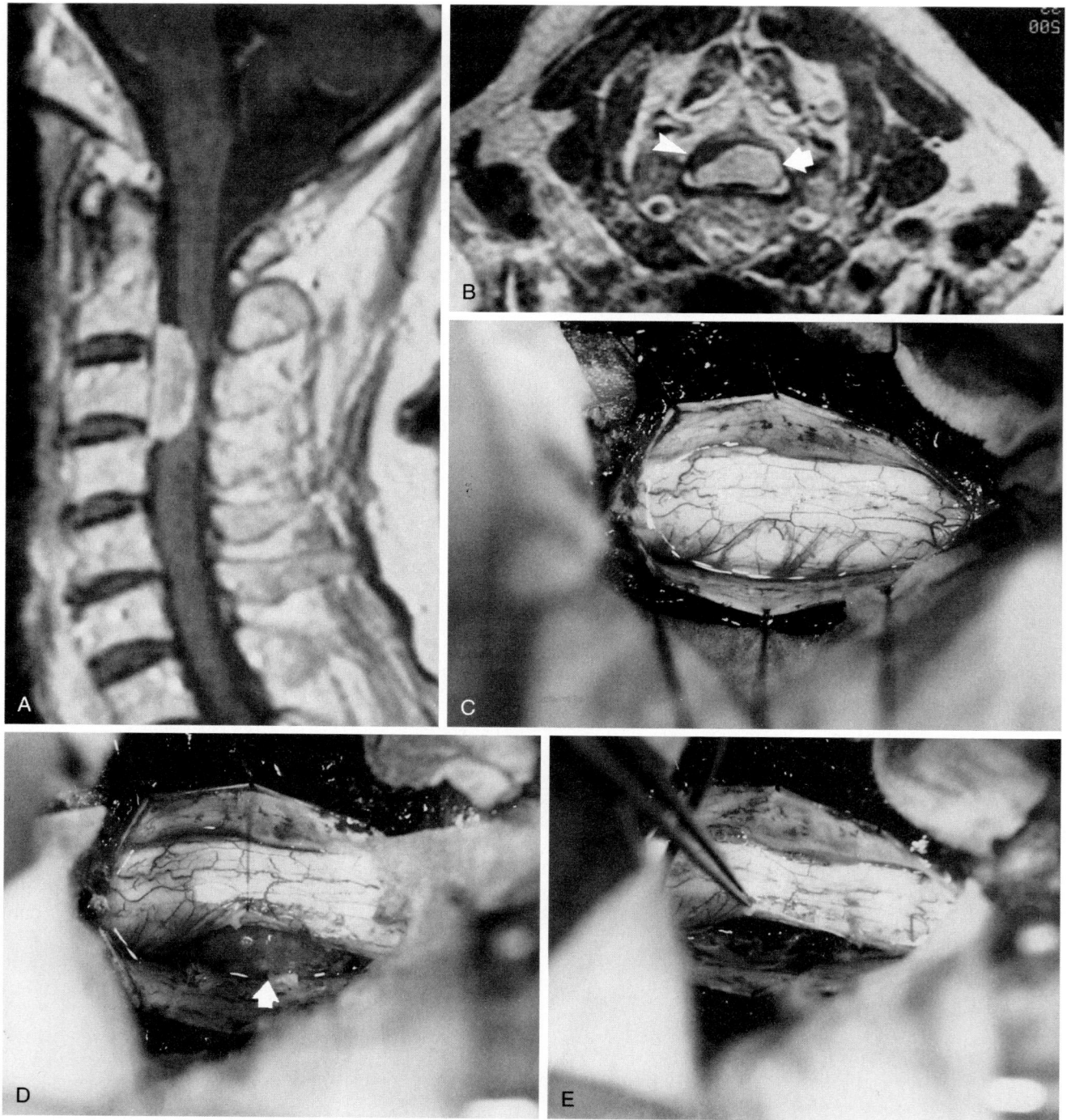

FIGURE 312–3. *A,* Gadolinium-enhanced MRI scan showing an upper cervical ventral meningioma. *B,* Axial MRI scan of the same lesion. *Arrow* indicates the enhancing tumor. *Arrowhead* demonstrates the compressed spinal cord. *C,* Intraoperative photograph showing the displacement of the spinal cord. *D,* Intraoperative photograph showing the tumor exposed after the pia has been opened and the dentate ligaments cut to rotate the spinal cord. Note the traction stitch on the dentate ligament. *Arrow* indicates tumor. *E,* Photograph of the cavity after resection.

are inclusion tumors and cysts that result from disordered embryogenesis.[20, 21] These lesions can occur throughout the spinal canal but are more common in the thoracolumbar and lumbar spine. They can be intramedullary or extramedullary. Associated anomalies such as metameric cutaneous lesions, sinus tracts, occult anterior or posterior rachischisis, or split cord malformations may be present.[20, 22] Inclusion tumors and cysts most often present as a mass lesion, but recurrent meningitis, tethered cord syndrome, or congenital deformity may represent the dominant clinical feature. In most cases, treatment consists of excision. A tethered spinal cord is released or a sinus tract is excised if necessary. In some cases, dense adherence of the lesion to neural structures precludes total extirpation.

Paragangliomas are rare tumors that originate from the neural crest origin and may arise from the filum terminale or cauda equina.[23] They are benign, nonfunctioning tumors and resemble extra-adrenal paraganglia (i.e., carotid body and glomus jugulare) histologically. Grossly, they appear as well-circumscribed vascular tumors that are indistinguishable clinically or radiographically from filum terminale ependymomas. Identification of dense core neurosecretory granules on electron microscopy establishes the diagnosis. Complete resection is usually possible. Cavernous malformations, hemangioblastomas, and ganglioneuromas may involve an intradural nerve root and present as an extramedullary mass lesion. Clinically, these tumors can manifest as nerve sheath tumors with early radicular symptoms. Ganglioneuromas often manifest as dumbbell tumors in pediatric patients. Subarachnoid hemorrhage has been associated with a nerve root cavernous malformation. These lesions are benign and are surgically removed. The involved nerve root is usually sacrificed, although occasionally it can be spared with small tumors.

Non-neoplastic lesions also manifest as extramedullary masses. Arachnoid cysts are a well-known example. They are most common in the thoracic spine dorsal to the spinal cord.[24] Intraspinal aneurysms are exceedingly rare. They usually occur in conjunction with arteriovenous malformations or coarctations of the aorta. Most isolated cases occur in the region of the foramen magnum and arise from the vertebral or posterior inferior cerebellar arteries. An anomalous vessel origin or course (i.e., kinking) is often described. Isolated spinal aneurysms have also been reported to arise from the anterior spinal artery, posterior spinal artery, and medullary arteries.[25] Most involve the anterior spinal artery. Patients with a spinal aneurysm can present with subarachnoid hemorrhage or compressive myelopathy. The definitive diagnosis is achieved with selective spinal angiography. Rarely, a herniated intervertebral disk transgresses the dura to occupy an intradural location.[26]

An inflammatory pathologic process such as sarcoidosis, tuberculoma, or subdural empyema occasionally manifests as an intradural mass lesion.[26, 27] Although spinal carcinomatous meningitis often complicates systemic cancer, secondary metastatic involvement of the spinal canal rarely manifests as a mass lesion. Malignant intracranial neoplasms that appose the subarachnoid space or ventricles are the most likely intracranial tumors to demonstrate cerebrospinal fluid (CSF) drop metastasis into the spinal subarachnoid space.[28] Systemic cancer gains access to the subarachnoid space through direct penetration of the dural root sleeve or, more commonly, through the choroid plexus.[29, 30] Surgical removal of a significant secondary neoplastic deposit may be appropriate in some cases.

Clinical Features

The clinical features of most extramedullary tumors reflect a slow-growing intraspinal mass. Specific clinical presentations are variable and are largely determined by tumor location (i.e., local pain and signs of compression of adjacent neural structures). Upper cervical and foramen magnum tumors are often located ventrally and become symptomatic with suboccipital pain and distal arm weakness with atrophy and clumsiness of the intrinsic hand muscles.[15] The cause of this well-known syndrome is uncertain but most likely results from venous insufficiency. Increased intracranial pressure and hydrocephalus rarely occur with extramedullary tumors at any level but are most common with upper cervical tumors.[31] This syndrome is probably caused by elevation of CSF protein, which impairs CSF flow and absorption. Segmental motor weakness and long tract signs are hallmarks of midlevel and lower cervical tumors. Asymmetrical early signs and symptoms are typical, reflecting the predominantly lateral location of most intradural tumors. A Brown-Séquard type of syndrome characterized by dysfunction of the corticospinal tract, posterior column, and contralateral spinothalamic tract dysfunction is common. Rarely, schwannomas present with subarachnoid hemorrhage.[32]

Long-tract complaints dominate the clinical presentation of thoracic tumors. The corticospinal tracts seem particularly vulnerable. Early signs of stiffness and fatigability eventually give way to spasticity. Weakness, especially dorsiflexion of the ankle and big toe, usually begins distally. Dorsal midline tumors may cause a sensory gait ataxia from bilateral compression of the posterior columns. Bowel and bladder function is not significantly impaired until late in the patient's clinical course. Ependymomas of the filum terminale most frequently manifest with back pain followed at variable intervals by asymmetrical radiation to both legs. Worsening pain on recumbency, an important clinical feature of extramedullary tumors, is most commonly associated with large cauda equina tumors.

Diagnostic Imaging

An intradural pathologic process is diagnosed with magnetic resonance imaging (MRI). Signal abnormalities, CSF capping, and spinal cord or cauda equina displacement identify most extramedullary masses on a technically adequate, nonenhanced MRI study. Lipomas, neurenteric cysts, dermoids or epidermoids, arachnoid cysts, or a vascular pathologic process can be diagnosed on the basis of MRI characteristics alone. Gadolinium enhancement markedly increases the sensitivity of MRI, particularly for small tumors.

On T1-weighted images, most intradural tumors are isointense or slightly hypointense with respect to the spinal cord. On T2-weighted images, nerve sheath tumors are more likely to be hyperintense to the spinal cord than are meningiomas, but exceptions exist. On both T1- and T2-weighted images, the signal intensity of cauda equina tumors usually is increased with respect to CSF. Small cauda equina tumors, however, are easily overlooked on nonenhanced images.[33]

Almost all spinal cord tumors demonstrate some degree of contrast enhancement. Meningiomas (see Figs. 312–2 and 312–3) typically exhibit intense uniform enhancement, although nonenhanced calcifications or intratumoral cysts occasionally occur. Enhancement of the adjacent dura (i.e., dural tail) strongly supports the diagnosis of meningioma.[34] Although most nerve sheath tumors and filum ependymomas demonstrate uniform uptake of contrast media, heterogeneous enhancement from intratumoral cysts, hemorrhage, or necrosis is common. A peritumoral hypointense rim is often present around meningiomas and corresponds with a well-formed peritumoral CSF space.[17]

Myelography and postmyelographic computed tomography (myelography-CT) are rarely used to evaluate intradural pathology. Nevertheless, the spatial resolution of a myelography-CT remains superior to that of MRI. When a tumor is closely applied to the surface of the spinal cord and whether it is intra- or extramedullary is equivocal on MRI, its location can be better resolved on myelography-CT. The intra- or extradural distribution of a paraspinal or dumbbell tumor is also better resolved with myelography-CT.

Treatment

Nerve Sheath Tumors. The treatment of benign nerve sheath tumors is complete surgical excision. In almost all cases, resection can be accomplished through a standard posterior laminectomy with partial or complete unilateral facetectomy as needed.[35, 36] Hemilaminectomy and unilateral facetectomy are options that can reduce postoperative pain and preserve spinal stability.[37] Recurrences are rare after gross total resection. Because these tumors grow slowly, subtotal resection is an option if neurologic deterioration is anticipated after complete resection. The rate of clinical recurrences after subtotal resection is 50%.[7] Most nerve sheath tumors are dorsal or dorsolateral to the spinal cord and are well visualized after the dura is opened. Ventral tumors may require section of a dentate ligament to achieve adequate visualization. Lumbar tumors may be covered by the cauda equina or conus medullaris. The nerve roots must be separated to provide adequate visualization. It is often possible to approach these tumors on one side of the cauda equina rather than approaching portions on either side of the cauda equina. This strategy permits a safe vector of traction to pull the tumor away from the cauda equina toward the lateral canal wall.

Once exposure is adequate, the correct plane of dissection (directly on the tumor surface) must be identified. The arachnoid membrane usually adheres to the tumor surface tightly. This is the fenestrated arachnoid layer, which separately ensheaths each dorsal and ventral nerve root within the subarachnoid space.[38] This layer is incised sharply and reflected off the surface of the tumor. The tumor capsule is cauterized to diminish its vascularity and to shrink the volume of the tumor. Tumor removal requires identification and division of the proximal and distal nerve root where the origin of the tumor attaches. With large tumors, this site may not be immediately apparent. Internal decompression with a laser or ultrasonic aspirator is used in such cases. The nerve root of origin usually must be sacrificed to remove the tumor. Occasionally, some fascicles of the nerve root may be preserved, especially with smaller tumors. The corresponding intradural nerve root, however, can usually be preserved because the fenestrated arachnoid sheaths allow anatomic separation of the dorsal and ventral nerve roots to a point just distal to the dorsal root ganglion. In a typical tumor of dorsal root origin, for example, it is possible to preserve the ventral root, which is tightly adherent to the ventral tumor surface.

Dumbbell extension through the nerve root sleeve, however, usually necessitates resection of the entire spinal nerve.[38] This resection rarely causes a significant deficit, even at cervical and lumbar enlargement levels. Presumably, the function of this root has already been compensated for by adjacent roots. A tumor with a very proximal origin may be partially embedded in the epipial tissue or may elevate the pia to occupy a subpial location. In such cases, the interface between the tumor and spinal cord may be difficult to develop. It may then be necessary to resect a segment of the pia to remove the tumor completely.

Significant tumor extension into the paraspinal region through an enlarged foramen increases the surgical considerations (see Fig. 312–1C). Surgical approaches are influenced by the surgeon's preference, size and location of the paraspinal tumor component, and intradural tumor extension. Preoperative determination of intradural tumor extension is particularly important. Although MRI adequately identifies various tumor components and relationships to both intraspinal and paraspinal structures, myelography-CT provides greater spatial resolution and more sensitive identification of intradural involvement of dumbbell tumors.

The cervical paraspinal region is difficult to access anteriorly because of the narrow confines of the neck and the numerous neurovascular structures such as the brachial plexus, descending lower cranial nerves, and vertebral artery. The mandible and skull base musculoskeletal attachments further limit upper cervical exposure. Fortunately, most cervical dumbbell tumors can be completely removed through an extended posterior exposure. A midline incision and standard laminectomy permit safe removal of both intra- and epidural intraspinal tumor components. Complete unilateral facetectomy allows paraspinal access up to 4 cm from the lateral dural margin.[36] The vertebral artery is consistently displaced anteromedially and is separated from the tumor capsule by periosteum and an extensive venous plexus. Some authors, however, prefer the anterolateral approach for cervical schwannomas below C2 because the facet is preserved and the vertebral artery can be controlled early.[39]

Although the destabilizing effects of unilateral cervical facetectomy cannot be predicted individually, a unilateral laminectomy may reduce the risk of instability.[37]

Unilateral laminectomy is not advised, however, if intraspinal exposure will be compromised. Alternatively, fusion of the contralateral intact facet joint with a lateral mass plate is an option.[36] Paraspinal extension from thoracic tumors can cause a large mass in the cavity. Standard posterior approaches provide inadequate exposure to the anterior paraspinal region. An anterior transpleural or extrapleural thoracotomy permits excellent visualization of the paraspinal region. Intraspinal access is more limited, however, and the spinal cord is not visualized until most of the tumor has been removed. Because of negative intrathoracic pressure and chest tube drainage, postoperative CSF pleural fistulas can occur if intradural exposure is required. A combination of both anterior and posterior exposures, either staged or consecutive, can be used. Thoracoscopic procedures may be useful for tumors located peripherally within the intercostal nerves or those that extend from the neural foramen into the chest without intradural extension.[40]

The lateral extracavitary approach is useful as a single-stage operation in cases that require concomitant complex exposure of intraspinal and paraspinal compartments.[41, 42] This exposure is achieved through a hockey stick incision and allows the surgeon to work on either side of the mobilized paraspinal muscles. The superficial thoracic scapular muscles (i.e., trapezius, rhomboid) are detached at the midline and rotated laterally with the skin flap to expose the longitudinally oriented paraspinal muscles. These muscles are mobilized off the posterior spinal elements and ribs. Rib resection and depression of the pleura provide extensive extrapleural paraspinal exposure lateral to the paraspinal muscles. Intraspinal exposure is obtained through a standard laminectomy medial to the paraspinal muscles. Circumferential stabilization, although rarely necessary after removal of dumbbell thoracic tumors, can also be performed through this exposure. CSF fistulas are not a significant problem because the pleural cavity is not entered.

Lumbar dumbbell tumors are also well exposed through the lateral extracavitary approach.[41, 42] At this level, the thoracodorsal fascia is incised in line with the skin incision and elevated laterally with the skin flap. Paraspinal tumor components in the lumbar spine are buried deep within the psoas muscle. Such components are difficult to remove safely through a retroperitoneal exposure because it is difficult to distinguish the tumor margins from the overlying elongated and blanched fibers of the psoas muscle. The lumbar nerve roots and their branches, including the femoral nerve, course through the psoas muscle. They are difficult to identify and subject to injury during retroperitoneal dissection of the psoas muscle.

The lateral extracavitary approach allows the tumor to be followed from the foramen into the psoas muscle. All dissection proceeds out on the surface of the tumor with minimal disruption of the psoas muscle. The nerves can be identified proximally, further minimizing the risk of neurologic injury. Intraspinal and intradural tumor extension can be managed easily through a laminectomy. The modest risk of instability after unilateral lumbar facetectomy probably does not justify a routine concomitant fusion procedure.

Dumbbell sacral tumors usually require both anterior and posterior exposures, which can be staged or performed simultaneously with the patient in a lateral position.[43]

Severe long-term adverse sequelae of surgical excision of schwannomas are rare. Unlike patients with neurofibromas, the life expectancy of patients with schwannomas parallels that of the general population.[7] Symptomatic arachnoiditis and cystic myelopathy may occur in 6% of patients within a few years after tumor removal.[7] More than half report some long-term local or radiating pain, but less than 10% seek medical attention.[7]

Meningiomas. Complete surgical removal is the treatment of choice for spinal meningiomas and can be achieved more than 90% of the time.[11] Favorable features relative to intracranial meningiomas include less difficult requirements for ventral exposure, absence of bony involvement because of the well-defined spinal epidural space, lack of venous sinus or major blood vessel involvement, and the presence of a peritumoral hypointense rim on MRI.[17, 38] Despite these favorable features, the recurrence rate of spinal meningiomas 10 years after gross total or nearly total removal is 10% to 15%.[44]

Posterior laminectomy provides adequate exposure in most cases. Unilateral laminectomy and facetectomy can be used for eccentrically located or ventral tumors. Large ventral tumors may also be approached satisfactorily through standard posterior exposures because the tumors have already retracted the spinal cord. Suture retraction on a divided dentate ligament or a noncritical dorsal root provides additional ventral exposure (see Fig. 312–3D). Depression of the paraspinal muscle mass with table-mounted retractors further facilitates ventral access. Alternatively, a costotransversectomy or lateral extracavitary approach can be used for ventral thoracic tumors.[41] The extreme lateral approach as described by Sen and Sekhar[45] is used when the tumor has a significant ventral component above the foramen magnum.

Despite these modifications, direct visualization of the entire tumor–spinal cord interface of ventrally located tumors may not be possible. Nevertheless, an arachnoid layer is almost invariably reflected over the central surface of the tumor. This plane is easily developed by gentle traction on the tumor away from the spinal cord. If a peritumoral hypointensity is not seen on MRI, blood vessels may be adherent to the surface of the tumor, but the pia is always intact.[17] *En plaque* meningiomas tend to be associated with a significant amount of arachnoid scarring, rendering surgery more difficult.[16]

Anterior approaches for intradural pathologic processes have been described.[46] Although they may be appropriate for small tumors and vascular lesions, these approaches are impractical and unnecessary for most intradural pathologic processes. These exposures are unfamiliar and provide limited intraspinal access.

The large postoperative dead space can create problems with CSF fistulas, particularly with meningiomas that require resection of the ventral dural origin when approached anteriorly. The epidural venous plexus is more developed ventrally and further enlarged with ventral dural tumor attachments. These vessels may cause troublesome bleeding during anterior exposures.

Various strategies can be used for tumor removal. Dorsal and dorsolateral meningiomas are delivered away from the spinal cord with traction on the open dural margins. A circumscribing excision of the dural origin completes the resection. For lateral and ventral tumors, the arachnoid over the exposed portion of the tumor is incised and reflected so that the dissection can proceed directly on the tumor's surface. The rostral and caudal poles of the tumor should be identified. Small cottonoid pledgets can be placed in the lateral canal gutters on either side of the tumor to minimize blood spillage into the subarachnoid space.

The exposed tumor surface is then cauterized to diminish the tumor's vascularity and to shrink its mass. Large tumors are bisected and debulked through a central trough. The tumor segment opposing the spinal cord is delivered into the resection cavity with gentle traction and surface dissection. The remaining dural base tumor is amputated from the dural attachment. The attachment is then coagulated extensively. Alternatively, the dural base can be excised and replaced with a thoracodorsal fascia patch graft. Blood and debris are irrigated from the subarachnoid space with warm saline. Arachnoid adhesions that hold the spinal cord in a deformed position are divided. These maneuvers may diminish the risk of postoperative complications—such as spinal cord tethering, arachnoiditis, delayed syrinx formation, and hydrocephalus—which occasionally complicate the removal of extramedullary tumors. Patching the dura with fascia lata may be necessary in certain circumstances.[16] Rarely, a spinal meningioma extends through a dural nerve root sleeve to present as a dumbbell tumor. The techniques for removal are similar to those already described for nerve sheath tumors. The nerve root at that level is usually sacrificed, but the risk of deficit after sacrifice is minimal, even with spinal meningiomas.

Management of the dural base is the most controversial aspect of treating spinal meningiomas. Options include excision of the dural origin with patch graft reconstruction or extensive in situ coagulation. Solero and colleagues[13] found no significant difference in recurrence rates between these two maneuvers. After complete resection, long-term recurrence rates have ranged between 3% and 23%.[8, 11, 13, 16] Therefore, management of the dural base is determined by practical considerations. Removal of dorsal and dorsolateral meningiomas is facilitated by excision of the dural base. Tumors of the ventral half of the canal, however, are amputated flush with the dura. The dural origin is then coagulated extensively.

Filum Terminale Ependymomas. The role of surgery for filum terminale ependymomas depends on the size of the tumor and its relationship to the surrounding roots of the cauda equina. Gross total en bloc resection should be attempted when possible. It can usually be accomplished for small and moderate tumors that remain well circumscribed within the fibrous coverings of the filum terminale and easily separable from the nerve roots of the cauda equina. Typically, a portion of uninvolved filum terminale is present between the tumor and spinal cord. The afferent and efferent filum segments must be amputated to remove the tumor. Internal decompression can increase the risk of CSF dissemination and therefore is not used for small and moderate-sized tumors. Recurrences after successful en bloc resection are rare.

Large ependymomas of the filum terminale, however, can be difficult to resect surgically. Typically, they are present for many years and are associated with a risk of being disseminated via the CSF. When a large cauda equina mass is identified, the entire neuraxis should be evaluated by MRI before surgical treatment. These tumors may become enormous within the capacious thecal sac before they are diagnosed. These unencapsulated, pliable neoplasms can insinuate among the nerve roots and within the arachnoid sheaths of the cauda equina, compartmentalized by innumerable arachnoid septa. They can also spread as contiguous tumor sheaths along the arachnoid septa, which act as a scaffolding for surface growth. CSF dissemination may have already occurred because of their location in the subarachnoid space. In such cases, tumor removal is necessarily piecemeal and almost always subtotal. Indeed, dense tumor attachments to the roots of the cauda equina are associated with significant risks of postoperative deficits because so much manipulation would be required for tumor resection. In these cases, subtotal removal aimed at diminishing the tumor bulk is all that can be accomplished. Even when piecemeal gross total removal is achieved, a recurrence rate of at least 20% can be anticipated.[18, 19, 47]

If a total or nearly total piecemeal removal has been achieved, patients can be followed with serial gadolinium-enhanced MRI, which provides some insight into the natural history of the tumor. Biologically aggressive tumors, which are more common in the younger population, demonstrate early tumor recurrence and can be treated with radiation therapy. If significant tumor burden is present after the initial surgery, however, particularly in the case of known CSF dissemination, postoperative radiation therapy is the primary adjunctive treatment modality. Postoperative radiation therapy is delayed if a piecemeal total or nearly total removal has been accomplished. In these cases, tumor recurrences can be treated with repeat surgery and followed by radiation therapy. Although the response of spinal cord ependymomas to radiation therapy is unpredictable, some evidence suggests that it offers long-term control.[48] This response, however, cannot be predicted individually. Because prior radiation therapy markedly increases the morbidity rate of future surgical prospects, it is typically delayed if further surgery may be contemplated.

INTRAMEDULLARY TUMORS

A wide variety of pathologic processes can arise from or secondarily involve the spinal cord as mass lesions.

Primary glial tumors account for at least 80% of intramedullary tumors in most series[49–53] and include astrocytomas, ependymomas, and less common glial neoplasms such as gangliogliomas, oligodendrogliomas, and subependymomas (see Table 312–1). Hemangioblastomas account for 3% to 8% of intramedullary neoplasms.[54] Inclusion tumors and cysts, metastases, nerve sheath tumors, neurocytomas, and melanocytomas account for most of the remaining intramedullary mass lesions. Metastatic involvement of the spinal cord accounts for fewer than 5% of intramedullary spinal cord tumors. Lung and breast are the most common primary tumor sites.

Clinically and radiographically, non-neoplastic processes may present as intramedullary mass lesions. Examples include inflammatory conditions such as bacterial abscess, tuberculoma, inflammatory pseudotumor, sarcoidosis, multiple sclerosis, viral or parainfectious myelitis, paraneoplastic involvement, or an intermediate entity between multiple sclerosis and acute disseminated encephalomyelitis.[26, 55–57] An acute or subacute clinical course, characteristic of systemic involvement, further suggests the diagnosis. These conditions are associated with an acute or subacute my-

elopathy that advances rapidly over several hours to a few days but rarely longer. With demyelinating disease, the course occasionally is chronic and progressive or recurring. Operative intervention in such patients should be undertaken with caution because tiny biopsy specimens tend to yield a nonspecific, inflammatory response and rarely provide the diagnosis or determine the medical treatment. Advances in imaging and microsurgical techniques have allowed surgery to evolve rapidly into the primary or even definitive treatment modality for most benign intramedullary neoplasms in adults.

Incidence and Etiology

Astrocytomas. About 3% of central nervous system astrocytomas arise within the spinal cord (Fig. 312–4).[1] These tumors occur at any age but seem most prevalent in the first three decades of life. By far, they are the most common pediatric intramedullary spinal cord tumor. They compose about 90% of intramedullary tumors in patients younger than 10 years and about 60% of adolescent intramedullary neoplasms. Almost 60% of these tumors occur in the cervical and cervicothora-

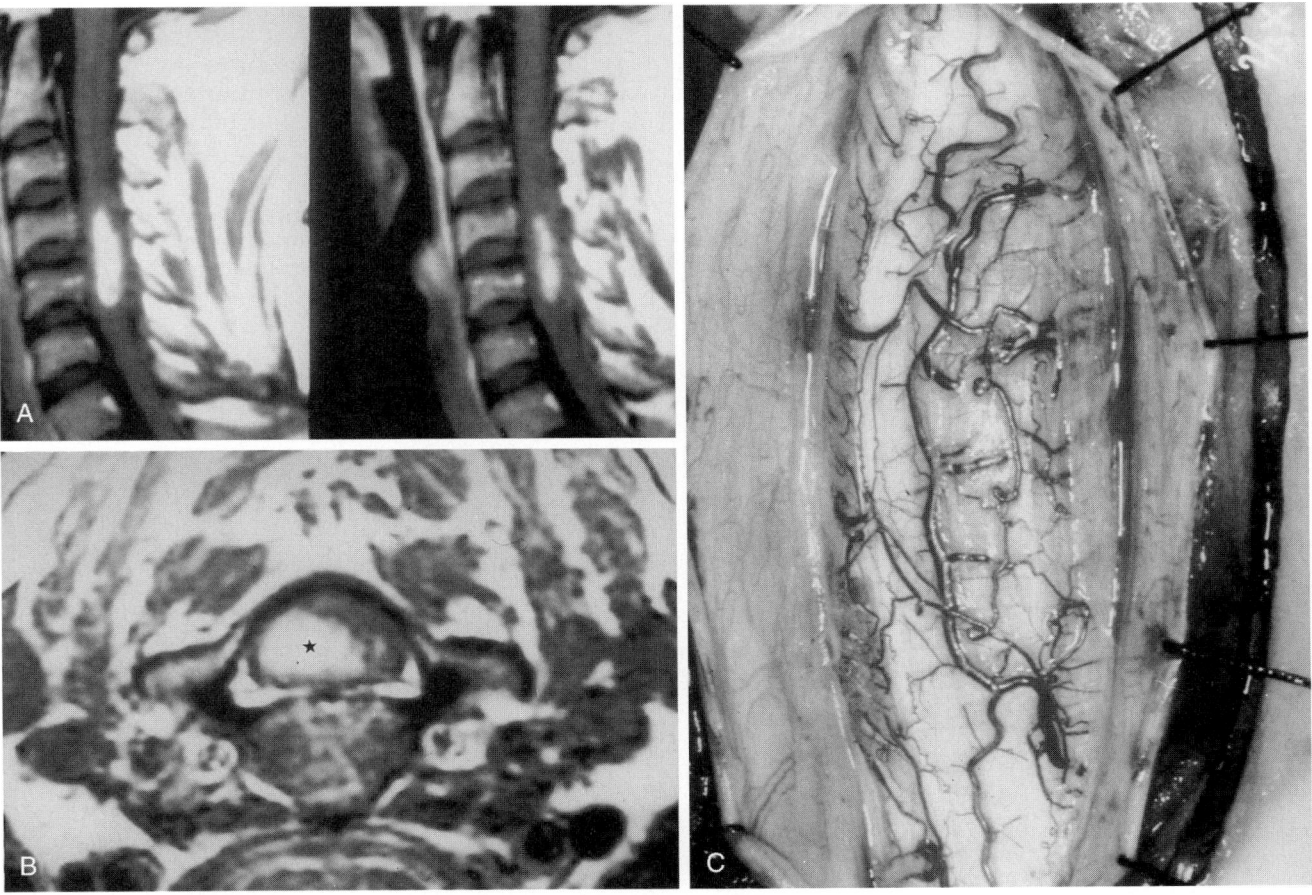

FIGURE 312–4. *A*, T1-weighted MRI scans with gadolinium showing an intramedullary astrocytoma with patchy enhancement with irregular borders. *B*, Axial MRI scan of the same lesion. *Asterisk* indicates enhancing tumor. *C*, Intraoperative photograph showing the enlarged spinal cord. The dural sutures maintain the exposure.

cic region,[50] and 20% have associated syringes.[58] Thoracic, lumbosacral, or conus medullaris locations are less common. Filum terminale examples are rare. There is an association between NF1 and intramedullary astrocytomas.[59]

Spinal cord astrocytomas are a heterogeneous group with respect to histologic features, gross characteristics, biologic features, and natural history. They include low-grade fibrillary and pilocytic astrocytomas, malignant astrocytomas and glioblastomas, gangliogliomas, and the rare oligodendrogliomas. Most are grade I or II fibrillary astrocytomas. Juvenile pilocytic astrocytomas and gangliogliomas are more common among the pediatric population. The designation of a pilocytic astrocytoma in an adult usually reflects an abundance of pilocytic features, which occur as secondary structures in an otherwise typical fibrillary astrocytoma.[3] Whether these pilocytic features have prognostic significance is unclear. About 25% of adult astrocytomas are malignant (Fig. 312–5).[50, 60]

Ependymomas. Ependymomas are the most common intramedullary tumors in adults.[61] They occur throughout life but are most common in the middle adult years. Men and women are equally affected. Approximately 65% have associated syringes, particularly when cervical locations are involved.[58] There is an association between NF2 and intramedullary ependymomas.[59] Most sporadic ependymomas also manifest mutations in the NF2 gene.[62] A variety of histologic subtypes may be encountered. The cellular ependymoma is the most common variety, but epithelial, tanycytic (fibrillar), subependymoma, myxopapillary, or mixed examples can occur. Almost all are histologically benign.[3, 50, 52, 60, 63] Although unencapsulated, these glial-derived tumors are usually well circumscribed and do not infiltrate adjacent spinal cord tissue (Fig. 312–6).

Hemangioblastomas. Hemangioblastomas account for 3% to 8% of intramedullary tumors.[54] Fifteen to 25% are associated with von Hippel–Lindau's syndrome, an autosomal dominant trait with incomplete penetrance and incomplete expression.[54] These tumors arise at any age but are rare in early childhood. Associated syringes are common.[58] Hemangioblastomas are benign tumors of vascular origin. They are sharply circumscribed but not encapsulated. Almost all have a pial attachment. Most are located dorsally or dorsolaterally (Fig. 312–7).

Miscellaneous Pathologic Processes. Inclusion tumors and cysts are rarely intramedullary. Lipomas are the most common dysembryogenic lesion and account for about 1% of intramedullary tumors (Fig. 312–8). They enlarge and produce symptoms in the early and middle adult years through increased fat deposition in metabolically normal fat cells. Because they occupy a subpial location, they are considered juxtamedullary. Metastases account for fewer than 5% of intramedullary tumors, probably because of the small size of the spinal cord and its remote vascular accessibility to hematogenous tumor emboli.[64] Lung and breast are the most common primary tumor sites. Melanocytomas, melanomas, fibrosarcomas, and primitive neuroectodermal tumors can also arise in an intramedullary location.[26, 65] The appearance of radiation necrosis can mimic an intramedullary tumor, but a history of radiation therapy to the appropriate level is needed to confirm its diagnosis.[66] Cavernous malformations, amyloid angiopathy, and other unusual intramedullary vascular lesions can also manifest as an intramedullary mass (Fig. 312–9).[56, 67]

Clinical Features

The clinical features of intramedullary spinal cord tumors are variable. Early symptoms are usually nonspe-

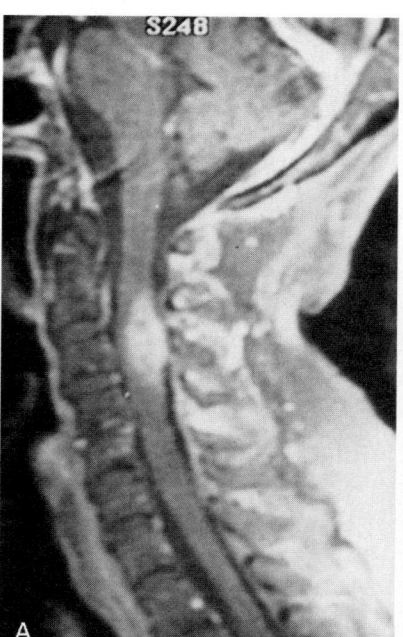
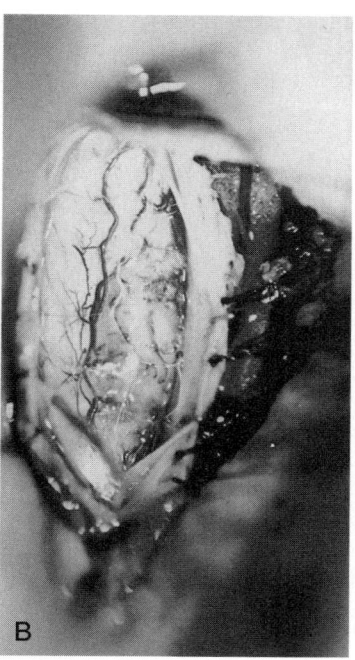

FIGURE 312–5. *A*, T1-weighted sagittal MRI scan with contrast showing a malignant intramedullary astrocytoma breaking through the dorsal surface of the spinal cord. *B*, Intraoperative photograph showing that the pial margin has been compromised.

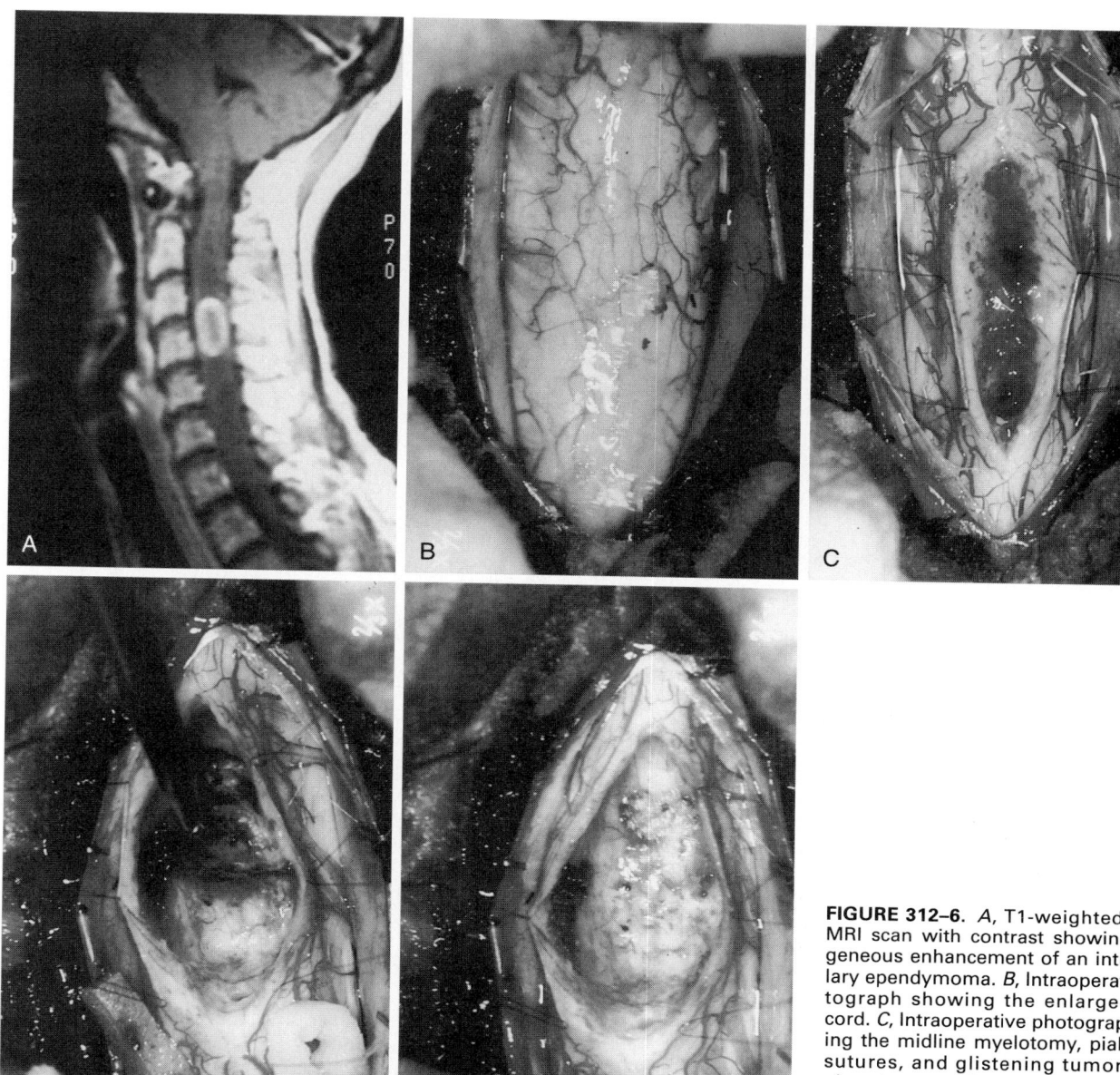

FIGURE 312–6. *A*, T1-weighted sagittal MRI scan with contrast showing homogeneous enhancement of an intramedullary ependymoma. *B*, Intraoperative photograph showing the enlarged spinal cord. *C*, Intraoperative photograph showing the midline myelotomy, pial traction sutures, and glistening tumor. *D*, The plane between the tumor and spinal cord is developed for gross total resection. *E*, After resection, a piece of Surgicel is placed for hemostasis.

cific, and their progression may be subtle. Symptoms are often present 3 to 4 years before diagnosis.[49, 53] The course of malignant or metastatic neoplasms is much-briefer, in the range of several weeks to a few months.[49, 53] Intratumoral hemorrhage can cause an abrupt deterioration, a presentation most often associated with ependymomas. In adults, pain and weakness are the most frequent presenting symptoms of intramedullary spinal cord tumors.[49, 50, 53, 68, 69] The pain typically localizes to the level of the tumor and is rarely radicular. The distribution and progression of the symptoms are related to the tumor's location. Upper extremity symptoms predominate with cervical neoplasms. Thoracic tumors produce spasticity and sensory disturbances. Numbness is a common complaint and typically begins distally in the legs and progresses proximally. Tumors of the lumbar enlargement and conus medullaris often become symptomatic with back and leg pain. The leg pain may be radicular. Urogenital and anorectal dysfunction tend to occur early.

Diagnostic Imaging

Gadolinium-enhanced MRI is the procedure of choice for preoperative evaluation of an intramedullary tumor.[70] Spinal cord enlargement and tumor enhancement are the characteristic findings. On T1-weighted images, most intramedullary tumors are isointense or slightly hypointense to the surrounding spinal cord.[70] On T1-weighted images, spinal cord enlargement is

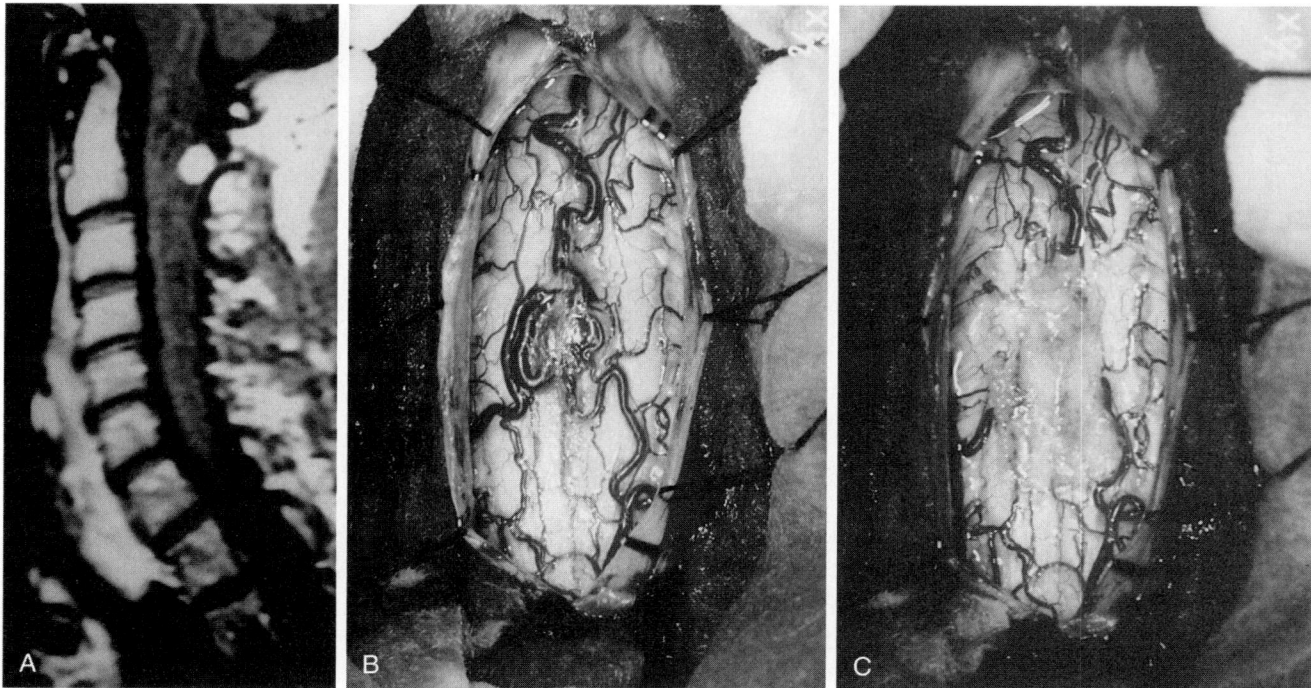

FIGURE 312–7. *A,* Sagittal MRI scan showing the dorsal location of an enhancing hemangioblastoma. *B,* Intraoperative photograph showing the tumor at the surface of the spinal cord. *C,* Intraoperative photograph of the tumor bed after resection.

often ill defined. Because most tumors are hyperintense to the spinal cord on T2-weighted images, they are the most sensitive for tumor identification.[70] Almost all intramedullary neoplasms demonstrate contrast uptake. Ependymomas usually demonstrate uniform contrast enhancement and are symmetrically located within the spinal cord (see Fig. 312–6A). Polar cysts are found in most cases, particularly in cervical and cervicothoracic locations.[58] Heterogeneous enhancement from intratumoral cysts or necrosis can be seen with ependymomas.

The appearance of astrocytomas on MRI is much more variable. On contrast-enhanced MRI, these tumors tend to be less well defined than ependymomas because of their irregular margins. Contrast uptake may be minimal, uniform, or patchy (see Figs. 312–4A and B).[70] Heterogeneous uptake and patchy irregular margins are common with astrocytomas because of intratumoral cysts or necrosis. Despite the characteristic pattern of astrocytomas on MRI, their appearance on MRI overlaps with that of other tumors, precluding competent histologic diagnosis of tumor type based on MRI characteristics alone.

The appearance of inflammatory conditions on MRI is variable and probably related to etiology.[56] Acute multiple sclerosis plaque, for example, usually demonstrates focal homogeneous contrast enhancement confined to white matter. There is minimal, if any, spinal cord enlargement. Patchy contrast enhancement over several spinal cord segments is more characteristic of viral or parainfectious myelitis. Leptomeningeal enhancement can be seen with lymphomas, metastases, and bacterial, fungal, or tuberculous myelitis.[70] Radiation necrosis may appear as a ring-enhancing lesion on T1-weighted images. High-intensity signal on T2-weighted images and spinal cord enlargement make the differentiation of radiation necrosis from intramedullary tumor difficult.[66]

Treatment

The role of surgery in the management of intramedullary spinal cord tumors has evolved considerably. Once used for diagnosis alone, surgery now represents the most effective treatment for benign, well-circumscribed tumors.[49–53, 60, 68] Most intramedullary spinal cord neoplasms are low-grade lesions; therefore, long-term tumor control or cure with preservation of neurologic function can be achieved in most patients with microsurgical removal alone.[49–53, 60, 68]

The most important factor in determining the surgical objective is the plane between the tumor and the spinal cord. This interface can be assessed accurately only through an adequate myelotomy that extends over the entire rostrocaudal extent of the tumor (see Fig. 312–6C). Although the presence of a syrinx may improve the chances of achieving gross total resection, it cannot be used as an independent predictor of outcome.[58] Benign tumors such as ependymomas and hemangioblastomas, although unencapsulated, are noninfiltrative lesions that typically display a distinct plane. Gross total removal is the treatment of choice in such cases (see Fig. 312–6E). Astrocytomas are more variable. Although some benign astrocytomas are well

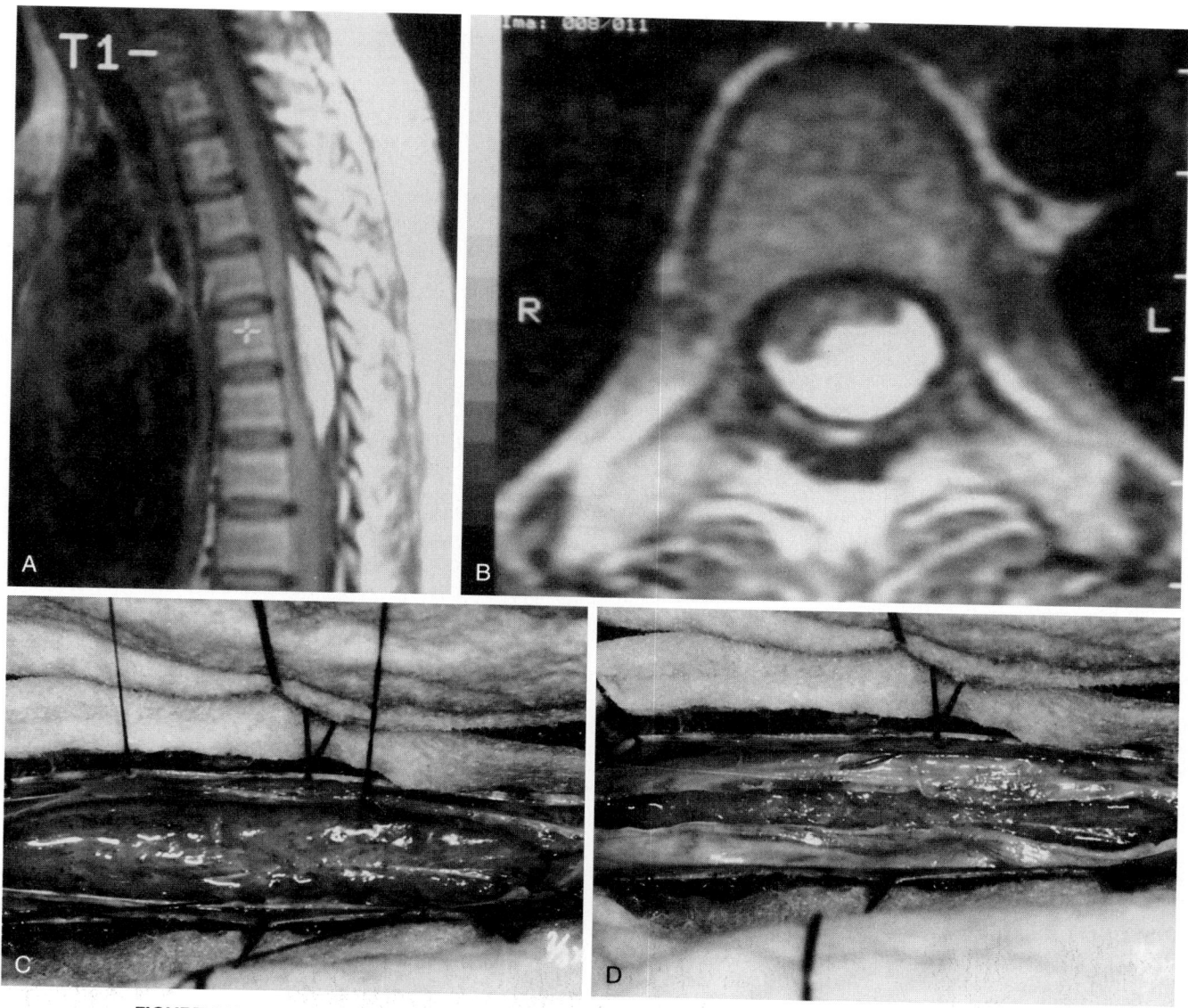

FIGURE 312–8. *A,* T1-weighted sagittal MRI scan without contrast showing the high-intensity signal from a dorsal lipoma. *B,* Axial MRI scan of the same lesion. *C,* Intraoperative photograph showing the lipoma at the surface of the spinal cord. *D,* Intraoperative photograph showing the tumor bed after resection.

circumscribed and allow gross total resection, most exhibit variable infiltration into the surrounding spinal cord (see Fig. 312–6E). This infiltration is often reflected in a gradual transition zone between the tumor and spinal cord. More peripheral dissection beyond what is clearly tumor tissue risks damaging neurologic function by resecting infiltrative yet functionally viable spinal cord parenchyma. Thus, the surgical objective for spinal cord astrocytomas remains unclear. Specifically, a definitive correlation between the extent of resection and tumor control has not been established.[50, 58, 69] Preservation of neurologic function, rather than complete tumor resection, is the more prudent treatment objective in such cases. Therefore, tumor removal is limited to tissue that is clearly distinguishable from the surrounding spinal cord. The extent of tumor removal therefore varies.

Management of less common intramedullary mass lesions is also dictated by the nature of the interface between the tumor and spinal cord. Metastatic spinal cord tumors, for example, usually present as a well-circumscribed focal mass amenable to gross total resection. Intramedullary lipomas are inclusion tumors that result from disordered embryogenesis, probably the defective cleavage of germ cell layers. They are not true neoplasms but probably enlarge slowly through continued fat deposition of metabolically normal cells. Gross total resection is impossible because these lesions insinuate into functional spinal cord tissue at their margins. In most cases, conservative internal decompression results in long-term clinical stabilization (see Fig. 312–8D).

Intraoperative biopsy can be useful in certain circumstances but should not be used as the sole criterion

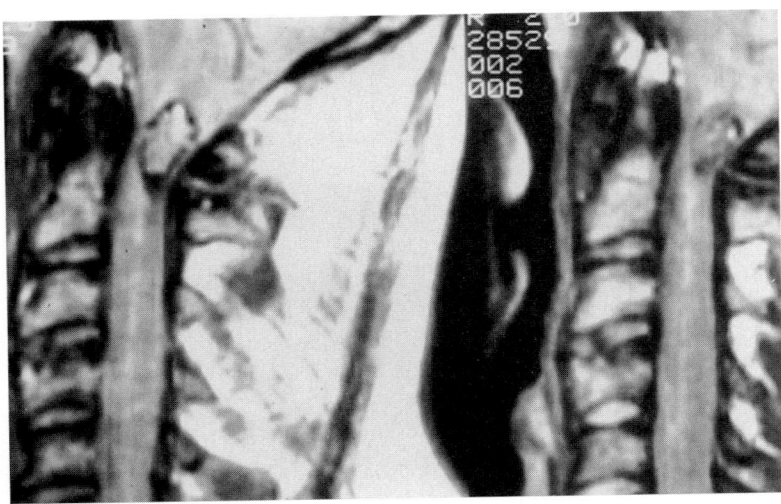

FIGURE 312–9. T2-weighted MRI scans showing an intramedullary cavernous malformation with its characteristic dark ring of hemosiderin.

dictating the surgical objective. First, interpretation of tiny biopsy fragments often is inaccurate or nondiagnostic and may consist of only peritumoral gliosis that can be interpreted erroneously as an infiltrating astrocytoma. Second, it is difficult, if not impossible, to assess the nature of the tumor–spinal cord interface accurately through a tiny myelotomy. Biopsy results, however, can sometimes be particularly helpful. Identification of a histologically malignant tumor, for example, independently signals an end to the procedure because surgery does not benefit malignant intramedullary neoplasms.[50, 71, 72] When the tumor–spinal cord interface is not apparent, confident histologic identification of an ependymoma reassures the surgeon that a plane must exist and that surgical removal should continue.

Surgical Technique. After intubation and perioperative administration of steroids and antibiotics, the patient is turned to the prone position. A Mayfield skull clamp is used for cervical and upper thoracic lesions. Neck flexion and head elevation (i.e., military prone) reduce the spinal curvature at these levels. Sensory and motor evoked potentials are monitored throughout the procedure.[73, 74] Sensory potentials disappear after a midline myelotomy and do not predict postoperative motor function. Subdural and epidural motor evoked potentials can be monitored in 60% of patients and provide real-time feedback. A 50% decline in the amplitude of motor evoked potentials can be an indication of a new, permanent postoperative weakness.[74]

A midline incision and subperiosteal bony dissection are carried out. A standard laminectomy, which should extend at least one segment above and below the solid tumor component, is performed. The facets are preserved. In adults, delayed instability rarely follows laminectomy for intramedullary tumor removal. Although laminoplasty may be a reasonable option,[49, 68] it is unnecessary in adults. Strict hemostasis must be secured before the dura is opened to prevent ongoing blood contamination of the dependent microsurgical field. Wide, moist, cottonoid wall-offs cover the exposed muscles. Oxidized cellulose (Surgicel, Johnson &

Johnson, Arlington, Tex) is spread generously over the lateral gutters to prevent contamination of blood in the operative field.

The dura is opened in the midline and tented laterally to the muscles with sutures, and the operating microscope is brought into the field (see Fig. 312–4C). The arachnoid is opened separately. The spinal cord is inspected for surface abnormalities. Some authors have commented that even during a first operation, arachnoid scarring and pial tethering can complicate the resection, and their presence predicts a poor functional outcome.[58, 68] In our experience, this phenomenon is rare. Most glial tumors cause only localized spinal cord enlargement. The spinal cord may be rotated. Occasionally, the overlying spinal cord may be thinned or even made transparent by a large or eccentrically located tumor or polar cyst. Ultrasonography is useful for tumor localization and to ensure adequate bony exposure.[75] Malignant neoplasms can replace surface spinal cord tissue or fungate through the pia into the subarachnoid space, or both (see Fig. 312–5B). Most hemangioblastomas arise from the dorsal half of the spinal cord with a visible pial attachment (see Fig. 312–7B).

A standard midline myelotomy is performed through the posterior median septum. The dorsal midline can be estimated accurately by noting the midpoint between the dorsal nerve root entry zones bilaterally. Small veins that exit from the septum also assist in establishing the midline. Midline crossing vessels in the pia are cauterized and divided. The pia is a robust, glistening white membrane with longitudinal striations. It must be incised sharply with a microknife or scissors. The myelotomy should extend over the entire rostrocaudal extent of the tumor. The myelotomy is deepened by spreading the posterior columns gently with microforceps or dissectors.

The tumor is first encountered in the area where the spinal cord is enlarged maximally. The dissection continues on the surface of the tumor until the entire rostrocaudal extent has been identified. Polar cysts are entered and drained when present. Once the entire dorsal extent of the tumor has been identified, 6–0 pial traction sutures are placed (see Fig. 312–6C). Small mosquito clamps on the sutures provide constant superior and lateral retraction of the spinal cord.

The technique of tumor removal is determined by the surgical objective and by the gross and histologic characteristics and size of the tumor. If no plane is apparent between tumor and surrounding spinal cord, the tumor is likely infiltrative. A biopsy is obtained to establish a histologic diagnosis. If an infiltrating or malignant astrocytoma is identified and consistent with the intraoperative findings, further tumor removal is unwarranted. In most cases, however, a reasonably well-defined benign glial tumor is identified. Ependymomas have a smooth, reddish gray glistening tumor surface that is sharply demarcated from the surrounding spinal cord (see Fig. 312–6C). Variable blood vessels cross the surface of the tumor, distinguishing these tumors from astrocytomas, which rarely display these surface characteristics. Traction on the surface of the tumor is used against the countertraction provided by the pial sutures, allowing the dissection plane to be developed (see Fig. 312–6D). Small feeding blood vessels and fibrous adhesions between the spinal cord and tumor are cauterized and divided. Large tumors may require internal decompression with an ultrasonic aspirator or laser. Once the tumor has been debulked significantly, the lateral and ventral margins can be dissected. The ventral tumor margin is developed by applying traction to a tumor pole, perpendicular to the long axis of the spinal cord. Feeding arteries from the anterior spinal artery are easily identified, cauterized, and divided.

Most benign astrocytomas present various degrees of circumscription. About a third of adult patients have benign, infiltrative tumors without an identifiable tumor mass. Biopsy for diagnosis is the only option for these patients. Occasionally, an astrocytoma may be so well developed as to mimic an ependymoma. Nevertheless, astrocytomas rarely have a plane as well defined as that of ependymomas. Dissection on the surface of an astrocytoma usually develops laminated pseudoplanes. Decompression is achieved with an ultrasonic aspirator or laser and proceeds systematically from the center of the tumor radially to the surface. Although most astrocytomas do not have a clean plane, the tumor is often a different color than the spinal cord. Surgeons must rely on their own judgment and experience. If gross tumor is easily identified, continued removal is reasonable. Changes in motor potentials or uncertainty about the spinal cord tumor interface should terminate the attempt at resection.

Removal of hemangioblastomas is facilitated by excising the pial attachment as part of the tumor mass. After the surface vessels have been cauterized, an incision is circumscribed around the pial base. The portion of the tumor buried within the spinal cord is easily dissected and delivered by applying traction to the pial base. A small polar myelotomy can improve visualization of larger tumors. These neoplasms cannot be decompressed internally, but cauterizing the surface shrinks the tumor to a more manageable size.

After an intramedullary tumor has been removed, the resection bed is inspected and bleeding points are controlled with warm saline or oxidized cotton. Pial traction sutures are removed to allow the spinal cord to assume its normal position. The myelotomy is not closed. The dura is usually closed primarily, although a dural patch graft may prevent dorsal tethering of the spinal cord at the operative site—a potential cause of postoperative morbidity. An autologous fascia lata or thoracodorsal fascia patch graft can be used. The remainder of the wound is closed in standard fashion. Meticulous closure techniques are especially important for reoperations or a previously irradiated spine, both of which are associated with a high risk of postoperative CSF fistula.

Early mobilization is encouraged to prevent complications of recumbency such as deep venous thrombosis and pneumonia. Paretic patients are particularly vulnerable to thromboembolic complications. Subcutaneous heparin (5000 units twice daily) is started on the second postoperative day. Orthostatic hypotension occasionally occurs after upper thoracic and cervical intramedullary neoplasms have been removed. This problem is usually self-limiting and can be managed with liberalization of fluids and gradual mobilization. A posterior fossa syndrome occasionally follows the removal of a high cervical intramedullary neoplasm. Such lesions are effectively managed with steroids, although a spinal tap may be required to rule out meningitis. CSF fistulas are managed aggressively to prevent meningitis. An early return to the operating room for wound revision is recommended to prevent this complication.

Despite confident gross total resection, benign intramedullary tumors present a continued risk of recurrence. These patients warrant long-term clinical and radiographic follow-up. Early postoperative MRI (6 to 8 weeks after surgery) establishes the completeness of resection and serves as a baseline against which further studies can be compared. Serial gadolinium-enhanced MRI studies are obtained annually because a radiographic tumor recurrence usually precedes clinical symptoms.

Outcome of Surgical Treatment. The immediate results of surgery are related primarily to the patient's preoperative status and tumor location.[49, 50, 53, 60, 68] Most patients note sensory loss soon after surgery, most likely as a result of the midline myelotomy, transient edema, or vascular compromise. These complaints are more subjective than objective and can be significant even when little or no objective deficit is present. They usually resolve within 3 months.[68] Additional surgical morbidity is directly related to the patient's preoperative status, the location of the tumor, and the presence of spinal cord atrophy and arachnoid scarring.[49,50,53,58,68] Patients with major or long-standing deficits rarely recover significantly, and their condition is likely to worsen after surgery. If preoperative symptoms have been present only a brief time, patients are more likely to improve, even if they had a significant preoperative deficit, particularly those with ependymomas.[68] Thoracic lesions have been correlated with a decline in postoperative function,[49, 51, 68, 76] perhaps due to the relatively tenuous blood supply in this region. Spinal cord atrophy and arachnoid scarring may indicate chronic spinal cord compression and predict poor functional outcomes.[58, 68] Preservation, rather than restoration, of neurologic function is the reasonable expectation for intramedullary tumor surgery. Minimally symptomatic patients with intramedullary tumors derive the greatest benefit and the least risk from surgery.[50, 53, 68] This relationship underscores the importance of early diagnosis and aggressive initial treatment before an objective deficit appears. It is equally important during follow-up because periodic evaluation by MRI will most likely demonstrate evidence of tumor recurrence before a clinical recurrence becomes apparent.

Long-term outcome and risk of recurrence primarily depend on the tumor's histologic characteristics and, with the exception of malignant neoplasms and many low-grade astrocytomas, on the completeness of the original resection. Gross total removal of benign intramedullary ependymomas more consistently cures or controls tumors long term than does subtotal resection and radiation therapy.[49, 52, 60, 68, 77] Nevertheless, these tumors are friable and often adhere to the spinal cord, particularly at their polar regions. These features may preclude total microscopic resection. Long-term follow-up with periodic clinical evaluation and gadolinium-enhanced MRI is mandatory because of the continued risk of tumor recurrence. Depending on the patient's age and critical circumstances, reoperation may be undertaken if a tumor recurrence is clearly established on MRI. The evidence supporting postoperative radiation after subtotal resection is difficult to interpret because it is largely based on studies with small patient populations, limited follow-up periods, and inadequate or no matched controls treated without radiation therapy.[53] Despite these limitations, the data accumulated from these series suggest that radiation may be beneficial after subtotal resection. We recommend adjuvant radiation for malignant ependymomas and the rare benign lesion that cannot be resected completely.

The optimal treatment strategy for astrocytomas is less clear. With the exception of high-grade gliomas, which all authors agree do not benefit from surgery and progress rapidly, low-grade intramedullary spinal cord astrocytomas have been difficult to evaluate because they are rare and biologically variable. Age appears to be the most significant prognostic factor. Pediatric astrocytomas are associated with a particularly indolent behavior, which is partly explained by their predominantly benign histologic characteristics (90%) and high percentage of juvenile pilocytic astrocytomas and gangliogliomas.[69, 78, 79] The influence of extent of resection on outcome remains controversial. Although some authors have found that gross total resection influences outcome,[49, 51] other authors find no such relationship.[50, 69]

Despite numerous interrelated factors that may correlate with clinical behavior, such as age of presentation, histologic features, and extent of resection, it is usually impossible to predict outcome for a given astrocytoma. In adults, however, astrocytomas usually pursue a progressive course. Parameters that predict which patients will benefit from aggressive resection have not been identified. We strive for gross total resection if it can be achieved safely because a surgical cure is possible in a small subgroup of patients.[51, 69] Lesions with favorable histologic features may lend themselves to more complete resection. If resection is subtotal only, radiation therapy may be given, although the data on its efficacy for low-grade tumors are inconclusive. Recurrence within the irradiated volume after radiation therapy occurs in approximately 50% of patients, and there is little agreement about the dose-response relationship.[50, 69, 78, 80, 81]

We do not routinely administer radiation therapy after subtotal resection for several reasons. It complicates the prospects for future surgery, efficacious doses may be higher than the accepted tolerance of the spinal cord, and it has been associated with an increased incidence of spinal deformity and secondary malignancy.[76, 80–82] Instead, we follow patients clinically and with serial MRI. Depending on the clinical circumstances, repeat surgery is offered at the time of a clinical recurrence, which is often several years after radiographic recurrence. Radiation therapy may then be considered depending on the time of recurrence and the degree of resection accomplished. Surgery plays only a diagnostic role in patients who harbor malignant intramedullary astrocytic neoplasms. Radical resection does not prolong survival and is associated with a high rate of surgical morbidity.[50, 51, 53] Radiation therapy is recommended for these patients, but their average survival is poor—6 to 12 months.[49–51, 72, 81]

CONCLUSIONS

The treatment of intradural spinal cord tumors remains a gratifying area of neurosurgery because most spinal neoplasms are benign. Advances in the sensitivity of imaging modalities and refinement of microsurgical skills have allowed microsurgical resection to be viewed as definitive treatment in most cases. Early diagnosis and aggressive definitive treatment, when possible, optimize the management of these neoplasms.

REFERENCES

1. Sloof JL, Kernohan JW, McCarthy CS: Primary Intramedullary Tumors of the Spinal Cord and Filum Terminale. Philadelphia, WB Saunders, 1964.
2. Nittner K: Spinal meningiomas, neurinomas and neurofibromas, and hourglass tumours. In Vinken PH, Bruyn GW (eds): Handbook of Clinical Neurology. New York, North Holland/America, Elsevier, 1976, pp 177–322.
3. Russell DS, Rubenstein LJ: Pathology of Tumors of the Nervous System. Baltimore, Williams & Wilkins, 1989.
4. Halliday AL, Sobel RA, Martuza RL: Benign spinal nerve sheath tumors: Their occurrence sporadically and in neurofibromatosis types 1 and 2. J Neurosurg 74:248–253, 1991.
5. Kernohan JW, Sayre GP: Tumors of the Central Nervous System, Fascicle 35. Washington D.C., Armed Forces Institute of Pathology, 1952.
6. Purcell SM, Dixon SL: Schwannomatosis: An unusual variant of

neurofibromatosis or a distinct clinical entity? Arch Dermatol 125:390–393, 1989.

7. Seppala MT, Haltia MJ, Sankila RJ, et al: Long-term outcome after removal of spinal schwannoma: A clinicopathological study of 187 cases. J Neurosurg 83:621–626, 1995.

8. Levy WJ, Latchaw J, Hahn JF, et al: Spinal neurofibromas: A report of 66 cases and a comparison with meningiomas. Neurosurgery 18:331–334, 1986.

9. Seppala MT, Haltia MJ, Sankila RJ, et al: Long-term outcome after removal of spinal neurofibroma. J Neurosurg 82:572–577, 1995.

10. Seppala MT, Haltia MJ: Spinal malignant nerve-sheath tumor or cellular schwannoma? A striking difference in prognosis. J Neurosurg 79:528–532, 1993.

11. Roux F-X, Nataf F, Pinaudeau M, et al: Intraspinal meningiomas: Review of 54 cases with discussion of poor prognosis factors and modern therapeutic management. Surg Neurol 46:458–464, 1996.

12. Levy WJ Jr, Bay J, Dohn D: Spinal cord meningioma. J Neurosurg 57:804–812, 1982.

13. Solero CL, Fornari M, Giombini S, et al: Spinal meningiomas: Review of 174 operated cases. Neurosurgery 25:153–160, 1989.

14. Preston-Martin S, Monroe K, Lee PJ, et al: Spinal meningiomas in women in Los Angeles County: Investigation of an etiological hypothesis. Cancer Epidemiol Biomarkers Prev 4:333–339, 1995.

15. Stein BM, Leeds NE, Taveras JM, et al: Meningiomas of the foramen magnum. J Neurosurg 20:740–751, 1963.

16. Klekamp J, Samii M: Surgical results of spinal meningiomas. Acta Neurochir Suppl (Wien) 65:77–81, 1996.

17. Salpietro FM, Alafaci C, Lucerna S, et al: Do spinal meningiomas penetrate the pial layer? Correlation between magnetic resonance imaging and microsurgical findings and intracranial tumor interfaces. Neurosurgery 41:254–258, 1997.

18. Sonneland PR, Scheithauer BW, Onofrio BM: Myxopapillary ependymoma: A clinicopathologic and immunocytochemical study of 77 cases. Cancer 56:883–893, 1985.

19. Davis C, Barnard RO: Malignant behavior of myxopapillary ependymoma: Report of three cases. J Neurosurg 62:925–929, 1985.

20. Pang D: Split cord malformation. Part II. Clinical syndrome. Neurosurgery 31:481–500, 1992.

21. Agnoli AL, Laun A, Schonmayr R: Enterogenous intraspinal cysts. J Neurosurg 61:834–840, 1984.

22. Gregorios JB, Green B, Page L, et al: Spinal cord tumors presenting with neural tube defects. Neurosurgery 19:962–966, 1986.

23. Reyes MG, Torres H: Intrathecal paraganglioma of the cauda equina. Neurosurgery 15:578–582, 1984.

24. Nabors MW, Pait TG, Byrd EB, et al: Updated assessment and current classification of spinal meningeal cysts. J Neurosurg 68:366–377, 1988.

25. Moore DW, Hunt WE, Zimmerman JE: Ruptured anterior spinal artery aneurysm: Repair via a posterior approach. Neurosurgery 10:626–630, 1982.

26. McCormick PC, Stein BM: Miscellaneous intradural pathology. Neurosurg Clin N Am 1:687–699, 1990.

27. Fraser RA, Ratzan K, Wolpert SM, et al: Spinal subdural empyema. Arch Neurol 28:235–238, 1973.

28. Calvo FA, Hornedo J, de la Torre A: Intracranial tumors with risk of dissemination in neuroaxis. Int J Radiat Oncol Biol Phys 9:1297–1301, 1983.

29. Perrin RG, Livingston KE, Aarabi B: Intradural extramedullary metastasis: A report of 10 cases. J Neurosurg 56:835–837, 1982.

30. Olson ME, Chernik NL, Posner JB: Infiltration of the leptomeninges by systemic cancer: A clinical and pathologic study. Arch Neurol 30:122–137, 1974.

31. Feldmann E, Bromfield E, Navia B: Hydrocephalic dementia and spinal cord tumor: Report of a case and review of the literature. Arch Neurol 43:714–718, 1986.

32. Mills B, Marks PV, Nixon JM: Spinal subarachnoid haemorrhage from an "ancient" schwannoma of the cervical spine. Br J Neurosurg 7:557–579, 1993.

33. Epstein NE, Bhuchar S, Gavin R, et al: Failure to diagnose conus ependymomas by magnetic resonance imaging. Spine 14:134–137, 1989.

34. Quekel LG, Versteege CW: The "dural tail sign" in MRI of spinal meningioma. J Comput Assist Tomogr 19:890–892, 1995.

35. McCormick PC, Post KD, Stein BM: Intradural extramedullary tumors in adults. Neurosurg Clin N Am 1:591–608, 1990.

36. McCormick PC: Surgical management of dumbbell tumors of the cervical spine. Neurosurgery 38:294–300, 1996.

37. Sridhar K, Ramamurthi R, Vasudevan MC, et al: Limited unilateral approach for extramedullary spinal tumours. Br J Neurosurg 12:430–433, 1998.

38. McCormick PC: Anatomic principles of intradural spinal surgery. Clin Neurosurg 41:204–223, 1994.

39. Lot G, George B: Cervical neuromas with extradural components: Surgical management in a series of 57 patients. Neurosurgery 41:813–822, 1997.

40. Dickman CA, Apfelbaum RI: Thoracoscopic microsurgical excision of thoracic schwannoma: Case report. J Neurosurg 88:898–902, 1998.

41. Steck JC, Dietze DD, Fessler RG: Posterolateral approach to intradural extramedullary thoracic tumors. J Neurosurg 81:202–205, 1994.

42. McCormick PC: Surgical management of dumbbell and paraspinal tumors of the thoracic and lumbar spine. Neurosurgery 38:67–75, 1996.

43. McCormick PC, Post KD: Surgical approaches to the sacrum. In Doty JR, SS Rengachary (eds): Surgical Disorders of the Sacrum. New York, Thieme, 1994, pp 257–265.

44. Mirimanoff RO, Dosoretz DE, Linggood RM, et al: Meningioma: Analysis of recurrence and progression following neurosurgical resection. J Neurosurg 62:18–24, 1985.

45. Sen CN, Sekhar LN: An extreme lateral approach to intradural lesions of the cervical spine and foramen magnum. Neurosurgery 27:197–204, 1990.

46. Miller E, Crockard HA: Transoral transclival removal of anteriorly placed meningiomas at the foramen magnum. Neurosurgery 20:966–968, 1987.

47. Ilgren EB, Stiller CA, Hughes JT, et al: Ependymomas: A clinical and pathological study. Part II. Survival features. Clin Neuropathol 3:122–127, 1984.

48. Whitaker SJ, Bessell EM, Ashley SE, et al: Postoperative radiotherapy in the management of spinal cord ependymoma. J Neurosurg 74:720–728, 1991.

49. Cristante L, Herrmann HD: Surgical management of intramedullary spinal cord tumors: Functional outcome and sources of morbidity. Neurosurgery 35:69–76, 1994.

50. Cooper PR: Outcome after operative treatment of intramedullary spinal cord tumors in adults: Intermediate and long-term results in 51 patients. Neurosurgery 25:855–859, 1989.

51. Epstein FJ, Farmer JP, Freed D: Adult intramedullary astrocytomas of the spinal cord. J Neurosurg 77:355–359, 1992.

52. Epstein FJ, Farmer JP, Freed D: Adult intramedullary spinal cord ependymomas: The result of surgery in 38 patients. J Neurosurg 79:204–209, 1993.

53. McCormick PC, Stein BM: Intramedullary tumors in adults. Neurosurg Clin N Am 1:609–630, 1990.

54. Neumann HP, Eggert HR, Weigel K, et al: Hemangioblastomas of the central nervous system: A 10-year study with special reference to von Hippel-Lindau syndrome. J Neurosurg 70:24–30, 1989.

55. Jallo GI, Zagzag D, Lee M, et al: Intraspinal sarcoidosis: Diagnosis and management. Surg Neurol 48:514–521, 1997.

56. Lee M, Epstein FJ, Rezai AR, et al: Nonneoplastic intramedullary spinal cord lesions mimicking tumors. Neurosurgery 43:788–795, 1998.

57. Kepes JJ: Large focal tumor-like demyelinating lesions of the brain: Intermediate entity between multiple sclerosis and acute disseminated encephalomyelitis? A study of 31 patients. Ann Neurol 33:18–27, 1993.

58. Samii M, Klekamp J: Surgical results of 100 intramedullary tumors in relation to accompanying syringomyelia. Neurosurgery 35:865–873, 1994.

59. Lee M, Rezai AR, Freed D, et al: Intramedullary spinal cord tumors in neurofibromatosis. Neurosurgery 38:32–37, 1996.

60. McCormick PC, Torres R, Post KD, et al: Intramedullary ependymoma of the spinal cord. J Neurosurg 72:523–532, 1990.

61. Helseth A, Mørk SJ: Primary intraspinal neoplasms in Norway, 1955 to 1986: A population-based survey of 467 patients. J Neurosurg 71:842–845, 1989.

62. Birch BD, Johnson JP, Parsa A, et al: Frequent type 2 neurofibromatosis gene transcript mutations in sporadic intramedullary spinal cord ependymomas. Neurosurgery 39:135–140, 1996.

63. Mørk SJ, Løken AC: Ependymoma: A follow-up study of 101 cases. Cancer 40:907–915, 1977.

64. Costigan DA, Winkelman MD: Intramedullary spinal cord metastases: A clinicopathological study of 13 cases. J Neurosurg 62:227–233, 1985.

65. Deme S, Ang LC, Skaf G, et al: Primary intramedullary primitive neuroectodermal tumor of the spinal cord: Case report and review of the literature. Neurosurgery 41:1417–1420, 1997.

66. Yasui T, Yagura H, Komiyama M, et al: Significance of gadolinium-enhanced magnetic resonance imaging in differentiating spinal cord radiation myelopathy from tumor: Case report. J Neurosurg 77:628–631, 1992.

67. Schwartz TH, Chang Y, Stein BM: Unusual intramedullary vascular lesions: Report of two cases. Neurosurgery 40:1295–1301, 1997.

68. Hoshimaru M, Koyama T, Hashimoto N, et al: Results of microsurgical treatment for intramedullary spinal cord ependymomas: Analysis of 36 cases. Neurosurgery 44:264–269, 1999.

69. Sandler HM, Papadopoulos SM, Thornton AF Jr, et al: Spinal cord astrocytomas: Results of therapy. Neurosurgery 30:490–493, 1992.

70. Bourgouin PM, Lesage J, Fontaine S, et al: A pattern approach to the differential diagnosis of intramedullary spinal cord lesions on MR imaging. AJR 170:1645–1649, 1998.

71. Cohen AR, Wisoff JH, Allen JC, et al: Malignant astrocytomas of the spinal cord. J Neurosurg 70:50–54, 1989.

72. Kopelson G, Linggood RM: Intramedullary spinal cord astrocytoma versus glioblastoma: The prognostic importance of histologic grade. Cancer 50:732–735, 1982.

73. Adams DC, Emerson RG, Heyer EJ, et al: Monitoring of intraoperative motor-evoked potentials under conditions of controlled neuromuscular blockade. Anesth Analg 77:913–918, 1993.

74. Morota N, Deletis V, Constantini S, et al: The role of motor evoked potentials during surgery for intramedullary spinal cord tumors. Neurosurgery 41:1327–1336, 1997.

75. Epstein FJ, Farmer JP, Schneider SJ: Intraoperative ultrasonography: An important surgical adjunct for intramedullary tumors. J Neurosurg 74:729–733, 1991.

76. Brotchi J, Dewitte O, Levivier M, et al: A survey of 65 tumors within the spinal cord: Surgical results and the importance of preoperative magnetic resonance imaging. Neurosurgery 29:651–657, 1991.

77. Fischer G, Mansuy L: Total removal of intramedullary ependymomas: Follow-up study of 16 cases. Surg Neurol 14:243–249, 1980.

78. Rossitch E Jr, Zeidman SM, Burger PC, et al: Clinical and pathological analysis of spinal cord astrocytomas in children. Neurosurgery 27:193–196, 1990.

79. Epstein FJ, Farmer JP: Pediatric spinal cord tumor surgery. Neurosurg Clin N Am 1:569–590, 1990.

80. Garcia DM: Primary spinal cord tumors treated with surgery and postoperative irradiation. Int J Radiat Oncol Biol Phys 11:1933–1939, 1985.

81. Linstadt DE, Wara WM, Leibel SA, et al: Postoperative radiotherapy of primary spinal cord tumors. Int J Radiat Oncol Biol Phys 16:1397–1403, 1989.

82. O'Sullivan C, Jenkin RD, Doherty MA, et al: Spinal cord tumors in children: Long-term results of combined surgical and radiation treatment. J Neurosurg 81:507–512, 1994.

CHAPTER 313

Tumors of the Vertebral Axis: Benign, Primary Malignant, and Metastatic Tumors

MARTIN B. CAMINS ■ ARTHUR L. JENKINS III ■ ASH SINGHAL ■
RICHARD G. PERRIN

The treatment of bony lesions along the vertebral axis has unique considerations owing to their inaccessibility, the necessity of removing the entire lesion to decrease the risk of recurrence, the close proximity of these lesions to the spinal cord and nerve roots, the desire to prevent excessive intraoperative bleeding, and the need to assess for potential postoperative instability requiring stabilization, perhaps both anteriorly and posteriorly.

New, aggressive, and highly technical options for the treatment of these vertebral lesions are evolving rapidly.[1] Magnetic resonance imaging (MRI) has significantly improved visualization of these lesions and soft tissue extension. New instrumentation hardware to stabilize the spine both anteriorly and posteriorly allows for more radical and safer circumferential tumor resection.[2] Endovascular techniques and the cell-saver are now routinely used to decrease blood loss.[3, 4] With these techniques, the neurological function and life expectancy of these patients have been improved dramatically.[5] In the future, genetic therapies and immunotherapies will add to the armamentarium of clinicians treating patients with these lesions.

SIGNS AND SYMPTOMS

Tumors involving the spine may present with spinal cord compression and neurological deficits, mechanical instability, structural changes such as scoliosis or torticollis, and pain, or they may be clinically asymptomatic. Understanding the clinical syndromes that may be associated with spinal tumors assists clinicians in recognizing the presence and identifying the nature of such lesions. As imaging modalities become increasingly sensitive, more tumors are being found incidentally when patients are evaluated for trauma, herniated disks, and non-neurosurgical diagnoses. The indications for intervention in an asymptomatic patient are different from those in a symptomatic patient.

Pain is the most common initial symptom. However, it can be nonspecific and may lead to a delay in diagnosis. Unlike the spinal pain associated with myofascial syndromes, spondylosis, or diskogenic disease, the pain caused by a bone tumor is persistent and is often noticeable at rest or in bed at night. Local pain can result from bone destruction or a compression fracture. This pain is continuous and often requires narcotics to control. Local pain that is easily controlled with aspirin is most indicative of osteoid osteoma. The type of tumor that can cause significant local pain depends on the patient's age, social history, and genetic history, but it is most often a destructive metastatic lesion. Instability can cause mechanical back pain, and a tumor that involves a joint or undermines a vertebral body or posterior element can result in motion or weight-bearing pain. This should be a warning sign to promptly initiate a comprehensive workup. The severity of symptoms may be related to the degree of involvement, but this is not always the case. Scoliosis and torticollis tend to be the result of chronic involvement by slow-growing tumors, such as osteoid osteoma and osteoblastoma. They occur as a result of changes in the vertebral body, and in any case of new scoliosis or torticollis, a tumor should be suspected.

Physical examination may reveal local tenderness, swelling, or muscle spasm. A palpable mass may be present with posterior lesions. Neurological findings depend on the level and site of the lesion. Tumors are most commonly situated in the vertebral body, pedicle, facet, and posterior arch. Anterior tumors can cause compression of the anterior aspect of the spinal cord and may also produce a deficit through infarction of the anterior spinal artery. Lesions at the facets may cause pain during movement of the motion segment. Radicular symptoms can be caused by compression at the neural foramina.

RADIOLOGIC ASSESSMENT

The radiographic characteristics of both primary bone tumors and metastatic tumors to the extradural space are discussed later. Objectives in the radiologic evaluation of tumors in the extradural space are to (1) determine the anatomic alignment and stability, (2) delineate thecal sac impingement, and (3) determine the degree of vertebral body destruction or collapse. MRI has proved to be as efficacious as or, in many instances, superior to the traditional modalities of computed tomography (CT) and myelography with postmyelographic CT. Most of the primary bone tumors along the vertebral axis are relatively unusual, except for hemangiomas.[6] As expected, metastatic tumors are more common in the extradural space.

Routine radiographs provide an initial evaluation of the degree of kyphosis, scoliosis, collapse, lytic destruction, or subluxation of the spine. The workup of instability should include chest radiographs and flexion-extension films of the relevant spinal region with dynamic imaging studies. These plain radiographs can define the specific levels to be examined by additional imaging studies. Bone scanning, MRI, and CT often complement one another.[7–10] CT identifies blastic and lytic lesions and the extent of cortical destruction. Axial images should be supplemented by sagittal and three-dimensional reconstruction to assist in formulating a treatment plan: decompression and tumor resection, stabilization, and instrumentation.

An unenhanced MRI scan is ideal for delineating extradural tumors. The morphology of lesions of the vertebral body are well defined as low-intensity lesions surrounded by the higher intensity of normal fat-containing marrow on short TR images. On long TR-TE sequences, tumors are of high signal intensity. Short T1 inversion recovery sequences and gradient-echo sequencing also help in the initial evaluation. MRI is more sensitive to marrow abnormalities than is radionuclide bone scanning.[7] In some instances, very aggressive lesions not visible on bone scans are detected by MRI. MRI of the spine in two orthogonal planes is quite precise in demonstrating tumor impingement on the thecal sac. It is also helpful in distinguishing between benign osteoporotic collapse and neoplastic replacement in patients with vertebral body compression fractures. In osteoporotic collapse, the scan reveals preservation of normal bone marrow, whereas tumors replace the marrow.

The contrast agent gadolinium–diethylenetriamine pentaacetic acid (Gd-DTPA) can be helpful in detecting vertebral lesions, indicating areas of more active tumor for biopsy, and determining a patient's response to chemotherapy.

Spinal angiography is invaluable to define the vascularity of a tumor and helps determine whether endovascular embolization is necessary. When indicated, preoperative embolization with polyvinyl alcohol particles can significantly reduce the amount of intraoperative blood loss in tumors such as hemangiomas, aneurysmal bone cysts, and metastatic thyroid and renal cell tumors. Embolization minimizes the need for transfusion and allows the surgeon to perform a safer, more aggressive tumor resection.

LABORATORY STUDIES

Mandatory clinical laboratory tests should include a complete blood count, serum chemistry, and urinalysis.

Examination of the stool for occult blood should be performed. Additional testing that may be helpful includes serum and urine protein electrophoresis in patients with a suspected myeloma or plasmacytoma, serum prostate-specific antigen level, and carcinoembryonic antigen level. Metastasis to the liver is suggested by elevated transaminase levels. A urinalysis should be obtained to evaluate for occult blood and Bence Jones proteins.

CAUSE OF TUMORS

Primary tumors found within the spinal axis can be described according to the cell of origin (Table 313–1). The main categories are cartilaginous tumors, bony tumors, vascular tumors, plasma cell dyscrasias, tumors that arise from embryonic rests, and non-neoplastic reactive changes that present as spinal masses. These tumors can be divided into benign or malignant types, based on clinical progression, histopathologic signs of invasiveness and high mitotic character, and response to therapy. In addition to spontaneously arising tumors, some so-called primary tumors can result from exogenous influences.

Benign tumors tend to occur in younger patients in the posterior vertebral elements. Beyond the second decade, the majority of these bony tumors are malignant. Malignant tumors are more likely to be found in the vertebral body. Metastatic lesions, far more common in the adult population than are primary tumors, are extremely rare in the pediatric population. When metastatic tumors present in the spine (which is common, with an incidence of up to 70%), the vertebral body and pedicles are involved if the spread is hematogenous. Direct spread of tumors, such as Pancoast's tumors or paraspinal sarcomas, usually occurs along tissue planes into the neural foramen and surrounding bone. Primary soft tissue tumors that commonly result in spinal metastases include prostate, kidney, thyroid, lung, and breast tumors.

Cartilaginous tumors arise from the cartilage and

T A B L E 3 1 3 – 1 ■ **Primary Tumors of the Spine**

True Bone Tumors	Associated Bone Tumors
Osteogenic	Vascular
Osteoma	Hemangioma
Osteoid osteoma	Aneurysmal bone cyst
Osteoblastoma	Hemangiopericytoma
Osteosarcoma	Hemangioendothelioma
Osteoclastic	Angiolipoma
Giant cell tumor	Angiosarcoma
Chondroblastic	Notochord
Chondroma	Chordoma
Enchondroma	Marrow
Osteochondroma	Plasmacytoma
Chondroblastoma	Myeloma
Chondrosarcoma	Ewing's sarcoma
Fibroblastic	Adipose
Fibroma	Lipoma
Fibrosarcoma	Angiolipoma
Fibrous histiocytoma	

end cap of the joint capsule. Benign tumors arising from the chondroblast include enchondromas, chondroblastomas, and osteochondromas. A chondrosarcoma is a malignant tumor arising from the cartilage cell or precursor; the majority occur as a result of induction by radiation, other exogenous stimuli, or metabolic diseases of bone.

Bony tumors can arise from either osteoblasts or osteoclasts. Benign tumors that arise from osteoblasts include osteoid osteomas and osteoblastomas.[11] Malignant tumors arising from osteoblasts are osteosarcomas. Tumors that arise from osteoblasts are characterized by active ossification and often exuberant bone formation. These tumors are almost uniformly highly active on a bone scan. The primary tumor arising from osteoclasts is the giant cell tumor. This tumor results in active resorption of bone with propagation of the low-density soft tissue material.

Vascular tumors include benign tumors such as angiolipomas, hemangiomas, and hemangioendotheliomas.[12, 13] Hemangiomas of bone are the most common tumor of the spine, with many asymptomatic lesions found incidentally. Malignant tumors of the spine derived from vascular elements include angiosarcoma and hemangiopericytoma.

Plasma cell dyscrasias are tumors derived from bone marrow cell precursors. Disease processes that involve the spine include benign tumors such as amyloidomas and plasmacytomas or the very malignant multiple myelomas.

Tumors can result from remnants of embryonic cells that fail to follow normal developmental pathways. Chordomas result from a remnant of the notochord within the vertebral body. Ewing's sarcoma was initially thought to have a vascular cause, but it is now thought to be of neural or neuroepithelial origin and is grouped with primitive neuroectodermal tumors.[14]

Other masses can be non-neoplastic inflammatory reactions to trauma and other tumors. Aneurysmal bone cysts are believed to be a reaction to a nearby lesion, such as a tumor, that may have involuted (most commonly a giant cell tumor). Eosinophilic granulomas, now known better as Langerhans' cell histiocytosis, are the result of a non-neoplastic proliferation of the antigen-presenting cell within the bone, resulting in a lytic lesion.

OSTEOGENIC TUMORS

Osteoid Osteoma

Osteoid osteoma is a small, benign, self-limited, painful tumor that has little potential for growth. The distinguishing feature between it and osteoblastoma is size. Osteoid osteoma is always less than 1.5 cm. Between 10% and 25% of all osteoid osteomas occur in the spine.[1, 15, 16] More than half of the osteoid osteomas that occur in the spine are found in the lumbar region (59%), followed by the cervical (27%), thoracic (12%), and sacral (2%) regions.[1] In the majority of cases, they occur in the peripedicular region of the posterior arch; the anterior column is affected only 7% of the time.[16]

Rarely does the tumor involve the vertebral body, epidural space, or paravertebral soft tissue. This tumor rarely presents after age 30 years; the highest incidence is in the second decade, at an average age of 16.7 years.[17] Similar to osteoblastomas, the prevalence is much higher in males by a 2:1 to 4:1 ratio.[18]

Classically, the principal presenting complaint is back pain that gradually becomes continuous and localized to the site of the lesion. Pain is intensified by weight-bearing activity and is worse at night. In as many as half the patients, this nocturnal pain is relieved by the use of salicylates or nonsteroidal anti-inflammatory agents. This response is considered pathognomonic by some physicians. Radiculopathy develops if the tumor encroaches on the neural foramina. Local point tenderness is the most common sign. An antalgic scoliosis due to muscle spasms or resultant pelvic tilt occurs in as many as 70% of all cases of adolescent osteoid osteoma.[19] In these cases, the tumor is located in the posterior or middle column, with the gibbus directed away from the lesion. Cervical osteoid osteomas present with pain, torticollis, and limited range of motion.

In approximately 30% of cases, plain radiographs may not demonstrate the lesion because the radiolucent lesion is obscured by surrounding bone.[20] If there is extensive sclerosis, the location of the nidus may also be difficult to see. Plain films may show a lucent nidus with a small amount of calcium in the nidus.

The most sensitive screening examination is the technetium radionuclide bone scan (Fig. 313–1A). Even small lesions can be localized to a specific level by their "hot spots." Preoperative planning is assisted by obtaining cross-sectional imagery with either MRI or CT to confirm the precise location of the nidus (see Fig. 313–1B).[21, 22] These tumors routinely demonstrate a heterogeneous appearance on MRI.[23] On T1- and T2-weighted images, the calcification within both the nidus and the surrounding areas of sclerosis are of low signal intensity. With contrast, there may be intense enhancement within the vascular nidus.

Osteoid osteoma causes an intense inflammatory response in the surrounding tissues, along with a periosteal reaction and sclerosis of bone because of the production of prostaglandins by the tumor, which regresses after tumor resection. At surgery, the nidus appears as a punctiform spot with a reddish color that contrasts with the surrounding white bone. Rarely is isotope bone scanning or tetracycline bone labeling required during surgery to assist in locating the tumor.[24, 25] The appropriate surgical technique is to expose the lesion and curet the nidus, with the gradual excision of minimal reactive bone (see Fig. 313–1C). Patients can expect immediate and complete pain relief after surgical excision and slow improvement of scoliosis, if present. The results of newer techniques for percutaneous removal of the nidus are incomplete, owing to the short follow-up.[26, 27] Histologically, these tumors are characterized by a very vascular, fibrous connective tissue with a surrounding osteoid matrix. It may be calcified in an irregular fashion (see Fig. 313–1D).

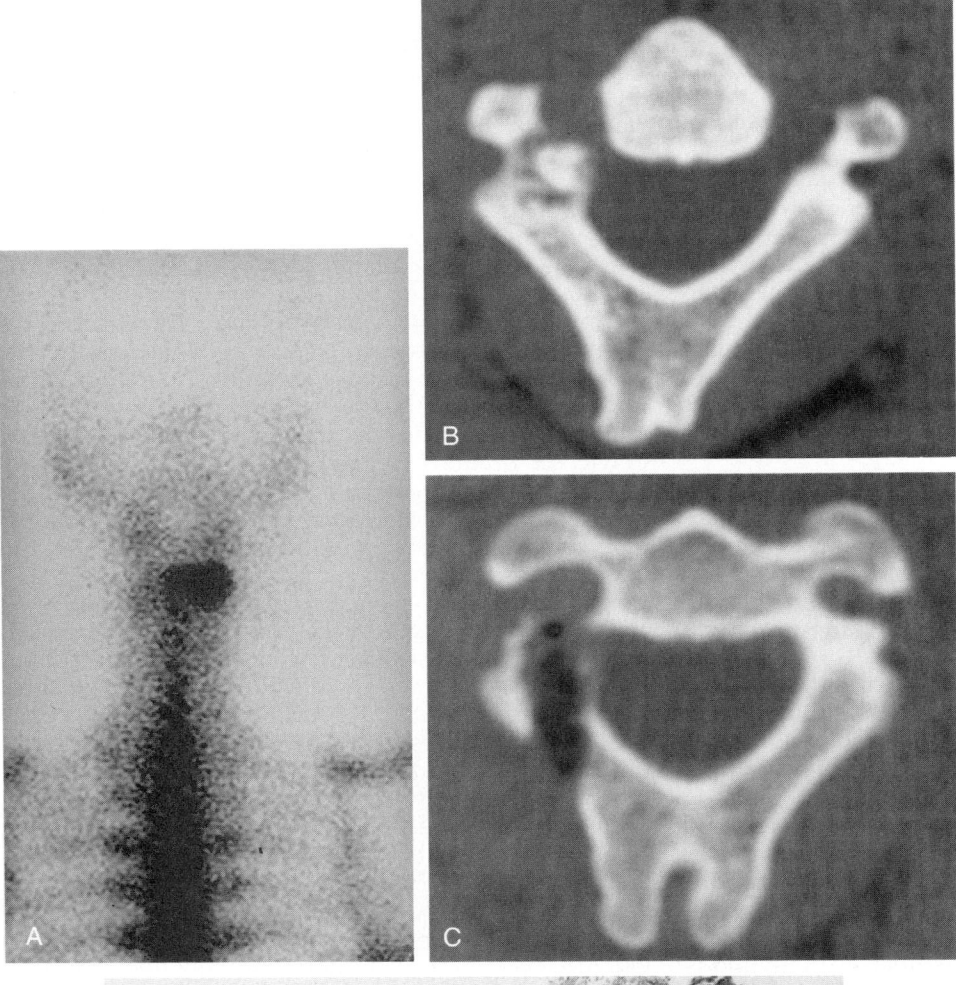

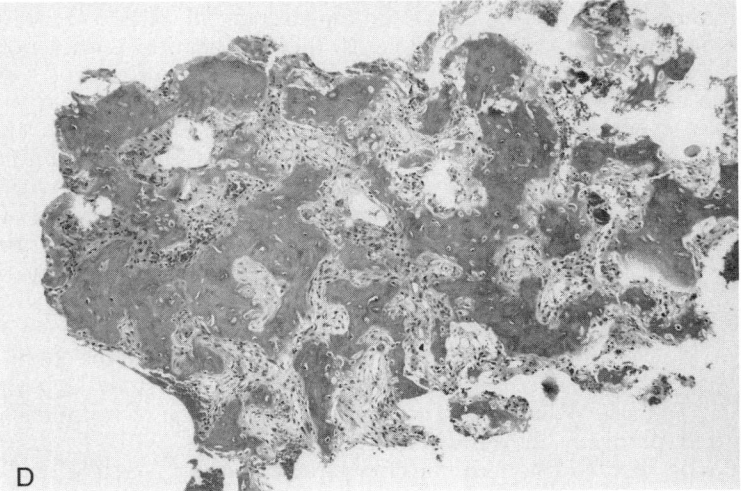

FIGURE 313–1. Osteoid osteoma at C2. *A,* Technetium bone scan demonstrates a focal area of high uptake of radionuclide in the upper cervical spine on the right, consistent with an osteoid osteoma. *B,* Computed tomographic scan of the cervical spine shows a small lucent defect in the anterior portion of the right lamina of C2, with calcification within it. The osteoid osteoma protrudes into the right intravertebral foramen at C2-3, causing narrowing of the foramen. *C,* Post-operative computed tomographic scan demonstrates the surgical path followed to excise the lesion. *D,* The entire lesion is encompassed in this low-power view. Fibrovascular stroma is interspersed between immature bone production, which is trabecular rather than lacelike. A few osteoclasts can be seen at the right at this power (×63).

Osteoblastoma

Osteoblastoma is an uncommon benign bone tumor, approximately four times less frequent than osteoid osteoma. It accounts for 1% of all primary bone tumors. The age of presentation overlaps with that of osteoid osteoma, with the majority of patients presenting between the ages of 10 and 25 years.[28-30] A plurality of all osteoblastomas occurs in the spine, with the sites evenly divided among the cervical, thoracic, and lumbar regions.[31] Like osteoid osteomas, osteoblastomas occur more frequently in multiple areas of the posterior elements, in the posterior elements and vertebral body, or in the adjacent vertebrae. Similar to osteoid osteomas, they may produce a continuous dull pain that is associated with paravertebral muscle spasms, causing torticollis or scoliosis. An epidural soft tissue component is frequently found. As a consequence, they are likely to cause a myelopathy by compression of the spinal cord.

Plain radiography and CT demonstrate a round or ovoid composite lesion between 1.5 and 6 cm with a surrounding thin cortex (Fig. 313–2A and B).[17] Expansion along the sclerotic rim may produce a poorly defined margin and soft tissue extension. This, as well as epidural extension, is visualized on MRI. If calcification or hemorrhage is present, the lesion is inhomogeneous on MRI. A thin rim of signal void may be observed due to the bony shell (see Fig. 313–2C). Corresponding to regions of vascularized stroma on long TR images, the lesion may be of high signal intensity. Osseous trabeculae are seen as irregular linear areas of signal void. Grossly, they are soft, granular, and very vascular. The sclerotic reaction around the tumor is less than that observed in osteoid osteomas. Histologically, osteoblastomas are similar to osteoid osteomas. A net-

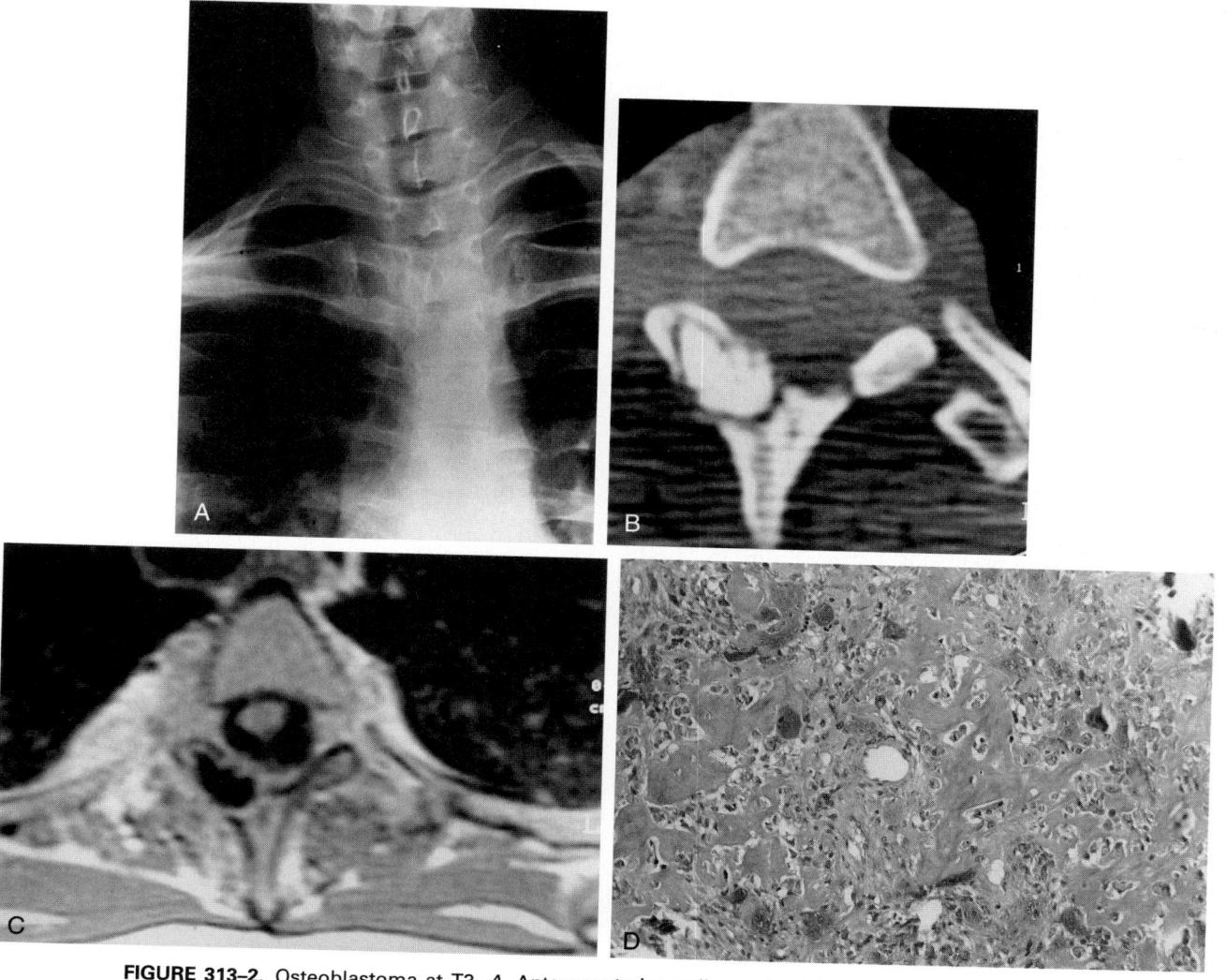

FIGURE 313–2. Osteoblastoma at T3. *A,* Anteroposterior radiograph of the thoracic spine reveals a focal sclerotic lesion at the T3 level. *B,* Axial computed tomographic scan of the vertebral body at T3 shows a focal sclerotic lesion within the lamina. *C,* Magnetic resonance imaging at the T3 level demonstrates a signal void, consistent with calcification. *D,* Medium-power view demonstrates bone matrix arranged in microtrabecular patterns, with many mononuclear cells of osteoblastic differentiation and fewer (but more prominent at this power) osteoclastic giant cells. At this magnification, osteoblastoma and osteoid osteoma are virtually identical (×157).

work of interlocking trabecular or woven bone lined with osteoblasts is seen within a fibrovascular stroma (see Fig. 313–2D).

En bloc surgical resection of the tumor is curative; however, incomplete resection of the tumor leads to a high probability of recurrence.[32] Aggressive surgical management is necessary, because these tumors are radioresistant, and they may recur as long as 9 years after surgery.[33] In some cases, stabilization and instrumentation may be necessary.

CARTILAGINOUS TUMORS

Enchondroma

Enchondromas (sometimes known as chondromas) are benign rests of hyaline cartilage within cancellous bone that result from failed migration of chondrocytes. Only about 1% of enchondromas occur in the spine, although they are more common in the setting of Ollier's syndrome (multiple enchondromatosis) or Maffucci's syndrome (multiple enchondromatosis and soft tissue hemangiomas).[34, 35] They can present from the first to sixth decade of life, although they are more common in the second and third decades. There may be a male predominance, although this is controversial. Patients are rarely symptomatic from isolated enchondromas of the spine. However, syndromic patients can develop a progressive and destabilizing deformity.

Enchondromas consist of hyaline cartilage surrounded by bone, usually in a blue matrix. There is no chondrocytic atypia, although there may be endochondral ossification. Myxoid features may be found in Maffucci's syndrome. There is a low incidence of malignant degeneration in spontaneous lesions, but in syndromic cases, it can reach 50%. Histologically, an active enchondroma may be difficult to differentiate from a low-grade chondrosarcoma.

Plain radiographs may demonstrate a lucency within the vertebral body, but the sensitivity for detection is low. Bone scans are positive if done during skeletal growth. CT and MRI can demonstrate the extent of the lesion and the lack of continuity with the disk space or cortical bone. CT may demonstrate the endochondral ossification as a smoke ring– or popcorn-shaped hyperdensity. Treatment for asymptomatic lesions is normally conservative; therapy for symptomatic lesions varies from curettage to resection with bone grafting and instrumentation. Malignant progression to chondrosarcoma must be verified by needle biopsy when suspected.

Osteochondroma

Despite being the most common benign bone tumor, only 3% of solitary and 7% of multiple osteochondromas occur within the spine (Fig. 313–3).[36, 37] Cases of multiple lesions are often transmitted by autosomal-dominant inheritance. Between 1843 and 1977, only 117 cases of symptomatic spinal osteochondromas were reported.[38] The peak incidence is in the third decade.

Males develop osteochondromas almost twice as often as females.[39] Osteochondromas have a predilection for the spinous process; involvement of the vertebral body is rare. The majority of cases occur in the cervical or upper thoracic spine; they are rarely found in the inferior thoracic or lumbar spine. Although pain is the most common symptom, radiculopathy or myelopathy seldom occurs because the majority of these lesions grow out of the spinal canal.[40]

Osteochondromas most likely arise through a process of endochondral ossification of aberrant cartilage of an epiphyseal growth plate resulting from trauma or a congenital defect. With progressive endochondral ossification, the tumor forms on a pedunculated stalk with a bony base and a cartilaginous cap. These tumors also routinely occur at the site of ligamentous insertions.

Plain films delineate the exostosis, and CT demonstrates the exact site of the tumor's attachment to adjacent bone. CT is also important in distinguishing a benign tumor from one that degenerates into an osteosarcoma or chondrosarcoma. Rapid growth of a lesion is an ominous sign, prompting suspicion of malignancy. On MRI, the cartilaginous cap is of increased signal intensity on long TR images, and the calcified bony base is of low signal intensity. The degree of thecal sac compression may best be defined on long TR or gradient-echo sequences.

When the diagnosis is in question, or when there is pain, a palpable mass, or neurological compromise, surgery should be considered. Surgery is usually curative, and because most tumors stop growing after closure of the epiphyseal plate during puberty, recurrence is rare. Malignant degeneration into chondrosarcoma occurs in 1% to 5% of solitary lesions and in 10% to 25% of patients with multiple hereditary exostoses.[2, 41]

VASCULAR TUMORS

Benign vascular tumors in the spinal column include hemangiomas and angiolipomas. Hemangiopericytomas are thought to be malignant.

Hemangioma

Intraosseous spinal hemangiomas are classified as benign vascular tumors.[31] A significant number of hemangiomas are incidentally discovered on routine radiographs and are asymptomatic.[42] They occur in up to 11% of autopsy cases in large series. Lesions that are symptomatic tend to be in the thoracic region, causing myelopathy by subperiosteal extension of the angiomatous tissue into the epidural space. Radicular pain may result from impingement on a nerve root. Other explanations for cord compression are an epidural hematoma secondary to the hemangioma or a compression fracture of the involved vertebral body.[43] Hemangiomas are slightly more common in women; they are solitary in 66% of cases and multiple in 34%. Significant paraspinal masses are occasionally seen.

Thickened vertical trabeculae visualized as parallel

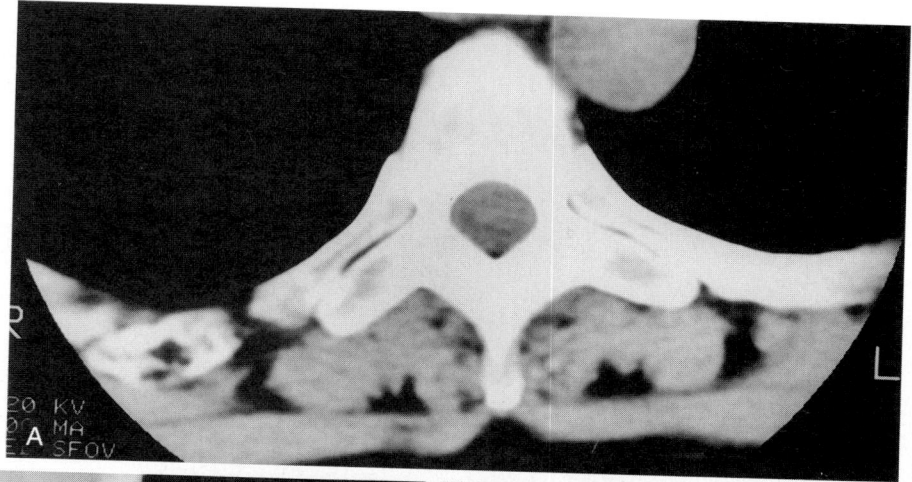

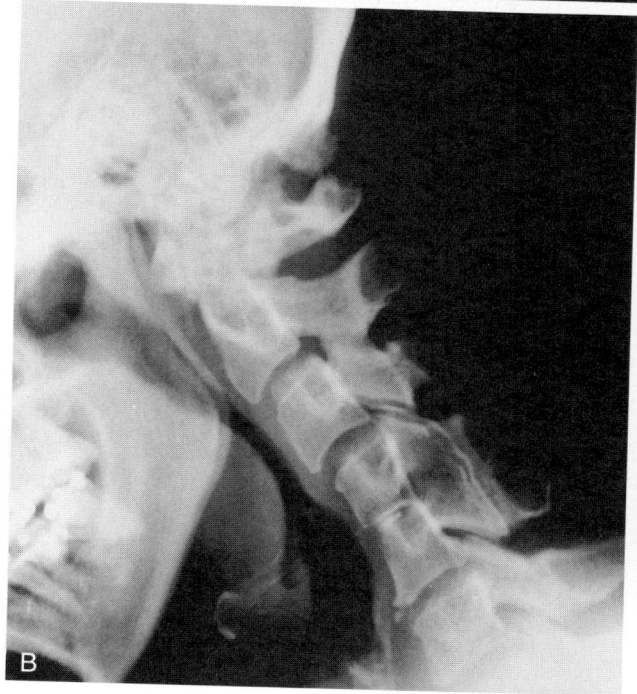

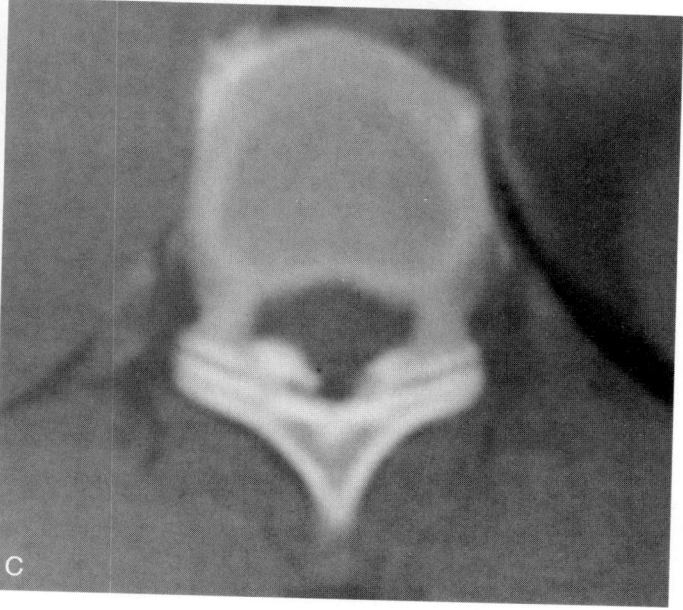

FIGURE 313–3. Osteochondroma. This patient with hereditary osteochondroma has multiple lesions involving the long bones. *A,* Ribs. *B,* Skull. *C,* Midthoracic spine at T6.

linear densities in the vertebral body are pathognomonic findings on plain films (Fig. 313–4*A*). On axial CT, the thickened vertical trabeculae surrounding dilated vascular spaces give the vertebral bodies a typical spotted honeycomb appearance (see Fig. 313–4*B*). Hemangiomas usually have increased signal intensity on both short TR and long TR images. The high signal reflects the adipose component of these lesions, not the hemorrhagic portion. MRI best demonstrates the paravertebral components or thecal sac compression (see Fig. 313–4*C*). Preoperative angiography is imperative to demonstrate the tumor blush that is usually fed by intercostal arteries. Endovascular embolization should complement surgical excision to minimize blood loss and thereby allow for a more aggressive resection (see Fig. 313–4*D* and *E*).[44, 45] If the arterial

supply to the cord arises from the tumor's feeding intercostal vessel, the procedure is terminated. Embolization is playing an increasingly important role because it may eliminate the need for surgery altogether in some cases. Blood recycling may limit the need for blood transfusions.

Although there have been recent reports of management using intralesional absolute alcohol, this procedure may have significant morbidity, including posttreatment Brown-Sequard syndrome.[46]

Symptomatic lesions, pain, or thecal sac compression can be managed by embolization, surgical resection, or radiotherapy (30 to 40 Gy).[47] The surgical technique employed depends on the location of the lesion. With a combined anterior and posterior approach, even circumferential lesions can be totally resected. Internal

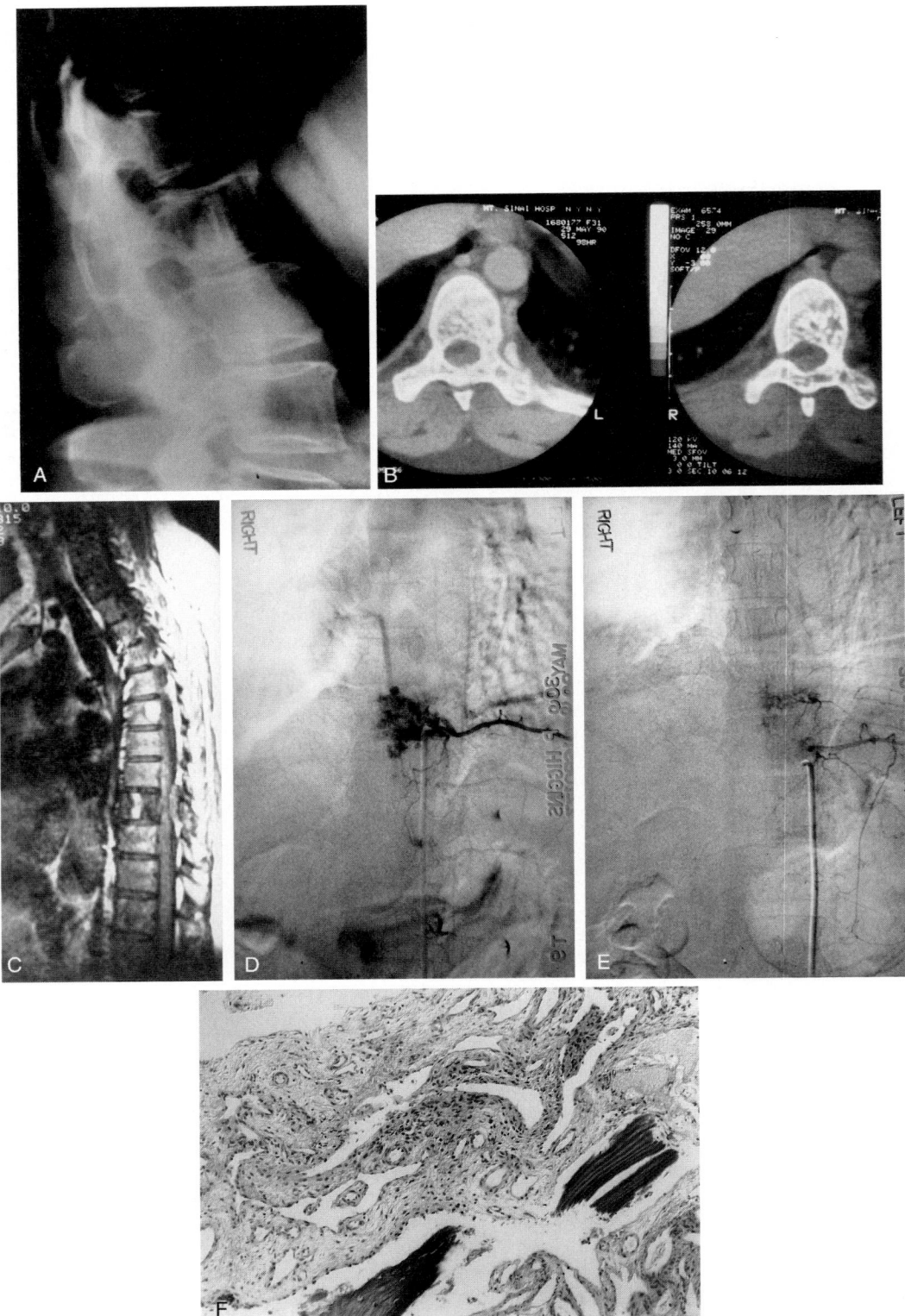

FIGURE 313–4. Hemangioma at T9. *A,* Lateral radiograph of the midthoracic spine reveals the characteristic vertical striations. *B,* Computed tomographic scan with the trabeculated honeycomb appearance of a hemangioma in a midthoracic vertebral body. A posterior epidural soft tissue lesion in the spinal canal is visualized compressing the thecal sac. *C,* T1-weighted sagittal magnetic resonance imaging scan of the thoracic spine demonstrates anterior involvement of the vertebral body and a posterior epidural mass compressing the thecal sac. *D* and *E,* Pre-embolization *(D)* and postembolization *(E)* selective angiography demonstrates almost complete obliteration of the intercostal arterial vascular supply to the tumor. *F,* Fragments of bone containing numerous simple vascular channels lined by flattened endothelium within loose, fibrous stroma (×125).

stabilization, instrumentation, and arthrodesis are employed in these cases.

Angiolipoma

Angiolipomas are lipomas with a significant vascular element. More than 60 tumors of this kind have been reported in the literature, with the majority presenting as extradural masses causing compression and neurological deficits.[48-50] They also extend outside the canal. Ten lesions have been reported in the literature as originating within the vertebral body. Although both infiltrating and noninfiltrating tumors have been identified, the infiltrating kind is more common. The Armed Forces Institute of Pathology reported that many of these tumors are actually hemangiomas with reactive fat surrounding the lesion, making the incidence of true angiolipomas even rarer than the literature implies.[51] The mesenchyma contains thin-walled blood vessels and large venous spaces. These tumors are distinct from hemangiomas with associated overgrowth of adipose tissue, which have occasionally been misidentified as angiolipomas. Although noninfiltrating lesions are not visible on plain radiographs, infiltrating tumors may show coarse trabeculation and bony erosion.[52] On CT and MRI, two thirds of these lesions have a fat density, and the other third has a soft tissue density. These tumors are curable after surgical resection.

NON-NEOPLASTIC REACTIVE MASSES

Aneurysmal Bone Cyst

Aneurysmal bone cyst is a rare, benign, hyperemic bony tumor of unknown origin.[53] Aneurysmal bone cysts account for 1.4% to 2.3% of primary bone neoplasms.[41, 54] Twelve percent of these tumors present in the spine, where they can cause low back pain in children. There may be a slight female predilection. They are destructive bony lesions that occur commonly in children and infrequently present in persons older than 30 years.[53] Aneurysmal bone cysts are most common in the cervical and thoracic spine. In 32% of cases, they may be associated with other lesions, including giant cell tumor, fibrous dysplasia, or chondroblastoma. In 60% of cases, the posterior elements are involved, and in 40% of these tumors, the vertebral arch is involved. They can bridge the disk space and invade adjacent vertebrae or involve the paraspinal soft tissue. Radicular pain results from neural foraminal encroachment, and long-tract signs occur with thecal sac compression.

Although aneurysmal bone cysts are benign, their growth pattern is characterized by rapid enlargement, bone destruction, and neurological compromise.

Gross pathologic features include an eggshell-thin cyst and a trabeculated cystic or hemorrhagic interior. Histopathologically, these benign growths are composed of large anastomosing cavernous spaces filled with blood. The solid portion of the tumor consists of

osteoid material intermixed with fibrous tissue (Fig. 313–5A). Benign osteoclast-like giant cells are seen in most cases, and a needle biopsy may lead to misdiagnosis.

Plain films demonstrate an expansile lytic lesion (see Fig. 313–5B) that can range in size from 2 to 9 cm. CT reveals extensive destruction of bone caused by tumor expansion and a trabeculated honeycomb appearance (see Fig. 313–5C). MRI exhibits paraspinal masses or epidural compression (see Fig. 313–5F). Multiple fluid-fluid levels and internal septation may be identified. Fluid levels are best seen on T2 magnified images.[53, 55, 56]

The combination of preoperative endovascular embolization and surgical curettage offers a complete cure with minimal blood loss (see Fig. 313–5F).[57] The majority of recurrences occur less than 6 months after the initial surgery. If a lesion recurs, radiotherapy should be considered after a more radical surgical procedure that will most likely require instrumentation and fusion.[58]

OTHER BENIGN TUMORS

Eosinophilic Granuloma

Eosinophilic granuloma is a non-neoplastic lesion that develops from abnormal growth of lipid-laden phagocytic histiocytes of the reticuloendothelial system.[59] It constitutes a variant of Langerhans' cell histiocytosis that occurs principally in children and adolescents.[60] There is a male predilection.[61] Ten percent to 15% of these lesions occur in the spine, usually in the thoracic or lumbar region.[62] A lesion in the vertebral body causes a wedge-shaped collagen that may result in spinal cord compression. Systemic symptoms, including fever and weight loss, may be present.

Grossly, these lesions appear cystic and hemorrhagic, with a yellowish brown appearance.[63] With time, they accumulate increased amounts of lipid and appear yellow. In later stages, they heal into gray fibrous lesions. The hallmark of these lesions is the presence of Langerhans' cells, and on electron microscopy, the key pathologic finding is Birbeck granules in the Langerhans' cell cytoplasm near the nucleus.[64] Even with complete vertebral body collapse, or vertebra plana (Fig. 313–6A), the areas of endochondral ossification are separate, and some degree of vertebral height recovery may occur.[65]

Plain radiographs demonstrate marginated lytic lesions with well-defined borders. Decreased signal intensity on T1-weighted images and increased intensity on T2-weighted images are demonstrated on MRI (see Fig. 313–6B).[66] A mild kyphosis on epidural impingment may also be seen. Rest and external immobilization are the most effective treatment.[67]

Two important prognostic factors—age and organ involvement—have been identified.[60] The mortality rate is higher in children younger than 2 years, and the prognosis is poor when the liver and bone marrow are involved.

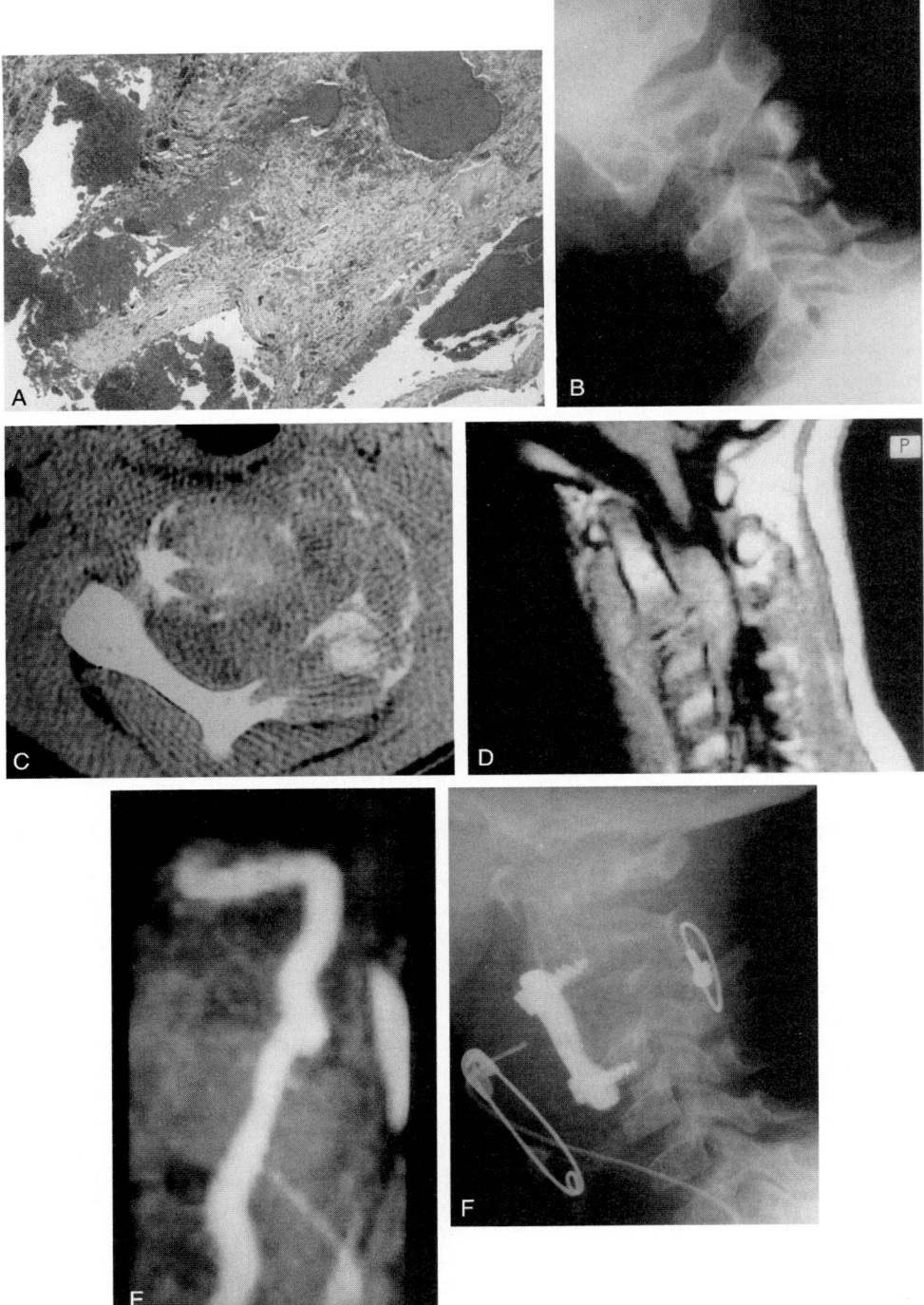

FIGURE 313–5. Aneurysmal bone cyst at C3. *A,* At this magnification, there are multiple sinusoidal channels filled with blood but no obvious endothelial lining. The solid tissue between the blood cells contains spindle-shaped fibroblasts, occasional multinucleated osteoclast-like giant cells, and occasional bone or osteoid trabeculae (×63). *B,* Preoperative lateral radiograph demonstrates destruction and collapse of the C3 vertebral body with anterior subluxation on this flexion view. *C,* Axial computed tomographic scan at C3 demonstrates destruction of the lamina, pedicle, and vertebral body with expansion of the cortex. *D,* Sagittal magnetic resonance imaging scan confirms the superior and inferior extent of the aneurysmal bone cyst on the left side, with displacement of the spinal cord to the right. *E,* Selective left vertebral angiogram demonstrates straightening and narrowing of the vertebral artery on the side ipsilateral to the tumor. There is no significant vascular pattern present. *F,* Lateral radiograph of the cervical spine demonstrates anterior and posterior stabilization.

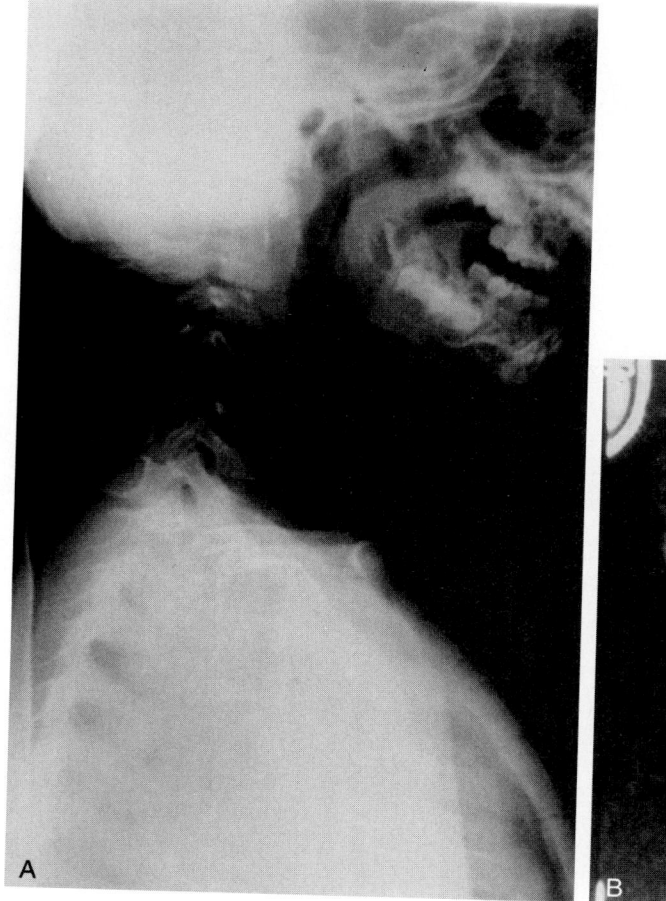
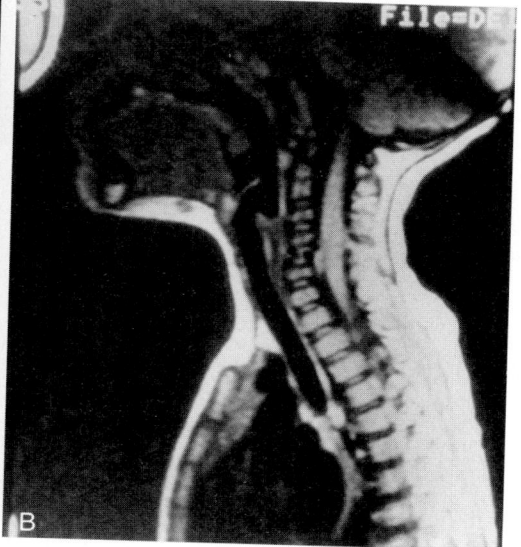

FIGURE 313–6. Eosinophilic granuloma at C5. *A,* Vertebra plana of C5 on this lateral radiograph is compatible with an eosinophilic granuloma. *B,* Sagittal T1-weighted magnetic resonance imaging scan demonstrates complete vertebral body collapse at C5.

MALIGNANT TUMORS

Osteosarcoma

Although osteosarcomas are one of the most common malignant bone tumors, they arise in the spine in less than 4% of cases.[68, 69] However, spread to the spine from osteosarcomas arising elsewhere is fairly common. In Dahlin's Mayo Clinic series, 62% of cases occurred in males and 38% in females.[41, 70] There is a peak incidence in the second decade of life, but in the spine, this tumor peaks in the third decade. This higher incidence in a younger population may be related to rapid bone growth, because the disease has a predilection for the metaphyseal areas of rapidly growing long bones. By the time a diagnosis is made, patients have often developed neurological deficits ranging from radiculopathy to paraplegia.[71] Paget's disease, osteochondroma, or radiotherapy may be predisposing factors in the older population.[72] A latent period of 5 to 25 years after irradiation may pass before the development of an osteosarcoma.

Plain radiographs demonstrate a mixture of sclerosis and osteolysis associated with an ossified soft tissue mass (Fig. 313–7A). MRI is superior to CT in demon-strating the extent of osteosarcoma within the marrow space (see Fig. 313–7B). On short TR sequences, the tumor appears to be of low signal intensity; on long TR sequences, there may be a combination of intensi-ties. MRI is sensitive for revealing the extent of soft tissue involvement, bone marrow infiltration, para-spinal soft tissue masses, and degree of epidural com-pression.[73–76] After the administration of contrast, osteo-sarcomas show immediate enhancement, distinguish-ing them from adjacent muscle, which only minimally enhances with gadolinium. Enhancement may demon-strate the more vascular portion of the tumor, whereas necrotic or sclerotic areas enhance poorly.[77] At the time of diagnosis of a spinal lesion, pulmonary metastasis is already present in 10% to 20% of cases and should be documented with chest CT.[78]

Gross inspection of these tumors reveals a firm, calcified mass. Microscopically, they are characterized by the presence of woven bone produced by malignant osteoblasts in a vascular stroma. The presence of oste-oid or bone may be extremely variable (see Fig. 313–7C). In the Mayo Clinic series, subcategorization based on documented histologic differentiation revealed 55% to be osteoplastic, 23% fibroplastic, and 22% chon-droplastic.[41]

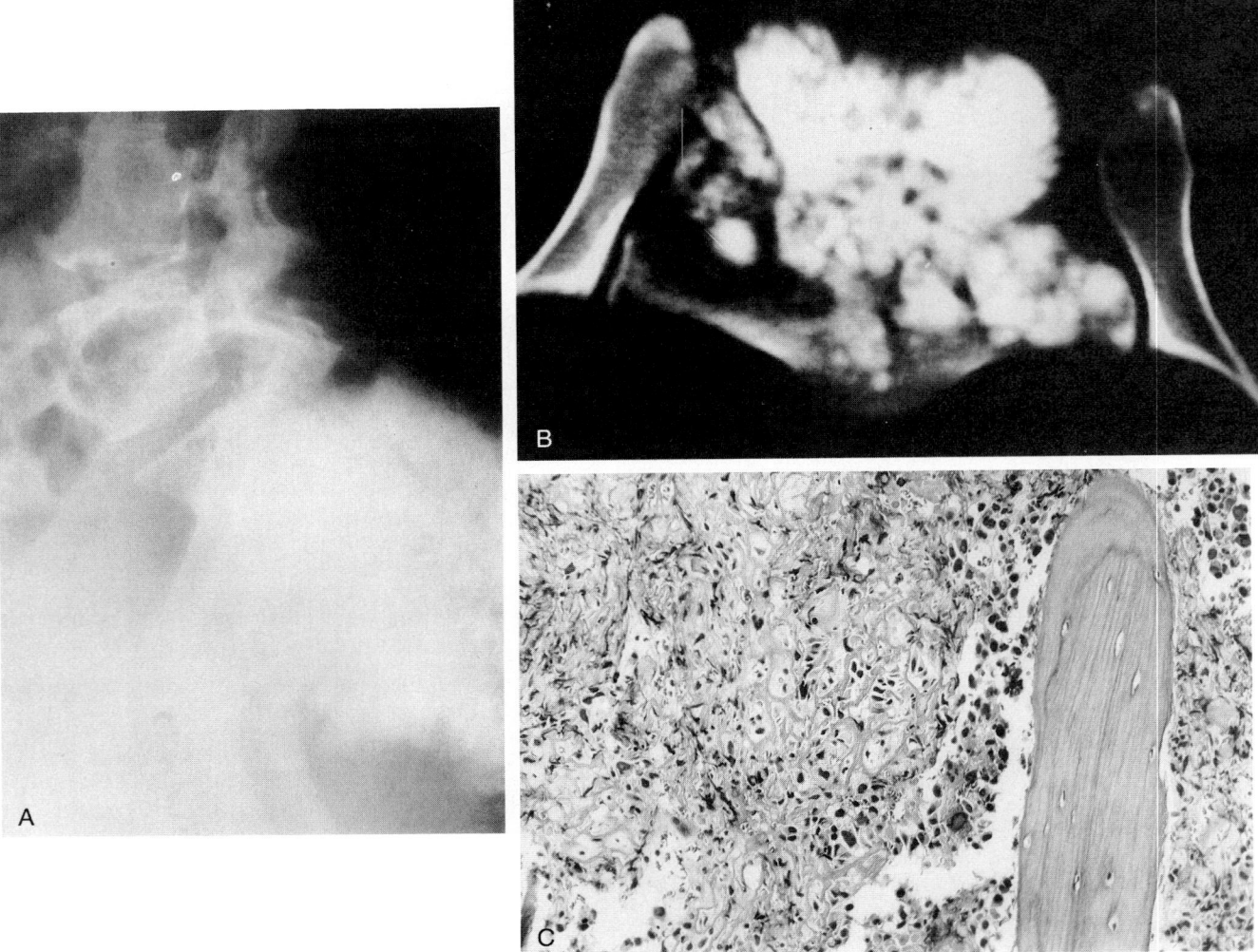

FIGURE 313–7. Osteosarcoma of the sacrum. *A,* Lateral radiograph of the lower lumbar spine and sacrum demonstrates a large sacral osteogenic sarcoma involving the entire sacrum. *B,* Computed tomographic scan demonstrates the extent of the anterior and posterior growth of the tumor. The spinal canal is obliterated. The tumor matrix has discrete areas of calcification and ossification. It is important to note that the lateral margins of the tumor do not extend beyond the sacroiliac joint. *C,* Pleomorphic tumor cells within delicate, lacelike osteoid streamers. The tumor permeates intertrabecular spaces and is seen on both sides of the mature bone trabecula on the right.

Aggressive anterior and posterior surgical intervention, together with systemic chemotherapy and radiation, improves long-term survival better than less extensive procedures and radiation do.[79] The median survival of patients with osteosarcomas of the spine is reportedly in the range of 6 to 10 months.[80] This may be attributed to the tumor's location, which frequently precludes complete resection with adequate margins. A combination of more radical surgical procedures (vertebrectomy), chemotherapy, and radiation may increase survival.[81, 82]

Chondrosarcoma

Chondrosarcomas are malignant hyalin-secreting tumors arising from cartilage. They can arise as primary tumors or secondarily from preexisting enchondromas or osteochondromas. Men are affected up to twice as frequently as women, with a peak incidence in the fifth and sixth decades.[83, 84] Less than 7% of all chondrosarcomas occur in the spine.[85] All areas of the vertebral column may be involved.[86] Most tumors occur on the lateral side of the vertebral body near the costotransverse junction and are thought to originate from the cartilaginous proximal end of the rib. In a Mayo Clinic report, almost half of 20 patients had neurological phenomena at the time of diagnosis.[70] Pain, either axial or radicular, is the most frequent symptom, and epidural compression may be present. Many times a palpable mass can be detected.

Plain radiographs are characterized by a lytic lesion with a calcified soft tissue mass (Fig. 313–8*A* and *B*).

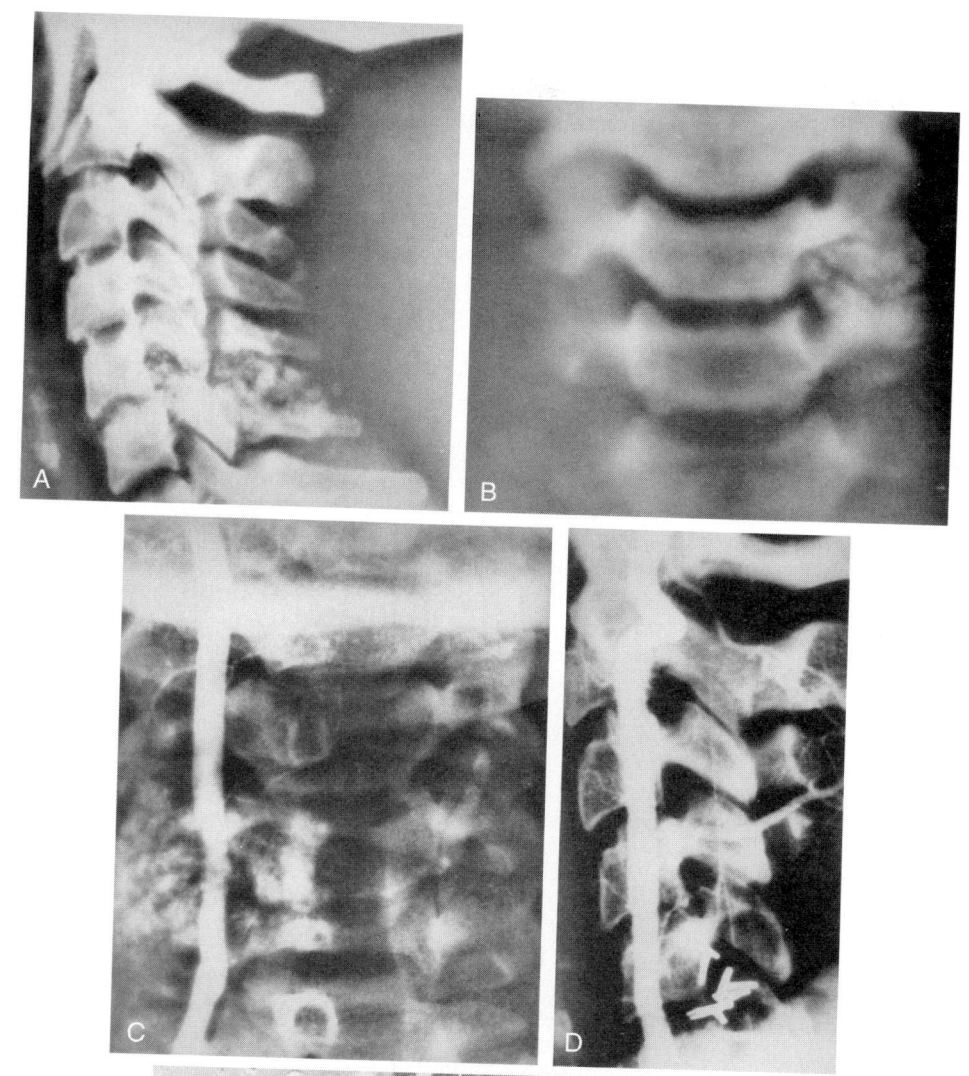

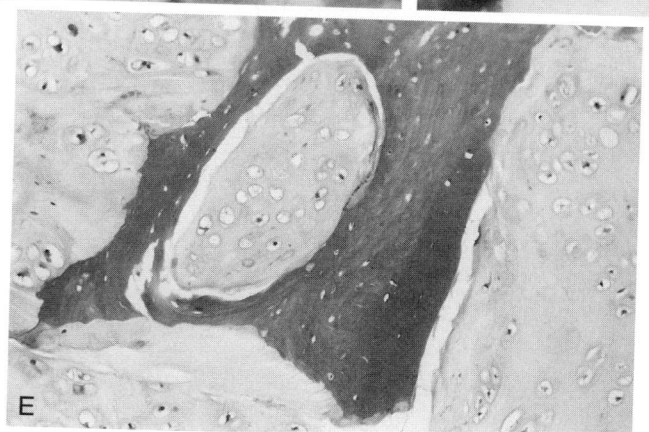

FIGURE 313–8. Chondrosarcoma at C5-6. *A* and *B,* Lateral radiograph *(A)* and frontal tomogram *(B)* demonstrate a calcified tumor arising in the vicinity of the appendages of the C5 and C6 vertebrae on the right side. *C* and *D,* Frontal preoperative *(C)* and lateral postoperative *(D)* vertebral angiograms of a patient with a chondrosarcoma. The preoperative arteriogram demonstrates a segmental narrowing of the vertebral artery. The postoperative angiogram confirms the preservation of the spinal branch of the vertebral artery, with no evidence of segmental narrowing. *E,* The moderately cellular hyaline cartilage matrix demonstrates a few enlarged nuclei in this low-grade chondrosarcoma. The absolute histologic confirmation of malignancy is demonstrated by its infiltrative behavior; the cartilage matrix is seen in a haversian canal (center), as well as in the medullary cavity (right) and outside the cortex (left) (×125).

The degree of calcification varies according to the differentiation of the tumor. CT and MRI are essential to evaluate the bony and soft tissue involvement. The signal intensity of chondrosarcomas on MRI is heterogeneous because of the combination of cartilage, calcification, soft tissue, and hemorrhage. When prominent areas of calcification are present, local areas of decreased signal intensity on long TR images are visualized. MRI may help in differentiating malignant chondrosarcomas from benign osteochondromas. Preoperative angiography and embolization are essential to decrease intraoperative blood loss, because these tumors may be extremely vascular (see Fig. 313–8C and D).

Long-term survival correlates with the grade of malignancy (see Fig. 313–8E).[87, 88] Low-grade tumors are predisposed toward long-term survival, whereas high-grade tumors are aggressive. In one series of 19 cases, the 5-year survival rate for chondrosarcomas of the spine was 21%.[86] In York's series of 21 patients, tumors recurred after 18 of 28 surgical procedures (64%).[84] A median disease-free interval of 12 months occurred in patients who underwent subtotal excision. The tumor recurrence rate was 20% in patients undergoing gross total resection, versus 69% in those who had subtotal resection. DNA flow cytometry offers additional prognostic information: polyploidy has been associated with a worse prognosis.[89, 90]

Radical surgical intervention to resect the tumor and any soft tissue mass is encouraged, because total excision is difficult, and recurrence and metastasis are common. In one series, the addition of radiotherapy prolonged the median disease-free interval from 16 months to 3.7 years, but this was not statistically significant.[84] Clinical tests have not demonstrated any effective chemotherapeutic agent.

Chordoma

Chordomas are rare primary malignant tumors that arise from the embryonal remnants of the notochord. The notochord, which forms the early fetal skeleton, extends from the clivus to the sacrum. The majority of tumors are in the sacrococcygeal region (48%) or spheno-occipital region (39%), where notochord rests also exist.[12] Because most tumors originate in the vertebral bodies, there may be notochord remnants there. Of the tumors that do not arise in the sacrum or clivus, half occur in the cervical region, with the remainder found in the lumbar (Fig. 313–9A) or thoracic region, in descending order of frequency.

Chordomas constitute less than 4% of all primary bone tumors.[91] These tumors are slow-growing, locally invasive neoplasms; pain is the most common symptom. There is a definite 2:1 male-female ratio. In children, there is a predilection for the sacrum. In adults, there is a peak incidence in the sixth decade. Complaints of patients with cervical chordomas include local pain due to nerve root or cord compression. A rectal mass may be palpable in sacral chordomas, and these patients may complain of constipation.[92]

Plain films demonstrate bone destruction, with areas of amorphous calcification. A large soft tissue mass and involvement of two or more adjacent vertebral bodies and the intervening disk are frequently seen.[93, 94] CT is best to delineate areas of osteolytic, osteosclerotic, or mixed areas of bone destruction (see Fig. 313–9B). MRI with Gd-DTPA enhancement provides the best imaging of epidural tumors (see Fig. 313–9C and D). Seventy-five percent of chordomas are isointense to the cord on short TR images, and 25% are hypointense. The lesions have high signal intensity on long TR images.[95, 96] Prominent enhancement is seen, as well as internal septations, cystic changes, and areas of hemorrhage.

Histologically, these tumors are composed of vacuo-lated physaliferous cells. These cells may be arranged in cords and contain abundant glycogen. Special stains can be used to demonstrate keratin and S-100 protein to further document this tumor.[97, 98] Fibrous septae divide the tumors into lobules, which may even be seen on gross examination.

Chordomas invade adjacent structures, have a high local recurrence rate, and may metastasize in as many as 30% of cases. Owing to anatomic limitations, including the proximity of the vertebral artery in cervical lesions, en bloc excision of a spinal chordoma is extremely difficult.

Aggressive surgical resection affords the best opportunity for prolonged survival. Fujita and colleagues described en bloc excision of cervical and thoracic lesions using a T-saw.[99] In selected cases, this technique allows en bloc resection with wide or marginal margins. In sacral disease, a sacrectomy should be performed above the highest level of involvement, because subtotal resection results in a greater probability of recurrence.[100] In lesions along the vertebral column, radical resection and stabilization using a combined anterior and posterior approach should be performed. Local recurrence is a significant problem and occurs as soon as 2 to 4 years after the initial treatment. These tumors are highly resistant to radiotherapy or chemotherapy. Proton and photon radiation has been reported to achieve a significant success rate in terms of local disease control.[101]

Ewing's Sarcoma

In 1921, Sir James Ewing first described this vascular tumor of bone consisting of round cells but devoid of osteoid production. It occurs in the nonsacral spine as a primary tumor in 3.5% to 14% of cases. It is the second most common primary malignant bone tumor after osteosarcoma. It usually presents in patients 15 to 25 years of age, and there is a higher incidence in males than in females.[102] It is frequently found in the spine as a metastasis. Chromosomal studies have revealed a unique reciprocal translocation: t(11;22), q(24;12).[34, 103] As occurs in a majority of bone tumors, there is a significant delay from the onset of symptoms to diagnosis.

These lesions present with pain localized to the neck or back. Point tenderness with swelling and a palpable mass is present in many patients. Plain films demonstrate the classic "onion peel" periosteal reaction. CT and MRI demonstrate the soft tissue paraspinal mass associated with this bony lesion (Fig. 313–10). CT can be used to guide a needle for a closed biopsy. Marrow invasion is demonstrated on MRI with a decreased signal intensity on the short TR image and an increased signal on the long TR image. Hemorrhage, calcification, or necrosis makes for an inhomogeneous appearance. MRI should also be used to determine a patient's response to chemotherapy. Because this lesion frequently metastasizes, interval radionuclide bone scans and computed tomographic scans of the chest should be performed.

In patients with significant or progressive neurologi-

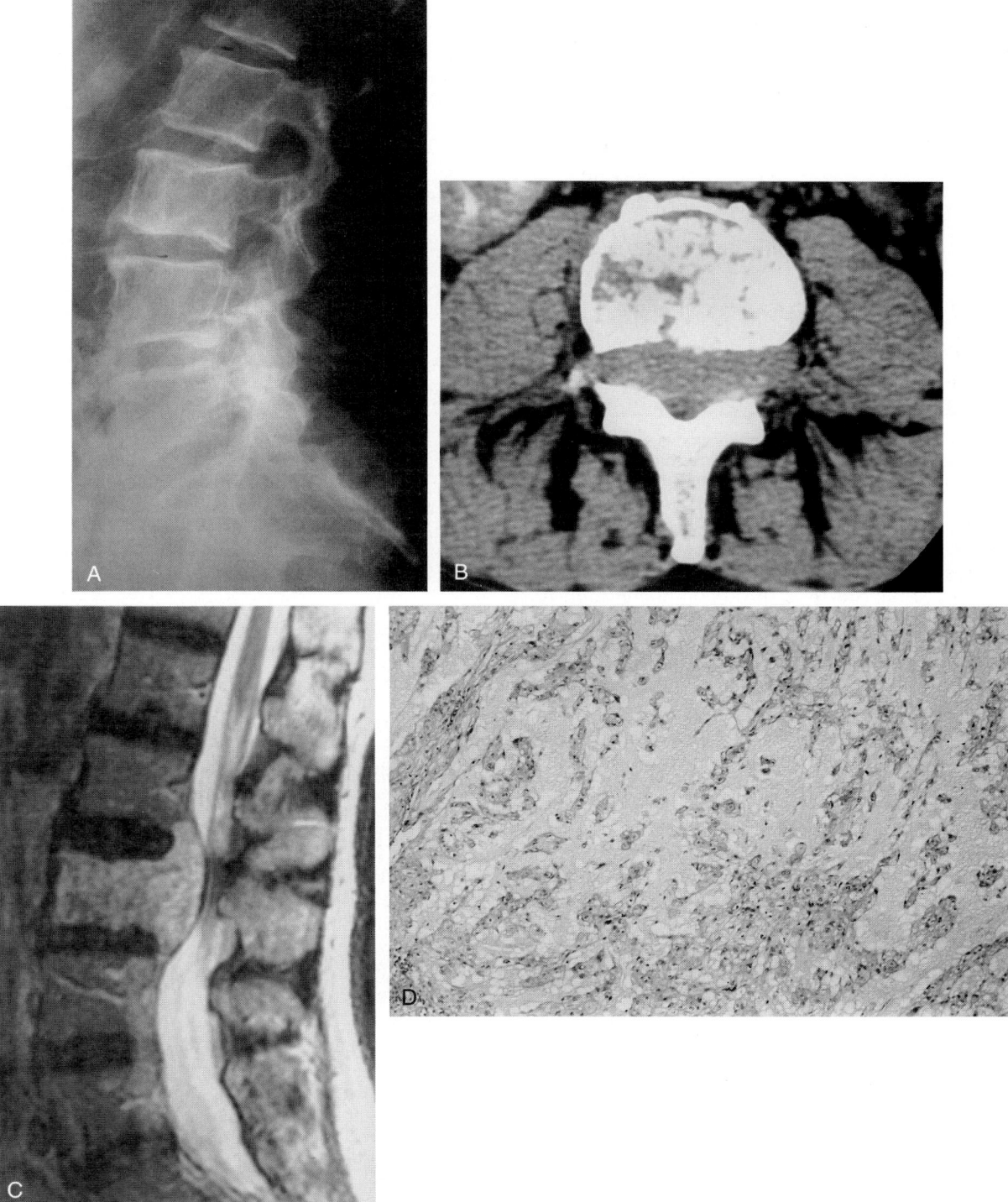

FIGURE 313–9. Chordoma at L3. *A,* Although the location is atypical, this bony lesion was proved histologically to be a chordoma. Lateral spine radiograph reveals subtle loss of the posterior cortex of the L3 vertebral body. *B,* Computed tomographic scan further demonstrates changes within the vertebral body and an epidural soft tissue mass. *C,* Sagittal T2-weighted magnetic resonance imaging (MRI) scan demonstrates an abnormal signal replacing the posterior portion of the L3 vertebral body. An anterior epidural tumor compresses and narrows the thecal sac. The L2-3 and L3-4 disk spaces are not affected. *D,* Axial T2-weighted MRI scan confirms significant pressure on the cauda equina.

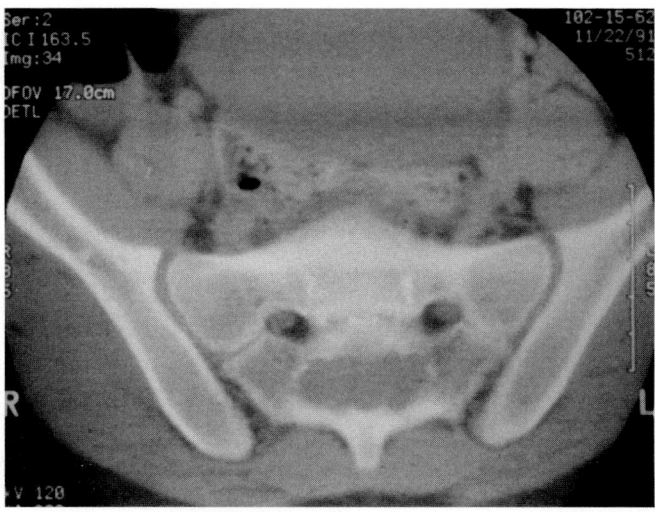

FIGURE 313–10. Ewing's sarcoma of the sacrum. Computed tomographic scan shows a large soft tissue mass within the sacrum and presacral region, obliterating the central canal.

cal deficits, induction chemotherapy should precede definitive surgical treatment. In the second Intergroup Ewing's Sarcoma Study, a protocol using high-dose intermittent vincristine, actinomycin, cyclophosphamide, and doxorubicin (Adriamycin) resulted in a higher remission rate than did a treatment protocol administering a moderate continuous dosage of the same drugs.[54, 104–106] Alternative treatment considerations include autologous bone marrow transplantation combined with radiotherapy and chemotherapy.[107, 108] Surgical resection can be tailored to reduce pain, decompress the thecal sac, and achieve spinal stability.[109, 110] Radiotherapy, 40 to 60 Gy, has been used as an adjunct to surgery, chemotherapy, or both.[111, 112] In Bradway and Pritchard's report from the Mayo Clinic, 13 of 19 patients with spinal Ewing's sarcoma died at an average of 33 months, and none lived longer than 5 years.[102, 113]

Giant Cell Tumor

Giant cell tumors are rare primary bone tumors. After the long bones (Fig. 313–11*A*), the sacrum is the most frequent site. They are frequently located in juxtametaphyseal areas of bone, where the osteoclastic response is associated with bone remodeling. Less than 5% occur in the nonsacral spine.[114] This lesion is the most frequent benign tumor to involve the sacrum. These growths are located primarily in the vertebral body, are locally invasive, and have a high possibility of recurring. Radicular pain is the most common presenting symptom. Women are affected more often than men, with a peak incidence in the second and third decades.

Jaffe correlated the aggressiveness of this tumor to the stromal cells, where ovoid cells with small nuclei are interspersed with multinucleated giant cells (see Fig. 313–11*B*).[114a] McInerney and Middlemiss divided these tumors into three grades, depending on the de-

gree of malignant features present.[115] Hypervascularity is characteristic, and preoperative angiography and possible embolization should be considered (see Fig. 313–11*C* and *D*).[116]

On plain radiographs, a lytic lesion with an expansile appearance is seen. The bone scan correlates with the findings on the CT of the sacrum (see Fig. 313–11*EF*). CT demonstrates a "soap bubble" vertebral expansion (see Fig. 313–11*F*). MRI best demonstrates the bony and soft tissue components of the lesion because the tumor displaces the normal high signal of the fat-containing marrow (see Fig. 313–11*G*).

Complete vertebrectomy with aggressive tumor resection is essential, because subtotal resections have a recurrence rate of up to 40%.[114, 117, 118] Radical resection of sacral tumors is difficult, if not impossible, because these osteophytic lesions destroy great portions of the sacrum and invade adjacent tissues. Unfortunately, radiotherapy is not effective in decreasing the recurrence rate and may increase the rate of sarcomatous degeneration.[119] Follow-up of these patients is essential not only because of local recurrence but also because of the high risk of lung metastasis.

PLASMA CELL DYSCRASIAS

Multiple myeloma and solitary plasmacytoma of bone represent a spectrum of plasma cell tumors, which are clonal B-cell tumors involving bone.[120] Multiple myeloma is by far the more common presentation (40% of all malignant spinal tumors) and consists of disseminated disease involving the marrow diffusely. In contrast, plasmacytoma consists of one or two foci without diffuse marrow involvement.

Solitary Plasmacytoma

Solitary plasmacytoma of bone accounts for only 3% of all plasma cell tumors and consists of one or sometimes two lesions. There is a 2:1 to 3:1 male-to-female predominance, and the average age of patients exceeds 50 years.[121, 122] Between one quarter and one half of all lesions occur in the spine. The thoracic spine is a common location, but lesions can appear anywhere and in anterior or posterior elements.[123] Clinical presentation is related to either local pain or the effect of root or cord compression.

Typically, radiography and CT reveal a lytic lesion, possibly with a cystic component. Sclerosis may be present. Immunoelectrophoresis of the urine and serum shows a monoclonal band, which resolves after definitive treatment.

Paraproteinemia, which can cause coagulopathy if severe, is present in a significant percentage of cases.[124] Bone scanning and skeletal survey radiography are performed to rule out additional lesions. MRI is an important adjunct owing to its sensitivity for finding additional foci.[125] Initially, a needle biopsy of the lesion should be performed, as well as a bone marrow biopsy to rule out multiple myeloma.

Radiotherapy is the first line of treatment for lesions not presenting with rapid neurological deterioration.[72]

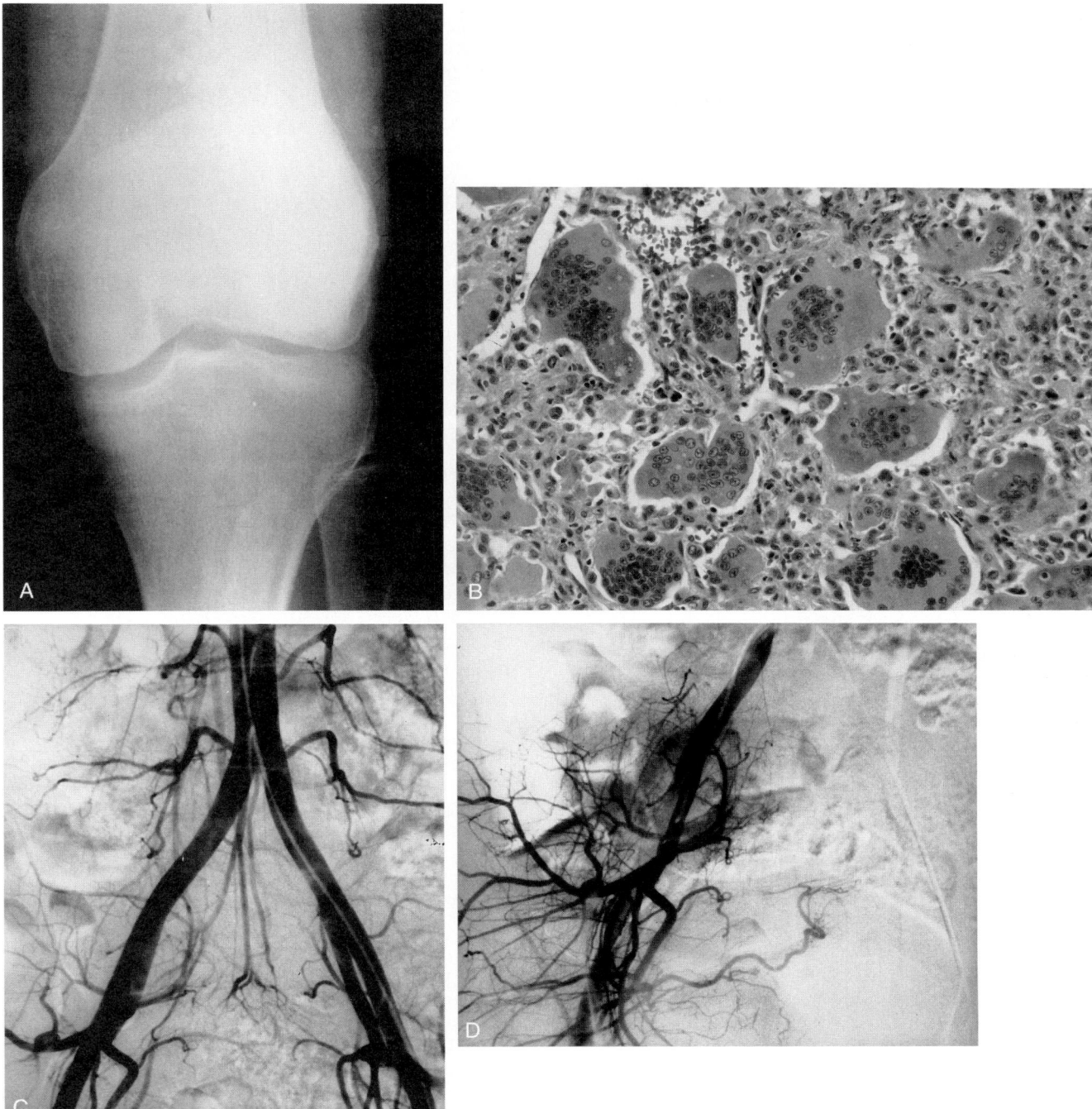

FIGURE 313–11. Giant cell tumor of the femur and sacrum. *A,* Giant cell tumor in the distal femur. *B,* Osteoclast-like giant cells are very large and have more nuclei than typical osteoclasts. They are arranged fairly uniformly in a background of round to polyhedral mononuclear cells, and the nuclei of the giant cells and the mononuclear cells appear virtually identical (×200). *C* and *D,* Preoperative *(C)* and postoperative *(D)* embolization angiography demonstrates a significant decrease in tumor neovascularity.

Illustration continued on following page

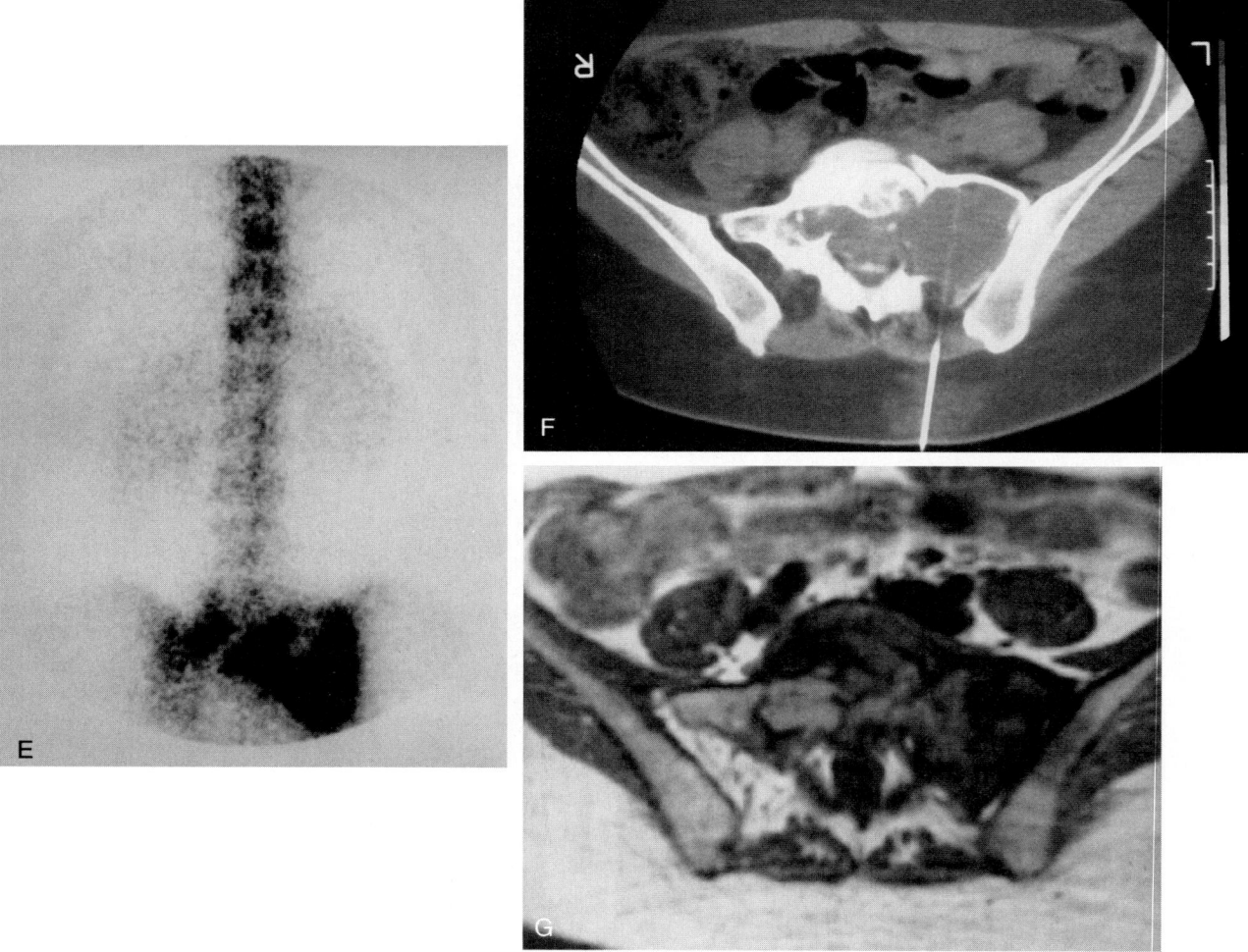

FIGURE 313–11. *Continued. E,* Technetium bone scan correlates with the findings on the lateral radiograph and computed tomographic scan of the sacrum. *F,* Computed tomography–guided needle biopsy of the sacral lesion attempts to obtain a histopathologic diagnosis. *G,* Axial magnetic resonance imaging scan of the sacrum demonstrates the extent of tumor destruction.

Local recurrence is rare when more than 45 Gy is given.[123, 126] Local control with radiotherapy is excellent, with rates up to 96% quoted in the literature and survival up to 11 years. About half of all patients have progressed to myeloma at 5 years from their initial diagnosis.

Surgical resection is performed for those lesions causing neural compression and significant neurological deterioration or bony instability. Complete resection and reconstruction with bone graft and instrumentation are the goals in plasmacytoma so that a cure can be achieved.[85, 127, 128] Subtotal tumor resection should be followed by radiotherapy and possibly chemotherapy. Paraprotein levels should be followed for evidence of recurrence or dissemination, and the presence of an immunoglobulin M component has been shown to predict progression to myeloma.[129]

Multiple Myeloma

The male-to-female prevalence is equal, and multiple myeloma patients are older at presentation (60 years) than are plasmacytoma patients. The annual incidence in the general population is approximately 0.002%.

Myeloma lesions (Fig. 313–12) can appear in any part of the spine but are not always symptomatic. Forty-five percent of all symptomatic lesions are in the spine.[15, 121] Back pain is a frequent first symptom, but neurological compromise often causes patients to seek medical attention.

The medical evaluation of a suspected myeloma patient should include urine and serum protein electrophoresis and 24-hour urine creatinine clearance. As a result of rapid progression of osteolysis, hypercalcemia is found in up to one third of patients. Plain radiographs demonstrate lytic lesions, compression fractures, and osteopenia. On MRI studies, the lesions are hyperintense on T2-weighted images; on T1-weighted images, they usually appear hypointense but may also appear hyperintense or isointense.[130, 131] Contrast enhancement can be used as a marker to determine success of treatment or progression of the disease. Care must be taken to obtain a noncontrast scan before the

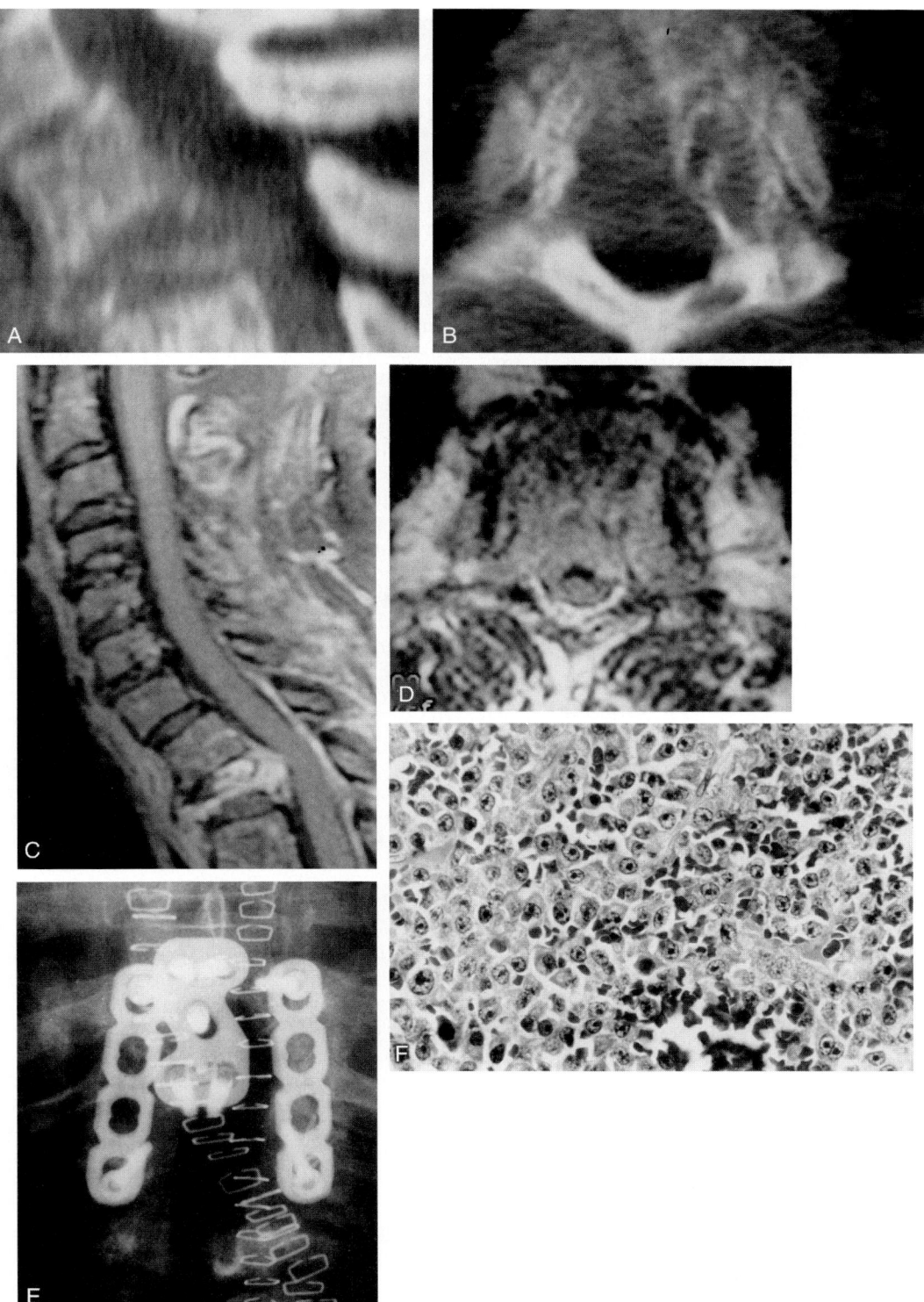

FIGURE 313–12. Multiple myeloma at T2. *A,* On this sagittal reconstruction computed tomographic scan, a destructive lesion is seen involving the T2 vertebra. It is associated with a pathologic vertebral compression fracture and epidural tumor extension into the adjacent spinal canal, obliterating the subarachnoid space and deforming the cord. *B,* On this axial computed tomographic scan, there is epidural tumor extension into the canal, with compression of the adjacent upper thoracic spinal cord. *C,* This sagittal magnetic resonance imaging (MRI) scan demonstrates collapse of the T2 vertebral body, with anterior compression of the spinal cord. *D,* Axial MRI scan demonstrates destruction of the T2 vertebral body, with compression of the thecal sac. *E,* Postoperative radiographs confirm axis plates posteriorly from T1 to T3 and a cervical spine locking plate anteriorly from T1 to T3. *F,* Plasmacytoid tumor cells with eccentric single and double nuclei, prominent nucleoli, and typical "clock-face" chromatin distribution (×400).

contrast injection to prevent underestimation of the degree of diffuse marrow involvement. Soft tissue extension, into either the spinal canal or the paraspinal regions, is commonly seen.

The hematologic workup is critical in myeloma patients. There is marrow suppression, usually with suppression of normal immunoglobulins, which can lead to anemia, neutropenia, and thrombocytopenia. There are oligoclonal bands on serum immunoelectrophoresis, and Bence Jones proteins are present in the urine. This can lead to a paraproteinemia, which may result in a significant coagulopathy. The presence of two or more significant findings (myeloma globulin >30 g/L, immunoglobulin A protein type, and Bence Jones protein excretion >50 mg/day) correlates with early progression of the disease and may distinguish patients requiring treatment from those who can be managed conservatively.[132] Later in the course of the disease, infections and renal failure are common.

Treatment in the absence of clinically significant cord compromise or spinal instability consists of irradiation and, in the case of multiple myeloma, chemotherapy as well.

Surgical intervention should be undertaken to decompress or stabilize the spine when the disease or its surgical treatment has created instability. As an alternative, a halo vest has been used successfully for patients with cervical myeloma during irradiation and chemotherapy to prevent neurological loss from instability, and it may promote stable bony reconstitution. Chemotherapy is a vital part of the treatment of myeloma patients, especially the alkylating agents: cyclophosphamide, melphalan, carmustine, and lomustine. Steroids are given concomitantly.

Prognosis is poor for multiple myeloma, with all published series describing less than 2.5 years median survival and 18% 5-year survival.[122] In addition, solitary plasmactyoma of bone has a 50% incidence of progression to multiple myeloma at 5 years, with most cases occurring within the first 2 years. When epidural compression is the presenting symptom, the median survival drops to less than 8 months, and when a patient with a known history of multiple myeloma presents with new epidural compression, median survival drops to 2 months. Poorer survival is associated with the presence of anemia, hypercalcemia, renal failure, multiple lesions, and hyperproteinuria.

SPINAL METASTASES

Metastatic tumors of the spine are a sinister manifestation of systemic cancer. Controversy continues concerning the relative merits of radiation, surgery, or a combination of these treatment options for patients with symptomatic spinal metastases.[133–135] Clarification of the indications for surgery and the evolution of various operative approaches and techniques have resulted in the refinement of surgical strategies for spinal metastases.

Incidence

Data from *SEER Cancer Statistics Review 1973–1991* reveal that the cancer incidence in the United States, for all sites combined, increased 31% and 15% for white males and females, respectively, and 34% and 18% for black males and females, respectively.[136] The rising overall cancer incidence and the improved life expectancy of cancer patients are likely to be associated with an increased incidence of spinal metastasis.

The majority of patients with systemic cancer develop skeletal secondary tumors, and the spine is most often involved.[137, 138] Spinal metastases are the most common tumors of the vertebral column. It is estimated that 5% to 10% of cancer patients develop symptomatic spinal metastases.[128, 139, 140]

Secondary tumors of the spine most commonly originate from primary cancers of breast, lung, and prostate, reflecting both the prevalence of these primary lesions and their predilection to metastasize to bone. Of patients with symptomatic spinal metastases, 10% present with an unknown primary tumor.[141–143] Half of these are subsequently found to harbor a lung cancer.[144]

Autopsy studies have shown that secondary tumors are distributed along the spinal axis in proportion to the bulk of the vertebrae: spinal metastases occur most frequently in any given lumbar vertebra and least often in any given cervical segment.[138] Clinically, however, symptomatic spinal metastases most often involve the thoracic spine.[142] Most patients with spinal metastases have disease confined to one or two adjacent vertebral levels, whereas up to 30% show evidence of neural compression at noncontiguous sites.[145, 146]

Spinal metastases are somewhat more common in males than in females (1.5:1).[145]

Classification

Tumors of the spine are conveniently classified by anatomic location (Table 313–2).[51, 139, 147–149] The vast majority of secondary spinal tumors occur extradurally. Extradural metastases are most commonly blood borne, either arterially or by venous spread along Batson's plexus.[150, 151] Less often, extradural metastases spread by direct extension and through the intervertebral foramina. Intradural extramedullary metastases are uncommon. These deposits are, for the most part, tertiary tumors that arise as seedlings from secondary cerebral tumors and gravitate through the cerebrospinal fluid to become entangled among the spinal nerve roots of the cauda equina.[148, 149, 152] Intramedullary spinal metastases are rarely encountered.[51, 147, 153, 154]

T A B L E 3 1 3 – 2 ■ **Anatomic Classification of Spinal Metastases**

TYPE	PERCENT
Extradural	95.0
Intradural extramedullary	4.5
Intramedullary	0.5

Data from references 2, 158, 182, 186.

SPINAL METASTASES

CLINICAL SYNDROME

PAIN

WEAKNESS

SENSORY LOSS

SPHINCTERS DYSFUNCTION

COMPLETE AND IRREVERSIBLE PARALYSIS

FIGURE 313–13. Clinical syndrome of spinal metastasis.

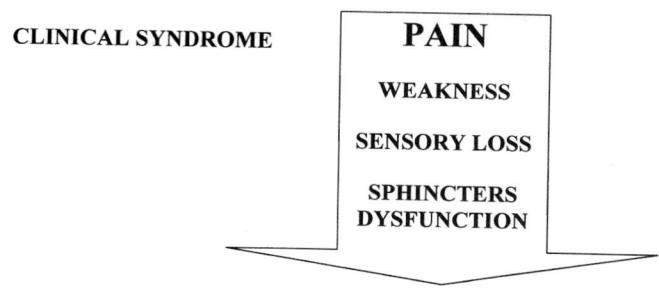

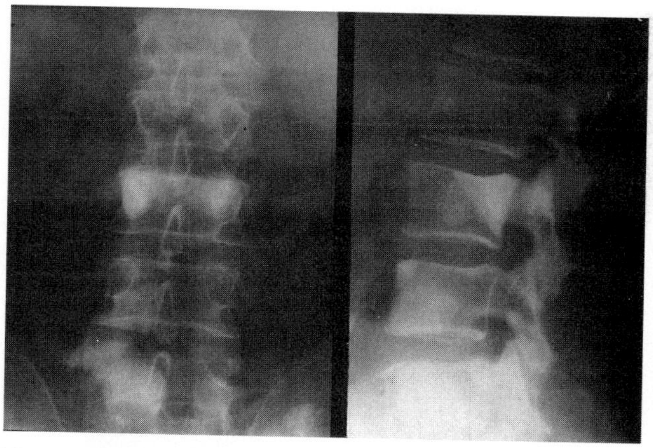

FIGURE 313–14. Osteosclerotic metastases from prostate cancer.

Symptoms and Signs

Spinal metastases produce a characteristic clinical syndrome (Fig. 313–13).[148, 155, 156] Pain is the earliest and most prominent feature in 90% of patients. A radicular neurological syndrome may accompany local back or neck pain. Palpation or percussion over the posterior spinous process at an afflicted level usually elicits local tenderness. If the pain is severe, burning, or dysesthetic in nature, the probability of intradural extramedullary spinal metastasis should be anticipated.[148] If the back or neck pain is aggravated by movement about the involved segment and relieved by immobilization, associated spinal instability should be suspected.[157]

Neck or back pain caused by degenerative disk or joint disease usually arises from the lower half of the cervical spine and low lumbar regions, is characterized by chronic exacerbations and remissions, and is generally relieved by rest and recumbency.[158] Pain caused by spinal metastasis may arise anywhere along the length of the spine (most often from the thoracic segments), tends to be constant and doggedly persistent, and is usually worse with recumbency, particularly at night.[151] Pain resulting from extradural spinal metastasis may be present for weeks or months before more blatant manifestations of spinal cord or nerve root compromise are apparent. Often, pain caused by spinal metastasis is initially attributed to a "slipped" disk, back strain, or muscle spasm.[159] It is axiomatic that a cancer patient with a new onset of neck or back pain harbors spinal metastasis until proved otherwise.

The median duration of symptoms before diagnosis is 2 to 4 months.[142, 145] Weakness, sensory loss, and sphincter dysfunction commonly occur after the onset of pain. The rate of clinical progression is variable. The natural history is one of relentless progression to complete and irreversible paraplegia unless timely treatment is undertaken.[141]

Investigations

Radiologic studies are performed for diagnosis, localization, staging, embolization, and follow-up of spinal metastases.

PLAIN FILMS

Plain radiographic studies should serve as the initial screening test. Anteroposterior and lateral radiographs of the spine demonstrate abnormalities in up to 90% of patients with symptomatic spinal metastases.[144, 160] Radiologic abnormalities are displayed at more than one level in one third of these patients.[80, 146] Sclerotic or blastic bony alteration may occur, typically with metastases arising from primary cancers of the prostate or breast (Fig. 313–14); however, lytic lesions account for the majority of plain film manifestations. Common plain film findings include pedicle erosion, paraspinal soft tissue shadow, vertebral collapse, and frank pathologic fracture-dislocation (Table 313–3).[142, 161, 162]

Among patients with symptomatic spinal metastases, 76% demonstrate pedicle erosion, producing a "winking owl" sign (Fig. 313–15).[161] Pedicle erosion is often associated with a paraspinal soft tissue shadow (Fig. 313–16). Further destruction of the vertebral body may result in a compression fracture (Fig. 313–17). Frank pathologic fracture-dislocation is seen most often in the cervical region, where the dependent position of the head, wide range of neck movement, and lack of rib cage supporting structure render the neck vulnerable to mechanical disruption (Fig. 313–18).[156]

TABLE 313–3 ■ **Common Plain Film Findings for Spinal Metastases***

	PERCENT
Pedicle erosion ('winking owl')	76
Paraspinal soft tissue shadow	23
Collapsed vertebra	22
Pathological fracture-dislocation	7

* Based on 101 consecutive patients with symptomatic spinal metastases.
From Krushelnycky, BW, Perrin, RG: Radiologic manifestations of spinal metastases. Paper presented at the 55th Annual Meeting of the Royal College of Physicians and Surgeons, Sep 25, 1986, Toronto.

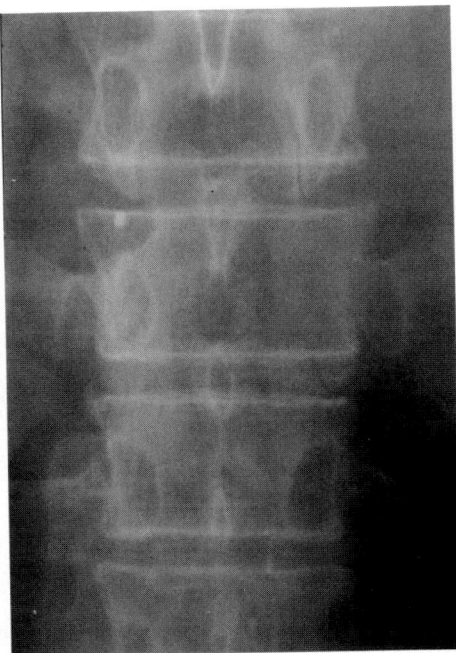

FIGURE 313–15. Pedicle erosion producing a "winking owl" sign.

MYELOGRAPHY

Myelography has been the standard method for establishing the level of and localizing spinal cord and nerve root compromise. Myelography helps distinguish among extradural, intradural extramedullary, and intramedullary spinal tumors. Analysis of cerebrospinal fluid obtained at lumbar puncture is essential when

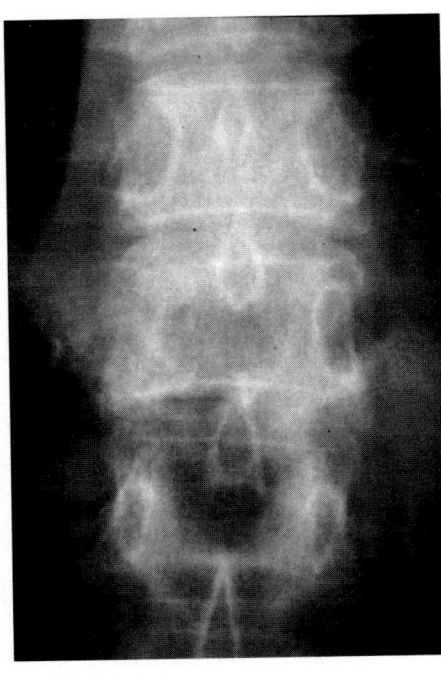

FIGURE 313–16. Paraspinal soft tissue shadow.

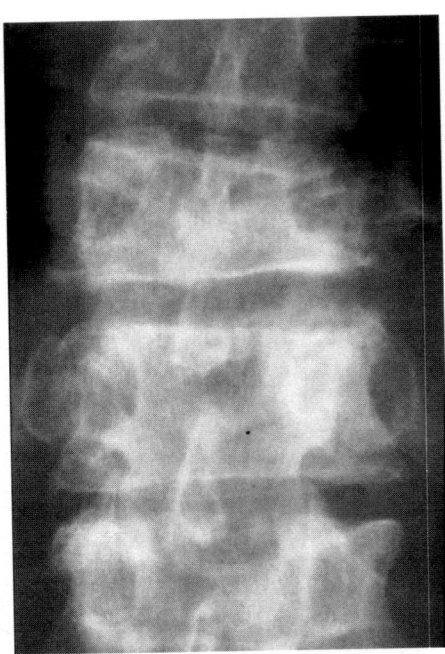

FIGURE 313–17. Compression fracture.

intradural extramedullary metastasis is suspected. If the level of a myelography block does not correspond to the clinical localization, or if multiple levels of tumor involvement are suspected beyond the area of complete block, a combination of lumbar and cisternal myelography studies may help demonstrate the extent of disease (Fig. 313–19).

Lumbar puncture performed in the presence of a complete cerebrospinal fluid block carries significant risk and may precipitate or hasten neurological deterioration in up to one quarter of patients.[163, 164]

COMPUTED TOMOGRAPHY

CT is useful principally to assess bony architecture and demonstrate the degree of bone destruction (Fig.

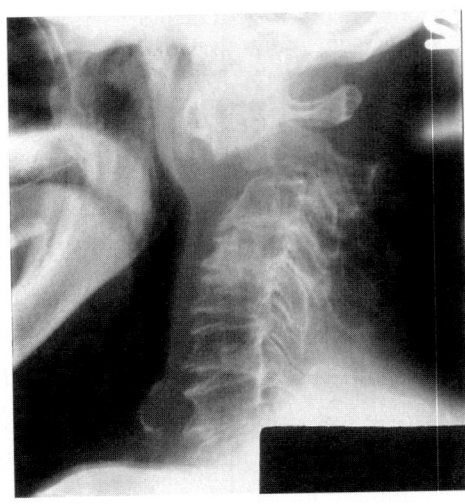

FIGURE 313–18. Pathologic fracture-dislocation.

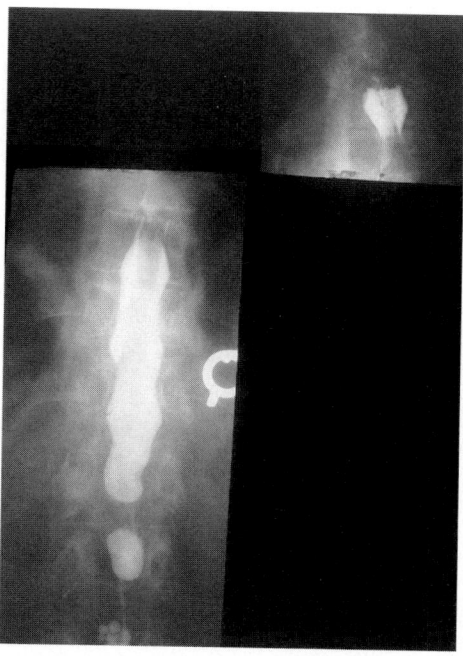

FIGURE 313–19. Combined lumbar and cisternal myelography delineates the extent of the compressing lesion.

313–20). The information provided should be used to determine the appropriate approach and techniques for surgical intervention. CT is especially informative if it is performed in conjunction with and immediately after myelography.[165, 166]

CT-guided needle biopsy has been advocated for spinal metastasis patients with no known primary tumor. However, this procedure is associated with a misdiagnosis rate as high as 20%.[167, 168]

MAGNETIC RESONANCE IMAGING

MRI has become the imaging modality of choice for spinal tumors.[95, 169–171] MRI can demonstrate the location, extent, and geometry of spinal tumors in transverse, sagittal, and coronal planes. The whole spine is readily surveyed to identify single, multiple contiguous, and multiple disparate levels of involvement (Fig. 313–21). Enhancement with Gd-DTPA permits visualization of intradural extramedullary and intramedullary metastases.[172, 173]

Some patients are unable to tolerate the MRI procedure because of claustrophobia or difficulty lying still for the duration of the examination. Further, there are contraindications to this procedure, including the presence of a cardiac pacemaker.

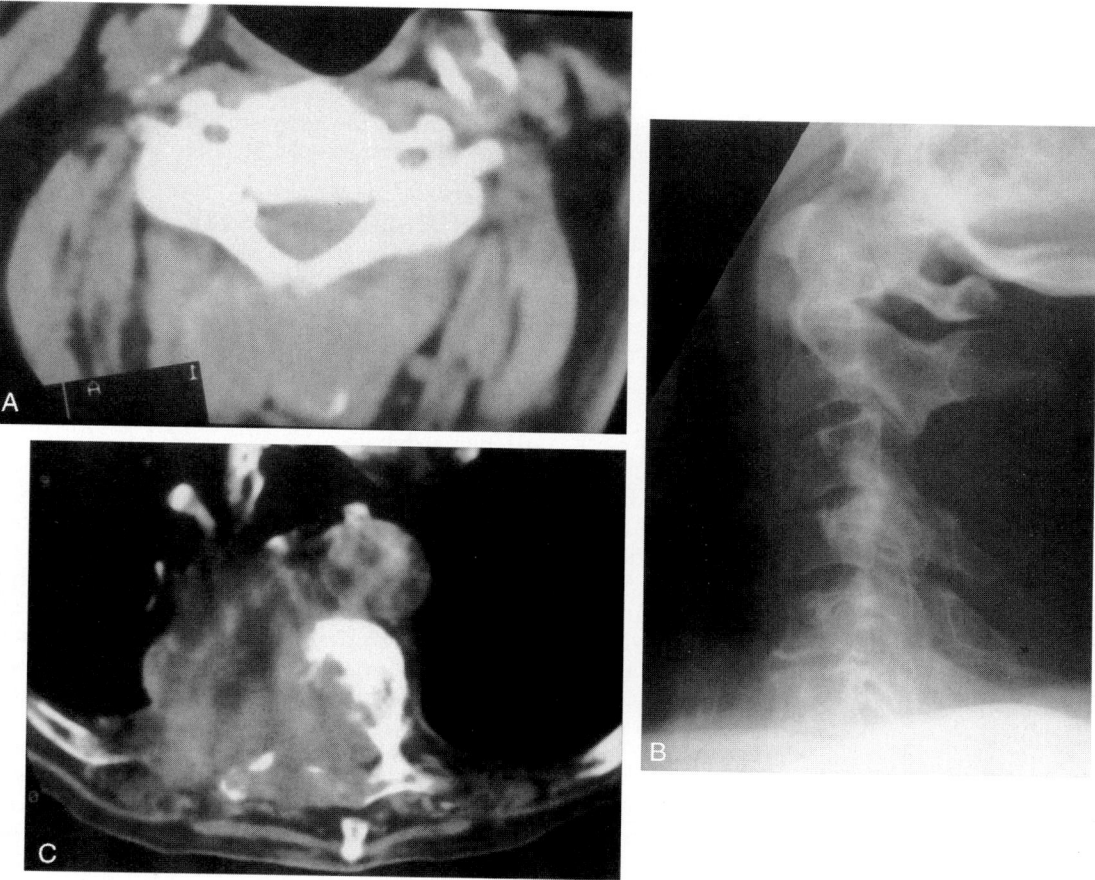

FIGURE 313–20. Computed tomographic scan *(A)* through C3 shows bone destruction corresponding to the plain film *(B)*. Computed tomographic scan *(C)* through the midthoracic spine demonstrates bone destruction.

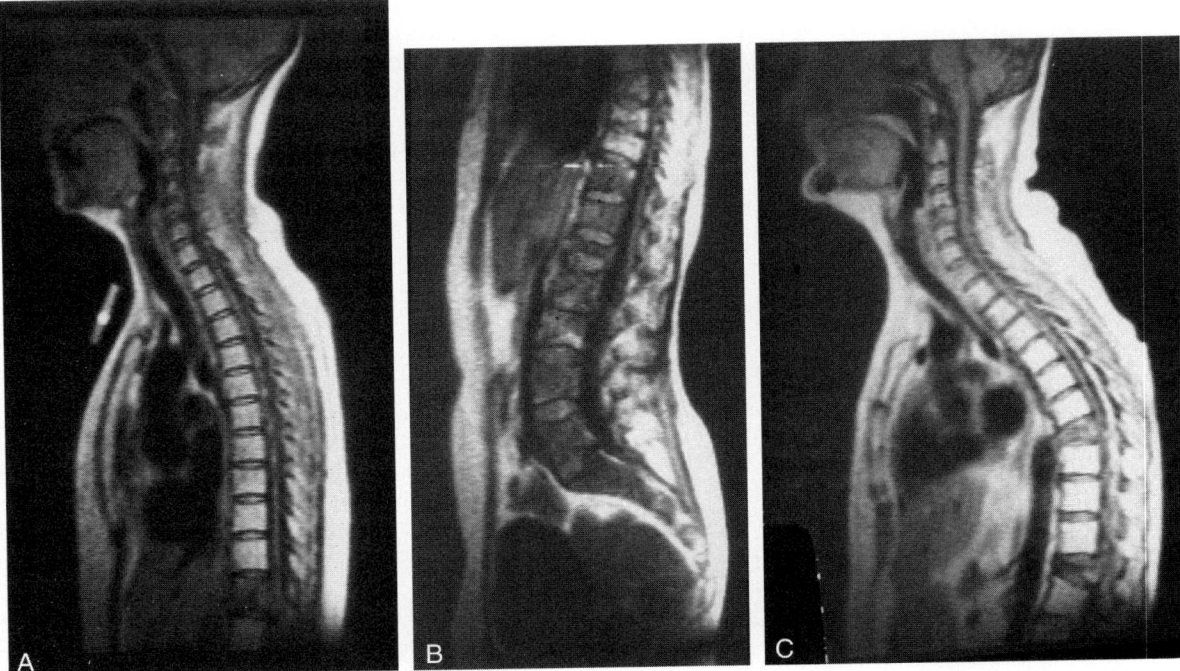

FIGURE 313–21. Magnetic resonance images show single *(A)*, multiple contiguous *(B)*, and multiple disparate *(C)* levels of involvement.

Although MRI is a sensitive method for displaying the presence, location, and extent of spinal tumors, CT provides a more reliable index of bone destruction.[5, 10, 109, 174]

BONE SCAN

Radionuclide bone scanning demonstrates bone pathology at an early stage but lacks specificity. Although bone scanning is more sensitive than plain radiographic studies in detecting spinal metastases, up to 30% of abnormalities displayed on bone scans of the spine are caused by benign disease.[7, 175, 176]

Management

The treatment of spinal metastasis is undertaken to relieve pain and preserve or restore neurological function. Rarely is it reasonable to anticipate a cure; palliation is the realistic treatment goal. Nevertheless, relief of pain and preservation or restoration of neurological function contribute immeasurably to the quality of a cancer patient's remaining life and often reduce the burden of care.

STEROIDS

Corticosteroids are a vital adjunct in the treatment of metastases causing spinal cord compression.[177–179] The improvement in neurological function after steroid administration, documented in both animal investigations and human studies, is attributed to a reduction of spinal cord edema near the compression site.[180, 181]

It is standard practice to give dexamethasone 10 mg intravenously when spinal cord compression is diagnosed and 4 mg every 6 hours thereafter, until definitive treatment (surgery or radiotherapy) is completed, after which the steroid regimen may be tapered.

RADIOTHERAPY VERSUS SURGERY

Therapeutic irradiation and surgery (decompression with or without stabilization) are the principal and complementary treatment options for patients with symptomatic spinal metastasis. The relative merits of therapeutic irradiation, surgery, or a combination of these treatment modalities have been the subject of extensive debate.[79, 139, 182, 183]

Irradiation is particularly effective for metastases of lymphoreticular origin, moderately effective for spinal metastases originating from breast or prostate tumors, and less effective for lung or melanoma metastases. Primary radiation treatment combined with "salvage" surgical decompression for spinal metastasis has become common practice. This approach is based in part on the disappointing results achieved in the past with the indiscriminate use of decompressive laminectomy. Retrospective analyses purporting to show that irradiation is as effective as surgery (with or without irradiation) in the treatment of spinal metastases are based on comparisons between therapeutic irradiation and simple laminectomy. It has become clear, however, that simple laminectomy is inadequate or inappropriate and is potentially harmful in most patients with spinal metastases. Simple laminectomy does not allow adequate decompression of the spinal cord and nerve roots in the majority of patients with extradural metastases and is appropriate only if the compressing mass is localized primarily about the dorsal surface of the dural sac. Laminectomy alone may also be deleterious because it aggravates or exacerbates mechanical instability.[184–186]

Elaboration of the posterolateral approach[156, 187, 188] and anterior exposures[79, 189–191] for decompression of the spinal cord and nerve roots, together with the evolution of spinal stabilization procedures (Table 313–4), has improved the outcome after surgery and supports the concept of initial (de novo) surgery for spinal metastasis.[79] Primary surgery avoids the high incidence of wound complications (up to 30%) attributed to operating through a radiation-saturated field.[108, 192]

Minimally invasive surgery promises to further reduce surgical morbidity.[193]

INDICATIONS FOR SURGERY

The indications for surgery in patients with symptomatic spinal metastases are listed in Table 313–5.

Failure of Radiotherapy. Most patients with symptomatic spinal metastases coming to surgery are referred after failure of radiotherapy. Typically, such patients suffer relapse during or recurrence after radiation

TABLE 313–4 ■ Posterior and Anterior Spinal Stabilization Devices and Techniques

METHOD	AUTHOR
Posterior	
Rib struts	Livingston & Perrin[142]
Interspinous wiring	Rogers[207]
Posterolateral facet fusion	Robinson et al[208, 209]
Dewar procedure	Davey et al[210]
Harrington rods	Harrington et al[211, 212]
San Francisco system	White et al[213]
Vermont system	Krag et al[214]
Roy-Camille plates	Roy-Camille et al[215]
Variable spine plating	Steffee et al[216]
Halifax clamp	Holness[217]
Luque rods/rectangle	Luque[218]
Contoured Luque	Ellis & Findlay[197]
Methyl methacrylate/ sublaminar wiring	Perrin
Lateral mass plates/transverse process hooks	York et al
Anterior	
Smith-Robinson	Robinson et al[208, 209]
Cloward	Cloward[219]
Corpectomy/iliac crest	Fielding et al[220]
Corpectomy/fibula	Conley et al[221]
Pins/methyl methacrylate	Scoville et al[222]
Double K-wire/methyl methacrylate	Sundaresan et al
Knodt rods/methyl methacrylate	Harrington[211, 212]
Metal prosthesis	Ono & Tada[223]
Wellesley wedge	Perrin et al
Chest tube/methyl methacrylate/locking plates	Gokaslan et al[198]

TABLE 313–5 ■ Indications for Surgery for Spinal Metastases

Failed radiotherapy
Diagnosis unknown
Pathologic fracture-dislocation
Rapid progression/far-advanced paraplegia

treatment. Surgical salvage is then entertained as a measure of last resort.

Unknown Diagnosis. Surgical intervention is indicated if a diagnosis other than spinal metastasis (e.g., disk protrusion, epidural abscess, hematoma) is suspected in a cancer patient.[159] In the 10% of patients with symptomatic spinal metastasis who present with an unknown primary tumor, spinal decompression may be diagnostic as well as therapeutic.

Pathologic Fracture-Dislocation. Approximately 10% of patients with symptomatic spinal metastases present with frank pathologic fracture-dislocation (see Fig. 313–18). The neurological compromise in such cases is the result of both compression of the spinal cord and nerve roots by metastatic tumor mass and distortion of the dural sac and its contents from spinal malalignment. Surgical treatment is required to relieve compression of the spinal cord and nerve roots and to restore and maintain alignment of the spinal column.[156]

Rapidly Progressing or Far-Advanced Paraplegia. Neurological deterioration that is rapidly progressing or far advanced represents a neurological emergency. Even if irradiation is considered appropriate, complete and irreversible paraplegia may supervene before any benefit of therapeutic irradiation is apparent. Surgical intervention is indicated in this circumstance to provide prompt and effective decompression of the spinal cord and nerve roots.

SURGICAL STRATEGIES

Surgical treatment for spinal metastasis must provide for both decompression of the spinal cord and the nerve roots and stabilization of the spinal column. Extradural metastases may already have caused instability of the spine by the time surgical treatment is undertaken. In addition, operative procedures providing adequate decompression of the spinal cord and nerve roots often aggravate or precipitate instability of the spinal column, making appropriate spinal reconstruction imperative.

ANTERIOR VERSUS POSTERIOR APPROACH

Surgery for spinal metastasis can be carried out from the front (anterior or anterolateral procedures) or from behind (posterior or posterolateral procedures). Each has its role, and no single approach is always applicable. Keeping in mind that surgical strategies must provide both decompression of the neural elements and stabilization of the structural support, the optimal ap-

SURGICAL STRATEGIES

FACTORS AFFECTING APPROACH

DECOMPRESSION
- **LOCATION OF TUMOR**
- **SPINAL LEVEL**

STABILIZATION
- *EXTENT OF DISEASE*
- **BONY INTEGRITY**

- **PATIENT DEBILITY**

FIGURE 313–22. Factors determining the surgical approach.

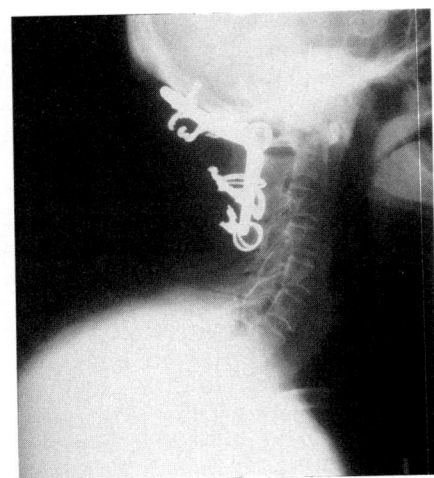

FIGURE 313–24. Steel rectangle fixation between the occiput and upper cervical segments.

proach is dictated by a number of interrelated factors (Fig. 313–22).[194, 195]

Location of Tumor. Intradural metastases are usually best approached through a wide laminectomy. A wide laminectomy also permits adequate decompression in the unusual circumstance of a spinal metastasis that involves only the posterior elements (see Fig. 313–20A and B). More often, however, spinal cord compression results from an anteriorly or laterally situated tumor mass or collapsed bone (see Fig. 313–20C). In such cases (and other factors being equal), an anterior or anterolateral approach may be the most appropriate route to achieve adequate decompression anteriorly.

Spinal Level. Spinal metastases occurring at the extreme ends of the vertebral column pose a particular challenge. Transoral and mandible-splitting techniques may provide adequate anterior exposure at the craniocervical junction. By the same token, combined anterior and posterior approaches may be used to achieve total sacrectomy.[196] However, the associated morbidity and lengthy postoperative convalescence are inconsistent with the basic aim of palliation for cancer patients with

a limited life expectancy. Further, although it is possible to achieve adequate spinal decompression from the front at the craniocervical junction and through staged surgeries at the lumbosacral region, anterior spinal reconstruction at these levels poses an enormous challenge. Consequently, the preferred initial approach at the rostral and caudal extremes of the spinal column is usually from behind. Stabilization may be achieved posteriorly at the craniocervical junction by sublaminar wiring to methyl methacrylate or a steel rectangle, and this fixation may be extended to the occiput (Figs. 313–23 and 313–24).[157, 197] Reconstruction at the lumbosacral junction involves instrumentation between lumbar laminae and the ilium on each side (Fig. 313–25). An anterior apparatus may then supplement the posteriorly applied device.

Extent of Involvement. Anterior or anterolateral spinal metastases involving one or two contiguous levels are usually best approached from the front (with the exception noted earlier). The anterior (or anterolateral) avenue provides the most direct access to the compressing lesion.[198] An anteriorly applied reconstruction prosthesis is most effective from a biomechanical point of view. Although anterior decompression procedures

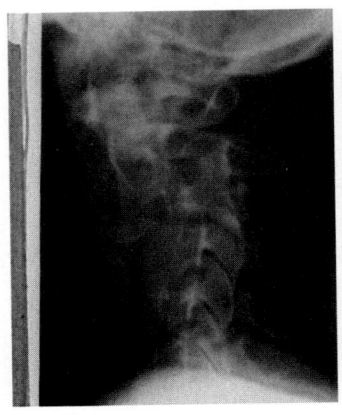
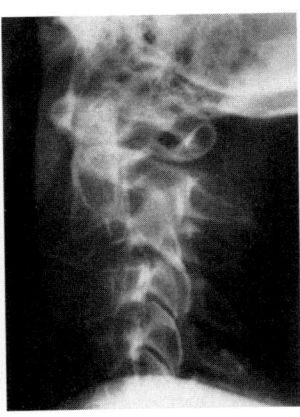
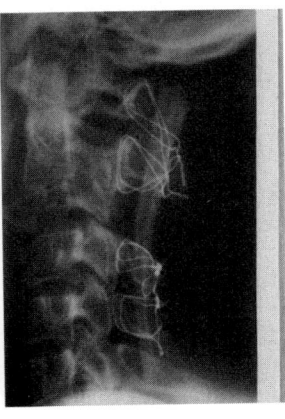

FIGURE 313–23. Pathologic fracture-dislocation managed with skeletal traction to produce realignment and posterior decompression with sublaminar wiring to rib struts for stabilization.

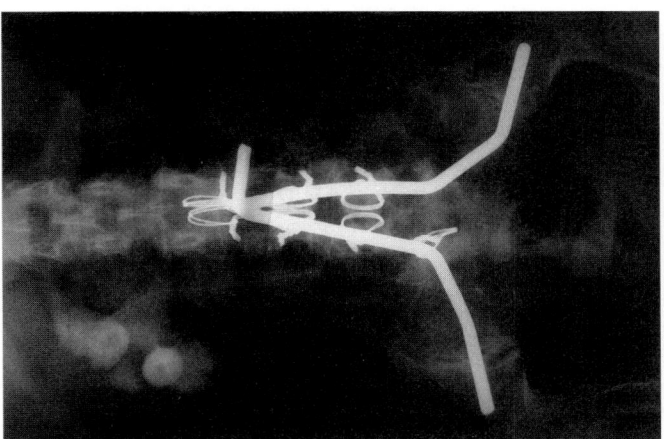

FIGURE 313–25. Pathologic fracture at L5 is managed with posterior decompression and instrumentation.

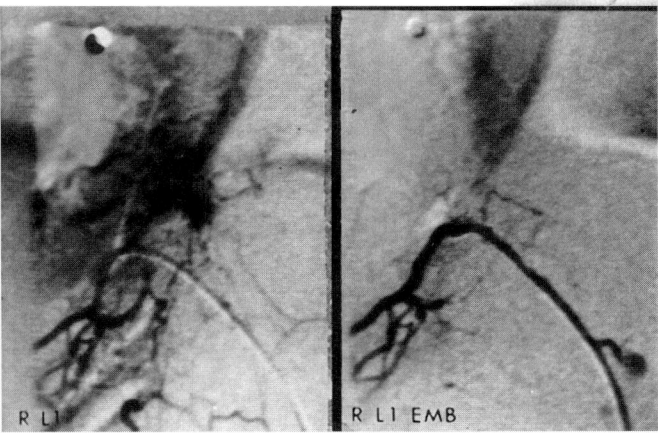

FIGURE 313–26. Spinal angiography before *(A)* and after *(B)* embolization of extradural metastases originating from hypernephroma.

extending across three or more vertebral segments are not impossible, fixation of an anterior construct in this circumstance is tenuous at best. In such cases, posterolateral decompression and posterior fixation may be more appropriate. Alternatively, if an anterior approach is undertaken, it is advisable to supplement an anteriorly applied reconstruction device with posterior spinal fixation.

Bone Integrity. The integrity of vertebral bodies adjacent to a decompressed segment must be sufficient to accept and anchor an anteriorly applied reconstruction apparatus. The vertebral bodies adjacent to a proposed anterior decompression site may be diseased to such a degree that fixation of a reconstruction prosthesis is impossible (see Fig. 313–21*B*). It then becomes necessary to consider posterolateral decompression followed by stabilization using a posterior construct secured by sublaminar wires.

Patient Debility. Local or systemic debility may influence the approach. Surgical exposure anteriorly through a radiation-saturated neck is accompanied by an increased risk of tracheoesophageal perforation and its associated consequences. The patient may be unable to tolerate the stress of a transthoracic or thoracoabdominal approach. Alternatively, lengthy spinal procedures performed with a midline incision through radiation-saturated skin and that include the installation of hardware in a cancer patient with impaired immunity and compromised nutrition carry a significant risk of wound complications.[108, 192]

It has been said, "When all you have is a hammer, everything looks like a nail." In other words, the optimal surgical strategy for patients with spinal metastases should not be biased by a surgeon's technical limitations; rather, it should be determined by the previously mentioned factors and then expertly executed.

EMBOLIZATION

Metastatic tumors of thyroid and renal cell origin are notoriously vascular. Preoperative embolization should be undertaken before direct surgical decompression to minimize the risk of catastrophic blood loss (Fig. 313–26).[199–202]

DECOMPRESSION

Laminectomy is usually appropriate for intradural metastases and may also suffice for epidural metastases involving only the posterior elements (see Fig. 313–20*A* and *B*). In most cases, however, decompression from behind requires a wide laminectomy with posterolateral extension to permit resection of the tumor-destroyed lateral elements and access to the vertebral body.[150] The tumor-destroyed vertebral body can then be systematically excavated. The dural sac and contents are decompressed by careful centrifugal displacement of the anterolateral epidural mass into the excavated vertebral body cavity before removal (Fig. 313–27). The posterolateral decompression may be applied bilaterally, resulting in effective circumferential decompression of the dural sac (see Fig. 313–27*D*).

Spinal decompression can be performed from the front by anterior access in the cervical and lower lumbar segments and through an anterolateral approach in the thoracic (transthoracic) and thoracolumbar (thoracoabdominal) regions (Fig. 313–28). In each case, the decompression is facilitated by initial resection of the intervertebral disks above and below the involved segment, followed by systematic excision of the vertebral body (corpectomy), including the posterior longitudinal ligament. Because the approach is directly anterior in the cervical and lower lumbar segments, the exposure permits decompression of the anterior dural sac and nerve root sleeves bilaterally. Between these areas, the approach is anterolateral through a thoracotomy to the thoracic spine and by thoracoabdominal exposure to the thoracolumbar region. Although the anterolateral approach permits excellent decompression of the anterior (thoracic and thoracolumbar) dural sac and ipsilateral nerve roots, the contralateral root sleeves are hidden from view. Attempted circumferential decom-

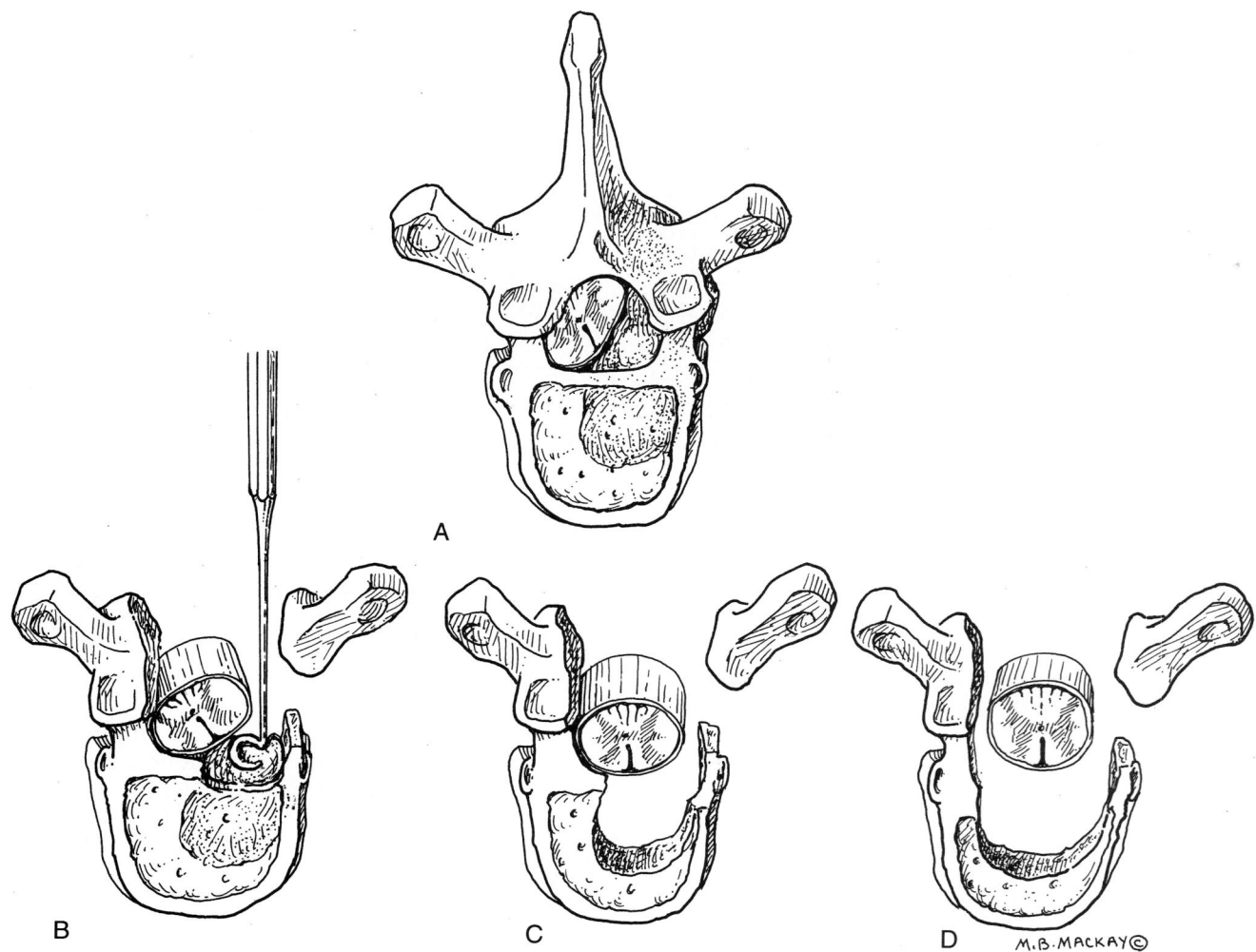

FIGURE 313–27. Diagrammatic representation of anterolateral extradural metastases *(A)* resected by posterolateral decompression *(B–D).*

pression of the dural sac runs the risk of inadvertent dural or nerve root injuries on the side not directly visualized.

STABILIZATION

Spinal reconstruction is undertaken to secure fixation that will remain rigidly in place during the patient's lifetime. A variety of methods, materials, and devices have been described. If prolonged survival is predicted, bone grafts may be used in anticipation of bony arthrodesis. However, the majority of patients with systemic cancer and symptomatic spinal metastases have a limited life expectancy. Consequently, a prosthetic reconstruction device may be more appropriate.

Stabilization from behind is secured with sublaminar wiring to suitable struts of bone, cement, steel rod or rectangle, or various other methods or devices (see Table 313–4). Fixation should, as a rule, be secured at a minimum of two levels above and two levels below the decompression defect (Fig. 313–29).

A number of anterior spinal reconstruction devices and techniques have been described (see Table 313–4). We prefer the individually tailored U-shaped stainless steel plate with interposed methyl methacrylate (Wellesley wedge) (Fig. 313–30).[203]

The variety of spinal stabilization alternatives available reflects the fact that no clearly superior technique has emerged.

Prognosis

Patients with spinal metastases constitute a heterogeneous group. This, together with the variability in data recording and results reporting, makes comparisons of published studies of questionable value.[204] One attempt at imposing some standardization stipulates that a "satisfactory result" has been achieved if a patient is ambulatory and continent 6 months after surgery[141]; another is the Frankel grading system.[205] It is generally agreed, however, that a number of factors contribute to determining the outcome after treatment (Table 313–6).

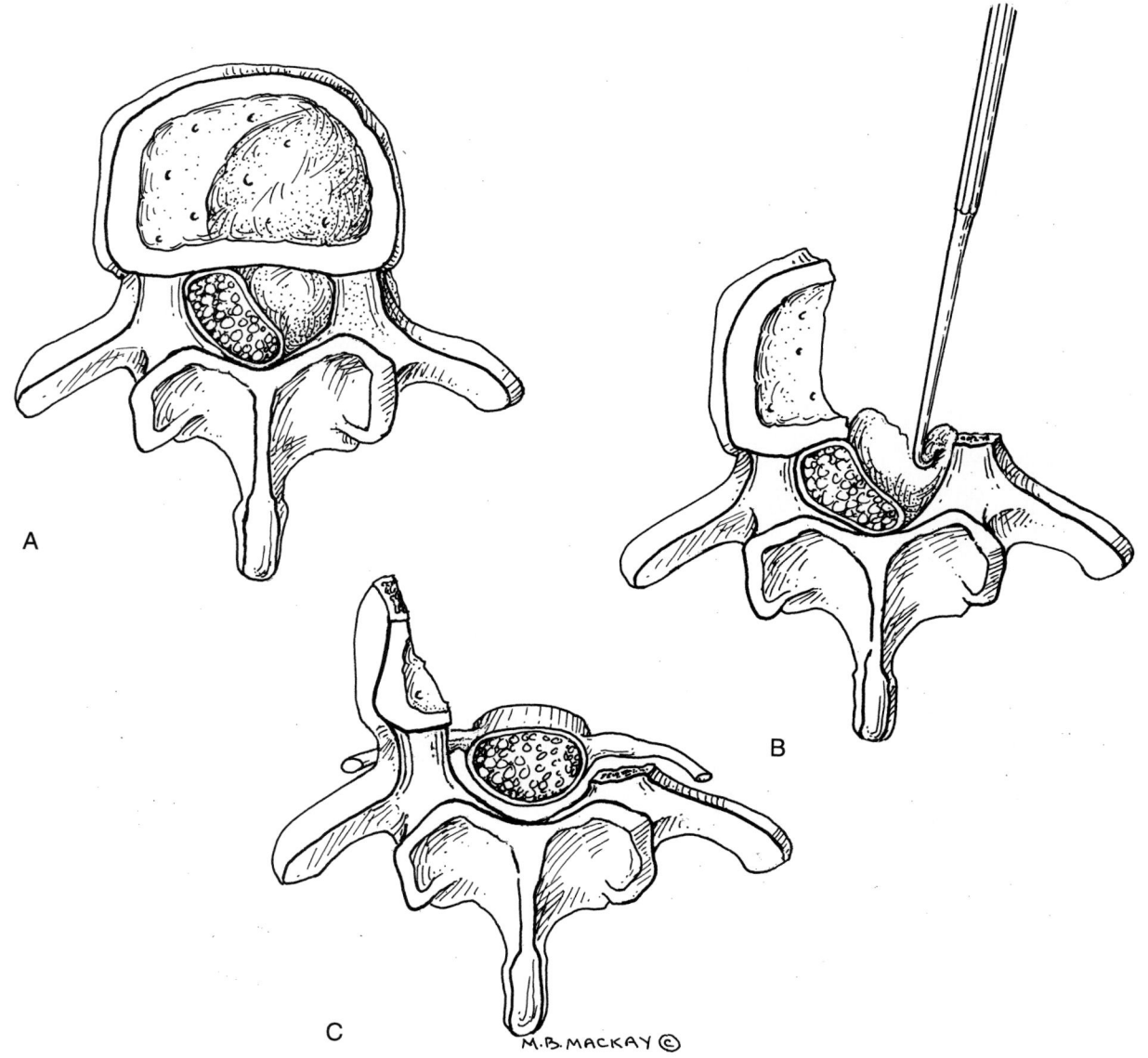

FIGURE 313–28. Diagrammatic representation of anterolateral extradural metastases *(A)* resected by anterior decompression *(B* and *C)*.

Degree of Deficit. The clinical condition at the time of surgery is the most important prognostic indicator. Patients who are walking at the time of surgery have the highest likelihood of maintaining ambulation. Patients who are paralyzed at the time of surgery have the worst outcome, with a less than 10% chance of recovering ambulation. Loss of bowel and bladder control is an ominous sign.

Duration of Symptoms. Long duration of symptoms with a slowly evolving neurological deficit is a relatively favorable sign. The abrupt onset of paraplegia may indicate vascular compromise with spinal cord infarction, in which case there is little chance of recovery.

Tumor Type. Biologic characteristics of the tumor, including rate of growth and sensitivity to radiation, determine the treatment options (surgery versus irradiation) and outcome. Metastatic lymphoma has a relatively favorable prognosis; metastatic carcinoma of the lung carries a poor prognosis.

Tumor Location. Intradural spinal metastases carry a dismal prognosis. Intradural extramedullary metastases characteristically produce a virulent clinical syndrome with rapid deterioration leading to a fatal outcome.

Advanced Disease. The degree of debility may determine the treatment options, including whether surgery is feasible at all and, if so, what approach is most suitable.

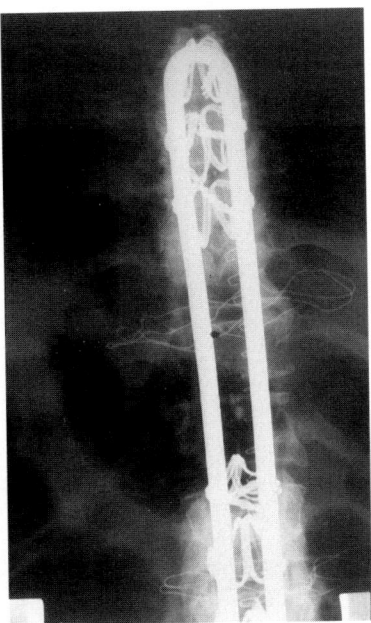

FIGURE 313–29. Sublaminar wiring to a steel rectangle.

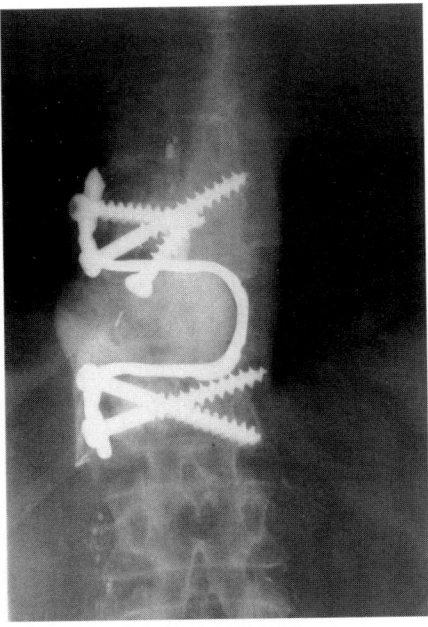

FIGURE 313–30. Radiograph showing anterior spinal reconstruction with the Wellesley wedge.

TABLE 313–6 ■ **Factors Determining Outcome of Treatment of Spinal Metastases**

Degree of deficit
Tumor type
Tumor location
Advanced disease
Surgical technique

SUMMARY

Metastatic tumors are by far the most commonly encountered spinal neoplasms. Successful surgical treatment of spinal tumors (including spinal metastases) must provide for both decompression of the spinal cord and nerve roots and stabilization of the spinal column. Recognition of this concept has stimulated the evolution of anterior and posterior approaches for spinal decompression, as well as various devices and techniques for spinal stabilization. The resulting refinement of surgical strategies and the promise of minimally invasive techniques have improved the outlook for patients with tumors of the spine.

Operative treatment for spinal metastasis should not be relegated to the realm of last-resort or salvage surgery. Therapeutic irradiation and surgery are complementary management options that should be applied in a setting of multidisciplinary cooperation among oncologists, radiotherapists, neurosurgeons, and orthopedic spine specialists.[206]

REFERENCES

1. Murphey MD, Andrews CL, Flemming DJ, et al: From the archives of the AFIP. Primary tumors of the spine: Radiologic-pathologic correlation. Radiographics 16:1131–1158, 1996.
2. Akeyson EW, McCutcheon IE: Single-stage posterior vertebrectomy and replacement combined with posterior instrumentation for spinal metastasis. J Neurosurg 85:211–220, 1996.
3. Ahuja A, Gibbons K: Endovascular therapy of central nervous system tumors. Neurosurg Clin N Am 5:541–545, 1994.
4. Dagi T, Schmidek H: Vascular tumors of the spine. In Sundaresan N, Schmidek HH, Schiller AI, Rosenthal DI (eds): Tumors of the Spine: Diagnosis and Clinical Management. Philadelphia, WB Saunders, 1990, pp 181–191.
5. Beltran J, Moto AM, Chakeres DW, et al: Tumors of the osseous spine: Staging with MR versus CT. Radiology 162:565–569, 1987.
6. Camins MB, Rosenblum B: Bony lesions of the cervical spine. In Camins MB, O'Leary PF (eds): Disorders of the Cervical Spine. Baltimore, Williams & Wilkins, 1992, pp 519–529.
7. Belliveau RE, Spencer RP: Incidence and sites of bone lesions detected by 99mTc polyphosphate scans in patients with tumors. Cancer 36:359–363, 1975.
8. Osborn AG: Diagnostic Neuroradiology. St Louis, Mosby–Year Book, 1994, p 936.
9. Sze G: Neoplastic disease of the spine and spinal cord. In Atlas SW (ed): Magnetic Resonance Imaging of the Brain and Spine, 2nd ed. Philadelphia, Lippincott-Raven, 1996, pp 1339–1385.
10. Zimmer WD, Berquist TH, McLeod RA, et al: Bone tumors: Magnetic resonance imaging versus computed tomography. Radiology 155:709–718, 1985.
11. Gitelis S, Schajowicz F: Osteoid osteoma and osteoblastoma. Orthop Clin North Am 20:313–325, 1989.
12. Bjornsson J, Wold L, Ebersold M, et al: Chordoma of the mobile spine: A clinicopathologic analysis of 40 cases. Cancer 71:735–740, 1993.
13. Shibata Y, Sugimoto K, Matsuki T, Nose T: Thoracic epidural angiolipoma—case report. Neurol Med Chir (Tokyo) 33:316–319, 1993.
14. Vlasak R, Sim F: Ewing's sarcoma. Orthop Clin North Am 27:591–603, 1996.
15. Ebersold MJ, Hitchon PW, Duff JM, Quast LM: Primary bone spinal lesions. In Benzel EC (ed): Spine Surgery: Techniques, Complication Avoidance, and Management, vol 1. New York, Churchill Livingstone, 1999, pp 663–677.
16. Levine A, Boriani S: Benign tumors of the cervical spine. In Clark C (ed): The Cervical Spine, 3rd ed. Philadelphia, Lippincott-Raven, 1998, pp 621–641.
17. Frassica FJ, Waltrip RL, Sponseller PD, et al: Clinicopathological

features of osteoma and osteoblastoma in children and adolescents. Orthop Clin North Am 27.3:559–574, 1996.

18. Jackson RP, Reckling FW, Mantz FA: Osteoid osteoma and osteoblastoma. Clin Orthop 128:303–313, 1977.

19. Raskas D, Graziano J, Herzenberg J, et al: Osteoid osteoma and osteoblastoma of the spine. J Spinal Disord 5:204–211, 1992.

20. Errico T, Cooper PR: A new method of thoracic and lumbar body replacement for spinal tumors: Technical note. Neurosurgery 32:678, 1989.

21. Gamba JL, Martinez S, Apple J, et al: CT of axial skeletal osteoid osteomas. AJR Am J Roentgenol 142:769–772, 1984.

22. Omojola MF, Cockshott P,, Beatty EG: Osteoid osteoma: An evaluation of diagnostic modalities. Clin Radiol 32:199–204, 1981.

23. Glass RB, Poznanski AK, Fisher MR, et al: Case report, MR imaging of osteoid osteoma. J Comput Assist Tomogr 10:1065–1067, 1986.

24. Ayala AG, Murray JA, Erling MA, et al: Osteoid osteoma: Intraoperative tetracyline fluorescence demonstration of the nidus. J Bone Joint Surg 68:747–751, 1986.

25. Lee DH, Malawer MM: Staging and treatment of primary and persistent osteoid osteoma: Evaluation of intraoperative nuclear scanning, tetracycline fluorescence, and tomography. Clin Orthop 281:229–238, 1992.

26. Campanacci M, Buggieri P, Gasbarrini A, et al: Osteoid osteoma: Direct visual identification and intralesional excision of the nidus with miminal removal of bone. J Bone Joint Surg Br 81: 814–820, 1999.

27. Labbe JL, Clement JL, Dupace B, et al: Percutaneous extraction of vertebral osteoma under computerized tomography guidance. Eur Spine J 4:368–371, 1995.

28. Amacher A: Spinal osteoblastoma in children and adolescents. Childs Nerv Syst 1:29–32, 1985.

29. Boriani S, Capanna R, Donati D, et al: Osteoblastoma of the spine. Clin Orthop 278:37–45, 1992.

30. Nemotot O, Moser R, Vandam B, et al: Osteoblastoma of the spine: A review of 75 cases. Spine 15:1272–1280, 1990.

31. Huvos A: Bone Tumors: Diagnosis, Treatment and Prognosis. Philadelphia, WB Saunders, 1979.

32. Schwartz H, Pinto M: Osteoblastomas of the cervical spine. J Spinal Disord 3:179–182, 1990.

33. Tucker AS, Aramsri B, Hughes CR: Roentgenographic diagnosis of spinal tumors. AJR Am J Roentgenol 78:54–65, 1957.

34. Lane J, Cammisa FJ, Glasser D: Benign cartilage tumors of the spine. In Sundaresan N, Schmidek HH, Schiller AL, Rosenthal DI (eds): Tumors of the Spine: Diagnosis and Clinical Management. Philadelphia, WB Saunders, 1990, pp 146–148.

35. Scarborough M, Moreau G: Benign cartilage tumors. Orthop Clin North Am 27:583–589, 1996.

36. Albrecht S, Crutchfield J, SeGall G: On spinal osteochondromas. J Neurosurg 77:247–252, 1992.

37. Karian JM, DeFilipp G, Buchheit WA, et al: Vertebral osteochondroma causing spinal cord compression. Neurosurgery 14:483–484, 1984.

38. Govender S, Parbhoo A: Osteochondroma with compression of the spinal cord. J Bone Joint Surg Br 81:667–669, 1999.

39. Fiumara E, Scarabino T, Guglielmi G, et al: Osteochondroma of the L-5 vertebra: A rare cause of sciatic pain. J Neurosurg (Spine 2) 91:219–222, 1999.

40. Moriwaka F, Hozen H, Nakane K, et al: Myelopathy due to osteochondroma. J Comput Assist Tomogr 14:128–130, 1990.

41. Dahlin DC, Unni KK: Bone Tumors. Springfield, IL, Charles C Thomas, 1986, pp 19–32, 228–229.

42. Fox M, Onofrio B: The natural history and management of symptomatic and asymptomatic vertebral hemangiomas. J Neurosurg 78:36–45, 1993.

43. Yochum T, Lile R, Schultz G, et al: Acquired spinal stenosis secondary to an expanding thoracic vertebral hemangioma. Spine 18:299–305, 1993.

44. De Cristofaro R, Biagini R, Boriani S, et al: Selective arterial embolization in the treatment of aneurysmal bone cyst and angioma of bone. Skeletal Radiol 21:523–527, 1992.

45. Ng VWK, Clifton A, Moore AJ: Preoperative endovascular embolization of a vertebral haemangioma. J Bone Joint Surg Br 79: 808–811, 1997.

46. Niemeyer T, McClellan J, Webb J, et al: Brown-Sequard syndrome after management of vertebral hemangioma with intralesional alcohol. Spine 24:1845–1847, 1999.

47. Bremmes R, Hauge H, Sagsveen R: Radiotherapy in the treatment of symptomatic vertebral hemangiomas: Technical case report. Neurosurgery 39:1054–1058, 1996.

48. Rubin G, Gornish M, Sandbank J, et al: Spinal extradural angiolipoma: Case report and review of the literature. Spine 17: 719–724, 1992.

49. Trabulo A, Cerqueira L, Monteiro J, et al: Spinal angiolipomas revisited: Two case reports. Acta Neurochir (Wien) 138:1311–1319, 1996.

50. Weill A, Melancon D, DelCarpio R, et al: Angiolipoma of the central nervous system. Rev Neurol (Paris) 147:285–292, 1991.

51. Murphey M, Fairbairn K, Parman L, Baxter K: From the archives of the AFIP. Musculoskeletal angiomatous lesions: Radiologic-pathologic correlation. Radiographics 15:893–917, 1995.

52. Kuroda S, Abe H, Akino M, et al: Infiltrating spinal angiolipoma causing myelopathy: Case report. Neurosurgery 27:315–318, 1990.

53. Papagelopoulos P, Currier B, Shaughnessy W, et al: Aneurysmal bone cyst of the spine: Management and outcome. Spine 23: 621–628, 1998.

54. Biesicker J, Marcove R, Huvos A, Mike V: Aneurysmal bone cyst: A clinicopathological study of 66 cases. Cancer 26:615–625, 1970.

55. Jansen J, Terwey B, Rama B, Markakis E: MRI diagnosis of aneurysmal bone cyst. Neurosurg Rev 13:161–166, 1990.

56. Kransdorf M, Sweet D: Aneurysmal bone cyst: Concept, controversy, clinical presentation, and imaging. AJR Am J Roentgenol 164:573–580, 1995.

57. Misasi N, Sadile F: Selective arterial embolization in orthopaedic pathology: Analysis of long term results. Chir Organi Mov 76: 311–316, 1991.

58. Cybulski G, Anson J, Gleason T, et al: Aneurysmal bone cyst of the thoracic spine: Treatment by excision and segmental stabilization with Luque rods. Neurosurgery 24:273–276, 1989.

59. Arcomano JP, Barnett JC, Wunderlich WO: Histiocystosis. AJR Am J Roentgenol 85:663–679, 1961.

60. Tomita T: Special considerations in surgery of pediatric spine tumors. In Sundaresan N, Schmidek HH, Schiller AL, Rosenthal DI (eds): Tumors of the Spine: Diagnosis and Clinical Management. Philadelphia, WB Saunders, 1990, pp 258–271.

61. Silberstein M, Sundaram M, Akbarnia B, et al: Eosinophilic granuloma of the spine. Orthopedics 8:267–274, 1985.

62. Dickinson L, Farhat S: Eosinophilic granuloma of the cervical spine. A case report and review of the literature. Surg Neurol 57–63, 1991.

63. Ladisch S, Jaffe E: The histiocytoses. In Pizzo P, Poplack D (eds): Principles and Practice of Pediatric Oncology, 2nd ed. Philadelphia, JB Lippincott, 1993, p 617.

64. Velez-Yanguas M, Warrier R: Langerhans' cell histiocytosis. Orthop Clin North Am 27:615–623, 1996.

65. Seimon L: Eosinophilic granuloma of the spine. J Pediatr Orthop 1:371–376, 1981.

66. De Schepper A, Ramon F, Van Marck E: MR imaging of eosinophilic granuloma: Report of 11 cases. Skeletal Radiol 22:170, 1993.

67. Green N, Robertson W, Kilroy A: Eosinophilic granuloma of the spine with associated neural deficit. J Bone Joint Surg 62: 1198–1202, 1980.

68. Huvos A: Osteogenic sarcoma of bones and soft tissue in older patients: A clinicopathologic analysis of 117 patients older than 60 years. Cancer 57:1442–1449, 1986.

69. Vander Griend R: Osteosarcoma and its variants. Orthop Clin North Am 27:575–581, 1996.

70. Sim FH, Frassica FJ, Wold LE, et al: Chondrosarcoma of the spine: Mayo Clinic experience. In Sundaresan N, Schmidek HH, Schiller AL, Rosenthal DI (eds): Tumors of the Spine: Diagnosis and Clinical Management. Philadelphia, WB Saunders, 1990, pp 155–162.

71. Dreghorn C, Newman R, Hardy G, et al: Primary tumors of the axial skeleton: Experience of the Leeds Regional Bone Tumor Registry. Spine 15:137–140, 1990.

72. McLain R, Weinstein J: Solitary plasmacytomas of the spine: A review of 84 cases. J Spinal Disord 2:69–74, 1989.

73. Miller T, Abdelwahab I, Hermann G, et al: Vertebral osteosarcoma. Skeletal Radiol 21:277–279, 1992.

74. Hall T, Kangarloo H: Magnetic resonance imaging of the musculoskeletal system in children. Clin Orthop 244:119–130, 1989.

75. Redmond OM, Stack JP, Dervan PA, et al: Osteosarcoma: Use of the MR imaging and MR spectroscopy in clinical decision making. Radiology 172:811–815, 1989.

76. Sundaram M, McGuire MH, Herbold DR: Magnetic resonance imaging of osteosarcoma. Skeletal Radiol 16:23–29, 1987.

77. Erlemann R, Reiser MF, Peters PE, et al: Musculoskeletal neoplasms: Static and dynamic Gd-DTPA–enhanced MR imaging. Radiology 171:767–773, 1989.

78. Sundaresan N, Schiller AL, Rosenthal DI: Osteosarcoma of the spine In Sundaresan N, Schmidek HH, Schiller AL, Rosenthal DI (eds): Tumors of the Spine: Diagnosis and Management. Philadelphia, WB Saunders, 1990, pp 128–145.

79. Sundaresan N, Steinberger A, Moore F, et al: Indications and results of combined anterior-posterior approaches for spine tumor surgery. J Neurosurg 85:438–446, 1996.

80. Spiegel D, Richardson W, Scully S, Harrelson J: Long-term survival following total sacrectomy with reconstruction for the treatment of primary osteosarcoma of the sacrum. J Bone Joint Surg Am 81:848–855, 1999.

81. Kawahara N, Tomita K, Fujita T, et al: Osteosarcoma of the thoracolumbar spine: Total en bloc spondylectomy. J Bone Joint Surg Am 79:453, 1997.

82. Stener B, Gunterberg B: High amputation of the sacrum for extirpation of tumors: Principles and technique. Spine 3:351–366, 1978.

83. Shives T, McLeod R, Unni K, et al: Chondrosarcoma of the spine. J Bone Joint Surg Am 71:1158–1165, 1989.

84. York JE, Berk R, Fuller G, et al: Chondrosarcoma of the spine: 1954–1997. J Neurosurg (Spine) 90:73–78, 1999.

85. Cahill D: Surgical management of malignant tumors of the adult bony spine. South Med J 89:653–665, 1996.

86. Camins MB, Duncan A, Smith J, et al: Chondrosarcoma of the spine. Spine. 3:202–209, 1978.

87. Cammisa FP Jr, Glasser DB, Lane JM: Chondrosarcoma of the spine: Memorial Sloan-Kettering Cancer Center experience. In Sundaresan N, Schmidek HH, Schiller AL, Rosenthal DI (eds): Tumors of the Spine: Diagnosis and Clinical Management. Philadelphia, WB Saunders, 1990.

88. Lee F, Mankin H, Fondren G, et al: Chondrosarcoma of bone: An assessment of outcome. J Bone Joint Surg Am 81:326–338, 1999.

89. Kreicbergs A, Boquist L, Borssen B, et al: Prognostic factors in chondrosarcoma: A comparative study of cellular DNA content and clinicopathologic features. Cancer 50:577, 1982.

90. Kreicbergs A, Soderberg G, Zetterberg A: The prognostic significance of nuclear DNA content in chondrosarcoma. Anal Quant Cytol 4:271, 1980.

91. Krol G, Sundaresan N, Deck M: Computed tomography of axial chordomas. J Comput Assist Tomogr 7:286–289, 1983.

92. York JE, Kaczaraj A, Abi-Said D, et al: Sacral chordoma: 40 year experience at a major cancer center. Neurosurgery 44:74–80, 1999.

93. Ducou le Pointe H, Brugieres P, Chevalier X, et al: Imaging of chordomas of the mobile spine. J Neuroradiol 18:267–276, 1991.

94. Firooznia H, Pinto RS, Lin JP, Zausner J: Chordoma: Radiologic evaluation of 20 cases. AJR Am J Roentgenol 127:797–805, 1976.

95. Sze G: Magnetic resonance imaging in the evaluation of spinal tumors. Cancer 67:1229–1241, 1991.

96. Sze G, Uichanco LS, Brant-Zawadzki M, et al: Chordomas: MR imaging. Radiology 166:187–191, 1988.

97. Sundaresan N, Krol G, Hughes J: Primary malignant tumors of the spine. In Youmans J (ed): Neurological Surgery, vol 5, 3rd ed. Philadelphia, WB Saunders, 1990, pp 3548–3573.

98. Sundaresan N, Rosenthal DI, Schiller AL, et al: Chordomas. In Sundaresan N, Schmidek HH, Schiller AL, Rosenthal DI (eds): Tumors of the Spine: Diagnosis and Clinical Management. Philadelphia, WB Saunders, 1990, pp 192–213.

99. Fujita T, Kawahara N, Matsumoto T, Tomita K: Chordoma in the cervical spine managed with en bloc resection Spine 24:1848–1851, 1999.

100. Stener B: Complete removal of vertebrae for extirpation of tumors: A 20 year experience. Clin Orthop 245:72–82, 1989.

101. Catton C, O'Sullivan B, Bell R, et al: Chordoma: Long-term follow-up after radical photon irradiation. Radiother Oncol 41:67–72, 1996.

102. Bradway J, Pritchard D: Ewing's tumor of the spine. In Sundaresan N, Schmidek HH, Schiller AL, Rosenthal DI (ed): Tumors of the Spine: Diagnosis and Clinical Management. Philadelphia, WB Saunders, 1990, pp 235–239.

103. Turc-Carel C, Aurias A, Mugneret F, et al: Chromosomes in Ewing's sarcoma: An evaluation of 85 cases of remarkable consistency of (t11;22) (q24;q12). Cancer Genet Cytogenet 32:229–238, 1988.

104. Burgert E, Nesbit M, Garnsey L, et al: Multimodal therapy for the management of nonpelvic, localized Ewing's sarcoma of bone: Intergroup study IESS-11. J Clin Oncol 8:1514–1524, 1990.

105. Evans R, Nesbit M, Askin F, et al: Multimodal therapy for the management of localized Ewing's sarcoma of pelvic and sacral bone: A report from the second intergroup study. J Clin Oncol 9:1173–1180, 1991.

106. Oberlin O, Patte C, Demeocq F, et al: The response to initial chemotherapy as a prognostic factor in localized Ewing's sarcoma. Eur J Cancer Clin Oncol 21:463–467, 1985.

107. Barbieri E, Emiliani E, Zini G, et al: Combined therapy of localized Ewing's sarcoma of bone: Analysis of results in 100 patients. Int J Radiat Oncol Biol Phys 19:1165–1170, 1990.

108. Heller M, McBroom RJ, MacNab T, et al: Treatment of metastatic disease of the spine with posterolateral decompression and Luque instrumentation. Neuroorthopedics 2:70–74, 1986.

109. Karnaze MG, Gado MH, Sartor KJ, et al: Comparison of MR and CT myelography in imaging the cervical and thoracic spine. AJR Am J Roentgenol 150:397–403, 1988.

110. Sudanese A, Toni A, Ciaroni D, et al: The role of surgery in the treatment of Ewing's sarcoma. Chir Organi Mov 75:217–230, 1990.

111. Pilepich M, Vietti T, Nesbit M, et al: Ewing's sarcoma of the vertebral column. Int J Radiat Oncol Biol Phys 7:27–31, 1981.

112. Sharafuddin M, Haddad F, Hitchon P, et al: Treatment options in primary Ewing's sarcoma of the spine: Report of seven cases and review of the literature. Neurosurgery 30:610–619, 1992.

113. Grubb M, Currier B, Pritchard D, Ebersold M: Primary Ewing's sarcoma of the spine. Spine 19:309–313, 1994.

114. Campanacci M, Boriani S, Giunti A: Giant cell tumors of the spine. In Sundaresan N, Schmidek HH, Schiller AL, Rosenthal DI (eds): Tumors of the Spine: Diagnosis and Management. Philadelphia, WB Saunders, 1990.

114a. Jaffee HL: Tumors and Tumorous Conditions of the Bones and Joints. Philadelphia, Lea & Febiger, 1958, p 230.

115. McInerney DP, Middlemiss JH: Giant cell tumor of bone. Skeletal Radiol 2:195–204, 1978.

116. Verhagen W, Bartels R, Schaafsma HE, deJong T: A giant cell tumor of the sacrum or a soft tissue giant cell tumor. Spine 23:1609–1611, 1998.

117. Sim FH, MacDonald D, McLeod R, et al: Giant cell tumors of the spine and sacrum: Mayo Clinic experience. In Sundaresan N, Schmidek HH, Schiller AL, Rosenthal DI (eds): Tumors of the Spine: Diagnosis and Clinical Management. Philadelphia, WB Saunders, 1990, pp 173–180.

118. Yan S, Xu Q, Lin J: Diagnosis and treatment of giant cell tumor in the thoracic spine. J Surg Oncol 40:128–131, 1989.

119. Dahlin DC: Giant cell tumor of the vertebrae above the sacrum. Cancer 39:1350–1356, 1997.

120. Boos M, Goytan M, Fraser R, Aebi A: Solitary plasma-cell myeloma of the spine in an adolescent. J Bone Joint Surg Br 79:808–811, 1997.

121. Kempin S, Sundaresan N: Disorders of the spine related to plasma cell dyscrasias. In Sundaresan N, Schmidek HH, Schiller AL, Rosenthal DI (eds): Tumors of the Spine: Diagnosis and Clinical Management. Philadelphia, WB Saunders, 1990, pp 214–225.

122. Weinstein J, McLain R: Tumors of the spine. In Rothman R, Simeone F (eds): The Spine, vol 2. Philadelphia, WB Saunders, 1992, pp 1279–1318.

123. Frassica D, Frassica F, Schray M, et al: Solitary plasmacytoma of bone: Mayo Clinic experience. Int J Radiat Oncol Biol Phys 16:43–48, 1989.

124. Meis J, Butler J, Osborne B, et al: Solitary plasmacytomas of

bone and extramedullary plasmacytomas: A clinicopathologic and immunohistochemical study. Cancer 59:1474–1485, 1987.

125. Mouloupoulos L, Dimopoulos M, Weber D, et al: Magnetic resonance imaging in the staging of solitary plasmacytoma of bone. J Clin Oncol 11:1311–1315, 1993.
126. Liebross R, Ha C, Cox J, et al: Solitary bone plasmacytoma: Outcome and prognostic factors following radiotherapy. Int J Radiat Oncol Biol Phys 41:1063–1067, 1998.
127. Shikata J, Yamamuro T, Mikawa Y, et al: Instrumentation surgery for primary tumors of the spine. Arch Orthop Trauma Surg 108:144–149, 1989.
128. Sundaresan N, Galicich JH, Bains MS, et al: Vertebral body resection in the treatment of cancer involving the spine. Cancer 53:1393–1396, 1984.
129. Cervoni L, Celli P, Salvati M, et al: Solitary plasmacytoma of the spine: Relationship of IgM to tumor progression and recurrence. Acta Neurochir (Wien) 135:122–125, 1995.
130. Rahmouni A, Divine M, Mathieu D, et al: Detection of multiple myeloma involving the spine: Efficacy of fat-suppression and contrast enhanced MR imaging. AJR Am J Roentgenol 160:1049–1052, 1993.
131. Rahmouni A, Divine M, Mathieu D, et al: MR appearance of multiple myeloma of the spine before and after treatment. AJR Am J Roentgenol 160:1053–1057, 1993.
132. Weber D, Dimopoulos M, Mouloupoulos L, et al: Prognostic features of asymptomatic multiple myeloma. Br J Haematol 97:810–814, 1997.
133. Chade HO: Metastatic tumors of the spine and spinal cord. In Vinken PJ Bruyn GW (eds): Handbook of Clinical Neurology, vol 20. Amsterdam, Elsevier North-Holland, 1976, pp 415–433.
134. Maranzano E, Latini P, Checcaglini F, et al: Radiation therapy in metastatic spinal cord compression. Cancer 76:1311–1317, 1989.
135. Sundaresan N, DiGiacinto GV, Hughes JE, et al: Treatment of neoplastic spinal cord compression: Results of a prospective study Neurosurgery 29:645–650, 1991.
136. Ries LAG, Miller BA, Hankey BF, et al (eds): SEER Cancer Statistics Review, 1973–1991. NIH Pub. No. 94–2789. Bethesda, MD, National Cancer Institute, 1994.
137. Clain A: Secondary malignant disease of bone. Br J Cancer 19:15–29, 1965.
138. Willis RA: The Spread of Tumor in the Human Body, 3rd ed. London, Butterworths, 1952.
139. Barron KD, Hirano A, Araki S, et al: Experiences with metastatic neoplasms involving the spinal cord. Neurology (Minneap) 9:91–106, 1959.
140. Galasko CSB: Skeletal metastases and mammary cancer. Ann R Coll Surg Engl 50:3–28, 1972.
141. Botterell EH, Fitzgerald GN: Spinal cord compression produced by extradural malignant tumors. Can Med Assoc J 80:791–796, 1959.
142. Livingston KE, Perrin RG: Neurosurgical management of spinal metastases. J Neurosurg 49:839–843, 1978.
143. MacDonald DR: Clinical manifestations. In Sundaresan N, Schmidek H, Schiller A, et al (eds): Tumors of the Spine: Diagnosis and Clinical Management. Philadelphia, WB Saunders, 1990, pp 6–21.
144. Stark RJ, Henson RA, Evans SJW: Spinal metastasis: A retrospective survey from a general hospital. Brain 105:189–213, 1982.
145. Gilbert RW, Kim H, Posner JB: Epidural spinal cord compression from metastatic tumor: Diagnosis and treatment. Ann Neurol 3:40–51, 1978.
146. Van der Sande JJ, Kroger R, Boogerd W: Multiple spinal epidural metastases: An unexpectedly frequent finding. J Neurol Neurosurg Psychiatry 53:1001–1003, 1990.
147. Edelson RN, Deck MDF, Posner IB: Intramedullary spinal cord metastases: Clinical and radiographic findings in nine cases. Neurology 22:1222–1231, 1972.
148. Perrin RG, Livingston KE, Aarabi B: Intradural extramedullary spinal metastasis. J Neurosurg 45:835–837, 1982.
149. Rogers L, Heard G: Intrathecal spinal metastases (rare tumors). Br J Surg 45:317–320, 1958.
150. Batson OV: Role of vertebral veins in metastatic processes. Ann Intern Med 16:38–45, 1942.
151. Galasko CSB: The anatomy and pathways of skeletal metastases. In Weiss L, Gilbert HA (eds): Bone Metastasis. Boston, GK Hall, 1981, pp 49–63.
152. West CGH: Spinal subarachnoid metastatic spread from non-neuraxial primary neoplasm. J Neurosurg 51:251–253, 1979.
153. Jellinger K, Kothbauer P, Sunder-Plassman E, et al: Intramedullary spinal cord metastases. J Neurol 220:31–41, 1979.
154. Murphy KC, Feld R, Evans WK, et al: Intramedullary spinal cord metastases from small cell carcinoma of the lung. J Clin Oncol 1:99–106, 1983.
155. Black P: Spinal metastasis: Current status and recommended guidelines for management. Neurosurgery 5:726–745, 1979.
156. Perrin RG, Livingston KE: Neurosurgical treatment of pathological fracture-dislocation of the spine. J Neurosurg 52:330–334, 1980.
157. Perrin RG, Livingston KE: Pathological fracture-dislocation of the cervical spine. In Tator CH (ed): Early Management of Acute Spinal Cord Injury. New York, Raven Press, 1982, pp 365–372.
158. Bryne TN, Waxman SG (eds): Spinal Cord Compression: Diagnosis and Principles of Management. Contemporary Neurology, Series 33. Philadelphia, FA Davis, 1990.
159. Goodkin R, Carr BI, Perrin RG: Herniated lumbar disc disease in patients with malignancy. J Clin Oncol 5:667–671, 1987.
160. Rodichok LD, Harper GR, Ruckdeschel JC, et al: Early diagnosis of spinal epidural metastases. Am J Med 70:1181–1188, 1981.
161. Perrin RG: Beware the winking owl [cover illustration]. J Neurosurg 48, 1978.
162. Perrin RG, McBroom RJ: Metastatic tumors of the cervical spine. Clin Neurosurg 37:740–755, 1989.
163. Eaton LM, Craig WM: Tumors of the spinal cord: Sudden paralysis following lumbar puncture. Mayo Clin Proc 15:170, 1940.
164. Hollis PH, Malis LI, Zappulla RA: Neurological deterioration after lumbar puncture below complete spinal subarachnid block. J Neurosurg 64:253–256, 1986.
165. Fink II, Garra BS, Zabell A, et al: Computed tomography with metrizamide myelography to define the extent of spinal canal block due to tumor. J Comput Assist Tomogr 8:1072–1075, 1984.
166. Helweg-Larsen S, Wagner A, Kjaer L, et al: Comparison of myelography combined with post myelographic spinal CT and MRI in suspected metastatic disease of the spinal canal. J Neurooncol 13:231–237, 1992.
167. Bommer KK, Ramzy I, Mody D: Fine-needle aspiration biopsy in the diagnosis and management of bone lesions. Cancer 81:148–156, 1997.
168. Dupuy DE, Rosenberg AE, Punyaratabandhu T, et al: Accuracy of CT-guided needle biopsy of musculoskeletal neoplasms. Am J Radiol 171:759–762, 1998.
169. Hagenau C, Grosh W, Currie M, et al: Comparison of spinal magnetic resonance imaging and myelography in cancer patients. I. Clin Oncol 5:1663–1669, 1987.
170. Jaekla KA: Neuroimaging for central nervous system tumors. Semin Oncol 18:150–157, 1991.
171. Sze G, Krol G, Zimmerman RD, et al: Malignant extradural spinal tumors: MR imaging with Gd-DTPA. Radiology 167:217–223, 1988.
172. Lim V, Sobel DE, Zyroff J: Spinal cord pial metastases: MR imaging with gadopentetate dimeglumine. AJR Am J Roentgenol 155:1077–1084, 1990.
173. Sze G, Abramson A, Krol G, et al: Gadolinium-DTPA in the evaluation of intradural extramedullary spinal disease. AJR Am J Roentgenol 50:911–921, 1988.
174. Colman LK, Porter BA, Redmond J, et al: Early diagnosis of spinal metastases by CT and MR studies. J Comput Assist Tomogr 12:423–426, 1988.
175. O'Mara RE: Bone scanning in osseous metastatic disease. JAMA 229:1915, 1974.
176. Portenoy RK, Galer BS, Salamon O, et al: Identification of epidural neoplasm: Radiography and bone scintigraphy in the symptomatic and asymptomatic spine. Cancer 64:2207–2213, 1989.
177. Cantu RC: Corticosteroids for spinal metastases. Lancet 2:912, 1968.
178. Delattre JY, Arbit E, Thaler HT, et al: A dose response study of dexamethasone in a model of spinal cord compression caused by epidural tumor. J Neurosurg 70:920–925, 1989.
179. Posner JB, Howieson J, Cvitkovic E: "Disappearing" spinal cord compression: Oncolytic effects of glucocorticoids (and other chemotherapeutic agents) on epidural metastases. Ann Neurol 2:409–413, 1977.

180. Ushio Y, Posner JB, Kim JH, et al: Experimental spinal cord compression by epidural neoplasm. Neurology 27:422–429, 1977.

181. Ushio Y, Posner R, Kim JH, et al: Treatment of experimental spinal cord compression caused by epidural neoplasms. J Neurosurg 47:380–390, 1977.

182. Gilbert H, Apuzzo M, Marshall L, et al: Neoplastic epidural spinal cord compression: A current perspective. JAMA 240: 2771–2773, 1978.

183. Young RE, Post EM, King GA: Treatment of spinal epidural metastases: Randomized prospective comparison. J Neurosurg 53:741–748, 1980.

184. Brice J, McKissock W: Surgical treatment of malignant extradural spinal tumors. BMJ 1:1341–1344, 1965.

185. Findlay GEG: Adverse effects of the management of malignant spinal cord compression. J Neurol Neurosurg Psychiatry 47: 761–768, 1984.

186. Findlay GEG: The role of vertebral body collapse in the management of malignant spinal cord compression. J Neurol Neurosurg Psychiatry 50:151–154, 1987.

187. Perrin RG, McBroom RJ: Surgical treatment of spinal metastases: The posterolateral approach. In Sundaresan N, Schmidek H, Schiller A, et al (eds): Tumors of the Spine: Diagnosis and Clinical Management. Philadelphia, WB Saunders, 1990, pp 305–315.

188. York JE, Garrett MD, Walsh L, et al: Combined chest wall resection with vertebrectomy and spinal reconstruction for the treatment of Pancoast tumors. J Neurosurg (Spine 1) 91:74–80, 1999.

189. Darling GE, McBroom RJ, Perrin RG: Modified anterior approach to the cervical thoracic junction. Spine 20:1519–1521, 1995.

190. Gokaslan ZL, Walsh GL: "Trap door" exposure of the cervicothoracic junction. Neurosurg Oper Atlas 8:253–260, 1998.

191. Walsh GL, Gokaslan ZL, McCutcheon IE, et al: Anterior approaches to the thoracic spine in patients with cancer: Indications and results. Ann Thorac Surg 64:1611–1618, 1997.

192. Martenson JA, Evans RG, Lie MR, et al: Treatment outcome and complications in patients treated for malignant epidural spinal cord compression. J Neurooncol 3:77–84, 1985.

193. Rosenthal D, Marquardt G, Lorenz R, et al: Anterior decompression and stabilization using a microsurgical endoscopic technique for metastatic tumors of the thoracic spine. J Neurosurg 84:565–572, 1996.

194. Dohn DF: Thoracic spinal cord compression: Alternative surgical approaches and basis of choice. Clin Neurosurg 27:611–623, 1980.

195. Perrin RG, McBroom RJ: Anterior versus posterior decompression for symptomatic spinal metastasis. Can J Neurol Sci 14: 75–80, 1987.

196. Gokaslan ZL, Romsdahl MM, Kroll SS, et al: Total sacrectomy. Neurosurg Oper Atlas 7:11–20, 1998.

197. Ellis PM, Findlay IM: Craniocervical fusion with contoured Luque rod and autogenic bone graft. Can J Surg 37:50–54, 1994.

198. Gokaslan ZL, York JE, Walsh GL, et al: Transthoracic vertebrectomy for metastatic spinal tumors. J Neurosurg 89:599–609, 1998.

199. Bhojraj SY, Dandaivate AV, Ramakantan R: Preoperative embolization, transpedicular decompression and posterior stabilization for metastatic disease of the thoracic spine causing paraplegia. Paraplegia 30:292–299, 1992.

200. Broaddus WC, Grady MD, Delashaw JB, et al: Preoperative superselective arteriolar embolization: A new approach to enhance resectability of spinal tumors. Neurosurgery 27:755–759, 1990.

201. Roscoe JM, McBroom RJ, St Louis E, et al: Preoperative embolization in the treatment of osseous metastases from renal cell carcinoma. Clin Orthop 238:302–307, 1989.

202. Tindal S, Perrin RG: Anesthesia for surgical management of spinal metastases. Probl Anesth 5:80–90, 1991.

203. Perrin RG, McBroom RJ: Spinal fixation after anterior decompression for symptomatic spinal metastasis. Neurosurgery 22: 324–327, 1988.

204. Sorenson PS, Borgesen SE, Rohde K: Metastatic epidural spinal cord compression: Results of treatment and survival. Cancer 65: 1502–1508, 1990.

205. Frankel HL, Hancock DO, Hyslop G, et al: The value of postural reduction in the initial management of closed injuries of the spine with paraplegia and tetraplegia. Paraplegia 7:179–192, 1969.

206. Hayes F, Thompson E, Hvizdala E, et al: Chemotherapy as an alternative to laminectomy and radiation in the management of epidural tumor. J Pediatr 104:221–224, 1984.

207. Rogers YA: Treatment of fracture-dislocation of the cervical spine. J Bone Joint Surg 24:245–258, 1942.

208. Robinson RA, Smith GW: Anterolateral cervical disc removal and interbody fusion for cervical disc syndrome. Bull Johns Hopkins Hosp 96:223–224, 1955.

209. Robinson RA, Southwick WO: Surgical approaches to the cervical spine. Am Acad Orthop Surg 17:299–330, 1960.

210. Davey JR, Rorabeck CH, Bailey SJ, et al: A technique of posterior cervical fusion for instability of the cervical spine. Spine 10: 722–728, 1985.

211. Harrington KD: Anterior cord decompression and spinal stabilization for patients with metastatic lesion of the spine. J Neurosurg 61:107–117, 1984.

212. Harrington PR, Dickson JH: Spinal instrumentation in the treatment of severe progressive spondylolisthesis. Clin Orthop 117: 157–163, 1976.

213. White AH, Zucherman JF, Hsu K: Lumbosacral fusions with Harrington rods and intersegmental wiring. Clin Orthop 203: 185–190, 1986.

214. Krag MH, Beynnon BD, Pope MH, et al: An internal fixator for posterior applications to short segments of the thoracic, lumbar or lumbosacral spine: Design and testing. Clin Orthop 203: 75–98, 1986.

215. Roy-Camille R, Roy-Camille M, Demeulenaere C: Osteosynthesis of thoraco-lumbar spine fractures with metal plates screwed through the vertebral pedicles. Reconstr Surg Traumatol 15:2, 1976.

216. Steffee AD, Biscup RS, Sitkowski DJ: Segmental spine plates with pedicle screw fixation: A new internal fixation device for disorders of the lumbar and thoracolumbar spine. Clin Orthop 203:45–53, 1986.

217. Holness RO: Posterior stabilization with an interlaminar clamp in cervical injuries: Technical note and review of the long term experience with the method. Neurosurgery 14:318–322, 1984.

218. Luque ER: Interpeduncular segment fixation. Clin Orthop 903: 54–57, 1986.

219. Cloward RB: The anterior approach for ruptured cervical discs. J Neurosurg 15:602–614, 1958.

220. Fielding W, Pyle RN, Fietti VG: Anterior cervical vertebral body resection and bone-grafting for benign and malignant tumors. J Bone Joint Surg Am 61:251–253, 1979.

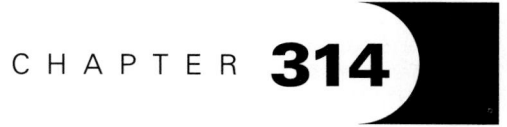

Approach to the Patient and Diagnostic Evaluation

ALLAN D.O. LEVI

Despite substantial improvements in emergency, diagnostic, and surgical care, spinal trauma continues to present a challenging spectrum of conditions for neurosurgeons to manage. When spinal trauma causes a spinal cord injury (SCI), the emotional and financial toll inflicted on individuals and their families is enormous. Since the 1970s, improvements in the quality of care delivered partially reflect the recognition that centers of excellence that focus on the acute treatment and rehabilitation of spinal cord–injured patients are best equipped to deal with the magnitude of services required by these patients.

EPIDEMIOLOGY

Incidence

Typically, SCIs occur in males at the peak of their productive lives. Each year in the United States, the incidence of traumatic SCI is approximately 10,000 new cases,[1] with a prevalence of 191,000 cases. The prevalence of SCIs is increasing steadily because survival during both the acute and chronic stages of the disease has improved. The amount spent on the treatment of SCIs in the United States is approximately $5.6 billion each year and is rising annually.[2] The cost of caring for the individual spinal cord–injured patient is directly related to the level of the SCI and to the patient's age, with the highest costs associated with older quadriplegic patients who are dependent on respirators.[2]

Etiology

Most spinal injuries result from high-speed motor vehicle accidents. Falls, recreational injuries, violent crimes, and work-related injuries are other important contributors. SCIs from violence are increasing dramatically, as

manifested by the proportion of individuals injured by assault. These injuries include penetrating injuries, such as gun and knife wounds. In the 1990s, sports-related injuries, which include football, horseback riding, and hockey-related injuries, received media attention.[3, 4] Recreational injuries from jet skis, snowmobiles, and parachuting are a constant source of newly injured patients. With the desire for extreme speed on land and water and in the air, we expect new recreational activity-related injuries to emerge from activities such as snowboarding, driving small watercraft, and so on.

PREVENTION

Preventive programs, which encourage children and young adults to modify risky behaviors, have the greatest potential for reducing the incidence of SCIs. These programs include but are not limited to the *Think First* program sponsored by the American Association of Neurological Surgeons and the Congress of Neurological Surgeons and its predecessor, the *Feet First, First Time* program, initially developed in northern Florida, which encourages water enthusiasts to jump feet first into unknown waters. Driver education courses and the arrest of drivers who are under the influence of drugs or alcohol should help avoid these tragic injuries. Finally, regulation of handguns and assault weapons, which have resulted in intentional and accidental injuries, could further reduce the number of injuries.

NEUROLOGIC LEVEL AND COMPLETENESS OF INJURY

An accurate determination of both the level and completeness of an SCI is critical when following patients after injury and also permits a comparison among patients, a critical component of any research. The Frankel grading system[5] was one of the initial classification schemes applied to SCI and bears some similarities to the more current American Spinal Injury Association and the International Medical Society of Paraplegia (ASIA/IMSOP) impairment scale. Frankel subdivided injuries as follows: (A) complete loss of motor-sensory function below level of lesion, (B) complete motor paralysis with some sensory preservation (includes sacral sparing), (C) retained motor function but useless, (D) retained useful motor function, and (E) recovery (free of neurologic symptoms). Since the 1980s, ASIA/IMSOP has developed and revised the current standard of SCI classification.[6] Components of the assessment include definitions of the neurologic level (motor and sensory), completeness of injury, the zone of partial preservation, determination of total motor and sensory scores and, finally, the ASIA/IMSOP impairment scale (Fig. 314–1).

The respective motor and sensory levels are the most caudal segment of the spinal cord with normal sensory and motor function on both sides of the body. In the new ASIA scoring system, the motor level is determined by identifying the most caudal key muscle with at least grade 3 power. The remaining cephalad key muscle groups must have grade 5 strength.[6] The key muscle groups for the upper extremities include elbow flexors (C5), wrist extensors (C6), elbow extensors (C7), finger flexors (C8), and finger adductors (T1). In the lower extremities, the key muscle groups include hip flexors (L2), knee extensors (L3), ankle dorsiflexors (L4), long toe extensor (L5), and ankle plantar flexors (S1).

The difference between a complete and incomplete injury relies on the detection of any evidence of neurologic function distally, including preservation of perineal sensation (sacral sparing). Assessment of sacral sensation is tremendously important because it may be the only evidence of neurologic function distal to an injury. Pathologically, many SCIs are characterized by a peripheral rim of preserved white matter around an area of central necrosis with or without hemorrhage. The retained white matter may be the neuroanatomic substrate carrying laterally placed sacral spinothalamic fibers and, thus, sensation from the perineum. The completeness of injury has important implications in determining prognosis because few patients with a neurologically complete injury recover useful function.[7, 8] According to ASIA guidelines, *tetraplegia* is the

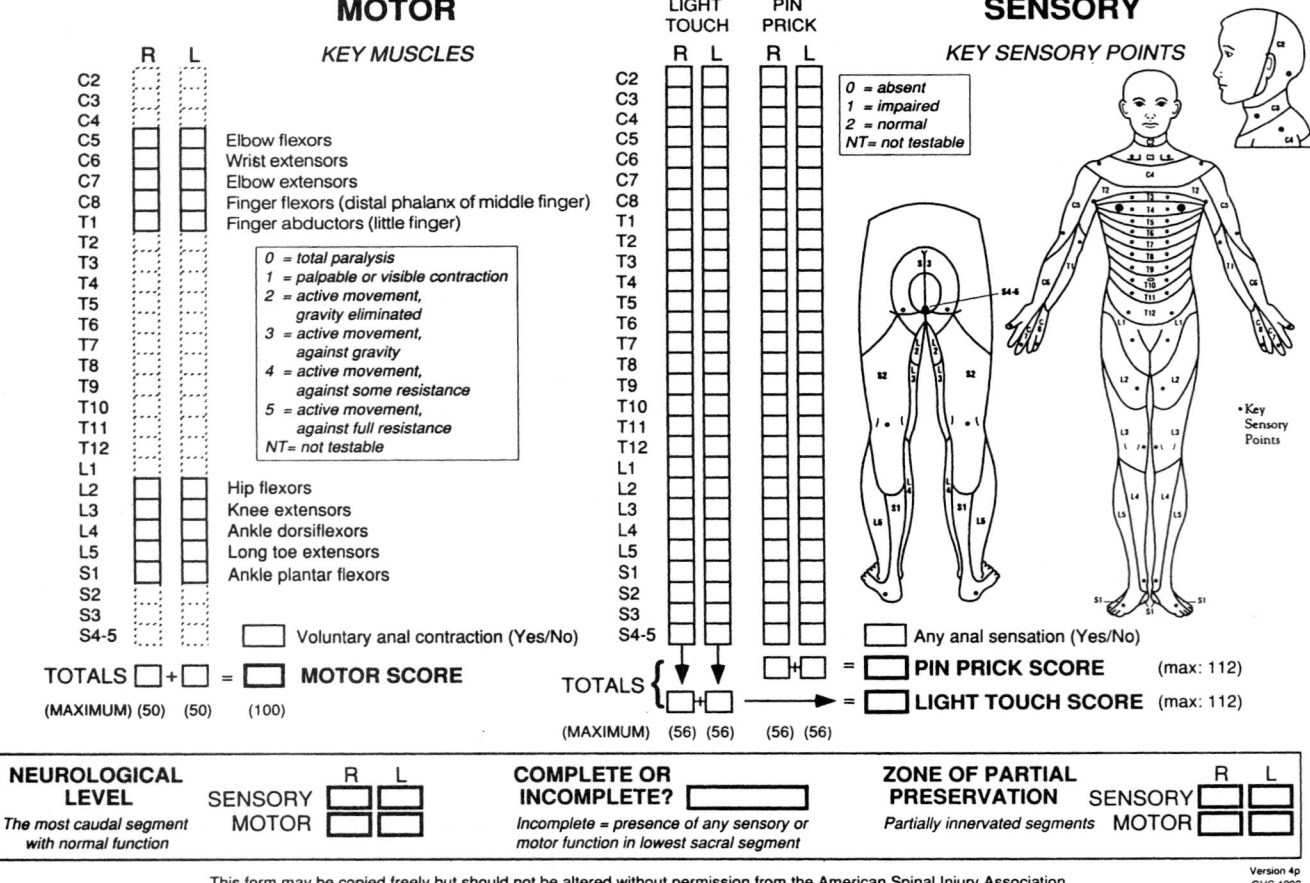

FIGURE 314–1. Neurologic examination as recommended by American Spinal Injury Association and the International Medical Society of Paraplegia (ASIA/IMSOP) for the assessment of spinal cord injury.

preferred term for describing patients with impaired motor or sensory function involving the spinal cord from T1 and above.

SPINAL CORD SYNDROMES

The following section focuses on the numerous discrete syndromes that have been described to characterize the clinical presentation of certain SCIs, all of which are predicated on an accurate knowledge of spinal cord anatomy. Patients with a complete loss of neurologic function distal to the level of the SCI, including the loss of sacral sensation, are deemed functionally complete. Functionally incomplete patients cover a wide spectrum of neurologic dysfunction.

Bell's Cruciate Paralysis

Cruciate paralysis was first described as a new clinical entity by Bell[9–12] and is characterized by weakness or paralysis of the hands and arms with relative preservation of lower extremity strength. Bell's cruciate paralysis is a syndrome observed after cervicomedullary injuries, the most common of which are C2 fractures.[13] A strikingly similar presentation may be seen in patients with a lower cervical injury, which has been referred to as *acute central cervical SCI*. Although the clinical presentations of these two syndromes are often indistinguishable, the location of the lesion in the corticospinal tract presumably differs in the two syndromes.[9, 10] The explanation for the pathophysiology of the dissociated strength in the upper and lower extremities assumes that the injury is localized within a somatotopically organized corticospinal tract. Evidence has challenged the assumptions that underlie the pathophysiologic basis of this disorder.[7]

The basis for the clinical presentation was thought to be midline damage to the rostral portion of the pyramidal decussation (Fig. 314–2). The injury could selectively ablate the fibers of the corticospinal tract subserving hand and arm function[12] and spare the corticospinal tract fibers decussating at a lower level that supply leg function. Wallenberg[14] first proposed that the corticospinal fibers subserving arm function decussate at a higher level within the cervicomedullary junction than those subserving the legs. He described a case of "hemiplegia cruciata" in which a patient had both ipsilateral arm and contralateral leg weakness. He presumed that such a peculiar presentation could occur only if a unilateral injury to the cervicomedullary junction could impinge on the recently crossed corticospinal arm fibers and the uncrossed leg fibers. The view that the level at which the arm fibers within the corticospinal tract decussate is higher than the level of leg fibers suggests that this tract was organized somatotopically at the cervicomedullary junction.

Acute Central Cervical Spinal Cord Injury

Acute central cervical SCI was first described by Schneider and associates.[15] The injuries typically occur

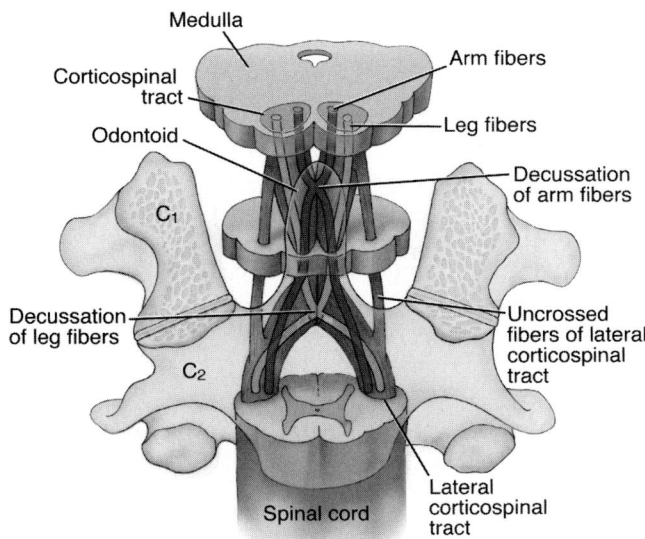

FIGURE 314–2. Diagram illustrating Bell's hypothesis that arm and leg fibers of the corticospinal tract decussate within the medullary pyramid at different levels. The corticospinal tract fibers that supply the arms are thought to decussate at a more rostral and central level than the leg fibers. Consequently, a localized injury at this level could theoretically produce the clinical picture of disproportionate weakness of the upper versus the lower extremities. (From Marano SR, Calica AB, Sonntag VKH: Bilateral upper extremity paralysis [Bell's cruciate paralysis] from a gunshot wound to the cervicomedullary junction. Neurosurgery 18:642–644, 1986.)

in patients who have sustained a hyperextension injury with inbuckling of the ligamentum flavum, compressing the spinal cord within an area of preexisting cervical spine stenosis. The clinical manifestations are similar, if not identical, to those of cruciate paralysis.[15, 16] As with cruciate paralysis, the proposed pathophysiologic mechanism is based on a somatotopically organized corticospinal tract, where an area of central cord injury involves the medially placed fibers of the tract within the posterolateral funiculus. The medially placed corticospinal fibers were presumed by Foerster[17] to represent specifically those subserving arm and hand function. Thus, injury to these medially placed fibers theoretically could result in relatively greater upper extremity weakness.

No neuroanatomic evidence, however, has ever supported the view that the corticospinal tract is organized somatotopically.[18] Nonetheless, the theory has prevailed and found its way into many neuroanatomic texts.[19, 20] An alternative hypothesis is that the clinical syndrome consisting of relatively greater hand and arm weakness than leg weakness can occur when an injury involves the corticospinal tract anywhere from the level of the medulla to the cervical enlargement. Such an injury may reflect that the main function of the corticospinal tract is to subserve fine motor movements to the distal musculature, especially those of the upper limbs. Leg movements and locomotor activity may be preserved because primarily other fiber tracts within the spinal cord, including the rubrospinal or vestibulospinal tracts, can mediate these functions.

Brown-Séquard Syndrome

The Brown-Séquard syndrome was first described in 1850. It is characterized by a physiologic hemisection of the spinal cord.[21] Thus, patients present with ipsilateral paralysis, ipsilateral loss of proprioception, and contralateral pain and temperature loss. This syndrome is uncommon as an isolated finding and may occur with other evidence of SCI or nerve root (or both) or brachial plexus injury. It is most often associated with cervical spine injuries and less frequently with thoracic lesions. The syndrome carries a relatively good prognosis for recovery. When the deficit occurs as a result of a penetrating injury, however, the recovery is somewhat less favorable.

Anterior Spinal Cord Syndrome

The anterior spinal cord syndrome is characterized by a physiologic ventral section of the spinal cord that spares the posterior columns. Patients present with motor paralysis and pain and temperature loss but are spared proprioception and vibration sense. It occurs with hyperflexion and axial-loading injuries as well as with central disk herniations, "teardrop fractures," and compression fractures that compromise the ventral aspect of the spinal canal. Although it is tempting to invoke blockage of the anterior spinal artery as part of the pathophysiology, it has yet to be demonstrated as an important component of the syndrome. Most incomplete injuries tend to recover over time, but the anterior cord syndrome has a less favorable prognosis.

Conus Medullaris Syndrome

Typically, the conus medullaris is found between the spinal levels of T11 and L2. This area of the spinal cord is prone to injury because its location at the thoracolumbar junction represents a transition zone between the relatively stiff thoracic spine, which is stabilized by the rib cage, and the lumbar spine. These patients typically present with symptoms of both upper and lower motor root findings. During the acute phase, paralysis of lower extremities, flaccid rectal tone, and urinary retention are found. During the chronic phase, evidence of atrophy and hyperreflexia is prominent. The deficits tend to be symmetrical. The prognosis for recovery of bladder and bowel function is relatively poor.

Cauda Equina Syndrome

A cauda equina syndrome represents an injury to the nerve roots arising from the conus medullaris and can be seen with a fracture or acute disk herniation extending from L2 and below. Patients present with asymmetrical paralysis, sensory loss, and areflexia, including loss of bowel and bladder control. In the case of an acute central disk herniation, prompt decompres-

sion is thought to improve the potential for the recovery of bowel and bladder function.[22] Some patients present with only autonomic dysfunction; thus, a high index of suspicion is required.

Spinal Shock

Significant confusion arises when the term *spinal shock* is used after SCI. The misunderstanding regarding its use stems from multiple causes. First, many physicians use the terms *spinal shock* and *neurogenic shock* interchangeably. *Neurogenic shock,* however, refers to a condition categorized by hypotension and bradycardia resulting from interruption of the sympathetic nervous system pathways within the spinal cord. The incidence of significant neurogenic shock increases with injuries above T6 because unopposed vagal tone slows the heart and creates lower systemic vascular resistance, resulting in venous pooling. The condition responds to the administration of fluids or colloids, or both, and occasionally requires the use of pressors. Neurogenic shock is distinct from hypovolemic shock, which occasionally occurs concomitantly in the multitrauma patient with an SCI who has evidence of external or internal bleeding.

Spinal shock encompasses a number of different neurologic manifestations with various time courses. Traumatic injuries to the spinal cord interrupt or temporarily damage a number of descending and ascending pathways. The most common initial presentation of a complete SCI with respect to reflex and autonomic function is a period of areflexia and flaccidity. This phase is gradually replaced by hypertonia, exaggerated reflexes and, in many cases, spasticity. The transition may last days to weeks. The immediate onset of hyperreflexia and spasticity is uncommon, and its presence is a bad prognostic sign. The period of transition in reflex and autonomic function is often referred to as *spinal shock.* Motor and sensory loss is also subject to change within the first few hours after a SCI. When such function rapidly recovers in the absence of confounding variables such as alcohol, drugs, or a closed head injury, spinal shock of the motor-sensory system is presumed to have resulted.

The bulbocavernosus reflex is monitored by performing a rectal examination and pinching the glans penis or by tugging on the Foley catheter in a male or a female. Involuntary contraction of the rectal sphincter indicates a positive reflex. The presence of this reflex implies the lack of supraspinal input to the sacral outflow and is suggestive of a complete spinal injury. During the early postinjury period, the bulbocavernosus reflex may be absent and suggests the continued presence of spinal shock. The bulbocavernosus reflex tends to be one of the earliest reflexes to recover from spinal shock.

A voluntary contraction of the sphincter during digital rectal examination or the presence of rectal sensation, or both, supports the presence of a communication between the lower spinal cord and supraspinal centers; thus the potential for further motor or sensory recovery is favorable. In some complete spinal cord injuries, rectal tone is maintained. In the absence of any other signs of spinal cord function, the presence of rectal tone in itself does not indicate an incomplete injury.

PROGNOSTIC FACTORS FOR RECOVERY

Clinicians use the neurologic examination, age, and the appearance of the spinal cord on magnetic resonance imaging (MRI) as well as other clinical data to guide patients and their families on the expected outcome for a specific injury. For any traumatic SCI, it is important to ascertain whether the patient has a functionally complete or incomplete neurologic deficit. The distinction is important because the prognosis for neurologic recovery differs for these two conditions. Patients with no evidence of motor or sensory function below the spinal column injury are considered to have functionally complete injuries. Patients with no voluntary motor control and only slight sensory preservation in their lowest sacral dermatomes or some anal tone are still considered to have incomplete injuries. Functionally, patients with complete cervical injuries that remain complete within the first 24 hours of admission are unlikely to regain significant ambulatory function (1% to 3%).[23, 24] In contrast, most patients who enter the hospital with an incomplete neurologic injury attain some degree of recovery. The level and degree of an incomplete injury also provide important prognostic information. Cervical injuries have a higher potential for recovery than do thoracic or thoracolumbar injuries. The less severe the SCI, the more likely it is that the patient will recover.[25]

Most SCIs occur in males, with more than half being in the 16- to 30-year age group. The prognosis for recovery is inextricably linked to age. Younger patients fare much better than their older counterparts in terms of regaining neurologic function after an SCI.[26] The two most important potential neurologic explanations are the capacity of the "young" spinal cord to function with major deficiencies in the neural circuitry as well as the possibility of some spontaneous regeneration of the central nervous system after injury.[27] The reverse also appears to be true. It is well recognized that patients with stable incomplete injuries may lose function as they age. This change may reflect the loss of the last few functioning neurons within the damaged spinal cord.[28] Neuronal loss is a normal part of the aging process for both the brain and the spinal cord, and the clinical deterioration observed after SCI may be likened to the postpolio syndrome.

MRI after SCI allows the spinal cord to be visualized in a noninvasive manner. The images provide immediate feedback about the degree of spinal cord compression and information about the stability of the spinal column through an assessment of the integrity of the ligaments, disks, and surrounding soft tissues. In addition, intramedullary hemorrhage is easily discerned and provides important prognostic information. Intramedullary hemorrhage is more commonly observed after neurologically complete injuries and signifies a worse neurologic and functional outcome.[29, 30]

PREHOSPITAL MANAGEMENT

Advances in emergency care include the recognition by emergency personnel that any trauma patient with multiple injuries could have a spinal column injury. SCIs are frequently associated with head injuries, which compound the difficulties associated with the initial assessment. All patients who sustain significant trauma should be presumed to have a SCI, and measures to prevent further injury should be instituted at the first possible opportunity.[31] Initial immobilization of the cervical spine with a hard collar is a priority during extrication. Rotation or angulation of any portion of the spine must be avoided.

Establishment and maintenance of an airway by the fastest and safest method are then required. For injuries above C4, apnea can ensue rapidly because of the functional loss of both intercostal and diaphragmatic muscles. Rapid intubation via a nasotracheal route or an orotracheal route with in-line stabilization is optimal. Typically, patients with cervical and high thoracic injuries present with neurogenic shock, which manifests as hypotension and bradycardia. The cardiac and circulatory manifestations stem from interruption of the sympathetic nervous pathways within the spinal cord and the resultant unopposed vagal tone. To increase the circulating volume effectively, intravenous access in the field permits fluid resuscitation of the patient. The potential for causing secondary damage to the spinal cord can also be reduced by adhering to a protocol of resuscitation that ensures adequate oxygenation and control of blood pressure to ensure perfusion of oxygenated blood to the traumatized spinal cord.[32]

Appropriate immobilization of the injured spine, transportation of patients on backboards, and their rapid evacuation to a level I trauma center have improved the outcome of spinal injuries by reducing the risk of iatrogenic SCIs in patients with unstable fractures. Placing the rare individual with a preexisting degenerative spinal deformity who sustains spinal trauma in a supine position can aggravate the SCI. For example, patients with ankylosing spondylitis may have significant preexisting cervical kyphosis or a C-shaped thoracic curvature. Angulation of the fracture can increase if patients who are normally stooped forward are forced into the supine position. This action can increase such patients' neurologic deficit. In these rare circumstances, patients must be transported in their position of comfort. Placing them in a flat position, such as on a backboard, should not be attempted. Turning the patient may be required to prevent the aspiration of vomitus and can be performed safely by three or four individuals using a "logrolling" technique.

EMERGENCY ROOM MANAGEMENT

Traction

Cervical traction is an important adjunct in the management of cervical fractures and dislocations (Fig.

314–3). Cervical traction can realign and stabilize the spine. Realignment of a cervical dislocation is one of the fastest methods of increasing the diameter of the spinal canal.[33, 34] Gardner-Wells tongs (Codman and Shurtleff, Inc., Randolph, Mass) can be applied under local anesthesia and attached to weights. In selected circumstances, the tongs can be used to apply manual traction. Inappropriate or excessive traction can be disastrous for patients and thus must always be applied after baseline imaging has been obtained. Traction also should be followed by a careful neurologic examination and serial imaging of the cervical spine. Recently, Grant and colleagues[35] demonstrated the relative safety of "closed reduction in cervical spine injuries" as evidenced by the low incidence of neurologic deterioration.

Absolute contraindications for the application of traction include occipitoatlantal dislocations and concomitant open skull fractures. Traction must be applied carefully in patients with ankylosing spondylitis because even small increments of weight can result in overdistraction. Weights should be added in 5- to 10-pound increments. The total maximal weight applied should be individualized, with larger weights required for lower cervical injuries in patients with muscular necks. Muscle relaxants and the reverse Trendelenburg position may facilitate reduction. Slight flexion or extension also can facilitate reduction of the fracture. Overdistraction of a fracture or disk space, neurologic worsening, or increasing pain require immediate reduction of the weight applied.

Considerable controversy exists regarding the role of pretraction MRI in patients with cervical fracture-dislocations. Although traction and realignment of the spine can cause an acute disk herniation with neurologic deterioration,[36, 37] this complication is rare in awake patients. On imaging studies, disk herniations have been documented after reduction,[38] but the significance of such herniations is uncertain.[39] Most neurosurgeons believe that prompt restoration of the diameter of the spinal canal plays an important role in neurologic recovery after SCI.[33] Administration of traction in patients with significant facet-fracture dislocations and neurologically complete injuries should be attempted before cervical MRI is performed. An iatrogenically dislodged disk caused by realigning the dislocated spine is rare.[35] In most institutions, this risk does not justify the time and risk of transporting a patient with an unreduced cervical spine to obtain a prereduction cervical MRI study. In selected patients who are neurologically intact or who have incomplete injuries, the information added by a prereduction MRI scan can justify its use.

Pharmacotherapy

The concepts of primary and secondary SCI are important principles in understanding the pathophysiology and role of pharmacotherapeutic agents in the emergent treatment of SCIs. The primary injury mechanism results from a mechanical insult that occurs at the time of impact and includes acute compression, impaction, distraction, laceration, and shear.[40] Secondary injuries occur after the initial injury and account for some of the progressive pathologic changes associated with an SCI.[40] A number of drugs have been tested in the laboratory, but only a few of these agents have progressed to clinical trials to evaluate their efficacy. Five randomized controlled trials of pharmacotherapy for acute SCI have been conducted, focusing on the therapeutic effect of either steroids or gangliosides.

Steroids. A number of studies have shown improved neurologic recovery in animals with SCIs that have received either dexamethasone or methylprednisolone.[32, 41-44] Initially, steroid treatment held promise as a potential therapeutic agent for its putative role in reducing white matter edema and inflammation. Current evidence, however, suggests that the major mechanism of action is reducing the effects of secondary injury and, in particular, the destructive effects of lipid peroxidation on cell membranes.[45] Other actions include improving spinal cord blood flow, enhancing the postinjury activity of Na^+/K^+-ATPase, and facilitating the recovery of extracellular calcium ions.[32, 46]

The first North American Spinal Cord Injury Study (NASCIS I) examined low- (100 mg) and high-dose (1000 mg) methylprednisolone given for 10 days. Unfortunately, this trial lacked a control group, and no significant difference in outcome was found except for an increased number of wound infections among patients in the high-dose group.[47]

The second (NASCIS II) trial was a prospective, randomized, double-blind, multicenter trial that demonstrated improved neurologic outcomes after 6 weeks, 6 months, and 12 months in patients who had received a regimen of methylprednisolone, which included a bolus dose of 30 mg/kg and a maintenance dose of 5.4 mg/kg/hr for 23 hours.[48] The improvements in motor and sensory scores associated with the administration of methylprednisolone were observed only if the drug was given within 8 hours of injury when compared with naloxone or a placebo. Some of the criticisms of this study relate to difficulties in randomization, analysis of benefit limited to small subgroups within the larger study, and lack of replication of results by completely independent group of investigators, among others.[49, 50] However, the administration of methylprednisolone is believed to reduce the amount of secondary injury that occurs after SCI, and this protocol has become an important tool in the treatment of SCI in most North American centers.

Published in 1997, the NASCIS III study compared the dosage of methylprednisolone used in the NASCIS II protocol with a longer dosing regimen (48 hours) and with a 21-aminosteroid.[51] The 21-aminosteroids (lazaroids) represent a new class of steroids that are potent inhibitors of lipid peroxidation and lack much of the glucocorticoid activity of many of the traditional steroid compounds. The results of this study suggest that when patients are seen within 3 hours of their injury, they should receive a bolus dose of methylprednisolone (30 mg/kg) followed by 23 hours of treatment (5.4 mg/kg). Patients seen between 3 and 8 hours

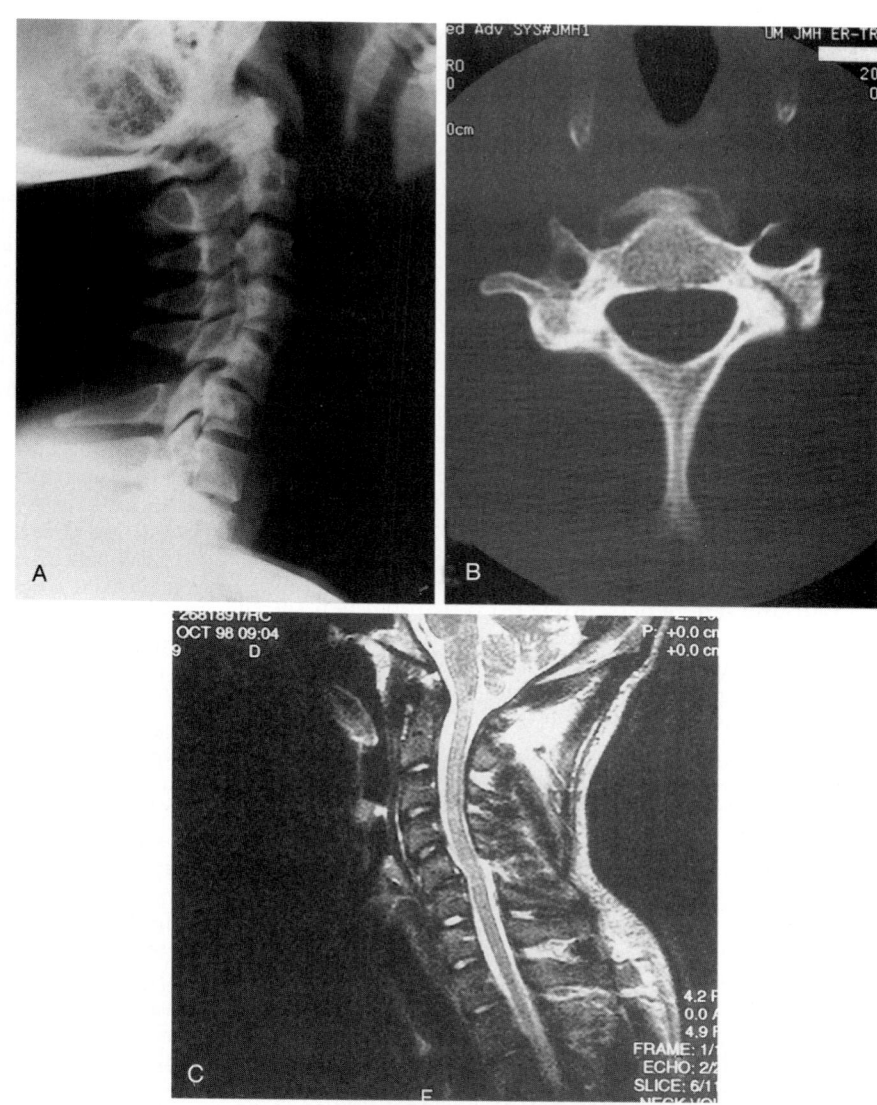
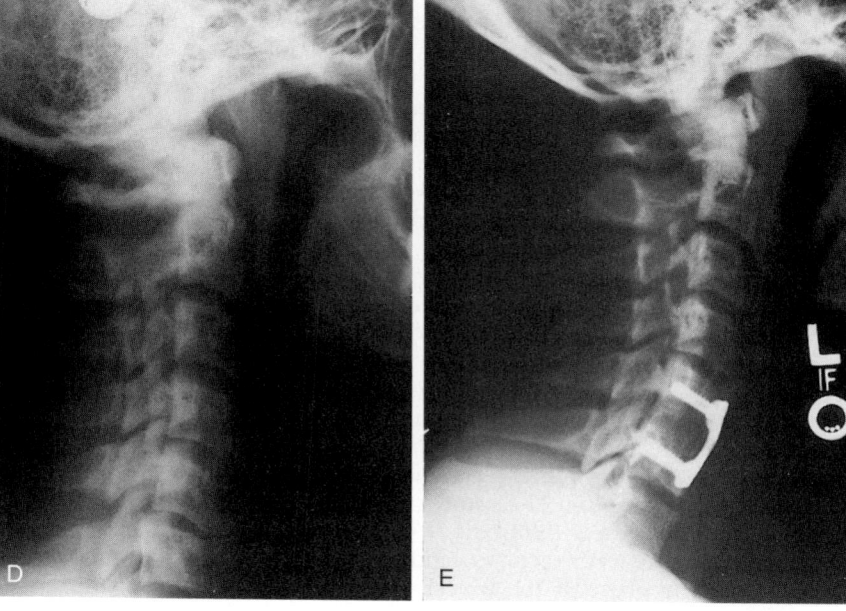

FIGURE 314–3. *A,* Lateral cervical spine radiograph demonstrating a C5–6 facet-fracture subluxation with perched facets producing a kyphotic deformity. *B,* Computed tomographic scan showing a fracture involving the left C5–6 facet. *C,* Magnetic resonance imagining (MRI) scan showing a bulging disk at the level of the subluxation with some degree of spinal cord compression. *D,* The patient was placed in traction (30 lb) with partial reduction of the deformity. *E,* Stabilization was performed via an anterior cervical approach with diskectomy and fusion using autograft and a Synthes (Synthes Spine, Paoli, Pa) plate. One-year follow-up lateral radiograph showing good alignment and an osseous union of autograft with the adjacent vertebral bodies.

should receive the same bolus followed by a longer dosing regimen (48 hours). The complications from 48 hours of treatment included a significant increase in severe sepsis and pneumonia.

Gangliosides. These agents consist of a complex sialic acid containing glycosphingolipids, which are present in high concentrations in neural membranes. These compounds are involved in a variety of cell surface phenomena such as cell substrate binding and receptor functions.[52] Since 1985, basic research has demonstrated that these compounds can (1) promote the survival of neurons in cell culture; (2) increase the number, length, and branching of neuronal processes in cell culture; and (3) improve functional recovery after a variety of traumatic and ischemic insults to the peripheral and central nervous systems. A limited number of animal studies have examined the role of gangliosides after SCI and found only a modest effect on the regeneration of serotonergic neurons.[53] A prospective, randomized, double-blind, single-center study found a beneficial effect on functional neurologic outcomes when the ganglioside GM1 was administered within 72 hours of a human SCI.[54] A multicenter trial is now being conducted to test both high and low concentrations of the drug.

IMAGING

The ability to image the spinal column and the spinal cord after trauma has improved considerably since the 1980s. The standard protocol for "clearing" the cervical spine in the traumatized patient remains a lateral radiograph that includes the first thoracic level, anteroposterior views, and open-mouthed odontoid views. The majority of significant cervical pathology requiring neurosurgical intervention is detected using these standard films.[55] However, significant fractures, particularly pure ligamentous injuries, can be missed with these views alone.[56] Hence, supplementary films of the cervical spine are often required. In selected injuries without a neurologic deficit, cervical flexion-extension views are obtained. These views may uncover a significant subluxation that would not be detectable on a neutral lateral spine radiograph. If the patient's ability to flex and extend the neck is severely limited, imaging obtained after a few days could help rule out significant ligamentous pathology.

High-resolution computed tomography (CT) with uniplanar and three-dimensional reconstructions has largely replaced tomography for diagnosing fractures of the spinal elements. When C2 fractures involve the odontoid, CT with sagittal and coronal reconstructions helps delineate the fracture's location, orientation, and degree of displacement, all of which have important implications for determining the likelihood of healing and for surgical planning. The safety of placing transarticular screws is aided by using thin-cut computed tomographic scans with reconstructions in the sagittal plane and in the plane of the trajectory of the screw.[57] A small C2 pars interarticularis and an aberrant high-

riding vertebral artery are two relative contraindications for transarticular screw placement (Fig. 314–4).

MRI is a valuable noninvasive tool for imaging the spine and related structures after an injury. Some of the most important advantages of MRI relate to its ability to image soft tissue injuries, including muscles, ligaments, and disks. The importance of MRI in diagnosing atlantoaxial instability is illustrated by the evaluation of a patient with a bursting-type fracture of the C1 ring (Jefferson's fracture). Indirect evidence of a transverse ligament rupture previously relied on measurements of the combined C1 lateral mass displacement relative to the lateral lips of the superior articular surface of C2 on an open-mouthed view (Spence's rule).[58] Similarly, the atlantodental interval has been used to detect an incompetent transverse ligament indirectly.[59] Currently, with high-resolution MRI (1.5 tesla), the transverse ligament and its attachments can be identified directly and their integrity assessed.[60]

MRI can also be used to assess ligamentous instability. D'Alise and colleagues[61] obtained MRI scans of the cervical spine in 121 intubated, post-traumatic obtunded or comatose patients; 25.6% of the patients had significant soft tissue injuries and 6.6% of the patients required surgical stabilization. MRI was the first study to detect significant ligamentous injury (Fig. 314–5). In many cases, a limited study, which included a gradient-echo sequence, could be used to "clear" the spine.

Other important applications of MRI in the setting of spinal trauma include detecting the presence of a hematoma within the spinal canal or spinal cord. Fortunately, significant hematomas, which compress the spinal cord after trauma, are uncommon except in the setting of ankylosing spondylitis, in which it should be sought diligently.[62] Intramedullary hemorrhage associated with SCI is commonly observed and is a negative predictor of a good outcome. Most importantly, MRI assists in defining the relationships among the fractured spinal column, spinal cord, and nerve roots in a noninvasive manner (Fig. 314–6). The degree of spinal canal compromise in relationship to the spinal cord and nerve roots is best assessed with this imaging modality.

The possible drawbacks of MRI relate to the time required to transfer patients to the specialized quarters required for housing the large-bore magnets. In most trauma centers, MRI is available within the same building, and nearby staff can run the machine for the length of time required for the imaging. The patients must be screened for any possible contraindication, such as metallic foreign bodies. All equipment, including traction, tongs, and weights, must be compatible with MRI.

TREATMENT

Surgery versus External Orthosis

There are several broad indications for surgery after spinal trauma: (1) deformity correction, (2) stabilization of the spine, and (3) decompression of neurologic elements. For cervical fractures, some deformities can sim-

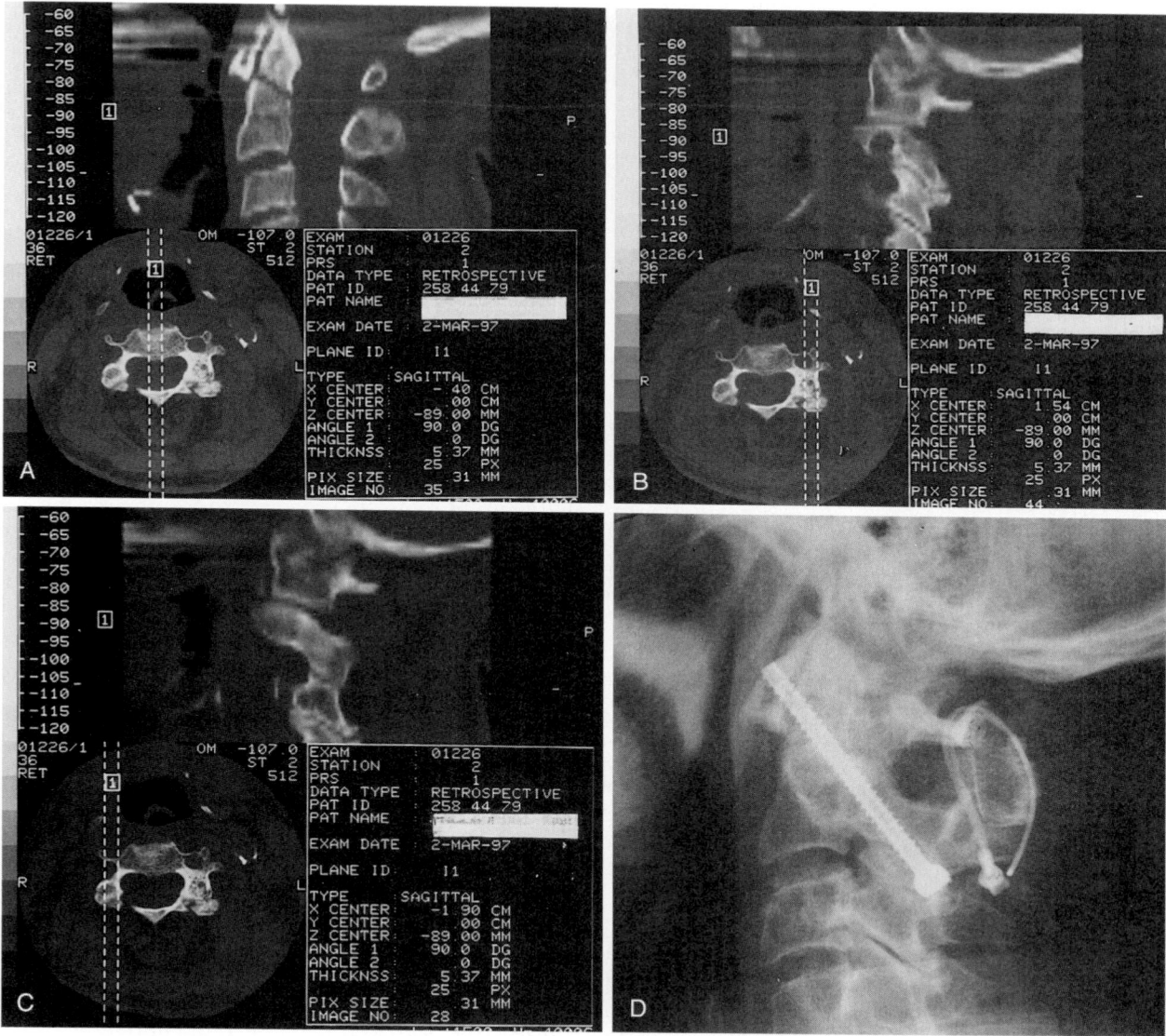

FIGURE 314–4. A 70-year-old woman sustained a type II odontoid fracture and an anterior arch fracture of C1 after a motor vehicle accident. *A*, Sagittal reconstruction showing the fracture at the base of the dens. A thin sagittal cut laterally along the trajectory of the screw shows a high-riding vertebral artery foramen on the left (*B*) that passes dangerously close to the anticipated placement of the transarticular screw. *C*, On the right, the size of the pars interarticularis is adequate and the position of the vertebral artery foramen is not aberrant. *D*, Postoperative lateral cervical radiograph showing the location of the single screw as well as posteriorly placed iliac crest bone graft and a Sonntag cable construct.

ply be corrected by the application of cervical traction, which is followed by an external orthosis (such as halo immobilization) or surgical stabilization to maintain the desired alignment.[33] Surgical approaches for deformity correction a priori are necessary when a traumatic herniated disk is present and realignment of the spine without prior disk removal may compress the spinal cord further, or when locked or fractured facets preclude external reduction.[37] Occasionally, late recognition of a cervical fracture can result in a malaligned fusion. In thoracic and lumbar fractures, deformity correction often requires surgical intervention. At surgery, various combinations of bone graft material and instru-

mentation can be used to maintain alignment. Failure to correct significant deformity can lead to future neurologic compromise,[63] abnormal posture, respiratory complications, or chronic pain.

An important indication for surgery in the setting of spinal trauma is an "unstable" fracture. Unstable fractures result from the loss of the normal relationship between adjacent vertebrae so that under physiologic loading, neurologic damage, progressive deformity, or intractable pain ensues.[64] Since the 1980s, major advances in surgical instrumentation have facilitated the stabilization of some of the most difficult spinal fractures.[57] An implicit advantage of immediate surgical

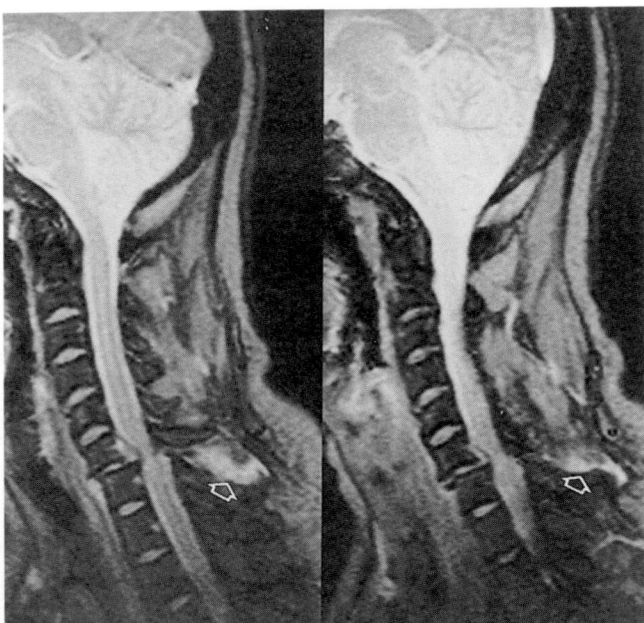

FIGURE 314–5. A 45-year-old woman was "cleared" in the emergency department after cervical spine radiography and computed tomography (*CT*) failed to demonstrate a fracture or subluxation. On admission, the patient's Glasgow Coma Scale score was 11 and she had significant facial fractures. One week after admission, she presented with weakness in her hands. MRI (gradient-echo sequence) demonstrated anterior subluxation of C6 on C7 with tearing of the posterior longitudinal ligament from the posterior aspect of the C6 vertebral body without definite disk herniation. Signal intensity within the C6–7 interspinous ligaments (*arrows*) increased, and the spinal canal was significantly narrowed, resulting in spinal cord compression.

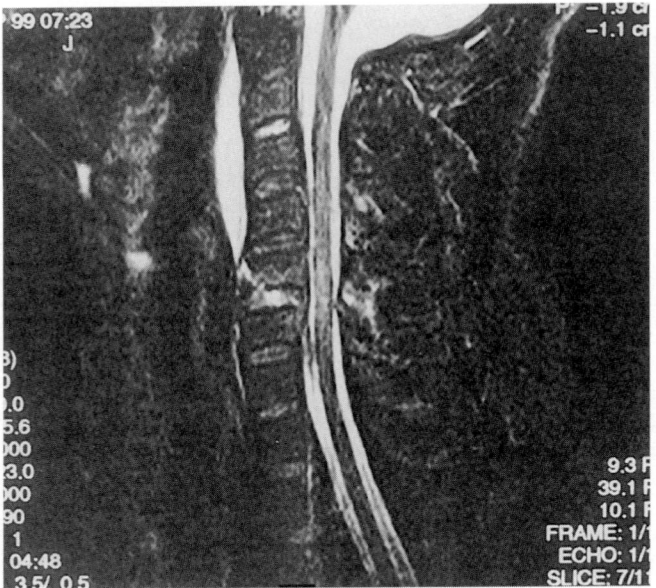

FIGURE 314–6. A 25-year-old man sustained a hyperflexion injury and presented with incomplete tetraparesis. His ASIA score was C. Sagittal T2-weighted MRI scan shows increased signal intensity of the cervical spinal cord without hemorrhage opposite a teardrop fracture involving the body of C5. The disk space is disrupted and edema is apparent at C5–6.

stabilization is the possibility of early mobilization of patients and the potential for reducing the complications associated with prolonged bed rest.[65]

The decompression of neurologic elements, either by realigning the spinal column or by elevating vertebral bone fragments or disk, appears a logical approach to improve the neurologic outcomes associated with spinal injuries. Yet, the value of surgically decompressing neurologic elements in spinal trauma is controversial. There are two major issues in the literature. First, does the decompression of injured neural tissue ultimately improve neurologic outcomes in patients with SCIs? Second, how does the timing of surgery influence outcome? It is convenient to distinguish between functionally complete and incomplete neurologic injuries because the potential for neurologic recovery associated with complete and incomplete injuries appears to be vastly different, independent of any specific management decisions. Patients with no evidence of motor or sensory function below the spinal column injury are considered to have functionally complete injuries. Patients with functionally incomplete injuries cover a wide spectrum of neurologic dysfunction that ranges from no voluntary motor function below the level of injury and minor residual sensory function to only minimal neurologic dysfunction that may allow unlimited ambulation.

An understanding of the potential benefits of surgically decompressing the spinal cord after spinal trauma should be derived from both laboratory and clinical research. There are a number of animal models for initiating and maintaining a predetermined level of spinal cord compression. In most instances, a laminectomy is performed and a deforming force is applied to the spinal cord. The rate, force, and duration of compression are varied so that the degree of injury imparted to the spinal cord can be quantified. Several well-investigated models of injury include the weight-drop method developed by Allen[66] during the early part of the 20th century, the rapid inflation of extradural balloons,[67] and the application of modified aneurysm clips.[68]

Although all the models are imperfect simulations of human SCI, a few basic observations have been found consistently. The force of impact and the duration of compression appear to be important predictors of neurologic recovery in several different animal models and types of injuries, although in most studies the duration of compression is too short to be considered clinically significant.[68, 69] Guha and colleagues[70] demonstrated a benefit from decompressing the spinal cord as long as it was 4 hours after mild injury in rats. No benefit, however, appears to be derived from delayed decompression when large forces are used to compress the spinal cord. In summary, some experimental data support the claim that surgical decompression of the injured spinal cord, particularly with lesser injuries, improves neurologic outcome.

In an analysis of the older clinical literature, it is important to note that the diagnostic and therapeutic tools available to surgeons for the management of patients with SCIs have changed substantially since the

1970s. With the advent of CT and MRI, surgeons can specifically assess the degree of neural compression in a patient. The adequacy of the decompression can also be evaluated. Before the 1970s, surgical procedures designed to decompress neural elements after spinal trauma were essentially limited to laminectomy. This procedure is valuable only in those rare cases when a posteriorly projecting piece of bone or posteriorly located hematoma compresses the spinal cord. Morgan and associates[71] quelled the initial enthusiasm[72] for decompressive laminectomies by demonstrating that most patients deteriorated or showed no neurologic improvement afterward. A laminectomy also increases the risk of destabilizing the spine, thereby inducing a post-traumatic kyphotic deformity.[73]

Among contemporary series, a number of retrospective reports and case studies have confirmed that patients who sustain complete cervical SCIs have only a small chance of neurologic recovery and that their potential for regaining ambulation is less than 3%.[23, 24, 44, 74, 75] Variables that can confound an assessment for a complete injury include the presence of an associated head injury, alcohol or drug intoxication, multiple associated injuries, and spinal shock as demonstrated by the absence of a bulbocavernosus reflex on admission. Categorizing some of these patients as having complete injuries may account for some of the unexpected recoveries that have been reported.

The role of surgical decompression in patients with complete SCIs remains controversial. The number of patients who demonstrate significant neurologic improvement remains low with all treatment modalities, including both nonsurgical and surgical approaches. Consequently, it is impossible to ascribe a direct role to surgery in the occasional patient with a complete injury who improves functionally after surgical decompression. Heiden and colleagues,[24] for example, retrospectively analyzed 199 patients with complete cervical injuries, 61% of whom underwent surgical decompression. No patients in the surgical group recovered ambulatory function. Of the 78 patients who were managed nonsurgically, however, two were ambulatory at a later follow-up examination. At the other end of the spectrum, in another retrospective series by Levi and associates,[23] 53 patients with complete injuries were managed surgically on either an early (<24 hours) or a delayed basis (>24 hours). On later follow-up, 3.8% of the patients were ambulatory when both groups were combined.

The timing of spinal cord decompression after trauma in patients with complete SCIs is another unresolved issue. With certain cervical fracture-subluxations, the spinal cord can be decompressed rapidly using traction. The traction must be performed in combination with serial radiography or fluoroscopy and clinical examination of the patient. When this treatment was applied to a small series of patients examined retrospectively, the few patients with complete injuries who underwent reduction in a timely fashion were those who tended to achieve significant recoveries.[33] In contrast, no significant differences in neurologic outcomes were identified in a cohort of patients who underwent either early or delayed surgical decompression[23]; however, the former approach promoted earlier transfer to rehabilitation and consequently was less costly. Advocates of delayed surgery have suggested that early surgery increases medical complications.[24, 75]

Finally, as an offshoot of the NASCIS II trial, a retrospective review of neurologic outcome was analyzed with respect to performance and timing of surgery.[76] There were no significant differences in the neurologic outcomes of patients treated surgically or nonsurgically. However, when surgery was performed within 25 hours of injury or more than 200 hours after injury, neurologic recovery appeared to improve. The potential for provoking injury to the spinal cord by operating during the immediate phase of injury (1 to 8 days), which is associated with white matter edema and the pathologic correlates of secondary injury, was suggested as the explanation for this finding.

Whether prompt surgical decompression ultimately results in functional improvement in patients with complete neurologic injuries will remain unanswered until a randomized, prospective, double-blind study is performed. However, given the amalgamated knowledge from numerous retrospective studies, it appears that prompt surgical decompression of the spinal cord in patients with complete injuries benefits few patients.

The role of decompressive surgery is also unclear in patients with incomplete injuries. A number of retrospective studies have suggested that decompression, even when delayed, can improve the degree of neurologic function in patients with incomplete injuries.[15, 74, 77, 78] This finding is consistent with experimental studies that have documented improvement in rats with less severe SCIs after decompression.[70] Unlike many patients with functionally complete SCIs,[23] many patients with incomplete injuries improve over time even without surgical treatment, particularly those with syndromes such as acute central cervical SCI or cruciate paralysis.[13, 15, 79] Thus, the improvement in incomplete injuries after surgery should not be attributed to surgery when, in fact, it reflects the natural history of the disease. Clarifying this dilemma could be accomplished only by designing a study on the role of decompressive surgery in incomplete injuries that contains a control group of untreated patients. Most surgeons in North America believe so strongly that decompressive surgery benefits incomplete injuries that a clinical trial including a nonoperated cohort of incomplete patients is unlikely.

Because the role of surgical decompression in incomplete SCIs has never undergone randomized, prospective, double-blind testing, rigorous evidence supporting this procedure is still lacking. However, a large literature supports the benefits of prompt surgical decompression after a variety of other central nervous system insults, including mass lesions after traumatic brain injuries. The bulk of evidence suggests that decompression of the spinal cord in patients with incomplete injuries, through external reduction using traction, operative decompression, or both, is beneficial. Persistent compression of the spinal cord is thought to increase the risk of secondary changes in the spinal cord over time. In one retrospective study, the incidence of syringomyelia on MRI was significantly increased in patients with persistent spinal cord compression.[63] This reasoning, combined with other well-established indications for spinal surgery after trauma, dictates an operative approach for many patients with incomplete SCIs.

The management of patients with traumatic injuries who initially present with a neurologic deficit that substantially improves or completely resolves by the time the patient is examined by the attending surgeon is particularly complex. A fracture associated with cruciate paralysis should be managed according to the presence or absence of instability, because most patients lack significant compression at this spinal cord level after cervical traction. Patients with acute central cervical SCI often have a significant degree of cervical spinal stenosis but lack an overt fracture or instability. One can make a logical argument for operative decompression in patients with significant cervical compression who have reached a plateau in neurologic recovery, who are exhibiting neurologic deterioration, or who have the potential to injure the cervical spine repetitively.

Another complex management issue arises in patients, particularly athletes, who present with transient neurologic disturbances, such as quadriparesis, after sustaining a high-velocity impact injury to the cervical spine. Most of these individuals improve within 24 hours of injury, although some may take as long as 5 days to regain complete neurologic function.[80, 81] Plain films, CT, and dynamic radiography often fail to disclose a fracture or overt instability. MRI, particularly T2-weighted images, may confirm the presence of a spinal cord contusion. Often, a concomitant finding in these patients is single or multilevel cervical spinal stenosis.[80, 82]

In patients who are neurologically intact after spinal trauma, surgeons should be guided primarily by the principles of correcting deformities and repairing the instability associated with the vertebral injury.

Management of Penetrating Spinal Cord Injuries

Violence as a cause of SCI is increasing, as is the number of penetrating injuries of the spinal column. Gunshot wounds can be divided into military (high-velocity injuries) and civilian (low-velocity injuries). The victims tend to be young men. The spinal cord or cauda equina may be injured by either the bullet or bone fragments adjacent to the path of the bullet. With high-velocity missiles, the percussive effect of the missile causes the injury.

Initial treatment in the field requires stabilizing the injured segment of the spinal column as with any spinal trauma. After the victim has been resuscitated, a careful neurologic evaluation is performed. Careful inspection of entry and possible exit sites is coupled with imaging studies to determine the exact trajectory of the bullet. The initial evaluation includes CT and plain radiography to localize the bullet and bone fragments. MRI also

is occasionally performed. If a ferromagnetic missile fragment is present, myelography followed by myelography-CT may be indicated. Associated injuries are common and can include both vascular and visceral injuries. The presence of a visceral injury can increase the risk of infection. In a review by Romanick and associates,[83] missiles that penetrated the colon were associated with a higher risk of spinal infection.[84] All injuries should be treated with prophylactic broad-spectrum intravenous antibiotics.

Absolute indications for surgery include cerebrospinal fluid fistula and neurologic deterioration in a patient who had been stable. Relative indications for surgery include removal of the missile fragment or decompression of the spinal cord and nerve roots. The value of removing a bullet fragment compressing the spinal cord or nerve roots is unknown. With respect to recovery after bullet removal, patients with conus and cauda equina injuries typically fare better than those with complete cervical and thoracic injuries.[85] The benefit of removal, however, is complicated by the retrospective nature of most studies.[86] The potential delayed benefits include a reduced incidence of abscess, spinal cord syrinx, and arachnoiditis. Potential negative features include the possibility of iatrogenic instability induced by removing the lamina of a spinal column that might have already sustained an anterior column injury.

The role of steroids in the management of penetrating trauma has not been studied prospectively. Both NASCIS II and NASCIS III trials[48, 51] excluded such injuries. A number of retrospective reviews have documented the lack of benefit of steroids on neurologic outcome in penetrating trauma.[86–88] Given the somewhat increased risk of cerebrospinal fluid fistula and infection in this setting, methylprednisolone is not recommended for open wounds associated with SCI.

Management in the Intensive Care Unit

After SCI, each of the vital systems is profoundly affected. A systematic approach must be taken to evaluate and treat each potential complication. Early and late complications occur, and the degree of involvement of each system is usually correlated with the level and severity of injury.

RESPIRATORY SYSTEM

Respiratory complications are a major source of morbidity and mortality after SCI. An 18% to 30% mortality rate is reported in patients with tetraplegia.[89, 90] Most cervical SCIs occur below C4; consequently, the phrenic nerves continue to innervate the diaphragm. However, the respiratory system is often severely affected, particularly after a cervical injury, because paralysis of the intercostal muscles and accessory muscles of respiration varies. Loss of abdominal muscle tone and ileus also reduce the mechanical efficiency of breathing.

In general, there is a grace period during which patients with cervical injuries maintain their respiratory status. However, 24 to 48 hours after admission, respiratory failure often ensues. Preparation for such events should be undertaken early so that if intubation is required it can be performed with stabilization using in-line traction. It is often supplemented by fiberoptic intubation using a bronchoscope. Measurements of arterial blood gases, negative inspiratory force, and forced vital capacity may provide a method to detect respiratory failure early. Additional injuries such as rib fractures, hemothorax, and so on can accelerate this respiratory deterioration.

The most common complications include atelectasis, pneumonia, pulmonary embolus, pulmonary edema, and adult respiratory distress syndrome. In addition to difficulty with taking deep breaths and coughing, patients are often unable to clear airway secretions. Accumulation of secretions, mucous plugs, or both can cause respiratory failure. Prevention includes respiratory treatment with bronchodilators, frequent pulmonary toilet, respiratory therapy, increasing airway humidity, intubation, and mechanical ventilation, including continuous positive airway pressure. The use of the Roto-Rest bed (Midmark Corporation, Versailles, Ohio) significantly decreases pulmonary complications associated with SCI,[89, 91] improving pulmonary blood flow and reducing the incidence of pulmonary emboli.

Pulmonary infections frequently complicate SCIs. Within days of admission, the normal flora of the oral cavity contains increasing numbers of nosocomial organisms. Hospital-acquired pulmonary infections are heralded by fever, increased white cells both in the sputum and within the peripheral blood, and changes on chest radiographs. After appropriate cultures have been obtained, broad-spectrum antibiotic therapy should be instituted.

Most patients can be disconnected or "weaned" from the ventilator after they have been stabilized medically, which usually means treatment of pulmonary infections, re-establishment of euvolemia, enhancement of respiratory muscle function through respiratory therapy, and nutritional supplementation to offset the high caloric requirements of the trauma. Initially, weaning the intermittent mandatory ventilation rate is followed by weaning the positive airway pressure. With prolonged periods of ventilation (more than 2 weeks) or multiple failed extubations, tracheostomy should be considered. The likelihood of requiring a tracheostomy increases with a high SCI, preexisting pulmonary disease, and the age of the patient. Tracheostomy effectively reduces the physiologic dead space. Northrup and colleagues[92] have demonstrated that a tracheostomy can be performed before anterior cervical instrumentation of the spine with a low risk of infection. If early surgery for stabilization is advocated, few patients undergo a tracheostomy before anterior cervical stabilization surgery.

CARDIOVASCULAR SYSTEM

The typical patient with SCI without associated vascular or visceral injuries presents to the emergency department with a mean arterial blood pressure of 80 mm Hg and a heart rate of 65 beats per minute.[93]

The patient's blood pressure may respond to volume resuscitation, but these patients often require low-dose pressor therapy. Aggressive medical management, including volume expansion and maintenance of mean arterial blood pressure above 85 mm Hg, is thought to enhance neurologic outcome by maximizing spinal cord perfusion at the injury site and thus reducing the likelihood of secondary injury.[40] Invasive hemodynamic monitoring demonstrates a normal cardiac index with a low systemic vascular resistance. In elderly patients with SCI, careful attention to volume replacement is required to avoid precipitating heart failure.

GASTROINTESTINAL SYSTEM

Hypoactive bowel sounds and impaired peristalsis are common accompaniments of SCI resulting from the lack of sympathic modulation. To avoid gastric and small bowel dilatation, it is wise to delay enteral feeding. If gastric distention impairs respiratory function, a nasogastric tube is indicated. Most cervical injuries require nasogastric suction because of impaired bowel motility, air swallowing that produces gastric distention, and respiratory compromise due to paralysis of intercostal muscles.

Patients with SCIs are at a high risk of developing gastric and duodenal stress ulcers. The use of steroids compounds the risk of significant gastrointestinal hemorrhage. At a minimum, all patients with SCIs should receive an H_2-blocker to prevent this dreaded complication. The reported risk of gastrointestinal hemorrhage in the NASCIS II study was 3% for the control group and 4.5% for the methylprednisolone group.[48]

URINARY SYSTEM

During the period of spinal shock that follows a cervical or thoracic SCI, the urinary bladder is atonic and flaccid. Over time it becomes an upper motor neuron bladder with a small capacity. Initially, an indwelling Foley catheter is placed. After 3 to 4 days, the patient is switched to intermittent bladder catheterization to keep urinary volumes at less than 500 mL. Urinary tract infections are common. If the patient develops a fever, urine cultures must be obtained. Antibiotics are selected based on culture sensitivities. Patients with SCIs above T6 may also develop autonomic dysreflexia if the bladder becomes overdistended. Sometimes with catheterization, sympathetic overactivity—and thus headaches, hypertension, sweating, and reduced body temperature—results. Long-term complications include chronic infections, obstructive uropathy, and renal calculi, which can progress to renal failure if left untreated.

INTEGUMENT

The spinal cord–injured patient is extremely susceptible to developing decubitus. Frequent log rolling is invaluable in preventing deterioration of the skin. The Roto-Rest bed[91] can reduce the incidence of skin breakdown by preventing pressure on a single area from frequent turning. The DuoDerm patch (Convatel, Princeton, NJ) is useful in both preventing and treating superficial or grade 1 pressure sores in paralyzed patients. Rotational flaps are reserved for SCI patients with deeper pressure sores that require tissue coverage.

THROMBOEMBOLIC COMPLICATIONS

SCI patients are at high risk of lower extremity venous thromboembolism, which may be manifested by deep vein thrombosis in the lower or upper extremities that causes leg swelling or pulmonary embolism. Prevention includes the administration of subcutaneous heparin, usually 5000 units subcutaneously twice daily or more. Lovenox (Rohrer, Collegeville, Pa) has been shown to reduce the risk of thrombotic complications effectively. Treatment of pulmonary emboli or above-knee deep vein thrombosis requires heparinization. Should there be a contraindication to heparinization, an inferior vena cava filter should be placed.

RESEARCH

SCI research is an absolute priority of the National Institutes of Health. Models of SCI, mechanisms of secondary injury, treatment of the acute phase of SCI, and the development of transplantation strategies to repair the damaged spinal cord are ongoing across North America and around the world. The treatment arms of the research can be divided into two categories: agents that can be given during the acute phase of injury and those that may limit secondary injury mechanisms or promote regeneration. Two of the most promising drugs, methylprednisolone and GM1, have yielded only modest results. The effects of methylprednisolone, which is used in almost all major SCI centers, is under closer scrutiny.[50] Drugs of the future include neurotrophins, which can promote the survival and regeneration of injured nerve cells; drugs that prevent the inflammatory response to SCI[94]; and drugs that prevent apoptotic cell death.[95] In the transplantation arena, cellular therapies to treat chronic injuries are important. Cells of interest include Schwann cells, olfactory ensheathing glia, embryonic spinal cord cells, and neural progenitor cells (stem cells). Antibodies that neutralize the inhibitory proteins within myelin have also demonstrated promise. Strategies that combine a number of these treatments are most likely to have a beneficial effect in the future.

CONCLUSIONS

Despite the enormous advances in the diagnosis and treatment of spinal fractures since the 1970s, a number of questions regarding the most appropriate management of patients with traumatic spinal fractures remain unanswered. Only a few aspects of the surgical management of spinal trauma have been raised in this chapter. It is clear, however, that a number of issues remain unresolved. Technologic advancements in spinal instrumentation and pharmacotherapeutics will continue in the 21st century. Both neurosurgeons and orthopedic surgeons must work together to test the efficacy and cost-effectiveness of some of the newer treatment modalities because determining both the best possible treatment and how to contain costs will be part of the management equation in the future. Outcome assessment should be at the forefront of all new ideas. Only through a critical and open-minded analysis of our treatment strategies will we be able to provide the best care for patients whose lives often are changed forever by their injury and the rapid sequence of events associated with acute hospitalization.

REFERENCES

1. Harvey C, Rothschild BB, Asmann AJ, et al: New estimate of traumatic SCI prevalence: A survey-based approach. Paraplegia 28:537–544, 1990.
2. Berkowitz M: Assessing the socioeconomic impact of improved treatment of head and spinal cord injuries. J Emerg Med 11(Suppl 1):63–67, 1993.
3. Torg JS, Naranja RJ Jr, Pavlov H, et al: The relationship of developmental narrowing of the cervical spinal canal to reversible and irreversible injury of the cervical spinal cord in football players. J Bone Joint Surg Am 78:1308–1314, 1996.
4. Tator CH, Carson JD, Edmonds VE: Spinal injuries in ice hockey. Clin Sports Med 17:183–194, 1998.
5. Frankel HL, Hancock DO, Hyslop G, et al: Value of postural reduction in initial management of closed injuries of the spine with paraplegia and tetraplegia. Paraplegia 7:179–192, 1969.
6. Maynard FM Jr, Bracken MB, Creasy G, et al: International Standards for Neurological and Functional Classification of Spinal Cord Injury: American Spinal Injury Association. Spinal Cord 35:266–274, 1997.
7. Levi AD, Tator CH, Bunge RP: Clinical syndromes associated with disproportionate weakness of the upper versus the lower extremities after cervical spinal cord injury. Neurosurgery 38:179–185, 1996.
8. Maynard FM, Reynolds GG, Fountain S, et al: Neurological prognosis after traumatic quadriplegia: Three-year experience of California Regional Spinal Cord Injury Care System. J Neurosurg 50:611–616, 1979.
9. Schneider RC, Crosby EC, Russo RH, et al: Traumatic spinal cord syndromes and their management. Clin Neurosurg 20:424–492, 1973.
10. Schneider RC, McGillicuddy JE: Concomitant craniocerebral and spinal trauma with special reference to the cervicomedullary region. In Vinken PJ, Bruyn GW (eds): Injuries of the Brain and Skull: Handbook of Clinical Neurology. Amsterdam, North Holland, 1976, pp 149–152.
11. Bell HS: Paralysis of both arms from injury of the upper portion of the pyramidal decussation: "Cruciate paralysis." J Neurosurg 33:376–380, 1970.
12. Bell HS: Cruciate paralysis. In Vinken PJ, Bruyn GW (eds): Injuries of the Spine and Spinal Cord: Handbook of Clinical Neurology. Amsterdam, North Holland, 1976, pp 391–392.
13. Dickman CA, Hadley MN, Pappas CTE, et al: Cruciate paralysis: A clinical and radiographic analysis of injuries to the cervicomedullary junction. J Neurosurg 73:850–858, 1990.
14. Wallenberg A: Anatomischer Befund in einem als "acute Bulbärraffection (embolie der Art. cerebellar post. inf. sinsistr?)" beschrieben Falle. Arch Psychiatr 34:923–959, 1901.
15. Schneider RC, Cherry G, Pantek H: The syndrome of acute central cervical spinal cord injury, with special reference to the mechanisms involved in hyperextension injuries of cervical spine. J Neurosurg 11:546–577, 1954.
16. Marano SR, Calica AB, Sonntag VKH: Bilateral upper extremity paralysis (Bell's cruciate paralysis) from a gunshot wound to the cervicomedullary junction. Neurosurgery 18:642–644, 1986.
17. Foerster O: Symptomatologie der erkrankungen des rücken-

marks und seiner wurzeln. In Bumke U, Foersters (eds): Handbook of Neurology. Berlin, Spring-Verlag, 1936, p 83.

18. Landau WM: Cruciate paralysis [letter]. Neurosurgery 19:676, 1986.

19. Crosby EC, Humphrey T, Lauer EW: Correlative Anatomy of the Nervous System. New York, Macmillan, 1962, pp 118, 490, 1076.

20. DeJong RN: The Neurological Examination: Incorporating the Fundamentals of Neuroanatomy and Neurophysiology, 2nd ed. New York, Hoeber-Harper, 1958, p 1076.

21. Brown-Séquard CE: Course of Lectures on the Physiology and Pathology of the Central Nervous System. Philadelphia, Collins, 1860.

22. Shapiro S: Cauda equina syndrome secondary to lumbar disc herniation. Neurosurgery 32:743–747, 1993.

23. Levi L, Wolf A, Rigamonti D, et al: Anterior decompression in cervical spine trauma: Does the timing of surgery affect the outcome? Neurosurgery 29:216–222, 1991.

24. Heiden JS, Weiss MH, Rosenberg AW, et al: Management of cervical spinal cord trauma in Southern California. J Neurosurg 43:732–736, 1975.

25. Tator, CH: Spine-spinal cord relationships in spinal cord trauma. Clin Neurosurg 30:479–494, 1983.

26. Cifu DX, Seel RT, Kreutzer JS, et al: A multicenter investigation of age-related differences in lengths of stay, hospitalization charges, and outcomes for a matched tetraplegia sample. Arch Phys Med Rehabil 80:733–740, 1999.

27. Inoue T, Kawaguchi S, Kurisu K: Spontaneous regeneration of the pyramidal tract after transection in young rats. Neurosci Lett 247:151–154, 1998.

28. Wang D, Bodley R, Sett P, et al: A clinical magnetic resonance imaging study of the traumatised spinal cord more than 20 years following injury. Paraplegia 34:65–81, 1996.

29. Schaefer DM, Flanders AE, Osterholm JL, et al: Prognostic significance of magnetic resonance imaging in the acute phase of cervical spine injury. J Neurosurg 76:218–223, 1992.

30. Kulkarni MV, McArdle CB, Kopanicky D, et al: Acute spinal cord injury: MR imaging at 1.5 T. Radiology 164:837–843, 1987.

31. Karbi OA, Caspari DA, Tator CH: Extrication, immobilization and radiologic investigation of patients with cervical spine injuries. CMAJ 139:617–621, 1988.

32. Young W: Secondary CNS injury. J Neurotrauma 5:219–221, 1998.

33. Hadley MN, Fitzpatrick BC, Sonntag VKH, et al: Facet fracture-dislocation injuries of the cervical spine. Neurosurgery 30:661–666, 1992.

34. Fehlings MG, Rao SC, Tator CH, et al: The optimal radiologic method for assessing spinal canal compromise and cord compression in patients with cervical spinal cord injury. Part II. Results of a multicenter study. Spine 24:605–613, 1999.

35. Grant GA, Mirza SK, Chapman JR, et al: Risk of early closed reduction in cervical spine subluxation injuries. J Neurosurg 90: 13–18, 1999.

36. Eismont FJ, Arena MJ, Green BA: Extrusion of an intervertebral disc associated with traumatic subluxation or dislocation of cervical facets: Case report. J Bone Joint Surg Am 73:1555–1560, 1991.

37. Doran SE, Papadopoulos SM, Ducker TB, et al: Magnetic resonance imaging documentation of coexistent traumatic locked facets of the cervical spine and disc herniation. J Neurosurg 79: 341–345, 1993.

38. Selden NR, Quint DJ, Patel N, et al: Emergency magnetic resonance imaging of cervical spinal cord injuries: Clinical correlation and prognosis. Neurosurgery 44:785–793, 1999.

39. Vaccaro AR, Falatyn SP, Flanders AE, et al: Magnetic resonance evaluation of the intervertebral disc, spinal ligaments, and spinal cord before and after closed traction reduction of cervical spine dislocations. Spine 24:1210–1217, 1999.

40. Tator CH, Fehlings MG: Review of the secondary injury theory of acute spinal cord trauma with emphasis on vascular mechanisms. J Neurosurg 75:15–26, 1991.

41. Braughler JM, Hall ED: Correlation of methylprednisolone levels in cat spinal cord with its effect on ($Na^+ + K^+$)-ATPase, lipid peroxidation, and alpha motor neuron function. J Neurosurg 56: 838–844, 1982.

42. Ducker TB, Hamit HF: Experimental treatments of acute spinal cord injury. J Neurosurg 30(6):693–697, 1969.

43. Green BA, Kahn T, Klose KJ: A comparative study of steroid therapy in acute experimental spinal cord injury. Surg Neurol 13:91–97, 1980.

44. Hansebout RR, Kuchner EF, Romero-Sierra C: Effects of local hypothermia and of steroids upon recovery from experimental spinal cord compression injury. Surg Neurol 4:531–536, 1975.

45. Hall ED, Yonkers PA, Andrus PK, et al: Biochemistry and pharmacology of lipid antioxidants in acute brain and spinal cord injury. J Neurotrauma 9(Suppl 2):S425–S442, 1992.

46. Lewin MG, Hansebout RR, Pappius HM: Chemical characteristics of traumatic spinal cord edema in cats: Effects of steroids on potassium depletion. J Neurosurg 40:65–75, 1974.

47. Bracken MB, Collins WF, Freeman DF, et al: Efficacy of methylprednisolone in acute spinal cord injury. JAMA 251:45–52,1984.

48. Bracken MB, Shephard MJ, Collins WF, et al: A randomized, controlled trial of methylprednisolone or naloxone in the treatment of acute cervical cord injury: Results of the Second National Acute Spinal Cord Injury Study. N Engl J Med 322:1405–1411, 1990.

49. Shapiro SA: Methylprednisolone for spinal cord injury [letter to the editor]. J Neurosurg 77:324–327, 1992.

50. Nesathurai S: Steroids and spinal cord injury: Revisiting the NASCIS 2 and NASCIS 3 trials. J Trauma 45:1088–1093, 1998.

51. Bracken MB, Shephard MJ, Holford TR, et al: Administration of methylprednisolone for 24 or 48 hours or tirilazad mesylate for 48 hours in the treatment of acute spinal cord injury: Results of the Third National Acute Spinal Cord Injury Randomized Controlled Trial. National Acute Spinal Cord Injury Study. JAMA 277:1597–1604, 1997.

52. Rodden FA, Wiegandt H, Bauer BL: Gangliosides: The relevance of current research to neurosurgery. J Neurosurg 74:606–619, 1991.

53. Commissiong JW, Toffano G: The effect of GM₁ ganglioside on ceruspinal, noradrenergic, adult neurons and on fetal monoaminergic neurons transplanted into the transected spinal cord of the adult rat. Brain Res 380:205–215, 1986.

54. Geisler FH, Dorsey FC, Coleman WP: Recovery of motor function after spinal-cord injury—a randomized placebo-controlled trial with GM₁ ganglioside. N Engl J Med 324:1829–1838, 1991.

55. MacDonald RL, Schwartz ML, Mirich D, et al: Diagnosis of cervical spine injury in motor vehicle crash victims: How many x-rays are enough? J Trauma 30:392–397, 1990.

56. Fazl M, LaFebvre J, Willinsky RA, et al: Posttraumatic ligamentous disruption of the cervical spine, an easily overlooked diagnosis: Presentation of three cases. Neurosurgery 26:674–678, 1990.

57. Paramore CG, Dickman CA, Sonntag VKH: The anatomical suitability of the C1–C2 complex for transarticular screw fixation. J Neurosurg 85:221–224, 1996.

58. Spence KF Jr, Decker S, Sell KW: Bursting atlantal fracture associated with rupture of the transverse ligament. J Bone Joint Surg Am 52:543–549, 1970.

59. Fielding JW, Cochran GVB, Lawsing JF 3rd, et al: Tears of the transverse ligament of the atlas: A clinical and biomechanical study. J Bone Joint Surg Am 56:1683–1691, 1974.

60. Dickman CA, Greene KA, Sonntag VKH: Injuries involving the transverse atlantal ligament: Classification and treatment guidelines based upon experience with 39 injuries. Neurosurgery 38: 44–50, 1996.

61. D'Alise MD, Benzel EC, Hart BL: Magnetic resonance imaging evaluation of the cervical spine in the comatose or obtunded trauma patient. J Neurosurg 91:54–59, 1999.

62. Foo D, Rossier AB: Post-traumatic spinal epidural hematoma. Neurosurgery 11:25–32, 1982.

63. Abel R, Gerner HJ, Smit C, et al: Residual deformity of the spinal canal in patients with traumatic paraplegia and secondary changes of the spinal cord. Spinal Cord 37:14–19, 1999.

64. Panjabi MM, Thibodeau LL, Crisco JJ 3rd, et al: What constitutes spinal instability? Clin Neurosurg 34:313–339, 1988.

65. Wilberger J: Diagnosis and management of spinal cord trauma. J Neurotrauma 8(Suppl 1):S21–S30, 1991.

66. Allen AR: Remarks on the histopathological changes in the spinal cord due to impact: An experimental study. J Nerv Ment Dis 41: 141–147, 1914.

67. Tarlov IM, Klinger H: Spinal cord compression studies: Time limits for recovery after acute compression in dogs. Arch Neurol Psych 71:271–290, 1954.

68. Rivlin AS, Tator CH: Effect of duration of acute spinal cord compression in a new acute cord injury model in the rat. Surg Neurol 10:39–43, 1978.

69. Dolan EJ, Tator CH, Endrenyi L: The value of decompression for acute experimental spinal cord compression injury. J Neurosurg 53:749–755, 1980.

70. Guha A, Tator CH, Endrenyi L, et al: Decompression of the spinal cord improves recovery after acute experimental spinal cord compression injury. Paraplegia 25:324–339, 1987.

71. Morgan TH, Wharton GW, Austin GN: The results of laminectomy in patients with incomplete spinal cord injuries. Paraplegia 9:14–23, 1971.

72. Covalt DA, Cooper IS, Hoen TI: Early management of patients with spinal cord injury. JAMA 151:89–94, 1953.

73. Malcom BW, Bradford DS, Winter RB, et al: Post-traumatic kyphosis: A review of forty-eight surgically treated patients. J Bone Joint Surg Am 63:891–899, 1981.

74. Benzel EC, Larson SJ: Functional recovery after decompressive operation for thoracic and lumbar spine fractures. Neurosurgery 19:772–778, 1986.

75. Marshall LF, Knowlton S, Garfin SR, et al: Deterioration following spinal cord injury: A multicenter study. J Neurosurg 66:400–404, 1987.

76. Duh MS, Shepard MJ, Wilberger JE, et al: The effectiveness of surgery on the treatment of acute spinal cord injury and its relation to pharmacological treatment. Neurosurgery 35:240–249, 1994.

77. Benzel EC, Larson SJ: Functional recovery after decompressive spine operation for cervical spine fractures. Neurosurgery 20:742–746, 1987.

78. Bohlman HH, Anderson PA: Anterior decompression and arthrodesis of the cervical spine: Long-term motor improvement. Part I. Improvement in incomplete traumatic quadraparesis. J Bone Joint Surg Am 74:671–682, 1992.

79. Braakman R: Some neurological and neurosurgical aspects of injuries of the lower cervical spine. Acta Neurochir (Wien) 22:245–260, 1970.

80. Bailes JE, Hadley MN, Quigley MR, et al: Management of athletic injuries of the cervical spine and spinal cord. Neurosurgery 29:491–497, 1991.

81. Zwimpfer TJ, Bernstein M: Spinal cord concussion. J Neurosurg 72:894–900, 1990.

82. Torg JS, Pavlov H, Genuario SE, et al: Neurapraxia of the cervical spinal cord with transient quadriplegia. J Bone Joint Surg Am 68:1354–1370, 1986.

83. Romanick PC, Smith TK, Kopaniky DR, et al: Infection about the spine associated with low-velocity-missile injury to the abdomen. J Bone Joint Surg Am 67:1195–1201, 1985.

84. Venger BH, Simpson RK, Narayan RK: Neurosurgical intervention in penetrating spinal trauma with associated visceral injury. J Neurosurg 70:514–518, 1989.

85. Cybulski GR, Stone JL, Kant R: Outcome of laminectomy for civilian gunshot injuries of the terminal spinal cord and cauda equina: Review of 88 cases. Neurosurgery 24:392–397, 1989.

86. Simpson RK Jr, Venger BH, Narayan RK: Treatment of acute penetrating injuries of the spine: A retrospective analysis. J Trauma 29:42–46, 1989.

87. Heary RF, Vaccaro AR, Mesa JJ, et al: Steroids and gunshot wounds to the spine. Neurosurgery 41:576–584, 1997.

88. Levy ML, Gans W, Wijesinghe HS, et al: Use of methylprednisolone as an adjunct in the management of patients with penetrating spinal cord injury: Outcome analysis. Neurosurgery 39:1141–1149, 1996.

89. Reines HD, Harris RC: Pulmonary complications of acute spinal cord injuries. Neurosurgery 21:193–196, 1987.

90. Silver JR, Gibbon NO: Prognosis in tetraplegia. Br Med J 4:79–83, 1968.

91. Green BA, Green KL, Klose KJ: Kinetic therapy for spinal cord injury. Spine 8:722–728, 1983.

92. Northrup BE, Vaccaro AR, Rosen JE, et al: Occurrence of infection in anterior cervical fusion for spinal cord injury after tracheostomy. Spine 20:2449–2453, 1995.

93. Vale FL, Burns J, Jackson AB, et al: Combined medical and surgical treatment after acute spinal cord injury: Results of a prospective pilot study to assess the merits of aggressive medical resuscitation and blood pressure management. J Neurosurg 87:239–246, 1997.

94. Bethea JR, Castro M, Keane RW, et al: Traumatic spinal cord injury induces nuclear factor-kappaB activation. J Neurosci 18:3251–3260, 1998.

95. Emery E, Aldana P, Bunge MB, et al: Apoptosis after traumatic human spinal cord injury. J Neurosurg 89:911–920, 1998.

CHAPTER 315

Cervical Spine Trauma

ARTHUR L. JENKINS III ■ DENNIS G. VOLLMER ■ MARC E. EICHLER

Acute injuries of the spine and spinal cord are among the most common causes of severe disability and death after trauma.[1-4] For this reason, the evaluation and treatment of trauma to the spine, spinal cord, and nerve roots demand a systematic approach that is integrated into the overall management of the traumatized patient. Early diagnosis of injury, preservation of spinal cord function, and maintenance or restoration of spinal alignment and stability are the keys to successful management. The creation of spinal cord rehabilitation centers, the evolution of multidisciplinary trauma teams, the development of modern methods of cervical fusion and stabilization, and the recent recognition by the public and policy makers of the importance of injury prevention have led to marked advances in the management of patients with spine and spinal cord injuries. A great deal of research is focused on the treatment of spinal cord–injured patients, and in our lifetimes we may see the demise of the dogma that spinal cord injury is permanent.

HISTORICAL CONSIDERATIONS

The Edwin Smith surgical papyrus, written 5000 years ago, describes spinal cord injuries as ailments not to be treated.[5] Such pessimistic views survived until the "golden era" of Greece, when more modern teachings in medicine were introduced. Hippocrates is credited with much of the advancement in the treatment of spinal injuries. His method of achieving vertebral reduction and alignment by the application of axial distraction while an anterior force is applied to the spine was used for centuries.

During the first half of the 20th century, many of the modern methods for treating patients with spinal cord injury were developed. The introduction of radiology brought about a greater understanding of the pathophysiology of vertebral fractures by allowing clinicians to visualize the lesion and the results of treatment over time. This led to advances in both conservative and operative management of patients with spinal injuries.

The development of methods of skeletal traction to reduce dislocation and maintain alignment of cervical spine fractures until healing occurs is one such advance. Cervical traction by means of a halter device was described by Taylor in 1929.[6] Although he did not publish his own work, Hepburn was one of the progenitors of the tongs form of cervical traction[7]; he influenced Crutchfield, who modified and popularized the technique.[8] This technique and device were improved later by Gardner.[9] Long-term skeletal traction and maintenance of alignment were advanced by the halo orthosis of Nickel and colleagues in 1968.[10]

Current concepts of spinal cord rehabilitation were pioneered in the 1940s by Guttmann at the Stoke Mandeville Hospital in Great Britain.[11] Before this time, the mortality rate for patients with spinal cord injury was 80% to 90% within the first year. Most patients developed pressure sores or urinary sepsis that led to death. Guttmann reduced cervical spine fractures through the use of traction and postural reduction, revolutionized nursing techniques, and introduced a comprehensive program of rehabilitation.[11-14] The dramatic decrease in mortality and morbidity achieved by these methods reversed the perception that the conditions of such patients were hopeless and made surgical stabilization of the traumatized spine both logical and practical.[12] As rehabilitation programs focus more and more on increasing the mobility of patients with spinal cord injury, the maintenance of alignment becomes even more critical.

Rogers established the modern principles of cervical fusion when he recommended operating under traction, reducing the fracture if necessary, fixing the spine with wires around the spinous processes, and then performing a fusion.[15] Interspinous wiring techniques originally developed by Rogers remained the principal stabilization techniques in cervical spine trauma for decades.[15, 16] Roy-Camille pioneered the development of lateral mass plates and screws, which provide rigid posterior fixation for patients with cervical spinal cord injuries but do not require intact spinous processes or laminae for fixation.[17, 18]

In the 1930s, otolaryngologists were regularly approaching the front of the cervical vertebrae to remove huge osteophytes that made swallowing difficult. It was not until the 1950s, however, after Smith and Robinson reported anterior disk removal and fusion through this approach, that orthopedists and neurosurgeons became interested.[19] In 1958, Cloward gave an oral presentation (that was later published in 1961) on his circular graft anterior cervical fusion procedure.[20] This was followed by Bailey and Badgley's report of an anterior cervical graft done for multiple-level fusions.[21]

Over the past 2 decades, there has been a greater emphasis on research and a marked renewal of interest in the treatment of spine and spinal cord injuries. The development of spinal cord injury centers and the upgrading of emergency rooms so that they are better equipped to care for multiply injured patients have significantly improved the care of those with spine or spinal cord injuries.[3, 12, 22, 23] Improvements in the transportation of trauma patients to medical facilities by paramedical personnel and the evolution of the multidisciplinary trauma team concept to optimize the acute care of multiply injured patients have significantly reduced mortality from injuries to the cervical spine and spinal cord.[3, 24–26]

Recent technologic innovations and the increased availability of neuroimaging techniques such as magnetic resonance imaging (MRI) and computed tomography (CT) have also contributed significantly to improvements in patient management and outcome after these injuries.[27, 28] The spinal cord injury suffered by actor Christopher Reeve focused attention on this field and resulted in dramatic increases in funding, with concomitant breakthroughs in stem cell research and other potential treatments for this condition.

The past 2 decades have also seen a rapid expansion in the surgical armamentarium for the treatment of traumatic cervical spine instability and spinal cord compression.

Finally, one of the most significant recent advances in the field is the recognition by the public and by policy makers of the importance of injury prevention. Educational efforts targeting school-age children have been shown to have an influence on the behaviors that increase the risk of spinal injury.

EPIDEMIOLOGY

Accidents are the fourth leading cause of death in the United States after heart disease, cancer, and stroke, accounting for about 50 deaths per 100,000 population each year.[29] Early traumatic deaths tend to be due to exsanguination, whereas delayed traumatic deaths (those happening more than 1 hour after arrival at the hospital) tend to be due to severe neurological compromise.[30] Traumatic spinal cord injury statistics vary by the source and the population base, and the numbers differ depending on whether the sample area covers regions such as Pennsylvania (5.3 new cases per 100,000)[31] or Mississippi (9.3 new cases per 100,000).[30] Many of these studies point out different injury prevalences for different groups based on race, age, and gender. In addition, concomitant drug or alcohol use tends to lead to more severe injuries, increased length of hospital stay, and increased cost of hospitalization.[30–35]

Spinal cord injuries tend to occur in young individuals (second or third decade), although a second peak exists in the elderly population.[31] Young males are affected 3 to 20 times more often than females,[31, 36, 37] although in the 85 and older population, the male-female ratio appears to be equal.[31] A high proportion of these injuries is associated with complete neurological deficit.[36, 37] Estimates of the number of patients living with spinal cord injuries in the United States alone range from 185,000 to 400,000. According to DeVivo and colleagues, about 2000 U.S. hospital beds are necessary each year to care for these patients.[38] Of the approximately 14,000 people who sustain spinal cord injuries annually, 4200 die before reaching the hospital, and an additional 1500 patients die during the initial hospitalization.[39]

Whereas cervical spine fractures represent approximately 20% to 30% of all spine fractures, cervical spinal cord injuries represent approximately half of all spinal cord injuries. Fortunately, only 10% to 30% of spinal trauma results in spinal cord injury.[40] Cervical spinal cord injuries result in severe disability and profound socioeconomic impact. In 1990, the total economic cost of spinal cord injury was estimated to be $4 billion in direct costs and $3.4 billion in lost wages.[41] The cost of caring for a spinal cord–injured patient depends partially on the level involved. A high cervical spine injury (C4 and above) costs an average of $549,000 in the first year and $98,000 per year after that. A lower cervical spine–injured patient incurs $355,000 in direct costs in the first year and $40,000 per year after that. A 25-year-old man with a high cervical cord injury is likely to incur lifetime costs of more than $2.1 million, with a life expectancy of about 30 years if he is spontaneously breathing or 15 years if he is ventilator dependent.[42]

Motor vehicle accidents cause between 35% and 45% of all spinal cord injuries.[31, 42] The cervical region is the segment of the spine most frequently injured in automobile accidents, especially among those who do not wear shoulder- and lap-belt restraints.[43, 44] The National Crash Severity Study found that in accidents in which a vehicle was damaged severely enough to be towed from the scene, 1 in 300 occupants sustained a severe neck injury.[44] The incidence of neck injury increases to 1 in 14 for occupants ejected from the car. In this study, projections of the number of fatalities related to cervical injuries indicated that 20% of all car deaths include severe or fatal cervical spine injuries. Alker and colleagues found that 21% of 146 traffic accident autopsies showed radiologic evidence of cervical spine injury,[45] and Bucholz and associates reported that of 100 fatally injured motor vehicle crash victims, 24% had cervical fractures or fracture-dislocations.[46]

The biomechanics of the cervical spine and head in a motor vehicle accident explains the high incidence of injury. The forward momentum of the skull is not checked, because there is no good head restraint system available commercially. As the body (restrained by the seat belt) is slowed by the decelerating car, the head pitches forward at a high rate of angular velocity and is then jerked back when the neck has no more room to bend or when the head strikes an object such as the windshield or an airbag. These rapid changes in angular momentum cause fractures of various parts of the spine and ligaments.

The spectrum of injury severity in vehicular trauma ranges from minor neck spasms to quadriplegia and death.[44, 47] Numerous variables relating to the type and severity of the crash, the type of vehicle, and the use of safety restraints have an impact on the frequency and severity of spinal injury.[44, 48, 49] For individuals wearing seat belts, the type of restraint may dictate the resultant spinal injury. The three-point lap and shoulder belt is associated with cervical injury by several mechanisms. Free movement of the cervicothoracic junction allows a hyperflexion-distraction force to produce cervical spine fractures, dislocations, or subluxations.[49, 50] If the victim should slide under the crossed chest restraint, the chin may be caught and the neck forcibly hyperextended, causing different injury patterns.[49, 51] Injury patterns in airplane crashes are similar, with a 25% incidence of associated cervical spine fractures in plane crash fatalities.[52]

Athletic injuries result in between 5% and 10% of all spinal cord injuries, with most injuries occurring in the cervical spine. Football has the most spinal cord injuries among all the organized sports activities (cheerleading is second), and there has been a dramatic decrease in the incidence and severity of football injuries. Each year, 1.5 million high school students play football; the overall incidence of severe injury has dropped to 8 per 100,000, and the incidence of spinal cord injury is 4 per 100,000.[53, 54] The fatality rate has dropped to less than 1 per year from 25 to 30 per year in the 1970s. This is the result of changes in the rules of the game, improved equipment, and better medical management. Other contact sports, such as rugby and ice hockey, have high incidences of spinal cord injury, and the prevalence and severity of degenerative changes in the cervical spine are increasing.[55-60] These contact sports have not yet experienced the dramatic improvement seen in football, and more must be done to make these sports safer for participants. Soccer, a sport that one would expect to have a high incidence of cervical trauma due to the technique of "heading" the ball, has a very low incidence of injury, with most injuries occurring as a result of goal frames tipping over and striking people on the head.[54] Alpine skiing has seen a decrease in the rate of severe injuries from 5 to 6 per 1000 skiing days to 3 per 1000 skiing days. Only 0.1% of these are cervical spine injuries; of these, one third result in neurological injury or death.[61-64]

Pediatric spinal trauma has an annual incidence of 1.8 per 100,000 population, with 80% of injuries occurring in patients older than 10 years.[65] Pediatric cervical spine injuries have a bimodal pattern. Whereas 73% of all injuries in patients younger than 18 years occur at C4 or lower, between 70% and 87% of injuries in those younger than 8 years occur at C3 or higher. In comparison, there is an 85% incidence of lower cervical spine injuries in adults. The higher the level of injury, the more likely it is to be fatal, with a 71% to 100% mortality from atlanto-occipital dislocation,[65-68] a 17% incidence of death from C1 injuries, and only a 3.7%

mortality from injuries at C4.[65] Sixty percent of pediatric cervical spine injuries result in fracture without neurological compromise, whereas spinal cord injury without radiographic abnormality (SCIWORA)—a state in which a neurological injury is clinically apparent without a radiographic correlate—occurs in about 20% of pediatric spinal injuries.[69, 70] SCIWORA is usually a complete injury (75%) and has a poor prognosis for recovery. The incidence of violence-induced cervical spine injury has doubled over the last 20 years, accounting for almost 10% of all injuries.

The increased incidence of high cervical spine injury in younger pediatric patients is likely due to differences in the anatomy of the head and cervical spine in children.[69, 71, 72] Young children have a larger head compared with the rest of the body, unossified synchondrosis of the dens, and less complete ossification of the other bones of the spine. This results in a higher center of gravity for the head-neck complex and more strain on the upper cervical ligaments and vertebrae. This is dramatized by the high incidence of fatal occipitoatlantal dislocation in young pediatric patients involved in motor vehicle accidents (10 of 14 fatal in one study).[68] A recent trend is the incidence of occipitocervical dislocation in pediatric airbag injuries.[73, 74] This is thought to be due to the airbag being targeted toward the chest and head of an average adult. More reports are coming in of children and other short-statured people receiving catastrophic injuries as a result of airbag deployment directly at the head, even in cases of accidental inflation or low-speed collisions.[74] The correct use of safety seats, "smart" cars that can detect lighter passengers and shut off the airbags, and even airbags with adjustable direction and force may reduce the incidence of injury and death from this otherwise lifesaving device.

ACUTE CARE OF CERVICAL SPINE INJURIES

Prehospital Management

Because motor vehicle accidents, falls, and trauma related to sports commonly result in cervical spine injuries, all accident victims must be assumed to have an unstable spine until proved otherwise. Increased awareness of the need for spinal immobilization before extrication and transport, coupled with a high index of suspicion while handling the patient, can prevent further cord damage and has been associated with a marked decline in complete spinal cord lesions.[75] Gillingham[76] and Giesler and associates[77] both reported on vertebral injuries made worse by well-intentioned but faulty first aid at the accident scene.

Proper care of a person with a suspected cervical spine or spinal cord injury must begin at the accident site with adequate immobilization of the head and neck, along with attention to the first priorities of trauma resuscitation: airway, breathing, and circulation.[78] Because aspiration and shock are the primary causes of death in spinal cord injury victims before they arrive in the emergency room, respiratory and circulatory management at the scene of the accident is critical. If the airway is adequate on initial assessment, the patient's head should be immobilized and secured. Supplemental oxygen should be administered by facemask or nasal cannula. If the airway is compromised, an airway must be obtained without cervical flexion or extension, because these movements could induce or potentiate neurological injury.

Commonly, airway difficulty after trauma is the result of prolapse of the tongue or airway obstruction with blood, secretions, or foreign bodies. Often, the airway can be established using a chin-lift or jaw-thrust technique that brings the tongue forward. The mouth should always be checked for debris and cleared either manually or with suction. In a semiconscious or unconscious patient, an oropharyngeal or nasopharyngeal airway should be gently inserted, if indicated. The esophageal obturator airway can be placed in an unconscious patient who has suffered respiratory arrest, but it is contraindicated in patients with an intact gag reflex. More recently, the use of a layrngeal mask airway has been effective.[79-81] If a satisfactory airway and ventilation cannot be established or maintained with manual techniques or an oropharyngeal or nasopharyngeal airway, endotracheal intubation is required. Gentle manual traction can be applied in line with the axial skeleton to accomplish intubation. Axial traction should not be overly vigorous, because even moderate traction can produce serious vertebral distraction and the associated risks of neurological injury.[82] Although a blind nasal intubation technique is frequently advocated in this situation, it is contraindicated in the presence of basilar skull fracture, which can be deduced from the presence of raccoon's eyes, significant craniofacial trauma, or clear fluid in the nose or nasal secretions.

Respiratory insufficiency should be suspected in all patients with cervical cord injuries. Hypoventilation can result from paralysis of the intercostal muscles, which leaves the patient breathing by use of the diaphragm alone. High cervical cord injury, such as in a patient with no arm function, may cause paralysis of one or both phrenic nerves, resulting in both intercostal and diaphragmatic paralysis. Inadequate ventilation in a quadriplegic or quadriparetic patient is another indication for early intubation.

Assessment of circulation can be difficult in cases of acute trauma. Although hypotension is usually a consequence of hypovolemia or cardiac dysfunction, hypotension in a spinal cord–injured patient may be the result of a loss of sympathetic tone, with decreased peripheral vascular resistance secondary to the neurological injury.[83, 84] This results in venous pooling and decreased cardiac preload, which is exacerbated by lack of a reflex, sympathetically mediated tachycardia. Unlike patients with hypotension from acute blood loss, these patients may appear to be well perfused peripherally, with pink, warm extremities.

Regardless of the presumed cause of the hypotension, intravenous access should be gained rapidly. Initial therapy should follow routine protocols of intravascular volume expansion; Trendelenburg positioning, if required; and military antishock trouser placement, if necessary. In the past, neurological deterioration has been reported in spine-injured patients in association with inflation of antishock trousers. Newer designs have decreased the likelihood of inadvertent spine motion during inflation.[85]

Spinal shock occurs with loss of cardiosympathetic antagonism of vagal input, with resultant bradycardia despite concomitant hypotension and profound loss of intravascular tone and venous pooling. Volume expansion counteracts this shock to some extent by increasing cardiac output through the Starling mechanism, but intravenous agents such as atropine and other inotropes may be required. If spinal shock does not respond appropriately to these measures, continued inadequate intravascular volume should be suspected.

After the patient's airway, breathing, and circulation have been ensured, a rapid head-to-toe second survey should be performed. Motor and sensory deficits may provide clues to level of injury, and scalp injuries may suggest cervical spine injuries and their possible mechanisms. Cervical tenderness and obvious deformity are also important clues.

Extrication of a patient with a suspected spinal injury requires immobilization of the neck and maintenance of normal axial alignment of the body. Except in the presence of extreme circumstances, such as fire, no patient should be moved before rigorous spinal stabilization is achieved. Soft cervical collars allow complete neck movement in all directions and should not be used.[86, 87] Instead, if a patient is seated in a vehicle or is in some other position making access difficult, a rigid cervical collar can be placed for some support. While still in the vehicle, the patient should be immobilized on a half-backboard for removal from the vehicle. In all cases, the patient should be placed in the supine position on a long backboard as soon as possible. Immobilization should then be obtained by securing sandbags or plastic intravenous bags alongside the head and neck with tape passed from one edge of the backboard, across the forehead, to the other edge of the backboard.[88, 89] This method allows free movement of the jaw and lower face for easy airway control.

The half-backboard or long backboard may not be suitable for extrication of all patients after injury. Other suitable alternatives are the Kendrick extrication device, which is a close-fitting jacket with extensions behind and on both sides of the head and neck, or the scoop sledge stretcher.[90] Pediatric patients also present unique problems with regard to immobilization. Because of the proportions of a young child, immobilization on a standard backboard may result in neck flexion. The use of specially designed pediatric backboards can minimize this problem.[91]

If the patient is found in the water and has a suspected spinal injury, all efforts should be made to keep the patient floating on the surface, with support for the head and neck. The common error of carrying the patient to dry ground usually allows the head to dangle unsupported. Instead, extrication from the water can be accomplished relatively easily by securing the floating patient to a long board while he or she is still in the water.

A motorcyclist, bicyclist, or athlete may be found at an accident scene with a helmet still in place. In-line traction should be applied for removal, with a second rescuer supporting the head and neck. If the helmet cannot be removed easily, it can be left in place during transport as long as the patient's airway is not compromised.

For sports injuries, it is now appreciated that only the faceplate of a helmet needs to be removed to obtain airway access; the rest of the helmet can be removed later, preventing any manipulation before evaluation of the injury.[92, 93] The helmet should be removed only to perform cardiopulmonary resuscitation. Before transport, the patient must be secured and fastened to the transport device and be able to withstand complete inversion without loss of immobilization. During transport, the patient may be confined to a small space, making many medical interventions difficult. Therefore, these difficulties must be anticipated and prevented. The immobilization device must be prevented from breaking free within the vehicle in the event of an accident or unstable transport conditions. Given the frequency and increased morbidity of early pulmonary problems in multitrauma patients, facility for the treatment of regurgitation and the prevention of aspiration must be available at all times during transport. If there is a question about the adequacy of the airway, intubation should be performed before the patient is loaded for transport, because intubation in close quarters is often difficult and hazardous.

Acute Evaluation and Management in the Emergency Room

Initial emergency room management of a patient with a suspected spinal injury should involve the same thorough evaluation afforded any multitrauma patient. A period of stable vital signs after trauma does not imply the absence of serious injury, regardless of the time that has elapsed since the accident. One should not focus exclusively on the spinal cord injury until other injuries have been diagnosed or ruled out. Although the potential for spinal injury must be kept in mind, the strict rules of immobilization must not prevent lifesaving maneuvers from being performed expeditiously.

Respiratory complications are common after cervical spinal cord injuries, and the incidence increases markedly if other bodily injuries are present. Further, all cervical spinal cord lesions have the potential to develop ascending levels of dysfunction because of increasing spinal cord hemorrhage or edema. Therefore, respiratory decompensation can occur at any time during the early stages of resuscitation. Because relative hypoxia can further damage an injured cord, all patients, regardless of the level of their injury, should receive supplemental oxygen. Respiratory function should be reassessed frequently, and intubation performed as necessary.

As in the field, maintenance of blood pressure within normal limits is critical. If the blood pressure remains low despite resuscitation with intravenous fluids, a pressor such as dopamine (which is advantageous in terms of renal perfusion but has a significant incidence of tachyphylaxis when given with phenytoin [Dilantin] and should be avoided in cases of concomitant significant head injury) should be started and titrated to effect. A Foley catheter should be placed to monitor urinary output and to prevent bladder distention in case the patient has neurogenic urinary retention from a spinal cord injury.

A full skeletal x-ray series, including the chest and pelvis, should be performed as indicated (see the section on radiologic evaluation). This is especially important in a neurologically impaired patient, because 11% of fractures associated with head or spinal cord injury are missed in the initial assessment, and an unconscious, confused, or neurologically impaired patient may have abdominal pathology that is obscured by the neurological injury.[94] In addition, cervical spine fractures are often associated with fractures elsewhere in the spinal axis.

Disruption of sympathetic nerve function at T8 or above is frequently associated with hypothermia. Euthermia should be restored by external warming, warmed intravenous fluids, and heated inspired air if the patient is intubated.

If the patient must be transported rapidly to the operating room for lifesaving surgery, anteroposterior and lateral radiographs of the cervical spine must be obtained. If possible, the thoracolumbar area should also be imaged in the emergency room, before the patient is moved to the operating room. If there is any question about a cervical or thoracolumbar spine injury, the patient should remain immobilized in the operating room, if possible. This can cause decubitus ulcer formation, so if the remainder of the spinal axis can be cleared, it should be. Further studies such as oblique films or CT can be performed after the patient is medically stabilized.

If the patient is stable on arrival in the emergency room and emergent surgical intervention is not required, the patient can be assessed from a multisystem viewpoint, and the vertebral column and spinal cord can be investigated in an orderly fashion. In awake and alert patients, a full neurological examination can be carried out, and the presence or absence of spinal cord injury can be determined definitively. In combative or unconscious patients, a spinal injury must be assumed to be present until specifically ruled out. These patients present special difficulties, especially during transportation and positioning for special procedures, such as CT or angiography. All diagnostic studies should be carried out with the patient secured in the initial immobilization device, if possible.

Injury to the spinal cord occurs because of stretching, crushing, vascular compromise, or compression. Certain types of injury mechanisms are more likely to be associated with specific neurological findings on clinical examination (Fig. 315–1). Spinal cord hemisection leading to Brown-Sequard syndrome usually re-

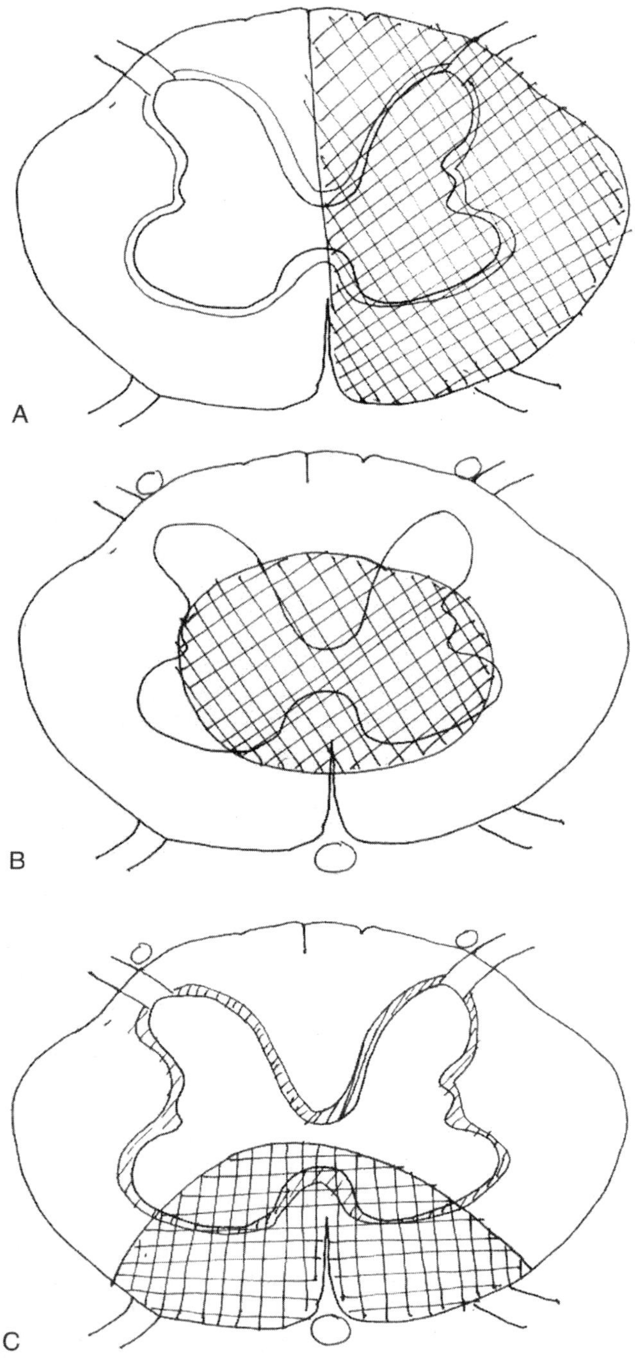

FIGURE 315–1. Spinal cord injury syndromes. *A*, Hemicord syndrome (Brown-Sequard syndrome) causes loss of pain and temperature sensation caudal to the lesion with preserved light touch (anterior spinothalamic tract). There is proprioceptive loss and motor paralysis below the lesion. *B*, Central cord syndrome is caused by compression of the spinal cord, resulting in venous infarction of the center of the cord (the vascular watershed region of the cord). Motor weakness is predominant in the upper extremities, with less effect in the lower extremities. There are varying degrees of sensory disturbance below the lesion, with sphincter dysfunction. *C*, Anterior cord syndrome is caused by compression or injury to the anterior spinal artery. It consists of motor and sensory loss below the lesion, with intact posterior column function (loss of pain and temperature sensation caudal to the lesion, but preservation of joint position sense and two-point discrimination).

sults from penetrating trauma but may also be seen after trauma with epidural cord compression.[94] On clinical examination, one finds contralateral dissociated sensory loss—that is, loss of pain and temperature sensation caudal to the lesion—with preserved light touch owing to redundant ipsilateral and contralateral axonal pathways (anterior spinothalamic tract). Ipsilaterally, one finds proprioceptive loss and motor paralysis below the lesion. Among the incomplete spinal cord syndromes, Brown-Sequard has the best prognosis, with approximately 90% of patients regaining the ability to ambulate independently and control sphincter function.[95]

After acute hyperextension injury, often in patients with preexisting congenital spinal stenosis, central cord syndrome may be evident.[96] Patients with this syndrome present with greater motor weakness in the upper extremities than in the lower extremities. Varying degrees of sensory disturbance occur below the level of the lesion, and sphincter dysfunction is commonly found. Only about half of these patients eventually recover enough neurological function in the lower extremities to ambulate independently.[95, 97–99] Recovery of upper extremity function is also poor, and fine motor control is usually absent. Bowel and bladder control is frequently recovered.

In patients who experience vertical compression or hyperflexion injuries, an anterior cord syndrome, also known as the anterior spinal artery syndrome, may occur.[100] Cord infarction in the vascular territory supplied by the anterior spinal artery is the proposed mechanism. In these patients, motor and sensory loss is evident below the lesion in the presence of intact posterior column function. This leads to a dissociated sensory loss, with loss of pain and temperature sensation caudal to the lesion but preservation of joint position sense and two-point discrimination. Anterior cord syndrome has the poorest prognosis of the incomplete spinal cord injuries. Only 10% to 20% of patients recover functional motor control and the ability to ambulate.[95]

Many treatments have been advocated over the past 3 decades to treat experimental acute spinal cord injury, including hypothermia, hyperbaric oxygen, electromagnetic fields, immobilization, and different classes of drugs given shortly after injury, such as intravenous lidocaine, melatonin, steroids (e.g., dexamethasone, methylprednisolone), and opiate antagonists such as naloxone.[23, 101–108] Although several earlier studies suggested that glucocorticoids or naloxone was ineffective in the treatment of acute spinal cord injury, other studies demonstrated beneficial effects.[102, 109–111] The second National Acute Spinal Cord Injury Study (NASCIS 2) revealed in a prospective, randomized, double-blind study that high-dose methylprednisolone was associated with improved neurological outcome in spinal cord–injured patients compared with placebo or naloxone.[112] This was followed by NASCIS 3, which compared 24- and 48-hour treatment with methylprednisolone with 24-hour treatment with tirilizad, a 21-aminosteroid antioxidant.[22] The results were then stratified by interval between injury and initiation of treatment. The study concluded that if treatment could be initiated within 3 hours after injury, a total of 24 hours of methylprednisolone should be given. If therapy was initiated within 3 to 8 hours of injury, 48 hours of methylprednisolone should be given. If the treatment could not be started within 8 hours of injury, steroids were of no benefit. Although there continue to be methodologic questions about the study (e.g., there was no placebo control group), it remains the most complete and definitive article on the subject. Despite the continued debate about the science behind the subject, this is considered the standard of care in most parts of North America (Fig. 315–2).

If, during assessment in the emergency room, an acute spinal cord injury is documented, treatment with methylprednisolone should be initiated without delay. To be effective, methylprednisolone must be started within 8 hours of injury and should be given as an initial intravenous bolus of 30 mg/kg administered over 15 minutes. This is followed 45 minutes later by a 5.4 mg/kg per hour continuous infusion of methylprednisolone. If the treatment is initiated less than 3 hours after injury, it continues over the next 23 hours. If the treatment starts more than 3 but less than 8 hours after injury, the infusion continues for 47 hours (for a total of 48 hours).

Other pharmacologic agents that have shown promise in the setting of acute spinal cord injury include calcium channel blockers such as nimodipine, modulators of excitotoxicity such as phencyclidine or dextrorphan, and blockers of lipid peroxidation and membrane destruction such as 21-aminosteroids and GN1 gangliocyte.[113–119] Unfortunately, at this time, only methylprednisolone has been shown to benefit patients, and even the long-term outcomes for patients treated with methylprednisolone are questionable.[120, 121]

After diagnostic cervical spine films are obtained, unstable or displaced spinal column injuries should be treated initially with cervical traction. The use of skull tongs to reduce fracture-dislocation and maintain alignment of cervical spine fractures is now routine in most centers. In patients with complete or incomplete injuries of the cord, one of the aims of management is immediate prevention of further neurological damage to the cord and nerve roots. This is accomplished by restoration of vertebral alignment and early immobilization of the vertebral column. The tongs used by physicians in the early 20th century to provide cervical traction in patients with fractures were first described by Crutchfield in 1938.[8]

Application of the most commonly used type, Gardner-Wells tongs, is straightforward and requires local anesthesia and aseptic preparation of the skin at the site of application by shaving and scrubbing with a cleansing agent. These tongs consist of a rigid semicircle that follows the coronal contour of the calvaria. A threaded hole on each end accommodates a screw for advancement of the skull fixation points through the skin into the calvaria. One of the cone-shaped points has a self-contained, spring-loaded indicator of the amount of compressive force exerted by the pin. Both pins tilt upward to avoid the danger of the tongs' being pulled out with increasing traction weight. The insertion site is usually 2 cm cephalad to the pinna, in line with the tragus, to allow for straightaway axial traction (Fig. 315–3). However, initial placement of the Gardner-Wells tongs can be altered to treat specific fracture-dislocations. Anterior placement of the tongs to produce hyperextension of the head along with distraction may be needed in cases of hyperflexion injuries, whereas management of unilateral or bilateral locked facets may require a more posterior placement of the tongs to produce slight flexion as an aid in reduction. After the entry point of the pins has been determined, the skin should be infiltrated with local anesthesia down to the galea. The pins are then tightened by hand until the indicator on the spring-loaded pin protrudes 1 mm. This indicates approximately 30 pounds of compressive force against the skull. At 24 hours after tong application, the spring-loaded pin should be retightened if the indicator is no longer protruding 1 mm. Thereafter, the pins should not be retightened.

The amount of weight to be applied with tong traction varies with the level of injury and the amount of suspected ligamentous disruption. Minimal weight should be used initially to avoid overdistraction and the possibility of neurological deterioration. As a gen-

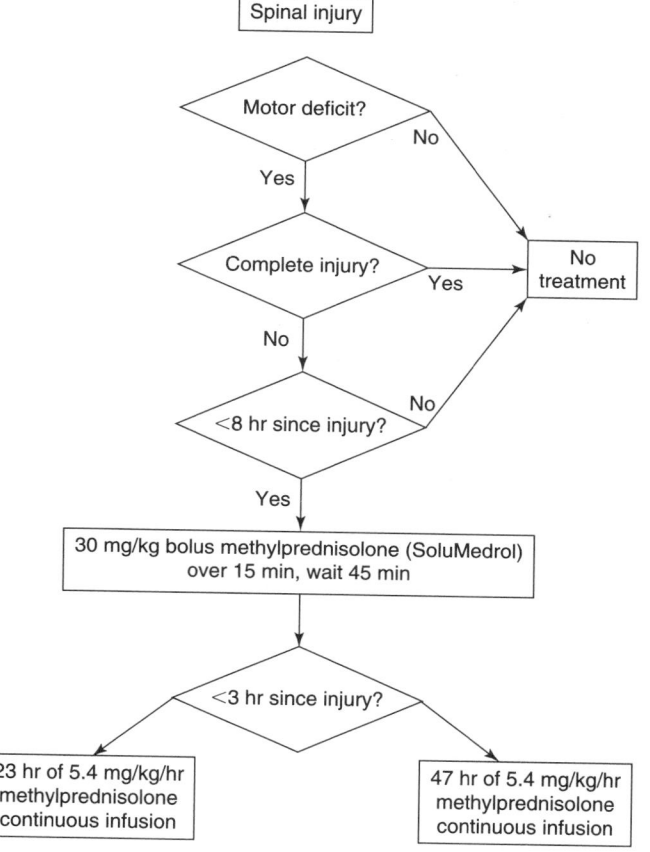

FIGURE 315–2. Protocol for management of spinal cord injury as dictated by the results of the National Acute Spinal Cord Injury Study III.[22]

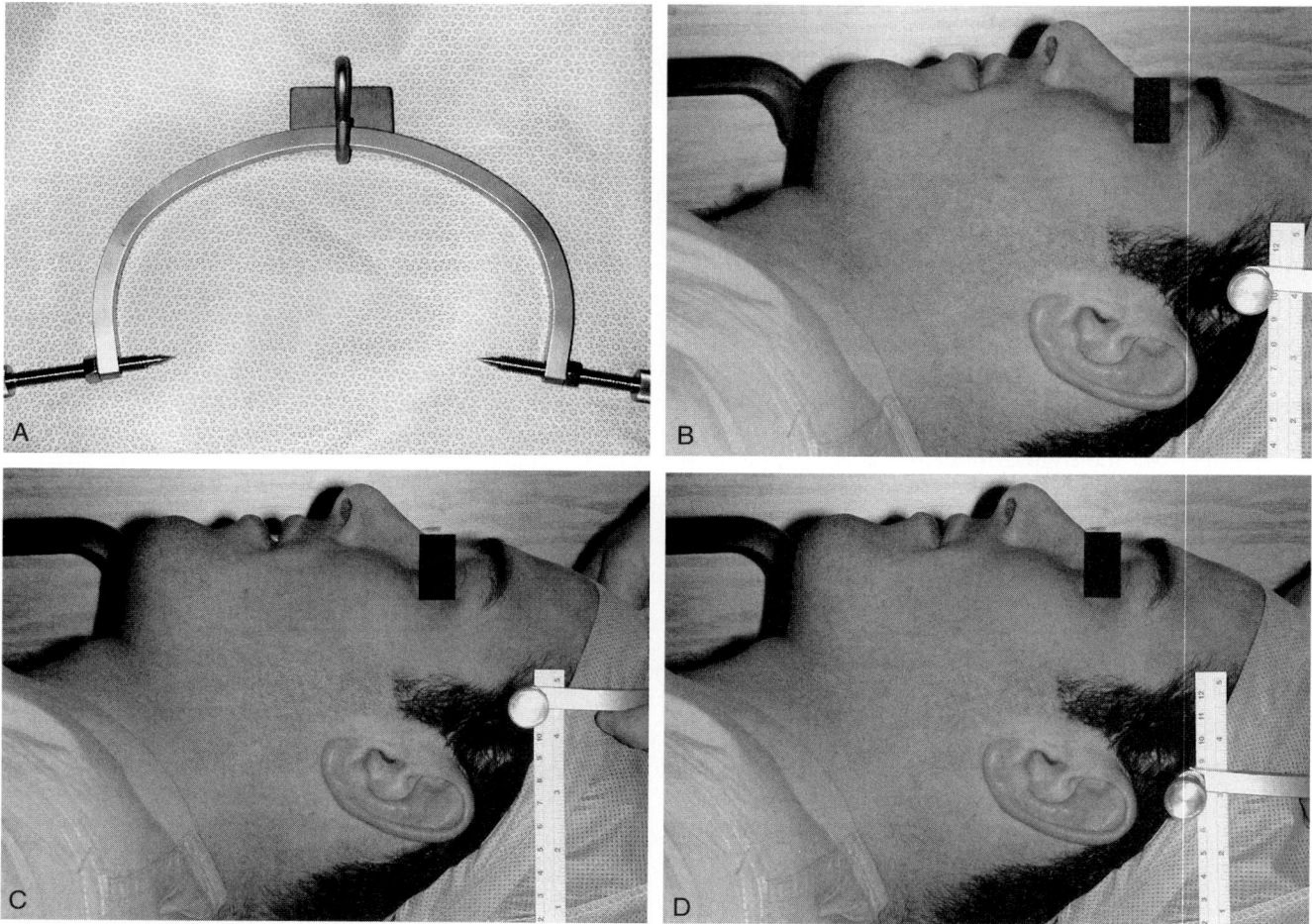

FIGURE 315–3. Proper tong placement techniques. *A,* Gardner-Wells tongs. *B,* Placement for neutral traction is 2 cm anterior and 2 cm above the anterior pinna. *C,* Placement for induction of flexion to counteract a jumped facet, or to counter an overextension injury, is 2 cm above the anterior pinna. *D,* Placement for induction of extension to counteract an odontoid fracture that reduces in extension, or to counteract cranial settling, is 2 cm above and 4 cm anterior to the anterior pinna.

eral rule, a maximum of 5 pounds per vertebral level between the fracture level and the occiput (e.g., 25 pounds at C5) is used initially for attempted reduction. Weights can be added in 5-pound increments, but serial lateral radiographs should be obtained with each incremental increase in weight to avoid overdistraction. Muscle spasms can make reduction significantly more difficult but can be treated with muscle relaxants and sedation. Muscle relaxants and sedatives should be administered slowly and cautiously. Clouding of the patient's neurological examination can occur with sedatives, and a marked reduction in paraspinous muscle tension may be observed with muscle relaxants, resulting in overdistraction without a significant change in the applied weight of traction.

Complications of cervical traction include overdistraction with or without subsequent neurological worsening, tong dislocation, pin site infection, and skull penetration. The main disadvantage of tongs and traction for definitive therapy has been the necessity of confining the patient to bed until bony fusion occurs, a process usually requiring 8 to 12 weeks. For this

reason, there has been a trend over the last decade toward initial realignment by tong traction followed by early operative stabilization through either an anterior or a posterior approach. Alternatively, long-term immobilization is achieved with the halo orthosis, which allows earlier mobilization of patients.

Radiologic Evaluation

After the primary survey, neurological examination, and external assessment of the spine, the next step in identifying specific spinal injuries is a radiologic evaluation. The diagnostic studies performed should be chosen to provide maximal information in a relatively short time. Imaging modalities include plain radiography, fluoroscopy, CT with multiplanar reconstructions and with or without myelography, and MRI.

PLAIN RADIOGRAPHY

Plain films are the foundation of spinal imaging for trauma patients suspected of having a cervical spine injury. Given the potentially devastating consequences of a misdiagnosis, a low threshold for ordering cervical films and a high index of suspicion for injury must exist. A cervical spine series is indicated in all trauma patients who present with localized pain, deformity, crepitus or edema, altered mental status, neurological dysfunction, or head injury. In addition, patients with multiple trauma or those whose mechanisms of injury suggest the potential for cervical spine injury should undergo cervical spine radiography.

A complete cervical spine series consists of a lateral cervical projection, an anteroposterior view, an open-mouth view of the odontoid, and oblique films.[122, 123] Pillar, swimmer, and flexion-extension views are additional films that can be considered, if needed, to more fully demonstrate the extent of injury.[123, 124] The optimal plain film evaluation of the cervical spine depends on the patient's clinical condition and neurological status and the type and magnitude of injury.

Ideally, trauma patients should receive initial radiologic examination while still immobilized on the original stretcher or backboard. The overall condition of the patient dictates the type of radiologic evaluation to be performed. Generally, patients can be divided into two groups: those with less severe or less acute injuries, and those with obviously severe injuries. A less severely injured patient is typically conscious, alert, and able to cooperate and has nonspecific signs and symptoms relative to the cervical spine, with or without other, relatively minor coexisting injuries. These patients should undergo the basic three-view radiologic examination of the cervical spine. A severely injured patient may be unconscious or have obvious signs of craniocervical trauma with or without neurological abnormalities, frequently has severe or life-threatening systemic injuries, and may have hemodynamic or respiratory instability. The clinical condition of these patients usually requires that the routine cervical spine examination be modified and limited to only lateral and anteroposterior projections. In all cases, a minimum of two views of the cervical spine, preferably in perpendicular planes, should be obtained.

The cross-table lateral cervical view should be the first film obtained in the cervical spine series, and in cases of multiple trauma, this film should precede all others. This projection is accurate in revealing posttraumatic abnormalities approximately 70% to 83% of the time.[122, 123, 125–130] With the addition of the anteroposterior and open-mouth views, however, the sensitivity is markedly improved.[122, 125, 126, 131, 132]

The initial cross-table lateral view should be done without applying traction in the event of atlanto-occipital or atlantoaxial dissociation, because minimal traction in this setting may lead to neurological damage.[133] However, the lateral radiograph should never be considered adequate unless all seven cervical vertebrae are visualized. In order to visualize the C7-T1 interspace on the lateral projection, depression of the patient's shoulders by pulling down on both arms may be required. This maneuver should not be applied if atlanto-occipital, atlantoaxial, or other significantly destabilizing cervical spine abnormalities are apparent on the

initial view. In some patients, the swimmer's view is required to provide visualization of the cervicothoracic junction.

The cross-table lateral view should be evaluated for alignment, bony abnormalities, disk space abnormalities, and soft tissue injuries. Although careful evaluation of the bony anatomy is of primary importance, close attention should also be paid to soft tissue details, because abnormal soft tissue swelling in the craniocervical region may be the most prominent sign of a subtle Jefferson's, dens, or hangman's fracture on plain radiography. Further, prevertebral soft tissue swelling may be the only radiologic sign in 30% to 40% of patients presenting with an acute central cord syndrome after a hyperextension injury of the cervical spine.[134, 135]

The anteroposterior view, although useful for evaluating the lower five cervical vertebrae and the upper thoracic vertebrae, is limited superiorly by superimposition of the mandible and occiput. For this reason, the upper cervical spine is not well visualized. The superior and inferior end plate, uncinate processes, joints of Luschka, and lateral cortical margins can easily be evaluated. However, superimposition of lateral masses makes evaluation of the bases of the facet joints difficult. The spinous processes are well visualized as a vertical row in the midline, and widening of any two spinous processes or rotation of spinous processes with respect to others may indicate a hyperflexion injury or facet dislocation. The trachea is also well visualized on the anteroposterior view by an air shadow in the midline. Lateral displacement of this air shadow may indicate hematoma or edema secondary to trauma.

The open-mouth view provides an anteroposterior projection of the upper cervical spine. Because of the opening of the mouth, the mandible is no longer superimposed on C1 and C2, which can now be well visualized. From this view, one can evaluate the coronal alignment of the atlas and axis, in which the dens should be centered between the lateral masses of the atlas. In addition, fractures of the atlas and axis, notably Jefferson's fractures or fractures of the dens, can be evaluated. However, the open-mouth view has limitations, especially in trauma patients with facial injuries who are unable to open their mouths and in patients requiring intubation, because the endotracheal tube often obscures the view of the atlas and axis. The occipital bone and the teeth may also obscure the region of the odontoid process on this projection.

Oblique cervical spine films are helpful for visualizing the uncinate processes of the vertebral bodies, laminae, pedicles, intervertebral foramina, articular masses, and interfacetal joints. Because the vertebral bodies obscure the articular masses and interfacetal joints on the opposite side, oblique films must be obtained from each side.

The pillar view is specifically designed to provide direct visualization of individual lateral masses. In addition, the integrity of the dens can be evaluated in patients who will not or cannot cooperate with the open-mouth view. Miller and coworkers advocate inclusion of the pillar view in all evaluations of the cervical spine after trauma.[136] However, the pillar view requires significant rotation of the patient's head. Therefore, it should be used only for those patients suspected of having articular mass fractures based on previous cervical spine views.

The swimmer's or Twining projection is designed to visualize the cervicothoracic junction in patients whose shoulder density obscures the lower cervical segments on the cross-table lateral view. Optimal positioning for this projection requires the patient to be rotated slightly off true lateral, with one upper extremity abducted 180 degrees and extended cranially and the other upper extremity extended posterocaudally. Although the swimmer's view may provide good visualization of the lower cervical vertebrae, it is often difficult to obtain in a severely injured patient.

Flexion-extension radiography may be useful to evaluate ligamentous integrity in patients with a suspected injury but without evidence of bony abnormality on a complete cervical spine series. Flexion-extension radiography is usually obtained with plain lateral radiography, but it can also be done by means of fluoroscopy. In either case, this study is absolutely contraindicated in patients with a neurological deficit or clear evidence of fracture or instability and should not be performed on disoriented, uncooperative, or intoxicated patients. The patient should simply be instructed to flex and extend his or her neck as far as possible and to stop if it becomes painful. The physician should never attempt to increase the patient's range of motion. Although flexion-extension radiography can be used in the setting of acute trauma, it is often reserved for patients with known fractures or ligamentous injuries with subluxation to assess spinal stability after treatment. In addition, because inadequate studies are often obtained in the acute setting due to muscle spasm and pain that limits spinal range of motion (up to 33% in some series), several authors have stated that there is no real benefit of flexion-extension radiography in the acute setting.[137–140]

Despite precautions, false-negative interpretations of cervical spine films have led to secondary injuries, and false-positive interpretations have led to unnecessary hospitalization and inappropriate application of traction devices.[141, 142] Familiarity with certain difficult portions of the cervical spine series, as well as certain conditions that lend themselves to misinterpretation, helps prevent errors. Some of the more common conditions include preexisting congenital anomalies (e.g., atlanto-occipital fusion), ligamentous laxity in children, and degenerative disease in adults, which is probably the most common cause of misdiagnosis of acute traumatic subluxation or fracture. Atlanto-occipital fusion and the often associated congenital fusion of C2 and C3 commonly cause atlantoaxial laxity because of greater stresses to this area, resulting from the block formation above or below. Atlantoaxial joint space widening may be seen in these circumstances but does not necessarily point to the presence of instability. Congenital abnormalities of the dens are not common, but if they occur, they may be difficult to differentiate from acute fracture. Anomalies of the dens such as os odontoideum,

whether congenital or acquired, are often confused with acute fractures and may or may not show abnormal translational motion on flexion-extension films.[138, 143] The incidence of radiographic patency of the synchondrosis of the dens with C2 is inversely dependent on age but may still be visible in patients in their 20s. Ligamentous laxity and shallow facet joints at C2-3 and C3-4 allow pseudosubluxation at these levels. Pseudosubluxation is often mistaken for acute injury. Further, ligamentous laxity and incomplete ossification in children allow as much as two thirds of the anterior arch of C1 to appear to be above the tip of the dens in the lateral projection.[144] This physiologic characteristic of infants and young children is often misinterpreted as atlantoaxial subluxation. Finally, degenerative disease of the cervical spine in adults, characterized by calcification of the anterior longitudinal ligament, flattening of the vertebral body, disk space narrowing with possible ligamentous laxity and subluxation, and facet arthrosis, can be confused with acute traumatic changes of the cervical spine. However, the presence of other degenerative changes, absence of fractures, and absence of soft tissue swelling should provide clues as to the chronic nature of the changes.

COMPUTED TOMOGRAPHY

At the present time, CT is the tomographic method of choice for the evaluation of acute spinal trauma.[145] Thin-section CT should be used to further evaluate areas of obvious or suspected cervical spine injury identified on plain radiography.[76, 145–148] CT is also indicated if the plain film study is inconsistent with the patient's clinical condition, in injuries resulting in neurological deficit, in fractures of the posterior arch of the cervical canal, and in every fracture with suspected retropulsion of bone fragments into the canal.[26, 149] Computed tomographic evaluation should usually precede dynamic flexion-extension films or angiography if these studies are indicated.

An exception to the rule of proceeding directly to CT after demonstration of an injury on initial cervical spine films may be the case of a patient with a fracture-dislocation or other significant subluxation with an acute neurological deficit. In these patients, every attempt should be made to reduce the malalignment early and thereby effect a decompression of the neural elements.[3, 26] Traction should be applied by means of Gardner-Wells tongs or a similar device, and reduction should be monitored by means of fluoroscopy or frequent plain film examination. After alignment has been restored or an inability to effect reduction has been established, CT or, in some cases, MRI is performed.

With CT, bone is imaged in exquisite detail, with clear demonstration of even small cortical disruptions, and bony encroachment in the canal can easily be seen. This is particularly useful for C1 and C2 fractures, because the precise fracture subtype is often difficult to discern on plain films.[150–152] Combination fractures involving both the atlas and the axis are difficult to identify without computed tomographic images, and axial views are particularly useful to evaluate vertebral body and posterior element injuries.[150, 152] Newer reformatting techniques that provide images in sagittal, coronal, or oblique planes can be performed without additional radiation exposure and are helpful to evaluate fractures that are not well visualized on plain radiography.[134] The recent availability of three-dimensional reformatted computed tomographic imaging has provided better visualization of complex cervical spine fractures.[130] However, this technique is still limited by the time required for such images to be obtained. Although CT is the tomographic technique of choice for evaluating acute spinal trauma, plain film tomography has some advantages. Plain tomography provides multisegmental spatial display in either the coronal or the sagittal plane and generally has sharper resolution than that of reformatted CT. Because plain tomography is oriented parallel to the longitudinal axis of the spinal column, it demonstrates axially oriented fractures (i.e., type II or III dens fractures) more clearly and more reliably than CT does. Fractures parallel to the axial scan plane may be entirely missed by CT. Rotational alignment is easily evaluated by CT, but other subluxations can be appreciated only if sagittal or coronal reconstructions are obtained. Movement of the patient can result in a sagittal reconstruction that appears to be malaligned. Despite these shortcomings, the advantages of CT far outweigh its disadvantages, and plain film radiography, combined with CT when indicated, is the current standard for radiologic evaluation of acute cervical spine injuries.

One recent development is use of the computed tomographic scan to "clear" either the C1-2 complex or the C7-T1 juncture. Many multitrauma patients are unable to cooperate or to tolerate studies such as openmouth or swimmer's views. Because many of these patients get computed tomographic scans of the head, chest, and abdomen anyway to rule out other injuries, it has become the protocol at many trauma institutions to scan the areas most likely to result in inadequate plain radiographic studies. In intubated and paralyzed patients, the sagittal and coronal reconstructions are usually free of motion artifact and give an excellent view of the alignment of the bodies in multiple planes. This is a good but by no means perfect option for intubated multitrauma patients who may be going to the operating room for other problems, giving the neurosurgeon the opportunity to get a good look at the areas in question. Limitations of this application of CT are the inability to achieve the resolution afforded by plain films and the possibility of missing fractures that run parallel to the axial plane. Patients in whom this is performed should be considered only conditionally cleared and at the earliest convenience should get formal plain radiographs.

MYELOGRAPHY

Intrathecal administration of water-soluble contrast medium, followed by plain radiography or CT, provides visualization of the spinal cord silhouette, subarachnoid space, and nerve roots. It demonstrates intramedullary and extramedullary mass lesions, obstruction of cerebrospinal fluid flow, root avulsions, dural tears, and, with delayed CT images, post-traumatic syringomyelia.[153, 154] However, very little direct information can be obtained about the intrinsic pathology of the cord in the setting of acute injury.

In the context of trauma, CT after intrathecal administration of contrast has largely supplanted the plain film myelography examination, because less patient movement is required. If CT–myelography is performed in patients with cervical injuries, the contrast may be introduced through the lateral C1-2 approach, further minimizing motion of the patient.

The studies can usually be performed rapidly and with low morbidity; patient access is better in the CT scanner than in the MRI scanner, and scanning times are shorter. However, myelography is an invasive procedure with specific complications, including the risk of direct spinal cord injury with the lateral C1-2 approach, intraspinal hemorrhage, and adverse reactions to the contrast agent. In addition, the value of the information obtained for the guidance of acute management decisions has been questioned. Thus, the role of plain film myelography or postmyelographic CT in the evaluation of acute traumatic cervical spine injuries remains controversial, and it is often reserved for institutions where acute MRI capabilities are limited.

MAGNETIC RESONANCE IMAGING

MRI is being used increasingly in the acute evaluation of injuries of the cervical spine and spinal cord. Technical improvements in spinal imaging, reductions in scanning time, and increased availability of life-support equipment and traction devices compatible with high-field magnets have increased the utility and safety of these examinations in trauma patients. Because the spinal cord and surrounding structures can be visualized directly and noninvasively by MRI, it has begun to replace postmyelography CT in the evaluation of cord compression and other intraspinal traumatic lesions. Spinal epidural hematomas, intramedullary hematomas, spinal cord contusions, encephalomalacia, and spinal cord edema are usually but not always well visualized with MRI; the longitudinal alignment of the vertebral bodies, the alignment of the facet joints, and the condition of the intervertebral disks are more difficult to see.[27, 155–161] Edema and hemorrhages within surrounding paraspinal soft tissues can also be seen on MRI. The vertebral arteries can be seen as columns of signal void; this provides valuable information if fractures or dislocations involve the transverse foramina. MRI can also directly delineate disruption of some ligamentous structures in the cervical spine that cannot be visualized by other radiologic techniques, such as the transverse ligament at C1-2.[156, 161, 162] Changes in spinal cord signal characteristics on MRI, such as those that may be caused by hematomas, contusions, and edema, have been correlated with the severity of neurological injury and eventual outcome.[161] Finally, MRI is more sensitive in detecting soft tissue swelling and blood around ligamentous structures—a subtle marker for trauma.[163]

Along with these many advantages, there are some problems associated with the use of MRI in cases of acute cervical spine trauma. These shortcomings include poor visualization of bony pathology, with frequent inability to demonstrate small cortical fractures or fragments; difficulty in obtaining good film quality in the setting of restless, acutely injured patients; and problems caring for unstable patients in the confines of the equipment. In addition, lack of access to facilities and a shortage of on-site technical personnel limit its use in the trauma setting at many institutions. Despite these problems, MRI is becoming the modality of choice for imaging cervical spine injuries characterized by spinal canal involvement or those that produce a clinical neurological deficit.

CLASSIFICATION OF CERVICAL SPINE INJURY

Universally accepted classifications for acute cervical spine fractures or dislocations do not exist. Some classifications focus on neurological injury without analysis of bony or soft tissue injury.[164, 165] Others subdivide injuries according to specific bony or soft tissue abnormalities without considering the pattern or mechanism of injury.[3, 166] Still others focus on the presumed mechanism but ignore the neurological component of injury. From both a conceptual and a clinical standpoint, it seems most appropriate and useful that the mechanism of injury be the basis for dividing cervical spine injuries into classes.[123, 141, 167]

Biomechanical studies and autopsy or cadaver experiments have established the fundamental relations among injury mechanism, force vectors, and the resulting osseous and ligamentous injuries of the spine.[168–175] In such controlled laboratory experiments, pure force vectors such as flexion, extension, vertical compression (axial load), lateral flexion, rotation, or a combination of forces (e.g., simultaneous flexion and rotation) have been shown to produce specific injuries. Clinically, however, the causative (vector) force of acute cervical spine injury can be inferred only on the basis of historical, physical, and radiologic evidence, because the mechanisms of injury are certainly not controlled. Further, in all probability, the injury is a result of multiple simultaneous forces with one predominant force vector rather than a single pure force. The probable mechanisms of cervical spine injury suggested by controlled laboratory models may nonetheless be applied reasonably to the injuries seen clinically because of the close pathologic and radiologic similarity of experimental and clinical lesions. Therefore, one can assume that clinically acute cervical spine injuries are the result of either predominant or pure vector forces similar to those demonstrated in experimental models.[176]

TWO- AND THREE-COLUMN CONCEPTS

The two-column concept of the spine is an aid to defining stability in the thoracolumbar spine.[87, 177–179]

The anterior column is made up of the anterior longitudinal ligament, vertebral body, intervertebral disk, and posterior longitudinal ligament; the posterior column consists of all the skeletal and ligamentous structures posterior to the posterior longitudinal ligament. This concept has been invaluable in understanding the pathophysiology of injuries occurring as a result of flexion, extension, and other forces on the cervical spine. More recently, Denis's redefinition of this column concept to include a third, middle spinal column has added substantially to our understanding of the biomechanics of injury and to the definitions of instability after cervical spine trauma.[180] The middle column consists of the posterior one third of the vertebral body, the annulus fibrosus, and the posterior longitudinal ligament; the posterior column is formed by the posterior neural arch, spinous process, and articular processes and their corresponding ligamentous capsules. Although the three-column concept was designed specifically for thoracolumbar fractures, such two- or three-column models are helpful in further redefining the biomechanics of cervical spine injury as well.

Hyperflexion is caused by forceful forward rotation of the head, which is usually limited by the chin striking the chest wall. Such movement applies distraction forces to the posterior elements and compression forces to the vertebral body and disk (anterior column). Depending on the degree of force, there can be ligamentous damage and bony involvement, including subluxations, bilateral facet dislocations, and compression or avulsion fractures.

Simultaneous flexion and rotation involves flexion with the head being slightly rotated at the outset. Such forces tend to produce partial disruption of the annulus, posterior ligaments, and capsule of the facet joint, resulting in unilateral dislocation of the facet on the side opposite the direction of rotation.[181] Unilateral facet dislocation may be associated with an impaction fracture of the articular masses of the dislocated facet joint, but such a fracture is usually not a major component of the injury.

Hyperextension injuries involve a force vector applied to the face or forehead, with the head being rotated backward. Simultaneous distraction of the anterior column and compression of the posterior elements occur, exactly the reciprocal of the hyperflexion injury. Hyperextension mechanisms can produce injuries such as avulsion fractures of the anterior arch of the atlas, teardrop fractures, posterior arch atlas fractures, laminar fractures, hyperextension fracture-dislocations, and hangman's fractures (traumatic spondylolisthesis).

In extension-rotation injuries, the principal force is either pure hyperextension, with the head already having rotated, or simultaneous rotation and extension caused by an eccentric force vector. This mechanism often results in a pillar fracture.

Vertical compression (axial loading) occurs with forces applied to the top of the head with the cervical spine in a neutral position. Such a force is transmitted through the skull and occipital condyle to the cervical spine, resulting in burst-type fractures. In the atlas, this results in a classic Jefferson's burst fracture; in the lower cervical spine, this produces bursting of the vertebral body (i.e., failure in compression of the anterior and middle columns). Lateral flexion injuries of the cervical spine occur with forces applied to the side of the head that cause translation or canting of a vertebra in the coronal plane.[182, 183] Lateral flexion is rarely seen as a principal vector but commonly occurs in association with another force vector such as rotation or vertical compression. If it does occur as an isolated mechanism of injury, it results in the uncinate process fracture. Atlanto-occipital and atlantoaxial disassociation, odontoid fractures, and torticollis result from combinations of forces; their causes and pathophysiology are enigmatic, and their mechanisms are poorly understood.

CERVICAL SPINE STABILITY

The abstract concept of spinal stability can often be difficult to understand and apply to actual clinical situations. To define stability of the spine, several factors must be considered, including the mechanism of injury, the magnitude and direction of forces applied to the spine, the radiologic appearance of the lesion, the anatomic structures involved, and the neurological status of the patient. Clinically, stability of the cervical spine implies three things: (1) that there will not be excessive displacement or deformity under physiologic loading; (2) that deformity or abnormal displacement will not develop during the healing process; and (3) that compression or injury of the neural elements is not present and will not occur over time with the application of physiologic loads.

The principal goals in the management of potential spinal instability are the prevention of secondary neurological injury and the provision of an optimal environment for the recovery of any existing neurological injury—one that prevents further neural injury or pain. The achievement of these goals requires an understanding of the bony and ligamentous pathology, the nature of neural tissue injury, and the healing processes that can be expected. In one review, 10% of patients developed new signs or symptoms of cervical spinal cord compression during the emergency room evaluation or during the acute phase of hospitalization.[16] These findings underscore the importance of recognizing spinal instability and taking appropriate measures to immobilize the spine and protect the spinal cord and nerve roots. If stability cannot be ensured, it is safer to assume that the spine is unstable until it can be shown otherwise.

The unique architecture and wide range of motion of the occipitoatlantoaxial region differentiate this area from the rest of the cervical spine. Upper cervical spine instability caused by injuries to the occipitocervical junction, atlas, or axis is determined by the integrity of the interrelated bony and ligamentous structures of the craniovertebral junction. Stability at the craniovertebral junction is provided by an inner and outer set of ligaments. The inner ligaments include the paired alar ligaments, apical ligament, vertically oriented cruci-

form ligament, and tectorial membrane. The outer ligaments are the articular capsules, anterior and posterior atlanto-occipital membranes, and nuchal ligament.[184] Werne, in a detailed analysis of the ligamentous stability of this region, concluded that hyperflexion is prevented by skeletal contact between the anterior margin of the foramen magnum and the odontoid, and that hyperextension and vertical translation are controlled by the tectorial membrane.[185] Lateral bending was thought to be controlled by the alar ligaments. He concluded that the tectorial membrane and the alar ligaments were the most important structures for maintaining stability, because sectioning of these ligaments led to atlanto-occipital dislocation.

Various anatomic structures have been implicated in maintaining stability in the lower cervical spine. Both Bailey and Bedbrook believed that the disk and associated anterior and posterior longitudinal ligaments were the most important structures for stability in the lower cervical spine.[186–189] Experimental work done by both Roaf and Munro supports these observations.[173, 190]

More recent work by White and Panjabi provided additional information on the ligaments' role in maintaining cervical spine stability.[87] From their observations using cadavers, they concluded that the loss of function of either all the anterior or all the posterior bony or ligamentous elements of the spine could render the lower cervical spine unstable. Further, they determined that horizontal and angular displacement between vertebrae did not exceed 2.67 mm and 10.7 degrees, respectively, before complete failure of the motion segment. Based on these data, in conjunction with other concepts of stability, they devised a graded checklist system for determining instability in the lower cervical spine.[174] Points are assigned if anterior or posterior column destruction is present, if the sagittal angulation is greater than 11 degrees, if sagittal plane translation is more than 3.5 mm, if a positive stretch test or cord damage is present, if a patient demonstrates root damage or disk narrowing, or if it is anticipated that the patient will place great stress on the cervical spine. A patient scoring more than 5 points is considered to have an unstable lower cervical spine. However, it is possible for patients with lower scores to have spinal instability and for patients with higher scores to be clinically asymptomatic. For this reason, there is no substitute for repeat examinations to identify potential spinal instability. These authors also recognized that flexion-extension radiography is hazardous for patients with significant ligamentous instability and suggested the so-called stretch test as a safer alternative.[174] For this evaluation, traction is applied to the cervical spine by a head halter or skeletal fixation; the traction is increased until one third of the body weight or 33 kg is reached or evidence of instability is found. Lateral cervical spine films should be obtained after each weight increase and examined for evidence of instability, which is defined as an increase in disk space height greater than 1.7 mm or a greater than 7.5-degrees change in angulation between the pretraction and post-traction vertebral position.

RESTORATION OF SPINAL STABILITY

Medical Management with Spinal Orthoses

After the acute stage of cervical spine injury, both immediate and long-term immobilization may be obtained with a number of spinal orthotic devices. These devices can be used to reduce or eliminate motion at an unstable vertebral segment and may be required to allow healing of bony and ligamentous injuries, reduce pain, correct deformity, and protect the adjacent spinal cord. The support and immobilization provided by orthotic devices vary widely, and the clinician must decide which type of device is most likely to achieve the specific treatment goals. More rigid forms of spinal orthosis control the position of the spine by the application of external forces. When used for the treatment of spinal instability, the orthosis must perform functions that would normally be accomplished by the spinal column and its associated supporting structures. Less rigid orthoses may be used for less severe injuries,

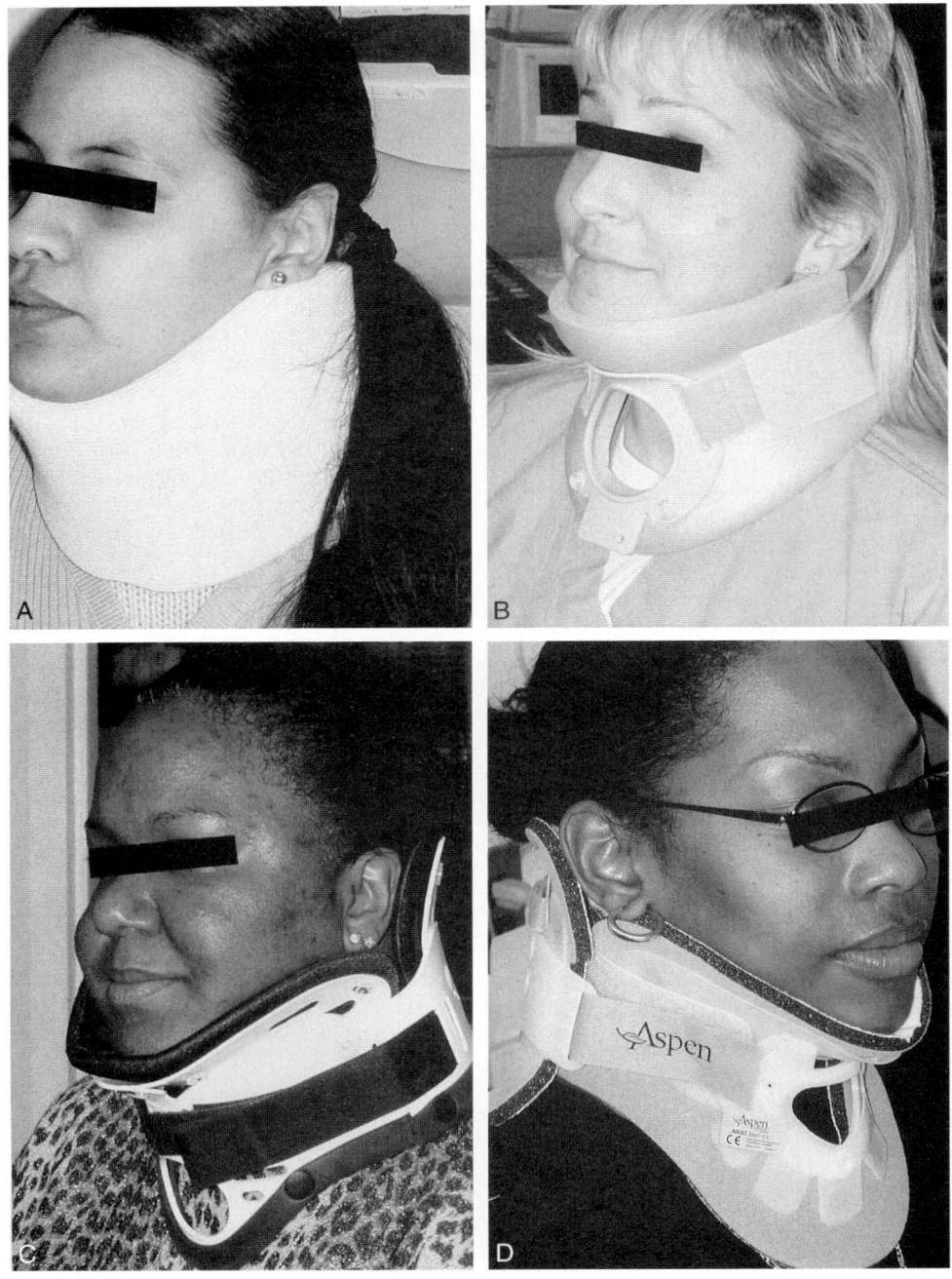

FIGURE 315–4. Spinal orthoses. *A,* Soft collar. *B,* Philadelphia collar. *C,* Miami-J. *D,* Aspen.

Illustration continued on following page.

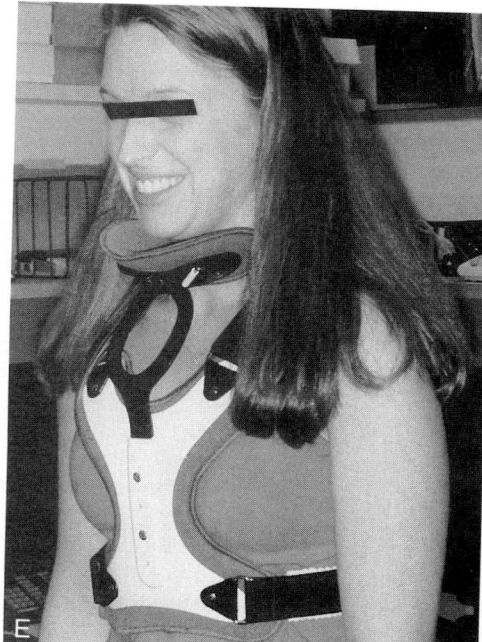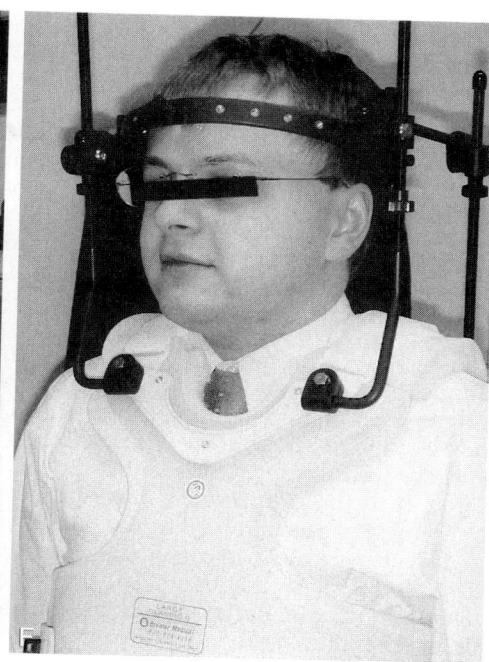

FIGURE 315–4 *Continued. E, Minerva. F, Halo.*

such as sprains, or for patients with musculoskeletal pain of a spinal origin. In these cases, the orthotic device is not responsible for the structural integrity of the vertebral column but rather is used to assist the spinal column and axial musculature during the treatment period.

Cervical orthoses have been categorized into four distinct types: collars, poster-type orthoses, cervicothoracic devices, and halo orthoses (Fig. 315–4). Cervical collars include the soft collar and the Philadelphia collar. The soft collar is of limited benefit for patients with cervical spine injuries and provides minimal limitation of axial rotation, extension, flexion, or lateral bending. The Philadelphia collar provides significantly more limitation of cervical motion than a soft collar, especially with respect to flexion-extension, but it is ineffective in limiting axial rotation and lateral bending. Poster-type orthoses provide more rigid support for the cervical spine and provide three-point fixation using the mandible, occiput, and shoulder or upper thorax. These poster-type orthoses include the Gilford orthoses and the sterno-occipital mandibular immobilization brace. Three-point fixation with these devices provides increased cervical segment immobilization compared with cervical collars. These devices limit flexion-extension to a greater degree than the Philadelphia collar but do not restrict axial rotation or lateral bending. Cervicothoracic braces provide more rigid immobilization than the Philadelphia collar or the poster-type devices. Devices such as the Yale orthosis and the Minerva jacket are effective in limiting cervical spine flexion-extension and axial rotation, and they provide some restriction of lateral bending. The new thermoplastic Minerva body jacket, a modification of the old plaster jacket, appears to limit cervical spine snaking better than even the halo orthosis.

Halo vests are the most reliable devices designed to control motion of the cervical spine and are the standard devices against which all other orthoses are compared. They limit flexion and extension, axial rotation, and lateral bending of the upper cervical spine, levels that are poorly immobilized by other devices. The halo cannot eliminate all motion of the cervical spine, but it significantly limits motion from the occiput through C3.[191, 192] The newer halo vests are easily applied and have been used for the acute reduction and immobilization of cervical spine injuries. Newer, nonmagnetic materials used in the construction of these halo devices allow MRI of the patient's head or spine while in the halo orthosis.

Halo vests have been recommended for the treatment of displaced atlas fractures, odontoid fractures (particularly type II fractures), most axis fractures, and combination C1-2 fractures, as well as for postoperative immobilization after surgical fusion of certain cervical spine injuries. The Philadelphia collar and poster-type orthoses have been advocated in the treatment of nondisplaced or minimally displaced C1 and C2 fractures and minimal body or spinous process fractures of the cervical spine; postoperatively, they provide short-term flexion and extension immobilization for such procedures as anterior cervical diskectomies with fusion. Cervicothoracic orthoses such as the Yale orthosis and the Minerva jacket are acceptable alternatives to the halo orthosis for middle and lower cervical spine injuries. In some instances, they provide better immobilization of the cervical spine than the halo vest, such as in controlling snaking of the spine.

Surgical Management

The goals of surgical treatment of cervical spine fractures include reduction of malalignment, decompression of the neural elements, and restoration of spinal stability. As a general rule, surgery is indicated if these objectives cannot be achieved by nonoperative means. There are several controversial issues with regard to surgical intervention in the management of trauma to the cervical spine. These controversies range from general questions about the relative value of surgical treatment to specific technical questions such as the choice of allograft or autologous bone grafting or plate fixation versus wire. Most important are the issues of the value of surgical decompression and the timing of such an operative procedure.

If progressive neurological deterioration is observed subsequent to an initial injury, there is little argument about the appropriateness of acute operative intervention to treat ongoing cord compression. There has been, however, considerable debate regarding the timing of surgery in the context of a stable deficit.[193, 194] Theoretically, early decompression and stabilization decrease ongoing secondary injury to the spinal cord and result in better neurological outcome. Proponents of early surgery also cite the beneficial physiologic effects of early patient mobilization and the shorter duration of acute hospitalization. Unfortunately, the importance of secondary injury in the overall morbidity of spinal cord injury has not been quantitated, and the dimensions of the "window of opportunity," during which early surgical treatment will have an enhanced effect, are unknown.

Advocates of late surgery emphasize that most neurological damage occurs at the moment of injury and cite the increased vulnerability of a recently traumatized cord, which could negate the benefits of early operation.[195–198] Further, they suggest that early operation on a polytraumatized patient may be associated with increased morbidity.[195, 198]

No prospective study has adequately addressed this important issue. A widely cited multicenter analysis by Marshall and colleagues examined the frequency of neurological worsening in 283 patients with acute spinal cord injury.[198] Neurological worsening was observed in 4.9% of patients overall during hospitalization. In patients with cervical cord injury, worsening was observed only in patients who underwent surgery within 5 days of injury. None of the patients operated on 6 or more days after injury deteriorated. Although the numbers are small, the implication is that early surgery is hazardous in ways that later surgery (>6 days after injury) is not. A report by Heiden and co-workers came to similar conclusions.[133]

A corollary argument involves the issue of surgery for patients with complete deficits associated with deformation but not complete anatomic disruption of the spinal cord. Is there a significant possibility of reversing such a deficit by acute or hyperacute surgical decompression? If so, how soon after injury does decompression need to be accomplished, and how do we recognize patients who are likely to benefit? Is there a role for late decompression at the time of internal fixation for patients with complete injuries? Benzel and Larson reported "substantial" recovery of root function in 15 of 25 patients with complete cervical myelopathy who underwent root decompression at the time of stabilization, compared with no significant recovery in 10 similar patients who underwent fusion without decompression.[194]

In patients who are neurologically intact, there are fewer questions regarding the timing of surgery, although the possibility of a period of increased spinal cord vulnerability during early surgery may also be relevant in these cases. However, whether neurologically intact patients with radiologic evidence of cord compression require early decompression is controversial. Again, the data regarding these issues are insufficient to allow rational decision making.

The increased availability of internal fixation systems for the cervical spine has resulted in a dramatic increase in the number of patients treated with these implants. The overall frequency of surgical treatment for unstable cervical spine injuries has also increased. Whether these operative methods have resulted in improved patient outcomes compared with more traditional methods, such as recumbent therapy or use of the halo vest or other external orthoses, has never been fully evaluated.

Prolonged recumbent therapy with cervical tong traction is clearly associated with forms of morbidity such as deep venous thrombosis, atelectasis and pneumonia, decubitus ulcers, and loss of lean body mass, all of which may be benefited by early mobilization. Also, the cost of such treatment has become prohibitive. As an alternative, the halo orthosis has increased early patient mobility and decreased length of hospitalization. Liabilities of the halo apparatus include the potential for loss of alignment or reduction, which results from the midcervical spine's tendency to snake in the halo and the halo's inability to provide traction forces. Similarly, the occurrence of nonunion or fibrous union with this form of therapy must be considered. Local problems with infection, loosening of pin sites, and disfigurement from scarring in the forehead are occasionally observed. The problems of respiratory compromise and cutaneous pressure associated with the vest portion of the apparatus have been decreased with improvements in design and the use of lighter materials. These issues are still relevant in elderly and debilitated patients, however. The degree of healing and subsequent stability of ligamentous injuries treated nonoperatively is unclear.

As a result of the foregoing concerns, the trend is to treat unstable injuries of the cervical spine operatively. The morbidity of operation must be weighed against that of alternative therapies. Although issues of cost may be relevant to policy makers, it is our opinion that the surgeon must view patient well-being as the chief consideration when deciding whether and how to intervene operatively.

The indications for surgical treatment of specific cervical spine fractures or dislocations are often not clear-cut. Nonetheless, there is evidence that surgical stabilization of these injuries results in decreased hospitalization and a more rapid institution of rehabilitation in spinal cord–injured patients. Surgical approaches for cervical spine trauma can generally be divided into anterior and posterior approaches.

ANTERIOR APPROACHES

Anterior approaches to the traumatized cervical spine are usually undertaken when there is neurological compromise secondary to ventral compression or when there is loss of anterior column integrity. The incision and soft tissue dissection are identical to those used for the anterior treatment of degenerative disk disease and are familiar to neurosurgeons.

Anterior plate fixation may be employed to enhance the stability of the spine and in some cases may eliminate the need for additional postoperative stabilization with a halo orthosis. Two main types of anterior cervical plates are currently available: those in which the screws lock to the plate (e.g., Synthes Anterior Cervical Spine Locking Plate) and those in which they do not (e.g., Aesculap ABC dynamic plate). The advantage of the former is that the screws maintain rigid alignment of the bone grafts; however, settling is not compensated for, and if it occurs, it is a result of the lower screws being driven down in the lower vertebral body. The dynamic plates, which allow vertical translocation but prevent lateral and anteroposterior translocation, permit the bone graft to collapse or telescope into the bodies, which reduces the likelihood of the screws loosening as the construct matures.

Additional anterior procedures include anterior screw fixation of the odontoid process. This procedure has been used for the treatment of type II odontoid fractures, especially in patients at high risk for nonunion. There is some controversy regarding whether to place one or two screws in the odontoid process and whether the procedure should be undertaken in cases of long-standing nonunion. Biplane fluoroscopy is essential for the performance of this procedure.

POSTERIOR APPROACHES

Surgical stabilization and fusion of the cervical spine after trauma are most commonly accomplished through a posterior approach. This approach is indicated for the treatment of dorsal compression of the neural elements and for failure of the posterior column structures with preservation of anterior column integrity (e.g., posterior ligamentous instability or locked facets irreducible by nonoperative methods). Posterior approaches allow an extensive exposure so that several segments can be exposed and stabilized. The approach is a familiar one to neurosurgeons and is associated with minimal morbidity. Treatment of instability of the craniovertebral or cervicothoracic junction is most easily accomplished through a posterior exposure. Application of onlay bone graft to decorticated posterior elements is straightforward.

Posterior approaches have some significant disadvantages for the treatment of cervical trauma that must be weighed when formulating a treatment plan. First, one cannot adequately deal with ventrally located compressive pathology from a dorsal approach. For example, burst fractures or traumatic disk herniations with cord compression must be decompressed anteriorly. Second, posterior reduction of certain dislocations, such as bilateral locked facets, has the potential to displace disk material into the canal and iatrogenically induce cord compression. Third, turning the patient to the prone position for surgery may carry additional risks in highly unstable injuries. Finally, posterior approaches for stabilization will prove inadequate if the anterior column is incapable of supporting axial loads. Nonetheless, for many traumatic injuries of the cervical spine, a posterior procedure allows adequate stabilization with minimal morbidity.

Several choices of internal fixation are currently available. These include a number of posterior wiring techniques, screw fixation methods, laminar clamps, rods segmentally fixed to the spine with wires or cables, and screw-plate systems. The use of wire to provide internal fixation to the cervical spine has a long history and is quite adaptable. Wires can be applied to the spinous processes and facets and in the sublaminar position. The chief disadvantages of wire fixation include wire breakage; the risks associated with their placement, especially in the sublaminar position; and their ability to function only as a tension band. More recently, multistrand cables have been introduced; they may be somewhat easier to handle in certain situations, have greater tensile strength, and have improved fatigue strength.

Occipitocervical fusion is usually performed by the posterior approach, although anterior approaches have been described. Occipitocervical fusion using a fibular graft after trauma to the craniocervical region was first described by Foerster in 1927.[199] Since that time, a number of innovations, including stabilizing wires, methyl methacrylate, and craniocervical instrumentation, have been described. Braided wire or stainless steel cables, which can be passed through the occipital bone and then extradurally to the foramen magnum and beneath the laminae of the atlas or axis on either side, have been used to achieve occipitocervical fusion. Wertheim and Bohlman,[200] Cone and Turner,[201] Robinson and Southwick,[202] and Grantham and associates[203] used bone graft wedged against the posterior aspect of the occiput and the posterior arch of C1. More recently, the use of methyl methacrylate to supplement fusions of the craniocervical junction has been advocated.[204, 205] Several authors have described fixation devices using Y-shaped or T-shaped plates that are molded to fit the occipitocervical contour.[17, 206, 207] Screws can be placed through the plates into the occiput with bicortical purchase and into the spinous processes of C2. Sublaminar wires can then be passed around the axis, afixing the plate to C2. Other authors have advocated the use of U-shaped Luque rods contoured to the occipitocervical region or Luque rectangles for internal fixation in patients with occipitocervical instability.[208–210]

Posterior transarticular screw fixation may be used across the atlantoaxial articulations as a posterior method for treating atlantoaxial instability.[211] This provides a very rigid construct that resists displacement in all planes. The technical demands of this procedure, however, are greater than those of more traditional posterior wiring techniques. The use of C-arm fluoroscopy is mandatory to ensure proper screw placement. The chief risk of this technique is vertebral artery injury.

Segmental posterior fixation with wires or cable and steel or titanium rods or loops is used mainly for occipitocervical fixation or long, multisegment posterior fixation. It is less frequently useful in the context of acute trauma when fusion of one or two motion segments is required. The use of sublaminar wires in the cervical spine, although controversial in general, must be even more carefully considered after trauma, because cord swelling further increases the susceptibility to injury.

Laminar clamps (e.g., Halifax clamps) are straightforward to apply in cases of posterior ligamentous instability affecting a single motion segment.[212] Design changes appear to have reduced the problem of instrumentation dislodgment or loosening. Although we have limited experience with laminar clamps, they appear to be useful in carefully selected cases.

Plates that are affixed to the lateral masses with screws are useful to provide internal fixation when laminar or spinous process fractures or prior laminectomy precludes the use of other methods. These devices provide rigid posterior fixation that may be applied across one or more motion segments. Fixation can be extended to C2 or T1 by placing screws into the pedicle. The primary risk of this type of fixation is injury to the nerve root or vertebral artery from improperly placed or overly long screws.

SPECIFIC LESIONS AND THEIR TREATMENTS

Occipital Condyle Fractures

Occipital condyle fractures are relatively uncommon injuries that are often found in association with fractures of the atlas. They most often cause occipitocervical pain rather than neurological symptoms, although lower cranial nerve palsies have been reported. Occipital condyle fractures were first described in 1817 by Bell.[213] The most common clinical presentation of patients with occipital condyle fractures is loss of consciousness or cranial nerve damage. This injury is probably often overlooked and is not obvious on plain films; the diagnosis requires a high index of suspicion. The lesion is usually apparent on CT, especially with coronal reconstruction, or with conventional tomography.

Condyle fractures are classified into three types. Type I fractures result from axial loading of the skull onto the atlas, similar to the mechanism that produces Jefferson's fractures. These lesions are characterized by comminution of the occipital condyle, with minimal or no displacement of fragments into the foramen magnum. The ipsilateral alar ligament may be torn; however, spinal stability is maintained by the intact tectorial membrane and contralateral alar ligament. Type II fractures occur as part of a basilar skull fracture. Axial CT usually reveals a linear fracture extending through

the condyle and into the foramen magnum. These are stable injuries, with both the alar ligaments and the tectorial membrane remaining intact. Type III condyle fractures are avulsion fractures of the occipital condyle by the alar ligament. The mechanism of injury is usually rotation, lateral bending, or a combination of the two. As avulsion of the occipital condyle occurs, the contralateral alar ligament and tectorial membrane may be disrupted. Therefore, type III fractures are potentially unstable and may require craniocervical fusion.

Atlanto-occipital Dislocations

Although atlanto-occipital dislocation is common in autopsy series of motor vehicle accident victims, this injury has been reported infrequently in clinical material and, until relatively recently, was thought to be rare. Improvements in prehospital management, notably in spine immobilization, have resulted in increased numbers of patients arriving at emergency rooms alive. Because of the high degree of instability of these injuries and the great potential for neurological worsening with the application of standard measures to manage an unstable cervical spine, the clinician must maintain a high level of suspicion for this lesion.

These injuries are probably produced by distraction forces, which may be coupled with other force vectors. The striking of a pedestrian by a motor vehicle is a common mechanism for this injury. Clinically, these patients may present with complete quadriplegia and respiratory arrest at the scene, or they may be neurologically normal. Cranial nerve palsies are occasionally observed. Severe occipitocervical pain may be described.

The diagnosis of occipitocervical dislocation on plain lateral cervical spine films may be difficult. This injury is manifest on the lateral projection as an increased distance between the clivus and the tip of the dens, or as either anterior or posterior displacement of the skull relative to the upper cervical spine. Wholey and colleagues concluded that there was a constant distance between the rostral tip of the dens and the basion.[214] This distance measured approximately 5 mm in adults and up to 20 mm in children. Powers and associates applied these same criteria to randomly selected cervical spine radiographs and found that 85% of the normal radiographs fell outside of the measurements originally proposed by Wholey.[215] Powers and his colleagues proposed an index that would be independent of x-ray magnification artifacts: the ratio of the distance between the basion (tip of the clivus) and the posterior arch of the atlas, divided by the distance from the posterior margin of the foramen magnum to the anterior arch of the atlas. Atlanto-occipital dislocation is suggested by a ratio greater than 1.0. The normal population has a ratio of 0.7 ± 0.09. This index is useful primarily in the diagnosis of the more common anterior atlanto-occipital dislocation.

Cervical traction is contraindicated in atlanto-occipital dislocation because it may worsen distraction and produce medullary injury. Levine and Edwards advocated the immediate application of a halo vest to partially stabilize the injury and allow respiratory management.[216] Most patients require operative stabilization, either with atlanto-occipital fusion or, more commonly, with occipitocervical fusion.

Atlas Fractures

Fractures of the atlas account for approximately 5% to 10% of cervical spine injuries.[155, 204] The anatomy of the atlas vertebra makes it susceptible to specific mechanisms of injury, notably axial compression and direct fracture of the posterior arch. Atlas fractures frequently occur in combination with fractures of the occipital condyle or C2. Four basic fracture patterns are seen: posterior arch fracture, lateral mass fracture, Jefferson's fracture, and horizontal fracture of the anterior arch.

Posterior arch fractures are thought to be produced by compression-hyperextension forces resulting in fracture of the posterior arch at the occiput or the spinous process of C2. These fractures must be differentiated from congenital anomalies of the posterior arch and from Jefferson's fractures. To visualize the latter, CT is usually required. If they occur in isolation, these are stable injuries that can be treated symptomatically in a cervical orthosis.

Lateral mass fracture of C1 is the result of axial loading coupled with lateral bending. These lesions are usually diagnosed on the open-mouth view, where there is asymmetry of the lateral masses of the atlas. CT generally clarifies the diagnosis. These fractures may be associated with lateral mass fractures of C2 or with condyle fractures. If there is minimal lateral displacement (<2 mm) of the lateral mass, treatment with a cervical orthosis may suffice. Greater degrees of displacement or comminution may require treatment with a halo orthosis or recumbent traction.

Jefferson's fracture, first described in 1920, is a bursting fracture of the C1 ring by axial compression (Fig. 315–5).[217] In this injury, there is bilateral spreading of the lateral masses with failure of both the anterior and posterior arches. Although these fractures are not generally associated with neurological deficit, they are considered unstable, and immobilization in a halo orthosis is usually advocated. If there is lateral displacement of the lateral masses totaling 7 mm or more from their normal location, it is presumed that transverse ligament disruption has occurred. CT can occasionally confirm this event if there has been an avulsion of the bony attachment of the ligament. MRI may also allow visualization of the integrity of the transverse ligament. If severe displacement of the lateral masses has occurred, treatment with recumbent traction has been recommended; traction is more effective at maintaining reduction than is a halo vest, which cannot provide axial distraction. Forty-one percent of Jefferson's fractures are associated with an additional fracture of C2.

The fourth type of atlas fracture is a transverse fracture of the anterior arch. These are thought to be avulsions produced by the superior attachment of the longus colli. They are uncommon injuries that, if seen in isolation, would be expected to heal in a cervical orthosis.

Axis Fractures

The anatomy of the second cervical vertebra is unique, leading to a number of unique patterns of injury. Fractures of the axis can be subdivided into fractures of the odontoid process, fractures of the lateral masses, so-called traumatic spondylolisthesis or hangman's fractures, and miscellaneous or combined fractures.

ODONTOID FRACTURES

Fractures of the odontoid process of the axis account for approximately 7% to 14% of cervical spine fractures.[151, 152] Neurological deficits are uncommon with odontoid fractures, and patients usually complain of occipital or high cervical pain. If nondisplaced, these fractures can readily be missed on lateral cervical radiography, so careful examination of the open-mouth view is essential. Likewise, because the fracture line is in the plane of the image, these lesions may be difficult to appreciate on axial CT, and coronal or sagittal reconstruction may be required. Odontoid fractures are most commonly classified according to the three-tiered scheme of Anderson and D'Alonzo (Fig. 315–6; Table 315–1).[218]

Type I fractures involve an avulsion of the distal odontoid process. This is thought to occur by a mechanism of rotation and lateral flexion that causes an avulsion of the attachment of one of the alar ligaments. Type I fractures are relatively uncommon injuries and can most often be treated in a cervical collar.

Type II fractures are characterized by a fracture line through the base of the odontoid process. This is the most common pattern, accounting for approximately 60% to 90% of odontoid fractures. A variant of the type II fracture in which comminuted fragments at the base of the odontoid process interfere with closed reduction

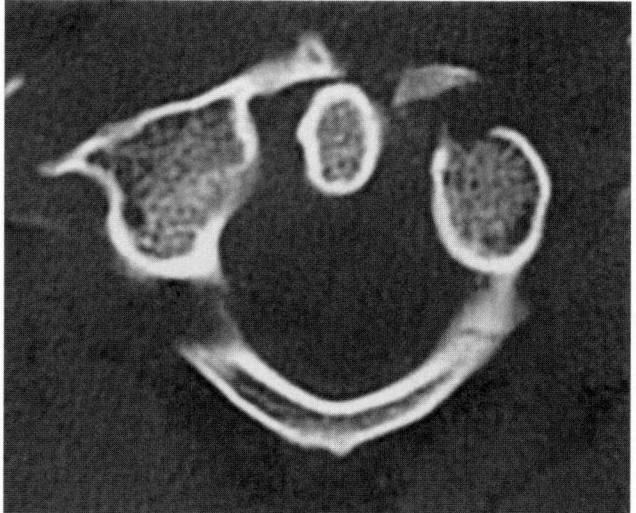

FIGURE 315–5. Nondisplaced Jefferson's fracture.

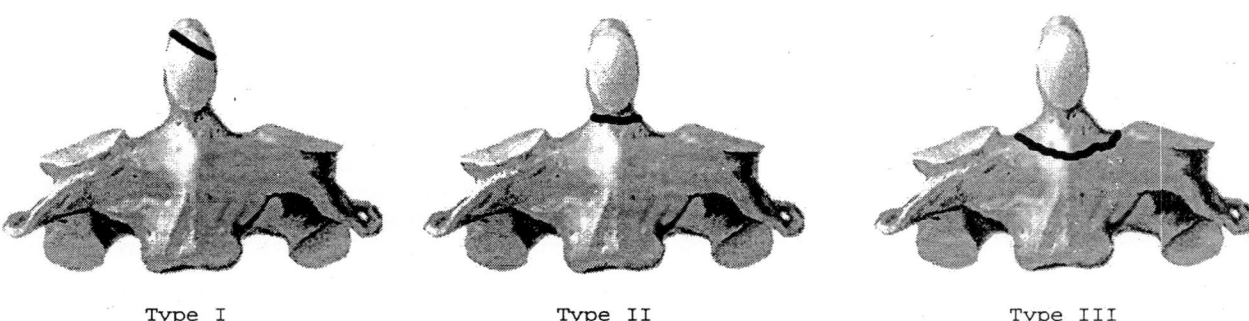

Type I	Type II	Type III

FIGURE 315–6. Odontoid fracture classification.

and subsequent healing has been described by Hadley and associates and termed a type IIA fracture.[219]

In addition, the angle of the fracture line is important in determining the type of treatment indicated. The angles are oblique sloping up, oblique sloping down, and straight lateral. Treatment with an anterior odontid screw, in experienced hands, can be performed with low morbidity, high efficacy, and minimal loss of mobility.[220] This treatment should be reserved for patients with oblique-down and transverse fracture angles and for those with intact transverse ligaments.

Type II fractures are treated with immobilization for 12 or more weeks in a halo orthosis. However, rates of nonunion with this form of treatment range from 25% to 63%. This is thought to be related to a relative lack of blood supply to the distal odontoid.

Several studies have attempted to define risk factors for nonunion in type II fractures.[143, 151, 221] Although there is no clear consensus, the following may be associated with higher nonunion rates: increased age (especially older than 65 years), greater degrees of dens displacement (especially >6 mm), and posterior displacement. Patients with nonunion and those who are at high risk of nonunion are treated surgically. Current surgical options include posterior fusion with internal fixation by means of a variety of atlantoaxial wiring

techniques or transarticular C1-2 screw fixation. Anterior osteosynthesis by means of transodontoid lag screw placement is another alternative if the transverse ligament is known to be intact. The two screw fixation techniques mentioned are of particular value if there is an associated fracture of the posterior C1 arch.

Type III fractures pass into the body of the axis. These fractures generally heal well if treated with external immobilization in a halo vest for approximately 12 weeks.

LATERAL MASS FRACTURES

Fractures of the lateral mass of the axis occur as a result of an axial loading mechanism similar to that producing lateral mass fractures at C1 (Fig. 315–7).

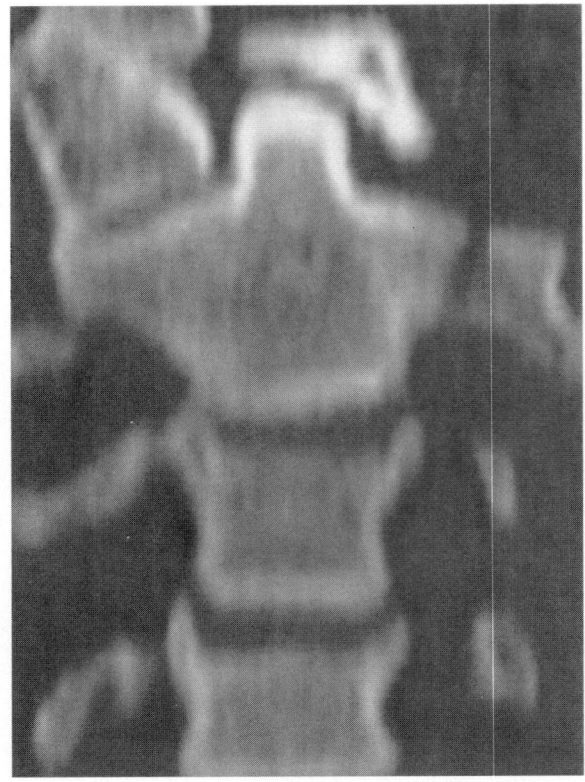

FIGURE 315–7. C2 lateral mass fracture in a 50-year-old unrestrained man whose head struck the windshield. He was neurologically intact but had other injuries.

T A B L E 3 1 5 – 1 ■ **Classification of Odontoid (Dens) Fractures**

Type I
Through tip of dens, not involving neck or transverse ligament
Oblique fracture, most likely unilateral alar ligament avulsion
May result in os odontoideum through resorption of lower portion
  from avascular necrosis

Type II
Through neck of dens, lower, not including body of C2
Transverse and alar ligaments still attached to tip
Anterior-posterior subluxation with possible compromise of canal
  by fragment

Type III
Fracture includes body of C2
Transverse and alar ligaments still attached to tip
Anterior-posterior subluxation with possible compromise of canal
  by fragment

From Anderson LD, D'Alonzo RT: Fractures of the odontoid process of the axis. J Bone Joint Surg Am 56: 1663–1674, 1974.

Indeed, these two types of fractures are often seen in combination. Lateral mass fractures of C2 are most often treated with a cervical collar, although marked compression deformity or comminution may require reduction of the displacement by axial traction and halo vest use.

TRAUMATIC SPONDYLOLISTHESIS

Traumatic spondylolisthesis of C2, the so-called hangman's fracture, is another common injury pattern affecting the axis (Fig. 315–8; Table 315–2). These injuries involve a bilateral fracture through the pars interarticularis or pedicles. The fracture line may cross the superior articular surface or encroach onto the axis body. Commonly, there is subluxation of C2 on C3, with concomitant disruption of ligamentous attachments and instability. Treatment is predicated on the degree of this ligamentous injury. Four radiologic patterns have been described as an aid to management.[216] Type I injuries, which can frequently be treated with immobilization in a rigid collar, are fractures in which there is no angulation of C2 relative to C3 and less than 3 mm of anterior translation. Type II injuries demonstrate both significant angulation (>11 degrees) and translation (>3.5 mm). Type III injuries are uncommon; they consist of high degrees of angulation and displacement in which there is a concomitant unilateral or bilateral facet dislocation of C2-3. The fourth pattern has been termed type IIA by Levine and Edwards; these fractures exhibit no significant translation but high degrees of angulation at C2-3 (Fig. 315–9).[216]

Hangman's fractures are infrequently associated with neurological injury, and most are successfully treated nonoperatively. Most type I fractures can be treated with a Philadelphia collar. Type II, IIA, and III fractures that can be reduced satisfactorily are treated in a halo orthosis. Anterior fusion with plate fixation

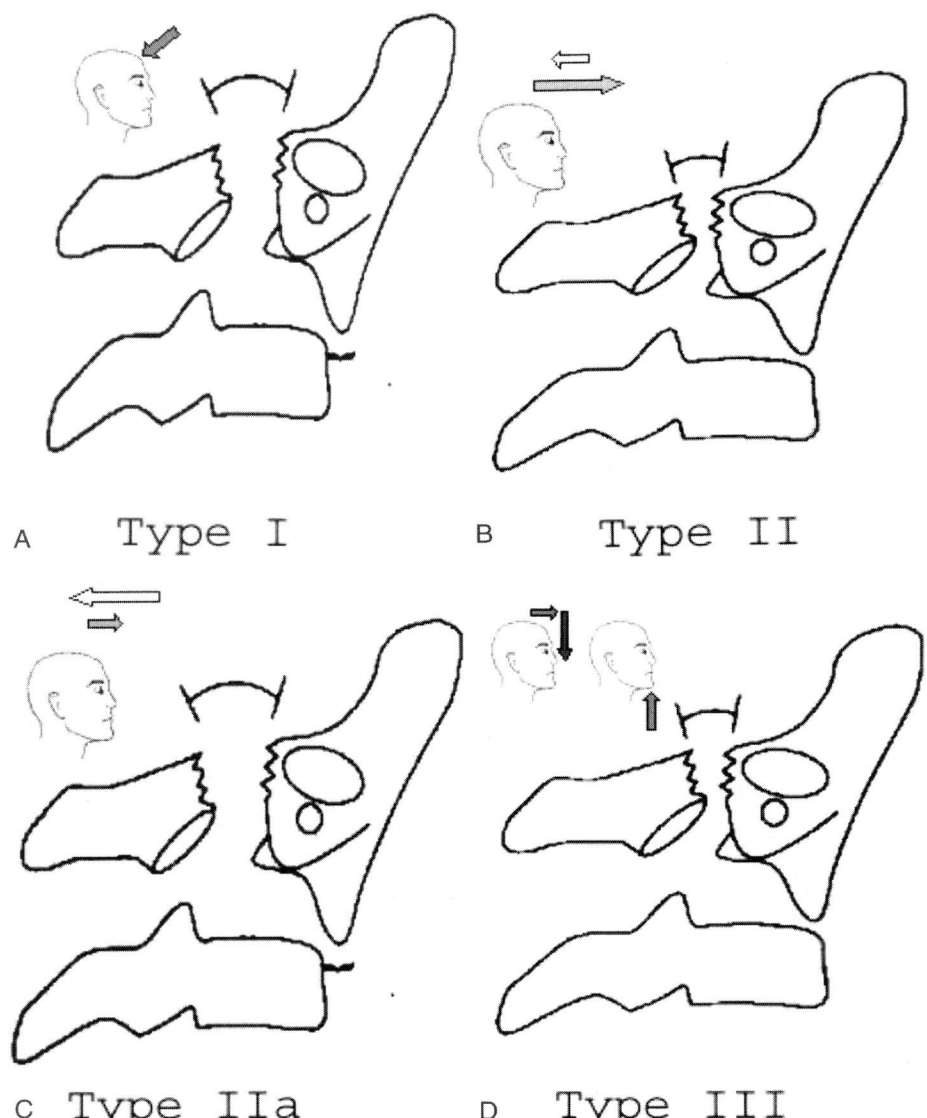

FIGURE 315–8. *A–D*, Hangman's fracture classification: types I, II, IIA, and III.

TABLE 315–2 ■ **Classification of Hangman's Fractures**

Type I

Levine & Edwards classification
Hyperextension and axial loading
Pars fracture, ≤2 mm dislocation
Stable fracture

Type II

Pars fracture, disruption of posterior longitudinal ligament, C2-3 disk disruption, possible anterior longitudinal ligament disruption or avulsion from C3
Unstable fracture
Angulation, distraction of fragments
Usually due to rebound flexion after extension
Reduces in light traction

Type IIA

Levine & Edwards classification
More force in flexion than extension; possible posterior distraction force involved
Same as type II, but less displacement and more angulation
Increases displacement and angulation in traction

Type III

Initial disruption of C2–3 facet capsules, then pars fracture after dislocated
Flexion followed by compression
"Traumatic spondylolisthesis of axis"
Also caused by submental traction injury causing severe extension (judicial hanging)

From Levine AM, Edwards CC: The management of traumatic spondylolisthesis of the axis. J Bone Joint Surg Am 67:217–226, 1985.

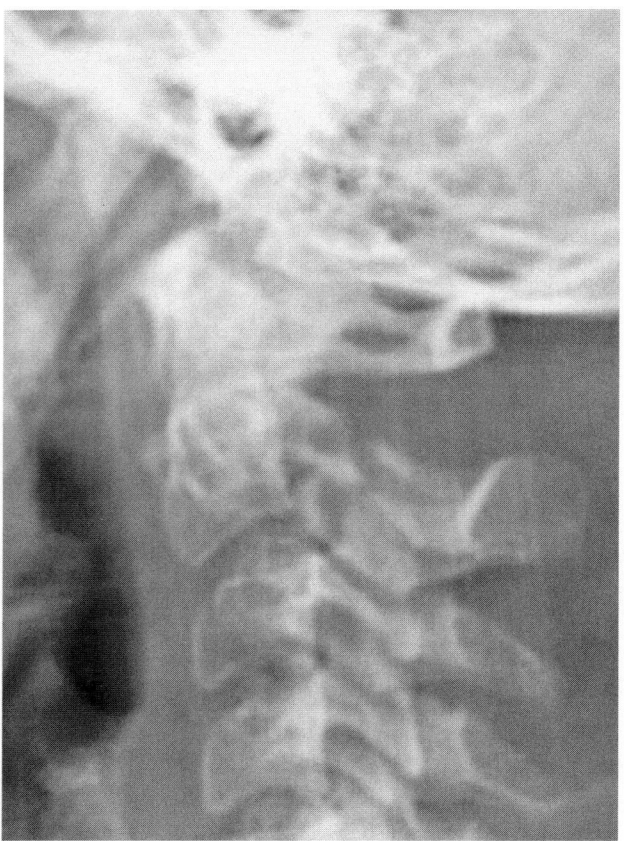

FIGURE 315–9. Hangman's fracture type IIA.

has been recommended for significant angulation at C2-3 that is not correctable by a halo orthosis.[222, 223]

ATLANTOAXIAL COMBINATION FRACTURES

Because of the complex anatomic interrelations of the atlas and axis vertebrae and the forces involved in fractures of this region, contiguous injuries are not uncommon. Dickman and colleagues described 25 patients with acute combination fractures of C1 and C2; these injuries accounted for 43% of the acute atlas fractures and 16% of the acute axis fractures treated at their institution during the study period.[150] Neurological injury is more common in this setting than it is with isolated fractures of either the atlas or the axis. Several patterns of injury are seen. Atlas fractures are variable, including posterior arch fractures, Jefferson's fractures, and lateral mass fractures. These lesions may be seen in various combinations with type II or type III odontoid fractures, hangman's fractures, or miscellaneous C2 fractures (Figs. 315–10 and 315–11).

Treatment of combination fractures must be individualized. Frequently, halo immobilization is sufficient. If an axis ring fracture is combined with a type II odontoid fracture, surgical fusion may be considered. Transarticular C1-2 fixation may be appropriate if a posterior atlas ring fracture is present, especially if the integrity of the transverse ligament is in doubt. With marked comminution of C1, occipitocervical fusion may need to be considered.

The high incidence of combination fractures of C1 and C2 mandates careful evaluation of any craniocervical fracture before treatment is planned. Combination fractures require close follow-up with radiologic monitoring if optimal results are to be obtained.

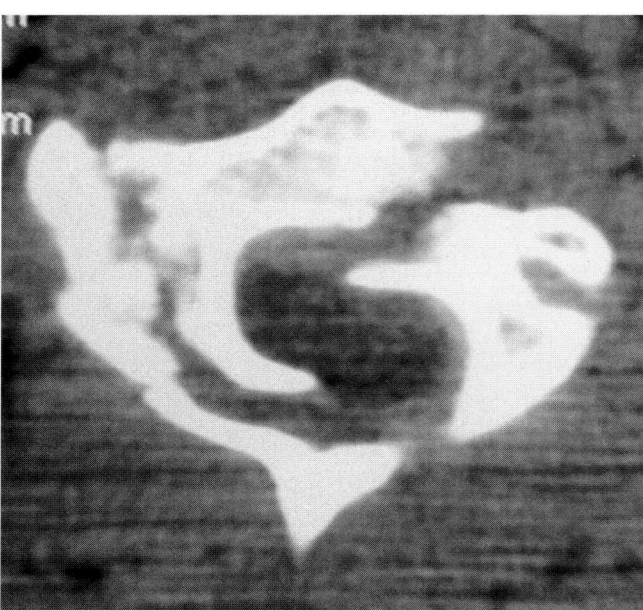

FIGURE 315–10. C2 body fracture.

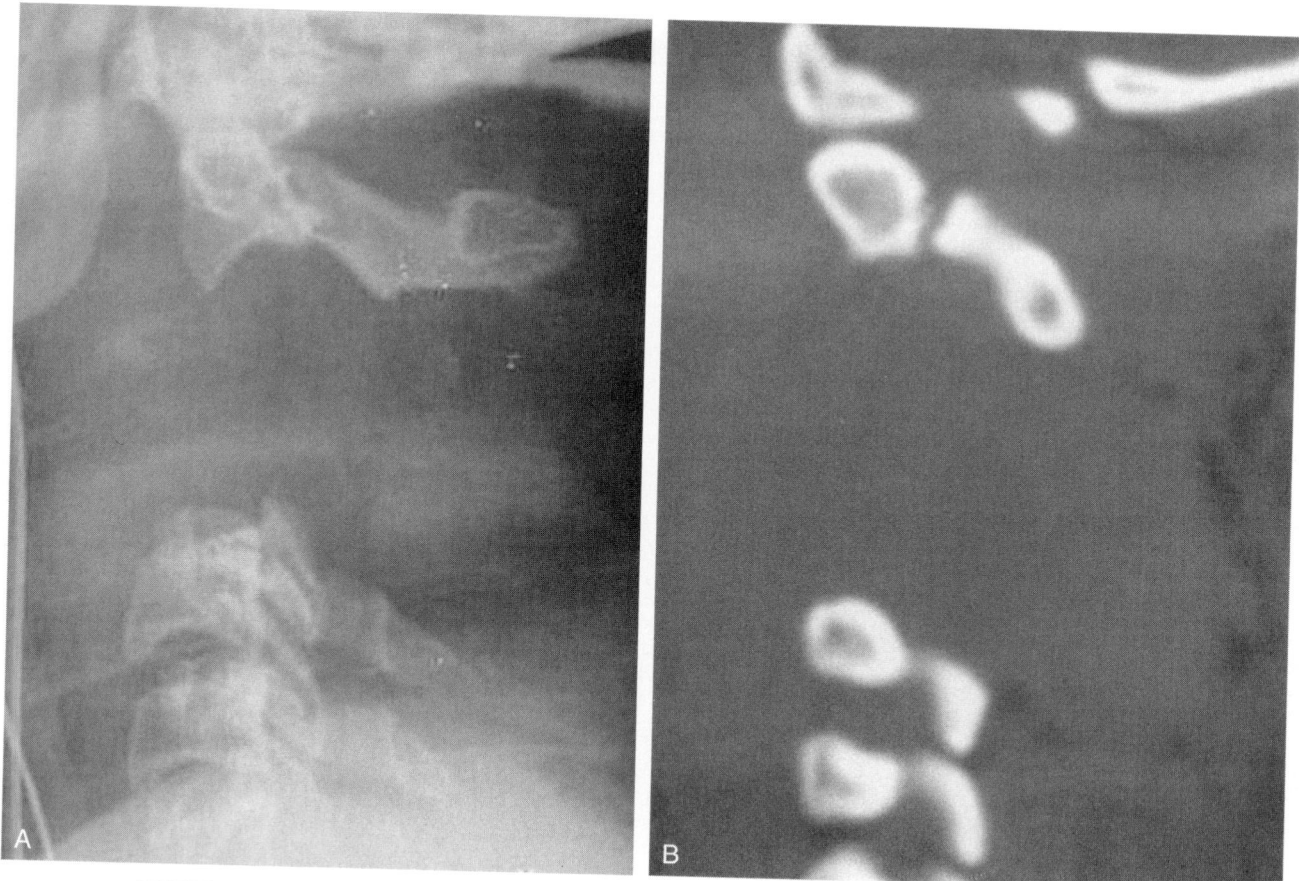

FIGURE 315–11. Ligamentous disruption of C2 on C3 in a 22-year-old driver who was unresponsive in the field. He was resuscitated but remained quadriparetic until he expired. The lateral radiograph (A) appeared to show a pure ligamentous injury, but the sagittal computed tomographic reconstruction (B) showed an associated hangman's fracture. The likely mechanism is unusually violent flexion (causing disruption of posterior ligaments), followed by hyperextension (causing disruption of anterior elements and fracture of the C2 pars interarticularis). The pars fracture likely happened with the hyperextension, or the posterior elements would have stayed with the lower cervical spine instead of staying with the C2 body. By the Allen criteria, this would also be classified as a DF 4 (see Table 315–3).

Subaxial Fractures and Dislocations

Fractures and dislocations of the cervical vertebrae below C2 are considered together because the vertebral anatomy is similar from level to level, and fracture patterns are likewise similar. The most common levels affected are C5 and C6. Some of the more common injury patterns include simple compression fractures, burst fractures, teardrop fractures, unilateral and bilateral locked facets, hyperflexion injuries, and clay shoveler's fractures. These were broken down into a classification system by Allen and coworkers in 1982, based on the presumed fracture mechanism (Table 315–3).[167]

COMPRESSION FRACTURES

Compression fractures of the cervical spine are common injuries. They are the result of a mechanism involving flexion and axial loading with failure of the anterior column. By definition, the middle column is intact and there is no compromise of the central canal.

These fractures are probably more common in association with osteoporosis and degenerative spondylosis with loss of the cervical lordotic curve. Treatment of these lesions is usually symptomatic, consisting of immobilization in a cervical collar.

BURST FRACTURES

Burst fractures of the cervical spine are produced primarily by axial forces, which may be combined with a flexion force. These fractures result in failure of the anterior, middle, and posterior columns, often with retropulsion of bone into the canal (Fig. 315–12). These fractures are often treated surgically if they are neurologically incomplete. Immobilization in a halo orthosis may be reasonable for patients with complete quadriplegia.

TEARDROP FRACTURES

Teardrop fractures are hyperflexion injuries characterized by a small chip of bone off the anterior inferior

T A B L E   3 1 5 – 3 ■ **Classification of Subaxial Cervical Fractures and Dislocations**

Compressive Flexion (CF)
1. Blunting of anterior end plate
2. Anterior wedge fracture
3. Linear oblique nondisplaced fracture
4. Linear oblique slightly displaced (<3 mm) fracture
5. Splaying of posterior elements, disruption of posterior longitudinal ligament

Compressive Extension (CE)
1. Unilateral posterior arch fracture, with or without rotatory subluxation
2. Bilateral arch fracture (frequently multiple)
3. Bilateral facet fractures
4. Bilateral arch fractures with partial vertebral body width displacement
5. Dissociation of posterior and anterior elements, full-thickness defect

Vertical Compression (VC)
1. Increased cupping of one end plate (central end plate failure)
2. Increased cupping of both end plates, minimal displacement of fracture lines
3. Fractured centrum, retropulsion of bone

Distractive Flexion (DF)
1. Splayed spinous processes
2. Unilateral jumped facet
3. Bilateral jumped facet
4. Floating vertebrae

Distractive Extension (DE)
1. Failure of anterior longitudinal ligament or disk annulus; also failure of center of body; no translocation or spondylolisthesis
2. All three ligaments failed, posterior spondylolisthesis of upper body (may appear normal in flexion or neutral position)

Lateral Flexion (LF)
1. Asymptomatic unilateral arch and body fracture
2. Displaced asymmetrical compression fracture

From Allen BL Jr, et al: A mechanistic classification of closed, indirect fractures and dislocations of the lower cervical spine. Spine 7:1–27, 1982.

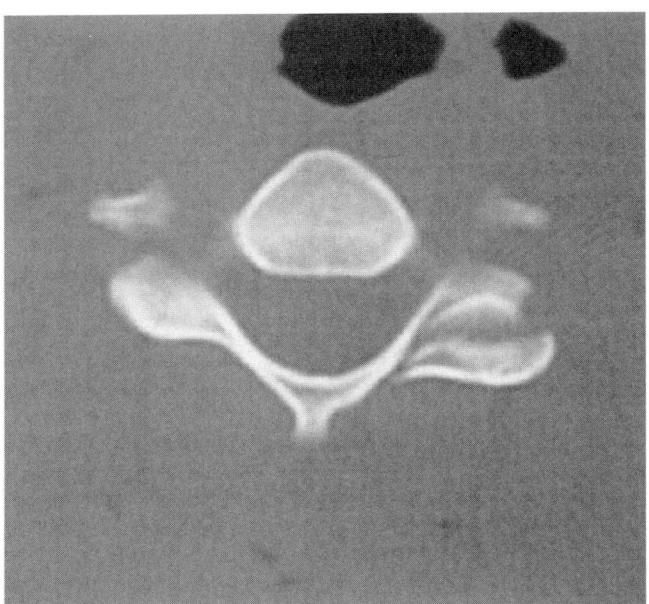

FIGURE 315–12. C5 lateral mass fracture with laminar fracture.

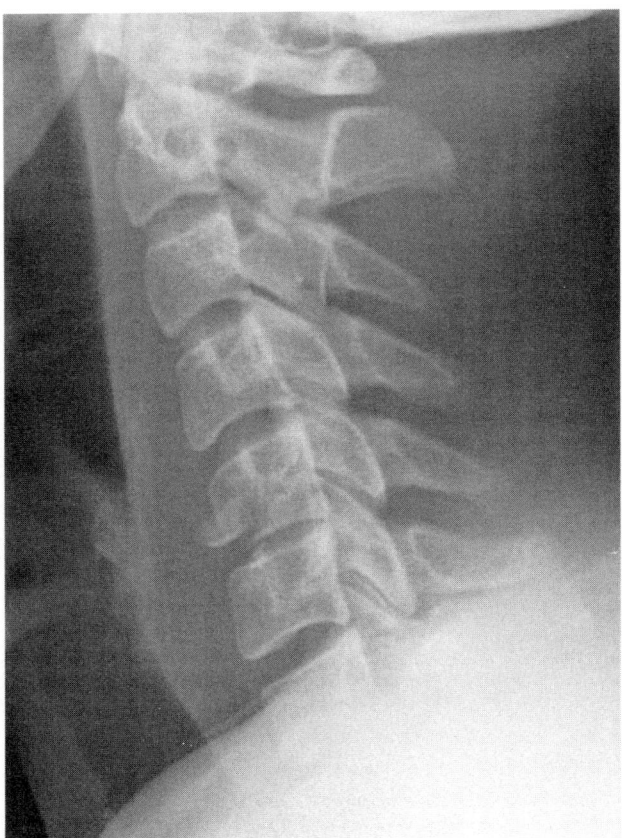

FIGURE 315–13. Teardrop fracture of C5.

aspect of the vertebral body (Fig. 315–13). Patients frequently, but not always, have severe neurological injury. Treatment includes management in a halo orthosis or surgical stabilization and fusion. A more severe injury with flexion and axial loading is the burst fracture.

UNILATERAL FACET DISLOCATIONS

Unilateral facet dislocation is often produced by a flexion-rotation mechanism. In this injury, the facet joints at one level are dislocated such that the inferior articular process of the upper vertebra locks anterior to the superior process of the lower vertebra. Plain radiography demonstrates a characteristic appearance. On the lateral projection, there is anterolisthesis of the upper vertebra, usually measuring less than 25% of the anteroposterior dimension of the body. There is also a rotary component such that, on a given lateral film, the segment of the spine either above or below the distal location appears rotated. Similarly, a malalignment of the spinous processes is seen in the anteroposterior projection. Unilateral locked facets may or may not be associated with spinal cord injury. The initial management of these unstable injuries is tong traction with an attempt at reduction. If closed reduction can be accomplished, most surgeons recommend halo immobilization. Many authors have advocated MRI in patients who are neurologically intact before reduction is attempted. Failure of closed reduction is usually considered an indication for operative reduction; in this case, the facets are drilled until they can be realigned under direct vision. Fusion and internal fixation by a variety of methods are then employed.

BILATERAL FACET DISLOCATIONS

Bilateral locked facets occur by a hyperflexion mechanism in which the posterior ligaments are disrupted sufficiently to allow both facet complexes to dislocate (Fig. 315–14). These injuries are commonly associated with neurological involvement. Plain lateral radiography demonstrates a subluxation of 25% or more of the vertebral body, often with a marked angular deformity. These injuries are highly unstable but can frequently be reduced by closed techniques. However, surgical stabilization is usually advocated after reduction.

HYPEREXTENSION INJURIES

Hyperextension spinal injuries, including hyperextension dislocation, hyperextension fracture-dislocation, and laminar fractures, are common in elderly patients with spondylosis but may also be seen in younger patients who sustain high-velocity injuries.[96] Hyperextension injuries usually result from a pure or predominantly backward force delivered to the cervical spine as a result of a force impacting the mandible, face, or forehead or an abrupt deceleration injury in which the head and spine are thrown into hyperextension. Radiographically, posterior laminar fractures with avulsion of the anterior longitudinal ligament and retrolisthesis of the vertebral body may be seen. However,

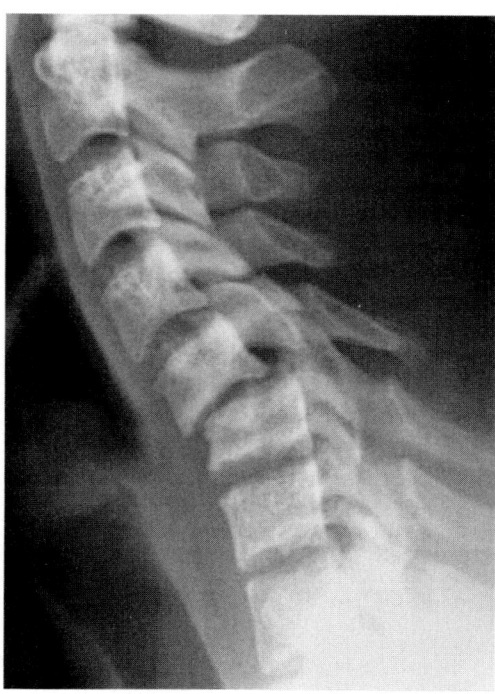

FIGURE 315–14. Bilateral jumped facets of C5-6.

the radiologic diagnosis of this injury may be difficult. Because the spine may return to its normal position after being dislocated posteriorly, the bony cervical spine may appear normal in alignment despite a severe spinal injury. However, close examination of the lateral cervical spine film may reveal diffuse prevertebral soft tissue swelling, widening or asymmetry of the disrupted intervertebral disk with a small vacuum sign, irregularity or horizontal fractures of the vertebral end plates, or small avulsion fractures of the anterior inferior margin of the vertebrae. Neurological examination may reveal no associated neurological damage to the spinal cord or nerve roots, or it may demonstrate significant neurological injury such as the central cord syndrome, which is often seen in elderly patients with cervical stenosis after a fall leading to hyperextension of the cervical spine.

Extension injuries that do not manifest instability, such as an isolated laminar fracture, do not require surgical intervention. Laminar fractures are best seen in the lateral projection on plain cervical spine films. CT is indicated in patients who have or are suspected of having a laminar fracture on plain films in order to confirm the diagnosis and determine the position of fragments relative to the spinal cord. The laminar fracture is usually stable, because the anterior column and interfacetal joints are intact. However, in the presence of neurological deficit secondary to cord involvement by laminar fragments, the laminar fracture should be considered unstable.

Hyperextension dislocation and hyperextension fracture-dislocation injuries are both considered unstable cervical spine injuries. Hyperextension dislocation may cause disruption of the intervertebral disk and displacement of the vertebra above this disk posteriorly. Both the anterior longitudinal ligament and the posterior longitudinal ligament may be disrupted. Posterior dislocation of the vertebra may result in compression of the spinal cord against the posterior arch of the spine and the ligamenta flava. Varying degrees of neurological deficit may occur, from transient weakness to complete quadriplegia. Often the spine returns to its normal position after being dislocated posteriorly, making radiologic diagnosis difficult. A triad of signs is usually present, including soft tissue injury to the middle face or forehead, some degree of acute central cervical cord syndrome, and diffuse prevertebral soft tissue swelling on a lateral cervical spine film in which the cervical vertebrae appear to be aligned normally. Hyperextension fracture-dislocation is also an unstable injury. Disruption of the anterior longitudinal ligament and fractures of the subjacent articular mass lead to forward translation of the vertebral body. This injury is often misinterpreted as being caused by a hyperflexion mechanism. Both hyperextension dislocation and hyperextension fracture-dislocation must be surgically stabilized, usually with an anterior approach.

CLAY SHOVELER'S FRACTURES

The classic clay shoveler's fracture is an avulsion of the spinous process of C7, although this term is often applied to the fracture of any cervical spinous process in the absence of other fracture. The most common mechanism is a direct blow to the posterior elements, but avulsion associated with a violent flexion mechanism is another possibility. These are stable fractures, although they may be painful. Care must be taken to rule out less obvious but more serious ligamentous or bony injuries, particularly if this fracture involves spinous processes above C6.

Spinal Cord Injury without Radiographic Abnormality

As the name implies, SCIWORA is an entity in which there are clinical signs of cervical cord damage in the absence of radiologic evidence of vertebral fracture or dislocation. The mechanism for such injuries in adults was initially postulated to be either hyperflexion-dislocation with immediate reduction by muscular action or temporary prolapse of the cervical disk after forcible flexion.[178, 208, 224] However, other authors have convincingly demonstrated that the most likely injury mechanism in adults is hyperextension superimposed on preexisting cervical spondylosis.[96, 135, 164, 225] The neurological picture is predominantly that of an acute central cord syndrome.[98, 99, 135, 225, 226]

Using cadavers, Taylor demonstrated that the ligamenta flava of the cervical spine bulge forward into the canal during hyperextension, producing a marked narrowing of the sagittal canal diameter and cord injury.[226] Additionally, shortening and therefore thickening of the cord during hyperextension as the spinal column shortens may further exacerbate the crowding of intraspinal contents during hyperextension. Taylor and Blackwood also postulated that during hyperextension sprain, the anterior longitudinal ligament can rupture and permit retrolisthesis of the upper segment, leading to cord compression.[135] Elastic recoil of the paraspinous muscles then results in spontaneous reduction of the displacement, giving a normal appearance on radiology. Support for this mechanism was provided by both cadaver and radiologic studies.

More recently, a similar phenomenon has been described in pediatric patients.[227-236] The mechanisms of injury noted in these cases included hyperextension, flexion, repetitive flexion-extension, longitudinal distraction, and direct crush injury.[228, 230, 231, 234, 237-239] Several anatomic features of the cervical spine in children account for an increased susceptibility to cord injury. These include more horizontally oriented articulating facet surfaces; forward wedging of the anterior portion of the vertebral body, which facilitates anterior slipping between adjacent bodies; and increased elasticity and redundancy of the interspinous ligaments, posterior joint capsules, and cartilaginous end plates.[240-242] In addition, the relatively underdeveloped cervical musculature of infants and young children, combined with the disproportionate weight of the head, creates an increased susceptibility to flexion-extension forces.[236, 243]

In the pediatric syndrome of SCIWORA, the lesion often involves complete cord transection, anterior cord syndromes, or severe incomplete cord syndromes.[228, 230, 234] This probably explains the generally poorer prognosis in pediatric patients with this syndrome compared with adults, because central cord syndrome is usually associated with good recovery, but complete cord transection or anterior cord syndromes have a more sinister prognosis.

REFERENCES

1. Bohlman H: Complications of treatment of fractures and dislocations of the cervical spine. In Epps C (ed): Complications of Orthopaedic Surgery. Philadelphia, JB Lippincott, 1985, pp 897–918.
2. Bohlman H, Ducker T, Lucas J: Spine and spinal cord injuries. In Rothman R, Simeone F (eds): The Spine. Philadelphia, WB Saunders, 1982, pp 661–757.
3. Bohlman HH: Acute fractures and dislocations of the cervical spine: An analysis of three hundred hospitalized patients and review of the literature. J Bone Joint Surg Am 61:1119–1142, 1979.
4. Bolesta M, Bohlman H: Late complications of cervical fractures and dislocations and their surgical treatment. In Frymoyer J (ed): The Adult Spine: Principles of Practice. New York, Raven Press, 1991, pp 1107–1126.
5. Breasted J: The Edwin Smith surgical papyrus. In Wilkins R (ed): Neurosurgical Classics. New York, Johnson Reprint Corp, 1965, pp 1–5.
6. Taylor A: Fracture dislocation of the cervical spine. Ann Surg 90:321–340, 1929.
7. Parney I, Allen P, Petruk K: Howard H. Hepburn and the development of skull tongs for cervical spine traction. Neurosurgery 47:1430–1432, discussion 1432–1433, 2000.
8. Crutchfield W: Treatment of injuries of the cervical spine. J Bone Joint Surg 20:696–704, 1938.
9. Gardner WJ: The principle of spring-loaded points for cervical traction: Technical note. J Neurosurg 39:543–544, 1973.
10. Nickel V, Perry J, Garrett A, Heppenstall M: The halo: A spinal skeletal traction fixation device. J Bone Joint Surg Am 50:1400–1409, 1968.
11. Guttmann L: Management of paralysis. Br Surg Pract 6:445–466, 1949.
12. Bedbrook GM: Spinal injuries with tetraplegia and paraplegia. J Bone Joint Surg Br 61:267–284, 1979.
13. Bracken MB, Hildreth N, Freeman DH Jr, Webb SB: Relationship between neurological and functional status after acute spinal cord injury: An epidemiological study. J Chronic Dis 33:115–125, 1980.
14. Guttmann L, Frankel H: The value of intermittent catheterization in the early management of traumatic paraplegia and tetraplegia. Paraplegia 4:63–84, 1966.
15. Rogers W: Treatment of fracture-dislocation of the cervical spine. J Bone Joint Surg Am 24:245–258, 1942.
16. Rogers W: Fractures and dislocations of the cervical spine: An end-result study. J Bone Joint Surg Am 39:341–376, 1957.
17. Roy-Camille R, Mazel C: Stabilization of the cervical spine with posterior plates and screws. In Camins M, O'Leary P (eds): Disorders of the Cervical Spine. Baltimore, Williams & Wilkins, 1992, pp 577–591.
18. Roy-Camille R, Saillant G, Mazel C: Internal fixation of the unstable cervical spine by a posterior osteosynthesis with plates and screws. In TCSRSE Committee (ed): The Cervical Spine, 2nd ed. Philadelphia, JB Lippincott, 1989, pp 390–403.
19. Smith GW, Robinson RA: The treatment of certain cervical-spine disorders by anterior removal of the anterior vertebral disc and interbody fusion. J Bone Joint Surg Am 40:607–623, 1958.
20. Cloward R: Treatment of acute fractures and fracture-dislocations of the cervical spine by vertebral-body fusion: A report of 11 cases. J Neurosurg 18:201–209, 1961.
21. Bailey R, Badgley C: Stabilization of the cervical spine by anterior fusion. J Bone Joint Surg Am 41:565–594, 1960.
22. Bracken MB, Shepard MJ, Holford TR, et al: Administration of methylprednisolone for 24 or 48 hours or tirilazad mesylate for 48 hours in the treatment of acute spinal cord injury: Results of the Third National Acute Spinal Cord Injury Randomized Controlled Trial. National Acute Spinal Cord Injury Study. JAMA 277:1597–1604, 1997.

23. Ducker TB: Treatment of spinal-cord injury. N Engl J Med 322:1459–1461, 1990.
24. Reiss S, Raque GH Jr, Shields CB, Garretson HD: Cervical spine fractures with major associated trauma. Neurosurgery 18:327–330, 1986.
25. Shackford SR, Mackersie RC, Hoyt DB, et al: Impact of a trauma system on outcome of severely injured patients. Arch Surg 122:523–527, 1987.
26. Sonntag VK, Hadley MN: Nonoperative management of cervical spine injuries. Clin Neurosurg 34:630–649, 1988.
27. Chakeres DW, Flickinger F, Bresnahan JC, et al: MR imaging of acute spinal cord trauma. AJNR Am J Neuroradiol 8:5–10, 1987.
28. Mirvis SE, Geisler FH, Jelinek JJ, et al: Acute cervical spine trauma: Evaluation with 1.5-T MR imaging. Radiology 166:807–816, 1988.
29. Yashon D: Spinal Injury. Norwalk, CT: Appleton-Century-Crofts, 1986.
30. Peng R, Chang C, Gilmore D, Bongard F: Epidemiology of immediate and early trauma deaths at an urban level I trauma center. Am Surg 64:950–954, 1998.
31. Fabio A, Weiss H, Forjoh S, et al: Head and Spinal Cord Injuries in Pennsylvania, 1995–98. Pittsburgh, Center for Violence and Injury Control, Department of Emergency Medicine, Allegheny University of the Health Sciences, 1998.
32. Becker BE, DeLisa JA: Model spinal cord injury system: Trends and implications for the future. Arch Phys Med Rehabil 80:1514–1521, 1999.
33. DeVivo MJ, Krause JS, Lammertse DP: Recent trends in mortality and causes of death among persons with spinal cord injury. Arch Phys Med Rehabil 80:1411–1419, 1999.
34. Nobunaga A, Go B, Karunas R: Recent demographic and injury trends in people served by the model spinal cord injury care systems. Arch Phys Med Rehabil 80:1372–1382, 1999.
35. Stover S, Whiteneck G, DeLisa J: Spinal Cord Injury: Clinical Outcome from the Model Systems. Gaithersburg, MD, Aspen, 1995.
36. Green BA, Gabrielsen MA, Hall WJ, et al: Analysis of swimming pool accidents resulting in spinal cord injury. Paraplegia 18:94–100, 1980.
37. Hall J, Burke D: Diving injury resulting in tetraplegia. Med J Aust 1:171, 1978.
38. DeVivo MJ, Fine PR, Maetz HM, Stover SL: Prevalence of spinal cord injury: A reestimation employing life table techniques. Arch Neurol 37:707–708, 1980.
39. Kraus JF, Franti CE, Riggins RS, et al: Incidence of traumatic spinal cord lesions. J Chronic Dis 28:471–492, 1975.
40. Hu R, Mustard CA, Burns C: Epidemiology of incident spinal fracture in a complete population. Spine 21:492–499, 1996.
41. Tator C: Epidemiology and general characteristics of the spinal cord injured patient. In Benzel E, Tator C (eds): Contemporary Management of Spinal Cord Injury. Park Ridge, IL, American Association of Neurological Surgeons, 1995, pp 9–20.
42. NSCIC: Spinal Cord: Facts and Figures at a Glance. Survey of Model Systems Spinal Cord Injury Rehabilitation Centers. Birmingham, AL, National Spinal Cord Injury Statistical Center, 2000.
43. Ersmark H, Lowenhielm P: Factors influencing the outcome of cervical spine injuries. J Trauma 28:407–410, 1988.
44. Huelke DF, Mendelsohn RA, States JD, Melvin JW: Cervical fractures and fracture-dislocations sustained without head impact. J Trauma 18:533–538, 1978.
45. Alker GJ Jr, Oh YS, Leslie EV: High cervical spine and craniocervical junction injuries in fatal traffic accidents: A radiological study. Orthop Clin North Am 9:1003–1010, 1978.
46. Bucholz RW, Burkhead WZ, Graham W, Petty C: Occult cervical spine injuries in fatal traffic accidents. J Trauma 19:768–771, 1979.
47. Cloward R: Acute cervical spine injuries. Clin Symp 32:132, 1980.
48. Kraus J, Franti C, Riggins R: Neurologic outcome and vehicle and crash factors in motor vehicle related spinal cord injury. Neuroepidemiology 1:223–238, 1982.
49. Huelke DF, O'Day J, Mendelsohn RA: Cervical injuries suffered in automobile crashes. J Neurosurg 54:316–322, 1981.
50. Taylor TK, Nade S, Bannister JH: Seat belt fractures of the cervical spine. J Bone Joint Surg Br 58:328–331, 1976.
51. Saldeen T: Fatal neck injuries caused by use of diagonal safety belts. J Trauma 7:856–862, 1967.
52. Lillehei KO, Robinson MN: A critical analysis of the fatal injuries resulting from the Continental flight 1713 airline disaster: Evidence in favor of improved passenger restraint systems. J Trauma 37:826–830, 1994.
53. Mueller FO: Fatalities from head and cervical spine injuries occurring in tackle football: 50 years' experience. Clin Sports Med 17:169–182, 1998.
54. Mueller FO, Cantu RC: Seventeenth Annual Report Fall 1982–Spring 1999. Chapel Hill, NC, National Center for Catastrophic Sport Injury, 2000.
55. Scher A: Rugby injuries to the cervical spine and spinal cord: A 10-year review. Clin Sports Med 17:195–206, 1998.
56. Scher AT: Premature onset of degenerative disease of the cervical spine in rugby players. S Afr Med J 77:557–558, 1990.
57. Berge J, Marque B, Vital JM, et al: Age-related changes in the cervical spines of front-line rugby players. Am J Sports Med 27:422–429, 1999.
58. Secin FP, Poggi EJ, Luzuriaga F, Laffaye HA: Disabling injuries of the cervical spine in Argentine rugby over the last 20 years. Br J Sports Med 33:33–36, 1999.
59. Tator CH, Carson JD, Edmonds VE: Spinal injuries in ice hockey. Clin Sports Med 17:183–194, 1998.
60. Wetzler MJ, Akpata T, Albert T, et al: A retrospective study of cervical spine injuries in American rugby, 1970 to 1994. Am J Sports Med 24:454–458, 1996.
61. Kip P, Hunter RE: Cervical spinal fractures in alpine skiers. Orthopedics 18:737–741, 1995.
62. Levy AS, Smith RH: Neurologic injuries in skiers and snowboarders. Semin Neurol 20:233–245, 2000.
63. Prall J, Winston K, Brennan R: Spine and spinal cord injuries in downhill skiers. J Trauma 39:1115–1118, 1995.
64. Sacco D, Sartorelli D, Vane D: Evaluation of alpine skiing and snowboarding injury in a northeastern state. J Trauma 44:654–659, 1998.
65. Nitecki S, Moir C: Predictive factors of the outcome of traumatic cervical spine fracture in children. J Pediatr Surg 29:1409–1411, 1994.
66. Eleraky MA, Theodore N, Adams M, et al: Pediatric cervical spine injuries: Report of 102 cases and review of the literature. J Neurosurg 92(1 Suppl):12–17, 2000.
67. Rekate H, Theodore N, Sonntag VK, Dickman CA: Pediatric spine and spinal cord trauma: State of the art for the third millennium. Childs Nerv Syst 15:743–750, 1999.
68. Shamoun JM, Riddick L, Powell RW: Atlanto-occipital subluxation/dislocation: A "survivable" injury in children. Am Surg 65:317–320, 1999.
69. Brockmeyer D: Pediatric spinal cord and spinal column trauma. Presented at Neurosurgery: On-Call, American Association of Neurological Surgeons/Congress of Neurological Surgeons, 2001.
70. Kriss VM, Kriss TC: SCIWORA (spinal cord injury without radiographic abnormality) in infants and children. Clin Pediatr (Phila) 35:119–124, 1996.
71. Baker C, Kadish H, Schunk JE: Evaluation of pediatric cervical spine injuries. Am J Emerg Med 17:230–234, 1999.
72. Kokoska ER, Keller MS, Rallo MC, Weber TR: Characteristics of pediatric cervical spine injuries. J Pediatr Surg 36:100–105, 2001.
73. Giguere JF, St-Vil D, Turmel A, et al: Airbags and children: A spectrum of C-spine injuries. J Pediatr Surg 33:811–816, 1998.
74. Maxeiner H, Hahn M: Airbag-induced lethal cervical trauma. J Trauma 42:1148–1151, 1997.
75. Gunby I: New focus on spinal cord injury. JAMA 245:1201–1206, 1981.
76. Gillingham J: The problem of head and spinal injuries: Prevention of the second accident. Med Sci Law 10:104–109, 1970.
77. Giesler W, Wynne-Jones M, Jousse A: Early management of the patient with trauma to the spinal cord. Med Serv J Can 22:512–523, 1966.
78. Yashon D, White R: Injuries of the vertebral column and spinal cord. In Feiring (ed): EH Brock's Injuries of the Brain and Spinal Cord and Their Coverings. New York, Springer, 1974, pp 668–743.
79. Moller F, Andres AH, Langenstein H: Intubating laryngeal mask airway (ILMA) seems to be an ideal device for blind intubation in case of immobile spine. Br J Anaesth 85:493–495, 2000.

80. Schuschnig C, Waltl B, Erlacher W, et al: Intubating laryngeal mask and rapid sequence induction in patients with cervical spine injury. Anaesthesia 54:793–797, 1999.

81. Waltl B, Waltl B, Leitgeb J, et al: Tracheal intubation and cervical spine excursion: Direct laryngoscopy vs intubating laryngeal mask. Anaesthesia 56:221–226, 2001.

82. Bivins HG, Ford S, Bezmalinovic Z, et al: The effect of axial traction during orotracheal intubation of the trauma victim with an unstable cervical spine. Ann Emerg Med 17:25–29, 1988.

83. Meyer G, Berman I, Doty D, et al: Hemodynamic responses to acute quadriplegia with or without chest trauma. J Neurosurg 34:168–177, 1971.

84. Troll GF, Dohrmann GJ: Anaesthesia of the spinal cord–injured patient: Cardiovascular problems and their management. Paraplegia 13:162–171, 1975.

85. Rockwell D, Butler AB, Keats TE, Edlich RF: An improved design of the pneumatic counter-pressure trousers. Am J Surg 143:377–379, 1982.

86. Johnson RM, Hart DL, Simmons EF, et al: Cervical orthoses: A study comparing their effectiveness in restricting cervical motion in normal subjects. J Bone Joint Surg Am 59:332–339, 1977.

87. White A, Panjabi M: Clinical Biomechanics of the Spine. Philadelphia, JB Lippincott, 1990.

88. Dunford J: Spinal column trauma. In Baxt W (ed): Trauma: The First Hour. Norwalk, CT, Appleton-Century-Croft, 1984, pp 171–219.

89. Podolsky S, Baraff LJ, Simon RR, et al: Efficacy of cervical spine immobilization methods. J Trauma 23:461–465, 1983.

90. Chesnut R, Marshall L: Early assessment, transport, and management of patients with post-traumatic spinal instability. In Cooper P (ed): Management of Post-traumatic Spinal Instability. Park Ridge, IL, American Association of Neurological Surgeons, 1990, pp 1–17.

91. Boswell H, Dietrich A, Shiels WE, et al: Accuracy of visual determination of neutral position of the immobilized pediatric cervical spine. Pediatr Emerg Care 17:10–14, 2001.

92. Gastel JA, Palumbo MA, Hulstyn MJ, et al: Emergency removal of football equipment: A cadaveric cervical spine injury model. Ann Emerg Med 32:411–417, 1998.

93. Waninger KN: On-field management of potential cervical spine injury in helmeted football players: Leave the helmet on! Clin J Sports Med 8:124–129, 1998.

94. Rumana C, Baskin D: Brown-Sequard syndrome produced by cervical disc herniation: Case report and literature review. Surg Neurol 45:359–361, 1996.

95. Greenberg M: Incomplete spinal cord injuries. In Greenberg M (ed): Handbook of Neurosurgery, 2nd ed. Lakeland, FL, Greenberg Graphics, 1991, pp 495–496.

96. Hughes J, Brownell B: Spinal-cord damage from hyperextension injury in cervical spondylosis. Lancet 1:687–690, 1963.

97. Dai L, Jia L: Central cord injury complicating acute cervical disc herniation in trauma. Spine 25:331–335, discussion 336, 2000.

98. Schneider R, Cherry G, Patek H: The syndrome of acute central cervical spinal cord injury: With special reference to the mechanisms involved in hyperextension injuries of cervical spine. J Neurosurg 11:546–577, 1954.

99. Schneider R, Thompson J, Bebin J: The syndrome of acute central cervical spinal cord injury. J Neurol Neurosurg Psychiatry 21:216–227, 1958.

100. Lifeso RM, Colucci MA: Anterior fusion for rotationally unstable cervical spine fractures. Spine 25:2028–2034, 2000.

101. Black P, Markowitz R: Experimental spinal cord injury in monkeys: Comparison of steroids and local hypothermia. Surg Forum 22:409–411, 1971.

102. Ducker TB, Hamit HF: Experimental treatments of acute spinal cord injury. J Neurosurg 30:693–697, 1969.

103. Faden AI, Jacobs TP, Holaday JW: Opiate antagonist improves neurologic recovery after spinal injury. Science 211:493–494, 1981.

104. Faden AI, Jacobs TP, Mougey E, Holaday JW: Endorphins in experimental spinal injury: Therapeutic effect of naloxone. Ann Neurol 10:326–332, 1981.

105. Fujimoto T, Nakamura T, Ikeda T, Takagi K: Potent protective effects of melatonin on experimental spinal cord injury. Spine 25:769–775, 2000.

106. Kaptanoglu E, Tuncel M, Palaoglu S, et al: Comparison of the effects of melatonin and methylprednisolone in experimental spinal cord injury. J Neurosurg 93(1 Suppl):77–84, 2000.

107. Taskiran D, Tanyalcin T, Sozmen EY, et al: The effects of melatonin on the antioxidant systems in experimental spinal injury. Int J Neurosci 104:63–73, 2000.

108. Ducker TB, Salcman M, Daniell HB: Experimental spinal cord trauma. III. Therapeutic effect of immobilization and pharmacologic agents. Surg Neurol 10:71–76, 1978.

109. Brodkey JS, Richards DE, Blasingame JP, Nulsen FE: Reversible spinal cord trauma in cats: Additive effects of direct pressure and ischemia. J Neurosurg 37:591–593, 1972.

110. Smith AJ, McCreery DB, Bloedel JR, Chou SN: Hyperemia, CO_2 responsiveness, and autoregulation in the white matter following experimental spinal cord injury. J Neurosurg 48:239–251, 1978.

111. Wallace MC, Tator CH: Failure of naloxone to improve spinal cord blood flow and cardiac output after spinal cord injury. Neurosurgery 18:428–432, 1986.

112. Bracken MB, Shepard MJ, Collins WF, et al: A randomized, controlled trial of methylprednisolone or naloxone in the treatment of acute spinal-cord injury: Results of the Second National Acute Spinal Cord Injury Study. N Engl J Med 322:1405–1411, 1990.

113. Anderson DK, Braughler JM, Hall ED, et al: Effects of treatment with U-74006F on neurological outcome following experimental spinal cord injury. J Neurosurg 69:562–567, 1988.

114. Bose B, Osterholm JL, Kalia M: Ganglioside-induced regeneration and reestablishment of axonal continuity in spinal cord-transected rats. Neurosci Lett 63:165–169, 1986.

115. Faden AI, Simon RP: A potential role for excitotoxins in the pathophysiology of spinal cord injury. Ann Neurol 23:623–626, 1988.

116. Fehlings MG, Tator CH, Linden RD: The effect of nimodipine and dextran on axonal function and blood flow following experimental spinal cord injury. J Neurosurg 71:403–416, 1989.

117. Lehmann J, Sills M, Tsai C, et al: Dextromethorphan modulates the NMDA-type receptor-associated ion channel by binding to its closed state. In Cavalheiro E (ed): Frontiers in Excitatory Amino Acid Research. New York, Allan R Liss, 1988, pp 571–578.

118. Martinez-Arizala A, Rigamonti DD, Long JB, et al: Effects of NMDA receptor antagonists following spinal ischemia in the rabbit. Exp Neurol 108:232–240, 1990.

119. Steinberg GK, Saleh J, Kunis D: Delayed treatment with dextromethorphan and dextrorphan reduces cerebral damage after transient focal ischemia. Neurosci Lett 89:193–197, 1988.

120. Hurlbert RJ: Methylprednisolone for acute spinal cord injury: An inappropriate standard of care. J Neurosurg 93(1 Suppl):1–7, 2000.

121. Short DJ, El Masry WS, Jones PW: High dose methylprednisolone in the management of acute spinal cord injury—a systematic review from a clinical perspective. Spinal Cord 38:273–286, 2000.

122. Gulli R, Spaite D, Simon R: The spine. In Gulli R, Spaite D, Simon R (eds): Emergency Orthopedics. Norwalk, CT, Appleton & Lange, 1989, pp 96–104.

123. Harris JH Jr, Edeiken-Monroe B, Kopaniky DR: A practical classification of acute cervical spine injuries. Orthop Clin North Am 17:15–30, 1986.

124. Gehweiler JA, Osborne RL Jr, Becker RF: The Radiology of Vertebral Trauma. Philadelphia, WB Saunders, 1980.

125. Blahd WH Jr, Iserson KV, Bjelland JC: Efficacy of the posttraumatic cross table lateral view of the cervical spine. J Emerg Med 2:243–249, 1985.

126. Gerrelts BD, Petersen EU, Mabry J, Petersen SR: Delayed diagnosis of cervical spine injuries. J Trauma 31:1622–1626, 1991.

127. Mace SE: Emergency evaluation of cervical spine injuries: CT versus plain radiographs. Ann Emerg Med 14:973–975, 1985.

128. Shaffer MA, Doris PE: Limitation of the cross table lateral view in detecting cervical spine injuries: A retrospective analysis. Ann Emerg Med 10:508–513, 1981.

129. Streitwieser DR, Knopp R, Wales LR, et al: Accuracy of standard radiographic views in detecting cervical spine fractures. Ann Emerg Med 12:538–542, 1983.

130. Wojcik WG, Edeiken-Monroe BS, Harris JH Jr: Three-dimensional computed tomography in acute cervical spine trauma: A preliminary report. Skeletal Radiol 16:261–269, 1987.

131. Doris PE, Wilson RA: The next logical step in the emergency radiographic evaluation of cervical spine trauma: The five-view trauma series. J Emerg Med 3:371–385, 1985.

132. Ross S, Schwab CW, David ET, et al: Clearing the cervical spine: Initial radiologic evaluation. J Trauma 27:1055–1060, 1987.

133. Heiden JS, Weiss MH, Rosenberg AW, et al: Management of cervical spinal cord trauma in southern California. J Neurosurg 43:732–736, 1975.

134. Edeiken-Monroe B, Wagner LK, Harris JH Jr: Hyperextension dislocation of the cervical spine. AJR Am J Roentgenol 146:803–808, 1986.

135. Taylor A, Blackwood W: Paraplegia in cervical injuries with normal radiographic appearance. J Bone Joint Surg Br 30:245–248, 1948.

136. Miller MD, Gehweiler JA, Martinez S, et al: Significant new observations on cervical spine trauma. AJR Am J Roentgenol 130:659–663, 1978.

137. Brady WJ, Moghtader J, Cutcher D, et al: ED use of flexion-extension cervical spine radiography in the evaluation of blunt trauma. Am J Emerg Med 17:504–508, 1999.

138. Dwek JR, Chung CB: Radiography of cervical spine injury in children: Are flexion-extension radiographs useful for acute trauma? AJR Am J Roentgenol 174:1617–1619, 2000.

139. Pollack CJ, Hendey G, Martin D, et al: The utility of flexion-extension radiographs of the cervical spine in blunt trauma: Data from the National Emergency X-radiography Utilization Study (NEXUS). Acad Emerg Med 8:488, 2001.

140. Wang JC, Hatch JD, Sandhu HS, et al: Cervical flexion and extension radiographs in acutely injured patients. Clin Orthop 365:111–116, 1999.

141. Galli R, Spaite D, Simon R: In Galli R, Spaite D, Simon R (eds): Emergency Orthopedics. Norwalk, CT, Appleton & Lange, 1989, pp 106–134.

142. Reid D, Henderson R, Saboe L, Miller JD: Etiology and clinical course of missed spine fractures. J Trauma 27:980–986, 1987.

143. Ekong CE, Schwartz ML, Tator CH, et al: Odontoid fracture: Management with early mobilization using the halo device. Neurosurgery 9:631–637, 1981.

144. Cattell HS, Filtzer DL: Pseudosubluxation and other normal variations in the cervical spine in children: A study of one hundred and sixty children. J Bone Joint Surg Am 47:1295–1309, 1965.

145. Keene JS, Goletz TH, Lilleas F, et al: Diagnosis of vertebral fractures: A comparison of conventional radiography, conventional tomography, and computed axial tomography. J Bone Joint Surg Am 64:586–594, 1982.

146. Cacayorin ED, Kieffer SA: Applications and limitations of computed tomography of the spine. Radiol Clin North Am 20:185–206, 1982.

147. Ghoshhajra K, Rao KC: CT in spinal trauma. J Comput Tomogr 4:309–318, 1980.

148. Maravilla KR, Cooper PR, Sklar FH: The influence of thin-section tomography on the treatment of cervical spine injuries. Radiology 127:131–139, 1978.

149. Brant-Zawadzki M, Miller EM, Federle MP: CT in the evaluation of spine trauma. AJR Am J Roentgenol 136:369–375, 1981.

150. Dickman CA, Hadley MN, Browner C, et al: Neurosurgical management of acute atlas-axis combination fractures: A review of 25 cases. J Neurosurg 70:45–49, 1989.

151. Hadley MN, Dickman CA, Browner CM, et al: Acute axis fractures: A review of 229 cases. J Neurosurg 71(5 Pt 1):642–647, 1989.

152. Hadley MN, Dickman CA, Browner CM, et al: Acute traumatic atlas fractures: Management and long term outcome. Neurosurgery 23:31–35, 1988.

153. Allen RL, Perot PL Jr, Gudeman SK: Evaluation of acute non-penetrating cervical spinal cord injuries with CT metrizamide myelography. J Neurosurg 63:510–520, 1985.

154. Cooper PR, Cohen A, Rosiello A, et al: Posterior stabilization of cervical spine fractures and subluxations using plates and screws. Neurosurgery 23:300–306, 1988.

155. Betz RR, Gelman AJ, DeFilipp GJ, et al: Magnetic resonance imaging (MRI) in the evaluation of spinal cord injured children and adolescents. Paraplegia 25:92–99, 1987.

156. Goldberg AL, Rothfus WE, Deeb ZL, et al: The impact of magnetic resonance on the diagnostic evaluation of acute cervicothoracic spinal trauma. Skeletal Radiol 17:89–95, 1988.

157. Hackney DB, Asato R, Joseph PM, et al: Hemorrhage and edema in acute spinal cord compression: Demonstration by MR imaging. Radiology 161:387–390, 1986.

158. Kadoya S, Nakamura T, Kobayashi S, et al: Magnetic resonance imaging of acute spinal cord injury: Report of three cases. Neuroradiology 29:252–255, 1987.

159. Kalfas I, Wilberger J, Goldberg A, et al: Magnetic resonance imaging in acute spinal cord trauma. Neurosurgery 23:295–299, 1988.

160. Pan G, Kulkarni M, MacDougall D, et al: Traumatic epidural hematoma of the cervical spine: Diagnosis with magnetic resonance imaging. J Neurosurg 68:798–801, 1988.

161. Schaefer D, Flanders A, Northrup B, et al: Magnetic resonance imaging of acute cervical spine trauma. Spine 14:1090–1095, 1989.

162. McArdle CB, Crofford MJ, Mirfakhraee M, et al: Surface coil MR of spinal trauma: Preliminary experience. AJNR Am J Neuroradiol 7:885–893, 1986.

163. White P, Seymour R, Powell N: MRI assessment of the prevertebral soft tissues in acute cervical spine trauma. Br J Radiol 72:818–823, 1999.

164. Marar BC: Hyperextension injuries of the cervical spine: The pathogenesis of damage to the spinal cord. J Bone Joint Surg Am 56:1655–1662, 1974.

165. Norrell H: Fractures and dislocations of the spine. In Rothman R, Simeone F (eds): The Spine. Philadelphia, WB Saunders, 1975, pp 529–566.

166. Norton W: Fractures and dislocations of the cervical spine. J Bone Joint Surg Am 44:115–139, 1962.

167. Allen BL Jr, Ferguson RL, Lehmann TR, et al: A mechanistic classification of closed, indirect fractures and dislocations of the lower cervical spine. Spine 7:1–27, 1982.

168. Bauze RJ, Ardran GM: Experimental production of forward dislocation in the human cervical spine. J Bone Joint Surg Br 60:239–245, 1978.

169. Beatson T: Fractures and dislocations of the cervical spine. J Bone Joint Surg Br 45:21, 1963.

170. Gosch HH, Gooding E, Schneider RC: An experimental study of cervical spine and cord injuries. J Trauma 12:570–576, 1972.

171. Maiman DJ, Yoganandan N: Biomechanics of cervical spine trauma: Clinical neurosurgery. In Proceedings of the Congress of Neurological Surgeons. Baltimore, Williams & Wilkins, 1989, pp 543–570.

172. Marar BC: The pattern of neurological damage as an aid to the diagnosis of the mechanism in cervical-spine injuries. J Bone Joint Surg Am 56:1648–1654, 1974.

173. Roaf R: A study of the mechanics of spinal injuries. J Bone Joint Surg Br 42:810–823, 1960.

174. White AA III, Johnson RM, Panjabi MM, et al: Biomechanical analysis of clinical stability in the cervical spine. Clin Orthop 109:85–96, 1975.

175. Yoganandan N, Sances A, Maiman DJ, et al: Experimental spinal injuries with vertical impact. Spine 11:855–860, 1986.

176. Sypert G: Management of lower cervical spinal instability. In Wilkins R (ed): Neurosurgery Update II: Vascular, Spinal, Pediatric, and Functional Neurosurgery. New York, McGraw-Hill, 1991, pp 234–244.

177. Holdsworth F: Fractures, dislocations, and fracture-dislocations of the spine. J Bone Joint Surg Am 52:1534–1551, 1970.

178. Lloyd S: Fracture dislocation of the spine. Med Rec 71:465–470, 1907.

179. Panjabi M, White A, Johnson R: Cervical spine mechanics as a function of transection of components. J Biomech 8:327–336, 1975.

180. Denis F: The three column spine and its significance in the classification of acute thoracolumbar spinal injuries. Spine 8:817–831, 1983.

181. Braakman R, Vinken PJ: Unilateral facet interlocking in the lower cervical spine. J Bone Joint Surg Br 49:249–257, 1967.

182. Evans DK: Anterior cervical subluxation. J Bone Joint Surg Br 58:318–321, 1976.

183. Rothman R, Simeone F: The Spine. Philadelphia, WB Saunders, 1975.

184. Fielding J, Burstein A, Frankel V: The nuchal ligament. Spine 1:3–14, 1976.

185. Werne S: Studies in spontaneous atlas dislocation. Acta Orthop Scand Suppl 23:1–50, 1957.

186. Bailey R: Observation of cervical intervertebral disk lesions in fractures and dislocations. J Bone Joint Surg Am 45:461–470, 1963.

187. Bedbrook G: Are cervical spine fractures ever unstable? J West Pac Orthop Assoc 6:729, 1969.

188. Bedbrook G: Closed injuries of the cervical spine and spinal cord extension-rotation injuries. Proc Veterans Admin Spinal Cord Injury Conf 19:58–59, 1973.

189. Bedbrook G: Compression, flexion and extension injuries of the cervical spine with tetraplegia. Proc Veterans Admin Spinal Cord Injury Conf 19:628, 1973.

190. Munro D: The factors that govern the stability of the spine. Paraplegia 3:219–228, 1966.

191. Wolf J, Johnson R: Cervical orthoses. In TCS Society (ed): The Cervical Spine. Philadelphia, JB Lippincott, 1983, pp 54–61.

192. Hartman JT, Palumbo F, Hill BJ: Cineradiography of the braced normal cervical spine: A comparative study of five commonly used cervical orthoses. Clin Orthop 109:97–102, 1975.

193. Benzel EC, Larson SJ: Recovery of nerve root function after complete quadriplegia from cervical spine fractures. Neurosurgery 19:809–812, 1986.

194. Benzel EC, Larson SJ: Functional recovery after decompressive spine operation for cervical spine fractures. Neurosurgery 20:742–746, 1987.

195. Braakman R, Penning G: Injuries of the cervical spine. In Vinken P, Bruyn G, Braakman R (eds): Handbook of Clinical Neurology: Injuries of Spine and Spinal Cord. Amsterdam, North Holland, 1976, pp 334–335.

196. Cheshire DJ: The stability of the cervical spine following the conservative treatment of fractures and fracture-dislocations. Paraplegia 7:193–203, 1969.

197. Guttmann L: The conservative management of closed injuries of the vertebral column resulting in damage to the spinal cord and spinal roots. In Vinken P, Bruyn G, Braakman R (eds): Handbook of Clinical Neurology: Injuries of the Spine and Spinal Cord. Amsterdam, North Holland, 1975, pp 285–306.

198. Marshall LF, Knowlton S, Garfin SR, et al: Deterioration following spinal cord injury: A multicenter study. J Neurosurg 66:400–404, 1987.

199. Foerster O: Die Leitungsbahnen des Schmerzgefühls und die chirurgische Behandlung der Schmerz-zustände. Berlin, Urban & Schwarzenberg, 1927.

200. Wertheim SB, Bohlman HH: Occipitocervical fusion: Indications, technique, and long-term results in thirteen patients. J Bone Joint Surg Am 69:833–836, 1987.

201. Cone W, Turner W: The treatment of fracture-dislocations of the cervical vertebrae by skeletal traction and fusion. J Bone Joint Surg 19:584–602, 1937.

202. Robinson R, Southwick W: Surgical approaches to the cervical spine. In American Academy of Orthopaedic Surgeons: Instructional Course Lectures. St Louis, CV Mosby, 1960, pp 299–330.

203. Grantham SA, Dick HM, Thompson RC Jr, et al: Occipitocervical arthrodesis: Indications, technic and results. Clin Orthop 65:118–129, 1969.

204. Brattstrom H, Granholm L: Atlanto-axial fusion in rheumatoid arthritis: A new method of fixation with wire and bone cement. Acta Orthop Scand 47:619–628, 1976.

205. Grob D, Dvorak J, Gschwend N, et al: Posterior occipito-cervical fusion in rheumatoid arthritis. Arch Orthop Trauma Surg 110:38–44, 1990.

206. Cooper PR, Cohen W: Evaluation of cervical spinal cord injuries with metrizamide myelography–CT scanning. J Neurosurg 61:281–289, 1984.

207. Heywood AW, Learmonth ID, Thomas M: Internal fixation for occipito-cervical fusion. J Bone Joint Surg Br 70:708–711, 1988.

208. Crooks F, Birkett A: Fractures and dislocations of the cervical spine. Br J Surg 31:252–265, 1944.

209. Itoh T, Tsuji H, Katoh Y, et al: Occipito-cervical fusion reinforced by Luque's segmental spinal instrumentation for rheumatoid diseases. Spine 13:1234–1238, 1988.

210. MacKenzie AI, Uttley D, Marsh HT, et al: Craniocervical stabilization using Luque/Hartshill rectangles. Neurosurgery 26:32–36, 1990.

211. Barbour J: Screw fixation and fractures of the odontoid process. S Aust Chir 5:20–24, 1971.

212. Cybulski GR, Stone JL, Crowell RM, et al: Use of Halifax interlaminar clamps for posterior C1-C2 arthrodesis. Neurosurgery 22:429–431, 1988.

213. Bell C: Surgical observations. Middlesex Hosp J 4:469–470, 1817.

214. Wholey M, Bruwer A, Baker H: The lateral roentgenogram of the neck. Radiology 71:350–356, 1958.

215. Powers B, Miller M, Kramer R, et al: Traumatic anterior atlanto-occipital dislocation. Neurosurgery 4:12–17, 1979.

216. Levine AM, Edwards CC: The management of traumatic spondylolisthesis of the axis. J Bone Joint Surg Am 67:217–226, 1985.

217. Jefferson G: Fracture of the atlas vertebra: Report of four cases, and a review of those previously recorded. Br J Surg 7:407–422, 1920.

218. Anderson LD, D'Alonzo RT: Fractures of the odontoid process of the axis. J Bone Joint Surg Am 56:1663–1674, 1974.

219. Hadley MN, Browner CM, Liu SS, et al: New subtype of acute odontoid fractures (type IIA). Neurosurgery 22(1 Pt 1):67–71, 1988.

220. Subach BR, Monroe MA, Haid RW, et al: Management of acute odontoid fractures with single-screw anterior fixation. Neurosurgery 45:812–819, discussion 819–820, 1999.

221. Dunn ME, Seljeskog EL: Experience in the management of odontoid process injuries: An analysis of 128 cases. Neurosurgery 18:306–310, 1986.

222. Caspar W, Barbier DD, Klara PM: Anterior cervical fusion and Caspar plate stabilization for cervical trauma. Neurosurgery 25:491–502, 1989.

223. Tuite GF, Papadopoulos SM, Sonntag VK: Caspar plate fixation for the treatment of complex hangman's fractures. Neurosurgery 30:761–764, discussion 764–765, 1992.

224. Cramer F, McGowan F: The role of the nucleus pulposus in the pathogenesis of so called "recoil" injuries of the spinal cord. Surg Gynecol Obstet 79:516–521, 1944.

225. Alexander EJ, Davis CJ, Field C: Hyperextension injuries of the cervical spine. Arch Neurol Psychiatry 79:146–150, 1958.

226. Taylor A: The mechanism of injury to the spinal cord in the neck without damage to the vertebral column. J Bone Joint Surg Br 33:543–547, 1951.

227. Ahmann PA, Smith SA, Schwartz JF, et al: Spinal cord infarction due to minor trauma in children. Neurology 25:301–307, 1975.

228. Burke DC: Traumatic spinal paralysis in children. Paraplegia 11:268–276, 1974.

229. Burke DC: Spinal cord trauma in children. Paraplegia 9:1–14, 1971.

230. Cheshire DJ: The paediatric syndrome of traumatic myelopathy without demonstrable vertebral injury. Paraplegia 15:74–85, 1977.

231. Glasauer FE, Cares HL: Traumatic paraplegia in infancy. JAMA 219:38–41, 1972.

232. Hasue M, Hoshino R, Omata S: Cervical spine injuries in children. Fukushima J Med Sci 20:115–123, 1974.

233. Kewalramani LS, Kraus JF, Sterling HM: Acute spinal-cord lesions in a pediatric population: Epidemiological and clinical features. Paraplegia 18:206–219, 1980.

234. Pang D, Wilberger J: Spinal cord injury without radiographic abnormalities in children. J Neurosurg 57:114–129, 1982.

235. Scher A: Cervical spinal cord injury without evidence of fracture or dislocation: An assessment of the radiological features. S Afr Med J 50:962–965, 1976.

236. Sherk HH, Schut L, Lane JM: Fractures and dislocations of the cervical spine in children. Orthop Clin North Am 7:593–604, 1976.

237. Dunlap J, Morris M, Thompson R: Cervical-spine injuries in children. J Bone Joint Surg Am 40:681–686, 1958.

238. Glasauer FE, Cares HL: Biomechanical features of traumatic paraplegia in infancy. J Trauma 13:166–170, 1973.

239. Papavasiliou V: Traumatic subluxation of the cervical spine during childhood. Orthop Clin North Am 9:945–954, 1978.

240. Bailey D: The normal cervical spine in infants and children. Radiology 59:712–719, 1952.

241. Sullivan C, Bruwer A, Harris L: Hypermobility of the cervical spine in children: A pitfall in the diagnosis of cervical dislocation. Am J Surg 95:636–640, 1958.

242. Townsend E, Rowe M: Mobility of the upper cervical spine in health and disease. Pediatrics 10:567–573, 1952.

243. Towbin A: Spinal injury related to the syndrome of sudden death ("crib-death") in infants. Am J Clin Pathol 49:562–567, 1968.

CHAPTER 316

Hyperextension and Hyperflexion Injuries of the Cervical Spine

SETH M. ZEIDMAN

Sprain of the cervical spine is one of the most common spinal injuries following motor vehicle accidents. This type of injury results from a combination of hyperextension and hyperflexion forces with or without applied rotation.[1] These injuries involve the soft tissue structures that surround the cervical spine and can be termed *musculoligamentous cervical sprain* or *strain*. A *sprain* is defined as a soft tissue injury in which individual fibers of the supporting ligament or ligaments are torn or stretched, but the major ligament or ligaments are left intact. The diagnosis excludes fractures or dislocations of the cervical spine as well as intervertebral disk herniation.

Automobile accidents account for the majority of cervical soft tissue injuries. Flexion-extension injuries occur more commonly secondary to rear-impact collisions, which account for more than 40% of all vehicular accidents.[2] Because patients with soft tissue injuries have few physical findings, these injuries are frequently the cause of prolonged disability and litigation. Soft tissue injuries are, however, associated with a wide variety of symptoms, including pain, paresthesias, and headache. The lack of physical findings in association with the high frequency of litigation can make patients with these injuries difficult to diagnose and treat.

HISTORY

Hyperflexion-hyperextension injuries associated with railroad accidents were described in Victorian times.[3, 4] Crowe introduced the term *whiplash* in 1928[5]; he subsequently tried to de-emphasize the use of the term by stating that whiplash "describes only the manner in which a head was moved suddenly to produce a sprain in the neck."[6] Despite Crowe's later emphasis on cervical spine sprain, the term *whiplash* gained rapid and widespread application to a variety of clinical syndromes resulting from automobile accidents. Although *whiplash* is used to describe the mechanism of injury in hyperflexion-hyperextension injuries, it is not a medical diagnosis and does not describe a pathologic condition. It has acquired a connotation of disability among

patients and frequently prejudices a clinician when informed by a patient that the problem is "whiplash." Alternative terms such as *acceleration-deceleration injury* and *cantilever injury* have been suggested, but they have not found favor with either clinicians or the general public.

Despite its unsavory reputation, whiplash has attracted considerable scientific inquiry, and research has dispelled many of the myths and concerns about whiplash. Multiple studies indicate that chronic neck pain after whiplash is not typically psychogenic and that psychological distress is often secondary to the pain. Several scientifically rigorous studies have demonstrated that cervical zygapophyseal joint pain is the most common basis for chronic neck pain after hyperflexion-hyperextension injury.[7, 8] However, controlled diagnostic blocks are necessary to definitively diagnose the condition.

Controversies surrounding hyperflexion-hyperextension have focused on what constitutes the injuring event, the nature of the injury, and the legitimacy of ascribing symptoms to the injury. An impressive body of knowledge exists defining the biomechanics, pathology, and mechanisms producing hyperflexion-hyperextension or so-called whiplash injury.[9, 10]

MECHANISM OF INJURY

The mechanism of all vehicular hyperflexion-hyperextension injuries derives from Newton's first law of motion, which states that "bodies in motion will remain in motion while those at rest will remain at rest unless external forces act upon them." The energy absorbed by the vehicle and its contents increases as a square of the velocity, so that doubling the speed quadruples the energy that must be absorbed. Although modern vehicles are outfitted with safety equipment and support structures designed to absorb the energy of an impact, some portion of the kinetic energy associated with a motor vehicle accident must be transmitted to the occupants. Hyperflexion-hyperextension injury is an inertial response of the body to the forces delivered to it, during which the head and neck undergo an excursion but do not suffer a direct blow. This feature distinguishes whiplash from the other injuring events associated with a motor vehicle accident.

Whether the struck vehicle is totally stopped or moving at a slower rate of speed than the striking vehicle, the body of the injured person is suddenly thrust forward in relation to the head and neck. The initial forces are applied through the vehicle via the seat. Because the head has no direct support, in almost all cases it is extended until it stops, or strikes the headrest. This hyperextension force places stress on the anterior muscles, disk annulus, and anterior longitudinal ligament.

The second force occurs when the initial energy is dissipated and the car stops accelerating. This could be caused by striking an object in front of the vehicle or simply by reaching the point at which maximal excursion occurs. In this part of the event, the head is still unrestrained relative to the body, which should be restrained by the seat belt. The hyperflexion movement stresses or injures posterior structures.

Before 1953, it was hypothesized that the major injuring event in a rear-end collision was forced neck flexion.[11] Research by Severy and colleagues concluded that hyperextension, rather than flexion, was the major injuring force.[12] They used anthropomorphous dummies as well as human volunteers to define the forces generated in experimental rear-end collisions. Accelerometers and high-speed motion-picture techniques provided the investigators with a complete picture of the movement of the body during and immediately after the crash.

At the time of impact, the front car accelerates, and as it does, it imposes acceleration forces on the driver and passengers. The front car reaches the peak rate of speed early, before the occupant is affected. The upper torso is pushed by the seat and accelerates at a rate approximating that of the car. The shoulders reach their peak rate of speed next, and the head reaches its peak last and with greater magnitude than the other parts. It is a continuation of the backward deflection and rotation that produces hyperextension. Head deflection continues until maximal extension occurs. After peak acceleration is reached, the rate of change declines, and the original position is resumed as deflection into flexion follows.

Hohl demonstrated that head action continues until a maximal extension of 122 degrees is reached, which is well beyond the physiologic range of motion of 60 to 75 degrees.[13] Macnab observed that when the head is thrown forward by virtue of its forward acceleration, the force applied stops when the chin hits the chest.[14] Experimental studies also demonstrate that when the head is thrown laterally, lateral flexion movement stops once the head hits the shoulder. In an individual with a healthy cervical spine, this movement is within physiologic limits, and lateral acceleration of the head does not produce significant damage to the neck. In extension-acceleration injuries, however, nothing stops the backward movement until the occiput hits the posterior chest wall. This degree of extension is far beyond the normal range of movement, which explains why extension-acceleration injuries produce more significant damage than other range-of-movement injuries do.

In 1970, Patrick used both volunteers and human cadavers to study hyperflexion and extension injuries.[15] He showed that considerably greater inertial forces can be sustained without injury in the hyperflexion mode than in the hyperextension mode, with maximal angle being the critical factor. McKenzie and Williams confirmed that the forces and the bending movements most likely to cause injury reach their maximum during hyperextension and are of greatest magnitude in the low cervical spine region.[16, 17] Panjabi and colleagues reported that the maximal forces occurring during flexion-extension injuries produce extension, and that these forces are greatest in the C5-6 region.[18] Wickstrom and coworkers demonstrated that the size of the head and neck influences the severity of injury.[19] Patrick's studies also illustrated the value of head restraints in the prevention of injury.[15]

Severy and associates demonstrated that the vertical acceleration of a car struck in the rear by another vehicle moving at 20 miles per hour was 11.7 g downward, followed by 1.0 g upward.[12] The force of the impact elevated the occupants' position by about 3 inches relative to the seat. This vertical component of force is an important consideration in the design of headrests. It was thought that headrests would significantly reduce the incidence of cervical spine injuries when they (or restraints) became mandatory in cars built in the United States after 1969; however, investigators have shown that headrests have reduced the number of cervical spine strain injuries in rear-impact collisions by only 14%.

Several studies have demonstrated relationships between the tendency for injury and both the location of the occupant in the car and the speed of impact. The most severe hyperextension injuries occur at a speed at which the force applied to the seat back by the torso is just below that required to cause the seat back to yield. With greater-impact velocities, the force applied to the seat may be sufficient to cause it to incline to a point at which the forces on the head and neck are more nearly in line with the long axis of the body; a traction rather than an acceleration strain is applied to the neck, and this decreases the danger of hyperextension. In 1969, Cornell Aeronautical Laboratory of Cornell University (Ithaca, NY) analyzed all passenger cars involved in rear-end impacts from July 1968 to evaluate seat failure and the occurrence of flexion-torsion (extension) injuries. The study demonstrated that flexion-torsion (extension) injuries occur with less frequency when the front seat of the automobile fails by bending or breaking.[20]

At speeds of 15 miles per hour, the driver can dampen the acceleration force of impact by bracing against the steering wheel; this maneuver puts the driver in less danger of injury than the front-seat passenger. If the speed of the striking vehicle on impact is greater than 20 miles per hour, the pelvis of the front-seat passenger slides forward in the seat, and the torso reclines. The position of the torso helps prevent hyperextension injury to the head and neck. Because the steering wheel prevents the trunk of the driver from reclining, the driver is at increased risk of hyperextension injury when impact occurs at that speed. Front-seat occupants have a higher incidence of neck injury than do rear-seat passengers in rear-end collisions.

Even new vehicles equipped with airbags do not completely eliminate spinal injury in vehicle trauma. Blacksin cited early patterns of specific airbag-related injury.[21] Significant injury may still occur in frontal collisions even if airbags inflate, and deployment usually does not occur in rear-end collisions. In various side collisions, or when the head or trunk is rotated in relation to the direction of force, other lateral structures can be damaged. The history of the trauma provides valuable information. From an examination of all the forces to the spine in vehicular injury, Severy and associates showed that higher-speed, higher-energy trauma often results in severe structural damage to the spine, pelvis, and extremities.[12] Victims often receive spinal cord injury from the instability created by such trauma. Lower-speed trauma results in more soft tissue and structural support injury.

Many of the initial hypotheses regarding the mechanism of injury need to be reconsidered, because recent experimental work has shown that the movements of the head during a rear-end collision are more complex than previously suspected. Research has illustrated that axial compression and coupled movements resulting in double curvatures of the spine are important and potentially damaging components of cervical spine movement during impact.[18]

Cadaver experiments have demonstrated that the lower cervical spine is thrust upward and forward on impact. The cervical spine is compressed from below, and the lower cervical segments are extended while the upper segments are relatively flexed. As a result, the cervical spine assumes an S shape during the first 50 to 75 msec after impact; after this brief period, segments are progressively thrown backward into extension.[22]

PATHOLOGY

Although animal and cadaver pathology is not totally applicable to the human subject, experiments with animals and cadavers have been invaluable in defining the pathologic mechanisms of these injuries. Severy and associates used animals and cadavers to demonstrate that when muscle injuries occur, they vary from minor tears of the sternocleidomastoid muscle to partial avulsion of the longus colli.[12] Retropharyngeal hemorrhage, laryngeal hyperemia, hemorrhage beneath the posterior longitudinal ligament, and paraspinous muscle hemorrhage were observed. Any tear of the longus colli was associated with a retropharyngeal hematoma and with damage to the cervical sympathetic nerves and the esophagus. The authors reported that brain damage, in addition to spinal cord and nerve root injury, also occurred. Soft tissue injuries

may include articular facet capsular strains, tearing of the interspinous ligaments, and stretching of the longitudinal ligaments. Wickstrom and coworkers used primates to show that the severity of pathologic changes is directly related to the degree of acceleration.[19] They also demonstrated that the injury is most often localized to C4-7, with a smaller area of concentration at C1-2.

Significant information about spinal trauma is provided by acceleration-deceleration injuries. Macnab demonstrated that disk avulsion and variable tears of sternocleidomastoid and longus colli muscles occurred in monkeys in experimental crash conditions.[23, 24] Wickstrom and coworkers reported some brain injury and disk damage as a result of this type of injury.[19]

Several factors suggest that the cause of pain has a scientific basis. Barnsley and colleagues showed that cervical zygapophyseal joints were routinely injured and symptomatic in more than half of their study group, and destruction and degeneration of the joints also occurred.[25] Zygapophyseal trauma is a cause of significant long-term pain. Muscle tear and hemorrhage are occasionally visible on acute magnetic resonance imaging (MRI). Facet fracture also may occur from the extremes of motion in flexion and extension.

Joint capsular injuries, together with cartilage and joint tears, have been demonstrated. Bogduk elegantly described block techniques to localize the joints involved; his studies showed that the medial nerve branch block can provide information in cases in which pain is difficult to pinpoint.[7] Jonsson and associates found that there is clear chronicity in a high percentage of cases.[26] The incidence of surgical injury was 2 in 50 cases for posterior ligamentous trauma and 8 in 50 cases for substantial diskogenic pain requiring diskectomy and fusion.

Although studies from 1994 emphasized compression as the principal injury force exerted on the cervical spine, this does not mean that compressive fractures are the expected injury.[27] Axial compression causes abnormal modes of extension. This is evident when extension occurs about an abnormally high axis of rotation and the vertebrae rotate without translation. The rotation of the vertebrae results in abnormal separation of the anterior elements of the neck and abnormal patterns of compression posteriorly.

The anterior structures at risk are the esophagus, anterior longitudinal ligament, anterior cervical muscles, odontoid process, and intervertebral disks. These structures can fail under tension, resulting in muscle, ligament, or disk tears or avulsion of the disk from the vertebral body. The odontoid process bears the weight of the head in extension and may fracture as a consequence. The posterior structures at risk are the spinous processes and the zygapophyseal joints. When extension occurs around an elevated axis of rotation, the zygapophyseal joints do not glide across their supporting articular surfaces. Instead, the inferior articular processes are driven into the superior articular facets, which results in compression fractures of the articular cartilage or the subchondral bone, hemarthroses, or tears in the intra-articular menisci.

When the cervical spine recoils into flexion, compressive forces are applied to the anterior elements of the neck, and tensile forces are applied to the posterior elements. Because they are designed to bear compressive loads, the vertebral bodies are unlikely to fail in compression, but the posterior elements of the spine are susceptible to failure in tension. Under tension, the capsules of the zygapophyseal joints, the ligamenta flava, and the posterior cervical musculature are susceptible to failure.

CLINICAL PRESENTATION

Acceleration-deceleration injury creates a varied but somewhat consistent group of complaints and physical findings. The direction and force of impact affect the nature and extent of injury. The symptoms are dominated by pain in the neck and headache. The second most common symptom is pain in the shoulder girdle, followed by paresthesias and weakness in the upper limbs. Less common and irregularly reported symptoms include dizziness, visual disturbances, and tinnitus. Headache is present in a majority of cases because of cervical muscle injury and intracranial contrecoup injury, which accompanies the acceleration-deceleration force. Loss of consciousness and direct head concussion can occur, especially in side and head-on collisions, but practitioners must be aware that brain injury can occur in adults without direct blows to the head.

Some unusual complaints include hemifacial numbness, unilateral visual disturbance, and auditory symptoms. Recognition of potential nonskeletal symptoms is essential when neurological consultation may be required. When animal studies are considered, this complex is much more understandable, because many studies document the concussion-like effects of the brain injury associated with hypermotion forces. Practitioners must be prepared to understand and treat these symptoms.

SYMPTOMS

Neck Pain

Most complaints occur within 24 hours of injury and include neck pain, stiffness, and motion loss. Neck pain is the most common complaint following cervical spine strain. Neck pain associated with cervical sprain is reported immediately in the 15% to 30% of patients examined in hospital emergency rooms. In nearly half of patients, the symptoms are delayed for more than 24 hours, and on follow-up, at least 60% of patients report stiffness and pain. The pain is perceived over the back of the neck and is either dull or aching in quality. Movement of the neck exacerbates the pain, which may be quite sharp. Neck pain is frequently associated with neck stiffness or restricted movement. Pain may radiate to the head, shoulder, arm, or interscapular region.

Headache

Occipital headache is the second most common complaint. The pain is typically reported to be occipital or suboccipital, radiating anteriorly into the temporal or orbital regions. Some authors have suggested that headache results from concussion, but they provide no convincing evidence to support this opinion. The headache may also derive from cervical sources. Intracranial causes of headache such as hemorrhage or other concurrent injury should be considered and systematically excluded, in addition to cervical causes. It is likely that during the chronic phase of injury the majority of headaches will be cervical in origin. Reassurance and headache relief are often the only appropriate treatment.

Low Back Pain

Some of the later symptoms that can develop include low back pain and upper extremity pain that is nonspinal in origin. Shoulder harness injuries can result in impingement syndrome. Although it has a low incidence, lumbar disk herniation can occur because of traumatic forces across the lumbar spine, especially in lap belt–only vehicles. Emergency treatment focuses on emergency complaints. The gradual development of additional symptoms is most often the result of the patient becoming aware of these symptoms as severe pain lessens with treatment and as use of the injured part increases with postaccident activity.

Arm Pain, Chest Pain, and Paresthesia

Various paresthesias, which are usually subjective, are also common complaints after acceleration-deceleration injury. Radiating pain or numbness in the upper extremities, or both, is sometimes described and can be associated with a poor prognosis for recovery. Cervical spine pain with a radicular component to distal sites may occur secondary to stimulation or irritation of deep somatic nerve endings found in joints, bone, and outer layers of a disk itself. Injuries to disk and ligamentous structures and to joints of the cervical spine may produce pain by stimulating somatic nerve endings. C fibers have nerve endings in facet joint capsules, outer layers of the annulus fibrosus, and anterior and posterior longitudinal ligaments. Innervation of bone travels with the vascular supply. Based on the pathologic changes demonstrated in primate studies, it is probable that with distortion of soft tissue structures (e.g., disks, longitudinal ligaments, joint capsules), hyperextension-hyperflexion injuries stimulate the C fibers and produce a pain syndrome.

Temporomandibular Joint Pain

Many patients with flexion-extension injuries develop signs and symptoms of temporomandibular joint disease. Epstein reported an association between headache, neck pain, and ear-related complaints and temporomandibular joint disease.[28] In hyperextension injuries, the mechanism of injury to the masticatory structure is believed to be rapid and excessive opening of the mouth, which may occur because the lower jaw does not keep up with the head movement during injury. This jaw opening results in stretching of the ligaments and other soft tissues and may cause intracapsular signs and symptoms as well as muscular pain.

Chrisman and Gervais reported otolaryngologic symptoms, with tinnitus being the most common complaint in 25% of patients with such injuries.[29] Also, dysphasia can develop in association with a retropharyngeal hematoma.[30]

Disk Herniation

Although acute disk herniation from a hyperextension injury is seldom seen, patients with ongoing neck pain and paresthesia, especially that associated with radicular pain to the shoulder or upper extremity, must be differentiated from patients with cervical disk herniation. A patient with an acutely herniated disk usually has radicular pain in the upper extremities and may have focal muscle weakness and dermatomal sensory loss in the upper extremity or hand. In acute cervical disk herniation, lateral flexion of the head toward the side of the pain usually increases radicular pain, because this motion aggravates the irritated nerve root by further decreasing the size of the intervertebral foramen. The sternocleidomastoid muscle and portions of the trapezius muscle are more likely to be inflamed and therefore more focally tender to palpation in patients with hyperextension injuries. MRI is frequently the most reliable method of excluding disk herniation in a patient with chronic neck and radicular pain. In the initial evaluation of patients after hyperextension injury, it is important to obtain the details of the accident, such as whether seat belts or head restraints (whether fixed or adjustable) were used, the position of the vehicle, the manufacturer of the vehicle, the direction of impact to the vehicle, and the speed of the striking vehicle. The time of onset and the location of pain help determine the severity of the injury and the prognosis for recovery.

Memory and Concentration Difficulties

Disturbances of memory or concentration are common among patients with whiplash but are not widely appreciated in the general community. Headache and mentation problems following a concussion can present a confusing picture that frustrates the patient and the doctor. It is easy to understand that loss of memory and difficulty with thought processes are frightening. The psychological trauma is aggravated when the doctor treats the patient with a high degree of skepticism. Whether these injuries may cause cerebral dysfunction remains a subject of controversy. In separate studies, Ettlin and Radanov and their respective coworkers evaluated questionnaires completed by patients who had sustained this type of injury.[31, 32] Both groups found evidence of some cognitive impairment and concluded that the impairment had some effect on the predicted outcome. Although MRI studies of the head and brainstem auditory evoked potentials were normal in all these patients, electroencephalographic findings were abnormal in 30% to 50% of injured patients. However, the mild overall slowing of waveforms found in 10% to 15% of normal subjects casts doubt on the significance of these findings.

PROGNOSIS

Symptoms after whiplash-associated injuries are common. Most patients recover within weeks to months, with little clinically significant recovery occurring after 1 to 2 years following injury. Studies indicate that more than 25% of patients experience ongoing symptoms, with approximately one third of these symptoms being severe, constant, or both. Despite the association of multiple factors with outcome, our ability to predict outcome in individual patients remains limited and deserves further study and refinement. Injury severity appears to be important but is often difficult to quantify. Acceleration-hyperextension injuries present a perplexing problem for the clinician who must evaluate them and formulate an accurate prognosis. The incidence of litigation on the part of injured parties is high, and the intensity of complaints is usually accompanied by few, if any, objective findings. Greenfield and Ilfeld reported that shoulder pain, arm pain, and hand pain equate with a prognosis of slower recovery and that upper back and intrascapular pain is associated with even longer periods of recovery and more intensive treatments. The average length of treatment reported was about 7 weeks, with 37% of patients remaining asymptomatic after this period.

In 1990, Gargan and Bannister[33] carried out one of the longest follow-up studies of whiplash injuries, based on a report by Norris and Watt[34] of 61 consecutive patients with soft tissue injuries of the neck seen between September 1977 and May 1980. Gargan and Bannister reviewed 43 of the same 61 patients 8 to 12 years after injury. Twelve percent were free of discomfort and considered their recovery complete. Work and leisure activities were not affected in the 45% who continued to have mild symptoms. Work and leisure activities were affected in 28% with severe symptoms, and these patients required analgesics, orthoses, or physical therapy. Of the patients with severe problems, 12% lost their jobs and continued their use of analgesics, orthoses, and other therapies.[35]

The incidence of disk degeneration appears to increase following hyperextension injuries to the cervical spine. The rate of degenerative disk disease is well illustrated by Hohl, who followed 146 patients for 4 years after hyperextension injury.[13] He found that 25% of patients 30 to 40 years old and 39% of patients 40 to 50 years old developed degenerative disk disease after hyperextension injury. The frequency of degenerative changes in uninjured, asymptomatic patients in the same age groups should be no greater than 6% and 25%, respectively. Although Hohl found no statistical correlation between the development of postinjury degenerative changes and the continuation of symptoms, Gargan and Bannister concluded that preexisting degenerative changes, no matter how slight, did appear to affect the prognosis.[13, 33, 35–37]

EFFECT OF LITIGATION

The effect of litigation is the most controversial aspect of hyperextension injuries, and litigation can influence the long-term prognosis. When a patient's chronic neck pain is not relieved by any mode of treatment or within a reasonable time, the physician is inclined to assume that the patient may be seeking personal gain by litigation or that the patient is "neurotic." In contrast to the evidence in support of painful, organic lesions in whiplash patients, there is little more than speculation and anecdote to suggest that symptoms are due to "litigation neurosis." The issue is complicated, because some authors contend that exaggerated complaints of pain and injury are made to secure financial gain.

In 1956, Gotten assessed 100 patients with "whiplash injury" after the settlement of litigation.[38] Of the 100 patients studied, 88 recovered after their litigation was settled; of these, 54 had no residual symptoms, and 34 had minor symptoms not requiring therapy. Twelve patients continued to have severe symptoms. Gotten concluded from this study that the potential for personal gain was a powerful instrument in influencing recovery from whiplash injury. This study has been criticized because it was conducted with a nonvalidated questionnaire administered by a single individual. Gotten contacted only 100 of 219 potential subjects, and because no data from a control group were included in the evaluation, the natural tendency for patients to improve spontaneously in the first few months after injury was not considered. Finally, many of the conclusions are based on anecdotes and opinions of the interrogator administering the questionnaire.

Mendelson analyzed 10 long-term studies of chronic pain and injury and observed that all included a significant proportion of patients who continued to manifest symptoms and remain unemployed, despite the settlement of legal claims.[39] In another comprehensive study, Hohl found that 43% of 146 patients followed for 5 years or longer still had significant permanent disability.[13]

In 1966, Macnab reviewed 575 patients with various acceleration injuries sustained in motor vehicle accidents. None of the patients with forward flexion or lateral flexion strains had significant symptoms lasting more than a few weeks.[23] Of 266 patients with extension-acceleration injuries, more than 45% continued to have symptoms 2 or more years after the settlement of litigation. Macnab made two important observations based on the data from these patients: (1) if these symptoms were only neurotic manifestations, it was unclear why a patient would become neurotic if his or her head were thrown backward but not if it were thrown forward or from side to side; and (2) many patients had associated injuries, including broken wrists, sprained ankles, and similar injuries, that

healed and returned to normal function within the expected time. Macnab questioned why a patient's traumatic neurosis should be confined solely to the neck and not involve continued disability from other injuries sustained at the same time.[23]

We need to dispel the notion that litigation or neurosis drives these symptoms. Our knowledge of pain generation in the spine is too great to simply dismiss pain as unfounded or for secondary gain. Long-term follow-up series all support the fact that symptoms resolve with a combination of time, exercise, and treatment in the majority of patients. Symptoms may extend beyond 12 months regardless of treatment in up to 30% of whiplash victims. Many researchers have demonstrated conclusively that litigation settlement has little effect on symptom resolution despite the older, widely held theory of the "green poultice." Physicians should provide treatment to these patients without prejudice.

Several well-done follow-up studies of whiplash patients reported that the likelihood of chronic symptoms following whiplash injury is entirely independent of litigation.[34, 40, 41] Formal study of litigation or compensation neurosis unearths little evidence in support of the concept but reveals a plethora of reports demonstrating that no difference exists between the recovery of compensation versus noncompensation patients.

No real evidence supports the idea that either malingering for financial gain or preexisting psychosocial factors contribute in any significant way to the natural history of whiplash injury. The unavoidable conclusion is that the majority of whiplash injuries cause organic lesions in genuine patients.

Several studies suggest that patients with more severe injuries are more likely to file compensation claims and have continued symptoms, irrespective of litigation status. These same patients may develop a chronic pain state, and the stress and anxiety of the litigation process itself may complicate and exacerbate their condition. Early settlement, if feasible, may shorten the duration of symptoms and simplify management of the injury. Improvement after the conclusion of litigation does not necessarily represent compensation neurosis but may reflect improvement after the accompanying stress and anxiety are relieved.

IMAGING

Radiographic examination of the cervical spine does not provide additional information unless a major disruption of ligament structures is present, as occurs in more severe injuries. It has been suggested that loss of a normal cervical lordosis indicates muscle spasm, although this loss occurs normally. Studies demonstrate that almost 17% of the normal adult population has some degree of straightening or reversal of cervical lordosis; the supine position and the "military" or "chin-on-chest" position physiologically reverse normal cervical lordosis. It is clear from these studies that a simple reversal of cervical lordosis cannot be reliably interpreted as a sign of neck injury.

MRI of the cervical spine in patients with hyperextension injuries can be of some benefit, in addition to ruling out an acutely herniated intervertebral disk. Although MRI does not show actual muscle tears, it can demonstrate a mass with signal characteristics of recent hemorrhage in the retropharyngeal fascial space. Ligamentous disruptions can also be seen on occasion. The studies of Shea and Panjabi and their respective colleagues demonstrate that the maximal forces during hyperextension injuries are at C4-7; C6-7 receives the greatest impact from these forces and is therefore the most likely site of ruptured anterior longitudinal ligaments and other structures.[18, 42]

TREATMENT

Although many symptoms have been ascribed or attributed to hyperflexion-hyperextension injury, pain is the only one that is commonly and systematically treated, and no clear consensus exists on the treatment of acute neck sprain. The Quebec Task Force on Whiplash-Associated Disorders attempted to synthesize the medical literature available up to September 1993; however, it was unable to provide any meaningful conclusions, stating that the evidence was "sparse and generally of unacceptable quality." Positive articles were so few that even a meta-analysis was not feasible. The task force eventually issued a consensus statement on management, but the risk of consensus is that unproven and ineffective therapies are endorsed and become entrenched as conventional and approved.[43]

Random studies contrasting early mobilization and exercises with orthosis and rest showed a significantly greater reduction in pain and stiffness in the actively treated group at both 4 and 8 weeks. Caution is needed when attempting to draw a valid conclusion about the efficacy of conservative treatment in patients with whiplash injury, however. It appears that "rest makes rusty," whereas active interventions tend to be more effective.[44] When a patient is seen within a few days of an acute cervical strain, however, it seems likely that immobilization of the cervical spine and soft tissue would be helpful to relieve discomfort and allow healing. Cervical traction and vigorous manipulation of the supine would tend to aggravate the situation, and for this reason, use of a soft collar is preferable. Prevention of hyperextension by means of an orthosis is particularly important in a patient with cervical spondylosis and superimposed cervical spine strain, to prevent further damage to nerve roots.

The administration of analgesics, anti-inflammatory drugs, or both and the use of a soft collar that is removed every few hours to allow gentle self-mobilization of the neck are a reasonable compromise to immobilization. As the patient improves, increased activity can be restored. Adequate analgesics should be prescribed for a defined period and with proper precautions. A period of 3 to 6 weeks of intermittent soft collar immobilization and appropriate pharmacologic treatment should resolve most mild to moderate sprains of the cervical spine. It is imperative for the physician to reassure these patients and to stress that

no evidence of fracture, spinal cord damage, or herniated disk exists. The physician should also emphasize that the problem will resolve in a short time, with a return to normal functional activity. One of the most important elements of treatment is to avoid giving patients with this array of problems notions of iatrogenic disability.

Patients with neurological signs and imaging evidence of disk herniation should be evaluated for possible surgical therapy. Surgery is sometimes recommended for patients with continued neck pain after the failure of conservative treatment. In some cases, myelography and diskography have led to surgical procedures such as diskectomy and fusion. The success rate of surgical procedures for neck pain in the absence of radicular pain is uniformly poor and in my opinion has no place in the treatment of acute or chronic cervical spine strain.

A patient with chronic pain syndrome several months after injury is a greater challenge. The cause of discomfort and disability is difficult to determine during this period, and litigation is often involved. At this stage, immobilization is not a factor; rather, the patient should be encouraged to perform range-of-motion exercises and to use traction and other modes of physical therapy. The use of a collar or other methods of immobilization should be discouraged, because prolonged restriction of motion is likely to increase the pain as well as the patient's sense of disability.

In summary, several factors are important in the treatment of whiplash injury:

1. The patient should avoid prolonged immobilization if neither bony nor ligamentous instability is present. Simple analgesics or nonsteroidal anti-inflammatory agents may be used to provide analgesia while the patient undergoes natural recovery, but with the knowledge that the efficacy of these drugs may be no greater than that of placebos.

2. The patient should avoid the prolonged use of habit-forming medications such as carisoprodol (Soma) and hydrocodone (Vicodin). For a number of reasons, these medications, especially when used in combination, create a roadblock to recovery. There is no evidence to justify the use of tranquilizers or tricyclic antidepressants.

3. Prolonged modality-type treatments, especially massage and manipulation, should be avoided in whiplash injury, although both can be beneficial in early, abbreviated courses.

4. In the first 8 weeks after injury, patients with acute neck pain after a hyperflexion-hyperextension injury can be successfully treated with rest and analgesia, but a more rapid resolution of pain might be achieved by the use of ice and passive mobilization. A home exercise program offers just as much chance of rapid resolution and a greater chance of being pain free within 2 years.

5. Traction, electromagnetic therapy, hard collar, transcutaneous electrical nerve stimulation, ultrasound, neck school, spray and stretch, and laser therapy should not be used in the treatment of acute neck pain after hyperextension-hyperflexion injury.

6. If a cost-effective and successful outcome is the goal, a combination of exercise rehabilitation and home treatment, such as mild analgesics and nonsteroidal anti-inflammatory drug therapy, has an extremely high rate of pain reduction and return of function. Expectations of recovery by both the doctor and the patient must be clearly stated and understood early in the treatment course, however.

LONG-TERM OUTCOME

Most patients with vehicular trauma–related pain are successfully treated and have resolution of their symptoms within 6 to 9 months; the rest have a positive resolution by 1 year. Several large series suggest that 15% to 30% of patients with acceleration-deceleration injuries have residual symptoms and pain for years and perhaps permanently. Conditioning and preaccident spinal health may contribute to persistent pain. Severity of disk and ligament injury in a perpetually mobile anatomic structure is the most likely explanation for chronic pain.

CONCLUSION

Motorized transportation and recreational activities that emphasize speed and contact may result in whiplash trauma to the spine. Although seldom life threatening, these injuries are responsible for physician visits and for the consumption of health care dollars. Whiplash patients continue to demand skilled diagnosis, management, and support. Treatment goals include spinal cord and neural protection, pain control, and restoration of function.

Clearly, cases of whiplash that involve "litigation neurosis" and even frank malingering do occur. Immediate dismissal of a patient's complaints as litigation neurosis, however, is a certain recipe for disaster and is unfair to the patient. Studies by Mendelson, Hohl, and Macnab all demonstrated that injuries persist after litigation is settled.[13, 23, 24, 39, 45] Chronic pain syndrome is also seen in patients not involved in litigation.

The term *whiplash* should not be used as a diagnosis. Rather, the diagnosis should be acute cervical strain or sprain or soft tissue injury, particularly because the general public associates whiplash injury with lasting disability and litigation. Treatment of chronic cervical spine strain syndrome requires that the physician provide strong reassurance to the patient, use physical therapy wisely, and scrupulously avoid iatrogenic contribution to the patient's problems.

REFERENCES

1. Grauer JN, Panjabi MM, Cholewicki J, et al: Whiplash produces an S-shaped curvature of the neck with hyperextension at lower levels. Spine 22:2489–2494, 1997.
2. Freeman MD, Croft AC, Rossignol AM, et al: A review and methodologic critique of the literature refuting whiplash syndrome. Spine 24:86–96, 1999.
3. Caplan EM: Trains, brains, and sprains: Railway spine and the origins of psychoneuroses. Bull Hist Med 69:387–419, 1995.
4. Harrington R: The "railway spine" diagnosis and Victorian responses to PTSD. J Psychosom Res 40:11–14, 1996.
5. Crowe: 1928.
6. Newman PK: Whiplash injury. BMJ 301:395–396, 1990.
7. Bogduk N: The anatomical basis for spinal pain syndromes. J Manipulative Physiol Ther 18:603–605, 1995.
8. Bogduk N, Teasell R: Whiplash: The evidence for an organic etiology. Arch Neurol 57:590–591, 2000.
9. Bogduk N, Yoganandan N: Biomechanics of the cervical spine. Part 3. Minor injuries. Clin Biomech 16:267–275, 2001.
10. Davis CG: Rear-end impacts: Vehicle and occupant response. J Manipulative Physiol Ther 21:629–639, 1998.
11. Gay J, Abbott K: Common whiplash injuries of the neck. JAMA 152:1698–1704, 1953.
12. Severy DM, Mathewson JH, Bechtol CO: Controlled automobile rear-end collisions: An investigation of related engineering and medical phenomena. Can Serv Med J 11:727, 1955.
13. Hohl M: Soft tissue injuries of the neck. Clin Orthop 109:42–49, 1975.
14. MacNab I: Acceleration injuries to the cervical spine. J Bone Joint Surg Am 46:1797, 1964.
15. Patrick LM: Studies of hyperextension and hyperflexion injury in volunteers and human cadavers. In Gurdjian ES, Thomas LM (eds): Neckache and Backache: Proceedings Workshop of the American Association of Neurological Surgeons and the National Institutes of Health. Springfield, IL, Charles C Thomas, 1970, pp 92–107.
16. McKenzie JA, Williams JF: The dynamic behaviour of the head and cervical spine during "whiplash." J Biomech 4:477–490, 1971.
17. Williams JF, McKenzie JA: The effect of collision severity on the motion of the head and neck during "whiplash." J Biomech 8: 257–259, 1975.
18. Panjabi MM, Cholewicki J, Nibu K, et al: Simulation of whiplash trauma using whole cervical spine specimens. Spine 23:17–24, 1998.
19. Wickstrom JK, Martinez JL, Rodriguez R Jr: Hyperextension and hyperflexion injuries to the head and neck of primates. In Gurdjian ES, Thomas LM (eds): Neckache and Backache: Proceedings Workshop of the American Association of Neurological Surgeons and the National Institutes of Health. Springfield, IL, Charles C Thomas, 1970, pp 108–117.
20. Kihlberg JK: Flexion-Torsion Neck Injury in Rear Impacts. Buffalo, NY, Cornell Aeronautical Laboratory, 1969.
21. Blacksin MF: Patterns of fracture after air bag deployment. J Trauma 35:840–843, 1993.
22. Panjabi MM, Nibu K, Cholewicki J: Whiplash injuries and the potential for mechanical instability. Eur Spine J 7:484–492, 1998.
23. Macnab I: Whiplash injuries of the neck. Manit Med Rev 46: 172–174, 1966.
24. Macnab I: The "whiplash syndrome." Orthop Clin North Am 2: 389–403, 1971.
25. Barnsley L, Lord SM, Wallis BJ, Bogduk N: The prevalence of chronic cervical zygapophysial joint pain after whiplash. Spine 20:20–25, discussion 26, 1995.
26. Jonsson H, Cesarini K, Sahlstedt B, Rauschning W: Findings and outcome in whiplash-type neck distortions. Spine 19:2733–2743, 1994.
27. Pettersson K, Hildingsson C, Toolanen G, et al: MRI and neurology in acute whiplash trauma: No correlation in prospective examination of 39 cases. Acta Orthop Scand 65:525–528, 1994.
28. Epstein JB: Temporomandibular disorders, facial pain and headache following motor vehicle accidents. J Can Dent Assoc 58: 488–489, 493–495, 1992.
29. Chrisman OD, Gervais RF: Otologic manifestations of the cervical syndrome. Clin Orthop 24:34, 1962.
30. McKay DC, Christensen LV: Whiplash injuries of the temporomandibular joint in motor vehicle accidents: Speculations and facts. J Oral Rehabil 25:731–746, 1998.
31. Ettlin TM, Kischka U, Reichmann S, et al: Cerebral symptoms after whiplash injury of the neck: A prospective clinical and neuropsychological study of whiplash injury. J Neurol Neurosurg Psychiatry 55:943–948, 1992.
32. Radanov BP, Di Stefano G, Schnidrig A, et al: Cognitive function-

ing after common whiplash: A controlled follow-up study. Arch Neurol 50:87–91, 1993.

33. Gargan MF, Bannister GC: Long-term prognosis of soft-tissue injuries of the neck. J Bone Joint Surg Br 72:901–903, 1990.

34. Norris SH, Watt I: The prognosis of neck injuries resulting from rear-end vehicle collisions. J Bone Joint Surg Br 65:608–611, 1983.

35. Gargan M, Bannister G: Soft tissue injuries to the neck. BMJ 303:786, 1991.

36. Gargan MF, Bannister GC: The rate of recovery following whiplash injury. Eur Spine J 3:162–164, 1994.

37. Hohl M: Soft tissue neck injuries—a review. Rev Chir Orthop Reparatrice Appar Mot 76(Suppl 1):15–25, 1990.

38. Gotten N: Survey of 100 cases of whiplash injury after settlement of litigation. JAMA 162:865, 1956.

39. Mendelson G: Not "cured by a verdict": Effect of legal settlement on compensation claimants. Med J Aust 2:132–134, 1982.

40. Maimaris C, Barnes MR, Allen MJ: "Whiplash injuries" of the neck: A retrospective study. Injury 19:393–396, 1988.

41. Pennie B, Agambar L: Patterns of injury and recovery in whiplash. Injury 22:57–59, 1991.

42. Shea M, Wittenberg RH, Edwards WT, et al: In vitro hyperextension injuries in the human cadaveric cervical spine. J Orthop Res 10:911–916, 1992.

43. Spitzer WO, Skovron ML, Salmi LR, et al: Scientific monograph of the Quebec Task Force on Whiplash-Associated Disorders: Redefining "whiplash" and its management. Spine 20(8 Suppl):1S–73S, 1995.

44. Peeters GG, Verhagen AP, de Bie RA, Oostendorp RA: The efficacy of conservative treatment in patients with whiplash injury: A systematic review of clinical trials. Spine 26:E64–E73, 2001.

45. Mendelson G: Follow-up studies of personal injury litigants. Int J Law Psychiatry 7:179–188, 1984.

Treatment of Occipital C1 Injury

DEREK A. TAGGARD ■ VINCENT C. TRAYNELIS

Trauma to components of the occipitoatlantal segment of the craniovertebral junction is common, contributing to approximately 25% of all cervical spine injuries. Associated fractures of the axis frequently occur. The clinical relevance of these injuries has increased markedly over the last few decades. This is due in part to enhanced emergency medical response services and resuscitation. Moreover, advances in imaging modalities have made the diagnosis of craniovertebral junction injury easier and perhaps more common.

Historically, diagnosis of an occipital condyle fracture (OCF) has been uncommon, as they are rarely visible on plain radiographs. Bell provided the first case report of an OCF in 1817.[1] This case was memorable because the patient was well until, at discharge, he reached down to "take up his bundle" and died suddenly. Acute compression of the medulla by the fracture fragment was thought to have caused his demise. In the current era, the common use of computed tomography (CT) as a diagnostic tool in patients with significant craniovertebral trauma has enhanced our ability to diagnose this injury. OCFs are becoming an increasingly common diagnosis.[2, 3]

The craniovertebral junction is often injured in patients who die following trauma to the head or neck.[4–6] Atlanto-occipital dislocation (AOD) is associated with 6% to 8% of all traumatic fatalities.[5, 6] One autopsy series conducted on victims of motor vehicle accidents noted that 9 of 26 patients with cervical spine injuries had sustained AOD, making it the leading injury to the cervical spine in that review.[6] Although frequently fatal, AOD can be expected to account for about 1% of presenting traumatic cervical spine injuries.[7–9] Reports of successful management of AOD with good neurological recovery emphasize the importance of prompt diagnosis and management.

In 1920, Jefferson described the various atlantal fractures through a review of 42 previously reported cases and 4 of his own.[10] The atlas is particularly vulnerable to forces of axial compression. Among cervical spine fracture series, the incidence of traumatic atlantal injuries ranges from 5% to 13%.[9, 11–15] Associated cervical injuries, particularly at C2 and, to a lesser extent, the subaxial spine, are common.[12, 16–18] Neurological morbidity from isolated C1 fractures is rare, and conservative management is generally appropriate for these injuries.

ANATOMY AND BIOMECHANICS

Two separate groups of ligaments maintain the craniovertebral articulation (Fig. 317–1). The articular capsular ligaments, the anterior and posterior atlanto-occipital ligaments, and two lateral atlanto-occipital ligaments attach the cranium to the atlas (C1). The anterior atlanto-occipital ligament is a continuation of the anterior longitudinal ligament, and the posterior atlanto-occipital ligament spans the posterior border of the foramen magnum and the posterior atlantal arch. The cruciate ligament (a longitudinally oriented structure associated with the transverse ligament of the atlas) also contributes to the stability of this articulation.

In addition to the ligaments attaching the skull to the atlas, the cranium is secured directly to the axis. Stability across the craniovertebral junction is provided primarily by this second set of ligaments. These ligaments include the apical dental ligament, the alar ligaments, the tectorial membrane, and the ligamentum nuchae.[19, 20] The apical dental ligament and the ligamentum nuchae contribute only slightly to the stability of the craniovertebral junction.

The alar ligaments are paired structures, each of which has atlantal and occipital components. These ligaments connect the tip of the odontoid to the occipital condyles and the lateral masses of the atlas, respectively.[21] The alar ligaments are the main restraints for axial rotation, with each ligament specifically restricting contralateral axial rotation. Axial rotation across the atlanto-occipital segment is minimal (4.4 to 5.9 degrees), compared with the atlantoaxial articulation (31 to 33 degrees). Isolated incompetence of the alar ligaments results in axial rotation of 10.5 degrees across O-C1 and 33 to 37 degrees across C1-2.[21] This amounts to a 29% increase in axial rotation across O-C1. To a lesser degree, the alar ligaments also limit lateral flexion.[19]

The tectorial membrane (also called the occipitoaxial ligament) runs from the dorsal surface of the odontoid to insert on the ventral surface of the foramen mag-

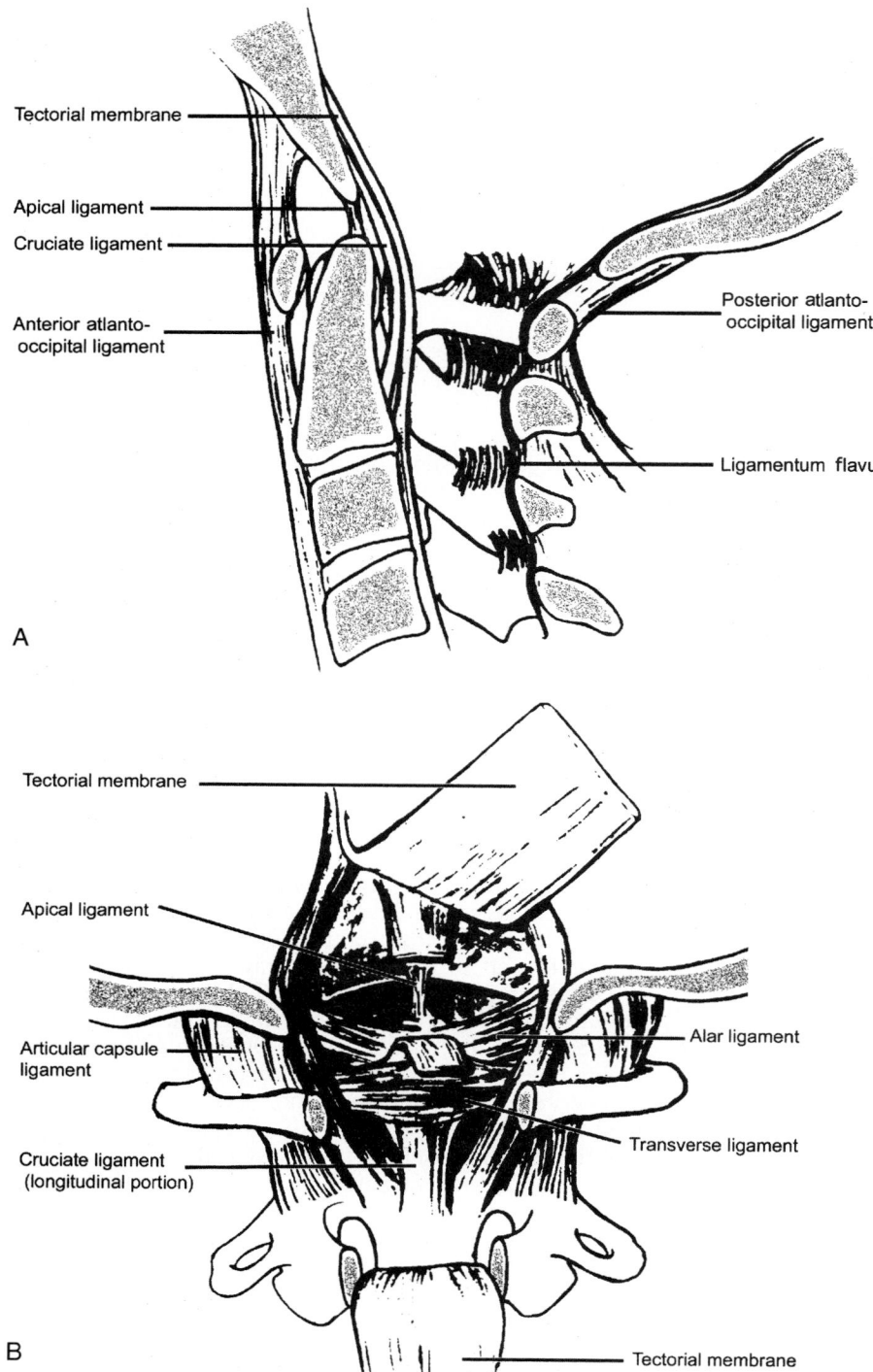

FIGURE 317–1. Lateral *(A)* and posterior *(B)* views of the craniovertebral junction's ligamentous anatomy. Note that the cruciate ligament is composed of horizontal fibers (transverse ligament) and vertical fibers. The tectorial membrane, the rostral extent of the posterior longitudinal ligament, has been sectioned and reflected in *(B)* to allow visualization of deeper structures. © 2000 University of Iowa.

num. It is a continuation of the posterior longitudinal ligament.[22, 23] The tectorial membrane resists hyperextension.[19] If the tectorial membrane is incompetent, contact between the posterior arch of the atlas and the occiput will limit hyperextension.[24, 25] Flexion is restricted by contact of the odontoid process with the anterior foramen magnum.[19]

OCCIPITAL CONDYLE FRACTURES

Clinical Presentation

The clinical presentation of patients with OCFs is variable. Subjects with a preserved sensorium may complain of pain and tenderness in the posterior occipitocervical region.[26] From a neurological standpoint, patients may be intact or have profound deficits, including lower cranial nerve palsies and varying degrees of hemi- or quadriparesis. Frequently, patients with OCF have concomitant head injuries.[3, 27, 28]

The proximity of numerous neurovascular structures to the occipital condyles explains many of the symptoms encountered with this injury. Structures at risk include the brainstem, lower cranial nerves, and venous and arterial vessels. At the base of the occipital condyle, on its anteromedial portion, is the hypoglossal canal. More medially, within the foramen magnum, are the cervicomedullary junction and the vertebral arteries. The jugular foramen is just lateral to the condyle and contains cranial nerves IX, X, and XI, as well as the jugular vein.

Lower cranial nerve palsies occur in nearly a third of patients with OCF.[29] Among patients with such deficits, approximately two thirds have acute deficits, and the rest develop lower cranial nerve dysfunction in a delayed manner.[29] Delayed palsies may occur secondary to bone fragment migration or fibrous tissue proliferation producing an insidious, progressive compression of the lower cranial nerves.[30, 31] Alternatively, progressive edema within the cranial nerves may account for a delayed presentation.[32]

Diagnostic Evaluation

OCFs may be associated with other injuries of the craniovertebral junction but are more commonly isolated injuries.[26–28] As with AOD, the presence of a retropharyngeal hematoma may be the only clue on a plain film that serious craniovertebral insult has occurred. Plain radiographs are inadequate to diagnose an OCF. Tomography or, more commonly, CT provides definitive diagnostic images.[3, 27, 28, 33] Fourteen of 15 cases of OCF at a single institution were diagnosed using bone windows of the head computed tomographic scan, and none were diagnosed on plain radiographs.[33]

Anderson and Montesano proposed an OCF classification scheme in 1988 based on CT morphology, probable mechanisms of injury, and potential for instability (Fig. 317–2).[28] Axial loading produces comminution of

the occipital condyle, with little or no displacement of fragments into the foramen magnum. Such a fracture is classified as type I and is potentially unstable because the ipsilateral alar ligament may be incompetent.[34] However, if the tectorial membrane and contralateral alar ligament are preserved, sufficient ligamentous support may remain to preserve stability. Type II fractures occur as an extension of a linear basilar skull fracture through the occipital condyle. Stability is maintained by intact alar ligaments and tectorial membrane. Excessive loading in rotation or lateral bending can result in condylar avulsion, or a type III OCF. A computed tomographic scan of a type III fracture is presented in Figure 317–3. Similar to type I fractures, the potential for instability exists, particularly because these fractures may be associated with increased load on the tectorial membrane.

Treatment

As an alternative to the radiographic classification of Anderson and Montesano, Tuli and coworkers proposed a management-based classification scheme.[29] Using this method, one first determines whether the condyle is nondisplaced (type I) or displaced (type II). Isolated type I OCFs do not require immobilization. Type II fractures are further subdivided based on demonstration of O–C1-2 instability by conventional radiographic or computed tomographic criteria or evidence of ligamentous disruption on magnetic resonance imaging (MRI). Suggested treatment for stable fractures with intact ligaments (type IIA) is immobilization in a hard collar. If instability or ligamentous disruption is detected, the fracture is classified as type IIB and treated with either a halo vest or internal fixation. Surgical intervention is rare, and conservative management of all isolated OCFs is generally supported, even in cases of brainstem compression with neurological injury.[29, 35]

Outcome assessments are difficult owing to the limited number of cases discussed in the literature, the lack of clinical follow-up in some series, and the variability of fracture descriptions and treatment approaches. In general, patients make reasonable neuro-

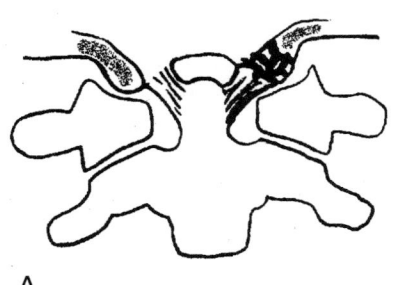 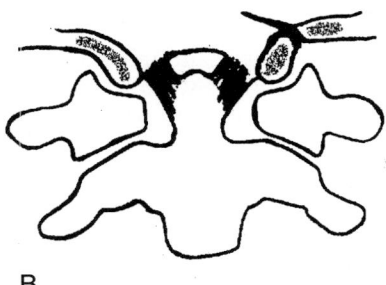 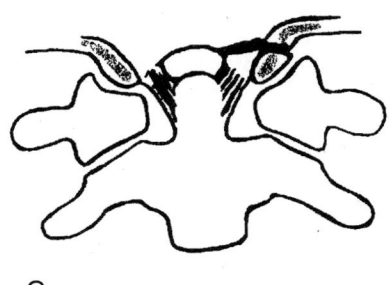

A   **B**   **C**

FIGURE 317–2. Anderson and Montesano's classification of occipital condyle fractures.[28] Comminuted fractures of the condyle with minimal or no displacement of bone fragments are type I fractures *(A)*. Type II fractures *(B)* result from extension of a linear basilar skull fracture into the occipital condyle. A condylar avulsion is a type III fracture *(C)*. © 2000 University of Iowa.

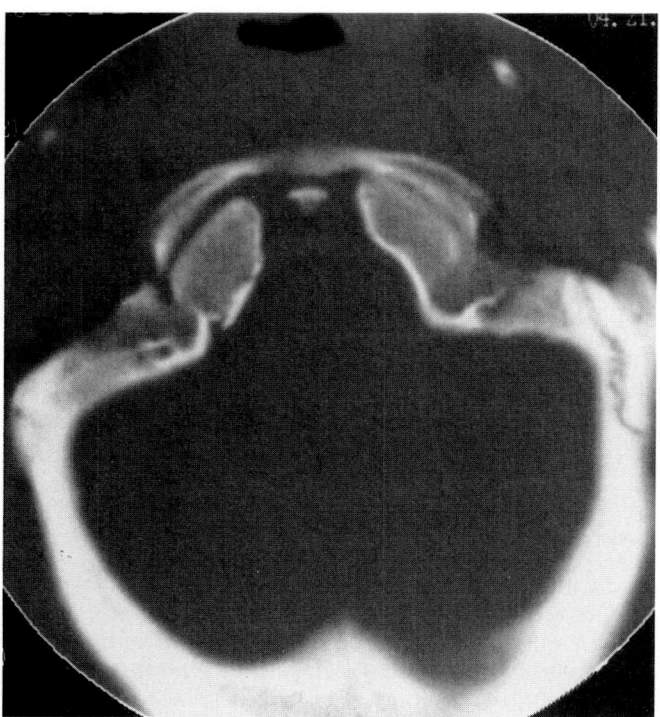

FIGURE 317–3. Axial computed tomographic scan of a type III occipital condyle fracture with minimal displacement of the condyle into the foramen magnum. The outline of the anterior arch of C1 can be seen anterior to the occipital condyles.

logical recoveries, though not necessarily complete.[32, 35] The prognosis of cranial nerve paralysis with a delayed presentation is more favorable than that of an acute presentation.[36] Consistent with other bony injuries, the fractures usually heal well with a conservative approach.

ATLANTO-OCCIPITAL DISLOCATION

Mechanisms of Injury

AOD occurs following complete or near-complete disruption of the ligamentous structures between the occiput and the upper cervical spine. Extreme forces in hyperextension, hyperflexion, or lateral flexion, or in combination, can result in this injury.[37] The most prominent force responsible for producing AOD is hyperextension, resulting in rupture of the tectorial membrane.[24, 36, 38–40] Incompetence of the alar ligaments and tectorial membrane allows for anterior dislocation of the cranium with respect to the upper cervical spine.[19] Other authors have suggested that hyperflexion forces may also be involved in some cases of AOD,[37] based on the observation that the posterior elements of C1 and C2 are commonly separated in the setting of AOD. Another theory focuses on damage to the alar ligaments through extreme lateral flexion.[41–43]

Type I and type II odontoid fractures may result in weakening or disruption of the alar and apical ligaments, as well as compromise of the tectorial membrane.[37] Loss of these supporting structures could substantially weaken the attachment of the skull to the spine, placing an individual at risk for AOD. Interestingly, AOD has been reported to occur in conjunction with type I odontoid fractures.[44]

Children appear to have a greater predisposition for AOD than adults do.[7, 36, 37] This observation may be related to the relatively high incidence of automobile-pedestrian accidents, immaturity of the craniovertebral junction, or both.[19, 37, 45] Several factors contribute to the relative instability of the pediatric craniovertebral junction compared with that of the adult. Before skeletal maturity, the articular plane between the occipital condyles and the atlas is horizontal, and the fossa of the superior facet of C1 is relatively shallow.[45, 46] As the atlanto-occipital segment matures, the mass of the condyles increases, and they become more deeply seated in the superior facets of the atlas. The result of this transition is a more vertically oriented articulation that improves its biomechanical stability. Additionally, the relative stiffness of ligamentous structures increases as one nears adolescence, further enhancing stability.[20, 46] The net effect of these maturational steps is a more stable O-C1 articulation. Finally, the young child's head is disproportionately larger in relation to the rest of the body compared with the adult condition. This may biomechanically predispose to AOD.

Clinical Presentation

High-speed motor vehicle accidents or pedestrian–motor vehicle accidents are the most common causes of AOD.[7, 37] Many other organ systems are at high risk for injury with such high-energy impacts, so a thorough evaluation by a multidisciplinary trauma unit is indicated. Associated head and facial injuries are frequent. Further, patients with craniovertebral injuries have a greater than 25% incidence of noncontiguous spinal fractures.[47]

The clinical examination is commonly confounded by coexistent head injury. Thus, it can be difficult to ascertain which neurological deficits are directly attributable to AOD. Nonetheless, it is known that the brain, brainstem, cranial nerves, spinal cord, and cervical nerve roots may suffer either primary or secondary injury in association with AOD. Conversely, a patient with AOD may be neurologically intact at the time of presentation.[34, 43, 44]

The high mortality rate of AOD is likely related to brainstem injury that occurs at the time of dislocation.[42] Cardiovascular instability and respiratory irregularities are common with brainstem dysfunction, the effects of which are probably magnified in multitrauma patients. Further, patients with complete injures at the cervicomedullary junction or cervical cord above the phrenic nerve likely succumb to respiratory arrest in the field. Another brainstem finding is decerebrate posturing, but again, this may be at least partially attributed to severe head injury. Rarely, a patient's presentation may be consistent with cruciate paralysis.[44] Ocular bobbing is a particularly ominous sign in these patients.[7]

Both cranial and upper cervical nerve root injuries

may occur. The abducent nerve is the most commonly injured cranial nerve, and this tends to occur in patients with coexistent head injury.[38, 41, 43] The lower cranial nerves, IX through XII, are the next most frequently involved. Injury to this latter group may occur as a result of stretching or avulsion when the skull base is separated from the upper cervical spine.[38] Denervation of the carotid bodies due to bilateral cranial nerve IX injuries may result in severe hypertension. Avulsion or stretching of upper cervical roots may result in radiculopathies that must be distinguished from damage to the brachial plexus.[43] Patients who survive AOD can develop pain or deficit in the distribution of the greater occipital nerve.[41]

A high cervical spinal cord injury may cause quadriparesis or quadriplegia; however, patients who survive AOD more commonly present with hemiparesis.[37] Such lateralized findings may result from unilateral pyramidal injury, although more rostral structures in the brainstem may also be involved. A crossed sensory deficit, such as that seen with Brown-Séquard syndrome, may also be present.[42] Quadriplegia is usually associated with complete sensory loss.

Vascular structures are at risk for injury during AOD. Namely, the anterior spinal, vertebral, or carotid arteries may be damaged.[8, 41, 48-50] Particularly in cases of significant subluxation, the vertebral arteries may be sacrificed by compression. In some instances, deficits result solely from vascular compromise and not mechanical damage to the cord.[48] Dissection or thrombosis may result from intimal tears that can be asymptomatic or produce posterior circulation infarctions. Angiography can be an important adjunct in the evaluation and treatment of these injuries.

Diagnostic Evaluation

Frankly obvious vertical displacement of the skull from the cervical spine can yield dramatic plain radiographic findings (Fig. 317–4). However, the alterations due to AOD may be subtle or even absent on initial films.[41-44] Thus, when alignment of bony structures appears to be preserved, one must appreciate suggestive indicators that dislocation has occurred. Moreover, it is important to recognize the essential role of CT in detailing the pathologic findings and the supportive role of MRI.

As with other cervical injuries, an increase in the prevertebral soft tissue shadow should raise the suspicion of serious spinal injury. In the case of AOD, a retropharyngeal hematoma is invariably present (see Fig. 317–4). In a review of 12 cases of AOD, the upper limit of normal prevertebral soft tissue was found to be 15 mm.[51] Laceration of the posterior pharyngeal wall can result in retropharyngeal emphysema.[36, 47] Commonly, the interval between the posterior elements of the atlas and the axis is increased.[37] Several different criteria can be applied to plain lateral cervical radiographs to secure the diagnosis of AOD.

Wackenheim's line can be used to examine the relationship of the occiput, atlas, and axis in the anteroposterior dimension (Fig. 317–5A). The line is drawn as a caudal extension of the posterior surface of the

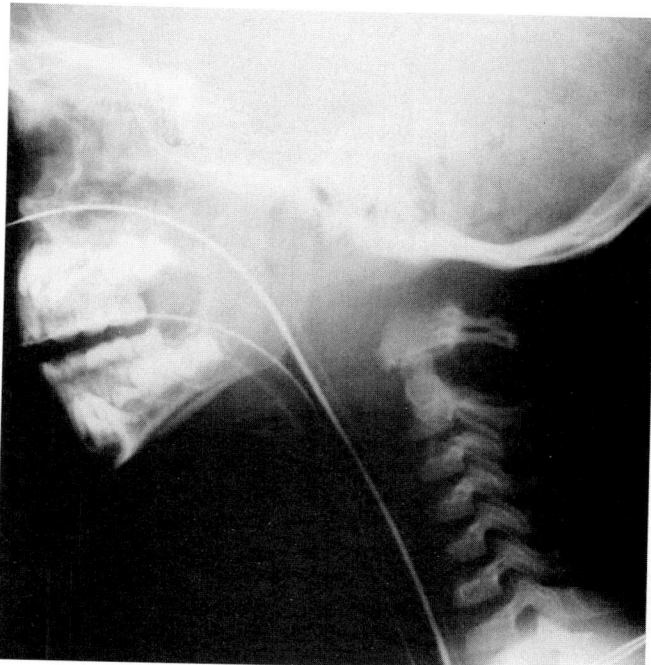

FIGURE 317–4. Lateral radiograph of a 4-year-old boy with atlanto-occipital dislocation. Note the gross separation of the occipital condyles from the atlas, the widening of the posterior elements of C1 and C2, and the abnormal amount of soft tissue anterior to the craniovertebral junction.

clivus in the midsagittal plane.[52] If the sphenoidal portion of the clivus is not straight, the dorsum sellae is ignored and only the lower portion is considered. The basilar line of Wackenheim normally lies tangential to the posterior tip of the odontoid process. With anterior displacement of the occiput relative to the atlantoaxial segment, the line intersects the dens. The line does not intersect any portion of the odontoid process in the case of posterior displacement of the skull. In a normal individual, the relationship between the skull base and the atlantoaxial segment is not altered by flexion or extension.

AOD is simple to diagnose if the distance between the odontoid apex and the basion is grossly increased (see Fig. 317–5B). The upper limit of normal of this distance is controversial. Wholey and colleagues reviewed 600 lateral cervical radiographs and noted that this relationship remained relatively constant in the normal spine.[53] The middle half of the rostral odontoid should lie directly beneath the basion and an average of 5 mm from it. This distance increases to 10 mm in infants. Separation beyond these measurements is abnormal.[52, 53] Measurement of the dens-basion interval should be made with the head in the neutral position, because flexion and extension may alter the distance.[52] The applicability of the dens-basion line was challenged following a review of 100 adult and 50 pediatric cervical spine radiographs in which 85% of individuals exceeded the proposed limits.[8] Powers and associates found no significant difference in the dens-basion distance in children and adults and stated that the mea-

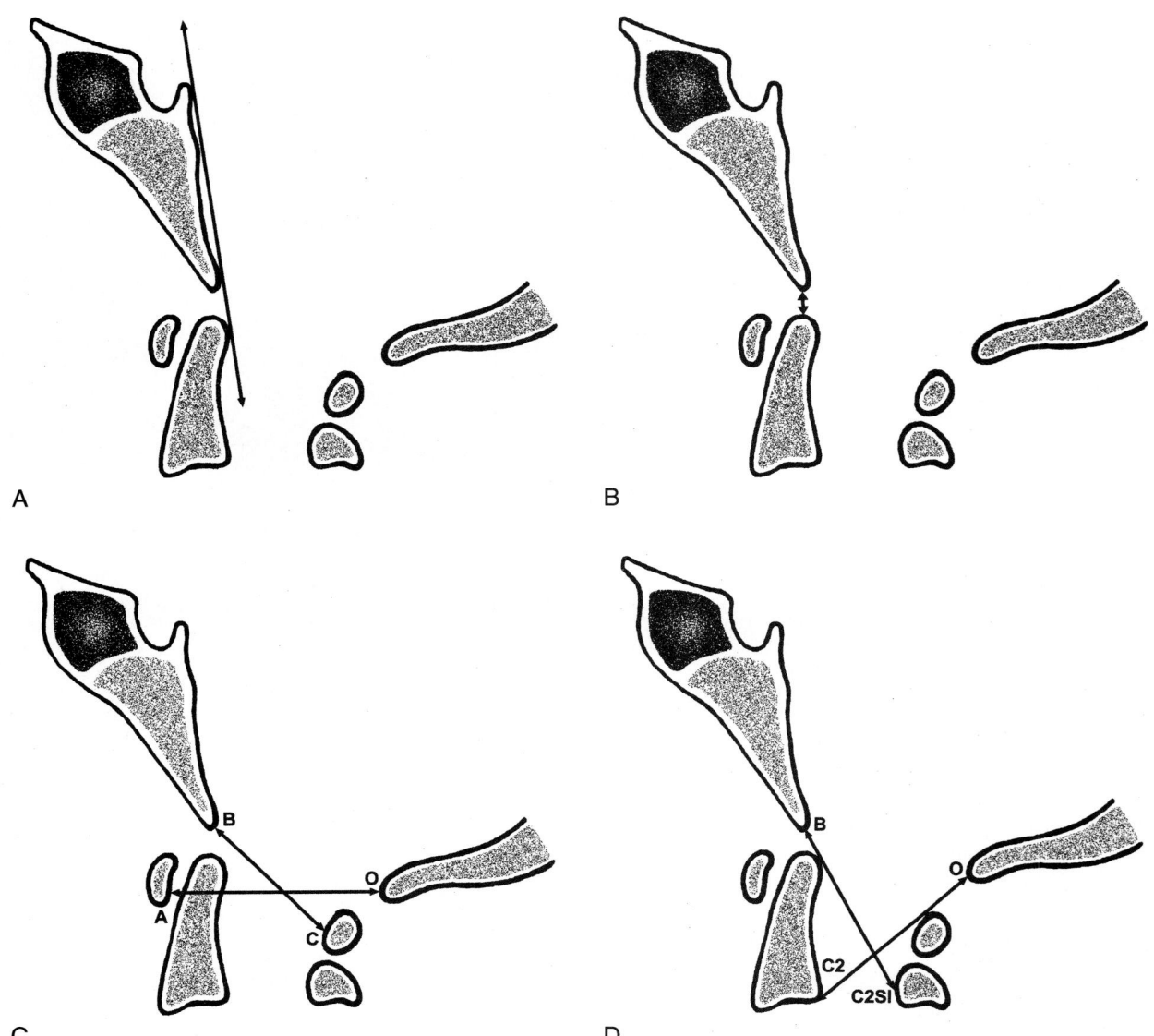

FIGURE 317–5. Schematic diagrams of the craniovertebral junction relationships. The basilar line of Wackenheim *(A)* is drawn as a caudal extension of the clivus and should tangentially intersect the tip of the dens in a normal individual. The dens-basion relationship *(B)* should measure 5 mm in an adult and up to 10 mm in infants. The Powers ratio *(C)* is defined as the distance between the basion (B) and inner surface of the posterior arch of C1 (C) divided by the distance from the opisthion (O) to the inner surface of the anterior arch of C1 (A). The BC/OA ratio in a normal subject is 0.77; a ratio greater than 1.0 indicates atlanto-occipital dislocation. Alteration of the relationships defined by the X-line method *(D)* may indicate atlanto-occipital dislocation. The line between the basion (B) and midpoint of the C2 spinolaminar line (C2Sl) should tangentially intersect the dens. The line defined by the opisthion (O) and the posteroinferior edge of the axis body (C2) should cross the rostral limit of the C1 spinolaminar line. © 2000 University of Iowa.

surement averaged 9 ± 3.6 mm (SD).[8] Based on these observations, these authors estimated that 50% of patients with known AOD might fall within the range spanned by the normal population.

This dissatisfaction with the dens-basion line motivated Powers and associates to define normal craniovertebral relationships using the ratio of two measurements (see Fig. 317–5C).[8] One measurement is the distance between the basion (B) and the inner aspect of the posterior atlantal arch (C), and the other denotes the distance between the opisthion (O) and the inner aspect of the anterior atlantal arch (A). These authors reported a mean BC/OA ratio in normal subjects of 0.77 and suggested that a value greater than 1.0 indicates AOD.[8] Appropriate use of this ratio requires one to accurately identify the opisthion and midpoint of the posterior atlantal arch, which can be difficult. Use of this ratio may be inappropriate in the setting of congenital anomalies or if the atlas is fractured. Additionally, if the occiput is dislocated posteriorly or purely longitudinally, a value greater than 1.0 may be obtained.[51, 54, 55]

In an effort to further improve the sensitivity of plain lateral radiographs in detecting AOD, the X-line method was developed by Lee and coworkers (see Fig. 317–5D).[51] The first line is the distance between the basion and the midpoint of the C2 spinolaminar line (BC2Sl), and the second is the distance from the opisthion to the posteroinferior edge of the axis body (C2O). In those older than 5 years, the BC2Sl should tangentially intersect the posterosuperior aspect of the dens in normal individuals. The C2O line should tangentially cross the most rostral edge of the C1 spinolaminar line. Although one of these relationships may be improperly aligned in normal subjects, alteration of both these relationships should lead one to be highly suspicious of AOD. The originators of the X-line method found it to be more sensitive than the Powers ratio and the dens-basion line as described by Wholey.[53] However, appropriate use of this method requires a normal atlantoaxial relationship—a segment that can be abnormal in more than half the cases of AOD.[37]

Another simple measurement is based on the relationship between the occipital condyle and the atlas. Although not detailed in adult subjects, this interval has been studied in children aged 1 to 15 years. In this group, the interval between the superior facet of C1 and the occipital condyle should not be greater than 5 mm.[54] Either a lateral or an anteroposterior projection can be used to assess this interval.

Certainly, AOD may be obvious without the application of a ratio or the determination of an interval as measured on cervical radiographs. Although each of the aforementioned methods was developed to improve the accuracy of diagnosis, none is sufficiently sensitive to warrant its independent use. Suspicion of AOD requires further imaging. High-resolution CT is an accurate means of diagnosing AOD,[37, 51] and it should include sagittal and coronal reconstructed images. The rim of the foramen magnum and the atlantal arch may produce a "double shadow" effect.[56] The sensitivity of CT can be further enhanced by the administration of intrathecal contrast.[24, 49] MRI can also be useful to evaluate soft tissue structures.

As previously discussed, a significant amount of ligamentous destruction is associated with AOD. CT and, to a lesser degree, plain radiographs can allow one to infer the degree of ligamentous injury when avulsion induces bony damage. The best means of assessing ligamentous and other soft tissue injury is MRI.[57] In a limited number of cases, the diagnosis of AOD has been made solely by MRI findings.[7] An MRI scan of a patient with AOD is presented in Figure 317–6. Adipose tissue, characterized by high-intensity signal, typically surrounds the anterior foramen magnum and rostral odontoid. Replacement of this bright signal with intermediate- to low-intensity signal may be consistent with edema associated with rupture of the adjacent ligaments if AOD is present. Further, edema may be appreciated adjacent to the occipital

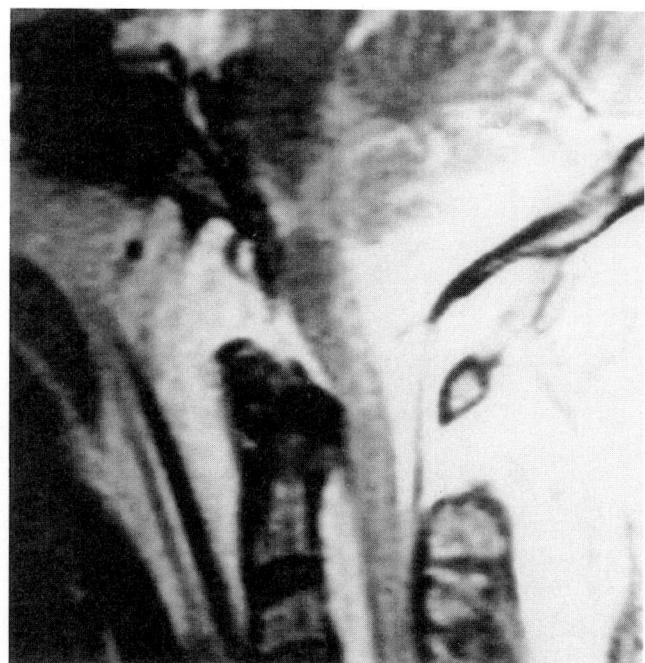

FIGURE 317–6. Sagittal T2-weighted magnetic resonance imaging scan of a patient with atlanto-occipital dislocation. Note the hematoma posterior to the dens, as well as the abnormal relationship between the basion and the odontoid tip.

condyles or lateral masses of C1 in the setting of articular capsular ligament disruption. Acute hemorrhage may be better visualized through techniques that magnify T2 effects, such as TE prolongation or small flip angles. Spinal cord signal abnormalities can be correlated with the clinical examination, and vertebral artery injury or thrombosis may be discovered.[40]

Three specific types of AOD can easily be classified according to the appearance on plain radiographs (Fig. 317–7).[37] A type I dislocation consists of anterior displacement of the occiput with respect to the atlas. Type II is primarily a longitudinal distraction with separation of the occiput from the atlas. Type III AOD exists when the occiput is dislocated in a posterior direction relative to C1. Additionally, rotatory AOD has been described.[7]

Treatment

Maintaining an awareness of the possibility of AOD is critical to making the diagnosis and appropriately treating the patient. A thorough initial evaluation and resuscitation are paramount to obtaining a successful outcome. Adequate pulmonary dynamics and circulatory support, while maintaining the cervical spine in the neutral position, are essential. Delay in providing appropriate respiratory support can lead to secondary ischemic injury to both the brain and the spinal cord. Patients with respiratory distress or who need airway protection should be intubated or, if necessary, have a surgical airway secured through cricothyroidotomy or tracheotomy. In addition to cardiopulmonary support

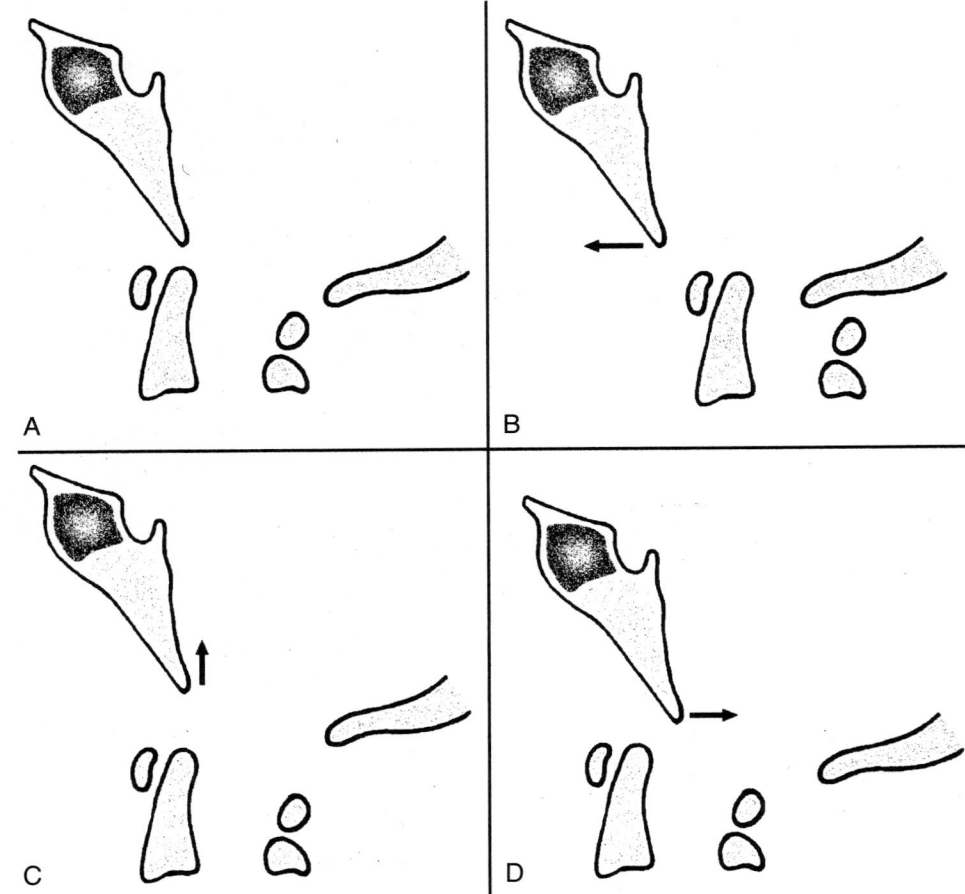

FIGURE 317–7. Classification system of atlanto-occipital dislocation as proposed by Traynelis and coworkers.[37] The normal craniovertebral junction is represented in *(A)*. Type I dislocation *(B)* occurs when the occiput is displaced anteriorly relative to the atlas. Separation of the occiput from the atlas by longitudinal distraction *(C)* results in type II dislocations. Type III dislocations represent posterior displacement of the occiput relative to the atlas *(D)*. © 2000 University of Iowa.

and spinal immobilization, the medical therapy of patients who may have a spinal cord injury includes intravenous methylprednisolone.[58, 59]

A patient with neurological compromise and an extra-axial hematoma, which can occur with AOD,[7] should be strongly considered for emergent decompressive procedures. A posterolateral approach with partial resection of the occipital condyle and, if needed, the lateral mass of C1 can be used for anterior hematomas.[57] Hematomas causing posterior compression may be easily exposed through a laminectomy and posterior occipital craniectomy. It should be noted, however, that surgical hematomas are rare in the setting of AOD.

Controversy exists regarding the use of traction in patients with AOD. Because AOD is a highly unstable injury, some authors have concluded that traction should not be used.[7, 34, 42, 55] However, many such patients have been successfully managed with this maneuver.[8, 38, 39, 41, 43, 44, 49, 50, 60] One must always strive to protect the patient from the onset of new or the worsening of existing neurological deficits. Recognition of the type of dislocation (type I, II, or III, as described

earlier) has been suggested as a means of guiding this decision.[37] Application of traction to a patient with a type II dislocation is contraindicated, because the pathology is primarily a result of longitudinal distraction, which would only be worsened by traction. Even in rotatory subluxations, small amounts of traction have resulted in a dangerous amount of distraction.[7]

Consideration of traction is best reserved for cases of type I (anterior), type III (posterior), and lateral AOD associated with neurological deficit.[37, 60] Application of traction in these situations may serve to decompress the neural elements by realigning the bony structures. Rapid resolution of marked neurological deficits has been documented in such patients treated with traction.[39, 44, 50] A reasonable approach to patients with only minor malalignment or slight neurological deficits is to attempt manual realignment with fluoroscopic guidance. Thus, the use of traction is reserved for cases of grossly abnormal alignment accompanied by significant neurological deficit. The use of fluoroscopy during the initial application of traction in patients with AOD is strongly recommended.

If the decision is made to proceed with traction, application of a halo ring allows optimal manipulation of the traction vector. Total weight of 5 pounds or less is typically sufficient; excessive weight should be avoided. Frequent clinical and radiographic monitoring is essential. Neurological worsening or an increase in distraction or subluxation should prompt a reduction or discontinuation of the traction. Once the end point of improved neurological status or radiographic realignment has been achieved, traction can be reduced to 1 to 2 pounds, or it can be discontinued and the patient immobilized in a halo vest.

As an injury primarily of ligamentous disturbances with severe instability, AOD frequently heals poorly with strictly conservative measures. Although external immobilization in a halo vest has been used successfully to treat this injury, others have reported difficulty in maintaining reduction.[7, 39, 41, 61] It is generally held that this injury is definitively treated with posterior fusion once the patient is medically stable.[7, 34, 37, 61–63] In fact, Dickman and colleagues recommend bypassing traction and performing acute internal reduction and fixation.[7]

The operative exposure for fusion is through a posterior route. Rigid internal fixation should be employed.[7, 61] Although the mobility of the cervical spine may be reduced up to 50%,[64] fusion of the occiput to at least C2 is required. The fusion has been extended to the level of the upper thoracic spine in high-level quadriplegics,[65] but instrumentation of such a large spinal segment may be unnecessary to keep the head erect owing to the spasticity that occurs after a complete spinal cord injury.

Whether due to immediate neurological devastation or other organ system trauma, AOD remains a highly lethal injury. However, patients surviving 48 hours after the traumatic event may have a good outcome. Up to one quarter of surviving patients are ultimately intact neurologically, and in another quarter, only minor neurological deficits remain.[37]

ATLAS FRACTURES

Mechanisms of Injury

Jefferson hypothesized that axial loading was the primary force responsible for C1 fractures.[10] He argued that impaction of the head into the spine would result in multiple fractures of the atlantal ring (classically at four sites), with lateral displacement of the lateral masses. Further refinements of this argument have been made as a result of experimental studies and clinical observations.

The atlas is structurally and functionally unique when compared with the other vertebrae. It is essentially a pair of lateral masses connected by two thin arches of bone—one anteriorly and the other posteriorly. The lengths and cross-sectional anatomy of the anterior and posterior arches are different.[66] Whereas symmetry is conserved about the midsagittal plane, asymmetry is the rule when a coronal plane is applied to the atlas. The anterior arch is shorter than the posterior arch, and both are weakest at the transition point between arch and lateral mass; for the posterior arch, this is the site of the vertebral artery groove. The anterior arch is weakest in the axial plane, and the posterior arch in the sagittal plane. The result is that unequal stresses act on the two arches to cause a variety of fracture patterns, depending on the ultimate force and vector of impaction, craniospinal posture, and physical properties of the spine, such as age.

Compression of the atlas while the neck is hyperextended is likely to result in fractures of the posterior arch. The posterior arch is struck by the occiput or the C2 spinous process and fails in tension.[66]

The ligamentous structure of critical importance in fractures of the atlas is the transverse ligament. It maintains the anatomic relationship between the odontoid and the anterior arch of C1. Atlantal fractures produced by axial loading with and without extension commonly result in injury to the transverse ligament. Avulsion at the site of bony insertion is more common than failure of the midsubstance of the ligament.[67] Injury at either site results in a functionally incompetent structure. As would be expected, the resulting instability is greatest in flexion.[66] Further, failure of the transverse ligament is related to the amount of lateral displacement of the lateral masses.[15, 66] The location of the ligamentous disruption becomes relevant when considering treatment options. Purely ligamentous (i.e., midsubstance) rupture is more difficult to heal with immobilization alone than is an adequately reduced bony avulsion.

Clinical Presentation

In patients who are alert and coherent, complaints of neck pain or stiffness are common. Frequently, patients localize pain to the suboccipital region.[14, 18] This may be due to damage either to the suboccipital nerve of C1 as it courses over the posterior arch or to the greater occipital nerve, which arises from the sensory roots of C2 and passes inferior to the posterior arch and lateral mass junction. Dysphagia may accompany retropharyngeal hematoma formation. Posterior fossa stroke or transient ischemic attack may result from vertebral artery damage.

Motor vehicle accidents are the most commonly reported cause of atlantal fractures.[11, 12, 14, 17, 18, 68] Falls are generally cited as the second most common mechanism,[11, 12, 17, 68] followed by diving injuries.[17, 68] Landells and Van Peteghem defined the biomechanical forces associated with 13 of 35 patients in their series of atlas fractures.[16] Axial loading was the most common mechanism (nine patients). A direct blow to the neck and a fall on the back of the head each occurred twice.

When an isolated C1 fracture is present, neurological deficit is extremely rare.[12, 16, 68] This is thought to be the case because isolated atlantal fractures rarely result in significant canal compromise. When deficit is present, it is nearly always secondary to an associated fracture. Of all associated fractures, the atlas is the most commonly involved. Fractures involving both the atlas and the axis, referred to as complex atlantoaxial fractures, have rates of neurological injury ranging from 12% to 37%.[12, 16, 18] Neurological deficit may also arise from associated closed head injury, which accompanies atlantal fractures in approximately 20% of cases.[12, 68]

Diagnostic Evaluation

Fractures of the atlas can involve the anterior arch, posterior arch, or lateral masses. Landells and Van Peteghem proposed a classification system based on fracture location (Fig. 317–8).[16] Type I fractures are limited to a single arch, either posterior or anterior; isolated anterior arch fractures are rare. Both arches are fractured in a type II injury. One would not expect lateral displacement of the lateral masses in a type I fracture because one arch remains intact; however, this may occur in a type II fracture. Type III fractures involve primarily the lateral mass, although the fracture line may extend into a single arch. The full extent of atlantal injury may not be fully appreciated on standard radiographs. CT is indicated to further delineate fracture details and to look for other occult injuries of the craniovertebral junction.

Landells and Van Peteghem reported on 35 atlantal fractures, noting that type I fractures (*n* = 16) were more common than type II fractures (*n* = 13). Type I fractures (predominantly posterior ring) were much more likely to be associated with axial or subaxial injury and were thus associated with greater neurological morbidity.[16] However, isolated posterior arch fractures are not usually associated with neurological morbidity.[68] Levine and Edwards had nearly identical findings in their series of 34 patients.[68] This later series also noted that a lateral mass fracture may be accompanied by a fracture of the posterior arch on the contralateral side, allowing for unilateral displacement of the fractured lateral mass. Additionally, the prevertebral soft tissue was significantly wider in patients with complex atlantoaxial fractures or type II or type III fractures compared with isolated posterior arch fractures.[68]

In addition to the fracture details of an atlantal injury, the extent of ligamentous injury is critical in determining appropriate treatment. Generally, if the transverse ligament is intact, an atlantal fracture is considered stable. In cases of transverse ligament incompetence, an isolated C1 fracture is considered unstable. Spence and associates, using cadaveric specimens of the craniovertebral junction, cut the anterior and posterior atlantal arches to simulate a C1 burst fracture.[15] Tension was then applied in the lateral direction until the ligament was torn. The study concluded that rupture of the transverse ligament was highly likely if the total lateral displacement of the lateral masses was greater than 6.9 mm. When applied to an open-mouth odontoid radiograph, this measurement should be revised to 8.1 mm, based on the 18% magnification that occurs with standard x-ray techniques.[69] Bony avulsion of the ligament insertion site may be visualized on CT. MRI may also prove helpful in assessing for evidence of ligamentous damage.

Identification of an atlantal fracture must raise the

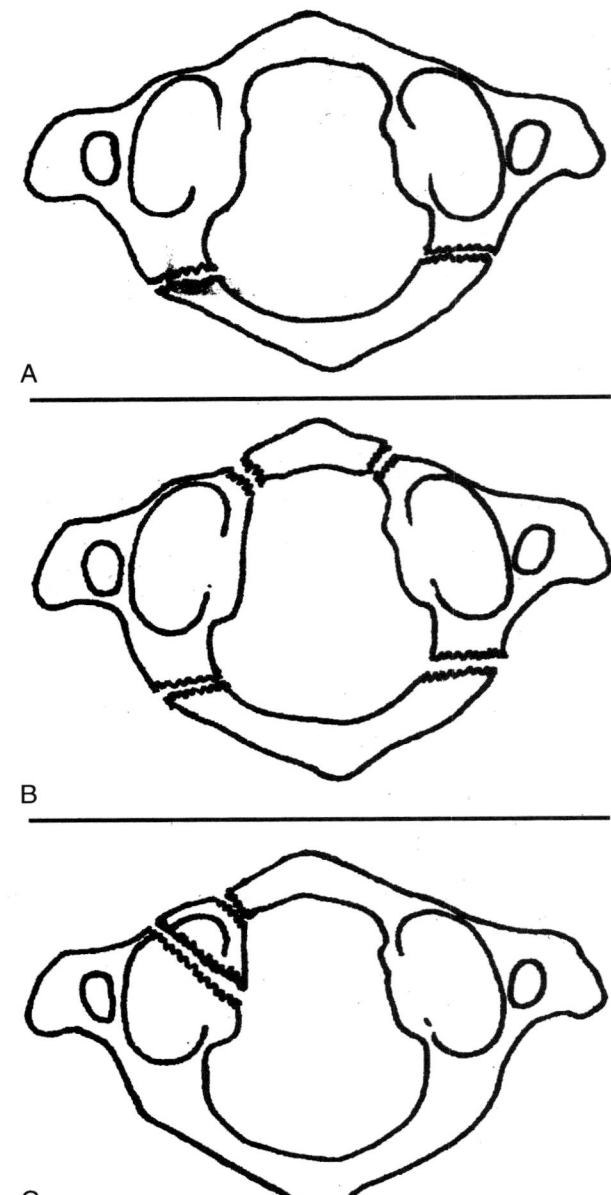

FIGURE 317–8. Classifications of atlantal fractures as proposed by Landells and Van Peteghem.[16] Fractures limited to one arch, most commonly the posterior, constitute a type I fracture *(A)*. A type II fracture *(B)* includes the classic Jefferson's fracture and involves both arches. Fracture of the lateral atlantal mass is classified as type III *(C)* and may or may not include fracture of an arch. © 2000 University of Iowa.

possibility of another fracture. Fractures of the subaxial cervical spine occur in approximately 10% to 20% of cases.[12, 16, 17] Nearly half of C1 fractures are accompanied by fractures of C2; these are termed complex atlantoaxial fractures (Fig. 317–9).[12, 16, 17, 68] The most common associated C2 injury is a type II odontoid fracture, followed by a type III odontoid fracture and a hangman's fracture. As mentioned previously, neurological morbidity is increased and is usually related to the associated fracture.[12, 16, 18]

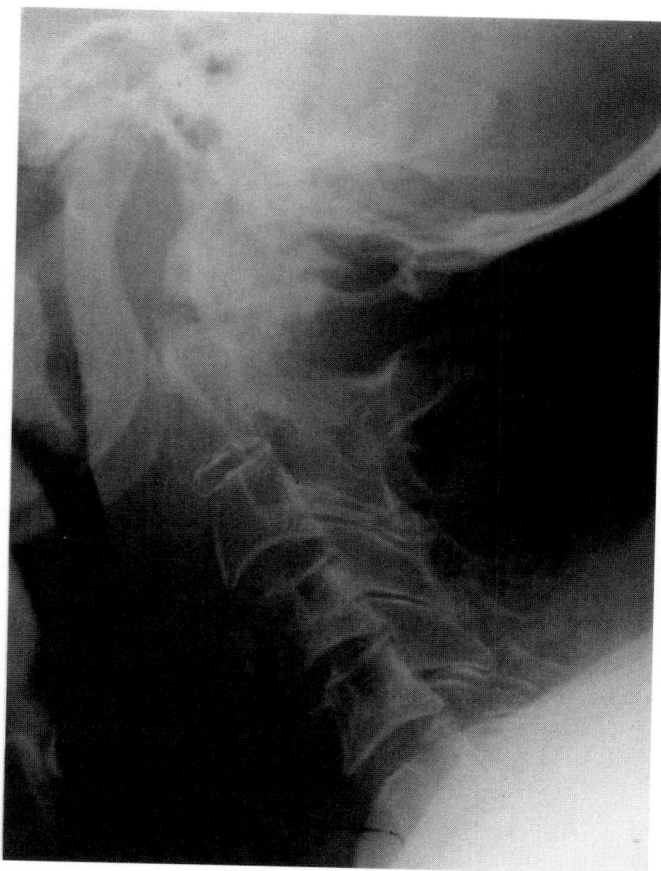

FIGURE 317–9. Lateral cervical radiograph showing a complex atlantoaxial fracture. Fracture of the posterior ring can be seen, as well as a posteriorly displaced type II odontoid fracture.

Treatment

Conservative management is the predominant theme in the treatment of atlantal fractures. More than 90% of C1 fractures, even including complex atlantoaxial fractures, achieve successful fusion with nonoperative strategies.[12, 16, 68] The status of the transverse ligament is a key element in determining appropriate therapy for isolated atlantal fractures. If the ligament is competent, simple external immobilization, such as a semirigid cervical collar for 6 to 8 weeks, generally proves adequate. In this situation, treatment failure is rare.[12, 17, 18]

Rupture of the transverse ligament or avulsion of its insertion site increases the complexity of the injury, resulting in an unstable fracture. Isolated atlantal fractures that are thought to be unstable can generally be treated successfully with halo vest immobilization, usually for 8 to 12 weeks.[12, 69] Surgical intervention can be reserved for nonunion of the fracture or the presence of atlantoaxial instability after an adequate trial of nonoperative management.[13, 14, 16, 69] Some authors have reported early surgery for unstable injuries, particularly in the setting of midsubstance disruption, with successful results.[18, 69]

Management of complex atlantoaxial injuries is based primarily on the type of C2 fracture.[68, 70, 71] Still, the majority of patients are appropriately treated nonoperatively. Reviewing 25 complex atlantoaxial fractures, Dickman and colleagues reported that 20 of 21 patients achieved fusion with either a sternal-occipital-mandibular immobilizer or halo vest immobilization after a median duration of 12 weeks.[70] Four patients had early surgery based on a displaced type II odontoid fracture.

If atlantoaxial instability persists after 8 to 12 weeks' external immobilization in a halo vest due to ligamentous incompetence or fracture nonunion, an operative procedure may be prompted.[13, 68] The benefit of such an approach is that the axial injury may also fuse, thus avoiding surgical morbidity altogether. Further, it can be argued that if the C1 injury is allowed to heal, the occiput does not need to be incorporated into the fusion, thus maintaining the motion segment at O-C1.

Early surgical intervention is valid when the incidence of fracture nonunion is high (e.g., type II odontoid fracture displaced >6 mm)[72] or reduction cannot be maintained because of gross instability.[70, 71] This more aggressive approach has the benefit of likely avoiding halo vest immobilization and may reduce the overall period of convalescence.[71] The operative approach must be tailored to the individual patient. If a posterior route is selected, the occiput will likely need to be incorporated into the construct if the C1 injury is unstable.[70] Alternatively, C1-2 transarticular screws may be used in the setting of an unstable C1 injury to preserve O-C1 motion.[73] Guiot and Fessler operated on 10 patients with complex atlantoaxial fractures with a 100% fusion rate.[71] Eight patients received odontoid screw fixation, two of whom required additional posterior fixation, and two were treated through a posterior route alone.

As a whole, these patients tend to have good outcomes. Reported fusion rates with conservative therapy are excellent. This appears to be true even if the C1 fracture is unstable or if a complex atlantoaxial injury is present. Some patients have chronic neck or suboccipital pain or limited neck movement. Once fracture union is documented, one should obtain dynamic radiographs to ensure that no instability due to ligamentous injury exists despite bony healing.

REFERENCES

1. Bell C: Surgical observations. Middlesex Hosp J 4:469–470, 1817.
2. Blacksin MF, Lee HJ: Frequency and significance of fractures of the upper cervical spine detected by CT in patients with severe neck trauma. AJR Am J Roentgenol 165:1201–1204, 1995.
3. Link TM, Schuierer G, Hufendiek A, et al: Substantial head trauma: Value of routine CT examination of the cervicocranium. Radiology 196:741–745, 1995.
4. Alexander EJ, Davis CHJ, Field CH: Hyperextension injuries of the cervical spine. Arch Neurol Psychiatry 79:146–150, 1958.
5. Bucholz RW, Burkhead WZ, Graham W, et al: Occult cervical spine injuries in fatal traffic accidents. J Trauma Inj Infect Crit Care 19:768–771, 1979.
6. Alker GJ Jr, Oh YS, Leslie EV: High cervical spine and craniocervical junction injuries in fatal traffic accidents: A radiological study. Orthop Clin North Am 9:1003–1010, 1978.
7. Dickman CA, Papadopoulos SM, Sonntag VK, et al: Traumatic

occipitoatlantal dislocations [review]. J Spinal Disord 6:300–313, 1993.

8. Powers B, Miller MD, Kramer RS, et al: Traumatic anterior atlanto-occipital dislocation. Neurosurgery 4:12–17, 1979.

9. Bohlman HH: Acute fractures and dislocations of the cervical spine: An analysis of three hundred hospitalized patients and review of the literature. J Bone Joint Surg Am 61:1119–1142, 1979.

10. Jefferson G: Fracture of the atlas vertebra: Report of four cases and a review of those previously recorded. Br J Surg 7:407–422, 1920.

11. Fowler JL, Sandhu A, Fraser RD: A review of fractures of the atlas vertebra [review]. J Spinal Disord 3:19–24, 1990.

12. Hadley MN, Dickman CA, Browner CM, et al: Acute traumatic atlas fractures: Management and long term outcome. Neurosurgery 23:31–35, 1988.

13. Lipson SJ: Fractures of the atlas associated with fractures of the odontoid process and transverse ligament ruptures. J Bone Joint Surg Am 59:940–943, 1977.

14. Sherk HH, Nicholson JT: Fractures of the atlas. J Bone Joint Surg Am 52:1017–1024, 1970.

15. Spence KF Jr, Decker S, Sell KW: Bursting atlantal fracture associated with rupture of the transverse ligament. J Bone Joint Surg Am 52:543–549, 1970.

16. Landells CD, Van Peteghem PK: Fractures of the atlas: Classification, treatment and morbidity. Spine 13:450–452, 1988.

17. Lee TT, Green BA, Petrin DR: Treatment of stable burst fracture of the atlas (Jefferson fracture) with rigid cervical collar. Spine 23:1963–1967, 1998.

18. Kesterson L, Benzel E, Orrison W, et al: Evaluation and treatment of atlas burst fractures (Jefferson fractures). J Neurosurg 75:213–220, 1991.

19. Werne S: Studies in spontaneous atlas dislocation. Acta Orthop Scand Suppl 23:1–150, 1957.

20. White AA III, Panjabi MM: The clinical biomechanics of the occipitoatlantoaxial complex. Orthop Clin North Am 9:867–878, 1978.

21. Dvorak J, Schneider E, Saldinger P, et al: Biomechanics of the craniocervical region: The alar and transverse ligaments. J Orthop Res 6:452–461, 1988.

22. Wiesel S, Kraus D, Rothman RH: Atlanto-occipital hypermobility. Orthop Clin North Am 9:969–972, 1978.

23. Wiesel SW, Rothman RH: Occipitoatlantal hypermobility. Spine 4:187–191, 1979.

24. Cohen A, Hirsch M, Katz M, et al: Traumatic atlanto-occipital dislocation in children: Review and report of five cases [review]. Pediatr Emerg Care 7:24–27, 1991.

25. Harris MB, Duval MJ, Davis JA Jr, et al: Anatomical and roentgenographic features of atlantooccipital instability. J Spinal Disord 6:5–10, 1993.

26. Desai SS, Coumas JM, Danylevich A, et al: Fracture of the occipital condyle: Case report and review of the literature. J Trauma Inj Crit Care 30:240–241, 1990.

27. Spencer JA, Yeakley JW, Kaufman HH: Fracture of the occipital condyle. Neurosurgery 15:101–103, 1984.

28. Anderson PA, Montesano PX: Morphology and treatment of occipital condyle fractures. Spine 13:731–736, 1988.

29. Tuli S, Tator CH, Fehlings MG, et al: Occipital condyle fractures [review]. Neurosurgery 41:368–376, 1997.

30. Bolender N, Cromwell LD, Wendling L: Fracture of the occipital condyle. AJR Am J Roentgenol 131:729–731, 1978.

31. Orbay T, Aykol S, Seckin Z, et al: Late hypoglossal nerve palsy following fracture of the occipital condyle. Surg Neurol 31:402–404, 1989.

32. Urculo E, Arrazola M, Arrazola M Jr, et al: Delayed glossopharyngeal and vagus nerve paralysis following occipital condyle fracture: Case report. J Neurosurg 84:522–525, 1996.

33. Noble ER, Smoker WR: The forgotten condyle: The appearance, morphology, and classification of occipital condyle fractures. AJNR Am J Neuroradiol 17:507–513, 1996.

34. Levine AM, Edwards CC: Traumatic lesions of the occipitoatlantoaxial complex. Clin Orthop 239:53–68, 1989.

35. Young WF, Rosenwasser RH, Getch C, et al: Diagnosis and management of occipital condyle fractures. Neurosurgery 34:257–260, 1994.

36. Bucholz RW, Burkhead WZ: The pathological anatomy of fatal atlanto-occipital dislocations. J Bone Joint Surg Am 61:248–250, 1979.

37. Traynelis VC, Marano GD, Dunker RO, et al: Traumatic atlanto-occipital dislocation: Case report. J Neurosurg 65:863–870, 1986; erratum in J Neurosurg 66:789, 1987.

38. Fruin AH, Pirotte TP: Traumatic atlantooccipital dislocation: Case report. J Neurosurg 46:663–666, 1977.

39. Page CP, Story JL, Wissinger JP, et al: Traumatic atlantooccipital dislocation: Case report. J Neurosurg 39:394–397, 1973.

40. Zampella EJ, Duvall ER, Langford KH: Computed tomography and magnetic resonance imaging in traumatic locked-in syndrome. Neurosurgery 22:591–593, 1988.

41. Gabrielsen TO, Maxwell JA: Traumatic atlanto-occipital dislocation; with case report of a patient who survived. Am J Roentgenol Radium Ther Nucl Med 97:624–629, 1966.

42. Pang D, Wilberger JE Jr: Traumatic atlanto-occipital dislocation with survival: Case report and review. Neurosurgery 7:503–508, 1980.

43. Woodring JH, Selke AC Jr, Duff DE: Traumatic atlantooccipital dislocation with survival. AJR Am J Roentgenol 137:21–24, 1981.

44. Eismont FJ, Bohlman HH: Posterior atlanto-occipital dislocation with fractures of the atlas and odontoid process. J Bone Joint Surg Am 60:397–399, 1978.

45. Englander O: Non-traumatic occipito-atlanto-axial dislocation. Br J Radiol 15:341–345, 1942.

46. Gilles FH, Bina M, Sotrel A: Infantile atlantooccipital instability: The potential danger of extreme extension. Am J Dis Child 133:30–37, 1979.

47. Alker GJ, Oh YS, Leslie EV, et al: Postmortem radiology of head neck injuries in fatal traffic accidents. Radiology 114:611–617, 1975.

48. Lee C, Woodring JH, Walsh JW: Carotid and vertebral artery injury in survivors of atlanto-occipital dislocation: Case reports and literature review [review]. J Trauma Inj Infect Crit Care 31:401–407, 1991.

49. Watridge CB, Orrison WW, Arnold H, et al: Lateral atlantooccipital dislocation: Case report. Neurosurgery 17:345–347, 1985.

50. Evarts CM: Traumatic occipito-atlantal dislocation. J Bone Joint Surg Am 52:1653–1660, 1970.

51. Lee C, Woodring JH, Goldstein SJ, et al: Evaluation of traumatic atlantooccipital dislocations. AJNR Am J Neuroradiol 8:19–26, 1987; see comments.

52. Wackenheim A: Roentgen Diagnosis of the Craniovertebral Region. Berlin, Springer-Verlag, 1974.

53. Wholey JH, Bruwer AJ, Baker HLJ: The lateral roentgenogram of the neck (with comments on the atlanto-odontoid-basion relationship). Radiology 71:350–356, 1958.

54. Kaufman RA, Carroll CD, Buncher CR: Atlantooccipital junction: Standards for measurement in normal children. AJNR Am J Neuroradiol 8:995–999, 1987.

55. Kaufman RA, Dunbar JS, Botsford JA, et al: Traumatic longitudinal atlanto-occipital distraction injuries in children. AJNR Am J Neuroradiol 3:415–419, 1982.

56. Van den Bout AH, Dommisse GF: Traumatic atlantooccipital dislocation. Spine 11:174–176, 1986.

57. Papadopoulos SM, Dickman CA, Sonntag VK, et al: Traumatic atlantooccipital dislocation with survival. Neurosurgery 28:574–579, 1991.

58. Bracken MB, Shepard MJ, Collins WF, et al: A randomized, controlled trial of methylprednisolone or naloxone in the treatment of acute spinal-cord injury: Results of the Second National Acute Spinal Cord Injury Study. N Engl J Med 322:1405–1411, 1990; see comments.

59. Bracken MB, Shepard MJ, Holford TR, et al: Administration of methylprednisolone for 24 or 48 hours or tirilazad mesylate for 48 hours in the treatment of acute spinal cord injury: Results of the Third National Acute Spinal Cord Injury Randomized Controlled Trial. National Acute Spinal Cord Injury Study. JAMA 277:1597–1604, 1997.

60. Jevtich V: Traumatic lateral atlanto-occipital dislocation with spontaneous bony fusion: A case report. Spine 14:123–124, 1989.

61. Belzberg AJ, Tranmer BI: Stabilization of traumatic atlanto-occipital dislocation: Case report [review]. J Neurosurg 75:478–482, 1991.

62. Collalto PM, DeMuth WW, Schwentker EP, et al: Traumatic at-

lanto-occipital dislocation: Case report. J Bone Joint Surg Am 68: 1106–1109, 1986.

63. Montane I, Eismont FJ, Green BA: Traumatic occipitoatlantal dislocation. Spine 16:112–116, 1991.

64. Parke WW: Applied anatomy of the spine. In Rothman RH, Simeone FA (eds): The Spine, 2nd ed. Philadelphia, WB Saunders, 1982, pp 18–51.

65. Zigler JE, Waters RL, Nelson RW, et al: Occipito-cervico-thoracic spine fusion in a patient with occipito-cervical dislocation and survival. Spine 11:645–646, 1986.

66. Panjabi MM, Oda T, Crisco JJ III, et al: Experimental study of atlas injuries. I. Biomechanical analysis of their mechanisms and fracture patterns. Spine 16(10 Suppl):S460–S465, 1991.

67. Segal LS, Grimm JO, Stauffer ES: Non-union of fractures of the atlas. J Bone Joint Surg Am 69:1423–1434, 1987.

68. Levine AM, Edwards CC: Fractures of the atlas. J Bone Joint Surg Am 73:680–691, 1991.

69. Heller JG, Viroslav S, Hudson T: Jefferson fractures: The role of magnification artifact in assessing transverse ligament integrity. J Spinal Disord 6:392–396, 1993.

70. Dickman CA, Hadley MN, Browner C, et al: Neurosurgical management of acute atlas-axis combination fractures: A review of 25 cases. J Neurosurg 70:45–49, 1989.

71. Guiot B, Fessler RG: Complex atlantoaxial fractures. J Neurosurg 91(2 Suppl):139–143, 1999.

72. Hadley MN, Browner C, Sonntag VK: Axis fractures: A comprehensive review of management and treatment in 107 cases. Neurosurgery 17:281–290, 1985.

73. McGuire RA Jr, Harkey HL: Primary treatment of unstable Jefferson's fractures. J Spinal Disord 8:233–236, 1995.

CHAPTER 318

Treatment of Axis Fractures

JULIE E. YORK ■ PAUL KLIMO ■ RONALD I. APFELBAUM

The incidence of cervical spine trauma in the United States exceeds 7000 cases per year, and approximately 20% of these injuries involve the C2 vertebra.[1-3] Most of the injuries are sustained in motor vehicle accidents or falls. It has been estimated that more than 25% of patients with acute C2 fractures die at the scene of the accident; however, neurological morbidity tends to be low among survivors.[4] Axis fractures are most often categorized as odontoid fractures involving the dens, traumatic bilateral spondylolisthesis of the pars interarticularis (hangman's fracture), or miscellaneous axis fractures. This chapter outlines the management of axis fractures.

ANATOMIC AND BIOMECHANICAL CONSIDERATIONS

The axis is often described as a transitional vertebra. The weight of the cranium is transferred through the occipital condyles and lateral masses of C1 to the lateral masses of C2. From there, the weight is transferred anteriorly to the body of C2 and down the spine to the more uniform vertebral bodies of the lower cervical vertebrae.

The unique anatomic features of the atlantoaxial region permit more rotary motion than any other spinal segment while protecting critical neurovascular structures. Special adaptations at this level include the absence of an intervertebral disk at C1-2 and the presence of substantially weaker ligamentous structures relative to those at lower spinal levels. For example, the ligamentum flavum is replaced by a thin, relatively weak atlantoaxial membrane, and the capsular ligaments are relatively lax. The spinal canal is more capacious at C1-2 than anywhere else, and the spinal cord is located close to the instantaneous axis of rotation, which minimizes distortion of the spinal cord during rotation.[5] The odontoid process of C2 is held within the anterior compartment of the C1 ring by the strong transverse ligament. This configuration prevents anteroposterior translation that could potentially injure the spinal cord. All these adaptations permit significant rotation of C1 on C2, which accounts for 50% of the normal rotation possible within the cervical spine.

ODONTOID FRACTURES

Odontoid fractures are the most common type of axis fracture and carry significant risk for a potentially catastrophic spinal cord injury related to atlantoaxial instability.[6] These fractures are usually classified by the method of Anderson and D'Alonzo (Fig. 318–1; Table 318–1).[7] Type I fractures involve the tip of the odontoid and are extremely rare. Type II fractures, which occur across the neck of the odontoid just above the body of C2, are the most common type. These fractures cause instability and are associated with the potential for spinal cord compression from excessive anteroposterior translation. All patients with type II fractures require treatment. Type III fractures occur through the cancellous body of the axis; most heal with external immobilization because the healing potential of this region is excellent.[2, 7–15]

Type I Fractures

Type I fractures account for less than 1% of odontoid fractures and are rarely addressed in the literature. The rarity of this injury precludes a detailed analysis of management and outcome. These injuries are typically considered stable because the fracture is high enough on the dens so that the transverse ligament remains intact. This opinion, however, has been challenged.[16, 17] Several authors suggest that type I odontoid fractures are unstable and should be considered a manifestation of atlanto-occipital dislocation.[18, 19] We recommend obtaining detailed imaging studies, including plain radiographs, computed tomography, or magnetic resonance imaging, to characterize the fracture completely. Flexion-extension films can be used to assess stability and guide management.

Type II Fractures

Type II fractures, in which the fracture passes through the base of the odontoid, are the most common. A subtype, termed type IIA, describes a comminuted fracture involving the base of the odontoid.[20] This subset is thought to be unstable. It heals poorly with immobilization, and early surgical intervention is therefore recommended.

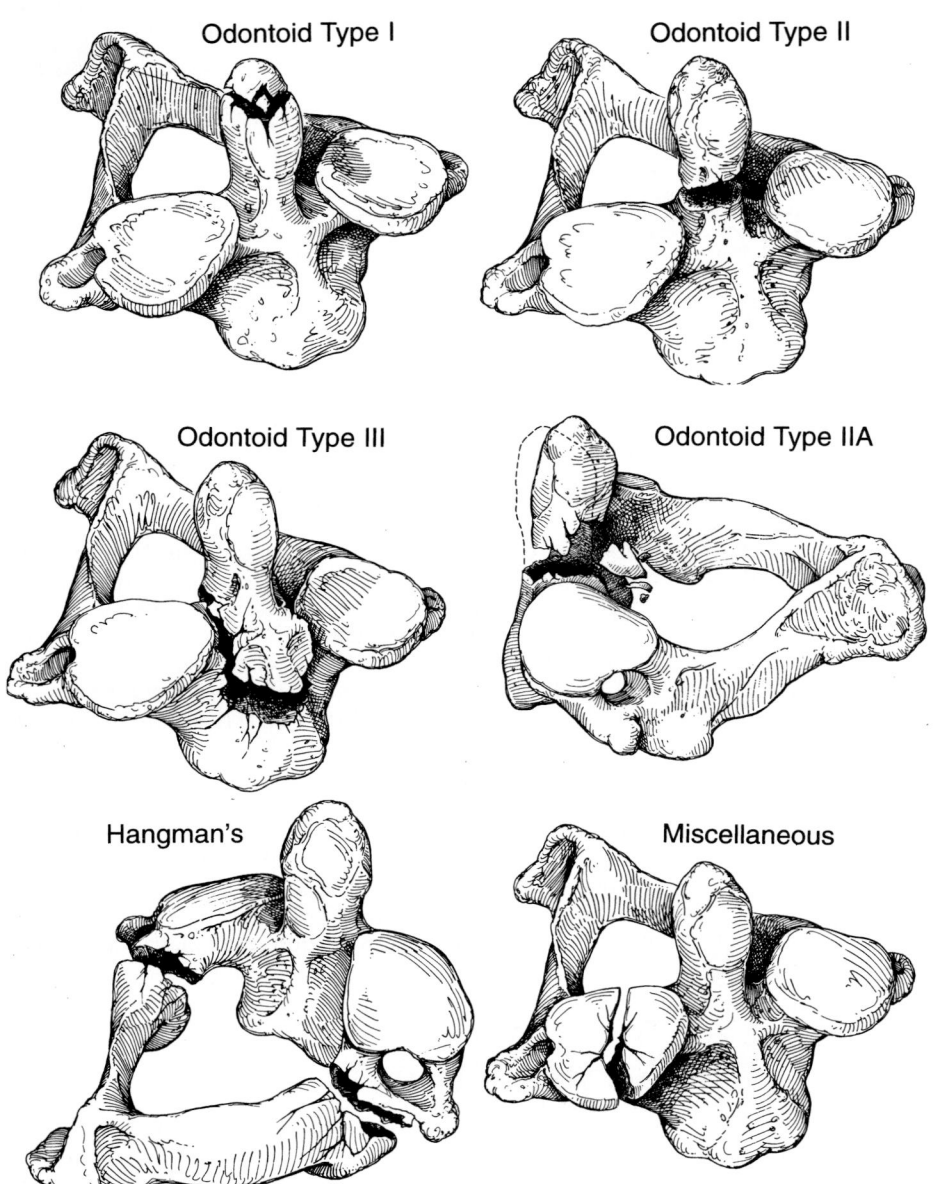

Odontoid Type I   Odontoid Type II

Odontoid Type III   Odontoid Type IIA

Hangman's   Miscellaneous

FIGURE 318–1. Artist's depiction of the major axis fracture types: odontoid fracture types I, II, IIA, and III; hangman's fracture; and miscellaneous axis fractures. (From Greene KA, Dickman CA, Marciano FF, et al: Acute axis fractures. Spine 22:1843–1852, 1997; *type I* from Sonntag VKH, Dickman CA: Treatment of upper cervical spine injuries. In Rea GL [ed]: Neurosurgical Topics Series, Park Ridge, IL, American Association of Neurological Surgeons, 1993; *types II, III, hangman's and miscellaneous* from Hadley MN, Browner C, Sonntag VKH: Miscellaneous fractures of the second cervical vertebra. BNI Quarterly 1:34–39, 1985; *type IIA,* from Hadley MN, Browner CM, Liu SS, et al: New subtype of acute odontoid fractures [type IIA]. Neurosurgery 22:67–71, 1988.)

TABLE 318–1 ■ **Anderson and D'Alonzo's Classification System of Odontoid Fractures**

FRACTURE	FEATURE
Type I	Small oblique avulsion fracture of the superior third of the odontoid
Type II	Fracture at the junction of the dens and the C2 body
Type IIA	Comminuted fracture involving the base of the odontoid
Type III	Fracture that extends into the body of C2 and courses through one or both of the superior articular processes

Modified from Anderson LD, D'Alonzo RT: Fractures of the odontoid process of the axis. J Bone Joint Surg Am 56:1663–1674, 1974.

Historically, the management of type II odontoid fractures has been controversial. Either external immobilization or internal fixation has been advocated to stabilize these fractures. Some authors recommend a period of external immobilization for all patients and reserve surgery for those who fail to achieve a satisfactory bony union. Other authors advocate operative management as the primary treatment modality. Based on an extensive literature search and critical review of the data, it is evident that no consensus exists for the treatment of type II odontoid fractures.[21, 22]

NONSURGICAL MANAGEMENT

Johnson and coworkers[23] demonstrated the superiority of the halo vest over conventional braces for external immobilization of the cervical spine. The halo vest restricts up to 75% of upper cervical spine motion, compared with 45% with conventional braces. The lack of total immobilization may explain the fusion failure rates associated with these devices. There are, however, drawbacks to halo vest immobilization,[7, 10, 16, 24] and the economic and social issues of external bracing must be considered as well. The halo vest greatly restricts patients' activities, usually precludes them from working, requires ongoing medical care, and may be associated with a number of complications, such as pin-site infections, skin deterioration, and skull perforation. Further, even after several months of immobilization, a significant number of patients may still require surgical treatment. Reported nonunion rates with external bracing alone range from 27% to 75%.[2, 8–10, 12–16, 25–33] The high rate of nonunion has prompted an effort to identify specific patient and fracture characteristics that might help guide treatment.

Seybold and Bayley[34] reviewed the functional outcome of patients with dens fractures based on the patient's age and type of fracture. They documented an overall fusion rate of 65% for patients with type II odontoid fractures treated with halo immobilization and found no statistically significant difference in the rate of fusion for patients younger than 60 years and for those older than 60 years. Further, the degree of displacement did not significantly affect the rate of fusion.

Greene and colleagues[35] reviewed their experience with 340 acute axis fractures. They identified two categories of unstable type II fractures that should be seriously considered for early surgical fusion. The first category was composed of patients with dens displacement of 6 mm or greater—the single most significant factor associated with nonunion after nonoperative treatment. The second category was composed of patients with comminuted dens fractures.[20]

In an earlier review by Hadley and coworkers[12] of the initial 107 patients in this group, there was a high incidence of failure after nonsurgical management of patients with more than a 6-mm offset of the odontoid in any direction. They found a 67% nonunion rate in patients with 6-mm or greater subluxation, compared with a 9% nonunion rate in patients with lesser degrees of subluxation. Neither the patient's age nor the direc-

tion of subluxation correlated with the risk of nonunion. In an additional review of 229 patients from this same group, there were similar results.[2]

Bettini and colleagues[32] reviewed 17 patients treated with either a halo or a Minerva brace and found an overall successful fusion rate of 71%. Displacement greater than 2 mm was associated with fusion failure.

Dunn and Seljeskog[9] studied 59 patients with type II odontoid fractures and found that patients older than 65 years had a high risk of nonunion with conservative management. Patients whose odontoid was displaced posteriorly were less likely to heal. The reported rate of nonunion was 70% in patients with retrolisthesis, compared with 30% in patients with anterolisthesis.

Apuzzo and colleagues[26] reported an 88% nonunion rate for patients with more than a 4-mm subluxation, compared with 16% for patients with less than a 4-mm displacement. They also observed a higher rate of nonunion among patients older than 40 years. They concluded that external immobilization was appropriate for all nondisplaced type II odontoid fractures, but patients with fractures displaced more than 4 mm were candidates for early surgical fusion. Their patients were treated with a variety of cervical collars and braces, many of which provided less stability than a halo brace.

In all these reviews (Table 318–2), it appears that greater offset implies greater instability and therefore a lower likelihood of healing when treatment consists of external immobilization alone. It is important to realize that these measurements of offset are essentially a random sampling of any given patient's condition. It would be dangerous to have such unstable patients flex or extend their necks to provide a true measurement of maximal offset. Some patients might therefore appear to have a minimal offset if the radiograph "catches" them in an aligned position. Nonetheless, their instability places them at high risk for failure of conventional immobilization treatment. For example, the alignment of the patient in Figure 318–2A is fairly good, predicting a good chance of healing with immobilization. This patient, however, was grossly unstable, as shown in a radiograph obtained a short time later (see Fig. 318–2B).

T A B L E 3 1 8 – 2 ■ Factors Associated with Nonunion of Type II Odontoid Fractures Treated Conservatively

AUTHOR AND YEAR	NO. OF PATIENTS	NONUNION RATE (%)	SIGNIFICANT FACTORS
Anderson & D'Alonzo, 1974[7]	49	36	None specified
Apuzzo et al, 1978[26]	45	33	Age >40 yr, displacement >4 mm
Ekong et al, 1981[10]	17	41	Age ≥55 yr, displacement >4–6 mm
Hadley et al, 1985[12]	40	26	Not age, displacement >6 mm
Clark & White, 1985[8]	106	32	Not age, displacement >5 mm
Dunn & Seljeskog, 1986[9]	88	24	Age >65 yr, posterior displacement
Hanssen & Cabanela, 1987[77]	42	50	Age >72 yr, posterior displacement
Schweigel, 1987[33]	47	10	Not age, not displacement
Hadley et al, 1989[2]	65	28	Not age, displacement ≥6 mm
Ryan & Taylor, 1993[78]	35	77	Posterior displacement
Seybold & Bayley, 1998[34]	37	29	Not age, displacement unknown
Greene et al, 1997[35]	88	28	Displacement ≥6 mm

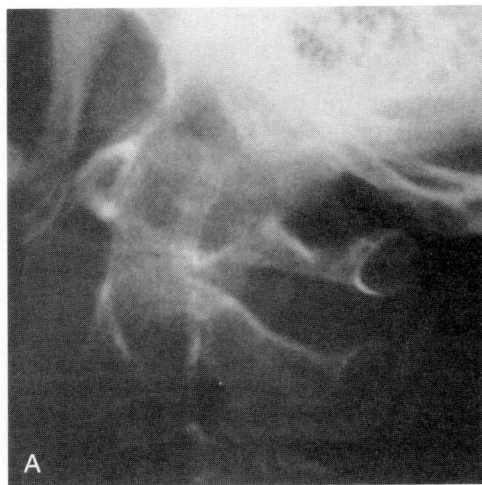
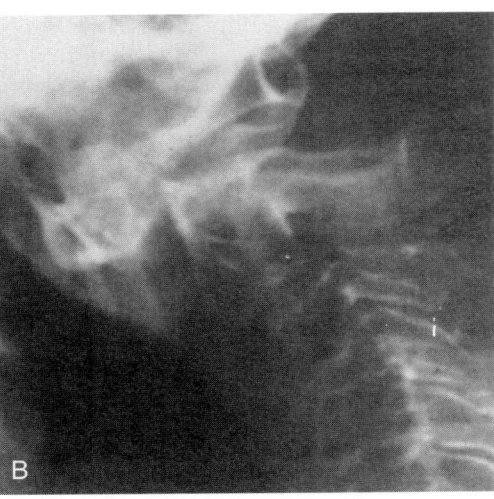

FIGURE 318–2. Patient with a type II odontoid fracture after a fall. *A,* Initial lateral cervical spine radiograph demonstrating normal alignment. *B,* Subsequent radiograph demonstrating more than 1 cm anterolisthesis. The patient was managed with anterior odontoid screw fixation.

SURGICAL MANAGEMENT

In 1985 Clark and White[8] compared immobilization with operative management in their series of 96 patients with type II odontoid fractures. Eighteen patients were untreated, and three patients were placed in a cervical collar. These 21 patients had a 100% nonunion rate. Thirty-eight patients were managed in a halo device, with a 34% nonunion rate. Thirty-four patients underwent operative stabilization (26 posterior, 8 anterior), with a nonunion rate of 6%. Based on this experience, Clark and White recommended operative intervention as the primary treatment modality.

Greene and coworkers[35] recommended early surgical intervention for patients whose axis fractures could not be maintained by external orthoses, those with ruptured transverse ligaments, those with 6 mm or more of dens displacement, and those with comminuted dens fractures.

Obviously, surgical treatment is not without risk, including the general risks inherent to all operations and the specific risks of potential injury to structures in the operative area. Surgical stabilization can be accomplished with either an anterior or a posterior approach. Traditionally, posterior atlantoaxial bone and wire fusion in conjunction with external immobilization has been the standard surgical treatment for odontoid fractures. Traynelis[4] reviewed the published literature on the treatment of type II odontoid fractures and reported an overall successful fusion rate of 64% for posterior bone and wire fusion techniques. The surgical rates of mortality and morbidity were approximately 2% each. Complications included loss of reduction and the development of new neurological deficits.

Numerous case series have advocated other surgical approaches, including posterior fusion with Halifax clamp fixation, posterior C1-2 transarticular screw fixation, and anterior odontoid screw placement.[36–39] Posterior C1-2 fusion, whether achieved with bone and wire fusion, Halifax clamp fixation, or transarticular screws, stabilizes the C1-2 complex at the expense of eliminating normal atlantoaxial rotatory motion. Loss of rotatory motion at C1-2, which accounts for 50% of the normal cervical rotatory excursion, is usually noticeable to patients.[40]

In contrast to external immobilization and posterior C1-2 fusion, direct screw fixation of the odontoid provides immediate stabilization and promotes bone healing while preserving normal C1-2 motion. Nakanishi,[41] in 1980 in the Japanese literature, and Bohler,[42, 43] who in 1982 independently reported his experience dating to 1968, first reported placement of an odontoid fixation screw. Subsequently, other authors reported success with the technique.[44, 45] Because most early techniques involved extensive dissection of the neck and significant potential morbidity, the approach was not widely adopted. More recently, a more refined approach associated with excellent outcomes has been described.[5, 38, 46–48]

Veres and associates[49] reported a fusion rate of 86% in 53 patients, ranging from 15 to 83 years old. Rainov and colleagues[50] reported a fusion rate of 100% in 30 patients, but there were complications in 12%, including persistent neck pain and decreased range of motion. Etter and coworkers[46] retrospectively reviewed 19 patients and reported a successful fusion rate of 79%.

The senior author of this chapter (RIA) has been involved in developing an approach that employs specially designed instrumentation (Aesculap Instrument Co., South San Francisco, CA) to allow reliable and relatively easy placement of anterior odontoid fixation screws in a minimally invasive manner under fluoroscopic guidance. The results have been excellent and the morbidity low.[5, 51] This technique is described later.

We recently reviewed the surgical outcome of 147 patients who underwent anterior odontoid screw fixation at two institutions.[51a] Patients had either recent (<6 months; *n* = 129) or chronic (>18 months; *n* = 18) odontoid fractures. There were 138 patients with type II fractures and 9 patients with type III fractures. Overall, anatomic bony fusion was successful in 77%. Nonanatomic bony fusion occurred in 3%, fibrous union in 9%, and nonunion in 11%. Separate analysis of the recent and chronic groups demonstrated an 88% fusion rate for patients with recent fractures, compared with a 25% fusion rate for those with chronic fractures. Chi-squared analysis of the effect of sex, age, fracture type, fracture orientation, degree of odontoid displacement, and number of screws placed (one or two) revealed that only fracture orientation significantly affected anatomic bony fusion. Fractures with an anterior oblique orientation were significantly more likely to result in nonanatomic fusion, fibrous union, or nonunion than were posterior oblique and horizontal fractures. Postoperatively, 14 patients had hardware complications. The two most common hardware failures were screws that pulled out ($n = 5$) and backed out ($n = 4$). Screws backed out when the odontoid screw did not fully engage the distal cortex of the odontoid tip. Screws pulled out of the body of C2 exclusively in patients who had fractures that extended into the body of C2. Although these fractures were recognized preoperatively, at surgery, the surgeon judged that the vertebral body would still provide an acceptable substrate for fusion. Based on our current results, we no longer recommend this procedure for patients with evidence of comminuted fractures of the C2 body.

INDICATIONS FOR ANTERIOR ODONTOID SCREW FIXATION

Most patients with acute type II odontoid fractures are considered good candidates for odontoid screw fixation. As addressed later, a subset of patients with acute type III fractures may also be candidates for this procedure. Disruption of the transverse ligament is an absolute contraindication to anterior odontoid screw placement, whereas severe osteopenia and fractures that slope obliquely and anteriorly are relative contraindications. Concerns about the integrity of the transverse ligament can be addressed with magnetic resonance imaging.[52] Osteopenia is often present in elderly patients with odontoid fractures. Although it is not an absolute contraindication, the holding power of the bone needs to be assessed at surgery. If it is questionable, an external orthosis should be used. Our own success rate did not change when analyzed as a function of patients' age—an indirect indicator of possible osteopenia. Obliquely anteriorly sloping fractures may allow the dens to slide anteriorly along the fracture line as the lag screw pulls it inferiorly. This situation seldom occurs with acute fractures because the irregular bone surfaces engage and lock together, but it can be a problem with fractures that are a few weeks to several months old.

Our experience suggests that up to 6 months between fracture and treatment is not detrimental to obtaining a successful fusion. Patients with long-standing or chronic nonunion of the odontoid process, including os odontoideum, are seldom good candidates for this procedure. For most patients with chronic nonunion of the odontoid process, and for all patients with disrupted transverse ligaments, posterior C1-2 fusion with transarticular screw fixation is preferable.

Type III Fractures

Type III odontoid fractures can usually be managed nonoperatively. Exceptions to this rule include patients who have ruptured transverse ligaments and those in whom immobilization fails to maintain alignment. The former require posterior C1-2 fusion, whereas the latter can often be managed effectively with anterior screw fixation if the fracture does not involve comminution of the C2 body.

Greene and colleagues[35] reported their results from 75 patients with type III odontoid fractures. Six patients underwent early surgical fusion because a halo vest failed to maintain alignment. The nonunion rate among the 69 patients treated nonoperatively was very low—only one patient failed conservative management. Anderson and D'Alonzo[7] reported similar results.

ANTERIOR ODONTOID SCREW FIXATION: SURGICAL TECHNIQUE

The procedure has been described in detail elsewhere.[51] Patients are positioned supine with a folded sheet behind the shoulders to permit neck extension during the procedure (Fig. 318–3). Gentle halter traction is applied. If the patient's fracture reduces with extension, the head is placed in an extended position; if not, a neutral position is initially used, with a support placed behind the patient's head. Head positioning is monitored with lateral C-arm fluoroscopy. If available, a second C-arm unit greatly facilitates the procedure. It is positioned for anteroposterior (transoral) odontoid viewing, using a radiolucent (plastic or cork) mouth prop.

To achieve a trajectory low enough for proper screw placement, the cervical spine is approached through a low cervical incision (at approximately C5-6). A standard approach to the anterior cervical spine is used, followed by placement of a modified Caspar retractor system beneath the bellies of the longus colli muscles. The prevertebral space is then opened to the C2 region, and an angled retractor is inserted into the space to create a tunnel up to C2, through which the remainder of the procedure is completed (Fig. 318–4A and B).

Under biplanar fluoroscopic guidance, a Kirschner wire (K-wire) is positioned on the anteroinferior lip of C2 at the exact entrance site desired for the fixation screw. An 8-mm hollow drill is placed over the K-wire and rotated by hand to create a shallow trough in the body of C3 and to incise the C2-3 annulus without cutting into the C2 body (see Fig. 318–4C and D). The drill guide system is placed over the K-wire. The outer guide tube has spikes that are impacted into the body of C3 to anchor the guide system. The tube also permits the C2-3 complex to be manipulated relative to the C1-odontoid complex for precise realignment of the spine. In patients with retrolisthesis of the odontoid, the support behind the patient's head is removed at this juncture. As the patient's head is extended, the alignment is maintained by exerting downward pressure on the C2-3 complex. In this manner, alignment is perfected while the neck is extended as needed to obtain the proper drill trajectory. The drill guide system is then used, and a drill is passed up through the body of C2 to the fracture site (Fig. 318–5). Before the odontoid process is engaged, the alignment can be further opti-

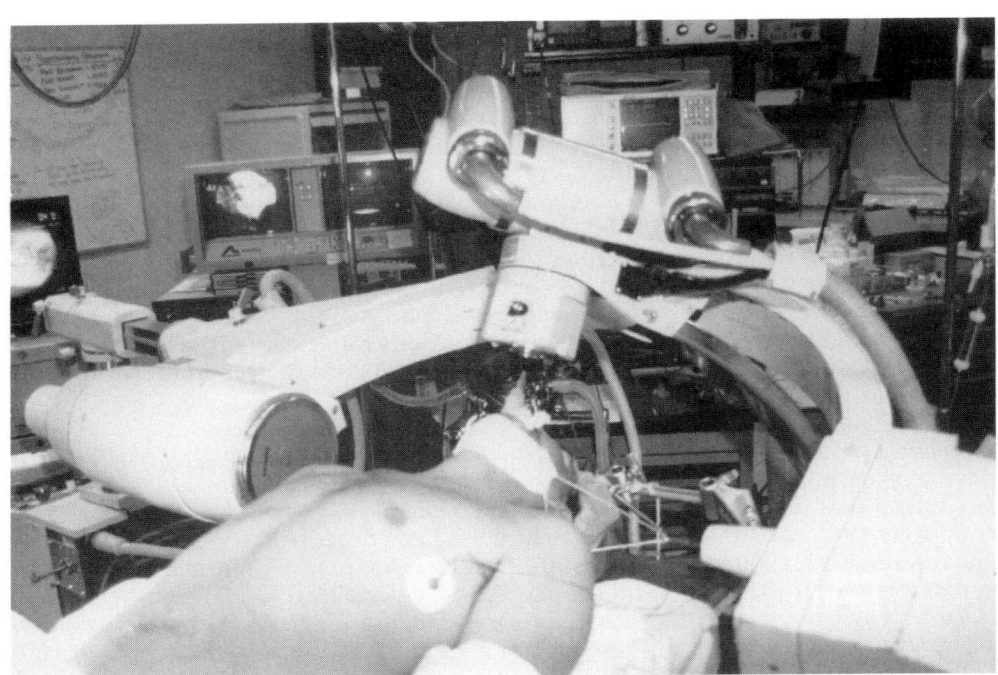

FIGURE 318–3. Patient positioned on the operating table. A folded sheet is placed under the shoulders to increase neck extension in this patient, whose fracture was reduced during extension. Two C-arm fluoroscopic units are used for anteroposterior (transoral) and lateral fluoroscopic imaging.

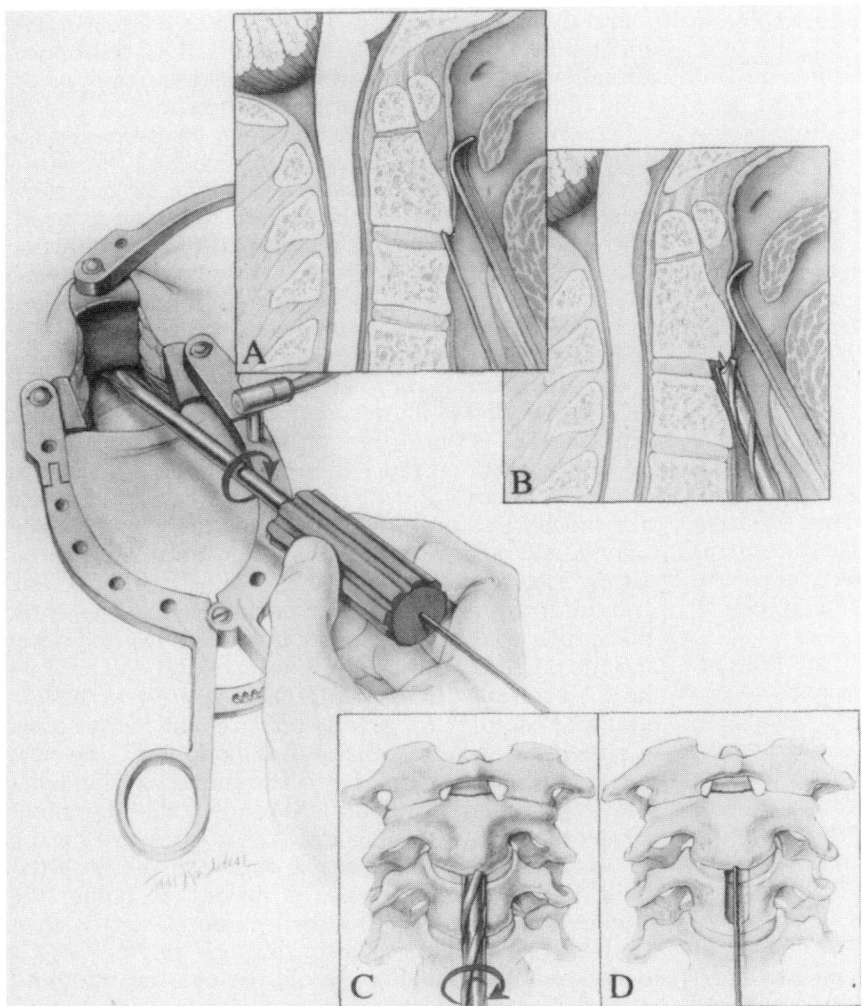

FIGURE 318–4. *A,* After retractors have been placed properly, the Kirschner wire (K-wire) is inserted as described in the text. *B–D,* A hollow-handled drill manipulated over the K-wire creates a shallow trough in the body of C3 and incises the C2-3 annulus. (From Apfelbaum RI: Anterior screw fixation of odontoid fractures. In Camins MB, O'Leary PF [eds]: Disorders of the Cervical Spine. Baltimore, Williams & Wilkins, 1992, pp 603–608.)

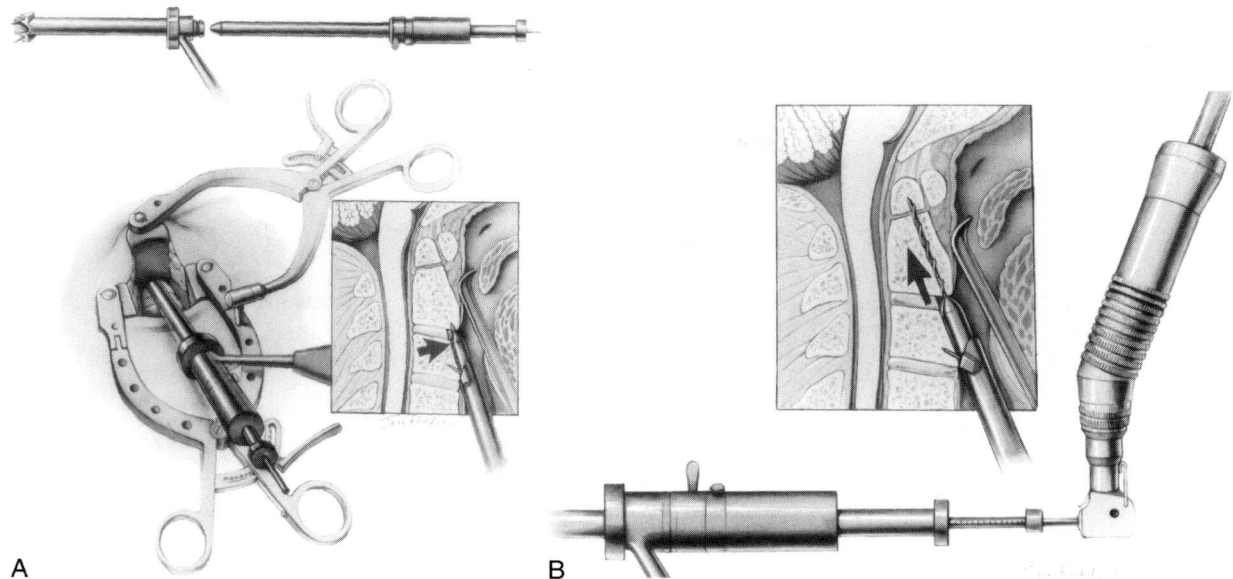

FIGURE 318–5. *A*, The drill guide system consists of inner and outer tubes that are mated and then placed over the Kirschner wire (K-wire). The spikes on the outer guide tube are impacted into C3 to stabilize the system. *B*, The K-wire is removed and replaced with the drill, which is fluoroscopically guided to the apex of the odontoid after the fracture is reduced. A pilot hole is drilled through the apical cortex of the odontoid. (From Apfelbaum RI: Anterior screw fixation of odontoid fractures. In Camins MB, O'Leary PF [eds]: Disorders of the Cervical Spine. Baltimore, Williams & Wilkins, 1992, pp 603–608.)

mized by manipulating the C2-3 complex relative to the odontoid-C1 complex by exerting either downward or upward pressure on the handle of the guide tube as necessary.

After satisfactory alignment is obtained, the pilot hole is drilled to and through the apex of the odontoid. If the distal cortex is not penetrated by the drill, screw placement may be difficult or impossible. Because the angle of drilling is coaxial with the long axis of the odontoid, penetration into the spinal canal toward the spinal cord is unlikely. Frequent biplanar imaging controls the drilling process. The pilot hole is then tapped, and a lag screw is inserted through the guide tube using a special screwdriver with an internal retaining spring to hold the screw (Fig. 318–6). The image with the drill in its final position is saved and compared with the live image. An identical position can thereby be achieved when tapping and placing the screw. Stabilization can be confirmed by flexing the patient's neck under fluoroscopic guidance.

The procedure is repeated if a second screw is to be placed. A lag screw is placed for the first screw to draw the odontoid down toward the body of C2. If a second screw is used, it can be fully threaded.

Standard wound closure is achieved with absorbable interrupted sutures in the sternocleidomastoid fascia, platysma, and subcutaneous layers, followed by adhesive strips on the skin. A cervical collar is seldom required unless bone density is a concern.

After the screw is placed, the fractures are immediately stabilized, and there is a very high rate of bony fusion, with minimal risk of morbidity. If not otherwise impaired by their injury, patients can return to normal activity within a few days. Given the availability of this procedure, many patients opt for early surgery if informed of all the issues in the management of odontoid fractures.

TRAUMATIC SPONDYLOLISTHESIS

Hanging has been a means of execution for hundreds of years.[53–55] Initially, the noose was placed around the individual's neck, and death resulted from asphyxiation or, in some cases, decapitation. It was later discovered that placing the knot in a submental position was a more efficient means of execution. Wood-Jones[56] first described the cervical spine injury caused by the submental method. In a letter to *Lancet* in 1913, he presented five victims who had suffered instantaneous death with the knot placed in a submental position. All five victims had identical lesions in the cervical vertebrae: "the posterior arch of the axis is snapped clean off and remains fixed to the third vertebra, while the atlas, the odontoid process, and the anterior arch of the axis remain fixed to the skull" (see Fig. 318–1).

Not until 1954 did Grogono[57] first notice the resemblance of a fracture-dislocation of the axis in a 45-year-old woman involved in a motor vehicle accident to the injury illustrated by Wood-Jones. Garber[58] later classified the fracture as "traumatic spondylolisthesis of the axis." Finally, in 1965, Schneider and colleagues[59] published the first definitive report exclusively on what they termed a "hangman's fracture." Since then, the terms hangman's fracture and traumatic spondylolisthesis have been used interchangeably. The hangman's

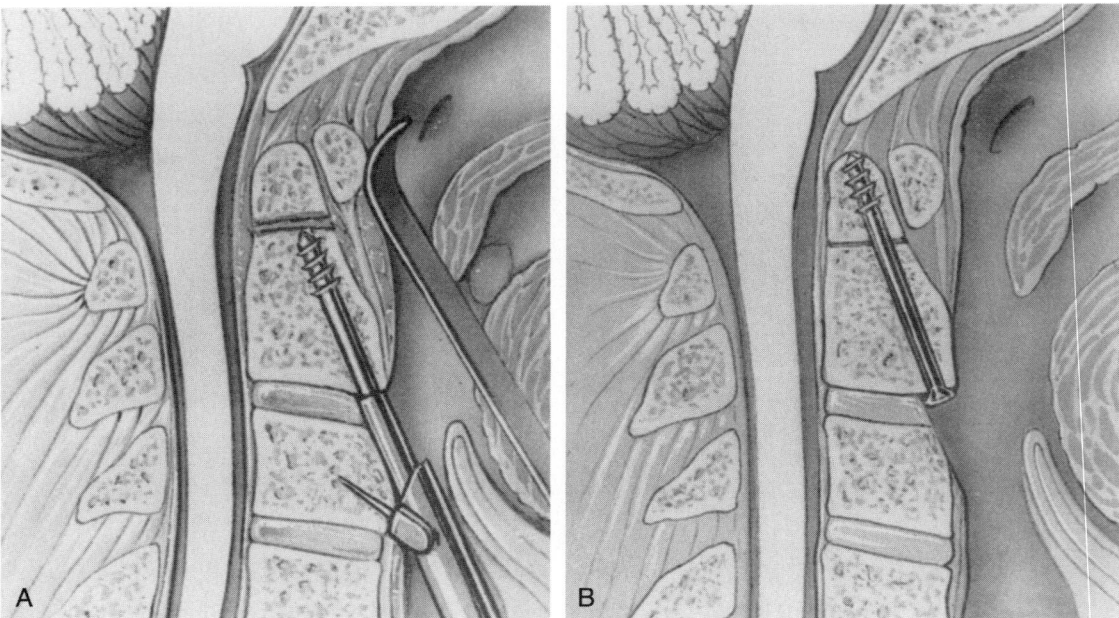

FIGURE 318–6. The screw is inserted through the guide tube and advanced through the pilot hole. (From Apfelbaum RI: Anterior screw fixation of odontoid fractures. In Camins MB, O'Leary PF [eds]: Disorders of the Cervical Spine. Baltimore, Williams & Wilkins, 1992, pp 603–608.)

fracture is now described as bilateral fractures through the pars interarticularis of C2.

Mechanism of Injury

Contemporary hangman's fractures are usually caused by hyperextension and axial compression. The classic scenario is that of an unrestrained motor vehicle passenger being thrown forward and hitting the windshield with his or her head, causing both hyperextension and compression.[59] Several series have reported facial trauma in a distribution that supports hyperextension as the underlying mechanism.[60–64]

In their classic paper, Schneider and colleagues[59] described how the combined forces of hyperextension and axial loading produce the hangman's fracture. They proposed that with sudden hyperextension and axial loading, the weight of the head is transmitted through the occipital condyles and C1-2 lateral masses bilaterally to converge at the base of the axis. These forces pass through the weakest part of the axis, namely, the pars interarticularis. Hyperextension first stresses the anterior supporting structures while compressing the posterior bony facets until the pars interarticularis fractures. With continued extension, the anterior longitudinal ligament and disk rupture. The classic hyperextension mechanism has been supported by autopsy studies; however, flexion can produce the same lesion.[64–67]

Four classification systems have been proposed for hangman's fractures. In 1981, two groups led by Effendi[68] and Francis[63] published classification systems. Levine and Edwards's[65] modification of the Effendi grading scale followed in 1985, and White and Panjabi[40] provided their own unique classification in 1990.

The most commonly used grading system is that of Levine and Edwards (Table 318–3).

According to the classification system of Levine and Edwards,[65] fractures are divided into categories based on their degree of displacement and angulation. Type I fractures are the result of hyperextension and axial loading strong enough to fracture the pars interarticularis but not strong enough to compromise the anterior or posterior longitudinal ligaments. These fractures are nonangulating and involve less than 3 mm of displacement. Type II fractures are due to a combination of initial hyperextension followed by flexion and axial compression. They include fractures that are significantly angulated and can also be displaced. Type III injuries display both severe angulation and displacement with unilateral or bilateral facet dislocations at C2-3.

TABLE 318–3 ■ Levine and Edwards' Classification of Traumatic Spondylolisthesis of the Axis

FRACTURE	FEATURE
Type I	Fracture of the pars interarticularis with <3 mm displacement and no angulation
Type II	Fracture of the pars interarticularis with >3 mm displacement and significant angulation
Type IIA	Fracture of the pars interarticularis with <3 mm displacement and significant angulation
Type III	Fracture of the pars interarticularis with unilateral or bilateral facet dislocation at C2-3

Modified from Levine AM, Edwards CC: The management of traumatic spondylolisthesis of axis. J Bone Joint Surg Am 67:217–226, 1985.

Management

The basic principles guiding the management of hangman's fractures have not changed since they were first described by Schneider and colleagues.[59] Of their eight cases, only one required surgical stabilization for increased subluxation after halter traction. They concluded that most fractures could be treated conservatively if alignment was corrected and the neck was immobilized.

Among the papers by Effendi and associates,[68] Levine and Edwards,[65] and Francis and coworkers,[63] 32%, 6%, and 5.6% of their patients, respectively, required surgical stabilization. Hadley and colleagues[2] reported that none of their 25 patients required either early or late surgical intervention. In contrast, Cornish[66] advocated early surgical stabilization for traumatic spondylolisthesis. Of his 14 patients, 8 were treated with early anterior fusion, and 2 more required surgical stabilization after initial conservative management failed.

Several authors have proposed treatment algorithms for the management of hangman's fractures based on fracture characteristics. Greene and coworkers[35] recommended managing type I fractures (nondisplaced or minimally displaced fractures) with a halo vest, hard cervical collar, or other external immobilization. A Philadelphia collar provides adequate stability to achieve fusion of minimally displaced fractures.[69, 70] Greene and coworkers[35] also advocated halo immobilization for type II and III fractures but stressed the need for frequent radiographic studies in patients with type III fractures to evaluate alignment and fusion. If there is significant disk or ligamentous injury at C2-3, the likelihood of instability at that level is high, and stabilization with fusion should be considered.

Most authors agree that there are few indications for surgery. In general, poor reduction and nonunion are the most common reasons to operate.[71–73] If surgery is required, stabilization can be achieved by a posterior fusion of C1-2 or an anterior fusion of C2-3, because the instability is between C1 and the anterior component of C2 and the posterior component of C2 and the lower cervical spine. The anterior approach may be preferable because it spares C1-2 rotation. Success with direct screw fixation between anterior and posterior elements of C2 using pedicle screws without fusing adjacent segments has been described.[74–76]

MISCELLANEOUS AXIS FRACTURES

Miscellaneous axis fractures are defined as nonodontoid, nonhangman's fractures. Benzel and coworkers[76] reviewed the fracture patterns of 15 patients with C2 vertebral body fractures and defined a new anatomic classification system. Type I body fractures were defined as coronally oriented vertebral fractures through the posterior aspect of the C2 vertebral body. Four possible mechanisms of injury were described for this type of injury. Type II C2 vertebral body fractures were sagittally oriented, caused by axial loading to the point of failure. A third type of C2 body fracture, a horizontal

fracture, was the same as that described by Anderson and D'Alonzo[7] as a type III odontoid fracture. The goal of this new classification system was to correlate the mechanism of injury with biomechanical principles to assist in the clinical management. Specific treatment recommendations, however, were not discussed in the article.

Greene and coworkers[35] described their management of 63 patients with acute miscellaneous fractures. The only patient treated with early surgery had a lateral mass fracture associated with 5-mm subluxation of C2 on C3. The remaining patients were managed nonoperatively with external immobilization, and only one of these patients required surgery for nonunion. This patient had been placed in a halo vest with immobilization for 15 weeks. Overall, their nonunion rate for miscellaneous axis fractures managed nonoperatively was 1.6%.

CONCLUSIONS

The management of patients with axis fractures depends on the characteristics of the fracture. Typically, patients with stable type I and type III odontoid fractures, hangman's fractures, and miscellaneous fractures do well with nonoperative management. Frequent radiographic studies are required to ensure proper alignment and fusion.

Options for the management of type II odontoid fractures are either nonoperative treatment or early surgical intervention. Nonunion rates in conservatively treated adults with type II odontoid fractures have been well documented. They are, however, quite variable, with no consensus on the extent that age and displacement influence healing rates. Because of the high nonunion rates associated with nonoperative treatment, we recommend surgical management with direct anterior odontoid screw fixation for type II odontoid fractures within 6 months of injury. It is an effective and safe method that confers immediate stability, preserves C1-2 rotation, and provides optimal conditions for bony fusion.

REFERENCES

1. Bracken MB, Freeman DH Jr, Hellenbrand K: Incidence of acute traumatic hospitalized spinal cord injury in the United States, 1970–1977. Am J Epidemiol 113:615–622, 1981.
2. Hadley MN, Dickman CA, Browner CM, et al: Acute axis fractures: A review of 229 cases. J Neurosurg 71:642–647, 1989.
3. Huelke DF, O'Day J, Mendelsohn RA: Cervical injuries suffered in automobile crashes. J Neurosurg 54:316–322, 1981.
4. Traynelis VC: Evidence-based management of type II odontoid fractures. Clin Neurosurg 44:41–49, 1997.
5. Apfelbaum RI: Anterior screw fixation of odontoid fractures. In Camins MB, O'Leary PF (eds): Disorders of the Cervical Spine. Baltimore, Williams & Wilkins, 1992, pp 603–608.
6. Crockard HA, Heilman AE, Stevens JM: Progressive myelopathy secondary to odontoid fractures: Clinical, radiological, and surgical features. J Neurosurg 78:579–586, 1993.
7. Anderson LD, D'Alonzo RT: Fractures of the odontoid process of the axis. J Bone Joint Surg Am 56:1663–1674, 1974.
8. Clark CR, White AA III: Fractures of the dens: A multicenter study. J Bone Joint Surg Am 67:1340–1348, 1985.
9. Dunn ME, Seljeskog EL: Experience in the management of odon-

toid process injuries: An analysis of 128 cases. Neurosurgery 18: 306–310, 1986.

10. Ekong CE, Schwartz ML, Tator CH, et al: Odontoid fracture: Management with early mobilization using the halo device. Neurosurgery 9:631–637, 1981.

11. Fujii E, Kobayashi K, Hirabayashi K: Treatment in fractures of the odontoid process. Spine 13:604–609, 1988.

12. Hadley MN, Browner C, Sonntag VKH: Axis fractures: A comprehensive review of management and treatment in 107 cases. Neurosurgery 17:281–290, 1985.

13. Maiman DJ, Larson SJ: Management of odontoid fractures. Neurosurgery 11:471–476, 1982.

14. Pepin JW, Bourne RB, Hawkins RJ: Odontoid fractures, with special reference to the elderly patient. Clin Orthop 193:178–183, 1985.

15. Ryan MD, Taylor TK: Odontoid fractures: A rational approach to treatment. J Bone Joint Surg Br 64:416–421, 1982.

16. Pointallart V, Lopez Orta A, Freitas J, et al: Odontoid fractures: Review of 150 cases and practical application for treatment. Eur Spine J 3:282–285, 1995.

17. Chiba K, Fujimura Y, Toyama Y, et al: Treatment protocol for fractures of the odontoid process. J Spinal Disord 9:267–276, 1996.

18. Eismont FJ, Bohlman HH: Posterior atlanto-occipital dislocation with fractures of the atlas and odontoid process. J Bone Joint Surg Am 60:397–399, 1978.

19. Scott EW, Haid RW Jr, Peace D: Type I fractures of the odontoid process: Implications for atlanto-occipital instability. Case report. J Neurosurg 72:488–492, 1990.

20. Hadley MN, Browner CM, Liu SS, et al: New subtype of acute odontoid fractures (type IIA). Neurosurgery 22:67–71, 1988.

21. Alexander JT, Haid RW Jr: Upper cervical spine trauma: Outcome assessment. Clin Neurosurg 44:305–313, 1997.

22. Keller RB: Outcomes research in orthopaedics. J Am Acad Orthop Surg 1:122–129, 1993.

23. Johnson RM, Hart DL, Simmons EF, et al: Cervical orthoses: A study comparing their effectiveness in restricting cervical motion in normal subjects. J Bone Joint Surg Am 59:332–339, 1977.

24. Schiess RJ, DeSaussure RL, Robertson JT: Choice of treatment of odontoid fractures. J Neurosurg 57:496–499, 1982.

25. Althoff B: Fracture of the odontoid process: An experimental and clinical study. Acta Orthop Scand Suppl 177:1–95, 1979.

26. Apuzzo ML, Heiden JS, Weiss MH, et al: Acute fractures of the odontoid process: An analysis of 45 cases. J Neurosurg 48: 85–91, 1978.

27. Blockey NJ, Purser DW: Fractures of the odontoid process of the axis. J Bone Joint Surg Br 38:794–817, 1956.

28. Dickson H, Engel S, Blum P, et al: Odontoid fractures, systemic disease and conservative care. Aust N Z J Surg 54:243–247, 1984.

29. Hentzer L, Schalimtzek M: Fractures and subluxations of the atlas and axis: A follow-up study of 20 patients [Danish]. Nord Med 85:772–775, 1971.

30. Schatzker J, Rorabeck CH, Waddell JP: Fractures of the dens (odontoid process): An analysis of thirty-seven cases. J Bone Joint Surg Br 53:392–405, 1971.

31. Wilson TAS, McWhorter JM: Atlantoaxial injuries. In Camins MB, O'Leary PF (eds): Diseases of the Cervical Spine. Baltimore, Williams & Wilkins, 1992, pp 285–291.

32. Bettini N, Cervellati S, Di Silvestre M, et al: The nonsurgical treatment of fractures of the dens epistrophei. Chir Organi Mov 76:17–24, 1991.

33. Schweigel JF: Management of the fractured odontoid with halo-thoracic bracing. Spine 12:838–839, 1987.

34. Seybold EA, Bayley JC: Functional outcome of surgically and conservatively managed dens fractures. Spine 23:1837–1846, 1998.

35. Greene KA, Dickman CA, Marciano FF, et al: Acute axis fractures: Analysis of management and outcome in 340 consecutive cases. Spine 22:1843–1852, 1997.

36. Aldrich EF, Weber PB, Crow WN: Halifax interlaminar clamp for posterior cervical fusion: A long-term follow-up review. J Neurosurg 78:702–708, 1993.

37. Dickman CA, Sonntag VKH, Papadopoulos SM, et al: The interspinous method of posterior atlantoaxial arthrodesis. J Neurosurg 74:190–198, 1991.

38. Geisler FH, Cheng C, Poka A, et al: Anterior screw fixation of

39. Marcotte P, Dickman CA, Sonntag VKH, et al: Posterior atlanto-axial facet screw fixation. J Neurosurg 79:234–237, 1993.

40. White AA, Panjabi MM: Clinical Biomechanics of the Spine. Philadelphia, JB Lippincott, 1990.

41. Nakanishi T: Internal fixation of odontoid fracture. Orthop Trauma Surg 23:399–406, 1980.

42. Bohler J: Fractures of the odontoid process. J Trauma 5:386–391, 1965.

43. Bohler J: Anterior stabilization for acute fractures and non-unions of the dens. J Bone Joint Surg Am 64:18–27, 1982.

44. Borne GM, Bedou GL, Pinaudeau M, et al: Odontoid process fracture osteosynthesis with a direct screw fixation technique in nine consecutive cases. J Neurosurg 68:223–226, 1988.

45. Lesoin F, Autricque A, Franz K, et al: Transcervical approach and screw fixation for upper cervical spine pathology. Surg Neurol 27:459–465, 1987.

46. Etter C, Coscia M, Jaberg H, et al: Direct anterior fixation of dens fractures with a cannulated screw system. Spine 16:S25–S32, 1991.

47. Jenkins JD, Coric D, Branch CL Jr: A clinical comparison of one- and two-screw odontoid fixation. J Neurosurg 89:366–370, 1998.

48. Montesano PX, Anderson PA, Schlehr F, et al: Odontoid fractures treated by anterior odontoid screw fixation. Spine 16:S33–S37, 1991.

49. Veres R, Casey ATH, Crockard HA, et al: Acute fractures of the odontoid process: A critical analysis of anterior screw fixation in 53 cases. Paper presented at the 64th Annual Meeting of the American Association of Neurological Surgeons, 1996, Minneapolis, Minn.

50. Rainov NG, Heidecke V, Burkert W: Direct anterior fixation of odontoid fractures with a hollow spreading screw system. Acta Neurochir (Wien) 138:146–153, 1996.

51. Apfelbaum RI: Anterior Screw Fixation of Odontoid Fractures (Aesculap Scientific Info 24). Tuttlingen, Germany, Aesculap AG, 1992.

51a. Apfelbaum RI, Lonser RR, Veres R, et al: Direct anterior screw fixation for recent and remote odontoid fractures. J Neurosurg 93(2Supp):227–236.

52. Dickman CA, Mamourian A, Sonntag VKH, et al: Magnetic resonance imaging of the transverse atlantal ligament for the evaluation of atlantoaxial instability. J Neurosurg 75:221–227, 1991.

53. Haughton S: Judicial hanging. Lancet 1:629, 1913.

54. de Zouche Marshall JJ: Judicial hanging. Lancet 1:639–640, 1913.

55. Haughton S: On hanging, considered from a mechanical and physiological point of view. Philosophical Magazine and Journal of Science 3:23–34, 1866.

56. Wood-Jones F: The ideal lesion produced by judicial hanging. Lancet 1:53, 1913.

57. Grogono B: Injuries of the atlas and axis. J Bone Joint Surg Br 36:397–410, 1954.

58. Garber JN: Abnormalities of the atlas and axis vertebrae—congenital and traumatic. J Bone Joint Surg Am 46: 1782–1791, 1964.

59. Schneider RC, Livingston KE, Cave AJ, et al: "Hangman's fracture" of the cervical spine. J Neurosurg 22:141–154, 1965.

60. Seljeskog EL, Chou SN: Spectrum of the hangman's fracture. J Neurosurg 45:3–8, 1976.

61. Pepin JW, Hawkins RJ: Traumatic spondylolisthesis of the axis: Hangman's fracture. Clin Orthop 157:133–138, 1981.

62. Coric D, Wilson JA, Kelly DL Jr: Treatment of traumatic spondylolisthesis of the axis with nonrigid immobilization: A review of 64 cases. J Neurosurg 85:550–554, 1996.

63. Francis WR, Fielding JW, Hawkins RJ, et al: Traumatic spondylolisthesis of the axis. J Bone Joint Surg Br 63:313–318, 1981.

64. Fielding JW, Francis WR Jr, Hawkins RJ, et al: Traumatic spondylolisthesis of the axis. Clin Orthop 239:47–52, 1989.

65. Levine AM, Edwards CC: The management of traumatic spondylolisthesis of the axis. J Bone Joint Surg Am 67:217–226, 1985.

66. Cornish BL: Traumatic spondylolisthesis of the axis. J Bone Joint Surg Br 50:31–43, 1968.

67. DeLorme TL: Axis-pedicle fractures. J Bone Joint Surg Am 49: 1472, 1967.

68. Effendi B, Roy D, Cornish B, et al: Fractures of the ring of the

axis: A classification based on the analysis of 131 cases. J Bone Joint Surg Br 63:319–327, 1981.

69. Lee KS, Kelley DL, Alexander E, et al: Satisfactory treatment of hangman's fractures without the halo apparatus [abstract]. Neurosurgery 21:120–121, 1987.

70. Grady MS, Howard MA, Jane JA, et al: Use of the Philadelphia collar as an alternative to the halo vest in patients with C-2, C-3 fractures. Neurosurgery 18:151–156, 1986.

71. An HS: Cervical spine trauma. Spine 23:2713–2729, 1998.

72. Tuite GF, Papadopoulos SM, Sonntag VKH: Caspar plate fixation for the treatment of complex hangman's fractures. Neurosurgery 30:761–765, 1992.

73. Barros TE, Bohlman HH, Capen DA, et al: Traumatic spondylolis-

thesis of the axis: Analysis of management. Spinal Cord 37: 166–171, 1999.

74. Ebraheim N, Rollins JR Jr, Xu R, et al: Anatomic consideration of C2 pedicle screw placement. Spine 21:691–695, 1996.

75. Borne GM, Bedou GL, Pinaudeau M: Treatment of pedicular fractures of the axis: A clinical study and screw fixation technique. J Neurosurg 60:88–93, 1984.

76. Benzel EC, Hart BL, Ball PA, et al: Fractures of the C-2 vertebral body. J Neurosurg 81:206–212, 1994.

77. Hanssen AD, Cabanela ME: Fractures of the dens in adult patients. J Trauma 27:928–934, 1987.

78. Ryan MD, Taylor TK: Odontoid fractures in the elderly. J Spinal Disord 6:397–401, 1993.

CHAPTER 319

Diagnosis and Management of Thoracic Spine Fractures

PARLEY W. MADSEN III ■ F. J. EISMONT ■ B. A. GREEN

The focus of this chapter is the management of patients with sustained thoracic spinal injuries at or below T1 and above T10. In this region, the spinal column is protected by the rib cage and the back and chest wall musculature. This protective cage of ribs and muscle strengthens the spinal column and shields the spinal cord from all but the highest velocity forces. Nonetheless, injury in this region of the thoracic spine is frequently associated with significant neurological deficit. The diagnosis of spinal fractures in this area is challenging, and fractures are difficult to detect, especially in patients who have sustained multiple injuries.[136] Although the thoracic spinal column is the most difficult to injure, the contained thoracic spinal cord is very susceptible to trauma and, when compared with other spinal regions, has the poorest prognosis for functional recovery. This chapter discusses the principles of management of thoracic spine fractures, including preservation of life, protection of neurological tissues, and restoration and maintenance of both spinal alignment and stability.

The exact regimen that will ensure the optimal clinical outcome has not been determined scientifically. In most areas of neurological trauma, significant controversy continues regarding the best approach for a given injury. We would like to emphasize that a solitary, scientifically validated treatment for treatment of thoracic fractures has not been delineated and that various management strategies have been used successfully by clinical teams skilled in their implementation. The material contained in this chapter represents the experience and the current protocols used by us in the treatment of patients with thoracic spine injury.

HISTORICAL PERSPECTIVE

The Egyptians were the first to diagnose and recommend a treatment for spine and spinal cord injuries involving the cervical spine, and Hippocrates described the clinical consequences of a thoracic spine injury and recommended a method of reducing the gibbus often associated with these injuries.[23] The pessimistic prognosis pronounced by the ancient Egyptians for a cervical spine dislocation with a complete spinal cord injury—"an ailment not to be treated"—remained the same at the time of Hippocrates. However, in the writings of Hippocrates, a racklike traction device called a *scamnum* was described, and its use was recommended to reduce the bony abnormalities of thoracic and lumbar spine fractures.[70, 108]

In the 7th century, Paulus of Aegina used the scamnum to reduce spinal fractures and then placed an external fixation device made of thin sheets of wood to secure the reduction. He was also the first clinician to suggest that laminar fragments pressing on the spinal cord were a source of pain and therefore advocated a laminectomy for débridement of the fracture site.[73] It is not certain that the operation recommended was ever actually performed during his career.[13]

Ambrose Paré was a 16th century French barber surgeon who, because of his observation of battlefield injuries, devised more effective treatments for a number of disorders, including thoracic spine fractures.[86] He was the first to describe the clinical symptoms of a thoracic spinal column and cord injury accurately, and his fascination with these lesions was revealed in a treatise on the management of "luxation" of the spine (as he described the deformities associated with trauma). Paré acknowledged the stability that the rib cage gave to the thoracic spinal column, and the significant differences between an anterior dislocation of the spine and a posteriorly displaced injury. Paré clearly outlined the neurological deficit that accompanied an anterior dislocation, pronounced it a "deadly" disorder without hope, and lamented the fact that he could "not through the belly, force it into its place."[24]

Although Paré was acquainted with the poor prognosis assigned these lesions in the writings attributed to Hippocrates, he advocated and described in detail surgical débridement of the injury site for the removal of the "splinters of the broken vertebrae which, driven in, press the spinal marrow in the nerves thereof." He believed that the pressure on the spinal cord was the cause of the patient's shortened life span.[14] He was also the first to use a metal orthosis constructed of lead sheets. This orthosis was not dissimilar to the modern thoracolumbosacral orthosis (TLSO) and was used to maintain the reduction of the vertebral bodies after extension and gentle manipulation of the deformity.[24]

Although there were isolated reports of "successful" surgery for spinal injuries before the mid-20th century (including the removal of a bullet from the thoracic spine in 1774 by Antoine Louis and the 1864 report of the recovery of neurological function in a patient rendered paralyzed by a fracture after a laminectomy), surgical treatment of spinal cord injuries was and is the subject of not insignificant debate.[14, 62, 73, 106] In 1839, Cooper was an advocate of surgical intervention for spinal injuries, whereas Bell's disdain in 1824 of surgery as additional iatrogenic injury was widely accepted: "Laying a patient upon his belly and by incision laying bare the bones of the spine, breaking up these bones and exposing the spinal marrow itself, exceeds all belief."[32, 73] Cushing reported that 80% of the soldiers fighting in World War I who suffered a spinal cord injury died within the first 2 weeks after the injury, and only those with a partial injury had any chance of survival. Cushing abandoned the surgical treatment of spinal injuries because of poor postoperative prognoses.[34] The prognosis for the spinal cord–injured patient remained dismal until the post–World War II era, and the generally accepted pessimistic outlook for the paraplegic patient was reflected in a 1924 report of the Medical Research Council as reported by Guttman: "The paraplegic patient may live for a few years in a state of more or less ill-health." These patients would succumb to the ravages of sepsis as a result of infections of the urinary tract or decubitus ulcers within 2 to 3 years of the initial injury.[73]

Bohler, in his textbook on the treatment of fractures, stressed that an early closed reduction of the fracture to anatomic position was necessary for a favorable outcome.[15] His teachings were widely accepted. Watson-Jones stated "perfect recovery is possible only if perfect reduction is insisted upon; even slight degrees of wedging of the vertebrae may cause persistent aching pain."[139] Nicoll demonstrated that this bias to obtain anatomic alignment was incorrect and without scientific basis when he reported his experience with coal miners with thoracolumbar fractures. He made no attempt at reduction of the bony abnormality, and many of his patients could return to heavy work after the fractures healed despite the abnormal alignment of the spinal column.[112]

Internal fixation of the thoracic spine began after World War II with the introduction of spinous process plates.[82] The debate regarding the use of surgical therapy permutated significantly toward nonsurgical management of these injuries when Guttmann demonstrated that postural reduction and meticulous attention to the medical care of this patient population could result not only in a nearly normal life span but also in a stable fusion of the injured spinal column.[73] He also demonstrated the effectiveness of a spinal cord injury center where intensive multidisciplinary care could be rendered to the spinal cord–injured patient. Munro, Bors, and Commar were simultaneously engaged in the establishment of spinal cord injury centers in the United States.[73] Before the introduction of the first effective internal fixation system by Harrington in the 1960s, surgical treatment did not offer the injured patient any significant gain in neurological function; rather, such treatment was often associated with a deterioration in function. This deterioration of function was associated with increased instability of the bony column by the removal of the posterior elements in a misguided attempt to "decompress" the injured cord.[110]

Although there are multiple devices now used for fixation of the unstable spine, the Harrington system (Zimmer-John & Associates, Warsaw, IN), with modifications by Moe and Edwards was, until recently, the "gold standard" to which all other systems were compared and upon which all other systems depended for approval for clinical use in the United States.[120] Despite increasingly more sophisticated internal fixation devices, there has not been a remarkable increase in the magnitude of the return of neural function after their use compared with that obtained with postural reduction championed by Guttmann, Frankel, and their coworkers. However, Krengel and colleagues reported that early stabilization and decompression of incomplete thoracic lesions was associated with improved neurological function when compared with historical controls.[61, 73, 89] This increase in neurological function may be related to the decompression technique, since Bohlman and coworkers demonstrated that anterior transthoracic decompression was more effective than conservative therapy or laminectomy for the return of ambulation in the patient with an incompletely injured thoracic spinal cord.[17, 19] There are also marginal data to suggest that early internal fixation is associated with decreased hospital stay, early initiation of rehabilitation, and the prevention of bony deformity.[20, 31] Although acknowledging that most American surgeons surgically remove bone or disk fragments that compress the spinal canal, Gaines and Humphreys also noted that the scientific soundness of this concept had not been proved in "matched sets of patients."[36, 44, 94, 113] Boerger concluded in a review of the literature that "surgical treatment of burst fractures in the belief that neurological improvement can be achieved is not justified."[14]

Only the upper portion of the thoracic spinal column that is affixed to the rib cage (T1-9) is considered in this chapter. The lower thoracic levels are addressed in Chapter 320, along with the upper lumbar levels to which they are functionally related.[16]

EPIDEMIOLOGY OF THORACIC SPINE INJURIES

In a large mutlicenter study, the T1-10 region accounted for 16% of spinal column fractures.[67] The most common injury to the thoracic spine is the wedge compression fracture; however, only 10% of thoracic vertebral body injuries are associated with a concurrent spinal cord injury. This compares with a 39% incidence of spinal cord injury in the injured cervical spine.[121] Tator re-

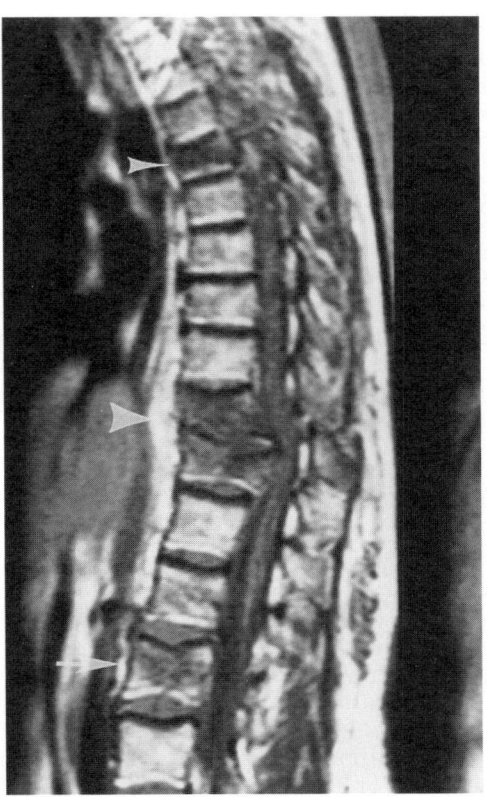

FIGURE 319–1. T1-weighted magnetic resonance imaging study of a patient suffering a complete spinal cord injury from a fracture-dislocation injury at the T10-T11 vertebral levels (*large arrowhead*). There are multiple noncontiguous fractures, including compression fractures at T5 (*small arrowhead*) and L2 (*arrow*).

downward-pointing spinous process. The center of gravity of the upright individual falls through the anterior body of T1, passes anteriorly to the thoracic spine, and falls through the midbody of T12 (Fig. 319–2).

In the upper levels of the thoracic spine, the facets are coronally oriented, whereas at the lower levels, they are sagittally oriented. These characteristics result in the facets of the upper thoracic levels rendering little resistance to rotational forces, while offering significant resistance to anterior translation. The opposite is seen in the lower thoracic levels where the more lumbar-like orientation of the facet joints limits rotation and has little resistive effect to translation. The facet joints also absorb compressive forces while offering resistance to flexion loading.

The thoracic spine is connected to the rib cage by body and transverse process articulations to individual ribs. The rib cage restricts the motion of the thoracic spinal column—especially extension, which is reduced by 70%. The effects of rib cage on flexion and lateral rotation are less prominent. The rib cage also adds stiffness to the spine, and experimental data have demonstrated a fourfold increase in the compression tolerance of the spinal column with an intact rib cage. The stabilization of the thoracic spine by the rib cage results

ported that 15% of all spinal cord injuries occur in the thoracic levels (T1-11), and Calenoff and colleagues reported that upper thoracic (T1-9) spinal cord injuries account for 16% of all spinal cord injuries.[26, 135] Roberts and Curtiss reported that 13 of 26 patients with traumatic paraplegia suffered fractures or dislocations located in the upper thoracic region.[124] This level of the spinal column is frequently involved when there are multiple noncontiguous fractures of the bony spinal column (Fig. 319–1).[125] As Rogers and associates reported, 17% of upper thoracic spine injuries result in paraplegia, and fractures in this region accounted for 33% to 50% of the primary fractures in all cases of multiple noncontiguous fractures.[71, 125, 135]

ANATOMIC AND BIOMECHANICAL CONSIDERATIONS

The thoracic spine consists of 12 vertebral bodies aligned with a prominent kyphotic curvature. These load-bearing elements of the spinal column are 2 to 3 mm lower in the anterior body height than in the posterior body height.[90] This is the primary cause of the normal kyphotic curve. There is also a dorsal arch that consists of relatively small pedicles, transverse processes, articulating facets, broad laminae, and a

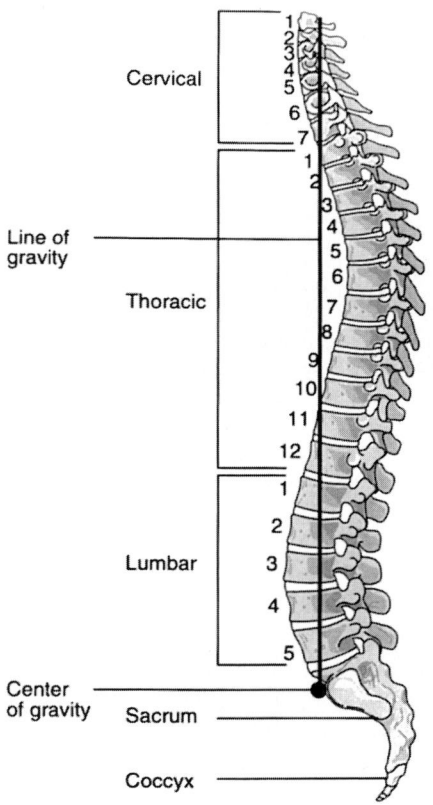

FIGURE 319–2. A schematic drawing of the spinal column with the center of gravity drawn. Note that the upper thoracic vertebral bodies (T1–T10) are posterior to the line of gravity. This causes a flexion moment to be placed upon this portion of the spinal column under normal conditions and is an important consideration when using fixation instrumentation to treat fractures of the thoracic bony column.

in an increased force being required to disrupt the spinal column at these levels compared with other regions of the spinal column.[143]

Normal motion of the thoracic spine is a function of multiple elements that constitute the thoracic spinal column and the associated rib cage. The rigidity of the rib cage and orientation of the facet joints have been addressed previously. The ribs limit the flexion and extension of the upper thoracic area, whereas the posterior elements also resist extension. Axial rotation, in contrast, is limited by the rib cage, ligamentum flavum, facet capsules, and the anterior and posterior longitudinal ligaments. Removal of the posterior elements also has significant effects on the motion of the thoracic spine. Hyperflexion is resisted by the rib cage, the annulus of the disk, the ligamentum flavum, and the posterior longitudinal ligament. The anterior longitudinal ligament and the rib cage resist extension.

The net result of the aforementioned anatomic considerations is that the mean of the range of flexion and extension at each segment in the upper thoracic spine is 4 degrees, whereas that of the middle thoracic spine is 6 degrees. The range of lateral bending is 6 degrees of motion per segment, whereas the range of axial rotation is 8 to 9 degrees (Fig. 319–3).[141] The rigidity of the midportion of the thoracic spine apparently places the midthoracic levels at increased risk for fracture. The upper thoracic and T10 levels are the most infrequently injured levels of the thoracic spine because they are protected by the adjacent, flexible cervical and thoracolumbar junctions (Fig. 319–4).[98]

SPINAL INSTABILITY

Clinical instability is the loss of the ability of the spine to maintain its pattern of displacement under physiologic loads so that there is no initial or additional neurological deficit, no major deformity, and no incapacitating pain.[142] Although this definition is very inclusive, it has rather limited utility to the clinician faced with the acutely injured patient. Various authors have tried to define stability and then recommend treatment based on the presumed injury mechanism. In 1949, Nicoll attempted to define stable versus unstable fractures using an anatomic classification based on an analysis of a series of 166 fractures or fracture-dislocations of the thoracolumbar spine. In his view, the major determinant of stability was the integrity of the interspinous ligament.[112] Holdsworth introduced the first modern classification of fractures and attempted to use radiography to identify specific patterns of spinal fractures associated with the development of early as well as the development of late instability.[81] This classification scheme is based on the two-column theory of spinal column stability and is essentially a biomechanical interpretation of the injury mechanisms determined by the review of plain radiography. The integrity of the posterior bony elements and the posterior ligamentous complex, including the interspinous and supraspinous ligaments and the ligamentum flavum, is the major determinant of stability. The flexion-rotation injury is the most unstable of spinal column injuries in this classification scheme because both the bony and the ligamentous elements of the posterior spinal column are compromised. Holdsworth acknowledged that this system was flawed and that it did not predict the presence of an unstable subset of compression fractures.[80]

There are experimental data that do not support the assertions by Nicoll or Holdsworth that disruption of the posterior ligamentous structures alone causes instability of the spinal column.[11, 81, 112] Denis modified the two-column theory of Holdsworth, dividing the anterior column into an anterior and a middle column, the latter consisting of the posterior longitudinal ligament and the posterior third of the vertebral body (Fig. 319–5).[39] He used computed tomography of the spinal col-

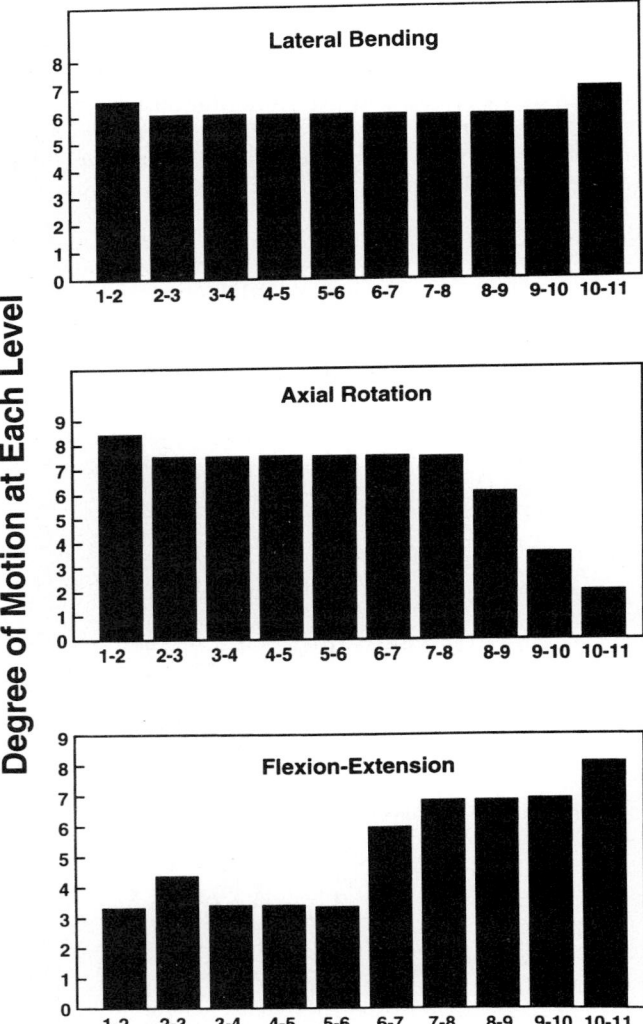

FIGURE 319–3. The degrees of motion of individual segments of the upper thoracic spine in lateral bending axial rotation and flexion-extension. (Adapted from Eismont FJ, Garfin SR, Abitol J: Thoracic and upper lumbar spine injuries. In Browner BD, Jupiter JB, Levine AM, et al (eds): Skeletal Trauma. Vol. I. Philadelphia, Saunders, 1993, p 731.)

Distribution of Frequency of Occurence of Thoracic Fractures

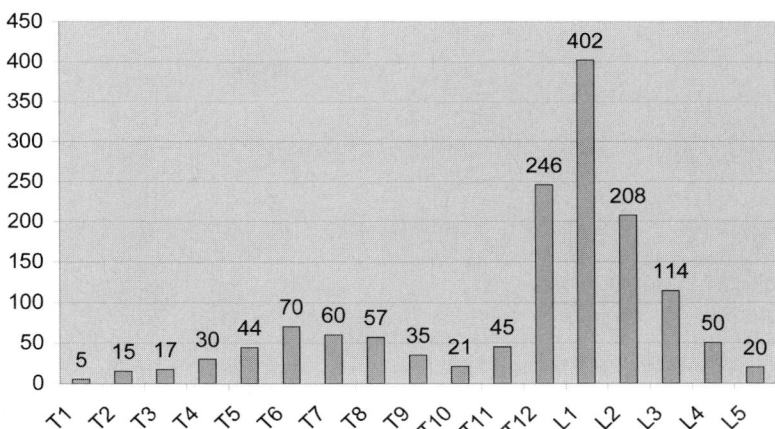

FIGURE 319–4. The distribution of thoracic fractures from T1-10 in a series of 1445 patients presenting with spinal fractures.[98]

umn injury to establish the integrity of the middle column. If what appears to be a compression fracture also has a disruption of the posterior vertebral body, it is actually a burst fracture. Using the computed tomographic images, the burst fracture is distinguished from the more common anterior wedge compression fracture by the continuity of the posterior cortical rim from one pedicle laterally, over the posterior vertebral body to the opposite pedicle (Fig. 319–6). The integrity of the middle column becomes the basis of a new classification of spinal stability, since an injury to the anterior and the middle or the posterior and the middle columns results in an "unstable" fracture.

Maiman and Pintar questioned the validity of this classification and based their objections on biomechanical considerations.[100] These authors cited experimental evidence that posterior ligamentous injury can occur

with a flexion-compression force on the spinal column before vertebral body failure occurs. They also objected to the use of static radiographs to assess the integrity of the ligamentous structures. McAfee and colleagues separated burst fractures into stable and unstable types; the latter type includes disruption of the ligamentous, or bony, posterior column.[104] James and associates also challenged the three-column theory and provided experimental data to suggest that the middle column adds little to the stability of the classic burst fracture.[84] Parker and associates agreed that the middle column is not directly related to the load transfer properties of the injured spine and concluded that the reliance of the three-column classification systems on the integrity of the middle column as the sole determinant of the necessity for surgical treatment results in many stable fractures being treated operatively.[114] James and coworkers also supported the assertion of Holdsworth that the posterior column is the "second crucial column."[81, 84]

Although Denis' three-column injury model of thoracic and lumbar fractures is widely accepted, two other classification systems address the shortcomings of this system. Both of these classification schemes are based on the mechanism of injury: (1) that of Ferguson and Allen reported in 1984 soon after the report of Denis and (2) that of Magerl, which was first published in 1991.[39, 58, 98, 99] Ferguson and Allen modified the three-column model (or regions as they preferred to refer to these anatomical areas) to analyze the effects of excessive loading that resulted in the failure of the spinal column. They used plain, tomographic, and computed tomographic imaging studies to assess the injury mechanism and then classified the resultant injury according to the mechanisms deduced from the findings on radiography of compression, tension, torsion, translation, or a combination of loading forces.[58] Their goal was to use the knowledge of the mechanism that resulted in the failure of the spinal column to guide the selection of the most appropriate method of reduction and the most efficacious type of fixation.[59]

The classification system of Magerl is also based on

Anterior Middle Posterior

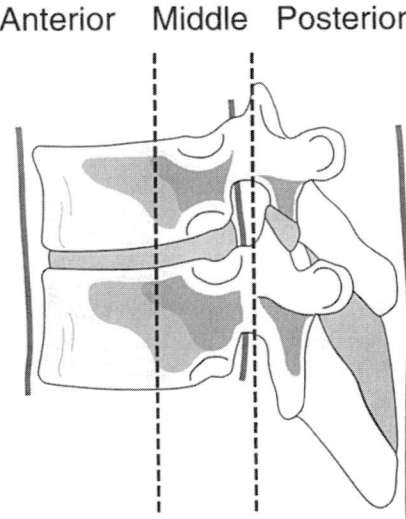

FIGURE 319–5. A diagrammatic representation of the three-column theory of spinal stability. Note that the middle column consists of the posterior portion of the vertebral body and the posterior longitudinal ligament.

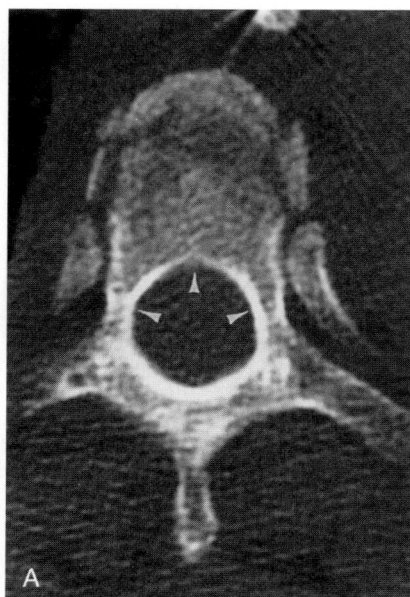 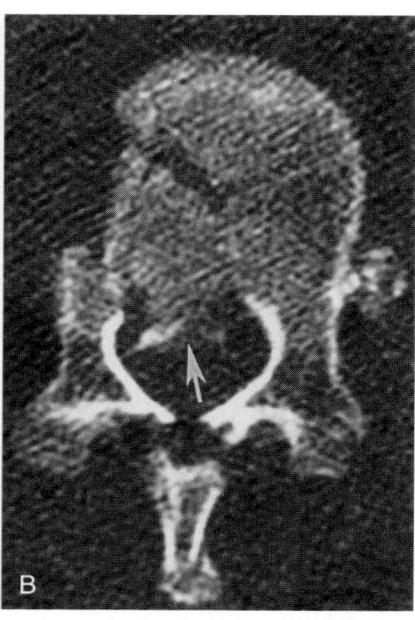

FIGURE 319–6. *A,* Computed axial tomography of a T5 compression fracture. *B,* Similar scan of a T10 burst fracture. Note the intact posterior wall of the vertebral body and the medial cortex of the pedicles in *A* (*arrowheads*) and the fragmentation of the posterior vertebral body (*arrow*) in *B.*

the mechanism of failure of the spinal column and is accepted, with modifications, as a research tool by the members of the major spine societies (Fig. 319–7).[66] This system is based on the two-column model of spinal fractures and on the three functions a stable spine should provide, as defined by Whitesides: ". . . withstand axial forces through the vertebral bodies, tension forces posteriorly, and rotational stress. . . ."[143] Inverting the functional definition of Whitesides, Magerl defines the types of injury patterns based on the pathomorphologic characteristics: type A, failure of the vertebral body in compression; type B, failure of the spinal column from a tensile injury moment; and type C, failure of the spinal column secondary to an axial torque. These types are ordered with increasing severity of the resultant spinal column injury and subdivided into groups according to the injury mechanisms.[98] The division into three groups is based on the morphologic features of the injury and the severity of the injury as it progresses through both the types and the groups, the most stable being the A1 fracture and the least stable, the C3.[98] Although the original classification contains further subdivisions, the simplified system reported by Gertzbein stops at the three by three grid (see Fig. 319–7).[66]

This system is also unique in that data from the whole of the spine are used to formulate the classes of fractures as opposed to previous classification systems that used data limited to the thoracolumbar spine.[37, 99] This system as modified by Gertzbein is simple and open ended. Compared with earlier classification systems, it provides promise both for research and for use as a guideline for fracture management.[66]

White and Panjabi suggested a systematic approach to the issue of instability and provided a checklist to determine stability.[142] They believed that this system was superior to other theories of instability, including that of Denis, because more variables are taken into consideration for the determination of stability.[39] Consideration of multiple variables, they believe, allows the prevention of overtreatment of stable injuries while protecting against neurological complications. Table 319–1 presents a checklist pertinent to the upper thoracic spine, and radiologic criteria are given in Figures 319–8 and 319–9. The patient is considered to have an unstable injury if the total score is 5 or greater.[142]

Although the determination of stability is difficult with only static radiographs, there are signs on plain radiography that should alert the clinician to the presence of instability (Fig. 319–10):[35, 53, 124]

- Displacement of the vertebrae, which implicates disruption of all three columns
- A widened interlaminar or interspinous distance seen with injury to the posterior ligaments and facet joints

T A B L E   3 1 9 – 1 ■ **Point System for Clinical Thoracic Spine Instability**

ELEMENT	POINT VALUE*
Anterior element destruction or malfunction	2
Posterior element destruction or malfunction	2
Costovertebral junction disruption	1
Radiographic criteria as previously described	4
1. Sagittal plane displacement >2.5 mm (2)	
2. Relative sagittal plane angulation	
>5 degrees (2)	
Spinal cord/cauda equina injury	2
Anticipated excessive loading	1

* Total points >5 = clinical instability.
Data from White AA, Panjabi M: Clinical Biomechanics of the Spine. 2nd ed. Philadelphia, JB Lippincott, 1990.

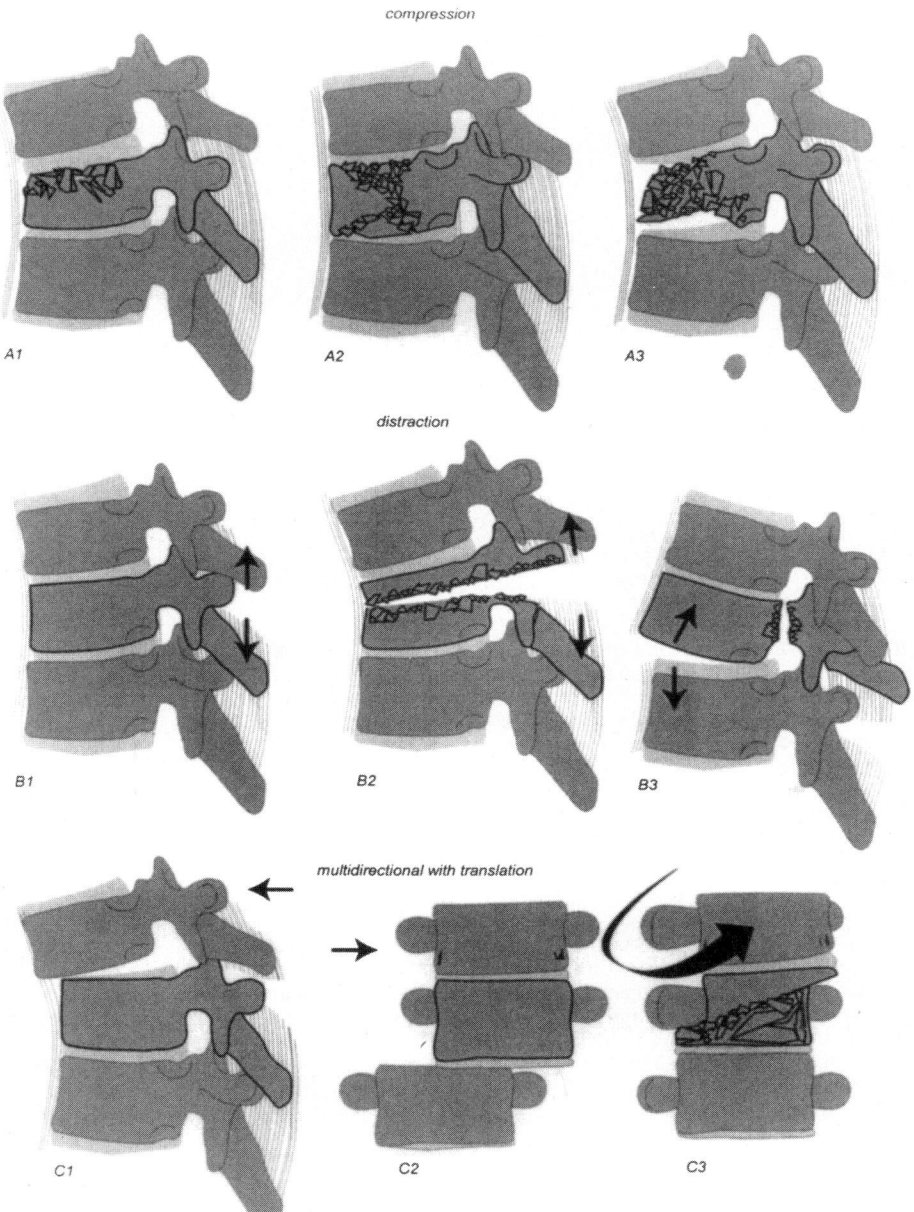

FIGURE 319–7. The fracture classification system as proposed by Magerl and coworkers and modified by Gertzbein. Fractures are divided into types according to major injury force: A(1-3), compression; B(1-3), distraction; and C(1-3), multidirectional with translation. Each type is subdivided into three groups (see text for details). The classification system is arranged in order of increasing severity: A1 is the most stable, whereas C3 is the least stable. The classification system can be used to determine the need for instrumentation and the optimal type of fixation. It represents a uniform method of classification of fractures for clinical research.[66, 98]

- An increased interpedicular distance, signaling injury to all three columns and seen with burst fractures
- A disrupted posterior vertebral body line, suggesting injury to the anterior and middle columns

The value of computed tomography in the assessment of bony injury has been validated by many investigators, including Denis and McAfee and coworkers.[39, 104] We use magnetic resonance imaging to assess the paraspinal soft tissues of the spinal column as well as the spinal cord parenchyma. It is also the imaging study of choice to assess residual spinal cord parenchyma compression by displaced intervertebral disk material, epidural hematoma, and so on.[12, 134]

MECHANISMS OF INJURY

Although considerable controversy exists regarding the surgical management of spinal column injuries, the majority of upper thoracic spinal column injuries associated with spinal cord injury are unstable because significant violence must be inflicted to injure the column in this region. Surgical therapy is undertaken to decompress the spinal cord and to stabilize the bony column to prevent additional injury to the cord in incomplete cord injuries and to allow early mobilization of patients with complete cord injury. The surgical therapy for an injured thoracic spine must take into account the injury force or forces that acted on the

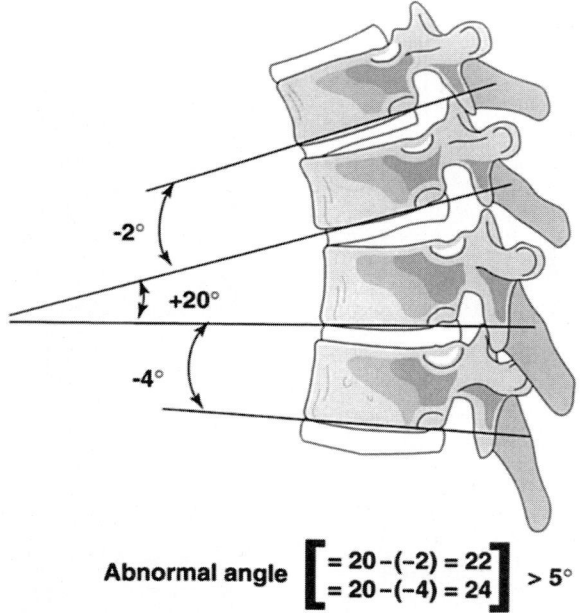

Abnormal angle $\left[\begin{array}{l} = 20 - (-2) = 22 \\ = 20 - (-4) = 24 \end{array}\right] > 5°$

FIGURE 319–8. The method of determination of the relative sagittal angulation at an interspace suspected of being unstable. If the angulation is more than 5 degrees greater than the angulation at either of the two adjacent interspaces, the spine should be considered unstable. This information is one of two radiologic tests that are a part of a point scoring system proposed to determine clinical instability of the thoracic spine (see Table 319–1). Lines are drawn on the inferior end plate of the vertebral body in question and the inferior end plates of the immediately superior and inferior vertebral bodies. In the diagram, the suspicious interval between two vertebral bodies is 20 degrees. The adjacent superior and inferior angulations are measured to be −2 and −4 degrees, respectively. Abnormal angulation and therefore a high suspicion for clinical instability are determined by a difference of 5 degrees or greater between the tested interspace and either of the adjacent vertebral bodies. For example, the differences in angulations are 22 and 24 degrees, respectively, in this example. Two points would be added to the scoring system outlined in Table 319–1.

bony column and the pattern of instability associated with the specific injury.

The forces responsible for a spinal column injury are generally accepted as compression, flexion, extension, rotation, shear, or distraction, or a combination thereof.[51, 91] Magerl and colleagues formulated a classification system by considering the pathomorphologic characteristics of the action of injury moments into three injury patterns: compressive, tensile, and axial torque, which correspond to the three injury types in the system: A, B, and C, respectively (see Fig. 319–7).[98]

The combination of plain radiographs, computed tomography, and magnetic resonance imaging allows definition of the bony and ligamentous injuries that have been inflicted. The information from these studies allows classification of the injury, identification of the unstable injuries, and selection of the proper instrumentation to stabilize the unstable spinal column elements adequately.

Compression. The normal kyphosis of the upper

thoracic spine results in an axial compression load being converted into an anterior flexion load to the vertebral body. The resultant fracture of the vertebral body is a wedge compression fracture; the same injury is produced by a flexion vector (Fig. 319–11).[51] Magerl classifies these fractures as types A1 to A3, depending on the injury pattern.[98]

Flexion. Compression and flexion loads produce an anterior force (flexion-compression), the most common load, on the anterior vertebral body and a simultaneous tensile force on the posterior column. The injury produced is an anterior wedge fracture with an intact posterior vertebral body and therefore an intact middle column. This fracture is stable and usually not associated with spinal cord injury. If the anterior vertebral body is compressed in excess of 50%, posterior ligamentous disruption or facet joint failure often occurs, rendering the injury unstable even in the absence of a fracture of the posterior column bony elements. A facet fracture or capsule injury can allow the superior body to sublux on the inferior body, resulting in a fracture-dislocation. The posterior elements are injured more frequently than is generally appreciated, and disruption of the posterior ligaments often occurs before failure of the vertebral body.[100] Severe injuries that compromise the posterior vertebral body in addition to the anterior vertebral body result in a distinctive pattern of fracture in which the superomedial portion of the

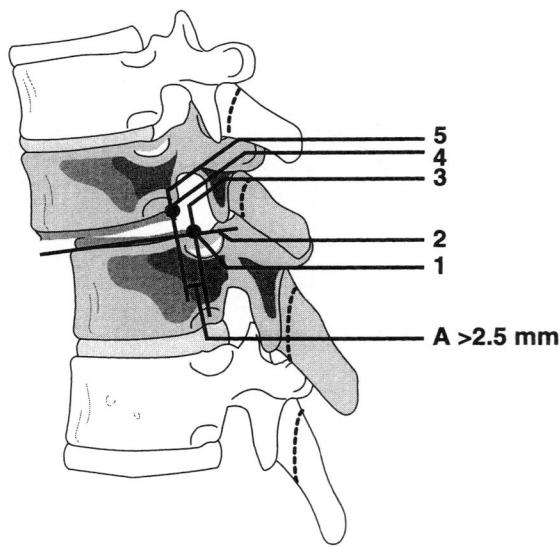

FIGURE 319–9. This diagram demonstrates a method of measuring sagittal plane displacement. Points are placed on the posterosuperior angle (1) of the caudal vertebral image and at the posteroinferior angle (4) of the superior vertebral body of the junction being evaluated. A line is drawn along the superior end plate (2) of the vertebra below the interspace being examined and a perpendicular line drawn to the line along the superior end plate that intersects point 1. A second line (5) perpendicular to the end plate line 2 that intersects point 4 is drawn. The linear distance between the perpendicular lines, defined as distance A, is measured. Instability is likely to be present when A is greater than 2.5 mm; two points are entered on the checklist (see Table 319–1).

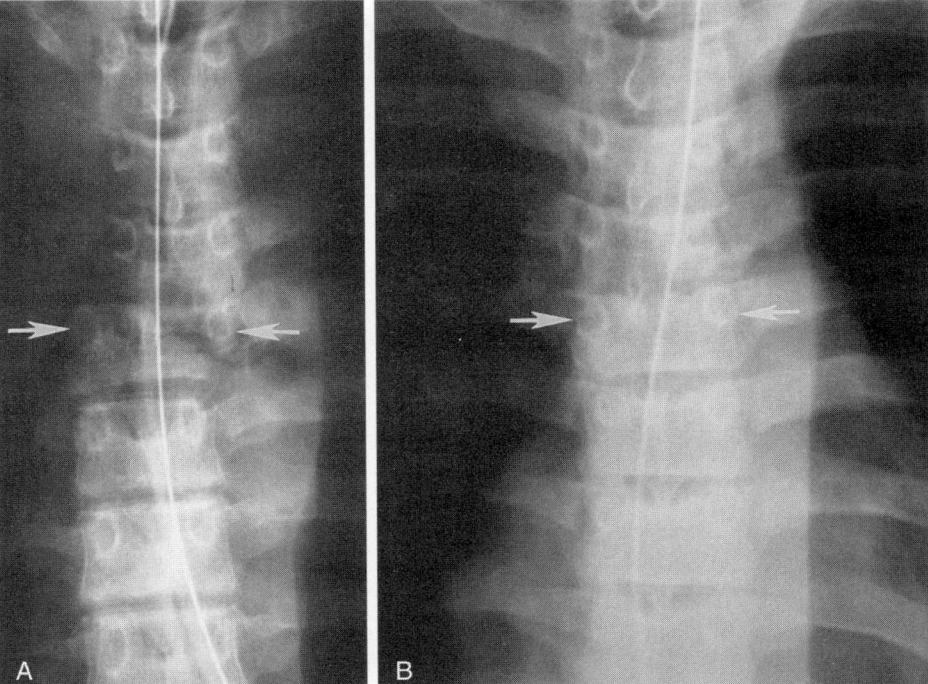

FIGURE 319–10. These are plain radiographs of two thoracic spine fractures: *A,* A fracture-dislocation injury at T7–T8 with comminution and displacement of the vertebral bodies. *B,* A burst fracture of the upper thoracic spine. Note the widened interpediculate distance (*arrows*) and the discontinuity in the alignment of the spinous processes in each of the images. These findings are static radiographic signs of a three column injury and therefore spinal column instability.

posterior vertebral body is fragmented from the remainder of the body; the fragment then rotates into the spinal canal, compromising the intracanalicular neural elements (see Fig. 319–11, A3). Although the resultant burst fracture is a type of compression fracture, the Magerl system differentiates between the stable burst fracture, type A3, which is similar to the more common wedge compression fracture, and the unstable burst fracture, type B1 or C1. The latter types of injuries are often associated with a spinal cord injury and are prone to long-term instability if not surgically reconstructed.

Flexion-Rotation. This combination of injury vectors produces an extremely unstable injury to the vertebral column (Fig. 319–12). The flexion load produces an anterior vertebral body compression fracture, whereas the rotational load disrupts the facet joints by fracturing the superior facet on one side and tearing the facet capsule on the other. In addition, the annulus may fail, the posterior ligaments are disrupted, and the posterior vertebral body may fracture, with retropulsion of bone into the canal.[91] The fracture-dislocation that results from this combination of load on a vertebral column

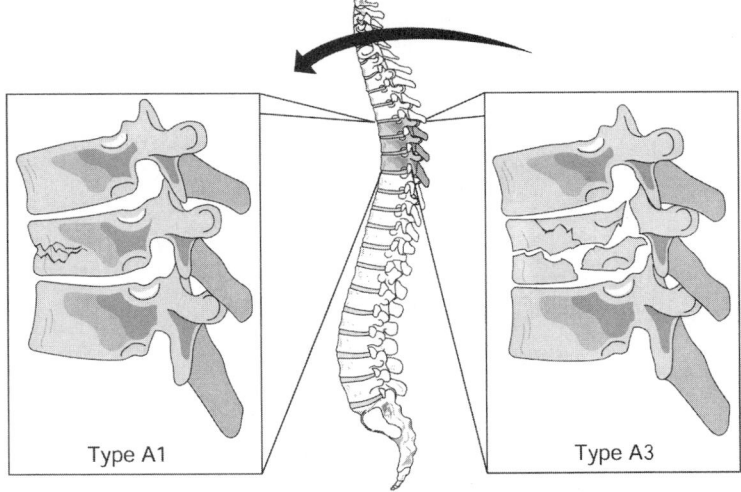

Type A1   Type A3

Flexion injury vector

FIGURE 319–11. A flexion injury vector causes anterior compression of the vertebral body. The resultant injury is usually a stable wedge compression fracture (Magerl type A1). If the tension on the posterior elements is sufficient and the ligamentous structures fail, an unstable compression fracture results. When there is axial loading in addition to the flexion vector, the posterior body fails in a characteristic manner, producing a burst fracture (Magerl type A3).

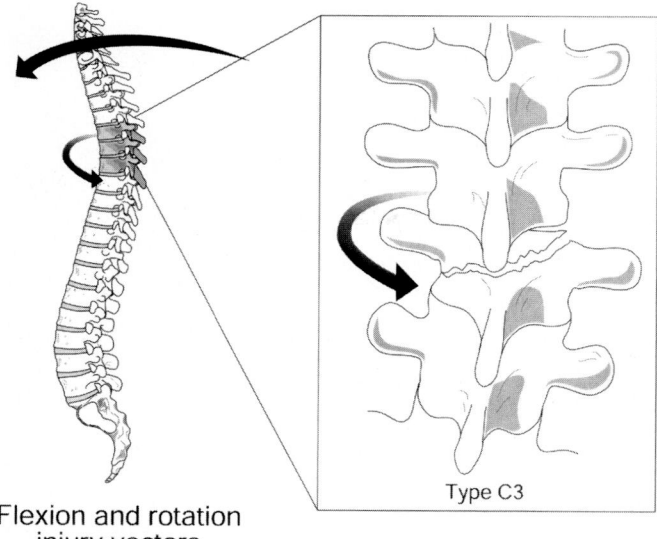

Flexion and rotation
injury vectors

FIGURE 319–12. The combination of flexion and rotation injury vectors is more likely to produce serious spinal column and cord injuries than those associated with a flexion injury vector only. This combination of injury vectors renders the posterior ligamentous structures and joint capsules incompetent and obliquely disrupts the anterior vertebral body and the associated disk. The injury pattern is classified as a Denis type D burst fracture or a Magerl type C3 injury.[39, 98]

was recognized by Holdsworth in his original paper as a highly unstable fracture that was "so constantly associated with paraplegia."[81] Magerl and associates classified this fracture as a aype C3, the most unstable fracture in their classification system.[98]

Shear. Shear forces can be directed in any direction along the longitudinal axis of the spine (Fig. 319–13). Roaf demonstrated that shear force can produce severe ligamentous disruption similar to that produced by the combination of flexion and rotation considered earlier.[123] The shear forces acting in a posterolateral direction cause the superior vertebral body to sublux anteriorly on the inferior vertebral body, with a complete spinal cord injury resulting from the movement of the vertebral bodies.[51] There have been occasions when the anterior movement of the superior body results in a disruption of the pars interarticularis or the pedicles, thereby "decompressing" the spinal cord and protecting it from serious injury.[126] The more common result of this load is an anterior spondylolisthesis; however, the anterior body can be displaced posteriorly or laterally on the inferior body. The Magerl classification of this fracture pattern is type C1.[98]

Flexion-Distraction. Although this type of injury was first described radiographically by Chance in 1948, the mechanism of injury was not defined until later.[28, 119] The injury is commonly associated with the use of seat belts and is now known as a seat-belt injury. Denis distinguished between the "seat-belt type" injuries, of

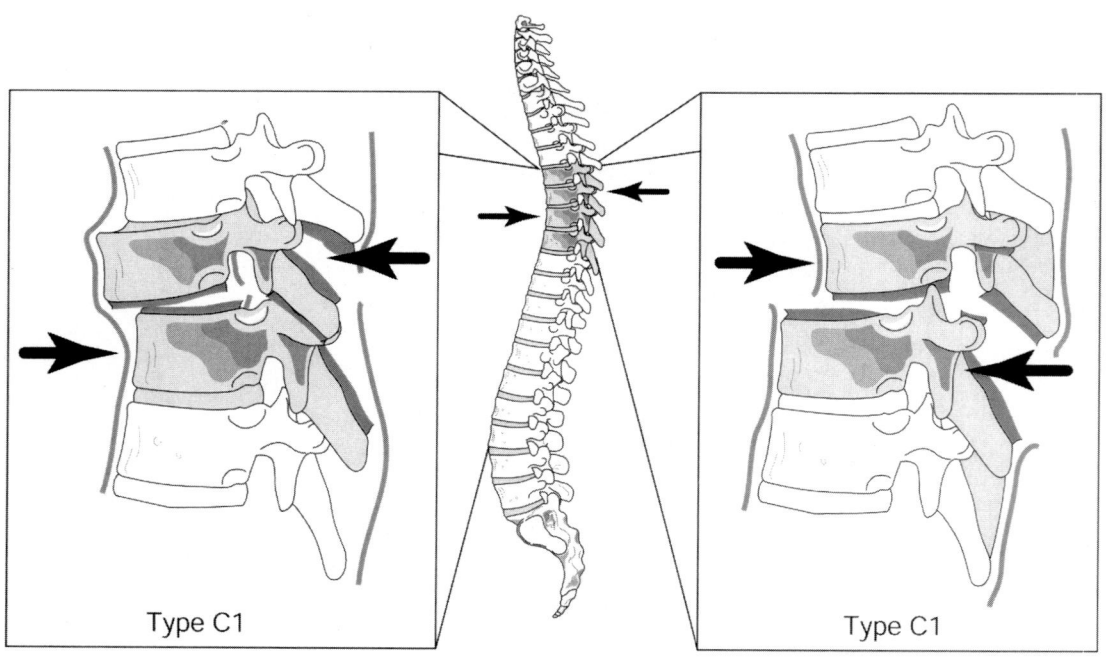

Shear injury vector

FIGURE 319–13. A shear injury is the result of injury vectors directed in opposite directions on different levels of a spinal column. The resultant injury is highly unstable because of the damage to all three columns of the spine. In addition to anterolisthseis and retrolithesis, displacement may be in a lateral direction, depending on the exact direction of the offending vectors. The resultant injury pattern is a Magerl type C1 fracture or a type C3 fracture if the injury vectors are in the coronal plane.[98]

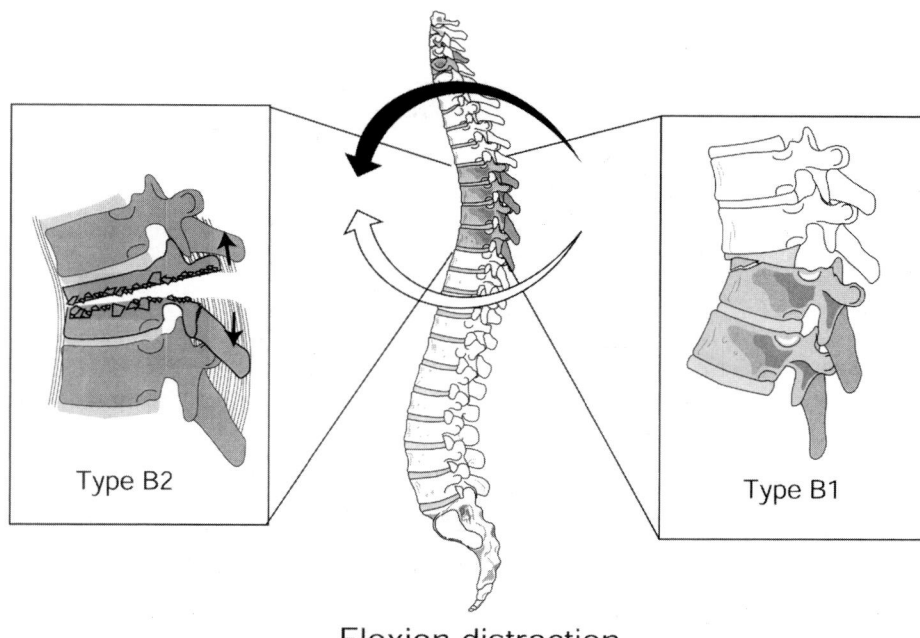

Flexion distraction
injury vector

FIGURE 319–14. The flexion-distraction injury vector is responsible for the seat belt injuries first described by Chance in 1948. Note that the axis of rotation is displaced anteriorly to the longitudinal axis of the bony column, and therefore the spinal column is under tension. In the upper thoracic spine, this injury vector can result in bilateral facet dislocation. The resultant injuries are classified as Magerl type B1 or B2 fractures.[98]

which the fracture described by Chance is only one, and the fracture-distraction injury, which is a subtype of the fracture-dislocation injury.[28, 39] Although the mechanism of injury is similar, that is, a flexion movement produces a tensile force on the posterior and middle columns acting on an axis of rotation that is translated anteriorly (by a seat belt holding the anterior abdominal wall to the seat) in both injuries, the latter injury is characterized by the failure of the anterior column, with disruption of the annulus and stripping of the anterior longitudinal ligament from the inferior vertebral body. The loss of the anterior column allows an anterior spondylolisthesis to occur. Although none of the fracture-dislocations of the flexion-distraction type occurred in the upper thoracic levels in the series reported by Denis, Eismont and associates stated that flexion-distraction can result in a bilateral facet dislocation in the thoracic spine (Fig. 319–14).[39, 51] The fracture described by Chance is designated a type B2 in the Magerl classification system, whereas the fracture-distractions involving ligamentous disruption of the posterior column are designated type B1.[98]

Extension. The vector in this injury is the opposite of the flexion vector acting on the trunk, resulting in forced posterior movement. Although the majority of the injuries resulting from this force are isolated fractures of the posterior elements (facet, lamina, or spinous process), if a severe force is applied, the anterior longitudinal ligament and annulus will fail, resulting in a highly unstable shear fracture, since retrolisthesis of the superior vertebral body on the inferior vertebral segment can occur.[104] Denis and Burkus reported 12 of these types of fractures, 7 of which were in the upper thoracic spine, in a report following Denis' original

paper (Fig. 319–15).[40] The Magerl classification of this fracture type is type B3.[98]

CLASSIFICATION OF THORACIC FRACTURES

There are many classification systems that have been proposed in an attempt to define the mechanism of injury, to determine fractures that are unstable, and to guide the surgeon in the type of instrumentation that is necessary for restoration of stability.[39, 58, 59, 99, 104] Although the most comprehensive classification may be that described by Magerl and colleagues, the system most universally used today is that of Denis, as discussed previously.[39, 58, 98] Although the title of the paper authored by Denis suggests that only thoracolumbar injuries are considered, the data presented include fractures of the upper thoracic region.[39] This system groups major injuries of the spinal column into four groupings, each with multiple subtypes. Unfortunately, although the author does break down the data by injury level and subtype, the raw data are not presented, which does not allow the determination of the number of subtypes occurring in the thoracic spine as opposed to those involving the lower thoracic and lumbar spine. The four major types of injuries are compression, burst, seat-belt type, and fracture-dislocation (Table 319–2).

Compression. This is the most frequently seen thoracic spine injury (42 of 80 thoracic fractures from Denis), but none of the patients with this fracture type in that series sustained a spinal cord injury.[104] In 41 of the 42 thoracic compression fractures in Denis' series,

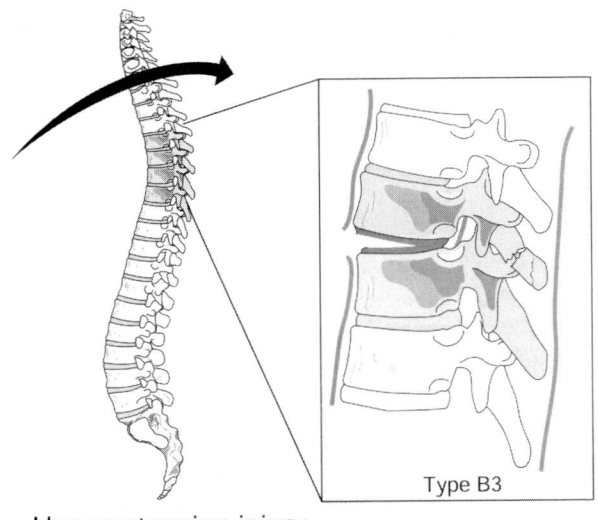

Hyperextension injury
vector

FIGURE 319–15. If an injury vector is posteriorly directed on the upper portion of the thoracic spine, the resultant hyperextension of the spinal column can cause failure of the anterior longitudinal ligament in tension and posterior elements in compression. The resultant injury can be highly unstable and is classified as a Magerl type B3 fracture.[98]

the vertebral body was fractured anteriorly, whereas the remaining fracture was lateral. Although Denis included four subtypes in his original paper, this classification system was dropped in a subsequent paper using the three-column classification to assess spinal stability of acute traumatic lesions.[40, 104]

Denis considers this type of injury to be stable, since the middle column by definition is intact.[16, 39] However, if the anterior vertebral body fracture reduces the anterior body height by 50% or greater, the possibility of posterior column failure, even with an intact middle column, is significant.[100] When the anterior body collapses, the middle column acts as a hinge, resulting in a tension force on the posterior ligamentous structures, which can result in their disruption. If the kyphotic deformity associated with this injury is greater than 30 degrees or if the patient has undergone a decompressive laminectomy, there is an increased incidence of a long-term deformity.[16] This would put the neural elements at risk; therefore, stabilization is recommended. A posterior fixation construct, with a universal segmental fixation system (which distracts the spi-

nal column), will correct the deformity and resist the failure that would otherwise be associated with axial loading of the injured spine.[51] The stable compression fractures are types A1 to A3 in the Magerl classification system (Fig. 319–11). The unstable compression fracture is classified as type B1, and a short posterior compression construct is recommended (see Fig. 319–14).[66, 98]

Burst Fracture. The burst fracture results from failure of the vertebral body under an axial load. Unlike the compression fracture, in which the posterior portion of the vertebral body remains intact, the middle column fails in a characteristic manner (see Fig. 319–6B). Denis listed the pathognomonics of this fracture: (1) comminution of the vertebral body, (2) increase of the interpedicular distance, (3) vertical fracture of the lamina, (4) retropulsion of the fractured posterior vertebral body into the canal, and (5) loss of posterior vertebral body height.[39] Neural deficits were seen in 47% of patients with this injury in the report by Denis; 10 of the 80 thoracic injuries in this series were of the burst type.[39] These injuries may be unstable and may need to have internal fixation applied surgically, especially if there is a posterior injury to the ligaments, facets, or the pars interarticularis or if there is an associated paralysis. The Magerl classification differentiates between the stable and unstable burst fractures: type A3 versus type B1.[98]

Seat-Belt Type Injuries. This group of injuries is the result of a flexion vector acting around an anteriorly placed axis of rotation. These injuries have been associated with the use of seat belts where the lower spine is fixed against the seat and the upper spine pivots around an axis anterior to the spine (see Fig. 319–14). This change in the axis of rotation results in the flexion vector, causing a distraction of the spine. The Magerl system classifies this lesion as a type B2 fracture. Both the Denis and original Magerl system subtype this fracture. All these injuries were seen in the lower thoracic and lumbar levels in the data presented by Denis and are therefore not considered further in this chapter.[37, 98]

Fracture-Dislocation. These fractures are characterized by failure of all the columns under compression, tension, rotation, shear, or extension. Denis described three subtypes of fracture-dislocation injuries (Fig. 319–16); 30 of the 80 upper thoracic injuries reported were of this type. Unfortunately, the author did not report the subtype of the injuries, so no determination can be

T A B L E 3 1 9 – 2 ■ **Major Types of Spinal Injuries and Column Involvement**

	FRACTURE TYPE			
COLUMN	**Compression**	**Burst**	**Seat-Belt**	**Fracture-Dislocation**
Anterior	Compression	Compression	Compression or none	Compression rotation shear
Middle	None	Compression	Distraction	Distraction rotation shear
Posterior	Distraction or none	None	Distraction	Distraction rotation shear

Data from Denis, F: The three-column spine and its significance in the classification of acute thoracolumbar spinal injuries. Spine 8:817, 1983.

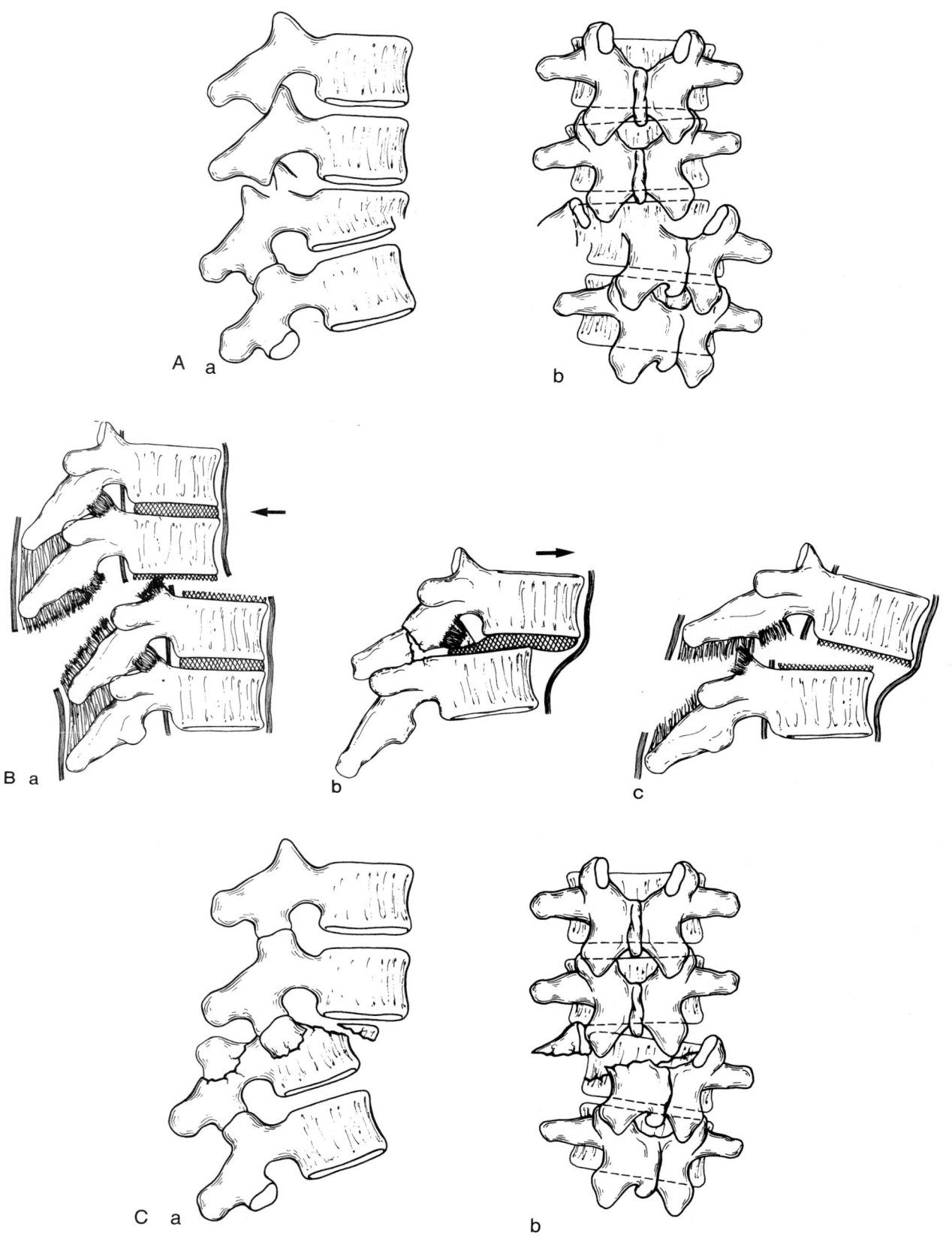

FIGURE 319–16. Illustrations of Denis classification of fracture-dislocation injuries. The major types are classified by the following capital letters. *A,* Type A: a flexion-rotation injury. *B,* Type B: a shear injury. *C,* Type C: disruption of the anterior column resulting in bilateral facet dislocation. Each of the major types has two to three subtypes according to the exact portion of the spinal-column that failed. (From Eismont FJ, Garfin SR, Abitol J: Thoracic and upper lumbar spine injuries. In Browner BD, Jupiter JB, Levine AM, et al. [eds]: Skeletal Trauma. Vol. I. Philadelphia, Saunders, 1993, p 758. Reprinted by permission.)

made as to the frequency of a fracture subtype occurrence in the upper thoracic region. This group of spinal column injuries is associated with the highest incidence of spinal cord lesions in Denis' series, and Bohlman and associates reported an 80% incidence of paraplegia with this type of thoracic fracture.[19, 39]

The type A fracture-dislocation is a flexion-rotation injury that was described by Holdsworth in miners who suffered a hyperflexion and rotation load on their spinal column as a result of mining accidents (see Fig. 319–12).[81] A fall from a height or a motor vehicle collision can also produce a similar injury. This is a Magerl type C3 fracture.[98]

The type B injuries are the result of shear vectors directed from the posterior to anterior spine, resulting in the subluxation of the superior body anteriorly, but vectors can be applied in the anterior to posterior direction, resulting in a retrolisthesis of the superior body (see Fig. 319–13). These injuries are unstable because of the damage to all three columns, and injury to the spinal cord is common. The former injuries can occasionally fracture the posterior elements, resulting in an "autolaminectomy" and a less severe spinal cord injury. The Magerl classification is type C1.[98]

Denis and Burkus reported 12 thoracic and lumbar injuries of the shear type in individuals who suffered the shear injury as a result of hyperextension of the spine secondary to lumberjacking or motor vehicle collision. All patients suffered a spinal cord injury: all except 1 was complete, and 7 of the 12 involved the upper thoracic spine.[39] The Magerl classification is type B3.[98]

Denis also described a third subtype, type C, which is a bilateral facet dislocation that superficially resembles the seat-belt type of flexion-distraction injury (see Fig. 319–14). In this case, the flexion-distraction force also injures the anterior column and hinders its ability to function as a hinge. Although the bony portion of the column fails and the anterior annulus is disrupted, the anterior longitudinal ligament is stripped from the anterior surface of the inferior body but is usually not torn.[39] Gellad and associates described 29 patients with this injury as the result of motor vehicle accidents, falls, objects falling on the victims, or bicycle accidents. None of the 29 patients had injuries in the upper thoracic spine and are therefore not considered further.[64] The Magerl classification for this type of fracture is type C3 because a rotational injury vector is involved.[98]

INITIAL MANAGEMENT OF A THORACIC SPINE INJURY

Initial management of the patient with thoracic spine injury begins in the field with the treatment of life-threatening injuries and the suspicion of a spinal cord injury in any multiply injured patient. A hard cervical collar and backboard must be used for safe transportation of the patient to a trauma center.

In the emergency department, the patient must be treated as though a spinal cord injury is present until this injury is ruled out. The initial management in the emergency department should follow the Advanced Trauma Life Support protocol of the American College of Surgeons.[3] Once the patient undergoes initial resuscitation, the integrity of all regions of the spinal column is assessed with plain radiographs of the cervical, thoracic, and lumbosacral spine.[3] High-speed helical computed tomography is used to visualize areas not imaged sufficiently well on plain films.

One must be cognizant of the possibility of a cervical injury or additional spinal fractures accompanying the thoracic fracture. Although the Advanced Trauma Life Support protocol includes high-dose methylprednisolone treatment for patients with spinal cord injury, the current assessment of the scientific basis for steroid use in spinal cord injury by the Section on Disorders of the Spine and Peripheral Nerves of the American Association of Neurological Surgeons and the Congress of Neurological Surgeons is that there is stronger evidence for complications than for positive clinical effect.[3, 20, 74] Steroids are therefore no longer used at our institutions.

A magnetic resonance imaging study or a computed tomography myelogram is needed to assess the bone and soft tissue injury accurately. This information is useful for the determination of the most appropriate subsequent therapy. Any neurological deficit secondary to a spinal cord injury is recorded using the American Spinal Injury Association Standard Classification of Spinal Cord Injury.[4] This information is valuable for the management of the patient, and the classification system is endorsed by the major spine societies for clinical spinal cord injury research.

SURGICAL VERSUS NONSURGICAL MANAGEMENT OF THORACIC INJURIES

The definitive management of thoracic spine injuries has long been the subject of serious debate. The deformity of the spinal column associated with thoracic lesions has fascinated physicians and surgeons since the beginning of recorded history. Starting with Ambroise Paré, both surgical and nonsurgical management of spine injuries has been advocated, but the ability to surgically treat the injured spine effectively awaited the development of aseptic technique, anesthesia, antibiotics, and effective treatment for shock. Before the introduction of the Harrington distraction system, internal fixation was generally ineffective, and the instability introduced by the laminectomies often performed increased the instability of the bony lesion.[20]

With the development of the Harrington distraction rods and continuing proliferation of internal fixation systems, there was, and continues to be, great enthusiasm for surgical therapy. Strong scientific evidence that spinal fractures are effectively managed nonoperatively, with bed rest and hospitalization tempers some of the enthusiasm for surgical management. The results reported by Frankel and colleagues remain the "gold standard" against which alternative treatments and final outcomes are measured; similarly excellent results are documented by Davies and associates using nonoperative therapy.[61, 89] Some series of thoracolumbar spine fractures show a slight trend toward better neurological improvement with surgical treatment, but the statistical significance is marginal. Neurological improvement of incomplete spinal cord lesions after anterior or posterior surgical decompression has been reported.[2, 41, 46, 48, 68, 88] Krengel and colleagues and Bohlman and associates specifically addressed incomplete lesion of the upper thoracic spine; the former groups advocated early treatment by posterior stabilization, whereas the latter group reported neurologic improvement after late anterior decompression. With late anterior decompression, Bohlman and associates reported an improvement of 2.0 Frankel grades per patient, whereas Krengel and colleagues reported an average recovery of 2.2 Frankel grades per patient attributable to early (less than 24 hours) stabilization after the initial injury.[19, 31] The number of patients in each group is small because this type of lesion represents less than 2% of all spinal injuries; definitive answers to the timing method of surgery await determination in a controlled study.

Neurological deterioration during nonoperative treatment can occur and is documented in 6 of 33 patients with burst fractures of the thoracic or thoracolumbar spine by Denis and coworkers. We conclude that surgical treatment is safer for this specific injury.[41] However, in the 371 patients in the population studies by Frankel and coworkers, there was only a 0.5% incidence of neurological deterioration with postural reduction and recumbency.[89] The lack of valid data hampers the determination of the most cost-effective method of treatment.

Although the bone deformity can be corrected with surgery, it is unclear whether this is clinically important.[36, 113] Nicoll noted no correlation between the degree of spinal deformity and the report of symptoms, whereas Soreff did find a significant correlation.[112, 129] McAfee and colleagues, in their review of delayed anterior decompression and fusion of thoracolumbar and lumbar injuries, found that patients with a residual kyphosis improve neurologically.[102] Edwards and Levine's data, in contrast, suggest that anatomical restoration is important for good long-term results.[49, 50] However, most authors agree that hospitalization time will be shortened with surgical stabilization in patients with paralysis.[31, 44, 60, 83] Mobilization and rehabilitation are facilitated with rigid surgical stabilization, and to date these remain the primary predictable advantages of early stabilization with instrumentation. Gaines and Humpreys felt that "the only absolute indication for surgical internal fixation of the spine" is when the spine is not likely to heal and is "generally associated with complete neurologic injury in which there is extremely poor or absent apposition of the fracture fragments."[62] We acknowledge that most surgeons in the United States would clear bone fragments from the injury site, but we also assert that the scientific basis for this proclivity is wanting. Boerger and associates, in a review of the literature, conclude that the surgical treatment of burst fractures in the hope that the patient will improve neurologically is not justified by the current scientific literature.[14] A large multicenter trial of spinal fractures finds little objective data that surgical management is preferable to nonoperative management. The study also documents a 3% complication rate in the nonoperative group, which is in stark contrast to the 25% complication rate in surgically managed patients.[67]

SURGICAL MANAGEMENT OF THORACIC INJURIES

There is no consensus regarding surgical therapy for an individual thoracic spine injury and, indeed, there are several equivalently efficacious treatment alternatives. Our philosophy is that good results can be obtained by more than one approach, but that there are several guidelines that may be of assistance in the selection of a particular approach to a given fracture.

Although there have been attempts to correlate the degree of kyphosis, percentage decrease in anterior vertebral body height, and amount of canal compromise from a retropulsed bone fragment with the degree of stability, no consensus exists. Most surgeons would agree with decompression and stabilization of neurologically incomplete spinal cord injuries, but consensus as to the exact procedure or procedures, the order, and the timing of the surgical intervention remains elusive. The role of surgery in patients with complete spinal cord injuries is more controversial. We aggressively treat complete lesions with posterior stabilization to facilitate transfer to the spinal cord rehabilitative center unless significant anterior column damage exists.

There are, however, recommendations based on several classification systems that offer the practitioner direction in the management of thoracic spinal fractures. Most of the schemes are based on the thoracolumbar junction but offer guidance in the determination of management. Gertzbein uses the simplified Magerl system to offer guidance for specific approaches to these fractures.[66] If type A injuries are treated surgically, a posterior distraction construct is needed for restoration, whereas type B injuries are often corrected with a short-segment compression construct. Type C injuries need a multilevel (two or more levels on either side of the injury) fixation system, and in some cases (because of severe instability), both anterior and posterior stabilization. Extrapolation from the Load-Sharing Classification scoring system developed by McCormack and associates helps the practitioner to assess the ability of the injured vertebral body to fuse before the fixation instrumentation fails. High scores are an indication of the necessity to address the injury with a reconstruction of the anterior column by an anterior approach (Fig. 319–17).[105]

Parker and colleagues select operative treatment for patients based on the presence of one or more of the following criteria: presence of a neurological lesion caused by the fracture, evidence of injury to all three of the spinal column segments, or translational displacement at the fracture site. Long posterior fixation systems

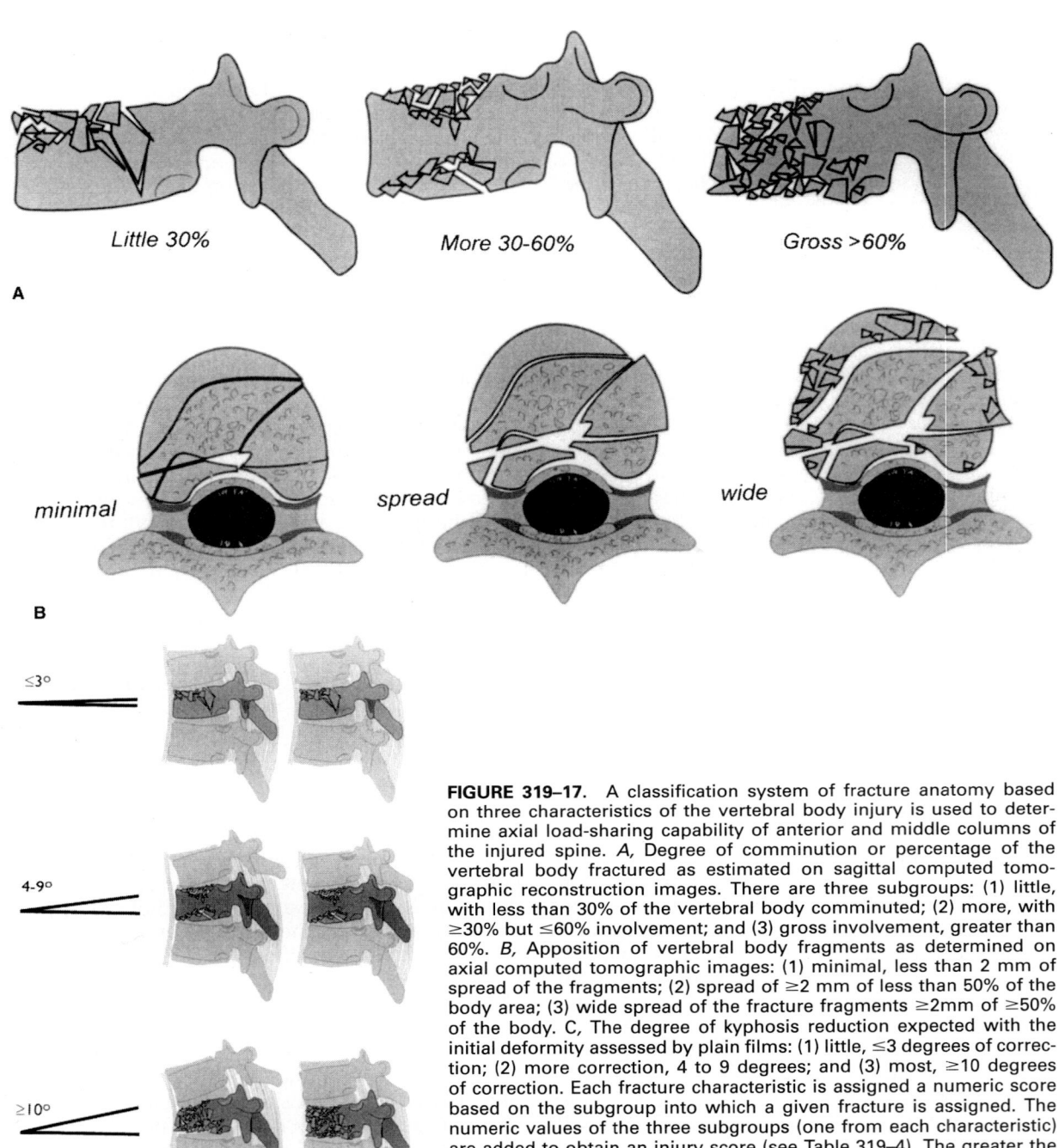

FIGURE 319–17. A classification system of fracture anatomy based on three characteristics of the vertebral body injury is used to determine axial load-sharing capability of anterior and middle columns of the injured spine. *A,* Degree of comminution or percentage of the vertebral body fractured as estimated on sagittal computed tomographic reconstruction images. There are three subgroups: (1) little, with less than 30% of the vertebral body comminuted; (2) more, with ≥30% but ≤60% involvement; and (3) gross involvement, greater than 60%. *B,* Apposition of vertebral body fragments as determined on axial computed tomographic images: (1) minimal, less than 2 mm of spread of the fragments; (2) spread of ≥2 mm of less than 50% of the body area; (3) wide spread of the fracture fragments ≥2mm of ≥50% of the body. *C,* The degree of kyphosis reduction expected with the initial deformity assessed by plain films: (1) little, ≤3 degrees of correction; (2) more correction, 4 to 9 degrees; and (3) most, ≥10 degrees of correction. Each fracture characteristic is assigned a numeric score based on the subgroup into which a given fracture is assigned. The numeric values of the three subgroups (one from each characteristic) are added to obtain an injury score (see Table 319–4). The greater the number, the less likely the injured vertebral body is to resist an axial load and the more likely a posterior, short-segment fixation construct is to fail.[105]

are used if the patient is unable to cooperate with postoperative bracing or has medical conditions that would interfere with reconstruction of the anterior column. Short-segment instrumentation is used posteriorly if there is a Load-Sharing Classification score of 6 or less (Table 319–3). Patients with a score of 7 or greater and no evidence of translation at the injury site are treated surgically using an anterior short segment fixator. Patients with translational displacement (all fracture-dislocations) are treated using the posterior approach with a staged anterior reconstruction. All patients with evidence of compression of neural tissue undergo decompression at the time of the initial surgery using a transpedicular approach for posterior devices or anterior decompression if an anterior fixator is placed.[114]

Mirza and associates offer specific treatments for spinal fractures based on the classification of McAfee and colleagues and the presence or absence of a neurological injury. The specific recommendations are based on the authors' collective experience and represent

TABLE 319–3 ■ **Scoring System for Quantitating the Ability of the Injured Vertebral Body to Share Axial Loading**

A: Comminution

	Little	More	Gross	
	<30%	≥30% and ≤60%	>60%	
Score	1	2	3	1–3

B: Apposition of fragments

	Minimal	Spread	Wide	
	Minimal	≥2 mm; <50%	≥2 mm; >50%	
Score	1	2	3	1–3

C: Deformity correction

	Little	More	Most	
	≤3°	4°–9°	≥10°	
Score	1	2	3	1–3
			Total score	3–9

The system assesses three characteristics of the injured spine: **A:** comminution of the vertebral body as estimated on sagittal CT reconstruction images; **B:** apposition or spread of the vertebral body fragments as assessed on an axial CT scan; and **C:** expected deformity correction that will be obtained with fixation instrumentation expressed as degrees of change in the kyphotic deformity. A numeric value is assigned for each characteristic (1–3) and added to determine the total that is related to the ability of the vertebral body to load-share (Fig. 319–17).[98]

more traditional, principally orthopedic, approaches to the treatment of spinal fractures. The recommendations are not scientifically validated (Table 319–4).[96, 104, 109]

Farcy and associates reported an algorithm for the treatment of thoracic fractures that is based on a sagittal index (SI) and an instability grade (IG) and used the algorithm in a prospective study.[57] The SI is defined as the measurement of segmental kyphosis at the injury level, which is then adjusted for the baseline sagittal contour (Table 319–5). The IG is based on the three-column theory of Denis and considers ligamentous damage in addition to bony element injury in the determination of instability (Fig. 319–5). One point is given for injury to bone and another point for injury to ligamentous structures associated with each column. A total disruption of the bony and ligamentous elements would result in an IG of 6 (Table 319–6). Based on a prospective study, the authors determined that a spinal injury with an SI of less than 25 degrees and an IG of less than 3 can be treated without surgery (Table 319–7).[55–57] Farcy and coworkers recommend that spinal injuries with an SI of greater than 25 degrees and less than 35 degrees or with an IG of greater than 3 but less than 5, or a combination of both, be treated with posterior reduction and instrumentation. A simultaneous anterior/posterior approach is recommended for an SI greater than 35 degrees or an IG greater than or equal to 5, or both.[57]

GENERAL PRINCIPLES

Electrophysiological monitoring of the spinal cord should be available intraoperatively, and intraoperative imaging, including ultrasound, is an important part of the surgical therapy. Baseline somatosensory evoked potentials and motor evoked potentials are obtained

TABLE 319–4 ■ **Treatment Guidelines as Identified by Mirza and Associates**

INJURY TYPE	SUGGESTED TREATMENT
Compression fracture	• Observation with followup, or prefabricated brace immobilization for 12 weeks
Burst fracture, stable	• Custom fitted orthosis or cast immobilization for 12 weeks • TLSO, L4 and above • TLSO or HTLSO, L5 and below • Hyperextension cast or brace, if kyphosis >15°
Burst fracture, unstable	• Surgical decompression and stabilization approach is controversial • Emergent posterior short-segment decompression and fusion, with immobilization in a custom TLSO for 12 weeks. • Delayed anterior decompression and fusion if the patient has residual cord compression in the setting of a neurologic deficit.
Flexion-distraction (Chance)	• Hyperextension cast, if osseous injury with no associated neurologic deficit and no abdominal injury (Chance injury). • Posterior short-segment stabilization and fusion, if associated neurologic injury or abdominal injury or when spinal injury is primarily ligamentous.
Fracture-dislocation	• Posterior long-segment surgical stabilization with pedicle screw fixation of two to three levels above and below the injury and fusion with local bone graft

TLSC, thoracolumbosacral orthosis; HTLSO, hip thoracolumbosacral orthosis.
Table modified from Mirza SK, Mirza AJ, Chapman JR, et al: Classification of thoracic and lumbar fractures: Rationale and supporting data. J Am Acad Orthop Surg 10:364, 2002.

TABLE 319-5 ■ Sagittal Index

	THORACIC VERTEBRAL LEVEL
Local kyphosis	X degrees
Baseline curve	5 degrees
Sagittal index (SI)	SI degrees = X degrees − 5 degrees

Adapted from Farcy JP, Weidenbaum M, Glassman SD: Sagittal index in management of thoracolumbar burst fractures. Spine 15:958, 1990.

TABLE 319-7 ■ Treatment of Spinal Fractures

TREATMENT	SAGITTAL INDEX	INSTABILITY GRADE
Brace	<15	<2
Closed reduction/cast	≥15 and <25	>1 and <3
Posterior instrumentation	≥25 and <35	≥3 and <5
Simultaneous anterior/posterior approach	≥35	≥5

Adapted from Farcy JP: Unstable fractures of the lumbar spine—discussion. Spinal Frontiers 3:4, 1996.

and spontaneous electromyography is performed, if appropriate and practical, before anesthesia. Perioperative prophylactic antibiotics are administered. Based on the results of the National Acute Spinal Cord Injury Study II, the methylprednisolone protocol was continued, or restarted as a prophylactic measure.[21] However, outcome data from patients who received the second dose of steroid show increased perioperative mortality with this second treatment, and the practice has now been discontinued.[38] Neurophysiological monitoring as a baseline, with the patient awake, starts with routine somatosensory evoked potentials. If the patient has a complete thoracic spinal cord injury, spinal cord monitoring is not continued in the lower extremities. It is used to monitor the upper extremities when an anterior transthoracic decompression is performed. Patients with unstable fractures are often intubated nasotracheally or orally while awake in a supine position and carefully "log-rolled" prone onto a four-post operating frame for posterior or posterolateral approaches or onto a radiolucent operating table into a lateral decubitus position for transthoracic or retroperitoneal approaches. This awake intubation technique is especially important in patients with incomplete deficits and with grossly unstable spinal columns.

Once the patient is properly positioned, the baseline neurological assessments are repeated to ensure that no deterioration has taken place. A nitrous-narcotic balanced anesthetic is usually given, because spinal cord monitoring is essential, since even low concentrations of inhalation anesthetic can significantly alter or obliterate the evoked waveforms.[25] In prone positioning, we prefer a Jackson table (Orthopaedic Systems, Inc., Union City, CA) or an Acromed Spinal Surgical Positioning Board (Depuy Acromed, Raynham, MA) and are careful to avoid malpositioning to eliminate brachial plexus injuries or meralgia paresthetica.

Proper positioning is critical to aid closed reduction of the spinal injury. To allow optimal positioning and to prevent injuries to the eyes, the Mayfield Skull Clamp (Ohio Medical Instrument Co., Cincinnati, OH) is used. A Cell Saver system (Haemonetics, Braintree, MA) is routinely used to minimize total blood loss, and hemostasis is maintained intraoperatively with powdered absorbable gelatin sponge (Surgifoam, Ethicon, Somerville, NJ) mixed with thrombin. Controlled hypotension is not recommended because of the deleterious effect of hypoperfusion on the compromised nervous system tissue. Sequential Compression Sleeves (Kendall Healthcare Products, Mansfield, MA) are also used intraoperatively to reduce the incidence of complications from venous stasis.

Any internal fixation devices that are used to align the spinal column must be viewed as a temporary construct that will universally fail if an adequate bone fusion does not occur. We use cadaveric grafts only in the reconstruction of anterior decompression defects and use autologous bone graft whenever possible. If an allograft or metal cage is placed to reconstruct the anterior bony column, bone salvaged from the vertebral body and rib taken at the time of the decompression is used for the fusion mass, and only rarely is it necessary to harvest additional autograft. In the fusion of the posterior constructs, autologous graft is harvested from the posterior iliac crests and is combined with facet arthrodesis and decortication of the transverse process, lamina, and pars interarticularis.

In the following sections, specific operative therapy is considered for fractures of the thoracic spine, including operative approaches, techniques, and specific instrumentation systems.

TABLE 319-6 ■ Instability Grade (IG)

	ANTERIOR COLUMN	MIDDLE COLUMN	POSTERIOR COLUMN
Bone	Anterior ²/₃ Vertebra*	Posterior ¹/₃ Vertebra*	Posterior Arch*
Ligament	Anterior longitudinal*	Posterior longitudinal*	Posterior complex*

* One point for injury to either bone or ligament in each column.
  0 = uninjured spine (maximum stability).
  6 = maximum injury to spine (maximum instability).
Adapted from Farcy JP, Weidenbaum M, Glassman SD: Sagittal index in management of thoracolumbar burst fractures. Spine 15:958, 1990.

POSTERIOR FIXATION DEVICES

Harrington Distraction Rods

Although Harrington introduced the distraction rod fixation system to treat postpolio scoliosis in 1949, the utility of this system to reduce and internally stabilize spinal fractures was soon realized.[43, 77, 120] This was the first effective internal fixation system that could reliably reduce and stabilize thoracic and lumbar spinal fractures. The good reduction of the deformity and long-term maintenance of the reduction were tempered by the 15.5% complication rate (Fig. 319–18).[22, 44, 49, 60, 107, 120] The Harrington system as introduced afforded poor control of a rotational instability, and the availability of more flexible fixation systems has largely replaced this system. We have found the powerful distraction force generated useful to reduce gross fracture-dislocation injuries.

Universal Segmental Fixation Systems

The Cotrel-Dubousset Instrumentation System (Medtronic, Memphis, TN) was developed to address the limited ability of the Harrington and Luque instrumen-

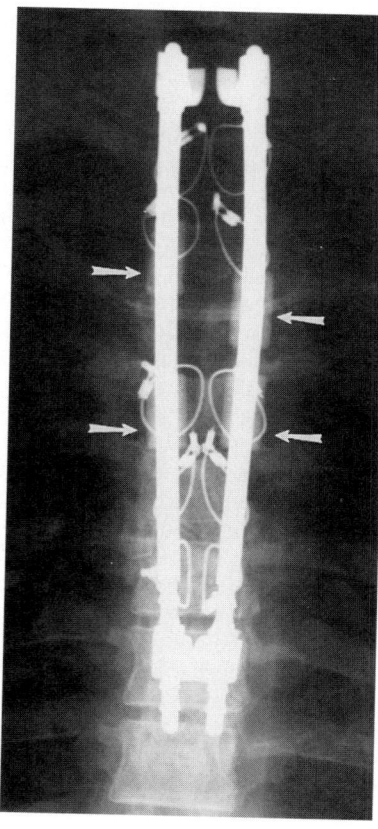

FIGURE 319–18. An anteroposterior plain radiograph of a Harrington rod construct that also employs Edward's sleeves (*arrows*) and Songer sublaminar cables. Note that the rod is inverted with the rachet area directed inferiorly because of the location of the superior hooks at the uppermost thoracic level. The combination of Edward's sleeves and the cables greatly enhances the rotary stability of the construct.

tation systems (Zimmer-Johns & Associates, Warsaw, IN) to correct scoliosis, in which the vertebral bodies are rotated and translated in multiple planes. The Harrington distraction rods do not attach to each vertebral body, and the resultant poor segmental fixation allows unopposed rotation of the vertebral bodies between the hook sites. This limitation in bone fixation also does not directly reduce rotatory translation or subluxation of vertebral bodies between the distal hooks and was the impetus for the development of the Cotrel-Dubousset instrumentation system. Cotrel and colleagues placed hooks at the extremes of the rod in a "claw" configuration to fix the rod to the spinal column.[33] The "claws" consisted of two hooks placed on the rostral and caudal surfaces of an individual vertebral-level lamina facing each other. Hooks placed on the intervening segmental levels and contouring of the rod are then used to position the vertebral bodies in any of the three dimensions or correct the local deformity. This type of bony anchorage allows either compression or distraction to be placed between the upper, intermediate, and lower vertebral levels. With parallel rods on either side of the spinous processes, reduction of an abnormal curvature could be accomplished and fixation of the spine held until the bony fusion matured. Pedicle hooks that are placed in the facet joint and abut the inferior edge of the pedicle were developed to obviate the necessity of placing hooks sublaminarly on the inferior surface of the instrumented lamina. Transverse process hooks were introduced as a replacement for the hooks placed sublaminarly on the superior laminar surface for the same reason. We prefer sublaminarly placed hooks in thoracic constructs that use hook fixation. The placement of cross-linked devices to lock the rods to each other, forming a rectangular construct, increases the stability of the construct and greatly increases the rotational stability of the instrumented spine, thus obviating another limitation of the Harrington distraction rod.[8, 33]

While Cotrel and colleagues were developing the Cotrel-Dubousset instrumentation systems, other groups were developing modifications to the Harrington distraction rods to increase the rotation stability.[6, 8, 132] Ashman and associates developed a cross-link to rigidly fix the rods together and had experimented with intermediate hooks on the Harrington distraction rods to allow more flexibility in the types of corrective forces that could be effected with this distraction system.[8] This initial work was incorporated in the development of the TSRH universal spine instrumentation system (Medtronic, Memphis, TN; Fig. 319–19). Asher and associates were also interested in improving the stability of fixation systems and independently developed a cross-link device for Luque rod sublaminar wire constructs.[88] Rather than use hooks for the bone interface in their device, Asher and associates based their efforts on refining the Luque-Galveston fixation described by Allen and Ferguson.[2, 7] This device was marketed as the Isola spinal system (Depuy Acromed, Raynham, MA) and eventually included hooks for bone interface as well (Fig. 319–20).

The universal instrumentation systems that incorpo-

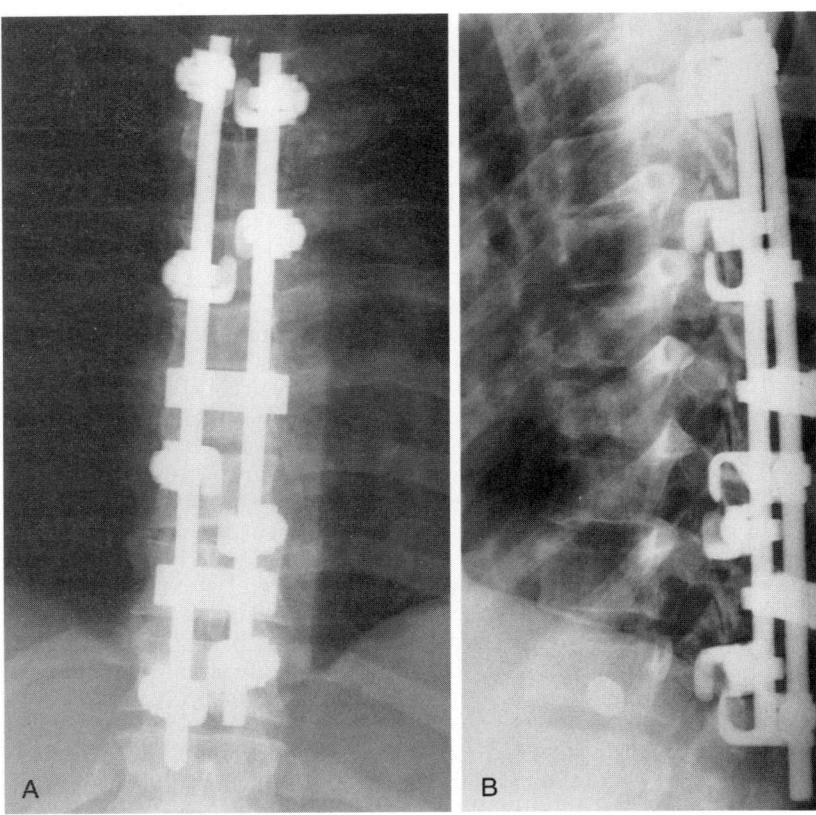

FIGURE 319–19. Anteroposterior (*A*) and oblique lateral (*B*) plain radiographs of a TSRH construct placed to stabilize a midthoracic fracture. Sublaminar hooks, rods, and cross-links were used.

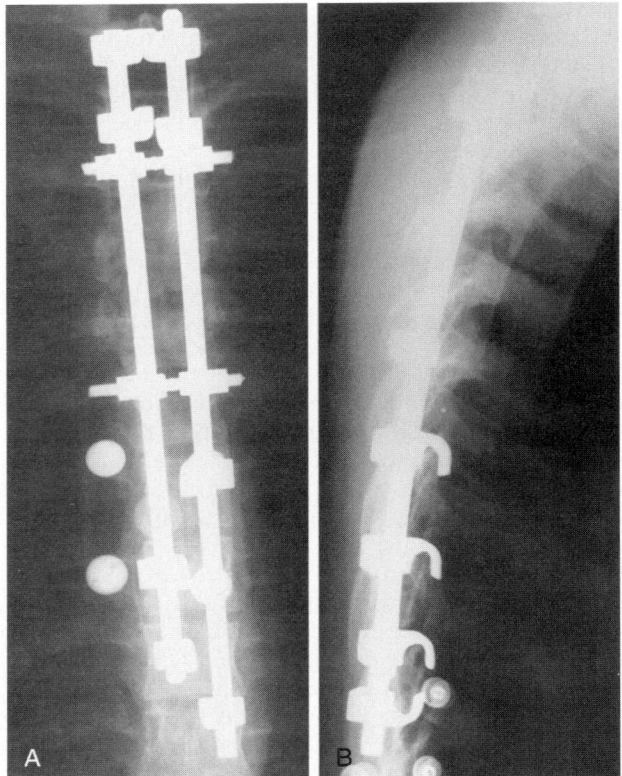

FIGURE 319–20. Plain radiographs of an Isola construct: Anteroposterior (*A*) and lateral (*B*) views of the sublaminar hooks, rods, and cross-links used to stabilize an upper thoracic fracture.

rate segmental fixation have largely replaced the Harrington distraction rod and the Luque rod constructs in the treatment of thoracic spine injuries, and these constructs can reduce fractures that otherwise could not be as successfully realigned with earlier fixation systems. This supplementary fixation is not without consequence, since additional manipulation of the injured spine is required to fit multiple hooks to the spine and rods compared with the single hooks placed at the extreme ends of the Harrington rods. Although the inventors of the systems report that the instrumented spine does not need an external orthosis, we use a TLSO routinely.[103] Another advantage of the universal fixation systems is the ability to use pedicle screws to affix the spine rigidly to the construct rods, but the usefulness of this type of fixation system in the upper thoracic region is limited because of the narrow mediolateral dimension of the thoracic pedicles.[133] Although there are clinicians using thoracic pedicle fixation for the length of the thoracic spine, we generally prefer hook fixation superior to T10 and inferior to T1. Unlike the lumbar level in which short-segment fixation has important clinical and functional consequences, the use of a segmental fixation construct with pedicle screw fixation in the thoracic region should be tempered because of the risk of spinal cord injury. When indicated, we also have used frameless stereotactic imaging systems (Steath Station, Medtronics, Denver, CO) to facilitate pedicle screw placement.

There are many recommendations regarding the length of the rods and the configuration of the hooks to be used in a construct to treat a given clinical situation.

Although Cotrel and associates first recommended that hooks be placed on the superior and inferior edges of the lamina at the caudal and rostral extent of the instrumentation, other authors (after additional clinical experience), recommended that these "claw" constructs incorporate two vertebral segments of increased biomechanical stability.[49, 87] Roach and associates experimentally confirmed that the pullout strength of a two-level construct was significantly greater compared with the single-level construct and noted that it is easier to insert the hooks in the two-level configuration.[122] There is no agreement about whether the construct should span two or three levels above or below the injured vertebral segment, or both.

Hooks can be placed in a variety of patterns. Figure 319–21A–C shows hooks similar to those originally recommended by Cotrel and Dubousset for the treatment of thoracolumbar fractures.[91] A short-segment compression fixation, as seen in Figure 319–21D, should be reserved for distraction injuries in which the posterior bony elements and the middle column are intact. Holt has advocated the pattern diagramed in Figure 319–21E, whereas Figures 319–21F and G are modifications.[91] The number of possible combinations of sublaminar, pedicular, and transverse process hook placement is large, and the pattern can and should be changed according to the clinical situation. The segmental fixation systems allow for a variety of corrective forces to be placed and for simultaneous compression

across the fracture site and distraction of the more distal element, with the patterns shown in Figure 319–21.

Surgical Technique. As previously stated, we prefer to place the patient prone on a four-post positioning system. This allows the patient to be in either a neutral or an extended position. These positioning devices also decrease the pressure on the abdomen and therefore the venous pressure. The decrease in venous pressure has positive effects on the perfusion of the spinal cord and decreases the blood loss. A subperiosteal dissection of the paraspinal muscles is effected to expose the spinous process, lamina, and transverse process at least three levels superior to and two levels inferior to the fracture site. The facet joints are identified and cleared of overlying soft tissue.

Sublaminar hooks facing cephalad require that the ligamentum flavum be stripped from the laminar surface with the appropriate instrument, although we frequently perform a laminotomy on the inferior lamina to ease hook placement and to prevent injury to the spinal cord (Fig. 319–22A). If a pedicle hook is used in place of a cephalad sublaminar hook, the superior facet of the joint to undergo instrumentation will have to be trimmed with an osteotome to allow proper engagement of the pedicle by the hook. Care must be taken not to remove too much of the facet because the remaining portion of the facet should cover the length of

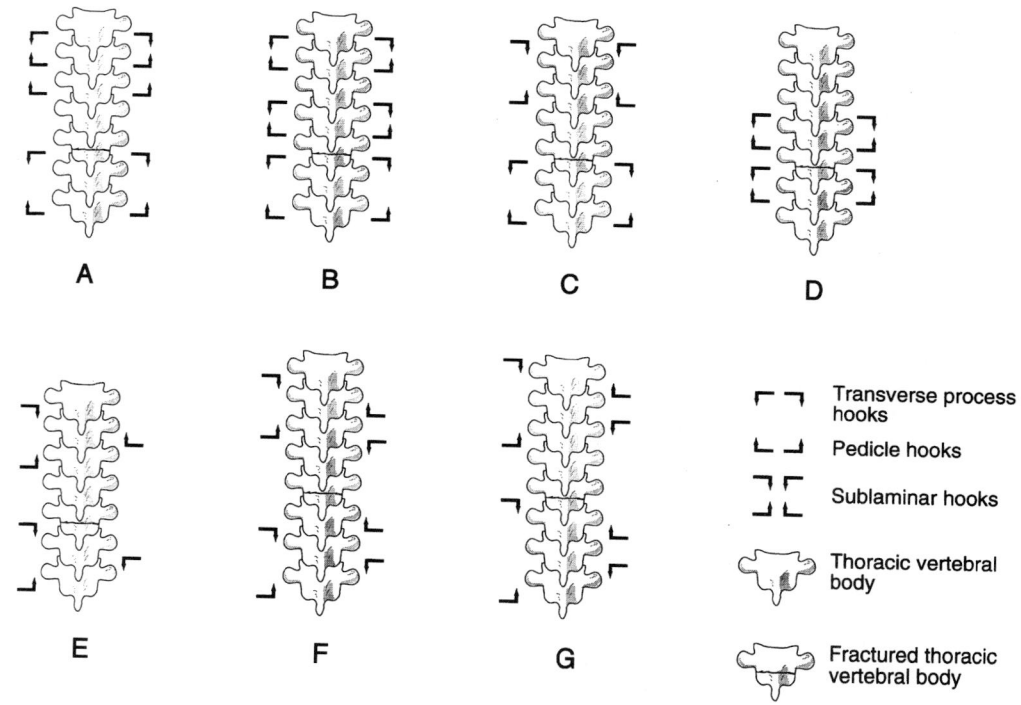

FIGURE 319–21. *A* through *G,* Many different hook placements have been used with universal instrumentation. The universal systems allow both distraction and compression to be placed at different levels with one construct. The patterns shown in *E* through *G* employ sublaminar hooks that are placed so that no level has two hooks directed in the same direction, thereby lessening the chance of iatrogenic narrowing of the spinal canal.

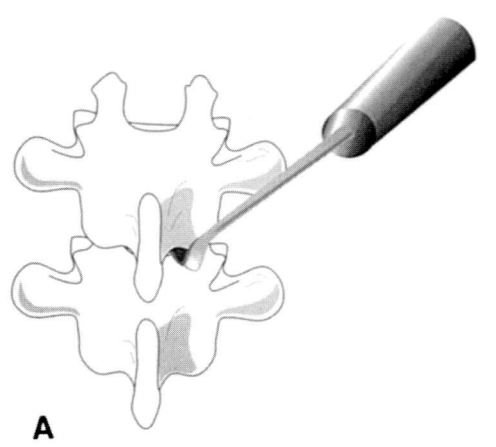

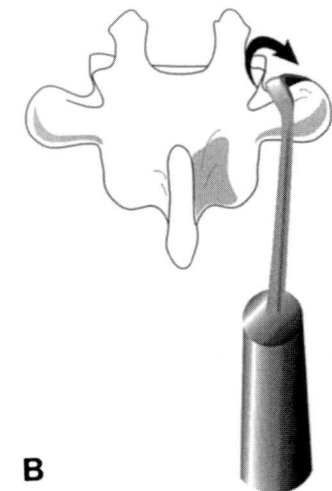

FIGURE 319–22. Unlike the placement of Harrington hooks or downward facing sublaminar hooks with a universal system, placement of upward facing sublaminar hooks or transverse process hooks does not necessarily require a laminotomy. Tools are available to elevate ligamentum flavum or soft tissue, respectively, allowing the upward facing sublaminar hook (*A*) and the transverse hook (*B*) to be placed without extensive bone work. Care must be taken to remove only the ligamentum flavum and to not place the tool intralaminarly.

the blade of the hook, once the hook is in place (Fig. 319–23). The recommended placement of the osteotomy site is 5 mm caudad to the transverse process and facet junction.[122] A transverse process hook may be substituted for a cephalad hook, and the same instrument that is used for stripping the ligamentum may be used to prepare the superior surface of the process for hook placement (see Fig. 319–22*B*). Care should be taken not to injure the lamina under which the hook is to be placed or the adjacent facet joints. It is also important to make certain the hook is in place under the anterior surface of the lamina and has not penetrated into the lamina. An intralaminar placement will significantly degrade the pullout strength of the hook. In the thoracic area, there is often no need to contour the rod because overcontouring the rod will result in loss of reduction of the fracture.

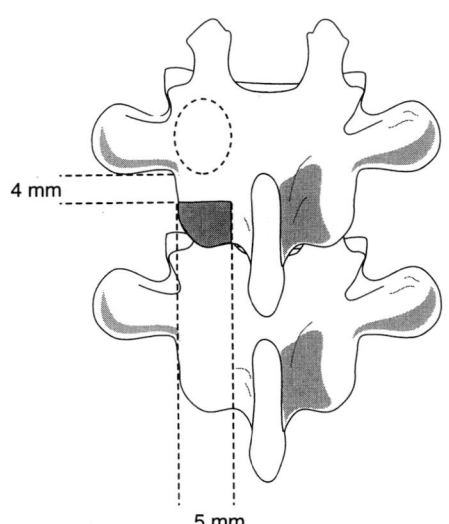

4 mm

5 mm

FIGURE 319–23. The extent of the facet and lamina resection necessary for a pedicle hook from a universal system to have the proper purchase. If too much of the lamina is removed, the hook may shift to a sublaminar position within the canal and may damage the neural contents of the canal.

Once the hooks are placed and the rods contoured for the final alignment of the spine, the hooks are connected to the rods and tightened sequentially in order to place the appropriately directed correctional force on the local vertebral segments. Two cross-linked devices should be placed to connect the rods, thereby creating a rectangular construct and increasing the rotatory stability of the construct, as discussed earlier. The cross-linked devices from each system should be placed on the rods with care to avoid the inadvertent dislodging of the previously placed hooks. The hook-to-rod connectors are then retightened after the cross-links are in place. A small laminotomy may also be performed at the fracture site to allow ultrasonographic intraoperative monitoring of the reduction of the fracture.

A posterolateral fusion with decortication of the facets, transverse process, and lamina (except for the lamina to which a hook is attached) and placement of autologous bone graft harvested from the posterior iliac crest are necessary; any construct will eventually fail without the development of an adequate fusion of the bony spinal column. Intraoperative plain x-ray films are necessary to verify that the fracture has been reduced and that the hooks are in the proper location. We routinely place patients in a TLSO but are inclined to discontinue this orthosis earlier than the usual 3- to 6- month postoperative interval when the construct extends at least three segments above and two segments below the fracture site.

POSTEROLATERAL DECOMPRESSION

Edwards and Levine demonstrated that there was a time-dependent inverse relationship between the amount of canal restoration and the interval from injury to surgical reduction by posterior instrumentation.[48] Although the data included fractures of the lower thoracic and lumbar spine, the spinal canal was restored an additional 32% if surgical reduction was performed within 2 days of injury, but only 23% when surgery was performed between 3 and 14 days from injury. If the posterior instrumentation was delayed more than 2 weeks, there was little to no improvement in the spinal canal diameter. With early surgery and therefore better surgical reduction, the need for a formal neural decompression is obviated.

The adequacy of reduction cannot be adequately assessed by plain radiographs. Although intraoperative myelography may be performed, evaluation of residual neural compression is difficult. Another intraoperative method of excluding neural compression by retained fracture fragments is spinal ultrasound, which is discussed later in this chapter.[52, 97] Other authors have suggested postoperative myelography and computed tomography, with an anterior decompression to remove residual compression.[63, 127]

If late operative treatment is required, posterolateral decompression may be indicated if significant residual compression remains after reduction with posterior instrumentation. This technique was originally described for thoracolumbar fracture treatment with Harrington distraction rod constructs.[54, 76] The advantage of this technique is that the anterior compression can be addressed at the time of posterior stabilization without a separate procedure.[47, 48, 54] The disadvantages include the removal of both additional posterior elements that may adversely affect long-term stability and the bone fragment that is causing the anterior compression "blindly," since the dura and neural elements obstruct direct visualization.[9]

Intraoperative ultrasound can obviate the latter disadvantage; Eismont and associates reported on the effectiveness of posterolateral decompression assessed intraoperatively with ultrasound.[52] In a series of 23 patients with thoracic or lumbar fractures, 12 required posterolateral decompression for continued compression of the neural elements. Of those 12 patients, 8 were evaluated by postoperative computed tomography and canal size was demonstrated to be adequately restored. The only treatment failure was a patient with a second area of compression that was not appreciated preoperatively. Garfin and colleagues also evaluated the effectiveness of posterolateral decompression performed in nine patients using postoperative computed tomography that revealed that only one patient had residual bone in the canal.[63] No patient experienced neurological deterioration because of the procedure.

Surgical Technique. Posterolateral decompression is performed at the time of posterior instrumentation and stabilization of a thoracic fracture. Preoperative computed tomography is performed to determine the side of maximal neural compression that will be used for the approach for decompression. Instrumentation is placed on the opposite side. A laminotomy is performed at the site of the maximal neural compression that is usually the area between the pedicles of the fractured vertebral body. This window is used for intraoperative ultrasound, and if an anterior bony fragment is seen to impinge on the neural elements, a posterolateral decompression can be started.

The laminotomy should be extended to the pedicle that will then be "cored" with a power bur, taking care not to penetrate the cortical margins (Fig. 319–24). The medial margin of the pedicle is then removed with a curette, taking care to not injure the exiting nerve root. A 1-cm trough is then cut into the vertebral body anterior to the medial portion of the pedicle and the compressing fragment undermined toward the vertebral body. Reverse angle curets and pituitary rongeurs can then be used to remove the compressing fragment. This can be done under ultrasonic guidance.

This technique allows lesions just lateral to the midline to be removed. If the ultrasound reveals lateral compression from the anterior body, the procedure can be repeated on the contralateral pedicle after pacing a rod construct on the decompressed side and removing the first construct. The superior disk can also be removed and bone graft impacted into the defect in the body and disk space. Instrumentation and posterolateral bony fusion are then completed.

ANTERIOR TRANSTHORACIC DECOMPRESSION AND FUSION

Anterior transthoracic decompression is used to treat fractures of the thoracic spine that impinge on the anterior canal and spinal cord. We use this approach for patients who are neurologically intact and have an incomplete spinal cord lesion or a fixed kyphotic deformity from previous spinal injury. In the thoracic area, this procedure (when combined with anterior grafting) may be the only treatment rendered, but the decrease in the strength of the reconstructed anterior spinal column after an anterior strut grafting may require posterior fusion and fixation for adequate stabilization of the spinal column. At this time, a concurrent injury to the posterior ligamentous or bony structures, or both, increases the necessity of posterior stabilization because there are no adequate anterior fixation devices for this circumferential lesion above T5.

Transthoracic decompression was first described for the treatment of tuberculosis of the spine in 1956 by Hodgson and Stock, who stated that "the region from C.6 to D.4 is reached without undue difficulty" through resection of a third rib.[79] Hodgson and Stock also advised using a rib resection above the level of the lesion in T4-12 lesions since "it is much easier to work downwards than upwards on the spine" and the rib was available for a reconstructive fusion. Although Chou and Selijeskog described transthoracic osteotomy for a variety of lesions, Eismont and associates credit Paul and colleagues with the first report of using this technique for decompression and fusion of a traumatic injury to the thoracic spine.[29, 51, 116] Bohlman and associates have published long-term results and details of the surgical techniques.[16, 19] In one review of acute injuries of the upper thoracic spine, eight patients were treated with transthoracic decompression and fusion for residual neural compression after spinal column and cord injuries. All eight patients had reached a plateau in their neurological recovery before the anterior decompression. After transthoracic decompression

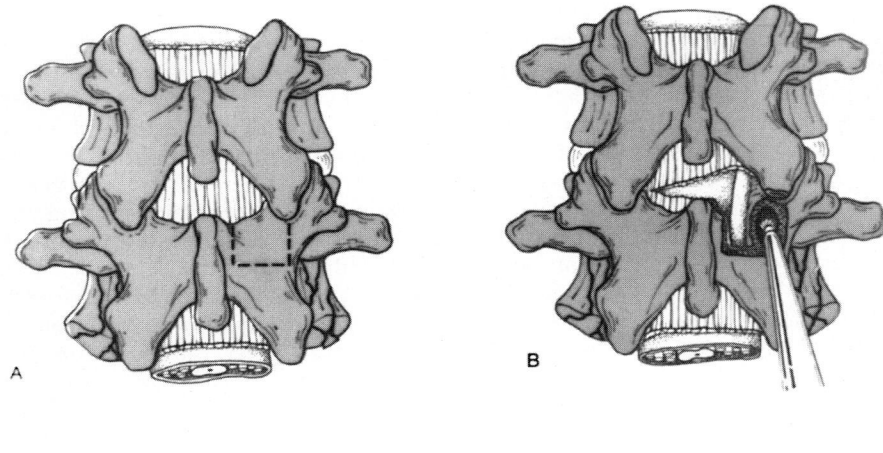

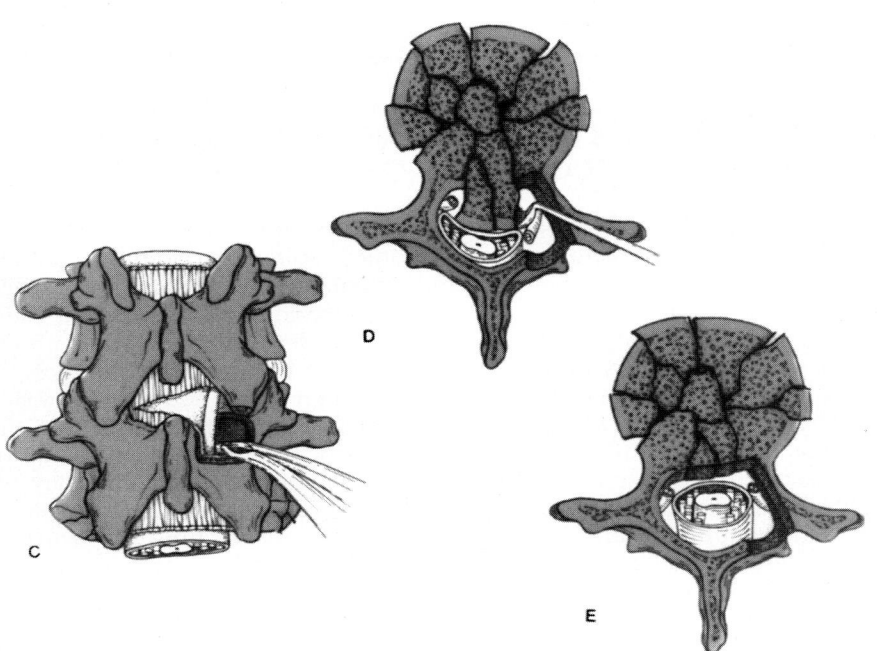

FIGURE 319–24. Posterolateral decompression of the spinal cord. *A,* The extent of the laminar resection is shown. Care is taken not to cut across the pars interarticularis. *B,* The ligamentum flavum is resected and the dura is exposed. A high-speed drill is then employed to remove bone lateral to the medial extent of the pedicle and caudally to the inferior extent of the pedicle. A hole is produced in the center of the pedicle, and the resection is carried anteriorly into the vertebral body. By leaving a circumferential rim of cortical bone, injury to the passing nerve root is avoided. *C,* A rongeur is used to remove the medial wall of the pedicle. *D,* A reverse-angle curet is used to remove the bone fragments from the spinal canal and push them into a hole created by the drill bur. *E,* The final result of a unilateral posterolateral transpedicular decompression is shown. It is possible to decompress slightly past the midline through a pedicle with this approach. (From Levine A, Eismont FJ, Garfin SR, Zigler JE: Spine Trauma. Philadelphia, Saunders, 1998. Used by permission.)

and fusion, five patients achieved independent ambulation, two recovered ambulatory status with assistive devices, and one gained increased motor function without recovering ambulatory status. All patients fused the anterior strut graft without instrumentation, but no data were given regarding initial or final angulation at the decompression site.[19]

Transthoracic decompression may cause destabilizing effects. Gurr and coworkers demonstrated that the spinal strength is markedly reduced after a corpectomy when compared with an intact spine in axial, flexion, or rotational loading. The addition of an anterior iliac graft still allowed three times the displacement with axial loading, whereas torsional stiffness was less than one third that of an intact spine.[72] Our experience with a variable length titanium cage (Synex, AO Synthes, Davos, Switzerland) has been positive, especially when combined with a rod-screw anterior fixation system (VentraFix, AO Synthes, Davos, Switzerland) (Fig. 319–

25). Uninstrumented anterior decompressions should be reserved for patients with a significant anterior canal compromise and minimal instability. Posterior fixation is necessary if the injury is unstable; we recommend the use of a TLSO.

Surgical Technique. For a lesion in the upper thoracic area, at T10 or above, a double-lumen endotracheal tube allows the collapse of the ipsilateral lung to enhance exposure. The spine can be exposed with the patient in either the left or the right lateral decubitus position. The left lateral decubitus position is most often used for the uppermost region of the thoracic spine, whereas the right lateral decubitus position is used for middle and lower thoracic regions. Either side can be used if necessary to obtain adequate exposure of the lesion.

An axillary roll is used to prevent a stretch palsy of the lower brachial plexus, and the superior arm is held

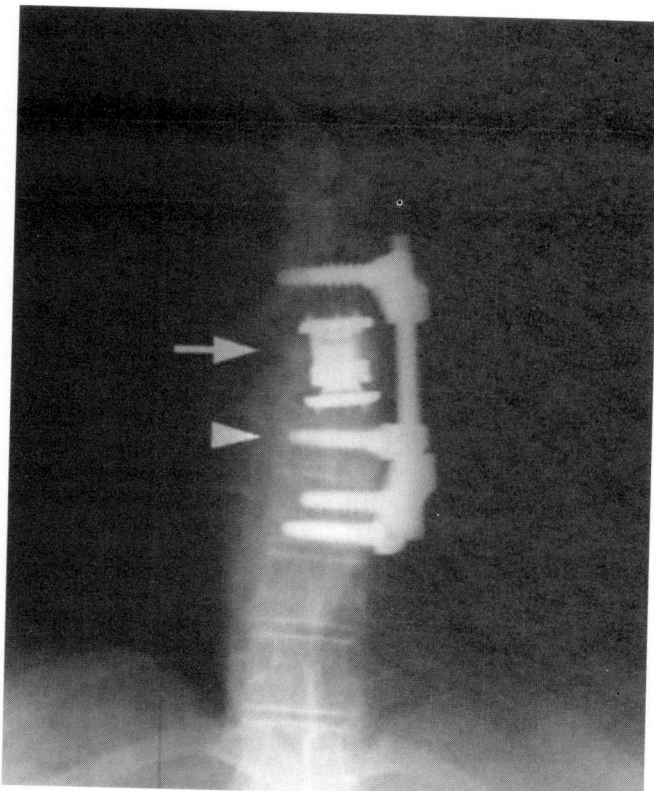

FIGURE 319–25. An x-ray showing a titanium cage, packed with salvaged vertebral body and rib, used to fill a defect in the anterior spinal column.

in a neutral position with an arm support, with the arm held in a forward flexion of no greater than 90 degrees at the shoulder to minimize risk of upper brachial plexopathy. Wide adhesive tape can be used to secure the position of the patient and should be placed at the level of the greater trochanter and across the shoulder. The tape should be securely affixed to the table. Some surgeons prefer to place a beanbag under the patient, but we are inclined not to because not using this device provides additional posterior exposure. This is an advantage in the rare incidence that simultaneous anterior decompression and posterior stabilization are necessary.[130] Care should be taken to prepare an adequate amount of skin: to the midline anteriorly, beyond the midline posteriorly, to just inferior to the axilla, to inferior to the iliac crest.

The skin incision is made over the rib one to two vertebral levels superior to the level of the lesion when dealing with lesions from T6-10. At the most superior thoracic levels, the skin incision should extend inferior to the tip of the scapula and halfway between the medial border of the scapula and the midline spinous processes (Fig. 319–26A and B). The incision should be extended to the subcutaneous tissues down to the deep fascia and muscles, which are divided in line with the skin incision. The rib to be resected is then stripped subperiosteally and divided with a rib cutter. The inner rib bed is divided to expose the chest cavity.

When exposing the uppermost levels in the thoracic

region, care should be taken not to injure the long thoracic nerve that runs in the midaxillary line from the axilla to the serratus anterior. It is preferable to detach the muscle from the anterior chest wall to avoid cutting the long thoracic nerve. With mobilization of the scapula by dividing the dorsal scapular muscles, rhomboids and trapezius, the third rib is more easily visualized and a greater area is visualized with the thoracotomy.

Once the ribs have been counted from inside the thoracic cavity and the level of the rib verified, a self-retaining retractor is then inserted over moist laparotomy sponges. With deflation of packing of the lung, the spine can be visually or tactually identified. The bony column is covered with a thin layer of parietal pleura. The proximal portion of the resected rib can be followed to the vertebral column where it inserts into the cephalic portion of the vertebral body of the same level. With this localization, the disk space or spaces can be identified and a spinal needle placed. A cross-table portable radiograph verifies the level.

The parietal pleura is then divided between the rib insertions on the vertebral body and the great vessels until one level superior and one level inferior to the injury levels are exposed. The segmental vessels are then identified in the middle of the vertebral body and are clamped, divided, and tied. An extraperiosteal dissection of the soft tissues overlying the vertebral body can be performed using dissectors or periosteal elevators. The dissection can be carried across the anterior midline of the vertebral body and a malleable retractor placed to protect the great vessels and the esophagus (see Fig. 319–26C).

The proximal portion of the rib inserting at the level of decompression has to be removed to expose the pedicle and neural foramen. The disk spaces immediately superior and inferior to the vertebrectomy site should be removed using a scalpel and rongeurs. A small periosteal elevator is useful for detaching the cartilaginous end plate, which can aid in the disk removal. An osteotome is then used to remove a portion of the vertebral body, taking care to leave the anteriormost portion of the vertebral body attached to the anterior longitudinal ligament, unlike the removal shown in Figure 319–26H. The dura can be exposed by using a power bur, rongeurs, curets, and osteotomes after first identifying the dura at the neural foramina following a partial resection of the pedicle (see Fig. 319–26D–G). The dissection should be extended across the full width of the canal until the pedicle on the distal side is identified. Measurements of the vertebral body width from the preoperative imaging studies are valuable. One should explore the superior disk space to verify that bone fragments attached to the annulus have been removed from the canal. If there is any question of residual bone fragments having penetrated the posterior longitudinal ligament, the ligament must be divided or a window cut to allow exploration of the epidural space.

The vertebrectomy site should be grafted to reconstruct the spinal column. Iliac crest can be harvested, but we use tibial allograft struts or titanium cages

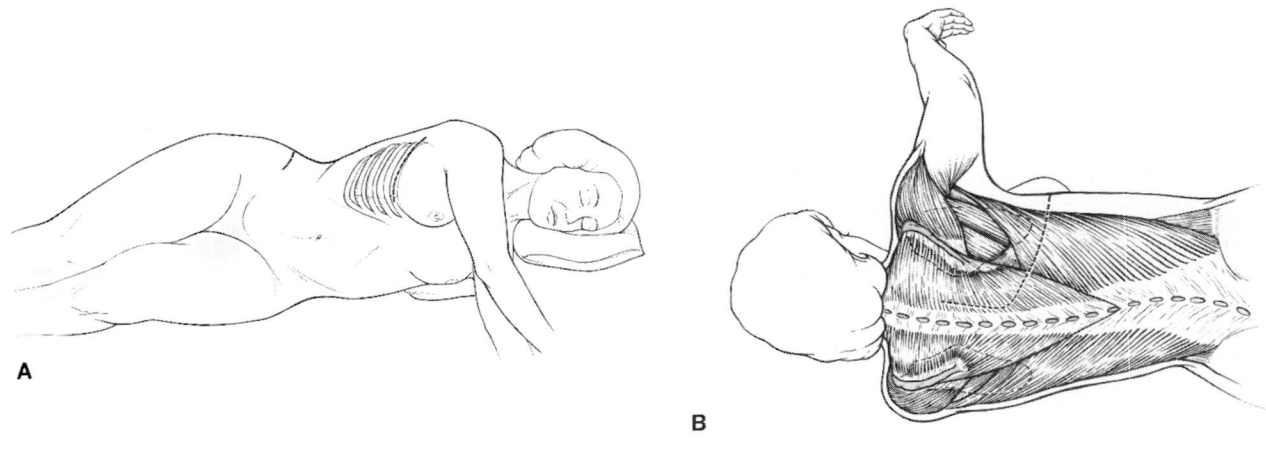

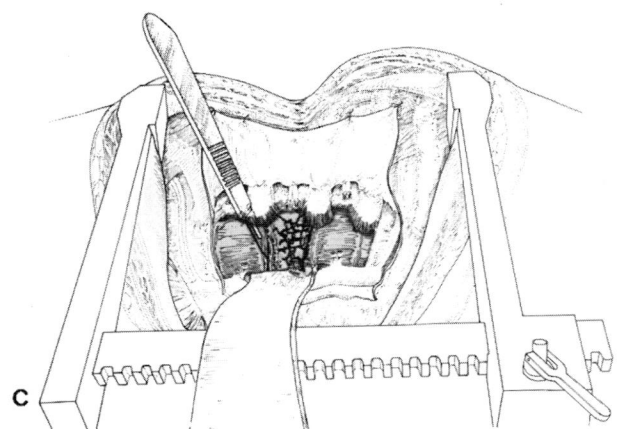

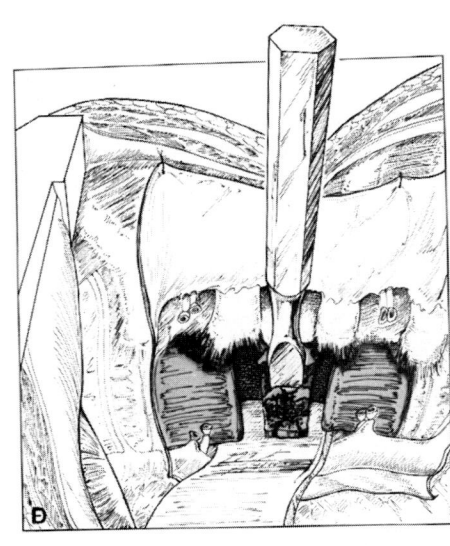

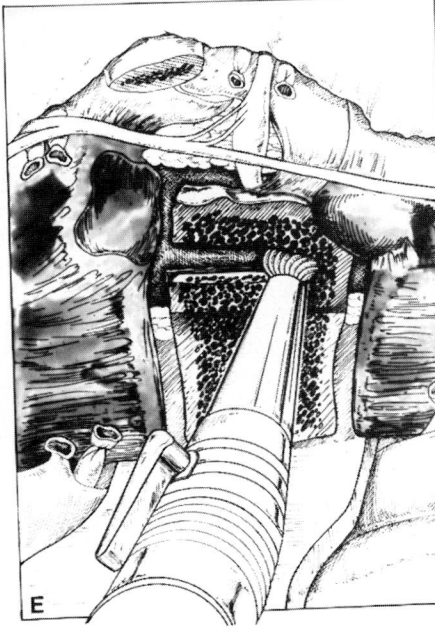

FIGURE 319–26. Demonstration of anterior transthoracic corpectomy and fusion. *A,* The patient is placed in the lateral decubitus position with the shoulder extended forward 90 degrees, with elbows straight and no abduction or adduction. An axillary roll is used as shown. The incision (*dotted line*) is made over the rib two levels above that of the vertebral body fracture. *B,* For exposure above the sixth rib, the posterior extent of the incision is carried cephalad halfway between the medial border of the scapula and the spinous processes. All the intervening muscles are divided and tagged down to the chest wall. *C,* After entering the thoracic cavity, the self-retaining chest retractor is inserted. The incision is made halfway between the anterior great vessels and the posterior neural foramina, and the segmental intercostal vessels are ligated serially. The vertebra to be excised plus the superior and inferior adjacent bodies are then exposed with an extraperiosteal dissection. A malleable retractor is placed on the opposite side of the spine and connected to the chest retractor with a clamp. The malleable retractor protects the great vessels during the corpectomy. Scalpel and rongeurs are used to remove the discs above and below the level of the vertebral fracture. *D,* An osteotome or chisel is used to excise the vertebral body to the level of the posterior cortex. Each cut with these instruments is made perpendicular to the floor, as long as cancellous bone is encountered. As soon as white cortical bone is encountered, these instruments should no longer be used. *E,* A high-speed bur can then be used to perforate the posterior cortex into the spinal canal. When neural compression is significant, a diamond-tipped bur can be used to minimize the chances of dural or neural injury.

Illustration continued on following page

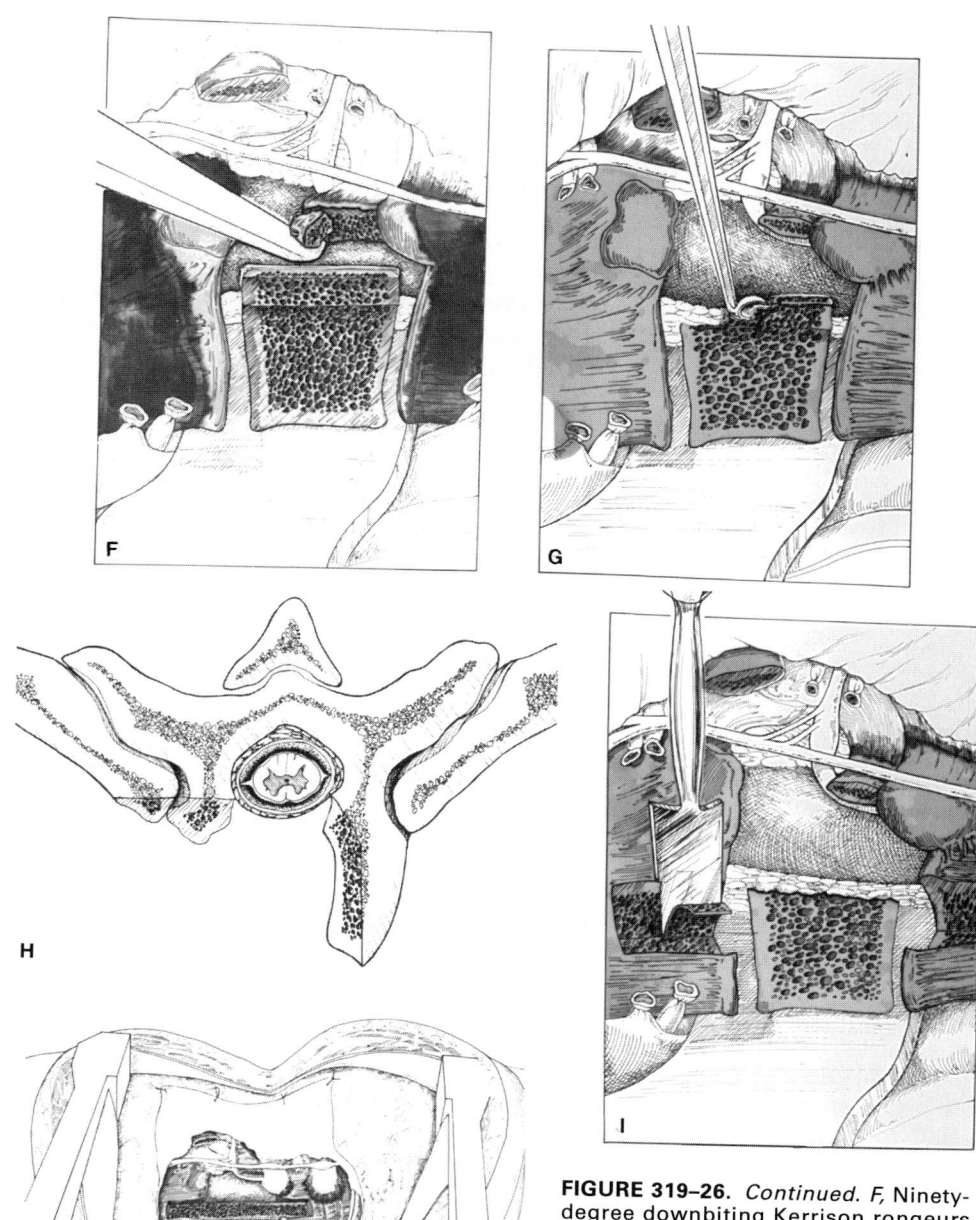

FIGURE 319–26. *Continued. F,* Ninety-degree downbiting Kerrison rongeurs are used to remove bone from the most superficial portion of the vertebral body. *G,* Reverse-angle curets are used to carefully remove bone projecting into the spinal canal. *H,* A transverse section of the vertebra shows the extent of the decompression, which is often underestimated intraoperatively. The resection should extend from one pedicle to the other. After completion of decompression, the dura should bulge anteriorly in a uniform fashion both from end plate to end plate and from pedicle to pedicle. If the dura does not bulge out, the surgeon should check for residual neural compression. There is an advantage to leaving more of the anterior vertebral body and associated anterior longitudinal ligaments intact. *I,* After the corpectomy and discectomies above and below the level of injury have been performed, a trough is made into the vertebral bodies above and below the corpectomy. If there is any osteoporosis, the trough should be cut through the cancellous bone up to the next intact end plate at the upper end of a cephalad vertebra and the lower end of a caudal vertebra. A ridge of bone should be preserved at the posterior aspect of the adjacent vertebrae to prevent the bone graft from migrating into the spinal canal. *J,* At the end of the decompression and fusion, there should be adequate space between the bone graft and dura and neural tissue to prevent iatrogenic neural compression. Three rib segments are used as the bone graft in this illustration, but a single large piece of iliac crest can be used and may provide a stronger anterior support. (From Eismont FJ, Garfin SR, Abitol J: Thoracic and upper lumbar spine injuries. In Browner BD, Jupiter JB, Levine AM, et al. [eds]: Skeletal Trauma. Vol. I. Philadelphia, Saunders, 1993, pp 780–783. Reprinted by permission.)

packed with salvaged fragments of the resected vertebral bodies and the resected rib from the thoracotomy site. If a tibial strut is used, the superior and inferior vertebral bodies are notched to lock the graft in place. More recently, a titanium cage (see Fig. 319–25) packed with salvaged vertebral body and rib has been used to fill the defect in the anterior spinal column. The cage can be expanded to engage the adjacent vertebral bodies and reduce kyphotic deformity. The space between the strut and the anterior longitudinal ligament is packed with salvaged autologous bone. A rib strut may also be used to fill the defect if there is minimal instability. There should be a space between the strut graft and the dura covering the neural elements; the graft should be locked in the superior and inferior vertebral bodies to prevent posterior migration in the spinal canal (see Figs. 319–26*I* and *J*).

Hemostasis should be obtained before closure and after the malleable retractor is removed. An attempt to close the parietal pleura should be made and a chest tube placed. A pleural catheter is also placed in the chest tube or through a separate percutaneous stab wound and is used for the delivery of local anesthetic to assist in postoperative pain control. Pericostal sutures are placed and tied after approximation of the ribs. The overlying tissues are closed in layers. Posterior stabilization and fusion should be performed if necessary to ensure stability of the spinal column. A custom-molded TLSO is recommended.

INTRAOPERATIVE SPINAL ULTRASOUND

Intraoperative ultrasound is a noninvasive technique for assessing the presence of a compressive mass that is not visualized directly. An anterior compressive mass is easily visualized from a posterior approach, which can be used to reduce, stabilize with a posterior fixation construct, and fuse an injured spine. Intraoperative ultrasound can be used to verify the reduction of a bony deformity and assess canal compromise during reduction or posterolateral decompression.[52, 63, 137] This technique has replaced intraoperative myelography in our institutions.[97]

Technique. We use a 7.5-MHz ultrasound unit, but there is evidence that a higher frequency machine (10 MHz) may be more suitable for spinal surgery. This frequency produces a superior image of the spinal cord and associated intradural structures and allows visualization of fine detail not resolved on the lower frequency machines.[69] Before intraoperative use of the ultrasound scanner, the transducer is placed in a sterile plastic sheath filled with a few ounces of lubricant. Care must be taken in placing the transducer into the lubricant to avoid air bubbles coming into contact with the transducers. The presence of air bubbles severely degrades the image quality. A laminectomy (or vertebrectomy in the case of an anterior approach) must be performed to produce at least a 1 × 1.5 cm opening. The surgical wound is filled with saline solution (Fig.

319–27) after hemostasis is assured and tissue debris is irrigated away. Blood and debris, as well as antibiotic solutions, will also degrade the image quality. Both transverse and sagittal images can be obtained by rotation of the transducer. Any fragment of bone, soft tissue density, or metallic fragment can be visualized, as can bone alignment. When used with posterolateral decompression, intraoperative ultrasound allows safe and adequate neural decompression from the posterior approach, which can be followed by fusion and stabilization without an additional surgical incision.

TREATMENT OF SPECIFIC INJURIES

Treatments of specific injuries as classified by Denis, with one modification, are discussed here.[39] Included are minor fractures, compression fractures, burst fractures, and fracture-dislocations. Also addressed are miscellaneous injuries, including soft tissue, disk, and gunshot injuries. Obviously, correct surgical treatment depends on accurate diagnosis. Accurate diagnosis is dependent on data garnered from the physical and neurological examinations, appropriate diagnostic studies, and proper imaging studies.[5, 10, 12, 75, 85, 116]

Minor Fractures

Spinous process fractures may occur as a result of direct trauma to the posterior spine, whereas violent

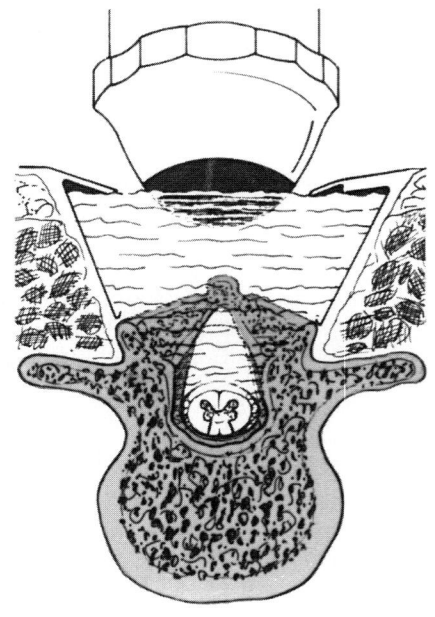

FIGURE 319–27. Intraoperative visualization of the neural elements is achieved with an ultrasound probe. A laminotomy is performed and the wound filled with sterile saline solution. The probe tip is then covered with a sterile barrier and a lubricant is used to conduct the ultrasound between the probe tip and the water bath. Any bubbles in the lubricant will significantly degrade the image. The patency of the canal can be verified or areas where corrective measures need to be taken can be identified at the time of operation. (From Eismont FJ, Garfin SR, Abitol J: Thoracic and upper lumbar spine injuries. In Browner BD, Jupiter JB, Levine AM, et al. [eds]: Skeletal Trauma. Vol. I. Philadelphia, Saunders, 1993, p 786. Reprinted by permission.)

muscular contraction or direct trauma can cause fractures of the transverse processes. Direct trauma can also cause a fracture of an articular process. Although each of these lesions in isolation can appear benign, the spinal column must be evaluated further to rule out additional injury. Computed tomography through the vertebral body in question, as well as through the adjacent vertebral body, is the most efficacious screening study. If these scans are normal, lateral flexion and extension plain radiographs are needed to exclude dynamic instability. With the exclusion of a major spine injury, the patient can be mobilized with impunity.

Compression Fractures

By definition, a compression fracture has a disrupted anterior and an intact middle column; the posterior column, however, may be intact or disrupted. The treatment of these injuries depends on the status of the posterior ligamentous structures, as well as on the integrity of the bony elements. As discussed earlier, the status of the anterior column can suggest the integrity of the posterior elements: A compression of greater than 40% of the anterior vertebral wall or a kyphotic deformity of greater than 25 degrees is often associated with ligamentous incompetency of the posterior elements. If the kyphosis is less than 25 degrees and the anterior body compression is less than 40%, the injury can be treated nonoperatively and the patient managed in a TLSO with minor activity restriction. The patient should be instructed to lie in the prone position and avoid lying in the supine position with a pillow under the head.

After 3 to 4 months in the orthosis, lateral upright flexion/extension films should be obtained with the patient out of the brace. If there is no excess motion and no progression of the deformity, the patient can be weaned from the orthosis and started with physical therapy to strengthen the muscles atrophied from disuse. The process of weaning may require several weeks. If there is abnormal motion, a progression of the deformity, or continued pain, the patient may be a candidate for surgical stabilization.

When the anterior column is compressed more than 40% or the kyphosis exceeds 25 degrees, surgical management is indicated.[67, 68] Consideration should be given to the force of the injury and the age of the patient in borderline cases. An elderly patient with osteoporosis who suffered a low-velocity injury would not necessarily undergo operation, whereas a young patient involved in a high-velocity injury would be considered for operation because of the possibility of posterior ligamentous injury.

If there is a possibility of a posterior ligamentous disruption with a severe compression fracture, our instrumentation system of choice is a posterior segmental fixation sytem. This allows distraction to be placed to reduce the flexion deformity. Although a compression system could be used if the middle column were intact, it would offer no advantage. Moreover, a compression system might cause an incompetent disk to herniate in the spinal canal. Although anterior decompression is not usually necessary in these injuries, destruction of the anterior column from an underlying disorder, as in severe osteoporosis and a high-velocity injury, may necessitate an anterior approach to reconstruct, graft, and possibly fix the anterior spinal column.

Burst Fractures

By definition, both the anterior and middle columns are disrupted in burst fractures, but the posterior column may or may not be injured. Some authors believe that the integrity of the posterior column is the determinant of stability in this type of vertebral injury.[84] Other important factors to consider in rendering treatment are the percentage of canal compromise, the degree of angulation, and the neurological status of the patient. No consensus exists regarding the treatment of burst fractures. We do not decompress lesions of the spine when there is less than a 40% spinal canal compromise and the patient is neurologically intact. If the degree of angulation of the kyphotic deformity is less than 25 degrees, the patient may be treated with a total-contact TLSO and allowed to ambulate. Upright radiographs are necessary to verify that the fracture is stable when the patient bears weight.[27]

If the canal compromise is greater than 40% and surgery is not performed, the patient may require treatment with bed rest for 3 to 6 weeks before being allowed to walk using a TLSO. The orthosis should be worn for at least 3 months in either situation. We obtain upright lateral radiographs on a regular basis to document that no interval increase in deformity has occurred. As with the recommendation for management of compression fractures, patients should be encouraged to lie in bed in the prone position and avoid the use of pillows when in the supine position. If the patient is unable to follow these recommendations, surgical treatment is indicated. Patients should be instructed to return for immediate re-evaluation if neurological deterioration occurs. Changes in motor function or bladder control or the development of paresthesias is reason for additional imaging studies.

After there is evidence of adequate healing of the vertebral fracture, the orthosis can be removed for flexion and extension lateral radiographs. If there is no motion at the fracture site, the patient can be weaned from the TLSO and physical therapy started. If, however, a neurological deficit develops or there is increasing angulation of the kyphosis, anterior decompression should be considered. Posterior instrumentation will be less satisfactory if 2 or 3 weeks have passed since the injury, and a posterolateral decompression may be necessary.

We believe that surgical therapy is preferred for burst fractures if the patient has a greater than 40% canal compromise, a greater than 25-degree kyphosis at the injury site, a neurological deficit, or a combination of these conditions. Potential neurological deficits from the injury include lower extremity motor and sensory abnormalities, decreased perineal sensation, and bowel and bladder dysfunction. A rectal examination should be performed, voluntary sphincter function documented, and bilateral perianal sensory function examined. The absence of the latter sensory and motor functions was found to correlate with a less favorable functional outcome and is the basis of the American Spinal Injury Association classification of a complete neurological injury.[4] The more neurologically intact the patient is, the more likely we are to recommend surgery to prevent deterioration from structural incompetence of the bony column and to alleviate continuing compression of neural tissues. A history of postinjury leg pain should be considered significant and would prompt us to consider surgical treatment.

Burst fractures can be reduced and stabilized from the posterior approach with any system that places the injured area in distraction. Although the Harrington distraction rod and associated variations were popular until the recent past, we favor the newer universal segmental fixation systems. With the use of a posterior fixation system, intraoperative ultrasound should be used to determine if posterolateral decompression is necessary. An alternative approach would be to obtain postoperative computed tomography to document adequate decompression. If a compressive lesion is found, anterior decompression should be undertaken. A compression construct should not be used without anterior decompression because the extent of the canal compromise may be increased.

Anterior decompression and fusion may be used to treat a burst fracture of a thoracic vertebral body, and there is at least one fixed-screw-and-plate system available for use as high as T5. The presence of significant posterior column disruption would be a contraindication for an anterior fixation device as the sole stabilization construct. We favor anterior decompression and fusion if the patient has an incomplete lesion, the presence of canal compromise with minimal kyphotic deformity, or significant comminution of the vertebral body with displacement of the disk material among the fractured vertebral body fragments. DeWald reported that burst fractures that were severely compressed preoperatively failed to reconstitute to a functional support structure after posterior reduction and fixation and failed to fuse.[42] Although DeWald did not provide a system to measure the amount of disruption of the vertebral body, he stated that "in a clinical situation it can almost be predicted which body will need anterior grafting by the amount of compression initially present."

The Load-Sharing Classification scoring system McCormack and associates described is a classification system that can be used to predict the load-sharing capabilities of the anterior column of spine fractures (see Fig. 319–17 and Table 319–3).[104, 113] Parker and associates use a modification of this system to assist in the identification of fractures that should be decompressed and fused anteriorly in addition to placement of a posterior hook and rod construct. The anterior procedure allows the anterior column to be properly reconstructed by placement of an adequate graft, thereby ensuring the ability of the column to load share while the fusion is maturing.

A burst fracture should not be treated with a laminectomy as the sole surgical procedure because of increased instability and increased neurological deficits associated with this procedure.[19, 22, 116, 121] Although a laminectomy may be indicated for decompression of a laminar fracture or to expose a dural tear, a posterolateral fusion and posterior instrumentation should also be effected to reestablish the stability of the spinal column. Internal fixation is vital because the laminectomy will significantly destabilize the otherwise intact posterior column.

Fracture-Dislocations

With fracture-dislocation injury, all three columns of the spine are disrupted and the spine is rendered very unstable. This is undoubtedly the reason for the high incidence of spinal cord injury associated with fracture-dislocation injuries. It is also the reason most fracture-dislocation injuries require surgical treatment. If after a fracture-dislocation injury of the spine, the patient has a normal neurological examination, the spine needs to be stabilized by internal fixation and fusion to prevent a spinal injury from occurring and to allow the patient to be rapidly mobilized. When the patient has an incomplete spinal cord injury from a fracture-dislocation injury to the spine, the spinal canal should be decompressed and the spine stabilized. Even the patient with a complete neurological deficit from a fracture-dislocation injury requires stabilization of the spine to minimize the length of the acute hospital stay and to begin rehabilitation promptly.

The exact surgical procedure performed depends on the nature of the neurological injury as well as the injury to the supporting spinal column. Patients with normal neurological examinations and those with incomplete spinal injuries should be intubated and positioned while awake. With the patient awake, the normal muscle tone helps splint the injured segments and prevent additional spinal cord injury while the patient is positioned. Most fracture-dislocations are treated with posterior fixation and fusion, necessitating prone positioning of the patient. After the patient is positioned, a rapid assessment of the neurological status is performed and, if satisfactory, the induction of anesthesia is begun.

Flexion-rotation injuries are associated with the highest incidence of early neurological deterioration and therefore should be managed with extreme care until the spinal column can be stabilized.[65] The anterior longitudinal ligament is usually intact in the fracture-dislocation injuries, and the flexion-rotation and flexion-distraction subtypes can be reduced and fixed with a posteriorly placed distraction rod construct. Unlike Harrington distraction rod constructs, the universal segmental systems do not need an additional compression rod because intermediate hooks can be placed in compression, while the overall construct is placed in distraction.[41] The "claw" hook constructs with these systems can fix the spine regardless of the competence of the ligamentous structures. A compression construct is not an effective method to secure anatomic reduction or stability of a flexion-rotation or flexion-distraction injury.

Within subtypes of fracture-dislocation injuries, the shear subtype is one of the most unstable injuries because all three columns are disrupted, including all associated supporting ligamentous structures. The hyperextension shear injuries were not included in the initial Denis classification but were reported as a new injury type.[38, 40] This fracture is classified as a Magerl B3 fracture. A long posterior construct of one of the universal segmental fixation systems, as discussed previously, is adequate for treating shear injuries.[66] We recommend a universal system for reduction and fixation, a posterolateral autograft fusion, and the use of a TLSO in the immediate postoperative period.

Although there is rarely a need for acute anterior decompression in fracture-dislocation injuries, a patient with an incomplete spinal cord injury and severe anterior disruption may warrant anterior decompression and grafting in addition to posterior instrumentation and fusion. The posterior approach is usually necessary because it is difficult to correct a significant deformity and to secure an adequate stabilization of the spine from an anterior procedure alone. However, expandable cages and anterior distraction devices help reduce the fractures at the time of graft placement. Occasionally, posterior treatment of a fracture-dislocation does not adequately decompress the spinal cord, and if the patient has an incomplete spinal cord injury, a secondary anterior procedure is necessary.[109, 114]

Miscellaneous Injuries

The diagnosis of a soft tissue injury involving the thoracic spine is made after excluding a bone fracture and neural element injury by a detailed history, physical and neurological examinations, and appropriate imaging. Treatment is symptomatic, with physical therapy and rapid mobilization after a short (2- to 3-day) period of bed rest. A nonsteroidal anti-inflammatory agent should be used as the primary pharmacologic agent in the treatment of these disorders. Prolonged bed rest, rigid immobilization, and chronic narcotic analgesics must be avoided. Persistent discomfort should be evaluated with flexion-extension lateral plain radiographs to exclude an unstable subluxation masked by muscular contraction in the immediate period after injury. A bone scan can help identify an occult fracture. Magnetic resonance imaging should be performed if the plain films are abnormal. Computed tomography can define bony detail.

Traumatic disk injuries are rare in the thoracic spine but are often associated with significant morbidity, including paralysis. The fact that the spinal cord nearly fills the spinal canal accounts for the frequency of associated injury with even a modest-sized disk protrusion. Symptoms associated with thoracic disk herniations include pain, paresthesias, and neurological deficits. The pain may involve the local trunk axially at the injury site or may radiate along a rib. Spinal cord injury is often associated with distal dysesthetic pain.

Neurological signs of myelopathy may be present,

or a recognized injury pattern like an anterior cord or Brown-Séquard syndrome may be present. Bladder function may be altered, and the patient may complain of urinary urgency or incontinence. Deep tendon reflexes may be normal or hyperreflexic, and the plantar responses may be extensor.

The presence of a thoracic disk herniation can be detected with a magnetic resonance study or myelography, followed by computed tomography. The latter without intradural contrast medium enhancement is not adequate to exclude a thoracic disk abnormality. Similarly, plain films are unlikely to be diagnostic.

The treatment of a symptomatic thoracic disk herniation is surgical. There are a number of potential approaches for treatment of these lesions, including transthoracic, transpedicular, and costotransversectomy. A standard laminectomy should not be used because the disk cannot be removed without manipulation of the spinal cord, and such manipulation can be associated with neurological deterioration. Logue reported neurological deterioration in 45% of patients undergoing thoracic disk excision from a standard laminectomy.[95] Reports of transthoracic, transpedicular, or costotransversectomy approaches documented that 80% to 90% of patients improve, whereas the remainder are unchanged.[92, 101, 115, 117] Bohlman and associates reviewed 19 patients undergoing surgical resection of a thoracic disk herniation (8 treated by a transthoracic opening and 11 undergoing a costotransversectomy). They preferred the transthoracic approach because the lesion and the neural structures were visualized more easily, and all patients with paralysis before surgery improved with this surgical treatment.[17]

The authors of literature concerning civilian gunshot wounds have advocated restraint in the surgical treatment of these injuries, regardless of the extent of neurological injury. Studies of patients with spinal cord injuries in conjunction with gunshot injuries failed to show any recovery of neurological function after primary treatment with a laminectomy.[78, 131, 138, 144] Stauffer and associates demonstrated that after primary treatment of gunshot wounds to the spine with a laminectomy, the incidence of spinal instability increased from 0% to 6%, the incidence of cerebrospinal fluid leakage increased from 0% to 6%, and the incidence of infection increased from 0% to 4% when compared with nonsurgical management.[131] In their study, Waters and Adkins failed to demonstrate any improvement in patients with complete thoracic spinal cord injury from gunshot wounds, and their data showed no significant difference in the development of late pain and sensation between surgically and nonsurgically managed patients.[138] The authors suggest that surgical treatment of patients with gunshot wounds to the thoracic spine be limited to patients in whom it can be demonstrated that there is neurological deterioration in the presence of neural compression. Instability of the spine is rarely associated with thoracic level gunshot wounds.

COMPLICATIONS

The availability of effective spinal instrumentation has allowed the stabilization of most spinal column injuries but not without risk of complications. Although many intraoperative complications can be avoided with careful planning, tailoring of the surgical approach to the individual patient, and intraoperative monitoring, these procedures are not free of risk. Certain complications—including death, deep venous thrombosis, and pulmonary embolism—are not unique to surgical treatment and therefore are not discussed here.

Neurological deterioration during or after surgery is a very serious complication that accompanies approximately 1% of operations for treatment of a spine injury.[30, 93, 111, 140] Overdistraction, inadvertent introduction of instrumentation into the spinal canal, overcompression, or loss of reduction can all be associated with neurological deterioration. Overdistraction has been associated with Harrington distraction rod constructs but is less of a concern with the universal segmental fixation systems that do not depend on the competence of ligamentous tissues. Compression can cause the herniation of a disk or bone fragment into the spinal canal, with resultant compression of the spinal cord. This injury can be minimized by using this type of construct only when the posterior vertebral body is intact and following anterior decompression and fusion/fixation, ventral decompression using intraoperative somatosensory monitoring, and use of intraoperative ultrasound. Hooks can compromise the spinal canal, and the close proximity of spinal cord to spinal canal does not leave much space for them. The use of pedicle and transverse hooks can reduce but not entirely obviate this complication. We have not experienced complications with carefully selected sublaminar hooks from any of the universal segmental fixation systems. The latter systems have all but eliminated the use of sublaminar wires for the stabilization of thoracic fractures.

We use intraoperative somatosensory monitoring during all surgical procedures in patients with sufficient neurological function to support the monitoring. Although somatosensory monitoring may not detect a local compromise of motor function, we have found it useful. Monitoring of the motor tracts is now possible and is used when available. The placement of hooks must be verified and altered if necessary. Removal of the instrumentation must be considered if the evoked potentials deteriorate or the patient cannot move muscles distal to the instrumented spinal segments on a wake-up test. The patient must be observed in the postoperative period for neurological deterioration. Loss of reduction, hematoma, spinal cord edema, or disk herniation may develop postoperatively and adversely affect the neurological examination of the patient. The deterioration in neurological function should be evaluated expeditiously with plain films and magnetic resonance imaging or with computed tomography and myelography.

Dural lacerations with associated cerebrospinal fluid leak may be the result of the initial injury or a complication of the surgical treatment. Identification of the tear may require removal of additional bone for direct visualization. A primary repair should be attempted, and a dural graft of fascia or allograft should be sutured into place if necessary. Commercial fibrin glue preparations (BioGlue, CyroLife, Kennesaw, GA) are used. A lumbar drain should be considered to reduce the intradural fluid pressure and to permit sealing of the dural repair. Postoperatively, patients are placed on bed rest for a minimum of 72 hours.

Infections can occur after spinal surgery, especially after a long surgical procedure for a complicated instrumentation placement. Superficial infections should be opened and débrided. The wound may be packed open or closed over drainage tubes. Antibiotics should be used. Deep infections should also be treated with aggressive irrigation and débridement. We attempt to keep the instrumentation and bone graft in place. Drainage tubes are left deep to the fascia for 7 to 10 days. If the infection persists, a second procedure can be tried, but occasionally the infection persists. The instrumentation and graft are normally left in place until the fusion is solid, and instrumentation may later need to be removed to eradicate the infection.

REFERENCES

1. Aebi M, Etter CHR, Kehl TH, et al: The internal skeletal fixation system. Clin Orthop 227:30, 1988.
2. Allen BL, Ferguson RL: The Galveston technique for L rod instrumentation of the scoliotic spine. Spine 7:276, 1982.
3. American College of Surgeons: Advanced Trauma Life Support Instructor Manual. Chicago, American College of Surgeons, 1993.
4. American Spinal Injury Association: Standards for Neurological and Functional Classification of Spinal Cord Injury. Chicago, American Spinal Injury Association, 1992.
5. Angtuaco EJC, Binet EF: Radiology of the thoracic and lumbar fractures. Clin Orthop 9:43, 1984.
6. Asher M, Carson W, Heining C, et al: A modular spinal linkage system to provide rotational stability. Spine 13:272, 1988.
7. Asher MA, Strippgen WE, Heining CF, et al: Isola spinal implant system: Principles, design, and applications. In An HS, Cotler JM (eds): Spinal Instrumentation. Baltimore, Williams, & Wilkins, 1992, pp 325–351.
8. Ashman RB: History and development of the TSRH system. In Ashman RB, Herring JA, Johnston CE, et al (eds): TSRH Universal Spinal Instrumentation. Dallas, Hundley & Associates, 1993, pp 1–7.
9. Balasubramanian K, Ranu HS, King AI: Vertebral response to laminectomy. J Biomech 21:813, 1978.
10. Bauer RB, Garfin SR, Northrup BE: Spinal trauma: An overview. In Garfin RR, Northrup BE (eds): Surgery for Spinal Cord Injuries. New York, Raven Press, 1993, pp 1–3.
11. Bedbrook GM: Stability of spinal fractures and fracture-dislocations. Paraplegia 9:23, 1971.
12. Berns DH, Blaser SI, Modic MT: MRI of the spine. Clin Orthop 244:78, 1989.
13. Bick EM: Source Book of Orthopaedics. Baltimore, Williams & Wilkins, 1948.
14. Boerger TO, Limb D, Dickson RA: Does "canal clearance" affect neurological outcome after thoracolumbar burst fractures? J Bone Joint Surg Br 82B:629, 2000.
15. Bohler L: The Treatment of Fractures. Baltimore, W Woods, 1935.
16. Bohlman HH: Treatment of fractures and dislocations of the thoracic and lumbar spine. J Bone Joint Surg Am 61:165, 1985.
17. Bohlman HH, Kirkpatrick JS, Delamarter RB, Leventhal M: Anterior decompression for late pain and paralysis after fractures of the thoracolumbar spine. Clin Orthop 300:24, 1994.
18. Bohlman HH, Zdelblick TA: Anterior excision of thoracic discs. J Bone Joint Surg Am 70:1038–1047, 1988.
19. Bohlman HH, Freehafer A, Dejak J: The results of treatment of acute injuries of the upper thoracic spine with paralysis. J Bone Joint Surg Am 67:360, 1985.
20. Braakman R, Fontijne WPJ, Zeegers R, et al: Neurological deficit

in injuries of the thoracic and lumbar spine: A consecutive series of 70 patients. Acta Neurochir 111:11, 1991.

21. Bracken MB, Shepard MJ, Collins WF, et al: A randomized, controlled trial of methylprednisolone or naloxone in the treatment of acute spinal-cord injury: Results of the Second National Acute Spinal Cord Injury Study. N Engl J Med 322:1405, 1990.
22. Bradford DS, Akbarnia BA, Winter RB, et al: Surgical stabilization of fracture and fracture-dislocation of the thoracic spine. Spine 2:185, 1977.
23. Breasted JH: The Edwin Smith Papyrus. Chicago, University of Chicago Press, 1930.
24. Brockbank W, Griffiths DL: Orthopaedic surgery in the sixteenth and seventeenth centuries. J Bone Joint Surg Br 30:556, 1948.
25. Calancie B, Klose KJ, Baier S, et al: Isoflurane-induced attenuation of motor evoked potentials caused by electrical motor cortex stimulation during surgery. J Neurosurg 74:897, 1991.
26. Callenoff L, Chessare JW, Rogers LF, et al: Multiple level spinal injuries: Importance of early recognition. AJR Am J Roentgenol 130:665, 1978.
27. Cantor JB, Lebwohl NH, Garvey T, Eismont FJ: Nonoperative management of stable thoracolumbar burst fractures with early ambulation and bracing. Spine 18:971, 1993.
28. Chance CQ: Note on a type of flexion fracture of the spine. Br J Radiol 21:452, 1948.
29. Chou SN, Seljieskog EL: Alternative surgical approaches to the thoracic spine. Clin Neurosurg 20:306, 1973.
30. Chozick BS, Toselli R: Complications of spinal instrumentation. In Benzel EC (ed): Spinal Instrumentation. Park Ridge, IL, American Association of Neurological Surgeons, 1994, pp 257–274.
31. Convery FR, Minteer MA, Smith RN: Fracture-dislocation of the dorsal lumbar spine: Acute operative stabilization by Harrington instrumentation. Spine 3:160, 1978.
32. Cooper A: The Lectures of Sir Astley Cooper on the Principles and Practice of Surgery, 5th ed. Philadelphia, Haswell, Barrington, & Haswell, 1839.
33. Cotrel Y, Dubousset J, Guillaumat M: New universal instrumentation in spinal surgery. Clin Orthop 227:10, 1998.
34. Cushing H: Care of head injuries and injuries to the spine and peripheral nerves in the forward hospitals. In Lynch C (ed): The Medical Department of the United States Army in World War, vol 11, Part 1. Washington, DC, U.S. Government Printing Office, 1927.
35. Daffner RH, Beeb ZL, Goldberg AK, et al: The radiologic assessment of post-traumatic vertebral stability. Skeletal Radiol 19:103, 1990.
36. Davies WE, Morris JH, Hill V: An analysis of conservative (nonsurgical) management of thoracolumbar fractures and fracture-dislocations with neural damage. J Bone Joint Surg Am 62:1324, 1980.
37. Dekutoski MB, Conlan ES, Salciccioli GG: Spinal mobility and deformity after Harrington rod stabilization and limited arthrodesis of thoracolumbar fractures. J Bone Joint Surg Am 75:168, 1993.
38. del Rosario Molano M, Broton JG, Bean JA, et al: Complications associated with the prophylactic use of methylprednisolone during surgical stabilization after spinal cord injury. J Neurosurg 96:267, 2002.
39. Denis F: The three-column spine and its significance in the classification of acute thoracolumbar spinal injuries. Spine 8:817, 1983.
40. Denis F, Burkus J: Shear fracture-dislocations of the thoracic and lumbar spine associated with forceful hyperextension (lumberjack paraplegia). Spine 17:156, 1992.
41. Denis F, Armstrong GWD, Searls K, et al: Acute thoracolumbar burst fractures in the absence of neurological deficit. Clin Orthop 189:142, 1984.
42. DeWald RL: Burst fractures of the thoracic and lumbar spine. Clin Orthop 189:150–161, 1984.
43. Dickson JH, Harrington PR, Erwin WD: Harrington instrumentation in the fractured, unstable thoracic and lumbar spine. Rex Med 69:91, 1973.
44. Dickson JH, Harrington PR, Erwin WD: Results of reduction and stabilization of the severely fractured thoracic and lumbar spine. J Bone Joint Surg Am 60:799, 1978.

45. Drummond D, Guadagni J, Keene JS, et al: Interspinous process segmental spinal instrumentation. J Pediatr Orthop 4:397, 1984.
46. Dunn HK: Anterior spine stabilization and decompression for thoracolumbar injuries. Orthop Clin N Am 17:113, 1986.
47. Durward QJ, Schweigel JF, Harrison P: Management of fractures of the thoracolumbar and lumbar spine. Neurosurgery 8:555, 1981.
48. Edwards CC, Levine AM: Early rod-sleeve stabilization of the injured thoracic and lumbar spine. Orthop Clin N Am 17:121, 1986.
49. Edwards CC, Levine AM: Complications associated with posterior instrumentation in the treatment of thoracic and lumbar injuries. In Garfin S (ed): Complications of Spine Surgery. Baltimore, Williams & Wilkins, 1989, pp 164–199.
50. Edwards CC, Levine AM, Weigel MC: Determinants of neurologic recovery following post-traumatic incomplete paraplegia. Orthop Trans 11:453, 1987.
51. Eismont FJ, Garfin SR, Abitol J: Thoracic and upper lumbar spine injuries. In Browner BD, Jupiter JB, Levine AM, et al (eds): Skeletal Trauma, vol I. Philadelphia, WB Saunders, 1993, pp 727–803.
52. Eismont FJ, Green BA, Berkowitz BM, et al: The role of intraoperative ultrasonography in the treatment of thoracic and lumbar fractures. Spine 9:782, 1984.
53. El-Khoury GY, Moore TE, Kathol M H: Radiology of the thoracic spine. Clin Neurosurg 38:261, 1990.
54. Erikson DL, Leider LL, Browno WE: One-stage decompression-stabilization for thoracolumbar fractures. Spine 2:53, 1977.
55. Farcy JP: Simultaneous anterior and posterior procedures for short segment spine pathology. Video tape 23112, Rosemont IL, American Academy of Orthopaedic Surgeons, 1993.
56. Farcy JP: Unstable fractures of the lumbar spine—discussion. Spinal Frontiers 3:4, 1996.
57. Farcy JP, Weidenbaum M, Glassman SD: Sagittal index in management of thoracolumbar burst fractures. Spine 15:958, 1990.
58. Ferguson RL, Allen BL: A mechanistic classification of thoracolumbar spine fractures. Clin Orthop 189:77, 1984.
59. Ferguson RL, Allen BL: An algorithm for the treatment of unstable thoracolumbar fractures. Orthop Clin N Am 17:105, 1986.
60. Flesch JR, Leider LL, Erickson DL, et al: Harrington instrumentation and spine fusion for unstable fractures and fracture-dislocation of the thoracic and lumbar spine. J Bone Joint Surg Am 59:143, 1977.
61. Frankel HL, Hancock DO, Huslop G, et al: The value of postural reduction in the initial management of closed injuries of the spine with paraplegia and tetraplegia. Paraplegia 7:179, 1969.
62. Gaines RW, Humphreys WG: A plea for judgement in management of thoracolumbar fractures and fracture-dislocations. Clin Orthop 189:36, 1984.
63. Garfin SR, Mowery CA, Guerra J, et al: Confirmation of the posterolateral technique to decompress and fuse thoracolumbar spine fractures. Spine 10:218, 1985.
64. Gellad RE, Levine AM, Joslyn JN, et al: Pure thoracolumbar facet dislocation: Clinical features and CT appearance. Radiology 161:505, 1986.
65. Gertzbein SD: Neurological deterioration in patients with thoracic and lumbar fractures after admission to the hospital. Spine 19:1723, 1994.
66. Gertzbein SD: Spine update: Classification of thoracic and lumbar fractures. Spine 19:626, 1994.
67. Gertzbein SD: Scoliosis Research Society: Multicenter spine fracture study. Spine 17:528, 1992.
68. Gertzbein SD, Court-Brown CM, Marks P, et al: The neurological outcome following surgery for spinal fractures. Spine 13:641, 1988.
69. Gooding GAW, Berger MS, Linkowski GD, et al: Transducer frequency considerations in intraoperative ultrasound of the spine. Radiology 160:273, 1986.
70. Griffiths DL, Brockbank W: Traction apparatus: The Vidian pictures. J Bone Joint Surg Br 31:313, 1949.
71. Gupta A, El Masri WS: Multilevel spinal injuries: Incidence, distribution, and neurological patterns. J Bone Joint Surg Br 71:692, 1989.
72. Gurr K, McAfee P, Shih C: Biomechanical analysis of anterior

and posterior instrumentation systems after corpectomy: A calf spine model. J Bone Joint Surg Am 70:1182, 1988.

73. Guttmann L: Spinal Cord Injuries: Comprehensive Management and Research. Oxford, Blackwell Scientific Publications, 1973.

74. Hadley MN: Guidelines for the management of acute cervical spine and spinal cord injuries: Pharmacological therapy after cervical spinal cord injury. Neurosurgery 50:S63, 2002.

75. Hachen HJ: Computed tomography of the spine and spinal cord: Limitation and applications. Paraplegia 19:155, 1981.

76. Hardaker WT, Cook WA, Friedman AH, et al: Bilateral transpedicular decompression and Harrington rod stabilization in the management of severe thoracolumbar burst fractures. Spine 17: 162, 1992.

77. Harrington PR: Instrumentation of spine instability other than spine scoliosis. S Afr J Surg 5:7, 1967.

78. Heiden JS, Weiss MH, Rosenberg AW, et al: Penetrating gunshot wounds of the cervical spine in civilians: Review of 38 cases. J Neurosurg 42:575, 1975.

79. Hodgson AR, Stock FE: Anterior spinal fusion: A preliminary communication on radical treatment of Pott's disease and Pott's paraplegia. Br J Surg 44:266, 1956.

80. Holdsworth FW: Fractures, dislocations, and fracture-dislocation of the spine. J Bone Joint Surg Am 52:1534, 1970.

81. Holdsworth FW: Fractures, dislocations, and fracture-dislocation of the spine. J Bone Joint Surg Br 45:6, 1963.

82. Holdsworth F, Harvey AG: Early treatment of paraplegia from fractures of the thoraco-lumbar spine. J Bone Joint Surg Br 33: 540, 1953.

83. Jacobs RR, Asher MA, Snider RK: Thoracolumbar spinal injuries: A comparative study of recumbent and operative treatment in 100 patients. Spine 5:463, 1980.

84. James KS, Wenger KH, Schiegel JD, et al: Biomechanical evaluation of the stability of thoracolumbar burst fractures. Spine 19: 1731, 1994.

85. Keene JS, Goletz TH, Lilleas F, et al: Diagnosis of vertebral fractures. J Bone Joint Surg Am 64:586, 1982.

86. Keynes G: Editor's introduction. In Keynes G (ed): The Apologie and Treatise of Ambroise Paré Containing the Voyages Made into Divers Places with Many of His Writings upon Surgery. London, Falcon, Educational Books, 1951.

87. Kling TF, Permutter J, Kauder H, et al: Early segmental stabilization of thoracolumbar spine fractures with neurologic deficits. Orthop Trans 9:121, 1986.

88. Kostuik JP: Anterior fixation for fractures of the thoracic and lumbar spine with or without neurologic involvement. Clin Orthop 189:103, 1984.

89. Krengel WF, Anderson PA, Henley MB: Early stabilization and decompression for incomplete paraplegia due to a thoracic-level spinal cord injury. Spine 18:2080, 1993.

90. Lauridsen KN, DeCarvalho A, Andersen AH: Degree of vertebral wedging of the dorso-lumbar spine. Acta Radiol Diagn 25: 29, 1984.

91. Lebwohl NH, Starr JK: Surgical management of thoracolumbar fractures. In Greenberg J (ed): Handbook of Head and Spine Trauma. New York, M. Dekker, 1993, pp 593–646.

92. Lesoin F, Leys D, Bouseaux M, et al: Thoracic disc herniation and Scheuermann's disease. Eur Neurol 26:145, 1987.

93. Levine AM, Edwards CC: Complications in the treatment of acute spinal injury. Orthop Clin N Am 17:183, 1986.

94. Lewis J, McKibbin B: The treatment of unstable fracture-dislocations of the thoraco-lumbar spine accompanied by paraplegia. J Bone Joint Surg 56B:603.

95. Logue V: Thoracic intervertebral disc prolapse with spinal cord compression. J Neurol Neurosurg Psychiatry 15:227, 1952.

96. Madsen PW, Baldwin N: Posterior thoracic and lumbar—combined/complex techniques. In Benzel EC (ed): Spinal Surgery: Techniques and Complication Avoidance and Management. Philadelphia, Churchill-Livingstone, 1999, pp 1085–1110.

97. Madsen PW, Eismont FJ: Intraoperative valuation: myelogram/ultrasound. In Garfin SR, Northrup BE (eds): Surgery for Spinal Cord Injuries. New York, Raven Press, 1993, pp 245–252.

98. Magerl F, Aebi M, Gertzbein SD, et al: A comprehensive classification of thoracic and lumbar injuries. Eur Spine J 3:184, 1994.

99. Magerl F, Harms J, Gertzbein SD, et al: A new classification of spinal fractures. Orthop Trans 15:728, 1991.

100. Maiman DJ, Pintar FA: Anatomy and clinical biomechanics of the thoracic spine. Clin Neurosurg 38:296, 1990.

101. Maiman DJ, Larson SJ, Luck E, et al: Lateral extracavitary approach to the spine for thoracic disc herniation: Report of 23 cases. Neurosurgery 12:178, 1984.

102. McAfee PC, Bohlman HH, Yuan HA: Anterior decompression of traumatic thoracolumbar fractures with inscomplete neurological deficit using a retroperitoneal approach. J Bone Joint Surg Am 67:673, 1985.

103. McAfee PC, Werner F, Glisson R: A biomechanical analysis of spinal instrumentation systems in thoracolumbar fractures: Comparison of traditional Harrington distraction instrumentation with segmental spinal instrumentation. Spine 10:204, 1985.

104. McAfee PC, Yuan H, Fredrickson B, et al: The value of computer tomography in thoracolumbar fractures. J Bone Joint Surg Am 65:471, 1983.

105. McCormack T, Karaikovic E, Gaines RW: The load-sharing classification of spine fractures. Spine 19:1741, 1994.

106. M'Donnell R: Case of fracture of the spine in which the operation of trephining was performed, with observation. Clin Orthop 189:3, 1984.

107. McEvoy RD, Bradford DS: The management of burst fractures of the thoracic and lumbar spine: Experience in 53 patients. Spine 10:631, 1983.

108. Mettler CC: History of Medicine. Philadelphia, Blakiston, 1947.

109. Mirza SK, Mirza AJ, Chapman JR, et al: Classification of thoracic and lumbar fractures: Rationale and supporting data. J Am Acad Orthop Surg 10:364, 2002.

110. Morgan TH, Wharton GW, Austin GN: The results of laminectomy in patients with incomplete spinal cord injury. Paraplegia 9:14, 1971.

111. Mueller WM, Larson SJ: Complications of spinal instrumentation. In Tarlov EC (ed): Complications of Spinal Surgery. Park Ridge, IL, American Association of Neurological Surgeons, 1991, pp 15–22.

112. Nicoll EA: Fractures of the dorso-lumbar spine. J Bone Joint Surg Br 31:376, 1949.

113. Osebold WR, Weinstein SL, Sprague BL: Thoracolumbar spine fractures: Results of treatments. Spine 6:13, 1981.

114. Parker JW, Lane JR, Karikovic EE, et al: Successful short-segment instrumentation and fusion for thoracolumbar spine fractures. Spine 25:1157, 2000.

115. Patterson RH, Arbit E: A surgical approach through the pedicle for protruded thoracic discs. J Neurosurg 48:768, 1978.

116. Paul RL, Michael RH, Dunn JE, et al: Anterior transthoracic surgical decompression of acute spinal cord injuries. J Neurosurg 43:299, 1975.

117. Perot PH, Munro DD: Transthoracic removal of midline thoracic disc protrusions causing spinal cord compression. J Neurosurg 31:452, 1969.

118. Purcel GA, Markolf KL, Dawson EG: Twelfth thoracic–first lumbar vertebral mechanical stability of fractures after Harrington-rod instrumentation. J Bone Joint Surg Am 63:71, 1981.

119. Rennie W, Mitchell N: Flexion dislocation fractures of the lumbar spine. J Bone Joint Surg Am 55:386, 1973.

120. Riebel GD, Yoo JU, Fredrickson BE, et al: Review of Harrington rod treatment of spinal trauma. Spine 18:479, 1993.

121. Riggins RS, Kraus JF: The risk of neurologic damage with fractures of the vertebrae. J Trauma 17:126, 1977.

122. Roach JW, Ashman RB, Allard RN: The strength of a posterior element claw at one versus two spinal levels. J Spinal Disord 3: 259, 1990.

123. Roaf R: A study of the mechanics of spinal injuries. J Bone Joint Surg Br 42:810, 1960.

124. Roberts JB, Curtiss PH: Stability of the thoracic and lumbar spine in traumatic paraplegia following fracture or fracture-dislocation. J Bone Joint Surg Am 52:1115, 1970.

125. Rogers F, Thayer C, Weinbert PE, et al: Acute injuries of the upper thoracic spine associated with paraplegia. AJR Am J Roentgenol 134:67, 1980.

126. Sasson A, Mozes G: Complete fracture-dislocation of the thoracic spine without neurologic deficit. Spine 12:67, 1987.

127. Schuman WP, Rogers JV, Sickler ME, et al: Thoracolumbar burst fractures: CT dimensions of the spinal canal relative to postsurgical improvement AJNR 6:337, 1985.

128. Scoliosis Research Society: Morbidity and Mortality Committee Report. Park Ridge, IL, Scoliosis Research Society, 1987.
129. Soreff J, Axdorph G, Bylund P, et al: Treatment of patient with unstable fractures of the thoracic and lumbar spine: A follow-up study of surgical and conservative treatment. Acta Orthop Scand 53:369, 1982.
130. Spencer DL, DeWald RL: Simultaneous anterior and posterior surgical approach to the thoracic and lumbar spine. Spine 4:29, 1979.
131. Stauffer ES, Wood RW, Kelly EG: Gunshot wounds in the spine: The effects of laminectomy. J Bone Joint Surg Am 61:389, 1979.
132. Sullivan JA, Carolla JJ, Wilkerson JA, et al: Laboratory testing of segmental spinal instrumentation versus traditional Harrington instrumentation for scoliosis treatment. Spine 7:265, 1982.
133. Sutherlin CE: Applications of TSRH instrumentation in trauma. In Ashman RB, Herring JA, Johnston CE, et al (eds): TSRH Universal Spinal Instrumentation. Dallas, Hundley & Associates, 1993, pp 115–134.
134. Tarr RW, Drolshagen LF, Kerner TC, et al: MR imaging of recent spinal trauma. J Comput Assist Tomogr 11:412, 1987.
135. Tator CH: Epidemiology and general characteristics of the spinal cord injured patient. In Benzel EC, Tator CH (eds): Contemporary Management of Spinal Cord Injury. Park Ridge, IL, American Association of Neurological Surgeons, 1994.
136. van Beck EJR, Been HD, Ponsen K, Maas M: Upper thoracic spinal fractures in trauma patients—a diagnostic pitfall. Injury 31:219, 2000.
137. Vincent KA, Benson DR, McGahan JP: Intraoperative ultrasonography for reduction of thoracolumbar burst fractures. Spine 14:387, 1989.
138. Waters RL, Adkins RH: The effects of removal of bullet fragments retained in the spinal canal: A collaborative study by the National Spinal Cord Injury Model Systems. Spine 16:934, 1991.
139. Watson-Jones R: Fracture and Joint Injuries, 3rd ed. Baltimore, Williams & Wilkins, 1943.
140. Wenger DR, Mubarak SJ: Managing complications of posterior spinal instrumentation and fusion. In Garfin SR, (ed): Complications of Spine Surgery. Baltimore, Williams & Wilkins, 1989, pp 127–143.
141. White AA, Panjabi MM: The basic kinematics of the lumbar spine: A review of past and current knowledge. Spine 3:12, 1979.
142. White AA, Panjabi M: Clinical Biomechanics of the Spine, 2nd ed. Philadelphia JB Lippincott, 1990.
143. Whitesides TE, Jr: Traumatic kyphosis of the thoracolumbar spine. Clin Orthop 128:78, 1997.
144. Yashon D, Jane JA, White RJ: Prognosis and management of spinal cord and cauda equina bullet injuries in sixty-five civilians. J Neurosurg 32:163, 1970.

CHAPTER 320

Diagnosis and Management of Thoracolumbar and Lumbar Spine Injuries

RUSS P. NOCKELS ■ JULIE YORK

Injuries to the thoracolumbar spine are the result of both anatomic spinal vulnerability and the accidental forces inherent in modern society. Each year, more than 50,000 patients sustain fractures of the thoracolumbar and lumbar spine in the United States. The immediate neurological damage that accompanies the bony destruction results in nearly 5000 cases of paraplegia per year.[1] The mechanisms and severity of these injuries reflect a mechanized and risk-taking culture, with common causes being motor vehicle accidents, falls, and direct blows to the back. These sudden decelerations and subsequent loading of the spine concentrate forces in the thoracolumbar and lumbar spine, where a zone of transition exists between the relatively immobile kyphosis of the thorax and the flexible lordosis of the lumbar region. Fortunately for neurosurgeons, the fracture patterns in these areas have been studied with regard to mechanism of damage, thereby identifying the work forces in play. A spectrum of treatment is available, depending on the severity of the injury, including recumbency, bracing, and surgery. The resulting guideline may provide long-term stability and protection of the neural structures. Early rehabilitation and the long-term prevention of progressive spinal deformity are the goals of any operative management. In the near future, the application of minimally invasive techniques and fusion biology may increase surgical success rates while minimizing operative morbidity.

INITIAL EVALUATION

Early recognition of spinal injury is the first step toward appropriate treatment; it is best when paramedics at the scene of an accident recognize that an individual may have a spinal injury. Basic tests of motor function and for the presence of spinal pain should be performed in the field. A patient suspected of having a spinal injury is placed on a transportation board in a neutral supine position and immobilized in a neck collar. There should be no further movement of the spine until the patient has been completely evaluated by a physician in the emergency room and radiographs have been examined. Stabilization of the patient's hemodynamics and airway takes initial precedence so that adequate oxygenation and perfusion of injured tissues can be maintained. In patients with neurological deficits, immediate peritoneal lavage or abdominal computed tomography (CT) is often advocated to rule out intra-abdominal injuries. Concurrent head injury, alcohol intoxication, and multiple injuries are common reasons for delay in the recognition of spinal injuries.[2]

A detailed history should be obtained, if possible, to ascertain the mechanism of injury and the relative force sustained. With respect to mode of injury, two groups of patients deserve special attention: individuals who fall from a height, and those injured as a result of lap seat belts.[3, 4] Individuals who fall or jump from a height often have hyperflexion injuries at the thoracolumbar region in association with pelvic and lower extremity fractures. Persons restrained by seat belts during motor vehicle accidents often have distraction injuries at the thoracolumbar junction. In these injuries, the presence of the seat belt moves the fulcrum of flexion from the center of the intervertebral disk to the anterior abdominal wall, so distraction becomes the primary force. The vertebrae can actually be pulled apart through the horizontal plane (Fig. 320–1).

Head injuries and extremity fractures commonly accompany vertebral fractures.[4] Although back pain is a reliable indicator of potential thoracolumbar injury, suspicion of occult injury needs to be highest in patients with altered sensorium, concomitant major injury, or masking neurological deficit.[5–7] Abdominal or urologic trauma can occur with lumbar fractures, particularly with seat belt–type injuries.[8] Concurrent direct injuries to adjacent intracavitary soft tissue structures must be considered, such as laceration of the renal capsule by a transverse process fracture between T10 and L1. In general, the more caudal the vertebral injury, the greater the biomechanical forces sustained; such injuries should prompt suspicion of occult severe injur-

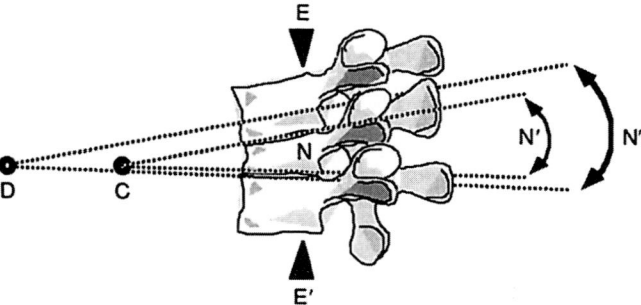

FIGURE 320–1. Effect of fulcrum position on spinal elements in a typical flexion injury. Note that as the distance between the fulcrum and the spine (points D and C) increases, so does the distractive force on the posterior elements (N″ versus N′). The presence of a seat belt in motor vehicle accidents shifts the fulcrum of flexion from the center of the intervertebral disk to the anterior abdominal wall, permitting this distraction to occur. In burst fractures, an additional compressive force (E and E′) acts on the vertebral body (N), resulting in failure of the middle column.

ies to the pelvis and sacrum. Likewise, 26% of sacral fractures and 8% of pelvic fractures have associated spinal fractures.[9] Overall 10% to 20% mortality has been reported for closed pelvic trauma.[10]

As early as possible, and no later than 8 hours after injury, patients with spinal cord injury should receive intravenous methylprednisolone 30 mg/kg in a bolus, followed by infusion at 5.4 mg/kg per hour for 48 hours. If the bolus is given within 3 hours of injury, the subsequent drip is necessary for only 23 hours. The results of the third National Acute Spinal Cord Injury Study (NASCIS III) demonstrated significantly better motor function and sensation at 6 months and 1 year in patients treated with this regimen compared with those given placebo.[11] Benefit was seen in patients with injuries initially considered to be neurologically complete, as well as in those believed to have incomplete lesions. Recently, the results of the NASCIS trials have been criticized, and some advocate methylprednisolone therapy as a treatment option.[12–14] The value of high-dose corticosteroids in cauda equina injuries has not been established. The relationship between the timing of surgical decompression and neurological outcome is widely debated owing to a lack of a randomized trial. Many researchers believe that because of the heterogeneity of the neural structures involved in thoracolumbar and lumbar fractures (i.e., conus medullaris and cauda equina), these injuries should be considered separately from cord injuries because they possess a greater capacity for spontaneous recovery.

Spinal Examination

In the spinal examination, the overlying skin should be inspected for abrasions or contusions by log-rolling the patient. General deviations from the normal curves, that is, thoracic kyphosis and lumbar lordosis, should be noted. Muscle spasm from pain flattens the spine, whereas fractures may cause a kyphotic deformity. Any lateral curvature or scoliosis is abnormal. The spine is

TABLE 320–1 ■ **Frankel Classification**

A. Complete loss of both motor and sensory function below a given level
B. Some preservation of sensation; complete motor paralysis
C. Motor useless; some motor function preserved, but insufficient to be useful
D. Motor useful; weak but useful motor function
E. Neurologically intact

The Frankel classification is based on motor function but is less specific and quantitative than the American Spinal Injury Association Motor Index Score (see Table 320–2).

palpated, and pain and tenderness are noted. A gibbous deformity or displaced or separated spinous processes are significant findings even in the absence of findings on plain radiographs.

Neurological Examination

The neurological examination is the most important and sensitive test for spinal cord injury. Any neurological deficit should be documented according to accepted classification schemes, such as the Frankel classification and the American Spinal Injury Association Motor Index (Tables 320–1 and 320–2).[15, 16] The initial examination may be difficult because of multiple trauma and spinal shock, and a determination of normal neurological function can never be accomplished in a hypotensive or hypoxic patient. Neurological examinations should be repeated and documented to serve as a reference for improvement or deterioration in the patient's neurological status over time.

A detailed neurological evaluation includes detection of a sensory level (if one is present), posterior column function, and any sacral sensory sparing. Muscle weakness is graded from 0 to 5. The abdominal skin reflex, bulbocavernosus (bulbospongiosus) reflex, superficial anal reflex, and Babinski's sign should be noted. A rectal examination to check tone and voluntary contracture is performed.

Although the distinction between complete and in-

TABLE 320–2 ■ **American Spinal Injury Association Motor Index Score**

RIGHT	KEY MUSCLE SEGMENT	LEFT
5	C5	5
5	C6	5
5	C7	5
5	C8	5
5	T1	5
5	L2	5
5	L3	5
5	L4	5
5	L5	5
5	S1	5
50	Total score	50

Each key muscle is graded as follows; 0, absent; 1, trace; 2, poor; 3, fair; 4, good; 5, normal. The grade values are put in the table and totaled. The score produced is used to compare admission, discharge, and follow-up status.

complete injuries has prognostic significance after the first 24 hours, one cannot rule out significant neurological potential in patients with so-called complete lesions immediately following injury. Spinal shock can last 24 to 48 hours, suppressing reflex activity below the lesion level. Some return of motor or sensory function below the level of the lesion suggests that sufficient anatomic substrate persists and some return of useful neurological function may occur. In addition to a sensory level, several other signs help localize the level of injury. Paralysis below the 10th thoracic level is indicated by Beevor's sign, which is cephalad movement of the umbilicus when the patient is asked to elevate his or her head in the supine position. This sign is due to paralysis of the lower abdominal muscles.

The relatively small size of the thoracolumbar canal in proportion to the conus medullaris results in neurological deficits that tend to be more severe for any given fracture type compared with lumbar injuries. However, an inconsistent relationship has been recognized between degree of canal compromise and neurological deficit.[17, 18] This is undoubtedly due, in part, to the dynamics of the injury at the instant of spinal deformation. The relative lack of axial loading in patients undergoing routine recumbent radiologic evaluation may also play a role. Fortunately, a common neurological syndrome resulting from contusion of the distal spinal cord spares some distal motor function and posterior column sensation of position and vibra-

tion. Obviously, radicular function must also be considered, especially when the neural foramen is compressed by the collapsed and retropulsed vertebrae. In general, thoracic nerve root function above T12 is not as critical as lower root function is.

Fractures of the thoracolumbar junction (T11-L2) can produce a mixture of cord and root syndromes.[19, 20] Such mixture occurs because the conus medullaris portion of the spinal cord, which contains the anterior horn cells of L5 to S5 as well as all the lumbar nerve roots as they pass down to their exit foramina, lies opposite the L1 vertebral body (Fig. 320–2). Complete damage of the sacral cord and nerve roots is manifested as no motor function or sensation below L1. The most common type of incomplete injury that occurs is complete sacral cord damage with variable sparing of the lumbar roots. Patients with this type of injury have complete bowel and bladder paralysis and sacral motor paralysis of the extremities; however, they retain some movement of the hips and knees and have preserved knee jerks and sensation in the lumbar dermatomes. The most common occult neurological injury is lower urinary tract dysfunction, which is best detected by serial urodynamics and is caused by autonomic dysfunction.[21] Incomplete sacral cord lesions are less common.

The cauda equina has a significant capacity for recovery. In one study, 12% of patients who were thought to have complete injuries on admission showed recov-

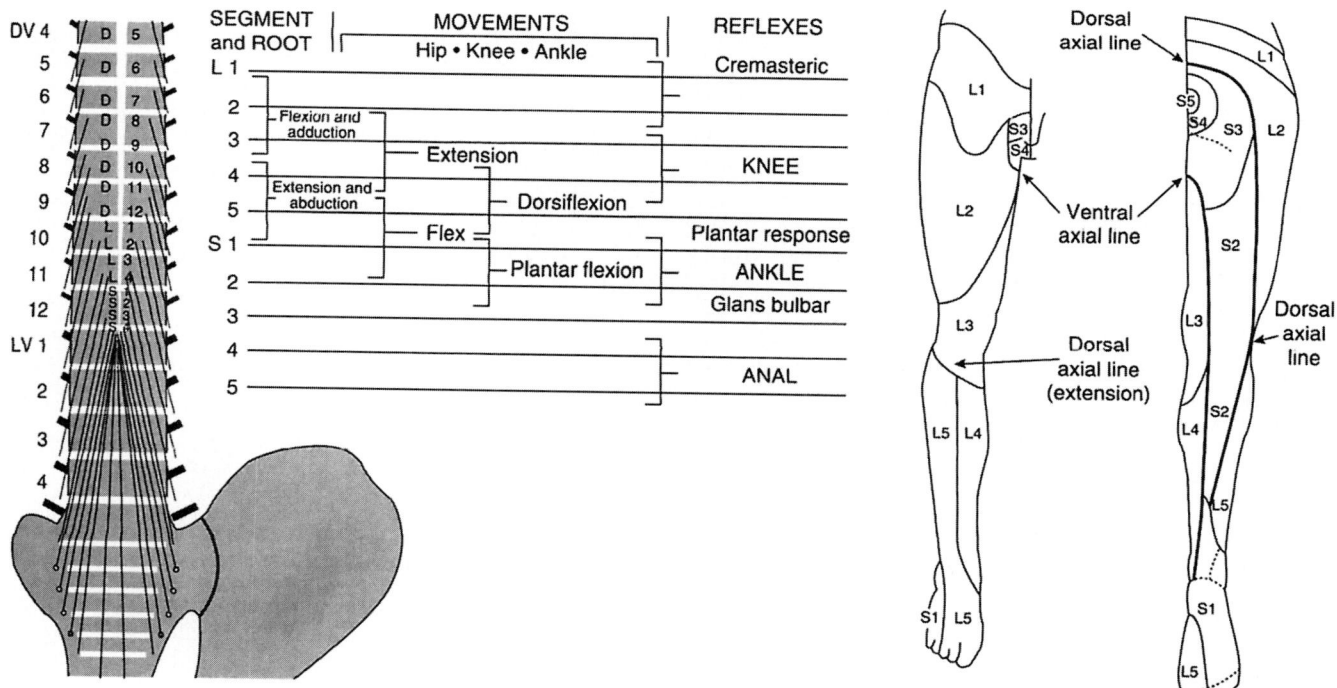

FIGURE 320–2. Anatomic relationship of the spinal cord, conus medullaris, and cauda equina to the bony anatomy of the spine. The conus, as well as all the lumbar nerve roots as they pass down to their exit foramina, lies opposite the L1 vertebral body. Injuries in this region can produce a mixture of cord and root syndromes. The segmental control of leg movements and reflexes is shown. The lumbar and sacral dermatomes are indicated. (From Holdsworth FW, Hardy KA: Early treatment of paraplegia from fractures of the thoracolumbar spine. J Bone Joint Surg Br 35:540–550, 1953.)

ery, and more than 75% of patients admitted with root-sparing and truly incomplete lesions showed useful recovery.[22]

Lower lumbar fractures may cause solitary or multiple radiculopathies. Massive disk herniations, fracture-dislocations, and burst fractures in the lumbar region can cause a cauda equina syndrome with variable paraparesis, asymmetrical saddle anesthesia, radiating pain, and sphincter disturbances.

Diagnostic Imaging

The most important initial radiographic examination is a complete spine series. Delayed recognition of a fracture might jeopardize remaining neurological function or worsen spinal malalignment. Relatively few significant injuries are missed when proper emergency spinal imaging protocols are followed.[5] Missed diagnoses are most common when imaging does not occur because of the need to treat other life-threatening injuries.[5, 6] A total of 5% to 20% of spinal fractures are multiple, and some (5% to 10.5%) may be at noncontiguous levels.[9, 23, 24] The lateral view is the best method for initial

localization of the fracture.[25, 26] An oblique spine view may be useful in defining facet and pars interarticularis fractures. In the lumbar spine, flexion and extension views help distinguish minor degrees of degenerative subluxation seen with disk disease from traumatic subluxations, but these views are contraindicated in the context of an obviously acute fracture. Lumbar fractures should prompt an anteroposterior radiograph of the pelvis.

Analysis of plain radiographs should proceed in an organized sequence. The physician assesses alignment on both lateral and frontal radiographs by identifying the margins of the vertebral bodies, spinolaminar line, articular pillars and their facet joints, interspinous distance, interpediculate distance, and position of the transverse processes. Abnormalities of alignment include disruption of the anterior or posterior vertebral body lines, disruption of the spinolaminar line, dislocated facets, rotation of spinous processes, and widening of the interpediculate distance. Kyphotic angulation and loss of lumbar lordosis are less important signs of an acute abnormality if they are not associated with misalignment or bony fractures. Disruption of

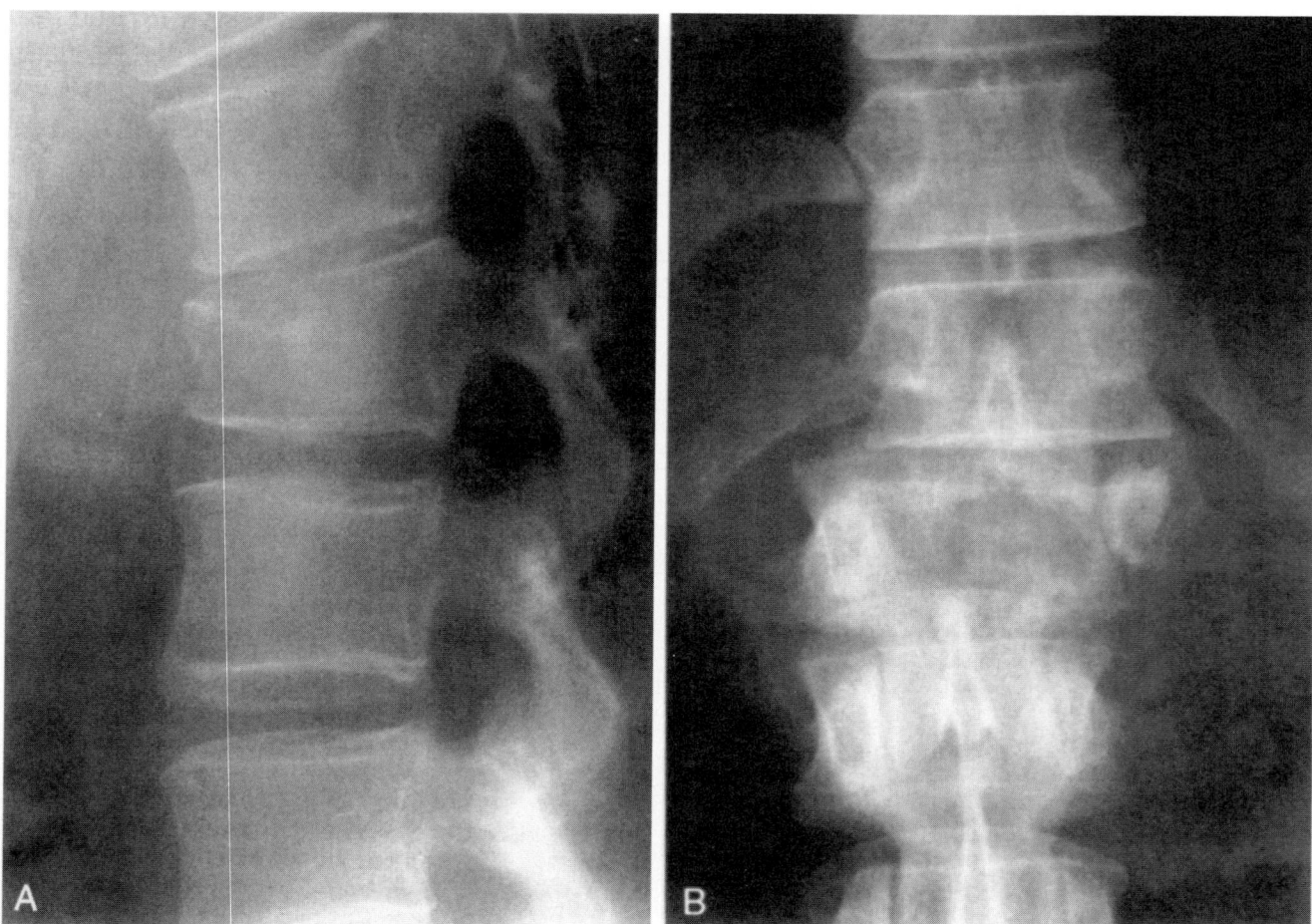

FIGURE 320–3. Plain radiographs in the evaluation of thoracolumbar trauma. *A,* Typical wedge compression fracture. Note the kyphotic angulation due to injury restricted to the anterior column of the spine. *B,* Increased interpediculate distance is demonstrated on an anteroposterior projection; this is typical of a burst fracture.

the posterior margin of the vertebral body line and widening of the interpediculate distance are important signs of vertebral disruption (Fig. 320–3). Nonosseous structures are more difficult to assess on plain radiographs. Narrowing of a disk space usually accompanies a flexion injury and is seen at the level above the fractured vertebra, but it is also common with degenerative disease. A more important finding is widening of the facet joint or even complete baring of the facets ("naked facets"). Either of these findings indicates that a severe posterior ligamentous injury has occurred as a result of distractive forces. These findings are almost always associated with widening of the interspinous distance, which should not be greater than 7 mm between adjacent segments.[27] Post-traumatic kyphosis is best determined by measuring a line through the superior end plate one level above and the inferior end plate one level below the injured segment.[28] Finally, soft tissue abnormalities are identified, including the presence of a paraspinal soft tissue mass and the loss of the psoas stripe.

Following the analysis of routine spine films, CT is performed on areas of suspected bony injury as determined by standard radiographs. Computed tomographic scanning best defines complex fractures and is essential for determining the involvement of the posterior elements and the degree of vertebral comminution (Fig. 320–4). The scan should include one full vertebra above and one full vertebra below the level of the fracture, with 3- or 5-mm-thick slices being used. Bone and soft tissue windows are imaged. Scout films are obtained to allow easy and rapid identification of all vertebrae. Fractures oriented in a horizontal plane (e.g., Chance fractures and compression fractures) may not

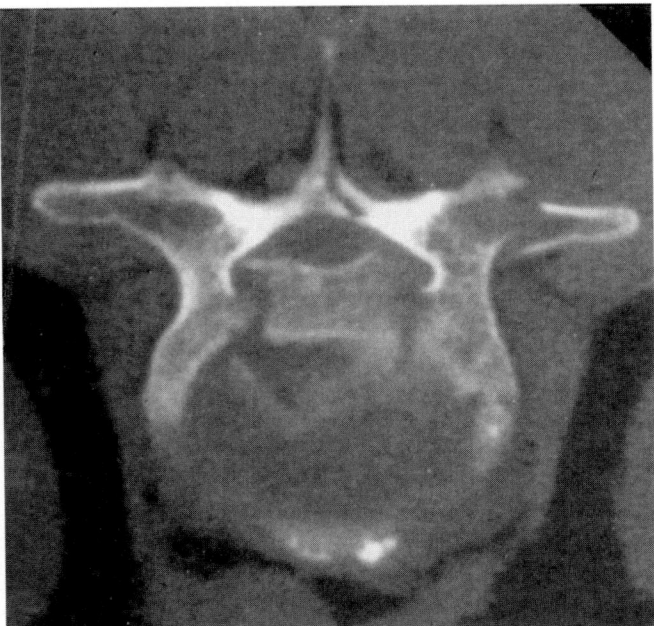

FIGURE 320–4. Axial computed tomography section through a typical burst fracture. The retropulsed bony fragment indicates failure of the middle column and distinguishes this injury from a wedge compression fracture.

be visualized with axial CT unless thin-cut (1 to 1.5 mm), high-resolution, contiguous sections are used. Sagittal reformation can be used to better define canal compromise and posterior element fractures.

When there is neurological deficit or when plain radiographs suggest canal compromise, myelography with CT or magnetic resonance imaging (MRI) must be used to obtain details of the neural compression. MRI has the advantage of better visualization of the cord and ligamentous injuries.[25, 29] High signal intensity is seen with parenchymal cord injury and edema, especially on T2-weighted and proton density–weighted images. Ligament disruptions, which must be inferred from CT, can sometimes be demonstrated with fat-suppressed T2-weighted sagittal imaging.[30] The anterior and posterior longitudinal ligaments are best seen on T1- and T2-weighted images, respectively. Disrupted ligaments are more easily identified than are intact ones. MRI also permits sagittal, axial, and coronal images to be obtained in a supine patient. The major disadvantages are that MRI-compatible mechanical ventilators and other life-support equipment must be used, and conscious patients with pain cannot be studied satisfactorily because of motion artifacts. Bony detail, such as the degree of vertebral body comminution, is marginally apparent on MRI.

ANATOMIC INFLUENCES

Anatomic features predispose the thoracolumbar junction to axial compression, flexion, and rotational injuries.[31, 32] First, the thoracolumbar junction (T11-L1) is situated between the rigid thoracic complex and the mobile lumbar spine. Thoracic fractures are stabilized by the rib cage and costotransverse and costovertebral ligamentous attachments by a factor of two to three.[33] Thus, rotational injuries are rare, and most osseous injuries are due to flexion and axial loading. Owing in large part to these mechanical differences between the lumbar and thoracic spine, stress concentration occurs at the thoracolumbar junction when the two regions undergo simultaneous deformation. Second, during axial loading, the thoracic spine deforms in kyphosis and the lumbar spine deforms in lordosis. Therefore, the thoracolumbar region may be exposed to pure compression. The resulting deformation may cause failure of the entire vertebral segment and compression of the spinal canal, especially when high rates of compression exist.[34] Finally, rotational forces are particularly effective in producing spine dislocations. The thoracic spine is protected from rotational strain by the ribs, and the lumbar spine is protected by inwardly directed articular processes. At the thoracolumbar junction, there is a predisposition for rotational injury because there is loss of rib support before there is effective reorientation of the facet joints from the thoracic frontal plane to the inwardly directed lumbar facets. This biomechanical rationale is validated by the fact that 60% of all fractures occur between T12 and L2, and about 90% are located between T11 and L4.[24, 35, 36]

The lower lumbar spine (L3-5) possesses several features that provide some protection against traumatic deformation. The vertebral bodies are larger, and there is more surrounding supportive musculature. The traumatic biomechanical forces that produce kyphotic deformity are less because the center of gravity lies close to the vertebral bodies in the erect position. For this reason, lower lumbar spine fractures are uncommon, constituting less than 4% of all spine fractures.[37, 38]

FRACTURE CLASSIFICATION

Although the factors discussed earlier predispose different levels of the spine to specific types of fractures, the processes by which the vertebral bodies, disks, and ligaments accommodate a sudden load are similar. This similarity results in fractures of an analogous nature occurring at various levels. Because of the high incidence of fractures at the thoracolumbar junction (T11-L1), most classification schemes have been defined at these levels.[36, 39] In 1963, Holdsworth postulated a two-column concept of the spine, with an anterior weight-bearing vertebral body and a posterior ligamentous complex.[40] Spinal instability was defined as rupture of the posterior ligamentous complex. This model, based on a large clinical experience and plain radiography, was an important first step toward an organized classification for fractures through which instability could be predicted. However, subsequent biomechanical data did not support this classification scheme.[41] Also, Holdsworth considered burst fractures to be stable despite clinical evidence that many were not.[36, 39]

In 1983, Denis[39] and McAfee and colleagues[36] independently postulated a three-column concept of spinal stability, to which most surgeons currently subscribe. This model is described in detail later. More recently, Magerl and colleagues proposed a classification scheme with three morphologic injury patterns (types A, B, and C) that result from three basic forces: compression, distraction, and rotation, respectively.[42, 43] These categories have been applied to all levels of the spine, with subcategories and subdivisions based on severity. The clinical usefulness of this model has yet to be assessed.

The three-column model of the spine is depicted in Figure 320-5. These regions include the anterior column (anterior half of the vertebral body, anterior half of the annulus fibrosus, and anterior longitudinal ligament), middle column (posterior half of the vertebral body, posterior half of the annulus fibrosus, and posterior longitudinal ligament), and the posterior column (supraspinous and infraspinous ligaments, ligamenta flava, articular processes, joint capsules, spinous processes, and laminae).

According to this model, instability occurs when there is injury to two or more columns. Because contiguous columns are commonly affected by the same injury, instability is heavily dependent on middle column failure.[44] For example, Denis identified four major spine injuries: compression fractures, burst fractures, seat belt–type injuries, and fracture-dislocations. Each of these can be distinguished by the middle column's

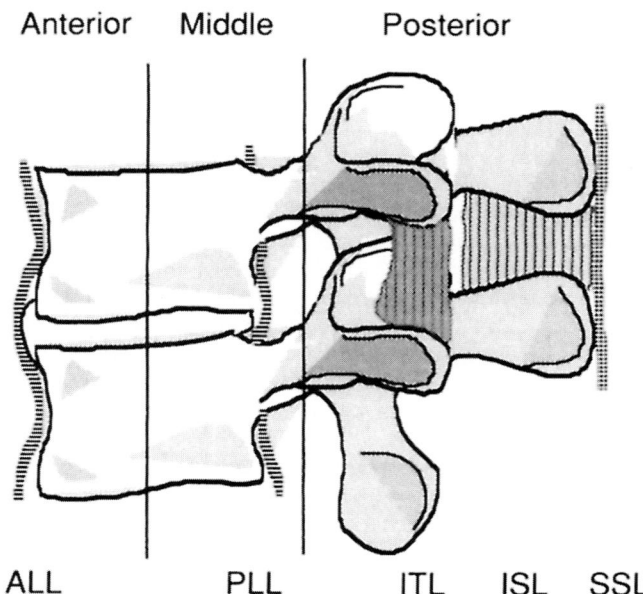

FIGURE 320–5. Denis's three-column model of the spine, consisting of anterior, middle, and posterior columns. The anterior column includes the anterior longitudinal ligament (ALL) and the anterior half of the annulus fibrosus. The middle column includes the posterior longitudinal ligament (PLL) and the posterior half of the annulus fibrosus. In addition to the bony anatomy depicted, the posterior column consists of the intertransverse ligaments (ITL), ligamenta flava, joint capsules, interspinous ligaments (ISL), and supraspinous ligaments (SSL).

mode of failure. According to Denis, instability can vary in magnitude and can be first degree (mechanical), second degree (neurological), or third degree (both mechanical and neurological). In contrast, McAfee defined six types of fractures (adding Chance fractures and subdividing burst fractures into stable and unstable types). In assessing stability, McAfee placed more emphasis on the integrity of the posterior column, so middle column failure was not synonymous with instability. Denis's and McAfee's classification schemes are summarized in Table 320-3. The end-stage deformity of the unstable spine common to all classification schemes is, as Whitesides and others have recognized, kyphosis.[45]

Major fractures involve the anterior and middle columns. Fractures of the transverse and spinous processes, isolated facet fractures, and traumatic spondylolisthesis are classified as minor fractures. They are rarely associated with neurological injury and are stable, except for bilateral pars interarticularis and bilateral pedicular fractures below L3, which may cause progressive deformity.

It is important to recognize that all classification schemes are intended to provide general guidelines in diagnosis. Other classification schemes include other features, such as neurological injury.[46] Magerl's classification emphasizes the mechanism of injury.[42, 43] In this scheme, the key forces that cause failure of the spine are matched with three categories of injury: compression (group A), distraction (group B), and axial torque (group C). The major effect in group A is damage to

TABLE 320–3 Comparison of Denis and McAfee Spinal Fracture Classification Schemes

FRACTURE TYPES		SPINAL COLUMN FAILURE			ASSESSMENT OF STABILITY	
Denis	McAfee	Anterior	Middle	Posterior	McAfee	Denis
Wedge compression	Wedge compression	F			Generally stable*	Stable†
Seat belt–type injury	Chance fracture		F	F	Generally stable	Unstable
	Flexion-distraction injury	F	F	F	Generally unstable	Unstable
Burst fracture	Stable burst fracture	F	F		Stable‡	Unstable§
	Unstable burst fracture	F	F	F	Unstable	Unstable
Fracture-dislocation	Translational injury	F	F	F	Unstable	Unstable

F, failure.
* Multilevel wedge compression fractures may require surgical therapy.
† Potential mechanical instability is seen with severe wedge fractures. This instability does not acutely threaten the neural elements.
‡ Potential mechanical instability.
§ Burst fractures are either neurologically unstable or both mechanically and neurologically unstable.

the vertebral body, which accounts for two thirds of all injuries to this area. Disruption in the transverse plane is the hallmark of group B injuries, and rotational injuries (group C) are most commonly superimposed on groups A and B. Subgroups define the degree of instability for each group. Stable compression fractures (group A1) are present in approximately 35% of injuries.

To guide proper management, thoracolumbar fractures are best viewed as belonging to a continuum of injury. For example, flexion forces, which commonly affect the thoracolumbar junction in deceleration-type injuries, produce increasing amounts of tissue disruption with increasing severity (see Fig. 320–1). The resulting fractures can be viewed as reflecting the spine's inherent capacity to absorb force as well as the eventual failure of the spine under these circumstances. A thoughtful assessment of the implications of the severity of these forces on both the bony and the ligamentous spinal components is invaluable in guiding successful management.

Wedge Compression Fractures

Wedge compression fractures are the most common vertebral injury, constituting 58% of major spinal fractures (Fig. 320–6).[39] Fracture and isolated failure of the anterior column under compression and flexion are present. Importantly, the middle column is not injured. As flexion forces become more severe, there may be a partial tension failure of the posterior column in distraction. Minimal and moderate wedge compression fractures with an intact posterior column affect only a single spinal column and are therefore considered stable. Severe compression fractures with disruption of the posterior ligamentous complex may exhibit mechanical instability as the spine buckles around the hinge of the middle column, resulting in kyphosis.

Burst Fractures

Burst fractures constitute 17% of major spinal fractures (Fig. 320–7).[39] Similar to wedge compression fractures, these fractures result from failure of the entire vertebral body (anterior and middle columns) because of the addition of axial compression loads to a flexion injury. This axial force is directed through the vertebral body, resulting in a loss of vertebral height. The resulting circumferential expansion of the vertebral body commonly causes bone fragments to retropulse into the spinal canal. Therefore, bony canal compression is found at the level of the pedicles, where the vertebral height is hardest to compress. In addition, fractures of the posterior elements are common.

Controversy surrounds the view that burst fractures are inherently unstable based on Denis's definition of two-column or greater injury. Many burst fractures are tolerated without neurological deficit and heal without progressive deformity. Fractures of the posterior elements, although common, are not universal, so McAfee and colleagues subdivided burst fractures into stable and unstable categories, based on the integrity of the posterior column.[36]

Seat Belt–Type Injuries

The spine is forced to rotate around a distant anterior point when the patient is retrained by a lap belt and a deceleration injury occurs. Seat belt–type injuries make up 6% of major spinal injuries (Fig. 320–8) and were first described by Chance in 1948.[3] The mechanism of injury is hyperflexion with distraction of the posterior spinal elements. The middle and posterior columns fail in distraction. These fractures are mechanically unstable in flexion (i.e., the spine may buckle around the hinge of the anterior column). However, this instability usually does not acutely threaten the neural elements. The classic Chance fracture is a horizontal fracture through the posterior arch and pedicles and extending into the posterior aspect of the vertebral body. The injury may involve more than one level, or it may be a purely ligamentous injury through the posterior longitudinal ligament and disk.

Fracture-Dislocations

Fracture-dislocations account for 20% of major spinal injuries (Fig. 320–9).[39] There is anterior and cranial

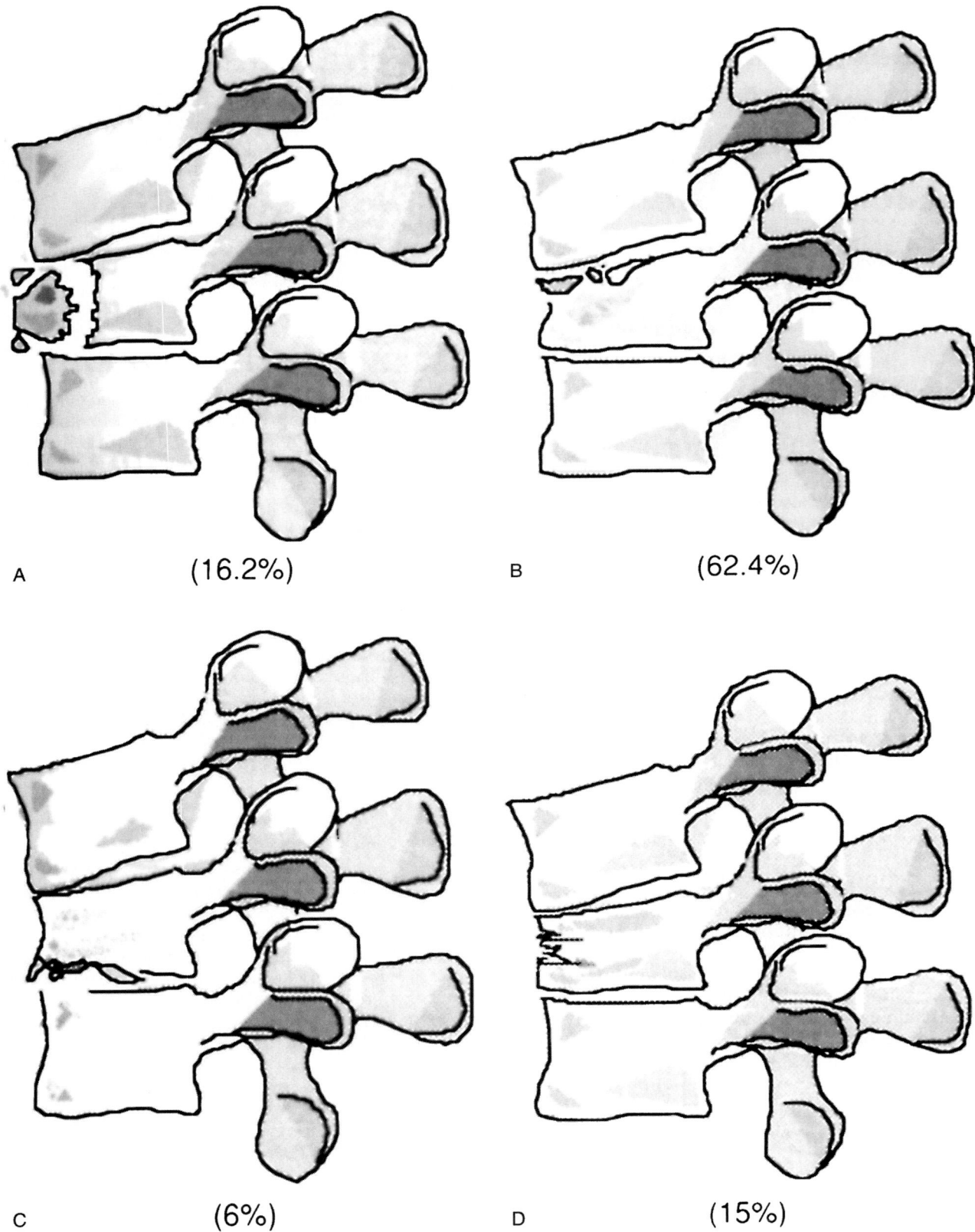

A   (16.2%)

B   (62.4%)

C   (6%)

D   (15%)

FIGURE 320–6. Four subtypes of wedge compression fractures and their relative frequency of occurrence, as defined by Denis. Type A: Fracture of both end plates and separation of the anterior body. Type B: Fracture of the superior end plate. Type C: Fracture of the inferior end plate. Type D: Fracture of the anterior vertebral body without involvement of the end plates. Note the absence of middle column involvement in all types.

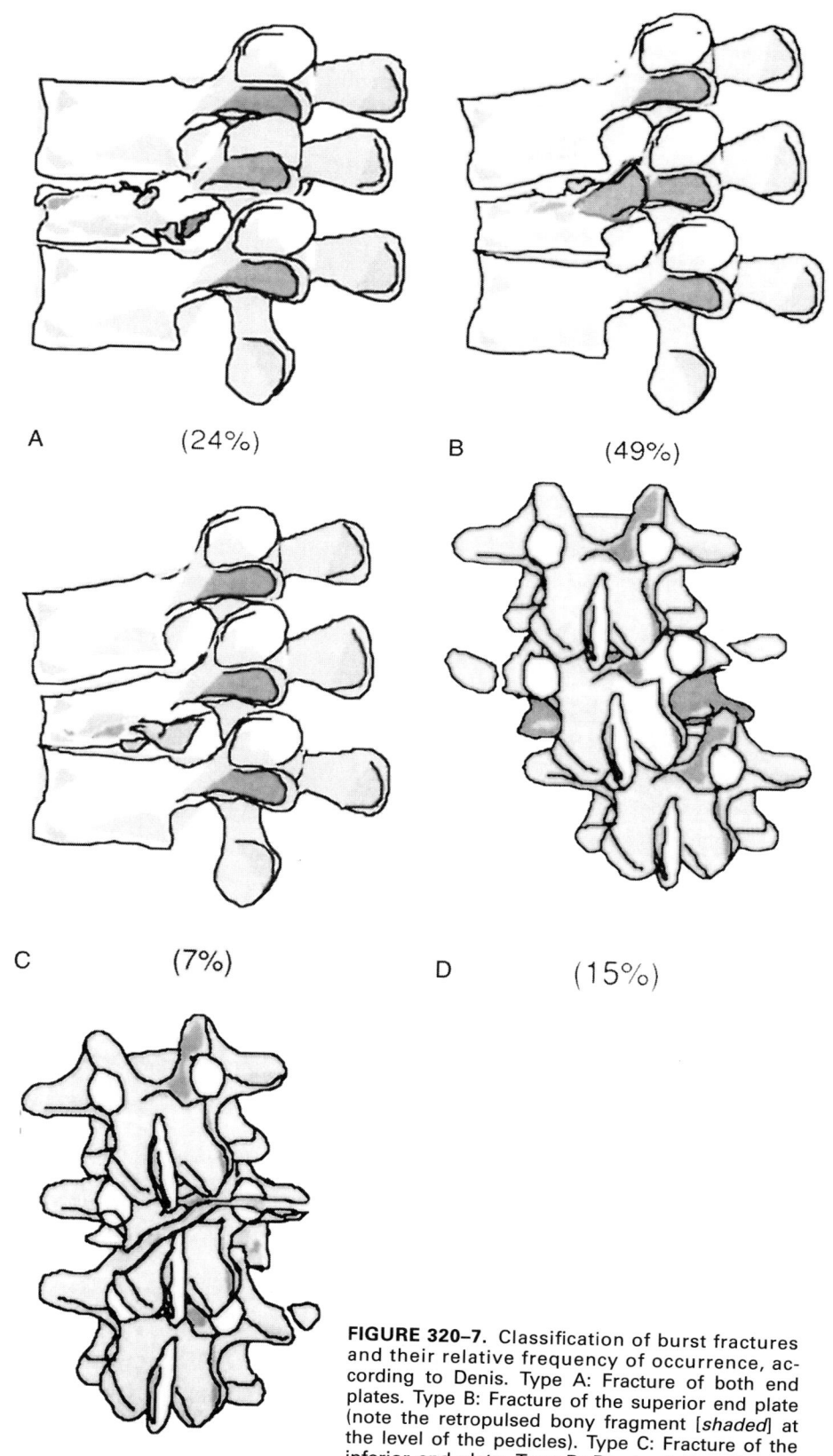

A   (24%)

B   (49%)

C   (7%)

D   (15%)

E   (5%)

FIGURE 320–7. Classification of burst fractures and their relative frequency of occurrence, according to Denis. Type A: Fracture of both end plates. Type B: Fracture of the superior end plate (note the retropulsed bony fragment [*shaded*] at the level of the pedicles). Type C: Fracture of the inferior end plate. Type D: Burst rotation. Type E: Burst lateral flexion. Note the increased interpedicuulate distance seen on the anteroposterior views (types D and E).

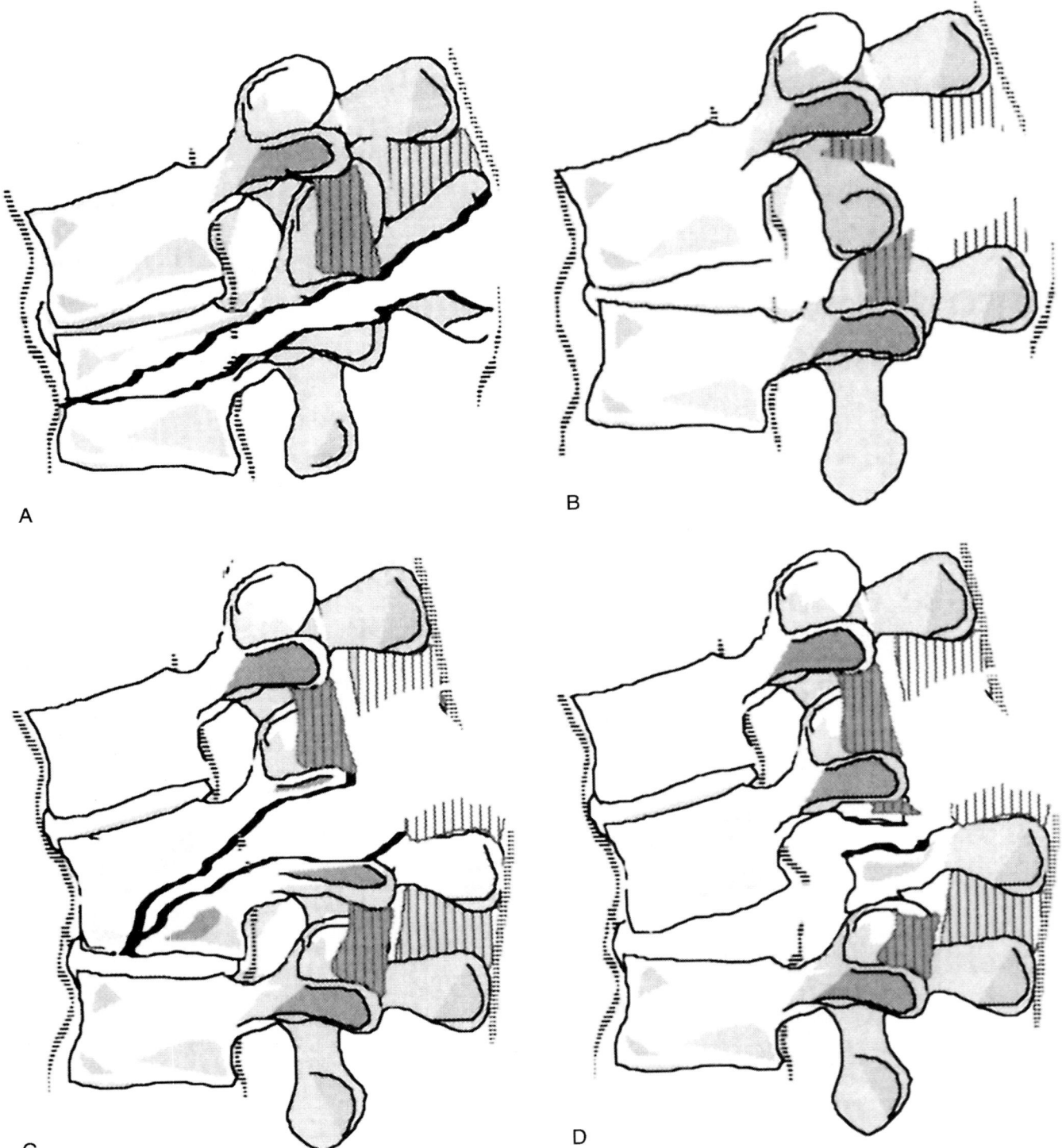

FIGURE 320–8. Classification of seat belt–type injuries, according to Denis. *A,* One-level seat belt–type injury through bone (Chance fracture). *B,* One-level seat belt–type injury through the ligaments. Note that only the anterior annulus and anterior longitudinal ligament are preserved. *C* and *D,* Two-level injuries. In *C,* the injury to the middle column is bony; in *D,* it is ligamentous.

displacement of the superior vertebral body with respect to the others, such that all three columns fail. Three subtypes have been defined, based on the mechanism of injury: flexion-rotation, flexion-distraction, and shear. Shear, or hyperextension, injuries are quite rare and have been described in lumberjacks struck across the midback by falling trees.[47] All ligamentous and supporting elements of the spine are disrupted in shear fractures, whereas flexion-rotation and flexion-distraction injuries usually involve preservation of the

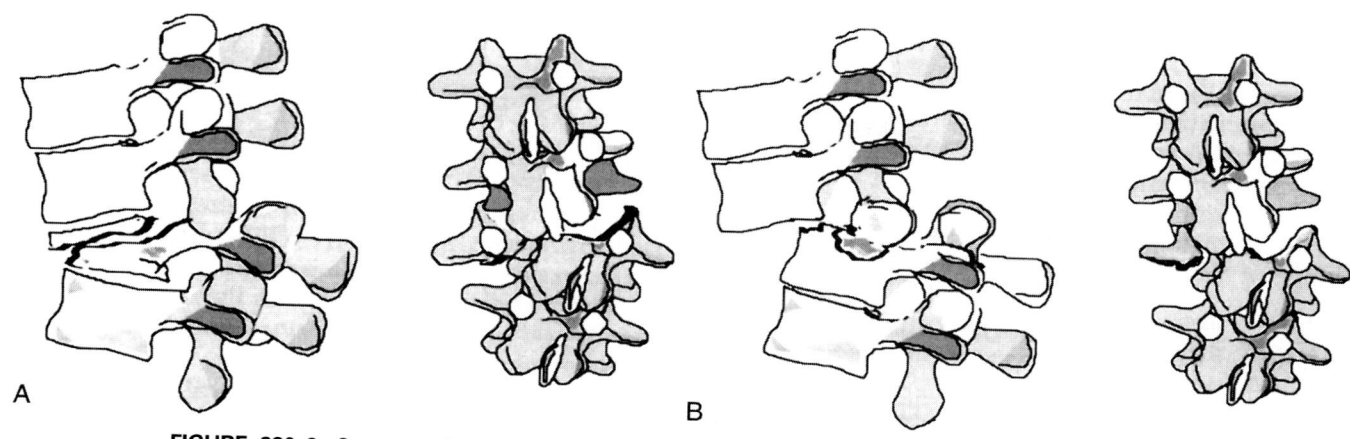

FIGURE 320–9. Common fracture-dislocation subtypes, according to Denis. Flexion-rotation–type injuries through the bone (slice fracture) *(A)* and through the disk *(B)*. Note the difference in rotation between involved spinal segments, which is best appreciated on anteroposterior views. In *B*, the only bony fracture is of the superior articular process. Not shown are fractures of the shear (posteroanterior) subtype, in which the superior segment is sheared off forward on top of the segment below; sometimes, a floating posterior arch remains. The frequency of dural tear and complete paraplegia is very high in this type of fracture.

anterior longitudinal ligament. If the dislocation has been reduced in the supine position, flexion-rotation and flexion-distraction injuries may be misidentified on radiographs as burst and seat belt–type injuries, respectively.

GENERAL MANAGEMENT PRINCIPLES

The goals of treatment are twofold: maximize neurological function and stabilize the fractured spine. Treatment aimed at maximizing neurological function allows early mobilization and rehabilitation while enhancing long-term quality of life. Stabilization is meant to minimize pain and subsequent deformity. Several means of achieving these goals exist, ranging from conservative therapy with bed rest and bracing to surgical intervention. Appropriate therapy must be individualized, based on the specific type of injury and its inherent stability, associated injuries, the likelihood of neurological improvement or loss, and the patient's wishes.

Initially, attention should be directed toward maintenance of spinal alignment and treatment of associated trauma, as previously discussed. The regimen for patients with unstable fractures should be full bed rest in full recumbency. Intermittent pneumatic compression stockings, in combination with low-dose subcutaneous heparin, are useful in preventing deep vein thrombosis. Patients with spinal cord injury require close surveillance to prevent medical complications (e.g., skin breakdown, pulmonary and urinary sepsis). Treatment includes frequent repositioning and vigorous pulmonary toilet. The bladder should be catheterized during the acute phase of the injury, followed by intermittent catheterization. Cystometrics and urodynamic studies are used to assess residual bladder function and are critical in evaluating many fractures.[21] A bowel regimen is instituted (e.g., stool softeners and enemas).

SURGICAL VERSUS NONOPERATIVE THERAPY FOR THORACOLUMBAR FRACTURES

Surgical therapy has been shown to decrease the length of the patient's hospital stay and the cost and to facilitate rehabilitation and earlier return to optimal function.[48–56] Traditional concerns about operative treatment, such as blood-borne infection and neural injury, have been minimized by autologous transfusion techniques and intraoperative somatosensory evoked potential monitoring, respectively.[57] In addition, modern spinal instrumentation systems have a low rate of hardware failure and a high associated arthrodesis rate.[56, 58, 59]

Not all fractures require operative treatment. Satisfactory results have been reported with nonoperative management in compression fractures and some burst fractures. The decision to operate should be based on (1) the stability of the fracture, (2) radiographic evidence of cord or cauda equina compression and its relationship to the patient's neurological examination, and (3) the patient's overall status. For example, some physicians believe that patients with multiple injuries and elderly patients require stabilization to benefit from early mobilization. Others report equally good results with or without surgery for burst fractures in neurologically intact patients. The following sections discuss fracture instability and neural compression, followed by a brief summary of the surgical indications for each major fracture type.

Fracture Instability and Indications for Fusion

The term *instability* is a vague one and is not synonymous with the need for surgery. Therefore, it is beneficial to consider instability as describing a spectrum of injuries and not to view it as an all-or-nothing phenomenon. Current classifications, such as Denis's and McAfee's, suggest that fracture stability can be determined by fracture pattern, and a consistent approach to fusion can be achieved by determining which columns are affected. The magnitude of fracture comminution may also be important in determining when anterior column damage is severe enough to require surgical stabilization. Many "unstable" fractures heal with external bracing (e.g., Chance fractures through vertebral elements) or prolonged bed rest. A well-fitted thoracolumbar orthosis can compensate for a 50% loss of stiffness at one level or 25% loss of stiffness at two levels, and it is especially suited for patients without ligamentous injuries.[60–62] Bed rest can be a successful treatment, with low complication rates, in carefully selected and closely monitored patients. Effective immobilization requires the use of kinetic beds, exercise, and deep vein thrombosis prophylaxis during recovery. Resorption of canal compromise occurs in 66% to 93% of patients in some series using bed rest as the sole treatment.[63] Late conversion to operative care is necessary in approximately 5% of these patients, mainly due to neurological deterioration.[64, 65] Nonoperative approaches to burst fractures are therefore best suited for neurologically intact patients without posterior column disruption. Prolonged recumbency and rigid bracing are effective in this group.[61, 62] Spinal fusion (arthrodesis) may be performed with or without implantable instrumentation, and references to "fusion" in the following discussion may also mean instrumentation and fusion. Instrumentation has been shown to reduce the incidence of pseudarthrosis, optimize spinal alignment, and provide immediate stability so that patients formerly treated with prolonged bed rest can be mobilized earlier.[66–70] For these reasons, the vast majority of surgeons prefer to use instrumentation for post-traumatic spinal instability.

Cord or Cauda Equina Compression and Indications for Surgical Decompression

The efficacy of decompressive surgery varies, depending on the level and degree of injury. Evidence exists from laboratory studies that ongoing compression of the injured spinal cord represents a potentially reversible form of secondary spinal cord injury.[71–76] Patients most likely to benefit from decompression have less complete cord injuries and tend to deteriorate with observation. In particular, patients with cauda equina or incomplete cord lesions have been shown to benefit even after long delays.[51, 77–82] Despite the generally improved outcome following decompressive surgery in these patients, the absolute significance of residual bone fragments in the canal and their relationship to the primary neural injury is controversial. Many studies fail to demonstrate a correlation between the degree of canal compromise at the thoracolumbar junction and neurological deficits, whereas others suggest that the higher the percentage of canal stenosis, the greater the probability of a neurological deficit.[36, 39, 83–90] In one study, stenosis rates of 35% or more at T11-12, 45% or more at L1, and 55% at L2 and below were significant factors for neurological deficit.[91] Thus, although decompression is advocated for patients with partial cord or cauda equina injuries, it is unclear what degree of canal compromise should be used to trigger such intervention in neurologically intact patients. Further, although some studies suggest that neurological recovery is related to the amount of canal decompression obtained with surgery, others fail to confirm this relationship.[48, 83, 86, 89, 90, 92, 93] Spontaneous remodeling of residual bony elements within the spinal canal after fracture healing has also been described.[63, 94] Therefore, the optimal surgical approach for decompression of incomplete cord or cauda equina injuries is controversial and is discussed in the section on surgical management of T1-10 and T11-L1 fractures.

The effect of the timing of decompressive surgery on neurological recovery also remains unclear. In the absence of a well-designed randomized, controlled clinical trial, acute decompression of the spinal canal should be considered a treatment option. Acutely injured patients can be treated by modern surgical methods without increasing the risk of patient mortality and morbidity.[55, 95] Improved neurological function has been reported with both early and late decompression.[51, 77, 80, 82] Most studies reporting the neurological recovery associated with late anterior decompression have not directly analyzed the significance of the timing of surgery. Some evidence exists to support early surgery (<8 hours after injury), particularly in patients with incomplete neurological injuries.[96]

There is some evidence that neurological recovery may be improved with early decompressive surgery.[77, 97, 98] Clohisy and associates compared the neurological outcomes in 11 patients treated with early decompression (48 hours after injury) and 9 patients treated with late surgery (average of 61 days after injury) for T12-L1 fractures.[91] Modified Frankel grades and American Spinal Injury Association Motor Index scores were significantly better for those treated with early surgery.

TREATMENT OF SPECIFIC FRACTURES

Wedge Compression Fractures

Most wedge compression fractures are treated with an external orthosis and heal uneventfully. However, fractures (1) with more than 50% loss of body height; (2) with more than 30 degrees of angulation; (3) that are multiple, with an aggregate deformity meeting criteria 1 and 2; or (4) in patients with prior laminectomies may cause progressive deformity, neurological deficits, or both (Fig. 320–10). In these situations, patients can be treated with fusion or an initial trial of bracing with follow-up radiographs. If the kyphotic deformity progresses or the patient's pain does not resolve, posterior fusion is recommended. Neurological deficits are less commonly associated with this type of fracture. When these deficits are present, the injury is often an incomplete cord lesion due to disk fragments and retropulsed bone, and surgical decompression is indicated.

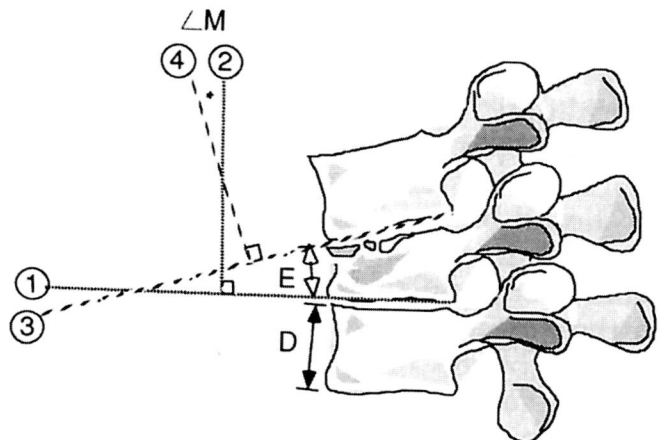

FIGURE 320–10. Method for measuring angulation and loss of vertebral height in thoracolumbar and lumbar fractures. The percentage of vertical height loss is expressed as (D − E/D) × 100. Angulation is measured by first drawing a line (1) parallel to the most caudal uninjured inferior vertebral end plate. A line perpendicular to line 1 is dropped (2). A line marking the most cranial uninjured inferior vertebral end plate (3) is similarly drawn, along with its respective perpendicular line (4). The angle (*) in degrees of kyphotic angulation (M) is given by lines 2 and 4.

Burst Fractures

When there is failure of the middle column—a feature that distinguishes wedge compression fractures from burst fractures—compression of the neural elements is often involved in the surgical decision-making process. Two factors have been studied: neurological deficit and degree of canal compromise. At T10, the majority of burst fractures are accompanied by complete neurological injury, and the major therapeutic consideration is stability. In the past, patients were treated conservatively, but many surgeons now advocate early posterior fusion, which has been shown to facilitate mobilization and the rehabilitation process. For neurologically intact patients with burst fractures between T11 and L4, good long-term outcomes have been reported with external bracing as the only form of treatment.[62] Short-segment surgical fixation may afford earlier pain relief and better kyphosis correction.[99] However, decompressive surgery for canal compromise has been recommended to avoid possible delayed neurological deterioration, although once again, there is little agreement over what degree of canal encroachment warrants surgery. For example, 50% canal compromise has been associated with neurological progression in one study but with good outcomes in another.[89, 100] Patients with lumbar burst fractures and incomplete neurological deficits can be expected to improve with time, with or without decompression, and surgical stabilization may not provide better resistance to progressive kyphosis compared with bracing alone.[101] Retropulsed bone fragments have been reported to resorb over time, suggesting that some patients with mild to moderate canal compromise may not require surgery acutely.[100]

At L5, nonoperative therapy has been advocated even for patients with root injuries and severe commi-

nution of bone.[102, 103] This conservative bias reflects the morbidity and pseudarthrosis rate seen with lumbosacral fusions performed in the past, as well as the difficulty of performing anterior decompression at this level. Improvements in lumbosacral fusion techniques may alter this philosophy.[104]

In summary, the management of burst fractures remains controversial, owing to the unpredictable relationship among post-traumatic canal compression, neurological deficit, and the likelihood of progressive deformity with surgery. At best, the decision to decompress and stabilize a burst fracture is based partly on the belief that neurological deficits are more likely to improve with acute reconstruction of the canal. Although unproven, decompression and reconstruction of the spinal canal appear to be indicated for patients with neurological deficits and moderate residual bone or disk fragments in the canal. Fusion is indicated for patients with mechanically unstable fractures. Acute instability, as defined by McAfee, is seen in burst fractures with (1) posterior element fractures, (2) kyphosis progressing 20 degrees or more, and (3) more than 50% loss of vertebral body height with facet joint subluxation.[54] For patients who are neurologically intact, success has been reported with the use of nonsurgical therapy and early or delayed surgery. Surgical therapy, if elected, may consist of fusion, or decompression and fusion, for appropriate patients. For patients with complete cord lesions, success has been reported with fusion or bracing. For patients with incomplete cord lesions and cauda equina lesions, early decompression and fusion are indicated.

Seat Belt–Type Fractures

Seat belt–type (flexion-distraction) injuries are unstable, but treatment depends on whether the injury is predominantly osseous or ligamentous. If the injury is osseous, management consists of bracing and careful radiographic follow-up. Flexion-distraction injuries resulting primarily in a ligamentous tearing injury heal less predictably and are best treated with posterior fusion and stabilization. Neurological deficits are rare, and decompressive surgery is usually not an issue.

Fracture-Dislocations

In general, all fracture-dislocations are unstable and require surgical therapy. Neurological deficits, 50% of which are complete, are seen in more than 75% of these injuries owing to collapse and distortion of the spinal canal.[39] Neural deficits are often associated with dural tears and exposed and avulsed nerve roots. Generally, posterior surgery with instrumentation is performed to realign the spine. Dural tears, which are more often on the dorsal dural surface, are exposed with laminectomy and repaired. A staged anterior decompression may be warranted if there are residual ventral fragments in the canal. Early anterior decompression of these injuries can be dangerous because of the likelihood of other associated visceral injuries.

SURGICAL APPROACH AND INSTRUMENTATION

When surgery is indicated, the operative approach and instrumentation used are determined by fracture location and fracture characteristics (neural compression, direction of canal compromise, instability). This section summarizes the surgical options for thoracolumbar fractures. L2-4 and L5 fractures are considered separately because of the different operative considerations.

T11-L1 Fractures

OPERATIVE APPROACH AND NEURAL DECOMPRESSION

Traumatic neural compression is almost always anterior. Hence, laminectomy has been abandoned except for the rare instance when there is infolding of a fractured lamina. Several techniques have been used to expose and decompress the anterior thoracolumbar and lumbar spine. These techniques fall into three general categories: anterior, posterolateral, and posterior approaches (Tables 320–4 and 320–5; Fig. 320–11).

With the transpedicular or posterior approach, a laminectomy or laminotomy is performed, and the medial portions of one or both facets and pedicles are removed with a high-speed drill. The surgeon then works lateral to the thecal sac to dissect fragments off the cord or to reimpact bone fragments anteriorly into the vertebral body. This approach is indicated when cord compression is accessible by this route and anterior strut grafting is not essential. Large midline retropulsed fragments are generally difficult to maneuver safely with this approach, analogous to the situation of large midline calcified disk herniations. Intraoperative ultrasonography is helpful in confirming neural decompression if visualization is poor.

The posterolateral approaches include the lateral extracavitary and costotransversectomy techniques.[105, 106] Both are performed with a posterior incision and require removal of various amounts of rib and transverse process to gain a lateral view of the vertebral body. The lateral extracavitary approach provides a better anterior exposure than the costotransversectomy does, allowing some visualization to the level of the opposite pedicle base, but its inherent morbidity is as high as 55%, owing to the extent of posterolateral exposure required.[107] With this approach, the surgeon dissects deep to the paravertebral muscles, which are elevated

TABLE 320–4 ■ **Comparison of Techniques for Neural Decompression at T10-L1**

APPROACH	TYPE	POSITION/ INCISION	INDICATIONS	CONTRAINDICATIONS	ADVANTAGES	DISADVANTAGES
Anterior	Transthoracic	Lateral decubitus/ thoracotomy	Incomplete cord or cauda equina injury with anterior compression	Posterior neural compression Polytrauma and medical complications are relative contraindications	Excellent anterior exposure Control of mediastinal vasculature	Extensive surgical procedure with morbidity of thoracotomy Staged posterior procedure may be necessary Requires diaphragm mobilization for access
Posterolateral	Costotrans- versectomy	Prone/paramedian	Incomplete cord or cauda equina injury with accessible anterolateral compression	Marked deformity and extensive vertebral body fractures with anterior neural compression are relative contraindications	Less surgery Posterior instrumentation performed simultaneously	Risk of incomplete decompression owing to limited exposure Anterior strut grafting is difficult
	Lateral extracavitary	Prone/"hockey stick"	Incomplete cord or cauda equina injury with anterior compression	Polytrauma and medical complications are relative contraindications	Anterior and posterior neural exposure Posterior instrumentation performed simultaneously Minimal risk of injury to visceral structures Minimal manipulation of diaphragm	Extension muscle dissection Difficult to visualize the ventral contralateral pedicle
Posterior	Laminectomy	Prone/midline	Posterior laminar fractures with incomplete cord or cauda equina injury, or with posterior epidural	Anterior neural compression	Less surgery Posterior dural tears easy to repair Posterior instrumentation performed simultaneously	Cord compression is almost always anterior May be destabilizing with anterior trauma
	Transpedicular	Prone/midline	Accessible anterior neural compression with incomplete cord or cauda equina injury	Marked deformity and extensive vertebral body fractures are relative contraindications	Less surgery Posterior instrumentation performed simultaneously Some access to lateral vertebral body	Risk of incomplete decompression due to limited exposure Risk of deformity without anterior strut grafting

TABLE 320–5 ■ Comparison of Anterior Techniques for Neural Decompression at L2–5

APPROACH	TYPE	POSITION/INCISION	INDICATIONS	CONTRAINDICATIONS	ADVANTAGES	DISADVANTAGES
Anterior	Retroperitoneal dissection	Lateral decubitus/ sympathectomy-type flank	Severe anterior neural compression and deformity at L2–5	Posterior neural compression	Excellent anterior exposure Avoids manipulation of diaphragm with thoracolumbar approach to L2 Avoids mobilization of iliac and hypogastric vessels Less risk of impotence	Risk of renal or ureteral injury L5 is difficult to visualize Variable exposure of L2
	Transabdominal retroperitoneal approach	Supine/paramedian abdominal	L4–5 fractures with severe anterior neural compression and deformity	Posterior neural compression		Less direct approach to vertebral body Exposure of L5 difficult without removal of moderate amounts of L4
	Transabdominal transperitoneal approach	Supine/paramedian abdominal	L4–5 fractures with severe anterior neural compression and deformity	Posterior neural compression	Optimal exposure of L4 and L5 vertebral bodies	Risk of impotence Requires mobilization of iliac and hypogastric vessels
Posterolateral	Lateral extracavitary approach	Prone/"hockey stick"	Lumbar fractures with severe anterior neural compression and deformity at L2–5		Minimal risk of injury to great vessels Anterior and posterior neural exposure Posterior instrumentation performed simultaneously	Extensive muscle dissection Visualization of the ventral contralateral pedicle difficult Visualization of L5 difficult Work must be carried out between lumbar nerve roots

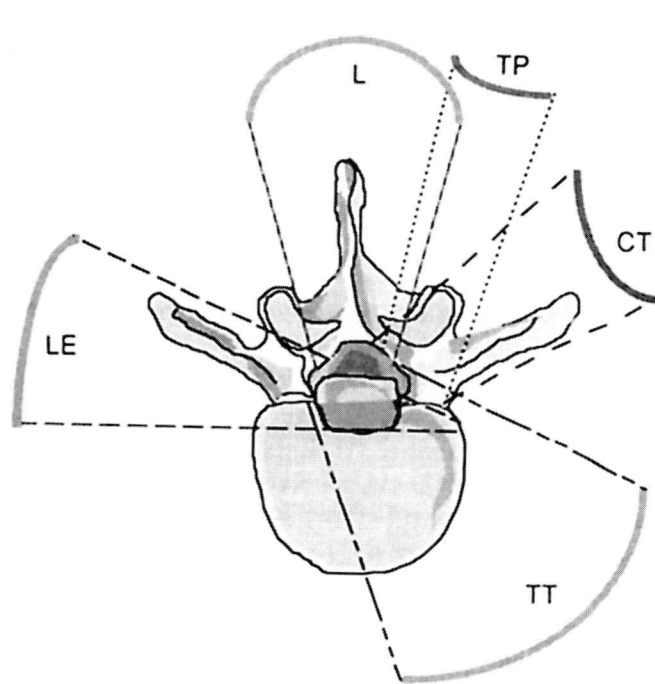

FIGURE 320–11. Schematic transverse section demonstrating the surgical approaches to the thoracic and lumbar spinal canal. Note that both the lateral extracavitary (LE) and transthoracic (TT) approaches can be extended into the vertebral bodies for the placement of anterior grafts. CT, costotransversectomy; L, laminectomy; TP, transpedicular.

and retracted medially. Neural decompression and vertebrectomy are performed, followed by strut grafting. The exposure with costotransversectomy is more limited, so decompression of large fragments compressing the cord and subsequent strut grafting may be difficult. Posterior instrumentation can be performed simultaneously through the same incision with both techniques.

Anterior approaches to T10 and T11 are performed through a standard thoracotomy incision with the patient placed in the lateral decubitus position.[4] The lung is retracted to expose the vertebral column. The parietal pleura, segmental vessels, and periosteum are mobilized off the fracture site. The disk spaces above and below are resected. The pedicle at the fracture site is identified, as it is an important landmark for locating the spinal canal. Cord decompression and vertebrectomy with bone strut grafting are performed. Exposure of T12 and L1 requires a thoracoabdominal approach that includes incising the diaphragm and mobilizing the viscera.

In addition to these three approaches, posterior instrumentation has been used to distract burst fractures in order to "indirectly" decompress the canal.[88, 90, 108–110] The use of this technique, called ligamentotaxis, was previously thought to be dependent on an intact posterior longitudinal ligament, which would reimpact bone fragments into the vertebral body following operative distraction. In fact, the fibers necessary for reduction of these bone fragments originate in the annulus of the superior vertebra in the midportion of the end plate of the spine.[111] There is clinical evidence that this annulotaxis is effective, although some believe that this technique results in incomplete decompression and risks neurological injury.

The advantages and disadvantages of the various approaches for neural decompression are reviewed in Tables 320–4 and 320–5 and Figure 320–11. In general, the approach selected should be the one that best addresses the pathology, with the expertise of the surgeon taken into account. The surgical management of burst fractures represents the most controversial area. For example, many believe that spinal realignment and the reduction of bone fragments with posterior distraction alone provide adequate neural decompression.[52, 86, 90, 112] Arguing that decompression with posterior instrumentation alone is incomplete, other surgeons have combined posterior distraction instrumentation with transpedicular decompression or posterolateral decompression.[54, 68, 113, 114] Advocates of the anterior approach believe that this technique provides reliable, if not superior, decompression.[51, 80, 109, 115] Anterior decompression, however, entails a greater magnitude of surgery and may be associated with ventral dural tears in up to 10% of cases; in addition, stabilization may require the placement of anterior implants or a staged posterior stabilization procedure.[115] Highly comminuted fractures of the vertebral body are best treated with either anterior surgery or combined anterior and posterior surgery; the loss of ventral column integrity in these injuries may lead to failure with posterior procedures alone.[59] The lateral extracavitary approach has the advantage of allowing direct anterior decompression and posterior instrumentation with a single incision, but it also carries a high morbidity.[107, 116] Figure 320–11 compares exposure for neural decompression using the lateral extracavitary approach with that using the direct anterior approach.

With regard to neurological recovery, no consistent differences have been established in the literature comparing posterior stabilization and indirect or direct decompression with anterior decompression.[117] The Scoliosis Research Society, which performed a large prospective study, found that anterior surgery was not more effective than posterior surgery in improving neurological outcome when neurological function was assessed with the Frankel or motor index scales, but there was a statistically significant difference when the Manabe scale was employed.[117, 118] In the subgroup of patients who deteriorated neurologically before surgery, greater neurological improvement was seen in the patients treated with anterior surgery compared with those treated nonoperatively and those in the overall surgically treated group. Anterior surgery was more beneficial in improving bladder function compared with posterior surgery.

POSTERIOR INSTRUMENTATION AND FUSION

In general, instability is treated with posterior instrumentation. In addition, spinal surgeons have a higher degree of comfort with posterior approaches to the spine. Posterior surgery for thoracolumbar injuries may be less time-consuming and less expensive and involve less blood loss than anterior surgery.[119] Rods are contoured to approximate the normal thoracic and lumbar curves. Compression and distraction are used to realign the spine by combating the forces leading to the deformity. For example, posterior implants should be configured to resist flexion and axial compression in unstable burst fractures. Therefore, distraction forces are used with caution in fracture-dislocations and are always avoided at the apex of the deformity. Pedicle screws, hooks, and, to a lesser degree, sublaminar wires are used for segmental vertebral attachment, with the choice depending on canal diameter, pedicle size, and the presence of posterior element fractures. Hooks are avoided immediately adjacent to the injury level. In the hierarchy of mechanical rigidity, pedicle screws are the most rigid, followed by hooks and sublaminar wires. In experienced hands, placement of lower thoracic pedicle screws (T9-12) carries little more risk than does placement of lumbar pedicle screws.[119] One should use the largest-diameter screw allowed by the pedicle and provide triangulation of the screws with appropriate cross-linking. In general, sublaminar wires and rods (Luque) should not be used in traumatic deformities because of the system's inability to resist axial compression and collapse of the fracture site due to sliding of the wires down the rod. Regardless of the type of instrumentation used, it will probably fail in the absence of a successful arthrodesis; therefore, strict surgical attention to soft tissue débridement, graft site decortication, and copious iliac or allograft bone grafting is imperative. A postoperative rigid orthosis is commonly used.

At the thoracolumbar junction, rods and pedicle screws are preferred. Pedicle screws are easier to insert in this location than in the remainder of the thoracic spine because of wider pedicle diameters. Screws fixate all three spinal columns as defined by Denis, and this biomechanical rigidity permits a short fusion length, which avoids greater immobilization of the lumbar spine.[120–124] Generally, at least two rostral and one caudal level should be engaged by pedicle fixation, with some authors noting adequate long-term stabilization with only a single motion segment instrumented on either side of the fracture or deformity.[125, 126] The fractured level need not be engaged, allowing for transpedicular decompression if indicated.[127] Biomechanically, a longer rostral segment combats the tendency to fail in kyphosis, and the combination of a hook and screw implant inferiorly likewise decreases the likelihood of screw pullout (Fig. 320–12). When local factors do not allow the placement of transpedicular instrumentation in the vertebra above the fracture, we generally substitute claw hooks for the upper transpedicular screws. The combination of an inferior laminar hook and a pedicle screw may help diminish the likelihood that the inferior construct will pull out in kyphotic failure.[128]

Regardless of the type of implant used, some loss of correction in the sagittal plane can be expected over time. Typically, this loss is slowly progressive and is less than 6 degrees of flexion at 1 year.[129] Highly comminuted vertebral body fractures that prevent load sharing of posteriorly placed fixation may require supplemental anterior instrumentation.[59] Hardware frac-

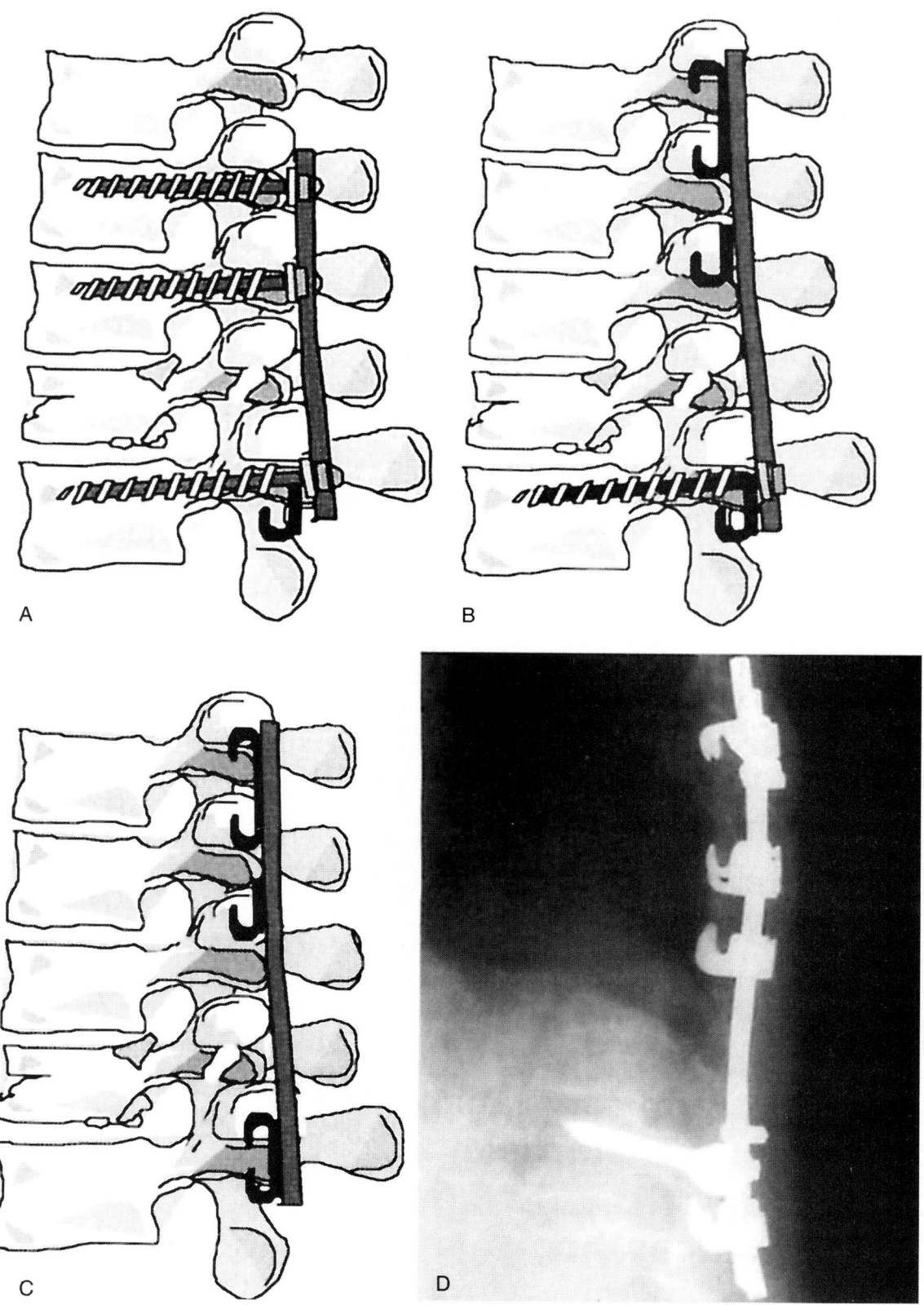

FIGURE 320–12. Posterior implant options illustrating a "two above–one below" pedicle screw construct *(A)* (note the inferior screw–laminar claw configuration), combination of hook-claw devices with a caudal pedicle screw *(B)*, and one without such a screw *(C)*. In general, the implants in *B* and *C* can also be limited to two segments above, although this limitation decreases their resistance to flexion deformity. A lateral radiograph *(D)* demonstrates the implant in *B*.

ture or removal worsens this phenomenon even if bony fusion has occurred.[130] Except in rare instances, this limited progressive kyphosis is to be expected and should be regarded as an asymptomatic radiographic finding.[131]

ANTERIOR INSTRUMENTATION AND FUSION

Instrumentation is usually recommended after anterior decompression for traumatic lesions. In the past, the anterior procedure was followed by a second-stage posterior fusion. This dual approach was used because of low fusion rates (e.g., 50% nonunion in one series) and the difficulty of maintaining correction after uninstrumented anterior surgery.[132] In some cases, this dual approach may no longer be necessary because of the development of anterior fixation devices.[80, 133–136] A combined anterior-posterior approach is still appropriate when posterior stabilization is planned in combination with anterior decompression or when sharing of the implant load is desired.[137] Anterior instrumentation has the advantages of avoiding a second-stage posterior fusion and fusing fewer segments.[67, 131] The initial devices were plates; subsequently, distraction devices were developed. These devices fall into the following categories: plates, rods secured outside the vertebral bodies, and interbody devices. A common form of anterior reconstruction involves the placement of an interbody spacer following vertebrectomy and supplemental anterolateral instrumentation (screws and plate or dual rod).[138] The clinical efficacy of these devices is comparable to that of posterior instrumentation systems.[10, 109] Because of the magnitude of surgery involved, anterior instrumentation should not be used unless anterior decompression is necessary or vertebral column failure is likely. In experienced hands, anatomic restoration of the injured vertebral segment is better with anterior reconstruction owing to the ability to directly distract the middle and anterior columns simultaneously.[124, 139] These devices are contraindicated in fracture-dislocations unless they are supplemented with posterior instrumentation. A thoracoabdominal approach is used, with incision of the diaphragm if necessary. A retropleural approach has been described by McCormick.[140]

Autologous bone graft is preferred at all sites of arthrodesis. In the anterior column, an iliac crest graft of sufficient length can usually be harvested from the patient to span two motion segments or one corrected height of a vertebral body. A cadaveric strut graft is a suitable replacement and may resist deformation better than iliac crest does because of its higher cortical bone content. A cadaveric fibular strut with cancellous bone harvested from the patient's rib or iliac crest can be used to combine axial strength with the osteoinductive potential of autograft. Similarly, excellent results have been achieved with a titanium mesh cylinder filled with a combination of autograft and allograft. Titanium cylinders are offered in several widths, and the largest implant possible should be used. Care must be taken so that the interbody device is well seated in the remaining end plates and is centered in the anterior column. Long-term studies describing ventral fusion rates are hampered by the difficulty of imaging a solid arthrodesis. Despite this shortcoming, structural allografts and titanium cylinders have high overall success rates.[141]

DEFORMITY CORRECTION

In addition to creating a safe environment for the neural elements and reducing fractured spinal elements, an attempt to surgically re-create the normal spinal mechanical axis should be made. Correcting any kyphotic or scoliotic deformity exposes adjacent segments to normal stresses in the healed spine and allows musculature to function at near optimal lengths with normal degrees of strain. Therefore, the implants must be of sufficient mechanical strength to maintain immediate reduction and tolerate postoperative bending forces. A well-designed implant also minimizes stress shielding of the fusion mass. To reduce and maintain correction of a kyphotic deformity, the construct length should extend two or more segments rostral to the injury.[117]

The degree to which a deformity is corrected depends on the force required, the ability of the bone to resist implant pullout, and the experience of the surgeon. Overdistraction of the injured neural elements is poorly tolerated during manipulation of the sagittal profile of the spine. Reduction of a deformity should never precede decompression of the spinal canal. Monoaxial screws are preferred to achieve greater transmission of corrective forces to the spine. A cantilever force may be applied following rigid fixation of the caudal screws. In this maneuver, the bent rod is closer to the idealized spinal configuration, and the rod is "persuaded" into the rostral screws. This achieves correction in the sagittal plane. It should be noted that the normal angulation across motion segments at the thoracolumbar junction nears 0 degrees.[142]

L2-4 Fractures

SURGICAL APPROACH AND NEURAL DECOMPRESSION

In general, low lumbar injuries are more stable than similar thoracolumbar fractures owing to the presence of iliolumbar ligaments and the stability afforded by the pelvic rim. The mobile nerves of the cauda equina lessen the likelihood of neurological injury. Therefore, the decision to treat is based on different criteria than for burst fractures of the thoracolumbar spine.

In the absence of neurological deficit, good results can be obtained with or without surgery for minimally comminuted fractures of the lower lumbar spine.[143] Fractures at L2-4 with neural compression can be approached posteriorly with laminectomy and transpedicular decompression. With severe neural compression, a retroperitoneal dissection through a flank incision is used.[144] Some surgeons advocate preoperative angiography to rule out the presence of a segmental artery contributing to the anterior spinal artery (e.g., artery of Adamkiewicz) in the planned operative exposure. An oblique straight or S-shaped incision from the tip of the 12th rib into the lower abdomen allows forward reflection of the peritoneum and abdominal contents. Mobilization of the psoas muscle and ligation of the lumbar segmental vessels allow access to the anterolateral aspect of the spine from L2 caudally. Vertebrectomy and strut grafting are performed, followed by instrumentation. Some surgeons have used the posterolateral extracavitary approach, as described previously, to expose the lateral vertebral bodies at L2-4. This approach is more challenging at L2-4 than at T11-12, because the nerve roots cannot be sacrificed to aid exposure. The surgical approaches to the lower lumbar vertebral bodies are reviewed in Figure 320–11 and Tables 320–4 and 320–5.

INSTRUMENTATION AND FUSION

Instrumentation should be aimed at minimizing the number of segments fused and maintaining physiologic lumbar lordosis. L3 fractures have the greatest tendency toward increasing kyphosis and loss of vertebral height in unoperated cases.[143] Long lumbar fusions and distractive forces should be avoided, because they may lead to a "flat back," sagittal imbalance, and often significant symptoms.[56, 145, 146] One method of decreasing fusion length with older Harrington-type systems was the "rod long, fuse short" technique, in which the rods were removed in a second operation, leaving a short-segment permanent arthrodesis. Facet degeneration occurred along the length of the instrumentation, however. With the popularization of pedicle screw fixation, these difficulties were avoided.[66, 109, 122, 123] Rods are contoured to a lordotic curve, and short-segment fusions (of two or three motion segments) are performed, usually two levels above and one below the injury. Distractive and compressive forces can then be applied to specific vertebral levels. In cases of severe misalignment, as in some seat belt–type injuries, controlled compression may correct the deformity. Alternatively, distraction can be applied in an attempt to reduce retropulsed bony fragments in burst fractures. The indications for anterior instrumentation are the same as those discussed for thoracolumbar fractures.

L5 Fractures

SURGICAL APPROACH AND NEURAL DECOMPRESSION

Conservative management is an option in neurologically intact patients, although some loss of vertebral height and lordosis may result.[146] Greater degrees of canal compromise are tolerated at this level. Most patients with low lumbar burst fractures can be treated nonoperatively with a custom-molded hyperextension thoracolumbar orthosis. A hip extension is required if the L5-S1 disk must be immobilized as well. Caution should be exercised in the case of a severely comminuted fractured vertebral body or if the fractured segments are widely separated, in which case surgical

reconstruction may be necessary. At L5, neural decompression can usually be managed posteriorly with laminectomy and unilateral or bilateral transpedicular decompression. Footed tamps can be used to reduce the fracture fragments. Rarely, anterior decompression is indicated with severe neural compression. This is best performed through a paramedian abdominal incision. Once the initial exposure is made through the anterior abdominal wall, the vertebrae can be reached through a transperitoneal or retroperitoneal route. The transperitoneal route provides a more extensive exposure, but because the spine is exposed directly from the front, the great vessels and hypogastric nerve plexus must be mobilized before the spine can be reached. This mobilization risks urogenital complications (e.g., impotence). With the retroperitoneal route, after incising the anterior abdominal wall, the surgeon dissects laterally in the retroperitoneal plane to reach the lumbar vertebrae. Some surgeons use a retroperitoneal approach to L5, as described for fractures at L2-4.

INSTRUMENTATION AND FUSION

For fractures at L5, sacral fixation is needed. Anterior instrumentation (e.g., plates) has been described, but it is extremely difficult to position at the lumbosacral joint. Therefore, posterior instrumentation with pedicle screws is preferred. Biomechanical studies suggest that sacral fixation is best obtained by directing the screws 45 degrees laterally into the ala or medially into the first pedicle. Poor fixation is provided by S2 pedicle screws.[147] Sacral sublaminar wiring can be used to reinforce the construct. Other techniques of lumbosacral instrumentation are still used successfully but are biomechanically inferior to pedicle screws. Postoperatively, patients are placed in a lumbosacral orthosis.

OUTCOMES AND COMPLICATIONS

Patients without neurological deficits can be expected to make excellent recoveries. The rate of return to previous work status, particularly for those whose duties do not involve great physical demands, may reach 90%.[63, 139, 148] Residual pain and preinjury levels of academic achievement seem to be the main determinants of level of post-traumatic employment in this group.[149] Those with neurological deficits have significant disability, although increasing numbers of paraplegics return to gainful employment. It is important to maintain rehabilitative support beyond the patient's acute recovery to guard against chronic infection, skin breakdown, and the disabling effects of spasticity. Long-term consequences such as kyphotic deformity or progressive syringomyelia are important considerations in the chronic care of these individuals. Any late deterioration in function should prompt imaging studies to assess the spinal canal for deformity, canal compromise, or cord pathology.

Both acute and long-term complications related to management may occur. Acute complications, particularly those stemming from immobilization, occur with

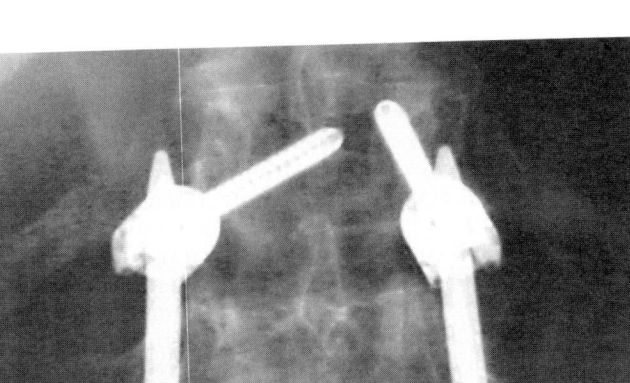

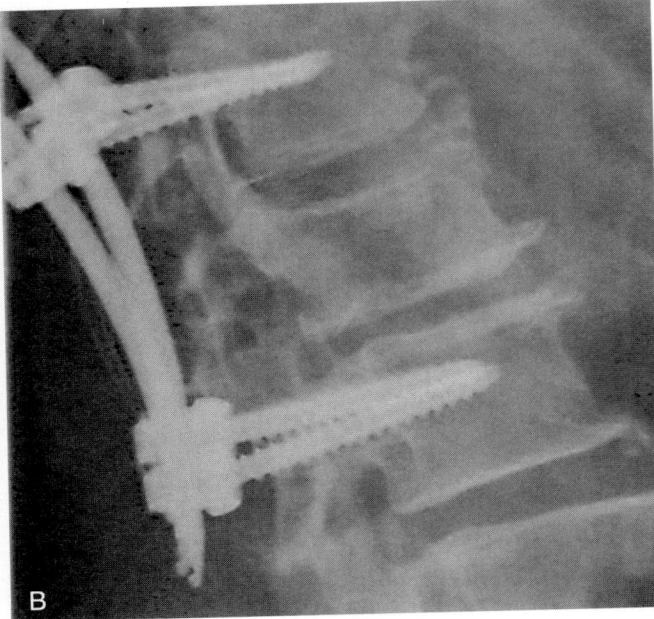

FIGURE 320–13. Anteroposterior and lateral radiographs of an L1 burst fracture treated percutaneously with posterior Sextant pedicle screws and rods.

near equal frequency in operated and nonoperated groups. Infections and implant complications are, of course, unique to operated patients and occur in 8% and 3%, respectively.[56] Mortality as a result of treatment is rare and usually occurs as a result of associated trauma or medical complications. Neurological deterioration can occur from neural traction, compression, or interruption of the vascular supply to the neural elements. The overall risk of neurological injury from posterior instrumentation is 1% to 3%; pedicle screws carry the highest risk of nerve injury.[150] Postoperative neurological deterioration may also occur from graft dislodgment, displaced hardware, or hemorrhage.

Intraoperative injury to the lung, major vessels, and viscera may occur during anterior vertebral exposure and reconstruction.[151] Dural tears may occur during decompression, and additional procedures may be required to stop postoperative cerebrospinal fluid leaks, such as the placement of a lumbar drain for 48 to 72 hours. Early implant failure is usually related to biomechanical factors, such as implant constructs without adequate bony attachment or insufficient implant length or rigidity to oppose postinjury forces.

Later hardware failure, including dislodgment or breakage, is usually related to pseudarthrosis and can be expected to occur in 20% of cases in the first 10 years postoperatively.[152] Pseudarthrosis may lead to progressive deformity, neural compromise, malunion, and pain. Hardware prominence with pain usually occurs in the rostral portion of the implant following progressive flexion deformity. Overall, a 9% surgical

revision rate over 5 years was noted in one large series.[153]

FUTURE MANAGEMENT

In the past several years, better implant design and concepts of rigid segmental fixation, applied in a balanced manner, have improved the care of patients with thoracolumbar injuries. Image guidance has been used to perform corpectomy with minimal tissue retraction and morbidity, although the technical difficulty of such procedures may limit their widespread use.[154, 155] Bone morphogenetic proteins, which have the potential to virtually eliminate pseudoarthroses, require further evaluation and refinement.[156] Some injuries may permit treatment with minimally invasive techniques, such as percutaneous screws and rods (Fig. 320–13).

REFERENCES

1. Graxier KL, Holbrook TL, Kelsey JL, et al: The Frequency of Occurrence, Impact, and Cost of Musculoskeletal Conditions in the United States. Chicago, American Academy of Orthopaedic Surgeons, 1984.
2. Bohlman HH: The neck. In D'Ambrosia RD (ed): Musculoskeletal Disorders: Regional Examination and Differential Diagnosis, 2nd ed. Philadelphia, JB Lippincott, 1985, pp 219–286.
3. Chance GO: Note on a type of flexion fracture of the spine. Br J Radiol 21:452, 1948.
4. Smith GR, Northrop CH, Loop JW: Jumper's fractures: Patterns of thoracolumbar spine injuries associated with vertical plunges. Radiology 122:657, 1977.

5. Meldon SW, Moettus LN: Thoracolumbar spine fractures: Clinical presentation and the effect of altered sensorium and major injury. J Neurotrauma 38:1110–1114, 1995.
6. Cooper C, Dunham CM, Rodriguez A: Falls and major injuries are risk factors for thoracolumbar fractures: Cognitive impairment and multiple injuries impede the detection of back pain and tenderness. J Trauma 38:692–696, 1995.
7. Holmes JF, Miller PQ, Panachek EA, et al: Epidemiology of thoracolumbar spine injury in blunt trauma. Acad Emerg Med 8:866–872, 2001.
8. Kauffler H, Hayes JT: Lumbar fracture-dislocations: A study of twenty-one cases. J Bone Joint Surg Am 48:788–795, 1966.
9. Albert TJ, Levine MJ, An HS, et al: Concomitant noncontiguous thoracolumbar and sacral fractures Spine 18:1285–1291, 1993.
10. Rubash HE, Steed DL, Mears DC: Fractures of the pelvic ring. Surg Rounds 5:16–30, 1982.
11. Bracken MB, Shepard MJ, Collins WF, et al: A randomized controlled trial of methylprednisolone or naloxone in the treatment of acute spinal-cord injury: Results of the Second National Acute Spinal Cord Injury Study. N Engl J Med 322:1405–1411, 1990.
12. Hurlbert RJ: The role of steroids in acute spinal cord injury: An evidence based analysis. Spine 26:S39–S46, 2001.
13. Bracken MB: Methylprednisolone and acute spinal cord injury: An update of the randomized evidence. Spine 26:S47–S54, 2001.
14. Fehlings MG, et al: Summary statement: The use of methylprednisolone in acute spinal cord injury. Spine 26:S55–S56, 2001.
15. Frankel H, Hancock D, Hyslop G, et al: The value of postural reduction in the initial management of closed injuries of the spine with paraplegia and tetraplegia. Paraplegia 7:179–192, 1969.
16. Lucas JT, Ducker TB: Motor classification of spinal cord injuries with mobility, morbidity, and recovery indices. Am Surg 45:151–158, 1979.
17. Mohanty SP, Venkatram N: Does neurologic recovery in thoracolumbar and lumbar burst fractures depend on the extent of canal compromise? Spinal Cord 40:295–299, 2002.
18. Vaccaro AR, Nachwalter RS, Klein GR, et al: The significance of thoracolumbar spinal canal size in spinal cord injury patients. Spine 26:371–376, 2001.
19. Holdsworth FW: Fractures, dislocations and fracture-dislocations of the spine. J Bone Joint Surg Am 52:1534–1551, 1970.
20. Holdsworth FW, Hardy A: Early treatment of paraplegia from fractures of the thoracolumbar spine. J Bone Joint Surg Br 35:540–550, 1953.
21. Watanabe T, Vaccaro AR, Kumon H, et al: High incidence of occult neurogenic bladder dysfunction in neurologically intact patients with thoracolumbar spinal injuries. J Urol 159:965–968, 1998.
22. Hardy AG: The treatment of paraplegia due to fracture-dislocations of the dorso-lumbar spine. Paraplegia 3:112–123, 1965.
23. Calenoff L, Chessare JW, Rogers LF, et al: Multiple level spinal injuries: Importance of early recognition. AJR Am J Roentgenol 130:665–699, 1978.
24. Post MJD: Radiographic Evaluation of the Spine: Current Advances with Emphasis on Computed Tomography. New York, Masson, 1980.
25. Brightman RP, Miller CA, Rea GI, et al: Magnetic resonance imaging of trauma to the thoracic and lumbar spine: The importance of the posterior longitudinal ligament. Spine 17:541–550, 1992.
26. Vaccaro AR, An HS, Lin S, et al: Noncontiguous injuries of the spine. J Spinal Disord 5:320–329, 1992.
27. Neumann P, Wang Y, Karrholm J, et al: Determination of interspinous distance in the lumbar spine: Evaluation of reference population to facilitate detection of severe trauma. Eur Spine J 8:272–278, 1999.
28. Kuklo TR, Polly DW, Owens BD, et al: Measurement of thoracic and lumbar fracture kyphosis: Evaluation of intraobserver, interobserver and technique variability. Spine 26:61–65, 2001.
29. Modic MT, Hardy RW, Weinstein MA, et al: Nuclear magnetic resonance of the spine: Clinical potential and limitation. Neurosurgery 15:583–592, 1984.
30. Lee HM, Kim HS, Kim DJ, et al: Reliability of magnetic resonance imaging in detecting posterior ligament complex injury in thoracolumbar spinal fractures. Spine 25:2079–2084, 2000.
31. Oxland TR, Lin RM, Panjabi MM: Three dimensional mechanical properties of the thoracolumbar junction. J Orthop Res 10:573–580, 1992.
32. White AA, Panjabi MM: Clinical Biomechanics of the Spine. Philadelphia, JB Lippincott, 1978.
33. Andriacchi T, Schultz A, Belytschko T, et al: A model for studies of mechanical interactions between the human spine and the rib cage. J Biomech 7:497–506, 1974.
34. Tran NT, Watson NA, Tencer AF, et al: Mechanism of the burst fracture in the thoracolumbar spine: The effect of loading rate. Spine 20:1984–1988, 1995.
35. Jefferson G: Discussion on spinal injuries. Proc R Soc Med 8:625–648, 1927.
36. McAfee PC, Yuan HA, Fredrickson BE, et al: The value of computed tomography in thoracolumbar fractures. J Bone Joint Surg Am 65:461–473, 1983.
37. Levine AM: The surgical treatment of low lumbar fractures. Semin Spine Surg 2:41–53, 1990.
38. Levine AM, Edwards CC: Low lumbar burst fractures: Reduction and stabilization using the modular spine fixation system. Orthopaedics 11:1427–1432, 1988.
39. Denis F: The three-column spine and its significance in the classification of acute thoracolumbar spinal injuries. Spine 8:817–831, 1983.
40. Holdsworth FW: Fractures, dislocations, and fracture-dislocations of the spine. J Bone Joint Surg Br 45:6–20, 1963.
41. Willen J, Lindahl S, Irstam L, et al: The thoracolumbar crush fracture: An experimental study on instant axial dynamic loading: The resulting fracture type and its stability. Spine 9:624–631, 1984.
42. Magerl F, Harms J, Gertzbein S: AO spinal fracture classification. Paper presented at the meeting of the American Spine International Fund, Oct 1989, Vale, CO.
43. Magerl F, Aebi M, Gertzbein SD, et al: A comprehensive classification of thoracic and lumbar injuries. Eur Spine J 3(4):184-201, 1994.
44. Panjabi MM, Oxland TR, Kifune M, et al: Validity of the three-column theory of thoracolumbar fractures: A biomechanic investigation. Spine 20:1122–1127, 1995.
45. Whitesides TE: Traumatic kyphosis of the thoracolumbar spine. Clin Orthop 128:78–92, 1977.
46. Rea GL, Zerick WR: The treatment of thoracolumbar fractures: One point of view. J Spinal Disord 8:368–382, 1995.
47. Denis F, Burkus K: Shear fracture-dislocations of the thoracic and lumbar spine associated with forceful hyperextension (lumberjack paraplegia). Spine 17:156–161, 1992.
48. Bradford DS, McBride GG: Surgical management of thoracolumbar spine fractures with incomplete neurologic deficits. Clin Orthop 218:201–216, 1987.
49. Davies WE, Morris JH, Hill V: An analysis of conservative (non-surgical) management of thoracolumbar fractures and fracture-dislocations with neural damage. J Bone Joint Surg Am 62:1324–1328, 1980.
50. Dickson JH, Harrington PR, Erwin WD: Results of reduction and stabilization of the severely fractured thoracic and lumbar spine. J Bone Joint Surg Am 60:799–805, 1978.
51. Dunn HK: Anterior spine stabilization and decompression for thoracolumbar injuries. Orthop Clin 17:113–118, 1986.
52. Jacobs R, Casey M: Surgical management of thoracolumbar spinal injuries. Clin Orthop 189:22–35, 1984.
53. Jelsma RK, Kirsch PT, Jelsma LF, et al: Surgical treatment of thoracolumbar fractures. Surg Neurol 18:156–166, 1982.
54. McAfee PC, Yuan HA, Lasda NA: The unstable burst fracture. Spine 7:365–373, 1982.
55. Tator CH, Duncan FG, Edmonds VE, et al: Comparison of surgical and conservative management in 208 patients with acute spinal cord injury. Can J Neurol Sci 14:60–69, 1987.
56. Rechtine GR, Cahill D, Chrin AM: Treatment of thoracolumbar trauma: Comparison of complications of operative versus nonperative treatment. J Spinal Disord 12:406–409, 1999.
57. Myer PR, Cotler HB, Gireesan GT: Operative neurological complications resulting from thoracic and lumbar spine internal fixation. Clin Orthop 237:125–131, 1986.
58. Chow GH, Nelson BJ, Gebhard JS, et al: Functional outcome of thoracolumbar burst fractures managed with hyperextension

casting or bracing and early mobilization. Spine 21:2170–2175, 1996.

59. Parker JW, Lane JR, Karaikovic EE, Gaines RW: Successful short segment instrumentation and fusion for thoracolumbar spine fractures: A consecutive 4½ year series. Spine 25:1157–1170, 2000.
60. Patwardhan AG, Siping L, Gavin T, et al: Orthotic stabilization of thoracolumbar injuries. Spine 15:654–661, 1990.
61. Oner FC, van Gills AP, Faber JA, et al: Some complications of common treatment schemes of thoracolumbar spine fractures can be predicted with magnetic resonance imaging: Prospective study of 53 patients with 71 fractures. Spine 27:629–636, 2002.
62. Cantor JB, Lebwohl NH, Garvey T, Eismont FJ: Nonoperative management of stable thoracolumbar burst fractures with early ambulation and bracing. Spine 18:971–976, 1993.
63. Mumford J, Weinstein JN, Spratt KF, Goel VK: Thoracolumbar burst fractures. Spine 18:955–970, 1993.
64. Weinstein JN, Collalto P, Lehman TR: Thoracolumbar "burst" fractures treated conservatively: A long-term follow-up. Spine 13:33–38, 1988.
65. Kinoshita H, Nagata Y, Ueda H, Kishi K: Conservative treatment of burst fractures of the thoracolumbar and lumbar spine. Paraplegia 31:58–67, 1993.
66. Dickman CA, Fessler RG, MacMillan M, et al: Transpedicular screw-rod fixation of the lumbar spine: Operative technique and outcome in 104 cases. J Neurosurg 77:860–870, 1992.
67. Esses SI, Botsford DJ, Wright R, et al: Operative treatment of spinal fractures with the AO internal fixator. Spine 16:S146–S150, 1991.
68. Hardaker WT, Cook WA, Friedman AH, et al: Bilateral transpedicular decompression and Harrington rod stabilization in the management of severe thoracolumbar burst fractures. Spine 17:152–161, 1992.
69. Lorenz M, Zindirck M, Schwaegler P, et al: A comparison of single-level fusions with and without hardware. Spine 16:S455–S458, 1991.
70. Rimoldi RL, Hu SS, Zigler JE, et al: The effect of surgical intervention on rehabilitation time in patients with thoracolumbar and lumbar spinal cord injuries. Paper presented at the 59th Meeting of the American Academy of Orthopaedic Surgeons, February 1992, Washington, DC.
71. Dolan EJ, Tator CH, Endrenyi L: The value of decompression for acute experimental spinal cord compression injury. J Neurosurg 53:749–755, 1980.
72. Rivlin AS, Tator CH: Effect of duration of acute spinal cord compression in a new acute cord injury model in the rat. Surg Neurol 10:39–43, 1978.
73. Dimar JR, Glassman SD, Raque GH: The influence of spinal canal narrowing and timing of decompression on neurologic recovery after spinal cord contusion in a rat model. Spine 24:1623–1633, 1999.
74. Zhang Y, Hillered L, Olsson Y: Time course of energy perturbation after compression trauma to the spinal cord: An experimental study in the rat using microdialysis. Surg Neurol 39:297–304, 1993.
75. Carlson GD, Minato Y, Okada A: Early time-dependent decompression for spinal cord injury: Vascular mechanisms of recovery. J Neurotrauma 14:951–962, 1997.
76. Delamarter RB, Sherman J, Carr JB: Pathophysiology of spinal cord injury: Recovery after immediate and delayed decompression. J Bone Joint Surg Am 77:1042–1049, 1995.
77. Benzel EC, Larson SJ: Functional recovery after decompressive operation for thoracic and lumbar spine fractures. Neurosurgery 19:772–778, 1986.
78. Bohlman HH, Freehafer A, Dejak J: The results of treatment of acute injuries to the upper thoracic spine with paralysis. J Bone Joint Surg Am 67:360–369, 1985.
79. Gertzbein SD, Court-Brown CM, Mark P, et al: The neurological outcome following surgery for spinal fractures. Spine 13:641–644, 1988.
80. Kaneda K, Abumi K, Fujiya M: Burst fractures with neurologic deficits of thoracolumbar-lumbar spine: Results of anterior decompression and stabilization with anterior instrumentation. Spine 9:788–795, 1984.
81. Maiman DJ, Sypert GW: Management of trauma of the thoracolumbar junction. Part II. Contemp Neurosurg 11: 1988.

82. McAfee PC, Bohlman HH, Yuan HA: Anterior decompression of traumatic thoracolumbar fractures with incomplete neurologic deficit using a retroperitoneal approach. J Bone Joint Surg Am 67:89–104, 1985.
83. Dall BE, Stauffer ES: Neurologic injury and recovery patterns in burst fractures at the T12 or L1 motor segment. Clin Orthop 233:171–176, 1988.
84. Fontinje WPJ, DeKlerk LWL, Braakman R, et al: CT scan prediction of neurological deficit in thoracolumbar burst fractures. J Bone Joint Surg Br 74:683–685, 1992.
85. Hashimoto T, Kaneda K, Abumi K: Relationship between traumatic spinal canal stenosis and neurologic deficits in thoracolumbar burst fractures. Spine 13:1268–1272, 1988.
86. Herndon W, Galloway D: Neurologic return versus cross-sectional canal area in incomplete thoracolumbar spinal cord injuries. J Trauma 28:680–683, 1988.
87. Keen JS, Fischer SP, Vanderby R, et al: Significance of acute post traumatic bony encroachment of the neural canal. Spine 14:799–802, 1989.
88. Starr JK, Hanley EN: Junctional burst fractures. Spine 17:551–557, 1992.
89. Trafton PG, Boyd C: Computed tomography of thoracic and lumbar spine injuries. J Trauma 24:506–515, 1984.
90. VanBuren RL, Wagner FC, Montesano PX: Management of thoracolumbar fractures with accompanying neurological injury. Neurosurgery 30:667–671, 1992.
91. Clohisy JC, Behrooz AA, Bucholz RD, et al: Neurologic recovery associated with anterior decompression of spine fractures at the thoracolumbar junction (T12–L1). Spine 17:S225–S330, 1992.
92. Schmidek H, Gomes F, Seligson D, et al: Management of acute unstable thoracolumbar fractures with and without neurological deficit. Neurosurgery 7:30–35, 1980.
93. Limb D, Shaw DI, Dickson RA: Neurologic injury in thoracolumbar burst fractures. J Bone Joint Surg Br 77:774–777, 1995.
94. De Klerk LW, Fontijne WP, Stijnen T, et al: Spontaneous remodeling of the spinal canal after conservative management of thoracolumbar burst fractures. Spine 23:1057–1060, 1998.
95. Wilberger JE: Diagnosis and management of spinal cord trauma. J Neurotrauma 8(Suppl 1):21–28, 1991.
96. Petitjean ME, Pointillart V, Daverat P: Administration of methylprednisolone or nimodipine or both versus placebo at the acute phase of spinal cord injury. J Neurotrauma 12:456, 1995.
97. Duh MS, Shepard MJ, Wilberger JE: The effectiveness of surgery on the treatment of acute spinal cord injury and its relation to pharmacological treatment. Neurosurgery 35:240–248, 1994.
98. Wiberg J, Hauge HN: Neurological outcome after surgery for thoracic and lumbar spine injuries. Acta Neurochir (Wien) 91:106–112, 1988.
99. Shen WJ, Liu TJ, Shen YS: Nonoperative treatment versus posterior fixation for thoracolumbar junction burst fractures without neurologic deficit. Spine 26:1038–1045, 2001.
100. Weinstein JN, Collalto P, Lehmann TR: Long-term follow-up of nonoperatively treated thoracolumbar spine fractures. J Orthop Trauma 1:152–159, 1987.
101. Knight RQ, Stornelli DP, Chan DPK, et al: Comparison of operative versus nonoperative treatment of lumbar burst fractures. Clin Orthop 293:112–121, 1993.
102. Court-Brown CW, Gertzbein SD: The management of burst fractures of the fifth lumbar vertebra. Spine 12:308–312, 1987.
103. Finn CA, Stauffer ES: Burst fracture of the fifth lumbar vertebra. J Bone Joint Surg Am 74:398–403, 1992.
104. An H, Vaccaro A, Colter J, et al: Low lumbar burst fractures: Comparison among body cast, Harrington rod, Luque rod, and Steffe plates. Spine 16:S440–S444, 1991.
105. Capener N: The evolution of lateral rhachotomy. J Bone Joint Surg Br 36:173–179, 1954.
106. Larson SJ, Holst RA, Hemmy DG, et al: Lateral extracavitary approach to traumatic lesions of the thoracic and lumbar spine. J Neurosurg 45:628–637, 1976.
107. Resnick DK, Benzel EC: Lateral extracavitary approach for thoracic and thoracolumbar spine trauma: Operative complications. Neurosurgery 43:796–802, 1998.
108. Crutcher JP, Anderson PA, King HA, et al: Indirect spinal canal decompression in patients with thoracolumbar burst fractures treated by posterior distraction rods. J Spinal Disord 4:39–48, 1991.

109. Esses SI, Botsford DJ, Kostuik JP: Evaluation of surgical treatment for burst fractures. Spine 15:667–672, 1990.
110. Gertzbein SD, Crowe PH, Fazl M, et al: Canal clearance in burst fractures using the AO Internal Fixator. Spine 17:558–560, 1991.
111. Fredrickson B, Mann K, Yuan H, et al: Reduction of the intracanal fragment in experimental burst fractures. Spine 13:267–271, 1988.
112. Fredrickson BE, Edwards WT, Rauschning W, et al: Vertebral burst fractures: An experimental, morphologic, and radiographic study. Spine 17:1012–1021, 1992.
113. Erickson DL, Leider LL, Brown WE: One-stage decompression-stabilization for thoracolumbar fractures. Spine 2:53–56, 1977.
114. Flesch JR, Leider LL, Erickson DL, et al: Harrington instrumentation and spine fusion for unstable fractures and fracture-dislocations of the thoracic and lumbar spine. J Bone Joint Surg Am 59:143–153, 1977.
115. Carl AL, Matsumoto M, Whalen JT: Anterior dural laceration caused by thoracolumbar and lumbar burst fractures. J Spinal Disorder 13:399–403, 2000.
116. Maiman DJ, Larson SJ, Benzel EC: Neurological improvement associated with late decompression of the thoracolumbar spinal cord. Neurosurgery 14:302–307, 1984.
117. Gertzbein SD: Scoliosis Research Society: Multicenter spine fracture study. Spine 17:528–540, 1991.
118. Manabe S, Tateischi A, Abe M, et al: Surgical treatment of metastatic tumors of the spine. Spine 14:41–47, 1989.
119. Danisa OA, Shaffrey CI, Jane JA, et al: Surgical approaches for the correction of unstable thoracolumbar burst fractures: A retrospective analysis of treatment outcomes. J Neurosurg 83:977–983, 1995.
120. Dick W: The "fixator interne" as a versatile implant for spine surgery. Spine 12:882–900, 1987.
121. McNamara MJ, Stephens GC, Spengler DM: Transpedicular short-segment fusions for the treatment of lumbar burst fractures. Spinal Disord 5:183–187, 1992.
122. Roy-Camille R, Saillant G, Mazel CH: Plating of thoracic, thoracolumbar, and lumbar injuries with pedicle screw plates. Orthop Clin 17:147–159, 1986.
123. Steffee AD, Biscup RS, Sitkowski DJ: Segmental spine plates with pedicle screw fixation: A new internal fixation device for disorders of the lumbar and thoracolumbar spine. Clin Orthop 203:45–53, 1986.
124. Schnee CL, Ansell LV: Selection criteria and outcome of operative approaches for thoracolumbar burst fractures with and without neurologic deficit. J Neurosurg 86:48–55, 1997.
125. Harms J, Stoltze D: The indications and principles of correction of post-traumatic deformities. Eur Spine J 1:142–151, 1992.
126. Silvestro C, Francaviglia N, Bragazzi R, et al: Near-anatomical reduction and stabilization of burst fractures of the lower thoracic or lumbar spine. Acta Neurochir (Wien) 116:53–59, 1992.
127. Viale GL, Silvestro C, Francaviglia N, et al: Transpedicular decompression and stabilization of burst fractures of the lumbar spine. Surg Neurol 40:104–111, 1993.
128. Yerby SA, Ehteshami JR, McLain RF: Offset laminar hooks decrease bending moments of pedicle screws during in situ contouring. Spine 22:376–381, 1997.
129. Benson DR, Burkus JK, Montesano PX, et al: Unstable thoracolumbar and lumbar burst fractures treated with the AO fixateur interne. J Spinal Disord 5:335–343, 1992.
130. Eysel P, Meinig G: Comparative study of different dorsal stabilization techniques in recent thoraco-lumbar spine fractures. Acta Neurochir (Wien) 109:12–19, 1991.
131. Leferink VJ, Nijboer JM, Zimmerman KW, et al: Thoracolumbar spinal fractures: Segmental range of motion after dorsal spondylodesis in 82 patients: A prospective study. Eur Spine J 11:2–7, 2002.
132. Malcolm BW, Bradford DS, Winter RB, et al: Post-traumatic kyphosis. J Bone Joint Surg Am, 63:891, 1981.
133. Haas N, Blauth M, Tscherne H: Anterior plating in thoracolumbar spine injuries: Indication, technique, and results. Spine 16:S100–S111, 1991.
134. Kostuik JP: Anterior spinal cord decompression for lesions of the thoracic and lumbar spine: Techniques, new methods of internal fixation, results. Spine 8:512–531, 1983.
135. Kostuik JP: Anterior fixation for burst fractures of the thoracic and lumbar spine with or without neurological involvement. Spine 13:286–293, 1988.
136. Schegel J, Yuan HA, Fredricksen B: Anterior interbody fixation devices. In Frymoyer JW (ed): The Adult Spine. New York, Raven Press, 1991, pp 1947–1959.
137. Dimar JR, Wilde PH, Glassman SD, et al: Thoracolumbar burst fractures treated with combined anterior and posterior surgery. Am J Orthop 25:159–165, 1996.
138. Van Loon JL, Slot GH, Pavlov PW: Anterior instrumentation of the spine in thoracic and thoracolumbar fractures: The single rod versus the double rod Slot-Zielke device. Spine 21:734–740, 1996.
139. Okuyama K, Abe E, Chiba M, et al: Outcome of anterior decompression and stabilization for thoracolumbar unstable burst fractures in the absence of neurologic deficit. Spine 21:620–625, 1996.
140. McCormick PC: Retropleural approach to the thoracic and thoracolumbar spine. Neurosurgery 37:908–914, 1995.
141. Finkelstein JA, Chapman JR, Mirza S: Anterior cortical allograft in thoracolumbar fractures. J Spinal Disord 12:424–429, 1999.
142. Oda T, Panjabi MM, Kato Y: The effects of pedicle screw adjustments on the anatomical reduction of thoracolumbar burst fractures. Eur Spine J 10:505–511, 2001.
143. Seybold EA, Sweeney CA, Fredrickson BE, et al: Functional outcome of low lumbar burst fractures: A multicenter review of operative and nonoperative treatment of L3-L5. Spine 24:2154–2161, 1999.
144. Westfall SH, Akbarnia BA, Merenda JJ, et al: Exposure of the anterior spine: Technique, complications, and results in 85 patients. Am J Surg 154:700–704, 1987.
145. LaGrone MO, Bradford DS, Moe JH, et al: Treatment of symptomatic flatback after spinal fusion. J Bone Joint Surg Am 70:569–580, 1988.
146. An HS, Simpson JM, Ebraheim NA, et al: Low lumbar burst fractures: Comparison between conservative and surgical treatments. Orthopedics 15:367–373, 1992.
147. Zindrick MR, Wiltse LL, Widell EH, et al: A biomechanical study of intrapeduncular screw fixation in the lumbosacral spine. Clin Orthop 203:99–111, 1986.
148. Kraemer WJ, Schemtisch EH, Lever J, et al: Functional outcome of thoracolumbar burst fractures without neurological deficit. J Orthop Trauma 10:541–544, 1996.
149. Tasdemiroglu E, Tibbs PA: Long-term follow-up results of thoracolumbar fractures after posterior instrumentation. Spine 20:1704–1708, 1995.
150. Scoliosis Research Society: Morbidity and Mortality Committee Report. Park Ridge, IL, Scoliosis Research Society, 1987.
151. Oskousian RJ Jr, Johnson JP: Vascular complications in anterior thoracolumbar spinal reconstruction. J Neurosurg 96(1 Suppl):1–5, 2002.
152. McAfee PC, Weiland DJ, Carlow JJ: Survivorship analysis of pedicle spinal instrumentation. Spine 16:S422–S427, 1991.
153. Knop C, Bastian L, Lange U, et al: Complications in the surgical treatment of thoracolumbar injuries. Eur Spine J 11:214–226, 2002.
154. Ohmori K, Kawaguchi Y, Kanamori M, et al: Image-guided anterior thoracolumbar corpectomy: A report of three cases. Spine 26:1197–1201, 2001.
155. Muhlbauer M, Pfisterer W, Eyb R, Knop E: Minimally invasive retroperitoneal approach for lumbar corpectomy and anterior reconstruction: Technical note. J Neurosurg 93(1 Suppl):161–167, 2000.
156. Laursen M, Hoy K, Hansen ES, et al: Recombinant bone morphogenic protein-7 as an intracorporeal bone growth stimulator in unstable thoracolumbar burst fractures in humans: Preliminary results. Eur Spine J 8:485–490, 1999.

CHAPTER 321

Sacral Fractures

NOEL I. PERIN

Sacral fractures occur in conjunction with pelvic fractures in patients with multiple injuries. Despite being relatively common, sacral fractures are frequently undiagnosed and treated inadequately. The number of sacral and pelvic fractures receiving treatment has increased, owing to improvements in the early evaluation and care of polytraumatized patients. However, as many as 49% of sacral fractures are not diagnosed during these patients' initial hospitalization. The most commonly missed sacral injury is a transverse fracture at S2.[1] Neurological deficits resulting from sacral injuries can also be overlooked in patients with multiple traumatic injuries. Because sacral fractures can be missed on routine radiographs of the spine and pelvis, the examiner's index of suspicion for such fractures is paramount in making a prompt and accurate diagnosis.

As reported by Malgaigne,[2] Richerand first recognized the injury in 1847 in a 53-year-old man who had fallen from a second-story window. In 1945, Bonnin[3] proposed the first classification system for fractures of the sacrum. In 1955, Macciocchi[4] reported a series of 52 cases. Numerous single case reports and small series have been published, and several reviews, including classification schemes, have appeared in the literature.[1, 5, 6]

This chapter reviews the relevant anatomy, pathophysiology, and classification of sacral fractures and provides an overview of the clinical presentation, diagnosis, and recommended treatment.

ANATOMY OF THE SACRUM

The sacrum is the most caudal fixed segment of the axial skeleton. The sacrum, or *sacred bone*, derives its name from the Greek *hieron osteon*. Use of the bone in sacrificial rites and its role in protecting the genitalia led to the word *hieron* being interpreted as "sacred" or "holy"; thus, the term *os sacrum* was coined by the Romans. The sacrum is a virtually motionless spinal segment that develops from five fused vertebrae. Each vertebra develops from three primary ossification centers giving rise to the anterior and posterior elements. The fibrocartilaginous disk between the last two sacral

vertebrae fuses at about 15 years of age; fusion continues in a cephalad direction until segmental fusion is complete around age 25. The sacrum sits like a keystone in the posterior arch of the pelvis and distributes load from the axial skeleton to the pelvis through the relatively immobile sacroiliac joints. Stability is enhanced by strong anterior and posterior ligamentous attachments between the sacrum and the pelvis.

The sacrum lies at a 40-degree angle from the horizontal at the lumbosacral junction. Thus, axial loads promote rotational stresses that are counteracted by the sacrotuberous and sacrospinous ligaments, which attach opposite the S4 foramina. The first sacral foramen has the largest diameter—the diameter of the foramina in the sacrum decreases from proximal to distal from S1 to S4. The diameter of the nerve root also decreases from one third of the foraminal diameter proximally to one sixth of the foraminal diameter distally; therefore, foraminal entrapment is less likely at the lower sacral levels.

PATHOPHYSIOLOGY AND CLASSIFICATION OF SACRAL FRACTURES

In discussions of stability, the sacrum and pelvis are considered one unit. The pelvic ring is a relatively rigid structure whose disruption requires discontinuity in at least two places. Discontinuity can occur as either a fracture or a ligamentous disruption. Gunterberg and coworkers[7] performed biomechanical studies of cadaveric specimens loaded to failure to evaluate pelvic stability after major amputation of the sacrum. Specimens resected below S2, sparing the sacroiliac joints, were stable. Specimens resected between S1 and S2 had one third of the sacroiliac joint resected, and stability was reduced 30%. Specimens resected 1 cm below the sacral promontory had half of the sacroiliac joint removed, and the load-to-failure strength was reduced 50%. Overall, the load to failure far exceeded the anticipated physiologic loads.

Bonnin's original classification divided sacral fractures into six categories[3]: (1) juxtailiac-marginal fractures; (2) fractures involving the S1 or S2 foramen with upward displacement of the lateral mass; (3) fractures through the sacral foramina, which separate the lateral mass from the body of the sacrum; (4) comminuted fractures of the upper sacrum; (5) avulsion fractures of the attachment of the sacrotuberous ligament; and (6) transverse fractures of the sacrum. Bonnin's classification delineates common fracture types but does not correlate the fracture with the mechanism of injury or aid in clinical evaluation and prognosis.

A number of classification systems for sacral fractures have been proposed since Bonnin's time. The goals of these classification schemes have been to correlate the observed fracture with the mechanism of injury and the clinical findings and to aid in treatment planning. In 1984, Schmidek and coworkers[6] proposed a classification based on the mechanism of injury and the resulting fracture pattern. They divided sacral fractures into those caused by direct trauma to the sacrum and those resulting from forces applied indirectly to the sacrum. Direct forces include penetrating injuries that result in open fractures, often accompanied by extensive pelvic visceral injuries. Penetrating injuries are usually stable if the sacrum and the sacroiliac joints above the S1 foramina are intact. Direct closed fractures are often caused by a hard fall onto the buttocks, causing low transverse-type fractures near the kyphos of the sacrum. Although such fractures usually occur through the foramina of S4, any of the lower three vertebrae can be involved. The distal fragment is often displaced anteriorly and may perforate the rectum in more severe cases. Because this part of the sacrum is not involved in the transmission of weight, these fractures are typically stable. Transverse fractures accounted for 5% to 10% of all sacral fractures in the series by Schmidek and colleagues.[6]

Indirect trauma to the sacrum follows injuries to the pelvic ring or lumbar spine. The mechanism, usually a flexion injury from a position of hip flexion with knee extension, causes traumatic spondylolisthesis through the S1 or S2 foramina, with forward displacement of the upper spinal segment. Typically, this type of injury occurs in younger patients before intersegmental ossification is complete. One fourth of transverse sacral fractures resulting from falls also have an associated thoracolumbar burst fracture. Thus, lower extremity motor weakness must prompt the examiner to look for associated spinal injuries. Lumbosacral fracture-dislocations are caused by mechanisms similar to those underlying high transverse sacral fractures, and they usually involve fracture of the S1 facet, with resultant instability.

Most fractures produced by indirect forces are vertical fractures of the sacrum, which almost always occur in conjunction with pelvic fractures. Schmidek and coworkers[6] classified these fractures into four fracture patterns: (1) lateral mass fractures (extending from the sacral notch through the ventral foramina), (2) juxta-articular fractures (lateral sacral mass fractures with fragments dissociated from the body of the sacrum), (3) cleaving fractures (vertically oriented fractures from the sacral notch through the sacrococcygeal region), and (4) avulsion fractures (along the convex margin of

the sacrum at the attachments of the sacrotuberous and sacrospinous ligaments). Combination fractures, with features of more than one pattern, may also occur. Although this scheme categorizes the different types of sacral fractures, it is cumbersome to remember and apply.

In 1988, Denis and colleagues[1] published a series of 236 sacral fractures and proposed a simplified classification scheme that categorizes sacral fractures based on the sacrum's division into three anatomic zones: zone I (alar region), zone II (foraminal region), and zone III (region of the central sacral canal). A zone II fracture can involve zone I but cannot extend into zone III, whereas a zone III fracture can involve zones I and II. In addition to being simple, this classification is relevant to the biomechanical forces applied to the sacrum and the probability of neural injury, and it aids in choosing among treatment options.[1]

Zone I fractures pass through the ala without damaging the foramina or central canal (Fig. 321–1). They are usually caused by lateral compression of the pelvis during pedestrian accidents in which the posterior sacroiliac ligaments remain intact and a portion of the ala is compressed anteriorly. Zone I fractures are stable by virtue of the intact posterior ligaments. Vertical shear injuries of the pelvis can produce more severe zone I fractures, with superior displacement of the ala and compression of the L5 nerve root between the fracture fragment and the L5 transverse process (Fig. 321–2). Wiltse and colleagues[8] named this mechanism of L5 root injury the *traumatic far-out syndrome*. Zone I fractures also include avulsion fractures at the bulbous enlargement of the sacrum adjacent to the S4 foramina, which is the point of attachment of the sacrospinous and sacrotuberous ligaments. A substantial degree of pelvic disruption occurs with avulsion fractures; therefore, the pelvis is often unstable.

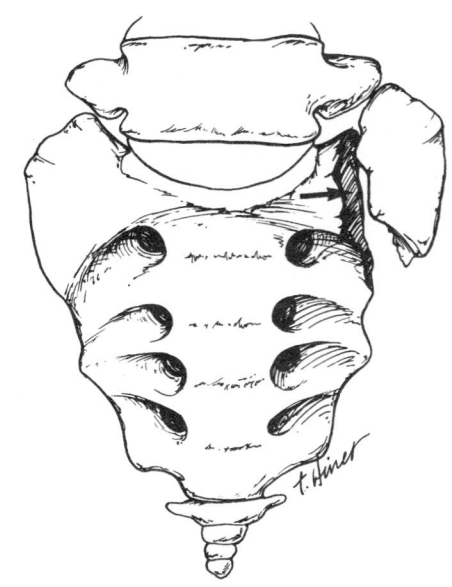

FIGURE 321–1. Zone I fracture (Denis classification) through the ala of the sacrum. *(arrow).*

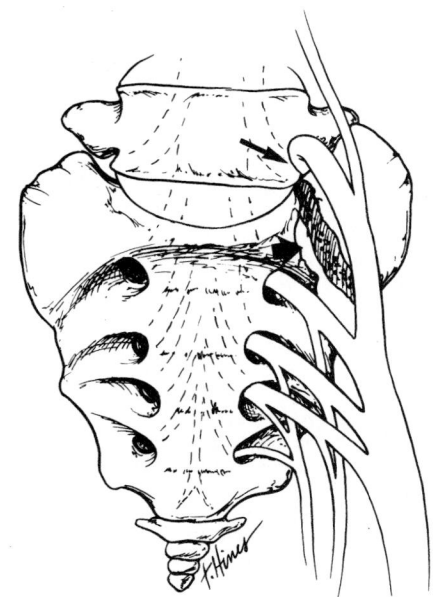

FIGURE 321–2. Zone I fracture (Denis classification) through the ala of the sacrum with upward displacement of the fracture fragment, trapping the L5 nerve root against the transverse process of L5 (traumatic far-out syndrome).

Zone II fractures involve one or several sacral foramina, but not the sacral canal (Fig. 321–3). They are often vertical shear fractures sustained by passengers involved in high-speed motor vehicle accidents, but they may also occur after lateral pelvic compression injuries such as those occurring in zone I fractures. Vertical shear injuries often involve zone II but may also involve zone III. Usually, they are part of an anteroposterior vertical fracture (double vertical fracture) of the pelvis. These fractures result from a significant

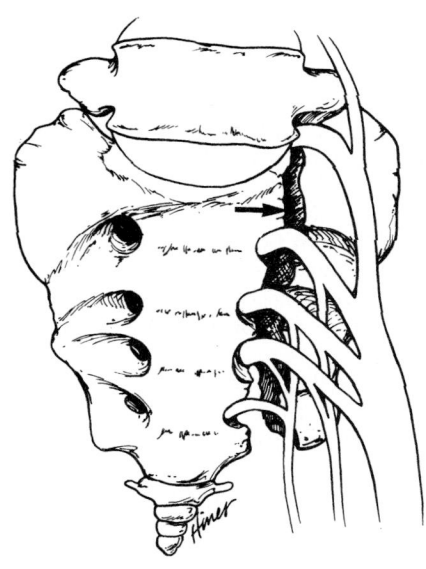

FIGURE 321–3. Zone II fractures (Denis classification) through the sacral foramina may involve one or several foramina.

transmission of force through one leg or on one side of the pelvis. Vertical shear injuries are uniformly unstable, and the degree of disruption of the sacroiliac joint correlates with both the degree of pelvic instability and the likelihood of neurological deficit.[6] Neurological injuries occur in 28% to 54% of zone II fractures.[1, 6]

Zone III fractures involve the sacral canal medial to the foramina and may involve zones I and II (Fig. 321–4). This group includes vertical shear injuries, high and low transverse fractures, and traumatic lumbosacral fracture-dislocations (or traumatic spondylolisthesis of L5 on S1). The transverse sacral fracture, also called the suicidal jumper's fracture,[9] commonly follows a fall from a height. This fracture typically crosses S2-3, just below the level of the sacroiliac joints, with anteroinferior displacement of the upper sacral segment. These transverse fractures account for 5% to 10% of sacral fractures and are frequently accompanied by neurological injury.[6, 9] Fractures in zone III are associated with a high incidence of bilateral nerve root damage and cauda equina dysfunction.

Certain features correlate with a high risk of instability: sacroiliac joint disruption, sacrospinous and sacrotuberous avulsion fractures, high transverse and bilateral sacral fractures, and vertical shear fractures. In contrast, lumbosacral fracture-dislocations are highly unstable during flexion.

CLINICAL PRESENTATION

Clinical suspicion is essential for an early diagnosis of sacral fracture. Sacral fractures can produce neurological deficits, which may be easily overlooked in patients with multiple traumatic injuries. The high incidence of sacral fractures associated with pelvic injuries should prompt a search for their presence when there is significant pelvic pathology.

Posterior pelvic fractures are associated with an increased risk of uncontrolled hemorrhage and death. Thus, these fractures are often immobilized and stabilized urgently to control pain and bleeding, typically by external fixation techniques performed after initial resuscitation.

In hemodynamically stable patients, the presence of pain, swelling, ecchymosis, open wounds, tenderness to palpation over the sacrum, or a palpable deformity should alert the examiner to the possibility of sacral injury. Deficits in lower extremity motor function may be observed—namely, weakness in eversion and plantarflexion of the foot (S1) and hip extension (S2). Motor deficits associated with isolated sacral fractures are usually minor because most lower extremity motor control arises cephalad to sacral fractures. The superior gluteal nerve can be injured, causing weakness of hip abduction and internal rotation. Much of the sacral innervation is associated with urogenital and anal sphincter control, as well as with perineal sensation. The second through fifth sacral roots innervate the muscles responsible for anal sphincter tone, anal wink, and bulbocavernosus reflex and also provide the parasympathetic input to the inferior hypogastric plexus.

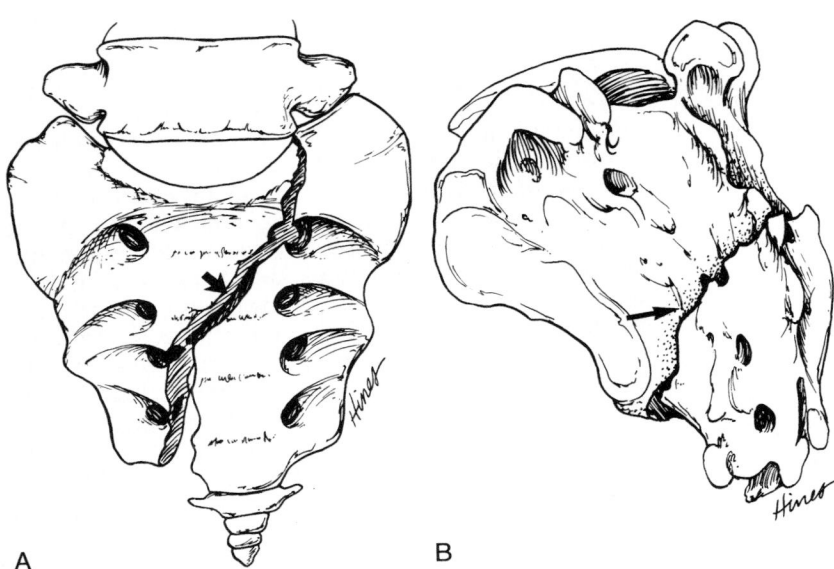

FIGURE 321–4. *A,* Zone III oblique fracture. *B,* Zone III transverse fracture. Zone III fractures involve the sacral canal medial to the foramina and can involve zones I and II. They include vertical shear fractures, high and low transverse fractures, and traumatic lumbosacral fracture-dislocations.

S2 is the main constituent of the pudendal nerve, which, with S3 and S4 branches, supplies the striated muscles of the internal and external anal sphincters. Parasympathetic innervation via pelvic splanchnic afferent nerves carries sensation for the awareness of bladder filling, and efferent fibers control both bladder detrusor and rectal contractions. Sympathetic innervation from S2 and S3 sympathetic ganglia controls contraction of the urethral and anal sphincters.

The incidence of neural injury in an unselected series of pelvic fractures was 0.75% to 11%. In Denis and coworkers' series of 236 sacral fractures, 49 patients (21%) had neurological deficits.[1] Five patients with deficits also had associated thoracolumbar fractures with paraparesis. The likelihood of neurological injury is increased in unstable pelvic and sacral fractures. In addition to immediate neurological deficits, delayed neurological injuries can follow callus formation and untreated spinal instability. Some patients with cauda equina syndrome may recover bowel and bladder function if the S2 and S3 nerve roots are preserved unilaterally.

The Denis three-zone classification system can be useful in anticipating neurological deficits associated with sacral fractures. Zone I fractures are rarely associated with neurological injuries. In the series by Denis and coworkers,[1] 5.9% of patients with zone I fractures presented with neurological deficits. Of these patients, 86% had L5 root lesions due to proximal displacement of the ala. Some patients with zone I injuries were impotent from pelvic or pudendal nerve injuries associated with bladder or urethral tears. In patients with zone II fractures, nerve root injuries can be expected if displacement is present. Denis and coworkers[1] found that 28% of fractures of this type were associated with neurological deficits. Neurological deficits in zone II fractures correlate strongly with ipsilateral disruption of the sacroiliac joint.[6] In displaced zone I and II fractures, the traumatic far-out syndrome,[8] with L5 nerve

root injury caused by cephalad displacement of the lateral mass of the sacrum and L5 nerve root compression against the L5 transverse process, may be a cause of radicular deficits. Fifty-seven percent of patients with zone III fractures had associated neurological deficits; of these patients, 76% had bowel or bladder impairment or both.[1]

DIAGNOSTIC IMAGING

The sacrum is poorly visualized on standard anteroposterior radiographs of the pelvis because of the orientation of the sacrum at the lumbosacral junction. In one series,[10] 49% of sacral fractures were not diagnosed during the initial hospitalization, including 24% of patients with neurological deficits referable to these fractures. Only 30% had appropriate radiographic studies that confirmed the fracture and explained the neurological deficit.[1] Therefore, unless a high degree of clinical suspicion is entertained, many sacral fractures will be missed on initial trauma radiographs. Certain findings on anteroposterior pelvic radiographs should arouse suspicion: (1) fracture of a lower lumbar transverse process, (2) significant anterior pelvic ring fracture without an identifiable posterior pelvic lesion, (3) asymmetry of the sacral notch, (4) clouding of the radiating trabecular pattern in the lateral sacral mass, or (5) irregularity of the arcuate lines of the upper three sacral foramina.

For patients with clinical signs of sacral injury or suspicious findings of anteroposterior pelvic films, or both, an appropriate imaging protocol includes a true anteroposterior sacral radiograph, performed with the x-ray beam directed 30 degrees cephalad (Ferguson's view), and a lateral sacral radiograph that includes the entire coccyx. Thin-cut computed tomographic scanning of the sacrum with reformatting is the most useful modality for evaluating complex sacral fractures and patients with neurological injuries.[10] Sagittal computed tomographic reconstructions are especially helpful for diagnosing transversely oriented fractures and for evaluating the sacroiliac joint.

Myelography can be useful for evaluating an injury at S1 and lumbosacral dislocation. This modality can show nonfilling of the nerve roots associated with transverse fractures and cauda equina nerve root avulsions associated with traumatic meningoceles. Myelography, however, is of limited use in evaluating neurological deficits caused by sacral fractures because the thecal sac ends at S2 and because the incidence of associated foraminal and extraforaminal nerve root injuries is high.

The value of magnetic resonance imaging in the evaluation of sacral fractures with neural injury has not been well defined. Many patients with multiple traumatic injuries are not candidates for magnetic resonance imaging because they are hemodynamically unstable or need mechanical ventilation. In addition, the external fixators used to stabilize pelvic fractures can cause a metallic artifact that obscures visualization of the neural elements. Sacral insufficiency fractures are even less frequently diagnosed, owing to the lack of an adequate history of trauma, minimal displacement of fracture fragments, and technical difficulties associated with interpreting radiographs of osteopenic bone. In such cases, radionuclide bone scanning is a sensitive test and produces a characteristic H-shaped pattern of uptake.

MANAGEMENT

The management of sacral fractures remains controversial, despite an improved understanding of the anatomy and mechanisms of injury. No controlled study of treatment protocols has been undertaken, and the available information comes from case reports and small series. A sacral fracture, however, needs to be managed in the context of the patient's general condition. The associated life-threatening injuries often encountered in patients with sacral fractures take precedence during early management. Therefore, early operative intervention for a sacral fracture can be constrained by these considerations. Loss of stability and the presence of neurological deficits are the primary considerations in the decision to operate. Sometimes, reduction and stabilization of an unstable pelvis (including the sacrum) may be a priority during resuscitation in an effort to control retroperitoneal hemorrhage and pain. Presacral or retroperitoneal bleeding occurs from injury to the internal iliac vessels and the presacral venous plexus.

Early treatment in patients with suspected sacral and pelvic fractures includes immobilization and military antishock trousers applied acutely. During transportation, intravascular volume resuscitation, external pelvic fixation, and fracture reduction should be instituted. Evacuation of retroperitoneal hematoma and pelvic exploration are contraindicated unless continuing and exsanguinating hemorrhage is present. An intra-abdominal or anterior approach to fresh sacral fractures, with evacuation of tamponading retroperitoneal blood, is fraught with the risk of causing uncontrollable hemorrhage.

Stability of sacral fractures can be defined crudely as the ability of the fractured sacrum to bear physiologic loads without further displacement. Certain fracture patterns are more likely to be associated with instability: disruption and displacement of the sacroiliac joints; vertical sacral fractures, especially those associated with shear; and sacrotuberous and sacrospinous ligamentous rupture or avulsion. Many sacral fractures can be successfully managed conservatively with bed rest and pelvic immobilization. Most surgical approaches involve posterior neural decompression with skeletal reduction and internal fixation.

Sacral fractures without prior trauma are a common source of lower back pain in elderly osteopenic women. In their early stages, these fractures are difficult to detect radiologically. Bone scans can detect such fractures and should be obtained when there is a high degree of suspicion. Sacral insufficiency fractures in zone II are oriented vertically, paralleling the sacroiliac joints. They are managed conservatively with bed rest and treatment of the osteoporosis.

Most zone I fractures (according to Denis's three-zone classification) are stable and cause no neurological injury. They are treated symptomatically, and early mobilization is possible. If the fracture is unstable and associated with an anterior pelvic fracture or disruption, anterior pelvic fixation or plating is required. When a vertical shear pattern of injury involves zone I, II, or III with proximal and posterior migration of the hemipelvis, the pelvic injury is life threatening and requires emergent treatment. Skeletal traction and external pelvic fixation reduce hemorrhage and facilitate the patient's management, but no external frame or anterior plate fixation adequately stabilizes a displaced posterior injury. In patients with L5 nerve root injuries caused by trapping from a superiorly displaced lateral mass of the sacrum, reduction of the fracture may decompress the nerve root adequately. For vertical shear injuries that are inherently unstable, early traction on the ipsilateral leg with or without manipulation may reduce the fracture. Reduction may be difficult to achieve if displacement is greater than 2 cm and the deformity has been present for more than 72 hours. In such cases, open reduction and internal fixation should be performed. Posterior fixation of the sacrum is performed indirectly by stabilizing the posterior pelvis, and reduction of the sacral pelvic injury may decompress the neural elements. Posterior tension banding using double cobra plates or threaded rod assemblies connects the posterior iliac crests posterior to the sacrum, providing immediate stability; this method may be used in conjunction with anterior fixation or plating.

For patients with zone II injuries and radiculopathy caused by foraminal stenosis, bed rest has been recommended as the first line of treatment. Foraminal compression of the L5 root with the lateral far-out syndrome, with ankle dorsiflexion weakness and persistent sciatic pain or plantarflexion weakness due to trapping of the S1 nerve root, may require early nerve root decompression. Sacral laminectomy and foraminotomy of the involved roots are the procedures of choice. If the fracture is stable with sciatic pain but without neurological deficit, bed rest for 1 month is the treatment of choice. If the radiculopathy fails to resolve after a month or recurs and foraminal stenosis persists, the patient should be offered the option of surgery. If the fracture is unstable and the patient is in pain, an anterior external fixator may provide relief.

By definition, zone III fractures are vertical or transverse sacral fractures and often involve the central canal, with a higher incidence of neurological deficits. Low transverse fractures commonly occur through the S4 sacral segment and do not compromise spinal or pelvic stability. Consequently, they are treated symptomatically. High transverse fractures and vertical sacral fractures through zone III are usually unstable and require internal or external stabilization. Decompression of the sacral canal and nerve roots, with or without reduction of the displaced fragments and fixation, may be indicated in the presence of neurological deficits. Simple transverse fractures can compress the roots of the cauda equina at the level of the fracture; high-resolution computed tomography with reformatting is necessary to identify the level of compression. We recommend early decompression of the sacral canal in patients with cauda equina injury in an effort to restore neurological function to the bowel, bladder, and sexual organs. Although severely displaced fractures can crush or lacerate the nerve roots beyond recovery, we recommend exploration and decompression because even unilateral preservation of the S2-4 roots permits the restoration of function.

SUMMARY

Sacral fractures are a poorly understood and inadequately treated condition, despite their common occurrence in patients with multiple traumatic injuries. Diagnosis is difficult, owing to their poor visualization on radiographs. Sacral fractures are commonly encountered in two groups of patients: those with multiple traumatic injuries and those with osteopenia. No controlled treatment options have been established yet; therefore, treatment of these complex injuries remains controversial.

REFERENCES

1. Denis F, Davis S, Comfort T: Sacral fractures: An important problem. Retrospective analysis of 236 cases. Clin Orthop 227: 67–81, 1988.
2. Malgaigne JF: Treatise on Fracture. Philadelphia, JB Lippincott, 1959.
3. Bonnin J: Sacral fractures and injuries to the cauda equina. J Bone Joint Surg 27:113–127, 1945.
4. Macciocchi B: Le fatture isolate del sacro. G Med Milit 10:787–791, 1955.
5. Sabiston CP, Wing PC: Sacral fractures: Classification and neurological implications. J Trauma 26:1113–1115, 1986.
6. Schmidek HH, Smith DA, Kristiansen TK: Sacral fractures. Neurosurgery 15:735–746, 1984.
7. Gunterberg B, Romanus B, Stener B: Pelvic strength after major amputation of the sacrum: An experimental study. Acta Orthop Scand 47:635–642, 1976.
8. Wiltse LL, Guyer RD, Spencer CW, et al: Alar transverse process impingement of the L5 spinal nerve: The far-out syndrome. Spine 9:31–41, 1984.
9. Roy-Camille R, Saillant G, Gagna G, Mazel C: Transverse fracture of the upper sacrum: Suicidal jumper's fracture. Spine 10:838–845, 1985.
10. Fishman EK, Magid D, Brooker AF, Siegelman SS: Fractures of the sacrum and sacroiliac joint: Evaluation by computerized tomography with multiplanar reconstruction. South Med J 81: 171–177, 1988.

SECTION

XI

Trauma

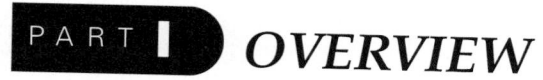
Modern Neurotraumatology: A Brief Historical Review

LAWRENCE F. MARSHALL ■ SHARON B. MARSHALL ■ M. SEAN GRADY

Neurotraumatology has an ancient and proud history spanning several continents, including the Americas, Europe, and Australia. A recent review provides an eloquent description of the experience in Peru,[1] beautifully illustrating the intellect and courage of the earliest "neurosurgeons" and that of their patients. Readers interested in this historical experience are also referred to Walker's classic text[2] and to the work of Courville and Abbott[3] and Campillo.[4] Two other particularly interesting achievements are Gama's modeling of concussion in 1830[5] and Denny-Brown and Russell's landmark experimental studies of concussion.[6] The focus in this chapter, however, is limited to the last 50 years in order to put neurotraumatology into better perspective in the early 21st century (Table 322–1).

It is important to emphasize that aside from McKissick's pioneering attempts to develop rational decision making for the treatment of intracerebral hemorrhage, no area of neurological surgery—or, for that matter, most of medicine—has focused as heavily on using laboratory and clinical research to provide rational and evidence-based treatment for an extremely complex and major public health problem. Contributions to our understanding of the pathophysiology and mechanisms that underlie brain injury have come from many disciplines, including neuropathology, bioengineering, neurochemistry, neurophysiology, intensive care, neurology, psychology, psychiatry, epidemiology, statistics, public health and public policy, and, most recently, genetics. It is somewhat sobering, however, to realize that the greatest advance in the reduction of brain injury was the introduction of lap and shoulder belts for motor vehicle passengers. This simple device, which costs less than $20 for each installation, has done more to prevent serious injury and death than any other advance. As with other major epidemic diseases, prevention of brain injury is better than treatment, but unfortunately, it tends to receive less attention.

BEGINNINGS OF MODERN NEUROTRAUMATOLOGY

The history of neurotraumatology in the last half century includes the pioneering observations on intracranial pressure (ICP) from Janny and colleagues[7] and Lundberg's[8] description of the continuous recording of ventricular fluid pressure. Lundberg's observation that pressure waves appeared to be spontaneous changes in ICP was the first clear demonstration of the types of perturbations that were possible. It provided us with some understanding of the mechanisms by which ICP could suddenly and rapidly increase. Of particular note was the A wave, also known as a "plateau" wave; it was characterized by an increase in ICP from 25 to 75 mm Hg that, if left untreated, could persist for approximately 5 to 20 minutes. Lundberg theorized that A waves were caused by increases in cerebral vascular volume because of dilatation of the vasculature. Later, Rosner and Becker[9] suggested that plateau waves reflected the brain's normal compensatory response to a reduction in brain perfusion, but it became clear that such waves in the face of compromised brain compliance could result in dangerous and potentially fatal rises in ICP.

Langfitt and coworkers[10, 11] expanded on Lundberg's initial observations regarding the mechanisms by which intracranial hypertension occurred. In a series of papers, they provided substantial evidence that loss of autoregulation and increases in intravascular volume played a significant role in intracranial hypertension.

Concurrently, Klatzo,[12] in a number of pioneering experiments, described mechanisms by which increased water content in the brain (brain edema) came about and introduced the terms *vasogenic* and *cytotoxic edema* to describe different mechanisms of extracellular and intracellular edema.

Investigations of cerebral blood flow and metabo-

TABLE 322-1 ■ Major Events in Modern Neurotraumatology

1. Continuous recording of intracranial pressure
2. Recognition of relationship between acute brain swelling and head injury
3. Identification of characteristics of cerebral blood flow changes in acute, severe head injury
4. Characterization of pattern of brain damage in humans
5. Recognition of volume-pressure relationships and their influence on treatment
6. Development of Glasgow Coma Scale
7. Development of Glasgow Outcome Scale
8. First well-designed, multicenter, multinational outcome study of acute, severe head injury
9. Improved outcome with aggressive treatment of acute head injury
10. Recognition of the influence of secondary insults on outcome
11. Sedation and metabolic depression used as a treatment for acute brain injury
12. Introduction of computed tomography (CT)
13. Improved mortality and morbidity in extra-axial hematomas
14. Creation of Traumatic Coma Data Bank: patterns of severe brain injury, outcome, influence of age, neurobehavioral observations, results of CT, new classification of head injury
15. Multicenter collaborative trials of pharmacologic therapies for acute traumatic brain injury
16. Development of American and European Brain Injury Consortia
17. Development of guidelines for the treatment of acute, severe brain injury
18. Development of models of experimental head injury in primates and nonprimates
19. Characterization of basic mechanisms in acute head injury and new concepts in pathophysiology of brain damage
20. Characterization of neurobehavioral sequelae of mild, moderate, and severe head injury
21. Recognition of spectrum of head injury
22. Development of adjunctive monitoring techniques: jugular oxygen saturation, brain tissue oxygen measurements, quantitative pupillometry
23. Investigation of genetics and the brain's response to injury

lism have also been important in furthering our understanding of the pathophysiology of acute brain injury. More than 25 years ago, Overgaard and Tweed[13] first described the relationship between cerebral blood flow and metabolism in brain-injured humans. Bruce and associates,[14] Obrist and colleagues,[15] and Bouma and coworkers[15–19] collaborated to provide us with new insights into the role of cerebral ischemia in head injury, providing much of the impetus for the maintenance of cerebral perfusion.

Central to the development of new therapeutic approaches to severe head injury were the pioneering studies of Stritch[20] and Adams and colleagues,[21–25] describing the neuropathology of brain damage in both human and animal models. The demonstration of unique patterns of initial impact injuries in the white matter, the finding of progressive changes, and the demonstration of ischemic changes in association with intracranial hypertension were essential to our understanding of the neuropathology and to our altered approaches to therapy.

The intense research in experimental and clinical head injury led to the development of a number of scientifically based hypotheses about intracranial hypertension and brain damage in humans and provided the foundation for the development of more rational approaches to treating acute brain injury. For the first time, a unified series of theories had been developed to explain the mechanisms by which intracranial hypertension (aside from that associated with mass lesions) could occur in patients with acute head injury. These seminal observations on intracranial hypertension were augmented by the work of Marmarou and coworkers[26] and Miller,[27] who improved our understanding of the Monro-Kellie doctrine, which describes the relationship between volume and pressure in the head. More recently, using the technique of diffusion-weighted imaging, Marmarou and colleagues provided convincing evidence that at least in the earliest stages of acute head injury, cytotoxic edema appears to be the major factor responsible for intracranial hypertension.[28, 29]

CLINICAL ADVANCES

Jennett and colleagues in Glasgow (particularly Teasdale, Miller, and Bond) deserve enormous credit for their contributions to the modernization of neurotraumatology. They developed now universally applied scales for classifying brain injury severity (Glasgow Coma Scale) and for measuring the outcome of brain injury weeks or months after the primary insult (Glasgow Outcome Scale).[30, 31] The development of these simple scales to assess the severity of injury in a logical manner and to classify outcome was immensely important, because they set the stage for modern clinical head injury research. They provided a reliable scheme for grading patients by injury severity and permitted the comparison of outcomes among patients in one unit and among patients treated in different neurosurgical units. In addition, because of its simplicity, the Glasgow Coma Scale (GCS) became a useful triage tool for grading injuries as mild (GCS score of 13 to 15), moderate (GCS score of 9 to 12), or severe (GCS score of 3 to 8). The GCS score was developed primarily as a predictive tool, not as a management tool, and certain additional vital information must be collected, such as the alertness of patients with less serious injuries and the status of the pupils, to sharpen the accuracy of predicted outcomes. However, the systematic application of these scales is the basis for longitudinal assessment in all modern clinical head injury research.

The multinational study of head injury outcome led by Jennett in Glasgow, working with Braakman in Rotterdam and with Heiden, Weiss, and colleagues in Los Angeles, began the systematic investigation of the outcome of severe head injury.[32] Several years later, Becker, working at the Medical College of Virginia, and Miller, working first in Glasgow and then also at the Medical College of Virginia, described their experience with the first rational attempt to establish an early diagnosis of intracranial mass lesions and intracranial hypertension and to apply systematic measures of care to those patients.[33] Their study transcended the revolutionary transition from angiography and ventriculography to modern neurodiagnostic imaging and has had a tremendous impact on modern neurotraumatology. They convincingly demonstrated that the logical application of their "treatment guidelines" had a significantly favorable impact on the outcome of severe brain injury.

An additional contribution of the Virginia group was the identification of the profound influence of "secondary insults."[34] They showed that the presence of hypercapnia, hypoxia, or hypotension was associated with significantly worse outcomes. These observations were extremely important, because they provided a sound rationale for the involvement of emergency medical services personnel in the early evaluation and treatment of patients with acute brain injury. At the time of these observations, many patients with acute head injury were transported facedown in police wagons, with no attempt to protect their airway or support their blood pressure. Chesnut and colleagues,[35] reporting on the experience of the Traumatic Coma Data Bank, overwhelmingly demonstrated that hypotension before or at the time of hospital arrival was associated with a significant increase in mortality and morbidity in patients with severe head injury, confirming the observations made by the Virginia group more than a decade earlier.

Shapiro and associates[36] used hypnotics, particularly pentobarbital, to treat head injury in patients with intractable intracranial hypertension. The logic behind the use of barbiturates was twofold. First, it was clear that these drugs reduced cerebral blood volume and thus would assist in controlling ICP. Second, given the embarrassment of cerebral blood flow that often characterized severe head injury, as demonstrated by Bruce and coworkers,[14] it seemed logical that the use of sedation would reduce metabolic demand and perhaps allow for better coupling of flow and metabolism.

COMPUTED TOMOGRAPHY

The introduction of computed tomography (CT) revolutionized medicine, particularly neurosurgery. Its most dramatic initial application was in head injury; previously, angiography, which often took several hours to perform, was the primary means of diagnosing an intracranial mass lesion in a head-injured patient. Although the initial CT scanners were slower and produced poorer-quality images than those we have today, there is little question that the widespread availability of CT dramatically reduced mortality, particularly in less severely injured patients with intracranial mass lesions. Seelig and coworkers,[37] in a landmark paper, described a dramatic reduction in mortality among patients with acute subdural hematomas when surgery was performed in the first 4 hours after injury. This, coupled with Bricolo and Pasut's[38] report of a dramatic reduction in mortality from extradural hematomas, confirmed the enormous importance of the rapid diagnosis of intracranial mass lesions made possible by CT.

TRAUMATIC COMA DATA BANK

Murray Goldstein, who later became the director of the National Institute on Neurological Diseases and Stroke (NINDS), was the primary force behind the development of the Traumatic Coma Data Bank (TCDB) and the Stroke Data Bank. His wisdom in applying techniques that today seem primitive but in the 1970s were novel and not yet proved should not be underestimated. The TCDB was a collaborative effort by the NINDS; its Office of Biometry and Field Studies, led by Weiss and Kunitz; and the four initial centers, led by Becker and Miller (Richmond, Virginia), Jane (Charlottesville, Virginia), Grossman and Eisenberg (Galveston, Texas), and Marshall (San Diego, California).[39–41] It became one of the most fruitful collaborations in clinical neurosurgery. Besides applying computerized techniques for the collection of head injury data, the TCDB provided an opportunity to collect data over many years, allowing for some extremely important longitudinal observations. For example, the relationship between shock and hypoxia and the clinical course and outcome in severe head injury became clear.[42–45] Perhaps most important, the relationships among different events that occurred over a short period could be captured and analyzed in a systematic way with data from multiple centers. Simple concepts such as centralized interpretation of computed tomographic scans and the recording of hourly vital sign data, including ICP; the development of a scale to measure the intensity of therapy; and the development of a CT-based classification[46] of severe head injury were all products of this landmark collaboration. The impact of the TCDB is still being felt today, because almost all clinical trials of new pharmacologic therapies for head injury are based on the TCDB's data collection instruments.[41] Also noteworthy was the collaborative relationship among the neurosurgeons, the NINDS, and the research nurses who were such an integral part of the TCDB. Such collaborative relationships have become the hallmark of many neurosurgical units throughout the world, and they had their origins in the TCDB.

CLINICAL TRIALS, CONSORTIA, AND GUIDELINES

As publications from the TCDB were disseminated and its work became more widely known, neurosurgeons, government agencies, and pharmaceutical companies became increasingly interested in the treatment of brain injury. A number of novel therapies, including tirilazad, pegorgotein, nimodipine, and hypothermia, have all undergone at least one clinical trial.[47–50] Although none of these trials has resulted in a successful new therapy for brain injury, much has been learned from the systematic application of the data collection techniques pioneered by Jennett and Teasdale and the TCDB investigators. This rational approach to evidence gathering and the widespread use of double-blind, randomized trials are among the most important legacies of head injury research in the second half of the 20th century.

An additional consequence of these initial trials was the creation of the Acute Brain Injury Consortium in the United States[51] and the European Brain Injury Consortium,[52] with centers in Israel as well. These consortia have developed specific protocols for the management of head-injured patients and have provided a systematic structure for the conduct of clinical trials so that treatments that have been appropriately tested in the laboratory can be rapidly transferred to the bedside for clinical trial. These organizations are playing a vital role in the further development of treatment strategies for brain-injured patients and will undoubtedly continue to assist in the development of guidelines for head injury care. Such guidelines have in fact been promulgated by the Brain Trauma Foundation and the American Association of Neurological Surgeons,[53, 54] as well as by the European Brain Injury Consortia. These guidelines have provided neurosurgeons and intensivists throughout the world with a series of logical strategies for patient management. Although such guidelines represent the consensus at the time they were drafted, they must be viewed as living documents that will surely be amended as laboratory and clinical investigations develop new information.

EXPERIMENTAL MODELS AND TRANSLATIONAL RESEARCH

Critical to the development of many hypotheses describing neurochemical and pathologic alterations in head-injured patients were the models developed by Marmarou and his group at the Medical College of Virginia[55, 56] and by Gennarelli and associates working at the University of Pennsylvania.[57] These experimental models have been enormously useful in improving our understanding of the neuropathologic consequences of brain injury and have allowed us to study, under controlled circumstances, a host of neurochemical alterations that appear to be important in human brain injury.

An important feature of neurotrauma research is the strong collaboration between basic scientists and myriad investigators in other areas. A large number of basic scientists, working in collaboration with neurosurgeons, have attempted to unravel the extremely complex physiologic and neurochemical mechanisms of brain injury.[58, 59] It is important to recognize that the similarities among some aspects of head injury, stroke, and aneurysmal subarachnoid hemorrhage have resulted in cross-fertilization in these fields. For example, the observations made almost 20 years ago that excitatory amino acids were neurotoxic in models of acute focal brain ischemia led to the application of therapies for acute brain injury based on the excitatory amino acid hypothesis.[60]

An example of elegant translational research comes from the observations of Becker's group at the University of California–Los Angeles, led by Hovda in the laboratory. These researchers have begun to systematically characterize abnormalities of metabolism, particularly hyperglycolysis, and how they relate to other pathophysiologic processes that occur early in acute brain injury.[61–63] By applying positron emission tomography and other modern imaging techniques, a better understanding of these complex interrelationships is being developed in humans.

NEUROPSYCHOLOGY AND THE SPECTRUM OF HEAD INJURY

It is important to acknowledge the role of pioneering neuropsychologists with an interest in head injury, such as Levin, Barr, Kreutzer, and Ruff, in the development of tools to measure and potentially treat the sequelae of brain injury.[64–66] Their work, following the initial development of the Glasgow Outcome Scale by Jennett (a neurosurgeon) and Bond (a neurosurgeon-psychiatrist),[32] has given us better tools to measure cognitive function. They have also illustrated the difficulty in determining what characterizes human function, because our efforts to measure actual disability and impairment still fall short. It will take imaginative efforts to unravel the almost incomprehensible complexity of human behavior and move us to the next step in ameliorating acute brain injury.

Significant progress has also been made in the recognition of the spectrum of head injury. Rimel and colleagues[67, 68] and many others, particularly Levin,[65] have emphasized the neurobehavioral sequelae of not only severe injury but also minor and moderate head injury. These observations were critical, because patients with minor head injuries were often thought to be malingering if their symptoms persisted for more than a few weeks. It is now apparent that a small but not insignificant percentage of patients with minor head injury (defined as a transient loss of consciousness) will have persistent sequelae, often for years.

MONITORING TECHNIQUES

Recent developments in adjunctive monitoring techniques are also worthy of mention. Jugular oxygen saturation, which has been used for more than a decade,[69] has provided useful information about global brain oxygenation and extraction.[70] However, it has a number of pitfalls, including varying results if both internal jugular veins are sampled and the possibility that changes in brain oxygen saturation may not truly represent adverse or positive changes in brain metabolism.[71] In part because of this concern, monitoring of brain tissue oxygen pressure has become increasingly prevalent in academic units, and it has been demonstrated that such measurements are useful as a predictive tool with regard to outcome and can also be useful in guiding critical care.[72] Another approach to monitoring is the introduction of quantitative pupillometry. In preliminary studies, this technology has demonstrated a strong correlation between changes in pupil size and reactivity and changes in ICP.[73] Much more work needs to be done to confirm these observations, but if this technology is demonstrated to be useful, it would permit noninvasive monitoring of many patients who are not candidates for other monitoring methods because their injuries are not severe or for whom monitoring is not available.

GENETICS

In the 21st century, no review of the recent history of neurotraumatology would be complete without at least a brief mention of the potential influence of genetic factors in characterizing the brain's vulnerability to injury and the outcome of such injury.[74] There are a number of reports of poor outcome and perhaps selective brain vulnerability in those who carry the Apo4E allele. The mechanism by which this genetic susceptibility occurs is not understood, but it emphasizes the increasingly recognized role of genetic expression—in terms of both the patient's own genetic profile and the factors expressed following injury—in the outcome of acute brain injury. It is safe to say that modern molecular biology and molecular genetics will have a profound influence on how we view head injury and its therapy in the future. But it is also important to remember that the basic principles of neurotrauma care, which include adequate oxygenation of the injured brain, adequate blood pressure, early evacuation of intracranial mass lesions, and attention to modern principles of critical care, will not be replaced by the manipulation of growth factors or of the human genome.

REFERENCES

1. Marino R, Portillo MC: Pre-conquest Peruvian neurosurgeons—a study of Inca and pre-Columbian trephination and the art of medicine in ancient Peru. Neurosurgery 47:940–950, 2000.
2. Walker AE: A History of Neurological Surgery. Baltimore, Williams & Wilkins, 1951.
3. Courville CB, Abbott: Cranial injuries of the pre-Columbian Incas. Bull Los Angeles Neurol Soc 7:107–130, 1942.
4. Campillo D: Neurosurgical pathology in prehistory. Acta Neurochir (Wien) 70:275–290, 1984.
5. Feinsod M: A flask full of jelly: The first in vitro model of concussive head injury, 1830. Neurosurgery 50:386–391, 2002.
6. Denny-Brown D, Russell WR: Experimental cerebral concussion. Brain 64:93–164, 1941.
7. Janny P, Joan JP, Janny L: A statistical approach to long-term monitoring of intracranial pressure. In Brock M, Dietz H (eds): Intracranial Pressure. Berlin, Springer-Verlag, 1972, pp 59–64.
8. Lundberg N: Continuous recording and control of ventricular fluid pressure in neurosurgical practice. Acta Psychiatr Neurol Scand Suppl 149:1–193, 1960.
9. Rosner MJ, Becker DP: Origin and evolution of plateau waves: Experimental observations and a theoretical model. J Neurosurg 60:312–324, 1984.
10. Langfitt TW, Tannanbaum HM, Kassell NF: The etiology of acute brain swelling following experimental head injury. J Neurosurg 24:47–56, 1966.
11. Langfitt TW, Weinstein JD, Kassell NF: Cerebral vasomotor paralysis produced by intracranial hypertension. Neurology 15:632–641, 1965.
12. Klatzo I: Neuropathological aspects of brain edema. J Neuropathol Exp Neurol 26:1–141, 1967.
13. Overgaard J, Tweed W: Cerebral circulation after head injury. Part I. Cerebral blood flow and its regulation after closed head injury with emphasis on clinical correlations. J Neurosurg 41:531–541, 1974.
14. Bruce DA, Langfitt TW, Miller JD, et al: Regional cerebral blood flow, intracranial pressure, and brain metabolism in comatose patients. J Neurosurg 38:131–144, 1973.
15. Obrist WD, Langfitt TW, Jaggi JL, et al: Cerebral blood flow and metabolism in comatose patients with acute head injury. J Neurosurg 61:241–253, 1984.
16. Bouma GJ, Mulzelaar JP, Choi SC, et al: Cerebral circulation and metabolism after severe traumatic brain injury: The elusive role of ischemia. J Neurosurg 75:685–693, 1991.
17. Bouma GJ, Muizelaar JP, Stringer WA, et al: Ultra-early evaluation of regional cerebral blood flow in severely head injured patients using xenon-enhanced computerized tomography. J Neurosurg 77:360–368, 1992.
18. Bouma GJ, Muizelaar JP, Bandoh K, Marmarou A: Blood pressure and intracranial pressure-volume dynamics in severe head injury: Relationship with cerebral blood flow. J Neurosurg 77:15–19, 1992.
19. Bouma GJ, Muizelaar JP: Cerebral blood flow, cerebral blood volume, and cerebrovascular reactivity after severe head injury. J Neurotrauma 9(Suppl 1):S333–S348, 1992.
20. Strich S: Diffuse degeneration of the cerebral white matter in severe dementia following head injury. J Neurol Neurosurg Psychiatry 19:163–185, 1956.
21. Adams JH, Graham DI, Scott G, et al: Brain damage in fatal non-missile head injury. J Clin Pathol 33:1132–1145, 1980.
22. Adams JH, Mitchell DE, Graham DI, Doyle D: Diffuse brain damage of immediate impact type. Brain 100:489–502, 1977.
23. Adams JH, Mitchell DE, Graham DI, et al: Diffuse axonal injury due to non-missile injury in humans: An analysis of 45 cases. Ann Neurol 12:557–563, 1982.
24. Adams JH: Head injury. In Adams JH, Corsellis JAN, Duchen LW (eds): Greenfield's Neuropathology, 4th ed. London, Edward Arnold, 1984, pp 85–124.
25. Graham DI, Adamas JH, Doyle D: Ischemic brain damage in fatal non-missile head injuries. J Neurol Sci 39:213–234, 1978.
26. Marmarou A, Shulman K, LaMorgese J: Compartmental analysis of compliance of outflow resistance of the cerebrospinal fluid system. J Neurosurg 43:523–534, 1976.
27. Miller JD: Clinical aspects of intracranial pressure-volume relationships. In McLaurin RL (ed): Head Injuries. New York, Grune & Stratton, 1976, pp 239–245.
28. Marmarou A, Fatouros PP, Barzo P, et al: Contribution of edema and cerebral blood volume to traumatic brain swelling in head injured patients. J Neurosurg 93:183–193, 2000.
29. Barzo P, Marmarou A, Fatouros P, et al: Contribution of vasogenic and cellular edema to traumatic brain swelling measured by diffusion-weighted imaging. J Neurosurg 87:900–907, 1997.
30. Teasdale G, Jennett B: Assessment of coma and impaired consciousness: A practical scale. Lancet 2:81–84, 1974.
31. Jennett B, Teasdale G, Galbraith S, et al: Severe head injuries in three countries. J Neurol Neurosurg Psychiatry 40:291–298, 1977.
32. Jennett B, Bond M: Assessment of outcome after severe brain damage: A practical scale. Lancet 1:480–484, 1975.
33. Becker DP, Miller JD, Ward JD, et al: The outcome from severe head injury with early diagnosis and intensive management. J Neurosurg 47:497–502, 1977.
34. Miller JD, Sweet RC, Narayan R, Becker DP: Early insults to the injured brain. JAMA 240:439–442, 1978.
35. Chesnut RM, Marshall LF, Klauber MR, et al: The role of secondary brain injury in determining outcome from severe head injury. J Trauma 34:216–222, 1993.
36. Shapiro HM, Whyte SR, Loeser J: Barbiturate-augmented hypothermia for reduction of persistent intracranial hypertension. J Neurosurg 40:90–100, 1979.
37. Seelig JM, Becker DP, Miller JD, et al: Traumatic acute subdural hematoma: Major mortality reduction in comatose patients treated within four hours. N Engl J Med 304:1511–1518, 1981.
38. Bricolo AP, Pasut ML: Extradural hematoma toward zero mortality: A prospective study. Neurosurgery 14:8–11, 1984.
39. Foulkes MA, Eisenberg HM, Jane JA, et al: The Traumatic Coma Data Bank: Design, methods, and baseline characteristics. J Neurosurg 75:S8–S13, 1991.
40. Foulkes MA: Neurosurgical data bases. J Neurosurg 75:S1–S7, 1991.

41. Marshall LF, Becker D, Bowers SA, et al: The National Traumatic Coma Data Bank. Part I. Design, purpose, goals and results. J Neurosurg 59:276–284. 1983.

42. Marmarou A, Anderson RL, Ward JD, et al: NINDS Traumatic Coma Data Bank: Intracranial pressure monitoring methodology. J Neurosurg 75:S21–S27, 1991.

43. Marmarou A, Anderson RL, Ward JD, et al: Impact of ICP instability and hypotension on outcome in patients with severe head trauma. J Neurosurg 75:S59–S66, 1991.

44. Marshall LF, Gautille T, Klauber MR, et al: The outcome of severe closed head injury. J Neurosurg 75:S28–S36, 1991.

45. Vollmer DG, Torner JC, Jane JA, et al: Age and outcome following traumatic coma: Why do older patients fare worse? J Neurosurg 75:S37–S49, 1991.

46. Marshall LF, Marshall SB, Klauber MR, et al: A new classification of head injury based on computerized tomography. J Neurosurg 75:S14–S20, 1991.

47. Marshall LF, Maas AI, Marshall SB, et al: A multicenter trial on the efficacy of using tirilazad mesylate in cases of head injury. J Neurosurg 91:737–743, 1999.

48. Young B, Runge JW, Waxman KS, et al: Effects of pegorgotein on neurologic outcome of patients with severe head injury: A multicenter, randomized controlled trial. JAMA 276:538–543, 1996.

49. European Study Group on Nimodipine in Severe Head Injury: A multicenter trial of the efficacy of nimodipine on outcome after severe head injury. J Neurosurg 80:797–804, 1994.

50. Clifton GL, Miller ER, Choi SC, et al: Lack of effect of induction of hypothermia after acute brain injury. N Engl J Med 344:556–563, 2001.

51. Marmarou A, American Brain Injury Consortium in Head Trauma: In Miller LP, Hayes RL (eds): Basic Preclinical Directions. New York, Wiley & Sons, 2001, pp 371–384.

52. Teasdale GM, Braakman R, Cohadon F, et al: The European Brain Injury Consortium: Nemo solus satis sapit—nobody knows enough alone. Acta Neurochir (Wien) 139:797–803, 1997.

53. Bullock R, Chesnut RM, Clifton G, et al: Guidelines for the management of severe head injury. J Neurotrauma 13:643–734, 1996.

54. Brain Trauma Foundation, American Association of Neurological Surgeons, Joint Section on Neurotrauma and Critical Care: Guidelines for the management of severe head injury. J Neurotrauma 13:641–734, 1996.

55. Marmarou A, Shima K: Comparative studies of edema produced by fluid-percussion injury with lateral and central modes of injury in cats. Adv Neurol 52:233–236, 1990.

56. Marmarou A, Abd-Elfatta Foda M, van den Brink W, et al: A new model of diffuse brain injury in rats. Part I. Pathophysiology and biomechanics. J Neurosurg 80:291–300, 1994.

57. Gennarelli TA, Thibault LE, Adams JH, et al: Diffuse axonal injury and traumatic coma in the primate. Ann Neurol 12:564–574, 1982.

58. Jenkins LW, Moszyniski K, Lyeth BG, et al: An increased vulnerability of the mildly traumatized rat brain to cerebral ischemia: The use of controlled secondary ischemia as a research tool to identify common or different mechanisms contributing to mechanical and ischemic brain injury. Brain Res 477:211–224, 1989.

59. Lenzlinger PM, Saatman KE, Raghupathi R, Mcintosh TK: Overview of basic mechanisms underlying neuropathological consequences of head trauma. In Miller LP, Hayes RL (eds): Basic Preclinical Directions. New York, Wiley & Sons, 2001, pp 371–384.

60. Morris GF, Juul N, Bullock R, et al: Failure of the competitive N-methyl-D-aspartate antagonist selfotel (CGS 19755) in the treatment of severe head injury: Results of two phase III clinical trials. J Neurosurg 91:737–743, 1999.

61. Andersen BJ, Marmarou A: Isolated stimulation of glycolysis following traumatic brain injury. In Hoff JT, Betz AL (eds): Intracranial Pressure VII. Berlin, Springer-Verlag, 1989, pp 575–580.

62. Bergsnider MA, Hovda DA, Shalmon E, et al: Cerebral hyperglycolysis following severe traumatic brain injury in humans: A positron emission tomography study. J Neurosurg 86:241–251, 1997.

63. Vespa P, Prins M, Ronne-Engstrom E, et al: Increase in extracellular glutamate caused by reduced cerebral perfusion pressure and seizures after human traumatic brain injury: A microdialysis study. J Neurosurg 89:971–982, 1998.

64. Levin HS, Benton AL, Grossman RG: Neurobehavioral Consequences of Closed Head Injury. New York, Oxford University Press, 1982.

65. Levin HS, Mattis S, Ruff RM, et al: Neurobehavioral outcome following minor head injury: A three center study. J Neurosurg 66:234–243, 1987.

66. Ruff RM, Young D, Gautille T, et al: Verbal learning deficits following severe head injury: Heterogeneity in recovery over 1 year. J Neurosurg 75:S50–S58, 1991.

67. Rimel RW, Giodani B, Barth JT: Disability caused by minor head injury. Neurosurgery 9:221–228. 1981.

68. Rimel RW, Giodani B, Barth JT: Moderate head injury: Completing the clinical spectrum of brain trauma. Neurosurgery 11:344–351, 1982.

69. Dearden NM: Jugular bulb venous oxygen saturation in the management of severe head injury. Curr Opin Anest 4:279–286, 1991.

70. Robertson CS: Desaturation episodes after severe head injury: Influence on outcome. Acta Neurochir (Wien) 59:98–101, 1993.

71. Stochetti N, Paparella A, Bridelli F, et al: Cerebral venous oxygen saturation studied with bilateral samples in the internal jugular vein. Neurosurgery 34:38–44, 1994.

72. Van Santbrink H, Maas AR, Avezaat CJJ: Continuous monitoring of partial pressure of brain tissue oxygen in patients with severe head injury. Neurosurgery 38:21–31, 1996.

73. Taylor WR, Chen JW, Meltzer H, et al: Quantitative pupillometry: A new technology. Normative data and preliminary observations in patients with acute head injury. Technical note. J Neurosurg 98:205–213, 2003.

74. Teasdale G, Nicoll JAR, Murray G, Fidees M: Association of apolipoprotein E polymorphism with outcome after head injury. Lancet 350:1069–1071, 1997.

Cellular Basis of Injury and Recovery from Trauma

LUCA LONGHI ■ KATHRYN E. SAATMAN ■ RAMESH RAGHUPATHI ■ PHILIPP M. LENZLINGER ■ M. SEAN GRADY ■ TRACY K. MCINTOSH

Traumatic brain injury (TBI) is associated with primary injury (due to the biomechanical effects of the impact) and with secondary or delayed molecular events that are initiated minutes after the injury and last up to several months.[1] Traumatic injury itself induces alterations in gene expression and the up-regulation and release of several mediators that interact in a complex network leading to cell dysfunction, death, or recovery. The extended nature of these cascades offers the opportunity to implement therapeutic strategies aimed at blocking degeneration or improving repair and promoting plasticity and regeneration.[2] Animal models of TBI recapitulate features of human head injury, allowing investigation of the mechanisms underlying post-traumatic damaging and reparative processes at cellular and molecular levels.[3, 4] This chapter summarizes the most relevant mechanisms associated with central nervous system (CNS) injury and repair.

CALCIUM ENTRY INTO INJURED CENTRAL NERVOUS SYSTEM CELLS

TBI disrupts brain calcium (Ca^{2+}) homeostasis, leading to secondary damage.[5] An increase in Ca^{2+} flux has been documented in several experimental models of TBI such as lateral fluid percussion (FP) brain injury[6] and weight-drop brain injury.[7] Calcium entry into neural cells may occur through membrane-associated receptors and channels. Trauma-induced depolarization leads to an increase in intracellular Ca^{2+} via voltage-sensitive Ca^{2+} channels. Antagonism of these channels—using Ca^{2+} channel blockers such as (S)-emopamil or the omega-conopeptide SNX-111—has been shown to be associated with a reduction of post-traumatic Ca^{2+} accumulation and attenuation of regional cerebral blood flow reductions, brain edema, and motor and cognitive deficits in a rat model of lateral FP injury, suggesting a role for Ca^{2+} in secondary post-traumatic brain damage.[8–10] Nimodipine, which blocks L-type voltage-sensitive Ca^{2+}, has been shown to be protective in models of cerebral ischemia.[11] However, when administered 24 hours after injury to severely head-injured patients, no significant clinical benefit was observed, except in a subgroup of patients with subarachnoid hemorrhage.[12]

Calcium may enter traumatized cells using the excitatory amino acid receptors.[2] The release or increase of excitatory amino acid neurotransmitters glutamate and aspartate and the activation of specific glutamate receptors are well-characterized events in both experimental and clinical TBI.[13–16] Trauma-induced alterations in membrane potential may be responsible, in part, for the release of excitatory amino acids via an alteration in the sodium-potassium (Na^+-K^+) transmembrane ratio.[17] Excitatory amino acids bind receptors that are ubiquitous in the brain, and several types of receptors have been described (for review, see reference 18). One subtype of receptors is activated by the glutamate analog N-methyl-D-aspartate (NMDA) and gates monovalent (Na^+) and divalent (Ca^{2+}) cations. Regulation of NMDA receptors is achieved through a magnesium (Mg^{2+})-dependent voltage block and by binding of glycine, polyamines, and zinc (Zn^{2+}) to specific receptor sites. A second subtype of glutamate receptors, activated by α-amino-3-hydroxy-5-methyl-4-isoxazole propionic acid and by kainate, consists of monovalent cation channels whose activation occurs in a voltage-independent manner. The third family of glutamate receptors, the so-called metabotropic receptors, consists

Competitive Antagonism
- 2-amino-5-phosphovaleric acid (APV)
- carbozypiperazin-4-yl)-propyl-1-phosphanate (CPP)
- CP101 606
- selfotel

Noncompetitive Antagonism
- phencyclidine (PCP)
- dizocilpine (MK-801)
- magnesium
- aptiganel
- remacemide hydrochloride
- dexanabinol
- ketamine
- dextrorphan and dextromethorphan

NMDA receptor

Modulation of Glycine or Polyamine Binding Sites
- ifenprodil
- eliprodil
- indole-2-carboxylic acid (I2CA),
- kyruneate
- 6-cyano-7-nitroquinoxaline-2,3-dine (CNQX)

Presynaptic Inhibition of Glutamate Release
- riluzole
- lubeluzole

FIGURE 323–1. Therapeutic strategies and compounds investigated following experimental traumatic brain injury to antagonize the excitotoxic pathway at the level of the *N*-methyl-D-aspartate (NMDA) receptor and to reduce glutamate release.

of G-protein–coupled receptors whose activation leads to a release of stored or bound intracellular Ca^{2+}. Excessive levels of excitatory amino acids can cause cell death through two distinct mechanisms: an acute increase in Na^+ and chlorine (Cl^-), leading to cell swelling, and an increase in the intracellular Ca^{2+} concentration.[19] Antagonism of excitatory amino acid receptors has been successful in the experimental setting (for review, see references 2, 20). Figure 323–1 illustrates the strategies used to antagonize excitotoxicity at the level of the NMDA glutamate receptor and to reduce glutamate release. However, the clinical application of these strategies in TBI has produced rather discouraging results.[21–23]

CALCIUM-MEDIATED INTRACELLULAR EFFECTS

Post-traumatic elevation of intracellular free calcium may precipitate an attack on the cellular membrane by activating phospholipases A_2 and C, resulting in the release of free fatty acids and diacylglycerol.[24, 25] Dhillon and colleagues[26] reported that the duration and extent of the increase in free fatty acids following lateral FP brain injury in rats were associated with the severity of the injury. Increases in brain free fatty acids can lead to secondary damage through blood-brain barrier breakdown and the formation of cerebral edema[27] and, indirectly, through the generation of prostaglandins, thromboxanes, and leukotrienes (cyclooxygenase and lipoxygenase products from arachidonic acid), which may affect cerebral blood flow and blood-brain barrier permeability. In addition, during the process of prostaglandin synthesis from arachidonic acid, reactive oxygen species are generated.[28] Intracellular free radicals such as superoxide anion, hydrogen peroxide, nitric oxide, and peroxinitrite are generated through several pathways, including the conversion

of xanthine dehydrogenase to xanthine oxidase, the activation of nitric oxide synthase, and cyclooxygenases. In addition, reactive oxygen species may be released by the mitochondria due to Ca^{2+}-mediated disorganization of the inner mitochondrial membrane and subsequent disruption of the electron transport chain.[29] Because reactive oxygen species appear to contribute to the pathology of CNS injury,[30] blocking their formation represents an important neuroprotective strategy. The formation of reactive oxygen species leads to peroxidative destruction of the cell membrane, proteins, and DNA.[30] Under physiologic conditions, reactive oxygen species are removed by endogenous antioxidants, including superoxide dismutases (SODs), glutathione peroxidase, and catalase. Therefore, increasing endogenous antioxidative mechanisms may have therapeutic value. When transgenic mice overexpressing the cytosolic copper-zinc SOD and the mitochondrial manganese SOD were subjected to weight-drop brain injury, they showed attenuated edema, lesion volume, and neurological motor deficits compared with their wild-type littermates.[31, 32] The free radical scavenger polyethylene glycol–conjugated SOD or tirilazad mesylate, a 21-aminosteroid inhibitor of free radical–mediated lipid peroxidation, has been tested in experimental TBI but did not produce significant benefits in head-injured patients.[33, 34]

Reactive oxygen species, released following TBI, can induce DNA strand breaks.[35] DNA single-strand breaks have been observed in the ipsilateral cortex as early as 30 minutes after controlled cortical impact (CCI) brain injury with imposed secondary hypoxic injury in rats. Single-strand breaks were maximal in the cortex and hippocampus at 6 hours after injury and were observed to last at least 72 hours. In contrast, double-strand breaks were first observed 2 hours after injury in the ipsilateral cortex, peaked at 24 hours in both the cortex and the hippocampus, and were reduced to baseline levels at 72 hours.[36] The tumor suppressor gene *p53* is up-regulated following DNA damage and can lead to DNA repair, cell growth arrest, or apoptosis.[37] Up-regulation of p53 mRNA and protein has been observed following experimental brain injury in rats.[38, 39] However, although brain-injured p53 knockout (-/-) mice showed attenuated motor deficits, no histologic protection (lesion volume and cell loss) was observed when compared with their wild-type littermates,[40] suggesting that the role of p53 in TBI-induced cell damage is complex. Up-regulation of the *p53* gene may activate pathways leading to cell death (i.e., pro-apoptotic production of Bax protein family) or cell survival (i.e., growth arrest and DNA damage-inducible gene [*GADD45*]).[41, 42]

Polyadenosine diphosphate-ribose polymerase (PARP) is a nuclear enzyme that has been proposed to play a role in DNA repair, particularly following oxidative DNA damage. Normally, DNA strand breaks activate PARP, which then binds to the nicked DNA and uses the oxidized form of nicotinamide adenine dinucleotide (NAD^+) as substrate to form polyadenosine diphosphate-ribose (PAR). This process continues until a critical PAR chain length is reached; then PARP is released from DNA, allowing other repair enzymes to complete the repair process. Activation of PARP may also lead to consumption of NAD, adenosine triphosphate reduction, and subsequent death associated with energy failure.[43] Lateral FP brain injury in the rat has been reported to activate PARP by 30 minutes after injury.[44] Studies of TBI involving either PARP-deficient mice or post-traumatic inhibition of PARP have demonstrated an attenuation of functional deficits[45] and a reduction in cortical damage[46] following experimental TBI, suggesting that the energy consumption associated with PARP activation may be deleterious.

CALPAIN ACTIVATION AND CYTOSKELETAL PROTEOLYSIS

Calpains are nonlysosomal cysteine proteases, ubiquitous in the CNS, that are activated by increased intracellular free calcium. There are two isoforms of calpain: m-calpain, with millimolar sensitivity to calcium in vitro, and μ-calpain, with micromolar sensitivity to calcium in vitro.[47] Activated calpains may cause the proteolysis of many cellular proteins, including cytoskeletal proteins such as spectrin, microtubule-associated proteins (MAP1B, MAP2, tau), neurofilament proteins, and tubulin (for review, see reference 48). Proteolytic activity of calpains has been observed as early as 15 minutes after injury in rats subjected to CCI brain injury or impact-acceleration brain injury.[49–51] Saatman and coworkers,[52] using an antibody that recognizes calpain-specific spectrin breakdown products, observed evidence of calpain-mediated spectrin proteolysis in the ipsilateral hemisphere as early as 90 minutes after injury and lasting up to 7 days following lateral FP injury in rats. Calpain-mediated spectrin breakdown products were found initially in axons and dendrites and later in neuronal perikarya before neuronal cell death, suggesting that calpains participate in

processes leading to cell death.[52] These experimental data are consistent with a recent study by McCracken and associates[53] in which significant degradation of neurofilament proteins and increased levels of calpain-mediated spectrin breakdown products were detected within the corpus callosum in humans who died 11 to 300 hours following blunt head injury.

Because calpains are ubiquitous in the brain and have many downstream targets, strategies aimed at blocking calpain activity are promising. Direct or indirect antagonism of calpain activation following experimental TBI has been shown to attenuate behavioral deficits and histologic damage, suggesting that this may be a promising therapeutic target.[54–59]

MITOCHONDRIA

It has been suggested that experimental and clinical TBI results in mitochondrial dysfunction and damage.[60, 61] Mitochondria play a central role in cellular energy production, and their dysfunction following TBI may lead to cell damage or death through several mechanisms. Xiong and colleagues,[61] studying CCI brain injury in rats, documented a decreased (nearly 50%) state 3 respiratory rate, P/O ratio, and respiratory control index as early as 1 hour after injury and lasting for 14 days. The authors also reported an increase in the amount of mitochondrial Ca^{2+}, particularly in the injured hemisphere, starting 6 hours after injury. Intramitochondrial Ca^{2+} accumulation impairs the electron transport chain, leading to reduced adenosine triphosphate production and the generation of reactive oxygen species, which can lead to cell death through energy failure and oxidative damage. The reduction of the capacity for oxidative metabolism following TBI remains a major topic of investigation, because providing adequate blood flow, glucose, and oxygen may not be sufficient to ensure adequate adenosine triphosphate for the brain. Restoring the oxidative metabolism in the mitochondria may provide a way to increase energy production and spare the neurons from damage or death caused by energy failure.

Mitochondrial Ca^{2+} loading is also responsible for a nonselective increase in the permeability of the inner mitochondrial membrane, called mitochondrial permeability transition megapore.[62] This process is responsible for the post-traumatic mitochondrial swelling that may lead to mitochondrial membrane rupture. Cyclophilins are proteins that constitute the mitochondrial permeability transition, and their inhibition using cyclosporin A is a promising therapeutic strategy in CNS injury. In fact, cyclosporin A has been shown to attenuate behavioral deficits, mitochondrial dysfunction, axonal injury, and lesion volume and to increase hippocampal plasticity following experimental TBI.[58, 63–67] These studies suggest that mitochondria may play a main role in the progression of secondary damage following TBI, both in the soma and in the axons, and may represent the final common pathway following excitotoxicity, Ca^{2+} overload, oxidation, energy failure, and apoptosis.

IMMEDIATE EARLY GENES

The increase in the intracellular Ca^{2+} concentration activates protein kinase C and calmodulin kinase, which phosphorylate transcription factors, which induce *jun* and *fos* mRNAs. Following experimental brain injury, bilateral increases in *c-fos*, *c-jun* and *junB* mRNA have been observed in the cortex and hippocampus as early as 5 minutes after injury, with a return to control values by 24 hours.[68–70] These experimental data were confirmed by the analysis of human brain tissue removed during surgical procedures following head injury, which showed positive immunoreactivity for immediate early genes in 67% of patients.[71, 72] The significance of the induction of immediate early genes is not completely understood, because these transcription factors up-regulate both genes that are implicated in cell death and those that are associated with cell survival.[73]

TRAUMATIC AXONAL INJURY

Diffuse axonal injury is one of the most important types of brain damage that can occur as a result of nonmissile head injury.[74] The biomechanical pathogenesis of axonal injury involves acceleration and deceleration of the brain. This type of injury has been shown to produce coma in the absence of impact to the brain.[75] Initially, it was believed that axons were torn at the moment of injury, but subsequent observations led to the conclusion that primary axotomy (occurring at the moment of injury) occurs only in the most severe cases; the majority of axons undergo a secondary, progressive axotomy associated with intra-axonal perturbations, cytoskeletal alterations (e.g., neurofilament compaction, microtubule loss or misalignment), impaired axoplasmic transport, and ultimately axonal disconnection (for review, see reference 76). More recent studies suggest that there may be multiple phenotypes or distinct pathways resulting in traumatic secondary axotomy.[77] Whereas some axons appear to undergo progressive swelling over time, others seem to maintain their caliber despite compaction of the neurofilament cytoskeleton.[77] In the first scenario, mild injury results in subtle alterations in axolemma permeability that are not detectable using tracers such as horseradish peroxidase and a submicromolar increase in axonal Ca^{2+} concentration. This is followed by activation of Ca^{2+}-calmodulin targets such as calcineurin, contributing to cytoskeletal misalignment, which in turn causes impaired axonal transport and accumulation of organelles.[78–82] In the second scenario, Povlishock and colleagues hypothesized that moderate or severe injury produces an increase in axolemma permeability (observed by 5 minutes after injury using the tracer horseradish peroxidase)[83] and allows a massive Ca^{2+} influx, followed by calpain activation, which is shown by the presence of spectrin breakdown products in injured axons by 15 minutes after injury.[84] In these axons, neurofilament compaction occurs by 5 to 15 minutes after injury; this may be due to dephosphorylation or calpain-mediated proteolysis of neurofilament sidearms, because spectrin breakdown products and neurofilament compaction have been shown to colocalize in the same injured axons.[84] Increased axonal Ca^2 is also followed by mitochondrial swelling, release of cytochrome *c*, and activation of caspase 3, which may further contribute to the cytoskeletal derangements observed in experimental models of traumatic axonal injury.[81] The final result in these pathways is axonal disconnection, followed by the downstream degeneration of the axonal segment, as shown schematically in Figure 323–2.

The finding that the majority of traumatically injured axons appear to undergo a secondary, delayed axotomy means that there may be a therapeutic window somewhere in the pathways involved in the progression of damage. Table 323–1 summarizes the studies performed analyzing the therapeutic strategies

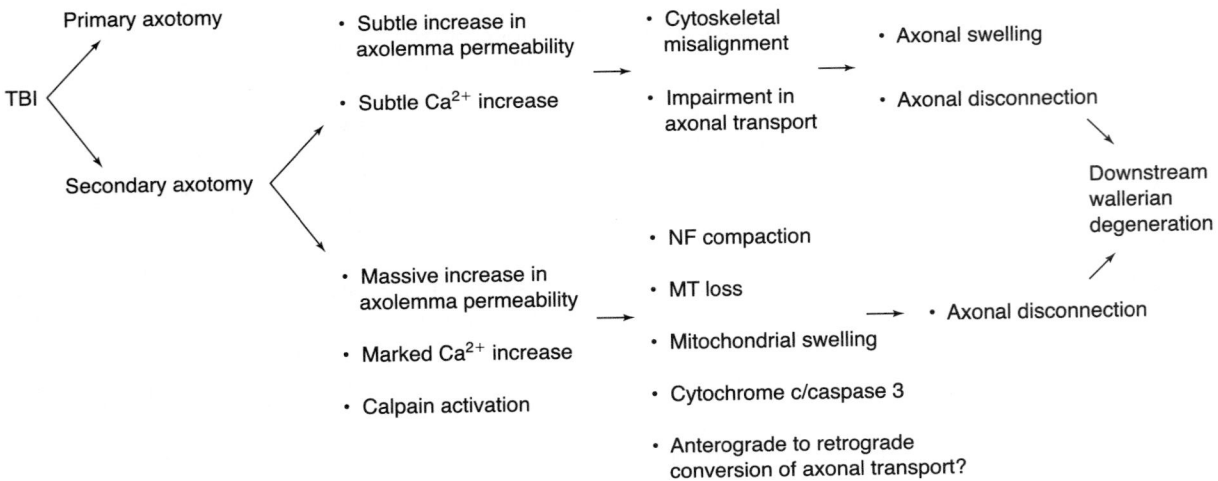

FIGURE 323–2. Schematic representation of the processes leading to axotomy following traumatic brain injury (TBI). MT, microtubule; NF, neurofilament.

T A B L E   3 2 3 – 1 ■ Studies Investigating Potential Therapeutic Strategies for Traumatic Axonal Injury

MODEL	TREATMENT	TIME POSTINJURY	OUTCOME	TIME OF EVALUATION	AUTHOR
CCI	Hypothermia 32°C	10–25 min	↓ NF breakdown products	24 hr	Marion & White, 1996[87]
CCI	21-aminosteroid	10–40 min	↓ NF breakdown products	24 hr	Marion & White, 1996[87]
IA	Hypothermia 32°C (rewarming = 90 min)	Immediately and 1 hr	↓ APP-positive axons	24 hr	Koizumi & Povlishock, 1998[86]
IA	Hypothermia 32°C (rewarming = 90 min)	Immediately	↓ SBDPs ↓ RMO-14 positive axons	3 hr	Buki et al, 1999[57]
IA	CsA	30 min	↓ SBDPs ↓ RMO-14 positive axons ↓ APP-positive axons	24 hr	Buki et al, 1999[58]
IA	Hypothermia 32°C (rewarming = 90 min)	Immediately	↑ Improved behavior ↓ APP-positive axons	1 wk	Koizumi & Povlishock, 2001[85]
IA	Hypothermia 32°C (rewarming < 20 min)	Immediately	↑ APP-positive axons (compared with 90 min rewarming)	24 hr	Suehiro & Povlishock, 2001[89]
IA	Hypothermia 32°C (rewarming < 20 min + CsA)	Immediately	↓ APP-positive axons (compared with < 20 min rewarming)	24 hr	Suehiro & Povlishock, 2001[89]
IA	Hypothermia 32°C (rewarming < 20 min + FK-506)	Immediately	↓ APP-positive axons (compared with < 20 min rewarming)	180 min	Suehiro et al, 2001[88]

APP, amyloid precursor protein; CCI, controlled cortical impact brain injury; CsA, cyclosporin A; IA, impact acceleration brain injury; NF, neurofilament; RMO-14, antibodies directed toward the rod domain of neurofilaments-M; SBDP, spectrin breakdown degradation products.

employed in animal models of traumatic axonal injury.[57, 58, 85–89]

INFLAMMATION AND CYTOKINES

TBI results in acute opening of the blood-brain barrier, which allows the entry of circulating leukocytes into the injured brain.[90] These cells (neutrophils and activated macrophages) may release reactive oxygen species, causing cellular damage, and inflammatory cytokines, which have been implicated in post-traumatic neuropathologic damage or recovery. Post-traumatic inflammation has been documented in both clinical and experimental TBI and is associated with the up-regulation of intercellular adhesion molecules such as ICAM-1, which is involved in vascular adhesion and transendothelial migration of leukocytes,[91, 92] and with the up-regulation and release of cytokines, such as tumor necrosis factor-α (TNF-α),[93, 94] and various interleukins, such as IL-1, IL-6, IL-10, and IL-12.[93, 95]

Initially, pharmacologic strategies were developed to antagonize cytokine production or activity, based on the hypothesis that the cytokines contributed to the secondary post-traumatic damage. Shohami and associates[96] showed that the administration of pentoxifylline (immediately after injury) to rats subjected to weight-drop brain injury reduced the levels of TNF-α at 4 hours after injury in the injured cortex, reduced the brain water content in the injured hemisphere at 24 hours, and attenuated neurological deficits over a 2-week period in comparison with a control group of injured rats. In the same study, the authors tested the effect of a physiologic blockade of TNF-α with a TNF binding protein and obtained similar positive results

in terms of brain water content and neurological deficits. In addition, the group treated with TNF binding protein showed reduced cell loss in the CA2 and CA3 regions of the ipsilateral hippocampus at 2 weeks after injury. In a subsequent study,[97] the ability of the compound dexanabinol (a cannabinoid known to block the NMDA receptor) to inhibit TNF-α production was tested. The compound was administered 5 minutes after injury, resulting in a reduced brain TNF-α protein level at 4 hours, attenuated motor neurological deficits over 2 weeks, reduced brain water content at 24 hours, and hippocampal cell loss at 2 weeks. These data suggest that an acute blockade of TNF-α production or activity may be helpful following TBI.

IL-1β mRNA has been shown to increase in the injured hemisphere of rats subjected to lateral FP injury from 1 to 6 hours after injury[98]; using the same model, IL-1 protein levels increased by 8 hours after injury and returned to baseline levels at 18 hours.[99] Systemic administration of the antagonist of IL-1β receptor by 15 minutes after injury for 1 week resulted in attenuated cognitive deficit (at 2 days after injury) and in reduced cell loss at 1 week in the cortex and hippocampus ipsilateral to the injury.[100] These data suggest a detrimental role of IL-1 following TBI. However, more recent work investigating cytokines such as TNF and IL-6 following TBI, using genetically engineered mice, suggests that the inflammatory response may play a dual role in the injury and recovery from trauma.

In conclusion, there is extensive evidence of a major inflammatory response to head trauma. However, little is known about its effects in the acute and chronic stages of TBI pathology, and further research is warranted to develop novel approaches in the therapy of TBI.

APOPTOSIS

Apoptotic cell death has been reported to occur in both the acute and the chronic post-traumatic period in experimental TBI[101–103] and, more recently, in tissue from human head-injured patients.[104] Apoptosis is triggered by intracellular or extracellular signals that converge to activate a specific group of cysteine proteases called caspases. Caspase 8 and caspase 9 are considered initiator caspases, and caspase 3 is thought to be the executioner caspase (for review, see references 105–107). Following experimental TBI, an increase in caspase 3 mRNA was observed in the ipsilateral cortex (by 4 hours and up to 72 hours after injury) and hippocampus (at 24 hours after injury).[108] Caspase 3–like activity is increased in the injured cortex by 6 hours after injury, peaks at 24 hours, and persists (at a lower extent) at 72 hours.[109] In addition, in the injured cortex, activated caspase 3 was localized in neurons, astrocytes, and oligodendrocytes, with predominance in the neurons.[110]

Pharmacologic inhibition of caspase 3 with the compound *N*-benzyloxycarbonyl-Asp-Glu-Val-Asp-fluoromethyl ketone gave different results. When administered 30 minutes before and 6 and 24 hours after lateral FP injury in rats, it reduced post-traumatic apoptosis at 3 days after injury and improved neurological recovery over a 2-week period.[108] When administered for 72 hours following CCI brain injury in rats, it reduced apoptotic neurons at 24 hours after injury and attenuated hippocampal cell loss and lesion volume at 3 weeks after injury, although functional outcome was unaffected.[109]

Caspase activation is under the control of the *Bcl-2* family of genes, including pro-apoptotic factors such as Bak, Bim, Bad, and Bax and anti-apoptotic factors Bcl-2 and Bcl-xl, whose function is related to cytochrome *c* release from mitochondria.[111] An imbalance in the expression of one of these groups of genes may exacerbate or reduce the extent of cell death following neuronal injury.[111] The *Bcl-2* gene family may play an important role in controlling cell survival following CNS injury, and an increase in *Bcl-2* mRNA and Bcl-2 protein was observed following experimental and clinical TBI.[104, 112] In contrast, Raghupathi and coworkers (unpublished data) observed that Bcl-2 immunoreactivity was decreased in the injured cortex and injured hippocampus by 2 hours following lateral FP injury, whereas Bax mRNA and protein were increased, suggesting that changes in the Bax–Bcl-2 ratio could participate in the process leading to the post-traumatic pattern of apoptosis in the injured cortex and hippocampus. Overexpression of Bcl-2 in transgenic mice subjected to CCI brain injury led to reduced lesion volume and attenuated hippocampal cell loss at 1 week after injury in comparison with their wild-type littermates.[113, 114] Kaya and associates[38] observed a translocation of Bax into the nuclei of neurons destined to die of apoptosis in the ipsilateral hemisphere 48 hours after injury. The role of Bax was also investigated by Carbonell and colleagues,[115] who observed that as early as 10 minutes following lateral FP brain injury, Bax

(−/−) mice showed fewer damaged neurons than did wild-type injured mice in the hippocampus but not in the cortex, suggesting that Bax is involved in mediating acute post-traumatic hippocampal neuronal damage. Because the hippocampus contains a high concentration of excitatory amino acid receptors, these results might be explained by an increased resistance to excitotoxicity due to the suppression of Bax.

Intracellular targets of activated caspase 3 are proteins involved in DNA repair, such as DNA-dependent protein kinase and PARP, or involved in DNA fragmentation, such as DNA fragmentation factor (DFF)-45.[109] An additional intracellular target of caspase 3 is actin, which is degraded in the parietal cortex (24 hours after injury), hippocampus (during the first week), and thalamus (by 24 hours and up to 3 weeks after injury). Degradation of actin (together with hyperpolymerization) is supposed to reduce its protective function toward DNA fragmentation.[116] Downstream from caspase activation, in fact, DNA fragmentation is mediated by a heterodimeric protein composed of 40- and 45-kDa subunits. These subunits have been named DFF-40 (or caspase-activated DNase) and DFF-45 (or inhibitor of caspase-activated DNase). During apoptosis, caspase 3 is believed to cleave DFF-45, dissociating it from DFF-40 and inducing a transformation of DFF-40 into a large protein complex with DNase activity.[117–119] Regional changes of DFF-40 and DFF-45 have been documented in lateral FP brain injury, where a decrease in DFF-45–like proteins in rat cortex was observed in the cytosolic and nuclear fraction during the first 24 hours following injury.[120] In the hippocampus, DFF-40 was found to be reduced in the cytosolic fraction and increased in the nuclear fraction at 2 and 24 hours following injury, suggesting a translocation from cytoplasm to nucleus during apoptosis.[120] Further studies are warranted on the complex pathways associated with post-traumatic cell death.

RECOVERY FROM TRAUMA

Plasticity, the ability of the brain to change its function and structure in response to stimuli, plays a major role in mediating the recovery from a CNS injury (for an excellent review related to postinjury functional recovery and strategies for potential treatment, see reference 121). Functional plasticity is evident in animal models of TBI. For example, although rats subjected to lateral FP brain injury demonstrate progressive tissue loss with concomitant ventriculomegaly in the hemisphere ipsilateral to injury, motor function improves over the weeks and months following TBI.[122, 123] Patients with head injury also show functional recovery despite atrophic changes in the brain.[124] In order to understand the pattern of behavioral recovery following CNS injury, the functional recovery of rats subjected to a specific unilateral lesion of the sensorimotor area of the cortex has been analyzed. The observed recovery of motor function is attributed to compensatory functional and structural mechanisms (e.g., an increase in the synapse-neuron ratio during the first month after injury) occurring in other regions of the brain.[125, 126]

CYTOKINES

It has already been shown that cytokines such as TNF-α and IL-1β, up-regulated following TBI, may play a detrimental role and that their antagonism may reduce post-traumatic damage. However, more recent work performed with genetically engineered mice has added information about the complexity of the post-traumatic inflammatory response. When knockout mice for the *TNF* gene were subjected to CCI brain injury and compared with their wild-type littermates, they exhibited attenuated cognitive deficits and motor dysfunction during the first week after injury. Wild-type mice subjected to mild TBI showed marked recovery over time, whereas TNF (-/-) mice displayed persistent motor deficits up to 4 weeks after injury. A significantly larger injury cavity was also observed in TNF (-/-) mice at 2 and 4 weeks after injury, suggesting that although this cytokine may be deleterious during the acute postinjury period, it may have a beneficial role in long-term behavioral recovery and tissue repair in the more chronic period after brain injury.[127]

IL-6 is a cytokine known to be up-regulated following clinical and experimental TBI.[94, 128] In studies performed 3 days following CNS injury, IL-6 knockout mice showed a reduced recruitment of astrocytes and monocytes or macrophages at the site of injury[129] and a greater cell loss in the injured cortex compared with their wild-type littermates. In addition, over the 2 weeks after injury, IL-6 (-/-) mice showed less cellular infiltration, neovascularization, and more necrosis.[130] In contrast, overexpression of IL-6 was associated with greater cellular infiltration, restoration of normal-appearing tissue, and neovascularization, suggesting that IL-6 plays a role in the healing of the brain.[130]

Reactive gliosis occurs following TBI, and this process has been considered a major obstacle to axonal regrowth following injury. However, it has been shown that astrocytes might contribute to the restoration of ionic homeostasis, buffer excitatory amino acid toxicity, and provide energetic substrate to the neurons.[131] In addition, activated astrocytes release cytokines and trophic factors, such as transforming growth factor-β, nerve growth factor (NGF), basic fibroblast growth factor (bFGF), and platelet-derived growth factor, and up-regulate their receptors, providing a permissive substratum for neuritic extension (for review, see reference 132).

GROWTH FACTORS

Four major classes of neurotrophins have been characterized in mammals—NGF, brain-derived neurotrophic factor, neurotrophin-3, and neurotrophin-4—plus additional non-neuronal trophic factors such as bFGF, glial-derived neurotrophic factor, insulin-like growth factor, ciliary neurotrophic factor, epidermal growth factor, and vascular endothelial growth factor (for review, see reference 133). Schematically, among the neurotrophins, several classes of receptors have also been identified, including the low-affinity receptor p75[NTR], which is a target for all the neurotrophins, and the tyrosine kinase (trk) receptors, which are divided into trk A (specific target for NGF), trk B (specific for brain-derived neurotrophic factor and neurotrophin-4) and trk C (specific for neurotrophin-3).[134] Neurotrophins mediate several types of intercellular communication and have been shown to act as (1) retrogradely transported, target-derived factors that influence afferent neurons; (2) locally released paracrine factors affecting both neurons and non-neuronal cells; (3) autocrine factors acting on the same cells that produce and release them; and (4) endocrine factors that are transported through the bloodstream.[135] In astrocytes, NGF expression is up-regulated by bFGF, IL-1, glutamate agonists, reactive oxygen species, high potassium, ischemia, and TBI.[136]

Several studies have analyzed the temporal course of the expression and level of growth factors in response to an insult to the brain. Following CNS injury, there is reportedly an increase in mRNA and protein expression for bFGF during the first week after injury in macrophages, neurons, astrocytes, and vascular endothelial cells, which suggests a bFGF-mediated role in the reparative attempt following injury.[137, 138]

Recent studies have reported a marked increase in NGF mRNA and NGF protein concentration in the acute post-traumatic period following TBI in both experimental animals and human patients.[139, 140] In a recent comparison of gene expression for NGF and its trk A receptor between injured TUNEL-positive cortical neurons and uninjured ones, O'Dell and coworkers[141] showed that at 12 hours after injury, a reduction in NGF mRNA in the injured pyramidal neurons occurs, whereas the gene expression of the trk A receptor is unchanged. These data provide a rationale for NGF administration following TBI. Several laboratories have reported that the intraparenchymal or intracerebroventricular administration of NGF attenuates cognitive deficits and cholinergic cell loss in the forebrain following FP brain injury and CCI brain injury in rats.[142-144] In a comprehensive review, Sofroniew and coauthors[136] recently summarized the neuroprotective mechanisms underlying NGF. Administration of NGF and other growth factors may regulate the intrinsic capacity of neurons to regenerate transected axons through the hostile extracellular environment of the injured adult CNS. In the adult spinal cord, the infusion of NGF and other growth factors stimulates the regrowth of fibers of receptor-expressing sensory neurons across the peripheral-central nervous system border in a manner that does not occur in the absence of this growth factor, suggesting that NGF can help these axons overcome environmental cues that inhibit axon elongation in the CNS.[145] Administration of other trophic factors can also be neuroprotective. Dietrich and colleagues[146] reported that acute administration of bFGF could attenuate cortical cell loss following lateral FP brain injury in rats. McDermott and coworkers,[147] using the same model, demonstrated that delayed intraparenchymal administration of bFGF, beginning 24 hours after injury, can significantly improve post-traumatic cognitive deficits in the rat. However, the diversity of cells responding to neurotrophin signaling may lead to a variety of undesirable or unwanted effects in patients and animals, including hypophagia, weight loss, sprouting of sensory fibers, and Schwann cell migration and proliferation in the subpial space surrounding the brainstem, leading to hyperalgesia[148] and ultimately precluding the clinical application of these compounds. An optimal delivery system for neurotrophins (using viral vectors or genetically modified cells) should be the object of investigation to ensure a constant release of trophic factors to a targeted area without the adverse effects related to systemic or intracerebroventricular administration.

NEURONAL REGENERATION

Regeneration of injured neurons is a multifactorial process involving many steps, including (but not limited to) survival of injured neurons, regeneration-associated gene expression, expression of permissive or inhibitory matrix molecules for growth cone activity, axonal regeneration, remyelination of axons, and functional synapse formation on the surface of targeted neurons.[149] Axonal disconnection appears to be followed by a limited regenerative attempt in the adult CNS, even though the axons may regenerate in the embryonic CNS and in the adult peripheral nervous system. This selective shutdown of axonal regeneration can be explained, in part, by intrinsic properties of neurons in the adult CNS and extrinsic environmental factors affecting axonal outgrowth. Two major pathways have been identified as being responsible for the inhibition of axonal regeneration: scar formation in and around the injury site, and the presence of myelin surrounding the axons. The molecular basis of this inhibition has been hypothesized to be dependent in part on the molecules chondroitin sulfate proteoglycan, tenascin, and semaphorin-3A, which are up-regulated in the scar and inhibit axonal regeneration.[150–152]

Myelin contains inhibitors of axonal regrowth such as myelin-associated glycoprotein, NI 35, and NI 250 (Nogo). The *Nogo* gene encodes for Nogo A, present in oligodendrocytes.[153–155] The extracellular domain Nogo-66 has been shown to bind a specific neuronal receptor,[156] and it has been hypothesized that this interaction regulates neural plasticity and regeneration following injury. Recently, administration of the monoclonal antibody IN-1 directed against Nogo A has been shown to induce the regeneration of transected spinal cord axons after 2 weeks[157] and to enhance functional recovery over a 5-week period following experimental spinal cord injury.[158] In addition, in a model of unilateral corticospinal tract lesions, the administration of IN-1 was followed 2 weeks postinjury by neurite outgrowth with sprouting of fibers that crossed the midline and established synaptic contacts, suggesting that CNS fibers can sprout and form new synapses in a growth-permissive environment.[159] These studies suggest that the modulation of Nogo activity might be a promising therapeutic strategy following CNS injury.

In addition to the extrinsic modulation of axonal regeneration, it has been shown that intrinsic neuronal factors can affect plasticity. Embryonic neurons transplanted in the adult CNS show neurite outgrowth, suggesting that there is an intrinsic difference between embryonic and adult neurons that cannot be explained by environmental differences alone. Recently, Condic[160] reported that fourfold overexpression of human integrins (receptors mediating axonal extension in embryonic and adult life) in adult cultured rat neurons was able to promote a robust neurite outgrowth in a medium containing low levels of growth-promoting molecules, suggesting that the intrinsic contribution to regeneration may be as important as the environmental one.

TBI appears to be followed by regenerative efforts and the increased expression of several growth-related proteins. Christman and associates[161] subjected cats to FP injury and observed that, following the initial phase of neurofilament damage, at 14 days after injury there was an increase in growth-associated protein 43 (GAP-43) immunoreactivity in the axons, coupled with sprouting. These sprouts formed junctional complexes and were surrounded by a thin myelin sheet. These data suggest a sustained regenerative attempt by injured axons, characterized by axonal cytoskeletal change and up-regulation of growth-associated proteins. Several proteins associated with normal development and regeneration, such as GAP-43, microtubule-associated protein 1B (MAP-1B), and polysialylated neural cell adhesion molecule (PSA-NCAM), have been observed to change following traumatic CNS injury. The re-expression of PSA-NCAM in the adult brain is associated with the reappearance of a developmental state, which has been hypothesized to occur following CNS trauma.[162] To investigate the regenerative pathways following TBI at the molecular level, Emery and coworkers[163] recently evaluated the expression of GAP-43, MAP-1B, and PSA-NCAM following lateral FP brain injury in rats and observed an increase in MAP-1B immunoreactivity and its phosphorylated isoform at 24 hours after injury; this returned to control levels within 1 week, except in the thalamus, where increased expression persisted for 2 months. PSA-NCAM was increased by 48 hours after injury and persisted for up to 2 weeks bilaterally in the dentate gyrus of the hippocampus, whereas GAP-43 was increased at 48 and 72 hours after injury bilaterally in the cortex and hippocampus. These data suggest that there may be a transient increase in developmentally expressed proteins in the traumatically injured brain that can be exploited to increase synaptic plasticity.

NEUROGENESIS AS SELF-REPAIR MECHANISM

The presence of endogenous neural progenitor cells resident within the CNS and the possibility of regulating their number and fate are of great interest. Stem cells are found in the adult mammalian brain,[164] and they can be found in the subventricular zone, dentate gyrus, white matter, and frontal and temporal cortex.[165, 166] The rate of proliferation of these cells can be modulated by several factors, such as stress (negatively) and exercise, activity, and enriched environment (positively).[167, 168] To evaluate the effect of TBI on neurogenesis in the adult brain, Dash and colleagues[169] subjected rats to CCI brain injury and observed an increase in the production of new granule neurons in the dentate gyrus of the hippocampus. The rate of production of new cells was maximal at 3 and 7 days and returned to the basal level by day 14 postinjury. These data suggest that neuronal replacement may be a viable therapeutic approach. In this regard, fetal cortical tissue, transplanted 24 hours after injury (alone or coupled with NGF infusion), has been observed to survive in the injured brain and to attenuate behavioral deficits and histologic damage, including hippocampal cell loss.[170–172] However, practical and ethical issues related to the use of fetal tissue have prompted researchers to look for other cell populations that are safe, available in an appropriate amount, and suitable for genetic manipulation to deliver therapeutic agents. Human cell lines such as neuroteratocarcinoma cells, differentiated ex vivo in neuronal-like cells, have been observed to (safely) survive in the injured brain,[173, 174] attenuate neurological motor deficit in a model of middle cerebral artery occlusion in rats,[175] and improve neurological recovery (over a 24-week postimplantation period) in a phase I clinical trial in patients 6 months after ischemic stroke.[176] In addition, progenitor cells, which can migrate into a damaged area of the brain and differentiate in neuronal and astroglial cells, have been used in a post-trauma transplantation paradigm. Recently, transplantation of hippocampal progenitor cells derived from embryonic rat hippocampus, retrovirally transduced to release NGF, 24 hours after lateral FP brain injury in rats led to attenuation of behavioral and cognitive deficits and hippocampal cell loss at 1 week after injury.[177] Mouse C17-2 embryonic stem cells have been shown to survive in the injured mouse brain for 12 weeks after CCI brain injury, to attenuate behavioral deficits, and to differentiate, expressing neuronal and astrocytic markers (Riess, unpublished data). Finally, bone marrow stromal cells, an accessible source of autologous progenitor cells, have been successfully transplanted into the injured brain, improving functional outcome and expressing neuronal and glial markers.[178] Further studies are warranted to characterize the signals that regulate cell proliferation, migration, and differentiation before the clinical evaluation of this therapeutic strategy.

These studies suggest that in addition to the degenerative cascades activated following TBI, an effort by the brain to repair itself and to recover and regenerate may underlie the limited functional recovery observed in animal models and clinically in patients. There is increasing evidence to refute the old dogma that brain cannot regenerate, and recent progress has been made with potentially useful resources such as neural and stem cells, transplantation and gene therapy. However,

further studies are warranted to determine which molecular signals regulate neurogenesis in the adult brain, the migration of newly generated cells, and the differentiation of transplanted or endogenous progenitor cells toward a specific phenotype. Further work is also warranted at the molecular level to investigate the extrinsic and intrinsic bases of neuronal regeneration in order to develop novel therapeutic strategies that could shift potentially aberrant compensatory mechanisms in the direction of plasticity and recovery. The complexity and heterogeneity of a disease such as TBI make it unlikely that the simplistic attenuation of a single deleterious pathway or the enhancement of a regenerative one will be translated into a successful treatment. Certainly, a multifactorial approach is warranted, and understanding the proper time of intervention will be crucial to our ability to antagonize the multiple pathogenic cascades and to correctly stimulate appropriate structural and functional recovery.

REFERENCES

1. Graham DI, Gennarelli TA: Pathology of brain damage after head injury. In Reilly P, Bullock R (eds): Head Injury, 4th ed. New York, Arnold Publishing, 1997, pp 133–153.
2. McIntosh TK, Juhler M, Wieloch T: Novel pharmacologic strategies in the treatment of experimental traumatic brain injury. J Neurotrauma 15:731–769, 1998.
3. Laurer HL, McIntosh TK: Experimental models of brain trauma. Curr Opin Neurol 12:715–721, 1999.
4. Povlishock JT, Hayes RL, Michel ME, et al: Workshop on animal models of traumatic brain injury. J Neurotrauma 11:723–732, 1994.
5. McIntosh TK, Saatman KE, Raghupathi R: Calcium and the pathogenesis of traumatic CNS injury: Cellular and molecular mechanisms. Neuroscientist 3:169–175, 1997.
6. Fineman I, Hovda DA, Smith M, et al: Concussive brain injury is associated with a prolonged accumulation of calcium: A ^{45}Ca autoradiographic study. Brain Res 624:94–102, 1993.
7. Shapira Y, Yadid G, Cotev S, et al: Accumulation of calcium in the brain following head trauma. Neurol Res 11:169–172, 1989.
8. Berman RF, Verweu BH, Muizelaar JP: Neurobehavioral protection by the neuronal calcium channel blocker ziconotide in a model of traumatic diffuse brain injury in rats. J Neurosurg 93:821–828, 2000.
9. Okiyama K, Smith DH, Thomas MJ, et al: Evaluation of a novel calcium channel blocker, (S)-emopamil, on regional cerebral edema and neurobehavioral function after experimental brain injury. J Neurosurg 77:607–615, 1992.
10. Samii A, Badie H, Fu K, et al: Effects of an N-type calcium channel antagonist (SNX 111; ziconotide) on calcium-45 accumulation following fluid-percussion injury. J Neurotrauma 16:879–892, 1999.
11. Fox AP, Nowycky MC, Tsien RW: Single-channel recordings of three types of calcium channels in chick sensory neurones. J Physiol 394:173–200, 1987.
12. A multicenter trial of the efficacy of nimodipine on outcome after severe head injury. The European Study Group on Nimodipine in Severe Head Injury. J Neurosurg 80:797–804, 1994.
13. Faden AI, Demediuk P, Panter SS, et al: The role of excitatory amino acids and NMDA receptors in traumatic brain injury. Science 244:798–800, 1989.
14. Katayama Y, Becker DP, Tamura T, et al: Massive increases in extracellular potassium and the indiscriminate release of glutamate following concussive brain injury. J Neurosurg 73:889–900, 1990.
15. Nilsson P, Hillered L, Ponten U, et al: Changes in cortical extracellular levels of energy-related metabolites and amino acids following concussive brain injury in rats. J Cereb Blood Flow Metab 10:631–637, 1990.
16. Alessandri B, Doppenberg E, Zauner A, et al: Evidence for

time-dependent glutamate-mediated glycolysis in head-injured patients: A microdialysis study. Acta Neurochir Suppl (Wien) 75:25–28, 1999.

17. Obrenovitch TP, Urenjak J: Altered glutamatergic transmission in neurological disorders: From high extracellular glutamate to excessive synaptic efficacy. Prog Neurobiol 51:39–87, 1997.

18. Dingledine R, Borges K, Bowie D, et al: The glutamate receptor ion channels. Pharmacol Rev 51:7–61, 1999.

19. Choi DW: Glutamate neurotoxicity and diseases of the nervous system. Neuron 1:623–634, 1988.

20. Laurer HL, McIntosh T: Pharmacologic therapy in traumatic brain injury: Update on experimental treatment strategies and recent findings. Curr Pharm Des 7:1505–1516, 2001.

21. Maas AI, Steyerberg EW, Murray GD, et al: Why have recent trials of neuroprotective agents in head injury failed to show convincing efficacy? A pragmatic analysis and theoretical considerations. Neurosurgery 44:1286–1298, 1999.

22. Morris GF, Bullock R, Marshall SB, et al: Failure of the competitive N-methyl-D-aspartate antagonist Selfotel (CGS 19755) in the treatment of severe head injury: Results of two phase III clinical trials. The Selfotel Investigators. J Neurosurg 91:737–743, 1999.

23. Reinert MM, Bullock R: Clinical trials in head injury. Neurol Res 21:330–338, 1999.

24. Alessandri B, Doppenberg E, Zauner A, et al: Evidence for time-dependent glutamate-mediated glycolysis in head-injured patients: A microdialysis study. Acta Neurochir Suppl (Wien) 75:25–28, 1999.

25. Shohami E, Shapira Y, Yadid G, et al: Brain phospholipase A_2 is activated after experimental closed head injury in the rat. J Neurochem 53:1541–1546, 1989.

26. Dhillon HS, Carman HM, Zhang D, et al: Severity of experimental brain injury on lactate and free fatty acid accumulation and Evans blue extravasation in the rat cortex and hippocampus. J Neurotrauma 16:455–469, 1999.

27. Unterberg A, Wahl M, Hammersen F, et al: Permeability and vasomotor response of cerebral vessels during exposure to arachidonic acid. Acta Neuropathol(Berl) 73:209–219, 1987.

28. Kontos HA: George E. Brown memorial lecture: Oxygen radicals in cerebral vascular injury. Circ Res 57:508–516, 1985.

29. Tymianski M, Tator CH: Normal and abnormal calcium homeostasis in neurons: A basis for the pathophysiology of traumatic and ischemic central nervous system injury. Neurosurgery 38:1176–1195, 1996.

30. Shohami E, Beit-Yannai E, Horowitz M, et al: Oxidative stress in closed-head injury: Brain antioxidant capacity as an indicator of functional outcome. J Cereb Blood Flow Metab 17:1007–1019, 1997.

31. Mikawa S, Kinouchi H, Kamii H, et al: Attenuation of acute and chronic damage following traumatic brain injury in copper, zinc-superoxide dismutase transgenic mice. J Neurosurg 85:885–891, 1996.

32. Sullivan PG, Bruce-Keller AJ, Rabchevsky AG, et al: Exacerbation of damage and altered NF-kappaB activation in mice lacking tumor necrosis factor receptors after traumatic brain injury. J Neurosci 19:6248–6256, 1999.

33. Marshall LF, Maas AI, Marshall SB, et al: A multicenter trial on the efficacy of using tirilazad mesylate in cases of head injury. J Neurosurg 89:519–525, 1998.

34. Young B, Runge JW, Waxman KS, et al: Effects of pegorgotein on neurologic outcome of patients with severe head injury: A multicenter, randomized controlled trial. JAMA 276:538–543, 1996.

35. Love S: Oxidative stress in brain ischemia. Brain Pathol 9:119–131, 1999.

36. Clark RSB, Chen M, Kochanek PM, et al: Detection of single- and double-strand DNA breaks after traumatic brain injury in rats: Comparison of in situ labeling techniques using DNA polymerase I, the Klenow fragment of DNA polymerase I, and terminal deoxynucleotidyl transferase. J Neurotrauma 18:675–689, 2001.

37. Evan G, Littlewood T: A matter of life and cell death. Science 281:1317–1322, 1998.

38. Kaya SS, Mahmood A, Li Y, et al: Apoptosis and expression of p53 response proteins and cyclin D1 after cortical impact in rat brain. Brain Res 818:23–33, 1999.

39. Napieralski JA, Raghupathi R, McIntosh TK: The tumor-suppressor gene, p53, is induced in injured brain regions following experimental traumatic brain injury. Brain Res Mol Brain Res 71:78–86, 1999.

40. Tomasevic G, Raghupathi R, Oga M, et al: Experimental TBI in mice lacking the tumor suppression p53 gene [abstract]. J Neurotrauma 16:999, 1999.

41. Artuso M, Esteve A, Bresil H, et al: The role of the ataxia telangiectasia gene in the p53, WAF1/CIP1(p21)- and GADD45-mediated response to DNA damage produced by ionising radiation. Oncogene 11:1427–1435, 1995.

42. Miyashita T, Reed JC: Tumor suppressor p53 is a direct transcriptional activator of the human bax gene. Cell 80:293–299, 1995.

43. Berger NA: Poly (ADP-ribose) in the cellular response to DNA damage. Radiat Res 101:4–15, 1985.

44. LaPlaca MC, Raghupathi R, Verma A, et al: Temporal patterns of poly (ADP-ribose) polymerase activation in the cortex following experimental brain injury in the rat. J Neurochem 73:205–213, 1999.

45. Whalen MJ, Clark RS, Dixon CE, et al: Reduction of cognitive and motor deficits after traumatic brain injury in mice deficient in poly (ADP-ribose) polymerase. J Cereb Blood Flow Metab 19:835–842, 1999.

46. LaPlaca MC, Zhang J, Raghupathi R, et al: Pharmacologic inhibition of poly (ADP-ribose) polymerase is neuroprotective following traumatic brain injury in rats. J Neurotrauma 18:369–376, 2001.

47. Hamakubo T, Kannagi R, Murachi T, et al: Distribution of calpains I and II in rat brain. J Neurosci 6:3103–3111, 1986.

48. Wang KK: Calpain and caspase: Can you tell the difference? Trends Neurosci 23:20–26, 2000.

49. Buki A, Siman R, Trojanowski JQ, et al: The role of calpain-mediated spectrin proteolysis in traumatically induced axonal injury. J Neuropathol Exp Neurol 58:365–375, 1999.

50. Kampfl A, Posmantur R, Nixon R, et al: Mu-calpain activation and calpain-mediated cytoskeletal proteolysis following traumatic brain injury. J Neurochem 67:1575–1583, 1996.

51. Pike BR, Zhao X, Newcomb JK, et al: Regional calpain and caspase-3 proteolysis of alpha-spectrin after traumatic brain injury. Neuroreport 9:2437–2442, 1998.

52. Saatman KE, Bozyczko-Coyne D, Marcy V, et al: Prolonged calpain-mediated spectrin breakdown occurs regionally following experimental brain injury in the rat. J Neuropathol Exp Neurol 55:850–860, 1996.

53. McCracken E, Hunter AJ, Patel S, et al: Calpain activation and cytoskeletal protein breakdown in the corpus callosum of head-injured patients. J Neurotrauma 16:749–761, 1999.

54. Saatman KE, Murai H, Bartus RT, et al: Calpain inhibitor AK295 attenuates motor and cognitive deficits following experimental brain injury in the rat. Proc Natl Acad Sci U S A 93:3428–3433, 1996.

55. Saatman KE, Zhang C, Bartus RT, et al: Behavioral efficacy of posttraumatic calpain inhibition is not accompanied by reduced spectrin proteolysis, cortical lesion, or apoptosis. J Cereb Blood Flow Metab 20:66–73, 2000.

56. Saatman KE, Bareyre FM, Grady MS, et al: Acute cytoskeletal alterations and cell death induced by experimental brain injury are attenuated by magnesium treatment and exacerbated by magnesium deficiency. J Neuropathol Exp Neurol 60:183–194, 2001.

57. Buki A, Koizumi H, Povlishock JT: Moderate posttraumatic hypothermia decreases early calpain-mediated proteolysis and concomitant cytoskeletal compromise in traumatic axonal injury. Exp Neurol 159:319–328, 1999.

58. Buki A, Okonkwo DO, Povlishock JT: Postinjury cyclosporin A administration limits axonal damage and disconnection in traumatic brain injury. J Neurotrauma 16:511–521, 1999.

59. Posmantur R, Kampfl A, Siman R, et al: A calpain inhibitor attenuates cortical cytoskeletal protein loss after experimental traumatic brain injury in the rat. Neuroscience 77:875–888, 1997.

60. Verweij BH, Muizelaar JP, Vinas FC, et al: Impaired cerebral mitochondrial function after traumatic brain injury in humans. J Neurosurg 93:815–820, 2000.

61. Xiong Y, Gu Q, Peterson PL, et al: Mitochondrial dysfunction

and calcium perturbation induced by traumatic brain injury. J Neurotrauma 14:23–34, 1997.

62. Bernardi P: Mitochondrial transport of cations: Channels, exchangers, and permeability transition. Physiol Rev 79:1127–1155, 1999.

63. Albensi BC, Sullivan PG, Thompson MB, et al: Cyclosporin ameliorates traumatic brain-injury-induced alterations of hippocampal synaptic plasticity. Exp Neurol 162:385–389, 2000.

64. Okonkwo DO, Buki A, Siman R, et al: Cyclosporin A limits calcium-induced axonal damage following traumatic brain injury. Neuroreport 10:353–358, 1999.

65. Scheff SW, Sullivan PG: Cyclosporin A significantly ameliorates cortical damage following experimental traumatic brain injury in rodents. J Neurotrauma 16:783–792, 1999.

66. Sullivan PG, Thompson M, Scheff SW: Continuous infusion of cyclosporin A postinjury significantly ameliorates cortical damage following traumatic brain injury. Exp Neurol 161:631–637, 2000.

67. Riess P, Bareyre FM, Saatman KE, et al: Effects of chronic, postinjury cyclosporin A administration on motor and sensorimotor function following severe, experimental traumatic brain injury. Neurosurgery 51:1043–1052, 2002.

68. Raghupathi R, Welsh FA, Lowenstein DH, et al: Regional induction of c-fos and heat shock protein-72 mRNA following fluid-percussion brain injury in the rat. J Cereb Blood Flow Metab 15:467–473, 1995.

69. Raghupathi R, McIntosh TK: Regionally and temporally distinct patterns of induction of c-fos, c-jun and junB mRNAs following experimental brain injury in the rat. Brain Res Mol Brain Res 37:134–144, 1996.

70. Yang K, Mu XS, Xue JJ, et al: Increased expression of c-fos mRNA and AP-1 transcription factors after cortical impact injury in rats. Brain Res 664:141–147, 1994.

71. Dutcher SA, Underwood BD, Walker PD, et al: Patterns of immediate early gene mRNA expression following rodent and human traumatic brain injury. Neurol Res 21:234–242, 1999.

72. Whitfield PC, Pickard JD: Expression of the immediate early genes c-fos and c-jun after head injury in man. Neurol Res 22:138–144, 2000.

73. Herdegen T, Skene P, Bahr M: The c-jun transcription factor—bipotential mediator of neuronal death, survival and regeneration. Trends Neurosci 20:227–231, 1997.

74. Adams JH, Doyle D, Ford I, et al: Diffuse axonal injury in head injury: Definition, diagnosis and grading. Histopathology 15:49–59, 1989.

75. Gennarelli TA, Thibault LE, Adams JH, et al: Diffuse axonal injury and traumatic coma in the primate. Ann Neurol 12:564–574, 1982.

76. Maxwell WL, Povlishock JT, Graham DL: A mechanistic analysis of nondisruptive axonal injury: A review. J Neurotrauma 14:419–440, 1997; erratum in J Neurotrauma 14:755, 1997.

77. Stone JR, Singleton RH, Povlishock JT: Intra-axonal neurofilament compaction does not evoke local axonal swelling in all traumatically injured axons. Exp Neurol 172:320–331, 2001.

78. Persechini A, Cronk B: The relationship between the free concentrations of Ca^{2+} and Ca^{2+}-calmodulin in intact cells. J Biol Chem 274:6827–6830, 1999.

79. Eyer J, Leterrier JF: Influence of the phosphorylation state of neurofilament proteins on the interactions between purified filaments in vitro. Biochem J 252:655–660, 1988.

80. Pettus EH, Povlishock JT: Characterization of a distinct set of intra-axonal ultrastructural changes associated with traumatically induced alteration in axolemmal permeability. Brain Res 722:1–11, 1996.

81. Buki A, Okonkwo DO, Wang KK, et al: Cytochrome c release and caspase activation in traumatic axonal injury. J Neurosci 20:2825–2834, 2000.

82. Povlishock JT, Stone JR: Traumatic axonal injury. In Miller LP, Hayes RL (eds): Head Trauma: Basic, Preclinical, and Clinical Directions. New York, John Wiley & Sons, 2001, pp 281–302.

83. Povlishock JT, Marmarou A, McIntosh T, et al: Impact acceleration injury in the rat: Evidence for focal axolemmal change and related neurofilament sidearm alteration. J Neuropathol Exp Neurol 56:347–359, 1997.

84. Buki A, Siman R, Trojanowski JQ, et al: The role of calpain-mediated spectrin proteolysis in traumatically induced axonal injury. J Neuropathol Exp Neurol 58:365–375, 1999.

85. Koizumi H, Povlishock JT: Early posttraumatic hypothermia provides persisting axonal protection and improves behavioral outcome. Brain Res (in press).

86. Koizumi H, Povlishock JT: Posttraumatic hypothermia in the treatment of axonal damage in an animal model of traumatic axonal injury. J Neurosurg 89:303–309, 1998.

87. Marion DW, White MJ: Treatment of experimental brain injury with moderate hypothermia and 21-aminosteroids. J Neurotrauma 13:139–147, 1996.

88. Suehiro E, Singleton RH, Stone JR, et al: The immunophilin ligand FK506 attenuates the axonal damage associated with rapid rewarming following posttraumatic hypothermia. Exp Neurol 172:199–210, 2001.

89. Suehiro E, Povlishock JT: Exacerbation of traumatically induced axonal injury by rapid posthypothermic rewarming and attenuation of axonal change by cyclosporin A. J Neurosurg 94:493–498, 2001.

90. Soares HD, Hicks RR, Smith D, et al: Inflammatory leukocytic recruitment and diffuse neuronal degeneration are separate pathological processes resulting from traumatic brain injury. J Neurosci 15:8223–8233, 1995.

91. Carlos TM, Clark RS, Franicola-Higgins D, et al: Expression of endothelial adhesion molecules and recruitment of neutrophils after traumatic brain injury in rats. J Leukoc Biol 61:279–285, 1997.

92. Whalen MJ, Carlos TM, Kochanek PM, et al: Soluble adhesion molecules in CSF are increased in children with severe head injury. J Neurotrauma 15:777–787, 1998.

93. Fan L, Young PR, Barone FC, et al: Experimental brain injury induces differential expression of tumor necrosis factor-alpha mRNA in the CNS. Brain Res Mol Brain Res 36:287–291, 1996.

94. Shohami E, Novikov M, Bass R, et al: Closed head injury triggers early production of TNF alpha and IL-6 by brain tissue. J Cereb Blood Flow Metab 14:615–619, 1994.

95. Morganti-Kossman MC, Lenzlinger PM, Hans V, et al: Production of cytokines following brain injury: Beneficial and deleterious for the damaged tissue. Mol Psychiatry 2:133–136, 1997.

96. Shohami E, Bass R, Wallach D, et al: Inhibition of tumor necrosis factor alpha (TNFalpha) activity in rat brain is associated with cerebroprotection after closed head injury. J Cereb Blood Flow Metab 16:378–384, 1996.

97. Shohami E, Gallily R, Mechoulam R, et al: Cytokine production in the brain following closed head injury: Dexanabinol (HU-211) is a novel TNF-alpha inhibitor and an effective neuroprotectant. J Neuroimmunol 72:169–177, 1997.

98. Fan L, Young PR, Barone FC, et al: Experimental brain injury induces expression of interleukin-1 beta mRNA in the rat brain. Brain Res Mol Brain Res 30:125–130, 1995.

99. Taupin V, Toulmond S, Serrano A, et al: Increase in IL-6, IL-1 and TNF levels in rat brain following traumatic lesion: Influence of pre- and post-traumatic treatment with Ro5 4864, a peripheral-type (p site) benzodiazepine ligand. J Neuroimmunol 42:177–185, 1993.

100. Sanderson KL, Raghupathi R, Saatman KE, et al: Interleukin-1 receptor antagonist attenuates regional neuronal cell death and cognitive dysfunction after experimental brain injury. J Cereb Blood Flow Metab 19:1118–1125, 1999.

101. Conti AC, Raghupathi R, Trojanowski JQ, et al: Experimental brain injury induces regionally distinct apoptosis during the acute and delayed post-traumatic period. J Neurosci 18:5663–5672, 1998.

102. Newcomb JK, Zhao X, Pike BR, et al: Temporal profile of apoptotic-like changes in neurons and astrocytes following controlled cortical impact injury in the rat. Exp Neurol 158:76–88, 1999.

103. Rink A, Fung KM, Trojanowski JQ, et al: Evidence of apoptotic cell death after experimental traumatic brain injury in the rat. Am J Pathol 147:1575–1583, 1995.

104. Clark RS, Kochanek PM, Chen M, et al: Increases in Bcl-2 and cleavage of caspase-1 and caspase-3 in human brain after head injury. FASEB J 13:813–821, 1999.

105. Bredesen DE: Apoptosis: Overview and signal transduction pathways. J Neurotrauma 17:801–810, 2000.

106. Eldadah BA, Faden AI: Caspase pathways, neuronal apoptosis, and CNS injury. J Neurotrauma 17:811–829, 2000.

107. Raghupathi R, Graham DI, McIntosh TK: Apoptosis after traumatic brain injury. J Neurotrauma 17:927–938, 2000.

108. Yakovlev AG, Knoblach SM, Fan L, et al: Activation of CPP32-like caspases contributes to neuronal apoptosis and neurological dysfunction after traumatic brain injury. J Neurosci 17:7415–7424, 1997.

109. Clark RS, Kochanek PM, Watkins SC, et al: Caspase-3 mediated neuronal death after traumatic brain injury in rats. J Neurochem 74:740–753, 2000.

110. Beer R, Franz G, Srinivasan A, et al: Temporal profile and cell subtype distribution of activated caspase-3 following experimental traumatic brain injury. J Neurochem 75:1264–1273, 2000.

111. Graham SH, Chen J, Clark RS: Bcl-2 family gene products in cerebral ischemia and traumatic brain injury. J Neurotrauma 17:831–841, 2000.

112. Clark RS, Chen J, Watkins SC, et al: Apoptosis-suppressor gene bcl-2 expression after traumatic brain injury in rats. J Neurosci 17:9172–9182, 1997.

113. Nakamura M, Raghupathi R, Merry DE, et al: Overexpression of Bcl-2 is neuroprotective after experimental brain injury in transgenic mice. J Comp Neurol 412:681–692, 1999.

114. Raghupathi R, Fernandez SC, Murai H, et al: BCL-2 overexpression attenuates cortical cell loss after traumatic brain injury in transgenic mice. J Cereb Blood Flow Metab 18:1259–1269, 1998.

115. Carbonell WS, Morrison RM, Kinoshita Y, et al: Bax is necessary for hippocampal, but not cortical, neuron damage 10 minutes after traumatic brain injury [abstract]. J Neurotrauma 16:1000, 1999.

116. Bareyre FM, Raghupathi R, Saatman KE, et al: DNase I disinhibition is predominantly associated with actin hyperpolymerization after traumatic brain injury. J Neurochem 77:173–181, 2001.

117. Enari M, Sakahira H, Yokoyama H, et al: A caspase-activated DNase that degrades DNA during apoptosis, and its inhibitor ICAD. Nature 391:43–50, 1998; erratum in Nature 393:396, 1998.

118. Liu X, Zou H, Slaughter C, et al: DFF, a heterodimeric protein that functions downstream of caspase-3 to trigger DNA fragmentation during apoptosis. Cell 89:175–184, 1997.

119. Liu X, Li P, Widlak P, et al: The 40-kDa subunit of DNA fragmentation factor induces DNA fragmentation and chromatin condensation during apoptosis. Proc Natl Acad Sci U S A 95:8461–8466, 1998.

120. Zhang C, Raghupathi R, Saatman KE, et al: Regional and temporal alterations in DNA fragmentation factor (DFF)–like proteins following experimental brain trauma in the rat. J Neurochem 73:1650–1659, 1999.

121. Schallert T, Leasure JL, Kolb B: Experience-associated structural events, subependymal cellular proliferative activity, and functional recovery after injury to the central nervous system. J Cereb Blood Flow Metab 20:1513–1528, 2000.

122. Pierce JE, Smith DH, Trojanowski JQ, et al: Enduring cognitive, neurobehavioral and histopathological changes persist for up to one year following severe experimental brain injury in rats. Neuroscience 87:359–369, 1998.

123. Smith DH, Chen XH, Pierce JE, et al: Progressive atrophy and neuron death for one year following brain trauma in the rat. J Neurotrauma 14:715–727, 1997.

124. Levin HS: Neurobehavioral Recovery from Head Injury. New York, Oxford University Press, 1985, pp 281–299.

125. Jones TA: Multiple synapse formation in the motor cortex opposite unilateral sensorimotor cortex lesions in adult rats. J Comp Neurol 414:57–66, 1999.

126. Whishaw IQ: Loss of the innate cortical engram for action patterns used in skilled reaching and the development of behavioral compensation following motor cortex lesions in the rat. Neuropharmacology 39:788–805, 2000.

127. Scherbel U, Raghupathi R, Nakamura M, et al: Differential acute and chronic responses of tumor necrosis factor–deficient mice to experimental brain injury. Proc Natl Acad Sci U S A 96:8721–8726, 1999.

128. Kossmann T, Hans V, Imhof HG, et al: Interleukin-6 released in human cerebrospinal fluid following traumatic brain injury may trigger nerve growth factor production in astrocytes. Brain Res 713:143–152, 1996.

129. Penkowa M, Moos T, Carrasco J, et al: Strongly compromised inflammatory response to brain injury in interleukin-6–deficient mice. Glia 25:343–357, 1999.

130. Swartz KR, Liu F, Sewell D, et al: Interleukin-6 promotes post-traumatic healing in the central nervous system. Brain Res 896:86–95, 2001.

131. Pellerin L, Magistretti PJ: Glutamate uptake into astrocytes stimulates aerobic glycolysis: A mechanism coupling neuronal activity to glucose utilization. Proc Natl Acad Sci U S A 91:10625–10629, 1994.

132. Ridet JL, Malhotra SK, Privat A, et al: Reactive astrocytes: Cellular and molecular cues to biological function. Trends Neurosci 20:570–577, 1997.

133. Huang EJ, Reichardt LF: Neurotrophins: Roles in neuronal development and function. Annu Rev Neurosci 24:677–736, 2001.

134. Abe K: Therapeutic potential of neurotrophic factors and neural stem cells against ischemic brain injury. J Cereb Blood Flow Metab 20:1393–1408, 2000.

135. Mufson EJ, Kroin JS, Sendera TJ, et al: Distribution and retrograde transport of trophic factors in the central nervous system: Functional implications for the treatment of neurodegenerative diseases. Prog Neurobiol 57:451–484, 1999.

136. Sofroniew MV, Howe CL, Mobley WC: Nerve growth factor signaling, neuroprotection, and neural repair. Annu Rev Neurosci 24:1217–1281, 2001.

137. Gomez-Pinilla F, Cotman CW: Transient lesion-induced increase of basic fibroblast growth factor and its receptor in layer VIb (subplate cells) of the adult rat cerebral cortex. Neuroscience 49:771–780, 1992.

138. Logan A, Frautschy SA, Gonzalez AM, et al: A time course for the focal elevation of synthesis of basic fibroblast growth factor and one of its high-affinity receptors (flg) following a localized cortical brain injury. J Neurosci 12:3828–3837, 1992.

139. DeKosky ST, Goss JR, Miller PD, et al: Upregulation of nerve growth factor following cortical trauma. Exp Neurol 130:173–177, 1994.

140. Goss JR, O'Malley ME, Zou L, et al: Astrocytes are the major source of nerve growth factor upregulation following traumatic brain injury in the rat. Exp Neurol 149:301–309, 1998.

141. O'Dell DM, Raghupathi R, Crino PB, et al: Traumatic brain injury alters the molecular fingerprint of TUNEL-positive cortical neurons in vivo: A single-cell analysis. J Neurosci 20:4821–4828, 2000.

142. Dixon CE, Flinn P, Bao J, et al: Nerve growth factor attenuates cholinergic deficits following traumatic brain injury in rats. Exp Neurol 146:479–490, 1997.

143. Sinson G, Voddi M, McIntosh TK: Nerve growth factor administration attenuates cognitive but not neurobehavioral motor dysfunction or hippocampal cell loss following fluid-percussion brain injury in rats. J Neurochem 65:2209–2216, 1995.

144. Sinson G, Perri BR, Trojanowski JQ, et al: Improvement of cognitive deficits and decreased cholinergic neuronal cell loss and apoptotic cell death following neurotrophin infusion after experimental traumatic brain injury. J Neurosurg 86:511–518, 1997.

145. Ramer MS, Priestley JV, McMahon SB: Functional regeneration of sensory axons into the adult spinal cord. Nature 403:312–316, 2000.

146. Dietrich WD, Alonso O, Busto R, et al: Posttreatment with intravenous basic fibroblast growth factor reduces histopathological damage following fluid-percussion brain injury in rats. J Neurotrauma 13:309–316, 1996.

147. McDermott KL, Raghupathi R, Fernandez SC, et al: Delayed administration of basic fibroblast growth factor (bFGF) attenuates cognitive dysfunction following parasagittal fluid percussion brain injury in the rat. J Neurotrauma 14:191–200, 1997.

148. Blesch A, Grill RJ, Tuszynski MH: Neurotrophin gene therapy in CNS models of trauma and degeneration. Prog Brain Res 117:473–484, 1998.

149. Horner PJ, Gage FH: Regenerating the damaged central nervous system. Nature 407:963–970, 2000.

150. Davies SJ, Fitch MT, Memberg SP, et al: Regeneration of adult axons in white matter tracts of the central nervous system. Nature 390:680–683, 1997.

151. Letourneau PC, Condic ML, Snow DM: Interactions of devel-

oping neurons with the extracellular matrix. J Neurosci 14:915–928, 1994.

152. Pasterkamp RJ, Giger RJ, Ruitenberg MJ, et al: Expression of the gene encoding the chemorepellent semaphorin III is induced in the fibroblast component of neural scar tissue formed following injuries of adult but not neonatal CNS. Mol Cell Neurosci 13:143–166, 1999.

153. Chen MS, Huber AB, van der Haar ME, et al: Nogo-A is a myelin-associated neurite outgrowth inhibitor and an antigen for monoclonal antibody IN-1. Nature 403:434–439, 2000.

154. Goldberg JL, Barres BA: Nogo in nerve regeneration. Nature 403:369–370, 2000.

155. GrandPre T, Nakamura F, Vartanian T, et al: Identification of the Nogo inhibitor of axon regeneration as a Reticulon protein. Nature 403:439–444, 2000.

156. Fournier AE, GrandPre T, Strittmatter SM: Identification of a receptor mediating Nogo-66 inhibition of axonal regeneration. Nature 409:341–346, 2001.

157. Brosamle C, Huber AB, Fiedler M, et al: Regeneration of lesioned corticospinal tract fibers in the adult rat induced by a recombinant, humanized IN-1 antibody fragment. J Neurosci 20:8061–8068, 2000.

158. Merkler D, Metz GA, Raineteau O, et al: Locomotor recovery in spinal cord–injured rats treated with an antibody neutralizing the myelin-associated neurite growth inhibitor Nogo-A. J Neurosci 21:3665–3673, 2001.

159. Blochlinger S, Weinmann O, Schwab ME, et al: Neuronal plasticity and formation of new synaptic contacts follow pyramidal lesions and neutralization of Nogo-A: A light and electron microscopic study in the pontine nuclei of adult rats. J Comp Neurol 433:426–436, 2001.

160. Condic ML: Adult neuronal regeneration induced by transgenic integrin expression. J Neurosci 21:4782–4788, 2001.

161. Christman CW, Salvant JB Jr, Walker SA, et al: Characterization of a prolonged regenerative attempt by diffusely injured axons following traumatic brain injury in adult cat: A light and electron microscopic immunocytochemical study. Acta Neuropathol(Berl) 94:329–337, 1997.

162. Daniloff JK, Levi G, Grumet M, et al: Altered expression of neuronal cell adhesion molecules induced by nerve injury and repair. J Cell Biol 103:929–945, 1986.

163. Emery DL, Raghupathi R, Saatman KE, et al: Bilateral growth-related protein expression suggests a transient increase in regenerative potential following brain trauma. J Comp Neurol 424:521–531, 2000.

164. Gage FH: Mammalian neural stem cells. Science 287:1433–1438, 2000.

165. Arsenijevic Y, Villemure JG, Brunet JF, et al: Isolation of multipotent neural precursors residing in the cortex of the adult human brain. Exp Neurol 170:48–62, 2001.

166. Palmer AM, Marion DW, Botscheller ML, et al: Traumatic brain injury–induced excitotoxicity assessed in a controlled cortical impact model. J Neurochem 61:2015–2024, 1993.

167. Gould E, Tanapat P, McEwen BS, et al: Proliferation of granule cell precursors in the dentate gyrus of adult monkeys is diminished by stress. Proc Natl Acad Sci U S A 95:3168–3171, 1998.

168. Kempermann G, van Praag H, Gage FH: Activity-dependent regulation of neuronal plasticity and self repair. Prog Brain Res 127:35–48, 2000.

169. Dash PK, Mach SA, Moore AN: Enhanced neurogenesis in the rodent hippocampus following traumatic brain injury. J Neurosci Res 63:313–319, 2001.

170. Sinson G, Voddi M, McIntosh TK: Combined fetal neural transplantation and nerve growth factor infusion: Effects on neurological outcome following fluid-percussion brain injury in the rat. J Neurosurg 84:655–662, 1996.

171. Soares H, McIntosh TK: Fetal cortical transplants in adult rats subjected to experimental brain injury. J Neural Transplant Plast 2:207–220, 1991.

172. Soares HD, Sinson GP, McIntosh TK: Fetal hippocampal transplants attenuate CA3 pyramidal cell death resulting from fluid percussion brain injury in the rat. J Neurotrauma 12:1059–1067, 1995.

173. Muir JK, Raghupathi R, Saatman KE, et al: Terminally differentiated human neurons survive and integrate following transplantation into the traumatically injured rat brain. J Neurotrauma 16:403–414, 1999.

174. Philips MF, Muir JK, Saatman KE, et al: Survival and integration of transplanted postmitotic human neurons following experimental brain injury in immunocompetent rats. J Neurosurg 90:116–124, 1999.

175. Saporta S, Borlongan CV, Sanberg PR: Neural transplantation of human neuroteratocarcinoma (hNT) neurons into ischemic rats: A quantitative dose-response analysis of cell survival and behavioral recovery. Neuroscience 91:519–525, 1999.

176. Kondziolka D, Wechsler L, Goldstein S, et al: Transplantation of cultured human neuronal cells for patients with stroke. Neurology 55:565–569, 2000.

177. Philips MF, Mattiasson G, Wieloch T, et al: Neuroprotective and behavioral efficacy of nerve growth factor–transfected hippocampal progenitor cell transplants after experimental traumatic brain injury. J Neurosurg 94:765–774, 2001.

178. Mahmood A: Intracranial bone marrow transplantation after traumatic brain injury improves functional outcome in adult rats. J Neurosurg 94:589–595, 2001.

CHAPTER 324

Clinical Pathophysiology of Traumatic Brain Injury

MARIKE ZWIENENBERG-LEE ■ J. PAUL MUIZELAAR

Many factors contribute to the disability caused by head injury. In the past decade it has become clear that much of the neuronal damage following severe head injury does not occur instantaneously but rather evolves over several hours after impact.[1-6] Traditionally, a distinction is made between primary and secondary brain injury. Primary brain injury refers to pathologic processes that arise as an immediate and direct result of trauma. Secondary brain injury refers to cellular damage, set into motion by the initial injury, that develops over hours to days after the initial traumatic insult. Secondary injury is of particular importance to the neurosurgeon because the process is open to therapeutic intervention.

Another commonly used term is *secondary insults*.[7] This refers to factors aggravating primary or secondary injuries, such as hypoxia, hypotension, raised intracranial pressure (ICP), and cerebral ischemia. Secondary insults are common, particularly after severe head injury. Miller and colleagues developed a system to detect and quantify secondary insults.[8, 9] Variables studied were ICP, cerebral perfusion pressure (CPP), arterial blood pressure, arterial oxygenation, jugular venous oxygen saturation, and presence of pyrexia, tachycardia, and bradycardia. Severity of insult was divided into three grades. One hundred twenty-four patients with severe, moderate, and minor head injury were monitored for these insults, and 90% of them were found to have one or more insults, with 50% of patients sustaining at least one insult at the highest grade. In the severely injured group, 67 of 68 patients suffered from secondary insults, compared with 7 of 36 and 3 of 20 in the moderate and minor head injury groups, respectively. Patients studied during transport within the hospital sustained secondary insults in approximately 50% of cases. Moreover, it was found that these patients were likely to suffer from further severe insults upon return to the intensive care unit.[7] Of all the data collected, five factors were found to be consistently related to poor outcome: arterial hypotension, reduced CPP, raised ICP, hypoxemia, and pyrexia.[9]

Mortality from severe head injury has decreased slightly between 1980 and the present (Fig. 324-1). In-creased recognition of the mechanism of secondary brain injury, as well as avoidance of secondary insults to the brain by optimizing cerebral perfusion and oxygenation, is probably responsible for most of the improvement in outcome. Advances have been made predominantly in the areas of prehospital care, resuscitation, and radiologic diagnosis (i.e., rapid diagnosis of intracranial mass lesions).[10] In addition, data indicating that early and aggressive surgical and medical treatment of intracranial mass lesions, raised ICP, and decreased CPP improves outcome have been provided, although no such treatment has been tested in a randomized, controlled clinical trial, in part because of ethical considerations.[11-15] Further improvements in therapy and outcome depend largely on the attainment of a better understanding of the basic pathophysiology of head injury.

In this chapter, the pathogenesis of closed head injury and the effect of trauma on cerebral metabolism and circulation are discussed. Basic concepts of therapeutic intervention are explained. Penetrating head injury is described in Chapter 331, and specific medical and surgical management of head injury is discussed in Chapters 326 to 328.

MECHANISMS OF BRAIN INJURY

The extent and type of primary brain injury resulting from head injury depend on the physical mechanisms

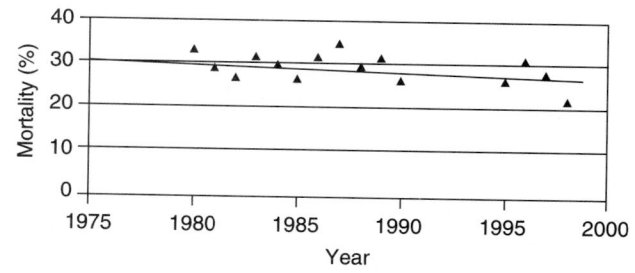

FIGURE 324-1. Mortality from severe head injury after 6 months at the Medical College of Virginia.

involved. Components include the nature of the force (contact or inertial loading), the type of injury (rotational, translational, or angular), and the magnitude and duration of the impact. A contact force to the head results when the head is prevented from moving after the impact. An inertial force occurs upon acceleration or deceleration of the head and results from differential motion of the brain relative to the skull. A contact force may initiate this type of injury.

Goldsmith defined three physical processes causing head injury[16]:

1. Collision of the head with a solid object at an appreciable velocity.
2. An impulsive load producing sudden motion of the head without significant physical contact.
3. A static or quasi-static load compressing the head with gradual force.

The first mechanism of injury causes brain injury through a combination of contact and inertial forces.[17] The second mechanism results in pure inertial loading to the head, but it is seldom the sole mechanism of injury; it may play a role in less severe head injuries, such as concussion, but it is almost always accompanied by some impact to the head in more severe head injuries.[18] The third mechanism involves a contact force, but the speed of impact is minimal or zero. The contribution of inertial forces can thus be ignored, because brain damage is caused by gradually increasing contact forces trapping the head against a rigid structure.

Contact forces result in focal injuries, either locally or remote from the impact. Examples are coup contusions and skull fractures. When the main component of inertial loading is translational acceleration, focal injuries such as contusions, intracerebral hematomas, and subdural hematomas result. When rotational acceleration is a significant component of the inertial force, concussions and diffuse axonal injury (DAI) are the result. Rotational injury is especially harmful because rotation damages not only the cortical surface but also the deep structures of the brain.

A combination of translational and rotational acceleration—angular acceleration—is the most common form of inertial injury. The mechanical and physical properties of the head and neck favor this type of injury (Fig. 324–2). The center of angulation is located in the middle or lower cervical spine, and the head's center of gravity bends around it. The magnitude of the rotational component depends on the distance between the center of gravity and the center of angulation: the smaller the distance, the larger the rotational component of angulation.[19]

Other mechanical components determining the extent of brain injury are the magnitude and duration of the injury. In an experimental model of angular acceleration, the influence of the duration of the acceleration force, the time to peak acceleration, and the magnitude of acceleration was tested. A threshold value of magnitude was established: below the threshold, the impact resulted in concussion, and above the threshold, subdural hematoma occurred.[20] The study

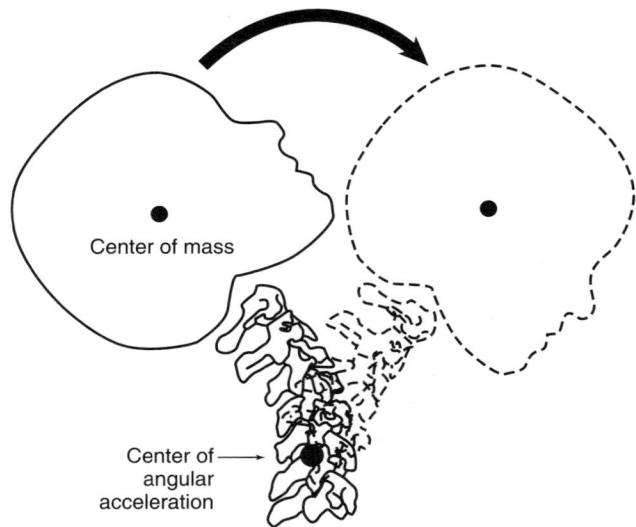

FIGURE 324–2. Mechanism of angular acceleration: Interaction of head and neck.

also revealed that a low magnitude of acceleration with a long duration resulted in DAI, due to propagation of the forces deep within the brain. In contrast, a brief, high-velocity impact resulted in tearing of superficial vessels such as the bridging veins and pial vessels, causing subdural hematoma. The former mechanism is typically seen with motor vehicle collisions, whereas the latter type of acceleration occurs in falls in which the head strikes a broad, hard surface or in assaults in which inertial loading is the predominant mechanism.[20, 21]

CLASSIFICATION OF HEAD INJURY

There are many ways to classify traumatic brain injury. Two widely used clinical methods are classification based on the severity of head injury and classification based on anatomic findings.

The Glasgow Coma Scale (GCS; Table 324–1) is universally accepted for grading the clinical severity of head injuries and other neurological causes of impaired consciousness.[22] In the era before computed tomography (CT), the scale was used to identify those patients who required contrast studies to detect intracranial collections of blood. The GCS is a valuable tool for ongoing clinical assessment and detection of neurological deterioration. A major limitation of the scale is that accurate scoring is not always possible. Today, many patients arrive in the hospital unresponsive owing to sedation and neuromuscular blockade, and the postresuscitation score cannot be determined until pharmacologic agents are actively antagonized or metabolized. In addition, intubation and orbital swelling interfere with accurate scoring. In one study, at least one component of the GCS could not be accurately scored in 38% of patients, and a GCS score could not be assigned in almost 50% of patients because of these confounding variables.[23]

TABLE 324–1 ■ Scoring System of the Glasgow Coma Scale

TEST	SCORE
Eye Opening (E)	
Spontaneous	4
To verbal command	3
To pain	2
None	1
Best Motor Response (M)	
Obeys commands	6
Localization of painful stimulus	5
Flexion-withdrawal response to pain	4
Abnormal flexion response to pain (decorticate rigidity)	3
Extension response to pain (decerebrate rigidity)	2
None	1
Best Verbal Response (V)	
Oriented conversation	5
Disoriented conversation	4
Inappropriate words	3
Incomprehensible sounds	2
None	1
Maximum Score (E + M + V)	15

A persistent misconception about the GCS, sustained by equating abnormal flexion with decorticate rigidity and extensor response with decerebrate rigidity, is that the type of motor response corresponds to the level of the lesion in the (mid) brain or brainstem, as in the Sherrington preparations.[24, 25] However, Greenberg and coworkers showed that in head injury, the GCS is related to the severity of injury at any site in the brain: absent motor response or decerebrate motor posturing can occur with severe, purely cortical, or hemispheric lesions.[26]

The head injury severity scale is based primarily on the GCS score (Table 324–2). The scale is less widely used but provides a relatively straightforward way of assessing head injury.[27]

Classification of brain injury into focal and diffuse injury (Table 324–3) is done according to anatomic criteria. The introduction of CT and magnetic resonance imaging led to the development of a system of injury classification based on neuroimaging; its main purpose is identifying risk factors associated with raised ICP, secondary deterioration, and poor outcome.

TABLE 324–2 ■ Head Injury Severity Scale

INJURY CATEGORY	GCS SCORE
Minimal	15, no loss of consciousness (LOC) or amnesia
Mild	14, or 15 plus amnesia or brief LOC or impaired alertness or memory
Moderate	9–13 or LOC ≥5 min or focal neurological deficit
Severe	5–8
Critical	3–4

Adapted from Stein S: Classification of head injury. In Narayan RK, Wilberger JE, Povlishock JT (eds): Neurotrauma. New York, McGraw-Hill, 1996, pp 31–41.

TABLE 324–3 ■ Focal versus Diffuse Injury

FOCAL INJURIES	DIFFUSE INJURIES
Contusions	Concussion
Fracture	Diffuse axonal injury
Coup	Moderate
Contrecoup	Severe
Herniation	
Intermediate	
Gliding	
Hematomas	
Epidural	
Subdural	
Intracerebral	

The National Institutes of Health Traumatic Coma Data Bank introduced a classification of head injury based on initial CT findings (Table 324–4).[28] This classification is used in clinical trials investigating new treatments for severe head injury. Eisenberg and colleagues showed a correlation between CT appearance, mortality, outcome, and frequency of raised ICP for some of the CT characteristics present after severe head injury (e.g., compression of the basal cisterns, presence of subarachnoid hemorrhage, midline shift).[29]

FOCAL AND DIFFUSE BRAIN INJURY

Intracranial lesions from a closed head injury can be categorized into focal or diffuse injuries (see Table 324–3). Focal injuries comprise the traumatic intracranial hematomas and contusions. Concussion and DAI are the components of diffuse injury.

Brain Contusion

In brain contusion, there is subpial extravasation of blood and swelling of the affected area. If the lesion

TABLE 324–4 ■ Classification of Head Injury Based on Initial Computed Tomography Findings

CATEGORY	DEFINITION
Diffuse injury I	No visible intracranial pathology
Diffuse injury II	Cisterns present with midline shift 0–5 mm and/or: Lesion densities present No high- or mixed-density lesion >25 cc May include bone fragments and foreign bodies
Diffuse injury III (swelling)	Cisterns compressed or absent with midline shift 0–5 mm; no high- or mixed-density lesion >25 cc
Diffuse injury IV	Midline shift >5 mm; no high- or mixed-density lesion >25 cc
Evacuated mass lesion	Any lesion surgically evacuated
Nonevacuated mass lesion	High- or mixed-density lesion >25 cc, not surgically evacuated

From Marshall L, Bowers S, Klauber M: A new classification of head injury based on computerized tomography. J Neurosurg 75:514–520, 1991.

is severe, the brain area may be necrotic, soft, and hemorrhagic. When the pia mater is torn, the lesion is termed a *laceration*, although the distinction between a contusion and a laceration may not be clear. Contusions usually have a characteristic distribution, affecting the frontal poles, the orbital gyri, the cortex above and below the sylvian fissures, the temporal poles, and the lateral and inferior aspects of the temporal lobes.

Fracture contusions are typically the result of direct contact injuries and underlie a skull fracture.[30] Coup contusions occur at the site of impact in the absence of a fracture; contrecoup contusions occur in the brain diametrically opposite the point of impact. Herniation contusions occur in areas where the medial parts of the temporal lobe make contact with the free edge of the tentorium, or where the cerebellar tonsils make contact at the foramen magnum. Intermediary contusions are single or multiple lesions in the deepest structures of the brain, including the corpus callosum, basal ganglia, hypothalamus, and brainstem.[31] Gliding contusions are focal hemorrhages in the cortex and the adjacent white matter of the superior margins of the cerebral hemispheres. These injuries are due to rotation, unlike the contusions mentioned earlier, which are the result of contact of the brain surface with bony protuberances.[31]

Contusion or laceration may result in focal neurological deficits, depending on the area involved. Subsequent hemorrhage, possibly related to the presence of coagulopathy, and swelling often accompany these lesions, accounting for delayed deterioration and secondary injury during the first days after the impact. Adams and colleagues developed a method of quantifying cerebral contusions in humans (the contusion index) caused by nonmissile head injury.[32, 33] They found that contusions are most severe in the frontal and temporal lobes, that there is no correlation between the severity of contusions and the nature of the injury, that contusions are more severe in patients who have a skull fracture in comparison to those who do not, that contusions are more severe in patients who do not experience a lucid interval than in those who do, and that contusions are less severe in patients with DAI than in those without DAI. In addition, they challenged the concept of contrecoup contusion as the most severe injury.

Traumatic Intracranial Hematoma

The formation of intracranial hematomas is the most important treatable cause of death and disability following head injury of any severity. The most important risk factor for the presence of an intracranial hematoma is a skull fracture (Table 324–5). In approximately half the patients with severe head injury and skull fracture, a sizable intracranial hematoma is present.[9, 34] Three types of traumatic intracranial hematomas can be distinguished: epidural, subdural, and intracerebral.

EPIDURAL HEMATOMA

Epidural hematomas result from tearing of dural or skull vessels caused by deformation of the skull or

TABLE 324–5 ■ **Relationship between Skull Fracture and Intracranial Hematoma in Patients with Severe, Moderate, and Minor Head Injury**

INJURY	HEMATOMA ON CT	NO HEMATOMA	TOTAL
Severe (GCS 8)			
Fracture	74 (44%)	94 (56%)	168
No fracture	43 (32%)*	91 (68%)	134
Moderate (GCS 9–12)			
Fracture	49 (29%)	118 (71%)	167
No fracture	25 (8%)†	299 (92%)	324
Minor (GCS 13–15)			
Fracture	42 (10%)	391 (90%)	433
No fracture	27 (1%)‡	2549 (99%)	2576
Totals	260	3542	3802

* P <0.05
† P <0.001
‡ P <0.0001.
CT, computed tomography; GCS, Glasgow Coma Scale.
Data from Miller J, Piper I, Jones P: Pathophysiology of head injury. In Narayan RK, Wilberger JE, Povlishock JT (eds): Neurotrauma. New York, McGraw-Hill, 1996, pp 61–69.

fracture (in 85% of cases). Epidural hematomas can occur at all ages but are seen primarily in patients younger than 50 years.[35–37] In published patient series, usually no more than 10% of patients are older than 50 years.[35, 38]

Acute epidural hematoma with significant mass effect is not a common complication of head injury, occurring in only about 2% of patients admitted to the hospital with any type of head injury[39] and accounting for 5% to 15% of fatal head injuries.[40] In adults, the incidence of epidural hematoma is lower than that of subdural and intracerebral hematoma. In pediatric patients, however, epidural hematoma is the most frequent post-traumatic intracranial hematoma. The abundant diploic and dural vascularization in infants and young children is thought to account for this higher incidence, notwithstanding the tight adherence of dura to the inner table of the skull.[41]

Most epidural hematomas occur over the convexity of the cerebral hemisphere, in the territory of the middle meningeal artery. Tearing of the artery due to a temporoparietal fracture of the skull results in arterial hemorrhage into the epidural space (>50% of the cases). Separation of dura and bone is thought to occur at the time of injury, with subsequent bleeding in the preformed epidural space, rather than stripping of the dura of the inner table of the skull with progressive enlargement of the clot.[42]

Zimmerman and Bilaniuk reviewed 45 patients with epidural hematomas.[43] They classified epidural hematomas into three types, based on CT criteria. Type I (acute) hematomas are characterized by a lucent "swirl" (unclotted blood) in a dense hematoma. These hematomas have been called hyperacute extradural hematomas by some. Type II (subacute) hematomas are solid clots, and type III (chronic) hematomas are mixed-density or lucent hematomas with a contrast-enhanced membrane. In type I hematomas (58%), the interval between trauma and CT was less than 24 hours (most within 2 to 8 hours); in type II hematomas (31%), between 12 hours and 4 days; and in type III hematomas (11%), 7 to 20 days.

The classic clinical course of a patient harboring an epidural hematoma, first described by Jacobson in 1886,[44] is an initial loss of consciousness after trauma, followed by recovery (lucid interval), and then (as the blood clot enlarges) a rapid progression of neurological symptoms: obtundation, contralateral hemiparesis, ipsilateral oculomotor nerve paresis, decerebrate rigidity, arterial hypertension, cardiac arrhythmias, respiratory disturbances, and, finally, apnea and death. The development of these symptoms is dependent on the size of the hematoma[45] and the presence of associated intracranial lesions.[46, 47] Patients who are in coma from the time of impact are more likely to have signs of DAI.[46, 48] The presence of associated intradural lesions affects outcome: Haselsberger and colleagues demonstrated that patients with a pure epidural outcome fared significantly better than those with associated intradural lesions; 70% and 44% of patients, respectively, had a good recovery.[49]

A significant proportion of the morbidity and mortality of epidural hematomas is due to delayed diagnosis and treatment, which is often attributed to a so-called atypical presentation. However, epidural hematomas more often present in atypical rather than typical fashion (i.e., the triad of a lucid interval, contralateral hemiparesis, and dilatation of the ipsilateral pupil). For example, the "lucid interval," which is described in many textbooks as a typical or classic presentation of epidural hematoma, occurs in only 14% to 21% of cases and may also be found in patients harboring subdural hematomas[50] or in patients with mild head injuries complicated by meningitis. In another series of 80 consecutive cases of epidural hematoma, the incidence of a lucid interval was far less than 20%; only five cases were described.[36] Patients exhibiting the classic lucid interval usually have pure epidural hematomas with higher hematoma volumes and CT signs of active bleeding.[45, 51] In summary, between 8% and 24% of patients have no loss of consciousness, 23% to 44% are unconscious from the time of injury, 20% to 28% regain consciousness after a brief coma, and 14% to 21% of patients who were initially awake deteriorate into coma.[35, 37, 52–54]

The "classic" contralateral hemiparesis results from direct pressure on the underlying motor cortex and is seen only with epidural hematomas occurring in the frontotemporal region (70% to 80% of cases).[37, 55] Hemiparesis, however, may also be ipsilateral and occurs when the opposite cerebral peduncle is pressed against the tentorial edge, classically called Kernohan's notch. In contrast, patients with frontal or occipital clots present with drowsiness followed directly by bilateral decerebrate rigidity rather than contralateral hemiparesis. Dilatation of the ipsilateral pupil, the last component of the classic triad, occurs in less than 50% of cases.[51, 56, 57]

Epidural hematomas in the posterior fossa are a rare finding. Of all post-traumatic intracranial mass lesions, only 5% are found in the posterior fossa.[58, 59] Of these, epidural hematomas are the most prevalent.[60, 61] Epidural hematomas in the posterior fossa deserve particular attention because these patients may remain conscious until late in the evolution of the hematoma and then suddenly lose consciousness, become apneic, and die. In addition, these hematomas often extend into the supratentorial compartment, thereby stripping the dura overlying the transverse sinus, which may be a difficult-to-handle source of bleeding.[9]

SUBDURAL HEMATOMA

Subdural hematomas may be of venous or arterial origin. Most frequently, these hematomas result from the tearing of a bridging vein between the cerebral cortex and a draining venous sinus. Subdural hematomas are usually classified as acute, subacute, or chronic, but there is no uniformity of nomenclature.[31, 62, 63] Attempts to age the hematomas histologically have been unsuccessful. In general, a subdural hematoma is classified as acute when the hematoma is composed of clot and blood (up to 48 hours after injury), as subacute when there is a mixture of clotted blood and fluid (between 2 and 14 days after injury), and as chronic when the hematoma is fluid (usually >14 days after injury)[31] (Table 324–6). Subdural hematomas may also be classified based on the time they become clinically evident after injury. In that case, an acute subdural hematoma is less than 3 days old, a subacute subdural hematoma is 3 to 21 days old, and a chronic subdural hematoma is more than 21 days old. CT can also provide another classification: acute hematomas are hyperdense, subacute hematomas are hyper- to isodense, and chronic hematomas are hypodense with respect to the adjacent brain.

Acute Subdural Hematoma

Fifty percent to 60% of acute post-traumatic hematomas are subdural hematomas. The average age of patients harboring subdural hematomas is greater than the age of patients with epidural hematomas. Acute subdural hematomas are twice as common after injuries that involve a sudden movement of the head, such as falls or assaults, than after injuries caused by more gradual movement, such as motor vehicle collisions.[38] In a study of pure acute subdural hematomas, it was found that in 72% of patients, head injury was produced by a fall or assault, and in only 24% was the

TABLE 324–6 ■ **Classification of Subdural Hematomas**

TYPE	DAYS AFTER INJURY	CONSISTENCY
Acute	0–2	Clot and blood
Subacute	2–14	Mixture of clotted and fluid blood
Chronic	>14	Fluid blood

cause a motor vehicle collision.[20] Acute subdural hematoma may also occur (sometimes after relatively minor trauma) in patients given anticoagulants and in those with coagulopathies.[64, 65]

Most acute subdural hematomas result from venous vascular injury that is produced by strain forces at the brain surface. Two distinct varieties exist.[66] The first type of hematoma, produced by contact forces, is associated with contusions or lacerations. The hematoma is the result of bleeding from a small vessel into the subdural space and is most common at the temporal pole. The complex of subdural hematoma and damaged and necrotic brain is termed *burst lobe*. The second type of hematoma is located over the cerebral convexity and is produced by inertial forces tearing the bridging veins.[20, 66] The underlying brain damage in this type of injury is usually milder than that in the first type. Extremely rapid deterioration, as in the case of classic epidural hematoma, may accompany these lesions, especially when there is surface artery rupture. Despite the relatively minor underlying brain damage, the speed of hematoma development is usually so rapid that unless the hematoma is rapidly evacuated,[67] the prognosis for these patients is not much better than for those in the first group.

Cerebral ischemia is an important component of brain injury caused by subdural hematoma. Postmortem studies have shown signs of ischemic damage in two thirds of the patients who died from subdural hematoma.[68] Ischemic damage has also been found in experimental subdural hematoma.[69] The mechanism and onset of ischemic damage remain elusive. Brain compression by the hematoma, resulting in impairment of the microcirculation, may be an important component. In a small series of five patients with acute subdural hematomas and low GCS scores (≤ 5), Verweij and colleagues found ICP between 40 and 80 mm Hg, CPP between 10 and 60 mm Hg, low jugular venous oxygen saturation (40% to 60%), and low cerebral blood flow (CBF) measured with laser Doppler immediately before hematoma evacuation.[70] All these values became more normal with removal of the bone flap, opening of the dura, and actual hematoma removal. Evidence of brain compression resulting in ischemia was reported by Schroder and colleagues[71]; in two patients with acute subdural hematomas, preoperative CBF was in the ischemic range (<18 mL/100 g per minute), and cerebral blood volume (CBV) was approximately half of normal, with recovery to more normal values immediately after surgery.

Even after operative decompression, the prognosis of subdural hematoma is still poor in many cases. It is thought that the coexisting brain damage (DAI, contusion, laceration) is mainly responsible for the poor outcome. In a subset of patients, however, compression of the microcirculation and resulting low CBF may explain the poor clinical condition and outcome. Patients who deteriorate after a lucid interval (i.e., patients who "talk and die") are likely candidates for this process of injury.[71] The resulting ischemia without (severe) physical brain damage may explain why timely clot evacuation (within 4 hours) results in much better outcome than does delayed hematoma removal.[72]

Chronic Subdural Hematoma

The presentation and pathophysiology of chronic subdural hematoma are quite different from those of acute subdural hematoma. Neurological symptoms and brain dysfunction are purely the result of brain compression, because there is usually no trauma causing significant primary injury or initiating secondary injury. Tanaka and colleagues suggested that chronic subdural hematomas might induce neurological dysfunction primarily through mechanical distortion of central brain regions such as the thalamus, with a secondary influence on remote regions due to transneural depression.[73] Their findings revealed that the effect of subdural hematoma on CBF and ICP is not a major cause of neurological dysfunction. These hematomas typically occur in the elderly, the very young, or those with prior brain atrophy. They usually evolve over weeks, and sometimes only minor previous head injury is noted; in many cases, no history of head injury can be obtained. Precipitating factors are chronic alcoholism, epilepsy, coagulopathy, and the use of anticoagulants.

In most cases, chronic subdural hematoma results from tearing of a bridging vein. The predilection of bridging veins to be disrupted in the subdural rather than the subarachnoid space is thought to be due to the lack of outer reinforcement of the bridging veins there. In the subdural space, the veins lack the support of the arachnoid trabeculae and are thus more fragile. The initial subdural hemorrhage is small in most cases and, owing to the venous origin of the hematoma, is not usually associated with a sudden or steep increase in ICP. In addition, the wide sulci and atrophic brain allow for some enlargement before the onset of significant neurological symptoms. In acute subdural hematoma, displacement of the brain resulting in a midline shift greater than 10 mm is usually associated with elevated ICP, often greater than 50 mm Hg. In patients suffering from chronic subdural hematoma, however, normal pressure has been observed in the presence of a midline shift as large as 20 mm. Owing to the slow expansion of the hematoma, the period of spatial compensation is probably long enough to cause considerable distortion of the brain before there is a significant rise in ICP.

Membrane formation around the hematoma is a characteristic feature of chronic subdural hematoma and is thought to be due to a nonspecific inflammatory response of the highly vascular inner dural layer to the presence of blood products, fibrin, and fibrin degradation products in the subdural cavity.[74] The avascular arachnoid has a much lower reaction potential than the inner dural layer. Consequently, the inner capsule of a chronic subdural hematoma has no significant vascularization.[75]

Secondary enlargement of a chronic subdural hematoma is common. The precise cause of this enlargement is unknown. Gardner proposed that the membrane around the hematoma acts as an osmotic membrane, with cerebrospinal fluid (CSF) diffusing into the hyperosmotic hematoma.[76] Zollinger and Gross also proposed an osmotic mechanism for enlargement of the hematoma.[77] They thought that flow across the membrane was the result of an increase of osmotic pressure from a breakdown of hemoglobin molecules in red cells. Weir, however, could not find a significant increase in osmolality of the hematoma with increasing age, nor were there any significant differences between the osmolality of blood and hematoma.[78] Sato and Suzuki used light and electron microscopy to examine the capsules of chronic subdural hematomas in 33 cases and found that in patients with neurological deficits, capillary endothelial cells in the capsule had many cytoplasmic protrusions and fenestrations, suggesting high permeability of the capillary wall.[79] Observations of Yamashima and Yamamoto revealed that gap junctions frequently form between adjacent endothelial cells.[80] Numerous blood components, including red blood cells and plasma, can be seen squeezing or spilling into the interstitial space of the outer membrane. It is no longer thought that an osmotic mechanism plays a significant role in hematoma enlargement. Either repeated microhemorrhages from the neocapillary network in the outer membrane or abnormally high vascular permeability is thought to be responsible for hematoma enlargement.[75, 81]

INTRACEREBRAL HEMATOMA

Intracerebral hematomas account for approximately 20% of all intracranial hematomas.[82] The hematomas are usually associated with extensive lobar contusions, from which they are often indistinguishable.[83, 84] The amount of blood in a lesion determines whether the lesion is classified as a hematoma or a contusion. If blood accounts for at least two thirds of the lesion, it is classified as an intracerebral hematoma. The remaining lesions are described as disrupted tissue with areas of microscopic hemorrhage.[85] A hemorrhagic mass should be considered an intracerebral hematoma when there is a homogeneous collection of blood with relatively well-defined margins. Multiple intracerebral hematomas are found in approximately 20% of cases.[86]

Intracerebral hematomas are caused primarily by direct rupture of intrinsic cerebral vessels (a small parenchymal artery in most cases) and therefore often arise from contusions. The hematomas tend to form in the inferior frontal and temporal lobes, as do most cerebral contusions.[58, 82, 83, 87, 88] In about 2% of cases, the hematoma is located within the basal ganglia and the internal capsule. Intracerebral hematomas are commonly seen in head injuries in which force is applied to the head over a small area, such as missile injuries, perforating wounds, and depressed skull fractures.[89] In a series of 400 consecutive cases of civilian depressed skull fracture, 28 patients harboring intracranial hematomas were found. Sixty-one percent of these hematomas were intracerebral.[90] Patients on long-term anticoagulant therapy are at increased risk of developing intracerebral hematomas, even after mild head injury.[89]

Diffuse Brain Injury

Diffuse brain injury is the most common type of head injury. There are several gradations of diffuse brain injury (see Table 324–3). They form a continuum that ranges clinically from concussion to persistent post-traumatic coma.[91]

CONCUSSION

Concussion is the mildest form of diffuse injury and is thought to be due to rotational acceleration of the head, in the absence of significant contact injury. A classic cerebral concussion results in a transient loss of consciousness followed by a rapid return to a normal state of alertness. However, repeated concussion may result in permanent neurological impairment.[92] The pathophysiology of concussion is not as well understood as that of DAI. Cairns related the disturbances of consciousness to lesions in the brainstem and diencephalon.[93] However, more recent investigations suggest that injury almost never occurs exclusively in the brainstem; in most cases, the cerebral hemispheres are affected as well.[94]

DIFFUSE AXONAL INJURY

DAI results from more severe angular or rotational acceleration. Shear and tensile forces acting on the axons during acceleration and deceleration are thought to cause this type of injury. DAI is believed to be responsible for the severely impaired neurological function in patients without gross parenchymal contusions, lacerations, or hematomas. It was first described by Strich in 1956, who reported a series of patients with severe post-traumatic dementia and found "diffuse degeneration of the white matter."[95] Subsequently, this injury has been referred to as shearing injury, diffuse damage to the white matter of the immediate-impact type, and diffuse white matter shearing injury, but DAI is the preferred description.[3, 94, 96–98]

DAI is most often associated with coronal or lateral acceleration injury, which produces the most severe DAI.[99] Acceleration in the oblique plane is also associated with DAI, but the injury is usually less severe. Sagittal acceleration only occasionally produces DAI.

Histologic findings consist of axonal swelling, disruption of the axons, "retraction balls" (the swollen proximal ends of the severed axons), and punctate hemorrhages in the pons, midbrain, and corpus callosum.[100] Many of these abnormalities, including axonal severing, are not present initially but develop over the course of several hours or days after injury.[101] In some cases it is difficult to distinguish axonal damage resulting from the initial shearing of the axons from damage caused by the subsequent biochemical and metabolic processes. Evidence from animal studies has revealed that axonal injury is often secondary or delayed, and there is some confirmation of this in humans.[101, 102] These findings have important implications for treatment: delayed severing due to biochemical cascades may be prevented with pharmacologic treatment

T A B L E   3 2 4 – 7 ▪ **Neuropathologic Classification of Diffuse Axonal Injury**

GRADE	LOCALIZATION OF LESION
I	Axonal injury of parasagittal white matter of cerebral hemispheres
II	Grade I plus focal lesion in corpus callosum
III	Grade II plus focal lesion in cerebral peduncle

From Adams JH, Doyle D, Ford I, et al: Diffuse axonal injury in head injury: Definition, diagnosis and grading. Histopathology 15:49–59, 1989.

after the injury, whereas nothing can be done to prevent anatomic damage from the initial mechanical "snapping."

Punctate hemorrhages, or Strich hemorrhages, are usually associated with severe DAI.[100] They occur in the area of maximal acceleration force on the brain and result from rupture of small cerebral vessels. Strich hemorrhages are most commonly found in the corpus callosum, walls of the third ventricle (hypothalamus, columns of the fornix, and anterior commissure), internal capsule, basal ganglia, dorsolateral brainstem, and superior cerebellar peduncles.

The extent and location of axonal injury are important determinants of functional recovery. Adams and colleagues used a primate model of traumatic brain injury and developed a grading system of DAI based on neuropathologic findings (Table 324–7).[3] A higher grade of DAI is related to deeper and more prolonged coma, as well as more severe residual deficit.

TRAUMATIC SUBARACHNOID HEMORRHAGE AND CEREBRAL VASOSPASM

The centripetal theory of Ommaya and Gennarelli holds that lesion depth is dependent on the force of injury.[103] Accordingly, traumatic subarachnoid hemorrhage (SAH) results from relatively severe injury to the brain: High angular acceleration of long duration is necessary to produce a strain that causes rupture of the superficial vessels in the subarachnoid space, especially at the base of the skull.

SAH is common after severe head injury. In a study from the National Institutes of Health Traumatic Coma Databank, it was identified in 39% of 753 patients with severe head injury.[29] This, however, is almost certainly an underestimate, because the resolution of neuroimaging has improved since the databank report. The occurrence of cerebral arterial spasm (vasospasm) after severe head injury has long been recognized.[104] It is thought that intradural bleeding that extends into the CSF spaces (subarachnoid, intraventricular, and subdural hemorrhage) plays a role in the pathogenesis of post-traumatic arterial spasm.[105] The distribution of traumatic SAH, as visualized on CT, is different from the distribution seen after aneurysmal SAH. Unlike aneurysmal SAH, traumatic SAH is not limited to cis-

terns surrounding the circle of Willis but extends to supratentorial regions and interhemispheric fissures. In addition, CT-detected SAH disappears very early with the traumatic type and more gradually with the aneurysmal type.[106]

Vasospasm can be demonstrated by either cerebral angiography or transcranial Doppler ultrasonography and occurs in approximately 25% to 40% of patients with head injury.[105] Similar to aneurysmal SAH–associated vasospasm, the arteries typically affected by post-traumatic vasospasm are the large cerebral arteries, such as the supraclinoid internal carotid artery, middle cerebral artery, anterior cerebral artery, and basilar artery. The time course of traumatic SAH–associated vasospasm also resembles that of aneurysmal vasospasm, first occurring 2 or more days after injury, peaking about 2 weeks after injury, and resolving after 3 weeks.

Pathophysiologically, vasospasm is an important post-traumatic secondary insult. Macpherson and Graham found a significant correlation between angiographic arterial narrowing and postmortem ipsilateral ischemic hemispheric damage.[104] In addition, several studies of severely head-injured patients showed low CBF values in combination with increased transcranial Doppler velocities, indicating that vasospasm is associated with impaired cerebral perfusion.[107, 108] However, Fukuda and colleagues reported that unlike aneurysmal SAH, in which all low-density areas on computed tomographic scans corresponded to vascular territories, low-density areas in patients with traumatic SAH were rarely associated with vascular territories. Instead, the low-density areas contained deep-seated or gliding contusions.[106] As discussed in detail later, vasospasm of the large intracranial arteries is accompanied by an increase in CBV, due to compensatory dilatation of the vessels in the microcirculation. Reduced CBF in the presence of increased CBV thus supports the diagnosis of large artery spasm. Schroder and colleagues simultaneously evaluated early CBF and CBV in seven patients with severe head injury.[109] These patients were selected from a larger series of 51 patients because they exhibited both nonischemic and ischemic (CBF <18 mL/100 g per minute) areas on stable xenon-CT measurements. Both CBF and CBV were significantly lower in the ischemic zones, indicating that in the early phase after injury, compromise of the microvasculature is the cause of ischemia, rather than vasospasm of the larger conductance vessels. No simultaneous studies have been performed at a later stage (i.e., when the highest incidence of vasospasm is expected).

In an earlier study, Martin and colleagues, using CBF and transcranial Doppler measurements, identified three different circulatory stages after severe head injury: phase I (hypoperfusion), phase II (hyperemia), and phase III (vasospasm).[108] The following parameters were evaluated (Table 324–8): CBF; transcranial Doppler velocity in the middle cerebral artery; hemispheric index, calculated as the ratio of middle cerebral artery and internal carotid artery velocity; arteriovenous oxygen difference ($AVDO_2$); and cerebral metabolic rate of oxygen ($CMRO_2$). Phase I occurs on the day of injury

TABLE 324-8 ■ **Circulatory Phases after Severe Head Injury**

PHASE	DAYS AFTER INJURY	CBF (ML/100 G/MIN)	AVDO₂ (VOL %)	CMRO₂ (ML/100 G/MIN)	V(MCA) (CM/SEC)	HI
Hypoperfusion	0	Low (32.2 ± 2)	Normal (5.4 ± 0.5)	Depressed (1.77 ± 0.18)	Normal (56.7 ± 2.9)	Normal (1.67 ± 0.11)
Hyperemia	1–3	Relatively increased (46.8 ± 3)	Decreased (3.8 ± 0.1)	Depressed (1.49 ± 0.82)	Increased (86 ± 3.7)	Normal/increased (2.41 ± 0.1)
Vasospasm	14–15	Decreased (35.7 ± 3.8)	Increased (5.9 ± 0.1)	Depressed (1.46 ± 0.65)	Increased (96.7 ± 6.3)	Increased (2.87 ± 0.22)

AVDO₂, arteriovenous difference of oxygen; CBF, cerebral blood flow; CMRO₂, cerebral metabolic rate of oxygen; HI, hemispheric index; V(mca), middle cerebral artery velocity.

(day 0) and is defined by a low CBF, normal middle cerebral artery velocity, normal hemispheric index, and normal AVDO₂. The CMRO₂ is approximately 50% of normal during this phase and remains depressed during the second and third phases. In phase II (relative hyperemia phase, days 1 to 3), CBF increases, AVDO₂ falls, middle cerebral artery velocity rises, and hemispheric index remains less than 3. In phase III (vasospasm phase, days 4 to 15), there is a fall in CBF, a further increase in middle cerebral artery velocity, and a pronounced rise in the hemispheric index.

The cause of post-traumatic vasospasm is unknown. Mechanisms similar to those in aneurysmal SAH–associated vasospasm are thought to be involved. Recent research in aneurysmal SAH–associated vasospasm suggested an important role for endothelium and its mediators.[110–120] Endothelium-mediated hyperreactivity of vascular smooth muscle due to a release of endothelins or an imbalance between the production of endothelium-derived relaxing factor (EDRF) and prostacyclin, on the one hand, and endothelium-derived contracting factors (endothelins and thromboxane A₂), on the other hand, may play a pivotal role in traumatic SAH–associated vasospasm.

INTRAVENTRICULAR HEMORRHAGE

As many as 25% of patients with severe head injury have intraventricular hemorrhage (IVH). The occurrence of IVH usually requires a very large force to the head and is generally a sign of severe head injury. Occasionally, IVH after mild head injury is reported.[121] The severity of the injury is reflected in the poor prognosis. Of the 32 patients with traumatic IVH studied by Hashimoto and colleagues, 20 died.[122] Intraparenchymal and basal ganglia hemorrhages are frequently accompanied by hemorrhage that continues into the ventricles.[123, 124]

Postmortem examination of 32 patients revealed that primary IVH (IVH in the absence of major intraparenchymal hemorrhage as revealed on CT) is most often caused by tearing of a subependymal vein in the fornix, septum pellucidum, or choroid plexus.[122] Tearing of the subependymal veins is thought to occur through the generation of a negative pressure when an impact along the sagittal diameter of the skull deforms the

skull by increasing the minor axis, increasing ventricular diameter.[123]

Acute hydrocephalus is uncommon after traumatic IVH. LeRoux and colleagues reported that only 4 of 43 patients with traumatic IVH required ventricular drainage for acute hydrocephalus.[124]

NORMAL PHYSIOLOGY OF CEREBRAL METABOLISM AND CIRCULATION

Disturbances of CBF and metabolism appear to play an important role in aggravating brain injury. Head injury interferes with both the supply and the metabolic conversion of substrates, which are well matched under normal circumstances.

Cerebral Metabolism

Cell metabolism involves the consumption of adenosine triphosphate (ATP) during work and the ensuing consumption of metabolic substrates to resynthesize ATP from adenosine diphosphate (ADP). ATP is generated in both cytosol (via glycolysis) and mitochondria (via oxidative phosphorylation).

Glucose is the sole energy substrate of the brain, unless there is ketosis. The presence of oxygen determines whether glucose is metabolized aerobically or anaerobically. Under normal circumstances, 95% of the energy requirement of the brain comes from the aerobic conversion of glucose to water and carbon dioxide (CO_2). ATP generation is highly efficient: glycolysis and subsequent oxidative phosphorylation result in the generation of 38 molecules of ATP for each molecule of glucose:

$$1 \text{ glucose} + 6 \text{ O}_2 + 38 \text{ ADP} + 38 \text{ Pi} \rightarrow$$
$$6 \text{ CO}_2 + 44 \text{ H}_2\text{O} + 38 \text{ ATP}$$

In the absence of oxygen, conversion of glucose takes place by anaerobic glycolysis, but energy production is much less efficient: two molecules of ATP and two molecules of lactate are generated for each molecule of glucose:

$$1 \text{ glucose} + 2 \text{ ADP} + 2 \text{ Pi} \rightarrow 2 \text{ lactate} + 2 \text{ ATP}$$

Two terms are common in reference to metabolic

turnover of glucose and oxygen: the cerebral metabolic rate of oxygen ($CMRO_2$) and the cerebral metabolic rate of glucose (CMRG). Under normal circumstances, in awake adults the $CMRO_2$ is approximately 3.3 mg/100 g brain per minute[125] and the CMRG is 5.5 mg/100 g per minute.[126] The lactate-oxygen index (LOI) is sometimes used as a measure of the ratio of the amount of glucose metabolized anaerobically to the amount metabolized aerobically ($LOI = -AVDL/AVDO_2$), although it does not accurately reflect the stoichiometry of glucose metabolism. AVDL is the arteriovenous difference of lactate, and $AVDO_2$ is the arteriovenous difference of oxygen.[126] Both are calculated by subtracting the jugular venous blood content ($SjvO_2$) from the systemic arterial blood content (SaO_2), followed by a correction for hemoglobin oxygen carrying capacity in the latter ($AVDO_2 = [SaO_2 - SjvO_2] \times 1.34 \times Hb + [PaO_2 - PjvO_2] \times 0.0031$).[127] In addition, Bergsneider and colleagues recently proposed a metabolic ratio ($MR = CMRO_2/CMRG$) to compare the amount of oxygen versus glucose utilization. CMRG was obtained by 2-fluoro-2-deoxy-D-glucose (FDG)–positron emission tomography. Reference values of metabolism are summarized in Table 324–9. The global arteriovenous difference of glucose (AVDG) has been estimated at 9.6 mL/dL[127] but requires careful interpretation because reliable AVDG values are difficult to obtain; the absolute AVDG value is near or within the accuracy limits of plasma glucose levels of most clinical laboratories.[128]

Of the total energy generated, 50% is used for interneuronal communication, generation, release, and uptake of neurotransmitters (synaptic activity); 25% is used for maintenance and restoration of ion gradients across the cell membrane; and the remaining 25% is used for molecular transport, biosynthesis, and other as yet unidentified processes.[129, 130] Most of the energy generated is consumed by neurons. Glial cells that make up almost 50% of the brain have a much lower metabolic rate than neurons and account for less than 10% of total cerebral energy expenditure.[130] Compared with other organs, the metabolic demand of the brain is high; the brain accounts for only 2% to 3% of total body weight and does not do any mechanical work, yet it receives 20% of all cardiac output.

TABLE 324–9 ■ **Normal Values of Parameters of Cerebral Metabolism and Circulation in Healthy Adults**

PARAMETER	VALUE
$CMRO_2$	3.3 ± 0.4 mL/100 g/min
CBF (mixed [sub] cortical flow)	54 ± 12 mL/100 g/min
$AVDO_2$	6.7 ± 0.8 mL/dL
CMRG	5.5 ± 1.1 mg/100 g/min
AVDG	9.6 ± 1.7 mL/dL
LOI	0.06 ± 0.03
MR	0.49 ± 0.07 mg O_2/mg glucose

AVDG, arteriovenous difference of glucose; $AVDO_2$, arteriovenous difference of oxygen; CBF, cerebral blood flow; CMRG, cerebral metabolic rate of glucose; $CMRO_2$, cerebral metabolic rate of oxygen; LOI, lactate-oxygen index; MR, metabolic ratio.

Regulation of Cerebral Blood Flow

The reserves of glucose and glycogen within the astrocytes of the brain are limited, and there is no significant storage capacity for oxygen. Therefore, the brain depends on a continuous blood flow to supply the glucose and oxygen it requires. In general, substrate availability is determined by three factors: concentration of substrate in blood, flow volume, and rate of substrate passage across the blood-brain barrier. The brain possesses several mechanisms to ensure substrate availability, both under normal circumstances and at times of physiologic stress.

Usually the brain is able to maintain an adequate supply of substrates by regulation of CBF. CBF increases with vasodilatation and decreases with vasoconstriction. Caliber changes take place mainly in the so-called cerebral resistance vessels (i.e., arterioles with a diameter of 30 to 300 μm).[131] Control of CBF by adjustments in vessel caliber is commonly referred to as *autoregulation* of blood flow.[132] In humans, several mechanisms, active under different circumstances, have been described.

METABOLIC AUTOREGULATION

CBF is functionally coupled to cerebral metabolism, changing proportionally with increasing or decreasing regional or global metabolic demands. Thus, the brain is able to precisely match local CBF to local metabolic needs. Because 95% of the energy in the normal brain is generated by oxidative metabolism, $CMRO_2$ is considered a sensitive measure of cerebral metabolism. The relation between CBF and metabolism is expressed in the Fick equation: $CMRO_2 = CBF \times AVDO_2$. Global $CMRO_2$ is thus obtained by multiplying global CBF by global $AVDO_2$.

In general, the brain responds to alterations in metabolism by changes in flow and thus has a tendency to keep $AVDO_2$ relatively constant. Examples of increasing metabolic demand are seizures and fever, when a proportional increase in CBF is observed. Decreased metabolic demand, and consequently diminished CBF, is observed in the case of anesthesia or deep coma.

PRESSURE AUTOREGULATION

Another important physiologic property of the cerebral circulation is the maintenance of a constant supply of substrates at the level set by metabolism. According to Poiseuille's equation, $CBF = k (CPP \times d^4)/(8 \times l \times v)$, in which k is constant, CPP is cerebral perfusion pressure, d is vessel diameter, l is vessel length, and v is blood viscosity. Changes in CPP (i.e., arterial hypotension or increases in ICP) will be followed by changes in CBF unless diameter regulation takes place. This type of autoregulation is termed *pressure autoregulation* and is the type of autoregulation referred to in most papers on autoregulation after head injury.

In humans, the limits of pressure autoregulation range from 40 to 150 mm Hg of perfusion pressure.

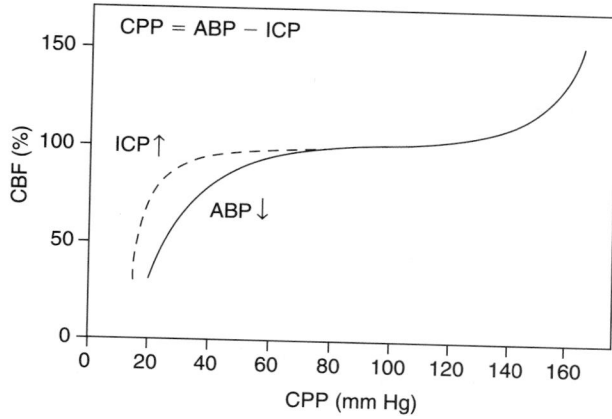

FIGURE 324–3. Pressure autoregulation in humans.

Beyond these limits, vessel caliber follows flow passively, leading to collapse of vessels at low pressure and forced dilatation, or *pressure breakthrough*, at high pressures (Fig. 324–3).

It has been suggested that defining autoregulation as constancy of CBF in spite of changes in CPP may be too strict, because under normal circumstances, small changes in CBF occur during CPP changes, even within the limits of autoregulation. Therefore, it may be more appropriate to define autoregulation in terms of cerebrovascular resistance (CVR)—that is, the change in CVR (calculated as CPP/CBF) that occurs in response to a given change in CPP.[133] Pressure autoregulation is considered intact if $0 < \Delta\% \text{ CPP}/\Delta\% \text{ CVR} < 2$.[134–136]

VISCOSITY AUTOREGULATION

According to Poiseuille's equation, CBF can vary with changes in the viscosity of blood. Blood viscosity changes with variations in hematocrit, gamma globulin, and fibrinogen components of plasma protein. Increased viscosity increases CVR $(8 \times 1 \times v/d^4)$. By means of diameter adjustment (viscosity autoregulation), CVR is decreased, and CBF can be kept constant.

THEORIES ON AUTOREGULATION

It is not clear what mechanism couples regional CBF to regional metabolism, nor are the exact mechanisms behind pressure and viscosity autoregulation known. It is likely that a similar mechanism is involved in all three types of autoregulation, but this has not yet been unraveled. Recently, the vascular endothelium has received much attention in both pressure and metabolic autoregulation, and investigators have been able to elucidate some of the underlying mechanisms.

Vasoactive metabolites released from the active nerve cell are thought to be responsible for metabolic coupling. This concept is already more than a century old. As early as 1890, Roy and Sherrington stated, "The chemical products of cerebral metabolism contained in the lymph, which bathes the walls of the arterioles of the brain, can cause variations in the caliber of the cerebral vessels. In the reaction the brain possesses an intrinsic mechanism by which its vascular supply can be varied locally in correspondence with local variations of functional activity."[136a] The identity of these vasoactive agents is not known. Agents that are directly influenced by local energy metabolism, such as CO_2, H^+, O_2, adenosine, and the ions K^+ and Ca^{2+}, have been proposed.[131, 137, 138] However, there are problems with each of these compounds as a sole factor.[130]

The vascular endothelium plays an important role in maintaining the normal physiologic function of the blood vessel wall by releasing relaxing and contracting factors. EDRF–nitric oxide (NO) is the primary mediator of endothelin-dependent relaxation.[139] The role of EDRF-NO in autoregulation is controversial.[140, 141] Most authors think that its main role is maintenance of basal CBF. Garthwaite and colleagues showed, however, that EDRF-NO may mediate a functional coupling of metabolism and CBF in certain types of neural activation.[142] They found that glutamate activation of the *N*-methyl-D-aspartate (NMDA) receptor causes a calcium-dependent release of a substance with properties similar to that of EDRF-NO. The observed vasodilatation after glutamate activation was inhibited by administration of both an NMDA antagonist and an NO synthase inhibitor, suggesting coupling of neuronal activation and CBF through EDRF-NO release.

Goadsby and colleagues simultaneously studied cerebral neuronal activity and local blood flow in cats by the induction of spreading depression (a wave of depolarization).[143] Neuronal activity and CBF in the parietal cortex were measured simultaneously. It was found that intravenous administration of *N*G-nitro-L-arginine methyl ester (1-NAME), a potent NO synthase inhibitor, resulted in a complete blockade of the hyperemia associated with spreading depression but did not cause a change in either resting cell firing or spreading depression–evoked increases in firing rate.

The observation that removal of the endothelium in canine femoral arteries significantly reduced the contractions generated in response to various vasoconstrictors and hypoxia was the first indication that endothelium mediates not only relaxation of the underlying smooth muscle but also vasoconstriction. Evidence accumulated over the years has established a central role for endothelium-dependent vasoconstriction in both peripheral and cerebral circulation. The observation that rapid elevation of transmural pressure triggers vasoconstriction (Bayliss effect) and that this response is prevented by removal of the endothelium led to the idea that pressure autoregulation may be endothelium mediated.[144, 145] Two major endothelium-derived contracting factors can be identified: thromboxane A_2 and endothelin.[141]

Martainez-Orgado and colleagues evaluated the influence of endothelial factors on pressure autoregulation in a recent study.[146] Middle cerebral arteries from 3- to 4-day-old piglets were cannulated, and diameter changes after transmural pressure variation were measured. Segments with endothelium showed vasodilatation during pressure decrease and vasoconstriction during pressure increase. Segments without endothelium responded passively to pressure change. Their results suggested an endothelium-dependent autoregulatory mechanism, with involvement of NO and K-Ca channels in vasodilatation during transmural pressure decrease and mediation of vasoconstriction by endothelin-1 (through endothelin A receptors) and prostanoids during pressure increase.

CARBON DIOXIDE REACTIVITY

Vascular caliber and CBF are also responsive to changes in arterial CO_2, a mechanism commonly referred to as CO_2 reactivity. CBF changes 2% to 3% for each mm Hg of $PaCO_2$, within the range of 20 to 60 mm Hg. Hypercarbia (hypoventilation) results in vasodilatation and higher CBF, and hypocarbia (hyperventilation) results in vasoconstriction and lower CBF. Autoregulation is a compensatory or adaptive response, adjusting CBF to metabolism, but CO_2 reactivity is fundamentally different. With CO_2 variation, vessel caliber changes and CBF follow passively. The vessels respond not to changes in $PaCO_2$ but to the pH in the perivascular space. CO_2 can cross the blood-brain barrier freely, thus changing the pH. But over 20 to 24 hours, with a constant new level of $PaCO_2$, the pH in blood and the perivascular space and the diameter of cerebral blood vessels return to baseline.[147] With CO_2 reactivity, changes in CBF are compensated for by changes in $AVDO_2$, so that a constant supply of substrates is maintained at the level set by metabolism ($CMRO_2$). In contrast, a constant $AVDO_2$ is a common feature of metabolic, pressure, and viscosity autoregulation; CBF is tuned to metabolism, and therefore $AVDO_2$ can be kept constant.

Cerebral Blood Flow and Cerebral Blood Volume

Alterations in vascular caliber not only affect the perfusion of the brain but also cause a change in the total intravascular blood volume, or CBV. CBV is considered a major determinant of ICP. The relationship between CBF and CBV can be characterized by the equation $CBV = CBF \times MTT$, in which MTT is the mean transit time of the blood through the cerebral vasculature.

CBV is determined by the diameter of the vascular bed; with increasing diameter, CBV increases, and vice versa. Vessels with a diameter between 30 and 300 μm, due to their relatively large number and fairly large size, probably contain most of the intracranial blood volume. Caliber alterations in these vessels take place mainly in the arterioles (200 μm). The diameter of the venules remains more or less constant.[131]

CEREBRAL CIRCULATION AND METABOLISM AFTER SEVERE HEAD INJURY: MECHANISMS OF SECONDARY INJURY

Traumatic and ischemic brain injury sets into motion a destructive cascade of neurochemical processes. Key features of this cascade are increased anaerobic energy generation, release of excitatory amino acid neurotransmitters and oxygen free radicals, and derangement of ion homeostasis, particularly that of calcium.

The effect of severe head injury on cerebral metabolism and circulation is complex and not completely understood. Certain basic concepts can be recognized, however, and these are discussed in the following paragraphs.

Disturbances of Cerebral Metabolism

The $CMRO_2$ in comatose patients is typically reduced from a normal value of 3.2 mL/100 g per minute to between 1.2 and 2.3 mL/100 g per minute. ATP generation from oxidative metabolism is impaired by either low supply (low CBF or hypoxia) or dysfunctional processing (mitochondrial failure). Under these circumstances, ATP is generated from glucose by the anaerobic glycolytic pathway. Parameters of increased anaerobic conversion are lactate production and an increased metabolic ratio ($MR = CMRG/CMRO_2$) or LOI, or hyperglycolysis. Evidence of hyperglycolysis occurring after severe head injury has been provided in several animal studies, and Bergsneider and colleagues identified post-traumatic hyperglycolysis in six patients with severe head injury.[128, 148–152]

Cerebral acidosis occurs frequently after severe head injury. Many investigators have found increased tissue and CSF lactate concentrations in patients with severe head injury. Although lactic acid is a by-product of anaerobic glycolysis, it may have some protective effect. Acidosis shifts the oxygen dissociation curve to the right, so that oxygen can be extracted more completely from hemoglobin. In addition, acidosis optimizes the pH for glycolysis and causes vasodilatation of blood vessels, thereby maximizing the available (collateral) blood flow. Despite these potential protective effects, functional recovery of tissue in the presence of high lactate and H^+ levels is usually poor. The exact cause of cellular damage due to the accumulation of lactate is still unknown. Mechanisms may be intracellular pH decrease, electrolyte disturbances, and delayed reversal of decreased CBF.[153, 154] Lactic acidosis may also denature vital proteins.[155]

In the past, increased anaerobic glycolytic turnover was attributed mainly to impaired oxygen supply. This idea was supported by the work of Vink and colleagues, who investigated mitochondrial function after severe head injury and found it unaffected.[156] However, they used a calcium-free medium in these experiments. More recent investigations in both experimental animals and head-injured patients suggest that mitochondrial function is impaired after severe head injury, which may explain the observed decrease in $AVDO_2$ and increase in anaerobic glycolytic turnover. However, findings that the initial increases in CSF lactate return to normal 12 hours after injury (i.e., before the onset of relative hyperemia and low $AVDO_2$) argue that the most common cause of CSF lactic acidosis is still cerebral ischemia.[157] It is thought that the mitochondrial damage is calcium mediated and that calcium interferes with mitochondrial respiratory chain–linked functions.

Disturbances of Cerebral Blood Flow

CEREBRAL ISCHEMIA

Ischemia, defined as CBF that is inadequate to meet the metabolic demands of the brain, is an important mechanism of secondary injury in patients with severe head injury. Ischemic brain damage is common; in autopsy findings of patients who died after severe head injury, histologic damage indicative of cerebral ischemia was seen in 80% of cases.[158] Bouma and colleagues found ischemia (defined as CBF <18 mL/dL with high AVDO$_2$ values) in 20% to 33% of patients with severe head injury within 4 to 12 hours of injury.[159] Ischemia was associated with a poor prognosis. Of the intracranial lesions, acute subdural hematoma and diffuse cerebral swelling were most often associated with ischemia. Experimental data suggest that the brain becomes more vulnerable to ischemia after a head injury, whereas similar ischemic insults are well tolerated under normal circumstances.[2] Common metabolic and biochemical derangements or abnormal neurotransmitter-receptor interactions, which reach a lethal threshold when the insults are combined, may explain this increased vulnerability.[138]

Under circumstances of declining CBF (due to failure of pressure autoregulation or severe hypotension), the brain can initially protect itself from ischemia and maintain metabolic supply by increasing extraction of the required oxygen from the available blood flow. Clinically, this results in an increased AVDO$_2$. Maximal oxygen extraction capacity is reached when AVDO$_2$ is approximately double its normal value ($\pm$13 mL/100 mL).[138] When CBF declines further, neuronal dysfunction occurs. Initially, this results in reduction of synaptic function (50% of the energy expenditure of the brain), but further lowering of CBF causes membrane failure, sodium-potassium pump arrest, cell swelling and dysfunction, and finally cell death. In an ischemia-occlusion model, the CBF threshold at which these changes occur was 18 mL/100 g per minute.[160] After severe head injury, however, it is more likely to be 20 mL/100 g per minute.[161] The resultant cell damage depends on both the duration and the amount of CBF depression (Fig. 324–4).

Ischemic, dysfunctional, and irreversibly damaged brain can also be defined in terms of CBF, AVDO$_2$, and CMRO$_2$. Langfitt and Obrist suggested three hypothetical states of brain dysfunction after head injury: brain regions that are irreversibly damaged, brain regions that are dysfunctional, and ischemic brain (Table 324–10).[162]

IMPAIRED CEREBROVASCULAR REACTIVITY

It is generally thought that cerebrovascular reactivity and autoregulation are disturbed after severe head injury. It should be mentioned that this may not always apply, and may not apply equally, to the different

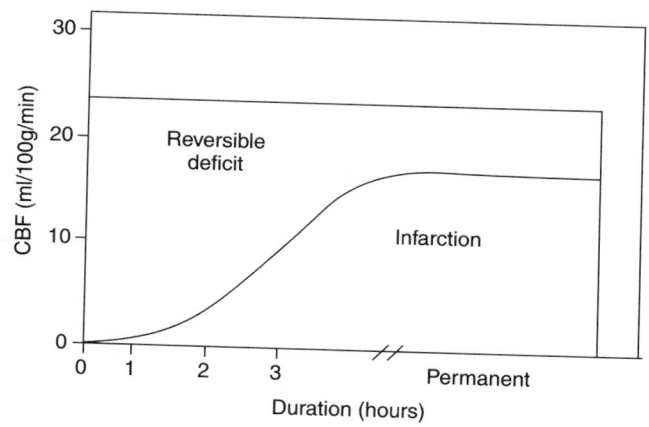

FIGURE 324–4. Cerebral blood flow and neuronal dysfunction.

mechanisms of cerebrovascular regulation.[138] In clinical studies of CBF, disturbed vascular reactivity is usually confined to certain areas and is not a generalized phenomenon.[163–166] Moreover, preserved CO$_2$ reactivity in the presence of impaired pressure autoregulation has frequently been observed, a phenomenon sometimes referred to as dissociation of CO$_2$ reactivity and pressure autoregulation.[163, 167, 168]

Metabolic Autoregulation

In comatose patients, CMRO$_2$ is typically reduced from a normal value of 3.3 mL/100 g per minute to approximately 2.1 mL/100 g per minute.[169] This is not always accompanied by a proportional decrease in CBF (metabolic coupling). In many studies in both adults and children, it has been found that CMRO$_2$ and CBF are uncoupled after severe head injury, particularly in the first 24 hours after injury.[136, 170–172] Normal metabolic coupling is maintained in approximately 45% of those suffering severe head injury.[171]

Uncoupling of CBF and CMRO$_2$ occurs when CBF exceeds CMRO$_2$, a phenomenon termed *luxury perfusion* or *hyperemia*. Obrist and colleagues defined luxury perfusion or hyperemia in comatose head-injured patients as CBF greater than 33 mL/100 g per minute; CBF between 33 and 55 mL/100 g per minute represents relative hyperemia, and CBF greater than 55 mL/100 g per minute is absolute hyperemia.[171] These limits were based on findings that in patients with GCS scores between 3 and 7 after acute head injury, CMRO$_2$

TABLE 324–10 ■ **Three Hypothetical States of Brain Dysfunction Following Head Injury**

FUNCTIONAL STATE	CBF	AVDO$_2$	CMRO$_2$
Irreversible damage	Low	Low	Very low
Dysfunctional but recoverable tissue	Low	Normal	Low
Ischemic brain	Low	High	Low

AVDO$_2$, arteriovenous difference of oxygen; CBF, cerebral blood flow; CMRO$_2$, cerebral metabolic rate of oxygen.

is approximately half of normal (i.e., 1.6 mL/100 g per minute), so a CBF value more than half normal suggests uncoupling of metabolism and flow. Absolute hyperemia has been defined as a value more than 2 standard deviations above the mean CBF found in head-injured patients. Likewise, an AVDO$_2$ value less than 4 has been considered a threshold value for uncoupling, with CBF exceeding metabolic demand. Hyperemia is thought to be most prevalent between 1 and 5 days after injury.[173, 174]

Pathophysiologically, the concept of hyperemia is important, particularly because a relationship among hyperemia, increased ICP, and diffuse cerebral swelling has been suggested.[171, 175] These studies were based on CBF (not CBV) determinations, and owing to the complex relationship between CBF and CBV, CBF may not accurately reflect CBV. In more recent work by Bouma and coworkers, CBV was significantly increased in a number of patients with increased ICP (>20 mm Hg). However, increased CBV was not consistently found in patients with CT evidence of diffuse swelling, suggesting that apart from vascular engorgement, other factors (cytotoxic edema) must play a role.[176] Yet in patients with acute subdural hematoma, raised ICP, and cerebral ischemia, CBV was actually half its normal value, arguing against the vascular engorgement explanation for severely increased ICP with acute trauma. Also, in pediatric head injury, it has been found that hyperemia may be a less common cause of increased ICP and diffuse cerebral swelling than previously thought.[177]

It should be noted that luxury perfusion is defined in terms of oxidative metabolism (CMRO$_2$). Based on the above-mentioned studies, and because "normal" cerebral metabolism is primarily oxidative in nature, it has been assumed that total cerebral metabolism is depressed after severe head injury. In fact, CBF is functionally coupled to CMRG.[178, 179] Therefore, increased CBF is not necessarily "luxury" but may occur in response to increased glucose turnover or hyperglycolysis and should thus be considered an appropriate response.[128, 180] As suggested by Bergsneider and colleagues, the metabolic state of the brain should be defined differentially in terms of glucose and oxygen metabolism.[128] This is particularly important, because certain therapeutic modalities, such as hyperventilation, may affect "luxury" CBF that is not in fact luxury but essential for ATP generation.

Pressure Autoregulation

Several authors have investigated pressure autoregulation after severe head injury.[136, 167, 168, 181, 182] Enevoldsen and Jensen found that autoregulation is usually intact during the first few days after head injury and is temporarily dysfunctional, with no apparent effect on outcome.[167] Another study found that pressure autoregulation was always intact during the first 36 hours and absent in 50% of patients between 36 and 96 hours after injury.[168] Overgaard and Tweed related autoregulatory capacity to clinical outcome and found that patients had a better outcome when autoregulation was

intact during the first week after injury. However, no such correlation could be found after the first week of injury.[181]

Bouma and colleagues performed autoregulation tests in 117 severely head-injured patients.[182] The tests consisted of xenon-133 CBF measurements before and after the administration of phenylephrine (an α-adrenergic agonist that does not affect cerebral vessels)[183–185] to increase mean arterial blood pressure or trimethaphan camsylate (a ganglion blocker without effect on cerebral vessels)[186] to decrease mean arterial blood pressure. Autoregulation was defined as intact if the percent change in CBF per percent change in CVR was between 0 and 2.[134–136] A total of 158 autoregulation tests were performed on 117 adult patients. Autoregulation was intact in 51% of the patients, but no specific temporal pattern or relation to clinical status could be determined.

The cause of defective pressure autoregulation is unknown. Based on a clinical study, it has been suggested that brainstem lesions damaging a brainstem autoregulatory center may be responsible.[167] Muizelaar and colleagues studied multimodality evoked potentials in severely head-injured children and could not find a relation between the status of autoregulation and the site of the lesion as indicated by multimodality evoked potential abnormalities.[136] Autoregulation was defective in 15 of the 37 children studied.

Endothelial damage may be responsible for the perturbation of pressure autoregulation. In experimental brain injury, endothelial lesions are often present with severe ischemia or trauma.[187] Oxygen radicals that are generated after injury may in part cause the endothelial damage.[188, 189] Impairment of vascular reactivity can be prevented by the administration of oxygen radical scavengers.[190, 191]

Viscosity Autoregulation

Few studies have specifically evaluated the status of viscosity autoregulation after severe head injury.[192, 193] The phenomenon known as viscosity autoregulation was first suggested by Muizelaar and coworkers following observations in cats.[194] In a subsequent study in humans, they evaluated the response of CBF to bolus administration of mannitol. In the group with intact pressure autoregulation, 5 of 28 patients showed a more than 10% increase in CBF following mannitol administration. In the group with defective pressure autoregulation, CBF increased by more than 10% of baseline in 11 of 14 patients. Thus, in a total of 16 of 42 cases (38%), viscosity autoregulation appeared to be defective. ICP decreased by more than 10% in 24 of 28 (86%) in the first group and in only 5 of 11 (36%) in the second group (Table 324–11).[135] These findings suggest a close correlation between the response of CBF and ICP to mannitol and the status of viscosity autoregulation. Regardless, the response is always beneficial.

Carbon Dioxide Reactivity

CO$_2$ reactivity is usually preserved after severe head injury. It may be low early after injury, but in most

TABLE 324–11 ■ Changes in Intracranial Pressure (ICP) and Cerebral Blood Flow (CBF) Larger than 10% of Baseline after Mannitol Administration

RESPONSE	AUTOREGULATION INTACT		AUTOREGULATION DEFECTIVE	
	Number	Percent	Number	Percent
Decreased ICP	24	86	5	36
Decreased CBF	5	18	11	79
No. of cases	28		14	

Data from Muizelaar JP, Lutz HA, Becker DP: Effect of mannitol on ICP and CBF and correlation with pressure autoregulation in severely head-injured patients. J Neurosurg 61:700–706, 1984.

cases, it returns to a normal 3% change per mm Hg CO_2 by 24 hours after injury.[167, 168, 171, 181, 195–197] In experimental studies, temporarily reduced CO_2 reactivity has been observed, but it returns to normal within a few hours.[198] Patients with severely impaired CO_2 reactivity usually die or are left with severe neurologic deficits.[171, 181] The pathologic mechanisms leading to disturbed CO_2 regulation are poorly understood. Free radicals may play a role; it has been shown in a cat model that the administration of free radical scavengers prevents loss of vasoresponsivity following injury.[198]

Marion and colleagues determined CO_2 vasoresponsivity in 17 patients with severe closed head injuries using stable xenon-enhanced CT.[173] Hemispheric, lobar, basal ganglia, and midbrain CBF values before and after P_{CO_2} reduction were used to determine CO_2 reactivity. CO_2 reactivity was expressed as the percent change in CBF per mm Hg P_{CO_2}. These authors reported similar findings of global CO_2 reactivity, but more importantly, they found that regional CO_2 reactivity was different from global reactivity in at least one area in all but one patient. In some cases, the difference was as large as 50%, particularly in patients with subdural hematomas or diffuse cerebral contusions. These findings have important clinical implications that are discussed later.

Cerebral Blood Flow, Cerebral Blood Volume, Arteriovenous Difference in Oxygen, and Autoregulation

The status of autoregulation determines the effect of certain treatment modalities, particularly those used to control ICP or CPP. As discussed previously, CBF is influenced by vascular diameter, blood viscosity, and CPP, whereas CBV is determined by vascular diameter only. With this in mind, alterations in CBF, CBV (ICP), and $AVDO_2$ in response to a variety of physiologic and pathologic conditions can be understood (Table 324–12). A decrease in cerebral metabolism results in a coupled decrease in CBF obtained by vasoconstriction (metabolic autoregulation). CBV decreases because of reduced vascular diameter, and $AVDO_2$ remains constant because CBF is tuned to metabolic demand ($CMRO_2 = CBF \times AVDO_2$). A reduction in CPP (mean

arterial blood pressure − ICP) leads to compensatory vasodilatation, or pressure autoregulation, when the latter mechanism is intact. CBF thus remains the same, but CBV increases because of the larger vascular diameter. Again, metabolism and CBF are matched, and $AVDO_2$ stays the same. In the third situation, CPP decreases under circumstances of defective autoregulation. In this scenario, CBF and CBV follow the decrease in perfusion pressure passively. $AVDO_2$ increases, because CBF is no longer adequate to meet the metabolic demand. A reduction of blood viscosity, as obtained with mannitol administration, results in vasoconstriction (intact viscosity autoregulation), reduced CBV, unchanged or slightly increased CBF, and normal $AVDO_2$. When this mechanism is defective, however, reduced blood viscosity does not induce a vascular response: CBF increases, CBV remains the same, and $AVDO_2$ decreases. Hypocapnia leads to a reduction in CBV due to vasoconstriction, and this has been the rationale for the use of hyperventilation to control ICP. However, owing to the vasoconstriction, CBF is also decreased and accompanied by increased oxygen extraction ($AVDO_2$) when CBF is insufficient to meet the metabolic demand. In the last example, the differential effect of large artery vasospasm on macro- and microcirculation is illustrated. When the large arteries are narrowed because of vasospasm, compensatory vasodilatation of the microcirculation may occur in response to the reduced perfusion pressure, thereby leading to high CBV in the presence of normal or reduced CBF.

Raised Intracranial Pressure

Raised ICP is a common complication of severe head injury and constitutes one of the main treatment problems. Approximately 50% of patients with intracranial mass lesions and up to 33% of those with diffuse injuries have persistently high ICP.[199] Sustained ICP elevation is usually associated with a poor progno-

TABLE 324–12 ■ Status of CBF, CBV, and $AVDO_2$ under Various Clinical Conditions

FEATURE WITH PRIMARY REDUCTION	CBF	CBV (ICP)	$AVDO_2$
$CMRO_2$ (within physiological limits)	⇓	⇓	=
CPP (autoregulation intact)	=	⇑	=
CPP (autoregulation defective)	⇓	⇓	⇑
Blood viscosity (autoregulation intact)	=	⇓	=
Blood viscosity (autoregulation defective)	⇑	=	⇓
$Paco_2$ (hyperventilation)	⇓	⇓	⇑
Large cerebral artery diameter (cerebral vasospasm)	⇓	⇑	⇑

$AVDO_2$, arteriovenous difference of oxygen; CBF, cerebral blood flow; CBV, cerebral blood volume; $CMRO_2$, cerebral metabolic rate of oxygen; CPP, cerebral perfusion pressure.

sis.[199–202] Mortality from severe head injury is related to the level of ICP elevation.[203]

By definition, ICP is the CSF pressure, which in turn is defined as the pressure that must be exerted against a needle introduced into the CSF space to prevent the escape of fluid.[204] Four parameters describe the static and dynamic CSF pressure: (1) the rate of CSF production, (2) the variable compliance given by the exponential relationship of CSF pressure to volume, (3) the outflow resistance, and (4) the intradural sinus pressure.[205]

The Monro-Kellie doctrine states that the total volume of the intracranial contents (CBV, CSF, and brain parenchyma) is constant. An increase in one of the three compartments must be accompanied by an equal decrease in one of the other compartments; otherwise, ICP will increase.[206–207a] As long as these volume compensations are sufficient, ICP remains relatively constant (compensated state), in the range of 8 to 10 mm Hg above the atmospheric level.[208] However, at a certain volume, this volume-buffering capacity is exhausted, resulting in an exponential pressure rise with any further volume addition (Fig. 324–5). Marmarou and coworkers noted that when this curve is plotted on a semilogarithmic scale, a straight line is the result (Fig. 324–6).[205] The slope of this line is defined as the pressure-volume index (PVI) and represents the amount of volume that must be added to or withdrawn from the craniospinal axis to increase or decrease ICP 10-fold:

$$PVI = \Delta V \div (\log ICPi/ICPo)$$

Change in volume is represented by ΔV, ICPo is the pressure before volume change, and ICPi is the pressure after volume change. Thus, PVI is a measure for the compliance ($\Delta V/\Delta P$) or tightness of the brain. Brain compliance can be estimated by injecting or withdrawing small quantities of fluid into or from the CSF space with simultaneous recording of ICP. This involves repeated injections of 2 to 3 mL in the CSF space, usually through lumbar infusion.

The normal PVI is 26 ± 4 mL[209]: 26 mL of volume raises ICP from 1 to 10 mm Hg, but the same volume also raises ICP from 10 to 100 mm Hg. Conversely, a change in volume of only 6.4 mL is required to increase ICP from 10 mm Hg (normal) to the treatment threshold of 20 mm Hg, indicating the sensitivity of ICP to

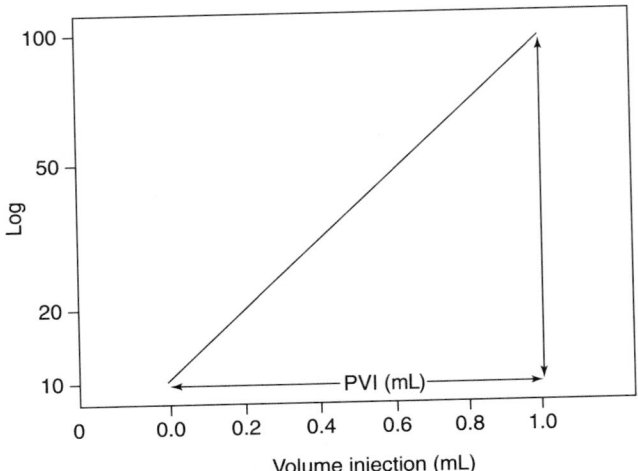

FIGURE 324–6. Relation between pressure and volume plotted on a semilogarithmic scale.

volume changes.[210, 211] Another measure of brain compliance is the volume-pressure ratio (VPR). The VPR describes the slope of the pressure-volume curve at a given level of ICP and is defined as the change in ICP achieved by a 1-mL bolus addition of CSF volume.[212, 213] The relationship with PVI under steady-state circumstances is as follows: $VPR = Po/(0.434\ PVI)$.[214]

The precise sequence of events leading to ICP elevation and the exact contribution of each of the components remain elusive. The following five pathways of intracranial volume increase were distinguished by Marmarou[214]: (1) CSF system, (2) CBV, (3) blood-brain barrier damage–associated edema (vasogenic edema), (4) neurotoxic edema, and (5) ischemic edema.

CSF components (CSF resistance to outflow and absorption) account for approximately one third of ICP elevation. This component can increase substantially in patients with SAH owing to increased outflow resistance as a result of blockage of the arachnoid villi. The remaining two thirds is attributed to a vascular component: increased blood volume (pathway 2) and increased tissue water (vasogenic, neurotoxic, and ischemic edema—pathways 3, 4, and 5).[215] Neurotoxic and ischemic edema are thought to be of cellular origin. Edema due to blood-brain barrier damage is thought to be of extracellular origin.

CBV is determined by the total diameter of the cerebrovascular bed. The cerebral veins contain most of the total blood volume, but their diameter and volume are relatively constant. Approximately 20 mL of blood (i.e., one third the total CBV) is located in the cerebral resistance vessels (15 to 300 μm). Because most autoregulatory and CO_2-dependent diameter variations take place in these vessels, CBV is determined mainly by their diameter. Typically, the diameter varies between 80% and 160% of baseline, resulting in volume changes between 64% and 256% of baseline. With a baseline CBV of 20 mL in the resistance vessels, CBV ranges from 13 mL (maximal vasoconstriction) to 51 mL (maximal vasodilatation). Given a PVI of 26, a change from maximal vasoconstriction to maximal va-

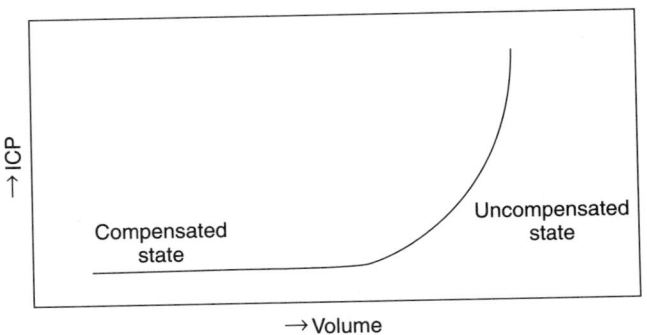

FIGURE 324–5. The exponential pressure-volume curve.

sodilatation would be accompanied by an almost 29-fold change in ICP, if other regulatory mechanisms (CSF outflow) were no longer operant.

Klatzo categorized cellular edema into neurotoxic and ischemic edema.[215a] Ischemic edema is thought to be related primarily to the disturbance of cellular osmoregulation that results from ionic pump failure. Neurotoxic edema is thought to be caused by excessive release of excitatory amino acids, loss of calcium and potassium homeostasis, and generation of free radicals.

In a series of experiments at the Medical College of Virginia, Barzo and colleagues investigated the role of vasogenic and cellular edema in a rodent model of diffuse brain injury. Using diffusion-weighted magnetic resonance imaging to determine the apparent diffusion coefficient and T1 sequencing to map total brain water, they found a biphasic development of vasogenic and cellular edema. The apparent diffusion coefficient increased with vasogenic edema and decreased with cytotoxic edema. Initially (i.e., in the first 40 minutes), an increase in the apparent diffusion coefficient was observed, consistent with an increase in extracellular fluid. This increase in extracellular volume is thought to be the result of blood-brain barrier compromise. Total water content was increased slightly 1 hour postinjury. Forty to 60 minutes postinjury, however, the apparent diffusion coefficient started to decrease, reaching a minimum in the second week after injury. Total brain water remained increased. These results suggest delayed intracellular fluid accumulation or cellular edema. No distinction between neurotoxic and ischemic edema could be made.

Secondary Displacement of the Brain

Any discrete, expanding intracranial mass lesion can lead to brain herniation or shift of brain tissue through existing rigid openings in the dura and skull, thereby causing brain compression and raised ICP. Displacement of the brain by expanding lesions and raised ICP are important mechanisms of secondary injury. Brain herniation occurs in five major patterns, and each is associated with a more or less specific clinical pattern (Table 324–13).[89]

SUBFALCINE (CINGULATE) HERNIATION

Mass lesions in the anterior or middle fossa may result in herniation of the cingulate gyrus under the free edge of the falx cerebri. Usually this is asymptomatic. If the herniation is severe, however, the pericallosal arteries may be compressed, resulting in unilateral or bilateral frontal infarcts in their region of distribution. Clinically, this may result in paresis of one or both legs.

LATERAL (UNCAL) TENTORIAL HERNIATION

Uncal herniation is caused by mass lesions in the lateral middle fossa or temporal lobe that displace the medial edge of the uncus and hippocampal gyrus medially over the ipsilateral edge of the tentorium cerebelli. The uncus and the hippocampus thus herniate in the space between the midbrain and the tentorial edge, resulting in compression of the midbrain from side to side and elongation of its anterior-posterior diameter. The ipsilateral cerebral peduncle and the oculomotor nerve are compressed, resulting in the classic syndrome of uncal herniation, which consists of contralateral hemiparesis, decreased consciousness (possibly due to distortion or deafferentation of the upper part of the reticular-activating system), and ipsilateral pupillary dilatation. In some cases, the herniation may cause compression of the contralateral cerebral peduncle against the tentorium and result in ipsilateral hemiparesis (Kernohan's notch). In these cases, the contralateral oculomotor nerve may also be stretched.

Ritter and colleagues recently suggested that a decrease in brainstem blood flow may be a cause of mydriasis after severe head injury.[216] They performed CBF measurements in the brainstems of 162 patients with severe head injuries and correlated these findings with pupillary responses. In patients with bilateral nonreactive pupils, the brainstem blood flow was significantly lower than that in patients with responsive pupils. The role of compression cannot be ruled out based on these data, and third nerve or brainstem compression may be the primary mechanism of mydriasis in many cases. However, the most important finding is that pupil dilatation may be an indicator of

TABLE 324–13 ■ **Sites of Brain Herniation Structures Involved, and Resulting Clinical Symptoms**

SITE OF HERNIATION	STRUCTURES INVOLVED	CLINICAL SYMPTOMS
Subfalcine (cingulate)	Cingulate gyrus Pericallosal arteries	Leg weakness
Lateral (uncal)	Oculomotor nerve Cerebral peduncle Posterior cerebral artery	Ptosis Ipsilateral mydriasis Contralateral hemiparesis Decreased consciousness
Posterior (tectal)	Superior colliculi	Bilateral ptosis Upward gaze paralysis
Central (axial)	Perforating branches from basilar artery	Depressed consciousness Impaired eye movement
	Midbrain, pons, medulla Reticular formation	Respiratory irregularity, apnea Hypertension Bradycardia
Tonsillar	Medulla	Apnea

brainstem ischemia and should be treated accordingly (i.e., rapid restoration of CPP and CBF).

POSTERIOR (TECTAL) HERNIATION

Posterior or tectal herniation may occur in patients who have purely frontal or occipital lesions or in those who have bilateral lesions, such as bilateral chronic subdural hematoma. Under these circumstances, the medial temporal structures do not herniate in between the tentorium and midbrain; rather, they herniate posteriorly or on both sides, thereby compressing the quadrigeminal plate at the level of the superior colliculi. Clinically, this results in findings resembling Parinaud's syndrome. The patient has bilateral ptosis and upward gaze paralysis in the presence of an initially preserved pupillary response.

CENTRAL (AXIAL) HERNIATION

Central or axial herniation is defined as a downward shift of the entire brainstem toward the foramen magnum. Because of this downward herniation, the brainstem is elongated in its anterior-posterior diameter, and stretching of the central perforating branches of the basilar artery may occur. This stretching is thought to produce ischemia and hemorrhage, the latter occasionally resulting from reversal of the displacement by operative decompression. Impaired consciousness has been related to this axial displacement. The Cushing response (arterial hypertension, bradycardia, and respiratory irregularity) has also been related to brainstem ischemia. However, brainstem blood flow is not always decreased in the presence of a Cushing response.[217] Moreover, so-called Cushing variant responses (tachycardia or systolic hypotension with absence of the classic Cushing triad) should not give one a false sense of security in the presence of posterior fossa lesions.

TONSILLAR HERNIATION

Prolapse of the cerebral tonsils through the foramen magnum can occur with either supra- or infratentorial masses or with generalized increased ICP. Tonsillar herniation causes obliteration of the cisterna magna and compression of the medulla oblongata, the latter resulting in apnea. The shape and size of the tentorial opening determine whether signs of tentorial or tonsillar herniation predominate with supratentorial mass lesions. When the opening is small, major symptoms are usually tentorial in nature; when the opening is large, tonsillar herniation may occur without any preceding signs of tentorial herniation.

SIGNIFICANCE OF EXTRACRANIAL INJURY

Systemic Hypotension and Arterial Hypoxia

Hypoxia and hypotension directly interfere with cerebral oxygenation. In a large study from the Traumatic Coma Databank, it was shown that single observations of systolic blood pressure less than 90 mm Hg and hypoxia (PaO$_2$ <60 mm Hg) in the prehospital arena were major predictors of a poor outcome.[218] Systemic injury leading to hypoxia and hypotension is common among head-injured patients. Thirty-five percent of 717 patients with severe closed head injury from the Traumatic Coma Databank had a systolic blood pressure below 90 mm Hg upon arrival in the emergency room, associated with a 150% increase in mortality.[6] In the intensive care unit, a blood pressure less than 90 mm Hg was observed in 29% of patients.[219] These patients had a poorer outcome relative to patients without hypotension. The injured brain's poor tolerance of hypotension is probably related to impaired pressure autoregulation.

Many patients with severe traumatic brain injury are hypoxic immediately after the insult. Causes of hypoxia vary from hypoventilation, airway obstruction, or aspiration to hemothorax or pneumothorax. Hypoxia that develops within the first 24 to 48 hours after injury is often due to lung contusions, atelectasis, fat emboli, pneumonia, or adult respiratory distress syndrome. Hypoxia is associated with increased morbidity and mortality. In a study of 225 patients, hypoxia was present in 35%; 50% of these patients died—more than twice the number of patients without hypoxia.[220] In the Traumatic Coma Databank study, the mortality rate was also nearly twice as high among hypoxic patients—50% versus 27%. It should be noted, however, that hypoxia alone adds very little to mortality; it is the combination of ischemia and hypoxia that appears to be responsible for increased mortality. Similarly, in experimental traumatic brain injury, it has been found that hypoxia alone has little effect on neurological status and brain energy metabolism. Widespread edema, ischemia, and poor outcome are found in animals subjected to a combination of brain injury and hypoxia.[221, 222] Hypoxia not only interferes directly with substrate supply but may also produce additional secondary injury by causing an increase in ICP. In the presence of hypoxia, CBF is increased (vasodilatation) to maintain CMRO$_2$. In normal adults, a PO$_2$ of 40 mm Hg increases CBF by 35%.[223] At a PO$_2$ of 35 mm Hg, CBF is increased by 70%. An increase in the volume of the cerebrovascular compartment may increase ICP significantly, particularly when brain compliance (PVI) is low. A more detrimental CBF response to hypoxia has been found in a cat model of fluid percussion injury: higher levels of injury (>2 atmospheres) severely impaired cerebrovascular reactivity, with an actual CBF decrease in response to hypoxia in some animals.[224]

Other Causes of Secondary Cerebral Damage

PYREXIA

Because fever causes cerebral metabolism to increase by 10% to 13% per degree Centigrade, it may cause significant secondary brain injury when metabolic autoregulation is disrupted and CBF does not increase proportionally. In animal models, temperatures above 39°C were associated with more severe histologic brain injury than were temperatures below 39°C.[225] In humans, pyrexia is one of the most significant predictors of mortality.[8]

ANEMIA

Hemoglobin is the oxygen carrier in the blood. Therefore, anemia interferes with the blood's oxygen-carrying capacity and can contribute to secondary brain injury. Again, the compensatory mechanism for reduced oxygen is an increase in CBF. Normovolemic hemodilution in normal individuals increases CBF by 19%.[226] Similar to its responses to hypoxia, the cerebral vasculature may not dilate sufficiently to provide adequate CBF, and ischemia may occur. Gopinath and colleagues identified anemia as one of the correctable causes of jugular venous desaturation.[227]

HYPERGLYCEMIA

Hyperglycemia is related to the severity of injury and correlates with a poorer outcome in patients with head injury.[228, 229] Increased production in the liver is mainly responsible for the increased glucose levels after injury. In experimental brain injury, an association between injury severity and plasma glucose levels was demonstrated.[230] The authors suggested that systemic hyperglycemia may be due to the sympathoadrenal response to injury. It is thought that the poorer outcome is due to the increased availability of glucose, which is metabolized anaerobically by the ischemic cells, with the resultant production of lactate. Lactate and acidosis appear to play an important role in causing secondary cell damage.[157, 231] Robertson and colleagues investigated the effects of glucose alimentation in a group of 21 severely head-injured patients randomized to either glucose infusion or saline. They found no significant increase in plasma or CSF levels of glucose but found an increased CSF lactate concentration in patients who received glucose alimentation.[232] The buffer tromethamine counteracts acidosis and has been effective in experimental brain injury.[233] However, no effect could be demonstrated in humans.[234]

INJURY TO THE SCALP AND SKULL

A large scalp laceration may cause significant hemorrhage. In young children, arterial hypotension may result if the bleeding is severe, but in adults, this is rare. Scalp injuries are a potential source of secondary injury to the brain, particularly because intracranial infections may arise from them.

Trauma to the skull results in a skull fracture when the force of deformation exceeds the skull's tolerance to strain. Three categories of skull injury are recognized: linear fractures, depressed fractures, and penetrating or perforating injuries. The type of injury is related to the nature of the impact. A depressed skull fracture results when strain is concentrated immediately beneath the impact, and all the energy is deposited locally in the bone. Small objects with a surface area of less than 2 square inches usually cause this type of injury when they strike the skull.[16] In the case of linear skull fractures, the energy is deposited over a wide surface area and absorbed along the fracture line during propagation of the fracture away from the point of impact.[235] Penetrating or perforating injury usually involves the high-energy impact of a small object on the skull.

Basilar skull fractures are caused by direct impact to the occiput, mastoid prominence, or supraorbital area; impact to the facial bones; or stress waves propagated from a site remote from the impact. The thin basilar skull is especially susceptible to the last type of injury.[17]

The brain damage associated with linear skull fractures depends on the degree of acceleration or deceleration of the head on impact. Severe fracturing of the skull may occur with crushing injuries, but there may be relatively minor brain injury because of the minimal, insignificant motion of the brain within the skull. Components determining the pattern of linear skull fractures are bone density, local thickness, and presence of sutures.

BASIC CONCEPTS OF THERAPY FOR SEVERE HEAD INJURY

The emphasis in this chapter has been on the cerebral circulation and metabolism. Thus, therapeutic concepts involving these aspects are discussed.

Intracranial Pressure Management

There is considerable evidence that high ICP is associated with poor outcome and that aggressive treatment reduces mortality and improves outcome after severe head injury. Treatment of raised ICP by reducing CBV has long been a cornerstone of head injury management. However, as can be concluded from the previous discussion, measures for treating ICP should be evaluated in light of their effect on CBF.

Hypocapnia (hyperventilation) reduces ICP by means of vasoconstriction and consequently improves CPP. However, net CBF is decreased, owing to the fact that vessel diameter in Poiseuille's equation is to the fourth power. In a randomized clinical trial, it was shown that preventive hyperventilation provided no residual benefit, and there was a suggestion that long-term outcome might be adversely affected. This may be due to CBF reduction to ischemic levels.[236] Moreover, it was shown that the cerebral vessels become unresponsive to CO_2 changes 24 hours after the institution of hypocapnia. Its rapid effect on ICP, however, is a great advantage in the situation of acute neurological deterioration (e.g., in the presence of an expanding mass lesion before evacuation can take place) and should be reserved for these situations.

There are two methods by which ICP reduction with vasoconstriction does not affect CBF. The first involves lowering the blood viscosity. As can be deduced from Poiseuille's equation, lowering the blood viscosity by itself leads to vasoconstriction, provided viscosity autoregulation is intact. With impaired autoregulation, lowering viscosity results in an increase in CBF but no decrease in ICP. However, this effect can be used to maintain CBF under vasoconstriction with hypocapnia. The effect of mannitol on ICP is thought to be mediated in part by lowering the blood viscosity.[135, 237] The second method involves increasing CPP, which can be done by raising the blood pressure. This method requires intact autoregulation: increased CPP leads to vasoconstriction (reduction of vascular diameter, CBV, and ICP), with the net CBF remaining constant.[136]

Generally, treatment is started when ICP reaches 20 mm Hg. Any interpretation of ICP must be combined with clinical features and a computed tomographic scan, because it is possible to have transtentorial herniation at an ICP of 15 mm Hg in the presence of a mass lesion. Conversely, with diffuse brain swelling, adequate CPP can be maintained despite a high ICP of 30 mm Hg. As a general rule, however, ICP of 20 mm Hg is an indication to initiate therapy.[238]

CEREBROSPINAL FLUID DRAINAGE

CSF drainage is an effective method of lowering ICP. The basis of CSF drainage is the Monro-Kellie doctrine.[206, 207] CSF drainage may be particularly useful under circumstances of a tight brain (low PVI or exponential part of the pressure-volume curve), although the small size of the ventricles at this stage may prevent adequate drainage.

SEDATIVES

Sedatives depress cerebral metabolism. In addition, they prevent ICP elevations associated with noxious stimuli.

MANNITOL ADMINISTRATION

As mentioned earlier, a major effect of mannitol is reduction of blood viscosity. Depending on the autoregulatory status, this results in either vasoconstriction and reduction of ICP with preserved CBF (intact autoregulation) or unaffected ICP with increased CBF (defective autoregulation).

HYPERVENTILATION

Hyperventilation reduces ICP by vasoconstriction and reduces CBF, which may be at critical ischemic levels in certain parts of the brain.[239] Therefore, hyperventilation ($P_{CO_2} <30$) should not be instituted prophylactically. In cases in which Pa_{CO_2} must be reduced to extremely low levels, hyperventilation can be combined with mannitol; this improves CBF by reducing blood viscosity.[237] AVDO$_2$ measurement by jugular venous oximetry is useful in these situations because it determines how much vasoconstriction CBF will allow.[227]

Cerebral Perfusion Pressure Management

The rationale behind CPP therapy is expressed in Poiseuille's equation, its effect depending on the status of autoregulation. Although the effect of CPP therapy has not been investigated in a randomized, controlled clinical trial, several studies suggest that CPP of 70 to 80 mm Hg is the threshold below which there may be significant risk of poor outcome to patients, particularly if CPP falls further.[11, 15] A recent study of almost 400 patients confirmed previous observations that CPP below 60 mm Hg is potentially hazardous in adults but failed to demonstrate that higher CPP was beneficial.[240] Maintenance of adequate CPP is critical in patients with defective autoregulation.[241] If autoregulation is defective, the cerebrovascular system becomes pressure passive; CBF decreases linearly with CPP and may reach ischemic levels. In patients with intact autoregulation, decreased CPP may also be detrimental; a decrease in CPP results in vasodilatation but leads to increased ICP and brain stiffness at the same time.

Increasing CPP under circumstances of intact autoregulation is thought to cause vasoconstriction and reduced ICP. However, Bouma and coworkers did not find this expected ICP decrease.[241] They argued that this might be due to the small effect of autoregulatory vasoconstriction (maximum 8% to 10% of baseline diameter) or to the fact that the bulk of CBV is contained in vessels smaller than those in which autoregulation takes place. At one end of the spectrum, increased CPP may result in pressure breakthrough; at this point, vasoconstriction is maximal, and a further increase in CPP will cause forced distention of the vessel wall, with a subsequent increase in CBV and enhanced edema formation. In contrast, lowering the mean arterial blood pressure can cause considerable increases in ICP. Therefore, part of the effect of inducing arterial hypertension may be the prevention of hypotension.

Increased CPP seems somewhat beneficial because of its effect on PVI in patients with intact autoregulation. The PVI tends to be higher when CPP is increased. Reduction of the diameter of the cerebrovascular compartment is thought to contribute to the increased brain compliance at increased CPP. The increased transmural pressure (leading to stiffening of the brain) is offset by this vasoconstriction. In patients with defective autoregulation, however, higher transmural pressure is not offset by arteriolar vasoconstriction and is consequently transmitted to the distal parts of the brain, leading to forced vascular distention in the microcirculation and stiffening of the brain.[241]

Hemoglobin, Hematocrit, and Blood Viscosity

To ensure optimal cerebral oxygenation, CPP, hemoglobin, and oxygen saturation should be optimized; vessel diameter should be maximized; and viscosity should be maintained in the low range. Hematocrit and viscosity are inversely related, and a balance must be established to ensure optimal oxygenation. If the hematocrit is too high, viscosity increases. If the hematocrit is too low, the oxygen carrying capacity of blood decreases. A hematocrit in the range of 30 to 35 is considered optimal; below 30, the oxygen carrying capacity falls without a significant change in viscosity, and above 35, viscosity increases disproportionately to the oxygen carrying capacity. Mannitol has a beneficial influence on blood viscosity, mainly through its effect on erythrocyte volume and hematocrit, but also through its effect on erythrocyte deformability.[242]

Brain Protection

When oxygen delivery cannot be improved sufficiently, brain protection can be offered by decreasing $CMRO_2$. The use of barbiturates for the treatment of severe head injury is based on several mechanisms by which they appear to exert cerebral protective and ICP-lowering effects: alterations in vascular tone, suppression of metabolism, and inhibition of free radical lipid peroxidation. The most important effect relates to the coupling of CBF to regional metabolic demands in such a manner that the lower the metabolic requirements, the less the CBF and related CBV. Barbiturate therapy is usually instituted when other measures to control ICP fail. In a case series of 25 patients with ICP greater than 40 mm Hg, Marshall and colleagues reported not only ICP control with barbiturates but also improvement in outcome.[201, 243] Of the patients in whom ICP control was achieved, 50% had a good recovery, whereas 83% of the patients in whom barbiturates failed to control ICP died. Prophylactic barbiturate therapy was also tested, but it failed to improve neurological outcome.[244] However, 54% of the barbiturate-treated patients were hypotensive, compared with 7% of the controls, but this trial was conducted before the present emphasis on maintaining CPP was recognized.

Hypothermia produces a balanced reduction in energy production and use and decreases $CMRO_2$ and CBF proportionately. Current protocols for hypothermia are cooling to 32°C to 33°C within 6 hours of injury, with maintenance of this temperature reduction for 24 to 48 hours. Two pilot clinical trials showed an improvement in neurological outcome.[245, 246] However, in a recent multicenter trial, an overall improvement in outcome could not be demonstrated.[246a] Only a subset of patients showed a clear benefit from hypothermia. Hypothermia to 33°C has also been shown to be effective for refractory high ICP and to improve outcome under those conditions. Side effects of hypothermia are cardiac arrhythmias and coagulation disorders, which were reported following cooling to 32°C to 33°C. Further, it is difficult to detect infection because of the lack of warning signs (spiking, elevated temperature).

CONCLUSIONS

Knowledge of cerebral metabolism and circulation under both normal and pathologic circumstances is essential for optimizing the therapy of severe head injury. It provides the clinician with useful tools to determine whether a certain treatment will be beneficial for the individual patient and allows tailored therapy. A better understanding of the pathophysiology has resulted in a modest improvement in the outcome of patients with severe head injuries.

An effort by both basic and clinical scientists to identify mechanisms of injury and then implement this knowledge in clinical trials continues. Pharmacologic brain protection and attempts to intervene in the cascade of biochemical events occurring after injury have shown some beneficial effects in phase II trials, but to date, no compound has clearly shown efficacy when tested in multicenter phase III clinical trials. Thorough testing of particular mechanisms or treatments in multiple experimental brain injury models, carefully conducted phase II trials to transfer knowledge from animal experiments to the human situation, custom-made clinical trials studying a subset of individuals out of the heterogeneous head-injured population, and a continuous effort to improve clinical trial design and evaluation are the challenges for the future.

REFERENCES

1. Povlishock JT, Becker DP, Cheng CL, Vaughan GW: Axonal change in minor head injury. J Neuropathol Exp Neurol 42: 225–242, 1983.
2. Jenkins LW, Moszynski K, Lyeth BG, et al: Increased vulnerability of the mildly traumatized rat brain to cerebral ischemia: The use of controlled secondary ischemia as a research tool to identify common or different mechanisms contributing to mechanical and ischemic brain injury. Brain Res 477:211–224, 1989.
3. Adams JH, Doyle D, Ford I, et al: Diffuse axonal injury in head injury: Definition, diagnosis and grading. Histopathology 15: 49–59, 1989.
4. Hovda DA, Becker DP, Katayama Y: Secondary injury and acidosis. J Neurotrauma 9(Suppl 1):S47–S60, 1992.
5. Katayama Y, Becker DP, Tamura T, Hovda DA: Massive increases in extracellular potassium and the indiscriminate release of glutamate following concussive brain injury. J Neurosurg 73: 889–900, 1990.
6. Chesnut RM, Marshall LF, Klauber MR, et al: The role of secondary brain injury in determining outcome from severe head injury. J Trauma 34:216–222, 1993.
7. Andrews PJ, Piper IR, Dearden NM, Miller JD: Secondary insults during intrahospital transport of head-injured patients. Lancet 335:327–330, 1990.
8. Jones PA, Andrews PJ, Midgley S, et al: Measuring the burden of secondary insults in head-injured patients during intensive care. J Neurosurg Anesthesiol 6:4–14, 1994.
9. Miller J, Piper I, Jones P: Pathophysiology of head injury. In Narayan RK, Wilberger JE, Povlishock JT (eds): Neurotrauma. New York, McGraw-Hill, 1996, pp 61–69.
10. Klauber MR, Marshall LF, Toole BM, et al: Cause of decline in head-injury mortality rate in San Diego County, California. J Neurosurg 62:528–531, 1985.
11. Rosner MJ, Rosner SD, Johnson AH: Cerebral perfusion pressure: Management protocol and clinical results. J Neurosurg 83: 949–962, 1995; see coments.
12. Rosner MJ: Introduction to cerebral perfusion pressure management. Neurosurg Clin N Am 6:761–773, 1995.
13. Rosner MJ: Role of cerebral perfusion pressure in acute brain trauma [letter; comment]. Crit Care Med 24:1274, discussion 1275–1276, 1996.
14. Cortbus F, Jones PA, Miller JD, et al: Cause, distribution and significance of episodes of reduced cerebral perfusion pressure following head injury. Acta Neurochir (Wien) 130:117–124, 1994.
15. McGraw C: A cerebral perfusion pressure greater than 80 mm Hg is more benificial. In Hoff J, Betz A (eds): Intracranial Pressure, vol. VII. Berlin, Springer-Verlag, 1989, pp 839–841.
16. Goldsmith W: The physical processes producing head injury. In

Head Injury Conference Proceedings. Philadelphia, JB Lippincott, 1966.

17. Gennarelli T, Meaney D: Mechanisms of primary head injury. In Wilkins R, Rengachary S (eds): Neurosurgery. New York, McGraw-Hill, 1996.

18. McLean AJ: Brain injury without head impact? J Neurotrauma 12:621–625, 1995.

19. Halliday A: Pathophysiology. In Marion D (ed): Traumatic Brain Injury. New York, Thieme Medical, 1999, pp 29–38.

20. Gennarelli TA, Thibault LE: Biomechanics of acute subdural hematoma. J Trauma 22:680–686, 1982.

21. Adams J, Graham D, Murray L: Diffuse axonal injury due to nonmissile injury in humans: An analysis of 45 cases. Ann Neurol 12:557–563, 1992.

22. Teasdale G, Jennet B: Assessment of coma and impaired consciousness: A practical scale. Lancet 2:81–84, 1974.

23. Gale J, Dikmen S, Wyler A: Head injury in the Pacific Northwest. Neurosurgery 12:487–491, 1983.

24. Denny-Brown D: Selected Writings of Sir Charles Sherrington. Oxford, Oxford University Press, 1979.

25. Eccles J, Gibson W: Sherrington, His Life and Thought. Berlin and Heidelberg, Springer International, 1979.

26. Greenberg RP, Stablein DM, Becker DP: Noninvasive localization of brain-stem lesions in the cat with multimodality evoked potentials: Correlation with human head-injury data. J Neurosurg 54:740–750, 1981.

27. Stein S: Classification of head injury. In Narayan RK, Wilberger JE, Povlishock JT (eds): Neurotrauma. New York, McGraw-Hill, 1996, pp 31–41.

28. Marshall LF, Marshall SB, Klauber MR, et al: The diagnosis of head injury requires a classification based on computed axial tomography. J Neurotrauma 9(Suppl 1):S287–S292, 1992.

29. Eisenberg HM, Gary HE Jr, Aldrich EF, et al: Initial CT findings in 753 patients with severe head injury: A report from the NIH Traumatic Coma Data Bank. J Neurosurg 73:688–698, 1990.

30. Teasdale G, Mathew P: Mechanism of cerebral concussion, contusion, and other effects of head injury. In Youmans J (ed): Neurological Surgery, 4th ed. Philadelphia, WB Saunders, 1996.

31. Graham D: Neuropathology of head injury. In Narayan RK, Wilberger JE, Povlishock JT (eds): Neurotrauma. New York, McGraw-Hill, 1996, pp 43–59.

32. Adams JH, Scott G, Parker LS, et al: The contusion index: A quantitative approach to cerebral contusions in head injury. Neuropathol Appl Neurobiol 6:319–324, 1980.

33. Adams JH, Doyle D, Graham DI, et al: The contusion index: A reappraisal in human and experimental non-missile head injury. Neuropathol Appl Neurobiol 11:299–308, 1985.

34. Miller JD: Minor, moderate and severe head injury. Neurosurg Rev 9:135–139, 1986.

35. Cordobaes F, Lobato RD, Rivas JJ, et al: Observations on 82 patients with extradural hematoma: Comparison of results before and after the advent of computerized tomography. J Neurosurg 54:179–186, 1981.

36. Heiskanen O: Epidural hematoma. Surg Neurol 4:23–26, 1975.

37. Reale F, Delfini R, Mencattini G: Epidural hematomas. J Neurosurg Sci 28:9–16, 1984.

38. Marshall L, Gautille T, Klauber M: The outcome of severe closed head injury. J Neurosurg 75:S28–S36, 1991.

39. Lindenberg R: Trauma of meninges and brain. Pathol Nerv Syst 2:1705–1765, 1971.

40. Maloney A: Clinical and pathological observations in fatal head injuries—a five-year study of 172 cases. Br J Surg 56:23, 1969.

41. Gallagher JP, Browder EJ: Extradural hematoma: Experience with 167 patients. J Neurosurg 29:1–12, 1968.

42. Teasdale G: Traumatic acute intracranial hematoma: Comment. In Palmer J (ed): Manual of Neurosurgery. New York, Churchill Livingstone, 1996, p 544.

43. Zimmerman RA, Bilaniuk LT: Computed tomographic staging of traumatic epidural bleeding. Radiology 144:809–812, 1982.

44. Jacobson W: On middle meningeal hemorrhage. Guy's Hosp Rep 43:147–308, 1886.

45. Lobato RD, Rivas JJ, Cordobes F, et al: Acute epidural hematoma: An analysis of factors influencing the outcome of patients undergoing surgery in coma. J Neurosurg 68:48–57, 1988.

46. Sahuquillo-Barris J, Lamarca-Ciuro J, Vilalta-Castan J, et al: Epidural hematoma and diffuse axonal injury [letter]. Neurosurgery 17:378–379, 1985.

47. Seelig J, Marshall L, Toutant S: Traumatic acute epidural hematoma: Unrecognized high lethality in comatose patients. Neurosurgery 15:617–620, 1984.

48. Sakas DE, Bullock MR, Teasdale GM: One-year outcome following craniotomy for traumatic hematoma in patients with fixed dilated pupils. J Neurosurg 82:961–965, 1995.

49. Haselsberger K, Pucher R, Auer L: Prognosis after acute subdural or epidural hemorrhage. Acta Neurochir (Wien) 90:111–116, 1988.

50. Brink Wvd, Zwienenberg M, Zandee S, et al: The prognostic importance of the volume of traumatic epidural and subdural haematomas revisited. Acta Neurochir (Wien) 141:1–6, 1999.

51. Rivas JJ, Lobato RD, Sarabia R, et al: Extradural hematoma: Analysis of factors influencing the courses of 161 patients. Neurosurgery 23:44–51, 1988.

52. Jamieson K, Yelland J: Extradural hematoma: Report of 167 cases. J Neurosurg 29:13–23, 1968.

53. Kvarnes T, Trumpy J: Extradural hematoma: Report of 132 cases. Acta Neurochir (Wien) 41:223–231, 1978.

54. Cooper P: Acute traumatic intracranial hematomas. In Wilkins R, Rengachary S (eds): Neurosurgery. New York, McGraw-Hill, 1985, pp 1657–1666.

55. Hooper R: Observations on extradural hematoma. Br J Surg 47:71–87, 1959.

56. Bricolo A, Pasut L: Extradural hematoma: Toward zero mortality. A prospective study. Neurosurgery 14:8–12, 1984.

57. Kuday C, Uzan M, Hanci M: Statistical analysis of the factors affecting the outcome of extradural hematomas: 115 cases. Acta Neurochir (Wien) 131:203–206, 1994.

58. Rivano C, Borzone M, Carta F, Michelozzi G: Traumatic intracerebral hematomas: 72 cases surgically treated. J Neurosurg Sci 24:77–84, 1980.

59. Wright RL: Traumatic hematomas of the posterior cranial fossa. J Neurosurg 25:402–409, 1966.

60. Zuccarello M, Pardatscher K, Andrioli GC, et al: Epidural hematomas of the posterior cranial fossa. Neurosurgery 8:434–437, 1981.

61. Ciembroniewicz J: Epidural hematomas of the posterior fossa: Review of the literature with addition of three cases. J Neurosurg 22:465–473, 1965.

62. Jennett B, Teasdale G (eds): Management of Head Injuries. Philadelphia, Davis, 1981.

63. Bullock R, Teasdale G: Surgical management of traumatic intracranial hematomas. In Braakman R (ed): Handbook of Clinical Neurology, vol 15. Amsterdam, Elsevier, 1990, pp 249–298.

64. Wintzen AR, de Jonge H, Loeliger EA, Bots GT: The risk of intracerebral hemorrhage during oral anticoagulant treatment: A population study. Ann Neurol 16:553–558, 1984.

65. Kawamata T, Takeshita M, Kubo O, et al: Management of intracranial hemorrhage associated with anticoagulant therapy. Surg Neurol 44:438–442, discussion 443, 1995.

66. Jamieson K, Yelland J: Surgically treated traumatic subdural hematomas. J Neurosurg 37:137–149, 1972.

67. Seelig J, Becker D, Miller J: Traumatic acute subdural hematoma: Major mortality reduction in comatose patients treated within four hours. N Engl J Med 304:1511–1518, 1981.

68. MacPherson P, Graham D: Correlation between angiographic findings and the ischemia of head injury. J Neurol Neurosurg Psychiatry 41:122–127, 1977.

69. Miller J, Bullock R, Graham D: Ischaemic brain damage in a model of acute subdural hematoma. Neurosurgery 27:433–439, 1988.

70. Verweij B, Vinas F, Muizelaar J: Hyperacute measurement of intracranial pressure, cerebral perfusion pressure, jugular venous oxygen saturation, and laser Doppler flowmetry, before and during removal of traumatic acute subdural hematoma. J Neurosurg 95:569–572, 2001.

71. Schroder ML, Muizelaar JP, Kuta AJ: Documented reversal of global ischemia immediately after removal of an acute subdural hematoma: Report of two cases. J Neurosurg 80:324–327, 1994.

72. Seelig JM, Greenberg RP, Becker DP, et al: Reversible brain-stem dysfunction following acute traumatic subdural hematoma: A

clinical and electrophysiological study. J Neurosurg 55:516–523, 1981.

73. Tanaka A, Nakayama Y, Yoshinaga S: Cerebral blood flow and intracranial pressure in chronic subdural hematomas. Surg Neurol 47:346–351, 1997.

74. Apfelbaum R, Guthkelch A, Shulman K: Experimental production of subdural hematomas. J Neurosurg 40:336–346, 1974.

75. Markwalder T: Chronic subdural hematomas: A review. J Neurosurg 54:637–645, 1981.

76. Gardner W: Traumatic subdural hematoma with particular reference to the latent interval. Arch Neurol Psychiatry 27:847–858, 1932.

77. Zollinger R, Gross R: Traumatic subdural hematoma, an explanation of the late onset of pressure symptoms. JAMA 103:245–249, 1934.

78. Weir B: The osmolality of subdural hematoma fluid. J Neurosurg 34:528–533, 1971.

79. Sato S, Suzuki J: Ultrastructural observations of the capsule of chronic subdural hematoma in various clinical stages. J Neurosurg 43:569–578, 1975.

80. Yamashima T, Yamamoto S: Clinical pathological classification of chronic subdural hematoma. Zentralbl Neurochir 46:304–314, 1985.

81. Goodman J: Pathophysiology. In Marion D (ed): Traumatic Brain Injury. New York, Thieme Medical, 1999, pp 143–154.

82. Zimmerman RA, Bilaniuk LT, Gennarelli T, et al: Cranial computed tomography in diagnosis and management of acute head trauma. AJR Am J Roentgenol 131:27–34, 1978.

83. Gudeman SK, Kishore PR, Miller JD, et al: The genesis and significance of delayed traumatic intracerebral hematoma. Neurosurgery 5:309–313, 1979.

84. Ribas G, Jane J: Traumatic contusions and intracerebral hematomas. In Jane J, Anderson D, Torner J, Young W (eds): Central Nervous System Trauma Status Report 1991. New York, MA Liebert, 1992, pp S265–S278.

85. Becker D, Doberstein C, Hovda D: Craniocerebral trauma: Mechanisms, management, and the cellular response to injury. In Current Concepts. Kalamazoo, Mich, UpJohn, 1994.

86. Chesnut R, Servadei F: Surgical treatment of post-traumatic mass lesions. In Marion D (ed): Traumatic Brain Injury. New York, Thieme Medical, 1999, pp 81–99.

87. Baratham G, Dennyson WG: Delayed traumatic intracerebral haemorrhage. J Neurol Neurosurg Psychiatry 35:698–706, 1972.

88. McLaurin RL: Epilepsy and contact sports: Factors contraindicating participation. JAMA 225:285–287, 1973.

89. Miller J, Becker D: Pathophysiology of head injury. In Youmans J (ed): Neurological Surgery, 2nd ed. Philadelphia, WB Saunders, 1982, pp 1896–1937.

90. Miller JD, Jennett WB: Complications of depressed skull fracture. Lancet 2:991–995, 1968.

91. Gennarelli T: Cerebral concussion and diffuse brain injuries. In Cooper P (ed): Head Injury. Philadelphia, Williams & Wilkins, 1983, pp 137–158.

92. Kelly JP, Nichols JS, Filley CM, et al: Concussion in sports: Guidelines for the prevention of catastrophic outcome. JAMA 266:2867–2869, 1991.

93. Cairns H: Disturbances of consciousness with lesions of the brain stem and diencephalon. Brain 75:109–146, 1952.

94. Adams J, Mitchell D, Graham D, Doyle D: Diffuse brain damage of immediate impact type: Its relationship to "primary brain stem damage" in head injury. Brain 100:489–502, 1977.

95. Strich S: Diffuse degeneration of the cerebral white matter in severe dementia following head injury. J Neurol Neurosurg Psychiatry 19:163–185, 1956.

96. Peerless SJ, Rewcastle NB: Shear injuries of the brain. Can Med Assoc J 96:577–582, 1967.

97. Adams J: Pathology of nonmissile head injury. Neuroimaging Clin N Am 1:397–410, 1991.

98. Zimmerman R, Bilaniuk L, Gennarelli T: Computed tomography of shearing injuries of the cerebral white matter. Radiology 127:393–396, 1978.

99. Gennarelli TA, Thibault LE, Adams JH, et al: Diffuse axonal injury and traumatic coma in the primate. Ann Neurol 12:564–574, 1982.

100. Strich S: Shearing of nerve fibers as a cause of brain damage due to head injury: A pathological study of twenty cases. Lancet 2:443–448, 1961.

101. Povlishock JT, Jenkins LW: Are the pathobiological changes evoked by traumatic brain injury immediate and irreversible? Brain Pathol 5:415–426, 1995.

102. Povlishock JT, Christman CW: The pathobiology of traumatically induced axonal injury in animals and humans: A review of current thoughts. J Neurotrauma 12:555–564, 1995.

103. Ommaya AK, Gennarelli TA: Cerebral concussion and traumatic unconsciousness: Correlation of experimental and clinical observations of blunt head injuries. Brain 97:633–654, 1974.

104. Macpherson P, Graham DI: Arterial spasm and slowing of the cerebral circulation in the ischaemia of head injury. J Neurol Neurosurg Psychiatry 36:1069–1072, 1973.

105. Martin NA, Doberstein C, Alexander M, et al: Posttraumatic cerebral arterial spasm. J Neurotrauma 12:897–901, 1995.

106. Fukuda T, Hasue M, Ito H: Does traumatic subarachnoid hemorrhage caused by diffuse brain injury cause delayed ischemic brain damage? Comparison with subarachnoid hemorrhage caused by ruptured intracranial aneurysms. Neurosurgery 43:1040–1049, 1998.

107. Lee JH, Martin NA, Alsina G, et al: Hemodynamically significant cerebral vasospasm and outcome after head injury: A prospective study. J Neurosurg 87:221–233, 1997.

108. Martin NA, Patwardhan RV, Alexander MJ, et al: Characterization of cerebral hemodynamic phases following severe head trauma: Hypoperfusion, hyperemia, and vasospasm. J Neurosurg 87:9–19, 1997.

109. Schroder ML, Muizelaar JP, Fatouros PP, et al: Regional cerebral blood volume after severe head injury in patients with regional cerebral ischemia. Neurosurgery 42:1276–1280, discussion 1280–1281, 1998.

110. Pierre LN, Davenport AP, Katusic ZS: Blockade and reversal of endothelin-induced constriction in pial arteries from human brain. Stroke 30:638–643, 1999.

111. Sobey CG, Faraci FM: Subarachnoid haemorrhage: What happens to the cerebral arteries? Clin Exp Pharmacol Physiol 25:867–876, 1998.

112. Zimmermann M, Seifert V: Endothelin and subarachnoid hemorrhage: An overview. Neurosurgery 43:863–875, discussion 875–876, 1998.

113. Zimmermann M: Endothelin in cerebral vasospasm: Clinical and experimental results. J Neurosurg Sci 41:139–151, 1997.

114. Caner HH, Kwan AL, Arthur A, et al: Systemic administration of an inhibitor of endothelin-converting enzyme for attenuation of cerebral vasospasm following experimental subarachnoid hemorrhage. J Neurosurg 85:917–922, 1996.

115. Zimmermann M, Seifert V, Leoffler BM, et al: Prevention of cerebral vasospasm after experimental subarachnoid hemorrhage by RO 47-0203, a newly developed orally active endothelin receptor antagonist. Neurosurgery 38:115–120, 1996.

116. Zimmermann M, Seifert V: [Prevention of cerebral vasospasms after experimental subarachnoid hemorrhage by the endothelin receptor antagonist RO 47-0203.] Zentralbl Neurochir 57:143–149, 1996.

117. Zuccarello M, Romano A, Passalacqua M, Rapoport RM: Decreased endothelium-dependent relaxation in subarachnoid hemorrhage-induced vasospasm: Role of ET-1. Am J Physiol 269(Pt 2):H1009–H1015, 1995.

118. Roux S, Leoffler BM, Gray GA, et al: The role of endothelin in experimental cerebral vasospasm. Neurosurgery 37:78–85, discussion 85–86, 1995.

119. Hirose H, Ide K, Sasaki T, et al: The role of endothelin and nitric oxide in modulation of normal and spastic cerebral vascular tone in the dog. Eur J Pharmacol 277:77–87, 1995; erratum in Eur J Pharmacol 284:335–336, 1995.

120. Seifert V, Leoffler BM, Zimmermann M, et al: Endothelin concentrations in patients with aneurysmal subarachnoid hemorrhage: Correlation with cerebral vasospasm, delayed ischemic neurological deficits, and volume of hematoma. J Neurosurg 82:55–62, 1995.

121. Karavelis A, Sirmos C: Primary post-traumatic intraventricular hemorrhage. J Neurosurg Sci 39:253–256, 1995.

122. Hashimoto T, Nakamura N, Ke R, Ra F: [Traumatic intraventricular hemorrhage in severe head injury.] No Shinkei Geka 20:209–215, 1992.

123. Fujitsu K, Kuwabara T, Muramoto M, et al: Traumatic intraventricular hemorrhage: Report of twenty-six cases and consideration of the pathogenic mechanism. Neurosurgery 23:423–430, 1988.

124. LeRoux PD, Haglund MM, Newell DW, et al: Intraventricular hemorrhage in blunt head trauma: An analysis of 43 cases. Neurosurgery 31:678–684, discussion 684–685, 1992.

125. Kety S, Schmidt C: The nitrous oxygen method for quantitative determination of cerebral blood flow in man. J Clin Invest 27:476–483, 1948.

126. Gibbs E, Lennox W, Nims L, Gibbs F: Arterial and cerebral venous blood: Arterial-venous differences in man. J Biol Chem 144:325–332, 1942.

127. Rowe G, Maxwell G, Castillo C: A study in man of cerebral blood flow and cerebral glucose, lactate and pyruvate metabolism before and after eating. J Clin Invest 38:2154–2158, 1959.

128. Bergsneider M, Hovda DA, Shalmon E, et al: Cerebral hyperglycolysis following severe traumatic brain injury in humans: A positron emission tomography study. J Neurosurg 86:241–251, 1997; see comments.

129. Astrup J: Energy-requiring cell functions in the ischemic brain: Their critical supply and possible inhibition in protective therapy. J Neurosurg 56:482–497, 1982.

130. Siesjo BK: Cerebral circulation and metabolism. J Neurosurg 60:883–908, 1984.

131. Kontos HA, Wei EP, Navari RM, et al: Responses of cerebral arteries and arterioles to acute hypotension and hypertension. Am J Physiol 234:H371–H383, 1978.

132. Lassen N: Cerebral blood flow and oxygen consumption in man. Physiol Rev 39:183–238, 1959.

133. Heistad D, Kontos H: Cerebral circulation. In Sheperd J, Abboud F (eds): Handbook of Physiology, sec 2, vol 3. Bethesda, Md, American Physiologic Society, 1983, pp 137–182.

134. Bouma GJ, Muizelaar JP: Relationship between cardiac output and cerebral blood flow in patients with intact and with impaired autoregulation. J Neurosurg 73:368–374, 1990.

135. Muizelaar JP, Lutz HA, Becker DP: Effect of mannitol on ICP and CBF and correlation with pressure autoregulation in severely head-injured patients. J Neurosurg 61:700–706, 1984.

136. Muizelaar JP, Ward JD, Marmarou A, et al: Cerebral blood flow and metabolism in severely head-injured children. Part 2. Autoregulation. J Neurosurg 71:72–76, 1989.

136a. Roy CS, Sherrington CS: On the regulation of the blood supply of the liver. J Physiol 11:85–108, 1890.

137. Kuschinsky W, Wahl M: Local chemical and neurogenic regulation of cerebral vascular resistance. Physiol Rev 58:656–689, 1978.

138. Bouma G: Cerebral Circulation after Severe Head Injury: A Clinical Study [thesis]. Amsterdam, University of Amsterdam, 1993.

139. Furchgott RF, Zawadzki JV: The obligatory role of endothelial cells in the relaxation of arterial smooth muscle by acetylcholine. Nature 288:373–376, 1980.

140. Tanaka K: Is nitric oxide really important for regulation of the cerebral circulation? Yes or no? Keio J Med 45:14–27, 1996.

141. Davies MG, Hagen PO: The vascular endothelium: A new horizon. Ann Surg 218:593–609, 1993.

142. Garthwaite J, Charles SL, Chess-Williams R: Endothelium-derived relaxing factor release on activation of NMDA receptors suggests role as intercellular messenger in the brain. Nature 336:385–388, 1988.

143. Goadsby PJ, Kaube H, Hoskin KL: Nitric oxide synthesis couples cerebral blood flow and metabolism. Brain Res 595:167–170, 1992.

144. Rubanyi GM: Endothelium-dependent pressure-induced contraction of isolated canine carotid arteries. Am J Physiol 255(Pt 2):H783–H788, 1988.

145. Rubanyi GM, Freay AD, Kauser K, et al: Mechanoreception by the endothelium: Mediators and mechanisms of pressure- and flow-induced vascular responses. Blood Vessels 27:246–257, 1990.

146. Martainez-Orgado J, Gonzaalez R, Alonso MJ, et al: Endothelial factors and autoregulation during pressure changes in isolated newborn piglet cerebral arteries. Pediatr Res 44:161–167, 1998.

147. Muizelaar JP, van der Poel HG, Li ZC, et al: Pial arteriolar vessel diameter and CO$_2$ reactivity during prolonged hyperventilation in the rabbit. J Neurosurg 69:923–927, 1988.

148. Andersen B, Marmarou A: Isolated stimulation of glycolysis following traumatic brain injury. In Hoff J, Betz A (eds): Intracranial Pressure, vol. VII. Berlin, Springer-Verlag, 1989, pp 575–580.

149. Andersen BJ, Marmarou A: Post-traumatic selective stimulation of glycolysis. Brain Res 585:184–189, 1992.

150. Inglis F, Kuroda Y, Bullock R: Glucose hypermetabolism after acute subdural hematoma is ameliorated by a competitive NMDA antagonist. J Neurotrauma 9:75–84, 1992.

151. Sunami K, Nakamura T, Ozawa Y, et al: Hypermetabolic state following experimental head injury. Neurosurg Rev 12(Suppl 1):400–411, 1989.

152. Yoshino A, Hovda DA, Kawamata T, et al: Dynamic changes in local cerebral glucose utilization following cerebral contusion in rats: Evidence of a hyper- and subsequent hypometabolic state. Brain Res 561:106–119, 1991.

153. Paljarvi L: Brain lactic acidosis and ischemic cell damage: A topographic study with high resolution light microscopy of early recovery in a rat model of severe complete ischemia. Acta Neuropathol (Berl) 64:89–98, 1984.

154. Brain injury: Neurochemical aspects. In Central Nervous System Trauma Status Report. Bethesda, Md, National Institutes of Health, 1985.

155. Kalimo H, Rehncrona S, Soderfeldt B: Brain lactic acidosis and ischemic cell damage. 2. Histopathology. J Cereb Blood Flow Metab 1:313–327, 1981.

156. Vink R, Head VA, Rogers PJ, et al: Mitochondrial metabolism following traumatic brain injury in rats. J Neurotrauma 7:21–27, 1990.

157. De Salles AA, Muizelaar JP, Young HF: Hyperglycemia, cerebrospinal fluid lactic acidosis, and cerebral blood flow in severely head-injured patients. Neurosurgery 21:45–50, 1987.

158. Adams J, Graham D: The pathology of blunt head injury. In Critchley M, O'Leary J, Jennet B (eds): Scientific Foundation of Neurology. London, W Heineman, 1972, pp 488–491.

159. Bouma GJ, Muizelaar JP, Choi SC, et al: Cerebral circulation and metabolism after severe traumatic brain injury: The elusive role of ischemia. J Neurosurg 75:685–693, 1991.

160. Jones T: Thresholds of focal cerebral ischemia in awake monkeys. J Neurosurg 54:773–782, 1981.

161. Schroder ML, Muizelaar JP, Kuta AJ, Choi SC: Thresholds for cerebral ischemia after severe head injury: Relationship with late CT findings and outcome. J Neurotrauma 13:17–23, 1996.

162. Langfitt T, Obrist W: Cerebral blood flow and metabolism after intracranial trauma. In Krayenbuhl H (ed): Progress in Neurological Surgery. Basel, S Karger, 1981, pp 10, 14–48.

163. Bruce DA, Langfitt TW, Miller JD, et al: Regional cerebral blood flow, intracranial pressure, and brain metabolism in comatose patients. J Neurosurg 38:131–144, 1973.

164. Cold GE, Jensen FT, Malmros R: The effects of PaCO$_2$ reduction on regional cerebral blood flow in the acute phase of brain injury. Acta Anaesthesiol Scand 21:359–367, 1977.

165. Cold GE, Jensen FT, Malmros R: The cerebrovascular CO$_2$ reactivity during the acute phase of brain injury. Acta Anaesthesiol Scand 21:222–231, 1977.

166. Enevoldsen EM, Jensen FT: Reproducibility of regional cerebral blood flow measurements in acute severe head injury. J Neurosurg 49:366–377, 1978.

167. Enevoldsen EM, Jensen FT: Autoregulation and CO$_2$ responses of cerebral blood flow in patients with acute severe head injury. J Neurosurg 48:689–703, 1978.

168. Fieschi C, Battistini N, Beduschi A, et al: Regional cerebral blood flow and intraventricular pressure in acute head injuries. J Neurol Neurosurg Psychiatry 37:1378–1388, 1974.

169. Robertson C: Nitrous oxide saturation technique for CBF measurement. In Narayan RK, Wilberger JE, Povlishock JT (eds): Neurotrauma. New York, McGraw-Hill, 1996, pp 487–501.

170. Muizelaar JP, Marmarou A, DeSalles AA, et al: Cerebral blood flow and metabolism in severely head-injured children. Part 1. Relationship with GCS score, outcome, ICP, and PVI. J Neurosurg 71:63–71, 1989.

171. Obrist WD, Langfitt TW, Jaggi JL, et al: Cerebral blood flow and metabolism in comatose patients with acute head injury:

Relationship to intracranial hypertension. J Neurosurg 61:241–253, 1984.

172. Lassen NA: The luxury-perfusion syndrome and its possible relation to acute metabolic acidosis localised within the brain. Lancet 2:1113–1115, 1966.

173. Marion DW, Darby J, Yonas H: Acute regional cerebral blood flow changes caused by severe head injuries. J Neurosurg 74:407–414, 1991.

174. Zane C, Khanna R, Martin N: Patterns of cerebral blood flow and transcranial Doppler ultrasound velocities following head injury [abstract]. J Neurosurg 76:399A, 1992.

175. Bruce DA, Alavi A, Bilaniuk L, et al: Diffuse cerebral swelling following head injuries in children: The syndrome of "malignant brain edema." J Neurosurg 54:170–178, 1981.

176. Bouma GJ, Muizelaar JP, Fatouros P: Pathogenesis of traumatic brain swelling: Role of cerebral blood volume. Acta Neurochir Suppl (Wien) 71:272–275, 1998.

177. Zwienenberg M, Muizelaar J: Severe pediatric head injury: The role of hyperemia revisited. J Neurotrauma 16:937–943, 1999.

178. Cox SB, Woolsey TA, Rovainen CM: Localized dynamic changes in cortical blood flow with whisker stimulation corresponds to matched vascular and neuronal architecture of rat barrels. J Cereb Blood Flow Metab 13:899–913, 1993.

179. Gonzalez MF, Sharp FR: Vibrissae tactile stimulation: (14C) 2-Deoxyglucose uptake in rat brainstem, thalamus, and cortex. J Comp Neurol 231:457–472, 1985.

180. Hovda DA, Lee SM, Smith ML, et al: The neurochemical and metabolic cascade following brain injury: Moving from animal models to man. J Neurotrauma 12:903–906, 1995.

181. Overgaard J, Tweed WA: Cerebral circulation after head injury. 1. Cerebral blood flow and its regulation after closed head injury with emphasis on clinical correlations. J Neurosurg 41:531–541, 1974.

182. Bouma GJ, Muizelaar JP: Cerebral blood flow, cerebral blood volume, and cerebrovascular reactivity after severe head injury. J Neurotrauma 9(Suppl 1):S333–S348, 1992.

183. Allen GS, Gross CJ: Cerebral arterial spasm. Part 7. In vitro effects of alpha adrenergic agents on canine arteries from six anatomical sites and six blocking agents on serotonin-induced contractions of the canine basilar artery. Surg Neurol 6:63–70, 1976.

184. Allen GS: Cerebral arterial spasm. Part 8. The treatment of delayed cerebral arterial spasm in human beings. Surg Neurol 6:71–80, 1976.

185. Hoff JT, Harper M, Sengupta D, Jennett B: Effect of alpha-adrenergic blockade on response of cerebral circulation to hypocapnia in the baboon. Lancet 2:1337–1339, 1972.

186. Taylor P: Ganglionic stimulating and blocking agents. In Gilman AG, Goodman L, Rall T (eds): The Pharmacological Basis of Therapeutics. New York, Macmillan, 1985, pp 215–235.

187. Wei EP, Dietrich WD, Povlishock JT, et al: Functional, morphological, and metabolic abnormalities of the cerebral microcirculation after concussive brain injury in cats. Circ Res 46:37–47, 1980.

188. Ignarro L, Byrns R, Wood K: Pharmacological and biochemical properties of endothelium-derived relaxing factor (EDRF): Evidence that EDRF is closely related to nitric oxide (NO) radical. Circulation 74(Suppl 2):287, 1986.

189. Beckman J, Beckman T, Chen J, et al: Apparent hydroxyl radical production by peroxynitrite: Implications for endothelial injury from nitric oxide and superoxide. Proc Natl Acad Sci U S A 87:1620–1624, 1990.

190. Ellis EF, Dodson LY, Police RJ: Restoration of cerebrovascular responsiveness to hyperventilation by the oxygen radical scavenger N-acetylcysteine following experimental traumatic brain injury. J Neurosurg 75:774–779, 1991.

191. Kontos HA, Wei EP: Oxygen-dependent mechanisms in cerebral autoregulation. Ann Biomed Eng 13:329–334, 1985.

192. Hudak ML, Koehler RC, Rosenberg AA, et al: Effect of hematocrit on cerebral blood flow. Am J Physiol 251(Pt 2):H63–H70, 1986.

193. Hudak ML, Jones MD Jr, Popel AS, et al: Hemodilution causes size-dependent constriction of pial arterioles in the cat. Am J Physiol 257(Pt 2):H912–H917, 1989.

194. Muizelaar JP, Wei EP, Kontos HA, Becker DP: Cerebral blood flow is regulated by changes in blood pressure and in blood viscosity alike. Stroke 17:44–48, 1986.

195. Cold GE, Jensen FT: Cerebral autoregulation in unconscious patients with brain injury. Acta Anaesthesiol Scand 22:270–280, 1978.

196. Enevoldsen EM, Cold G, Jensen FT, Malmros R: Dynamic changes in regional CBF, intraventricular pressure, CSF pH and lactate levels during the acute phase of head injury. J Neurosurg 44:191–214, 1976.

197. Messeter K, Nordstreom CH, Sundbearg G, et al: Cerebral hemodynamics in patients with acute severe head trauma. J Neurosurg 64:231–237, 1986.

198. Zimmerman R, Muizelaar J, Wei E, Kontos H: Acute cerebral arteriolar responses following cold injury. In Cervos-Navarro J, Ferszt R (eds): Stroke and Microcirculation. New York, Raven Press, 1987, pp 303–309.

199. Becker DP, Miller JD, Ward JD, et al: The outcome from severe head injury with early diagnosis and intensive management. J Neurosurg 47:491–502, 1977.

200. Marmarou A, Anderson R, Ward J: The Traumatic Coma Databank: Monitoring of ICP. In Hoff J, Betz A (eds): Intracranial Pressure, vol. VII. New York, Springer-Verlag, 1989, pp 549–551.

201. Marshall LF, Smith RW, Shapiro HM: The outcome with aggressive treatment in severe head injuries. Part II. Acute and chronic barbiturate administration in the management of head injury. J Neurosurg 50:26–30, 1979.

202. Marshall LF, Gautille T: Large and small "holes" in the brain: Reversible or irreversible changes in head injury. Acta Neurochir Suppl (Wien) 51:300–301, 1990.

203. Miller JD: Physiology of trauma. Clin Neurosurg 29:103–130, 1982.

204. Cohadon F, Castel J, Nouillant A: Volume pressure relationship in clinical and experimental condition of raised ICP. In Lundberg N, Ponten U, Brock M (eds): Intracranial Pressure, vol. II. Berlin, Springer-Verlag, 1975, pp 107–110.

205. Marmarou A, Shulman K, Rosende RM: A nonlinear analysis of the cerebrospinal fluid system and intracranial pressure dynamics. J Neurosurg 48:332–344, 1978.

206. Kellie G: On death from cold, and on congestions of the brain: An account of the appearances observed in the dissection of two of three individuals presumed to have perished in the storm of 3rd November 1821; with some reflections on the pathology of the brain. Trans Med Chir Soc Edinb 84–169, 1824.

207. Monro A: Observations on the structure and function of the nervous system. Edinburgh, Creech and Johnson, 1823, p 5.

207a. Kellie G: An account of the appearances observed in the dissection of two of the three individuals presumed to have perished in the storm of the third, and whose bodies were discovered in the vicinity of Seith on the morning of the 4th November 1821 with some reflections on the pathology of the brain. Trans Med Chir Sci Edinburgh 1:84–169, 1824.

208. Ekstedt J: CSF hydrodynamic studies in man. 2. Normal hydrodynamic variables related to CSF pressure and flow. J Neurol Neurosurg Psychiatry 41:345–353, 1978.

209. Shapiro K, Marmarou A, Shulman K: Characterization of clinical CSF dynamics and neural axis compliance using the pressure-volume index. I. The normal pressure-volume index. Ann Neurol 7:508–514, 1980.

210. Yoshihara M, Bandoh K, Marmarou A: Cerebrovascular carbon dioxide reactivity assessed by intracranial pressure dynamics in severely head injured patients. J Neurosurg 82:386–393, 1995; see comments.

211. Marmarou A: Increased intracranial pressure in head injury and influence of blood volume. J Neurotrauma 9(Suppl 1):S327–S332, 1992.

212. Miller JD, Garibi J, Pickard JD: Induced changes of cerebrospinal fluid volume: Effects during continuous monitoring of ventricular fluid pressure. Arch Neurol 28:265–269, 1973.

213. Miller JD, Pickard JD: Intracranial volume pressure studies in patients with head injury. Injury 5:265–268, 1974.

214. Marmarou A: Pathophysiology of intracranial pressure. In Narayan RK, Wilberger JE, Povlishock JT (eds): Neurotrauma. New York, McGraw-Hill, 1996, pp 413–428.

215. Marmarou A, Maset AL, Ward JD, et al: Contribution of CSF

and vascular factors to elevation of ICP in severely head-injured patients. J Neurosurg 66:883–890, 1987.

215a. Klatzo I: Presidential address: Neuropathological aspects of brain edema. J Neuropathol Exp Neurol 26:1–14, 1967.

216. Ritter AM, Muizelaar JP, Barnes T, et al: Brain stem blood flow, pupillary response, and outcome in patients with severe head injuries. Neurosurgery 44:941–948, 1999.

217. Rowan JO, Teasdale G: Brain stem blood flow during raised intracranial pressure. Acta Neurol Scand Suppl 64:520–521, 1977.

218. Chesnut RM, Marshall SB, Piek J, et al: Early and late systemic hypotension as a frequent and fundamental source of cerebral ischemia following severe brain injury in the Traumatic Coma Data Bank. Acta Neurochir Suppl (Wien) 59:121–125, 1993.

219. Piek J, Chesnut RM, Marshall LF, et al: Extracranial complications of severe head injury. J Neurosurg 77:901–907, 1992.

220. Miller J, Becker D: Secondary insults to the injured brain. J R Coll Surg 27:292–298, 1982.

221. Ishige N, Pitts LH, Hashimoto T, et al: Effect of hypoxia on traumatic brain injury in rats. Part 1. Changes in neurological function, electroencephalograms, and histopathology. Neurosurgery 20:848–853, 1987.

222. Ishige N, Pitts LH, Pogliani L, et al: Effect of hypoxia on traumatic brain injury in rats. Part 2. Changes in high energy phosphate metabolism. Neurosurgery 20:854–858, 1987.

223. Kety S, Schmidt C: The effects of altered arterial tensions of carbon dioxide and oxygen on cerebral oxygen consumption of normal young man. J Clin Invest 27:484–492, 1948.

224. Lewelt W, Jenkins LW, Miller JD: Effects of experimental fluid-percussion injury of the brain on cerebrovascular reactivity of hypoxia and to hypercapnia. J Neurosurg 56:332–338, 1982.

225. Dietrich WD, Alonso O, Halley M, Busto R: Delayed posttraumatic brain hyperthermia worsens outcome after fluid percussion brain injury: A light and electron microscopic study in rats. Neurosurgery 38:533–541, 1996.

226. Paulson OB, Parving HH, Olesen J, Skinhoj E: Influence of carbon monoxide and of hemodilution on cerebral blood flow and blood gases in man. J Appl Physiol 35:111–116, 1973.

227. Gopinath SP, Robertson CS, Contant CF, et al: Jugular venous desaturation and outcome after head injury. J Neurol Neurosurg Psychiatry 57:717–723, 1994.

228. Young B, Ott L, Dempsey R, et al: Relationship between admission hyperglycemia and neurologic outcome of severely brain-injured patients. Ann Surg 210:466–472, discussion 472–473, 1989.

229. Lam AM, Winn HR, Cullen BF, Sundling N: Hyperglycemia and neurological outcome in patients with head injury. J Neurosurg 75:545–551, 1991.

230. Rosner MJ, Newsome HH, Becker DP: Mechanical brain injury: The sympathoadrenal response. J Neurosurg 61:76–86, 1984.

231. Sieber FE, Traystman RJ: Special issues: Glucose and the brain. Crit Care Med 20:104–114, 1992.

232. Robertson CS, Goodman JC, Narayan RK, et al: The effect of glucose administration on carbohydrate metabolism after head injury. J Neurosurg 74:43–50, 1991.

233. Rosner MJ, Becker DP: Experimental brain injury: Successful therapy with the weak base, tromethamine, with an overview of CNS acidosis. J Neurosurg 60:961–971, 1984.

234. Wolf AL, Levi L, Marmarou A, et al: Effect of THAM upon outcome in severe head injury: A randomized prospective clinical trial. J Neurosurg 78:54–59, 1993.

235. Yoganandan F, Pintar A Jr: Biomechanics of skull fracture. J Neurotrauma 12:659–668, 1995.

236. Muizelaar JP, Marmarou A, Ward JD, et al: Adverse effects of prolonged hyperventilation in patients with severe head injury: A randomized clinical trial. J Neurosurg 75:731–739, 1991.

237. Muizelaar JP, Wei EP, Kontos HA, Becker DP: Mannitol causes compensatory cerebral vasoconstriction and vasodilation in response to blood viscosity changes. J Neurosurg 59:822–828, 1983.

238. Chesnut R: Treating raised intracranial pressure in head injury. In Narayan RK, Wilberger JE, Povlishock JT (eds): Neurotrauma. New York, McGraw-Hill, 1996, pp 445–469.

239. Skippen P, Seear M, Poskitt K, et al: Effect of hyperventilation on regional cerebral blood flow in head-injured children. Crit Care Med 25:1402–1409, 1997.

240. Juul N, Morris G, Marshall S, Marshall L: Intracranial hypertension and cerebral perfusion pressure: Influence on neurological deterioration and outcome in severe head injury. J Neurosurg 92:1–6, 2000.

241. Bouma GJ, Muizelaar JP, Bandoh K, Marmarou A: Blood pressure and intracranial pressure—volume dynamics in severe head injury: Relationship with cerebral blood flow. J Neurosurg 77:15–19, 1992.

242. Burke AM, Quest DO, Chien S, Cerri C: The effects of mannitol on blood viscosity. J Neurosurg 55:550–553, 1981.

243. Marshall LF, Smith RW, Shapiro HM: The outcome with aggressive treatment in severe head injuries. Part I. The significance of intracranial pressure monitoring. J Neurosurg 50:20–25, 1979.

244. Ward JD, Becker DP, Miller JD, et al: Failure of prophylactic barbiturate coma in the treatment of severe head injury. J Neurosurg 62:383–388, 1985.

245. Clifton GL, Allen S, Barrodale P, et al: A phase II study of moderate hypothermia in severe brain injury. J Neurotrauma 10:263–271, discussion 273, 1993.

246. Marion DW, Obrist WD, Carlier PM, et al: The use of moderate therapeutic hypothermia for patients with severe head injuries: A preliminary report. J Neurosurg 79:354–362, 1993; see comments.

246a. Clifton GL, Miller ER, Choi SC, et al: Lack of effect of induction of hypothermia after acute brain injury. N Engl J Med 344:556–563, 2001.

247. Marshall L, Bowers S, Klauber M: A new classification of head injury based on computerized tomography. J Neurosurg 75:S14–S20, 1991.

CHAPTER 325

Mild Head Injury in Adults

FRANCO SERVADEI ■ GLEN S. MERRY

The term *minor head injury* was used in a paper by Rimel and colleagues[1] in 1981 to describe the extent of injury in patients with a Glasgow Coma Scale (GCS) score of 13 to 15 on admission, a loss of consciousness (LOC) for less than 20 minutes, and a required hospital stay of less than 48 hours. Since then, many other methods for defining a head injury as minor or mild have been suggested (Table 325–1).

These patients constitute the vast majority of head injury admissions (80% according to Kraus and Nourjah[2, 3] and Stiell and coworkers[4]). Only a small subgroup of such patients harbors potentially lethal intracranial lesions, and most or all of these cases are salvageable with early diagnosis and proper treatment. In the last 20 years, many papers dealing with the diagnosis and management of mild or minor head injuries have been produced in various parts of the world. The diffusion of computed tomography (CT) scanners beyond a few sophisticated hospitals[5] has significantly changed the population of head-injured patients admitted to neurosurgical units. There has been a marked increase in the number of patients admitted in a noncomatose state. Miller and colleagues[6] showed that a more liberal CT policy led to a shift in the proportion of hematomas detected in noncomatose patients—from 42% in 1981 to 62% in 1989. There is still a lack of consensus on the indications for performing CT in patients with minor or mild head injuries. A recent paper based on two consecutive prospective studies found that the use of CT can be safely limited to those patients who have certain clinical findings.[7] Conversely, another paper also based on a prospective study and published the same year concluded that CT cannot be excluded in patients with minor head injuries and completely normal neurological examinations on admission.[8]

Why should neurosurgeons be involved in mild head injury management? Mildly head-injured patients who are found on early CT to have intracranial lesions currently constitute a significant percentage of head injury admissions to busy neurosurgical units.[9, 10] The impact of an effective mild head injury management program on the overall outcome of brain-injured patients can be demonstrated by studying a hypothetical area of 1 million people with only one neurosurgical unit. In this area, there will be approximately 2000 head injury admissions, including about 200 comatose patients.[11, 12] Given a mortality rate of 30% for patients with moderate to severe head injuries, as reported in recent studies,[13–16] an unrealistic[17] 10% decrease in severe head injury mortality (due to better and more sophisticated care, new drug therapies) will save 20 lives per year in this area. If we hypothesize that 2% of patients admitted with mild head injuries are harboring potentially lethal post-traumatic lesions, in the same area, more than 30 lives will be saved by early diagnosis and proper management. Ultimately, effective treatment of mildly head-injured patients will produce better results in terms of overall outcome than would increasing the elaborate medical management of severe head injuries in a few sophisticated institutions.[18] This is the reason why neurosurgeons need to take a leadership role in the process of organizing the care of patients with mild head injuries, even though in most parts of the world they deal with only select cases.

The neurosurgical community has already provided guidelines to peripheral hospitals for minor head injury management.[19–24] The aim of these guidelines is early intracranial hematoma detection with the use of CT, even in patients with few or no clinical symptoms. Almost all mildly head-injured patients can be treated without morbidity or mortality if hematoma evacuation (when indicated) occurs before there is clinical deterioration.[25, 26] The identification of these few cases requires organization and cooperation with other physicians (accident and emergency doctors, surgeons, neurologists, radiologists). Indeed, early management of these patients in peripheral hospitals is usually in the hands of emergency physicians. Thus, accident and emergency physicians need to know which patients can be sent home safely after select investigations. A minority of patients need admission to a hospital. Questions that arise include which hospital, and for how long?

DEFINITION

Table 325–1 demonstrates some published definitions of mild or minor head injury. The terms *mild* and

TABLE 325-1 ■ **Definitions of Minor or Mild Head Injury**

AUTHOR	TERMINOLOGY	GCS SCORE	CLINICAL DATA	RADIOLOGY
Rimel et al[1]	Minor	13–15	LOC < 20 min, hospital stay < 48 hr	—
Miller et al,[10] Teasdale et al,[43] Poon et al[109]	Minor	15	Fully conscious	—
Miller & Jones,[63] Miller[64]	Minor	13–14 (scale up to 14)	—	—
Jeret et al,[31] Lee et al[41]	Mild	15	LOC/amnesia	—
Borczuk,[60] Dacey et al,[30] Harad & Kerstein,[55] Shackford et al,[44] Feuerman et al,[58] Stein[23] & Ross	Minor—mild	13–15	LOC/amnesia	—
Culotta et al,[52] Ingebrigtsen et al[62]	Mild	13–15	As above, plus absence of focal neurological deficits	Skull fracture
Servadei et al[38]	Minor—low risk	13–15	Brief LOC or →	—
Mohanty et al[61]	Minor	15	Absence of neurological deficits	—
Gomez et al,[28] Hsiang et al[33]	Mild	13–15	With or without LOC	—

GCS, Glasgow Coma Scale; LOC, loss of consciousness.

minor have been used to identify a similar population. Teasdale[27] defined a minor head injury as occurring in a patient who is oriented and alert, corresponding to a GCS score of 15; those with a mild head injury have a GCS score of 13 to 14. This definition was not adopted by subsequent authors, and confusion was added by the combination of more than one parameter in the definition. Some papers exclude those patients deteriorating within 4 hours of injury,[28] thus eliminating most of the complicated cases and altering the calculation of risk factors. Other authors exclude patients with gunshot wounds and penetrating injuries.[29–31] These patients have a much higher incidence of intracranial hematomas. Therefore, the inclusion or exclusion of these cases is relevant for statistical comparison.

A patient with a mild head injury complicated by an intracranial lesion has more severe sequelae and disability compared with a patient with an uncomplicated injury. According to Williams and associates,[32] this justifies excluding these injuries from being classified as mild. However, we believe that criteria for inclusion in a particular category have to be based on one parameter alone. In this case, the only reliable parameter is the GCS score on admission. Patients with admission GCS scores of 13, 14, or 15 have, in our opinion, minor or mild head injuries. Any other clinical, radiologic, or surgical finding is an added risk factor that does not change the classification.

STUDY TYPE

Only a few published papers contain prospective studies.[4, 7, 30, 31, 33–42] Some papers were partly prospective and partly retrospective,[43, 44] whereas Miller and colleagues[10] presented a prospective data collection examined retrospectively. All the remaining studies were retrospective.

DEMOGRAPHICS

Epidemiology

A number of studies determined the epidemiology of all head injuries. The annual estimated incidence in the United States and European countries is 200 to 300 patients per 100,000 population.[11, 12]

In 1991, 1.5 million noninstitutionalized U.S. civilians sustained head injuries. These injuries caused LOC but were not severe enough to cause death or long-term institutionalization. It is estimated that in 1991, 381,000 brain-injured patients sought no medical care; 221,000 were treated in clinics and offices, 543,000 were treated in emergency departments, and 392,000 were admitted to hospitals.[45] Other reports[2, 4, 46] estimate that about 350,000 patients require hospital treatment for mild head injury each year in the United States, representing 80% of all patients admitted to hospitals for head injury.

It is also estimated that about 1 million recently head-injured patients go to hospitals each year in the United Kingdom, one fiftieth of the population.[47–49] Of these, 800,000 patients have minor or mild head injuries, and 80,000 of them are admitted to hospitals.[50] Head injury causes 10% of new accident and emergency admissions in the United Kingdom and accounts for about 25% of all emergency observation ward admissions, with 96% of patients admitted for less than 24 hours.[48] The incidence of minor head injury in Sweden has been reported at 5000 per million population per year.[51]

In spite of the different data, which can probably be explained by different methods of data collection (e.g., all patients seen in emergency departments versus patients admitted), the phenomenon of mild head injury causes a significant number of visits to emergency departments and a substantial number of hospital admissions in both the United States and Europe.

Causes

Table 325–2 shows the incidence of the most frequent causes of trauma in various published series of mildly head-injured patients. Assaults can cause from 1% to 56% of injuries, road traffic accidents from 17% to 68%, and falls (with or without alcohol consumption) from 8% to 63%. Culotta and associates[52] showed a relation between severity of injury (based on GCS

T A B L E 3 2 5 – 2 ■ **Main Causes of Mild Head Injuries Worldwide**

AUTHOR	ASSAULT (%)	RTA/MVC (%)	FALL (%)	OTHER (%)	COUNTRY
Nagy et al[34]	50	31	11		US
Chan et al[35]	16	26	46		Hong Kong
Miller et al[10]	19	20	54		UK
Gomez et al[28]	23	36	35	Pedestrian, 5	Spain
Arienta et al[57]	6	42	31		Italy
Stiell et al[41]	17	43	23	Pedestrian, 7	Canada
Murshid[56]	5	37	53		Saudi Arabia
Voss et al[71]	56	17	13	Pedestrian, 8	South Africa
Servadei et al[38]	1	68	25		Italy
Borczuk[60]	25	35	30	Pedestrian, 7	US
Shackford et al[44]	8	57	21	Pedestrian, 7	US
Lee et al[41]	<2	52	8	Pedestrian, 38	Taiwan
Harad & Kerstein[55]	19	44	19	Pedestrian, 14	US
Jeret et al[3]	31	56	63		US
Duus et al[59]	18	34	22	Sports, 10	Denmark
Miller & Jones[63]	20	27	41	Sports, 7	UK
Dacey et al[30]	9	60	20		US
Rimel et al[1]	10	46	23	Sports, 18	US

MVC, motor vehicle crash; RTA, road traffic accident.

score on admission) and cause of trauma, with assaults being more frequent in patients with more severe injury.

Causes of trauma also influence the rate of hospital admission (with motor vehicle crashes causing most admissions)[45] and are also age related (with falls being more frequent in the elderly).[29]

Age

Because risk factors for hematoma development differ in children and adults,[35, 53] it is crucial to know the age of patients included in reported series. No age range was reported by several authors.[23, 40, 46, 54, 55] In one paper, the mean age was 17 years, with a range from 1 month to 89 years; 300 of 633 patients (47%) were younger than 10 years.[56] Shackford and colleagues reported a mean age of 27 years with a range from 2 months to 90 years.[44] Other papers have included (or have studied separately) only patients older than 3 years,[7] 6 years,[57] 10 years,[30, 33] 13 years,[49] 14 years[8, 38, 52] 16 years,[4, 41, 58–60] or 18 years.[31, 61] The mean age varies, according to the inclusion criteria, from 17 to 37 years.[4, 31, 34, 38, 41, 44, 57, 59, 62] The relationship between severity of trauma (GCS score) and mean age was studied in two papers,[33, 52] with no significant differences found; the mean age ranged from 33 to 40 years in the different GCS categories (13, 14, 15). Obviously, conclusions about risk factors in studies containing a significant number of children may differ from conclusions drawn in studies including only adults.

Gender

The percentage of males in the reported series varied from 54% to 74%.* The proportion of females increased with age, so that 72% of patients age 30 years or younger were male, whereas 62% of those older than

70 years were female.[28] According to Culotta and associates,[52] the percentage of males remained nearly the same (64% to 67%) among patients having various GCS scores.[13–15]

Substance Abuse

A substantial number of patients presenting with mild head injuries have consumed alcohol. Nagy and coworkers[34] reported that 247 of 1170 patients (21%) were intoxicated on admission, 91% due to alcohol consumption. Of 1555 patients tested, 780 (50%) had positive blood alcohol concentration (BAC) tests on admission. In the vast majority of positive cases (80%), the BAC was greater than 0.10 mL/dL.[44] In two studies, the BAC on admission was greater than 0.01 g/dL in 51%[30] and 43%[1] of patients. Other series have reported similar data.[52, 59, 63]

In the clinical assessment of a mild head injury, the effect of alcohol should be taken into account in determining the severity of injury. Serial clinical examinations are essential in these circumstances. The late detection of an intracranial hematoma in an intoxicated patient is, unfortunately, a common occurrence. We agree with published guidelines[21, 24] that whenever there is a doubt about the clinical assessment of such patients, a computed tomographic scan must be obtained.

Other Injuries

The presence of associated injuries has received little attention in the literature. Miller[64] found facial injuries in 11% of patients, limb injuries in 7%, thoracic or abdominal injuries in 6%, and spinal injuries in 5%.

CLINICAL AND RADIOLOGIC PARAMETERS

Glasgow Coma Scale

The GCS score is the standard method of evaluating patients with mild head injuries, even if the only scores

---

* See references 4, 9, 30, 31, 34, 38, 41, 44, 55–57, 59, 62.

used are 13, 14, and 15.[1] Table 325–3 shows the percentage of different GCS scores in various studies. Patients admitted with a GCS score of 13 account for 2% to 9%, those with a score 14 for 4% to 28%, and those with a score of 15 for 63% to 94% in adult series. Even if these series contain only patients admitted to hospitals, the number of patients admitted in a relatively asymptomatic state (GCS score of 15) overwhelms other categories.

Marion and Carlier[65] showed in a multicenter survey that there are important differences in how, when, and by whom the initial GCS score is obtained. The conclusion of this study was that we need to know this information before comparing different reports. Admis-

T A B L E   3 2 5 – 3 ■ **Relationship between GCS Score on Admission and Presence of Intracranial Lesion or Need for Surgery in Mildly Head-Injured Patients**

AUTHOR AND YEAR	STUDY TYPE	NO. OF CASES		NO. HAVING CT	INTRACRANIAL LESION PRESENT (%)	CRANIOTOMY REQUIRED (%)
Dacey et al, 1986[30]	Prospective	GCS 13–15	610	68	5	3
Feurmann et al, 1988[58]	Retrospective	GCS 13	34 (9%)	21	62	3
		GCS 14	103 (28%)	49	41	3
		GCS 15	236 (63%)	59	34	0.8 (ICP excluded)
Stein & Ross, 1990[23]	Retrospective	GCS 13	62 (9%)	62	40	11
		GCS 14	142 (22%)	142	22	6
		GCS 15	454 (69%)	454	13	4 (igroma, ICP included)
Shackford et al, 1992[44]	Prospective	GCS 13	221 (8%)	200	33	
		GCS 14	646 (23%)	512	18	4.2
		GCS 15	1899 (69%)	1454	15	(GCS 13–15) (ICP included)
Stein & Ross, 1992[46]	Retrospective	GCS 13	120 (8%)	120	37	3.7
		GCS 14	301 (19%)	301	24	(GCS 13–15)
		GCS 15	1117 (73%)	1117	6.5	(ICP included)
Harad & Kerstein, 1992[55]	Retrospective	GCS 13	11 (4%)	11	27	
		GCS 14	40 (13%)	40	23	3.6
		GCS 15	251 (83%)	251	17	(GCS 13–15) (ICP excluded)
Borczuk, 1995[60]	Retrospective	GCS 13	40 (3%)	40	27	7.5
		GCS 14	197 (13%)	197	18	3.6
		GCS 15	1211 (84%)	1211	6	0.08
Servadei et al, 1995[38]	Prospective	GCS 13	47 (5%)			GCS 13–15
		GCS 14	110 (13%)	196	36	0.6
		GCS 15	702 (82%)			GCS 13–15 (ICP excluded)
Gomez et al, 1996[28]	Retrospective	GCS 13	45 (2%)	39	67	27
		GCS 14	88 (4%)	58	55	4.5
		GCS 15	2351 (94%)	90	41	0.6 (ICP included, only 1 patient)
Culotta et al, 1997[52]	Retrospective	GCS 13	176 (5%)	173	28	4.5
		GCS 14	796 (24%)	755	16	1.6
		GCS 15	2398 (71%)	2179	4	0.4
Hsiang et al, 1997[33]	Prospective	GCS 13	45 (4%)	43	58	20
		GCS 14	138 (10%)	115	35	5.1
		GCS 15	1177 (86%)	683	18	2.2
Holmes et al, 1997[36]	Prospective	GCS 14	264	264	13	1.5 (ICP included)
Miller et al, 1997[37]	Prospective	GCS 15	2143	2143	13	0.2 (ICP excluded)
Nagurney et al, 1998[29]	Retrospective	GCS 14–15	age > 60 yr 318(19%)	318	18	3
		GCS 14–15	age < 60 yr 1331(81%)	1331	8	1.3 (ICP excluded)
Murshid, 1998[56]	Retrospective	GCS 13	11 (2%)	11	72	50
		GCS 14	8 (1%)	8	62	16.6
		GCS 15	614 (97%)	112	15	0.6 (CSDH included ICP excluded)
Nagy et al, 1999[34]	Prospective	GCS 15	1170	1170	3	0.3 (ICP excluded)

CSDH, chronic subdural hematoma; CT, computed tomography; GCS, Glasgow Coma Scale; ICP, intracranial pressure monitoring.

sion GCS score was reported in most papers on mild head injuries.* Only four studies recorded when this assessment was made: within 6 to 24 hours of injury[10] or within 24 hours.[7, 31, 58] The assessment was made by neurosurgeons,[28, 33, 56] emergency physicians,[35, 38] trauma surgeons,[34, 52, 61] neurologists,[31] or "junior doctors."[59] It was repeated by nursing personnel every 15 minutes,[56] every hour,[30] or every 2 hours.[38] We believe that a reliable assessment should be made on admission by a physician and repeated at least every hour for the first 24 hours by nursing personnel.

Timing of the First Computed Tomographic Scan

The timing of the initial computed tomographic scan is important. It has been shown that 14% to 20% of patients admitted with a diffuse brain injury may develop a mass lesion.[66] This change is likely to occur within 12 to 24 hours after injury.[67, 68] Thus, the danger is particularly evident when patients with mild head injuries undergo CT very early.[69, 70]

Indications for Obtaining a Computed Tomographic Scan

There is wide variation in the indications for obtaining a computed tomographic scan in the published series. One approach is to scan the vast majority of mildly head-injured patients, with the only indication being LOC or a period of post-traumatic amnesia (PTA).[23, 31, 34, 37, 46, 62] Another approach is to scan a patient only in the presence of clinical deterioration[10, 30, 41, 59] and a focal neurological deficit.[71]

Some investigators have suggested a combination of clinicoradiologic parameters, such as CT for all patients with a GCS score of 13 or 14 or a skull fracture. In patients with a GCS score of 15, the decision is left to the discretion of the admitting neurosurgeon.[33, 35] Another combination is based on the presence of a skull fracture, persistent headache or vomiting, or clinical deterioration.[38] Purely clinical indications for CT are mild head injury with PTA or LOC; focal neurological deficits; presence or persistence of vomiting, nausea, or headache; intoxication; a serious injury mechanism[7, 28, 29, 42, 54]; or Masters' criteria.[29, 60]

A prospective study in seven Canadian emergency departments showed significant variation in the rate of ordering CT in mildly head-injured patients, from as low as 16% to as high as 70% of admitted patients. All cases of initially missed hematomas (five) occurred at institutions with high rates of CT use, demonstrating that frequent use of CT does not necessarily translate to a high detection rate. Further, there was significant heterogeneity in the ordering of CT among staff physicians, even in the same institution.[4] An American multicenter study also showed different indications in the various centers.[44]

The lack of consensus on indications for obtaining a computed tomographic scan in mildly head-injured patients has generated a series of reports that are difficult to compare. For example, Duus and coworkers[59] reported that in a series of 1876 patients admitted following mild head injury, only 27 (1.4%) underwent CT, with the sole indication for scanning being the presence of clinical deterioration. Nine patients had intracranial hematomas. These patients represented 0.5% of the total population but 33% of those undergoing CT. Stein and Ross[46] studied 1538 mildly head-injured patients with CT and found that 209 (13.5%) had "abnormal" scans. Thus, the difference in the number of intracranial lesions in similar populations is due to the large number of patients harboring intracranial abnormalities who do not deteriorate. Our indications for obtaining a computed tomographic scan are listed later.

Definition of Abnormal Computed Tomographic Scan

The usual end point in clinical series of head-injured patients is patient outcome. The outcome in recent studies of severe head injury was determined after 6 months using the Glasgow Outcome Score (GOS).[72] However, only a few papers refer to GOS,[9, 10, 33, 38, 63] and others study only mortality.[6, 31, 44, 52, 57] The combination of mortality and GOS has not been used as a study end point. This is because in a population of mildly head-injured patients, the percentage of poor results is low, and the statistical study of risk factors is extremely difficult. The vast majority of clinical studies have related the clinicoradiologic findings to the presence or absence of CT "abnormalities." Unfortunately, the definition of "abnormalities" is inconsistent in the various papers. A common definition includes all intracranial post-traumatic hematomas and depressed fractures, in addition to traumatic subarachnoid hemorrhage, intraventricular hemorrhage, linear fractures, a form of brain edema or swelling, and pneumocephalus.[23, 31, 36, 37, 46, 60] Stein and Ross[46] reported that in a study of 209 "abnormal scans," 82 cases (39%) had "diffuse swelling." Because "diffuse swelling" is not defined, it is difficult to accept that these scans can be included in the group of abnormal computed tomographic scans that includes intracranial post-traumatic hematomas.

We agree with a series of studies that considered abnormal computed tomographic scans to be those demonstrating an intracranial post-traumatic lesion,* excluding diffuse edema and linear skull fractures and, in a few cases, even traumatic subarachnoid hemorrhage.[9, 10, 35, 43]

There have also been attempts to separate lesions that are relevant in terms of medical and surgical treatment from "incidental" findings. Shackford and colleagues[44] defined an "abnormal scan" as an examination showing any abnormality, whether related to trauma or not; a "positive scan" as one showing an acute pathologic state in the brain or skull; and a "relevant positive scan" as one showing acute changes

---

* See references 28, 30, 31, 33, 35, 38, 52, 56, 58, 59, 61.

* See references 9, 10, 28, 30, 33, 35, 39, 43, 57, 61, 71.

of the contents of the skull, excluding isolated linear and basilar fractures. The key point is to relate the risk factors not to the presence of lesions but to significant intracranial hematomas, which are those hematomas requiring close CT monitoring and possibly surgical evacuation.

Intracranial Abnormalities and Lesion Type

In 1992, an estimated 270,000 computed tomographic scans were ordered for head injuries by emergency departments in the United States, and of these, 96% to 99% were normal.[4] Thus, the search for patients harboring intracranial lesions is expensive and probably requires a better target than "all mildly head-injured patients." In Table 325–3 we report the incidence of abnormal computed tomographic scans in studied populations. Unfortunately, as stated previously, the definition of "abnormal" varies. The other key factor is the percentage of computed tomographic scans obtained in the overall population. The percentage of patients studied with CT in Table 325–3 was 11%[30] to 100%.[23, 34, 36, 37, 46, 55, 60] When there is a selective policy, the rate of computed tomographic scanning is obviously higher in patients with a GCS score of 13 or 14.[28, 33, 38, 44] Taking into consideration only those reports (see Table 325–3) in which a computed tomographic scan was obtained in the vast majority of patients, the rate of intracranial abnormalities ranged from 27% to 40% with an admission GCS score of 13, from 16% to 24% with a score of 14, and from 3% to 15% with a score of 15. One can conclude that patients with a GCS score of 13 have a risk similar to that of patients with moderate head injuries[73, 74] and should not be considered to have mild head injuries. Further, patients with a GCS score of 15 have an exceedingly small risk of having an intracranial lesion[43]; these patients need a separate pathway.

Voss and coworkers[71] studied 323 patients with a GCS score of 15 who were seen in the emergency room, sent home, and subsequently readmitted because of clinical complaints. CT after the second admission showed 87 abnormalities (27%). The conclusion was that patients who return to the hospital after discharge have a higher percentage of intracranial lesions and need a computed tomographic scan. Jeret and associates[31] used a stepwise discriminant function analysis to relate CT and clinical findings. No single item or combination of items could be used to classify 95% of patients into either normal or abnormal CT groups.

In Table 325–4 we report the distribution of various lesions (including only intracranial hematomas and depressed fractures) on CT studies. In studies on unselected populations with mild head injuries, epidural hematomas occur in 4% to 28%, subdural hematomas in 10% to 31%, contusions and intraparenchymal hematomas in 37% to 69%, and depressed fractures in 3% to 17%. In the two studies on a selected population of patients admitted to neurosurgery departments,[9, 10] epidural hematomas increased to about 50%. Epidural hematomas are the lesions that most frequently require operation in these series.

Surgery

Table 325–3 shows the rate of surgical interventions. Some papers explicitly exclude intracranial pressure monitoring from the group of surgical procedures,[28, 34, 37, 38, 55, 56, 58] whereas others include it.[23, 36, 44, 46] In the remaining studies, this parameter is not reported.[33, 52, 60] We believe that intracranial pressure monitoring is indicated in severe head injuries[75] and in selected cases of moderate head injuries.[74, 75] No published guidelines contain indications for intracranial pressure monitoring in mildly head-injured patients.

There is a strong relationship between a decreasing GCS score and an increasing number of surgical procedures (see Table 325–3).

Dacey and associates[30] noted that 9 of 12 surgically treated patients had right-sided masses. This may indicate that our reliance on language functions to assess the level of consciousness after head injury in relatively alert patients may limit the early detection of right-sided lesions.

Only a small percentage of patients harboring intracranial lesions had an operation (see Table 325–4). Determining the indications for surgical treatment in patients without symptoms or clinical signs is a challenge for neurosurgeons. The indiscriminate conservative treatment of the past, when these patients did not undergo CT, must be changed to a deliberate choice between surgery and repeat CT examinations. This problem has been extensively studied for epidural hematomas, and guidelines have been developed for when to operate on occult intracranial hematomas. In the absence of clinical symptoms, hematomas with a thickness of less than 15 mm,[76–78] a volume of less than 30 cc,[78] and a midline shift of less than 5 mm[77, 78] can safely be managed conservatively. An important risk factor is the presence of a heterogeneous clot or a lucent swirl within an area of high density on CT,[79, 80] because these signs are related to active bleeding and hematoma enlargement. The most important factor in deciding in favor of nonsurgical management is, in our opinion, the time from injury to hematoma detection. One paper confirmed previous findings[81] about the timing of hematoma enlargement: in a study of 160 patients with epidural hematomas that were managed conservatively, 37 demonstrated an increase in hematoma size. Mean time to enlargement was 8 hours from injury and 5 hours from the first computed tomographic scan.[82] In no case did the hematoma increase after 36 hours. Guidelines for conservative treatment of epidural hematomas must also contain indications for repeat CT, especially in the first 12 hours after injury.[83]

Similar indications for surgery based on CT data (e.g., hematoma thickness and midline shift) have been published for occult subdural hematomas.[84, 85] An interesting finding is the possibility of hematoma reabsorption in the case of small, acute, thin subdural clots. The mechanism appears to be that the hematoma spreads over a larger surface, making it invisible on CT but detectable on magnetic resonance imaging (MRI).[86] This reabsorption occurs mainly in hematomas de-

TABLE 325–4 ■ Lesion Type and Surgical Findings

	CT LESION				SURGICAL LESION			
AUTHOR AND YEAR	Epidural Hematoma	Subdural Hematoma	Contusion/ Intraparenchymal Hematoma	Depressed Fracture	Epidural Hematoma	Subdural Hematoma	Contusion	Depressed Fracture
Dacey et al, 1986[30]		33						
Feurmann et al, 1988[58]	7 (16%)	8 (18%)	30 (66%)	—	1	3	1	3
Stein & Ross, 1990[23]	9 (14%)	7 (11%)	37 (58%)	11 (17%)	3	3	0	—
Shackford et al, 1992[44]	64 (14%)	97 (21%)	272 (59%)	29 (6%)	30 craniotomies + ICP monitoring			
Stein & Ross, 1992[46]	18 (14%)	12 (10%)	82 (65%)	14 (11%)	82 craniotomies			29
Borczuk, 1995[60]	10 (8%)	34 (28%)	71 (58%)	8 (6%)	58 craniotomies + ICP monitoring			
Servadei et al, 1995[38]	13 (28%)	5 (10%)	29 (62%)	—	11 craniotomies			—
Gomez et al, 1996[28]	21 (24%)	27 (31%)	32 (37%)	7 (8%)	3	1	1	—
Culotta et al, 1997[52]	27 (12%)	67 (30%)	132 (58%)	—	8	11	3	7
Holmes et al, 1997[36]	4 (13%)	8 (26%)	19 (61%)	—	31 craniotomies			—
Hsiang et al, 1997[33]	16 (19%)	22 (26%)	46 (55%)	—	2	2	0	—
Miller et al, 1997[37]	4 (4%)	27 (24%)	78 (69%)	3 (3%)	42 craniotomies			—
Nagurney et al, 1998[29]		Age >60 yr, 31 / Age <60 yr, 48			Age <60 yr, 8	Age >60 yr, 15 / Age <60 yr, 10	Age >60 yr, 1 / Age <60 yr, 1	3
*Servadei et al, 1993[9]	49 (44%)	6 (5%)	41 (36%)	17 (15%)	21 (52%)	1 (3%)	5 (13%)	Age <60 yr, 9
*Miller et al, 1990[10]					98 (54%)	35 (19%)	27 (15%)	13 (32%) / Combination 18 (10%)

*Selected series collected in neurosurgical department. CT, computed tomography; ICP, intracranial pressure.

tected within 3 hours of injury.[67] Repeat CT must be planned in the case of nonoperative treatment of acute subdural hematomas.

Parenchymal post-traumatic damage occurs frequently in patients with mild head injuries, but the need for surgical evacuation is rare (see Table 325–4). Management of brain contusion in mildly head-injured patients has received very little attention in the neurosurgical literature. It looks as if no advancement has been made since 1768, when Pott wrote: "an intracerebral hematoma can be present in the absence of clinical deterioration. It may therefore be difficult to decide what to do."[87] Clinical deterioration as recently defined,[88] such as a drop of at least 2 points in the GCS score or the appearance of pupillary abnormalities or focal neurological deficits, is still, in our opinion, the principal indication for surgery in these cases. Radiologic signs of cisterns, compression, and increasing hematoma size on follow-up CT[67, 68, 89] are also indications for surgery.

In conclusion, nonsurgical management of intracranial hematomas requires expertise and close collaboration between neurosurgeons and neuroradiologists.

Clinical Deterioration

Neurological deterioration (defined as an increase in a preexisting neurological deficit, the development of a new focal sign, or a 2-point decrease in GCS score)[88] is more frequent in patients with GCS scores of 13 or 14.[28] The causes of clinical deterioration are surgical masses,[9, 41] seizures, or hyponatremia.[41] In the case of deterioration caused by mass lesions, whenever it occurs early (within 4 to 6 hours of injury), the intracranial hematomas are usually extracerebral,[9] whereas late deterioration is usually related to evolving parenchymal damage.[9, 41]

RISK FACTORS

It is critical to identify those few patients at risk of developing intracranial hematomas. An anonymous mail survey was conducted on a random sample of 300 members of the Canadian Association of Emergency Physicians. The vast majority (85%) responded that they did not agree with the recommendation of ordering a computed tomographic scan on every patient with a minor head injury. Fifty-two percent of the responders said that they would require guidelines for obtaining a CT scan to be 100% sensitive for identifying lesions necessitating neurosurgical intervention.[90] With this aim, all the previously reported demographics and clinical and radiologic parameters have been related to the presence of intracranial post-traumatic lesions to determine which group among the vast population of mildly head-injured patients seen in emergency departments can be identified as at "higher risk." Most of the premises that allow a valid comparison among different papers are not fulfilled: the definition of mild or minor head injury differs, the causes of injury vary significantly, only a few papers consider children and adults separately (and the age limit is different), indications for CT are varied, and the timing of the first computed tomographic scan is spread over at least 24 hours. Of particular importance is the lack of consensus concerning the definition of the end point of any study of risk factors ("abnormal CT"). We cannot expect to have similar results if we compare studies of an unspecified number of children with indications for CT based on LOC and a broad definition of abnormal CT[23, 46] with studies of adult populations with a selective policy for performing CT and the presence of intracranial post-traumatic lesions in each abnormal scan.[28, 33]

Age

Hsiang and coworkers[33] reported that all deaths in patients with GCS scores of 15 occurred in the elderly (older than 65 years) and were due to expanding subdural hematomas.

Two groups of patients younger (1324 patients) or older (377 patients) than 65 years admitted to the hospital after minor head injury (GCS 13 to 14; scale up to 14) were compared with regard to clinical and radiologic parameters. Patients older than 65 were found to have an equal sex ratio; falls accounted for more than 75% of cases, alcohol was commonly involved in males, and the presence of intracranial hematomas was higher. The conclusion was that an increased demand to perform CT to detect intracranial hematomas at an early stage and prevent avoidable mortality would come largely from the older age group.[91]

Most papers[29, 31, 33, 41, 57, 60] confirm that the elderly have an increased risk of developing intracranial hematomas that becomes statistically significant over the age of 60 to 65 years. However, it is unlikely that there is a specific age threshold above which the risk suddenly increases. The underlying pattern is of a gradual, progressive increase in intracranial complications that becomes notable and clinically relevant at about 60 years of age.

Gender

A number of papers studied the effect of gender on the risk of developing an intracranial lesion. Lee[41] and Jeret[31] and their respective colleagues found no difference in the rate of abnormal CT and clinical deterioration. In contrast, Edna[92] showed that the male-female ratio was 2.3:1 in all series but 8:1 in patients with acute intracranial hematomas. In one report,[30] patients requiring surgical intervention were more likely to be male. In summary, there is no indication that gender has a significant influence on outcome in patients with mild head injuries.

Race

Only Jeret and colleagues[31] demonstrated an increased risk of hematoma in whites. Abnormal CT findings were observed in 21 of 152 white patients (14%), in 38 of 463 black patients (8%), and in 2 of 69 Hispanic patients (3%).

Causes

Pedestrians struck by cars and patients who have been assaulted are at substantially increased risk of hematoma development and of poorer outcome.[31, 44, 55, 60] The risk of readmission after discharge and the need for a neurosurgical procedure were significantly higher in cases of penetrating injury.[71]

Patients who have been assaulted and those with gunshot wounds are more likely to need intracranial surgery, which is only partly explained by the increased incidence of depressed skull fractures.[55] Be-

cause the rate of injuries due to assaults varies widely in the published series (see Table 325–2), the calculation of the risk factors both for intracranial lesions and for surgical procedures in various parts of the world, and even in the same country, may lead to different conclusions.

Focal Neurological Deficits

The indication for CT was limited to neurological deterioration in a series of 1873 Danish patients. Subsequently, both the rate of neurological deterioration and the number of computed tomographic scans were related to the presence of an abnormal neurological examination. Among the 1828 patients with normal neurological examinations, there were only 22 cases of clinical deterioration (1.2%). Among the 45 patients with abnormal neurological examinations, 5 patients deteriorated (11%).[59]

Lee and coworkers[41] also related clinical deterioration and focal motor weakness on admission. All 15 patients with abnormal neurological examinations on admission deteriorated.

In a multicenter series of 2766 patients admitted with a CGS score of 13 to 15, 2112 had normal neurological examinations. Surgical intervention was required in 59 patients in this group (2.8%), whereas it was required in 51 of 647 patients (7.8%) with abnormal neurological examinations.[44]

Patients presenting with focal neurological deficits, in spite of a normal level of consciousness, are immediately identified in the emergency room as being at higher risk for intracranial hematoma. Nevertheless, it cannot be assumed that a computed tomographic scan will be obtained.[93] A study conducted in Scotland in 183 patients who presented at the first hospital with normal consciousness and subsequently required surgery for an intracranial hematoma showed that one third had a neurological deficit when first seen.[10]

The incidence of intracranial hematomas in patients with mild injuries and focal neurological deficits[29, 41, 58, 59, 60, 71] is high enough that some of the recently published guidelines[21, 24] exclude these patients from the group classified as having minor head injuries. We believe that the level of consciousness is the only way to classify patients according to the GCS. Although these injuries are "mild," the risk of an intracranial hematoma means that CT must be performed promptly.

Headache, Vomiting, Nausea, and Seizures

Conflicting results have been published concerning the significance of headache, vomiting, and nausea as risk factors for hematoma development. Some authors have found no relationship between these symptoms and the presence of intracranial traumatic lesions.[31, 33, 35, 39, 94] Others have shown a significant relationship between headache, vomiting,[7, 59] and nausea and an increased frequency of intracranial lesions,[10, 34, 60] clinical deterioration,[41] and skull fractures.[34, 95]

Miller and associates[37] studied a series of 1873 patients admitted within 2 hours of injury with a GCS score of 15. All patients underwent CT. Among 841 patients with headache, nausea, vomiting, or clinical signs of depressed fracture, 90 (11%) were found to have intracranial lesions. In the absence of these symptoms, lesions were present in only 48 of 1032 (3.7%). No neurosurgical operations were performed in patients with no risk factors. The authors concluded that, using the four clinical criteria for head injury, 65% sensitivity and 63% specificity would be achieved in detecting patients with abnormal computed tomographic scans. There would be 100% sensitivity, however, for detecting patients who required surgical intervention.[37] Unfortunately, this study did not specify the patients' age (i.e., the number of children) or the causes of trauma. Their suggestion concerning the use of clinical criteria to determine indications for neuroradiologic examinations is not new. In 1987, Masters and colleagues[42] suggested clinical criteria for obtaining a skull radiograph and a computed tomographic scan. Their data on 4068 patients enrolled prospectively showed that the chance of missing an occult intracranial hematoma in the low-risk group of patients (as defined only by clinical parameters), omitting x-ray examination, would be no higher than 8.5 in 10,000 cases. As in previous studies,[96, 97] there were no intracranial injuries in the low-risk group of patients.[42]

With the increasing use of CT in patients with mild head injuries in the past decade, we have learned that occasional patients may harbor significant intracranial lesions without showing clinical symptoms.[8, 9, 54, 55] Holmes and coworkers[36] prospectively studied 264 patients admitted with a GCS score of 14 to determine the utility of Miller's[37] criteria to select those patients who required CT. The use of these criteria would have resulted in missing 17 of 35 abnormal scans and 2 of 4 patients who required craniotomies.[36]

The presence of seizures was studied in an unselected (no age limit) series of 633 patients. Twenty-five (4%) had a generalized convulsion within 24 hours of injury, and 17 of these patients (68%) were younger than 15 years. A computed tomographic scan was obtained in 14 patients and was positive in 3 (21%), but no surgical treatment was necessary.[56]

Loss of Consciousness and Post-traumatic Amnesia

The occurrence of a transient LOC or a period of amnesia has been used to differentiate a brain injury from a scalp bruise or a skull injury. The duration of PTA has been accepted for many years as an index of brain injury severity.[98] In a large study of fully conscious patients, it was estimated that a history of altered consciousness increased the risk of traumatic intracranial hematoma by a factor of five, that is, from 1 in 31,370 to 1 in 6663.[43] However, the absolute risk remained quite small.

LOC is a difficult variable to quantify, because qualified witnesses are usually not available. Whenever an attempt was made to investigate the presence of LOC, a large number of patients (26% to 82%) presented with

a "questionable" LOC.[33, 34, 60] The variable "questionable LOC" as opposed to "confirmed LOC" was not related to the presence of intracranial lesions.[60] Using LOC or amnesia as a criterion for CT would have missed 2 patients who required surgical intervention and 27 with positive scans.[60] A paper by Hsiang and colleagues[33] raised concerns[99] about the use of LOC or PTA as the only indication for CT, a concern that had also been noted in other reports.[23, 46, 62] As already stated,[33, 60] this variable is important, but it is difficult to collect reliable information. Unfortunately, the detection of asymptomatic hematomas is complex. The best results are probably obtained by combining different clinical and radiologic parameters and not by relying on a debatable variable.

Mental Status

The forward and reverse digit span and object recall were not significantly different in patients with normal and abnormal computed tomographic scans.[31] In patients with an admission GCS score of 15 and a normal mental status examination (a patient with a score of 15 can have memory deficits), the chance of developing a serious complication is exceedingly small.[58]

Glasgow Coma Scale and Clinical Factors

In Table 325–3 we reported the incidence of both intracranial abnormalities and surgical indications as related to the GCS score on admission. There is a straightforward relationship between GCS score and the risk of intracranial hematoma, with patients having a score of 13 being at higher risk. Further, these patients harbor lesions that are similar to those found in moderately head-injured patients (GCS score 9 to 12).[73, 74] For this reason, patients with admission GCS scores of 13 have recently been included by some investigators in the moderately head-injured group.[21, 24, 73]

The clinical assessment is usually made on admission. However, admission to an accident and emergency observation ward does not ensure accurate or frequent neurological examinations.[49] A written questionnaire was sent to all 63 Norwegian hospitals treating head injury in 1996. Only 9 of 63 (14%) had established criteria for admission, 34 of 63 (54%) did not use coma scales to assess the level of consciousness, 46 of 63 (73%) did not perform routine radiologic investigation, and only 32 of 63 (51%) had established routines for repeated assessment. In these hospitals, mildly head-injured patients were assessed every hour.[100] Thus, even in a well-organized health care system like Norway's, the clinical surveillance of mildly head-injured patients is far from optimal. Elsewhere, Shackford and coworkers[44] showed that only 70% of patients admitted had frequent neurological assessments, and Livingston and associates[101] reported serial neurological examinations in as few as 50% of patients. The problem therefore relates not to hospital admission but to the mechanism for clinical follow-up.

Skull Fracture

A debate persists about the significance of skull fracture as a risk factor for intracranial hematoma in mildly head-injured patients. Initially in the United Kingdom[19, 43, 102, 103] and subsequently in other countries such as Italy,[21, 38, 39, 57] Spain,[28, 70] South Africa,[71] and Hong Kong,[33, 35] the presence of a skull fracture was included as a principal risk factor in any protocol for mild head injury management. In contrast, the presence of only a brief period of LOC or PTA was taken as an indication for CT by most American authors.[7, 23, 34, 36, 37, 44, 46, 60] This attitude may reflect the availability of CT scanners in different areas of the world. In Canada, however (where CT is readily available in most hospitals), a survey mailed to 300 members of the Canadian Association of Emergency Medicine showed that 85% of responders did not agree with the recommendation by some experts that a computed tomographic scan of the head be ordered for all patients with mild or minor head injuries.[90]

As already discussed in the section on clinical factors, when we wish to select patients for CT, most clinical indicators appear to be inadequate. The use of an objective parameter such as the presence or absence of skull fracture has been examined extensively by many authors.

The presence of a linear skull fracture in an adult patient correlates with a risk of developing an intracranial hematoma that is 3 to 175 times greater* than in the absence of a skull fracture. Because the risk of hematoma is not zero in patients without fractures, a skull radiograph is indicated in adults with mild head injury only when CT is not readily available. In fact, a recent meta-analysis[104] concluded that the estimated sensitivity of a radiographic finding of skull fracture for the diagnosis of intracranial hematomas is 0.38, with a corresponding specificity of 0.95.

A paper published by Masters and coworkers[42] in 1987 summarized radiologists' opinions. In four different studies,[42, 96, 97, 105] fractures were detected in the low-risk group of patients at a rate of 0.4% to 1.6%. In these patients, there were no intracranial injuries. Therefore, the conclusion was that skull radiographs should be avoided in this group. In the moderate-risk group (which encompasses the vast majority of patients admitted to hospital care), intracranial hematomas were found in 3 of 47 patients (6.4%) with skull fractures and in 7 of 1081 (0.65%) without skull fractures. Therefore, the risk of hematoma in moderate-risk patients is 10 times greater in the presence of skull fracture,[42] in accordance with previously reported series.

In conclusion, the presence of a skull fracture increases the risk of intracranial hematoma in adult patients. However, skull radiographs are of value only when CT is not available.

Coagulopathy

With the increased use of anticoagulant therapy in the elderly population, it has become more common to admit mildly head-injured patients on such treatment.

In the review by Volans,[106] among mildly head-injured patients on anticoagulant therapy, the risk of developing an intracranial hematoma increased in fully oriented patients from 1 in 7866 to 1 in 800, and in confused patients from 1 in 180 to 1 in 18; in those fully oriented with a fracture, the risk increased from 1 in 45 to 1 in 4, and in confused patients with a fracture, from 1 in 5 to 1 in 2. Saab and colleagues[47] reported a 10-fold increase in the risk of developing intracranial hematomas in patients on anticoagulants. They suggested that all mildly head-injured patients on anticoagulants be admitted to the hospital for neurological observation and international normalized ratio (INR) determination. An INR greater than 2 increases the risk of hematoma. It has been shown that up to one third of patients on anticoagulants do not have sufficient indications for this treatment; in these cases, anticoagulant therapy can be suspended immediately. In all other patients, a computed tomographic scan should be obtained, even in the presence of mild symptoms such as headache. Whenever a hematoma is detected, reversal of anticoagulant therapy should be arranged. Borczuk[60] and Arienta and associates[57] confirmed these findings, showing that the number of abnormal scans was doubled in patients on anticoagulant therapy.

A coagulopathy can also follow a mild injury. Selladurai and coworkers[107] showed in a subset of 43 patients admitted with a GCS score of 13 to 15 that all 11 patients who had poor outcomes had moderate to severe fibrin degradation product scores.

Indications for Obtaining a Computed Tomographic Scan

Following are some of the different recommendations for performing CT:

1. GCS score of 13, 14, or 15 with an abnormal mental status.[58]
2. GCS score of 15 with skull fracture at any age.[43, 71, 103]
3. GCS score of 13, 14, or 15 with LOC.[23, 34, 46, 62]
4. Mandatory for patients with GCS score of 13.[44]
5. Any one or more of the following: (a) focal neurological deficits; (b) basilar skull fracture; (c) scalp injury; (d) age older than 60 years.[60]
6. GCS score of 13, 14, or 15 in adults with skull fracture.[28, 38, 57]
7. GCS score of 15 if one of the following is present: nausea, vomiting, headache, clinical signs of depressed skull fracture,[37, 41] short memory deficits, intoxication, age older than 60 years, trauma above the clavicles.[7]
8. Only in the case of clinical deterioration.[40, 59]

These varying recommendations have led to controversy and clinical confusion. The establishment of a consistent policy is the main reason to develop a coherent, risk-based approach to classification.

Unfortunately, neither clinical nor radiologic risk factors will be able to identify all mildly head-injured patients who will develop an intracranial hematoma. Indeed, 29 patients (16%) in a series of 183 who devel-

---

* See references 9, 10, 28, 30, 33, 35, 39, 43, 57, 61, 71.

oped intracranial hematoma and were admitted with a GCS score of 15 presented with no skull fracture and no clinical signs (including LOC) when first seen.[10]

Our Suggestions for Obtaining a Computed Tomographic Scan

First, an accurate neurological examination based on the GCS and including testing of the patient's state of alertness and orientation, pupillary size and response, motor power, and vital signs must be performed. Information on the mechanism of injury, the type of injury, and previous medical history (including current therapies) should be collected. If available, a qualified witness should be questioned to determine the presence or absence of LOC at the scene of the injury.

Patients younger than 60 years; not receiving any kind of anticoagulant therapy; with trauma not due to assault or gunshot wound; and with a GCS score of 15 without LOC or PTA, diffuse headache, vomiting, or neurological deficits can be classified in the emergency room as having a "low-risk mild head injury."[108] The risk of an intracranial hematoma requiring surgical evacuation in these cases is less than 1 in 1000, and the cost-benefit ratio is strongly against any radiologic examination. Patients can be sent home with written recommendations about the onset of symptoms (e.g., headache, vomiting, drowsiness) that require a prompt return to the hospital.

Patients with a GCS score of 15 but with LOC or PTA, diffuse headache, or vomiting are classified as having a "medium-risk mild head injury." In these patients, the risk of a surgical hematoma is 1 to 3 in 100. A computed tomographic scan of the head must be obtained as soon as possible and should include bone windows. In the case of a normal computed tomographic scan, the patient can be safely discharged, except if there is a skull fracture or an associated coagulopathy. These patients should be admitted to the hospital for at least 24 hours, with consideration of a repeat computed tomographic scan before discharge, because the risk of a delayed hematoma is higher in this group. In the case of an abnormal post-traumatic computed tomographic scan, a neurosurgeon must be contacted (via video link, whenever possible). Decisions concerning transfer to a neurosurgical unit, repetition of the computed tomographic scan, and indications for surgery are issues for neurosurgical consultation. If CT is not readily available in the admitting hospital, an adult patient should have a skull radiograph; if this shows a fracture, the patient should be moved to the "high-risk" category and undergo a computed tomographic scan, even if this requires transfer to another hospital.

Patients with admission GCS scores of 14 or 15 but with skull fractures or neurological deficits are defined as having a "high-risk mild head injury." The risk of an intracranial hematoma is 6 to 10 in 100. In these patients, a computed tomographic scan must be obtained immediately. If on-site CT is not available, the patient should be transferred to a hospital where it is. Irrespective of the neurological presentation, patients having other risk factors (e.g., coagulopathy, drug or alcohol consumption, previous neurosurgical procedures, epilepsy, gunshot wound or assault, age older than 60 years) are included in the high-risk category.

In patients with admission GCS scores of 13, the risk of intracranial hematoma and the possibility of needing a surgical procedure are similar to the rates in patients with moderate head injuries (GCS score 9 to 12), and they should be managed as such.

Clinical deterioration related to an epidural hematoma occurs mainly in the first 6 hours after injury.[69, 81] In a series of delayed epidural hematomas, only 2 of 31 (6%) appeared in mildly head-injured patients. All these patients could be identified as being at risk by the presence of a skull fracture on admission.[109] The risk of missing a delayed hematoma is overwhelmed by the benefits of early hematoma detection. A computed tomographic scan should be obtained as soon as possible, preferably within 4 hours of injury. Most cases of delayed epidural hematomas are identified on admission as small collections that subsequently enlarge.[69] The detection and interpretation of the importance of small collections and other findings (e.g., lucent areas within the hematoma and the presence of air) require expertise, and the scans of these patients should be reviewed by a neurosurgeon (even by video link), because transfer may be needed even if there is no indication for immediate operation. In areas where neurosurgery is centralized, early transfer can be life saving, because any subsequent clinical deterioration or hematoma enlargement will occur where the patient can be treated promptly with surgery.

In conclusion, Teasdale and colleagues'[43] expectation that "CT scanning of all head injured patients in coma or alert with a skull fracture should achieve early detection of at least 95% of intracranial hematomas" is close to reality. Other expectations, such as that mortality for "pure" epidural hematoma could be as low as zero,[25] are also feasible.[38] The achievement of these results requires joint efforts involving neurosurgeons, emergency physicians, radiologists, and, in some areas of the world, neurologists, general surgeons, and, on occasion, orthopedic surgeons.

OUTCOME

Only a few studies have applied the GOS[72] at 6 months to a population of mildly head-injured patients. Unfavorable outcomes (including death, persistent vegetative state, and severe disability) are reported in 0.2% to 3.4% of cases in the published series.[6, 31, 33, 38, 44, 63]

In many areas of the world, neurosurgery facilities are centralized. Thus, outcome studies in mildly head-injured patients should include referral area studies. Mortality is very low, and it should be almost totally avoidable with early diagnosis and prompt treatment. In one study,[9] the mortality in the neurosurgical center was zero, but the referral area mortality was 1.8%.

GUIDELINES FOR MANAGEMENT

Neurosurgeons have produced guidelines for mild head injury management. The first attempt was made in the early 1980s by a group of British neurosurgeons,[19] and another group of British neurosurgeons has updated these guidelines (Table 325–5).[20] This second set of guidelines takes into account Teasdale and colleagues'[43] observation that patients who are fully conscious (GCS score of 15), when indicated,[19] should have skull radiographs. If a fracture is not shown, they are sent home with printed instructions. In the case of

---

TABLE 325–5 ■ Guidelines for the Initial Management of Head Injuries

Indications for Skull Radiographs after Recent Head Injury*

Oriented patient:
1. History of LOC or amnesia
2. Suspected penetrating injury
3. CSF or blood loss from nose or ear
4. Scalp laceration (to bone or >5 cm long), bruise, or swelling
5. Violent mechanism of injury
6. Persisting headache or vomiting
7. In a child, fall from a significant height or onto a hard surface, tense fontanelle, suspected nonaccidental injury

Patient with impaired consciousness or neurological signs: always, unless urgent CT is performed or transfer to neurosurgery is arranged

Indications for Admission to a General Hospital
1. Skull fracture or suture diastasis
2. Persisting neurological signs or symptoms
3. Difficulty in assessment (drugs, alcohol, epilepsy, attempted suicide)
4. Lack of responsible adult to supervise patient
5. Other medical condition (coagulopathy)
6. All patients with impaired consciousness

Indications for Consultation with a Neurosurgeon or Urgent CT
1. Coma persisting after resuscitation
2. Deteriorating consciousness or progressive neurological signs
3. Skull fracture with any of the following: confusion or worse impairment of consciousness, epileptic seizure, neurological symptoms and signs
4. Open injury, depressed compound fracture of skull vault, fracture of base of skull, penetrating injury

Additional conditions requiring urgent CT within 2–4 hr of admission:
1. Skull fracture or seizure
2. Confusion or neurological signs persisting after initial assessment and resuscitation
3. Unstable systemic state precluding transfer to neurosurgery
4. Diagnosis uncertain
5. Tense fontanelle or suture diastasis in children

Intracranial Abnormalities Suggesting Need for Urgent Neurosurgical Management
1. High- or mixed-density intracranial lesion (size and site)
2. Shift of midline
3. Obliteration of third ventricle
4. Relative dilatation of lateral ventricle
5. Obliteration of basal cisterns
6. Intracranial air
7. Subarachnoid or intraventricular hemorrhage

Additional indications for referral to a neurosurgical unit after CT
1. Abnormal CT
2. Normal CT, but clinical progress unsatisfactory

---

*Skull radiographs are not necessary when CT is performed. CSF, cerebrospinal fluid; CT, computed tomography; LOC, loss of consciousness.
From Bartlett J, Kett-White R, Mendelow AD, et al: Guidelines for the initial management of head injuries. Br J Neurosurg 12:349–352, 1998.

TABLE 325–6 ■ Guidelines for the Management of Minor Head Injuries in Adults

Group 0: patients having a GCS score of 15 on admission with dizziness or pain in the impact area and possible scalp contusion, without LOC or amnesia, diffuse headache, or vomiting
Group 1: patients having a GCS score of 15 on admission, who have LOC or amnesia, vomiting, or diffuse headache
Group 2: patients with an admission GCS score of 14

Group 0
No radiologic examination.
Patients can be sent home with an information sheet after at least 6 hr of observation.
Patients with risk factors* always need CT.

Group 1
Radiologic examination is necessary.
If CT is readily available, it should be performed. If CT is negative, the patient can be discharged. If CT shows post-traumatic intracranial lesions, a neurosurgical consultation is mandatory (CT video links with neurosurgical units are useful).
If CT is not available, a skull radiograph must be obtained. If it is positive for a vault fracture, CT is required, even if this means transfer to another hospital. If the skull radiograph is negative, there should be a 24-hr period of observation before discharge.
For patients with risk factors* (particularly coagulopathy), the first CT is always mandatory, even in the absence of skull fracture, and a second negative CT is required before discharge.

Group 2
CT is always performed. Clinical observation is indicated until the patient becomes neurologically intact.
In the presence of intracranial lesions, a neurosurgical consultation is mandatory.
As in group 1, negative CT should be followed by a second CT before discharge in the case of risk factors.*

---

*Relevant risk factors are coagulopathy, chronic alcoholism, drug abuse, epilepsy, previous neurosurgical treatment, and disabled elderly patients. CT, computed tomography; GCS, Glasgow Coma Scale; LOC, loss of consciousness.
From Study Group on Head Injury of the Italian Society for Neurosurgery: Guidelines for minor head injured patients' management in adult age. J Neurol Sci 40:11–15, 1996.

---

a skull fracture, an urgent computed tomographic scan is obtained. If the scan is negative, the patient is observed in the hospital until recovery is complete. If the scan is positive, a neurosurgical consultation is obtained.[43, 103] A similar set of guidelines has been published by Italian neurosurgeons (Table 325–6).[21] These guidelines have been adopted in France[22] and Spain (R. Lobato, J. Sauquillo, personal communication). They have also been published in Argentina[110] and take into account previously published guidelines by Italian authors.[38, 57] A recent addition to these guidelines involves patients who have sustained mild head injuries and have associated risk factors for the development of delayed epidural hematomas (skull fracture or GCS score <15); these patients must be admitted to the hospital for neurological observation, even if the first computed tomographic scan is normal.[70, 109]

Guidelines for mild head injury from the United States are based on clinical factors, excluding any role for skull radiographs (Tables 325–7 to 325–9). Recently published Scandinavian guidelines (Fig. 325–1)[24] are a combination of previously reported European and American guidelines.

TABLE 325-7 ■ Recommendations for Obtaining Skull Radiographs after Head Trauma

Low-Risk Group

Possible findings

Asymptomatic, headache, dizziness, scalp hematoma, scalp laceration, scalp contusion or abrasion, absence of moderate-risk or high-risk criteria

Recommendations

Observation alone: discharge patients with head injury information sheet (listing subdural precautions) and a second person to observe them

Moderate-Risk Group

Possible findings

History of change of consciousness at the time of injury or subsequently, history of progressive headache, alcohol or drug intoxication, unreliable or inadequate history of injury, age younger than 2 yr (unless injury very trivial), post-traumatic seizure, vomiting, post-traumatic amnesia, multiple trauma, serious facial injury, signs of basilar fracture, possible skull penetration or depressed fracture, suspected physical child abuse

Recommendations

Extended close observation (watch for signs of high-risk group)
Consider CT and neurosurgical consultation
Skull series may (rarely) be helpful if positive, but do not exclude intracranial injury if normal

High-Risk Group

Possible findings

Depressed level of consciousness not clearly due to alcohol, drugs, or other causes; focal neurological signs; decreasing level of consciousness; penetrating scalp injury or palpable depressed fracture

Recommendations

Patients are candidates for neurosurgical consultation, emergency CT, or both

CT, computed tomography.
From Masters SJ, McClean PM, Arcarese JS, et al: Skull x-ray examinations after head trauma. N Engl J Med 316:84-91, 1987.

OTHER INVESTIGATIONS

Computed tompgraphic scanning of the head is the examination of choice in mildly head-injured patients in the acute phase. Nevertheless, other examinations have been suggested, including MRI, single photon emission computed tomography (SPECT), and positron emission tomography (PET), for patient management, especially in the subacute-chronic phase.

TABLE 325-8 ■ Recommendations for Patients with Low-Risk Head Injuries

1. Every patient with a history of PTA/LOC should undergo CT
2. GCS score of 13 indicates higher risk; treat as a moderate head injury
3. GCS score of 14-15: normal CT predicts good outcome; patient can usually be sent home[21]

CT, computed tomography; GCS, Glasgow Coma Scale; LOC, loss of consciousness; PTA, post-traumatic amnesia.
From Stein SC, Ross SE: The value of computed tomographic scans in patients with low-risk head injuries. Neurosurgery 26:638-640, 1990.

TABLE 325-9 ■ Clinical Utility of Computed Tomography and Neurological Examination in the Management of Patients with Mild Head Injuries

1. CT is recommended for all patients with MHI, because 1 in 5 will have an acute lesion detectable by the scan
2. CT should be *mandatory* for a patient with MHI *and* a GCS score of 13, because 1 in 3 will have an acute lesion, and 1 in 10 will require craniotomy
3. Patients with MHI and *abnormal* results on NEx should be admitted, because 1 in 5 will require some form of treatment
4. Patients with MHI and *positive* findings on CT should be admitted, because 1 in 4 will require treatment
5. Patients with MHI who have *abnormal* results on NEx and *positive* findings on CT should be admitted to an ICU, because 2 in 5 will require treatment, and 1 in 4 will require either ICP monitoring or craniotomy
6. Patients with MHI who have *normal* results on NEx and *negative* findings on CT have a very small risk of requiring treatment (1 in 50) and no risk of requiring craniotomy
7. Admission to the hospital does not guarantee skilled neurological observation
8. *Reliable* patients with MHI who have *normal* results on NEx and *negative* findings on CT can be discharged from the emergency room, provided there is a mechanism for follow-up

CT, computed tomography; GCS, Glasgow Coma Scale; ICP, intracranial pressure; ICU, intensive care unit; MHI, mild head injury; NEx, neurological examination.
From Shackford SR, Ward SL, Ross SE, et al: The clinical utility of computed tomographic scanning and neurologic examination in the management of patients with minor head injuries. J Trauma 33:385-394, 1992.

Magnetic Resonance Imaging

The use of MRI in the acute phase is so rare that van der Naalt and coworkers[111] defined "early" MRI as an examination obtained within 1 to 3 months of injury. They studied 67 patients with moderate and mild head injuries with CT and MRI; this examination revealed lesions in 25% of patients with normal computed tomographic scans on admission. In this study, frontal lesions on early MRI and duration of PTA were related to outcome. A similar study[112] was performed in 20 patients admitted following mild injuries (GCS score 13 to 15, no subsequent deterioration, LOC <20 minutes) with normal computed tomographic scans. MRI performed within 4 days of injury showed abnormalities compatible with diffuse axonal injury in the white matter of 6 patients (30%). Tokutomi and associates[113] performed MRI within 28 days of injury in a series of 44 mildly head-injured (GCS score 13 to 15) patients. Only one patient (2%) had an abnormal signal in the corpus callosum. In those with moderate head injuries, this abnormal signal was present in 3 of 31 patients (10%), and it was present in 17 of 45 (38%) with severe head injuries. The conclusion was that an abnormal MRI signal within the corpus callosum following closed head injury is related to trauma severity. In a study performed later (1 to 3 months after trauma), 90% of adolescents and adults admitted with mild to moderate head injuries had parenchymal changes on MRI.[114]

The utility of a new technique—fluid-attenuated inversion recovery (FLAIR)—was investigated in 56 cases of moderate to mild head injuries 1 to 36 days after

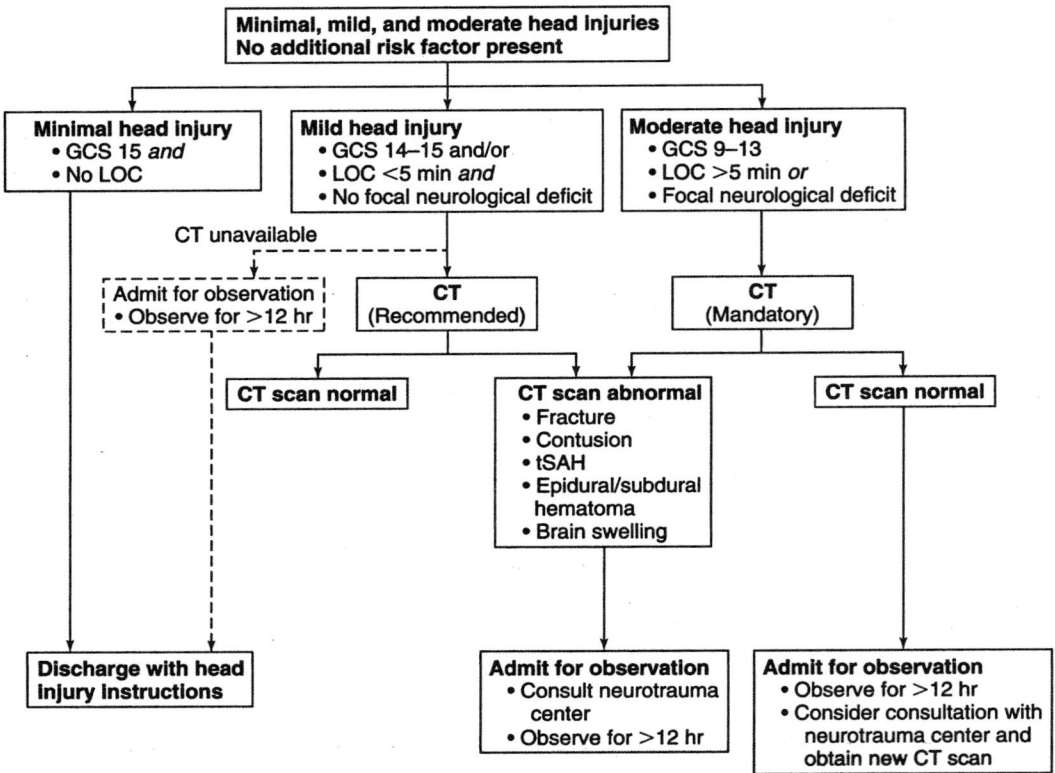

FIGURE 325–1. Patient management as suggested by a group of Scandinavian neurosurgeons.[24] CT, computed tomography; GCS, Glasgow Coma Scale; LOC, loss of consciousness; tSAH, traumatic subarachnoid hemorrhage.

injury. In all cases, the sensitivity of FLAIR images was equal or superior to that of conventional spin-echo images. In particular, some cortical contusions and corpus callosum lesions were seen only on sagittal FLAIR images.[115]

We believe that the use of MRI in the acute phase of mild traumatic brain injury is rarely justified. However, when there are neurological abnormalities in spite of a normal computed tomographic scan, MRI can demonstrate areas of contusion without a hemorrhagic component that are not visible on CT. We agree with Shackford and Wald[116] that in no case has MRI actually changed the management of the patient.

Single Photon Emission Computed Tomography

A significant number of reports have been published on the use of SPECT for the long-term evaluation of mildly head-injured patients. Only a limited number of authors have used this examination in the acute-subacute phase. In mild head injuries, SPECT brain perfusion imaging is more sensitive than other examinations (CT and MRI), according to Nedd and coworkers.[117] Reports on the use of SPECT in patients with mild or moderate head injuries have several problems[118]: the small number of cases reported, the lack

of correlation between abnormal findings and clinical status, the lack of follow-up studies and treatment evaluation, nonspecificity, and difficulty in interpreting abnormal results.

Gonçalves and associates[119] studied 14 head-injured patients with some kind of focal neurological deficits but with normal CT and MRI. Technetium-99m HM-PAO SPECT showed changes in cerebral perfusion in areas correlated with neurological abnormalities. Nedd and colleagues[117] compared SPECT and CT in 16 patients admitted for mild to moderate head injuries. SPECT showed intraparenchymal differences in regional cerebral blood flow more often than did CT. Further, in several patients, the area of involvement was larger on SPECT than on CT. Other studies[120, 121] demonstrated that SPECT shows areas of decreased regional cerebral blood flow in patients with normal CT or MRI. Abdel-Dayem and colleagues[118] reported 228 patients with mild to moderate head injuries studied with SPECT. The most interesting finding was that of 41 patients who had mild traumatic head injury without LOC and with normal computed tomographic scans, 28 had abnormal SPECT studies. In contrast with previous reports, the sites of abnormality were more frequently located in the basal ganglia and thalamus. Interestingly, according to the current guidelines for mild head injury, these patients usually do not undergo CT and probably are not even admitted to the hospital.

Positron Emission Tomography

Fluorodeoxyglucose technique with PET (FDG-PET) was used in the evaluation of local cerebral metabolic rates of glucose in mildly head-injured patients.[122] Unfortunately, only single case studies followed this promising paper. In a series of 28 patients admitted following severe head injury, the use of FDG-PET demonstrated that hyperglycolysis occurs both regionally and globally.[123] Nine patients who had neuropsychological sequelae following mild head injury and almost normal nonfunctional neuroimaging (CT and MRI) were studied with FDG-PET. In all nine patients, there was a positive correlation between neuropsychological testing and PET pathology, which was located predominantly in the frontal and frontotemporal regions.[124] Jansen and colleagues[125] used PET with cobalt-55 isotope, a calcium tracer that enables imaging of ischemic tissue. They studied five patients with moderate head injury and demonstrated a focal cobalt-PET uptake that extended well beyond the morphologic abnormalities shown by CT and MRI. In conclusion, PET is still a research tool limited to a few select cases of mild head injury.

ACKNOWLEDGMENTS

We wish to thank Graham Teasdale, University Department of Neurosurgery, Institute of Neurological Sciences, Glasgow, and Lawrence F. Marshall, Division of Neurological Surgery, University of California, San Diego Medical Center, for their valuable contributions in preparing the manuscript.

REFERENCES

1. Rimel RW, Giordani B, Barth JT, et al: Disability caused by minor head injury. Neurosurgery 9:221–228, 1981.
2. Kraus J, Nourjah P: The epidemiology of mild head injury. In Levin HS, Eisenberg HM, Benton AL (eds): Mild Head Injury. New York, Oxford University Press, 1989, pp 8–22.
3. Kraus J, Nourjah P: The epidemiology of mild, uncomplicated brain injury. J Trauma 28:1637–1643, 1988.
4. Stiell IG, Wells GA, Vandemheen K, et al: Variation in ED use of computed tomography for patients with minor head injury. Ann Emerg Med 30:14–22, 1997.
5. Servadei F: Computed tomographic examination in minor head injury [letter]. Lancet 21:788, 1991.
6. Miller JD, Jones PA, Dearden NM, et al: Progress in the management of head injury. Br J Surg 79:60–64, 1992.
7. Haydel MJ, Preston CA, Mills TJ, et al: Indications for computed tomography in patients with minor head injury. N Engl J Med 343:100–105, 2000.
8. Vilke GM, Chan TC, Guss DA: Use of a complete neurological examination to screen for significant intracranial abnormalities in minor head injury. Am J Emerg Med 18:159–163, 2000.
9. Servadei F, Vergoni G, Nasi MT, et al: Management of low-risk head injuries in an entire area: Results of an 18-month survey. Surg Neurol 39:269–275, 1993.
10. Miller JD, Murray LS, Teasdale GM: Development of a traumatic intracranial hematoma after a "minor" head injury. Neurosurgery 27:669–673, 1990.
11. Kraus J, Romer C, Holst H, et al: Prevention, Critical Care and Rehabilitation of Neurotrauma. Stockholm, WHO Collaborating Centers for Neurotrauma, Karolinska Institute, 1995.
12. Jennett B: Epidemiology of head injury. J Neurol Neurosurg Psychiatry 60:362–369, 1996.
13. Marshall LF, Gautille T, Klauber M, et al: The outcome of severe closed head injury. J Neurosurg 75:S28–S36, 1991.
14. Murray LS, Teasdale GM, Murray GD, et al: Head injuries in four British neurosurgical centres. Br J Neurosurg 13:564–569, 1999.
15. Murray LS, Teasdale GM, Murray GD, et al: Does prediction of outcome alter patient management? Lancet 341:1487–1491, 1993.
16. Murray GD, Teasdale GM, Braakman R, et al: The European Brain Injury Consortium survey of head injuries. Acta Neurochir (Wien) 141:223–236, 1999.
17. Maas AIR, Steyerberg EW, Murray GD, et al: Why have recent trials of neuroprotective agents in head injury failed to show convincing efficacy? A pragmatic analysis and theoretical considerations. Neurosurgery 44:1286–1298, 1999.
18. Klauber MR, Marshall LF, Luerssen TG, et al: Determinants of head injury mortality: Importance of the low risk patient. Neurosurgery 24:31–36, 1989.
19. Briggs M, Clarke P, Crockard A, et al: Guidelines for initial management after head injury in adults. BMJ 288:983–985, 1984.
20. Bartlett J, Kett-White R, Mendelow AD, et al: Guidelines for the initial management of head injuries. Br J Neurosurg 12:349–352, 1998.
21. Study Group on Head Injury of the Italian Society for Neurosurgery: Guidelines for minor head injured patients' management in adult age. J Neurol Sci 40:11–15, 1996.
22. Lapierre F, Societe Francaise de Neurochirurgie: Guide-lines concernant les traumatismes craniens legers de l'adulte. Neurochirurgie 44:55–56, 1998.
23. Stein SC, Ross SE: The value of computed tomographic scans in patients with low-risk head injuries. Neurosurgery 26:638–640, 1990.
24. Ingebrigtsen T, Romner B, Kock-Jensen C: Scandinavian guidelines for initial management of minimal, mild, and moderate head injuries. J Trauma 48:760–766, 2000.
25. Bricolo AP, Pasut L: Extradural hematoma: Toward zero mortality. Neurosurgery 14:8–11, 1984.
26. Servadei F, Vergoni G, Staffa G, et al: Extradural haematomas: How many deaths can be avoided? Protocol for early detection of haematoma in minor head injuries. Acta Neurochir (Wien) 133:50–55, 1995.
27. Teasdale GM: Head injury. J Neurol Neurosurg Psychiatry 58:526–539, 1995.
28. Gomez PA, Lobato RD, Ortega JM, et al: Mild head injury: Differences in prognosis among patients with a Glasgow Coma Scale score of 13 to 15 and analysis of factors associated with abnormal CT findings. Br J Neurosurg 10:453–460, 1996.
29. Nagurney JT, Borczuk P, Thomas SH: Elder patients with closed head trauma: A comparison with nonelder patients. Acad Emerg Med 5:678–684, 1998.
30. Dacey RG, Alves WM, Rimel RW, et al: Neurosurgical complications after apparently minor head injury. J Neurosurg 65:203–210, 1986.
31. Jeret JS, Mandell M, Anziska B, et al: Clinical predictors of abnormality disclosed by computed tomography after mild head trauma. Neurosurgery 32:9–16, 1993.
32. Williams DH, Levin HS, Eisenberg HM: Mild head injury classification. Neurosurgery 27:422–428, 1990.
33. Hsiang JNK, Yeung T, Yu ALM, et al: High-risk mild head injury. J Neurosurg 87:234–238, 1997.
34. Nagy KK, Joseph KT, Krosner SM, et al: The utility of head computed tomography after minimal head injury. J Trauma 46:268–270, 1999.
35. Chan KH, Mann KS, Yue CP, et al: The significance of skull fracture in acute traumatic intracranial hematomas in adolescents: A prospective study. J Neurosurg 72:189–194, 1990.
36. Holmes FJ, Baier ME, Derlet RW: Failure of the Miller criteria to predict significant intracranial injury in patients with a Glasgow Coma Scale score of 14 after minor head trauma. Acad Emerg Med 4:788–792, 1997.
37. Miller EC, Holmes JF, Derlet RW: Utilizing clinical factors to reduce head CT scan ordering for minor head trauma patients. J Emerg Med 15:453–457, 1997.
38. Servadei F, Ciucci G, Loroni L, et al: Diagnosis and management of minor head injury: A regional multicenter approach in Italy. J Trauma 39:696–701, 1995.

39. Servadei F, Ciucci G, Morichetti A, et al: Skull fracture as a factor of increased risk in minor head injuries. Surg Neurol 30: 364–369, 1988.
40. Rosenorn J, Duus B, Nielsen K, et al: Is a skull x-ray necessary after milder head trauma? Br J Neurosurg 5:135–139, 1991.
41. Lee ST, Liu TN, Wong CW, et al: Relative risk of deterioration after mild closed head injury. Acta Neurochir (Wien) 135:136–140, 1995.
42. Masters SJ, McClean PM, Arcarese JS, et al: Skull x-ray examinations after head trauma. N Engl J Med 316:84–91, 1987.
43. Teasdale GM, Murray G, Anderson E, et al: Risks of acute traumatic intracranial haematoma in children and adults: Implications for managing head injuries. BMJ 300:363–367, 1990.
44. Shackford SR, Ward SL, Ross SE, et al: The clinical utility of computed tomographic scanning and neurologic examination in the management of patients with minor head injuries. J Trauma 33:385–394, 1992.
45. Sosin DM, Sniezek JE, Thurman DJ: Incidence of mild and moderate brain injury in the United States, 1991. Brain Injury 10:47–54, 1996.
46. Stein SC, Ross SE: Mild head injury: A plea for routine early CT scanning. J Trauma 33:11–13, 1992.
47. Saab M, Gray A, Hodgkinson D, et al: Warfarin and the apparent minor head injury. J Accid Emerg Med 13:208–209, 1996.
48. MacLaren RE, Ghoorahoo HI, Kirby NG: Use of an accident and emergency department observation ward in the management of head injury. Br J Surg 80:215–217, 1993.
49. Brown SR, Raine C, Robertson CE, et al: Management of minor head injuries in the accident and emergency department: The effect of an observation ward. J Accid Emerg Med 11:144–148, 1994.
50. Hutchinson PJA, Kirkpatrick PJ, Addison J, et al: The management of minor traumatic brain injury. J Accid Emerg Med 15: 84–88, 1998.
51. Carlsson GS: Head injuries in a population study. Acta Neurochir Suppl (Wien) 36:13–15, 1986.
52. Culotta VP, Sementilli ME, Gerold K, et al: Clinicopathological heterogeneity in the classification of mild head injury. Neurosurgery 38:245–250, 1996.
53. Mann KS, Chan KH, Yue CP: Skull fractures in children: Their assessment in relation to developmental skull changes and acute intracranial hematomas. Childs Nerv Syst 2:258, 1986.
54. Stein SC, Spettell C, Young G, et al: Limitations of neurological assessment in mild head injury. Brain Injury 7:425–430, 1993.
55. Harad FT, Kerstein MD: Inadequacy of bedside clinical indicators in identifying significant intracranial injury in trauma patients. J Trauma 32:359–363, 1992.
56. Murshid WR: Management of minor head injuries: Admission criteria, radiological evaluation and treatment of complications. Acta Neurochir (Wien) 140:56–64, 1998.
57. Arienta C, Caroli M, Balbi S: Management of head-injured patients in the emergency department: A practical protocol. Surg Neurol 48:213–219, 1997.
58. Feuerman T, Wackym PA, Gade GF, et al: Value of skull radiography, head computed tomographic scanning, and admission for observation in cases of minor head injury. Neurosurgery 22: 449–453, 1988.
59. Duus BR, Boesen T, Kruse KV, et al: Prognostic signs in the evaluation of patients with minor head injury. Br J Surg 80: 988–991, 1993.
60. Borczuk P: Predictors of intracranial injury in patients with mild head trauma. Ann Emerg Med 25:731–736, 1995.
61. Mohanty SK, Thompson W, Rakower S: Are CT scans for head injury patients always necessary? J Trauma 31:801–805, 1991.
62. Ingebrigtsen T, Romner B: Routine early CT-scan is cost saving after minor head injury. Acta Neurol Scand 93:207–210, 1996.
63. Miller JD, Jones PA: The work of a regional head injury service. Lancet 18:1141–1144, 1985.
64. Miller JD: Minor, moderate and severe head injury. Neurosurg Rev 9:135–139, 1986.
65. Marion DW, Carlier PM: Problems with initial Glasgow Coma Scale assessment caused by prehospital treatment of patients with head injuries: Results of a national survey. J Trauma 36: 89–95, 1994.
66. Servadei F, Murray GD, Penny K, et al: The value of the "worst"
67. computed tomographic scan in clinical studies of moderate and severe head injury. Neurosurgery 46:70–77, 2000.
67. Servadei F, Nanni A, Nasi MT, et al: Evolving brain lesions in the first 12 hours after head injury: Analysis of 37 comatose patients. Neurosurgery 37:899–907, 1995.
68. Yamaki T, Hirakawa K, Ueguchi T, et al: Chronological evaluation of acute traumatic intracerebral haematoma. Acta Neurochir (Wien) 103:112–115, 1990.
69. Smith HK, Miller JD: The danger of an ultra early computed tomographic scan in a patient with an evolving intracranial hematoma. Neurosurgery 29:258–260, 1991.
70. Riesgo P, Piquer J, Botella C, et al: Delayed extradural hematoma after mild head injury: Report of three cases. Surg Neurol 48:226–231, 1997.
71. Voss M, Knottenbelt JD, Peden MM: Patients who reattend after head injury: A high risk group. BMJ 311:1395–1398, 1995.
72. Jennett B, Bond M: Assessment of outcome after severe brain damage. Lancet 1:480–485, 1975.
73. Stein SC, Ross SE: Moderate head injury: A guide to initial management. J Neurosurg 77:562–564, 1994.
74. Fearnside M, McDougall P: Moderate head injury: A system of neurotrauma care. Aust N Z J Surg 68:58–64, 1998.
75. Bullock R, Teasdale G: Surgical management of traumatic intracranial hematomas. In Braakman R (ed): Handbook of Clinical Neurology: Head Injury, vol 13. New York, Elsevier Science, 1990, pp 249–298.
76. Servadei F, Faccani G, Roccella P, et al: Asymptomatic extradural haematomas: Results of a multicenter study of 158 cases in minor head injury. Acta Neurochir (Wien) 96:39–45, 1989.
77. Pozzati E, Tognetti F: Spontaneous healing of acute extradural haematomas: Study of twenty-two cases. Neurosurgery 16:696–700, 1986.
78. Chen TY, Wong CW, Chang CN, et al: The expectant treatment of "asymptomatic" supratentorial epidural haematomas. Neurosurgery 32:176–179, 1993.
79. Hamilton M, Wallace C: Nonoperative management of acute epidural hematoma diagnosed by CT: The neuroradiologist's role. AJNR Am J Neuroradiol 13:853–859, 1992.
80. Zimmerman RA, Bilaniuk LT: Computed tomographic staging of traumatic epidural bleeding. Radiology 144:809–812, 1982.
81. Knuckey NW, Gelbard S, Epstein MH: The management of asymptomatic epidural hematomas: A prospective study. J Neurosurg 70:392–396, 1989.
82. Sullivan TP, Jarvik JG, Cohen WA: Follow-up of conservatively managed epidural haematomas: Implications for timing of repeat CT. AJNR Am J Neuroradiol 20:107–113, 1999.
83. Procaccio F, Stocchetti N, Citerio G, et al: Guidelines for the treatment of adults with severe head trauma. J Neurosurg Sci 44:1–10, 2000.
84. Mathew P, Olouch-Olunyaa DL, Condon BR, et al: Acute subdural hematoma in the conscious patient: Outcome with initial nonoperative management. Acta Neurochir (Wien) 121:100–108, 1993.
85. Croce MA, Dent DL, Menke PG, et al: Acute subdural hematoma: Nonsurgical management in selected patients. J Trauma 36:820–827, 1994.
86. Polman CH, Gijsberg CJ, Heimans CJ, et al: Rapid spontaneous resolution of an acute subdural hematoma. Neurosurgery 19: 446–448, 1986.
87. Galbraith S, Teasdale G: Predicting the need for operation in the patient with an occult traumatic intracranial hematoma. J Neurosurg 55:75–81, 1981.
88. Morris GF, Juul N, Bowers Marshall S, et al: Neurological deterioration as a potential alternative endpoint in human clinical trials of experimental pharmacological agents for treatment of severe traumatic brain injuries. Neurosurgery 43:1369–1374, 1998.
89. Marshall LF, Marshall SB, Klauber MR, et al: A new classification of head injury based on computed tomography. J Neurosurg 75(Suppl):S14–S20, 1991.
90. Graham ID, Stiell IG, Laupacis A, et al: Emergency physicians' attitudes toward and use of clinical decision rules for radiography. Acad Emerg Med 5:134–140, 1998.
91. Pentland B, Jones PA, Roy CW, et al: Head injury in the elderly. Age Ageing 15:193–202, 1986.

92. Edna TH: Acute traumatic intracranial haematoma and skull fracture. Acta Chir Scand 149:449–451, 1983.
93. Chandler WF: Comment to Miller JD: Development of a traumatic intracranial hematoma after a "minor" head injury. Neurosurgery 27:673, 1990.
94. Ando S, Otani M, Moritake K: Clinical analysis of post-traumatic vomiting. Acta Neurochir (Wien) 119:97–100, 1992.
95. Nee PA, Hadfield JM, Yates DW, et al: Significance of vomiting after head injury. J Neurol Neurosurg Psychiatry 66:470–473, 1999.
96. Masters SJ: Evaluation of head trauma: Efficacy of skull films. AJR Am J Roentgenol 135:539–547, 1980.
97. Royal College of Radiologists: Costs and benefits of skull radiography for head injury: A national study by the Royal College of Radiologists. Lancet 2:791–795, 1981.
98. Dikmen SS, Levin HS: Methodological issues in the study of mild head injury. J Head Trauma Rehabil 8:30–37, 1993.
99. Stein SC: High-risk minor head injury [letter]. J Neurosurg 88:613, 1998.
100. Ingebrigtsen T, Rommer B: Management of minor head injuries in hospitals in Norway. Acta Neurol Scand 95:51–55, 1997.
101. Livingston DH, Loder PA, Koziol J, et al: The use of CT scanning to triage patients requiring admission following minimal head injury. J Trauma 31:483–489, 1991.
102. Mendelow AD, Teadsdale G, Jennett B, et al: Risks of intracranial haematoma in head injured adults. BMJ 287:1173–1176, 1983.
103. Cranshaw J, Hughes G, Clancy M: Computerised tomography and acute traumatic head injury: Time for change? J Accid Emerg Med 13:80–85, 1996.
104. Hofman PAM, Nelemans P, Kemerink GJ, et al: Value of radiological diagnosis of skull fracture in the management of mild head injury: Meta-analysis. J Neurol Neurosurg Psychiatry 68:416–422, 2000.
105. Balasubramaniam S, Kapadia T, Campbell J, Jackson TL: Efficacy of skull radiography. Am J Surg 142:366–369, 1981.
106. Volans AP: The risk of minor head injury in the warfarinised patient. J Accid Emerg Med 15:159–161, 1998.
107. Selladurai BM, Vickneswaran M, Duraisamy S, et al: Coagulopathy in acute head injury—a study of its role as a prognostic indicator. Br J Neurosurg 11:398–404, 1997.
108. Servadei F, Teasdale G, Merry G: Defining acute mild head injury in adults: A proposal based on prognostic factors, diagnosis and management. J Neurotrauma 18:657-664, 2001.
109. Poon WS, Poon CYS, Li AKC: Traumatic extradural hematoma of delayed onset is not a rarity. Neurosurgery 30:681–686, 1992.
110. Tomei G, Brambilla GL, Delfini R, et al: Guias para el manejo de los pacientes adultos con traumatismo encelocraneano leve. Medicina Intensiva 15:99–104, 1999.
111. Van der Naalt J, Hew JM, van Zomeren AH, et al: Computed tomography and magnetic resonance imaging in mild to moderate head injury: Early and late imaging related to outcome. Ann Neurol 46:70–78, 1999.
112. Mittl RL, Grossman RI, Hiehle JF, et al: Prevalence of MR evidence of diffuse axonal injury in patients with mild head injury and normal head CT findings. AJNR Am J Neuroradiol 15:1583–1589, 1994.
113. Tokutomi T, Hirohata M, Miyagi T, et al: Posttraumatic edema in the corpus callosum shown by MRI. Acta Neurochir Suppl (Wien) 70:80–83, 1997.
114. Levin HS, Amparo E, Eisenberg HM, et al: Magnetic resonance imaging and computerized tomography in relation to the neurobehavioral sequelae of mild and moderate head injuries. J Neurosurg 66:706–713, 1987.
115. Ashikaga R, Araki Y, Ishida O: MRI of head injury using FLAIR. Neuroradiology 39:239–242, 1997.
116. Shackford SR, Wald SL: Acute care of mild head injury. In Marion DW (ed): Traumatic Brain Injury. New York, Thieme, 1999, pp 155–163.
117. Nedd K, Sfakianakis G, Ganz W, et al: ^{99m}Tc-HMPAO SPECT of the brain in mild to moderate traumatic brain injury patients: Compared with CT—a prospective study. Brain Inj 6:469–479, 1993.
118. Abdel-Dayem HM, Abu-Judeh H, Kumar M, et al: SPECT brain perfusion abnormalities in mild or moderate traumatic brain injury. Ciln Nucl Med 23:309–317, 1998.
119. Gonçalves JM, Vaz R, Cerejo A, et al: HM-PAO SPECT in head trauma. Acta Neurochir Suppl (Wien) 55:11–13, 1992.
120. Fumeya A, Ito K, Yamagiwa O, et al: Analysis of MRI and SPECT in patients with acute head injury. Acta Neurochir Suppl (Wien) 51:283–285, 1990.
121. Holman BL, Zimmerman RE, Johnson KA, et al: Computer-assisted superimposition of magnetic resonance and high-resolution technetium-99m-HMPAO and thallium-201 SPECT images of the brain. J Nucl Med 32:1478–1484, 1991.
122. Humayun MS, Presty SK, Lafrance ND, et al: Local cerebral glucose abnormalities in mild closed head injured patients with cognitive impairments. Nucl Med Commun 10:335–344, 1989.
123. Bergsneider M, Hovda DA, Shalmon E, et al: Cerebral hyperglycolysis following severe traumatic brain injury in humans: A positron emission tomography study. J Neurosurg 86:241–251, 1997.
124. Ruff RM, Crouch JA, Troster AI, et al: Selected cases of poor outcome following a minor brain trauma: Comparing neuropsychological and positron emission tomography assessment. Brain Inj 8:297–308, 1994.
125. Jansen HML, van der Naalt J, van Zomeren AH, et al: Cobalt-55 positron emission tomography in traumatic brain injury: A pilot study. J Neurol Neurosurg Psychiatry 60:221–224, 1996.

CHAPTER **326**

Initial Resuscitation and Patient Evaluation

GRANT SINSON ■ PATRICK M. REILLY ■ M. SEAN GRADY

EARLY PATHOPHYSIOLOGIC CONSIDERATIONS: SECONDARY INSULTS

The initial goal in the management of severe head injury is to halt any ongoing injury and prevent the onset of additional injury. These "secondary injuries" are defined as "physiological events that can occur within minutes, hours, or days after the primary injury and can lead to further damage of nervous tissue, prolonging and/or contributing to permanent neurological dysfunction"[1](Fig. 326–1). The most obvious source of additional injury relates to mass effect on the brain due to either hemorrhage or brain edema.

The incidence of intracranial hemorrhage after traumatic brain injury (TBI) varies greatly with the severity of injury and the definition used for the presence of hemorrhage. For instance, 44% of patients with a severe injury and a skull fracture have an intracranial hematoma, but this excludes small hemorrhagic contusions.[2] Neural injury from hemorrhage results from direct compression of the brain, increased intracranial pressure (ICP), decreased cerebral perfusion pressure (CPP), and eventually infarction or herniation. In the presence of large hematomas, outcome correlates with the amount of neural injury present before surgical evacuation.[3] Subdural hematoma results from tearing of surface vessels or rupture of bridging veins. Because the inertial forces that can result in subdural hematoma are similar to the forces that cause diffuse axonal injury, these injuries commonly occur together. An epidural hematoma is often seen in conjunction with a skull fracture in the temporal region, where the skull can be quite thin and the middle meningeal artery is present in the underlying dura. Epidural hematomas may oc-

cur without any damage to the underlying brain; therefore, the damage correlates directly with the amount of blood and the duration of the mass effect before evacuation. Intraparenchymal hemorrhages range from small contusions that are clinically silent to large hematomas that require evacuation. All intraparenchymal hematomas result in some reaction by the surrounding brain. Breakdown of the blood-brain barrier results in vasogenic edema in the brain immediately adjacent to the hemorrhage. In patients with many contusions or diffuse brain swelling, this edema can become significant. There is also evidence for the release of the excitotoxic neurotransmitter glutamate into the penumbra around these areas of hemorrhage.[4]

Brain swelling after TBI is classified as vasogenic or cytotoxic edema. Vasogenic edema results from a

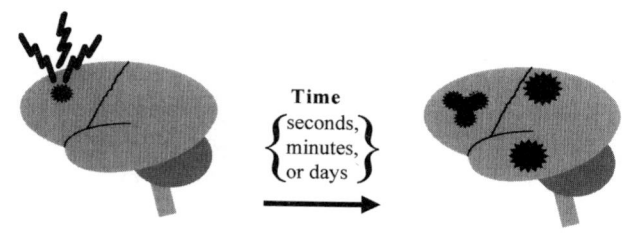

Primary injury　　　　**Secondary injury**

FIGURE 326–1. With severe traumatic brain injury, the primary injury results in some permanent neural damage. This primary injury may be diffuse or focal, but it is often a combination of injury types. Cascades of different mechanisms of secondary injury begin immediately after the primary injury and may continue for days. This secondary injury may occur adjacent to the primary injury or at remote sites.

breakdown of the blood-brain barrier, followed by a flow of fluid into the extracellular spaces. Cytotoxic edema is due to swelling of neurons, glia, or both. Classically, most of the edema after TBI was thought to be related to vasogenic mechanisms. After injury, there is an early but self-limited opening of the blood-brain barrier. In areas of brain contusion, this opening is more prolonged, and in patients with multiple contusions, this can result in massive edema and increased ICP. Recent evidence using diffusion-weighted magnetic resonance imaging suggests that cytotoxic edema may play a larger role in post-TBI edema than was previously appreciated. Barzo and colleagues showed decreased water diffusion as early as 45 minutes after experimental TBI.[5] This is consistent with increased intracellular edema and remains significant for 2 weeks after injury. When the majority of the edema is hemispheric and unilateral, falcine or tentorial herniation occurs, resulting in compression of either the pericallosal arteries or the posterior cerebral artery, respectively. Further swelling results in tonsilar herniation, compression of the brainstem, and death.

An additional source of secondary injury relates to decreased oxygen delivery to the brain. Adams and coworkers studied the brains of human victims of TBI and identified the presence of ischemia in 40% of these patients and evidence of raised ICP in 70%.[6] This suggests either that the injured brain is more sensitive to minor levels of ischemia or that patients have episodes of ischemia that are not documented. Data from the Traumatic Coma Data Bank demonstrated that 35% of patients with severe TBI had at least one episode of hypotension (systolic blood pressure <90 mm Hg) or hypoxia (PaO_2 <60 mm Hg).[7] Mortality increased 150% in those patients with episodes of hypotension compared with those without. Shackford and associates also identified autopsy evidence of secondary brain injury in 66% of patients who died from their head injuries.[8] Measurement of venous oxygen saturation in the jugular bulb permits the identification of cerebral ischemia when the oxygen saturation falls below 50 mm Hg. Using this technology, 39% of patients with severe TBI were found to have had at least one episode of jugular bulb desaturation, and these episodes correlated with higher mortality.[9]

Autoregulation normally maintains cerebral blood flow (CBF) constant, despite CPP that ranges between 50 and 150 mm Hg. There is an uncoupling of autoregulation after TBI that results in the brain's increased susceptibility both to ischemia from low CPP (with decreased CBF) and to raised ICP from high CPP (with increased CBF). Experimental TBI results in CBF falling proportionally when CPP falls below 80 mm Hg.[10] CBF less than 18 mL/100 g per minute correlates with poor outcome after human TBI.[11] There is a period of hypoperfusion early after injury when even patients who have a good outcome have low CBF.[11, 12] During days 1 to 3 after injury, either normal or high CBF can be present and is often accompanied by a lower metabolic rate of oxygen termed *relative* or *absolute hyperemia*, respectively.[12] These CBF changes after TBI are also tied to treatment; the loss of autoregulation allows

some control of CBF by blood pressure management, and the persistence of carbon dioxide (CO_2) reactivity of the cerebral vasculature permits adjustment of CBF by changing ventilatory parameters.

A number of cellular mechanisms of injury have also been identified. Many of these processes occur over hours to days after the primary injury, but their role in delayed neuronal injury suggests that they may provide targets for early therapies in the future. Changes in cerebral metabolism appear to occur in both oxidative metabolism and the rate of glycolysis. Bergsneider and colleagues showed that a relative increase in glucose metabolism (hyperglycolysis) occurs and persists for many days after TBI.[13] They demonstrated a relative increase in gylcolysis compared with the cerebral metabolic rate of oxygen in six patients with severe TBI using glucose uptake studies with positron emission tomography. The mechanism for lowering the cerebral metabolic rate of oxygen in the days following TBI is not known; however, Verweij and coworkers showed a decrease in oxidative metabolism at the level of the mitochondria in both a cortical impact model of TBI and operative specimens from human victims of TBI.[14]

The production of superoxide and hydroxyl radical in the minutes after brain injury contributes to cellular injury.[15] These are produced by the arachidonic acid cascade, mitochondrial leak, infiltrating white blood cells, and release of catalytically reactive iron from ferritin, transferrin, or hemoglobin.[16] Lipid peroxidation triggered by these radicals blocks phospholipid-dependent enzymes, increases membrane permeability, and can lead directly to membrane destruction. Free radical formation can also contribute to the release of glutamate.[17] Glutamate stimulates neuronal depolarization by activating three different classes of receptors: the *N*-methyl-D-aspartate receptor, the metabotropic receptor, and the kainate and amino-3-hydroxy-5-methyl-4-isoxazole propionate family of receptors. Glutamate overstimulation of these receptors can cause neuronal depolarization, swelling, and eventually death.[18] Activation of these receptors all contribute to the eventual rise in intracellular calcium. High calcium levels can be buffered initially by adjusting levels in the endoplasmic reticulum and mitochondria and by binding substances such as phosphates.[19–21] Continued elevation of intracellular calcium results in the activation of numerous proteases, including phospholipases, nucleases, and superoxide dismutase. New technology has permitted microdialysis studies in human victims of TBI. Bullock and colleagues demonstrated levels of excitatory amino acids up to 50 times normal in patients with severe TBI.[4] The magnitude of these elevations was greatest in patients with contusions or those who suffered secondary ischemic events.

Ultrastructural evaluation of neurofilament staining in the white matter after brain injury classically shows "retraction balls," which represent axons that have damaged neurofilaments and impaired axonal transport but remain intact, or axons that have undergone axotomy. Evidence suggests that this axonal damage and breakdown of the cytoskeleton may be due to

TABLE 326–1 ■ Secondary Cerebral Insults

Clinical Treatment Targets
Hemorrhage: intra-axial, subdural, epidural
Cerebral edema
Increased intracranial pressure
Ischemia: hypotension
Ischemia: hypoxia

Possible Future Treatment Targets
Diffuse axonal injury
Vasospasm
Apoptosis
Free radicals
Excitotoxicity
Mitochondrial dysfunction
Cytoskeletal damage

activation of the protease calpain.[22] In rodent models of TBI, inhibition of calpain resulted in improved neurological outcomes.[23, 24] Neuronal death after TBI was previously attributed to cell swelling and necrosis. Rink and associates first showed evidence of apoptosis after TBI in an animal model, and this has been confirmed in human specimens.[25–27] This important observation suggests that neuronal death after TBI may not be a passive, irreversible cascade of destructive events; rather, in some cell populations, it may be a complex sequence of events driven by the activation of specific genes. Blocking apoptosis with nerve growth factor results in neurological improvements after experimental TBI.[28] As additional examples of these molecular mediators are identified, blocking their detrimental effects will be the target of new treatments that will likely be most efficacious when applied during the prehospital or initial evaluation component of patient care (Table 326–1).

BIOMECHANICAL CONSIDERATIONS IN TRAUMATIC BRAIN INJURY

The forces actually experienced by the bone and soft tissue of the head during TBI are classified as either *contact* or *inertial loading*. Contact forces occur during an impact to the head, and damage occurs when the strain limits of the tissue (usually the skull) is exceeded. The most pure form of contact injury results in a skull fracture that can have varying degrees of underlying brain injury, depending on the degree of tissue displacement. These injuries can be associated with depressed skull fractures, epidural hematomas, and coup contusions. Before the widespread use of computed tomography (CT), skull x-rays were a useful screening test for intracranial hematoma, because the presence of a fracture significantly increases the chance of hematoma development.[29, 30]

Inertial loading of the head can result from impact or from impulsive loading that then causes rapid acceleration and deceleration and subsequent tissue strain. Increasing the duration or the magnitude of the acceleration results in increased strain. Tolerance curves based

on strain correlate with the degree of axonal injury.[31, 32] The variables contributing to the calculation of strain are peak angular acceleration and maximal changes in angular velocity.[32] With a moderate duration of acceleration, the periphery of the brain experiences the highest degree of strain, which can tear bridging veins and result in subdural hematoma.[33] If the duration of the acceleration is increased, the elevated strains penetrate deeper in the brain and result in diffuse axonal injury[34] (Fig. 326–2). The most common clinical situation involving inertial injury is a high-speed motor vehicle accident. There are often components of both contact and inertial forces, resulting in more severe injuries. The removal of direct head impact from a rotational injury necessitates doubling the rotational velocity to reproduce the injury seen with a rotational injury produced by direct head impact.[35, 36]

Penetrating trauma to the head is most commonly the result of gunshot wounds. The potential for injury depends on a number of variables: trajectory, velocity, mass, and shape. The actual kinetic energy of the projectile can be calculated as follows:

$$\text{Kinetic energy} = (\text{mass} \times \text{velocity}^2)/2$$

Consequently, a rifle with a muzzle velocity of 2000 feet/second has a much greater potential for tissue damage than does a .44 Magnum handgun with a muzzle velocity of 1350 feet/second, despite the weight of the .44-caliber bullet being greater than that of many rifle bullets. When the bullet enters tissue, its energy dissipation varies with the size of the bullet and how rapidly it decelerates. Bullets with hollow noses are designed to flatten on impact, resulting in a more rapid deceleration and therefore a more rapid transfer of kinetic energy. In many cases, the skull absorbs the majority of the energy of a low-velocity projectile, resulting in little or no penetration into the brain. The bullet traverses the path of least resistance, which in the case of a tangential trajectory, can result in the bullet traveling some distance in the subgaleal

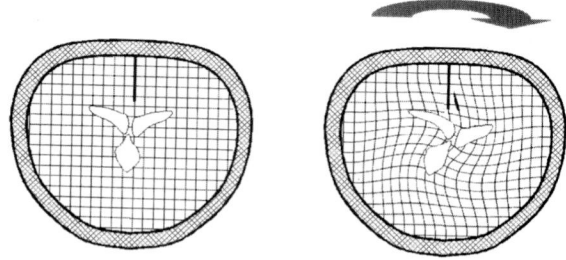

FIGURE 326–2. Tissue strains can be measured using finite element modeling. A model of the brain is constructed using orthogonal grids. Each element within the grid can be assigned biomechanical properties that approximate those of the tissue being modeled. On the *left*, a model has been made with different biomechanical regions to represent the bone, cerebrospinal fluid, falx cerebri, and brain tissue. The model is then subjected to rotational acceleration injury to identify regions of the brain at risk for strains that may be greater than the known tolerance of normal tissue.

space and never penetrating the skull. Entrance wounds are usually small and round and often have a blackened area of burn at their periphery. Owing to the significant energy dissipated when a bullet enters the skull, there is often insufficient energy to result in an exit wound in most civilian injuries. However, penetrating the skull causes the bullet to tumble, which causes additional energy dissipation into the surrounding brain. If there is enough energy to result in an exit wound, the site is usually much larger because of the energy released from the tumble and the additional slowing of the projectile.

PREHOSPITAL MANAGEMENT

The goal of all prehospital management is to remove victims of trauma from hostile injury environments and place them in environments where they become patients. All this must be done without worsening the effects of the primary injury. This desire to minimize additional injury has led to abandonment of the "scoop and run" concept of getting victims to a hospital setting. It has been replaced by an approach that safely removes victims from accident scenes and transports them to the hospital while simultaneously stabilizing them medically. Implementation of this approach varies considerably among countries and among different geographic regions within the same country.

Wilmink and coworkers reviewed 737 motor vehicle accidents and found that 90 (12%) involved victim entrapment that required extrication.[37] They recommend a target of less than 30 minutes for the release of such victims but emphasize that uncontrolled release is indicated only if there is an immediate threat to the victim's life. Siegel and colleagues studied 144 victims of motor vehicle accidents, and 102 (71%) were extricated at the scene.[38] In their cohort, brain injury occurred in 51% of patients requiring extrication but in only 35% of those not extricated. Although expertise in safely extricating patients is crucial, there is considerable evidence that the level of rescuers' medical training and the timeliness of transport to an appropriate hospital also impact patient outcomes.

Klauber and associates followed patient outcomes in San Diego as paramedic services and a helicopter transport system were implemented between 1979 and 1981.[39] The number of deaths at the scene declined 28%, the number of patients declared dead on arrival at the hospital declined 68%, and mortality rates for hospitalized patients did not change. Also during this time, the percentage of patients transported by police declined from 15% to less than 5%. This same region underwent reorganization in 1984 to designate five adult trauma centers. Shackford and colleagues reviewed the care of major trauma victims before and after this regionalization of trauma care.[40] They reported suboptimal care in 32% of patients before regionalization, compared with 4.2% after regionalization; the percentage of preventable deaths dropped from 13.6% to 2.7% during the same period. Colohan and coworkers prospectively compared head injury

mortality in two different emergency medical service environments: New Delhi, India, and Charlottesville, Virginia.[41] The overall mortality rate was 11% in New Delhi versus 7.2% in Charlottesville. The mortality rates for victims with severe injuries (Glasgow Coma Scale [GCS] motor score of 1 to 4) and those with minimal injuries (GCS motor score of 6) were similar at both centers. Those patients with moderate injuries (GCS motor score of 5) had a mortality of 12.5% in New Delhi, compared with 4.8% in Charlottesville. This dramatic difference is attributed to the differences in prehospital emergency services. In New Delhi, 2.7% of victims received first aid administered by paramedical personnel or police before arriving at the hospital, whereas in Charlottesville, 84.3% were attended to by paramedics and transported by ambulance. These differences in transportation were also reflected in the percentage of patients admitted to the hospital within 1 hour of being injured: 6.9% in New Delhi, versus 50.2% in Charlottesville. In regions where air transport is a feasible means of decreasing transport time to the trauma center, reductions in predicted mortality as high as 52% have been reported.[42]

The level of management that can be delivered in the prehospital setting varies with the training of the emergency medical system response team. Adding a physician to the response team is not always practical or possible, yet doing so has been shown to improve the delivery of care.[43, 44] Baxt and Moody compared outcomes in victims of blunt trauma who were transported by helicopter accompanied by a flight nurse and a paramedic versus similar patients transported by helicopter accompanied by a flight nurse and a physician.[44] Those patients treated by the nurse-physician team had a mortality rate 35% lower than predicted based on the severity of their injuries.

It is difficult to attribute improved outcomes in patients treated in the prehospital setting to a specific intervention; however, as with outcomes based on hospital data, prevention of hypoxia and hypotension appears to be vital.[45, 46] Gentleman showed that the incidence of hypoxia or hypotension on arrival at the hospital could be decreased from 30% to 12% by simple improvements in prehospital airway management, including an increased use of intubation and mechanical ventilation.[47] Prehospital intubation in patients with a GCS score less than 9 was shown to improve outcome after evaluating 1092 patients.[48] Adequate resources must be available to include paramedics or physicians in the emergency response group who are capable of intubating patients in the prehospital setting. Efforts to train basic emergency medical technicians to perform prehospital intubation safely have had disappointing results.[49, 50] Resnick and colleagues followed 37 patients with severe TBI and prolonged raised ICP.[51] Only one of eight patients with prehospital hypotension had a good outcome, and this was significantly worse than those patients without prehospital hypotension. When a GCS score is determined in the prehospital setting, it can be useful as a comparison with the score in the emergency department. Winkler and coworkers demonstrated that patients whose GCS did not improve between the prehospital evaluation and the initial hospital evaluation had worse outcomes.[52]

GENERAL TRAUMA RESUSCITATION

Trauma Team

Organization of a trauma response group should comply with the standards outlined by the American College of Surgeons Committee on Trauma.[53] Additionally, most local governments have guidelines for the level of care that must be available at specific medical centers. The composition and organization of the trauma response team vary with the resources available and with the volume of traumas treated at each medical center. The goal of this group is to pick up where the transport team left off in the process of transitioning the victim into a patient, treating the primary injuries, and preventing additional injury. A center with few trauma cases may assess and resuscitate these patients in a general "code room" within the emergency department or, in some cases, an available operating room. Because of the different needs of trauma patients compared with other medical codes, most trauma centers use a designated trauma area within the emergency department. Immediate access to a ventilator, operative instruments, unmatched O negative packed red blood cells, and plain radiographs is necessary. Prompt availability of a CT scanner, preferably within the emergency department, is essential.

Regardless of who is on the trauma team, all participants must strictly follow universal precautions. This includes a fluid-impervious gown, mask, eye shield, head covering, and gloves. Lead gowns can also be worn to permit plain radiographs to be taken without interrupting the evaluation. The risk of patients having human immunodeficiency virus (HIV) or hepatitis is higher in trauma patients than in nontrauma patients in the emergency department.[54] Tardiff and colleagues studied patients who died from trauma in New York City. Overall, 7.2% were HIV positive, and 20.8% of patients 35 to 44 years old were HIV positive.[55] Kelen and associates tested all patients visiting an inner-city emergency department in Baltimore and found that 24% were infected with at least one of the following: HIV, hepatitis B virus, or hepatitis C virus.[56]

In the "vertical" approach, a single physician carries out the initial evaluation of a trauma patient, with support from nursing, respiratory therapy, radiology, and laboratory personnel and the blood bank. In contrast, the "horizontal" approach uses multiple physicians, each performing specific components of the evaluation simultaneously. Obviously, the horizontal approach requires additional physician resources, but it increases the speed of the evaluation and stabilization of a severely injured trauma victim. The trauma team leader assigns portions of the evaluation to specific individuals. These assignments are best done in advance; if, however, they are done during the evaluation, they must be clear and specific, to minimize confusion. Aspects of the initial assessment that may be given to other members of the team include airway management, intravenous access, or the primary survey. Nursing support is vital to assist in each step of the process. One individual should also be responsible for recording rapidly received data onto the trauma flow sheet. Additional support may be needed from a social worker to communicate with family members, a security guard to minimize the presence of unnecessary people in the trauma area, a secretary to call consultants, and a messenger service to assist with patient or resource transport.

Primary Survey

The primary survey provides the initial opportunity for evaluating and stabilizing a trauma patient. During the survey, the ABCDEs of trauma care are addressed. Although these steps are generally presented in a sequential fashion, many of them can be performed simultaneously.

A, for Airway. Airway management requires both an initial evaluation and constant vigilance throughout resuscitation to keep the airway unobstructed. It is commonly stated that a speaking patient has an adequate airway, but this does not obviate the need for this step. Foreign bodies such as gastric contents or dentures can quickly compromise the airway in an otherwise stable patient. Soft tissue swelling from facial, mandibular, or tracheal injury should be assessed, and a low threshold for intubation in these patients can prevent the need for emergency tracheostomy or cricothyrotomy. The presence of neurological deficits may result in airway compromise simply because the patient's level of consciousness is inadequate for him or her to protect the airway. To control the airway, a jaw thrust or chin lift may initially be helpful. A definitive airway should be obtained if there is any question of the patient's ability to maintain his or her own airway.[57] Endotracheal intubation is generally preferred in trauma victims, owing to the risk of intracranial placement in patients with facial fractures; this is an uncommon complication, however.[58]

B, for Breathing. Breathing is usually assessed by the same member who examined the airway. Adequate oxygen delivery and CO_2 release are confirmed at this stage. Jugular venous distention or tracheal shift may represent increased intrathoracic pressures. The chest wall is exposed and inspected to confirm symmetrical and adequate movement. The chest is auscultated to assess breath sounds. The presence of flail chest, tension pneumothorax, or open pneumothorax is identified and treated. Patients should receive supplemental oxygen and be monitored for adequate oxygenation with pulse oximetry.

C, for Circulation and Control of Hemorrhage. Within seconds, the patient's level of consciousness, skin color, and pulse are assessed. These signs can be nonspecific, but the presence of a radial artery pulse confirms a systolic blood pressure of at least 80 mm Hg. External hemorrhage should be identified and controlled with manual pressure. In some instances, a pneumatic splint can be useful. Intravenous access with at least two large-bore lines is obtained, in conjunction with obtaining the following laboratory tests: type and crossmatch, pregnancy test, coagulation studies, hemoglobin, platelet count, electrolytes, drug screen, and alcohol level. Warmed Ringer's lactate is the initial crystalloid, but uncrossmatched O negative packed red blood cells should be available for early use in patients with significant blood loss. Blood pressure measurement and placement of an electrocardiographic monitor are sometimes not done until the secondary survey; however, this can be important information, and if personnel permit, this is an excellent time to incorporate them into the evaluation.

D, for Disability. This is the first time the patient's neurological status is specifically considered. In a patient with an altered level of consciousness and no evidence of hypoxia or hypotension, a traumatic central nervous system (CNS) injury should be assumed. Two types of evaluations of disability have been advocated for this portion of the survey. The AVPU mnemonic is: Alert, arouses to Verbal or Painful stimuli, or is Unresponsive. The GCS is an alternative that can be performed rapidly during this portion of the examination. Knowledge of the GCS facilitates communication between the primary trauma team and the neurosurgical consultants and can correlate with patient outcome.[59, 60] The examination consists of three parts: evaluation of eye opening, assessment of motor activity, and response to verbal stimuli (Table 326–2). Examiners who are familiar with the GCS can often obtain the score during earlier portions of the evaluation. Eye opening, verbal response, and motor activity are simply documented during airway assessment and placement of intravenous access, which provide both the verbal and the painful stimuli necessary to apply the scale. Most patients with possible cervical spine injur-

ies have been put in rigid cervical collars before transport to the hospital, but adequate immobilization should be confirmed at this time.

E, for Exposure and Environmental control. This part of the evaluation requires the removal of all clothing, often with heavy scissors, to permit further examination. Owing to the risks of hypothermia, once the examination is done, the patient should be covered with warm blankets to prevent further cooling.

Other Elements. Some physicians also include F, for Foley catheter, and G, for gastric tube, in the primary survey. A Foley catheter should be inserted in all victims of severe trauma. Because of the risk of urethral injury, the catheter should not be placed if there is blood at the urethral meatus, a high-riding prostate on rectal examination in a male patient, a known or suspected pelvic fracture, or scrotal or perineal ecchymosis. In these instances, a retrograde urethrogram should be done before catheter placement. A gastric tube is used to decompress the stomach and decrease the risk of aspiration. In patients with significant facial fractures or when there is suspicion of a fracture in the floor of the frontal fossa, an oral gastric tube should be used to prevent intracranial placement. Other adjuvants to the primary assessment include plain anteroposterior (AP) radiographs of the chest and pelvis and a lateral cervical spine film. These studies should not be obtained, however, if doing so would impair the initial survey and resuscitation.

Secondary Survey

This portion of the examination should be done only if the primary survey and resuscitation have been completed and the patient's vital signs have stabilized. In short, this is a head-to-toe examination that includes a re-evaluation of important aspects of the primary survey. The first portion of the survey is obtaining a history using the AMPLE mnemonic: Allergies, Medications, Past medical history/Pregnancy, Last meal, and Events relating to the injury. If patients are unable to provide this information, it should be sought from family members or from emergency medical personnel.

The examination begins at the head with close palpation of the scalp and head for fractures, lacerations, or contusions. The eyes are checked for visual acuity, pupillary size and reactivity, ocular motility, and hemorrhage and to remove contact lenses. The face is examined for areas of ecchymosis or leakage of spinal fluid from the ears or nose. Confirmation of an appropriate airway is also performed at this time.

The neck is inspected for a midline trachea, significant edema, or jugular venous distention. Palpation may identify crepitation, cervical carotid artery pulses, and posterior cervical pain or the presence of a spinous process step-off. Evaluation for spine pain or a step-off through the entire spinal column must be done during the secondary survey when the patient is stable enough to be turned using the log-roll technique. Radiographic evaluation of the cervical spine includes a lateral film that visualizes down to the C7-T1 junction, an AP view,

TABLE 326–2 ■ **Glasgow Coma Scale**

Motor Score

Obey verbal commands	6
Localize to painful stimuli	5
Withdrawal to painful stimuli	4
Flexion (decorticate) posturing to painful stimuli	3
Extension (decerebrate) posturing to painful stimuli	2
No motor response	1

Verbal Score

Oriented and conversing	5
Conversing but disoriented	4
Inappropriate words	3
Incomprehensible sounds	2
No verbal response	1
Intubated	T

Eye Score

Open spontaneously	4
Open to verbal stimuli	3
Open to painful stimuli	2
No eye opening	1
Total Score	**3–15**

and an open-mouth study of the odontoid. Auscultation of the carotid arteries may identify a bruit, which suggests a carotid artery dissection. The thoracic region is reinspected for adequate ventilatory movement and breath sounds. Distant heart sounds may suggest cardiac tamponade. If an AP chest radiograph has not yet been obtained, it should be done at this time.

Examination of the abdomen includes inspection, palpation, and auscultation. A significant injury can be present in a patient with a normal examination, and a patient with a head injury may have an abdominal examination that is quite limited. Adjuvant diagnostic tests include abdominal ultrasonography, peritoneal lavage, and CT. The choice of test depends on availability, physician experience, and the need for other emergent operative interventions.

The pelvis and perineum are inspected for obvious injury. The rectal examination and AP radiograph of the pelvis should have been performed during the primary survey. Female patients should have a vaginal examination for the presence of blood or lacerations. The extremities are evaluated for contusion, laceration, deformity, and appropriate distal arterial pulses.

The last portion of the secondary survey is a more detailed neurological assessment. At a minimum, this should include repeat GCS determination, pupillary examination, and gross examination of sensation and movement in the extremities. Applying a mildly painful stimulus (such as nail bed pressure) to all four extremities permits the evaluation of sensation, movement, ability to vocalize, and ability to localize.

The most common adjuvant test at this point is CT of the head, chest, or abdomen. In some cases, angiography is also required to evaluate for major vascular injury. At this time, laboratory evaluations should be available, and subspecialists can be consulted.

General guidelines for urgent neurosurgical consultation during the primary or secondary survey include open depressed skull fracture, open head injury with visible brain tissue, lateralizing neurological signs (unilateral third cranial nerve palsy, decerebrate or decorticate posturing, hemiparesis, or hemiplegia), a GCS score less than 13, or head CT findings of hemorrhage or cerebral edema. In these instances, a focused neurosurgical evaluation is appropriate and should be performed simultaneously with the ongoing general survey already outlined.

NEUROLOGICAL ASSESSMENT

History

Gathering relevant history concerning a patient's neurological status may be somewhat different from gathering general trauma information. During the neurological assessment, information can be obtained from people who witnessed the injury, medical personnel at the scene, family members, or police officers. Specific details of the mechanism of injury may change the neurosurgeon's index of suspicion that a significant neurological injury is present. For instance, the speed

limit, the amount of damage the car sustained, the severity of injuries to other people involved in the accident, the patient's location in relation to the vehicle (driver or passenger, inside or thrown from the vehicle), and the presence of airbags or seatbelts all influence the evaluation of the possible forces the victim was subjected to during the accident. Because these data affect the patient's general trauma care, emergency room personnel or traumatologists have often gathered it already.

Other information is available from a patient's early neurological examination. The accuracy of these data should be critically evaluated by considering the source; however, useful information can be obtained concerning the progression of a patient's neurological functioning. Witnesses may be able to describe seizure activity, an awake but confused state, flaccid unconsciousness, focal weakness, or posturing. It is not uncommon to be told that a patient was "posturing" at the scene of the injury, but this cannot be taken at face value. Although some emergency medical teams have an excellent understanding of neurological signs, other movements are often misinterpreted as posturing. A detailed description of what they saw usually permits one to determine the validity of the claim. The report of a patient who is initially lucid but deteriorates into coma suggests an 80.5% chance of a focal mass lesion being present on computed tomographic scans.[61] The lack of improvement in the GCS between the initial prehospital evaluation and the first emergency room score correlates with a worse outcome.[52] This type of history can be obtained while donning the appropriate gear to follow universal precautions before performing a more detailed neurological examination.

Examination

The general evaluation outlined earlier is typically performed by a trauma team before or during the initial neurosurgical evaluation of a patient with a possible TBI. Because of the close relationship between the CNS and the control of vital functions, the neurosurgeon must be aware of ongoing efforts to assess and treat the patient's ABCs. Maintaining an airway and adequate blood oxygenation is straightforward, but the appropriate blood CO_2 level is somewhat controversial. The therapeutic use of hyperventilation is discussed in more detail later, but during the early evaluation of a trauma victim, the patient's CO_2 should be maintained in the low-normal range. For each unit elevation of CO_2, the CBF increases 2% to 4%.[62] In a patient who is not adequately ventilating, CO_2 retention can cause cerebrovascular dilatation, which may increase ICP if there is already a mass lesion or diffuse edema. Consequently, one should have a low threshold for instituting mechanical ventilation to minimize the chance of hypercarbia in a patient suspected of having a moderate or severe head injury. This beneficial effect of low CO_2 levels on ICP has resulted in hyperventilation being used empirically in patients at risk for severe head injury. This technique became so widespread that respiratory therapists and paramedics often gently hyperventilated patients during transport to improve ICP and prevent hypercarbia. This can result in very low CO_2 levels. Muizelaar and coworkers performed a prospective, randomized study of empirical hyperventilation in head injury patients and demonstrated worse outcomes in those who were hyperventilated.[63] During the initial evaluation of these patients, an arterial CO_2 of 30 to 35 mm Hg should be targeted and confirmed with arterial blood gases.

Blood pressure management in trauma victims usually involves correction of hypotension due to some form of shock. Hypotension accompanied by bradycardia should alert the neurosurgeon to the possibility of neurogenic shock associated with a spinal cord injury. In this case, the hypotension should be treated with pressors rather than aggressive volume expansion after other potential sources of occult hemorrhage have been ruled out. Hypovolemic hypotension can also occur from blood loss due to head injury. Laceration of a major intracranial artery from penetrating trauma may cause a tremendous blood loss. Although this type of bleeding is generally easily identified, the rather brisk bleeding that can occur from scalp lacerations of the galeal blood vessels is often overlooked. This underscores the need for the neurosurgeon to closely examine the head for lacerations and any ongoing hemorrhage. Do not assume that this has been done during the general secondary survey. When significant scalp bleeding is identified, the use of Rainey clips can rapidly stop the bleeding and permit further examination before definitively repairing the laceration.

The Cushing response occurs as a late event from raised ICP and herniation. Described by Cushing in 1901, the response includes hypertension, bradycardia, and respiratory irregularity.[64] The respiratory changes are rarely seen clinically, because all these patients should be mechanically ventilated at this point in their care. Deviation from the more typical hypotension and tachycardia seen in trauma patients should alert the trauma team that significant intracranial hypertension may be the cause.

Assessing neurological status is difficult when a patient is intubated and paralyzed. It is therefore important to have a clear understanding of the indications the traumatologists are using to decide when and how to pharmacologically paralyze and intubate patients with possible neurological injuries. This discussion should take place before any patient resuscitation. When it is necessary to proceed with intubation, a short-acting paralytic such as vecuronium or succinylcholine should be used. If possible, the neurosurgeon should be given a chance to evaluate the patient before intubation. This evaluation should include only the determination of an accurate GCS score (including motor focality), because the remainder of the examination can be done after intubation. When the patient has been intubated before the neurosurgeon's evaluation, the other aspects of the examination should still be performed as outlined. Often the pupillary examination can be done in a medicated patient.

The secondary survey of the head is sometimes inadvertently ignored during the trauma evaluation: the traumatologists and the neurosurgeon both think that the other is doing it. Hair that is matted down with vomitus, blood, or other fluids can hide entrance wounds or significant lacerations. Lacerations should be assessed for the presence of foreign bodies, bony step-offs, or injured brain. The ears should be checked for blood or cerebrospinal fluid (CSF) behind the tympanic membrane or within the ear canal itself. The presence of otorrhea should also be noted. Ecchymosis over the mastoid region (Battle's sign) or unilateral facial weakness may suggest a basilar skull fracture. Periorbital ecchymosis (raccoon eyes) is also associated with skull fracture.

Numerous injury scales have been developed to permit the rapid evaluation of a patient's neurological status. The GCS has become the standard because of its ease of application and its usefulness in communicating a patient's status among the various specialties involved in treatment decisions.[65] All three categories of the GCS can be assessed in approximately 30 seconds. While approaching the patient, observe for spontaneous eye opening, then address the patient with a greeting and a simple command and note his or her verbal, eye opening, and motor response. If the patient is not responsive enough to permit completion of a score at this point, proceed to painful stimuli with a sternal rub, supraorbital pressure, or nipple pinch. A verbal and eye opening score can then be given. If a motor score has not yet been assigned, peripheral painful stimuli should be applied using a reflex hammer to provide nail bed pressure. Before assessing the GCS, one should confirm that the patient is not hypotensive or pharmacologically paralyzed, both of which prevent accurate scoring. The score that has the most prognostic importance is referred to as the postresuscitation GCS, which is obtained after the patient's airway and hemodynamic status have been stabilized.

Patients who are intubated cannot be given verbal scores; consequently, the sum of the motor and eye opening scores are followed by a "T" to provide this information. For example, an intubated patient with spontaneous eye opening (4) and localizing to painful stimuli (5) would be given a GCS score of 9T. When assigning a score, the best response should be used; thus, a patient with decerebrate posturing on the left and decorticate posturing on the right would be given a motor score of 3. This type of focality is not formally a part of the GCS, but it should be noted, because early signs of herniation due to a mass lesion are generally unilateral. Also, it is important to reassess the GCS as the resuscitation continues, because deterioration may suggest ongoing secondary injury that requires emergent treatment. Although the entire GCS should be evaluated, at a minimum, the motor score must be documented; this portion of the examination is the most reproducible and carries the most prognostic information.[66]

Like the GCS, the pupillary examination should be part of the initial neurological assessment. Independent of the GCS, the patient's age and pupillary findings have great prognostic significance.[66, 67] The pupils are also easily reexamined during resuscitation to identify neurological worsening. A unilateral dilated pupil that does not react to light (or does so very slowly) in a trauma patient should be considered caused by ipsilateral temporal lobe herniation until proved otherwise. If third nerve function is completely lost, the eye will deviate inferiorly and laterally. Other causes of unilateral pupil dilatation are direct trauma to the eye and a drug reaction. Therefore, this sign must be interpreted in the context of the patient's complete examination. An optic nerve injury may result in an ipsilateral unreactive or dilated pupil, but the pupil in the contralateral eye should respond to light (an afferent pupillary defect or Marcus Gunn pupil). Bilateral dilated pupils are more difficult to interpret and may result from hypoxia, hypotension, or bilateral third nerve dysfunction. Unilateral pupil constriction is often accompanied by mild ptosis when Horner's syndrome is present. Bilateral pupillary constriction may be a drug response (especially if narcotics were given) or represent a pontine lesion.

In an era of high-resolution magnetic resonance imaging and computed tomographic scans, herniation syndromes and radiographic herniation are often confused. The importance of radiographic herniation varies with its acuity; for example, a slow-growing brain tumor may cause significant tonsillar herniation in a patient with no neurological deficits. It is the presence of a clinical herniation syndrome that has great significance in trauma patients. The most common syndrome is uncal tentorial herniation, which is due to medial herniation of the uncus and parahippocampal gyrus between the tentorial notch and the midbrain. This may be caused by an ipsilateral mass lesion such as an epidural hematoma or from temporal lobe edema or hemorrhage. The clinical manifestation of this syndrome is usually from direct compression of the ipsilateral third cranial nerve and the ipsilateral cerebral peduncle, resulting in ipsilateral pupillary enlargement and contralateral hemiparesis. In some cases, this may also cause compression of the posterior cerebral artery and result in an occipital lobe infarction if it is not rapidly corrected (Fig. 326–3). Kernohan's notch effect occurs if the uncal herniation results in ipsilateral pupillary dilatation and *ipsilateral* hemiparesis due to pressure on the *contralateral* cerebral peduncle that is pushed up against the contralateral tentorial edge.[68] Therefore, the side of the pupillary findings is more useful when localizing the side of the uncal herniation. If the herniation is untreated, third nerve compression will progress and affect eye motility, with lateral and inferior eye deviation, and hemiparesis will become decerebrate posturing. This represents the functional disconnection of the cerebral cortex from the brainstem as demonstrated by Sherrington, who was able to reproduce decerebrate posturing in animals by transecting the brainstem at the intercollicular level.[69]

Tonsillar herniation results if there is continued supratentorial downward compression or if there is a primary posterior fossa mass. The cerebellar tonsils are forced downward through the foramen magnum, resulting in medullary compression. Clinically, this compression causes rapid loss of respiratory drive and

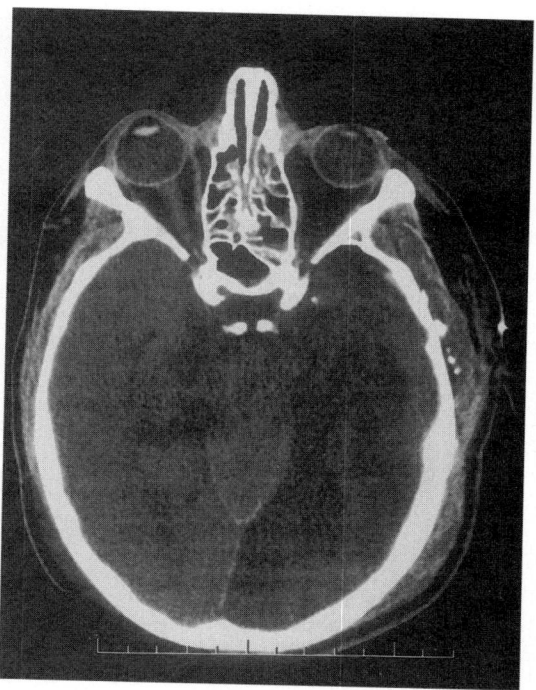

FIGURE 326–3. This 25-year-old man suffered a minor head injury 3 weeks earlier. He then had a dirt bike accident and was reported to be moving nonpurposefully at the scene. His initial examination revealed a Glasgow Coma Scale score of 3 and bilateral unreactive pupils. The initial computed tomographic scan showed an acute left-sided subdural hematoma and left hemisphere edema. Despite immediate evacuation and decompression, his follow-up computed tomographic scan demonstrated bilateral posterior cerebral artery infarcts consistent with bilateral uncal herniation.

irreversible brainstem damage if it is not immediately decompressed. Both uncal and tonsillar herniation can result in brainstem hemorrhage that is located in the midline (Duret's hemorrhage) (Fig. 326–4), which can be differentiated from the superficial dorsal midbrain hemorrhage associated with diffuse axonal injury (Fig. 326–5).[70]

In the acute stages of TBI, the deep tendon reflexes are not particularly useful for assessing the degree of injury, because they may be absent for reasons unrelated to the trauma and can also persist after brain death. The oculocephalic and oculovestibular reflexes evaluate brainstem function. In an unconscious patient, the oculocephalic reflex is assessed by rapidly rotating the head in the horizontal plane. In response, the eyes should move conjugately in the opposite direction ("doll's eyes"), suggesting intact tegmental structures in the pons and midbrain. Cold caloric (oculovestibular) testing can be done to further evaluate the brainstem. In a comatose patient, the head is placed at 30 degrees, and 30 mL of ice water is used to irrigate the ear canal. A patient with an intact oculovestibular reflex will have conjugate eye deviation toward the side being stimulated. Rarely do such findings play a role in decision making during the assessment of an acutely injured patient, so these reflexes are seldom tested in this setting. Additionally, a doll's eyes test should not

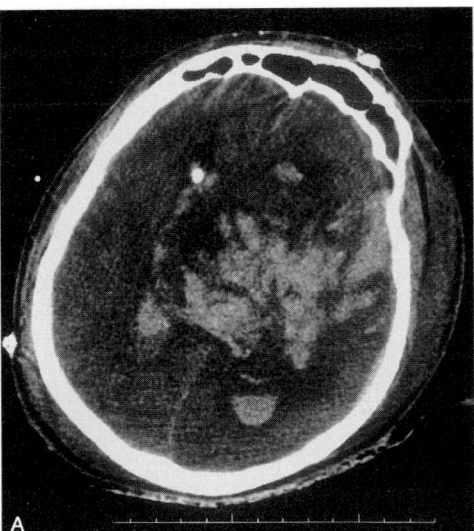 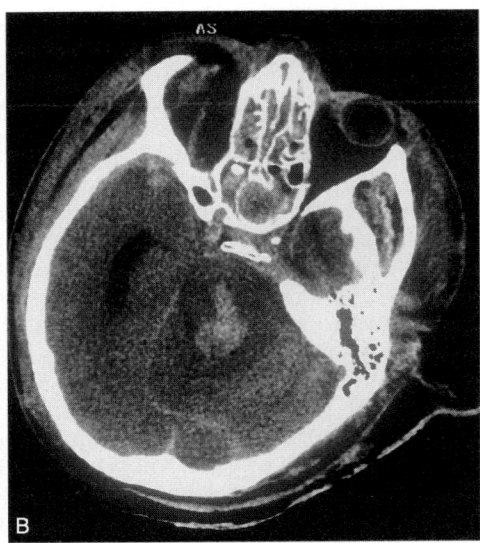

FIGURE 326–4. This young man was struck by a bus near the hospital. In the emergency department, he had a Glasgow Coma Scale score of 3 and bilateral unreactive pupils. *A*, Computed tomographic scan shows massive supratentorial contusion and hemorrhage. *B*, Hemorrhage into the brainstem is consistent with Duret's hemorrhage of uncal herniation.

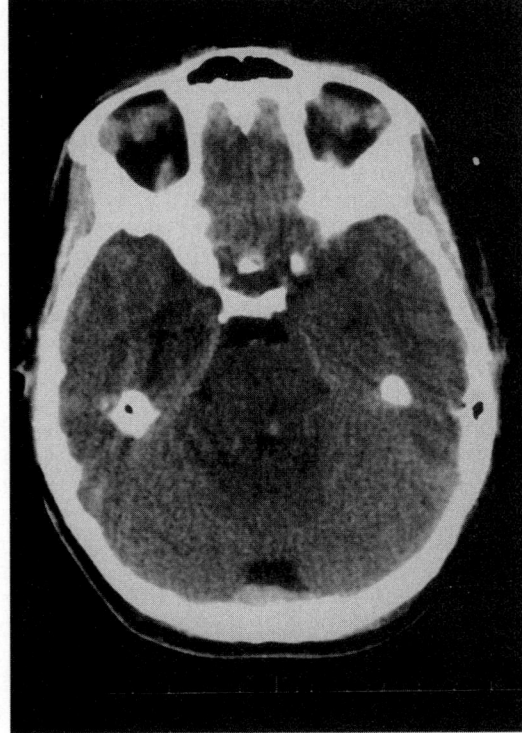

FIGURE 326–5. This 15-year-old girl was thrown from her horse and struck the top of her head. She was wearing a helmet. She had bilaterally reactive pupils and a Glasgow Coma Scale score of 4. Computed tomographic scan shows a dorsal midbrain hemorrhage, which is one of the hallmarks of diffuse axonal injury.

be done in a patient at risk for a cervical spine injury, which includes all patients with acute moderate or severe TBIs. An exception is when determining brain death; however, because most of these patients have received medications that complicate this determination (i.e., paralytics), this examination is often deferred until the medication has been metabolized.

Radiographic Evaluation

Since its introduction into clinical use in the early 1970s, CT has completely changed the practice of evaluating victims of head trauma. Modern computed tomographic scans offer an outstanding view of the components of the various pathologies associated with head injury: acute blood, bone, brain parenchyma, air, CSF, and most foreign bodies. No other test provides this degree of information, and the study can be performed in minutes. Obtaining the head computed tomographic scan concludes the initial evaluation; the patient generally proceeds from the CT scanner to either the operating room for surgical treatment or the intensive care unit for medical treatment targeting the pathology seen on the scan. The specific indications for these treatments are discussed in accompanying chapters.

If computed tomographic scans of other parts of the body (e.g., chest, abdomen, neck) are necessary, the head should be scanned first. A noncontrast study with 1.5-mm cuts in the posterior fossa and 5-mm cuts through the remainder of the head can be screened while the technician is preparing for the other scans. If a surgical lesion is found, these other scans are stopped, and the patient is immediately taken to the operating room. The head scan includes a tremendous amount of information that should not be overlooked by the initial reader. This requires availing oneself of all the scans and the different windowing. The brain-bone interface can be difficult to interpret without subdural windowing, and in some cases, manual windowing at the workstation can clarify a questionable finding (Fig. 326–6). The presence and location of acute hemorrhage and associated mass effect should be documented. Brain edema with loss of the basal cisterns and attenuation of the gray-white junction is evaluated (see Fig. 326–6). Any skull fractures with comminuted or depressed fragments are also assessed (Fig. 326–7). Finally, the ventricular system is viewed for hydrocephalus or the presence of midline shift.

Before the widespread availability of CT, plain skull radiographs played an important role in head trauma. A skull fracture seen on plain films significantly increases the risk of there being an important intracranial hematoma.[29] When there is a linear nondisplaced fracture parallel to the plane of the computed tomographic scan, a plain film may be more sensitive in identifying it. However, this is uncommon, and often the lateral scout film done as part of the computed tomographic scan provides the same information. Consequently, the time spent obtaining a plain skull film is probably better spent preparing the patient for CT. One instance when plain films may be used is in patients with severe abdominal or thoracic injuries that preclude hemodynamic resuscitation. These patients may require immediate surgical intervention before computed tomographic scanning, and plain radiographs of the skull can be taken in the operating room. If these have positive findings or there is physical or neurological evidence of a head injury, a ventriculostomy and air ventriculogram can be done in the operating room.[71] The ventriculostomy is performed in a standard fashion, and the opening pressure is measured. If the pressure is greater than 15 cm CSF, 10 mL of CSF is drained and replaced with 10 cc of air. An AP skull film is then done and evaluated for ventricular shift or effacement, which suggests an extra-axial hematoma.

CT has almost entirely replaced cerebral angiography in the evaluation of TBI. However, angiography remains superior to any other method for evaluating the cerebral vasculature. Intracranial vascular occlusion or dissection is rare after blunt trauma, but it should be considered in patients with focal neurological deficits that cannot be explained by the injuries seen on computed tomographic scans. The deficit occurs acutely, and there may be a lucid interval between the trauma and the deterioration.[72] In contrast, traumatic intracranial aneurysms generally become symptomatic days to weeks after the trauma; therefore, angiography is not usually indicated during the initial evaluation of these patients.[73] Exceptions are made in patients with brisk epistaxsis or a mechanism of injury that suggests a vascular injury. Examples include skull base fractures in patients with significant subarachnoid hemorrhage or penetrating trauma that requires surgical decompression or débridement. Continued refinement of CT-angiography and magnetic resonance angiography techniques may further limit the use of formal angiography, but formal angiography also permits the application of various endovascular techniques to treat some of these vascular injuries.

The application of magnetic resonance technology in the acute phase remains limited. Magnetic resonance imaging provides excellent visualization of hematomas and diffuse axonal injury, but fractures are more difficult to assess (Fig. 326–8). Other magnetic resonance techniques such as diffusion imaging and spectroscopy have proved to be important research tools in understanding the pathophysiology of brain injury and may be of benefit in determining long-term prognosis.[5, 74, 75] Unfortunately, the time necessary to perform a scan and problems related to the compatibility of the equipment used to support these patients (e.g., ventilators,

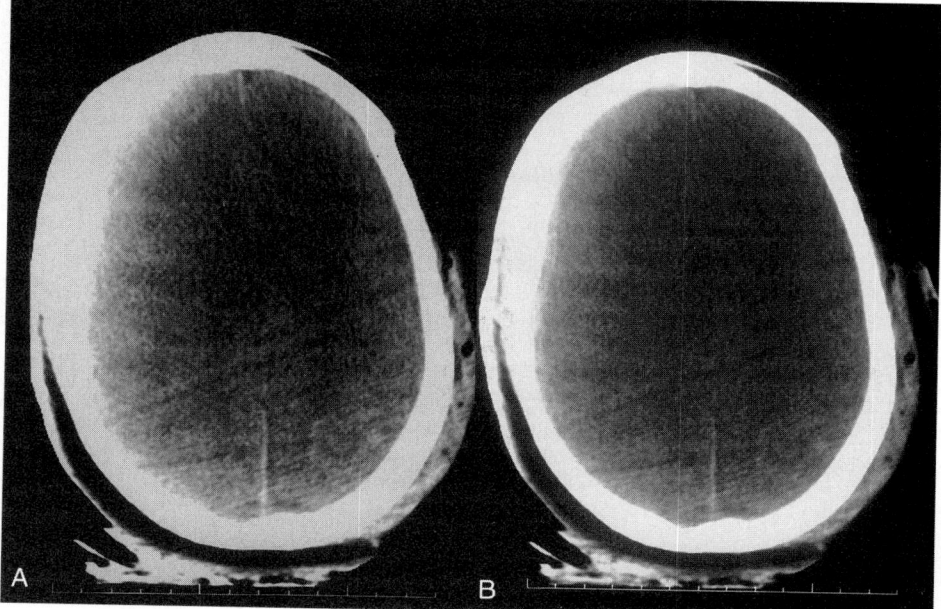

FIGURE 326–6. This young woman was found in the street and presumed to have been struck by a motor vehicle. The time of the injury was not known. Her Glasgow Coma Scale score was 3, and she had bilateral unreactive pupils. *A*, Normal brain windows demonstrate diffuse swelling and loss of the gray-white junction. Bone artifact prevents accurate evaluation of a subdural hematoma. *B*, Subdural windowing clearly shows a right subdural hematoma.

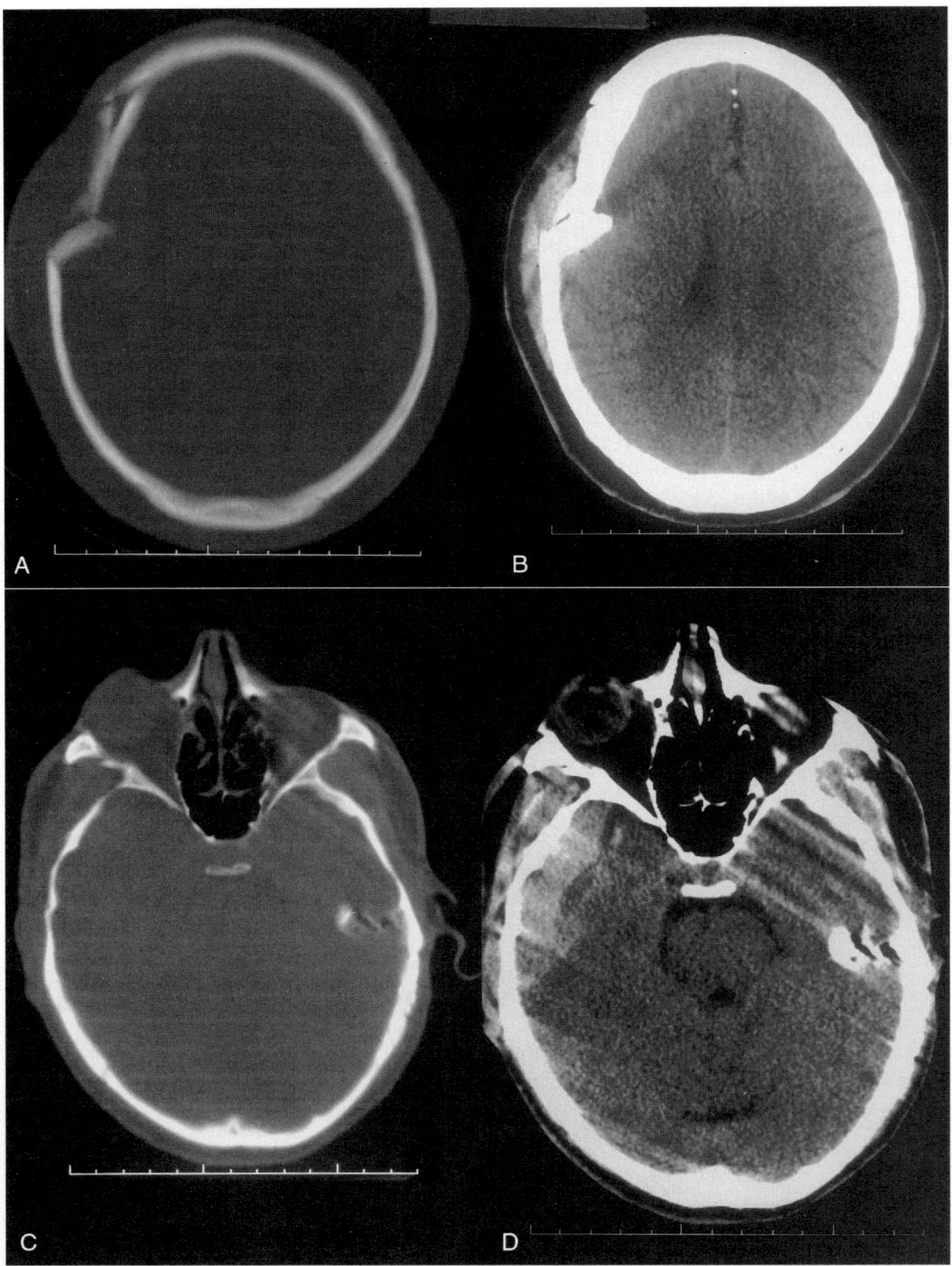

FIGURE 326–7.   *A,* Bone windows show a comminuted, depressed right skull fracture in a 30-year-old man struck by a hammer. His Glasgow Coma Scale (GCS) score was 14. *B,* In the same patient, the brain window demonstrates minimal hemorrhage associated with the fracture. *C,* This 26-year-old man was in a motor vehicle accident and presented with a GCS score of 14 and a slightly enlarged right pupil. The bone window reveals a right temporal skull fracture. *D,* In the same patient, the fracture was associated with a large epidural hematoma that was emergently evacuated.

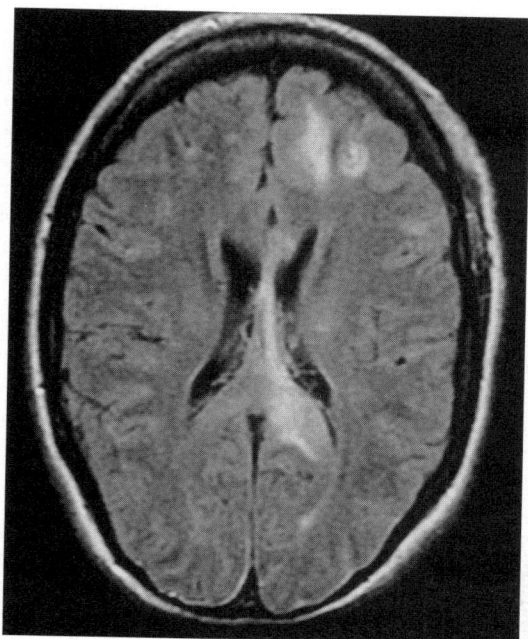

FIGURE 326–8. This 35-year-old woman was in a high-speed motor vehicle accident. Her Glasgow Coma Scale score was 4, and the initial computed tomograpic scan showed only a small frontal contusion. This FLAIR magnetic resonance imaging scan demonstrates signal abnormality in the corpus callosum, fornix, and septum, which is consistent with severe diffuse axonal injury. She remained in a vegetative state.

intravenous pumps, hemodynamic monitors, ICP monitors) with the strong magnetic fields prevent the widespread use of the technique.

NEUROLOGICAL CONSIDERATIONS AND ACUTE MANAGEMENT

Triage

The care of severely injured trauma victims often brings two different surgical subspecialists, the neurosurgeon and the traumatologist, together in a tense situation wherein everyone's goals appear to conflict. Understanding the goals of the traumatologist and maintaining appropriate communication can improve the efficiency of the process. The secondary survey is sometimes summarized as "tubes and fingers in every orifice."[76] This may conceptualize the general surgery scope of the examination, but in evaluating the CNS, much of the data gathered during this portion of the examination does not require that degree of invasiveness. This bias can also be seen in general trauma literature, which states that "most cerebral injuries are not of the highest priority."[77] Gutman and colleagues evaluated the incidence of intracranial mass lesions and severe abdominal injuries and concluded, "in MVA [motor vehicle accident] victims who are less than 30 years old, are hypotensive, and tachycardic, the diag-

nosis and emergent treatment of severe torso injury should take precedence over measures designed to detect and treat intracranial mass lesions."[78] Such statements oversimplify a very difficult situation.

Acosta and coworkers reviewed the 900 trauma patients who died in their institution over an 11-year period.[79] Deaths within 1 hour of admission were most commonly due to CNS or thoracic vascular injuries, and deaths within 72 hours were mostly due to CNS injury. A CNS injury was the cause of death in 44% of all the trauma deaths. Seelig and associates reviewed 82 cases of acute subdural hematoma and found a mortality rate of 30% for patients operated on within 4 hours of injury, compared with a mortality of 90% in those operated on after 4 hours.[3] The work of Wilberger and colleagues shows a similar trend.[80] These studies emphasize the importance of the rapid assessment and treatment of intracranial mass lesions. Although the physical examination may reveal fractures or overt signs of herniation, it is not very sensitive for identifying specific intracranial pathology. Harad and Kerstein reviewed 302 trauma patients thought to be at low risk for intracranial injury (GCS score of 13 to 15) and found that 18% had abnormal computed tomographic scans and 4% required neurosurgical intervention.[81] Advanced trauma life-support guidelines suggest a goal of 30 minutes between injury and computed tomographic scan.[76] This may be difficult to achieve, however, because transport time cannot be controlled. Using a horizontal approach to rapidly perform the initial assessment and resuscitation can minimize the time between admission and computed tomographic scan. Timesaving approaches should be sought in conjunction with the trauma surgeons. For example, to prepare the patient for CT, contrast material is often given through the nasogastric tube to improve visualization of the abdominal portion of the scan. In a patient that the neurosurgeon suspects has an intracranial mass lesion (based on mechanism of injury or neurological signs), contrast administration should not slow down the patient's transport to the CT scanner. If necessary, the contrast material can be given after the head scan and before the abdominal scan; or if the head scan shows a surgical hematoma, the contrast is not necessary at all, because the patient will be going straight to the operating room.

It is also important for the neurosurgeon to realize that more than half of all patients with severe head injuries have additional major injuries.[82] Miller and coworkers reviewed the incidence of other injures in these patients and found pelvis or long bone fracture in 32%, major chest injury in 23%, facial fracture in 22%, abdominal visceral injury in 7%, and spinal cord injury in 2%.[82] The incidence of cervical spine injuries in patients with head injury is 1.2% to 7.8%.[83–86] The highest incidence is in patients with a GCS score of 8 or less.[83] Consequently, in-line stabilization should be performed during intubation of these patients to minimize cervical spine movement.[87] Orthopedic injuries in these patients often require operative fracture fixation, but the risk of intraoperative hypotension or hypoxia can be as high as 16% and 11%, respectively; therefore, fixation should not be done acutely if possible.[88]

Oxygenation and Ventilation

A single episode of hypoxia (PaO$_2$ <60 mm Hg) increases a patient's chance of having a poor outcome after a severe head injury.[7, 89] Initially, patients should be rapidly intubated using a short-acting paralytic agent.[57] Adequate oxygenation should be confirmed with arterial blood gas measurement and monitored with pulse oximetry. Thiagarajan and associates were able to improve jugular venous oxygen saturation in head-injured patients by increasing the PaO$_2$ to greater than 200 mm Hg.[90] Menzel and coworkers also increased the PaO$_2$ to 441 ± 88 mm Hg by increasing the FiO$_2$ to 100% in 12 patients.[91] They demonstrated improved parenchymal PO$_2$ and an attenuation of the increased brain lactate seen in a control group with PaO$_2$ of 136 ± 22 mm Hg. These studies suggest that raising the FiO$_2$ empirically may improve oxygen delivery, but this has not yet been correlated with improvements in outcome.

CO$_2$ diffuses into the brain, where carbonic anhydrase produces protons, resulting in a lower pH that has a profound vasodilatory effect.[92] This tight coupling of CO$_2$ and CBF permits modulation of flow by manipulation of the ventilatory rate.[62] Low CBF occurs early after severe brain injury.[93] Hyperventilation during this period can result in ischemia, as measured by xenon-enhanced CT,[94] and in jugular venous desaturation in humans[95, 96] and loss of CA3 hippocampal neurons in experimental animals.[97] Empirical hyperventilation to a PaO$_2$ of 25 mm Hg has been shown by Muizelaar and colleagues to worsen outcome after severe head injury.[63] Alternatively, hypercarbia results in significant increases in ICP. Diringer and coworkers evaluated the impact of milder hyperventilation to a PaO$_2$ of 30 mm Hg.[98] They measured the effect of this mild hyperventilation on CBF, cerebral blood volume, cerebral metabolic rate of oxygen, and oxygen extraction fraction and found no impairment in cerebral metabolism. In the acute setting, without a monitor of cerebral ischemia (i.e., jugular venous catheter), the PCO$_2$ should be maintained between 30 and 35 mm Hg. In a patient who is acutely deteriorating, as evidenced by signs of herniation, more aggressive hyperventilation can be done after other methods of lowering ICP have been tried (sedation, paralysis, mannitol, CSF drainage) while preparing to transport the patient for computed tomographic scanning or to the operating room.

Hemodynamics

Miller and colleagues were the first to draw attention to the frequency and detrimental effects of hypotension after TBI.[82] The Traumatic Coma Data Bank showed a 150% increased risk of mortality for patients who had at least one episode of hypotension (systolic blood pressure <90 mm Hg) between the time of their injury and completion of resuscitation compared with patients without hypotension.[7, 99] Low systemic blood pressure results in additional cerebral ischemia and further rises in ICP.[100] The CPP is defined as the difference between the mean arterial pressure and the ICP. Rosner and associates reported excellent outcomes using a treatment paradigm aimed at maintaining the CPP greater than 70 mm Hg.[101] They enrolled patients with GCS scores of 7 or less and reported a mortality rate of 29%. Of the survivors, 80% had favorable outcomes. Chan and coworkers showed that episodes of jugular venous desaturation were associated with CPP values falling below 70 mm Hg.[102] Kiening and colleagues demonstrated that maintaining the CPP greater than 60 mm Hg prevented or reversed drops in parenchymal PO$_2$.[103]

More recently, two studies raised questions about how aggressively the CPP should be maintained. Robertson and associates performed a randomized trial comparing an ICP-targeted treatment protocol with a CBF-targeted protocol in 189 patients.[104] In the ICP group, the CPP was kept above 50 mm Hg, and hyperventilation was used to control ICP; in the CBF group, the CPP was kept above 70 mm Hg, and no hyperventilation was used. When hyperventilation was used, a jugular venous catheter was placed to monitor for ischemia. There was no significant difference in patient outcome: 49% of the ICP-targeted group and 40% of the CBF-targeted group had favorable outcomes at 6 months. Ten percent of the patients developed adult respiratory distress syndrome, and 83% of those patients were in the CBF-targeted group, suggesting that aggressive CPP management may increase the risk for that syndrome. Juul and colleagues performed a retrospective evaluation of data from a multicenter study of an N-methyl-D-aspartate receptor antagonist for the treatment of severe head injury.[105] The study enrolled 427 patients and analyzed the impact of CPP and ICP on outcome. As shown previously, they found that an ICP greater than 20 mm Hg correlated with neurological deterioration and increased mortality. There was no independent correlation with outcome when the CPP was greater than 60 mm Hg. When the CPP was less than 60 mm Hg, the ICP was almost always greater than 20 mm Hg; therefore, CPP less than 60 mm Hg could not be separated out as an independent variable. These data emphasize the importance and efficacy of treating raised ICP and point out the need to be cautious when aggressively targeting CPP.

During acute resuscitation, the systolic blood pressure should be maintained greater than 100 mm Hg using volume. Hypotension without tachycardia should alert the trauma team to a possible spinal cord injury resulting in neurogenic shock. Except in the presence of spinal cord injury, pressors are rarely used during the acute resuscitation. Failure of the hypotension to resolve with volume requires immediate evaluation by the general surgeon to rule out occult bleeding. Measuring the central venous pressure or placing a pulmonary artery catheter can provide important information, but this is usually not done until the patient has undergone a computed tomographic scan or been taken to the operating room and then to the intensive care unit.

Medications

Mannitol is an osmotic diuretic that rapidly lowers ICP. It decreases the water content of the brain, although this does not appear to be the primary mechanism that impacts ICP.[106, 107] Acutely, mannitol increases CBF by volume expansion and decreased blood viscosity, which permits cerebral vasoconstriction, resulting in lower ICP.[108–110] Serum osmolarity should be checked and maintained below 320 mOsm to prevent acute tubular necrosis.[111] If a patient has overt signs of herniation or there is a high index of suspicion that a head injury is present, and the patient is hemodynamically stable, a bolus of 0.5 to 1.0 g/kg mannitol should be administered. Because of the diuretic effects, a Foley catheter must be in place, and volume replacement should be given to maintain euvolemia.

The effectiveness of phenytoin in preventing post-traumatic seizures was evaluated with a randomized trial involving 404 patients.[112] Those receiving phenytoin had a 3.6% rate of seizures during the first week, compared with 14.2% in the placebo group. After the initial week, there was no reduction in seizure frequency in the treatment group. Based on these results, phenytoin is given for the first week after injury. Rapid infusion of intravenous phenytoin can cause cardiac arrhythmia and hypotension, especially in patients with known cardiovascular disease.[113–115] Fosphenytoin has fewer cardiovascular side effects.[116] Given the danger of hypotension in these patients, the phenytoin loading dose is generally not administered until the patient has been fully resuscitated and is hemodynamically stable.

The prophylactic use of barbiturates after head injury was evaluated in a randomized study of 53 patients by Ward and colleagues.[117] There was no difference in outcome, but the treatment group had a much higher incidence of hypotension. Bullock and coworkers recommend the use of barbiturates to treat refractory ICP in patients who are hemodynamically stable.[89] Owing to the detrimental effects of barbiturates on blood pressure and their sedating effects, which make it impossible to perform a neurological examination, they are not used during acute resuscitation. The newer general anesthetic propofol has a neuroprotective mechanism by acting as a GABA receptor antagonist.[118] This agent is being used more frequently owing to its short half-life and ease of administration,[119, 120] but the role of propofol in head-injured patients remains to be fully studied.

The use of steroids for TBI remains controversial. Bullock and coworkers reviewed the literature and recommended that steroids not be used in this setting.[89] Alderson and Roberts performed a meta-analysis of this data and concluded that although the data did not support a significant beneficial effect of steroids, there was a modest positive trend.[121] Amid this controversy, a large multicenter trial has been initiated in Europe and plans to enroll 10,000 to 20,000 patients.[122, 123]

Hypertonic saline infusion has also been evaluated as a means of both volume resuscitation and ICP control.[124–133] Its ease of administration and beneficial effects on ICP warrant additional study and comparison to current practices.[134]

Invasive Procedures

A number of scenarios require neurosurgical intervention before the patient goes to the intensive care unit or, in some cases, even before a computed tomographic scan. If a patient has life-threatening chest or abdominal injuries that prevent hemodynamic stabilization, thoracotomy or laparotomy may be necessary either in the trauma resuscitation area or in the operating room before a head computed tomographic scan can be done. If there is a high index of suspicion that a head injury is also present, a ventriculostomy should be placed through a frontal twist drill hole. If the ICP is greater than 15 cm CSF, an air ventriculogram should be done, as discussed earlier. The AP skull film evaluates for midline shift, which, if present, warrants a craniotomy while the other surgery is ongoing. If the ICP is not high, the ventriculostomy is connected to a pressure transducer to permit ICP monitoring during the remainder of the case.[135] If there is a lower index of suspicion that a head injury is present, but no neurological examination or computed tomographic scan can be done expediently, an intraparenchymal pressure transducer should be placed to check and monitor the ICP. In either situation, a computed tomographic scan should be obtained as soon as the patient is able to leave the operating room.

These same principles should be considered for patients taken to the operating room for general or orthopedic emergency procedures after a head scan has been done. If the computed tomographic scan shows evidence of acute hemorrhage or edema, the ICP should be monitored while the patient is under general anesthesia, regardless of the initial neurological examination. Also, consideration should be given to delaying the procedure if it is not urgent.[88] Narayan and colleagues recommend monitoring ICP in all patients with a GCS score of 3 to 8 and an abnormal computed tomographic scan.[136] Patients with a GCS score of 3 to 8 and a normal computed tomographic scan should also be monitored until a neurological examination can be done.[137] Those patients with a GCS score greater than 8 and a normal computed tomographic scan may also be considered for monitoring if the mechanism of injury is severe enough to place them at risk for delayed hemorrhage. In patients with abnormal computed tomographic scans who require an ICP monitor, a ventriculostomy is placed; an intraparenchymal fiberoptic monitor is placed if the scan is normal.

With the increased availability and speed of CT, the indications for exploratory bur holes have become limited. Andrews and associates demonstrated the usefulness of this technique in patients with clinical signs of herniation.[138] Their results also point out that an acute hematoma cannot always be adequately decompressed through a bur hole, and this technique may miss intraparenchymal or contralateral hemorrhages. Every effort should be made to obtain a computed tomographic scan; however, when a scan cannot be done and there are focal signs of tentorial herniation, bur holes should be considered.[138] Frontal, temporal, and parietal bur holes should be placed, and the incisions should be made to permit conversion to a large question-mark trauma craniotomy, if necessary. A computed tomographic scan should still be performed as soon as possible.

Laboratory Tests

As discussed earlier, both serum osmolality and arterial blood gases should be assessed during the initial resuscitation. The other tests most critical to a head injury are the coagulation studies: prothrombin time, partial thromboplastin time, and platelet count. Stein and co-workers reviewed 253 head injury patients and found that 49% developed new or progressive lesions on serial computed tomographic scans.[139] The risk of progression was 31% in patients with normal coagulation studies, compared with 85% in patients with at least one abnormal clotting study on admission. Fresh frozen plasma or platelet transfusions should be strongly considered to correct abnormalities in this group of patients.

CONCLUSIONS

Study of the pathophysiology of TBI has demonstrated that applying the basic principles of trauma resuscitation can minimize secondary brain injury. The primary goals of current therapy are preventing hypoxia and hypotension, maintaining low normocarbia, rapidly assessing and decompressing mass lesions, and controlling ICP. When possible, emergency medical technicians should begin these actions in the prehospital setting. In the emergency department, the traumatologist and neurosurgeon must develop an organized approach to evaluating and treating these patients while respecting each other's primary goals, which may appear to conflict. As early as possible, a neurological assessment including GCS, motor focality, and pupillary examination should be performed. The next priority is to obtain a head computed tomographic scan while continuing to ensure adequate oxygenation, ventilation, and perfusion.

Further research into the specific pathophysiologic mechanisms responsible for the neuronal sensitivity to secondary injury will lead to treatments that are most efficacious when given early after the primary injury. TBI remains a heterogeneous disease, and this early treatment will require early differentiation among different pathophysiologic mechanisms. For example, a patient with a GCS score of 6 due to diffuse axonal injury may require treatment directed at preventing further damage to the neuronal cytoskeleton. A patient with a similar neurological examination who has multiple contusions with surrounding edema and increased ICP may benefit from treatment that stabilizes mitochondrial function and calcium-mediated excitotoxicity. Integrating these approaches into current treatment paradigms is the challenge in the future treatment of TBI.

REFERENCES

1. Kelly DF, Doberstein C, Becker DP: General principles of head injury management. In Narayan RK, Wilberger JE, Povlishock JT (eds): Neurotrauma. New York, McGraw-Hill, 1996, pp 71–101.
2. Teasdale GM, Murray G, Anderson E, et al: Risks of acute traumatic intracranial haematoma in children and adults: Implications for managing head injuries. BMJ 300:363–367, 1990.
3. Seelig JM, Becker DP, Miller JD, et al: Traumatic acute subdural hematoma: Major mortality reduction in comatose patients treated within four hours. N Engl J Med 304:1511–1518, 1981.
4. Bullock R, Zauner A, Woodward JJ, et al: Factors affecting excitatory amino acid release following severe human head injury. J Neurosurg 89:507–518, 1998.
5. Barzo P, Marmarou A, Fatouros P, et al: Contribution of vasogenic and cellular edema to traumatic brain swelling measured by diffusion-weighted imaging. J Neurosurg 87:900–907, 1997.
6. Adams J, Graham D, Murray L, et al: Diffuse axonal injury due to nonmissile head injury in humans: An analysis of 45 cases. Ann Neurol 12:557–563, 1982.
7. Chesnut RM, Marshall LF, Klauber MR, et al: The role of secondary brain injury in determining outcome from severe head injury. J Trauma 34:216–222, 1993.
8. Shackford SR, Mackersie RC, Davis JW, et al: Epidemiology and pathology of traumatic deaths occurring at a level I trauma center in a regionalized system: The importance of secondary brain injury. J Trauma 29:1392–1397, 1989.
9. Gopinath SP, Robertson CS, Contant CF, et al: Jugular venous desaturation and outcome after head injury. J Psychiatry Neurosci 57:717–723, 1994.
10. Lewelt W, Jenkins LW, Miller JD: Autoregulation of cerebral blood flow after experimental fluid percussion injury of the brain. J Neurosurg 53:500–511, 1980.
11. Bouma GJ, Muizelaar JP, Choi SC, et al: Cerebral circulation and metabolism after severe traumatic brain injury: The elusive role of ischemia. J Neurosurg 75:685–693, 1991.
12. Martin NA, Patwardhan RV, Alexander MJ, et al: Characterization of cerebral hemodynamic phases following severe head trauma: Hypoperfusion, hyperemia, and vasospasm. J Neurosurg 87:9–19, 1997.
13. Bergsneider M, Hovda DA, Shalmon E, et al: Cerebral hyperglycolysis following severe traumatic brain injury in humans: A positron emission tomography study. J Neurosurg 86:241–251, 1997.
14. Verweij BH, Muizelaar JP, Vinas FC, et al: Mitochondrial dysfunction after experimental and human brain injury and its possible reversal with a selective N-type calcium channel antagonist (SNX-111). Neurol Res 19:334–339, 1997.
15. Hall ED, Andrus PK, Yonkers PA: Brain hydroxyl radical generation in acute experimental head injury. J Neurochem 60:588–594, 1993.
16. Thomas CE, Morehouse LA, Aust SD: Ferritin and superoxide-dependent lipid peroxidation. J Biol Chem 260:3275–3280, 1985.
17. Pellegrini-Giampietro DE, Cherici G, Alesiani M, et al: Excitatory amino acid release and free radical formation may cooperate in the genesis of ischemia-induced neuronal damage. J Neurosci 10:1035–1041, 1990.
18. Olney JW: Glutamate-induced retinal degeneration in neonatal mice: Electron microscopy of the acutely evolving lesion. J Neuropathol Exp Neurol 28:455–474, 1969.
19. Auerbach S, Young W: Total phosphate determination in brain tissues: A method for regional determination of total phosphate in rat brain. Cent Nerv Syst Trauma 4:53–61, 1987.
20. Kumar K, Goosmann M, Krause GS, et al: Ultrastructural and ionic studies in global ischemic dog brain. Acta Neuropathol (Berl) 73:393–399, 1987.
21. Young W: The role of calcium in spinal cord injury. Cent Nerv Syst Trauma 2:109–114, 1985.
22. Saatman KE, Bozyczko-Coyne D, Marcy V, et al: Prolonged

calpain-mediated spectrin breakdown occurs regionally following experimental brain injury in the rat. J Neuropathol Exp Neurol 55:850–860, 1996.

23. Saatman KE, Murai H, Bartus RT, et al: Calpain inhibitor AK295 attenuates motor and cognitive deficits following experimental brain injury in the rat. Proc Natl Acad Sci U S A 93:3428–3433, 1996.

24. Saatman KE, Zhang C, Bartus RT, et al: Behavioral efficacy of posttraumatic calpain inhibition is not accompanied by reduced spectrin proteolysis, cortical lesion, or apoptosis. J Cereb Blood Flow Metab 20:66–73, 2000.

25. Ng I, Yeo TT, Soong R, et al: Young Investigator's Award: Induction of apoptosis following traumatic head injury in humans. Ann Acad Med Singapore 28:363–365, 1999.

26. Clark RS, Kochanek PM, Chen M, et al: Increases in Bcl-2 and cleavage of caspase-1 and caspase-3 in human brain after head injury. FASEB J 13:813–821, 1999.

27. Rink A, Fung K-M, Trojanowski JQ, et al: Evidence of apoptotic cell death after experimental traumatic brain injury in the rat. Am J Pathol 147:1575–1583, 1995.

28. Sinson G, Perri B, Trojanowski JQ, et al: Improvement of cognitive deficits and decreased cholinergic neuronal cell loss and apoptotic cell death following neurotrophin infusion after experimental traumatic brain injury. J Neurosurg 86:511–518, 1997.

29. Mendelow AD, Teasdale G, Jennett B, et al: Risks of intracranial haematoma in head injured adults. BMJ (Clin Res Ed) 287:1173–1176, 1983.

30. Teasdale E, Cardoso E, Galbraith S, et al: CT scan in severe diffuse head injury: Physiological and clinical correlations. J Neurol Neurosurg Psychiatry 47:600–603, 1984.

31. Ryan GA, Vilenius AT: Field and analytic observations of impact brain injury in fatally injured pedestrians. J Neurotrauma 12:627–634, 1995.

32. Margulies SS, Thibault LE: A proposed tolerance criterion for diffuse axonal injury in man. J Biomech 25:917–923, 1992.

33. Gennarelli TA, Thibault LE: Biomechanics of acute subdural hematoma. J Trauma 22:680–686, 1982.

34. Gennarelli TA, Thibault LE, Adams JH, et al: Diffuse axonal injury and traumatic coma in the primate. Ann Neurol 12:564–574, 1982.

35. Ommaya AK, Hirsch AE: Tolerances for cerebral concussion from head impact and whiplash in primates. J Biomech 4:13–21, 1971.

36. Ommaya AK, Hirsch AE, Flamm ES, et al: Cerebral concussion in the monkey: An experimental model. Science 153:211–212, 1966.

37. Wilmink AB, Samra GS, Watson LM, et al: Vehicle entrapment rescue and pre-hospital trauma care. Injury 27:21–25, 1996.

38. Siegel JH, Mason-Gonzalez S, Dischinger PC, et al: Causes and costs of injuries in multiple trauma patients requiring extrication from motor vehicle crashes. J Trauma 35:920–931, 1993.

39. Klauber MR, Marshall LF, Toole BM, et al: Cause of decline in head-injury mortality rate in San Diego County, California. J Neurosurg 62:528–531, 1985.

40. Shackford SR, Hollingworth-Fridlund P, Cooper GF, et al: The effect of regionalization upon the quality of trauma care as assessed by concurrent audit before and after institution of a trauma system: A preliminary report. J Trauma 26:812–820, 1986.

41. Colohan AR, Alves WM, Gross CR, et al: Head injury mortality in two centers with different emergency medical services and intensive care. J Neurosurg 71:202–207, 1989.

42. Baxt WG, Moody P: The impact of a rotorcraft aeromedical emergency care service on trauma mortality. JAMA 249:3047–3051, 1983.

43. Singbartl G: Significance of preclinical emergency treatment for the prognosis of patients with severe craniocerebral trauma. Anasth Intensivther Notfallmed 20:251–260, 1985.

44. Baxt WG, Moody P: The impact of a physician as part of the aeromedical prehospital team in patients with blunt trauma. JAMA 257:3246–3250, 1987.

45. Kokoska ER, Smith GS, Pittman T, et al: Early hypotension worsens neurological outcome in pediatric patients with moderately severe head trauma. J Pediatr Surg 33:333–338, 1998.

46. Stocchetti N, Furlan A, Volta F: Hypoxemia and arterial hypotension at the accident scene in head injury. J Trauma Injury Infect Crit Care 40:764–767, 1996.

47. Gentleman D: Causes and effects of systemic complications among severely head injured patients transferred to a neurosurgical unit. Int Surg 77:297–302, 1992.

48. Winchell RJ, Hoyt DB: Endotracheal intubation in the field improves survival in patients with severe head injury: Trauma Research and Education Foundation of San Diego. Arch Surg 132:592–597, 1997.

49. Bradley JS, Billows GL, Olinger ML, et al: Prehospital oral endotracheal intubation by rural basic emergency medical technicians. Ann Emerg Med 32:26–32, 1998.

50. Sayre MR, Sakles JC, Mistler AF, et al: Field trial of endotracheal intubation by basic EMTs. Ann Emerg Med 31:228–233, 1998.

51. Resnick DK, Marion DW, Carlier P: Outcome analysis of patients with severe head injuries and prolonged intracranial hypertension. J Trauma 42:1108–1111, 1997.

52. Winkler JV, Rosen P, Alfry EJ: Prehospital use of the Glasgow Coma Scale in severe head injury. J Emerg Med 2:1–6, 1984.

53. American College of Surgeons Committee on Trauma: Resources for Optimal Care of the Injured Patient: 1999. Chicago, American College of Surgeons, 1999.

54. Nagachinta T, Gold CR, Cheng F, et al: Unrecognized HIV-1 infection in inner-city hospital emergency department patients. Infect Control Hosp Epidemiol 17:174–177, 1996.

55. Tardiff K, Marzuk PM, Leon AC, et al: Human immunodeficiency virus among trauma patients in New York City. Ann Emerg Med 32:151–154, 1998.

56. Kelen GD, Green GB, Purcell RH, et al: Hepatitis B and hepatitis C in emergency department patients. N Engl J Med 326:1399–1404, 1992.

57. Redan JA, Livingston DH, Tortella BJ, et al: The value of intubating and paralyzing patients with suspected head injury in the emergency department. J Trauma 31:371–375, 1991.

58. Rosen CL, Wolfe RE, Chew SE, et al: Blind nasotracheal intubation in the presence of facial trauma. J Emerg Med 15:141–145, 1997.

59. Gennarelli TA, Champion HR, Copes WS, et al: Comparison of mortality, morbidity, and severity of 59,713 head injured patients with 114,447 patients with extracranial injuries. J Trauma 37:962–968, 1994.

60. Marshall LF, Gautille T, Klauber MR, et al: The outcome of severe closed head injury. J Neurosurg 75:S28–S36, 1991.

61. Lobato RD, Rivas JJ, Gomez PA, et al: Head-injured patients who talk and deteriorate into coma: Analysis of 211 cases studied with computerized tomography. J Neurosurg 75:256–261, 1991.

62. Fortune JB, Bock D, Kupinski AM, et al: Human cerebrovascular response to oxygen and carbon dioxide as determined by internal carotid artery duplex scanning. J Trauma 32:618–627, 1992.

63. Muizelaar JP, Marmarou A, Ward JD, et al: Adverse effects of prolonged hyperventilation in patients with severe head injury: A randomized clinical trial. J Neurosurg 75:731–739, 1991.

64. Cushing H: Concerning a definite regulatory mechanism of the vasomotor center which controls blood pressure during cerebral compression. Johns Hopkins Hosp Bull 12:290–292, 1901.

65. Teasdale G, Jennett B: Assessment of coma and impaired consciousness: A practical scale. Lancet 2:81–84, 1974.

66. Choi SC, Narayan RK, Anderson RL, et al: Enhanced specificity of prognosis in severe head injury. J Neurosurg 69:381–385, 1988.

67. Braakman R, Gelpke GJ, Habbema JD, et al: Systematic selection of prognostic features in patients with severe head injury. Neurosurgery 6:362–370, 1980.

68. Kernohan JW, Woltman HW: Incisura of the crus due to contralateral brain tumor. Arch Neurol Psychiatry 21:274, 1929.

69. Sherrington CS: Decerebrate rigidity and reflex coordination of movements. J Physiol 22:319, 1898.

70. Strich SJ: Cerebral trauma. In Blackwood W, Corsellis JAN (eds): Greenfield's Neuropathology. Chicago, Year Book Medical Publishers, 1976, pp 327–360.

71. Kaufmann GE, Clark K: Emergency frontal twist drill ventriculostomy: Technical note. J Neurosurg 33:226–227, 1970.

72. Morgan MK, Besser M, Johnston I, et al: Intracranial carotid artery injury in closed head trauma. J Neurosurg 66:192–197, 1987.

73. Uzan M, Cantasdemir M, Seckin MS, et al: Traumatic intracranial carotid tree aneurysms. Neurosurgery 43:1314–1320, 1998.

74. Sinson G, Bagley LJ, Cecil KM, et al: The use of magnetic resonance studies to evaluate neuronal damage after traumatic brain injury. Paper presented to the American Association of Neurological Surgeons, Apr 1998, Philadelphia.

75. Bagley LJ, McGowan JC, Grossman RI, et al: Magnetization transfer imaging of traumatic brain injury. J Magn Reson Imaging 11:1–8, 2000.

76. American College of Surgeons Committee on Trauma: Advanced Trauma Life Support for Doctors. Chicago, American College of Surgeons, 1997.

77. Schwartz GR, Price DP: Management issues in the initial treatment of patients with severe trauma. In Schwartz GR (ed): Principles and Practice of Emergency Medicine. Philadelphia, Lea & Febiger, 1992, pp 924–935.

78. Gutman MB, Moulton RJ, Sullivan I, et al: Relative incidence of intracranial mass lesions and severe torso injury after accidental injury: Implications for triage and management. J Trauma 31:974–977, 1991.

79. Acosta JA, Yang JC, Winchell RJ, et al: Lethal injuries and time to death in a level I trauma center. J Am Coll Surg 186:528–533, 1998.

80. Wilberger JE, Harris M, Diamond DL: Acute subdural hematoma: Morbidity and mortality related to timing of operative intervention. J Trauma 30:733–736, 1990.

81. Harad FT, Kerstein MD: Inadequacy of bedside clinical indicators in identifying significant intracranial injury in trauma patients. J Trauma Injury Infect Crit Care 32:359–361, 1992.

82. Miller JD, Sweet RC, Narayan R, et al: Early insults to the injured brain. JAMA 240:439–442, 1978.

83. Hills MW, Deane SA: Head injury and facial injury: Is there an increased risk of cervical spine injury? J Trauma Injury Infect Crit Care 34:549–553, 1993.

84. O'Malley KF, Ross SE: The incidence of injury to the cervical spine in patients with craniocerebral injury. J Trauma Injury Infect Crit Care 28:1476–1478, 1988.

85. Gbaanador GB, Fruin AH, Taylon C: Role of routine emergency cervical radiography in head trauma. Am J Surg 152:643–648, 1986.

86. Kennedy FR, Gonzalez P, Beitler A, et al: Incidence of cervical spine injury in patients with gunshot wounds to the head. South Med J 87:621–623, 1994.

87. Majernick TG, Bieniek R, Houston JB, et al: Cervical spine movement during orotracheal intubation. Ann Emerg Med 15:417–420, 1986.

88. Jaicks RR, Cohn SM, Moller BA: Early fracture fixation may be deleterious after head injury. J Trauma Injury Infect Crit Care 42:1–5; discussion 5–6, 1997.

89. Bullock R, Chesnut RM, Clifton G, et al: Guidelines for the management of severe head injury. J Neurotrauma 13:639–734, 1996.

90. Thiagarajan A, Goverdhan PD, Chari P, et al: The effect of hyperventilation and hyperoxia on cerebral venous oxygen saturation in patients with traumatic brain injury. Anesth Analg 87:850–853, 1998.

91. Menzel M, Doppenberg EM, Zauner A, et al: Increased inspired oxygen concentration as a factor in improved brain tissue oxygenation and tissue lactate levels after severe human head injury. J Neurosurg 91:1–10, 1999.

92. Kontos HA, Raper AJ, Patterson JL: Analysis of vasoactivity of local pH, PCO_2 and bicarbonate on pial vessels. Stroke 8:358–360, 1977.

93. Bouma GJ, Muizelaar JP: Cerebral blood flow, cerebral blood volume, and cerebrovascular reactivity after severe head injury. J Neurotrauma 9:S333–S348, 1992.

94. Stringer WA, Hasso AN, Thompson JR, et al: Hyperventilation-induced cerebral ischemia in patients with acute brain lesions: Demonstration by xenon-enhanced CT. AJNR Am J Neuroradiol 14:475–484, 1993.

95. Cruz J, Miner ME, Allen SJ, et al: Continuous monitoring of cerebral oxygenation in acute brain injury: Assessment of cerebral hemodynamic reserve. Neurosurgery 29:743–749, 1991.

96. Sheinberg M, Kanter MJ, Robertson CS, et al: Continuous monitoring of jugular venous oxygen saturation in head-injured patients. J Neurosurg 76:212–217, 1992.

97. Forbes ML, Clark RS, Dixon CE, et al: Augmented neuronal death in CA3 hippocampus following hyperventilation early after controlled cortical impact. J Neurosurg 88:549–556, 1998.

98. Diringer MN, Yundt K, Videen TO, et al: No reduction in cerebral metabolism as a result of early moderate hyperventilation following severe traumatic brain injury. J Neurosurg 92:7–13, 2000.

99. Marmarou A, Anderson RL, Ward JD, et al: Impact of ICP instability and hypotension on outcome in patients with severe head trauma. J Neurosurg 75:S59–S66, 1991.

100. Rosner MJ, Daughton S: Cerebral perfusion pressure management in head injury. J Trauma Injury Infect Crit Care 30:933–940, 1990.

101. Rosner MJ, Rosner SD, Johnson AH: Cerebral perfusion pressure: Management protocol and clinical results. J Neurosurg 83:949–962, 1995.

102. Chan KH, Miller JD, Dearden NM, et al: The effect of changes in cerebral perfusion pressure upon middle cerebral artery blood flow velocity and jugular bulb venous oxygen saturation after severe brain injury. J Neurosurg 77:55–61, 1992.

103. Kiening KL, Unterberg AW, Bardt TF, et al: Monitoring of cerebral oxygenation in patients with severe head injuries: Brain tissue pO_2 versus jugular vein oxygen saturation. J Neurosurg 85:751–757, 1996.

104. Robertson CS, Valadka AB, Hannay HJ, et al: Prevention of secondary ischemic insults after severe head injury. Crit Care Med 27:2086–2095, 1999.

105. Juul N, Morris GF, Marshall SB, et al: Intracranial hypertension and cerebral perfusion pressure: Influence on neurlogical deterioration and outcome in severe head injury. J Neurosurg 92:1–6, 2000.

106. Clasen RA, Cooke PN, Pandolfi S, et al: Hypertonic urea in experimental cerebral edema. Arch Neurol 12:424–434, 1965.

107. Hartwell RC, Sutton LN: Mannitol, intracranial pressure, and vasogenic edema. Neurosurgery 32:444–450; discussion 450, 1993.

108. Mendelow AD, Teasdale GM, Russell T, et al: Effect of mannitol on cerebral blood flow and cerebral perfusion pressure in human head injury. J Neurosurg 63:43–48, 1985.

109. Muizelaar JP, Lutz HA, Becker DP: Effect of mannitol on ICP and CBF and correlation with pressure autoregulation in severely head-injured patients. J Neurosurg 61:700–706, 1984.

110. Rosner MJ, Coley I: Cerebral perfusion pressure: A hemodynamic mechanism of mannitol and the postmannitol hemogram. Neurosurgery 21:147–156, 1987.

111. Feig PU, McCurdy DK: The hypertonic state. N Engl J Med 297:1444–1454, 1977.

112. Temkin NR, Dikmen SS, Wilensky AJ, et al: A randomized, double-blind study of phenytoin for the prevention of post-traumatic seizures. N Engl J Med 323:497–502, 1990.

113. Randazzo DN, Ciccone A, Schweitzer P, et al: Complete atrio-ventricular block with ventricular asystole following infusion of intravenous phenytoin. J Electrocardiol 28:157–159, 1995.

114. Donovan PJ, Cline D: Phenytoin administration by constant intravenous infusion: Selective rates of administration. Ann Emerg Med 20:139–142, 1991.

115. Earnest MP, Marx JA, Drury LR: Complications of intravenous phenytoin for acute treatment of seizures: Recommendations for usage. JAMA 249:762–765, 1983.

116. Browne TR: Fosphenytoin (Cerebyx). Clin Neuropharmacol 20:1–12, 1997.

117. Ward JD, Becker DP, Miller JD, et al: Failure of prophylactic barbiturate coma in the treatment of severe head injury. J Neurosurg 62:383–388, 1985.

118. Hollrigel GS, Toth K, Soltesz I: Neuroprotection by propofol in acute mechanical injury: Role of GABAergic inhibition. J Neurophysiol 76:2412–2422, 1996.

119. Matta B, Menon D: Severe head injury in the United Kingdom and Ireland: A survey of practice and implications for management. Crit Care Med 24:1743–1748, 1996.

120. Stewart L, Bullock R, Rafferty C, et al: Propofol sedation in severe head injury fails to control high ICP, but reduces brain metabolism. Acta Neurochir Suppl (Wien) 60:544–546, 1994.

121. Alderson P, Roberts I: Corticosteroids in acute traumatic brain injury: Systematic review of randomised controlled trials. BMJ 314:1855–1859, 1997.

122. Newell DW, Temkin NR, Bullock R, et al: Corticosteroids in acute traumatic brain injury. BMJ 316:396, 1998.
123. Roberts I: Design of CRASH trial: Trial is best way to elucidate effectiveness of corticosteroids in acute severe head injury. BMJ 319:1069, 1999.
124. Simma B, Burger R, Falk M, et al: A prospective, randomized, and controlled study of fluid management in children with severe head injury: Lactated Ringer's solution versus hypertonic saline. Crit Care Med 26:1265–1270, 1998.
125. Qureshi AI, Suarez JI, Bhardwaj A, et al: Use of hypertonic (3%) saline/acetate infusion in the treatment of cerebral edema: Effect on intracranial pressure and lateral displacement of the brain. Crit Care Med 26:440–446, 1998.
126. Hartl R, Ghajar J, Hochleuthner H, et al: Hypertonic/hyper-oncotic saline reliably reduces ICP in severely head-injured patients with intracranial hypertension. Acta Neurochir Suppl (Wien) 70:126–129, 1997.
127. Anderson JT, Wisner DH, Sullivan PE, et al: Initial small-volume hypertonic resuscitation of shock and brain injury: Short- and long-term effects. J Trauma Injury Infect Crit Care 42:592–600, 1997.
128. Mattox KL, Maningas PA, Moore EE, et al: Prehospital hypertonic saline/dextran infusion for post-traumatic hypotension: The USA Multicenter Trial. Ann Surg 213:482–491, 1991.
129. Vassar MJ, Perry CA, Holcroft JW: Analysis of potential risks associated with 7.5% sodium chloride resuscitation of traumatic shock. Arch Surg 125:1309–1315, 1990.
130. Vassar MJ, Perry CA, Gannaway WL, et al: 7.5% Sodium chloride/dextran for resuscitation of trauma patients undergoing helicopter transport. Arch Surg 126:1065–1072, 1991.
131. Vassar MJ, Fischer RP, O'Brien PE, et al: A multicenter trial for resuscitation of injured patients with 7.5% sodium chloride: The effect of added dextran 70. The Multicenter Group for the Study of Hypertonic Saline in Trauma Patients. Arch Surg 128:1003–1011; discussion 1011–1013, 1993.
132. Vassar MJ, Perry CA, Holcroft JW: Prehospital resuscitation of hypotensive trauma patients with 7.5% NaCl versus 7.5% NaCl with added dextran: A controlled trial. J Trauma Injury Infect Crit Care 34:622–632; discussion 632–633, 1993.
133. Wade CE, Grady JJ, Kramer GC, et al: Individual patient cohort analysis of the efficacy of hypertonic saline/dextran in patients with traumatic brain injury and hypotension. J Trauma Injury Infect Crit Care 42:S61–S65, 1997.
134. Clark RS, Kochanek PM: Pass the salt? Crit Care Med 26:1161–1162, 1998.
135. Valadka AB, Narayan RK: Emergency room management of the head-injured patient. In Narayan RK, Wilberger JE, Povlishock JT (eds): Neurotrauma. New York, McGraw-Hill, 1996, pp 119–135.
136. Narayan RK, Kishore PR, Becker DP, et al: Intracranial pressure: To monitor or not to monitor? A review of our experience with severe head injury. J Neurosurg 56:650–659, 1982.
137. O'Sullivan MG, Statham PF, Jones PA, et al: Role of intracranial pressure monitoring in severely head-injured patients without signs of intracranial hypertension on initial computerized tomography. J Neurosurg 80:46–50, 1994.
138. Andrews BT, Pitts LH, Lovely MP, et al: Is computed tomographic scanning necessary in patients with tentorial herniation? Results of immediate surgical exploration without computed tomography in 100 patients. Neurosurgery 19:408–414, 1986.
139. Stein SC, Young GS, Talucci RC, et al: Delayed brain injury after head trauma: Significance of coagulopathy. Neurosurgery 30:160–165, 1992.

CHAPTER 327

Critical Care Management of Traumatic Brain Injury

CLAUDIA ROBERTSON

The damage to the brain that occurs after traumatic injury is usually divided into two general types: primary and secondary (Fig. 327–1). The primary injury occurs before the patient arrives at the hospital and cannot be modified by the treating physicians. The severity of the primary injury, however, can be classified and quantified for prognostic purposes, and the primary injury often initiates a cascade of secondary injury processes that evolve over the first few postinjury days. In addition, the traumatized brain is exquisitely sensitive to ischemia, and secondary ischemic insults can damage the brain further. Pharmacologic treatment of these secondary injury processes and modern emergency and critical care management to prevent secondary ischemic insults are the primary goals in the early treatment of traumatic brain injury.

The science of the pharmacologic treatment of these secondary injury processes is still in its infancy. Although a large number of injury mediators have been identified in experimental studies, treatment with agents that block these known injury mediators has not been demonstrated to improve neurological outcome in clinical studies. Corticosteroids, calcium channel blockers, free radical scavengers, N-methyl-D-aspartate receptor antagonists, and hypothermia have all been tested in large multicenter clinical trials, without significant improvement in outcome.

As a result, the outcome of severe head injury depends to a large extent on anticipation, recognition, and early treatment of secondary ischemic insults. Intensive care monitoring offers the opportunity to rapidly identify and treat the post-traumatic insults that may impair ultimate recovery. Modern intensive care management techniques attempt to provide the optimal environment for the injured brain to recover. Several studies have suggested that with aggressive emergency and critical care treatment, the mortality rate after severe head injury can be decreased.[1-4]

HISTORY OF HEAD TRAUMA MANAGEMENT

Coma Data Banks

Systematic, multicenter efforts to study the management of traumatic brain injury began in the 1970s. Initially, this work took the form of observational studies. Two large databases of prospectively collected clinical information resulted from this early interest.

The International Data Bank, which consists of prospectively collected clinical information from 1000 comatose patients from three centers in Scotland, the Netherlands, and the United States, was reported in 1979.[5] These investigators developed simple but practical scales for the assessment of coma (Glasgow Coma Scale [GCS]; Table 327–1) and the assessment of neurological outcome (Glasgow Outcome Scale; Table 327–2) and presented some of the early work on the factors that determine outcome after neurological injury.[6, 7] It was apparent from these studies that the outcome after severe head injury is often dependent on the severity and type of the primary injury.

The Traumatic Coma Data Bank (TCDB) consists of prospectively collected clinical data from 1030 comatose patients from four centers in the United States.[8] Because of this study (initially reported in 1991) and work from other head injury centers, the critical role of prehospital insults such as hypoxia and hypotension, the importance of prompt evacuation of intracranial mass lesions, and the importance of intracranial hypertension were more clearly identified.[9-11] In addition, a new classification of primary injury based on computed tomography (CT) findings was developed from the TCDB data.[12]

Head Injury Guidelines

In 1996, a task force supported by the Brain Injury Foundation published evidence-based guidelines for the management of severe head injury.[13] The most important finding of the task force was that little of the current critical care management of severe head injury is based on well-designed randomized clinical trials. As a result, there are few standards (accepted principles that reflect a high degree of clinical certainty). Most of the task force's recommendations were guidelines (management strategies that reflect a moderate degree of clinical certainty) or options (management strategies for which there is unclear clinical certainty). The following three standards were proposed:

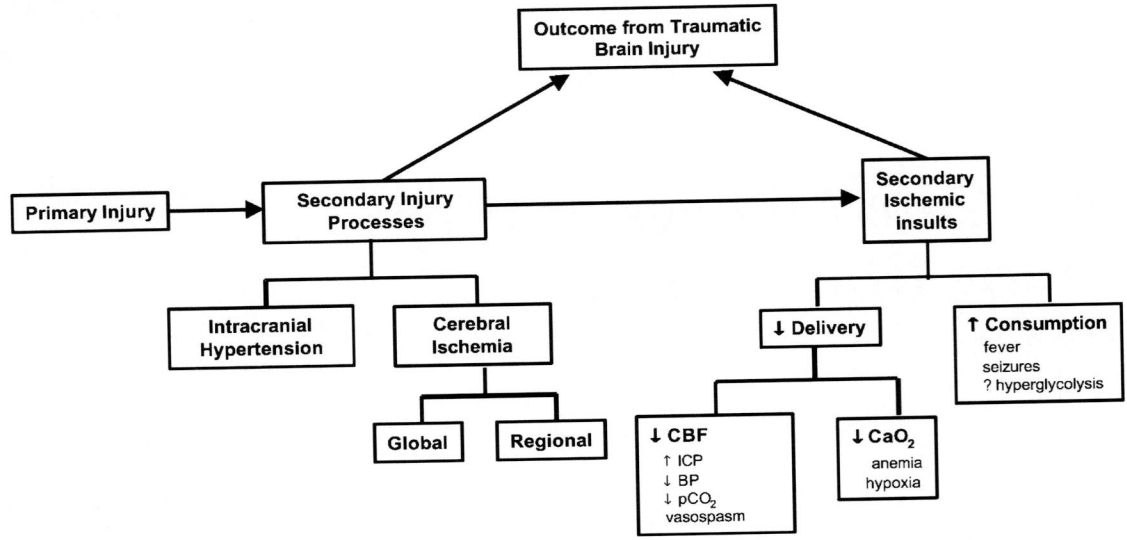

FIGURE 327–1. The outcome after traumatic brain injury is determined by a number of factors, including the type and severity of the primary injury. The primary injury then initiates secondary injury processes and causes the injured brain to be more susceptible to secondary ischemic insults. BP, blood pressure; Cao₂, arterial oxygen concentration; CBF, cerebral blood flow; ICP, intracranial pressure; pCO₂, partial pressure of carbon dioxide.

1. In the absence of intracranial hypertension, chronic hyperventilation should be avoided.

2. The use of glucocorticoids is not recommended for improving outcome or reducing intracranial pressure (ICP) in patients with severe head injury.

3. Prophylactic use of phenytoin, carbamazepine, or phenobarbital is not recommended for preventing late post-traumatic seizures.

The following eight guidelines were supported by prospective clinical studies:

1. All regions in the United States should have organized trauma care systems.

2. Hypotension (systolic blood pressure <90 mm Hg) and hypoxia (arterial oxygen partial pressure [Po_2] <60 mm Hg) should be avoided or, if unavoidable, should be corrected immediately.

3. ICP monitoring is appropriate in patients with severe head injury and abnormal computed tomographic scans or in those with normal computed tomographic scans and adverse factors such as age older than 40 years, hypotension, or decerebrate posturing.

4. ICP treatment should be initiated at an upper threshold of 20 to 25 mm Hg.

5. The use of prophylactic hyperventilation (arterial carbon dioxide partial pressure [Pco_2] <35 mm Hg) during the first 24 hours after severe head injury should be avoided.

6. Mannitol is effective for control of ICP after severe head injury. Limited data suggest that intermittent doses may be more effective than continuous infusion. Effective doses range from 0.25 to 1 g/kg.

7. High-dose barbiturate therapy may be considered in hemodynamically stable, salvageable patients with intracranial hypertension refractory to maximal medical and surgical ICP-lowering therapies.

8. Enteral or parenteral nutrition should be used to replace 140% of resting energy expenditure in nonparalyzed patients and 100% of resting energy expenditure in paralyzed patients by the seventh day after injury, using formulas in which at least 15% of calories is provided by protein.

The European Brain Injury Consortium also developed guidelines for the management of traumatic brain injury, based on consensus and expert opinion rather than clinical evidence.[14] Despite the different approaches in developing the guidelines, the actual recommendations in the U.S. and European versions are quite similar.

Whether the introduction of such guidelines has really altered the care of head-injured patients is debatable. Follow-up surveys suggest that the guidelines have made physicians more aware of the management principles contained therein. However, the most important consequence may have been to point out the

TABLE 327–1 ■ **Glasgow Coma Scale for Assessment of Coma and Impaired Consciousness**

EYE OPENING	BEST MOTOR RESPONSE	BEST VERBAL RESPONSE
4 = Spontaneous	6 = Obeying	5 = Oriented
3 = To speech	5 = Localizing	4 = Confused
2 = To pain	4 = Withdrawing	3 = Inappropriate
1 = None	3 = Flexing	2 = Incomprehensible
	2 = Extending	1 = None
	1 = None	

From Teasdale G, Jennett B: Assessment of coma and impaired consciousness. Lancet 2:81–84, 1974.

TABLE 327-2 ■ Glasgow Outcome Scale for Assessment of Outcome

SUMMARY	GLASGOW OUTCOME SCALE	EXTENDED GLASGOW OUTCOME SCALE
Asleep or awake, nonsentient	1 = Dead 2 = Persistent vegetative state	1 = Dead 2 = Persistent vegetative state
Conscious but dependent	3 = Severe disability	3 = Lower severe disability 4 = Upper severe disability
Independent but disabled	4 = Moderate disability	5 = Lower moderate disability 6 = Upper moderate disability
May have mild residual effects	5 = Good recovery	7 = Lower good recovery 8 = Upper good recovery

From Jennett B, Bond MR: Assessment of outcome after severe brain damage. Lancet 1:480–484, 1975; Wilson JT, Pettigrew LE, Teasdale GM: Structured interviews for the Glasgow Outcome Scale and the extended Glasgow Outcome Scale: Guidelines for their use. J Neurotrauma 15:573–585, 1998.

many deficits in our knowledge base about the management of traumatic brain injury.

Multicenter Clinical Trials

Laboratory studies have provided a better understanding of the basic mechanisms of secondary injury to the brain following trauma. Anticholinergic agents, corticosteroids, calcium channel antagonists, free radical scavengers, N-methyl-D-aspartate receptor antagonists, bradykinin antagonists, and moderate hypothermia have all been studied in experimental head injury models and been found to have beneficial effects. A number of potentially beneficial therapies derived from these laboratory studies have been tested in phase III clinical trials. To date, only nimodipine has been demonstrated to have a beneficial effect on outcome, and this occurred only in a subgroup of patients with traumatic subarachnoid hemorrhage.[15] As reported by Bullock and colleagues,[16] a number of pitfalls may be encountered when taking a treatment from the laboratory to a successful clinical trial.

One of the most challenging problems in traumatic brain injury is the heterogeneity of the clinical disorder. Most patients have a combination of focal and diffuse injuries, although some have primarily diffuse injuries and others may have only focal mass lesions. The basic mechanisms of these injuries are very different. In addition, hypotension, hypoxia, or both may complicate the picture in some patients. Other systemic injuries and complications associated with trauma, such as adult respiratory distress syndrome and sepsis, may also interact with the brain injury in determining the final outcome. A drug therapy directed at a single basic mechanism of injury may not benefit all patients. Trials directed at subgroups of patients who are most likely to benefit from the drug's action may be the best approach. Nimodipine may be the best example of this approach.

Another challenging problem in clinical trials is that the beneficial effect of a drug may be very small. Corticosteroids illustrate this problem. Although they have been used for many years in the treatment of traumatic brain injury, no benefit has been demonstrated, despite numerous clinical trials. Alderson and Roberts[17] re-

viewed all clinical trials of corticosteroid use in head injury published through March 1996. A total of 2073 randomized patients in 13 clinical trials was analyzed. The pooled odds ratio for a corticosteroid effect on outcome was 0.91, and the pooled absolute risk reduction was 1.8%. Thus, any effect, if present, is very small and would require a large number of patients to demonstrate it. Under these circumstances, a large simple trial might be the only way to demonstrate efficacy.

The greatest apparent improvements in the outcome of head-injured patients have occurred as a result of better prehospital, emergency room, and critical care management, not from pharmacologic manipulation of the primary injury. The major changes that have contributed to this improved outcome are organized prehospital care and faster transport to dedicated trauma centers, rapid resuscitation, prompt identification and evacuation of surgical hematomas, and better critical care management.

PATHOPHYSIOLOGY OF TRAUMATIC BRAIN INJURY

Primary Brain Injury

Two pathologic processes are uniquely characteristic of trauma: diffuse axonal injury (DAI) and contusion and hematoma formation. Diffuse injures are more common. In the TCDB series, 56% of patients with severe closed head injury had a diffuse injury, and 42% had a focal mass lesion. However, the mortality rate is generally higher with a focal lesion than with a diffuse injury—39% versus 24%.[8]

DIFFUSE AXONAL INJURY

Histopathologic findings of DAI have been observed in 25% of patients who die of traumatic brain injury.[18] When more sensitive indicators of axonal injury, such as β-amyloid immunohistochemistry, are used, as many as 90% of patients who die of traumatic brain injury have DAI changes.[19] Current thought about the development of DAI is that axotomy may not be complete immediately after the trauma. Secondary, or delayed, axotomy may predominate in many circumstances. Secondary axotomy begins with an impairment of axoplasmic transport that is initiated, depending on the severity of the injury, by either focal cytoskeletal misalignment or axolemmal permeability change with concomitant cytoskeletal collapse. These focal axonal changes are related to the focal impairment of axoplasmic transport, which in turn triggers the progression of reactive axonal change, leading to disconnection. With mild injury, deafferentation may lead to an adaptive neuroplastic recovery, whereas in more severe injury, a disordered or maladaptive neuroplastic reorganization occurs, consistent with the enduring morbidity associated with severe injury.[20, 21]

DAI is primarily a pathologic diagnosis, with microscopic damage scattered throughout the brain, but clinical correlations have been described. Traumatic loss of consciousness for less than 6 hours is considered a concussion and is usually associated with amnesia for the events related to the injury. Traumatic coma lasting longer than 6 hours is usually attributed to DAI. Three levels of severity, based on clinical criteria, are recognized: (1) mild DAI—coma of 6 to 24 hours' duration, (2) moderate DAI—coma lasting more than 24 hours without decerebrate posturing, and (3) severe DAI—coma lasting more than 24 hours with decerebrate posturing or flaccidity. Severe DAI has a 50% mortality.[22]

HEMATOMA AND CONTUSION

Subdural hematoma is the most common focal intracranial lesion, occurring in 24% of patients with severe closed head injury in the TCDB series.[8] The hematoma is between the dura and the brain, usually resulting from a torn bridging vein between the cortex and the draining sinuses. An acute subdural hematoma, identified within 72 hours after trauma, usually appears on CT as a high-density, homogeneous, crescent-shaped mass paralleling the calvaria (Fig. 327–2). However, up to 10% of acute subdural hematomas may be isodense with brain because of the low hemoglobin content.[23]

The mortality rate in patients with subdural hematomas is high—50% in the TCDB series.[9] Several factors are significantly related to outcome in patients with subdural hematomas, including age, time from injury to treatment, presence of pupillary abnormalities, GCS or motor score on admission, immediate coma or lucid interval, CT findings, postoperative ICP, and type of surgery.[24] The following CT findings are particularly predictive of outcome: hematoma thickness, midline shift, and presence of underlying brain swelling or contusions.[25, 26] The survival rate is 50% for patients with subdural hematomas approximately 18 mm thick and with a midline shift of 20 mm. Survival sharply decreases to 0% when the midline shift is more than 25 mm.[25] A large midline shift that cannot be accounted for by the volume of subdural blood is associated with a poor outcome. Survival decreases from 50% when the midline shift exceeds the hematoma thickness by 3 mm, reaching 25% when the midline shift exceeds the hematoma thickness by 5 mm.[25] The presence of associated cerebral contusions significantly worsens the prognosis for subdural hematoma.[26]

Subdural hematomas cause brain damage by increasing ICP and by shifting brain structures. Reductions in cerebral blood flow (CBF) below ischemic thresholds[27] and marked reductions in cerebral oxygenation[28, 29] have been observed preoperatively and are rapidly reversed by surgical evacuation of the hematoma. The presence of blood in the subdural space may also have direct toxic effects, but experimental studies have not consistently demonstrated this mechanism.[30] The primary treatment of a subdural hematoma is prompt surgical evacuation; the greater the delay between injury and surgery, the more severe the ischemic damage. Small subdural hematomas in patients who are not in coma can be managed nonsurgically, but most require prompt surgical evacuation.[31] Several studies reported a decrease in the mortality or morbidity of patients who undergo early evacuation of subdural hematomas.[1, 22, 32]

Epidural hematomas, or collections of blood between the skull and the dura, are less common. Epidural hematomas occurred in 6% of patients with severe closed head injuries in the TCDB series.[8] Whereas patients with subdural hematomas are usually immediately comatose, only one third of patients with epidural hematomas are unconscious from the time of injury, one third have a lucid interval, and one third are never unconscious.[33] An epidural hematoma is almost always associated with a skull fracture (91% of the time in adults and 75% in children).[34] The blood comes from torn dural vessels, usually arterial, from the fractured skull bone, or occasionally from torn venous sinuses. On CT (see Fig. 327–2), an epidural hematoma is characterized by a biconvex, uniformly hyperdense lesion. Associated brain lesions are less common than with subdural hematomas. Epidural hematomas may also develop in a delayed fashion[35] or on the contralateral side after evacuation of an initial epidural hematoma.[36]

The outcome of patients with epidural hematomas depends on their neurological status at the time of surgery. The mortality rate varies: 0% for patients who are not in coma, 9% for obtunded patients, and 20% for patients in deep coma. The following parameters were found to be significantly related to outcome: age, time from injury to treatment, immediate coma or lucid interval, presence of pupillary abnormalities, GCS or motor score on admission, CT findings (hematoma volume, degree of midline shift, signs of active hematoma bleeding, associated intradural lesion), and postoperative ICP.[37]

The primary treatment of epidural hematomas is prompt surgical evacuation. Small epidural hematomas in asymptomatic patients may resolve spontaneously and not require surgery. The following criteria predict the eventual need for surgical evacuation of asymptomatic epidural hematomas: volume (>30 mL for supratentorial hematomas; >10 mL for infratentorial hematomas), thickness greater than 15 mm, midline shift greater than 5 mm, or presence of other intracranial lesions.[38, 39]

Intracerebral blood can take the form of a hematoma

CATEGORIES OF DIFFUSE INJURY

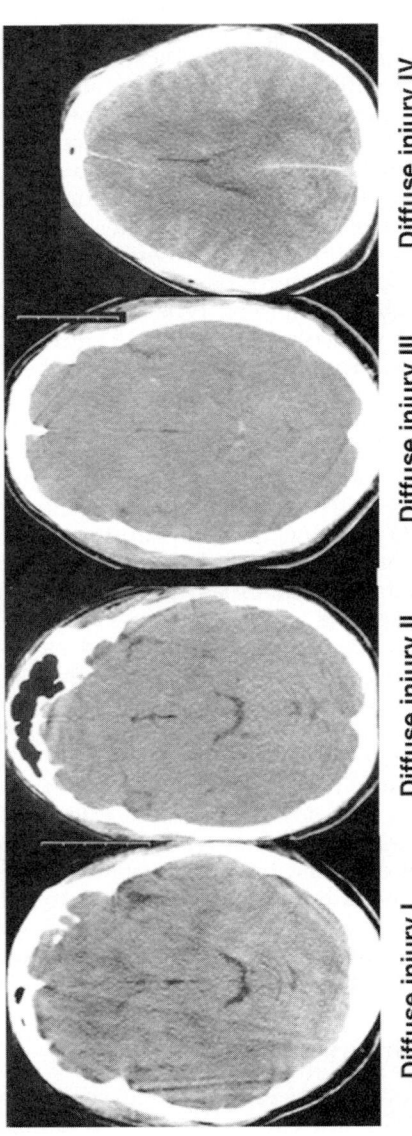

Typical CT scan appearance

Diagnostic criteria:	Diffuse injury I	Diffuse injury II	Diffuse injury III	Diffuse injury IV
Hematoma >25 mL?	no	no	no	no
Any abnormalities?	no	yes	yes	yes
Compression of brainstem cisterns?	no	no	yes	yes
Midline shift >5 mm?	no	no	no	yes
Incidence (overall 56%)	7%	24%	21%	4%
Mortality rate (overall 24%)	10%	14%	34%	56%

TYPES OF HEMATOMAS

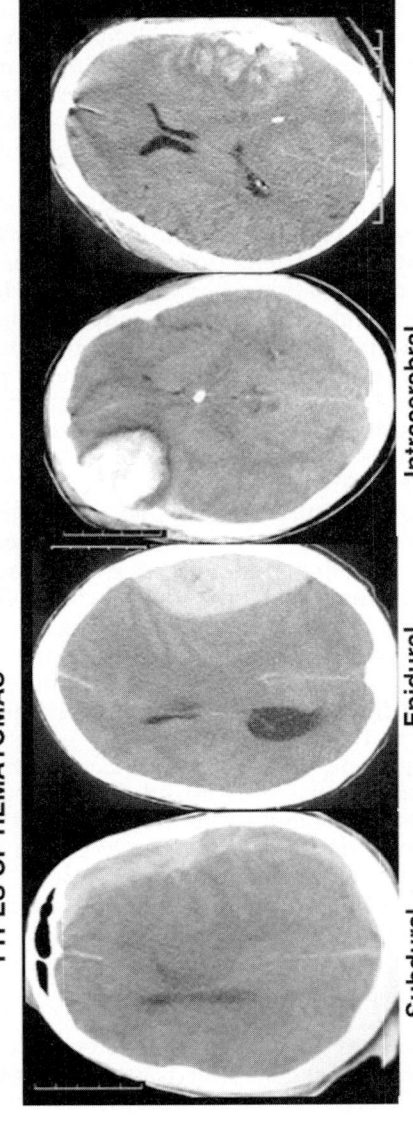

Typical CT scan appearance

Diagnostic criteria:	Subdural Hematoma	Epidural Hematoma	Intracerebral Hematoma	Contusion
Incidence (overall 42%)	24%	6%	10%	3%
Mortality rate (overall 39%)	50%	18%	27%	

FIGURE 327–2. Categorization of primary brain injury. (Traumatic Coma Data Bank categories from reference 12.)

or a contusion. Intracerebral hematomas are more common, occurring as the primary lesion in 10% of the severe closed head injuries in the TCDB series.[8] Occasionally, it may be difficult to differentiate a traumatic intracerebral hematoma from a spontaneous hemorrhage; however, the presence of an associated contusion, fracture, or air-fluid level in the sinus helps identify the hematoma as traumatic. A zone of surrounding hypodensity denotes contusion or edema.

Most intracerebral hematomas are visualized as hyperdense mass lesions (see Fig. 327–2). They are usually located in the frontal and temporal lobes and can be detected by CT immediately after the trauma. However, delayed intracerebral hematomas may also manifest during the hospital course. A delayed hematoma is one that is seen on a repeat computed tomographic scan within 24 to 48 hours of the injury or operation but was not present on the initial scan. Commonly, a delayed hematoma is associated with clinical deterioration. In one series, 19% of patients with severe head injuries who neurologically deteriorated after admission to the hospital had large delayed intracerebral hematomas.[40] Factors that determine the outcome in patients with intracerebral hematomas include GCS, hematoma volume, and occurrence of hypoxia.[41]

Hemorrhagic contusions were present as the primary lesions in 3% of severe closed head injuries in the TCDB series.[8] Single contusions are located either below or opposite the region of impact. Contusions appear as heterogeneous areas of brain necrosis, hemorrhage, and infarct representing mixed-density lesions on CT.[42] Multiple focal contusions have a "salt and pepper" appearance on CT. Ischemia may play a role in the pathogenesis of contusions, and regional CBF values averaging 17.5 ± 4.0 mL/100 g per minute have been measured in pericontusional tissue.[43]

CLASSIFICATION OF INJURY

A number of injury severity schemes have been developed for predicting mortality after trauma and other critical illnesses. In general, these schemes have been developed in other patient populations and do not accurately predict outcome in neurologically injured patients. Rocca and coworkers[44] studied 70 patients with traumatic brain injury and found that the GCS was superior to the Acute Physiology Score, the Simplified Acute Physiology Score (SAPS), and the Therapeutic Intervention Scoring System. More recently, Alvarez and colleagues[45] studied 401 patients with traumatic brain injury and compared the predictive ability of the Acute Physiology and Chronic Health Evaluation (APACHE II), SAPS II, Mortality Probability Models (MPM II), and GCS. The MPM II system provided a good estimation of mortality. SAPS II and APACHE II systems did not calibrate well, and the logistic regression model containing the GCS as an independent variable and developed in this group of patients was not as well calibrated as the MPM II.

Schemes that are good at predicting outcome after traumatic brain injury generally include age, severity of injury, and type of injury. For the severity of injury

scale, the GCS—either the sum score or, for comatose patients, the motor score alone—is used. For the type of injury, a classification that separates focal and diffuse injuries is typically used. A new classification of head injury based on information obtained in the initial computed tomographic scan was described from the TCDB data.[12] This scheme used the status of mesencephalic cisterns, the amount of midline shift, and the presence or absence of surgical masses. The diffuse injury category included all patients with no mixed- or high-density lesions greater than 25 mL. Diffuse injuries were divided into four subgroups: type I, all head injuries with no visible pathology; type II, all diffuse injuries with cisterns present and less than 5 mm shift; type III, all diffuse injuries with compressed or absent cisterns but less than 5 mm shift; and type IV, all diffuse injuries with more than 5 mm midline shift. Examples of these diffuse injury categories are shown in Figure 327–2. The category of mass lesions, which included all patients with mixed- or high-density lesions greater than 25 mL, was divided into those with the mass surgically evacuated (including subdural, epidural, and intracerebral hematomas) and those with nonevacuated mass lesions.

This classification scheme provides a good assessment of the risk of intracranial hypertension and of a fatal outcome. Patients with type I diffuse injuries had the lowest mortality rate, at 10%; those with types II, III, and IV had mortality rates of 14%, 34%, and 56%, respectively. The mortality rate for those with evacuated hematomas was 39%. One criticism of this classification scheme is that all evacuated hematomas are included in a single category, but the mortality rate is quite different for the different types of hematomas. Probably the most descriptive scheme at present is the TCDB classification, but with evacuated mass lesions divided into the three major hematoma types.

Secondary Brain Injury

Trauma initiates secondary injury processes in the brain that evolve during the early phase of hospitalization. Vascular changes are prominent and well described and can lead to additional brain injury if CBF is inadequate. Cellular processes are initiated that may lead to cell edema and cell death. Finally, inflammatory processes are initiated and can result in late vascular and cellular effects. These processes are manifested clinically by the development of intracranial hypertension and cerebral ischemia.

TRAUMATIC BRAIN SWELLING AND INTRACRANIAL HYPERTENSION

Brain edema, vascular engorgement, or both may be responsible for the brain swelling that accompanies severe traumatic brain injury. Although the relative contribution of these two entities to the swelling process is controversial, there is increasing evidence that edema plays the predominant role. In experimental models of brain trauma, the water content of the brain is increased, but the cerebral blood volume is decreased, suggesting that edema is the major component of brain swelling after trauma.[46] Clinical studies using magnetic resonance imaging techniques to quantify water and blood content have confirmed these experimental findings in humans.[47]

Brain edema can be vasogenic (due to opening of the blood-brain barrier) or cellular. Most experimental evidence, including recent data using diffusion-weighted imaging techniques to differentiate types of edema formation, suggests that the early, immediate increase in brain water content after trauma is probably vasogenic, whereas the gradual increase in water content that occurs during the first few days after injury is cellular.[48, 49]

The clinical manifestation of brain swelling is intracranial hypertension, which develops in 50% of patients in coma caused by severe head injury. It is a misconception that ICP is always low after operative evacuation of large intracranial hematomas; in fact, intracranial hypertension occurs in 50% to 70% of patients after evacuation of such hematomas.[3, 50] This postoperative intracranial hypertension may be due to a postoperative hematoma, either at the site of the operation or at a new site; progressive swelling of focal contusions; diffuse brain swelling; and other systemic complications. The incidence of intracranial hypertension is greater after evacuation of an intracerebral hematoma (71%) than after evacuation of a subdural or epidural hematoma (39%).[3] In patients with no mass lesions, elevated ICP has been observed to occur during hospitalization in 30% to 80% of patients.[3, 51]

The association between severity of intracranial hypertension and poor outcome after head injury is well recognized. In one series, 77% of patients with ICP less than 15 mm Hg had a favorable outcome, compared with only 43% of patients with ICP greater than 15 mm

Hg.[52] Miller and associates[53] reported that the mortality rate increased from 18% to 92%, and the frequency of good outcomes decreased from 74% to 3%, in patients with normal ICP compared with those whose ICP could not be reduced below 20 mm Hg. Similarly, Saul and Ducker[4] reported a 69% mortality rate in patients with ICP greater than 25 mm Hg, compared with a 15% mortality rate if ICP remained less than 25 mm Hg.

The relationship between elevated ICP and poor outcome is not simply a reflection of the severity of the initial neurological injury. Severe intracranial hypertension can result in secondary injury to the brain through ischemia, produced by a reduction in cerebral perfusion pressure (CPP), and it can also distort and compress the brainstem. Although no randomized clinical trial has addressed this issue, several clinical series have suggested that reducing ICP to less than 20 mm Hg reduces mortality after severe head injury.[1-4]

EFFECT OF TRAUMA ON CEREBRAL VASCULATURE

Many investigators have studied CBF after traumatic brain injury and emphasized various patterns. A few studies closely examined the evolution of traumatic brain injury over time with serial measurements of CBF.[54, 55] These serial studies in particular have helped develop the overall picture of postinjury changes in CBF (Table 327–3).

Martin and coworkers[54] described a phasic pattern of cerebral hemodynamic changes in 125 severely head-injured patients with GCS scores less than 8 who were studied prospectively with intravenous xenon-133 CBF measurements and cerebral metabolic or transcranial Doppler evaluations. An early hypoperfusion phase occurred during the first 24 hours after injury and was

T A B L E 3 2 7 – 3 ■ **Summary of CBF Patterns during the Evolution of Severe Head Injury**

	CBF PATTERN			
	Hypoperfusion (<35 mL/100 g/min)	**Hyperemia (>55 mL/100 g/min)**	**Vasospasm**	**Chronic State**
Hemodynamic findings				
CBF	Decreased	Increased	Normal–decreased	Normal–decreased, but appropriate for CMRO2
Flow velocity	Decreased	Increased, normal hemispheric index	Increased, high hemispheric index	Normal–decreased
AVDO2	Increased	Decreased	Normal–increased	Normal
SjvO2/PbtO2	Decreased	Increased	Normal–decreased	Normal
Typical timing of CBF pattern	First 12–24 hr after injury	Days 1–3	Days 5–14	After day 14
Incidence of CBF pattern	≈65% transient ≈15% persistent	≈25% transient ≈15% persistent	≈50%	
Consequences of CBF findings	Additional injury from ischemia More susceptible to secondary ischemic insults	Some studies suggest an association with intracranial hypertension	Additional injury from ischemia	

AVDO2, arteriovenous difference in oxygen; CBF, cerebral blood flow; CMRO2, cerebral metabolic rate of oxygen; PbtO2, brain tissue oxygen tension; SjvO2, jugular venous oxygen saturation.
Data from references 54–56, 59, 301.

characterized by low CBF and normal middle cerebral artery (MCA) flow velocity. This was followed by a hyperemic phase that occurred in about 40% of patients between postinjury days 1 and 3; CBF was transiently increased, with a rapidly rising MCA flow velocity but a normal hemispheric index. Later (postinjury days 4 to 15), a vasospasm phase occurred with low-normal CBF values, a high MCA flow velocity, and an elevated hemispheric index. Bouma and colleagues[56] found global or regional CBF values less than 18 mL/100 g per minute in 31% of head-injured patients when the CBF evaluation was done within 6 hours of injury, suggesting that most of the severe ischemia occurs soon after injury.

These CBF patterns, which have been described primarily with global CBF measurements, can also occur regionally. Hypoperfusion, in particular, can occur in brain surrounding a focal contusion or underlying a subdural hematoma. Schroder and associates[43] observed regional CBF values averaging 17.5 mL/100 g per minute in pericontusional brain. McLaughlin and Marion[57] observed that CBF values in contused and pericontusional brain were significantly lower than those in the rest of the brain. Focal hyperemia has been observed in 38% of patients, particularly in tissue adjacent to intraparenchymal or extracerebral focal lesions.[58]

EFFECT OF CEREBRAL BLOOD FLOW ABNORMALITIES ON OUTCOME

Although no studies have demonstrated that monitoring CBF improves outcome after severe head injury, many studies have demonstrated a close relationship between CBF abnormalities (hypoperfusion, hyperemia, vasospasm) and poor neurological recovery. This relationship may simply indicate that abnormal CBF is a marker of more severe injury, but in many of these studies, CBF is an independent predictor of outcome, even when adjustments for the usual measures of injury severity are applied (Table 327–4).

Hypoperfusion

CBF studies using the xenon-133 method or the nitrous oxide (N_2O) saturation method have described the prognostic value of global CBF measurements. Obrist and coworkers[59] found that 45% of patients had CBF values below normal; however, because the arteriovenous oxygen difference ($AVDO_2$) remained normal, the low CBF was thought to be appropriate for the reduced cerebral metabolic requirements. Although this observation may be true in the chronic stages of head injury, some studies suggest that a low CBF, particularly during the first few hours after head injury, is a poor prognostic finding. Robertson and associates[55]

T A B L E 3 2 7 – 4 ■ **Selected Studies Demonstrating a Relationship between CBF Patterns and Poor Outcome after Severe Head Injury**

AUTHOR	NUMBER OF PATIENTS	DEFINITION OF CBF PATTERN	INCIDENCE OF CBF PATTERN (%)	ASSOCIATION OF CBF PATTERN AND OUTCOME
Hypoperfusion				
Jaggi et al, 1990[302]	96 adults	[133]Xe CBF < normal values	45	No relation when all patients were examined; in patients with reduced CBF, outcome poorer with lower CBF
Robertson et al, 1992[55]	102 adults	N_2O CBF < normal values	25	Patients with reduced CBF had significantly worse outcome, even when adjusted for other factors
Bouma et al, 1992[56]	35 adults	Xe CT rCBF <18 mL/100 g/min	31	Regional or global CBF <18 mL/100 g/min associated with poor outcome
Gopinath et al, 1994[64]	112 adults	$SjvO_2$ <50%	39	One desaturation doubled, and multiple desaturations increased by 14-fold, the risk of poor outcome
Kelly et al, 1997[60]	54 adults	[133]Xe CBF <33 mL/100 g/min	13	Low CBF associated with poorer outcome
Hyperemia				
Bruce et al, 1973[69]	22 adults	[133]Xe CBF > normal values	25	Mortality 2-fold higher in patients with elevated CBF
Obrist et al, 1979[68]	36 adults	[133]Xe CBF > normal values	25	Mortality higher in patients with elevated CBF
Vasospasm				
Lee et al, 1997[77]	152 adults	FV >120 cm/sec, HI >3, decreased CBF	42	Outcomes poorer when hemodynamically significant vasospasm present
Zurynski et al, 1995[303]	50 adults	High FV, decreased CBF	40	Outcomes poorer when vasospasm diagnosed

CBF, cerebral blood flow; FV, flow velocity; HI, hemispheric index; N_2O, nitrous oxide; rCBF, regional cerebral blood flow; $SjvO_2$, jugular venous oxygen saturation; ^{133}Xe CBF, [133]xenon cerebral blood flow; Xe CT, stable xenon enhanced computed tomography.

described several hemodynamic patterns from serial measurements of CBF and observed that patients with reduced CBF any time during the first 7 days after injury had a higher mortality rate, and there was a poorer recovery among survivors. Kelly and colleagues[60] found that patients with CBF values less than 33 mL/100 g per minute had a higher incidence of evacuated intracranial hematomas and had worse outcomes than patients with higher flows. Using the thermal diffusion CBF method, Sioutos and coauthors[61] found a CBF value less than 18 mL/100 g per minute in one third of the patients monitored. Low CBF persisted throughout the monitoring period in those with poor neurological outcomes, whereas in patients who recovered, the CBF increased.

A low regional CBF has an equally poor prognosis. Data from intracarotid xenon techniques in the 1980s showed that regional CBF values of less than 20 mL/100 g per minute occurred in 61% of patients who died or were severely disabled.[62] More recently, with the availability of stable xenon CT scanning, it has been observed that about one third of patients with severe traumatic brain injury have regional or global CBF in the ischemic range (<18 mL/100 g per minute) within the first 6 hours after injury.[56] The occurrence of ischemia was significantly related to a poor outcome. Early reductions in CBF within 4 hours after trauma occurred more commonly in patients with multiple bihemispheric contusions.[63]

Methods of continuous CBF monitoring have associated transient hypoperfusion, manifested by a reduction of jugular venous oxygen saturation ($SjvO_2$) below 50%, with a poor neurological outcome. $SjvO_2$, monitored in 116 patients with severe head injury, was reduced below 50% at least once in 39% of the patients.[64] When adjusted for injury severity, one episode of jugular desaturation was associated with a twofold increased risk of a poor outcome, and multiple episodes of jugular desaturation were associated with a 14-fold increased risk of a poor outcome.

Hyperemia and Intracranial Hypertension

Hyperemia has been associated with both intracranial hypertension and with a poor neurological outcome. Defined as above-normal CBF, hyperemia has been observed to occur in 20% of adults with severe head injury. If severely headinjured patients with CBF values in the normal range are considered to have "relative hyperemia," because CBF is higher than that needed to meet the reduced metabolic requirements associated with coma, then 55% of severely head-injured adults have hyperemia.[59] It is even more common in children, with up to 88% having normal or elevated CBF.[65]

The association between hyperemia and intracranial hypertension is particularly common in children but has also been observed in adults. Bruce and coworkers[51] found elevated CBF in children with diffuse brain swelling and intracranial hypertension. Obrist and associates[59] found a strong relationship between CBF and ICP in a series of 75 patients with severe head injury. Seventy-seven percent of patients with a normal or

elevated CBF had intracranial hypertension, compared with only 23% of patients with a reduced CBF. Kelly and colleagues[66] found that the incidence of intracranial hypertension was slightly higher when the CBF was elevated than when it was reduced: 32% versus 22%. Other investigators have found no relationship between hyperemia and ICP. Muizelaar and coauthors,[65] studying a group of 32 children, found that 67% of the patients with normal or elevated CBF had intracranial hypertension, compared with 100% of those with reduced CBF. Robertson and coworkers[55] also found no relationship between CBF pattern and intracranial hypertension.

Numerous studies have associated elevated CBF and outcome (see Table 327–4). Overgaard and Tweed[67] reported a good outcome in only 1 of 12 patients with an elevated CBF. In a study of 36 patients, the mortality rate was 67% in patients with an elevated CBF, compared with 9% in those with a normal CBF and 27% in those with a reduced CBF.[68] In a study of 22 patients, the mortality rate was 80% in those with an elevated CBF, 40% in those with a reduced CBF, and 47% in those with a normal CBF.[69] In contrast, other studies have found elevated CBF to be associated with a relatively good outcome.[55] Focal hyperemia has also been thought to be associated with a favorable outcome.[58] Sometimes hyperemia is defined by a low $AVDO_2$ or a high $SjvO_2$, because this finding suggests a CBF in excess of cerebral metabolic requirements. In terms of prognosis, however, the finding of an elevated $SjvO_2$ describes a wide spectrum of outcomes.[70] A high $SjvO_2$ predicts a poor outcome if it is caused by a low cerebral metabolic rate of oxygen ($CMRO_2$); in contrast, if high CBF is the cause of the elevated $SjvO_2$, it often predicts a favorable outcome.

Vasospasm

The TCDB study reported the occurrence of subarachnoid hemorrhage in 39% of patients with severe head injury, although more recent studies have reported a higher frequency, probably because of the improved resolution of modern CT scanners.[11] Angiographic evidence of cerebral vasospasm reportedly occurs in 19% of patients with moderate to severe head injury.[71–73] With transcranial Doppler studies, the incidence of cerebral vasospasm is approximately 30%.[74, 75]

The incidence of ischemic injury due to vasospasm is more difficult to estimate because the neurological signs of ischemia are superimposed on the neurological deficits of the traumatic injury, but a few studies suggest that cerebral vasospasm may be an important cause of evolving injury in some patients. Chan and colleagues[76] studied the relationship between an increased flow velocity and the development of cerebral infarction on CT in 121 patients. They found that of 23 patients who developed a mean flow velocity greater than 100 cm/second, 4 developed an infarction in the territory of the involved cerebral vessel.

Lee and coworkers[77] reported a significant relationship between vasospasm and a poor neurological outcome in 152 patients, even after adjusting for injury severity. This was particularly true if the transcranial Doppler findings were associated with reduced CBF. Other studies found no relationship between an elevated flow velocity after traumatic brain injury and outcome.[78]

Secondary Ischemic Insults

Evidence that secondary insults can cause additional damage after traumatic brain injury is both experimental and clinical. In the fluid percussion injury model, 6 minutes of forebrain ischemia (bilateral carotid occlusion with hypotension) significantly increased hippocampal neuronal loss compared with either traumatic injury or ischemia alone.[79] In the controlled cortical impact injury model, bilateral carotid occlusion significantly increased the contusion volume and hippocampal neuronal loss compared with either traumatic injury or ischemia alone.[80]

Clinical studies have demonstrated an association between the occurrence of secondary insults and poor neurological outcome. Jones and coworkers[81] reported that secondary insults occurred in 91% of 124 patients studied with a computerized detection system. The duration of hypotensive, febrile, and hypoxic insults was significantly associated with mortality. Gopinath and associates[64] observed that the occurrence of secondary insults severe enough to result in desaturation of jugular venous blood was significantly related to poor neurological outcome. Even when adjusted for other confounding factors, such as age, type of injury, and neurological status, the occurrence of one episode of jugular desaturation was associated with a twofold increase in the risk of a poor neurological outcome, and the occurrence of multiple episodes of jugular desaturation was associated with a 14-fold increase.

The major reason that the traumatized brain is so sensitive to secondary insults is that the regulatory processes that normally preserve CBF during reductions in blood pressure, arterial P_{O_2}, and hemoglobin concentration are dysfunctional after trauma. Therefore, the goal must be to optimize cerebral perfusion in the traumatized brain.

CAUSES

Any pathophysiologic process that impairs cerebral energy metabolism can cause a secondary ischemic insult after head injury. As shown in Figure 327–1, these processes can be divided into two general categories: those that decrease cerebral delivery of energy substrates, and those that increase cerebral energy consumption.

Cerebral oxygen delivery is the product of CBF and arterial oxygen content (CaO_2). CBF is normally closely regulated by cerebral metabolic rate and can also be affected by CPP and arterial P_{CO_2}. However, in disease states, CBF can be uncoupled from metabolic rate and can be higher or lower than normal. CaO_2 is calculated from the arterial oxygen saturation and hemoglobin concentration and is normally around 20 mL/dL (9 μmol/mL). Both hypoxia and anemia can reduce CaO_2.

Cerebral oxygen consumption, or $CMRO_2$, has a normal value of 3.4 mg/100 g per minte (1.5 μmol/g per minute). Numerous conditions are known to alter the $CMRO_2$. Head injury, anesthesia, and hypothermia are known to decrease $CMRO_2$, while fever and seizures increase it.[59, 82–88] Recent studies using fluorodeoxyglucose positron emission tomography to study glucose metabolism after severe head injury suggest that the cerebral metabolic rate of glucose may be elevated regionally, and perhaps even globally, at times when the $CMRO_2$ is normal or reduced.[89] This "hyperglycolysis" may indicate mitochondrial damage and the brain's inability to metabolize oxygen normally. If energy metabolism is dependent on glucose metabolism, then energy failure due to glucose depletion is another possible cause of secondary ischemic insults after severe head injury.

NEUROLOGICAL INTENSIVE CARE MONITORING

The two most important secondary injury processes that can be monitored, anticipated, and treated in the intensive care unit are intracranial hypertension and cerebral ischemia. In addition, secondary ischemic insults can be anticipated and prevented or detected early and treated before they are severe enough to injure the brain.

To accomplish these goals, severely head-injured patients should have ICP monitoring, preferably by ventriculostomy, and monitoring of cerebral perfusion, often with jugular bulb oximetry (with or without brain tissue P_{O_2}). In addition, head-injured patients should have close monitoring of systemic parameters, including electrocardiogram, heart rate, blood pressure, temperature (rectal), and fluid intake and output. An arterial catheter is usually indicated to continuously monitor blood pressure and to provide easy access for blood sampling; it is also required if pressor agents are needed to maintain adequate blood pressure. Severely head-injured patients should be routinely monitored with pulse oximetry and capnography to avoid unrecognized hypoxemia or changes in ventilation. A central venous catheter and, in certain circumstances, a Swan-Ganz catheter may be needed to judge volume status. A Foley catheter is necessary for accurate measurement of urine output.

Neurological Status

To assess the neurological status of the patient, evaluation of mental status and cranial nerve, pupillary, and motor functions should be included in the periodic neurological examination whenever possible. This helps determine whether there is improvement, deterioration, or no change in the patient's clinical condition. A 24-hour record of the patient should be available on one sheet, such as that described by Clifton and Grossman,[90] and should include information regarding vital signs and laboratory values. Computerized information systems are becoming more widespread in intensive care units and can markedly reduce the burden of such record keeping.

Intracranial Hypertension

ICP cannot be reliably estimated from any clinical feature after severe head injury. Clinical symptoms of raised ICP, such as headache, nausea, and vomiting, are impossible to elicit in comatose patients. Papilledema is uncommon after head injury, even in patients with intracranial hypertension.[91] In one study, although 54% of patients had increased ICP, only 3.5% had papilledema on funduscopic examination. Other neurological signs, including pupillary dilatation and decerebrate posturing, can occur in the absence of intracranial hypertension. CT signs of brain swelling, such as midline shift and compressed basal cisterns, are predictive of raised ICP, but intracranial hypertension can occur without these findings.[92]

MONITORING TECHNIQUES

Recording of cerebrospinal fluid (CSF) pressure was initially performed through lumbar puncture in the late 1800s. Continuous pressure recordings of ICP were first reported in 1951 by Guillaume and Janny.[93] In 1960, Lundberg reported the results of ventricular catheter pressure recordings in 143 patients with various neurosurgical diagnoses.[94] This was a landmark work that emphasized both the safety and the importance of ICP monitoring.

Although several new types of monitors have been marketed, the ventriculostomy catheter remains the preferred device for monitoring ICP and is the standard against which all new monitors are compared. The ventriculostomy catheter is positioned with its tip in the frontal horn of the lateral ventricle and is coupled by fluid-filled tubing to an external pressure transducer that can be reset to zero and recalibrated against an external standard. The ventriculostomy catheter provides the most reliable measurement of ICP throughout the normal and pathologic ranges. In addition, it allows treatment of elevated ICP by intermittent drainage of CSF. However, the risk of ventriculitis and intracranial hemorrhage is highest with ventriculostomy,[95] and proper placement of the catheter tip in the lateral ventricle can be difficult in patients with small, compressed ventricles.

When the ventricle cannot be cannulated, alternative devices can be used. A number of nonfluid-coupled devices have become available for ICP monitoring and have replaced the subarachnoid bolt as an alternative to ventriculostomy in most institutions. The microsensor transducer[96] and the fiber-optic transducer[97] are the most widely available devices. These miniature pressure transducer–tipped catheters can be inserted in the subdural space or directly into brain tissue. Their main advantage is the ease of insertion, especially in patients with compressed ventricles. They provide more reliable measures of ICP than subarachnoid bolts and fluid-coupled catheters in the subdural space because they have no lumen to become obstructed. The

transducers, however, cannot be reset to zero after they are inserted into the skull, and they exhibit drift over time.[98]

For surgical patients, the ICP monitor can be inserted at the end of the surgical procedure. Those who do not require surgery are immediately transferred to the intensive care unit after the initial computed tomographic scan, and an ICP monitor is inserted there. A pressure tracing should display the pulsatile nature of the ICP. A dampened tracing may not be a reliable measure of ICP.

ICP monitoring is continued for as long as treatment of intracranial hypertension is required, typically 3 to 5 days. A secondary rise in ICP has been observed 3 to 10 days after injury in 30% of patients with intracranial hypertension,[99] due to the development of a delayed intracerebral hematoma, cerebral vasospasm, or systemic factors such as hypoxia or hypotension. Souter and colleagues[100] have associated an increase in the blood leukocyte count with late intracranial hypertension.

COMPLICATIONS

The two major complications of ICP monitoring are ventriculitis and hemorrhage. Infection may be confined to the skin wound, but in 1% to 10% of cases, ventriculitis occurs. Most studies have found a higher rate of infection in ventriculostomy-monitored patients than in those monitored with subarachnoid bolts or subdural catheters.[95, 101] In most studies, the rate of infection is directly related to the duration of monitoring, with very few infections in patients monitored for less than 3 days. The practice of replacing the ventriculostomy catheter after 5 days, if continued monitoring is required, has been recommended on the basis of these studies. Another study, however, demonstrated that most ventriculostomy-related infections occurred in the first week and were thus presumably due to contamination at the time of catheter insertion.[102] An analysis of data from the TCDB study also suggested that there was no benefit in exchanging ventriculostomy catheters at 5-day intervals.[103] The best strategy for reducing the risk of ventriculitis associated with ICP monitoring is to minimize the duration of monitoring. No controlled studies have demonstrated the ability of prophylactic antibiotics to reduce the incidence of ventriculostomy-related infections, but prophylactic treatment with an antibiotic having gram-positive coverage is common.

The second major complication of ICP monitoring is intracerebral hemorrhage. Although the risk of hemorrhage is low (1% to 2%), it is an important complication to recognize and treat.[95] Patients with coagulopathies are at a greater risk of developing this complication.

NORMAL VALUES

Normally, resting ICP is less than 10 mm Hg. Transient elevations of ICP occur normally with straining, coughing, or the Trendelenburg position. A sustained ICP greater than 20 mm Hg is clearly abnormal. An

ICP between 20 and 40 mm Hg is considered moderate intracranial hypertension. An ICP greater than 40 mm Hg represents severe, usually life-threatening intracranial hypertension.[104] These guidelines for determining the severity of intracranial hypertension assume a normal blood pressure. When a temporal mass lesion is present, however, herniation can occur at ICP values less than 20 mm Hg.[105]

Different authors have recommended treatment of ICP greater than 15, 20, or 25 mm Hg. There are no studies that clearly establish one of these values as the most appropriate threshold for treatment. Marmarou and associates[106] observed an increasingly worse outcome with greater durations of ICP higher than 20 mm Hg, and Contant and coworkers[107] observed a worse outcome with greater durations of ICP higher than 25 mm Hg. Both the American and the European head injury guidelines recommend treatment of ICP greater than 20 to 25 mm Hg.[13, 14]

INDICATIONS FOR MONITORING

Monitoring of ICP can result in serious complications and is therefore indicated only in those patients at significant risk of developing intracranial hypertension. Patients who are particularly at risk include those with GCS scores of 8 or less after resuscitation and abnormal computed tomographic scans, and those with GCS scores of 8 or less and normal computed tomographic scans but adverse features such as age older than 40 years, systolic blood pressure of 90 mm Hg or less, or motor posturing.[95] Some studies have shown that comatose patients without these adverse features may also have transiently elevated ICP, suggesting that all patients with GCS scores of 8 or less should have ICP monitoring.[108] Patients with GCS scores greater than 8 might be considered for ICP monitoring if they require treatment that would not allow serial neurological examinations,[109] such as prolonged anesthesia for surgery to treat multiple injuries or prolonged pharmacologic paralysis for ventilatory management, or if they require a treatment that might raise ICP, such as positive end-expiratory pressure (PEEP). A severe coagulopathy is the only major contraindication to ICP monitoring.

Cerebral Ischemia

As with intracranial hypertension, there are no reliable clinical findings for cerebral ischemia. The neurological signs caused by brain injury usually obscure any focal findings that might be caused by secondary ischemia. Therefore, cerebral perfusion must be monitored to detect secondary cerebral ischemia after traumatic brain injury.

The ideal monitor for cerebral ischemia after traumatic brain injury does not exist. This ideal monitor would give information about regional CBF, because there can be marked regional differences after trauma; it would also give continuous information, because CBF evolves over time after injury. The available techniques fall under two general categories—those that

monitor cerebral perfusion or blood flow, and those that monitor CBF adequacy.

CEREBRAL PERFUSION

Cerebral Perfusion Pressure

The simplest measure of cerebral perfusion is CPP, which is calculated by subtracting the ICP from the mean arterial blood pressure. The normal lower limit of autoregulation for CPP is 50 mm Hg. In severely head-injured patients, the ability to autoregulate may be impaired, and CBF may be inadequate even with CPP values greater than 50 mm Hg. CPP can be reduced through either decreases in blood pressure or increases in ICP. For equivalent levels of CPP, cerebral perfusion is impaired more by reductions in blood pressure than by increases in ICP.[110] CPP monitoring is widely available and convenient, but a limitation is that only ischemia caused by increased ICP or decreased blood pressure is assessed.

Transcranial Doppler Flow Velocity

Transcranial Doppler ultrasonography uses a pulsed ultrasonic signal in the 2-MHz range that is transmitted through thin areas of the skull. Blood flow volume and flow velocity are not synonymous. However, flow volume is directly proportional to flow velocity and can be determined by multiplying the velocity by the cross-sectional area of the vessel insonated. Because transcranial Doppler measures flow velocity in the arteries at the circle of Willis, and because the radius of the vessel is not generally known and the collateral blood flow is variable, transcranial Doppler ultrasonography cannot provide quantitative data on regional tissue perfusion.

Several studies assessing the relationship between peak flow velocity and changes in CBF have suggested that changes in MCA flow velocity can be used as an indicator of relative changes in blood flow. Kofke and associates,[111] investigating the relationship between MCA flow velocity and CBF assessed by stable xenon CT during balloon test occlusion of the carotid artery in 31 patients, found a significant correlation in the alteration of flow detected by the two methods. More recently, changes in MCA flow velocity and changes in CBF observed with stable xenon CT in patients with various intracranial pathologies, including eight with closed head injury, have shown a close correlation.[112]

During arterial spasm, flow velocity increases through the narrowed segment in proportion to the reduction in the vessel's diameter. Severe vasospasm, with a greater than 50% reduction in vessel diameter, is associated with flow velocity greater than 200 cm/second.[113] However, an increase in flow velocity may also reflect hyperemia, which is a frequent post-traumatic event. To differentiate between these two hemodynamic phenomena in the absence of direct CBF measurements, the MCA–extracranial internal carotid artery flow velocity ratio, also known as the Lindegaard or hemispheric index, has been measured. In the presence of hyperemia, raised flow velocity in both extracranial and intracranial vessels does not alter the ratio; however, in vasospasm, flow velocity is high only in the intracranial vessels, resulting in a high hemispheric index. The mean hemispheric index in normal individuals is 1.76 ± 0.1, and pathologic values suggestive of vasospasm are generally greater than 3.[114]

Cerebral Blood Flow

Recently, new technologies have made measurement of CBF more feasible in critically ill patients. Measurement of global CBF by the classic Kety-Schmidt technique, using N_2O as the diffusible indicator, can be performed at the bedside with minimal expense and equipment. Instruments for measuring regional CBF using the stable xenon-enhanced CT technique are commercially available. However, both these measurements of CBF are intermittent and require the patient to be hemodynamically stable during the time required for the measurements. Therefore, transient reductions in CBF or reductions in CBF in acutely unstable patients are difficult to document with these technologies.

The original CBF technique developed by Kety and Schmidt is based on the Fick principle, which states that the amount of a substance taken up by any organ per unit of time equals the quantity delivered by the arterial blood minus the quantity carried away by the venous blood. This technique assumes that the tracer substance completely diffuses into the brain, reaches equilibrium, and is not metabolized. Traditionally, 15% N_2O is administered for 15 minutes, and arterial and venous N_2O concentration is measured in blood samples drawn at intervals after administration. CBF is related to the area between the arterial and venous N_2O saturation curves. Most other techniques of measuring CBF use some derivation of the Kety-Schmidt technique.

The stable xenon CT method relies on the radiodensity of xenon, its inertness, and its rapid diffusion into tissues. An initial noncontrast scan helps in choosing the levels for CBF measurement. Baseline scans, usually at four levels, are followed by multiple scans at each of the four levels at 1-minute intervals during inhalation of 28% to 33% xenon. The baseline scans are subtracted from the subsequent xenon scans to provide quantitative enhancement values in Hounsfield units. Clearance curves proportional to brain xenon concentration and arterial concentrations from an end-tidal analyzer are converted into CT enhancement units. The blood flow is then calculated from the Kety-Schmidt equation for each CT voxel. Studies in normal volunteers have indicated that xenon at a concentration of 30% has an effect on cerebral hemodynamics, causing arterial vasodilatation and enhancement of CBF.[115, 116] This probably occurs as a result of an increase in metabolism and a vasodilatory effect of xenon. Some studies have observed a small increase in ICP averaging 6.9 ± 7.7 mm Hg during xenon CT CBF measurements,[117] but others have not.[118]

Two methods for continuously measuring local CBF are now commercially available—the thermal diffusion method, and the laser Doppler method. Both methods are invasive, requiring the probe to be placed on the surface of the brain at surgery. Both methods measure CBF in only a small volume of brain, which may or may not be representative of the whole brain. However, the continuous nature of the measurements gives a dynamic picture of brain perfusion. Although there is extensive documentation of the reliability of these methodologies in the laboratory, there is limited experience in the intensive care unit.[61, 119, 120] However, especially for patients undergoing craniotomy, these may be practical methods for monitoring CBF postoperatively.

Thermal diffusion flowmetry uses heat transfer as a tracer in the measurement of blood flow. The sensor consists of two gold disks embedded in a 3-mm Silastic leaf. One disk is heated slightly above brain temperature (to a maximum of 44°C), and the other is neutral. The probe is laid on the surface of the brain. The temperature difference between the two disks is monitored and converted to blood flow in milliliters per 100 g per minute by the monitor using a digital display. Carter and Atkinson[121] modified a thermal sensor described by Brawley[122] and were able to quantitate the flow measured by the thermal sensor. They derived a mathematical formula by comparing the thermal diffusion CBF with the xenon-133 CBF[123] and further confirmed the reliability through comparison with hydrogen clearance.[124]

Figure 327–3 (left) shows the close relationship between thermal diffusion CBF values and regional CBF values measured by the stable xenon CT technique (Robertson and Valadka, unpublished data). Because the thermal diffusion probe measures local CBF, these values do not have a good correlation to global CBF in a disorder such as traumatic brain injury, in which there is regional heterogeneity of flow (see Fig. 327–3, right). Gopinath and colleagues[125] compared thermal diffusion CBF to global CBF values measured by the N_2O saturation technique in a group of 35 patients with severe head injury. As expected, the thermal diffusion CBF, which is a measure of cortical flow, was significantly higher than the global CBF, which is a mixture of gray and white matter flow. However, there was a close correlation between the two measures over time, and a change in the thermal diffusion CBF reliably predicted a change in global CBF. These studies suggest that thermal diffusion flowmetry gives an accurate measure of local CBF under the probe and is a reasonable estimate of trend changes in global CBF.

Laser Doppler flowmetry is a technique in which CBF is measured indirectly from the magnitude of frequency shift of monochromatic light by a moving column of blood. The laser light is directed at the region of interest through a small probe that illuminates about 1 mm^3 of tissue. With this high spatial resolution, it is designed primarily for measuring flow in capillaries. The photons penetrate the translucent capillary wall and are scattered by the moving red blood cells; their frequencies are shifted according to the Doppler principle. A photodetector collects the scattered light, analyzes the signal to calculate the flow velocity, and reports the flow in milliliters per 100 g per minute using certain calibration factors. Flow

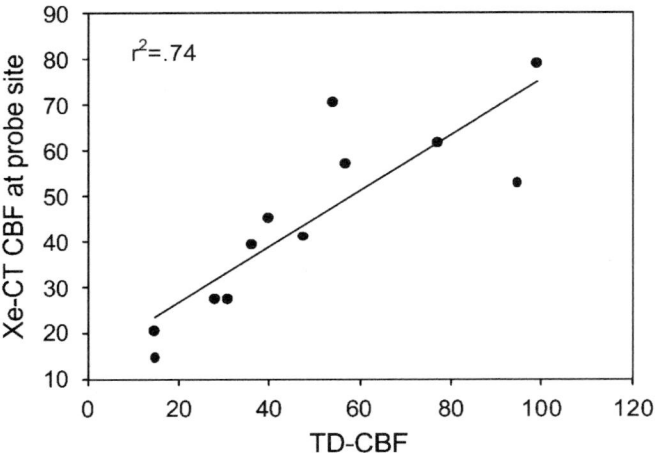
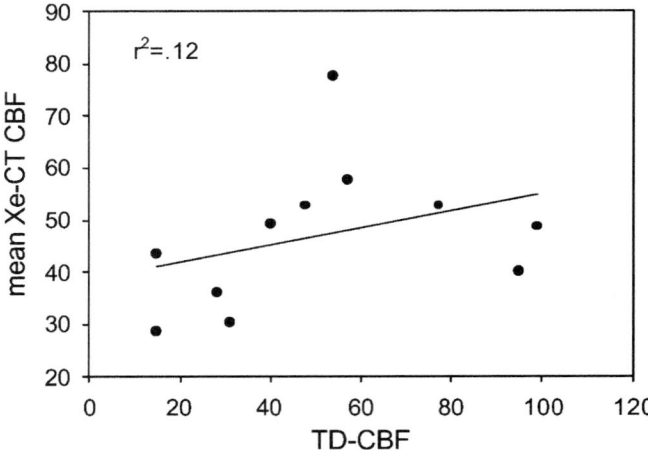

FIGURE 327–3. Cerebral blood flow (CBF) measured with a thermal diffusion probe is closely related to CBF measured by the xenon-computed tomography (CT) technique in a region of interest at the site of the CBF probe *(left)*, but not to average cortical CBF measured by the xenon CT technique *(right)*. (From unpublished data of Robertson and Valadka.)

estimated by laser Doppler compares favorably with more established CBF measurements.[126] However, proper placement of the probe is a strong determinant of the success of the monitoring. The most accurate recordings are made when the probe is in direct contact with the region of interest but away from obviously visible vessels that will bias the capillary flow. The pial vessels on the cortical surface are best avoided by inserting the probe about 2 to 3 mm into the brain parenchyma. The most useful application of laser Doppler flowmetry is in continuous monitoring of CBF in the intensive care unit. The high temporal resolution allows the detection of transient hemodynamic events, although the information is about relative changes in local CBF.

CEREBRAL BLOOD FLOW ADEQUACY

Measures of cerebral oxygenation, such as $SjvO_2$ or brain tissue PO_2, have been used in place of quantitative CBF measurements because they indicate the adequacy of CBF relative to cerebral metabolic requirements. Because cerebral metabolic requirements may be reduced after traumatic brain injury, normal CBF values may not apply. When CBF is low (25 to 30 mL/100 g per minute), it can be difficult to decide whether this is an appropriate response to lower cerebral metabolic requirements or whether the brain is hypoperfused. A measure of cerebral oxygenation can be helpful in making this distinction. If the brain is hypoperfused, oxygen extraction will be increased, and $SjvO_2$ will be reduced. If CBF is appropriate for the brain's metabolic requirements, $SjvO_2$ will be normal. Often this information is more clinically useful than are absolute CBF values.

Jugular Venous Oxygen Saturation

The nonlinear relationship between $SjvO_2$ and CBF in 100 head-injured patients is illustrated in Figure

327–4. The sequence of cerebrovascular changes in a head-injured patient with global cerebral ischemia is similar to that described in normal subjects.[127] Initially, increasing oxygen extraction compensates for the reduced CBF, and there is no effect on cerebral metabolism (Fig. 327–5). At this stage, $SjvO_2$ is decreased, and $CMRO_2$ is unchanged. As CBF decreases further, the brain can no longer compensate fully by increasing oxygen extraction, so $CMRO_2$ falls and cerebral lactate production increases.

The major difference from normal subjects is that after a head injury, CBF can be decreased at less severe reductions in CPP. Lewelt and coworkers[128] showed in a fluid percussion injury model that autoregulation was severely impaired after both low-level and high-level injuries. Normally, CBF is constant until CPP falls below 60 mm Hg. After the fluid percussion injury, CBF decreased proportional to CPP, as CPP fell below 80 mm Hg. Chan and associates[129] described similar

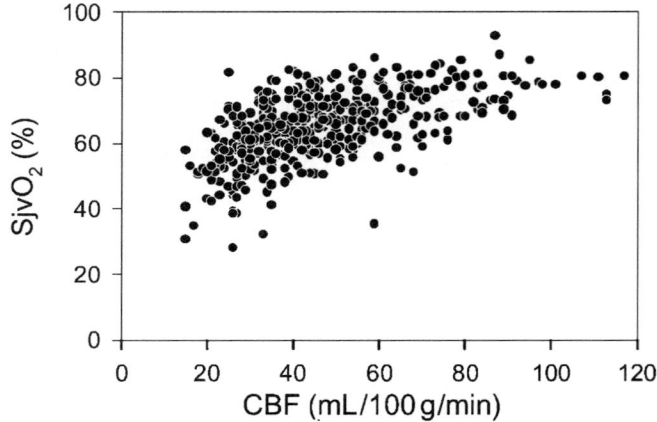

FIGURE 327–4. Nonlinear relationship between jugular venous oxygen saturation ($SjvO_2$) and cerebral blood flow (CBF). (Data from reference 127.)

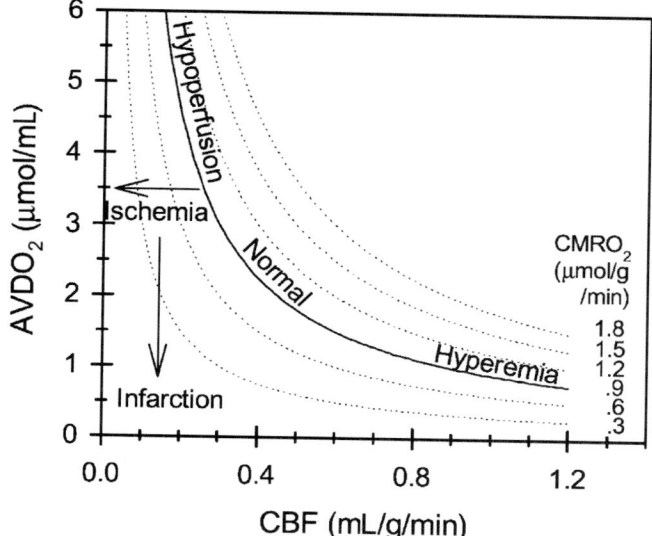

FIGURE 327–5. Changes in the cerebral arteriovenous oxygen difference (AVDO₂) as cerebral blood flow (CBF) falls. Initially, the decrease in CBF is compensated by increasing oxygen extraction (hypoperfusion). As CBF falls beyond the ability of the brain to compensate, cerebral metabolic rate of oxygen (CMRO₂) decreases (ischemia). If the CBF remains low for long enough, the tissue will become irreversibly injured (infarction). (From Robertson CS, Narayan RK, Gokaslan Z, et al: Cerebral arteriovenous oxygen difference as an estimate of cerebral blood flow in comatose patients. J Neurosurg 70:222–230, 1989.)

findings in patients with head injury; MCA flow velocity, measured by transcranial Doppler, and SjvO₂ decreased as CPP was reduced below 70 mm Hg.

Historical Aspects. When SjvO₂ was first sampled in the 1930s and 1940s, the jugular bulb was directly punctured by a needle inserted 1 cm below and anterior to the mastoid process.[130] More recently, placement of an internal jugular vein catheter, similar to the type used for central venous pressure monitoring but directed cephalad into the jugular bulb, has allowed repetitive sampling of SjvO₂ without repeated needle punctures.[59, 127, 131–133] Currently, the development of in vivo reflectance oximetry using fiber-optic catheters has allowed continuous monitoring of SjvO₂ without the need to sample blood, except for calibration purposes.[134–136]

Initial experiences with these types of monitors placed in the jugular bulb were unsatisfactory. However, the performance of newer catheters is much improved.[137–139] Figure 327–6 shows the close relationship between the catheter and blood sample measurement of SjvO₂ using one of these catheters.

Side of Catheterization. Early studies suggested that either jugular bulb would provide similar SjvO₂ information in most normal people. However, as early as 1945,[140] it was observed that in patients with focal lesions, there may be a significant difference in the oxygen saturation obtained in the right and left jugular bulbs. This occurs because there is often incomplete mixing of cerebral venous blood before the sagittal sinus divides into the right and left transverse sinuses.

Studies comparing bilateral measurements of SjvO₂ or comparing SjvO₂ to oxygen saturation in the confluence of the cerebral sinuses clearly show that when there are focal lesions after traumatic brain injury, there may be significant differences in the oxygen saturation measured in the left and right jugular bulbs.[141, 142] If the monitoring strategy is to use SjvO₂ as a monitor of global oxygenation, cannulating the dominant jugular vein is logical, because it will be most representative of the whole brain. However, if the strategy is to identify the most abnormal oxygen saturation, the recommendations of Metz and coworkers[142] should be followed.

Normal Values. Gibbs and colleagues[130] studied 50 normal young males and observed that their SjvO₂ ranged from 55% to 71% (mean, 61.8%). This is lower than normal mixed venous oxygen saturation, indicating that the brain normally extracts oxygen more completely from arterial blood than do many other organs. Simultaneous measurements of oxygen saturation in the jugular bulb and in the pulmonary artery clearly

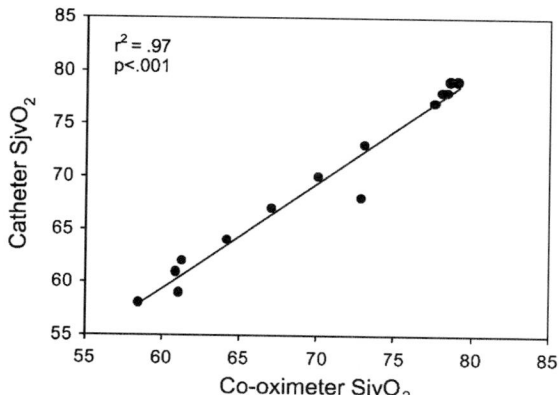

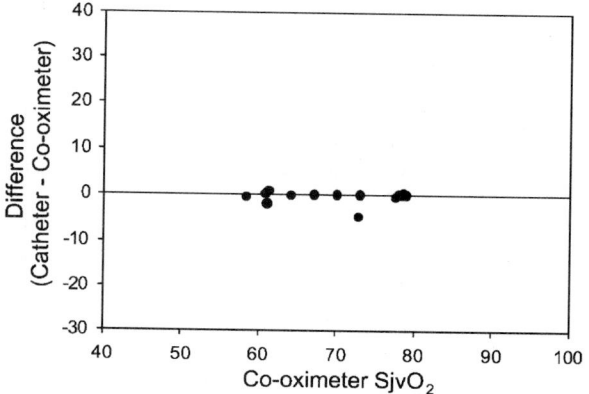

FIGURE 327–6. Bland-Altman plots of oximetry catheter data, showing good performance of the newer-generation jugular venous oxygen saturation (SjvO₂) catheter. (From Howard L, Gopinath SP, Uzura M, et al: Evaluation of a new fiberoptic catheter for monitoring jugular venous oxygen saturation. Neurosurgery 44:1280–1285, 1999.)

show that $SjvO_2$ cannot be predicted from mixed venous oxygen saturation.[143]

In head-injured patients, the average $SjvO_2$ is higher than normal, and the range for $SjvO_2$ is considerably wider than in normal subjects. In a series of 116 patients with continuous measurement of $SjvO_2$ for the first 5 to 10 days after a severe head injury, $SjvO_2$ averaged 68.1% ± 9.7% (range, 32% to 96%) in 1329 measurements. Jugular venous oxygen partial pressure averaged 37 ± 7 mm Hg (range, 22 to 85 mm Hg).[64]

Experimental studies have extensively examined the ischemic thresholds for CBF. Only a few studies have examined the $SjvO_2$ threshold associated with the depletion of energy stores in animals and with loss of consciousness or electroencephalographic changes during anoxia in normal humans. A summary of these studies is shown in Figure 327–7. From these studies, it appears that normal brain metabolism can be altered at $SjvO_2$ values less than 50% but that values less than 20% are required for irreversible ischemic injury.

Brain Tissue Po₂

The major limitation of $SjvO_2$ as a monitor of CBF adequacy is that regional ischemia cannot be identified. In circumstances such as brain trauma, when regional differences in CBF may occur, brain tissue Po_2 as a monitor of cerebral oxygenation may have an important advantage. The catheters for monitoring brain tissue Po_2 have only recently become available, but early studies suggest that this may become an important advance in brain monitoring.[144–147] Normal values for brain tissue Po_2 are 20 to 40 mm Hg, and

critical reductions are 8 to 10 mm Hg. Hoffman and coworkers[148] found that brain tissue Po_2 in patients with ischemia demonstrated by single photon emission CT averaged 10 ± 5 mm Hg, compared with 37 ± 12 mm Hg in normal brain. Valadka and colleagues[149] found that the likelihood of death following a severe head injury increased with a longer duration of brain tissue Po_2 less than 15 mm Hg and with any occurrence of brain tissue Po_2 less than 6 mm Hg. Kiening and associates[150] correlated serial measurements of both $SjvO_2$ and brain tissue Po_2 and found that an $SjvO_2$ of 50% in general correlates with a brain tissue Po_2 of 8.5 mm Hg.

Near-Infrared Spectroscopy

Measurements of cerebral oxygen saturation using near-infrared spectroscopy have been performed in head-injured patients.[151] However, a number of problems must be solved before this technology can be recommended for routine clinical use. The oxygen saturation measurements are not quantitative, and the importance of scalp contribution to the measurements is controversial. In adults, the contribution of extracerebral tissues to the signal is dependent on the separation of the light source and the sensor, as well as on the area of the skull monitored. One study suggested that with optode separations of less than 4 cm, extracerebral tissues may contribute the majority of the signal.[152] In head-injured patients, the presence of intracranial blood in the form of extracerebral collections or contusions can interfere with the measurements. The absorbance of near-infrared light by extravascular blood

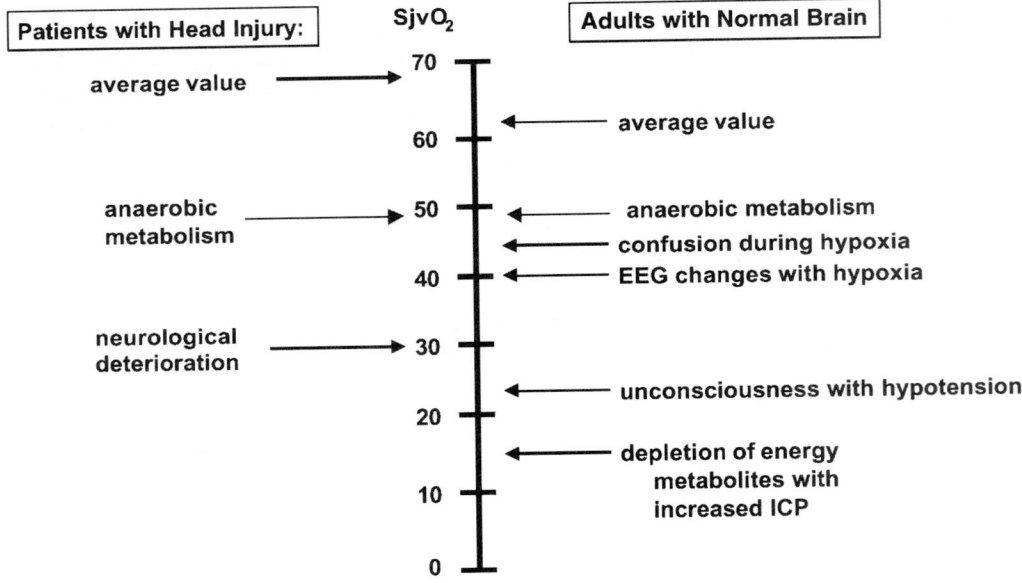

FIGURE 327–7. Thresholds for jugular venous oxygen saturation (SjvO₂) obtained from experimental and clinical studies. When the data were reported for oxygen content rather than SjvO₂, the SjvO₂ was calculated for a hemoglobin concentration of 10 g/dL. EEG, electroencephalogram; ICP, intracranial pressure. (Data from references 330–335.)

has been used to identify intracranial hematomas in head-injured patients.[153]

SUMMARY OF MONITORING OPTIONS

It is clear from the description of the available devices that none is ideal in the head injury setting. No single monitor gives continuous high-resolution regional CBF information. At present, a reasonable strategy is to use intermittent measurements of regional CBF, preferably by the stable xenon CT method, to obtain information about whether regional abnormalities of flow exist. If there are no hypoperfused regions, a global monitor, such as SjO_2, should suffice. If there are significant regional abnormalities of flow, it may be better to use brain tissue PO_2 or one of the local CBF probes as a local monitor of the hypoperfused area, in addition to a global monitor such as SjO_2.

Figure 327–8 illustrates how this strategy might be used to identify and guide the treatment of focal ischemia after a head injury. This patient was initially admitted with a subdural hematoma (see Fig. 327–8, left scan), which was evacuated promptly on arrival at the hospital. At surgery, a brain tissue PO_2 catheter was placed near contused brain underlying the evacuated hematoma. Initially, the brain tissue PO_2 was normal, but over postinjury hours 36 to 46, it gradually decreased to 5 mm Hg, with no change in any other physiologic parameters. Note that the SjO_2, which is a measure of global oxygenation, remained low-normal (~55%), despite the very low brain tissue PO_2, and that CPP was 65 to 70 mm Hg. Placing the patient on 100% oxygen raised the brain tissue PO_2 to 15 mm Hg (see Fig. 327–8, top graph). A computed tomographic scan (see Fig. 327–8, middle scan) showed increased swelling around the contusion, and a stable xenon computed tomographic scan showed a large area with regional CBF values less than 10 mL/100 g per minute at the contusion site. The patient was started on dopamine, and later phenylephrine was added to increase blood pressure. As CPP increased with this treatment, the brain tissue PO_2 returned to normal (see Fig. 327–8, bottom graph), and a repeat stable xenon computed tomographic scan (see Fig. 327–8, right scan) showed significant improvement in CBF.

In this case, the progressive focal ischemia in the area of the contusion could have been suspected based on the changing appearance of the computed tomographic scan; however, stable xenon CT and brain tissue PO_2 provided a convenient way to grasp the severity and extent of the ischemia, and the latter also provided a good method for following the effectiveness of treatments applied in the intensive care unit. The challenge with this monitoring strategy is to place the local monitor in an area of the brain that is vulnerable to developing ischemia.

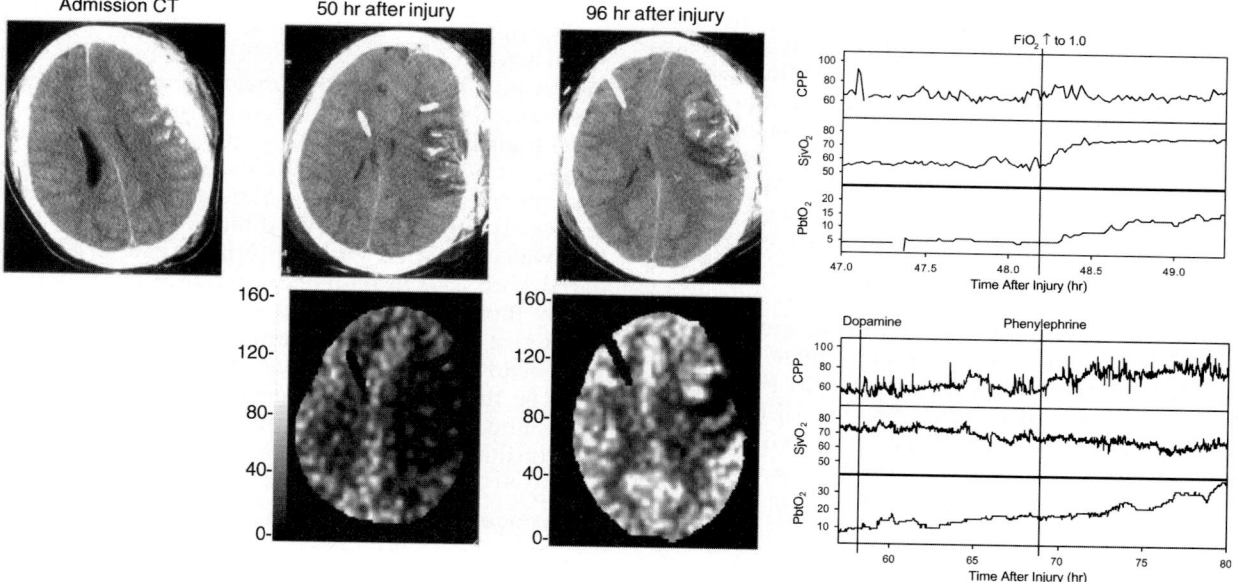

FIGURE 327–8. Example of focal ischemia identified and treated based on the oxygen partial pressure (PO_2) of brain tissue. This patient was admitted with a subdural hematoma *(left scan)*, which was evacuated promptly on arrival at the hospital. A brain tissue PO_2 catheter was placed near the contused brain underlying the evacuated hematoma. Initially, the brain tissue PO_2 was normal, but over postinjury hours 36 to 46, it gradually decreased to 5 mm Hg. Note that the jugular venous oxygen saturation (SjO_2), which is a measure of global oxygenation, remains low-normal despite the very low brain tissue PO_2; cerebral perfusion pressure (CPP) is 65 to 70 mm Hg. Placing the patient on 100% oxygen raised the brain tissue PO_2 to 15 mm Hg *(top graph)*. Computed tomography (CT) *(middle scan)* shows increased swelling around the contusion, and xenon CT shows a large area with regional cerebral blood flow values less than 10 mL/100 g per minute at the contusion site. The patient was started on dopamine, and later phenylephrine was added to increase blood pressure. As CPP increased with this treatment, the brain tissue PO_2 increased *(bottom graph)*, and repeat xenon CT *(right scan)* shows significant improvement in CBF.

Figure 327–9 outlines some areas of management that can be individualized based on knowledge of CBF or cerebral oxygenation. Much more work is needed to determine whether these changes will make a difference in outcome. However, Miller and coworkers[154] suggest that treatment of intracranial hypertension is more successful if it is directed at the underlying physiologic abnormalities.

Secondary Ischemic Insults

Secondary ischemic insults are global and usually transient. Therefore, a global but continuous measure of CBF adequacy, such as SjvO$_2$, is useful for monitoring for secondary insults. In addition, physiologic variables that are common causes of secondary ischemic insults should be monitored (Fig. 327–10).

CEREBRAL CAUSES

Intracranial Hypertension

Intracranial hypertension was the most common cause of jugular venous desaturation in a prospective study of 116 patients with severe head injury,[64] accounting for 44% of the total number of episodes. As discussed earlier, ICP should be monitored, preferably by ventriculostomy.

Seizures

Seizures can dramatically increase the cerebral metabolic rates of both oxygen and glucose. In rats whose seizures were induced by bicuculline, CMRO$_2$ was increased by 150% to 250%.[86] If CBF is marginal or uncoupled from cerebral metabolic rate, ischemia can occur during the seizure.

Seizures occur in approximately 15% of patients with head injury.[155] Because patients are often sedated and pharmacologically paralyzed to treat intracranial hypertension, clinical monitoring is not helpful. For this reason, continuous electroencephalographic monitoring may be useful for this high-risk group of patients.[156] Seizures are not a common cause of jugular venous desaturation, but as illustrated in Figure 327–10, they can significantly reduce SjvO$_2$ if CBF is unable to meet the increased cerebral metabolic requirements. Increases in extracellular glutamate have also been reported during post-traumatic seizures.[157]

SYSTEMIC CAUSES

Hypotension

Autoregulation is the ability of the brain to maintain a normal CBF over a wide range of blood pressures, normally from a mean blood pressure of 50 to 150 mm Hg. After a traumatic brain injury, the cerebral vasculature can lose the ability to autoregulate completely, causing the CBF to rise and fall with the blood pressure; alternatively, the lower limit of autoregulation, which is normally 50 mm Hg, can be shifted to a higher pressure. The consequence is that low blood

pressures that are normally tolerated without sequelae can result in cerebral ischemia after a traumatic brain injury. Lewelt and colleagues[128] showed in a fluid percussion injury model that autoregulation was severely impaired after both low-level and high-level injuries. In the cat, CBF is normally constant until CPP falls below 60 mm Hg. After the fluid percussion injury, CBF decreased proportionally to CPP below 80 mm Hg. Chan and associates[129] described similar findings in patients with head injury; MCA flow velocity measured by transcranial Doppler and SjvO$_2$ decreased as CPP was reduced below approximately 70 mm Hg.

Hypotension is common at the time head-injured patients are admitted to the hospital. The TCDB study of 717 patients[10] reported that 35% had a systolic blood pressure less than 90 mm Hg on arrival in the emergency room. Hypotension on admission increased the mortality rate by 150%. Miller and Becker[158] found in a group of 225 patients that a systolic blood pressure of less than 95 mm Hg on arrival in the emergency room was associated with a twofold increase in the mortality rate.

Hypotension is also common during hospitalization and is associated with a worse outcome. In another TCDB study,[159] 29% of patients had a systolic blood pressure of less than 90 mm Hg during their intensive care unit stay, which was associated with a significantly worse outcome. In a prospective study in which SjvO$_2$ was monitored in 116 patients,[64] hypotension was the third most common cause of jugular venous desaturation, accounting for 10% of the episodes. Marmarou and colleagues[106] analyzed 428 patients whose ICP, mean arterial pressure, and CPP were recorded hourly; the proportion of time that mean arterial pressure was less than 80 mm Hg was significantly related to poor neurological outcome. Pietropaoli and coworkers[160] observed in a study of 53 patients undergoing early surgery for traumatic intracranial hematomas that intraoperative hypotension (systolic blood pressure <90 mm Hg) was associated with a mortality rate of 82%, compared with 25% in patients without hypotension.

For these reasons, blood pressure is a particularly important physiologic parameter to monitor after severe head injury. Usually, an arterial catheter is indicated so that blood pressure can be monitored continuously, and the goal should be a mean arterial pressure greater than 80 to 90 mm Hg.

Hypocapnia

Induced hyperventilation constricts cerebral blood vessels, reducing global CBF and cerebral blood volume. The effect of changes in arterial PCO$_2$ on cerebral vessels is mediated by the change in pH induced in the extracellular fluid.[161] Carbon dioxide (CO$_2$) reactivity is preserved in most patients with severe head injury,[162] so hyperventilation can rapidly lower ICP through the reduction in cerebral blood volume. The effects of hyperventilation on ICP are immediate, but the duration of the effect is brief because the pH of the brain, at least in normal individuals, soon equilibrates to the lower arterial PCO$_2$ level. Hyperventilation clearly re-

CBF PATTERN

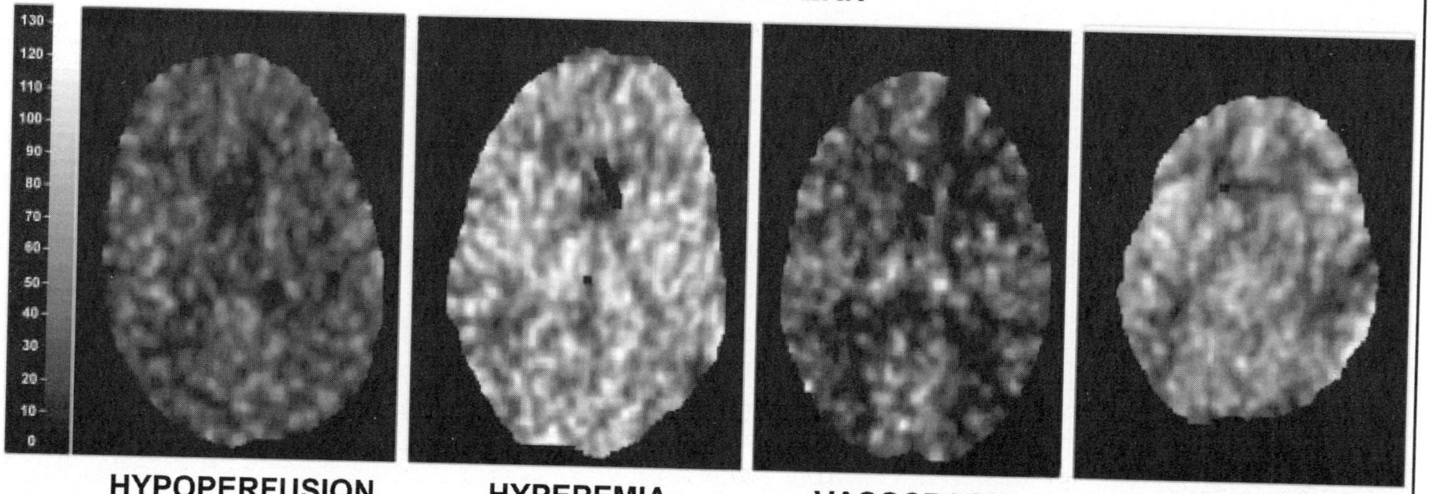

	HYPOPERFUSION	HYPEREMIA	VASOSPASM	CHRONIC STATE
MANAGEMENT IF ICP IS NORMAL:				
BP/CPP management	Optimize CPP (>70-80 mm Hg may be needed)	Normal CPP (50 mm Hg) may be adequate	Optimize CPP (>70-80 mm Hg may be needed)	Normal CPP
MANAGEMENT IF ICP IS INCREASED:				
BP/CPP management	Optimize CPP (>70-80 mm Hg may be needed)	Normal CPP (50 mm Hg) may be adequate and may reduce edema formation. High CPP (> 70-80 mm Hg) may reduce ICP if pressure autoregulation curve is shifted to the right	Optimize CPP (>70-80 mm Hg may be needed)	
Hyperventilation	Avoid	May hyperventilate ensuring that $SjvO_2$ does not fall <50 mm Hg	Avoid	
Mannitol	May be more effective than hypnotic agents if edema is cause of increased ICP. Decreases ICP if autoregulation intact, but increases CBF if autoregulation is impaired			
Barbiturate coma	May be effective if ICP is refractory and CO_2 reactivity is intact. May be more effective than mannitol if vascular engorgement is cause of increased ICP			

FIGURE 327-9. Summary of therapeutic decisions in which cerebral blood flow (CBF) information has implications for management of the individual head-injured patient. BP, blood pressure; CO_2, carbon dioxide; CPP, cerebral perfusion pressure; ICP, intracranial pressure; $SjvO_2$, jugular venous oxygen saturation. (From references 185, 187, 274, and 336.)

CEREBRAL CAUSES:	Example of SjvO₂ Tracings
Decreased oxygen delivery: Intracranial hypertension ---overall incidence in head injury = 50% ---incidence as a cause of secondary insults = 44% ---monitor = ventriculostomy ---therapeutic goal = ICP < 20-25 mm Hg	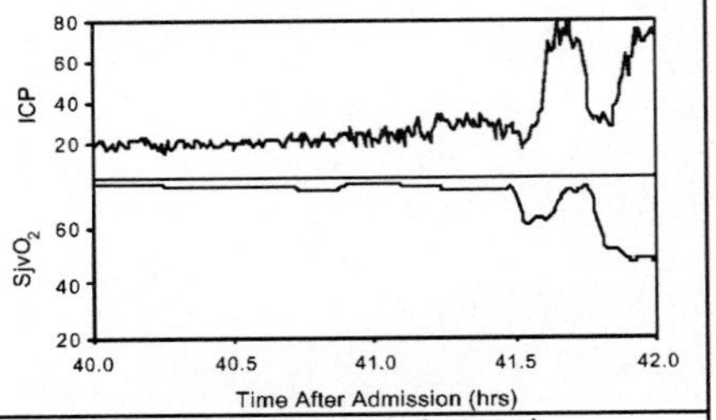
Increased oxygen consumption: Seizures ---overall incidence in head injury = 15% ---incidence as a cause of secondary insults < 1% ---monitor = clinical examination and EEG ---therapeutic goal = no seizures	(arrows indicate seizures)

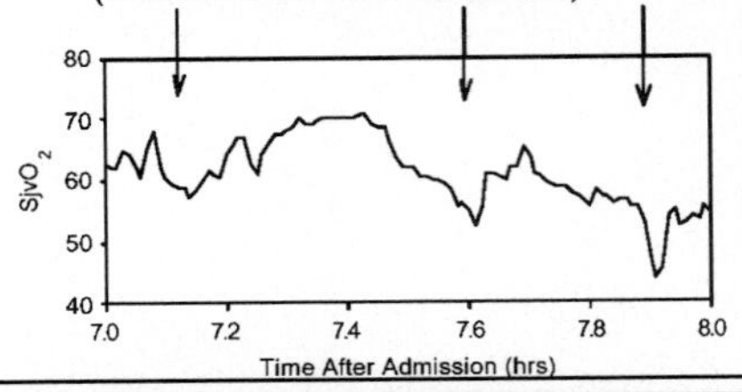

SYSTEMIC CAUSES:	Example of SjvO₂ Tracings
Decreased oxygen delivery: Hypotension ---overall incidence in head injury = 35% in ER = 29% in ICU ---incidence as a cause of secondary insults = 10% ---monitor = arterial catheter ---therapeutic goal = MAP > 80-90 mm Hg	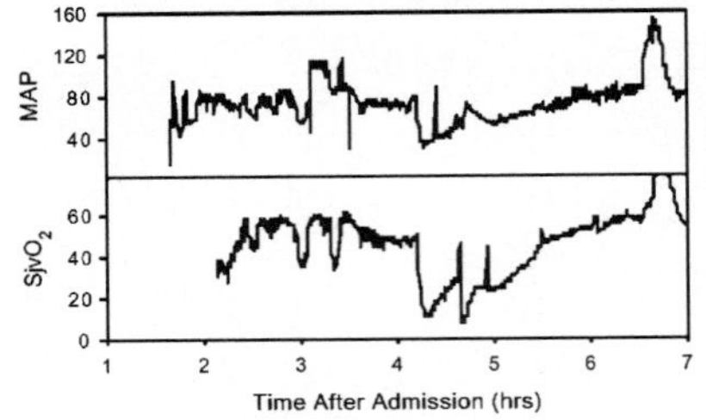
Hypocapnia ---overall incidence in head injury = 45% ---incidence as a cause of secondary insults = 36% ---monitor = end-tidal CO_2 ---therapeutic goal = end-tidal CO_2 35-40 mm Hg	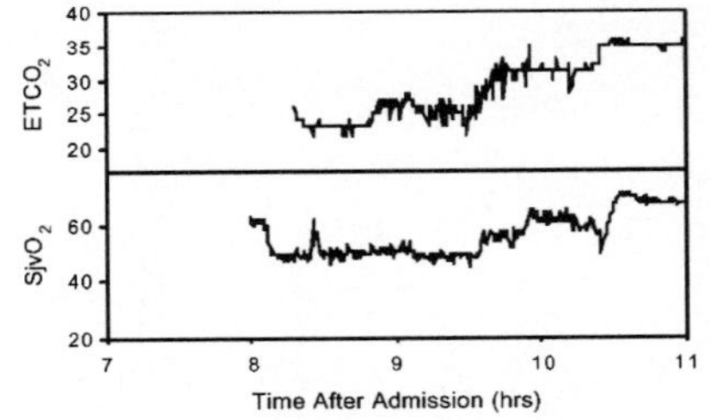
Hypoxia ---overall incidence in head injury = 19-35% in ER = 28% in ICU ---incidence as a cause of secondary insults = 8% ---monitor = pulse oximeter ---therapeutic goal = SaO_2 > 95%	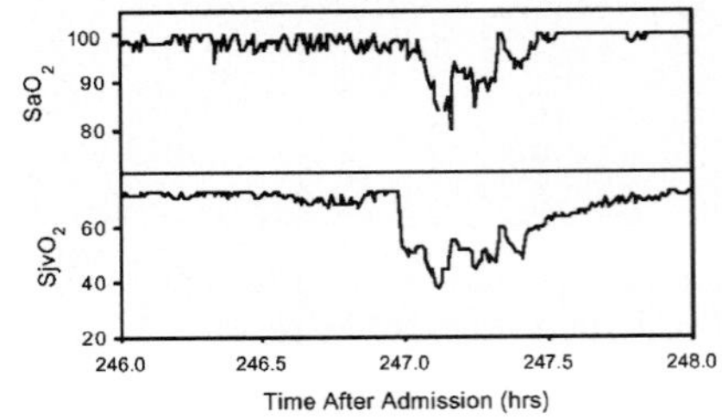
Increased oxygen delivery: Fever ---overall incidence in head injury =65% ---incidence as a cause of secondary insults < 1% ---monitor = rectal (± brain) temperature ---therapeutic goal = 37°C	

FIGURE 327–10. Physiologic parameters to monitor for secondary ischemic insults. CO_2, carbon dioxide; EEG, electroencephalogram; ER, emergency room; $ETCO_2$, end-tidal carbon dioxide concentration; ICP, intracranial pressure; ICU, intensive care unit; MAP, mean arterial pressure; SaO_2, oxygen concentration in arterial blood; $SjvO_2$, jugular venous oxygen saturation. (From references 10, 64, 158, and 159.)

duces ICP, but this potentially beneficial effect is at the expense of cerebral perfusion. Whether hyperventilation can actually result in cerebral ischemia in head-injured patients is controversial. However, several studies suggest that excessive hyperventilation after severe head injury can cause a secondary ischemic insult. In a prospective study in which $SjvO_2$ was monitored in 116 patients with severe head injury, hypocapnia was the second most common cause of jugular venous desaturation, accounting for 36% of the episodes.[64]

If areas of the brain that are marginally perfused have impaired CO_2 reactivity, hyperventilation might constrict the normal areas of the brain and actually improve perfusion to the marginally perfused areas. This has been termed the *inverse steal response*.[163] Cold[164, 165] conducted 45 paired studies of regional CBF before and after hyperventilation during days 1 to 3 after injury in 27 comatose patients and did not find this phenomenon. When the PCO_2 was reduced from 36 to 26 mm Hg, the proportion of regions with oligemia, defined as regional CBF less than 20 mL/100 g per minute, increased from 5% to 16%. Similarly, the proportion of regions with severe oligemia (regional CBF <15 mL/100 g per minute) increased from 0.1% to 0.3%. A low hemispheric CBF before hyperventilation predisposed to this increased frequency. Stringer and colleagues[166] measured regional CBF before and after hyperventilation in 12 patients with acute brain lesions using xenon CT. In five of the patients, hyperventilation induced ischemic levels of regional CBF in apparently normal regions of the brain. Five of the patients had ischemic areas that demonstrated the inverse steal response, that is, increases in regional CBF with hyperventilation.

End-tidal CO_2 is a convenient way to continuously estimate arterial PCO_2. In head-injured patients without pulmonary disease, end-tidal CO_2 correlates well with arterial PCO_2.[167] With pulmonary insufficiency, there may be large gradients between end-tidal CO_2 and arterial PCO_2, and arterial blood gases should be monitored instead. In the absence of intracranial hypertension, the goal should be to maintain a normal arterial PCO_2, carefully avoiding both hypo- and hypercapnia.

Hypoxia

Normally, a decrease in arterial PO_2 is compensated for by increases in CBF and does not result in a decrease in overall cerebral oxygen delivery, unless the hypoxia is very severe. At a fraction of inspired oxygen (FiO_2) of 0.10 (corresponding to a PO_2 of 40 mm Hg), CBF in normal adults is increased by 35%.[168] At an FiO_2 of 0.09 (PO_2 of 35 mm Hg), CBF is increased by 70%.[169] The increase in cerebral blood volume that results from the cerebral vasodilatation can markedly increase ICP, especially if intracranial compliance is decreased.[170] Nevertheless, the increase in CBF prevents cerebral ischemia from occurring.

Lewelt and colleagues[171] showed that traumatic brain injury impairs this normal CBF response to hypoxia. In a fluid percussion head injury model in cats,

a 1- to 2-atmosphere impact resulted in mild impairment of the cerebral vasodilator response to hypoxia. After an impact greater than 2 atmospheres, the cerebral vasodilator response to hypoxia was severely impaired; some animals had decreases in CBF in response to hypoxia. It is likely that this is one of the mechanisms whereby hypoxia increases the severity of traumatic injuries.

Pulmonary complications that can result in hypoxia are common after severe head injury. On a patient's arrival in the emergency room, hypoxia can be due to hypoventilation, obstruction of the airway, aspiration, or hemo- or pneumothorax. Hypoxia that persists after the initial resuscitation or develops within the first 24 to 48 hours after injury can be due to lung contusion, atelectasis, fat emboli, pneumonia, or adult respiratory distress syndrome. Piek and coworkers[159] reported that in the TCDB studies, pneumonia developed as a complication during hospitalization in 41% of patients, and pulmonary insufficiency occurred in 28%.

Several studies have investigated the effects of hypoxia after traumatic brain injury. In a prospective study in which $SjvO_2$ was monitored in 116 patients,[64] hypoxia was the fourth most common cause of jugular desaturation, accounting for 8% of the episodes. An example of this is illustrated in Figure 327–10. In a study of 225 patients, hypoxia, which was present in 35% of patients, increased the mortality rate from 24% to 50%; hypercarbia, present in 8% of patients, increased the mortality rate to 67%.[158] In another study, there was a 20% increase in the number of patients left vegetative or dead when the initial PO_2 was less than 60 mm Hg or the patient was apneic.[172] In the TCDB studies, the occurrence of hypoxia on admission significantly increased the mortality rate to 50%, compared with 27% for patients without hypoxia. The association remained significant when adjusted for age, diagnosis, GCS score, pupillary reactivity, and the presence of other causes of secondary injury, but hypoxia had less effect on outcome than did systemic hypotension.[10]

Pulmonary complications during the hospital course have also been associated with worse neurological outcomes. In the TCDB studies, the occurrence of pneumonia during hospitalization was significantly associated with an unfavorable outcome.[159]

Pulse oximetry is widely available and is a convenient way to monitor systemic oxygenation in patients with severe head injuries. The goal should be to maintain arterial oxygen saturation greater than 95%.

Anemia

The cerebrovascular effects of anemia have been studied extensively in normal experimental animals and normal humans. Until the decrease in CaO_2 is extreme, the primary mechanism for compensation for the decrease in CaO_2 is an increase in CBF.[173] In normal humans, normovolemic hemodilution sufficient to decrease the hematocrit by 26% resulted in a 19% increase in CBF.[174] As a consequence of the compensatory increase in CBF, $SjvO_2$ stays relatively constant with a normovolemic reduction in hemoglobin concentration. Only when the increase in CBF is no longer able to compensate for the reduction in CaO_2 does $SjvO_2$ decrease.

After head injury, however, the cerebral vasculature may not be capable of dilating in response to the drop in CaO_2, and ischemia may occur. DeWitt and associates[175] compared the effects of an acute hemorrhage of 30% of the total blood volume, followed by resuscitation with blood or hetastarch (hydroxyethylstarch), in normal cats and in cats with moderate fluid percussion injuries. The animals with head injuries had significantly lower blood pressure, CBF, and cerebral oxygen delivery than did the uninjured animals. Additionally, after head injury, the increase in CBF that results from anemia can increase ICP.

Hemoglobin concentration should be measured at least daily during the early phase after injury. In patients with multiple injuries, more frequent monitoring is often indicated.

Fever

Fever increases the body's metabolic rate by approximately 10% to 13% per degree Celsius. The effect of fever on $CMRO_2$ has been studied in neonatal pigs.[82] Increasing temperature from 38°C to 42°C increased CBF by 97% and $CMRO_2$ by 65%.

In experimental studies, moderate hyperthermia (39°C) results in more severe brain damage after fluid percussion injury,[176] and moderate hypothermia is protective.[177–179] Jones and colleagues[81] found a significant relationship between fever and poor neurological outcome.

Recently, it has been recognized that measuring rectal temperature alone may significantly underestimate the actual brain tissue temperature. In a study of seven neurosurgical patients, the temperatures of the lateral ventricle, epidural space, tympanic membrane, and rectum were measured.[180] More recently, intracranial temperature has been recorded in neurosurgical patients with a temperature probe incorporated into a standard ventriculostomy ICP monitor or with a separate temperature probe.[181–184] In these studies, intracranial temperature was 0.5°C to 2.0°C higher than body temperature (Fig. 327–11).

NEUROLOGICAL INTENSIVE CARE MANAGEMENT

Approaches to the Management of Traumatic Brain Injury

The traditional approach to the management of brain-injured patients is to control ICP using a stair-step approach, adding or subtracting therapies as needed. Traditionally, the therapies are added in an order that reflects the risk of complications associated with each therapy. Recently, however, several groups have advocated different overall approaches to the management of traumatic brain injury. These approaches are based on an understanding of certain aspects of the pathophysiology of traumatic brain injury and on favorable clinical experiences with these approaches. None of these approaches has strong clinical data to support its superiority over the others.

One approach, called CPP management, has been advocated by Rosner and coworkers.[185] It is based on a concept called the vasodilatory cascade, diagrammed in Figure 327–12. According to this hypothesis, a reduction in CPP—either a decrease in blood pressure or an

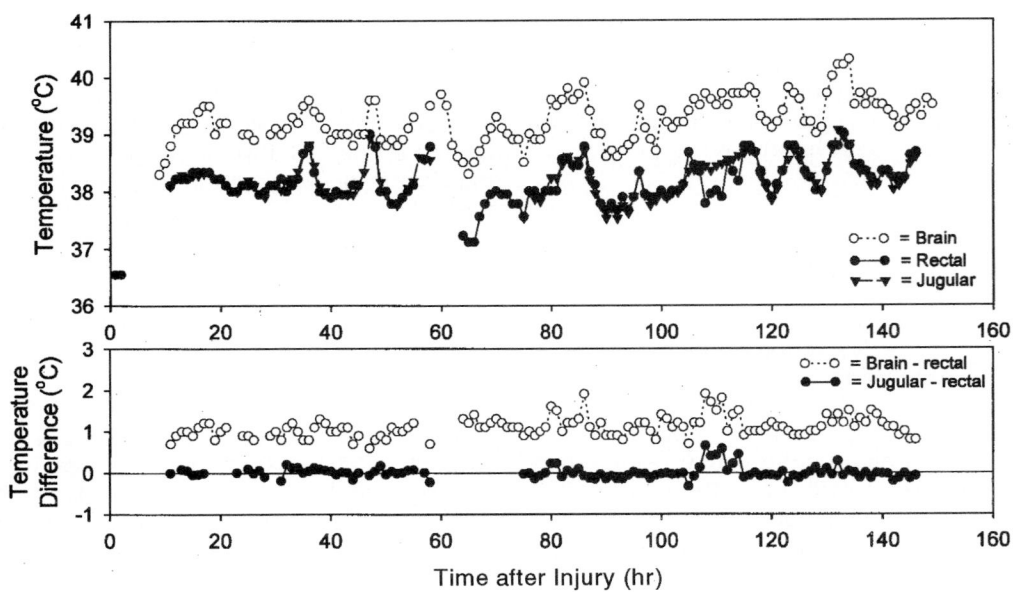

FIGURE 327–11. Example of brain temperature measurements in a patient with severe head injury. (From Rumana CS, Gopinath SP, Uzura M, et al: Brain temperature exceeds rectal temperature in head-injured patients. Crit Care Med 26:562–567, 1998.)

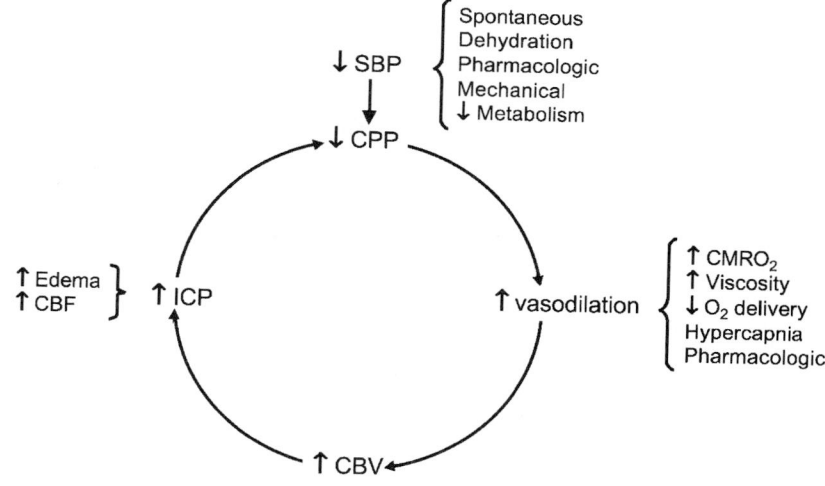

FIGURE 327–12. The vasodilatory cascade. CBF, cerebral blood flow; CBV, cerebral blood volume; $CMRO_2$, cerebral metabolic rate of oxygen; CPP, cerebral perfusion pressure; ICP, intracranial pressure; O_2, oxygen; SBP, systolic blood pressure. (From Rosner MJ, Rosner SD, Johnson AH: Cerebral perfusion pressure: Management protocol and clinical results. J Neurosurg 83:949–962, 1995.)

increase in ICP—stimulates the cerebral vessels to dilate in an attempt to maintain CBF. This is the normal autoregulatory response to a decrease in CPP. Because the increase in cerebral blood volume that accompanies vasodilatation further reduces CPP, this sets up a cycle that leads to ever-reducing CPP. An increase in blood pressure breaks the cycle and reduces ICP. In a clinical series of 158 patients admitted to the hospital with GCS scores less than 7, mortality was 29%, and 59% of patients achieved a good recovery or had only moderate disability by 6 months after injury.[185] This approach has been widely adapted, and it was included in the 1996 head injury guidelines as an option.[13]

A recent randomized clinical trial evaluated a treatment strategy that is similar but not identical to the CPP management approach.[186] This trial compared a CBF-targeted strategy with a conventional ICP-targeted strategy in the initial management of acute traumatic brain injury. The CBF-targeted treatment, in which CPP was kept at 70 mm Hg or greater and hyperventilation was not used, reduced the incidence of secondary ischemic events by approximately 50%. However, this treatment strategy also increased the incidence of adult respiratory distress syndrome fivefold and did not improve long-term neurological outcome. One interpretation of this study is that the beneficial effect of the CBF-targeted treatment was offset by systemic complications associated with maintaining blood pressure at an elevated level.

Another approach, called the Lund therapy, emphasizes a reduction in microvascular pressures to minimize edema formation in the brain (Fig. 327–13). The goals of this approach are to preserve a normal colloid osmotic pressure (by infusion of albumin and red blood cells), reduce capillary hydrostatic pressure by reducing systemic blood pressure (with metoprolol and clonidine), and reduce cerebral blood volume by vasoconstricting precapillary resistance vessels (using low-dose thiopental and dihydroergotamine). Treatments that would favor increasing transcapillary filtration of fluid

are avoided, including CSF drainage, high-dose (to burst suppression) barbiturates, osmotic diuretics, and high CPP. Decompressive craniectomy, which can also increase edema formation, is reserved as a last resort after all other treatments have failed. A detailed description of this approach is given in two recent publications, including a report of a clinical series in which mortality was reduced to 8% and 80% of patients had a good recovery or only moderate disability 6 months postinjury after institution of these measures.[187, 188]

A final approach has been to try to match the treatment to the underlying pathophysiology. In this approach, it is emphasized that traumatic brain injury is heterogeneous, and each individual patient has a predominant pathophysiologic pattern. In addition, it recognizes that the pathophysiology of traumatic brain injury evolves over time, and treatment that is appropriate in the first few hours after injury may not necessarily be optimal 2 to 3 days after injury.

All these approaches have some physiologic basis for their use, but no studies have demonstrated the superiority of any one approach, and caution should be used when comparing the results of these clinical

$$Jv = K_f[(P_c - P_i) - \sigma(\pi_p - \pi_i)]$$

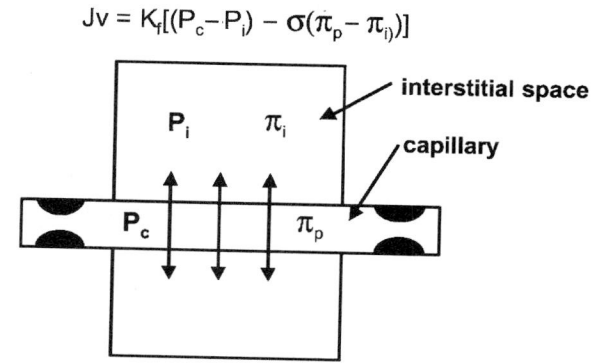

FIGURE 327–13. Forces that govern edema formation in the brain.

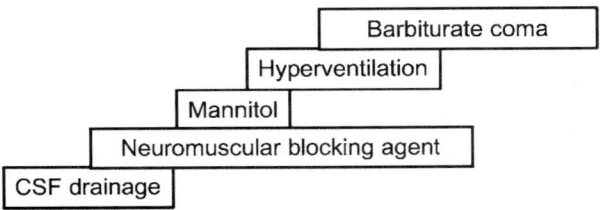

FIGURE 327–14. Traditional stair-step treatment of intracranial hypertension. CSF, cerebrospinal fluid.

series, which may not be comparable. It seems logical that individualized therapy based on underlying pathology would be the most successful. For example, in the first few hours after injury, when hypoperfusion is prominent, attention to maintaining adequate CPP may be beneficial. Later, when edema, resulting in intracranial hypertension, becomes the predominant pathophysiology, a strategy to minimize cerebral hydrostatic pressures may be beneficial. Much more work needs to be done to clarify these issues. For the purpose of this text, the traditional approach is described (Fig. 327–14), but differences in the various approaches are outlined in Table 327–5.

General Measures to Minimize Intracranial Hypertension and Improve Cerebral Perfusion

In all patients with severe head injury, simple measures should be taken to minimize systemic factors that can cause or aggravate intracranial hypertension and that impair cerebral perfusion. Commonly recommended practices include elevation of the head 15 to 30 degrees, sedation, airway protection or controlled ventilation, seizure prophylaxis, and treatment of systemic hypertension and fever when present. In addition, general supportive care should be given, including appropriate fluid and electrolytes, nutritional support, and prophylaxis for gastric ulceration and thromboembolism.

VENOUS OUTFLOW RESISTANCE

Elevating the head of the bed and keeping the head in a neutral position to minimize compression of venous return from the brain were standard practices for the management of ICP. However, the ideal head position for patients with head injuries has been disputed in recent years. Rosner and Coley advocated keeping the patient's head flat, as part of an overall treatment program intended to maximize CPP.[189, 190] Other studies showed a reduction in ICP without a reduction in either CPP or CBF in most patients when the head was elevated to 30 degrees.[191–193] In 22 patients with severe head injury, elevation of the head to 30 degrees reduced ICP and blood pressure without changing CPP or CBF in most patients.[192] Meixensberger and associates[193] observed that elevating the head 30 degrees reduced ICP and increased CPP but did not change brain tissue Po$_2$. Therefore, unless the patient is hypovolemic and head elevation results in hypotension, the reduction in ICP afforded by 15 to 30 degrees of head elevation is probably advantageous. If head elevation is used, it is im-

T A B L E   3 2 7 – 5 ■ **Management Approaches to Head-Injured Patients**

	MANAGEMENT APPROACH			
TREATMENT	**Traditional**	**CPP Management**	**Lund Therapy**	**Individualized Therapy**
Head position	15°–30° elevation	Flat	Flat	Whatever position gives best CPP and ICP
Sedation	Morphine + lorazepam	None	Low-dose thiopental	Morphine + lorazepam
Treatment of systemic hypertension	Treat SBP >160 mm Hg using labetalol	No	Metoprolol + clonidine	Ischemia/hypoperfusion pattern: don't treat Adequate perfusion: may treat with labetalol
Nutritional support	Yes, avoid hyperglycemia	No	Yes, avoid hyperglycemia	Yes, avoid hyperglycemia
Neuromuscular blockade	Yes	Yes	No	Yes
Hyperventilation	Yes	No	No	Ischemia/hypoperfusion pattern: don't use Adequate perfusion: may use
CSF drainage	Yes	Yes	No	Yes
Osmotherapy	Yes	Yes	No	Hypoperfusion/edema pattern: yes Hyperemia/vascular engorgement pattern: no
Barbiturate coma	Yes	No	No	Hypoperfusion/edema pattern: no Hyperemia/vascular engorgement pattern: yes

CPP, cerebral perfusion pressure; CSF, cerebrospinal fluid; ICP, intracranial pressure; SBP, systolic blood pressure.
From references 154, 185, 187, 304.

portant to remember that both the ICP and the blood pressure transducers should be zeroed at the same level, that is, at the level of the foramen of Monro.[189]

In multiple trauma patients, abdominal injury may be present, and increased intra-abdominal pressure may impede venous return from the brain, decrease blood pressure, and increase ICP. Experimental and clinical studies suggest that abdominal decompression can significantly improve control of ICP when abdominal compartment syndrome is present.[194, 195]

SEDATION AND ANALGESIA

Sedative and analgesic drugs blunt the effect of routine nursing care on ICP. In general, the benzodiazepines cause a coupled reduction in $CMRO_2$ and CBF, with no effect on ICP; the narcotics have no effect on $CMRO_2$ or CBF but have been reported to increase ICP in some patients.[196, 197] A combination of morphine and lorazepam is a frequently used regimen that is well tolerated and provides good sedation and analgesia.

In choosing a sedative agent for a head-injured patient, it is important to avoid drugs with hypotensive side effects (Table 327–6). Hypovolemia predisposes to hypotensive side effects of sedatives, and this should be remedied before administering sedative agents. Propofol has the advantage of a short half-life, which allows intermittent neurological examination, but it is a potent systemic vasodilator and can cause hypotension that exceeds the reduction in ICP, so that CPP can be significantly reduced.[198]

SYSTEMIC HYPERTENSION

Systemic hypertension associated with head injury is common and is characterized by a systolic blood pressure increase that is greater than the diastolic increase. It is associated with a hyperdynamic state, including tachycardia and increased cardiac output. Systemic hypertension is associated with sympathetic hyperactivity.[199] It is unwise to reduce systemic blood pressure in patients with hypertension associated with untreated intracranial mass lesions, because cerebral perfusion is being maintained by the higher blood pressure. Treatment of systemic hypertension (systolic blood pressure >160 mm Hg) during the postoperative course after a head injury is recommended by many neurosurgeons. Because autoregulation is frequently impaired after severe head injury, systemic hypertension may increase CBF and ICP[200] and may exacerbate cerebral edema.[201] However, this is a controversial issue, and others have emphasized the importance of maintaining CPP, even at the expense of a higher ICP.[190, 202]

If hypertension is treated in a head-injured patient, the choice of antihypertensives is important (Table 327–7). Systemic hypertension often resolves with sedation. If antihypertensive drugs are required, vasodilating drugs, including hydralazine, nicardipine, and nitroprusside, consistently increase ICP.[203, 204] Sympathomimetic-blocking antihypertensive drugs, such as beta-blocking drugs (propanolol, esmolol, labetalol) or centrally acting α-receptor agonists (clonidine, alpha-methyldopa), are preferred because they reduce blood pressure without affecting ICP.[199] The effects of labetalol and hydralazine on ICP and CBF in hypertensive head-injured patients have been compared.[205] Although both drugs reduced blood pressure by approximately 20 mm Hg, ICP increased from 16 ± 1 to 24 ± 1 mm Hg with hydralazine but did not significantly change with labetalol. The increase in ICP with hydralazine was accompanied by an increase in CBF and a decrease in cerebrovascular resistance and $AVDO_2$. In addition, the systemic cardiovascular abnormalities resolved with labetalol but were exaggerated with hydralazine. Agents with a short half-life have an advantage when the blood pressure is labile.

AIRWAY PROTECTION AND CONTROLLED VENTILATION

Patients in coma cannot protect their airways and should be intubated to prevent aspiration and airway

T A B L E 327–6 ■ Cerebrovascular Effects of Sedative and Analgesic Agents

DRUG	INITIAL IV DOSE	MAINTENANCE DOSE	EFFECT ON BP	EFFECT ON ICP	EFFECT ON CBF
Benzodiazepines[305–308]					
Diazepam	0.1–0.2 mg/kg		Decrease	No change	Decrease
Lorazepam	0.04 mg/kg		Decrease	No change	Decrease
Midazolam	0.025–0.35 mg/kg	0.05–5 μg/kg/min	Decrease	No change or decrease	Decrease
Narcotics[196,197,809–312]					
Morphine	2–5 mg	2–5 mg/hr	Decrease	Increase	No change
Fentanyl	25–50 mg	50–100 μg/hr	Decrease	Increase	No change
Alfentanil	10–15 μg/kg	0.5–3 μg/kg/min	Decrease	Increase	No change
Sufentanil	0.2–0.6 μg/kg	0.01–0.05 μg/kg/min	Decrease	Increase	No change
Others[313,314]					
Propofol	1–2 mg/kg	5–50 μg/kg/min	Decrease	Decrease	Decrease
Etomidate	0.3–0.4 mg/kg		Decrease	Decrease	Decrease

BP, blood pressure; CBF, cerebral blood flow; ICP, intracranial pressure; IV, intravenous.

T A B L E   3 2 7 – 7 ■ **Cerebrovascular Effects of Antihypertensive Agents**

DRUG	LOADING DOSE	MAINTENANCE DOSE	EFFECT ON ICP	EFFECT ON CBF
Sympathetic Blocking Agents[199,315–317]				
Labetalol	5–20 mg	2–3 mg/min	No change	No change
Esmolol	500 μg/kg	50–200 μg/kg/min	No change	No change
Propranolol	1–3 mg	3–8 mg/hr	No change	No change
Clonidine		0.1–0.3 mg q12h PO	No change	No change
Trimethaphan		1–15 mg/min	No change	No change
Vasodilating Agents[203,204,318]				
Nicardipine		5–15 mg/hr	Increase	Increase
Nifedipine		10–20 mg q8h	Increase	Increase
Nitroprusside		0.5–10 μg/kg/min	Increase	Increase
Hydralazine		10–25 mg q4h	Increase	Increase

CBF, cerebral blood flow; ICP, intracranial pressure; PO, by mouth.

obstruction. Respiratory dysfunction, reported by clinical observations and measured by abnormal blood gas values, is common after head injury. In a series of 225 patients with severe head injury, hypoxia ($PO_2 < 60$ mm Hg) was seen on admission to the hospital in 35% of patients, and hypercarbia was present in 8%.[158] Kohi and associates[206] found that 36% of 67 comatose head-injured patients had either hypoxia ($PO_2 < 65$ mm Hg) or severe respiratory dysfunction requiring mechanical ventilation on admission. In another study, 9% of 363 patients admitted in coma due to head injury were hypoxic (cyanotic or $PO_2 < 60$ mm Hg) on admission.[207] In the TCDB studies, hypoxia was present in 19% of comatose head-injured patients upon arrival in the emergency room.[10] Pneumonia developed as a complication during hospitalization in 41%, and pulmonary insufficiency occurred in 28%.[159]

Following experimental impact and missile head injury, an increasing duration of apnea has been observed with increasing severity of brain injury.[208, 209] Immediate deaths in these models are usually caused by apnea. There is little information on apnea after human head injury, probably because the actual impact is typically not observed. Apnea at the scene of the accident, lasting for 3 and 12 minutes, respectively, was reported in two patients who eventually recovered well with the early institution of cardiopulmonary resuscitation and artificial ventilation.[210] Pfenninger and colleagues[211] measured arterial blood gases before resuscitation at the scene of the accident (6 to 21 minutes after injury) in 33 patients with head injuries. An elevated PCO_2, suggesting apnea or hypoventilation, was strongly correlated with severity of injury in these patients. These studies suggest that apnea probably occurs in human head injury similar to that observed in experimental models.

North and Jennett[212] examined the breathing patterns in 227 spontaneously breathing patients with neurosurgical diagnoses, most commonly trauma. Sixty percent of the patients had some type of breathing abnormality, including periodic respirations, tachypnea, and irregular breathing. All 12 patients with medullary lesions had abnormal breathing patterns, and 8 of these had irregular breathing. In contrast, periodic breathing was not correlated with any particular anatomic site of neurological injury.

Treatment of these ventilatory abnormalities during the acute phase after injury consists of controlled ventilation to prevent rapid changes in PCO_2. Sedation and occasionally paralysis may be necessary to control ventilation. Hypoxia and hypercarbia can dramatically raise ICP. Patients with severe head injury can have periodic episodes of hypoventilation that precipitate episodes of intracranial hypertension; controlled ventilation helps prevent these episodes. Early tracheostomy in patients who remain ventilator dependent has been shown to reduce the length of stay in the intensive care unit.[213]

FEVER

Fever is common during recovery from a head injury. In experimental studies, postinjury fever worsens the outcome from fluid percussion injury.[176] Fever is a potent cerebral vasodilator and can raise ICP. In addition, fever can raise cerebral metabolic requirements. Elevated rectal temperatures should be treated with antipyretics, cooling blankets, or both. Infectious causes of fever should be investigated with appropriate cultures and treated with antibiotics.

SEIZURES

The risk of post-traumatic seizure is approximately 15% with severe head injury.[155] The risk of seizures is related to the severity of injury. In a study of 4541 patients with head injuries, the standardized incidence ratio for developing seizures was 1.5 after mild injuries, with no increase over the expected number after 5 years; 2.9 after moderate injuries; and 17.0 after severe injuries. In the multivariate analysis, significant risk factors for later seizures were brain contusion with subdural hematoma, skull fracture, loss of consciousness or amnesia for more than 1 day, and age 65 years or older.[214]

The use of anticonvulsants to prevent seizures is

controversial. Although seizures can dramatically increase the cerebral metabolic rate, there is no clear relationship between the occurrence of early seizures and a worse neurological outcome.[215] Young and co-workers[216] found no difference in the incidence of seizures with prophylactically administered phenytoin. Tempkin and colleagues[217] reported results from a double-blind study in which 404 severely head-injured patients randomly received phenytoin or placebo for 1 year. Phenytoin reduced the incidence of seizures during the first week but not thereafter. Therefore, it is reasonable to give all severely head-injured patients in the emergency room phenytoin 15 mg/kg intravenously at a rate that does not exceed 25 mg/minute, followed by a daily maintenance dose adjusted to keep plasma levels in the therapeutic range. If no early seizures occur, phenytoin can be tapered and discontinued after 1 week.

Other General Measures

THROMBOEMBOLISM PROPHYLAXIS

Venous thromboembolism is a common complication after major trauma, with an observed incidence as high as 58% if prophylaxis is not used.[218] In the general trauma population, risk factors for thromboembolism include spinal cord injury; pelvic, femur, or tibia fracture; surgery; blood transfusion; and older age.[218] In some studies, head injury is also a risk factor.[219, 220]

Both venous compression devices and low-dose heparin are effective in reducing the risk of thromboembolism and subsequent pulmonary embolism. Dennis and associates[219] found that the incidence of thromboembolism decreased from 8.98% to 2.9% with prophylactic treatment. Both low-dose heparin and sequential venous compression prophylaxis were equally effective in this study. Because traumatic brain injury may be a relative contraindication to anticoagulation, sequential compression devices are preferred by many.[221] The use of prophylactic vena cava filters in high-risk patients is controversial, and this type of prophylaxis has long-term consequences that are probably not outweighed by the small increase in protection against pulmonary embolism.[220, 222]

GASTRIC ULCER PROPHYLAXIS

Stress ulcers are a common complication in critically ill patients. Endoscopic evidence of mucosal damage can appear within 24 hours of a severe brain injury, and 17% of these early erosions can progress to clinically significant hemorrhage.[223] The major risk factor for the development of gastric bleeding is the severity of the brain lesion.[223] Other common risk factors in trauma patients include burns greater than 25% of body surface area, respiratory failure, hypotension, sepsis, jaundice, peritonitis, coagulopathy, and hepatic failure.[224]

The mechanism of stress ulceration is not completely understood, but increased gastric acidity plays a major role. Studies have suggested that intracranial injury, particularly involving the diencephalon and brainstem, results in increased production of gastrin and gastric acid.[225–227] In a study of high-risk postoperative neurosurgical patients, the major risk factors were a gastric pH less than 4 and a high daily volume of gastric output.[228]

Prevention of stress ulceration has traditionally been directed at neutralization of gastric acid or reduction of gastric acid production with H_2 blockers. Both methods have been shown to be effective in reducing the incidence of gastric bleeding, but the administration of antacids, which is most effective if titrated to stomach pH, is more time-consuming.[228, 229] H_2 blockers, however, can have central nervous system effects that may be troublesome in neurosurgical patients.

One potential side effect common to both these preventive strategies is an increase in the risk of nosocomial pneumonia, probably as a result of aspiration of colonized gastric secretions. When gastric pH is greater than 4, bacterial colonization of the stomach occurs. This may result in an increase in the incidence of nosocomial pneumonia, although the data are conflicting. Sucralfate, which is a complex of sucrose, sulfates, and aluminum hydroxide, is an alternative that does not work by decreasing gastric acidity; rather, it strengthens the gastric mucosa and increases mucosal blood flow. Sucralfate has been demonstrated to be at least as effective as antacids in preventing clinical gastric bleeding.[229]

PROPHYLACTIC ANTIBIOTICS

In a study of post-traumatic bacterial meningitis, the incidence of meningitis was found to be 18% and 9% when associated with otorrhea and rhinorrhea, respectively, compared with 0.38% in the absence of a CSF leak.[230] Tenney[231] found a higher risk of infection with rhinorrhea than with otorrhea. The organisms causing post-traumatic meningitis are evenly divided between gram-positive and gram-negative organisms.[232] The efficacy of prophylactic antibiotics in patients with traumatic CSF fistula is controversial. Antibiotics are recommended only when symptoms or signs of meningitis develop.

NUTRITIONAL SUPPORT

Patients with severe head injury are hypermetabolic and catabolic, similar to patients with multiple trauma.[233] A number of studies have measured protein and caloric requirements in head-injured patients.[234] In these studies, caloric expenditure after traumatic brain injury averages 140% of normal resting energy expenditure, based on age, gender, and body size. Resting energy expenditure (REE) can be calculated from the Harris Benedict equation:

$$\text{REE (men)} = 66.47 + 13.75 \times \text{weight [kg]} + 5.00 \times \text{height [cm]} - 6.76 * \text{age [years]}$$

$$\text{REE (women)} = 655.10 + 9.56 \times \text{weight [kg]} + 1.85 \times \text{height [cm]} - 4.68 * \text{age [years]}$$

For a 70-kg, 25-year-old man, normal resting energy

expenditure is 1700 kcal/day. The projected caloric expenditure is 2400 kcal/day. In patients who are paralyzed or in barbiturate coma, caloric expenditure is 100% to 120% of normal resting levels. The average nitrogen loss for a head-injured patient is 0.2 g/kg per day, or 14 g/day in a 70-kg man. This is two to three times the normal fasting nitrogen loss and can result in a 10% decrease in lean body mass in 1 week.

These projected losses should be replaced, preferably with enteral feedings, beginning as soon as possible, but certainly within 72 hours after injury. The goal should be to gradually increase feedings and be at full caloric replacement by the end of the first week after injury. As the rate of enteral feedings is increased, maintenance fluids should be decreased to maintain a balance between total fluid input and output.

Enteral feedings are preferable to parenteral feedings because gut integrity is better maintained, which may reduce the risk of sepsis.[235, 236] If gastric emptying is impaired, feeding via jejunal tube is usually successful.[237, 238] In the more chronic phase, percutaneous gastrostomies are a safe and effective method of establishing a permanent route for enteral feeding and are less costly than open gastrostomies.[239]

MANAGEMENT OF FLUID AND ELECTROLYTES

Electrolyte abnormalities are common in patients with head injuries, occurring at least once during the hospital course of 59% of the TCDB patients.[159] Abnormalities in sodium, both hyponatremia and hypernatremia, are among the most common. Hyperglycemia is also common and is part of the stress response to injury. Meticulous attention should be paid to fluid administration and fluid balance.

Maintenance Fluids

After resuscitation, maintenance fluids, usually 0.9% normal saline, should be given at 35 mL/kg per day.

Additional fluids may be needed to replace fluid losses from nasogastric aspiration or other drains.

Hyponatremia Syndromes

The differential diagnosis of hyponatremia in head trauma patients usually consists of two entities—the syndrome of inappropriate antidiuretic hormone secretion (SIADH) and cerebral salt wasting (Fig. 327–15). The diagnosis of SIADH requires the following: hyponatremia (serum sodium < 135 mEq/L), hypo-osmolarity (serum osmolarity < 280 mOsm/L), urine osmolarity greater than serum osmolarity, and inappropriately high urine sodium (>40 mEq/L). Patients with SIADH are normovolemic or slightly volume expanded. In contrast, patients with salt-wasting syndrome are hypovolemic. Cerebral salt wasting also results in a high urine sodium (>40 mEq/L). The volume status is the critical clinical distinction between the two syndromes. SIADH is caused by enhanced secretion of antidiuretic hormone (ADH), and cerebral salt wasting is caused by elevated levels of circulating natriuretic factors, possibly including atrial natriuretic factor.

For SIADH, fluid restriction is the primary treatment. Limiting fluid intake to 800 to 1000 mL/day results in a steady rise in serum sodium concentration. If fluid restriction is impractical, which is often the case in critically ill patients, demeclocycline is an alternative. Demeclocycline is an antibiotic that inhibits ADH's action on the collecting duct of the kidney, producing a water diuresis. For patients with severe hyponatremia or significant symptoms, such as seizures or increased ICP, hypertonic (3%) saline may be administered slowly. Concomitant administration of furosemide can reduce the risk of producing hypervolemia and also increase the free water diuresis.

For salt-wasting syndrome, replacement of intravascular volume with normal saline is the initial treatment.

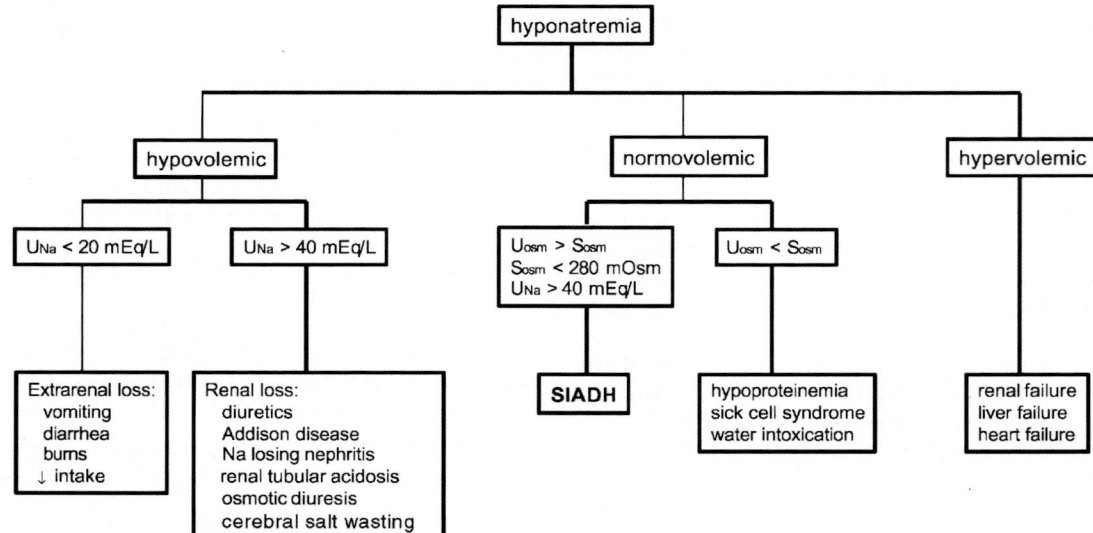

FIGURE 327–15. In head-injured patients, most hyponatremia can be attributed to either cerebral salt wasting or the syndrome of inappropriate antidiuretic hormone secretion (SIADH).

Sodium deficits then continue to be replaced with normal or hypertonic saline. Sodium losses in the urine may be replaced in the more chronic phase with enterally administered salt tablets.

Hypernatremia: Diabetes Insipidus

Diabetes insipidus occurs when there are inadequate circulating quantities of ADH, which results in an inability to concentrate urine. The free water loss causes a hypovolemic hypernatremia. Diabetes insipidus generally results from disruption of the hypothalamic-hypophyseal axis, which in a patient with severe brain injury is usually a grave prognostic sign.

Mild to moderate forms of diabetes insipidus can be treated with water replacement. However, in head-injured patients, administration of large volumes of free water may exacerbate intracranial hypertension. In this circumstance, intravenous administration of aqueous desmopressin acetate 2 to 4 μg decreases free water clearance for 8 to 12 hours. This dose can be repeated as needed.

Hypernatremia in a patient with severe intracranial hypertension is a particularly difficult problem. Correction of the hypernatremia can significantly exacerbate the intracranial hypertension, so it should be done slowly over 48 hours.

Hyperglycemia

Hyperglycemia has been associated with poor neurological outcome after traumatic brain injury.[240, 241] Part of this association is because hyperglycemia is a usual feature of the stress response to injury and simply reflects the occurrence of a severe injury. However, experimental studies show that hyperglycemia can worsen the outcome from a traumatic injury, especially when a secondary insult occurs.[242, 243] Therefore, part of the association may be hyperglycemia's tendency to exacerbate the secondary injury process.

Hyperglycemia should be avoided during the early postinjury period. Maintenance and replacement intravenous fluids should be glucose free if possible. Blood glucose levels should be checked periodically, and glucose concentrations greater than 200 mg/dL should be treated with appropriate doses of insulin.

Timing of Surgery for Other Injuries

Patients with severe head injuries often have other systemic injuries that require surgical procedures. If the systemic injury is life-threatening, the surgical procedure is needed emergently. However, controversy often arises about the timing of surgery for injuries that are not immediately life-threatening. One common example is a femur fracture. Early surgery is recommended for femur fractures to minimize pulmonary complications, primarily fat emboli. However, intraoperative hypotension can significantly worsen the neurological consequences of brain trauma,[160] and many recommend postponing nonemergent surgery for several days until intracranial hypertension has resolved.[244]

McKee and coworkers[245] compared a group of head-injured patients with multiple trauma that included femur fractures with a similar group without femur fractures. There was no difference in outcome, and the authors concluded that their practice of early fixation of femur fractures did not increase morbidity or mortality. Poole and colleagues[246] reported similar findings after retrospectively analyzing a group of 114 patients with head injuries and femur or tibia fractures. Early surgery did not increase morbidity of the head injury, nor did it reduce the risk of pulmonary complications. Both pulmonary and intracranial complications were related primarily to the severity of the brain injury and not to the timing of the orthopedic surgery. Kalb and associates[247] observed that head-injured patients operated on within the first 24 hours after injury for fixation of an orthopedic injury required more fluid resuscitation and blood product transfusions than did similar patients operated on after 24 hours. However, there was no difference in the long-term neurological outcome. These studies suggest that with meticulous attention to the management of blood pressure, fluid resuscitation, and ICP, surgical procedures for other injuries can often be performed safely.

Treatment of Intracranial Hypertension

Surgical lesions should always be ruled out by CT whenever severe intracranial hypertension develops unexpectedly, when intracranial hypertension is accompanied by clinical neurological deterioration, or when intracranial hypertension is refractory to medical management. For patients with sustained ICP greater than 20 to 25 mm Hg despite the general measures described previously, specific measures are added in a stepwise fashion until ICP is controlled (see Fig. 327–14).

PHARMACOLOGIC PARALYSIS

Data from the TCDB suggest that routine paralysis of all patients with severe head injury increases the risk of pulmonary complications and prolongs the intensive care unit stay.[248] However, ICP raised by agitation, posturing, or coughing should be prevented by narcotics and nondepolarizing muscle relaxants that do not alter cerebrovascular resistance (Table 327–8). A reasonable regimen is morphine and lorazepam for analgesia and sedation and cisatracurium or vecuronium as a muscle relaxant, with the dose titrated by twitch response to stimulation.[249, 250] Although the neurological status cannot be closely monitored while the patient is paralyzed, the muscle relaxants can be withheld once a day, usually before morning rounds, to perform a brief neurological examination.

One complication of neuromuscular blockade that has received little attention in patients with traumatic brain injury is critical illness myopathy and neuropathy. Weakness in critically ill patients can be categorized into three general syndromes (Fig. 327–16). The first, critical illness myopathy, was initially described in 1977,[251] and numerous cases have been reported since then.[252] The syndrome seems to occur most com-

TABLE 327–8 ■ **Cerebrovascular Effects of Muscle Relaxants**

DRUG	INTUBATION DOSE (MG/KG)	MAINTENANCE DOSE (MG/HR)	DURATION OF EFFECT (MIN)	EFFECT ON BP	EFFECT ON ICP	EFFECT ON CBF
Depolarizing[319,320]						
Succinylcholine	1		5–10	No change	Increase	Increase
Nondepolarizing[321–329]						
D-Tubocurarine	0.5	1.5–2	150	Decrease	Increase	Increase
Metocurine	0.4	7	150	Decrease	No change	No change
Pancuronium	0.1	4–8	120	Increase	No change	No change
Atracurium	0.5	20–50	30–45	Decrease or no change	No change	No change
Vecuronium	0.1	4–10	45–60	No change	No change	No change
Doxacurium	0.05	0.35–2.1	100–120	No change	No change	No change
Pipecuronium	0.1		120–150	No change	No change	No change

BP, blood pressure; CBF, cerebral blood flow; ICP, intracranial pressure.

monly in patients with asthma who require mechanical ventilation for status asthmaticus and who receive a combination of corticosteroids and neuromuscular blocking agents. β₂-Agonists, methylxanthines, and aminoglycosides may also play a role in the development of this syndrome. Second, prolonged neuromuscular blockade can occur with neuromuscular blocking agents, particularly in patients with kidney or liver dysfunction, and in patients who also receive aminoglycosides.[253] Finally, an acute polyneuropathy has been observed in patients with sepsis and multiple organ syndrome.[254] There is considerable overlap in these typical syndromes, and a combined myopathy-neuropathy may occur. Patients with traumatic brain injury who are given neuromuscular blocking agents to control ICP are at high risk for these syndromes, but the symptoms are often difficult to separate from the symptoms of their neurological injuries.[255] In the proper setting, however, an electromyogram and a muscle and nerve biopsy can be helpful in distinguishing weakness due to these syndromes from weakness due to the brain injury.

The underlying mechanisms of these syndromes are not known, but the association with neuromuscular blocking agents and critically ill patients is strong. Recommendations to minimize the risk of these complications include limiting the use of neuromuscular blocking agents, limiting the dose of neuromuscular blocking agents by train-of-four monitoring, measuring creatine phosphokinase daily while neuromuscular blocking agents are given, and stopping the neuromuscular blocking agents at least once a day to observe motor response.[253]

HYPERVENTILATION

The relationship of hyperventilation and global CBF was examined in a series of 171 head-injured patients during the first 10 days after injury.[256] Of 1212 CBF measurements in these patients, 132 (11%) were less

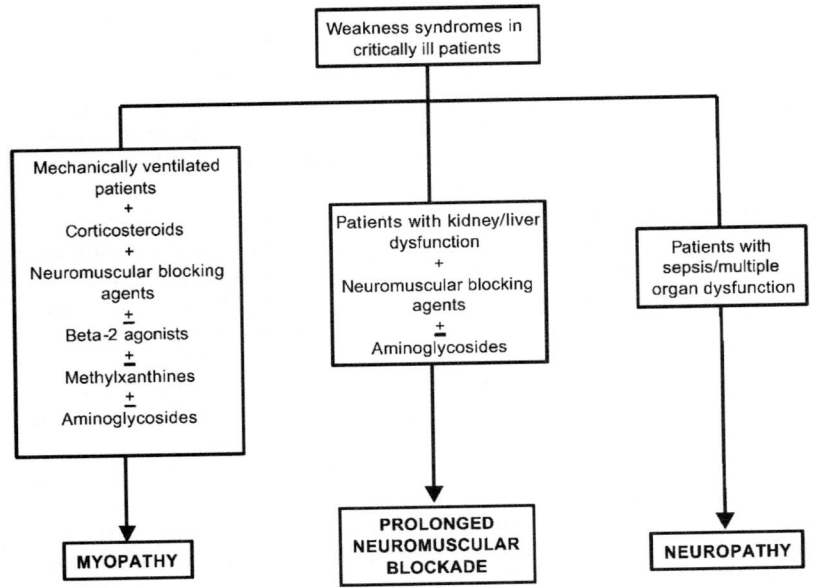

FIGURE 327–16. Weakness syndromes in critically ill patients.

than 25 mL/100 g per minute. Of the 132 low CBF values, 71 (54%) were appropriately reduced relative to the lower $CMRO_2$, and 61 (46%) were associated with increased oxygen extraction, increased cerebral lactate production, or both, suggesting a relative inadequacy of perfusion. The incidence of inadequate CBF steadily increased as the Pco_2 decreased; it was 2%, 4%, 8%, and 23% when the arterial Pco_2 was greater than 30, 25 to 30, 20 to 25, and less than 20 mm Hg, respectively. The incidence of inadequate CBF was twice as high during the first 24 hours than on any other day (8%, compared with 4%). The incidence was higher in patients with reduced CBF (11%) than in those with normal or elevated CBF (2%).

Routine hyperventilation (arterial Pco_2 of 20 to 25 mm Hg) was shown to have a detrimental effect on outcome in one randomized trial.[257] The authors of this study recommended using hyperventilation only in patients with intracranial hypertension rather than routinely in all head-injured patients. In general, arterial Pco_2 should not be reduced to less than 25 mm Hg unless $SjvO_2$ is monitored to make certain that ischemia is not being produced.

In patients who have been chronically hyperventilated, abruptly returning the arterial Pco_2 to normal can result in a dramatic increase in ICP. Muizelaar and colleagues[258] showed, in an experimental study, that this phenomenon occurred after 24 hours of hyperventilation and was associated with vasodilatation of cerebral vessels as the CSF pH equilibrated at the new lower Pco_2 level. Hyperventilation should be withdrawn over several days to avoid this increase in ICP.

CEREBROSPINAL FLUID DRAINAGE

Although removal of 1 mL of CSF normally does not change ICP by more than 1 to 2 mm Hg, in patients with elevated ICP, drainage of 1 to 2 mL of CSF through the ventriculostomy catheter can temporarily lower ICP. This modality can be an important adjunct for lowering ICP.[259] However, as the brain becomes more swollen, the ventricles collapse, less CSF is available for drainage, and the effectiveness of this modality is reduced.

DEHYDRATION AND OSMOTHERAPY

Before a method for measuring ICP became available, dehydration therapy was common in the management of head-injured patients. Normovolemia does not result in an increased rate of intracranial hypertension, and it eliminates severe electrolyte abnormalities and renal failure.[260] Fluid overload, however, should be avoided. Fluid restriction may be necessary in cases of hyponatremia caused by SIADH.

The osmotic diuretic mannitol is given as an intravenous infusion of 0.25 to 1 g/kg and maximally reduces ICP within 10 minutes of administration. The reduction in ICP usually persists for 3 to 4 hours. Serum osmolarity appears to be optimal when raised to 300 to 320 mOsm and should be kept below 320 mOsm to avoid side effects of therapy such as hypovolemia, hyperos-

molarity, and renal failure. Loop diuretics, such as furosemide, decrease CSF production and increase serum osmolarity by increasing free water clearance by the kidney. Given along with mannitol, furosemide (0.7 mg/kg) results in a greater (62% versus 57%) and more sustained (5 hours versus 2 hours) decrease in ICP than mannitol alone.[261]

Hypertonic saline has also been used to raise the serum sodium concentration to 145 to 155 mmol/L and lower ICP.[262, 263] Serial measurement of brain water using spin-echo T2-weighted magnetic resonance imaging demonstrates a significant reduction in brain water content in a freeze lesion after infusion of 7.5% saline.[264]

BARBITURATE COMA

Barbiturate coma is another treatment modality that has been used to lower ICP in head-injured patients.[52, 265, 266] In addition to lowering ICP, extracellular concentrations of lactate and excitatory amino acids are reduced after treatment with barbiturates.[267] Barbiturates are protective during periods of cerebral hypoxia.[268] Although routine use of barbiturates in unselected patients has not been consistently effective in reducing morbidity or mortality after severe head injury,[269, 270] a randomized multicenter trial demonstrated that instituting barbiturate coma in patients with refractory intracranial hypertension resulted in a twofold greater chance of controlling ICP.[271]

Because of the hypotensive complications associated with barbiturates and because the neurological examination cannot be performed during treatment, barbiturate coma is usually reserved for patients with intracranial hypertension resistant to other modalities. Pentobarbital is given in both loading and maintenance doses. The loading dose is 10 mg/kg, given over 30 minutes, followed by 5 mg/kg each hour for three doses. This typically provides a therapeutic level after the fourth dose. The maintenance dose is 1 to 2 mg/kg per hour, adjusted so that either the serum level is in the therapeutic range of 30 to 50 μg/mL or the electroencephalogram has a burst suppression pattern. Winer and colleagues[272] reported that plasma and CSF pentobarbital levels do not accurately reflect the physiologic effects of pentobarbital and recommended monitoring the electroencephalogram instead of pentobarbital levels. Pulmonary wedge pressure and cardiac output are monitored in all patients. Hypotension caused by pentobarbital is treated first with volume replacement and then with dopamine if necessary. Laboratory studies suggest that for the treatment of hypotension associated with barbiturate coma, volume resuscitation may be better than dopamine.[273] In these studies, dopamine infusion increased cerebral metabolic requirements and partially offset the beneficial effects of barbiturates on metabolism.

The mechanism of ICP reduction by barbiturates is not entirely clear but is thought to be hemodynamic because of the immediate effect on ICP. Studies by Nordstrom[84] and Messeter[274] and their coworkers suggested that the reduction in ICP with barbiturates is closely tied to the retention of CO_2 reactivity by the brain. Studies by Cruz[275] showed that outcomes are significantly worse in patients whose $SjvO_2$ is reduced to less than 45% with the initiation of barbiturate coma. Complications during the treatment of intracranial hypertension with barbiturate coma reportedly include the following: hypotension in 58%, hypokalemia in 82%, respiratory complications in 76%, infections in 55%, hepatic dysfunction in 87%, and renal dysfunction in 47%.[276]

In a study of 67 patients in barbiturate coma for refractory intracranial hypertension, the most consistent cerebral effect was a reduction in $CMRO_2$ by an average of 31%.[277] The change in $CMRO_2$ with the loading dose of pentobarbital was closely related to the pretreatment value ($n = 67$, $r^2 = 0.65$, $P < 0.001$). In the 30 patients with a good ICP response to pentobarbital infusion, pretreatment $CMRO_2$ and $AVDO_2$ were greater, and $CMRO_2$ and $AVDO_2$ decreased more with the loading dose of pentobarbital, than in the patients with partial or no ICP response. The outcome was significantly better in the patients with a good or partial ICP response to pentobarbital, with 21% having a good recovery or only moderate disability at 3 months postinjury, compared with 100% of nonresponders experiencing a persistent vegetative state or death.

In summary, barbiturate coma can be useful for acutely reducing ICP in selected patients. Patients with overwhelmingly severe injuries are not likely to benefit, partly because their $CMRO_2$ is already markedly reduced by the injury, and partly because their outcome is already predetermined by the injury. Patients with systemic hypotension are not likely to have a good response, because hypotension limits the amount of barbiturates that can be given.

OTHER TREATMENTS

Corticosteroids have been used to reduce the edema associated with head injury, but several randomized, double-blinded clinical trials failed to demonstrate a beneficial effect of steroids.[278–281] Although most neurosurgeons have discontinued the routine use of steroids in head-injured patients because of these studies, the successful trial of methylprednisolone in spinal cord injury has led to renewed interest in the use of steroids in head injury.

Mild hypothermia has been used to reduce ICP after head injury. A decrease in temperature to 34°C has been observed to control ICP in patients refractory to other methods of treatment.[282] In experimental studies, hypothermia improves outcome from fluid percussion injury.[177, 178, 283] Studies have suggested that hypothermia improves the outcome after severe head injury,[284] and a randomized multicenter trial of hypothermia to 33°C for 48 hours after head injury was recently completed and is under analysis.

The role of decompressive surgical procedures remains controversial. Anecdotal reports, such as the one by Gower and associates,[285] in which the mortality rate for refractory intracranial hypertension was reduced from 82% to 40% with the addition of subtemporal decompression, have led to renewed interest in the procedure. In a recent case-controlled study, Polin and colleagues[286] reported improved outcomes for a selected group of patients with diffuse brain swelling undergoing bilateral frontal decompressive craniectomy. A favorable outcome was observed in 46% of patients undergoing surgery within 48 hours of admission.

Treatment of Cerebral Ischemia

The goal of therapy is to optimize oxygen delivery to the brain. Oxygen delivery is dependent on two parameters: oxygen content of the blood and CBF. Both these parameters can be manipulated to a certain degree after traumatic brain injury.

Oxygen content of the blood can be increased by ensuring an adequate hemoglobin concentration and by increasing arterial PO_2. The optimal hemoglobin concentration for tissue oxygenation is approximately 10 g/dL.[287] A lower hemoglobin concentration reduces the oxygen carrying capacity of the blood more than it improves viscosity. A higher hemoglobin concentration reduces viscosity and CBF even though it increases oxygen carrying capacity.

Increasing arterial PO_2 after hemoglobin is nearly 100% saturated increases arterial oxygen content by only a small amount—that is, by the amount of oxygen dissolved in the blood. However, if tissues are ischemic, even small increases in oxygen content can be important. As the example in Figure 327–8 illustrates, simply increasing FiO_2 can significantly increase brain tissue PO_2. Menzel and coworkers[288] observed an increase in brain tissue PO_2 and a decrease in extracellular lactate concentration in the brain, measured by microdialysis, when patients with very low baseline brain tissue PO_2 were placed on 100% oxygen. The reduction in lactate accumulation with this therapy suggests that the increase in brain tissue PO_2 alters ischemic cerebral metabolism favorably. Given the relatively small effect observed and the potential for toxicity with inspiring 100% oxygen, this approach to improving oxygenation needs further investigation.

The most effective way to improve ischemic metabolism is to increase CBF, which is dependent on CPP. After traumatic brain injury, the brain may require a higher than normal CPP to perfuse the brain adequately. CPP should be increased by both reducing elevated ICP and raising blood pressure. Often blood pressure is the easier parameter to manipulate. Measurement of central venous pressure (CVP) or, in some cases, insertion of a Swan-Ganz catheter to measure pulmonary wedge pressure (PWP) should be done to make certain that intravascular volume is adequate. If blood pressure still needs to be increased after an adequate intravascular volume is assured, a pressor agent can be added.

There are few studies that compare the effectiveness of the various pressor agents in increasing CBF. Table 327–9 summarizes some of these studies, most of which were done in normal experimental preparations. All the agents listed raise blood pressure via sympathomi-

TABLE 327-9 ■ **Effect of Inotropic and Pressor Agents on Cerebral Hemodynamics**

DRUG	RECEPTOR					EFFECT IN NORMAL BRAIN		
	α_1	α_2	β_1	β_2	DA_1, DA_2	MAP	ICP	CBF
Dopamine, <2 μg/kg/min					+++	No change	No change	No change or decrease
Dopamine, 2–6 μg/kg/min			+++	+		Increase	No change or increase	Increase
Dopamine, 7–20 μg/kg/min	++	++				Increase	No change or increase	Decrease or increase
Phenylephrine	+++	0	0	0	0	Increase	No change	No change
Norepinephrine	++++	++++	+++	0	0	Increase	No change	No change
Epinephrine	++++	+++	++++	++	0	Increase	No change	No change

CBF, cerebral blood flow; ICP, intracranial pressure; MAP, mean arterial pressure.
Data from Von Essen C, Zervas NT, Brown DR, et al: Local cerebral blood flow in the dog during intravenous infusion of dopamine. Surg Neurol 13: 181–188, 1980; Myburgh JA, Upton RN, Grant C, et al: A comparison of the effects of norepinephrine, epinephrine, and dopamine on cerebral blood flow and oxygen utilisation. Acta Neurochir Suppl (Wien) 71: 19–21, 1998.

metic actions. Dopamine has the most complex actions and is the most variable among the different studies. In very low doses dopamine can actually reduce CBF. At intermediate doses it increases CBF, and at higher doses the effect is again to decrease CBF.[289] Myburgh and coworkers[290] compared the effects of equal doses of norepinephrine, epinephrine, and dopamine on CBF and ICP. At doses greater than 20 μg/kg per minute, dopamine increased ICP, and at doses greater than 60 μg/kg per minute, dopamine increased CBF. Norepinephrine and epinephrine at similar doses did not have a significant effect on either CBF or ICP.

In patients with cerebral ischemia, however, results may be different. Areas of ischemia are likely to have lost the ability to autoregulate, and blood flow may be more dependent on CPP. It might be expected that any agent that increases CPP will improve CBF, especially in ischemic areas. Darby and colleagues[291] studied CBF before and after raising blood pressure from 90 to 111 mm Hg with dopamine in 13 patients with suspected vasospasm. The dopamine infusion increased regional CBF in more than 90% of the regions where CBF was less than 25 mL/100 g per minute at baseline. Dopamine also unexpectedly reduced regional CBF in one third of the nonischemic territories. Although dopamine is the most widely used pressor agent in the setting of hypotension and shock, it may not be the best agent for induced hypertension as a treatment of cerebral ischemia. Pressor drugs such as norepinephrine or phenylephrine may have more predictable effects on CBF, although there may also be more systemic ischemic complications with these agents.

Treatment of Secondary Ischemic Insults

HYPOTENSION

The treatment of hypotension in a head-injured patient is similar to that in any other critically ill trauma patient, except that the goal is to provide a CPP that is adequate for the injured brain. Initially, the intravascular volume should be assessed, and if it is low, volume should be added. A central venous pressure monitor

or, in some cases, a Swan-Ganz catheter is appropriate to assess intravascular volume. Low intravascular volume should be treated with infusion of crystalloids, colloids, or blood, as appropriate for the clinical situation. Most studies show no advantages of colloid over crystalloid resuscitation in experimental head injury. Experimentally, hypertonic saline allows the replacement of intravascular volume with less increase in ICP than does saline or dextran.[292] In one multicenter study of hypertonic saline for resuscitation of trauma patients, the head-injured patients treated with hypertonic saline had a significantly better rate of survival to discharge.[293] If volume replacement does not provide adequate blood pressure, inotropic and pressor agents should be used (Fig. 327–17).

The underlying cause of the hypotension must be sought and treated. Hypotension in adults is only occasionally caused by head injury alone, and another mechanism should be sought.[294] Blood loss from another injury, an associated spinal cord injury, cardiac contusion or tamponade, and tension pneumothorax are other causes of hypotension to consider.

HYPOCAPNIA

Hypocapnia in ventilated patients can be corrected easily by reducing the minute ventilation. Sedation may be required to prevent spontaneous hyperventilation. If the hypocapnia has been present for more than 6 hours, the correction should be done slowly, perhaps no more than 1 torr/hour, to prevent the ICP from increasing.

HYPOXIA

The treatment of hypoxia is similar to that in other critically ill trauma patients. Increasing FiO_2 often improves oxygenation. When pulmonary edema is present, oxygen supplementation may not be sufficient to improve arterial Po_2. The addition of PEEP may increase functional residual capacity and improve ventilation perfusion mismatch. As a result, PEEP may allow the inspired oxygen concentration to be de-

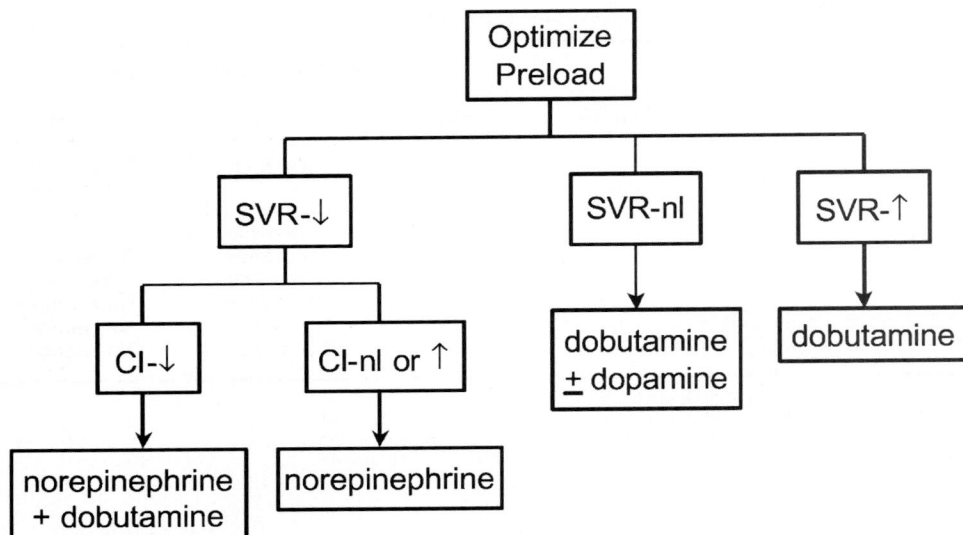

FIGURE 327–17. Treatment of hypotension. CI, cardiac index; SVR, systemic vascular resistance.

creased, reducing the potential for oxygen toxicity. However, PEEP can have adverse effects on ICP and on blood pressure. PEEP can raise ICP by increasing intrathoracic pressure, central venous pressure, and cerebral venous pressure. In addition, by decreasing venous return to the heart, blood pressure can be reduced. The combined effect on ICP and blood pressure is a reduction in cerebral perfusion.

The severity of PEEP's effect on ICP depends on both intracranial and pulmonary compliance. In patients with normal intracranial compliance, ICP does not change significantly, because the brain is able to compensate for the increased cerebral venous blood volume caused by the increase in intrathoracic pressure. In contrast, when intracranial compliance is decreased, even small increases in cerebral venous pressure induced by PEEP may cause dangerous increases in ICP. Apuzzo and associates[295] studied the effects of PEEP in 25 head-injured patients. ICP increased in 12 patients, all of whom had decreased intracranial compliance. CPP decreased to less than 60 mm Hg in 50% of the patients with increased ICP. Shapiro and Marshall found that 6 of 12 head-injured patients had a 10 mm Hg increase in ICP with the addition of 4 to 8 cm PEEP.[52] In most cases, elevating the patient's head reduces the effect of high airway pressures on ICP.[296]

The extent to which any given amount of PEEP is transmitted to the venous system also depends on the severity of the pulmonary injury. When the lungs are poorly compliant, exposure to PEEP does not usually cause marked increases in venous pressure or in ICP.[297, 298]

Removal of PEEP must also be judicious. Sudden removal may precipitate a sudden increase in central blood volume, arterial blood pressure, and CPP, resulting in an increase in ICP.[297, 299]

For each patient, maintaining adequate oxygenation is the most important consideration, so PEEP is often necessary. It is important to keep mean airway pressure at a minimum by using the smallest amount of PEEP necessary to maintain oxygenation at a safe FiO_2 and by using intermittent mandatory ventilation. The intermittent mandatory ventilation rate is adjusted to the patient's ventilatory requirements to minimize the number of mechanical breaths and allow the patient to breathe spontaneously. Reductions in blood pressure are treated by volume expansion or with dopamine, if necessary.

ANEMIA

Anemia can be easily remedied by transfusing packed red blood cells. The optimal hematocrit for improving oxygen delivery after head injury is not clear. Studies that examined the relationship between CBF and hematocrit demonstrated that CBF and tissue oxygen delivery increase as hematocrit and viscosity decrease, until hematocrit falls to 33%. Below a hematocrit of 33%, tissue oxygen delivery decreases.[287] In normal adults, adequate oxygen carrying capacity is usually met by a hemoglobin concentration of 7 g/dL or a hematocrit of 21% when the intravascular volume is normal. However, because cerebral vascular responses are impaired after traumatic brain injury, it cannot be assumed that the same hematocrit will be adequate in a head-injured patient.

FEVER

Fever in a head-injured patient should be treated with acetaminophen and a cooling blanket if necessary. A search for the cause of the fever should be undertaken, and treatment with appropriate antibiotics should begin if an infectious cause is found. This effort should not delay treatment of the fever, however. Remember that brain temperature is often 1°C to 2°C higher than rectal temperature during fever spikes.

SEIZURES

In a head-injured patient who is actively convulsing, the seizure activity should be arrested immediately.

Diazepam 5 to 10 mg intravenously, or lorazepam 2 to 3 mg intravenously, is given initially to stop the seizure. The action of these drugs is short-lived, and the seizures may recur if other antiepileptics are not given. Intravenous phenytoin should be administered at 25 mg/minute until a loading dose of 15 to 20 mg/kg has been given. Maintenance doses of phenytoin, 300 to 400 mg/day, are given to prevent subsequent seizures.

CEREBRAL VASOSPASM

Symptomatic vasospasm after traumatic brain injury is treated similarly to vasospasm after subarachnoid hemorrhage. Nimodipine may be effective in reducing the neurological consequences of vasospasm after head injury. It is not clear that the beneficial effect of nimodipine after head injury is due to an effect on vasospasm. However, the only subgroup of head-injured patients that has been found to benefit are those with subarachnoid hemorrhage.[15]

Hypervolemic hemodilution and induced hypertension are the primary therapies for vasospasm. The patient should be volume expanded. Usually a Swan-Ganz catheter is indicated to optimize cardiac output. If the patient is still symptomatic after volume expansion, a pressor agent should be added to raise blood pressure. The choice of pressor agents is controversial, as discussed earlier in relation to the treatment of secondary ischemia. Information about cardiac output, obtained from the Swan-Ganz catheter, can be helpful in making this decision. If cardiac output is normal or elevated, a pressor agent such as phenylephrine or norepinephrine is likely to be more effective in raising blood pressure. If cardiac output is reduced, dopamine may be a better choice, but it must be remembered that dopamine has been observed to have an unpredictable effect on CBF in some studies.[289, 291]

REFERENCES

1. Becker DP, Miller JD, Ward JD, et al: The outcome from severe head injury with early diagnosis and intensive management. J Neurosurg 47:491–502, 1977.
2. Bowers SA, Marshall LF: Outcome in 200 consecutive cases of severe head injury treated in San Diego County: A prospective analysis. Neurosurgery 6:237–242, 1980.
3. Miller JD, Becker DP, Ward JD, et al: Significance of intracranial hypertension in severe head injury. J Neurosurg 47:503–516, 1977.
4. Saul TG, Ducker TB: Effect of intracranial pressure monitoring and aggressive treatment on mortality in severe head injury. J Neurosurg 56:498–503, 1982.
5. Jennett B, Teasdale G, Braakman R, et al: Prognosis of patients with severe head injury. Neurosurgery 4:283–289, 1979.
6. Jennett B, Bond MR: Assessment of outcome after severe brain damage. Lancet 1:480–484, 1975.
7. Teasdale G, Jennett B: Assessment of coma and impaired consciouness. Lancet 2:81–84, 1974.
8. Foulkes M, Eisenberg HM, Jane JA, et al: The Traumatic Coma Data Bank: Design, methods, and baseline characteristics. J Neurosurg 75(Suppl):S8–S13, 1991.
9. Marshall LF, Gautille T, Klauber MR, et al: The outcome of severe closed head injury. J Neurosurg 75(Suppl):S28–S36, 1991.
10. Chesnut RM, Marshall LF, Klauber MR, et al: The role of secondary brain injury in determining outcome from severe head injury. J Trauma 34:216–222, 1993.
11. Eisenberg HM, Gary HE Jr, Aldrich EF, et al: Initial CT findings in 753 patients with severe head injury. J Neurosurg 73:688–698, 1990.
12. Marshall LF, Marshall SB, Klauber MR, et al: A new classification of head injury based on computerized tomography. J Neurosurg 75:S14–S20, 1991.
13. Brain Trauma Foundation, American Association of Neurological Surgeons, Joint Section on Neurotrauma and Critical Care: Guidelines for the management of severe head injury. J Neurotrauma 13:641–734, 1996.
14. Maas AIR, Dearden M, Teasdale GM, et al: EBIC guidelines for management of severe head injury in adults. Acta Neurochir (Wien) 139:286–294, 1997.
15. Harders A, Kakarieka A, Braakman R: Traumatic subarachnoid hemorrhage and its treatment with nimodipine: German tSAH Study Group. J Neurosurg 85:82–89, 1996.
16. Bullock MR, Lyeth BG, Muizelaar JP: Current status of neuroprotection trials for traumatic brain injury: Lessons from animal models and clinical studies. Neurosurgery 45:207–220, 1999.
17. Alderson P, Roberts I: Corticosteroids in acute traumatic brain injury: A systematic review of randomized trials. BMJ 314:1855–1859, 1997.
18. Adams JH, Graham DI, Gennarelli TA: Head injury in man and experimental animals: Neuropathology. Acta Neurochir Suppl (Wien) 32:S15–S30, 1983.
19. Gentleman SM, Roberts GW, Gennarelli TA, et al: Axonal injury: A universal consequence of fatal closed head injury. Acta Neuropathol (Berl) 89:537–543, 1995.
20. Maxwell WL, Povlishock JT, Graham DI: A mechanistic analysis of nondisruptive axonal injury. J Neurotrauma 14:419–440, 1997.
21. Povlishock JT, Christman CW: The pathobiology of traumatically induced axonal injury in animals and humans: A review of current thought. J Neurotrauma 12:555–564, 1995.
22. Gennarelli TA, Spielman GM, Langfitt TW, et al: Influence of the type of intracranial lesion on outcome from severe head injury: A multicenter study using a new classification system. J Neurosurg 56:26–32, 1982.
23. Smith WP, Batnitzky S, Rengachary SS: Acute isodense subdural hematomas: A problem in anemic patients. Am J Radiol 136:543–546, 1981.
24. Servadei F: Prognostic factors in severely head injured adult patients with acute subdural haematomas. Acta Neurochir (Wien) 139:279–285, 1997.
25. Zumkeller M, Behrmann R, Heissler HE, et al: Computed tomographic criteria and survival rate for patients with acute subdural hematoma. Neurosurgery 39:708–712, 1996.
26. Massaro F, Lanotte M, Faccani G, et al: One hundred and twenty-seven cases of acute subdural haematoma operated on: Correlation between CT scan findings and outcome. Acta Neurochir (Wien) 138:185–191, 1996.
27. Schroder ML, Muizelaar JP, Kuta AJ: Documented reversal of global ischemia immediately after removal of an acute subdural hematoma. J Neurosurg 80:324–327, 1994.
28. Gopinath SP, Cormio M, Ziegler J, et al: Intraoperative jugular desaturation during surgery for traumatic intracranial hematomas. Anesth Analg 83:1014–1021, 1996.
29. Doppenberg EM, Watson JC, Broaddus WC, et al: Intraoperative monitoring of substrate delivery during aneurysm and hematoma surgery: Initial experience in 16 patients. J Neurosurg 87:809–816, 1997.
30. Duhaime AC, Gennarelli LM, Yachnis A: Acute subdural hematoma: Is the blood itself toxic? J Neurotrauma 11:669–678, 1994.
31. Croce MA, Dent DL, Menke PG, et al: Acute subdural hematoma: Nonsurgical management of selected patients. J Trauma 36:820–826, 1994.
32. Seelig JM, Becker DP, Miller DP, et al: Traumatic acute subdural hematoma: Major mortality reduction in comatose patients treated within four hours. N Engl J Med 304:1511–1518, 1981.
33. Jamieson KG, Yelland JDN: Extradural hematoma: Report of 167 cases. J Neurosurg 29:13–23, 1968.
34. Jennett B, Teasdale G, Galbraith S, et al: Severe head injuries in three countries. J Neurol Neurosurg Psychiatry 40:291–298, 1977.
35. Di RA, Ellis SJ, Landes C: Delayed epidural hematoma. Neuroradiology 33:253–254, 1991.

36. Dharker SR, Bhargava N: Bilateral epidural haematoma. Acta Neurochir (Wien) 110:29–32, 1991.

37. Servadei F: Prognostic factors in severely head injured adult patients with epidural haematomas. Acta Neurochir (Wien) 139:273–278, 1997.

38. Chen TY, Wong CW, Chang CN, et al: The expectant treatment of "asymptomatic" supratentorial epidural hematomas. Neurosurgery 32:176–179, 1993.

39. Wong CW: The CT criteria for conservative treatment—but under close clinical observation—of posterior fossa epidural haematomas. Acta Neurochir (Wien) 126:124–127, 1994.

40. Clifton GL, Grossman RG, Makela ME, et al: Neurological course and correlated computerized tomography findings after severe closed head injury. J Neurosurg 52:611–624, 1980.

41. Choksey M, Crockard HA, Sandilands M: Acute traumatic intracerebral haematomas: Determinants of outcome in a retrospective series of 202 cases. Br J Neurosurg 7:611–622, 1993.

42. Zimmerman RA, Bilaniuk LT, Dolinskas C, et al: Computed tomography of acute intracerebral hemorrhagic contusion. J Comput Assist Tomogr 1:271–279, 1977.

43. Schroder ML, Muizelaar JP, Bullock MR, et al: Focal ischemia due to traumatic contusions documented by stable xenon-CT and ultrastructural studies. J Neurosurg 82:966–971, 1995.

44. Rocca B, Martin C, Viviand X, et al: Comparison of four severity scores in patients with head trauma. J Trauma 29:299–305, 1989.

45. Alvarez M, Nava JM, Rue M, et al: Mortality prediction in head trauma patients: Performance of Glasgow Coma Score and general severity systems. Crit Care Med 26:142–148, 1998.

46. Kita H, Marmarou A: The cause of acute brain swelling after the closed head injury in rats. Acta Neurochir Suppl (Wien) 60:452–455, 1994.

47. Marmarou A, Barzo P, Fatouros P, et al: Traumatic brain swelling in head injured patients: Brain edema or vascular engorgement? Acta Neurochir Suppl (Wien) 70:68–70, 1997.

48. Barzo P, Marmarou A, Fatouros P, et al: Contribution of vasogenic and cellular edema to traumatic brain swelling measured by diffusion-weighted imaging. J Neurosurg 87:900–907, 1997.

49. Barzo P, Marmarou A, Fatouros P, et al: Biphasic pathophysiological response of vasogenic and cellular edema in traumatic brain swelling. Acta Neurochir Suppl (Wien) 70:119–122, 1997.

50. Miller JD, Sweet RC, Narayan RK, et al: Early insults to the injured brain. JAMA 240:439–442, 1978.

51. Bruce DA, Raphaely RC, Goldberg AI, et al: Pathophysiology, treatment, and outcome following severe head injury in children. Childs Brain 5:174–191, 1979.

52. Marshall LF, Smith RW, Shapiro HM: The outcome with aggressive treatment in severe head injuries. Part I. Significance of intracranial pressure monitoring. J Neurosurg 50:20–25, 1979.

53. Miller JD, Butterworth J, Gudeman SK, et al: Further experience in the management of severe head injury. J Neurosurg 54:289–299, 1981.

54. Martin NA, Patwardhan RV, Alexander MJ, et al: Characterization of cerebral hemodynamic phases following severe head he trauma: Hypoperfusion, hyperemia, and vasospasm. J Neurosurg 87:9–19, 1997.

55. Robertson CS, Contant CF, Gokaslan ZL, et al: Cerebral blood flow, arteriovenous oxygen difference, and outcome in head injured patients. J Neurol Neurosurg Psychiatry 55:594–603, 1992.

56. Bouma GJ, Muizelaar JP, Stringer WA, et al: Ultra-early evaluation of regional cerebral blood flow in severely head-injured patients using xenon-enhanced computerized tomography. J Neurosurg 77:360–368, 1992.

57. McLaughlin MR, Marion DW: Cerebral blood flow and vasoresponsivity within and around cerebral contusions. J Neurosurg 85:871–876, 1996.

58. Sakas DE, Bullock MR, Patterson J, et al: Focal cerebral hyperemia after focal head injury in humans: A benign phenomenon. J Neurosurg 83:277–284, 1995.

59. Obrist WD, Langfitt T, Jaggi J, et al: Cerebral blood flow and metabolism in comatose patients with acute head injury: Relationship to intracranial hypertension. J Neurosurg 61:241–253, 1984.

60. Kelly DF, Kordestani RK, Martin NA, et al: Cerebral blood flow as a predictor of oucome following traumatic brain injury. J Neurosurg 86:633–641, 1997.

61. Sioutos PJ, Orozco JA, Carter LP, et al: Continuous regional cerebral cortical blood flow monitoring in head-injured patients. Neurosurgery 36:943–950, 1995.

62. Overgaard J, Molsdal C, Tweed TA: Cerebral circulation after head injury. Part 3. Does reduced regional cerebral blood flow determine recovery of brain function after blunt head injury? J Neurosurg 55:63–74, 1981.

63. Marion DW, Darby J, Yonas H: Acute regional cerebral blood flow changes caused by severe head injuries. J Neurosurg 74:407–414, 1991.

64. Gopinath SP, Robertson CS, Contant CF, et al: Jugular venous desaturation and outcome after head injury. J Neurol Neurosurg Psychiatry 57:717–723, 1994.

65. Muizelaar JP, Marmarou A, DeSalles AA, et al: Cerebral blood flow and metabolism in severely head-injured children. Part 1. Relationship with GCS score, outcome, ICP, and PVI. J Neurosurg 71:63–71, 1989.

66. Kelly DF, Kordestani RK, Martin NA, et al: Hyperemia following traumatic brain injury: Relationship to intracranial hypertension and outcome. J Neurosurg 85:762–771, 1996.

67. Overgaard J, Tweed WA: Cerebral circulation after head injury. Part 4. Functional anatomy and boundary-zone flow deprivation in the first week of traumatic coma. J Neurosurg 59:439–446, 1983.

68. Obrist WD, Gennarelli TA, Segawa H, et al: Relation of cerebral blood flow to neurological status on outcome in head-injured patients. J Neurosurg 51:292–300, 1979.

69. Bruce DA, Langfitt TW, Miller JD, et al: Regional cerebral blood flow, intracranial pressure, and brain metabolism in comatose patients. J Neurosurg 38:131–144, 1973.

70. Cormio M, Valadka AB, Robertson CS: Elevated jugular bulb oxygen saturation after severe head injury. J Neurosurg 90:9–15, 1999.

71. Wilkins RH, Odom GL: Intracranial arterial spasm associated with craniocerebral trauma. J Neurosurg 32:626–633, 1970.

72. Suwanweh C, Suwanweh N: Intracranial arterial narrowing and spasm in acute head injury. J Neurosurg 26:314–323, 1972.

73. MacPherson P, Graham DI: Correlation between angiographic findings and the ischemia of head injury. J Neurol Nurosurg Psychiatry 41:192–197, 1978.

74. Martin NA, Doberstein C, Zane C: Posttraumatic cerebral arterial spasm: Transcranial Doppler ultrasound, cerebral blood flow, and angiographic findings. J Neurosurg 77:575–583, 1992.

75. Weber M, Grolimund P, Seiler RW: Evaluation of posttraumatic cerebral blood flow velocities by transcranial Doppler ultrasonography. Neurosurgery 27:106–112, 1990.

76. Chan KH, Dearden NM, Miller JD: The significance of posttraumatic increase in cerebral blood flow velocity: A transcranial Doppler ultrasound study. Neurosurgery 30:697–700, 1992.

77. Lee JH, Martin NA, Alsina G, et al: Hemodynamically significant cerebral vasospasm and outcome after head injury: A prospective study. J Neurosurg 87:221–233, 1997.

78. Steiger HJ, Aaslid R, Stooss R, et al: Transcranial Doppler monitoring in head injury: Relations between type of injury, flow velocities, vasoreactivity, and outcome. J Neurosurg 34:79–85, 1994.

79. Jenkins LW, Moszynski D, Lyeth BG, et al: Increased vulnerability of the mildly traumatized rat brain to cerebral ischemia: The use of controlled secondary ischemia as a research tool to identify common or different mechanisms contributing to mechanical and ischemic brain injury. Brain Res 477:211–224, 1989.

80. Cherian L, Goodman JC, Robertson CS: Secondary ischemia causes increased brain injury after controlled cortical impact injury in rats. J Neurotrauma 13:371–383, 1996.

81. Jones PA, Andrews PJD, Midgley S, et al: Measuring the burden of secondary insults in head-injured patients during intensive care. J Neurosurg Anesthesiol 6:4–14, 1994.

82. Busija DW, Leffler CW, Pourcyrous M: Hyperthermia increases cerebral metabolic rate and blood flow in neonatal pigs. Am J Physiol 255:H343–H346, 1988.

83. Croughwell N, Smith LR, Quill T, et al: The effect of temperature on cerebral metabolism and blood flow in adults during cardiopulmonary bypass. J Thorac Cardiovasc Surg 103:549–554, 1992.

84. Nordstrom CH, Messeter K, Sundbarg G, et al: Cerebral blood

flow, vasoreactivity, and oxygen consumption during barbiturate therapy in severe traumatic brain lesions. J Neurosurg 68: 424–431, 1988.

85. Marion DW, Obrist WD, Carlier PM, et al: The use of moderate therapeutic hypothermia for patients with severe head injuries: A preliminary report. J Neurosurg 79:354–362, 1993.

86. Meldrum BS, Nilsson B: Cerebral blood flow and metabolic rate early and late in prolonged seizures induced in rats by bicuculline. Brain 99:523–542, 1976.

87. Michenfelder JD, Milde JH: The relationship among canine brain temperature, metabolism, and function during hypothermia. Anesthesiology 75:130–136, 1991.

88. Pierce EC, Lambertsen CJ, Deutsch S, et al: Cerebral circulation and metabolism during thiopental anesthesia and hyperventilation in man. J Clin Invest 41:1664–1671, 1962.

89. Bergsneider M, Hovda DA, Shalmon E, et al: Cerebral hyperglycolysis following severe traumatic brain injury in humans: A positron emission tomography study. J Neurosurg 86:241–251, 1997.

90. Clifton GL, Grossman RG: Technical flow: Flowsheet for the neurosurgical intensive care units. Neurosurgery 11:280–283, 1982.

91. Selhorst JB, Gudeman SK, Butterworth JF, et al: Papilledema after acute head injury. Neurosurgery 16:357–363, 1985.

92. Kishore PRS, Lipper MH, Becker DP, et al: The significance of CT in head injury: Correlation with intracranial pressure. AJNR Am J Neuroradiol 2:307–311, 1981.

93. Guillaume J, Janny P: Manometrie intracranienne continue: Interet de la methode et premiers resultats. Rev Neurol 84:131–142, 1951.

94. Lundberg N: Continuous recording and control of ventricular fluid pressure in neurosurgical practice. Acta Psychiatr Neurol Scand 149(Suppl 36):1–193, 1960.

95. Narayan RK, Kishore PRS, Becker DP, et al: Intracranial pressure: To monitor or not to monitor? A review of our experience with severe head injury. J Neurosurg 56:650–659, 1982.

96. Gopinath SP, Robertson CS, Contant CF, et al: Clinical evaluation of a miniature strain-gauge transducer for monitoring intracranial pressure. Neurosurgery 36:1137–1141, 1995.

97. Chambers IR, Mendelow AD, Sinar EJ, et al: A clinical evaluation of the Camino subdural screw and ventricular monitoring kits. Neurosurgery 26:421–423, 1990.

98. Czosnyka M, Czosnyka Z, Pickard JD: Laboratory testing of three intracranial pressure microtransducers: Technical report. Neurosurgery 38:219–224, 1996.

99. Unterberg A, Kiening K, Schmiedek P, et al: Long-term observations of intracranial pressure after severe head injury: The phenomenon of secondary rise of intracranial pressure. Neurosurgery 32:17–24, 1993.

100. Souter MJ, Andrews PJ, Pereirinha MR, et al: Delayed intracranial hypertension: Relationship to leukocyte count. Crit Care Med 27:177–181, 1999.

101. North B, Reilly P: Comparison among three methods of intracranial pressure recording. Neurosurgery 18:730–732, 1986.

102. Kanter RK, Weiner LB: Ventriculostomy-related infections. N Engl J Med 311:987, 1984.

103. Holloway KL, Barnes T, Choi S, et al: Ventriculostomy infections: The effect of monitoring duration and catheter exchange in 584 patients. J Neurosurg 85:419–424, 1996.

104. Lundberg N, Troupp H, Lorin H: Continuous recording of the ventricular fluid pressure in patients with severe acute traumatic brain damage: A preliminary report. J Neurosurg 22:581–590, 1965.

105. Andrews BT, Chiles BW III, Oslen WL, et al: The effect of intracerebral hematoma location on the risk of brain stem compression and on clinical outcome. J Neurosurg 69:518–522, 1988.

106. Marmarou A, Anderson RL, Ward JD, et al: Impact of ICP instability and hypotension on outcome in patients with severe head injury. J Neurosurg 75:S59–S64, 1991.

107. Contant CF, Robertson CS, Gopinath SP, et al: Determination of clinically important thresholds in continuously monitored patients with head injury [abstract]. J Neurotrauma 10(Suppl 1):S57, 1993.

108. O'Sullivan MG, Statham PF, Jones PA, et al: Role of intracranial pressure monitoring in severely head-injured patients without signs of intracranial hypertension on initial computerized tomography. J Neurosurg 80:46–50, 1994.

109. Teasdale G, Galbraith S, Jennett B: Operate or observe? ICP and the management of the "silent" traumatic intracranial hematoma. In Shulman K (ed): Intracranial Pressure IV. Berlin, Springer-Verlag, 1980, pp 35–38.

110. Miller JD, Stanek A, Langfitt TW: Concepts of cerebral perfusion pressure and vascular compression during intracranial hypertension. Prog Brain Res 35:411–432, 1971.

111. Kofke WA, Brauer P, Policare R, et al: Middle cerebral artery blood flow velocity and stable xenon-enhanced computed tomographic blood flow during balloon test occlusion of the internal carotid artery. Stroke 26:1603–1606, 1995.

112. Brauer P, Kochs E, Werner C, et al: Correlation of transcranial Doppler sonography mean flow velocity with cerebral blood flow in patients with intracranial pathology. J Neurosurg Anesthesiol 10:80–85, 1998.

113. Newell DW, Winn HR: Transcranial Doppler in cerebral vasospasm. Neurosurg Clin N Am 1:316–328, 1990.

114. Lindegaard KF, Nornes H, Bakke SJ, et al: Cerebral vasospasm diagnosis by means of angiography and blood velocity measurements. Acta Neurochir (Wien) 100:12–24, 1989.

115. DeWitt DS, Fatouros PP, Wist AO, et al: Stable xenon versus radiolabeled microsphere cerebral blood flow measurements in baboons. Stroke 20:1716–1723, 1989.

116. Gur D, Yonas H, Jackson DL, et al: Measurement of cerebral blood flow during xenon inhalation as measured by the microspheres method. Stroke 16:871–874, 1985.

117. Ploughmann J, Astrup J, Pederson J, et al: Effect of stable xenon inhalation on intracranial pressure during measurement of cerebral blood flow in head injury. J Neurosurg 81:822–828, 1994.

118. Marion DW, Crosby K: The effect of stable xenon on ICP. J Cereb Blood Flow Metab 11:347–350, 1991.

119. Dickman CA, Carter LP, Baldwin HZ, et al: Continuous regional cerebral blood flow monitoring in acute craniocerebral trauma. Neurosurgery 28:467–472, 1991.

120. Lam JM, Hsiang JN, Poon WS: Monitoring of autoregulation using laser Doppler flowmetry in patients with head injury. J Neurosurg 86:438–445, 1997.

121. Carter LP, Atkinson JR: Cortical blood flow in controlled hypotension as measured by thermal diffusion. J Neurol Neurosurg Psychiatry 36:906–913, 1973.

122. Brawley BW: The pathophysiology of intracerebral steal following carbon dioxide inhalation, an experimental study. Scand J Clin Lab Invest Suppl 102:13B, 1968.

123. Carter LP, Erspamer RJ, Bro WJ: Cortical blood flow thermal diffusion vs. isotope clearance. Stroke 12:513–518, 1981.

124. Gaines C, Carter LP, Crowell RM: Comparison of local cerebral blood flow determined by thermal and hydrogen clearance. Stroke 14:66–69, 1983.

125. Gopinath SP, Valadka A, Contant CF, et al: Relationship between cortical and global cerebral blood flow in patients with head injury. Neurosurgery 44:1273–1279, 1998.

126. Fukuda O, Endo S, Kuwayama N, et al: The characteristics of laser-Doppler flowmetry for the measurement of regional cerebral blood flow. Neurosurgery 36:358–364, 1995.

127. Robertson CS, Narayan RK, Gokaslan Z, et al: Cerebral arteriovenous oxygen difference as an estimate of cerebral blood flow in comatose patients. J Neurosurg 70:222–230, 1989.

128. Lewelt W, Jenkins LW, Miller JD: Autoregulation of cerebral blood flow after experimental fluid percussion injury of the brain. J Neurosurg 53:500–506, 1980.

129. Chan KH, Miller JD, Dearden NM, et al: The effect of changes in cerebral perfusion pressure upon middle cerebral artery blood flow velocity and jugular bulb venous oxygen saturation after severe brain injury. J Neurosurg 77:55–61, 1992.

130. Gibbs EL, Lennox WG, Nims LF, et al: Arterial and cerebral venous blood: Arterial-venous differences in man. J Biol Chem 144:325–332, 1942.

131. Cruz J: Continuous versus serial global cerebral hemometabolic monitoring: Applications in acute brain trauma. Acta Neurochir Suppl (Wien) 42:35–39, 1988.

132. Garlick R, Bihari D: The use of intermittent and continuous recordings of jugular venous bulb oxygen saturation in the unconscious patient. Scand J Clin Lab Invest Suppl 188:47–52, 1987.

133. Robertson CS, Grossman RG, Goodman JC, et al: The predictive value of cerebral anaerobic metabolism with cerebral infarction after head injury. J Neurosurg 67:361–368, 1987.

134. Andrews PJD, Dearden NM, Miller JD: Jugular bulb cannulation: Description of a cannulation technique and validation of a new continuous monitor. BMJ 67:553–558, 1991.

135. Cruz J: Combined continuous monitoring of systemic and cerebral oxygenation in acute brain injury: Preliminary observations. Crit Care Med 21:1225–1232, 1993.

136. Sheinberg M, Kanter MJ, Robertson CS, et al: Continuous monitoring of jugular venous oxygen saturation in head-injured patients. J Neurosurg 76:212–217, 1992.

137. Ritter AM, Gopinath SP, Contant C, et al: Evaluation of a regional oxygen saturation catheter for monitoring SjvO2 in head injured patients. J Clin Monit 12:285–291, 1996.

138. Souter MJ, Andrews PJD: Validation of the EdsLab dual lumen oximetry catheter for continuous monitoring of jugular bulb oxygen saturation [abstract]. J Neurotrauma 12:471, 1995.

139. Howard L, Gopinatb SP, Uzura M, et al: Evaluation of a new fiberoptic catheter for monitoring jugular venous oxygen saturation. Neurosurgery 44:1280–1285, 1999.

140. Gibbs EL, Lennox WG, Gibbs FA: Bilateral internal jugular blood: Comparison of A-V differences, oxygen-dextrose ratios and respiratory quotients. Am J Psychiatry 102:184–190, 1945.

141. Stocchetti N, Paparella A, Bridelli F, et al: Cerebral venous oxygen saturation studied using bilateral samples in the jugular veins. Neurosurgery 34:38–44, 1994.

142. Metz C, Holzschuh M, Bein T, et al: Monitoring of cerebral oxygen metabolism in the jugular bulb: Reliability of unilateral measurements in severe head injury. J Cereb Blood Flow Metab 18:332–343, 1998.

143. Croughwell ND, White WD, Smith LR, et al: Jugular bulb saturation and mixed venous saturation during cardiopulmonary bypass. J Card Surg 10:503–508, 1995.

144. Dings J, Meixensberger J, Roosen K: Brain tissue pO2-monitoring: Catheter stability and complications. Neurol Res 19:241–245, 1997.

145. Charbel FT, Hoffman WE, Misra M, et al: Cerebral interstitial tissue oxygen tension, pH, HCO3, CO2. Surg Neurol 48:414–417, 1997.

146. Kiening KL, Hartl R, Unterberg AW, et al: Brain tissue pO2-monitoring in comatose patients: Implications for therapy. Neurol Res 19:233–240, 1997.

147. Zauner A, Doppenberg E, Woodward JJ, et al: Multiparametric continuous monitoring of brain metabolism and substrate delivery in neurosurgical patients. Neurol Res 19:265–273, 1997.

148. Hoffman WE, Charbel FT, Edelman G: Brain tissue oxygen, carbon dioxide, and pH in neurosurgical patients at risk for ischemia. Anesth Analg 82:582–586, 1996.

149. Valadka A, Gopinath SP, Contant CF, et al: Critical values for brain tissue PO2 to outcome after severe head injury. Crit Care Med 26:1576–1581, 1998.

150. Kiening KL, Unterberg AW, Bardt TF, et al: Monitoring of cerebral oxygenation in patients with severe head injuries: Brain tissue PO2 versus jugular vein oxygen saturation. J Neurosurg 85:751–757, 1996.

151. Kirkpatrick PJ, Smielewski P, Czosnyka M, et al: Near-infrared spectroscopy use in patients with head injury. J Neurosurg 83:963–970, 1995.

152. Harris DN, Cowans FM, Wertheim DA, et al: NIRs in adults—effects of increasing optode separation. Adv Exp Med Biol 345:837–840, 1994.

153. Gopinath SP, Robertson CS, Grossman RG, et al: Near-infrared spectroscopic localization of intracranial hematomas. J Neurosurg 79:43–47, 1993.

154. Miller JD, Piper IR, Dearden NM: Management of intracranial hypertension in head injury: Matching treatment with cause. Acta Neurochir Suppl (Wien) 57:152–159, 1993.

155. Jennett B: Epilepsy after Nonmissile Head Injuries, 2nd ed. London, Heineman, 1975, pp 1–179.

156. Vespa PM, Nenov V, Nuwer MR: Continuous EEG monitoring in the intensive care unit: Early findings and clinical efficacy. J Clin Neurophysiol 16:1–13, 1999.

157. Vespa P, Prins M, Ronne-Engstrom E, et al: Increase in extracellular glutamate caused by reduced cerebral perfusion pressure

and seizures after human traumatic brain injury: A microdialysis study. J Neurosurg 89:971–982, 1998.

158. Miller JD, Becker DP: Secondary insults to the injured brain. J R Coll Surg Edinb 27:292–298, 1982.

159. Piek J, Chesnut RM, Marshall LF, et al: Extracranial complications of severe head injury. J Neurosurg 77:901–907, 1992.

160. Pietropaoli JA, Rogers FB, Shackford SR, et al: The deleterious effects of intraoperative hypotension on outcome in patients with severe head injuries. J Trauma 33:403–407, 1992.

161. Kontos HA, Raper AJ, Patterson JL Jr: Analysis of vasoactivity of local pH, pCO2, and bicarbonate on pial vessels. Stroke 8:358–360, 1977.

162. Cold GE: Cerebral blood flow in acute head injury: The regulation of cerebral blood flow and metabolism during the acute phase of head injury, and its significance for therapy. Acta Neurochir Suppl (Wien) 49:1–64, 1990.

163. Lassen NA, Palvolgyi R: Cerebral steal during hypercarbia and the inverse reaction during hypocapnea observed by the 133xenon technique in man. Scand J Clin Lab Invest 102(Suppl): D, 1968.

164. Cold GE: Measurements of CO2 reactivity and barbiturate reactivity in patients with severe head injury. Acta Neurochir (Wien) 98:153–163, 1989.

165. Cold GE: Does acute hyperventilation provoke cerebral oligemia in comatose patients after acute head injury? Acta Neurochir (Wien) 96:100–106, 1989.

166. Stringer WA, Hasso AN, Thompson JR, et al: Hyperventilation-induced cerebral ischemia in patients with acute brain lesions: Demonstration by xenon CT. AJNR Am J Neuroradiol 14:475–484, 1993.

167. Kerr ME, Zempsky J, Sereika S, et al: Relationship between arterial carbon dioxide and end-tidal carbon dioxide in mechanically ventilated adults with severe head trauma. Crit Care Med 24:785–790, 1996.

168. Kety S, Schmidt CF: The effects of altered arterial tensions of carbon dioxide and oxygen on cerebral oxygen consumption of normal young man. J Clin Invest 27:484–492, 1948.

169. Cohen PJ, Alexander SC, Smith TC, et al: Effects of hypoxia and normocarbia on cerebral blood flow and metabolism in conscious man. J Appl Physiol 23:183–189, 1967.

170. Siesjo BK, Carlsson C, Hagerdal M, et al: Brain metabolism in the critically ill. Crit Care Med 4:283–294, 1976.

171. Lewelt W, Jenkins LW, Miller JD: Effects of experimental fluid-percussion injury of the brain on cerebrovascular reactivity to hypoxia and to hypercapnia. J Neurosurg 56:332–338, 1982.

172. Eisenberg H, Cayard C, Papinicolaou A, et al: The effects of three potentially preventable complications on outcome after severe head injury. In Ishii S, Nagai H, Brock M (eds): Intracranial Pressure V. Berlin, Springer-Verlag, 1983, pp 549–553.

173. Borgstrom L, Johannsson H, Siesjo BK: The influence of acute normovolemic anemia on cerebral blood flow and oxygen consumption of anesthetized rats. Acta Physiol Scand 93:505–514, 1975.

174. Paulson OB, Parving HE, Olesen J, et al: Influence of carbon monoxide and of hemodilution on cerebral blood flow and blood gases in man. J Appl Physiol 35:111–116, 1973.

175. DeWitt DS, Prough DS, Taylor CL, et al: Reduced cerebral blood flow, oxygen delivery, and electroencephalographic activity after traumatic brain injury and mild hemorrhage in cats. J Neurosurg 76:812–821, 1992.

176. Dietrich WD, Alonso O, Halley M, et al: Delayed posttraumatic brain hyperthermia worsens outcome after fluid percussion brain injury: A light and electron microscopic study in rats. Neurosurgery 38:533–541, 1996.

177. Clifton GL, Jiang JY, Lyeth BG, et al: Marked protection by moderate hypothermia after experimental traumatic brain injury. J Cereb Blood Flow Metabol 11:114–121, 1991.

178. Dietrich WD, Alonso O, Busto R, et al: Post-traumatic brain hypothermia reduces histopathological damage following concussive brain injury in the rat. Acta Neuropathol (Berl) 87:250–258, 1994.

179. Lyeth BG, Jiang JY, Liu S: Behavioral protection by moderate hypothermia initiated after experimental traumatic brain injury. J Neurotrauma 10:57–64, 1993.

180. Mellergard P, Nordstrom CH: Epidural temperature and possi-

ble intracerebral temperature gradients in man. Br J Neurosurg 4:31–38, 1990.

181. Sternau LL, Thompson C, Dietrich WD, et al: Intracranial temperature observations in the human brain [abstract]. J Cereb Blood Flow Metab 11(Suppl 2):123, 1991.

182. Verlooy J, Heytens L, Veeckmans G, et al: Intracerebral temperature monitoring in severely head injured patients. Acta Neurochir (Wien) 134:76–78, 1995.

183. Mellergard P: Intracerebral temperature in neurosurgical patients: Intracerebral temperature gradients and relationships to consciousness level. Surg Neurol 43:91–95, 1995.

184. Rumana CS, Gopinath SP, Uzura M, et al: Brain temperature exceeds rectal temperature in head-injured patients. Crit Care Med 26:562–567, 1998.

185. Rosner MJ, Rosner SD, Johnson AH: Cerebral perfusion pressure: Management protocol and clinical results. J Neurosurg 83:949–962, 1995.

186. Robertson CS, Valadka AB, Hannay HJ, et al: Prevention of secondary insults after severe head injury. Crit Care Med 27:2086–2095, 1999.

187. Eker C, Asgeirsson B, Grande PO, et al: Improved outcome after severe head injury with a new therapy based on priniciples for brain volume regulation and preserved microcirculation. Crit Care Med 26:1881–1886, 1998.

188. Grande PO, Asgeirsson B, Nordstrom CH: Physiologic principles for volume regulation of a tissue enclosed in a rigid shell with application to the injured brain. J Trauma 42:S23–S31, 1997.

189. Rosner MJ, Coley IB: Cerebral perfusion pressure, intracranial pressure, and head elevation. J Neurosurg 65:636–641, 1986.

190. Rosner M: Cerebral perfusion pressure: Link between intracranial pressure and systemic circulation. In Wood JH (ed): Cerebral Blood Flow. New York, McGraw-Hill, 1987, pp 425–448.

191. Durward QJ, Amacher AL, Del Maestro RF, et al: Cerebral and cardiovascular responses to changes in head elevation in patients with intracranial hypertension. J Neurosurg 59:938–944, 1983.

192. Feldman Z, Kanter MJ, Robertson CS, et al: Effect of head elevation on intracranial pressure, cerebral perfusion pressure, and cerebral blood flow in head-injured patients. J Neurosurg 76:207–211, 1992.

193. Meixensberger J, Baunach S, Amschler J, et al: Influence of body position on tissue-pO_2, cerebral perfusion pressure and intracranial pressure in patients with acute brain injury. Neurol Res 19:249–253, 1997.

194. Bloomfield GL, Ridings PC, Blocker CR, et al: Effects of increased intra-abdominal pressure upon intracranial and cerebral perfusion pressure before and after volume expansion. J Trauma 40:941–943, 1996.

195. Bloomfield GL, Dalton JM, Sugerman HJ, et al: Treatment of increasing intracranial pressure secondary to the acute abdominal compartment syndrome in a patient with combined abdominal and head trauma. J Trauma 39:1168–1170, 1995.

196. de Nadal M, Ausina A, Sahuquillo J, et al: Effects on intracranial pressure of fentanyl in severe head injured patients. Acta Neurochir Suppl (Wien) 71:10–12, 1998.

197. Albanese J, Viviand X, Potie F, et al: Sufentanil, fentanyl, and alfentanil in head trauma patients: A study on cerebral hemodynamics. Crit Care Med 27:407–411, 1999.

198. Pinaud M, Lelausque JN, Chetanneau A, et al: Effects of Diprivan on cerebral blood flow, intracranial pressure and cerebral metabolism in head injured patients. Ann Fr Anesth Reanim 10:2–9, 1991.

199. Robertson CS, Clifton GL, Taylor AA, et al: Treatment of hypertension associated with head injury. J Neurosurg 59:445–460, 1983.

200. Enevoldsen EM, Jensen JT: Autoregulation and CO_2 responses of cerebral blood flow in patients with severe head injury. J Neurosurg 48:689–703, 1978.

201. Durward QJ, Del Maestro RF, Amacher AL, et al: The influence of systemic arterial pressure and intracranial pressure on the development of cerebral vasogenic edema. J Neurosurg 59:803–809, 1983.

202. Changaris DG, McGraw CP, Richardson JD, et al: Correlation of cerebral perfusion pressure and Glasgow Coma Scale to outcome. J Trauma 27:1007–1013, 1987.

203. Cottrell JE, Patel K, Turndorf H, et al: Intracranial pressure changes induced by sodium nitroprusside in patients with intracranial mass lesions. J Neurosurg 48:329–331, 1978.

204. Overgaard J, Skinhoj E: A paradoxical cerebral hemodynamic effect of hydralazine. Stroke 6:402–404, 1975.

205. Gokaslan ZL, Villareal C, Robertson CS, et al: Treating hypertension in neurosurgical patients [abstract no. 12]. Congress of Neurological Surgeons Abstracts, 1991.

206. Kohi YM, Mendelow AD, Teasdale GM, et al: Extracranial insults and outcome in patients with acute head injury—relationship to the Glasgow Coma Scale. Injury 16:25–29, 1984.

207. Price DJE, Murray A: Influence of hypoxia and hypotension on recovery from head injury. Injury 3:218–224, 1972.

208. Levasseur JE, Patterson JL, Ghatak JR, et al: Combined effect of respirator-induced ventilation and superoxide dismutase in experimental brain injury. J Neurosurg 71:573–577, 1989.

209. Carey ME, Sarna GS, Farrell JB, et al: Experimental missile wound to the brain. J Neurosurg 71:754–764, 1989.

210. Levine JE, Becker D, Chun T: Reversal of incipient brain death from head injury apnea at the scene of accidents. N Engl J Med 301:109, 1979.

211. Pfenninger EG, Ahnefeld FW, Kilian J, et al: Behavior of blood gases in patients with craniocerebral trauma at the accident site and at the time of admission to the clinic. Anesthetist 36:570–576, 1987.

212. North JB, Jennett S: Abnormal breathing patterns associated with acute brain damage. Arch Neurol 31:338–344, 1974.

213. Armstrong PA, McCarthy MC, Peoples JB: Reduced use of resources by early tracheostomy in ventilator-dependent patients with blunt trauma. Surgery 124:763–766, 1998.

214. Annegers JF, Hauser WA, Coan SP, et al: A population-based study of seizures after traumatic brain injuries. N Engl J Med 338:20–24, 1998.

215. Lee ST, Lui TN, Wong CW, et al: Early seizures after severe closed head injury. Can J Neurol Sci 24:40–43, 1997.

216. Young B, Rapp RP, Norton NA, et al: Failure of prophylactically administered phenytoin to prevent early posttraumatic seizures. J Neurosurg 58:231–235, 1983.

217. Tempkin NR, Dikmen SS, Wilensky AJ, et al: A randomized, double-blind study of phenytoin for the prevention of posttraumatic seizures. N Engl J Med 323:497–502, 1990.

218. Geerts WH, Code KI, Jay RM, et al: A prospective study of venous thromboembolism after major trauma. N Engl J Med 331:1601–1606, 1994; see comments.

219. Dennis JW, Menawat S, Von Thron J, et al: Efficacy of deep venous thrombosis prophylaxis in trauma patients and identification of high-risk groups. J Trauma 35:132–138, 1993.

220. Rogers FB, Shackford SR, Wilson J, et al: Prophylactic vena cava filter insertion in severely injured trauma patients: Indications and preliminary results. J Trauma 35:637–641, 1993.

221. Hammond FM, Meighen MJ: Venous thromboembolism in the patient with acute traumatic brain injury: Screening, diagnosis, prophylaxis, and treatment issues. J Head Trauma Rehabil 13:36–50, 1998.

222. Spain DA, Richardson JD, Polk HC Jr, et al: Venous thromboembolism in the high-risk trauma patient: Do risks justify aggressive screening and prophylaxis? J Trauma 42:463–467, 1997.

223. Kamada T, Fusamoto H, Kawano S, et al: Gastrointestinal bleeding following head injury: A clinical study of 433 cases. J Trauma 17:44–47, 1977.

224. Lu WY, Rhoney DH, Boling WB, et al: A review of stress ulcer prophylaxis in the neurosurgical intensive care unit. Neurosurgery 41:416–425, 1997.

225. Bowen JC, Fleming WH, Thompson JC: Increased gastrin release following penetrating central nervous system injury. Surgery 75:720–724, 1974.

226. Idjadi F, Robbins R, Stahl W, et al: Prospective study of gastric secretion in stressed patients with intracranial injury. J Trauma 11:686, 1971.

227. Nevton L, Greer J, Eiseman B: Gastric secretory response to head injury. Arch Surg 101:200–204, 1970.

228. Chan KH, Lai ECS, Tuen H, et al: Prospective double-blind placebo-controlled randomized trial on the use of ranitidine in preventing postoperative gastroduodenal complications in high-risk neurosurgical patients. J Neurosurg 82:412–417, 1995.

229. Tryba M: Sucralfate versus antacids of H₂ blockers for stress ulcer prophylaxis: A meta-analysis on efficacy and pneumonia rate. Crit Care Med 19:942–949, 1991.

230. Lau YL, Kenna AP: Posttraumatic meningitis in children. Injury 17:407–409, 1986.

231. Tenney JH: Bacterial infection of the central nervous system in neurosurgery. Neurol Clin 4:91–114, 1986.

232. Baltas I, Tsoulfa S, Sakellariou P, et al: Posttraumatic meningitis: Bacteriology, hydrocephalus, and outcome. Neurosurgery 35:422–426, 1994.

233. Clifton GL, Robertson CS, Grossman RG, et al: The metabolic response to severe head injury. J Neurosurg 60:687–696, 1984.

234. Clifton GL, Robertson CS, Choi SC: Assessment of nutritional requirements of head injured patients. J Neurosurg 64:895–901, 1986.

235. Jenkins M, Gottschlich M, Alexander JW, et al: Effect of immediate enteral feeding on the hypermetabolic response following severe burn injury. JPEN J Parenter Enteral Nutr 13(Suppl 1):128, 1989.

236. Inoue S, Epstein MD, Alexander JW: Prevention of yeast translocation across the gut by a single enteral feeding after burn surgery. JPEN J Parenter Enteral Nutr 13A:565–571, 1989.

237. Graham TW, Zadrozny DB, Harrington T: Benefits of early jejunal hyperalimentation in the head-injured patient. Neurosurgery 25:729–735, 1989.

238. Kirby DF, Clifton GL, Turner H, et al: Early enteral nutrition after brain injury by percutaneous endocopic gastrojejunostomy. JPEN J Parenter Enteral Nurt 15:298–302, 1991.

239. Harbrecht BG, Moraca RJ, Saul M, et al: Percutaneous endoscopic gastrostomy reduces total hospital costs in head-injured patients. Am J Surg 176:311–314, 1998.

240. Young B, Ott L, Dempsey R, et al: Relationship between admission hyperglycemia and neurologic outcome of severely brain-injured patients. Ann Surg 210:466–472, 1989.

241. Lam AM, Winn HR, Cullen BF, et al: Hyperglycemia and neurological outcome in patients with head injury. J Neurosurg 75:545–551, 1991.

242. Cherian L, Goodman JC, Robertson CS: Hyperglycemia increases brain injury caused by secondary ischemia after cortical impact injury in rats. Crit Care Med 25:1378–1383, 1997.

243. Cherian L, Hannay HJ, Vagner G, et al: Hyperglycemia increases neurological damage and behavioral deficits from post-traumatic secondary ischemic insults. J Neurotrauma 15:307–322, 1998.

244. Meixensberger J, Roosen K: Clinical and pathophysiological significance of severe neurotrauma in polytraumatized patients. Langenbecks Arch Surg 383:214–219, 1998.

245. McKee MD, Schemitsch EH, Vincent LO, et al: The effect of a femoral fracture on concomitant closed head injury in patients with multiple injuries. J Trauma 42:1041–1045, 1997.

246. Poole GV, Miller JD, Agnew SG, et al: Lower extremity fracture fixation in head-injured patients. J Trauma 32:654–659, 1992.

247. Kalb DC, Ney AL, Rodriguez JL, et al: Assessment of the relationship between timing of fixation of the fracture and secondary brain injury in patients with multiple trauma. Surgery 124:739–744, 1998.

248. Hsiang J, Chesnut RM, Crisp CB, et al: Early, routine paralysis for ICP control in severe head injury: Is it necessary? Crit Care Med 22:1471–1476, 1994.

249. Lauer KK, Connolly LA, Schmeling WT: Opioid sedation does not alter intracranial pressure in head injured patients. Can J Anaesth 44:929–933, 1997.

250. Schramm WM, Jesenko R, Bartunek A, et al: Effects of cisatracurium on cerebral and cardiovascular hemodynamics in patients with severe brain injury. Acta Anaesthesiol Scand 41:1319–1323, 1997.

251. MacFarlane I, Rosenthal F: Severe myopathy after status asthmaticus. Lancet 2:615–616, 1977.

252. Douglass JA, Tuxen DV, Horne M, et al: Myopathy in severe asthma. Am Rev Respir Dis 148:817–819, 1992.

253. Nates JL, Cooper DJ, Day B, et al: Acute weakness syndromes in critically ill patients—a reappraisal. Anaesth Intensive Care 25:502–513, 1997.

254. Zochodne DW, Bolton CF, Wells GA, et al: Critical illness polyneuropathy. Brain 110:819–842, 1987.

255. Latronico N, Rasulo FA, Recupero D, et al: Acute quadriplegia with delayed onset and rapid recovery. J Neurosurg 88:769–772, 1998.

256. Hayes C, Robertson CS, Narayan RK, et al: The effect of hyperventilation on cerebral blood flow in head injured patients [abstract no. 1271]. American Association of Neurological Surgeons Abstracts, 1992.

257. Muizelaar JP, Marmarou A, Ward JD, et al: Adverse effects of prolonged hyperventilation in patients with severe head injury: A randomized clinical trial. J Neurosurg 75:731–739, 1991.

258. Muizelaar JP, van der Poel HG, Li ZC, et al: Pial artery diameter and CO₂ reactivity during prolonged hyperventilation in the rabbit. J Neurosurg 69:923–927, 1988.

259. Ghajar JB, Hariri R, Patterson RH: Improved outcome from traumatic coma using only ventricular CSF drainage for ICP control. Adv Neurosurg 21:173–177, 1993.

260. Robertson CS, Clifton GL, Grossman RG: Oxygen utilization and cardiovascular function in head-injured patients. Neurosurgery 15:307–314, 1984.

261. Pollay M, Fullenwider C, Roberts A, et al: Effect of mannitol and furosemide on blood-brain osmotic gradient and intracranial pressure. J Neurosurg 59:945–950, 1983.

262. Hartl R, Ghajar J, Hochleuthner H, et al: Hypertonic/hyper-oncotic saline reliably reduces ICP in severely head-injured patients with intracranial hypertension. Acta Neurochir Suppl (Wien) 70:126–129, 1997.

263. Qureshi AI, Suarez JI, Bhardwaj A, et al: Use of hypertonic (3%) saline/acetate infusion in the treatment of cerebral edema: Effect on intracranial pressure and lateral displacement of the brain. Crit Care Med 26:440–446, 1998.

264. Bacher A, Wei J, Grafe MR, et al: Serial determinations of cerebral water content by magnetic resonance imaging after an infusion of hypertonic saline. Crit Care Med 26:108–114, 1998.

265. Rea GL, Rockswold GL: Barbiturate therapy in uncontrolled intracranial hypertension. Neurosurgery 12:401–404, 1983.

266. Lee MW, Deppe SA, Sipperly ME, et al: The efficacy of barbiturate coma in the management of uncontrolled intracranial hypertension following neurosurgical trauma. J Neurotrauma 11:325–331, 1994.

267. Goodman JC, Valadka AB, Gopinath SP, et al: Lactate and excitatory amino acids measured by microdialysis are decreased by pentobarbital coma in head-injured patients. J Neurotrauma 13:549–556, 1996.

268. Smith AL: Barbiturate protection in cerebral hypoxia. Anesthesiology 47:285–290, 1977.

269. Schwartz ML, Tator CH, Rowed DW, et al: The University of Toronto Head Injury Treatment Study: A prospective, randomized comparison of pentobarbital and mannitol. Can J Neurol Sci 11:434–440, 1984.

270. Ward JD, Becker DP, Miller JD, et al: Failure of prophylactic barbiturate coma in the treatment of severe head injury. J Neurosurg 62:383–388, 1985.

271. Eisenberg HM, Frankowski RF, Contant CF, et al: High-dose barbiturate control of elevated intracranial pressure in patients with severe head injury. J Neurosurg 69:15–23, 1988.

272. Winer JW, Rosenwasser RH, Jimenez F: Electroencephalographic activity and serum and cerebrospinal fluid pentobarbital levels in determining the therapeutic endpoint during barbiturate coma. Neurosurgery 29:739–742, 1991.

273. Sato M, Niiyama K, Kuroda R, et al: Influence of dopamine on cerebral blood flow, and metabolism for oxygen and glucose under barbiturate administration in cats. Acta Neurochir (Wien) 110:174–180, 1991.

274. Messeter K, Nordstrom CH, Sundbarg G, et al: Cerebral hemodynamics in patients with acute severe head trauma. J Neurosurg 64:231–237, 1986.

275. Cruz J: Adverse effects of pentobarbital on cerebral venous oxygenation of comatose patients with acute traumatic brain swelling: Relationship to outcome. J Neurosurg 85:758–761, 1996.

276. Schalen W, Messeter K, Nordstrom CH: Complications and side effects during thiopentone therapy in patients with severe head injuries. Acta Anaesthesiol Scand 36:369–377, 1992.

277. Cormio M, Gopinath SP, Valadka AB, Robertson CS: Cerebral hemodynamic effects of pentobarbital coma in head injured patients. J Neurotrauma 16:927–936, 1999.

278. Cooper PR, Moody S, Clark WK, et al: Dexamethasone and severe head injury: A prospective double-blind study. J Neurosurg 51:307–316, 1979.

279. Dearden NM, Gibson JS, McDowal DG, et al: Effect of high-dose dexamethasone on outcome from severe head injury. J Neurosurg 64:81–88, 1986.

280. Gudeman S, Miller J, Becker D: Failure of high-dose steroid therapy to influence intracranial pressure in patients with severe head injury. J Neurosurg 51:301–306, 1979.

281. Saul T, Ducker T, Saleman M, et al: Steroids in severe head injury: A prospective, randomized clinical trial. J Neurosurg 54:596–600, 1981.

282. Shiozaki T, Sugimoto H, Taneda M, et al: Effect of mild hypothermia on uncontrollable intracranial hypertension after severe head injury. J Neurosurg 79:363–368, 1993; see comments.

283. Bramlett HM, Green EJ, Dietrich WD, et al: Posttraumatic brain hypothermia provides protection from sensorimotor and cognitive behavioral deficits. J Neurotrauma 12:289–298, 1995.

284. Marion DW, Penrod LE, Kelsey SF, et al: Treatment of traumatic brain injury with moderate hypothermia. N Engl J Med 336:540–546, 1997.

285. Gower DI, Lee KS, McWhorter JM, et al: Role of subtemporal decompression in severe closed head injury. Neurosurgery 23:417–422, 1988.

286. Polin RS, Shaffrey ME, Bogaev CA, et al: Decompressive bifrontal craniectomy in the treatment of severe refractory posttraumatic cerebral edema. Neurosurgery 41:84–94, 1997.

287. Kee DB, Wood JH: Rheology of the cerebral circulation. Neurosurgery 15:125–131, 1984.

288. Menzel M, Doppenberg EMR, Zauner A, et al: Increased inspired oxygen concentration as a factor in improved brain tissue oxygenation and tissue lactate levels after severe human head injury. J Neurosurg 91:1–10, 1999.

289. Von Esson C, Zervas NT, Brown DR, et al: Local cerebral blood flow in the dog during intravenous infusion of dopamine. Surg Neurol 13:181–188, 1980.

290. Myburgh JA, Upton RN, Grant C, et al: A comparison of the effects of norepinephrine, epinephrine, and dopamine on cerebral blood flow and oxygen utilisation. Acta Neurochir Suppl (Wien) 71:19–21, 1998.

291. Darby JM, Yonas H, Marks EC, et al: Acute cerebral blood flow response to dopamine-induced hypertension after subarachnoid hemorrhage. J Neurosurg 80:857–864, 1994.

292. Grunner WP, Merlotti JG, Barrett J, et al: Resuscitation from hemorrhagic shock: Alteration of the intracranial pressure after normal saline, 3% saline, and dextran-40. Ann Surg 204:686–692, 1986.

293. Vassar MJ, Fisher RP, O'Brien PE, et al: A multicenter trial for resuscitation of injured patients with 7.5% sodium chloride: The effect of added dextran-70. Arch Surg 128:1003–1011, 1993.

294. Illingworth G, Jennett B: The shocked head injury. Lancet 2:511–514, 1965.

295. Apuzzo ML, Weiss MH, Petersons V, et al: Effects of positive end-expiratory pressure ventilation on intracranial pressure in man. J Neurosurg 46:227–232, 1977.

296. Frost EA: Effect of positive end-expiratory pressure on intracranial pressure and compliance in brain-injured patients. J Neurosurg 47:195–200, 1977.

297. Aidinis AJ, Lafferty J, Shapiro HM: Intracranial responses to PEEP. Anesthesiology 45:275–286, 1976.

298. Huseby JS, Luce JM, Cary JM, et al: Effects of positive end-expiratory pressure on intracranial pressure in dogs with intracranial hypertension. J Neurosurg 55:704–705, 1981.

299. Papo I, Caruselli G: The effects on intracranial pressure of stopping controlled ventilation in patients with severe head injury. Neurochirurgia 21:157–163, 1978.

300. Wilson JT, Pettigrew LE, Teasdale GM: Structured interviews for the Glasgow Outcome Scale and the Extended Glasgow Outcome Scale: Guidelines for their use. J Neurotrauma 15:573–585, 1998.

301. Bouma GJ, Muizelaar JP, Choi SC, et al: Cerebral blood flow and metabolism after severe traumatic brain injury: The elusive role of ischemia. J Neurosurg 75:685–693, 1991.

302. Jaggi JL, Obrist WD, Gennarelli TA, et al: Relationship of early cerebral blood flow and metabolism to outcome in acute head injury. J Neurosurg 72:176–182, 1990.

303. Zurynski YA, Dorsch NW, Pearson I: Incidence and effects of increased cerebral blood flow velocity after severe head injury: A transcranial Doppler ultrasound study. I. Prediction of posttraumatic vasospasm and hyperemia. J Neurol Sci 134:33–40, 1995.

304. Grande PO, Asgeirsson B, Nordstrom C: Aspects on the cerebral perfusion pressure during therapy of a traumatic head injury. Acta Anaesthesiol Scand Suppl 110:36–40, 1997.

305. Tateishi A, Maekawa T, Takeshita H, et al: Diazepam and intracranial pressure. Anesthesiology 54:335–337, 1981.

306. Cotev S, Shalit MN: Effects of diazepam on cerebral blood flow and oxygen uptake after head injury. Anesthesiology 43:117–122, 1975.

307. Griffin JP, Cottrell JE, Shwiry B, et al: Intracranial pressure, mean arterial pressure, and heart rate following midazolam or thiopental in humans with brain tumors. Anesthesiology 60:491–494, 1984.

308. Larsen R, Hilfiker O, Radle J, et al: The effects of midazolam on the general circulation, the cerebral blood flow, and cerebral oxygen consumption in man. Anaesthetist 30:18–21, 1981.

309. Moyer JH, Pontius R, Morris G, et al: Effect of morphine and N-allylnormorphine on cerebral hemodynamics and oxygen metabolism. Circulation 15:379–384, 1957.

310. Sperry RJ, Bailey PL, Reichman MV, et al: Fentanyl and sufentanil increase intracranial pressure in head trauma patients. Anesthesiology 77:416–420, 1992.

311. Moss E, Powell D, Gibson RM, et al: Effects of fentanyl on intracranial pressure and cerebral perfusion pressure during hypocapnia. Br J Anaesth 50:779–784, 1978.

312. Marx W, Shah N, Long C, et al: Sufentanil, alfentanil, and fentanyl: Impact on cerebrospinal fluid pressure in patients with brain tumors. J Neurosurg Anesthesiol 1:3–7, 1989.

313. Pinaud M, Lelausque J-N, Chetanneau A, et al: Effect of propofol on cerebral hemodynamics and metabolism in patients with brain trauma. Anesthesiology 73:404–409, 1990.

314. Moss E, Powell D, Gibson RM, et al: Effect of etomidate on intracranial pressure and cerebral perfusion pressure. Br J Anaesth 51:347–352, 1979.

315. Van Aken H, Puchstein C, Schweppe ML, et al: Effect of labetalol on intracranial pressure in dogs with and without intracranial hypertension. Acta Anaesthesiol Scand 26:615–619, 1982.

316. Bunegin L, Albin MS, Gelineau EF: Effect of esmolol on cerebral blood flow during intracranial hypertension and hemorrhagic hypovolemia [abstract]. Anesthesiology 67:A424, 1987.

317. Asgeirsson B, Grande PO, Nordstrom CH, et al: Effects of hypotensive treatment with alpha 2-agonist and beta 1-antagonist on cerebral haemodynamics in severely head-injured patients. Acta Anaesthesiol Scand 39:347–351, 1995.

318. Griffin JP, Cottrell JE, Hartung J, et al: Intracranial pressure during nifedipine-induced hypotension. Anesth Analg 62:1078–1082, 1983.

319. Stirt JA, Grosslight KR, Bedford RF, et al: "Defasciculation" with metocurine prevents succinylcholine induced increases in intracranial pressure. Anesthesiology 67:50–53, 1987.

320. Lanier WL, Milde JH, Michenfelder JD: Cerebral stimulation following succinylcholine in dogs. Anesthesiology 64:551–559, 1986.

321. Tarkkanen L, Laitinen L, Johansson G: Effects of D-tubocuranine on intracranial pressure and thalamic electrical impedance. Anesthesiology 40:247–251, 1975.

322. Vesely R, Hoffman WE, Gil KSL: Cerebrovascular effects of curare and histamine in the rat [abstract]. Anesthesiology 65:A336, 1986.

323. Lanier WL, Milde JH, Michenfelder JD: The cerebral effects of pancuronium and atracurium in halothane anesthetized dogs. Anesthesiology 63:587–597, 1985.

324. Griffin JP, Litwak B, Cottrell JE, et al: Intracranial pressure, mean arterial pressure, and heart rate after rapid paralysis with atracurium in cats. Can Anaesth Soc J 32:618–621, 1985.

325. Minton MD, Stirt JA, Bedford RF, et al: Intracranial pressure after atracurium in neurosurgical patients. Anesth Analg 64:1113–1116, 1985.

326. Rosa G, Orfei P, Sanfilippo M, et al: The effects of atracurium besylate (Tracrium) on intracranial pressure and cerebral perfusion pressure. Anesth Analg 65:381–384, 1986.

327. Rosa G, Sanfilippo M, Viardi V, et al: Effects of vecuronium

bromide on intracranial pressure and cerebral perfusion pressure. Br J Anaesth 58:437–440, 1986.

328. Rosa G, Sanfilippo M, Orfei P, et al: The effects of pipecurium bromide on intracranial pressure and cerebral perfusion pressure. J Neurosurg Anesthesiol 3:253–257, 1991.

329. Stirt JA, Maggio W, Haworth C, et al: Vecuronium: Effect on intracranial pressure and hemodynamics in neurosurgical patients. Anesthesiology 67:570–573, 1987.

330. Sutton LN, McLaughlin AC, Dante S, et al: Cerebral venous oxygen content as a measure of brain energy metabolism with increased intracranial pressure and hyperventilation. J Neurosurg 73:927–932, 1990.

331. Meyer JS, Gotoh F, Ebihara S, et al: Effects of anoxia on cerebral metabolism and electrolytes in man. Neurology 15:892–901, 1965.

332. Lennox WG, Gibbs FA, Gibbs EL: Relationship of unconsciousness to cerebral blood flow and to anoxemia. Arch Neurol Psych 34:1001–1013, 1935.

333. Sapire KJ, Gopinath SP, Farhat G, et al: Cerebral oxygenation during warming after cardiopulmonary bypass. Crit Care Med 25:1655–1662, 1997.

334. Gopinath SP, Cormio M, Ziegler J, et al: Intraoperative jugular desaturation during surgery for traumatic intracranial hematomas. Anesth Analg 83:1014–1021, 1996.

335. Cruz J: On-line monitoring of global cerebral hypoxia in acute brain injury: Relationship to intracranial hypertension. J Neurosurg 79:228–233, 1993.

336. Muizelaar JP, Lutz HA, Becker DP: Effect of mannitol on ICP and CBF and correlation with pressure autoregulation in severely head-injured patients. J Neurosurg 61:700–706, 1984.

CHAPTER 328

Surgical Management of Traumatic Brain Injury

SUJIT S. PRABHU ■ ALOIS ZAUNER ■ M. R. ROSS BULLOCK

The management of traumatic brain injury continues to be a challenge for neurosurgeons worldwide. The complexity of the injury, which is usually associated with trauma to other organ systems, makes decisions about medical or surgical management critical to patient outcome. Gennarelli and coworkers showed that the overall mortality is three times higher in trauma patients with head injury than in those without intracranial trauma.[1] Their study also showed that among head-injured patients, the cause of death was attributed to brain injury in 67.8% of patients, extracranial injuries in 6.6%, and both cranial and extracranial trauma in 25.6%. Severity of head injury still remains the strongest predictor of overall outcome in multiply traumatized individuals.[1–3] The quality of prehospital and emergency room care is an extremely important determinant of outcome in trauma patients, and the components of this care are described in the ATLS publications and in recent guidelines from the American College of Surgeons and the Brain Trauma Foundation.[4] They form the basis for certification of hospitals as level 1, 2, or 3 trauma centers throughout the United States; availability of neurosurgical care within 30 minutes of arrival in the emergency room is one of the prerequisites for level 1 certification.

In the past, many neurosurgeons regarded surgery for post-traumatic intracranial hematomas as unrewarding. This pessimism was based on the belief that outcome is determined principally by the magnitude of the initial injury and frequently remains poor despite optimal surgery. Although the mortality rate after severe head injury remains high at 30% to 35%, it is consistently falling in those centers that treat brain injury frequently and aggressively. In the Traumatic Coma Data Bank series, only 37% of comatose patients underwent surgery for the removal of intracranial hematomas.[5] Even though improvements in early resuscitation, diagnosis, and emergent surgical treatment of head injury victims may be reaching a plateau in terms of further reducing mortality and morbidity, refinements in critical care continue to offer new avenues for enhancing outcome. The decision to operate depends on the patient's neurological status, imaging findings, and extent of extracranial injury.

As mentioned earlier, about one third of patients who sustain severe head injuries are candidates for craniotomy. Hence, a majority of patients are managed by conservative means, usually directed at reducing intracranial pressure (ICP). At the Medical College of Virginia, we have developed a "staircase" of therapeutic steps to optimally treat elevated ICP (Fig. 328–1). The early, aggressive management of ICP by surgical or medical means is directed primarily at optimizing cerebral blood flow (CBF) and preventing cerebral ischemia and the consequent irreversible neurological deficits and mortality (Fig. 328–2A). Uncal herniation with midbrain compression and Duret's hemorrhages of the brainstem are postmortem findings in patients who succumb to untreatable intracranial hypertension (see Fig. 328–2B). Management decisions in individual patients must take into account a number of factors, such as extracranial injuries, the age of the patient, preexisting conditions, and the presence of associated intracerebral contusions or hemisphere swelling. In patients with intraparenchymal lesions such as contusions and intracerebral hematomas, management decisions are more complex and difficult, given the risk of coagulopathy and bleeding.

CONSERVATIVE MANAGEMENT

About two thirds of patients with severe head injury have no significant mass lesion on the initial computed tomographic scan. At least 80% demonstrate high ICP, and in the majority who die, high ICP is the cause of death.[6–9] For this reason, ICP monitoring and ICP-directed intensive care therapy are advocated for all patients older than 40 years whose Glasgow Coma Scale (GCS) score remains 8 or lower at 6 or more hours after injury. In patients younger than 40, ICP monitoring can be based on the status of the basal cisterns as demonstrated on a good-quality computed tomographic scan. Effaced cisterns are associated with high ICP in more than 70% of cases and mandate ICP monitoring. In patients younger than 40 with patent cisterns, a normal computed tomographic scan, and

Staircase ICP Control Algorithm - Medical College of Virginia - 2000

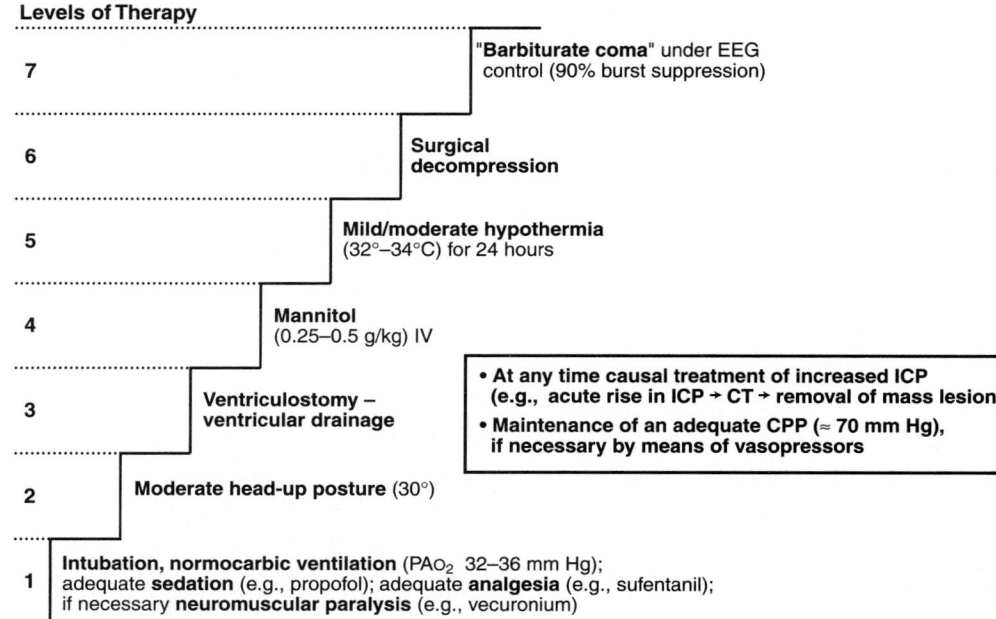

Levels of Therapy

7 — "**Barbiturate coma**" under EEG control (90% burst suppression)

6 — **Surgical decompression**

5 — **Mild/moderate hypothermia** (32°–34°C) for 24 hours

4 — **Mannitol** (0.25–0.5 g/kg) IV

3 — **Ventriculostomy –** **ventricular drainage**

- At any time causal treatment of increased ICP (e.g., acute rise in ICP → CT → removal of mass lesion)
- Maintenance of an adequate CPP (≈ 70 mm Hg), if necessary by means of vasopressors

2 — **Moderate head-up posture** (30°)

1 — **Intubation, normocarbic ventilation** (PAo₂ 32–36 mm Hg); adequate **sedation** (e.g., propofol); adequate **analgesia** (e.g., sufentanil); if necessary **neuromuscular paralysis** (e.g., vecuronium)

FIGURE 328–1. Algorithm used at the Medical College of Virginia for the stepwise management of elevated intracranial pressure.

the absence of hypoxic or ischemic episodes, ICP monitoring can be deferred and a repeat computed tomographic scan obtained in 6 to 12 hours.[8] Among the most difficult neurotrauma patients to manage are those whose GCS scores are between 8 and 14 and who have mass lesions of intermediate size. Often they are restless, combative, uncooperative, or intoxicated, making the GCS assessment very difficult. In such circumstances, it is usually best to intubate, sedate, and ventilate the patient in an intensive care setting and carry out ICP monitoring. If the ICP is persistently greater than 20 to 25 mm Hg, surgical evacuation is indicated even for small mass lesions, because associated brain swelling is extremely common.

Some recent studies have provided guidelines for the management of subdural and extradural hematomas in the relatively uncommon situation of a fully conscious patient. Nonoperative management should be considered only if the patient is fully conscious, the extra-axial mass lesion is the single dominant lesion (i.e., there are no multiple contusions or potentially significant contralateral mass lesions, which may be preventing midline shift), and there are no features of mass effect, such as midline shift greater than 3 mm, or basal cistern effacement.[10] If these criteria are met in a conscious patient with an acute subdural hematoma less than 10 mm at its thickest point, conservative treatment has been shown to be successful in most cases.[11] Similarly, deep-seated tentorial or interhemispheric subdural hematomas (Fig. 328–3) and small extradural hematomas in a stable, conscious patient often do not require surgical evacuation. When doubt exists, however, and when consciousness is depressed, the neurosurgeon should always monitor ICP or remove mass lesions in such patients.

INDICATIONS FOR THE EVACUATION OF INTRACRANIAL HEMATOMAS

In general, all acute traumatic extra-axial hematomas at least 1 cm thick and containing more than 40 mL of blood warrant urgent surgical evacuation. Temporal lobe hematomas (Fig. 328–4) are especially likely to cause brainstem compression at low ICPs with little midline shift and should be evacuated.

Surgical removal is always indicated in the presence of a mass lesion when there is a decline in the patient's level of consciousness, the development of new focal signs, and severe and worsening headache, nausea, or vomiting. In unconscious, noncommunicating, or sedated and ventilated patients, surgical evacuation is always indicated when there is a decline in the neurological status (this may be indicated only by the development of brainstem signs) and a sustained increase in ICP (e.g., >25 mm Hg). An urgent computed tomographic scan to evaluate the progression of the intracranial hematoma and brain swelling should be done, and a blood gas analysis should be performed to exclude the onset of hypoxemia, if appropriate. An increase in the size of an intracranial hematoma on computed tomographic scan is also an indication for surgical removal.[12]

In those patients who require operative intervention, urgent and rapid evacuation of the mass lesion ensures the best outcome, because ischemic brain damage is dependent on the duration of ischemia.

PREOPERATIVE PREPARATION

In general, cranial surgery should not be performed until a stable blood pressure and adequate lung func-

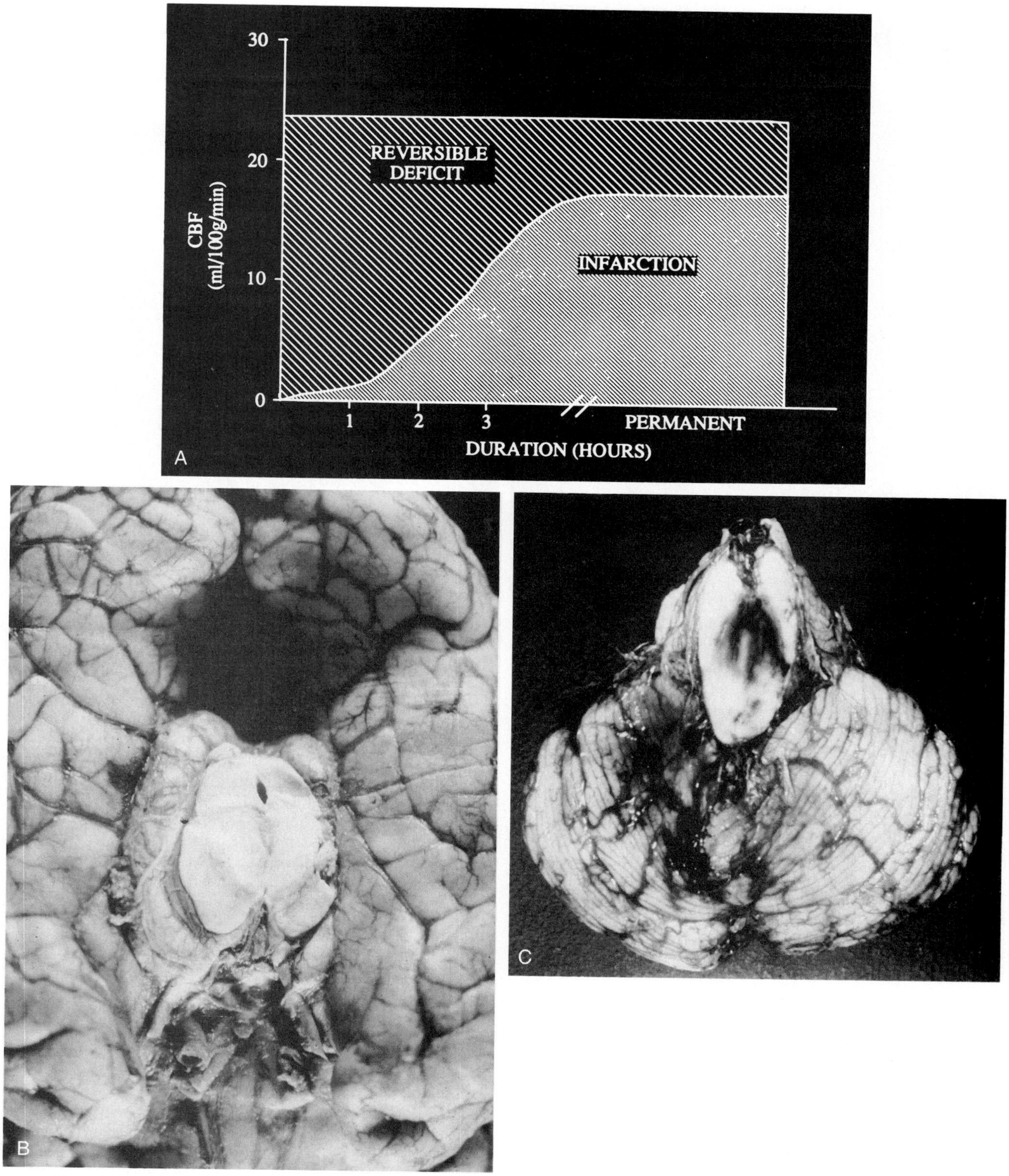

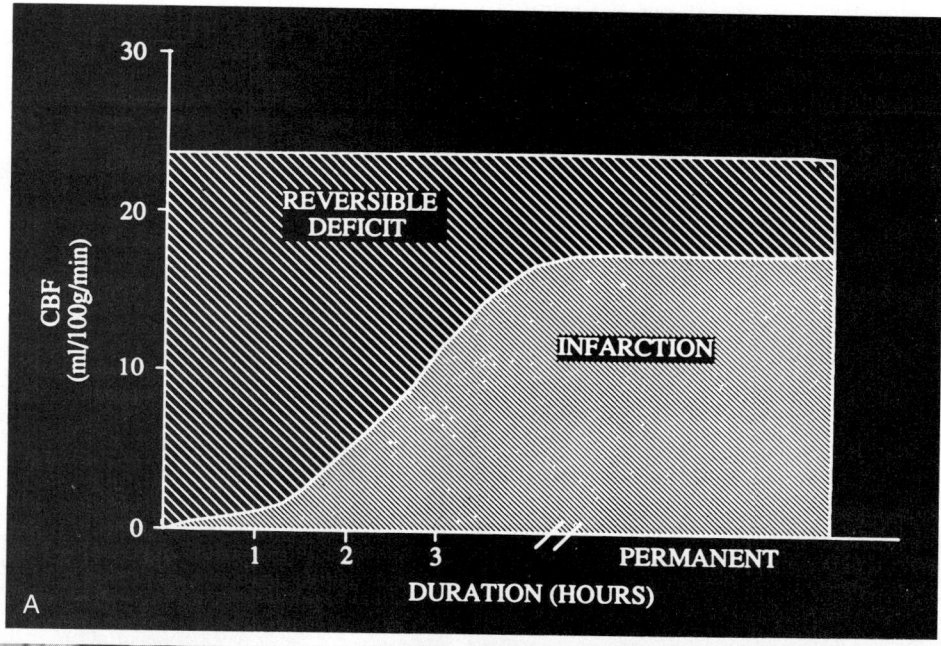

FIGURE 328–2. *A,* Illustration showing the importance of maintaining cerebral blood flow above 20 mL/100 g per minute to prevent permanent neurological deficits. Aggressive management of severe head injury can optimize the area of reversible deficit and prevent cerebral ischemia and infarction. *B,* Postmortem photograph of the midbrain at the level of the tentorium showing compression of the midbrain from uncal herniation. *C,* Postmortem photograph showing the brainstem and cerebellum with Duret's hemorrhages in the brainstem (pons and medulla) from downward traction of the midline blood vessels supplying the brainstem, resulting in hemorrhagic infarctions.

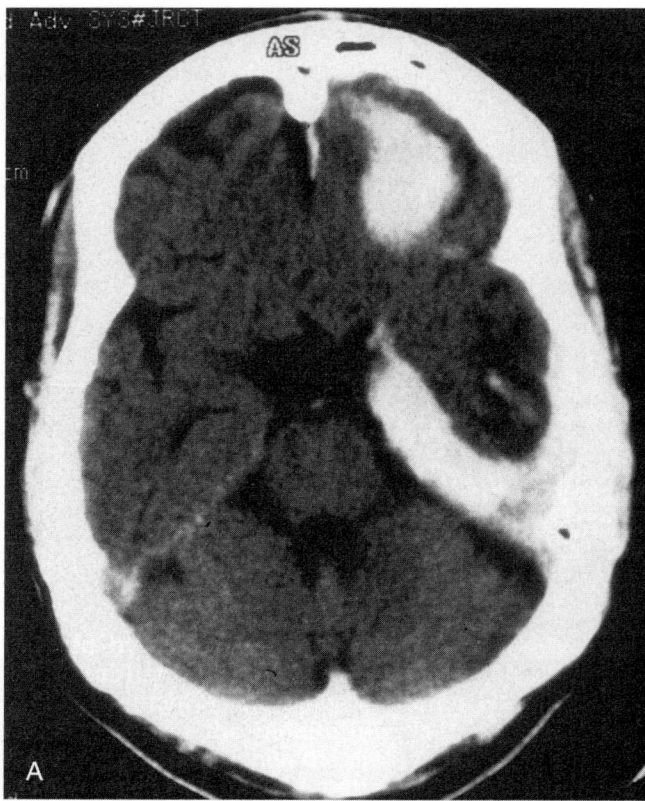

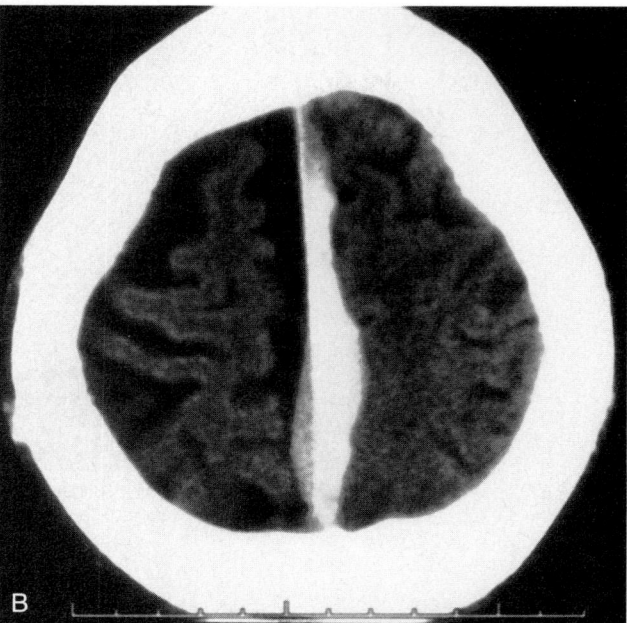

FIGURE 328–3. Axial computed tomographic scan of a subdural hematoma under the left tentorial margin *(A)* with no evidence of mass effect and another in the interhemispheric region *(B)*. Both these mass lesions were treated conservatively.

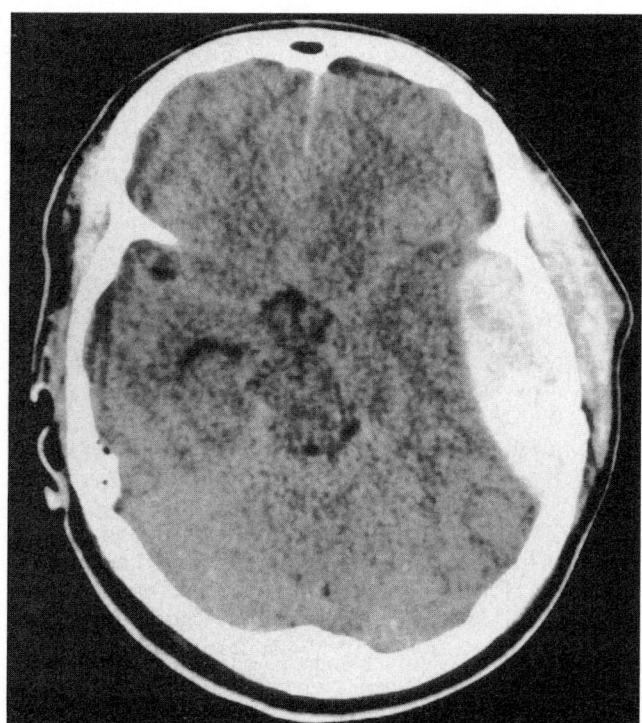

FIGURE 328–4. Axial computed tomographic scan of a left temporal extradural hematoma with mass effect. These lesions are known to cause acute deterioration in conscious patients.

tion, confirmed by radiographs and blood gas analysis, have been achieved. However, in a patient who is comatose, particularly if there has been a documented deterioration in the level of consciousness or the development of focal signs (e.g., dilated pupils), removal of the hematoma is a matter of great urgency. The patient should be intubated and hyperventilated if this has not already been done, and mannitol 1 g/kg should be given immediately as the patient is taken to the operating room.

Before or during preparation for craniotomy, the following checklist should be completed:

1. Blood sent to the laboratory for:
   a. Crossmatching (at least 2 units of packed red cells)
   b. Coagulation studies
      i. Prothrombin index
      ii. Partial thromboplastin time
      iii. Platelet count
   c. Blood gas analysis
   d. Routine full blood count and electrolytes
2. Radiographs of chest and cervical spine (or keep the cervical spine immobilized in a collar)
3. Consent for surgery
4. Foley catheter in the bladder
5. Two large-bore peripheral intravenous lines, or one peripheral and one central line (maintaining central venous pressure >5 cm H_2O)
6. Arterial catheter

7. Protection of both eyes from fluid and pressure
8. Adequately secured cuffed endotracheal tube
9. Both lower extremities placed in sequential compression devices to minimize the risk of deep vein thrombosis
10. Antibiotics and anticonvulsants given before surgery

Figure 328–5 shows how a patient is positioned for a craniotomy. In general, the head is placed on a horseshoe or doughnut headrest; turned to the opposite side, avoiding any constriction of the neck veins; and elevated above the level of the heart. A sandbag placed beneath the ipsilateral shoulder makes turning the head easier and also relaxes the tissues in the neck. The pressure points should be carefully padded. Unless deterioration is rapid, the scalp should be shaved and prepared as for any other neurosurgical procedure.

Strict attention to anesthetic techniques is vital to avoid hypercarbia and further elevation of ICP. All inhalation anesthetics have a potential cerebral vasodilator effect and therefore may increase ICP. They also lower cerebral metabolism, with the exception of nitrous oxide (N_2O); thus, a beneficial dissociation of CBF and cerebral metabolic rate of oxygen ($CMRO_2$) may occur.[13–15]

Nitrous oxide was used widely in the past to maintain anesthesia, and its rapid action allows easy control of the depth of anesthesia. However, because there is evidence that N_2O may increase ICP due to vasodilatation, and because the interaction of N_2O with volatile and intravenous anesthetics is complex, N_2O should be avoided in surgery after acute central nervous system trauma. Similarly, the use of halothane has decreased in recent years for surgery on intracranial lesions, although it may be safe in low concentrations (approximately 0.5%). Halothane uncouples CBF and $CMRO_2$ in a dose-dependent manner, producing cerebral vasodilatation and a decline in $CMRO_2$.[15] Enflurane, like halothane, is a cerebral metabolic depressant but has weaker vasodilatory properties. Because of its potential effects on ICP and the risk of inducing seizures, high concentrations of enflurane should be avoided in neurosurgical patients. Sevoflurane and desflurane have cerebrovascular effects similar to those of enflurane and should be avoided. Isoflurane produces a moderate increase in CBF and a pronounced beneficial decrease in cerebral metabolism. Because of its depressive effect on cerebral metabolism, isoflurane may be neuroprotective and is a more desirable anesthetic for neurosurgical procedures.

Intravenous anesthetics also cause a decrease in CBF and $CMRO_2$ due to their depressant effect on cerebral metabolism. Propofol's metabolic effect on cerebral metabolism is similar to that of barbiturates and may

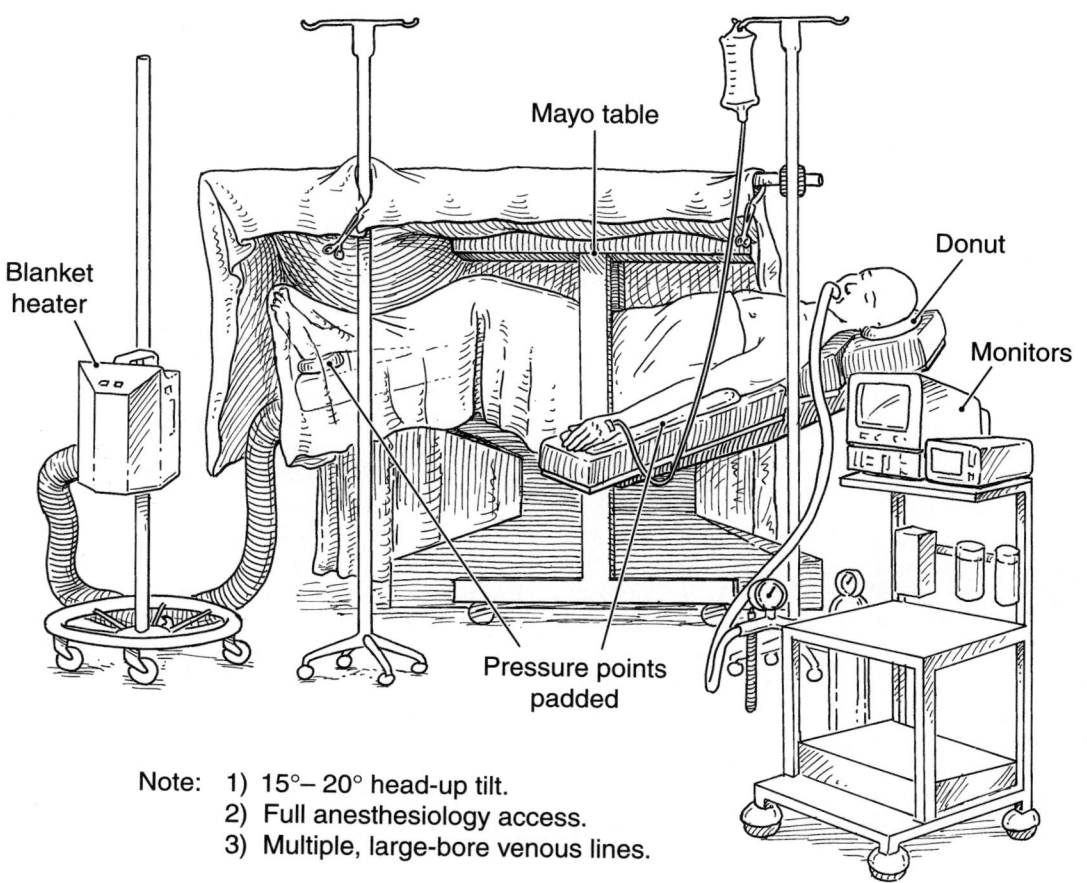

Note: 1) 15°– 20° head-up tilt.
       2) Full anesthesiology access.
       3) Multiple, large-bore venous lines.

FIGURE 328–5. Patient position and setup in the operating room for the performance of a craniotomy.

decrease ICP.[16] This drug is very useful in neurosurgical patients for sedation and as an anesthetic, provided hypotension is prevented. Barbiturates (thiopental, pentobarbital) produce a potent dose-dependent reduction in CBF, CMRO$_2$, and ICP, as well as a burst suppression pattern on electroencephalogram (at about a 40% decrease in CBF). Barbiturates also attenuate the cerebral vasodilatation produced by volatile anesthetics.[17] Etomidate has metabolic effects similar to those of barbiturates, and both may be used for "cerebral protection" and to control brain swelling intraoperatively after traumatic brain injury.[18] Benzodiazepine derivatives (midazolam) are also useful as induction or supplemental drugs during anesthesia in neurosurgical patients with traumatic brain injury.

Narcotic analgesics (morphine, fentanyl, sufentanil) have modest depressive effects on CBF and CMRO$_2$, and in most circumstances, they have only a minimal effect on the ICP. They should generally be avoided or used in small amounts in anesthesia for acute central nervous system trauma, owing to their long duration of action and the availability of other agents.[19]

The use of nondepolarizing muscle relaxants (tubocurarine, pancuronium, atracurium, vecuronium) changes CBF and ICP only minimally if respiration is well controlled. If succinylcholine is used, a small dose of a nondepolarizing muscle relaxant should be given before its administration to prevent an ICP rise with fasciculation.[20]

VENTRICULOSTOMY

A ventriculostomy catheter serves two basic purposes. It is the "gold standard" method for measuring ICP, and it provides cerebrospinal fluid drainage to lower ICP. The procedure can be done at the bedside under local anesthesia and is a quick and effective method of reducing raised ICP.

After shaving of the scalp and sterile surgical preparation, the patient's head is placed supine. A small incision (less than an inch) is made in the midpupillary line, 4 cm from the midline and 2 cm in front of the coronal suture on the right side (Fig. 328–6A). The incision is carried down to the underlying bone, and the periosteum is elevated. If the coronal suture cannot be felt easily under the scalp, a distance of approximately 10 cm is measured upward from the superior orbital margin posteriorly, in the midpupillary plane. Next, a twist drill is used to make an opening in the skull perpendicular to the plane of the skull. The twist drill hole is cleaned of any bony fragments using a small curet, and the underlying dura is pierced with a blunt stylet. A ventriculostomy catheter is placed using the standard landmarks—in the mediolateral plane, aiming at the medial canthus of the ipsilateral eye (see Fig. 328–6B), and in the anteroposterior plane, aiming at the tragus of the ipsilateral ear (see Fig. 328–6C). A distinct "popping " sensation is felt as one reaches the frontal horn of the lateral ventricle; the tip of the ventricular catheter is then advanced approximately 5 to 7 cm from the surface of the skull, at the opening of the foramen of Monro of the ipsilateral frontal horn. The ventriculostomy catheter is tunneled for a few centimeters in the subgaleal space (see Fig. 328–6D) and brought out through a separate stab incision. It is then secured firmly to the skin with sutures and connected to the pressure transducer system.

The standard landmarks may be altered in patients with intracranial mass lesions because of the associated brain swelling, resulting in slit-like ventricles, and because of the shift of the ventricles due to mass-producing lesions. No more than three passes for the ventricles should be tried before intraparenchymal pressure monitoring devices (e.g., the Codman or Camino transducer-tipped device) are placed.

For the placement of intraparenchymal monitoring devices, the twist drill opening is made as described earlier. Following the opening of the dura with a blunt stylet, the transducer tip is directly placed in the brain parenchyma at a distance of 2 to 3 cm. The catheter is then tunneled under the skin. For these devices, a fixation bolt may be useful (see Fig. 328–6E).

A ventriculostomy catheter is placed before leaving the operating room in all patients with an initial GCS score of 8 or less, because at least 80% of these patients develop raised ICP requiring treatment.[6, 7, 21] It may also be placed under direct vision, before closure of the bone flap.

At the Medical College of Virginia, the ventriculostomy catheter is placed through a triple-lumen bolt, along with a microdialysis probe and a tissue sensor measuring oxygen, carbon dioxide, and pH. Such multiparameter monitoring is being evaluated and may provide evidence of harmful effects such as ischemia, hypoxia, seizures, and excessive toxic mediators.[22, 23]

EXPLORATORY BUR HOLES

In the modern CT era, neurosurgeons seldom need to use exploratory bur holes; however, every neurosurgeon should be familiar with the procedure and be prepared to proceed to a full craniotomy, because acute traumatic hematomas cannot be dealt with adequately through bur holes.

The patient is placed supine with the head preferably in a head holder, which also gives wide access the both sides (Fig. 328–7B). The whole head is shaved, prepared, and draped to allow access to frontal, parietal, and temporal areas. The bur holes typically are placed on the side of localizing neurological findings—ipsilateral to a dilated pupil, contralateral to the most abnormal motor response, and ipsilateral to a skull fracture. It must be stressed that none of these signs is absolute, and if no hematoma is found on the suspected side, the other side should be explored in all cases. Initially, a bur hole is placed in the temporal region 2.5 cm above the zygomatic arch (see Fig. 328–7A). Following a diagnosis of either an acute subdural or extradural hematoma or no hematoma, two additional bur holes can be appropriately placed in the parietal and frontal regions. The skin incisions must be made in such a manner that if a formal craniotomy is

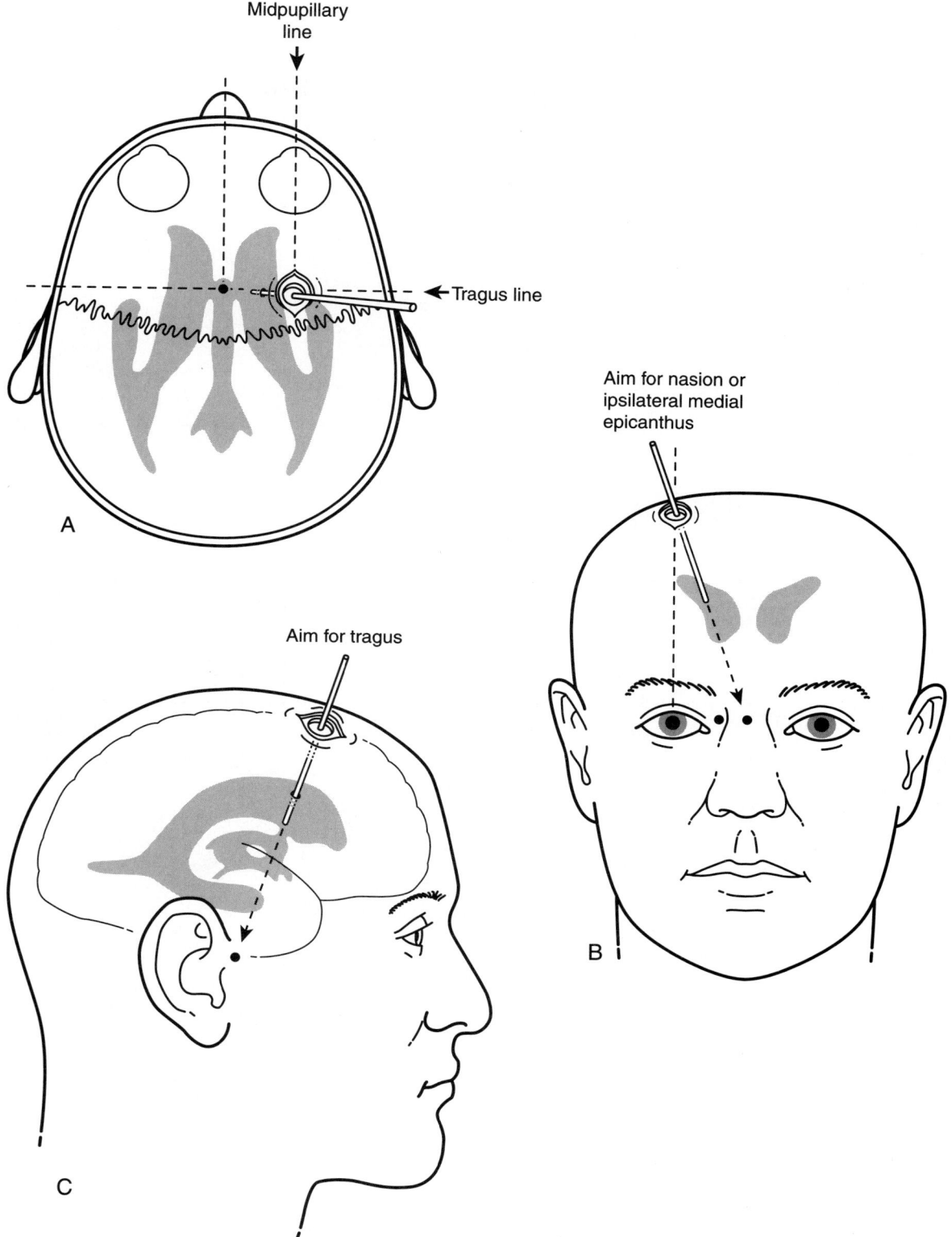

FIGURE 328–6. Schematic representation of landmarks used for ventriculostomy catheter placement. *B*, In the mediolateral plane, one should aim for the ipsilateral medial canthus. *C*, In the anteroposterior plane, one should aim for the ipsilateral tragus.

Illustration continued on following page

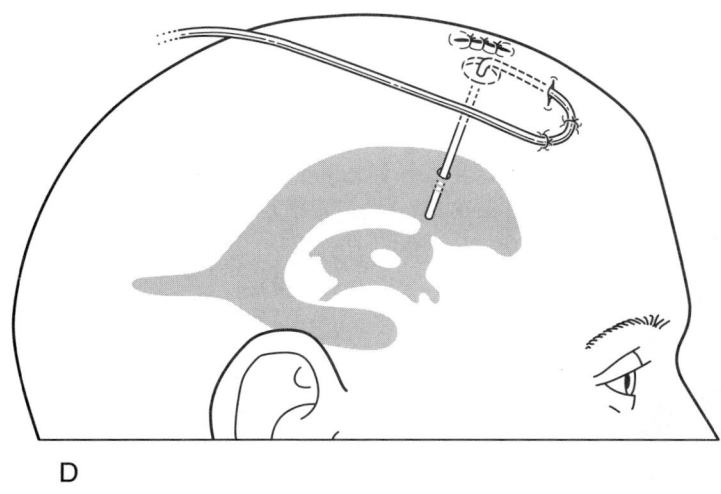

D

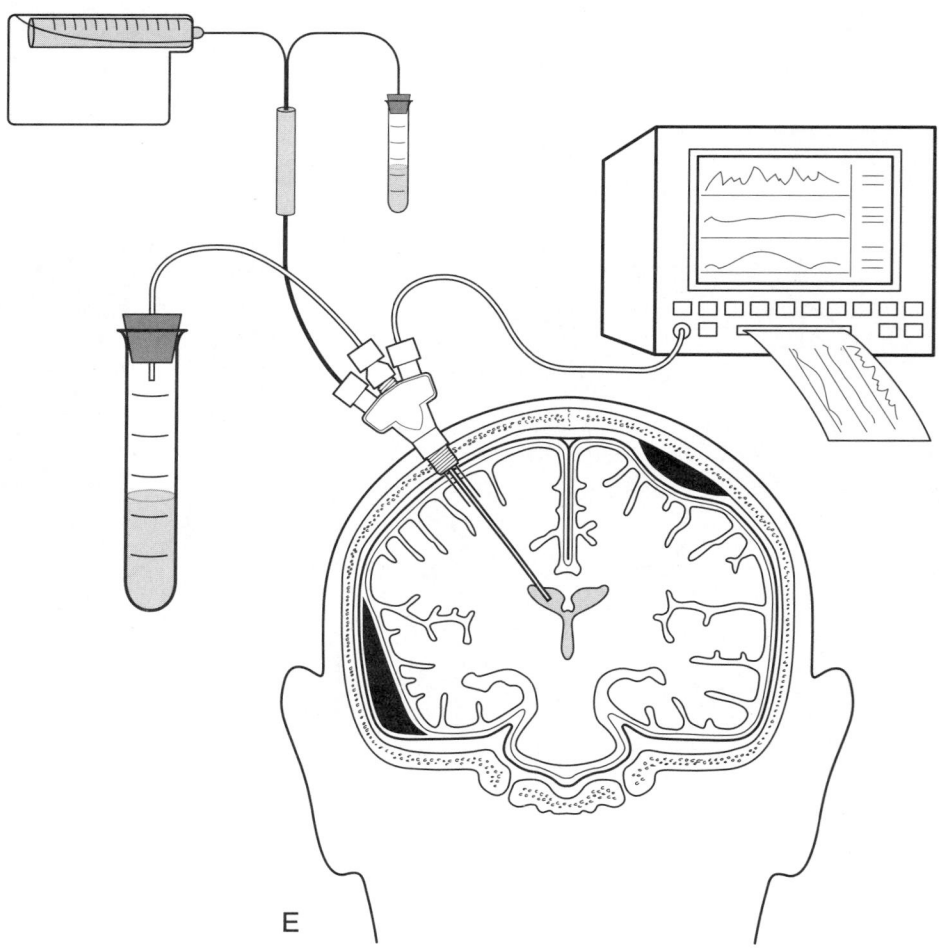

E

FIGURE 328–6. *Continued. E,* Triple-lumen bolt with the ventriculostomy catheter, microdialysis probe, and multiparametric probe (recording tissue pH, P_{O_2}, and P_{CO_2}).

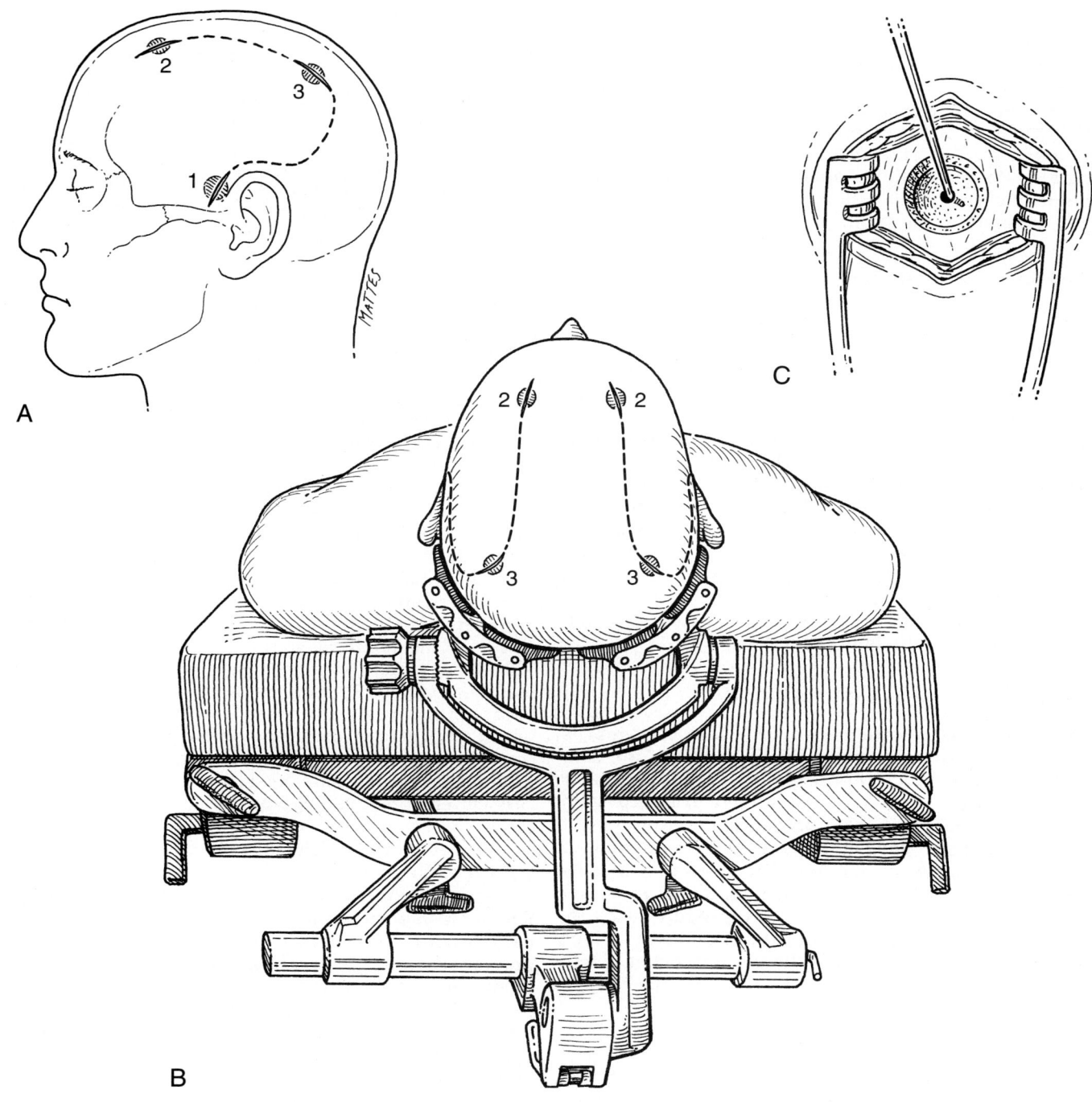

FIGURE 328–7. Placement of exploratory bur holes should begin in the temporal fossa, ipsilateral to the suspected lesion. The patient is positioned in a subdural head holder, exposing both sides of the scalp.

required, they can be joined to form the skin flap (see Fig. 328–7A).

SUPRATENTORIAL HEMATOMA

Rationale for Use of a Large Craniotomy

There is a high incidence of temporal and frontal contusions and tearing of midline bridging veins in trau-matic brain injury associated with mass lesions requir-ing a craniotomy. Because adequate decompressive operations may require débridement of these lesions, the frontal and temporal lobes (especially the poles) should be accessible in the field of exposure. The infe-rior part of the frontal lobe should also be accessible down to the floor of the anterior fossa, because the orbital gyri are frequently involved. About 30% to 40% of acute subdural hematomas are the result of tearing of the parasagittal midline bridging veins, and once the tamponade effect of the blood clot is released following a craniotomy, these veins start bleeding and can be better visualized if the craniotomy is close to the midline. However, the craniotomy should be carefully sited no closer than 1.5 to 2 cm from the midline to avoid inadvertent tearing of the sagittal sinus and parasagittal granulations, which are especially vulnerable in the elderly, in whom the dura is usually thin and adherent to the skull.

Craniotomy Technique

SCALP INCISION

The skin incision is started about 1 cm in front of the tragus at the zygomatic arch and then curved backward and upward above the auricle to reach the midline; it is then carried forward to the frontal region and curved across the midline just behind the hairline (Fig. 328–8A). In balding patients, the frontal part of the incision may be carried into the forehead, but it should be closed with 5–0 nylon suture for a good cosmetic result. Hemostasis of the skin margins is obtained with Raney clips. Then, using a Bovie cutting diathermy, an incision is made in the superficial temporal fascia and in the temporalis muscle down to the bone, close to the margin of the skin opening. The myocutaneous flap is reflected inferiorly and secured.

RAPID TEMPORAL DECOMPRESSION

In a patient who is herniated or whose condition is deteriorating from an intracranial hematoma, the temporal end of the incision is rapidly opened, and a bur hole is placed. This opening is then extended with Leksell rongeurs to form a limited craniectomy about 3 cm in diameter (see Fig. 328–8A). If the hematoma is in the subdural space, the dura is opened in a cruciate manner, and the underlying hematoma is promptly evacuated (see Fig. 328–8B). This procedure helps reduce ICP before completion of the craniotomy, which can then be completed more slowly, with better hemostasis.

BONE FLAP

Multiple bur holes are placed in the parietal and frontal regions (see Fig. 328–8A). Using a Kerrison bone punch, the bur holes are enlarged and undermined to allow a Penfield no. 3 to slide between the dura and the inner aspect of the bone flap, gently separating the dura from the skull. Special care is needed at this stage near the sagittal sinus. Joining the burr holes completes the craniotomy opening. The bone flap is fashioned so that its medial margin is at least 1.5 to 2 cm from the midline. If greater medial exposure is needed, it can be safely carried out with Leksell ronguers under direct vision. Further exposure of the middle fossa is obtained using Leksell rongeurs to remove parts of the lateral sphenoid wing and temporal bone in a piecemeal fashion, as needed for temporal tip access.

DURAL OPENING

A no. 15 blade knife is used to open the dura low over the frontal and temporal regions, with the base on the sagittal sinus, to avoid damage to the parasagittal bridging veins (see Fig. 328–8C). Care is taken to protect the underlying brain with a cottonoid patty if indicated. The opening can be extended in a *U* shape as needed. This opening provides safe access to the areas along the midline as well as the middle and frontal fossae (see later).

EPIDURAL HEMATOMA

In 1990, Pickard and coworkers showed that the surgical management of post-traumatic epidural hematoma is one of the most "cost-effective" of all surgical procedures in terms of quality of life and years preserved.[24] Epidural hematomas are located primarily in the temporal (see Fig. 328–4) and temporoparietal regions and are usually caused by tears of the anterior or posterior divisions of the middle meningeal artery, with an associated linear fracture of the skull. The bleeding sometimes occurs from the veins. The deformation of the skull is probably responsible for initiating the process of dural stripping. As the hematoma enlarges, the dura is progressively stripped from the inner table. The blood in the epidural space is usually clotted (Fig. 328–9). Sometimes, depressed skull fractures overlying the major venous sinuses are associated with epidural hematomas. Posterior fossa epidural hematomas, which often extend above and below the tentorium, account for approximately 5% to 10% of these lesions.[25, 26] Epidural hematomas are one of the most urgent neurosurgical emergencies, and prompt evacuation is indicated.

The preoperative checklist is carried out as described earlier, and the patient is positioned as shown in Figure 328–5. The scalp incision and the craniotomy flap are fashioned to provide complete exposure of the hematoma using the preoperative computed tomographic scan as a guide. A frontotemporoparietal craniotomy is usually carried out, depending on where the clot is situated. If neurological deterioration has been rapid, an initial bur hole is placed over the thickest part of the clot as seen on computed tomographic scan, and a small craniectomy is carried out to decompress the clot and promptly reduce ICP.

Following the skin incision, hemostasis is obtained with the help of Raney clips, or multiple curved hemostatic forceps are applied to the galeal layer and "turned over" the scalp. Multiple bur holes are then placed with a craniotome, and a craniotomy opening is completed; the size of the opening is based on measurements taken from the computed tomographic scan and is made large enough to encompass the clot in the craniotomy. The blood, which is usually clotted, is removed with the help of suction, irrigation, and cup forceps (see Fig. 328–9). The bleeding source, which is usually a branch of the middle meningeal artery, can usually be controlled with bipolar diathermy. Occasion-

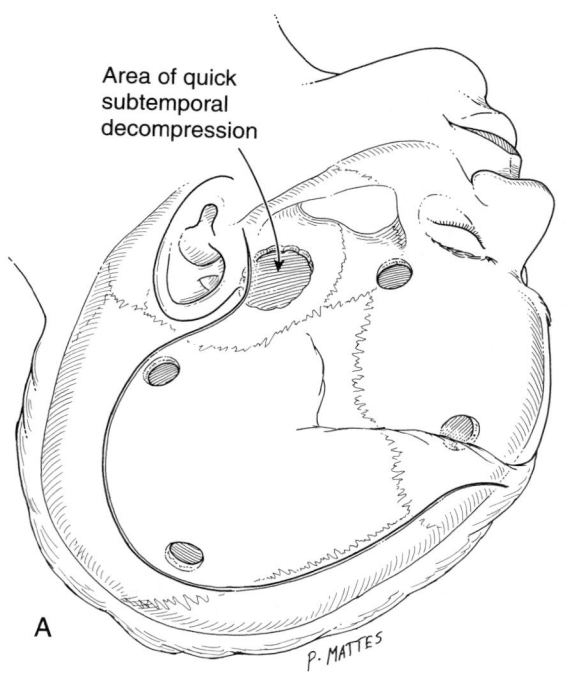

Area of quick
subtemporal
decompression

P. MATTES

A

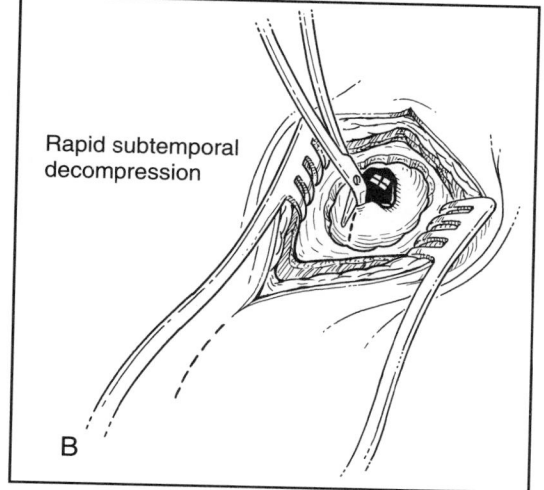

Rapid subtemporal
decompression

B

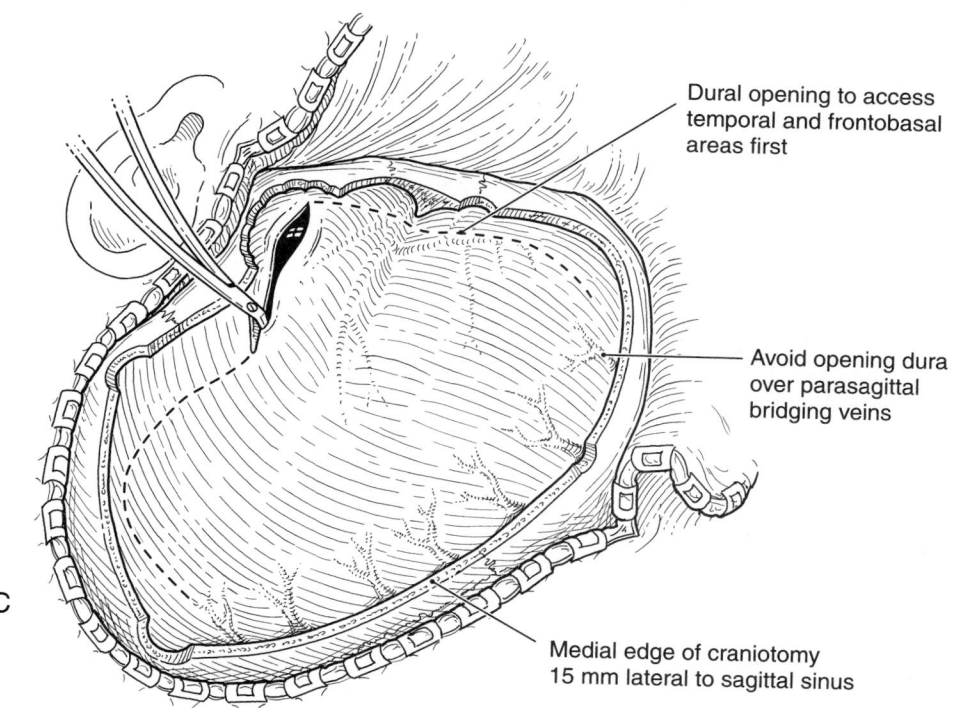

Dural opening to access
temporal and frontobasal
areas first

Avoid opening dura
over parasagittal
bridging veins

Medial edge of craniotomy
15 mm lateral to sagittal sinus

C

FIGURE 328–8. *A,* Schematic of a standard trauma craniotomy showing a large skin flap marked out with bur hole placements. *B,* Rapid temporal decompression is carried out if there is significant deterioration in the clinical condition of a patient with mass effect. *C,* Extent of the dural opening to visualize the midline bridging veins and expose the temporal and frontal lobes.

Illustration continued on following page

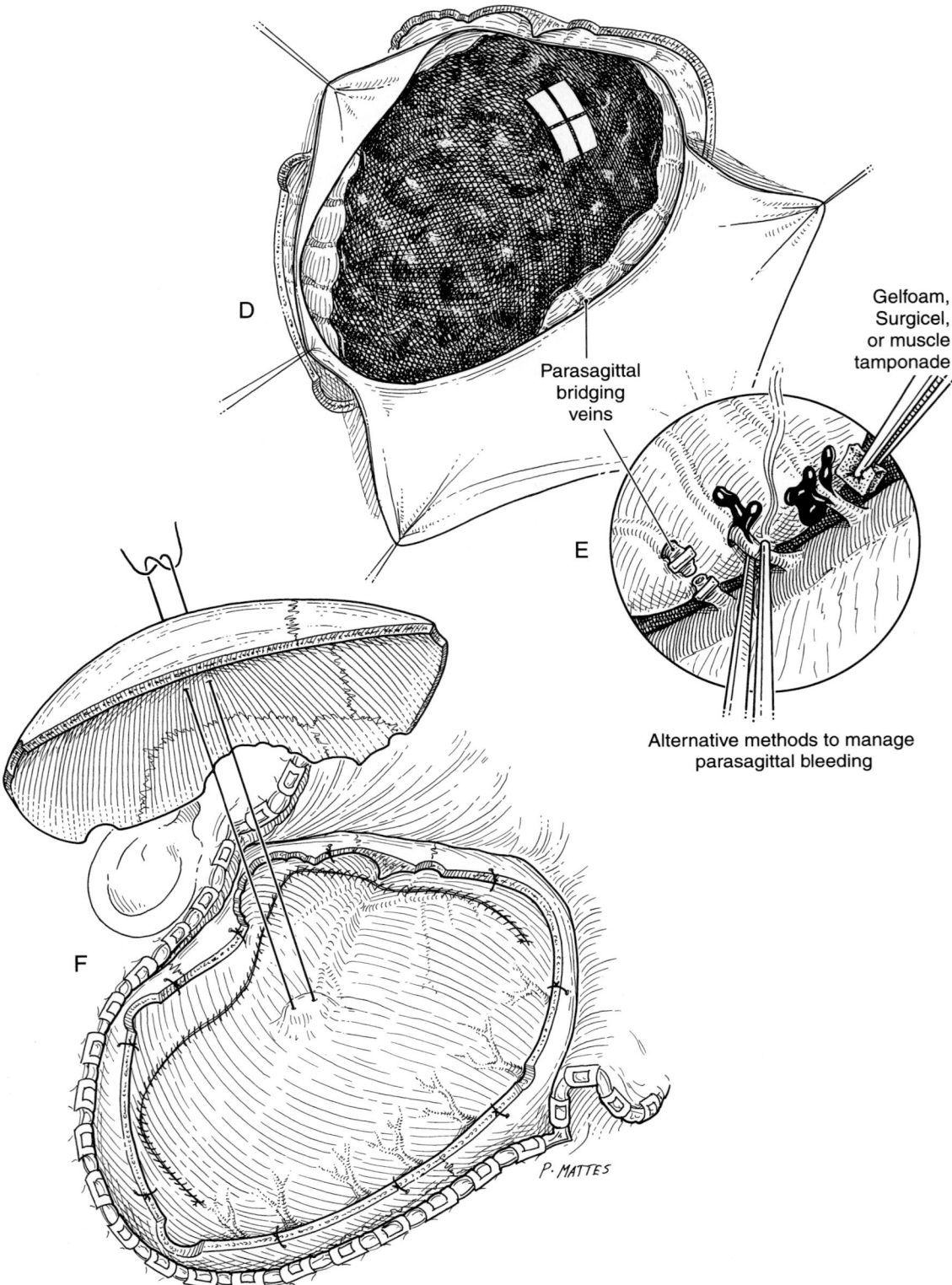

FIGURE 328–8. *Continued. E,* Bipolar diathermy of the bridging veins at the sagittal sinus. Weck clips can also be applied in these situations, as shown. An attempt is made to close the dura in a watertight fashion. *F,* Dural tack-up sutures are placed around the periphery, with a central tack-up suture in the middle of the craniotomy flap.

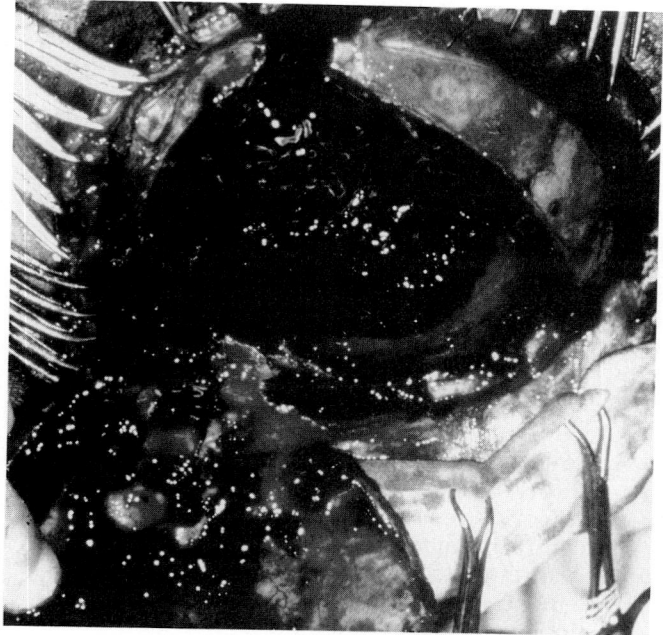

FIGURE 328–9. Intraoperative photograph showing a large, clotted acute epidural hematoma.

Fig. 328–8*F*). Central dural tack-up sutures are also placed in the bone flap to obliterate the central dead space under the bone flap (see Fig. 328–8*F*). The bone flap is then replaced, preferably using a miniplate system. Bur hole covers should always be placed over the frontal bur holes for the best cosmetic result. A 3.5-mm vacuum drain (medium hemovac) is placed under the galeal layer. The superficial temporal fascia and then the galea are approximated using 2–0 Dexon or similar suture. Skin staples are placed on the skin margins, the wound is dressed, and a head bandage is placed.

Sometimes, intracerebral hematomas are seen underlying extradural hematomas. Following evacuation of the extradural hematoma, if the underlying dura feels tense, a limited opening is made in the dura; using gentle suction and bipolar diathermy, any hematoma is removed. A larger dural opening must be made if persistent subdural bleeding is seen. A ventriculostomy may be needed in unconscious patients, especially if an intraparenchymal mass lesion is present (see later).

ally, the main trunk of the middle meningeal artery is bleeding due to a fracture involving the petrous bone. In these cases, the foramen spinosum can be packed with bone wax or a combination of bone wax and Surgicel. After evacuation of the hematoma, meticulous hemostasis is obtained in the epidural space with Surgicel and Gelfoam, and bone wax is applied to the bone edges. Dural tacking sutures are placed at 2.5-cm intervals in a circumferential fashion using 4–0 silk (see

ACUTE SUBDURAL HEMATOMA

Despite major advances in modern head injury management, patients who develop acute subdural hematomas have a worse prognosis than any other group of head-injured patients, with mortality reported to be between 50% and 60% in various series.[27–30] Acute subdural hematomas are due to bleeding from contused, lacerated cortex; torn bridging veins; or a torn cortical blood vessel. Approximately 50% of patients have associated intracranial lesions, including contusions, hematomas, or cortical lacerations, with the majority occurring in the frontal and temporal lobes (Fig.

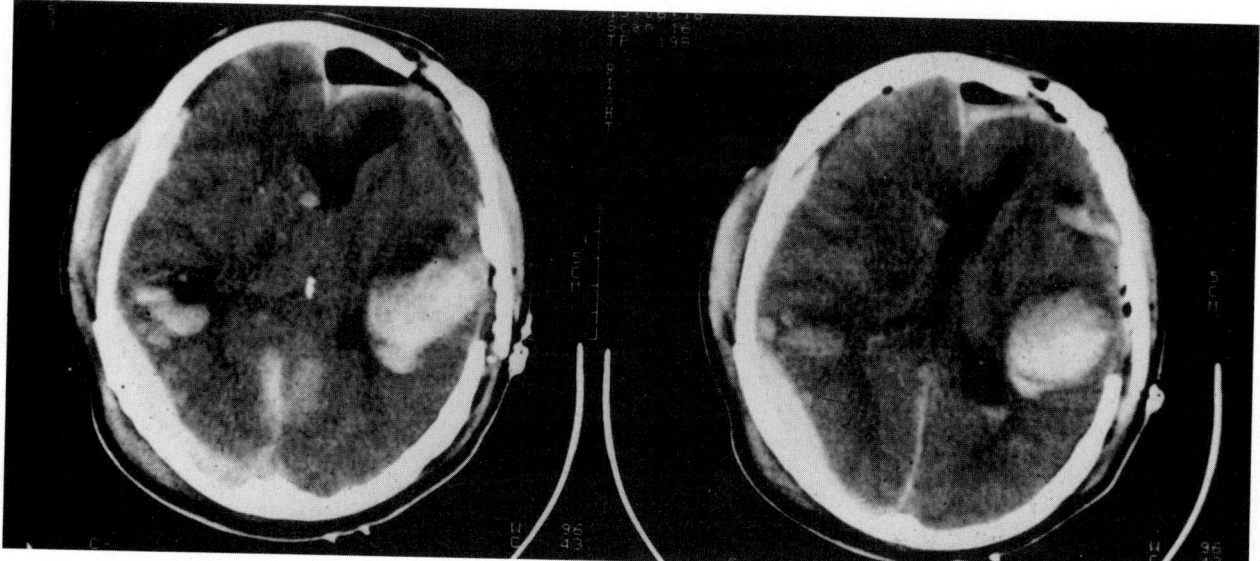

FIGURE 328–10. Computed axial tomogram showing multiple intracranial masses, including a subdural hematoma in the left frontal and parafalcine regions (which was operated on), a small epidural hematoma in the right posterior parietal region, and multiple intracerebral contusions.

328–10). The important predictors of outcome include age, admission GCS score, pupillary responsiveness, ICP, and the presence of hypotension and hypoxia. Age is probably the most significant factor in the prediction of outcome. In a retrospective study, 34 patients older than 65 years were compared with a similarly treated younger patient population (33 patients aged 18 to 40 years); mortality rates were more than four times higher in the older patients than in the younger group.[31] Recently, it has also been shown that the primary underlying brain injury is as important as the subdural clot itself in dictating outcome, emphasizing the need for postoperative ICP control.[32, 33]

Acute subdural hematomas are frequently an important and potentially lethal complication of anticoagulant treatment.[34] They are usually large and can be part of a coexistent chronic subdural hematoma (Fig. 328–11). In a recent study of 68 consecutive patients with warfarin-related intracranial hemorrhages, Mathiesen and associates reported that traumatic hematomas were found in 26 patients.[34] The hematomas were subdural in 23 patients (acute in 10 and chronic in 13), epidural in 1, and intraparenchymal associated with contusions in 2. The mortality was 79% in the group with traumatic intracranial hemorrhages. However, lower mortality rates of 48% and 16% have been reported following warfarin-related intracranial hemorrhages.[35, 36]

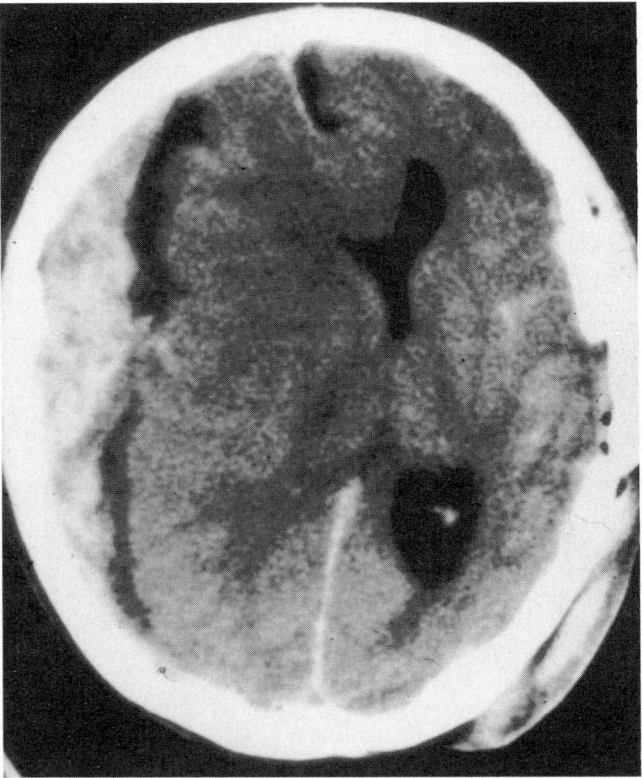

FIGURE 328–11. Axial computed tomographic scan showing a large frontoparietal acute-on-chronic subdural hematoma with significant midline shift in a patient on warfarin.

Craniotomy Technique

Following a decision to evacuate a subdural hematoma, the emergency preoperative workup and positioning of the patient are as described earlier. A large frontotemporoparietal craniotomy (described earlier) is generally required to adequately remove an acute subdural hemtoma and to address underlying parenchymal injuries. After a generous dural opening (see Fig. 328–8C), the clot is carefully removed with irrigation, suction, and cup forceps. The subdural space should be widely inspected for additional hematoma, bleeding, and surface contusions. Intracerebral hematomas underlying an acute subdural hematoma sometimes present on the surface and can be surgically removed through a limited corticotomy. Obtaining and maintaining hemostasis at the postoperative site are the most difficult and most important aspects of trauma neurosurgery. Frequently, these patients are coagulopathic with thrombocytopenia, making hemostasis especially difficult to maintain.[37]

Bleeding points on the cortical surface are cauterized with bipolar diathermy. Sometimes, two surgeons with two bipolar instruments are needed to do this. Occasionally, a bridging vein is clearly avulsed, and it can be easily cauterized with bipolar diathermy (see Fig. 328–8E). When bleeding is directly from the sinus wall, however, the use of bipolar diathermy is contraindicated because it will only enlarge the opening. In these situations, it is best to use Gelfoam, Surgicel, or Avitene and gentle tamponade with a cottonoid patty to stop the oozing. A muscle patch about 15 by 15 mm helps in these situations. Gentle irrigation and suction are applied to wash any additional clots from under the dural margins. Care must be taken during these maneuvers to prevent any additional bleeding.

If there are large areas of focal brain contusions, they should be removed with gentle suction and the use of bipolar diathermy, as demonstrated in Figure 328–14G. If diffuse oozing is persistent throughout hematoma evacuation, the anesthesiologist should be asked to send a fresh set of coagulation studies (prothrombin time, partial thromboplastin time, platelet count, and INR), and a simple in vitro clotting time is determined. Five to 10 units of fresh frozen plasma or up to 5 to 10 packs of platelet concentrate may be needed. After the clot is evacuated and hemostasis is obtained, closure of the dura is considered. Dural tackup sutures are first placed as described for epidural hematomas, and usually, a dural augmentation procedure (duraplasty) is done, unless the dura can be closed easily and brain swelling is considered unlikely. This is followed by routine closure of the craniotomy using miniplates and bur hole covers. Whenever there is significant or anticipated intracerebral swelling (Fig. 328–12), a dural substitute is placed loosely over the swollen brain and sewn to the dural margins. In these situations, the bone flap is not replaced. The patient is then treated medically for raised ICP as previously described. The bone flap can be replaced in 6 weeks to 2 months. If there is any evidence of brain swelling and the patient's preoperative GCS score was 8 or

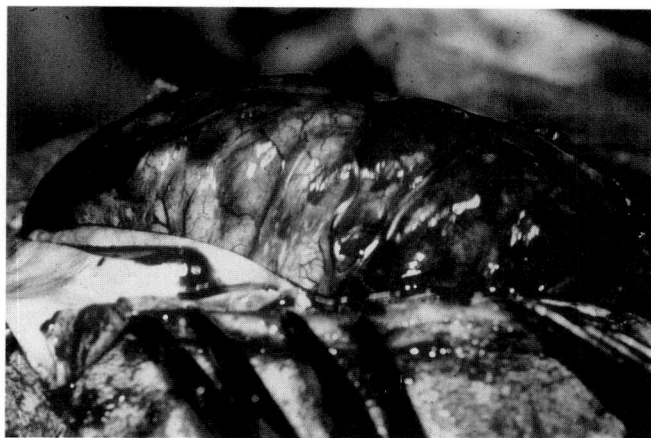

FIGURE 328–12. Fulminant cerebral swelling seen after evacuation of an acute subdural hematoma.

lower, a ventriculostomy catheter is placed either ipsilateral or contralateral to the craniotomy site before closure.

INTRACEREBRAL HEMATOMA AND CEREBRAL CONTUSION

Almost all patients with severe head injury, and about 25% of those with moderate injuries, demonstrate surface contusions and small intracerebral hematomas on computed tomography. However, only about 25% of trauma craniotomies are performed primarily for space-occupying contusional intracerebral hematomas.

Intracerebral hematomas and contusions generally do not require surgical evacuation unless there is significant mass effect or intracranial hypertension. They resorb in 4 to 6 weeks by macrophage phagocytosis and gliosis. The majority of intraparenchymal lesions occur in the temporal and frontal lobes, due to the brain impacting against the skull. Parietal and occipital lobe hematomas are much less common and are usually due to direct impact, as in assaults.[38–41] At least 25% of patients with intracranial mass lesions show clinical or radiologic worsening in the first 2 to 3 days after injury. In patients with cerebral contusions and hematomas, perilesional swelling and enlargement of bleeding are the norms rather than the exceptions, as shown in Figure 328–13. Accordingly, computed tomographic scans should be repeated at least daily over the first 3 days after injury, unless ICP is monitored and remains low. Associated subdural and epidural hematomas are encountered in a large number of patients.

In a patient with an intracerebral hematoma or contusion and a worsening neurological condition, high ICP, or mass effect on computed tomographic scan, a bifrontal craniotomy sometimes has to be performed. This procedure provides a large area of decompression; in addition, the underlying contused and hemorrhagic tissue can be more readily visualized and removed if necessary. This type of bifrontal decompressive craniec-

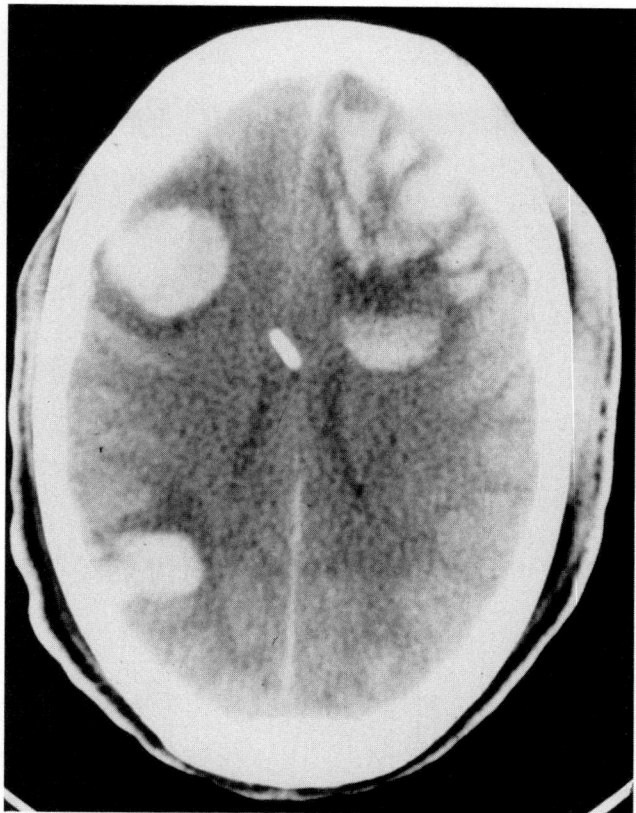

FIGURE 328–13. Axial computed tomographic scan showing an acute subdural hematoma in the right temporal region with bifrontal intracerebral contusions. There is significant midline shift to the left. An incidental left temporal arachnoid cyst is also seen.

tomy can also be performed over areas of maximal hemispheric swelling. Decompressive bifrontal craniectomy for intractable ICP in the absence of mass lesions is controversial; however, two recent studies showed better outcomes when the procedure was performed before irreversible ischemic brain damage resulted.[42, 43]

The preoperative workup and positioning of the patient are as described earlier. For a bifrontal craniotomy, the patient is placed supine on the operating table with the head resting on a doughnut device (Fig. 328–14). A bicoronal incision is marked out behind the hairline, starting low at the level of the zygoma (see Fig. 328–14A). In the temporal region, the incision is first carried down to the galea; above the superior temporal line, the incision is carried down to the bone. Raney clips are then applied to the skin margins for hemostasis. A Bovie monopolar cutting diathermy is used to incise the superficial temporal fascia and the temporalis muscle, taking special care to avoid possible injury to the facial nerve by remaining above the zygoma at the inferior end of the incision. Using a combination of periosteal elevators and monopolar diathermy to separate the periosteum from the skull, a myocutaneous flap is reflected as low as possible anterior to the supraorbital margins and the sphenoid wing in the temporal region. The scalp flap is then pulled

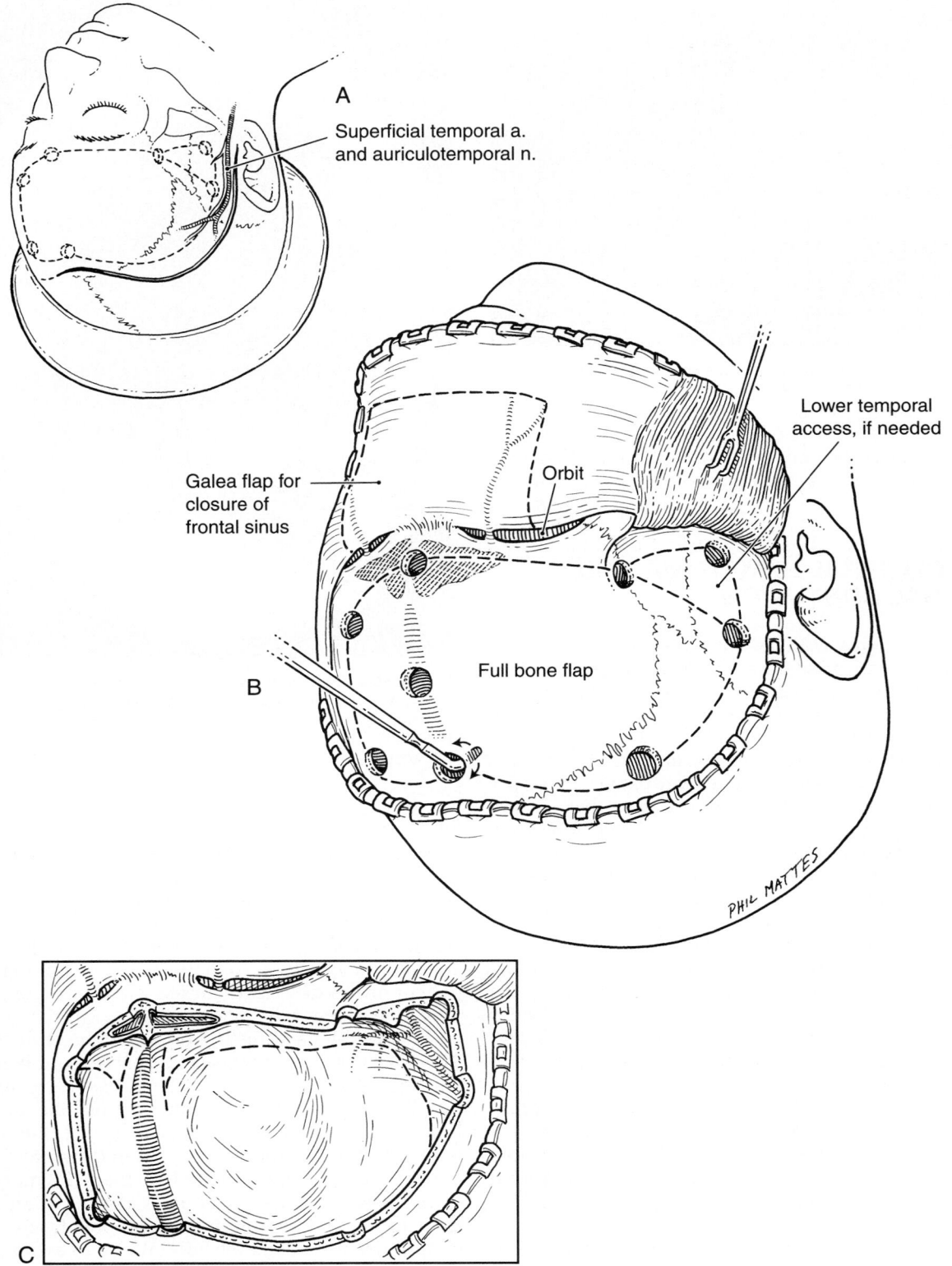

FIGURE 328–14. Schematic showing a bifrontal craniotomy. Following the scalp incision, multiple bur holes are placed, especially in relationship to the superior sagittal sinus. Following the large craniotomy opening, the dura is opened down to the frontobasal regions *(C)*.

Illustration continued on following page

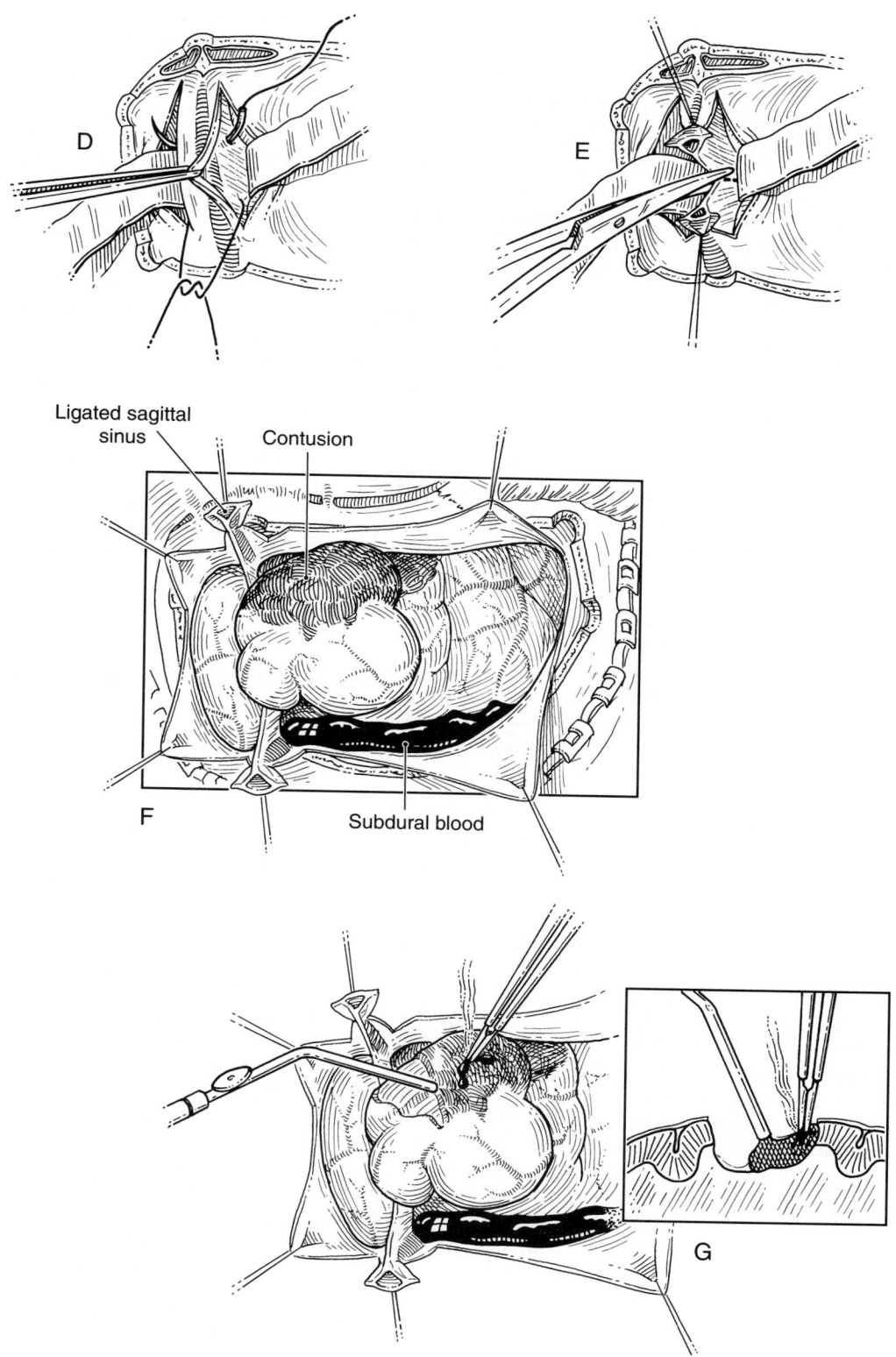

FIGURE 328–14. *Continued.* If required, the anterior aspect of the sagittal sinus is ligated close to the crista galli (*D–F*). The surface contusions and hemorrhages are then evacuated using a combination of suction and bipolar diathermy (*G*).

down and secured. Using a high-speed drill, multiple bur holes are placed in the temporal and frontal regions (see Fig. 328–14*B*). A Kerrison's punch and a curved curet are then used to enlarge the bur holes and undermine the inferior aspect to allow a Penfield no. 3 to slide into a plane between the dura and the inner aspect of the skull (see Fig. 328–14*B*). The dura is gently stripped over the midline sinus. Following this, a cutting craniotome blade is used to perform the craniotomy cuts, again keeping low in the frontal and temporal areas. The last cut of the craniotomy should be the one carried over the midline sagittal sinus region, to minimize bleeding. The superior sagittal sinus must be completely freed from the crista galli to the cephalad bur hole, and extra bur holes may be needed. Bone wax is applied to the bony margins, and strips of Surgicel or Gelfoam are placed around the craniotomy margins and over the bleeding points from the sagittal sinus. Dural tack-up sutures are placed around the margins of the craniotomy site using 4–0 silk suture. The dura is then opened with the flaps based toward the sagittal sinus (see Fig. 328–14*C*). Care is taken during the dural opening to protect the underlying brain and parasagittal draining veins with cottonoid patties. If there are bifrontal contusions or an acute subdural hematoma, or if frontobasal access is required, the most proximal superior sagittal sinus is double-ligated and cut (see Fig. 328–14*D* to *F*). Using bipolar diathermy, the pia mater and superficial vessels are cauterized over the cortical area with the most damage, swelling, and contusion. The pia mater is opened with a no. 15 knife blade, and a subpial plane is developed, if possible, to minimize bleeding. Using gentle suction and bipolar diathermy, the contused and hemorrhagic areas are removed (see Fig. 328–14*G*). Gentle retraction of the surrounding brain adjacent to the cavity is created with a hand-held malleable retractor. If there is significant swelling of the brain, a frontal or temporal "polectomy" can be carried out to minimize the pressure effects of postoperative brain swelling. The areas of the frontal lobe most prone to hemorrhagic contusions are the inferior orbital aspects of the gyrus-rectus and inferior frontal gyrus; in the temporal regions, it is the tips of the lobe. Following adequate decompression, hemostasis is obtained in the surgical bed with Surgicel; gentle tamponade can be maintained with cotton balls soaked in saline or half-strength hydrogen peroxide. The dura is then closed in a watertight fashion using 4–0 silk sutures. If there is significant brain swelling, the dura should be left open and a dural patch graft sutured to the margins of the dural edges. In this situation, the bone flap should also be left out. A central tack-up suture is also placed in the dura. If the bone flap is to be replaced, it is done using a miniplate system. Bur hole covers are placed over the frontal bur hole openings to improve the cosmetic appearance. The wound is then closed as described earlier. A ventriculostomy catheter is usually placed before closure if brain swelling is present or anticipated or if the patient is in a coma.

Traumatic intracerebral hematomas are also known to develop 24 to 72 hours after the initial injury. When a patient presents with a traumatic intracerebral hematoma and has not deteriorated or developed a new neurological deficit since the injury, the decision to remove the hematoma is controversial. Sometimes, delayed intracerebral hematomas do not manifest with changes in ICP; hence, the neurological condition of the patient should be closely monitored, and ICP monitoring is advocated if the patient is not obeying commands. A high degree of suspicion is necessary, because early identification and treatment of these lesions, which appear to enlarge after the initial computed tomographic scan, may prevent later neurological deterioration and thus improve outcome.

In a study reported by Bullock and colleagues, ICP monitoring failed to predict a rise in ICP in 17% of those with low ICP initially.[44] Five of the 30 patients who had ICP monitors suddenly deteriorated or died 6 to 11 days after injury, with features of high ICP clinically or at postmortem examination. Using near-infrared spectroscopy, Gopinath and coworkers were able to make an early diagnosis of delayed intracranial hematomas, resulting in a favorable outcome in 67% of the patients.[45]

POSTERIOR FOSSA HEMATOMA

Diagnosis

The posterior fossa is an uncommon site for intracranial hematomas, but that location may account for 3% to 5% of hematomas seen on computed tomographic scans. The clinical progress is usually silent and slow, but deterioration can be sudden and rapidly fatal if not treated promptly, owing to obstructive hydrocephalus. Such hematomas are usually associated with occipital skull fractures. The majority of patients who develop posterior fossa lesions have sustained direct occipital trauma, usually from a fall backward, from a blow to the head, or in association with a motor vehicle accident. Signs of occipital trauma are evident in more than 80% of patients and include scalp abrasions, lacerations, hematomas, and open fractures. An epidural hematoma is the most common posterior fossa lesion that requires surgery (Fig. 328–15), followed by subdural and intracerebellar hematomas, respectively. Infratentorial epidural hematoma is most often due to lateral sinus injury, but injury to sinuses deep at the skull base may be more frequent than is commonly realized.[46] Occipital fractures extend into the petrous bones in more than one third of cases, resulting in significant hearing loss (mostly sensorineural) in 20% of cases and facial nerve injury in 9% of cases.[46]

Procedure

The patient is taken to the operating room as urgently as possible, in view of the risk of obstructive hydro-

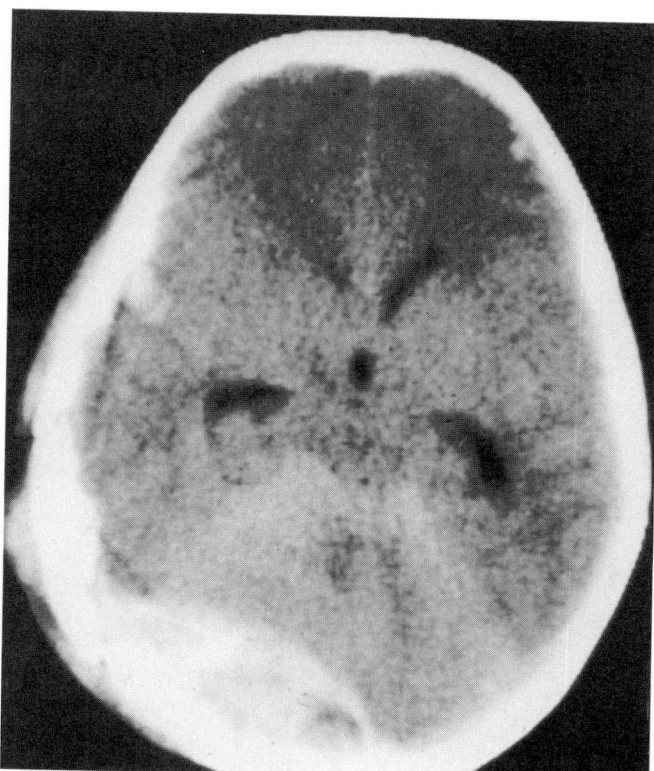

FIGURE 328–15. Axial computed tomographic scan showing a posterior fossa extradural hematoma with early dilatation of the ventricular system.

cephalus. Placement of a right frontal ventriculostomy is mandatory before surgery for any posterior fossa traumatic lesion. The head is fixed in a Mayfield three-point fixation device (Fig. 328–16*A*). After turning the patient to the prone position and fixing the head to the head holder, the head end of the bed is raised so that the head is slightly above the level of the heart. The head is then flexed forward to expose the occipital region optimally. A midline incision is carried out, and the occipital bone is exposed widely and bilaterally. Using a high-speed drill, multiple bur holes are placed above and below the transverse sinus (see Fig. 328–16*B*). If an extradural hematoma is present, the dura will already be separated from the underlying bone by the clot, and the craniotomy is then completed (see Fig. 328–16*C*). Because the dura is already stripped from the inner table of the bone, posterior fossa epidural hematomas are amenable to a craniotomy rather than the usual craniectomy. However, careful bone removal over the venous sinuses is necessary, and this should be performed last. A clear separation of the underlying bone from the sinuses is achieved with the help of a Penfield no. 3 instrument. The extradural hematoma is then gently removed with the help of cup forceps and suction. Any bleeding over the dura should be meticulously controlled, especially if it arises from the venous sinuses. A combination of Surgicel, Gelfoam, and Avitene, and sometimes a "muscle patch," can be employed to stop the bleeding. After hemostasis over the

dural surface is achieved, multiple dural tacking sutures are placed along the craniotomy margin at 20-mm intervals and centrally through the middle of the bone flap using 4–0 silk. The bone flap is then secured using cranial miniplates or 3–0 wire. The wound is closed in layers using 2–0 Dexon to the muscle layer and the subcutaneous tissues. A 3–0 subcuticular stitch is used for skin closure. A vacuum drain system is always advisable.

When a posterior fossa subdural hematoma is large, necessitating surgery, major bleeding should be anticipated; large-bore lines should be placed, and cross-matched blood should be available in the operating room. The initial bur holes over the cerebellar convexities should be widened to a large craniectomy with the help of Leksell rongeurs or a high-speed bur. A small dural opening is then created, and part of the underlying clot is aspirated to reduce the pressure rapidly in the posterior fossa. Bone removal should include the rim of the foramen magnum inferiorly and go up to the edge of the transverse sinus superiorly, to allow identification and control of bleeding from the sinus or from torn bridging veins over the superior cerebellar surface. The dura is opened in a cruciate manner (see Fig. 328–16*D*). The hematoma is then removed with the help of gentle suction (see Fig. 328–16*E*); if the underlying cerebellar surface appears contused, it is gently aspirated, and hemostasis is established with bipolar diathermy. In cases of cerebellar swelling, a dural substitute graft is used to achieve a wide decompression. If significant swelling is foreseen, the posterior arch of the atlas can also be removed as part of the bony decompression.

In cases of post-traumatic intracerebellar hematoma, the initial craniectomy and the dural opening should be large (as described for subdural hematoma), to maximize the decompressive effect. Initially, the cerebellar surface overlying the hematoma is subjected to diathermy through a small dural opening, and a blunt needle (e.g., a Dandy cannula) is passed into the cerebellar hemisphere to aspirate some clot and partly decompress the cerebellar hemisphere. Subsequently, the wide durotomy is completed, the clot cavity is entered, and hemostasis is obtained after clot removal as for any other intracerebral hematoma. Almost all posterior fossa mass lesions swell markedly in the first few post-injury days, making a wide decompression and augmentation duraplasty mandatory. Delayed cranioplasty is seldom necessary.

When preparing a patient with a posterior fossa hematoma for emergency craniotomy, the most important goals are avoiding hypotension and hypoxia, treating intracranial hypertension, and assessing and treating coagulopathy. Seizure prophylaxis is indicated in most patients as well, owing to coexistent supratentorial injuries. A ventriculostomy catheter is always placed first for cerebrospinal fluid drainage in patients with post-trauamtic surgical lesions. To avoid the rare possibility of upward herniation after placement of the ventriculostomy, some authorities advise slower cerebrospinal fluid drainage, but as soon as the posterior fossa is decompressed, this risk is removed.[47]

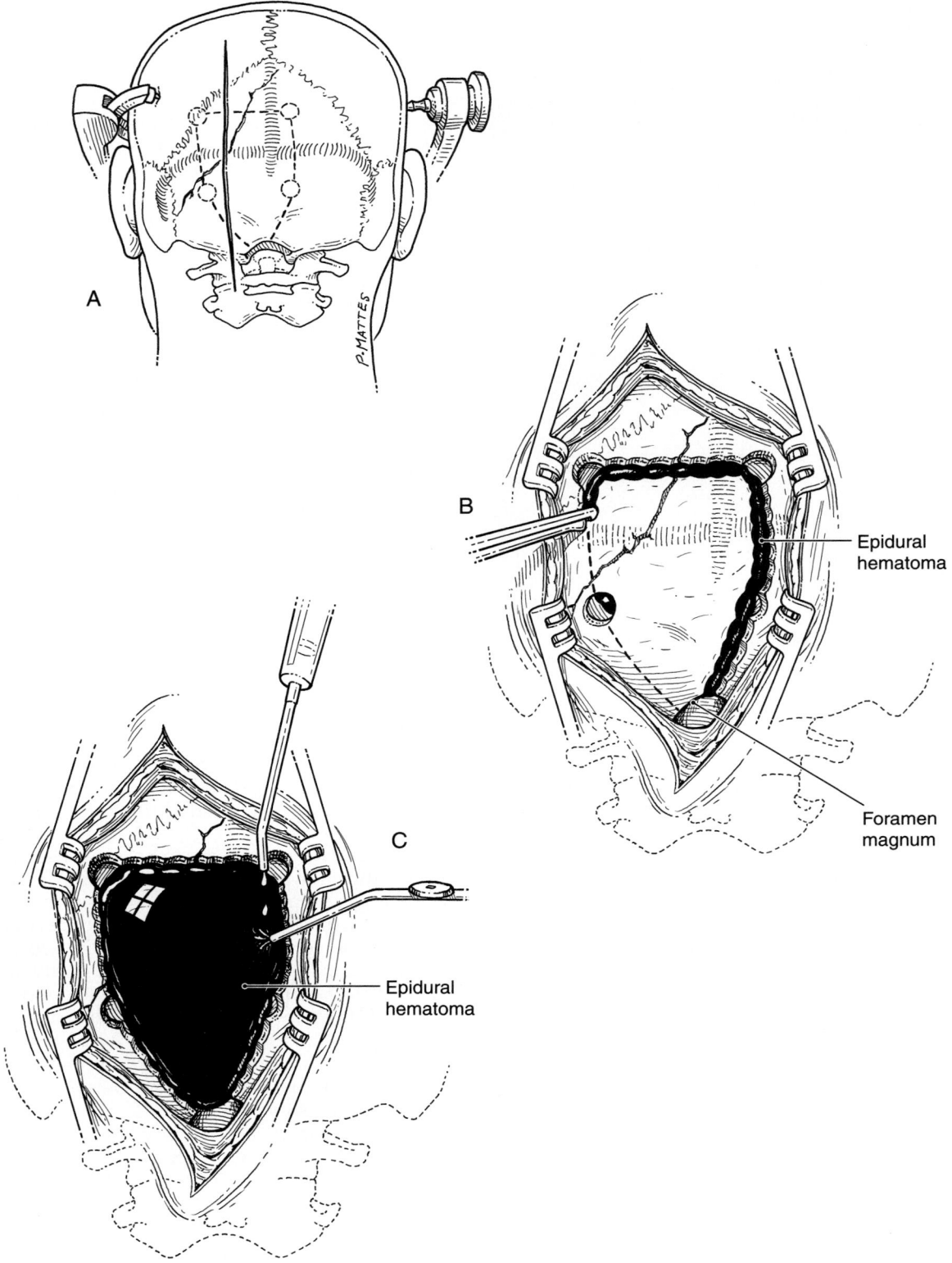

FIGURE 328–16. Schematic of a posterior fossa craniotomy for evacuation of an acute extradural hematoma *(C)* and a subdural hematoma *(E)*. The head is fixed in Mayfield pins, and a wide craniotomy is carried out both above and below the transverse sinus.

Illustration continued on following page

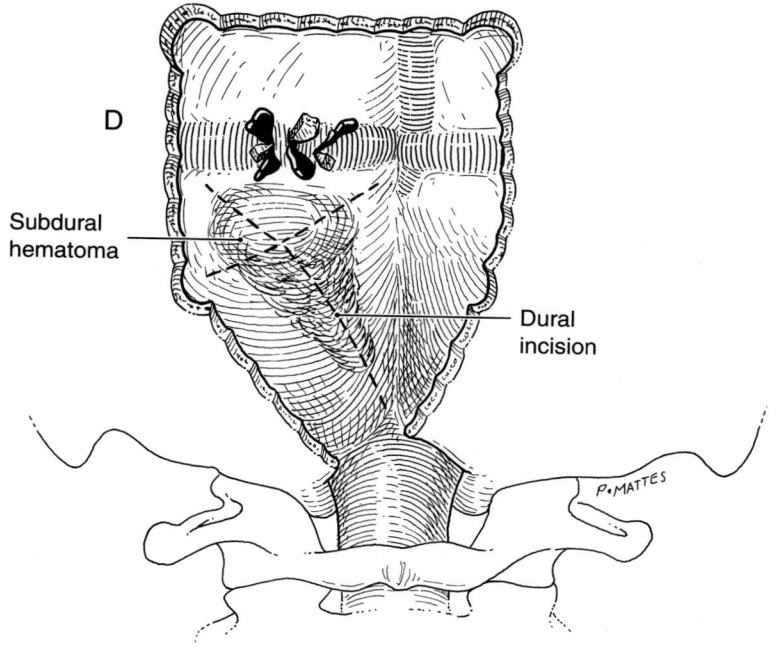

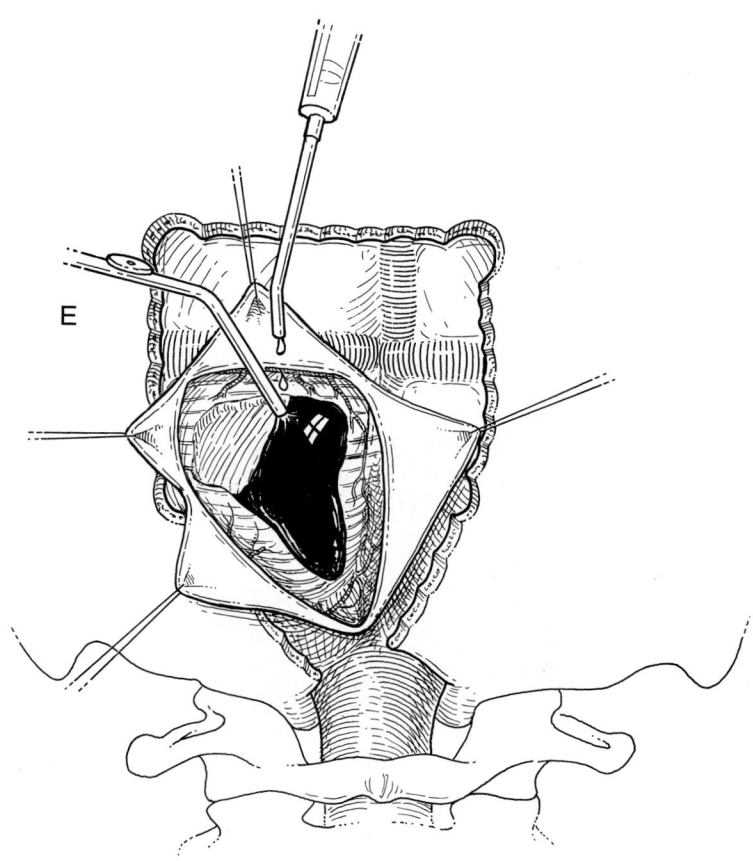

FIGURE 328–16. *Continued*

DEPRESSED SKULL FRACTURE

Depressed skull fractures are commonly seen in children (Fig. 328–17). Traditionally, surgery for depressed skull fractures is indicated if (1) the depth of the depressed fragments of the fracture is equal to or greater than the width of the surrounding bone; (2) the fracture occurs over cosmetic areas, such as the forehead; (3) the fracture is of a compound variety; and (4) there is a significant underlying intracranial hematoma that requires surgery.

Procedure

The patient is placed on the operating table with the head resting on a doughnut device and elevated above the level of the heart. If the scalp is lacerated, the incision can be extended to include the laceration in a lazy *S* fashion; a linear incision may also be appropriate. The incision should be planned carefully to expose the entire fracture adequately and include excision of any ragged, devitalized scalp tissue or contamination (Fig. 328–18*A*). A bur hole is placed at the edge of the fracture, and the underlying dura is exposed (see Fig. 328–18*B*). A Leksell rongeur or Kerrison punch is used to take small bites of bone around the fracture to free the underlying fragments (see Fig. 328–18*C* and *D*). Besides being depressed, the fragments often tend to slide under the edge of the fracture margins; these fragments are carefully elevated with a Penfield no. 3 instrument and removed, to prevent any fragments being driven down into the brain. During this process, care must be taken not to apply any downward pressure on the underlying dura and brain. Often, a dural tear with an underlying cerebral contusion is present. Once all the bone fragments are taken off the defect, they may be fitted together like a jigsaw puzzle and held together with miniplates if the fracture is clean. The underlying dura is inspected carefully for any tears, which are sutured primarily or grafted. If an underlying subdural or intracerebral hematoma is present, the dura is widely opened (see Fig. 328–18*E*), and

the underlying hematoma is gently evacuated with the help of suction and bipolar diathermy. Careful hemostasis is obtained using bipolar diathermy and Surgicel (see Fig. 328–18*F*). The dural edges are then approximated in a watertight fashion using 4–0 silk sutures. Sometimes, the underlying dura is lacerated and may have to be replaced with a synthetic dural substitute such as Duraguard (bovine pericardium) (see Fig. 328–18*G*). The fractured bone fragments held together with miniplates are then placed over the defect and secured to the edges of the bone with a miniplate and screw system. The scalp layers are closed as described earlier. When the wound is heavily contaminated or more than 24 hours old, bone fragments should not be placed primarily. Delayed cranioplasty 1 to 2 months later can be performed with a titanium mesh, acrylic, or titanium sheet prosthesis.

COMPOUND SINUS INJURY

In patients with compound frontal sinus injuries, careful attention must be paid to fractures involving both the anterior and posterior walls. Nondepressed fractures through only the posterior wall of the frontal sinus generally do not warrant surgical repair other than scalp closure. When the force is significant enough to penetrate the anterior and posterior tables, the probability of delayed infection is very high.[48] Such fractures necessitate intracranial exploration and repair, as detailed later. This should be done within a few days of injury, especially when there has been penetration by a sharp object. Wooden objects are notorious for delayed sepsis, even years after apparently trivial injuries. This approach is also appropriate for delayed anterior fossa cerebrospinal fluid leaks.

Procedure

Repair of the fracture requires a bicoronal craniotomy. To minimize retraction on the frontal lobes, in the majority of patients it is prudent to administer mild hyperventilation to a $PaCO_2$ of 30 to 35 mm Hg and a bolus of intravenous mannitol 1 g/kg at the onset of surgery. The patient is placed supine on the operating table with the head immobilized in a three-pin Mayfield head holder, held in extension (Fig. 328–19*A*). A bicoronal scalp flap is marked out about 15 mm behind the hairline (see Fig. 328–19*A*). The coronal flap is elevated to the supraorbital rim and the zygomatic arches. A vascularized galeal flap based on the reflected scalp margin is created for placement over the sinus defect (see Fig. 328–19*B*). Multiple bur holes are then made, including those over the sagittal sinus in the midline (see Fig. 328–14*B*), to safely reflect the underlying dura with the help of a Penfield no. 3 instrument and curved curets. The craniotomy is then completed as usual by joining the bur holes using a craniotome. The craniotome cuts over the sagittal sinus are performed last. The entire frontal air sinus is then exenterated by stripping out the mucosa. If there are any depressed fragments of the anterior or posterior

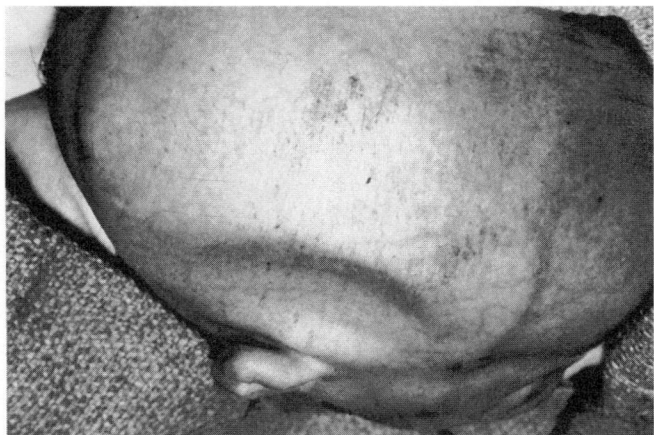

FIGURE 328–17. Photograph showing a closed depressed skull fracture above the right auricle.

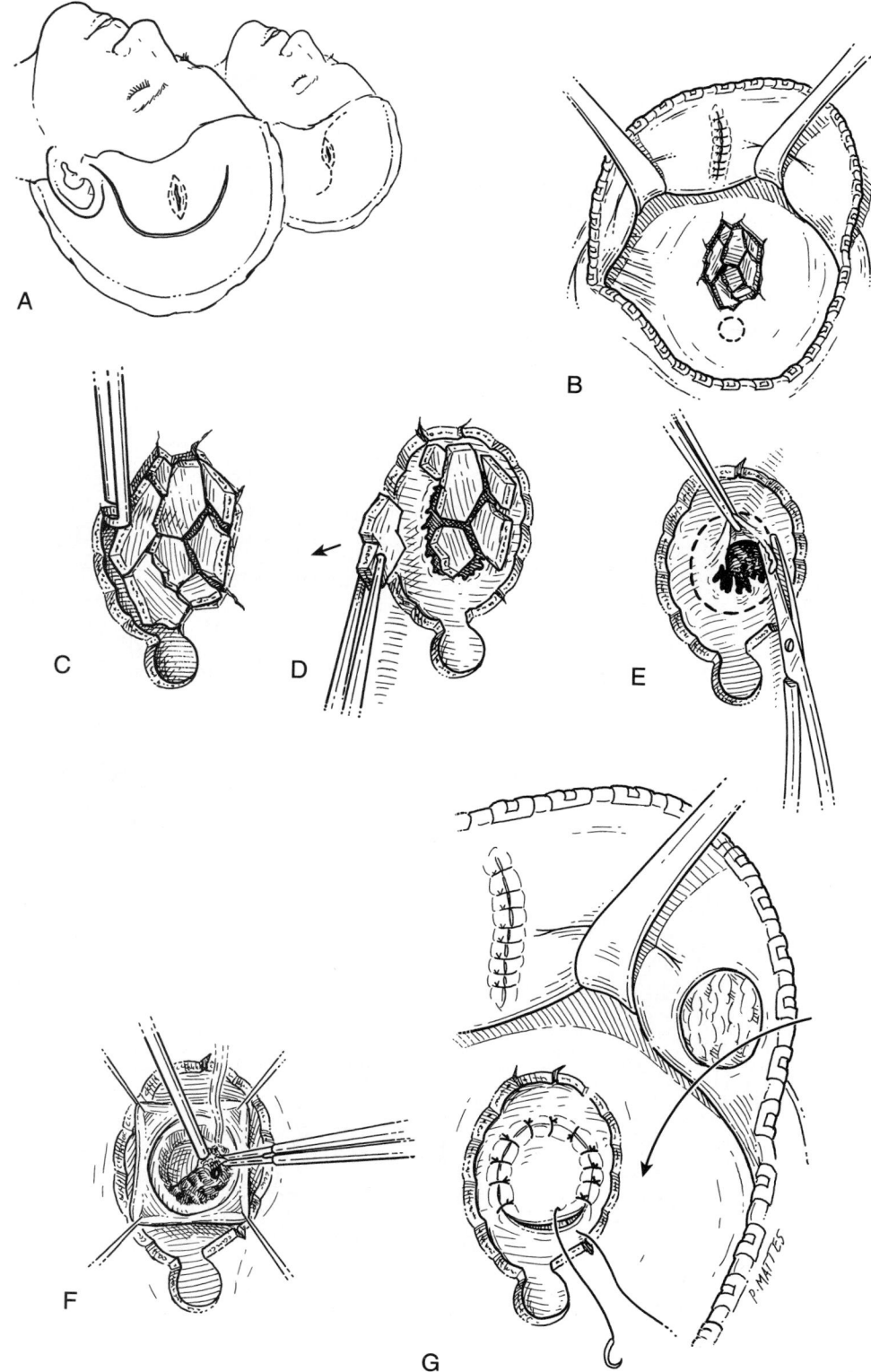

FIGURE 328–18. Schematic showing elevation of a depressed skull fracture. A lazy *S* incision is made, incorporating the scalp laceration. A bur hole is then placed at the margins of the fracture, and the bone fragments are gently elevated. A dural patch graft may be required in some instances *(G)*.

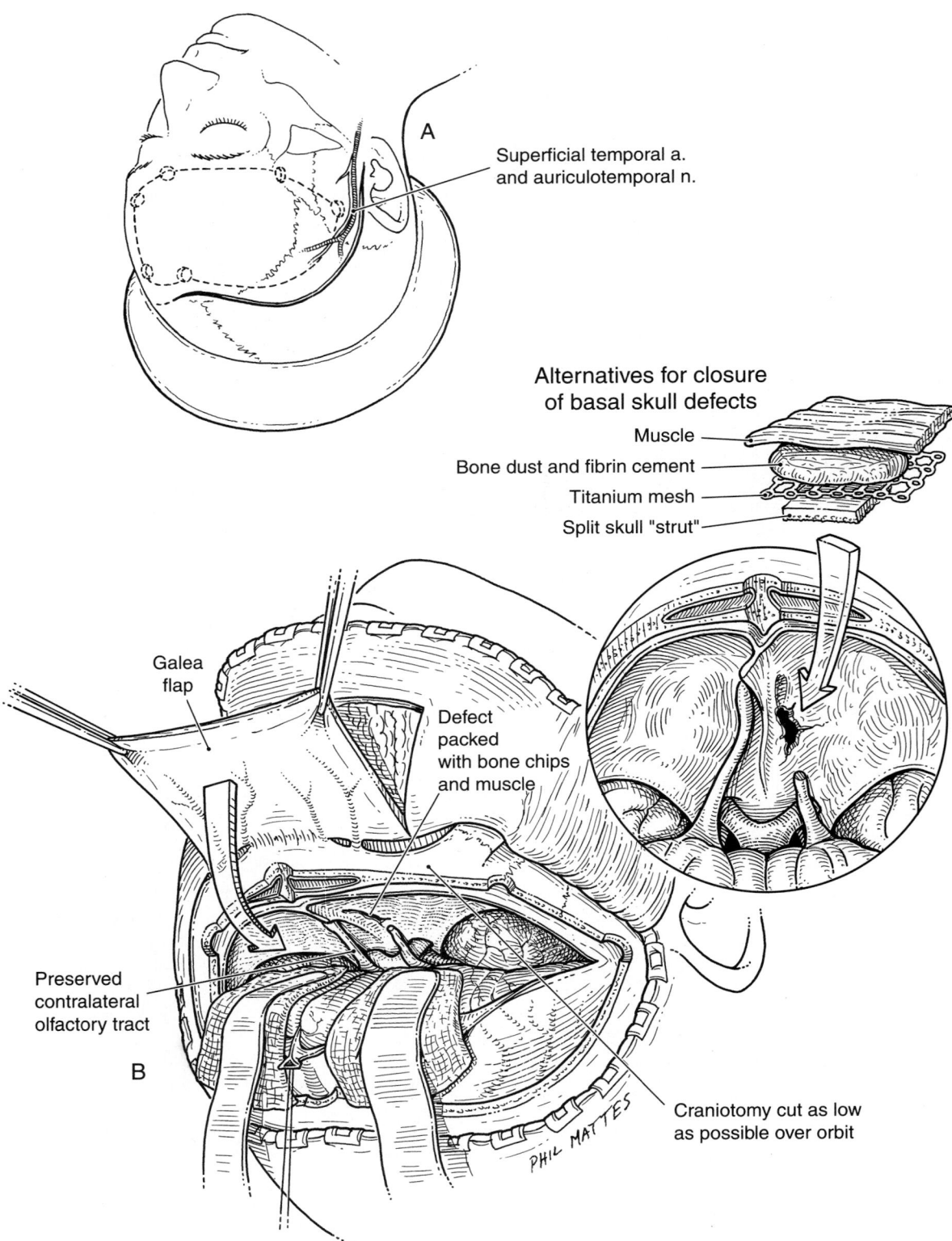

Superficial temporal a. and auriculotemporal n.

Alternatives for closure of basal skull defects

Muscle

Bone dust and fibrin cement

Titanium mesh

Split skull "strut"

Galea flap

Defect packed with bone chips and muscle

Preserved contralateral olfactory tract

B

Craniotomy cut as low as possible over orbit

PHIL MATTES

FIGURE 328–19. Schematic of a bicoronal approach to repair fractures involving the frontal sinus and anterior skull base. After cranializing the frontal sinus, a vascularized galeal flap is placed over the sinus *(B)*.

Illustration continued on following page

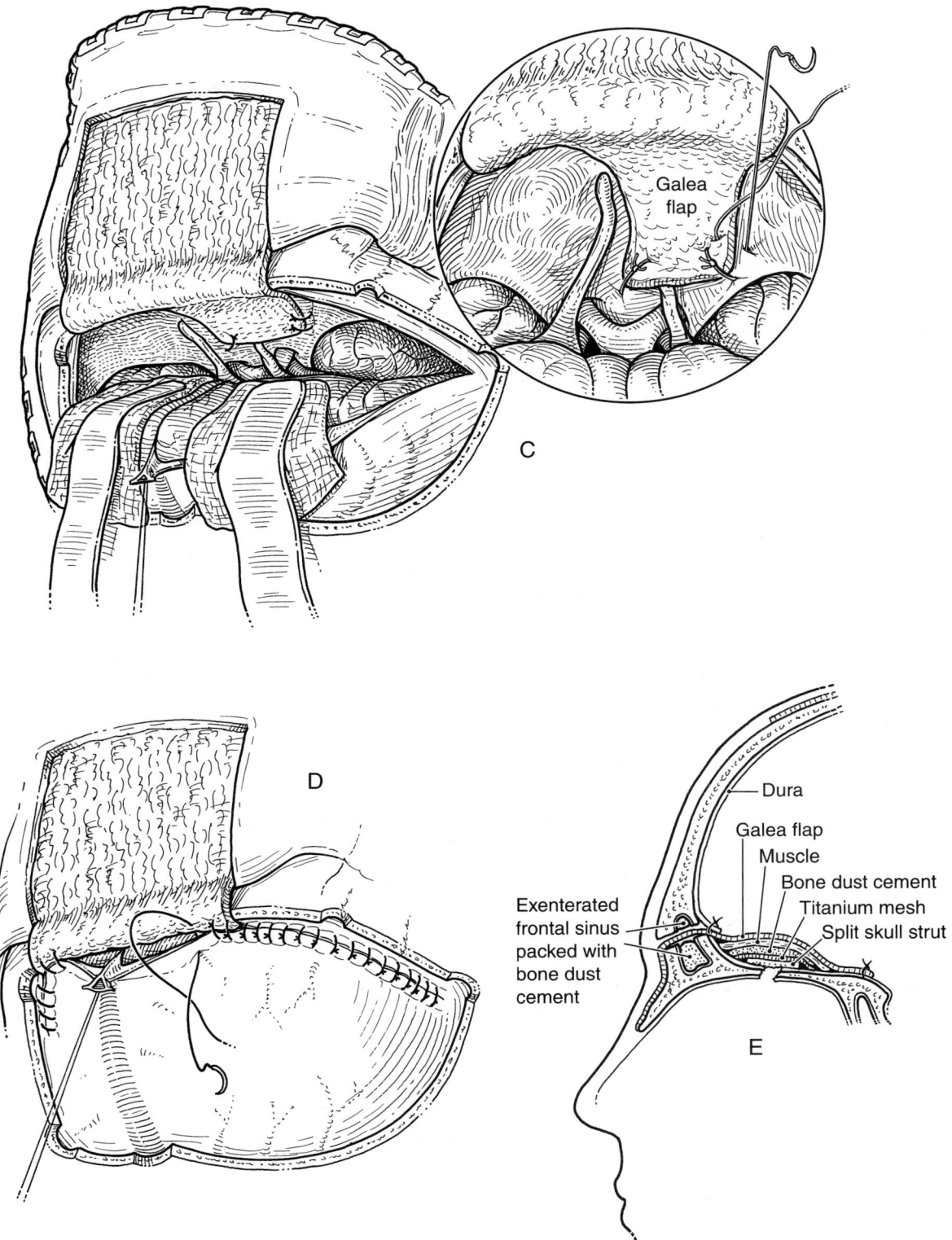

FIGURE 328–19. *Continued.* If defects in the ethmoid bone are seen, a combination of a split skull "strut" graft, titanium mesh, bone dust, and fibrin, including muscle, can be used to further reinforce the defect *(B)*. A sagittal section following the repair is shown *(E)*.

sinus wall, they are elevated or removed. The sinus mucosa is best removed with curets and cup forceps, as well as cauterized with monopolar diathermy, to avoid future mucocele formation.[49] The dura is opened as shown in Figure 328–19B, and the underlying brain is débrided of any necrotic, contused tissue; it is closed in a watertight fashion using 4–0 sutures after meticulous hemostasis has been obtained (see Fig. 328–19D). A vascularized pericranial flap is then placed over the cranialized frontal sinus (see Fig. 328–19B and C). If fractures of the floor of the frontal fossa, including the ethmoid bones, are seen, further reinforcements can be placed over the defect, including a fascia lata graft or fibrin glue; for large defects, titanium mesh can be fixed in place using small screws (see Fig. 328–19E). A piece of inner table of skull from the craniotomy can also be used, and a paste made of bone dust kept at the time of the craniotomy and fibrin glue can be used to seal the leak in the base of the skull. The fragments of the anterior table of the frontal sinus are repaired with miniplates, and the craniotomy flap is replaced and fixed to the adjacent bone using miniplates and screws. The pericranial flap is closed in layers, and a pressure dressing applied. For all patients with a documented cerebrospinal fluid fistula or dural laceration underlying the frontal sinus, a 3- to 5-day period of lumbar or ventricular drainage is instituted.[50]

DEPRESSED FRACTURE OVER A VENOUS SINUS

A depressed skull fracture that is closed, has no mass effect, and does not require repair for cosmetic reasons should not be elevated if overlying a venous sinus. The choice of treatment depends on the neurological condition of the patient, the site of venous sinus involvement, and the degree of venous flow compromise. If a major sinus occlusion results in raised ICP with deteriorating neurological status, urgent fracture elevation and sinus repair with restoration of blood flow is required.[51] Kapp and associates, in a report of 78 Vietnam War casualties injured by missiles, ligated the anterior 50% of the superior sagittal sinus in 27 patients, with only one death (4%).[52] Injuries of the posterior half of the sagittal sinus were associated with a 24% mortality rate. Principles concerning the transverse sinuses are more difficult to define, because their contribution to the venous drainage of the supra- and infratentorial spaces is variable and bilateral. Determining transverse sinus dominance is critical, because many individuals have significant asymmetry, with the right side being dominant. If the superior sagittal sinus drains unilaterally into the right transverse sinus, ligation at this site would be disastrous. Unless urgently addressed, occlusion of the torcular or a dominant transverse or sigmoid sinus will result in the rapid development of sustained intracranial hypertension and often death. If, however, the superior sagittal sinus drains bilaterally or through the uninvolved sinus, ligation may be safe. Preoperative angiography or magnetic resonance angiography should be used

whenever possible to assist in making this determination.

Any operative procedure involving the sinuses should have the personnel and materials in place to deal with potentially severe hemorrhage. The most important aspect of such procedures is to ensure that the patient's head is elevated above the level of the heart on the operating table, so that bleeding and the risk of air embolism are minimized (Fig. 328–20C). The head end of the table should be easily maneuverable. In this way, the venous pressure can be lowered to decrease hemorrhage and raised to prevent air embolism. A gentle Valsalva's maneuver may be helpful to judge this. All precautions should be taken to prevent venous obstruction in the neck by avoiding extremes of flexion and rotation of the head on the shoulders. A right atrial catheter should always be inserted for aspiration should an air embolism occur, and an esophageal stethoscope should be used by the anesthesiologist.[53] At least 2 to 4 units of packed cells should be available in the operating room.

A curvilinear or large horseshoe incision is made over the involved sinus to maximize the exposure (see Fig. 328–20A and B). To decompress the sinus from any depressed bone fragments, sufficient bone is removed around the margins of the sinus using Leksell rongeurs (see Fig. 328–20D). This allows proximal and distal control of the sinus. Long (~25 mm) aneurysm clips or vascular "bulldog" clamps are kept ready to temporarily occlude the sinus and parasagittal veins if necessary, and a variety of Weck clips are kept ready to occlude the sinus if necessary. The sinus can be directly sutured using continuous suture (see Fig. 328–20D). An onlay graft using fascia lata can also be used (see Fig. 328–20D). Sometimes, if the tear involving the sinus is significant, temporary diversion of the sinus blood can be achieved using a Kapp-Gielchinsky shunt. This shunt can be inflated at either end after being introduced into the lumen of the venous sinus, during which time an anastomosis of the venous sinus can be carried out using a saphenous vein patch or dural patch. If temporary distal venous sinus occlusion is going to be carried out, it is advisable to measure ICP during occlusion. If the pressure rises more than 20 mm Hg, mannitol should be used and hyperventilation increased until venous flow is rapidly restored. Following successful repair of the venous sinus, hemostasis is achieved, and the depressed bone fragments can be replaced using a miniplate system.

CHRONIC SUBDURAL HEMATOMA

With chronic subdural hematomas, the trauma is minimal or even unrecognized in one third of cases.[54] A subdural hematoma is considered chronic when it is discovered 3 weeks or more after the initiating injury. Post-traumatic subdural fluid collections are reported to occur in about 6% of head-injured patients, and 5% of patients with persistent subdural fluid collections develop chronic subdural hematomas.[55, 56] The majority of patients are elderly, demented, or chronic alcoholics,

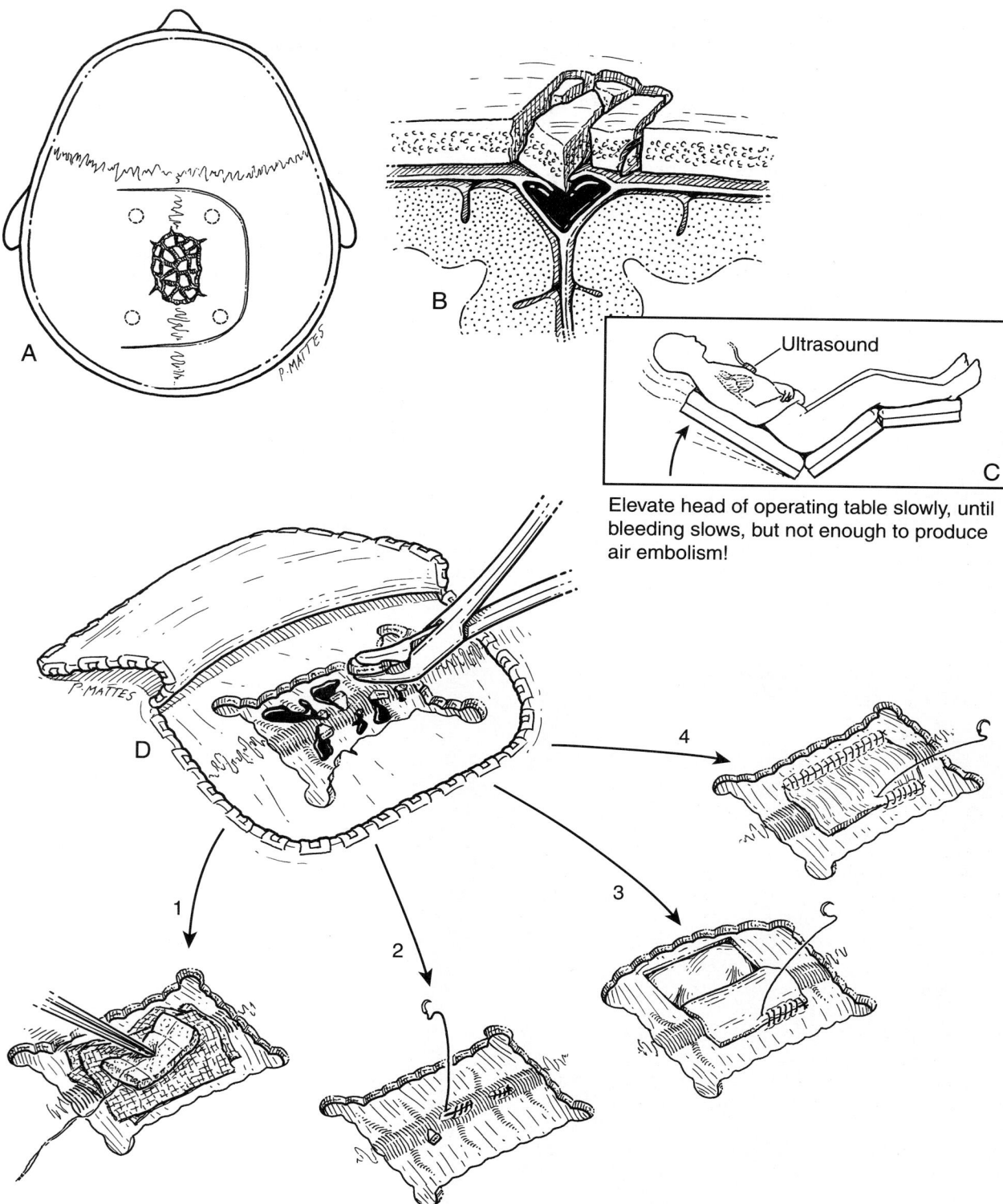

Elevate head of operating table slowly, until bleeding slows, but not enough to produce air embolism!

Alternative methods for sagittal sinus injury

FIGURE 328–20. Schematic showing elevation of a depressed skull fracture over a venous sinus and repair. Care is taken to elevate the depressed fragments overlying the sinus with Leksell rongeurs. *D,* Bleeding from the sinus can be stopped with gentle tamponade (1) and repaired after inserting a shunt (2) by directly suturing the defect (3) or by using an onlay patch graft (4).

and cerebral atrophy is the most important predisposing factor. This explains the amazingly high mortality rates of 15% to 20% reported in some series.[54, 57] The lesions are bilateral in 15% to 20% of cases (Fig. 328–21). The symptoms and signs of chronic subdural hematoma are variable and nonspecific. The classic presentation of a post-traumatic chronic subdural hematoma includes two phases. The first phase is the traumatic event, which is usually minor. After its dissipation and a silent period of variable length, the second phase begins with the onset of delayed clinical manifestations, usually consisting of headaches, decline in mental function, and motor deficits. Coagulopathy and anticoagulant therapy may accelerate this presentation in many cases.

Chronic subdural hematomas can be of differing densities on computed tomography and can also result in significant mass effect requiring urgent evacuation (Fig. 328–22). The mechanisms for the early development and enlargement of chronic subdural hematomas are not yet fully understood. In a recent review of more than 800 acute subdural hematomas, including those treated nonoperatively, hematomas less than 10 mm in maximal thickness always resolved spontaneously, whereas those greater than 10 mm thick evolved into chronic subdural hematomas.[11] Rupture of the bridging veins as they cross the subdural space from the cortex

to the sagittal sinus may form the basis of the lesion, but tearing of small arterial adhesions may also be a factor. Various theories have been put forward to explain the enlargement of the subdural collection once it forms, including an osmotic theory, with fluid passing from the cerebrospinal fluid to the hematoma because of a difference in oncotic pressure and the fragility of the neocapillaries in the outer membranes, resulting in microhemorrhages, subsequent accumulation of fluid, and excessive fibrinolytic activity in the outer membrane.[58-66] Weir and Gordon found that subdural fluid contained low fibrinogen and high fibrin degradation product concentrations in 25 cases of chronic subdural hematoma.[67] These products are known to have anticoagulant effects and could inhibit platelet aggregation.

The aim of surgical treatment is to achieve sufficient drainage of the hematoma fluid to eliminate the procoagulant fibrin degradation products, collapse the hematoma cavity, and encourage resorption of the hematoma membranes. For this reason, washing out of the cavity seems to be associated with the best surgical results.

Spontaneous regression of chronic subdural hematomas occurs when the fluid volume and membrane thickness are not too large. Initial nonoperative management is advocated for chronic subdural hematomas

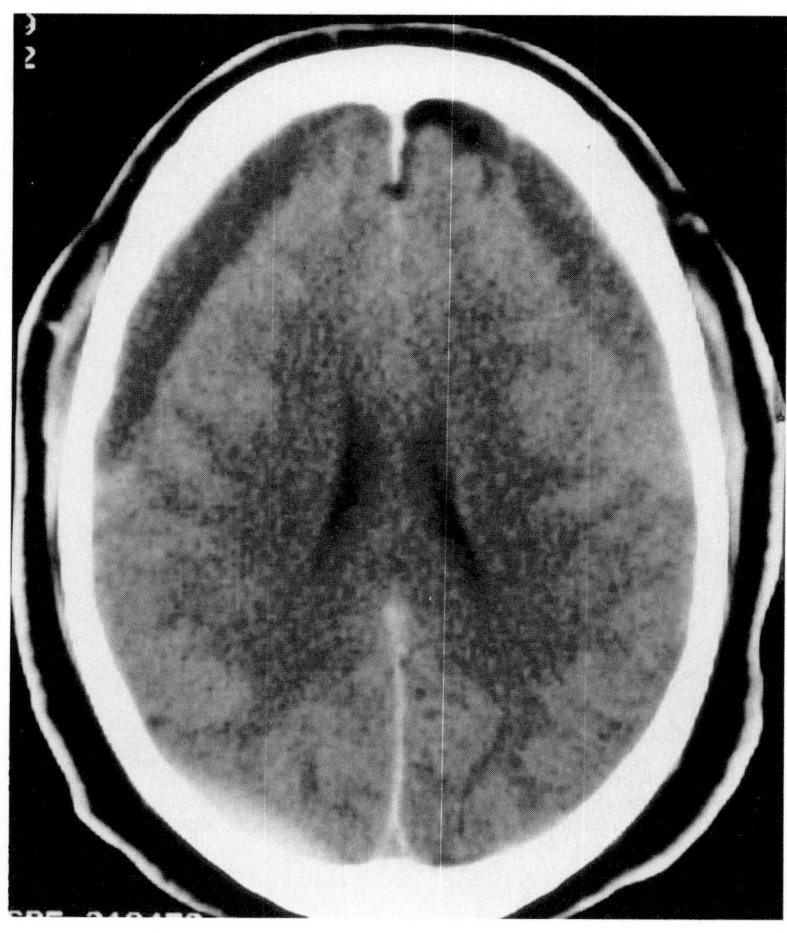

FIGURE 328–21. Axial computed tomographic scan showing a bilateral subdural collection.

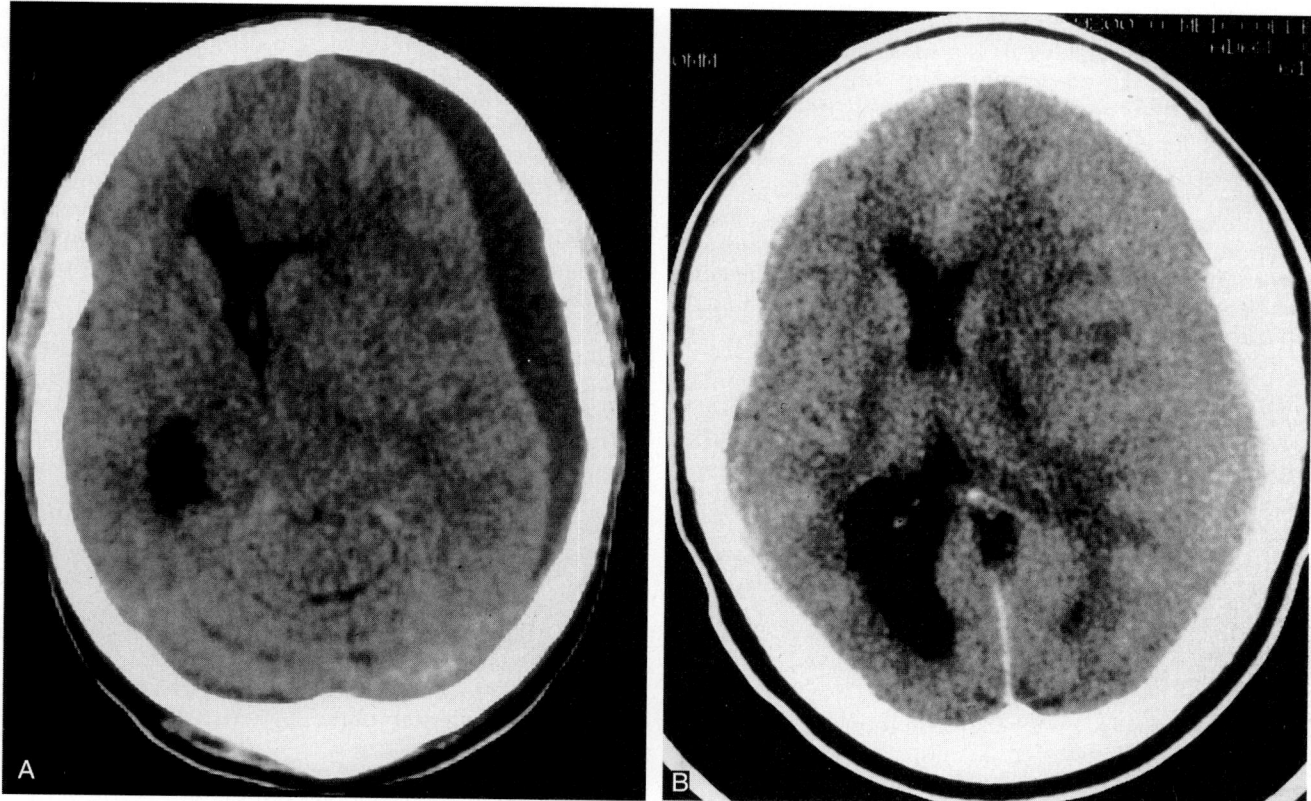

FIGURE 328–22. Axial computed tomographic scans showing chronic subdural collections of varying densities. *A*, The collection is hypodense. *B*, The collection appears isodense relative to the brain. These collections are associated with significant midline shift.

that are small, lack mass effect, and evolve slowly. The surgical treatment of choice in chronic subdural hematomas is still controversial. Methods advocated include steroid treatment alone, drainage via one or two bur holes, twist drill craniostomy and drainage, and craniotomy and placement of a subduroperitoneal shunt.

Bur Hole Drainage

This is the most widely used method for the drainage of chronic subdural hematomas. Many studies have shown the efficacy of this procedure, but the rate of recurrences requiring a second operation is 2% to 18.5%.[68–71]

In patients who are not agitated, and especially in those who are very frail with multiple medical problems, the bur hole drainage procedure can be carried out under local anesthesia using 1% lidocaine (Xylocaine). The patient is positioned with the head in a subdural head holder (see Fig. 328–7*B*). The bur holes are usually placed over the thickest part of the hematoma as seen on computed tomographic scans. The incisions in the scalp are made so that they can be incorporated into a craniotomy flap if required (see Fig. 328–7*A*). After making the skin incision and separating the underlying periosteum, a single bur hole is placed. The underlying dura is subjected to diathermy,

and a cruciate opening is made in the dura to release the subdural fluid slowly. This maneuver prevents rapid shifts of the underlying brain. The second bur hole is then made, the dura is opened, and a soft Silastic irrigation catheter (e.g., a Becker ventriculostomy catheter) is guided over a Penfield no. 3 into the subdural space (not into the brain). The subdural fluid collection is then gently washed out with at least 400 mL of warm normal saline. After this, the drainage catheters are tunneled under the skin and secured. Meticulous hemostasis is obtained at the dural margins, and the wound is closed in layers using 2–0 Dexon in the galea and staples at the skin margins. The subdural catheters are then connected to closed drainage bags without suction and kept at the level of the head to facilitate drainage. The patient is usually kept flat in bed for 24 to 48 hours.

Twist Drill Drainage

The advantage of this procedure is that it can be done at the bedside quickly in frail, medically unfit, or very elderly individuals. Several studies have shown this to be a safe and efficacious procedure.[57, 72, 73] With the patient under local anesthesia, a single twist drill hole is made over the most prominent part of the subdural collection based on computed tomographic scans. A ventriculostomy catheter is then carefully guided into the subdural space and tunneled several centimeters away from the twist drill site. The catheter is then connected to a closed drainage bag. Initially, the fluid is drained slowly for about 30 minutes to 1 hour.

Craniotomy

Craniotomy is reserved for patients in whom subdural hematoma has recurred and in whom the underlying membranes prevent adequate re-expansion of the cerebral hemisphere. The mortality rate is high, and acute subdural bleeding often follows this procedure.

Shunting

A subdural hematoma can be drained into the peritoneum, a procedure that is usually carried out in infants and children and rarely in adults with multiple recurrences.[74] Complications of this procedure include focal edema of the underlying brain, delayed re-expansion of the cerebral hemisphere, epileptic seizures, bleeding, and subdural tension pneumocephalus.

Cranioplasty

In modern practice, the most common indication for cranioplasty is following decompressive craniectomy for raised ICP. It is usually carried out 6 to 8 weeks after the initial procedure, assuming the patient has made a full recovery from the initial injury. In the interim, the patient is protected in a "hockey helmet" against any direct injury to the cranial defect.

Usually, the autologous bone flap harvested and frozen after the initial surgery is used, giving good cosmetic results. The bone flap remains intact and sterile in a −70°C freezer for many months. Autoclaving of the bone before use may be indicated; however, this can reduce the viability of the graft. Others have advocated storing the bone flap in the patient's own abdominal subcutaneous tissues to preserve better bone viability.[75] Materials such as methyl methacrylate and titanium mesh can be used as substitutes when the bone is heavily comminuted or contaminated.[76, 77] For large, cosmetically important defects, the use of casts, models, and computed tomography–based reconstruction technology can improve the appearance of the defect, but this is much more expensive and labor intensive.

The patient is placed supine, with the head on a doughnut device, turned to the opposite side, and elevated above the level of the heart. To maximize intracranial relaxation, the patient is given mannitol and mildly hyperventilated. The patient is also given prophylactic antibiotics at least an hour before the procedure. The previous craniotomy incision is reopened. Dissection in the subgaleal plane is carried out and may be facilitated by first infiltrating the space with saline to open the planes and lifting the galea from the underlying dura. Dissection is done with an upward lifting motion of the skin margins (Fig. 328–23D). The back of the blade or the scalpel blade handle is best used during this procedure. The entire flap is then

dissected off the underlying dura. The bony margins of the craniotomy opening are exposed using a periosteal elevator and curved curet while protecting the underlying dura, which can be friable. Meticulous hemostasis is obtained with the help of monopolar and bipolar diathermy to prevent postcranioplasty hematomas, which are common and predispose to infection. If the patient's own bone flap is used, a miniplate system is used to fix it to the margins of the defect. Bur hole covers are placed over the frontal holes for improved cosmesis (see Fig. 328–23A). If methyl methacrylate is used, great care must be taken, because the polymerized state is reached with the generation of an exothermic reaction; thus, the curing cement may cause devastating thermal injury to the brain if it is allowed to cure in contact with the cortex. Therefore, it is best to place the material in a plastic bag and mold it to the underlying defect using copious amounts of cold normal saline (see Fig. 328–23B); it is removed from the patient for the final hardening stages to avoid any thermal injury to the underlying structures. This process can be carried out over a piece of wet gauze to protect the brain. The molded methyl methacrylate is then removed, and the outer surfaces are smoothed with a high-speed drill. This is then fixed to the skull margins with a miniplate system. Alternatively, titanium mesh can be used after trimming the edges to fit the craniotomy defect (see Fig. 328–23C). It too can be fixed to the bone edges with miniplate screws. A subgaleal drain is inserted (and left in place for 14 days), and the flap is closed using 2–0 Dexon in the galea and staples at the skin margins. The head is then wrapped in the usual manner.

COMPLICATIONS

Bleeding

Recurrent hematomas are common after surgery for traumatic intracranial lesions and may jeopardize the outcome. Routine evaluation of coagulation parameters is mandatory, either pre- or intraoperatively, and transfusion of fresh frozen plasma, platelet concentrate, and, rarely, specific coagulation factors may be needed; these should be given even when coagulation parameters or platelet counts are borderline. Intraoperatively, meticulous hemostasis is mandatory and may take 30 to 60 minutes or more to achieve. Bipolar diathermy (and sometimes two surgeons with bipolars) is necessary. Final hemostasis should be achieved at an arterial Pa_{CO_2} of 35 to 40 mm Hg, and Valsalva's maneuver should be done before closing the craniotomy to avoid delayed venous bleeding when the patient emerges from anesthesia.

Arterial bleeding during the craniotomy can usually be stopped after the source has been visualized, although it may be necessary to extend the craniotomy by nibbling away more bone. Rarely, profuse bleeding may arise from a laceration of the carotid artery at the base of the skull. Packing with muscle may be temporarily successful in controlling this bleeding, but

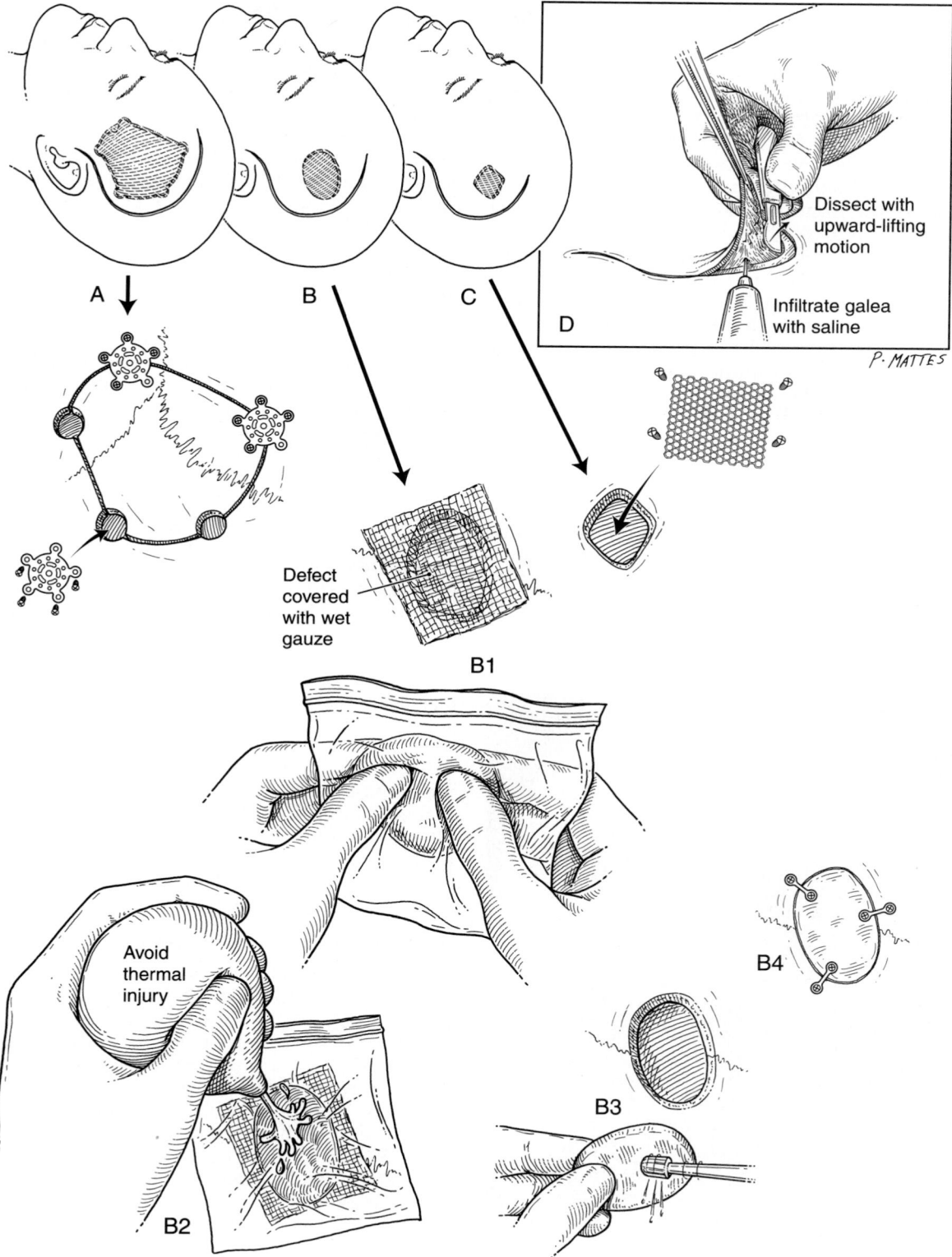

FIGURE 328–23. Schematic showing a cranioplasty involving a craniotomy defect. Infiltrating the galea with saline helps in dissection of the tissue planes (D). The defect can be closed using the patient's own bone (A), methyl methacrylate mold (B), or titanium mesh (C). When using methyl methacrylate, the initial molding can be done in a plastic bag; then the defect is covered with a copious amount of irrigation to overcome the exothermic reaction.

angiography and intra-arterial balloon occlusion are usually needed. The management of arterial injuries is discussed in greater detail elsewhere in this text. Increasing the head-up tilt can usually control venous bleeding from the brain. If this is not successful, the possibility of raised intrathoracic pressure due to pneumothorax should be considered. Bleeding from the large venous sinuses was discussed earlier in the section on depressed skull fracture.

Diffuse oozing from the brain and dura is the most common source of major blood loss during craniotomy and contributes to the cytokine-mediated hyperemia that always follows trauma. If this occurs, thrombocytopenia, a qualitative platelet defect, or disseminated intravascular coagulation should be excluded.[44, 78, 79] It may be necessary to give fresh frozen plasma before the results of coagulation studies are available. Coagulation studies should be repeated after craniotomy, because platelet counts fall to their lowest levels on the second or third day.[44]

Acute Brain Swelling

Fulminant brain swelling is one of the most dreaded complications in neurosurgery and represents a pathophysiologic entity that is not yet fully understood (Fig. 328–24).[80–82] Different components, such as vasogenic and cytotoxic edema, reactive hyperemia, and vascular

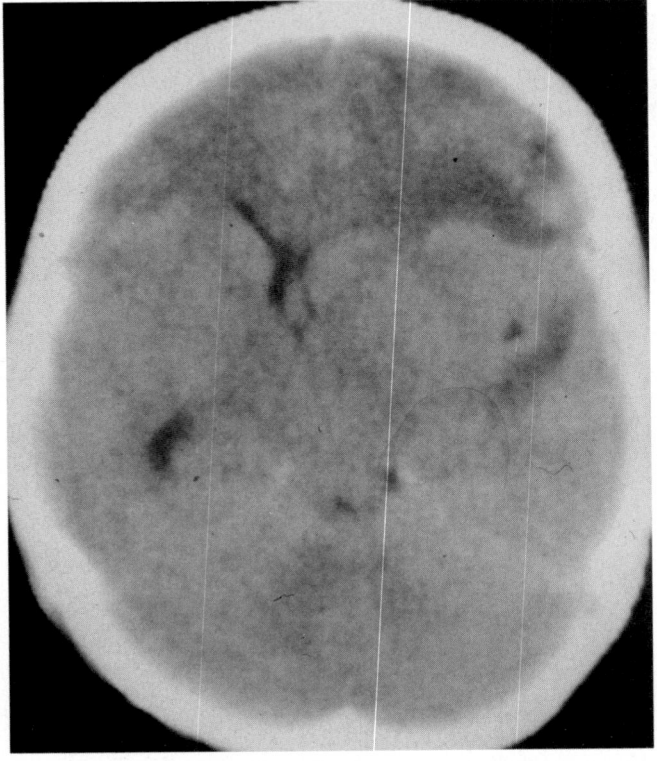

FIGURE 328–24. Axial computed tomographic scan showing diffuse brain swelling bifrontally and also involving the left temporal fossa. The basal cisterns are obliterated, and there is evidence of early hydrocephalus with dilatation of the temporal horns.

engorgement, are probably the main factors.[28, 83] It has been reported in up to one fifth of patients with acute subdural hematoma (Fig. 328–25).[81] When fulminant brain swelling occurs intraoperatively, the endotracheal tube position should be reassessed and an arterial blood gas analysis performed; Pao_2 should be maintained above 100 mm Hg and $Paco_2$ reduced to about 25 mm Hg. The head of the operating table should be elevated, and rotation of the patient's head and neck minimized. Marked arterial hypertension should be controlled, because these patients do not autoregulate their cerebral vasculature. Even modest hypotension must be avoided, however, given that drops in blood pressure typically result in significant increases in ICP. Thus the mean arterial blood pressure of about 70 to 80 mm Hg should be maintained.[84, 85] As these maneuvers are carried out, further narcotic sedation, muscle relaxants, and mannitol should be given and a ventriculostomy attempted for cerebrospinal fluid drainage. The possibility of occult bleeding from an evolving ipsilateral intracerebral hematoma or a contralateral hematoma must be excluded. Intraoperative ultrasonography, if available, should be performed, and contralateral bur holes can be placed.[86] In cases that remain refractory to these measures, pentobarbital coma can be initiated with a 10 mg/kg intravenous bolus given over 20 to 30 minutes. Alternatively, the short-acting general anesthetic agents etomidate and propofol can be used to effectively reduce ICP. When hypotension is a concern, a short course of etomidate is preferable over propofol or pentobarbital, because the latter two agents are more likely to significantly lower blood pressure. The use of cerebral protectants for managing refractory intracranial hypertension is discussed further in Chapter 327. Closure can usually be achieved by removing the bone flap, enlarging the bony defect, and making a large duraplasty. It is often necessary to resect part of the temporal or frontal lobe to achieve closure in these circumstances. After surgery, a computed tomographic scan should be performed urgently and may occasionally show a new clot in a remote site.

Postcraniotomy Hematoma

Intracranial hematomas develop under the previous craniotomy in approximately 3% to 7% of head injuries (Fig. 328–26).[38, 78, 80, 87] However, intracranial hematomas remote from the operation site have also been reported (Fig. 328–27). Of 850 patients who underwent craniotomy for evacuation of a traumatic intracranial mass, 59 (6.9%) developed second hematomas at the initial operation site that required another operation.[88] Of these, 39 had epidural hematomas, 12 had intracerebral hematomas, and 8 had mixed epidural and subdural hematomas.

Reaccumulation rates range from 7.8% in a series of extradural hematomas reported by Lobato and colleagues[81] to 61% of acute subdural hematomas drained by bur holes about 30 years ago.[81, 89] In the older neurosurgical literature, higher rates of recurrence for acute subdural hematoma were almost always due to the use of bur holes instead of craniotomy for evacuation; bur holes did not allow adequate visualization of the source of bleeding or complete removal of the hema-

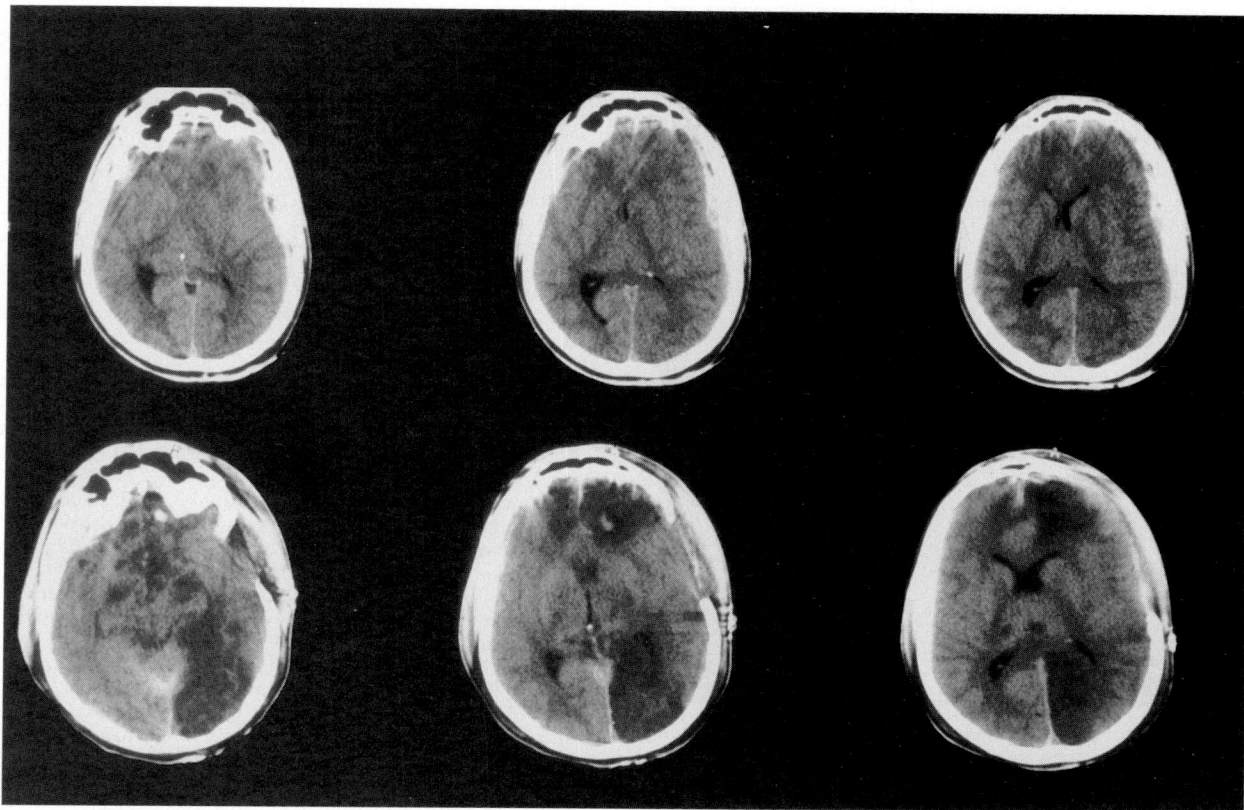

FIGURE 328–25. Axial computed tomographic scans of a patient who underwent evacuation of an acute subdural hematoma involving the left frontoparietal region. The patient developed fulminant intraoperative brain swelling, and the bone flap was left out. The patient was then treated medically, and a computed tomographic scan 2 days later showed significant swelling of the ipsilateral hemisphere, with the development of ischemic areas in the distribution of the anterior and posterior cerebral arteries.

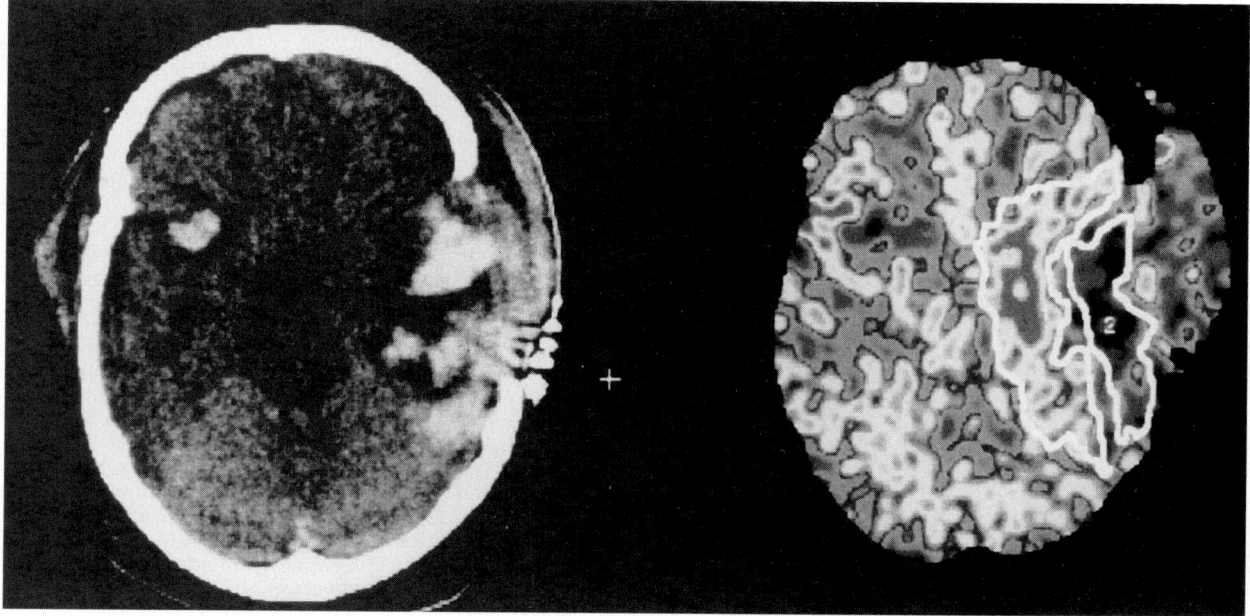

FIGURE 328–26. Axial computed tomographic scan showing a postoperative intracerebral hematoma that developed under the craniotomy site. A xenon-133 blood flow study shows impaired blood flow at the site.

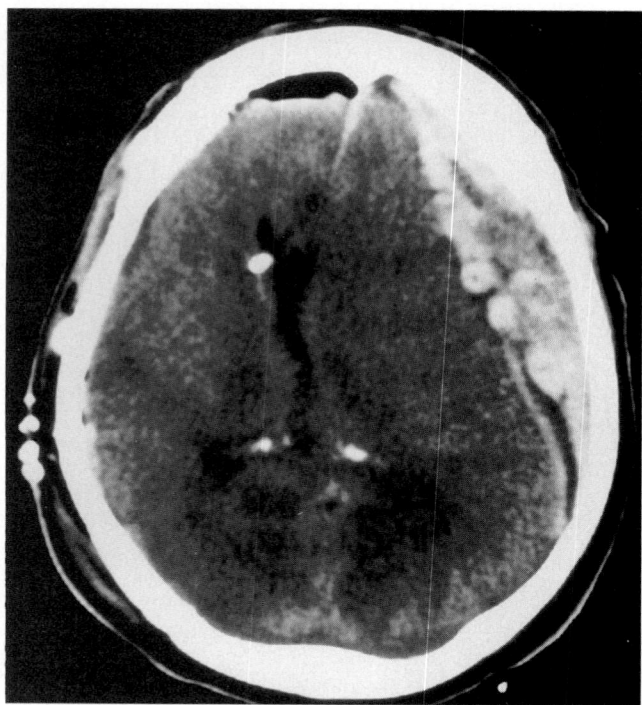

FIGURE 328–27. Axial computed tomographic scan showing development of an acute subdural hematoma on the contralateral side of the craniotomy. Also note the ventriculostomy catheter in the right frontal horn.

toma.[38, 41, 80, 82, 89] Delayed intracerebral hematomas may be the result of hypoxic, hypotensive, and coagulation defects seen in these patients.[38, 78, 80]

CONCLUSION

For surgery to positively affect outcome, head injuries must be identified early, and mass lesions must be promptly evacuated. Optimal care of patients with multiple injuries, including neurotrauma, is complex. Neurosurgical involvement is required not only for the management of intracranial mass lesions but also for the detection, monitoring, and management of raised ICP; to educate prehospital, emergency room, and intensive care unit personnel; to provide guidance and prognostic information to families; and to coordinate nursing and rehabilitation.

REFERENCES

1. Gennarelli TA, Champion HR, Sacco WJ, et al: Mortality of patients with head injury and extracranial injury treated in trauma centers. J Trauma 29:1193–1202, 1989.
2. Pal J, Brown R, Fleiszer D: The value of the Glasgow Coma Scale and Injury Severity Score: Predicting outcome in multiple trauma patients with head injury. J Trauma 29:746–748, 1989.
3. Vollmer DG, Torner JC, Jane JA: Age and outcome following traumatic coma: Why do older patients fare worse? J Neurosurg 75:S37–S49, 1991.
4. Bullock R, Chestnut RM, Clifton G, et al: Guidelines for the management of severe head injury. J Neurotrauma 13:643–734, 1996.
5. Eisenberg H, Jane JA, Marmarou A, et al: The Traumatic Coma Data Bank: Design methods and baseline characteristics. J Neurosurg 75:S8–S13, 1991.
6. Albericho AM, Ward JD, Choi SC, et al: Outcome after severe head injury, relationship to mass lesions, diffuse injury, and ICP course in pediatric and adult patients. J Neurosurg 67:648–656, 1987.
7. Marmarou A, Andersin RL, Ward JD, et al: NINDS Traumatic Coma Data Bank: Intracranial pressure monitoring methodology. J Neurosurg 75:S21–S27, 1991.
8. Narayan RK, Kishore PRS, Becker DP, et al: Intracranial pressure: To monitor or not to monitor? J Neurosurg 56:650–659, 1982.
9. Miller JD, Becker DP, Ward JD, et al: Significance of intracranial hypertension in severe head injury. J Neurosurg 47:503–516, 1977.
10. Bullock R, Teasdale G: Head injuries—surgical management of traumatic intracerebral hematomas. In Braakman R (ed): Handbook of Clinical Neurology, vol 57. Amsterdam, Elsevier, 1990, pp 249–298.
11. Mathew P, Oluoch-Olunya DL, Condon BR, et al: Acute subdural hematoma in the conscious patient: Outcome with initial nonoperative management. Acta Neurochir (Wien) 121:100–108, 1993.
12. Galbraith S, Teasdale G: Predicting the need for operation in the patient with an occult traumatic intracranial hematoma. J Neurosurg 55:75–81, 1981.
13. Lam A, Mayberg T: Use of nitrous oxide in neuroanesthesia: Why bother? J Neurosurg Anesthesiol 4:290–294, 1992.
14. Boarini DJ, Kassell NF, Coester H, et al: Comparison of systemic and cerebrovascular effects of isoflurane and halothane. Neurosurgery 15:400–409, 1984.
15. Eintrei C, Leszniewski W, Carlsson C: Local application of 133-xenon for measurement of regional cerebral blood flow (rCBF) during halothane, enflurane, and isoflurane anesthesia in humans. Anesthesiology 63:391–394, 1985.
16. Pinaud M, Lelausque JN, Chetanneau A, et al: Effects of propofol on cerebral hemodynamics and metabolism in patients with brain trauma. Anesthesiology 73:404–409, 1990.
17. Kassell NF, Hitchon PW, Gerk MK, et al: Alterations in cerebral blood flow, oxygen metabolism, and electrical activity produced by high dose sodium thiopental. Neurosurgery 7:598–603, 1980.
18. Dearden NM, McDowell DG: Comparison of etomidate and althesin in the reduction of increased intracranial pressure after head injury. Br J Anaesth 57:361–368, 1985.
19. Albanese J, Viviand X, Potie F, et al: Sufentanil, fentanyl, and alfentanil in head trauma patients: A study on cerebral hemodynamics. Crit Care Med 27:407–411, 1999.
20. Minton MD, Grosslight K, Stirt JA, et al: Increases in intracranial pressure from succinylcholine: Prevention by prior nondepolarizing blockade. Anesthesiology 65:165–169, 1986.
21. Miller JD, Dearden NM, Piper IR, et al: Control of intracranial pressure in patients with severe head injury. J Neurotrauma 9(Suppl 1):S317–S326, 1992.
22. Zauner A, Doppenberg E, Soukup J, et al: Extended neuromonitoring: New therapeutic opportunities? Neurol Res 20:S85–S90, 1998.
23. Zauner A, Doppenberg EM, Woodward JJ, et al: Continuous monitoring of cerebral substrate delivery and clearance: Initial experience in 24 patients with severe acute brain injuries. Neurosurgery 41:1082–1091, 1997.
24. Pickard JD, Bailey S, Sanderson H, et al: Steps towards cost-benefit analysis of regional neurosurgical care. BMJ 301:629–635, 1990.
25. Holzschuh M, Schuknect B: Traumatic epidural hematomas of the posterior fossa: 20 new cases and a review of the literature since 1961. Br J Neurosurg 3:171–180, 1989.
26. Bozbuga M, Izgi N, Polat G, et al: Posterior fossa epidural hematomas: Observations on a series of 73 cases. Neurosurg Rev 22:34–40, 1999.
27. Wilberger JE, Harris M, Diamond DL: Acute subdural hematoma: Mortality, morbidity and operative timing. J Neurosurg 74:212–218, 1991.

28. Becker DP: Acute subdural hematomas. In Vigourox RP (ed): Neurotraumatology. Vienna, Springer-Verlag, 1986, pp 51–95.

29. Miller JD, Butterworth JF, Gudeman SK, et al: Further experience in the management of severe head injury. J Neurosurg 54:289–299, 1981.

30. Marshall LF, Gautille T, Klauber MR, et al: The outcome of severe closed head injury. J Neurosurg 75(Suppl):S28–S36, 1991.

31. Howard MA III, Gross AS, Dacey RG Jr, et al: Acute subdural hematomas: An age-dependent clinical entity. J Neurosurg 71:858–863, 1989.

32. Massaro F, Lanotte M, Faccani G, et al: One hundred and twenty-seven cases of acute subdural hematoma operated upon: Correlation between CT findings and outcome. Acta Neurochir (Wien) 138:185–191, 1996.

33. Ko RK, Akdemir H, Oktem IS, et al: Acute subdural hematoma: Outcome and outcome prediction. Neurosurg Rev 20:239–244, 1997.

34. Mathiesen T, Benediktsdottir K, Johnson H, et al: Intracranial traumatic and non-traumatic hemorrhagic complications of warfarin treatment. Acta Neurol Scand 91:208–214, 1995.

35. Wintzen AR, Tijssen JGP: Subdural hematoma and oral anticoagulant therapy. Arch Neurol 39:69–72, 1982.

36. Mattle H, Kohler S, Huber P, et al: Anticoagulation-related intracranial extracerebral hemorrhage. J Neurol Neurosurg Psychiatry 52:829–837, 1989.

37. Resnick DK, Marion DW, Darby JM: The effect of hypothermia on the incidence of delayed traumatic intracerebral hemorrhage. Neurosurgery 34:252–255, 1994.

38. Gudeman SK, Kishore PR, Miller JD, et al: The genesis and significance of delayed traumatic intracerebral hematoma. Neurosurgery 5:309–313, 1979.

39. Rivano C, Borzone M, Carta F, et al: Traumatic intracerebral hematomas: 72 cases surgically treated. J Neurosurg Sci 24:77–84, 1980.

40. Jamieson KG, Yelland JDN: Traumatic intracerebral hematoma: Report of 63 surgically treated cases. J Neurosurg 37:528–532, 1972.

41. Sprick C, Bettag M, Bock WJ: Delayed traumatic intracranial hematomas: Clinical study of seven years. Neurosurg Rev 12(Suppl 1):228–230, 1989.

42. Guerra WK-W, Gaab MR, Dietz H, et al: Surgical decompression for traumatic brain swelling: Indications and results. J Neurosurg 90:187–196, 1999.

43. Polin RS, Shaffrey ME, Bogaev CA, et al: Decompressive bifrontal craniectomy in the treatment of severe refractory posttraumatic cerebral edema. Neurosurgery 41:84–94, 1997.

44. Bullock R, Golek J, Blake G: Traumatic intracerebral hematoma—which patients should undergo surgical evacuation? CT scan features and ICP monitoring as a basis for decision making. Surg Neurol 33:181–187, 1989.

45. Gopinath SP, Robertson CS, Contant CF, et al: Early detection of delayed traumatic intracranial hematomas using near-infrared spectroscopy. J Neurosurg 83:438–444, 1995.

46. Young HA, Schmidek HH: Complications accompanying occipital skull fracture. J Trauma 22:914–920, 1982.

47. Cuneo RA, Caronna JJ, Pitts L, et al: Upward transtentorial herniation: Seven cases and a review of the literature. Arch Neurol 36:618–623, 1979.

48. Sataloff RT, Sariego J, Myers DL, et al: Surgical management of the frontal sinus. Neurosurgery 15:593–596, 1984.

49. Donald PJ, Bernstein L: Compound frontal sinus injuries with intracranial penetration. Laryngoscope 88:225–231, 1978.

50. Cooper PR: Depressed skull fracture. In Apuzzo MLJ (ed): Brain Surgery Complication Avoidance and Management. New York, Churchill Livingstone, 1993, pp 1273–1282.

51. Kapp JP, Gielchinsky I: Management of combat wounds of the dural venous sinuses. Surgery 71:913–917, 1972.

52. Kapp JP, Gielchinsky I, Deardourff SL: Operative techniques for management of lesions involving the dural venous sinuses. Surg Neurol 7:330–342, 1977.

53. Albin MS, Carroll RG, Maroon JC: Clinical considerations concerning detection of venous air embolism. Neurosurgery 3:380–384, 1978.

54. Cameron M: Chronic subdural hematoma: A review of 114 cases. J Neurol Neurosurg Psychiatry 41:834, 1987.

55. French BN, Cobb CA, Corkill G, et al: Delayed evolution of posttraumatic subdural hygroma. Surg Neurol 9:145–148, 1978.

56. Ohno K, Suzuki R, Masaoka H, et al: Chronic subdural hematoma preceded by persistent traumatic subdural fluid collection. J Neurol Neurosurg Psychiatry 50:1694–1697, 1987.

57. Hubschmann OR: Twist drill craniostomy in the treatment of chronic and subacute subdural hematomas in severely ill and elderly patients. Neurosurgery 6:233–236, 1980.

58. Gjerris F, Sorensen S: Colloid osmotic and hydrostatic pressures in chronic subdural hematomas. Acta Neurochir (Wien) 54:53–60, 1980.

59. Rabe EF, Young GF, Dodge PR: The distribution and fate of subdurally instilled human serum albumin in infants with subdural collections of fluid. Neurology 14:1020–1028, 1964.

60. Weir B: The osmolality of subdural hematoma fluid. J Neurosurg 34:528–533, 1971.

61. Weir B: Oncotic pressure of subdural fluids. J Neurosurg 53:512–515, 1980.

62. Friede RL: Incidence and distribution of neomembranes of dura mater. J Neurol Neurosurg Psychiatry 34:439–446, 1971.

63. Friede RL, Schachenmayr W: The origin of subdural neomembranes. II. Fine structure of neomembranes. Am J Pathol 92:69–78, 1978.

64. Labadie EL, Glover D: Local alterations of hemostatic-fibrinolytic mechanisms in reforming subdural hematomas. Neurology 25:669–675, 1975.

65. Ito H, Yamamoto S, Komai T, et al: Role of local hyperfibrinolysis in the etiology of chronic subdural hematoma. J Neurosurg 45:26–31, 1976.

66. Ito H, Komai T, Yamamoto S: Fibrinolytic enzymes in the lining walls of chronic subdural hematoma. J Neurosurg 48:197–200, 1978.

67. Weir B, Gordon P: Factors affecting coagulation: Fibrinolysis in chronic subdural fluid collections. J Neurosurg 58:242–246, 1983.

68. Kotwica Z, Brzezinski J: Chronic suubdural hematoma treated by burr holes and closed drainage: Personal experience in 131 patients. Br J Neurosurg 5:461–465, 1991.

69. Hamilton MG, Frizzell JB, Tranmer BI: Chronic subdural hematoma: The role for craniotomy reevaluated. Neurosurgery 33:67–72, 1993.

70. Matsumoto K, Akagi K, Abekura M, et al: Recurrence factors for chronic subdural hematomas after burr-hole craniostomy and closed system drainage. Neurol Res 21:277–280, 1999.

71. Smely C, Madlinger A, Scheremet R: Chronic subdural hematoma—a comparison of two different treatment modalities. Acta Neurochir (Wien) 139:818–825, 1997.

72. Carlton CK, Saunders R: Twist drill craniotomy and closed system drainage of chronic and subacute subdural hematomas. Neurosurgery 13:153–159, 1983.

73. Tabaddor K, Shulman K: Definitive treatment of chronic subdural hematoma by twist-drill craniostomy and closed-system drainage. J Neurosurg 46:220–226, 1977.

74. Markwalder TM: Chronic subdural hematomas: A review. J Neurosurg 54:637–645, 1981.

75. Kreider GN: Repair of cranial defect by a new method. JAMA 64:1024, 1920.

76. Malis LI: Titanium mesh and acrylic cranioplasty. Neurosurgery 25:351–355, 1989.

77. Prolo DJ, Hara H, Ichinose Y: The use of bone grafts and alloplastic materials in cranioplasty. Clin Orthop 268:270–278, 1991.

78. Kaufman HH, Moake JL, Olson JD, et al: Delayed and recurrent hematomas related to disseminated intravascular clotting and fibrinolysis in head injury. Neurosurgery 7:445–449, 1980.

79. Greenberg J, Cohen WA, Cooper PR: The "hyper-acute" extra-axial intracranial hematoma: Computed tomographic findings and clinical significance. Neurosurgery 17:48–56, 1985.

80. Ninchoji T, Emara K, Shimoyama I, et al: Traumatic intracerebral hematomas of delayed onset. Acta Neurochir (Wien) 71:69–90, 1984.

81. Lobato RD, Rivas JJ, Cordobes F, et al: Acute epidural hematoma: An analysis of factors influencing the outcome of patients undergoing surgery in coma. J Neurosurg 68:48–57, 1988.

82. Tindall GT, Payne NS, O'Brien MS: Complications of surgery for subdural hematoma. Clin Neurosurg 23:465–482, 1976.

83. Kobrine AJ, Timmons E, Rajjoub JK, et al: Demonstration of massive traumatic brain swelling within 20 minutes after injury. J Neurosurg 46:256–258, 1977.

84. Bouma GJ, Muizellar JP, Bandoh K, et al: Blood pressure and intracranial pressure-volume dynamics in severe head injury: Relationships with cerebral blood flow. J Neurosurg 77:15–19, 1992.

85. Rosner MJ: Pathophysiology and management of increased intracranial pressure. In Andrews BT (ed): Neurosurgical Intensive Care. New York, McGraw-Hill, 1993, pp 57–112.

86. Andrews BT, Bederson JB, Pitts LH: Use of intraoperative ultrasonography to improve the diagnostic accuracy of exploratory burr holes in patients with traumatic tentorial herniation. Neurosurgery 24:345–347, 1989.

87. Stone JL, Rifai MHS, Sugar O, et al: Subdural hematomas. I. Acute subdural hematoma: Progress in definition, clinical pathology, and therapy. Surg Neurol 19:216–231, 1983.

88. Bullock R, Hanemann CO, Murray L, et al: Recurrent hematomas following craniotomy for traumatic intracranial mass. J Neurosurg 72:9–14, 1990.

89. Richards T, Hoff T: Factors affecting survival from acute subdural hematoma. Surgery 75:253–258, 1974.

CHAPTER 329

Sequelae of Traumatic Brain Injury

RONALD RUFF

Neuropsychological deficits commonly accompany traumatic brain injury (TBI). However, the extent of these deficits varies significantly among individuals. The variations depend on a host of factors, including the nature and severity of the brain trauma, the primary cerebral system involved, the extent and severity of comorbid medical complications, and a range of neuromedical treatments. In addition, preinjury variables such as cognitive strengths and weaknesses, personality traits, and psychosocial resources also serve as mediators in the neurobehavioral sequelae of TBI. Despite the multiplicity of factors that can contribute to post-TBI status, there are a number of neuropsychological deficits that are commonly observed after TBI in adults. The most common residua of TBI are listed in Table 329–1.

This chapter addresses the key issues involved in the neuropsychological evaluation of adult TBI. The first section introduces a theoretical framework that is based on a patient-oriented approach. In the second section, the various components of neurocognitive assessment are highlighted, along with their theoretical underpinnings. The third section reviews the emotional sequelae that follow TBI, and in the fourth section, the challenges specific to mild TBI are elucidated.

DISCIPLINE-SPECIFIC SEQUELAE VERSUS PATIENT-ORIENTED APPROACH

What we observe is not nature itself, but nature exposed to our method of questioning.
—WERNER HIESENBERG

Clinicians examining TBI patients are basically trained as scientists; thus, as empiricists their knowledge is based on specific observations. However, it is important to recognize that these observations are, as a rule, embedded in discipline-specific schemas. Given that each clinician is trained in discipline-specific schemas, information that is congruent with the particular schema is processed more quickly and is also viewed as more relevant. Over time, the skill of a specialized diagnostician is to attend, with a high degree of acuity, to these discipline-specific symptom complexes, ignoring those outside the boundaries of the discipline, in order to achieve a discipline-specific diagnosis. For example, for a neurosurgeon, the neurological symptoms and signs make up the core, and emotional dysfunctions are relegated to the periphery. However, a clinical psychologist or psychiatrist focuses on the emotional symptoms because the psychological status is viewed by these disciplines as essential. A cognitive psychologist or neuropsychologist places cognition in the center, and on the basis of neurocognitive assessments relates his or her findings to TBI. Although there is nothing wrong with this specialization, it does present inherent limitations:

1. Disciplines have evolved in a more or less arbitrary fashion. There are reasonable traditions that train health care professionals in various disciplines; however, no conceptual model exists by which these disciplines can integrate their knowledge base. Indeed, clinicians depend on specified jargon within their discipline; this jargon evolves and with time distinguishes or separates the disciplines even further.

2. It is rather naive to assume that the observations from disciplines will fall together like the pieces of a puzzle, without an a priori conceptual model. Within the philosophy of science, this simplistic assumption has been labeled as atomistic, and the pitfalls of the atomistic assumptions have, of course, been pointed out for centuries. Among the analogies used, the question is posed, "What would happen if you placed strings of wool on the floor? Would you expect to come back the next day and find a rug?" Similarly, two-dimensional strings of data across disciplines that are scattered among a multitude of journals will not weave themselves into a three-dimensional understanding without a conceptual integration.

3. Given the insight from philosophy of science, the limit of side-by-side data collection that fills our journals each year becomes evident. However, what is even more tragic is if we expect our patients who are brain-injured to integrate discipline-specific information that is provided by the different specialists. Why should patients be responsible for sorting through the jargon to arrive at a meaningful integration? Do we, in a sense, make our patients responsible for the integration, when we have not made an effort to achieve a multidisciplinary approach to their problems?

TABLE 329–1 ■ **Intrapersonal and Interpersonal Sequelae of TBI**

INTRAPERSONAL		INTERPERSONAL	
Physical	**Cognitive**	**Emotional**	**Psychosocial**
Motor Paralysis or hemiparesis, gait disturbances, reduced motor speed, and coordination	**Attention** Altered consciousness, disorientation, hemi-inattention, distractibility and reduced capacity for multitasking	**Irritability** Mild to severe agitation and frustration, anger, overt hostility	**Isolation** Loss of family, divorce, loss of friends at school or work, feelings of alienation
Sensory Deficits Blindness, field cuts, diplopia Deafness, reduced hearing capacity Partial or total loss of smell (anosmia) Changes in tolerance to sound, light, and heat	**Memory** Global amnesia, varying degrees of post-traumatic amnesia, anterograde memory difficulty; may involve the processing of verbal or nonverbal material, or both	**Emotional Lability** Mood swings, alternating pessimism-optimism, silliness **Depression** Suicidal ideation, loss of hope, helplessness, sadness, grief; brief or long lasting	**Dependence** May require 24-hr supervision, or reliance on others for assistance in activities of daily living **Status Change** Loss of vocational identity and financial loss; reliance on state support
Headache Occasional, intermittent, or constant pain	**Language-Communication** Dysarthria, aphasia, anomia, subtle communication deficits	**Denial** Ranging from anosognosia to impaired mental and emotional acceptance	**Sexual Adjustment** Disinhibition, hyper-sexuality, insensitivity or indifference to others, decreased libido, or a combination
Energy Level Anergia, increased fatigue and reduction of energy toward the end of the day	**Visuospatial** Disorientation, lack of spatial mapping ability, and nonverbal cognitive deficits	**Paranoia** Loss of trust in others, increased suspiciousness, or overt paranoia	**Drug and Alcohol Use** Infrequent to frequent use for self-medication; decreased tolerance due to TBI effects or medications, or both
Seizure Disorder Ranging in severity and frequency; often limited to early recovery stages	**Problem Solving** General intellectual deficits, poor judgment, decreased abstraction, perseverative tendencies, concreteness, and problems shifting cognitive sets		

To address these issues I have chosen the constructivist approach, which is based on the formative work of Piaget,[1, 2] the contemporary theory of self-organization,[3] and the study of evolving knowledge by Popper[4] and Campbell.[5] Constructivism, as a philosophy of science, largely rejects the notion that knowledge is based on scientific positivism and also rejects the atomistic assumption. Instead, an approach is used that assumes that realities are basically a dynamic human invention, as opposed to empiricism, which views reality as a stable and knowable "truth." Constructivism views knowledge as inherently flawed, or potentially fallible, and revisions and modifications are best viewed in terms of their present viability. This approach provides the freedom to postulate a viable construct that can be used as a system to explain the phenomena observed and reported by our TBI patients.

SUMMARY

On the basis of this constructivistic approach, it is my premise that the sequelae of TBI are best understood if we transcend our own disciplines by making a conscious decision to examine how our patients live inside an injured brain and face their day-to-day problems. Thus, our discipline-specific schemas should be inte-grated with a holistic patient-based approach so that we are not trapped in reductionism. Patients do not experience just physical or emotional or cognitive problems, but all three, as all three areas are affected by the TBI. These three domains overlap to some extent, yet all three are part of the intrapersonal dynamic (Fig. 329–1.) This model is a construct that allows clinicians to evaluate the interactions among the factors influencing the TBI patient's status. This model does not negate or replace discipline-specific measures; however, it does promote an attitude that information outside one's own discipline is not relegated to "noise." The neurosurgeon, neuropsychologist, and other health care professionals must work across disciplines, as opposed to perpetuating static parallel approaches. Such an interaction is no doubt best achieved if the TBI patient's symptoms and disabilities are the central focus.

NEUROCOGNITIVE SEQUELAE

I think, therefore I am.

—RENÉ DESCARTES

Given our model (see Fig. 329–1), the patient's cognitive residua need to be understood as a series of inter-

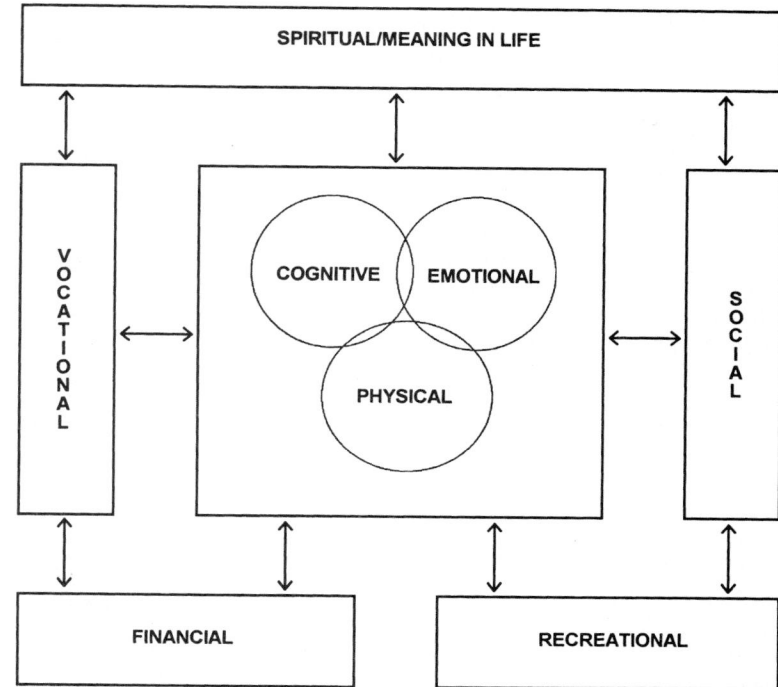

FIGURE 329–1. Intrapersonal and interpersonal dimensions affected by traumatic brain injury (TBI).

actions among the intrapersonal and interpersonal dimensions. Having constructed this global approach, this section focuses on human cognition and TBI. Cognition is, of course, also a construct that has been subdivided into multiple components, with multiple interactions among them. For an overview of the various cognitive domains that are typically evaluated for TBI patients, see Table 329–2.

Value of Neuropsychological Testing

Various cognitive functions are evaluated according to scientifically based criteria that are the underpinnings

TABLE 329–2 ■ **Cognitive Domains in Neuropsychology**

DOMAIN	FUNCTIONS
Sensory perceptual	Processing sensory input in auditory, visual, and tactile modalities
Motor abilities	Processing motor output; manual motor speed and dexterity
Attention	Processing information according to arousal-alertness, selective focusing, capacity, and speed
Memory and learning	Encoding, storage, and retrieval of information
Language	Communicating by receiving and expressing verbal information
Spatial and constructional abilities	Processing and manipulating spatial information; copying of geometric designs
Executive functioning	Modulating cognitive processes to solve problems and achieve goals
Intelligence	Balance between assimilation and accommodation

of psychometrics. The standards set by the American Psychological Association for psychological tests[6] include the criteria of (1) standardization, (2) reliability, (3) validity, and (4) normative values. To exemplify these criteria, a classic neurological "test" is discussed under each of these sections. The selected test is the commonly used task of having the patient serially subtract the number 7, starting from 100 (i.e., serial 7 or 100 − 7).

STANDARDIZATION

Standardization refers to the principle that allows two qualified examiners to administer a test in the exact same manner so that the results are more or less identical. Conversely, standardization is not achieved if most clinicians who use the same task vary the parameters. For example, having observed various clinicians administer the 100 − 7 task, I have noted great variation. No consistency emerges for how much time was given. When should the test be discontinued? Should the patient be made aware of errors, and so on? To avoid confusion regarding test administration, the principle of standardization ensures that the test is administered in exactly the same way among clinicians. Thus, standardization provides the benefit that any two examiners will administer the same test in the exact same manner so that the results are more or less independent of the examiner. Moreover, no variations are allowed for recording the patients' responses. Thus, the subtraction of 7s from 100 could be standardized, with respect to the exact instructions provided to each patient, the time that is allowed, the cues (if any) that are given, and the setpoint at which the test should be discontinued.

RELIABILITY

Reliability evaluates the consistency of a patient taking the test at two different time intervals, with various factors potentially playing a role. Reliability needs to be established before a test is published by administering the test to the same individuals on two occasions and determining the degree to which a positive correlation exists. The American Psychological Association[6] recommends that the correlation coefficient should be equal to or greater than 0.8 for reliability to be deemed satisfactory. In addition to the test-retest technique, there are also split-half reliability techniques. The split-half procedure is applicable for a test that has a range of items that can be separated into two comparable halves to assess whether both halves evaluate the behavior in a consistent manner. Two equivalent versions of the same test can also be used to establish reliability. If we return to our 100 − 7 task, do we know how reliable it is? It becomes obvious that if the test is not standardized, it cannot be reliable. Moreover, the 100 − 7 task should not be considered a "test" if there is significant fluctuation among the scores reported by a neurologist, a psychiatrist, and a neurosurgeon. However, a reliability study of the 100 − 7 task is easily conceptualized by having 100 normal participants take a standardized 100 − 7 test on two occasions or along with an alternative version (e.g., 100 − 9).

VALIDITY

Validity refers to "what" the test measures, and "how well" it achieves its aim. Going back to our example, what cognitive function is the 100 − 7 task actually capturing? For example, is subtracting 7s from 100 a test of oral arithmetic? Is it a measure of attention? Is it a measure of speed of information processing? Is it designed to evaluate a combination of functions? More important, what conclusions will be reached based on this test? For example, if someone makes three mistakes before he or she reaches 51, can one state with a reasonable degree of certainty that this individual has cognitive difficulties?

As a rule, the more agreement that exists for a specific concept, the easier it is to establish validity. For example, the construct of memory is fairly straightforward in that a patient is given a set of stimuli, which is followed by an interference interval, after which the patient is asked to recall, recognize, or retrieve the stimuli presented earlier. In contrast, the concept of intelligence is far less clearly spelled out because almost everyone has a different concept for what they consider "an intelligent individual." Is a patient who is academically or financially successful more intelligent than an individual who has finished only 7 years of education or one who has not held a job consistently? Obviously, there is not only one form of intelligence, and in many individuals psychological factors can prevent an individual from achieving certain successes.

For psychometric validity to be established, various methods can be used, such as content-related validity, criterion-related validity, and construct-related validity.

Content validity involves a systematic examination of the test content by experts to determine whether the behavioral domain that is to be measured is adequately represented by the test items. Content validity tends to go beyond face validity by theoretical and systematic examination of the behavior that is to be examined. For example, if we consider the 100 − 7 task to be an oral arithmetic test, one would carefully evaluate the relevant course syllabi and academic textbooks to consider the grade level at which an individual should be able to perform the task. Given the variation of oral arithmetic, one would also want to evaluate the educational achievements and descriptions of oral arithmetic and determine whether indeed 100 − 7 (i.e., a subtraction) is a representative task that would cover the range of what is considered oral arithmetic (i.e., addition, division, multiplication). Thus, subject matter experts should opine whether they agree that the 100 − 7 is a representative test of oral arithmetic.

Criterion-related validation procedures determine the effectiveness of a test in predicting an individual's performance in specific activities. Again, returning to the 100 − 7 task, does the result of this particular measure predict mathematical aptitude? In the context of a neurological examination, does the 100 − 7 task reliably capture the individual's cerebral integrity?

A commonly used technique is *concurrent validity*, which can compare two independent test measures with each other. Specific to our example, can the 100 − 7 test predict the score on another oral arithmetic test?

Finally, *construct-related validity* refers to the examination of how well a measure captures a theoretical construct or trait, that is, does the 100 − 7 test capture oral arithmetic capacities? How well does it capture the psychological construct of sustained attention? Techniques used can include factor analysis, internal consistency, and convergent and discriminant analyses.[7, 8]

It should also be noted that no test can be valid if it is not reliable. However, reliability does not ensure that a test is valid. Reliability could be established for the 100 − 7 task by administering it to 100 individuals along with an alternative version, the 100 − 9 test. If the reliability coefficients fell at greater than or equal to 0.8, the two test forms are reliable. Next, the degree to which these tests are valid for a particular theoretical construct needs to be evaluated. If a decision is made that this test captures arithmetic, to establish the concurrent validity, one would give a standardized arithmetic test and find the degree to which performance on the 100 − 7 test is representative of oral calculation. Obviously, a challenge exists for a test that attempts to be valid for multiple functions.

NORMATIVE VALUES

Normative values typically provide education-, age-, and gender-sensitive distributions. A primary benefit of testing is that most cognitive functions are normally distributed and thus yield themselves to generalizations. For example, if a memory task is administered to men between the ages of 16 and 25 with educational stratifications, and these individuals do not have a premorbid history of neurological or psychiatric illnesses, their scores, if distributed normally, can provide powerful predictions for the overall population with the same demographic characteristics. Based on the randomized sampling, if 100 or 150 of this subgroup are examined in North America, it is reasonable to conclude that the results would be more or less similar to the data that could be obtained if we examined all men in the same age brackets across the United States and Canada. Thus, the statistical concept of normal distribution allows for powerful generalizations, which at the same time are a reasonable estimate of an individual's baseline or premorbid functioning.

Returning to our example of subtracting 7s from 100, ask yourself what "normative standards" are being used. For example, if a 27-year-old male TBI patient makes three mistakes before he reaches 51, is this considered to be a score that falls within the normal range or is it in the deficient or seriously deficient range? In the absence of normative values, these estimates are just good guesses. However, given psychometric standards, exact percentiles could easily be established that compare a TBI patient to a demographically matched cohort.

Assessment of Cognitive Functions

GENERAL COGNITIVE AND INTELLECTUAL ABILITIES

Historically, intelligence was conceptualized as a single function that fueled all the cognitive activities. Over time, numerous definitions of intelligence have been proposed. However, as mentioned earlier, no generally agreed upon concept of intelligence has emerged in the literature. Thus, Boring[9] stated in a classic historical treatise that the best definition is that intelligence is what the intelligence test measures. Intelligence tests were basically designed to evaluate the academic potential of children in order to determine whether their grades fell into line with their potential. For example, if a student was doing poorly, the question was raised whether this was primarily due to a cognitive limitation versus some emotional or motivational factors. Thus, the intelligence quotient (IQ) captures multiple cognitive abilities that are summarized in a single score, and this score does not have a high degree of specificity to identify the cerebral region that is disturbed.

Since TBI frequently affects a variety of underlying cerebral functions, it can, in more severe cases, diminish IQ scores. Within the field of neuropsychology, the Wechsler Adult Intelligence Scale—III (WAIS-III)[10] is the most commonly used measure. The particular strength of the WAIS-III is its subtests, which can describe specific language, visuospatial, or performance capacities. A composite score can reveal a Verbal IQ as well as a Performance IQ, and the two can be combined into a Full-Scale IQ.

Both the Verbal and Performance IQs are composed of multiple subtests, each of which captures function-specific cognitive domains. Among the verbal subtests, there are measures that focus on remote memory by asking standardized questions of learned material typically acquired through education and reading. Comprehension is evaluated by posing specific situations within a social context for which the patient needs to respond with appropriate solutions. Another subtest uses word definitions to evaluate the level of vocabulary, and abstraction is addressed by having the patient provide the common feature that combines two words. For the Performance IQ, examples of subtests include Picture Completion, in which the patient is asked to identify items missing from a picture that would logically appear there. On the Block Design subtest, red and white blocks need to be arranged to match a specific design. Overall, there are seven verbal and seven performance subtests in the WAIS-III.

The primary value of the WAIS-III for neuropsychology are the subtests because they facilitate function-specific descriptions that are sensitive to specific brain regions. A substantial difference between the Verbal and Performance IQs (typically 20 points or more) can have implications relative to which hemisphere is more compromised.[11, 12] The verbal subtests are sensitive to various language disturbances. The performance subtests represent fluid tasks, requiring adaptive abilities that are more readily affected by right hemisphere dysfunction.[13]

Two typical misconceptions should definitely be avoided by non-neuropsychologists:

1. The first misconception is that reduction in IQ represents a rollback or regression in mental age. For example, if a 24-year-old individual with a preinjury IQ of 140 suffers a TBI and thereafter has an IQ of 70, it should not be suggested to the patient's family that he is now functioning at a 12-year-old level. TBIs do not systematically "roll back" intellectual abilities. Instead, there is typically a diffuse or uneven pattern of compromise across the various cognitive domains.

2. A second misconception is the belief that a reduction in IQ is, in itself, a powerful predictor of the degree of cerebral dysfunction. This notion is flawed because the pattern of deficits among the subtests (or cognitive domains) is far more critical. For example, a patient may have a low IQ of 80 that is primarily due to motor or perceptual difficulties that compound a range of performances and therefore lead to a "reduction" of the overall IQ. Conversely, a high IQ of 120, in itself, does not mean that there has not been a reduction in cognition. Indeed, there can be a deficit in visuospatial construction that affects one subtest in particular. Averaging can cancel out a dip within a profile. In short, the concept of intelligence (particularly the Full-Scale IQ) has limited application in neuropsychology.

LANGUAGE FUNCTIONS

Language disorders have classically been subdivided into expressive and receptive difficulties. Expressive language is frequently compromised by frontal lobe problems (dysfluency, Broca's aphasia, or motor aphasia). If comprehension is also affected (e.g., fluent or Wernicke's aphasia) and an expressive aphasia is also present, the classification of global aphasia is typically made. Benson[14] proposed a variety of aphasias that can interfere with the programming of verbal sequences such as repetition and retrieval defects (i.e., conduction aphasia). The memory- or retrieval-based language disturbances are typically referred to as amnestic or anomic aphasia.

Although global aphasia appears to be an uncommon sequela of TBI,[15] word finding difficulty (dysnomia) is more common.[16] Defective performance on a task of visual confrontation naming has been found to be particularly common, occurring in about 40% of a consecutive series of patients with a variety of levels of TBI severity in a study by Levin and colleagues.[17] Recovery of language dysfunction after TBI largely occurs within 6 to 9 months of the injury.[1, 18] However, if patients are (very) severely aphasic (global aphasics), the expectation of recovery is rather bleak. Thompsen[19] reported that 84 of 90 initially aphasic TBI patients remained significantly aphasic 2.5 years after injury. Dysarthria has also shown a tendency to persist over time.

The Verbal Fluency Test is one of the more sensitive measures for evaluating a patient's ability to generate as many words as possible, either beginning with the same letter of the alphabet or with a category prompt. One of the most frequently used verbal fluency measures is the Benton Controlled Oral Word Association Test (COWAT).[20, 21] According to the Controlled Oral Word Association Test, verbal fluency is reduced in most TBI patients.[22, 23] Indeed, blood flow studies in normal individuals have demonstrated that word fluency is localized in the left dorsolateral prefrontal cortex.[24] The components that play a role in word fluency have been discussed by Ruff and associates.[25]

VISUOSPATIAL, VISUOCONSTRUCTUAL, AND VISUOPERCEPTUAL ABILITIES

The category of visuospatial, visuoconstructual, and visuoperceptual abilities includes a variety of nonverbal skills that are particularly affected in TBI patients with right hemisphere damage. The more common dysfunctions include constructional problems that affect, for example, the drawing of shapes and visuospatial integration required in relating spatial objects to one another. (For a general overview of many of these deficits, the interested reader is referred to Benton.[26]) The visuospatial performance tests of the WAIS-III are frequently affected in TBI.[12] In particular, the Digit Symbol subtest of the WAIS-III tends to be highly sensitive to brain dysfunction, regardless of lesion location, and relies on a number of visuospatial abilities. Constructional praxis is typically measured by having the patient copy a complex geometric figure. The missing parts and distortions found thereafter indicate deficits.[27] Studies of facial recognition performance in TBI patients have been few, although Levin and colleagues[28] found deficient performances in more than

one quarter of their sample of TBI patients who had been unconscious for more than a few minutes.

ATTENTION AND CONCENTRATION

Attention and concentration difficulties are among the most striking neuropsychological sequelae after TBI. Although numerous studies have documented these attentional deficits by using a range of tests,[29–32] no generally accepted theoretical framework has emerged within neuropsychology that allows us to differentiate the various attentional deficits. Based on a review of the neurophysiologic, cognitive, and neuropsychological literature,[33] we proposed for such a division a framework that separates attention into the following three subdivisions: (1) arousal-alertness and sustained attention, (2) selective attention, (3) energetic aspects of attention that encompass concepts such as effort, resource allocation, and speed of processing.

Arousal. The drive state that enhances all behavior is referred to as *arousal*. Two physiologic states that are typically distinguished are phasic changes, which occur very fast and are often under voluntary control, and tonic changes, which occur slowly and are more or less involuntary.[34, 35] Thus, if a TBI patient with reduced arousal is acutely stimulated by a loud noise, there can be a quick alertness to the surrounding condition. However, if a patient is unable to respond to such signals, the phasic aspect of arousal is affected.[36] In contrast, tonic changes of awareness affect overall human performance on a more subtle basis. These changes are typically accompanied by metabolic changes, and many factors can influence tonic arousal.[37, 38] For example, sleep deprivation, heat, or even high levels of chronic anxiety or depression can lower the level of arousal and can have a negative impact on attention. The opposite has been observed when TBI patients have been given stimulant drugs (e.g., methylphenidate [Ritalin]) or incentives.

Selective Attention. The ability to set priorities in information processing is referred to as *selective attention*. TBI patients are frequently less able to set priorities, and during a conversation may be distracted by a concurrent noise in the room. When selective attention is functionally optimal, distractions play a minimal role. The two forms of selective attention are automatic detection and controlled search.[39, 40] Automatic detection is based on overlearned selection mechanisms, whereas controlled search demands a conscious awareness, and the individual has to put effort into the selection process. TBI patients can be affected differently in both types of selective attention. For example, if other individuals are talking in the background while the patient is having a conversation with a therapist, increased concentration is required to eliminate the distraction of the background voices (i.e., controlled search). However, if the other individuals in the room are all speaking in other languages, and the patient speaks only English, the patient can more easily focus on his or her conversation in English (i.e., automatic detection). Thus, the nature of the distracters influences selective attention.

Effort and Resource Allocation. In order to determine the patient's overall available mental energy, effort and resource allocation need to be assessed by a neuropsychologist. Mental energy can vary significantly within a day, and many patients fatigue toward the end of the day. This often leads to a decline in cognitive functioning at that time of day. In severe cases, in which patients become nonfunctional, this is called *sundowning.*

LEARNING AND MEMORY

Memory is typically defined as a covert process that, as a result of perceived past experiences, permits the subject to demonstrate overt changes from baseline behavior. From a testing standpoint, memory can easily be operationalized by (1) presenting a set of stimuli; (2) introducing a delay, with or without interference; and (3) requesting recall or recognition of the information presented. In this context, learning and memory tasks are distinguishable because, in the former, the examiner provides implicit or explicit feedback. Thus, a learning curve over trials can be evaluated, whereas memory usually is evaluated with a single presentation of stimuli material that then has to be recalled.

Squire[41] proposed a useful division between declarative memory and procedural memory. Declarative memory refers to the information that needs to be recalled and declared after presentation, for example, remembering names or short stories. Procedural memory refers to the acquisition of motor or mental skills, such as learning to use a wheelchair or the nondominant hand for eating or learning typing skills. For example, an amnestic patient improved his performance during repeated daily testing on the mirror-tracing task, despite his inability to remember the same testing from prior sessions.[42] Thus, procedural memory can be spared, even in individuals who suffer from severe amnesia. There are different neuroanatomic substrates to procedural and declarative memory. Declarative memory requires the integration of the dorsomedial nucleus of the thalamus and the temporal-hippocampal-amygdaloid structures.[41] In contrast, procedural memory is not necessarily localized. However, it does require the integrity of various subcortical structures (e.g., basal ganglia) as well as the associative cortex.[43]

Despite the theoretical advances made in this area, the neuropsychological test procedures that are currently available focus primarily on declarative memory, whereas there are virtually no sophisticated normative test batteries available for procedural memory. We frequently see the separation between these two memory types in rehabilitation. Physical therapists, relying primarily on procedural memory, can frequently demonstrate significant gains even in amnestic patients. Speech therapists, in contrast, rely primarily on declarative memory and are all too often unable to elicit significant gains in the same patients.

Neuropsychologists and experimental scientists also frequently separate memory into short-term and long-term components. Short-term memory typically refers to the ability to hold on to information in storage after an interference delay of seconds to minutes following the presentation of stimuli. Typical measurements for short-term memory include having individuals repeat a paragraph that was read to them or redraw a geometric figure that they just copied.[44, 45]

Long-term memory, which spans both recent and remote events, can last from hours to years. Thus, problems with long-term memory can affect the recall before injury (retrograde amnesia) as well as after the TBI (anterograde amnesia). However, the focus of neuropsychological testing is on the patient's capacity at the time of testing when the task is to recall information after a few seconds (short term) and after a delay of 15 to 30 minutes (long term).

Clinically, it is most useful to evaluate learning because recovery can be facilitated by relearning. Within the verbal modality, a series of words is typically presented to the TBI patient, and he or she is asked to learn this list over repeated trials. Examples that capture such measures include the Rey Auditory Verbal Learning Test,[45] the Buschke Selective Reminding Test,[46] and the California Verbal Learning Test.[47] Far fewer tests are available to evaluate learning in the visuospatial mode. Examples include the Ruff-Light Trail Learning Test,[48] in which dots are connected with lines in order to learn a 15-step pathway across multiple trials. For both the memory and learning tests, alternative forms have been developed to establish learning as well as memory across multiple trials. By determining if the verbal or visuospatial learning is more accessible, more effective interventions can be implemented.

EXECUTIVE FUNCTIONING

Executive functioning refers to a set of flexible regulatory and effector processes that, in turn, modulate other cognitive processes in the refinement of achieving goal-directed activities. According to Lezak,[45] executive functioning addresses the "how" and "whether" a particular behavior occurs, to which one might add a "when" and "under what conditions" the behavior takes place. TBI patients are most susceptible to frontal lobe damage, and thus they may have a range of deficits among the various components of executive functioning. However, there is still no clear understanding of executive functioning and how the frontal lobe works. We do know that the frontal lobes maintain rich reciprocal connections, not only with the brainstem and limbic system but also with the sensory association and motor regions of the cortex.[49] By means of these subcortical connections, the frontal regions have significant influence on flexibility as well as modulation of arousal, attention, and emotional function.[50] Frontal lobe functions play a role in strategies for learning, storage of information, and motor planning. Further, it appears that the frontoreticular system, in conjunction with the thalamic relays, constitutes a system that allows for selective attention to a variety of stimuli. These composite functions are necessary for executive function.

Classic measures that evaluate frontal lobe functions include the Wisconsin Card Sorting Test.[45, 51, 52] In this measure, an individual is given two identical decks of 64 cards, with a number (one, two, three, or four) of geometric shapes printed on them (triangle, star, cross, circle) in one of four colors (red, green, yellow, or blue). Four stimuli or key cards are presented to the individual, who is asked to match similar but not identical cards according to a principle. The task is to figure out the correct categories, and the examiner provides no further clues except to state whether the placement of the card is correct or incorrect. Thus, rule finding and problem solving are evaluated by this test.

Another set of measures for executive functioning focuses on reaching a solution to a problem that is within the behavioral repertoire of a patient. Tests of self-directed, continuous response include verbal fluency tests as well as figural fluency tests. In the verbal fluency test (Controlled Oral Word Association Test), the patient is asked to generate as many words as he or she can that begin with a specific letter of the alphabet.[20] In the nonverbal fluency test (Ruff Figural Fluency Test), the patient is asked to draw different figures by connecting two or more dots within a configuration of multiple dots.[53] As mentioned earlier, blood flow studies have shown increased left dorsolateral activities during verbal fluency.[24] Conversely, figural fluency is most compromised after right prefrontal lobe damage.[54]

Other popular measures of frontal lobe functioning evaluate inhibition. These include tests such as the Porteus Maze[55, 56] and the Color Word Naming Test by Stroop.[57] A classic neuropsychological test that is sensitive to the sequencing of complex behavior is the Trail Making Test,[58] that requires the patient to attend to digit and alphabet sequencing simultaneously. In Part A, 25 numbers that are randomly placed on a page are connected with a line in numerical order. In Part B, 25 numbers and letters need to be connected, alternating between each, in numerical and alphabetical order. Abstraction and attribute identification have also been considered part of executive functioning and are typically examined by the Similarities subtest of the WAIS-III[59] and the earlier mentioned Wisconsin Card Sorting Test.

SENSORY PERCEPTUAL AND PSYCHOMOTOR-VISUOMOTOR FUNCTIONING

The neuropsychological examination must evaluate the extent of visual and auditory deficits in order to compensate and adjust the testing procedures. Hemi-inattention or neglect will, of course, affect a range of neurocognitive tests, and the compounding effects need to be sorted out.

A neuropsychological test battery also will include tests to evaluate motor and visuomotor capacities. Some tests require graphomotor skills, whereas others require bimanual dexterity. Thus, motor-based deficits

need to be differentiated from the cognitive domains evaluated by these tests.

Motor speed is typically evaluated according to the Finger Tapping Test that assesses rapid movement of the index finger on either hand, in alternating 10-second intervals. Eye-hand coordination is measured with the Grooved Pegboard Test by having the patient insert metal pegs into rotated slots with either hand. Age- and gender-stratified norms allow for quantifications of both hands separately.[45, 60]

Estimate of Premorbid Cognitive Functioning

An estimate of preinjury cognitive functioning is particularly relevant for patients with mild to moderate TBI because the effects of their injuries can be determined most accurately if the degree of impairment is based on a comparison between the premorbid and current abilities. The greatest impediment in determining preinjury functioning is that this information usually has to be collected retrospectively. Thus, it is critical that when diagnosing the effects of brain injury on cognition for patients with milder TBI, the following questions be answered:

1. Is there a decline of functioning between the estimated premorbid level and the present functioning level?
2. Does this decline represent a worsening of a preexisting weakness, or is it a distinctly new symptom?

The typical sources available to clinicians for evaluating premorbid functioning include the patient interview and interviews with those familiar with the patient before and after the accident (spouses, friends, family, employers). Review of pre- and postmorbid patient records can also be helpful, particularly if they include academic grades, test performances, and job evaluations that describe the type of employment as well as advances and promotions.

Mental ability deficits can obviously affect vocational aptitude, interpersonal skills, and emotional functioning. Thus, a clear estimate of an individual's premorbid cognitive functioning can provide the neuropsychologist with the nature and extent of changes to current functioning. The key questions that clinicians need to address specific to cognitive functioning follow:

- What were the strengths and weaknesses in the individual's preinjury cognitive functioning? Among the weaknesses, were there particular cognitive disabilities such as dyslexia or attention deficit hyperactivity disorder?
- Was there a preinjury history of serious alcohol or substance abuse that led to an impairment in cognition?
- Were there any medical illnesses that compromised cognition before the TBI?
- Were significant emotional or psychosocial problems evident that compromised cognitive development (e.g., prolonged periods of depression, social withdrawal, antisocial traits)?

• What role has education played with respect to cognitive development? For example, is the patient an overachiever, or an underachiever? Did the individual lack educational opportunities? Did noncognitive factors such as finances, illness, family difficulties (e.g., parents divorced) affect the educational level attained?

In addition to a clinical interview, there are three approaches to answering these questions.

NORMATIVE VALUES

Neuropsychological assessment derives an indirect estimate of preinjury functioning levels according to normative values for specific tests. Since normative test data are obtained for each test measure from a group of individuals who have no history of neurological or psychiatric illnesses, these scores serve as an indirect baseline representing a distribution of the expected or "normal" preinjury functioning levels. As normative values are typically stratified according to gender, age, and education, a TBI patient can be compared with a matched premorbid estimate. Thus, estimates of each individual's premorbid level of functioning may often provide unique insights into the real impact of the injury.

In the literature, an effort has been made to estimate premorbid intelligence beyond a comparison of normative values on a specific test. For example, Nelson[61] estimated premorbid IQ based on the National Adult Reading Test (NART). Crawford[62] used the National Adult Reading Test in combination with demographic variables. Obviously, in TBI patients who have, for example, diplopia, visual field deficits, word-finding difficulties, or even dyslexia, reading tests are clearly limited.

One of the more commonly used estimates of intelligence was introduced by Barona and colleagues[63] and relies on age, gender, race, education, occupation, geographic region of the participants' residence, and handedness. It should be noted that none of these estimates of premorbid intelligence are very powerful. However, they provide the best possible estimates to date.

PERFORMANCE AND PATTERN ANALYSIS

If the neurocognitive deficits are not severely reduced across all functions, the most powerful estimate of premorbid levels is an analysis and comparison within the neuropsychological test battery.[45] Since a neuropsychological test battery assesses multiple domains, an analysis of strengths and weaknesses within the cognitive profile provides strong indicators of preinjury functioning levels. One technique that is commonly used is the best performance analysis, which examines the highest functioning levels in the profile as an indication of preserved functioning (if indicated). Thus, the strengths within an individual profile can, in some cases, be used as an estimate of the patient's baseline functioning, against which current weaknesses can be viewed.

The analysis of best performances among the various subtests of the WAIS-III has been studied in neurologically impaired populations. Subtests in which TBI patients maintain or hold preinjury scores are termed *hold* subtests. Other subtests that are more vulnerable to the effects of a TBI are termed *do not hold* subtests. Formulas have been proposed to calculate the ratio between the hold and the do not hold subtests (i.e., subtests that are more resistant versus those that are more vulnerable to the effects of TBI). For example, Gonen[64] suggested that the Block Design and Digit Symbol subtests are least resistant (do not hold) to diffuse cerebral damage, whereas the Information and Comprehension subtests were most resistant (hold) to diffuse nonlateralized damage. Even more established is the notion that the Vocabulary subtest represents the single best indicator of premorbid verbal intellectual endowment.[65] However, when applied with TBI patients, a seasoned neuropsychologist will need to determine the degree to which moderator variables such as motor slowing, visual field cut, neglect, dysnomia, and reduced motor skills play a role. Such analyses are usually referred to as pattern analysis, which can be combined with the best performance analysis to provide a benchmark for premorbid estimation.

Pattern analyses depend on the body of literature that, for various causes, has established a type of cognitive deficit that is typically demonstrated.[45] For example, we know that in patients with mild TBI, sustained and selective attention, memory and learning, and executive functioning are particularly compromised.[66] Therefore, given this expected pattern, we can evaluate the extent to which those specific cognitive deficits have been compromised in a particular patient, with the remaining portions of the test profile, such as sensory perception, motor functioning, intelligence, and so on being relatively preserved. Further strength can also be added to the best performance in pattern analysis if neuropsychological tests are repeated over time. The hold tests obviously should remain stable, whereas the do not hold measures should show a gradual improvement over time. Indeed, if such trends across testing are documented, the reliability of the premorbid estimates gains strength.

REVIEW OF SCHOOL RECORDS

Scholastic records often do not provide an accurate estimate of premorbid mental or neurocognitive functioning. Multiple factors other than cognition influence school performances. For example, a high achiever can receive high grades with average neurocognitive ability, whereas a student with motivational difficulties can obtain poor grades despite average or superior cognitive function. Thus, it is essential when reviewing school records to consider, for example, phases of rebellion during the teenage years or to evaluate whether the individual was an underachiever with average cognitive abilities. In short, it must be strongly emphasized, particularly with physicians who have seriously pursued academics, that grades do not necessarily correlate with cognitive abilities.

If education has been successfully pursued, this can positively affect neuropsychological functioning. In other words, good grades are more powerful predictors than bad grades. Successful completion of higher education can lead to higher performances on specific neuropsychological tests.[45] Indeed, Zarit and associates[67] concluded that education can influence performance to the extent that poorly educated but cognitively intact individuals may perform more poorly on tests of memory and learning than better educated individuals with mild impairment. Thus, it is essential that test norms be stratified according to education to deal with the potent and pervasive influence of education on neuropsychological functioning.

SUMMARY

Cognition is clearly one of the most sensitive measures of the integrity of the central nervous system. Thus, the most sophisticated evaluation of cognition that we can muster is frequently indicated, particularly for patients with moderate to mild sequelae. Cognitive evaluation is also a requirement for more severely injured individuals if one wants to delineate their recovery over time. The estimation of pre-existing cognitive functioning is essential in determining the extent to which the current cognitive deficits play a role. A seasoned neuropsychologist can tease out pre-existing strengths and weaknesses and determine the extent to which these are still reflective within the current neuropsychological test profile. Moreover, analyzing the test profiles and the interaction among the various functions is critical. For example, how does a short-term memory deficit affect the scores on long-term memory? The neuropsychologist needs to analyze the interactions among the various cognitive domains. These interactions include a comparison between pre-injury and postinjury functioning and, of course, interactions among the emotional, physical, and situational factors (see Fig. 329–1).

The neurosurgeon plays a key role in delineating what decisions need to be made based on the neuropsychological evaluation. As a rule, tests should be administered to answer a question. If the referral question is rather vague, most likely the report will represent a fairly global delineation of cognitive strengths and weaknesses. There is nothing "wrong" with this, if the clinician is primarily interested in having the neuropsychologist provide documentation of the patient's level of cognitive functioning at a given time. This may serve as a baseline on which subsequent testing can ascertain the degree of potential recovery. Psychometric classifications do have advantages over the typical clinical evaluations given by neurologists and neurosurgeons. They include t and z scores or percentile ranks that are based on comparisons with normative samples of individuals matched for gender, age range, and educational level. Thus, subtler improvements can be recognized, for example, if a patient's sustained attention score fell in the 7th percentile initially and improves to the 25th percentile after a 3-month interval. Such gains are not typically captured by having someone subtract 7 from 100 without specific normative benchmarks. It is implicitly expected that the neuropsychologist should also evaluate the effect of premorbid factors, such as substance abuse or emotional turmoil, that may affect the postinjury adjustments. These questions need to be specified. Neurocognitive testing, in itself, does not address these questions.

EMOTIONAL SEQUELAE

. . .I could never slip back into my former innocence when I believed my losses were all correctable. . .
— CLAUDIA OSBORN (TBI SURVIVOR)

Emotional disturbances after TBI are common and often have a major impact on the patient and his or her family.[68] Although the assessment of the physical and cognitive status of TBI patients is of critical importance, too little attention is paid to the emotional sequelae. For example, symptoms of depression and anxiety are frequently encountered after moderate to severe TBI.[69] Psychological disturbances after TBI may (1) represent a reaction to the acquired deficits and limitations, (2) be directly related to damages to the cerebral systems that serve the emotional functions, or (3) be a combination of both.[70]

The emotional sequelae of TBI are divided into two categories. The first represents the organically based alteration of the patient's emotional functioning and depends on the site of cerebral damage and the amount of time that has passed since the onset of the disorder. Difficulty with anger control is one of the most common residua of organically based emotional difficulties. In more severe cases, lack of initiation, lability, and being overly emotional are sequelae frequently attributed to organic causes.

The second category is composed of those psychological disturbances that represent a reaction to the circumstances that the TBI has caused in the individual's life. Living inside an injured brain can result in emotional turmoil that is difficult to understand and empathize with as an individual who has not suffered TBI. This is most succinctly described in a personal account by a physician[71]:

I am most lonely and isolated when I am with my friends. The person they look for doesn't live here any more, and I don't know how to establish new, and equal, relationships. I don't seek life which is quiescent or predictable; I do want to be able to cope with the unexpected. (p 217)

The one feeling that was readily identifiable was the consuming depression that followed each jolt of memory about the permanence of my injuries. The trigger was invariably related to my desire to do medicine. (p 126)

I, who had been easily stirred by music, art, drama, books, nature and poetry, felt nothing when I heard a Puccini aria or viewed a spectacular landscape. I did not delight in the beautiful or thrill to the magnificent or feel awe at the wondrous. Nor was I aware, apart from the complaints of others, that my capacity for enjoyment was dampered. Nor did I mind. (p 123)

Assessment of Emotional Functioning

Numerous tests have been developed to evaluate psychological functioning, but few tests focus specifically on the behavioral effects of TBI. Since most personality tests are validated on a range of patients with psychopathologic conditions, it is frequently difficult to determine the extent of the validity for TBI patients who suffer from psychological problems in addition to extensive neuropathology. The questionnaires that are most commonly used for TBI populations are reviewed in the following sections.

KATZ ADJUSTMENT SCALE, REVISED[72]

Although the Katz Adjustment Scale, Revised (KAS-R) can be filled out by the patient, a form completed by the relatives is particularly useful for patients with more severe TBI in the earlier stages. The psychosocial issues that are dealt with are, of course, particularly relevant if the TBI patients have returned to live with their families. The relative scale consists of five inventories, and in the first inventory questions address the patient's adjustment to sleep, fears, quality of speech, and preoccupations. The second scale addresses socially expected activities, such as helping with household chores, going to parties, and so on. The third scale deals with expectations for performance in social activities, and the fourth and fifth scales evaluate how the TBI patient spends his or her free time (e.g., specific leisure activities such as watching television, shopping, or playing cards). Katz and Lyerly suggest three major factors: (1) social obstreperousness, composed of problems with belligerence, verbal expansiveness, negativism, or general psychopathology; (2) acute psychoticism with items that cluster around anxiety, bizarreness, and hyperactivity; and (3) withdrawal and depression, which encompass items of withdrawal and helplessness.[73] Fordyce and coworkers[74] showed differences between the scores obtained during the first 6 months after a TBI and those obtained an average of 25 months after injury. Hinkledy and Corrigan[75] found a similar pattern, particularly that belligerence scores are often higher in the earlier stages. That is not to say that 2 to 4 years after injury patients do not continue to have problems with belligerence and negativism,[76] yet typically they are less severe.

NEUROBEHAVIORAL RATING SCALE

The Neurobehavioral Rating Scale (NBRS)[77] is a 27-item scale that was developed specifically for TBI patients. The responses are rated along a seven-point scale. Four factors have been proposed that, again, can vary in severity when TBI patients are examined at different times. Factors include (1) cognition and energy, (2) meta cognition (higher order cognition such as self-reflection, thinking about thinking, and so on), (3) somatic anxiety, and (4) language. The item clusters, particularly under factors 2 and 4, were able to differentiate milder TBI patients from those with more severe damage.

PORTLAND ADAPTABILITY INVENTORY[68, 78]

The Portland Adaptability Inventory (PAI) provides a systematic record of maladaptations that interfere with a TBI patient's ability to resume family and social activities. The first factor evaluates temperament and emotionality according to items that assess irritability, aggression, anxiety, agitation, depression, delusions and hallucinations, paranoid and abnormal suspiciousness, and levels of initiative. A second factor focuses on activities of social behavior and is composed of questions about significant relationships, residence, social contacts, self-care, work and school, leisure activities, driving, inappropriate social interactions, law violations, and alcohol and drug use. A third major factor looks at physical capacities and addresses items on ambulation, use of hands, sensory status for audition and vision, dysarthria, and aphasia. The Portland Adaptability Inventory has a demonstrated efficacy for outcome predictions, with respect to which TBI patients in rehabilitation would be successful in their vocational outcomes.[79]

Neurosurgeon's Role in Evaluating Emotional Status

The following guidelines may assist the neurosurgeon in evaluating the emotional status of a patient.

EXAMINATION OF MOTIVATIONAL CAPACITY

Recovery subsequent to TBI is based on two factors, the first, biologic and neurochemical repair, can also be called spontaneous recovery. This is limited to the first year or two after injury; most recovery occurs relatively early. The second factor is based on relearning, which is effortful and has no time restrictions. Relearning does require motivation, and thus it is essential to examine the motivational capacity of a TBI patient. Indeed, in the early stages, when the repair process is most pronounced, patients are most motivated to work on their recovery. However, once a plateau begins to emerge for spontaneous recovery, a negative effect on motivation can occur because patients realize that they will not return to preinjury functioning levels. At this juncture, motivational difficulties and problems of acceptance can lead to depression and elevated anxiety. Thus, it is essential for the treating physician to evaluate the patient's motivational capacities carefully.

Motivation is, to a large degree, idiosyncratic. TBI can result in apathy and a diminished sense of motivation. Given the changed status, it can be helpful to ask patients about their likes and dislikes, what they do for fun, and what makes them upset or angry. However, such an evaluation should avoid the message that the patient is in total "control" over the degree of the recovery. Indeed, unrealistic expectations deflate motivation. There are patients whose volitional incompetence prevents them from providing the necessary motivation toward relearning. Conversely, if there is a motivation that can be established on the basis of a realistic awareness and goal-setting, relearning and an effortful engagement in the rehabilitation process can be guided more efficiently.

EXAMINING CAPACITY FOR SELF-AWARENESS

TBI can lead to a defective self-awareness of varying degree. Again, there is a brain-based denial and a psychologically based denial, as well as an interaction between the two. The lack of awareness will, of course, interfere directly with the acceptance of a problem. The motivation for change is sabotaged if one does not accept the problem to begin with. For example, if a patient is abusing alcohol subsequent to TBI but denies it, he or she will be poorly motivated to alter behavior.

TBI patients can lack awareness of their *physical status*. For example, they may have inaccurate body images, distorted perceptions, or a feeling of being "intact" when they are actually impaired. Patients can also lack an awareness of their *environmental* or *situational* context. This can be examined by questions about the time of day, season of the year, or current events. *Social awareness* can be differentially affected subsequent to TBI. Some patients, despite reasonably normal cognitive and physical functioning, lack normal adult self-consciousness. As a result, they can be poorly groomed or their behavior can be childish, crude, selfish, nonempathetic, and without feelings for others. This information can be gathered by observing the patients and interviewing family members about the patient's social awareness. If there are problems, limit-setting, structure, and consistency can facilitate a more socially appropriate behavior, particularly if it is provided along with needed emotional support.

The greater the severity of the TBI, the greater the brain-based contributions to personality and emotional changes. Neurosurgeons should evaluate the potential for depression (e.g., sleep disturbances, appetite changes, altered libido, mood fluctuations, thoughts of death or suicide), as depression is the most common emotional sequelae of TBI, followed by anxiety.[80] Chronic anxiety can interact with a depressed mood and can fuel depression, and vice versa. If deficits are elaborated with an excessive degree of detail, obsessive-compulsive traits need to be evaluated.[68] Finally, TBI patients should be questioned regarding irritability, restlessness, and low tolerance for frustration. Based on the examination outlined here, referral questions can be more specifically directed.

ESTIMATING PREMORBID EMOTIONAL FUNCTIONING

Neither brain-based nor reactive emotional changes occur in a vacuum; they are usually rooted in pre-existing personality structures. It is essential for the neuropsychologist or neuropsychiatrist to differentiate between disorders on Axis II (according to the Diagnostic and Statistical Manual of Mental Disorders–IV [DSM-IV]), which represents long-standing personality characteristics, and Axis I, which represents acute emotional states. There is a paucity of literature regarding the evaluation of Axis II diagnoses in TBI populations.

Nonetheless, the clinician is faced with estimating pre-injury emotional status in order to answer the following questions:

- Did the patient suffer from a psychiatric illness before the accident, such as an affective disorder, depression, schizophrenia, personality disorder, or post-traumatic stress disorder?
- In the absence of psychiatric illness, did the individual have a vulnerable personality style before the accident, such as insecurity, grandiosity, obsessive-compulsive traits, overachievement, and so forth?
- How would the clinician have expected this individual to react emotionally to the TBI? What were the key defense mechanisms by which such a crisis would have been handled?

The documentation of pre-existing psychiatric illnesses, particularly if hospitalization was involved, is relatively easy to evaluate in the medical records. However, it is typically advantageous to contact treating physicians and health care providers to receive more detailed information. The procedural difficulties involved in the estimation of premorbid functioning in the absence of documented psychiatric history are similar to those of evaluating premorbid cognitive abilities.

To capture both premorbid and postmorbid traits, the Millon Clinical Multi-Axial Inventory (MCMI-III)[81] is particularly useful because multiple factors address both Axis I and Axis II according to the DSM-IV. Such a separation with this relatively short test (175 questions) can be most valuable. However, with all personality questionnaires, including the Minnesota Multiphasic Personality Inventory-2 (MMPI-2), it is most difficult to differentiate the extent to which present symptoms influence the patient's perception in reporting of past personality characteristics. Specific to the Minnesota Multiphasic Personality Inventory-2, TBI patients tend to show an elevation of depression and schizophrenia. Indeed, Cullum[70] concluded, subsequent to his systematic analysis of patients who had right cerebrovascular accidents versus those who had left cerebrovascular accidents for whom depression and especially schizophrenia scales were elevated, that any measure of psychological status in patients with neurological disorders requires a readjustment of the traditional framework. The framework for psychodiagnostic tests is traditionally based on psychopathology, not neuropathology. Reinterpretations are required to avoid potentially misleading interpretations. Thus, it is essential that the computer-generated reports be subjected to clinical review and revisions tailored to the TBI patient's unique symptom complex. A clinician should address the following areas:

- Family history
- Psychiatric and psychotherapeutic treatments, including medications
- Psychiatric history of family members
- Drug and alcohol history
- Treatment for addictive behavior
- Near-death experiences or accidents

- Abusive relationships, including sexual and physical assaults
- Parent-child dynamics, with description of father, mother, and siblings
- Legal and criminal involvement in litigation
- Current spouse and partnership history

There are a few caveats regarding pre-existing emotional risk factors. Research has suggested that many TBI patients exhibited premorbid antisocial behavior. Ruff and associates[82] described four individuals with pre-existing personality traits that colored their outcome subsequent to mild TBI. In one of these cases, grandiosity and narcissistic features resulted in a poor outcome after mild TBI. In a second case, a pre-existing borderline feature of recurrent depression exemplified how those traits can compound the outcome subsequent to mild TBI. In a third patient, who was an overachiever with perfectionistic tendencies, the awareness of multiple deficits subsequent to mild TBI resulted in elevated stress levels. Finally, in a fourth case, the unmet pre-existing dependency needs, combined with the previous signs of post-traumatic stress, were exacerbated and resulted in a particularly poor outcome after mild TBI.

Three more personality characteristics are particularly vulnerable to mild TBI. First, individuals with histrionic personality characteristics do exhibit attention-seeking behavior. These emotional traits typically color the postmorbid symptom presentation, and such individuals are likely to add a dramatic flavor in order to capture the attention of the clinician. Such individuals may also shift, or replace old symptoms with new ones, particularly if the clinician appears to have found some effective treatments. Their style of symptom description is typically impressionistic and lacks detail.

A second premorbid personality style that needs to be recognized is characterized by a somatoform presentation, particularly in patients who have preinjury polysymptomatic histories that include pain, gastrointestinal, sexual, and pseudoneurological problems. Their emotional reaction to TBI may be compounded by these pre-existing symptoms, and therefore an effort should be made to tease apart the pre- and postmorbid symptoms.

The third patient type that is important to identify is one who, before the TBI, suffered from a post-traumatic stress disorder (PTSD). Even when prior traumas did not include a concussion (as concussions do not usually overlap with a post-traumatic stress disorder diagnosis), prior traumatic experiences such as rape, assault, or other near-death experiences can lead to a cumulative stress reaction. These individuals tend to be more intensely fearful, helpless, disorganized, and agitated; this can impede recovery and impair social and occupational functioning. For an overview of premorbid personality characteristics and their influence on symptom presentation, see Table 329–3.[99]

TABLE 329–3 ■ Vulnerable Preinjury Personality Styles

STYLE	PREMORBID PSYCHOLOGICAL TRAITS	POSTMORBID REACTIONS
Overachiever	Sense of self derived from driven accomplishments, which is frequently accompanied by obsessive-compulsive traits	Catastrophic reaction if drop in performance is perceived
Dependency	Excessive need to be taken care of, frequently leading to submissive behavior and fear of separation	Paralyzed by symptoms, if a critical erosion of independence occurs
Borderline personality characteristics (not disorder)	Pattern of instability in interpersonal relationships and self-image with fear of rejection or abandonment	Exacerbation of personality disorganization, including despair, panic, impulsivity, instability, and self-destructive acts
Insecurity	Weak sense of self, which can include shame, guilt, and dependency needs	Magnification of symptoms
Grandiosity	Overestimation of abilities and inflating accomplishments; can include need for admiration and lack of empathy	Minimization or denial of symptoms; if failure results, crash of self-esteem can result in catastrophic reaction
Antisocial behavior	Tendency to be manipulative or deceitful, temperamental, impulsive and irresponsible; lacks sensitivity to others	Possible exaggeration or malingering; increased risk taking, irritability; takes little responsibility for recovery
Hyperactivity	Restless, unfocused, and at times disorganized	Attentional difficulties and impulsivity may be compounded; possible oppositional behavior
Depression	Mood fluctuations dominated by negative affect	Increase of depressive symptoms, despondency
Histrionic style	Emotionality and attention-seeking behavior	Dramatic flavor to symptom presentation, blaming behavior
Somatic orientation	Preoccupation with physical well-being, reluctance to accept psychological conflicts	Endorsement of multiple premorbid physical symptoms intermixed with new or changing TBI residua
Post-traumatic stress disorder	Prior stressors produced an emotional reaction of fear and helplessness	Decreased coping ability, cumulative effect of traumas with exaggerated reaction to current crisis

TBI, traumatic brain injury.
From Ruff RM, Richardson AM: Mild traumatic brain injury. In Sweet J (ed): Forensic Neuropsychology: Fundamentals and Practice. Amsterdam, Swets and Zeitlinger, 1999, pp 315–338.

To address such pre-existing emotional risk factors, several sources of information are available. The most important is the clinical interview, which is the primary mode by which premorbid emotional functioning can be determined. Because TBI may affect the accuracy of a patient's ability to report his or her history, individuals familiar with the patient before and after the accident can add valuable information.

SUMMARY

The enduring emotional and behavioral problems subsequent to TBI frequently pose the greatest challenges, not only for the patients but also for family members. It should be noted that for patients and family members, the focus on psychological issues is most difficult. Regrettably, emotional problems are all too often expressed via physical complaints such as gastrointestinal problems, headaches, or even pseudoneurological symptoms and seizure disorders. It is difficult for most individuals to discuss their emotional problems openly in the limited framework of a clinical consultation with their physician, when there is only time to address one or two of their physical symptoms. The challenge of evaluating premorbid emotional characteristics thus takes multiple sessions. More importantly, a rapport and trust among the patient, the family members, and the clinician is vital.

In the context of TBI, there are distinct challenges. Severe TBI can limit the individual's cognitive ability to be an accurate historian. If, for example, a patient has a remote memory difficulty, word-finding difficulties, or inattention to detail, this can interfere with his or her ability to articulate pre- or postmorbid emotional difficulties accurately. A second component that needs to be addressed is that, subsequent to TBI, patients and families go through different stages: shock and denial, followed by anger and depression. For many, these are followed by awareness and acceptance. In severe cases, however, I have found that families who were told by neurosurgeons that the patient may or may not survive considered it a miracle if the patient did survive. Given that one "miracle" had occurred, they were prone to expect a second miracle in the form of full recovery. In this context, many family members and patients will view their present difficulties through "rose-colored glasses." Other family members may blame the patient; for example, if the patient had gone to church or had not drunk alcohol, he or she never would have had a head injury. Thus, an estimate of premorbid functioning may be skewed by present emotional reaction or the phase of recovery that the historian is in, and the clinician needs to understand the context in which the information is retrieved. Finally, in obtaining a pre- or postmorbid emotional history, it is important to note that family members can share the patient's personality pathology, for example, excessive alcohol consumption or sociopathology. In the context of a dysfunctional family, it becomes difficult to have family members describe the pathology of the TBI patient when it overlaps with their own. Families have different styles and

rules, with varying degrees and tendencies of denial. There are also some families who are closed and are not willing to consider psychological resources, or who do not focus on an introspective evaluation. Such families may view emotional problems as a nonissue, that is, certain psychopathologies can "blind" the historian, a challenge that is not unique to TBI patients.

Biases of the clinicians also typically play a part in the evaluation of emotional difficulties. Some clinicians are wedded to the notion that premorbid personality characteristics are basically exacerbated by brain damage. For example, impulsivity, anger outbursts, and antisocial traits are viewed as amplified pre-existing traits. This is not always the case, however. Prigatano[83] identified two types of causative factors responsible for personality disturbances: (1) disturbances of perception, thinking, or judgment that are the root of psychological problems and (2) psychosocial situations that become powerful determinants in psychological disturbances, particularly in patients with severe TBI. Agreement exists in the literature that damage to specific brain regions can lead to certain predictable personality disorders. For example, damage disconnecting the frontal lobe from the limbic system can result in emotional symptoms that are novel to the patient.[84] Trauma can also lead to new behaviors such as dependency, passivity, irresponsibility, and so on. Individual psychotherapy can be effective in further teasing out and comprehending the premorbid dispositions of the patients and how they have changed, as well as what new postmorbid difficulties have occurred that can affect the recovery process.

MILD TRAUMATIC BRAIN INJURY SEQUELAE

Since the great majority of all TBIs are mild, it is essential to come to terms with evaluating the neurobehavioral residua of these patients. It has been estimated that each year in the United States alone, a minimum of 1 million individuals sustain mild TBI.[85] The key challenges faced by both neurosurgeons and neuropsychologists are (1) discrepant diagnostic criteria, (2) lack of conclusive objective evidence based on neuroimaging, and (3) coming to terms with the role the examiner's viewpoint or bias plays in sorting through the subjective symptoms.

Strengths and Limits of the Glasgow Coma Scale

Since its introduction in 1974, the Glasgow Coma Scale (GCS)[86] has served the international neurosurgical community well in classifying the severity of TBI. However, the GCS is geared toward rating more severe TBIs. Its strength, as well as its weakness, is the fact that the assessment is time-dependent. Its strength is that it can be used for triaging, and its weakness is that the actual time of administration is relatively arbitrary. In the diagnosis of mild TBI, the GCS is often administered after the passing of the acute symptoms of loss of consciousness (LOC) and post-traumatic amnesia (PTA). For example, in an individual who has sustained an LOC of 5 to 10 minutes and to whom the first GCS is administered 0.5 hour after injury, the GCS will be 15 and indistinguishable from the score of an individual who has never sustained an LOC. Especially for patients who have a transient alteration of consciousness or a brief PTA that lasts a few minutes, the GCS is usually administered too late and therefore lacks sensitivity.

If a neurosurgeon or a neuropsychologist needs to evaluate a patient 3 or 4 hours after an accident, and the GCS is 15, it is important that an alternative standardized tool be used to evaluate the potential for mild TBI. An alternative tool for diagnosing mild TBI has been published by the American Congress of Rehabilitation Medicine[87] and is primarily based on an estimate of the duration of LOC and PTA. The following four inclusion criteria have been identified, of which at least *one* must be manifested:

- Any period of loss of consciousness; LOC should not exceed 30 minutes
- Any loss of memory for events immediately before and after the accident; however, PTA should not persist longer than 24 hours
- Any alteration of mental state at the time of accident (e.g., feeling dazed, disoriented, or confused)
- Focal neurological deficit or deficits that may or may not be transient

Psychiatrists in the DSM-IV have proposed a research definition for postconcussional disorders that suggests the criteria to be used for mild TBIs. The established DSM-IV criteria that have been suggested include the following:

- A period of unconsciousness lasting more than 5 minutes
- A period of PTA that lasts more than 12 hours subsequent to closed head injury
- A new onset of seizures or marked worsening of pre-existing seizure disorders that occur within the first 6 months

In an attempt to improve diagnostic accuracy in patients with mild TBI, we use the GCS scores when available, if they are obtained at the appropriate time intervals (early stages for mild TBI patients). For retrospective analysis to determine the extent of LOC and PTA, the Galveston Orientation and Amnesia Test (GOAT)[88] is used. The GOAT is a standardized tool

that can be used retrospectively, as well as being a time-dependent measure. However, when the GOAT is administered retrospectively, the following additional instructions need to be added: "When answering the questions regarding your accident, please rely on your own independent recall, without supplementing or adding information that you have learned from others since you had the accident." The test items that are particularly relevant to determining PTA are the questions regarding the first event after the accident and the last event before the accident that can be recalled. Based on the GOAT, the mild TBI population is divided into one of the three types noted in Table 329–4.[89]

The three subtypes are based on the recognition that mild TBIs can have a substantial range, and a finer tuning could prove to be advantageous. Type I is consistent with the American Congress of Rehabilitation Medicine (ACRM) definition. Type III corresponds with the DSM-IV definition, and type II bridges the two discrepant definitions. Based on a study with these three types in a sample of 76 outpatients, we found that the distribution was reasonably balanced: type I, 33%; type II, 33%; and type III, 34%. However, neither the neuropsychological data nor psychological symptoms differed significantly across the three subtypes.[90] Given this finding, combined with the arbitrary nature of the subdivisions, my colleagues and I proposed as the next step a more refined scaling for mild TBI modeled on the GCS. We developed the California Concussion Scale, which proposes a unique 3- to 15-point scale for patients with mild TBI and a GCS score of 13, 14, or 15 (Fig. 329–2). This scale does not replace the GCS, but rather captures a greater differentiation for the heterogeneity that exists among the mild TBI population. The time has come to establish more uniform mild TBI diagnoses across disciplines. The time has also come to view definitions as constructs that must be sensitive for those thousands of patients for whom we are forced to rely on retrospective symptom presentation.

For those of us who have retrospectively evaluated a patient's reported LOC and PTA, there does emerge a certain clinical experience and confidence. Initially, I focused primarily on LOC; however, over the years I have relied more on PTA. Indeed, the memory gap, as a rule, precedes the impact by a few seconds, and most patients with LOC or PTA will not recall the main impact or acceleration-deceleration forces that resulted in the injury to the brain. I listen for a "gap" in the detailed information that the patients provide about

TABLE 329–4 ■ Classifications for Mild Traumatic Brain Injury

	TYPE I	TYPE II	TYPE III
LOC	Altered state or transient loss	Definite loss with time unknown or <5 min	Loss 5–30 min
PTA	1–60 sec	60 sec–12 hr	>12 hr–24 hr
Neurological symptoms	One or more	One or more	One or more

LOC, loss of consciousness; PTA, post-traumatic amnesia.
From Ruff R: Discipline specific approach vs. individual care. In Varney N, Roberts R (eds): Mild Head Injury: Causes, Evaluation, and Treatment. Mahway, NJ, Lawrence Erlbaum, 1999, pp 99–113.

The California Concussion Scale (CCS) is a practical rating for the severity of mild traumatic brain injury where the post-traumatic amnesia does not exceed 24 hours and the loss of consciousness is less than 30 minutes. For more severe cases of traumatic brain injury the utilization of the Glasgow Coma Scale is recommended. The CCS is a retrospective scale and should not be administered to a patient who is in post-traumatic amnesia.

Post-traumatic amnesia (PTA)	Estimated duration_____	Rel. Code 1, 2, 3*
Greater than 24 hours†		0
Greater than 12 hours but less than 24 hours		1
Greater than 1 hour but less than 12 hours		2
Greater than 15 minutes but less than 1 hour		3
Greater than 1 minute but less than 15 minutes		4
Transient amnesia with a loss of memory for events immediately before or after the accident lasting less than 1 minute		5
No post-traumatic amnesia (continuous recall of events)		6

Loss of Consciousness (LOC)	Estimated duration_____	Rel. Code 1, 2, 3*
Greater than 30 minutes†		0
Greater than 5 minutes but less than 30 minutes		1
Less than 5 minutes or definite loss of consciousness with duration unknown		2
Altered mental state (e.g., transient loss of consciousness, disoriented, confused)		3
No loss of consciousness		4

Focal neurological signs (permanent or temporary)	Rel. Code 1, 2, 3*
Four or more signs	1
Three signs	2
Two signs	3
One sign	4
No neurological signs	5

TOTAL CCS SCORE _____

(from 3 to 15)

*Reliability: 1 = Reliable documentation by health care provider
2 = Questionable and inconsistent documentation
3 = Unreliable
†Greater impairment indicates a moderate to severe brain injury; thus, do not use CCS alone.

FIGURE 329–2. California Concussion Scale.

the events before and after the PTA. No doubt, we are navigating somewhat murky water when asking a patient to determine the length of PTA. Within the window of PTA, which typically is longer than LOC, the question of whether a patient has sustained an LOC is difficult for any patient with mild TBI to answer. In other words, if I cannot remember a half-hour period, how could I know whether I had LOC during that period? No doubt, many patients have falsely denied or endorsed a brief LOC because of a lack of memory.

Evaluating Outcome in Mild Traumatic Brain Injury

Given the data from a three-center study,[91] it has become evident that most individuals with a single, un-complicated mild TBI have a good outcome. When tested at baseline, 1, and 3 months, most patients demonstrated cognitive deficits in the first weeks after the trauma. Three months after the accident, the patients as a group did not significantly deviate from a noninjured control group.

It has been estimated that approximately 80% to 90% of all patients with mild TBI enjoy a favorable recovery.[85, 92, 93] Thus, methods need to be developed by which the clinician can predict the 10% to 20% of patients with mild TBI who will have a poor outcome or fall into the so-called miserable minority.[89]

It has been recognized in the literature that the static imaging techniques (computed tomography [CT] and magnetic resonance imaging [MRI]) lack sufficient sensitivity for diagnosing the microscopic damage in the form of diffuse axonal injuries that can occur in mild TBI. Some inroads have been made using functional neuroimaging techniques. In a study of patients with mild TBI who fall within the miserable minority, all nine patients with significant neurocognitive residua also demonstrated positive positron emission tomography (PET) findings.[94] Single photon emission computed tomography (SPECT) studies have found similar sensitivity, and these dynamic techniques frequently show damage to the frontotemporal regions.[95] At this time, however, it is generally recognized that the functional neuroimaging techniques for the diagnosis of mild TBI are experimental and, indeed, this has been explicitly formulated in a statement published by the Academy of Neurology.[96]

Given the current state of objective neuroimaging techniques, which are viewed as inconclusive, mild TBI needs to be diagnosed on the basis of PTA and LOC.[97] The GCS, the GOAT, and other techniques have shown insufficient sensitivity to capture the miserable minority, and thus more refined techniques need to be researched. In the interim, the neurocognitive symptoms that exist after a mild TBI can be most effectively captured by a neuropsychological evaluation.

The term *postconcussional disorder* refers to acquired physical, emotional, or cognitive symptoms that occur as a direct consequence of cerebral concussion.[98] Among the more frequent physical problems are headaches, fatigue, sleep disorders, and vertigo. Less common residua include nausea, numbness, vision problems, hearing problems (e.g., tinnitus and hyperacusis). Seizure disorders are rare; however, alcohol intolerance is fairly common. Typical emotional residua include irritability (aggression with little or no provocation), anxiety, depression, and affective lability. Somewhat less frequent emotional symptoms include personality changes (social inappropriateness), apathy, and lack of spontaneity. The most pronounced cognitive impairments include difficulties with attention (concentration, shifting focus of attention), performing simultaneous or multiple cognitive tasks, and memory and learning problems. Less frequently, declines occur in the executive functions (problem solving, avoiding perseverations) and general slowing and information processing.

It may be useful to use the term *acute postconcussional disorder* for patients who complain of residua within the first 3 months versus *chronic* for those with persistent residua after 3 months. Regrettably, the miserable minority is primarily composed of individuals whose postconcussional disorders persist for years. Note that the problem areas endorsed are similar when compared with more severely injured TBI patients (see Table 329–1).

Differential Diagnosis

For neuropsychologists, it remains a challenge to determine if the sequelae of the miserable minority patients are (1) neurogenic; (2) psychogenic; (3) due to comorbid medical complications such as cervical injuries, vestibular problems, and so on; (4) reflective of premorbid psychological problems; or (5) associated with financial gain. As mentioned earlier, epidemiologic data suggest that at least 1 million individuals sustain a mild TBI each year in the United States alone, and thus the 10% to 20% of these patients who fall within the miserable minority compose a sample of 100,000 to 200,000 per year.

Neurogenic. For a neurogenic diagnosis to become probable, it is advisable to administer an extensive neuropsychological battery. If, according to pattern analysis, attention, memory, short-term memory, learning, and executive functioning are affected in an individual whose other neurocognitive performances fall within the intact ranges, diagnostic certainty is enhanced. It is also important to note the existence of pre-existing neurological illnesses such as prior concussions, substance abuse, seizure disorders, or even aging (i.e., older than age 40). These factors can render an individual more vulnerable to the effects of mild TBI. The reason for this is based on the model of neuronal reserve, which is depleted by these neurological factors. Such depletion renders an individual far more vulnerable to the effects of a mild TBI.

Psychogenic. A psychogenic diagnosis becomes reasonably probable if a patient suffers from a catastrophic reaction and as a consequence the overall neurocognitive profile has deteriorated substantially across all domains. The presence of an Axis I or an Axis II diagnosis, or both, in the absence of neurocognitive deficits, supports a psychogenic diagnosis. Severe clinical depression, somatization, and hysterical reactions subsequent to a mild TBI are flags for a differential diagnosis of psychogenic origin.

Comorbid Medical Complications. Symptoms such as cervical pain, vestibular problems, excessive fatigue, and medication effects can interfere with a good outcome. Typically, repeated testing across time can substantially assist in this differentiation, particularly if there is an improvement that can be linked to the decline of comorbid medical symptoms.

Premorbid Problems. The potential premorbid cognitive and emotional contributions to the mild TBI residua have been discussed in detail, and the effect on personality style and symptom presentation have been summarized in Table 329–5.[100]

Secondary Gain. Since many TBI patients seek assistance through litigation, the effects of secondary gain need to be considered. A host of specific tests have been developed to detect malingering and symptom magnification, based on the forced-choice format. A profile analysis within the battery can determine a level of consistency that is sufficient for the data to yield reasonable validity. Some of the indirect clinical indicators that can be flagged are summarized in Table 329–5.

Among the patients with mild TBI who fall into the miserable minority, a combination of neurogenic, psychogenic, and comorbid interactions is by far the most common presentation. It can be extremely challenging to differentiate among the potential contributors that can compound a symptom presentation and

TABLE 329-5 ■ **Potential Indicators of Insufficient Effort**

Premorbid Indicators
Antisocial personality traits
Borderline personality disorder
Prior incapacitating injuries
Prior claims for injury
Poor work record or job satisfaction
Intolerable life conflicts

Behavioral Indicators during Examination
Uncooperative or inconsistent cooperation
Suspicious, aloof
Ill at ease, unfriendly
Evasive

Test Performance
Frequently responds with "I don't know"
Missed random items in a test comprising items with
  increasing difficulty
Easily gives up on more difficult items
Spurious results (e.g., unexplained outlier)
Inconsistent profile within test battery or between tests across
  battery
Malingering-like performance on direct measures of
  malingering

Patient's Presenting Postmorbid Complaints
Description of events surrounding accident in great detail
Endorsement of an unusually large number of symptoms
Absurd or preposterous reporting of symptoms
Nonselectivity of physical, emotional, or cognitive symptoms
Overidealized functioning or lack of reasonable difficulties
  before accident
Inconsistencies in symptom reporting itself

Reported or Observed Activities of Daily Living
Engaged in activities not consistent with reported deficits
Discrepant capacity between work and recreation
Refuses employment with partial disability

For Personal Injury Litigants
Significant financial stressors
Resistance or lack of seeking reasonable remedies
Lack of reasonable follow-through on available treatments
Attributing all life's problems to accident
Blaming others for all life's problems
Seeking unnecesssary examinations and treatments without
  consulting experts

From Ruff RM, Wylie T, Tennant W: Malingering and malingering-like aspects of mild closed-head injury. J Head Trauma Rehabil 8:60–73, 1993.

also to determine the interactions among the physical, emotional, and psychological sequelae.

Beyond a Discipline-Specific Approach

As stated earlier in the section "Discipline-Specific Sequelae Versus Patient-Oriented Approach," every clinician has a certain focus. Symptoms that fall within each clinician's discipline are highlighted, and the others are frequently regarded as "noise." If one wishes to understand the miserable minority, it is essential that the approach transcend one's own discipline in order to grasp the patient's changed life. To achieve this, the model shown in Figure 329–1 is used to elicit combinations of multiple interactions that can lead to dysfunction.

The goal of this constructed model is to illustrate the clinical need to bridge the gap between isolated observations. Most patients will not do us the favor of having problems in only one discipline; rather, they present with a range of symptoms. The patient-oriented approach addresses interactions among the physical, emotional, and cognitive symptoms. For example, a patient may be deeply depressed because of family problems, and this can lead to sleepless nights, which can, in turn, affect concentration and attention. Another patient may have a neck injury that interferes with sleep, leading to similar attentional difficulties. Yet another individual may present with neurologically based attention problems that can lead to a strong emotional reaction, insecurity, and vocational difficulties, which can, in turn, lead to financial stressors and finally to depression. The model shown in Figure 329–1 demonstrates the intrapersonal dynamic among the emotional, cognitive, and physical domains. Moreover, it addresses the interpersonal dynamic, based on the individual's interactions with his or her social and recreational network. It is also dependent on vocation and financial components. One's meaning in life or spiritual direction can provide direction and focus, and its absence can contribute to poor outcome. Thus, interpersonal issues such as loss of employment, which affects finances and limits one's recreational outlets and social life, can also negatively influence the intrapersonal dimensions. This patient-oriented approach does not replace discipline-based patient care, but it goes beyond each clinician's particular viewpoint to offer a greater chance of understanding the miserable minority.

SUMMARY

Neurosurgeons and neuropsychologists, together with other health care professionals, must standardize a diagnostic framework specific for mild TBI. These definitions must incorporate different durations of LOC, PTA, and neurological symptoms. A scale similar to the GCS has been proposed in this chapter, namely, the California Concussion Scale (see Fig. 329–2).

Given that 10% to 20% of patients with mild TBI present with chronic difficulties, it would be ideal if predictors in the emergency room could be developed, which would allow us to identify patients who most likely will recover versus those with a poor outcome. The miserable minority is composed of patients who suffer from different constellations of symptoms, not one unified postconcussive "syndrome." Some patients suffer from primarily neurological difficulties. For others, emotional issues are the driving force. No doubt in most cases, there exists a combination of physical, emotional, and cognitive symptoms, which interact and sustain multiple dysfunctional interactions. Therefore, various diagnostic constellations need to be systematically studied for the various subpopulations that compose the miserable minority.

Continued research is called for in the area of dynamic neuroimaging. The initial studies with positron emission tomography and single photon emission computed tomography have demonstrated a far greater sensitivity than have computed tomography and magnetic resonance imaging. Given that only 10% to 20% of the population with mild TBI have a poor outcome, large samples are called for to evaluate the sensitivity of dynamic neuroimaging.

At this time, clinical determinations and interpretations are the basis for deciding whether the patient's problems are neurogenic, psychogenic, influenced by comorbid medical complications, associated with financial gain, primarily influenced by premorbid issues, or any combination of these. As if this was not complicated enough, the post-traumatic symptoms fluctuate because patient recovery is a moving target. I have observed that while a patient is in a phase of positive recovery, symptoms are to a degree not as "real" because the patient has the expectation that there will be a full recovery. However, a plateau represents a decline to the patient, and a "new" challenge emerges of adjusting to the permanent residua. Some individuals are more able to cope with accepting these multiple layers of difficulties over time. In the future, clinicians must become more sensitive to these various phases of recovery in order to provide the patient with the needed information so that they can accurately determine the extent of the improvement over time. Although significant advances have been made in the field of mild TBI since the mid-1980s, we are only beginning to unravel the complexity involved in diagnosing this condition, and much work is needed for establishing efficacious treatments for the various symptom constellations.

REFERENCES

1. Piaget J: The Construction of Reality in the Child. New York, Basic Books, 1954.
2. Piaget J: Psychology and Epistemiology: Toward a Theory of Knowledge. New York, Viking, 1970.
3. Mahoney M: Human Change Processes. New York, Basic Books, 1991.
4. Popper K: Objective Knowledge: An Evolutionary Approach. London, Oxford University Press, 1972.
5. Campbell D: Evolutionary epistemology. In Schlipp P (ed): The Philosophy of Karl Popper, vol. 14 [I and II]. La Salle, Ill, Open Court, 1974, pp 416–463.
6. American Psychological Association: Standards for Educational and Psychological Testing. Washington, D.C., American Psychological Association, 1985.
7. Campbell D: Recommendation for the APA Test Standards regarding construct, trait and discriminant validity. Am Psychol 15:546–553, 1960.
8. Anastasi A: Psychological Testing, 6th ed. New York, Macmillan, 1988.
9. Boring E: A History of Experimental Psychology, 2nd ed. New York, Appleton-Century-Crofts, 1957.
10. Wechsler D: WAIS-III: Manual. New York, Psychological Corporation, 1996.
11. Bigler E, Steinman D, Newton J: Clinical assessment of cognitive deficit in neurological disorder. II. Cerebral Trauma. Clin Neuropsychol 3:13–18, 1981.
12. Russell E: Three patterns of brain damage on the WAIS. J Clin Neuropsychol 35:611–620, 1979.
13. Cullum C, Steinman D, Bigler E: Relationship between fluid and crystallized cognitive functions using Category Test and WAIS scores. Int J Clin Neuropsychol 6:172–174, 1984.
14. Benson F: Aphasia. In Heilman KM, Valenstein E (eds): Clinical Neuropsychology, 3rd ed. New York, Oxford University Press, pp 17–36.
15. Heilman K, Safran A, Geshwind N: Closed head trauma and aphasia. J Neurol Neurosurg Psychiatry 34:265–269, 1971.
16. Sarno M: Verbal impairment after closed head injury. J Nerv Ment Dis 172:475–479, 1984.
17. Levin H, Grossman R, Kelly P: Aphasic disorder in patients with closed head injury. J Neurol Neurosurg Psychiatry 39:1062–1070, 1976.
18. Newcombe F, Fortuny L: Problems and perspectives in the evaluation of psychological deficits after cerebral lesions. Int Rehab Med 1:182–192, 1979.
19. Thompsen I: Late outcome of very severe blunt head trauma: A 10–15 year second follow-up. J Neurol Neurosurg Psychiatry 47:260–268, 1984.
20. Benton A, Hamsher K deS, Sivan A: Multilingual Aphasia Examination. Iowa City, AJA Associates, 1994.
21. Ruff R, Light R, Parker S, Levin H: Controlled Oral Word Association Test: Reliability and updated norms. Arch Clin Neuropsychol 11:329–338, 1996.
22. Ruff R, Evans R, Marshall L: Impairment of verbal and figural fluency following traumatic head injury. Arch Clin Neuropsychol 1:87–101, 1986.
23. Gruen A, Frankle B, Schwartz R: Word fluency generation skills of head-injured patients in an acute trauma center. J Commun Disord 23:163–170, 1990.
24. Warkentin S, Risberg J, Nilsson A, et al: Cortical activity during speech production: A study of regional cerebral blood flow in normal subjects performing a word fluency task. Neuropsychiatry Neuropsychol Behav Neurol 4:305–316, 1991.
25. Ruff R, Light R, Parker S, Levin H: The psychological construct of word fluency. Brain Language 57:394–405, 1997.
26. Benton A: Visuoperceptual, visuospatial, and visuoconstructional disorders. In Heilman K, Valenstein E (eds): Clinical Neuropsychology. New York, Oxford University Press, 1985, pp 151–185.
27. Bigler E: Diagnostic clinical neuropsychology (revised ed). Austin, University of Texas Press, 1988.
28. Levin H, Grossman R, Kelly P: Impairment of facial recognition after closed head injuries of varying severity. Cortex 13:119–130, 1977.
29. Oddy M, Humphrey M, Uttley M: Subjective impairment and social recovery after closed head injury. J Neurol Neurosurg Psychiatry 41:611–616, 1978.
30. Rutherford W, Merret J, McDonald J: Symptoms at one year following concussion from minor head injuries. Injury 10:226–230, 1979.
31. Van Zomeren A, Van den Burg W: Residual complaints of patients two years after severe head injury. J Neurol Neurosurg Psychiatry 48:21–28, 1985,.
32. Gronwall D, Wrightson P: Memory and information processing capacity after closed head injury. J Neurol Neurosurg Psychiatry 44:889–895, 1981.
33. Niemann H, Ruff R, Kramer J: An attempt towards differentiating attentional deficits in traumatic brain injury. Neuropsychol Rev 6:11–46, 1996.
34. Pribram K, McGuinness D: Arousal, activation and effort in the control of attention. Psychol Rev 82:116–149, 1975.
35. Skinner J, Yingling C: Central gating mechanisms that regulate event-related potentials and behavior: A neural model for attention. In Desmedt J (ed): Attention, Voluntary Contraction and Event-Related Cerebral Potentials: Progress in Clinical Neurophysiology, vol. 1, Karger, Basel, 1977, pp 30–69.
36. Walter W, Cooper R, Aldridge V, et al: Contingent negative variation: An electrical sign of sensorimotor association and expectancy in the human brain. Nature 203:380–384, 1964.
37. Posner M: Psychology of attention. In Gazzaniga M, Blakemore C (eds): Handbook of Psychobiology. New York, Academic Press, 1975, pp 441–480.
38. Parasuraman R: Vigilance, arousal and the brain. In Gale A, Edwards J (eds): Physiological Correlates of Human Behaviour, vol. 2: Attention and Performance. New York, Academic Press, 1983, pp 35–55.
39. Shiffrin R, Schneider W: Short-term store: Organized active memory. Paper presented at the Midwestern Psychological Association, 1977, Chicago.

40. Schneider W, Shiffrin R: Controlled and automatic human information processing. I. Detection, search and attention. Psychol Rev 84:1–66, 1977.

41. Squire L: Memory and Brain. New York, Oxford University Press, 1987.

42. Milner B: Les troubles de la memoire accompagnant des lésions hippocampiques bilatérales. In Physiologie de L'hippocampe. Paris, Centre National de la Recherche Scientifique, 1962, pp 257–272.

43. Butters N, Salmon D, Cullum C, et al: Differentiation of amnestic and demented patients with the Wechsler Memory Scale—Revised. Clin Neuropsychol 2:133–148, 1988.

44. Wechsler D: Wechsler Memory Scale—Revised manual. New York, Psychological Corporation, 1987.

45. Lezak M: Neuropsychological Assessment, 3rd ed. New York, Oxford University Press, 1995.

46. Buschke H, Fuld P: Evaluating storage, retention, and retrieval in disordered memory and learning. Neurology 11:1019–1025, 1974.

47. Delis D, Kramer J, Kaplan E, Ober B: California Verbal Learning Test Manual. New York, Psychological Corporation, 1987.

48. Ruff R, Allen C: Ruff-Light Trail Learning Test: Professional Manual. Odessa, Fla, Psychological Assessment Resources, 1999.

49. Stuss D, Benson D: Neuropsychological studies of the frontal lobes. Psychol Bull 95:3–28, 1984.

50. Thompson R: Introduction to Physiological Psychology. New York, Harper & Row, 1976.

51. Berg EA: A simple objective treatment for measuring flexibility in thinking. J Gen Psychol 39:15–22, 1948.

52. Heaton RK, Grant I, Matthews CG: Comprehensive norms for an expanded Halstead-Reitan battery: Demographic corrections, research findings, and clinical applications. Odessa, Fla, Psychological Assessment Resources, 1991.

53. Ruff R: Ruff Figural Fluency Test: Professional Manual. Odessa, Fla, Psychological Assessment Resources, 1996.

54. Ruff R, Allen CC, Farrow CE, et al: Figural fluency: Differential impairment in patients with left vs. right frontal lobe lesions. Arch Clin Neuropsychol 9:41–45, 1994.

55. Porteus S: The Maze Test and Clinical Psychology. Palo Alto, Pacific Books, 1959.

56. Porteus S: Porteus Maze Test: Fifty Years' Application. New York, Psychological Corporation, 1965.

57. Perret E: The left frontal lobe of man and the suppression of habitual response in verbal categorical behavior. Neuropsychologia 12:323–330, 1974.

58. Reitan R, Davidson L: Clinical Neuropsychology: Current Status and Applications. New York, Winston/Wiley, 1974.

59. Wechsler D: Wechsler Memory Scale III: Manual. New York, Psychological Corporation, 1997.

60. Ruff R, Parker S: Gender- and age-specific changes in motor speed and eye-hand coordination in adults: Normative values for the Finger Tapping and Grooved Pegboard Test. Percept Mot Skills 76:1219–1230, 1993.

61. Nelson H: The National Adult Reading Test (NART): Test Manual. Windsor, Berks, UK, NFER-Nelson, 1982.

62. Crawford J: Current and premorbid intelligence measures in neuropsychological assessment. In: Crawford JR, Parker DM, McKinlay WW (eds): A Handbook of Neuropsychological Assessment. Hove, UK: Lawrence Erlbaum, 1992.

63. Barona A, Reynolds C, Chastain R: A demographically based index of pre-morbid intelligence for the WAIS-R. J Clin Psychol 52:885–887, 1984.

64. Gonen J: The use of Wechsler's deterioration quotient in cases of diffuse and symmetrical cerebral atrophy. J Clin Psychol 26:174–177, 1970.

65. Yates A: The validity of some psychological tests of brain damage. Psychol Bull 51:359–379, 1954.

66. Varney N, Roberts R: The Evaluation and Treatment of Mild Traumatic Brain Injury. London, Lawrence Erlbaum, 1999.

67. Zarit S, Miller N, Kahn R: Brain function, intellectual impairment and education in the aged. J Am Geriatr Soc 26:58–67, 1978.

68. Lezak M: Subtle sequelae of brain damage: Perplexity, distractibility, and fatigue. Am J Phys Med 57:9–15, 1978.

69. Cullum CM, Bigler ED: Short-form MMPI findings in patients with predominantly lateralized cerebral dysfunction: Neuropsychological and CT-derived parameters. J Nerv Ment Dis 176:332–342, 1988.

70. Cullum C: Cerebral imaging and emotional correlations. In: Bigler E, Yeo R, Turkheimer E (eds): Neuropsychological Function and Brain Imaging. New York, Plenum Press, 1989.

71. Osborn C: Over My Head. Kansas City, Kan, Andrews McMeel, 1998.

72. Katz M, Lyerly S: Methods for measuring adjustment and social behavior in the community. I. Rationale, description, discriminative validity and scale development. Psychol Rep 13:503–535, 1963.

73. Grant I, Alves W: Psychiatric and psychosocial disturbances in head injury. In Levin HS, Grafman J, Eisenberg HM (eds): Neurobehavioral Recovery from Head Injury. New York, Oxford University Press, 1987.

74. Fordyce D, Roueche J, Prigatano G: Enhanced emotional reactions in chronic head trauma patients. J Neurol Neurosurg Psychiatry 46:620–624, 1983.

75. Hinkledy N, Corrigan J: The structure of head-injured patients' neurobehavioral complaints: A preliminary study. Brain Injury 4:115–134, 1990.

76. Klonoff P, Snow W, Costa L: Quality of life in patients two to four years after closed head injury. Neurosurgery 19:735–743, 1986.

77. Levin H, High W, Goethe K, et al: The Neurobehavioral Rating Scale assessment of the behavioural sequelae of head injury by the clinician. J Neurol Neurosurg Psychiatry 50:183–193, 1987.

78. Lezak M, O'Brien KP: Longitudinal study of emotional, social, and physical changes after traumatic brain injury. J Learn Disabil 32:456–463, 1988.

79. Malec J, Smigielski J, DePompolo R: Goal attainment scaling and outcome measurement in post-acute brain injury rehabilitation. Arch Phys Med Rehabil 72:138–143, 1991.

80. Lezak M: Subtle sequelae of brain damage: Perplexity, distractability, and fatigue. Am J Phys Med 57:9–15, 1978.

81. Millon T: Millon Clinical Multiaxial Inventory—III (Manual). Minneapolis, National Computer Systems, 1994.

82. Ruff R, Camenzuli L, Mueller J: Miserable Minority: Emotional risk factors that influence the outcome of a mild traumatic brain injury. Brain Inj 10:551–565, 1996.

83. Prigatano G: Neuropsychological rehabilitation after brain injury. Baltimore, Johns Hopkins Press, 1986.

84. Alexander M: The role of neurobehavioral syndromes in the rehabilitation and outcome from head injury. In Levin HS, Grafman J, Eisenberg HM (eds): Neurobehavioral Recovery from Head Injury. Oxford, Oxford University Press, 1987, pp 191–205.

85. Kay T, Newman B, Cavallo M, et al: Toward a neuropsychological model of functional disability after mild traumatic head injury. Neuropsychology 6:371–384, 1992.

86. Teasdale G, Jennett B: Assessment of coma and impaired consciousness: A practical scale. Lancet 2:81–84, 1974.

87. American Congress of Rehabilitation Medicine, Mild Traumatic Brain Injury Committee: Definition of mild traumatic brain injury. J Head Trauma Rehab 8:86–87, 1993.

88. Levin H, O'Donnell V, Grossman R: The Galveston Orientation and Amnesia Test: A practical scale to assess cognition after head injury. J Nerv Ment Dis 167:675–684, 1979.

89. Ruff R: Discipline specific approach vs. individual care. In: Varney N, Roberts R (eds): Mild Head Injury: Causes, Evaluation and Treatment. Mahwah, NJ, Lawrence Erlbaum, 1999, pp 99–113.

90. Ruff R, Jurica P: In search of a unified definition for mild traumatic brain injury. Brain Inj 13:943–952, 1999.

91. Levin H, Mattis S, Ruff R, et al.: Neurobehavioral outcome of minor head injury: A three center study. J Neurosurg 66:234–243, 1987.

92. Wong J, Regennitter R, Barrios F: Base rate and simulated symptoms of mild head injury among normals. Arch Clin Neuropsychol 9;441–426, 1994.

93. Binder L, Rohling M, Larrabee G: A review of mild head trauma. Part I. Meta-analytic review of neuropsychological studies. J Clin Exp Neuropsychol 19:421–431, 1997.

94. Ruff R, Crouch J, Tröster A, et al: Selected cases of poor outcome following a minor brain trauma: Comparing neuropsychological and positron emission tomography assessment. Brain Inj 8:297–308, 1994.
95. Varney N, Bushnell D, Nathan M, et al: NeuroSPECT correlates of disabling mild head injury: Preliminary findings. J Head Trauma Rehab 10:18–28, 1995.
96. American Academy of Neurology, Therapeutics and Technology Assessment Subcommittee: Assessment of brain SPECT. Neurology 46:278–285, 1996.
97. Alexander M: Mild traumatic brain injury: Pathophysiology, natural history, and clinical management. Neurology 45:1253–1260, 1995.
98. Alves W, Colohan A, O'Leary T, et al: Understanding posttraumatic symptoms after minor head injury. J Head Trauma Rehab 1:1–12, 1986.
99. Ruff RM, Richardson AM: Mild traumatic brain injury. In Sweet J (ed): Forensic Neuropsychology: Fundamentals and Practice. Amsterdam: Swets and Zeitlinger, 1999, pp 315–338.
100. Ruff RM, Wylie T, Tennant W: Malingering and malingering-like aspects of mild closed-head injury. J Head Trauma Rehab 8:60–73, 1993.

CHAPTER 330

Traumatic Cerebrovascular Injury

J. PAUL ELLIOTT ■ DAVID W. NEWELL

Vascular injury is an important and increasingly recognized cause of neurological deficit following trauma. Injuries are best described with respect to both anatomic region of interest and mechanism of injury. Injury to the great vessels in the thoracic cavity, the cervical vessels, and the intracranial vasculature can all result in a variety of neurological deficits, depending on the specific vessel injured. The mechanism of traumatic injury—that is, whether penetrating or nonpenetrating (blunt)—is critical in determining the appropriate diagnostic and treatment regimens. This chapter reviews the anatomic and mechanistic considerations relevant to the clinical presentation, diagnosis, treatment options, complications, and outcome of cerebrovascular injuries.

HISTORICAL BACKGROUND

The often dramatic nature of cervical and cranial penetrating injuries has been referred to throughout the records of Western and Eastern civilizations. Because significant experience with such injuries was gained during wartime, modern treatment principles have evolved largely from military experience.

A policy of mandatory surgical exploration for all penetrating injuries of the neck was initially adopted and considered standard.[1, 2] More recently, many penetrating cervical vascular injuries have been successfully treated nonoperatively after a detailed diagnostic evaluation.[3] Penetrating cranial injuries were once generally considered to be unsurvivable, but débridement of devitalized brain, dural and calvarial reconstruction, and use of effective antimicrobials have improved survival. As a result, there has been an increase in the subsequent presentation of related intracranial vascular injuries.

It was not until 1872 that the first specific reference was made to a nonpenetrating (blunt) vascular injury. In that case, carotid artery thrombosis following blunt neck trauma resulted in cerebral infarction.[4] At autopsy, an intimal tear in the proximal common carotid artery was found to be the cause. To this day, nonpenetrating vascular injuries are significantly underdiagnosed.

One of the unanticipated consequences of the development of computed tomography (CT) was that it replaced angiography as the primary diagnostic test following head trauma. Indirectly, this technologic advancement resulted in underdiagnosis of blunt vascular injury. Thus, it is critical that a high clinical suspicion for blunt vascular injury be maintained, because the sequelae of vascular injury often present in a delayed fashion, and the manifestations of traumatic brain injury often obscure more subtle clinical deficits. A thorough understanding of the epidemiology, anatomy, and mechanisms of injury is advisable.

EPIDEMIOLOGY AND MECHANISMS OF INJURY

Penetrating Cerebrovascular Injury

Consistent with other types of trauma, penetrating cerebrovascular injury affects primarily young males. The majority of penetrating vascular injuries result from gunshot wounds (GSWs) or knife wounds. The mechanism of injury is dependent on the population affected. Military injuries often involve high-velocity weapons or shrapnel, where the blast effect may cause vessel wall injury without direct contact by the projectile. Civilian injuries are more commonly caused by low-velocity weapons or knives with direct vessel wall injury.

It is useful to divide penetrating vascular injuries into those that are or are not associated with blood flow compromise. Flow compromise can occur when there is transection of the vessel or when injury to the vessel lumen results in stenosis or occlusion. Stenosis or occlusion may result from vessel wall hematoma, dissection, or false aneurysm or from external compression by a soft tissue hematoma. Emboli formation and thrombosis may also occur and lead to the development of neurological deficits.

Although penetrating neck injuries are not uncommon, very few involve the major arteries supplying the brain. In a report of 274 penetrating neck injuries, 4% involved the carotid artery, and 1% involved the vertebral artery (VA).[5] The higher incidence of penetrating injury to the carotid artery reflects its greater anterior exposure and size, and possibly the lack of protective bone around it. Carotid artery injuries usually involve the common rather than the internal carotid artery (ICA).[6-8] Traumatic injuries to the external carotid artery and its branches that do not cause a hematoma are rarely diagnosed; they are well tolerated neurologically unless there is preexisting cerebrovascular disease.

Penetrating VA injury is much less common than penetrating carotid artery injury and is often asymptomatic.[9] These injuries are usually caused by GSWs. When symptomatic, they may present with an expanding neck mass or vertebrobasilar ischemia.[10]

Traumatic arteriovenous fistulas are rare lesions and result from GSWs in military populations and from stab wounds or low-caliber GSWs in civilians. A study from the Vietnam era demonstrated involvement of only 8 ICAs and 6 VAs among 558 arteriovenous fistulas and false aneurysms identified.[11] When the carotid artery is involved, it usually communicates with the jugular vein. A VA arteriovenous fistula most often involves a vessel segment in the foramen transversarium in communication with the surrounding vertebral venous plexus. VA arteriovenous fistulas often have multiple feeding and draining channels.

Only 3% of GSWs with intracranial penetration result in traumatic intracranial aneurysms.[12] Their presentation is often delayed.

Nonpenetrating (Blunt) Cerebrovascular Injury

Penetrating trauma was thought to account for more than 95% of all cerebrovascular injuries in the past, but it appears that blunt cerebrovascular injury (BCVI) may account for one third or more of all cases. BCVI may involve both the carotid and vertebral arteries and is caused by direct forces to the neck as well as by stretching, tearing, and compressive mechanisms. Virtually any mechanism involving acute hyperextension, flexion, or rotation of the neck can result in blunt injury to the carotid artery (Fig. 330–1). Specific anatomic features of the ICA make it vulnerable to blunt injury. The C1-3 vertebral body transverse processes lie just dorsal to the ascending cervical ICA. The petrous ICA is also vulnerable to injury by the surrounding bone as it traverses the carotid canal in the petrous portion of the temporal bone and then turns to traverse the foramen lacerum. Skull base fractures in this region may result in formation of a pseudoaneurysm.

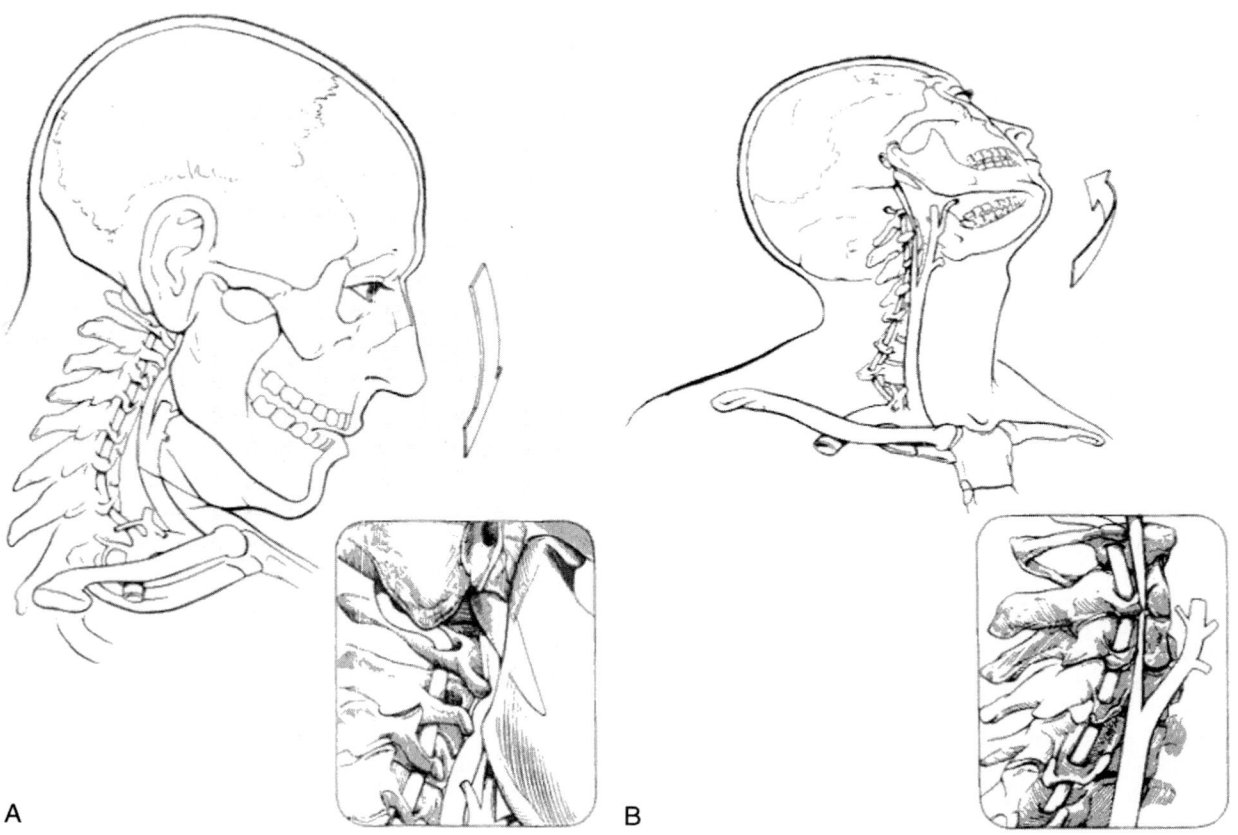

A   B

FIGURE 330–1. *A*, Cervical hyperflexion produces direct compression of the artery between the mandible and the upper cervical vertebrae, which may result in intimal disruption or mural hematoma. *B*, Cervical hyperextension-rotation stretches the internal carotid artery across the transverse processes of the second and third cervical vertebrae, causing intimal disruption. (From Aelenock GB, Kazmers A, Whitehouse WM Jr, et al: Extracranial ICA dissections: Noniatrogenic traumatic lesions. Arch Surg 117:437, 1982.)

The majority of blunt vascular injuries are attributed to motor vehicle crashes,[13-18] but other mechanisms such as motorcycle accidents, falls, near hangings, snow sports mishaps, and biking accidents play a significant role.[19, 20] Vascular injuries from apparently trivial trauma may occur secondary to predisposing arterial or bony abnormalities.

BLUNT CAROTID ARTERY INJURY

Incidence

The true incidence of blunt carotid injury (BCI) is difficult to ascertain. Lack of diagnosis secondary to early fatality, absent or delayed symptoms, and coincident morbidity such as head injury all contribute to a falsely low incidence.

Until recently, the available literature has been dominated by case reports. Yamada and colleagues identified only 51 cases of BCI in the literature before 1967, including the original case report by Verneuil in 1872.[21] Krajewski and Hertzer documented an additional 44 cases occurring before 1980.[22] During the 1980s, 75 new cases were reported, and 309 additional cases were reported from 1990 to 1995, including larger series.[13]

In addition to an increase in the absolute number of reported BCIs, an increase in BCIs relative to penetrating carotid injuries has been documented over time, rising from 27% to 38%.[17, 23-26] It is also noteworthy that the overall incidence of BCIs suffered by blunt trauma victims appears to be increasing. Several multicenter reviews suggested that BCI occurs in 0.08% to 0.17% of all blunt trauma victims admitted to a hospital.[17, 27-29] Several single-center studies reported an even higher incidence. Fabian reported an overall incidence of BCI in 0.33% of all blunt trauma admissions, with the motor vehicle accident cohort sustaining a 0.67% incidence of BCI.[13] Other publications reported a similarly high incidence of 0.24% to 0.31% of all blunt trauma patients.[16, 30] Although the reported incidence is undoubtedly increasing because of more aggressive diagnostic testing, significant percentages of patients in recent reports are symptomatic.[13] This suggests that the true incidence may be increasing.

Classification by Mechanism

In 1974 Crissey and Bernstein identified four fundamental mechanisms of BCI.[31] Type I injuries, which account for a minority of BCIs, result from a direct blow to the neck. They appear to be more common in elderly patients with advanced atherosclerotic disease and relatively noncompliant and calcified vessels that crack easily on impact. Although not part of the original description, another type of direct-blow injury involves acute cervical hyperflexion in motor vehicle accidents or falls, with the artery being compressed between the mandible and the vertebral prominences[32] (see Fig. 330–1A). Seat-belt injuries, strangulation injuries, and near hangings may injure the common or internal carotid artery by a similar direct-blow mechanism.[33, 34] A prominent styloid process has also been implicated as a direct cause of carotid artery injury,

resulting in pseudoaneurysms in as many as 30% of cases.[35, 36]

Type II injuries are the most common and result from hyperextension of the neck and contralateral rotation of the head; they often occur during motor vehicle accidents (see Fig. 330–1B). Because the lateral articular processes and pedicles of the upper three cervical vertebrae project anteriorly, the overlying distal cervical ICA is prone to stretch injury during cervical hyperextension.[37] Further, the ICA is adherent to the periosteum where it enters the carotid canal at the skull base. With hyperextension of the neck, the carotid canal and artery are elevated, and the artery can be stretched across the lateral articular processes of C1 through C3, resulting in injury. Rotation at the atlantoaxial joint may result in anterior movement of the contralateral C1 lateral mass, exacerbating the stretch injury.

There is considerable debate about the role played by rotation. Batnitzky and colleagues pointed out that bilateral injuries are not uncommon.[38] This would be unlikely if unilateral rotation was linked to the contralateral vessel injury. Increased age, with its associated vessel tortuosity and stiffness and decreased cervical spine mobility, may be protective for this type of vessel injury. Conversely, tethering of the ICA by depressed sternal fracture fragments[39] or inflammatory adherence secondary to previous pharyngeal infection[40] may increase the risk of injury.

Type III injuries result from intraoral trauma. They are most commonly reported in children who have fallen with hard objects in their mouths, such as pencils.[41-44]

Type IV injuries are associated with basilar skull fractures, most commonly involving the sphenoid or petrous bone, which result in arterial laceration.[45, 46] This type of injury can also occur as the intracranial ICA enters the dura just medial to the anterior clinoid process. Brain displacement may stretch the vessel at this point where it is tethered by the dura. Depending on the degree of injury, a carotid cavernous fistula or intracranial hemorrhage may ensue.[47]

BLUNT VERTEBRAL ARTERY INJURY

Until recently, few studies have focused on VA injury following blunt trauma, so it is difficult to estimate its true incidence. Many cases of blunt vertebral injury (BVI) likely remain asymptomatic or result in subtle neurological deficits that go undetected. Therefore, without aggressive diagnostic screening, BVIs are underdiagnosed.

Age and sex were initially thought to distinguish a cohort of patients at increased risk for BVI. Initial reports identified women aged 30 to 50 years with VA dissections who were seemingly distinct from the patient group experiencing BVI.[48, 49] However, subsequent reports identified the majority of BVIs in the typical trauma population.[50-55]

Cervical spine injury appears to have a specific association with BVI. High-speed motor vehicle crashes and falls account for the majority of cervical spine fractures and may account for the majority of VA injuries as well. Although BVI was initially thought to occur principally with upper cervical fractures, angiographic screening of cervical fractures has documented a significant coincidence of BVI with all types of spinal injuries: 40% of lateral dislocations,[52] 46% of midcervical fractures with facet injury,[50] and 88% of fractures involving the foramen transversarium.[51]

An understanding of VA anatomy in relation to the cervical spine helps explain these injury patterns. In contrast to the carotid arteries, the VAs demonstrate considerable asymmetry. An autopsy study by Thomas and colleagues revealed that 1.8% of right and 3.1% of left VAs do not communicate with the basilar artery, with an overall 15% rate of VA hypoplasia.[56] These variations are usually of no clinical significance, but they become important when the dominant VA is injured.

The first portion of the VA is rarely injured from blunt trauma, possibly owing to its mobility and lack of any surrounding bone. However, the second portion of the VA, which ascends through the transverse foramina of the upper six cervical vertebrae, is frequently injured when cervical fractures involve the foramen.[50, 51] The third portion of the VA curves posteriorly behind the lateral mass of the atlas and lies in the groove on the upper surface of the posterior arch of the atlas. Because of the high frequency of cervical fractures and ligamentous injuries in this region, as well as stretching and compression at the atlantoaxial and atlanto-occipital joints during head rotation, this segment of the VA extending from C2 to the dura is particularly prone to injury during blunt trauma[48, 57] (Fig. 330–2). Variations in this intricate anatomy may explain BVI in patients with mechanisms involving head rotation and seemingly minor traumatic components.[53]

FINAL COMMON PATHWAY IN BLUNT CEREBROVASCULAR INJURY

Regardless of the specific mechanism of injury, the final common pathway of blunt vascular injury is usually intimal disruption. The resulting exposure of thrombogenic subendothelial collagen promotes platelet aggregation and increases the potential for embolization, partial thrombosis with low flow, or complete thrombosis. An intimal tear may predispose to arterial dissection with progressive narrowing of the lumen and ultimately distal thrombosis or vessel occlusion. A pseudoaneurysm may also form. An increase in pseudoaneurysm size may be accompanied by compression and occlusion of the parent vessel lumen, platelet thromboembolism, or pseudoaneurysm rupture. Extracranial or intracranial hemorrhage, as well as the formation of an arteriovenous fistula, may result.[58]

TRIVIAL MECHANISMS OF BLUNT CEREBROVASCULAR INJURY

Numerous reports in the literature document vascular injury in association with seemingly trivial trauma. By definition, spontaneous dissection occurs in the absence of known causative factors and may account for 2.5% of primary strokes.[59] There is likely a continuum extending from spontaneous events (which may be truly spontaneous or may be a delayed presentation from previous minor trauma) to injuries associated with minor or major trauma. Several risk factors have been reported in association with spontaneous dissection, including hypertension, Marfan's syndrome, fibromuscular dysplasia, syphilis, arteriopathies, and Erdheim's cystic medial necrosis.[60] It is possible that true spontaneous vascular injury is exceedingly rare,

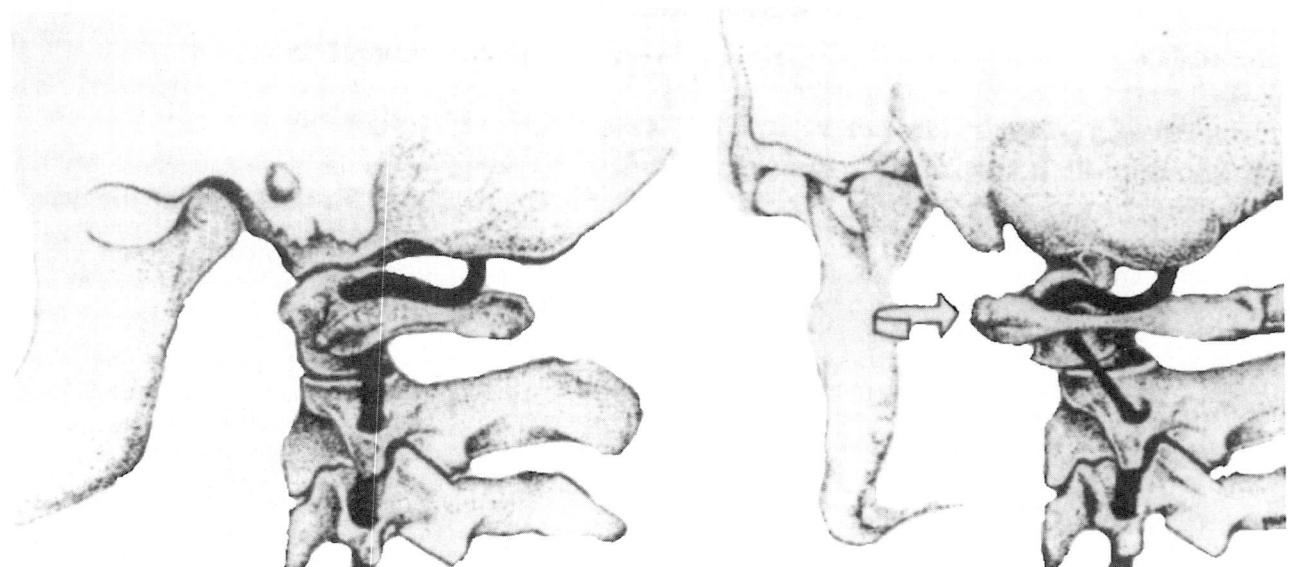

FIGURE 330–2. Stretching of the vertebral artery between C1 and C2 due to rotation in extension. (From Barnett HJM: Progress toward stroke prevention: Robert Wartenberg lecture. Neurology 30: 1212–1225, 1980.)

and known risk factors simply increase the likelihood of injury secondary to trivial mechanisms.[61, 62] Patients often fail to report these so-called trivial events, considering them insignificant.[63]

Traumatic Aneurysm

Traumatic aneurysms occur based on location-specific mechanisms. Cervical traumatic arterial aneurysms are rare. In a series of 2000 head injuries in which diagnosis involved angiography, only 1 case was identified.[64] They usually result from penetrating trauma (Fig. 330–3) but may also be associated with blunt mechanisms.[65] Pathologic evaluation usually shows a false aneurysm with the wall partially composed of hematoma.

Traumatic aneurysms at the skull base are also rare. When located in the petrous or cavernous portion of

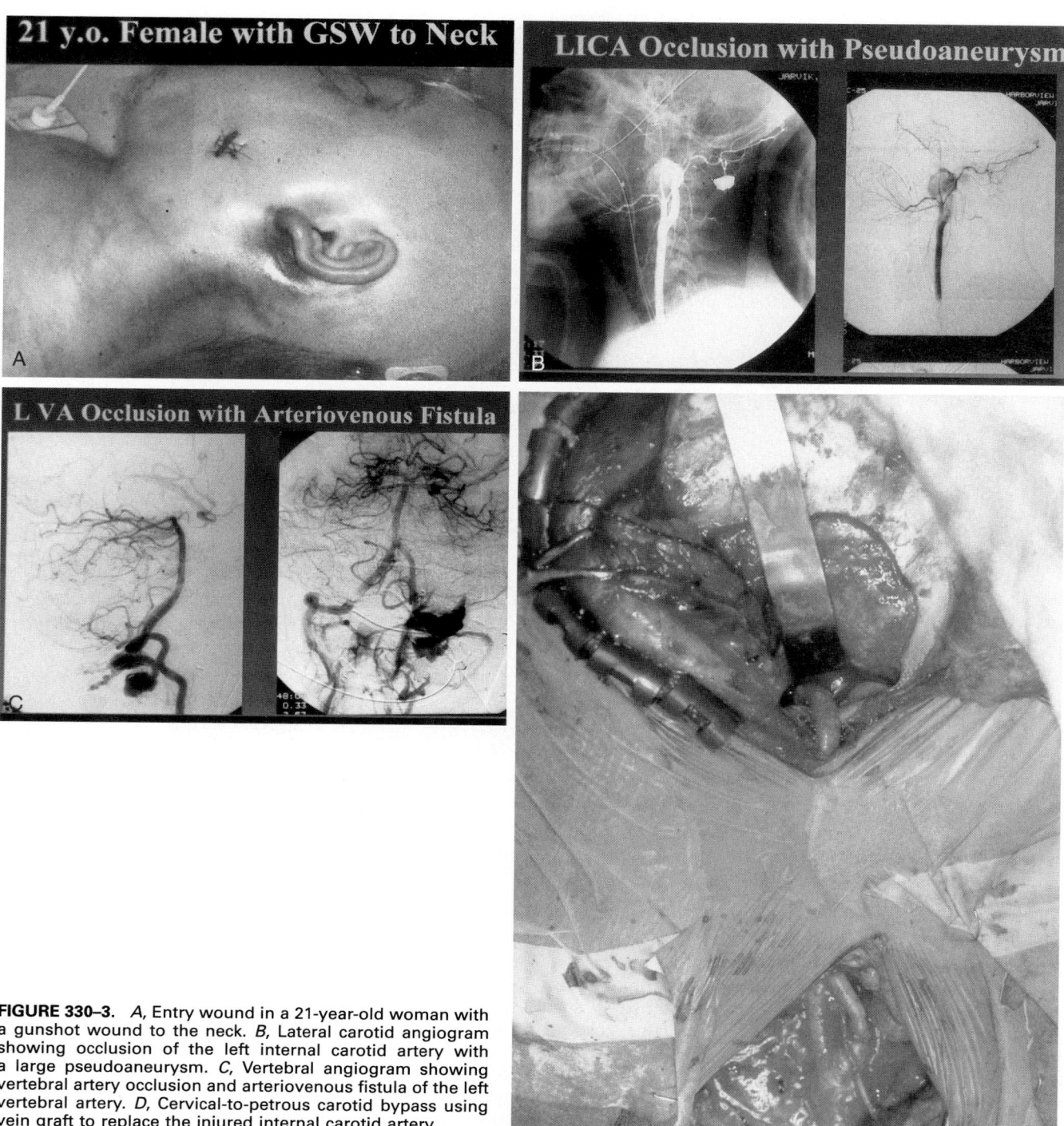

FIGURE 330–3. *A,* Entry wound in a 21-year-old woman with a gunshot wound to the neck. *B,* Lateral carotid angiogram showing occlusion of the left internal carotid artery with a large pseudoaneurysm. *C,* Vertebral angiogram showing vertebral artery occlusion and arteriovenous fistula of the left vertebral artery. *D,* Cervical-to-petrous carotid bypass using vein graft to replace the injured internal carotid artery.

Illustration continued on following page

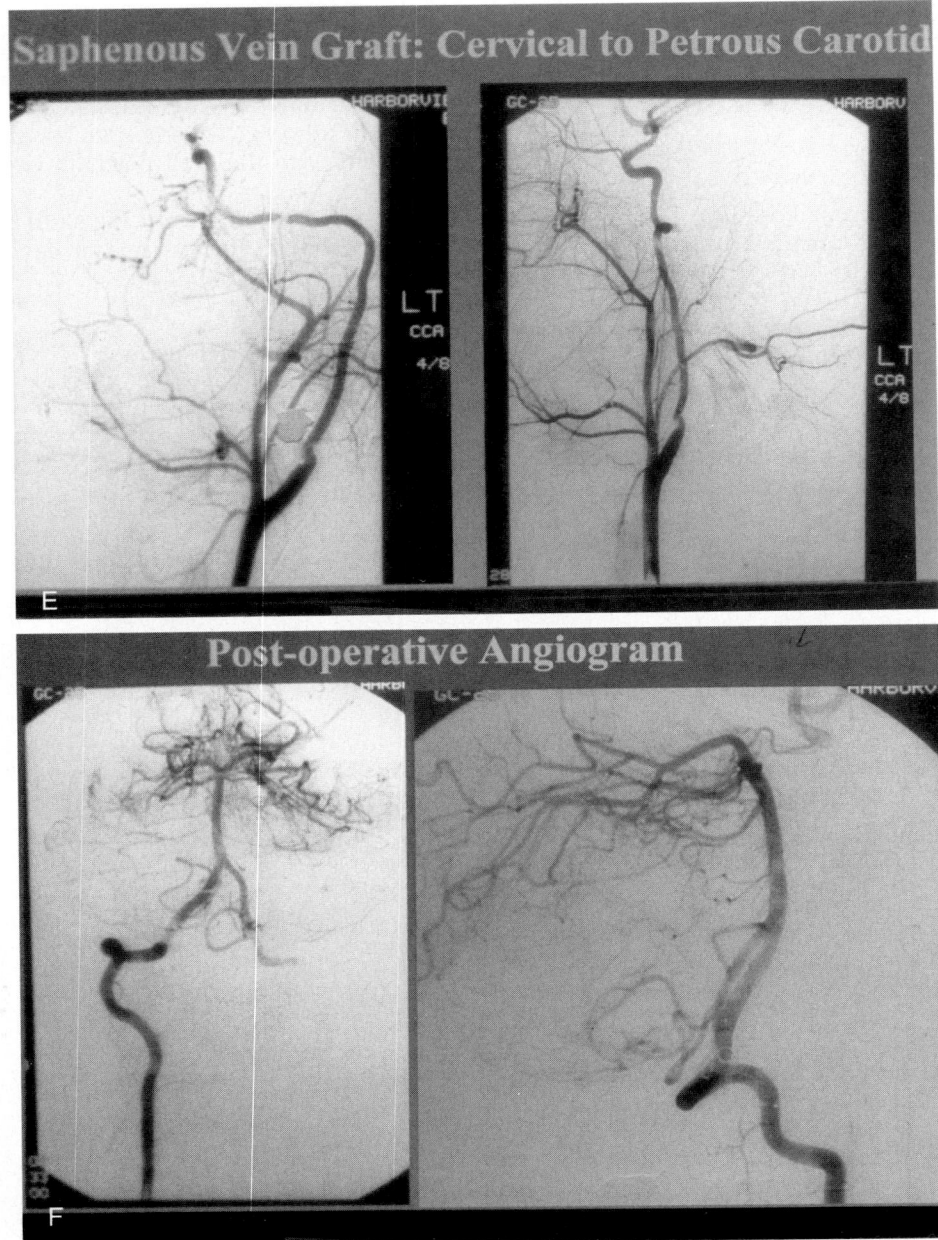

FIGURE 330–3 *Continued. E,* Postoperative carotid artery angiogram showing the saphenous vein replacement graft from the cervical to petrous internal carotid artery. *F,* Postoperative vertebral artery angiogram showing the results of operative ligation of the left vertebral artery.

the ICA, they are usually associated with basilar skull fractures, with pathology showing false aneurysms. Like traumatic vascular injuries of the carotid and vertebral arteries, their incidence may be underestimated.

Traumatic intracranial aneurysms are also very rare. Although trauma is the most common cause of subarachnoid hemorrhage, traumatic aneurysms account for only 1% of aneurysms associated with subarachnoid hemorrhage.[66] These aneurysms most commonly occur with penetrating injury (Fig. 330–4) or vascular injury associated with a contiguous cranial fracture. Pathology may demonstrate a true or false aneurysm.

Direct contusion of the vessel wall from contact with a contiguous structure is thought to cause the injury—for example, the carotid artery against the skull base, the anterior cerebral artery against the falx, or the middle cerebral artery against the sphenoid wing. In rare cases, significant energy imparted from a blunt injury mechanism, combined with a predisposing anatomic configuration, results in a traumatic aneurysm in the posterior fossa.[67] Traumatic aneurysm formation via a blunt mechanism may represent a continuum of injury. Energy transfer, in combination with predisposing factors (anatomic variation, fibromuscular dysplasia, athero-

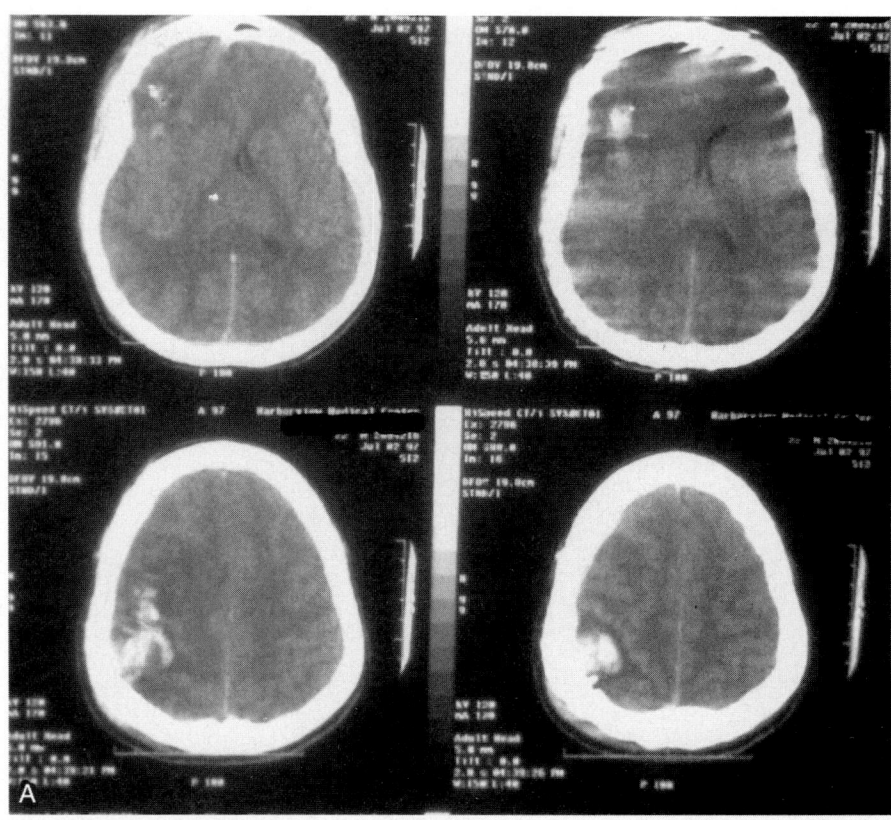

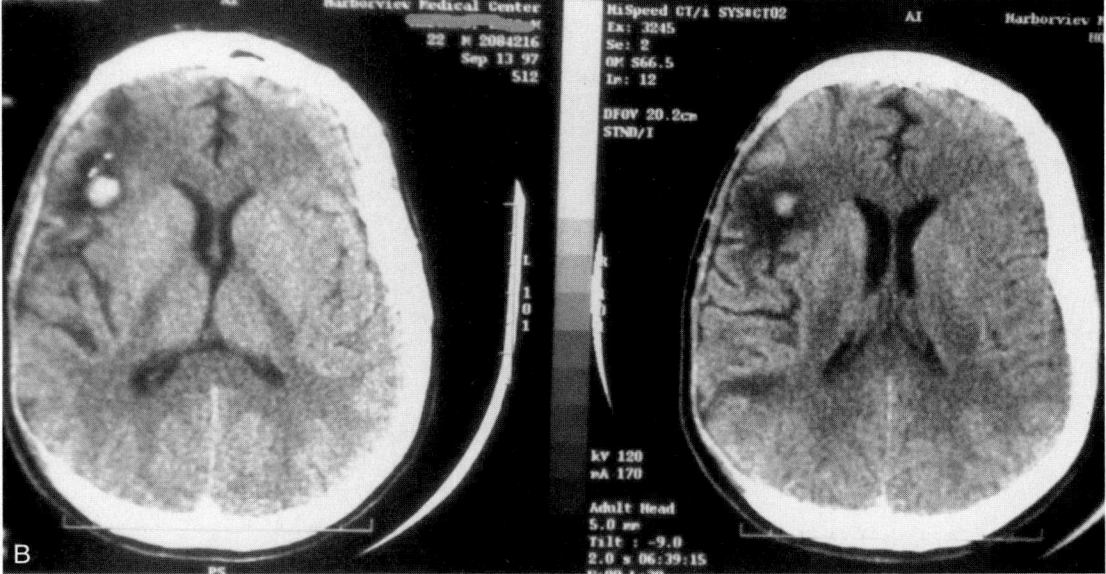

FIGURE 330–4. *A,* Initial computed tomographic scans of a 22-year-old man with a gunshot wound to the head and bone fragments from the subfrontal, supraorbital region. *B,* Upon his return for cranioplasty, a high-density lesion was noted in the middle cerebral artery region, which on angiograms proved to be a pseudoaneurysm of a branch of the middle cerebral artery.

Illustration continued on following page

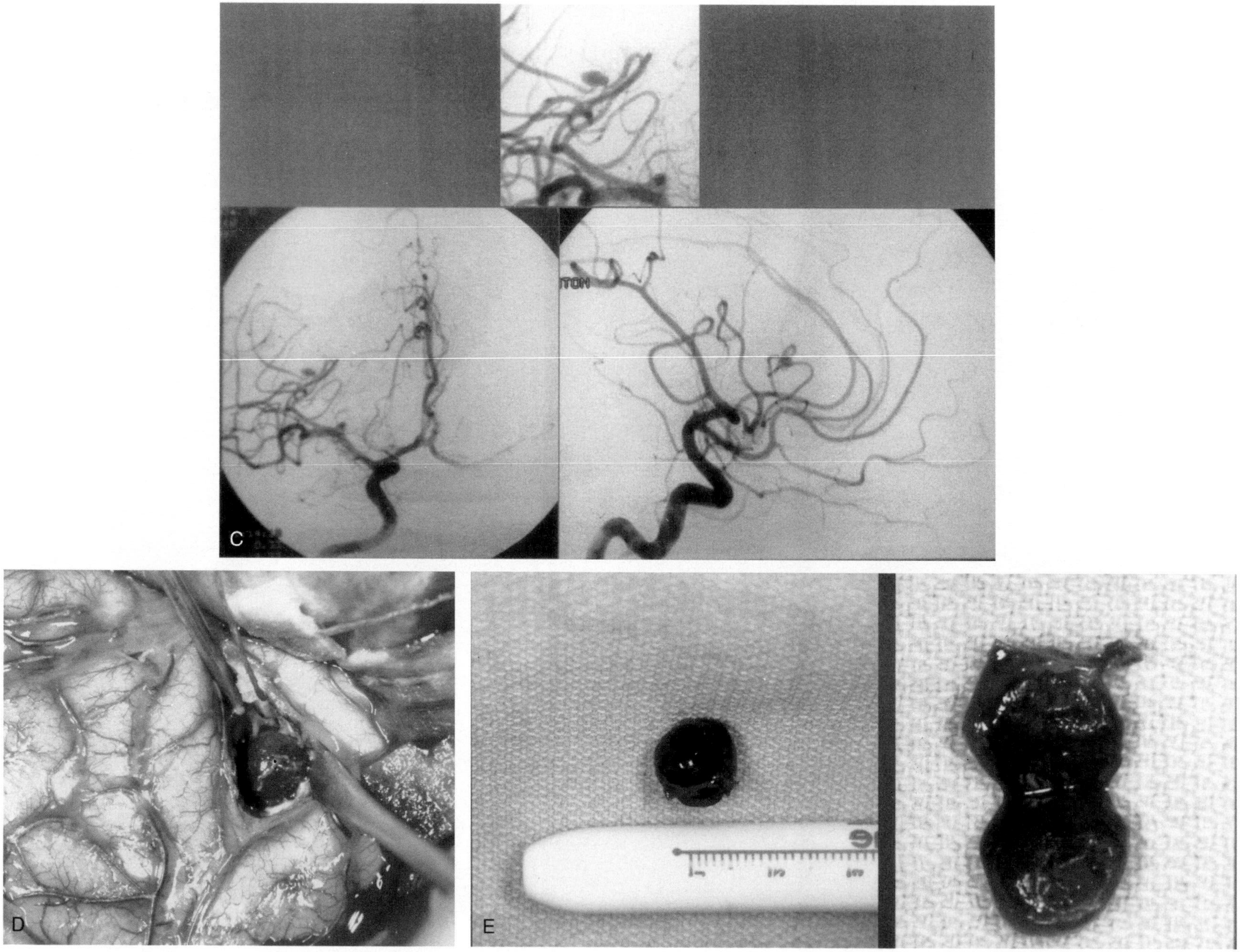

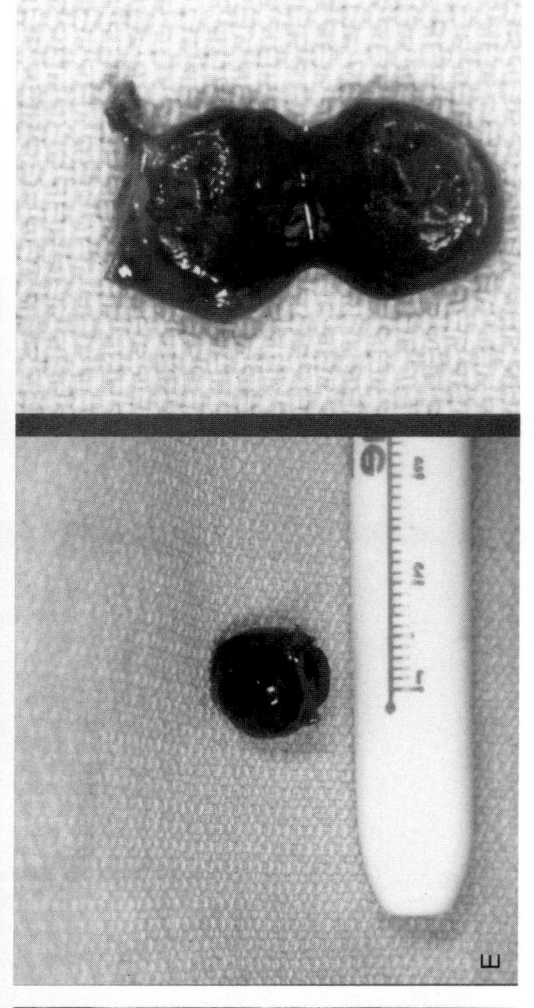

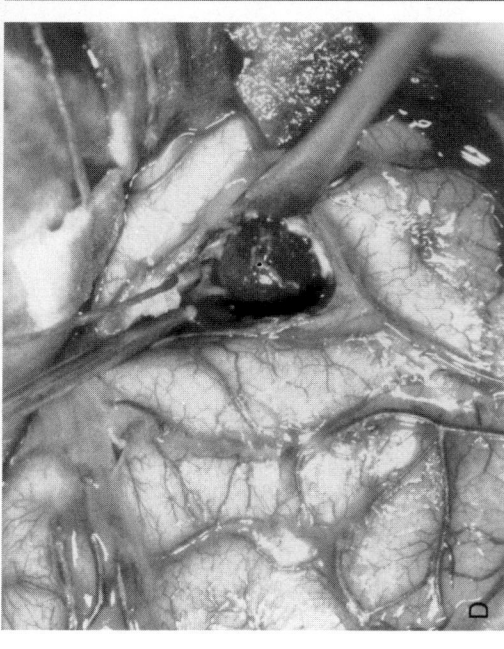

FIGURE 330-4 *Continued. C,* Angiograms showing pseudoaneurysm of the middle cerebral artery. *D,* Intraoperative photograph showing exposure of the pseudoaneurysm. *E,* Surgical specimen after pseudoaneurysm resection.

sclerosis), may result in dissection, aneurysm formation, or vessel disruption.

Carotid Cavernous Fistula

Carotid cavernous fistulas, because of their distinctive clinical presentation, have been widely studied. They are covered in depth in Chapter 139. A carotid cavernous fistula occurs when the ICA or one of its branches ruptures within the multiseptated cavernous sinus and communicates with the venous channels. This may involve the meningohypophysial or other small branches or may involve a laceration of the ICA. A false aneurysm within the cavernous sinus that does not communicate directly with the venous structure may also occur without resulting in the typical clinical presentation of a carotid cavernous fistula.

Carotid cavernous fistulas occur principally in young men following trauma.[68] They usually result from significant head injury, often with a basilar skull fracture. A minority of cases seemingly occur spontaneously in older women without documented trauma.

Intracranial arteriovenous fistulas involving vessels other than the carotid artery and cavernous sinus are extremely rare. There have been documented cases resulting from penetrating injury, including depressed skull fractures. Spontaneous resolution is uncommon, and early diagnosis and treatment are important.

Venous Sinus Laceration and Occlusion

The overall incidence of dural sinus injury has been reported to be as high as 12% in penetrating cranial trauma during wartime, compared with approximately 1% to 4% in civilian populations, where blunt trauma is more prevalent.[69] Venous sinus laceration is usually associated with a depressed skull fracture or GSW. It may be accompanied by brain contusion or hemorrhage. When the laceration is open, there may be catastrophic and fatal exsanguination. When it is closed, there may be delayed development of a symptomatic venous epidural hematoma. Isolated traumatic venous sinus occlusion may also result from a depressed skull fracture or edema or bleeding from extension of thrombus from damaged emissary veins.[70]

CLINICAL PRESENTATION

The clinical manifestations of vascular injury depend on the mechanism of injury, the anatomy affected, and the existence of collateral circulation and associated injuries. Diagnostic considerations are based on clinical manifestations as well as screening in the context of known high-risk injury mechanisms and patterns. Both penetrating and blunt injury mechanisms are reviewed with respect to their typical clinical presentations.

Penetrating Injury

Penetrating neck injuries may be associated with vascular injury. Clear vascular injury is accompanied by active pulsatile bleeding or expanding hematoma. These dramatic cases are rarely difficult to diagnose. The majority of patients suffering knife wounds, GSWs, or other projectile injuries to the neck may present with nothing more than an apparent entry wound with or without an exit wound. Any structure accessible from the neck may be injured, including the vascular structures, trachea, esophagus, recurrent laryngeal nerve, thoracic duct, and spinal cord. Patients may present with ongoing hemorrhage, expanding hematoma, hemoptysis, dysphonia, crepitation, hematemesis, dysphagia, or neurological deficit.[3]

Nonpenetrating (Blunt) Injury

GENERAL CONSIDERATIONS

The hallmarks of BCVI are delayed presentation and delayed diagnosis. The latent period between injury and clinical symptoms results from the biologic factors discussed earlier. Immediate transection or vessel occlusion at the site of injury is rare. The time between injury and the development of vessel occlusion or thrombosis is variable. The majority of neurological symptoms referable to vascular injury present more than 10 hours after injury, with 23% to 50% becoming symptomatic more than 1 day after injury.[20, 22, 26, 71, 72] In one large series, mean time to diagnosis was 58 hours.[13]

The majority of patients with BCVI have multisystem trauma, and initial attention is often focused on life-saving treatments.[18] It may be difficult to identify subtle neurological changes in this early resuscitation period. Coexisting head injuries may further limit the detection of subtle neurological deficits early in their progression.

BLUNT INTERNAL CAROTID ARTERY INJURY

When the presenting signs and symptoms of BCI are not masked by traumatic brain injury or multisystem injury, they most often include pain, Horner's syndrome, or a variable degree of hemisensory hemiplegia and dysphasia, accompanied by an altered level of consciousness.

Traumatic cervical vascular injury should be considered in the differential diagnosis of post-traumatic neck pain and headache. Pain is associated with a significant percentage of carotid artery dissections and may reflect mural hemorrhage or vessel wall dissection. It may involve the neck, ear, face, or periorbital region. In a report including both spontaneous and traumatic carotid artery injury, pain was the initial symptom in 74% of patients; the majority had pain for several days before the onset of neurological deficits.[73]

Oculosympathetic paresis, commonly referred to as partial Horner's syndrome, is another common presentation following traumatic carotid artery injury. Damage to the cervical carotid artery by traumatic or spontaneous mechanisms disrupts the periarterial sympathetic plexus in as many as 50% of patients.[73–76] Pupillary asymmetry with ptosis and miosis is evident on examination. In contradistinction to the large, minimally reactive pupil secondary to brain herniation, with BCI, the larger pupil is reactive and the smaller pupil is abnormal. Cervical carotid artery injury should be ruled out ipsilateral to the smaller, abnormally reactive pupil. In a minority of cases, the external carotid plexus may also be injured, resulting in anhidrosis.

Unilateral traumatic occlusion of the ICA may be asymptomatic or result in infarction of the ipsilateral hemisphere. This depends not only on embolic phenomena but also on collateral circulation. Absence of a normal anterior communicating artery increases the risk of infarction. The typical clinical presentation with inadequate collateral flow includes a depressed level of consciousness and contralateral hemiplegia. A patient with normal collateral flow may be asymptomatic or may manifest ICA occlusion with a normal level of consciousness and contralateral sensorimotor deficits in the arm, face, and leg (in decreasing order of severity). When the ICA supplying the dominant hemisphere is affected, there may be global aphasia.

Bilateral traumatic ICA occlusion is rare. Patients may present in coma with deficits attributed to a brain injury, resulting in delayed diagnosis. Of three patients with bilateral traumatic carotid artery occlusion, two presented in coma and died, and the other presented with a normal examination but progressed to aphasia and hemiplegia within 4 hours, surviving with permanent deficits.[77] An additional 20 patients with significant bilateral carotid artery lesions were diagnosed by the same authors. Fifteen patients presented with neurological deficits, and the other five progressed to significant deficits within 48 hours. Hemiparesis and coma were the two most common signs.

BLUNT VERTEBRAL ARTERY INJURY

Cervical VA injury often remains asymptomatic. Cervical VA occlusions are less likely than carotid artery occlusions to result in neurological deficits. Protection is afforded by the rich anastomosis of muscular branches in the upper cervical region and the potential for retrograde flow from one VA to the distal occluded VA through the vertebrobasilar junction. Pain is not uncommon following traumatic VA dissection, occurring primarily in the posterior cervical and occipital regions.[48, 49, 57, 78, 79] When it occurs, vertebrobasilar ischemia may result in a combination of ipsilateral cranial nerve or cerebellar deficits and contralateral sensorimotor deficits.

VA injury may also result in embolic stroke. This may include the lateral medullary (Wallenberg's) syndrome, which variably includes ipsilateral facial and contralateral body analgesia, Horner's syndrome, and ataxia. Cerebellar edema following stroke can result in obstruction of the fourth ventricle and hydrocephalus, or brainstem compression and herniation. When embolic stroke results in a unilateral posterior cerebral artery (PCA) stroke, there is resultant contralateral homonymous hemianopsia (Fig. 330–5); bilateral PCA infarction leads to cortical blindness (Anton's syndrome). Brainstem stroke from perforator compromise may also occur and is typically identified by its pattern of

crossed deficits involving ipsilateral cranial nerve palsies and contralateral hemiparesis.

Although both carotid and VA injury can present with subarachnoid hemorrhage, it is more common with VA injury. VA rupture may be fatal and is often associated with head and neck extension.[80] An association with alcohol intoxication may be due to decreased reaction time and muscle relaxation at the craniovertebral junction.[80, 81]

Traumatic Intracranial Artery Injury

Traumatic intracranial artery injury is rare. Presentation follows the expected clinical patterns. Middle cerebral artery occlusion results from embolization much more commonly than from direct injury. A stroke in this distribution involves contralateral hemiparesis and hemisensory loss, generally affecting the face and arm and sparing the leg. Broca's (motor) aphasia may be present if the dominant hemisphere is involved. There may be a resultant visual field deficit or Wernicke's dysphasia. Nondominant middle cerebral artery infarcts may result in hemineglect, hemianopsia, or other parietal lobe deficits. Infarctions of the entire distribution can lead to significant swelling and intracranial pressure problems. Infarctions involving two thirds or more of the middle cerebral artery territory have a 17% mortality, with the majority of deaths due to brain edema. One half result in permanent severe disabilities.[82]

Vascular injury affecting the anterior cerebral artery alone is unusual. It usually presents with motor and, to a lesser degree, sensory deficits in the contralateral leg and foot. Mutism and neuropsychological deficits may also be manifest.

Basilar artery occlusions have a varied presentation, depending on collateral circulation, and may range from no symptoms to coma. Emboli that pass the posterior inferior cerebellar artery (PICA) tend to lodge rostrally in the distal basilar artery at its terminal bifurcation into the paired PCAs. Unilateral occlusion of the PCA may result in contralateral homonymous hemianopsia, with macular sparing. Metamorphopsia (visual distortion of objects) or palinopsia (persistence of an image after it has left the visual field) may also be manifest.[83] Occlusion of combinations of the numerous small penetrating branches near the top of the basilar artery supplying the thalamus and midbrain may result in devastating strokes with bilateral oculomotor nerve palsies and coma.

Other Cerebrovascular Injuries

Carotid cavernous fistulas usually occur in the cavernous or cerebral segment of the ICA, typically secondary to a basilar skull fracture that lacerates the artery. Increased pressure in the superior ophthalmic vein results in conjunctival hyperemia and chemosis. Exophthalmos, ophthalmoplegia, and orbital pain are common features. There is often a cephalic bruit and a palpable thrill over the orbit. These lesions are rarely life threatening but can severely compromise visual

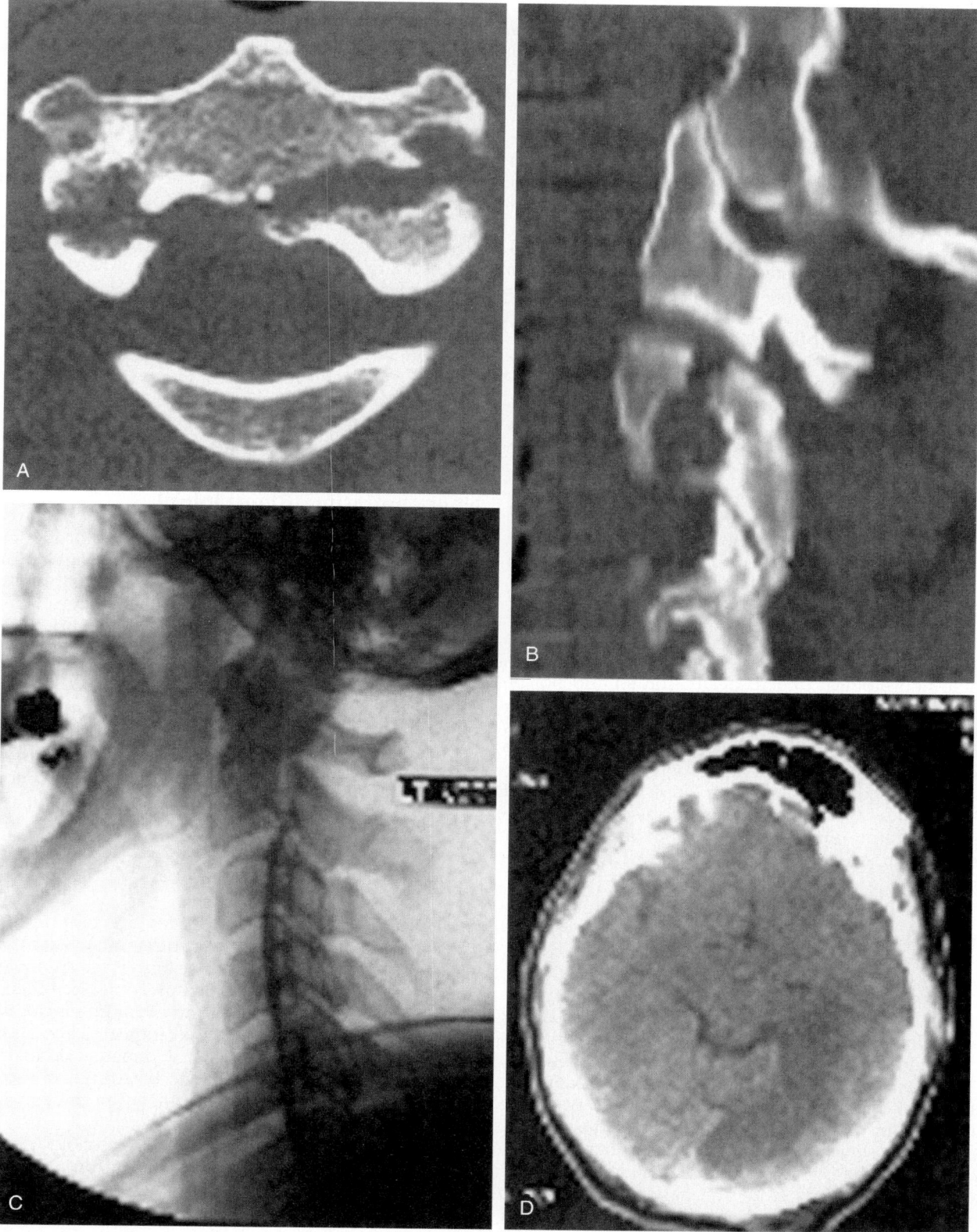

FIGURE 330–5. *A,* Initial axial computed tomographic scan through C2 in a patient who suffered a cervical fracture in a motor vehicle accident. The fracture involves the left foramen transversarium of C2. *B,* Sagittal reconstructions further demonstrate involvement of the left foramen transversarium. *C,* Vertebral angiography demonstrates vertebral artery occlusion at the level of the C2 fracture. *D,* Head computed tomographic scan before the institution of anticoagulation demonstrates left posterior cerebral artery territory infarct. Physical examination demonstrated a homonymous visual field deficit. Owing to the size of the infarct, the patient was treated with aspirin only. The visual field deficit improved but persisted.

function. An uncommon but potentially life-threatening consequence of BCI is epistaxis. Typically, this is a manifestation of an ICA pseudoaneurysm at the skull base. Massive hemorrhage can occur, even weeks after the injury.[84, 85]

The sequelae of venous sinus occlusion depend on its location. Often, occlusion of the anterior superior sagittal sinus or a nondominant transverse sinus is asymptomatic. Occlusion of the posterior sagittal sinus or dominant transverse sinus is often associated with significant elevation in intracranial pressure and, depending on the architecture of the draining cortical veins and their involvement, neurological deficit or venous infarction.[86, 87] Spastic paraparesis of the legs may result from injury to the middle third of the sagittal sinus, and cortical blindness occasionally accompanies injury to the posterior third.[88] Sinus injury may present in a subacute fashion after trauma with complaints of persistent headache, vomiting, papilledema, ataxia, or confusion.[70, 86] Dural arteriovenous fistula may be a late sequela of sinus injury.[89]

DIAGNOSTIC EVALUATION

General Considerations

Diagnostic evaluation should be pursued to rule out cerebrovascular injury when there is suspicion of injury based on clinical symptoms and signs or mechanism of injury. Because delayed diagnosis may result in irreversible neurological deficit, evaluation should not be delayed unnecessarily. Prompt diagnosis of BCVI depends on a high index of suspicion and a cooperative, multidisciplinary trauma team. Arteriography is the gold standard for the diagnosis of vascular lesions, yielding information relevant to injury location and collateral flow. The role of arteriography in both penetrating and blunt injury is reviewed. In addition, other potentially useful noninvasive modalities are discussed.

Penetrating Injury

The risk of injury to the major vessels, their branches, and surrounding structures is dependent on the anatomic site of the penetrating injury. Mandatory surgical neck exploration for all penetrating cervical injuries was recommended in the past.[1, 2] Recent re-evaluation has demonstrated the efficacy of a selective diagnostic strategy.[3] Although unstable patients require emergent exploration for diagnosis and treatment, stable patients may undergo selective diagnostic testing based on injury location. The cervical region is divided into three zones: zone I extends from the base of the neck to the cricoid cartilage, zone II extends from the cricoid cartilage to the angle of the mandible, and zone III comprises the area cephalad to the angle of the mandible. Patients with zone I injuries with or without symptoms undergo angiography and esophageal studies (esophagoscopy and esophageal contrast studies). Those with zone II injuries go to the operating room if

symptomatic and are observed if asymptomatic. Patients with zone III injuries undergo angiography if symptomatic, with possible subsequent surgery, and are observed if asymptomatic.

Diagnostic evaluation for transcervical GSWs is controversial. Emergent neck exploration with a low threshold for performing a bilateral exploration has been advocated.[90] Among 41 patients, 22 (54%) had confirmed vascular injuries, in addition to a multitude of other visceral injuries. Some, however, recommend careful clinical examination combined with angiography and selective endoscopy and esophagography.[91] The nonsurgical approach detected a 48% incidence of vascular injuries in 33 patients, a rate similar to that detected with mandatory surgical exploration.

Transcranial GSWs may be associated with acute or delayed vascular injury. Early angiography is performed if the bullet trajectory crosses a vascular territory or if there is unexpected or uncontrolled bleeding. Delayed angiography may also be indicated to rule out late pseudoaneurysm development.

Nonpenetrating (Blunt) Injury

Important signs of BCVI include a cervical bruit, neurological deficits incongruous with the findings on brain CT, and CT demonstration of an intracranial infarct or delayed or atypical intracranial hemorrhage. A thorough initial neurological examination and frequent repeat examinations are critical to the localization of potential BCVIs. Similarly, an initial head CT should be followed by sequential CT examinations when the patient fails to improve neurologically, even if the initial head CT was negative. Arteriography is currently the diagnostic test of choice for symptomatic or suspected blunt vascular injury. Other noninvasive modalities may ultimately prove useful either alone or in combination.

CEREBRAL ANGIOGRAPHY

Standard angiographic techniques are employed for the study of both cervical and intracranial vasculature to assess traumatic injury. Because it is an invasive procedure involving a complex physiologic milieu, cerebral angiography in the setting of trauma is not without risk. When arteriography is indicated for another reason (e.g., assessment of a widened mediastinum or embolization of active pelvic bleeding), it may be reasonable to assess cervical vascular injury in the same setting.

Possible serious complications of angiography include stroke, vascular occlusion or rupture, and renal impairment. In elective evaluations of nontrauma patients, cerebrovascular angiography is associated with approximately a 1% to 2% risk of significant complication and a 1% risk of significant renal toxicity. Although specific data are lacking, these risks are presumed to be greater in trauma patients, who may experience shock as well as other pathophysiologic insults. Data assessing angiography's sensitivity and specificity for the diagnosis of traumatic vascular injury are also lacking.

Recently, dynamic helical CT has replaced angiography for the evaluation of potential thoracic aortic injuries following blunt trauma. The benefits of angiography for the diagnosis of cerebrovascular injury must therefore be great enough to justify its use despite the associated risks. It is important to accurately determine the risks of angiography in the setting of trauma, as well as the diagnostic efficacy of noninvasive techniques used alone or in combination.

NONINVASIVE TECHNIQUES

Duplex Doppler

Duplex Doppler scanning combines real-time B-mode ultrasound imaging with pulsed Doppler flow detection. Although it is the screening test of choice for extracranial carotid atherosclerotic disease and for many peripheral vascular structures, its efficacy in screening for traumatic vascular injury is not well defined.

A comparison of duplex Doppler to arteriography in a dog model of experimental vascular injury found duplex Doppler to be more sensitive and arteriography to be more specific.[92] Although duplex Doppler has been promoted by some as the principal screening test for blunt traumatic vascular injury, the supporting data are not conclusive and are limited to individual cases or small series.[27–29, 93] Lesions at the skull base, such as traumatic pseudoaneurysms, appear to be underdiagnosed by duplex ultrasonography.[27] Duplex Doppler may also miss injuries that initially show little luminal compromise but later progress. Conversely, ultrasonography may prove useful in specific injuries, such as direct blows to the neck. It may also be useful for following up a known lesion, especially if a baseline examination was obtained. The ultimate accuracy can be significantly affected by the technician's expertise.

Computed Tomography–Angiography

Most multisystem trauma patients require CT. This makes the potential use of computed tomography–angiography (CTA) for the identification of cervical vascular injuries attractive. Potential lesions can be visualized in the context of associated brain injuries, facial or basilar skull fractures, or cervical spine injuries. It is noninvasive, has a relatively short examination time, and requires less dye than arteriography, and resulting data sets can be manipulated in three dimensions.[94] CTA also has good sensitivity and specificity for the identification of carotid dissection[95, 96] and good correlation with arteriography for atherosclerotic stenosis and occlusion.[97, 98]

For the diagnosis of vascular injury in the setting of trauma, however, CTA has several shortcomings.[99] Imaging of the entire carotid and vertebral systems with a slice thickness and pitch adequate for sufficient sensitivity is not practical, and the option of limited evaluation of high-risk areas remains suboptimal.[96] Although three-dimensional CT appears to approach arteriography in terms of lesion demonstration, it may underestimate the degree of stenosis.[100] Evaluation of the petrous and cavernous portions of the ICA is suboptimal because of local bone artifact. Finally, the timing of contrast administration is critical to the success of CTA and may be suboptimal in the setting of acute trauma.

Magnetic Resonance Angiography

In theory, magnetic resonance angiography (MRA) has the greatest potential to replace arteriography as the diagnostic modality of choice for traumatic vascular injury. It is noninvasive, does not require contrast administration, and has a relatively short acquisition time. Data sets can be manipulated to allow visualization of the vessels from any angle. Imaging of the brain with diffusion-weighted sequences at the same setting also allows for identification of ischemic infarction, which may influence the choice of treatment for the injured vessel.[101]

Several preliminary studies have shown MRA to be useful in the setting of trauma.[77, 102] In the specific setting of cervical spine injury, a greater than 20% incidence of unilateral VA injury or occlusion was demonstrated.[54, 55] One of these patients ultimately died from a related cerebellar hemorrhagic infarct.

However, MRA is not without disadvantages. There is a lack of timely availability at many institutions. In addition, many ventilatory and orthopedic external fixation devices are incompatible with the use of MRA, obviating its utility in severely injured multisystem trauma patients. In addition, pseudoaneurysms may be difficult to detect with MRA alone, owing to turbulence.[103]

Transcranial Doppler Ultrasonography

The development of transcranial Doppler ultrasonography, in which ultrasound waves penetrate the skull, has enhanced noninvasive cerebrovascular diagnostic capabilities.[104, 105] Although transcranial Doppler is used primarily to detect vasospasm after subarachnoid hemorrhage, it can also detect emboli and assess normal flow velocities after trauma. It has been used successfully to detect both air and non-air emboli.[106, 107] Detection and prevention of emboli are important, given their documented relationship to postoperative neuropsychological deficits following coronary artery bypass.[108] The high incidence of intracranial microemboli in the middle cerebral artery downstream from ICA dissections was reported by Srinivasan and colleagues, who found a significant correlation between the presence of emboli and clinical manifestations of stroke.[109] It is possible that emboli detection with transcranial Doppler may ultimately prove useful as part of a screening program for the identification of BCVI, especially in combination with other noninvasive studies such as MRA.

Venous Sinus Injury

Diagnostic considerations for vascular sinus injury are guided by the presence of a penetrating injury or depressed skull fracture in proximity to a major venous sinus or by symptoms consistent with sinus occlusion that cannot be explained by other causes. Although head CT may show focal hyperdensity in an occluded sinus, MRA allows better visualization of the entire venous system. However, MRA may be difficult to obtain in the acute trauma setting. Angiography may therefore be indicated for diagnosis.

Summary

At this time, there is no single noninvasive modality that can match cerebral arteriography in diagnosing BCVI. Although many flow-limiting dissections, pseudoaneurysms, occluded arteries, and arteriovenous fistulas can be reliably detected with noninvasive modalities, their diagnostic sensitivity and specificity have not been clearly delineated. It is likely that future strategies will employ a combination of noninvasive modalities in the majority of situations, reserving angiography for the most demanding circumstances.

SCREENING FOR BLUNT CEREBROVASCULAR INJURY

It is widely believed that traumatic cerebrovascular injuries are so rare that screening is not practical. One report of 24 patients with BCIs, all with neurological symptoms at the time of diagnosis, concluded, "there was no reliable means to suspect this injury prior to neurologic or CT abnormalities."[110] There is increasing evidence, however, that BCVI is much more common than previously believed, with an incidence approaching 1% of blunt trauma admissions.[13, 19]

Fortunately, several injuries help identify BCVI. Eight asymptomatic carotid injuries were identified by screening patients with basilar skull fractures involving the carotid canal.[111] The recognized association between cervical spine fractures and VA injuries has also prompted screening. Angiography in patients with facet injuries or fractures involving the foramen transversarium demonstrated a 46% incidence of BVI.[50] Similarly, an 88% angiographic incidence of BVI was identified in patients with transverse process fractures that extended into the foramen transversarium.[112]

One study delineated a screening strategy based on both injury mechanism and physical and radiographic findings.[113] Angiography demonstrated BCVI in 27% of patients screened. The following factors were associated with BCVI: hyperextension or hyperflexion injuries, coma (Glasgow Coma Scale score <8), diffuse axonal injury of the brain, cervical spine fracture, petrous bone fracture, and Le Fort fracture.

GRADING OF BLUNT CEREBROVASCULAR INJURY

The goal of a grading system is to aid treatment and prognosis. This has been challenging, because BCVI comprises such a heterogeneous group of lesions. Fakhry and colleagues classified BCI according to the arteriographic appearance, noting the presence of spasm, "mural wrinkling," intimal dissection without narrowing, intimal dissection with narrowing, occlusion, and transection.[114] Fabian and colleagues subsequently proposed a simplified system for treatment purposes using categories of partial injury or complete transection.[13] The complete transections were treated either surgically or with interventional endovascular techniques, whereas the partial transections were generally treated with anticoagulation. In the Western Trauma Association multicenter review of BCI, Cogbill and associates concluded that "stratification of injuries by type, location, and neurologic presentation are essential to the development of rational treatment strategies."[27] Subsequently, Biffl and coworkers developed a grading scale that broadly categorizes lesions as nonhemodynamically significant injuries (grade I), potentially hemodynamically significant injuries (grade II), pseudoaneurysms (grade III), occlusions (grade IV), and transected vessels (grade V); these grades appear to have prognostic and therapeutic implications.[20]

TREATMENT OF BLUNT CEREBROVASCULAR INJURY

The optimal management of BCVI remains controversial. The goal in treating BCVI is to avoid the development or progression of neurological deficits by preventing embolization or thrombosis. Potential management strategies include observation, surgical treatment, anticoagulation, and endovascular techniques.

Although observation may be advisable in select cases of asymptomatic BCVI (especially when treatment is contraindicated by systemic injuries), the natural history of untreated symptomatic BCVI includes the potential for significant morbidity and mortality. Yamada and colleagues identified a 30% mortality associated with BCI, with 42% of survivors suffering severe, permanent neurological deficits.[21] Perry and coworkers came to a similar conclusion, reporting a 23% mortality and 54% morbidity among 17 patients with BCI.[71] More recent multicenter reviews confirmed these results, demonstrating 21% to 33% mortality and 33% to 64% morbidity.[27, 28] Early diagnosis and treatment of symptomatic lesions are imperative. The proper treatment of asymptomatic lesions identified through screening paradigms is less clear.

Surgical Treatment

Surgical treatment of BCVIs has been supplanted to a significant degree by anticoagulation and endovascular therapies, including occlusion and stent placement. In certain emergent situations, when angiography is not possible, it may be necessary to expose the carotid or vertebral arteries for ligation or, in select situations, to repair injured vessels using sutures or grafts (autologous or prosthetic). Other situations may call for vascular bypass (see Fig. 330–3). Technical details of the surgical exposure of the carotid and vertebral arteries and neurovascular bypass are covered in Chapters 97 and 102.

CAROTID ARTERY

The foundation of surgical treatment of carotid artery injuries evolved from military experience and was based on penetrating trauma. After the Korean War, most carotid injuries were explored and repaired. However, the possible danger associated with repair of the injured carotid artery in the setting of neurological deficit was also recognized.[7, 115, 116] Concern about possible conversion of ischemic brain to hemorrhagic stroke resulted in the use of artery ligation in many situations.

In 1982, Brown and coworkers reported a greater potential for neurological improvement associated with revascularization (65%) compared to ligation (13%).[117] Other authors reached similar conclusions.[46, 118] Although outcome was generally poor regardless of treatment in patients presenting in coma, patients with less severe neurological deficits appeared to do better after repair than did those treated with ligation (85% versus 50% good outcome).[118]

Experience with penetrating trauma appears to have influenced the initial treatment of BCI. Early surgical treatment for BCI in patients with transient ischemic attacks, evolving strokes, and mild complete neurological deficits was supported by Krajewski and Hertzer.[22] They reported an 86% rate of severe, permanent neurological sequelae or death in patients managed nonoperatively, compared with 53% in those undergoing arterial reconstruction. Perry and coworkers had poor results in all patients treated with ligation or nonoperatively, compared with a 75% good neurological outcome in those having arterial repair.[71]

Appropriateness is also dependent on injury type. A direct blow to the neck usually has no associated intracranial injury and may be amenable to direct repair, whereas distal ICA injuries at the skull base are often inaccessible.[25] This latter type of BCI may be effectively treated with extracranial-intracranial bypass combined with carotid artery occlusion (see Fig. 330–3).[119, 120] With advancing technology, more and more BCIs are amenable to early anticoagulation followed by endovascular treatment when indicated.

VERTEBRAL ARTERY

Early series of VA injuries, composed predominantly of penetrating injuries, recommended surgical treatment. A combined proximal and distal ligation was recommended by Meier and colleagues in any patient with a VA injury, a normal contralateral VA, and no demonstrable extracranial branches to the spinal cord.[121] Reid and Weigelt similarly recommended proximal and distal ligation for VA injuries. Their mortality rate associated with VA injury was 4.7%.[9]

Over the past decade, treatment emphasis has shifted toward use of anticoagulation and endovascular techniques. But proximal VA ligation remains an option when active hemorrhage is problematic or when large pseudoaneurysms or arteriovenous fistulas cannot be embolized.[122] Although unilateral VA ligation is usually well tolerated, an autopsy study by Thomas and colleagues demonstrated that 1.8% of right and 3.1% of left VAs do not communicate with the basilar artery.[56] Angiography is therefore recommended before ligation whenever clinically possible.

Nonsurgical Treatment

ANTICOAGULATION

Fabian and coworkers demonstrated improved neurological outcome when patients were fully anticoagulated with heparin following BCI.[13] Forty-seven of 67 patients with BCIs were treated with systemic anticoagulation. Improved neurological outcome was demonstrated in patients presenting with both minor and major neurological deficits. Heparin was identified as the only independent factor associated with improved neurological outcome. Other authors agreed on the benefit of heparinization in improving neurological outcome when vascular injuries were diagnosed early.[20, 27, 28, 113] However, some authors still dispute the value of early heparinization.[111, 123] Although early anticoagulation appears to decrease neurological deficits when instituted early, many injuries progress anatomically on repeat angiography. Definitive treatment, including the use of endovascular stenting or occlusion, remains controversial.

Patients with BCVIs are prone to complications from anticoagulation because of their multiple associated injuries, particularly of the head and face. They are also at risk for spontaneous hemorrhage of the retroperitoneum or gastrointestinal tract. Although Fabian and coworkers reported improved neurological outcome with early heparinization, morbidity and mortality were adversely affected by bleeding complications.[13] Bleeding complications were decreased by Biffl and colleagues from 54% to 18% by lowering the dose of heparin (partial thromboplastin time, 50 to 60 seconds).[124] It remains unclear whether antiplatelet agents will afford the benefits of heparinization while decreasing treatment risk.

ENDOVASCULAR TREATMENT

Endovascular Stenting

Coronary and large central arteries have been successfully treated with endovascular techniques, including stents,[125] but stenting of the carotid artery for atherosclerotic disease[126] and trauma is still under investigation,[127–129] although it can be effective in restoring normal carotid artery architecture (Fig. 330–6). Coldwell and associates reported successful treatment of both carotid dissections and pseudoaneurysms following trauma.[129] Sixteen of 18 carotid stents placed in 14 patients were patent on follow-up arteriography. Three patients suffered complications related to treatment. Two patients had stent thrombosis (one with cerebral infarction), and one patient developed tran-

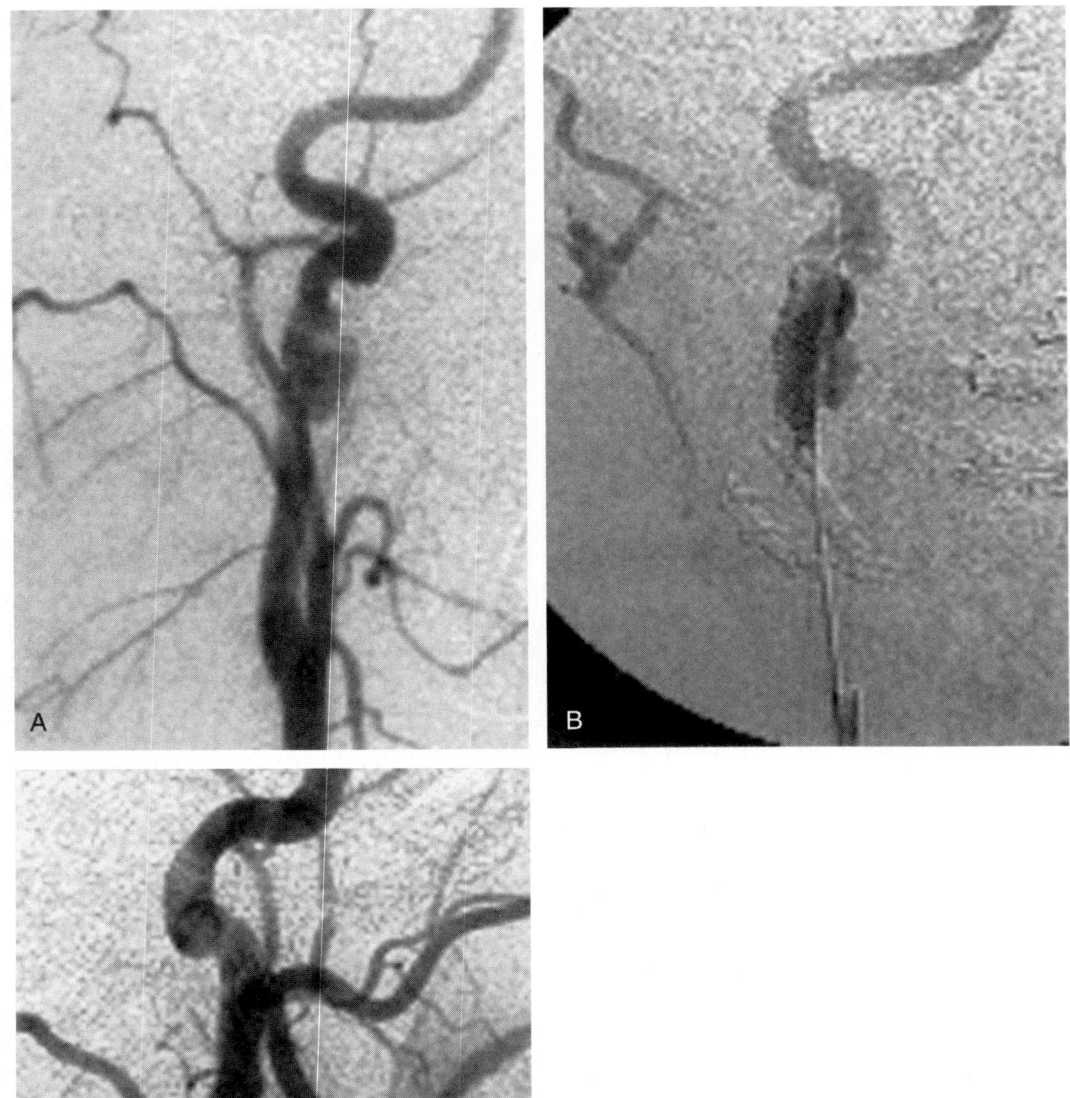

FIGURE 330–6. *A,* Initial screening carotid angiogram of a 21-year-old man involved in a motor vehicle accident. His injuries included a minor traumatic brain injury, C1 fracture, and ipsilateral mandible fracture. Carotid pseudoaneurysm was diagnosed and initially treated with heparin (partial thromboplastin time, 50). He remained neurologically stable with no infarct on head computed tomography. *B,* Follow-up angiography 1 week later demonstrates increased pseudoaneurysm size. He was treated with an endovascular stent and placed on warfarin (Coumadin) for 3 months. *C,* Angiography 3 months after stent placement demonstrates normal internal carotid artery anatomy. Aspirin was continued for an additional 3 months. The patient made a full recovery.

sient ischemic attacks. All complications were associated with early cessation of or inadequate anticoagulation. Although antiplatelet therapy may be adequate following stenting for atherosclerotic carotid disease,[126] it appears that anticoagulation may be required, at least in the early post-treatment period, after stenting for traumatic vascular injury. Optimal patient selection and optimal use, timing, and duration of anticoagulation remain to be determined.

Selective Arterial Embolization

Whereas stenting is more commonly used in the carotid artery, selective arterial embolization has been used in the VA as an alternative to surgical ligation. Kobernick and Carmody first described this technique to treat blunt transection of the VA.[130] As stenting technology improves, it will likely make VA preservation possible in many cases.

CONCLUSIONS

Many questions remain to be answered regarding the natural history, diagnosis, and optimal treatment of traumatic cerebrovascular injury. BCVI, in particular, appears to be underdiagnosed, and optimization of cost-effective screening strategies is required. The specific roles of surgery, anticoagulation, and endovascular therapies remain to be determined.

REFERENCES

1. Fogelman MJ, Stewart RD: Penetrating wounds of the neck. Am J Surg 91:581–599, 1956.
2. Fitchett VH, Pomerantz M, Butsch DW, et al: Penetrating wounds of the neck: A military and civilian experience. Arch Surg 99:307–314, 1969.
3. Biffl WL, Moore EE, Degmar H, et al: Selective management of penetrating neck trauma based on cervical level of injury. Am J Surg 174:678–682, 1997.
4. Verneuil M: Contusions multiples; delire violent; hemiplegie a droite, signes de compression cerebrale. Bull Acad Natl Med (Paris) 36:46–56, 1872.
5. Jones RF, Terrell JC, Salyer KE: Penetrating wounds of the neck: An analysis of 274 cases. J Trauma 7:228–237, 1967.
6. Pierce W, Whitehill T: Carotid and vertebral arterial injuries. Surg Clin North Am 68:705–723, 1988.
7. Cohen CA, Brief D, Mathewson C Jr: Carotid artery injuries: An analysis of eighty-five cases. Am J Surg 120:210–214, 1970.
8. Karlin RM, Marks C: Extracranial carotid artery injury: Current surgical management. Am J Surg 146:225–227, 1983.
9. Reid JDS, Weigelt JA: Forty-three cases of vertebral artery trauma. J Trauma 28:1007–1012, 1988.
10. Golueke P, Sclafani S, Phillips T, et al: Vertebral artery injury—diagnosis and management. J Trauma 27:856–865, 1987.
11. Rich NM, Hobson RW, Collins GJ: Traumatic arteriovenous fistulas and false aneurysms: A review of 558 lesions. Surgery 78:817–828, 1975.
12. Levy ML, Rezai A, Masri LS, et al: The significance of subarachnoid hemorrhage after penetrating craniocerebral injury: Correlations with angiography and outcome in a civilian population. Neurosurgery 32:532–540, 1993.
13. Fabian TC, Patton JH Jr, Croce MA, et al: Blunt carotid injury: Importance of early diagnosis and anticoagulant therapy. Ann Surg 223:513–525, 1996.
14. Hellner D, Thie A, Lachenmayer L, et al: Blunt trauma lesions of the extracranial internal carotid artery in patients with head injury. J Craniomaxillofac Surg 21:234–238, 1993.
15. Mokri B: Traumatic and spontaneous extracranial internal carotid artery dissections. J Neurol 237:356–361, 1990.
16. Parikh AA, Luchette FA, Valente JF, et al: Blunt carotid artery injuries. J Am Coll Surg 185:80–86, 1997.
17. Ramadan F, Rutledge R, Oller D, et al: Carotid artery trauma: A review of contemporary trauma center experiences. J Vasc Surg 21:46–56, 1995.
18. Welling RE, Saul TJ, Tew JM Jr, et al: Management of blunt injury to the internal carotid artery. J Trauma 27:1221–1226, 1987.
19. Biffl WL, Moore EE, Ryu RK, et al: The unrecognized epidemic of blunt carotid arterial injuries: Early diagnosis improves neurologic outcome. Ann Surg 228:462–470, 1998.
20. Biffl WL, Moore EE, Offner PJ, et al: Blunt carotid arterial injuries: Implications of a new grading scale. J Trauma 47:845–853, 1999.
21. Yamada S, Kindt GW, Youmans JR: Carotid artery occlusion due to nonpenetrating injury. J Trauma 7:333–342, 1967.
22. Krajewski LP, Hertzer NR: Blunt carotid artery trauma: Report of two cases and review of the literature. Ann Surg 191:341–346, 1980.
23. Rubio PA, Ruel GJ Jr, Beall AC Jr, et al: Acute carotid artery injury: 25 years' experience. J Trauma 14:967–973, 1974.
24. Fry RE, Fry WJ: Extracranial carotid artery injuries. Surgery 88:581–587, 1980.
25. Richardson JD, Simpson C, Miller FB: Management of carotid artery trauma. Surgery 104:673–680, 1988.
26. Fabian TC, Georges SM, Croce MA Jr, et al: Carotid artery trauma: Management based on mechanism of injury. J Trauma 30:953–963, 1990.
27. Cogbill TH, Moore EE, Meissner M, et al: The spectrum of blunt injury to the carotid artery: A multicenter perspective. J Trauma 37:473–479, 1994.
28. Davis JW, Holbrook TL, Hoyt DB, et al: Blunt carotid artery dissection: Incidence, associated injuries, screening, and treatment. J Trauma 30:1514–1517, 1990.
29. Martin RF, Eldrup-Jorgensen J, Clark DE, et al: Blunt trauma to the carotid arteries. J Vasc Surg 14:789–795, 1991.
30. Punjabi AP, Plaisier BR, Haug, RH, et al.: Diagnosis and management of blunt carotid artery injury in oral and maxillofacial surgery. J Oral Maxillofac Surg 55:1388–1396, 1997.
31. Crissey MM, Bernstein EF: Delayed presentation of carotid intimal tear following blunt craniocervical trauma. Surgery 75:543–549, 1974.
32. Zelenock GB, Kazmers A, Whitehouse WM Jr, et al: Extracranial internal carotid artery dissections: Noniatrogenic traumatic lesions. Arch Surg 117:425–432, 1982.
33. Baik S, Uku JM, Joo KG: Seat-belt injuries to the left common carotid artery and left internal carotid artery. Am J Forensic Med Pathol 9:38–39, 1988.
34. Chedid MK, Deeb ZL, Rothfus WE, et al: Major cerebral vessels injury caused by a seatbelt shoulder strap: Case report. J Trauma 29:1601–1603, 1989.
35. Mokri B, Piepgras DG, Houser OW: Traumatic dissections of the extracranial internal carotid artery. J Neurosurg 68:189–197, 1988.
36. Sundt TM Jr, Pearson BW, Piepgras DG, et al: Surgical management of aneurysms of the distal extracranial internal carotid artery. J Neurosurg 64:169–182, 1986.
37. Zelenock G, Kazmers A, Whitehouse W, et al: Extracranial internal carotid artery dissections. Arch Surg 117:425–432, 1982.
38. Batnitzky S, Price HI, Holden RW, et al: Cervical internal carotid artery injuries due to blunt trauma. AJNR Am J Neuroradiol 4:292–295, 1983.
39. Hughes JT, Brownell B: Traumatic thrombosis of the internal carotid artery in the neck. J Neurol Neurosurg Psychiatry 31:307–314, 1968.
40. Boldrey E, Maass L, Miller RR: Role of atlantoid compression in etiology of internal carotid thrombosis. J Neurosurg 13:127–139, 1956.
41. Melio FR, Jones JL, Djang WT: Internal carotid artery thrombosis in a child secondary to intraoral trauma. J Emerg Med 14:429–433, 1996.
42. Pitner SE: Carotid thrombosis due to intraoral trauma. N Engl J Med 274:764–767, 1966.
43. Moriarty KP, Harris BH, Benitez-Marchand K: Carotid artery thrombosis and stroke after blunt pharyngeal injury. J Trauma 42:541–543, 1997.
44. Woodhurst WB, Robertson WD, Thompson GB: Carotid injury due to intraoral trauma: Case report and review of the literature. Neurosurgery 6:559–563, 1980.
45. Carter DA, Mehelas TJ, Savolaine ER, et al: Basal skull fracture with traumatic polycranial neuropathy and occluded left carotid artery: Significance of fractures along the course of the carotid artery. J Trauma 44:230–235, 1998.
46. Unger SW, Tucker WS Jr, Mrdeza MA, et al: Carotid arterial trauma. Surgery 87:477–487, 1980.
47. Janon EA: Traumatic changes in the internal carotid artery associated with basal skull fractures. Radiology 96:55–59, 1970.
48. Hinse P, Thie A, Lachenmayer L: Dissection of the extracranial vertebral artery: Report of four cases and review of the literature. J Neurol Neurosurg Psychiatry 54:863–869, 1991.
49. Mas JL, Bousser MG, Hasboun D, et al: Extracranial vertebral

artery dissections: A review of 13 cases. Stroke 18:1037–1047, 1987.

50. Willis BK, Greiner F, Orrison WW, et al: The incidence of vertebral artery injury after midcervical spine fracture or subluxation. Neurosurgery 34:435–442, 1994.

51. Woodring JH, Lee C, Duncan V: Transverse process fractures of the cervical vertebrae: Are they insignificant? J Trauma 34:797–802, 1993.

52. Parent AD, Harkey HL, Touchstone DA, et al: Lateral cervical spine dislocation and vertebral artery injury. Neurosurgery 31:501–509, 1992.

53. Showalter W, Esekogwu V, Newton KI, et al: Vertebral artery dissection. Acad Emerg Med 4:991–995, 1997.

54. Friedman D, Flanders A, Thomas C, et al: Vertebral artery injury after acute cervical spine trauma: Rate of occurrence as detected by MR angiography and assessment of clinical consequences. AJR Am J Roentgenol 164:443–449, 1995.

55. Vaccaro AR, Klein GR, Flanders AE, et al: Long-term evaluation of vertebral artery injuries following cervical spine trauma using magnetic resonance angiography. Spine 23:789–795, 1998.

56. Thomas GI, Anderson KN, Hain RF, et al: The significance of anomalous basilar artery communications in operations on the heart and great vessels. Surgery 46:747–757, 1959.

57. Josien E: Extracranial vertebral artery dissection: Nine cases. J Neurol 239:327–330, 1992.

58. Kaplan SS, Ogilvy CS, Gonzalez R, et al: Extracranial vertebral artery pseudoaneurysm presenting as subarachnoid hemorrhage. Stroke 24:1397–1399, 1993; see comments.

59. Bogousslavsky J, Despland PA, Regli F: Spontaneous carotid dissection with acute stroke. Arch Neurol 44:137–140, 1987.

60. O'Sullivan RM, Graeb DA, Nugent RA, et al: Carotid and vertebral artery trauma: Clinical and angiographic features. Australas Radiol 35:47–55, 1991.

61. Eachempati SR, Sebastian MW, Reed RL II: Posttraumatic bilateral carotid artery and right vertebral artery dissections in a patient with fibromuscular dysplasia: Case report and review of the literature. J Trauma 44:406–409, 1998.

62. Young PH, Smith KR Jr, Crafts DC, et al: Traumatic occlusion in fibromuscular dysplasia of the carotid artery. Surg Neurol 16:432–437, 1981.

63. Trosch RM, Hasbani M, Brass LM: "Bottoms up" dissection. N Engl J Med 320:1564–1565, 1989.

64. El Gindi S, Salama M, Tawfik E, et al: A review of 2000 patients with craniocerebral injuries with regard to intracranial hematomas and other vascular complications. Acta Neurochir (Wien) 48:237–244, 1979.

65. Solheim K: Common carotid artery aneurysm after blunt trauma. J Trauma 19:707–709, 1979.

66. Holmes B, Harbaugh RE: Traumatic intracranial aneurysms: A contemporary review. J Trauma 35:855–860, 1993.

67. Schuster JM, Santiago P, Elliott JP, et al: Acute traumatic posteroinferior cerebellar artery aneurysms: Report of three cases. Neurosurgery 45:1465–1468, 1999.

68. Love L, Marsan RE: Carotid cavernous fistula. Angiology 25:231–236, 1974.

69. Meier U, Gartner F, Knopf W, et al: The traumatic dural sinus injury: A clinical study. Acta Neurochir (Wien) 119:91–93, 1992.

70. Taha JM, Crone KR, Berger TS, et al: Sigmoid sinus thrombosis after closed head injury in children. Neurosurgery 32:541–546, 1993.

71. Perry MO, Snyder WH, Thal ER: Carotid artery injuries caused by blunt trauma. Ann Surg 192:74–77, 1980.

72. Mokri B, Piepgras DG, Sundt T, et al: Extracranial internal carotid artery aneurysms. Mayo Clin Proc 57:310–321, 1982.

73. Sturzenegger M: Spontaneous internal carotid artery dissection: Early diagnosis and management in 44 patients. J Neurol 242:231–238, 1995.

74. Mokri B, Sundt TM Jr, Houser OW, et al: Spontaneous dissection of the cervical internal carotid artery. Ann Neurol 19:126–138, 1986.

75. Biousse V, D'Anglejan-Chatillon J, Massiou H, et al: Head pain in non-traumatic carotid artery dissection: A series of 65 patients. Cephalalgia 14:33–36, 1994.

76. Hart RG, Easton JD: Dissections of cervical and cerebral arteries. Neurol Clin 1:155–182, 1983.

77. Gouny P, Nowak C, Smarrito S, et al: Bilateral thrombosis of the internal carotid arteries after a closed trauma: Advantages of magnetic resonance imaging and review of the literature. J Cardiovasc Surg (Torino) 39:417–424, 1998.

78. Stahmer SA, Raps EC, Mines DI: Carotid and vertebral artery dissections. Emerg Med Clin North Am 15:677–698, 1997.

79. de Bray JM, Penisson-Besnier I, Dubas F, et al: Extracranial and intracranial vertebrobasilar dissections: Diagnosis and prognosis. J Neurol Neurosurg Psychiatry 63:46–51, 1997.

80. Asai T, Kataoka K, Uejima T, et al: Traumatic laceration of the intracranial vertebral artery causing fatal subarachnoid hemorrhage: Case report. Surg Neurol 45:566–569, 1996.

81. Miyazaki T, Kojima T, Chikasue F, et al: Traumatic rupture of intracranial vertebral artery due to hyperextension of the head: Reports on three cases. Forensic Sci Int 47:91–98, 1990.

82. Heinsius T, Bogousslavsky J, Van Melle G: Large infarcts in the middle cerebral artery territory: Etiology and outcome patterns. Neurology 50:341–350, 1998.

83. Cohen SM: Clinical manifestations and evaluation of patients with ischemic cerebrovascular disease. In Rutherford RB (ed): Vascular Surgery. Philadelphia, WB Saunders, 1995, pp 1474–1480.

84. Chen D, Concus AP, Halbach VV, et al: Epistaxis originating from traumatic pseudoaneurysm of the internal carotid artery: Diagnosis and endovascular therapy. Laryngoscope 108:326–331, 1998.

85. Lee JP, Wang AD: Epistaxis due to traumatic intracavernous aneurysm: Case report. J Trauma 30:619–622, 1990.

86. Kinal ME: Traumatic thrombosis of dural venous sinuses in closed head injury. J Neurosurg 27:142–145, 1967.

87. Kapp JP, Gielchinsky I, Deardourff SL: Operative techniques for management of lesions involving the dural venous sinuses. Surg Neurol 7:339–342, 1977.

88. Rish BL: The repair of dural venous sinus wounds by autogenous venorrhaphy. J Neurosurg 35:392–395, 1971.

89. Feldman RA, Hieshima G, Giannotta SL, et al: Traumatic dural arteriovenous fistula supplied by scalp, meningeal, and cortical arteries: Case report. Neurosurgery 6:670–674, 1980.

90. Hirshberg A, Wall MJ, Johnston RH, et al: Transcervical gunshot injuries. Am J Surg 167:309–312, 1994.

91. Demetriades D, Theodorou D, Asensio J, et al: Transcervical gunshot injuries: Mandatory operation is not necessary. J Trauma 40:758–760, 1996.

92. Panetta TF, Hunt JP, Buechter KJ, et al: Duplex ultrasonography versus arteriography in the diagnosis of arterial injury: An experimental study. J Trauma 33:627–636, 1992.

93. Fry WR, Dort JA, Smith RS, et al: Duplex scanning replaces arteriography and operative exploration in the diagnosis of potential cervical vascular injury. Am J Surg 168:693–696, 1994.

94. Nagler RM, Braun J, Daitzman M, et al: Spiral CT angiography: An alternative vascular evaluation technique for head and neck microvascular reconstruction. Plast Reconstr Surg 100:1697–1702, 1997.

95. Leclerc X, Godefroy O, Salhi A, et al: Helical CT for the diagnosis of extracranial internal carotid artery dissection. Stroke 27:461–466, 1996.

96. Egelhof T, Jansen O, Winter R, et al: CT angiography in dissections of the internal carotid artery: Value of a new examination technique in comparison with DSA and Doppler ultrasound [German]. Radiologe 36:850–854, 1996.

97. Link J, Brossman J, Grabener M, et al: Spiral CT angiography and selective digital subtraction angiography of internal carotid artery stenosis. AJNR Am J Neuroradiol 17:89–94, 1996.

98. Simeone A, Carriero A, Armillota M, et al: Spiral CT angiography in the study of the carotid stenoses. J Neuroradiol 24:18–22, 1997.

99. Biffl WL, Moore EE, Mestek M: Patients with blunt carotid and vertebral artery injuries [letter]. J Trauma 47:438–439, 1999.

100. Papp Z, Patel M, Ashtari M, et al: Carotid artery stenosis: Optimization of CT angiography with a combination of shaded surface display and source images. AJNR Am J Neuroradiol 18:759–763, 1997.

101. Moseley ME, Cohen Y, Mintorovitch J: Early detection of regional cerebral ischemia in cats: Comparison of diffusion- and T2-weighted MRI and spectroscopy. Magn Reson Med 14:330–346, 1990.

102. Bok APL, Peter JC: Carotid and vertebral artery occlusion after blunt cervical injury: The role of MR angiography in early diagnosis. J Trauma 40:968–972, 1996.

103. Laitt RD, Lewis TT, Bradshaw JR: Blunt carotid arterial trauma. Clin Radiol 51:117–122, 1996.

104. Aaslid R, Markwalder TM, Nornes H: Noninvasive transcranial Doppler ultrasound recording of flow velocity in basal cerebral arteries. J Neurosurg 57:769–774, 1982.

105. Aaslid R: Developments and principles of transcranial Doppler. In Newell DW, Aaslid R (eds): Transcranial Doppler. New York, Raven Press, 1992, pp 1–8.

106. Padayachee TS, Parsons S, Theobald R, et al: The detection of microemboli in the middle cerebral artery during cardiopulmonary bypass: A transcranial Doppler ultrasound investigation using membrane and bubble oxygenators. Ann Thorac Surg 44: 298–302, 1987.

107. Spencer MP, Thomas GI, Nicholls SC, et al: Detection of middle cerebral artery emboli during carotid endarterectomy using transcranial Doppler ultrasonography. Stroke 21:415–423, 1990.

108. Pugsley W, Klinger L, Paschalis C: Microemboli and cerebral impairment during cardiac surgery. Vasc Surg 24:34–43, 1990.

109. Srinivasan J, Newell DW, Sturzenegger M, et al: Transcranial Doppler in the evaluation of internal carotid artery dissection. Stroke 27:1226–1230, 1996.

110. Carrillo EH, Osborne DL, Spain DA, et al: Blunt carotid artery injuries: Difficulties with the diagnosis prior to neurologic event. J Trauma 46:1120–1125, 1999.

111. Eachempati SR, Vaslef SN, Sebastian MW, et al: Blunt vascular injuries of the head and neck: Is heparinization necessary? J Trauma 45:997–1004, 1998.

112. Woodring JH, Lee C, Duncan V: Transverse process fractures of the cervical vertebrae: Are they insignificant? J Trauma 34: 797–802, 1993.

113. Biffl WL, Moore EE, Offner PJ, et al: Optimizing screening for blunt cerebrovascular injuries. Am J Surg 178:517–522, 1999.

114. Fakhry SM, Jaques PF, Proctor HJ: Cervical vessel injury after blunt trauma. J Vasc Surg 8:501–508, 1988.

115. Bradley EL III: Management of penetrating carotid injuries: An alternative approach. J Trauma 13:248–255, 1973.

116. Ledgerwood AM, Mullins RJ, Lucas CE: Primary repair vs ligation for carotid artery injuries. Arch Surg 115:488–493, 1980.

117. Brown MF, Graham JM, Feliciano DV, et al: Carotid artery injuries. Am J Surg 144:748–753, 1982.

118. Liekweg WG Jr, Greenfield LJ: Management of penetrating carotid arterial injury. Ann Surg 188:587–592, 1978.

119. D'Alise MD, Vardiman AB, Kopitnik TA Jr, et al: External carotid-to-middle cerebral bypass in the treatment of complex internal carotid injury. J Trauma 40:452–455, 1996.

120. Vishteh AG, Maricano FF, David CA, et al: Long-term graft patency rates and clinical outcomes after revascularization for symptomatic traumatic internal carotid artery dissection. Neurosurgery 43:761–768, 1998.

121. Meier DE, Brink BE, Fry WJ: Vertebral artery trauma: Acute recognition and treatment. Arch Surg 116:236–239, 1981.

122. Demetriades D, Theodorou D, Asensio J, et al: Management options in vertebral artery injuries. Br J Surg 83:83–86, 1996.

123. Colella JJ, Diamond DL: Blunt carotid injury: Reassessing the role of anticoagulation. Am Surg 62:212–217, 1996.

124. Biffl WL, Moore EE, Elliott JP, et al: Blunt cerebrovascular injuries. Curr Probl Surg 36:507–599, 1999.

125. Ryu R: Endovascular stents and clinical applications: The state of the art. Appl Radiol 26(Suppl):63–70, 1997.

126. Higashida RT: Carotid interventions: PTA and stenting. J Vasc Interv Radiol 12:84–88, 1998.

127. Bernstein SM, Coldwell DM, Prall JA, et al: Treatment of traumatic carotid pseudoaneurysm with endovascular stent placement. J Vasc Interv Radiol 8:1065–1068, 1997.

128. Duke BJ, Ryu RK, Coldwell DM, et al: Treatment of blunt injury to the carotid artery by using endovascular stents: An early experience. J Neurosurg 87:825–829, 1997.

129. Coldwell DM, Novak Z, Ryu RK, et al: Treatment of posttraumatic internal carotid arterial pseudoaneurysms with endovascular stents. J Trauma 48:470–472, 2000.

130. Kobernick M, Carmody R: Vertebral artery transection from blunt trauma treated by embolization. J Trauma 24:854–856, 1984.

CHAPTER 331

Bullet Wounds to the Brain among Civilians

MICHAEL E. CAREY

EFFECTS OF WOUNDING

The Physical Substrate

A missile (e.g., a bullet) causes damage by depositing energy within tissue; it crushes tissue directly in its path and sets up pressure waves that can cause damage beyond its path. Missile trajectory is a major consideration in the lethality of an intracranial missile—a crushed brainstem is simply incompatible with life. A missile traveling faster than the speed of sound when it impacts tissue causes a sonic wave to radiate outward from the point of impact. This sonic wave has an extremely high pressure but lasts only microseconds and is not thought to cause tissue damage. The moving missile also displaces tissue radially from its path, which creates low-pressure waves within the tissue. These low-pressure waves are not as intense as the sonic wave, but they last milliseconds and cause damage adjacent to the wound track and also at a considerable distance from it.[1]

A missile fired into a cerebral hemisphere many centimeters from the brainstem causes brainstem effects, including apnea.[2-5] Besides these immediate effects, intracranial bleeding may further compromise the brain. Later effects of brain wounding include brain edema[6] and possibly infection. Other factors such as hypotension and hypoxia may also impair brain function.

Skull Fractures

Skull fractures are commonly associated with brain wounding. The greater the missile energy of deposit, the more extensive the skull fracturing. Fractures may be around the bullet entry site or remote from it, including the orbital roof. Fractures are more frequent with contact wounds.[7]

The Bullet Track

Freytag's[7] autopsy series of 254 people who died from bullet wounds to the brain indicated a single missile

This review is condensed from "Civilian Brain Wounds from Bullets," *Neurosurgery Quarterly* 10:1–41, 2000.

track in 82%; the remainder had multiple tracks throughout the brain from internal ricochets. Thirty-one of Kirkpatrick and Di Maio's[8] 42 autopsy cases also had a single wound track, and 11 exhibited intracerebral ricochets. Freytag[7] believed that most brain wound tracks corresponded to bullet diameter and were uniform throughout their length. High-velocity bullets produced uniformly large tracks, and such wounds were associated with a ring of ischemic tissue around the wound canal, with a zone of small hemorrhages outside the ischemic ring. She postulated that the ischemia resulted from sudden tissue compression associated with temporary cavity formation when the bullet passed.

Kirkpatrick and Di Maio's[8] studies on fixed brains indicated that bullet tracks were not uniform but varied in size and shape according to the amount of energy transferred from the moving missile to the brain. More kinetic energy is transferred to surrounding brain where the missile undergoes greatest slowing, such as when the bullet tumbles and presents its long axis to the flight path. Brain tissue in the region of slowing is thrust farther radially from the missile track; consequently, the missile track cavity is larger in this area. Contact wounds were associated with both large and small tracks. Gas from propellant combustion appeared to exhibit little effect on the brain wound; apparently, scalp and skull dissipated any effects of the gas jet. These investigators postulated that the dividing line between low- and high-velocity wounds was a bullet speed of 1500 feet/second, because a marked increase in brain wound severity occurred when the bullet muzzle velocity was 2000 feet/second or higher.

Mechanism of Death

Thirty-nine of Kirkpatrick and Di Maio's[8] 42 fatal cases showed signs of increased intracranial pressure evidenced by basifrontal contusions, tentorial grooves on the uncus, or cerebellar tonsillar coning caused by forcible, temporary displacement of brain tissue against bone or dural ridges by the brief but severe increase in intracranial pressure associated with bullet passage.

Freytag[7] noted that cerebellar tonsillar herniation was frequently seen in supratentorial wounds, and medullary contusions were often seen adjacent to the cerebellar tonsils. When the cerebellar tonsils became contused, hemorrhagic, and swollen from transient impaction against the foramen magnum, they could compress the medulla and cause respiratory arrest.

Freytag[7] believed that transient brainstem axial distortion from supratentorial overpressure might also cause respiratory paralysis leading to death. She emphasized that respiratory paralysis was often the cause of death from brain wounds, and she likened the traumatic respiratory dysfunction to concussive unconsciousness.

Kirkpatrick and Di Maio[8] noted cerebellar tonsillar hemorrhage in only 2 of their 42 fatal brain wound cases but essentially agreed with Freytag[7] concerning the cause of death, because the volume of grossly damaged brain was often trivial.

Experimental studies confirm Freytag's hypothesis. When anesthetized cats received a 2-mm pellet missile into the right cerebral hemisphere, local tissue destruction was minimal. The probability of fatal apnea, however, rose with increasing energy deposit within the brain, even though the brainstem was not directly involved: if 0.9 J were deposited, 14% of animals became fatally apneic; with 1.4 J, 40% had fatal apnea; when 2.4 J were deposited, 67% sustained fatal apnea.[5]

Koszyca and colleagues[9] studied the distribution of axonal damage throughout the brain immunohistologically in 14 individuals who died shortly after sustaining brain wounds. Using amyloid precursor protein as a marker for axonal damage, they determined that a brain missile wound caused widespread axon injury, particularly in the brainstem. They inferred that such brainstem axon destruction could be responsible for missile-induced apnea.

DEMOGRAPHICS AND RELATED DATA

Men are far more likely to be victims of brain gunshot wounds (GSWs) than are women, with the peak incidence usually in the third and fourth decades (Table

T A B L E 3 3 1 – 1 ■ **Demographics of Civilian Brain Gunshot Wounds in 31 Studies**

AUTHOR	YEAR	NO. IN SERIES	DURA PENETRATED	KNOWN ATTEMPTED HOMICIDE	KNOWN ATTEMPTED SUICIDE	KNOWN ACCIDENT	MALE	FEMALE	AGE
Goodman & Kalsbeck[10]	1965	23	19	—	23	—	22	1	19–71 yr
Yashon et al[11]	1972	154	105	—	—	—	119	35	16–66 yr
Byrnes et al[12]	1974	93	93	—	—	—	89	4	1st–8th decade
Lillard[13]	1978	83	83	59	15	9	68	15	29–64 yr
Hernesniemi[14]	1979	90	90	—	78	—	87	3	12–81 yr
Sherman et al[15]	1980	79	79	—	27	—	64	15	1st–8th decade
Brandt et al[16]	1983	23	18	5	16	2	—	—	—
Shoung et al[17]	1985	56	56	15	35	6	47	9	5–78 yr
Suddaby et al[18]	1987	49	49	1	43	4	43	6	8–92 yr
Clark et al[19]	1986	76	76	41	35	—	67	9	—
Kaufman et al[20]	1986	143	136	82	61	—	118	25	1st–9th decade
Nagib et al[21]	1986	55	55	29	21	5	50	5	5–77 yr
Cavaliere et al[22]	1988	178	178	43	126	9	150	28	2–89 yr
Mancuso et al[23]	1988	40	40	—	—	—	37	3	5–70 yr
Selden et al[24]	1988	67	67	—	65	—	58	9	8–87 yr
Sarnaik et al[25]	1989	14	14	—	—	—	—	—	1–12 yr
Miner et al[26]	1990	33	33	3	11	17	23	10	8 mo–15 yr
Grahm et al[27]	1990	100	93	24	63	3	84	16	8 mo–87 yr
Benzel et al[28]	1991	120	120	59	32	12	96	24	4 mo–77 yr
Levi et al[29]	1991	31	31	10	14	7	27	4	8–65 yr
Siccardi et al[30]	1991	314	314	78	217	—	278	36	1st–9th decade
Aldrich et al[31]	1992	151	151	—	—	—	124	27	—*
Helling et al[32]	1992	89	89	34	42	11	81	8	13–73 yr
Shaffrey et al[33]	1992	62	62	—	37	—	54	8	10–72 yr
Deshmukh et al[34]	1992	107	107	107	0	0	90	17	15–45 yr†
Kennedy et al[35]	1993	192	192	—	~10	—	—	—	—
Levy et al[36]	1994	190	190	170	17	3	169	21	2–47 yr
Pikus & Ball[37]	1995	35	35	2	33	—	31	4	17–80 yr
Stone et al[38]	1995	480	230	450	27	—	432	48	1.5–82 yr
Freytag[7]‡	1963	254	254	85	147	21	—	—	—
Kirkpatrick & Di Maio[8]‡	1978	42	42	15	26	—	36	6	2nd–6th decade
Total		3423	3101	1312	1221	109	2544	396	3rd–4th decade

*146 of 151 were older than 16 years.
†Encompasses "most brain injuries."
‡Autopsy studies.

331–1). GSWs in those older than 50 years are often self-inflicted by depressed or infirm people attempting to end their lives. Suicides were most frequent in those 50 to 60 years of age, homicides predominated in the 20- to 30-year age group, and accidents occurred in children and teenagers.[7]

Whether more GSWs result from homicide or suicide reflects the mores of the report's country of origin. Almost all cases in Hernesniemi's[14] Finnish series and Siccardi and coworkers'[30] series from Genoa, Italy, were suicide attempts. These European reports contrast with those from the United States, where guns and gang warfare are common. In Levy and associates'[36] series of 190 patients admitted to Los Angeles County Hospital, 170 were homicide attempts and only 17 were suicide attempts. The single exception to assaults being rarer in European studies is Byrnes and colleagues'[12] report from Northern Ireland, where most if not all cases were homicide attempts resulting from the ongoing civil war. Hunting accidents may account for a large portion of cases in rural areas.[39] Miner and co-workers'[26] data indicate that most children are wounded accidentally. Startlingly, however, one third of the children in that series, all older than 10 years, attempted suicide using an unsecured handgun in the home.

Race

Whites, especially men, attempt suicide more often than blacks; blacks attempt homicide more frequently than whites. For instance, 86% of the attempted suicides in Clark and coworkers'[19] series occurred in whites, and 78% of the attempted homicides occurred in blacks. Naturally, all racial data must be interpreted in the context of the racial composition of the community the hospital serves.

Suicide and the Side of Bullet Entry

Ninety-seven of 147 suicide victims in Freytag's[7] autopsy study shot themselves in the right temple, 14 in the left temple, and 21 in the forehead. Clinical studies show the same trends. Goodman and Kalsbeck[10] stated that the bullet entered the right side four times as often as the left. Sherman,[15] Kaufman,[20] and Seldon[24] and their coauthors noted a right-sided entry in 68%, 64%, and 63% of suicide attempts, respectively. Miner and colleagues'[26] study of 33 children reported a right-sided entry in all 11 suicide attempts.

Age and Outcome

Sherman and associates[15] noted that 70% of patients older than 60 died, but in those 21 to 40 years of age, mortality was only 15%. In Kaufman and coworkers'[20] series, survival was better for those in the first decade and poor after age 40 years. Suddaby and colleagues,[18] studying .22-caliber brain wounds, stated that those younger than 40 years had a slightly better outcome, and Narayan and associates[40] noted that increasing age

was a powerful negative prognostic factor for those with a Glasgow Coma Scale (GCS) score greater than 5. Investigators, including Benzel,[28] Hernesniemi,[14] Kennedy,[35] Lillard,[13] Shaffrey,[33] and their associates could not correlate age with outcome.

Bullet Caliber

Bullet calibers were not always known, but some investigators thought that increasing bullet caliber positively correlated with a fatal outcome[10, 13, 17, 41]; others could not support this relationship.* Yashon and associates,[11] for instance, documented both nonfatal and fatal brain wounds caused by bullets from .22 to .45 caliber.

Clearly, even the smallest-caliber bullet commonly used today is quite capable of inflicting a fatal brain wound because its energy of deposit is high enough to severely damage the brainstem either by a direct hit or indirectly from cerebellar pressure coning, axial displacement, or axon tearing, irrespective of trajectory. This mitigates against finding a correlation between bullet caliber and mortality in the clinical setting.

Bullet caliber should not be thought of as synonymous with bullet energy. For example, the M-16 rifle uses about a .25-caliber bullet, but the M-16 bullet has much more energy than a .45-caliber bullet.

Circumstances

Some investigators[18, 24, 37] have observed high mortalities (51% to 84%) in series largely comprising attempted suicides, which they attributed to the proximity of the gun to the head. Over distances commonly employed, however, a bullet loses only a small fraction of its muzzle velocity, so the distance of the gun from the head is of small import.[8] Further, gas from propellant combustion has little effect on the brain wound.[8]

Mortality differences between attempted suicide and homicide may reflect bullet trajectory. Suicide attempts usually involve a bullet trajectory into or near the thalamus, basal ganglia, or upper brainstem. Unless the homicide attempt is "execution" style, the bullet trajectory may be more random within the brain and miss vital brain centers. Random trajectories may explain why accidental brain wounds often have a lower mortality. Siccardi and colleagues,[30] commenting on the equivalent mortalities of assaults and suicide attempts in their series, believed that most assaults were really premeditated homicide attempts. Taking careful aim ensured that assault and attempted suicide wounds produced equally severe brain wounds and equal mortalities.

Alcohol and Drugs

A few investigators[7, 10, 19, 20, 34, 37, 41] have cited alcohol and illegal drugs as contributing factors to GSWs, but up to 90% of GSW victims are not routinely screened for alcohol or drugs,[34] so their exact importance is unknown. Although alcohol seems to have some rele-

---

*See references 7, 11, 14, 21, 24, 26, 27, 29–31, 33, 37.

vance to brain wounds in civilians, it does not appear to be the major factor accounting for the current epidemic of brain GSWs in the United States. A glance at any newspaper shows that drugs and their trade are far more important. Alcohol and illegal drugs should be looked for in all GSW victims.

VIGOR OF FIELD AND HOSPITAL RESUSCITATION

A sea change in the vigor of field resuscitative measures occurred in the 1970s and 1980s as civilian communities around the world emulated U.S. Army resuscitation and evacuation techniques pioneered in World War II and the Korean War and perfected in Vietnam in the late 1960s. The need for a military-like rapid evacuation scheme was the underlying theme of several reports.[12, 28, 41] Others reported the results for the brain wounded after such evacuation systems had been instituted in civilian communities.[20, 26, 27, 29, 36, 38]

Raimondi and Samuelson[41] in 1970 stated that only 2 of 89 GSW victims transferred to Cook County Hospital in Chicago had been tracheotomized, and none had an endotracheal tube in place before or during transport. They documented a decline in neurological status in these patients during transport: 45 of 89 brain-wounded patients were "alert," and 6 were posturing when initially seen at outlying hospitals. Only 36 were still alert upon arrival at Cook County Hospital, and 22 were decerebrate or decorticate.

Such neurological deterioration during transport is in direct contrast to the highly sophisticated and vigorous field resuscitation techniques implemented in the 1970s and 1980s. For example, in 1974, Byrnes and coworkers[12] from Belfast stated that initial therapy after wounding usually occurred within minutes. Field medical workers took great care to maintain the patient's airway, often using intubation. Patients were quickly admitted to the hospital, where controlled respiration was often used; blood was liberally replaced to combat hypotension. Other reports also indicated the development of programs ensuring vigorous field resuscitation and rapid transport to a neurosurgical center.[20, 24, 26, 27, 29, 36] Stone and colleagues[38] found that 17% of patients improved with resuscitation, and 18% worsened. These changes for better or worse were highly predictive of ultimate outcome.

EFFECT OF HYPOTENSION AND HYPOXIA ON MORTALITY

Concomitant hypotension, systolic blood pressure (SBP) less than 90 mm Hg, and hypoxia adversely affect the outcome from closed head injury.[42, 43] One would anticipate that they adversely affect the outcome from brain GSW as well.

Hypotension and Brain Wounding

Byrnes and coworkers[12] observed that patients with penetrating brain wounds often had an SBP less than 90 mm Hg from concomitant bleeding, and 72% of these patients died. Of those with SBP from 90 to 150 mm Hg, 41% died, but if the SBP were greater than 150 mm Hg, 93% died. Post-traumatic hypertension may reflect intracranial hypertension, presaging death.

In Suddaby and associates'[18] series, the mortality for patients with an admission SBP less than 90 mm Hg was 80%. If the SBP was between 90 and 150 mm Hg, 52% died, and if it was greater than 150 mm Hg, mortality was 61%. These mortality differences were not significant. Kaufman and coworkers[20] reported SBP less than 90 mm Hg in 33% of 48 survivors and in 58% of 95 patients with fatal wounds. They concluded that although hypotension was more common in those with fatal wounds, its presence did not preclude survival.

In Aldrich and colleagues'[31] series, SBP less than 90 mm Hg occurred in 44 of 103 patients early in the course of their treatment. Whereas 84% of hypotensive patients died, so did 76% of those not in shock. These differences were not significant, and no clear-cut effect of hemorrhagic hypotension on survival following brain wounding could be discerned.

Hypoxia and Brain Wounding

The occurrence of hypoxia after brain wounding has been difficult to study, because patients who are truly hypoxic from their wounds may be intubated in the field, and their initial transient hypoxia may be undocumentable. In the hectic, early minutes when the brain-wound victim presents to the emergency department, blood gas or pulse oximetry values may not be obtained before intubation and oxygenation. If hypoxia occurs from loss of respiratory effort because of the brain wound, death may result. Stone and colleagues[38] noted a 75% mortality in brain-wounded patients with apnea or respiratory depression.

Byrnes and coworkers[12] in 1974 were among the earliest to stress the importance of maintaining oxygenation and providing an airway by intubation in the field. They stressed that brain-wounded patients often had partial airway obstructions from inhaled blood or aspirated gastric contents, which could lead to raised $PaCO_2$, lowered PaO_2, and increased intracranial pressure (ICP). They were strong proponents of endotracheal intubation and controlled ventilation using muscle relaxants or anesthesia, if necessary. They observed that any deterioration was usually attributed to inadequate ventilation rather than intracranial hematoma formation.

Kaufman and associates[20] noted that only 10% of brain-wound survivors (5 of 48) were hypoxic on admission (PaO_2 <65 mm Hg), whereas 29% of those who died (28 of 95) had low PaO_2.

In Grahm and colleagues'[27] study, 6 of 79 brain-wounded patients who were intubated had GCS improvement, and 4 of these patients were eventually discharged home; this represented 10% of the surviving patients. They concluded that preventing secondary injury from hypoxia (and, by inference, hypotension) would improve overall outcome following brain wounding.

TIME BETWEEN INJURY AND ADMISSION

Intuitively, one might expect that the mortality from GSWs of the brain might be reduced with speedy admission to the hospital. Among Raimondi and Samuelson's[41] 150 patients with craniocerebral wounds, those admitted at a mean postinjury time of 2.5 hours had a 25% mortality, whereas those who entered, on average, 5.5 hours after wounding had a 34% mortality, an insignificant difference. Lillard[13] believed that a shorter interval between wounding and surgery should be an important factor in decreasing mortality, but paradoxically, his data showed that the time from injury to definitive therapy averaged 2.8 hours for fatalities and 5.9 hours for survivors. Hubschmann and colleagues[44] concluded that rapid transport of brain-wound victims to the hospital uncovered a class of patients with severe injuries who could be maintained for a while with sophisticated care but who had no real hope of survival.

In Byrnes and coworkers'[12] Northern Ireland series, 63 of 93 brain-wounded patients arrived at the hospital within 30 minutes; 23 of 64 operated patients were in the operating room within 2 hours of hospital admission, and another 23 (46 total) were there within 4 hours. Despite these heroic efforts, 53 of 93 patients died, a 57% mortality. Like Hubschmann, Byrnes explained the high hospital mortality by wound severity and by the exceptionally rapid transport of moribund patients to the hospital.

In conclusion, although an occasional person may be helped by quick transportation to a hospital, data do not support the contention that rapid evacuation to a hospital significantly lowers mortality for large numbers of brain GSW victims.

NUMBER WOUNDED VERSUS NUMBER OPERATED ON

Freytag,[7] in her autopsy study, noted that 63% of all brain GSW victims were dead on arrival at the hospital, 27% died within 24 hours, and only 10% lived more than a day. Hernesniemi[14] commented that neurosurgeons see only the "tip of the iceberg." In his series of 111 penetrating brain wounds (mostly suicide attempts), only 16 underwent craniotomy—18% of all those arriving alive at the hospital.

Kaufman and associates[20] ascertained that 71% of all victims of brain GSWs were dead at the scene, another 14% died within 5 hours, 13% died between 5 and 48 hours, and less than 2% survived longer than 48 hours. Of 143 patients admitted to their hospital, only 28 underwent craniotomy. They noted that very few patients with low GCS scores underwent brain débridement and wondered whether a "self-fulfilling prophecy" of doom had been effected by withholding care from such patients.

In Grahm and coworkers'[27] series, all brain-wound victims, even those with GCS scores of 3 to 5, received vigorous resuscitation in the field; expedited transport to the hospital, usually within minutes; and vigorous in-hospital care. Despite this aggressive approach, only 43 of 93 brain-wounded patients underwent craniotomy. Of those admitted, 49 were not surgical candidates owing to their poor neurological status or because they could not be resuscitated. The operative mortality was 10 of 43 (23%), and the overall mortality of those admitted was 59 of 93 (63%). Because all patients received the same aggressive care irrespective of GCS score, Grahm concluded that the deaths that occurred were inevitable and not the result of a "self-fulfilling prophecy."

EVALUATION OF THE BRAIN-WOUNDED PATIENT

Much of the literature from World War II and the Korean War concerning specific neurological signs that determine the viability of brain-wounded patients and the surgeon's decision to operate is vague. In the early 1960s, however, McNealy and Plum[45] set forth specific neurological criteria to evaluate brainstem viability. I used these criteria in Vietnam in 1968–1969 and found them to be accurate predictors of clinical outcome.[46, 47] The GCS[48] has largely replaced McNealy and Plum's system.

Level of Consciousness

Goodman and Kalsbeck[10] noted that all patients who were comatose and demonstrated severe neurological impairment failed to survive, no matter what treatment was used. They used a three-step system: confusion (0% mortality), responsive with deficit (60% mortality), and comatose (100% mortality). Subsequently, four- and five-step clinical scores were used to rank brain-wound victims.[11–15, 17, 28, 41, 44] All showed that the chance of survival following a GSW to the brain decreased with brainstem compromise, denoted by decreasing level of consciousness and motor release phenomena.

Clark and associates[19] were the first to rank civilian GSW victims by the GCS and noted that all 33 severely wounded patients who were not considered for surgery had a GCS score of 3 or 4. Table 331–2 shows the correlation of various GCS scores with mortality.

Controversy exists whether the admission or postresuscitation GCS score better predicts outcome. Grahm and colleagues[27] concluded that the postresuscitation GCS score was the best outcome predictor, but Aldrich and coworkers[31] found that the initial GCS score was a stronger predictor.

If the GCS continues to be the method used to indicate level of neurological function and the criterion on which neurosurgical decision making is based, it is imperative that emergency medical technicians and emergency room physicians provide absolutely accurate GCS scores before any intubation and induced paralysis. Neurosurgeons must stress the importance of accurate GCS determinations and teach emergency

TABLE 331–2 ■ **Overall Mortality for 460 Patients Based on Glasgow Coma Scale Score**

GLASGOW COMA SCALE SCORE	NO. LIVED	NO. DIED	% MORTALITY
12 or 13–15	97	3	3
9–11 or 12	44	8	15
6–8	30	43	59
3–5	15	220	94
Total	186	274	60

Data from references 20–24, 27, 29, 30, and Michael DB: Gunshot wounds to the head. Contemp Neurosurg 17 : 1–5, 1995; Michael's unpublished GCS data were received via personal communication, May 21, 1996.

TABLE 331–3 ■ **Pupillary Size, Equality, and Reactivity versus Level of Consciousness**

	LEVEL OF CONSCIOUSNESS			
PUPILS	Alert	Drowsy	Responds to Pain	Deep Coma
Normal	24	11	7	5
Unequal	2	5	10	4
Fixed, dilated	0	2	7	16
	26	18	24	25
Died	3	6	19	25
% Mortality	12	33	79	100

room physicians and ambulance paramedics how to do this test.

Motor Release Findings

Although the level of consciousness, reflecting integrity of the brainstem reticular activating system, is the predominant feature of all coma scores, postural changes may be seen with compromise of the reticular activating system because it is close to ascending and descending tracks controlling posture. Analysis of 231 patients revealed that 220 designated as decorticate, decerebrate, or flaccid to painful stimuli died (95% mortality).[11–13, 15, 17, 28, 41, 44] Only 10 of 15 patients with motor release findings in Sherman and coworkers'[15] study died; however, and Miner and associates[26] reported two children with decerebrate posturing who recovered with only moderate disabilities. They opined that in children, decorticate or decerebrate posturing after a brain wound does not inevitably mean a poor outcome. Nevertheless, in GSW victims, decorticate or decerebrate posturing or no response to pain carries an extremely poor prognosis.

Pupillary Findings

A fairly good correspondence exists between level of consciousness and pupillary findings, because both the reticular activating system and the third nerve nuclei are in the midbrain (Table 331–3).

The fact that Byrnes and coworkers[12] had five comatose patients with brain wounds who had normal pupils (20% of all those in coma) vitiates the predictive value of pupillary findings for death. Pupillary findings are not as reliable as coma in predicting a fatal outcome.

Hubschmann and colleagues[44] found that the only consistently reliable variables predicting outcome were level of consciousness and the presence of motor release phenomena (decorticate or decerebrate posturing or flaccidity). Pupillary inequality provided no additional prognostic information.

Grahm and coworkers[27] also found that the pupillary reaction was equivocal in predicting outcome. In their series, 95% of patients with GCS scores of 3 to 5

had no pupillary reaction. In groups with higher GCS scores, about 50% had impaired ocular findings. They believed that ocular dysfunction confirmed severe brain injury in comatose patients, but in more awake patients, lack of pupillary response usually represented injury to the orbit, globe, anterior visual apparatus, or cranial nerves.

Suddaby and associates[18] noted that unequal pupils were not necessarily associated with a poor outcome, but fixed and dilated or midrange pupils presaged death. Kaufman and colleagues[20] observed that if both pupils responded, 30 of 38 patients (79%) survived; if one pupil responded, 4 of 8 (50%) lived; but only 1 of 70 patients (1%) with nonreactive pupils survived. In Stone and coworkers'[38] series, only 4% of patients with fixed, dilated pupils survived, and three quarters were vegetative. Pupillary reactivity but not size was a significant ($P < 0.05$) predictor of outcome, but GCS score was a far more powerful outcome predictor ($P < 0.001$).

Bilaterally fixed pupils, whether midrange or dilated, are an ominous prognostic sign, but unequal pupils are less predictable. Some patients with fatal traumatic coma may have normally reacting pupils. Pupillary findings are not as reliable as level of consciousness and motor release signs in predicting outcome.

IMAGING STUDIES

Plain Skull Radiographs

Skull radiographs can suggest the missile trajectory, including whether the missile crossed the midsagittal or coronal planes; document indriven bone; show the extent of skull fractures, including suture diastasis; and demonstrate intracerebral air or fluid in the sinuses.

Angiography

Raimondi and Samuelson[41] made extensive use of angiography to define the presence, location, and, in some cases, nature of intracranial lesions, such as contrecoup injury, damage to arteries or dural sinuses, epidural hematomas, and false aneurysms. Hubschmann and colleagues[44] did not use angiography and contended that in most cases, any significant hematomas or masses caused by necrotic brain that would have been identified by angiography would be encountered and evacuated during brain débridement. No unsuspected hematoma was missed among their 45 operated patients. They cautioned, however, that sudden deterioration in postoperative patients might be caused by bleeding from a traumatic aneurysm, and such patients should undergo arteriography expeditiously.

Benzel and coworkers[28] reported on 120 brain-wounded patients evaluated by computed tomographic scans. Two patients suddenly deteriorated and died after surgical débridement due to middle cerebral artery infarction. An additional patient developed a traumatic middle cerebral artery pseudoaneurysm that was treated successfully. In all three cases, the missile had traversed the middle cerebral artery complex, and the authors concluded that if the missile trajectory includes the sylvian region, angiography is warranted because of the possibility of the development of a late traumatic pseudoaneurysm amenable to clipping or an arterial dissection or thrombosis that could be treated by surgical bypass.

Levy and associates[49] documented an overall 1% incidence of traumatic pseudoaneurysm following bullet wounding and a 3.2% incidence when subarachnoid hemorrhage was demonstrated by computed tomography (CT).

Computed Tomography

The preoperative computed tomographic scan can delineate depressed skull fractures; intraparenchymal bone fragments; the missile track; epidural, subdural, intraparenchymal, intraventricular, and subarachnoid hemorrhage; cerebral edema or hyperemia; brain shifts; the presence or absence of basilar cisterns; intracranial or parenchymal air; ischemia; evidence of a carotid cavernous fistula; ventricular dilatation; and metal and bone fragments. Postoperatively, it can detect retained bone and metal fragments, cerebral edema, brain shifts, intracranial air, brain abscess, and sometimes pseudoaneurysm.[15, 17, 18, 49, 50]

MISSILE TRACK

In 1978, using surgical and autopsy data, Lillard[13] showed that patients with one lobe injured by a bullet had a 23% mortality. If the bullet crossed the midsagittal plane, 40% of patients died; if it crossed the midcoronal plane, 53% died; and if both midcoronal and midsagittal planes were crossed, 75% died. Lillard was the first to analyze mortality in terms of missile track, and he believed that the missile track must be correlated with missile size, because in three of his cases, a small .22-caliber bullet (low energy of deposit) crossed both sagittal and coronal planes, but the patients did well. This point is rarely emphasized by those discussing CT-determined missile tracks and mortality. Shoung and colleagues[17] and others extended the track concept using CT (Table 331–4).

In most series, unilateral lobe injury is associated with 20% to 30% mortality. If the missile crosses the midsagittal or midcoronal plane or the sagittal, coronal, or horizontal midventricular plane, mortality tends to be two- to four-fold higher. If it crosses both sagittal and coronal planes, mortality is close to 100%.

TRANSVENTRICULAR INJURIES

Transventricular injuries, unilateral or bilateral, as demonstrated by CT, have high mortality and morbidity. Nagib and coworkers[21] reported that 5 of 6 patients with ventricular injury died, as did 14 of Levi and colleagues'[29] 22 patients (64%) and 88% in Aldrich and coauthors'[31] large series. In Cavaliere and associates'[22] study, 117 of 119 patients with massive intraventricular hemorrhage died. Grahm and colleagues'[27] patients with bihemispheric injuries and transventricular penetration had dismal outcomes: 90% dead, 10% neurologically devastated. Even unilateral hemisphere wounds with ventricular injury had a poor prognosis; only

TABLE 331–4 ■ **Percent Mortality as a Function of Extent of Brain Involvement Determined by Bullet Track Visualized on Computed Tomography**

AUTHOR	ONE LOBE	ONE LOBE OR UNILATERAL MULTIPLE LOBES, UNSPECIFIED	UNILATERAL MULTIPLE LOBES	CROSS MID-SAGITTAL PLANE	CROSS MID-CORONAL PLANE	CROSS BOTH PLANES	CROSS HORIZONTAL MIDVEN-TRICULAR PLANE	CROSS SAGITTAL, HORIZONTAL, CORONAL PLANES
Shoung et al[17]	20			50	80	92		
Kaufman et al[20]		36		85				
Nagib et al[21]	0		35	83				
Cavaliere et al[22]	76		93	98				
Selden et al[24]	45			80	88	100		
Grahm et al[27]		28		79				
Levi et al[29]	20		68	65				
Siccardi et al[30]	77		92	96				
Stone et al[38]		26		60				
Miner et al[26]		23		80				
Shaffrey et al[33]				68			76	9

those without transventricular wounds had satisfactory outcomes.

MIDLINE SHIFT

Suddaby and coworkers'[18] review showed that patients with midline shift tended to have poorer outcomes. Kaufman and associates[20] observed that any midline shift of 10 mm or greater was associated with a mortality of more than 50%. They also noted that those with bihemispheral injuries often did not show midline displacement because of the bilateral swelling. In Aldrich and colleagues'[31] series, 43 of 89 patients had a midline shift greater than 3 mm, and almost 80% of these patients died. Shaffrey and coauthors,[33] in contrast, could not correlate the extent of midline shift with mortality.

MISSILE FRAGMENTATION

Nagib and coworkers[21] noted that the presence of bone and metal fragments away from the bullet's path, even as a single radiographic finding, carried a uniformly bad prognosis. Six of seven such patients died, and the seventh was devastated. The deleterious effects of missile fragmentation were confirmed by Levy and colleagues.[36]

COMPRESSED CISTERNS

This phenomenon occurred in 61 of 89 patients, and 85% of those with compressed cisterns died.[31]

INTRACRANIAL BLEEDING

The incidence of epidural bleeding is low following brain wounding, but the occurrence of other types of intracranial bleeding varies widely: subdural hematomas, 3%[29] to 56%[36]; intracerebral hematomas, 4%[32] to 37%[32]; intraventricular hemorrhage, 1%[32] to 56%[32]; and subarachnoid hemorrhage, 9%[38] to 78%.[31] Reconciling these reported frequencies is difficult, because some investigators may have noted only clinically significant collections (e.g., Suddaby's[18] subdural and intracerebral clots that required surgical evacuation); others may have counted *any* occurrence of a particular type of intracranial bleeding seen on CT. Further, some investigators may have relied on chart reports instead of personally reviewing all computed tomographic scans. Shoung's[17] and Levy's[49] groups reported primarily CT studies, and one assumes that all scans were reviewed by the authors. Even so, the reported incidence of subarachnoid blood varied almost by a factor of two—Shoung reporting 59% and Levy 31%.

SUBARACHNOID HEMORRHAGE

Several studies document that subarachnoid hemorrhage following brain wounding is associated with significantly increased mortality and morbidity. Levy and colleagues[49] evaluated the computed tomographic scans of 100 consecutive brain-wounded patients and ascertained that 31 had subarachnoid hemorrhage. All these patients had angiograms, and a traumatic aneurysm was found in one. Of 28 who died, 19 (68%) had subarachnoid hemorrhage, whereas only 12 of 72 survivors (17%) did (χ^2, $P < 0.005$). Stone and coauthors[38] stated that 65% of patients with subarachnoid hemorrhage died, whereas Aldrich's group[31] noted an 81% mortality for this condition. Neither the group led by Shaffrey[33] nor Pikus and Ball[37] found subarachnoid blood to be significantly related to mortality. Why subarachnoid hemorrhage may contribute to poor outcome is unclear. Possibly it reflects injury severity or contributes to secondary vasospasm, further impairing the injured brain.

CLINICAL AND IMAGING PREDICTORS OF MORTALITY

Several investigators have related multiple clinical and CT findings to mortality using statistical techniques.[31, 33, 36–38] In every analysis, GCS score is the paramount predictor of mortality, but pupillary defects also rank high. Among CT findings, bihemispheric wounding, ventricular injury, intracerebral hemorrhage, and possibly subarachnoid hemorrhage are important predictors of mortality.

ADJUNCTIVE THERAPY

Tetanus Prophylaxis and Antibiotics

Tetanus prophylaxis should always be given to patients with brain wounds. I recommend using antibiotics for patients with open wounds and continuing them for 5 to 7 days after brain débridement.

Steroids

Because available evidence indicates that glucocorticoids have no effect on traumatized brain, there is little point in using them for brain GSW victims. Further, steroids may cause hyperglycemia, which is known to adversely affect damaged brain.[51]

Prophylactic Anticonvulsants

Some evidence shows that prophylactic anticonvulsants decrease the incidence of seizures during the first postinjury week but not thereafter.[51, 52] This beneficial effect must be weighed against the fact that seizures occur in only 4% to 25% of severely head-injured patients (not just GSW patients) within a week of brain injury, and anticonvulsants may impair neural recovery.[53, 54]

Prophylactic anticonvulsants were used in only about one quarter of the GSW series reviewed, and even in centers where they were frequently used, they were omitted in as many as 10% of patients in Sherman's study[15] and in more than 75% of those in Lillard's.[13] Clark's[19] and Benzel's[28] groups used anticonvulsants only if the brain-wounded patient began having seizures.

Intracranial Pressure Monitoring

Sixteen groups indicated that ICP monitoring was used to determine cerebral perfusion pressure in at least some patients.* For instance, 35 of 157 GSW victims in Aldrich's[31] series were monitored. Mean ICP was 31 mm Hg for the 13 who lived and 62 mm Hg for fatalities. That analysis indicated that next to the GCS score, ICP was the most important outcome predictor. Thus, measuring ICP in comatose brain-wounded patients may have some utility. Among 33 brain-wounded children, Miner and colleagues[26] monitored ICP in 18. Nine of these patients died; eight had ICP greater than 40 mm Hg. Of the nine monitored patients who lived, three had ICP less than 20 mm Hg, two had ICP less than 30 mm Hg with medical treatment, and four had ICP greater than 40 mm Hg. Two of the four patients with ICP greater than 40 mm Hg ended up with severe disabilities, and two had moderate disabilities.

Barbiturate Coma

Most investigators over the last decade have not resorted to the use of barbiturate coma for those with GSWs to the brain. Cited instances are fragmentary and incidental and do not provide a sense of barbiturate coma's effectiveness.[21, 25, 26, 36, 38] Because it is used only in those who are severely decompensated with persistently elevated ICP, who would be expected to have high mortality and morbidity, it may be impossible to judge the efficacy of this treatment short of a rigorously controlled, multicenter study.

Summary

Although the use of tetanus prophylaxis and antibiotics appears sound, prophylactic anticonvulsants, ICP monitoring, and barbiturate coma are of uncertain value for GSW management; otherwise, they would have been widely adopted. Kaufman and associates[55] documented the widespread lack of uniform treatment for brain wounds among American neurosurgeons.

SURGERY

A neurosurgeon cannot possibly influence the two major effects accounting for damage following missile wounding: missile trajectory and energy deposit causing low-pressure waves. The latter may damage diencephalic and brainstem structures even if the missile does not. Hypoxia and hypotension must be prevented or promptly treated by field or hospital resuscitation teams, usually before the neurosurgeon arrives. The neurosurgeon's job is to determine whether the victim is a surgical candidate and, if so, to evacuate significant hematomas or swollen, hemorrhagic, or edematous brain and prevent infection by appropriate wound care.

Goals of Surgery

Traditional surgical goals as enumerated succinctly by Byrnes and coworkers[12] include (1) arrest hemorrhage, (2) evacuate intracerebral hematoma, (3) débride devitalized brain, (4) remove bone and metal fragments to prevent infection, (5) repair the dura, and (6) ensure adequate scalp cover. Some neurosurgeons today would agree only on arresting hemorrhage, evacuating major intracerebral hematomas, and ensuring adequate scalp cover as primary goals.

Timing of Surgery

Usually, surgery for brain wounds is done sooner rather than later, especially if a large mass is seen on CT. A delay in patient admission or the need to treat other life-threatening injuries sometimes delays brain débridement.

Selection for Surgery

In many reports, specific criteria for surgery were not provided, even when the author was a neurosurgeon.[10-14, 19, 20, 23, 24, 41] For Hubschmann and colleagues,[44] whether a patient was brought to surgery was determined by "the presence or lack of a significant mass lesion and the potential for neurologic recovery." Patients selected for surgery had lesser neurological deficits or were suspected of having intracranial mass lesions.

After McNealy and Plum's[45] 1962 elucidation of brainstem reflexes to evaluate brainstem viability, Sherman and coworkers[15] reported that surgery was performed on all who could speak or follow simple commands and on comatose patients who maintained brainstem reflexes and had respirations. Apneic patients without brainstem reflexes were excluded from surgery. At Kaufman's[20] institution, the decision whether to operate was based on the patient's clinical status, the presence or absence of a space-occupying mass, and the bullet's energy and trajectory. Very few severely injured patients underwent surgery. Shoung's group[17] undertook surgery as quickly as possible before clinical deterioration occurred but withheld it from decerebrate or flaccid patients. For Grahm and associates,[27] if after resuscitation a patient had two intact neurological signs, motor movements (e.g., reactive pupils; intact corneal, cough, or gag reflex) plus spontaneous respirations, he or she was taken to surgery.

After its development in 1974, surgeons began basing surgical decisions on the GCS. Cavaliere and colleagues[22] operated only on patients with a GCS score of 6 or greater. At Siccardi's[30] hospital, neurosurgeons required a GCS score of 4.

Helling and associates[32] noted that those with mass lesions tended to be operated on earlier, but neurosurgeons were less aggressive in patients with poor GCS

---

*See references 12, 13, 15, 17, 20, 21, 24–31, 33, 36, 38.

scores. Stone and coworkers[38] used the postresuscitation GCS score plus "hemodynamic stability" as the primary criteria for surgery. Hemodynamically stable patients in the following groups underwent débridement: (1) GCS score of 3 with reactive pupils, (2) GCS score of 4 to 7 without fixed dilated pupils, (3) GCS score of 8 to 15 with intracranial bone fragments or clot. All other patients got supportive care and were re-evaluated for surgery if improvement occurred.

Levy and coauthors'[36] 1994 series of 190 patients was unique because it focused on patients with GCS scores of 3, 4, and 5. Most were operated on if they were normotensive with reactive pupils, but a few patients with unreactive pupils were also operated on.

Number of Patients Undergoing Surgery

The number of operated patients is invariably fewer than the total number of GSW victims presenting to a hospital. The most common reason for not operating on a brain-wounded person is a depressed neurological status indicating severe brainstem compromise. Also, brain wounds caused by bullets entering through the face and penetrating the base of the skull often are not operated on if the patient is doing well. Other reasons for not operating range from respecting the obvious intent of a suicide attempt, following the wishes of the next of kin, and failure to recognize that a bullet has indeed penetrated the brain.[20, 27, 36, 38, 44]

Surgical Mortality

Statistics for overall surgical mortality are hard to evaluate because the level of consciousness, reflecting brainstem function, has such an overwhelming influence on mortality. Surgical mortality is best understood when coupled with a specific clinical grade, as demonstrated in Table 331–5.

The surgical mortality in patients with GCS scores of 12 to 15 is low (3%), and death may occur from an untoward event such as meningitis or pulmonary embolus. Surgical mortality rises with diminishing GCS score or level of consciousness, because these states signify compromise of vital brainstem structures that may not be reversed by brain débridement. Chi-square analysis reveals no relationship between brain débridement and mortality for those with GCS scores

greater than 5: GCS score 12 to 15, $\chi^2 = 0.49$ (1 df), $P > 0.05$; GCS score 9 to 11, $\chi^2 = 0.08$ (1 df), $P > 0.05$; GCS score 6 to 8, $\chi^2 = 0.67$ (1 df), $P > 0.05$. Clearly, however, if these patients had not undergone surgery, many would have died from brain infections.

For patients with GCS scores of 3 to 5 reported by the authors represented in Table 331–5, only 4 of 413 nonoperated patients (1%) lived, whereas 7 of 35 patients (20%) who were operated on lived ($\chi^2 = 48.79$ [1 df], $P < 0.05$). At first glance, this seems to indicate that surgery was beneficial for these critically injured individuals, but in reality, this result may be spurious, because all unoperated patients were expected to die. They may have had no or minimal care, which assured their death. Any who lived may have done so by chance. Although surgery appears to increase survival for patients with GCS scores of 3 to 5, the dismal ramifications of this are considered in the outcome section.

Types of Surgery

Throughout the years, neurosurgeons have proposed various débridement techniques to achieve better outcomes. These techniques have varied from "minimal" to "conservative" to "standard" to "radical." Because these are subjective terms, readers must make their own evaluations of the various débridement techniques.

MINIMAL

Shoung[17] and Suddaby[18] and their colleagues used a restrictive surgical approach. The entrance and exit sites were débrided, but no attempt was made to retrieve missile fragments unless they were easily accessible. Dura was closed with a graft, if needed. Shoung monitored ICP and provided continuous external ventricular drainage in comatose patients. Suddaby did not give prophylactic antibiotics but provided general support. Levi and coworkers[29] gave only local wound care in 16 patients with either punctate entrance wounds or penetration through the skull base and no evidence of an intracranial lesion on CT. If the GCS score was less than 8, subdural ICP monitoring was also used. Craniectomy was done on only three patients who had extensive entrance wounds or protruding brain. Necrotic tissue and debris were removed, followed by a watertight dural closure.

CONSERVATIVE

Raimondi and Samuelson[41] recommended conservative débridement along the missile track. If the angiogram did not reveal a hematoma adjacent to the missile, it was left in place. Blood clots and any accessible missile or foreign body were removed. No intracranial foreign body was approached through uninjured cerebral tissue. Yashon and coauthors[11] recommended only necessary superficial débridement. The bullet was removed only when it was eminently accessible. Hubschmann and colleagues[44] removed bone fragments and necrotic

TABLE 331–5 ■ **Surgical Mortality for Patients Based on Glasgow Coma Scale Scores**

GLASGOW COMA SCALE SCORE	NO. LIVED	NO. DIED	% MORTALITY
12 or 13–15	61	2	3
9–11 or 12	29	5	15
6–8	18	26	59
3–5	7	28	80
Total	115	61	35

Data from references 20, 22, 23, 27, 30.

tissue but made no attempt to remove the bullet if it was located in a vital area or if removal was technically too difficult.

STANDARD

Byrnes and coworkers[12] removed bone and, when accessible, metal fragments, but these were not sought if removal would require dissection through normal tissue. The dura was closed. Lillard[13] débrided the dura and opened it to allow irrigation and suction débridement of underlying cerebral tissue and the missile track. After superficial débridement and removal of bone fragments and other foreign material, the wound track was irrigated by catheter until no further bone fragments or necrotic material returned. Large cerebral incisions were avoided, and no attempt was made to retrieve inaccessible missile fragments. Sherman and associates[15] removed foreign material (e.g., metal and bone fragments, dirt, hair, powder granules) and evacuated extra-axial and intra-axial hematomas. They débrided necrotic brain and soft tissues and achieved an adequate dural and soft tissue closure. Kaufman and coauthors[20] believed that devitalized tissue should be débrided, hematomas evacuated, accessible missile and bone fragments removed, meticulous hemostasis achieved, and the dura closed. Clark and colleagues[19] carefully explored the wound and removed intracranial hematomas, depressed or indriven bone fragments, hair, and other foreign bodies. Necrotic brain was débrided. The bullet or fragments were removed only when accessible through an approach not involving uninjured cerebral tissue. The dura was closed meticulously with or without a fascial or pericranial graft. Siccardi and coworkers[30] débrided necrotic brain, removed readily accessible indriven bone fragments and foreign bodies, evacuated hematomas, achieved accurate hemostasis, and performed watertight dural closure. Occasionally, they used ICP monitoring. Levy and coworkers[36] evacuated mass lesions and débrided necrotic tissue and bony fragments at entrance and exit sites. Only superficial or local bone fragments were débrided. Deep parenchymal fragments and those not readily accessible were not removed. Dural lacerations were repaired primarily or by fascial grafts. Aggressive hemostasis was obtained. Miner and associates[26] removed all devitalized tissue and accessible foreign bodies.

RADICAL

Grahm and colleagues[27] débrided dural entrance and exit sites, which were opened widely to allow complete access to the underlying damaged brain. Necrotic brain, hematomas, and accessible missile and bone fragments were removed. The bullet track was followed to its exit site, if possible. An ICP monitor was placed, and the dura was closed; antibiotics were given. Stone and associates[38] irrigated the missile track by a catheter. Brain around the track was débrided by suction until viable tissue was seen. The track was palpated by finger to locate foreign bodies. Although

complete removal of indriven bone was considered ideal, no attempt was made to remove inaccessible bone fragments. The dura was closed. Postoperative ICP monitoring was used if the GCS score was less than 8. Ventriculostomies were placed if the ventricle was penetrated or if ventricular hemorrhage was present.

SUMMARY

Shoung's[17] and Suddaby's[18] patients and most of Levi's[29] patients (those with punctate skull entrance wounds) clearly had minimal treatment. Although the groups led by Raimondi,[41] Yashon,[11] and Hubschmann[44] recommended a "conservative" approach, their surgical approaches were not much different from "standard" techniques. Similarly, Stone's group[38] advocated aggressive surgery, but their surgical description did not differ significantly from that of those doing "standard" débridements, especially Lillard.[13] Thus, despite their claims of being "conservative" or "radical," most surgeons, except for the minimalists, do approximately the same thing when débriding the brain following a missile wound. Grahm's[27] approach seems the most radical.

I favor visualization and thorough débridement of the missile track, with removal of necrotic brain back to normal-appearing brain. I rarely follow a missile track through the falx. The amount of tissue débrided can be greater in noneloquent brain areas, but in any case, enough damaged brain should be removed so that postoperative brain edema does not cause brainstem compromise. All possible indriven bone should be removed. Visual inspection of the track searching for bone is supplemented by digital palpation to locate indriven bone fragments that may be held up around blood vessels. Following small bone fragments into the thalamus or basal ganglia is not recommended. Metallic fragments are removed if readily accessible. Inaccessible, mobile metallic fragments within a ventricle should be removed at a second procedure. A watertight dural closure is highly recommended. A dural graft is often necessary, and autologous temporal fascia or pericranium should suffice. The scalp should be closed over the exposed dura without tension using scalp advancement or relaxing incisions, if necessary.

Aggressive versus Less Aggressive Surgery and Therapy

Several investigators[20, 32, 38] have raised the issue of whether a more aggressive strategy might improve the outcome of those with brain wounds. An "aggressive" strategy has many facets, including resuscitation in the field and emergency ward, the clinician's decision for or against surgical débridement, the actual extent of débridement, and the amount and type of postoperative care. Grahm and coworkers'[27] patients had vigorous preoperative resuscitation and the most radical surgery, yet the surgical mortality in this series, 23%, was similar to that reported by several investigators with decidedly more conservative débridement philosophies: Raimondi (16%),[41] Lillard (33%),[13] Hubschmann (22%),[44] and Benzel (28%).[28] Stone,[38] whose patients apparently received vigorous resuscitation in the field and the hospital receiving area and who may have had an aggressive surgical approach, had a surgical mortality of 21%, little different from Raimondi's[41] 16% mortality from the same institution 25 years earlier.

Because most surgical patients with GCS scores greater than 8 live and most with scores of 5 or below die (see Table 331–5), perhaps the best way to evaluate the efficacy of conservative, standard, or radical surgery (or any adjunctive drug therapy) is to examine mortality for patients with GCS scores of 6 to 8, because their lives hang in the balance (Table 331–6).

Mortalities for the four investigators claiming "standard" brain débridements ranged from 42% to 67%. Grahm,[27] who favored radical surgery, and Levi,[29] who did minimal brain débridement on most patients, reported mortalities of 25% and 20%, respectively. The number of patients with GCS scores of 6 to 8 in their series was quite small, so it is difficult to say that the aggressive surgery per se lowered the mortality rate.

Whereas some investigators believe that radical surgery might make a difference in mortality, others believe that except for wounds with associated intracranial hemorrhage, surgery or its extent makes little difference in survival. Yashon and coauthors[11] stated, "We have not separated surgical from nonsurgical deaths because we do not believe that surgical therapy *per se* was the predominant factor in survival except where a significant space occupying lesion was present." Byrnes and coworkers[12] concluded, "Survival depends more on airway control with mechanical ventilation than any other factor," and Clark and associates[19] lamented, "In spite of sophisticated preadmission, perioperative, and postoperative care, it is somewhat frustrating to note our general lack of improvement in the morbidity or mortality rates associated with civilian craniocerebral gunshot wounds. . . . The most important factors for prognostication are the GCS and factors related to the wound such as the presence of intracranial hematomas, ventricular injury or bihemispheric injury." Benzel's group[28] noted that Hubschmann's[44] and Kaufman's[20] mortality figures were similar despite a "conservative" and "aggressive" approach, implying that a more aggressive surgical approach may not change the ultimate outcome. They also suggested that an aggressive approach may help selected patients, such as those with intracranial mass lesions. They did not equate aggressiveness with surgery alone but felt that aggressive medical management could also be efficacious at times.

In conclusion, the telling factors in brain wounding are missile energy of deposit and trajectory. Although prevention or treatment of hypoxia and hypotension would appear to give damaged brain a greater chance for survival and the patient a better neurological recovery, the effect of such treatment on mortality is equivocal. Neither vigorous resuscitation, early admission, nor radical surgery appears to diminish mortality.

SPECIFIC PROBLEMS RELATED TO BRAIN WOUNDING

Cerebral Contusions

Brain wounding usually produces cortical contusions near the bullet entrance and exit sites. Autopsy studies[7, 8] show that remote contusions may be present in the white matter; in the basal ganglia close to the wound canal; in the cortex away from the wound track, particularly at the base of the brain; on the convexity; and on the medial surfaces of the cerebral hemispheres. These contusions arise from the high ICP generated by the bullet as it displaces tissue radially away from its track. Contusions noted from autopsy studies are probably more extensive than those found in nonfatal cases. Shaffrey and colleagues[33] noted that contusions in excess of 20% of the brain's normal volume dramatically increase mortality.

Intracranial Hematomas

Intuitively, one might expect brain GSWs to be associated with large amounts of intracranial bleeding, which would cause severe neurological decompensation and require neurosurgical evacuation. Further, if intracranial bleeding occurred often, one might expect prompt, vigorous surgery to have an important bearing on mortality.

Surprisingly, a large amount of intracranial bleeding

T A B L E   3 3 1 – 6 ■ Effects of Resuscitation and Type of Surgery on Mortality of Patients with Glasgow Coma Scale Scores of 6 to 8

AUTHOR	FIELD RESUSCITATION	HOSPITAL RESUSCITATION	TYPE OF SURGERY	NO. OF PATIENTS	% SURGICAL MORTALITY
Hubschmann et al[44]*	ND	V	S	7	43
Kaufman et al[20]	V	V	S	11	55
Grahm et al[27]	V	V	R	8	25
Benzel et al[28]	ND	V	S	12	42
Levi et al[29]†	V	V	M	5	20
Siccardi et al[30]	ND	V	S	12	67

*Hubschmann's four-grade clinical score converted to Glasgow Coma Scale.
†L. Levi, Personal communication, November 28, 1995.
M, minimal surgery; ND, not described; R, radical surgery; S, standard surgery; V, very aggressive.

is uncommon. Freytag's[7] autopsy data on 160 patients revealed "no or only insignificant amounts of blood within the wound canal." No mention was made of intracranial blood clots in the 82 individuals who lived for a period of time before succumbing. Kirkpatrick's and Di Maio's[8] autopsy study did not even discuss the presence of intracerebral or intraparenchymal hematoma.

It is possible that autopsy series do not record significant intracranial bleeding because death comes too quickly. Patients evaluated by neurosurgeons have lived longer than those constituting an autopsy series and might be more likely to have developed intracranial hematomas.

A brain-wounded individual may be expected to have several types of intracranial bleeding (e.g., a small subdural hemorrhage near the entrance site, clot within the missile track, and some subarachnoid hemorrhage as well). From reports, it is often difficult to know which (if any) blood collection was the most clinically important, and occurrence rates are disparate. In earlier surgical and autopsy studies, "significant" intracranial clots occurred in only 2% of Yashon's[11] and 11% of Hubschmann's[44] 187 cases but in 44% of Raimondi's[41] 150 patients. Among CT studies, significant intracranial bleeding was seen in 13% of Suddaby's[18] cases compared with 51% of Clark's.[19]

Only Sherman[15] and Aldrich[31] defined the volumes of "significant" intracranial hematomas: greater than 20 mL at surgery and greater than 15 mL by CT, respectively. Although a 15- or 20-mL clot in the temporal or posterior fossa might be clinically significant (i.e., contributing to neurological deterioration), similar clots in the frontal or occipital lobes might have no clinical significance. One investigator might consider an intracranial clot "significant" if it causes a shift on CT, but another might consider it "significant" only if it is associated with such neurological depression that clot evacuation is deemed necessary. Further, authors advocating the creation of more advanced trauma evacuation systems might be more likely to report the occurrence of "significant" clots responsive to expeditious neurosurgical treatment in order to make their case.

Patients with intra- or extra-axial hemorrhages and mass effect or subarachnoid hemorrhage often fare poorly compared with patients without these findings. Although the presence of mass lesions documented by CT was more likely to lead to early surgery,[18, 32] the evacuation of such blood was not always beneficial. The surgical mortality of patients with large intraparenchymal clots ranged from 50% to 78%.[18, 22–24, 30]

Five of six patients with intraventricular hemorrhage in Nagib's[21] study succumbed. Cavaliere[22] concluded that intraventricular hemorrhage was associated with high mortality (98%), but subdural or epidural hemorrhage was less lethal.

Benzel[28] had four comatose patients with intracerebral hematomas who unexpectedly survived. Two with small clots made satisfactory recoveries, and two with large hematomas remained vegetative.

In future studies, a "significant" intracranial hematoma should be defined both radiologically and clinically. Hematomas (or brain swelling) might be considered "clinically imperative" as opposed to just radiologically "significant" if they mandate surgery because of their mass effect. "Significant" intracranial bleeding may be present in up to 50% of patients, but clinically imperative clots requiring surgical evacuation occur in about 10% to 15% of all patients. Following removal of such clots, mortality can be expected to remain in excess of 50%.

Brain Swelling and Edema

Brain swelling and edema are not serious issues in the usual nonfatal brain wound. Only Lillard[13] reported serious postdébridement swelling that required additional surgery. Suddaby[18] and Levi[29] treated brain-wounded individuals with simple skin closure, doing minimal if any brain débridement. Experimental missile wounding indicates that mild vasogenic brain edema occurs only along the missile track.[6]

In fatal cases, the situation may be somewhat different, presumably because of loss of cerebral blood flow autoregulatory control. In Freytag's[7] autopsy series, 71 of 94 people who did not die immediately had brain edema with or without compressive hemorrhage in the midbrain and upper pons; 46 had midbrain and pontine edema. Kirkpatrick and Di Maio[8] noted cerebral edema (or brain swelling) in 15% of individuals, often in those who died quite acutely. The edema could not be related to missile velocity, size of permanent cavity, or survival duration.

Vascular Injuries

Only a few investigators have reported whether intracranial bleeding came from arteries or veins. Concomitant arterial vascular injury may lead to major brain infarctions, causing damage far more extensive than that made by the bullet, and pseudoaneurysm formation.[25, 28, 44] Goodman and Kalsbeck's[10] study of 22 brain wounds noted three superior sagittal sinus injuries. Clark's group[19] observed major vascular injuries in 13 of 76 patients: eight venous, five arterial. Mancuso and coworkers[23] recorded major subdural or intracerebral hemorrhage in 13 of 40 patients (3 venous, 10 arterial), but Grahm[27] noted a large venous subdural hematoma in only 1 of 43 operated patients. Benzel and associates[28] believed that 3 of 67 deaths were associated with vascular injuries: 2 from delayed middle cerebral artery infarcts, and 1 from intraoperative hemorrhage from a superior sagittal sinus tear. They successfully diagnosed and treated an additional patient who developed a middle cerebral artery pseudoaneurysm. One patient in Pikus and Boll's[37] series had bilateral carotid cavernous fistulas, presumably because of temporal bone injury.

Cerebral arteriography should be done if a bullet has passed near the leash of middle cerebral vessels because of the likelihood of arterial injury, occlusion, or pseudoaneurysm formation. Angiography should also be considered when the bullet traverses the medial temporal bone, because the carotid artery may be injured.

Wounds near the major venous sinuses should be treated with utmost respect; minor bone depressions adjacent to major sinuses should be left alone. If surgical exploration is undertaken, the surgeon must have a well-thought-out plan to arrest sinus bleeding, which may be ferocious.

Ventricular Wounds

Ventricular wounds carry a high mortality because of their proximity to vital diencephalic structures. Before CT, these injuries could be shown only at surgery or autopsy. Cushing[56] and later Schwartz and Rhoulhac[57] stated that ventricular injuries had a high mortality, although Wannamaker's[58] data from Korea failed to confirm this. In 1986, Clark and colleagues,[19] using both CT and surgical visualization, reiterated the lethality of ventricular injury from bullets: 90% of their patients with ventricular wounds had a poor outcome, whereas only 24% of those without such wounds did poorly.

Other investigators reporting high mortalities following ventricular wounding include Levi (64%),[29] Stone (60%),[38] Kaufman (86%),[20] Nagib (83%),[21] and Shaffrey (70%).[33] Grahm[27] thought that patients with ventricular injuries did so poorly that even those with GCS scores as high as 6 to 8 should not undergo surgical débridement.

Posterior Fossa Wounds

Few posterior fossa wounds are reported in surgical series because most brain wounds have an anterior entry. Being close to brainstem structures, posterior fossa wounds are particularly deadly, and patients with these wounds usually do not reach the neurosurgeon. Lillard[13] counted five posterior fossa wounds in his series of 83 cases and implied that these patients did poorly. Hubschmann[44] reported one late death from an undiagnosed posterior fossa wound. Selden and coauthors,[24] studying suicide patients, stated that when a bullet came to rest in the posterior fossa, death was inevitable. Because most suicide attempts have a frontal, temporal, or basifrontal bullet entry site, any such bullet finding its way into the posterior fossa directly or by ricochet would more than likely damage vital brainstem or vascular structures. Stone,[38] however, noted four nonfatal posterior fossa wounds among 150 patients who underwent brain débridement. They attributed surgical success in these patients to rapid, generous cerebellar débridement in patients in whom the bullet spared the brainstem.

Disseminated Intravascular Coagulation

Several authors have commented on the occurrence of disseminated intravascular coagulation (DIC) after brain wounding.[15, 20, 33, 37] In an experimental model of brain wounding, Awasthi and associates[59] showed that fibrinogen levels, platelets, and platelet aggregates decreased significantly 120 minutes after a brain wound.

At Kaufman's[20] hospital, GSW victims were screened for DIC by six tests: activated partial thromboplastin time, thrombin time, prothrombin time, fibrinogen level, fibrin split products, and platelet count. Among nonsurvivors, 49 of 52 (94%) had at least one abnormal test, but so did 30 of the 42 survivors (71%). Kaufman suggested that the tendency to develop DIC is related to the volume of tissue damaged, with resultant release of tissue thromboplastin. Because DIC may be related to the severity of brain injury, measurements of coagulation abnormalities have been used as mortality predictors. Among Shaffrey's[33] 62 patients, mortality was 80% for those with coagulopathy and 7% for those without. Polin's[60] and Shaffrey's[33] groups recommended that the readily available prothrombin time, partial thromboplastin time, and platelet count tests be done on all GSW victims on hospital entry. In their experience, coagulopathy, as indicated by a single abnormality in prothrombin time or activated partial thromboplastin time, within the first day of admission was significantly related to mortality.

Levy and colleagues[36] excluded patients with DIC from their analysis of patients with GCS scores of 3 to 5 because DIC by itself is associated with such a high mortality. Other investigators may also have summarily excluded brain-wounded patients with DIC from analysis, so this phenomenon may be underreported.

DIC may occur after brain wounding, but its manifestation as an abnormal laboratory test is far more frequent than as a complication during brain débridement. DIC is seen most often in patients with severely damaged brains who are not surgical candidates. When DIC does occur during brain débridement, the result is usually catastrophic.

COMPLICATIONS FOLLOWING BRAIN DÉBRIDEMENT

Table 331–7 presents postdébridement complications observed by 20 investigators. Of 764 patients, 115 had complications (15%), and 25 (3%) died from those complications.

Brain infections (meningitis, cerebritis, brain abscess) were the most common complications, despite the stated or presumed use of antibiotics by most surgeons, Suddaby[18] excepted. Brain infections resulted in a 29% mortality. Cerebrospinal fluid leaks occurred as frequently as brain infections, but death from this complication was rare (3%). Wound and bone flap infections accounted for 14% of the complications. Occasionally they led to deep brain infections and disability or death.

Postoperative brain swelling may result if too little brain is débrided, so this complication and hemorrhage should be kept in mind if early neurological deterioration occurs. CT can delineate this. Reopening the wound for further brain débridement or hemorrhage evacuation is necessary if the neurological status worsens and a mass lesion is evident. Hydrocephalus usually occurs later in the postoperative course.

T A B L E 3 3 1 – 7 ■ Summary of Postoperative Complications in 764 Patients

TYPE	COMPLICATIONS RELATED TO BRAIN	NO. DIED	COMPLICATIONS NOT RELATED TO BRAIN	NO. DIED
Brain infections, all	34	10		
Cerebrospinal fluid leak	34	1		
Wound/flap infection	17	0		
Postoperative brain hemorrhage	8	1		
Hydrocephalus	9	0		
Postdébridement brain swelling	7	0		
Traumatic pseudoaneurysm	3	1		
Middle cerebral artery occlusion	2	2		
Subdural hygroma	1	0		
Disseminated intravascular coagulation	3	3		
Respiratory problems			7	4
Pulmonary embolism			2	2
Gastrointestinal bleeding			1	0
Tracheal bleeding			1	1
	118*	18	11	7

*Some patients had more than one complication. Data from references 10–16, 18, 19, 21, 23, 25–29, 32, 37, 41, 44.

Though occurring infrequently, traumatic pseudoaneurysm and occlusion of major intracranial blood vessels had a 60% lethality. Hubschmann's[44] and Benzel's[28] admonition to consider angiography if the missile passes near the middle cerebral artery complex should be remembered so that the diagnosis can be made before catastrophe occurs.

Complications not directly related to the brain were probably underreported, especially nonfatal ones such as pneumonitis. Considering the number of patients who underwent great physiologic stress, the lack of gastrointestinal bleeding is remarkable, as is the infrequency of pulmonary embolism among patients who were bedridden for extended periods.

RETAINED BONE AND MISSILES: SUBSEQUENT BRAIN INFECTION

During the Vietnam War, removal of all indriven bone fragments identified on preoperative radiographs was an army medical policy, because prior war experiences had shown their infective potential.[61] Sometimes multiple operations were required for their removal. No attempt was made, however, to remove inaccessible metal fragments, because past experience indicated that these were unlikely to cause late infection.

In contrast, civilian neurosurgeons became interested in the infective potential of retained metal within the brain, but most have not directly addressed late infections from retained bone. Because many civilian neurosurgeons did and do quite modest brain débridements compared with those done by neurosurgeons in Vietnam, it can be surmised that civilian neurosurgeons often left (and leave) bone within the brain. Despite this fact, the occurrence of late infections has been less than 5% (see Table 331–7) in civilians, regardless of any retained bone or metal. This low rate probably reflects the rapid neurosurgical care afforded brain-wounded civilians. Devitalized brain is removed, and the dura and skin are closed relatively quickly, decreasing the chance of external bacterial contamination. Large doses of antibiotics are also usually given.

Civilian neurosurgeons in general have never addressed the late infective potential of indriven bone in a systematic way. Several authors[11, 13, 15, 18, 21, 29] have noted postdébridement infections and, by statement or inference, retained bone fragments. The cause of these infections was either not stated or ascribed to other complications, such as cerebrospinal fluid and sinus injury, rather than to the retained bone. Mancuso and colleagues[23] concluded that metal fragments were less infective than bone but thought that retained metal could be a source of infection even years later. They stated that neither their experience nor the literature led to definite conclusions concerning the removal of metal fragments and recommended that any decision to reoperate be made on a case-by-case basis.

Although this civilian experience may have relevance to military situations when evacuation is speedy and treatment occurs quickly, it does not apply if definitive treatment occurs days after wounding, when an open brain wound with indriven bone fragments can be colonized by bacteria.

The availability of CT scanning and ultrasonography has given neurosurgeons more flexibility concerning indriven bone or metal than pre-CT neurosurgeons enjoyed. One can quickly determine whether unremoved bone or metal is lying quietly within the brain and should be left alone or whether such a collection is the nidus of an infection and must be removed.

ASSOCIATED WOUNDS

Sophisticated trauma centers are now widespread, resulting in lower morbidity and mortality from somatic wounds. By inference, such facilities might be thought to lower mortality for those with brain wounds. Review of many series[11–16, 18, 20–22, 26–30, 38, 41, 44] indicates, however, that rapid evacuation of brain-wounded individuals and prompt neurosurgical débridement do not lead to appreciably lower mortality. The greatest benefit of prompt care to the brain wounded in trauma centers is derived from the care of associated life-threatening wounds. In contrast to wounded soldiers, however, the usual brain-wounded civilian does not have such wounds. Clark and colleagues,[19] for instance, noted that among their 76 brain-wounded patients, only 3 of 46 deaths (7%) were caused by body wounds. They concluded that trauma centers may not provide a great reduction in brain-wound mortality. Only about 10% of the civilian brain wounded receive additional body wounds, and most of these associated wounds are not life threatening.[10–13, 19, 23, 28, 30] Clark's conclusion, unfortunately, stands.

OUTCOME FOLLOWING BRAIN GUNSHOT WOUNDS

The patient's neurological condition at the time of hospital presentation or operation is the major determinant of long-term outcome. Early attempts at patient outcome stratification for civilian GSWs were based on various clinical descriptions, such as Lillard's.[13] In the mid-1970s, these were gradually replaced by the Glasgow Outcome Score (GOS),[62] which is currently widely used. Kaufman and coworkers[63] pointed out that most disabilities in GSW victims were related to focal brain damage that caused cognitive impairments and motor deficits.

Among the series reviewed, Nagib,[21] Grahm,[27] Aldrich,[31] Levi,[29] and Michael (see the footnote in Table 331–2) present the most comparable data, because all wounds penetrated the brain, patients were primarily adults having GCS scores from 3 to 15, the authors used similar GCS and GOS stratifications, and they included all patients whether operated on or not (Table 331–8).

The overall story is quite grim, moderated only by a more favorable outlook for the 21% of patients (74 of 349) presenting with or achieving favorable GCS scores of 9 to 15 before surgery. Of the 349 patients, 231 (66%) were neurologically devastated by their brain wounds at the time of admission (GCS score 3 to 5). Of these patients, 93% died, and none had a good outcome; only 1% were left with moderate disabilities, and 6% had severe disabilities or remained in a persistent vegetative state. Among 44 patients with GCS scores of 6 to 8, 14 (32%) made a satisfactory recovery (GOS good to moderate), 10 (23%) were severely disabled, and 20 (45%) died.

Little question exists that prompt and aggressive resuscitation and appropriate surgical care should be given to patients with GCS scores of 9 to 15, because few die and three quarters of the survivors make a satisfactory recovery. More than half of patients with GCS scores of 6 to 8 live, and almost a third have a satisfactory outcome, so these patients also deserve neurosurgical treatment.

For the last decade, however, neurosurgeons have been wrestling with the terrible problem of what to do with GSW victims whose GCS scores are 3 to 5, because their prognosis for survival and for a subsequent functional life is so poor. Several investigators have explored this issue. Levy and coworkers[36] and Stone and associates[38] showed that without surgery, death is a virtual certainty for these patients: 242 of 246 unoperated patients died. Among the 60 patients in Levy's[36] series who had GCS scores of 3 to 5 and were operated on, 75% died or remained in a persistent vegetative state, only 3% survived with moderate disabilities, and none made a good recovery (Table 331–9).

Kaufman[20] did not match GCS with GOS but reported that 83 of 86 patients with GCS scores of 3 to 5 died. Of the three survivors, one was working (good outcome), one was caring for himself (moderate disability), and one required only occasional assistance (moderate disability) (my estimates of disability).

Available data indicate that death for those with GCS scores of 3 to 5 is all but inevitable without operation, so it is probable that all the survivors represented in Table 331–9 underwent surgery, though it is difficult to discern this. Some of Levi's[29] patients may have had only superficial wound débridement and scalp closure, because he advocates minimal surgery for brain wounds unless the brain frankly extrudes. Table 331–9

T A B L E 3 3 1 – 8 ■ **Outcome as a Function of Glasgow Coma Scale Score**

GLASGOW COMA SCALE SCORE	GLASGOW OUTCOME SCALE					
	Dead	Persistent Vegetative State	Severe Disability	Moderate Disability	Good Outcome	TOTAL
9–15	7	0	10	25	32	74
6–8	20	0	10	11	3	44
3–5	215	6	8	2	0	231
Total	242	6	28	38	35	349

Data from references 21, 27, 29, 31, and Michael (see footnote to Table 331–2).

T A B L E   3 3 1 – 9 ■ **Outcome of Patients with Glasgow Coma Scale Scores of 3 to 5, Operated and Unoperated**

AUTHOR	DEATH	PERSISTENT VEGETATIVE STATE	SEVERE DISABILITY	MODERATE DISABILITY	GOOD OUTCOME	
Kaufman et al[20]	83	—	—	2	1	
Nagib et al[21]	26	1	1	1	—	
Grahm et al[27]	54	3	1	—	—	
Levi et al[29]	16	1	3	—	—	
Aldrich et al[31]	116	1	5	1	—	
Michael*	3	—	1	—	—	
Levy et al[36]	160	8	14	4	—	
Total	458 (90%)	14 (3%)	25 (5%)	9 (2%)	1 (0.2%)	507 (100%)

*See footnote to Table 331–2.

indicates that 93% of GCS score 3 to 5 patients died or remained in a persistent vegetative state; the chance of making a good recovery was vanishingly small (0.2%), and only about 2% recovered with only moderate disability. The remaining 5% who lived were severely disabled. Analysis of 67 patients from Levy's[36] and Siccardi's[30] data who *definitely* underwent surgery reveals that 66% died, 31% were in a persistent vegetative state or had severe disability, and only 3% were left with moderate disability; no patient had a good outcome. Whether operated on or not, the terrible prognosis of patients with GCS scores of 3 to 5 remains the same. Similarly, the dilemma facing neurosurgeons also remains, because a rare patient does make a reasonable recovery.

WHO SHOULD BE OPERATED ON?

Historically, this has been one of the most difficult decisions a neurosurgeon faces: Which brain-wounded patients can be helped by surgery? In 1964, Goodman and Kalsbeck[10] observed that comatose patients fail to survive. Raimondi and Samuelson[41] did not operate on comatose or decorticate patients. Similarly, Cavaliere's group[22] operated only on patients with GCS scores of at least 6.

Hubschmann and colleagues[44] in 1979 recommended that all alert or obtunded patients and those responsive to pain undergo brain débridement. They suggested that decorticate, decerebrate, or unresponsive patients undergo CT scanning. If a clot was found, it should be removed. If no clot was found, the patient should be watched and considered for surgery 24 to 48 hours later if clinical improvement occurred. Benzel and coauthors[28] concurred with Hubschmann but recommended that deeply comatose patients be considered for surgery on a case-by-case basis. Some comatose patients should be aggressively treated medically to see if they might improve and warrant surgery. Hernesniemi[14] believed that nothing should be done for unconscious patients who had attempted suicide. Shoung and colleagues[17] recommended that patients who were decerebrate or flaccid on admission not be considered surgical candidates. If, however, CT

showed an expansive lesion (hematoma or contusion), presumably in a nondecorticate or nondecerebrate individual, decompressive surgery should be performed early, before clinical deterioration occurred.

Clark,[19] Mancuso,[23] and Siccardi[30] and their coworkers stated that surgery was not indicated for GCS score 3 patients. Additionally, Clark[19] thought that those with intracranial hematomas or ventricular or bihemispheric injury would not benefit from surgery.

Nagib and associates[21] opined that no surgery should be undertaken for patients with GCS scores of 3 to 5 with unilateral multilobe injuries or with bihemispheric wounds, especially if the missile had fragmented and scattered. Comatose patients who had unilateral multilobar injuries with scattering of bone and metal fragments were also not operated on. This opinion was reinforced if the patient had attempted suicide.

Grahm and coauthors[27] concluded that patients with postresuscitation GCS scores of 3 to 5 should undergo surgery only if they have a significant hematoma demonstrated on CT. Those with GCS scores of 6 to 8 should be operated on only if they have a hematoma or a unilateral nondominant hemisphere wound that does not involve the ventricle. If a GCS score 6 to 8 patient has a bihemispheric wound or a unilateral dominant hemisphere, multilobe wound with or without ventricular penetration, no surgery is advised because of the poor functional outcome expected. All patients with a GCS score greater than 8 deserve aggressive surgery.

Levi and coworkers[29] stated that GCS score 3 and 4 patients were beyond help, but GCS score 5 patients deserve surgery, because one of five such patients in their series survived and was only moderately disabled. Siccardi and associates[30] stated that surgery on patients with GCS scores of 4 or 5 was "controversial and unsettled."

Levy's group[36] analyzed many factors in patients with GCS scores of 3 to 5, using linear and logistic models to predict outcome. They concluded that such patients were unlikely to benefit from surgery. If, however, such a patient had responsive pupils, no missile fragmentation, no subarachnoid hemorrhage, and no bihemispheric injury or ventricular involvement on CT, surgery might be considered. They thought that very few GCS score 3 to 5 patients merit vigorous medical or surgical care.

Stone and colleagues[38] would operate on GCS score 3 patients if they were hemodynamically stable and if they had pupillary reactions on admission or after intubation and mannitol. They recommended operating on normotensive GCS score 4 to 7 patients if their pupils reacted or if their pupils were fixed and dilated but they had a motor response.

The issue of patients with GCS scores of 3 to 5 was discussed collectively by Kaufman, Levy, and Stone.[64] Levy reiterated his stance that patients with admission GCS scores of 3, 4, or 5 are not likely to benefit from operative intervention. Although survival is enhanced, good outcomes are not achieved. Patients presenting with admission GCS scores of 3, 4, or 5 without radiologic evidence of subarachnoid hemorrhage, ventricular involvement, or fragmentation in the presence of reactive pupils should be followed closely. If spontaneous improvement occurs, surgery might be considered. Stone restated his position that hemodynamically stable GCS score 3 patients with reactive pupils either on admission or after intubation and mannitol be operated on. Normotensive GCS score 4 to 6 patients with reactive pupils or those with fixed pupils but a motor response could also undergo brain débridement. Stone reported two "good" (GOS 4 or 5) recoveries among 27 GCS score 3 to 5 patients. This percentage of good recoveries is at variance with results reported by other investigators. Stone's original paper included patients with nonpenetrating head wounds, and in that paper, Stone made the salient point that frontal lobe wounds were less devastating. Perhaps these two survivors had nonpenetrating or frontal lobe wounds and their low GCS scores resulted from a recoverable concussion rather than from intrinsic brain damage. Both Levy and Stone concluded that a cooperative clinical trial would be necessary to settle the issue of how best to handle patients with GCS scores of 3 to 5.

Kaufman ended the discussion by stating that bioethical concerns must govern any proposed treatment of GCS score 3 to 5 patients. He outlined a utilitarian approach based on outcome, a virtue-based ethical approach founded on the "caring bond and the public trust," and a communitarian ethical approach based on what is reasonable for the patient and does not harm others. Kaufman stated that the physician, in deciding what to do with the severely brain wounded, must consider the patient, the family and friends, and society. He reiterated the traditional role of the physician as the patient's advocate and also the primary injunction *primum non nocere.* He concluded that society as a whole should develop better guidelines for the care of such patients.

The problems inherent in the treatment of GSW patients with GCS scores of 3 to 5 are too complex and technical for society to grapple with, and I do not see a political groundswell to convene a national committee to consider this issue. Consequently, neurosurgeons must use their best judgment now and probably for the foreseeable future. With outcome data on more than 500 such patients gathered from the world's literature (see Table 331–9), there is no need for cooperative studies. Among 507 patients with GCS scores of 3 to 5, 90% died, and 8% were left in a persistent vegetative state or severely disabled. Only 2% were only moderately disabled, and just one person (0.2%) had a good outcome.

Thus, surgery for these patients involves an extremely high postoperative mortality and at least four to six times more poor outcomes than satisfactory ones. The probability of a good outcome is vanishingly small. These data, whether considered from a utilitarian, virtue-based, or communitarian-based ethic or with regard to the Hippocratic dictum *primum non nocere,* indicate that surgical débridement should not be undertaken for brain-wounded patients with such low GCS scores. The vast majority will die, and of those who live, far more will be left devastated than will be helped to lead a reasonable life.

Table 331–8 indicates that the mortality of patients with GCS scores of 6 to 8 approaches 50%, but almost a third of survivors achieved a satisfactory outcome. Thus, ample justification exists to treat this group of patients medically and surgically. Because almost half of this group currently dies despite best surgical efforts, however, the question arises: Do all such patients deserve surgery? In 1998, we reviewed brain-wound patients at Charity Hospital, New Orleans (unpublished data). Of 16 patients with GCS scores of 6 to 8, nine lived and seven died. Some GCS score 6 patients made good recoveries, and some GCS score 8 patients died, sometimes from untoward complications. Therefore, it may be difficult to sort out this group concerning expected survivors. This implies that all patients with GCS scores of 6 to 8 deserve aggressive care. To my knowledge, no study specifically evaluating surgical mortality and outcome in these patients exists. Such a study would be useful, because it might clarify surgical indications and expected ultimate outcomes for brain-wounded patients with GCS scores of 6 to 8.

SEIZURES AFTER WOUNDING: USE OF POSTOPERATIVE ANTICONVULSANTS

Although some investigators consider seizures a complication, I do not, because seizures are to be expected following a traumatic cortical injury. None of the studies discussed in this review were designed to evaluate the occurrence of seizures after craniocerebral missile wounding, so the reported seizure incidence is likely grossly underreported. Further, follow-ups were often short, and many survivors were lost to follow-up; many authors did not include this topic in their studies. Thus, it is difficult to draw conclusions concerning the incidence of postwounding seizures in civilians.

No consensus exists on the use of anticonvulsants after brain wounding, but considering that prophylactic anticonvulsants are not beneficial beyond the first week following severe brain injury (studied mostly in those with closed head injuries),[51] their use does not seem indicated, except possibly in the immediate postwounding period. All patients in Grahm and colleagues'[27] series were placed on prophylactic anticonvulsants for an indeterminate period, whereas Miner and associates[26] continued anticonvulsants in children for 6 months postoperatively. Levi's group[29] put their patients on "prophylactic" anticonvulsants for 1 year. Benzel and coworkers[28] gave anticonvulsants only to those who had seizures.

Of the 50 patients followed by Sherman and coauthors[15] for longer than 2 years, 21 (42%) had seizures, and 20 of these had been placed on anticonvulsants shortly after hospital admission. Stone and colleagues[38] stated that all patients in their series received anticonvulsants routinely from shortly after admission through the postoperative period. None of their patients had seizures before discharge, but by 1 year, the seizure incidence was at least 21%. Lillard[13] noted that only 20 patients had been placed on anticonvulsants at admission, and he thought that any "prophylactic" effect of anticonvulsants was problematic. All four patients in Pikus and Ball's[37] series who developed seizures had been placed on prophylactic anticonvulsants.

SUGGESTIONS FOR THE FUTURE

Future descriptive studies will tell how particular neurosurgery services are faring in the treatment of brainwounded patients, but more focused clinical studies analyzing the favorable and adverse factors affecting the outcome in patients with GCS scores of 6 to 8 would be more useful. Realistic surgical criteria for these patients should be developed, but because such patients constitute only about 12% of the brain wounded, a cooperative study may be needed. If the reader is not convinced by this analysis of the futility of treating patients with GCS scores of 3 to 5, further outcome work evaluating this group should be undertaken.

It would be useful if several neurosurgical centers tried minimal brain débridement for civilians with GSWs to the brain, because civilians are generally treated within a few hours of wounding. Levi's[29] and Suddaby's[18] groups seem to have had reasonable results with this method. It would be helpful if others could confirm this method's usefulness.

Future authors should carefully delineate and categorize their brain-wound populations. Important issues are obfuscated if patients with wounds that do not penetrate the dura are included in data dealing with penetrating brain wounds. Likewise, if the brain is injured by a few flecks of indriven bone (a "penetrating" injury) but not by the missile itself, the outcome will be vastly improved, because the energy of deposit within the brain is much less and the bullet's trajectory within the brain is not a factor. Such cases should also be separated in data presentation. Patients actually undergoing surgery should be clearly indicated, preferably in some form of chart (see, e.g., Cavaliere[22] and Siccardi[30]), so that any future reviewer does not have to do a detailed reanalysis to find out how many of the reported patients actually had surgery.

Presurgical GCS scores (whether pre- or postresuscitation) and surgical outcomes, including mortality and complications, should also be documented. Until better systems are devised, the GCS and GOS are useful ways to present the patient's clinical condition before treatment and the eventual outcome. If other systems are used, their GCS equivalents should be given. If patients with all GCS ranges are being studied, all GCS or GOS categories should be presented. A four-level GCS stratification has been most commonly used, but in light of the dilemma of what to do with low–GCS score patients, it will be particularly important to provide mortality and outcome data for each GCS grade individually for GCS scores of 8 and below. This will aid future analyses of prognosis and treatment efficacy for these severely damaged patients.

ACKNOWLEDGMENTS

I give great thanks to my wife, Dr. Betty Oseid, who spent many hours reading this manuscript and made many helpful suggestions. Similarly, I thank Elizabeth Hulbert, my secretary, who typed the many iterations of this manuscript. Diane Lane in our neurosurgical laboratory and William Johnson in the department of biometry provided invaluable help as well.

REFERENCES

1. French RW, Callender GR: Ballistic characteristics of wounding agents. In Beyer JC (ed): Wound Ballistics. Washington, DC, Office of the Surgeon General, Department of the Army, 1972, pp 91–141.
2. Horsley V: The destructive effects of small projectiles. Nature 50:104–108, 1894.
3. Webster JE, Gurdjian ES: Acute physiological effects of gunshot and other penetrating wounds of the brain. J Neurophysiol 6:255–262, 1943.
4. Crockard HA, Johns L, Levett J, et al: "Brainstem" effects of experimental cerebral trauma. In Popp J, Bourke RS, Nelson LR, et al (eds): Neural Trauma. New York, Raven Press, 1979, pp 19–25.
5. Carey ME, Sarna GS, Farrell JB, et al: Experimental missile wound to the brain. J Neurosurg 71:754–764, 1989.
6. Carey ME, Sarna GS, Farrell JB: Brain edema following an experimental missile wound to the brain. J Neurotrauma 7:13–20, 1990.
7. Freytag E: Autopsy findings in head injuries from firearms. Arch Pathol 76:215–225, 1963.
8. Kirkpatrick JB, Di Maio V: Civilian gunshot wounds of the brain. J Neurosurg 49:185–198, 1978.
9. Koszyca B, Blumbers PC, Manavis J, et al: Widespread axonal injury in gunshot wounds to the head using amyloid precursor protein as a marker. J Neurotrauma 15:675–683, 1998.
10. Goodman JM, Kalsbeck J: Outcome of self-inflicted gunshot wounds of the head. J Trauma 5:636–642, 1965.
11. Yashon D, Jane JA, Martonffy D: Management of civilian craniocerebral bullet injuries. Ann Surg 38:346–351, 1972.
12. Byrnes DP, Crockard HA, Gordon DS, et al: Penetrating craniocerebral missile injuries in the civil disturbances in Northern Ireland. Br J Surg 61:169–176, 1974.
13. Lillard PL: Five years experience with penetrating craniocerebral gunshot wounds. Surg Neurol 9:79–83, 1978.
14. Hernesniemi J: Penetrating craniocerebral gunshot wounds in civilians. Acta Neurochir (Wien) 49:199–205, 1979.
15. Sherman WD, Apuzzo MLJ, Heiden JS, et al: Gunshot wounds to the brain—a civilian experience. West J Med 132:99–105, 1980.
16. Brandt F, Roosen K, Weiler G, et al: Die neurochirurgische Behandlung von Kopfschussverletzungen. Neurochirurgia 26:164–171, 1983.

17. Shoung HM, Sichez JP, Pertuiset B: The early prognosis of craniocerebral gunshot wounds in civilian practice as an aid to the choice of treatment: A series of 56 cases studied by computerized tomography. Acta Neurochir (Wien) 74:27–30, 1985.

18. Suddaby L, Weir B, Forsyth C: The management of .22 caliber gunshot wounds of the brain: A review of 49 cases. Can J Neurol Sci 14:268–272, 1987.

19. Clark WC, Muhlbauer MS, Watridge CB, et al: Analysis of 76 civilian craniocerebral gunshot wounds. J Neurosurg 65:9–14, 1986.

20. Kaufman HH, Makela ME, Lee KF, et al: Gunshot wounds to the head: A perspective. Neurosurgery 18:689–695, 1986.

21. Nagib MG, Rockswold GL, Sherman RS, et al: Civilian gunshot wounds to the brain: Prognosis and management. Neurosurgery 18:533–537, 1986.

22. Cavaliere R, Cavenago L, Siccardi D, et al: Gunshot wounds of the brain in civilians. Acta Neurochir (Wien) 94:133–136, 1988.

23. Mancuso P, Chiaramonte I, Passanisi M, et al: Craniocerebral gunshot wounds in civilians: Report on 40 cases. J Neurosurg Sci 32:189–194, 1988.

24. Selden BS, Goodman JM, Cordell W, et al: Outcome of self-inflicted gunshot wounds of the brain. Ann Emerg Med 17:247–253, 1988.

25. Sarnaik AP, Kopec J, Moylan P, et al: Role of aggressive intracranial pressure control in management of pediatric craniocerebral gunshot wounds with unfavorable features. J Trauma 29:1434–1437, 1989.

26. Miner ME, Ewing-Cobbs L, Kopaniky DR, et al: The results of treatment of gunshot wounds to the brain in children. Neurosurgery 26:20–25, 1990.

27. Grahm TW, Williams FC, Harrington T, et al: Civilian gunshot wounds to the head: A prospective study. Neurosurgery 27:696–700, 1990.

28. Benzel EC, Day WT, Kesterson L, et al: Civilian craniocerebral gunshot wounds. Neurosurgery 29:67–72, 1991.

29. Levi L, Linn S, Feinsod M: Penetrating craniocerebral injuries in civilians. Br J Neurosurg 5:241–247, 1991.

30. Siccardi D, Cavaliere R, Pau A, et al: Penetrating craniocerebral missile injuries in civilians: A retrospective analysis of 314 cases. Surg Neurol 35:455–460, 1991.

31. Aldrich EF, Eisenberg HM, Saydjari C, et al: Predictors of mortality in severely head-injured patients with civilian gunshot wounds: A report from the NIH traumatic coma data bank. Surg Neurol 38:418–423, 1992.

32. Helling TS, McNabney WK, Whittaker CK, et al: The role of early surgical intervention in civilian gunshot wounds to the head. J Trauma 32:398–401, 1992.

33. Shaffrey ME, Polin RS, Phillips CD, et al: Classification of civilian craniocerebral gunshot wounds: A multivariate analysis predictive of mortality. J Neurotrauma 9(Suppl 1):S279–S285, 1992.

34. Deshmukh VD, Laneve L, Fallon WF: Violent brain injuries by gunshot in Duval County, Florida, 1989–1991 [letter]. Arch Neurol 49:588, 1992.

35. Kennedy F, Gonzales P, Dang C, et al: The Glasgow Coma Scale and prognosis in gunshot wounds to the brain. J Trauma 35:75–77, 1993.

36. Levy ML, Masri LS, Lavine S, et al: Outcome prediction after penetrating craniocerebral injury in a civilian population: Aggressive surgical management in patients with admission Glasgow Coma Scale scores of 3, 4, or 5. Neurosurgery 35:77–85, 1994.

37. Pikus HJ, Ball PA: Characteristics of cerebral gunshot injuries in the rural setting. Neurosurg Clin N Am 43:611–620, 1995.

38. Stone JL, Lichtor T, Fitzgerald LF: Gunshot wounds to the head in civilian practice. Neurosurgery 37:1104–1112, 1995.

39. Morrow PL, Hudson P: Accidental firearm fatalities in North Carolina 1976–1980. Am J Public Health 76:1120–1123, 1986.

40. Narayan RK, Contant CF, Russell KD, et al: Gunshot wounds to the head; lessons from a 9 year civilian experience. Paper presented at the Scientific Program, 60th Annual Meeting of the American Association of Neurological Surgeons, 1992, San Francisco, p 367.

41. Raimondi AJ, Samuelson GH: Craniocerebral gunshot wounds in civilian practice. J Neurosurg 32:647–653, 1970.

42. Chestnut RM, Marshall LF, Klauber MR, et al: The role of secondary brain injury in determining outcome from severe head injury. J Trauma 34:216–222, 1993.

43. Miller JD, Becker DP: Secondary insults to the injured brain. J R Coll Surg Edinb 27:292–298, 1982.

44. Hubschmann O, Shapiro K, Baden M, et al: Craniocerebral gunshot injuries in civilian practice—prognostic criteria and surgical management: Experience with 82 cases. J Trauma 19:6–12, 1979.

45. McNealy DE, Plum F: Brainstem dysfunction with supratentorial mass lesions. Arch Neurol 7:10–32, 1962.

46. Carey ME, Young HF, Mathis JL: The neurosurgical treatment of craniocerebral missile wounds in Vietnam. Surg Gynecol Obstet 135:386–390, 1972.

47. Carey ME, Young HF, Rish BL, et al: Followup study of 103 American soldiers who sustained a brain wound in Vietnam. J Neurosurg 41:542–549, 1974.

48. Teasdale G, Jennett B: Assessment of coma and impaired consciousness, a practical scale. Lancet 2:81–84, 1974.

49. Levy ML, Rezai A, Masri L, et al: The significance of subarachnoid hemorrhage after penetrating craniocerebral injury: Correlations with angiography and outcome in a civilian population. Neurosurgery 32:532–540, 1993.

50. Cooper PR, Maravilla K, Cone J: Computerized tomographic scan and gunshot wounds of the head: Indications and radiographic findings. Neurosurgery 4:373–380, 1979.

51. Brain Trauma Foundation: Guidelines for the Management of Severe Head Injury. Joint initiative of the Brain Trauma Foundation, the American Association of Neurological Surgeons, and the Joint Section on Neurotrauma and Critical Care, 1995.

52. Temkin NR, Dikmen SS, Wilensky AJ, et al: A randomized double-blind study of phenytoin for the prevention of post traumatic seizures. N Engl J Med 323:497–502, 1990.

53. Watson CW, Kennard MA: The effect of anticonvulsant drugs on recovery of function of following cerebral cortical lesions. J Neurophysiol 8:221–231, 1945.

54. Brailowsky S, Knight RT, Efron R: Phenytoin increases the severity of cortical hemiplegia in rats. Brain Res 376:71–77, 1986.

55. Kaufman HH, Schwab K, Salazar AM: A national survey of neurosurgical care for penetrating head injury. Surg Neurol 36:370–377, 1991.

56. Cushing H: A study of a series of wounds involving the brain and its enveloping structures. Br J Surg 5:558–684, 1914.

57. Schwartz HG, Roulhac GE: Penetrating wounds of the cerebral ventricles. Ann Surg 127:58–74, 1948.

58. Wannamaker GT: Transventricular wounds of the brain. J Neurosurg 11:151–160, 1954.

59. Awasthi D, Rock WA, Carey ME, et al: Coagulation changes after an experimental missile wound. Surg Neurol 36:441–446, 1991.

60. Polin RS, Shaffrey ME, Philips CD, et al: Multivariate analysis and prediction of outcome following penetrating head injury. Neurosurg Clin N Am 43:689–699, 1995.

61. Martin J, Campbell TH: Early complications following penetrating wounds of the skull. J Neurosurg 3:58–73, 1946.

62. Jennett B, Bond M: Assessment of outcome after severe brain damage. Lancet 1:480–484, 1975.

63. Kaufman HH, Levin HS, High WM, et al: Neurobehavioral outcome after gunshot wounds to the head in adult civilians and children. Neurosurgery 16:754–758, 1985.

64. Kaufman HH, Levy ML, Stone JL, et al: Patients with Glasgow Coma Scale scores 3, 4, 5 after gunshot wounds to the brain. Neurosurg Clin N Am 43:701–714, 1995.

CHAPTER 332

Craniofacial Trauma

JOSEPH S. GRUSS ■ RICHARD G. ELLENBOGEN ■ MICHAEL F. WHELAN

Major facial injuries in adults usually result from motor vehicle accidents, personal altercations, and industrial trauma. The institution of lower speed limits and compulsory seat belt laws in various parts of the world has led to a relative decrease in the overall incidence of facial injuries. However, the organization of regional trauma centers and rapid air transport systems has contributed to improved survival rates in patients with extensive multisystem trauma associated with complex craniomaxillofacial injuries, resulting in an increase in the number of severe facial injuries requiring treatment. Conventional techniques of investigation and treatment have proved to be inadequate in this group of patients. Our experience with more than 2000 such cases has resulted in the evolution of a method of managing complex facial injuries based on the principles of reconstructive craniofacial surgery.

Multiple facial fractures in polytraumatized patients are distinguished by the severity of the bony injury. The majority of these fractures, particularly in the midface, are unstable and often have multiple comminuted segments. Areas of bone may be sufficiently damaged to preclude any form of fixation, or they may actually be missing, having been lost through large skin or mucosal lacerations. Gross instability in the craniofacial skeleton predisposes to massive soft tissue swelling and potential problems with swallowing and upper airway obstruction. In the absence of adequate fixation, the skeletal framework tends to collapse, and the overlying soft tissues become atrophic, scarred, and constricted.

Conventional techniques of fracture management are inadequate in the treatment of these complex facial injuries. Standard radiographs fail to demonstrate the degree of comminution or bone loss. Attempts at closed reduction or internal wire suspension of these comminuted areas result in eventual bony collapse and soft tissue shrinkage. External fixation techniques maintain the position of mandibular segments but cannot maintain the position of comminuted midfacial bony segments. The inability to stabilize these midfacial segments results in rapid soft tissue shrinkage and makes secondary bone correction difficult or impossible.

Management of complex facial trauma aims to restore and maintain the normal anatomy of the craniofacial skeleton, thereby minimizing the secondary problems of massive edema, bony collapse, and soft tissue shrinkage. Comprehensive clinical examination, computed tomography, and selective radiographic views are used to establish the severity and extent of facial fractures. Operative treatment of facial injuries is performed as early as possible. Craniofacial surgical techniques are used in the complete exposure of the facial skeleton and anatomic reduction of fracture segments. Rigid internal fixation, using a combination of lag screws, compression plates, and miniplates, provides optimal stability in the reconstructed skeletal framework. This reestablishes a normal craniofacial skeletal anatomy and maintains soft tissue expansion during the healing phase. Comminuted or missing bone is replaced by immediate bone grafting. These techniques allow the repair of even the most severe injury in one stage and prevent the development of secondary deformity.

PRIORITIES IN TREATMENT

In any patient with severe facial trauma, it is essential to check carefully for any associated injuries, both locally in the head and neck region and in the other body systems. The priorities of resuscitation and treatment dictate that maintenance of a patent airway, control of hemorrhage, and management of neurosurgical, thoracic, and abdominal trauma take precedence over the management of facial injuries and fractures. However, in many patients, management of facial injuries and fractures can be coordinated with the repair of trauma to other systems, facilitating more rapid treatment and rehabilitation. Whenever possible, facial injuries are treated early, particularly when neurosurgical exploration is contemplated. Careful extension of the neurosurgical incisions and approaches following the completion of intracranial repair allows the synchronous repair of orbital and midfacial injuries.

In patients with head injuries, intracranial pressure monitoring allows the safe, early repair of facial fractures. It is essential not to delay the repair of facial injuries until a patient has fully recovered from a head injury, as young patients may take many weeks to months to recover. Failure to repair facial fractures within a 2-week period will result in a severe, established deformity that is often impossible to correct secondarily. In children, early exploration is essential, because fracture sites tend to adhere much more rapidly, owing to the increased osteogenic potential of the periosteum and more rapid bone healing.

With careful coordination among members of the trauma team, facial injuries can be repaired during initial trauma care. It is not uncommon in our institution to repair intra-abdominal, neurosurgical, orthopedic, and facial injuries on the day of admission, under the same anesthetic. The early repair of facial injuries is facilitated by the use of rigid internal fixation techniques that allow the anesthetist adequate control of the airway without the need for intermaxillary fixation.

SPECIAL CONSIDERATIONS

Airway Management

Patients with major craniofacial injuries are at particular risk of developing upper airway obstruction. A variety of causative factors have been identified (Table 332–1). Most commonly, facial fractures predispose to supraglottic obstruction. Foreign bodies such as dentures, teeth, or fracture fragments may become displaced and occlude the airway.

Mandibular or midfacial fractures are frequently associated with massive swelling and ecchymosis in the pharynx, hypopharynx, and laryngeal region, out of all proportion to the extent of external swelling. Bleeding from the nasal cavity or from intraoral lacerations may cause sudden airway obstruction due to the lodging of blood clots in the laryngotrachea. Comminuted, unstable fractures of the mandible result in loss of support in the hypomandibular complex and consequent ptosis and retroposition of the tongue.

Other injuries commonly associated with facial trauma may cause airway obstruction. In particular, head injuries or cervical spine fractures can result in vocal cord paralysis. Direct tracheobronchial injuries

TABLE 332–1 ■ Causes of Upper Airway Obstruction

ANATOMIC LOCATION	CAUSATIVE FACTORS
Supraglottic	Foreign body—dentures, teeth, fracture fragments, vomitus, mucus
	Pharyngeal/laryngeal swelling
	Massive hemorrhage
	Glossoptosis
Glottic	Spasm
	Edema
	Paralysis—head injury, spinal cord injury, recurrent laryngeal nerve palsy
Infraglottic	Tracheobronchial injury—laceration, disruption, edema

must be suspected in the presence of penetrating neck wounds or subcutaneous emphysema.

Initial establishment and maintenance of an adequate airway is mandatory. Some form of artificial airway is indicated in patients with respiratory obstruction, inability to clear secretions, a need for artificial ventilation, or unconsciousness. An oropharyngeal airway or endotracheal tube is generally used.

Continued management of the airway is facilitated by the use of rigid internal fixation techniques (Fig. 332–1). In repairing midfacial or mandible injuries, the orotracheal tube can be pushed to the side, allowing temporary intermaxillary fixation to establish the correct occlusion. Following rigid internal fixation of the mandible and midface, the intermaxillary fixation is released. This allows endotracheal intubation to be maintained postoperatively until a patent airway is ensured.

The use of rigid internal fixation in the treatment of facial fractures has obviated the need for tracheostomy in many patients. Remaining indications for tracheostomy include massive soft tissue trauma and panfacial fractures associated with bilateral condylar neck fractures. In the latter situation, continued intermaxillary fixation is required to maintain the position of the mandible in relation to the midface and skull base. Tracheostomy may also be needed in multiple trauma patients for the subsequent management of head injury, chest trauma, or spinal cord injury.

Massive Hemorrhage

Severe primary hemorrhage resulting from facial injuries is uncommon. Massive soft tissue trauma, particularly scalp avulsions, and direct penetrating injuries to the facial, internal maxillary, or external carotid vessels can lead to considerable blood loss. Hemorrhage is usually effectively controlled by pressure or direct ligation of bleeding vessels.

Midfacial fractures can cause hemorrhage from sources that are less accessible and more difficult to control. Significantly displaced fractures of the maxilla may disrupt the internal maxillary artery, and nasoethmoidal fractures predispose to avulsions of posterior ethmoidal or sphenopalatine vessels. Patients who present with epistaxis and bleeding from the oral cavity are at risk for aspiration or airway problems. Brisk epistaxis may respond to packing of the anterior nose with petrolatum gauze. If this is unsuccessful, a posterior nasal pack is indicated. A Foley catheter is carefully guided though the nasal cavity into the mouth. The balloon is inflated with air rather than water, to prevent aspiration in the event of rupture, and then lodged in the nasopharynx. Failure to control hemorrhage with these techniques necessitates urgent operative intervention. The facial fractures are reduced, and the external carotid artery or, preferably, the internal maxillary artery is ligated. Alternatively, the bleeding site can be accurately localized by angiography, and hemostasis can be obtained using selective arterial embolization.

Ocular Injury

Direct injury to the eyeball should be suspected in all patients with orbital fractures or lacerations to the eyelids and periorbital tissues. In a prospective study of 49 patients with orbital fractures, Jabaley and coworkers reported a 29% incidence of ocular injury.[1] A careful history and physical examination are required, and all findings should be documented before the institution of fracture treatment. If there is any question about the status of the globe, ophthalmologic consultation is indicated.

Orbital fractures and periorbital lacerations without direct ocular injury are generally pain free, and other eye symptoms are usually absent. The presence of pain, decreased vision, and spots before the eyes is highly suggestive of trauma to the globe itself. Under these circumstances, a detailed examination and determination of visual acuity are mandatory. Injuries that may require immediate ophthalmologic treatment or result in permanent sequelae include corneoscleral lacerations, lens dislocation, major hyphema, acute glaucoma, and retinal detachment.

Initial blindness is a rare occurrence in orbital trauma. Major globe rupture is frequently the cause and generally necessitates enucleation of the globe. There are reports of patients sustaining blunt trauma who present with normal vision that is progressively lost. Causative factors include intraneural hemorrhage or edema in the optic nerve or displaced fractures through the optic canal. Initial management consists of serial assessment of visual acuity, funduscopy, and computed tomographic scans to visualize the optic canal and orbit. Anderson and coworkers recommend a trial of megadose steroids, using dexamethasone 3 to 5 mg/kg per day.[2] Failure of medical treatment or radiographic demonstration of fracture fragments impinging on the optic nerve is an indication for surgical decompression.

Cerebrospinal Fluid Rhinorrhea

The discharge of cerebrospinal fluid (CSF) into the nasal cavity implies a defect in the pia-arachnoid and a resulting communication between the subarachnoid space and the external environment. The decreased thickness of bone in the basal skull region and the close adherence of the pia-arachnoid to the base of the anterior fossa and cribriform plate predispose to direct laceration of the dura by displaced fracture fragments. Midface injuries, including Le Fort II and III and nasoethmoidal fractures, are commonly implicated. The resulting fracture lines extend to the cribriform plate and the ethmoid or sphenoid sinuses, all of which are frequent sites of CSF fistula. Fractures that involve the posterior wall of the frontal sinus are similarly at risk of tearing the pia-arachnoid.

Clinically, CSF leaks should be actively searched for in patients with craniofacial or high midfacial fractures. Clear or serosanguineous nasal discharge, anosmia, or a salty taste in the mouth is highly suggestive. Lateral skull films and computed tomographic scans may dem-

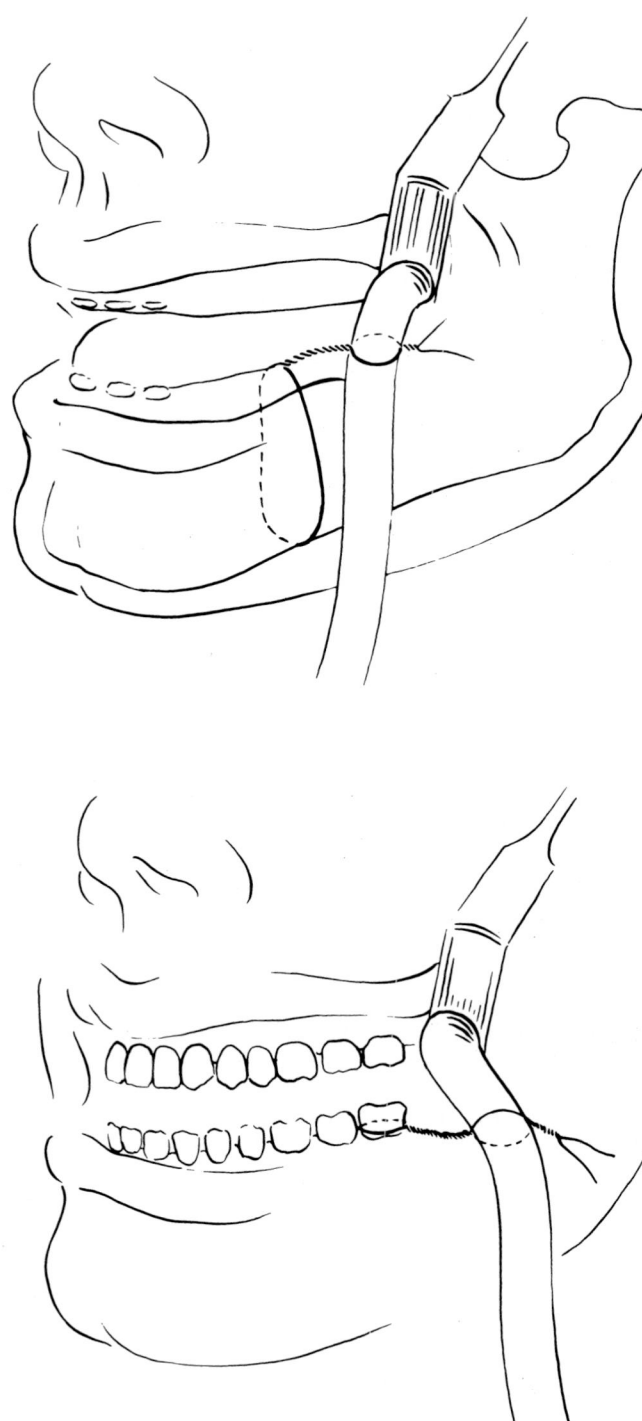

FIGURE 332–1. Intraoperative airway management using rigid wiring of the endotracheal tube to the mandible. *A,* In a patient with adequate dentition, 24- or 26-gauge wire is rigidly wired to a posterior molar tooth. The wire is twisted, leaving a braid 2 to 3 cm long so that the tube can be repositioned in the mouth. The wire is then rigidly fixed to the endotracheal tube—preferably an armor tube. *B,* In a patient with an edentulous mandible or a young child whose teeth are inadequate for fixation, a circummandibular wire is placed around the mandible and then fixed to the tube in a similar fashion.

onstrate pneumocephalus or air-fluid levels in the frontal sinus. The diagnosis is confirmed by collecting the nasal discharge and a concomitant blood sample and submitting both for laboratory investigation. CSF is differentiated from serum by its low protein concentration and can be further distinguished from normal nasal secretions by the presence of glucose but no mucin.

Morgan and associates reviewed 300 patients with severe facial fractures and reported a 35% incidence of CSF rhinorrhea.[3] Spontaneous cessation of flow was observed in 66% of cases by the 10th day. Factors that predispose to persistent CSF leaks include significantly displaced fractures that interfere with dural approximation and increased CSF pressures that exceed the tensile strength of healing tissue.

Most CSF fistulas close spontaneously, particularly following accurate open reduction of facial fractures. The patient's neurological status is continuously monitored, and measures are introduced to minimize increased intracranial pressure. Persistence of CSF leak beyond the first postinjury week requires neurosurgical consultation and more aggressive investigation and treatment. Metrizamide can be injected into the lumbar subarachnoid space and its course followed by computed tomography of the head to precisely localize the CSF fistula. Surgical exploration and obliteration of the fistula by a dural patch graft may be necessary in selected patients.

Infection

Despite excellent vascular perfusion of facial soft tissues, there is some risk of infection in more severe craniofacial injuries, particularly in fractures of the mandible. The anatomic situation of the mandible is such that most fractures occurring through the body or parasymphyseal region, even with slight displacement, must be considered compound. These fractures are initially contaminated through tears in the closely adherent intraoral mucosa, by teeth in the fracture line, or by compound external wounds.

Factors predisposing to infection of the facial fracture site are as follows.

Local Factors
1. Poor oral hygiene, gingivitis, pyorrhea
2. Devitalized, fractured, or abscessed teeth in the area of the fracture
3. Hematoma or lymphatic stasis near the fracture site
4. Foreign bodies in the wound
5. Severe soft tissue injury
6. Destruction of periosteum
7. Devitalized bone sequestra
8. Delayed or inadequate fracture immobilization

General Factors
1. Age
2. Malnutrition
3. Disease (e.g., diabetes, blood dyscrasia)

Infection is a potentially serious complication resulting in increased morbidity, disability, and prolonged hospitalization. Undesirable consequences include nonunion, osteomyelitis, and extension of infection to adjacent anatomic sites, such as the neck or temporomandibular joint.

Some factors, such as age or constitutional disease, are obviously beyond the control of the surgeon. However, local predisposing factors can be effectively treated to decrease the incidence of infection. Measures to reduce the bacterial contamination in open wounds and in the oral cavity should be instituted immediately. Facial lacerations must be adequately irrigated and débrided, and all foreign bodies or clearly devitalized tissue must be meticulously removed. A good oral hygiene program consisting of frequent use of mouthwash, brushing of teeth, and dental prophylaxis to remove clearly devitalized or loose teeth fragments can significantly decrease intraoral bacterial counts.

Early definitive treatment of fractures is an extremely important preventive measure. Experimental studies and clinical observations at the maxillofacial surgical unit of the University of Basel have confirmed that fracture instability promotes infection, and rigid stabilization is an efficient prophylaxis against it.[4] Anatomic reduction and rigid internal fixation of facial fractures serve to minimize edema, lymphatic stasis, and the risk of secondary infection, even in the presence of bacterial contamination. An equally important consideration is the preservation of adequate blood supply to the bone fragments. Viable, well-perfused soft tissue cover is required over the fracture site, and intact periosteum is preserved whenever possible. This is of particular significance in badly displaced fractures, in fractures through an edentulous mandible, or in the presence of circumscribed butterfly fragments. Under these circumstances, the major blood supply to bone through nutrient vessels is diminished or absent, and the survival of osteogenic cells is contingent on a vascularized periosteal envelope.

Prophylactic antibiotics are indicated in all compound fractures.[5] Closed facial fractures, in contrast, are associated with a relatively low incidence of infection. In our institution, only patients with compound fractures are treated prophylactically. For this purpose, we use cephalosporins, administered parenterally as a bolus 1 hour preoperatively, and then repeated every 6 hours for 48 hours.

Occlusion

Occlusion describes the contact of the masticating and incising surfaces of the maxillary and mandibular teeth. A basic knowledge of normal occlusion and the ability to recognize malocclusal patterns are necessary for the accurate diagnosis and management of facial fractures.

The adult dentition is composed of 32 teeth divided into four equal quadrants. Within each quadrant, the arrangement of teeth from medial to lateral is as follows: central incisor; lateral incisor; canine; first and second premolars; first, second, and third molars. Maxillary and mandibular fracture lines can be precisely localized and described by relating them specifically to the teeth involved.

The maxillary dentition should overlap the mandibular dentition in three separate ways during normal occlusion.

1. *Overjet* describes the horizontal overlap of the maxillary incisors, located labial (or anterior) to the mandibular incisors.

2. *Overbite* describes the vertical overlap, whereby the incisal edge of the maxillary incisors lies 2 to 3 mm below the edge of the mandibular incisors.

3. The maxillary arch is wider than the mandibular arch. The upper premolar and molar teeth, therefore, overlap the corresponding mandibular dentition on the buccal (or lateral) aspect by a distance of one cusp.

The dental occlusion further defines the normal skeletal relationship between the maxilla and mandible. Angle's classification describes these skeletal patterns, based on the occlusion of the first maxillary molar to the first mandibular molar.

An initial assessment of the patient's occlusion is critical in the evaluation of facial fractures. An anterior open-bite deformity characterized by an increased gap between the upper and lower central incisors is indicative of a rotated, impacted maxillary fracture or bilateral condylar neck fractures. Unilateral posterior open bites are associated with unilateral condylar neck fractures. Posterior crossbite should alert the examining physician to the presence of collapsed, comminuted vertical fractures of the maxilla or displaced parasymphyseal fractures of the mandible.

Reestablishment and maintenance of premorbid occlusion are the keystones to accurate reduction of facial fractures. In an unconscious or anesthetized patient, the wear facets on corresponding teeth serve as a guide to the premorbid articulations between the maxillary and mandibular dentition. Care is taken to ensure that the midline interval between the two central incisors of the maxillary and mandibular arches is realigned, that the maxillary teeth overlap the mandibular teeth, and that the resulting bite is stable. This establishes the correct skeletal relationship between the maxilla and the mandible.

SOFT TISSUE INJURY

Basic wound management in the head and neck differs little from that applied to wounds in other areas. Optimal results are obtained following primary wound closure. However, in a polytraumatized patient, facial wound closure can be delayed for 24 to 36 hours, pending stabilization of the patient's general condition. The wounds are cleansed, hemostasis is obtained, and occlusive moist gauze dressings are applied. Favorable wound healing can be expected because of excellent vascular perfusion to the scalp and face.

All facial wounds, whether destined for immediate or delayed repair, must be thoroughly irrigated with copious amounts of sterile isotonic saline. Foreign bodies and dirt are removed, and minimal débridement of clearly devitalized tissue is performed.

Accidental Tattoo

Multiple small dirt particles, pigment, and foreign bodies may become embedded in the depths of healing wounds or abrasions. It is best to remove all such foreign material before the onset of wound healing and epithelialization. Failure to do so results in permanent, unattractive discoloration in the skin, which is difficult to treat secondarily.

Adequate anesthesia is first obtained. Scrubbing the wound with a stiff, sterile brush and soap is usually effective in removing most tattooing foreign bodies. Isolated, deeply embedded particles occasionally require excision. Care must be taken to preserve the deep dermal layers and prevent secondary scarring.

Laceration

Lacerations are the most common form of facial soft tissue injury. These range from simple lacerations associated with penetrating trauma to complex stellate lacerations resulting from blunt injuries. In all cases, initial management consists of cleaning, irrigation, and meticulous removal of foreign matter. Ragged or severely contused wound edges are conservatively excised to provide perpendicular skin edges. Clearly devitalized tissue is débrided, regardless of its previous location or importance.

The primary objective in repairing these injuries is to return displaced structures to their original anatomic positions. Landmarks are identified on either side of an irregular wound and precisely approximated. This facilitates the suturing of intervening wound edges in the position they occupied relative to one another before the injury. Irregularities in the lip margin, eyebrow, eyelid, or nostril can thus be avoided.

Avulsion Flap

The avulsion flap is an extensively undermined laceration caused by sharp tangential trauma. Soft tissues are sheared off in the plane of least resistance, usually through the subgaleal or subfascial loose areolar tissue. Vascular perfusion of the flap depends on the size and substance of the pedicle and the integrity of communications between subdermal and facial vascular networks. Despite the degree of undermining and the presence of an almost circumferential wound, avulsion flaps in the head and neck generally remain visible.

Adequate blood supply to the avulsion flap is first confirmed by the presence of capillary refill and dermal bleeding. Only clearly devitalized tissue and the beveled skin edges are excised, and closure is performed in the same manner as for simple lacerations. Suction drains are consistently used to minimize dead space beneath the flap.

Tissue Loss

Facial soft tissue injuries, regardless of severity, are rarely associated with actual loss of tissue. The size of the cutaneous defect is often more apparent than real.

The governing principle in treating such injuries is to first replace surviving tissues in their correct anatomic position. The defect can then be properly displayed and assessed in terms of the tissue lost.

Reconstruction of the defect is performed in a manner that does not distort adjacent anatomic structures. If the recipient site is adequately vascularized, application of split skin grafts promotes rapid healing and leaves conditions suitable for subsequent definitive repair. Primary reconstruction is mandatory only when exposed bone or cartilage renders the recipient site unsuitable for grafting, and vascularized soft tissue cover is required to prevent further necrosis or desiccation of these structures.

Regional Considerations

The goal of soft tissue repair in the head and neck is to effectively restore both function and appearance. The proximity of many complex and vital underlying structures requires a careful, systematic physical examination to rule out occult injury to these parts. Injuries to the eyelids, nose, or perioral region commonly transect composite tissue layers. Meticulous approximation of the mucosal lining, muscular or cartilaginous supporting structures, and the cutaneous cover is necessary to meet the functional requirements in these areas.

EYELIDS

Assessment
1. Rule out injury to the globe.
2. Examine extraocular muscle movements and the ability to elevate the upper lid and appose both lids.
3. With penetrating injuries to the medial canthal region, suspect avulsion of the medial canthus and possible injury to the lacrimal duct.

Repair
1. Superficial lacerations require simple skin closure only.
2. Penetrating injuries to the upper lid demand exploration. Division of the levator palpebrae or superior rectus muscles should be repaired primarily.
3. Full-thickness lacerations through the lid require repair in layers with careful approximation of the lid margin to prevent notching.

EARS

1. Lacerations are repaired by repositioning the cartilage and suturing the skin only.
2. Partial-thickness abrasions require occlusive moist dressings.
3. Cutaneous defects are skin grafted if the perichondrium is intact.
4. In the presence of exposed cartilage or complete avulsion of an auricular segment, immediate plastic surgery consultation is indicated.

NOSE

Assessment
1. Determine the extent of injury to the cutaneous cover and the cartilaginous framework.

2. Use a nasal speculum to rule out septal hematoma and assess mucosal injury.

Repair
1. Septal hematomas must be immediately evacuated through a small mucosal incision to prevent cartilage necrosis and resorption.
2. For injuries penetrating all layers of the nose, the mucous membrane lining is repaired first.
3. Torn nasal cartilages are realigned under direct vision, and their position is maintained by accurate repair of mucosa and overlying skin.
4. Packing of the nasal cavity with petrolatum gauze maintains the position of the cartilaginous fragments.

LIPS

Assessment
1. Determine the depth of the lacerations and the integrity of the orbicularis oris muscle sphincter.
2. Examine the extent of intraoral injuries.

Repair
1. Initial repair demands precise approximation of the vermilion border.
2. The lip is then closed in layers, suturing the orbicularis muscle first, followed by the oral mucosa and skin.

FACIAL NERVE

Assessment
1. Suspect injury to the nerve branches with penetrating trauma to the lateral facial region.
2. Clearly document nerve function before the infiltration of local anesthetic.
3. Observe the symmetry of facial animation with spontaneous expression and with active maneuvers to test the muscles of facial expression.

Repair
1. Anterior to an imaginary vertical line extending down from the lateral canthus of the eye, facial nerve injuries do not require repair. The plexus-like arrangement of multiple terminal branches in this area and the proximity of their target muscles promote spontaneous reanimation.
2. More proximal nerve lacerations, and injuries to either the frontal or the marginal mandibular branches, necessitate formal exploration and primary nerve repair.

PAROTID GLAND AND DUCT

Assessment
1. Injury should be suspected with penetrating wounds to the lateral cheek.
2. Inspection of the wound depths may reveal lacerated glandular tissue or clear fluid discharge.
3. Duct injury must be ruled out by diagnostic probing. A polyethylene catheter is introduced intraorally through the duct orifice, adjacent to the second upper molar, and threaded in a retrograde fashion toward the wound.

Repair

1. Lacerations of the parotid gland do not require direct repair, provided there is no associated ductal obstruction.

2. Lacerations of the parotid duct necessitate reanastomosis of the several duct ends over an intraluminal Silastic catheter. The catheter is maintained as a splint until the repair is healed.

CRANIOFACIAL FRACTURES

High-velocity accidents may cause profound injury to the bones of the skull and face. These combined injuries of the cranium and face—craniofacial in the true sense of the word—are a challenge to even the most energetic and well-trained reconstructive surgeon.

The number of patients surviving the initial trauma has increased, and surgeons are now often called on to treat patients with complex craniofacial injuries. This requires a synthesis of neurosurgical techniques and techniques derived from reconstructive craniofacial surgery that have been successfully applied to the treatment of complex facial injuries. The management of concomitant frontal sinus injury is still controversial but remains a key element in the treatment of these injuries.

The correct management of coexistent midfacial fractures is crucial. The classic patterns of midfacial fractures occurring in the lines of weakness of the face as originally described by Le Fort are rarely encountered in clinical practice. The great majority of maxillary fractures consist of combinations and permutations of Le Fort–type fractures. To add another dimension of complexity to these fractures, injury patterns following high-speed motor vehicle accidents are often associated with a significant component of comminution of the maxilla. The aim of treating combined injuries of the cranium and face is the correct anatomic restoration of the maxilla in relation to the cranial base above and the mandible below and the reconstruction of any associated craniofacial, naso-orbitoethmoidal, and zygomatic fractures. The plethora of techniques described for the management of these injuries attests to the fact that controversy and confusion still surround their treatment.

Pathogenesis and Classification

The frontal, ethmoid, and sphenoid bones form a major complex at the junction of the midfacial skeleton and the cranial base. The involvement of this complex and the adjacent buttresses of the facial skeleton establishes the pattern of craniofacial injury.[6–11] Combined injuries of the cranium and face may be isolated to the cranio-orbital and ethmoid region or extend to involve the midface and mandible.

CENTRAL CRANIOFACIAL FRACTURES

Force directed over the frontonasal region creates a central fracture.[6] The fracture lines involve the fronto-nasomaxillary and perhaps the frontoethmoidal vomerine buttresses, then extend to enter the frontal sinus and ethmoid complex. These fractures involve nasal, vomer, maxillary, ethmoid, and frontal bones. The infraorbital rim is often interrupted, and the medial wall of the orbit may be severely comminuted. If the frontal sinus is large, it may absorb a large proportion of the force, and the posterior wall may remain intact without exposure of the dura, even when there is severe comminution of the anterior wall. If the sinus is small, fractures may occur in the posterior table. With small linear cracks in the posterior wall, the dura may be intact, but with more significant disruption, the dura is commonly injured, resulting in CSF leak. If the sinus is rudimentary or the fractures are outside the sinus, large linear or segmental fractures occur, with involvement of the superior orbital rim and orbital roof. These fractures are often impacted and difficult to reduce, even with extended open reduction techniques.

LATERAL CRANIOFACIAL FRACTURES

Force applied to the frontozygomatic area causes fractures in the lateral face and cranium. The fracture lines cross the frontozygomaticomaxillary buttress and extend to involve the greater wing of the sphenoid.[6] Fractures of this type commonly involve maxillary, zygomatic, frontal, and sphenoid bones. An ipsilateral Le Fort III pattern is often present in association with a contralateral Le Fort II fracture. In some cases, the adjacent parietal and temporal bones are also involved.

The supraorbital margin is frequently damaged, and there may be extension into the lateral aspect of the frontal sinus.[10] The lateral orbit wall and the orbit floor are outwardly displaced, causing orbital dystopia and enophthalmos. In some cases, the lateral orbital wall is severely comminuted. Orbital fat is then displaced into the temporal fossa.

COMBINED CENTRAL AND LATERAL FRACTURES

With marked force, fractures involving both the central and the lateral skull and face may be produced. Profound instability and dislocation are present. These injuries have a high probability of extension into the anterior, middle, or, rarely, posterior fossa.

Early Approaches to Repair

Following World War II and during the ensuing decades, combined injuries of the cranium and face were treated in a different manner than they are today. The surgical repair was directed primarily (and sometimes singularly) toward management of the central nervous system. Clotted peridural blood was evacuated, brain and dura were débrided, and depressed cranial bone was elevated.

The repair of facial fractures was deferred to a second operation, particularly when coma was present. A limited amount of periosteum was elevated, for fear of interrupting the blood supply to the craniofacial bones. Comminuted segments, particularly those of frontal bones, were discarded. Great lengths were taken to remove the muscosal lining of the frontal sinus, and methods were developed to obliterate the sinus and nasofrontal duct.

Bone grafting was seldom considered, and defects in forehead contour were repaired at secondary and tertiary procedures. Foreign substances such as methyl methacrylate were often used in the reconstruction of the frontal bone.

Current Principles of Management

Once life-support systems have been established and the initial general examination has been completed, attention is directed to identification and management of the craniofacial injury.[12-16]

CLINICAL EXAMINATION

The hallmarks of craniofacial fractures are instability and deformation. Marked mobility of the fracture sites is thus a major clue to the presence of a craniofacial injury. The severity of the bony injury in the cranio-orbital region may be underestimated in the presence of marked soft tissue swelling and ecchymosis, and this may lead to inadequate or incorrect treatment and result in secondary deformity. Lacerations, particularly over the frontonasal ethmoid region, may communicate directly with the intracranial cavity.

The characteristic instability and deformation reflect the severe dislocation of the fractured segments over a broad area. Centrally, the naso-orbitoethmoid infrastructure is comminuted. Nasal projection is lost, and traumatic telecanthus is present. A similar loss of contour is often palpable in the frontal region. The orbital and zygomatic regions are flattened, accompanied by protrusion of the globe of the eye, owing to migration of the greater wing of the sphenoid and a blow-in fracture of the orbital roof. More laterally, a step-off along the supraorbital ridge may be noted.

RADIOGRAPHIC STUDIES

High-resolution computed tomography became available in 1980. It offers greater detail than that possible with conventional computed tomographic scanning techniques. By choosing a wide or narrow "window," one can program the computer for bone or soft tissue, respectively.[11] The higher mode of imaging is able to disclose what would otherwise be occult fractures. More recently, three-dimensional tomography has been used to facilitate diagnosis and treatment planning.

SURGICAL TECHNIQUES

Optimally, a patient with craniofacial injuries undergoes treatment within 12 to 48 hours. When possible, the maxillofacial and craniofacial repairs are accomplished at the time of neurosurgical exploration.

General health statistics (trauma scores), age, and the absence of neurological deficits are used to determine whether patients can tolerate surgical intervention, even in the presence of coma. Mannitol, hyperventilation, barbiturates, and intracranial pressure monitoring provide control.

The neurosurgical procedures are accomplished, and then the fractures of the skull and facial skeleton are reduced (Figs. 332–2 to 332–7). With the use of sharp instruments, the periosteum is elevated widely. Broad expanses of bone are exposed, and the actual fracture pattern is assessed by direct inspection. Only then is the final surgical plan formulated. The fragments of bone are wired together or stabilized using plates and screws.[12, 14–17] Bone, including the anterior table of the frontal sinus, is preserved for use in the subsequent repair.

Primary bone grafting offers a means of repairing comminuted areas or osseous deficits in the face or cranium, based on techniques learned from congenital craniofacial surgery (Fig. 332–8).[12–16] Split skull and, occasionally, split rib grafts are used to accomplish the reconstruction in most patients. Splitting the intact skull provides bone for small to medium-sized defects. Splitting the neurosurgical bone flap provides a larger source of cranial bone. Split rib grafts, in combination with split skull grafts, may be needed for reconstruction of extensive and multiple craniofacial defects.

REPAIR OF FRONTAL SINUS

The management of frontal sinus fractures depends on the type of fracture (site and displacement), whether the fracture is open or closed, and the presence or absence of a CSF leak.[8, 9, 16, 18, 19] Closed, undisplaced fractures of the anterior wall are observed. Open or depressed fractures are explored through a bicoronal incision. Foreign bodies and mucosal shreds are meticulously removed, and copious irrigation is used. The anterior wall is reconstructed. No attempt is made to occlude or drain the nasofrontal duct.[18, 19] Coexisting linear undisplaced fractures of the posterior wall without CSF leak are left alone, and just the anterior wall is reconstructed. Displaced and comminuted fractures of the posterior wall are usually associated with dural injury. The posterior wall is removed to provide access for neurosurgical repair, and only the anterior wall is subsequently reconstructed.

With concomitant injury to the floor, the potential for blockage of the nasofrontal duct and subsequent mucocele formation is accentuated. In addition, severe injuries to the floor, with comminution and bone loss, result in direct communication between the nasal cavity and the frontal sinus and intracranial cavity when the posterior wall is injured. It is essential to separate the nasal cavity from the frontal sinus and intracranial cavity to minimize the risk of ascending infection. Separation can be accomplished by bone grafting, vascularized soft tissue flaps, or, preferably, a combination of both.

Our current technique is to place split calvarial grafts, calvarial bone paste and chips, or iliac cancellous bone along the injured floor. Separate plugs of bone can be inserted into the nasofrontal ducts. The posterior wall is removed to "cranialize" the sinus. A

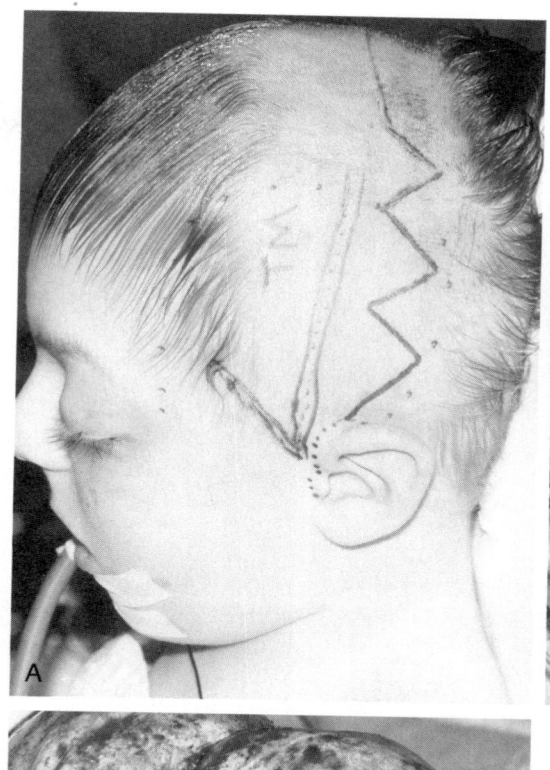

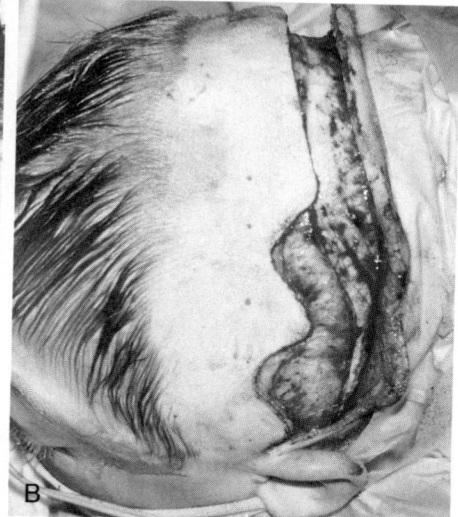

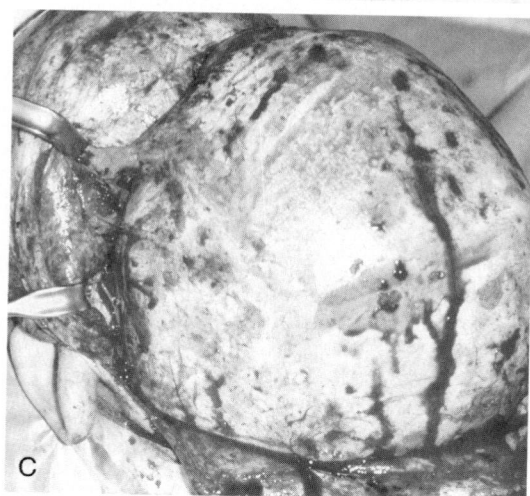

FIGURE 332–2. *A*, Modern approach for craniofacial surgery using a zigzag incision to hide the coronal scar. Whenever possible, the incision should be placed behind the level of the ear, and the anterior and posterior branches of the superficial temporal artery should be preserved. If necessary, the incision can be extended in the preauricular or postauricular region to increase exposure, although this is rarely necessary. *B*, When an approach to the region of the pterion and lateral orbit is needed, and exposure of the zygomatic arch is not necessary, the temporalis muscle can be left attached to the scalp flap. Shown is the incision through the pericranium behind the temporalis muscle, which is raised together with the scalp flap, so as not to disturb its position in relation to the scalp. *C*, The entire coronal incision is shown, with excellent visualization of the whole skull and temporal region, the lateral and superior orbital region, and the region of the pterion and sphenoid. The temporalis muscle, which is attached to the skull flap, is not disturbed; it can be seen between the two retractors. Once the surgery is completed, the scalp flap is simply repositioned; nothing needs to be done to the temporalis muscle. This prevents the common postsurgical complication of temporal hollowing due to atrophy of the temporalis muscle.

vascularized soft tissue flap of pericranium or, preferably, a galeal frontalis flap is funneled into the sinus and sutured to the dura posteriorly to provide a vascularized curtain between the nasal and intracranial cavities.[20]

SEQUENCE OF REPAIR

A sequential approach is often necessary in the presence of craniofacial trauma (Fig. 332–9). The extent of injury, suggested by clinical examination and radiographic studies, is confirmed by wide periosteal evaluation and exposure of all the fractured segments. The repair is completed using the following sequence.[8, 9, 13]

If there is no loss of cranial bone, first stabilize the cranial vault with rigid interosseous and miniplate fixation. The facial complex is then reattached to the reconstituted cranial vault.

When portions of cranial bone are missing or when massive cranial comminution is present, a reverse order of fixation is used. First, the midface and mandible are repaired. The reconstituted facial complex is then reattached to the residual cranial vault. The amount of missing frontal, ethmoid, and sphenoid bone can then be assessed. Split rib or split cranial grafts are used to reconstruct the cranial vault.

With associated maxillary, mandibular, or combined maxillary and mandibular fractures, the normal occlusion is first established. Maxillary and mandibular fractures are repaired whenever possible with rigid internal fixation using plates and screws. Following completion of the craniofacial repair, the intermaxillary fixation can be released, thus facilitating airway management with endotracheal intubation in patients with head injury, cervical spine fracture, or polytrauma. Tracheostomy is needed only following prolonged intuba-

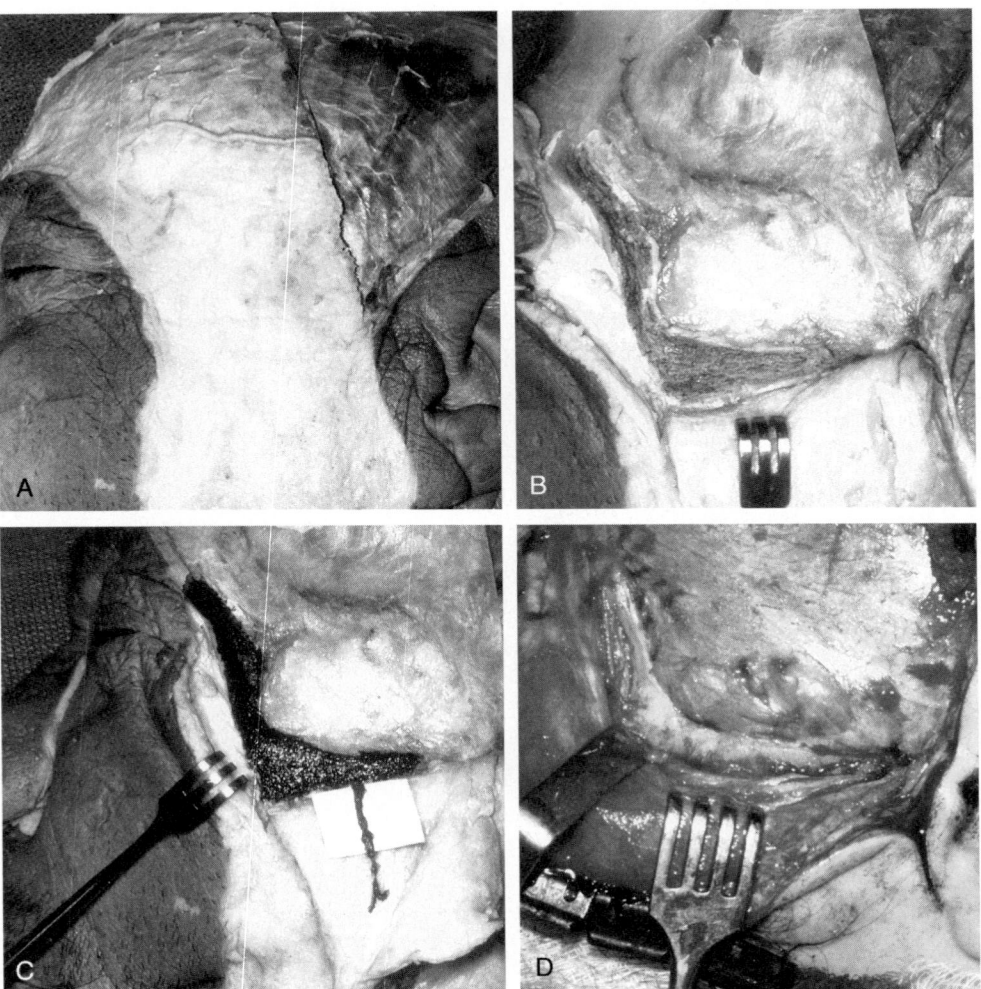

FIGURE 332–3. When an approach to the zygomatic arch is needed, the temporalis muscle has to be dissected on the surface, which requires a proper understanding of the anatomy in this region. *A,* The different fascial layers in the face and temporal region. The superficial layer is composed of the superficial temporoparietal fascia, through which the superficial temporal artery runs. Below the zygomatic arch, this is contiguous with the superficial musculoaponeurotic system fascia and then continues into the neck as the platysma. The superficial temporoparietal fascia is continuous with the galea in the scalp. Below this is the true deep fascia over the temporalis muscle, which can be seen glistening white and is contiguous with the pericranium. *B,* The correct level of dissection is to the deep temporal fascia overlying the temporalis muscle between the fascia and the superficial temporoparietal fascia. This leads the surgeon down to the lateral orbital wall and zygomatic arch. Approximately 1/2 to 1 cm above the zygomatic arch, the fascial attachment of the temporalis muscle is incised, thus incising the periosteum over the arch as well and lifting it with the flap. Just above the arch is the temporal fat pad, which needs to be visualized and preserved as far as possible to ensure that one is in the correct plane of dissection. *C,* This dissection shows the relationship of the frontal branch of the facial nerve to the fascial layers. The frontal branch of the facial nerve is protected by the superficial temporoparietal fascia, which is raised with the flap. The nerve usually lies above or within the superficial temporal fascia, and as long as the dissection is carried down along the deep temporal fascia, the nerve is always preserved. *D,* This exposure obtained in a live patient shows the complete dissection of the lateral orbit and the zygomatic arch, without disturbing the temporalis muscle, and the preservation of the frontal branch of the facial nerve. If further access is needed, an anterior craniotomy can be performed. The temporalis muscle can be lifted up in one piece and then carefully stretched and reattached to bone at the end of the procedure to prevent atrophy.

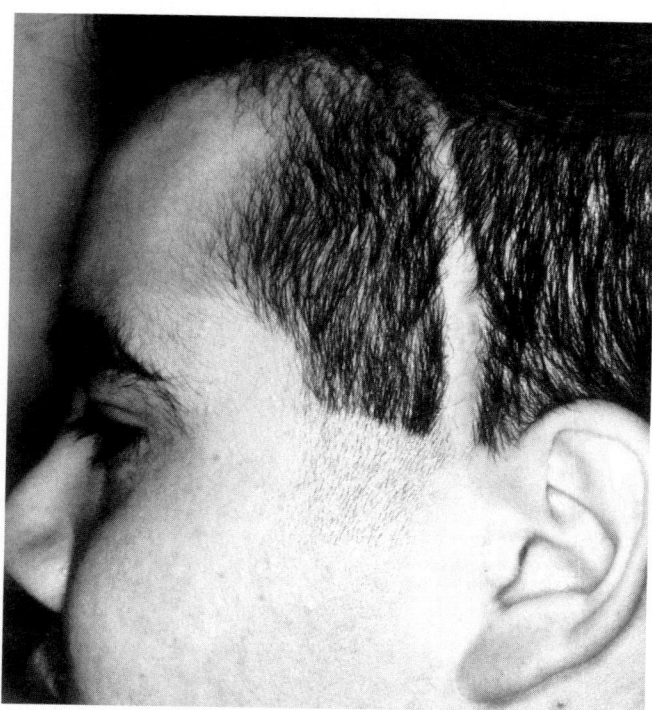

FIGURE 332–4. Older, straight-line coronal incisions such as this one are usually visible, particularly in male patients. This incision was also made too far forward, damaging the superficial temporal artery.

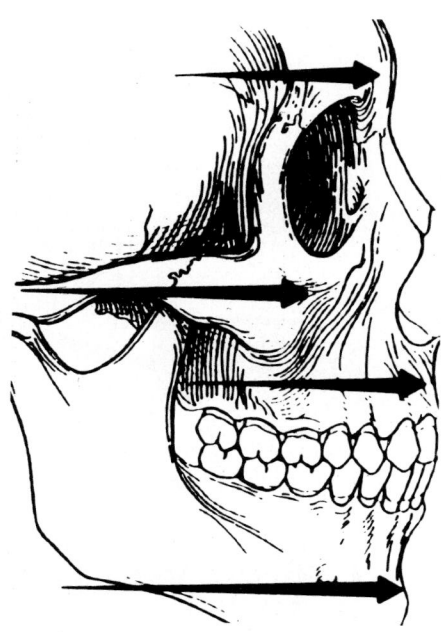

FIGURE 332–6. When repairing complex craniofacial injuries, adequate projection of the cranium and face must be accomplished by careful repair of the frontal, zygomatic, maxillary, and mandibular buttresses.

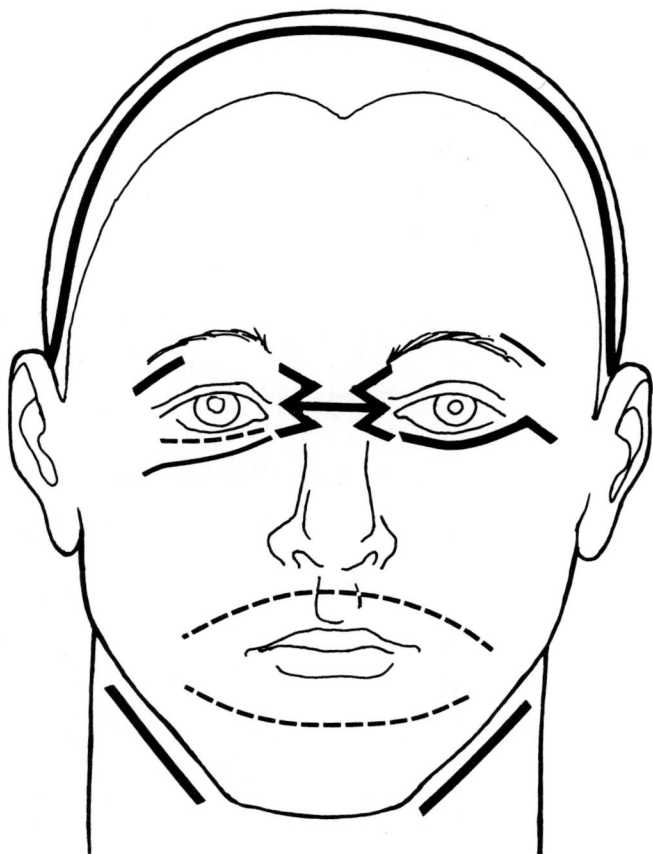

FIGURE 332–5. Combination approach to the craniofacial skeleton. The older straight-line coronal incision *(above)* is combined with other incisions *(below)* and incisions inside the mouth and in the neck. In complex craniofacial injuries, all these incisions are linked subperiosteally to provide visualization of the craniofacial skeleton.

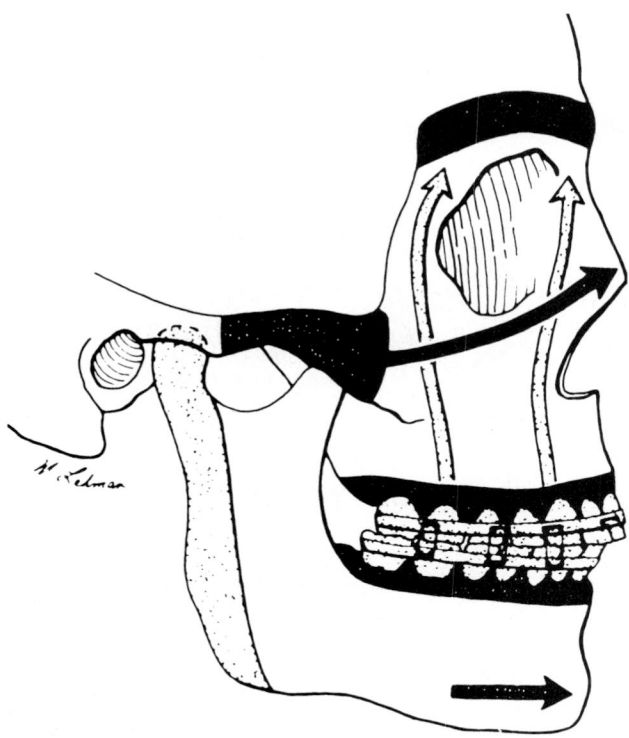

FIGURE 332–7. Areas of buttress, both transverse and longitudinal, that need to be restored in complex craniofacial injuries. Areas needing more rigid fixation include the frontal buttress, zygomatic arch, maxilla, and mandible. This will restore the correct facial projection and height.

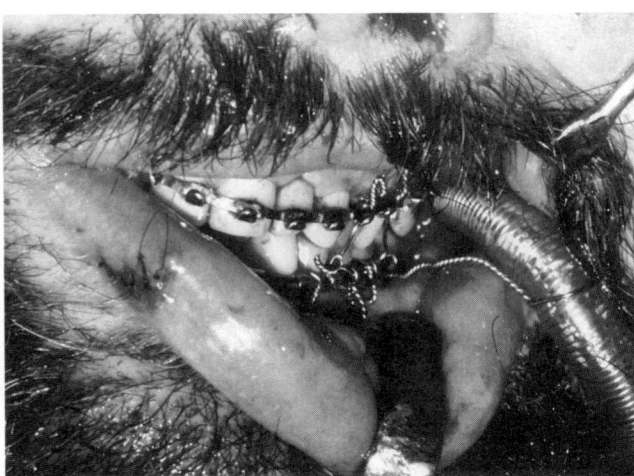

FIGURE 332–9. Close-up showing adequate application of intermaxillary fixation with the armor tube passing intraorally behind the posterior molar teeth. Twisted braid and wire can be seen.

tion, in patients with coma, or in those with other injuries such as associated bilateral condylar neck fractures that are not amenable to open reduction, in which case intermaxillary fixation has to be retained. External fixation devices are almost never needed.[13–15, 21, 22]

TECHNICAL PROBLEMS AND PITFALLS

Based on our experience in treating these complex cases, certain technical problems and potential pitfalls have surfaced (Figs. 332–10 to 332–25).[8, 9]

Inadequate reconstruction of the supraorbital ridge commonly leads to flatness in this region. Using a full-

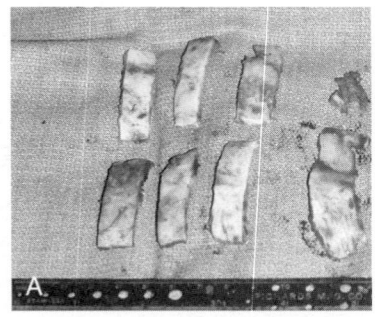

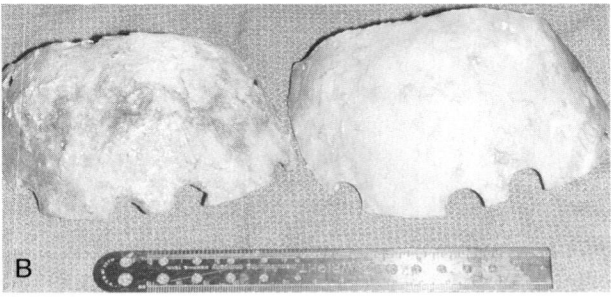

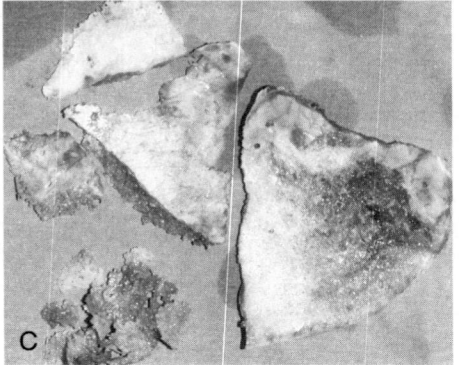

FIGURE 332–8. Methods of harvesting cranial bone graft for craniofacial reconstruction. *A,* Large amounts of split cranial bone graft strips can be harvested from the outer table. *B,* When a neurosurgical bone flap is available, it can be carefully split into inner and outer tables, providing a large source of potential reconstruction material. *C,* Frontal bone flap split into inner and outer tables. A large amount of cancellous bone can then be harvested from the diploë and used to seal off the frontal sinus and anterior cranial fossa.

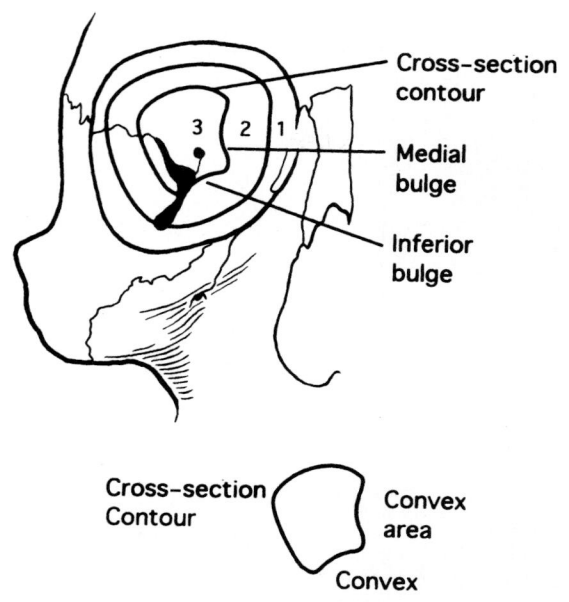

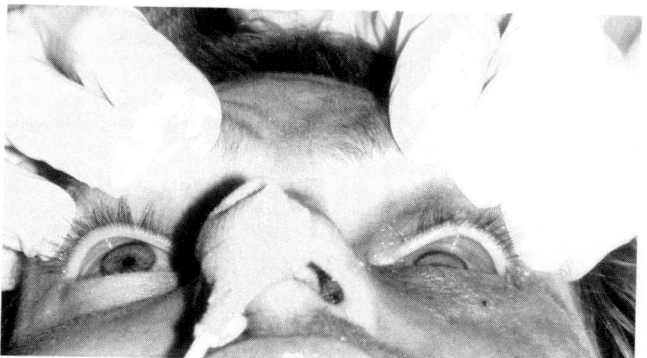

FIGURE 332–12. Patient with acute enophthalmos on the left side. This type of injury is caused by orbital blow-out fractures with enlargement of the orbital volume.

FIGURE 332–10. Orbital reconstruction is a key element in the management of all craniofacial injuries, and the orbital anatomy must be understood. The orbit is not a simple cone but has characteristic bulges that cause postglobal constriction in the orbit and maintain the position of the globe. There is a medial bulge from the ethmoid bone and an inferior bulge from the maxillary sinus. The thicker outer area of the orbit (1) is rarely comminuted, and the inner orbital apex (3) is rarely fractured. Most fractures involve the thinner area in zone 2. Injuries involving zone 3 may lead to superior orbital fissure syndrome or orbital apex syndromes, with involvement of structures passing through the superior orbital fissure or optic canal. When the orbit is reconstructed, the surgeon's goal is to reconstruct the correct anatomy and the correct bulges to restore correct eyeball position.

thickness rib graft or stacking bone grafts in layers prevents this.

Injury to the orbital roof may result in isolated fractures, comminuted fractures, or areas of bony destruction or loss. Concomitant loss of the posterior wall of the frontal sinus results in direct communication between the anterior cranial fossa and the orbit. The orbital roof should always be reconstructed in this situation to separate the two cavities. When the poste-

rior wall of the frontal sinus is intact, it is not necessary to reconstruct small defects of the orbital roof; however, failure to reconstruct larger defects may lead to herniation and entrapment of orbital contents and possible enophthalmos and diplopia.[23-25]

When a total loss of the supraorbital rim is reconstructed with bone grafts, it is difficult to obtain perfect symmetry with the uninvolved orbit. Exophthalmos and downward displacement of the ocular globe may occur if excess bone is inadvertently used, especially when concomitant reconstruction of the orbital roof has been performed. Care must be taken to contour the supraorbital rim and roof correctly and prevent overcorrection of the deformity.

True orbital dystopia may be difficult to recognize clinically when it is associated with combined injuries of the cranio-orbital region, midface, and orbitozygomatic complex, particularly when there is severe soft tissue and bony injury. Failure to recognize and correct it adequately at the time of the initial reconstruction may result in an established orbital dystopia that is extremely difficult to correct with secondary surgery. The key to reestablishment of the orbital position is adequate exposure and reconstruction of the zygomatic arch and lateral orbital rim and wall. This produces an intact outer facial frame with the correct facial projection and width. The inner facial frame, composed of orbital rims and the nasoethmoid region, can be recon-

Text continued on page 5260

FIGURE 332–11. A, Sagittal view through the orbit shows the relationship of the eyeball to the critical inframedial bulge behind the eyeball, which maintains the eyeball position. Fractures occurring behind the axis of the globe tend to cause globe positional changes in an anteroposterior and inferior direction. B, Loss of the inframedial bulge following fracture produces sinking in of the eye, or enophthalmos.

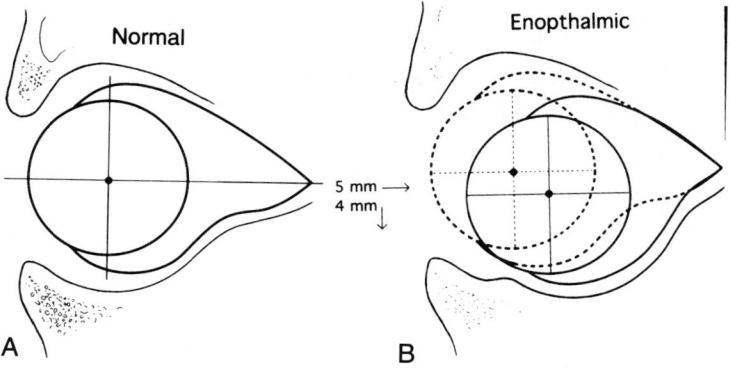

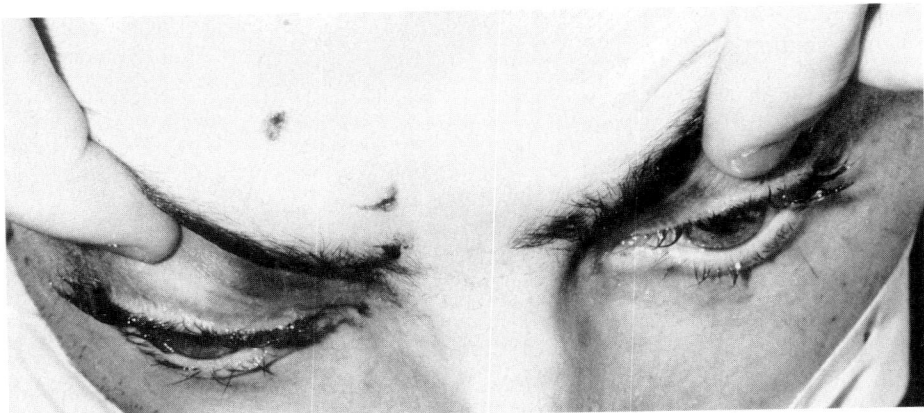

FIGURE 332–13. Blow-in fractures of the orbital walls and rim can lead to proptosis. This blow-in fracture of the orbital roof led to decreased orbital volume and acute exophthalmos.

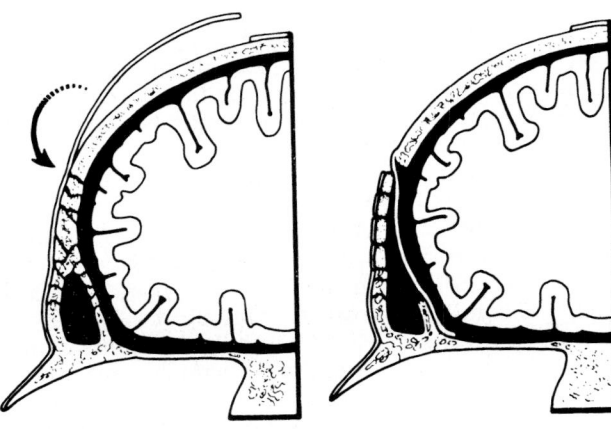

FIGURE 332–14. When fractures of the frontal sinus involve the posterior table and floor, drainage problems may occur. The frontal sinus should be separated from the cranial cavity by means of a soft tissue flap—either a pericranial flap or a galea-frontalis flap—and the rest of the sinus can be obliterated using bone graft.

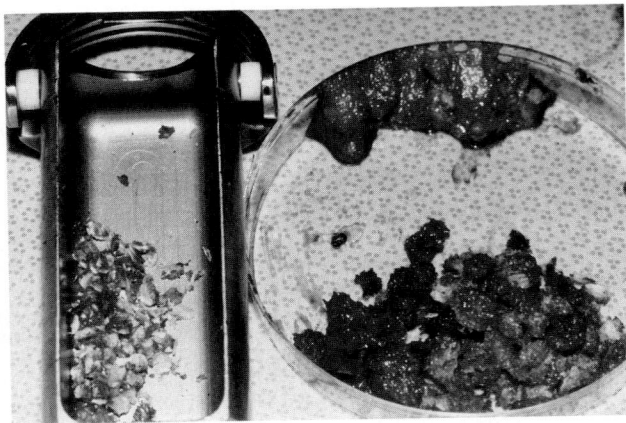

FIGURE 332–15. A large amount of bone material is available from the neurosurgical bone flap. On the left are multiple bone chips that have been ground up in the bone mill. On the right are bone dust and cancellous bone chips that have been harvested from the diploë of the skull and during the drilling of bur holes. All this bone material can be mixed together to form excellent material for sealing off the frontal sinus or anterior cranial fossa.

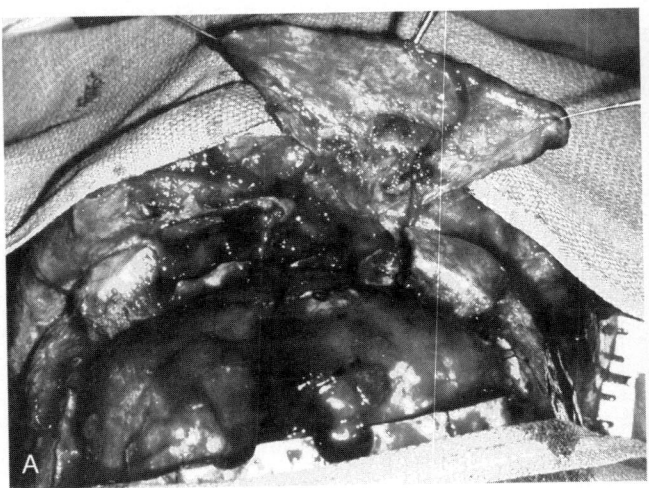
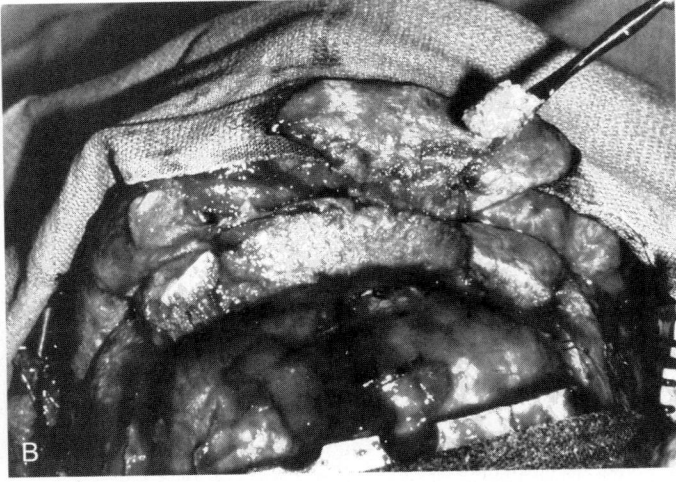

FIGURE 332–16. *A,* Patient with a complex craniofacial injury involving the anterior and posterior wall and the floor of the frontal sinus, as well as a facial fracture. One can see the open frontal sinus after débridement and a galea-frontalis flap ready to be used for sealing off the dura and frontal sinus. *B,* The frontal sinus is packed off with bone material.

Figure continues on following page

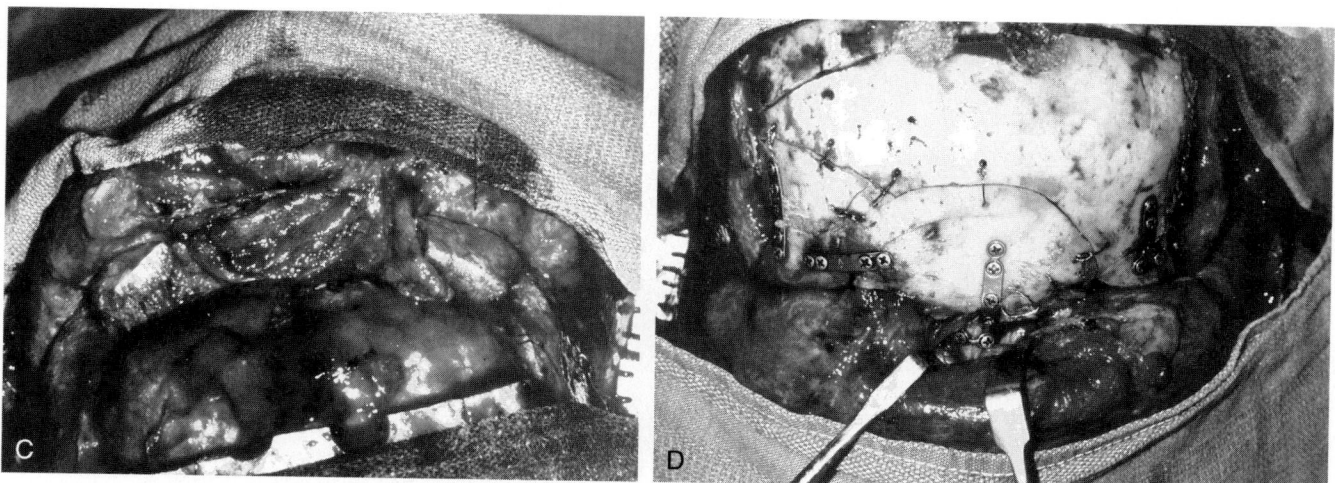

FIGURE 332–16 *Continued. C,* The galea-frontalis flap is turned over the frontal sinus and sutured to the dura to seal off the anterior cranial fossa from the frontal sinus. *D,* The bone flap is replaced and rigidly fixed in place with plates and screws.

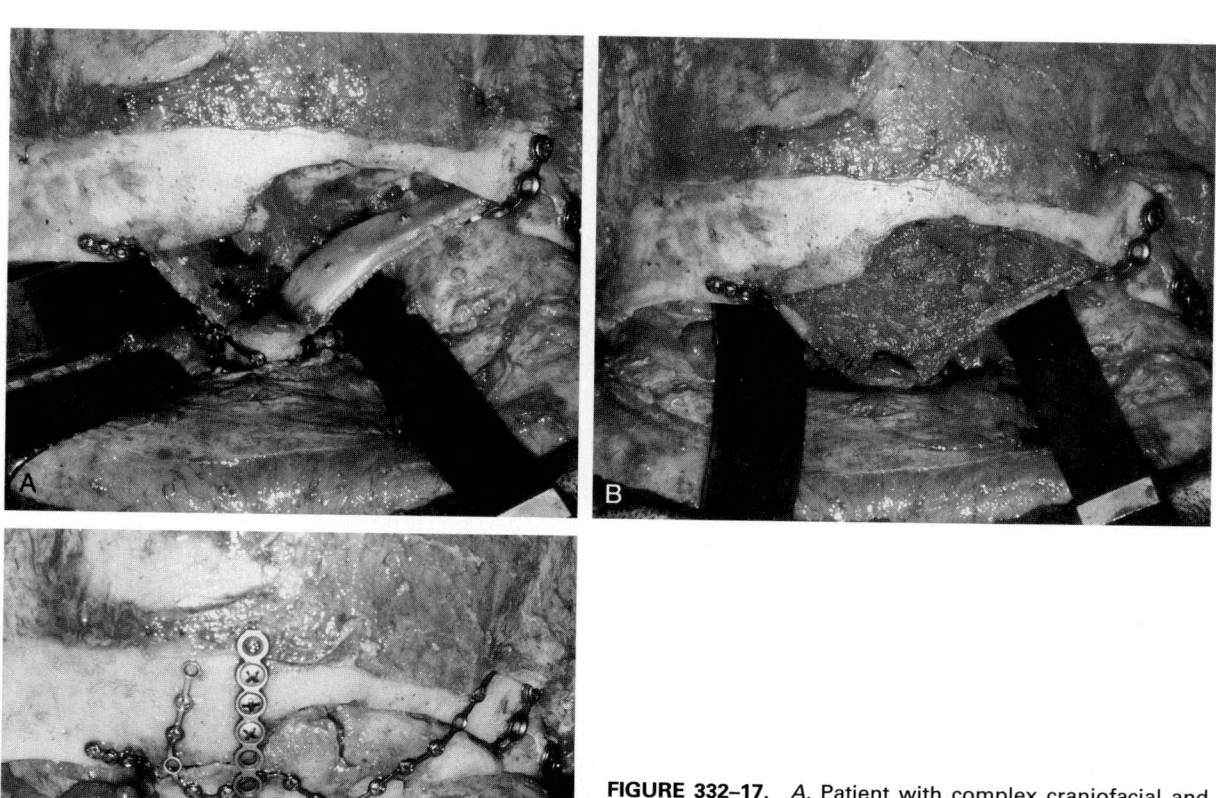

FIGURE 332–17. *A,* Patient with complex craniofacial and frontal sinus injuries, including complete loss of the orbital roof and floor of the frontal sinus. Walls of the frontal sinus and orbital roof are being reconstructed with split cranial bone graft rigidly fixed in place. *B,* The frontal sinus is completely obliterated with cancellous bone and bone paste. *C,* The anterior wall of the frontal sinus and nasal glabella region is repaired with primary bone grafting, and a nasal bone graft is inserted to complete the reconstruction. All bone grafts are rigidly fixed in place with small plates and screws.

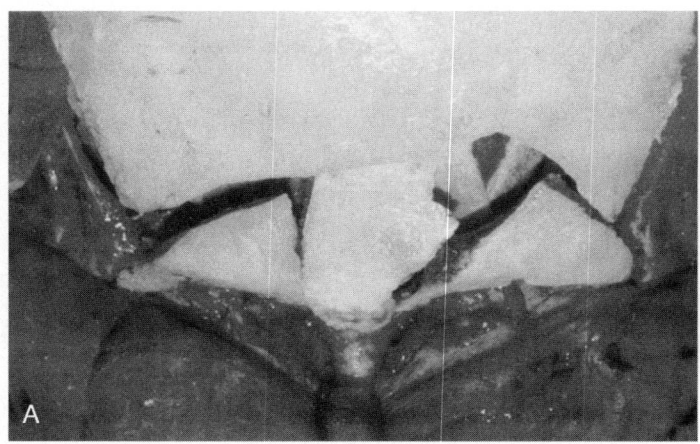

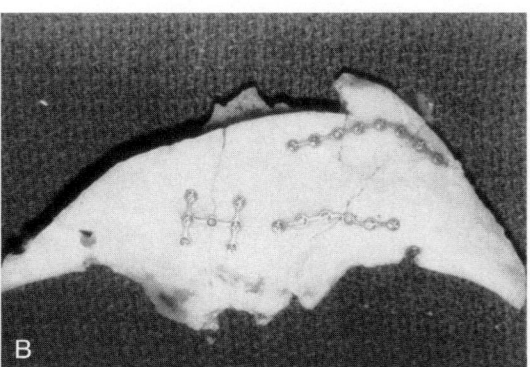

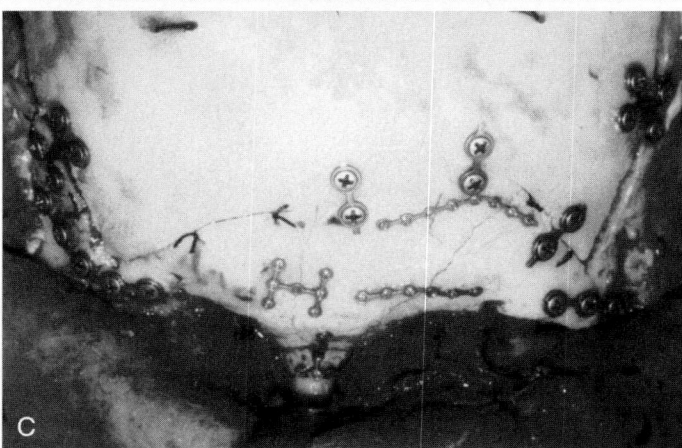

FIGURE 332–18. In complex craniofacial fractures, all the comminuted bone can be removed with the bone flap. *A,* Complex frontal orbital facial injury with comminuted fractures extending across the entire frontal region. *B,* All these fracture segments can be removed with the frontal bone flap and reassembled on a back table or while the neurosurgeon is completing the neurosurgical portion of the repair. *C,* Once the neurosurgical repair is complete, the entire complex can be replaced in one piece, saving time and facilitating repair.

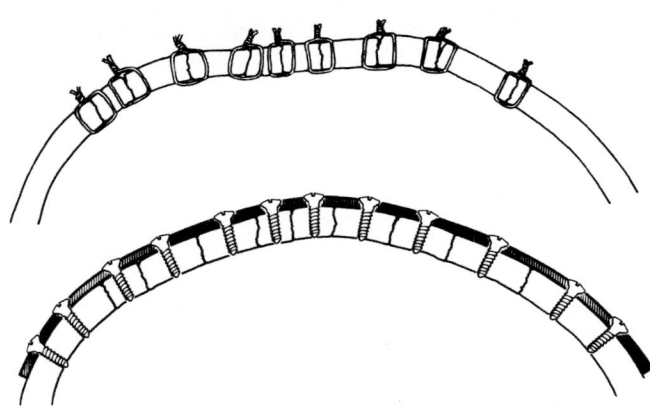

FIGURE 332–19. With comminuted fractures of the frontal bone, it is difficult to maintain the correct contour and shape of the bone simply by using interosseous wiring. An advantage of a plate and screws is that the plate can be contoured to the exact shape of the skull and frontal bone, and then each fragment can be lagged to the plate with an individual screw, thus maintaining a perfect contour and preventing the soft tissue forces from collapsing the bone.

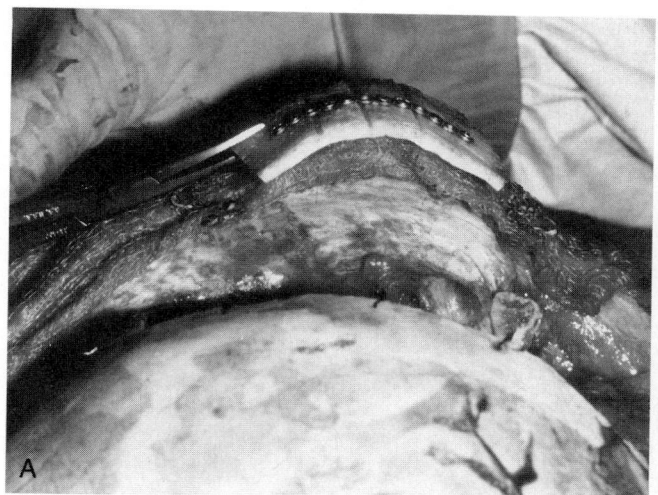

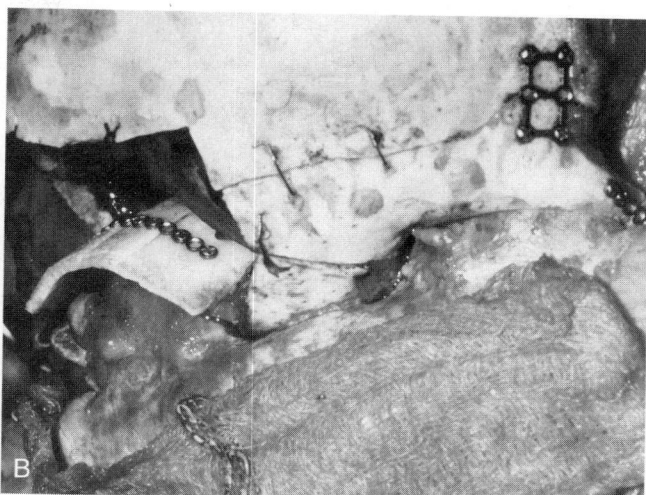

FIGURE 332–20. Surgical methods of obtaining correct orbital roof contour in reconstruction. *A,* Complete orbital roof reconstruction with cranial bone graft and greenstick osteotomies on the superior surface and careful bending of the bone to the correct shape of the supraorbital region and orbital roof, held in place with miniplates and screws. *B,* The completed orbital roof reconstruction has adequate contour to prevent vertical globe positioning.

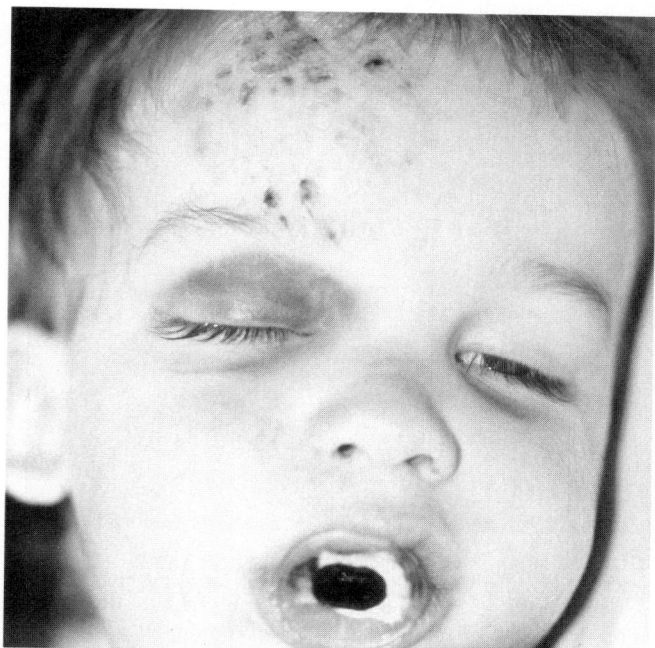

FIGURE 332–21. Orbital roof fracture in the pediatric population is one of the most commonly missed injuries. Young patients often present to the emergency department with bruising and swelling in the orbital and supraorbital regions. One must have a high index of suspicion for orbital roof fractures in this age group.

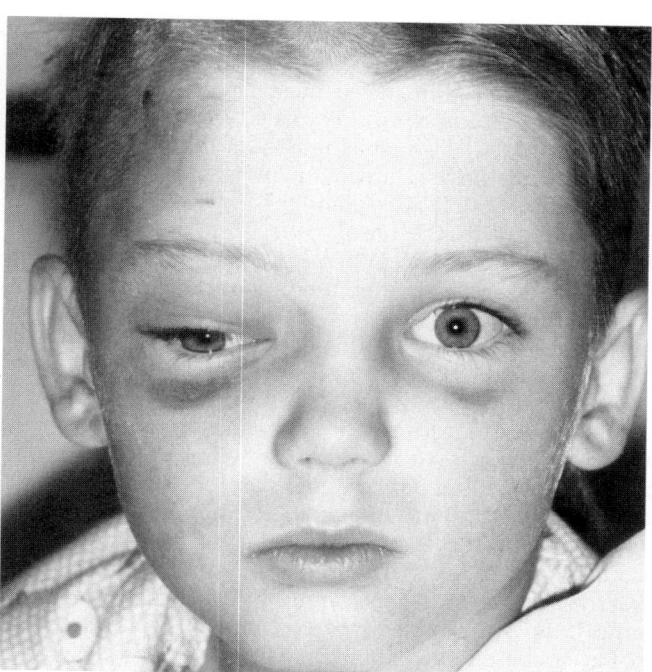

FIGURE 332–22. Four-year-old boy with severe, displaced orbital roof fracture and obvious vertical globe dystopia, with intracranial involvement.

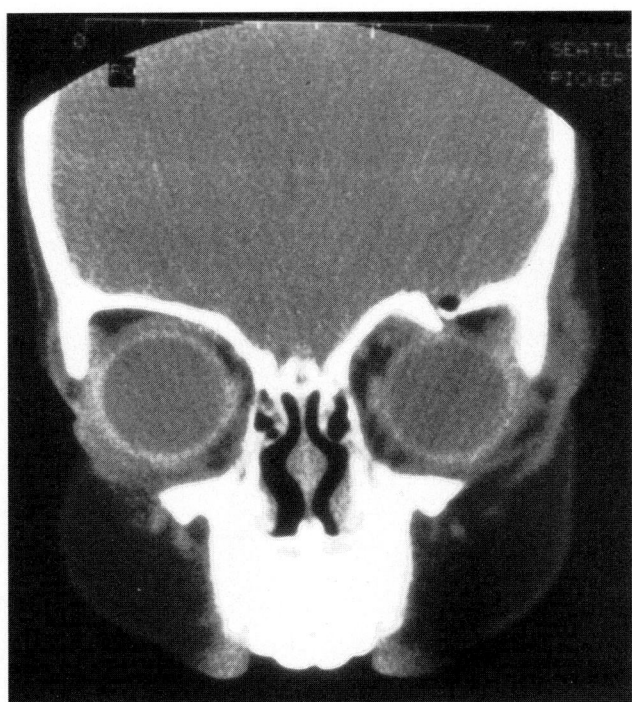

FIGURE 332–23. Displaced orbital roof fracture in a 2-year-old child. This fracture needs to be carefully reduced to prevent post-treatment morbidity.

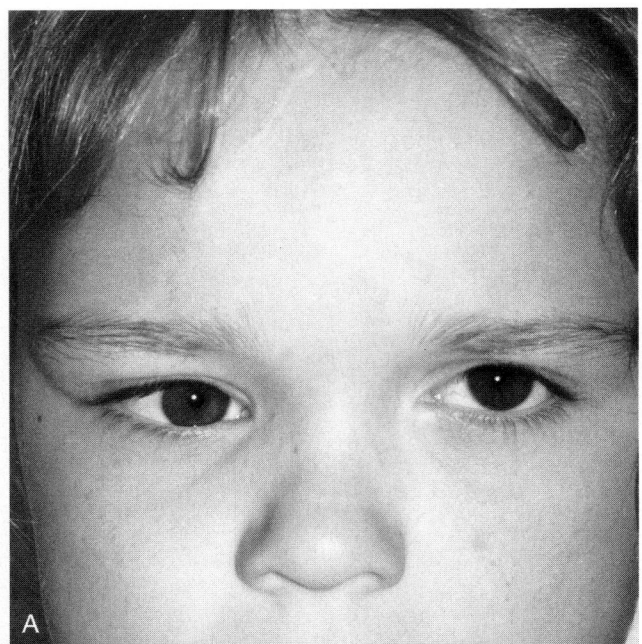

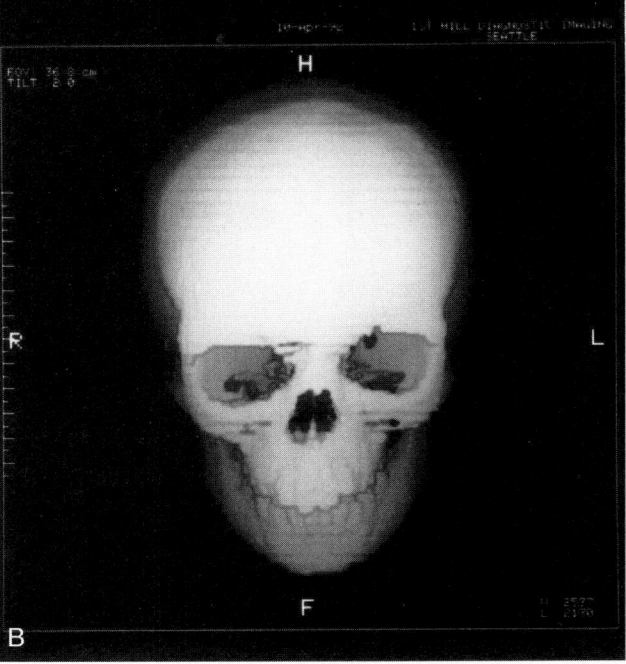

structed within this outer facial frame, resulting in exact repositioning of the displaced orbit.[26–31]

Severe injuries in the nasoglabellar region may result in significant bony destruction or loss of the glabella or nasal bones or both. Glabellar loss is reconstructed with bone grafts; the nasal bone is then reattached to this rebuilt bony base. When both the glabella and the nasal bones are lost, glabellar reconstruction is combined with immediate bone graft reconstruction of the nose. The nasal bone graft is attached to the glabellar graft and cantilevered as necessary.[14–16]

The frontocranial region is under the influence of minimal muscular forces; thus, meticulous interosseous wire fixation can produce a stable reconstruction in many cases. Maintenance of the correct convex contour is difficult with interosseous wiring alone when extensive comminution is present in the frontal and fronto-orbital regions. Long miniplates or microplates can be exactly contoured to the shape of the skull to maintain contour and minimize late collapse. Individual fragments can be fixed to the plate using specially designed miniscrews that are 3 to 4 mm in length, to prevent them from entering the cranial cavity and damaging the dura.

PANFACIAL INJURIES

Panfacial injuries are true craniofacial injuries involving fractures of the cranium, midface, and mandible (Fig. 332–26).[15, 32–34] Treatment of these injuries involves

FIGURE 332–24. Failure to adequately reduce a displaced orbital roof fracture in a young child leads to progressive dystopia of the whole orbit, as it remodels in response to the injury. *A*, Five-year-old girl with an undiagnosed orbital roof fracture in infancy. Note that she now has a true orbital dystopia with malposition of not just the globe but the whole orbit, as evidenced by the canthal attachments. This is a difficult problem to treat, because the entire orbit has to be moved upward using a combined intracranial-extracranial approach. *B*, In response to a simple displaced orbital roof fracture, the whole orbit is pushed in a downward direction.

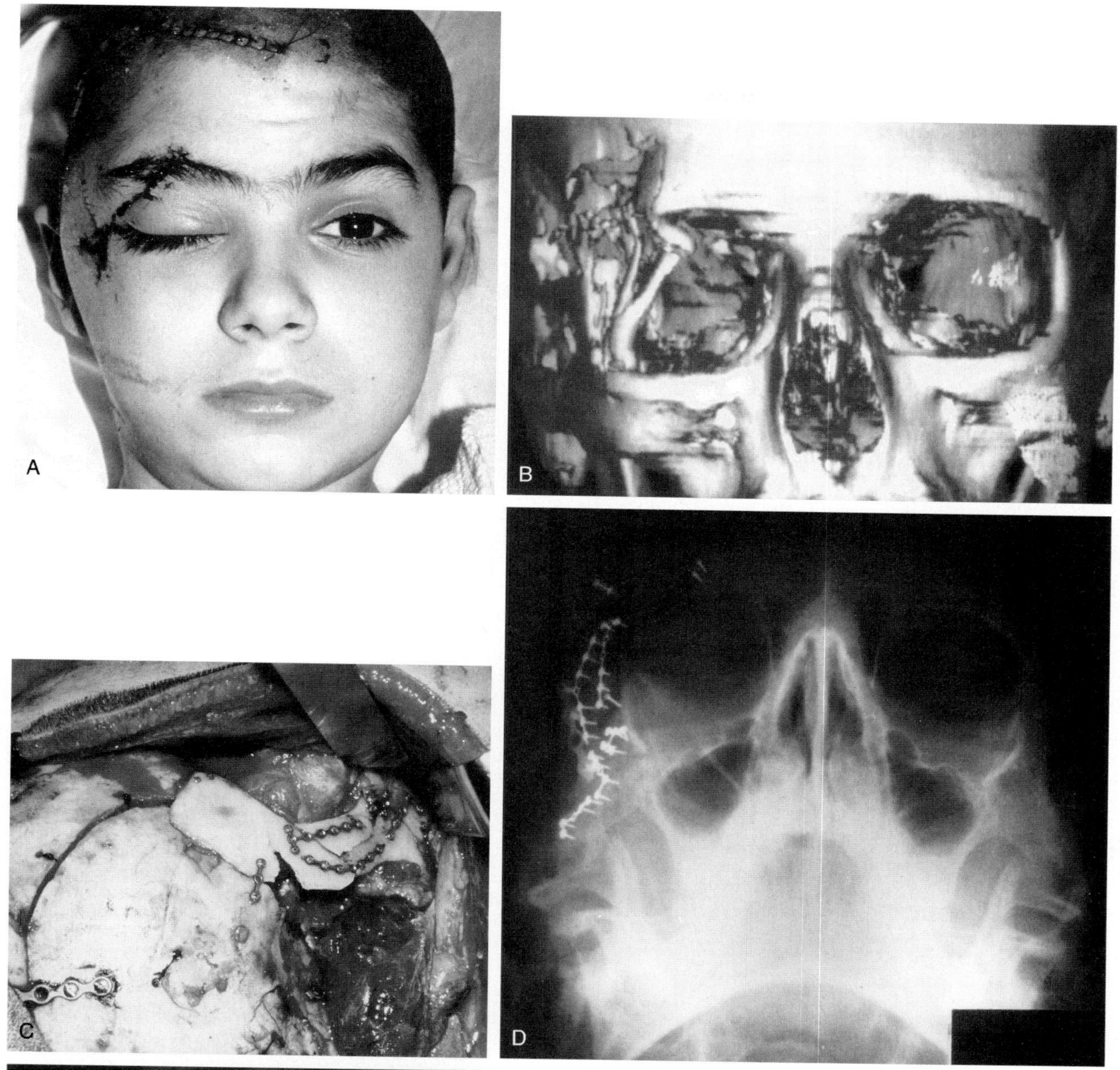

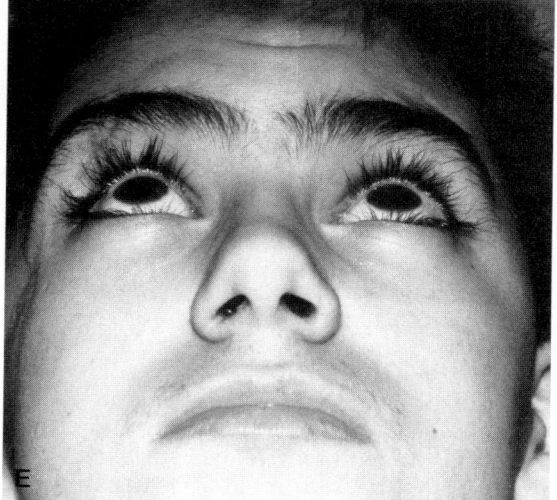

FIGURE 332–25. *A*, Five-year-old boy kicked in the head by a horse, resulting in lateral orbit and skull injuries. *B*, Three-dimensional computed tomographic scan illustrates the complex injury of the skull, orbital roof, and lateral orbit. Note the blow-in fracture with marked reduction in intraorbital volume. *C*, Primary bone reconstruction using inner table skull is performed in the orbital roof, supraorbital margin, lateral orbit, and zygoma. All bone grafts are rigidly fixed in place with microplates and screws. Once this is done, the soft tissue is reattached, including the midfacial soft tissue and the lateral canthal tendon. *D*, Postoperative radiograph shows extensive primary reconstruction. *E*, Final results 5 years later, with perfect restoration of orbital contour and eye position. Combined reconstruction at the time of neurosurgical exploration is the ideal way to handle these cases.

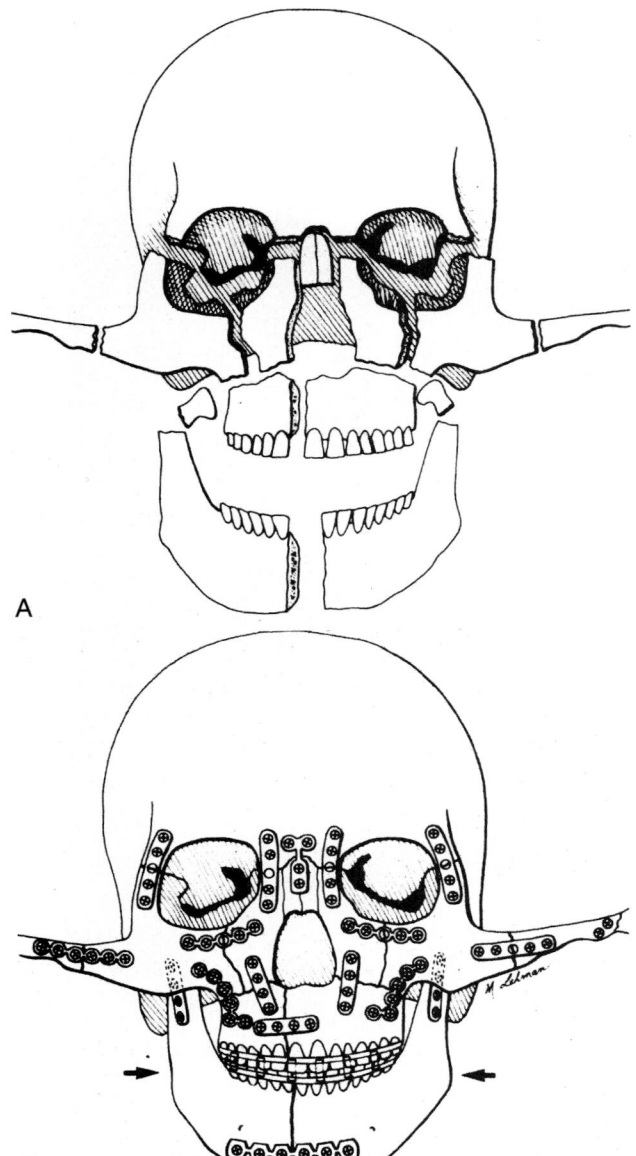

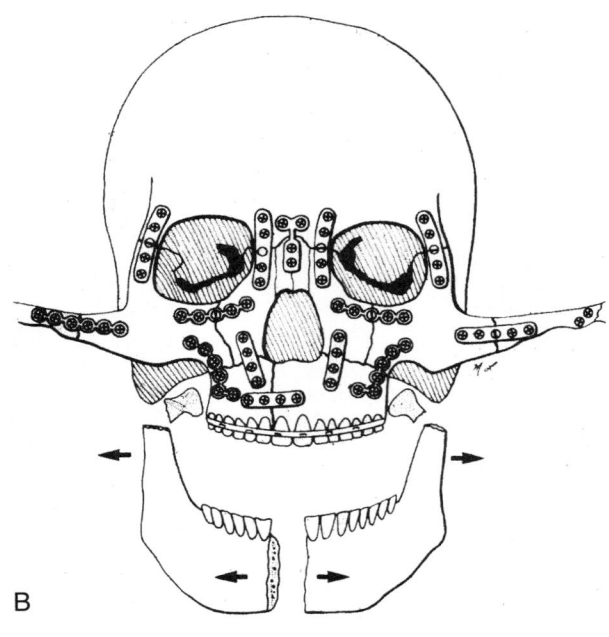

FIGURE 332–26. *A,* With panfacial fractures, all relationships to the skull base and mandible are lost, particularly when there are sagittal splitting fractures of the palate and parasymphyseal and bilateral condylar neck fractures of the mandible. The major problem here is restoring the correct facial width. *B,* The most accurate way to perform reconstruction is by using the zygomatic arch. The lateral and upper facial skeleton is reconstructed first, restoring the correct upper facial width, which can be related to the correct width of the maxilla. Once the correct width is related to the base of the skull, the mandibular width can be determined and reconstruction completed. *C,* It is important to reconstruct the correct width of the mandible by pushing in at the angles of the mandible before applying the strong parasymphyseal region plate. In complex injuries such as this, one or both condylar necks need to be reconstructed as well, achieving a complete three-dimensional reconstruction of the face. When injuries also involve the frontal bone, the frontal buttress is stabilized first, before reconstruction of the upper facial skeleton.

a coordinated repair of the frontal bar, zygomatic arches, central midface, and mandible. The understanding of certain factors relating to the repair of these regions is crucial to facilitate a comprehensive repair.

Mandible Plating

Compression or reconstruction plate fixation of mandibular fractures, resulting in rigid internal fixation, and miniplate and bone graft fixation of the maxillary buttresses, combined with mandibular fixation, have significantly improved the intraoperative and postoperative management of these patients. Intraoperatively, the oral reinforced-armor endotracheal tube can be pushed to the side, lateral to the posterior molar teeth, and interdental fixation can be applied. Once the maxillary and mandibular stabilization has been completed,

the interdental wires can be released, and the endotracheal tube can be left in place until the patient no longer requires airway management. The interdental wires can be replaced, if necessary, but in the great majority of patients who undergo rigid maxillary and mandibular repair, subsequent interdental fixation is not required, and the need for tracheostomy is thus obviated. This type of airway management facilitates the care of polytrauma patients and those with head injuries or cervical spine fractures. Only if Le Fort fractures are associated with bilateral condylar neck fractures is it essential to maintain interdental fixation following the repair, and in these patients, a tracheostomy is usually needed. Rigid internal fixation of both the maxilla and the mandible allows early removal of interdental fixation, if used, often at a maximum of 3 to 4 weeks following repair. In an edentulous patient,

CHAPTER 333

Traumatic Cerebrospinal Fluid Fistulas

ROBERT J. BUCHANAN ■ ADAM BRANT ■ LAWRENCE F. MARSHALL

CLASSIFICATION AND EPIDEMIOLOGY

Cerebrospinal fluid (CSF) fistulas are caused by a breach in the arachnoid, dura, and skull. The most common cause of CSF leaks is head trauma, with the remainder attributed to postoperative or spontaneous mechanisms.[1-4] Fractures of the skull base are relatively common, and their frequency increases as more force is applied to the head during an accident. The fact that the dura is firmly adherent to the skull base makes it vulnerable to laceration by the fractured bone. The incidence of basal skull fracture from nonpenetrating head trauma is in the range of 7% to 15.8%, with associated CSF fistulas occurring in 2% to 20.8% of cases.[2, 5-7] One paper reported the breakdown of post-traumatic fistulas as 80% cranionasal and 20% cranioaural, with the latter having a better chance of spontaneous closure.[8] A report of fractures of the sella turcica documented CSF fistulas in 53% of patients.[9] The Traumatic Coma Data Bank,[7a] in a prospective series of 753 patients with severe head injuries, reported that 25% had basilar skull fractures. The frequency of fractures in patients with severe head injuries is very high, and because of their serious clinical conditions, their CSF leaks may go undiagnosed. The incidence of fistulas in these patients is most likely higher than reported. Penetrating injuries to the head also cause CSF fistulas. Three studies of penetrating injuries quoted the rate of leakage as 7% to 10%, with an increased rate if the ventricle was violated.[10-12] Given these percentages, it is important to have a high degree of suspicion that a patient may have a CSF fistula.

CSF leaks can be divided into two categories: early and delayed. Early leaks present within a week of injury, and delayed leaks may occur weeks to years after the injury. Most CSF leaks (70%) present within 48 hours of injury, and 98% are clinically obvious by 3 months.[1, 2, 6, 7, 13] Okada and coworkers reported CSF rhinorrhea in two patients whose head trauma occurred 10 and 30 years before the leak.[14] It is important to elicit a good history, because leaks that are initially thought to be spontaneous may be caused by a traumatic event in the distant past. Delayed leaks can be caused by increasing intracranial pressure, lysis of a blood clot, necrosis of tissue overlying a dural defect, or resolution of soft tissue edema.[15] Seventy percent of post-traumatic fistulas resolve without treatment within 7 days; most of the remaining fistulas resolve within 6 months. Rhinorrhea can recur after healing (unlike otorrhea, which almost never returns).

Another classification used for spontaneous fistulas that is also germane to traumatic leaks is whether the leak is under high or low pressure. Head trauma patients, both those with and those without evidence of intracranial hemorrhage, can develop hydrocephalus. It is important to keep this in mind when evaluating CSF fistulas in this population, because the hydrocephalus must be treated before the leak can be effectively repaired.[16, 17]

PATHOPHYSIOLOGY

The route of egress of CSF is commonly dictated by the location of the injury in relation to the bone and underlying meninges. Post-traumatic fistulas are frequently multiple and quite complex. In theory, any linear skull fracture can cause a leak; however, if the scalp is intact, the egress of CSF is impossible. The terms *otorrhea* and *rhinorrhea* are defined as CSF dripping from the ear and nose, respectively, and patients can present with one or the other or sometimes both. Otorrhea is often caused by a temporal bone fracture, and rhinorrhea is commonly caused by a fracture in the frontal, ethmoid, or sphenoid bones; however, there are routes by which CSF can reach a site of egress that is not near the fracture site.

The base of the skull and its sinuses are the primary routes of CSF leakage. CSF follows the path of least resistance, producing otorrhea through the mastoid air cells or middle ear and rhinorrhea through the paranasal sinuses. Fractures of the cribriform-ethmoid junction and through the ethmoid bone itself are the most frequent causes of rhinorrhea.[18] The lateral aspect of the cribriform plate, where the anterior ethmoidal artery creates a natural dehiscence, is especially vulnerable.[19] Fracture of the cribriform plate can also present as tearing of the eye.[20] Avulsion of the olfactory fibrils from their insertion sites in the cribriform plate can also cause rhinorrhea in the absence of a fracture. When the posterior wall of the frontal sinus is fractured, CSF tracks through the nasolacrimal duct into and out of the nose. A fracture in the middle cranial fossa involving the sphenoidal sinus also causes rhinorrhea. If the tympanic membrane remains intact, CSF leaking through a temporal bone fracture may track through the eustachian tube and then through the throat and nose. This is called *otorhinorrhea*. Most temporal bone fractures (70% to 90%) are parallel to the long axis of the petrous ridge and may damage the ossicle bones, resulting in conductive hearing loss. The fracture may also damage the seventh cranial nerve and the geniculate ganglion. A less common pattern is a transverse temporal bone fracture, which can be associated with complete loss of eighth cranial nerve function (vestibular dysfunction and sensorineural hearing loss). Transverse fractures are more commonly associated with seventh cranial nerve deficits than are longitudinal fractures. Because longitudinal fractures are more common than transverse fractures, the absolute number of CSF fistulas occurring in association with these fractures is higher; however, the percentage of otorrhea seen with both types of fractures is similar.[21] CSF fistulas that are less likely to remit spontaneously are those in which dura is trapped by the sharp edges of the fracture or in which the meninges are impaled by bony spicules.

CLINICAL PRESENTATION

History

The first step in diagnosis is eliciting a thorough history. Patients who are able to communicate often complain of tearing eyes, nasal discharge, a salty taste and dripping in the back of the throat, and fullness in the ear accompanied by some degree of hearing loss. The salty taste is due to the sodium chloride content of CSF. If the tympanic membrane is disrupted, the CSF drips out of the ear. A large volume of fluid flowing out of the nose or ear during a change in head position (reservoir sign) may indicate that a CSF-filled sinus has drained all at once.[22] Patients often complain of leaking in the morning when they are shaving, eating, or sitting on the commode. Headaches often accompany CSF fistulas and may be either high-pressure or low-pressure types. A high-pressure headache is described as a steady buildup of pain that is relieved by fluid drainage. This pattern repeats over time. Patients with low-pressure headaches report that their pain is position dependent and is least troublesome when they are in a recumbent position. Recurrent episodes of headache, fever, and meningitis should also alert the physician to look for a CSF fistula in a patient with a history of head trauma.

Other symptoms can point the astute clinician to the fracture site. Patients who complain of a loss of taste and smell often have fractures of the cribriform plate and fovea ethmoidalis. Cooper stated that if a patient does not have anosmia, it is unlikely that the fistula is coming from the cribriform plate.[23] If there is a complaint of imbalance, dizziness, hearing loss, or facial muscle dysfunction, a fracture in the temporal bone is likely. An uncommon but significant symptom of visual change may point to a fracture in the posterior ethmoids, tuberculum sellae, or sphenoidal sinus.

Physical Examination

On examination, patients may have periorbital ecchymosis (raccoon sign) or a palpable depression in the forehead, which points to a fracture in the anterior fossa. Patients with head injuries and periorbital hematomas are at a greater risk of unobserved dural tear and delayed CSF leakage.[24] Battle's sign—ecchymosis of the scalp over the mastoid process—indicates a petrous ridge fracture. The ear must be examined to determine whether the tympanic membrane is intact and to look for evidence of bubbles or an air-fluid level behind it. If it is ruptured, evidence of a flow of blood and fluid may be seen. It is important to remember that if the patient has a swollen brain, the leak may not be immediately evident because the swelling may act to tamponade the meningeal and bony defect.

Leakage of clear CSF should be obvious if the volume is large, but low-volume or intermittent fistulas may be overlooked. It may be necessary to have the patient initiate Valsalva's maneuver or flex at the waist and neck to see the flow of CSF. In a patient who is unable to cooperate and does not have intracranial hypertension, careful bilateral compression of the jugular veins may help produce the leak.

A thorough neurological examination can also provide valuable localizing information. Anosmia most likely points to the anterior cranial fossa at or near the cribriform plate. As described earlier, abnormal function of the seventh and eighth cranial nerves indicates a fracture of the temporal bone. Deficits in vision or visual fields (optic nerve) and facial sensory loss (first division of the trigeminal nerve) localize to the anterior fossa. A fracture involving the foramen rotundum in the middle cranial fossa could produce a characteristic pattern of facial sensory loss in the second division of the trigeminal nerve.

Hypothesizing that a fracture and CSF fistula are ipsilateral to the nostril producing rhinorrhea is accurate only 77% of the time. In one review, 5 of 21 patients had rhinorrhea from the nostril contralateral to site of the fracture and leakage.[25] Before the advent of more definitive diagnostic tests, neurosurgeons planning operative intervention had to rely on the fact that the fistula and rhinorrhea were most commonly on the same side.[2]

Meningitis

Meningitis is a relatively common and dangerous sequela of CSF fistulas. The overall risk of meningitis caused by traumatic CSF leaks is approximately 25%. Acute leaks are associated with a 20% incidence of meningitis; in delayed fistulas, this climbs to 57%.[1, 16, 26–31] The mortality rate for meningitis caused by traumatic CSF leaks has been reported to be 10%.[32] High-flow leaks and those associated with increased intracranial pressure are associated with lower rates of meningitis.

The most common organism cultured is pneumococcus, but multiorganism infections, often with anaerobes, are not uncommon.

Pneumocephalus

Pneumocephalus is seen in 20% to 30% of patients with post-traumatic CSF fistulas.[1, 2, 33] The presence of intracranial air indicates that there is an open communication and should be considered a form of CSF fistula. Pneumocephalus places the patient at an increased risk for meningitis. Very small volumes of air (<1 to 2 cc) are frequently seen after head trauma and usually resolve without treatment. However, larger volumes of air often indicate a substantial likelihood of a persistent site of open communication that requires neuroimaging. Tension pneumocephalus is a serious complication that has been reported as a patient's presenting condition.[25]

IDENTIFICATION AND LOCALIZATION OF THE FISTULA

Simple Bedside Tests

If clear fluid is leaking from the patient's nose or ear, the diagnosis is easy and straightforward. However, if the fluid is blood tinged or appears to be mixture of CSF and nasal discharge, a simple test can be done. The fluid is placed on a piece of filter paper or on an absorbent cloth, such as a handkerchief or pillowcase. If CSF is present, a target sign will form as the CSF content of the fluid migrates farther out in a ringlike pattern. The final product looks like a bull's-eye, with the thicker blood or mucus in the center and the lighter-colored, thinner CSF migrating beyond the inner ring.

Historically, glucose oxidase papers have been used to effectively eliminate the presence of CSF from a fluid sample. These test strips turn positive at relatively low levels of glucose—greater than 20 mg/100 mL. It is known that nasal secretions contain approximately 10 mg/100 mL of glucose; however, they can elicit false-positive reactions. Also, lacrimal gland secretions and nasal mucus have reducing substances that may cause a positive reaction with glucose concentrations as low as 5 mg/dL. Therefore, a negative glucose strip test eliminates the possibility of a CSF leak, but because of the test's high sensitivity, a positive result cannot be clinically interpreted.

Laboratory Tests

If a small volume of fluid (0.5 to 1 mL) can be collected, it can be sent to the laboratory for a quantitative measurement of the glucose content. If the glucose concentration in the fluid is 0.5 to 0.67 that of the serum glucose concentration, the fluid is most likely CSF. Of course, it is important to take into account clinical conditions that may alter the level of glucose in the CSF and serum. Some institutions also measure the fluid for chloride concentration; if it is greater than 110 mEq/L, the fluid is most likely CSF.

Another test that is quite specific is to measure the fluid's level of β2-transferrin. Transferrin is a polypeptide involved in ferrous ion transport. β1-transferrin is found in serum, tears, nasal secretions, and saliva. β2-Transferrin is a protein found only in CSF, perilymph, and vitreous humor.[34] It accounts for 15% of the total transferrin in CSF. Given its presence in the vitreous humor, it is important to evaluate a trauma patient for an eye injury with an open globe before interpreting the β2-transferrin results. A small volume of fluid (<1 mL) is necessary for the test. Qualitative detection of β2-transferrin is performed by agarose gel electrophoresis, and results are available in 3 hours.[35] It is a highly specialized test that not every medical center can perform. It is the most sensitive and specific test to date; however, one study indicated that there can be false-positive results.[36]

Neuroimaging Techniques

Many neurotrauma patients have plain skull radiographs or computed tomographic scans with bone windows during their workups. By examining these for evidence of a basilar skull fracture or an air-fluid level in the paranasal sinuses, the clinician can begin to localize possible areas of dural laceration. It should be understood that the use of skull radiographs alone is associated with a high failure rate of localization.

Fine-cut (3-mm) computed tomographic scans in both the coronal and axial planes can locate the fistula in more than 50% of cases. A fracture involving the middle ear, sphenoidal sinus, ethmoidal sinus, or cribriform plate is best seen in a coronal image. The frontal sinus and fractures of it are best visualized on axial images. Ikeda and colleagues used three-dimensional computed tomographic reconstructions to reveal the bony defects in cases of rhinorrhea.[37] When the site of the leak cannot be found by closely scrutinizing the computed tomographic images, the use of radioactive and nonradioactive tracers can provide the diagnosis in the majority of cases. The use of intrathecal and intraventricular substances such as methylene blue, fluorescein, and iodinated materials has fallen out of favor with most neurosurgeons because of the neurotoxicity and level of invasiveness (ventriculography).[38, 39] Another tracer dye used by some neurosurgeons is indigo carmine. Unlike fluorescein, indigo carmine can be seen with the unaided eye and may be useful in localizing a CSF fistula intraoperatively. Indigo carmine is also a safer choice because it does not have any overt toxicity.

When fine-cut computed tomographic scanning does not reveal the defect, the decision must be made to proceed to contrast cisternography or radionuclide cisternography. For patients with active leaks, the use of water-soluble contrast agents such as iopamidol, iohexol, or metrizamide identifies the fistula 46% to

81% of the time.[1, 40–42] Metrizamide is a nonionic, triiodinated, water-soluble compound used since the early 1970s. A baseline computed tomographic scan is obtained before infusion of the contrast material. The contrast material is then injected into the subarachnoid space, and the prone patient is placed in Trendelenburg's position for 4 minutes to allow the contrast material to make its way throughout the subarachnoid space and into the basal cisterns. The table is then brought back into a neutral position, the patient's head is extended slightly, and another computed tomographic scan is performed.[42] The clinician examines it for evidence of contrast material leaking through a fracture or into a sinus. Studies have shown that metrizamide computed tomography–cisternography can localize the leak in 76% to 100% of cases. It is much more accurate in active leaks than inactive leaks, where the sensitivity drops to 60%.[40, 43]

Fistulas that are intermittent can be investigated by radionuclide cisternography. In this technique, a radiolabeled compound is injected into the subarachnoid space and allowed to circulate up into the cisterns and ventricles. Today, the two most commonly employed compounds are technetium 99–labeled albumin (half-life of 6 hours) and indium 111–labeled pentetic acid (DTPA; half-life of 2.8 days).[44–46] This method has also been used to identify CSF–pleural fistulas.[47] The technique involves the placement of cotton pledgets along areas thought to be harboring a fistula. The usual areas targeted are the anterior and posterior roof of the nose, the sphenoethmoid recess, the middle meatus, and the posterior end of the inferior turbinate. Active leaks usually contaminate the pledgets within 0.5 to 2 hours. A slow or intermittent leak can be detected by leaving the pledgets in place for 6 to 48 hours. It is necessary to check for isotope contamination periodically and then replace the pledgets if none is found. The presence of low levels of contamination must be viewed with suspicion, because it may result from isotope secretion from the nasal mucosa, active transport from the CSF, leakage by the olfactory nerves, or passive lymphatic drainage. These processes increase over time, and if low levels are measured 5 hours after isotope installation, these mechanisms should be suspected. Calculation of the radioactive index (RI) ratio can improve the accuracy of weakly positive tests. The RI ratio equals the RI of the pledget divided by the RI of 1 mL of the patient's blood. The radioactivity is measured in radioactive counts per minute. An RI ratio of less than 0.3 is considered normal. Studies have revealed that the RI ratio should be 1.5 or greater to reflect the presence of a leak. If the anterior nasal pledget is positive, the site of the fistula is most likely the anterior ethmoidal roof or cribriform plate. When the posterior nasal or sphenoethmoidal pledget is stained, the leak might be coming from the posterior ethmoidal or sphenoidal sinus. A positive pledget from the middle meatus indicates a frontal sinus leak, and a positive pledget in the inferior turbinate points to a fistula from the eustachian tube.[1, 48–50] In a 1994 review article examining the utility of radionuclide cisternography, Eljamel reported a 70% accuracy rate for locating active rhinorrhea but only a 28% accuracy rate for inactive or intermittently active leaks.[51] If the leak is high flow and high volume, it is difficult to get meaningful results because of fast oversaturation of the pledgets and gross staining of the surrounding tissues.

Magnetic resonance imaging is not used universally to localize CSF leaks. Because of the length of time needed to perform the study and the poor resolution of bone, its utility is limited. Another factor is the lack of an acceptable intrathecal contrast substance for use in magnetic resonance imaging. In a study using heavily T2-weighted images (a technique called magnetic resonance cisternography), a fistula in the sphenoidal sinus was successfully isolated; this was a leak that computed tomographic cisternography had failed to identify.[52] With more experience and new magnetic resonance imaging sequences, this technique may someday be more mainstream.

Direct nasal endoscopy often allows visualization of fistulas from the ethmoid bone, cribriform plate, and sphenoid bone. Endoscopy provides a means of diagnosis, but it is also employed for the surgical treatment of leaks (described in the next section).

MANAGEMENT AND TREATMENT

Infection Prophylaxis

The use of prophylactic antibiotics in patients with basilar skull fractures and CSF fistulas remains controversial. In most studies, the frequency of infection following basilar fracture without a fistula in patients with severe head injury is low. However, the Traumatic Coma Data Bank reported a higher rate of 8.7%. There has been only one prospective, double-blind, randomized trial examining antibiotic prophylaxis in CSF fistulas.[53] Those authors found that meningitis occurred in none of the patients on antibiotics and in only 1 of 26 patients given placebo. It was the authors' recommendation that prophylactic antibiotics not be used routinely.

The risk of meningitis depends on many factors, including a delayed onset of CSF leakage, an increased duration of CSF leakage, the site of the fistula, and any concomitant infection. Brodie performed a meta-analysis of six studies that examined post-traumatic CSF leaks, including rhinorrhea and otorrhea, over a 25-year period.[54] Only 2.5% of patients receiving prophylactic antibiotics developed meningitis, versus 10% of patients who received no antibiotics. This paper also showed that patients with post-traumatic fistulas lasting longer than 7 to 10 days had an 8- to 10-fold increased risk of developing meningitis; similar conclusions have been reached in many studies. One paper even reported that traumatic fistula patients who received prophylactic antibiotics had a significantly greater incidence of meningitis.[24] Overall, routine antibiotics are no longer used in traumatic leaks.[55, 56]

The fact that basilar fractures allow direct communication between the "outside world" and the subarachnoid space should always be kept in mind. In our experience, we have seen two cases of fulminant basilar meningitis with sterile ventricular fluid samples that showed no pleocytosis. We now realize that negative ventricular fluid cannot be relied on to exclude a diagnosis of meningitis. There is a 2.6 times greater rate of intracranial infection with a basilar fracture when a ventricular catheter is used.[57] Wyler and Kelly advocate the use of prophylactic antibiotics when indwelling catheters are used.[58] They found the infection rate with catheters to be 10%; with antibiotics, this rate decreased by two thirds. The risk of infection is considerably lower with lumbar catheters.[59] Therefore, the use of ventricular catheters in this population must have a sound clinical indication.

Nonoperative Treatment

Patients with fistulas are kept head-up in bed. The angle can be anywhere from 30 to 70 degrees, depending on convention. Awake patients are warned against maneuvers that would cause sudden increases in intracranial pressure, such as nose blowing, coughing, and sneezing. Patients should routinely be placed on a bowel regimen, including laxatives and stool softeners, to avoid unnecessary straining. Because most leaks stop on their own, we wait 96 hours before proceeding to the next step—an external lumbar drain. Mincy found that 35% of leaks stopped in 24 hours, 68% in 48 hours, and 85% by 1 week without intervention.[60] If the leak does not stop, we place a lumbar external drainage system in those patients without any contraindications.[16] If a ventricular catheter has been placed—for example, for intracranial pressure monitoring—the drip chamber is placed at a level that ranges from the external ear to the shoulder. We allow 3 to 4 days for the leak to resolve. If the leak does not stop, we begin operative planning.

Operative Treatment

Patients who have failed nonoperative treatment are considered for definitive operative treatment, which consists mainly of intracranial (intra- and extradural) and extracranial (extradural and endoscopic) procedures. The choice of procedure depends on the location and severity of the injury. Patients who have enlarging pneumocephalus, persistent CSF leaks, or meningitis need urgent surgical repair. It is our practice to explore and repair those leaks that continue beyond 1 week. Meningitis must be eradicated before surgical closure of the fistula. We take a more aggressive approach when treating patients with significant pneumocephalus, defined as greater than 2 cc of persistent intracranial air. Pneumocephalus often represents the presence of a large dural tear, which is unlikely to heal spontaneously and is associated with a higher incidence of meningitis. If the patient has a significantly larger amount of intracranial air on repeat scanning, operation must be seriously considered. Early operation is justified if the patient has a large volume of intraparenchymal or intraventricular air.

We routinely repair dural fistulas during operations required for other traumatic brain injuries. Delayed leaks and those associated with extensive fractures of the frontal fossa and high-energy missile wounds are unlikely to heal spontaneously and usually require early surgery. High-volume leaks through the sella turcica and petrous bone usually do not heal spontaneously and may be best treated with early exploration.

The intracranial procedure chosen depends on the anatomic location of the CSF leak. Before incision, the patient is given steroids, anticonvulsant, mannitol, and prophylactic antibiotics. If the patient has a lumbar drain in place, this can be used to drain CSF as needed to obtain good brain relaxation and minimize the degree of brain retraction.

The frontal fossa can be approached by both intradural and extradural routes. If the fistula was localized to one side of the anterior fossa preoperatively, a unilateral exposure can be carried out. If there are bilateral frontal fractures or if the site of the leak was not localized, the prudent approach is to fashion a bicoronal skin flap and a bilateral bone flap. When exposing the anterior fossa, it is important to fashion the bone flap very low, to clearly visualize the floor. This often causes violation of the frontal sinus. If this happens, the mucosa of the sinus must be exenterated, and the sinus should be plugged with muscle, Gelfoam, or fat. The instruments used for this part of the operation should be considered contaminated and discarded from the operative field. Closure of the sinus with a pericranial flap is carried out in the usual fashion.

The extradural technique can successfully treat leaks, although it has limitations. During the exposure, the dura is often torn, creating yet another breach in the meninges, which makes identification of the "original" traumatic CSF fistula more difficult. Technically, closure of the dural defect can be more difficult extradurally, and permanent closure rates are lower than with intradural repairs. The intradural approach provides superb exposure of the entire frontal fossa all the way back to the lateral aspects of the sphenoid wings and to the anterior clinoid processes. The dura should be opened far anteriorly, which requires that the anterior part of the sagittal sinus be ligated and cut. The falx must also be cut to provide full exposure, and part of it may be used for dural graft material to repair the fistula. On close examination, the site of the leak can often be visualized or palpated. The identification of a parenchymal brain contusion may point to the region of the dural leak. Many times, the brain is adherent to or herniated through a dural fistula. Often, multiple leaks can be visualized on the frontal floor, and care must be taken to close all of them.[61] The operating microscope should be used if an injury cannot be easily found by the naked eye. If the operation has been delayed and the patient has had multiple episodes of meningitis, the operating microscope often allows visualization of leaks on the scarred floor. Another technique that can be used to visualize the bony defect, described by Ray and Bergland,[62] is the use of positive pressure ventilation. Specially designed tubes seal the nares and posterior pharynx, allowing the field, which is filled with saline, to be examined for bubbles coming from the fistula. Once located, the fistula should be packed with a plug of abdominal fat. This should then be covered with a dural flap or free patch graft. A patch graft can also be obtained from autologous pericranium, temporalis fascia, or fascia lata. Commercially obtained lyophilized dura can also be used; however, it is a second choice to autologous materials.

There are times when a discrete fistula cannot be found. In these cases, the entire floor of the anterior fossa needs to be covered with a large pericranial graft. It is important that the graft reach all the way to the limbus sphenoidale and cover both cribriform plates completely. Again, pericranium and fascia lata are superior to cadaveric or synthetic dura. The availability of fibrin glue appears to have improved the success of operative closure and is strongly recommended in fistula closure. Lumbar drainage is used postoperatively to minimize fistula recurrence.

An exploration of the middle fossa and sometimes the posterior fossa is necessary to locate and treat fistulas coming from a fractured petrous bone. The exploration is begun extradurally, but caution must be used to avoid damaging the facial nerve by causing excessive traction on the geniculate ganglion. Leaks from the posterior aspects of the middle fossa are the easiest to approach extradurally. Most leaks are found and treated extradurally by the techniques described earlier. We have also found fibrin glue to be helpful in dural repair and fistula closure, particularly in the middle fossa, where bone disruption is occasionally severe.[63, 64]

Extracranial approaches are often performed in conjunction with an otolaryngologist. Some leaks coming from the frontal sinus, cribriform plate and adjacent ethmoidal labyrinth, sphenoidal sinus, oval window, and petrous bone can be approached extracranially. The decision to use an endoscopic approach should be made only after careful analysis of the neuroimaging studies. The common practice of otolaryngologists is to inject an intrathecal dye, such as fluorescein, 30 minutes before surgery. This allows the fluorescein-stained CSF, which is a bright green-yellow color, to be seen coming from the fistula. Frontal sinus fractures through the posterior wall are repaired by the frontal osteoplastic sinusotomy technique.[65] This approach employs an eyebrow or coronal scalp incision. A fistula of the cribriform plate or ethmoidal labyrinth is approached through a medial orbital incision. The orbital contents are dissected posteriorly in a subperiorbital plane. The ethmoidal labyrinth is entered through the lacrimal bone and the lamina papyracea. A complete ethmoidectomy is then performed. The dural defect is identified and repaired with a mucoperiosteal flap. The sphenoidal sinus is approached via a trans-septosphenoid approach, which employs either a transnasal or a sublabial route. The petrous bone is approached and repaired through a mastoidectomy. This approach spares the cochlea and seventh and eighth nerve function.

An endoscopic approach has been successful in closing CSF fistulas and cephaloceles in 86% to 100% of cases.[66–68] The use of nasal endoscopy also eliminates the need for manipulation of the brain and the associated complications, such as anosmia. The technique is well suited for the repair of fistulas caused by fractures of the sphenoidal sinus. Once the sphenoidotomy is performed and the fistula is located, a fat graft is harvested from the abdomen. It is placed over the defect and sealed with fibrin glue. The face of the sphenoidal and ethmoidal recess is then firmly packed with Gelfoam or Surgicel. The repair of the ethmoid roof and cribriform plate is done much like the sphenoid repair. Care must be taken to remove all remaining mucosa from the graft recipient site. A turbinate graft is harvested from the contralateral nasal cavity and cleaned of all its mucosa as well. This turbinate graft can be placed on the intracranial or extracranial side of the defect. Once the graft is placed, the site is covered with fibrin glue. Many surgeons also employ removable supports, such as balloons or nasal tampons, to provide further structural support to the repair. Once again, lumbar drainage is continued postoperatively to help seal the fistula.

Operative care of a patient who has facial fractures and a CSF fistula must be individualized. A CSF fistula is not a contraindication to proceeding with the reduction of facial fractures. Often, a CSF leak closes spontaneously once the facial fractures are reduced. It is thought that the fracture reduction aids in healing the leak. For a stable patient, repair of the fistula at the time of reduction of the facial fractures is optimal; however, in an unstable patient, a delayed approach is certainly defensible.[31, 32]

THE FUTURE

The availability of tissue glue, coupled with the development of improved flexible endoscopy, will alter the surgical management of traumatic CSF fistulas in the foreseeable future. As three-dimensional imaging techniques also improve, resulting in better fistula localization, it is likely that minimally invasive techniques will become routine for closing CSF leaks. In the interim, careful analysis of the clinical data and radiologic studies provide sufficient information for successful closure of these leaks in the great majority of patients using intracranial and present endoscopic techniques.

REFERENCES

1. Park JI, Strelzow VV, Friedman WH: Current management of cerebrospinal fluid rhinorrhea. Laryngoscope 93:1294, 1983.
2. Lewin W: Cerebrospinal fluid rhinorrhea in closed head injuries. Br J Surg 42:1, 1954.
3. Raaf J: Post-traumatic cerebrospinal fluid leaks. Arch Surg 95: 648, 1967.
4. Spetzler RF, Zabramski JM: Cerebrospinal fluid fistula. Contemp Neurosurg 8:1, 1986.
5. Brawley BW, Kelly WA: Treatment of basal skull fractures with and without CSF fistula. J Neurosurg 26:57, 1967.
6. Brisman R, Hughes JE, Mount LA: Cerebrospinal fluid rhinorrhea. Arch Neurol 22:245, 1966.
7. Cooper P: Cerebrospinal fluid fistulas and pneumocephalus. In Barrow DL (ed): Complications and Sequelae of Head Injury: Neurosurgical Topics. Park Ridge, IL, AANS, 1992, pp 1–12.

7a. Eisenberg HM, Gary HE, Aldrich EF, et al: Initial CT findings in 753 patients with severe head injury. A report from the INH Traumatic Coma Data Bank. J Neurosurg 73(5):6881, 1990.

8. Arabi B, Leibrock LG: Neurosurgical approaches to cerebrospinal fluid rhinorrhea. Ear Nose Throat J 71:300, 1992.

9. Ceviker N, Baykaner K, Keskil S, et al: Sella turcica fractures in a trauma series and their clinical significance. Surg Neurol 44:28, 1995.

10. Meirowsky AM, Caveness WF, Dillon JD et al: Cerebrospinal fluid fistulas complicating missile wounds of the brain. J Neurosurg 54:44, 1981.

11. Aarabi B: Causes of infections in penetrating head wounds in the Iran-Iraq war. Neurosurgery 25:923, 1989.

12. Taha JM, Haddad FS, Brown JA: Intracranial infection after missile injuries to the brain: Report of 30 cases from the Lebanese conflict. Neurosurgery 29:864, 1991.

13. Lowe F, Pertuiset B, Cahumier EE, et al: Traumatic, spontaneous, and postoperative CSF rhinorrhea. In Symon L (ed): Advances and Technical Standards in Neurosurgery. Vienna, Springer-Verlag, 1984, pp 169–207.

14. Okada J, Tsuda T, Takasugi S, et al: Unusually late onset of cerebrospinal fluid rhinorrhea after head trauma. Surg Neurol 35:213, 1991.

15. McCormack B, Hunt CE, Sofer S: Extracranial repair of cerebrospinal fluid fistulae: Techniques and results in 37 patients. Neurosurgery 27:412, 1998.

16. Leech PJ, Patterson R: Conservative and operative management for cerebrospinal leakage after closed head injury. Lancet 1:1013, 1973.

17. Omaya AK: Spinal fluid fistulae. Clin Neurosurg 23:363, 1975.

18. Johnson RT, Dutt P: On dural laceration over paranasal and petrous air sinuses. Br J Surg 1:141, 1947.

19. Calcaterra TC: Diagnosis and management of ethmoid cerebrospinal rhinorrhea. Otolaryngol Clin North Am 18:99, 1985.

20. Joshi KK, Crockard HA: Traumatic cerebrospinal fluid fistula simulating tears: Case report. J Neurosurg 49:121, 1978.

21. Hicks GW, Wright JW, Wright JW III: Cerebrospinal fluid otorrhea. Laryngoscope 90(Suppl 25):1, 1980.

22. Kaufman B, Nulsen FE, Weiss MH, et al: Acquired spontaneous nontraumatic normal-pressure cerebrospinal fluid fistulas originating from the middle fossa. Radiology 122:379, 1977.

23. Cooper PR: Skull fracture and traumatic cerebrospinal fluid fistulas. In Cooper PR (ed): Head Injury, 3rd ed. Baltimore, Williams & Wilkins, 1993, p 115.

24. Choi D, Spann R: Traumatic cerebrospinal fluid leakage: Risk factors and the use of prophylactic antibiotics. Br J Neurosurg 10:571, 1996.

25. Hubbard JL, McDonald TJ, Pearson BW: Spontaneous cerebrospinal fluid rhinorrhea: Evolving concepts in diagnosis and surgical management based on the Mayo Clinic experience from 1970 through 1981. Neurosurgery 16:14, 1985.

26. Lewin W: Cerebrospinal fluid rhinorrhea in nonmissile head injuries. Clin Neurosurg 12:237, 1966.

27. Jamieson KG, Yelland JDN: Surgical repair of the anterior fossa because of rhinorrhea, aerocele, or meningitis. J Neurosurg 39:328, 1973.

28. Flanagan JC, McLachlan DL, Shannon GM: Orbital roof fractures: Neurological and neurosurgical considerations. Ophthalmology 87:325, 1980.

29. Westmore GA, Whittam DE: Cerebrospinal spinal fluid rhinorrhoea and its management. Br J Surg 69:489, 1982.

30. Koso-Thomas AK, Harley EH: Traumatic cerebrospinal fluid fistula presenting as recurrent meningitis. Otolaryngol Head Neck Surg 112:469, 1995.

31. Daly DT, Lydiatt WM, Ogren FP, et al: Extracranial approaches to the repair of cerebrospinal fluid rhinorrhea. Ear Nose Throat J 71:311, 1992.

32. Marentette LJ, Valentino J: Traumatic anterior fossa cerebrospinal fluid fistulae and craniofacial considerations. Otolaryngol Clin North Am 24:151, 1991.

33. Bakay L, Glausauer FE: Head Injury. Boston, Little, Brown, 1980, p 280.

34. Costantino PD, Janecka IP: Cranial-base surgery. In Bailley B (ed): Head and Neck Surgery—Otolaryngology, 2nd ed. Philadelphia, Lippincott-Raven, 1998, pp 1848–1853.

35. Ryall RG, Peacock MK, Simpson DA: Usefulness of beta 2-transferrin assay in the detection of cerebrospinal fluid leaks following head injuries. J Neurosurg 77:737, 1992.

36. Sloman AJ, Kelly RH: Transferrin allelic variants may cause false positives in the detection of cerebrospinal fluid fistulae. Clin Chem 39:1444, 1993.

37. Ikeda S, Watanbe T, Sato M: Two cases of recurrent bacterial meningitis following traumatic cerebrospinal fluid rhinorrhea. Brain Dev 21:76, 1999.

38. Evans JP, Keegan HR: Danger in the use of intrathecal methylene blue. JAMA 174:856, 1960.

39. Mahaley MS, Odom GL: Complication following intrathecal injection of fluorescein: Case report. J Neurosurg 25:298, 1968.

40. Schaefer SD, Diehl JT, Briggs WH: The diagnosis of CSF rhinorrhea by metrizamide CT scanning. Laryngoscope 90:871, 1980.

41. Colquhoun IR: CT cisternography in the investigation of cerebrospinal fluid rhinorrhea. Clin Radiol 47:403, 1993.

42. Ahmadi J, Weiss MH, Segall HD, et al: Evaluation of cerebrospinal fluid rhinorrhea by metrizamide computed tomographic cisternography. Neurosurgery 16:54, 1985.

43. Chow JM, Goodman D, Mafee MF: Evaluation of CSF rhinorrhea by computerized tomography with metrizamide. Otolaryngol Head Neck Surg 100:99, 1989.

44. Kirchner FR, Proud GO: Method of identification and localization of cerebrospinal fluid, rhinorrhea, and otorrhea. Laryngoscope 70:921, 1960.

45. Jacobson I, Maran AG: Localization of cerebrospinal fluid rhinorrhea. Arch Otolaryngol 93:79, 1971.

46. McKusick KA, Malmud LS, Kordela PA, et al: Radionucleotide cisternography: Normal values for nasal secretion of intrathecally injected ^{111}In-DTPA. J Nucl Med 14:933, 1973.

47. Krasnow AZ, Collier BD, Isitman AT, et al: The use of radionucleotide cisternography in the diagnosis of pleural–cerebrospinal fluid fistulae. J Nucl Med 30:120, 1989.

48. Staab EV, Shirkhoda A: Cerebrospinal fluid scanning. Clin Nucl Med 6:103, 1981.

49. Spetzler RF, Wilson CB: Management of recurrent CSF rhinorrhea of the middle and posterior fossa. J Neurosurg 49:393, 1978.

50. McCormack BM, Cooper PR, Persky M, et al: Extracranial repair of cerebrospinal fluid fistulas: Technique and results in 37 patients. Neurosurgery 27:412, 1990.

51. Eljamel MS: Fractures of the middle third of the face and cerebrospinal fluid rhinorrhea. Br J Neurosurg 8:289, 1994.

52. Nakayama Y, Tanaka A, Ueno Y, et al: Spontaneous cerebrospinal fluid leakage detected by magnetic resonance cisternography—case report. Surg Neurol 39:251, 1999.

53. Klastersky J, Sadeghi M, Brihaye J: Antimicrobial prophylaxis in patients with rhinorrhea or otorrhea: A double-blind study. Surg Neurol 6:111, 1976.

54. Brodie HA: Prophylactic antibiotics for posttraumatic cerebrospinal fluid fistulae: A meta-analysis. Arch Otolaryngol Head Neck Surg 123:749, 1997.

55. Ignelzi RJ, VanderArk GD: Analysis of the treatment of basilar skull fractures with and without antibiotics. J Neurosurg 43:75, 1975.

56. Dagi TF, Meyer FB, Poletti CA: The incidence and prevention of meningitis after basilar skull fracture. Am J Emerg Med 3:295, 1983.

57. Luerssen TG, Chestnut RM, van Berkum CM, et al: Post-traumatic cerebrospinal fluid infections in the Trauma Coma Bank: The influence of the type and management of ICP monitors. In Avezaat CJJ (ed): Intracranial Pressure VIII. Rotterdam, Springer-Verlag, 1991, p 42.

58. Wyler AR, Kelly WA: The use of antibiotics with external ventriculostomies. J Neurosurg 37:185, 1972.

59. Vourc'h G: Continuous cerebrospinal fluid drainage by indwelling spinal catheter. Br J Anaesth 35:118, 1963.

60. Mincy JE: Posttraumatic cerebrospinal fluid fistula of the frontal fossa. J Trauma 6:618, 1966.

61. Laun A: Traumatic cerebrospinal fluid fistulas in the anterior and middle fossae. Acta Neurochir (Wien) 60:215, 1982.

62. Ray BS, Bergland RM: Cerebrospinal fluid fistula: Clinical aspects, techniques of localization, and methods of closure. J Neurosurg 30:399, 1969.

63. Shaffrey CI, Spotnitz WD, Shaffrey ME, et al: Neurosurgical applications of fibrin glue: Augmentation of dural closure in 134 patients. Neurosurgery 26:207, 1991.

64. Sierra DH, Nissen AJ, Welch J: The use of fibrin glue in intracranial procedures: Preliminary results. Laryngoscope 100:360, 1990.

65. Calcaterra TC: Extracranial surgical repair of cerebrospinal rhinorrhea. Ann Otol 89:108, 1980.

66. Mattox DE, Kennedy DW: Endoscopic management of cerebrospinal fluid leaks and cephaloceles. Laryngoscope 100:857, 1990.

67. Dodson EE, Gross CW, Swerdloff JL, et al: Transnasal endoscopic repair of cerebrospinal fluid rhinorrhea and skull base defects: A review of 29 cases. Otolaryngol Head Neck Surg 111:600, 1994.

68. Lanza DC, O'Brien DA, Kennedy DW: Endoscopic repair of cerebrospinal fluid fistulae and cephaloceles. Laryngoscope 106:1119, 1996.

CHAPTER 334

Diagnosis and Management of Seventh and Eighth Cranial Nerve Injuries Due to Temporal Bone Fractures

W. LEE WARREN ■ J. BRAD BELLOTTE ■ JAMES E. WILBERGER

A common yet frequently overlooked associated injury in head trauma patients is the temporal bone fracture. These injuries occur most frequently after motor vehicle accidents,[1] and up to 25% of patients with temporal bone fractures have associated facial nerve dysfunction.[2] Many complications of these injuries can be prevented or treated most effectively if the injury is diagnosed early. Neurosurgeons involved in the care of patients with head injuries must be aware of the spectrum of injuries that can occur to the temporal bone, their associated complications, and the proper diagnostic and therapeutic procedures to be used in order to effectively manage these injuries. Temporal bone fractures frequently cause injury to the facial, auditory, or vestibular nerves. This chapter addresses the assessment of patients with suspected temporal bone trauma, the classification of temporal bone fractures, and the diagnosis and management of cranial neuropathies secondary to these injuries.

ASSESSMENT OF THE PATIENT WITH SUSPECTED TEMPORAL BONE INJURY

Resuscitation and Clinical Examination

Patients with head injuries should be thoroughly evaluated for evidence of temporal bone trauma as early as possible after the overall evaluation is performed to detect and stabilize any life-threatening injuries. The details of the accident, such as the type of forces applied to the skull, can lead to an increased index of suspicion for temporal bone trauma. In the alert patient, symptoms such as tinnitus, vertigo, or hearing loss can be clues to the presence of temporal bone injury. Consultation with a neurotologist or otolaryngologist is beneficial in the management of some sequelae of temporal bone fractures and should be sought as early as possible.

Common signs of temporal bone fracture are hemotympanum, cerebrospinal fluid (CSF) otorrhea or rhinorrhea, retromastoid ecchymosis (Battle's sign), ruptured tympanic membrane, bleeding from the ear, nystagmus, facial weakness, and a deformed osseous canal. Common symptoms include a sense of fullness in the ear, hearing loss, tinnitus, otalgia, dysequilibrium, and vertigo. The examiner should look for these signs and symptoms, and any abnormalities should be carefully documented. A standard grading scale for facial nerve dysfunction such as that of House and Brackmann (Table 334–1) is helpful to improve interobserver reliability of the facial nerve examination over time. Any evidence of seventh or eighth nerve dysfunction should lead to appropriate neurophysiologic testing such as electroneurography or auditory brain stem responses.

The ear canal should be cleaned with sterile cotton applicators and carefully examined to discover bony step-offs, lacerations, hemotympanum, CSF, and perforations of the tympanic membrane. If the patient is alert, facial nerve function can be evaluated easily by having the patient open and close the eyes and bare the teeth. Even in a patient with depressed mental status, the facial grimace to pain and the flaring of the nostrils with respirations can give the examiner insight into the function of the facial nerve. Facial symmetry at rest is not a reliable indicator of nerve continuity or function; movement of the facial muscles must be seen to verify the nerve's integrity. Hearing can also be screened in the alert patient with voice and the tuning fork tests of Weber and Rinne. Because early intervention greatly improves outcome in some types of traumatic facial nerve injuries, it is critical to clearly establish in the record the initial status of facial nerve function.[1]

Radiographic Evaluation

After the initial examination, imaging studies should be obtained to document and better define the temporal bone fracture. High-resolution computed tomography (CT) has replaced plain skull radiographs as the

TABLE 334–1 ■ **House-Brackmann Scale of Facial Nerve Dysfunction**

GRADE	FUNCTION	DESCRIPTION
1	Normal	Normal function in all areas
2	Mild dysfunction	Slight weakness on close inspection
3	Moderate dysfunction	Obvious but not disfiguring
4	Moderate to severe dysfunction	Obvious weakness or disfiguring asymmetry
5	Severe dysfunction	Barely perceptible motion
6	Total paralysis	No movement

procedure of choice because of its ability to demonstrate the anatomy of the cranial base clearly.[3] The ability to look at the temporal bone in thin sections (1.0 and 1.5 mm) and in axial and coronal planes is vital to understanding the complex nature and course of these fractures (Fig. 334–1). Three-dimensional reconstructions are also sometimes helpful. Holland found that 10-mm computed tomographic sections missed half of temporal bone fractures revealed by 1.5-mm cuts.[4] The sensitivity of CT for detection of facial discontinuity or impingement by bony spicules, as well as that for detecting ossicular chain disruption, approaches 100%.[4]

Magnetic resonance imaging, with its inability to demonstrate bony details, is of little value in the acute setting after temporal bone trauma.

Evaluation of Auditory and Vestibular Function

Patients with temporal bone fractures frequently have injury to their auditory and vestibular apparatus. Proper diagnosis and management of these problems requires tests of hearing and balance. The function of the cochleovestibular system should be documented as early as possible after the trauma. Air conduction and pure-tone bone conduction testing, along with speech discrimination, are performed as early as is practical. Brain stem auditory evoked potential testing can be of value in estimating the hearing level in patients with a depressed level of consciousness or coma. Rotatory testing and electronystagmography are of value in the patient with vestibular complaints (such as dizziness or dysequilibrium).

ANATOMY AND CLASSIFICATION OF TEMPORAL BONE FRACTURES

A number of authors have devised classification systems to describe various types of temporal bone fractures. The standard method used is to divide the fractures into *transverse, longitudinal,* and *mixed types.* These terms describe the fracture relative to the long axis of the petrous ridge, which lies along a 45-degree angle to the midsagittal axis of the skull. These descriptions of temporal bone fractures arose from experiments performed in the 1940s using direct blows to cadaver skulls.[5] Later investigators used whole cadavers to simulate the forces experienced by victims of motor vehicle accidents. These experiments showed that most frac-

tures do not fall into one category, but rather tend to combine the elements of the various types.[2, 6, 7] As neuroimaging techniques such as high-resolution CT have evolved, it has become apparent that temporal bone fractures take on a number of complex morphologic features. This has led to the development of other, more clinically relevant schemes for describing temporal bone fractures.

Longitudinal Temporal Bone Fractures

According to studies using the standard classification system, approximately 80% to 90% of temporal bone fractures are longitudinal, 10% to 20% are transverse, and 8% to 10% are bilateral.[8, 9] Longitudinal fractures usually result from blunt trauma to the temporal or parietal region of the head.[10] The fracture thus starts in the squamous temporal bone and runs parallel to the external auditory canal (EAC). Some fractures extend anterior to the EAC, tearing the skin in the canal as well as the tympanic membrane. These patients may have bloody otorrhea, hemotympanum, a bony step-off in the EAC, or a combination of these conditions. Fractures that originate posterior to the EAC run through the mastoid air cells, sparing the tympanic membrane but frequently tearing small emissary veins from the sigmoid sinus, producing retromastoid ecchymosis (Battle's sign). The appearance of this bruising may be delayed 24 to 48 hours.[10]

Whether they originate anterior or posterior to the EAC, the longitudinal fractures extend anteromedially, passing through the middle ear (Fig. 334–2). This frequently leads to disruption of the ossicular chain and conductive hearing loss (and often a concomitant sensorineural hearing loss due to cochlear concussion).[11] Passing anterior and lateral to the otic capsule, the fractures reach the eustachian tube, foramen lacerum, or foramen ovale. Usually terminating in the middle fossa or sphenoid bone, these fractures can extend into the carotid canal, jugular fossa, temporomandibular joint, or anterior fossa or cross the clivus to extend into the opposite side, producing a bilateral fracture (Fig. 334–3).[12] Approximately 20% to 30% of longitudinal temporal bone fractures produce facial nerve paralysis, usually due to geniculate ganglion disruption.[10, 13]

Transverse Temporal Bone Fractures

Far less common than the longitudinal variety, temporal bone fractures make up 10% to 20% of temporal

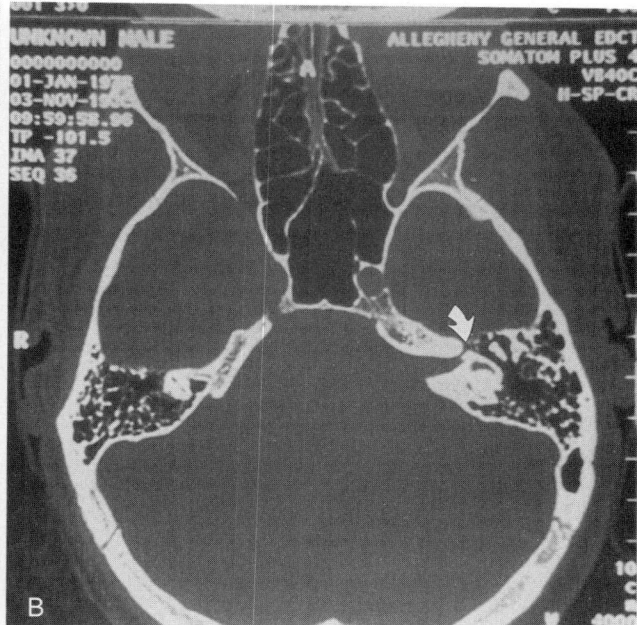

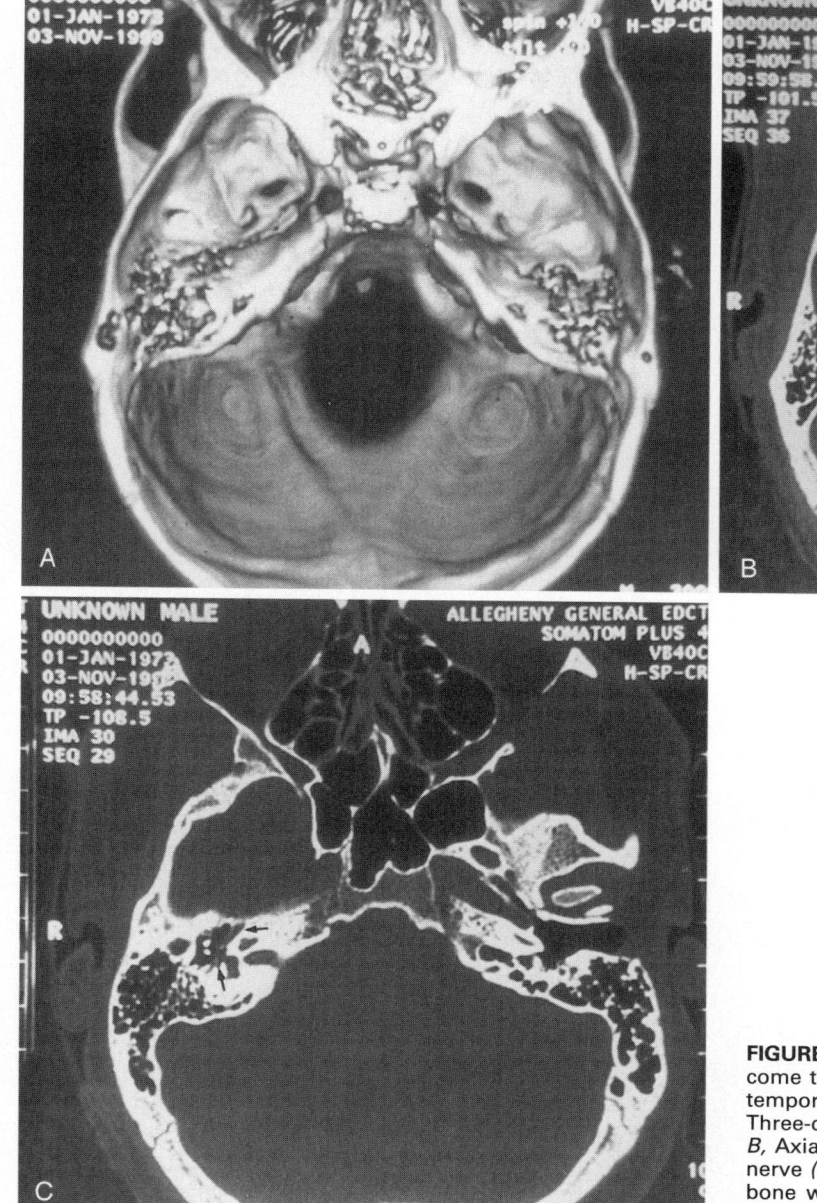

FIGURE 334–1. Modern computed tomography (CT) has become the standard imaging technique for the evaluation of temporal bone trauma because of its high resolution. *A*, Three-dimensional axial reconstruction of the cranial base. *B*, Axial bone window demonstrates the genu of the facial nerve *(curved arrow)* in the petrous temporal bone. *C*, Axial bone window demonstrating the horizontal portion of the facial nerve *(arrows)*.

bone fractures and are transverse to the long axis of the petrous temporal bone.[8, 9] These fractures are usually produced by a blow to the occipital or mastoid region of the skull, although occasionally transverse fractures are seen after frontal trauma. Transverse temporal bone fractures are associated with a higher incidence of other central nervous system injuries than is the longitudinal pattern because of the much higher degree of force required to produce them. Intracerebral hemorrhage, epidural hematoma, and *contrecoup* brain contusions are commonly seen in patients with transverse temporal bone fractures.

The fracture typically begins in the foramen magnum or jugular fossa and crosses the posterior aspect of the temporal bone at a right angle to its long axis (Fig. 334–4). Most commonly, the fracture then passes into the otic capsule, disrupting the cochlear and vestibular labyrinthine components, and travels into the fallopian canal along its tympanic portion to the geniculate ganglion. Occasionally, the fracture will travel medial to the otic capsule and through the internal auditory canal to extend into the middle fossa. Conversely, the fracture may pass lateral to the otic capsule to extend into the middle fossa by way of the middle ear.

Because of their medial course, transverse fractures are associated with less external evidence of their presence than is seen with longitudinal fractures. The tym-

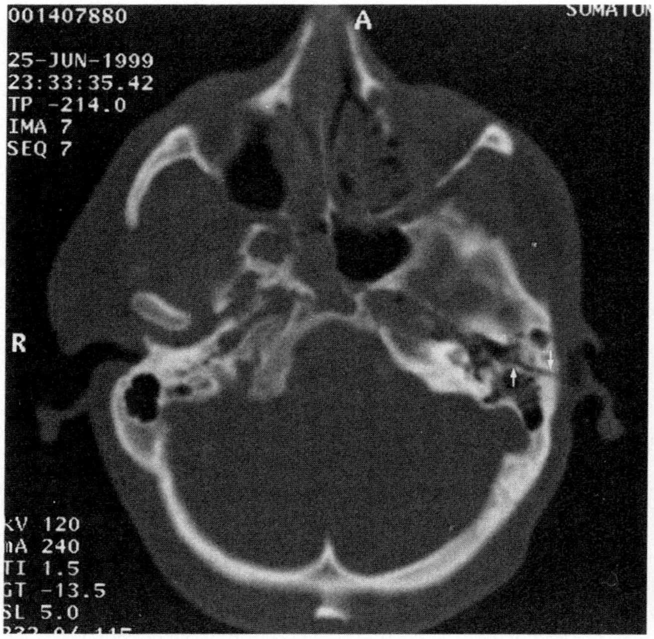

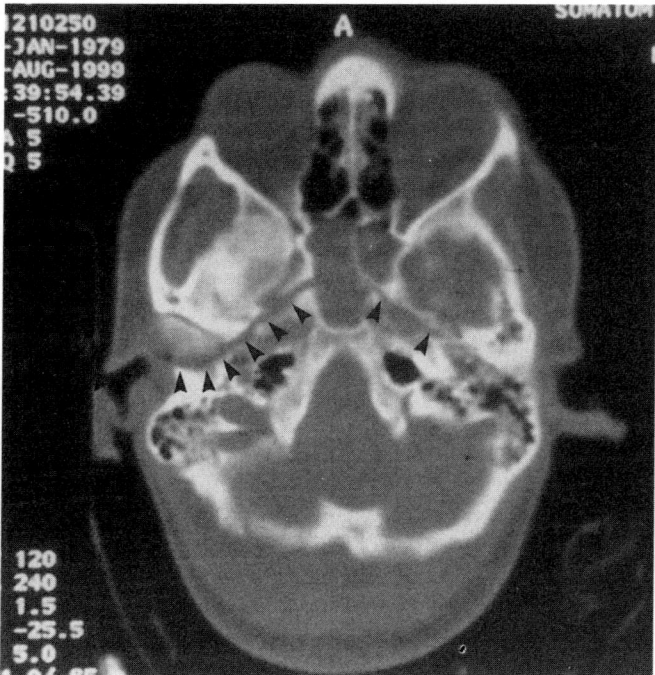

FIGURE 334–2. Axial computed tomographic scan bone window demonstrating longitudinal fracture of the temporal bone *(arrows)*.

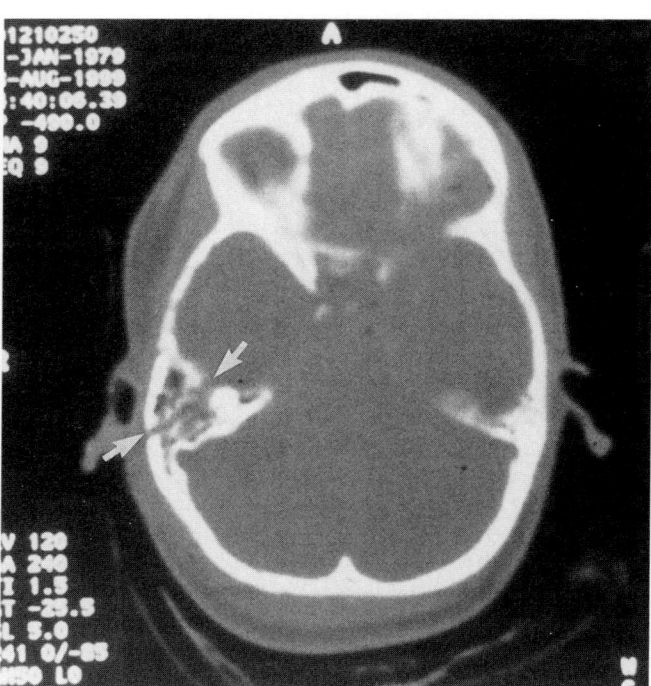

FIGURE 334–4. Axial computed tomographic scan bone window demonstrating transverse temporal bone fracture *(arrows)*.

FIGURE 334–3. Axial computed tomographic scan bone window demonstrates longitudinal temporal bone fracture extending through both carotid canals and crossing anterior to the clivus *(arrowheads)*, producing bilateral fractures. This 20-year-old woman died as a result of massive cerebral infarction after dissection and subsequent thrombosis of both internal carotid arteries.

panic membrane and EAC are usually spared, making hemotympanum and CSF otorrhea relatively infrequent.[2] Vertigo, severe sensorineural hearing loss, and nystagmus are commonly present because of disruption of the internal auditory canal. CSF rhinorrhea is also seen frequently. Approximately 50% of patients with transverse temporal bone fractures present with facial paralysis, with the nerve usually injured in the geniculate ganglion or in the tympanic segment superior to the oval window.[14]

Mixed Fracture Patterns

Temporal bone fractures are classically described as falling neatly into either longitudinal or transverse varieties; however, high-resolution CT has shown that the most common fracture has elements of both types. This knowledge has led to the classification of some fractures as *mixed* or *oblique* types relative to their slanting course across the petrous pyramid. In clinical practice, many patients present with features of both longitudinal and transverse fractures. These patients are usually found to have oblique fractures.[15, 16]

Other Classifications of Temporal Bone Fractures

The fact that modern imaging technology has revealed flaws in the traditional classification of temporal bone fractures has led some authors to develop other, more clinically relevant schemes. Classically described longitudinal fractures usually spare the otic capsule, whereas transverse fractures are associated with its disruption. Fisch described fractures that cross the otic capsule and cause loss of inner ear function.[17] Those fractures that do not disrupt the otic capsule are now referred to as *otic-sparing fractures*.[20] Fisch pointed out that otic capsule–disrupting fractures were much more likely to produce facial nerve or inner ear dysfunction and other complications than were otic-sparing fractures, a finding also verified by others.[1, 19] This distinction becomes important in making decisions regarding the management of facial nerve dysfunction after temporal bone fractures,[18] that is, otic-disrupting fractures are more likely to disrupt the facial nerve anatomically, making operative decompression and repair necessary. Facial nerve dysfunction after otic-sparing fracture is frequently from reversible nerve contusion. Further, since otic-disrupting fractures usually cause irreversible hearing loss, the translabyrinthine approach to repair of the facial nerve is more reasonable. Thus, knowledge of the fracture's path relative to the otic capsule provides assistance in decision-making and operative planning.

Yanagihara and associates have proposed an alternative classification scheme for temporal bone fractures. They attempted to correlate the anatomy of the fracture with neurotologic and surgical findings.[20] The fractures are divided into four types based on their course through the temporal bone. Type 1 fractures travel across the mastoid process. If the fracture reaches the EAC, it is type 2, and those reaching the pyramidal or horizontal portion of the seventh nerve are type 3 fractures. Type 4 fractures travel across the tegmen of the middle ear and the antrum and involve the geniculate ganglion. Type 4 fractures are further divided into types 4a and 4b depending on whether the inner ear and internal auditory canal are spared or involved, respectively. The type 4b fracture corresponds to the classically described transverse fracture.

Yanagihara found the type 2 fracture to be most common. Type 1 and type 2 fractures are associated with facial palsy only, resulting from injury of the mastoid and pyramidal portions of the nerve. Hemotympanum is frequently seen in these fractures and resolves spontaneously. Type 3 fractures are associated with disruption of the ossicular chain and profound conductive or mixed hearing loss, as well as facial nerve injury at the level of the geniculate ganglion. Bloody otorrhea from tearing of skin in the EAC or rupture of the tympanic membrane is common in types 2 and 3. Type 4 fractures injure the facial nerve from the labyrinthine to the pyramidal segment, creating dry eye because of lost input to the greater superficial petrosal nerve. Type 4a fractures produce conductive hearing loss, and type 4b fractures are associated with sensorineural hearing loss and nystagmus.

Penetrating Temporal Bone Trauma

The vast majority of temporal bone fractures are the result of blunt trauma, with penetrating injuries composing less than 10% of most series.[1, 8] The most common penetrating injury to the temporal bone is the gunshot wound, although at our institution we have seen temporal bone fractures from golf balls, tree branches, arrows, and other materials. The increasing prevalence of handgun violence in the United States has led to predictions that gunshot wounds will surpass motor vehicle accidents as the leading cause of injury-related mortality by the early part of the 21st century.[21]

- Gunshot wounds to the temporal bone may present with features of neck injury or head injury, or both. They usually produce comminuted or mixed fracture types.[22] CT allows assessment of the middle structures, cochlea, labyrinth, and facial nerve and determines the presence of bullet fragments, hematoma, pneumocephalus, and so forth. Up to 75% of patients with these injuries have facial nerve involvement, 60% have hearing loss, and about 30% have vascular injuries (usually carotid artery or sigmoid sinus). Given the high incidence of vascular injury associated with temporal bone fractures, carotid angiography is indicated in these patients. The venous phase should be examined also because many patients have injuries to the transverse or sigmoid sinus. CSF leak, vestibular dysfunction, and other cranial neuropathies are also seen frequently in patients who survive the injury.[21, 23–25] More than 30% of patients with gunshot wounds to the temporal bone require craniotomy for major intracranial injuries.[22]

COMPLICATIONS OF TEMPORAL BONE FRACTURES

Cerebrospinal Fluid Fistula

Leakage of CSF complicates up to one third of temporal bone fractures.[1, 16, 26] When the fracture tears the dura, CSF leaks into the tympanomastoid space. If the tympanic membrane has been disrupted, otorrhea occurs (Fig. 334–5). If the membrane is intact, the fluid can leak down the eustachian tube into the nasopharynx, leading to rhinorrhea.

The diagnosis of CSF fistula is frequently made based on the history and clinical examination. In a patient with a known temporal bone fracture, clear fluid gushing from the nose or running out the ear is pathognomonic for CSF fistula. However, if the drainage is intermittent or slight, the diagnosis can be difficult to establish firmly. In addition, patients with severe allergic rhinitis can have copious nasal secretions that can be confused with CSF. The "halo" sign is a clear ring around a bloody center on absorbent paper or cotton gauze and if present can imply the presence of CSF. Attempts to demonstrate the leak can be aided by the Valsalva maneuver or jugular vein compression and by flexing the neck of the sitting patient to facilitate rhinorrhea.

Glucose oxidase papers are a relatively nonspecific indicator of the presence of CSF, producing positive test results in up to 75% of normal nasal discharge specimens. However, they are nearly 100% sensitive in detecting the presence of glucose in the fluid; thus,

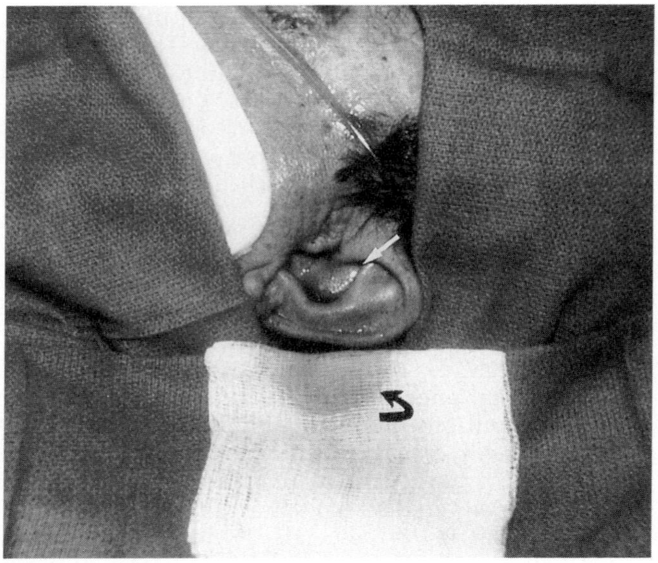

FIGURE 334–5. This 64-year-old man suffered a complex temporal bone fracture during an altercation. Photograph demonstrates cerebrospinal fluid fistula that presented as profuse otorrhea. Note fluid flowing from the ear canal *(white arrow)* and onto sponge *(curved black arrow)*.

false-negative results are rare.[27] If enough fluid can be obtained, laboratory determination of the glucose concentration can be helpful. A concentration of greater than 30 mg/dL is highly indicative of CSF leak, unless the sample is contaminated by blood. If the diagnosis remains in doubt, some laboratories are capable of performing immunoassays for the presence of the CSF-specific substance β_2-transferrin. This test, although rarely needed, is diagnostic for CSF.

The role of prophylatic antimicrobial agents in patients with CSF fistula has not been firmly established. Early reports argued empirically for the use of antibiotics to prevent meningitis.[28] However, most studies in the literature fail to show a significant benefit in preventing meningitis from prophylactic antibiotics.[1, 29–31] Some data exist that indicate that the preventive use of these agents may even be harmful, for at least two reasons. First, the antibiotics chosen are often given in inappropriately low doses or are agents with poor CSF penetration. A number of reports exist of patients developing meningitis while receiving prophylaxis with an antibiotic to which the organism was sensitive because of inadequate CSF concentrations of the drug. Also, the normal flora of the nasopharynx is eliminated by prophylactic antibiotic use, creating an environment for colonization with more virulent organisms.[32, 33]

The vast majority of post-traumatic CSF fistulas close spontaneously within 2 weeks of the trauma.[1, 34] Bed rest, elevating the head 30 degrees, stool softeners, and occasionally fluid restriction are used as conservative treatments. In profuse or longer lasting leaks, continuous lumbar subarachnoid drainage can be helpful.[1, 31, 35]

Indications for surgical repair of post-traumatic CSF fistula include persistence beyond 2 weeks, persistent

or enlarging pneumocephalus, and meningitis. Meningitis should be cleared with antibiotics before surgical therapy. The usual choice for surgical closure of a CSF fistula is the subtemporal-extradural approach. The dura can sometimes be closed primarily but more frequently requires a dural substitute graft, such as fascia, temporalis muscle, or commercially available grafting materials. If the patient has lost hearing in the ipsilateral ear, the temporal bone air cells may be obliterated and packed with fat, along with eustachian tube ligation.

Life-Threatening Hemorrhage

Temporal bone fractures that disrupt the EAC or tympanic membrane usually produce hemorrhage from the ear. Other causes include a penetrating foreign body, an extrinsic laceration resulting in the presence of blood in the ear, and concussive laceration of the tympanic membrane. The ear and EAC should be gently cleaned with a sterile suction catheter or cotton-tipped applicators to locate the source of the bleeding. Packing the lateral EAC with sterile gauze will tamponade most forms of post-traumatic ear hemorrhage.

Rarely, a temporal bone fracture can result in life-threatening hemorrhage.[22, 36] Injury to the petrous carotid artery can produce communication into the middle ear and result in rapid and fatal exsanguination. When rapid hemorrhage from the ear is encountered, the EAC should be packed with gauze, and the patient should be taken urgently for angiography and vessel occlusion via balloon occlusion or embolization. Intracranial epidural or subdural hemorrhage can occur because of arterial or venous injury after temporal bone fracture. Although usually diagnosed on the initial computed tomographic scan during the resuscitation phase, these hemorrhages can produce serious morbidity or death if not recognized and properly managed.

Impaired Hearing

Twenty to 80% of patients with temporal bone fractures demonstrate some degree of hearing loss.[1, 2, 31, 35] About half of patients with longitudinal fractures have conductive loss, whereas essentially all patients with transverse fractures have partial or complete sensorineural losses.[2] As described earlier, the fracture can disrupt hearing at any point in the anatomic circuitry. Patients with known or suspected temporal bone fractures should have their hearing evaluated as soon as possible, preferably beginning during the initial resuscitation. Patients with an altered level of consciousness may be tested using auditory evoked potentials, although disruption of the EAC or blood in the middle ear can make the results less reliable.

Conductive Hearing Loss

Injury to the auricle, EAC, tympanic membrane, or ossicular chain can result in conductive hearing loss, that is, the sound waves from the environment cannot be transmitted normally to the inner ear because of anatomic disruption of the conductive system. In the case of hemotympanum, the hearing loss gradually improves over time as the clot is resorbed. More lasting or permanent deficits result from tympanic membrane rupture or disruption of the ossicular chain.

The majority of tympanic membrane perforations heal without treatment if no infection occurs.[37] The patient must be instructed to avoid getting water into the ear canal to decrease the risk of infection. Antibiotic prophylaxis or topical medications are not needed in the absence of infection. Long-term sequelae of tympanic membrane rupture are rare but include cholesteatoma from implantation of squamous epithelium from the EAC into the middle ear. This diagnosis should be considered in a patient with new or worsening conductive hearing loss years after a closed head injury.[38]

Approximately 80% of patients with conductive hearing loss will improve spontaneously, although an initial loss greater than 50 dB rarely returns to normal.[35] Conductive hearing loss greater than 30 dB persisting beyond three months in a patient with an intact tympanic membrane is highly suspicious for ossicular chain disruption.[31, 35] An otolaryngologist should be consulted for consideration of ossicular chain reconstruction. Surgical therapy is usually carried out 3 to 6 months following the injury to ensure the lack of spontaneous recovery. The most common finding is incostapedial joint dislocation, followed by incus dislocation and fracture of the stapedial arch.[7, 8] The results for surgical reconstruction of the ossicular chain are quite good, with improvement of hearing to an air-bone gap around 10 dB in most patients.[2]

Sensorineural Hearing Loss

Some degree of hearing loss is common in patients with head injuries, even in the absence of temporal bone fracture. Up to 25% of adults and 16% of children have high-frequency sensorineural hearing loss after skull trauma.[9, 31, 39] Any trauma to the cochlea, cochlear nerve, or central auditory pathways produces sensorineural loss. The organ of Corti and the hair cells of the cochlea are damaged by the acceleration and deceleration from the trauma, and the inner ear membranes may also be displaced. Bleeding into the cochlea may lead to fibrosis and osteogenesis as well.[40]

The prognosis for recovery of significant sensorineural hearing loss is poor. Most authors recommend amplification with a hearing aid.[31, 35] Patients should be carefully evaluated for correctable aspects of conductive hearing loss before they are offered amplification. Tinnitus is a frequent finding in patients with post-traumatic sensorineural hearing loss; it usually improves or resolves in the weeks after the injury. Persistent tinnitus sometimes can be masked with amplification using a hearing aid.

Vestibular Dysfunction

Most patients with head injuries, and virtually all patients with temporal bone fractures, complain of some degree of balance disturbance. The most frequent finding is transient, nonspecific dizziness in the days to weeks after the trauma. True vertigo is characterized by vestibular dysfunction and is nearly always accompanied by nystagmus.[35] A number of patients have transient episodic vertigo, with symptoms of sudden rapid motion, which occur for several weeks to a few months after injury. These symptoms are generally self-limited and have no permanent sequelae. This problem has been termed *labyrinthine* or *vestibular concussion.* Diagnostic testing such as electronystagmography or magnetic resonance imaging can be valuable in the workup of a patient with post-traumatic vestibular dysfunction to identify or exclude central lesions.

Otic capsule–disrupting temporal bone fractures result in severe vertigo, frequently leading to profound nausea and vomiting. Nystagmus, with the fast component beating away from the injured ear, is always seen in these patients. Although the vertigo usually diminishes over a few days, complete resolution can require months. Permanent balance disturbances are uncommon but can be seen in elderly patients, vision-impaired individuals, or those with bilateral vestibular dysfunction.

Benign paroxysmal positional vertigo, or cupulolithiasis, is a form of positional dizziness. It is characterized by episodes of vertigo, which last from several seconds to 1 minute and are brought on by rapid head motion, usually with a 10- to 15-second delay in onset. The symptoms demonstrate reproducibility with certain head positions as well as fatigability with repeated head motion. Benign paroxysmal positional vertigo tends to be episodic and is characterized by months of symptom-free intervals interspersed with recurrent vertigo attacks that can last for days. The prevailing theory of benign paroxysmal positional vertigo is that there is traumatic dislocation of calcium carbonate crystals from the macula of the utricle or saccule, which fall against the cupula of the posterior semicircular canal and stimulate it. This results in an exaggerated response to motion. Treatment is with vestibular suppressants and an exercise program designed to enhance compensatory mechanisms. When conservative therapy fails, treatment is with denervation of the semicircular canals by vestibular nerve sectioning.

A syndrome of episodic vertigo lasting several hours and associated with hearing loss, tinnitus, and perceived pressure in the ear is occasionally seen after temporal bone trauma. This problem often presents several years after the injury and is due to hydrops of the endolymphatic system. Pathologically, there is increased fluid pressure in the endolymphatic compartment of the inner ear. The treatment of post-traumatic endolymphatic hydrops includes dietary salt restriction, vestibular suppressants, and occasionally surgical drainage.[41]

Leakage of the perilymph from the inner to the middle ear can cause hearing loss or vestibular dysfunction. Although rather uncommon, perilymphatic fistula should be in the differential diagnosis for all cases of post-traumatic hearing or balance problems after head injury.[42–50] This fistula is usually via the round window but occasionally is through the oval window after subluxation of the stapes or otic capsule fracture.[47, 50] The hearing loss is sensorineural, but occasionally coexisting ossicular chain disruption or tympanic membrane perforations produces an additional conductive loss. The vertigo is relatively nondescript and is not consistently reproducible but may sometimes be revealed by vigorous exercise or the Valsalva maneuver. The definitive diagnosis of perilymph fistula requires a high index of suspicion. A fistula test involves increasing the ear canal pressure with a pneumatic otoscope, which may elicit vertigo and nystagmus. Serial audiograms and electronystagmography are sometimes helpful, but the definitive diagnosis is made by surgical exploration and evaluation of the oval and round windows. If perilymph is collected in the middle ear, it can be positively identified by β_2-transferrin analysis.[51] Fascia, muscle, or other autologous or allograft material can be used to repair the fistula.

Facial Nerve Injury

EPIDEMIOLOGY

The facial nerve is the second most frequently injured cranial nerve in head-injured patients, after the sixth nerve. Seventh nerve palsy complicates up to 3% of all head injuries.[52] Facial palsy can be complete or partial or unilateral or bilateral[53] and can occur immediately or in a delayed fashion. Practically all cases of posttraumatic facial palsy occur in the setting of temporal bone fractures. Conversely, only 3% to 25% of temporal bone fractures produce facial nerve injury.[1, 2, 31, 54] Approximately 20% to 30% of longitudinal temporal bone fractures produce facial nerve paralysis.[10, 13] The transverse fracture more commonly causes seventh nerve dysfunction, producing a deficit in about 50% of cases.[14] Adults are much more likely to suffer facial palsy after temporal bone fracture than are children, possibly because of decreased ossification in children's skulls.[31, 55]

ANATOMY AND PATHOPHYSIOLOGY OF TRAUMATIC FACIAL NERVE PALSY

The facial nerve must traverse approximately 30 mm through the fallopian canal of the temporal bone. This bony entrapment places the nerve at risk for injury when the temporal bone is fractured. The labyrinthine portion of the nerve is the most commonly injured segment.[17] This 2.5 mm wide and 6 mm long portion of the nerve extends from the fundus of the internal auditory canal to the first genu and includes the geniculate ganglion. More than 90% of traumatic facial nerve injuries are located in the perigeniculate region.[13]

Facial nerve dysfunction can be caused by a hematoma within the nerve, anatomic disruption, contusion, or an impinging bony fragment.[13, 17, 56] In longitudinal fractures, the nerve is more likely to be in continuity than in transverse fractures; nerve disruption is most frequently seen in the latter type. Transverse fractures

usually pass through the labyrinthine segment proximal to the geniculate ganglion, resulting in severe nerve injury. Conversely, longitudinal fractures extend through the upper tympanic segment of the nerve, being deflected anteriorly by the otic capsule. Thus, the fracture often passes though the geniculate ganglion and along the greater superficial petrosal nerve. The perigeniculate region of the facial nerve, being tethered by the greater superficial petrosal nerve, is susceptible to stretch injury. The internal auditory canal and descending mastoid portions of the facial nerve are less common sites of injury, except in gunshot injuries, which frequently affect the distal portions of the nerve.[13] In patients with any sign of preauricular or facial trauma and coexisting facial nerve dysfunction, extracranial nerve injury should be suspected and the cheek and parotid regions should also be evaluated.

DIAGNOSIS AND EVALUATION OF TRAUMATIC FACIAL NERVE PALSY

The initial examination of every patient with a potential head injury must include an assessment of facial nerve function. This is because the best hope for recovery of function in certain types of facial nerve injury is rapid diagnosis and proper surgical treatment. The examiner should seek to determine the timing of onset of facial weakness (i.e., immediate or delayed), whether the injury is partial or complete, and the location of the injury relative to the geniculate ganglion.

Facial weakness or paralysis from the time of initial presentation usually indicates a direct nerve injury (i.e., from tearing, stretching, or actual discontinuity of the nerve) that is unlikely to resolve spontaneously. Although it is sometimes difficult to determine facial nerve function in an unconscious patient or in patients with trauma and swelling of the face, the documentation of any facial function immediately after injury is of considerable therapeutic and prognostic significance. The recognition of delayed-onset facial palsy is important because the vast majority of these patients will recover fully.[57] Delayed paralysis may develop at any time during the first 2 weeks after trauma and may progress to complete palsy. It is seen most commonly after the first 72 hours. Delayed facial palsy is usually due to an increase in pressure on the nerve within the bony canal resulting from hemorrhage or edema. The presence of any residual motion ensures the integrity of the perineurium and indicates a good prognosis for recovery. The determination of whether paralysis is due to a blockage of impulses along a nerve in continuity or is the result of disruption of the nerve must be made as early as possible. Electrophysiologic testing can provide objective data to help in making this distinction, whereas radiographic studies and topographic methods of assessing the location of the injury along the nerve's course assist in planning the surgical approach.

The percutaneous nerve excitability test compares the electrical stimulus-response thresholds of the normal and injured sides. A hand-held electrical nerve stimulator is used, allowing this test to be performed on a daily basis at the patient's bedside when necessary. The electrode is placed on the skin over the main trunk of the facial nerve as it exits the stylomastoid foramen. The stimulus-response threshold for facial twitching on the normal side is first determined and is generally between 3 and 7 mA. The procedure is then repeated on the affected side, and the two thresholds are compared. The test's usefulness is limited in the early postinjury period by the fact that electrical excitability is preserved in the distal portion of a transected nerve for 72 to 96 hours after injury.[59] Thus, even a nerve that is proximally transected will respond to stimulation early; subsequent wallerian degeneration will produce a difference in the stimulation thresholds between the normal and affected sides of at least 3.5 mA.[54] The test is somewhat subjective in that the examiner must determine the response of the facial nerve and can be misled by stimulation of other muscles in the face (i.e., the masseter muscle).

Evoked electromyography, or electroneurography (ENOG), provides an alternative and objective measure of facial nerve function.[17, 60] This test uses supramaximal transcutaneous stimulation of the nerve, with electrodes in the facial muscles used to record the amplitude of the compound action potentials generated by the stimulus. Results are expressed as a percentage of the amplitude on the normal side, with greater than 90% reduction indicative of severe neural degeneration. ENOG provides an objective and quantitative assessment of the degree of injury to the nerve.[2] However, it is more expensive and more difficult to perform, and the instruments are more cumbersome compared with those for the percutaneous nerve excitability test. ENOG is also inaccurate in the first 3 to 4 days after injury.

Topographic localization of the facial nerve injury relative to the geniculate ganglion helps to determine the surgical approach. High-resolution temporal bone CT may suggest the location of the lesion by demonstrating the disruption of the fallopian canal. The greater superficial petrosal nerve leaves the facial nerve at the geniculate ganglion to innervate the lacrimal gland; thus, lesions at or proximal to the ganglion impair lacrimation. This provides the basis for Schirmer's test, which can quantitate the amount of tearing. Litmus paper is placed on the conjunctiva of each lower eyelid; the wetting of the paper of one side is compared with that of the other after 5 minutes. A normal lacrimal gland will wet 2 to 3 cm of the litmus paper, whereas a denervated gland may wet no more than a few millimeters. The nerve to the stapedius muscle departs from the main trunk of the facial nerve in the facial canal; a hypersensitivity to sound (hyperacusis) indicates injury to this nerve. In a patient with normal lacrimation on the side of facial paresis and hyperacusis, the injury is localized beyond the geniculate ganglion. An objective measure of the integrity of the stapedial reflex is impedance testing, but this is not possible in a patient with impaired hearing. The chorda tympani branch also leaves the nerve in the facial canal and provides taste sensation to the anterior two thirds of the tongue. Although taste testing is possible, it is difficult and of limited usefulness in the trauma patient. Another function-based topographic test of facial nerve function is salivary flow measurement. Although accurate, it is difficult to perform and labor-intensive; thus, it is rarely used in this setting.[61]

MANAGEMENT OF THE PATIENT WITH A FACIAL NERVE INJURY

Controversy exists regarding which patients require surgical intervention, and the proper timing of such surgery.[5, 13, 17, 20, 52, 62–64] Approximately 90% of patients with delayed onset of facial paralysis or those who have facial paresis only will fully recover spontaneously or have minimal dysfunction at 6 months after injury.[65] Thus, conservative therapy is indicated in the majority of patients. Medical management includes short-term oral corticosteroid therapy to reduce edema of the nerve within the fallopian canal. In patients with complete facial paralysis, treatment decisions are based on timing of onset, nature of the injury (i.e., blunt versus penetrating), and electrophysiologic testing.

The literature indicates that surgical intervention is warranted in patients with penetrating injury or in those in whom radiography demonstrates an obviously discontinuous fallopian canal, with immediate complete facial paralysis. There is disagreement regarding the timing of surgery, with some authors advocating immediate exploration and débridment,[57] whereas others recommend waiting 21 days and operating if ENOG demonstrates nerve degeneration.[22] The role of surgery in patients with delayed facial paralysis is even more controversial. Some authors endorse surgical exploration and decompression when ENOG indicates complete absence of nerve excitability or a greater than 90% reduction of summating potential.[2, 59, 66] Given the good prognosis for spontaneous recovery in patients with delayed paralysis, however, many authors argue for conservative therapy.[62, 63] Most agree that surgical exploration is indicated in patients with total facial paralysis who demonstrate no functional recovery or electrophysiologic evidence of reinnervation potentials at 8 to 12 months after injury.

The hearing status and site of injury to the facial nerve dictate the surgical approach chosen. If adequate cochlear reserve is present, the intratemporal segments of the nerve can be adequately exposed by combining the transmastoid and middle fossa approaches. Most longitudinal fractures injure the nerve in the perigeniculate region, and the nerve is best examined in this location using the middle fossa approach to unroof the internal auditory canal, geniculate ganglion, and the tympanic and labyrinthine segments of the nerve. Common findings are bony spicules embedded in the nerve, contusion, and intraneural hematoma. Removal of hematoma and bone fragments facilitates nerve regeneration.[13, 56, 59, 67] Significant temporal lobe swelling or contusion can make this approach difficult or impossible. In the patient with a deaf ear on the side of the facial paralysis, the translabyrinthine approach can be used to expose the entire intratemporal facial nerve.

However, this approach is not appropriate in an ear with salvageable hearing.

The nerve sheath should be left intact if possible. Severely contused or disrupted nerves require grafting to provide a conduit for regeneration of the motor neurons. Resection of the damaged portion with end-to-end anastomosis is appropriate if the resulting nerve is under no tension. The sural or greater auricular nerves are good choices for interpositional grafts if the fresh ends cannot be primarily reapproximated. The nervous tissue should be carefully handled with micro-instruments. The operating microscope provides superior lighting and magnification to loupes. Precise end-to-end anastomosis should be accomplished using 9–0 or 10–0 monofilament suture.[68] Facial nerve grafting, when successful, can require up to 2 years for full regeneration. Patients should be counseled that even under ideal circumstances, forehead weakness and some degree of facial synkinesis are to be anticipated. The results of interposition grafting, however, are superior to those of other techniques (i.e., cross-facial anastomoses, and hypoglossal-facial nerve anastomoses).[61]

For all patients with facial paralysis, the protection of the eye from exposure keratitis is vital. This exposure to the environment in an eye incapable of closing on its own can lead to blindness. Artificial tears, ointment, and taping of the eyelids in the closed position at night are usually sufficient. However, for patients with severe or prolonged exposure, insertion of a gold weight into the upper eyelid will keep the eye closed and protected from the environment. Temporary tarsorrhaphy is also occasionally used to narrow the palpebral fissure.

REFERENCES

1. Brodie HA, Thompson TC: Management of complications from 820 temporal bone fractures. Am J Otol 18:188–197, 1997.
2. Nosan DK, Benecke JE Jr, Murr AH: Current perspective on temporal bone trauma. Otolaryngol Head Neck Surg 117:67–71, 1997.
3. Yeakley JW: Temporal bone fractures. Curr Probl Diagn Radiol 28:65–98, 1999.
4. Holland BA, Brant-Zawadzki M: High-resolution CT of temporal bone trauma. AJR Am J Roentgenol 143:391–395, 1984.
5. Gurdjian ES: Re-evaluation of the biomechanics of blunt impact injury of the head. Surg Gynecol Obstet 140:845–850, 1975.
6. Travis LW, Stalnaker RL, Melvin JW: Impact trauma of the human temporal bone. J Trauma 17:761–766, 1977.
7. Hough JV: Restoration of hearing loss after head trauma. Ann Otol Rhinol Laryngol 78:210–226, 1969.
8. Adegbite AB, Khan MI, Tan L: Predicting recovery of facial nerve function following injury from a basilar skull fracture [see comments]. J Neurosurg 75:759–762, 1991.
8. Cannon CR, Jahrsdoerfer RA: Temporal bone fractures: Review of 90 cases. Arch Otolaryngol 109:285–288, 1983.
9. Tos M: Course of and sequelae to 248 petrosal fractures. Acta Otolaryngol (Stockh) 75:353–354, 1973.
10. Hough JV, Stuart WD: Middle ear injuries in skull trauma. Laryngoscope 78:899–937, 1968.
11. Lindsay JR, Zajtchuk J: Concussion of the inner ear. Ann Otol Rhinol Laryngol 79:699–709, 1970.
12. Griffin JE, Altenau MM, Schaefer SD: Bilateral longitudinal temporal bone fractures: A retrospective review of seventeen cases. Laryngoscope 89:1432–1435, 1979.
13. Coker NJ, Kendall KA, Jenkins HA, et al: Traumatic intratemporal facial nerve injury: Management rationale for preservation of function. Otolaryngol Head Neck Surg 97:262–269, 1987.
14. Coker NJ, Knox GW: Temporal Bone Injuries. In Narayan RK, Wilberger JE, Povlishock JT (eds): Neurotrauma. New York, McGraw-Hill, 1996, pp 253–262.
15. Aguilar EA, Yeakley JW, Ghorayeb BY, et al: High resolution CT scan of temporal bone fractures: Association of facial nerve paralysis with temporal bone fractures. Head Neck Surg 9:162–166, 1987.
16. Ghorayeb BY, Yeakley JW, Hall JW, et al: Unusual complications of temporal bone fractures. Arch Otolaryngol Head Neck Surg 113:749–753, 1987.
17. Fisch U: Facial paralysis in fractures of the petrous bone. Laryngoscope 84:2141–2154, 1974.
18. Kelly KE, Tami TA: Temporal bone and skull base trauma. In Jackler RK, Brackmann DE (eds): Neurotology. St. Louis, Mosby-Year Book, 1994, pp 1127–1147.
19. Pollak AM, Pauw BK: Temporal bone histopathology: Residents' quiz: Otogenic pneumococci meningitis after transverse temporal bone fracture during childhood. Am J Otolaryngol 12:56–58, 1991.
20. Yanagihara N, Murakami S, Nishihara S: Temporal bone fractures inducing facial nerve paralysis: A new classification and its clinical significance [see comments]. Ear Nose Throat J 76:79–80, 83–76, 1997.
21. Qiu WW, Yin SS, Pate WE, et al: Neurotologic evaluation of facial nerve paralysis caused by gunshot wounds. Ear Nose Throat J 78:270–272, 274, 276 passim, 1999.
22. Duncan NO, Coker NJ, Jenkins HA, et al: Gunshot injuries of the temporal bone. Otolaryngol Head Neck Surg 94:47–55, 1986.
23. Atchison J, Lett ED, Cozart R, et al: Gunshot wound to the face causing unilateral facial nerve injury. Tenn Med 91:361–363, 1998.
24. Haberkamp TJ, McFadden E, Khafagy Y, et al: Gunshot injuries of the temporal bone. Laryngoscope 105:1053–1057, 1995.
25. Sabin SL, Lee D, Har-el G: Low velocity gunshot injuries to the temporal bone. J Laryngol Otol 112:929–933, 1998.
26. Nageris B, Hansen MC, Lavelle WG, et al: Temporal bone fractures. Am J Emerg Med 13:211–214, 1995.
27. Gadenholt H: The reaction of glucose-oxidase test paper in normal nasal secretions. Acta Otolaryngol (Stockh) 58:271–272, 1964.
28. Lewin W: Cerebrospinal fluid rhinorrhea in closed head injuries. Br J Surg 42:1–18, 1954.
29. Eljamel MS: Antibiotic prophylaxis in unrepaired CSF fistulae. Br J Neurosurg 7:501–505, 1993.
30. Klastersky J, Sadeghi M, Brihaye J: Antimicrobial prophylaxis in patients with rhinorrhea or otorrhea: A double-blind study. Surg Neurol 6:111–114, 1976.
31. Lee D, Honrado C, Har-El G, et al: Pediatric temporal bone fractures. Laryngoscope 108:816–821, 1998.
32. Ignelzi RJ, VanderArk GD: Analysis of the treatment of basilar skull fractures with and without antibiotics. J Neurosurg 43: 721–726, 1975.
33. Romig DA, Voth DW, Liu C, et al: Bacterial flora and infection in patients with brain injury. J Neurosurg 38:710–716, 1973.
34. Tos M: Post-traumatic cerebrospinal fluid otorrhoea. ORL J Otorhinolaryngol Relat Spec 35:30–35, 1973.
35. Hickham MJ, Cote DN: Temporal bone fractures. J La State Med Soc 147:527–530, 1995.
36. Pollanen MS, Deck JH, Blenkinsop B, et al: Fracture of temporal bone with exsanguination: Pathology and mechanism. Can J Neurol Sci 19:196–200, 1992.
37. Griffin WL Jr: A retrospective study of traumatic tympanic membrane perforations in a clinical practice. Laryngoscope 89:261–282, 1979.
38. McKennan KX, Chole RA: Post-traumatic cholesteatoma. Laryngoscope 99:779–782, 1989.
39. Zimmerman WD, Ganzel TM, Windmill IM, et al: Peripheral hearing loss following head trauma in children. Laryngoscope 103:87–91, 1993.
40. Makishima K, Sobel SF, Snow JB Jr: Histopathologic correlates of otoneurological manifestations following head trauma. Laryngoscope 86:1303–1314, 1976.
41. Clark SK, Rees TS: Posttraumatic endolymphatic hydrops. Arch Otolaryngol 103:725–726, 1977.
42. Bellucci RJ: Traumatic injuries of the middle ear. Otolaryngol Clin N Am 16:633–650, 1983.
43. Emmett JR, Shea JJ: Traumatic perilymph fistula. Laryngoscope 90:1513–1520, 1980.

44. Emmett JR, Staab EV, Fischer ND: Perilymph fistulas secondary to gunshot wound: Localization with a radioactive pharmaceutical. Arch Otolaryngol 103:98–102, 1977.

45. Glasscock ME, Hart MJ, Rosdeutscher JD, et al: Traumatic perilymphatic fistula: How long can symptoms persist? A follow-up report. Am J Otol 13:333–338, 1992.

46. Glasscock ME, McKennan KX, Levine SC: Persistent traumatic perilymph fistulas. Laryngoscope 97:860–864, 1987.

47. Goodhill V: Labyrinthine membrane ruptures in sudden sensorineural hearing loss. Proc R Soc Med 69:565–572, 1976.

48. Goodhill V: Sudden deafness and round window rupture. Laryngoscope 81:1462–1474, 1971.

49. Goodhill V, Brockman SJ, Harris I, et al: Sudden deafness and labyrinthine window ruptures: Audio-vestibular observations. Ann Otol Rhinol Laryngol 82:2–12, 1973.

50. Lyos AT, Marsh MA, Jenkins HA, et al: Progressive hearing loss after transverse temporal bone fracture. Arch Otolaryngol Head Neck Surg 121:795–799, 1995.

51. Skedros DG, Cass SP, Hirsch BE, et al: Beta-2 transferrin assay in clinical management of cerebral spinal fluid and perilymphatic fluid leaks. J Otolaryngol 22:341–344, 1993.

52. Adegbite AB, Khan MI, Tan L: Predicting recovery of facial nerve function following injury from a basilar skull fracture [see comments]. J Neurosurg 75:759–762, 1991.

53. Holla SP, Smith RR, Sanford RA: Bilateral traumatic facial paralysis. Neurosurgery 6:290–292, 1980.

54. Chang CY, Cass SP: Management of facial nerve injury due to temporal bone trauma. Am J Otol 20:96–114, 1999.

55. Liu-Shindo M, Hawkins DB: Basilar skull fractures in children. Int J Pediatr Otorhinolaryngol 17:109–117, 1989.

56. Lambert PR, Brackmann DE: Facial paralysis in longitudinal temporal bone fractures: A review of 26 cases. Laryngoscope 94:1022–1026, 1984.

57. McKennan KX, Chole RA: Facial paralysis in temporal bone trauma. Am J Otol 13:167–172, 1992.

58. McGovern FH: Facial nerve injuries in skull fractures: Recent advances in management. Arch Otolaryngol 88:536–542, 1968.

59. Adkins WY, Osguthorpe JD: Management of trauma of the facial nerve. Otolaryngol Clin N Am 24:587–611, 1991.

60. Kartush JM, Lilly DJ, Kemink JL: Facial electroneurography: Clinical and experimental investigations. Otolaryngol Head Neck Surg 93:516–523, 1985.

61. Glasscock ME, Wiet RJ, Jackson CG, et al: Rehabilitation of the face following traumatic injury to the facial nerve. Laryngoscope 89:1389–1404, 1979.

62. Adour KK, Boyajian JA, Kahn ZM, et al: Surgical and nonsurgical management of facial paralysis following closed head injury. Laryngoscope 87:380–390, 1977.

63. May M: Trauma to the facial nerve. Otolaryngol Clin North Am 16:661–669, 1983.

64. Rosenwasser RH, Liebman E, Jimenez DF, et al: Facial reanimation after facial nerve injury. Neurosurgery 29:568–574, 1991.

65. Turner JW: Facial palsy in closed head injuries: The prognosis. Lancet 6:756–757, 1944.

66. Alford BR, Sessions RB, Weber SC: Indications for surgical decompression of the facial nerve. Laryngoscope 81:620–635, 1971.

67. Fisch U: Management of intratemporal facial nerve injuries. J Laryngol Otol 94:129–134, 1980.

68. Coker NJ: Management of traumatic injuries to the facial nerve. Otolaryngol Clin N Am 24:215–227, 1991.

CHAPTER **335**

Rehabilitation and Prognosis after Traumatic Brain Injury

PAUL T. DIAMOND ■ KIMBERLY J. STEWART

HISTORY

The practice of traumatic brain injury (TBI) rehabilitation began toward the end of World War I. Before this, head trauma often resulted in death. However, with significant advances in neurosurgical techniques under the leadership of Harvey Cushing, survival among U.S. soldiers sustaining brain injuries during combat increased to about 65%.[1] This large number of head injury survivors prompted significant expansion in military hospital–based rehabilitation programs.[2] Whereas only 16 U.S. military hospitals offered general rehabilitation services in 1918, this number had increased to 46 facilities within 1 year. With the end of the war, most of these programs were discontinued.[2] However, interest in the clinical practice of rehabilitation persisted, and in the 1920s, medical organizations such as the American Medical Association Council on Physical Therapy and the American Society of Physical Therapy Physicians were formed. In 1926, Dr. John Stanley Coulter initiated the first continuing education program in physical medicine at Northwestern University Medical School. Dr. Frank Krusen, who coined the term *physiatrist*, formed the first residency training program in physical medicine at the Mayo Clinic in 1936.[3]

With the advent of World War II, the United States, along with countries such as Great Britain and the Soviet Union, developed specialized hospital-based brain injury rehabilitation programs.[2] These units adopted a broad, multidisciplinary approach geared toward the complex, multiple needs of brain-injured patients and included physical therapy, speech therapy, psychotherapy, and vocational retraining. Again, after the war, many of these specialty units closed.[2] However, the importance of rehabilitative care after injury continued to be recognized. Dr. Howard A. Rusk, an internist who had worked at the Army Air Corps Convalescent and Rehabilitation Services at Jefferson Barracks during World War II, is credited with demonstra-

ting the superiority of aggressive rehabilitation of soldiers compared with the more common strategy of passive convalescence. His work was reportedly so impressive that it led to the expansion of general rehabilitation programs to all Army Air Corps hospitals. Rusk went on to establish the Institute of Rehabilitation Medicine at the New York University Medical Center and is now recognized as the "father" of rehabilitation medicine. In 1947, the current specialty of physical medicine and rehabilitation was formally established.[3]

It was not until the early 1970s that specialty programs geared toward the rehabilitation of brain trauma victims began to be reestablished.[2] This renewed focus on TBI rehabilitation has been attributed to the growing number of head injuries caused by motor vehicle accidents.[2] One of the first units established was at the Rancho Los Amigos Hospital near Los Angeles. The cognitive rehabilitation protocols developed at Rancho Los Amigos are the basis of many programs today.[2] In the late 1970s, day and residential treatment programs for persons with TBI became available. In 1977, the first residential program for postacute TBI opened at the Center for Comprehensive Services in Carbondale, Illinois. A year later, one of several day treatment programs for postacute TBI was developed by Ben-Yishay at New York University.[2]

Today, TBI remains a significant cause of adult disability, directly impacting the lives of millions of Americans, their family members, and their communities. Of all injuries, TBI is the most likely to result in permanent disability or death.[4] It affects all age groups but is the leading cause of long-term disability and death among young adults and children.[5] Of the estimated 1.5 million to 2 million persons who incur TBIs annually, the majority are seen and treated in the nation's emergency departments and then released.[5] An estimated 300,000 persons are hospitalized annually, and 70,000 to 90,000 sustain long-term disabilities.[5] Somewhere between 2.5 million and 6.5 million Americans are currently living with disabilities resulting from TBI.[5] The economic cost is thought to approach $40 billion annually; the health and psychosocial impact on the injured and their caregivers is devastating.[4]

ASSESSMENT OF PATIENTS WITH TRAUMATIC BRAIN INJURY

TBI may result in an array of impairments, disabilities, and handicaps. The World Health Organization has defined impairment as "any loss or abnormality of psychological, physiological, or anatomical structure or function."[6] Examples include a hemiparetic arm, a spastic lower extremity, or a visual field cut. Disability is "any restriction or lack of ability to perform an activity within the range considered normal for a human being."[6] Examples of impairments include inability to dress oneself, walk, type at a keyboard, or operate a motor vehicle. Handicap is "a disadvantage for a given individual, resulting from an impairment or a disability that limits or prevents the fulfillment of a role that is normal for that individual."[6] Unlike impairment or disability, a handicap is imposed by society. For example, if an individual's place of employment is not wheelchair accessible, an employee who cannot ambulate has a handicap that impedes his or her ability to return to work.

A comprehensive rehabilitation program starts with a detailed assessment to define all impairments, disabilities, and handicaps that have resulted from the brain injury. A full psychosocial and employment history, along with a detailed neurological examination, neurocognitive assessment, and functional evaluation, enables the rehabilitation team to develop a treatment plan and define the therapeutic goals. Numerous functional and neurocognitive assessment tools have been developed to measure motor and cognitive functioning and monitor response to rehabilitation.

Functional Assessment

Several functional assessment measures are commonly used in clinical practice to describe functional status, monitor response to therapies, and assess long-term outcome.

The Glasgow Outcome Scale (GOS) has been used for almost 30 years and has been the most commonly used tool in TBI outcome research.[7] The five GOS groups are broadly defined (Table 335–1), however, and because of this, the GOS is not suitable to document the response to a given rehabilitation intervention or to closely monitor recovery.

The Barthel Index (BI) was developed in the mid-1960s to score and track improvement in functional status in patients receiving rehabilitation.[8] The BI is a 100-point scale with 10 categories in which the examiner rates the patient's ability to perform various self-care activities, ambulate, ascend and descend stairs, and maintain bowel and bladder continence. The BI is commonly used as a functional assessment measure in clinical trials in conjunction with neurological outcome

T A B L E 3 3 5 – 1 ■ **Glasgow Outcome Scale**

OUTCOME	DESCRIPTION
Good recovery	Resumption of normal daily activities independently
Moderate disability	Impairments or disabilities persist, but with adaptive or assistive equipment, worksite modifications, or other compensatory strategies; the individual remains functionally independent
Severe disability	Impairments or disabilities persist, and assistance of others is required to perform daily activities
Persistent vegetative state	Unresponsive with sleep-wake cycles
Death	Patient does not survive

From Jennett B, Bond MR: Assessment of outcome in severe brain damage: A practical scale. Lancet 1:480–484, 1975.

measures to document therapeutic response. However, a significant limitation of the BI is that it does not measure cognitive-linguistic or psychosocial functioning. Therefore, although the BI is well suited for orthopedic or deconditioned patients, it is less effective in assessing and monitoring recovery in individuals with TBI and associated neurocognitive or behavioral deficits.

The Functional Independence Measure (FIM) was developed in 1987 to measure functional status and monitor recovery during rehabilitation.[9] Its six main categories are self-care, mobility, communication, sphincter control, locomotion, and social cognition; within these categories are 18 separate items that are scored on a scale from 1 (total assistance) to 7 (complete independence) (Table 335–2). In addition to a total score, motor and cognitive subscores can be calculated. The FIM has been shown to have high interrater reliability[10] and is now the most widely used functional assessment tool in rehabilitation medicine.[11] The FIM is typically administered on admission to acute inpatient rehabilitation programs and again on discharge. It can also be used to monitor weekly progress.

The Disability Rating Scale (DRS) was designed specifically for head trauma patients as a tool to monitor disability from coma through community reentry.[12] The DRS takes only a few minutes to complete and, unlike the FIM, is simple to administer. Patients are scored on eye opening, verbalization, motor response, cognitive ability to perform self-care tasks, overall functional dependence on others, and employability. A total score (ranging from 0 [no disability] to 30 [death]) is calculated and reflects the level of disability. The DRS is particularly useful during the postacute phase of TBI recovery, when progress is measured less frequently than during acute inpatient rehabilitation. For example, it may be administered monthly during day treatment or prevocational training to assess recovery and level of functioning.

The Rancho Los Amigos Levels of Cognitive Functioning Scale (RLAS)[13] is commonly used as a qualitative and descriptive tool for TBI patients (Table 335–3).

T A B L E   3 3 5 – 2 ■ **Functional Independence Measure: Subscales and Domains**

MOTOR DOMAINS				COGNITIVE DOMAINS	
Self-Care	**Sphincter Control**	**Transfers**	**Locomotion**	**Communication**	**Social Cognition**
Eating Bathing Dress upper Dress lower Toileting	Bladder Bowel	Bed Toilet Tub	Walking Stairs	Comprehension Expression	Social interaction Problem solving Memory

From Hanger CV, Hamilton BB: Uniform Data Set for Medical Rehabilitation. Buffalo, Research Foundation, State University of New York, 1987.

Ratings are subjective and have not been shown to have prognostic significance. Also, patients may progress from level to level, may have characteristics of more than one level at a given time, or may skip levels altogether. As such, the RLAS is generally not viewed as a functional assessment measure. It can be used to convey a broad description of the patient at a given point in his or her recovery or to assign patients to selected rehabilitation protocols. For example, TBI patients at levels I through III are considered to be in coma and may qualify for enrollment in a coma stimulation protocol. However, most acute inpatient rehabilitation units limit TBI admissions to patients at levels IV and above.

Another assessment tool, popular for both its ease of administration and its prognostic significance, is the Galveston Orientation and Amnesia Test (GOAT).[14] The GOAT is a brief, structured interview that assesses both orientation and recall of events and helps identify when the patient is no longer suffering from post-traumatic amnesia (PTA). A score of 75 or more (out of 100 total points) for more than 2 consecutive days signifies that the patient no longer has PTA and can recall day-to-day events. As is discussed later, length of PTA has been shown to correlate with long-term outcome.

Neurocognitive Assessment

Neuropsychological testing helps develop an accurate picture of the person's level of cognitive, emotional,

T A B L E   3 3 5 – 3 ■ **Rancho Los Amigos Levels of Cognitive Functioning Scale**

LEVEL	DESCRIPTION
I	No response
II	Generalized response
III	Localized response
IV	Confused/agitated
V	Confused/inappropriate
VI	Confused/appropriate
VII	Automatic/appropriate
VIII	Purposeful/appropriate

From Hagen C, Malkmus D, Durham P: Levels of cognitive functions. In Rehabilitation of Head-Injured Adult: Comprehensive Physical Management. Dowrey, CA, Professional Staff Association, Rancho for Los Amigos Hospital, 1979.

and interpersonal functioning, including areas of spared ability or compensatory strength. Test results can be used to estimate an individual's ability to perform functional activities and can also help determine the most effective means of increasing learning based on the areas of spared cognitive functioning. Neuropsychological test results are often an integral part of the initial TBI rehabilitation assessment. They are also a useful tool for monitoring progress throughout the rehabilitation and recovery process.

Neuropsychological testing uses standardized test instruments with established reliability (ability to consistently obtain the same results) and validity (extent to which the test measures what it purports to measure) based on a normative sample. Interpretation of results includes adjustments for age, educational level, linguistic and cultural backgrounds, and current cognitive status. Component cognitive processes include attention, memory, new learning, executive functioning, visual-spatial skills, language, behavior, and emotional adjustment. Testing of these cognitive domains includes assessment of subdomains within each area. For example, attention includes several distinct processes that can be assessed individually and that affect one's ability to perform a given functional task successfully. The different levels of attention include focused, sustained, divided, selective, and alternating. Memory evaluation should include assessment of verbal, visual-spatial, recognition, and short-term and long-term components. Executive functioning includes inhibitory and interference control, problem solving and planning, fluency, mental flexibility, and self-awareness. It is important to have caregivers provide corroborating data to compare with the patient's self-report, owing to the lack of deficit awareness in this population. Commonly used neuropsychological tests in TBI are summarized in Table 335–4.

Results of neuropsychological testing are often used to draw conclusions about an individual's ability to function safely and independently in the community and perform certain complex functional tasks such as driving. However, numerous investigators have questioned the validity of assuming that performance on written neuropsychological tests translates to performance in real-life settings.[33, 34] This is known as the *ecological validity* of a given test. Thus, decisions regarding when an individual is capable of resuming high-risk activities after TBI, such as driving or operating

TABLE 335–4 ■ **Common Neuropsychological Assessment Tools for Traumatic Brain Injury**

Attention
Wechsler Adult Intelligence Scale III: Digit Span, Digit-Symbol Coding, Symbol Search, Arithmetic, Letter-Number Sequencing[15]
Trail Making Test[16,17]
Conners' Continuous Performance Test[18]
Paced Auditory Serial Addition Test[19]

Memory/Learning
Wechsler Memory Scale III[20]
California Verbal Learning Test II[21]
Rey Complex Figure—Recall and Recognition[22]
Benton Visual Retention Test—Revised[23]
Tactual Performance Test—Memory and Localization[24]
Recognition Memory Test[25]
Rivermead Behavioral Memory Test[26]

Executive Functions
Stroop Color and Word Test[27,28]
Wisconsin Card Sorting Test[29]
Rey Complex Figure—Copy[22]
Controlled Oral Word Association Test[30]
Category Test[17,24]

Behavior
Neurobehavioral Rating Scale[31]
Neurobehavioral Functioning Inventory[32]

heavy machinery, are generally based on a combination of neuropsychological test performance, history taking and examination, and observational assessments by a driving trainer or job coach.

Assessment of Prognosis

After severe TBI, it is important to draw a distinction between prognosis and outcome prediction. Prognosis is used by the rehabilitation specialist to set realistic goals for the rehabilitation program and to begin to educate family caregivers about appropriate expectations for recovery and long-term needs. However, too many independent variables affect outcome in TBI to allow a definitive prediction of the extent of recovery in any given patient. Generally, when the rehabilitation specialist assesses functional prognosis in a TBI patient, he or she considers (1) baseline characteristics unique to the individual (e.g., age, premorbid function, presence of caregiver support), (2) initial injury severity or pattern and time course of recovery (e.g., initial Glasgow Coma Scale score, length of coma, duration of PTA), and (3) neurological and functional findings on clinical evaluation.

INDIVIDUAL BASELINE CHARACTERISTICS

Premorbid function is extremely important when establishing rehabilitation goals and prognosis after TBI.[35] For example, if an individual with a previous neurological injury and functional impairment at baseline sustains a new TBI, the therapeutic goal of a comprehensive rehabilitation program is at best to return the individual to his or her baseline level of function. Psychosocial background and presence of a supportive family are also considered strong factors in recovery.[36] Substance abuse has been associated with a worse outcome.[35, 37] A recent study using quantitative magnetic resonance imaging (MRI) demonstrated that, after controlling for injury severity, greater brain atrophy developed in TBI survivors with a history of substance abuse compared with TBI survivors who were not substance abusers.[38]

Older age is associated with lower rates of survival following TBI.[39–44] Functional prognosis is also considered worse in older individuals with TBI. For example, an early study of older adults found that less than 5% with severe brain injury achieved good recovery.[39] More recently, Katz and Alexander found prolonged PTA and worse functional outcome following severe TBI in persons older than 40 years.[45] Zafonte's group observed that age in combination with PTA contributed to a regression model predicting discharge FIM and DRS scores following acute inpatient rehabilitation.[46] In this model, prolonged PTA and advanced age correlated with a worse outcome. Another study, based on data from the National Institute on Disability and Rehabilitation Research TBI Model Systems Program, compared the outcomes of patients older than 55 years with those of patients 18 to 50 years of age. The older group required longer stays in acute inpatient rehabilitation and incurred higher total rehabilitation charges.[47] However, although discharge DRS scores and RLAS levels were lower in the older group, no significant differences were observed between groups in final discharge FIM or discharge disposition. Other studies have also demonstrated the ability of older adults to make significant functional gains and recovery following severe TBI.[48, 49] Although younger age is associated with better prognosis after TBI, it has been suggested that children younger than 6 years may have worse motor and cognitive outcomes.[50]

Gender may also be related to outcome following TBI. Both the prevalence of TBI and the subsequent mortality rates are greater in males than in females.[51–60] Groswasser and colleagues found better functional outcomes in female TBI patients receiving acute inpatient rehabilitation and suggested that progesterone may exert a neuroprotective effect.[61] Findings in an animal model study by Roof and Hall suggested that estrogen may play a role in maintaining adequate cerebral perfusion acutely following TBI.[62] Igarashi's group found gender-specific patterns of neuronal protection in a TBI mouse model.[63] In contrast, a recent meta-analysis of gender differences in TBI found that outcome was worse for females than for males in 85% of the measured variables; however, this report was limited by the small number of TBI outcome studies addressing gender differences.[63a] Additional studies of gender differences in TBI outcome are warranted.

MEASURES OF INJURY SEVERITY

Most patients who require acute inpatient rehabilitation following TBI have had severe injuries, defined as initial Glasgow Coma Scale scores of 3 to 8, although some with moderate injuries (scores of 9 to 12) may also be admitted. Among patients who sustain severe TBIs and remain in comas longer than 6 hours, 50% to 60% survive.[64–66] In initial survivors, it is believed that the majority of neurological recovery occurs within the first 6 months of the injury.[67] Motor recovery typically plateaus earliest, whereas certain neurocognitive domains may demonstrate recovery for up to a year or longer. In their oft-cited work, Jennett and Teasdale demonstrated that by 12-month follow-up, 50% of severe TBI survivors had attained good recovery, 31% had moderate disability, 16% had severe disability, and 3% were in a vegetative state.[68]

Patients in comas or persistent vegetative states for prolonged periods have been shown to have worse outcomes.[69–73] For example, among comatose patients at 2 weeks after injury, Bricolo and colleagues found that 13% had achieved good recovery at 1-year follow-up, 18% had moderate disability, 31% had severe disability, 8% were in a persistent vegetative state, and 30% had died.[69] A study by Braakman and coworkers observed that among patients who remained in a persistent vegetative state at 1 month after injury, 10% achieved some level of independence by 1 year, 26% were severely disabled, 11% remained in a persistent vegetative state, and 51% had died.[71] Groswasser and Sazbon looked specifically at the outcomes of patients who regained consciousness after more than 1 month.[74] Of 134 patients with severe TBI and prolonged coma, 54% regained consciousness. Among these individuals, almost half were independent in terms of self-care at long-term follow-up, and 11% had returned to competitive employment.

The duration of PTA has also been shown to correlate with prognosis for functional recovery.[45, 46, 75] Katz and Alexander found that in patients admitted for acute inpatient rehabilitation following TBI, 80% achieved good recovery at 12-month follow-up if the duration of PTA did not exceed 2 weeks.[45] When PTA ranged from 2 to 4 weeks, 60% achieved good recovery and 40% had moderate disability. When PTA exceeded 12 weeks, no patients achieved good recovery, 73% had moderate disability, and 27% had severe disability. In patients who experienced PTA beyond 24 weeks, only 12% achieved moderate disability, and the remaining 88% had severe disability. Zafonte and coworkers found that duration of PTA was correlated with other more detailed measures of functional outcome, including total FIM and DRS scores at the time of discharge from the acute inpatient rehabilitation service.[46]

CLINICAL AND LABORATORY EVALUATION

Fundamental to the assessment of prognosis following severe TBI is a functional evaluation of the patient. Ability to actively participate in therapies and achieve early functional gains is probably the most valued indicator of a favorable prognosis among rehabilitation specialists. It is one of the fundamental criteria used in determining whether a patient is a candidate for admission to an acute inpatient rehabilitation program.

Numerous investigators have studied the relationship between certain clinical findings and outcome following TBI. Pupillary response has been identified as an important indicator of prognosis following TBI.[64, 76–80] In one study of patients with abnormal pupillary responses following TBI, only 12% achieved good recovery at 12-month follow-up.[78] Another study found a mortality rate of 87% in TBI patients with nonreactive pupils.[79] In contrast, 50% of patients with intact pupillary responses achieved good recovery or moderate disability.[80] Impaired oculocephalic reflex has also been shown to correlate with a poor outcome.[64, 76]

Although not often obtained, evoked potentials have been shown to correlate with both time course of recovery[81] and TBI outcome.[36, 81–84] In contrast, findings on computed tomographic scans, taken alone, have not been particularly useful in predicting functional outcome following TBI.[36]

A number of studies have found correlations between late findings on MRI and clinical outcome, but there is limited support for the use of early standard MRI techniques to predict outcome.[85–89] In patients with brainstem TBI, Shibata and coworkers demonstrated that early abnormalities on T1-weighted and T2-weighted images in the deep dorsal brainstem were associated with a worse outcome than were lesions in the ventral or superficial dorsal brainstem.[87] Another study using a regression model found that frontal lesions detected on early MRI (1 to 3 months after injury), along with frontotemporal atrophy on late MRI (6 to 12 months after injury) and PTA, were predictive of a poor outcome.[89] A study using gradient-echo MRI to detect small regions of hemorrhage found that abnormalities at 3 months after TBI were correlated with outcome at 1 year.[90]

Recent MRI advances, such as diffusion- and perfusion-weighted imaging techniques and functional MRI, may lead to an increased role for neuroimaging in TBI outcome assessment in the future.[91] A study using diffusion-weighted MRI within a few days of severe TBI identified lesions not visualized on T2-weighted MRI.[92] Another study using perfusion-weighted MRI found that TBI patients with areas of decreased cerebral blood volume in otherwise normal-appearing areas of the brain had poorer clinical outcomes than did patients without similar abnormalities.[88] A preliminary functional MRI study in patients with TBI found differences in activation patterns in the prefrontal and parietal areas between patients with good performance of a planning task and those with poor performance.[93] There is significant interest in pursuing further research on the use of functional MRI to establish prognosis as well as to guide rehabilitation interventions following TBI.

THE REHABILITATION CONTINUUM

Thirty years ago, Walker summarized the findings of an international symposium on TBI rehabilitation held in Goteborg, Sweden, in which attendees discussed strategies to optimize the rehabilitation of individuals with TBI.[94] The importance of early intervention, comprehensive or total rehabilitation of the individual, family involvement, social adjustment within the home and community, and vocational retraining were all emphasized. The rehabilitative principles they discussed in 1972 continue to form the foundation of TBI rehabilitation today. When discussing rehabilitation, it is helpful to think of it as multifaceted. The central components include (1) prevention of the sequelae of disuse (e.g., contracture, deconditioning), (2) restoration of function (e.g., neuromuscular re-education), (3) accommodation (e.g., adaptive and assistive equipment prescription), (4) diagnosis and management of associated complications (e.g., heterotopic ossification), and (5) education.

TBI rehabilitation occurs in two basic models: the medical model and the postacute or community-based model. The full continuum of TBI rehabilitation services refers to the availability of both acute and subacute TBI rehabilitation services (medical model), as well as an array of postacute TBI programs. Early intervention occurs while the patient is still in intensive care and is focused on preventing the complications of immobility, such as deconditioning, contracture, and skin breakdown. Patients are mobilized, positioned appropriately in bed, and splinted as appropriate. Mobilization, therapeutic exercise, and early self-care retraining continue on the acute neurosurgical ward. When clinically stable, the TBI patient is discharged to an appropriate level of continued rehabilitation care, depending on his or her functional and neurocognitive deficits and overall rehabilitation needs.

Medical Model

ACUTE INPATIENT REHABILITATION

Acute inpatient rehabilitation for severe TBI typically occurs on a Medicare-designated rehabilitation unit that is either based in the acute care facility or exists in a freestanding rehabilitation hospital. Care is provided by a multidisciplinary team that generally includes a physician with expertise in rehabilitation medicine, physical therapist, occupational therapist, speech language pathologist, psychologist, rehabilitation nurse, case manager, recreational therapist, and nutritionist. Patients are evaluated by all disciplines on admission, and a treatment plan and therapeutic goals are established. The team then meets on a weekly basis to review progress toward goals, establish new goals, and determine length of stay. During the acute phase of recovery, care focuses on mobility, basic self-care skills, and orientation. The physical therapist focuses on therapeutic exercise, bed mobility, transfers, wheelchair management and propulsion, and gait training. The occupational therapist provides self-care retraining, functional upper extremity kinetic activities, and cognitive-perceptual assessment and retraining. The speech language pathologist does a cognitive and linguistic evaluation, evaluates swallowing function, and provides speech treatment, dysphagia therapy, and cognitive rehabilitation. The psychologist, who may have a background in either rehabilitation psychology

or neuropsychology, performs cognitive and behavioral assessments, provides supportive therapy for both the patient and family caregivers, and helps design effective strategies for implementing therapeutic plans. The recreational therapist focuses on leisure skills activities and, in conjunction with the occupational therapist, often supervises community outings. The rehabilitation treatment plan needs to consider the patient's RLAS level, neurocognitive strengths and weaknesses, and behavioral responses. During the early stages of recovery, when the patient is confused, agitated, and disoriented, rehabilitation may be more appropriately provided in a quiet, one-on-one therapeutic setting. Little can be done at this stage to retrain cognitive functioning. Rather, highly structured activities, limited stimulation, and close physician and nursing supervision are indicated. As arousal, alertness, and self-awareness increase, more structured cognitive therapies can be implemented.[95]

Caregivers are actively involved in the rehabilitation process, receive education on TBI and the needs of the injured family member, and receive training before the patient is discharged. Usually, an overnight activities-of-daily-living suite is available, and the primary caregiver spends a night in the rehabilitation unit caring for the patient before his or her discharge to ensure that appropriate care will continue after the patient returns home. A home safety evaluation can also be performed by the physical or occupational therapist before discharge so that recommendations regarding home adjustments or modifications to increase patient safety and function can be made.

Medicare requires that an acute rehabilitation unit be architecturally distinct. Rehabilitation services must be provided a minimum of 3 hours per day, 5 days per week, by a multidisciplinary team through a coordinated plan of care.[96] Medicare also sets guidelines for admission to and continued stay within the unit. In general, an appropriate candidate for admission requires 24-hour nursing care and close physician supervision, has the ability to actively participate and progress at a reasonable rate in the rehabilitation program, and has realistic therapeutic goals representing significant practical improvement that could not be readily achieved in a less intensive rehabilitation setting. If a patient's functional progress significantly slows or plateaus, the therapeutic goals have been met or can be met in a less intensive rehabilitation setting, or the patient is no longer capable of participating in the acute rehabilitation program, the patient is discharged either home or to a more appropriate level of care. Length of stay in the acute rehabilitation unit following TBI typically does not exceed 3 to 4 weeks. In general, most third-party payers have adopted guidelines similar to Medicare's but require precertification before admission for acute inpatient rehabilitation, as well as weekly recertification reviews. In our experience, third-party payers typically deny acute inpatient rehabilitation for TBI patients with neurocognitive deficits alone (i.e., in the absence of impaired mobility or self-care skills).

The Balanced Budget Act of 1997 mandated that

reimbursement for acute inpatient rehabilitation care be transitioned to a prospective payment system. Reimbursement now falls under Medicare's prospective payment system, replacing the previous diagnosis-related group–exempt, reasonable cost–based system under which rehabilitation units and hospitals had previously been paid.[97] Under this system, diagnostic groups fall under specific rehabilitation impairment categories (RICs), one of which is TBI. Within the TBI RIC, patients are further classified by FIM–functional-related guidelines (FIM-FRGs) based on admission motor and cognitive FIM scores. The FIM-FRGs were specifically developed to characterize severity of impairment for use in a prospective payment system for inpatient rehabilitation.[98] Reimbursement is determined by the patient's assigned RIC and FIM-FRG and is adjusted for specific hospital variables such as overall payer mix, region, and patient acuity levels. The prospective payment system for acute inpatient rehabilitation necessitates early assessment of TBI patients to ensure assignment to the correct FIM-FRG. The intended goal is to provide appropriate reimbursement based on level of impairment and rehabilitation needs while encouraging the cost-effective use of resources. The long-term financial impact on providers of acute inpatient rehabilitation services and on quality of care has not been determined.

SUBACUTE INPATIENT REHABILITATION

Subacute rehabilitation for TBI has been defined as nursing and rehabilitation care for patients who are unable to participate in a more intensive rehabilitation setting.[99] Generally, these services are provided at a skilled level of care within a nursing facility. TBI patients with severe impairments that limit their capacity to respond and make measurable progress on an acute inpatient rehabilitation service may be referred for interim skilled care. Length of stay in a subacute unit is typically measured in months rather than weeks. As recovery from TBI occurs, patients may demonstrate increased participation in therapies and more rapid functional gains. At this stage, patients may be reconsidered for a more intensive acute inpatient rehabilitation program geared toward preparing the patient to return home and reenter the community.

Postacute, Community-Based Model

Malec and Basford provide a detailed description of postacute brain injury rehabilitation services and outcomes.[99] Unlike the medical model of rehabilitation, which focuses on maintenance of medical stability, physical rehabilitation, and early neurocognitive and behavioral treatments, postacute rehabilitation emphasizes cognitive and behavioral therapies and community reintegration. Close medical follow-up and routine care of the patient are generally turned over to the primary care physician. Community-based residential programs, also known as transitional rehabilitation services, provide a structured, homelike environment for the treatment of patients with significant neurocogni-

tive or behavioral impairments. Care is typically holistic and includes cognitive and behavioral therapies, prevocational and vocational training, sheltered workshops, leisure skills retraining, and therapeutic community outings.

For patients who can be safely cared for in the home environment by designated caregivers, comprehensive neurological day treatment programs have been designed to essentially replicate the intensity of an acute inpatient rehabilitation program but allow the patient to return home in the evenings. These postacute services provide physical, occupational, speech, and recreational therapies with a team-directed approach, but unlike acute inpatient rehabilitation, they typically focus on independent living skills and community reentry.

Many TBI programs also offer adaptive driving assessments and retraining, vocational evaluation and training, and return-to-work programs with on-site job coaches. Other services include individual outpatient therapies and home care services. In general, if a patient is not homebound, he or she is encouraged to participate in outpatient therapies because of the availability of a fully equipped therapeutic gym and a more regular, intensive therapy program. Not infrequently, patients are initially prescribed home care therapies in conjunction with a home safety evaluation, followed by a transition to outpatient therapies when appropriate. The availability of postacute rehabilitation services and community-based programs varies considerably by community.

SPECIAL CONSIDERATIONS IN TRAUMATIC BRAIN INJURY REHABILITATION

Cognitive Rehabilitation

Impairment of cognitive function is a common cause of disability following TBI.[100] Cognitive rehabilitation (CR) can be viewed as an assortment of procedures that fit into four categories: restorative, compensatory, environmental, and behavioral.[101] Restorative techniques purport to restore component cognitive processes that underlie specific problems (e.g., attention). Compensatory techniques teach patients to work around the disability to increase their everyday functioning using new skills and aids such as a memory notebook. Environmental changes help shape the surroundings to maximize the person's performance. Behavioral approaches use reinforcement and feedback to maximize the speed, extent, and level of learning or adaptation.

A National Institutes of Health consensus conference on TBI rehabilitation observed that despite the existence of numerous CR strategies, programs, and interventions, limited data exist to support their effectiveness.[102] However, the Brain Injury Interdisciplinary Special Interest Group of the American Congress of Rehabilitation Medicine recently authored a comprehensive report on CR that provided evidence-based recommendations for the use of CR in clinical practice.[100] This group concluded that support exists for the use of several forms of CR for persons with TBI, directed toward remediation of attention, memory, functional communication, and executive functioning. Techniques such as vanishing cues, errorless learning, and immediate feedback have been advocated for use in CR.[103, 104]

Owing to the heterogeneous nature of TBI, no single set of strategies will work with every person; therefore, program development and treatment planning must be individually tailored to each patient's needs.[105] Sohlberg and Mateer recommended an integrative neuropsychological approach that considers the individual's cognitive, emotional, and behavioral needs while employing a variety of therapeutic strategies.[106] For treatment to be effective, rehabilitation staff members need to be well trained in the neurocognitive and neurobehavioral sequelae of brain injury so they do not mistakenly attribute cognitive deficits to volitional behaviors.[105] Forming a therapeutic alliance among the patient, team, and family is essential for successful treatment.[105]

One of the leading CR models is the REAL (Rehabilitation for Everyday Adaptive Living) approach, which is a patient-centered community reentry program.[101] The tenets of the REAL program include the following: (1) focus on the disability or handicap, (2) identify and train adaptive behaviors using the patient's strengths, (3) involve the patient and family, (4) assess and use the most effective learning style of the patient, (5) use a team approach, and (6) evaluate the impact of the intervention. This program is noted for its focus on functional tasks, which are more applicable to everyday life (versus exercises in the gym), and for its generalization to real-world settings.

Certain strategies employed in TBI CR take advantage of preserved cognitive domains to improve functional skills. For example, despite profound impairments in declarative or fact-based memory, procedural memory may be relatively preserved following severe brain trauma.[107, 108] Proponents of using computer-based virtual reality in CR suggest that this approach takes advantage of preserved procedural learning skills to retrain functional skills.[109] Several investigators have begun to examine the use of virtual reality technology for both neurocognitive assessment and cognitive retraining following TBI.[105, 109–113] Factors that may limit the clinical benefit of CR include lack of generalization to nontreatment settings and poor maintenance of gains across time.[101] It has been suggested that virtual reality–based CR may be an effective strategy for improving the generalization and transfer of functional skills to the real world.[109]

Behavior Management

Neurobehavioral problems such as impulsivity, reduced frustration tolerance, verbally threatening or physically aggressive behavior, disinhibition, inappropriate social behavior, attention seeking, manipulative behavior, changes in emotional expression, decreased initiation, and decreased insight are common following TBI.[101]

Behavior management is the investigation and control of factors that affect behavior, which include the brain injury, the person, and the environment. The premise is to use observable, verifiable, and reproducible methods to decrease undesirable behaviors and increase adaptive behaviors.[114] Behavior management plans also help track functional change, program accountability, and treatment outcome.

Behavioral approaches incorporate teaching new skills and manipulating the environment to help TBI patients maximize their adaptive functioning. However, there is no single set of principles that works with all patients. Each program needs to be tailored to the individual and his or her unique needs, including physiologic, cognitive, environmental, medical, social, financial, and family issues. The challenge for the treatment team is to help these individuals learn new behaviors despite their somatic, cognitive, and neurobehavioral difficulties. Consistency is the key to a successful behavioral management plan.[114] This is also the greatest obstacle in most treatment settings. Every member of the treatment team needs to adhere to the behavior plan if it is to become successful. Therefore, training the staff in the guidelines for proper implementation and monitoring is imperative. Ethically, the programs should focus on client benefit versus program convenience. Each program must consider the rights and dignity of patients when developing treatment strategies.[105]

Behavior management uses several techniques to teach new skills and shape behavior. Most behavioral programs begin by using the "A-B-C" method of identifying the "antecedents" and "consequences" that surround the maladaptive "behavior" manifested by the patient.[114] Antecedents, or stimuli, include external and internal factors that precipitate the maladaptive behavior (e.g., too much stimulation, time of day, an irritating person, pain, fatigue). Consequences include either positive or negative events that occur after the behavior is demonstrated (e.g., avoidance of treatment, attention). The A-B-C model involves having staff document all antecedents and consequences that occur surrounding the identified behavior in order to develop hypotheses regarding why this behavior is occurring, under what circumstances, and how it benefits the patient. After these theories are narrowed down to one hypothesis (e.g., the patient becomes aggressive to avoid physical therapy), specific behavioral principles can be applied to decrease the maladaptive behavior and replace it with a more adaptive and positive response.[114]

Owing to short-term memory impairment and the tendency for concrete thinking processes in TBI patients, the consequences of behavioral programs must be meaningful, immediate, and obvious.[105] When the goal is to increase a behavior, positive reinforcement is often the most effective method, or consequence. Social reinforcement such as praise is often the most powerful form of positive reinforcement. Material reinforcement such as money or food is useful in promoting positive behavior and is often used in setting up a "token economy." In terms of decreasing an undesirable behavior, "time out" is useful for attention seeking and aggression.[101]

Family involvement is essential to the effectiveness of any behavioral program.[101, 105] Having the family understand how the injury has changed the person both biologically and psychosocially is crucial to promote recovery. Family involvement also promotes generalization and maintenance of positive behaviors and emotional adjustment. This is often the most difficult part of this process and is why many behaviors reemerge after traditional therapy is discontinued.

Mild Traumatic Brain Injury

The majority of TBIs are classified as mild, which is generally defined as loss of consciousness not exceeding 20 minutes, a Glasgow Coma Scale score of 13 to 15, less than 48 hours of hospitalization, and negative radiologic findings.[115] It is now recognized that despite the use of the term *mild* to characterize this type of head injury, it may be associated with a constellation of neurocognitive, somatic, and psychiatric symptoms known as *postconcussion syndrome*.[57] Common symptoms include memory impairment (50% to 60% of cases), poor attention or concentration (40%), headache (55% to 75%), decreased energy (65%), dizziness (40%), insomnia (40%), depression or irritability (65%), and anxiety (55%).[116] Many individuals with mild TBI are symptom free within 1 month, and most have returned to baseline within 3 to 12 months. However, for some, a prolonged period of disability may ensue.[117] A study by Rimel's group revealed an unemployment rate of 34% at 3 months following mild head injury among those employed premorbidly. Executives and professionals had the highest return-to-work rates (83% to 100%), compared with about 60% among skilled and unskilled laborers.[57]

Key to the management of persons who sustain mild TBI are education and reassurance of both the patient and the caregiver about the kinds of symptoms and impairments to look for in postconcussion syndrome.[115, 117] Close follow-up, along with a detailed clinical history, is important to identify symptom onset and overall impact on the individual's ability to function at home, at work, and in the community. Sometimes, subtle neurocognitive or behavioral changes associated with mild head injury may prove quite devastating, disrupting relationships or compromising job performance. Once these issues have been identified, further assessment, such as neuropsychological testing, may be indicated. A rehabilitation program including cognitive remediation, training in compensatory strategies, and supportive psychotherapy can then be prescribed.[115] Often, when job performance is affected, the rehabilitation professional obtains a detailed job description and makes specific recommendations about temporary modifications to work assignments or the job site to maximize job performance.

Postacute Complications

Numerous complications can occur during the rehabilitation and recovery phase following severe TBI. Medical management and rehabilitation intervention for these complications are a primary function of TBI rehabilitation. Some examples of common post-TBI complications and a brief overview of management options are presented here.

SPASTICITY

Spasticity can be managed through a variety of physical modalities, medications, and procedures. Treatment is indicated when it interferes with function, is associated with pain, interferes with hygiene or local skin care, or could result in significant contracture.[118] Commonly used modalities to treat spasticity include range-of-motion and stretching exercises, heat and cold, serial casting, and electrical stimulation. Oral medication options include centrally acting agents such as baclofen, tizanidine, diazepam, and clonidine, as well as dantrolene sodium, an agent that acts peripherally at the muscle.[119–121] Intrathecal baclofen has also been used successfully to treat spasticity following TBI.[122] Other treatment options include motor point or nerve blocks, botulinum toxin injection, dorsal rhizotomy, and orthopedic surgical procedures such as muscle transfers and selective lengthening.[121, 123]

HETEROTOPIC OSSIFICATION

Heterotopic ossification (HO) is defined as the formation of mature lamellar bone in soft tissues and occurs in 11% to 76% of adult TBI patients.[72, 124, 125] Although its cause is unknown, patients with spasticity, prolonged coma (>2 weeks), long bone fractures, and decreased range of motion appear to be at increased risk.[126] The hip and knee are the most commonly affected sites, but HO can involve the shoulder, elbow, and nonjoint sites.[118, 127, 128] HO typically presents 1 to 3 months after injury; the onset can be insidious or mimic thrombophlebitis.[118] Early detection is possible with triple-phase bone scan, but HO is typically diagnosed clinically by loss of range of motion in conjunction with an elevated alkaline phosphatase level. Plain films may not show evidence of HO for 4 to 6 weeks following onset.[129] HO cannot be reversed; therefore, treatment is limited to prophylaxis against further HO formation. Typically, etidronate disodium (Didronel) is used once HO is detected, but it is not used for general prophylaxis in all TBI patients.[130–132] Once initiated, therapy is generally continued for a total of 6 to 9 months.[130, 132] Range-of-motion exercise is continued to maintain existing motion at the joint. Some clinicians ask that therapists not perform vigorous ranging beyond the end range because of the theoretical concern that an inflammatory response and further HO could be precipitated. Once HO has fully matured (12 to 18 months after onset), patients can be referred for surgical excision if the loss of range of motion has resulted in significant functional deficits.[118]

NEUROPSYCHIATRIC DISORDERS

Neuropsychiatric disorders following TBI are common and have been well described.[133] Major depression has been reported to occur in 10% to 77% of TBI patients, depending on the study cited.[134, 135] Depression has been shown to negatively impact functional recovery, and the importance of early diagnosis and treatment has been acknowledged.[134] Anxiety disorder is estimated to occur in about 30% of TBI patients, and aggression or agitation has been reported in 35% to 96% of patients during the acute recovery period.[135] Delirium should always be ruled out as a cause of neuropsychiatric symptoms in TBI patients. Diagnosis and treatment of psychiatric disorders in this patient population are complicated by TBI-associated neurocognitive and neurobehavioral changes. It is therefore important that a neuropsychiatrist be available to assist the rehabilitation team in caring for a TBI patient.

OTHER COMPLICATIONS

An array of other medical complications associated with TBI has been described.[136] These include skin breakdown, contracture, gastrointestinal ulcer, hypertension, deep vein thrombosis, infection, neurogenic bladder, hepatic dysfunction, endocrine abnormalities, post-traumatic epilepsy, and reflex sympathetic dystrophy. The prevalence of complications in the postacute phase of recovery from TBI underscores the need for close medical supervision during the early components of the rehabilitation program.

TRAUMATIC BRAIN INJURY MODEL SYSTEMS PROGRAM

In 1987, the U.S. Department of Education's National Institute on Disability and Rehabilitation Research established the TBI Model Systems Program. It was established to support advances in the treatment and outcome of individuals with TBI.[137] Currently, approximately 15 centers are funded in the United States. Each center has demonstrated that it offers the full continuum of TBI rehabilitation services, has an adequate volume of TBI patients to make a meaningful contribution to the national TBI database, and is capable of conducting research activities that support the priorities of the TBI model system initiative. Data from the institute's national TBI database have resulted in numerous publications on TBI outcome research. New trends in TBI rehabilitation research will be directed toward the development and assessment of new and innovative rehabilitation interventions to improve outcome.

REFERENCES

1. Gurdjian ES: Head Injury from Antiquity to the Present with Special Reference to Penetrating Head Wounds. Springfield, IL, CC, Thomas, 1973.
2. Boake C: A history of cognitive rehabilitation of head-injured patients, 1915 to 1980. J Head Trauma Rehabil 4:1–8, 1989.
3. The History of Physiatry (1999). http://www.physiatry.org/start/index.html.
4. National Center for Injury Prevention and Control, Centers for Disease Control and Prevention. www.cdc.gov/ncipc/dacrrdp/tbi.htm.
5. Rehabilitation of Persons with Traumatic Brain Injury: NIH Consensus Conference. JAMA 282:974–983, 1999.
6. World Health Organization: International Classification of Impairments, Disabilities, and Handicaps: A Manual of Classification Relating to the Consequences of Disease. Geneva, World Health Organization, 1980.
7. Jennett B, Bond MR: Assessment of outcome in severe brain damage: A practical scale. Lancet 1:480–484, 1975.
8. Mahoney FI, Barthel DW: Functional evaluation: The Barthel Index. Paper presented at the annual meeting of the Rehabilitation Section, Baltimore City Medical Society, 1965, pp 61–63.
9. Granger CV, Hamilton BB: Uniform Data Set for Medical Rehabilitation. Buffalo, Research Foundation, State University of New York, 1987.
10. Hamilton BB, Laughlin JA, Fiedler RC, Granger CV: Interrater reliability of the 7-level functional independence measure (FIM). Scand J Rehab Med 26:115–119, 1994.
11. Ditunno JF: Functional assessment measures in CNS trauma. J Neurotrauma 9(Suppl 1):301–305, 1992.
12. Rappaport M, Hall KM, Hopkins K, et al: Disability rating scale for severe head trauma: Coma to community. Arch Phys Med Rehabil 63:118–123, 1982.
13. Hagen C, Malkmus D, Durham P: Levels of cognitive functions. In Rehabilitation of Head-Injured Adult: Comprehensive Physical Management. Downey, CA, Professional Staff Association, Rancho Los Amigos Hospital, 1979.
14. Levin H, O'Donnell V, Grossman R: The Galveston Orientation and Amnesia Test. J Nerv Ment Dis 167:675–684, 1979.
15. Wechsler D: Wechsler Adult Intelligence Scale III. San Antonio, TX, Psychological Corporation, 1997.
16. Reitan RM: The validity of the Trail Making Test as an indicator of organic brain damage. Percept Mot Skills 9:127–130, 1958.
17. Reitan RM, Wolfson D: Category Test and Trail Making Test as measures of frontal lobe functions. Clin Neuropsychologist 9:50–55, 1995.
18. Conners CK, Multi-Health Systems Staff: Conner's Continuous Performance Test. Toronto, Multi-Health System, 1995.
19. Gronwall D: Paced auditory serial addition task: A measure of recovery from concussion. Percept Mot Skills 44:367–373, 1977.
20. Wechsler D: Wechsler Memory Scale III. San Antonio, TX, Psychological Corporation, 1997.
21. Delis DC, Kramer JH, Kaplan E, Ober BA: California Verbal Learning Test: Adult Version. San Antonio, TX, Psychological Corporation, 1987.
22. Rey A: L'Examen psychologique dan les cas d'encephalopathie traumatique. Arch Psychol 28:286–340, 1941.
23. Benton AL: Revised Visual Retention Test, 4th ed. New York, Psychological Corporation, 1974.
24. Reitan RM, Wolfson D: The Halstead-Reitan neuropsychological test battery: Theory and clinical interpretation. Tucson, AZ, Neuropsychology Press, 1993.
25. Warrington EK: Recognition Memory Test. Windsor, England, National Foundation for Educational Research, 1984.
26. Wilson BA, Cockburn J, Baddeley AD: The Rivermead Behavioral Memory Test. Bury St Edmunds, England, Thames Valley Test Company, 1985.
27. Golden JC: Stroop Color and Word Test. Chicago, Stoelting, 1978.
28. Stroop JR: Studies of interference in serial verbal reaction. J Exp Psychol 18:643–662, 1935.
29. Heaton RK: Wisconsin Card Sorting Test. Odessa, FL, Psychological Assessment Resources, 1981.
30. Spreen O, Denton AL: Neurosensory Center Comprehensive Examination for Aphasia (NCCEA). Victoria, University of Victoria Neuropsychology Laboratory, 1977.
31. Levin HS, Mattis S, Ruff RM, et al: Neurobehavioral outcome following minor head injury: A three center study. J Neurosurg 66:234–243, 1987.
32. Kreutzer J, Seel R, Marwitz J: The Neurobehavioral Functioning Inventory. San Antonio, TX, Psychological Corporation, 1999.

33. Burgess PW, Alderman N, Evans J, et al: The ecological validity of tests of executive function. J Int Neuropsychol Soc 4:547–558, 1998.

34. Goldberg E, Podell K: Adaptive decision making, ecological validity, and the frontal lobes. J Clin Exp Neuropsychol 22: 56–68, 2000.

35. DeLisa JA, Gans BM: Rehabilitation Medicine. Philadelphia, Lippincott-Raven, 1998.

36. Mack A, Horn L: Functional prognosis in traumatic brain injury. Phys Med Rehabil: State Art Rev 3:13–26, 1989.

37. Sparadeo F, Gill D: Effects of prior alcohol use on head injury recovery. J Head Trauma Rehabil 4:75–82, 1989.

38. Barker LH, Bigler ED, Johnson SC, et al: Polysubstance abuse and traumatic brain injury: Quantitative magnetic resonance imaging and neuropsychological outcome in older adolescents and young adults. J Int Neuropsychol Soc 5:593–608, 1999.

39. Heiskanen H, Sipponen P: Prognosis of severe brain injury. Acta Neurol Scand 46:343, 1970.

40. Amacher AL, Bybee DE: Toleration of head injury by the elderly. Neurosurgery 20:954, 1979.

41. Sosin DN, Sacks JJ, Smith SM: Head injury–associated deaths in the US from 1979–1986. JAMA 282:2251, 1989.

42. Pennings JL, Bachulis BL, Simons CT, Slazinski T: Survival after severe brain injury in the aged. Arch Surg 128:787, 1993.

43. Herneasniemi J: Outcome following head injuries in the aged. Acta Neurochir (Wien) 49:67, 1979.

44. Jennett B, Teasdale G, Braakman R, et al: Predicting outcome in individual patients after severe head injury. Lancet 1:1031, 1976.

45. Katz DI, Alexander MP: Predicting course of recovery and outcome for patients admitted to rehabilitation. Arch Neurol 51:661–670, 1994.

46. Zafonte RE, Mann NR, Millis SR, et al: Posttraumatic amnesia: Its relation to functional outcome. Arch Phys Med Rehabil 78: 1103–1106, 1997.

47. Cifu DX, Kreutzer JS, Marwitz JH, et al: Functional outcomes of older adults with TBI: A prospective, multicenter analysis. Arch Phys Med Rehabil 77:883–888, 1996.

48. Reeder K, Rosenthal M, Lichtenberg P, et al: Impact of age on functional outcome following traumatic brain injury. J Head Trauma Rehabil 11:22, 1996.

49. Saywell RM Jr, Woods JR, Rappaport SA, Allen TL: The value of age and severity as predictors of costs in geriatric head injury trauma patients. J Am Geriatr Soc 37:625, 1989.

50. Kriel RL, Krach LE, Panser LA: Closed head injury: Comparison of children younger and older than 6 years of age. Pediatr Neurol 5:296–300, 1989.

51. Silver JM, Yudofsky SC, Hales RE: Neuropsychiatry of traumatic brain injury. In Kraus JF, Sorenson SB (eds): Epidemiology. Washington, DC, American Psychiatric Press, 1994, pp 3–41.

52. Diamond PT: Brain injury in the commonwealth of Virginia: An analysis of central registry data, 1988–1993. Brain Inj 10: 413–419, 1996.

53. Cohadon F, Richer E, Castel JP: Head injuries: Incidence and outcome. J Neurol Sci 103(Suppl):S27–S31, 1991.

54. Kraus JF, Black MA, Hessol N, et al: The incidence of acute brain injury and serious impairment in a defined population. Am J Epidemiol 119:186–201, 1984.

55. Levie L, Linn S, Revach M, et al: Head trauma in northern Israel: Incidence and types. Neuroepidemiology 9:278–284, 1990.

56. Marshall LF, Decker DP, Bowers SA, et al: The National Traumatic Coma Data Bank. Part 1. Design, purpose, goals, and results. J Neurosurg 59:276–284, 1983.

57. Rimel RW, Giordani D, Darth JT, et al: Disability caused by minor injury. Neurosurgery 9:221–228, 1981.

58. Rimel RW, Giordani B, Barth JT, et al: Moderate head injury: Completing the clinical spectrum of brain trauma. Neurosurgery 11:344–351, 1982.

59. Wang CC, Schoenberg BS, Li SC, et al: Brain injury due to head trauma: Epidemiology in urban areas of the People's Republic of China. Arch Neurol 43:570–572, 1986.

60. Mackenzie EJ, Edelstein SL, Flynn JP: Hospitalized head-injured patients in Maryland: Incidence and severity of injuries. Md Med J 38:725, 1989.

61. Groswasser Z, Cohen M, Keren O: Female TBI patients recover better than males. Brain Inj 12:805–808, 1998.

62. Roof RL, Hall ED: Estrogen-related gender difference in survival rate and cortical blood flow after impact acceleration head injury in rats. J Neurotrauma 17:1155–1169, 2000.

63. Igarashi T, Huang T, Noble LJ: Regional vulnerability after traumatic brain injury: Gender differences in mice that overexpress human copper, zinc, superoxide dismutase. Exp Neurol 172:332–341, 2001.

63a. Farace E, Olves WM: Do women fare worse: A meta-analysis of gender differences in outcome after traumatic brain injury. J Neurosurg 93:539–545, 2001.

64. Braakman R, Gelpke GJ, Habbema JDF, et al: Systematic selection of prognostic features in patients with severe head injury. Neurosurgery 6:362–370, 1980.

65. Jennett B, Teasdale G, Braakman R, et al: Prognosis in series of patients with severe head injury. Neurosurgery 4:283–289, 1979.

66. Miller JD, Butterworth JF, Gudeman SK, et al: Further experience in the management of severe head injury. J Neurosurg 54: 289–299, 1981.

67. Whyte J, Hart T, Laborde A, Rosenthal: Rehabilitation of the patient with traumatic brain injury. In DeLisa JA, Gans BM, Rosenthal M, et al (eds): Rehabilitation Medicine, Principles and Practice. Philadelphia, Lippincott-Raven, 1998.

68. Jennett B, Teasdale G: Management of Head Injuries. Philadelphia, FA Davis, 1981, pp 1191–1239.

69. Bricolo A, Turazzi S, Feriotti G: Prolonged posttraumatic unconsciousness: Therapeutic assets and liabilities. J Neurosurg 52: 625, 1980.

70. Pitts LH: San Francisco General Hospital Medical Center Head Injury Data Bank. Cited in Bartowski M, Lovely MP: Prognosis in coma and the persistent vegetative state. J Head Trauma Rehabil 1:1, 1986.

71. Braakman R, Jennett WB, Minderhoud JB: Prognosis of the post traumatic vegetative state. Acta Neurochir (Wien) 95:49, 1988.

72. Sazbon L, Najenson T, Tartakovsky M, et al: Widespread periarticular new-bone formation in long-term comatose patients. J Bone Joint Surg Br 63:120–125, 1981.

73. Levin HS, Saydjari C, Eisenberg HM, et al: Vegetative state after closed-head injury: A Traumatic Coma Data Bank report. Arch Neurol 48:580, 1991.

74. Groswasser Z, Sazbon L: Outcome in 134 patients with prolonged posttraumatic unawareness. J Neurosurg 72:81–84, 1990.

75. McMillian T, Jongen M, Greenwood R: Assessment of posttraumatic amnesia after severe closed head injury: Retrospective or prospective? J Neurol Neurosurg Psychiatry 60:422–427, 1996.

76. Becker D, Miller JD, Ward JD, et al: The outcome from severe head injury with early diagnosis and intensive management. J Neurosurg 47:491–502, 1977.

77. Levin HS, Grossman RG, Rose JE, Teasdale G: Long-term neuropsychological outcome of closed head injury. J Neurosurg 50: 412–422, 1979.

78. Warren JB, Peck EA: Factors which influence neuropsychological recovery from severe head injury. J Neurosurg Nurs 16: 248–252, 1984.

79. Pondagg W: Disseminated intravascular coagulation related to outcome in head injury. Acta Neurochir (Wien) 28(Suppl):98–102, 1979.

80. Levin HS, Eisenberg HM: Neuropsychological outcome of closed head injury in children and adolescents. Childs Brain 5: 281–292, 1979.

81. Greenberg RP, Becker DP, Miller JD, Mayer DJ: Evaluation of brain function in severe human head trauma with multimodality evoked potentials. J Neurosurg 47:163–177, 1977.

82. Judson JA, Cant BR, Shaw NA: Early prediction of outcome from cerebral trauma by somatosensory evoked potentials. Crit Care Med 18:363–368, 1990.

83. Rappaport M: Evoked potential and head injury in a rehabilitation setting. In Miner M, Wagner K (eds): Neurotrauma: Treatment, Rehabilitation and Related Issues. Boston, Butterworths, 1986, pp 189–194.

84. Narayan RK, Greenberg RD, Miller JD, et al: Improved confidence of outcome prediction in severe head injury. J Neurosurg 54:751–762, 1981.

85. Levin HS, Williams DH, Eisenberg HM, et al: Serial MRI and neurobehavioral findings after mild to moderate closed head injury. J Neurol Psychiatry 55:255–262, 1992.

86. Levin HS, Benavidez DA, Verger-Maestre K, et al: Reduction of corpus callosum growth after severe traumatic brain injury in children. Neurology 54:647–653, 2000.

87. Shibata Y, Matsumura A, Meguro K, et al: Differentiation of mechanism and prognosis of traumatic brain stem lesions detected by magnetic resonance imaging in the acute stage. Clin Neurol Neurosurg 102:124–128, 2000.

88. Garnett MR, Cadoux-Hudson T, Styles P: How useful is magnetic resonance imaging in predicting severity and outcome of traumatic brain injury? Curr Opin Neurol 14:753–757, 2001.

89. Van der Naalt J, Hew JM, van Zomeren AH, et al: Computed tomography and magnetic resonance imaging in mild to moderate head injury: Early and late imaging related to outcome. Ann Neurol 46:70–78, 1999.

90. Grados MA, Slomine BS, Gerring JP, et al: Depth of lesion model in children and adolescents with moderate to severe traumatic brain injury: Use of SPGR MRI to predict severity and outcome. J Neurol Neurosurg Psychiatry 70:350–358, 2001.

91. Azouvi P: Neuroimaging correlates of cognitive and functional outcome after traumatic brain injury. Curr Opin Neurol 13:665–669, 2000.

92. Jones DK, Dardis R, Ervine M, et al: Cluster analysis of diffusion tensor magnetic resonance images in human head injury. Neurosurgery 47:306–313, 2000.

93. Cazalis F, Feydy A, Granon S, et al: Prefrontal activation after traumatic brain injury (TBI): An fMRI study with a Tower of London task [abstract]. J Int Neuropsychol Soc 6:379, 2000.

94. Walker AE: Summary for the international symposium on rehabilitation in head injury. Scand J Rehabil 4:154–156, 1972.

95. Mills VM, Cassidy JW, Katz DI: Neurologic Rehabilitation: A Guide to Diagnosis, Prognosis, and Treatment Planning. Boston, Blackwell Science, 1997.

96. Med Manual, 211, Inpatient Hospital Stays. http://hr.cch.com/primesrc/bin/hig.

97. Centers for Medicare and Medicaid Services (CMS), HHS: Medicare program; prospective payment system for inpatient rehabilitation facilities: Final rule. Fed Reg 66:41315–41430, 2001.

98. Stineman MG, Escarce JJ, Goin JE, et al: A case-mix classification system for medical rehabilitation. Med Care 32:366–379, 1994.

99. Malec JF, Basford JS: Postacute brain injury rehabilitation. Arch Phys Med Rehabil 77:198–207, 1996.

100. Cicerone KD, Dahlberg C, Kalmar K, et al: Evidence-based cognitive rehabilitation: Recommendations for clinical practice. Arch Phys Med Rehabil 81:1596–1615, 2000.

101. Ponsford J: Traumatic Brain Injury: Rehabilitation for Everyday Adaptive Living. Hillsdale, NJ, Lawrence Erlbaum, 1995.

102. National Institutes of Health: Rehabilitation of persons with traumatic brain injury. NIH Consensus Statement 16:1–41, 1998.

103. Glisky EL, Schacter DL, Tulving E: Learning and retention of computer-related vocabulary in amnesic patients: Method of vanishing cues. J Clin Exp Neuropsychol 8:292–312, 1986.

104. Baddeley AD, Wilson BA, Watts FN: Handbook of Memory Disorders. Chichester, England, Wiley, 1995.

105. Christensen A-L, Uzzell BP: Brain Injury and Neuropsychological Rehabilitation: International Perspectives. Hillsdale, NJ, Lawrence Erlbaum, 1994.

106. Sohlberg MM, Mateer CA: Cognitive Rehabilitation: An Integrative Neuropsychological Approach. New York, Guilford Press, 2001.

107. Richardson JTE: Clinical and Neuropsychological Aspects of Closed Head Injury, 2nd ed. Hove, UK, Psychology Press, 1999.

108. Timmerman ME, Brouser WH: Slow information processing after very severe closed head injury: Impaired access to declarative knowledge and intact application and acquisition of procedural knowledge. Neuropsychologia 37:467–478, 1999.

109. Rizzo AA, Buckwalter JG: Virtual reality and cognitive assessment and rehabilitation: The state of the art. In Riva G (ed): Virtual Reality in Neuro-Psycho-Physiology. Amsterdam, IOS Press, 1997.

110. Rizzo AA, Buckwalter JG, McGee JS, et al: Virtual environments for assessing and rehabilitating cognitive/functional performance. Presence 10:359–374, 2001.

111. Wilson PN, Foreman N, Staunton D: Virtual reality, disability and rehabilitation. Disabil Rehabil 19:213–220, 1997.

112. Zhang L, Abreu B, Masel B, et al: Virtual reality in the assessment of selected cognitive function after brain injury. Am J Phys Med Rehabil 80:597–604, 2001.

113. Gengenfelder J, Schultheir M, Al-Shihabi T, et al: Divided attention and driving: A pilot study using virtual reality technology. J Head Trauma Rehabil 17:26–37, 2002.

114. Jacobs HE: Behavior Analysis Guidelines and Brain Injury Rehabilitation: People, Principles, and Programs. New York, Aspen, 1993.

115. Barth JT, Macciocchi SN, Diamond PT: Mild head injury: Current research and clinical issues. In Rosenthal M, Griffith ER, Kreutzer JS, Pentland B (eds): Rehabilitation of the Adult and Child with Traumatic Brain Injury, 3rd ed. Philadelphia, FA Davis, 1999, pp 471–478.

116. McAllister TW: Mild traumatic injury and the post concussive syndrome. In Silver JM, Yudofsky SC, Hales RE (eds): Neuropsychiatry of Traumatic Brain Injury. Washington, DC, American Psychiatric Press, 1994, pp 357–392.

117. Barth JT, Diamond R, Errico A: Mild head injury and post concussion syndrome: Does anyone really suffer? Clin Electroencephalogr 27:183–186, 1996.

118. Bontke CF, Boake C (eds): Principles of brain injury rehabilitation. In Braddom RL, Buschbacher RM, Dumitru D, et al (eds): Physical Medicine and Rehabilitation. Philadelphia, WB Saunders, 1996, 1027–1051.

119. Meythaler JM, Guin-Renfroe S, Johnson A, Brunner RM: Prospective assessment of tizanidine for spasticity due to acquired brain injury. Arch Phys Med Rehabil 82:1155–1163, 2001.

120. Katz RT: Management of spastic hypertonia after stroke. J Neuro Rehab (Suppl 1):S5–S12, 1991.

121. Nooy DV, Elovic E: Advances in the Management of Spasticity. Edison, NJ, JFK Johnson Rehabilitation Institute, 1997.

122. Meythaler JM, Guin-Renfroe S, Grabb P, Hadley MN: Long-term continuously infused intrathecal baclofen for spastic-dystonic hypertonia in traumatic brain injury: 1-year experience. Arch Phys Med Rehabil 80:13–19, 1999.

123. Mayer NH: Functional management of spasticity after head injury. J Neuro Rehab 5(Suppl 1):S1–S4, 1991.

124. Garland DE, Blum CE, Waters RL: Periarticular heterotopic ossification in head-injured adults. J Bone Joint Surg Am 62:143–1146, 1980.

125. Garland DE: Clinical observations on fractures and heterotopic ossification in the spinal cord and traumatic brain injured populations. Clin Orthop 233:86–101, 1988.

126. Buschbacher R: Heterotopic ossification: A review. Crit Rev Phys Med Rehabil 4:199, 1992.

127. Citta-Pietrolungo TJ, Alexander MA, Steg NL: Early detection of heterotopic ossification in young patients with traumatic brain injury. Arch Phys Med Rehabil 73:258–262, 1992.

128. Hurvitz EA, Mandac BR, Davidoff G, et al: Risk factors for heterotopic ossification in children and adolescents with severe traumatic brain injury. Arch Phys Med Rehabil 73:459–462, 1992.

129. Pittenger DE: Heterotopic ossification. Orthop Rev 20:33–39, 1991.

130. Gennarelli TA: Subject review: Heterotopic ossification. Brain Inj 2:175, 1988.

131. Rogers RC: Program idea: Heterotopic calcification in severe head injury: A prevention program. Brain Inj 2:169, 1988.

132. Spielman G, Gennarelli TA, Rogers CR: Disodium etidronate: Its role in preventing heterotopic ossification in severe head injury. Arch Phys Med Rehabil 64:539, 1983.

133. Silver JM, Yudofsky SC, Hales RE (eds): Neuropsychiatry of Traumatic Brain Injury. Washington, DC, American Psychiatric Press, 1994.

134. Rosenthal M, Christensen BK, Ross TP: Depression following traumatic brain injury. Arch Phys Med Rehabil 79:90–103, 1998.

135. Robinson RG, Jorge R: Mood disorders. In Silver JM, Yudofsky SC, Hales RE (eds): Neuropsychiatry of Traumatic Brain Injury. Washington, DC, American Psychiatric Press, 1994, pp 219–250.

136. Rosenthal M, Griffith ER, Kreutzer JS, Pentland B: Rehabilitation of the Adult and Child with Traumatic Brain Injury, 3rd ed. Philadelphia, FA Davis, 1999.

137. National Institute on Disability and Rehabilitation Research: http://www.ed.gov/offices/OSERS/NIDRR/, 2002.

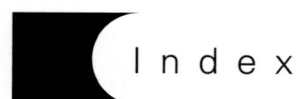

Index

Note: Page numbers followed by f indicate illustrations; those by a b, boxes; those by a t, tables.

ABC system, of cervical spine anterior
  screw-plate fixation, 4630t, 4635–4636,
  4636f
ABCDEs, 5087–5088
Abdomen, trauma assessment of, 5089
Abducens nerve, 29, 316, 316f, 1899, 1974
  examination of, 266
    pediatric, 3173–3174
  injury to, in atlanto-occipital dislocation,
    4929
  paresis of, 317, 318t, 320, 320f
Abortion, CNS transplantation tissue from,
  2833, 2835
Abscess
  epidural. See Epidural abscess; Pyogenic
    infection, spinal.
  tuberculous, 1443
Absolute alcohol wash, for cerebral palsy,
  3731
ABT-627, as angiogenesis antagonist, 779t
Abulia, 285
  in frontal lobe tumors, 830
Abuse, reporting obligations in, 411
Academic practice, legal issues regarding,
  409–410
Accessory nerve, 1973–1974
Acetaminophen, for pain, 2959
Acetazolamide
  for brain edema, 802
  for elevated intracranial pressure, 1429
  for infantile posthemorrhagic
    hydrocephalus, 3411
Acetyl coenzyme A, synthesis of, 1483t
Acetylcholine, in action potential, 3814
Achilles tendonitis, vs. distal tibial nerve
  entrapment, 3936
Achondroplasia, 3362–3371
  apnea in, 3363–3364
  cervicomedullary compression in,
    3364–3365
    decompression of, 3367–3368
      outcome of, 3369
      ventriculostomy for, 3367
  craniovertebral region, 3343, 3344f
  epidemiology of, 3362–3363
  genetics of, 3362–3363
  hydrocephalus in, 3365–3366, 3398
  intracranial pressure in, 3365–3366
  jugular bulb dehiscence in, 3364
  medical complications of, 3363–3364,
    3363t
  neurologic complications of, 3363t
  neurologic vs. orthopedic aspects of,
    3366
  psychosocial problems in, 3363
  reproduction in, 3363
  spinal stenosis in, 3365, 3366–3367
    decompression of, 3368–3369
      outcome of, 3369–3370
    recurrence of, 3370–3371, 3370f, 3371f
Acid-base metabolism, 123–126, 125f
Acidosis, cerebral, in head injury, 5050
Acoustic meatus, internal, 36f, 40f
Acoustic neuroma, 1147–1164. See also
  Brainstem, glioma of.

Acoustic neuroma (Continued)
  arterial involvement in, 1159, 1159t
  cerebellopontine angle
    anatomic distortions in, 1158–1159,
      1158t
    auditory tests in, 335f–336f
    treatment of, 1163–1164, 1163f
  diagnosis of, 1149–1150, 1149f, 1152,
    1153f
  facial nerve distortions in, 1158–1159,
    1158t, 1159t
  features of, 1147, 1147f
  historical review of, 1147–1150, 1148f,
    1149f
  in pregnancy, 872
  intracanalicular, 1162–1163, 1163f
  magnetic resonance imaging of, 1149,
    1149f
  pathology of, 1152–1153, 1154f
  posterior fossa anatomic variations in,
    1158–1159, 1158t
  radiosurgery for, 1154–1155, 4055–4056,
    4059f
    complications in, 574
    linac, 4112
    vs. microsurgery, 1164, 4056, 4057t,
      4058t
  surgery for, 1154–1158, 1158t
    complications of, 1161–1162
      avoidance of, 570–571
    cranial nerve preservation in,
      1160–1161
    evolution of, 1150–1152
    facial nerve monitoring during,
      1159–1160
    facial nerve paralysis after, 1161
    headache after, 1162
    middle fossa approach to, 1155
    morbidity in, 1161–1162
    mortality in, 1161
    neurophysiologic monitoring during,
      1160
    outcome in, 1164
    posterior fossa intradural approach to,
      925–926
    suboccipital approach to, 1156–1158,
      1156f–1158f
    translabyrinthine approach to,
      1148–1149, 1155–1156
  treatment of, 1147, 1150
    tumor size and, 1162–1164, 1163f
  venous involvement in, 1159, 1159t
  vs. facial nerve schwannoma, 1147,
    1147f, 1148f
  vs. meningioma, 1153
  vs. peripheral schwannoma, 1153, 1154f
Acoustic radiation, 9
Acoustic reflex, hearing assessment with,
  334, 335f–336f
Acquired immunodeficiency syndrome
  (AIDS)
  neuropathy in, 3841
  primary central nervous system
    lymphoma in, 1069–1070, 1071f

Acquired immunodeficiency syndrome
  (AIDS) (Continued)
  pyogenic spinal infections in, 4363–4364
    differential diagnosis of, 4371
    medical management of, 4379
  reporting obligations in, 411–412
  systemic lymphoma in, 1070, 1072
Acromegaly
  carpal tunnel syndrome in, 3890
  diagnosis of, in pregnancy, 868
  dopamine agonists for, 1193
  growth hormone excess and, 1189, 1190
  neuropathy in, 3843
  radiation therapy for, 1193, 4035–4036
  radiosurgery for, 4062
  recurrence of, 1193–1194
  somatostatin analogs for, 1192–1193
  surgery for, 1176
Actin, in axonal regeneration, 197
Actinomyces israelii, spinal infection with,
  4295
Actinomycin, for Ewing's sarcoma, 4850
Actinomycosis, spinal, 4385
Action potential, 73
  calcium, 219, 220, 222–224
  conductance changes during, 220–221,
    221f
  electrodiagnostic testing of, 3851–3852,
    3851f
  generation of, 220–221, 221f
  glial, 221
  ion currents in, 219
  maintenance of, 224–225
  motor unit, polyphasic nature and,
    3856–3857, 3856f
  muscle fiber, spontaneous, peripheral
    nervous system abnormalities with,
    3856, 3856t
  neuronal, 3813, 3813f, 3814b
  repolarization of, 220, 224–225
  sodium, 220–222
Adamantinoma, pituitary, 1207
Adaptive development, 3170, 3170t
Adductor reflex testing, pediatric, 3180
Adenoassociated viruses
  as central nervous system gene therapy
    vector, 4166–4167
  as vectors, 818
Adenocarcinoma, paranasal sinus, 1312
Adenohypophysis, morphology of,
  1171–1172
Adenoid cystic carcinoma, paranasal sinus,
  1312, 1313f
Adenoma, pituitary. See Pituitary
  adenoma.
Adenosine
  for pain, 2966
  in cerebral autoregulation, 1475
  in cerebral blood flow–metabolism
    coupling, 1489
Adenosine triphosphate, 119–120
  after brain injury, 2455–2456
  generation of, 118–119, 119f
  in cerebral metabolism, 1479, 1482
  in focal cerebral ischemia, 134, 134f
  in neurons, 1486

Behavioral therapy, pain treatment with, 2966
  regression of benefit in, 2940–2941
Bell's cruciate paralysis, 4871, 4871f
Bence Jones protein, in multiple myeloma, 4854
BendMeister rod bender, 4659f, 4660
Benedikt's syndrome, 273
Benton Controlled Oral Word Association Test (COWAT), 5186
Benzel-Kesterson interspinous wiring modification, 4645, 4647f
Benzodiazepines, 1508
  for dystonia, 2796
  for pain, 2966
  in intracranial pressure management, 5127, 5127t
  in pregnancy, 2422
Beriberi, neuropathy in, 3844
Bernard-Horner syndrome, in nerve plexus injury, 3970
Bethanechol, for multiple sclerosis, 1455t
Biceps reflex testing, pediatric, 3180
Biglycan, 4230
Bilharziosis, spinal, 4390
Bing's sign, 268
Bioartificial materials, for central nervous system repair, 4163
Biochemical markers, for neoplastic meningitis, 1232
Biomechanics
  of atlantoaxial joint, 4187, 4188
  of axis, 4939
  of cervical spine, 4187–4190, 4193–4194, 4432
  of craniovertebral junction, 3333–3334
  of facet joints, 4185
  of internal spinal fixation, 4592–4596, 4593f, 4594f
  of intervertebral disk, 4185–4186
  of lumbar spine, 4191, 4714–4715
  of pediatric atlantoaxial joint, 3537–3538, 3538f
  of pediatric atlanto-occipital joint, 3528–3529
  of pediatric spinal injury, 3515–3516
  of spinal cord injury without radiographic abnormality, 3516
  of spine, 4181–4199, 4586, 4587f, 4588–4589
  of spondylolisthesis, 4543–4547
  of thoracic spine, 4190–4191, 4953–4954, 4953f–4955f
  of thoracic spine fixation, 4195–4198
  of thoracic spine fractures, 4192, 4195–4198
  of thoracic spine posterior procedures, 4694–4695
  of vertebrae, 4184–4185
Biopsy
  complications in, 573, 573t
  endoscopic, 3430
  in frameless stereotactic surgery, 945–946
  in pyogenic spinal infection, 4369, 4370f
  muscle, 3963–3964
  of pineal region tumors, 1014–1016, 1014f, 1014t
  of third ventricle tumors, 1248–1249
  peripheral nerve, 3837, 3838t, 3962–3963
  surgical navigation in, 945–946
Birbeck granules, in eosinophilic granuloma, 4843
Birth history, 3169–3170
Birth trauma, 3481–3486

Birth trauma *(Continued)*
  brachial plexus injury in, 3488–3495, Brachial plexus, obstetric injury to
  epidural hematoma in, 3483–3484, 3483f
  incidence of, 3481
  intracranial hemorrhage in, 3483–3485, 3483f–3486f
  posterior fossa subdural hematoma in, 3484–3485, 3485f, 3486f
  risk factors for, 3481
  scalp injury in, 3481–3482
  subdural hematoma in, 3484, 3484f
Bisphosphonates, in bone metabolism, 4233
Bisulfan, for ependymoma, 1048t
Bithermal caloric test, 344–345, 344f
Biventral lobule, 30f, 33f
Bladder
  anatomy of, 357–358, 357f, 358f
  autonomic receptors in, 358, 358f
  distention of, 364
  dysfunction of, in cerebral palsy, 3728, 3732, 3744–3745
  filling dysfunction of, 364–365, 365f
  neuromuscular function of, 363
  reflex contraction of, 377
  storage dysfunction of, 364–365, 365f
    treatment of, 378–379
  storage function of, 363
  voiding dysfunction of, 365
Bladder outlet resistance, 359
Bladder outlet retention, treatment of, 379–380
Blastocyst, development of, 4239, 4240f
Blastomycosis
  cranial destruction in, 430, 430f
  spinal, 4388f, 4389
Bleomycin, for craniopharyngioma, 1219, 3683–3684
Blepharospasm, 2729
Blindness
  in trigeminal schwannoma, 1345, 1345f
  monocular, 2541, 2542f
    optic nerve lesions, 2542, 2542f
  patient positioning and, 612–614
  prone positioning and, 603–604
Blink response, pediatric, 3173
Blood pressure. *See also* Arterial pressure.
  in cervical spine trauma, 4888, 4889
  in intracerebral hemorrhage, 1740
  in pregnancy, 2421
  in stroke, 1500–1501
  in trauma, 5090
Blood transfusion, 2829
Blood vessels, lumbar spine and, surgical anatomy of, 4706
Blood viscosity
  hypothermia effects on, 1532
  in head injury, 5058–5059
Blood-brain barrier, 153–170
  adherens junctions in, 157
  amino acid transport across, 160–161, 160t, 161f
  anatomic, 159
  capillaries of, 154
  cell biology of, 154–159, 155f
  contrast media penetration of, 164
  diseases affecting, 163–167
  disruption of, in chemotherapy, 879
  drug delivery across, 15–18, 16f
  endothelial cells forming, 153–154
  functional, 159
  gap junctions in, 157
  glucose transport across, 154, 159–160, 159f

Blood-brain barrier *(Continued)*
  GLUT-1 in, 158–159
  glutamate transport across, 161–162
  γ-glutamyltranspeptidase in, 158, 161
  immune cell passage through, 890
  in aging, 166–167
  in brain injury, 166
  in brain tumors, 164–165, 165t
  in cerebral edema, 165–166
  in cerebral ischemia, 166
  in cerebral metabolism, 1487
  in chemotherapy, 878
  in epilepsy, 166
  in experimental allergic encephalomyelitis, 164
  in hypertension, 166
  in immune response, 673
  in multidrug resistance, 162–163
  in multiple sclerosis, 164
  in radiation injury, 166
  in stress, 166
  inflammation effects on, 163–164
  ion transport across, 162
  ketone body transfer across, 1485
  lipoprotein transport across, 162
  macromolecular passage through, 154–155
  markers of, 157–159
  maturation of, 158
  microenvironmental influences on, 157–159
  morphology of, 154–155, 155f
  neurotransmitter transport in, 154, 161–162
  opening of
    chemotherapy delivery via, 153
    for brain edema, 802–803
  pediatric, 3462
  pericytes in, 153
  perivascular glia in, 153
  permeability of, 154, 155f
    cellular mechanisms of, 163
    disease effects on, 11–15
    lipophilicity and, 15, 16f
    to nucleosides, 158
    to nucleotides, 157–158
  physiology of, 791–792, 792f
  protective metabolic function of, 161
  receptor-mediated transport across, 163
  regulation of, astrocytes in, 109–110
  tight junctions in, 156–157, 159f
  transcellular endocytosis in, 159f
  transcellular lipophilic pathway in, 159f
  transcytosis through, 163
  transendothelial pathways of, drug delivery via, 159, 159f
  transport across, 156, 159–163, 159f
Blood–cerebrospinal fluid barrier, 791–792, 792f
Blood-tumor barrier, 17
Bmp4, 53t
Bobble-head doll syndrome, in suprasellar cysts, 3294
Bohlman triple-wire technique, 4645–4646, 4647f–4648f
Bone
  abnormalities of, head shape and, 3300
  anatomy of, 4227–4229, 4228f, 4613–4614
  biochemistry of, 4614–4615
  calcium in, 4231
  cancellous, 4227–4229, 4228f, 4613–4614
  cellular elements of, 4229, 4230f, 4614
  cortical, 4227, 4228f, 4613
  formation of, 4231–4233, 4231f, 4232t, 4613
    in spondyloarthropathies, 4460

Cortex (*Continued*)
area of functional deficit of, 2438
contusions of, bullet wounds and, 5234
developmental anomalies of,
classification of, 2492
eloquent, seizure control in, 2635
epileptogenic lesions of, 2437–2438
surgical history of, 2442–2443
epileptogenic zone of, 2438–2439
function of, testing of, 264–265, 264f,
264t
functional deficit zone of, surgical
history of, 2442–2443
insular, 2933
irritative zone of, 2436
surgical history of, 2440–2442, 2441f
mapping of, 2531–2538
patient selection in, 2531
motor, stimulation mapping of, 2534
neuronal development in, 79f
seizure onset zone of, 2436–2437, 2437f
sensory, 2931–2932
functional magnetic resonance
imaging of, 2519
stimulation mapping of, 2534
patient selection in, 2531
somatosensory area of, 2932, 2933f
somatosensory evoked potential
mapping of, 2533–2534, 2534f
spinothalamic tract and, 2927, 2930f
stimulation mapping of, seizures during,
2533
structure localization in, before surgery,
2531–2532, 2532f
symptomatogenic zone of, 2435–2436
surgical history of, 2439–2440
tumors of, resection of, 2537
vascular malformations in, resection of,
2537
zones of, 2435–2438
Cortical dysgenesis
magnetic resonance imaging of, 2491
magnetic resonance spectroscopy of,
2497
vs. tumor, 2492, 2492f
Cortical dysplasia
in epileptic resection, 2577–2578
in extratemporal lobe epilepsy, 2598
magnetic resonance imaging of, 2485
non–balloon cell focal, magnetic
resonance imaging of, 2493–2494,
2494f
Corticobasal degeneration, 2715
positron emission tomography of,
2761–2762
vs. Parkinson's disease, 2735
Corticospinal tract
decussation of, 4871, 4871f
in lower urinary tract function, 362
Corticosteroids
epidural injections of, 2973–2976, 2975t.
See also Epidural steroid injections.
for aneurysmal subarachnoid
hemorrhage, 1822
for brain edema, 801–802, 5134
for brain metastases, 1078
for bullet wounds, 5230
for chronic inflammatory demyelinating
polyradiculoneuropathy, 3840
for glial tumors, 870
for intracerebral hemorrhage, 1740
for medulloblastoma, 3644
for pain, 2959
for primary central nervous system
lymphoma, 1072

Corticosteroids (*Continued*)
for primitive neuroectodermal tumors,
1003
for pseudotumor cerebri, 1429
for pyogenic spinal infection, 4376
for sarcoidosis, 1438–1439
for spinal cord compression, 4047
for spinal cord injury, 4874, 4876
for spinal metastases, 4858
for therapeutic injections, 2970
for traumatic brain injury, 5097
for tumor-associated edema, 13–14
intracranial pressure and, 188
osteoporosis from, 4235
pseudotumor cerebri from, 1423, 1425
Corticostriatal projection, functional
organization of, 2683–2685
Corticosubthalamic projection, 2690
Corticotrophin-releasing hormone test, in
Cushing's disease, 1196
Cortisol, measurement of, 1196
Costotransversectomy, 640
for thoracic disk herniation, 4981
vs. other techniques, 4758, 4758t
Costovertebral triangle, 4765–4766
Cotrel-Dubousset rod–multiple hook
construct, in lumbar spine fixation,
4734, 4734f
Cotrel-Dubousset rod-screw plate
in occipitocervical fusion, 4661, 4663f
in thoracic spine fixation, 4969–4972,
4970f–4972f
Coumarin, in pregnancy, 2423
Court proceedings
in child abuse, 3509–3510, 3510t
in life-sustaining treatment refusal, 415
^{11}C-PK 11195, glial marking by, 1609
Cranial fixation, complications of, 562–563
Cranial nerves
examination of, 265–267
I. *See* Olfactory nerve.
II. *See* Optic nerve.
III. *See* Oculomotor nerve.
in acoustic neuroma, 1159, 1159t
in craniovertebral junction tumors, 4800
in skull base surgery, 1266
inferior petrosal sinus and, 1302, 1302f
injury to
after skull base surgery, 572
in atlanto-occipital dislocation,
4928–4929
IV. *See* Trochlear nerve.
IX. *See* Glossopharyngeal nerve.
monitoring of, in ependymoma surgery,
3630–3631
palsy of
glomus jugulare tumor embolization
and, 1300–1301
glomus jugulare tumors and,
1305–1306
in basilar trunk aneurysms, 2037
in sarcoidosis, 1435–1436
pediatric basilar skull fracture and,
3467–3468
pediatric, examination of, 3173–3176
posterior circulation aneurysm and, 1976
preservation of, in acoustic neuroma
surgery, 1160–1161
schwannoma of
magnetic resonance imaging of,
459–460, 460f
radiologic features of, 837
V. *See* Trigeminal nerve.
VI. *See* Abducens nerve.
VII. *See* Facial nerve.

Cranial nerves (*Continued*)
VIII. *See* Vestibular-auditory nerve.
X. *See* Vagus nerve.
XI. *See* Spinal accessory nerve.
XII. *See* Hypoglossal nerve.
Cranial neuralgia, 3018t
Cranial neuropathy, 318t
Cranial settling, 4571
Craniectomy, historical aspects of,
3159–3161, 3161f–3163f
Craniocervical junction
acquired abnormalities of, 4569–4583
metastases to, 4860
osseous relationships at, 519
rheumatoid arthritis of
radiologic features of, 4574,
4574f–4577f
surgical indications for, 4574–4575,
4578
treatment of, 4578–4580, 4579f–4581f
seronegative spondyloarthritis of,
4580–4581, 4582f, 4583f
Craniofacial anomalies
historical aspects of, 3155–3164
in utero compression and, 3301
Craniofacial resection, for paranasal sinus
tumors, 1318–1320, 1320f–1322f
Craniofacial syndromes, 3315–3329. *See
also* specific type, e.g., Crouzon's
syndrome.
evaluation of, 3316–3317
fibroblast growth factor receptor
mutations in, 3315–3316
functional matrix theory of, 3315
historical aspects of, 3315–3316, 3316f
hydrocephalus in, 3398–3399
radiography of, 3317, 3317f
surgery for, 3321–3329
complications of, 3328–3329
distraction osteogenesis in, 3327–3328
Le Fort III osteotomy in, 3326–3327
monoblock osteotomy in, 3327, 3328f
psychological considerations in, 3318
timing of, 3317–3318
Craniofacial trauma, 5245–5266
airway management in, 5246, 5246t,
5247f
avulsion flap in, 5249
central fractures in, 5251
combined central and lateral fractures
in, 5251
comminuted fracture in, 5260f
ears in, 5251
eyelids in, 5251
facial nerve in, 5251
fractures in, 5251–5262
classification of, 5251
clinical examination of, 5252
radiography of, 5252
treatment of, 5252–5262
bone flap in, 5260f
bone graft in, 5252, 5256f
bone material for, 5258f–5259f
frontal sinus repair in, 5252–5253
galea-frontalis flap in, 5258f–5259f
historical approaches to, 5251–5252
priorities in, 5245–5246
sequence of, 5253, 5256, 5256f
surgical, 5252, 5253f–5256f
technical problems in, 5256–5257,
5257f–5263f, 5262
hemorrhage in, 5246–5247
infection in, 5248
laceration in, 5249
lateral fractures in, 5251

Death (*Continued*)
  determination of, 415
  diagnosis of, 393–394
Débridement
  for postoperative spinal infection, 4384
  for pyogenic spinal infection, 4375–4376,
    4376f, 4378
  for spinal tuberculosis, 4387
  of bullet wounds, 5236–5237, 5237t
Decompression
  for cervical degenerative disease,
    4409–4428
  for cubital tunnel syndrome, 3909–3910
  for degenerative spondylolisthesis,
    3581–3583
  for failed back syndrome, 4337–4339
  for lumbar fracture, 5004–5005
  for pyogenic spinal infection, 4374–4375,
    4379
  for spinal cord injury, 4878–4880
  for spinal metastases, 4858–4862,
    4860f–4863f
  for spinal stenosis, 3368–3369
  for spinal tuberculosis, 4387
  for thoracic disk herniation, 4981
  for thoracic spine fracture, 4972–4978,
    4974f–4977f, 4980
  for thoracolumbar scoliosis, 4562
  for thoracolumbar spine fracture,
    5000–5002, 5000t, 5001f, 5001t
  microvascular, of trigeminal nerve,
    3005–3014
  neurovascular, for vertigo, 2909
  of cauda equina compression, 4998
  of cervicomedullary compression,
    3367–3368
  of spinal cord compression, 4998
  of ulnar nerve entrapment, 3909–3910
  of vertebral arteries, 1700, 1702, 1703,
    1705f, 1709
  stereotactic, for craniopharyngioma,
    1216
  thoracic spine
    anterior, 4973–4978, 4974f–4977f
    posterolateral, 4972–4973
  transoral, for upper cervical spine,
    4751–4752, 4752f
  transthoracic, 4974, 4975–4978, 4975f
Decorin, 4230–4231
Deep brain stimulation, 3026–3027
  chronic pain treatment with, 3119–3129,
    3123
    complications of, 3128–3129
    electrode implantation in, 3125–3126
    functional magnetic resonance
      imaging in, 3122
    generator implantation in, 3126
    head frame for, 3123
    hemorrhage in, 3128, 3128t
    historical aspects of, 3119–3120
    mechanisms of, 3121–3122
    microelectrode recording in, 3124
    outcomes in, 3126–3128, 3127t, 3128t
    paresthesia-producing targets in,
      3121–3122, 3122t
    patient selection in, 3120–3121, 3121t
    periaqueductal gray targets in, 3121,
      3121t, 3122, 3125, 3125f
    periventricular gray targets in, 3121,
      3121t, 3122, 3125
    procedure in, 3126–3127
    site selection in, 3121, 3121t, 3122t
    stimulation trial in, 3125
    target selection in, 3123, 3124
    technique of, 3122–3126

Deep brain stimulation (*Continued*)
  for Parkinson's disease, 2662, 2662f
  movement disorder treatment with,
    2803–2825. *See also* specific target,
    e.g., Globus pallidus, internal.
    atlases in, 2808–2809
    basal ganglia targeting in, 2804
    clinical validation in, 2809
    complications of, 2822–2824
    computed tomography in, 2808
    coordinates in, 2809, 2809f
    costs of, 2825
    electrode implantation in, 2810, 2811f,
      2812–2813, 2812f
    electrophysiologic studies in, 2813,
      2814f–2816f, 2815–2817
    generators in, 2817–2819, 2818f, 2824
    indications for, 2819–2820
    lesion targeting in, 2805–2810
    magnetic resonance imaging in,
      2804–2805, 2806f–2808f, 2807–2808
    microadjustments in, 2815–2817
    microrecording in, 2813, 2815, 2815f
    parallel processing model and, 2819
    patient selection in, 2819–2820
    radiography in, 2804
    results of, 2820–2822
    side-effects of, 2824
    software for, 2810
    target localization in, 2819, 2824
    ventriculography in, 2804, 2805–2807,
      2805f
    vs. ablation, 2824
    vs. neural grafts, 2824
  seizure outcome with, 2579
  vs. thalamotomy, 2780
Deep hypothermic circulatory arrest,
  1528–1537, 2108
  cannulation sites in, 1534
  cerebral ischemia pathophysiology and,
    1532
  complications in, 1536
  for posterior circulation aneurysms,
    2000, 2002
  history of, 1528
  in aneurysm treatment, 1511, 1528–1529,
    1529f–1531f, 1531, 1807
  indications for
    anatomic factors in, 1528–1529,
      1529f–1531f, 1531
    patient-related factors in, 1531–1532,
      1531t
  medical evaluation before, 1533–1534
  neuroanesthetic management in,
    1534–1535
  patient preparation for, 1534
  results of, 1536–1537
  surgical management in, 1535–1536
  technical preparations before, 1533
  techniques for, 1533–1536
Deep tendon reflexes
  in peripheral neuropathy, 3833
  testing of, 3824–3825
Deep venous thrombosis, 563–564
Degenerative disease
  neuronal, 4315t–4316t, 4319–4321, 4320f
  spinal, 4147–4148
    cervical. *See* Cervical disk disease.
    lumbar. *See* Lumbar disk disease.
    thoracic. *See* Thoracic disk herniation.
    vs. pyogenic infection, 4371
Degenerative spondylolisthesis
  pathogenesis of, 4545–4546, 4545f, 4546f
  treatment of, 4551–4553, 4552f
Dehydration, intracranial hypertension
  treatment by, 5133

Dejerine-Sottas disease, 536, 537f
Delirium, 286
  after traumatic brain injury, 5296
Delivery
  brachial plexus injury in, 3488–3495. *See
    also* Brachial plexus, obstetric injury
    to.
  epidural hematoma in, 3483–3484, 3483f
  in neoplastic disease, 873
  intracranial hemorrhage in, 3483–3485,
    3483f–3486f
  intraparenchymal hemorrhage in, 3485
  posterior fossa subdural hematoma in,
    3484–3485, 3485f, 3486f
  scalp injury in, 3481–3482
  skull fracture in, 3482–3483, 3482f
  subdural hematoma in, 3484, 3484f
  traumatic. *See also* Birth trauma; Brachial
    plexus, obstetric injury to.
  vertex, brachial plexus injury in, 3488,
    3489f
Delta, 53t
Dementia, 285–286
  colloid cyst and, 3688
  Lewy body
    apoptosis in, 2710
    clinical features of, 2712
    forms of, 2708–2709
    neuritic Alzheimer's disease changes
      in, 2712
    pathology of, 2712–2713
    substantia nigra pars compacta in,
      2706f
  positron emission tomography of,
    484–485
  thalamic, strategic infarcts and, 1609
Demyelination, 3961, 3961f
  imaging of, 541, 543f
  in multiple sclerosis, 1450–1451
  in sensory nerve action potential, 3853,
    3853f
  primary, 3962
  radiation-induced, 854
  secondary, 3962
  segmental, 3962
  urologic disorders in, 375
  vertigo in, 2902
Dendrite(s), 72f, 73
  antigen presentation by, 893
  structure of, 77
Denervation
  prolonged, 201
  urologic disorders in, 375
Denervation hypersensitivity, in cerebral
  vasospasm, 1849
Dens
  aplasia-hypoplasia of, 3341
  fracture of. *See also* Odontoid fracture.
    imaging of, 519, 519f
Dentate gyrus, 26f, 27, 2486, 2487f
Dentate ligament, 3060, 3060f
  in cordotomy, 3063, 3066f
  triangular processes of, 36f
Dentate tubercle, 31f
Dentatorubropallidoluysian atrophy,
  2718–2719, 2740
Dentition, in craniofacial trauma,
  5248–5249
2-Deoxyglucose, in positron emission
  tomography, 480, 481t, 482
Dependency
  definition of, 3783–3784
  in traumatic brain injury response, 5193t
Depolarization, 3813, 3813f
Depolarizing potentials, 228

Endothelium-derived relaxing factor. *See*
Nitric oxide.
Endothoracic fascia, 4674
Endotracheal tube, complications of,
patient positioning and, 609–610
Endovascular occlusion
for cerebral vasospasm, 1547
for spinal aneurysmal bone cyst, 4843
for spinal hemangioma, 4841, 4842f
historical considerations in, 1464–1465
of aneurysms, 1803–1806, 2057–2074,
2121. *See also* Aneurysms,
embolization of; Aneurysms,
endovascular occlusion of.
of brain tumors, 862–864
Engle Class, 242t
Enkephalin receptors, in striatum, 2687
Enlimomab, in ischemia protection, 1522
Enophthalmos, orbital blow-out fracture
and, 5257f
Entacapone, for Parkinson's disease, 2733
Enteric infection, after myelomeningocele
repair, 3223
Enterocolitis, necrotizing, after
myelomeningocele repair, 3223
Enterogenous cyst. *See* Neurenteric cyst.
Enteroviruses, myelitis from, 4311, 4312t
Enthesis, 4580
Enthesitis, in spondyloarthropathies, 4460
Enthesopathies, 4475–4487. *See also*
Posterior longitudinal ligament,
ossification of.
anatomy and physiology in, 4479–4480
Environment control, 5088
Environmental awareness, after traumatic
brain injury, 5192
Eosinophilic granuloma
craniovertebral junction, 4809
spinal, 4296t, 4297–4298, 4355, 4837,
4843, 4845f
pediatric, 3567, 3591, 3592f
Ependyma, 97
Ependymal cells, 49, 83, 93
Ependymal cyst
histopathologic classification of, 664–665,
664t
vs. neurenteric cyst, 1229
Ependymoblastoma, 669
Ependymoma, 1043–1048, 4296t
anaplastic, 664–665, 664t
cause of, 1044
chemotherapy for, 1048, 1048t
classification of, 664–665, 664t,
1044–1045, 1045t
diagnosis of, 1044–1046
epidemiology of, 1044
filum terminale, 4296t, 4300–4301
treatment of, 4824
fourth ventricle, 3624, 3625, 3626f, 3627
gene alterations in, 751t
imaging of, 525, 525f
immunohistology of, 1046
in pregnancy, 872
light microscopy of, 1045–1046
locations of, 1043
magnetic resonance imaging of, 453,
454f, 1046
metastatic, 527, 528f
myxopapillary, 665, 701
pediatric, 3623–3634, 3697
chemotherapy for, 3631–3632, 3632f,
3703
complications of, 3628–3631
dissemination of, 3626
epidemiology of, 3623

Ependymoma (*Continued*)
genetic factors in, 3623
grading of, 3624
hydrocephalus in, 3626–3627
imaging of, 3625–3626, 3625f, 3626f,
3626t, 3699
neurophysiologic monitoring in,
3630–3631
pathology of, 3623–3624, 3624f
quality of life after, 3634
radiation therapy for, 3631, 3631t
recurrent, 3634
signs/symptoms of, 3624–3625, 3625t
surgery for, 3627–3628, 3628f
survival in, 3632–3634, 3633f, 3633t
treatment of, 3626–3628
platelet-derived growth factor in, 730
posterior fossa, 3624, 3630
proliferation markers for, 700–701
radiation therapy for, 1047–1048
radiologic features of, 840
rates of, 1044
recurrence of, 1043
resection of, 1043, 1047
spinal cord, 4040, 4302, 4826, 4827f
MIB-1 labeling index for, 701, 701t
radiation therapy for, 4042, 4043,
4043t
surgery for, 4043
treatment of, 4828
third ventricular, 1246
treatment of, 1046–1048
ultrastructure of, 1046
variants of, 1045, 1045t
ventricular, MIB-1 labeling index for,
700–701, 700t
Ephrins, 80
Epiblast, 47, 4239, 4240f, 4241
Epidemiology, 235–259. *See also* Diagnostic
tests; Outcomes assessment.
analytic studies in, 249–253
case reports/series in, 248–249
case-control studies in, 249
cohort studies in, 249–250
common biases in, 247, 248t
cross-sectional surveys in, 249
descriptive cohort studies in, 249
descriptive studies in, 247–249
diagnosis studies in, 250
dose-escalation studies in, 251
individual studies in, 248–249
interventional studies in, 251–252
medical literature assessment in, 257–259
meta-analysis in, 252–253
natural history studies in, 250–251
observational studies in, 249–251
population correlation studies in,
247–248
randomized, controlled studies in,
251–252
study designs in, 247–253, 247t
Epidermal growth factor, 726
in central nervous system repair, 4160
Epidermal growth factor receptor
in brain tumors, 726–727
in gliomas, 715
Epidermoid cyst, 1207, 1223–1224,
3690–3691, 3690f, 3691f, 4259–4260
cerebellopontine angle, retrosigmoid
approach to, 927
congenital, 4317
imaging of, 1224, 1225f
orbital, 1374
pial, 3689
radiologic features of, 838–839

Epidermoid cyst (*Continued*)
skull, 1385–1386, 1386f
pediatric, 3718–3719
vs. trigeminal schwannoma, 1348
Epidural abscess. *See also* Pyogenic
infection, spinal.
clinical presentation of, 4366
incidence of, 4363–4364
magnetic resonance imaging of, 4379,
4380f
myelitis in, 4313
neurological deficit in, 4373–4374
outcome of, 4381, 4382f
pain in, 4291, 4293, 4293f
pediatric, 3566
postdiskography, 4384
treatment of, 4378–4379, 4380f
Epidural catheters, infections from,
4384–4385
Epidural hematoma, 5042–5043
after arterial bypass, 2117
delivery and, 3483–3484, 3483f
evacuation of, 5154, 5157, 5157f
in mild head injury, 5070, 5071t
in traumatic brain injury, 5083, 5106,
5107f
magnetic resonance imaging of, 469
pediatric, head injury and, 3475–3476,
3475f, 3476t, 3477
postoperative, 936, 937f
spinal cord compression in, 523, 524f
treatment of, 5146
Epidural scar, postoperative, 580
Epidural space
abscess of, pain from, 4291, 4293, 4293f
infection of, imaging of, 540, 540f
Epidural steroid injections, 2974–2976
approaches to, 2976
contraindications to, 2974, 2975t
fluoroscopy in, 2973–2974
indications for, 2974, 2975t
interlaminar, 2975
limitations of, 2974, 2975t
outcomes in, 2976
rationale for, 2974
transforaminal, 2975–2976
Epilepsy. *See also* Seizures.
area of functional deficit in, 2438
as chronic illness, 2565, 2567f
blood-brain barrier in, 166
brain mapping in, 2511, 2557
cavernous malformations in, 2314
cerebellar ganglioglioma in, 2578
chemical-shift imaging of, 2496–2497,
2497f
classification of, 2463–2464, 2464t
clinical features of, 2526–2527
cognitive outcome in, 2571
corpus callosotomy for, 2578–2579
cortical zones in, 2435–2439
epileptogenic, 2438–2439
irritative, 2436
seizure onset, 2436–2437, 2437f
symptomatogenic, 2435–2436
cost of, 2565
cryptogenic, 2461
death rate in, 2576
deep brain stimulation for, 2579
definition of, 2461–2462, 2525
developmental disorders and, magnetic
resonance imaging of, 2491–2495,
2492f–2494f
diagnosis of, 2461–2467
complications of, 2575
electrode-based, 2529–2530

Hyperventilation *(Continued)*
in pediatric head injury, 3474–3475
in traumatic brain injury, 5120, 5122f, 5123
intracranial pressure and, 187, 5058
Hypervolemia, for cerebral vasospasm, 1855
Hypoadrenalism, in pediatric craniopharyngioma, 3675
Hypocapnia
in traumatic brain injury, 5120, 5122f, 5123, 5135
intracranial pressure reduction by, 5057
treatment of, 5135
Hypochondroplasia, genetics of, 3362
Hypoesthesia, 3821
Hypoglossal nerve
dysfunction of, glomus jugulare tumors and, 1305
examination of, 267
pediatric, 3176
vagus nerve stimulator implantation and, 2643
Hypoglossal triangle, 33f
Hypogonadism, prolactinoma and, 1185
Hypokalemia, surgery and, 550
Hypometabolism
contralateral hemisphere, stroke and, 1607–1608
in stroke recovery, 1609
Hyponatremia, after subarachnoid hemorrhage, 1829–1830
Hyponatremia syndrome, in traumatic brain injury, 5130–5131, 5130f
Hypoparathyroidism, posterior longitudinal ligament ossification in, 4476
Hypophonia, subthalamic nucleus stimulation for, 2821
Hypophosphatemia, in altered consciousness, 295
Hypophyseal artery, superior, 19, 1896, 1898
aneurysm of, 1904
Hypophysectomy, 3030
Hypopituitarism
in pregnancy, 2429
transsphenoidal surgery and, 1182
Hypotension
in altered consciousness, 295
in bullet wounds, 5226
in cervical spine trauma, 4888, 4889
in head injury, 1551–1552
in pregnancy, 2423–2424
in trauma, 5090
in traumatic brain injury, 5096, 5120, 5122f
treatment of, 5135, 5136f
intraoperative, outcome in, 1551–1552
systemic, 1528
in extracranial head injury, 5056–5057
Hypothalamic sulcus, 14f
Hypothalamus, 13
after brain death, 398
arteriovenous malformation of, 2243
glioma of, pediatric, 3596
injury to, transsphenoidal surgery and, 569, 1181–1182
pituitary adenoma of, 1174
sarcoidosis of, 1436
stimulation of, 2854
Hypothermia
brain death and, 398
brain protection with, 5059
coma from, 294

Hypothermia *(Continued)*
in aneurysm treatment, 1807
in giant arteriovenous malformation surgery, 2273
in intracranial hypertension treatment, 5134
in ischemia protection, 1521, 1532
intracranial pressure and, 189
protective. *See* Deep hypothermic circulatory arrest.
side effects of, 1532–1533, 1533t
Hypothyroidism
in pediatric craniopharyngioma, 3675
neuropathy in, 3843
Hypotonia, pediatric, 3178
Hypovolemia, after aneurysmal subarachnoid hemorrhage, 1829
Hypoxia
in bullet wounds, 5226
in extracranial head injury, 5056–5057
in infantile posthemorrhagic hydrocephalus, 3408
in traumatic brain injury, 5122f, 5123, 5135–5136
myelination delay from, 64
pediatric tolerance for, 3462
radiomarkers for, 1609
treatment of, 5135–5136
Hysteria, conversion, pediatric, 3568

Idarubicin, for ependymoma, 1048t
Ifosfamide, for ependymoma, 1048, 1048t
Iliac crest, posterior, bone graft harvest from, 4605–4606, 4606f
IM862
angiosuppressive therapy with, 783
as angiogenesis antagonist, 779t
Image cytometry, in tumor proliferation marking, 694–695
Image-guided spinal navigation, 4743–4756
clinical applications of, 4747–4753
fluoroscopic, 4754–4755, 4755f
for anterior thoracolumbar surgery, 4752–4753, 4754f
for cervical spine screw fixation, 4748–4751, 4751f, 4752f
for pedicle fixation, 4747–4748, 4748f–4750f
for transoral surgery, 4751–4752, 4752f
pitfalls of, 4753–4754
principles of, 4743–4747, 4744f–4746f
Immobilization, after cervical spine trauma, 4887, 4888–4889
Immune modulation, of tumors, 821
Immune response, 674–675, 675f
adaptive, 674
antigenic determinants in, 675–676
blood-brain barrier in, 12
effector function in, 673, 680–681, 681f
for brain targets, 681–683
historical perspective on, 673–674
in central nervous system, 673–685
initiation of, 679–680
site-specific features of, 683–685, 683f, 684f
T cells in, 677–679, 678f
Immune system
astrocytoma evasion of, 891
in cerebral vasospasm, 1847
Immune-associated antitumor effect, in gene transfer, 818–819
Immune-inflammatory network, 675
in neurodegenerative disorders, 684

Immunoblastic sarcoma. *See* Central nervous system, primary lymphoma of.
Immunoblot, 753, 753f
Immunocompromise
primary central nervous system lymphoma in, 1067, 1069, 1070f
pyogenic spinal infections in, 4363–4364
differential diagnosis of, 4371
medical management of, 4379
outcome of, 4381
Immunogenicity, of bone grafts, 4616t, 4617
Immunoglobulin
for chronic inflammatory demyelinating polyradiculoneuropathy, 3840
for Guillain-Barré syndrome, 3839
Immunoglobulin G, blood-brain barrier transcytosis of, 163
Immunoglobulin superfamily, in malignant glioma, 763
Immunology, central nervous system inflammation and, 4155
Immunosuppressants, in focal cerebral ischemia, 135
Immunosuppression, tumor-induced, 681, 892
Immunotherapy
autoimmune disease and, 894
for brain tumors, 891–895
immunization site in, 893–894
Impairment, 3783
IN-1 antibody, in neuron regeneration, 204, 5032
Incidentaloma, 1170
Inclusion tumor, 3689–3690, 3689t
Incontinence
in cerebral palsy, 3727, 3728, 3732, 3744–3745
in multiple sclerosis, 1452
in occult spinal dysraphism, 3259, 3259f
urinary. *See* Urinary incontinence.
Index test, 497
Individual studies, 248–249
Indomethacin, pseudotumor cerebri from, 1424
Induction, 47–48, 48t
Industrial exposure, brain tumors and, 810
Infarction
choroidal artery, 1615
distal anterior cerebral artery, 1952
in stroke, 1622
magnetic resonance imaging of, 463–464, 465f, 466
middle carotid artery, 1615
periventricular hemorrhagic, 3407, 3407f
pons, 273
spinal cord, 4310–4311, 4310t
imaging of, 537, 539f
Infection. *See also* specific infection.
after skull base surgery, 572
after spinal surgery, 4383–4384, 4518–4519, 4982
brain tumors and, 810
extravascular, aneurysm from, 2101, 2102
in ankylosing spondylitis, 4459
in bullet wounds, 5236
in carotid atherosclerosis, 1613
in cerebral venous thrombosis, 1723
in cerebrospinal fluid shunt, 3419–3424. *See also* Cerebrospinal fluid shunt, infection of.
in craniofacial surgery, 3328–3329
in craniofacial trauma, 5248

Palmar grasp, in cerebral palsy, 3725, 3726t

Palsy, pressure, patient positioning and, 610–612, 612t

Pan plexus, injury to, 3821f

Pancoast's syndrome, intralaminar thalamotomy for, 3077

Pancreas, carcinoma of, thoracic endoscopic sympathectomy for, 4762–4763

Pancreatitis, chronic, celiac plexus block for, 2983

Pancuronium, 1508

Panfacial injury, 5262–5266, 5264f
treatment of, 5265–5266

Pannus, rheumatoid, 4570

PaO$_2$, in cerebral blood flow regulation, 551, 1478, 1478f

Papaverine
for cerebral vasospasm, 1854, 1856, 1856f, 1857
in anterior communicating artery aneurysm surgery, 1936

Papez circuit, limbic system and, 2854

Papilledema, 305–306, 306f
in brain tumors, 828–829
in increased intracranial pressure, 183
in pseudotumor cerebri, 1419, 1420f–1423f

Papilloma, choroid plexus. See Choroid plexus, papilloma of.

Paracentral lobule, 25

Paracentral ramus, 24, 24f

Parachute response testing, 3182

Paraganglia, tumors of, 1678

Paraganglioma
filum terminale, 666–667
skull, 1396–1397, 1397f
spinal cord, 4821
vascular supply to, 860t

Parahippocampal gyrus, 12f, 15f, 18f, 25, 26f, 2486, 2487f

Paralysis
acute, 4310–4311, 4310t
anesthesia positioning and, 611
pediatric intramedullary tumor surgery and, 3713
pharmacologic, in traumatic brain injury, 5131–5132, 5132t
succinylcholine and, 270

Paramedian fissure, 29

Paramedian nuclei, 33f

Paranasal sinus(es)
adenocarcinoma of, 910, 911f, 1312
adenoid cystic carcinoma of, 1312, 1313f
injury to, 425, 426f
metastases to, 1313, 1315f
neuroendocrine carcinoma of, 1312–1313
chemoradiation therapy for, 1327, 1328f–1329f
osteoma of, 1383, 1384f
squamous cell carcinoma of, 1312
transitional (schneiderian) carcinoma of, 1312

Paranasal sinus tumors, 1311–1330
adjuvant therapy for, 1326–1327
chemotherapy for, 1327, 1328f–1329f
classification of, 1317, 1318t
computed tomography of, 1316f, 1317
diagnosis of, 1315–1317
epidemiology of, 1311–1312
Epstein-Barr virus and, 1312
extension of, 1315–1316
histologic distribution of, 1313–1315, 1315t

Paranasal sinus tumors (Continued)
magnetic resonance imaging of, 1317, 1317f, 1318f
occupational hazards and, 1311, 1311t
outcome in, 1327
pathogenesis of, 1311–1312
pathology of, 1312–1315, 1313f–1315f, 1313t–1315t
radiation therapy for, 1327, 1328f–1329f
rhinoscopy of, 1315, 1316f
surgery for, 1318–1326
complications of, 1326, 1326t
craniofacial resection in, 1318–1320, 1320f–1322f
lateral approaches to, 1323f–1325f, 1324–1326
orbitectomy in, 1322–1323, 1323f
treatment of, 1317–1318, 1318t, 1319f

Paraneoplastic cerebellar degeneration, 832

Paraneoplastic disorders, 832–833

Paraneoplastic syndrome
neuropathy in, 3845
vertigo in, 2902

Paraolfactory gyrus, 25

Paraolfactory sulcus, 25

Paraplegia
from spinal metastases, 4859
hereditary spastic, 4319
patient positioning and, 615–616

Paraproteinemia
in multiple myeloma, 4854
in plasmacytoma, 4850, 4852

Parasagittal region, meningioma of
diagnosis of, 1268, 1268f, 1269f
surgical approach to, 1276, 1277f, 1278
results of, 1278, 1279t, 1280

Parasagittal sinus, surgical complications of, 1258

Parasellar region
anatomy of, 1266
surgery on, visual evoked potentials during, 2544
surgical anatomy of, 918–919, 919f, 920f
tumors of, frontotemporal approach to, 918–919, 919f

Parasitic infection
myelitis from, 4312t, 4313
spinal, 4390

Parasomina, vs. seizure, 2466

Parasympathetic nervous system, in lower urinary tract function, 361–362, 362f

Parasympathomimetic agents, for bladder retention, 377

Paraterminal gyrus, 24f, 25

Parathyroid hormone, in bone metabolism, 4231–4232

Paravermian fissure, 34

Parenchymal tumors, cranial
morbidity/mortality rates for, 566t
surgical complications in, 566–567, 566t, 567t

Paresis
acute, 4310–4311, 4310t
nerve root, after cervical laminectomy, 4425

Paresthesia, 3831
hyperextension-hyperflexion injury and, 4918

Parietal lobe, 4–5, 26f
hemorrhage of, 1738
inferior, 5
seizures in, 2591–2592
superior, 4
tumors of, 830–831
venous drainage of, 17, 28

Parietal lobule, superior, 4f

Parietal veins, 17

Parietooccipital artery, 23

Parietooccipital sulcus, 3, 10f, 22f, 24f, 26f

Parinaud's syndrome, 322–323, 1013
examination in, 3174

PARK2, in familial Parkinson's disease, 2711

Parkinson-dementia complex of Guam, 2716

Parkinsonism, 2703
causes of, 2703, 2703t
definition of, 2703, 2731
drug-related, 2716
dystonia with, 2678, 2721
experimental, positron emission tomography in, 492, 492f
pathophysiology of, 2673–2676, 2674f, 2675f
postencephalitic, 2715–2716
substantia nigra pars compacta in, 2706f
secondary, 2716–2717
signs of, modified testing for, 268
toxic, 2716
vascular, 2716

Parkinson's disease, 2704–2712, 2706f, 2731–2735
activation studies in, 2759–2760
age of onset in, 2732
akinetic-rigid type, 2707–2708
apoptosis in, 2710
bradykinesia in, 2732
brain-derived neurotrophic factor in, 2706
causes of, 2732
clinical presentation of, 2830
CNS transplantation for, 2830–2847. See also Fetal tissue transplantation.
cognitive impairment in, Lewy bodies and, 2709
deep brain stimulation for, 2733–2734, 2820
dementia with, Lewy bodies in, 2712–2713
diagnosis of, 2704, 2732t, 2746–2747
differential diagnosis of, 2734–2735, 2746–2747
dopamine transporter in, 2706
dopaminergic system in, 2704, 2706, 2706f
lesion type and, 2707–2708
drug-induced, 2735
dyskinesias in, 2733
extranigral systems in, 2708
familial, 2711–2712
family history of, 2732
fetal function in, positron emission tomography of, 2757–2758, 2758f
fetal tissue transplantation for, 2830–2843. See also Fetal tissue transplantation.
gait abnormalities in, 2732
gene therapy for, 817
idiopathic, 2704–2712
incidence of, 2704, 2704t
juvenile, 2710–2711, 2732
lesion pattern in, 2707–2708
Lewy bodies in, 2704, 2708–2709
medical therapy for, 2732–2733
misdiagnosis in, 2704, 2705t
motor functions in, pallidotomy effects on, 2791t
neuron degeneration in, 2710, 2711f
neuronal cell death in, 2708–2709

Postolivary sulcus, 29
Postoperative hyperperfusion syndrome, carotid endarterectomy and, transcranial Doppler ultrasonography of, 1550
Postpolio syndrome, 4319–4320
Post–subarachnoid hemorrhage vasculopathy. *See* Vasospasm.
Postsynaptic cell, 72f, 73
Postsynaptic potential
excitatory, 227–228, 228t
inhibitory, 227–228, 228t
Post-traumatic amnesia, in injury severity estimation, 5195–5196
Post-traumatic stress disorder, in traumatic brain injury response, 5193, 5193t
Postural instability, in Parkinson's disease, 2732
Posture
frog-leg, 3177
in ankylosing spondylitis, 4460, 4461f
pediatric, examination of, 3177
Potassium
astrocyte uptake of, 101, 102, 103f
equilibrium potential for, 3812
extracellular
after fluid pressure injury, 2456, 2456f, 2457f
after traumatic brain injury, 2454–2456, 2454f–2457f
in epileptiform activity, 2457, 2458f
in astrocytes, 1486
in cerebral blood flow–metabolism coupling, 1488–1489
in electrical synaptic transmission, 227
in extracellular homeostasis, 228, 229f, 230
in neuron excitability, 228, 230
in neurons, 3812, 3812t
resting membrane potential and, 218–219, 219f
Potassium channels, 220t, 224–225
glial, 225
in cerebral blood flow–metabolism coupling, 1489–1490
Potassium chloride, in glial cells, 2455
Potassium spatial buffering, 102, 104f, 228, 229f, 1486, 2455–2456, 2455f–2457f
Pou1f1, 54t
Precentral gyrus, 4f, 5, 6f, 24f
Precentral sulcus, 3, 4f
Precuneus, 24f, 25, 26f
Precursor cells
astrocyte, 98, 98f
glia-restricted, 98, 98f
neuroepithelial, 4159–4160
neuron-restricted, 98
Prednisone
for multiple sclerosis, 1454t
for optic neuritis, 309
for sarcoidosis, 1439
Preeclampsia, 2425
Prefrontal cortex, dorsolateral, in motor control, 2759
Pregabalin, for pain, 2965
Preganglionic fibers, 2981
Pregnancy
acoustic neuroma in, 872
anesthesia in, 873
aneurysms in, 2424–2426
angiomatous hemorrhage in, 2426–2427
anticoagulants in, 2422–2423
anticonvulsants in, 2422
antifibrinolytic agents in, 2424
antihypertensives in, 2423–2424

Pregnancy *(Continued)*
antiplatelet agents in, 2423
arterial occlusion in, 2427–2428, 2428t
arteriovenous malformations in, 2166, 2426–2427
brain tumors in, 867–874
breast cancer in, 872
carotid-cavernous fistula in, 2429
carpal tunnel syndrome in, 3890
cerebral hemorrhage in, 2166
cerebral ischemia in, 2427–2428, 2428t
cerebral vasospasm after, 2429
cerebrovascular disorders during, 2421–2429
choroid plexus papilloma in, 872
coma in, 295, 295t
confusion in, 295, 295t
craniotomy in, anesthesia for, 873
drug effects of, 2422–2424
ependymoma in, 872
folic acid supplementation in, 871
glial tumors in, 870–871, 870f
growth hormone–secreting adenoma in, 869
hemangioblastoma in, 872
imaging during, 2424
informed consent during, 409
intracranial aneurysm in, 1800–1801
lung cancer in, 872
mannitol in, 2423
medulloblastoma in, 872
melanoma in, 872
meningioma in, 871–872, 872f
metastases in, 872
metastatic choriocarcinoma in, 2428–2429
moyamoya in, 1720
nimodipine in, 2423
physiologic changes during, 2421–2422
pituitary adenoma in, 867–870, 869f
pituitary apoplexy in, 2429
primary brain lymphoma in, 872
prolactinoma in, 1188–1189
pseudotumor cerebri in, 872–873, 1430
stroke in, 2427–2428, 2428t
subarachnoid hemorrhage in, 2424–2426
surgery during, 2424
venous thrombosis in, 2428
Premamillary artery, 20
Premature infants
cerebral palsy and, 3723, 3724t, 3736
germinal matrix–intraventricular hemorrhage in. *See* Hydrocephalus, infantile posthemorrhagic.
subgroups of, 3405, 3405t
Premotor cortex, lateral, 2759
Preolivary sulcus, 29, 30f, 37
Prepyramidal fissure, 33f
Prepyriform cortex, 26f
Pressor agents, cerebral blood flow effects of, 5134–5135, 5135t
Pressure, 176
Pressure palsy, patient positioning and, 610–612, 612t
Pressure reactivity index, 182, 182f
Pressure-volume curve, 177, 177f, 182, 182f
Pressure-volume index, 177, 177f, 182, 182f
in intracranial compliance, 1504
in intracranial pressure, 5054, 5054f
Presynaptic cell, 72–73, 72f
Presynaptic terminal, 78
Prevalence, 236–237, 237t
Primary fissure, 31f, 35f
Primidone
in pregnancy, 2422
pharmacology of, 2470t, 2471

Primitive neuroectodermal tumors, 997–1007, 3639
biologic indicators in, 1006, 1006t
complications of, 1004
craniospinal irradiation in, 1005
grading of, 1004, 1004t
histopathologic classification of, 668–669, 668t
history of, 997
hydrocephalus management in, 1002–1003
incidence of, 997–998
insulin-like growth factors in, 729
magnetic resonance imaging of, 461, 461f
neurotrophins in, 729
outcome in, 1004–1007, 1006t
pathology of, 998–999, 998f–1000f
pediatric, 3697
pathology of, 3700
posterior fossa. *See* Medulloblastoma.
radiation therapy for, 4023
radiography of, 1000, 1001f–1003f, 1002
radiologic features of, 847, 848f, 849
signs/symptoms of, 1000
supratentorial, 997–998, 1031
imaging of, 1002f
outcome in, 1006
pediatric, 3699, 3700f
chemotherapy for, 3702
terminology for, 997, 1031
treatment of, 1002–1004
tumor factors in, survival and, 1006, 1006t
vs. medulloblastoma, 1032
Primitive node, 47
Primitive reflexes, in cerebral palsy, 3725, 3726t
Primitive streak, 47
development of, 4239, 4240f
regression of, 4241, 4242f
Prinomastat, angiosuppressive therapy with, 777
Proapoptotic genes, 719
Proatlas, segmentation abnormality of, 3338
Probability
in diagnosis, 235–238
post-test, 235–236, 236f
pretest, 235–236, 236f
Procarbazine, 881
for malignant glioma, 976
Progenitor cells
in central nervous system repair, 4159, 4160, 4161
transplantation of, 93, 94f
in neural regeneration, 5033
Progesterone receptors, in meningioma, 1108
Progressive pallidum atrophy, 2719–2720
Progressive supranuclear palsy
neurodegeneration in, 2714–2715
histologic features of, 2714
positron emission tomography of, 2761, 2762f
striatal neurons in, 2708
substantia nigra pars compacta in, 2706f
vs. Parkinson's disease, 2735
Prolactin
after pituitary surgery, 1191
in growth hormone–secreting pituitary adenoma, 1190
in meningioma, 1108
in pituitary adenoma, 1174–1175
in prolactinoma, 1185–1186

Prolactinoma, 1170
  clinical presentation of, 1185
  in pregnancy, 1188–1189
  laboratory studies for, 1185–1186
  macro-, 1185
    surgery for, 1188
  medical treatment of, 1186–1187
    in pregnancy, 1189
  micro-, 1185
    surgery for, 1187–1188
  radiation therapy for, 4036
  radiosurgery for, 4063
  surgery for, 1187–1189
    in pregnancy, 1189
    indications for, 1187, 1187t
    recurrence after, 1188
  tumor progression in, 1185
Proliferating cell nuclear antigen
  as tumor proliferation marker, 693–694
  in glioblastoma, 4097
  in meningioma, 1103, 1103f
Pronator syndrome, median nerve
    compression in, 3924–3925
Pronator teres muscle, median nerve
    entrapment at, 3924
Prone position, 597t, 600, 602–604, 602f
  complication avoidance in, 561–562
  dependent edema in, 563
  for craniotomy, 628–630, 629f
  in posterior cervical approach, 635–636
  orbital complications from, 576
Propionibacterium
  pyogenic spinal infections from, 4365
  shunt infection by, 3422–3423
Propofol, 1508
  cerebral physiology and, 551
  in craniotomy, 5149–5150
  in epilepsy surgery, 2621
  in ischemia protection, 1521
Proprioception
  pediatric, testing of, 3183–3184
  sensory nerve fibers in, 3809
Propriospinal multisynaptic ascending
    system, 2930
Proptosis, orbital tumors and, 1371
Prosencephalic vein, median, 3434
Prostaglandins
  in cerebral vasospasm, 1848–1849
  synthesis of, 2959
Prostate, transurethral resection of, for
    bladder outlet retention, 380
Prostatism, nocturia with, 365
Protease inhibitors, as angiogenesis
    antagonist, 776–777, 777t
Proteases
  in angiogenesis, 775t
  in apoptosis, 1519
  in axonal degeneration, 199
Protein
  as tumor antigens, 677
  phosphorylation of, in cell death, 127
  regulatory, in bone growth, 4614, 4614t
  synthesis of, in cell death, 132
Protein analysis, 752–753, 753f
Protein C, in cerebral venous thrombosis,
    1723
Protein kinase C system, in cerebral
    vasospasm, 1848
Protein truncation test, 753
Proteoglycans
  in axonal growth failure, 205
  in bone, 4230
  in malignant glioma, 762–763

Proton radiosurgery, 4123–4129
  evolving technology in, 4129
  historical perspective on, 4123
  physical principles of, 4123–4127,
    4124f–4126f
  technique of, 4128–4129
  treatment principles for, 4127–4128,
    4128f
  vs. linac radiosurgery, 4115–4116
Proto-oncogenes, 739
Protuberance, 29
Prourokinase, trials of, 1496
Psammoma bodies, 1101, 1101f
P-selectin, in cerebral ischemia, 140–141
Pseudallescheria boydii, infectious
    intracranial aneurysms from, 2102
Pseudarthrosis
  after scoliosis surgery, 4566
  complication avoidance in, 577
Pseudoaneurysms
  displacement artifact and, 1579f
  internal carotid artery, 1880, 1883f
  peripheral nerve involvement in, 3949
  traumatic, 2131, 5208, 5209f–5210f
    after débridement, 5237
Pseudobulbar palsy, medulloblastoma
    surgery and, 3645–3646
Pseudochondroplasia, atlantoaxial
    instability in, 3543
Pseudocoma, 293
Pseudoephedrine
  for bladder outlet incontinence, 380–381
  spontaneous intracerebral hemorrhage
    in, 1735
Pseudomeningocele
  brachial plexus injury with, 3491, 3491f
  cerebellar astrocytoma surgery and, 3659
  ependymoma surgery and, 3630
  postoperative, 564–565
  spinal surgery and, 574–576
Pseudomonas
  infectious aneurysms from, 2102
  pyogenic spinal infections from, 4365,
    4379f
Pseudoparkinsonism, arteriosclerotic,
    2716
Pseudopod, in craniopharyngioma, 3672,
    3672f
Pseudospondylolisthesis, 3580
Pseudotumor, orbital, 1376
Pseudotumor cerebri, 1419–1430
  causes of, 1419–1426
  cerebral venous drainage obstruction
    and, 1420–1422, 1424t
  clinical manifestations of, 1419,
    1420f–1423f
  complications of, 1426
  conversion from hydrocephalus to, 3400,
    3400f
  diagnosis of, 1426, 1427f, 1428
  endocrine dysfunction and, 1422, 1424t
  epidemiology of, 1419
  exogenous substances and, 1422–1425,
    1424t
  familial, 1426
  headache in, 1419
  imaging of, 1426, 1427f
  in pregnancy, 872–873
  lumbar puncture in, 1426
  metabolic dysfunction and, 1422, 1424t
  optic disk in, 1426, 1427f
  papilledema in, 1419, 1420f–1423f
  pathophysiology of, 1426
  systemic illness and, 1425–1426, 1425t

Pseudotumor cerebri (*Continued*)
  treatment of, 1429–1430
    during pregnancy, 1430
  venous hypertension and, 3398
Pseudoxanthoma elasticum, intracranial
    aneurysms in, 1773
Psuedopuberty, precocious, 1013
Psychiatric disorders
  after traumatic brain injury, 5296
  anterior capsulotomy for, 2859, 2859f
  anterior cingulotomy for, 2856–2857,
    2857f
  in epilepsy, 2573
  in failed back syndrome, 4337
  limbic leucotomy for, 2858–2859, 2858f
  neurosurgery for, 2853–2861
    anatomic basis for, 2854–2855
    approaches to, 2856–2861
    evaluation before, 2861
    historical perspective on, 2853–2854
    indications for, 2859–2860
    outcome in, 2860–2861
    patient selection in, 2855–2856
    repeat procedures in, 2860
    subcaudate tractotomy for, 2857–2858,
      2858f
Psychological disturbances
  after glomus jugulare tumor surgery,
    1308
  traumatic brain injury and, 5190–5191
  vs. multiple sclerosis, 1455
Psychological measurement, 385
Psychomotor function, after traumatic
    brain injury, 5188
Psychosocial problems, in achondroplasia,
    3363
Psychosocioeconomic syndrome, low back
    pain in, 4332
Psychosurgery, 2853
  politics of, 2660–2661
Ptc, 54t
PTCH/SMOH/SHH, 742–743
PTEN, in glioma, 716
PTEN/MMAC1/TEP1, 742
Pterion, 423–424, 423f
Ptosis, examination of, 266
Pudendal nerve, in lower urinary tract
    function, 362, 362f, 363f
Pulmonary edema
  in subarachnoid hemorrhage, 1826–1827,
    1869
  neurogenic, 1869
Pulmonary embolism, 563–564
Pulse repetition frequency, 1540
Pulvinar, thalamic, 10f, 11
Pumps, implantable
  complications of, 3140
  for intrathecal baclofen, 3749–3752,
    3749f, 3750f, 3753–3754
  for intrathecal drug infusion, 3136–3140,
    3137f–3139f
Pupil(s), 321–322, 322f, 323f
  abnormally large, 322, 322f
  abnormally small, 322, 323f
  dilation of, in brainstem lesions, 288,
    288f
  examination of, 266
  football, 288
  in bullet wounds, 5228, 5228t
  near-light dissociation of, 322
  oval, 288
  size of, 322
Pupillary defect, relative afferent, 302,
    304b

Surgical navigation (*Continued*)
 imaging in, 941
 in biopsy, 945–946
 in craniotomy, 942–945, 943f–945f, 945t
 intraoperative imaging in, 946
 multimodality imaging in, 946
 pointing devices in, 941
 registration in, 941
Sutures
 anomalies of
  head shape and, 3300
  historical aspects of, 3158, 3158f, 3159f
 coronal, 423f
 diastatic, 427
 lambdoid, 423f
 metopic, 431–432
 occipitomastoid, 423f
 ossification of, 3301
 premature fusion of, 3304–3305, 3305t
 prominent, in infants, 431–432
 squamosal, 423f
Swimmer's projection, in cervical spine
  radiography, 4894
Sylvian cistern, in aneurysm surgery, 1879
Sylvian fissure, 5–6, 6f
 anatomy of, 2608
 arachnoid cyst of, 3292–3293, 3293f
 arteriovenous malformation of,
  2237–2238, 2239f
 dissection of, 1933
 in craniometrics, 630–631
 localization of, 2531, 2532f
 posterior ramus of, 4, 4f
Sylvian fissure stem, 4f
Sylvian point, 14, 16
Sylvian triangle, 16
Sylvian vein, superficial, 17
Sympathectomy, 3028, 3093–3102
 approaches to, 3096
 historical aspects of, 3093–3094
 lumbar endoscopic, 3102, 3102f
 nomenclature in, 3094
 patient selection for, 3095–3096
 thoracic endoscopic, 3096–3102,
  4762–4765
  anatomic orientation for, 4763–4764,
   4764f
  care after, 3100
  closure in, 4764
  complications of, 3101–3102, 4765
  dissection in, 3099–3100, 3099f
  goals of, 4763
  indications for, 3096–3097, 4762–4763,
   4762t
  instruments for, 3098–3099
  intrathoracic anatomy in, 3098f, 3099
  outcome in, 3100–3101, 3100t, 3101t,
   4765
  ports for, 3099
  positioning for, 3097f, 3098, 3098f,
   4763, 4763f
  transection in, 4764, 4764f
  unilateral vs. bilateral, 3095t
Sympathetic block, paravertebral, in
  sympathetic-mediated pain, 3096
Sympathetic dystrophy, 3094
Sympathetic fiber bundles, 1899
Sympathetic nerve trunk, vagus nerve
  stimulator implantation and, 2643
Sympathetic nervous system
 afferent fibers of, 2981
 anatomy of, 2981
 blockade procedures in, 2981–2984
 efferent fibers of, 2981
 endoscopy of, 3093

Sympathetic nervous system (*Continued*)
 in lower urinary tract function, 361, 361f
 indications for, 2981–2982
Synapses, 71–73, 72f
 ensheathment of, 86
 in brain metabolism, 86
 transduction in, in post-traumatic
  epilepsy, 2451–2452, 2451f
Synaptic terminal, 72f, 73
Synaptic transmission, 226–228
 chemical, 227–228
 electrical, 226–227
Synaptogenesis
 in post-traumatic epilepsy, 2450–2451
 reactive, 3785
Synchondrosis, neural central, 3332
Syncope, 275
 neurocardiogenic, vs. seizure, 2466
Syndrome of inappropriate antidiuretic
  hormone secretion (SIADH)
 after aneurysmal subarachnoid
  hemorrhage, 1829–1830, 1830t
 in traumatic brain injury, 5130, 5130f
 vs. salt wasting, 1830
Synostosis
 bilateral coronal, surgery for, 3321
  after age three, 3322
  before age one, 3321–3322, 3322f,
   3323f
 coronal, deformational anterior
  plagiocephaly and, 3301f
 primary, vs. skull molding, 3301–3304
 sagittal, growth restriction in, 3315,
  3316f
 unilambdoid, vs. deformational
  plagiocephaly, 3302, 3302f, 3303f,
  3303t
Synovial cyst
 imaging of, 512, 513f–514f
 vs. lumbar disk disease, 4511, 4511f
Synovitis, in spondyloarthropathies, 4460
Synthes system, of cervical spine anterior
  screw-plate fixation, 4630t, 4632, 4632f
α-Synuclein, 2703
 in Lewy bodies detection, 2709
Synucleopathies, 2703–2714, 2703t
Syphilis
 congenital, endolymphatic hydrops in,
  350
 myelitis in, 4313
Syringocele, 3226
Syringohydromyelia
 imaging of, 533, 535f, 3356
 in Chiari malformation type II, 3351
Syringomyelia, 4315t, 4317
 cerebrospinal fluid obstruction and, 3393
 embryonic tissue transplantation for,
  4159
 endoscopy in, 3430–3431
 post-traumatic, 4308
 terminal, 3273–3274, 3273f
Syringomyelocele, 3226
Syrinx (syringes), in Chiari malformation
  type I, 3349, 3349f
Systemic lupus erythematosus
 chorea with, 2736
 pseudotumor syndrome in, 1425
Systolic blood pressure, in bullet wounds,
  5226

T cell receptor
 diversity of, 890
 peptide-MHC recognition by, 676

T cells
 active extravasation by, 682
 antigen presentation to, in brain tumor
  therapy, 887, 888f
 antigen receptors on, 675–676, 677
 antigen recognition by, 680
 arrest of, 682
 effector functions of, 680
 helper, 678
  in immune response initiation, 679
  in multiple sclerosis, 1450
 in immune response, 675, 675f
 in multiple sclerosis, 1450
 in perivascular space, 683
 MHC class II–restricted, 678, 679
 MHC class I–restricted, 678
 migrant, antigen presentation to, 682
 secreted factors of, 680
 selective adhesion of, 682
Tactile sensibility, pediatric, 3183
Taenia thalami, 12–13
Tamoxifen, for meningioma, 1110
Tamsulosin, for bladder outlet retention,
 380
Tapetum, 7f, 8f, 9
Tardy ulnar palsy, 3897, 3926
Tarlov cysts, 4511
Tarsal tunnel, 653
 tibial nerve surgery at, 655, 655f
Tarsal tunnel syndrome, 3935–3936
Tattoo, accidental, in craniofacial trauma,
 5249
Tauopathy, 2703, 2703t, 2714–2716
Taylor-Haughton lines, 631, 631f
Teardrop fractures, 4907–4908, 4908f
Technology, evaluation of, 253–254
Tectal beaking, in Chiari malformation
  type II, 3351
Tectal vein, 36f
Tectorial membrane, 4925–4926, 4926f
 hemorrhage in, spinal cord injury
  without radiographic abnormality
  and, 3521, 3522f
 pediatric, in atlanto-occipital dislocation,
  3529, 3531, 3531f
Tectum, 29, 3054
Tegmental pedunculopontine nucleus
 nigral projections to, 2693, 2694f, 2695
 pallidal projections to, 2693, 2694f, 2695
Tegmentum, 29, 3054, 3074
Tela choroidea, 13, 31f, 33f, 35f, 36f
Telangiectasia
 capillary. *See* Capillary telangiectasia.
 radiation-induced, 854
Telencephalon, in Chiari malformation
  type II, 3351, 3351f
Telovelar junction, 33f
Temozolomide, 882
Temperature
 in cerebral blood flow, 1504
 instability of, in deep hypothermic
  circulatory arrest, 1536
 pediatric, testing of, 3183
Temporal arteritis, 276t
Temporal artery
 inferior, 22–23, 22f
 superficial
  bypass with, for moyamoya, 1719,
   1719f, 1720f
  in middle cerebral artery aneurysm,
   1965, 1967f
  middle cerebral artery bypass with,
   1674, 2113, 2113f, 2114f
  superior cerebellar artery bypass with,
   2115

Tonic neck reflex
  in cerebral palsy, 3725, 3726t
  testing of, 3182
Tonsillar herniation, 826t, 827, 5055t, 5056, 5091, 5092f
  in Chiari malformation type I, 3349, 3350f
Tonsils, 31f, 32
  superior pole of, 33f
Topectomy, 2629–2633
  anesthesia for, 2632
  cortical stimulation during, 2632–2633
  electrocorticography during, 2632
  evaluation before, 2630–2632
  outcome in, 2633, 2633t
  patient selection for, 2629–2630
  principles of, 2632
  technique of, 2633
Topiramate, 2470t, 2472
Topoisomerase inhibitors, 882
Torcular Herophili
  meningioma of, 1276
  venous drainage of, 1266
Torticollis, 2729
  atlas assimilation in, 3340
  clinical forms of, 2891–2893, 2892f–2894f, 2895, 2896t
  craniovertebral junction abnormalities in, 3334
  rotatory, 2892, 2892f, 2896t
  spasmodic, 2891–2899
    electromyography of, 2895
    physiopathology of, 2891
    selective peripheral denervation for, 2897–2898
      indications for, 2895
    results of, 2898–2899, 2898t, 2899t
    surgical techniques for, 7–8, 2896t
  tumor-related, 4835
Touch, testing of, pediatric, 3183
Touch receptors, 73–74, 74f
Tourette's syndrome, obsessive-compulsive disorder in, 2854–2855
Toxins
  neuropathy from, 3832t, 3843–3844
  parkinsonism from, 2716
  peripheral nerve effects of, 3816
Tp53
  in cell cycle control, 820–821
  in gliomas, 950–951
  in malignant glioma, 969–970
Trace elements, in angiogenesis, 775t
Traction
  cervical, 4891–4892, 4892f, 4900
  peripheral nerve injury from, 3827
Traction response, testing of, 3182
Tractotomy, midbrain. *See* Midbrain, tractotomy of.
TRAIL, in astrocytoma immunotherapy, 894
Tramadol
  for diabetic neuropathy, 3838
  for failed back syndrome, 4336
  for pain, 2964
Tranexamic acid, in pregnancy, 2424
Transcranial Doppler ultrasonography, 1540–1555
  diagnosis with, 1543–1544, 1544f
  during carotid endarterectomy, 1548–1550
  examination techniques in, 1541–1543, 1541f–1543f, 1542t
  flow velocity recording in, 1543–1544
  historical aspects of, 1540–1541, 1542t
  neurosurgical applications of, 1545–1554

Transcranial Doppler ultrasonography (*Continued*)
  of aneurysms, 1548, 1549f
  of arteriovenous malformation, 1547–1548
  of brain death, 1553–1554
  of cerebral vasospasm, 1545–1546, 1545t, 1850–1851
  of cerebrovascular disease, 1554–1555
  of emboli, 1544
  of head injury, 1550–1552, 1551f
  of increased intracranial pressure, 1552–1553, 1553f
  of stroke, 1554–1555
  of subarachnoid hemorrhage, 1545–1546, 1545t
  predictive value of, 1547, 1548f
  principles of, 1541–1544, 1544f
Transcription factors, 51, 743–744, 4252–4253
Transferrin
  in cerebrospinal fluid fistula, 5269
  transcytosis of, through blood-brain barrier, 163
Transforming growth factor, in stroke, 142
Transforming growth factor-α, in brain tumors, 726
Transforming growth factor-β
  in astrocytoma treatment, 891, 892
  in bone, 4609, 4614–4615
  in brain tumors, 730–731
  in cerebral ischemia, 140
Transfusion reaction, 564
Transgenic mice, 714
Transient ischemic attacks, 1623–1624, 1624f
  carotid artery disease and, 1613, 1614–1615, 1614t
  definition of, 1495–1496
  in moyamoya, 1716
  magnetic resonance angiography of, 1576f
  positron emission tomography of, 2478
  presentation of, 1624
  single-photon emission computed tomography of, 2478
  stroke in, 1624
  thromboembolism and, 1623–1624, 1624f
Transitional (schneiderian) carcinoma, paranasal sinus, 1312
Transplantation, 2829, 2829t
  central nervous system, 2829–2847, 2829t
    adrenal medulla tissue in, 2831
    brain death and, 395–396, 395t, 403, 403t
    disease pathophysiology in, 2844
    gene therapy trials in, 2844–2845
    historical aspects of, 2829
    intracerebral, 2843
    neural cells in, 93, 94f
    neurotrophic factors in, 2843–2844
    Parkinson's disease treatment with, 2830–2843. *See also* Fetal tissue transplantation.
    porcine xenografts for, 2841
    retinal-pigmented epithelial cells for, 2841
    retroviral vectors in, 2845–2846, 2845t
    stem cells for, 2841, 2843
    terminology for, 2829, 2830t
    tissue sources for, 2841–2843
  embryonic tissue, 4158, 4159
  fetal tissue. *See* Fetal tissue transplantation.
  glial cellular, 4161–4163

Transplantation (*Continued*)
  inflammatory cell, 4164
Transtentorial herniation, 826
Transverse crest, 40f
Transverse ligament, in atlas fracture, 4933, 4934, 4935
Transverse sinus, thrombosis of, 1421
  magnetic resonance angiography of, 1597, 1597f
Trapezius muscle, pediatric, 3176
Trapidil, for meningioma, 1110
Trauma
  aneurysms from. *See* Aneurysms, traumatic.
  brain tumors and, 810–811
  cellular basis of, 5025–5033
  cerebral venous thrombosis from, 1723
  cerebrovascular. *See* Cerebrovascular injury, traumatic.
  cranial destruction in, 430
  craniofacial. *See* Craniofacial trauma.
  death due to, central nervous system injury and, 5095
  in pediatric lumbar disk herniation, 3560
  magnetic resonance imaging of, 469
  open, peripheral nerve injury in, 3820
  pediatric, surgery for, 3195–3196
  peripheral nerve injury in, evaluation of, 3819–3820
  positron emission tomography of, 2481
  recovery from, 5025–5033
  resuscitation for, 5087–5089
    primary survey in, 5087–5088, 5088t
    secondary survey in, 5088–5089
  single-photon emission computed tomography of, 2481
  spinal, 4148–4149, 4307–4308, 4308f
    cervical, 4885–4910
    lumbar, 4702–4704, 4731, 4732t
    thoracic, 4951–4982
  spondylolisthesis from, 3573–3574
  to brain. *See* Brain injury, traumatic.
Trauma team, 5087
Traumatic Coma Data Bank, 5019, 5103
Traumatic far-out syndrome, 5012
Traumatic spondylolisthesis, 4546
Treatment, legal obligations for, 408
Tremor
  action, 2729
  cerebellar, 2778–2779
  classification of, 2750
  definition of, 2729
  differential diagnosis of, 2750t
  environmental exposure and, 2750
  essential, 2731, 2750, 2776–2778
    deep brain stimulation for, 2820
    mechanism of, 2772f, 2776
    thalamotomy for, 2776–2777, 2777f, 2777t
    results of, 2777–2778
    ventral intermedius nucleus stimulation for, 2821
  in Parkinson's disease, 2732
  intention, 2750
  kinetic, 2750
  parkinsonian. *See* Parkinson's disease, tremor in.
  pediatric, assessment of, 3179–3180
  resting, 2729, 2750
  senile, 2750
  subthalamic nucleus stimulation for, 2822
  surgery for, 2748, 2750, 2803
  thalamotomy for, 2769–2780
    vs. thalamic deep brain stimulation, 2780